Knowles' NEOPLASTIC HEMATOPATHOLOGY

THIRD EDITION

Knowles'
NEOPLASTIC HEMATOPATHOLOGY

THIRD EDITION

EDITED BY

Attilio Orazi, MD, FRCPath

Professor of Pathology and Laboratory Medicine
Department of Pathology and Laboratory Medicine
Weill Cornell Medical College
Vice-Chair for Hematopathology and Director
Division of Hematopathology
Department of Pathology and Laboratory Medicine
New York–Presbyterian Hospital
New York, New York

Kathryn Foucar, MD

Professor
Department of Pathology
University of New Mexico Health Sciences Center
Albuquerque, New Mexico

Daniel M. Knowles, MD

David D. Thompson Professor and Chairman of
    Pathology and Laboratory Medicine
Weill Cornell Medical College
Chief Medical Officer
Weill Cornell Physician Organization
Pathologist-in-Chief
New York-Presbyterian Hospital, Weill Cornell
    Medical Center
New York, New York

Lawrence M. Weiss, MD

Senior Consultant Pathologist
Clarient, Inc.
Aliso Viejo, California

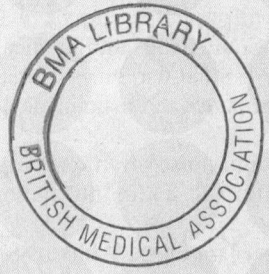

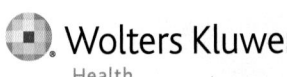 Wolters Kluwer | Lippincott Williams & Wilkins
Health
Philadelphia · Baltimore · New York · London
Buenos Aires · Hong Kong · Sydney · Tokyo

Acquisitions Editor: Ryan Shaw
Product Manager: Kate Marshall
Production Project Manager: David Saltzberg
Senior Manufacturing Coordinator: Beth Welsh
Marketing Manager: Alexander Burns
Designer: Stephen Druding
Production Service: SPi Global

Library of Congress Cataloging-in-Publication Data
Knowles neoplastic hematopathology / [edited by] Attilio Orazi, Kathryn Foucar. —Third edition.
    p. ; cm.
  Preceded by (work): Neoplastic hematopathology / edited by Daniel M. Knowles. 2nd ed. c2001.
  Includes bibliographical references and index.
  ISBN 978-1-60913-682-6
  I. Orazi, Attilio, editor of compilation. II. Foucar, Kathryn, editor of compilation.
  [DNLM: 1. Hematopoietic System—pathology. 2. Bone Marrow Diseases—pathology. 3. Hematologic Neoplasms—pathology. 4. Leukemia—pathology. 5. Lymphoproliferative Disorders—pathology. WH 140]
  616.4'1071—dc23

2013012016

With love and gratitude
to Marian, Daniel, Louise, and Tyler

—DMK

To Maria, my wife, and to Giulia and Rita, our daughters, for their love and support.
To my parents who by their example have given me the drive and discipline
to tackle all tasks with enthusiasm and determination.

—AO

To Elliott, Jim, Morgan, and Charlie Foucar

—KF

To my wife Tina and my daughters, Dina and Tessa

—LMW

Contributors

John Anastasi, MD
Associate Professor of Pathology, Assistant Director of Hematopathology, Department of Pathology, University of Chicago Medicine, Chicago, Illinois

Daniel A. Arber, MD
Professor and Vice Chair, Department of Pathology, Stanford University; and Medical Director of Anatomic Pathology and Clinical Laboratory Services, Stanford Hospital & Clinics, Lucile Packard Children's Hospital at Stanford, Stanford, California

Stefano Ascani, MD
Associate Professor, Institute of Pathology, Perugia University School of Medicine, Perugia, Italy; and Director, Surgical Pathology Unit in Terni, Santa Maria Hospital, Terni, Italy

Adam Bagg, MD
Professor, Department of Pathology and Laboratory Medicine, University of Pennsylvania; and Director, Hematology, Medical Director, Cancer Cytogenetics, Director, MRD Resource Laboratory, Department of Pathology and Laboratory Medicine, Hospital of the University of Pennsylvania, Philadelphia, Pennsylvania

Peter M. Banks, MD
Clinical Professor of Pathology, Department of Pathology and Laboratory Medicine, University of North Carolina—Chapel Hill, Chapel Hill, North Carolina

Carolina M. Barra, BS
PhD student, Inflammatory and Cardiovascular Disorders, Institut de Recerca Hospital del Mar, Barcelona, Spain

Todd S. Barry, MD, PhD
Medical Director and Hematopathologist, Spectrum Pathology, Mission Viejo, California

Françoise Berger, MD
Professor, Department of Hematopathology, Hospices Civils de Lyon, Lyon, France; and Chief, Department of Pathology, Centre Hospitalier Lyon-Sud, Pierre-Bénite, France

Gerald J. Berry, MD
Professor, Department of Pathology, Stanford University; and Director of Cardiac and Pulmonary Pathology, Stanford University Medical Center, Stanford, California

Michael J. Borowitz, MD, PhD
Professor, Departments of Pathology and Oncology, Johns Hopkins Medical Institutions; and Director, Division of Hematopathology, Department of Pathology, Johns Hopkins Hospital, Baltimore, Maryland

Richard D. Brunning, MD
Professor Emeritus, Department of Laboratory Medicine and Pathology, University of Minnesota, Minneapolis, Minnesota

Jerome S. Burke, MD
Adjunct Clinical Professor, Department of Pathology, Stanford University School of Medicine, Stanford, California; and Senior Pathologist, Department of Pathology, Alta Bates Summit Medical Center, Berkeley, California

Linda Cassis, PhD
Researcher, Inflammatory and Cardiovascular Disorders, Institut de Recerca Hospital del Mar, Barcelona, Spain

Andrea Cerutti, MD
Professor of Medicine, Department of Medicine, Division of Clinical Immunology, Mount Sinai School of Medicine, New York, New York; and Senior Icrea Research Professor, Inflammatory and Cardiovascular Disorders, Istitut de Recerca Hosital del Mar, Barcelona, Spain

Ethel Cesarman, MD, PhD
Professor, Department of Pathology and Laboratory Medicine, Weill Cornell Medical College; and Attending, Department of Pathology and Laboratory Medicine, New York–Presbyterian Hospital, New York, New York

Wing C. Chan, MD
Amelia and Austin Vickery Professor of Pathology, Department of Pathology and Microbiology, University of Nebraska Medical Center, Omaha, Nebraska

Karen L. Chang, MD
Director of Immunohistochemistry and Histology, Department of Pathology, Kaiser Permanente–Southern California, North Hollywood, California

Yi-Hua Chen, MD
Assistant Professor, Department of Pathology, Northwestern University Feinberg School of Medicine, Chicago, Illinois

Alejo Chorny, PhD
Postdoctoral Researcher, Department of Medicine, Division of Clinical Immunology, Mount Sinai School of Medicine, New York, New York

Montserrat Cols, PhD
Postdoctoral Researcher, Department of Medicine, Division of Clinical Immunology, Mount Sinai School of Medicine, New York, New York

James R. Cook, MD, PhD

Associate Professor, Department of Pathology, Cleveland Clinic Lerner College of Medicine; and Section Head, Molecular Hematopathology, Department of Molecular Pathology, Cleveland Clinic, Cleveland, Ohio

Magdalena Czader, MD, PhD

Associate Professor, Department of Pathology and Laboratory Medicine, Indiana University; and Director, Division of Hematopathology, Department of Pathology and Laboratory Medicine, Indiana University, Indianapolis, Indiana

David Czuchlewski, MD

Assistant Professor, Department of Pathology, University of New Mexico; and Associate Director, Molecular Diagnostics, Department of Pathology, University of New Mexico, Albuquerque, New Mexico

Joseph A. DiGiuseppe, MD, PhD

Director, Special Hematology Laboratory, Department of Pathology and Laboratory Medicine, Hartford Hospital, Hartford, Connecticut

Ahmet Dogan, MD, PhD

Professor, Department of Laboratory Medicine and Pathology, College of Medicine, Mayo Clinic; and Consultant, Department of Laboratory Medicine and Pathology, Mayo Clinic, Rochester, Minnesota

Ming-Qing Du, MB, PhD, FRCPath

Professor of Oncological Pathology, Department of Pathology, University of Cambridge; and Honorary Consultant of Molecular Pathology, Department of Histopathology, Cambridge University Hospitals NHS Foundation Trust, Addenbrooke's Hospital, Cambridge, United Kingdom

Scott Ely, MD, MPH

Associate Professor, Department of Pathology and Laboratory Medicine, Weill Cornell Medical College; and Attending Physician, Department of Pathology, New York–Presbyterian Hospital, New York, New York

Fabio Facchetti, MD, PhD

Full Professor, Department of Pathology, Brescia University, Brescia, Italy

Brunangelo Falini, MD

Full Professor of Haematology, Institute of Haematology, Perugia University School of Medicine; and Director, Haematology Unit, Renato Silvestrini Hospital, Perugia, Italy

Andrew L. Feldman, MD

Assistant Professor, Department of Laboratory Medicine and Pathology, College of Medicine, Mayo Clinic; and Consultant, Department of Laboratory Medicine and Pathology, Mayo Clinic, Rochester, Minnesota

Kathryn Foucar, MD

Professor, Department of Pathology, University of New Mexico Health Sciences Center, Albuquerque, New Mexico

Aharon G. Freud, MD, PhD

Chief Resident, Department of Pathology, Stanford University Medical Center, Stanford, California

Maurizio Gentile, BS

PhD Student, Inflammatory and Cardiovascular Disorders, Institut de Recerca Hospital del Mar, Barcelona, Spain

Ulrich Germing, MD

Vice Head, Department of Hematology, Oncology, and Clinical Immunology, Heinrich-Heine University Düsseldorf, Düsseldorf, Germany

Julia Turbiner Geyer, MD

Assistant Professor, Department of Pathology and Laboratory Medicine, Weill Cornell Medical College; and Assistant Attending, Department of Pathology and Laboratory Medicine, New York–Presbyterian Hospital, New York, New York

Kate E. Grimm, MD

Clinical Assistant Professor, Department of Pathology, Keck School of Medicine of the University of Southern California, Los Angeles, California; and Staff Hematopathologist, Department of Pathology, Clarient, Inc., Aliso Viejo, California

Cindy Gutzeit, PhD

Postdoctoral Researcher, Translational Immunology Unit, Department of Medicine, Solna, Karolinska Institutet, Stockholm, Sweden

Martin-Leo Hansmann, MD

Associate Professor, Department of Pathology, Frankfurt University; and Department of Pathology, Johann Wolfgang Goethe University, Frankfurt, Germany

Sylvia Hartmann, MD

Hematopathologist, Department of Pathology, Johann Wolfgang Goethe University, Frankfurt, Germany

Rana S. Hoda, MD, FIAC

Professor of Pathology, Department of Pathology and Laboratory Medicine, Weill Cornell Medical College; and Chief of Cytopathology, Department of Pathology and Laboratory Medicine, New York–Presbyterian Hospital, New York, New York

Hans-Peter Horny, MD

Professor of Pathology, Department of Pathology, Institute of Pathology, Munich, Germany

Dragan Jevremovic, MD, PhD

Assistant Professor, Department of Laboratory Medicine and Pathology, Division of Hematopathology, College of Medicine, Mayo Clinic; and Consultant, Department of Laboratory Medicine and Pathology, Division of Hematopathology, Mayo Clinic, Rochester, Minnesota

Michael G. Kharas, PhD

Assistant Member, Departments of Molecular Pharmacology and Chemistry, Sloan-Kettering Institute, New York, New York

Philip M. Kluin, MD

Professor in Oncological Pathology, Departments of Pathology and Laboratory Medicine, Academic Hospital Groningen, Department of Pathology and Medical Biology, Groningen University Medical Center, Groningen, The Netherlands

Daniel M. Knowles, MD

David D. Thompson Professor and Chairman of Pathology and Laboratory Medicine, Weill Cornell Medical College; Chief Medical Officer, Weill Cornell Physician Organization; and Pathologist-in-Chief, New York–Presbyterian Hospital–Weill Cornell Campus, New York, New York

Steven H. Kroft, MD
Professor, Department of Pathology, Medical College of Wisconsin; and Director of Hematopathology, Department of Pathology, Froedtert Memorial Lutheran Hospital, Milwaukee, Wisconsin

Ralf Küppers, PhD
Professor, Institute of Cell Biology (Cancer Research), University of Duisburg-Essen, Essen, Germany

Michelle M. Le Beau, PhD
Arthur and Marian Edelstein Professor, Department of Medicine, University of Chicago, Chicago, Illinois

Giuliana Magri, MD
Postdoctoral Researcher, Inflammatory and Cardiovascular Disorders, Institut de Recerca Hospital del Mar, Barcelona, Spain

Cynthia Magro, MD
Professor of Pathology and Laboratory Medicine, Director of Dermatopathology, Division of Dermatopathology, Weill Cornell Medical College, New York, New York

Tomer Mark, MD, MSc
Assistant Professor, Department of Medicine, Weill Cornell Medical College; and Assistant Attending, Department of Medicine, New York–Presbyterian Hospital, New York, New York

Yasodha Natkunam, MD, PhD
Associate Professor, Department of Pathology, Stanford University, Stanford, California

L. Jeffrey Medeiros, MD
Professor, Department of Hematopathology, The University of Texas; and Chair, Department of Hematopathology, The University of Texas MD Anderson Cancer Center, Houston, Texas

William G. Morice, MD, PhD
Associate Professor, Department of Laboratory Medicine and Pathology, College of Medicine, Mayo Clinic; and Chair, Division of Hematopathology, Department of Laboratory Medicine and Pathology, Mayo Clinic, Rochester, Minnesota

Angela R. Murray, MS
Laboratory Manager, Immunopathology Laboratory, New York-Presbyterian Hospital, Weill Cornell Medical Center, New York, New York

Shigeo Nakamura, MD
Professor and Chairman, Department of Pathology and Laboratory Medicine, Nagoya University; and Chief, Department of Pathology and Laboratory Medicine, Nagoya University Hospital, Nagoya, Japan

Beverly P. Nelson, MD
Associate Professor of Pathology, Department of Pathology, Northwestern University Feinberg School of Medicine; and Hematopathologist, Department of Pathology, Northwestern Memorial Hospital, Chicago, Illinois

Ruben Niesvizky, MD
Associate Professor, Department of Medicine, Weill Cornell Medical College; and Director, Multiple Myeloma Center, Department of Medicine, NewYork–Presbyterian Hospital, New York, New York

Grant Nybakken, MD, PhD
Hematopathology Fellow, Department of Pathology, Stanford University Medical Center, Stanford, California

Dennis P. O'Malley, MD
Adjunct Associate Professor, Department of Pathology, Division of Hematopathology, The University of Texas MD Anderson Cancer Center, Houston, Texas; and Pathologist, Department of Pathology, Clarient, Inc./GE Healthcare, Aliso Viejo, California

Koichi Ohshima, MD, PhD
Professor, Department of Pathology, Kurume University, Kurume, Japan

Attilio Orazi, MD, FRCPath
Professor of Pathology and Laboratory Medicine, Department of Pathology and Laboratory Medicine, Weill Cornell Medical College; and Vice-Chair for Hematopathology and Director, Division of Hematopathology, Department of Pathology and Laboratory Medicine, New York–Presbyterian Hospital, New York, New York

Karen J. Ouyang, PhD
Clinical Cytogenetics Fellow, Department of Medicine, Hematology/Oncology Section, University of Chicago, Chicago, Illinois

Christopher Y. Park, MD, PhD
Assistant Member, Human Oncology and Pathogenesis Program, Memoral Sloan-Kettering Cancer Center; and Assistant Attending Physician, Department of Pathology and Clinical Labs, Memorial Sloan-Kettering Cancer Center, New York, New York

Laura Pasqualucci, MD
Associate Professor, Institute for Cancer Genetics and Department of Pathology and Cell Biology, Columbia University, New York, New York

LoAnn Peterson, MD
Paul E. Steiner Research Professor of Pathology, Department of Pathology, Feinberg School of Medicine Northwestern University; and Director of Hematopathology, Department of Pathology, Northwestern Memorial Hospital, Chicago, Illinois

Stefano A. Pileri, MD, PhD
Full Professor of Pathology, Department of Haematology and Oncological Sciences "L. and A. Seràgnoli", University of Bologna; and Director, Unit of Haematopathology, Department of Oncology, Haematology, and Laboratory Medicine, St. Orsola Hospital, Bologna, Italy

Sonam Prakash, MBBS
Assistant Professor, Department of Pathology and Laboratory Medicine, Weill Cornell Medical College; and Assistant Attending Pathologist, Department of Pathology and Laboratory Medicine, New York–Presbyterian Hospital, New York, New York

Irene Puga, PhD
Associate Investigator, Inflammatory and Cardiovascular Disorders, Institut de Recerca Hospital del Mar, Barcelona, Spain

Kaaren K. Reichard, MD

Associate Professor of Pathology, Division of Hematopathology, Mayo Clinic, Rochester, Minnesota

Stefano Rosati, MD

Department of Pathology and Laboratory Medicine, Academic Hospital Groningen, Department of Pathology and Medical Biology, Groningen University Medical Center, Groningen, The Netherlands

Michele Renee Roullet, MD

Assistant Professor, Department of Pathology and Anatomy, Eastern Virginia Medical School; and Hematopathologist, Pathology Sciences Medical Group, Norfolk, Virginia

Jonathan Said, MD

Professor of Pathology, Department of Pathology, David Geffen School of Medicine at University of California, Los Angeles; and Chief, Anatomic Pathology, Department of Pathology and Laboratory Medicine, University of California, Los Angeles, Los Angeles, California

Karl Sotlar, MD

Assistant Professor, Institute of Pathology, University of Munich, Munich, Germany

Steven H. Swerdlow, MD

Professor of Pathology, Department of Pathology, University of Pittsburgh School of Medicine; and Director, Division of Hematopathology, Department of Pathology, University of Pittsburgh Medical Center–Presbyterian, Pittsburgh, Pennsylvania

Wayne Tam, MD, PhD

Associate Professor of Clinical Pathology and Laboratory Medicine, Weill Cornell Medical College; and Associate Attending Pathologist, NewYork–Presbyterian Hospital, New York, New York

Alexandra Traverse-Glehen, MD, PhD

Laboratory of Molecular Biology of the Cell, UFR Lyon-Sud—Charles Mérieux, Université Lyon 1, Hematopathology Department, Hospices Civils de Lyon, Lyon, France

Peter Valent, MD

Department of Medicine, Division of Hematology & Hemostaseology, Ludwig Boltzmann Cluster Oncology, Medical University of Vienna, Vienna, Austria

Michiel van den Brand, MD

Resident Pathologist, Department of Pathology, Radboud University Nijmegen Medical Centre, Nijmegen, the Netherlands

J. Han van Krieken, MD, PhD

Head of Department, Department of Pathology, Radboud University Nijmegen Medical Centre, Nijmegen, the Netherlands

James W. Vardiman, MD

Professor Emeritus of Pathology, Department of Pathology, University of Chicago Medicine, Chicago, Illinois

Y. Lynn Wang, MD, PhD

Associate Professor, Department of Pathology and Laboratory Medicine, Weill Cornell Medical College; and Director, Molecular Hematopathology Laboratory, Weill Cornell Medical College, New York, New York

Roger Warnke, MD

Ronald F. Dorfman Professor of Hematopathology, Emeritus Active, Department of Pathology, Stanford University School of Medicine, Stanford, California

Christopher David Watt, MD, PhD

Assistant Professor, Department of Pathology and Laboratory Medicine, University of Pennsylvania; and Associate Director, Molecular Pathology, Department of Pathology and Laboratory Medicine, Hospital of the University of Pennsylvania, Philadelphia, Pennsylvania

Lawrence M. Weiss, MD

Senior Consultant Pathologist, Clarient, Inc., Aliso Viejo, California

Andrew C. Wotherspoon, FRCPath

Consultant Histopathologist, Department of Histopathology, The Royal Marsden Hospital, London, United Kingdom

Ken H. Young, MD, PhD

Associate Professor, Department of Hematopathology, The University of Texas MD Anderson Cancer Center, Houston, Texas

Qian-Yun Zhang, MD, PhD

Associate Professor, Department of Pathology, University of New Mexico; and Medical Director, University Hospital Lab Hematology, University of New Mexico, TriCore Reference Laboratories, Albuquerque, New Mexico

Preface to the First Edition

Pathologists have traditionally experienced difficulty in diagnosing hematologic neoplasms. One factor that accounts for these difficulties is that malignant lymphoma and leukemia cells often exhibit cytomorphologic features that mimic those of normal differentiating hematolymphoid cells. A second and perhaps more significant factor for many years was the lack of knowledge and understanding of the hematopoietic and immune systems. This prevented pathologists from comprehending the origin and nature of hematologic neoplasms and their relation to the normal cellular components of the hematopoietic and immune systems. The unprecedented explosion of new scientific information concerning the hematopoietic and immune systems that has taken place during the past 20 years, however, has generated the scientific bases for the reliable and reproducible diagnosis and classification of most hematologic neoplasms.

Modern hematopathology began in the early 1970s soon after immunologists discovered that lymphocytes are divisible into two distinct subpopulations: B cells and T cells, which vary according to their differentiation process, anatomic localization, and functional properties and are distinguishable according to their differential expression of various surface membrane and cytoplasmic antigens and receptors. Pathologists soon discovered that many neoplastic lymphoid cells also express B- and T-cell–associated markers, presumptive evidence of their B- or T-cell origin. They also discovered that benign, reactive lymphoid proliferations are polyclonal (i.e., contain mixtures of B and T cells), whereas many non-Hodgkin lymphomas and lymphoid leukemias are monoclonal B-cell proliferations (i.e., contain a predominance of B cells that express only one immunoglobulin light chain class, either κ or λ). These discoveries led to the use of cell marker analysis (the routine classification of lymphoid neoplasms as B- or T-cell derived) as an adjunct to morphologic interpretation in the diagnosis of lymphoid neoplasia, encouraged the correlation of morphologic features with immunologic cell markers, and fostered the development of new terminology and classification schemes.

The second phase of modern hematopathology, the monoclonal antibody era, began in the early 1980s when an array of highly specific monoclonal antibodies that detect B-cell, T-cell, monocyte/macrophage, and myeloid lineage differentiation and subset-associated antigens became commercially available. During the same time, several comparatively inexpensive fluorescent-activated cell sorters that permit rapid, accurate, and objective analysis and sorting of cell populations also became available. In addition, several very sensitive immunohistochemical staining techniques, particularly the avidin–biotin-complex immunoperoxidase and alkaline phosphatase/antialkaline phosphatase methods, were developed, and the reagents were made available in a kit form for use in routine pathology laboratories. The combined commercial availability of sensitive and specific monoclonal antibodies and immunohistochemical reagents and affordable fluorescent-activated cell sorters resulted in the establishment of specialized hematopathology laboratories that routinely perform immunophenotypic analysis. The result has been an enormous collective experience with immunophenotypic analysis in the diagnosis and classification of hematologic neoplasms. This experience has allowed us to document the immunophenotypic profiles exhibited by nearly all the major clinicopathologic categories of hematologic neoplasia and to establish guidelines for their immunodiagnosis, resulting in a substantial improvement in diagnostic accuracy and greatly facilitating our understanding of the relation between malignant hematolymphoid cells and normal cells of the hematopoietic and immune systems.

The third and current phase of modern hematopathology, the molecular biology era, began in the mid-1980s. The development of the Southern blot hybridization technique, the cloning of the immunoglobulin and T-cell receptor genes, and the preparation and dissemination of the DNA probes that detect clonal rearrangements of these genes have provided pathologists with a sensitive, accurate, and objective method for determining the lineage and clonality of lymphoid neoplasms. This approach has allowed for the determination of the lineage of neoplasms that exhibit immature, ambiguous, and anomalous immunophenotypes; the determination of the monoclonal nature of lymphoid proliferations of an uncertain nature; and the detection of the clonal B- and T-cell populations that are undetectable by morphologic examination and/or by immunophenotypic analysis. The availability of many additional DNA probes and the development of DNA amplification techniques such as the polymerase chain reaction now allow us to routinely detect oncogenes, chromosomal translocations, and viral sequences as well, thereby facilitating the investigation of the pathogenesis of hematologic neoplasia.

Unfortunately, this sudden and rapid growth has generated a constantly changing and often confusing and conflicting literature. The rapid turnover of knowledge in hematopathology and the increasing reliance on new scientific techniques by hematopathologists have left many experienced pathologists (unfamiliar with the changing concepts and who are unable to perform these modern diagnostic techniques) uncomfortable in rendering definitive diagnostic opinions concerning hematolymphoid proliferations. Pathologists in training have often been discouraged from studying hematopathology for the same reasons. Furthermore, no single source of information that encompasses the morphologic, immunologic, and molecular aspects of hematolymphoid neoplasia has been available to pathologists (to guide them in daily practice) or to pathologists in training (to assist them in acquiring the basic tenets of knowledge of modern hematopathology) until now.

This book represents the first definitive textbook of modern hematopathology. It is aimed at providing a thorough overview of the morphologic, immunologic, and molecular genetic characteristics of the benign and malignant proliferations derived from the hematopoietic and immune systems. The volume begins with a review of our current understanding of the structural and functional characteristics of the hematopoietic and immune systems, followed by chapters that describe the currently available immunologic markers and their application in the flow cytometric and immunohistochemical analysis of hematologic neoplasms, the structure and function of the antigen receptor genes and oncogenes and their application in the diagnosis and classification of hematologic neoplasms, and an overview of the role of cytogenetics. Practical guidelines for the organization and operation of a hematopathology laboratory and for the technical evaluation of lymph node biopsies also are provided. The role of fine needle biopsy and imprint cytology in the diagnosis and classification of hematologic neoplasms is discussed next. These background chapters are followed by 21 chapters that describe in detail the benign, reactive lymphoid proliferations that stimulate malignant lymphoma, Hodgkin disease, each major clinicopathologic category of non-Hodgkin lymphoma, and the extranodal lymphoid hyperplasias and malignant lymphomas. This is followed by practical guidelines for the handling and cytochemical and immunohistochemical analysis of bone marrow specimens. The final chapters deal with bone marrow involvement by malignant lymphoma, the acute and chronic lymphoid and myeloid leukemias, the myeloproliferative disorders, histiocytic and dendritic cell proliferations, mast cell disease, and the splenic manifestations of hematolymphoid neoplasia.

This volume is a multiauthored text by necessity. The vast amount of information currently available that concerns the clinical and biologic aspects of the numerous and diverse categories of hematopoietic neoplasia precludes any one individual from successfully preparing a definitive, accurate, and up-to-date reference work on neoplastic hematopathology. For that reason, a sincere effort was made to select for the preparation of each chapter experts who have been closely associated with the growth and development of and who have made significant contributions to that particular aspect of hematopathology. The result is that the list of contributors to this textbook represents a veritable Who's Who in hematopathology. These are the very same investigators who have been largely responsible for the many exciting and important developments that have taken place in hematopathology during the past 20 years. Each expert has responded with excitement and enthusiasm for this project. I am grateful to them for their support of and participation in the preparation of *Neoplastic Hematopathology*.

Daniel M. Knowles, MD

Preface to the Second Edition

Since publication of the first edition in 1992, our knowledge in all facets of hematopathology (i.e., morphology, immunology, and molecular biology) has continued to grow unabated.

In 1992, a lack of consensus on lymphoma classification existed; the Working Formulation was the standard in the United States; and the Kiel classification was the standard in most European countries. However, as our conceptual understanding of newly as well as previously recognized lymphoma entities grew, it became increasingly obvious that both classifications had inherent deficiencies. For example, the Working Formulation categories were broadly defined to accommodate the classification of all lymphomas but did not permit the recognition and distinction of specific disease entities (i.e., mantle cell lymphoma, the low-grade extranodal B-cell lymphomas arising in mucosa-associated lymphoid tissue (MALT), and peripheral T-cell lymphomas). In addition to other shortcomings, the Kiel classification neglected to include extranodal lymphomas and failed to distinguish MALT lymphomas.

A group of 19 expert hematopathologists from the United States, Europe, and Asia, designating themselves the International Lymphoma Study Group (ILSG), began to meet informally in 1991 to exchange ideas and information concerning the lymphomas. In 1993, the ILSG undertook the task to reach consensus on a list of "real" lymphoma entities based upon a combination of clinical, morphologic, immunophenotypic, and molecular genetic characteristics. This consensus list was published in 1994 and designated the Revised European-American Lymphoma (REAL) classification, since it represented a revision of the current European and American lymphoma classifications. Shortly thereafter, the reproducibility and clinical utility of the REAL classification were validated in a multiobserver study of 1,300 cases of non-Hodgkin lymphoma gathered from several institutions around the world.

Since 1995, members of the American and European Hematopathology Societies have been collaborating on a new World Health Organization (WHO) classification of hematologic malignancies. The WHO classification employs an updated version of the REAL classification for the lymphomas and expands the tenets of the REAL classification to codify the myeloid and histiocytic neoplasms. The WHO classification will replace all existing classifications and thus represents the first classification of hematologic malignancies in which true international consensus has been achieved.

By the time the first edition of this book was published, four international white cell differentiation antigen workshops had taken place, and leukocyte antigens CD1 through CDw78 had been defined. Since then, two more workshops have been convened, leading to the further clarification of the structural and functional properties of these antigens and the expanded recognition of distinct leukocyte antigens through CD166. Thus, in the 8-year interval between the publication of the first and second editions of this book, the number of distinct monoclonal antibody–defined leukocyte antigens has doubled.

In 1992, immunophenotypic characterization of lymphoproliferative disorders involving solid tissues was most often performed by immunohistochemical staining of frozen tissue sections. Most monoclonal antibodies commercially available at that time were not immunoreactive in paraffin tissue sections; only a few antigens, principally CD3, CD15, CD20, CD30, CD43, and CD45, were detectable in paraffin tissue sections. However, during the past several years, a concerted effort by many investigators to prepare paraffin-reactive monoclonal antibodies has resulted in an explosion of new antibody reagents capable of detecting most of the additional leukocyte antigens that are critical to immunophenotypic analysis, including CD1a, CD4, CD5, CD8, CD10, and CD79α, in paraffin tissue sections. In addition, several investigators have developed heat-based antigen retrieval techniques capable of "unmasking" heretofore undetectable antigens in paraffin tissue sections. These techniques have further expanded the spectrum of paraffin-reactive monoclonal antibodies as well as enhanced the sensitivity and reproducibility of antigen detection in paraffin tissue sections. Finally, efficient, reliable automated immunohistochemical staining instruments have been introduced and widely accepted. As a consequence, at the present time, unlike in 1992, immunophenotypic characterization of the majority of lymphoproliferative disorders involving solid tissues are performed by the immunohistochemical staining of paraffin tissue sections, and, in many instances, by using automated instrumentation. These advances obviated the special requirements and technical difficulties associated with frozen tissue section immunohistochemistry, which has resulted in a marked expansion of the routine immunophenotypic analysis of hematologic malignancies.

By 1992, molecular characterization of the hematologic malignancies had become an established facet of hematopathology. However, the laborious, time-consuming, and relatively insensitive Southern blot technique restricted such studies to a few specialized laboratories. The introduction of simpler, more rapid, and far more sensitive polymerase chain reaction–based assays has resulted in a marked expansion of studies aimed at deciphering the molecular pathology of the hematologic malignancies. In addition, numerous significant discoveries in basic molecular biology have occurred since 1992. One example is the discovery of the *BCL-6* gene, a transcriptional repressor belonging to the POZ/Zinc finger family of transcriptional factors, which appears to play an important role in germinal center formation. Rearrangements of the *BCL-6* gene preferentially occur in diffuse large B-cell lymphomas where they may be associated with extranodal disease and a better prognosis. Another example is the discovery of the Kaposi sarcoma–associated herpes virus, also referred to as human herpesvirus-8, which is a novel gamma 2-herpesvirus present in virtually all Kaposi sarcoma lesions. This virus also has been found to be highly associated with an uncommonly occurring subset of unusual non-Hodgkin lymphomas referred to as *primary effusion lymphomas*, which appear to originate in the body cavities as an effusion in the absence of an identifiable tumor mass. The combination of these and other scientific discoveries and the ever-widening use of molecular biologic techniques in the study of hematologic malignancies have contributed significantly to our understanding of the role of molecular genetic lesions in the pathogenesis and the clinical and biologic behavior of hematologic malignancies.

Our enhanced knowledge and understanding of the morphologic, immunologic, and molecular genetic characteristics of the hematologic malignancies and the lesions that simulate them necessitated that this book be updated. That is precisely what we have done. This second edition represents a thorough revision and marked expansion of the first edition to reflect our increased knowledge and current concepts of hematopathology. Each chapter appearing in the first edition has been revised; indeed, nearly all of them have been entirely rewritten. The result is that this book represents the definitive textbook of modern hematopathology.

This book is aimed at providing a thorough overview of the morphologic, immunologic, and molecular genetic characteristics of the benign and malignant proliferations derived from the cellular elements that comprise the hematopoietic and immune systems. The book begins with a review of our current understanding of the structural and functional characteristics of the hematopoietic and immune systems, followed by chapters that describe the currently available immunologic markers and their application in the flow cytometric and immunohistochemical analysis of hematologic neoplasms, the normal histology and immunoarchitecture of the lymphoid organs, the structure and function of the antigen receptor genes and oncogenes and their application in the diagnosis and classification of hematologic neoplasms, and an overview of the role of cytogenetics. Practical guidelines for the organization and operation of a hematopathology laboratory and for the technical evaluation of lymph node biopsies also are provided. The role of fine needle biopsy and imprint cytology in the diagnosis and classification of hematologic neoplasms is discussed next. These background chapters are followed by 23 chapters that describe in detail the benign, reactive lymphoid proliferations that simulate malignant lymphoma, the atypical lymphoproliferative disorders, Hodgkin disease, the current classification of the non-Hodgkin lymphomas and Hodgkin disease, and the clinical significance of these classifications, each major clinicopathologic category of non-Hodgkin lymphoma, and the extranodal lymphoid hyperplasias and malignant lymphomas. This is followed by practical guides for the handling and cytochemical and immunohistochemical analysis of bone marrow specimens. The final chapters deal with bone marrow involvement by malignant lymphoma, acute and chronic lymphoid and myeloid leukemias, myeloproliferative disorders, histiocytic and dendritic cell proliferations, mast cell disease, and the splenic manifestations of hematolymphoid neoplasia.

This book is a multiauthored text by necessity. The vast amount of information concerning the clinical, pathologic, and biologic aspects of the numerous and diverse categories of hematopoietic neoplasia currently available precludes any one individual from successfully preparing a definitive, accurate, and up-to-date reference work on neoplastic hematopathology. For that reason, a sincere effort was made to select for the preparation of each chapter experts who have been closely associated with the growth and development, and who have made significant contributions to that particular aspect of hematopathology. The result is that the list of contributors represents a veritable Who's Who in hematopathology. These are the very same investigators who have been largely responsible for many of the exciting and important developments that have taken place in hematopathology during the past 25 years. Each expert responded with excitement and enthusiasm for this project. I am grateful to each of them for their support and participation in the preparation of the second edition of *Neoplastic Hematopathology*.

Daniel M. Knowles, MD

Preface to the Third Edition

Our understanding of the immunologic and the molecular biologic basis for the clinical and morphologic diversity of the hematologic malignancies has continued to grow unabated during the past decade. Indeed, that growth has accelerated. This, in turn, has helped up to further delineate the morphologic criteria that define distinct clinical pathologic entities. As a result, the 2008 WHO classification represents our most successful effort to date to bring clarity and understanding to the classification of the malignant neoplasms derived from hematopoietic cells. In the 8-year interval between the first and second editions of this textbook, the number of monoclonal antibody–defined leukocyte antigens doubled, reaching CD166. In the ensuing decade since the publication of the second edition, additional leukocyte differentiation antigen workshops have propelled us to CD350. The human genome has been successfully sequenced. Continued molecular technologic advances now allow us to rapidly sequence individual human malignancies. This is allowing us to identify novel therapeutic targets. The introduction of next-generation sequencing into the clinical laboratory over the next several years will usher in the era of personalized medicine. Each individual malignant neoplasm will be sequenced, its unique molecular signature delineated, and a therapeutic strategy tailored to that individual neoplasm will be developed and implemented, hopefully allowing us to cure more individuals who have cancer. The widespread adoption of the new WHO classification, the marked expansion of the monoclonal antibody panel used to characterize hematologic malignancies in daily practice, and the technologic explosion in molecular biology necessitate that this textbook be updated. That is precisely what I have done with the assistance of three of the foremost hematopathologists in the United States today, Drs. Attilio Orazi, Lawrence Weiss, and Kathy Foucar. Together, the four of us have reorganized this textbook, invited the most highly qualified individuals to contribute to this textbook, and have carefully read, edited, and reread every chapter contributed by them. We believe that the result is a completely revised third edition of this classic textbook of modern hematopathology, one that provides a thorough, up-to-date overview of the morphologic, immunologic, and molecular characteristics of the benign and malignant proliferations derived from the hematopoietic and lymphoid systems.

Daniel M. Knowles, MD

Acknowledgments

The opportunity to thank publicly those persons who have contributed substantially to one's professional development and career comes infrequently; therefore, I would like to take this opportunity to do precisely that. I wish to express my sincere appreciation to Dr. Henry Rappaport for his stimulating hematopathology lectures, which I attended as a medical student at the University of Chicago and which sparked my initial interest in hematopathology; to Dr. Henry Rappaport's surgical pathology faculty and house staff at the University of Chicago for inspiring me as a senior medical student to become a surgical pathologist; to Dr. Ralph Williams for introducing me to research during a medical student elective in his laboratory at the University of New Mexico, for assisting me in the preparation of my first abstract and paper, and for guiding me toward academic medicine; to Dr. Donald West King for accepting me into the pathology residency training program at the Columbia University College of Physicians and Surgeons and for providing an extraordinarily flexible training program that was a wonderful, nurturing environment, which allowed me to grow personally and professionally; to Drs. Raffaele Lattes, Nathan Lane, Marianne Wolff, and Karl Perzin for training me in surgical pathology and for establishing a superior standard of diagnostic excellence to which I shall always aspire; to the late Dr. Henry Kunkel, the finest scientific intellect I have ever known, and to his staff at the Rockefeller University for guiding my training in laboratory research; to Dr. Vittorio Defendi, Chairman of Pathology at the New York University, and Dr. Michael Shelanski, Chairman of Pathology at the Columbia University College of Physicians and Surgeons, for their friendship and uncompromising support while I was a member of their departments; to the other members of the International Lymphoma Study Group for making the annual scientific meetings intellectually stimulating and personally rewarding; to Dr. Robert Michaels and Dr. Antonio M. Gotto, former Deans, and Dr. Laurie Glimcher, the present Dean, of the Weill Cornell Medical College, and to Dr. David B. Skinner and Dr. Herbert Pardes, former Presidents, and Dr. Steve Corwin, current Chief Executive Officer, of New York–Presbyterian Hospital, for their generous support of me and the Department of Pathology and Laboratory Medicine; to all the Basic Science and Clinical Department Chairs at the Weill Cornell Medical College for their warm collegiality; and to my faculty for making our department better clinically and academically.

In addition, I wish to thank the numerous physicians with whom I have worked and collaborated during the past 35 years, but especially Drs. Riccardo Dalla-Favera, James Halper, Giorgio Inghirami, Pier Giuseppe-Pelicci, and Chang Yi Wang. I also thank all the fellows, residents, graduate students, technicians, and clerical staff who have worked for me during the past 35 years and who have helped my Hematopathology Laboratory grow and prosper. In this regard, I give special thanks to two of my former fellows: Dr. Ethel Cesarman, now a successful independent research scientist and colleague, whose intelligence and creativity has inspired our hematopathology group for the past 20 years, and Dr. Amy Chadburn, now a successful hematopathologist and former colleague, who oversaw the daily operation of our Hematopathology Laboratory for 20 years; to Angela Murray, our laboratory manager whose intelligence, enthusiasm, devotion, and hard work have been responsible for many of the successes of my laboratory during the past 25 years; to Gina Imperato, my Departmental Administrator, whose extraordinary abilities, dedication, and support have contributed so much to my success as Chairman of Pathology and Laboratory Medicine at the Weill Cornell Medical College; and to my office staff, whose presence makes each workday easier and more pleasant. I also thank Timothy Satterfield of Williams and Wilkins for convincing me to prepare the first edition of this textbook 20 years ago and the staff at Lippincott Williams & Wilkins for being so helpful during the preparation of all three editions of this textbook.

I wish to thank all the contributors to all three editions of this textbook for their time and effort in the preparation of their chapters and for being so tolerant of my editorial recommendations and revisions and my constant nagging to complete their chapters on schedule. This textbook owes its title, *Neoplastic Hematopathology*, to the highly acclaimed "Tutorial on Neoplastic Hematopathology," developed by Dr. Henry Rappaport, which has been successfully conducted annually for more than 40 years under the direction initially of Dr. Henry Rappaport, later Dr. Richard Brunning, and now me. I wish to pay my respects to all of the individuals who have taught in the Tutorial and thereby have contributed to my education and to that of thousands of others. Lastly, but most importantly, I express my deepest and most sincere gratitude to Marian, my wife, who graciously and unhesitatingly supported me while I labored on many evenings and weekends for so many years during the preparation of each edition of this textbook. I could not have completed any of the three editions of this textbook without her support and understanding.

Daniel M. Knowles

Three coeditors have been added for the third edition of this book. Each of these coeditors was influenced by giants in the field of hematopathology such as Drs. Henry Rappaport and Richard Brunning.

In addition, Attilio Orazi wishes to acknowledge that he owes much to those who taught him and influenced him the most, including Franco Rilke with whom he trained and Richard S. Neiman, for his mentoring and friendship. I wish to acknowledge my debt of gratitude to Daniel M. Knowles for inspiring me at many different levels and for offering me the privilege of participating in the creation of the third edition of "his" book. Finally, I wish to thank all of my colleagues in the Division of Hematopathology at Weill Cornell Medical College for their help, insights, and support during the preparation of this book.

Individual acknowledgments for Kathryn Foucar include Drs. Robert McKenna (first mentor), Robert Anderson (former Chair), Mary Lipscomb (former Chair), and Thomas Williams (current Chair). Over my 35 years of practice in hematopathology, I have had the privilege of working with many stellar faculty colleagues, and all of the hematopathology fellows and residents who I have trained over the years have added such an important dimension to my life.

Attilio Orazi, Kathryn Foucar, Lawrence M. Weiss

Contents

Chapter 1
The Hematopoietic System and Hematopoiesis

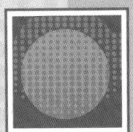

Christopher Y. Park • Michael G. Kharas

The hematopoietic system is a wonderfully complex biologic system, composed of numerous cell types that serve a countless number of roles with respect to organismal homeostasis. For example, the hematopoietic system is comprised of the red blood cells (RBCs) that carry oxygen to all the tissues of the body, the platelets that preserve volume by controlling bleeding, and the numerous cells of the innate and cellular immune systems (Fig. 1.1). These mature hematopoietic cells are the products of an intricate system of positive and negative control mechanisms that maintain homeostasis by regulating the ability of hematopoietic stem cells (HSCs) and lineage-committed progenitors to give rise to the cells that replenish postmitotic, terminally differentiated cells. This ability has evolved to allow rapid adaptation to environmental stress, probably best exemplified by the ability of the hematopoietic system to generate large numbers of cells in the setting of acute blood loss and infection. In some situations, this ability is compromised due to acquired genetic or epigenetic alterations, resulting in hematologic malignancies or inherited disorders of inappropriate or ineffective hematopoiesis. Thus, in many ways, disorders of the hematopoietic system can be viewed as a loss of homeostatic control, and understanding the mechanisms that regulate normal hematopoiesis will reveal many insights regarding the molecular pathways underlying the pathogenesis of hematologic disorders.

Because disorders of the hematopoietic system can be viewed as examples of abnormal hematopoiesis, it is imperative for medical professionals and researchers to understand the mechanisms that regulate normal hematopoiesis, which include a large number of cell-intrinsic factors such as transcriptional regulators and cell surface receptors, a variety of growth factors and cytokines, extracellular matrix proteins, and the stromal cells that make up the specialized bone marrow environment that supports HSC self-renewal, survival, and lineage commitment. Such knowledge will provide important clues to mechanisms of disease pathogenesis, provide novel methods for the diagnosis and detection of disease, as well as identify targets for therapy. For example, identifying aberrantly activated self-renewal pathways in hematologic cancers will allow for the development of novel therapies that target disease maintenance pathways. Similarly, elucidation of the cell-intrinsic pathways and extrinsic signals required for HSC self-renewal will allow investigators to develop methods to expand HSCs from autologous sources or induced pluripotent stem cells (iPSCs) induced to differentiate into HSCs *ex vivo*. Thus, patients who previously could not receive a therapeutic bone marrow transplant due to the absence of suitable donors or sufficient numbers of HSCs will have access to this life-saving treatment.

So how does the hematopoietic system maintain homeostasis when it is responsible for the production of more than 1 million mature cells per second over the lifetime of the average human adult? This requires a highly adaptable system of complex feedback mechanisms that maintain HSCs as well as allow them to give rise to appropriate hematopoietic cells in response to physiologic stress. In this chapter we will describe the factors that regulate normal HSC function as well as those

that help to give rise to the diversity of cell types that make up this dynamic system. We will discuss the important contributions of the numerous growth factors and cytokines that have long been appreciated to regulate hematopoiesis as well as emerging data that demonstrate that local, systemic, and nervous system inputs play important roles in regulating hematopoiesis. In addition, we will discuss how our understanding of HSC function and differentiation has influenced our view of the pathogenesis of hematologic disorders. Finally, it should be noted that our detailed understanding of hematopoiesis is the result of an enormous effort by a large group of scientists and is also a constantly evolving field. Thus, we apologize in advance to our colleagues for the work we could not cite or discuss due to space limitations.

ORGANIZATION OF THE HEMATOPOIETIC SYSTEM

The hematopoietic system is initiated and maintained by the HSC, which has the ability not only to give rise to all the different cell types of the hematopoietic system, but also to give rise to other HSCs for the lifetime of an organism through a process termed self-renewal. HSCs lie at the top of a hierarchically organized developmental system in which they give rise to progenitors that become increasingly lineage-restricted, or committed (Fig. 1.1). Of note, it is also worth emphasizing proper usage of the term HSC. Usage of this term can be confusing since investigators frequently use this term when referring to heterogeneous populations. As we will discuss later, such populations (e.g., human CD34+ cells, mouse Lin–Sca+c-Kit+ or LSK cells) represent immature hematopoietic populations that comprise a minority of HSCs. Thus, we prefer to use the term "hematopoietic stem/progenitor cells" (HS/PCs) to more accurately reflect the biologic heterogeneity represented in these cell populations. While some committed progenitors do have the ability to self-renew for short periods of time (days to weeks), HSCs are distinguished from progenitors by virtue of their ability to self-renew for long periods of time (months to years). Lineage-committed progenitors, sometimes also referred to as transit-amplifying cells, proliferate more rapidly than HSCs, and as such, they give to numerous progeny that continue to mature to generate terminally differentiated cells. Because of their enormous expansion potential, committed progenitors can give rise to the large number of cells required to reconstitute and maintain the various cellular components of the blood. It is now clear that HSCs give rise to short-term HSCs (defined in the mouse by their ability to give rise to lymphomyeloid reconstituted grafts for <6 months when transplanted into secondary hosts), multipotent progenitors (MPPs) (giving rise to lymphomyeloid cells for <16 weeks), common myeloid progenitors (CMPs), common lymphoid progenitors (CLPs), granulocyte-macrophage progenitors (GMPs), megakaryocyte-erythroid progenitors (MEPs), as well as single lineage restricted progenitors for T, B, natural

1

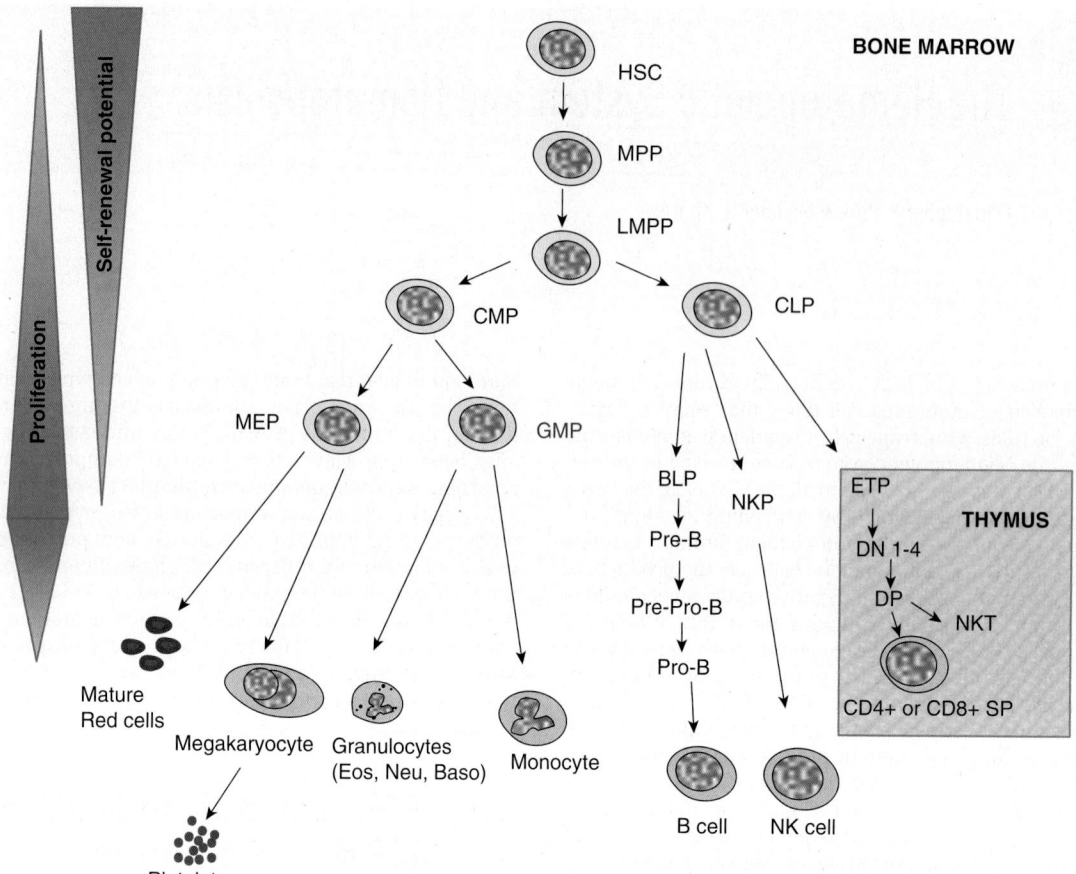

FIGURE 1.1. Hierarchy of hematopoiesis. Hematopoiesis is initiated by the hematopoietic stem cell (HSC), which gives rise to progenitors that exhibit increasing lineage restriction and decreased self-renewal with differentiation, ultimately giving rise to the postmitotic, terminally differentiated hematopoietic cells of the various lineages. While most hematopoietic development occurs in the bone marrow, T-cell development occurs in the thymus, which is seeded by a bone marrow–derived progenitor. MPP, multipotent progenitor; LMPP, lymphoid primed multipotent progenitor; CMP, common myeloid progenitor; CLP, common lymphoid progenitor; MEP, megakaryocyte-erythroid progenitor; GMP, granulocyte-macrophage progenitor; BLP, B-cell lymphoid progenitor; NKP, natural killer progenitor; ETP; early thymocyte progenitor; NKT, natural killer/T cells; Eos, eosinophils; Neu, neutrophils; Baso, basophils; NK cells, natural killer cells.

killer (NK), and dendritic cells (Fig. 1.1). While differentiated progenitors exhibit increasingly lineage restricted potential as well as loss of self-renewal capacity, one important exception to this basic rule is the memory lymphocyte, which has the capacity to persist for a lifetime, even after successive rounds of expansion and contraction when rechallenged with antigen.

Much of our knowledge regarding the functional and molecular properties of HSCs is based on studies of the mouse hematopoietic system due to the relative ease of performing transplantation studies using congenic models, which allow discrimination of donor and recipient cells based on differential expression of CD45 alleles (1). Unfortunately, studies with human HSCs have been limited by the lack of experimental models that allowed engraftment of immunologically incompatible human grafts in mouse hosts. Fortunately, our understanding of the organization and molecular mechanisms that regulate the human hematopoietic system has improved tremendously due to the development of experimental models allowing transplantation of human HSCs into immunodeficient mice. These studies demonstrate that while the mouse and human hematopoietic systems share many features, they also exhibit unique properties with respect to the molecular control of differentiation and the hierarchical organization of the hematopoietic systems. Equally important in improving our understanding of hematopoiesis was the development of *in vitro* assays that serve as important complementary techniques to study HSC biology. These *in vitro* assays allow assessment of lineage potential as well as surrogates of self-renewal such as the ability to serially

replate and form colonies, as well as the ability to form cells that can reconstitute transplanted recipients after long culture periods; however, these assays are limited by their inability to faithfully recapitulate all the elements of the endogenous hematopoietic microenvironment, and thus all *in vitro* studies must be interpreted with caution and confirmed by *in vivo* studies. In this chapter, we will refer to studies utilizing both mouse and human hematopoietic cells. In most cases, similar findings were observed in both systems, but we will highlight differences when relevant. As our understanding of hematopoiesis continues to evolve, it will be important to be aware of potential differences between humans and other model organisms and to confirm findings using human cells when experimentally possible (2).

IDENTIFICATION OF THE HEMATOPOIETIC STEM CELL

The first efforts to identify HSCs were inspired by the observation that death following radiation exposure is due to hematopoietic failure. This was experimentally confirmed by demonstrating that irradiated mice survive by either shielding the spleen during irradiation or by transplanting spleen or bone marrow cells following exposure to lethal doses (3–5). Later studies showed that radioprotection is not conferred by HSCs, but by more committed PCs that rapidly give rise to mature cells. Formal demonstration of the existence of HSCs was accomplished nearly a decade later by Till and McCullough, who showed that clonal hematopoietic cells can give rise to all the cells of the various myeloerythroid lineages (granulocytes, macrophages, red cells, megakaryocytes), that some of these cells possess the ability to generate more of themselves (now referred to as self-renewal), and that the spleens of these mice contained cells that could give rise to lymphocytes (6–10). It is interesting to note that while these studies relied on measuring the ability of transplanted cells to form colonies in the spleen (CFU-S) 10 days after transplantation into irradiated hosts, later studies showed that these spleen colony seeding cells actually represent committed progenitors, not HSCs (11–13). Nonetheless, these studies heralded the beginning of the fields of HSC biology and hematopoietic transplantation as it became clear that the ability to replace the hematopoietic systems of irradiated hosts could be therapeutically applied. These studies eventually led to the first successful human allogeneic bone marrow transplant performed by E. Donnell Thomas in 1956. His pioneering work in bone marrow transplantation resulted in his receipt of the Nobel Prize in Physiology or Medicine in 1990.

Although HSCs were shown to exist in the mid-1950s, it was not until the late 1980s that they were prospectively purified from mammals. While experiments using retrospective genetic marking techniques had provided evidence that HSCs existed (8,14), the only way to understand the specific contribution of these cells to transplantation biology, or even to show that self-renewal was limited to a specific cell type, was through their prospective separation. Moreover, limiting dilution analysis of transplanted mouse bone marrow cells determined that HSCs are rare, with early estimated HSC frequencies ranging from 1 in 10,000 to 1 in 100,000 cells in the bone marrow (1,15,16). Early experiments relied on techniques that physically separated cells based on differences in size and density (17,18), but then eventually relied primarily on differences in cell surface protein expression (19), which was only possible due to the advent of new technologies including the ability to generate monoclonal antibodies as well as the ability to identify cells by flow cytometry and separate cells using fluorescence activated cell sorting (FACS) based on the seminal work of Leonard Herzenberg (20,21). Irving Weissman et al. (22) then demonstrated that cells meeting all the functional criteria for HSCs could be isolated from the mouse bone marrow in 1988. This discovery was followed by the isolation of human HSCs, initially using *in vitro* systems, and then followed by *in vivo* experiments utilizing immunodeficient mouse models (discussed below in section "Developing Xenograft transplant models").

Taking advantage of improved flow cytometry techniques and the discovery of genes differentially expressed in immature hematopoietic cells versus their differentiated progeny, HSC activity has been increasingly purified in both the human and mouse systems. Initial attempts using flow cytometry relied on eliminating cells expressing markers of mature hematopoietic cells (the so-called lineage negative or Lin⁻ cell fraction) (23–30), and later studies identified other markers enriching HS/PCs including c-Kit (in mouse and humans) (30,31) and CD34 (in humans) (32). After decades of work, the mouse HSC can be purified at a frequency of approximately one in two cells and can initiate long-term hematopoiesis when transplanted into the same mouse strain (see Table 1.1 for frequencies of HSCs) (33,34). While all investigators do not use the same markers to identify HSCs, it is standard to isolate mouse HSCs from lineage low/negative cells (lacking Gr-1, Mac-1, Ter119, CD4, CD8, B220, CD3) that are also c-Kit⁺, Sca-1⁺, CD34⁻, CD150⁺ (SLAMf150), CD48⁻. Of note, additional markers have also been shown to enrich for HSCs including rhodamine-low Hoechst-negative, CD49bˡᵒ, Flkˡᵒ, Esam1⁺, Endoglin⁺, and others (35). Unfortunately, most of these markers have been validated for mouse HSCs and many do not similarly purify human HSCs. For example, human HSCs express CD34 and the FLT3

Table 1.1	FREQUENCY OF HEMATOPOIETIC STEM CELLS IN MOUSE BONE MARROW
Cell Population	**HSC Frequency**
Bulk bone marrow cells	<1:20,000
Lin⁻	~1:2,500
Lin⁻c-Kit⁺Sca-1⁺ (LSK)	~1:25
Lin⁻c-Kit⁺Sca-1⁺CD34⁻ (LSK34⁻)	~1:5
Lin⁻CD34+CD38⁻Rhoˡᵒʷ	~1:30
Lin⁻c-Kit⁺Sca-1⁺CD34⁻CD48⁻CD150⁺ (LSK34⁻)	~1:2

receptor, while mouse HSCs do not (36); similarly, mouse HSCs express CD150, whereas human HSCs do not (37).

DEVELOPING XENOGRAFT TRANSPLANT MODELS

The ability to perform transplants in histocompatible recipients helped facilitate the identification of HSCs in mouse, but such systems are not possible to study human HSCs *in vivo*. The development of immunodeficient mouse models has allowed xenogeneic transplantation to serve as a surrogate assay for human HSC activity. Such assays were first described in the 1980s with the severe combined immune deficient (SCID) and hu-SCID animal models (38), and further improved with the NOD/SCID, NOD/SCID/β_2 microglobulin null (39) NOD/SCID/IL2R gamma common chain null (NSG) (40–42), RAG2/IL2R gamma common chain null (43,44), and NOD/RAG2/IL2R gamma common chain null mice (45). Using these models, initial estimates of human hematopoietic repopulating activity, termed SCID-repopulating units, was estimated at 1 in 9.3×10^5 mononuclear cells (46), and 1 in 617 CD34⁺CD38⁻Lin⁻ cells (47). Purification of human cells engrafting immunodeficient mice resulted in progressively enriched HSCs characterized by expression of CD34 (42,48), followed by descriptions of CD34⁺CD38⁻ (47,49), Lin⁻CD34⁺CD38⁻ (47,50), and Lin⁻CD34⁺CD38⁻CD90⁺ immunophenotypes (51–53). These findings were followed by the finding that the combination of CD90 and CD45RA markers can distinguish between long-term and short-term engrafting cells (54). Most recently, investigators showed that long-term engrafting HSCs could be further enriched from Lin-CD34⁺CD38⁻CD90⁺CD45RA⁻ cells based on expression of the integrin CD49f, while CD90⁻CD49f⁻ cells could transiently repopulate hosts with lymphomyeloid grafts for up to 16 weeks, consistent with an MPP. Furthermore, they showed that as few as one in two cells present in this highly purified cell population could initiate long-term lymphomyeloid grafts when transplanted into NSG mice lacking T, B, and NK cells (see Table 1.2 for HSC frequencies in human bone marrow populations) (55).

Assays to Measure Hematopoietic Lineage Potential and Self-Renewal

Despite the early adoption of human bone marrow transplantation as a therapeutic modality, our understanding of the molecular mechanisms that regulate HS/PC function were severely hampered by the lack of experimental models to study human cells as well as the use of time-consuming and resource-intensive transplantation studies. Investigations of HS/PCs were greatly aided by the development of *in vitro* culturing techniques in the 1970s including the Whitlock-Witte culture and its variants, which used a combination of recombinant cytokines, semisolid support media including methylcellulose, and/or bone marrow

Table 1.2	FREQUENCY OF HEMATOPOIETIC STEM CELLS IN HUMAN BONE MARROW		
Cell Population	HSC Frequency	Assay System	Reference
Bulk bone marrow cells CD34+	1/1e6	SCID SCID/beige/XID NOD/SCID NOD/ SCIDIL2Rgamma null (NOG) mice	Wang et al. (46) Dick et al. (48) Shultz et al. (42)
Lin−CD34+CD90−	N/A	In vitro SCID-hu mice	McCune et al. (38) Murray et al. (52)
Lin−CD34+CD38−	~1:600	NOD/SCID	Bhatia et al. (47) Hogan (55a)
Lin−CD34+CD38−Rholow	~1:30	SCID	McKenzie et al. (55b)
Lin−CD34+CD38−CD90+CD45RA−	~1:10	NSG	Majeti et al. (54)
Lin−CD34+CD38−CD90+CD45RA−CD49fSPlo	~1:2	NSG	Notta et al. (55) Science et al. 2011

or fetal liver–derived stromal support cells, to allow for growth of hematopoietic colonies in vitro (56). Following culturing, the resulting cells could be assessed for reconstitution potential in transplantation assays, thereby allowing incorporation of an in vivo readout into these experiments. While in vitro assays are very convenient systems to characterize alterations in hematopoiesis and to support conclusions based on in vivo functional evaluation of HS/PCs, it should be stressed that these assays are primarily assays of PC function and that true HSC function can only be determined by in vivo transplantation assays, which are described below.

HSCs can be cultured long-term when cocultured with pre-established stromal layers, and the physical association of HSCs with stromal cells is presumed to be required to recapitulate HSC interactions with the bone marrow microenvironment (57). This method has been modified to assess the ability of hematopoietic cells to migrate and grow beneath the established stromal layer to form "cobblestone-area forming cells" (CAFCs) (58–60), which are presumed to recapitulate the interactions between HSCs and their specialized niche since CAFC frequency at different time points following culture initiation correlates well with different colony-forming activities using other assays including CFU (in culture), and CFU-S on day 12 (CFU-S-12), and marrow-repopulating activity. A similar in vitro culturing technique involves growing HSCs on stromal layers followed by the assessment of PC colony-forming ability, otherwise known as the long-term culture-initiating cell (LTC-IC) assay. Instead of scoring CAFC, the LTC-IC determines the presence of committed progenitors by replacing the culture medium after 5 to 6 weeks of culture with a semisolid medium such as methylcellulose and scoring for colonies arising 7 to 14 days later (61,62). This assay was used initially to assess human HSC growth in vitro (61), but was also useful to measure mouse HSC frequency and was modified to support lymphomyeloid progenitors (62). While the CAFC and LTC-IC assays are the only in vitro assays that have the ability to measure HS/PC frequencies as verified by long-term in vivo reconstitution experiments and can provide a basis for comparisons with long-term repopulating activity in radiosensitivity (63), or cytotoxicity (64) assays, their utility as predictors of HSC activity under all conditions is not clear, and in some cases, the two assays may generate conflicting results; this appears to depend on the specific stromal line used and the accessory cells (65–68). On balance, it is likely that these assays reflect the activity of immature hematopoietic cells, but they do not allow direct assessment of HSCs.

Colony-forming cell (CFC) assays, first described in the 1960s (69,70), and later modified for human hematopoiesis (71,72), evaluate the growth of individual HS/PC clones in semisolid agar—or defined methylcellulose-based culture media containing cytokines that support the growth of hematopoietic progenitors that can give rise to the erythroid, myeloid, lymphoid, and megakaryocytic lineages (73). The semisolid nature of the media prevents the migration of PCs, and thus the colonies are clonal, arising from single cells. These colonies represent the progeny from progenitors that can give rise to single, dual, or multiple lineages including erythroid-restricted burst-forming units-erythroid (BFU-E), which are presumed to arise from more immature cells than colony-forming units-erythroid (CFU-E), since they produce larger numbers of mature progeny. Additional types of colonies that describe the types of hematopoietic cells produced include megakaryocyte-restricted (CFU-Mk), colony-forming units-granulocytes (CFU-G), and colony-forming units-granulocytes/macrophages (CFU-GM). Some colonies contain granulocytes, erythrocytes, macrophages, and/or megakaryocytes (CFU-GEMM or CFU-mixed). These are usually measured 12 days after initiation of the culture and are presumed to arise from a primitive progenitor. Generation of B- and T-lymphocyte CFCs is more difficult than for the myeloid lineages and therefore typically requires specialized coculture systems (74,75), although a commercially available methylcellulose-based colony assay to measure pre-B cells is available. As the cellular composition of individual colonies can be determined on the basis of colony morphology, by cytologic evaluation of cells in individual colonies, or by flow cytometric evaluation of individual colonies, the lineage potential of individual HS/PCs can be readily assessed. As colonies are largely derived from PCs, serial replating assays using the progeny of cells generated in methylcellulose or liquid cultures can be used to reinitiate similar cultures sequentially. HSC-enriched populations can give rise to colonies during serial replatings in methylcellulose, and therefore gains and losses of HSC self-renewal can be estimated in this manner.

When the soft agar and methylcellulose colony assays were first developed, the concept that factor(s) could increase colony formation was postulated and they were named colony stimulating factors (CSFs) (69,70,76). Over the next two decades, the purification, cloning, and characterization of four different CSFs was accomplished including M-CSF, GM-CSF, G-CSF, and multi-CSF, with most of the cloning of the CSFs completed in the 1980s (IL-3). Both GM-CSF and G-CSF were found to be robust promoters of neutrophil development and activation, as well as mobilization of HSC/progenitors. Many laboratories over the years have utilized these factors for understanding myeloid development. Most importantly, these factors have become extraordinary therapies for treating neutropenic patients and mobilizing HSCs into the peripheral blood as a superior source of blood donor cells (77–80). Indeed, because of the ability to generate mobilized peripheral blood HS/PC grafts, the use of traditional bone marrow grafts for transplantation is now dwindling.

While myeloid and lymphoid cells develop from HSCs and MPPs, they require different external cues to execute their differentiation programs, and therefore different culture conditions are required to efficiently generate them in vitro. Development of lymphocytes in vitro can be achieved with specialized coculture systems (74,75). However, similar to the initial transplantation studies in which CFU-S were initially mistaken as initiated by HSCs (6), the cellular origins of colonies generated in these assays is not uniform. Colony types can be incorporated into a hierarchical scheme of hematopoiesis based on their lineage output, with multilineage colonies presumed to arise from the most immature cells and lineage-restricted colonies presumed to arise from lineage-restricted progenitors (81). However, since even the most highly purified HSCs can give rise to both multilineage and restricted colony types when cultured in methylcellulose, the colony assay is not necessarily reflective of *in vivo* potential. Moreover, these assays cannot efficiently promote significant self-renewal of HSCs since they cannot faithfully recapitulate all of the features of the bone marrow microenvironment. The relationships between distinct HS/PC populations identified based on cell surface marker expression and the CFU initiating cells has been determined for a subset of mouse erythroid progenitors (82), but these correlations have not been rigorously characterized for most mouse and human PC populations. Because of difficulties in defining human HSCs functionally using the serial transplantation assay, identification of candidate human progenitor populations has largely relied on *in vitro* assays. Using *in vitro* culturing conditions such as methylcellulose colony assays and stromal coculture models, investigators were able to identify candidate CLPs (83,84) as well as multiple myeloid progenitor populations including the CMP, GMP, and MEP (85). Finally, additional caution is required regarding identification of specific HS/PC populations using cell surface markers in genetically manipulated models since surface marker profiles may be altered under such conditions, thereby providing misleading conclusions from sorted cells.

Experimental demonstration of HSC activity requires long-term repopulation or reconstitution assays. This typically involves transplantation of cells into irradiated or otherwise compromised hosts, and in mice these experiments are aided by the presence of different alleles of the hematopoietic marker CD45, in which CD45.1 and CD45.2 represent donor and recipient alleles. Following transplantation, donor engraftment levels can be assessed by flow cytometry using the CD45 congenic marker as well as lineage markers, with long-term HSCs defined by their ability to give rise to myeloid lineage cells for at least 16 weeks posttransplant. Lymphoid cells are not considered good indicators of ongoing HSC contributions to the hematopoiesis since they can persist for long periods of time after their generation, especially through the generation of memory lymphocytes. In some cases, transplantation is performed in the presence of competitor bone marrow cells derived from mice with the same CD45 allele as the host, allowing the donor and competitor HSCs to be compared with respect to engraftment capacity (15,16), but it does not necessarily allow for direct quantification of HSC frequency or number. In order to calculate the frequency of competitive repopulating units (CRUs), the limiting dilution assay is used. In these experiments, test cells are titrated, transplanted into congenic hosts, and then the percentage of hosts that fail to engraft donor cells is determined. With a minimum of three different doses tested in which positive and negative recipients are present, a best-line fit can be generated by Poisson statistics to calculate the number of CRUs, or HSCs (86,87).

While all of the previously described assays can assess the ability of candidate HSC populations to reconstitute hosts, the most stringent test of stem cell activity is the serial transplantation assay (14). In this gold standard assay, cells from primary recipients are transplanted successively into irradiated recipients for up to a maximum of five to seven rounds (due to the finite self-renewal of normal HSCs) (88,89). However, it should be noted that transplantation itself stresses HSCs, with the process of transplantation being sufficient to induce HSC cell cycling that can last for at least 4 months after transplant (90). Indeed, recent studies suggest that transplantation into irradiated hosts is sufficient to affect HSC function by promoting a myeloid lineage bias (91). Thus, alternative methods to engraft donor cells without irradiation may become a more common strategy to evaluate HSC function, as both genetic mouse models (e.g., those mutant in c-Kit such as W/W^v) (92,93) and antibody-mediated conditioning regimens (94) also allow engraftment of transplanted HSCs. One caveat that warrants mentioning is that these assays, while assessing the presence

of self-renewing cells, also assume that the self-renewing cells mature normally. This may, in fact, not be the case for mutant cells in which downstream progenitors gain aberrant self-renewal or fail to mature normally (95). In such cases, readouts may be misleading and therefore more detailed evaluation of specific HS/PC populations may be required to determine the specific developmental stage at which functional defects manifest. Finally, it should be noted that noncompetitive transplants most closely mimic the clinical situation, and that competitive transplants may, in fact, yield misleading negative results, especially if the number of cells tested is small, or if test, transplanted HSCs are outcompeted, even though they were functional under normal, steady-state hematopoiesis prior to being harvested for transplantation studies (96).

Development of the Hematopoietic System

While the major site of hematopoiesis in the adult is the bone marrow, the major sites of hematopoiesis during embryonic development are in the yolk sac followed by the fetal liver. Thus, it is likely that factors that regulate HSCs are developmental stage and cell context dependent. Investigation of the factors that regulate HSCs in each site of hematopoiesis is likely to provide insight into the cell-intrinsic and cell-extrinsic factors that regulate HSC function. Some of the earliest discoveries in developmental hematopoiesis originated from studies performed in vertebrate model organisms including zebrafish, *Xenopus*, and chicken. For more thorough reviews on these developmental systems please refer to Refs. (97–100). Our understanding of early mammalian hematopoiesis is largely drawn from investigations in mice. Recent studies of *in vitro* directed hematopoietic differentiation from embryonic stem cells (ESCs) and iPSCs have also been an important source of information regarding the earliest commitment to the hematopoietic lineage, and this approach holds great promise as a tractable system for generating large numbers of HSCs *ex vivo*.

During mammalian embryonic development, blood cells arise in two phases (Fig. 1.2). During the first phase, also known as embryonic hematopoiesis, primitive erythrocytes and myeloid cells are generated in the yolk sac. This phase is followed by definitive hematopoiesis, which is defined by the emergence of definitive HSCs (dHSCs), which are capable of giving rise to all mature adult blood cell types (erythroid, myeloid, and lymphoid) as well as reconstituting multilineage hematopoiesis when transplanted into adult recipients. Thus, during embryonic hematopoiesis, committed blood precursors appear prior to dHSCs. This phenomenon is thought to reflect the needs of the developing embryo, since embryonic hematopoiesis allows the embryo to address its short-term need for proper oxygenation, while definitive hematopoiesis allows the organism to establish and maintain lifelong hematopoiesis. While this model makes evolutionary sense, it is not clear whether embryonic and definitive (adult) hematopoiesis occur independently or are initiated simultaneously from a common ancestor. While both models have been proposed, the latter would require one to hypothesize that the common ancestor is not detectable using standard transplantation assays since there is no experimental evidence of a multilineage HSC during early development.

The first evidence of blood formation in the mouse occurs in the yolk sac between E7.0 and 7.5 during mouse development (mouse gestation is ~21 days, with gestational day denoted with a preceding "E") as the extraembryonic mesoderm ingresses through the posterior primitive streak (101). While hematopoietic cells were first identified in the yolk sac in the late 19th century, it was not until the early 1970s that investigators were able to demonstrate the presence of hematopoiesis in the yolk sac using the novel *in vitro* hematopoietic assays developed at that time (102). Later, more stringent assays requiring regeneration of CFU-S *in vivo* were utilized to show that the yolk sac

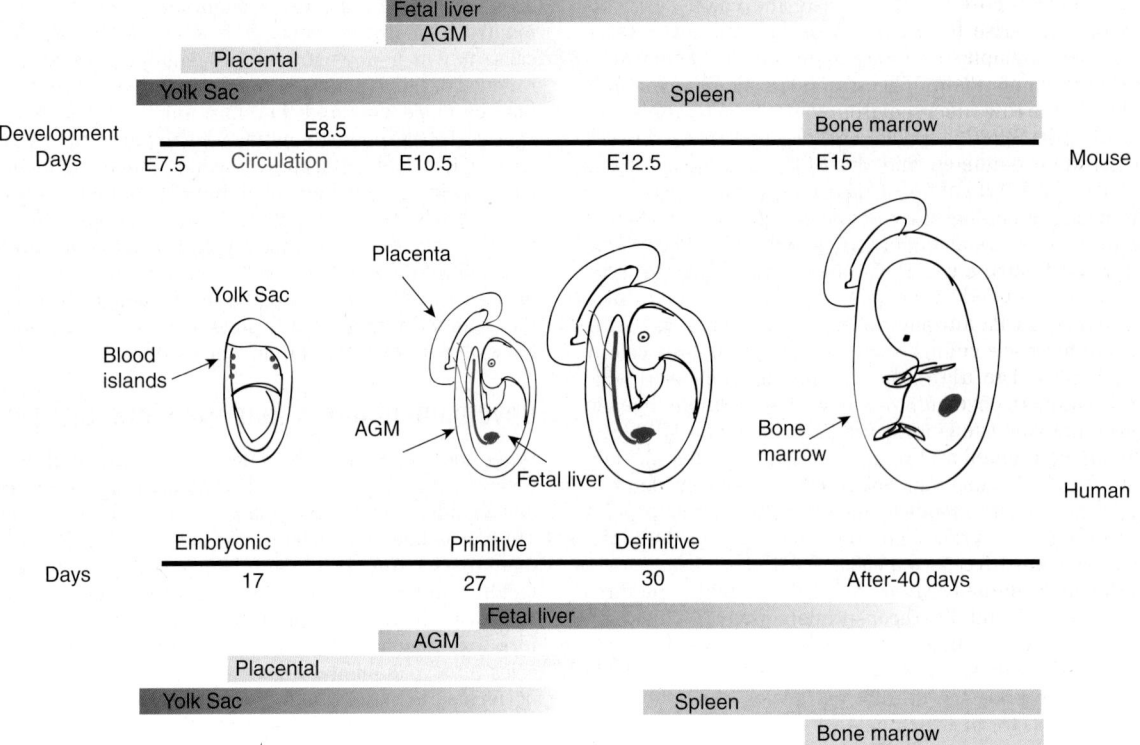

FIGURE 1.2. Developmental hematopoiesis in mouse and humans. The major sites of hematopoiesis shift during embryonic and fetal development with hematopoiesis starting in the yolk sac, then shifting to the aorto-gonado-mesonephros (AGM), then to the fetal liver, and then to the bone marrow. The *arrows* indicate the various sites of hematopoiesis based on the developmental stage. In the mouse, the developmental stage is designated based on the day postconception (E). *Colored boxes* indicate the different waves of hematopoiesis.

lacks CFU-S prior to E9.5 and that dHSCs are absent prior to E11.5 (103,104).

dHSCs form in the aorto-gonado-mesonephros (AGM) region, where they can be generated autonomously (103,104), and explants of AGM are able to initiate and expand dHSCs at E10.5 and E11.5, respectively (105). It is likely that the AGM is the major source of dHSCs since they cannot be initiated or expanded from other hematopoietic tissues (106,107), while AGM derived and AGM explants can be cultured in the presence of appropriate growth factors to give rise to a 150-fold expansion of dHSCs (108,109).

While the first blood cells arise from the wall of the aorta of the developing embryo, typified by the generation of RBCs and macrophages, the site of hematopoiesis shifts to the fetal liver later during development as dHSCs from the AGM region, placenta, and yolk sac (105,110) colonize the liver at E12.5 to establish definitive hematopoiesis in a process that likely requires $\beta1$ integrins (111,112). Once in the liver, dHSCs expand through the action of molecules that promote proliferation such as angiopoietin-like factors and the Sox17 transcription factor (113,114). At this point, HSCs can be detected experimentally using standard transplantation assays in adult animals.

The relationship between embryonic sites of hematopoiesis and adult hematopoiesis remains a source of controversy. While the presence of yolk sac hematopoiesis and AGM generation of dHSC activity strongly suggest that adult mammalian hematopoiesis originates in the embryo, this does not exclude the possibility that the yolk sac directly contributes to adult hematopoiesis and that embryonic ancestors of dHSCs are not detectable simply due to their inability to engraft adult recipients. Using such assays, dHSCs have also been identified outside of the AGM in the embryo (99,115).

The importance of the circulation in inducing early hematopoiesis has been the subject of intense investigation in recent years. The initial indication of a functional link between the

vascular system and hematopoiesis was shown in mouse mutant models. *Ncx-1* null mice fail to develop beating hearts but do develop erythrocytes and CFU-Cs in the yolk sac normally; however, their body lacks these progenitors, indicating that AGM hematopoietic activity depends on colonization by yolk sac cells (116). Similarly, *Rac1* mutant embryos exhibit impaired cell migration from the yolk sac to the body proper, which results in a similar phenotype (117). Together, these studies showed dissociation between the establishment of hematopoiesis in the yolk sac and the AGM, and they also showed that yolk sac–derived precursors colonize the AGM region.

The importance of mechanical stress generated by blood flow on endothelial cell function has been long appreciated (118). Endothelial cells respond to shear stress via expression of mechanoreceptors, resulting in the induction of specific genes, and one of the major products induced by such stress is nitric oxide (NO) (119). These observations led a number of groups to hypothesize that the physical forces generated by blood flow may induce hematopoietic cell formation from the endothelium lining the AGM region via NO signaling. Validation of this hypothesis involved experiments in which shear stress was recreated *in vitro*, resulting in both ESCs and AGM-derived cells up-regulating *Runx1* and *cellular myeloblastosis viral oncogene homolog (c-Myb)* with an accompanying increase in CFU-C production (120). These effects could be suppressed by addition of inhibitors of NO signaling (120,121). Additionally, evaluation of "silent-heart" zebrafish mutants that lack blood flow revealed that the number of Runx1+ and CD41+ HS/PCs was markedly reduced (121,122). The dependence of this phenotype on NO production was confirmed by treating with an NO donor, s-nitroso-*N*-acetylpenicillamine, which rescued the phenotype. Finally, mice lacking *nitric oxide synthase 3* (*Nos3*) demonstrated defects in AGM hematopoietic development, confirming these studies (121).

The intimate relationship between the vascular and hematopoietic systems has been appreciated for many years, leading some to propose that the endothelial and hematopoietic systems may arise from a common, bipotent progenitor called the hemangioblast. Indeed, early blood islands first appear as clusters of cells immediately surrounded by an outer endothelial lining (123,124). These blood islands eventually give rise to endothelial networks filled with blood, and these areas of blood formation encircle the yolk sac in a single, belt-like structure (125). While there was no experimental evidence of a hemangioblast in the developing embryo for more than a century, *in vitro* ESC blast colony assays finally provided the first evidence for such a cell (126–128). Subsequently, equivalent cells were identified in the mouse embryo within the posterior primitive streak, and these cells were also shown to give rise to smooth muscle cells, providing evidence for a tripotent progenitor (129). The difficulties in identifying a hemangioblast earlier during development is likely due to the fact that by the time the yolk sac is colonized by hemangioblasts, they have already committed to the endothelial and hematopoietic lineages.

While these studies provide evidence for a hemangioblast-like precursor in developing embryos, it is not clear whether endothelial cells can give rise to hematopoietic cells later during embryogenesis or to the adult hematopoietic system. Evidence for such hemogenic endothelium in the developing embryo has been supported by live imaging studies in which it was demonstrated that aortic endothelium in zebrafish (130,131), or AGM region cells in mouse (132) give rise to dHSCs directly. But what is the relationship between the hemangioblast and hemogenic endothelium? A recent study proposed that FLK1+ hemangioblasts generate hemogenic endothelium first, when they generate hematopoietic cells (133). While these studies demonstrate the presence of hemogenic endothelium, it is important to note that only a small subset of endothelial cells have this capacity. In the mouse yolk sac, it is estimated that <2% of total endothelial cells at E8.5 (134,135) and within the AGM at E10.5 exhibit this potential (136).

While hemogenic endothelium can generate multilineage HS/PCs in the yolk sac, AGM, and placenta, evidence for hemogenic endothelium in the fetal liver and bone marrow is lacking. While such cells may possess such potential, it is likely that the fates of hemogenic endothelium progeny may depend on their site of origin or developmental stage. For example, hemogenic endothelial cells within the yolk sac can give rise to MPPs *in vitro* (137), but they have limited capacity to do so when transplanted *in vivo* (103). In contrast, the multilineage precursors (dHSCs) from the AGM can repopulate neonatal and adult recipients. Overall, these observations support a model in which HSCs are born in the yolk sac and AGM and then migrate to subsequent sites of definitive hematopoiesis (i.e., the fetal liver and bone marrow).

In the mouse, HSCs leave the liver to colonize the bones by E17.5 and through the first 2 weeks of postnatal life. They are actively recruited by the chemokine CXCL12/SDF-1 through interactions with CXCR4 expressed on HSCs (138). In humans, liver hematopoiesis is established at approximately 23 days of gestation (139). Additional factors promote localization of HSC to the bone marrow in concert with CXCR4 such as prostaglandin E2 and Robo4 (140,141) or through effects independent of CXCR4 including c-Kit, the calcium-sensing receptor, and the transcription factor Egr1 (142–144). Once entering the specialized bone marrow niche in the bone marrow, HSCs remain in the niche through integrin-dependent interactions (145,146). However, a small percentage of HSCs flux out of the bone marrow into the circulation before returning to the bone marrow niche even during homeostatic hematopoiesis (147,148), which explains why the cellular composition of the adult bone marrow appears similar regardless of the bone marrow site sampled.

Late during embryonic development (e.g., third trimester in humans), hematopoiesis slowly shifts to the bone marrow and coincident with this transition, numerous other changes occur in the hematopoietic system. HSC expansion becomes attenuated and self-renewal decreases such that at the time of birth, the human hematopoietic system is maximally proliferative, allowing for expansion of the blood-forming capability of the maturing young human.

Characteristics of Hematopoietic Stem Cells

We now know that in addition to their properties of self-renewal and multilineage differentiation, HSCs exhibit other characteristics that distinguish them from lineage-committed progenitors and other hematopoietic cells. One of the most frequently described features of adult HSCs is their relative quiescence. Approximately 5% of total bone marrow HSCs are actively cycling (defined as S, G2, or M phases) at any given time during adult life as demonstrated by stains that distinguish the cell cycle status as well as pulse-labeling experiments that allow investigators to estimate the frequency at which HSCs undergo cell division (149–151). Interestingly, this characteristic of HSCs is established as rapidly as 4 weeks after birth, even though HSCs in the mouse fetal liver actively cycle with 95% to 100% of HSCs cycling with a cell cycle transit time of 10 to 14 hours (150,152). Using markers of cell division such as BrdU retention and histone 2B-green fluorescent protein dilution, bone marrow HSCs exhibit heterogeneity in their degree of quiescence (153,154) and appear to be composed of cells (5% to 10% of HSCs) that can be readily recruited into cell cycle as well as those that are relatively resistant to cycling. Estimations of division times suggest that dormant HSCs divide only once every 145 days or more and are enriched for long-term reconstitution potential. This has led to the hypothesis that the relatively dormant pool of HSCs may represent a reservoir of HSC activity only called upon to cycle during stress hematopoiesis. Interestingly, human HSCs appear to enter the cell cycle on average only once every 40 weeks (155), indicating a significant species difference in HSC cell cycling.

The importance of HSC quiescence is perhaps best exemplified by the poor performance of HSCs in the S-G2-M phases of the cell cycle to reconstitute recipients in transplantation studies, suggesting that cycling itself severely compromises adult HSC self-renewal (152,156). Other examples linking cell cycling to impaired HSC self-renewal are observed in mice lacking *p21* (157), *Gfi1* (158,159), and the thrombopoietin (TPO) receptor, *c-Mpl* (160). HSC self-renewal must also be maintained in other situations when HSCs undergo rapid expansion following bone marrow insult in the form of chemo-, radio-, or immunoablation (161,162), a point supported by the ability of single HSCs to long-term reconstitute the hematopoietic system of lethally irradiated recipients (163). While these studies indicate that cell cycling is a physiologic state in which HSCs may exhibit diminished self-renewal capacity, they also indicate that cycling does not, in and of itself, confer loss of self-renewal to HSCs. There is some suggestion that specific phases of the cell cycle may be particularly critical for maintaining HSC function since while fetal and adult HSCs divide at different frequencies, once they enter into the G1 phase of the cell cycle, both exhibit the same slow cell cycle transit rates compared to their more differentiated progeny (152). In addition, as noted previously, fetal liver and bone marrow HSCs possess the ability to undergo increased proliferation and expansion without exhaustion following marrow injury. Thus, HSC decisions to enter the cell cycle and the consequences of cell cycle entry appear to be context dependent, and likely depend on both cell-intrinsic and cell-extrinsic factors.

Due to the high turnover of the blood and the longevity of HSCs, it is important for HSCs to maintain themselves by avoiding senescence and maintaining a proper metabolic state. Consistent with this notion, HSCs exhibit elevated telomerase activity compared to committed progenitors and mature cells

(164). In addition, telomere erosion is associated with the decreased functional engraftment observed in aging HSCs or during serial transplantation of HSCs (90,165,166). Mice deficient in telomerase activity through deletion of the telomerase RNA component (Terc) exhibit progressive shortening of telomeres, reduced life span, decreased stress responsiveness, decreased hematopoietic cell proliferation, genetic instability, and increased spontaneous malignancies (167–169). *Terc* null mice showed decreased replating ability of CFU-GMs, reduced proliferative capacity of bone marrow cells, and reduced long-term reconstitution capacity and decreased serial replating capacity (90,170,171). Together, these data strongly suggest that telomere maintenance is critical for HSC maintenance.

HSCs also exhibit a unique metabolic state due to their relative quiescence as well as their presence in a hypoxic bone marrow microenvironment (172). Indeed, it is well established that HSCs cultured under hypoxic conditions exhibit better colony-forming and transplantation properties (173–175). However, as hypoxia also induces HSC quiescence (176,177), it is not clear whether the effects of hypoxia are independent of cell cycle kinetics/status. Moreover, mice lacking key metabolic enzymes including Lkb1 (178–180) and FoxO3 (181,182) experience significant HSC loss, indicating that HSCs are susceptible to cellular stressors, in particular, reactive oxygen species (ROS). Indeed, HSCs with lower levels of ROS retain higher reconstitution ability than those with higher levels of ROS, as assessed by staining with the ROS-sensitive substrate dihydro-dichlorofluorescein diacetate (183). Direct measurement of HSC mitochondrial activity has shown that HSCs have low mitochondrial activity and increased glycolysis; however, these changes in mitochondrial activity are thought to reflect the hypoxic environment (184). Such changes in mitochondrial metabolism have raised interest in the role of autophagy in HSC function. Consistent with this notion, LSK cells from mice deficient in *Atg7*, an essential component of the autophagosome, failed to reconstitute the hematopoietic system in lethally irradiated hosts (185). The loss of *Pten*, which induces constitutive phosphatidylinositol 3-kinase (PI3K)/Akt signaling, leads to HSC exhaustion (186,187), which can be restored by loss of p53 or p16^{Ink4a} (188). Thus, activation of HSC bioenergetic signaling through the PI3K/Akt/mTOR pathway is associated with increased HSC proliferation and exhaustion (189). In contrast, the loss of Akt signaling in *Akt1/Akt2* double knockout HSCs results in increased HSC quiescence and impaired differentiation, presumably by reducing ROS (190). Unfortunately, these data do not distinguish between mutational effects on HSC proliferation and loss of self-renewal, and thus whether or not HSC self-renewal depends on cell cycle status remains an open question.

Recent evidence suggests that HSCs possess unique DNA damage responses and DNA repair mechanisms that make them more stress tolerant. HSCs possess the ability to efflux drugs via ATP-dependent transporters such as the breast cancer resistance protein (Bcrp1, or Abcg2), presumably preventing HSCs from accumulating toxic molecules (191). HSCs have also developed mechanisms to cope with DNA damage. DNA double-stranded breaks that occur during the G$_0$ phase of the cell cycle in mice are p53 dependent (192) and immediately repaired by nonhomologous end-joining ability (193), which is more error prone than homologous recombination. Given the quiescent nature of HSCs, this is thought to lead to increased retention of mutations in HSCs (194). Paradoxically, this phenomenon is predicted to contribute to HSC senescence, apoptosis, and leukemic transformation since the acquired genetic changes through this DNA repair mechanism would be propagated to their progeny, thereby serving as the altered genetic context in which transforming events could occur (195–197). Interestingly, the DNA damage response appears to differ in human HSCs, which are sensitized to apoptosis after irradiation, leading to loss of damaged HSCs and improving maintenance of genomic integrity (198).

Regulators of HSC Function

While the determinants of HSC self-renewal are not completely understood, numerous cellular and molecular pathways, both cell-intrinsic and cell-extrinsic, have been implicated in HSC function. Cell-intrinsic pathways include cell cycle regulators, conserved developmental pathways, signal transduction pathways, epigenetic regulators, and RNA and posttranscriptional regulators. Because the number of factors that regulate HSC function is rather large, in this section we can only present some of the major pathways that regulate HSC function. We have attempted to provide a summary of experimentally validated HSC regulators (Table 1.3), but for a more complete discussion of these factors, we point the reader to a number of excellent reviews on this subject (35,199,200). Cell-extrinsic regulators of HSC function will be discussed within the broader context of the bone marrow microenvironment and its associated factors.

Cell Cycle Regulators

P53 and P21

Mice lacking *p53* show significant increase in HSC number as assessed by competitive reconstitution experiments using *p53*$^{-/-}$ bone marrow cells or purified LSK cells, as well as by cell surface immunophenotype (204,219). However, when more purified *p53*$^{-/-}$ HSCs were transplanted (Lin$^-$CD41$^-$CD150$^+$CD48$^-$), they showed lower levels of engraftment, consistent with reduced HSC function (219). This reduction in HSC potential is associated with relative loss of HSC quiescence (205). As cycling HSCs have been shown to possess decreased long-term reconstitution potential (220), it is possible that the increase in *p53*$^{-/-}$ HSC number and concomitant loss of engraftment capability may be due to increased cycling.

P21 is a cyclin-dependent kinase (Cdk) inhibitor that acts by binding to and inhibiting cyclin E/Cdk2 and cyclin D/Cdk4/6 complexes. Consistent with its negative regulatory role in cell cycle progression, mice deficient in p21 exhibit increased frequency of cycling HSC/progenitors as well as increased CFU frequency *in vitro* (157). However, when *p21* null HSC self-renewal was assessed through serial bone marrow transplants and multiple 5-fluorouracil (5-FU) treatments, they displayed an early exhaustion phenotype (157). While this led investigators to conclude that p21 is required to maintain HSC quiescence and hence self-renewal, more recent work using more highly purified HSCs (LSKCD48$^-$CD150$^+$) showed no differences in HSCs quiescence in *p21* null HSC (154). Another study confirmed a limited role for p21 in maintaining HSC quiescence during steady-state hematopoiesis, with *p21*-deficient HSCs showing a deficiency only in the context of competitive transplants using irradiated bone marrow cells (221).

Retinoblastoma

The retinoblastoma (Rb) family of transcriptional repressors, including *pRb*, *p107*, and *p130*, restricts cell cycle entry by repressing E2F-dependent transcription of positive cell cycle regulators including E-type cyclins. Rb proteins are regulated through phosphorylation events that alter their biologic activity, with hypophosphorylated Rb inhibiting entry into the G1 phase. Upon phosphorylation by cyclin dependent kinases such as the cyclin D-Cdk4/6 complex, Rb proteins are partially inactivated and cells are allowed to progress through G1. Subsequent phosphorylation by cyclin E-Cdk2 further inactivates Rb-mediated inhibition of E2F, resulting in G1 exit and entry into the S phase. In HSCs, a role for Rb in cell cycle regulation did not become evident until all family members were deleted, as *p130*-deficient mice did not exhibit a hematopoietic phenotype (222), *p107*-deficient mice only exhibited a mild myeloid hyperplasia (223), and *pRb*-deficient mice did not exhibit any defects in HSC self-renewal, although they did

Table 1.3	INTRINSIC CELLULAR REGULATORS OF HSCs			
Category	**HSC Phenotype**	**Genes**	**Details**	**Reference**
Cell cycle	Defect	Rb	Cell intrinsic/extrinsic effect	Walkley et al. (201)
				Walkley and Orkin (202)
		p21	Loss of quiescence/no phenotype	Cheng et al. (223a)
		p57	Quiescence and self-renewal	Zou et al. (203)
				Matsumoto et al. (223b)
	Improved	p53	Improved engraftment/loss of quiescence	TeKippe et al. (204)
				Dumble et al. (223c)
				Liu et al. (205)
		p27	Increased engraftment	Cheng et al. (223d.)
Conserved Developmental Pathways				
Notch pathway	None	Numb/NumbL, Notch1/2, Jagged1 (extrinsic)	Normal	Wilson et al. (223e)
TGF-β pathway	None	Tgfb2, Tgfbr1, Smad5	Tgfbr1 unresponsive to Tgfb1, mainly *in vitro* expansion defects otherwise normal	Langer et al. (223f)
				Larsson et al. (223g)
				Singbrant et al. (223h)
	Defect	Smad4, Tgfbr2 (extrinsic)	Defects in engraftment	Karlsson et al. (206)
Wnt/β-catenin pathway	Defect	Ctnnb1	Normal/defect depending on Mx1 vs. Vav-Cre insensitive to GS3b inhibitor expansion	Cobas et al. (207)
				Zhao et al. (208)
				Huang et al. (209)
	Defect	Wnt3a (extrinsic)	Defect in serial transplants (fetal liver)	Luis et al. (210)
Hedgehog pathway	None	Smo	Normal HSC	Gao et al. (211)
				Hofmann et al. (212)
	Improved	Gli	Increased engraftment	Merchant et al. (213)
Transcription and lineage transcription factors	Defect	Bmi1	Decreased engraftment	Park et al. (214)
				Iwama et al. (223i)
		Pbx1	Decreased developmental HSC	DiMartino et al. (223j)
				Boyarsky et al. (223k)
		c-Myc	Increased in phenotypic HSC with decreased engraftment and development	Baena et al. (223l)
				Laurenti et al. (223m)
				Wilson et al. (223n)
		Gfi1/Gfi1b	Myeloid differentiation defects alteration in HSC	Hock et al. (158)
				Khandanpour et al. (223o)
		Scl/Tal1	Increase in number of HS/PC differentiation	Mikkola et al. (223p)
				Curtis et al. (223q)
		IRF2	Defect in HSC	Sato et al. (223r)
Signaling pathways	Defect	FoxOs (FoxO1, FoxO3a, FoxO4)	Loss of quiescence	Tothova et al. (182)
				Miyamoto et al. (181)
		Pten	Increased cycling and exhaustion	
PI3K/AKT and metabolic sensing		mTORC1/mTORC2	Loss of self renewal	
		Lkb1	Loss of HSC	Gurumurthy et al. (180)
				Gan et al. (179)
				Nakada et al. (178)
Other signaling regulators		STAT5	Decreased engraftment	Li et al. (223s)
				Wang et al. (223t)
				Bradley et al. (223u)
				Bunting et al. (223v)
	Improved	Lnk	Increased engraftment	Takaki et al. (223w)
Epigenetic regulators	Defect	Dnmt1	Decreased lymphoid engraftment	Broske et al. (215)
	Improved	Dnmt3a	Improved engraftment	Challen et al. (216)
	Improved	Tet2	Increased engraftment and self renewal	Quivoron et al. (223x)
				Ko et al. (217)
				Moran-Crusio et al. (223y)
RNA-related binding proteins	Defect	Msi2	Decreased self renewal	Kharas et al. (293)
		Ott1/Spen	HSC defects and engraftment and differentiation	Ito et al. (40)
				Hope et al. (294)
				de Andres-Aguayo et al. (218)
		HuR (Elavl1)	Loss of HS/PC	Xiao et al., Niu et al. (223z,224)
				Ghosh et al. (224a)

exhibit a non–cell autonomous myeloid expansion (201,202). However, conditional loss of all three family members resulted in a lethal, cell-intrinsic myeloproliferative disorder that was associated with an increase in HSC number and proliferation, but markedly decreased self-renewal, as assessed by transplantation (224b). These studies indicate that Rb family members serve overlapping and redundant roles in maintaining HSC function.

Conserved Developmental Pathways

Notch

The Notch family consists of cell surface proteins that interact with members of the Jagged and Delta family of ligands on adjacent cells, including Jagged 1 and 2 as well as Delta 1, 3, and 4 (225). Upon Jagged or Delta binding, Notch is first cleaved in its extracellular domain by the TNF-α-converting enzyme, followed by cleavage of the intracellular domain by a γ-secretase complex. The cleaved intracellular domain is then competent for translocation into the nucleus, where it activates transcription by interacting with coactivators such as recombination signal binding protein for immunoglobulin kappa J region (RBP-jk, also known as CBF-1) and Mastermind-like (Maml) to induce transcription of targets such as *Hes1*, *Hes5*, *Hey1*, and *Notch1* itself (226,227). The critical role of this pathway in embryonic HSC development has been shown in mice lacking *Notch1*, *Jagged1*, and *Cbf-1* (228–230). Although the Notch1/2 receptors are expressed on HSCs, and Jagged/Delta are expressed on niche cells, the role for the Notch pathway in adult hematopoiesis remains controversial. Studies that have inhibited Notch signaling with a dominant negative Maml or deletion of CSL/RBP-Jk have produced conflicting results (231,232). In favor of a more limited role, mice that lack Notch1/2, Numb/L, or Jagged1 have normal HSC function even in stress-related settings. Additional studies suggest that HSCs are able to respond to Notch signaling, as *in vitro* stimulation can support expansion and supraphysiologic levels results in the loss of self-renewal *in vivo* (233–236).

TGF-β Family

The transforming growth factor-β (TGF) family of cytokines is large, consisting of 3 mammalian isoforms of TGF-β, approximately 20 isoforms of bone morphogenic protein (BMP), and activin. These family members play important roles in diverse developmental processes (237,238). In the bone marrow, both stromal cells and immature hematopoietic cells secrete TGF-β, suggesting that TGF-β may be part of a feedback loop that regulates HSC function (239). Early studies of TGF-β function showed that TGF-β1 and 3 exert antiproliferative effects on HS/PCs *in vitro* (240). Indeed, *ex vivo* treatment of LSK34$^-$ cells with TGF-β results in attenuation of mitogen-mediated Akt and Src activation, with attenuation of Akt signaling resulting in increased activation and nuclear accumulation of FoxO3a, which then negatively regulates ROS levels and maintains HSC quiescence *in vivo* (181,241). However, *in vivo* studies using mouse models deficient in components of the TGF-β signaling pathway suggest a more complex role of TGF-β in HSC biology. Deletion of *Tgf-β1* results in multiple developmental defects with most mice dying during embryonic development, and those that do survive develop an autoinflammatory condition leading to a wasting disease (242–244). Deletion of *TβRI* results in a similar autoimmune phenotype, but there is no evidence of alterations in HSC number, cell cycle distribution, or self-renewal. Similarly, deletion of downstream signaling components Smad1/Smad5 also results in normal HSC function. In contrast, when *TgfbR2* or *Smad4*, a downstream component of the TGF-β signaling pathway, is deleted, HSCs exhibit self-renewal defects during competitive transplantation assays (245). In the *Smad4*-deleted cells there was decreased expression of c-Myc and Notch-1 (206). One potential mechanism for TGF-β's effects may be its downstream target p57Kip2, a cell cycle inhibitor protein that has also shown to be essential for maintaining quiescence in HSCs (203,246).

WNT/β-Catenin

The Wnt proteins are soluble glycoproteins that exert a wide range of effects on both immature and mature hematopoietic cells (247). Originally identified as regulators of *Drosophila* development and named for the *Wingless* phenotype, these proteins activate this cell-signaling pathway by interacting with a cell surface receptor complex consisting of Frizzled (Fz) and its two coreceptors; Low Density Lipoprotein

Receptor-related Protein 5/6 (Lrp5/6). In the absence of Wnt stimulation, the transcription factor β-catenin remains inactivated, destabilized, and is degraded when it is sequestered in a cytoplasmic multimeric protein complex that consists of adenomatous polyposis coli (Apc), Axin1, and the kinases glycogen synthase kinase 3β (Gsk3β) and casein kinase 1 (Ck1). Sequential phosphorylation by these proteins allows for β-Trcp E3 ubiquitin ligase to recognize β-catenin and target it for proteasomal-mediated elimination. Without nuclear β-catenin, Wnt-responsive genes are bound and repressed by the T-cell factor/lymphoid enhancer factor (TCF/LEF) family of transcription factors. However, in the presence of Wnts, the Fz/Lrp5/6 protein complex recruits another scaffold called Dishevelled (Dvl) to the plasma membrane, resulting in the dissociation of the β-catenin-Axin complex, thus liberating β-catenin to translocate to the nucleus, bind to the TCF/LEF proteins, and activate Wnt-target genes such as *Cyclin D1* and *c-Myc*.

Although still controversial, Wnt protein has been shown to regulate HSC function in a number of contexts. *In vitro* treatment of LSK cells with Wnt5a induces expansion of *B-cell lymphoma gene-2* (*bcl2*)-transgenic LSK cells (247). Ectopic expression of a constitutively active form of β-catenin results in similar findings, with inhibition of the pathway by Axin1 overexpression decreasing HSC growth. A greater role for β-catenin in regulating hematopoietic differentiation was supported by experiments in which expression of a constitutively active β-catenin in lineage-committed myeloid and lymphoid progenitors conferred multilineage potential to these cells (248). The controversy concerning the role of β-catenin signaling stems from studies that failed to demonstrate a phenotype in mice lacking β-catenin (207,249,250). Additionally, overexpression of constitutively activated β-catenin resulted in a loss of HSCs (251,252). In contrast, experiments in which β-catenin was deleted or in which the canonical Wnt signaling inhibitor *Dickkopf1* (*Dkk*) was expressed by osteoblasts revealed impaired HSC self-renewal in reconstitution assays (208,253). Similarly, *Wnt3a$^{-/-}$* fetal liver HSCs showed a loss in self-renewal potential (210). The role of Wnt signaling has also been investigated through a series of gain-of-function studies. Treatment of mice with the GSK3 inhibitor CHIR-911 increased the reconstitution potential of both mouse and human HS/PCs in NOD/SCID mice (254). Activation of the Wnt/β-catenin pathway by inhibiting GSK3β and adding rapamycin to block growth factor signaling results in the maintenance of LT-HSCs in an *in vitro* culture system using both mouse and human HSCs (209). Moreover, deletion of β-catenin reverses this maintenance effect with the combined inhibitor treatment. Finally, HSCs from *Apc^{min}* mice carrying a mutated *Apc* gene with a premature stop codon predicted to exhibit increased Wnt signaling displayed increased reconstitution potential in competitive transplantations (255). In sum, it is clear that there is a role for β-catenin in HSC self-renewal and that the concentration and levels of activation dictate if there is a gain or a loss of self-renewal.

Hedgehog Pathway

The Hedgehog (Hh) family comprises three secreted proteins including Sonic hedgehog (Shh), Indian Hedgehog (Ihh), and Desert hedgehog (Dhh), which regulate numerous development processes by binding to receptors including Patched (Ptch1), which associates with and negatively regulates another cell surface protein, smoothened (Smo). Following Hh binding to Ptch1, Smo is released from Ptch1, allowing Smo to activate the glioblastoma (Gli) transcription factors, Gli1 and Gli2, which activate transcription of key target genes including *Cyclin D1*, *Cyclin E*, *c-Myc*, *platelet derived growth factor*, *Ptch1*, and *vascular endothelial growth factor* (*Vegf*) (254).

Several studies support a role for the Hh pathway in promoting HSC self-renewal. Ihh expression on human stromal cells promotes colony formation by human CD34+ cells (256), and Shh has been shown to promote proliferation of human CD34+ cord blood cells (257,258). Studies in mice have produced less consistent results, as fetal liver cells from Vav-Cre-driven deletion of *Smo* resulted in reduced reconstitution and colony formation in serially passaged colonies (259,260). Given this finding, it was unexpected to find increased numbers of HSCs in *Gli*1-deficient mice (213). In mice heterozygous for *Ptch1*, LSK numbers were increased, but they showed increased cycling and increased short-term reconstitution, consistent with progenitor expansion, but decreased reconstitution potential, supporting decreased HSC frequencies (254). Such a defect in long-term reconstitution was not observed when *Ptch1*+/− fetal liver cells were transplanted, although the significance of this finding to adult HSCs is not entirely clear (259). When *Smo* was conditionally deleted in adult mice using *Mx-Cre*, no changes in hematopoiesis were observed, either in the steady-state or under stress hematopoiesis as assessed by transplantation or 5-FU treatment (211,212); however, this may indicate that Hh signaling is only required during early development and dispensable during adult hematopoiesis. Additional studies utilizing appropriately timed deletions and highly purified HSCs will be required to clarify the role of the Hh pathway in HSC function.

Signal Transduction Pathways

PI3K Signaling Pathway

The PI3K pathway is an important signaling pathway that regulates cell proliferation, growth, and survival in numerous cellular contexts by integrating numerous upstream signals including growth factors, nutrients, and growth status (261). The pathway includes downstream regulators such as Akt and the mammalian target of rapamycin-1 (mTOR) kinase as well as negative regulators including phosphatase and tensin homolog (PTEN) and promyelocytic leukemia, which negatively regulate Akt activation. The mTOR kinase associates with two separate protein complexes mammalian target of rapamycin complex (mTORC1)/regulatory associated protein of MTOR, complex-1 (Raptor), and mTORC2/Rictor, which are nonredundant, regulated differently, and play distinct roles in HSCs. For example, tuberous sclerosis complex 1/2 can inhibit activation of mTorc1 and deletion of mTORC1/Raptor results in a loss of HSC regenerative capacity while loss of mTORC2 results in minimal alterations in HSC transplant capacity (262,263). Activated Akt also inhibits the activity of the Forkhead box protein O (FoxO) family of transcription factors, which are critical mediators of oxidative stress, by leading to their nuclear exclusion. In HSCs, activation of this pathway leads to dramatic phenotypes. Activation of the pathways through conditional deletion of *Pten* or activation with a constitutive AKT in adult HSC results in a rapid T-cell acute lymphoblastic leukemia (T-ALL) and myeloproliferative disorder (186,187,189, 190) which then quickly progresses to acute myeloid leukemia (AML) in the *Pten*-deficient animals (186). Additionally, analysis of HSCs (LSKFCD48−) in *Pten*-deficient mice showed that there was a threefold increase in cycling HSCs, suggesting that Pten acts to limit HSCs proliferation (186). While the mice initially experienced an increase in HSCs, over time the absolute number of HSCs actually decreased. Consistent with a loss of HSC reconstitution potential, *Pten*−/− HSCs transplanted into recipient mice did not persist. Rapamycin, an inhibitor of mTOR, eliminated the leukemia and rescued the HSC phenotype. Similarly, loss of mTORC1 could delay development of the leukemia and the loss of mTORC2 could reverse the effect on both the HSCs as well as T-ALL progression (262,263). Thus,

the downstream targets of the PI3K axis play a complex role in both normal HSC and leukemia biology.

The FoxO family of transcription factors integrates growth and stress signals to modulate metabolism, proliferation, and survival. In *Caenorhabditis elegans,* activation of the homologous factor DAF-16 can extend the lifespan as much as 50%. HSCs from mice deficient in *FoxO3a* differentiate normally but exhibit a marked stem cell exhaustion phenotype when challenged with serial transplants or with 5-FU treatment (181). Interestingly, when mice deficient in multiple family members including *FoxO1, FoxO3a,* and *FoxO4* are evaluated, they show a more severe hematopoietic defect, with triple null mice exhibiting early loss of HSCs in the bone marrow and a concomitant increase in extramedullary hematopoiesis associated with a myeloid expansion (182). Both *FoxO*-deficient mice show increased HSC cycling and higher levels of ROS in HSCs (181,182). Treatment of mice with the antioxidant N-acetyl L-cysteine (NAC) reversed many of the observed hematopoietic phenotypes. The deletion of FoxO family members extends the latency and maintains the leukemia stem cell (LSC), which provides additional evidence for FoxO's role in stem cell self-renewal (264). These data add additional complexity to the previously discussed proleukemic activity and negative regulatory function of Akt.

Lkb1

Lkb1 is an evolutionarily conserved regulator of cellular energy metabolism in eukaryotic cells and functions as the major upstream kinase that phosphorylates AMP-activated protein kinase (AMPK) and 12 other AMPK-related kinases (265–267). Several groups recently generated *Lkb1*-deficient mice and demonstrated that deletion of *Lkb1* results in severe pancytopenia and subsequent death (178–180). Evaluation of HSCs from these mice reveals that HSCs exhibit increased cell cycling, decreased survival, and eventual exhaustion. Transplantation of HSCs showed a marked reduction in reconstitution potential. The cell cycling and survival effects appeared to be specific for HSCs and was not observed in downstream progenitors, indicating a specific functional role of Lkb1 in HSCs, likely reflective of their unique metabolic state.

CDC42

The *cell division cycle 42* (Cdc42) protein is a GTPase associated with cell polarity (268–270). Recent studies indicate that Cdc42 expression is increased in HSCs during normal aging and required for HSC maintenance through its ability to regulate HSC polarity. Using mice deficient in *p50RhoGAP*, a selective inhibitor of *Cdc42* (*Cdc42GAP*−/− mice), the authors confirmed that the previously described aging phenotype (271) is also present in HSCs. Furthermore, they showed that Cdc42 is not asymmetrically distributed, but that it is diffusely distributed in the cell body of *Cdc42GAP*−/− HSCs. They then showed that pharmacologic inhibition of Cdc42 activity using a novel Cdc42 specific inhibitor, CASIN, reduced Cdc42 activity in aged HSC to levels comparable to young HSC, restored their polarity, and reversed age-related functional HSC phenotypes, including their decreased ability to reconstitute recipients in competitive transplants, myeloid lineage skewing, and cell polarity defects (272). Moreover, the "rejuvenation" phenotype was long lasting, persisting even through a second round of bone marrow transplantation. These data provide evidence supporting the notion that maintaining cell polarity is critical for HSC function, and provide a rationale for pharmacologic intervention to prevent HSC aging phenotypes. Whether or not such interventions may serve as preventative interventions for age-associated hematologic diseases including malignancies such as AML and the myelodysplastic syndromes (MDS) remains to be seen.

Epigenetic Regulators

Bmi1

B lymphoma Mo-MLV insertion region 1 homolog (Bmi1) is a member of the Polycomb Group gene family that functions in multimeric protein complexes to repress gene expression through addition of epigenetic marks at genetic loci. Bmi1 controls cell proliferation by repressing the *Ink4/Arf* locus, which encodes two structurally distinct proteins, the CDK-inhibitor p16^{Ink4a} and the tumor suppressor gene p19^{ARF} (273). Mice lacking *Bmi1* exhibit severe hematopoietic defects early in life with bone marrow failure due to a loss of HSCs (214,274). Consistent with loss of self-renewal capacity, HSCs transplanted from *Bmi1$^{-/-}$* bone marrow transiently reconstitute recipients. As expected, *Bmi-1* loss results in increased p16^{Ink4a} and p19^{ARF} protein expression, and retroviral reconstitution of immature hematopoietic cells with p16^{Ink4a} and p19^{ARF} is sufficient to induce growth arrest and cell death, respectively, *in vitro*. Deletion of *p16^{Ink4a}* or *p19^{ARF}* restores many of the defects observed in the *Bmi-1$^{-/-}$* bone marrow but combined deletion only partially rescued the loss of HSCs, indicating that Bmi-1 may exert effects on HSCs independently of its cell cycle targets (275).

DNA Methyltransferase

While evaluation of somatically mutated genes in hematologic malignancies has identified many genes that regulate HSC function, recent data also suggest that epigenetic factors play a major role in determining HSC function. Deletion of the maintenance DNA methylation enzymes results in marked pancytopenia and death due to loss of immature LSK cells (215). Hypomorphs of *Dnmt1* exhibit attenuated, but significant hematopoietic phenotypes, with reduced numbers of HS/PCs, decreased HSC self-renewal, and alterations in lineage potential with loss of lymphoid potential with concomitant aberrant expression of myeloid-erythroid genes in LSK cells. Loss-of-function mutants of the maintenance DNA methyltransferase *Dnmt3a* exhibit decreased HSC differentiation as well as HSC expansion. Examination of methylomes demonstrated that *Dnmt3a* null HSCs up-regulated HSC multipotency genes and down-regulated differentiation factors. In addition, their progeny exhibited global hypomethylation and incomplete repression of HSC-specific genes (216). Thus, the epigenome is highly dynamic during even the earliest stages of hematopoiesis and widespread loss of DNA methylation is a necessary step in lineage commitment.

RNA and Posttranscription Levels of Regulation

Approximately 2% of the genome is transcribed and encodes for proteins while approximately 40% of the genome is actively transcribed but not translated. The role for this vast number of non–protein-encoding RNAs that includes piwiRNAs, microRNAs, small nucleolar RNA (snoRNAs), and large noncoding RNAs remains largely unknown and provides an exciting direction for investigation. These various RNAs have vastly different functions from silencing genes to acting as transcriptional scaffolds for epigenetic regulators. Furthermore, RNA-binding proteins (RBPs) may functionally interact with these RNAs, and even compete for the same binding complementary seed sequences thereby modifying RNA function. In this chapter we will discuss microRNAs and select RBPs to highlight this emerging field.

microRNAs

MicroRNAs are small, 22 to 25 nucleotides long of RNA that do not encode for proteins, but are able to exert significant inhibitory effects by binding to the 3′UTRs of target mRNAs and inducing message degradation or inhibiting protein translation (276). Because miRNAs recognize their targets through perfect or imperfect base-pair complementary via a 6 to 8 nt "seed sequence," they can bind to numerous mRNA targets simultaneous. It is estimated that on average, each miRNA can bind to approximately 300 mRNA targets. Since there are over 1,000 unique miRNAs in humans, miRNAs are predicted to target more than 30% of transcripts in human cells (277). Recent studies have demonstrated that a number of miRNAs can regulate HSC function. miR-125 family members have been shown to regulate HSC self-renewal by blocking apoptosis (278–280). One additional effect of this block in apoptosis is skewing in HSC lineage bias since lymphoid-biased HSCs preferentially exhibited decreased apoptosis when miR-125b was ectopically expressed in mouse bone marrow cells (278). miR-29a was also shown to regulate self-renewal of hematopoietic progenitors, as expression of miR-29a was sufficient to induce aberrant self-renewal of mouse committed progenitors, but target genes for this miRNA were not definitively identified (281). Enforced expression of miR-155, a miRNA highly expressed in HSCs, results in the development of a hematologic disorder resembling a myeloproliferative neoplasm (MPN) (282). Other groups have shown that miRNAs are differentially regulated during hematopoietic development and that numerous miRNAs are differentially expressed in HSCs (279,283,284). miR-126 is also highly expressed in HSCs (285), and recent studies have shown that miR-126 regulates HSC self-renewal and expansion, but not cell cycling, in both mouse and human HSC by modulating activity of the PI3K pathway (286). Together, these data demonstrate that multiple miRNAs regulate HSC function and that their misexpression in hematologic malignancies makes them potential therapeutic targets.

RNA Binding Proteins

RBPs have been shown to regulate hematopoiesis and to be dysregulated in hematologic disorders. RBPs can function in a variety of biologic roles including the regulation of mRNA splicing, polyadenylation, mRNA export, mRNA stability, and translational control (287). Some of the best-studied RBPs are downstream mediators of the PI3K/mTOR pathway and include several elongation and initiation factors (eIFs such as eIF4G and eIF4E) that allow for specific sets of transcripts to be translated and to increase cell proliferation and growth (288). mTOR phosphorylates and blocks 4E-BP1, an inhibitor of EIF4G/E, thus resulting in translation initiation of target mRNAs (289). This pathway was shown to be critical in HSCs and leukemia-initiating cells because mTOR inhibitors could reverse the effects of constitutive PI3K/Akt activity (186,189).

Another set of RBPs have been more recently shown to be important for hematopoietic cells include splicing factors SF3B1, serine/arginine-rich splicing factor 2 (SRSF2), U2 small nuclear RNA auxiliary factor 1 (U2AF35), zinc finger (CCCH type), RNA-binding motif and serine/arginine rich-2 (ZRSR2), SF3A1, PRP40 pre-mRNA processing factor 40 homolog B (PRP40B), SF1, U2AF1, and U2AF65—all found to be commonly mutated or highly expressed in hematologic malignancies and disorders (290). Investigations of how these splicing factors alter hematopoietic development and their role in disease is only in its initial stages. Other RBPs control several aspects of RNA processing important for cell fate determination. For example, ELAVL1 (HuR) controls stability and export from the nucleus to the cytoplasm, and postnatal deletion of HuR reduces hematopoietic PC function and results in decreased engraftment in transplantation assays. Another RBP, Lin28b, possesses pleiotropic functions in HSCs and ESCs through its regulation of the processing of the Let7 family of miRNAs; however, it can also bind to mRNAs to alter their stability (291). Overexpression of Lin28b can reprogram adult

HS/PCs and increase the development of B-1a, marginal zone B cells, gamma/delta (γ/δ) T cells, and NK/T cells (292). Additionally, RBPs can regulate self-renewal. For example, Msi2 overexpression can increase HSC numbers, and deletion results in reduced self-renewal and engraftment of HSCs and MPPs (218,293,294). How expression of these RBPs is controlled and what pathways they regulate remain to be determined, but the pathways they activate are clearly multifunctional and have wide-ranging effects on metabolism, cell cycle control, and self-renewal (295).

Extrinsic Factors

Bone Marrow and the HSC Niche

HSCs depend on extrinsic signals for their function and the bone marrow provides a unique microenvironment to support adult hematopoiesis. Our understanding of the critical components that regulate hematopoiesis has expanded significantly in the past decade. As part of this discussion, we would like to review the anatomic composition of the bone marrow as well as the different specialized microenvironments within the bone marrow that control hematopoiesis.

Cortical bone is mainly composed of mineralized, calcified connective tissue, and the bony cavity is occupied by a 3D matrix of cancellous or spongy trabecular bone. Within the inner portions of the bone, or the medullary region, hematopoietic cells reside in a specialized microenvironment called the bone marrow, which is fed and penetrated by the vasculature via a nutrient artery and periosteal artery; the former connects to the central artery running along the bone while radial arteries connect to the latter (Fig. 1.3A) (296). The vasculature of the bone marrow follows a path from the arterioles to the capillaries, eventually leading into a plexus of venous sinuses, and the sinusoids or small vessels then drain into the longitudinal vein, followed by the nutrient vein that connects it to the systemic circulation (Fig. 1.3A). Thus, the bone marrow vasculature is organized similar to other peripheral tissues. While these architectural features of the bone are easy to identify morphologically, the areas of the bone marrow that maintain HSCs are less defined.

The "niche" is a general term used to describe the presumed local environment required to support HSC self-renewal and differentiation, but the cellular and molecular components that make up the niche are not completely understood. Schofield (11) first hypothesized the concept of a "niche" in the late 1970s and suggested that stromal components in the bone marrow regulate hematopoiesis. The niche is thought to provide HSCs with the factors required for their maintenance and activation through cell-cell interactions, extracellular matrix proteins, and other secreted regulators that modulate hematopoiesis during steady-state and stress conditions. The concept

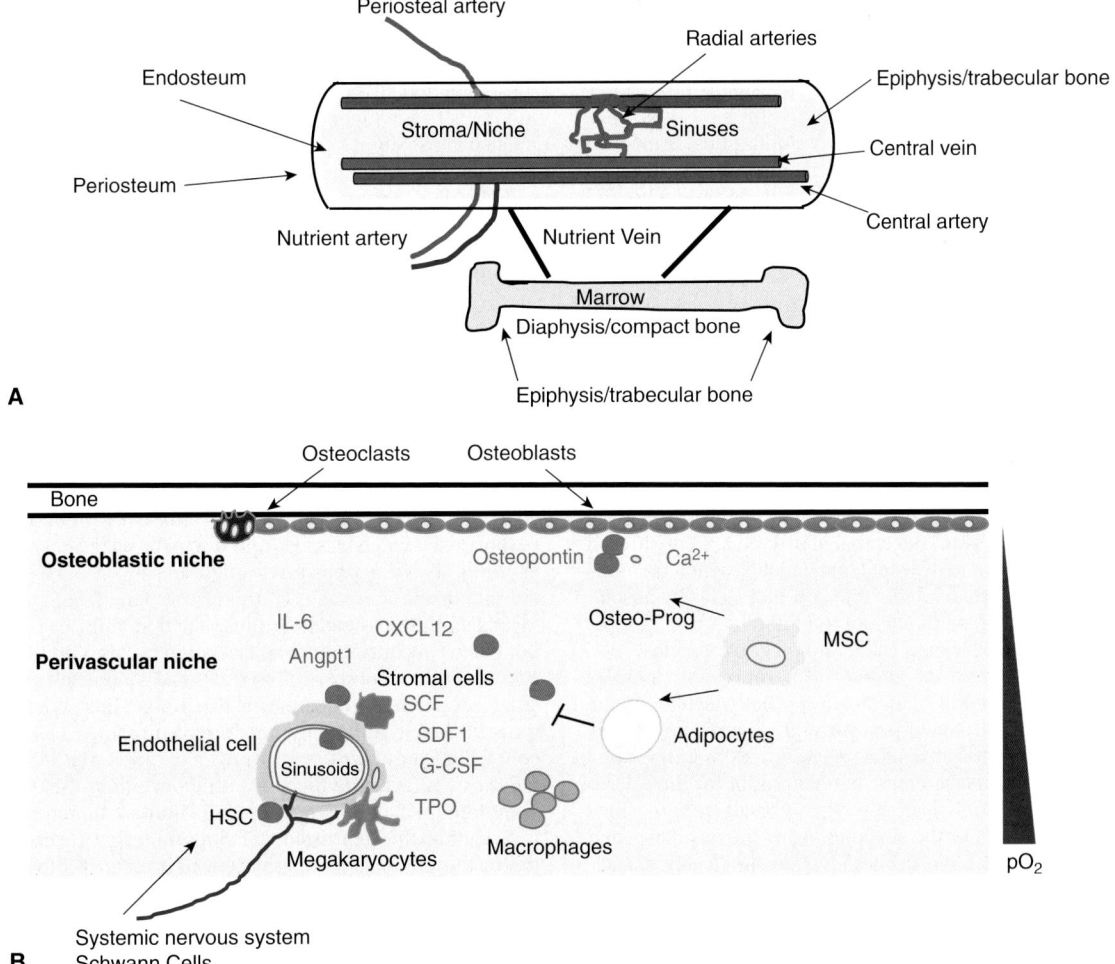

FIGURE 1.3. Hematopoietic niche in the bone marrow. A: Schematic of the physical structure and vasculature of the bone marrow. **B:** The hematopoietic "niche" contains numerous cell types that maintain HSCs through direct physical interactions or through the elaboration of secreted factors. Cytokines and regulators are in *red*. Oste-Prog, osteoblast progenitor; MSC; mesenchymal stem cell; HSC, hematopoietic stem cell.

of an architecturally definable HSC niche was supported by studies of other tissue systems, in particular in the gonads of other model systems including *Drosophila* and *Caenorhabditis elegans*, where interactions of germ cells with niche cells was demonstrated (297–299). We now know that several hematopoietic and nonhematopoietic cell types contribute to the HSC niche. Perhaps the best-described niche component is the endosteal cell layer that covers the trabecular bone and is made up of several cell types including osteoblasts, osteoclasts, and reticular cells (296). The location of specific cell types within the marrow has been investigated since as early as 1938 when mature hematopoietic cells were observed to be localized further away from the endosteum (300). While this led to a model that held that immature hematopoietic cells reside near the endosteum and move away as they differentiate, this model has been challenged by recent findings demonstrating the presence of endosteal and vascular HSC niches, which will be discussed in greater detail below.

What are these stromal components of the bone marrow that modulate hematopoiesis? These hematopoietic and non-hematopoietic components are collectively referred to as the "stroma" and have been described over the years as composed of a variety of cell types including mesenchymal stromal cells, osteoblasts, adipocytes, reticular stromal cells, neural cell types, endothelial cells, macrophages, and megakaryocytes (301,302). Unfortunately, as most of these stromal components have been described on the basis of morphologic, immunophenotypic, and/or functional differences definitive experimental evidence of their function and tissue/lineage origin have been frequently lacking. For example, reticular stromal cells are classified based on their appearance, but it is not clear from which lineage they are derived, and methods to isolate them have not been developed (303). Advances in identifying cell surface markers that mark specific stromal cell populations, improved animal genetic models of hematopoiesis, and *in vivo* imaging techniques have improved our understanding of the niche and its complexity. Currently, one of the prevailing models of the hematopoietic niche posits that there are two separate, distinct regions: the osteoblastic and perivascular niches. This is based on the observation that morphologically immature hematopoietic cells are enriched in these two areas of the bone marrow. However, this simplified scheme has been complicated by *in situ* live imaging studies suggesting that these niches might not be anatomically separate as once thought, especially in the calvarium, where direct live imaging studies of HSC interactions in the bone marrow are technically possible (304,305), and demonstrate that the blood vessels are often physically located in proximity to the endosteum. Nevertheless, cells physically associated with, or close to, the trabecular bone are considered to be part of the endosteal or osteoblastic niche, which includes osteoblasts and osteoclasts. Cells that are more closely associated with vascular sinusoids include endothelial cells, macrophages, mesenchymal stromal cells, and megakaryocytes.

The endosteal niche is thought to represent a relative hypoxic environment compared to the vascular niche (173,306). The overall partial pressure (pO_2) is approximately 55 mm Hg and the saturation of O_2 is close to 90% in the bone marrow, but these measurements do not account for the microenvironmental variation in local oxygen concentration, since the pO_2 drops rapidly as the distance from the capillary bed increases (307). HSCs have been shown to be closely associated with the areas that are poorly perfused (173,306,308). This continuum of oxygenation levels between the niches is thought to be functionally important for maintaining HSC quiescence, numbers, and function, as hypoxia limits the production of reactive oxygen radicals that inhibit HSC function (309). Mice with a mutant *Vegfa$^{\delta\delta}$* gene lacking the hypoxia inducible factor (HIF) binding element showed reduced HSC function and VEGFR1 expression is dependent on HIF1 (310,311).

Cells within the vascular niche respond to VEGF signaling by up-regulating CXCL12. Consistent with the importance of a hypoxic HSC niche, HSCs grown under hypoxic conditions *in vitro* exhibit improved growth, reduced cell cycling, and increased engraftment capability when transplanted into mice (312,313). Mice lacking *HIF1α* exhibit reduced quiescence in HSCs and decreased engraftment in transplants (314). Besides an effect on HSCs, deletion of HIF members in mice leads to a block in B-cell development and alters macrophage activation (315). Given the difference in oxygenation at the endosteal and vascular niches, the two likely serve different functions with respect to HSC maintenance (316) (see Fig. 1.3B for details on the different cells of the niche).

Mesenchymal Stromal Populations

Many of the nonhematopoietic components of the bone marrow are derived from mesenchymal stem cells (MSCs). Like HSCs, MSCs exhibit long-term self-renewal and possess multilineage potential, being able to differentiate into mesenchymal stromal cells, CXCL12-abundant reticular (CAR) cells, and adipocytes. Since MSCs and their progeny include cell types that have each been shown to have the capacity to maintain and regulate hematopoiesis, many investigators have developed methods to study their function. Of note, MSCs are thought to have broad therapeutic potential as a cellular regenerative therapy with the promise of efficacy in multiple organ systems and utility in various diseases [reviewed in (317,318)]. Perivascular MSCs contribute to the maintenance of HSC numbers and function and are characterized by Nestin positivity in mice and CD146 expression in humans (303,319). Current models hold that mesenchymal stromal cells are located at the sinusoids, tethering HSCs to the niche and providing migration and growth signals such as Angpt1, stem cell factor (SCF), and CXCL12 (303). Another subpopulation of MSCs, CXCL12 abundant reticular cells (CARs), are also critical for HSC maintenance, as depletion leads to a reduction in HSC number (320). These cells can signal through CXCR4 and are located between endothelial and osteoblastic cells (320). These CXCL12 expressing mesenchymal stromal cells can also retain and modulate the migration of HSC out of the marrow and into the circulation (320).

Systemic Nervous System

Sensory and autonomic fibers are found along the arterioles in the bone marrow and associate with a variety of cell types in both the osteoblastic and perivascular niches; thus, the nervous system can mediate direct effects on hematopoiesis in response to acute stressors and normal oscillations in circadian rhythms. These actions are thought to rely on the hypothalamic suprachiasmatic nucleus of the brain, which can stimulate the local secretion of catecholamines such as noradrenaline in the bone marrow during normal circadian cycles, and this activates β-adrenergic receptors (β2 and β3) on osteoblasts and perivascular mesenchymal stromal cells (303). Thus, normal oscillations in the circadian rhythms might provide a mechanism for controlling the migratory turnover of HSCs and even hematopoietic cells from the niche into the periphery (321–324). After stimulation of G-CSF or GM-CSF, human hematopoietic PCs up-regulate the expression of dopaminergic receptors resulting in the increased sensitivity to neurotransmitters that then alters the migration, proliferation, and engraftment into immunodeficient mice (325). Glial fibrillary acidic protein–positive Schwann cells wrapping around nerve fibers in the bone marrow provide signals to HSCs such as TGFβ, which is important for maintaining HSC quiescence and dormancy as previously discussed (245). They do so by activating the large reservoir of latent and inactive TGFβ produced by numerous cells present in the bone marrow, thereby maintaining HSCs (245).

Osteoblasts

MSCs can differentiate into osteoblasts, which are located in close physical proximity to HSCs. However, the functionally relevant osteoblasts that support HSC function may not represent the most mature osteoblasts that synthesize bone matrix, but may instead be composed predominantly of osteolineage PCs (301). Nonetheless, homing assays showed that the HSCs lodge in the bone marrow in close proximity to N-cadherin and Flamingo (Fmi) expressing osteoblasts and that cotransplantation of osteoblasts with HSCs improved overall engraftment (326–329).

Osteoblasts are thought to maintain HSCs through cell-cell contacts as well as their elaboration of secreted products. Initial reports of N-cadherins playing an important role in both HSCs and osteoblasts has been tempered by more recent reports utilizing a set of mouse lines that delete them within the osteoblastic niche and within HSCs (330–332). In contrast, preosteoblasts express N-cadherin and signal through noncanonical Wnt signaling via the interactions of Flamingo (Fmi) and Fz receptors that maintain HSC quiescence and maintenance within the niche. Thus, these conflicting results might be explained by this alternative signaling mechanism (329). Osteoblasts can also support hematopoietic cells by secreting multiple factors including CXCL12, SCF, IL-6, GM-CSF, Angpt1, and others. It remains unclear if specific factors secreted by osteoblasts are required for normal hematopoietic development. However, loss of osteopontin secreted from osteoblasts results in reduced HSC number and decreased migration away from the endosteum (333,334). Moreover, mice deficient in osteopontin demonstrated an increase in hematopoietic progenitors while osteopontin treatment resulted in reduced cycling of HSCs *in vitro* (333,334). Taken together, these studies suggest an inhibitory role for osteopontin on HS/PC.

Recent studies suggest that osteoblastic niche cells may directly contribute to the pathogenesis of hematologic disorders. Mice lacking Dicer, an enzyme required for microRNA biogenesis, specifically in the osteoblast lineage exhibited a reduction in HSCs and altered differentiation with ineffective hematopoiesis and morphologic evidence of dysplasia; some of the mice exhibited a progressive phenotype with the development of AML (335). Consistent with the concept that specific subsets of osteoblasts are critical for proper HSC homeostatic control, deletion of *Dicer* in more committed osteoblasts yielded no phenotype, indicating that only a specific subset of osteolineage cell types has significant ability to regulate hematopoiesis. Overall, these studies underscore the importance of proper interactions between the niche and the hematopoietic cells and suggest that modulation of niche function may become a therapeutically relevant strategy for the treatment of bone marrow–based disease in the future.

Adipocytes and Mature Hematopoietic Cells

Some established stromal cell lines have the ability to maintain limited self-renewal of HSCs, and as described previously, these may be used to assess HS/PC activity in *in vitro* experimental models such as LTC-IC and CAFC assays. One commonly used stromal line, OP9, is derived from the osteopetrotic mouse lacking CSF-1 (*op/op*) and can be differentiated into adipocytes under certain conditions. The supportive function of these stromal cells for HSCs becomes severely compromised once they show evidence of adipocytic differentiation, suggesting that adipocytes may negatively regulate HSCs (336,337). In support of this concept, vertebral bodies of the tail in mice contain higher proportions of adipocytes and decreased frequencies of HS/PCs compared to the thoracic portion of the vertebral column (336). Additionally, genetic or pharmacologic inhibition of adipocytic differentiation led to increased numbers of

immunophenotypically defined HSCs as well as their reconstitution capacity upon bone marrow transplant (336). Taken together, these data provide evidence for a negative role of adipocytes in HSC maintenance (336). As bone marrow adipocyte content increases with age, this raises the intriguing possibility that adipocytes may contribute to age-related changes in the hematopoietic system.

Hematopoietic cells that reside in the marrow may also contribute to the maintenance of HSCs. For example, deleting macrophages expressing CD169 or M-CSFR leads to increased mobilization of HSCs, supporting the notion that macrophages provide negative signals for HSC retention (338). While these signals could emanate directly from macrophages, it could also be mediated by other niche cell types such as osteoblasts, Nestin+ mesenchymal stromal cells, or sympathetic nerves. These studies also suggest that G-CSF's ability to stimulate macrophages relieves the negative feedback inhibition on HSCs and mobilizes them into blood. When the immune system becomes activated due to an infection, inflammatory signals from hematopoietic cells from both the innate and adaptive immune system can directly alter the self-renewal and differentiation potential of HSCs in the bone marrow (339). Proinflammatory cytokines such as IL-1, IL-6, IL-8, TNF, and type 1 and II interferons (IFNs) have pleiotropic effects on hematopoietic development (Table 1.4). For example, lipopolysaccharide (LPS) stimulation can result in TNF activation which inhibits HSC self-renewal. (340). During chronic infections, sustained levels of IFNγ can deplete HSCs by inducing increased HSC cycling and differentiation (341). Type 1 IFNs such as IFNα can increase Ly-6A/E (Sca-1) levels on hematopoietic cells, thereby confounding attempts to identify or prospectively separate HS/PCs based on immunophenotype in the mouse system (342).

Osteoclasts

Osteoclasts are derived from the monocyte lineage and are critical for resorption of the bone matrix. While these cells are activated in response to bone injury as well as in response to aberrant growth factor secretion in hematologic malignancies such as multiple myeloma (343), they are also required to create the complex meshwork and cavities within the bone marrow space during normal bone turnover and growth. Based on their essential role as bone remodelers, many predicted that osteoclasts would be an important component or regulator of the niche. However, osteoprotegerin-deficient mice exhibiting osteoporosis due to increased osteoclastogenesis and bone resorption showed a reduction in HS/PC mobilization. Also, mutant mice exhibiting defects in osteoclast development such as *op/op* mice, r*eceptor activator of nuclear factor κappa B ligand, (Rankl)*-deficient mice, and *c-Fos*-deficient mice demonstrated comparable or increased HS/PC mobilization with no apparent increase in HSC numbers (344). These results indicate that osteoclasts inhibit HSC maintenance and mobilization. Recent studies have attempted to link bone remodeling to HSC expansion (345,346). During the process of mineralizing bone, Ca^{2+} is increased near the endosteal surface, and this increase may signal to the calcium sensing receptors present on HSCs which are required for HSC self-renewal and engraftment (143).

Perivascular Niche Cells

Evidence for a perivascular HSC niche originated from studies of normal development and the observation that early hematopoietic cells arise from hemangioblasts and hemogenic endothelium. Supporting the absence of a requirement for an endosteal niche for HSC maintenance, HSCs reside in the yolk sac, AGM, or fetal liver in the developing embryo where no such niche is present. Imaging studies have shown that HSCs physically associate with endothelial cells and osteoblasts

Table 1.4	CYTOKINES REGULATING HEMATOPOIESIS			
Cytokines (Ligand)	Cognate Receptor	Sources	Target Cells	Biologic Activity
SCF/KitL	c-Kit	Perivascular niche cells/osteoblast cells	HSCs and progenitors	Increased proliferation/differentiation
TPO	MPL	Liver and stromal cells from bone marrow	HSC/HS/PC/Megakaryocytes	Promotes megakaryocyte and HSC proliferation and development
FLT3L	FLT3R	Stromal components	Myeloid progenitors and progenitor B cells	Progenitors proliferation and early maintains B-cell development and survival
M-CSF	M-CSFR	Stromal cell and macrophages	Monocytes, HSCs, myeloid progenitors	Alters myeloid differentiation and DCs
G-CSF	G-CSFR	Stromal cell and macrophages	Granulocytes, myeloid progenitors	Myeloid differentiation and DCs
GM-CSF	GM-CSFR	Stroma cells, endothelial cells, macrophages	Granulocytes, macrophages progenitors and erythroid progenitors	Increase proliferation
EPO	EPOR	Kidneys and endothelial cells	Erythroid progenitors	Maintains erythroid and RBC production
IL-3	IL-3R	T-lymphocytes, mast cells, and NK cells	Myeloid cells and lymphoid cells	Stimulates growth and survival
IL-4	IL-4R	Basophils, T cells	Monocytes, mast cells, and T cells	Commit monocytes toward DC lineage, TH2 skewing of T cells
IL-5	IL-5R	T cells	Eosinophils, B cells	Activation, proliferation
IL-6	IL-6R	Stromal cells, endothelial cells, T cells	Progenitors, myeloid progenitors	Activation, proliferation
IL-7	IL-7R	Stromal cells	Progenitor B and T cells	Proliferation and survival
IL-11	IL-11R	Stromal cells	Megakaryocytes	Megakaryocyte development
IL-13	IL-13R	NK, TH2-skewed T cells	Macrophages	Activation
IL-15	IL-15R	T cells	NK cells	Development of NK cells, stimulation of CD4 T cells
IFNγ	IFNγR	Macrophages, T cells, NK cells	T cells, macrophages	TH1-T-cells, macrophages, B-cell activation and development
IFNα	IFNαR	Plasmacytoid DCs	M1 macrophages, HSCs	Activation and development after infections

(304,347,348). Providing a supportive role for endothelial cells in HSC maintenance, hematopoietic cells can be maintained *in vitro* on endothelial-derived cell lines, and embryonic sources of endothelial cells can support adult HSCs (314). When HSCs are grown on transformed endothelial cells, they can maintain their ability to self-renew by up-regulating Notch ligands (314). Recent studies provide the best evidence for the importance of the perivascular niche. While it is known that osteoblasts, MSCs, and endothelial cells all express SCF, selective deletion of SCF in Nestin+ or osteoblasts showed no changes in HSCs numbers or activity; however, when SCF was deleted from perivascular, leptin receptor expressing cells or endothelial cells, the HSC compartment was greatly reduced (349). These studies indicate that one of the critical growth factors for HSC maintenance is expressed in cells that reside in the perivascular niche. While Leptin receptor expressing perivascular cells are similar to MSCs, they are unable to differentiate into osteoblasts, and thus it remains unclear how these stromal populations are related to the perivascular MSCs mentioned above (349). It should be noted, though, that in addition to SCF, endothelial cells secrete a variety of other cytokines known to regulate hematopoiesis as summarized in the Table 1.4.

Megakaryocytes

TPO is well known for its ability to promote megakaryocytic differentiation and platelet production by binding to its receptor, myeloproliferative leukemia (MPL) virus protooncogene, present on HS/PCs, and thus mice deficient in TPO have dramatically reduced megakaryocytes and platelets (350,351); however, TPO is also an important regulator of HSC cell cycle progression. In fact, mouse HSCs can be distinguished on the basis of c-Mpl expression and separated into quiescent (LSK34⁻ MPL⁺) and proliferative (LSK34⁺MPL⁺) forms (352). Megakaryocytes are mostly associated with sinusoids and may act as a sink for TPO in the stroma (352). Besides its ability to bind

to c-Mpl on megakaryocytes, TPO can initiate signals in HSCs and mediate quiescence (160,352). *c-Mpl*-deficient mice have reduced plasma cells, indicating that megakaryocytes can regulate other cell types within the niche, raising the prospect that megakaryocytes may indirectly regulate HSC function (350).

Migration, Trafficking, and Development from Secreted and Other Niche Components

One of the remarkable characteristics of the hematopoietic system is that at any given moment in time, samples taken from different sites of hematopoiesis are similar with respect to cellular composition. This is possible because HSCs are highly mobile cells, constantly exiting and reentering the bone marrow after traveling through the circulatory system, seeding sites conducive for hematopoiesis. But why should HSCs traffic normally? A number of models have been proposed. First, given the importance of an organism to be able to maintain hematopoietic output, migration of HSCs to multiple sites of hematopoiesis ensures that hematopoietic cell production is not reduced, even when a single hematopoietic site is injured. Second, HSC mobilization may allow for more rapid responses to immune challenge since the lymphatic circulation can be used by migrating HSCs and progenitors to migrate to peripheral tissues and secondary lymphoid organs where they can rapidly give rise to inflammatory cells locally through a process partially regulated by the sphingosine 1 phosphate receptor (147). Regardless of the evolutionary and biologic explanations for HSC trafficking, it is this property that allows clinical HSC transplantation possible, as HSC can migrate back to the bone marrow after a simple infusion of cells into the peripheral blood.

The earliest evidence for HSC migration was observed in rat parabiosis experiments, which involves connecting the circulation of one rat to that of another. When one of the rats was lethally irradiated, the hematopoietic cells from its nonirradiated partner reconstituted its damaged immune system

(353). These studies were followed by experiments in mice in which the peripheral blood of 200 donors was transplanted into irradiated recipients and shown to be able to reconstitute the recipient's immune system (354). More recent mouse parabiosis experiments using genetically marked animals have shown that HSCs constitutively circulate in the peripheral blood and can repopulate unconditioned bone marrow (355). While it had been assumed for some time that myeloablative conditioning may be required to eliminate HSCs from their niches, it appears that approximately 0.1% to 1% of all HSC niches are unoccupied at any given moment in time and therefore can be engrafted by circulating HSCs (356). Moreover, HSC egress from the bone marrow does not depend on alterations in HSC cell cycle status (148), indicating that this process is likely regulated. The mechanisms underlying this process are poorly understood.

As noted earlier, G-CSF is a widely used agent for mobilizing HS/PCs in the clinic. Although it is known that HSC mobilization following administration can occur as early as 5 days after treatment, the exact mechanism underlying this effect remains unclear since the target cell of G-CSF's action in the bone marrow has not been clearly identified (357,358). One would postulate that G-CSF directly binds to HS/PCs to drive mobilization, but it has long been thought to not require expression of the G-CSF receptor on the HS/PCs themselves (359). However, more recent studies demonstrated that functional G-CSF receptors are expressed on the surface of human and mouse HSCs (360). Besides this potential direct effect of G-CSF on HSCs, monocytic cells that express high levels of G-CSF receptor have been shown to be sufficient to drive mobilization, likely through the release of proteases that process CXCL12, c-Kit, or VCAM (309,361). However, this model has not been formally proven because it is unclear which proteases are essential for mobilization, as deletion of neutrophil serine proteases and metalloproteinase inhibitors had no effect on mobilization (362–364). Besides proteases, other factors may facilitate mobilization such as the stimulation of complement receptors C3a or C3 allowing for HS/PCs to become sensitive to G-CSF stimulation (365).

Despite these advances in our understanding of HSC migration, currently employed strategies to mobilize HSCs for autologous bone marrow transplants do not always succeed in collecting sufficient numbers of HSCs, and thus other strategies will be required to optimize such protocols. Secreted factors such as chemokines provide signals to hematopoietic cells to migrate, lodge, and engraft in the bone marrow, and therefore their manipulation may be useful. CXCR4 and its ligand CXCL12 are critical players that regulate HSC migration to the bone marrow. HSCs express CXCR4 and cells from the niche can provide CXCL12, which activates the Rac/Rho family of GTPases, to signal HSCs to migrate toward the endosteal niche (366). An antagonist to CXCR4 (AMD3100) has shown efficacy in inducing proliferation and mobilizing HS/PCs in mice, nonhuman primates, and in humans in a variety of clinical settings (367–369). Another clinically relevant factor that may increase HS/PC mobilization is parathyroid hormone (PTH). PTH initially was thought to act on HS/PCs by inducing signals from osteoblasts, but recent data suggest that this occurs, instead, through interactions with T cells (234,370–372). Other cytokines and factors known to be capable of mobilizing HSCs from the marrow include SCF, MIP-1α, Grob, IL-1, IL-3, IL-6, IL-7, IL-8, IL-1, and IL-12 (373–381).

Selectins are adhesion molecules expressed on endothelial cells that are critical for mediating recruitment of mature leukocytes to inflamed sites (382,383). Consistent with a similar function in mediating HS/PC migration to the marrow, homing was compromised in the absence of either E- or P-selectins (384). Integrins also play an important role in HSC migration, as inhibition of $\alpha 4$ integrins or VCAM-1 function results in markedly reduced HS/PC homing (385). Integrins including CD49d/CD29 ($\alpha 4 \beta 1$ or VLA-4), $\alpha 4 \beta 7$, and CD49b ($\alpha 2$) have

also been shown to regulate HSC homing to the bone marrow (386–390). Within the marrow, LFA-1 and VLA-4 promote the migration of HSCs toward osteoblasts (388,391).

Factors secreted by the niche such as BMP4 and angiopoietin-1 (Ang1) have been shown to be important in maintaining HSCs *in vitro* (392–394). Ang1 is also expressed by osteoblasts and binds to HSCs (394). Many products expressed from MSCs and osteoblasts have been shown to regulate HSC function. Tissue inhibitor of metalloproteinase-3 was shown to regulate HSC quiescence and fate determination as well as normal bone formation and maintenance (395,396). Agrin, a proteoglycan typically associated with the neuromuscular junction, supports hematopoietic progenitor proliferation, presumably by interacting with its receptor, α-dystroglycan, which is expressed on HSCs (397). However, transplantation of agrin-deficient HSCs demonstrated no defect in engraftment or reconstitution of the immune system.

Stem Cell Factor

SCF is produced by multiple cell types in the bone marrow niche, including osteoblasts, endothelial cells, and perivascular cells, and engages c-Kit on the surface of HSCs to initiate cell signals. SCF exists in two forms, membrane-bound and soluble, generated by proteolytic cleavage of SCF by a number of proteases including MMPs (398–400). The importance of this pathway in HSC maintenance has been demonstrated through a number of approaches. Mice with mutations in SCF (e.g. *Sl/Sld*, steel dickie mutants) or in c-Kit (e.g. *W/Wv*, white spotting mutant) exhibit reduced numbers of HSCs and decreased HSC function (401,402). Blocking SCF:c-Kit interactions with an antibody results in loss of HSCs (94). The importance of membrane-bound SCF was demonstrated by analyzing HSC function in mice lacking this form. These mice showed decreased HSC numbers and reduced ability to support HSCs following transplant (403). More recently, studies utilizing tissue-specific Cre-recombinase indicate that the predominant functional source of SCF in the bone marrow is the endothelial cells and/or the perivascular cells surrounding them, but not in osteoblastic lineage cells (349).

The Niche in Hematologic Disorders

Given the importance of the niche in regulating HSC homeostasis, it is not difficult to imagine that an altered niche may allow for the survival and maintenance of abnormal cells in hematopoietic disorders and malignancies. Emerging evidence indicates that many regulators of normal HSCs in the niche are co-opted by LSCs (404,405). Cytokines such as IL-6, IL-3, G-CSF, and GM-CSF increase proliferation of leukemic cells. CXCR4 is frequently increased on AML blasts, and anti-CD44 monoclonal antibody treatment decreases leukemic blast homing and engraftment (406,407). An attractive theory is that the hypoxic and low perfusion environment within the niche may provide a protection from classical chemotherapy (408). Antiangiogenic inhibitors also could be used as a therapy to prevent VEGF signaling to drive leukemia. Overall, developing inhibitors to disrupt the HSC and LSC interactions with the niche components could provide an additional therapeutic strategy for treating leukemias.

Hematopoietic Development
Hematopoietic Progenitors

The classical hematopoietic hierarchy held that MPPs differentiate into a CMP or a CLP, establishing the myeloid and lymphoid arms of the hematopoietic system (27,28,409). More recently this model has been amended to include another PC that reflects the recognition that there is also a hierarchy of multipotent progenitors. In humans this cell has been described as the multilymphoid progenitor (MLP), which has the potential to differentiate into the GMP or CLP; in mouse, they are referred to as early lymphoid progenitor or lymphoid primed multipotent progenitor (82,410–413). Markers for the MLP are CD34pos CD38neg Thy1lo CD45RApos. This more recent concept incorporates the idea that the lymphoid/myeloid switch occurs in progenitors downstream of the MPP and also loses its ability to differentiate into the megakaryocyte/erythroid lineages (414). Evidence for the existence of this progenitor comes from single-cell assays from sorted populations, lineage tracing, and myeloid potential being retained in thymocyte precursors (415,416). Although the mouse system is better defined, confusion remains regarding the exact lineage order and overall plasticity of human progenitors.

Transcriptional Factor Network

Extrinsic signals activate a set of lineage-specifying transcriptional modulators in HS/PCs. Extensive transcriptional profiling of functionally distinct populations within the hematopoietic hierarchy as well as numerous loss- and gain-of-function mouse models have revealed a set of critical regulators that dictate hematopoietic developmental fates (417,418). As one would expect, alterations in regulators of hematopoietic differentiation and self-renewal can lead to hematopoietic disorders and malignancies. Due to the large number and complex regulation of transcription factors and other modulators, this chapter will only highlight a small set.

One of the most critical transcriptional factors is Runx1, shown to be required for embryonic and fetal hematopoiesis, but not for adult hematopoiesis (314). However, Runx1 plays an important role in mediating proper megakaryocytic, B-cell, and T-cell development (314). One critical target of Runx1 is *Pu.1*, which can act as a master regulator of hematopoiesis by itself (419). As a member of the E-twenty six (ETS) family, deletion of this transcription factor leads to a block in the generation of CMPs and CLPs (420,421). PU.1 is expressed during many stages of hematopoietic development, but can also regulate a critical myeloid PC fate decision since high levels of expression skew progenitors toward the macrophage lineage while lower levels favor granulocyte differentiation (420,422). Consistent with its important role as a driver of myeloid differentiation, loss of *Pu.1* and its gene regulatory regions induces AML in mice (420).

Myeloid differentiation and commitment is also regulated by the transcription factor CEBPα, which is commonly deleted in AML and a critical driver of the CMP to GMP transition (423,424). Its potent activity as an inducer of myeloid fates is perhaps best illustrated by its ability to reprogram mature B or T cells into macrophages (425).

Another lineage program can be dictated through overexpression of GATA-1, which redirects CLPs into the megakaryocytic and erythroid lineages (425). Additional transcription factors such as growth factor independent 1 (GFI1) and interferon regulatory factor 8 (IRF8) can modulate the differentiation fate of myelocytes and granulocytes. Gfi-1 is required for terminal neutrophil differentiation, and deletion of *Irf8* results in fewer myeloid cells with an additional skewing toward granulocytes at the expense of macrophages (236,426,427). This complex interplay of transcriptional regulators is compounded by the general feature that the same set of transcription factors or gene expression programs tends to be reused to regulate cell fate in both immature and mature progenitors as well as in later stages of differentiation (417). Although there are many examples of this phenomenon, PU.1 has been shown to be important in HSC self-renewal, development of CMPs, and then again in the development of different dendritic cell (DC) subtypes (428,429).

Cytokines can coordinate transcriptional programs, which can then dictate a specific cell fate. Specific cytokines through signaling pathways can be connected to individual transcription factors. For example, when Mafb/c-Maf transcription factors were deleted, these mice demonstrated increased monocytic development and proliferation *in vitro* in the presence of only M-CSF and not other myeloid-specific cytokines. Interestingly, this cytokine specific proliferation was robust and did not result in transformation to leukemia (430). Additionally, this model illustrates the importance of understanding the role of transcription factors in the context of specific extrinsic signals.

Myelopoiesis

Monocytes and Macrophages

The innate immune system functions mainly through myeloid lineage cells that migrate throughout the body and provide the first line of defense for a variety of pathogens. The mononuclear phagocytic system (MPS) is comprised of a diverse set of cell types expressing different cell surface markers, levels of phagocytic and antigen-presenting activity, and gene expression profiles and includes monocytes, macrophages, and DCs (see Fig. 1.4 for the hierarchy of the MPS) (431). The MPS is essential for mediating the inflammatory response and interacting with the adaptive immune system.

Monocytes arise from GMPs and progress through several morphologically defined differentiation stages downstream of the GMP including the monoblast, promonocyte, and mature monocyte (432). Increased nuclear folding, the appearance of cytoplasmic granules, and an increasing cytoplasm to nuclear ratio characterize the basic developmental stages of monocytes. However, the appearance of mature monocytes can be quite heterogeneous based on their activation state. After developing in the bone marrow, monocytes migrate into the peripheral blood, where they represent about 10% of the total white blood cells in humans and circulate for as short as 3 hours to 3 days (433). Monocyte development depends on M-CSF, as mice lacking *Csf-1R* (M-CSFR) exhibit dramatically reduced monocytes (434–436). Although mature monocytes enter the periphery and have limited proliferation potential, they can undergo further differentiation into tissue-resident macrophages or inflammatory DCs, and thus monocytes can restore the pool of macrophages in specific tissues. While monocytes and macrophages are both capable of phagocytosing pathogens, producing cytokines to interact with the adaptive immune system, and presenting antigen via class II MHC to clear infections (432), they are less effective in doing so compared to macrophages or DCs.

While monocytes and their terminally differentiated counterparts share these activities, it is not clear that all monocytes serve similar physiologic functions. "Classical monocytes" that are involved in an infection are characterized by a Gr1/Ly6C^{high} cell surface phenotype and differentiate into DCs that secrete TNFα, ROS, and NOS (437). Some of these cells can also be described as myeloid suppressor cells that have the ability to inhibit immune cells recruited to clear tumor cells or respond to chronic infections (438). Nonclassical monocytes include Gr1/Ly6C^{low} cells, which are smaller, and express CX3CR1 and LFA-1, but lack CCR2 and L-selection expression and differentiate into the M2 subtype of macrophages (439). GM-CSF and IL-4 can drive differentiation toward the DC lineage, and M-CSF commits monocytes toward the macrophage lineage (440). As in mice, humans have a larger subset of monocytes with increased phagocytic activity and a smaller subset with the ability to expand rapidly. The larger subset is characterized by a CD14$^+$CD16$^-$ immunophenotype and expresses similar chemokines to the mouse equivalents, consistent with the cells defined as "classical monocytes" (437).

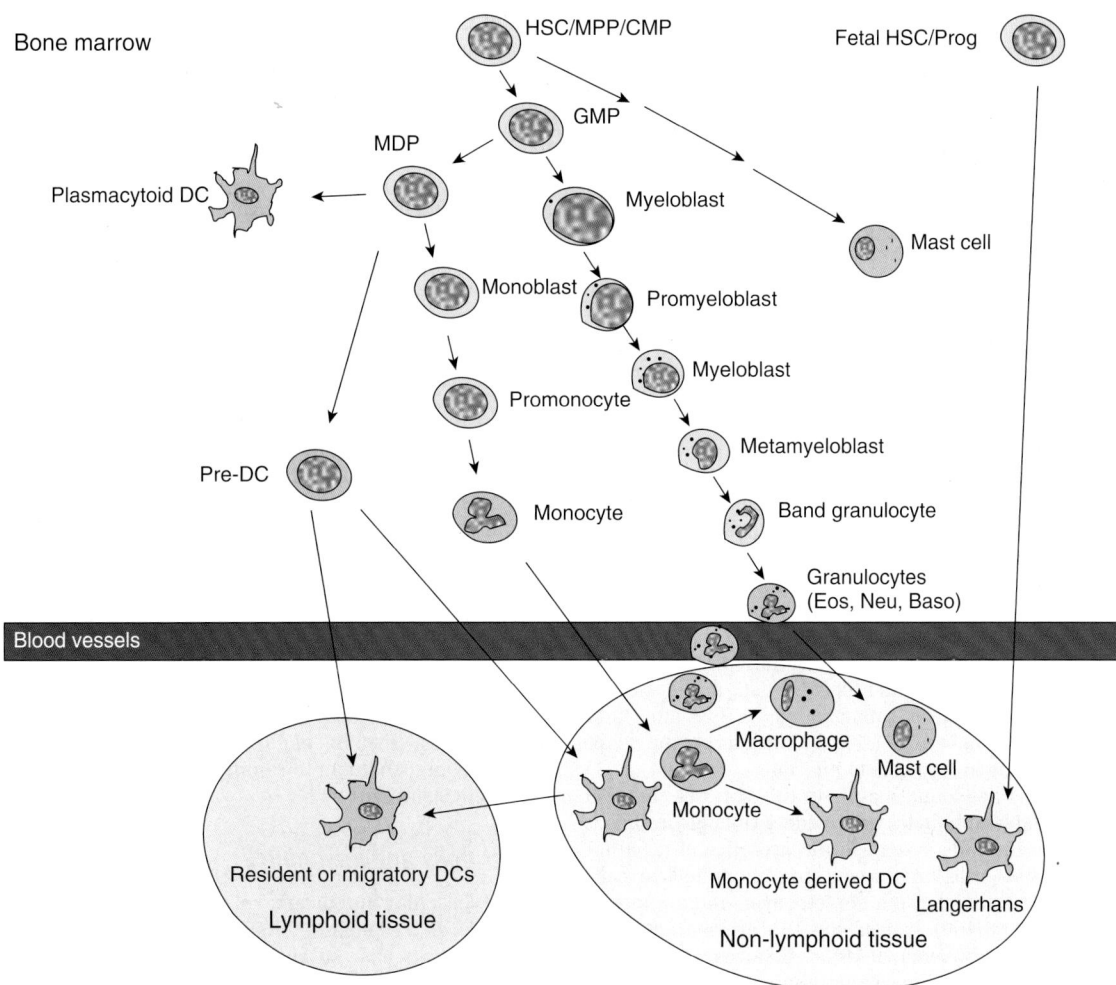

FIGURE 1.4. Hierarchy of the myeloid developmental program. Myeloid development can also be described in terms of cell surface marker antigens as well as the cytologic features of differentiating precursors. Once monocytes leave the bone marrow and enter peripheral sites, they differentiate into macrophages. Some myeloid lineages such as DCs may arise from more than one developmental pathway while others such as Langerhans cells can differentiate rapidly from immature hematopoietic cells without generating large numbers of identifiable intermediates. HSC, hematopoietic stem cell; MPP, multipotent progenitor; CMP, common myeloid progenitor; Prog, progenitor; GMP, granulocyte monocyte progenitor; MDP, monocyte plasmacytoid progenitor cell; DC, dendritic cell; Pre-DC, pre-dendritic cell; Eos, eosinophils; Neu, neutrophils; Baso, basophils. *Arrows* indicate order of differentiation and lineage relationship. Granules (*small black circles*) and changes in nuclear morphology are represented during maturation stages.

Once monocytes enter peripheral tissue, their designation depends on their tissue of residence. For example, microglia are macrophages of the nervous system, and Kupffer cells are macrophages found lining the sinusoids in the liver. Similar to monocytes, it is now recognized that macrophages can be divided into classes based on their function. These classes include the M1, M2, and tumor-associated macrophages (441–443). These macrophages are polarized based on the cytokines they secrete as well as their ability to induce specific T-helper responses (444,445). M1 macrophages show increased antigen-presenting ability and are activated by LPS or IFNγ, whereas M2 macrophages are closely associated with responses to parasites, wounds, tissue repair, and other anti-inflammatory responses (446,447). The M2 macrophages can be activated by IL-4 or IL-13. It should be emphasized that these different macrophage effector functions are not necessarily fixed and that the transition and conversion between these two types of macrophages may occur depending on the persistence of antigens or changes in the local cytokine environment. Additionally, tumor-associated macrophages, although phenotypically similar to M2 type macrophages, are functionally distinct. These macrophages suppress the immune response and can promote tumorigenesis (297,312).

Dendritic Cells

Historically, DCs were originally recognized as a unique cell type based on their "veiled" appearance characterized by their irregular shape and pseudopods. It is now clear that these cells can arise from diverse developmental pathways and serve critical roles in linking the innate and adaptive immune responses. Immature DCs are generally less spindle-shaped, while mature DCs contain increased lamellipodia (432,443,448). DCs are considered part of the MPS system and can be classified into four major groups based on their cellular derivation and function including the conventional or classical DCs (cDCs), plasmacytoid DCs, Langerhans DCs, and monocyte-derived DCs (mDCs) (449). A particular challenge in the DC field has been characterizing these different subsets of DC since markers expressed on the different DC populations rapidly change after activation. Moreover, DCs are rare and studies using expansion approaches to study their biology alter their fate and/or marker profile, making it especially challenging definitive conclusions about specific subtypes.

Pre-DC progenitors can develop into macrophages and cDCs, but these progenitors are not considered monocytes (450,451). These DCs can be either migratory or resident in lymph nodes or tissues (448,452,453). The migratory DCs can be further subdivided into interstitial DCs (CD11b⁺) or the CD11b⁻ CD103⁺ integrinαEβ7 DCs (454–456). Initially, migratory cDCs reside within the tissue where they exhibit a high phagocytic capacity. However, upon activation by antigenic challenge, they increase MHCII expression and migrate to lymph nodes where they present antigens to T cells. Unlike the migratory DCs, the lymphoid tissue–resident DCs are found within all secondary lymphoid organs and can be additionally subclassified based on CD4 and CD8 expression (457,458). Lymph node–resident DCs are presumed to be necessary for the surveillance of antigens circulating in the blood and entering the lymphatic system.

mDCs, described earlier in this section, are mainly resident in nonlymphoid organs (421,459,460). The mDCs are similar to cDCs in their ability to act as potent antigen-presenting cells. Also, the mDCs express markers CD11c, MHCII, CD209a, MAC3 and are negative for LyGC.

The search to identify the source of cells that produce high-level type 1 IFNs eventually led to the discovery of plasmacytoid pDCs in 1999 (461,462). This subset of DCs originates in the bone marrow and arises from a similar pre-DC progenitor that also produces cDCs (463,464). pDCs are generally long-lived and are usually found in the lymphatic system, where they can directly recognize viruses using toll-like receptors 7 and 9 (TLR7/9) and express CD45RA with low-level expression of CD11b/c or MHCII (465). Several markers can be used to identify pDCs including IL-T7 and BDCA-2 in humans and Siglec-H Bst2 in mice. Since pDCs can produce high concentrations of type 1 IFNs after viral infections, they are thought to be critical for triggering the adaptive immune response in response to infection.

Langerhans DCs are found mainly in the skin but can also migrate to regional lymph nodes to provide T-cell help and activate the adaptive immune system in the presence of a pathogen (466,467). These cells are derived from mononuclear cells during development, mainly from the fetal liver, and a minority from the yolk sac (468,469). Langerhans DCs are characterized by high Fcγ expression. Deletion of *M-Csfr* in mice leads to a loss of Langerhans cells (468). Remarkably, and unlike many hematopoietic cells, Langerhans cells have the ability to renew and can survive for long periods in the dermis. They are also known to express c-type lectins and are characterized by Birbeck granules (rod-shaped organelles), which can be identified by electron microscopy (470). Because these cells are rare, they have been difficult to isolate and study. However, novel mouse models that utilize a Langerin promoter specifically mark Langerhans cells *in vivo* and will provide key tools to further our understanding of this interesting DC population (471,472).

Granulocytes

Neutrophils, basophils, mast cells, and eosinophils are myeloid lineage cells that are collectively known as granulocytes based on the presence of cytoplasmic granules following staining by special cytologic and histologic stains. There are five morphologically defined stages of development that occur stepwise in the bone marrow: myeloblast, promyelocyte, myelocyte, metamyelocyte, and band form. Large myeloblasts containing nuclei with open chromatin, high nuclear to cytoplasmic ratios, and few cytoplasmic granules, give rise to promyelocytes characterized by a slightly decreased nuclear to cytoplasmic ratio and primary granules. As development continues, the cell becomes smaller, exhibits increased granulation, and undergoes increased packing and folding of the nucleus until it becomes the mature granulocyte (Fig. 1.4).

Neutrophils

Neutrophils, also known as polymorphonuclear leukocytes, develop in the bone marrow and are the most common cell in the peripheral blood (473). These cells comprise 70% of the blood in humans, but only approximately 20% in mice, and are characterized by a multilobed nucleus with neutral pink cytoplasmic staining. Neutrophils are potent first responders and effectors of the innate immune system that are produced in the bone marrow at a constant daily rate of 10¹¹ cells with a life span that varies from as short as 6 to 8 hours to 5 days (474–476). The morphologic development of neutrophils has been well-characterized downstream of the GMP. The primary azurophilic or myeloperoxidase-positive granules are the largest in the neutrophils. Secondary granules contain lactoferrin, and the third class of granules containing gelatinases and metalloproteinases arises during the band neutrophil stage (477).

Mature neutrophils can become captured through selectins expressed on endothelial cells lining the blood vessels and then adhere to them via integrin interactions (478–480). Migration across the endothelial cells and into the tissue is mediated by signals from bacterially derived factors and chemokines such as IL-8 that are released by other immune cells. Higher levels of IL-8 expression can lead to degranulation, while G-CSF can rapidly expand the population. Neutrophils can be attracted and activated through the interactions of other cells in the innate immune system including macrophages and DCs. The ability of neutrophils to phagocytize pathogens is further enhanced by their ability to use neutrophil extracellular traps, including fibers with proteases and chromatin that can bind bacteria (305,481,482). Neutrophils rely on NADPH oxidases to create enough ROS to destroy phagocytized bacteria. Neutrophils can also be engulfed by macrophages, which can serve as a mechanism to remove toxins or pathogens from the local environment.

Mast Cells and Basophils

Mast cells play important roles in both the innate immune and allergic responses. Although the developmental pathway for mast cells has not been settled, earlier studies suggesting that mast cells are derived from GMPs have been challenged by more recent work suggesting that the CMP or MPP has the potential to differentiate into a common, bipotential precursor that can give rise to basophils and mast cells (429,483). This is perhaps not a surprising finding since mast cells and basophils have similar appearances and have some overlapping functions. Mast cells are mainly found within tissues where they express the IgE receptor (FcεRI). Binding of this receptor initiates a rapid strong inflammatory response characterized by a release of inflammatory mediators including proteases, histamines, and lipids.

Mast cells remain immature in the periphery and terminally differentiate once they migrate to and reside in tissues. Critical growth and differentiation factors for mast cells include SCF in humans and IL-3 and SCF in mice (484). Mice lacking the SCF receptor c-Kit/CD117 are almost devoid of mast cells (485). β7 integrin expressed on mast cells was required for proper homing to the small intestine, but not required for any other tissue (486). β7 expression can distinguish the fate of the bipotent mast cell/basophil precursor with high expression associated with cells differentiating toward the mast cell lineage (487).

Like mast cells, basophils are involved in allergic responses and express the FcεRI receptor (488). Although fewer in number than mast cells and comprising only 0.5% of all immune cells, basophils account for the majority of IL-4 that is produced *in vivo* (489). Basophil granules appear bluish-black after staining with basophilic aniline dyes. Basophils are characterized by the surface marker phenotype c-Kit⁻, FcεRI⁺, CD11b⁺, IL-3Rʰⁱ (490). Basophils play a role in the defense against certain parasites, ticks, and in allergy models involving the skin (488). Most importantly, they can control the initiation of the Th2-dependent response through the secretion of IL-4 and other factors (491).

Eosinophils

The eosinophil is a key cellular component of the innate immune response to parasites and microbial infections and also actively coordinates the adaptive immune system (217). Eosinophils differentiate from the GMP, and like mast cells and other hematopoietic cells, they develop in the bone marrow and migrate to the periphery to become tissue-resident. These cells, named for their characteristic strong staining of their secondary granules by the acidic dye eosin, can release proteins such as major basic protein, toxins, and peroxidases after activation to stimulate other immune cells or to destroy parasites. Eosinophils can also contribute to T-cell-mediated responses through their expression of costimulatory molecules, cytokines, and presenting antigen via the MHCII. Cytokines including IL-3 and GM-CSF are able to stimulate eosinophils, but only IL-5 remains a specific regulator of activation (492). The critical role of IL-5 in eosinophil development was demonstrated in mice deficient in IL-5/eotaxin, which exhibited a near absence of eosinophils. These mice also exhibited reduced IL-13 production and defective TH2 responses (493).

Erythroid and Megakaryocyte Development

Erythropoiesis

The human bone marrow has the remarkable capacity to produce approximately 2 million RBCs per second. RBCs, only 6 to 8 μm in size, are characterized by a distinctive concave shape and circulate in the peripheral blood with a half-life of about 120 days while carrying oxygen bound to hemoglobin to tissues throughout the body. As described previously, human RBCs first arise in the yolk sac from hematopoietic progenitors as early as gestational day 19 and continue as early erythrocytes for as long as 9 weeks (103,494). Definitive erythropoiesis originates from the AGM then switches to the fetal liver followed by the bone marrow beginning between the fifth and sixth weeks of gestation. In addition to being produced in different anatomic sites during development, erythroid cells exhibit a number of other important differences compared with other hematopoietic cells, perhaps best exemplified by alterations in the types of hemoglobins produced due to the action of a set of transcription factors (495). Primitive erythroblasts are characterized by predominant expression of ($\zeta_2\varepsilon_2$) and ($\alpha_2\varepsilon_2$) hemoglobins and begin to express the ζ, ε, α, γ globin and minimal amounts of the β globin during the transition to definitive erythropoiesis. As fetal and adult erythropoiesis replaces embryonic erythropoiesis, ε hemoglobin is silenced and α, γ hemoglobins are highly expressed, eventually being replaced at birth by β globin (496). Adult erythrocytes are also generally smaller than fetal erythrocytes.

Erythroid development has been defined in a number of ways, including morphologic, functional, and now immunophenotypic. It has been appreciated for some time that erythroid development is characterized by stereotypic morphologic changes. After erythroid progenitors commit to the lineage, maturation is accompanied by condensation of the nucleus, decreasing in overall size and followed by the process of enucleation, which can take about 2 weeks to complete *in vitro*. Several rounds of division, increased ribosomal assembly, and synthesis of hemoglobin characterize the first cells during erythroid development named proerythroblasts. The basophilic erythroblast, polychromatic erythroblast, and orthochromatic erythroblast are sequential stages named according to their Wright-Giemsa–stained appearance that are associated with increasingly condensed nuclear chromatin and decreased size. The latter stages are defined by a more acidic cytoplasm, condensed chromatin, and the extrusion of the pyknotic nuclei. The nucleus becomes quickly phagocytized by macrophages

that are usually closely associated with erythroid progenitors (497,498). This immature RBC or reticulocyte is retained in the bone marrow for several days before it migrates into the periphery and fully matures into a RBC.

Erythroid intermediates have also been classified based on their activity in colony assays. BFU-E colonies arise from early, proliferative erythroid progenitors that rise to grapelike clusters of erythroid cells. These cells are developmentally upstream of progenitors that give rise to CFU-E, which are smaller colonies composed of more mature RBCs. While these progenitor types allow one to functionally identify erythroid progenitors with specific activity, unfortunately they do not allow their prospective separation.

Most recently, flow cytometric and FACS technology have allowed the identification of prospectively isolatable populations including the MEP, as previously discussed. Downstream of the MEP, flow cytometric markers can be used to capture a continuum of specific developmental changes characterized by increasing glycophorin-A expression and expression of specific blood antigens (A, B, O, and Rh). Transferrin receptor (CD71) expression is higher in earlier stages and then becomes reduced in the later stages of erythroid development. These trends can also be observed in mouse erythropoiesis, and combined with an additional mouse erythroid lineage marker Ter119, immature erythroid progenitors can be distinguished from proerythroblasts.

Like other hematopoietic lineages, cytokines play a major role in regulating the proliferation and survival of progenitors representing various stages of erythroid development. The most important cytokines that stimulate erythropoiesis are erythropoietin (EPO) and GM-CSF, whereas SCF, FLT3, and IL-3 can provide additional proliferative signals. EPO, predominantly synthesized by the renal peritubular cells in the kidneys, provides homeostatic and systemic control of red cell output in the bone marrow, as hypoxia sensed in the kidney via HIF signaling stimulates the secretion of EPO that stimulates blood production (499). EPO/EPOR stimulation of early erythroid progenitors leads to activation of JAK/STAT signaling, and in combination with the other cytokines activates PI3K signaling to allow expansion of erythroid progenitors (500).

The commitment and development of the erythroid lineage requires evolutionarily conserved transcription factors including GATA1/2, FOG-1, erythroid Krüppel-like factor (EKLF) (501,502). For example, deletion of *Eklf* blocks globin expression and loss of *Gata1* blocks differentiation at the proerythroblast stage (503,504). The importance of GATA1 in erythroid differentiation is exemplified by patients that harbor familial mutations in GATA1, who exhibit severe anemia and thrombocytopenia (505). Due to the wide variety of diseases characterized by defects in erythroid development, understanding the relationship among the erythroid transcription factors, globin genes, and epigenetic regulators is an important and exciting area of investigation and may provide exciting opportunities for novel therapies incorporating cellular engineering technologies.

Megakaryopoiesis

Platelets were first described as megakaryocyte derivatives during the early 20th century (506). Because megakaryocyte generate platelets, they are critical for maintaining hemostasis and thrombosis (507,508). Although megakaryocytes make up only a small fraction of all bone marrow cells, in humans they possess the capacity to produce platelets at a rate of approximately 1 million per second with one megakaryocyte being able to produce 1 to 3 thousand platelets; this results in approximately 1 trillion platelets in circulation at any given time (509,510). Besides their primary function as cellular clotting factors in response to tissue injury, platelets serve additional roles in both the innate and adaptive immune system. For example, platelets express P-selectin and costimulatory receptors such as CD40L and TLRs, which can participate in recruiting leukocytes to sites of injury and promoting the inflammatory response (511).

During development, megakaryocytes are first detected in the embryonic yolk sac, similar to erythroid cells. In the adult bone marrow, megakaryocytes are thought to arise from more than one developmental pathway, differentiating directly from HSCs/MPPs and bypassing the CMP (82), or from classically defined bipotent MEPs (424,508). TPO promotes the differentiation and expansion of megakaryocytes and leads to an increase in platelets.

After commitment to the megakaryocytic lineage, megakaryocytic progenitors undergo a series of rounds of DNA replication without cell division (endomitosis) in order to generate the unique morphology characteristic of mature megakaryocytes (512). This differentiation process can take approximately 6 to 10 days (512). In the early stages of this process, megakaryoblasts undergo rounds of proliferation, are 15 μm in size and 4N in DNA content, and exhibit basophilic staining. The promegakaryocyte stage is easily identified by increased numbers of granules that represent dense proteins in organelles specific for platelet production and contain peroxisomes (α, β, and γ) (513). In the final stage, megakaryocytes begin to produce platelets, are as large as 150 μM in size, and can be associated with as much as 64N ploidy. Interestingly, ploidy does not always correlate with the maturation and development of megakaryocytes (514). Terminally differentiated megakaryocytes exhibit increased nuclear folding and significantly increased size and generate lobulated projections. Such mature megakaryocytes, located in close proximity to marrow sinusoids and bone, rapidly shed platelets directly into the circulation via their projections that can extend through the sinusoidal endothelium, and the platelets can last up to 9 days in the circulation (515). Once the megakaryocytes stop producing platelets, they are denuded, become senescent, and undergo apoptosis and subsequent clearance by macrophage engulfment (516). Besides their distinct morphology, megakaryocytes express a variety of markers including CD31, CD41, CD42b and CD61, Gly Ib/IIB, and factors V and VII, with later stages expressing the von Willebrand factor (513,517). Platelets largely express the same markers present on mature megakaryocytes (517).

As discussed previously, the major cytokine that regulates megakaryopoiesis is TPO through interactions with its cognate receptor MPL. Deletion of this receptor in mice reduces platelet production dramatically, although not completely, suggesting there is a minor non-TPO-dependent pathway for platelet production present (350,455,518). TPO is mainly produced in the liver and bone marrow stromal cells. Platelets have the ability to bind soluble TPO in the periphery, effectively regulating overall levels in the blood and providing a negative feedback loop for TPO production (156,519–521). Other cytokines, while not necessary for platelet production, can stimulate megakaryocyte development including SCF, IL-3, IL-11, and GM-CSF (522). In addition, like other cell types, SDF1 (CXCL12) can cause increased migration and force megakaryocytes out of their niche in the bone marrow to provide local sources of platelets in other tissues such as the spleen (100,523).

Similar to erythropoiesis, megakaryocyte development relies on a set of key transcription factors. Deletion of GATA1 and FOG in megakaryocytes resulted in reduced megakaryocytes and platelet production (524,525). Mice deficient in NF-E2 exhibit a dramatic developmental block near the final stage of megakaryopoiesis before platelets are produced and result in the development of dysplastic megakaryocytes and thrombocytopenia (526).

Lymphopoiesis

While the exact ontogeny and marker expression of the lymphoid progenitor is somewhat controversial (see Hematopoietic Progenitor section), subsequent steps of development are more clearly defined. Both mature B cells and T cells possess the potential to be long-lived and maintained in a quiescent state like long-term HSCs. These seemingly dormant cells can rapidly proliferate following stimulation through their immune regulatory receptors.

B-Cell Development

B cells are central mediators of the adaptive immune system through their roles as immunoglobulin producers. They were originally named based on their discovery in the bursa of fabricius, a specialized organ found only in birds. In humans, B-cell development initially occurs in the fetal liver at 5 to 7 weeks gestation but eventually moves to the bone marrow when HSCs migrate there (527–529). B-cell development has been rigorously studied in an attempt to understand how they produce the impressive antibody diversity that is essential for effective adaptive immunity. The first committed B-cell progenitor is the pro-B cell, which is characterized by heavy chain rearrangement. This developmental stage is followed by the pre-B cell in which light chain rearrangements occur, and this stage is critical since improperly rearranged B-cell receptors cause the developing B cells to quickly undergo apoptosis. Productive B-cell antibody rearrangement results in IgM^{high} and IgD^{low} expressing immature B cells that then exit the bone marrow to enter the periphery and secondary lymphoid organs. The maturation of the B cells then continues after stimulation within these lymphoid organs. The early committed B-cell progenitors express CD10, then gains in CD19 expression following expression of V-PreB. Once the B cell matures, it also expresses CD10, CD19/CD22, CD24, and CD40. Overall, this complex developmental process is generally characterized by proliferative bursts followed by resting stages, marker alterations, and sensitivity to stromal interactions.

Specification of B cells requires a defined set of transcription factors including paired box protein 5 (Pax5), early B-cell factor 1, surrogate light chain (VpreB), Rag1 and Rag2, terminal deoxytidyl transferase (TdT), and others. Besides the role for these transcription factors, cytokines can also sustain B-cell development. Stromal cells provide important signals including TGFβ, CXCL12, FLT3L, and IL-7. Most importantly, IL-7 in mice sustains B-cell development *in vitro*, but only partially stimulates human B-cell precursors. Deletion of the common γ-chain of the IL-7 receptor results in the depletion of B cells, T cells, and NK cells in mice, but SCID patients with disruption of IL-7 are only deficient in T cells. Consequently, this reduced reliance on IL-7 has made it more challenging to study human B-cell development.

A more comprehensive description of B-cell development and function will be presented in Chapter 2.

T-Cell Development

T cells make up another major component of the adaptive immune system. These cells are named based on their origin and development in the thymus. T cells interact with components of both the adaptive and innate immune system and confer the ability to rapidly stimulate the cellular immune response against specific pathogens. While cytotoxic T-cell populations directly clear infections, regulatory T cells act as suppressors of the immune system, providing a way to control aberrant activation of the immune response and peripheral tolerance. Early T-cell lineage progenitor (ETPs) are initially established in the bone marrow from lymphoid progenitors. In mice, these T-cell precursors are classically defined by their surface immunophenotype, Lin^{low}, CD44, CD117^{+}, and CD35^{-}. In humans, ETPs express CD34^{high}, CD33^{low}, CD38^{low}, CD44, and IL-7Ra. These cells, destined to become T cells, then leave the bone marrow to enter the thymus. In humans, pre-T cells can be identified based on their expression of TdT, CD7, CD2, CD5, and IL-7R (530).

Lineage-tracing experiments demonstrate that ETP maintain their ability to differentiate into myeloid cells *in vitro,* but they rarely become myeloid (415,531). Efforts to understand early T-cell development have benefited greatly from many *in vitro* studies using stromal lines expressing DLL1, a Notch ligand, or cultures using cells derived from the thymus. Like other progenitors, cytokines such as IL-7 and FLT3 have shown an ability to sustain and also drive T-cell maturation. Perhaps not surprisingly, normal T-cell developmental pathways are commonly altered in T-cell neoplasms, best exemplified by the discovery of frequent Notch mutations in T-ALL. While the stages of T-cell development will be further discussed in Chapter 2, it is important to note that T cells mature through an intricate selection process that allows the generation of thymocytes that are able to recognize antigen in the context of MHC, while eliminating autoreactive T cells. Through this process, thymocytes that fail to produce productive T-cell receptors (TCRs) or that produce TCRs that are activated by autoantigens presented on thymic epithelial cells rapidly undergo apoptosis, while functional T cells are positively selected for and expanded.

Natural Killer Cells

NK cells bridge the innate and adaptive immune systems through their ability to rapidly respond to pathogens and provide tumor immunosurveillance (532,533). One of the most important features of NK cells is their ability to distinguish self from nonself. This is particularly relevant in cancer therapeutics where NK cells are considered a promising tool for immunotherapy due to their powerful antitumor sensing ability. NK cells can originate from multiple sites including the bone marrow, thymus, or even secondary lymphoid organs. NK cells require IL-15, which signals through CD122, for their development and survival. Additional cytokines can promote NK cell development including IL-21, FLT3L, and SCF. NK/T (NKT) cells develop from T-cell precursors in the thymus and closely resemble CD8+ cytotoxic T cells. During the emergence of double-positive T cells in the thymus, type 1 or invariant iNKTs respond to antigens expressing MHC class I–like CD1d and undergo a specific *TCR α* chain gene rearrangement expressing the semi-invariant TCR (Vα14–Jα18 in mice; Vα24–Jα18 in humans), while type 2 NKT express a more diverse set of TCR gene rearrangements. Like CD8+ T cells, NK cells express a variety of granules that are critical for target cell lysis and also secrete immunomodulatory levels of IFNγ. In contrast to CD8+ T cells that express CD3 on the surface, in mice NK cells express intracellular CD3 and can be further distinguished by the expression of NK1.1 and CD122. Several NK subsets express CD56high, CD16low or a CD56high, CD16high, with the former demonstrating a lower cytotoxic potential, but secrete more cytokines compared to the latter (530). The best identifier of NK cells is the expression of a specific transcription factor E4BP4 (E4 promoter-binding protein 4; also known as NFIL3) (532). Additionally, mice lacking *Id2* are completely devoid of NK cells (532). NK cells can be quickly stimulated or inhibited through a set of receptors called killer cell immunoglobulin-like receptor. Many of these receptors are specific for MHC I molecules, and if their target cells lack these interactions the NK cells can then be activated.

Aging, Dysregulated Hematopoiesis, Cellular Therapy, and Beyond

Hematopoiesis During Aging

Aging is associated with significant changes in the hematopoietic system, and these changes themselves are thought to contribute to many age-related diseases and conditions, largely through alterations in adaptive immunity. In the bone marrow, characteristic morphologic changes are visible, including decreased cellularity and a decreasing hematopoietic cell to adipose ratio. While the rate at which replacement of the bone marrow space by adipocytes does slow with age. After the age of 50, humans typically experience a 10% decline in cellularity with each decade after being born with nearly a 100% cellular marrow (534–536). In addition, the hematopoietic system exhibits marked alterations in cellular composition and function. Decreased red cell production and a greater propensity to anemia are common in the elderly (537,538). The immune system also undergoes numerous changes. The thymus involutes and T-cell production declines dramatically, resulting in decreased TCR repertoire usage and impaired cellular immunity (539–541). Studies in mice demonstrate that B-cell production declines with age (542–544), but the effect is less clear in humans (545,546). However, B cells from older patients do show decreased ability to undergo class switch recombination (547), suggesting a cell-intrinsic basis for the decreased humoral immunity observed in elderly individuals, although altered CD4+ T-helper cell function may also contribute to this decline (548). HSCs also exhibit a lineage bias, with preferential formation of granulocytes and monocytes (549–551).

The effects of aging on the innate immune system are less clear. While it has been reported that cells of the innate immune system including macrophages and neutrophils become increasingly activated with age, other studies have not identified such changes (552,553). The overall effect of these changes in the immune system is a decline in adaptive immunity as well as low-grade, chronic systemic inflammation that is thought to promote DNA damage and disease (554). These changes are also thought to increase the risk of infection as well as increase the risk of cancer and other age-associated disorders that have a major inflammatory component. Consistent with this view, age is strongly correlated with a number of hematopoietic disorders including MPNs, myelodysplastic syndrome, and acute myeloid leukemia (555,556). While these changes have been appreciated for some time, only more recently have investigators begun to connect these phenotypes to a combination of cell-intrinsic and cell-extrinsic factors, many of which directly affect HSC function.

Age-related changes in the hematopoietic system can be viewed as a reflection of a diminished capacity to maintain tissue homeostasis after tissue injury. Studies of HSCs from old mice show that the competitive repopulating capacity of HSCs is decreased compared to their young counterparts, even though HSCs defined by immunophenotype are increased in number (549–551,557,558). These age-related changes in HSC number and function were recently confirmed in humans as well (559,560). Despite these changes, old bone marrow is still capable of repopulating the blood system after serial transplantation (561,562), and in matched unrelated allogeneic stem cell transplants comparing old and young donors, the old marrow demonstrated equivalent neutrophil engraftment, but worse overall survival (563). But what molecular mechanisms drive the aging process in HSCs? Several mouse mutants defective in genomic maintenance pathways exhibit reductions in HSC number and function (196). It appears that during HSC aging, tumor suppressors including p53 and p16 are activated, leading to decreased cell cycling (197,564). Consistent with an important role in HSC aging, mice deficient in *p16^{INK4a}* exhibit increased numbers of HSCs, increased HSC cycling, and better reconstitution ability than wild-type HSCs than age-matched controls (275). These changes result in reduced cell cycling, presumably due to an accumulation of mutations caused by environmental stresses such as ROS.

Consistent with this hypothesis, aging HSCs exhibit increased numbers of γ-H2AX DNA foci (a marker of DNA damage) in both mouse and humans (36,196). Lymphoid-biased HSCs demonstrated increased differentiation and reduced self-renewal in mice that lack telomerase activity (mimicking DNA damage), providing a potential mechanism for the observed skewing toward the myeloid lineage by HSCs (565). This process was partially controlled by the basic leucine zipper transcription factor (BATF), ATF-like. Moreover, the accumulation of DNA damage and increased BATF expression are also observed in old human HSCs (36,566). Telomere erosion induces cellular senescence (567) and in the hematopoietic system, it appears that telomere shortening during normal aging may limit HSC self-renewal potential. Telomerase is expressed in HSCs in both the mouse fetal liver and adult bone marrow, and activity correlates with self-renewal capacity, as activity is reduced as HSCs differentiate to MPPs (164). Despite the presence of constitutive telomerase activity in HSCs, telomeres continue to shorten as HSCs divide (90,165,166).

A large body of evidence indicates that alterations in the lineage composition of mature hematopoietic cells is significantly determined at the level of the HSC, as myeloid-biased, lymphoid-biased, and myeloid-lymphoid balanced HSCs are present in both the mouse and human hematopoietic systems. Studies using single-cell HSC transplants showed that the clonal contribution to the different blood cell lineages varies significantly in young mice and can be stably maintained through serial transplants, indicating that the pool of HSCs represents distinct clonal subtypes with differing lineage and self-renewal potential (568–570). Moreover, the various HSCs with differing lineage biases can be prospectively isolated from mice based on differential expression of the cell surface marker CD150/SLAMf1, with SLAM^high HSCs exhibiting myeloid-biased differentiation (571). Consistent with this, SLAM^high HSCs expand during aging (571,572). Experimental demonstration of HSC clones with distinct functional capacity has not yet been shown in the human system. Moreover, lineage bias appears to be a relatively stable and intrinsic feature of HSCs, as the bias is maintained through serial transplantations (571). These alterations in HSC lineage bias results in concomitant changes in downstream lineage-committed progenitors, including decreased numbers of CLPs (573), including pre-B cells (543,574–576) and ETP (351). Age is also associated with decreased HSC self-renewal as assessed by the reduced ability of old HSCs to reconstitute hosts in the context of transplantation. This observation may partially explain why patients receiving grafts from younger donors experience better outcomes (563).

Although the lineage bias program is maintained during serial transplantation into young hosts (549), the mechanisms underlying the HSC myeloid bias during aging is not entirely clear. Given the associations among altered immune cell composition, chronic inflammation, and aging, some investigators have hypothesized that the changes in the hematopoietic system may be due to the generalized systemic changes observed in aging individuals including reductions in the amount of human growth hormone as well as increased circulating inflammatory cytokines including IL-6 and TNFα (577,578). Recent studies using barcoding methods to track the progeny of HSCs suggest that the lineage bias itself is determined by clonal expansion of specific types of HSC with intrinsic lineage bias (91); however, this bias may be cell-extrinsic, as this phenomenon was observed in irradiated hosts but not nonirradiated hosts. As aging is associated with myeloid bias and clonal hematopoiesis as assessed by X-inactivation studies, a recent study examined the presence of somatic mutations and identified mutations in the TET2 enzyme, a mutation frequently observed in myeloid disorders in the elderly (579). Therefore, many of the changes observed in the aging hematopoietic system are recapitulated by genetic lesions that promote leukemogenesis.

The potential role of the microenvironment in regulating HSC aging is also supported by experiments in which subcutaneous bone grafts from young or old mice demonstrated decreased repopulation of young cells into the old bone grafted onto young mice (580). In addition, coculture experiments using bone marrow–derived stromal cells derived from either young or old mice demonstrated the decreased capacity of old stroma to support hematopoietic PCs (581). Also supporting a potential role of the niche in regulating HSC lineage bias, myeloid- and lymphoid-biased HSCs respond differentially to the effects of TGF-β, which stimulates myeloid-biased HSCs to proliferate while inhibiting lymphoid-biased HSCs (582).

While the aging process may require cell-extrinsic as well as cell-intrinsic factors, recent evidence suggests that the aging process may be inhibited or even reversed by antiaging interventions through inhibition of the mTOR pathway with rapamycin (583) or by transient exposure to small molecule inhibitors of CDC42 (272). Whether or not these mechanisms are relevant to humans or can be targets of intervention through dietary, behavioral, or pharmacologic interventions will be an interesting area of investigation in the years to come.

HSC and the Development of Hematologic Malignancies

Because of the morphologic and immunophenotypic similarities between HSCs and blasts in acute leukemias, a number of investigators hypothesized that leukemias originating from immature hematopoietic cells may be derived from HSCs or early committed progenitors (409). Studies of human AML from John Dick et al. demonstrated that these blasts exhibit immunophenotypes consistent with those of human HSCs/committed progenitors also possess the unique capability to engraft immunodeficient mice (584–586). In addition, as in the normal hematopoietic system, the leukemia was hierarchically organized with cells expressing immature markers giving rise to more "mature" blasts, but not vice versa. Because the leukemia-initiating cells possess properties of normal HSCs including self-renewal, long-term engraftment ability, hierarchical organization, and the ability to reconstitute the various immunophenotypic components of the leukemia, these cells have also been referred to as leukemic stem cells (LSCs).

Subsequent studies of human AML have shown that LSCs may not be readily distinguished from leukemic progenitors solely on the basis of cell surface marker expression (587–589), but it still appears that LSC activity can be enriched based on immature hematopoietic markers or by using other techniques (590–593). While prospective separation of LSCs in AML remains an open area of investigation, these results do not diminish the importance of these studies, as they represent the first formal experimental demonstration of cancer stem cells, and they support the prevailing hypothesis that AML arises from immature hematopoietic cells. A number of investigators have attempted to identify the cells of origin in AML. Studies by several groups showed that ectopic expression of oncogenic fusion proteins was sufficient to transform purified mouse HSCs as well as committed progenitors as mature as the GMP; however, more differentiated cells were not transformable (594–597). Unfortunately, similar studies using human HS/PCs have not been performed due to technical difficulties genetically manipulating human cells in xenograft models. Nonetheless, such studies may be possible, as investigators have successfully established human models of induced leukemia in mice by ectopically expressing oncogenic fusion proteins in human CD34+ cells (598).

While these studies support a model in which AML arises from immature cells, they are limited in several respects. First, they rely on the introduction and nonphysiologic overexpression of oncogenic fusion proteins into HSCs or committed progenitors. That committed progenitors cannot be transformed may not be an unexpected finding since they already exhibit limited self-renewal capacity and are preprogrammed to give rise to differentiating cells thus limiting the time in which they can be transformed. Second, most human AMLs are likely the result of multiple genetic and epigenetic alterations (599–602), and thus experimental oncogenic transformation may not mimic leukemogenesis in human AML. While some studies have investigated cooperating mutations in mouse models of AML, these studies are in their early phases and it is unclear whether or not mouse models of AML can recapitulate the order of mutational acquisition in human AML.

Investigations of CML progression have been informative with respect to developing models of myeloid leukemogenesis. Studies of CML blast crisis reveal that the blasts exhibit an immunophenotype consistent with GMP (referred to as leukemic-GMP, or L-GMP), and L-GMPs are sufficient to transplant disease into immunodeficient mouse hosts (603). Combined with the observation that BCR-ABL expression is not sufficient for CML transformation of committed progenitors in mice (594), these results led to the hypothesis that the HSC is the cell that is altered during leukemogenesis and that its intrinsic self-renewal capacity allows it to retain changes and propagate them to their progeny over long periods of time, thereby increasing the chances for transformation (195).

The identification of somatic mutations in HSCs as well as their relative resistance to targeted or nonspecific therapies is consistent with a critical role of HSCs as the disease-initiating cell in various hematologic neoplasms including CML, MDS, and AML. While the discovery of small molecule inhibitors of the BCR-ABL kinase fusion protein including imatinib mesylate, dasatinib, and nilotinib has revolutionized the treatment of CML such that many patients now experience a near-normal quality of life and markedly improved overall survival (604–606), it is clear that these drugs are relatively ineffective in eliminating HSCs harboring the BCR-ABL translocation, as patients taken off therapy relapse rapidly (607–609). Investigation of HSCs from treated patients demonstrate that HSCs from these patients are sensitive to the induction of apoptosis by tyrosine kinase inhibitors, although these agents did exhibit potent antiproliferative effects (610–614). Similar findings have been observed in other myeloid disorders including treatment of 5q(del) MDS patients treated with lenalidomide (615) as well as JAK2 mutant MPN patients treated with selective JAK2 inhibitors (616). More recently, residual HSCs from AML patients were separated from AML blasts based on differential expression of cell surface proteins, and sequencing for mutations in the residual HSCs revealed the presence of somatic mutations in the HSCs that were identified in the resulting AML (599). When single-cell analysis was performed, the mutations present supported a clonal progression model since multiple mutations occurred in the HSCs of some AML patients. Together, these data indicate that while targeted inhibition of driver mutations in hematologic disorders may be an effective method of treating patients with significant alleviation of morbidity, curing these disorders will require a more detailed understanding of the disease-initiating cells in these disorders as well.

Cell Therapy

HSC transplants may be performed for many reasons including treatment of malignant hematologic diseases as well as reconstitution of the immune system of immunodeficient patients. However, depending on the type of leukemia and the age of the recipients, the probability of survival of the transplanted patients can vary drastically. Unfortunately, even though the first HSC transplants were performed more than 50 years ago, our understanding of why transplants fail to engraft or induce a potent graft versus leukemia (GVL) effect remains relatively poor despite advances in HLA matching, reducing immunologic rejection, and increased understanding of the immunologic basis of GVL. Moreover, transplanted patients are more susceptible to opportunistic infections during the vulnerable period of reconstitution (617) and many face the complications that are caused by chronic graft versus host disease.

While these complications are major clinical concerns, also limiting is the number and quality of histocompatible grafts composed of sufficient numbers of HSCs to effectively engraft patients. It is clear that improved methods to expand adult and umbilical cord blood HSCs could increase the probability that transplant candidates can find histocompatible grafts. Furthermore, the ability to generate HSCs from autologous sources holds the promise of providing immunologically matched grafts that can avoid the significant morbidity and mortality associated with allogeneic transplants.

Although much is known about the pathways that regulate the growth, self-renewal, and the survival of HSCs, no single factor has been identified that allows for long-term growth and expansion of HSCs *in vitro*. Nonetheless, experiments from a large number of groups provide information regarding potential methods to expand HS/PCs *ex vivo*. Some of the strategies to expand HS/PCs *ex vivo* utilize cytokine cocktails and other factors to promote HSC survival and/or self-renewal (e.g., TPO, SCF) (457,485). More recent examples include stimulating prostaglandin receptors and β-catenin activation by blocking GSK3β (139,209,428,429,618). Notch agonists in the presence of cocultured cells have been shown to enhance the growth of HS/PCs (236,619,620). An unbiased screen identified an aryl hydrocarbon agonist (e.g., SR1) as a compound that could expand HSCs, which was experimentally verified by its ability to enhance engraftment of umbilical cord blood; it is currently being tested clinically (426,621). Alternatively, novel technologic approaches using special bioreactors that dilute the negative feedback signals or provide exogenous transcription factors that promote self-renewal are all potential strategies that might expand HSCs (622). Future innovations in humanized xenograft models that allow for better engraftment, or artificially constructed niches grown *in vitro* or implanted *in vivo*, might allow for improved artificial environments to both model normal human hematopoiesis and expand HSCs.

The principle of using exogenous factors to promote self-renewal or reprogram cells has been demonstrated most elegantly by groundbreaking studies performed in the Yamanaka laboratory. Skin fibroblasts could be reprogrammed into induced iPSCs using a defined set of transcription factors (623–625). This discovery has led to one of the most exciting and burgeoning fields of research—cellular reprogramming (626). In addition to showing that skin cells can be converted to iPSCs, it has been shown that human peripheral blood cells can also be reprogrammed to iPSCs (624,627,628), thereby allowing potential antigen-specific immune cells or creating patient-derived cells that harbor mutations present in their cancers or normal tissues. This approach has already been used to reprogram cells from patients with defined genetic disorders of the hematopoietic system such as sickle cell anemia and metabolic disorders, as well as patients with hematologic malignancies (629,630). While the process of reprogramming from hematopoietic cells is not efficient currently, several groups have demonstrated that improvements in reprogramming efficiency can be achieved by directly reprogramming from HS/PCs (631). In fact, while peripheral blood B cells can be reprogrammed with an efficiency of <0.5%, HSCs can be reprogrammed with >15% efficiency when expressing the reprogramming factors *Oct4*, *Sox2*, c-*Myc*, and *Klf4* (631–633).

The standardization of culturing techniques and the ability to maintain large numbers of stable ESCs/iPSCs allows them to be more amenable to genetic manipulation. Moreover, the idea of using one's own cells to generate graft for transplant is especially appealing since matching the genetic background and minimizing immunologic rejection will lead to better therapeutic outcomes. However, this strategy will only be useful if it becomes possible to convert iPSCs into adult HSCs or other blood lineages. This has shown to be especially challenging in part due to the fact that the HSC field has been unable to develop conditions that can sustain or expand adult HSCs.

While *in vitro* differentiation of ESCs/iPSCs has successfully generated hematopoietic progenitors with limited potential as well as several mature cell types it is likely that efficient development of dHSCs from ESCs or iPSCs will require a better understanding of the molecular changes required for the emergence of dHSCs during embryogenesis. Nonetheless, conversion of a differentiated cell type to another without an embryonic intermediate allows for a therapeutic option without the need for relying on ESC or iPSC conversion. Examples of such a conversion include the direct differentiation of skin cells into neural cells or deletion of Pax5 in mature B cells that results in their conversion into functioning T cells, or overexpression of C/EBPα in B or T cells reprogramming these cells into macrophages. Understanding how to coax cells to convert from one lineage to another could provide novel strategies for therapy, and ultimately these approaches may lead to a future in which storing one's own primitive cells or a set of HLA-matched banked samples to create personalized platelets or RBCs for therapeutic benefit becomes commonplace.

References

1. Harrison DE. Competitive repopulation: a new assay for long-term stem cell functional capacity. *Blood* 1980;55(1):77–81.
2. Doulatov S, et al. Hematopoiesis: a human perspective. *Cell Stem Cell* 2012;10(2):120–136.
3. Jacobson LO, et al. Recovery from radiation injury. *Science* 1951;113(2940):510–511.
4. Lorenz E, et al. Modification of irradiation injury in mice and guinea pigs by bone marrow injections. *J Natl Cancer Inst* 1951;12(1):197–201.
5. Jacobson LO, et al. The role of the spleen in radiation injury and recovery. *J Lab Clin Med* 1950;35(5):746–770.
6. Till JE, McCulloch EA. A direct measurement of the radiation sensitivity of normal mouse bone marrow cells. *Radiat Res* 1961;14:213–222.
7. Siminovitch L, McCulloch EA, Till JE. The distribution of colony-forming cells among spleen colonies. *J Cell Physiol* 1963;62:327–336.
8. Becker AJ, McCulloch EA, Till JE. Cytological demonstration of the clonal nature of spleen colonies derived from transplanted mouse marrow cells. *Nature* 1963;197:452–454.
9. Wu AM, et al. A cytological study of the capacity for differentiation of normal hemopoietic colony-forming cells. *J Cell Physiol* 1967;69(2):177–184.
10. Wu AM, et al. Cytological evidence for a relationship between normal hemotopoietic colony-forming cells and cells of the lymphoid system. *J Exp Med* 1968;127(3):455–464.
11. Schofield R, The relationship between the spleen colony-forming cell and the haemopoietic stem cell. *Blood Cells* 1978;4(1–2):7–25.
12. Magli MC, Iscove NN, Odartchenko N. Transient nature of early haematopoietic spleen colonies. *Nature* 1982;295(5849):527–529.
13. Na Nakorn T, et al. Myeloerythroid-restricted progenitors are sufficient to confer radioprotection and provide the majority of day 8 CFU-S. *J Clin Invest* 2002;109(12):1579–1585.
14. Lemischka IR, Raulet DH, Mulligan RC Developmental potential and dynamic behavior of hematopoietic stem cells. *Cell* 1986;45(6):917–927.
15. Harrison DE, et al. Primitive hemopoietic stem cells: direct assay of most productive populations by competitive repopulation with simple binomial, correlation and covariance calculations. *Exp Hematol* 1993;21(2):206–219.
16. Szilvassy SJ, et al. Quantitative assay for totipotent reconstituting hematopoietic stem cells by a competitive repopulation strategy. *Proc Natl Acad Sci U S A* 1990;87(22):8736–8740.
17. Iscove N. Haematopoiesis. Searching for stem cells. *Nature* 1990;347(6289):126–127.
18. Iscove NN, et al. Human marrow cells forming colonies in culture: analysis by velocity sedimentation and suspension culture. *Ser Haematol* 1972;5(2):37–49.
19. Visser JW, et al. Isolation of murine pluripotent hemopoietic stem cells. *J Exp Med* 1984;159(6):1576–1590.
20. Herzenberg LA, et al. The history and future of the fluorescence activated cell sorter and flow cytometry: a view from Stanford. *Clin Chem* 2002;48(10):1819–1827.
21. Julius MH, Masuda T, Herzenberg LA. Demonstration that antigen-binding cells are precursors of antibody-producing cells after purification with a fluorescence-activated cell sorter. *Proc Natl Acad Sci U S A* 1972;69(7):1934–1938.
22. Spangrude GJ, Heimfeld S, Weissman IL. Purification and characterization of mouse hematopoietic stem cells. *Science* 1988;241(4861):58–62.
23. Coffman RL, Weissman IL. A monoclonal antibody that recognizes B cells and B cell precursors in mice. *J Exp Med* 1981;153(2):269–279.
24. Kina T, et al. The monoclonal antibody TER-119 recognizes a molecule associated with glycophorin A and specifically marks the late stages of murine erythroid lineage. *Br J Haematol* 2000;109(2):280–287.
25. Muller-Sieburg CE, Whitlock CA, Weissman IL. Isolation of two early B lymphocyte progenitors from mouse marrow: a committed pre-pre-B cell and a clonogenic Thy-1-lo hematopoietic stem cell. *Cell* 1986;44(4):653–662.
26. Coffman RL, Weissman IL. B220: a B cell-specific member of th T200 glycoprotein family. *Nature* 1981;289(5799):681–683.
27. Akashi K, et al. A clonogenic common myeloid progenitor that gives rise to all myeloid lineages. *Nature* 2000;404(6774):193–197.
28. Kondo M, Weissman IL, Akashi K. Identification of clonogenic common lymphoid progenitors in mouse bone marrow. *Cell* 1997;91(5):661–672.
29. Morrison SJ, et al. Identification of a lineage of multipotent hematopoietic progenitors. *Development* 1997;124(10):1929–1939.
30. Morrison SJ, Weissman IL. The long-term repopulating subset of hematopoietic stem cells is deterministic and isolatable by phenotype. *Immunity* 1994;1(8):661–673.
31. Ikuta K, Weissman IL. Evidence that hematopoietic stem cells express mouse c-kit but do not depend on steel factor for their generation. *Proc Natl Acad Sci U S A* 1992;89(4):1502–1516.
32. Civin CI, et al. Antigenic analysis of hematopoiesis. III. A hematopoietic progenitor cell surface antigen defined by a monoclonal antibody raised against KG-1a cells. *J Immunol* 1984;133(1):157–165.
33. Kiel MJ, et al. SLAM family receptors distinguish hematopoietic stem and progenitor cells and reveal endothelial niches for stem cells. *Cell* 2005;121(7):1109–1121.
34. Ema H, et al. Quantification of self-renewal capacity in single hematopoietic stem cells from normal and Lnk-deficient mice. *Dev Cell* 2005;8(6):907–914.
35. Warr MR, Pietras EM, Passegue E. Mechanisms controlling hematopoietic stem cell functions during normal hematopoiesis and hematological malignancies. *Wiley Interdiscip Rev Syst Biol Med* 2011;3(6):681–701.
36. Rube CE, et al. Accumulation of DNA damage in hematopoietic stem and progenitor cells during human aging. *PLoS One* 2011;6(3):e17487.
37. Larochelle A, et al. Human and rhesus macaque hematopoietic stem cells cannot be purified based only on SLAM family markers. *Blood* 2011;117(5):1550–1554.
38. McCune JM, et al. The SCID-hu mouse: murine model for the analysis of human hematolymphoid differentiation and function. *Science* 1988;241(4873):1632–1639.
39. Kollet O, et al. Beta2 microglobulin-deficient (B2m(null)) NOD/SCID mice are excellent recipients for studying human stem cell function. *Blood* 2000;95(10):3102–3105.
40. Ito M, et al. NOD/SCID/gamma(c)(null) mouse: an excellent recipient mouse model for engraftment of human cells. *Blood* 2002;100(9):3175–3182.
41. Yahata T, et al. Functional human T lymphocyte development from cord blood CD34+ cells in nonobese diabetic/Shi-scid, IL-2 receptor gamma null mice. *J Immunol* 2002;169(1):204–209.
42. Shultz LD, et al. Human lymphoid and myeloid cell development in NOD/LtSz-scid IL2R gamma null mice engrafted with mobilized human hemopoietic stem cells. *J Immunol* 2005;174(10):6477–6489.
43. Traggiai E, et al. Development of a human adaptive immune system in cord blood cell-transplanted mice. *Science* 2004;304(5667):104–107.
44. Gimeno R, et al. Monitoring the effect of gene silencing by RNA interference in human CD34+ cells injected into newborn RAG2-/- gammac-/- mice: functional inactivation of p53 in developing T cells. *Blood* 2004;104(13):3886–3893.
45. Brehm MA, et al. Parameters for establishing humanized mouse models to study human immunity: analysis of human hematopoietic stem cell engraftment in three immunodeficient strains of mice bearing the IL2rgamma(null) mutation. *Clin Immunol* 2010;135(1):84–98.
46. Wang JC, Doedens M, Dick JE. Primitive human hematopoietic cells are enriched in cord blood compared with adult bone marrow or mobilized peripheral blood as measured by the quantitative in vivo SCID-repopulating cell assay. *Blood* 1997;89(11):3919–3924.
47. Bhatia M, et al. Purification of primitive human hematopoietic cells capable of repopulating immune-deficient mice. *Proc Natl Acad Sci U S A* 1997;94(10):5320–5325.
48. Dick JE, et al. In vivo dynamics of human stem cell repopulation in NOD/SCID mice. *Ann N Y Acad Sci* 2001;938:184–190.
49. Mazurier F, et al. Rapid myeloerythroid repopulation after intrafemoral transplantation of NOD-SCID mice reveals a new class of human stem cells. *Nat Med* 2003;9(7):959–963.
50. Lansdorp PM, Sutherland HJ, Eaves CJ. Selective expression of CD45 isoforms on functional subpopulations of CD34+ hemopoietic cells from human bone marrow. *J Exp Med* 1990;172(1):363–366.
51. Baum CM, et al. Isolation of a candidate human hematopoietic stem-cell population. *Proc Natl Acad Sci U S A* 1992;89(7):2804–2808.
52. Murray L, et al. Enrichment of human hematopoietic stem cell activity in the CD34⁺Thy-1⁺Lin⁻ subpopulation from mobilized peripheral blood. *Blood* 1995;85(2):368–378.
53. Negrin RS, et al. Transplantation of highly purified CD34⁺Thy-1⁺ hematopoietic stem cells in patients with metastatic breast cancer. *Biol Blood Marrow Transplant* 2000;6(3):262–271.
54. Majeti R, Park CY, Weissman IL. Identification of a hierarchy of multipotent hematopoietic progenitors in human cord blood. *Cell Stem Cell* 2007;1(6):635–645.
55. Notta F, et al. Isolation of single human hematopoietic stem cells capable of long-term multilineage engraftment. *Science* 2011;333(6039):218–221.
55a. Hogan CJ. Differential long-term and multilineage engraftment potential from subfractions of human CD34+ cord blood cells transplanted into NOD/SCID mice. *Proc Natl Acad Sci* 2002;99:413–418.
55b. McKenzie JL, Takenaka K, Gan OI, et al. Low rhodamine 123 retention identifies long-term human hematopoietic stem cells within the Lin-CD34+CD38- population. *Blood* 2007;109:543–545.
56. van Os RP, Dethmers-Ausema B, de Haan G. In vitro assays for cobblestone area-forming cells, LTC-IC, and CFU-C. *Methods Mol Biol* 2008;430:143–157.
57. Dexter TM, Allen TD, Lajtha LG. Conditions controlling the proliferation of haemopoietic stem cells in vitro. *J Cell Physiol* 1977;91(3):335–344.
58. Ploemacher RE, et al. Wheat germ agglutinin affinity of murine hemopoietic stem cell subpopulations is an inverse function of their long-term repopulating ability in vitro and in vivo. *Leukemia* 1993;7(1):120–130.
59. Ploemacher RE, et al. Use of limiting-dilution type long-term marrow cultures in frequency analysis of marrow-repopulating and spleen colony-forming hematopoietic stem cells in the mouse. *Blood* 1991;78(10):2527–2533.
60. Ploemacher RE, et al. An in vitro limiting-dilution assay of long-term repopulating hematopoietic stem cells in the mouse. *Blood* 1989;74(8):2755–2763.
61. Sutherland HJ, et al. Characterization and partial purification of human marrow cells capable of initiating long-term hematopoiesis in vitro. *Blood* 1989;74(5):1563–1570.
62. Lemieux ME, et al. Characterization and purification of a primitive hematopoietic cell type in adult mouse marrow capable of lymphomyeloid differentiation in long-term marrow "switch" cultures. *Blood* 1995;86(4):1339–1347.
63. Down JD, et al. Variations in radiation sensitivity and repair among different hematopoietic stem cell subsets following fractionated irradiation. *Blood* 1995;86(1):122–127.

64. Wierenga PK, et al. Peripheral blood stem cells differ from bone marrow stem cells in cell cycle status, repopulating potential, and sensitivity toward hyperthermic purging in mice mobilized with cyclophosphamide and granulocyte colony-stimulating factor. *J Hematother Stem Cell Res* 2002;11(3):523–532.

65. Weaver A, Ryder WD, Testa NG. Measurement of long-term culture initiating cells (LTC-ICs) using limiting dilution: comparison of endpoints and stromal support. *Exp Hematol* 1997;25(13):1333–1338.

66. Mazini L, et al. Mature accessory cells influence long-term growth of human hematopoietic progenitors on a murine stromal cell feeder layer. *Stem Cells* 1998;16(6):404–412.

67. Koller MR, Manchel I, Smith AK. Quantitative long-term culture-initiating cell assays require accessory cell depletion that can be achieved by CD34-enrichment or 5-fluorouracil exposure. *Blood* 1998;91(11):4056–4064.

68. Denning-Kendall P, et al. Cobblestone area-forming cells in human cord blood are heterogeneous and differ from long-term culture-initiating cells. *Stem Cells* 2003;21(6):694–701.

69. Ichikawa Y, Pluznik DH, Sachs L. In vitro control of the development of macrophage and granulocyte colonies. *Proc Natl Acad Sci U S A* 1966;56(2):488–495.

70. Bradley TR, Metcalf D. The growth of mouse bone marrow cells in vitro. *Aust J Exp Biol Med Sci* 1966;44(3):287–299.

71. Moore MA, Williams N, Metcalf D. In vitro colony formation by normal and leukemic human hematopoietic cells: characterization of the colony-forming cells. *J Natl Cancer Inst* 1973;50(3):603–623.

72. Pike BL, Robinson WA. Human bone marrow colony growth in agar-gel. *J Cell Physiol* 1970;76(1):77–84.

73. Eaves CJ. Assays of hematopoietic progenitor cells. In: Beutler, et al., eds. *Hematology*. 5th ed. New York: McGraw-Hill, 1995:L22–L26.

74. Schmitt TM, Zuniga-Pflucker JC. Induction of T cell development from hematopoietic progenitor cells by delta-like-1 in vitro. *Immunity* 2002;17(6):749–756.

75. Whitlock CA, Witte ON. Long-term culture of B lymphocytes and their precursors from murine bone marrow. *Proc Natl Acad Sci U S A* 1982;79(11):3608–3612.

76. Bradley TR, Metcalf D, Robinson W. Stimulation by leukaemic sera of colony formation in solid agar cultures by proliferation of mouse bone marrow cells. *Nature* 1967;213(5079):926–927.

77. Welte K, et al. Purification and biochemical characterization of human pluripotent hematopoietic colony-stimulating factor. *Proc Natl Acad Sci U S A* 1985;82(5):1526–1530.

78. Nomura H, et al. Purification and characterization of human granulocyte colony-stimulating factor (G-CSF). *EMBO J* 1986;5(5):871–876.

79. Wong GG, et al. Human GM-CSF: molecular cloning of the complementary DNA and purification of the natural and recombinant proteins. *Science* 1985;228(4701):810–815.

80. Stanley ER Heard PM. Factors regulating macrophage production and growth. Purification and some properties of the colony stimulating factor from medium conditioned by mouse L cells. *J Biol Chem* 1977;252(12):4305–4312.

81. Knowles DM. *Neoplastic hematopathology*, 2nd ed. Philadelphia: Lippincott Williams & Wilkins, 2001.

82. Pronk CJ, et al. Elucidation of the phenotypic, functional, and molecular topography of a myeloerythroid progenitor cell hierarchy. *Cell Stem Cell* 2007;1(4):428–442.

83. Galy A, et al. Human T, B, natural killer, and dendritic cells arise from a common bone marrow progenitor cell subset. *Immunity* 1995;3(4):459–473.

84. Hao QL, et al. Identification of a novel, human multilymphoid progenitor in cord blood. *Blood* 2001;97(12):3683–3690.

85. Manz MG, et al. Prospective isolation of human clonogenic common myeloid progenitors. *Proc Natl Acad Sci U S A* 2002;99(18):11872–11877.

86. Taswell C. Limiting dilution assays for the determination of immunocompetent cell frequencies. I. Data analysis. *J Immunol* 1981;126(4):1614–1619.

87. Szilvassy SJ, et al. Isolation in a single step of a highly enriched murine hematopoietic stem cell population with competitive long-term repopulating ability. *Blood* 1989;74(3):930–939.

88. Harrison DE, Astle CM, Delaittre JA. Loss of proliferative capacity in immunohemopoietic stem cells caused by serial transplantation rather than aging. *J Exp Med* 1978;147(5):1526–1531.

89. Harrison DE, Astle CM. Loss of stem cell repopulating ability upon transplantation. Effects of donor age, cell number, and transplantation procedure. *J Exp Med* 1982;156(6):1767–1779.

90. Allsopp RC, Cheshier S, Weissman IL. Telomere shortening accompanies increased cell cycle activity during serial transplantation of hematopoietic stem cells. *J Exp Med* 2001;193(8):917–924.

91. Lu R, et al. Tracking single hematopoietic stem cells in vivo using high-throughput sequencing in conjunction with viral genetic barcoding. *Nat Biotechnol* 2011;29(10):928–933.

92. Waskow C, et al. Hematopoietic stem cell transplantation without irradiation. *Nat Methods* 2009;6(4):267–269.

93. Boggs DR, et al. Hematopoietic stem cells with high proliferative potential. Assay of their concentration in marrow by the frequency and duration of cure of W/Wv mice. *J Clin Invest* 1982;70(2):242–253.

94. Czechowicz A, et al. Efficient transplantation via antibody-based clearance of hematopoietic stem cell niches. *Science* 2007;318(5854):1296–1299.

95. Purton LE, Scadden DT. Limiting factors in murine hematopoietic stem cell assays. *Cell Stem Cell* 2007;1(3):263–270.

96. van Os R, Kamminga LM, de Haan G. Stem cell assays: something old, something new, something borrowed. *Stem Cells* 2004;22(7):1181–1190.

97. Bertrand JY, Traver D. Hematopoietic cell development in the zebrafish embryo. *Curr Opin Hematol* 2009;16(4):243–248.

98. Ciau-Uitz A, Liu F, Patient R. Genetic control of hematopoietic development in Xenopus and zebrafish. *Int J Dev Biol* 2010;54(6–7):1139–1149.

99. Cumano A, Godin I. Ontogeny of the hematopoietic system. *Annu Rev Immunol* 2007;25:745–785.

100. Avecilla ST, et al. Chemokine-mediated interaction of hematopoietic progenitors with the bone marrow vascular niche is required for thrombopoiesis. *Nat Med* 2004;10(1):64–71.

101. Silver L, Palis J. Initiation of murine embryonic erythropoiesis: a spatial analysis. *Blood* 1997;89(4):1154–1164.

102. Moore MA, Metcalf D. Ontogeny of the haemopoietic system: yolk sac origin of in vivo and in vitro colony forming cells in the developing mouse embryo. *Br J Haematol* 1970;18(3):279–296.

103. Medvinsky A, Dzierzak E. Definitive hematopoiesis is autonomously initiated by the AGM region. *Cell* 1996;86(6):897–906.

104. Muller AM, et al. Development of hematopoietic stem cell activity in the mouse embryo. *Immunity* 1994;1(4):291–301.

105. Kumaravelu P, et al. Quantitative developmental anatomy of definitive haematopoietic stem cells/long-term repopulating units (HSC/RUs): role of the aorta-gonad-mesonephros (AGM) region and the yolk sac in colonisation of the mouse embryonic liver. *Development* 2002;129(21):4891–4899.

106. de Bruijn MF, et al. Definitive hematopoietic stem cells first develop within the major arterial regions of the mouse embryo. *EMBO J* 2000;19(11):2465–2474.

107. Ottersbach K, Dzierzak E. The murine placenta contains hematopoietic stem cells within the vascular labyrinth region. *Dev Cell* 2005;8(3):377–387.

108. Robin C, et al. An unexpected role for IL-3 in the embryonic development of hematopoietic stem cells. *Dev Cell* 2006;11(2):171–180.

109. Taoudi S, et al. Extensive hematopoietic stem cell generation in the AGM region via maturation of VE-cadherin+CD45+ pre-definitive HSCs. *Cell Stem Cell* 2008;3(1):99–108.

110. Gekas C, et al. The placenta is a niche for hematopoietic stem cells. *Dev Cell* 2005;8(3):365–375.

111. Hirsch E, et al. Impaired migration but not differentiation of haematopoietic stem cells in the absence of beta1 integrins. *Nature* 1996;380(6570):171–175.

112. Potocnik AJ, Brakebusch C, Fassler R. Fetal and adult hematopoietic stem cells require beta1 integrin function for colonizing fetal liver, spleen, and bone marrow. *Immunity* 2000;12(6):653–663.

113. Kim I, Saunders TL, Morrison SJ. Sox17 dependence distinguishes the transcriptional regulation of fetal from adult hematopoietic stem cells. *Cell* 2007;130(3):470–483.

114. Zhang CC, et al. Angiopoietin-like proteins stimulate ex vivo expansion of hematopoietic stem cells. *Nat Med* 2006;12(2):240–245.

115. Dzierzak E, Speck NA. Of lineage and legacy: the development of mammalian hematopoietic stem cells. *Nat Immunol* 2008;9(2):129–136.

116. Lux CT, et al. All primitive and definitive hematopoietic progenitor cells emerging before E10 in the mouse embryo are products of the yolk sac. *Blood* 2008;111(7):3435–3438.

117. Ghiaur G, et al. Rac1 is essential for intraembryonic hematopoiesis and for the initial seeding of fetal liver with definitive hematopoietic progenitor cells. *Blood* 2008;111(7):3313–3321.

118. Lehoux S, Tedgui A. Cellular mechanics and gene expression in blood vessels. *J Biomech* 2003;36(5):631–643.

119. Niranjan B, et al. HGF/SF: a potent cytokine for mammary growth, morphogenesis and development. *Development* 1995;121(9):2897–2908.

120. Adamo L, et al. Biomechanical forces promote embryonic haematopoiesis. *Nature* 2009;459(7250):1131–1135.

121. North TE, et al. Hematopoietic stem cell development is dependent on blood flow. *Cell* 2009;137(4):736–748.

122. Murayama E, et al. Tracing hematopoietic precursor migration to successive hematopoietic organs during zebrafish development. *Immunity* 2006;25(6):963–975.

123. Sabin FR. Studies on the origin of blood vessels and of red corpuscles as seen in the living blastoderm of the chick during the second day of incubation. *Contrib Embryol* 1920;9:213–262.

124. Maximow A. The lymphocyte as a stem cell common to different blood elements in embryonic development and during the post-fetal life of mammals [Originally in German]. *Folia Haematol* 1909;8(1909):125–134.

125. Ferkowicz MJ, Yoder MC. Blood island formation: longstanding observations and modern interpretations. *Exp Hematol* 2005;33(9):1041–1047.

126. Choi K. Hemangioblast development and regulation. *Biochem Cell Biol* 1998;76(6):947–956.

127. Keller G. Embryonic stem cell differentiation: emergence of a new era in biology and medicine. *Genes Dev* 2005;19(10):1129–1155.

128. Kennedy M, et al. Development of the hemangioblast defines the onset of hematopoiesis in human ES cell differentiation cultures. *Blood* 2007;109(7):2679–2687.

129. Huber TL, et al. Haemangioblast commitment is initiated in the primitive streak of the mouse embryo. *Nature* 2004;432(7017):625–630.

130. Kissa K, Herbomel P. Blood stem cells emerge from aortic endothelium by a novel type of cell transition. *Nature* 2010;464(7285):112–115.

131. Bertrand JY, et al. Haematopoietic stem cells derive directly from aortic endothelium during development. *Nature* 2010;464(7285):108–111.

132. Boisset JC, et al. In vivo imaging of haematopoietic cells emerging from the mouse aortic endothelium. *Nature* 2010;464(7285):116–120.

133. Lancrin C, et al. Blood cell generation from the hemangioblast. *J Mol Med (Berl)* 2010;88(2):167–172.

134. Goldie LC, et al. Cell signaling directing the formation and function of hemogenic endothelium during murine embryogenesis. *Blood* 2008;112(8):3194–3204.

135. Nadin BM, Goodell MA, Hirschi KK. Phenotype and hematopoietic potential of side population cells throughout embryonic development. *Blood* 2003;102(7):2436–2443.

136. Hirschi KK. Hemogenic endothelium during development and beyond. *Blood* 2012;119(21):4823–4827.

137. Cumano A, Dieterlen-Lievre F, Godin I. Lymphoid potential, probed before circulation in mouse, is restricted to caudal intraembryonic splanchnopleura. *Cell* 1996;86(6):907–916.

138. Ma Q, et al. Impaired B-lymphopoiesis, myelopoiesis, and derailed cerebellar neuron migration in CXCR4 - and SDF-1-deficient mice. *Proc Natl Acad Sci U S A* 1998;95(16):9448–9453.

139. Tavian M, Peault B. Embryonic development of the human hematopoietic system. *Int J Dev Biol* 2005;49(2–3):243–250.

140. Hoggatt J, et al. Prostaglandin E2 enhances hematopoietic stem cell homing, survival, and proliferation. *Blood* 2009;113(22):5444–5455.

141. Smith-Berdan S, et al. Robo4 cooperates with CXCR4 to specify hematopoietic stem cell localization to bone marrow niches. *Cell Stem Cell* 2011;8(1):72–83.

142. Christensen JL, et al. Circulation and chemotaxis of fetal hematopoietic stem cells. *PLoS Biol* 2004;2(3):E75.

143. Adams GB, et al. Stem cell engraftment at the endosteal niche is specified by the calcium-sensing receptor. *Nature* 2006;439(7076):599–603.

144. Min IM, et al. The transcription factor EGR1 controls both the proliferation and localization of hematopoietic stem cells. *Cell Stem Cell* 2008;2(4):380–391.

145. Scott LM, Priestley GV, Papayannopoulou T. Deletion of alpha4 integrins from adult hematopoietic cells reveals roles in homeostasis, regeneration, and homing. *Mol Cell Biol* 2003;23(24):9349–9360.

146. Forsberg EC, Smith-Berdan S. Parsing the niche code: the molecular mechanisms governing hematopoietic stem cell adhesion and differentiation. *Haematologica* 2009;94(11):1477–1481.

147. Massberg S, et al. Immunosurveillance by hematopoietic progenitor cells trafficking through blood, lymph, and peripheral tissues. *Cell* 2007;131(5):994–1008.

148. Bhattacharya D, et al. Niche recycling through division-independent egress of hematopoietic stem cells. *J Exp Med* 2009;206(12):2837–2850.

149. Cheshier SH, et al. In vivo proliferation and cell cycle kinetics of long-term self-renewing hematopoietic stem cells. *Proc Natl Acad Sci U S A* 1999;96(6):3120–3125.

150. Bowie MB, et al. Hematopoietic stem cells proliferate until after birth and show a reversible phase-specific engraftment defect. *J Clin Invest* 2006;116(10):2808–2816.

151. Kiel MJ, et al. Haematopoietic stem cells do not asymmetrically segregate chromosomes or retain BrdU. *Nature* 2007;449(7159):238–242.

152. Nygren JM, Bryder D, Jacobsen SE. Prolonged cell cycle transit is a defining and developmentally conserved hemopoietic stem cell property. *J Immunol* 2006;177(1):201–208.

153. Wilson A, et al. Hematopoietic stem cells reversibly switch from dormancy to self-renewal during homeostasis and repair. *Cell* 2008;135(6):1118–1129.

154. Foudi A, et al. Analysis of histone 2B-GFP retention reveals slowly cycling hematopoietic stem cells. *Nat Biotechnol* 2009;27(1):84–90.

155. Catlin SN, et al. The replication rate of human hematopoietic stem cells in vivo. *Blood* 2011;117(17):4460–4466.

156. Orford KW, Scadden DT. Deconstructing stem cell self-renewal: genetic insights into cell-cycle regulation. *Nat Rev Genet* 2008;9(2):115–128.

157. Cheng T, et al. Hematopoietic stem cell quiescence maintained by p21cip1/waf1. *Science* 2000;287(5459):1804–1808.

158. Hock H, Hamblen MJ, Rooke HM, et al. Gfi-1 restricts proliferation and preserves functional integrity of haematopoietic stem cells. *Nature* 2004;431(7011):1002–1007.

159. Zeng H, et al. Transcription factor Gfi1 regulates self-renewal and engraftment of hematopoietic stem cells. *EMBO J* 2004;23(20):4116–4125.

160. Qian H, et al. Critical role of thrombopoietin in maintaining adult quiescent hematopoietic stem cells. *Cell Stem Cell* 2007;1(6):671–684.

161. Pawliuk R, Eaves C, Humphries RK. Evidence of both ontogeny and transplant dose-regulated expansion of hematopoietic stem cells in vivo. *Blood* 1996;88(8):2852–2858.

162. Iscove NN, Nawa K. Hematopoietic stem cells expand during serial transplantation in vivo without apparent exhaustion. *Curr Biol* 1997;7(10):805–808.

163. Osawa M, et al. Long-term lymphohematopoietic reconstitution by a single CD34-low/negative hematopoietic stem cell. *Science* 1996;273(5272):242–245.

164. Morrison SJ, et al. Telomerase activity in hematopoietic cells is associated with self-renewal potential. *Immunity* 1996;5(3):207–216.

165. Brummendorf TH, et al. Limited telomere shortening in hematopoietic stem cells after transplantation. *Ann N Y Acad Sci* 2001;938:1–7; discussion 7–8.

166. Notaro R, et al. In vivo telomere dynamics of human hematopoietic stem cells. *Proc Natl Acad Sci U S A* 1997;94(25):13782–13785.

167. Lee HW, et al. Essential role of mouse telomerase in highly proliferative organs. *Nature* 1998;392(6676):569–574.

168. Rudolph KL, et al. Longevity, stress response, and cancer in aging telomerase-deficient mice. *Cell* 1999;96(5):701–712.

169. Blasco MA, et al. Telomere shortening and tumor formation by mouse cells lacking telomerase RNA. *Cell* 1997;91(1):25–34.

170. Allsopp RC, et al. Telomerase is required to slow telomere shortening and extend replicative lifespan of HSCs during serial transplantation. *Blood* 2003;102(2):517–520.

171. Samper E, et al. Long-term repopulating ability of telomerase-deficient murine hematopoietic stem cells. *Blood* 2002;99(8):2767–2775.

172. Suda T, Takubo K, Semenza GL. Metabolic regulation of hematopoietic stem cells in the hypoxic niche. *Cell Stem Cell* 2011;9(4):298–310.

173. Cipolleschi MG, Dello Sbarba P, Olivotto M. The role of hypoxia in the maintenance of hematopoietic stem cells. *Blood* 1993;82(7):2031–2037.

174. Danet GH, et al. Expansion of human SCID-repopulating cells under hypoxic conditions. *J Clin Invest* 2003;112(1):126–135.

175. Ivanovic Z, et al. Simultaneous maintenance of human cord blood SCID-repopulating cells and expansion of committed progenitors at low O2 concentration (3%). *Stem Cells* 2004;22(5):716–724.

176. Hermitte F, et al. Very low O2 concentration (0.1%) favors G0 return of dividing CD34+ cells. *Stem Cells* 2006;24(1):65–73.

177. Shima H, et al. Acquisition of G(0) state by CD34-positive cord blood cells after bone marrow transplantation. *Exp Hematol* 2010;38(12):1231–1240.

178. Nakada D, Saunders TL, Morrison SJ. Lkb1 regulates cell cycle and energy metabolism in haematopoietic stem cells. *Nature* 2010;468(7324):653–658.

179. Gan B, Hu J, Jiang S, et al. Lkb1 regulates quiescence and metabolic homeostasis of haematopoietic stem cells. *Nature* 2010;468(7324):701–704.

180. Gurumurthy S, Xie SZ, Alagesan B, et al. The Lkb1 metabolic sensor maintains haematopoietic stem cell survival. *Nature* 2010;468(7324):659–663.

181. Miyamoto K, Araki KY, Naka K, et al. Foxo3a is essential for maintenance of the hematopoietic stem cell pool. *Cell Stem Cell* 2007;1(1):101–112.

182. Tothova Z, Kollipara R, Huntly BJ, et al. FoxOs are critical mediators of hematopoietic stem cell resistance to physiologic oxidative stress. *Cell* 2007;128(2):325–339.

183. Jang YY, Sharkis SJ. A low level of reactive oxygen species selects for primitive hematopoietic stem cells that may reside in the low-oxygenic niche. *Blood* 2007;110(8):3056–3063.

184. Simsek T, et al. The distinct metabolic profile of hematopoietic stem cells reflects their location in a hypoxic niche. *Cell Stem Cell* 2010;7(3):380–390.

185. Mortensen M, et al. The autophagy protein Atg7 is essential for hematopoietic stem cell maintenance. *J Exp Med* 2011;208(3):455–467.

186. Yilmaz OH, et al. Pten dependence distinguishes haematopoietic stem cells from leukaemia-initiating cells. *Nature* 2006;441(7092):475–482.

187. Zhang J, et al. PTEN maintains haematopoietic stem cells and acts in lineage choice and leukaemia prevention. *Nature* 2006;441(7092):518–522.

188. Lee JY, et al. mTOR activation induces tumor suppressors that inhibit leukemogenesis and deplete hematopoietic stem cells after Pten deletion. *Cell Stem Cell* 2010;7(5):593–605.

189. Kharas MG, et al. Constitutively active AKT depletes hematopoietic stem cells and induces leukemia in mice. *Blood* 2010;115(7):1406–1415.

190. Juntilla MM, et al. AKT1 and AKT2 maintain hematopoietic stem cell function by regulating reactive oxygen species. *Blood* 2010;115(20):4030–4038.

191. Challen GA, Little MH. A side order of stem cells: the SP phenotype. *Stem Cells* 2006;24(1):3–12.

192. Mohrin M, et al. Hematopoietic stem cell quiescence promotes error-prone DNA repair and mutagenesis. *Cell Stem Cell* 2010;7(2):174–185.

193. Branzei D, Foiani M. Regulation of DNA repair throughout the cell cycle. *Nat Rev Mol Cell Biol* 2008;9(4):297–308.

194. Blanpain C, et al. DNA-damage response in tissue-specific and cancer stem cells. *Cell Stem Cell* 2011;8(1):16–29.

195. Weissman I. Stem cell research: paths to cancer therapies and regenerative medicine. *JAMA* 2005;294(11):1359–1366.

196. Rossi DJ, et al. Deficiencies in DNA damage repair limit the function of haematopoietic stem cells with age. *Nature* 2007;447(7145):725–729.

197. Rossi DJ, Jamieson CH, Weissman IL. Stems cells and the pathways to aging and cancer. *Cell* 2008;132(4):681–696.

198. Milyavsky M, et al. A distinctive DNA damage response in human hematopoietic stem cells reveals an apoptosis-independent role for p53 in self-renewal. *Cell Stem Cell* 2010;7(2):186–197.

199. Bryder D, Rossi DJ, Weissman IL. Hematopoietic stem cells: the paradigmatic tissue-specific stem cell. *Am J Pathol* 2006;169(2):338–346.

200. Orkin SH, Zon LI. Hematopoiesis: an evolving paradigm for stem cell biology. *Cell* 2008;132(4):631–644.

201. Walkley CR, Shea JM, Sims NA, et al. Rb regulates interactions between hematopoietic stem cells and their bone marrow microenvironment. *Cell* 2007;129(6):1081–1095.

202. Walkley CR, Orkin SH. Rb is dispensable for self-renewal and multilineage differentiation of adult hematopoietic stem cells. *Proc Natl Acad Sci U S A* 2006;103(24):9057–9062.

203. Zou P, Yoshihara H, Hosokawa K, et al. p57(Kip2) and p27(Kip1) cooperate to maintain hematopoietic stem cell quiescence through interactions with Hsc70. *Cell Stem Cell* 2011;9(3):247–261.

204. TeKippe M, Harrison DE, Chen J. Expansion of hematopoietic stem cell phenotype and activity in Trp53-null mice. *Exp Hematol* 2003;31(6):521–527.

205. Liu Y, Elf SE, Miyata Y, et al. p53 regulates hematopoietic stem cell quiescence. *Cell Stem Cell* 2009;4(1):37–48.

206. Karlsson G, Blank U, Moody JL, et al. Smad4 is critical for self-renewal of hematopoietic stem cells. *J Exp Med* 2007;204(3):467–474.

207. Cobas M, Wilson A, Ernst B, et al. Beta-catenin is dispensable for hematopoiesis and lymphopoiesis. *J Exp Med* 2004;199(2):221–229.

208. Zhao C, Blum J, Chen A, et al. Loss of beta-catenin impairs the renewal of normal and CML stem cells in vivo. *Cancer Cell* 2007;12(6):528–541.

209. Huang J, et al. Maintenance of hematopoietic stem cells through regulation of Wnt and mTOR pathways. *Nat Med* 2012;18(12):1778–1785.

210. Luis TC, Weerkamp F, Naber BA, et al. Wnt3a deficiency irreversibly impairs hematopoietic stem cell self-renewal and leads to defects in progenitor cell differentiation. *Blood* 2009;113(3):546–554.

211. Gao J, Graves S, Koch U, et al. Hedgehog signaling is dispensable for adult hematopoietic stem cell function. *Cell Stem Cell* 2009;4(6):548–558.

212. Hofmann I, Stover EH, Cullen DE, et al. Hedgehog signaling is dispensable for adult murine hematopoietic stem cell function and hematopoiesis. *Cell Stem Cell* 2009;4(6):559–567.

213. Merchant A, Joseph G, Wang Q, et al. Gli1 regulates the proliferation and differentiation of HSCs and myeloid progenitors. *Blood* 2010;115(12):2391–2396.

214. Park IK, Qian D, Kiel M, et al. Bmi-1 is required for maintenance of adult self-renewing haematopoietic stem cells. *Nature* 2003;423(6937):302–305.

215. Broske AM, Vockentanz L, Kharazi S, et al. DNA methylation protects hematopoietic stem cell multipotency from myeloerythroid restriction. *Nat Genet* 2009;41(11):1207–1215.

216. Challen GA, Sun D, Jeong M, et al. Dnmt3a is essential for hematopoietic stem cell differentiation. *Nat Genet* 2012;44(1):23–31.

217. Ko KH, et al. GSK-3beta inhibition promotes engraftment of ex vivo-expanded hematopoietic stem cells and modulates gene expression. *Stem Cells* 2011;29(1):108–118.

218. de Andres-Aguayo L, Varas F, Kallin EM, et al. Musashi 2 is a regulator of the HSC compartment identified by a retroviral insertion screen and knockout mice. *Blood* 2011;118(3):554–564.

219. Chen J, et al. Enrichment of hematopoietic stem cells with SLAM and LSK markers for the detection of hematopoietic stem cell function in normal and Trp53 null mice. *Exp Hematol* 2008;36(10):1236–1243.

220. Passegue E, et al. Global analysis of proliferation and cell cycle gene expression in the regulation of hematopoietic stem and progenitor cell fates. *J Exp Med* 2005;202(11):1599–1611.

221. van Os R, et al. A Limited role for p21Cip1/Waf1 in maintaining normal hematopoietic stem cell functioning. *Stem Cells* 2007;25(4):836–843.

222. Cobrinik D, et al. Shared role of the pRB-related p130 and p107 proteins in limb development. *Genes Dev* 1996;10(13):1633–1644.

223. LeCouter JE, et al. Strain-dependent myeloid hyperplasia, growth deficiency, and accelerated cell cycle in mice lacking the Rb-related p107 gene. *Mol Cell Biol* 1998;18(12):7455–7465.

223a. Cheng T, Rodrigues N, Shen H, et al. Hematopoietic stem cell quiescence maintained by p21cip1/waf1. *Science* 2000b;287:1804–1808.

223b. Matsumoto A, Takeishi S, Kanie T, et al. p57 is required for quiescence and maintenance of adult hematopoietic stem cells. *Cell Stem Cell* 2011;9:262–271.

223c. Dumble M, Moore L, Chambers SM, et al. The impact of altered p53 dosage on hematopoietic stem cell dynamics during aging. *Blood* 2007;109:1736–1742.

223d. Cheng T, Rodrigues N, Dombkowski D, et al. Stem cell repopulation efficiency but not pool size is governed by p27(kip1). *Nat Med* 2000a;6:1235–1240.

223e. Wilson A, Ardiet DL, Saner C, et al. Normal hemopoiesis and lymphopoiesis in the combined absence of numb and numblike. *J Immunol* 2007;178:6746–6751.

223f. Langer JC, Henckaerts E, Orenstein J, et al. Quantitative trait analysis reveals transforming growth factor-beta2 as a positive regulator of early hematopoietic progenitor and stem cell function. *J Exp Med* 2004;199:5–14.

223g. Larsson J, Blank U, Helgadottir H, et al. TGF-beta signaling-deficient hematopoietic stem cells have normal self-renewal and regenerative ability in vivo despite increased proliferative capacity in vitro. *Blood* 2003;102:3129–3135.

223h. Singbrant S, Moody JL, Blank U, et al. Smad5 is dispensable for adult murine hematopoiesis. *Blood* 2006;108:3707–3712.

223i. Iwama A, Oguro H, Negishi M, et al. Enhanced self-renewal of hematopoietic stem cells mediated by the polycomb gene product Bmi-1. *Immunity* 2004;21:843–851.

223j. DiMartino JF, Selleri L, Traver D, et al. The Hox cofactor and proto-oncogene Pbx1 is required for maintenance of definitive hematopoiesis in the fetal liver. *Blood* 2001;98:618–626.

223k. Boyarsky G, Rosenthal N, Barrett E, et al. Effect of diabetes on Na(+)-H+ exchange by single isolated hepatocytes. *Am J Physiol* 1991;260:C167–C175.

223l. Baena E, Ortiz M, Martinez AC, et al. c-Myc is essential for hematopoietic stem cell differentiation and regulates Lin(–)Sca-1(+)c-Kit(–) cell generation through p21. *Exp Hematol* 2007;35:1333–1343.

223m. Laurenti E, Varnum-Finney B, Wilson A, et al. Hematopoietic stem cell function and survival depend on c-Myc and N-Myc activity. *Cell Stem Cell* 2008;3:611–624.

223n. Wilson A, Murphy MJ, Oskarsson T, et al. c-Myc controls the balance between hematopoietic stem cell self-renewal and differentiation. *Genes Dev* 2004;18:2747–2763.

223o. Khandanpour C, Sharif-Askari E, Vassen L, et al. Evidence that growth factor independence 1b regulates dormancy and peripheral blood mobilization of hematopoietic stem cells. *Blood* 2010;116:5149–5161.

223p. Mikkola HK, Klintman J, Yang H, et al. Haematopoietic stem cells retain long-term repopulating activity and multipotency in the absence of stem-cell leukaemia SCL/tal-1 gene. *Nature* 2003;421:547–551.

223q. Curtis DJ, Hall MA, Van Stekelenburg LJ, et al. SCL is required for normal function of short-term repopulating hematopoietic stem cells. *Blood* 2004;103:3342–3348.

223r. Sato T, Onai N, Yoshihara H, et al. Interferon regulatory factor-2 protects quiescent hematopoietic stem cells from type I interferon-dependent exhaustion. *Nat Med* 2009;15:696–700.

223s. Li G, Wang Z, Zhang Y, et al. STAT5 requires the N-domain to maintain hematopoietic stem cell repopulating function and appropriate lymphoid-myeloid lineage output. *Exp Hematol* 2007;35:1684–1694.

223t. Wang Z, Li G, Tse W, et al. Conditional deletion of STAT5 in adult mouse hematopoietic stem cells causes loss of quiescence and permits efficient nonablative stem cell replacement. *Blood* 2009;113:4856–4865.

223u. Bradley HL, Hawley TS, Bunting KD. Cell intrinsic defects in cytokine responsiveness of STAT5-deficient hematopoietic stem cells. *Blood* 2002;100:3983–3989.

223v. Bunting KD, Bradley HL, Hawley TS, et al. Reduced lymphomyeloid repopulating activity from adult bone marrow and fetal liver of mice lacking expression of STAT5. *Blood* 2002;99:479–487.

223w. Takaki S, Morita H, Tezuka Y, et al. Enhanced hematopoiesis by hematopoietic progenitor cells lacking intracellular adaptor protein, Lnk. *J Exp Med* 2002;195:151–160.

223x. Quivoron C, Couronne L, Della Valle V, et al. TET2 inactivation results in pleiotropic hematopoietic abnormalities in mouse and is a recurrent event during human lymphomagenesis. *Cancer Cell* 2011;20:25–38.

223y. Moran-Crusio K, Reavie L, Shih A, et al. Tet2 loss leads to increased hematopoietic stem cell self-renewal and myeloid transformation. *Cancer Cell* 2011;20:11–24.

223z. Xiao N, Jani K, Morgan K, et al. Hematopoietic stem cells lacking Ott1 display aspects associated with aging and are unable to maintain quiescence during proliferative stress. *Blood* 2012;119:4898–4907.

224. Niu C, Zhang J, Breslin P, et al. c-Myc is a target of RNA-binding motif protein 15 in the regulation of adult hematopoietic stem cell and megakaryocyte development. *Blood* 2009;114:2087–2096.

224a. Ghosh M, Aguila HL, Michaud J, et al. Essential role of the RNA-binding protein HuR in progenitor cell survival in mice. *J Clin Invest* 2009;119:3530–3543.

224b. Viatour P, et al. Hematopoietic stem cell quiescence is maintained by compound contributions of the retinoblastoma gene family. *Cell Stem Cell* 2008;3(4):416–428.

225. Radtke F, Fasnacht N, Macdonald HR. Notch signaling in the immune system. *Immunity* 2010;32(1):14–27.

226. Weber JM, Calvi LM. Notch signaling and the bone marrow hematopoietic stem cell niche. *Bone* 2010;46(2):281–285.

227. Schwanbeck R, et al. Notch signaling in embryonic and adult myelopoiesis. *Cells Tissues Organs* 2008;188(1–2): 91–102.

228. Kumano K, et al. Notch1 but not Notch2 is essential for generating hematopoietic stem cells from endothelial cells. *Immunity* 2003;18(5):699–711.

229. Robert-Moreno A, et al. Impaired embryonic haematopoiesis yet normal arterial development in the absence of the Notch ligand Jagged1. *EMBO J* 2008;27(13):1886–1895.

230. Robert-Moreno A, et al. RBPjkappa-dependent Notch function regulates Gata2 and is essential for the formation of intra-embryonic hematopoietic cells. *Development* 2005;132(5):1117–1126.

231. Duncan AW, et al. Integration of Notch and Wnt signaling in hematopoietic stem cell maintenance. *Nature Immunology* 2005;6(3):314–322.

232. Maillard I, et al. Canonical notch signaling is dispensable for the maintenance of adult hematopoietic stem cells. *Cell Stem Cell* 2008;2(4):356–366.

233. Chiang MY, et al. Divergent effects of supraphysiological Notch signals on leukemia stem cells and hematopoietic stem cells. *Blood* 2013;121(6):905–917.

234. Calvi LM, et al. Osteoblastic cells regulate the haematopoietic stem cell niche. *Nature* 2003;425(6960):841–846.

235. Karanu FN, et al. The notch ligand jagged-1 represents a novel growth factor of human hematopoietic stem cells. *J Exp Med* 2000;192(9):1365–1372.

236. Butler JM, et al. Endothelial cells are essential for the self-renewal and repopulation of Notch-dependent hematopoietic stem cells. *Cell Stem Cell* 2010;6(3):251–264.

237. Isufi I, et al. Transforming growth factor-beta signaling in normal and malignant hematopoiesis. *J Interferon Cytokine Res* 2007;27(7):543–552.

238. Singbrant S, et al. Canonical BMP signaling is dispensable for hematopoietic stem cell function in both adult and fetal liver hematopoiesis, but essential to preserve colon architecture. *Blood* 2010;115(23):4689–4698.

239. Ruscetti FW, Akel S, Bartelmez SH. Autocrine transforming growth factor-beta regulation of hematopoiesis: many outcomes that depend on the context. *Oncogene* 2005;24(37):5751–5763.

240. Goey H, et al. Inhibition of early murine hemopoietic progenitor cell proliferation after in vivo locoregional administration of transforming growth factor-beta 1. *J Immunol* 1989;143(3):877–880.

241. Yamazaki S, et al. TGF-beta as a candidate bone marrow niche signal to induce hematopoietic stem cell hibernation. *Blood* 2009;113(6):1250–1256.

242. Dickson MC, et al. Defective haematopoiesis and vasculogenesis in transforming growth factor-beta 1 knock out mice. *Development* 1995;121(6):1845–1854.

243. Yaswen L, et al. Autoimmune manifestations in the transforming growth factor-beta 1 knockout mouse. *Blood* 1996;87(4):1439–1445.

244. Kulkarni AB, et al. Transforming growth factor beta 1 null mutation in mice causes excessive inflammatory response and early death. *Proc Natl Acad Sci U S A* 1993;90(2):770–774.

245. Yamazaki S, et al. Nonmyelinating Schwann cells maintain hematopoietic stem cell hibernation in the bone marrow niche. *Cell* 2011;147(5):1146–1158.

246. Scandura JM, et al. Transforming growth factor beta-induced cell cycle arrest of human hematopoietic cells requires p57KIP2 up-regulation. *Proc Natl Acad Sci U S A* 2004;101(42):15231–15236.

247. Staal FJ, Luis TC. Wnt signaling in hematopoiesis: crucial factors for self-renewal, proliferation, and cell fate decisions. *J Cell Biochem* 2010;109(5):844–849.

248. Baba Y, et al. Constitutively active beta-catenin promotes expansion of multipotent hematopoietic progenitors in culture. *J Immunol* 2006;177(4):2294–2303.

249. Jeannet G, et al. Long-term, multilineage hematopoiesis occurs in the combined absence of beta-catenin and gamma-catenin. *Blood* 2008;111(1):142–149.

250. Koch U, et al. Simultaneous loss of beta- and gamma-catenin does not perturb hematopoiesis or lymphopoiesis. *Blood* 2008;111(1):160–164.

251. Kirstetter P, et al. Activation of the canonical Wnt pathway leads to loss of hematopoietic stem cell repopulation and multilineage differentiation block. *Nat Immunol* 2006;7(10):1048–1056.

252. Scheller M, et al. Hematopoietic stem cell and multilineage defects generated by constitutive beta-catenin activation. *Nat Immunol* 2006;7(10):1037–1047.

253. Fleming HE, et al. Wnt signaling in the niche enforces hematopoietic stem cell quiescence and is necessary to preserve self-renewal in vivo. *Cell Stem Cell* 2008;2(3):274–283.

254. Trowbridge JJ, Scott MP, Bhatia M. Hedgehog modulates cell cycle regulators in stem cells to control hematopoietic regeneration. *Proc Natl Acad Sci U S A* 2006;103(38):14134–14139.

255. Lane SW, et al. The Apc(min) mouse has altered hematopoietic stem cell function and provides a model for MPD/MDS. *Blood* 2010;115(17):3489–3497.

256. Kobune M, et al. Indian hedgehog gene transfer augments hematopoietic support of human stromal cells including NOD/SCID-beta2m-/- repopulating cells. *Blood* 2004;104(4):1002–1009.

257. Bhardwaj G, et al. Sonic hedgehog induces the proliferation of primitive human hematopoietic cells via BMP regulation. *Nat Immunol* 2001;2(2):172–180.

258. Chung UI, et al. Indian hedgehog couples chondrogenesis to osteogenesis in endochondral bone development. *J Clin Invest* 2001;107(3):295–304.

259. Dierks C, et al. Expansion of Bcr-Abl-positive leukemic stem cells is dependent on Hedgehog pathway activation. *Cancer Cell* 2008;14(3):238–249.

260. Zhao C, et al. Hedgehog signalling is essential for maintenance of cancer stem cells in myeloid leukaemia. *Nature* 2009;458(7239):776–779.

261. Chalhoub N, Baker SJ. PTEN and the PI3-kinase pathway in cancer. *Annu Rev Pathol* 2009;4:127–150.

262. Kalaitzidis D, et al. mTOR complex 1 plays critical roles in hematopoiesis and pten-loss-evoked leukemogenesis. *Cell Stem Cell* 2012;11(3):429–439.

263. Magee JA, et al. Temporal changes in PTEN and mTORC2 regulation of hematopoietic stem cell self-renewal and leukemia suppression. *Cell Stem Cell* 2012;11(3):415–428.

264. Sykes SM, et al. AKT/FOXO signaling enforces reversible differentiation blockade in myeloid leukemias. *Cell* 2011;146(5):697–708.

265. Alessi DR, Sakamoto K, Bayascas JR. LKB1-dependent signaling pathways. *Annu Rev Biochem* 2006;75:137–163.

266. Hardie DG. AMP-activated/SNF1 protein kinases: conserved guardians of cellular energy. *Nat Rev Mol Cell Biol* 2007;8(10):774–785.

267. Shackelford DB, Shaw RJ. The LKB1-AMPK pathway: metabolism and growth control in tumour suppression. *Nat Rev Cancer* 2009;9(8):563–575.

268. Florian MC, Geiger H. Concise review: polarity in stem cells, disease, and aging. *Stem Cells* 2010;28(9):1623–1629.

269. Etienne-Manneville S. Cdc42–the centre of polarity. *J Cell Sci* 2004;117(Pt 8):1291–1300.

270. Cau J, Hall A. Cdc42 controls the polarity of the actin and microtubule cytoskeletons through two distinct signal transduction pathways. *J Cell Sci* 2005;118(Pt 12):2579–2587.

271. Wang L, et al. Cdc42 GTPase-activating protein deficiency promotes genomic instability and premature aging-like phenotypes. *Proc Natl Acad Sci U S A* 2007;104(4):1248–1253.

272. Florian MC, et al. Cdc42 activity regulates hematopoietic stem cell aging and rejuvenation. *Cell Stem Cell* 2012;10(5):520–530.

273. Sherr CJ. The INK4a/ARF network in tumour suppression. *Nat Rev Mol Cell Biol* 2001;2(10):731–737.

274. Lessard J, Sauvageau G. Bmi-1 determines the proliferative capacity of normal and leukaemic stem cells. *Nature* 2003;423(6937):255–260.

275. Janzen V, et al. Stem-cell ageing modified by the cyclin-dependent kinase inhibitor p16INK4a. *Nature* 2006;443(7110):421–426.

276. Wu L, Belasco JG. Let me count the ways: mechanisms of gene regulation by miRNAs and siRNAs. *Mol Cell* 2008;29(1):1–7.

277. Doench JG, Sharp PA. Specificity of microRNA target selection in translational repression. *Genes Dev* 2004;18(5):504–511.

278. Ooi AG, et al. MicroRNA-125b expands hematopoietic stem cells and enriches for the lymphoid-balanced and lymphoid-biased subsets. *Proc Natl Acad Sci U S A* 2010;107(50):21505–21510.

279. O'Connell RM, et al. MicroRNAs enriched in hematopoietic stem cells differentially regulate long-term hematopoietic output. *Proc Natl Acad Sci U S A* 2010;107(32):14235–14240.

280. Guo S, et al. MicroRNA miR-125a controls hematopoietic stem cell number. *Proc Natl Acad Sci U S A* 2010;107(32):14229–14234.

281. Han YC, et al. microRNA-29a induces aberrant self-renewal capacity in hematopoietic progenitors, biased myeloid development, and acute myeloid leukemia. *J Exp Med* 2010;207(3):475–489.

282. O'Connell RM, et al. Sustained expression of microRNA-155 in hematopoietic stem cells causes a myeloproliferative disorder. *J Exp Med* 2008;205(3):585–594.

283. Georgantas RW III, et al. CD34+ hematopoietic stem-progenitor cell microRNA expression and function: a circuit diagram of differentiation control. *Proc Natl Acad Sci U S A* 2007;104(8):2750–2755.

284. Petriv OI, et al. Comprehensive microRNA expression profiling of the hematopoietic hierarchy. *Proc Natl Acad Sci U S A* 2010;107(35):15443–15448.

285. Gentner B, et al. Identification of hematopoietic stem cell-specific miRNAs enables gene therapy of globoid cell leukodystrophy. *Sci Transl Med* 2010;2(58):58ra84.

286. Lechman ER, et al. Attenuation of miR-126 activity expands HSC in vivo without exhaustion. *Cell Stem Cell* 2012;11(6):799–811.

287. Lunde BM, Moore C, Varani G. RNA-binding proteins: modular design for efficient function. *Nat Rev Mol Cell Biol* 2007;8(6):479–490.

288. Keene JD. RNA regulons: coordination of post-transcriptional events. *Nat Rev Genet* 2007;8(7):533–543.

289. Ma XM, Blenis J. Molecular mechanisms of mTOR-mediated translational control. *Nat Rev Mol Cell Biol* 2009;10(5):307–318.

290. Visconte V, et al. Emerging roles of the spliceosomal machinery in myelodysplastic syndromes and other hematological disorders. *Leukemia* 2012;26(12):2447–2454.

291. Viswanathan SR, Daley GQ. Lin28: a microRNA regulator with a macro role. *Cell* 2010;140(4):445–449.

292. Yuan J, et al. Lin28b reprograms adult bone marrow hematopoietic progenitors to mediate fetal-like lymphopoiesis. *Science* 2012;335(6073):1195–1200.

293. Kharas MG, et al. Musashi-2 regulates normal hematopoiesis and promotes aggressive myeloid leukemia. *Nat Med* 2010;16(8):903–908.

294. Hope KJ, et al. An RNAi screen identifies Msi2 and Prox1 as having opposite roles in the regulation of hematopoietic stem cell activity. *Cell Stem Cell* 7(1):101–113.

295. Cooper TA, Wan L, Dreyfuss G. RNA and disease. *Cell* 2009;136(4):777–793.

296. Travlos G. Histopathology of bone marrow. *Toxicol Pathol* 2006;34(5):566–598.

297. Mantovani A, et al. Macrophage polarization: tumor-associated macrophages as a paradigm for polarized M2 mononuclear phagocytes. *Trends Immunol* 2002;23(11):549–555.

298. Xie T, Spradling AC. decapentaplegic is essential for the maintenance and division of germline stem cells in the Drosophila ovary. *Cell* 1998;94(2):251–260.

299. Xie T, Spradling AC. A niche maintaining germ line stem cells in the Drosophila ovary. *Science* 2000;290(5490):328–330.

300. Weinbeck J, Weinbeck. Die Granulopese des Kindlichen Knockenmarkes und ihre reaktion auf infectionen. *Beitr Pathol Anat Allg Pathol* 1938;101:268–283.

301. Scadden DT. Rethinking stroma: lessons from the blood. *Cell Stem Cell* 2012;10(6):648–649.

302. Lymperi S, Ferraro F, Scadden DT. The HSC niche concept has turned 31. *Ann N Y Acad Sci* 2010;1192(1):12–18.

303. Méndez-Ferrer S, et al. Mesenchymal and haematopoietic stem cells form a unique bone marrow niche. *Nature* 2010;466(7308):829–834.

304. Lo Celso C, et al. Live-animal tracking of individual haematopoietic stem/progenitor cells in their niche. *Nature* 2009;457(7225):92–96.

305. Celebi B, Mantovani D, Pineault N. Effects of extracellular matrix proteins on the growth of haematopoietic progenitor cells. *Biomed Mater* 2011;6(5):055011.

306. Levesque JP, et al. Hematopoietic progenitor cell mobilization results in hypoxia with increased hypoxia-inducible transcription factor-1α and vascular endothelial growth factor A in bone marrow. *Stem Cells* 2007;25(8):1954–1965.

307. Harrison JS, et al. Oxygen saturation in the bone marrow of healthy volunteers. *Blood* 2002;99(1):394.

308. Parmar K, et al. Distribution of hematopoietic stem cells in the bone marrow according to regional hypoxia. *Proc Natl Acad Sci U S A* 2007;104(13):5431–5436.

309. Winkler IG, et al. Bone marrow macrophages maintain hematopoietic stem cell (HSC) niches and their depletion mobilizes HSCs. *Blood* 2010;116(23):4815–4828.

310. Rehn M, et al. Hypoxic induction of vascular endothelial growth factor regulates murine hematopoietic stem cell function in the low-oxygenic niche. *Blood* 2011;118(6):1534–1543.

311. Okuyama H, et al. Expression of vascular endothelial growth factor receptor 1 in bone marrow-derived mesenchymal cells is dependent on hypoxia-inducible factor 1. *J Biol Chem* 2006;281(22):15554–15563.

312. Schmieder A, et al. Differentiation and gene expression profile of tumor-associated macrophages. *Semin Cancer Biol* 2012;22(4):289–297.

313. Eliasson P, et al. Hypoxia mediates low cell-cycle activity and increases the proportion of long-term-reconstituting hematopoietic stem cells during in vitro culture. *Exp Hematol* 2010;38(4):301–310.e2.

314. Takubo K, et al. Regulation of the HIF-1α level is essential for hematopoietic stem cells. *Stem Cell* 2010;7(3):391–402.

315. Butler JM, et al. Endothelial cells are essential for the self-renewal and repopulation of Notch-dependent hematopoietic stem cells. *Cell Stem Cell* 2010;6(3):251–264.

316. Kiel MJ, Morrison SJ. Uncertainty in the niches that maintain haematopoietic stem cells. *Nat Rev Immunol* 2008;8(4):290–301.

317. Shi M, Liu ZW, Wang FS. Immunomodulatory properties and therapeutic application of mesenchymal stem cells. *Clin Exp Immunol* 2011;164(1):1–8.

318. Trounson A, et al. Clinical trials for stem cell therapies. *BMC Med* 2011;9:52.

319. Sacchetti B, et al. Self-renewing osteoprogenitors in bone marrow sinusoids can organize a hematopoietic microenvironment. *Cell* 2007;131(2):324–336.

320. Sugiyama T, et al. Maintenance of the hematopoietic stem cell pool by CXCL12-CXCR4 chemokine signaling in bone marrow stromal cell niches. *Immunity* 2006;25(6):977–988.

321. Alito AE, et al. Autonomic nervous system regulation of murine immune responses as assessed by local surgical sympathetic and parasympathetic denervation. *Acta Physiol Pharmacol Latinoam* 1987;37(3):305–319.

322. Scheiermann C, et al. Adrenergic nerves govern circadian leukocyte recruitment to tissues. *Immunity* 2012;37(2):290–301.

323. Méndez-Ferrer S, et al., Haematopoietic stem cell release is regulated by circadian oscillations. *Nature* 2008;452(7186):442–447.

324. Méndez-Ferrer S, Frenette PS. Galpha(s) uncouples hematopoietic stem cell homing and mobilization. *Cell Stem Cell* 2009;4(5):379–380.

325. Spiegel A, et al. Catecholaminergic neurotransmitters regulate migration and repopulation of immature human CD34+ cells through Wnt signaling. *Nat Immunol* 2007;8(10):1123–1131.

326. El-Badri NS, et al. Osteoblasts promote engraftment of allogeneic hematopoietic stem cells. *Exp Hematol* 1998;26(2):110–116.

327. Nilsson SK, Johnston HM, Coverdale JA. Spatial localization of transplanted hemopoietic stem cells: inferences for the localization of stem cell niches. *Blood* 2001;97(8):2293–2299.

328. Zhang J, et al. Identification of the haematopoietic stem cell niche and control of the niche size. *Nat Cell Biol* 2003;425(6960):836–841.

329. Sugimura R, et al. Noncanonical Wnt signaling maintains hematopoietic stem cells in the niche. *Cell* 2012;150(2):351–365.

330. Kiel MJ, et al. Hematopoietic stem cells do not depend on N-cadherin to regulate their maintenance. *Cell Stem Cell* 2009;4(2):170–179.

331. Hosokawa K, et al. Knockdown of N-cadherin suppresses the long-term engraftment of hematopoietic stem cells. *Blood* 2010;116(4):554–563.

332. Greenbaum AM, et al. N-cadherin in osteolineage cells is not required for maintenance of hematopoietic stem cells. *Blood* 2012;120(2):295–302.

333. Stier S, et al. Osteopontin is a hematopoietic stem cell niche component that negatively regulates stem cell pool size. *J Exp Med* 2005;201(11):1781–1791.

334. Nilsson SK, et al. Osteopontin, a key component of the hematopoietic stem cell niche and regulator of primitive hematopoietic progenitor cells. *Blood* 2005;106(4):1232–1239.

335. Raaijmakers MH, et al. Bone progenitor dysfunction induces myelodysplasia and secondary leukaemia. *Nature* 2010;464(7290):852–857.

336. Naveiras O, et al. Bone-marrow adipocytes as negative regulators of the haematopoietic microenvironment. *Nature* 2009;460(7252):259–263.

337. Kodama H, et al. Involvement of the c-kit receptor in the adhesion of hematopoietic stem cells to stromal cells. *Exp Hematol* 1994;22(10):979–984.

338. Chow A, et al. Bone marrow CD169+ macrophages promote the retention of hematopoietic stem and progenitor cells in the mesenchymal stem cell niche. *J Exp Med* 2011;208(2):261–271.

339. King KY, Goodell MA. Inflammatory modulation of HSCs: viewing the HSC as a foundation for the immune response. *Nat Rev Immunol* 2011;11(10):685–692.

340. Scumpia PO, et al. Cutting edge: bacterial infection induces hematopoietic stem and progenitor cell expansion in the absence of TLR signaling. *J Immunol* 2010;184(5):2247–2251.

341. Baldridge MT, et al. Quiescent haematopoietic stem cells are activated by IFN-gamma in response to chronic infection. *Nature* 2010;465(7299):793–797.

342. Snapper CM, et al. Induction of Ly-6A/E expression by murine lymphocytes after in vivo immunization is strictly dependent upon the action of IFN-alpha/beta and/or IFN-gamma. *Int immunol* 1991;3(9):845–852.

343. Ema H, Suda T. Two anatomically distinct niches regulate stem cell activity. *Blood* 2012;120(11):2174–2181.

344. Miyamoto K, et al. Osteoclasts are dispensable for hematopoietic stem cell maintenance and mobilization. *J Exp Med* 2011;208(11):2175–2181.

345. Kollet O, Dar A, Lapidot T. The multiple roles of osteoclasts in host defense: bone remodeling and hematopoietic stem cell mobilization. *Ann Rev Immunol* 2007;25:51–69.

346. Chan AS, et al. Id1 represses osteoclast-dependent transcription and affects bone formation and hematopoiesis. *PLoS One* 2009;4(11):e7955.

347. Celebi B, Mantovani D, Pineault N. Irradiated mesenchymal stem cells improve the ex vivo expansion of hematopoietic progenitors by partly mimicking the bone marrow endosteal environment. *J Immunol Methods* 2011;370(1–2):93–103.

348. Xie Y, et al. Detection of functional haematopoietic stem cell niche using real-time imaging. *Nature* 2008;457(7225):97–101.

349. Ding L, et al. Endothelial and perivascular cells maintain haematopoietic stem cells. *Nature* 2012;481(7382):457–462.

350. Alexander WS, et al. Deficiencies in progenitor cells of multiple hematopoietic lineages and defective megakaryocytopoiesis in mice lacking the thrombopoietic receptor c-Mpl. *Blood* 1996;87(6):2162–2170.

351. Solar GP, et al. Role of c-mpl in early hematopoiesis. *Blood* 1998;92(1):4–10.

352. Yoshihara H, et al. Thrombopoietin/MPL signaling regulates hematopoietic stem cell quiescence and interaction with the osteoblastic niche. *Cell Stem Cell* 2007;1(6):685–697.

353. Min H, Montecino-Rodriguez E, Dorshkind K. Reduction in the developmental potential of intrathymic T cell progenitors with age. *J Immunol* 2004;173(1):245–250.

354. Goodman JW, Hodgson GS. Evidence for stem cells in the peripheral blood of mice. *Blood* 1962;19:702–714.

355. Wright DE, et al. Physiological migration of hematopoietic stem and progenitor cells. *Science* 2001;294(5548):1933–1936.

356. Bhattacharya D, et al. Purified hematopoietic stem cell engraftment of rare niches corrects severe lymphoid deficiencies without host conditioning. *J Exp Med* 2006;203(1):73–85.

357. de Haan G, et al. The kinetics of murine hematopoietic stem cells in vivo in response to prolonged increased mature blood cell production induced by granulocyte colony-stimulating factor. *Blood* 1995;86(8):2986–2992.

358. Molineux G, et al. Transplantation potential of peripheral blood stem cells induced by granulocyte colony-stimulating factor. *Blood* 1990;76(10):2153–2158.

359. Liu F, Poursine-Laurent J, Link DC. Expression of the G-CSF receptor on hematopoietic progenitor cells is not required for their mobilization by G-CSF. *Blood* 2000;95(10):3025–3031.

360. Gibbs KD Jr., et al. Single-cell phospho-specific flow cytometric analysis demonstrates biochemical and functional heterogeneity in human hematopoietic stem and progenitor compartments. *Blood* 2011;117(16):4226–4233.

361. Christopher MJ, et al. Expression of the G-CSF receptor in monocytic cells is sufficient to mediate hematopoietic progenitor mobilization by G-CSF in mice. *J Exp Med* 2011;208(2):251–260.

362. Levesque JP, et al. Vascular cell adhesion molecule-1 (CD106) is cleaved by neutrophil proteases in the bone marrow following hematopoietic progenitor cell mobilization by granulocyte colony-stimulating factor. *Blood* 2001;98(5):1289–1297.

363. Levesque JP, et al. Disruption of the CXCR4/CXCL12 chemotactic interaction during hematopoietic stem cell mobilization induced by GCSF or cyclophosphamide. *J Clin Invest* 2003;111(2):187–196.

364. Levesque JP, et al. Characterization of hematopoietic progenitor mobilization in protease-deficient mice. *Blood* 2004;104(1):65–72.

365. Ratajczak J, et al. Mobilization studies in mice deficient in either C3 or C3a receptor (C3aR) reveal a novel role for complement in retention of hematopoietic stem/progenitor cells in bone marrow. *Blood* 2004;103(6):2071–2078.

366. Cancelas JA, Williams DA. Rho GTPases in hematopoietic stem cell functions. *Curr Opin Hematol* 2009;16(4):249–254.

367. Broxmeyer HE, et al. Rapid mobilization of murine and human hematopoietic stem and progenitor cells with AMD3100, a CXCR4 antagonist. *J Exp Med* 2005;201(8):1307–1318.

368. Costa LJ, et al. Growth factor and patient-adapted use of plerixafor is superior to CY and growth factor for autologous hematopoietic stem cells mobilization. *Bone Marrow Transplant* 2011;46(4):523–528.
369. DiPersio JF, et al. Phase III prospective randomized double-blind placebo-controlled trial of plerixafor plus granulocyte colony-stimulating factor compared with placebo plus granulocyte colony-stimulating factor for autologous stem-cell mobilization and transplantation for patients with non-Hodgkin's lymphoma. *J Clin Oncol* 2009;27(28):4767–4773.
370. Li JY, et al. PTH expands short-term murine hemopoietic stem cells through T cells. *Blood* 2012;120(22):4352–4362.
371. Brunner S, et al. Parathyroid hormone effectively induces mobilization of progenitor cells without depletion of bone marrow. *Exp Hematol* 2008;36(9):1157–1166.
372. Ballen K. Targeting the stem cell niche: squeezing blood from bones. *Bone Marrow Transplant* 2007;39(11):655–660.
373. Irhimeh MR, Fitton JH, Lowenthal RM. Fucoidan ingestion increases the expression of CXCR4 on human CD34+ cells. *Exp Hematol* 2007;35(6):989–994.
374. Kovach NL, et al. Stem cell factor modulates avidity of alpha 4 beta 1 and alpha 5 beta 1 integrins expressed on hematopoietic cell lines. *Blood* 1995;85(1):159–167.
375. Neben S, Marcus K, Mauch P. Mobilization of hematopoietic stem and progenitor cell subpopulations from the marrow to the blood of mice following cyclophosphamide and/or granulocyte colony-stimulating factor. *Blood* 1993;81(7):1960–1967.
376. Priestley GV, Ulyanova T, Papayannopoulou T. Sustained alterations in biodistribution of stem/progenitor cells in Tie2Cre+ alpha4(f/f) mice are hematopoietic cell autonomous. *Blood* 2007;109(1):109–111.
377. Pruijt JF, et al. Neutrophils are indispensable for hematopoietic stem cell mobilization induced by interleukin-8 in mice. *Proc Natl Acad Sci U S A* 2002;99(9):6228–6233.
378. Velders GA, Pruijt J, Verzaal P. Enhancement of G-CSF–induced stem cell mobilization by antibodies against the β2 integrins LFA-1 and Mac-1. *Blood* 2002;100:327–333.
379. King AG, et al. Rapid mobilization of murine hematopoietic stem cells with enhanced engraftment properties and evaluation of hematopoietic progenitor cell mobilization in rhesus monkeys by a single injection of SB-251353, a specific truncated form of the human CXC chemokine GRObeta. *Blood* 2001;97(6):1534–1542.
380. Pelus LM. Peripheral blood stem cell mobilization: new regimens, new cells, where do we stand. *Curr Opin Hematol* 2008;15(4):285–292.
381. Pelus LM, et al. Neutrophil-derived MMP-9 mediates synergistic mobilization of hematopoietic stem and progenitor cells by the combination of G-CSF and the chemokines GROβ/CXCL2 and $GRO\beta_T$/$CXCL2_{\Delta 4}$. *Blood* 2004;103:110–119.
382. Labow MA, et al. Characterization of E-selectin-deficient mice: demonstration of overlapping function of the endothelial selectins. *Immunity* 1994;1(8):709–720.
383. Frenette PS, et al. Susceptibility to infection and altered hematopoiesis in mice deficient in both P- and E-selectins. *Cell* 1996;84(4):563–574.
384. Frenette PS, et al. Endothelial selectins and vascular cell adhesion molecule-1 promote hematopoietic progenitor homing to bone marrow. *Proc Natl Acad Sci U S A* 1998;95(24):14423–14428.
385. Papayannopoulou T, et al. The VLA4/VCAM-1 adhesion pathway defines contrasting mechanisms of lodgement of transplanted murine hemopoietic progenitors between bone marrow and spleen. *Proc Natl Acad Sci U S A* 1995;92(21):9647–9651.
386. Voermans C, et al. Adhesion molecules involved in transendothelial migration of human hematopoietic progenitor cells. *Stem Cells* 2000;18(6):435–443.
387. Imai K, et al. Selective transendothelial migration of hematopoietic progenitor cells: a role in homing of progenitor cells. *Blood* 1999;93(1):149–156.
388. Peled A, et al. The chemokine SDF-1 activates the integrins LFA-1, VLA-4, and VLA-5 on immature human CD34(+) cells: role in transendothelial/stromal migration and engraftment of NOD/SCID mice. *Blood* 2000;95(11):3289–3296.
389. Wagers AJ, Weissman IL. Differential expression of alpha2 integrin separates long-term and short-term reconstituting Lin-/loThy1.1(lo)c-kit+ Sca-1+ hematopoietic stem cells. *Stem Cells* 2006;24(4):1087–1094.
390. Katayama Y, et al. Integrin alpha4beta7 and its counterreceptor MAdCAM-1 contribute to hematopoietic progenitor recruitment into bone marrow following transplantation. *Blood* 2004;104(7):2020–2026.
391. Papayannopoulou T, Nakamoto B. Peripheralization of hemopoietic progenitors in primates treated with anti-VLA4 integrin. *Proc Natl Acad Sci U S A* 1993;90(20):9374–9378.
392. Goldman DC, et al. BMP4 regulates the hematopoietic stem cell niche. *Blood* 2009;114(20):4393–4401.
393. Gomei Y, et al. Functional differences between two Tie2 ligands, angiopoietin-1 and -2, in regulation of adult bone marrow hematopoietic stem cells. *Exp Hematol* 2010;38(2):82–89.
394. Arai F, et al. Tie2/angiopoietin-1 signaling regulates hematopoietic stem cell quiescence in the bone marrow niche. *Cell* 2004;118(2):149–161.
395. Shen Y, et al. Tissue inhibitor of metalloproteinase-3 (TIMP-3) regulates hematopoiesis and bone formation in vivo. *PLoS One* 2010;5(9):e13086.
396. Nakajima H, et al. TIMP-3 recruits quiescent hematopoietic stem cells into active cell cycle and expands multipotent progenitor pool. *Blood* 2010;116(22):4474–4482.
397. Mazzon C, et al. The critical role of agrin in the hematopoietic stem cell niche. *Blood* 2011;118(10):2733–2742.
398. Heissig B, et al. Recruitment of stem and progenitor cells from the bone marrow niche requires MMP-9 mediated release of Kit-ligand. *Cell* 2002;109(5):625–637.
399. de Paulis A, Minopoli G, Arbustini E. Stem cell factor is localized in, released from, and cleaved by human mast cells. *J Immunol* 1999;163(5):2799–2808.
400. Longley BJ, et al. Chymase cleavage of stem cell factor yields a bioactive, soluble product. *Proc Natl Acad Sci U S A* 1997;94(17):9017–9021.
401. Brannan CI, et al. Steel-Dickie mutation encodes a c-kit ligand lacking transmembrane and cytoplasmic domains. *Proc Natl Acad Sci U S A* 1991;88(11):4671–4674.
402. Arguello F, et al. Incidence and distribution of experimental metastases in mutant mice with defective organ microenvironments (genotypes Sl/Sld and W/Wv). *Cancer Res* 1992;52(8):2304–2309.
403. Driessen RL, Johnston HM, Nilsson SK. Membrane-bound stem cell factor is a key regulator in the initial lodgment of stem cells within the endosteal marrow region. *Exp Hematol* 2003;31(12):1284–1291.
404. Lane SW, Scadden DT, Gilliland DG. The leukemic stem cell niche: current concepts and therapeutic opportunities. *Blood* 2009;114(6):1150–1157.
405. Lane SW, et al. Differential niche and Wnt requirements during acute myeloid leukemia progression. *Blood* 2011;118(10):2849–2856.
406. Tavor S, et al. CXCR4 regulates migration and development of human acute myelogenous leukemia stem cells in transplanted NOD/SCID mice. *Cancer Res* 2004;64(8):2817–2824.
407. Jin L, et al. Targeting of CD44 eradicates human acute myeloid leukemic stem cells. *Nat Med* 2006;12(10):1167–1174.
408. Takubo K, Suda T. Roles of the hypoxia response system in hematopoietic and leukemic stem cells. *Int J Hematol* 2012;95(5):478–483.
409. Reya T, et al. Stem cells, cancer, and cancer stem cells. *Nature* 2001;414(6859):105–111.
410. Lai AY, Kondo M. Asymmetrical lymphoid and myeloid lineage commitment in multipotent hematopoietic progenitors. *J Exp Med* 2006;203(8):1867–1873.
411. Yoshida T, et al. Early hematopoietic lineage restrictions directed by Ikaros. *Nat Immunol* 2006;7(4):382–391.
412. Adolfsson J, et al. Identification of Flt3+ lympho-myeloid stem cells lacking erythro-megakaryocytic potential a revised road map for adult blood lineage commitment. *Cell* 2005;121(2):295–306.
413. Doulatov S, et al. Revised map of the human progenitor hierarchy shows the origin of macrophages and dendritic cells in early lymphoid development. *Nat Immunol* 2010;11(7):585–593.
414. Mansson R, et al. Molecular evidence for hierarchical transcriptional lineage priming in fetal and adult stem cells and multipotent progenitors. *Immunity* 2007;26(4):407–419.
415. Bell JJ, Bhandoola A. The earliest thymic progenitors for T cells possess myeloid lineage potential. *Nature* 2008;452(7188):764–767.
416. Wada H, et al. Adult T-cell progenitors retain myeloid potential. *Nature* 2008;452(7188):768–772.
417. Novershtern N, et al. Densely interconnected transcriptional circuits control cell states in human hematopoiesis. *Cell* 2011;144(2):296–309.
418. Kee BL. A comprehensive transcriptional landscape of human hematopoiesis. *Cell Stem Cell* 2011;8(2):122–124.
419. Huang GP, et al. Ex vivo expansion and transplantation of hematopoietic stem/progenitor cells supported by mesenchymal stem cells from human umbilical cord blood. *Cell Transplant* 2007;16(6):579–585.
420. Rosenbauer F, et al. Acute myeloid leukemia induced by graded reduction of a lineage-specific transcription factor, PU.1. *Nat Genet* 2004;36(6):624–630.
421. León B, López-Bravo M, Ardavín C. Monocyte-derived dendritic cells formed at the infection site control the induction of protective T helper 1 responses against Leishmania. *Immunity* 2007;26(4):519–531.
422. Pello OM, et al. Role of c-MYC in alternative activation of human macrophages and tumor-associated macrophage biology. *Blood* 2012;119(2):411–421.
423. Jeannin P, Duluc D, Delneste Y. IL-6 and leukemia-inhibitory factor are involved in the generation of tumor-associated macrophage: regulation by IFN-gamma. *Immunotherapy* 2011;3(4 Suppl):23–26.
424. Luc S, Buza-Vidas N, Jacobsen SE. Delineating the cellular pathways of hematopoietic lineage commitment. *Semin Immunol* 2008;20(4):213–220.
425. Laiosa CV, Stadtfeld M, Graf T. Determinants of lymphoid-myeloid lineage diversification. *Annu Rev Immunol* 2006;24:705–738.
426. Boitano AE, et al. Aryl hydrocarbon receptor antagonists promote the expansion of human hematopoietic stem cells. *Science* 2010;329(5997):1345–1348.
427. Durand EM, Zon LI. Newly emerging roles for prostaglandin E2 regulation of hematopoiesis and hematopoietic stem cell engraftment. *Curr Opin Hematol* 2010;17(4):308–312.
428. Goessling W, et al. Prostaglandin E2 enhances human cord blood stem cell xenotransplants and shows long-term safety in preclinical nonhuman primate transplant models. *Cell Stem Cell* 2011;8(4):445–458.
429. Goessling W, et al. Genetic interaction of PGE2 and Wnt signaling regulates developmental specification of stem cells and regeneration. *Cell* 2009;136(6):1136–1147.
430. Aziz A, et al. MafB/c-Maf deficiency enables self-renewal of differentiated functional macrophages. *Science* 2009;326(5954):867–871.
431. Chow A, Brown BD, Merad M. Studying the mononuclear phagocyte system in the molecular age. *Nat Rev Immunol* 2011;11(11):788–798.
432. Auffray C, Sieweke MH, Geissmann F. Blood monocytes: development, heterogeneity, and relationship with dendritic cells. *Ann Rev Immunol* 2009;27(1):669–692.
433. Van Furth R. *Production and migration of monocytes and kinetics of macrophages. In mononuclear phagocytes biology of monocytes and macrophages.* Dordrecht: Kluwer Academic Publishers, 1992:3–12.
434. Dai XM, et al. Targeted disruption of the mouse colony-stimulating factor 1 receptor gene results in osteopetrosis, mononuclear phagocyte deficiency, increased primitive progenitor cell frequencies, and reproductive defects. *Blood* 2002;99(1):111–120.
435. Cecchini MG, et al. Role of colony stimulating factor-1 in the establishment and regulation of tissue macrophages during postnatal development of the mouse. *Development* 1994;120(6):1357–1372.
436. Wiktor-Jedrzejczak W, Gordon S. Cytokine regulation of the macrophage (M phi) system studied using the colony stimulating factor-1-deficient op/op mouse. *Physiol Rev* 1996;76(4):927–947.
437. Strauss-Ayali D, Conrad SM, Mosser DM. Monocyte subpopulations and their differentiation patterns during infection. *J Leukoc Biol* 2007;82(2):244–252.
438. Gama L, et al. Expansion of a subset of CD14highCD16negCCR2low/neg monocytes functionally similar to myeloid-derived suppressor cells during SIV and HIV infection. *J Leukoc Biol* 2012;91(5):803–816.
439. Auffray C, et al. Monitoring of blood vessels and tissues by a population of monocytes with patrolling behavior. *Science* 2007;317(5838):666–670.
440. Gordon S, Taylor PR. Monocyte and macrophage heterogeneity. *Nat Rev Immunol* 2005;5(12):953–964.
441. Martinez FO. Macrophage activation and polarization. *Front Biosci* 2008;13(13):453.
442. Mosser DM, Edwards JP. Exploring the full spectrum of macrophage activation. *Nat Rev Immunol* 2008;8(12):958–969.
443. Lawrence T, Natoli G. Transcriptional regulation of macrophage polarization: enabling diversity with identity. *Nat Rev Immunol* 2011;11(11):750–761.
444. Stine JT, et al. Divergent effects of interleukin-4 and interferon-γ on macrophage-derived chemokine production: an amplification circuit of polarized T helper 2 responses. *Blood* 1998;92(8):2668–2671.
445. Desmedt M, Rottiers P, Dooms H. Macrophages induce cellular immunity by activating Th1 cell responses and suppressing Th2 cell responses. *J Immunol* 1998;160(11):5300–5308.

446. Chakkalath HR, Titus RG. Leishmania major-parasitized macrophages augment Th2-type T cell activation. *J Immunol* 1994;153(10):4378–4387.
447. Anthony RM, et al. Memory T(H)2 cells induce alternatively activated macrophages to mediate protection against nematode parasites. *Nat Med* 2006;12(8):955–960.
448. Banchereau J, Steinman RM. Dendritic cells and the control of immunity. *Nature* 1998;392(6673):245–252.
449. Belz GT, Nutt SL. Transcriptional programming of the dendritic cell network. *Nat Rev Immunol* 2012;12(2):101–113.
450. Onai N, et al. Identification of clonogenic common Flt3+M-CSFR+ plasmacytoid and conventional dendritic cell progenitors in mouse bone marrow. *Nat Immunol* 2007;8(11):1207–1216.
451. Naik SH, et al. Development of plasmacytoid and conventional dendritic cell subtypes from single precursor cells derived in vitro and in vivo. *Nat Immunol* 2007;8(11):1217–1226.
452. Mellman I, Steinman RM. Dendritic cells: specialized and regulated antigen processing machines. *Cell* 2001;106(3):255–258.
453. Geissmann F, et al. Development of monocytes, macrophages, and dendritic cells. *Science* 2010;327(5966):656–661.
454. Belz GT, et al. Distinct migrating and nonmigrating dendritic cell populations are involved in MHC class I-restricted antigen presentation after lung infection with virus. *Proc Natl Acad Sci U S A* 2004;101(23):8670–8675.
455. Heath WR, Carbone FR. Dendritic cell subsets in primary and secondary T cell responses at body surfaces. *Nat Immunol* 2009;10:1237–1244.
456. Bedoui S, et al. Cross-presentation of viral and self antigens by skin-derived CD103+ dendritic cells. *Nat Immunol* 2009;10(5):488–495.
457. Antonchuk J, Sauvageau G, Humphries RK. HOXB4-induced expansion of adult hematopoietic stem cells ex vivo. *Cell* 2002;109(1):39–45.
458. Singh P, et al. Blockade of prostaglandin E2 signaling through EP1 and EP3 receptors attenuates Flt3L-dependent dendritic cell development from hematopoietic progenitor cells. *Blood* 2012;119(7):1671–1682.
459. Naik SH, et al. Intrasplenic steady-state dendritic cell precursors that are distinct from monocytes. *Nat Immunol* 2006;7(6):663–671.
460. Lundie RJ, et al. Blood-stage Plasmodium infection induces CD8+ T lymphocytes to parasite-expressed antigens, largely regulated by CD8alpha+ dendritic cells. *Proc Natl Acad Sci U S A* 2008;105(38):14509–14514.
461. Cella M, et al. Plasmacytoid monocytes migrate to inflamed lymph nodes and produce large amounts of type I interferon. *Nat Med* 1999;5(8):919–923.
462. Siegal FP, et al. The nature of the principal type 1 interferon-producing cells in human blood. *Science* 1999;284(5421):1835–1837.
463. Trinchieri G. Anti-viral activity induced by culturing lymphocytes with tumor-derived or virus-transformed cells. Identification of the anti-viral activity as interferon and characterization of the human effector lymphocyte subpopulation. *J Exp Med* 1978;147(5):1299–1313.
464. Pelayo R, et al. Derivation of 2 categories of plasmacytoid dendritic cells in murine bone marrow. *Blood* 2005;105(11):4407–4415.
465. Walasek MA, van Os R, de Haan G. Hematopoietic stem cell expansion: challenges and opportunities. *Ann N Y Acad Sci* 2012;1266:138–150.
466. Flores-Guzman P, et al. Comparative in vitro analysis of different hematopoietic cell populations from human cord blood: in search of the best option for clinically oriented ex vivo cell expansion. *Transfusion* 2012;53(3):668–678.
467. Kallinikou K, et al. Engraftment defect of cytokine-cultured adult human mobilized CD34(+) cells is related to reduced adhesion to bone marrow niche elements. *Br J Haematol* 2012;158(6):778–787.
468. Emond H, et al. Cotransplantation of ex vivo expanded progenitors with nonexpanded cord blood cells improves platelet recovery. *Stem Cells Dev* 2012;21(17):3209–3219.
469. Larbi A, et al. The HOXB4 homeoprotein promotes the ex vivo enrichment of functional human embryonic stem cell-derived NK cells. *PLoS One* 2012;7(6):e39514.
470. Nishino T, Osawa M, Iwama A. New approaches to expand hematopoietic stem and progenitor cells. *Expert Opin Biol Ther* 2012;12(6):743–756.
471. Celebi B, Mantovani D, Pineault N. Insulin-like growth factor binding protein-2 and neurotrophin 3 synergize together to promote the expansion of hematopoietic cells ex vivo. *Cytokine* 2012;58(3):327–331.
472. Ferreira MV, et al. Compatibility of different polymers for cord blood-derived hematopoietic progenitor cells. *J Mater Sci Mater Med* 2012;23(1):109–116.
473. Curtis KM, Gomez LA, Schiller PC. Rac1b regulates NT3-stimulated Mek-Erk signaling, directing marrow-isolated adult multilineage inducible (MIAMI) cells toward an early neuronal phenotype. *Mol Cell Neurosci* 2012;49(2):138–148.
474. Yang M, Shu LL, Cui Y. [The role of PDGF/PDGFR in the regulation of platelet formation]. *Zhongguo Shi Yan Xue Ye Xue Za Zhi* 2011;19(5):1097–1101.
475. Broxmeyer HE, et al. Angiopoietin-like-2 and -3 act through their coiled-coil domains to enhance survival and replating capacity of human cord blood hematopoietic progenitors. *Blood Cells Mol Dis* 2012;48(1):25–29.
476. Pourcher G, et al. Human fetal liver: an in vitro model of erythropoiesis. *Stem Cells Int* 2011;2011:405–429.
477. Yang J, et al. Enhanced self-renewal of hematopoietic stem/progenitor cells mediated by the stem cell gene Sall4. *J Hematol Oncol* 2011;4:38.
478. Nishino T, et al. Ex vivo expansion of human hematopoietic stem cells by garcinol, a potent inhibitor of histone acetyltransferase. *PLoS One* 2011;6(9): e24298.
479. Mortera-Blanco T, et al. Long-term cytokine-free expansion of cord blood mononuclear cells in three-dimensional scaffolds. *Biomaterials* 2011;32(35):9263–9270.
480. Migliaccio G, et al. Under HEMA conditions, self-replication of human erythroblasts is limited by autophagic death. *Blood Cells Mol Dis* 2011;47(3):182–197.
481. Fournier M, et al. HOXA4 induces expansion of hematopoietic stem cells in vitro and confers enhancement of pro-B-cells in vivo. *Stem Cells Dev* 2012;21(1): 133–142.
482. Hodby K, Pamphilon D. Concise review: expanding roles for hematopoietic cellular therapy and the blood transfusion services. *Stem Cells* 2011;29(9): 1322–1326.
483. Spanholtz J, et al. Clinical-grade generation of active NK cells from cord blood hematopoietic progenitor cells for immunotherapy using a closed-system culture process. *PLoS One* 2011;6(6):e20740.
484. Yuan Y, et al. Ex vivo amplification of human hematopoietic stem and progenitor cells in an alginate three-dimensional culture system. *Int J Lab Hematol* 2011;33(5):516–525.
485. Dahlberg A, Delaney C, Bernstein ID. Ex vivo expansion of human hematopoietic stem and progenitor cells. *Blood* 2011;117(23):6083–6090.
486. Gurish MF, et al. Intestinal mast cell progenitors require CD49dbeta7 (alpha-4beta7 integrin) for tissue-specific homing. *J Exp Med* 2001;194(9):1243–1252.
487. Arinobu Y, et al. Developmental checkpoints of the basophil/mast cell lineages in adult murine hematopoiesis. *Proc Natl Acad Sci U S A* 2005;102(50):18 105–18110.
488. Bashir Q, et al. Umbilical cord blood transplantation. *Clin Adv Hematol Oncol* 2010;8(11):786–801.
489. Kishore V, Eliason JF, Matthew HW. Covalently immobilized glycosaminoglycans enhance megakaryocyte progenitor expansion and platelet release. *J Biomed Mater Res A* 2011;96(4):682–692.
490. Cattoglio C, et al. High-definition mapping of retroviral integration sites defines the fate of allogeneic T cells after donor lymphocyte infusion. *PLoS One* 2010;5(12):e15688.
491. Sokol CL, Medzhitov R. Role of basophils in the initiation of Th2 responses. *Curr Opin Immunol* 2010;22(1):73–77.
492. Marturana F, Timmins NE, Nielsen LK. Short-term exposure of umbilical cord blood CD34+ cells to granulocyte-macrophage colony-stimulating factor early in culture improves ex vivo expansion of neutrophils. *Cytotherapy* 2011;13(3):366–377.
493. Tung SS, et al. Ex vivo expansion of umbilical cord blood for transplantation. *Best Pract Res Clin Haematol* 2010;23(2):245–257.
494. Pardanaud L, Yassine F, Dieterlen-Lievre F. Relationship between vasculogenesis, angiogenesis and haemopoiesis during avian ontogeny. *Development* 1989;105(3):473–485.
495. Dore LC, Crispino JD. Transcription factor networks in erythroid cell and megakaryocyte development. *Blood* 2011;118(2):231–239.
496. Kingsley PD, et al. "Maturational" globin switching in primary primitive erythroid cells. *Blood* 2006;107(4):1665–1672.
497. Chasis JA, Mohandas N. Erythroblastic islands: niches for erythropoiesis. *Blood* 2008;112(3):470–478.
498. Barbé E, et al. A novel bone marrow frozen section assay for studying hematopoietic interactions in situ: the role of stromal bone marrow macrophages in erythroblast binding. *J Cell Sci* 1996;109(Pt 12):2937–2945.
499. Wang GL, et al. Hypoxia-inducible factor 1 is a basic-helix-loop-helix-PAS heterodimer regulated by cellular O2 tension. *Proc Natl Acad Sci U S A* 1995;92(12): 5510–5514.
500. Constantinescu S, Ghaffari S, Lodish H. The erythropoietin receptor: structure, activation and intracellular signal transduction. *Trends Endocrinol Metab* 1999;10(1):18–23.
501. Martin D, et al. Expression of an erythroid transcription factor in megakaryocytic and mast cell lineages. *Nature* 1990;344(6265):444–447.
502. Miller IJ, Bieker JJ. A novel, erythroid cell-specific murine transcription factor that binds to the CACCC element and is related to the Krüppel family of nuclear proteins. *Mol Cell Biol* 1993;13(5):2776–2786.
503. Mancini E, et al. FOG-1 and GATA-1 act sequentially to specify definitive megakaryocytic and erythroid progenitors. *EMBO J* 2011;31(2):351–365.
504. Gutiérrez L, et al. Ablation of Gata1 in adult mice results in aplastic crisis, revealing its essential role in steady-state and stress erythropoiesis. *Blood* 2008;111(8):4375–4385.
505. Nichols KE, et al. Familial dyserythropoietic anaemia and thrombocytopenia due to an inherited mutation in GATA1. *Nat Genet* 2000;24(3):266–270.
506. Wright JH. The origin and nature of the blood plates. *Boston Med Surg J* 1906;154:643.
507. Geddis AE. Megakaryopoiesis. *Semin Hematol* 2010;47(3):212–219.
508. Kaushansky K. Historical review: megakaryopoiesis and thrombopoiesis. *Blood* 2008;111(3):981–986.
509. Stenberg PE, Levin J. Mechanisms of platelet production. *Blood Cells* 1989;15(1): 23–47.
510. Boilard E, Blanco P, Nigrovic PA. Platelets: active players in the pathogenesis of arthritis and SLE. *Nat Rev Mol Cell Biol* 2012;8(9):534–542.
511. Semple JW, Freedman J. Platelets and innate immunity. *Cell Mol Life Sci* 2010;67(4):499–511.
512. Vitrat N, et al. Endomitosis of human megakaryocytes are due to abortive mitosis. *Blood* 1998;91(10):3711–3723.
513. Schmitt A, et al. Of mice and men: comparison of the ultrastructure of megakaryocytes and platelets. *Exp Hematol* 2001;29(11):1295–1302.
514. Lefebvre P, et al. Ex vivo expansion of early and late megakaryocyte progenitors. *J Hematother Stem Cell Res* 2000;9(6):913–921.
515. Cohen JA, Leeksma CH. Determination of the life span of human blood platelets using labelled diisopropylfluorophosphonate. *J Clin Invest* 1956;35(9):964–969.
516. Zauli G, et al. In vitro senescence and apoptotic cell death of human megakaryocytes. *Blood* 1997;90(6):2234–2243.
517. Roth GJ, Yagi M, Bastian LS. The platelet glycoprotein Ib-V-IX system: regulation of gene expression. *Stem Cells* 1996;14(Suppl 1):188–193.
518. Murone M, Carpenter DA, de Sauvage JA. Hematopoietic deficiencies in c-mpl and TPO knockout mice. *Stem Cells* 1998;16(1):1–6.
519. Aghideh AN, et al. Platelet growth factors suppress ex vivo expansion and enhance differentiation of umbilical cord blood CD133+ stem cells to megakaryocyte progenitor cells. *Growth Factors* 2010;28(6):409–416.
520. Fielder PJ, et al. Human platelets as a model for the binding and degradation of thrombopoietin. *Blood* 1997;89(8):2782–2788.
521. Broudy VC, Lin NL, Sabath DF. Human platelets display high-affinity receptors for thrombopoietin. *Blood* 1997;89(6):1896–1904.
522. Kashiwakura I, et al. Effects of the combination of thrombopoietin with cytokines on the survival of X-irradiated CD34(+) megakaryocytic progenitor cells from normal human peripheral blood. *Radiat Res* 2002;158(2):202–209.
523. Hamada T, et al. Transendothelial migration of megakaryocytes in response to stromal cell-derived factor 1 (SDF-1) enhances platelet formation. *J Exp Med* 1998;188(3):539–548.
524. Maghdooni Bagheri P, De Ley M. Metallothionein in human immunomagnetically selected CD34(+) haematopoietic progenitor cells. *Cell Biol Int* 2011;35(1): 39–44.
525. Duchez P, et al. Thrombopoietin to replace megakaryocyte-derived growth factor: impact on stem and progenitor cells during ex vivo expansion of CD34+ cells mobilized in peripheral blood. *Transfusion* 2011;51(2):313–318.
526. Karlsson C, Larsson J, Baudet A. Forward RNAi screens in human stem cells. *Methods Mol Biol* 2010;650:29–43.
527. Ii M, et al. Synergistic effect of adipose-derived stem cell therapy and bone marrow progenitor recruitment in ischemic heart. *Lab Invest* 2011;91(4):539–552.

528. Domashenko AD, et al. TAT-mediated transduction of NF-Ya peptide induces the ex vivo proliferation and engraftment potential of human hematopoietic progenitor cells. *Blood* 2010;116(15):2676–2683.
529. Kawasaki H, Guan J, Tamama K. Hydrogen gas treatment prolongs replicative lifespan of bone marrow multipotential stromal cells in vitro while preserving differentiation and paracrine potentials. *Biochem Biophys Res Commun* 2010;397(3):608–613.
530. Blom B, Spits H. Development of human lymphoid cells. *Ann Rev Immunol* 2006;24(1):287–320.
531. Schlenner SM, et al. Fate mapping reveals separate origins of T cells and myeloid lineages in the thymus. *Immunity* 2010;32(3):426–436.
532. Vivier E, et al. Targeting natural killer cells and natural killer T cells in cancer. *Nat Rev Immunol* 2012;12(4):239–252.
533. Sun JC, Lanier LL. Natural killer cells remember: an evolutionary bridge between innate and adaptive immunity? *Eur J Immunol* 2009;39(8):2059–2064.
534. Hartsock RJ, Smith EB, Petty CS. Normal variations with aging of the amount of hematopoietic tissue in bone marrow from the anterior iliac crest. A study made from 177 cases of sudden death examined by necropsy. *Am J Clin Pathol* 1965;43:326–331.
535. Friebert SE, et al. Pediatric bone marrow cellularity: are we expecting too much? *J Pediatr Hematol Oncol* 1998;20(5):439–443.
536. Bain BJ. The bone marrow aspirate of healthy subjects. *Br J Haematol* 1996;94(1):206–209.
537. Guralnik JM, et al. Prevalence of anemia in persons 65 years and older in the United States: evidence for a high rate of unexplained anemia. *Blood* 2004;104(8):2263–2268.
538. Izaks GJ, Westendorp RG, Knook DL. The definition of anemia in older persons. *JAMA* 1999;281(18):1714–1717.
539. Steinmann GG. Changes in the human thymus during aging. *Curr Top Pathol* 1986;75:43–88.
540. Steinmann GG, Klaus B, Muller-Hermelink HK. The involution of the ageing human thymic epithelium is independent of puberty. A morphometric study. *Scand J Immunol* 1985;22(5):563–575.
541. Scollay RG, Butcher EC, Weissman IL. Thymus cell migration. Quantitative aspects of cellular traffic from the thymus to the periphery in mice. *Eur J Immunol* 1980;10(3):210–218.
542. Miller JP, Allman D. The decline in B lymphopoiesis in aged mice reflects loss of very early B-lineage precursors. *J Immunol* 2003;171(5):2326–2330.
543. Johnson KM, Owen K, Witte PL. Aging and developmental transitions in the B cell lineage. *Int Immunol* 2002;14(11):1313–1323.
544. Van der Put E, et al. Aged mice exhibit distinct B cell precursor phenotypes differing in activation, proliferation and apoptosis. *Exp Gerontol* 2003;38(10):1137–1147.
545. Rossi MI, et al. B lymphopoiesis is active throughout human life, but there are developmental age-related changes. *Blood* 2003;101(2):576–584.
546. Rego EM, et al. Age-related changes of lymphocyte subsets in normal bone marrow biopsies. *Cytometry* 1998;34(1):22–29.
547. Frasca D, et al. Aging down-regulates the transcription factor E2A, activation-induced cytidine deaminase, and Ig class switch in human B cells. *J Immunol* 2008;180(8):5283–5290.
548. Haynes L, Swain SL. Why aging T cells fail: implications for vaccination. *Immunity* 2006;24(6):663–666.
549. Rossi DJ, et al. Cell intrinsic alterations underlie hematopoietic stem cell aging. *Proc Natl Acad Sci U S A* 2005;102(26):9194–1999.
550. Sudo K, et al. Age-associated characteristics of murine hematopoietic stem cells. *J Exp Med* 2000;192(9):1273–1280.
551. Chambers SM, et al. Aging hematopoietic stem cells decline in function and exhibit epigenetic dysregulation. *PLoS Biol* 2007;5(8):e201.
552. Shaw AC, et al. Aging of the innate immune system. *Curr Opin Immunol* 2010;22(4):507–513.
553. Gomez CR, et al. Innate immunity and aging. *Exp Gerontol* 2008;43(8):718–728.
554. Franceschi C, et al. Inflammaging and anti-inflammaging: a systemic perspective on aging and longevity emerged from studies in humans. *Mech Ageing Dev* 2007;128(1):92–105.
555. Lichtman MA, Rowe JM. The relationship of patient age to the pathobiology of the clonal myeloid diseases. *Semin Oncol* 2004;31(2):185–197.
556. Deschler B, Lubbert M. Acute myeloid leukemia: epidemiology and etiology. *Cancer* 2006;107(9):2099–2107.
557. Morrison SJ, et al. The aging of hematopoietic stem cells. *Nat Med* 1996;2(9):1011–1016.
558. de Haan G, Nijhof W, Van Zant G. Mouse strain-dependent changes in frequency and proliferation of hematopoietic stem cells during aging: correlation between lifespan and cycling activity. *Blood* 1997;89(5):1543–1550.
559. Pang WW, et al. Human bone marrow hematopoietic stem cells are increased in frequency and myeloid-biased with age. *Proc Natl Acad Sci U S A* 2011;108(50):20012–20017.
560. Kuranda K, et al. Age-related changes in human hematopoietic stem/progenitor cells. *Aging Cell* 2011;10(3):542–546.
561. Harrison DE. Mouse erythropoietic stem cell lines function normally 100 months: loss related to number of transplantations. *Mech Ageing Dev* 1979;9(5–6):427–433.
562. Harrison DE. Long-term erythropoietic repopulating ability of old, young, and fetal stem cells. *J Exp Med* 1983;157(5):1496–1504.
563. Kollman C, et al. Donor characteristics as risk factors in recipients after transplantation of bone marrow from unrelated donors: the effect of donor age. *Blood* 2001;98(7):2043–2051.
564. Collado M, Blasco MA, Serrano M. Cellular senescence in cancer and aging. *Cell* 2007;130(2):223–233.
565. Mandal PK, Rossi DJ. DNA-damage-induced differentiation in hematopoietic stem cells. *Cell* 2012;148(5):847–848.
566. Wang J, et al. A differentiation checkpoint limits hematopoietic stem cell self-renewal in response to DNA damage. *Cell* 2012;148(5):1001–1014.
567. Sharpless NE, DePinho RA. Telomeres, stem cells, senescence, and cancer. *J Clin Invest* 2004;113(2):160–168.
568. Dykstra B, et al. Long-term propagation of distinct hematopoietic differentiation programs in vivo. *Cell Stem Cell* 2007;1(2):218–229.
569. Cho RH, Sieburg HB, Muller-Sieburg CE. A new mechanism for the aging of hematopoietic stem cells: aging changes the clonal composition of the stem cell compartment but not individual stem cells. *Blood* 2008;111(12):5553–5561.
570. Sieburg HB, et al. The hematopoietic stem compartment consists of a limited number of discrete stem cell subsets. *Blood* 2006;107(6):2311–2316.
571. Beerman I, et al. Functionally distinct hematopoietic stem cells modulate hematopoietic lineage potential during aging by a mechanism of clonal expansion. *Proc Natl Acad Sci U S A* 2010;107(12):5465–5470.
572. Muller-Sieburg CE, Sieburg HB. The GOD of hematopoietic stem cells: a clonal diversity model of the stem cell compartment. *Cell Cycle* 2006;5(4):394–398.
573. Min H, Montecino-Rodriguez E, Dorshkind K. Effects of aging on the common lymphoid progenitor to pro-B cell transition. *J Immunol* 2006;176(2):1007–1012.
574. Sherwood EM, et al. Senescent BALB/c mice exhibit decreased expression of lambda5 surrogate light chains and reduced development within the pre-B cell compartment. *J Immunol* 1998;161(9):4472–4475.
575. Stephan RP, Lill-Elghanian DA, Witte PL. Development of B cells in aged mice: decline in the ability of pro-B cells to respond to IL-7 but not to other growth factors. *J Immunol* 1997;158(4):1598–1609.
576. Stephan RP, Reilly CR, Witte PL. Impaired ability of bone marrow stromal cells to support B-lymphopoiesis with age. *Blood* 1998;91(1):75–88.
577. Cevenini E, et al. Age-related inflammation: the contribution of different organs, tissues and systems. How to face it for therapeutic approaches. *Curr Pharm Des* 2010;16(6):609–618.
578. De la Fuente M, Miquel J. An update of the oxidation-inflammation theory of aging: the involvement of the immune system in oxi-inflamm-aging. *Curr Pharm Des* 2009;15(26):3003–3026.
579. Busque L, et al. Recurrent somatic TET2 mutations in normal elderly individuals with clonal hematopoiesis. *Nat Genet* 2012;44(11):1179–1181.
580. Hotta T, et al. Age-related changes in the function of hemopoietic stroma in mice. *Exp Hematol* 1980;8(7):933–936.
581. Mauch P, et al. Decline in bone marrow proliferative capacity as a function of age. *Blood* 1982;60(1):245–252.
582. Challen GA, et al. Distinct hematopoietic stem cell subtypes are differentially regulated by TGF-beta1. *Cell Stem Cell* 2010;6(3):265–278.
583. Chen C, Liu Y, Zheng P. mTOR regulation and therapeutic rejuvenation of aging hematopoietic stem cells. *Sci Signal* 2009;2(98):ra75.
584. Lapidot T, et al. A cell initiating human acute myeloid leukaemia after transplantation into SCID mice. *Nature* 1994;367(6464):645–658.
585. Bonnet D, Dick JE. Human acute myeloid leukemia is organized as a hierarchy that originates from a primitive hematopoietic cell. *Nat Med* 1997;3(7):730–737.
586. Hope KJ, Jin L, Dick JE. Acute myeloid leukemia originates from a hierarchy of leukemic stem cell classes that differ in self-renewal capacity. *Nat Immunol* 2004;5(7):738–743.
587. Taussig DC, et al. Anti-CD38 antibody-mediated clearance of human repopulating cells masks the heterogeneity of leukemia-initiating cells. *Blood* 2008;112(3):568–575.
588. Sarry JE, et al. Human acute myelogenous leukemia stem cells are rare and heterogeneous when assayed in NOD/SCID/IL2Rgammac-deficient mice. *J Clin Invest* 2011;121(1):384–395.
589. Gibbs KD Jr, et al. Decoupling of tumor-initiating activity from stable immunophenotype in HoxA9-Meis1-driven AML. *Cell Stem Cell* 2012;10(2):210–217.
590. Gerber JM, et al. A clinically relevant population of leukemic CD34(+)CD38(−) cells in acute myeloid leukemia. *Blood* 2012;119(15):3571–3577.
591. Cheung AM, et al. Aldehyde dehydrogenase activity in leukemic blasts defines a subgroup of acute myeloid leukemia with adverse prognosis and superior NOD/SCID engrafting potential. *Leukemia* 2007;21(7):1423–1430.
592. Pearce DJ, Bonnet D. The combined use of Hoechst efflux ability and aldehyde dehydrogenase activity to identify murine and human hematopoietic stem cells. *Exp Hematol* 2007;35(9):1437–1446.
593. Pearce DJ, et al. Characterization of cells with a high aldehyde dehydrogenase activity from cord blood and acute myeloid leukemia samples. *Stem Cells* 2005;23(6):752–760.
594. Cozzio A, et al. Similar MLL-associated leukemias arising from self-renewing stem cells and short-lived myeloid progenitors. *Genes Dev* 2003;17(24):3029–3035.
595. Huntly BJ, et al. MOZ-TIF2, but not BCR-ABL, confers properties of leukemic stem cells to committed murine hematopoietic progenitors. *Cancer Cell* 2004;6(6):587–596.
596. Krivtsov AV, et al. Transformation from committed progenitor to leukaemia stem cell initiated by MLL-AF9. *Nature* 2006;442(7104):818–822.
597. Somervaille TC, Cleary ML. Identification and characterization of leukemia stem cells in murine MLL-AF9 acute myeloid leukemia. *Cancer Cell* 2006;10(4):257–268.
598. Barabe F, et al. Modeling the initiation and progression of human acute leukemia in mice. *Science* 2007;316(5824):600–604.
599. Jan M, et al. Clonal evolution of preleukemic hematopoietic stem cells precedes human acute myeloid leukemia. *Sci Transl Med* 2012;4(149):149ra118.
600. Walter MJ, et al. Clonal architecture of secondary acute myeloid leukemia. *N Engl J Med* 2012;366(12):1090–1098.
601. Patel JP, et al. Prognostic relevance of integrated genetic profiling in acute myeloid leukemia. *N Engl J Med* 2012;366(12):1079–1089.
602. Figueroa ME, et al. DNA methylation signatures identify biologically distinct subtypes in acute myeloid leukemia. *Cancer Cell* 2010;17(1):13–27.
603. Jamieson CH, et al. Granulocyte-macrophage progenitors as candidate leukemic stem cells in blast-crisis CML. *N Engl J Med* 2004;351(7):657–667.
604. Druker BJ, et al. Five-year follow-up of patients receiving imatinib for chronic myeloid leukemia. *N Engl J Med* 2006;355(23):2408–2417.
605. Cortes JE, et al. Nilotinib as front-line treatment for patients with chronic myeloid leukemia in early chronic phase. *J Clin Oncol* 2010;28(3):392–397.
606. Cortes JE, et al. Results of dasatinib therapy in patients with early chronic-phase chronic myeloid leukemia. *J Clin Oncol* 2010;28(3):398–404.
607. Mahon FX, et al. Discontinuation of imatinib in patients with chronic myeloid leukaemia who have maintained complete molecular remission for at least 2 years: the prospective, multicentre Stop Imatinib (STIM) trial. *Lancet Oncol* 2010;11(11):1029–1035.
608. Cortes J, et al. Front-line and salvage therapies with tyrosine kinase inhibitors and other treatments in chronic myeloid leukemia. *J Clin Oncol* 2011;29(5):524–531.
609. Rousselot P, et al. Imatinib mesylate discontinuation in patients with chronic myelogenous leukemia in complete molecular remission for more than 2 years. *Blood* 2007;109(1):58–60.
610. Jorgensen HG, et al. Nilotinib exerts equipotent antiproliferative effects to imatinib and does not induce apoptosis in CD34+ CML cells. *Blood* 2007;109(9):4016–4019.

611. Copland M, et al. Dasatinib (BMS-354825) targets an earlier progenitor population than imatinib in primary CML but does not eliminate the quiescent fraction. *Blood* 2006;107(11):4532–4539.

612. Graham SM, et al. Primitive, quiescent, Philadelphia-positive stem cells from patients with chronic myeloid leukemia are insensitive to STI571 in vitro. *Blood* 2002;99(1):319–325.

613. Konig H, et al. Enhanced BCR-ABL kinase inhibition does not result in increased inhibition of downstream signaling pathways or increased growth suppression in CML progenitors. *Leukemia* 2008;22(4):748–755.

614. Konig H, Holyoake TL, Bhatia R. Effective and selective inhibition of chronic myeloid leukemia primitive hematopoietic progenitors by the dual Src/Abl kinase inhibitor SKI-606. *Blood* 2008;111(4):2329–2338.

615. Tehranchi R, et al. Persistent malignant stem cells in del(5q) myelodysplasia in remission. *N Engl J Med* 2010;363(11):1025–1037.

616. Mullally A, et al. Physiological Jak2V617F expression causes a lethal myeloproliferative neoplasm with differential effects on hematopoietic stem and progenitor cells. *Cancer Cell* 2010;17(6):584–596.

617. Brunstein CG, Gutman JA, Weisdorf DJ. Allogeneic hematopoietic cell transplantation for hematologic malignancy: relative risks and benefits of double umbilical cord blood. *Blood* 2010;116(22):4693–4699.

618. North TE, et al. Prostaglandin E2 regulates vertebrate haematopoietic stem cell homeostasis. *Nature* 2007;447(7147):1007–1011.

619. Varnum-Finney B, Brashem-Stein C, Bernstein ID. Combined effects of Notch signaling and cytokines induce a multiple log increase in precursors with lymphoid and myeloid reconstituting ability. *Blood* 2003;101(5):1784–1789.

620. Milner LA, Kopan R, Martin DI. A human homologue of the Drosophila developmental gene, Notch, is expressed in CD34+ hematopoietic precursors. *Blood* 1994;83(8):2057–2062.

621. Zhang CC, et al. Angiopoietin-like 5 and IGFBP2 stimulate ex vivo expansion of human cord blood hematopoietic stem cells as assayed by NOD/SCID transplantation. 2008;111(7):3415–3423.

622. Csaszar E, et al. Rapid expansion of human hematopoietic stem cells by automated control of inhibitory feedback signaling. *Cell Stem Cell* 2012;10(2):218–229.

623. Takahashi K, Yamanaka S. Induction of pluripotent stem cells from mouse embryonic and adult fibroblast cultures by defined factors. *Cell* 2006;126(4):663–676.

624. Narita M, et al. Induction of pluripotent stem cells from adult human fibroblasts by defined factors. *Cell* 2007;131(5):861–872.

625. Okita K, Ichisaka T, Yamanaka S. Generation of germline-competent induced pluripotent stem cells. *Nature* 2007;448:313–317.

626. Daley GQ. Cellular alchemy and the golden age of reprogramming. *Cell* 2012;151(6):1151–1154.

627. Park IH, et al. Reprogramming of human somatic cells to pluripotency with defined factors. *Nature* 2007;451(7175):141–146.

628. Yu J, et al. Induced pluripotent stem cell lines derived from human somatic cells. *Science* 2007;318(5858):1917–1920.

629. Hanna J, et al. Treatment of sickle cell anemia mouse model with iPS cells generated from autologous skin. *Science* 2007;318(5858):1920–1923.

630. Park IH, et al. Disease-specific induced pluripotent stem cells. *Cell* 2008;134(5):877–886.

631. Eminli S, et al. Differentiation stage determines potential of hematopoietic cells for reprogramming into induced pluripotent stem cells. *Nat Genet* 2009;41(9):968–976.

632. Loh YH, et al. Generation of induced pluripotent stem cells from human blood. *Blood* 2009;113(22):5476–5479.

633. Hanna J, et al. Direct reprogramming of terminally differentiated mature B lymphocytes to pluripotency. *Cell* 2008;133(2):250–264.

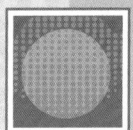

Chapter 2
The Immune System: Structure and Function

Andrea Cerutti • Giuliana Magri • Montserrat Cols • Linda Cassis • Cindy Gutzeit • Alejo Chorny • Maurizio Gentile • Carolina M. Barra • Irene Puga

 ## GENERAL PRINCIPLES

The immune system is composed of a series of highly integrated physical structures and biologic processes that protect our body against disease. This protection involves the recognition and clearance of foreign agents, also referred to as antigens, that range from toxic molecules to complex microorganisms, including viruses, bacteria, fungi, and parasites. In addition, the immune system recognizes and eliminates abnormal host cells capable of inducing inflammation or tumor growth (1). All these protective functions require a sophisticated system of "sensors" (receptors) that discriminate molecules associated with healthy cells from molecules associated with foreign, dead, or abnormal cells (2,3). Any perturbation of this discriminatory capacity can lead to the onset of autoimmunity, inflammation, or cancer (4). As exemplified by the epithelial surfaces that separate the sterile milieu of our body from the external environment, another remarkable property of our immune system relates to its ability to generate multiple layers of innate and adaptive defenses that have increasing specificity (5).

In both skin and mucosal organs, epithelial cells have a rapid turnover that permits the elimination of the microorganisms eventually adherent to the most superficial epithelial layers (6). Epithelial cells also secrete mucin proteins to form a highly dynamic mucus barrier that not only limits the invasion of mucosal organs by pathogenic microbes but also provides a nutrient-rich environment for commensal bacteria that colonize our intestine after birth (7). These bacteria provide essential digestive, metabolic, and immune functions and also form a highly competitive ecological niche that excludes pathogens. Of note, mucins not only facilitate the growth of commensals but also limit their adhesion to the apical surface of epithelial cells, which is an event that can cause inflammation (8).

Epithelial cells further limit microbial colonization by eliminating mucus-anchored microbes through the coordinated movement of apical cilia (9). Moreover, epithelial cells release acid secretions, toxic fatty acids, bile salts, proteases, and antimicrobial peptides that impose further restrictions on the number and quality of microbes associated with epidermal or mucosal surfaces (10). In addition to generating nonspecific protection mechanisms typically associated with the innate immune system, epithelial cells function as "facilitators" of certain specific responses of the adaptive immune system (11). In particular, epithelial cells transport specific antibody molecules, also known as immunoglobulins (Igs), from the lamina propria into the lumen of mucosal organs (12). These antibodies derive from plasma cells of the specific adaptive immune system and not only repel pathogens but also control the composition of the commensal microbiota (13). Thus, epithelial cells exert both nonspecific and specific protective functions that exemplify the multilayered nature of our immune system.

Innate and Adaptive Immune Responses

Pathogens usually invade our body through the skin or mucosal surfaces (8). When invasion occurs, the proper cells of our immune system known as leukocytes (commonly known as white blood cells) sense the presence of the intruding microbes and thereafter remove them by mounting protective responses characterized by a progressively increasing specificity. Leukocytes can be broadly subdivided into granulocytes (also known as polymorphonuclear leukocytes), monocytes, macrophages, dendritic cells (DCs), mast cells, and lymphocytes (Fig. 2.1). Granulocytes include neutrophils, eosinophils, and basophils, whereas lymphocytes are composed of natural killer (NK) cells, invariant NKT (iNKT) cells, T cells and B cells. While granulocytes, monocytes, macrophages, DCs, mast cells, and NK cells play essential roles in the innate immune system, T cells and B cells functionally belong to the adaptive immune system. iNKT cells occupy an intermediate position together with specific subsets of T and B cells, including $\gamma\delta$ T cells, peritoneal B-1 cells, and splenic marginal zone (MZ) B cells (14). Granulocytes, monocytes, macrophages, and DCs cooperate with soluble components of the innate immune system, such as complement proteins, to mount nonspecific protective responses that occur very rapidly but do not confer long-lasting protection (15). These responses promote the initial containment of invading microbes by inducing an inflammatory reaction that triggers the recruitment of granulocytes and monocytes from the circulation to the site of infection (16). Inflammation is functionally linked with the complement and coagulation cascades and begins with the secretion of cytokines and chemokines released by mucosal epithelial cells, vascular endothelial cells, interstitial macrophages, and interstitial DCs from the infected tissue (Tables 2.1 and 2.2). Inflammation is further amplified by cytokines and chemokines secreted by lymphocytes at a later stage of the immune response. In general, lymphocytes cooperate with the innate immune system to mount specific protective responses that occur more slowly but confer long-lasting protection.

Innate Immunity

Granulocytes, monocytes, macrophages, DCs, and NK cells promote innate immune responses by recognizing and responding to microbes through nonspecific germline-encoded pattern recognition receptors (PRRs) (2). Neutrophils are the first leukocytes that migrate from the circulation to the infection site (17). At this site, neutrophils remove dead cells and cellular debris and phagocytose and kill microbes. NK cells play a major role in the recognition and destruction of cells that are either infected by viruses or transformed by a neoplastic process (18). Monocytes contribute to the induction of inflammation but also differentiate to macrophages and DCs (19,20). Macrophages phagocytose microbes, dead cells, and cellular debris; kill engulfed pathogens; and induce inflammation (21). Furthermore, macrophages

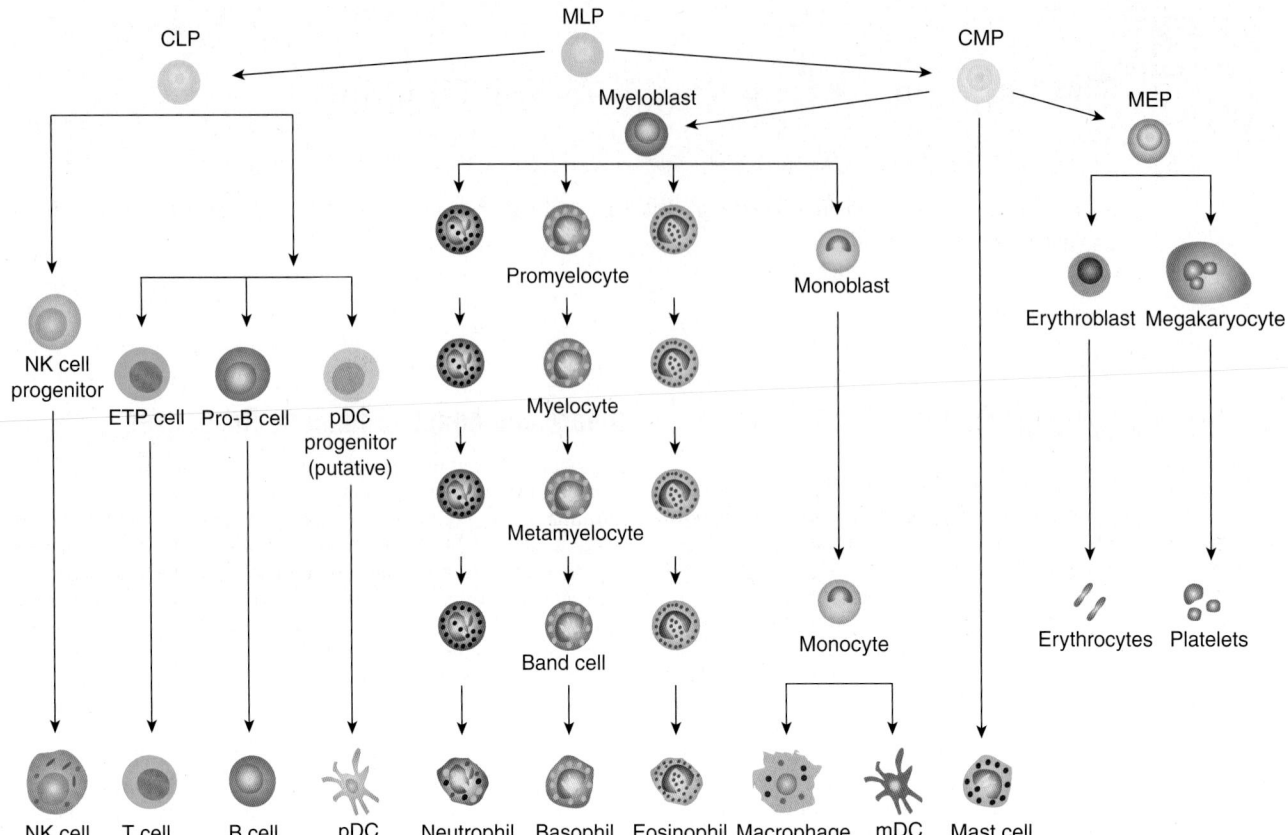

FIGURE 2.1. Immune cells and their origin from hematopoietic progenitors. Self-renewing multipotent progenitor (MLP) cells give rise to common lymphoid progenitor (CLP) cells and common myeloid progenitor (CMP) cells in the bone marrow. CLP cells further differentiate into NK-cell progenitors, T-cell progenitors (known as ETP cells), B-cell progenitors (pro-B cells), and putative plasmacytoid DC (pDC) progenitors that generate mature NK cells, T cells, B cells, and pDCs, respectively. Intermediate differentiation stages of T and B cells are not shown here because they are described in later figures. CMP cells differentiate into myeloblasts and megakaryocyte/erythrocyte progenitor (MEP) cells. Myeloblasts give rise to mature neutrophils, eosinophils, and basophils via sequential subset-specific differentiation stages that include promyelocytes, myelocytes, metamyelocytes, and band cells. Myeloblasts also give rise to monoblasts and monocytes, which further differentiate into macrophages and myeloid DCs (mDCs) in peripheral tissues. Mast cells derive from CMP cells through an autonomous differentiation pathway. Finally, MEP cells give rise to erythroblasts and megakaryoblasts that generate mature erythrocytes and platelets, respectively, through various intermediate stages not shown here because it is beyond the scope of this chapter.

present native antigen to B cells. In contrast, DCs internalize microbes to generate antigenic peptides that are presented to T cells in the context of major histocompatibility complex (MHC, defined as human leukocyte antigen [HLA] in humans) molecules (22). This process usually takes place after DC migration from the infection site to draining lymph nodes and leads to the activation of both T and B cells. DCs also promote the recruitment, activation, and maturation of multiple cells of the innate and adaptive immune systems, including T and B cells (23). There are two types of DCs: myeloid DCs (mDCs) are mainly involved in antigen presentation, whereas lymphoid or plasmacytoid DCs (pDCs) are predominantly implicated in antiviral responses (24). In addition, both mDCs and pDCs mediate immunostimulation. Finally, mast cells elicit inflammation and cooperate with eosinophils and basophils to induce the expulsion of parasites infesting mucosal organs (25,26).

Adaptive Immunity

T and B cells promote adaptive immune responses by recognizing microbes through specific somatically recombined antigen receptors known as T-cell receptor (TCR) and B-cell receptor (BCR), respectively. T cells can be further divided into $CD4^+$ T cells and $CD8^+$ T cells (27). Antigen-activated $CD4^+$ T cells differentiate into multiple antigen-specific T helper (T_H) effector cell subsets that enhance the recruitment and activation of granulocytes

and macrophages, collaborate with B cells to induce antibody production, and enhance the antimicrobial activity of epithelial cells (28). In contrast, antigen-activated $CD8^+$ T cells develop into cytotoxic T lymphocytes (CTLs) that specifically kill infected cells to prevent the spreading of invading microbes such as viruses throughout the body (29). Antigen-activated B cells differentiate into plasma cells that secrete antigen-specific antibody molecules belonging to the IgM, IgG, IgA, or IgE class (or isotype), each of which is associated with specific effector functions (30). These antibodies provide immune protection by neutralizing toxins and viruses, by inducing complement-mediated lysis of microbes, and by enhancing the phagocytic, killing, and inflammatory functions of granulocytes, monocytes, macrophages, NK cells, and mast cells. In addition, IgA antibodies interact with epithelial cells to generate mucosal immunity (31). Another remarkable feature of T- and B-cell responses is that they generate long-lived memory cells (32). These cells patrol both circulation and lymphoid organs for years after the initial infection and mount very rapid and robust anamnestic responses upon encountering antigen for a second time.

Immune Regulation

After encountering antigen, immature and mature lymphocytes can develop either immunity or tolerance (33). The latter is essential for the prevention of harmful immune responses

| Table 2.1 | COMMON CYTOKINES |

Cytokine	Function	Expression
IL-1	Immunoactivation, inflammation	Monocytes, macrophages, DCs, endothelial cells
IL-2	T-cell proliferation and activation, Treg cell expansion	Activated T cells
IL-3	Granulopoiesis, basophil activation	Activated T cells, mast cells
IL-4	T_H2-cell differentiation, B-cell activation, IgG and IgE class switching	T_H2 cells, basophils, eosinophils, mast cells
IL-5	Eosinophil activation and maturation	T_H2 cells, mast cells
IL-6	Inflammation, T_H17-cell differentiation, plasma cell differentiation, and survival	Monocytes, macrophages, DCs, endothelial cells
IL-7	Lymphopoiesis	Stromal cells
IL-8	Granulocyte recruitment, inflammation	Monocytes, macrophages, DCs, endothelial cells, epithelial cells
IL-9	Mast cell survival and activation	Mast cells, eosinophils, T_H9 cells
IL-10	Immunoregulation, IgG class switching, plasma cell differentiation	Monocytes, macrophages, DCs, Treg cells, Breg cells
IL-11	Hematopoiesis, osteoclast differentiation	Stromal cells, epithelial cells, endothelial cells, fibroblasts
IL-12	T_H1-cell differentiation	DCs, monocytes, macrophages
IL-13	Mucus secretion, inflammation, IgE class switching	T cells, mast cells, NK cells
IL-14	B-cell proliferation, inhibition of antibody production	Activated T cells
IL-15	NK- and T-cell proliferation	DCs, monocytes, macrophages, stromal cells
IL-16	$CD4^+$ T-cell migration	T cells
IL-17	Mucosal immunity, inflammation	T_H17 cells
IL-18	T_H1 cell differentiation, induction of IFN-γ, inflammation	DCs, monocytes, macrophages
IL-19	Inflammation	Monocytes, macrophages
IL-20	Epithelial cell regulation	Monocytes, epithelial cells
IL-21	B-cell and NK-cell proliferation, IgM, IgG and IgA production	T_H17 cells, T_{FH} cells
IL-22	Mucosal homeostasis and immunity	T_H17 cells, T_H22 cells
IL-23	T_H17-cell expansion and maintenance	DCs, macrophages
IL-24	Induction of TNF-α and IFN-γ, inflammation	NK cells, T cells, fibroblasts, melanocytes
IL-25	Induction of IL-4 and eotaxin, T_H2-cell activation and differentiation	Stromal cells, T cells
IL-26	Epithelial cell regulation (similar to IL-20)	T cells, NK cells
IL-27	Inflammation, mucosal immunity	DCs, macrophages, endothelial cells, plasma cells
IL-28	Antiviral responses (cooperates with IFN-β)	DCs (mDCs)
IL-29	Antiviral responses (similar to IL-28)	DCs (mDCs)
IL-30	Inflammation, mucosal immunity (subunit of IL-27)	DCs, macrophages
IL-31	Granulocyte and monocyte recruitment, inflammation	T_H2 cells, monocytes
IL-32	Induction of TNF, inflammation	NK cells
APRIL	B-cell activation, class switching, plasma cell differentiation and survival	DCs, macrophages, granulocytes, epithelial cells, endothelial cells
BAFF	B-cell survival, class switching, plasma cell differentiation	DCs, macrophages, granulocytes, epithelial cells, stromal cells
G-CSF	Myelopoiesis, granulocyte survival, and activation	Monocytes, macrophages, endothelial cells, fibroblasts
GM-CSF	Myelopoiesis, granulocyte and macrophage survival, and activation	Activated T cells, T_H17 cells, fibroblasts, endothelial cells, macrophages
IFN-α/β	Antiviral responses, DC maturation, immunoactivation	DCs (pDCs), broad expression
IFN-γ	T_H1-cell responses, macrophage activation, inflammation	T_H1 cells, NK cells, iNKT cells
TNF	DC maturation, immunoactivation, inflammation	Monocytes, macrophages, DCs, T cells, NK cells, iNKT cells, granulocytes
TGF-β	Immunoregulation, anti-inflammatory activity, IgA production	Treg cells

against antigens belonging to the host (self-antigens) and involves multiple regulatory mechanisms that vary with the stage of T- and B-cell development (34,35). In mature lymphocytes, key tolerogenic signals are provided by T-regulatory (Treg) and B-regulatory (Breg) cells (36,37). Lymphocytes require additional regulatory signals to control the magnitude of an immune response and induce its termination after the completion of antigen clearance. Such termination signals are generated by death-inducing and inhibitory immune receptors expressed on the surface of lymphocytes (38). Together with signals from anti-inflammatory cytokines, inhibitory immune receptors also negatively regulate the activation of the innate immune system.

Evolutionary Considerations

In complex multicellular organisms, the evolution of the immune system likely stemmed from the need to recognize the internal milieu, or self, and respond to its alterations in order to ensure the continuation of the species (39). Thus, the recognition of self has a primary importance in immunity, as it is this recognition that permits the immune system to sense the presence of alterations brought about by harmful internal or external stressors. The evolutionarily ancient innate arm of the immune system recognizes and responds to external danger signals from invading microbes by sensing nonself molecular patterns through nonspecific microbe recognition receptors, also known as PRRs (40). Many of these receptors also function as danger recognition receptors that mount protective responses after sensing internal danger signals from injured cells. The evolutionarily recent adaptive arm of the immune system further discriminates self from nonself in the context of antigen-presenting MHC molecules (41).

Given that the most ancestral function of the immune system relates to the recognition of self, it is not surprising that even protozoan organisms such as amoebae can internalize and degrade bacteria through a phagocytic process that does not induce self-digestion. These and other simple species discriminate self from nonself by utilizing PRRs (42), which mount

| | Table 2.2 | **COMMON CHEMOKINES** | | |

Name	Receptor	Expression	Target
XCL1 (lymphotactin)	XCR1	Thymus, CD8$^+$ T cells, NK cells, mast cells	NK cells, thymocytes
XCL2 (SCM1b)	XCR1	Thymus, CD8$^+$ T cells, NK cells, mast cells	NK cells, thymocytes
CCL1	CCR8	Activated T cells, monocytes	T cells, neutrophils
CCL2 (MCP-1)	CCR2	Endothelial cells, eosinophils	Activated T cells, DCs, monocytes, basophils
CCL3 (MIP-1α)	CCR1, CCR3, CCR5	T cells, B cells, DCs,	T cells, NK, DCs, eosinophils, monocytes, macrophages
CCL4 (MIP-1β)	CCR5	NK cells, T cells, B cells, DCs	T$_H$1 cells, DCs, monocytes, macrophages
CCL5 (RANTES)	CCR1, CCR5	Endothelial cells, epithelial cells	T$_H$1 cells, NK, DCs, eosinophils, monocytes, macrophages
CCL7 (MCP-3)	CCR1	Monocytes, fibroblasts	NK cells, immature DCs, eosinophils, monocytes
CCL8 (MCP-2)	CCR2	Fibroblast, neutrophils	Activated T cells, DCs, monocytes, basophils
CCL11 (eotaxin)	CCR3	Endothelial, epithelial cells	T$_H$2 cells, monocytes, eosinophils
CCL13 (MCP-4)	CCR2	Macrophages	Activated T cells, DCs, monocytes, basophils
CCL17 (TARC)	CCR4	Thymus, lung, intestine	DCs, thymocytes, T$_H$2 cells, NK cells
CCL19 (ELC)	CCR7	Broad expression in lymphoid tissues	B cells, naïve T cells, mature DCs
CCL20 (LARC)	CCR6	Broad expression in lymphoid tissues	B cells, memory T cells, immature DCs
CCL21 (SLC)	CCR7	Broad expression in lymphoid tissues	B cells, naïve T cells, T$_H$2 cells, DCs, eosinophils, monocytes
CCL22	CCR4	Lymph nodes, macrophages	DCs, thymocytes, T$_H$2 cells, NK cells
CCL25 (TECK)	CCR9	DCs, stromal cells, epithelial cells	DCs, thymocytes, macrophages
CCL27 (CTACK)	CCR10	Epithelial cells	T cells
CCL28 (MEC)	CCR10	Epithelial cells	T cells
CXCL1 (GROα)	CXCR2	Monocytes, fibroblasts, endothelial cells	Neutrophils, fibroblasts
CXCL2 (GROβ)	CXCR2	Monocytes, fibroblasts, endothelial cells	Neutrophils, fibroblasts
CXCL3 (GROγ)	CXCR2	Monocytes, fibroblasts, endothelial cells	Neutrophils, fibroblasts
CXCL5	CXCR2	Monocytes, platelets	Neutrophils, fibroblasts
CXCL6	CXCR1	Fibroblasts, monocytes, lymphocytes	Neutrophils
CXCL7	CXCR2	Monocytes, platelets	Neutrophils, fibroblasts
CXCL8 (IL-8)	CXCR1, CXCR2	Fibroblasts, monocytes, endothelial cells	Neutrophils
CXCL9 (MIG)	CXCR3	Monocytes, hepatocytes, endothelial cells	Activated T$_H$1 cells, NK, monocytes, eosinophils
CXCL10 (IP-10)	CXCR3	Monocytes, hepatocytes, endothelial cells	Activated T$_H$1 cells, NK, monocytes, eosinophils
CXCL11 (I-TAC)	CXCR3	Monocytes, hepatocytes, endothelial cells	Activated T$_H$1 cells, NK, monocytes, eosinophils
CXCL12 (SDF-1)	CXCR4	Stromal cells, FDCs, innate immune cells	B cells, plasma cells
CXCL13 (BCA-1)	CXCR5	Stromal cells, FDCs, innate immune cells	Germinal center B cells, T$_{FH}$ cells
CXCL16	CXCR6	DCs	T and NK cells
CXC3CL (fractalin)	CX3CR1	Endothelial cells, monocytes, microglia	T cells, NK, monocytes, neutrophils

protective responses against external pathogens by inducing the release of antimicrobial peptides (43). In metazoan organisms such as humans, immune coexistence strategies have allowed not only the preservation of self-tissues but also the establishment of complex commensal and symbiotic relationships with trillions of intestinal bacteria that are required for the health of the host (44).

Immune elimination strategies are nonetheless required for the containment and clearance of stressors, two conditions essential for the initiation of tissue repair. The archaic multimodular innate immune system removes stressors by orchestrating a close cooperation between phagocytes and various types of innate lymphocytes, including NK cells, B-1 cells, $\gamma\delta$ T cells, and iNKT cells. In addition to integrating and optimizing the effector functions of phagocytes, some of these innate lymphocytes and iNKT cells jump-start and fine-tune both innate and adaptive immune responses to provide quick protection (45). If innate mechanisms fail to clear the stressor, B and T cells of the adaptive immune system are recruited to optimize both clearing and healing processes (46). Of note, T and B cells discriminate self from nonself by utilizing MHC-restricted recognition systems such as TCR and BCR molecules, respectively, and work in concert with the innate immune system to promote protection, restore homeostasis, and induce memory.

Historical Remarks

Immunity originates from the Latin word *immunis* (*in* = no; *munus* = task, duty, burden), which was initially used by Titus Livy in his "History of Rome" to indicate servicemen who were exempt from active fighting. Among others, these individuals included doctors, architects, engineers, stonecutters, woodcutters, cooks, and shoemakers who were employed in the logistical support of the army for their specific skills. Coincidentally, individuals exempt from serving in battle were less exposed to infections caused by improperly healed wounds. The notion of exemption resulting from the professional specialization of an individual reemerged later with the use of the word *immunis* to designate diplomats who were exempt from taxes or imprisonment. Fascinatingly, also the medical term immunity implies the notions of exemption and specialization. Indeed, the immune system protects from infection through the induction of a highly specific biologic response.

Historical references to acquired specific immunity can be found in the fifth century BC from "The History of the Peloponnesian War," in which Thucydides reports that individuals who survived the Athenian plague were relatively unaffected by a second exposure and were able to nurse the sick and dying in recurrent epidemics. Chinese medical practitioners were reported to empirically inoculate smallpox virus into healthy individuals as early as in the 10th century AD, but this practice was not documented until the 17th century AD. However, in Chinese history, a peaceful replacement of a dynasty with another only rarely occurred, and this often determined the partial or complete loss of recorded accounts over previous scientific advances.

Some consider Edward Jenner as the founder of modern immunology. In 1798, Jenner reported that inoculation of humans with cowpox (or vaccinia) afforded protection against smallpox. In his practice as a physician in Gloucestershire,

England, Jenner observed that material from pustules of horses' hoofs was transmitted to the nipples of cows (Latin, *vaccae*) by farm workers. He observed that milkmaids who developed lesions on their hands and wrists after handling such cows were thereafter immune to smallpox infection. The term "vaccination" is derived from Jenner's deduction that inoculation with vaccinia conferred later protection to the organism that causes smallpox, and it is still used to describe methods of inducing immunity by inoculation. Although some cultural practices throughout the world reflected a pragmatic understanding of infection and immunity, there was little formal appreciation for specific immune mechanisms until after Robert Koch's identification of microorganisms as the cause of infectious disease. Koch's important observation that anthrax could be transmitted from a culture system to animals, reported in 1876, was followed shortly by Louis Pasteur's demonstration that vaccination could protect animals from infections such as cholera and anthrax.

These advances in the last part of the 19th century spurred investigations regarding specific mechanisms of microbial immunity in animals and humans. Based on their work at the Pasteur Institute, Emile Roux and Alexandre Yersin reported the purification of a soluble toxin from the supernatants of microbial cultures of diphtheria. At the Koch Institute, Emile von Behring and Shibasaburo Kitasato soon discovered that vaccination of animals with diphtheria or tetanus toxins led to the production of a humoral substance that inhibited the effect of the toxin and was therefore called "antitoxin." In the first 50 years of the 20th century, work on vaccines continued and led to the development of vaccines against yellow fever and pneumococcal disease. In 1928, Alexander Flemming serendipitously discovered that the bacterium *Penicillium rubens* exuded a substance with antibiotic properties, but it was not until 1942 that penicillin was purified and developed to treat bacterial infections. In 1930, Paul Ehrlich postulated the existence of immune bodies later referred to as antibodies that function as cellular receptors for specific antigens to which they bind directly. Ehrlich speculated that antibody engagement by a specific antigen results in antibody shedding from the cell surface.

Earlier theories proposed by Metchnikoff had suggested that phagocytes were the major cells responsible for immunity, but eventually "humoralists" such as Emil Adolf Von Behring, Emile Roux, and Jules Bordet independently demonstrated that immunity could be transferred from one individual to the other and that this transfer involved soluble factors corresponding to antibodies and complement. Nonetheless, "cellularists" such as Karl Landsteiner and Merrill Chase proved that cells also played an important role in immunity by showing that transfer of cells from guinea pigs immunized with *Mycobacterium tuberculosis* to healthy controls elicited an immune recall response that was not present in the control animals. In this manner, the dichotomy between antibody-mediated (immediate) and cell-mediated (delayed) immunity was established. By 1950, Svante Arrhenius coined the term antibody as the fundamental unit of immunity. Later studies led to the identification of the antibody structure and to the discovery that small lymphocytes initiate the immune response (47).

During the early 20th century, a variety of hypotheses were proposed to explain the extreme diversity and specificity of antibody formation in mammals. Linus Pauling and others proposed *instructive theories*, according to which the structure and specificity of an antibody was shaped by its physical interaction with a particular antigen. Niels Jerne posed the first *selection model* for antibody affinity and maturation (48). His work was followed by that of Frank Macfarlane Burnet and David Talmage, who explained immunologic memory as the cloning of two types of lymphocyte. One clone acts immediately to combat infection whilst the other is longer lasting,

remaining in the immune system for a long time, which results in immunity to that antigen. Then, Gustav Nossal and Joshua Lederberg showed that one B cell always produces only one antibody, which was the first formal evidence for the modern theory of clonal selection and expansion.

LYMPHOID ORGANS

Lymphoid organs are specialized tissues that foster the development and activation of lymphocytes. These organs can be classified as "primary," "secondary," or "tertiary." Primary lymphoid tissues are sites where lymphocytes develop from progenitor cells into functional and mature lymphocytes. During embryonic life, the yolk sac, the aorta-gonad mesonephros region, and the fetal liver are primary sites of hematopoiesis (49). In adults, primary lymphoid tissues are the bone marrow, where all lymphocyte progenitors reside and differentiate, and the thymus, where T cells undergo maturation and acquire functional competence. Secondary or peripheral lymphoid organs include lymph nodes, the spleen, and various mucosa-associated lymphoid tissues (MALTs). In secondary lymphoid tissues, lymphocytes interact with each other and with nonlymphoid cells to mount immune responses to antigen (50). Moreover, secondary lymphoid organs are important for the regulation of peripheral tolerance to control autoreactive lymphocytes that escape from central selection processes (51). Tertiary lymphoid organs are ectopic accumulations of lymphoid cells that frequently form at sites of chronic inflammation and during microbial infection, graft rejection, or autoimmune disease (52). After emerging from primary lymphoid organs, mature lymphocytes enter the general circulation and the lymphatic system. This latter is an essential component of the circulatory system and consists of an extensive network of lymphatic vessels that carry interstitial fluid (lymph), antigens, and DCs from peripheral tissues; lymphocytes from lymph nodes; and fat (chyle) from the digestive tract (53). Lymphatic ducts collect the content of lymphatic vessels and discharge it in the venous system.

Primary Lymphoid Organs

Bone Marrow

The bone marrow is a highly cellular and richly vascularized tissue located in the central cavities of axial and long bones. The main function of bone marrow is to provide specialized niches to guide and constrain the development of hematopoietic stem cells and progenitor cells as well as lineage-restricted immune cells (54). Bone marrow niches regulate cell renewal, differentiation, and quiescence by delivering contact-dependent and contact-independent signals through stromal cells, matrix components, and soluble factors. In addition to hematopoietic precursors, the bone marrow contains different types of nonhematopoietic stromal cells that include adipocytes, reticular cells, endothelial cells, fibroblasts, osteoblasts, osteoclasts, and mesenchymal cells. These stromal cells are essential to maintain the pool of stem cells and induce the differentiation of multipotent progenitor (MLP) cells to either lymphoid or erythroid-myeloid lineages, resulting in the formation of common lymphoid progenitor (CLP) and common myeloid progenitor (CMP) cells. CLP cells further differentiate into B and T cells (55). While B-cell development exclusively takes place in the bone marrow, T cells develop in the thymus.

Thymus

The thymus is a bilobed gland located in the upper anterior thorax of higher vertebrates and constitutes the primary lymphoid organ responsible for the production of a diverse

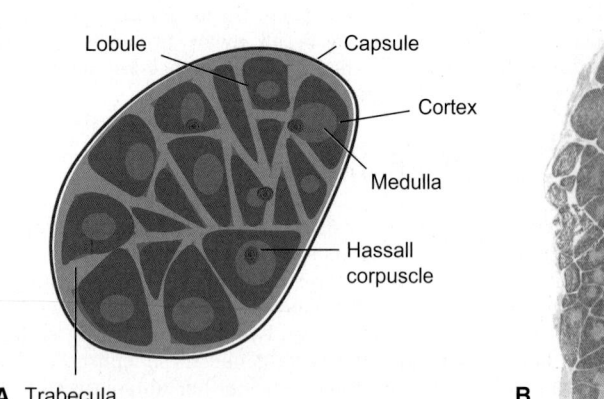
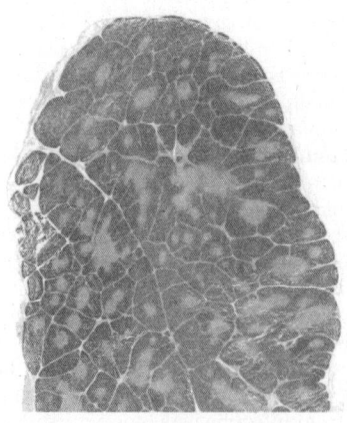
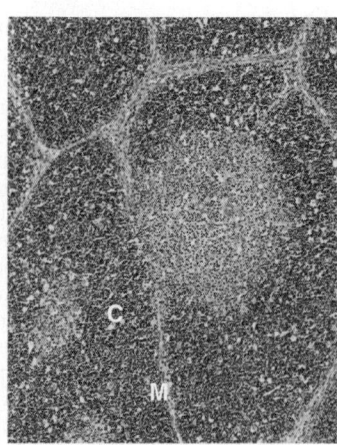

A Trabecula   **B**

FIGURE 2.2. Structure of the thymus. A: Diagram of the thymus showing trabecula emanating from a fibrous capsule that divides the organ into lobules composed of an outer cortex and an inner medulla. The medulla includes Hassall corpuscles formed of concentric layers of epithelial cells. **B:** Light micrographs of thymus sections stained by hematoxylin and eosin. The cortical tissue of thymic lobules appears dark because of numerous proliferating thymocytes interspersed with thymic cortical epithelial cells and macrophages. The medulla contains mature thymocytes, thymic medullary epithelial cells, macrophages, and DCs. C, cortex; M, medulla. Original magnification, ×1 (left micrograph) and ×10 (right micrograph). (Courtesy of Sergi Serrano, M.D., and Laura Comerma, M.D., Institut Hospital del Mar d'Investigacions Mèdiques)

repertoire of MHC-restricted and self-tolerant T cells (56). Thymic function is known to decline with age. After birth, the thymus starts a gradual process of involution or atrophy characterized by the replacement of lymphoid tissue with fat and reduced production of new T cells (57). Nearly 98% of the cells within the thymus are T cells (or thymocytes) at various stages of development (58). The remaining cells constitute the stromal microenvironment, a three-dimensional network mainly composed by thymic epithelial cells as well as DCs, macrophages, and endothelial cells (59). Structurally, the thymus consists of several lobules organized in the inner region or medulla and the outer compartment or cortex (Fig. 2.2). Bone marrow stem cell–derived T-cell precursors enter the thymus via large vessels located at the corticomedullary junction and later migrate to the subcapsular region of the thymic cortex. As developing T cells progress along different maturation stages, they further move through the cortex toward the medulla, and indeed the most mature T cells have medullary topography. Of note, the epithelial cells from the thymic cortex are functionally and phenotypically different from the epithelial cells from the thymic medulla and indeed support different stages of T-cell development (59). In general, T-cell development requires the correct patterning and organization of the thymic stroma, including epithelial cells, and indeed thymocytes need to closely interact with stromal cells throughout their various maturation stages in order to receive appropriate differentiation signals. Thus, it is not surprising that defects in the stromal matrix of the thymus can cause immunodeficiency and/or autoimmunity (58).

Secondary Lymphoid Organs

Lymph Nodes

Lymph nodes are encapsulated bean-shaped structures located at strategic positions along the lymphatic vasculature. Lymph nodes always develop at the same location along large veins and often at sites of blood vessel branching (50). A pivotal role in lymph node development is played by a unique subset of hematopoietic cells derived from fetal liver progenitors, called lymphoid tissue inducer cells (60). These cells interact with stromal organizer cells to produce homeostatic chemokines and express adhesion molecules required for the attraction and retention of additional lymphoid tissue inducer cells as well as

B cells, T cells, and DCs (61). Morphologically, the lymph node is divided in three compartments: the cortex, the paracortex, and the inner medulla (Fig. 2.3). A fibrous capsule and an underlying subcapsular sinus surround the cellular content of the lymph node. The cortex contains densely packed B cells, follicular dendritic cells (FDCs), and macrophages arranged into discrete clusters called primary follicles. Primary follicles are largely composed of naïve B cells that extensively migrate in search of cognate antigen. The interaction of B cells with antigen and T cells generates secondary follicles containing a germinal center that is replete with B cells that actively undergo proliferation, antibody class switching, and affinity maturation (62). The paracortex is located under the cortex and is the site for T-cell interaction with DCs. The medulla consists of medullary cords composed of packed lymphocytes and numerous plasma cells that actively secrete antibodies. Around the cords, medullary sinuses join efferent lymphatic vessels that collect lymphatic fluid from the node. Lymphocytes enter the lymph node by extravasation across high endothelial venules (50). Antigen and DCs enter the lymph node via afferent lymphatic vessels at multiple sites along the capsule. Eventually, filtered lymphatic fluid and immune cells leave the lymph node via a single efferent lymphatic vessel (63).

Spleen

The spleen functions as a blood-filtering system that removes aged erythrocytes, cellular debris, and antigen from the circulation (64). The spleen also plays a major role in the initiation of fast antibody responses against blood-borne pathogens by combining innate and adaptive immune pathways in a highly integrated way. This dual role of the spleen is reflected by its complex architecture. The highly specialized structure of the splenic venous system forms the red pulp and takes part in the removal of aged or defective blood cells and foreign elements from the bloodstream (64). The lymphoid compartment accounts for the white pulp, which consists of two separate compartments: the T-cell zone, also known as the periarteriolar lymphoid sheath (PALS), and the B-cell zone, which includes follicles surrounded by a large MZ (Fig. 2.4). The correct organization of the white pulp requires specific chemokines that attract T and B cells to appropriate lymphoid compartments. In humans, B-cell follicles are not separated from the MZ by marginal sinuses as in rodents, and the MZ can be divided into

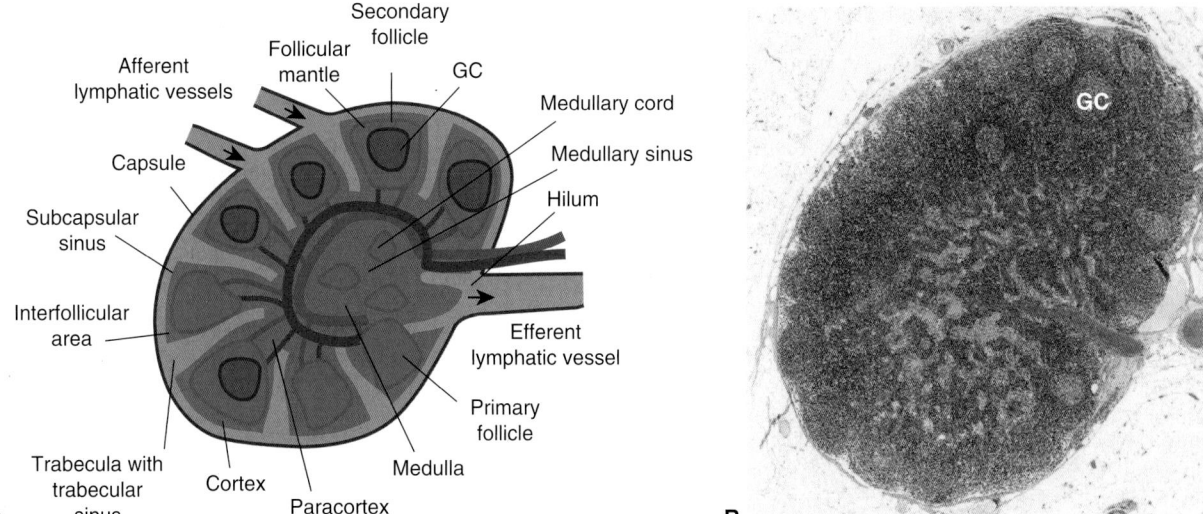

FIGURE 2.3. Structure of lymph nodes. A: Diagram of a lymph node with afferent lymphatic vessels that drain lymph from peripheral tissues into a subcapsular sinus running beneath a fibrous capsule. Trabecula emanating from the capsule contains trabecular (or cortical) sinuses that receive lymph from the subcapsular sinus. Trabecular tissue divides the organ into lobular compartments composed of cortex, paracortex, and medulla. The cortex contains B cells organized into primary follicles with no germinal center and secondary follicles with germinal center. Interfollicular areas separate follicles from each other and contain T cells interacting with DCs. The paracortex predominantly includes T cells and DCs. The medulla contains cords composed of plasma cells, B cells, and macrophages. Medullary cords are separated by vessel-like spaces named medullary sinuses that drain the lymph from cortical sinuses into an efferent lymphatic vessel. The hilum connects the lymph node with the efferent lymphatic vessel and arterial and venous vessels. **B:** Light micrograph of a lymph node section stained with hematoxylin and eosin. The germinal center (GC) contains large antigen-activated B cells and FDCs and therefore stains paler then the follicular mantle, which contains densely packed small naïve B cells. Numerous follicles are visible in the cortex. Original magnification, ×2. (Courtesy of Sergi Serrano, M.D., and Laura Comerma, M.D., Institut Hospital del Mar d'Investigacions Mèdiques)

an inner portion and outer portion, the latter being surrounded by a large perifollicular zone containing sialoadhesin-positive macrophages and neutrophils (65–67). In general, the white pulp is involved in the initiation of adaptive immune responses. In this context, the MZ plays a unique role, because it contains specialized MZ B cells that mount quick antibody responses to highly conserved antigens in the absence of help from T cells. In addition, the MZ is a site transited by B cells as they reach the general circulation (67).

Mucosal Lymphoid Tissue

Mucosal surfaces comprise various lymphoid structures collectively known as MALT (68). This secondary lymphoid organ can be further divided into functionally connected subregions, including the gut-associated lymphoid tissue (GALT), the nasopharynx-associated lymphoid tissue (NALT), and the bronchus-associated lymphoid tissue (BALT). The MALT is functionally divided into inductive sites, where antigens are sampled from the mucosal

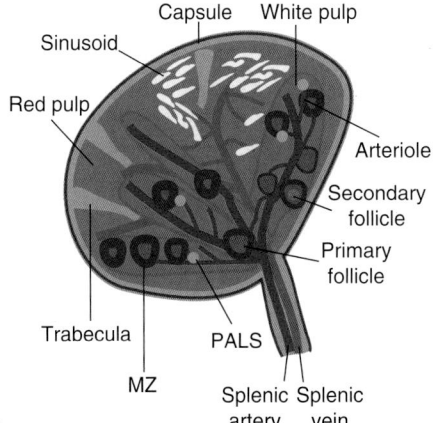
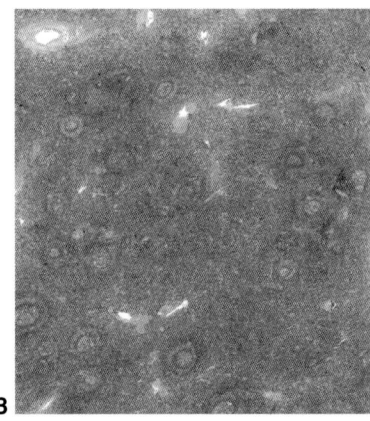
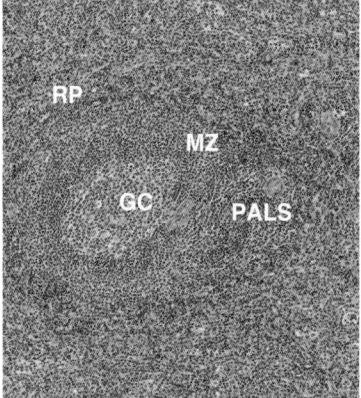

FIGURE 2.4. Structure of the spleen. A: Diagram of the spleen with trabecula that forms lobular compartments after emanating from a fibrous capsule. The splenic artery enters the organ and branches into arterioles that terminate in the red pulp. The white pulp includes lymphoid structures called periarteriolar lymphoid sheath (PALS), which are composed of T cells organized around a central arteriole. The white pulp also includes primary follicles with no germinal center and secondary follicles with a germinal center. Each follicle is surrounded by a large MZ that is in direct contact with the open circulation of the red pulp. Sinusoidal vessels drain blood from the red pulp into the venous system. **B:** Light micrographs of spleen sections stained with hematoxylin and eosin. The red pulp (RP) is filled with erythrocytes from circulating blood, whereas the white pulp contains numerous lymphoid follicles surrounded by a clear MZ area and with or without a germinal center (GC). The MZ contains constitutively activated B cells that are larger than the small naïve B cells lodged in the follicular mantle. Therefore, the MZ stains paler than the follicular mantle. Original magnification, ×2 (**left image**) and ×20 (**right image**). (Courtesy of Sergi Serrano, M.D., and Laura Comerma, M.D., Institut Hospital del Mar d'Investigacions Mèdiques)

surface and presented to naïve T and B cells, and effector sites, where immune cells exert their protective functions, including the release of cytokines and antibodies (13). The latter are predominantly secretory IgA (SIgA) molecules that translocate across epithelial cells through a process known as transcytosis and provide protection against commensal and pathogenic microbes. Although having an overall organization similar to that of systemic lymphoid organs, the MALT lacks efferent lymphatics and contains specialized subsets of DCs that sample antigen directly from the epithelial surface.

The GALT includes the inductive sites of Peyer patches, mesenteric lymph nodes, and isolated lymphoid follicles as well as the effector site of the lamina propria. Peyer patches develop during fetal life independently of gut colonization by bacteria and consist of large structures built on a stromal scaffold composed of several B-cell follicles separated by areas containing T cells and DCs. Usually, there are 30 Peyer patches in the small intestine, and each includes a specialized follicle-associated epithelium provided with unique microfold (M) cells capable of sampling antigen directly from the intestinal lumen. Unlike conventional intestinal epithelial cells, M cells lack microvilli and form large invaginations that contain lymphocytes and DCs. These and other DCs located in the subepithelial dome receive antigen from M cells and then migrate to perifollicular areas to initiate T- and B-cell responses, including IgA production (69). However, gut DCs can also sample antigen directly from the lumen by emanating cellular projections across epithelial cells. In Peyer patches, lymphoid follicles are characterized by an ongoing germinal center reaction that continuously drives IgA diversification and production (70).

Mesenteric lymph nodes range from 100 to 150 in number and lie between the layers of the mesentery. Like Peyer patches, mesenteric lymph nodes include lymphoid follicles with a continuously active germinal center reaction that generates IgA (13). Isolated lymphoid follicles are scattered throughout the intestine and represent another important site for IgA induction. These lymphoid structures consist of solitary B-cell clusters built on a scaffold of stromal cells, with a few interspersed T cells and more abundant perifollicular DCs. Unlike Peyer patches, which develop in the sterile fetal microenvironment, isolated lymphoid follicles develop after postnatal bacterial colonization of the intestine from smaller anlagen structures located at the base of intestinal villi known as cryptopatches. Similar to Peyer patches, isolated lymphoid follicles have a follicular epithelium composed of antigen-sampling M cells as well as a subepithelial area containing DCs. Finally, the intestinal lamina propria contains a nonorganized lymphoid tissue composed of dispersed lymphocytes, DCs, and plasma cells that secrete large amounts of IgA. In addition to serving as an IgA effector site for the containment of commensal bacteria and pathogens, the lamina propria has some IgA inductive function that becomes more evident in immunodeficiencies involving an impairment of the germinal center reaction (71–74).

The NALT consists of a set of lymphoid aggregates known as Waldeyer ring, which occupies strategic areas of the oropharynx and nasopharynx and includes pharyngeal tonsils (or adenoids) as well as tubal, palatine, and lingual tonsils (75). Finally, the BALT is composed of organized lymphoid aggregates located within the bronchial submucosa that mainly develop in response to infection or under chronic inflammatory conditions (76).

INNATE IMMUNE RESPONSES

Microbial Sensing

Vertebrates coexist with an extraordinary dense and diverse community of microorganisms. One of the most challenging tasks of the immune system is the discrimination between self and potential microbial invaders, which is an essential requisite to mount a proper immune response (77). Viruses, bacteria, fungi, and parasites are recognized by the innate immune system through invariant receptors known as PRRs (78). In contrast to somatically recombined antigen receptors such as BCR and TCR, which are highly diversified and recognize individual antigenic determinants with narrow specificity, germline-encoded PRRs have a broad reactivity for a large number of microbial molecules known as pathogen-associated molecular patterns (PAMPs) or microbe-associated molecular patterns (79). These highly conserved structural motifs are essential for microbial survival, which limits the appearance of mutants that could avoid immune recognition (15). The main bacterial and fungal signatures recognized by PRRs are cell wall components such as lipopolysaccharide (LPS), peptidoglycan, lipoteichoic acids, lipoproteins, and β-glucan. In contrast, the predominant viral signatures recognized by PRRs are nucleic acids such as single-strand RNA (ssRNA), double-strand RNA (dsRNA), and nonmethylated deoxyribocytidinephosphateguanosine (CpG) DNA. This is probably because viruses are composed of envelope and/or capsid structures that include molecules originating from the infected cells of the host (2).

Of note, PRRs cannot discriminate PAMPs from invasive pathogens and PAMPs from noninvasive commensals inhabiting our mucosal surfaces. Yet, the immune system attacks pathogens but tolerates commensals (80). It is actually remarkable that the massive microbial ecosystem that colonizes the intestinal mucosa shortly after birth establishes a homeostatic noninflammatory relationship with the immune system of the host (81). Such a relationship is highly mutualistic, because commensals utilize food-derived nutrients generated in the intestinal mucosa for their growth but at the same time help the intestinal mucosa to generate essential vitamins, digest fibers, and strengthen the local immune system. However, the immune system generates inflammatory responses when commensals become pathogenic as a result of changes in the local environment (8).

PRRs are expressed in different cellular compartments that provide individual PRRs with selective accessibility to specific microbial ligands (Fig. 2.5). PRRs with a transmembrane domain are located on the cell surface or in intracellular organelles, whereas PRRs with no transmembrane domain are positioned in the cytoplasm or released in the extracellular environment. PRRs are an essential component of the innate immune system, and their main protective functions include the induction of opsonization, complement activation, phagocytosis, inflammation, and immune cell maturation (82,83). In general, PRRs are mostly expressed by innate immune cells, stromal cells, endothelial cells, and epithelial cells, where they trigger the production of inflammatory tumor necrosis factor (TNF), interleukin (IL)-1β, and IL-6 cytokines that coordinate local and systemic immune responses. Locally, TNF and IL-1β enhance the recruitment of serum proteins and leukocytes by inducing vasodilation, increasing vascular permeability and activating vascular endothelial cells. Systemically, TNF, IL-1β, and IL-6 stimulate hepatocytes to produce acute-phase proteins that consist of soluble PRRs belonging to the pentraxin and collectin families (2).

Transmembrane Pattern Recognition Receptors

Toll-Like Receptors

These PRRs are type-I transmembrane proteins with an extracellular domain that binds PAMPs via a leucin-rich repeat region and an intracellular domain Toll-IL-1 receptor (TIR) domain that mediates downstream signal transduction. Ten Toll-like receptors (TLRs) have been identified so far in humans, both in cells of the innate immune system and in B cells (84). TLRs recognize lipids, lipoproteins, proteins, and nucleic acids derived from viruses, bacteria, fungi, and parasites. TLR1, TLR2, TLR4, TLR5, TLR6, and TLR11 localize on the cell surface, whereas TLR3,

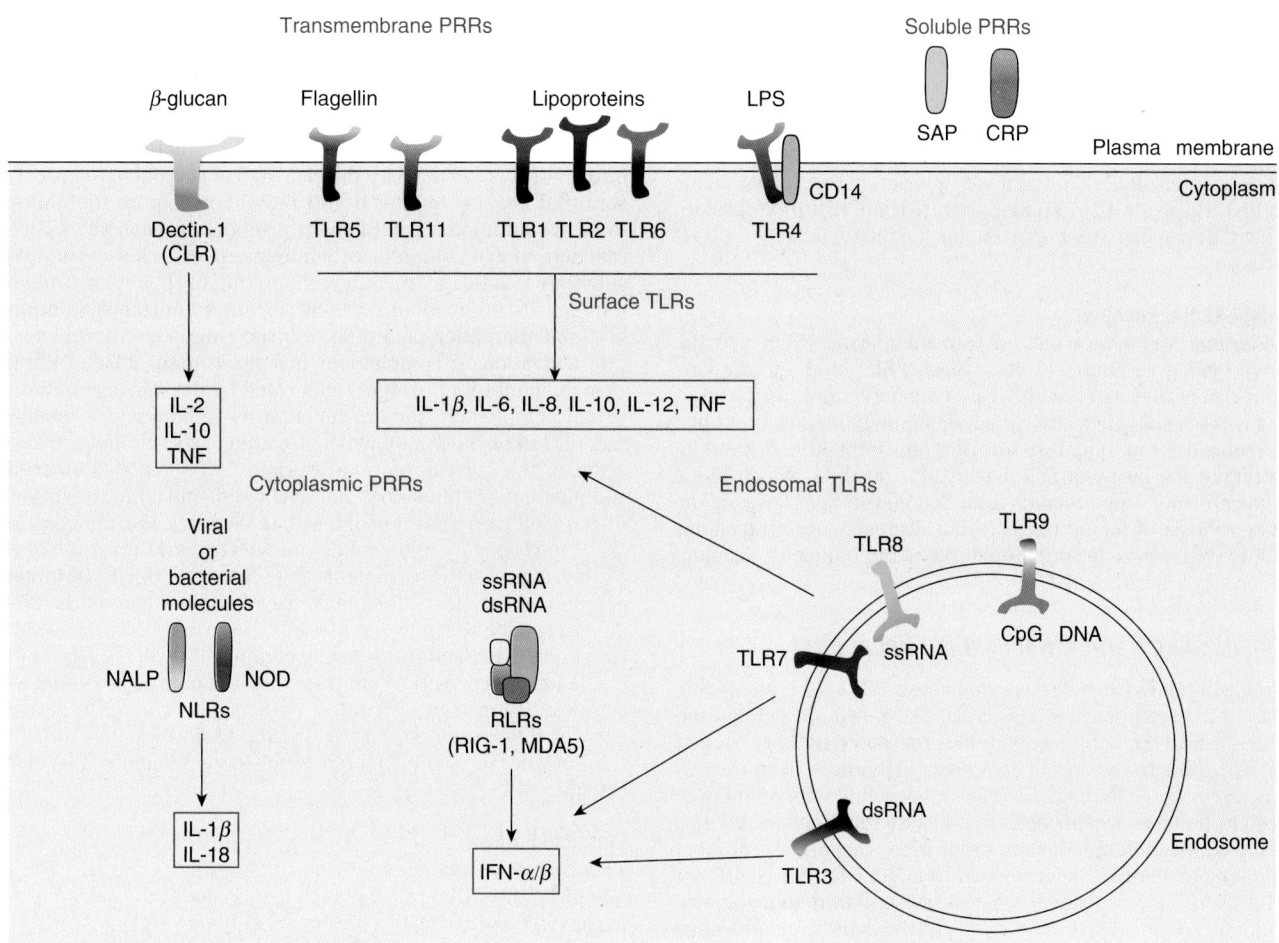

Transmembrane PRRs

Soluble PRRs

FIGURE 2.5. Mechanisms underlying microbial sensing. The immune response begins after the recognition of microbial intruders by PRRs belonging to the innate immune system. PRRs containing a transmembrane domain are positioned on the plasma membrane or in intracellular organelles such as endosomes. These transmembrane PRRs include Toll-like receptors (TLRs, from 1 to 11) and C-type lectin receptors (CLRs), including Dectin-1 and many other molecules. TLR1, TLR2, and TLR6 recognize bacterial lipoproteins, TLR4 and its co-receptor CD14 detect bacterial lipopolysaccharide (LPS), and TLR3 binds viral double-stranded RNA (dsRNA). In addition, TLR7 and TLR8 recognize viral single-stranded RNA (ssRNA), whereas TLR9 senses microbial CpG DNA. After interacting with microbial molecules, TLRs induce inflammatory cytokines such as IL-1β, IL-6, IL-8, IL-12, and TNF as well as anti-inflammatory cytokines such as IL-10. Moreover, TLR3, TLR7, TLR8, and TLR9 elicit the production of antiviral cytokines, including IFN-α and IFN-β (IFN-α/β). CLRs such as Dectin-1 induce the secretion of IL-2, IL-10, and TNF after recognizing β-glucan associated with fungi. PRRs with no transmembrane domain are composed of soluble and cytoplasmic PRRs. Soluble PRRs include serum amyloid P (SAP) and C-reactive protein (CRP), which recognize various carbohydrates associated with microbes. Cytoplasmic PRRs include NOD-like receptors (NLRs) such as NLR3 (or NALP) and NOD (nucleotide oligomerization domain) proteins, which induce the production of inflammatory cytokines such as IL-1β and IL-18 after recognizing various viral and bacterial molecules, including CpG DNA and muramyl dipeptide. Furthermore, cytoplasmic PRRs include retinoic acid–inducible gene 1–like receptors (RLRs) such as RIG-1 and MDA5, which trigger the production of antiviral IFN-α/β after sensing viral ssRNA and dsRNA, respectively.

TLR7, TLR8, and TLR9 localize in intracellular vesicles such as the endoplasmic reticulum, endosomes, lysosomes, and endolysosomes. Accordingly, extracellular TLRs recognize mainly lipids, lipoproteins, and proteins from extracellular microbes, whereas endosomal TLRs recognize nucleic acids. The compartmentalization of these intracellular TLRs prevents innate immune activation by host DNA, which is usually excluded from endolysosomes. This strategy prevents responses that could lead to the development of inflammation and autoimmunity. After recognizing specific cognate ligands, TLRs recruit TIR domain-containing adaptor proteins such as MyD88 and TRIF to initiate downstream signaling events that trigger activation of various transcription factors, including nuclear factor-kappa B (NF-κB). This pathway induces the generation and secretion of inflammatory cytokines (IL-1β, IL-6, IL-12, TNF), antiviral cytokines such as type-I interferons (IFN-α and IFN-β, hereafter referred to as IFN-α/β), chemokines, and antimicrobial peptides. In general, TLR signaling initiates an inflammatory response that

causes recruitment of neutrophils, activation of macrophages, and induction of IFN-stimulated genes that help the killing of intracellular pathogens, including viruses. In addition, TLR signaling promotes the maturation of DCs, which in turn initiate the adaptive immune response by presenting processed antigens to T cells and unprocessed antigens to B cells (85).

Surface TLRs. TLR4 was the first TLR ever identified and forms a receptor complex with MD2 and CD14 molecules to recognize LPS, a component of the outer membrane of Gram-negative bacteria. TLR2 detects lipopeptides, peptidoglycan, and lipoteichoic acid from Gram-positive or Gram-negative bacteria, lipoarabinomannan from mycobacteria, zymosan from fungi, lipoproteins from parasites, and a hemagglutinin protein from measles virus. TLR2 can also form heterodimers with TLR1 or TLR6 to recognize triacylated lipopeptides from Gram-negative bacteria or diacylated lipopeptides from Gram-positive bacteria. Finally, TLR5 recognizes flagellin, a monomeric protein that makes up the flagellum of bacteria. The function of TLR10 remains unclear.

Endosomal TLRs. TLR3 recognizes viral dsRNA, whereas TLR7 and TLR8 detect viral ssRNA, and TLR9 binds CpG DNA associated with viruses and bacteria. In addition to inducing NF-κB, endosomal TLRs activate interferon regulatory factor (IRF)-1, IRF-3, or IRF-7 and induce IFN-α and IFN-β expression, which are particularly important for the innate defense against viruses.

C-Type Lectin Receptors
Additional well-characterized transmembrane PRRs are the C-type lectin receptors (CLRs). These PRRs bind specific carbohydrates associated with viruses, bacteria, and fungi and in some cases activate intracellular signaling pathways that elicit microbicidal, inflammatory, and immunostimulating responses. Arguably, the best-characterized CLR is dectin-1, which binds β-glucan from fungi. Signals from dectin-1 not only trigger the phagocytosis of fungal particles but also activate intracellular killing via oxygen-dependent pathways and induce DC production of IL-2, IL-10, and TNF (86).

Cytoplasmic Pattern Recognition Receptors

Similar to endosomal TLRs, cytoplasmic PRRs such as nucleotide oligomerization domain (NOD)-like receptors (NLRs) and retinoic acid–inducible gene 1–like receptors (RLRs) function as intracellular sensors of molecular signatures from viruses and bacteria. NLRs include about 20 proteins with a common protein domain organization but diverse functions (87). NLRs of the NLRC subfamily (where C stands for caspase recruitment domain, or CARD) include NOD1 (or NLRC1) and NOD2 (or NLRC2) receptors, which recognize meso-diaminopimelic acid from the peptidoglycan of Gram-negative bacteria and muramyl dipeptide from both Gram-negative and Gram-positive bacteria through a leucin-rich repeat region. NLRs of the NLRP subfamily (where P stands for pyrin domain) include NALP3 (or NLR3), which interacts with the intracellular adaptor protein ASC and caspase-1 to form an intracellular signaling platform known as inflammasome. NLRs recognize various bacterial, viral, and danger molecules, including muramyl dipeptide, nonmethylated CpG DNA, dsRNA, and uric acid (88). NLRP proteins trigger the formation of inflammatory IL-1β and IL-18 cytokines from inactive intracellular pre-proteins that are cleaved via caspase-1 or caspase-5. Finally, RLRs include RIG-I and MDA5, which detect viral ssRNA containing 5′ triphosphate and viral dsRNA, respectively. These viral sensors activate NF-κB- and IRF-dependent signaling pathways that induce the expression of antiviral cytokines such as IFN-α/β and IFN-γ (89).

Soluble Pattern Recognition Receptors

Soluble PRRs are composed of different families of proteins, including collectins, ficolins, and pentraxins. The acute-phase proteins C-reactive protein (CRP) and serum amyloid P (SAP) belong to the pentraxin family and recognize a variety of microbes in the fluid phase (90). CRP binds phosphorylcholine (PC), a major constituent of C-type capsule polysaccharides from Pneumococcus. In addition, CRP binds many other pathogens, including fungi and yeast. SAP recognizes LPS, PC, and terminal mannose or galactose residues and therefore interacts with a wide range of bacteria and even viruses. Microbe-bound CRP and SAP proteins function as innate opsonins (as opposed to adaptive opsonins or antibodies) that enhance phagocytosis by interacting with FcγRs expressed on the surface of monocytes, macrophages, and neutrophils. In addition, CRP and SAP proteins contribute to the activation of all the major complement pathways.

Complement

The complement system consists of more than 30 proteins located in the circulation and on cell surfaces (91,92). These proteins are organized in hierarchical proteolytic cascades that initiate with the recognition of microbial surfaces. This initial event is followed by the cleavage of complement precursors that become activated and thereafter acquire the ability to cleave additional complement proteins. In each successive reaction, active complement components can cleave multiple substrates. In this manner, a reaction initially involving a small number of complement proteins becomes enormously amplified and thereafter generates a large complement response. The activation of complement has three main effects. First, many peptides and proteins generated by the cleavage of individual complement factors function as inflammatory mediators (or anaphylatoxins), which are able to recruit and activate cells of the innate immune system (93). Second, cleaved complement proteins coat the surface of intruding microbes to function as innate opsonins that facilitate the phagocytosis of microbes by neutrophils, monocytes, and macrophages expressing specific complement receptors. Third, terminal components of the complement cascade induce lysis of the targeted microbe through the assembly of a pore-forming structure known as membrane attack complex (MAC). Complement activation proceeds through three distinct pathways known as classical, lectin, and alternative pathways (Fig. 2.6). Although each of these pathways differs in the molecules that initiate the cascade, they all converge to the same effector molecules (94,95).

Classical Pathway
This pathway initiates following the binding of the C1q component of the C1 complex (which also includes the serine proteases C1r and C1s) to clusters of antibody (IgM or IgG) or pentraxin molecules complexed with antigen. However, C1q can also directly recognize distinct structures on microbial and apoptotic cells, independently of opsonins. C1q has six globular heads held together by a collagen-like tail. Binding of more than one globular head leads to a conformational change that permits C1q to activate C1r. This latter cleaves C1s to generate an active serine protease that cleaves C4 into a smaller C4a fragment and a larger C4b fragment. Covalent attachment of C4b to the microbial surface promotes the recruitment of C2 and its cleavage into C2a and C2b fragments by C1s. The serine protease C2a associates with C4b and remains attached to microbial surfaces to form the *classical C3 convertase*. Of note, the generation of C3 convertase constitutes the point of convergence of all complement activation pathways. C3 convertase cleaves C3 into the anaphylatoxin C3a and the opsonin C3b. While C3b undergoes rapid deposition on the surface of the microbe, C3a initiates a local inflammatory response by inducing chemotactic recruitment of neutrophils, monocytes, and macrophages. C3b also binds C3 convertase to form the *C5 convertase*, which cleaves C5 to generate C5a and C5b fragments. While C5a serves as an additional anaphylatoxin with powerful inflammatory activity, C5b induces assembly of the C6, C7, C8, and C9 fractions. The resulting terminal MAC generates a pore in the membrane of the microbe, ultimately leading to its death.

Lectin Pathway
This pathway requires mannose-binding lectin (MBL) and ficolins, which recognize carbohydrates associated with microbes. Similar to C1q, MBL has six sugar-binding heads that form a complex with MBL-associated serine protease-1 (MASP-1) and MASP-2, two proteases homologous to C1r and C1s, respectively. Activated MASP-1 and MASP-2 cleave C4 and C2 to generate the classical C3 convertase (C2bC4b).

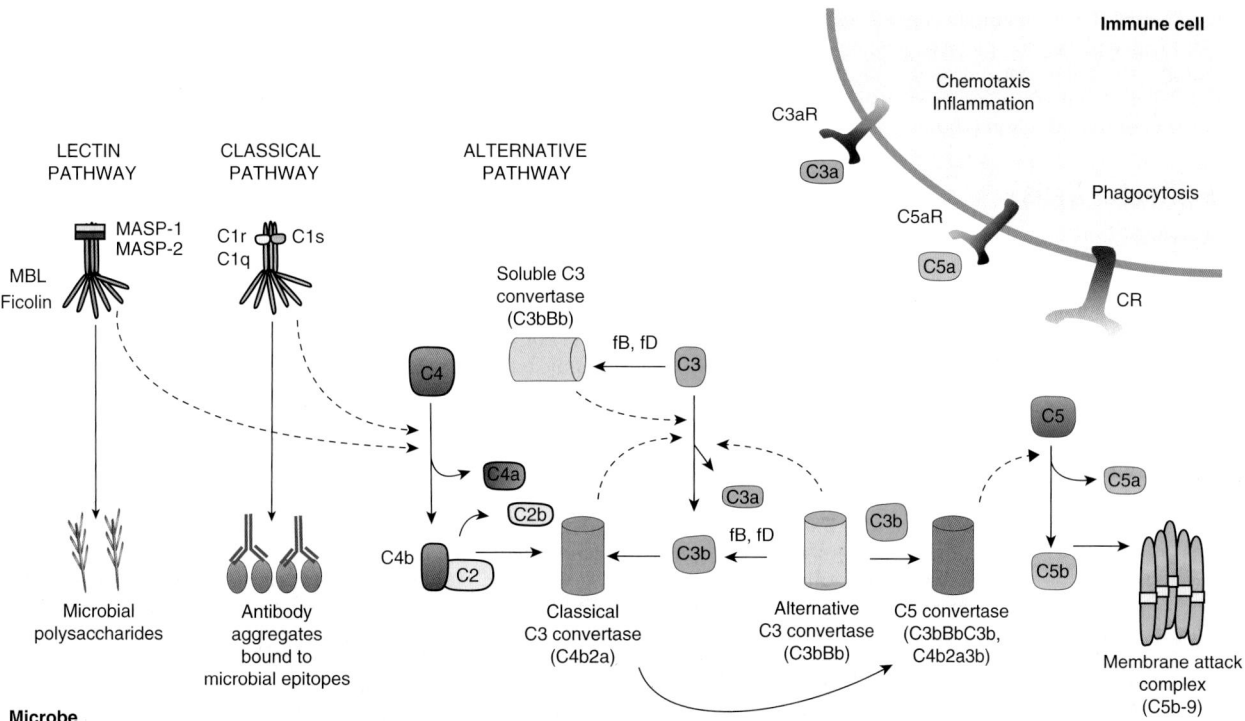

FIGURE 2.6. Complement pathways. In the classical pathway, interaction of C1q with IgM or IgG antibodies aggregated on microbial surfaces leads to the sequential activation of C1r and C1s. This latter cleaves C4 into C4a and C4b fragments and C2 into C2a and C2b fragments. The C4 and Cb2a fragments interact to form the classical C3 convertase. In the lectin pathway, classical C3 convertase is induced after interaction of mannan-binding lectin (MBL) or ficolin with polysaccharides on microbial surfaces. The ensuing activation of MBL-associated serine protease-1 (MASP-1) and MASP-2 leads to the cleavage of C4 and C2. In the alternative pathway, spontaneous hydrolysis of C3 is followed by interaction of C3 with factor B (fB) and factor D (fD), which leads to the formation of a C3bBb complex known as soluble C3 convertase. This enzyme cleaves C3 to generate C3a and C3b. Deposition of C3b on microbial surfaces mediates microbial opsonization and phagocytosis through the interaction of C3b with complement receptor 1 (CR1) on innate immune cells, including phagocytes. In addition, the interaction of microbe-bound C3b with fB, fD, and properdin (P) generates an alternative convertase that cleaves more C3 through an amplification pathway. Interaction of C3b with classical and alternative C3 convertase causes the assembly of C4bC2aC3b and C3bBbC3b complexes known as C5 convertase. This enzyme cleaves C5 into C5a and C5b fragments. Soluble C5a and C3a fragments function as anaphylotoxins that induce proinflammatory and chemotactic responses by binding to cognate receptors (C5aR and C3aR, respectively) on innate immune cells. In addition, microbe-bound C5b interacts with C6, C7, C8, and C9 to form a pore-forming C5b-C9 membrane attack complex (MAC) that causes osmotic lysis of the microbe. *Dashed arrows* indicate protein interactions causing protein cleavage, whereas *solid arrows* indicate protein assembly.

Alternative Pathway

This pathway involves a slow and continuous turnover of C3 to form C3b and C3a. While both classical and lectin pathways depend on the recognition of a pathogen by C1q or MBL, the alternative pathway is initiated by the spontaneous hydrolysis of C3. Although C3 is relatively inert in its native form, a small fraction of C3 is constantly hydrolyzed, exposing new binding sites. Hydrolyzed C3 (C3H$_2$O) binds to factor B (fB), which renders fB susceptible to cleavage by factor D (fD). The resulting *soluble C3 convertase* cleaves C3 into its active fragments C3a and C3b. After covalently binding microbial surfaces, some C3b interacts with fB, which allows its cleavage by fD. This process leads to the assembly of the *alternative C3 convertase*. Importantly, the alternative pathway can be amplified by any membrane-bound C3 convertase, regardless of its origin. Consequently, the alternative pathway usually accounts for up to 80% to 90% of total complement activation, even when this activation is initially triggered through a classical or lectin pathway.

Complement Regulation

Given its destructive nature, the complement pathway needs to be tightly regulated and confined to appropriate pathogenic surfaces to prevent damage to bystander healthy tissues (96). Both plasma and cell membranes contain complement regulator proteins that either prevent the assembly of the convertase complex or promote its dissociation. C1 esterase inhibitor (C1-INH) is a soluble regulator that inhibits several proteases of both classical and lectin complement pathways. In contrast, factor H (fH) is a soluble regulator of the alternative complement pathway. This protein interacts with C3b to competitively remove Bb from the alternative C3bBb convertase in a process known as decay acceleration. In addition, fH serves as a cofactor for the degradation of C3b to its inactive derivate iC3b by a factor I (fI) protein also known as C3b/C4b inactivator. Additional convertase regulators are expressed on the surface of healthy cells and include complement regulator 1 (CR1) and decay accelerating factor (DAF or CD55), which competitively remove Bb from C3bBb as fH does. Additional regulator proteins interfere with the formation of the MAC.

In addition to inducing effector innate immune responses, complement contributes to the resolution of inflammation by promoting the clearance of immune complexes and dying cells (97). In this regard, C1q binds to apoptotic cells and thereby tags them for elimination by resident macrophages. An insufficiency of this process resulting from deleterious C1q gene mutations predisposes to autoimmunity (98). Remarkably, complement is also involved in adaptive immune responses. Indeed, complement proteins associated with opsonized microbes interact with complement receptors on the surface of antigen-activated B cells to amplify signals emanating from the BCR (99). Furthermore, complement proteins trap and retain antigen on the surface of FDCs located in the germinal center of lymphoid follicles, which is a major inductive site for antibody diversification and production (100).

Innate Effector Cells

Granulocytes

Granulocytes are the largest population of leukocytes in the circulation and derive their name from the large number of dense granules present in their cytoplasm (101). Granulocytes are also called polymorphonuclear leukocytes because of the varying shapes of their indented nucleus and are composed of neutrophils, eosinophils, and basophils, which can be distinguished on the basis of the morphology of their nucleus and staining properties of their granules (102). Neutrophils constitute 50% to 60% of circulating leukocytes, whereas eosinophils and basophils account for 1% to 6% and 0.01% to 0.3% of circulating leukocytes, respectively. Each subset of granulocytes emerges from a CMP in the bone marrow, which sequentially gives rise to myeloblasts and subset-specific forms of promyelocytes, myelocytes, metamyelocytes, and band cells through a maturation process that requires multiple growth factors. Granulocyte colony-stimulating factor (G-CSF), granulocyte-macrophage colony-stimulating factor (GM-CSF), and IL-3 are required for the development of all granulocyte subsets, whereas eosinophils also need IL-5 (17,103). The number of granulocytes that

exit the bone marrow to enter the circulation greatly increases in response to inflammation. This process also stimulates the migration of circulating granulocytes into inflamed tissues through extravasation (16). After penetrating infected, inflamed, or injured tissues, granulocytes undergo degranulation and phagocytosis, two innate defensive mechanisms that promote inflammation, clearance, and digestion of foreign or necrotic material, and extracellular or intracellular killing of microbes and parasites (17,104). In addition to playing a central role in innate immunity, granulocytes regulate adaptive immunity, including cellular and humoral immune responses (14).

Extravasation

Granulocyte migration to inflamed tissues involves an initial phase of *chemoattraction* that is mediated by microbial attracting factors such as fMLP and by endothelial and macrophage attracting factors such as chemokines (CXCL1, CXCL3, CXCL5, CXCL8), complement proteins (C5a), and leukotriene B4 (16,17). The initial interaction of granulocytes with vascular endothelial cells constitutes the *rolling adhesion* (or *capture*) phase of leukocyte trafficking and is mediated by a low-affinity interaction of sialyl-Lewisx on granulocytes with E-selectins (CD62E) and P-selectins (CD62P) on endothelial cells lining blood vessels (Fig. 2.7). Microbial products such as LPS and inflammatory cytokines such as IL-1β, TNF, and CXCL8 (IL-8) from macrophages up-regulate endothelial expression of E-selectins and P-selectins, thereby inducing the slowing down of granulocytes and their brief adhesion to the endothelium of small blood vessels (17,105). During this rolling motion,

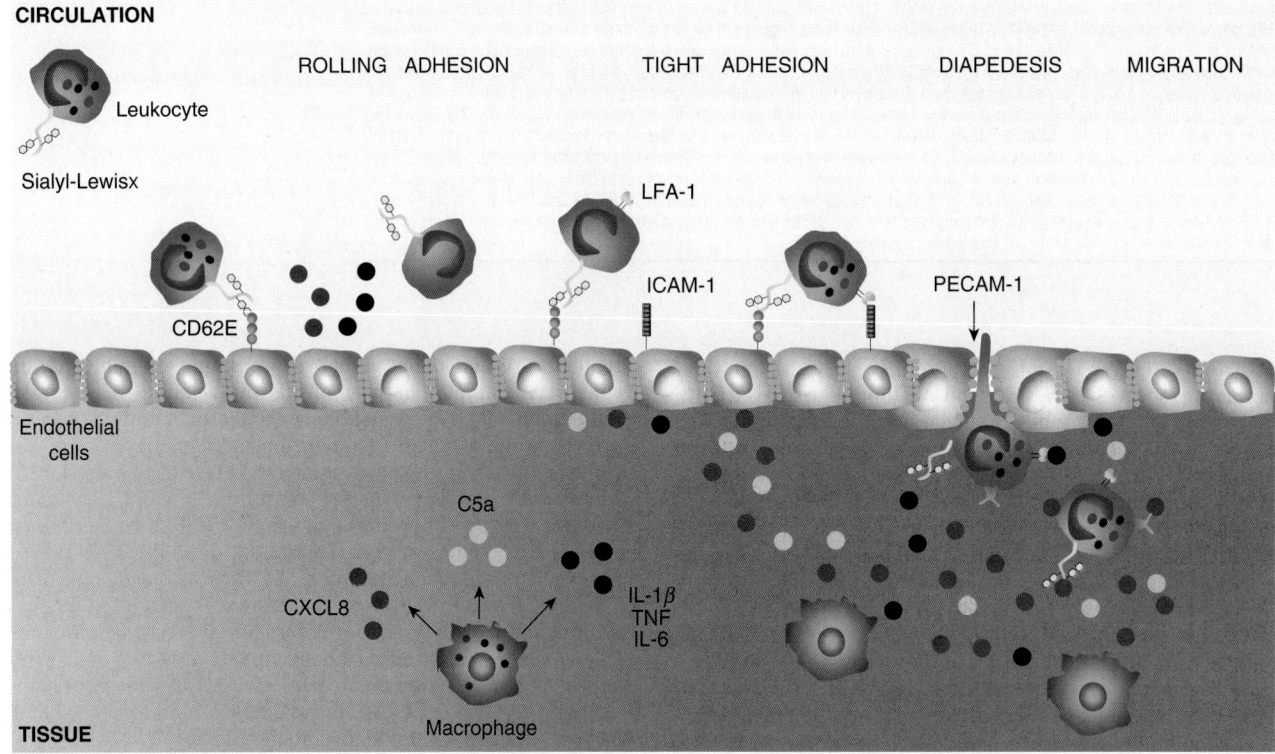

FIGURE 2.7. Extravasation of leukocytes. In infected or inflamed tissues, endothelial cells, macrophages, and other resident cells release chemoattracting factors such as CXCL8 and C5a, which recruit circulating leukocytes expressing sialyl-Lewis^x. In the *rolling adhesion* phase of extravasation, a reversible low-affinity interaction of sialyl-Lewis^x with CD62E (E-selectin) on endothelial cells slows down the motion of the circulating leukocyte. In addition to chemotactic factors, tissue cells release inflammatory cytokines such as IL-1β, TNF, and IL-6, which cooperate with microbial products to induce the activation of local leukocytes and endothelial cells. Activated endothelial cells up-regulate the expression of integrin complexes such as leukocyte functional adhesion-1 (LFA-1), whereas activated endothelial cells up-regulate the expression of intercellular adhesion molecule (ICAMs) such as ICAM-1. In the *tight adhesion* phase of extravasation, a high-affinity interaction between integrins and ICAM-1 causes the arrest of the rolling leukocyte, allowing its subsequent *diapedesis* across endothelial cells through a mechanism involving homotypic binding of platelet-endothelial cell adhesion molecule-1 (PECAM-1) molecules that are expressed on both leukocytes and endothelial cells. Chemoattractants and proteases (not shown) induce the final *migration* of the leukocyte into the tissue.

transitory bonds are formed and broken between selectins and their ligands. At the same time, IL-1β, TNF, CXCL8, and other chemokines up-regulate the expression of three distinct surface integrin complexes on rolling leukocytes (106). These complexes are composed of a common $\beta2$ chain (CD18) and an α chain corresponding to CD11a (leukocyte functional adhesion-1 [LFA-1] complex), CD11b (MAC-1 complex), or CD11c. The up-regulation of integrin expression switches granulocytes from a default low-affinity binding state to a high-affinity binding state, which characterizes the *tight adhesion* (or *tethering*) phase. In this phase, integrins bind intercellular adhesion molecule (ICAM) receptors called CD54 (ICAM-1) and CD102 (ICAM-2) on endothelial cells with high affinity, which causes the immobilization of granulocytes despite the shear forces of the ongoing blood flow. Binding of the integrin $\alpha4$ chain (CD49d)-$\beta1$ chain (CD29) complex on activated granulocytes to VCAM-1 (CD106) on activated endothelial cells further enhances the tethering phase of granulocyte transmigration (17). The final entry of granulocytes into the tissue involves a *diapedesis* (or *transmigration*) phase that requires the homotypic interaction of CD31 (or PECAM-1) on neutrophils with CD31 on endothelial cells. The subsequent penetration of granulocytes into the inflamed tissue also involves the opening of interendothelial junctions and the release of proteases to digest the basement membrane that separates the blood vessel from the extravascular space. Throughout each extravasation phase, granulocytes undergo locomotion, contraction, and pseudopod extension by reorganizing a broad array of cytoskeletal proteins, including actin, myosin, and gelsolin.

Respiratory Burst

After activation by microbial products, cytokines, or opsonins, neutrophils but also monocytes and macrophages increase their oxygen consumption to undergo a respiratory burst that generates toxic oxygen metabolites such as hydrogen peroxide and superoxide (107). The enzyme responsible for superoxide generation is the membrane-associated electron transport complex NADPH oxidase, which catalyzes the transfer of electrons from NADPH to oxygen in mitochondria (108). After the generation of hydrogen peroxide from superoxides and water by the enzyme superoxide dismutase, the enzyme myeloperoxidase produces hypochlorous acid, a potent oxidant that destroys amino acids, amines, thiols, thioesters, nucleotides, and other organic components of phagocytosed materials. Hypochlorous acid is the neutrophil component responsible for the greenish color and characteristic odor that occur when large numbers of neutrophils are present in microbial abscesses.

Neutrophils

The name neutrophil derives from staining characteristics on hematoxylin and eosin–stained histologic or cytologic preparations. Whereas basophils stain dark blue and eosinophils stain bright red, neutrophils stain a neutral pink (101). Circulating neutrophils include mature cells that contain a segmented nucleus divided into two to five lobes and immature cells (or band cells) that have a banded nucleus. Dense cytoplasmic granules are the hallmark of neutrophils and include primary (or azurophilic) granules containing myeloperoxydase, elastase, bactericidal and permeability-increasing protein, defensins, and cathepsin G; secondary (or specific) granules containing cationic proteins, lactoferrin, and cathelicidin; and tertiary granules containing gelatinase (17). In general, primary granules are more important for the digestion of phagocytosed material, whereas secondary and tertiary granules are more important for the induction of killing and the initiation of inflammation and immunity (101). Circulating neutrophils typically express CD15 (an adhesion molecule) and CD16 (FcγRIII, an IgG receptor), but little or no CD14 (a co-receptor for LPS). Neutrophils also express CD10 (neprylisin or neutral

endopeptidase), CD11b (integrin), CD13 (aminopeptidase N), CD16 (FcγRIII), CD32 (FcγRII), CD33 (adhesion molecule), CD64 (FcγRI), and CD89 (FcαRI) (103).

In the circulation, neutrophils have an average life span of about 5 to 6 days. These granulocytes are rapidly mobilized from the bone marrow and migrate from the circulation to sites of infection, injury, or inflammation as a first line of innate immune defense to eliminate microbes and necrotic cells (104). Neutrophil transmigration into tissues is a hallmark of acute inflammation and is regulated by complex signaling pathways emanating from microbial sensors as well as chemokine and cytokine receptors (103). In inflamed tissues, neutrophils survive for 1 or 2 days to exert their phagocytic and killing functions and then undergo apoptosis to be cleared by tissue macrophages. Phagocytosis is facilitated by signals from microbial PRRs and opsonin receptors, including complement receptors and IgG o IgA antibody receptors such as FcγRI, FcγRII, FcγRIII, and FcαRI molecules. The resulting phagosome undergoes fusion with a lysosome to allow the degradation of ingested material (108). Killing of microbes mostly occurs through an intracellular oxygen-dependent pathway that follows phagocytosis and involves the production of reactive oxygen species (ROS) through the enzyme nicotinamide adenine dinucleotide phosphate-oxidase (NADPH). A less efficient extracellular oxygen-independent pathway follows degranulation and involves the discharge of proteolytic enzymes and antimicrobial factors contained in granules, including proteases, lysozyme, defensins, cathelicidin (or LL-37), cationic proteins, and lactoferrin (107). In addition to undergoing degranulation, neutrophils form neutrophil extracellular traps, which are cellular projections capable of trapping and killing bacteria. These structures originate from an apoptotic process called NETosis and contain decondensed chromatin embedded with cytoplasmic and granular proteins with antimicrobial function, including proteases and cathelicidin (17,103,109).

In spite of having a brief half-life and lacking proliferative potential, neutrophils can synthesize and release chemokines (CCL3, CXCL8, CXCL12), inflammatory cytokines (IL-1β, IL-6, IL-8, TNF, vascular endothelial growth factor [VEGF]), and a heterogeneous set of mediators known as alarmins, which help the recruitment, activation, and differentiation of monocytes and DCs (103). While monocyte-derived macrophages complete the clearance of invading microbes and dead cells during the innate phase of the immune response, DCs initiate more specific adaptive immune responses by presenting processed antigens to T cells in draining lymph nodes. Neutrophils can also establish a direct crosstalk with DCs, NK cells, T cells, and B cells (103). In particular, neutrophils regulate both innate and adaptive arms of the immune response by releasing the anti-inflammatory cytokine IL-10 (110), which inhibits the activation of monocytes, macrophages, granulocytes, NK cells, DCs, and T cells. Furthermore, neutrophils enhance the humoral component of the adaptive immune response by releasing B-cell–activating factor of the TNF family (BAFF or BLyS) and its homologue proliferation-inducing ligand (APRIL), two powerful antibody-inducing factors of the TNF family that stimulate B cells (103,111,112).

Eosinophils

This granulocyte subset has bilobed nuclei and granules containing arginine-rich basic proteins that bind the acidic eosin stain with high affinity, which results in a red appearance. Granular proteins such as major basic protein, eosinophil peroxidase, eosinophil cationic protein, and eosinophil-derived neurotoxin exert cytotoxic activity on both parasites and host tissues upon their release by degranulation (113). Eosinophils also contain ribonuclease, deoxyribonucleases, collagenase, lipase, leukotrienes, and platelet-activating factor and show a surface phenotype characterized by the expression of CD16,

CD23 (FcεRII, a low-affinity IgE receptor), FcεRI (high-affinity IgE receptor), and CCR3 (eotaxin receptor), but not CD14 (114).

Eosinophils circulate in the blood for 8 to 12 hours, but are likely to survive for more extended periods in the thymus, intestine, ovary, uterus, bone marrow, spleen, and lymph nodes. The fact that these organs contain variable numbers of eosinophils in healthy individuals suggests that eosinophils play some important immunoregulatory role under homeostatic conditions (26). Consistent with this possibility, tissue-based eosinophils express MHC-II, CD80, and CD86 molecules involved in antigen presentation and release inflammatory and immunoregulatory cytokines such as IL-4, IL-6, IL-10, and IL-12 (114). Eotaxin-1 from epithelial cells regulates the migration of eosinophils to the intestinal lamina propria, suggesting that eosinophils serve a unique role in mucosal immunity (26). In healthy individuals, eosinophils also promote the long-term survival of plasma cells in the bone marrow through a mechanism involving the release of the cytokines APRIL and IL-6 (115). However, eosinophils are better known for their important role in cytotoxic responses against multicellular parasites such as helminths.

Eosinophils migrate to tissues affected by helminth infection in response to eotaxin-1 (CCL11) and eotaxin-2 (CCL24), two relatively broadly expressed chemokines that bind the eotaxin receptor CCR3 on eosinophils. IL-4, IL-5, and IL-13 from T$_H$2 cells and IL-3 and GM-CSF from T cells and myeloid cells further enhance the migration, activation, and differentiation of eosinophils at sites of infection (26,116). Eosinophils undergo degranulation after recognizing IgE antibodies bound to the surface of parasites. The resulting discharge of cytotoxic mediators allows the extracellular killing of parasites or their expulsion from the lumen of mucosal organs. By this mechanism, eosinophils remove pathogens that are too large to be engulfed by macrophages. Remarkably, IgE production involves B cells stimulated by T$_H$2 cells via IL-4 and eosinophils may further enhance this process by releasing their own IL-4 (117). Similar chemokines and cytokines promote the migration and activation of eosinophils in allergic disorders, which involves the abnormal production of IgE to environmental antigens known as allergens (26,116).

Basophils

This granulocyte subset usually has bilobed nuclei and large cytoplasmic granules containing heparin and other sulfated and carboxylated acidic proteins that bind the basic hematoxylin stain with high affinity, which results in a blue appearance (118). For decades, basophils have remained an enigmatic cell type due to the lack of proper markers for their identification and their short life span, which is estimated to be in the range of 1 to 2 days (119). It is now known that basophils express FcεRI, CD11b, and CD123 (IL-3R), but lack CD117 (or c-Kit), a molecule typically expressed by mast cells. Of note, mast cells are morphologically, phenotypically and functionally similar to basophils, but originate from a distinct precursor in the bone marrow under the influence of IL-3 (118). This cytokine also promotes the migration of basophils to sites of infection or inflammation and enhances the activation and maturation of basophils at these sites (120). Similar to eosinophils and mast cells, basophils play an important role in parasitic infections and allergies. Indeed, basophils bind IgE through FcεRI. Cross-linking of pre-bound IgE by parasitic antigens or allergens induces basophil degranulation, which leads to the release of powerful vasodilators like histamine (118). Activated basophils also express molecules involved in antigen presentation such as MHC-II, CD80 (B7-1), and CD86 (B7.2), and release inflammatory cytokines such as IL-6 and TNF, T$_H$2-inducing cytokines such as IL-4 and IL-10, and B-cell–stimulating cytokines such as BAFF (121). Activated basophils also express CD40 ligand, a membrane-bound B-cell–stimulating factor of the TNF family

structurally related to BAFF and APRIL. In addition to IgE, basophils bind IgD through an unknown receptor (122). IgD is secreted by plasmablasts from the upper respiratory mucosa, binds to respiratory microbes, and triggers basophil expression and secretion of antimicrobial, inflammatory, and antibody-inducing factors, including IL-1β, IL-4, IL-13, TNF, and BAFF (123). Thus, basophils may regulate the immune response to multiple types of antigens.

Monocytes and Macrophages
Monocytes

Monocytes derive from a common myeloid precursor in the bone marrow. This hematopoietic progenitor sequentially gives rise to myeloblasts, monoblasts, promonocytes, and monocytes through a maturation process that requires the growth factors M-CSF, GM-CSF, and IL-3 and takes place over the course of approximately 6 days (124,125). After leaving the bone marrow, monocytes enter the circulation to patrol the bloodstream for up to 3 days. In the presence of infection or inflammation, monocytes rapidly migrate to peripheral tissues through extravasation (126). Similar to granulocytes and other circulating leukocytes, monocytes extravasate in response to chemotactic factors and inflammatory cytokines released by infected or damaged tissues. As they adhere to and migrate through endothelial cells, monocytes initiate a series of changes that induce their differentiation into either macrophages or DCs (127). Macrophages are specialized in phagocytosis, digestion, and killing, whereas DCs are specialized in antigen presentation and immune activation (128). Remarkably, about half of monocytes accumulate in the red pulp of the spleen under homeostatic conditions instead of patrolling the circulation (128). These monocytes do not undergo macrophage or DC differentiation, but rather form a large reservoir of macrophage and DC precursors ready for deployment in case of infection or inflammation.

Circulating monocytes show morphologic heterogeneity and indeed include three phenotypically distinct subsets (20). Classical monocytes express high levels of CD14 but no CD16; intermediate monocytes express high levels of CD14 and low levels of CD16 and may develop from classical monocytes; and nonclassical monocytes express low levels of CD14 together with high levels of CD16 and may represent a more mature subset deriving from intermediate monocytes. Regardless of their maturation stage, monocytes also express low levels of CD4, CD11b, CD13, CD32, CD33, CD40, CD64, CD115 (M-CSFR), and the chemokine receptor CX3CR1 (20,129,130).

Monocytes are a central component of the innate immune system in that they can sense the presence of microbial molecules through a large array of PRRs and scavenger receptors (19). After stimulation by microbial products such as LPS or inflammatory cytokines such as type-II IFN (commonly known as IFN-γ) and TNF, monocytes promote the initial containment of intruding microbes by actively engulfing them through a process known as phagocytosis (131). While mediating phagocytosis, monocytes enhance their intracellular killing activity by undergoing a respiratory burst that results in the production of cytotoxic ROS. In addition, activated monocytes produce a plethora of mediators that activate both innate and adaptive arms of the immune system. Such mediators include inflammatory cytokines (IL-1β, IL-6, IL-12, TNF, and CXCL8), anti-inflammatory cytokines (IL-10), angiogenic factors (VEGF), proteases, complement fractions, and prostaglandins (131,132). Of note, intermediate monocytes have more pronounced phagocytic activity and produce more IL-1β and TNF in response to LPS (129), whereas nonclassical monocytes have poor phagocytic activity but produce more IL-12 (19).

Macrophages

Macrophages originate from the differentiation of monocytes in tissues and, together with neutrophils, constitute the most efficient population of phagocytes in our immune system (128). Similar to neutrophils, macrophages phagocytose foreign material, cellular debris, apoptotic cells, necrotic cells, tumoral cells, and intruding microbes as either stationary or mobile cells. However, while neutrophils play a dominant role at an early stage of infection or inflammation, macrophages become more important in later stages (20). Furthermore, while neutrophils survive in tissues for a few hours, macrophages can survive for up to several months. In addition to mediating phagocytosis, intracellular killing, and other key innate immune functions, macrophages activate the adaptive immune system by presenting processed or native antigens to T and B cells, respectively. However, it must be noted that macrophages are way less efficient antigen-presenting cells (APCs) than DCs. In general, macrophages express CD68 (a receptor for low-density lipoprotein) together with CD4, CD11b, CD11c, CD13, CD14, CD32, CD33, CD40, CD64, CD161, CD163 (scavanger receptor), and CD169 (a lectin highly expressed by MZ macrophages).

Similar to DCs, macrophages include different subsets that can be distinguished on the basis of their specific anatomical location. Thus, one can recognize histiocytes (interstitial connective tissue), alveolar macrophages (lung), peritoneal macrophages (peritoneum), osteoclasts (bone), microglia (brain), subcapsular macrophages (lymph nodes), tingible body macrophages (germinal centers of lymphoid follicles), Kupffer cells (liver), MZ macrophages (spleen), sinusoidal lining cells (spleen and liver), epithelioid cells (granulomas), giant cells (granulomas), and foam cells (atherosclerotic plaque) (127). Macrophages can be further classified on a functional basis. Classically activated macrophages (or M1 cells) are mostly generated by microbial products and IFN-γ, an inflammatory cytokine produced by NK cells and T_H1 cells, whereas alternatively activated macrophages (or M2 cells) predominantly require signals from IL-4 and IL-13, two inflammatory cytokines produced by T_H2 cells, basophils, eosinophils, and mast cells (20,128).

Macrophages sense the presence of pathogens and dead or dying cells through a huge variety of surface and intracellular PRRs, including TLRs, NLRs, RLRs, CLRs, and cysteine-rich scavenger receptors (128). In the presence of activating signals, macrophages undergo phagocytosis and then initiate the respiratory burst, which leads to the killing of phagocytosed microbes through the generation of ROS and nitric oxide. The production of this latter involves inducible nitric oxide synthase, an enzyme highly responsive to LPS, IFN-γ, and TNF. Activated macrophages also produce IL-12, IL-23, and TNF, which enhance innate immunity and trigger inflammation, partly by promoting the differentiation or expansion of inflammatory T_H1 and T_H17 cells producing IFN-γ and IL-17, respectively (133). Conversely, IFN-γ from T_H1 cells enhances the phagocytic, killing and inflammatory functions of macrophages (134,135). Activated macrophages also synthesize antimicrobial factors such as lysosome and diverse hydrolytic enzymes whose degradative activity does not require oxygen. Furthermore, activated macrophages up-regulate the expression of MHC-II, CD80 (B7.1), and CD86 (B7.2) molecules, which are required for the activation of antigen-specific T cells and the initiation of cellular and humoral responses. However, activated macrophages are less efficient than DCs in regard to their APC function. Importantly, M1 macrophages mediate most of the protective functions described so far, whereas M2 macrophages predominantly antagonize the activity of M1 macrophages (136). Indeed, M2 macrophages deliver immunoregulatory signals that dampen inflammation and attenuate antimicrobial and antitumor immune responses by releasing various anti-inflammatory and immunoregulatory factors, including the cytokine

IL-10 (128). Furthermore, M2 macrophages promote wound healing, tissue remodeling, and angiogenesis (134).

Dendritic Cells

DCs were first described by Ralph Steinman and Zanvil Cohn as a novel subset of adherent cells with an elongated and stellate morphology characterized by the presence of branched neuron-like cytoplasmic projections (or dendrites) that were not detected in canonical macrophages (137). Compared to macrophages, DCs have distinct morphology, phenotype, and functional features. While macrophages predominantly serve as resident phagocytes specialized in the engulfment and killing of microbes, DCs mostly function as highly motile sentinels that promptly activate the immune system after sensing the presence of microbes. In particular, DCs function as professional APCs that efficiently stimulate naïve T cells to initiate primary immune responses. Indeed, DCs process antigen and generate T-cell–stimulating peptide-MHC complexes more efficiently than any other APC type, including macrophages and B cells (23,138). Remarkably, DCs present not only processed antigens to T cells but also native antigens to B cells. In this manner, DCs functionally link the innate and adaptive immune systems.

The APC function of DCs varies in relationship to their maturation stage. Indeed, immature DCs can efficiently capture and present antigen, but do not simulate T cells as mature DCs do (22). This functional difference has a morphologic correlate in the formation of large projections called "veils" by immature DCs, whereas mature DCs form highly branched dendrites. Multiple subsets of functionally plastic DCs circulate in the peripheral blood and populate peripheral tissues, including preferential sites of antigen entry such as the skin and mucosal surfaces. Each DC subset has distinct morphologic, phenotypic, and functional features that determine the type and quality of the immune response (24,139). Cutaneous and mucosal surfaces contain a particularly prominent network of DCs because these tissues are inhabited by large communities of commensal bacteria and also serve as major portal sites for pathogen entry. Thus, cutaneous and mucosal DCs are needed not only to mount inflammatory responses against invasive pathogens but also to orchestrate noninflammatory responses against commensal bacteria (80).

Dendritic Cell Maturation

Hematopoietic progenitors located in the bone marrow give rise to circulating precursors of myeloid and lymphoid DCs that home to peripheral organs to generate immature DCs. Regardless of their myeloid or lymphoid lineage, immature DCs possess high endocytic and phagocytic capacity that permit antigen capture, but express low levels of MHC-II and costimulatory CD80 and CD86 molecules, which are required for the activation of T cells (140). Immature DCs migrate to sites of microbial infection or tissue damage in response to a large spectrum of inflammatory chemokines produced by local cells, including CCL3, CCL5, and CCL20 (141,142). At these sites, immature DCs recognize general molecular signatures associated with microbes through a broad array of germline-encoded PRRs, including TLRs and CLRs with endocytic function (143–145). Microbial recognition not only enhances the internalization of intruding microbes via pinocytosis and endocytosis but also triggers the release of immunostimulating and inflammatory cytokines (IL-6, IL-12, TNF, IFN-α/β) as well as antimicrobial factors (defensins, IFN-α/β) that limit the spread of the infection (23). Simultaneously, immature DCs undergo a maturation process characterized by the following series of coordinated events: (a) loss of endocytic and phagocytic receptors; (b) increased surface expression of MHC-II, CD80, and CD86 molecules; (c) changes in morphology, including formation of highly branched dendrites; and (d) activation of the antigen-processing machinery, including a shift in lysosomal compartments and increase in DC lysosome-associated membrane protein (DC-LAMP) expression. In addition, immature DCs (e) down-regulate their responsiveness to inflammatory CCL3, CCL5, and CCL20 chemokines through either down-regulation or desensitization of CCR1, CCR5, and CCR6 receptors, respectively, and (f) up-regulate their responsiveness to homeostatic CCL19 and CCL21 chemokines via up-regulation of the CCR7 receptor (140,146,147). Consequently, mature DCs move via the afferent lymphatics from peripheral sites of infection or inflammation to the T-cell areas of local draining lymph nodes or mucosa-associated lymphoid follicles (148). Here, mature DCs undergo cognate interaction with rare antigen-specific T cells to induce their activation and differentiation into effector T_H cells that orchestrate both cellular and humoral immune responses (149–151). Cognate DC-T-cell interaction involves the "instruction" of naïve T cells as to the nature and composition of antigen and the "priming" of naïve T cells by DC cytokines such as IL-6, IL-10, IL-12, IL-23, type-I IFN-α/β, and TGF-β (23). In addition to including phenotypically recognizable immature and mature differentiation stages, conventional DCs are composed of ontogenetically, morphologically, phenotypically, genotypically, and functionally distinct subsets of plasmacytoid (or lymphoid) and mDCs (24,152).

Lymphoid Dendritic Cells

Lymphoid DCs or pDCs are a unique DC subset that derives from a lymphoid progenitor. More than 40 years ago, rare leukocytes with plasma cell-like morphology and a hybrid T-cell-monocyte surface phenotype were identified in the paracortical areas of reactive lymph nodes and designated as either plasmacytoid T cells or plasmacytoid monocytes (153). It was later found that these leukocytes were poor stimulators of T cells, but could develop into immature DCs in response to IL-3 (154). Similar leukocytes were also detected in the circulation. These cells produced large amounts of IFN-α/β in response to viruses and were therefore defined as natural IFN-producing cells (155). Finally, plasmacytoid T cells, plasmacytoid monocytes, and natural IFN-producing cells were confirmed to correspond to the same cell type, which was defined as pDC (156). In humans, pDCs express the lymphoid molecule CD4, the IL-3 receptor CD123, the lectin receptor CD303 (or BDCA2), and the VEGF and semaphorin receptor CD304 (or BDCA4). Compared to conventional DCs of myeloid origin, pDCs lack the integrin CD11c and the LPS co-receptor CD14 but contain more microbial RNA sensors such as TLR3, TLR7, and TLR8 and more microbial DNA sensors such as TLR9 (156). When exposed to microbial nucleic acids, pDCs release large amounts of IFN-α/β, a type-I IFN that mediates immediate antiviral responses and activates both innate and adaptive immune systems by favoring the maturation of conventional DCs and the formation of effector T_H cells (157,158).

Myeloid Dendritic Cells

mDCs constitute the large majority of classical DCs and are thought to derive from monocytes. In humans, mDCs are present in the circulation and peripheral tissues and express CD4, CD11c, CD14, and HLA-II, but lack CD123, CD303, and CD304. Circulating mDCs can be further subdivided into mDC1 cells expressing the MHC-I–like molecule CD1c (or BDCA1) and high CD11c and mDC2 cells expressing the thrombomodulin CD141 (or BDCA3) and low CD11c (139). While mDC1 cells may serve as circulating precursors of Langherans cells, mDC2 cells may function as circulating precursors of interdigitating DCs lodged in the extrafollicular areas of lymph nodes. Unlike pDCs, which differentiate in response to IL-3, mDCs differentiate in response to GM-CSF. Depending on the cytokine milieu, the resulting mature mDCs can elicit the formation of different types of effector T_H cells (139).

Other Dendritic Cell Subsets

Similar to macrophages, conventional DCs can also be distinguished on the basis of their anatomical location. *Langerhans cells* and *dermal DCs* populate the epidermal and dermal layers of the skin, respectively, and show distinct morphology and phenotype (159,160). *Interstitial DCs* colonize the liver, kidney, heart, and other connective tissues and tend to be associated with vascular structures (161). Various types of *mucosal DCs* are found in the oral cavity, intestinal tract, respiratory tract, and urogenital tract. These cells develop from myeloid and lymphoid precursors in the blood and provide a sort of "frontline" sentinel system (70,161,162). In lymphoid tissues, the germinal center, which is the microenvironment that allows the generation of high-affinity antibody responses, contains *FDCs* and *germinal center DCs*. FDCs are distinct from conventional DCs, and indeed FDCs likely originate from a mesenchymal precursor (163,164). Thus, their inclusion among DC subsets only relates to their dendritic morphology. Notably, FDCs have the unique capacity to trap antigen in the form of immune complexes for long periods of time to facilitate the selection of germinal center B cells with high affinity for antigen (14,165). In contrast, germinal center DCs function as strong APCs for a subset of germinal center T cells specialized in the induction of B-cell activation, survival, proliferation, and differentiation (13,166). Antigen-capturing DCs that migrate from nonlymphoid sites and mucosal surfaces to afferent lymphatic vessels are recognized as *veiled DCs*. These cells migrate to lymph nodes through the afferent lymphatics to become *interdigitating DCs* in the T-cell areas of the paracortex. At this site, DCs initiate immune responses by establishing a cognate interaction with T cells (167). *Thymic DCs* are suggested to be involved in the negative selection of T cells (168). All these DC subsets show various phenotypic differences, but their circulating precursors, intermediate maturation stages, and functional differences have not been firmly established.

Natural Killer Cells

NK cells originate in the bone marrow from hematopoietic progenitor cells and are widespread throughout lymphoid and nonlymphoid tissues (18). They constitute 5% to 25% of human peripheral blood mononuclear cells and up to 5% of the whole lymphocyte population in secondary lymphoid tissues (169). Additionally, NK cells can be found throughout most nonlymphoid tissues, including the liver, lungs, and uterine mucosa. In humans, NK cells are conventionally defined as CD56$^+$CD3$^-$ lymphocytes. Based on the surface density of CD56, NK cells can be further divided into two subsets that display distinct phenotypic and functional properties. CD56^{dim} NK cells represent the vast majority of NK cells in the peripheral blood but are rare in lymph nodes, express high levels of CD16, and show strong cytotoxic activity (170). In contrast, CD56^{bright} NK cells are the predominant subset of NK cells in lymph nodes and have weak cytolytic activity but efficiently produce cytokines (170).

NK cells are important effector cells of the innate immune system and mainly mediate protective responses against viral and parasitic infections and against tumors (171). NK cells provide protection through two major effector mechanisms: (1) recognition and killing of target cells through the release of perforin and granzymes or the expression of death-inducing ligands and (2) activation and recruitment of other immune cell types through the secretion of cytokines and chemokines. NK cells kill infected or neoplastic cells by direct contact or antibody-dependent cell-mediated cytotoxicity (ADCC), which involves engagement of the CD16 receptor on NK cells by IgG bound on target cells (Fig. 2.8).

The main cytotoxic pathway utilized by NK cells involves the release of perforin and granzymes. These death-inducing

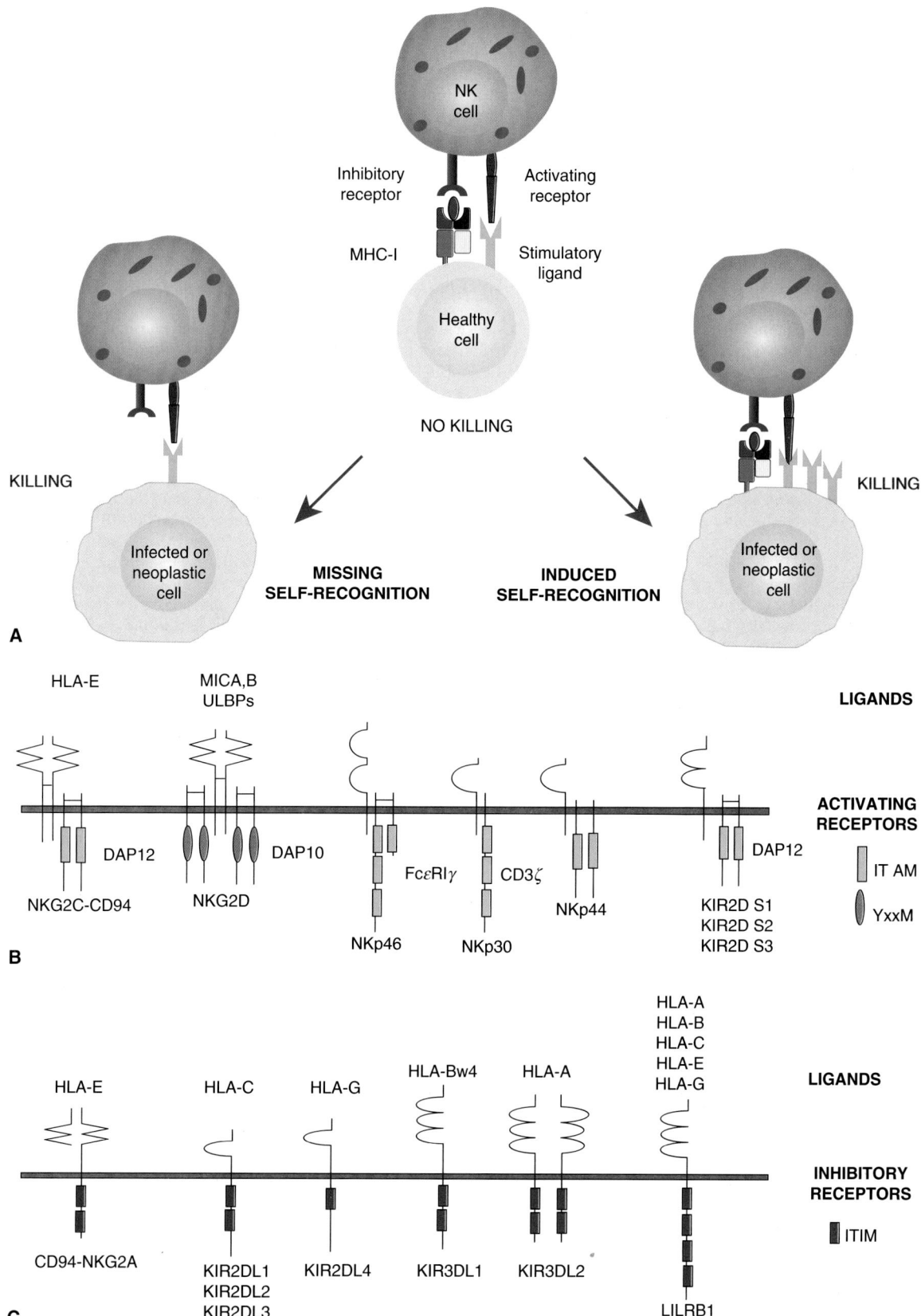

FIGURE 2.8. Activating and inhibitory NK-cell receptors. A: Schematic representation of the balance between inhibitory and activating signals that govern the function of NK cells. Healthy cells are protected against killing when signals delivered by activating receptors are counterbalanced by signals delivered by inhibitory receptors on NK cells. Infected or neoplastic cells are killed by NK cells following down-regulation of the expression of inhibitory ligands (missing self-recognition) or up-regulation of stimulatory ligands (induced self-recognition). **B:** Activating receptors on NK cells and some of their ligands. Activating receptors are associated with DAP10, DAP12, FcεRγ, or CD3ζ adaptor proteins containing one or more immunoreceptor tyrosine-based activating motif (ITAM) domains or an YxxM motif (where Y is tyrosine, x is any amino acid, and M is methionine). Many ligands for inhibitory receptors remain unknown. The names of the receptor and that of the adaptor are indicated below and on the right of the receptor complex, respectively. **C:** Inhibitory receptors on NK cells and their ligands. Inhibitory receptors belong to both killing inhibitory receptor (KIR) and leukocyte immunoglobulin-like receptor (LILR) families and contain one or more immunoreceptor tyrosine-based inhibitory motif (ITIM) domains.

proteins are stored in specific intracellular granules that are released through exocytosis upon target cell recognition by NK cells. Further mechanisms include the killing of target cells by TNF-related apoptosis-inducing ligand (TRAIL) or Fas ligand (FasL), two death-inducing TNF family members that engage death receptor (DR) or Fas (or CD95) molecules on target cells, respectively. NK cells have also been shown to recruit and activate other effector cells by releasing various chemokines and cytokines, including IFN-γ and TNF (170).

NK cells express different combinations of activating and inhibitory receptors that regulate the delivery of cytotoxic signals through complementary pathways. In other words, the outcome of an NK-cell response depends on the balance between activating and inhibitory signals generated by surface NK-cell receptors in response to cognate ligands expressed on the surface of a target cell. For instance, engagement of inhibitory receptors on NK cells by MHC-I ligands on healthy cells blocks activating signals simultaneously delivered by stimulatory ligands and thereby prevents the killing of healthy cells by NK cells. Conversely, down-regulation of MHC-I expression or up-regulation of stimulatory ligand expression renders infected or neoplastic cells susceptible to the killing activity of NK cells. The effector functions of NK cells are further regulated by cytokines such as IFN-α/β, IL-1β, IL-12, IL-18, and IL-15, which are released by neighboring immune cells (172).

NK cell–inhibitory receptors share a common signaling motif in their cytoplasmic region called immunoreceptor tyrosine-based inhibitory motif (ITIM). Engagement of an inhibitory receptor causes phosphorylation of the ITIM by Src family kinases, followed by docking of protein tyrosine phosphatases such as SHP-1 and SHP-2. These phosphatases deliver negative signals by dephosphorylating different intracellular substrates that vary in relationship to the particular array of activating receptors engaged on a given NK cell (173). Three different families of genes for inhibitory receptors have been identified and encode killer immunoglobulin-like receptors (KIRs), leukocyte immunoglobulin-like receptors (LILRs), and the CD94/NKG2 heterodimer. Each of these families also includes members that encode activating molecules whose physiologic role remains unclear. In general, each receptor exhibits a variegated expression pattern, leading to a complex combinatorial repertoire of NK-cell specificities for MHC-I molecules (173). The KIRs and LILRs family members recognize different alleles of HLA-A, HLA-B, and HLA-C molecules, whereas the CD94/NKG2 heterodimers bind the nonclassical MHC-I molecule HLA-E (174). This latter has a surface expression that changes in relationship to the binding of signal peptides derived from classical MHC-I molecules (174).

Activating NK-cell receptors lack ITIMs in their cytoplasmic domain, but have charged residues in their transmembrane domain that facilitate the recruitment of adaptor proteins with docking sites for downstream stimulatory signaling molecules. Most adaptor proteins, including FcεRγ, CD3ζ, and DAP12, have cytoplasmic domains with immunoreceptor tyrosine-based activation motifs (ITAMs) that mediate the recruitment of ZAP70 and/or Syk tyrosine kinases. In contrast, DAP10 has a transmembrane domain with an YxxM motif that mediates the recruitment of phosphatidylinositol 3-kinase (PI3-K) (175). In humans, NK-cell–activating receptors include CD16, which is a low-affinity receptor for the Fc portion of IgG1 and IgG3, NKG2D, and natural cytotoxicity receptors (NCRs) such as NKp30, NKp46, and NKp44.

The best-characterized NK-cell–activating receptor is NKG2D. This CLR family member is expressed on the surface of NK cells as a disulfide-linked homodimer and delivers intracellular signals by interacting with the adaptor protein DAP10 (176). NKG2D binds stress-inducible ligands that are distantly related homologues of MHC-I molecules. In humans, these molecules are composed of two families:

the MHC-I polypeptide–related chain (MIC) protein family, which includes MICA and MICB proteins, and the cytomegalovirus UL16-binding proteins (ULBPs). The expression of these NKG2D ligands increases after viral infection through a mechanism involving either induction by virus-associated proteins or induction by virus-induced cytokines such as IFN-α/β (177). Alternatively, the expression of NKG2D ligands augments after activation of the DNA damage response as a result of tumor transformation (177).

Mast Cells

Mast cells originate from a hematopoietic precursor distinct from the one that gives rise to basophils. While basophils predominantly patrol the circulatory system and migrate to tissues in the presence of infection or after immunization (178), mast cells are constitutively located in mucosal and connective tissues, where they acquire specific phenotypes (179). Because of their strategic position in the connective tissues of blood vessels and subepithelial areas of mucosal surfaces, mast cells are among the first immune cells that interact with environmental antigens, allergens, or toxins (180). Mast cells are long-lived cells that contain large cytoplasmic granules filled with pre-formed vasoactive mediators such as histamine and serotonin, anticoagulants such as heparin, and serine proteases such as tryptase (179). Mast cells also release newly formed vasoactive and inflammatory mediators such as prostaglandins and leukotrienes and secrete various cytokines. The phenotype of mast cells is distinct from that of basophils, in that mast cells express CD117 together with FcεRI and CD123 (179).

Similar to basophils, mast cells play an important role in parasitic infections and allergies (178). Indeed, mast cells bind IgE through FcεRI, and cross-linking of IgE by parasitic antigens or allergens induces mast cell degranulation. The resulting local vasodilation leads to an immediate transmigration of inflammatory cells such as neutrophils and macrophages from the circulation to the tissue. The lymphatic flow to and from the inflamed area is also augmented, which causes an increased delivery of tissue antigens to draining lymph nodes. Histamine, serotonin, prostaglandins, and leukotrienes trigger the contraction of smooth muscle fibers in both gut and bronchi, which facilitates the mechanical elimination of invading pathogens from these mucosal sites (179,181). It must be noted that mast cells are activated by a number of other factors in addition to IgE, including inflammatory cytokines. Mast cells are also involved in the amplification or suppression of both innate and adaptive immune responses (182). Indeed, activated mast cells can express MHC-II, CD80, and CD86 and release IL-4, IL-6, IL-10, IL-13, TNF, and TGF-β (179,181).

Innate Lymphoid Cells

In addition to NK cells, various subsets of innate lymphoid cells (ILCs) have been identified during the last decade (183). Common hallmarks of ILCs are the lymphoid morphology, the lack of rearranged antigen receptors, the absence of common lineage markers, and the requirement for a transcriptional factor known as inhibitor of DNA binding 2 (Id2). This last feature suggests that all ILCs derive from a common precursor (183). Two main subsets of ILCs have been described thus far: RORγt$^+$ ILCs and type-II ILCs.

RORγt$^+$ ILCs require the RORγt transcription factor for lineage specification and rely on IL-7 for their development and survival (184). These innate cells are essential for the formation of lymph nodes and Peyer patches during fetal development by interacting with lymphoid tissue organizer (LTo) cells (60). ILCs are also required for the formation of intestinal cryptopatches after postnatal colonization of the intestine by commensal bacteria (185). In adults, RORγt+ ILCs function as sentinels of lymphoid architecture that promote the repair of secondary lymphoid tissues (186). In addition to a role in lymphoid organogenesis and repair, RORγt+ ILCs expressing NK-cell receptors (NKR+RORγt+ ILCs) are found in the lamina propria of the intestinal mucosa, where they participate in intestinal homeostasis and mucosal immunity by releasing IL-22 (183). IL-22 is an important cytokine that acts directly on epithelial cells by promoting the release of antimicrobial factors such as β-defensins, RegIIIβ, and RegIIIγ, which are essential for the protection against gut pathogens (183).

Type-II ILCs or natural helper cells or nuocytes correspond to a recently identified subset of ILCs that require Id2 and IL-7 but not RORγt for their development and survival (184). In humans, type-II ILCs are present in several tissues, including lung, intestine, palatine tonsils, and peripheral blood. Type-II ILCs are functionally characterized by their ability to produce T_H2-associated cytokines such as IL-5 and IL-13 in response to IL-25 or IL-33, two cytokines produced by epithelial cells (183). Based on this ability, type-II ILCs participate in the immune response to helminth infections (187) and contribute to the pathogenesis of allergic disorders of the respiratory tract, including asthma (183). In addition, type-II ILCs play a critical role in the repair of the respiratory epithelium during influenza infection (188).

Links Between the Innate and Adaptive Immune Systems

Over the past decade, growing evidence shows that the innate and adaptive immune systems influence their activity by inducing a complex network of mutually regulating signals (189). Arguably, DCs provide the most prominent link between the innate and adaptive branches of our immune system. In addition to sensing the presence of invading microbes through innate antigen receptors called PRRs, DCs activate T and B cells by presenting processed or native antigen to adaptive antigen receptors called TCR and BCR, respectively. In addition, DCs release chemokines and cytokines that promote the recruitment, activation, and differentiation of T and B cells (190). Ultimately, the resulting effector T and B cells enhance the phagocytic, killing, and inflammatory functions of granulocytes, macrophages, and other effector cells of the innate immune system by secreting cytokines and antibodies, respectively. The molecular and cellular links that regulate the innate and adaptive phases of the immune response are discussed in the section describing antibody Fc receptors (FcRs) and iNKT cells.

Fc Receptors

Antibodies expressed by B cells function as transmembrane antigen receptors (or BCRs) or soluble effector molecules, depending on the stage of B-cell differentiation. Remarkably, B cells cooperate with the innate immune system by utilizing both transmembrane and secreted antibodies. Indeed, complement receptors enhance the activation of B cells by amplifying signals generated by the BCR in response to complement-opsonized microbes. Conversely, soluble antibodies enhance microbial recognition, clearance, and killing by activating the complement cascade (99,191). Soluble antibodies further regulate the function of the innate immune system by engaging specific FcRs (192). These molecules interact with the constant region (or Fc fragment) of soluble antibodies and belong to a group of surface glycoproteins known as multichain immune recognition receptors (MIRRs). By binding to antibody molecules, FcRs connect adaptive humoral responses to key regulatory and effector pathways of the innate and adaptive immune systems. Indeed, cross-linking of FcRs by secreted antibodies not only augments phagocytosis, respiratory burst, cytokine secretion, and ADCC in effector cells of the innate immune system but also decreases antibody production by B cells (193,194). Of note, there is a specific FcR for each class of antibodies (Table 2.3). Thus, IgG binds to FcγRI, FcγRII (A, B, and C), FcγRIII (A and B), and FcRn (195,196); IgA to FcαR and FcαRI (197,198); IgE to FcεRI and FcεRII (199–201); and IgM to FcμRI (192,202). The FcδR for IgD remains to be identified (203). Here we briefly discuss FcγRs due to their prominent importance in the activation of the innate immune system.

FcγRs belong to three distinct classes with distinct binding affinities for IgG. FcγRI (or CD64) binds IgG with higher affinity than FcγRII (or CD32) and FcγRIII (or CD16) (204–206). Of note, FcγRII can be further divided into A, B, and C types. All these FcRs can be further classified on the basis of their activating or inhibiting function. Indeed, FcγRI, FcγRIIA, FcγRIIC, and FcγRIII deliver powerful stimulating signals to monocytes, macrophages, DCs, granulocytes, and mast cells via an ITAM (173,207). In contrast, FcγRIIB transmits inhibitory signals to B cells and innate immune cells via an ITIM (173,208). In humans, the presence of multiple FcγRs mirrors the existence of four IgG subclasses, which bind FcγRs with different affinity and specificity (209). IgG also binds to the neonatal Fc receptor (FcRn), which is structurally related to MHC-I molecules (210). FcRn is expressed by various cell types, including leukocytes, trophoblasts, and some epithelial cells, and accounts for the half-life of extracellular IgG and for the active transport of maternal IgG to the fetus across the placenta (211–213). FcRn may also permit innate immune cells to present native IgG-opsonized

Table 2.3	Fc RECEPTORS

Name (CD)	Name (FcR)	Ligand	Affinity	Signaling	Expression	Function
CD89	FcαRI	IgA	Medium	ITAM	Phagocytes, eosinophils	Phagocytosis, cytotoxicity
—	Fcα/μR	IgA/IgM	—	—	Macrophages, B cells, mesangial cells	Endocytosis
CD64	FcγRI	IgG1,3,4	High	ITAM	Phagocytes, DCs	Phagocytosis
CD32	FcγRIIA	IgG3,1,2	Low	ITAM	Phagocytes	Phagocytosis, degranulation
CD32	FcγRIIB	IgG3,1,2,4	Low	ITIM	B cells, DCs, monocytes, macrophages	Termination of immune activation
CD32	FcγRIIC	IgG	Low	ITAM	Phagocytes, Langerhans cells	Phagocytosis, degranulation
CD16	FcγRIIIA	IgG	Low	ITAM	Phagocytes, NK cells, Langerhans cells	Cytotoxicity
CD16	FcγRIIIB	IgG1,3,2,4	Low	ITAM	Neutrophils	Degranulation
—	FcRn	IgG	High	—	Fetus, newborn gut	Maternal-fetal transfer of IgG
—	FcεRI	IgE	High	ITAM	Mast cells, basophils, eosinophils	Degranulation
CD23	FcεRII	IgE	Low	FcεRIγ	B cells	B-cell activation

antigens to B cells. Indeed, FcRn not only internalizes IgG-antigen complexes but also recycles these complexes to the cell surface (214,215).

The low affinity of many FcγRs for IgG is crucial to avoid the continuous activation of leukocytes by IgG molecules present in our circulation. An additional control layer relates to the activation threshold that each FcγR needs to achieve in order to deliver activating signals. Such signals also depend on a concentration threshold of circulating IgG, which is partly controlled by FcRn. Adaptor proteins containing ITAM or ITIM domains further regulate signals emanating from FcγRs (216). An important biologic aspect of FcγRs and FcRn relates to their ability to enhance adaptive immunity by regulating the uptake, processing, and presentation of antigen by DCs. Indeed, DCs can internalize IgG-bound antigen to an MHC compartment through FcγRs and subsequently present the processed antigen to T cells (209). Alternatively, DCs can internalize IgG-bound antigen to a non-MHC compartment through FcRn and subsequently present the unprocessed antigen to B cells (214). Finally, it is important to emphasize that regulatory signals from FcγRIIB inhibit not only antibody production by B cells but also innate immune responses mediated by macrophages, DCs, granulocytes, and mast cells (209). In this manner, FcγRIIB provides a powerful negative feedback signal that attenuates immunity and inflammation after IgG antibodies have cleared the intruding microbe.

iNKT Cells

Some lymphocytes of our immune system are strategically positioned at the interface between innate and adaptive immune responses in that they express somatically recombined receptors together with phenotypic and functional features typical of innate immune cells. These innate lymphocytes include iNKT cells, γδ T cells, splenic MZ B cells, and peritoneal B-1 cells (these cells are abundant in mice, but their existence in humans remains controversial). The phenotype, development, and functional features of these lymphocytes and their receptors will be described in the sections describing T-cell subsets and TI responses. iNKT cells express a somatically recombined but invariant TCR and recognize highly conserved lipid antigens such as α-galactosylceramide in the context of the MHC-I–like molecule CD1d (217–219). Due to their remarkable evolutionary conservation and distinct functional features, iNKT cells are thought to have an important nonredundant role in the immune response (220,221).

After exposure to CD1d-bound glycolipids presented by DCs, macrophages, or B cells, iNKT cells become activated and produce a variety of effector cytokines that play an important role in both immunity and pathology (222). In particular, iNKT cells rapidly release TNF-α, IFN-γ, IL-4, IL-13, and IL-17 that promote the differentiation of naïve T cells into various effector T_H cell types. In addition, iNKT cells secrete a vast array of chemokines that promote the activation and maturation of DCs. In this manner, iNKT cells regulate not only the formation of T follicular helper (T_{FH}) cells with B-helper and antibody-inducing functions but also the expansion of CTLs with killing function (45,218,223). Furthermore, iNKT cells can directly provide help to B cells to stimulate the induction of rapid waves of antibodies against microbes (224–226). This innate pathway integrates the slower antibody response induced by canonical T_{FH} cells.

ADAPTATIVE IMMUNE RESPONSES

The adaptive immune system includes T and B cells that mediate specific but temporally delayed responses after recognizing discrete antigen epitopes through somatically recombined receptors named TCR and BCR, respectively (39). Activation

signals from antigen receptors trigger the clonal expansion and differentiation of T and B cells into effector and memory lymphocytes that closely cooperate with each other and with cells of the innate immune system to generate protective immunity and long-lasting memory (227,228).

Antigen Recognition

Antigen Presentation

T cells develop protective responses against microbes without damaging self-tissues by recognizing antigens that have been processed by APCs in the context of cell surface MHC proteins (229). Engagement of the TCR by a peptide-MHC complex leads to the clonal expansion of antigen-specific T cells that subsequently differentiate into effector CD4+ T_H cells and CD8+ CTLs. Unlike T cells, B cells recognize native antigens that are either present in the fluid phase or exposed on the surface of macrophages, DCs, and FDCs (165). Engagement of the BCR by antigen is followed by antigen internalization and processing, which results in the formation of a peptide-MHC complex that is presented to T cells (230). The ensuing cognate T cell-B cell interaction generates T_H signals that induce the clonal expansion of antigen-specific B cells, followed by their differentiation into effector antibody-secreting plasma cells and memory B cells (231).

MHC Locus

The MHC locus is located in the short arm of chromosome 6, where it occupies about 3.5 kilobases. Based on their structure and properties, the products of MHC genes include class I and class II proteins that are recognized by different types of T cells (232). MHC-I molecules present antigens to CD8+ T cells, whereas MHC-II molecules present antigen to CD4+ T cells (233).

MHC-I molecules are heterodimers made up of one variable heavy-chain α of 44 to 47 kD and an invariant light chain of 12 kD called β2-microglobulin. The latter is associated with the α chain and is essential for the stability of the structure and for the binding of the peptide derived from the processed antigen. A stable expression of MHC-I on the cell surface is achieved only when the α chain, the β2-microglobulin, and the peptide are properly assembled. MHC-II molecules consist of two variable α and β chains of 32 to 34 and 29 to 32 kD, respectively, which form a peptide-binding domain. Like MHC-I molecules, MHC-II molecules require proper assembly of the α chain, β chain, and peptide to form a stable complex (234).

In humans, there are many different allelic forms of MHC genes, which implies that MHC molecules are highly polymorphic and bind a large variety of peptides. MHC polymorphism is determined only in the germline, and diversity is not generated through DNA recombination (235). Although there is a high degree of polymorphism, an individual can have six different MHC-I products and a few more MHC-II products, ranging from 10 to 20 (236). In humans, there are three loci defined as HLA-A, HLA-B, and HLA-C that encode MHC-I molecules and three loci defined as HLA-DP, HLA-DQ, and HLA-DR that encode MHC-II molecules.

The extracellular antigen-binding cleft present on an MHC molecule determines the type of peptide that binds to that MHC molecule, but each individual MHC molecule can bind different peptides. MHC-I molecules bind only short peptides of 8 to 11 amino acids, whereas MHC-II molecules are open at both ends and therefore can bind longer peptides of 13 to 30 amino acids. Antigenic peptides must have certain amino acids in specific positions—known as "anchor sites"—in order to successfully interact with MHC molecules (237). In addition, the TCR must recognize antigenic peptides in the context of specific amino acids within the MHC molecule in order to trigger an effective response (233,238).

In addition to class I and class II proteins, the MHC locus encodes class III proteins that are required for antigen presentation and include transporter associated with antigen presentation (TAP) and proteasome proteins. Class III proteins also include heat shock proteins and complement proteins (235).

Antigen Processing

MHC-I proteins are found on every nucleated cell of the body, and their function is to bind fragments of proteins expressed in the cytoplasm of a cell during infection or neoplastic transformation. The resulting MHC-I-peptide complex is inserted into the plasma membrane and presented to cytotoxic CD8$^+$ T cells (239). Healthy cells are ignored, while diseased cells expressing antigenic peptides are attacked and destroyed. Because MHC-I molecules present peptides derived from cytosolic proteins, the MHC-I pathway of antigen presentation is also called cytosolic or endogenous pathway. Although constitutively expressed on the cell surface, MHC-I molecules can undergo further up-regulation of their expression in response to immunostimulating cytokines (IFN-α, IFN-β, IFN-γ, TNF) delivered by the immune system in response to infection or neoplastic transformation (240,241). This strategy ensures a more effective killing of infected and tumor cells by CTLs. Of note, MHC-I can also serve as an inhibitory ligand for NK cells. Down-regulation of MHC-I expression by viruses and tumors authorizes the killing of infected or neoplastic cells by NK cells (173).

MHC-I proteins consist of a polymorphic α chain that is noncovalently linked with an invariant β2-microglobulin chain. MHC-I molecules bind peptides 8 to 10 amino acid in length mainly generated from degradation of cytosolic proteins by the proteasome (242). This intracellular structure includes catalytic elements such as low molecular mass polypeptide-1 (LMP-1) and LMP-7 proteins that process antigen for loading onto MHC-I molecules. In general, proteins committed to degradation by the proteasome require tagging by several copies of ubiquitin (243). However, some proteins can also undergo degradation via proteolytic enzymes contained in the endoplasmic reticulum. After their release from the proteasome, processed peptides are translocated into the lumen of the endoplasmic reticulum by an ATP-dependent transporter associated with a dimer composed of TAP1 and TAP2 subunits (Fig. 2.9). In the endoplasmic reticulum, newly synthesized α chain MHC-I-β2-microglobulin complexes are assembled and stabilized by endoplasmic reticulum chaperone proteins like tapasin (244). Additional chaperones like calreticulin and ERp57 further stabilize the MHC-I molecule. All these proteins form a peptide-loading complex that is released after the peptide binds to MHC-I. At this stage, the MHC-I complex leaves the endoplasmic reticulum and enters the Golgi network to reach the cell membrane via Golgi-derived vesicles (245).

Antigens that do not encounter appropriate MHC-I molecules are removed from the endoplasmic reticulum and redirected to the cytoplasm for destruction (246). Conversely, MHC-I molecules that do not bind peptides become unstable and either get degraded in the endoplasmic reticulum or are internalized in endosomal compartments and recycled to present endosomal peptides. Poorly understood mechanisms regulate the balance between translation, degradation, and presentation of peptides produced at a higher rate, as for example after viral infection. Transfer of peptides between adjacent infected or tumor cells through gap junctions and their presentation on MHC-I has been suggested to be a mechanism by which the immune system amplifies its response against infections or tumors (247).

MHC-II proteins are mainly expressed by professional APCs such as DCs. However, in addition, macrophages, B cells, and other cell types such as fibroblasts and endothelial cells can express MHC-II and become APCs after activation (232,248). Nevertheless, these APCs are usually less effective than DCs. APCs internalize extracellular antigens by endocytosis or pinocytosis, and therefore the MHC-II pathway of antigen presentation is also called endocytic or exogenous pathway. Antigen contained in early endosomes transits into late endosomes, which are highly acidic compartments that cleave antigen into immunogenic peptides through a broad array of proteolytic enzymes, including cathepsins. These peptides are loaded onto MHC-II molecules in a specialized endosomal compartment derived from the trans-Golgi network called MIIC. The resulting MHC-II-peptide complex is inserted into the plasma membrane and presented to CD4$^+$ T cells. Of note, APCs can up-regulate MHC-II expression in response to microbial products such as TLR ligands or immunostimulating cytokines such as IFN-α, IFN-β, IFN-γ, and TNF (249,250). In this manner, APCs enhance their ability to activate antigen-specific CD4$^+$ T cells.

MHC-II proteins are heterodimers that consist of two polymorphic α and β chains that bind peptides between 13 and 25 amino acid residues in length. In the endoplasmic reticulum, the α chain covalently links with the β chain and with a third protein called invariant chain or Ii. This protein occupies the peptide-binding site of MHC-II to stabilize the complex and avoid binding of irrelevant peptides. Vesicles containing MHC-II and Ii complexes transit through the trans-Golgi network to enter the endocytic pathway, where Ii is progressively removed from MHC-II by proteolysis, leaving a short fragment known as class II–associated invariant protein (CLIP) in the peptide cleft of MHC-II (Fig. 2.10). The acquisition of peptides by MHC-II takes place in the MIIC, a late endosomal compartment with a multilaminar structure derived from the fusion of antigen-containing late endosomes with MHC-II-containing vesicles derived from the trans-Golgi network (251). The acidic environment of MIIC and the molecule HLA-DM promote the replacement of CLIP on the cleft of MHC-II with the antigenic peptide. In activated B cells, binding of HLA-DO to HLA-DM may further modulate this exchange (252). Following removal of CLIP, the antigenic peptide binds to MHC-II to form a complex that is transported to the cell surface for insertion on the plasma membrane (253). Similar to MHC-I, only properly assembled MHC-II-peptide complexes can reach the plasma membrane.

In addition to the classical MHC-I and MHC-II pathways of antigen presentation, there are two alternative pathways that follow somewhat different rules. *Cross-presentation* is the process whereby APCs take up, process, and present extracellular antigens to CD8$^+$ T cells in the context of MHC-I molecules (254). This process may be important for the early priming of memory CD8$^+$ T cells by DCs in response to viral or tumor antigens. The precise mechanism regulating cross-presentation remains poorly understood. *Autophagy* is a process whereby intracellular contents are targeted to acidic vacuoles called autophagosomes for degradation (247). After processing by autophagy, cytosolic antigens such as foreign, tumoral but also autologous proteins are assembled on MHC-II molecules and presented to CD4$^+$ T cells. In this way, APCs can amplify the repertoire of antigens presented through the MHC-II pathway (255).

T-Cell Receptor Structure and Function

T cells recognize antigens through the TCR. While CD4$^+$ T cells recognize MHC-II-peptide complexes, CD8$^+$ T cells recognize MHC-I-peptide complexes. The TCR protein is composed of α and β chains in $\alpha\beta$ T cells and γ and δ chains in $\gamma\delta$ T cells covalently linked by disulfide bridges (Fig. 2.11). Here we briefly discuss the structure of the TCR from $\alpha\beta$ T cells, which is the best-studied and most abundant T-cell subset of our body. TCR β genes are composed of V, D, and J gene segments,

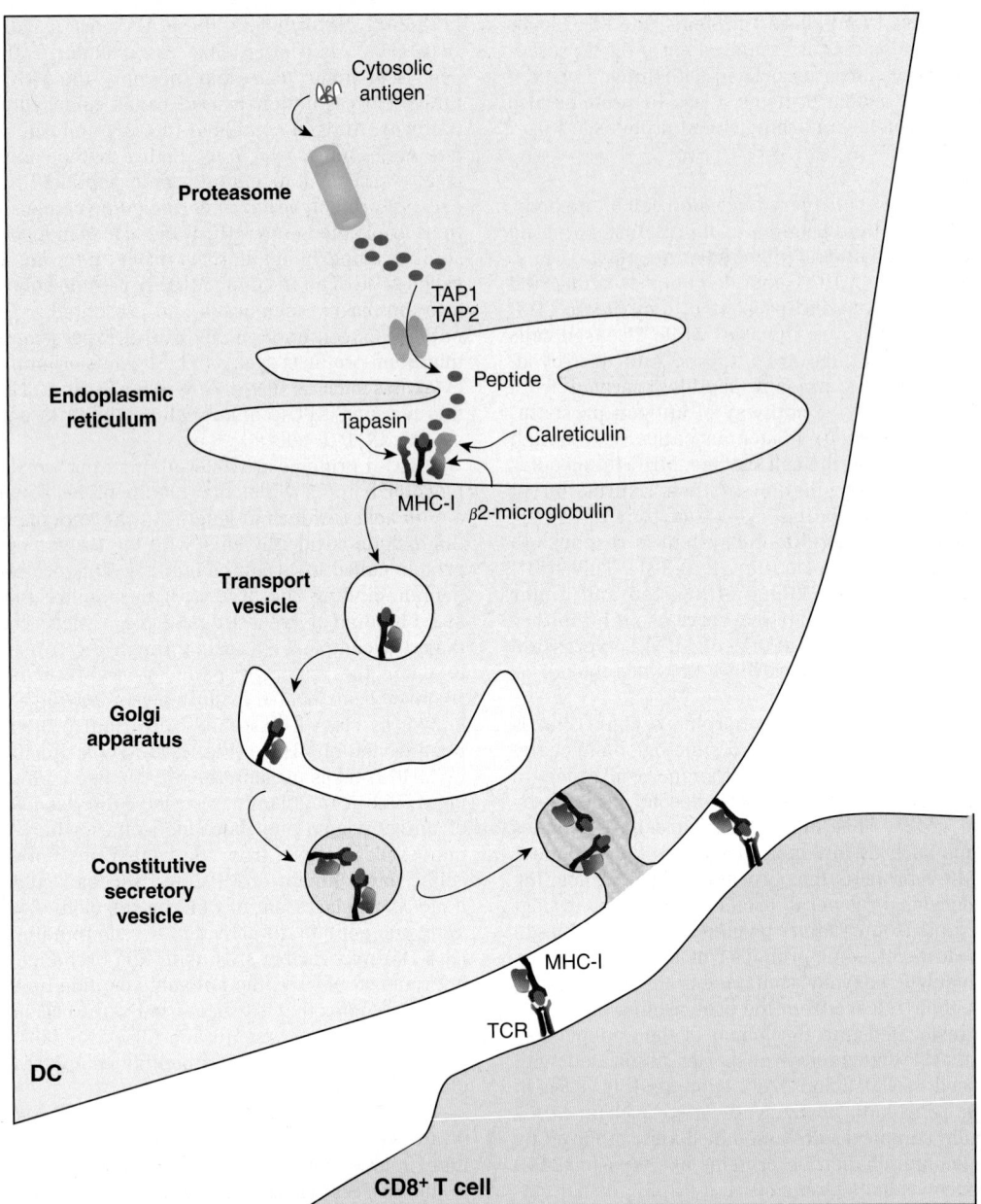

FIGURE 2.9. Endogenous MHC-I pathway of antigen presentation. In a DC, degradation of a cytosolic antigen from an intracellular pathogen by the proteasome generates peptides that are transported into the endoplasmic reticulum by a transporter associated with antigen presentation (TAP) proteins forming a TAP1-TAP2 complex. In the endoplasmic reticulum, peptides encounter MHC-I molecules that interact with β2-microglobulin to form a complex stabilized by two chaperones known as calreticulin and tapasin. When a peptide binds to MHC-I, the chaperones dissociate from MHC-I, and the resulting MHC-I-peptide complex is transported from the endoplasmic reticulum to the cell surface through a pathway including a transport vesicle, the Golgi apparatus, and a constitutive secretory vesicle. At this stage, the DC presents a MHC-I-peptide complex to the TCR of an antigen-specific CD8+ T cell to induce its activation.

whereas TCR α genes have only V and J gene segments that undergo somatic rearrangements during T-cell maturation. The specificity of each TCR molecule is determined by the combination of α and β chains. Both chains are characterized by a short cytoplasmic domain, a transmembrane domain anchored to the cell membrane through hydrophobic bounds, and an extracellular domain consisting of an antigen-binding variable (V) region and a constant (C) region. The V region contains three hypervariable domains called complementarity-determining region 1 (CDR1), CDR2, and CDR3 that mediate peptide recognition. Of these hypervariable regions, CDR3 is the most important to define the specificity of the TCR for a given peptide (256).

The TCR is noncovalently linked to a membrane-bound CD3 complex. This complex is composed of ε, γ, δ, and ζ subunits (or chains) that associate to form $\gamma\varepsilon$ and $\delta\varepsilon$ heterodimers and one $\zeta\zeta$ homodimer. The intracellular portion of each of these CD3 subunits contains an ITAM required for signal transduction. Each ε, γ, and δ chain includes a single ITAM, whereas the ζ chain contains three ITAMs. All these ITAMs contribute to the activation of T cells by antigen. Following engagement of the TCR by an MHC-peptide complex, CD3-associated ITAMs undergo tyrosine phosphorylation by members of the src-related protein tyrosine kinase family, including Lck and Fyn. This event leads to the recruitment of ZAP-70 kinase, which anchors itself to phosphorylated ITAMs of the

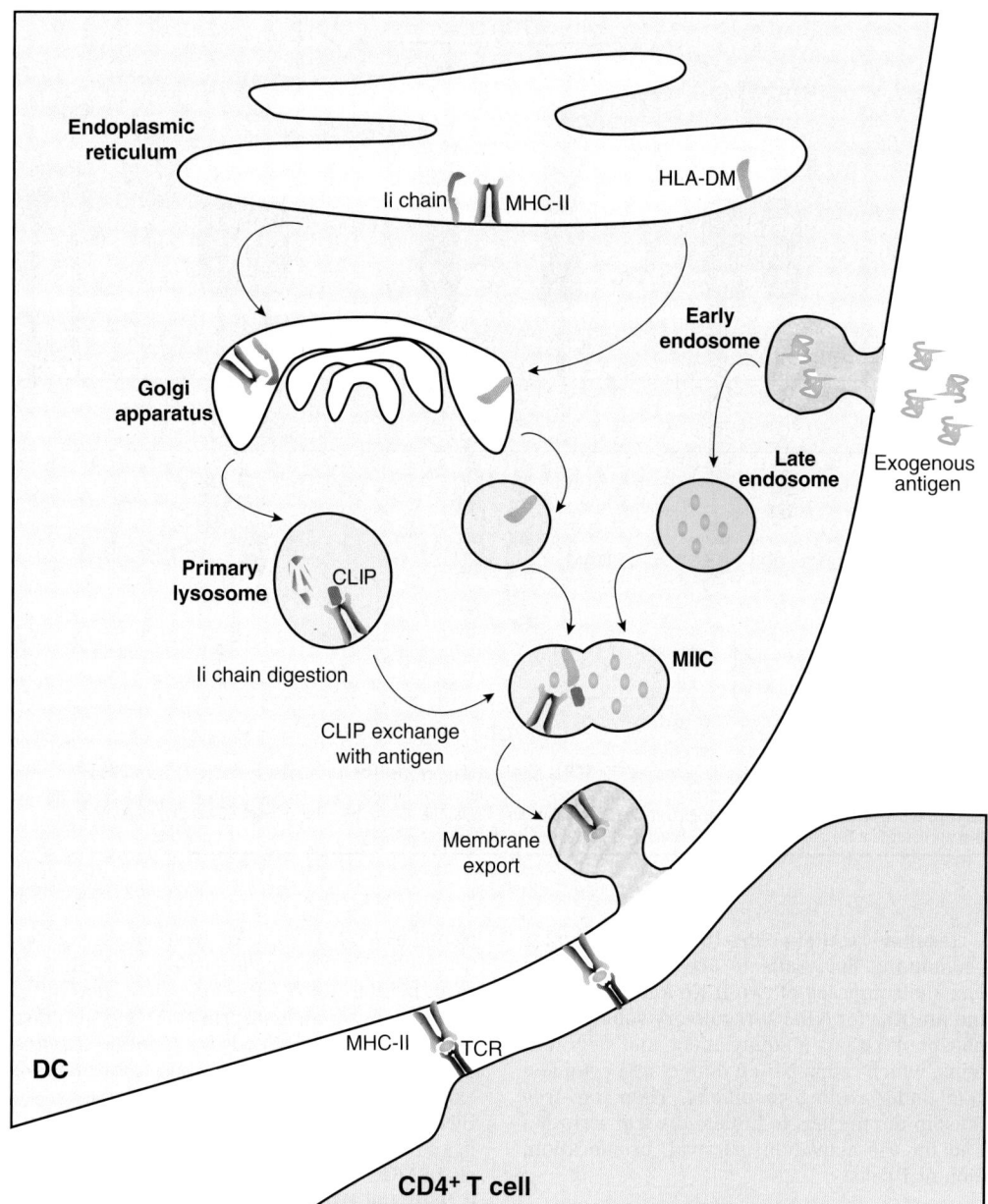

FIGURE 2.10. Exogenous MHC-II pathway of antigen presentation. DCs take up exogenous antigens from extracellular pathogens by pinocytosis or endocytosis through a pathway involving the sequential formation of early endosomes and highly acidic late endosomes. MHC-II synthesized in the endoplasmic reticulum is associated with an Ii chain that occupies the peptide-binding site. The MHC-II-Ii complex moves through the Golgi apparatus into primary lysosomes that progressively degrade the Ii chain through proteases. This process leaves the peptide-binding site of the MHC-II molecule occupied by a fragment of the Ii chain known as class-II–associated invariant protein (CLIP). Then, primary lysosomes fuse with antigen-containing late endosomes to form an MHC-II compartment known as MIIC. Proteases brought into the MIIC by primary lysosomes degrade antigen into peptides. At the same time, HLA-DM is delivered from the endoplasmic reticulum to MIIC, where HLA-DM facilitates the exchange of CLIP with antigenic peptides that bind to MHC-II molecules. DCs subsequently export the MHC-II-peptide complex to the plasma membrane and present this complex to the TCR of an antigen-specific CD4+ T cell to initiate its activation.

ζ chains through an Src homology 2 (SH2) domain. Activated ZAP-70 propagates signal transduction by catalyzing the phosphorylation of downstream transducers such as LAT (linker activator for T cells), TRIM (T-cell receptor interacting molecule), SLP-76, and Vav-1. These proximal events initiate the activation of multiple downstream signaling cascades involving extracellular signal-related kinase (ERK), NFAT, JNK, and NF-κB pathways, which ultimately lead to the activation of antigen-primed T cells (257).

The NF-κB pathway is essential for the activation, survival, proliferation, and differentiation of antigen-activated

T cells (258). Similar to BCR signaling, TCR signaling activates phospholipase C-gamma (PLC γ), which hydrolyzes the membrane-associated lipid phosphatidylinositol-4,5-biphosphate (PIP2) to generate inositol-1,4,5-trisphosphate (IP3) and diacylglycerol (DAG). While IP3 induces the release of intracellular calcium, DAG activates protein kinase C θ (PKCθ). This PKC family member activates a downstream NF-κB–activating signaling module that includes CARMA1, Bcl-10, and MALT1 (259). In particular, PKCθ phosphorylates the CARD of CARMA1, and thereafter CARMA1 interacts with the CARD domain of Bcl-10, a Bcl family member that binds MALT1

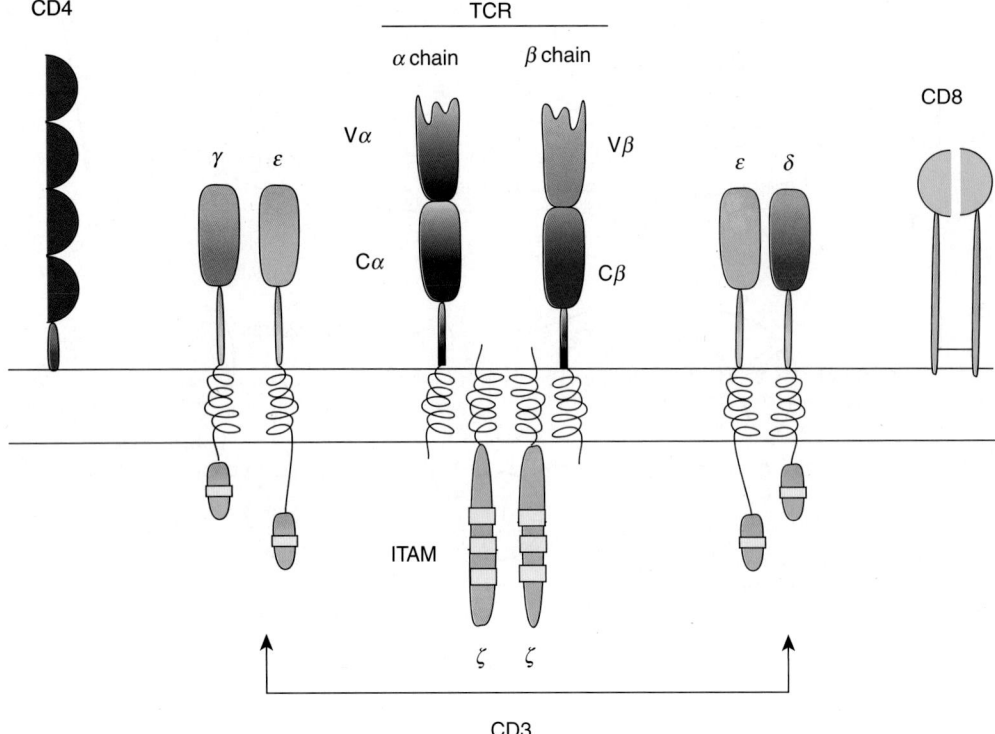

FIGURE 2.11. Structure of the TCR signaling complex. The TCR is composed of $\alpha\beta$ or $\gamma\delta$ chains that are noncovalently linked to CD3 signaling subunits, including $\gamma\varepsilon$ and $\delta\varepsilon$ heterodimers and $\zeta\zeta$ homodimer. The intracellular domain of each CD3δ, CD3ε, and CD3γ molecule contains one ITAM required for signal transduction. CD3ζ chain has three ITAMs. The TCR complex also includes CD4 or CD8 co-receptors that are needed for the interaction with MHC-II and MHC-I molecules, respectively, on APCs.

(260,261). The resulting CARMA1-Bcl-10-MALT1 complex moves to TCR-containing lipid rafts to activate IκB kinase (IKK), an oligoenzyme composed of two IKKα and IKKβ catalytic subunits and an IKKγ (or NEMO)-regulatory subunit. IKK catalyzes the phosphorylation, ubiquitylation, and degradation of IκB proteins, which retain NF-κB dimers in a cytoplasmic inactive state under resting conditions. Then, IκB-free NF-κB translocates to the nucleus to initiate the transcription of genes required for the activation, survival, proliferation, and differentiation of T cells.

DC-T-Cell Interaction

The sustained interaction of the TCR with an MHC-peptide complex causes the formation of an increasingly stable and organized area of intercellular contact known as immunologic synapse, which orchestrates TCR-mediated signal transduction (262). The immunologic synapse is structured in a bull's eye arrangement of supramolecular activation clusters (SMACs) that form within a few minutes after the initial contact of a T cell with an APC (Fig. 2.12). The central portion of the SMAC contains molecules of the TCR-CD3 complex, including CD4 or CD8 and PKCθ, whereas the peripheral portion of the SMAC contains the integrin adhesion molecule LFA-1 and talin (263). By stabilizing interactions that can last for 10 to 24 hours, the immunologic synapse plays a critical role in the optimal activation of T cells and in their adaptation to different levels and strengths of antigen receptor signaling. The affinity of the TCR for antigen strongly influences the quality of the T-cell response. Generally, the activation and proliferation of T cells involve a high-affinity interaction of the TCR with an MHC-bound peptide (264).

The activation requirements and type of response vary in different subsets of T cells. Naïve T cells continuously circulate

from the blood to secondary lymphoid organs to sample antigens presented by DCs in the context of MHC-II. Although necessary, binding of TCR by antigen is not sufficient to activate T cells. Indeed, antigen-primed T cells also need costimulatory signals that are provided by DCs after activation. DCs become activated in response to signals from microbial products, for example, TLR ligands, cytokines—for example, IFN-α, IFN-β, IFN-γ, and TNF—and/or T-cell molecules, for example, CD40 ligand. These signals induce DCs to express higher surface levels of MHC-II and T-cell costimulatory molecules such as B7.1 (CD80) and B7.2 (CD86) (265). In the absence of B7 costimulatory signals, antigen-activated T cells do not form a stable immunologic synapse and either die by apoptosis or become anergic (266).

Engagement of CD28 on T cells by B7.1 and B7.2 on activated DCs stimulates the activation, proliferation, and differentiation of antigen-primed T cells (267). Conversely, activated T cells up-regulate the expression of the TNF receptor (TNFR) family member CD40 ligand (CD40, or CD154), which engages CD40 on APCs. By inducing up-regulation of B7.1 and B7.2 expression, signals from CD40 enhance the maturation of DCs and the activation of T cells. Activated DCs also express CD70 and 4-1BBL (CD137L), which deliver additional costimulatory signals to T cells by engaging CD27 and 4-1BB (CD137) receptors, respectively (268). Of note, different subsets of T cells have distinct requirements for costimulatory signals. Indeed, compared to naïve T cells, effector and memory T cells require less costimulatory signals to become activated. For this reason, effector and memory T cells can be activated not only by professional APCs such as activated DCs but also by less specialized APCs such as activated macrophages and B cells.

In the presence of costimulatory signals, antigen-activated T cells secrete the cytokine IL-2 and up-regulate the expression of the IL-2 receptor (IL-2R), which delivers vigorous

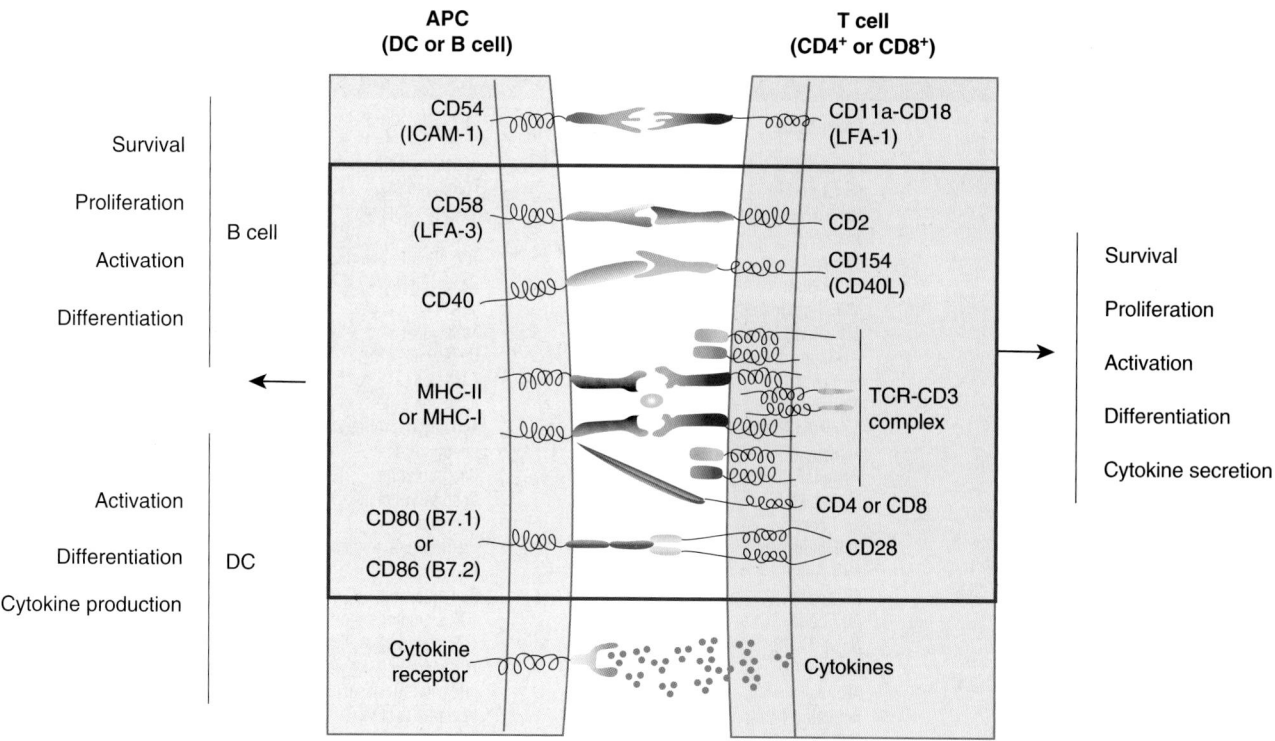

FIGURE 2.12. Composition of the immunologic synapse. Main molecular interactions in the immunologic synapse that connect an APC (DC or B-cell) with a T cell (CD4+ or CD8+). Such interactions are organized in a structure called SMAC. The center of the SMAC (central purple frame) includes interactions between the MHC-peptide complex and the TCR-CD3 complex as well as interactions between costimulatory accessory molecules such as CD80, CD86, CD40, CD58, and their cognate receptors/ligands, including CD28, CD40L, and CD2, respectively. The periphery of the SMAC includes interactions between the adhesion molecule ICAM-1 and the integrin complex LFA-1.

proliferation signals to mediate the expansion phase of a T-cell response (269). As discussed later, other cytokines different from IL-2 induce the differentiation of uncommitted CD4+ T cells into T_H1, T_H2, T_H17, and T_H22 effector cells or the differentiation of CD8+ T cells into CTLs. Importantly, the activation of T cells by DCs is regulated by negative feedback signals emanating from CTLA-4 (CD152), a CD28-related receptor that delivers powerful inhibitory signals after engaging B7.1 and B7.2 on DCs (270). These and other negative signals dominate the contraction phase of a T-cell response. Nevertheless, some antigen-specific T cells persist at the end of a primary response to generate a pool of quiescent long-lived memory T cells that undergo quick IL-2–dependent expansion after secondary exposure to antigen (271). This secondary response occurs more rapidly than a primary response, because memory T cells have less stringent requirements for antigen and costimulatory signals. As in a primary T-cell response, the initial expansion phase of a secondary T-cell response is followed by a contraction phase in which most antigen-activated T cells die by apoptosis.

T- and B-Cell Interaction

Activation of B cells by antigen involves the cognate interaction of antigen-presenting B cells with a specialized subset of CD4+ T cells known as T_{FH} cells (62). These T_{FH} cells provide helper signals to B cells such as cytokines and CD40L, a molecule essential for the initiation of the germinal center reaction and the induction of class-switched IgG, IgA, and IgE antibodies (272). Binding of antigen by the BCR is followed by antigen internalization and processing to form a peptide-MHC-II complex that is presented to T_{FH} cells in the context of a cognate interaction (230,273). Antigen binding to the BCR initiates a cascade of signaling events that are further detailed

in one of the following sections of this chapter. These events up-regulate the expression of MHC-II and costimulatory B7.1 and B7.2 molecules (274,275). The resulting activated B cells function as efficient APCs that provide key stimulatory signals to T_{FH} cells. B cells establish cognate interactions with T_{FH} cells in at least two areas of the lymphoid follicle: a first interaction occurs at the interface between the T-cell zone and the B-cell follicle (also known as T-B boundary), whereas a second interaction takes place in the germinal center. In all these cognate interactions, B cells form an immunologic synapse with T_{FH} cells expressing powerful B-cell–stimulating factors such as CD40L and the cytokines IL-4, IL-10, and IL-21 (276,277). These stimuli induce antigen-activated B cells to undergo proliferation; antibody affinity maturation through somatic hypermutation (SHM); class switching from IgM to IgG, IgA, or IgE; and differentiation to memory B cells or antibody-secreting plasma cells (62). The key role of CD40L-CD40 interaction is exemplified by cases of hyper-IgM syndrome (HIGM) caused by deleterious mutations of the genes encoding the CD40L or CD40 molecules (272). The resulting primary antibody deficiency is characterized by the absence of germinal centers in secondary lymphoid organs; severe reduction of class-switched IgG, IgA, and IgE antibodies; and impaired affinity maturation (278).

T Cells

General Principles

T cells include two genotypically distinct populations defined as $\alpha\beta$ T cells, which express an $\alpha\beta$ TCR, and $\gamma\delta$ T cells, which express a $\gamma\delta$ TCR (279). These T-cell populations can be further divided into phenotypically and functionally distinct subsets known as CD4+ T cells and CD8+ T cells (Table 2.4).

Table 2.4	COMMON T-CELL–SURFACE MOLECULES	
Name	**Expression**	**Function**
CD2 (LFA-2, CD58L)	All T cells	Adhesion, activation
CD3	All T cells	TCR signaling
CD4	MHC-II–restricted T cells, T_H cells, Treg cells	MHC-II co-receptor
CD5	All T cells	TCR signaling inhibitor
CD7	All T cells	Costimulation
CD8	MHC-I–restricted T cells	MHC-I co-receptor
CD9	Activated T cells	Adhesion
CD10	T-cell precursors	Unknown
CD11a (LFA-1)	All T cells	Adhesion
CD18	All T cells	Adhesion
CD25 (IL-2Rα)	Activated T cells, Treg cells	Activation, proliferation, immunoregulation
CD26	Activated T cells	Costimulation
CD27 (CD70R)	Medullary thymocytes, T-cell subsets	Costimulation
CD28	All T cells	Costimulation
CD29	All T cells	Adhesion
CD30	Activated T cells	Proliferation, apoptosis
CD43 (sialophorin)	All T cells	Adhesion
CD44	All T cells	Cell adhesion
CD45	All T cells	TCR signaling regulator
CD45RA	Naïve T cells	TCR signaling regulator
CD45RO	Memory T cells	TCR signaling regulator
CD49a	All T cells	Integrin that associates with CD29
CD54 (ICAM-1)	Activated T cells	Receptor for LFA-1
CD56 (N-CAM)	NKT cells	Adhesion
CD57	T_{FH} cells	Adhesion
CD58 (LFA-3, CD2R)	All T cells	Adhesion
CD62L (L-selectin)	Naïve and memory T cells	Adhesion, homing
CD69	Activated T cells	Activation
CD70 (CD27L)	Activated T cells	Costimulation
CD90 (Thy-1)	Thymocytes	Unknown
CD95 (Fas)	Activated T cells	Apoptosis
CD103 (integrin)	Mucosal T cells	Homing
CD154 (CD40L)	Activated T cells, T_{FH} cells, Treg cells	B-cell survival, activation, proliferation, class switching
CD185 (CXCR5)	Activated T cells, T_{FH} cells	Migration to the germinal center
CD278 (ICOS)	T_{FH} cells	Costimulation
CD279 (PD-1)	T_{FH} cells	TCR signaling inhibitor

$\alpha\beta$ T cells are by far the most frequent T cells in the immune system and include CD4+ and CD8+ T-cell subsets that are defined by the surface expression of either CD4 or CD8 co-receptors. CD4 and CD8 co-receptors are TCR-associated cell surface molecules that utilize their extracellular domain to bind invariant determinants of MHC molecules and their intracellular domain to amplify signals emanating from the TCR-CD3 complex (280,281).

$\gamma\delta$ T cells are a heterogeneous group of CD4+ and CD8+ T cells that are mostly located in epithelial barriers separating internal tissues from the external environment, including the skin, lung, and intestine. At these sites, $\gamma\delta$ T cells are thought to form a first line of rapid immune defense. Some $\gamma\delta$ T cells are also present in the peripheral blood and secondary lymphoid tissues. Compared to $\alpha\beta$ T cells, $\gamma\delta$ T cells express a less diversified TCR and therefore tend to recognize stereotyped antigens. Of note, the TCR repertoire of $\gamma\delta$ T cells strikingly differs in distinct anatomic sites, suggesting that $\gamma\delta$ T cells recognize ligands specifically expressed in infected or stressed cells present in specific sites (282,283).

CD4+ T cells are MHC-II–restricted lymphocytes that differentiate into T_H cells after recognizing extracellular antigens in association with MHC-II molecules. The CD4+ T-cell subset also includes Treg cells that are actively involved in the preservation of immune tolerance (36). In contrast to CD8+ T cells, CD4+ T cells are classically activated by extracellular antigens presented by professional APCs such as DCs. Proteins taken up by DCs through endocytosis or phagocytosis are subsequently processed to form a MHC II-peptide complex that is presented to the TCR on CD4+ T cells. Depending on the cytokine milieu in which antigen presentation takes place, CD4+ T cells differentiate into various T_H-cell effector subsets (28).

CD8+ T cells are MHC-I–restricted lymphocytes that differentiate into CTLs after encountering intracellular antigens in association with MHC-I molecules. These molecules typically upload short peptides that are generated in the cytoplasm of any cell type as a result of protein degradation by the proteasome. Therefore, CD8+ T cells are mainly activated by peptides derived from intracellular pathogens such as viruses (284). However, CD8+ T cells can also be activated by extracellular antigens in a process referred to as cross-priming, which is only mediated by DCs (285,286). CTLs kill infected or neoplastic cells that present antigenic peptides in association with MHC-I molecules. Killing occurs through the release of pore-forming perforin proteins that are stored in specific intracellular granules. Perforin forms channels on the membrane of the target cell, which allow death-inducing molecules such as granzymes A and B to enter the target cell. Alternatively, CTLs kill target cells by expressing FasL, a TNF family member that engages the death-inducing receptor Fas (or CD95) on target cells. Both these process initiate programmed cell death or apoptosis through the activation of the caspase pathway (287).

T-Cell Development

T cells arise from bone marrow-derived hematopoietic progenitors that migrate to the thymus. Their proliferation and maturation requires dynamic relocation of developing lymphocytes, named thymocytes, into the multiple environments of the thymus (288). Signals from nonhematopoietic stromal cells, including various types of thymic epithelial cells and mesenchymal fibroblasts, play a crucial role in the regulation of T-cell development and selection (289).

The process of T-cell maturation involves sequential developmental stages characterized by TCR gene recombination events, positive selection of T cells capable of recognizing self MHC molecules, and negative selection of T cells with excessive affinity for self antigens (Fig. 2.13). After entry in the thymus, progenitor cells named early thymic progenitors (ETPs) differentiate into double-negative (DN) thymocytes that are committed to the T-cell lineage (290). The initial phase of thymocyte development is highly dependent on stromal signals involving Notch receptor ligands, stem cell factor, fms-like tyrosine kinase 3 ligand, and IL-7. The latter promotes the survival, proliferation, and development of ETPs and their further progression through subsequent developmental stages (291). Recently, the Bcl-11b transcription factor has been involved in the commitment of ETPs to the T-cell lineage (292).

DN thymocytes express neither the TCR nor the CD4 or CD8 molecules and differentiate in the thymic cortex through a series of DN1, DN2, DN3, and DN4 developmental stages defined by specific expression patterns of surface CD117, CD25, and CD44 molecules (293,294). DN1 cells express CD117 and CD44 and progress to the DN2 stage by up-regulating CD25 expression in response to thymic environmental signals. At this stage, a recombinase machinery composed of recombination activation gene 1 (RAG1) and RAG2 endonucleases initiates

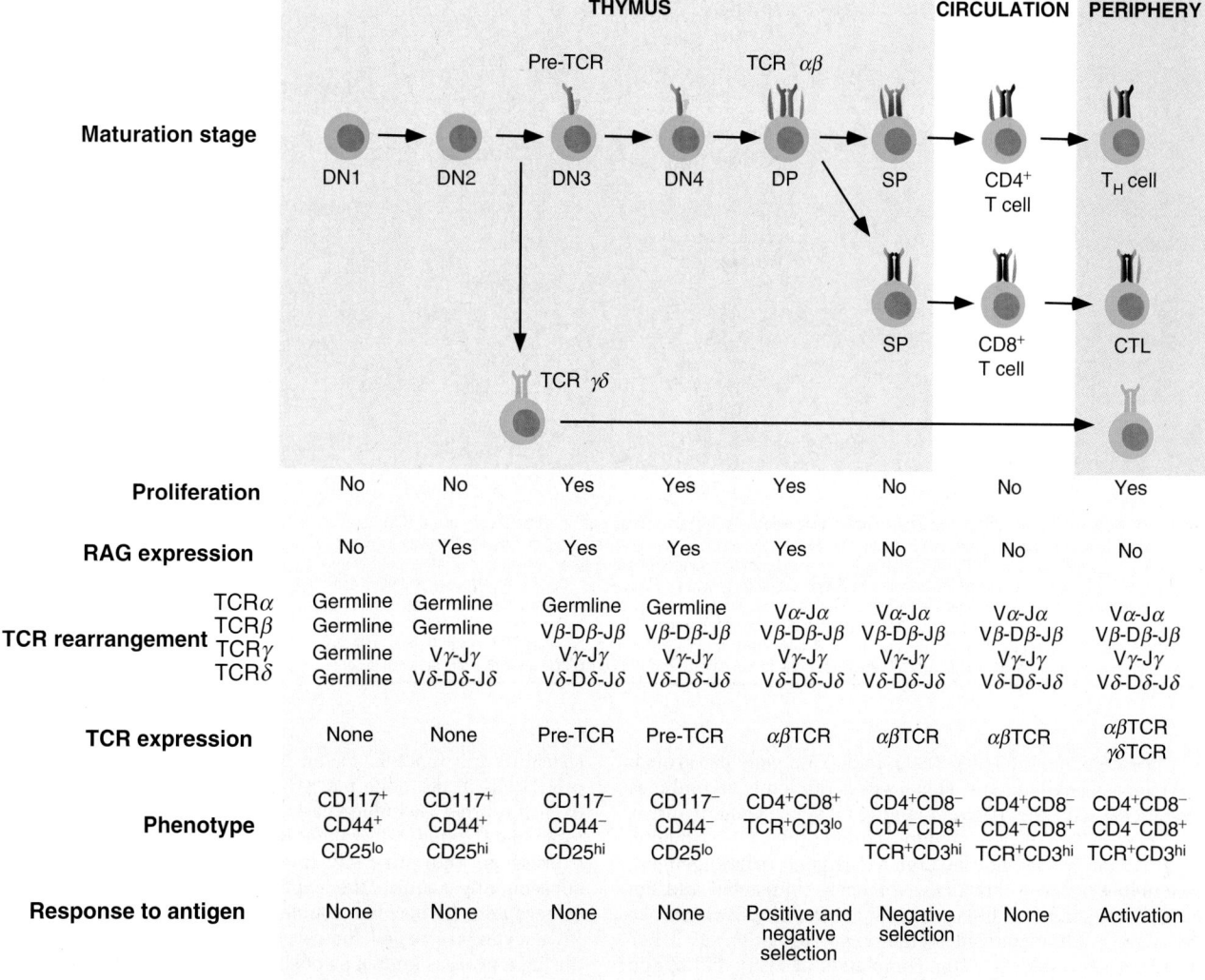

	DN1	DN2	DN3	DN4	DP	SP	CD4+ T cell / SP / CD8+ T cell	T_H cell / CTL
Proliferation	No	No	Yes	Yes	Yes	No	No	Yes
RAG expression	No	Yes	Yes	Yes	Yes	No	No	No
TCR rearrangement TCRα	Germline	Germline	Germline	Germline	Vα-Jα	Vα-Jα	Vα-Jα	Vα-Jα
TCRβ	Germline	Germline	Vβ-Dβ-Jβ	Vβ-Dβ-Jβ	Vβ-Dβ-Jβ	Vβ-Dβ-Jβ	Vβ-Dβ-Jβ	Vβ-Dβ-Jβ
TCRγ	Germline	Vγ-Jγ	Vγ-Jγ	Vγ-Jγ	Vγ-Jγ	Vγ-Jγ	Vγ-Jγ	Vγ-Jγ
TCRδ	Germline	Vδ-Dδ-Jδ	Vδ-Dδ-Jδ	Vδ-Dδ-Jδ	Vδ-Dδ-Jδ	Vδ-Dδ-Jδ	Vδ-Dδ-Jδ	Vδ-Dδ-Jδ
TCR expression	None	None	Pre-TCR	Pre-TCR	αβTCR	αβTCR	αβTCR	αβTCR γδTCR
Phenotype	CD117+ CD44+ CD25lo	CD117+ CD44+ CD25hi	CD117− CD44− CD25hi	CD117− CD44− CD25lo	CD4+CD8+ TCR+CD3lo	CD4+CD8− CD4−CD8+ TCR+CD3hi	CD4+CD8− CD4−CD8+ TCR+CD3hi	CD4+CD8− CD4−CD8+ TCR+CD3hi
Response to antigen	None	None	None	None	Positive and negative selection	Negative selection	None	Activation

FIGURE 2.13. Development of T cells in the thymus. Early thymic progenitor cells migrate from the bone marrow to the thymus, where they initiate the antigen-independent phase of T-cell development. In the thymic cortex, double-negative (DN) thymocytes lack both CD4 and CD8 and progress along DN1, DN2, DN3, and DN4 stages to become double-positive (DP) thymocytes that express both CD4 and CD8. At the DN2 to DN3 transition, thymocytes either give rise to a small population of γδ T cells that lack CD4 and CD8 or further develop into DN3, DN4, DP, and SP thymocytes. Each of these maturation stages is characterized by specific changes in proliferation, RAG expression, TCR gene recombination, TCR protein expression, surface phenotype, and responsiveness to antigen. DP thymocytes that recognize self-peptide–MHC complexes on cortical epithelial cells are positively selected and differentiate to SP cells, whereas DP thymocytes that do not receive survival signals from antigen (about 97%) are negatively selected and undergo death by apoptosis. After undergoing an additional round of negative selection in the thymic medulla, SP thymocytes generate CD4+ and CD8+ T cells that express a conventional αβ TCR. These CD4+ and CD8+ T cells further differentiate into effector T_H cells and CTLs, respectively, after encountering antigen in peripheral lymphoid tissues.

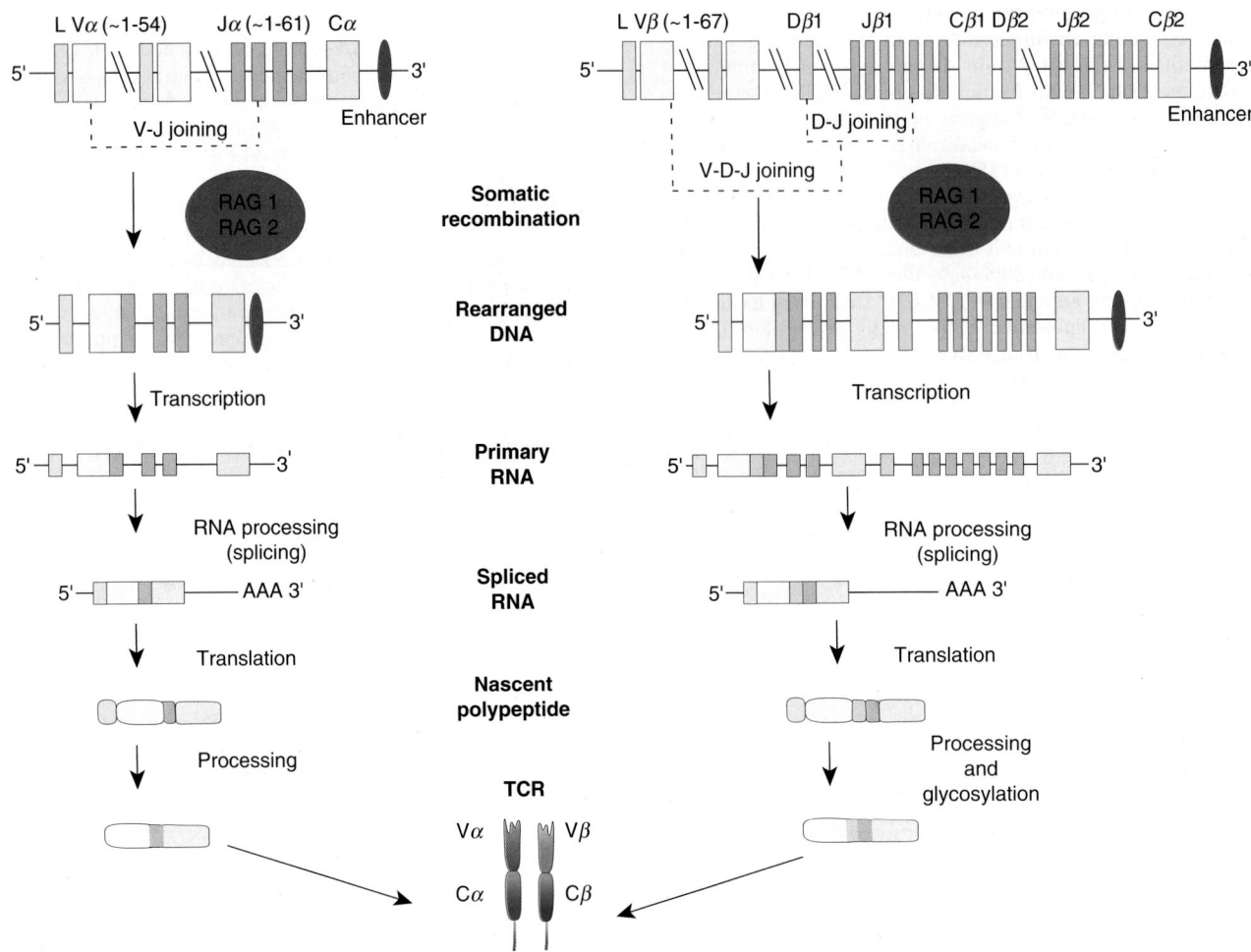

FIGURE 2.14. Mechanism underlying the generation of TCR molecules. The TCR loci include multiple cassettes of V and J (TCRα locus) and V, D, and J (TCRβ locus) gene segments that undergo random rearrangement during thymic T-cell development through a process involving RAG1 and RAG2 proteins. In the TCRα locus, a Vα gene segment rearranges with a Jα gene segment to generate a VαJα exon. Transcription of VαJα and subsequent splicing of VαJα mRNA to Cα mRNA generates a VαJα-Cα mRNA that is polyadenylated (AAA) and then translated into a mature TCRα chain protein. In the TCRβ locus, similar recombination and transcription events lead to the formation of VβDβJβ and Cβ mRNAs that undergo splicing and polyadenylation to generate a mature TCRβ chain protein. In each TCR locus, V gene transcription initiates at the level of a leader (L) sequence positioned upstream of each V segment. Ultimately, TCRα and β chain proteins are paired to generate a membrane-bound αβ TCR heterodimer. The formation of the γδ TCR heterodimer involves a similar mechanism.

the rearrangement of TCRγ, TCRδ, and TCRβ gene loci trough V(D)J gene recombination. This process randomly recombines variable (V), diversity (D), and joining (J) gene segments organized in each TCR locus as multiple families (Fig. 2.14). Of note, the TCRα locus does not undergo V(D)J gene rearrangement, presumably because this locus is densely compacted and not accessible to the recombinase machinery at the DN2 stage. The DN3 stage is characterized by the down-regulation of CD117 and CD44 expression and the completion of TCRγ, TCRδ, and TCRβ gene rearrangements, which leads to the formation of fully functional TCRγ, TCRδ, and TCRβ proteins. The transition from DN2 to DN3 developmental stages is also associated with the commitment of thymocytes toward an αβ or γδ lineage. This commitment depends on the strength of signals emanating from the newly assembled γδ TCR. A strong signal from γδ TCR results in the commitment of DN2 cells to γδ T cells, whereas a weak signal promotes the generation of αβ T cells (295,296).

In the DN3 stage, the newly rearranged TCRβ chain associates with the invariant pre-TCRα (pTα) chain and with CD3 molecules to form a pre-TCR complex that is analogous in structure and function to the pre-BCR complex expressed by pre-B cells in the bone marrow (297,298). Signals emanating from the pre-TCR induce cessation of TCRβ chain gene rearrangement, rapid cell proliferation, down-regulation of CD25 expression, and entry into the DN4 stage (299). Thymocytes subsequently acquire the expression of both CD4 and CD8 co-receptors to become double-positive (DP) cells. These DP thymocytes are tested for recognition of self-MHC molecules during a process known as positive selection (300). During this phase, DP thymocytes undergo productive rearrangement of the TCRα locus and eventually assemble a fully competent surface αβ TCR. Similar to the Igκ and Igλ light chain loci in B cells, the TCRα locus lacks D gene segments and undergoes productive rearrangement only after expression of a partner TCRβ chain. In addition, the TCRα locus lacks orientation, and the multiplicity of V and J gene segments allows successive gene rearrangements until positive selection or cell death occurs. Positive selection occurs in the thymic cortex and requires interaction of DP thymocytes expressing αβ TCR with epithelial cells presenting self-peptides in the context of MHC molecules.

This process leads to the selection of a few DP cells expressing a TCR with appropriate affinity for peptide-MHC complexes. All the DP thymocytes that do not receive survival signals from the TCR undergo programmed cell death (301,302).

The outcome of positive selection is ultimately the commitment of DP cells to a CD4 or CD8 lineage. DP cells selected by TCR interaction with MHC-I molecules develop into CD4⁻CD8⁺ single-positive (SP) thymocytes, whereas DP cells selected by TCR interaction with MHC-II molecules differentiate into CD4⁺CD8⁻ SP thymocytes (303,304). How the TCR specificity dictates the CD4 versus CD8 lineage choice is unclear, but it is now widely accepted that the kinetics of TCR signaling plays an important role in the determination of the fate of DP cells (305,306). In this kinetic signaling model, DP thymocytes first down-regulate the expression of CD8 and then express the IL-7 receptor. The subsequent lineage choice depends on the persistence of signals from MHC-engaged TCR molecules. If termination of CD8 expression does not result in the loss of TCR signals, the CD8 gene remains silent and intermediate CD4⁺CD8⁻ thymocytes fully commit to the CD4 lineage. In contrast, loss of TCR signals following termination of CD8 expression triggers activation of signaling via the IL-7 receptor. This event induces intermediate CD4⁺CD8⁻ thymocytes to down-regulate the expression of CD4, up-regulate the expression of CD8, and differentiate into mature CD8⁺ T cells (307).

Following positive selection, SP thymocytes migrate to the thymic medulla, where they undergo negative selection or clonal deletion. Negative selection eliminates potentially self-reactive T cells and is also referred to as central tolerance (308). During this process, thymocytes expressing a TCR with high affinity for a self-peptide are deleted by apoptosis, whereas thymocytes expressing a TCR with low affinity for a self-peptide receive rescue signals that block their death by neglect (309). In order to establish tolerance, antigens from various peripheral tissues are actively transcribed by epithelial cells, macrophages, and DCs populating the thymic medulla and presented to SP thymocytes in the context of MHC molecules (310,311). The resulting ectopic expression of tissue-restricted antigens, which is also known as promiscuous gene expression, seems to be promoted by a thymic protein called autoimmune regulator (AIRE). Consistent with this, AIRE-deficient mice do not express subsets of tissue-restricted antigens and develop organ-specific autoimmune diseases (312). Similarly, humans with deleterious mutations of the gene encoding AIRE develop a rare autoimmune disease known as autoimmune polyendocrinopathy-candidiasis-ectodermal dystrophy (313,314). Following negative selection, mature naïve T cells migrate toward postcapillary venules located at the corticomedullary junction and enter the general circulation to colonize secondary lymphoid organs (315).

T-Cell Responses

Naïve T cells continuously recirculate from the blood to T-cell areas of secondary lymphoid organs, where they screen the surface of local DCs for the presence of antigenic peptide-MHC complexes (316). In the presence of appropriate costimulatory signals, engagement of TCR by antigen causes extensive T-cell proliferation and differentiation of effector T cells and leads to the establishment of immunologic memory (317). Of note, certain molecules known as superantigens can simultaneously bind the Vβ domain of certain TCRs and the α chain of MHC-II to induce massive activation and proliferation of T cells regardless of their antigen specificity. By co-engaging TCR and MHC molecules in an unconventional manner, superantigens such as staphylococcal enterotoxins, tetanus shock syndrome toxin, and exfoliative dermatitis toxin cause massive activation of T cells, which is followed by overproduction of T-cell cytokines and systemic toxicity.

Primary T-cell responses are characterized by a well-defined sequence of functionally distinct phases. In the *expansion phase*, antigen-specific T cells undergo clonal proliferation and differentiate into T$_H$ cells and CTLs that carry out specific effector functions. T$_H$ cells release specific sets of cytokines that activate both innate and adaptive immune effector cells, whereas CTLs kill target cells expressing microbe (mostly virus)- or tumor-associated antigens (318). The expansion of T cells primarily involves IL-2 and IL-15, two growth-inducing cytokines secreted by activated T cells and innate immune cells, respectively (319). The differentiation of T cells into specific T$_H$-cell subsets requires a specific cytokine milieu and distinct sets of transcriptional factors that will be described in the section describing TH cell subsets. The expansion phase is followed by a *contraction phase* in which the majority of effector T cells die by apoptosis.

The few antigen-activated T cells left after the contraction phase develop into long-lived but functionally quiescent memory T cells (320). Compared to naïve T cells, memory T cells show more rapid and robust responses to antigenic stimulation, which renders them capable of conferring prompt protection upon secondary exposure to the same antigen. Memory T cells can be further distinguished into central memory and effector memory T-cell subsets that are characterized by distinct functional and homing properties (321). Central memory T cells have a CD62L^{hi}CCR7^{hi} phenotype, localize in secondary lymphoid tissues, and mainly produce IL-2 following TCR engagement by antigen. Effector memory T cells express a CD62L^{lo}CCR7^{lo} phenotype, localize in both secondary lymphoid and peripheral tissues, and promptly develop specific effector functions upon TCR engagement by antigen. While effector memory T cells provide an immediate line of immune defense at sites of pathogen entry, central memory T cells replenish and sustain the pool of effector T cells by undergoing rapid expansion and differentiation in secondary lymphoid organs (321).

T-Cell Effector Subsets

T$_H$ cells represent a heterogeneous population of CD4⁺ T cells that were originally identified for their ability to help B cells and enhance antibody-mediated immunity (322). Later, T$_H$ cells were also found to enhance cell-mediated immunity, including delayed-type hypersensitivity, which involves an inflammatory reaction characterized by the activation of macrophages by T$_H$ cells. In general, T$_H$ cells are essential to orchestrate adaptive immune responses, and their formation involves a cognate interaction between DCs and naïve CD4⁺ T cells lodged in draining lymph nodes. DC migration from peripheral tissues to draining lymph nodes is facilitated by chemokines and cytokines that are produced by local immune and stromal cells in response to intruding microbes (323). After establishing a cognate interaction with DCs, CD4⁺ T cells differentiate into distinct subsets of effector T$_H$ cells characterized by well-defined cytokine secretion patterns and effector functions. The typology of T$_H$-cell differentiation involves the production of polarizing cytokines by local immune and stromal cells and the expression of lineage-specifying transcription factors by antigen-activated CD4⁺ T cells. The differentiation of CD8⁺ T cells into effector CTLs is less complex and has been described in the section describing general principles of T cell biology.

The main subsets of T$_H$ cells include T$_H$1, T$_H$2, T$_H$17, T$_H$22, and T$_{FH}$ cells specializing in IFN-γ, IL-4, IL-17, IL-22, and IL-21 production, respectively. Recently T$_H$9 cells specialized in IL-9 production were also described, at least in mice. Furthermore, there are Treg cells specializing in TGF-β and IL-10 production. The development of T$_H$ and Treg cells is instructed by polarizing cytokines released by local immune cells. For instance, *T$_H$1* differentiation is promoted by IL-12, IFN-γ, and IFN-α, whereas T_H2 differentiation involves IL-4 (324–326). T_H2 cells undergo T_H9 differentiation in response to TGF-β and IL-4 (327–329), whereas TGF-β and IL-21 trigger T_H17 development (330–333). T_H22 differentiation involves IL-6 and TNF (334,335), whereas T_{FH} differentiation requires IL-21 (225,336–340).

In the absence of IL-6, TGF-β promotes the formation of peripheral *Treg* cells, also known as inducible iTreg cells to distinguish them from natural (or central) nTreg cells (330–333). iTreg and nTreg cells comparably suppress inflammatory T_H-cell responses, but have a distinct ontogeny. Importantly, T_H-cell–derived cytokines not only induce specific sets of effector functions but also suppress the emergence of alternative T_H differentiation fates. For example, IFN-γ from T_H1 cells suppresses the development of T_H2 and T_H17 cells, whereas IL-4 from T_H2 cells inhibits the emergence of T_H1 and T_H17 cells (341–345). In addition, TGF-β from Treg cells inhibits the induction of T_H1 and T_H2 cells (341–345).

The commitment of naïve CD4$^+$ T cells toward T_H or Treg cells occurs through a stepwise differentiation process that is regulated by specific transcription factors. During T_H1 differentiation, IFN-γ from TLR-activated NK cells and IFN-α from TLR-activated DCs activate signal transducer and activator of transcription (STAT)-1 in naïve CD4$^+$ T cells. STAT-1 up-regulates the expression of *Tbet*, a master regulator of T_H1 differentiation that induces early IFN-γ production and up-regulates IL-12R expression in T_H cells. Next, IL-12 from TLR-activated DCs or macrophages binds the IL-12R on T_H cells to induce the transcription factor STAT-4, which enhances IFN-γ production and sustains IL-12R expression by T_H cells (346–349). T_H2 differentiation involves the release of IL-4 by either naïve T_H cells in response to antigen or mast cells and basophils in response to microbial products. Binding of IL-4 to its receptor on T_H cells activates STAT-6, which in turn up-regulates *Gata3*, the master regulator of T_H2 differentiation. STAT-6 and Gata3 induce the secretion of copious amounts of IL-4, IL-5, and IL-13 by activated T_H2 cells (346,350–353). The differentiation of Treg cells requires *Foxp3*, a transcription factor induced by CD4$^+$ T cells in response to signals from antigen and IL-2. Induction of Foxp3 in iTreg cells also requires TGF-β and retinoic acid from DCs (354–356).

In the presence of IL-4, TGF-β stimulates T_H2 cells to express the transcription factors PU1 and IRF-4, thereby stimulating the conversion of T_H2 cells into T_H9 cells, at least in mice (357–359). In humans, T_H9 differentiation involves Gata3, whereas the role of PU1 and IRF-4 remains unknown. In the presence of IL-21, TGF-β induces *RORγt*, the master regulator of T_H17 differentiation. While TGF-β and IL-21 trigger T_H17 differentiation from naïve T_H cells, IL-1β, IL-6, and IL-23 enhance the expansion of already differentiated and memory T_H17 cells (360–363). Finally, T_{FH} differentiation requires the induction of the transcription factor *Bcl-6* by IL-21. In addition to promoting germinal center B-cell differentiation, Bcl-6 antagonizes T_H1, T_H2, and T_H17 differentiation and instead turns on a genetic program favoring T_{FH} differentiation (28,336,348,351,364–367). Of note, Tbet, Gata3, RORγt, Bcl-6, and Foxp3 proteins are both necessary and sufficient to induce T_H1, T_H2, T_H17, T_{FH}, and Treg polarization, respectively. It remains unclear whether a specific transcription factor regulates T_H22 differentiation, but some evidence points to the involvement of *AhR*, an aryl-hydrocarbon receptor that regulates gene transcription.

T$_H$-Cell Effector Functions

Effector T_H subsets (Fig. 2.15) are identified according to their inducing transcription factors and cytokine expression profiles (368).

T_H1 cells predominantly mediate adaptive immune responses against intracellular pathogens and contribute to the pathogenesis of inflammatory disorders by releasing IFN-γ, TNF, and IL-2 (369,370). While IFN-γ and TNF enhance the ability of macrophages and other nonspecific innate immune cells to phagocytose and destroy pathogens, IFN-γ and IL-2 augment the expansion and cytolytic function of CD8$^+$ T cells (371). In addition, IFN-γ enhances IgG2 and IgG3 production by B cells, at least in mice.

T_H2 cells mostly mediate immune responses against extracellular pathogens, including helminths, and contribute to the pathogenesis of allergic disorders by releasing IL-4, IL-5, and IL-13 (372–374). IL-4 stabilizes T_H2 polarization, provides an alternative pathway for macrophage activation, and induces B-cell production of IgG1 and IgE. In contrast, IL-5 triggers the mobilization, maturation, and recruitment of eosinophils. Finally, IL-13 elicits goblet cell differentiation, mucus secretion, and tissue repair (375–379).

T_H9 cells emerge from T_H2 progenitors, and therefore, it is not surprising that these cells contribute to the pathogenesis of allergic and inflammatory disorders through a mechanism involving the release of IL-9 (328,329,380).

T_H17 cells enhance adaptive immune responses against commensals and pathogens at mucosal sites and contribute to the pathogenesis of inflammatory disorders by releasing IL-17 (381–385). IL-17 is also known as IL-17A and represents the founding member of a cytokine family that also includes IL-17B, IL-17C, IL-17D, IL-17E (or IL-25), and IL-17F. Among its multiple functional effects, IL-17 enhances the recruitment and activation of neutrophils during the inflammatory phase of an immune response and promotes immunity and wound healing at mucosal sites and in the skin (386–392). T_H17 cells also produce IL-21, which is important for T_H17 differentiation and B-cell activation. Consistent with their key role in mucosal immunity, T_H17 cells further release IL-22 to enhance the expression of antimicrobial peptides by epithelial cells (393).

T_H22 cells play a key role in mucosal and cutaneous homeostasis by releasing IL-22 but not IL-17 (335,394). IL-22 is a member of the IL-10 cytokine family that stimulates the survival, differentiation, and antimicrobial activity of mucosal and cutaneous epithelial cells (395–397).

T_{FH} cells induce humoral immune responses against extracellular pathogens by releasing IL-21. Together with CD40L, IL-21 delivers survival, proliferation, and differentiation signals to B cells located at the T- and B-cell boundary and in the germinal center of lymphoid follicles (398–400). Early T_{FH} cells at the T- and B-cell border stimulate antigen-specific B cells to differentiate along one of two alternative pathways: an extra-follicular pathway that leads to the formation of IgM-secreting plasmablasts or a follicular pathway that leads to the differentiation of germinal center B cells. In the latter pathway, T_{FH} cells stimulate the survival, clonal expansion, selection, and differentiation of germinal center B cells, which give rise to either memory B cells or plasma cells expressing class-switched IgG, IgA, or IgE antibodies with high affinity for antigen (401,402). Of note, both germinal center T_{FH} cells and B cells require the transcription factor Bcl-6 to exert their functions and indeed the lack of Bcl-6 greatly impairs the antibody response to common protein antigens (366,367,403,404).

iTreg cells suppress polarized T_H cells through TGFβ and IL-10 (405,406). Together with nTreg cells, iTreg cells exert a tight control over immune responses against gut commensal bacteria to prevent the onset of local inflammatory tissue damage. In general, Treg cells are key negative regulators of adaptive immune responses and therefore play a primary function in immune tolerance and homeostasis (407). Consistent with this, Treg cells can inhibit the onset and development of autoimmune and inflammatory diseases (407). Treg cells exert their suppressive function not only by releasing TGF-β and IL-10 but also by inducing cell lysis, metabolic disruption, and inhibition of DC maturation and function (345,408–413). Remarkably, Treg cells also have some inductive functions. Indeed, Treg cells enhance intestinal immunity and homeostasis by

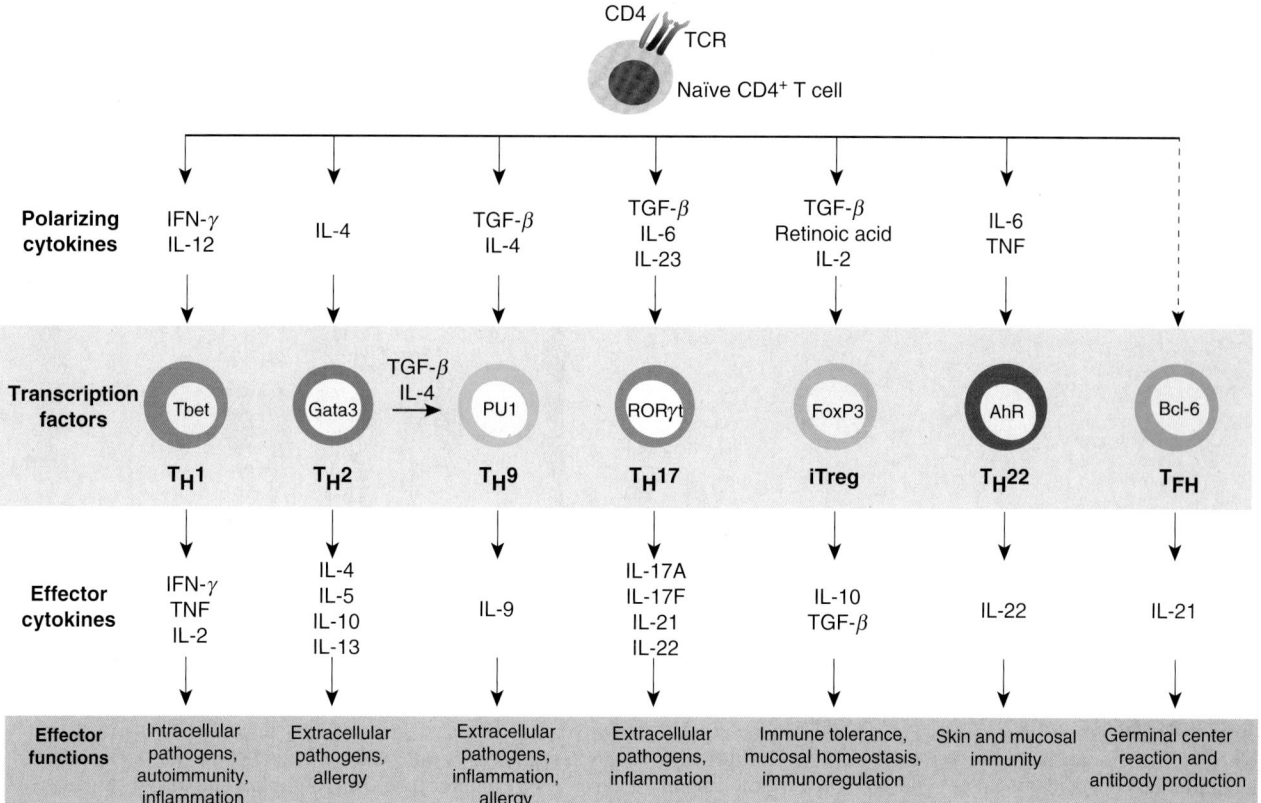

FIGURE 2.15. Development of effector T cells in the periphery. After activation by antigen, naïve CD4+ T cells can differentiate to multiple subsets of T_H cells that have specific effector functions. The differentiation of each T_H cell subset involves the induction of specific transcription factors by cytokines produced by innate immune cells and T cells. T_H1 cells require induction of the transcription factor T-bet by IL-12 and IFN-γ and secrete the effector cytokines IFN-γ, TNF, and IL-2, which promote immunity against intracellular pathogens and inflammation. T_H2 cells require induction of the transcription factor Gata3 by IL-4 and release the effector cytokines IL-4, IL-5, IL-10, and IL-13, which promote immunity against extracellular pathogens and allergic inflammation. T_H9 cells require induction of the transcription factor PU1 by IL-4 and TGF-β and secrete the effector cytokine IL-9, which promotes immunity against worms and inflammation. T_H17 cells require induction of the transcription factor RORγt (RORC in humans) by TGF-β and IL-6, undergo expansion in response to IL-23, and secrete the effector cytokines IL-17A, IL-17F, IL-21, and IL-22, which promote immunity against extracellular pathogens and inflammation. Inducible iTreg cells require induction of the transcription factor Foxp3 by TGF-β, retinoic acid, and IL-2 and secrete the inhibitory cytokines TGF-β and IL-10 to mediate immune tolerance, mucosal homeostasis, and immune suppression. T_H22 cells involve induction of the transcription factor AhR by IL-6 and TNF and secrete the effector cytokine IL-22 to promote homeostasis and immunity on both skin and mucosal surfaces. Finally, T_{FH} cells require induction of the transcription factor Bcl-6 by poorly understood signals and secrete the effector cytokine IL-21, which is important for the germinal center reaction and antibody production.

inducing B-cell production of IgA, an antibody isotype devoid of inflammatory activity (13). Indeed, TGF-β and IL-10 not only suppress inflammatory T_H cells but also stimulate B cells to switch from IgM to IgA. Finally, Treg cells optimize the affinity of systemic IgG responses by suppressing T_{FH} cells (414). In this manner, Treg cells limit the expansion of germinal center B cells with low affinity for antigen.

B Cells

General Principles

B cells are a subset of lymphocytes that play a key role in the humoral immune response. This response provides immune protection by producing Ig molecules commonly known as antibodies that target specific antigenic determinants (or epitopes) associated with intruding microbes. B cells were originally designated from the *b*ursa of Fabricius, which is the site of B-cell maturation in birds and chickens (415). This nomenclature turned out to be very appropriate, because the *b*one marrow is the major site of B-cell development in several mammalian species, including humans. In the bone marrow, precursors of B cells undergo a series of Ig gene modifications to generate an

antibody repertoire capable of recognizing any antigen present in the external environment (416,417). Mature B cells emerging from the bone marrow express primary IgM and IgD antibodies that serve as surface BCR molecules for antigen (Fig. 2.16) (418,419). After recognizing antigen through the BCR, mature B cells undergo a second wave of Ig gene modifications in secondary lymphoid organs. These modifications increase the affinity of B cells for antigen and enable B cells to express secondary IgG, IgA, and IgE antibodies that are provided with novel effector functions (420). Eventually, antigen-activated B cells become plasma cells that release large amounts of soluble antibodies in the circulation, tissues, and mucosal secretions (421). The development of appropriate antibody responses requires central and peripheral "checkpoint" mechanisms that ensure the generation of immune protection against foreign antigens whilst promoting tolerance against autologous antigens (422).

B-Cell Development

In humans, B cells develop from hematopoietic stem cells in the fetal liver during gestation and in the bone marrow after birth (423). Each newly generated B lymphocyte carries a transmembrane Ig receptor that is composed of two identical

FIGURE 2.16. Structure of the BCR signaling complex. The BCR is composed of two transmembrane IgH chains (μ, δ, γ, α, or ε,) and two IgL chains (κ or λ) that are held together by disulfide bonds. The BCR is noncovalently linked to Igα (CD79a) and Igβ (CD79b), two proteins that contain one cytosolic ITAM region for signal transduction. The BCR complex also includes CD19 (signaling threshold regulator), CD21 (complement receptor), and CD81 (costimulator) molecules that are needed for the amplification of BCR signaling. The CD22 molecule negatively regulates BCR signaling as FcγRIIB does (not shown here).

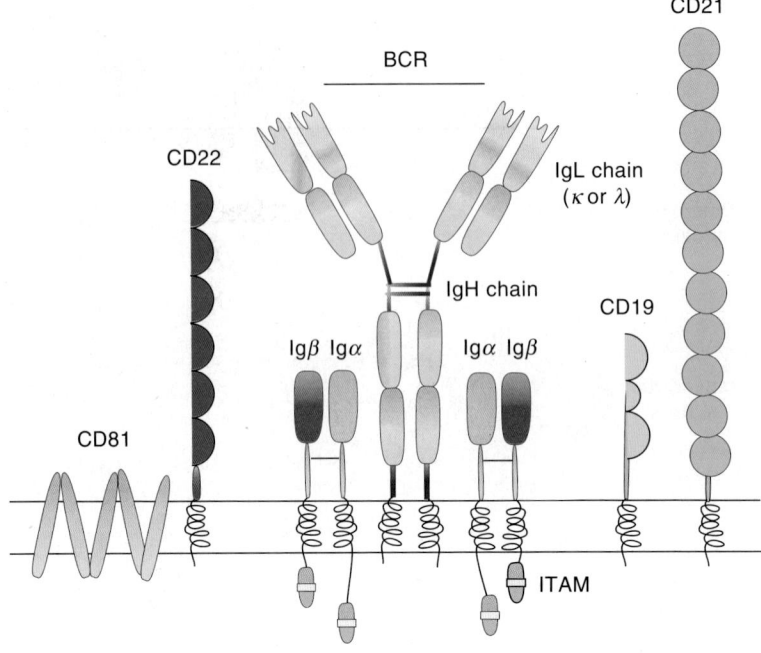

Ig heavy chain (H) molecules and two identical Ig light chain (L) molecules, which can be either Igκ or Igλ (424). The IgH and IgL chain molecules include an antigen-binding variable region encoded by recombined V_HDJ_H and V_LJ_L genes, respectively. The V, D, and J segments of these genes are organized in multiple families within the IgH and IgL loci, and their assembly into in-frame V_HDJ_H and V_LJ_L exons requires an antigen-independent diversification process known as V(D)J recombination (425,426). B-cell development proceeds through several intermediate stages (Figs. 2.17 and 2.18) that can be distinguished on the basis of the expression of various cell surface markers (Table 2.5) and ordered patterns of IgH and IgL chain gene rearrangement (427,428). Progression through these stages involves cross-talk between B-cell precursors and bone marrow stromal cells, which guide B-cell development through the expression of both membrane-bound and soluble growth and differentiation factors, including IL-7, fms-related tyrosine kinase 3 (FLT3) ligand, and thymic stromal lymphopoietin (TSLP) (429). Several transcription factors regulate the early steps of B-cell development, including the Pax5 protein (430).

V(D)J Recombination

Pro-B cells initially recombine D and J segments in the IgH locus to form a DJ segment that subsequently recombines with a V segment to assemble a complete V_HDJ_H gene (Fig. 2.19). These recombination events randomly target individual members of multiple V, D, and J gene families and require the induction of double-stranded DNA breaks in specific recombination signal sequences by a heterodimeric recombination activating gene (RAG) complex that includes RAG1 and RAG2 proteins (55,431). As discussed earlier, RAG1 and RAG2 recombinases are also required for the rearrangement of TCR gene segments, and indeed deleterious mutations of RAG1 or RAG2 lead to severe combined immunodeficiency (SCID), which is characterized by the lack of both B and T cells (432). The enzyme terminal deoxynucleotidyl transferase (TdT) increases the diversity of Ig genes by adding N-nucleotides at the DJ junction of a recombined V_HDJ_H exon (433). Productive V_HDJ_H recombination stops the expression of RAG proteins (426), leading to the transcription of the V_HDJ_H gene together with the constant (C) heavy chain gene μ (Cμ) gene to form a complete IgH chain (434). Subsequent assembly of the IgH chain with

surrogate invariant IgL proteins encoded by V-pre-B and λ5 gene segments is followed by transient surface expression of a pre-B-cell receptor (pre-BCR) complex that also includes invariant Igα and Igβ subunits with signaling function (435). Signals emanating from the pre-BCR are a critical checkpoint for B-cell development as they regulate the expansion of pre-B cells and their further differentiation into immature B cells (436). Immature B cells re-express RAG proteins to initiate the rearrangement of V and J segments from the IgL locus and form a complete Ig molecule (434). Of note, RAG proteins target the Igλ locus when the Igκ locus fails to generate an in-frame (or productive) VJ rearrangement. Assembly of the IgL chain with the IgH chain is followed by the expression of a fully competent IgM receptor which functions as a surface BCR (437).

Checkpoints and Transitional B Cells

Following Ig gene rearrangement, immature B cells that express an autoreactive BCR undergo receptor editing, which involves the replacement of the V segment in the recombined V_LJ_L gene with an upstream V segment through an RAG-mediated reaction (438). An immature B cell unable to edit its autoreactive BCR is eliminated by apoptosis through a process referred to as clonal deletion (422). After progressing through this tolerance checkpoint, immature B cells leave the bone marrow as transitional B cells that co-express IgM and IgD through a process of alternative splicing of a long RNA containing V_HDJ_H as well as Cμ and Cδ exons (203). Transitional B cells are typically short-lived and functionally immature and express high levels of the developmentally regulated molecules CD24 and CD38, but not the memory B-cell molecule CD27 (439). These transitional B cells become fully mature naïve B cells expressing unmutated V(D)J genes, IgM, IgD, and CD19, but not CD24, CD27, and CD38 after colonizing peripheral lymphoid organs. Here, stromal cells provide mandatory survival signals such as BAFF, which supports the maintenance of a highly diversified and fully functional repertoire of peripheral B cells (440,441).

B-Cell Responses

Naïve B cells undergo additional differentiation steps after encountering native antigens in secondary lymphoid organs such as spleen, lymph nodes, and MALT. Naïve B cells recognize and

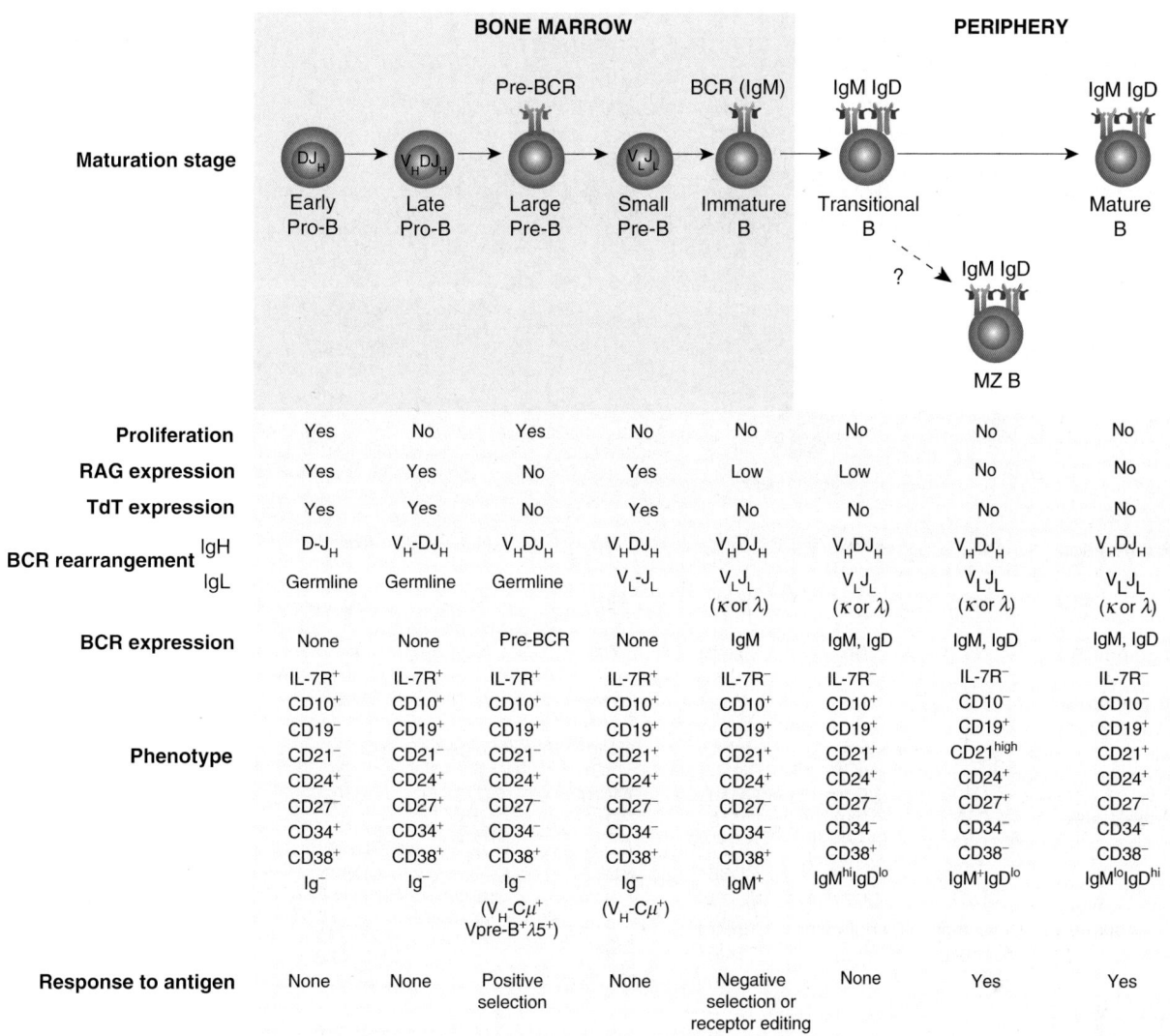

Maturation stage	Early Pro-B	Late Pro-B	Large Pre-B	Small Pre-B	Immature B	Transitional B		Mature B
Proliferation	Yes	No	Yes	No	No	No	No	No
RAG expression	Yes	Yes	No	Yes	Low	Low	No	No
TdT expression	Yes	Yes	No	Yes	No	No	No	No
BCR rearrangement IgH	D-J_H	V_H-DJ_H	$V_H DJ_H$	$V_H DJ_H$	$V_H DJ_H$	$V_H DJ_H$	$V_H DJ_H$	$V_H DJ_H$
IgL	Germline	Germline	Germline	V_L-J_L	$V_L J_L$ (κ or λ)	$V_L J_L$ (κ or λ)	$V_L J_L$ (κ or λ)	$V_L J_L$ (κ or λ)
BCR expression	None	None	Pre-BCR	None	IgM	IgM, IgD	IgM, IgD	IgM, IgD
Phenotype	IL-7R$^+$ CD10$^+$ CD19$^-$ CD21$^-$ CD24$^+$ CD27$^-$ CD34$^+$ CD38$^+$ Ig$^-$	IL-7R$^+$ CD10$^+$ CD19$^+$ CD21$^-$ CD24$^+$ CD27$^+$ CD34$^+$ CD38$^+$ Ig$^-$	IL-7R$^+$ CD10$^+$ CD19$^+$ CD21$^-$ CD24$^+$ CD27$^-$ CD34$^-$ CD38$^+$ Ig$^-$ (V_H-Cμ^+ Vpre-B$^+\lambda$5$^+$)	IL-7R$^+$ CD10$^+$ CD19$^+$ CD21$^+$ CD24$^+$ CD27$^-$ CD34$^-$ CD38$^+$ Ig$^-$ (V_H-Cμ^+)	IL-7R$^-$ CD10$^+$ CD19$^+$ CD21$^+$ CD24$^+$ CD27$^-$ CD34$^-$ CD38$^+$ IgM$^+$	IL-7R$^-$ CD10$^+$ CD19$^+$ CD21$^+$ CD24$^+$ CD27$^-$ CD34$^-$ CD38$^+$ IgM^{hi}IgD^{lo}	IL-7R$^-$ CD10$^-$ CD19$^+$ CD21^{high} CD24$^+$ CD27$^+$ CD34$^-$ CD38$^-$ IgM$^+$IgD^{lo}	IL-7R$^-$ CD10$^-$ CD19$^+$ CD21$^+$ CD24$^+$ CD27$^-$ CD34$^-$ CD38$^-$ IgM^{lo}IgD^{hi}
Response to antigen	None	None	Positive selection	None	Negative selection or receptor editing	None	Yes	Yes

FIGURE 2.17. Development of early B cells in the bone marrow. Early B-cell development occurs in an antigen-independent manner through phenotypically distinct differentiation stages characterized by specific Ig gene rearrangement events. Pro-B cells emerge from common lymphoid precursor cells and include early pro-B (or pre-pro-B) and late pro-B (or pro-B) cells that undergo DJ_H and V-DJ_H gene rearrangements, respectively. These DNA recombination events require RAG1 and RAG2 endonucleases and are associated with D gene diversification by nucleotide addition via the enzyme terminal deoxyribonucleotidyl transferase (TdT). Late pro-B cells differentiate to large pre-B cells that express a surface pre-BCR molecule composed of a V_H-Cμ IgH chain and a pseudo (or surrogate) IgL chain formed by the Vpre-B and λ5 proteins. Large pre-B cells with in-frame $V_H DJ_H$ rearrangements undergo positive selection and further differentiate to small pre-B cells, which down-regulate surface pre-BCR expression, contain cytoplasmic V_H-Cμ protein, and undergo V_L-J_L recombination via RAG proteins. Subsequent assembly of two IgH and two IgL chains leads to the formation of a surface BCR in immature B cells. In the presence of strong BCR signals from self-antigens, immature B cells undergo negative selection by clonal deletion. However, some autoreactive immature B cells can be rescued through receptor editing, which requires a new up-regulation of RAG protein expression. Then, immature B cells differentiate to transitional B cells that express both surface IgM and IgD through alternative splicing of a long $V_H DJ_H$-Cμ-Cδ mRNA. Transitional B cells exit the bone marrow and further differentiate to either mature naïve B cells or mature MZ B cells in secondary lymphoid organs. Naïve and MZ B cells initiate antibody production after differentiating to plasma cells in response TD or TI antigens, respectively.

internalize antigen by utilizing surface IgM and IgD receptors (230,418). Large antigens usually require the interaction of B cells with antigen-sampling macrophages and DCs located in the subcapsular sinus and paracortical areas of lymph nodes or in the MZ of the spleen, whereas small soluble antigens gain access to B cells after entering the follicle through a specialized transport system known as the follicular conduit network (442–446). This structure communicates with afferent lymphatic vessels and consists of collagen fiber cores surrounded by myofibroblast-like cells known as fibroblastic reticular cells (447–449). After receiving activating signals from the BCR, B cells downregulate the expression of surface IgD, process the internalized antigen to form an MHC-II-peptide complex, and migrate to the

boundary of the follicle with the T-cell zone, also known as the T-B border (165,399). There, B cells present antigen to T_{FH} cells, a professional B-cell helper subset of CD4$^+$ T cells that express CD40L and cytokines such as IL-4, IL-10, IL-21, and IFN-γ (277,450). These T_{FH} cells originate from naïve CD4$^+$ T cells recognizing antigen on IL-12-producing DCs (272,276,451). After establishing a cognate interaction with early T_{FH} cells, antigen-activated B cells differentiate along one of two alternative pathways (452). The extrafollicular pathway generates short-lived plasmablasts that secrete IgM (453), whereas the follicular pathway yields germinal center B cells known as centroblasts and centrocytes that mediate antibody diversification, selection, and production (Fig. 2.20) (62,454,455).

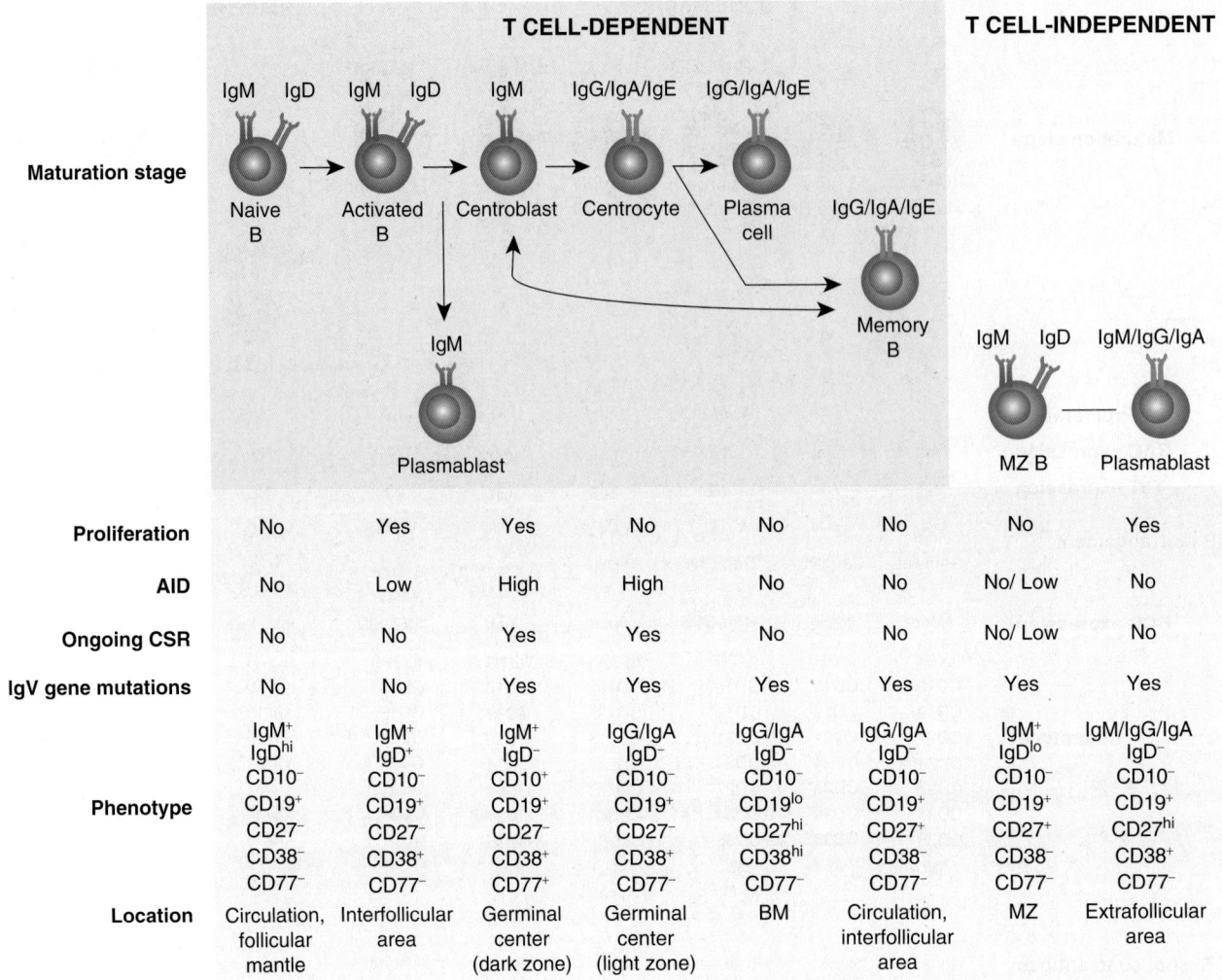

			T CELL-DEPENDENT				T CELL-INDEPENDENT	
Maturation stage	Naive B	Activated B	Centroblast	Centrocyte	Plasma cell	Memory B / Plasmablast	MZ B	Plasmablast
Proliferation	No	Yes	Yes	No	No	No	No	Yes
AID	No	Low	High	High	No	No	No/ Low	No
Ongoing CSR	No	No	Yes	Yes	No	No	No/ Low	No
IgV gene mutations	No	No	Yes	Yes	Yes	Yes	Yes	Yes
Phenotype	IgM+ IgDhi CD10− CD19+ CD27− CD38− CD77−	IgM+ IgD+ CD10− CD19+ CD27− CD38+ CD77−	IgM+ IgD− CD10+ CD19+ CD27− CD38+ CD77+	IgG/IgA IgD− CD10− CD19+ CD27− CD38+ CD77−	IgG/IgA IgD− CD10− CD19lo CD27hi CD38hi CD77−	IgG/IgA IgD− CD10− CD19+ CD27+ CD38− CD77−	IgM+ IgDlo CD10− CD19+ CD27+ CD38− CD77−	IgM/IgG/IgA IgD− CD10− CD19+ CD27hi CD38+ CD77−
Location	Circulation, follicular mantle	Interfollicular area	Germinal center (dark zone)	Germinal center (light zone)	BM	Circulation, interfollicular area	MZ	Extrafollicular area

FIGURE 2.18. Development of mature B cells in secondary lymphoid organs. Mature B cells progress along phenotypically and genotypically distinct stages of differentiation after encountering antigen in secondary lymphoid organs. Naïve B cells populate the MZ of lymphoid follicles and predominantly differentiate through a T-cell–dependent (TD) pathway that involves an antigen-driven cognate interaction with T_{FH} cells. Activated B cells emerging from this interaction either differentiate along an extrafollicular pathway that leads to the formation of short-lived IgM-secreting plasmablasts or enter the germinal center (GC) to become highly proliferating centroblasts. These cells undergo robust IgV gene SHM and, after completing class switching from IgM to IgG, IgA, or (very rarely) IgE, become noncycling centrocytes. Both SHM and class switching require the enzyme activation-induced cytidine deaminase (AID). Centrocytes further differentiate to either long-lived memory B cells, which recirculate, or long-lived antibody-secreting plasma cells, which migrate to the bone marrow. MZ B cells populate the MZ of the spleen and predominantly differentiate through a TI pathway that involves noncognate interaction with innate immune cells. MZ B cells express moderately mutated IgV genes and differentiate into plasmablasts that secrete IgM but also class-switched IgG and IgA antibodies.

Germinal Center Reaction

After increasing the expression of the chemokine receptor CXCR5, early T_{FH} cells and activated B cells move to the follicle in response to the chemokine CXCL13, a CXCR5 ligand produced by FDCs (456–458). Early T_{FH} cells become germinal center T_{FH} cells by entering a Bcl-6-dependent genetic program that is induced by signals present in the follicular environment (366,367). By expressing high levels of CD40L and IL-21, germinal center T_{FH} cells sustain the proliferation, differentiation, diversification, and selection of centroblasts and centrocytes (459–461). Similar to T_{FH} cells, these germinal center B cells express Bcl-6, a transcription factor essential for the maintenance and development of the germinal center reaction (455). Centroblasts undergo extensive clonal expansion in the dark zone of the germinal center, thereby pushing naïve IgM+IgD+ B cells to a peripheral area of the follicle called the MZ (455). Centroblasts undergo clonal expansion as well as SHM and class switch recombination (CSR), two Ig-diversifying processing that are highly dependent on the enzyme activation-induced cytidine deaminase (AID) (401,462–464). Then, centroblasts exit the cell cycle to become smaller and nondividing centrocytes that recognize native antigen trapped on the surface of FDCs using their newly hypermutated BCR (459–461,465,466). After binding antigen, centrocytes establish a cognate interaction with germinal center T_{FH} cells (338,459–461). This interaction mainly occurs in the light zone of the germinal center and contributes not only to the maintenance and selection of high-affinity and class-switched centrocytes but also to the differentiation of centrocytes into memory B cells or plasma cells (466–470). Centrocytes expressing a low-affinity BCR die by apoptosis and then are engulfed by resident phagocytes known as tingible body macrophages (450,455).

The typical structure of the germinal center is fully formed within approximately 2 weeks after immunization

Table 2.5	COMMON B-CELL–SURFACE MOLECULES

Name	Expression	Function
IgM	Immature, transitional, naïve, and MZ B cells, B-1 cells	BCR signaling, endocytosis
IgD	Immature, transitional, naïve, and MZ B cells, B-1 cells	BCR signaling, endocytosis
IgG	GC and memory B cells	BCR signaling, endocytosis
IgA	GC and memory B cells	BCR signaling, endocytosis
CD5	B-1 cells, activated B cells	BCR signaling inhibitor
CD9	Pre-B cells, MZ B cells, B-1 cells, plasma cells	Adhesion, migration
CD10	Developing B cells, GC centroblasts	Unknown
CD19	All B cells except plasma cells	BCR signaling amplifier
CD20	All B cells except early pro-B cells and plasma cells	Activation
CD21 (complement receptor 1)	Mature B cells	BCR signaling amplifier
CD22 (Siglec-2)	All B cells	BCR signaling inhibitor
CD23 (FcεRII)	Activated B cells, follicular mantle B cells	Activation
CD25 (IL-2Rα)	Activated B cells	Activation and proliferation
CD27 (CD70R)	MZ B cells, plasma cells, memory B cells	Differentiation
CD30	Some activated interfollicular B cells	Activation, regulation
CD32 (FcγRIIB)	Mature B cells	Inhibition of survival, activation, proliferation
CD35 (complement receptor 2)	Mature B cells	BCR signaling amplifier
CD38 (NAD glycohydrolase)	Transitional B cells, GC B cells, plasma cells	Activation
CD39 (ecto-ADPase)	Activated B cells	Adhesion
CD40	Mature B cells	Activation, proliferation, differentiation
CD43 (sialophorin)	Activated B cells, B-1 cells	Adhesion
CD45	All B cells	BCR signaling regulator
CD54 (ICAM-1)	Activated B cells	Adhesion
CD62L (L-selectin)	Circulating B cells	Adhesion
CD69	Activated B cells	Signal transduction
CD70 (CD27L)	Activated B cells	Stimulation
CD71 (transferrin receptor)	Proliferating and activated B cells	Activation, proliferation
CD72	All B cells except plasma cells	Regulation of activation and proliferation
CD73	Mature B cells	Unclear
CD75	Mature B cells	Adhesion
CD77	GC centroblasts	Apoptosis
CD79a,b (Igα,β)	All B cells	BCR signaling
CD80 (B7.1)	Activated B cells	Costimulation of T cells
CD81 (TAPA-1)	All B cells	BCR signaling amplifier
CD86 (B7.2)	GC and memory B cells	Costimulation of T cells
CD89 (FcαR)	Mature B cells	Activation, regulation
CD95 (Fas)	Activated B cells, GC B cells	Apoptosis
CD124 (IL-4Rα)	Mature B cells	Activation, differentiation, class switching
CD126 (IL-6Rα)	Activated B cells, plasma cells	Plasma cell differentiation
CD127 (IL-7Rα)	B-cell precursors	Development
CD138 (syndecan-1)	Plasma cells	Adhesion
CD150 (SLAM)	All B cells	Activation
CD267 (TACI)	MZ B cells, memory B cells, activated B cells	Class switching, antibody production
CD268 (BAFF-R, BR3)	Mature B cells	Survival, differentiation
CD269 (BCMA)	Plasma cells	Survival, antibody production

(455). Chemokine gradients mostly generated by FDCs mediate the positioning of centroblasts and centrocytes in the light and dark zones of the germinal center (471). In particular, an initial up-regulation of CXCR5 expression promotes the movement of centroblasts toward a CXCL13 gradient generated by FDCs in the dark zone of the germinal center. Subsequent up-regulation of CXCR4 expression and concomitant down-regulation of CXCR5 expression induces centrocytes to migrate toward a CXCL12 gradient generated by FDCs in the light zone of the germinal center (471). However, it must be emphasized that germinal center B cells can move both between and within the dark and light zones, indicating that the compartmentalization of the germinal center is less well defined than originally thought (460,461). Centroblasts and centrocytes express IgM or IgG or IgA together with CD19, CD27, CD38, and CD10, but not IgD and CD24. Of note, centroblasts also express CD77, whereas centrocytes do not (472,473). Furthermore, centroblasts and centrocytes contain highly mutated V(D)J genes, express the germinal center-associated transcription factor Bcl-6, and contain molecular footprints of ongoing CSR and SHM, including strong AID expression (455). Unlike naïve B cells from the follicular mantle, centroblasts and centrocytes lack the intracellular anti-apoptotic factor Bcl-2 and instead express intracellular Bcl-2 family members with proapoptotic activity (472,474,475). This feature renders germinal center B cells highly susceptible to apoptosis, which allows their elimination in the absence of engagement of BCR by high-affinity antigens. T_{FH} cells expressing FasL further increase the elimination of low-affinity germinal center B cells (476,477). Indeed, germinal center B cells up-regulate the expression of the death-inducing receptor Fas upon engagement of CD40 by CD40L on T_{FH} cells (478–481). In the presence of CD40 signaling, the death-inducing signals emanating from Fas are overridden by strong "rescue" signals generated by the BCR. This mechanism promotes the survival of germinal center B cells expressing a BCR with high affinity for antigen.

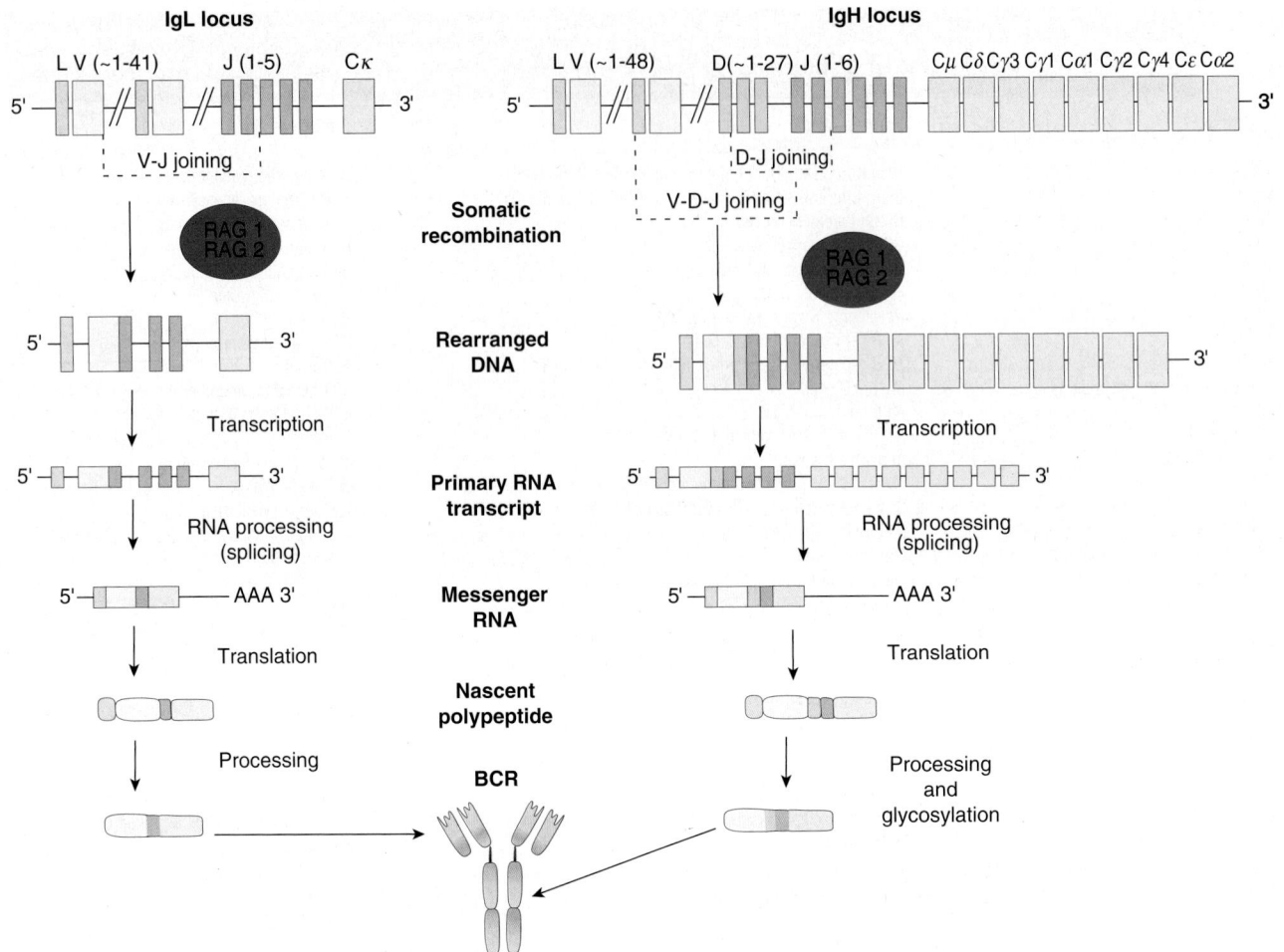

FIGURE 2.19. Mechanism underlying the generation of antibody molecules. The Ig loci include multiple cassettes of V, D, and J (IgH locus) and V and J (IgL loci termed Igκ and Igλ) gene segments that undergo random rearrangement during B-cell development in the bone marrow through a process involving RAG proteins. In the IgL loci, a V_L gene segment rearranges with a J_L gene segment to generate a $V_L J_L$ exon. Transcription of $V_L J_L$ and subsequent splicing of $V_L J_L$ mRNA to a Cκ or Cλ mRNA generates a $V_L J_L$-C_L mRNA that is polyadenylated and then translated into a mature IgL chain protein. In the IgH locus, similar recombination and transcription events lead to the formation of a $V_H D_H J_H$-C_H (Cμ in the earliest stages of B-cell differentiation) mRNA that undergoes splicing and polyadenylation to generate a mature IgH protein. In each Ig locus, V gene transcription initiates at the level of a leader (L) sequence positioned upstream of each V segment. Ultimately, two identical IgH and two identical IgL chain proteins are assembled to generate a membrane-bound heterotetrameric protein termed BCR.

Ig Diversification

Bone marrow B-cell precursors generate antigen recognition diversity by undergoing V(D)J gene recombination through an antigen-independent process that requires RAG proteins. Mature B cells emerging from the bone marrow further diversify their Ig genes through two antigen-dependent processes known as SHM and CSR (Fig. 2.21). These processes require AID, a DNA-editing enzyme strongly expressed by centroblasts and centrocytes (463,482). Although predominantly occurring in germinal center B cells engaged in a T-cell–dependent (TD) antibody response against protein antigens, CSR and SHM can also occur in extrafollicular B cells engaged in a T-cell–independent (TI) antibody response against carbohydrate or lipid antigens (483,484). While CSR diversifies the effector functions of an Ig molecule, SHM provides a structural substrate for the selection of Igs with higher affinity for antigen.

Class Switch Recombination

This process is an irreversible DNA recombination event that replaces the Cμ gene encoding the C_H region of the IgM molecule with the Cγ1, Cγ2, Cγ3, Cγ4, Cα1, Cα2, or Cε gene encoding the C_H region of IgG1, IgG2, IgG3, IgG4, IgA1, IgA2, or IgE, respectively (485,486). In humans, there also is a noncanonical form of CSR that replaces Cμ with Cδ and leads to the selective expression of IgD (123,203). CSR targets intronic switch (S) regions located upstream of each C_H gene and initiates with the germline transcription of a specific C_H gene in response to cooperative CD40L and cytokine signals (486,487). Cytokine signals are important to target specific C_H genes. Thus, while IL-4 and IL-13 preferentially activate Cγ4 and Cε, TGF-β predominantly induces Cα1 and Cα2 genes (69,488,489). Moreover, IL-4, IL-10, and IL-21 mostly target Cγ1, Cγ2, and Cγ3 genes (490–493). Germline transcription yields a primary transcript that encompasses the S region and its downstream C_H gene (494). Although later spliced into a noncoding germline, the primary transcript plays a central role in CSR (495). Indeed, this RNA physically associates with the template DNA strand of the targeted S region to form a stable DNA-RNA hybrid that becomes substrate of AID, a DNA-editing enzyme induced by CSR-inducing signals (463). AID deaminates cytosine residues on both DNA strands of the actively transcribed S region to generate multiple DNA lesions that are subsequently processed by a complex DNA repair machinery to form double-stranded DNA breaks (486). Fusion of double-stranded DNA breaks via the nonhomologous end-joining pathway induces looping-out deletion

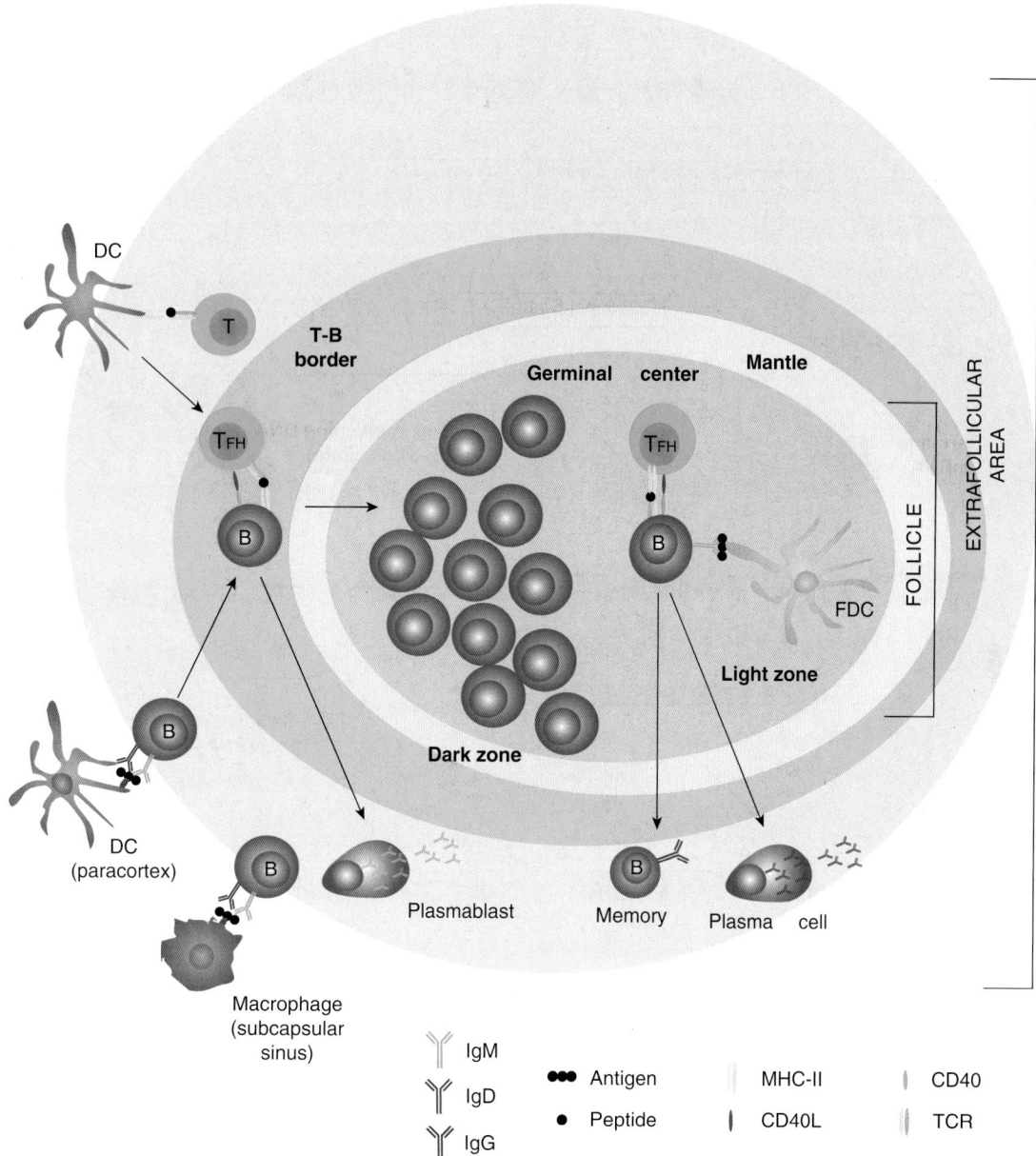

FIGURE 2.20. The germinal center reaction. Naïve B cells capture native antigen from subcapsular sinus macrophages and paracortical DCs through the BCR (both IgM and IgD molecules) and subsequently establish a cognate interaction with T$_{FH}$ cells located at the boundary between the follicle and the extrafollicular area (T-B border). After activation by T$_{FH}$ cells via CD40L and cytokines such as IL-21, B cells enter either an extrafollicular pathway to become short-lived IgM-secreting plasmablasts or a follicular pathway to become germinal center centroblasts. In the dark zone of the germinal center, centroblasts undergo extensive proliferation, express AID, and induce SHM and CSR from IgM to IgG, IgA, or IgE (the figure only shows IgG). After exiting the cell cycle, centroblasts differentiate into centrocytes that interact with FDCs located in the light zone of the germinal center. FDCs expose immune complexes containing native antigen to the BCR and centrocytes with low affinity for antigen die by apoptosis, whereas centrocytes with high affinity for antigen differentiate to long-lived memory B cells or plasma cells expressing high-affinity and class-switched antibodies. Memory B cells recirculate, whereas plasma cells migrate to the bone marrow.

of the intervening DNA with subsequent replacement of Cμ with a downstream C$_H$ gene. The resulting juxtaposition of the recombined VDJ gene with a Cγ, Cα, or Cε gene permits B cells to acquire an Ig with novel effector functions but identical specificity for antigen (486).

Somatic Hypermutation
This process introduces point mutations in the recombined V(D)J exons encoding the antigen-binding V region of an antibody (496,497). In the germinal center of secondary lymphoid follicles, these point mutations provide the structural correlate for the selection of high-affinity B cells by antigen exposed on

FDCs. During affinity maturation, the point mutations induced by AID mostly generate amino acid replacements in CDRs, which play a key role in the formation of the antigen-binding pocket formed by the V regions of IgH and IgL chains (486,497). SHM includes an initial phase that requires the mutagenic activity of AID, followed by a second phase that involves the error-prone repair of AID-induced mutations (498). Of note, these mutations preferentially target specific hotspots, including the DGYW motif, where D stands for G, A, or T nucleotides, Y for C or T nucleotides, and W for A of T nucleotides (497). Error-prone DNA repair is performed by members of a family of low-fidelity translesional DNA polymerases that recognize

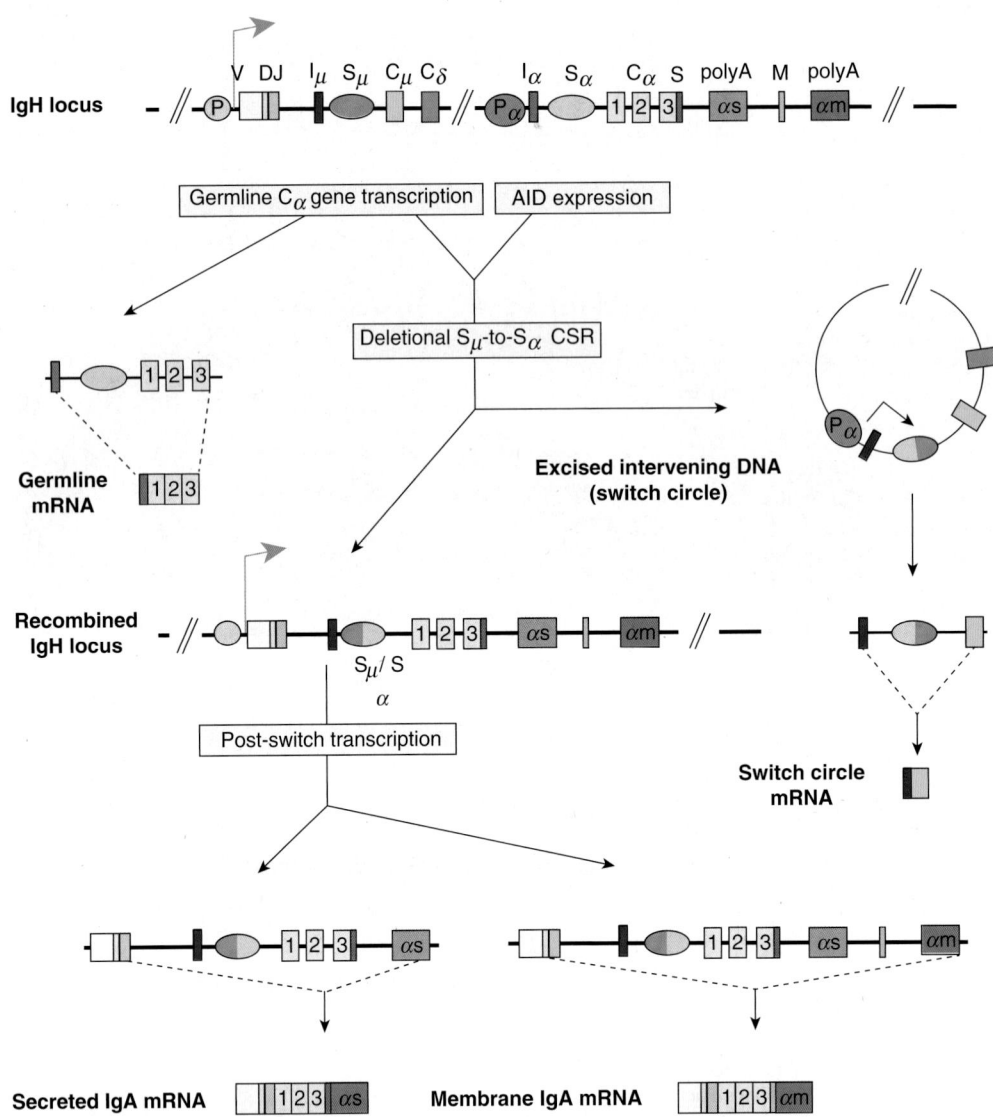

FIGURE 2.21. Mechanism underlying antibody class switching. The IgH locus contains a rearranged V_HDJ_H exon encoding the antigen-binding domain of an Ig. Following rearrangement of the IgL locus, B cells produce intact IgM and IgD through a transcriptional process driven by a promoter (P) upstream of V_HDJ_H (*blue arrow*). Production of downstream IgG, IgA, or IgE with identical antigen specificity but different effector function occurs through CSR. The diagram shows the mechanism of IgA CSR, but a similar mechanism underlies IgG and IgE CSR. Appropriate stimuli induce germline transcription of the $C\alpha$ gene from the promoter $(P\alpha)$ of an intronic α ($I\alpha$) exon (*black arrow*) through an intronic switch α ($S\alpha$) region located between $I\alpha$ and $C\alpha$ exons. In addition to yielding a sterile $I\alpha$-$C\alpha$ mRNA, germline transcription renders the $C\alpha$ gene substrate for AID an essential component of the CSR machinery. AID expression occurs following activation of B cells by helper signals from T_{FH} cells (in the TD pathway) or innate immune cells (in the TI pathway). By generating and repairing DNA breaks at $S\mu$ and $S\alpha$, the CSR machinery rearranges the IgH locus, thereby yielding a reciprocal deletional DNA recombination product known as $S\alpha$-$S\mu$ switch circle. This episomal DNA transcribes a chimeric $I\alpha$-$C\mu$ mRNA under the influence of signals that activate $P\alpha$. Postswitch transcription of the IgH locus generates mRNAs for both secreted and membrane IgA proteins. $C\alpha1$-3, exons encoding the $C\alpha$ chain of IgA; S, 3′ portion of $C\alpha3$ encoding the tailpiece of secreted IgA; M, exon encoding the transmembrane and cytoplasmic portions of membrane-bound IgA; αs, polyadenylation site for secreted IgA mRNA; αm, polyadenylation site for membrane-bound IgA mRNA.

DNA lesions and bypass them by inserting bases opposite to the lesion (499,500). Amino acid replacements brought about by SHM increase the affinity and fine specificity of an antibody, but do not modify the framework regions (FRs), which regulate the structural organization of Ig molecules. Similarly, SHM does not induce amino acid replacements in the promoter and intronic enhancer, which regulate the transcriptional activity of the Ig locus.

Plasma Cell and Memory B-Cell Differentiation

The germinal center reaction leads to the formation of long-lived antibody-secreting plasma cells that migrate to the bone marrow and memory B cells that enter the circulation

and lymphoid organs to screen peripheral lymphoid organs for the presence of antigen (32,501,502). Plasma cells accumulate IgM, IgG, IgA, or IgE in their cytoplasm and usually express mutated V(D)J genes, CD19, high levels of CD27 and CD38, but not IgD (except for some plasmablasts from the upper respiratory tract) or CD24 (502,503). Short-lived plasmablasts from extrafollicular areas or peripheral blood also express the proliferation molecule Ki-67 as well as some levels of surface Ig receptors (453). Instead, long-lived plasma cells from the bone marrow usually lack Ki-67 and surface Ig receptors, but typically express the syndecan-1 molecule, CD138. In the bone marrow, stromal cells, eosinophils, and megakaryocytes provide powerful survival signals to plasma cells, including the BAFF-related molecule APRIL (14,115,504). Memory B cells are critical to mount quick secondary humoral responses to recall antigens. In addition to entering the circulation, memory B cells form IgG-expressing extrafollicular aggregates and IgM-expressing follicle-like structures in draining lymph nodes (32,468). After a subsequent exposure to recall antigen, IgG-expressing memory B cells rapidly generate antibody-secreting plasmablasts, whereas IgM-expressing memory B cells initiate a secondary germinal center reaction. All these responses are characterized by rapid B-cell activation, proliferation, differentiation, and secretion of high-affinity antibodies (505). Memory B cells express mutated V(D)J genes, IgG, IgA, or (more rarely) IgM as well as CD19, CD24, and CD27, but not IgD or CD38 (506). The signals involved in the long-term survival of memory B cells remain unclear. Some studies point to antigen-independent polyclonal signals from B-cell–intrinsic TLRs, whereas others point to antigen-dependent signals involving T cells and basophils (14).

The differentiation of germinal center B cells into plasma cells and memory B cells involves a complex network of transcriptional regulators that include Bcl-6, Pax5, and B lymphocyte–induced maturation protein-1 (Blimp-1) (470,507). The transcription factor Bcl-6 was initially identified in B-cell lymphomas (508) and is required for the establishment and maintenance of germinal center B cells (509,510). The transcription factor Pax5 is essential for the development and function of naïve, germinal center, and memory B cells (511). In addition to activating a number of genes required for the germinal center reaction, Bcl-6 and Pax5 suppress expression of the plasma cell–inducing transcriptional repressor Blimp-1,

and therefore their functional inactivation is required for the differentiation of germinal center B cells into plasma cells (470). Up-regulation of Blimp-1 expression by a subset of germinal center B cells initiates plasma cell differentiation through a mechanism involving the suppression of Bcl-6 and Pax5 gene expression (470,512). In addition, Blimp-1 up-regulates the expression of X-box–binding protein (XBP)-1 and that of IRF-4, which is a transcription factor required for both CSR and plasma cell differentiation (507).

Antibody Structure and Function

The basic subunit of a transmembrane or secreted antibody is a pair of identical IgH and IgL chains that are connected by disulfide bonds to form a Y-shaped structure (Fig. 2.22) (424,513). Upon treatment with the proteolytic enzyme papain, antibodies are cleaved into a fragment antigen-binding (Fab) region and a fragment crystallizable (Fc) region. In the N-terminal portion of the Fab fragment, the IgH and IgL chains form a variable amino acid sequence termed V region, which mediates antigen binding. Each V region contains three hypervariable CDRs that interact directly with antigen and four relatively constant FRs that provide a structural scaffold for the Fab fragment of the antibody. In the carboxy-terminal portion of the Fc fragment, the IgH chains form the C_H region, which mediates the effector functions of an antibody. This C_H region not only activates the complement system but also binds various activating FcRs expressed by effector cells of the innate immune system, including monocytes, macrophages, DCs, granulocytes, and mast cells (192). The C_H region of an antibody can also bind inhibitory FcRs expressed by

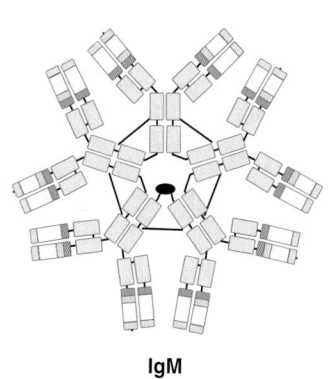

IgM

Ab class	H chain	L chain	Subclass	Structure
IgM	μ	κ, λ	-	Pentamer
IgD	δ	κ, λ	-	Monomer
IgG	$\gamma 1$	κ, λ	IgG1	Monomer
	$\gamma 2$		IgG2	Monomer
	$\gamma 3$		IgG3	Monomer
	$\gamma 4$		IgG4	Monomer
IgA	$\alpha 1$	κ, λ	IgA1	Monomer or
	$\alpha 2$		IgA2	dimer
IgE	ε	κ, λ	-	Monomer

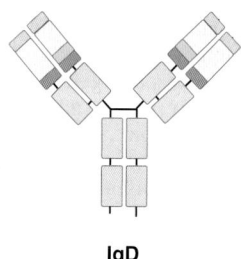

IgD

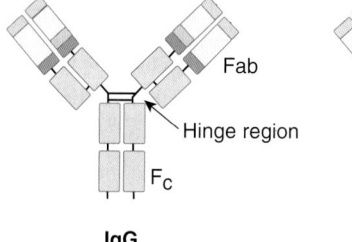

Fab

Hinge region

Fc

IgG

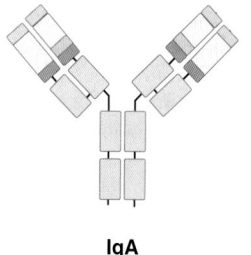

IgA

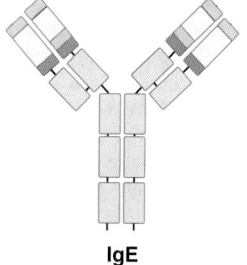

IgE

FIGURE 2.22. Structure of antibodies. Antibodies (or Igs) are heterotetrameric molecules composed of two identical IgH chains and two identical IgL chains that are held together by disulfide bonds (*black lines*). Each IgH chain contains a V region encoded by a $V_H DJ_H$ exon and a C region encoded by $C\mu$, $C\delta$, $C\gamma$, $C\alpha$, or $C\varepsilon$ exons, which determine the IgM, IgD, IgG, IgA, and IgE isotype (or class) of an antibody. $C\gamma$ and $C\alpha$ exons can be further divided into $C\gamma 1$, $C\gamma 2$, $C\gamma 3$, $C\gamma 4$, $C\alpha 1$, and $C\alpha 2$ exons, which determine the IgG1, IgG2, IgG3, IgG4, IgA1, and IgA2 subclass of an antibody. Similar to IgH chains, IgL chains contain a V region encoded by a $V_L J_L$ exon and a C region encoded by $C\kappa$ or $C\lambda$ exons. The hinge region connects the Fab fragment, which is the antigen-binding portion of the antibody, with the Fc fragment, which mediates the effector functions of the antibody. While IgD, IgG, and IgE antibodies are exclusively produced as monomeric molecules, IgM and IgA antibodies are produced as either monomeric or oligomeric molecules, including IgM pentamers and IgA dimers. Transmembrane IgM and IgA are always monomeric, whereas secreted IgM and IgA can be either monomeric (circulating IgA) or oligomeric (circulating IgM, mucosal IgM, and mucosal IgA).

B cells and cells of the innate immune system. Activating and inhibitory FcRs deliver powerful signals that enable antibody molecules to either amplify or terminate the humoral immune response (514).

General biologic functions shared by all antibodies include neutralization of microbes or toxins, opsonization, as well as complement-mediated destruction of microbes and infected or neoplastic cells. Additional functions such as antibody-dependent cell-mediated cytotoxicity (ADCC), translocation across mucosal epithelial cells, and expulsion of parasites are more specific to certain antibody classes. In humans, there are five antibody classes or isotypes named IgM, IgD, IgG, IgA, and IgE (495). Each class is associated with specific effector functions that are mainly determined by the C_H region (μ, δ, γ, α, or ε). IgG and IgA further include IgG1, IgG2, IgG3, IgG4, IgA1, and IgA2 subclasses.

IgM is expressed by pre-B, immature, transitional, and mature naïve B cells and serves as surface BCR (515,516). IgM is also released by plasmablasts emerging immediately after the activation of B cells by antigen, and indeed IgM antibodies are measured to diagnose the presence of an ongoing infection. However, IgM is also naturally released by subsets of B cells equivalent to mouse B-1 cells in the absence of immunization or infection (517). This natural or pre-immune IgM accounts for the majority of natural antibodies present in our circulation and provides a first line of protection at an early phase of infection by recognizing multiple phylogenetically conserved structures associated with microbes (518). In general, IgM antibodies have a rather low affinity but high avidity for antigen. Indeed, IgM antibodies are mostly unmutated but form pentameric and more rarely hexameric complexes that bind antigen with higher avidity than monomeric antibody molecules (519). In oligomeric IgM complexes, monomeric subunits are linked with each other by disulfide bonds and are further stabilized by a polypeptide joining (J) chain specifically produced by plasma cells (520). The main effector functions of IgM are neutralization, opsonization, and complement fixation. In addition, IgM binds to an Fcμ/α receptor expressed by B cells, macrophages, and mesangial cells that also binds IgA and promotes the endocytosis of antigen (198).

IgD is expressed by transitional and mature naïve B cells together with IgM and mainly functions as a surface BCR. Co-expression of surface IgM and IgD involves alternative splicing of a long pre-mRNA that contains VDJ, Cμ, and Cδ exons (521). After activation by antigen, B cells down-regulate the expression of IgD through a transcriptionally regulated mechanism. However, some B cells lodged in the human upper respiratory mucosa can undergo a poorly understood form of CSR from Cμ to Cδ that leads to the loss of IgM and the formation of plasmablasts that selectively secrete IgD (203). Structurally, IgD is characterized by a long hinge region that increases the flexibility of the antigen-binding Fab portion of IgD, allowing IgD to bind epitopes expressed at low density on microbes (122). The effector functions of IgD may include neutralization and opsonization, but not complement activation. Remarkably, some IgD-producing plasmablasts enter the circulation and release IgD molecules that bind an unknown receptor on the surface of various innate effector cells, including basophils (123). Cross-linking of IgD activates basophil release of antimicrobial, opsonizing, inflammatory, and B-cell–stimulating factors.

IgG is expressed by memory B cells as a surface BCR after the induction of class switching but is also released by class-switched plasma cells, representing the most abundant antibody isotype in our circulation (522). IgG is also abundant in mucosal secretions from the respiratory and urogenital tracts. IgG is composed of four IgG1, IgG2, IgG3, and IgG4 subclasses that are named in order of their abundance in the serum, IgG1 being the most abundant. All IgG subclasses are released as monomers that can easily perfuse tissues

to perform neutralization, opsonization, and complement fixation. IgG subclasses vary in the number of disulfide bonds, length of the hinge region, and degree and quality of glycosylation. These structural differences account for functional differences that relate to Fab flexibility, complement-fixing activity, and affinity for specific FcγRs (196,523). In general, IgG1 and IgG3 have more Fab flexibility, complement-fixing activity, and affinity for FcγRs than IgG2 and IgG4. FcγRs are composed of various FcγRI, FcγRII, and FcγRIII molecules that functionally link IgG with the innate immune system to enhance the phagocytosis of opsonized microbes and promote NK-cell–mediated ADCC of infected or tumoral cells (196,209). Of note, IgG also binds to FcγRIIB, an inhibitory receptor that contributes to the termination of an antibody response by delivering powerful negative feedback signals to B cells, including BCR-inhibiting signals (205). Together with FcγRIIB, some CLRs that bind carbohydrates associated with the Fc portion of IgG may account for the inhibitory activity that IgG has on the immune system (524). IgG further interacts with the FcRn on trophoblastic cells to cross the placenta and provide passive protection to neonates before their own immune system fully develops (13,514). Moreover, IgG interacts with TRIM21 (tripartite motif-containing protein 21), an intracellular high-affinity IgG receptor that conveys IgG-opsonized nonenveloped virions to the proteasome for intracellular antibody-mediated proteolysis (525).

IgA is expressed by memory B cells as a surface BCR after induction of class switching, but is also released by class-switched plasma cells in both circulation and mucosal secretions (31,526). IgA includes two IgA1 and IgA2 subclasses that are named in order of their abundance in the serum, IgA1 being more abundant than IgA2 (527). Circulating IgA is composed mostly of IgA1, whereas mucosal IgA encompasses both IgA1 and IgA2. Mucosal IgA1 and IgA2 are mostly dimeric and oligomeric, whereas circulating IgA1 is mostly monomeric. Of note, IgA2 is particularly abundant at sites heavily colonized by bacteria, including the distal intestinal tract and the female urogenital tract (69,70,526). This may relate to the fact that IgA2 has a shorter hinge region than IgA1 (528), which renders IgA2 less susceptible to degradation by proteases from mucosal bacteria that specifically target the hinge region of IgA1. Mucosal IgA polymers originate from the interaction of IgA monomers with the J chain, a polypeptide synthesized by plasma cells (529). In addition to assembling monomeric IgA, the J chain interacts with the polymeric immunoglobulin receptor (pIgR), an antibody-transporting protein expressed on the basolateral surface of mucosal epithelial cells. The pIgR shuttles IgA across epithelial cells through a transcytotic process that culminates in the translocation of a SIgA complex to the mucosal surface (12,530). This complex is composed of a secretory chain (SC) that originates from the endocytic cleavage of pIgR and confers mucophilic properties to SIgA. Remarkably, SIgA neutralizes toxins and pathogens without causing inflammation due to its inability to fix and activate the complement cascade (527). In addition, SIgA anchors commensal bacteria to the mucus, thereby impeding their adhesion to the apical surface of mucosal epithelial cells. Furthermore, SIgA promotes the establishment of a mutualistic host-microbe relationship by down-modulating the expression of proinflammatory epitopes on commensal bacteria (69,530–532). Moreover, SIgA mediates intracellular neutralization of microbial compounds with proinflammatory activity and facilitates the formation of a biofilm that favors the growth of commensals while attenuating that of pathogens (31). The function of circulating IgA is less clear. Monomeric IgA binds to high-affinity FcαRI (or CD89) as well as less characterized Fcα/Fcμ receptor, asialoglycoprotein receptor, and transferrin receptor (or CD71) on granulocytes, monocytes, macrophages, DCs, Kupffer cells, and mesangial cells and may thereby provide a second line of defense against microbes that breach the mucosal barrier (198,528).

IgE is expressed by memory B cells as a surface BCR after the induction of class switching, but is also released by class-switched plasma cells in both the circulation and in mucosal secretions (533). IgE is a very potent antibody isotype that triggers inflammatory reactions to airborne, dietary, or blood-borne allergens (534). Indeed, in spite of having a very small serum concentration and a very short half-life, IgE has high affinity for a powerful FcεRI expressed by mast cells, eosinophils, and basophils (200,535). Binding of FcεRI-associated IgE by high-affinity antigens triggers the discharge of pre-formed or newly formed inflammatory and antimicrobial mediators, including histamine, cationic proteins, cathelicidin, prostaglandins, leukotrienes, and proteases (534). In addition to mediating allergic reactions, IgE interaction with FcεRI provides immune protection against parasites, and indeed increased serum IgE levels correlate with the presence of worm infections (536). IgE is also produced under homeostatic conditions, perhaps to enhance the survival and optimize the protective function of mast cells, eosinophils, and basophils that populate mucosal surfaces (537). Consistent with this, binding of IgE to FcεRI is thought to deliver survival signals to mucosal mast cells in the absence of antigen (538). In addition, binding of FcεRI-associated IgE by low-affinity antigen may induce basophil and mast cell secretion of protective cytokines without eliciting degranulation (539). IgE also interacts with FcεRII (or CD23), a low-affinity receptor that modulates the activation of B cells and mediates IgE translocation across mucosal epithelial cells (534,540).

Pathways and Signals for Ig Production

Antibody responses to protein antigens require cognate interaction of follicular B cells with T_{FH} cells expressing CD40L (541). In spite of generating immune protection and memory, this TD pathway is relatively slow and needs to be integrated with a faster TI pathway that activates extrafollicular B cells through CD40L-like factors released by cells of the innate immune system, including BAFF and APRIL (542,543). These mediators cooperate with microbial BCR and TLR ligands to induce early CD40-independent antibody responses to highly conserved carbohydrate and lipid antigens (72,74,544,545).

TD Responses

Follicular naïve B cells, also known as B-2 cells, characteristically respond to TD protein antigens captured by macrophages and DCs. As discussed earlier, engagement of the BCR by antigen induces activating signals that cause antigen internalization, antigen processing, and B-cell cognate interaction with T_{FH} cells. By providing strong costimulatory signals via CD40L and cytokines such as IL-21, T_{FH} cells induce B cells to migrate to the germinal center, where they undergo clonal expansion, CSR, SHM, and antigen-driven selection (62). Ultimately, this TD pathway generates germinal center B cells that differentiate to either memory B cells or plasma cells producing protective IgG, IgA, and IgE antibodies with high affinity for antigen. Usually, TD antibody responses require 5 to 7 days, which is too much of a delay to control mucosal antigens and blood-borne pathogens. To compensate for this limitation, specialized subsets of extrafollicular B cells initiate more rapid antibody responses that target highly conserved microbial determinants.

TI Responses

Extrafollicular B cells strategically positioned at the mucosal interface and in the MZ of the spleen typically respond to TI carbohydrate and glycolipid antigens captured by macrophages and DCs (453,546,547). Such "frontline" B cells include B-1 cells and MZ B cells (67,517,548). In the mouse, B-1 cells

constitute a distinct lineage of self-renewing B cells that are produced during fetal life and are mostly localized in the peritoneal cavity, spleen, and intestine (517). B-1 cells generate innate (or "natural") adaptive immunity by spontaneously releasing polyspecific IgM but also IgA and IgG antibodies that provide a first line of defense against viral and bacterial infections (546). Recent work has identified a small subset of B cells functionally equivalent to mouse B-1 cells in the circulation of humans, but further studies are needed to confirm these findings (549). Similar to B-1 cells, MZ B cells express polyspecific antibodies that recognize TI antigens with low affinity, at least in mice (546). In humans, MZ B cells can also produce mono-specific antibodies to TI antigens (67). Classically, TI antigens are classified into type-1 (TI-1) antigens, which include microbial TLR ligands such as LPS, and type-2 (TI-2) antigens, which include bacterial cell wall polysaccharides. Additional TI antigens include microbial glycolipids recognized by MHC-I–like CD1 molecules expressed by MZ B cells (550). Both B-1 and MZ B cells are characterized by a state of active readiness that involves elevated expression of nonspecific TLRs (72,74,517,544) and poorly diversified BCR molecules capable of recognizing multiple microbial products (548,550). B-1 and MZ B cells also show elevated expression of the transmembrane activator and calcium-modulating cyclophilin-ligand interactor (TACI), a receptor that triggers CSR and antibody production in response to BAFF and APRIL (31,546). These CD40L-like factors are released by cells of the innate immune system such as macrophages, DCs, granulocytes, and epithelial cells after sensing the presence of microbes via TLRs (14,72,551–553).

In both mice and humans, B-1 cells express a phenotype that includes surface IgM, IgD, CD19, CD5, and CD43 (517). B-1 cells produce natural IgM antibodies to highly conserved antigens, but also mount IgM and IgA responses to intestinal commensal bacteria. Together with canonical IgA production via the TD pathway, production of IgA via alternative TI pathways is important to promote a homeostatic interaction between the host and the intestinal microbiota (442,554,555). MZ B cells populate the border between the white and red pulp of the spleen, but in humans they are also present in the peripheral blood (67,548). In humans, MZ B cells express moderately mutated V(D)J genes, high IgM, low IgD, CD19, CD24, CD27, the MHC-like molecule CD1c, and high levels of the complement receptor CD21, but not CD38 (67). In mice, MZ B cells have a similar phenotype, but their V(D)J genes are largely unmutated (548,550). In general, MZ B cells secrete IgM as well as IgG and IgA that recognize TI antigens with low affinity. However, MZ B cells can also mount high-affinity IgG responses to capsular polysaccharides, at least in humans (67,442,554,555). Remarkably, MZ B cells can also participate in TD antibody responses owing to their ability to capture antigen and shuttle from the MZ to the follicle, where they can deposit antigen on FDCs and even present antigen to T_{FH} cells (556,557).

BCR Signaling

Activating signals from the BCR are required for both TD and TI antibody responses. Binding of the BCR by antigen initiates a complex cascade of signaling events that lead to B-cell survival, activation, proliferation, and differentiation. BCR signal transduction requires Igα and Igβ (or CD79a and CD79b) heterodimers noncovalently associated with the transmembrane Ig receptor (558–560). These invariant Igα and Igβ subunits have a cytoplasmic tail that contains an ITAM domain (558,560). Antigen-induced aggregation of the BCR complex rapidly phosphorylates the ITAMs associated with Igα and Igβ through the activity of Src family kinases such as Lyn, Blk, and Fyn (561). This phosphorylation creates docking sites for the SH2-related tyrosine kinases Syk and Btk, which in turn promote the recruitment of B-cell linker protein (BLNK or SLP-65) and PLCγ2 (562). BLNK is important for the activation of the Ras-MAP (mitogen-activated protein) kinase pathway, whereas PLCγ2 breaks PIP$_2$ into IP$_3$ and DAG, two signaling intermediates that activate PKC by increasing intracellular free Ca^{2+}. All these early signaling events are further amplified by CD19, CD21 (a type-2 complement receptor or CR2), and CD81 (a tetraspanin molecule also known as TAPA-1) co-receptor molecules, which are associated with BCR, Igα, and Igβ to form the BCR receptor complex (563).

BCR signaling ultimately induces nuclear translocation of various transcription factors, including NF-κB, AP-1, and NFAT, which activate a host of genes involved in the survival, activation, proliferation, and differentiation of B cells. The nuclear translocation of NF-κB implicates PLCγ2 as well as other enzymes such as PI3K. By inducing DAG formation, PLCγ2 recruits and activates PKCθ, which in turn phosphorylates the scaffold protein CARMA1 to allow the formation of a signaling module that also contains Bcl-10 and MALT1 proteins (260,564). The CARMA1-Bcl-10-MALT1 complex activates IKK, an oligomeric enzyme that mediates the nuclear translocation of NF-κB (565). By phosphorylating the cytoplasmic inhibitor IκB, IKK tags IκB for ubiquitination and proteasome-mediated degradation (566), thereby enabling IκB-free NF-κB dimers to translocate from the cytoplasm to the nucleus. The nuclear translocation of AP-1 involves the Ras-MAP kinase pathway, which activates ERK to promote the generation of the Fos-Jun B heterodimer forming AP-1 (567). Finally, the nuclear translocation of NFAT involves calcium-mediated activation of calmodulin. This calcium sensor protein activates calcineurin, a phosphatase that dephosphorylates serine residues in the amino-terminal portion of NFAT, thereby inducing conformational changes that lead to the exposure of a nuclear localization signal required for the nuclear import of NFAT (568).

Given its central role in the activation of B cells, the BCR signaling pathway is negatively regulated by several inhibitory receptors, including CD22, FcγRIIB (or CD32), CD45, and PIR-B (569). These inhibitory receptors provide negative feedback signals that contribute to the termination of the B-cell response. A detailed discussion of these inhibitory receptors is beyond the scope of this chapter. Suffice to say that the cytoplasmic domain of CD22 contains an ITIM domain that recruits the SH2-containing phosphatase SHP-1 after engagement of CD22 by poorly understood sialic acid–containing ligands possibly associated with antigen (570). SHP-1 inhibits BCR signaling by dephosphorylating tyrosine residues in the ITAMs of both Igα and Igβ subunits (571). As described below, FcγRIIB delivers similar negative signals after binding IgG associated with opsonized antigen (196).

CD40 Signaling Pathway

In TD antibody responses, binding of CD40 on B cells by CD40L on T$_{FH}$ cells causes the recruitment of TNF receptor-associated factor 1 (TRAF1), TRAF2, TRAF3, TRAF5, and TRAF6 adaptor proteins to the cytoplasmic tail of CD40 (572–575). This event is followed by the activation of IKK, which triggers degradation of IκB and nuclear translocation of NF-κB. Signals from CD40 induce B-cell proliferation, survival, germinal center differentiation, class switching, and antibody production (480,576,577). Remarkably, CD40 provides a key survival signal for germinal center B cells that express BCR molecules with high affinity for antigen (578,579). In the absence of strong signals from BCR, CD40 cannot overdrive death-inducing signals emerging from Fas (or CD95), a death-inducing receptor induced on B cells by CD40 (580). The critical role of CD40-CD40L interaction in immunity is exemplified by the onset of HIGM in primary immunodeficient patients with deleterious mutations of the genes encoding CD40L or CD40 (581–583). These patients

develop recurrent infections due to a severe impairment of class switching and affinity maturation that is associated with a failure of antigen-activated B cells to differentiate into germinal center B cells.

TACI, BCMA, BAFF-R and TLR Signaling Pathways

In TI antibody responses, binding of TACI by BAFF or APRIL leads to the activation of MZ B cells and B-1 cells (577,584). BAFF and APRIL are structurally related molecules produced as transmembrane ligands or soluble trimers by DCs, monocytes, macrophages, neutrophils, eosinophils, basophils, FDCs, endothelial cells, epithelial cells, and stromal cells (112,543,545,551,553,585,586). TACI on B cells undergoes extensive crosslinking by high-order BAFF and APRIL oligomers that are released by innate immune cells in response to intruding microbes (542,577). The ensuing aggregation of TACI receptors activates NF-κB through a mechanism involving the recruitment of TRAF2, TRAF3, TRAF5, and TRAF6 to the cytoplasmic tail of TACI. This receptor further activates NF-κB by recruiting MyD88, an adaptor protein usually associated with TLRs (552). However, TACI interacts with MyD88 through a motif distinct from the canonical TIR motif of TLRs. Interaction of TACI or TLRs with MyD88 is followed by activation of IRAK-1 and IRAK-4 kinases, recruitment of TRAF6, induction of IKK via TAK1, and nuclear translocation of NF-κB. Although highly expressed by MZ and B-1 B cells, TACI and TLRs are also expressed by follicular B cells and therefore contribute to both TI and TD antibody responses. In addition to inducing class switching, antibody production, and plasma cell differentiation, TACI seems to regulate the size of the peripheral B-cell pool by either controlling the amount of BAFF available for signaling through BAFF-R or limiting the amount of TRAF available to transmit BAFF-R signals (587,588).

In addition to engaging TACI, both BAFF and APRIL interact with the B-cell maturation antigen (BCMA) receptor to promote plasma cell survival. BCMA is mostly expressed by antibody-producing plasmablasts and plasma cells, and its engagement by BAFF or APRIL causes NF-κB activation through a canonical TRAF-dependent pathway similar to that induced by CD40 and TACI (589).

Unlike APRIL, BAFF also engages BAFF receptor (BAFF-R or BR3), a protein widely expressed by B cells at any stage of differentiation, except plasma cells (589–591). BAFF-R is typically activated by soluble BAFF trimers that are continually released by innate immune cells and stromal cells under homeostatic conditions. Engagement of BAFF-R by BAFF elicits the recruitment of TRAF3, which is followed by the degradation of TRAF3 through a mechanism involving TRAF2, cellular inhibitor of apoptosis protein (c-IAP), and MALT1 (592,593). TRAF3 degradation causes activation of the enzyme NF-κB–inducing kinase (NIK) and induction of a noncanonical NF-κB pathway that up-regulates the expression of intracellular antiapoptotic Bcl-2 family proteins, including Bcl-2, Bcl-xL, and Mcl-1 (594). BAFF-R also triggers down-regulation of intracellular proapoptotic Bcl-2 family proteins, such as Bax, Bid, and Bad. Of note, this pathway may cooperate with survival signals from the BCR (591). In general, BAFF-R is essential for the survival of peripheral B cells, but some evidence indicates the additional involvement of BAFF-R in TI antibody production (551,595,596).

Cytokine Receptor Signaling Pathways

In humans, the major cytokines involved in the activation of mature B cells are IL-4, IL-6, IL-10, IL-21, and TGF-β (490,491,493,597,598). Signals from cytokine receptors cooperate with signals from BCR, CD40, TACI, BCMA, BAFF-R, and TLRs to induce optimal B-cell proliferation, survival, and differentiation, including CSR, SHM, and antibody production. Ligation of IL-4, IL-6, IL-10, and IL-21 receptors induces activation of Jak kinases that elicit phosphorylation, dimerization, and nuclear translocation of STAT proteins (599). While IL-6, IL-10, and IL-21 receptors activate STAT1 and STAT3, the IL-4 receptor activates STAT6. Finally, the TGF-β receptor has an intrinsic kinase activity that induces activation and nuclear translocation of SMAD transcription factors (600).

Primary Antibody Deficiencies

Primary antibody deficiencies mainly lead to recurrent infections by pyogenic bacteria and result from a broad variety of gene defects that directly or indirectly affect the function of B cells (601). Here we briefly review primary antibody deficiencies caused by gene defects affecting some of the main B-cell–stimulating pathways.

Agammaglobulinemia is characterized by the complete lack of peripheral B cells, severe antibody deficiency, and increased susceptibility to infections immediately after birth. The molecular defects underlying agammaglobulinemia are heterogeneous, but the majority of patients have deleterious X-linked mutations of the gene that encodes Btk. The resulting lack of BCR signaling blocks the development of B cells in the bone marrow at an early pro-B-cell stage (602). In addition to X-linked cases, there are autosomal recessive cases of agammaglobulinemia that are due to defects of genes encoding key components of the pre-BCR such as Cμ, λ5, Igα, and Igβ proteins.

SCID causes severe infections early in life and is frequently caused by X-linked mutations of the gene encoding the common γ chain (γc), a key signaling component of IL-2, IL-4, IL-7, IL-9, IL-15, and IL-21 receptors which is required for the development of T cells (603). Although retaining peripheral B cells, patients with X-linked SCID have impaired antibody production due to the lack of functional T cells. However, B-cell–intrinsic defects of IL-4 and IL-21 receptors may also play a role in the genesis of this antibody deficiency. Additional cases of SCID are characterized by mutations of genes encoding adenosine deaminase (ADA), which is required for the breakdown of toxic purines in both T and B cells, or RAG proteins, which are required for VDJ recombination in both T and B cells. In these cases, the antibody deficiency is due to the depletion and functional impairment of both T and B cells.

Selective IgA deficiency (SIgAD) is the most prevalent primary antibody deficiency, but its underlying molecular defect remains unknown (604). A large proportion of SIgAD patients remain asymptomatic, but some adult individuals develop mucosal infections and intestinal inflammation. Indeed, IgA not only neutralizes specific pathogens but also controls the composition and compartmentalization of the intestinal microbiota to mitigate the overall inflammatory tone of the intestine (162). This function explains why some patients with SIgA or other primary antibody deficiencies develop gut nodular lymphoid hyperplasia, a benign lymphoproliferative disorder that consists of multiple nodular lesions made up of lymphoid aggregates usually confined to the lamina propria of the small intestine. Nodular lymphoid hyperplasia is thought to originate from polyclonal activation of intestinal B cells by commensal bacteria that undergo aberrant expansion as a result of IgA deficiency. Indeed, the lack of IgA causes small bowel bacteria overgrowth syndrome. Over time, the lack of IgA can lead to the aberrant expansion of allergen-reactive, autoreactive, and clonal B cells that would otherwise be doomed to die. These abnormal B cells could contribute to the increased frequency of allergy, autoimmunity (celiac disease, hemolytic anemia, immune thrombocytopenic purpura), and B-cell tumors (mostly non-Hodgkin lymphoma) in IgA-deficient patients.

Common variable immunodeficiency (CVID) is the second most prevalent primary immunodeficiency and is characterized by hypogammaglobulinemia, impaired specific antibody responses to vaccines, and recurrent infections that mostly appear in adult age (605). In all CVID cases, the differentiation of B cells to plasma cells is impaired, but only in a minority of patients is the underlying molecular defect known. In approximately 8% of CVID cases, the gene encoding TACI is mutated, although mutations of BAFF-R and other B-cell–associated molecules such as CD19 and CD81 have also been described (601).

HIGM is a heterogeneous group of disorders characterized by recurrent infections that usually appear early in life. These infections are associated with lack of germinal centers, impaired CSR and SHM, and decreased IgG, IgA, and IgE production with normal or elevated IgM production. Mutations of genes encoding CD40L, CD40, or AID are the predominant cause of HIGM (606). Of note, IgG and IgA responses are not abrogated in mucosal surfaces, which relates to the presence of alternative CD40-independent pathways for B-cell activation (162).

IMMUNE REGULATION

The initiation of protective immune responses requires the induction of multiple activating signals for the stimulation of cells of the innate and adaptive immune systems. As the response progresses, these activating signals need to be bridled by regulatory signals to prevent an excessive activation of the immune system, terminate the immune response, and restore homeostasis. Key regulatory signals are provided by death-inducing receptors (DR) such as Fas and TNFR1, which limit the life span of activated immune cells by inducing apoptosis. Further regulatory signals are provided by a large family of inhibitory receptors that regulate the function of activating immune receptors with common ligand-binding properties but divergent signaling capacity (173). In addition to DR and inhibitory immune receptors, TGF-β and IL-10 receptors further contribute to the regulation of innate and adaptive immune responses (607,608). TGF-β and IL-10 are anti-inflammatory cytokines produced by activated innate immune cells, including DCs and macrophages located at the mucosal interface. TGF-β and IL-10 are also produced by Treg cells, a T-cell subset specialized in the control of effector T$_H$ cells. Recent evidence shows that also the B-cell compartment includes a subset of Breg cells specialized in IL-10 production.

Apoptosis

Cell death or survival results from a tightly regulated balance between proapoptotic and antiapoptotic signals. Apoptosis or programmed cell death is an evolutionarily conserved developmental program that controls cell growth and homeostasis (609). Apoptosis is essential to delete autoreactive lymphocytes specific for self-antigens, eliminate antigen-specific lymphocytes during the contraction phase of the immune response, and remove infected or neoplastic immune and nonimmune cells (610). Apoptosis involves a sequence of morphologic changes that include condensation of the cytoplasm, margination of nuclear chromatin, and formation of one or several membrane-bound apoptotic bodies containing cytoplasmic organelles and nuclear fragments (611,612). After "sensing" apoptotic cells through specific recognition receptors, neighboring phagocytes activate a clearing program that removes the apoptotic cell without triggering inflammation (613,614). In general, apoptosis follows either an INTRINSIC or an EXTRINSIC pathway (Fig. 2.23). These pathways can be distinguished on the basis of the origin of the death-inducing signal, but they all lead to the activation of specialized proteases called aspartic-acid cysteine proteases or caspases (615). The activity of these enzymes is negatively regulated by c-IAP molecules associated with cell surface receptors that enhance cell survival via the transcription factor NF-κB.

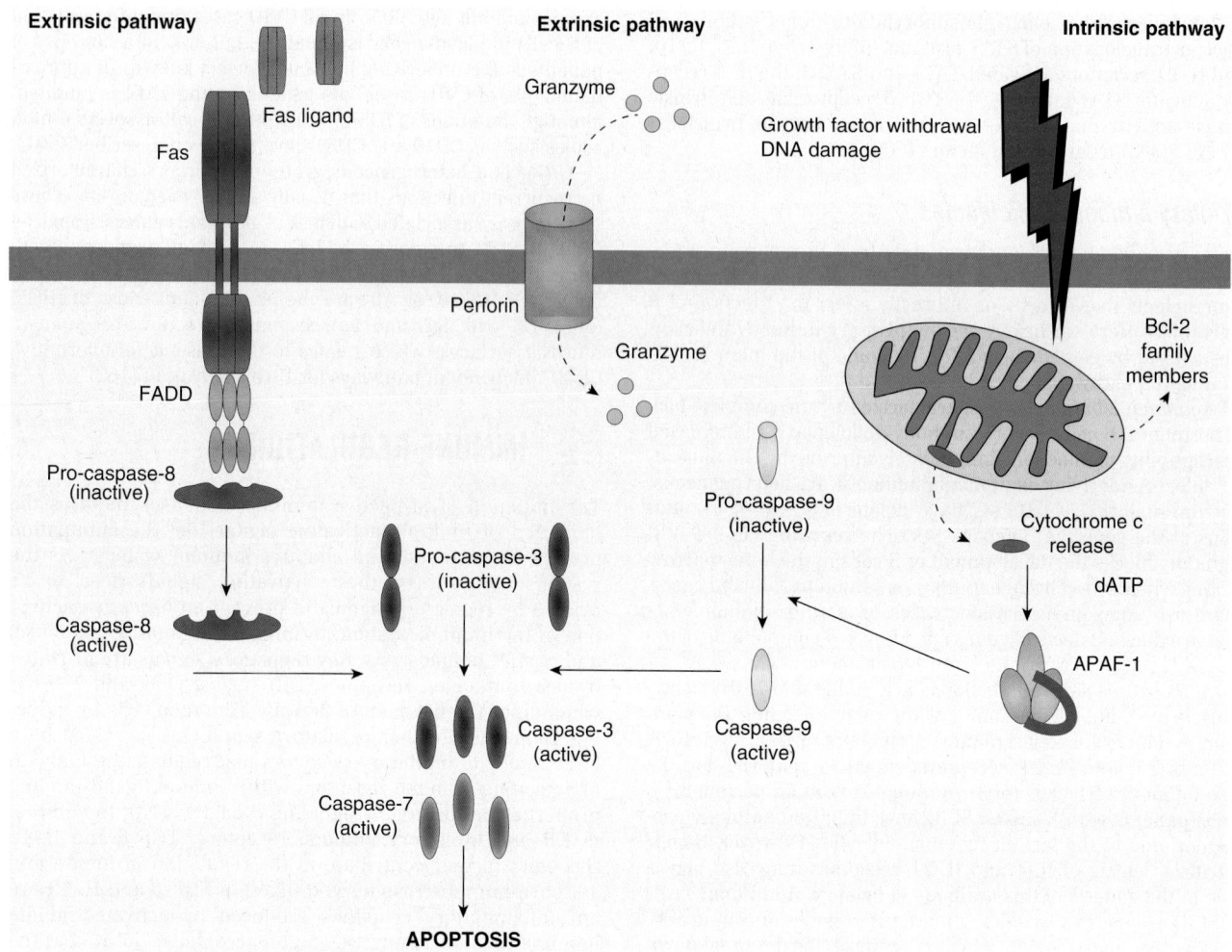

Extrinsic pathway   **Extrinsic pathway**   **Intrinsic pathway**

FIGURE 2.23. Extrinsic and intrinsic pathways of apoptosis. The Fas receptor and the perforin-granzyme system are prototypical players of the EXTRINSIC PATHWAY of apoptosis. After engagement by FasL trimers on activated T cells, Fas on B cells, T cells, and other cell types undergo oligomerization and recruit the adaptor protein FADD and the enzyme pro-caspase-8. Subsequent cleavage-dependent induction of active caspase-8 leads to the recruitment and activation of effector caspases-3 and -7 that trigger apoptosis. Perforin from NK cells and CTLs induces membrane pores that permit the entry of granzymes into target cells. Granzyme induces apoptosis by altering intracellular osmosis, activating effector caspases, or increasing outer mitochondrial membrane permeabilization. The INTRINSIC PATHWAY is controlled by antiapoptotic and proapoptotic proteins of the Bcl-2 family, which regulate the permeability of the mitochondrial membrane. Stressors such as DNA damage and growth factor withdrawal alter the balance between antiapoptotic and proapoptotic Bcl-2 family members, thereby inducing the release of cytochrome c and dATP from mitochondria and the subsequent activation of apoptotic protease-activating factor-1 (Apaf-1). This protein causes activation of caspase-9, which in turn triggers apoptosis by inducing effector caspase-3 and -7.

Caspases are a conserved family of enzymes that irreversibly commit a cell to die (616). The name caspase stems from the fact that these enzymes function as cysteine proteases that target their substrates at the level of an aspartate residue. Caspases are generally divided into initiator caspases, which include caspase-2, -8, -9, and -10 and effector caspases, which include caspase-3, -6, and -7. Initiator caspases have long pro-domains that contain the protein-protein interaction motif death effector domain (DED) or CARD, which promote interaction with upstream adaptor proteins. Effector caspases have a short pro-domain and are typically cleaved and activated by upstream initiator caspases. Most caspases become activated after proteolytic cleavage (617). Active effector caspases mediate the downstream execution steps of the apoptotic program by cleaving multiple cytoplasmic and nuclear proteins (618). To date, over 400 substrates have been identified, including poly ADP ribose polymerase (PARP), caspase-activated DNase (CAD), lamin, and focal adhesion kinase. Caspase-induced protein cleavage leads to cytoplasmic shrinkage, DNA fragmentation, and nuclear condensation. Caspases are subject to

transcriptional regulation and post-translational modifications (619). In addition, caspases are subjected to the regulatory activity of c-IAPs, which potently inhibit active caspases by conveying them into the proteasome pathway after ubiquitination (620).

NF-κB proteins form a family of transcription factors that regulate cell growth, activation, proliferation, differentiation, survival, and transformation (565,621). The NF-κB family includes p65 (or Rel-A), Rel-B, c-Rel, p50, and p52 signaling subunits as well as p100 precursor subunit. In resting cells, p65, p50, and c-Rel are complexed with inhibitory IκB proteins such as IκBα to form inactive cytoplasmic p50-p65, c-Rel-p65, and c-Rel-p50 dimers. Cell activation releases these dimers from IκB, thereby inducing translocation of active p50-p65, c-Rel-p65, and c-Rel-p50 complexes to the nucleus. Similar to IκB, the p100 protein functions as an inactive precursor of p52 in resting cells. Activation leads to the processing of p100, followed by the release of active p52, dimerization of p52 with Rel-B, and translocation of active p52-RelB dimers from the cytoplasm to the nucleus. Once in the nucleus, NF-κB dimers induce the transcription of target genes by binding to κB motifs located within NF-κB–responsive gene promoters. This binding involves a transactivation domain located in the carboxy-terminal portion of p65, c-Rel and Rel-B proteins. There are two pathways that mediate NF-κB activation (621): the classical or canonical pathway and the alternative or noncanonical pathway.

The *canonical NF-κB pathway* is induced by the vast majority of NF-κB–inducing stimuli, including BCR, TCR, several members of the TNFR family, TLRs, and IL-1R; in contrast, the noncanonical NF-κB pathway is induced by selected members of the TNFR family such as BAFF-R (622). Inducers of the canonical NF-κB pathway cause activation of a large IKK complex that contains two catalytic IKKα and IKKβ subunits and a regulatory IKKγ (or NEMO) subunit (623). IKK induces phosphorylation of inhibitory IκB proteins at two conserved amino-terminal serine residues, thereby targeting IκB for ubiquitination and proteasome-mediated degradation (566). Functional release of IκB unmasks a nuclear localization signal on NF-κB dimers, thereby permitting their translocation from the cytoplasm to the nucleus, where they transcriptionally activate a large set of NF-κB-responsive genes. One of these genes encodes IκBα. Once re-synthesized in the cytoplasm, IκBα moves back to the nucleus to bind DNA-associated NF-κB dimers, namely those containing p65. The ensuing release of NF-κB-IκBα complexes from DNA is followed by translocation of inactive NF-κB-IκBα complexes from the nucleus to the cytoplasm.

The alternative NF-κB pathway involves activation of IKKα by NIK, which is followed by IKKα-mediated phosphorylation of the precursor protein p100 (624). After its phosphorylation, p100 is proteolytically processed to form a p52 subunit that dimerizes with RelB (625). Then, p52-RelB dimers translocate from the cytoplasm to the nucleus, where they activate a specific set of NF-κB–responsive genes. In general, p52-RelB dimers predominantly activate genes involved in cell survival, whereas p50-p65, c-Rel-p65, and c-Rel-p50 dimers mostly activate genes involved in cell growth, activation, proliferation, and differentiation. However, this distinction is not absolute, as the canonical NF-κB pathway is also involved in cell survival.

Extrinsic Pathway

The extrinsic pathway of apoptosis initiates outside a cell, when conditions in the extracellular environment determine that a cell must die. Based on the triggering stimulus and nature of the components involved, at least two extrinsic apoptotic pathways can be identified: the first pathway involves cytotoxic effector proteins such as perforin and granzyme, whereas the second pathway involves death-inducing receptor proteins.

Perforins and granzymes are death-inducing proteins expressed by NK cells and CTLs, two subsets of effector lymphocytes that mediate defensive programs against transformed or infected cells (626). NK cells and CTLs contain specialized intracellular compartments known as secretory lysosomes that consist of membrane-bound organelles filled with cytolytic proteins (627–630). Perforins are calcium-dependent pore-forming proteins, whereas granzymes are serine proteases with a typical His-Asp-Ser catalytic triad. In humans, there are five granzymes that are defined as A, B, H, K, and M. The most extensively studied is granzyme B (631), which cleaves substrates at the level of aspartic acid residues and proteolytically activates a number of caspases. Granzyme B also promotes cell death via the mitochondrial pathway, and indeed its rapid death-inducing activity involves both proteolytic processing of caspase-3 and permeabilization of the mitochondrial outer membrane (632). Upon recognition of a target cell, NK cells and CTLs deposit the contents of secretory granules in the

immunologic synapse (633). By generating pores in the plasma membrane, perforins enable granzymes to enter the cell for the induction of apoptosis via effector caspases (634).

Death-inducing receptors include TNFR family proteins that have a broad range of biologic functions, including immune activation and regulation (635). In general, the TNFR family includes more than 20 proteins that share similar cysteine-rich extracellular domains (Fig. 2.24) and require ligand-induced trimerization to generate signal transduction (636). Remarkably, some members of the TNFR family such as TNFR-1 and Fas have a death domain (DD) in their cytoplasmic tail (637). This domain mediates activation of the apoptotic pathway and plays a crucial role in the negative regulation of the immune response, particularly in the context of Fas signaling. As for DD-less TNFR family members, some induce apoptosis by promoting autocrine production of TNF (this is the case of CD30, which can induce death signals via TNFR-1), whereas others inhibit apoptosis by blocking signals emerging from DD-containing receptors (this is the case of CD40, which inhibits apoptosis induced by Fas, at least in the presence of strong BCR co-signals).

TNFRs include TNFR-1 (CD120a), which is expressed by a broad spectrum of immune and nonimmune cells, and TNFR-2 (CD120b), which is mostly expressed by immune cells. TNFR-1 and TNFR-2 bind TNF, a pleiotropic inflammatory cytokine produced by macrophages, lymphocytes, fibroblasts, epithelial cells, and many other cell types in response to inflammation, infection, and other environmental stresses. TNFR-1 and TNFR-2 lack intrinsic enzymatic activity and thus deliver their signals by interacting with multiple adaptor proteins. These proteins activate complex signaling cascades that induce multiple and often conflicting functional effects. Here we only discuss death- and NF-κB–inducing signals. TNFR-1 contains a DD that promotes the recruitment of the adaptor protein TNFR-1–associated death domain (TRADD) (638). The resulting TNFR-1-TRADD complex interacts with the kinase RIP1 to form a seeding ground for the additional association of the Fas-associated death domain (FADD) adaptor protein (639). The resulting death-inducing signaling complex (DISC) elicits recruitment and proteolytic activation of pro-caspase-8, which initiates a caspase-3–dependent effector pathway leading to apoptosis (640). In addition to triggering apoptosis, TRADD elicits a powerful inflammatory pathway that involves NF-κB (641). Indeed, the TNFR-1-TRADD complex causes nuclear translocation of NF-κB by recruiting the adaptor protein TRAF2, which triggers the activation of IKK (642). Of note, TNFR-1 also activates other transcription factors, including AP-1. While TNFR-1 is well known for its role in apoptosis, inflammation, and lymphoid development, the role of TNFR-2 remains poorly understood. However, TNFR-2 recruits TRAF2 to activate NF-κB as TNFR-1 does.

Fas (or CD95) is broadly expressed by both immune and nonimmune cells, whereas its cognate ligand (FasL) is predominantly expressed by T cells and NK cells (643). Fas mostly induces apoptosis, but growing evidence points to an additional role for this molecule in cell activation and proliferation. Fas shows elevated expression on activated and germinal center B cells and has an essential role in the negative regulation of antibody production (644). Indeed, the germinal center reaction is associated with the elimination of B cells that have either suboptimal affinity for antigen or reactivity for self-antigen (autoreactive). This negative selection requires the engagement of Fas on B cells by FasL on T_FH cells. B cells that have high affinity for antigen are rescued from Fas-mediated apoptosis through a pathway that involves signals from BCR and CD40. The latter delivers survival signals by activating NF-κB and by up-regulating intracellular inhibitors of apoptosis such as c-IAPs, FLIP, and Bcl-xL proteins (645).

Binding of Fas by FasL leads to formation of a DISC complex composed of FADD and procaspase-8 (or FLICE),

FIGURE 2.24. TNF ligand and receptor superfamilies. These large groups of molecules mediate the proliferation, differentiation, and apoptosis of lymphocytes and other immune cell types. Members of the TNF ligand family have extracellular cysteine-rich domains required for the interaction with cognate receptors, whereas members of the TNFR family have cytosolic death domains and/or TRAF-binding domains required for signal transduction. Only some TNFR family members have death domains for the induction of apoptosis. LT, lymphotoxin α and lymphotoxin β; TRAIL, TNF-related apoptosis inducing ligand (TRAIL); RANK, receptor activator of nuclear factor-κB; OPG, osteoprotegerin; OPGL, osteoprotegerin ligand; TWEAK, TNF-related WEAK inducer of apoptosis; LIGHT, ligand for herpesvirus entry mediator; HVEM, herpesvirus entry mediator; NGF, nerve growth factor; NGFR, NGF receptor.

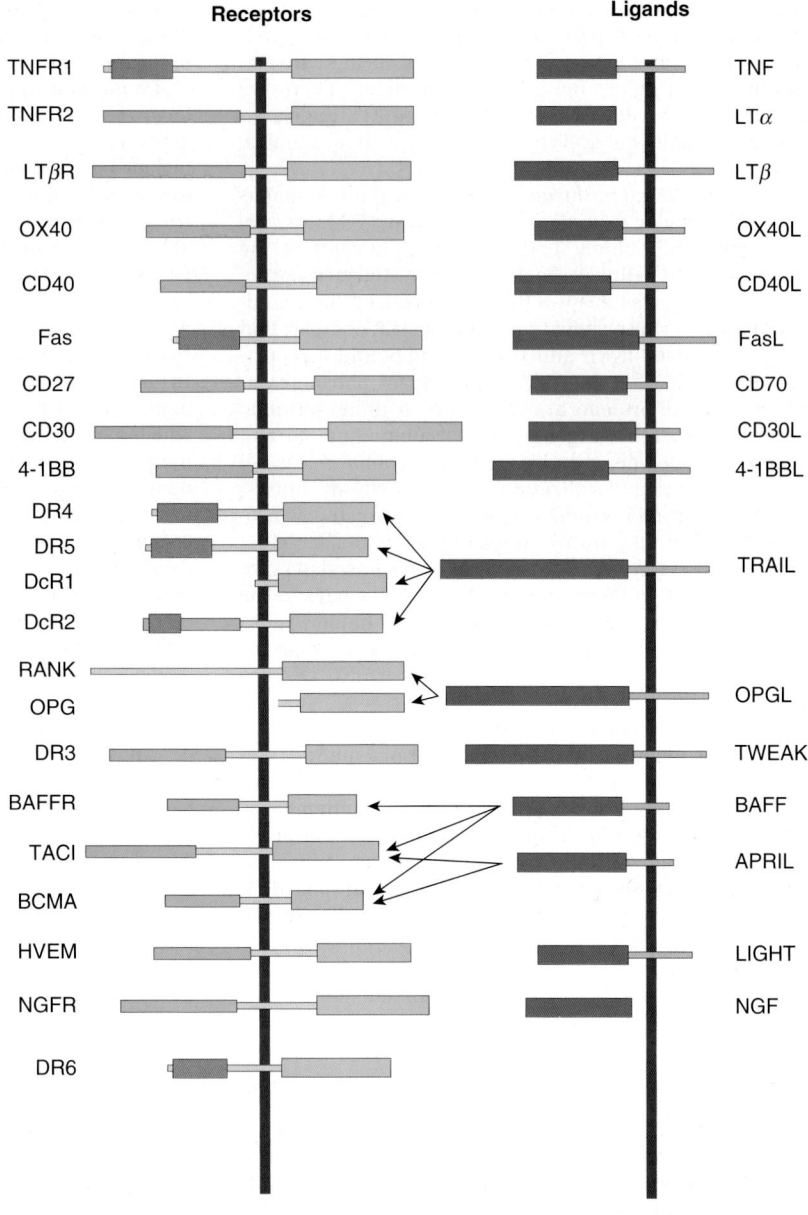

procaspase-10, and cellular FLICE inhibitory protein (c-FLIP), which is a negative regulator of procaspase-8 (646,647). Interactions between different components of the DISC complex are based on homotypic contacts: the DD of Fas interacts with the DD of FADD, whereas the DED of FADD interacts with the DED of procaspases-8 and c-FLIP (648). Activated caspase-8 causes activation of downstream effectors caspase-3 and -7, thereby leading to apoptosis. This process is modulated by three isoforms of c-FLIP termed long (L), short (S), and raji (R) (649). The short FLIP isoforms S and R block activation of procaspase-8 and apoptosis, whereas the isoform L has both antiapoptotic and proapoptotic functions (650). Interestingly, two cleavage products of c-FLIP enhance the activation of NF-κB by interacting with the IKK complex.

DR and decoy receptors (DCR) are mostly expressed by macrophages and DCs and bind TRAIL, a TNF superfamily member constitutively expressed by a broad range of cells, including cells from the spleen and prostate (651,652). TRAIL delivers apoptotic signals via death receptor 4 (DR4, or TRAIL-R1) and

DR5 (or TRAIL-R2) through a mechanism involving DISC formation (653). TRAIL also binds DCR1 and DCR2, which prevent the induction of apoptosis in different tumor cells, at least *in vitro*.

CD30 is expressed by some thymocytes, a subset of activated T and B cells, pancreatic exocrine cells, and decidual cells. CD30 is also highly expressed by malignant B cells from classical Hodgkin lymphoma (654) and malignant T cells from anaplastic large cell lymphoma. CD30 ligand (CD30L) is expressed on activated T cells, activated macrophages, B cells, neutrophils, eosinophils, and mast cells. Like other TNFR superfamily members, CD30 activates NF-κB through a mechanism involving recruitment of multiple TRAF adaptor proteins, including TRAF2 (655). Signals emanating from CD30 promote cell proliferation and survival, but also induce anti-proliferative responses and cell death, particularly in the thymus, where CD30 seems to enhance the negative selection of thymocytes (656). The mechanism underlying CD30-induced apoptosis remains poorly understood, but may involve induction of autocrine TNF (657).

Intrinsic Pathway

The intrinsic pathway of apoptosis involves receptor-independent intracellular signals that function in either a positive or negative manner. The intrinsic pathway is also called mitochondrial pathway due to the essential role of mitochondria in the delivery of death signals (658). This pathway becomes activated in response to stress stimuli such as DNA damage, chemotherapeutic agents, serum starvation, and UV radiation. By altering the permeability of the inner mitochondrial membrane, these and other stressants cause cytosolic release of two main groups of apoptotic proteins that are normally sequestered within mitochondria. The first group of mitochondrial apoptotic proteins consists of cytochrome *c*, Smac/DIABLO (659), and the serine protease HtrA2/Omi, which work in a caspase-dependent manner (660). Cytochrome *c* forms an apoptosome after binding and activating Apaf-1 and pro-caspase-9 (661). In this complex, active caspase-9 becomes an initiator caspase that further activates caspase-3 and caspase-7 effector caspases. Smac/DIABLO and HtrA2/Omi promote apoptosis by inhibiting c-IAP proteins (662). The second group of mitochondrial apoptotic proteins includes apoptosis-inducing factor (AIF), endonuclease G, and CAD, which partly work in a caspase-independent manner. The control of all these mitochondrial events occurs through members of the Bcl-2 family.

Bcl-2 proteins govern the permeability of the mitochondrial membrane and deliver either proapoptotic or antiapoptotic signals. The anti-apoptotic Bcl-2 family members Bcl-2, Bcl-XL, Bcl-w, Mcl-1, A1, and Bcl-B contain four BH domains (BH1-BH4) involved in protein-protein interaction and protect cells against apoptosis through their association with the outer mitochondrial membrane (663). The proapoptotic Bcl-2 members can be divided into two groups. Bax-like multidomain apoptotic proteins contain up to three BH domains (BH1-BH3) and include Bax, Bak, and Bok proteins, whereas BH3-only proteins contain only one BH3 domain and include Bik, Bid, Bad, Puma, Noxa, Bim, Hrk, and Bmf proteins (664). It is generally thought that Bcl-2 proteins form homo-dimers and hetero-dimers in which proapoptotic and antiapoptotic family members neutralize the activity of each other (665). Therefore, the intracellular balance between proapoptotic and antiapoptotic Bcl-2 proteins is critical to determine the fate of an individual cell (666). Some members of the TNFR family such as BAFF-R promote cell survival by shifting this intracellular balance toward antiapoptotic Bcl-2 proteins (594).

Inhibitory Immune Receptors

About 60 inhibitory immune receptors have been described thus far, including KIRs in NK cells, FcγRIIB in innate immune cells and B cells, CD22 and PIR-B in B cells, and CTLA-4 and PD-1 in T cells (173). Usually, inhibitory immune receptors undergo phosphorylation of cytoplasmic ITIM regions after recruiting Src tyrosine kinases in response to receptor engagement by a cognate ligand (38,667). ITIM phosphorylation leads to the activation of SH2 domain-containing phosphatases such as SHP-1, SHP-2, or SHIP, which terminate cell activation by dephosphorylating effector molecules induced by immune activating receptors. Although typically regulating ITAM-containing activating immune receptors, ITIM-containing inhibitory immune receptors can also suppress activating immune receptors that lack ITAM regions, including TLRs and cytokine receptors. Among inhibitory immune receptors, FcγRIIB is probably the best characterized.

FcγRIIB is a member of the FcγR family, which includes various cell surface molecules that bind the Fc portion of IgG, the most abundant antibody class in circulation (202,216). FcγRs include activating FcγRI, FcγRIIA, and FcγRIII receptors and the inhibitory FcγRIIB receptor, which display remarkable differences in structure, expression, IgG binding affinity, signaling activity, and function (196). FcγRIIB plays a key role in limiting the activation of B cells involved in IgG production and innate immune cells involved in IgG effector functions, including DCs, monocytes, and macrophages. The signaling cascade triggered by FcγRIIB is similar to that initiated by other ITIM-containing inhibitory immune receptors. When B cells are exposed to IgG-opsonized antigens, co-ligation of BCR and FcγRIIB results in the inhibition of ITAM-dependent signals emanating from the BCR through an ITIM-dependent mechanism that involves FcγRIIB (668). In this manner, FcγRIIB negatively regulates the survival, activation, proliferation, and differentiation of B cells that have already undergone IgG production (669,670). FcγRIIB utilizes a similar mechanism to inhibit the activation of innate immune cells by IgG-opsonized antigen via FcγRI, FcγRIIA, and FcγRIII.

Treg Cells and Breg Cells

Treg cells and more recently identified Breg cells provide additional mechanisms for the regulation of the magnitude and quality of the immune response. A detailed analysis of these cells goes beyond the scope of this chapter. As discussed earlier in the section "T-Cell Effector Subsets," natural and inducible Treg cells are subpopulations of T cells that regulate inflammatory responses, self-tolerance, and immune homeostasis through various mechanisms involving the production of immunosuppressive soluble factors such as IL-10 and TGF-β as well as the expression of membrane CTLA-4 and glucocorticoid-induced TNF receptor (GITR). Similar to Treg cells, Breg cells are a functional lymphocyte subset specialized in immune regulation (37). Indeed, Breg cells show numerical and functional defects in various autoimmune disorders and may therefore play a central role in the maintenance of immune tolerance (671,672). In addition, Breg cells regulate inflammation and indeed exert a protective activity against multiple sclerosis, arthritis, and colitis (673–675). In the presence of appropriate activating signals, multiple subsets of B cells can give rise to Breg cells, including MZ, transitional, and follicular B cells. In general, Breg cells express CD1d, produce large amounts of IL-10, and inhibit inflammation by interfering with signals emanating from inflammatory cytokines, including IL-1β (675).

SUMMARY AND CONCLUSIONS

The immune system includes a wide range of physical, cellular, and molecular elements that provide protection against infections. Innate immune responses by granulocytes, monocytes, macrophages, DCs, NK cells, and mast cells provide fast nonspecific protection but not memory by promoting recognition, engulfment, and killing of microorganisms. Adaptive immune responses by T cells and B cells provide slower but specific protection and long-term memory by generating CTLs and antibody-secreting plasma cells. These adaptive responses require the presentation of processed antigen to T cells by DCs as well as the presentation of native antigen to B cells by DCs and macrophages. During the past three decades, developments in immunology have elucidated the biology of specific hematologic neoplasms, such as the leukemias and lymphomas and of solid tumors such as renal cell carcinoma and melanoma. Vaccine strategies, which are being tried for diverse tumors such as multiple myeloma and melanoma, depend on antigen presentation and the coordinated response induced by DCs and T cells. Passive immunotherapies, based on the infusion of monoclonal antibodies to particular antigens or the delivery of cytokines, are engineered based on information regarding cell-surface antigens and their particular functions. Adaptive immunotherapies, by which autologous DCs, T cells, or other cells are cultivated and manipulated *ex vivo* to generate an expanded, tumor-reactive effector cell population, are based on principles of antigen recognition, tolerance, and cell-mediated cytotoxicity. Our understanding of the pathophysiology of specific neoplasms and our capacity to treat them effectively rests in our expanding knowledge of normal host defenses.

ACKNOWLEDGMENTS

We thank Sergi Serrano and Laura Comerma (Institut Hospital del Mar d'Investigacions Mèdiques) for providing photographic material.

References

1. Janeway CA Jr. Approaching the asymptote? Evolution and revolution in immunology. *Cold Spring Harb Symp Quant Biol* 1989;54(Pt 1):1–13.
2. Janeway CA Jr, Medzhitov R. Innate immune recognition. *Annu Rev Immunol* 2002;20:197–216.
3. Hoebe K, Janssen E, Beutler B. The interface between innate and adaptive immunity. *Nat Immunol* 2004;5:971–974.
4. Grivennikov SI, Greten FR, Karin M. Immunity, inflammation, and cancer. *Cell* 2010;140:883–899.
5. Gallo RL, Nakatsuji T. Microbial symbiosis with the innate immune defense system of the skin. *J Invest Dermatol* 2011;131:1974–1980.
6. Artis D. Epithelial-cell recognition of commensal bacteria and maintenance of immune homeostasis in the gut. *Nat Rev Immunol* 2008;8:411–420.
7. McAuley JL, Linden SK, Png CW, et al. MUC1 cell surface mucin is a critical element of the mucosal barrier to infection. *J Clin Invest* 2007;117:2313–2324.
8. Sansonetti PJ. War and peace at mucosal surfaces. *Nat Rev Immunol* 2004;4:953–964.
9. Shen L, Turner JR. Role of epithelial cells in initiation and propagation of intestinal inflammation. Eliminating the static: tight junction dynamics exposed. *Am J Physiol Gastrointest Liver Physiol* 2006;290:G577–G582.
10. Gallo RL, Hooper LV. Epithelial antimicrobial defence of the skin and intestine. *Nat Rev Immunol* 2012;12:503–516.
11. Nagler-Anderson C. Man the barrier! Strategic defences in the intestinal mucosa. *Nat Rev Immunol* 2001;1:59–67.
12. Mostov KE. Transepithelial transport of immunoglobulins. *Annu Rev Immunol* 1994;12:63–84.
13. Cerutti A, Chen K, Chorny A. Immunoglobulin responses at the mucosal interface. *Annu Rev Immunol* 2011;29:273–293.
14. Cerutti A, Cols M, Puga I. Activation of B-cells by non-canonical helper signals. *EMBO Rep* 2013;13:798–810.
15. Medzhitov R, Janeway CA Jr. Innate immunity: the virtues of a nonclonal system of recognition. *Cell* 1997;91:295–298.
16. Muller WA. Mechanisms of leukocyte transendothelial migration. *Annu Rev Pathol* 2011;6:323–344.
17. Borregaard N. Neutrophils, from marrow to microbes. *Immunity* 2010;33:657–670.
18. Caligiuri MA. Human natural killer cells. *Blood* 2008;112:461–469.
19. Serbina NV, Jia T, Hohl TM, et al. Monocyte-mediated defense against microbial pathogens. *Annu Rev Immunol* 2008;26:421–452.
20. Geissmann F, Manz MG, Jung S, et al. Development of monocytes, macrophages, and dendritic cells. *Science* 2010;327:656–661.
21. Adams DO, Hamilton TA. The cell biology of macrophage activation. *Annu Rev Immunol* 1984;2:283–318.
22. Sallusto F, Lanzavecchia A. The instructive role of dendritic cells on T-cell responses. *Arthritis Res* 2002; 4(Suppl 3):S127–S132.
23. Steinman RM, Hemmi H. Dendritic cells: translating innate to adaptive immunity. *Curr Top Microbiol Immunol* 2006;311:17–58.
24. Hashimoto D, Miller J, Merad M. Dendritic cell and macrophage heterogeneity in vivo. *Immunity* 2011;35:323–335.
25. Wedemeyer J, Tsai M, Galli SJ. Roles of mast cells and basophils in innate and acquired immunity. *Curr Opin Immunol* 2000;12:624–631.
26. Kita H. Eosinophils: multifaceted biological properties and roles in health and disease. *Immunol Rev* 2011;242:161–177.
27. Seder RA, Ahmed R. Similarities and differences in CD4+ and CD8+ effector and memory T-cell generation. *Nat Immunol* 2003;4:835–842.
28. Zhu J, Yamane H, Paul WE. Differentiation of effector CD4 T-cell populations (*). *Annu Rev Immunol* 2010;28:445–489.
29. Williams MA, Bevan MJ. Effector and memory CTL differentiation. *Annu Rev Immunol* 2007;25:171–192.
30. Elgueta R, de Vries VC, Noelle RJ. The immortality of humoral immunity. *Immunol Rev* 2010;236:139–150.
31. Cerutti A. The regulation of IgA class switching. *Nat Rev Immunol* 2008;8:421–434.
32. Dogan I, Bertocci B, Vilmont V, et al. Multiple layers of B-cell memory with different effector functions. *Nat Immunol* 2009;10:1292–1299.
33. Goodnow CC. Balancing immunity and tolerance: deleting and tuning lymphocyte repertoires. *Proc Natl Acad Sci U S A* 1996;93:2264–2271.
34. Xing Y, Hogquist KA. T-cell tolerance: central and peripheral. *Cold Spring Harb Perspect Biol* 2012;4:1–15.
35. Meffre E, Wardemann H. B-cell tolerance checkpoints in health and autoimmunity. *Curr Opin Immunol* 2008;20:632–638.
36. Josefowicz SZ, Lu LF, Rudensky AY. Regulatory T-cells: mechanisms of differentiation and function. *Annu Rev Immunol* 2012;30:531–564.
37. Mauri C, Bosma A. Immune regulatory function of B-cells. *Annu Rev Immunol* 2012;30:221–241.
38. Bolland S, Ravetch JV. Inhibitory pathways triggered by ITIM-containing receptors. *Adv Immunol* 1999;72:149–177.
39. Cooper MD, Alder MN. The evolution of adaptive immune systems. *Cell* 2006;124:815–822.
40. Akira S, Uematsu S, Takeuchi O. Pathogen recognition and innate immunity. *Cell* 2006;124:783–801.
41. Flajnik MF, Kasahara M. Comparative genomics of the MHC: glimpses into the evolution of the adaptive immune system. *Immunity* 2001;15:351–362.
42. Hoffmann JA, Kafatos FC, Janeway CA, et al. Phylogenetic perspectives in innate immunity. *Science* 1999;284:1313–1318.
43. Shafer WM. *Antimicrobial peptides and human disease*. Heidelberg, Germany: Springer, 2006.
44. Cooper MD, Herrin BR. How did our complex immune system evolve? *Nat Rev Immunol* 2010;10:2–3.
45. Issazadeh-Navikas S. NKT-cell self-reactivity: evolutionary master key of immune homeostasis? *J Mol Cell Biol* 2012;4:70–78.
46. Eason DD, Cannon JP, Haire RN, et al. Mechanisms of antigen receptor evolution. *Semin Immunol* 2004;16:215–226.
47. Gowans JL, McGregor GD, Cowen DM. Initiation of immune responses by small lymphocytes. *Nature* 1962;196:651–655.
48. Jerne NK. The natural-selection theory of antibody formation. *Proc Natl Acad Sci U S A* 1955;41:849–857.
49. Orkin SH, Zon LI. Hematopoiesis: an evolving paradigm for stem cell biology. *Cell* 2008;132:631–644.
50. Randall TD, Carragher DM, Rangel-Moreno J. Development of secondary lymphoid organs. *Annu Rev Immunol* 2008;26:627–650.
51. van de Pavert SA, Mebius RE. New insights into the development of lymphoid tissues. *Nat Rev Immunol* 2010;10:664–674.
52. Neyt K, Perros F, GeurtsvanKessel CH, et al. Tertiary lymphoid organs in infection and autoimmunity. *Trends Immunol* 2012;33:297–305.
53. Nicoll PA, Taylor AE. Lymph formation and flow. *Annu Rev Physiol* 1977;39:73–95.
54. Mercier FE, Ragu C, Scadden DT. The bone marrow at the crossroads of blood and immunity. *Nat Rev Immunol* 2012;12:49–60.
55. Busslinger M. Transcriptional control of early B-cell development. *Annu Rev Immunol* 2004;22:55–79.
56. Rodewald HR. Thymus organogenesis. *Annu Rev Immunol* 2008;26:355–388.
57. Lynch HE, Goldberg GL, Chidgey A, et al. Thymic involution and immune reconstitution. *Trends Immunol* 2009;30:366–373.
58. Anderson G, Jenkinson EJ. Lymphostromal interactions in thymic development and function. *Nat Rev Immunol* 2001;1:31–40.
59. Manley NR, Richie ER, Blackburn CC, et al. Structure and function of the thymic microenvironment. *Front Biosci* 2012;17:2461–2477.
60. Mebius RE. Organogenesis of lymphoid tissues. *Nat Rev Immunol* 2003;3:292–303.
61. Ruddle NH, Akirav EM. Secondary lymphoid organs: responding to genetic and environmental cues in ontogeny and the immune response. *J Immunol* 2009;183:2205–2212.
62. MacLennan IC. Germinal centers. *Annu Rev Immunol* 1994;12:117–139.
63. Drayton DL, Liao S, Mounzer RH, et al. Lymphoid organ development: from ontogeny to neogenesis. *Nat Immunol* 2006;7:344–353.
64. Mebius RE, Kraal G. Structure and function of the spleen. *Nat Rev Immunol* 2005;5:606–616.
65. Kraal G, Mebius R. New insights into the cell biology of the marginal zone of the spleen. *Int Rev Cytol* 2006;250:175–215.
66. Steiniger B, Timphus EM, Barth PJ. The splenic marginal zone in humans and rodents: an enigmatic compartment and its inhabitants. *Histochem Cell Biol* 2006;126:641–648.
67. Weill JC, Weller S, Reynaud CA. Human marginal zone B-cells. *Annu Rev Immunol* 2009;27:267–285.
68. Brandtzaeg P, Farstad IN, Johansen FE, et al. The B-cell system of human mucosae and exocrine glands. *Immunol Rev* 1999;171:45–87.
69. Cerutti A, Rescigno M. The biology of intestinal immunoglobulin A responses. *Immunity* 2008;28:740–750.
70. Chorny A, Puga I, Cerutti A. Innate signaling networks in mucosal IgA class switching. *Adv Immunol* 2010;107:31–69.
71. He B, Xu W, Santini PA, et al. Intestinal bacteria trigger T-cell-independent immunoglobulin A(2) class switching by inducing epithelial-cell secretion of the cytokine APRIL. *Immunity* 2007;26:812–826.
72. Xu W, Santini PA, Matthews AJ, et al. Viral double-stranded RNA triggers Ig class switching by activating upper respiratory mucosa B-cells through an innate TLR3 pathway involving BAFF. *J Immunol* 2008;181:276–287.
73. Xu W, Santini PA, Sullivan JS, et al. HIV-1 evades virus-specific IgG2 and IgA responses by targeting systemic and intestinal B-cells via long-range intercellular conduits. *Nat Immunol* 2009;10:1008–1017.
74. He B, Qiao X, Cerutti A. CpG DNA induces IgG class switch DNA recombination by activating human B-cells through an innate pathway that requires TLR9 and cooperates with IL-10. *J Immunol* 2004;173:4479–4491.
75. Kiyono H, Fukuyama S. NALT- versus Peyer's-patch-mediated mucosal immunity. *Nat Rev Immunol* 2004;4:699–710.
76. Holt PG, Strickland DH, Wikstrom ME, et al. Regulation of immunological homeostasis in the respiratory tract. *Nat Rev Immunol* 2008;8:142–152.
77. Medzhitov R. Recognition of microorganisms and activation of the immune response. *Nature* 2007;449:819–826.
78. Palm NW, Medzhitov R. Pattern recognition receptors and control of adaptive immunity. *Immunol Rev* 2009;227:221–233.
79. Aderem A, Ulevitch RJ. Toll-like receptors in the induction of the innate immune response. *Nature* 2000;406:782–787.
80. Macpherson AJ, Harris NL. Interactions between commensal intestinal bacteria and the immune system. *Nat Rev Immunol* 2004;4:478–485.
81. Sansonetti PJ. The innate signaling of dangers and the dangers of innate signaling. *Nat Immunol* 2006;7:1237–1242.
82. Kawai T, Akira S. The roles of TLRs, RLRs and NLRs in pathogen recognition. *Int Immunol* 2009;21:317–337.

83. Underhill DM. Collaboration between the innate immune receptors dectin-1, TLRs, and Nods. *Immunol Rev* 2007;219:75–87.
84. Kawai T, Akira S. Toll-like receptors and their crosstalk with other innate receptors in infection and immunity. *Immunity* 2011;34:637–650.
85. Takeda K, Kaisho T, Akira S. Toll-like receptors. *Annu Rev Immunol* 2003;21:335–376.
86. Kerrigan AM, Brown GD. Syk-coupled C-type lectins in immunity. *Trends Immunol* 2011;32:151–156.
87. Kufer TA, Sansonetti PJ. NLR functions beyond pathogen recognition. *Nat Immunol* 2011;12:121–128.
88. Elinav E, Strowig T, Henao-Mejia J, et al. Regulation of the antimicrobial response by NLR proteins. *Immunity* 2011;34:665–679.
89. Pichlmair A, Reis e Sousa C. Innate recognition of viruses. *Immunity* 2007;27:370–383.
90. Bottazzi B, Doni A, Garlanda C, et al. An integrated view of humoral innate immunity: pentraxins as a paradigm. *Annu Rev Immunol* 2010;28:157–183.
91. Muller-Eberhard HJ. Molecular organization and function of the complement system. *Annu Rev Biochem* 1988;57:321–347.
92. Ricklin D, Hajishengallis G, Yang K, et al. Complement: a key system for immune surveillance and homeostasis. *Nat Immunol* 2010;11:785–797.
93. Sturfelt G, Truedsson L. Complement in the immunopathogenesis of rheumatic disease. *Nat Rev Rheumatol* 2012;8:458–468.
94. Degn SE, Jensenius JC, Thiel S. Disease-causing mutations in genes of the complement system. *Am J Hum Genet* 2011;88:689–705.
95. Skattum L, van Deuren M, van der Poll T, et al. Complement deficiency states and associated infections. *Mol Immunol* 2011;48:1643–1655.
96. Zipfel PF, Skerka C. Complement regulators and inhibitory proteins. *Nat Rev Immunol* 2009;9:729–740.
97. Flierman R, Daha MR. The clearance of apoptotic cells by complement. *Immunobiology* 2007;212:363–370.
98. Lappegard KT, Christiansen D, Pharo A, et al. Human genetic deficiencies reveal the roles of complement in the inflammatory network: lessons from nature. *Proc Natl Acad Sci U S A* 2009;106:15861–15866.
99. Dempsey PW, Allison ME, Akkaraju S, et al. C3d of complement as a molecular adjuvant: bridging innate and acquired immunity. *Science* 1996;271:348–350.
100. Roozendaal R, Carroll MC. Complement receptors CD21 and CD35 in humoral immunity. *Immunol Rev* 2007;219:157–166.
101. Borregaard N, Cowland JB. Granules of the human neutrophilic polymorphonuclear leukocyte. *Blood* 1997;89:3503–3521.
102. Bainton DF, Farquhar MG. Origin of granules in polymorphonuclear leukocytes. Two types derived from opposite faces of the Golgi complex in developing granulocytes. *J Cell Biol* 1966;28:277–301.
103. Mantovani A, Cassatella MA, Costantini C, et al. Neutrophils in the activation and regulation of innate and adaptive immunity. *Nat Rev Immunol* 2011;11:519–531.
104. Nathan C. Neutrophils and immunity: challenges and opportunities. *Nat Rev Immunol* 2006;6:173–182.
105. Kennedy AD, DeLeo FR. Neutrophil apoptosis and the resolution of infection. *Immunol Res* 2009;43:25–61.
106. Schenkel AR, Mamdouh Z, Muller WA. Locomotion of monocytes on endothelium is a critical step during extravasation. *Nat Immunol* 2004;5:393–400.
107. Segal AW. How neutrophils kill microbes. *Annu Rev Immunol* 2005;23:197–223.
108. Nauseef WM. How human neutrophils kill and degrade microbes: an integrated view. *Immunol Rev* 2007;219:88–102.
109. Brinkmann V, Reichard U, Goosmann C, et al. Neutrophil extracellular traps kill bacteria. *Science* 2004;303:1532–1535.
110. Zhang X, Majlessi L, Deriaud E, et al. Coactivation of Syk kinase and MyD88 adaptor protein pathways by bacteria promotes regulatory properties of neutrophils. *Immunity* 2009;31:761–771.
111. Puga I, Cols M, Barra CM, et al. B-cell-helper neutrophils stimulate the diversification and production of immunoglobulin in the marginal zone of the spleen. *Nat Immunol* 2012;13:170–180.
112. Scapini P, Bazzoni F, Cassatella MA. Regulation of B-cell-activating factor (BAFF)/B lymphocyte stimulator (BLyS) expression in human neutrophils. *Immunol Lett* 2008;116:1–6.
113. Gleich GJ, Adolphson CR. The eosinophilic leukocyte: structure and function. *Adv Immunol* 1986;39:177–253.
114. Rothenberg ME, Hogan SP. The eosinophil. *Annu Rev Immunol* 2006;24:147–174.
115. Chu VT, Frohlich A, Steinhauser G, et al. Eosinophils are required for the maintenance of plasma cells in the bone marrow. *Nat Immunol* 2011;12:151–159.
116. Hogan SP, Rosenberg HF, Moqbel R, et al. Eosinophils: biological properties and role in health and disease. *Clin Exp Allergy* 2008;38:709–750.
117. Spencer LA, Weller PF. Eosinophils and Th2 immunity: contemporary insights. *Immunol Cell Biol* 2010;88:250–256.
118. Schroeder JT. Basophils: emerging roles in the pathogenesis of allergic disease. *Immunol Rev* 2011;242:144–160.
119. Ohnmacht C, Voehringer D. Basophil effector function and homeostasis during helminth infection. *Blood* 2009;113:2816–2825.
120. Min B, Brown MA, Legros G. Understanding the roles of basophils: breaking dawn. *Immunology* 2012;135:192–197.
121. Nakanishi K. Basophils are potent antigen-presenting cells that selectively induce Th2 cells. *Eur J Immunol* 2010;40:1836–1842.
122. Chen K, Cerutti A. New insights into the enigma of immunoglobulin D. *Immunol Rev* 2010;237:160–179.
123. Chen K, Xu W, Wilson M, et al. Immunoglobulin D enhances immune surveillance by activating antimicrobial, proinflammatory and B-cell-stimulating programs in basophils. *Nat Immunol* 2009;10:889–898.
124. Fogg DK, Sibon C, Miled C, et al. A clonogenic bone marrow progenitor specific for macrophages and dendritic cells. *Science* 2006;311:83–87.
125. Goasguen JE, Bennett JM, Bain BJ, et al. Morphological evaluation of monocytes and their precursors. *Haematologica* 2009;94:994–997.
126. Auffray C, Fogg D, Garfa M, et al. Monitoring of blood vessels and tissues by a population of monocytes with patrolling behavior. *Science* 2007;317:666–670.
127. Murray PJ, Wynn TA. Protective and pathogenic functions of macrophage subsets. *Nat Rev Immunol* 2011;11:723–737.
128. Galli SJ, Borregaard N, Wynn TA. Phenotypic and functional plasticity of cells of innate immunity: macrophages, mast cells and neutrophils. *Nat Immunol* 2011;12:1035–1044.
129. Grage-Griebenow E, Flad HD, Ernst M. Heterogeneity of human peripheral blood monocyte subsets. *J Leukoc Biol* 2001;69:11–20.
130. Auffray C, Fogg DK, Narni-Mancinelli E, et al. CX3CR1+ CD115+ CD135+ common macrophage/DC precursors and the role of CX3CR1 in their response to inflammation. *J Exp Med* 2009;206:595–606.
131. Auffray C, Sieweke MH, Geissmann F. Blood monocytes: development, heterogeneity, and relationship with dendritic cells. *Annu Rev Immunol* 2009;27:669–692.
132. Qu C, Edwards EW, Tacke F, et al. Role of CCR8 and other chemokine pathways in the migration of monocyte-derived dendritic cells to lymph nodes. *J Exp Med* 2004;200:1231–1241.
133. Krausgruber T, Blazek K, Smallie T, et al. IRF5 promotes inflammatory macrophage polarization and TH1-TH17 responses. *Nat Immunol* 2011;12:231–238.
134. Mosser DM, Edwards JP. Exploring the full spectrum of macrophage activation. *Nat Rev Immunol* 2008;8:958–969.
135. Wynn TA, Barron L. Macrophages: master regulators of inflammation and fibrosis. *Semin Liver Dis* 2010;30:245–257.
136. Biswas SK, Mantovani A. Macrophage plasticity and interaction with lymphocyte subsets: cancer as a paradigm. *Nat Immunol* 2010;11:889–896.
137. Steinman RM, Cohn ZA. Identification of a novel cell type in peripheral lymphoid organs of mice. I. Morphology, quantitation, tissue distribution. *J Exp Med* 1973;137:1142–1162.
138. Banchereau J, Steinman RM. Dendritic cells and the control of immunity. *Nature* 1998;392:245–252.
139. Ziegler-Heitbrock L, Ancuta P, Crowe S, et al. Nomenclature of monocytes and dendritic cells in blood. *Blood* 2010;116:e74–e80.
140. Banchereau J, Briere F, Caux C, et al. Immunobiology of dendritic cells. *Annu Rev Immunol* 2000;18:767–811.
141. Dieu MC, Vanbervliet B, Vicari A, et al. Selective recruitment of immature and mature dendritic cells by distinct chemokines expressed in different anatomic sites. *J Exp Med* 1998;188:373–386.
142. Viola A, Luster AD. Chemokines and their receptors: drug targets in immunity and inflammation. *Annu Rev Pharmacol Toxicol* 2008;48:171–197.
143. Blander JM, Medzhitov R. Toll-dependent selection of microbial antigens for presentation by dendritic cells. *Nature* 2006;440:808–812.
144. Figdor CG, van Kooyk Y, Adema GJ. C-type lectin receptors on dendritic cells and Langerhans cells. *Nat Rev Immunol* 2002;2:77–84.
145. Geijtenbeek TB, Torensma R, van Vliet SJ, et al. Identification of DC-SIGN, a novel dendritic cell-specific ICAM-3 receptor that supports primary immune responses. *Cell* 2000;100:575–585.
146. Forster R, Davalos-Misslitz AC, Rot A. CCR7 and its ligands: balancing immunity and tolerance. *Nat Rev Immunol* 2008;8:362–371.
147. Randolph GJ, Ochando J, Partida-Sanchez S. Migration of dendritic cell subsets and their precursors. *Annu Rev Immunol* 2008;26:293–316.
148. Miller MJ, Safrina O, Parker I, et al. Imaging the single cell dynamics of CD4+ T-cell activation by dendritic cells in lymph nodes. *J Exp Med* 2004;200:847–856.
149. Delamarre L, Pack M, Chang H, et al. Differential lysosomal proteolysis in antigen-presenting cells determines antigen fate. *Science* 2005;307:1630–1634.
150. Dudziak D, Kamphorst AO, Heidkamp GF, et al. Differential antigen processing by dendritic cell subsets in vivo. *Science* 2007;315:107–111.
151. Itano AA, McSorley SJ, Reinhardt RL, et al. Distinct dendritic cell populations sequentially present antigen to CD4 T-cells and stimulate different aspects of cell-mediated immunity. *Immunity* 2003;19:47–57.
152. Collin M, Bigley V, Haniffa M, et al. Human dendritic cell deficiency: the missing ID? *Nat Rev Immunol* 2011;11:575–583.
153. Lennert K, Remmele W. Karyometric research on lymph node cells in man. I. Germinoblasts, lymphoblasts & lymphocytes. *Acta Haematol* 1958;19:99–113.
154. Grouard G, Rissoan MC, Filgueira L, et al. The enigmatic plasmacytoid T-cells develop into dendritic cells with interleukin (IL)-3 and CD40-ligand. *J Exp Med* 1997;185:1101–1111.
155. Liu YJ. IPC: professional type 1 interferon-producing cells and plasmacytoid dendritic cell precursors. *Annu Rev Immunol* 2005;23:275–306.
156. Colonna M, Trinchieri G, Liu YJ. Plasmacytoid dendritic cells in immunity. *Nat Immunol* 2004;5:1219–1226.
157. Szabo G, Dolganiuc A. The role of plasmacytoid dendritic cell-derived IFN alpha in antiviral immunity. *Crit Rev Immunol* 2008;28:61–94.
158. Reizis B, Bunin A, Ghosh HS, et al. Plasmacytoid dendritic cells: recent progress and open questions. *Annu Rev Immunol* 2011;29:163–183.
159. Banchereau J, Thompson-Snipes L, Zurawski S, et al. The differential production of cytokines by human Langerhans cells and dermal CD14+ DCs controls CTL priming. *Blood* 2012;119:5742–5749.
160. Guilliams M, Henri S, Tamoutounour S, et al. From skin dendritic cells to a simplified classification of human and mouse dendritic cell subsets. *Eur J Immunol* 2010;40:2089–2094.
161. Iwasaki A. Mucosal dendritic cells. *Annu Rev Immunol* 2007;25:381–418.
162. Cerutti A, Cols M, Gentile M, et al. Regulation of mucosal IgA responses: lessons from primary immunodeficiencies. *Ann N Y Acad Sci* 2011;1238:132–144.
163. Klaus GG, Humphrey JH, Kunkl A, et al. The follicular dendritic cell: its role in antigen presentation in the generation of immunological memory. *Immunol Rev* 1980;53:3–28.
164. Mandel TE, Phipps RP, Abbot A, et al. The follicular dendritic cell: long term antigen retention during immunity. *Immunol Rev* 1980;53:29–59.
165. Batista FD, Harwood NE. The who, how and where of antigen presentation to B-cells. *Nat Rev Immunol* 2009;9:15–27.
166. Turley SJ, Fletcher AL, Elpek KG. The stromal and haematopoietic antigen-presenting cells that reside in secondary lymphoid organs. *Nat Rev Immunol* 2010;10:813–825.
167. Steinman RM. The dendritic cell system and its role in immunogenicity. *Annu Rev Immunol* 1991;9:271–296.
168. Steinman RM, Hawiger D, Nussenzweig MC. Tolerogenic dendritic cells. *Annu Rev Immunol* 2003;21:685–711.
169. Yokoyama WM, Kim S, French AR. The dynamic life of natural killer cells. *Annu Rev Immunol* 2004;22:405–429.
170. Cooper MA, Fehniger TA, Caligiuri MA. The biology of human natural killer-cell subsets. *Trends Immunol* 2001;22:633–640.

171. Moretta L, Bottino C, Pende D, et al. Human natural killer cells: their origin, receptors and function. *Eur J Immunol* 2002;32:1205–1211.
172. Vivier E, Tomasello E, Baratin M, et al. Functions of natural killer cells. *Nat Immunol* 2008;9:503–510.
173. Ravetch JV, Lanier LL. Immune inhibitory receptors. *Science* 2000;290:84–89.
174. Lopez-Botet M, Llano M, Navarro F, et al. NK cell recognition of non-classical HLA class I molecules. *Semin Immunol* 2000;12:109–119.
175. Lanier LL. Up on the tightrope: natural killer cell activation and inhibition. *Nat Immunol* 2008;9:495–502.
176. Raulet DH. Roles of the NKG2D immunoreceptor and its ligands. *Nat Rev Immunol* 2003;3:781–790.
177. Champsaur M, Lanier LL. Effect of NKG2D ligand expression on host immune responses. *Immunol Rev* 2010;235:267–285.
178. Galli SJ, Kalesnikoff J, Grimbaldeston MA, et al. Mast cells as "tunable" effector and immunoregulatory cells: recent advances. *Annu Rev Immunol* 2005;23:749–786.
179. Abraham SN, St John AL. Mast cell-orchestrated immunity to pathogens. *Nat Rev Immunol* 2010;10:440–452.
180. Frossi B, Gri G, Tripodo C, et al. Exploring a regulatory role for mast cells: 'MCregs'? *Trends Immunol* 2010;31:97–102.
181. Galli SJ, Tsai M. Mast cells in allergy and infection: versatile effector and regulatory cells in innate and adaptive immunity. *Eur J Immunol* 2010;40:1843–1851.
182. Galli SJ, Grimbaldeston M, Tsai M. Immunomodulatory mast cells: negative, as well as positive, regulators of immunity. *Nat Rev Immunol* 2008;8:478–486.
183. Spits H, Cupedo T. Innate lymphoid cells: emerging insights in development, lineage relationships, and function. *Annu Rev Immunol* 2012;30:647–675.
184. Klose CS, Hoyler T, Kiss EA, et al. Transcriptional control of innate lymphocyte fate decisions. *Curr Opin Immunol* 2012;24:290–296.
185. Tsuji M, Suzuki K, Kitamura H, et al. Requirement for lymphoid tissue-inducer cells in isolated follicle formation and T-cell-independent immunoglobulin A generation in the gut. *Immunity* 2008;29:261–271.
186. Scandella E, Bolinger B, Lattmann E, et al. Restoration of lymphoid organ integrity through the interaction of lymphoid tissue-inducer cells with stroma of the T-cell zone. *Nat Immunol* 2008;9:667–675.
187. Neill DR, Wong SH, Bellosi A, et al. Nuocytes represent a new innate effector leukocyte that mediates type-2 immunity. *Nature* 2010;464:1367–1370.
188. Monticelli LA, Sonnenberg GF, Abt MC, et al. Innate lymphoid cells promote lung-tissue homeostasis after infection with influenza virus. *Nat Immunol* 2011;12:1045–1054.
189. Iwasaki A, Medzhitov R. Regulation of adaptive immunity by the innate immune system. *Science* 2010;327:291–295.
190. Schreibelt G, Tel J, Sliepen KH, et al. Toll-like receptor expression and function in human dendritic cell subsets: implications for dendritic cell-based anti-cancer immunotherapy. *Cancer Immunol Immunother* 2010;59:1573–1582.
191. Fearon DT, Carter RH. The CD19/CR2/TAPA-1 complex of B lymphocytes: linking natural to acquired immunity. *Annu Rev Immunol* 1995;13:127–149.
192. Daeron M. Fc receptor biology. *Annu Rev Immunol* 1997;15:203–234.
193. Powell MS, Hogarth PM. Fc receptors. *Adv Exp Med Biol* 2008;640:22–34.
194. Nimmerjahn F, Ravetch JV. Fc-Receptors as regulators of immunity. *Advances in immunology* 2007;179–204.
195. Muta T, Kurosaki T, Misulovin Z, et al. A 13–amino-acid motif in the cytoplasmic domain of Fc gamma RIIB modulates B-cell receptor signalling. *Nature* 1994;369:340.
196. Ravetch JV, Bolland S. IgG Fc receptors. *Annu Rev Immunol* 2001;19:275–290.
197. Wines BD, Hogarth PM. IgA receptors in health and disease. *Tissue Antigens* 2006;68:103–114.
198. Monteiro RC, Van De Winkel JG. IgA Fc receptors. *Annu Rev Immunol* 2003; 21:177–204.
199. Nissim A, Jouvin MH, Eshhar Z. Mapping of the high affinity Fc epsilon receptor binding site to the third constant region domain of IgE. *EMBO J* 1991;10:101–107.
200. Kinet JP. The high-affinity IgE receptor (Fc epsilon RI): from physiology to pathology. *Annu Rev Immunol* 1999;17:931–972.
201. Grangette C, Gruart V, Ouaissi MA, et al. IgE receptor on human eosinophils (FcE-RII). Comparison with B-cell CD23 and association with an adhesion molecule. *J Immunol* 1989;143:3580–3588.
202. Ravetch JV. Fc receptors. *Curr Opin Immunol* 1997;9:121–125.
203. Chen K, Cerutti A. The function and regulation of immunoglobulin D. *Curr Opin Immunol* 2011;23:345–352.
204. Chappel MS, Isenman DE, Everett M, et al. Identification of the Fc gamma receptor class I binding site in human IgG through the use of recombinant IgG1/IgG2 hybrid and point-mutated antibodies. *Proc Natl Acad Sci U S A* 1991;88:9036–9040.
205. Takai T. Roles of Fc receptors in autoimmunity. *Nat Rev Immunol* 2002;2:580–592.
206. Bruhns P. Properties of mouse and human IgG receptors and their contribution to disease models. *Blood* 2012;119:5640–5649.
207. Wang AV, Scholl PR, Geha RS. Physical and functional association of the high affinity immunoglobulin G receptor (Fc gamma RI) with the kinases Hck and Lyn. *J Exp Med* 1994;180:1165–1170.
208. Pricop L, Redecha P, Teillaud JL, et al. Differential modulation of stimulatory and inhibitory Fc gamma receptors on human monocytes by Th1 and Th2 cytokines. *J Immunol* 2001;166:531–537.
209. Nimmerjahn F, Ravetch JV. Fc[gamma] receptors as regulators of immune responses. *Nat Rev Immunol* 2008;8:34–47.
210. Martin WL, West AP Jr, Gan L, et al. Crystal structure at 2.8 A of an FcRn/heterodimeric Fc complex: mechanism of pH-dependent binding. *Mol Cell* 2001;7:867–877.
211. Leach JL, Sedmak DD, Osborne JM, et al. Isolation from human placenta of the IgG transporter, FcRn, and localization to the syncytiotrophoblast: implications for maternal-fetal antibody transport. *J Immunol* 1996;157:3317–3322.
212. Wines BD, Powell MS, Parren PW, et al. The IgG Fc contains distinct Fc receptor (FcR) binding sites: the leukocyte receptors Fc gamma RI and Fc gamma RIIa bind to a region in the Fc distinct from that recognized by neonatal FcR and protein A. *J Immunol* 2000;164:5313–5318.
213. Story CM, Mikulska JE, Simister NE. A major histocompatibility complex class I-like Fc receptor cloned from human placenta: possible role in transfer of immunoglobulin G from mother to fetus. *J Exp Med* 1994;180:2377–2381.
214. Bergtold A, Desai DD, Gavhane A, et al. Cell surface recycling of internalized antigen permits dendritic cell priming of B-cells. *Immunity* 2005;23:503–514.
215. Dickinson BL, Badizadegan K, Wu Z, et al. Bidirectional FcRn-dependent IgG transport in a polarized human intestinal epithelial cell line. *J Clin Invest* 1999;104:903–911.
216. Hulett MD, Hogarth PM. Molecular basis of Fc receptor function. *Adv Immunol* 1994;57:1–127.
217. Barral P, Eckl-Dorna J, Harwood NE, et al. B-cell receptor-mediated uptake of CD1d-restricted antigen augments antibody responses by recruiting invariant NKT-cell help in vivo. *Proc Natl Acad Sci U S A* 2008;105:8345–8350.
218. Barral P, Polzella P, Bruckbauer A, et al. CD169(+) macrophages present lipid antigens to mediate early activation of iNKT-cells in lymph nodes. *Nat Immunol* 2010;11:303–312.
219. Silk JD, Hermans IF, Gileadi U, et al. Utilizing the adjuvant properties of CD1d-dependent NK T-cells in T-cell-mediated immunotherapy. *J Clin Invest* 2004; 114:1800–1811.
220. Kerzerho J, Yu ED, Barra CM, et al. Structural and functional characterization of a novel nonglycosidic type I NKT agonist with immunomodulatory properties. *J Immunol* 2012;188:2254–2265.
221. Godfrey DI, Pellicci DG, Patel O, et al. Antigen recognition by CD1d-restricted NKT T-cell receptors. *Semin Immunol* 2010;22:61–67.
222. Jordan MA, Baxter AG. The genetics of immunoregulatory T-cells. *J Autoimmun* 2008;31:237–244.
223. Joyce S, Girardi E, Zajonc DM. NKT cell ligand recognition logic: molecular basis for a synaptic duet and transmission of inflammatory effectors. *J Immunol* 2011;187:1081–1089.
224. Chang PP, Barral P, Fitch J, et al. Identification of Bcl-6-dependent follicular helper NKT-cells that provide cognate help for B-cell responses. *Nat Immunol* 2012; 13:35–43.
225. King IL, Mohrs K, Mohrs M. A nonredundant role for IL-21 receptor signaling in plasma cell differentiation and protective type 2 immunity against gastrointestinal helminth infection. *J Immunol* 2010;185:6138–6145.
226. Leadbetter EA, Brigl M, Illarionov P, et al. NK T-cells provide lipid antigen-specific cognate help for B-cells. *Proc Natl Acad Sci U S A* 2008;105:8339–8344.
227. Kalia V, Sarkar S, Gourley TS, et al. Differentiation of memory B and T-cells. *Curr Opin Immunol* 2006;18:255–264.
228. McHeyzer-Williams LJ, McHeyzer-Williams MG. Antigen-specific memory B-cell development. *Annu Rev Immunol* 2005;23:487–513.
229. Benacerraf B. Role of MHC gene products in immune regulation. *Science* 1981;212:1229–1238.
230. Lanzavecchia A. Antigen-specific interaction between T and B-cells. *Nature* 1985;314:537–539.
231. Claman HN, Chaperon EA, Triplett RF. Immunocompetence of transferred thymus-marrow cell combinations. *J Immunol* 1966;97:828–832.
232. Neefjes J, Jongsma ML, Paul P, et al. Towards a systems understanding of MHC class I and MHC class II antigen presentation. *Nat Rev Immunol* 2011;11:823–836.
233. Madden DR. The three-dimensional structure of peptide-MHC complexes. *Annu Rev Immunol* 1995;13:587–622.
234. Klein J, Sato A. The HLA system. First of two parts. *N Engl J Med* 2000;343: 702–709.
235. Horton R, Wilming L, Rand V, et al. Gene map of the extended human MHC. *Nat Rev Genet* 2004;5:889–899.
236. Kumanovics A, Takada T, Lindahl KF. Genomic organization of the mammalian MHC. *Annu Rev Immunol* 2003;21:629–657.
237. Del Val M, Schlicht HJ, Ruppert T, et al. Efficient processing of an antigenic sequence for presentation by MHC class I molecules depends on its neighboring residues in the protein. *Cell* 1991;66:1145–1153.
238. Garcia KC, Adams EJ. How the T-cell receptor sees antigen—a structural view. *Cell* 2005;122:333–336.
239. Moron G, Dadaglio G, Leclerc C. New tools for antigen delivery to the MHC class I pathway. *Trends Immunol* 2004;25:92–97.
240. Zhou F. Molecular mechanisms of IFN-gamma to up-regulate MHC class I antigen processing and presentation. *Int Rev Immunol* 2009;28:239–260.
241. Boehm U, Klamp T, Groot M, et al. Cellular responses to interferon-gamma. *Annu Rev Immunol* 1997;15:749–795.
242. Rock KL, Goldberg AL. Degradation of cell proteins and the generation of MHC class I-presented peptides. *Annu Rev Immunol* 1999;17:739–779.
243. Ciechanover A. The ubiquitin-proteasome proteolytic pathway. *Cell* 1994;79:13–21.
244. Ortmann B, Copeman J, Lehner PJ, et al. A critical role for tapasin in the assembly and function of multimeric MHC class I-TAP complexes. *Science* 1997;277:1306–1309.
245. Hammer GE, Shastri N. Construction and destruction of MHC class I in the peptide-loading complex. *Nat Immunol* 2007;8:793–794.
246. Hughes EA, Hammond C, Cresswell P. Misfolded major histocompatibility complex class I heavy chains are translocated into the cytoplasm and degraded by the proteasome. *Proc Natl Acad Sci U S A* 1997;94:1896–1901.
247. Vyas JM, Van der Veen AG, Ploegh HL. The known unknowns of antigen processing and presentation. *Nat Rev Immunol* 2008;8:607–618.
248. Geppert TD, Lipsky PE. Antigen presentation by interferon-gamma-treated endothelial cells and fibroblasts: differential ability to function as antigen-presenting cells despite comparable Ia expression. *J Immunol* 1985;135:3750–3762.
249. Cella M, Engering A, Pinet V, et al. Inflammatory stimuli induce accumulation of MHC class II complexes on dendritic cells. *Nature* 1997;388:782–787.
250. Rosa FM, Fellous M. Regulation of HLA-DR gene by IFN-gamma. Transcriptional and post-transcriptional control. *J Immunol* 1988;140:1660–1664.
251. Cresswell P. Assembly, transport, and function of MHC class II molecules. *Annu Rev Immunol* 1994;12:259–293.
252. Ting JP, Trowsdale J. Genetic control of MHC class II expression. *Cell* 2002; 109(Suppl):S21–S33.
253. Rocha N, Neefjes J. MHC class II molecules on the move for successful antigen presentation. *EMBO J* 2008;27:1–5.
254. Heath WR, Carbone FR. Cross-presentation in viral immunity and self-tolerance. *Nat Rev Immunol* 2001;1:126–134.
255. Munz C. Enhancing immunity through autophagy. *Annu Rev Immunol* 2009;27: 423–449.
256. Borg NA, Ely LK, Beddoe T, et al. The CDR3 regions of an immunodominant T-cell receptor dictate the 'energetic landscape' of peptide-MHC recognition. *Nat Immunol* 2005;6:171–180.
257. Smith-Garvin JE, Koretzky GA, Jordan MS. T-cell activation. *Annu Rev Immunol* 2009;27:591–619.

258. Baeuerle PA, Henkel T. Function and activation of NF-kappa B in the immune system. *Annu Rev Immunol* 1994;12:141–179.
259. Thome M. CARMA1, BCL-10 and MALT1 in lymphocyte development and activation. *Nat Rev Immunol* 2004;4:348–359.
260. Abbas AK, Sen R. The activation of lymphocytes is in their CARMA. *Immunity* 2003;18:721–722.
261. Cheng J, Montecalvo A, Kane LP. Regulation of NF-kappaB induction by TCR/CD28. *Immunol Res* 2011;50:113–117.
262. Grakoui A, Bromley SK, Sumen C, et al. The immunological synapse: a molecular machine controlling T-cell activation. *Science* 1999;285:221–227.
263. Bromley SK, Burack WR, Johnson KG, et al. The immunological synapse. *Annu Rev Immunol* 2001;19:375–396.
264. Huppa JB, Davis MM. T-cell-antigen recognition and the immunological synapse. *Nat Rev Immunol* 2003;3:973–983.
265. Guermonprez P, Valladeau J, Zitvogel L, et al. Antigen presentation and T-cell stimulation by dendritic cells. *Annu Rev Immunol* 2002;20:621–667.
266. Schwartz RH. T-cell anergy. *Annu Rev Immunol* 2003;21:305–334.
267. Acuto O, Michel F. CD28-mediated co-stimulation: a quantitative support for TCR signalling. *Nat Rev Immunol* 2003;3:939–951.
268. Watts TH. TNF/TNFR family members in costimulation of T-cell responses. *Annu Rev Immunol* 2005;23:23–68.
269. Boyman O, Sprent J. The role of interleukin-2 during homeostasis and activation of the immune system. *Nat Rev Immunol* 2012;12:180–190.
270. Teft WA, Kirchhof MG, Madrenas J. A molecular perspective of CTLA-4 function. *Annu Rev Immunol* 2006;24:65–97.
271. Dutton RW, Bradley LM, Swain SL. T-cell memory. *Annu Rev Immunol* 1998;16:201–223.
272. Banchereau J, Bazan F, Blanchard D, et al. The CD40 antigen and its ligand. *Annu Rev Immunol* 1994;12:881–922.
273. Davidson HW, Watts C. Epitope-directed processing of specific antigen by B lymphocytes. *J Cell Biol* 1989;109:85–92.
274. Lenschow DJ, Sperling AI, Cooke MP, et al. Differential up-regulation of the B7-1 and B7-2 costimulatory molecules after Ig receptor engagement by antigen. *J Immunol* 1994;153:1990–1997.
275. Siemasko K, Eisfelder BJ, Williamson E, et al. Cutting edge: signals from the B lymphocyte antigen receptor regulate MHC class II containing late endosomes. *J Immunol* 1998;160:5203–5208.
276. Vinuesa CG, Tangye SG, Moser B, et al. Follicular B helper T-cells in antibody responses and autoimmunity. *Nat Rev Immunol* 2005;5:853–865.
277. Crotty S. Follicular helper CD4 T-cells (TFH). *Annu Rev Immunol* 2011;29:621–663.
278. Kracker S, Gardes P, Mazerolles F, et al. Immunoglobulin class switch recombination deficiencies. *Clin Immunol* 2010;135:193–203.
279. Davis MM, Bjorkman PJ. T-cell antigen receptor genes and T-cell recognition. *Nature* 1988;334:395–402.
280. Liu S, Cerutti A, Casali P, et al. Ongoing immunoglobulin class switch DNA recombination in lupus B-cells: analysis of switch regulatory regions. *Autoimmunity* 2004;37:431–443.
281. Holler PD, Kranz DM. Quantitative analysis of the contribution of TCR/pepMHC affinity and CD8 to T-cell activation. *Immunity* 2003;18:255–264.
282. Carding SR, Egan PJ. Gammadelta T-cells: functional plasticity and heterogeneity. *Nat Rev Immunol* 2002;2:336–345.
283. Haas W, Pereira P, Tonegawa S. Gamma/delta cells. *Annu Rev Immunol* 1993;11:637–685.
284. Yewdell JW, Bennink JR. Immunodominance in major histocompatibility complex class I-restricted T lymphocyte responses. *Annu Rev Immunol* 1999;17:51–88.
285. Sigal LJ, Rock KL. Bone marrow-derived antigen-presenting cells are required for the generation of cytotoxic T lymphocyte responses to viruses and use transporter associated with antigen presentation (TAP)-dependent and -independent pathways of antigen presentation. *J Exp Med* 2000;192:1143–1150.
286. Bevan MJ. Cross-priming for a secondary cytotoxic response to minor H antigens with H-2 congenic cells which do not cross-react in the cytotoxic assay. *J Exp Med* 1976;143:1283–1288.
287. Barry M, Bleackley RC. Cytotoxic T lymphocytes: all roads lead to death. *Nat Rev Immunol* 2002;2:401–409.
288. Anderson MK. At the crossroads: diverse roles of early thymocyte transcriptional regulators. *Immunol Rev* 2006;209:191–211.
289. Takahama Y. Journey through the thymus: stromal guides for T-cell development and selection. *Nat Rev Immunol* 2006;6:127–135.
290. Matsuzaki Y, Gyotoku J, Ogawa M, et al. Characterization of c-kit positive intrathymic stem cells that are restricted to lymphoid differentiation. *J Exp Med* 1993;178:1283–1292.
291. Radtke F, Wilson A, Stark G, et al. Deficient T-cell fate specification in mice with an induced inactivation of Notch1. *Immunity* 1999;10:547–558.
292. Liu P, Li P, Burke S. Critical roles of Bcl11b in T-cell development and maintenance of T-cell identity. *Immunol Rev* 2010;238:138–149.
293. Godfrey DI, Kennedy J, Suda T, et al. A developmental pathway involving four phenotypically and functionally distinct subsets of CD3-CD4-CD8- triple-negative adult mouse thymocytes defined by CD44 and CD25 expression. *J Immunol* 1993;150:4244–4252.
294. Zuniga-Pflucker JC, Lenardo MJ. Regulation of thymocyte development from immature progenitors. *Curr Opin Immunol* 1996;8:215–224.
295. Haks MC, Lefebvre JM, Lauritsen JP, et al. Attenuation of gammadeltaTCR signaling efficiently diverts thymocytes to the alphabeta lineage. *Immunity* 2005;22:595–606.
296. Hayes SM, Li L, Love PE. TCR signal strength influences alphabeta/gammadelta lineage fate. *Immunity* 2005;22:583–593.
297. von Boehmer H. Unique features of the pre-T-cell receptor alpha-chain: not just a surrogate. *Nat Rev Immunol* 2005;5:571–577.
298. Fehling HJ, Krotkova A, Saint-Ruf C, et al. Crucial role of the pre-T-cell receptor alpha gene in development of alpha beta but not gamma delta T-cells. *Nature* 1995;375:795–798.
299. Ceredig R, Rolink T. A positive look at double-negative thymocytes. *Nat Rev Immunol* 2002;2:888–897.
300. Alam SM, Travers PJ, Wung JL, et al. T-cell-receptor affinity and thymocyte positive selection. *Nature* 1996;381:616–620.
301. Kisielow P, Miazek A. Positive selection of T-cells: rescue from programmed cell death and differentiation require continual engagement of the T-cell receptor. *J Exp Med* 1995;181:1975–1984.
302. Sebzda E, Mariathasan S, Ohteki T, et al. Selection of the T-cell repertoire. *Annu Rev Immunol* 1999;17:829–874.
303. Singer A, Bosselut R. CD4/CD8 coreceptors in thymocyte development, selection, and lineage commitment: analysis of the CD4/CD8 lineage decision. *Adv Immunol* 2004;83:91–131.
304. Taniuchi I, Ellmeier W, Littman DR. The CD4/CD8 lineage choice: new insights into epigenetic regulation during T-cell development. *Adv Immunol* 2004;83:55–89.
305. Sarafova SD, Erman B, Yu Q, et al. Modulation of coreceptor transcription during positive selection dictates lineage fate independently of TCR/coreceptor specificity. *Immunity* 2005;23:75–87.
306. Yasutomo K, Doyle C, Miele L, et al. The duration of antigen receptor signalling determines CD4+ versus CD8+ T-cell lineage fate. *Nature* 2000;404:506–510.
307. Singer A, Adoro S, Park JH. Lineage fate and intense debate: myths, models and mechanisms of CD4- versus CD8-lineage choice. *Nat Rev Immunol* 2008;8:788–801.
308. Hogquist KA, Baldwin TA, Jameson SC. Central tolerance: learning self-control in the thymus. *Nat Rev Immunol* 2005;5:772–782.
309. Nossal GJ. Negative selection of lymphocytes. *Cell* 1994;76:229–239.
310. Derbinski J, Schulte A, Kyewski B, et al. Promiscuous gene expression in medullary thymic epithelial cells mirrors the peripheral self. *Nat Immunol* 2001;2:1032–1039.
311. Derbinski J, Gabler J, Brors B, et al. Promiscuous gene expression in thymic epithelial cells is regulated at multiple levels. *J Exp Med* 2005;202:33–45.
312. Anderson MS, Venanzi ES, Chen Z, et al. The cellular mechanism of Aire control of T-cell tolerance. *Immunity* 2005;23:227–239.
313. Finnish-German APECED Consortium. An autoimmune disease, APECED, caused by mutations in a novel gene featuring two PHD-type zinc-finger domains. *Nat Genet* 1997;17:399–403.
314. Mathis D, Benoist C. A decade of AIRE. *Nat Rev Immunol* 2007;7:645–650.
315. McCaughtry TM, Wilken MS, Hogquist KA. Thymic emigration revisited. *J Exp Med* 2007;204:2513–2520.
316. Love PE, Bhandoola A. Signal integration and crosstalk during thymocyte migration and emigration. *Nat Rev Immunol* 2011;11:469–477.
317. Gattinoni L, Lugli E, Ji Y, et al. A human memory T-cell subset with stem cell-like properties. *Nat Med* 2011;17:1290–1297.
318. Bevan MJ. Helping the CD8(+) T-cell response. *Nat Rev Immunol* 2004;4:595–602.
319. Liao W, Lin JX, Leonard WJ. IL-2 family cytokines: new insights into the complex roles of IL-2 as a broad regulator of T helper cell differentiation. *Curr Opin Immunol* 2011;23:598–604.
320. Sallusto F, Lenig D, Forster R, et al. Two subsets of memory T lymphocytes with distinct homing potentials and effector functions. *Nature* 1999;401:708–712.
321. Sallusto F, Geginat J, Lanzavecchia A. Central memory and effector memory T-cell subsets: function, generation, and maintenance. *Annu Rev Immunol* 2004;22:745–763.
322. Sallusto F, Lanzavecchia A. Heterogeneity of CD4+ memory T-cells: functional modules for tailored immunity. *Eur J Immunol* 2009;39:2076–2082.
323. Zygmunt B, Veldhoen M. T helper cell differentiation more than just cytokines. *Adv Immunol* 2011;109:159–196.
324. Hsieh CS, Macatonia SE, Tripp CS, et al. Development of TH1 CD4+ T-cells through IL-12 produced by Listeria-induced macrophages. *Science* 1993;260:547–549.
325. Manetti R, Parronchi P, Giudizi MG, et al. Natural killer cell stimulatory factor (interleukin 12 [IL-12]) induces T helper type 1 (Th1)-specific immune responses and inhibits the development of IL-4-producing Th cells. *J Exp Med* 1993;177:1199–1204.
326. Kopf M, Le Gros G, Bachmann M, et al. Disruption of the murine IL-4 gene blocks Th2 cytokine responses. *Nature* 1993;362:245–248.
327. Wong MT, Ye JJ, Alonso MN, et al. Regulation of human Th9 differentiation by type I interferons and IL-21. *Immunol Cell Biol* 2010;88:624–631.
328. Dardalhon V, Awasthi A, Kwon H, et al. IL-4 inhibits TGF-beta-induced Foxp3+ T-cells and, together with TGF-beta, generates IL-9+ IL-10+ Foxp3(-) effector T-cells. *Nat Immunol* 2008;9:1347–1355.
329. Veldhoen M, Uyttenhove C, van Snick J, et al. Transforming growth factor-beta 'reprograms' the differentiation of T helper 2 cells and promotes an interleukin 9-producing subset. *Nat Immunol* 2008;9:1341–1346.
330. Bettelli E, Carrier Y, Gao W, et al. Reciprocal developmental pathways for the generation of pathogenic effector TH17 and regulatory T-cells. *Nature* 2006;441:235–238.
331. Mangan PR, Harrington LE, O'Quinn DB, et al. Transforming growth factor-beta induces development of the T(H)17 lineage. *Nature* 2006;441:231–234.
332. Veldhoen M, Hocking RJ, Atkins CJ, et al. TGFbeta in the context of an inflammatory cytokine milieu supports de novo differentiation of IL-17-producing T-cells. *Immunity* 2006;24:179–189.
333. Chen W, Jin W, Hardegen N, et al. Conversion of peripheral CD4+CD25- naive T-cells to CD4+CD25+ regulatory T-cells by TGF-beta induction of transcription factor Foxp3. *J Exp Med* 2003;198:1875–1886.
334. Duhen T, Geiger R, Jarrossay D, et al. Production of interleukin 22 but not interleukin 17 by a subset of human skin-homing memory T-cells. *Nat Immunol* 2009;10:857–863.
335. Trifari S, Kaplan CD, Tran EH, et al. Identification of a human helper T-cell population that has abundant production of interleukin 22 and is distinct from T(H)-17, T(H)1 and T(H)2 cells. *Nat Immunol* 2009;10:864–871.
336. Nurieva RI, Chung Y, Hwang D, et al. Generation of T follicular helper cells is mediated by interleukin-21 but independent of T helper 1, 2, or 17 cell lineages. *Immunity* 2008;29:138–149.
337. Vogelzang A, McGuire HM, Yu D, et al. A fundamental role for interleukin-21 in the generation of T follicular helper cells. *Immunity* 2008;29:127–137.
338. Linterman MA, Beaton L, Yu D, et al. IL-21 acts directly on B-cells to regulate Bcl-6 expression and germinal center responses. *J Exp Med* 2010;207:353–363.
339. Zotos D, Coquet JM, Zhang Y, et al. IL-21 regulates germinal center B-cell differentiation and proliferation through a B-cell-intrinsic mechanism. *J Exp Med* 2010;207:365–378.
340. Rankin AL, MacLeod H, Keegan S, et al. IL-21 receptor is critical for the development of memory B-cell responses. *J Immunol* 2011;186:667–674.
341. Harrington LE, Hatton RD, Mangan PR, et al. Interleukin 17-producing CD4+ effector T-cells develop via a lineage distinct from the T helper type 1 and 2 lineages. *Nat Immunol* 2005;6:1123–1132.
342. Park H, Li Z, Yang XO, et al. A distinct lineage of CD4 T-cells regulates tissue inflammation by producing interleukin 17. *Nat Immunol* 2005;6:1133–1141.

343. Yamane H, Zhu J, Paul WE. Independent roles for IL-2 and GATA-3 in stimulating naive CD4+ T-cells to generate a Th2-inducing cytokine environment. *J Exp Med* 2005;202:793–804.

344. Gorelik L, Fields PE, Flavell RA. Cutting edge: TGF-beta inhibits Th type 2 development through inhibition of GATA-3 expression. *J Immunol* 2000;165: 4773–4777.

345. Gorelik L, Constant S, Flavell RA. Mechanism of transforming growth factor beta-induced inhibition of T helper type 1 differentiation. *J Exp Med* 2002;195: 1499–1505.

346. Murphy KM, Reiner SL. The lineage decisions of helper T-cells. *Nat Rev Immunol* 2002;2:933–944.

347. Szabo SJ, Dighe AS, Gubler U, et al. Regulation of the interleukin (IL)-12R beta 2 subunit expression in developing T helper 1 (Th1) and Th2 cells. *J Exp Med* 1997;185:817–824.

348. Szabo SJ, Kim ST, Costa GL, et al. A novel transcription factor, T-bet, directs Th1 lineage commitment. *Cell* 2000;100:655–669.

349. Afkarian M, Sedy JR, Yang J, et al. T-bet is a STAT1-induced regulator of IL-12R expression in naive CD4+ T-cells. *Nat Immunol* 2002;3:549 557.

350. Kaplan MH, Schindler U, Smiley ST, et al. Stat6 is required for mediating responses to IL-4 and for development of Th2 cells. *Immunity* 1996;4:313–319.

351. Zheng W, Flavell RA. The transcription factor GATA-3 is necessary and sufficient for Th2 cytokine gene expression in CD4 T-cells. *Cell* 1997;89:587–596.

352. Zhu J, Cote-Sierra J, Guo L, et al. Stat5 activation plays a critical role in Th2 differentiation. *Immunity* 2003;19:739–748.

353. Amsen D, Blander JM, Lee GR, et al. Instruction of distinct CD4 T helper cell fates by different notch ligands on antigen-presenting cells. *Cell* 2004;117:515–526.

354. Hori S. Stability of regulatory T-cell lineage. *Adv Immunol* 2011;112:1–24.

355. Izcue A, Coombes JL, Powrie F. Regulatory lymphocytes and intestinal inflammation. *Annu Rev Immunol* 2009;27:313–338.

356. Lee HM, Bautista JL, Hsieh CS. Thymic and peripheral differentiation of regulatory T-cells. *Adv Immunol* 2011;112:25–71.

357. Chang HC, Sehra S, Goswami R, et al. The transcription factor PU.1 is required for the development of IL-9-producing T-cells and allergic inflammation. *Nat Immunol* 2010;11:527–534.

358. Ma CS, Tangye SG, Deenick EK. Human Th9 cells: inflammatory cytokines modulate IL-9 production through the induction of IL-21. *Immunol Cell Biol* 2010;88:621–623.

359. Noelle RJ, Nowak EC. Cellular sources and immune functions of interleukin-9. *Nat Rev Immunol* 2010;10:683–687.

360. Yang L, Anderson DE, Baecher-Allan C, et al. IL-21 and TGF-beta are required for differentiation of human T(H)17 cells. *Nature* 2008;454:350–352.

361. Lee WW, Kang SW, Choi J, et al. Regulating human Th17 cells via differential expression of IL-1 receptor. *Blood* 2010;115:530–540.

362. Wilson NJ, Boniface K, Chan JR, et al. Development, cytokine profile and function of human interleukin 17-producing helper T-cells. *Nat Immunol* 2007;8:950–957.

363. Maddur MS, Miossec P, Kaveri SV, et al. Th17 cells: biology, pathogenesis of autoimmune and inflammatory diseases, and therapeutic strategies. *Am J Pathol* 2012;181:8–18.

364. Hori S, Nomura T, Sakaguchi S. Control of regulatory T-cell development by the transcription factor Foxp3. *Science* 2003;299:1057–1061.

365. Ivanov II, McKenzie BS, Zhou L, et al. The orphan nuclear receptor RORgammat directs the differentiation program of proinflammatory IL-17+ T helper cells. *Cell* 2006;126:1121–1133.

366. Johnston RJ, Poholek AC, DiToro D, et al. Bcl6 and Blimp-1 are reciprocal and antagonistic regulators of T follicular helper cell differentiation. *Science* 2009;325:1006–1010.

367. Yu D, Rao S, Tsai LM, et al. The transcriptional repressor Bcl-6 directs T follicular helper cell lineage commitment. *Immunity* 2009;31:457–468.

368. Murphy KM, Stockinger B. Effector T-cell plasticity: flexibility in the face of changing circumstances. *Nat Immunol* 2010;11:674–680.

369. Constant SL, Bottomly K. Induction of Th1 and Th2 CD4+ T-cell responses: the alternative approaches. *Annu Rev Immunol* 1997;15:297–322.

370. Swain SL, McKinstry KK, Strutt TM. Expanding roles for CD4(+) T-cells in immunity to viruses. *Nat Rev Immunol* 2012;12:136–148.

371. Mosser DM. The many faces of macrophage activation. *J Leukoc Biol* 2003; 73:209–212.

372. Paul WE, Zhu J. How are T(H)2-type immune responses initiated and amplified? *Nat Rev Immunol* 2010;10:225–235.

373. Okoye IS, Wilson MS. CD4+ T helper 2 cells–microbial triggers, differentiation requirements and effector functions. *Immunology* 2011;134:368–377.

374. Anthony RM, Rutitzky LI, Urban JF Jr, et al. Protective immune mechanisms in helminth infection. *Nat Rev Immunol* 2007;7:975–987.

375. de Vries JE, Punnonen J, Cocks BG, et al. Regulation of the human IgE response by IL4 and IL13. *Res Immunol* 1993;144:597–601.

376. Herbert DR, Holscher C, Mohrs M, et al. Alternative macrophage activation is essential for survival during schistosomiasis and downmodulates T helper 1 responses and immunopathology. *Immunity* 2004;20:623–635.

377. Motoji T, Okada M, Takanashi M, et al. Induction of eosinophilic colonies by interleukin-5 on acute myeloblastic leukaemic cells. *Br J Haematol* 1990;74: 169–172.

378. Takatsu K, Tanaka K, Tominaga A, et al. Antigen-induced T-cell-replacing factor (TRF). III. Establishment of T-cell hybrid clone continuously producing TRF and functional analysis of released TRF. *J Immunol* 1980;125:2646–2653.

379. Wynn TA. IL-13 effector functions. *Annu Rev Immunol* 2003;21:425–456.

380. Angkasekwinai P, Chang SH, Thapa M, et al. Regulation of IL-9 expression by IL-25 signaling. *Nat Immunol* 2010;11:250–256.

381. Fossiez F, Djossou O, Chomarat P, et al. T-cell interleukin-17 induces stromal cells to produce proinflammatory and hematopoietic cytokines. *J Exp Med* 1996;183:2593–2603.

382. Khader SA, Bell GK, Pearl JE, et al. IL-23 and IL-17 in the establishment of protective pulmonary CD4+ T-cell responses after vaccination and during *Mycobacterium tuberculosis* challenge. *Nat Immunol* 2007;8:369–377.

383. Liang SC, Long AJ, Bennett F, et al. An IL-17F/A heterodimer protein is produced by mouse Th17 cells and induces airway neutrophil recruitment. *J Immunol* 2007;179:7791–7799.

384. Lin Y, Ritchea S, Logar A, et al. Interleukin-17 is required for T helper 1 cell immunity and host resistance to the intracellular pathogen Francisella tularensis. *Immunity* 2009;31:799–810.

385. Ye P, Rodriguez FH, Kanaly S, et al. Requirement of interleukin 17 receptor signaling for lung CXC chemokine and granulocyte colony-stimulating factor expression, neutrophil recruitment, and host defense. *J Exp Med* 2001;194:519–527.

386. Denning TL, Wang YC, Patel SR, et al. Lamina propria macrophages and dendritic cells differentially induce regulatory and interleukin 17-producing T-cell responses. *Nat Immunol* 2007;8:1086–1094.

387. Uematsu S, Fujimoto K, Jang MH, et al. Regulation of humoral and cellular gut immunity by lamina propria dendritic cells expressing Toll-like receptor 5. *Nat Immunol* 2008;9:769–776.

388. Zygmunt BM, Rharbaoui F, Groebe L, et al. Intranasal immunization promotes th17 immune responses. *J Immunol* 2009;183:6933–6938.

389. Pickert G, Neufert C, Leppkes M, et al. STAT3 links IL-22 signaling in intestinal epithelial cells to mucosal wound healing. *J Exp Med* 2009;206:1465–1472.

390. Happel KI, Dubin PJ, Zheng M, et al. Divergent roles of IL-23 and IL-12 in host defense against Klebsiella pneumoniae. *J Exp Med* 2005;202:761–769.

391. LeibundGut-Landmann S, Gross O, Robinson MJ, et al. Syk- and CARD9-dependent coupling of innate immunity to the induction of T helper cells that produce interleukin 17. *Nat Immunol* 2007;8:630–638.

392. Robinson MJ, Osorio F, Rosas M, et al. Dectin-2 is a Syk-coupled pattern recognition receptor crucial for Th17 responses to fungal infection. *J Exp Med* 2009; 206:2037–2051.

393. Liang SC, Tan XY, Luxenberg DP, et al. Interleukin (IL)-22 and IL-17 are coexpressed by Th17 cells and cooperatively enhance expression of antimicrobial peptides. *J Exp Med* 2006;203:2271–2279.

394. Eyerich S, Eyerich K, Pennino D, et al. Th22 cells represent a distinct human T-cell subset involved in epidermal immunity and remodeling. *J Clin Invest* 2009;119:3573–3585.

395. Wolk K, Kunz S, Witte E, et al. IL-22 increases the innate immunity of tissues. *Immunity* 2004;21:241–254.

396. Boniface K, Bernard FX, Garcia M, et al. IL-22 inhibits epidermal differentiation and induces proinflammatory gene expression and migration of human keratinocytes. *J Immunol* 2005;174:3695–3702.

397. Wolk K, Sabat R. Interleukin-22: a novel T- and NK-cell derived cytokine that regulates the biology of tissue cells. *Cytokine Growth Factor Rev* 2006;17:367–380.

398. Bentebibel SE, Schmitt N, Banchereau J, et al. Human tonsil B-cell lymphoma 6 (BCL6)-expressing CD4+ T-cell subset specialized for B-cell help outside germinal centers. *Proc Natl Acad Sci U S A* 2011;108:E488–E497.

399. Kerfoot SM, Yaari G, Patel JR, et al. Germinal center B-cell and T follicular helper cell development initiates in the interfollicular zone. *Immunity* 2011;34: 947–960.

400. Kitano M, Moriyama S, Ando Y, et al. Bcl6 protein expression shapes pre-germinal center B-cell dynamics and follicular helper T-cell heterogeneity. *Immunity* 2011;34:961–972.

401. Pape KA, Kouskoff V, Nemazee D, et al. Visualization of the genesis and fate of isotype-switched B-cells during a primary immune response. *J Exp Med* 2003; 197:1677–1687.

402. Toellner KM, Luther SA, Sze DM, et al. T helper 1 (Th1) and Th2 characteristics start to develop during T-cell priming and are associated with an immediate ability to induce immunoglobulin class switching. *J Exp Med* 1998;187:1193–1204.

403. Lee SK, Rigby RJ, Zotos D, et al. B-cell priming for extrafollicular antibody responses requires Bcl-6 expression by T-cells. *J Exp Med* 2011;208:1377–1388.

404. Nurieva RI, Chung Y, Martinez GJ, et al. Bcl6 mediates the development of T follicular helper cells. *Science* 2009;325:1001–1005.

405. Sakaguchi S, Sakaguchi N, Asano M, et al. Immunologic self-tolerance maintained by activated T-cells expressing IL-2 receptor alpha-chains (CD25). Breakdown of a single mechanism of self-tolerance causes various autoimmune diseases. *J Immunol* 1995;155:1151–1164.

406. Belkaid Y. Regulatory T-cells and infection: a dangerous necessity. *Nat Rev Immunol* 2007;7:875–888.

407. Sakaguchi S, Miyara M, Costantino CM, et al. FOXP3+ regulatory T-cells in the human immune system. *Nat Rev Immunol* 2010;10:490–500.

408. Vignali DA, Collison LW, Workman CJ. How regulatory T-cells work. *Nat Rev Immunol* 2008;8:523–532.

409. Asseman C, Mauze S, Leach MW, et al. An essential role for interleukin 10 in the function of regulatory T-cells that inhibit intestinal inflammation. *J Exp Med* 1999;190:995–1004.

410. Nakamura K, Kitani A, Strober W. Cell contact-dependent immunosuppression by CD4(+)CD25(+) regulatory T-cells is mediated by cell surface-bound transforming growth factor beta. *J Exp Med* 2001;194:629–644.

411. Cao X, Cai SF, Fehniger TA, et al. Granzyme B and perforin are important for regulatory T-cell-mediated suppression of tumor clearance. *Immunity* 2007;27: 635–646.

412. Deaglio S, Dwyer KM, Gao W, et al. Adenosine generation catalyzed by CD39 and CD73 expressed on regulatory T-cells mediates immune suppression. *J Exp Med* 2007;204:1257–1265.

413. Fallarino F, Grohmann U, Hwang KW, et al. Modulation of tryptophan catabolism by regulatory T-cells. *Nat Immunol* 2003;4:1206–1212.

414. Tsuji M, Komatsu N, Kawamoto S, et al. Preferential generation of follicular B helper T-cells from Foxp3+ T-cells in gut Peyer's patches. *Science* 2009;323: 1488–1492.

415. Cooper MD, Raymond DA, Peterson RD, et al. The functions of the thymus system and the bursa system in the chicken. *J Exp Med* 1966;123:75–102.

416. Alt FW, Blackwell TK, Yancopoulos GD. Development of the primary antibody repertoire. *Science* 1987;238:1079–1087.

417. Tonegawa S. Somatic generation of antibody diversity. *Nature* 1983;302:575–581.

418. Batista FD, Iber D, Neuberger MS. B-cells acquire antigen from target cells after synapse formation. *Nature* 2001;411:489–494.

419. Fu SM, Winchester RJ, Kunkel HG. Occurrence of surface IgM, IgD, and free light chains of human lymphocytes. *J Exp Med* 1974;139:451–456.

420. Maizels N. Immunoglobulin gene diversification. *Annu Rev Genet* 2005;39:23–46.

421. Manz RA, Hauser AE, Hiepe F, et al. Maintenance of serum antibody levels. *Annu Rev Immunol* 2005;23:367–386.

422. von Boehmer H, Melchers F. Checkpoints in lymphocyte development and autoimmune disease. *Nat Immunol* 2010;11:14–20.

423. Hardy RR, Hayakawa K. B-cell development pathways. *Annu Rev Immunol* 2001;19:595–621.

424. Edelman GM. Antibody structure and molecular immunology. *Science* 1973; 180:830–840.

425. Bassing CH, Swat W, Alt FW. The mechanism and regulation of chromosomal V(D)J recombination. *Cell* 2002;109(Suppl):S45–S55.
426. Schatz DG, Swanson PC. V(D)J recombination: mechanisms of initiation. *Annu Rev Genet* 2011;45:167–202.
427. Alt FW, Blackwell TK, DePinho RA, et al. Regulation of genome rearrangement events during lymphocyte differentiation. *Immunol Rev* 1986;89:5–30.
428. LeBien TW, Tedder TF. B lymphocytes: how they develop and function. *Blood* 2008;112:1570–1580.
429. Nagasawa T. Microenvironmental niches in the bone marrow required for B-cell development. *Nat Rev Immunol* 2006;6:107–116.
430. Nutt SL, Kee BL. The transcriptional regulation of B-cell lineage commitment. *Immunity* 2007;26:715–725.
431. Oettinger MA, Schatz DG, Gorka C, et al. RAG-1 and RAG-2, adjacent genes that synergistically activate V(D)J recombination. *Science* 1990;248:1517–1523.
432. Schwarz K, Gauss GH, Ludwig L, et al. RAG mutations in human B-cell-negative SCID. *Science* 1996;274:97–99.
433. Komori T, Okada A, Stewart V, et al. Lack of N regions in antigen receptor variable region genes of TdT-deficient lymphocytes. *Science* 1993;261:1171–1175.
434. Gellert M. V(D)J recombination: RAG proteins, repair factors, and regulation. *Annu Rev Biochem* 2002;71:101–132.
435. Melchers F. The pre-B-cell receptor: selector of fitting immunoglobulin heavy chains for the B-cell repertoire. *Nat Rev Immunol* 2005;5:578–584.
436. Herzog S, Reth M, Jumaa H. Regulation of B-cell proliferation and differentiation by pre-B-cell receptor signalling. *Nat Rev Immunol* 2009;9:195–205.
437. Davis AC, Shulman MJ. IgM—molecular requirements for its assembly and function. *Immunol Today* 1989;10:118–122; 127–128.
438. Goodnow C, Adelstein S, Basten A. The need for central and peripheral tolerance in the B-cell repertoire. *Science* 1990;248:1373–1379.
439. Chung JB, Silverman M, Monroe JG. Transitional B-cells: step by step towards immune competence. *Trends Immunol* 2003;24:342–348.
440. Gorelik L, Gilbride K, Dobles M, et al. Normal B-cell homeostasis requires B-cell activation factor production by radiation-resistant cells. *J Exp Med* 2003;198:937–945.
441. Minges Wols HA, Underhill GH, Kansas GS, et al. The role of bone marrow-derived stromal cells in the maintenance of plasma cell longevity. *J Immunol* 2002;169:4213–4221.
442. Balázs M, Martin F, Zhou T, et al. Blood dendritic cells interact with splenic marginal zone B-cells to initiate T-independent immune responses. *Immunity* 2002;17:341–352.
443. Carrasco YR, Batista FD. B-cells acquire particulate antigen in a macrophage-rich area at the boundary between the follicle and the subcapsular sinus of the lymph node. *Immunity* 2007;27:160–171.
444. Junt T, Moseman EA, Iannacone M, et al. Subcapsular sinus macrophages in lymph nodes clear lymph-borne viruses and present them to antiviral B-cells. *Nature* 2007;450:110–114.
445. Phan TG, Green JA, Gray EE, et al. Immune complex relay by subcapsular sinus macrophages and noncognate B-cells drives antibody affinity maturation. *Nat Immunol* 2009;10:786–793.
446. Sixt M, Kanazawa N, Selg M, et al. The conduit system transports soluble antigens from the afferent lymph to resident dendritic cells in the T-cell area of the lymph node. *Immunity* 2005;22:19–29.
447. Bajenoff M, Germain RN. B-cell follicle development remodels the conduit system and allows soluble antigen delivery to follicular dendritic cells. *Blood* 2009;114:4989–4997.
448. Pape KA, Catron DM, Itano AA, et al. The humoral immune response is initiated in lymph nodes by B-cells that acquire soluble antigen directly in the follicles. *Immunity* 2007;26:491–502.
449. Roozendaal R, Mempel TR, Pitcher LA, et al. Conduits mediate transport of low-molecular-weight antigen to lymph node follicles. *Immunity* 2009;30:264–276.
450. Vinuesa CG, Sanz I, Cook MC. Dysregulation of germinal centres in autoimmune disease. *Nat Rev Immunol* 2009;9:845–857.
451. Schmitt N, Morita R, Bourdery L, et al. Human dendritic cells induce the differentiation of interleukin-21-producing T follicular helper-like cells through interleukin-12. *Immunity* 2009;31:158–169.
452. Allen CD, Okada T, Cyster JG. Germinal-center organization and cellular dynamics. *Immunity* 2007;27:190–202.
453. MacLennan IC, Toellner KM, Cunningham AF, et al. Extrafollicular antibody responses. *Immunol Rev* 2003;194:8–18.
454. Berek C, Berger A, Apel M. Maturation of the immune response in germinal centers. *Cell* 1991;67:1121–1129.
455. Klein U, Dalla-Favera R. Germinal centres: role in B-cell physiology and malignancy. *Nat Rev Immunol* 2008;8:22–33.
456. Breitfeld D, Ohl L, Kremmer E, et al. Follicular B helper T-cells express CXC chemokine receptor 5, localize to B-cell follicles, and support immunoglobulin production. *J Exp Med* 2000;192:1545–1552.
457. Gunn MD, Ngo VN, Ansel KM, et al. A B-cell-homing chemokine made in lymphoid follicles activates Burkitt's lymphoma receptor-1. *Nature* 1998;391:799–803.
458. Schaerli P, Willimann K, Lang AB, et al. CXC chemokine receptor 5 expression defines follicular homing T-cells with B-cell helper function. *J Exp Med* 2000;192:1553–1562.
459. Allen CD, Okada T, Tang HL, et al. Imaging of germinal center selection events during affinity maturation. *Science* 2007;315:528–531.
460. Hauser AE, Junt T, Mempel TR, et al. Definition of germinal-center B-cell migration in vivo reveals predominant intrazonal circulation patterns. *Immunity* 2007;26:655–667.
461. Schwickert TA, Lindquist RL, Shakhar G, et al. In vivo imaging of germinal centres reveals a dynamic open structure. *Nature* 2007;446:83–87.
462. Kolar GR, Mehta D, Pelayo R, et al. A novel human B-cell subpopulation representing the initial germinal center population to express AID. *Blood* 2007;109:2545–2552.
463. Muramatsu M, Kinoshita K, Fagarasan S, et al. Class switch recombination and hypermutation require activation-induced cytidine deaminase (AID), a potential RNA editing enzyme. *Cell* 2000;102:553–563.
464. Toellner KM, Gulbranson-Judge A, Taylor DR, et al. Immunoglobulin switch transcript production in vivo related to the site and time of antigen-specific B-cell activation. *J Exp Med* 1996;183:2303–2312.
465. Liu YJ, Malisan F, de Bouteiller O, et al. Within germinal centers, isotype switching of immunoglobulin genes occurs after the onset of somatic mutation. *Immunity* 1996;4:241–250.
466. Victora GD, Schwickert TA, Fooksman DR, et al. Germinal center dynamics revealed by multiphoton microscopy with a photoactivatable fluorescent reporter. *Cell* 2010;143:592–605.
467. Avery DT, Deenick EK, Ma CS, et al. B-cell-intrinsic signaling through IL-21 receptor and STAT3 is required for establishing long-lived antibody responses in humans. *J Exp Med* 2010;207:155–171.
468. Blink EJ, Light A, Kallies A, et al. Early appearance of germinal center-derived memory B-cells and plasma cells in blood after primary immunization. *J Exp Med* 2005;201:545–554.
469. Phan TG, Paus D, Chan TD, et al. High affinity germinal center B-cells are actively selected into the plasma cell compartment. *J Exp Med* 2006;203:2419–2424.
470. Shapiro-Shelef M, Lin KI, McHeyzer-Williams LJ, et al. Blimp-1 is required for the formation of immunoglobulin secreting plasma cells and pre-plasma memory B-cells. *Immunity* 2003;19:607–620.
471. Allen CD, Ansel KM, Low C, et al. Germinal center dark and light zone organization is mediated by CXCR4 and CXCR5. *Nat Immunol* 2004;5:943–952.
472. Klein U, Tu Y, Stolovitzky GA, et al. Transcriptional analysis of the B-cell germinal center reaction. *Proc Natl Acad Sci U S A* 2003;100:2639–2644.
473. Phan RT, Dalla-Favera R. The BCL6 proto-oncogene suppresses p53 expression in germinal-centre B-cells. *Nature* 2004;432:635–639.
474. Liu YJ, Mason DY, Johnson GD, et al. Germinal center cells express bcl-2 protein after activation by signals which prevent their entry into apoptosis. *Eur J Immunol* 1991;21:1905–1910.
475. Liu YJ, Joshua DE, Williams GT, et al. Mechanism of antigen-driven selection in germinal centres. *Nature* 1989;342:929–931.
476. Martinez-Valdez H, Guret C, de Bouteiller O, et al. Human germinal center B-cells express the apoptosis-inducing genes Fas, c-myc, P53, and Bax but not the survival gene bcl-2. *J Exp Med* 1996;183:971–977.
477. Smith KG, Nossal GJ, Tarlinton DM. FAS is highly expressed in the germinal center but is not required for regulation of the B-cell response to antigen. *Proc Natl Acad Sci U S A* 1995;92:11628–11632.
478. Clark EA, Ledbetter JA. How B and T-cells talk to each other. *Nature* 1994;367:425–428.
479. Grammer AC, McFarland RD, Heaney J, et al. Expression, regulation, and function of B-cell-expressed CD154 in germinal centers. *J Immunol* 1999;163:4150–4159.
480. Kehry MR. CD40-mediated signaling in B-cells. Balancing cell survival, growth, and death. *J Immunol* 1996;156:2345–2348.
481. Rathmell JC, Townsend SE, Xu JC, et al. Expansion or elimination of B-cells in vivo: dual roles for CD40- and Fas (CD95)-ligands modulated by the B-cell antigen receptor. *Cell* 1996;87:319–329.
482. Honjo T, Kinoshita K, Muramatsu M. Molecular mechanism of class switch recombination: linkage with somatic hypermutation. *Annu Rev Immunol* 2002;20:165–196.
483. William J, Euler C, Christensen S, et al. Evolution of autoantibody responses via somatic hypermutation outside of germinal centers. *Science* 2002;297:2066–2070.
484. Weller S, Braun MC, Tan BK, et al. Human blood IgM "memory" B-cells are circulating splenic marginal zone B-cells harboring a prediversified immunoglobulin repertoire. *Blood* 2004;104:3647–3654.
485. Chaudhuri J, Alt FW. Class-switch recombination: interplay of transcription, DNA deamination and DNA repair. *Nat Rev Immunol* 2004;4:541–552.
486. Stavnezer J, Guikema JE, Schrader CE. Mechanism and regulation of class switch recombination. *Annu Rev Immunol* 2008;26:261–292.
487. Cerutti A, Schaffer A, Shah S, et al. CD30 is a CD40-inducible molecule that negatively regulates CD40-mediated immunoglobulin class switching in non-antigen-selected human B-cells. *Immunity* 1998;9:247–256.
488. Defrance T, Vanbervliet B, Briere F, et al. Interleukin 10 and transforming growth factor beta cooperate to induce anti-CD40-activated naive human B-cells to secrete immunoglobulin A. *J Exp Med* 1992;175:671–682.
489. Zan H, Cerutti A, Dramitinos P, et al. CD40 engagement triggers switching to IgA1 and IgA2 in human B-cells through induction of endogenous TGF-beta: evidence for TGF-beta but not IL-10-dependent direct S mu–>S alpha and sequential S mu–>S gamma, S gamma–>S alpha DNA recombination. *J Immunol* 1998;161:5217–5225.
490. Briere F, Servet-Delprat C, Bridon JM, et al. Human interleukin 10 induces naive surface immunoglobulin D+ (sIgD+) B-cells to secrete IgG1 and IgG3. *J Exp Med* 1994;179:757–762.
491. Coffman RL, Lebman DA, Rothman P. Mechanism and regulation of immunoglobulin isotype switching. *Adv Immunol* 1993;54:229–270.
492. Ozaki K, Spolski R, Feng CG, et al. A critical role for IL-21 in regulating immunoglobulin production. *Science* 2002;298:1630–1634.
493. Pene J, Gauchat JF, Lecart S, et al. Cutting edge: IL-21 is a switch factor for the production of IgG1 and IgG3 by human B-cells. *J Immunol* 2004;172:5154–5157.
494. Stavnezer J. Molecular processes that regulate class switching. *Curr Top Microbiol Immunol* 2000;245:127–168.
495. Stavnezer J. Antibody class switching. *Adv Immunol* 1996;61:79–146.
496. Wagner SD, Neuberger MS. Somatic hypermutation of immunoglobulin genes. *Annu Rev Immunol* 1996;14:441–457.
497. Odegard VH, Schatz DG. Targeting of somatic hypermutation. *Nat Rev Immunol* 2006;6:573–583.
498. Di Noia JM, Neuberger MS. Molecular mechanisms of antibody somatic hypermutation. *Annu Rev Biochem* 2007;76:1–22.
499. Lehmann AR, Niimi A, Ogi T, et al. Translesion synthesis: Y-family polymerases and the polymerase switch. *DNA Repair (Amst)* 2007;6:891–899.
500. Peled JU, Kuang FL, Iglesias-Ussel MD, et al. The biochemistry of somatic hypermutation. *Annu Rev Immunol* 2008;26:481–511.
501. Dilosa RM, Maeda K, Masuda A, et al. Germinal center B-cells and antibody production in the bone marrow. *J Immunol* 1991;146:4071–4077.
502. Shapiro-Shelef M, Calame K. Regulation of plasma-cell development. *Nat Rev Immunol* 2005;5:230–242.
503. Radbruch A, Muehlinghaus G, Luger EO, et al. Competence and competition: the challenge of becoming a long-lived plasma cell. *Nat Rev Immunol* 2006;6:741–750.

504. Winter O, Moser K, Mohr E, et al. Megakaryocytes constitute a functional component of a plasma cell niche in the bone marrow. *Blood* 2010;116:1867–1875.
505. Tarlinton D. B-cell memory: are subsets necessary? *Nat Rev Immunol* 2006;6:785–790.
506. Berkowska MA, Driessen GJ, Bikos V, et al. Human memory B-cells originate from three distinct germinal center-dependent and -independent maturation pathways. *Blood* 2011;118:2150–2158.
507. Calame KL, Lin K-I, Tunyaplin C. Regulatory mechanisms that determine the development and function of plasma cells. *Annu Rev Immunol* 2003;21:205–230.
508. Ye BH, Lista F, Lo Coco F, et al. Alterations of a zinc finger-encoding gene, BCL-6, in diffuse large-cell lymphoma. *Science* 1993;262:747–750.
509. Dent AL, Shaffer AL, Yu X, et al. Control of inflammation, cytokine expression, and germinal center formation by BCL-6. *Science* 1997;276:589–592.
510. Ye BH, Cattoretti G, Shen Q, et al. The BCL-6 proto-oncogene controls germinal-centre formation and Th2-type inflammation. *Nat Genet* 1997;16:161–170.
511. Cobaleda C, Schebesta A, Delogu A, et al. Pax5: the guardian of B-cell identity and function. *Nat Immunol* 2007;8:463–470.
512. Turner CA Jr, Mack DH, Davis MM. Blimp-1:a novel zinc finger-containing protein that can drive the maturation of B lymphocytes into immunoglobulin-secreting cells. *Cell* 1994;77:297–306.
513. Schroeder HW Jr, Cavacini L. Structure and function of immunoglobulins. *J Allergy Clin Immunol* 2010;125:S41–S52.
514. Heyman B. Regulation of antibody responses via antibodies, complement, and Fc receptors. *Annu Rev Immunol* 2000;18:709–737.
515. Kehry M, Ewald S, Douglas R, et al. The immunoglobulin mu chains of membrane-bound and secreted IgM molecules differ in their C-terminal segments. *Cell* 1980;21:393–406.
516. Fuentes-Panana EM, Bannish G, Monroe JG. Basal B-cell receptor signaling in B lymphocytes: mechanisms of regulation and role in positive selection, differentiation, and peripheral survival. *Immunol Rev* 2004;197:26–40.
517. Baumgarth N. The double life of a B-1 cell: self-reactivity selects for protective effector functions. *Nat Rev Immunol* 2011;11:34–46.
518. Ehrenstein MR, Notley CA. The importance of natural IgM: scavenger, protector and regulator. *Nat Rev Immunol* 2010;10:778–786.
519. Czajkowsky DM, Shao Z. The human IgM pentamer is a mushroom-shaped molecule with a flexural bias. *Proc Natl Acad Sci U S A* 2009;106:14960–14965.
520. Brandtzaeg P, Prydz H. Direct evidence for an integrated function of J chain and secretory component in epithelial transport of immunoglobulins. *Nature* 1984;311:71–73.
521. Preud'homme JL, Petit I, Barra A, et al. Structural and functional properties of membrane and secreted IgD. *Mol Immunol* 2000;37:871–887.
522. Shakib F, Stanworth DR. Human IgG subclasses in health and disease. (A review). Part II. *Ric Clin Lab* 1980;10:561–580.
523. Pan Q, Hammarstrom L. Molecular basis of IgG subclass deficiency. *Immunol Rev* 2000;178:99–110.
524. Nimmerjahn F, Ravetch JV. Divergent immunoglobulin g subclass activity through selective Fc receptor binding. *Science* 2005;310:1510–1512.
525. Mallery DL, McEwan WA, Bidgood SR, et al. Antibodies mediate intracellular immunity through tripartite motif-containing 21 (TRIM21). *Proc Natl Acad Sci U S A* 2010;107:19985–19990.
526. Fagarasan S, Kawamoto S, Kanagawa O, et al. Adaptive immune regulation in the gut: T-cell-dependent and T-cell-independent IgA synthesis. *Annu Rev Immunol* 2010;28:243–273.
527. Macpherson AJ, McCoy KD, Johansen FE, et al. The immune geography of IgA induction and function. *Mucosal Immunol* 2008;1:11–22.
528. van Egmond M, Damen CA, van Spriel AB, et al. IgA and the IgA Fc receptor. *Trends Immunol* 2001;22:205–211.
529. Brandtzaeg P, Baekkevold ES, Morton HC. From B to A the mucosal way. *Nat Immunol* 2001;2:1093–1094.
530. Suzuki K, Fagarasan S. How host-bacterial interactions lead to IgA synthesis in the gut. *Trends Immunol* 2008;29:523–531.
531. Chen K, Cerutti A. Vaccination strategies to promote mucosal antibody responses. *Immunity* 2010;33:479–491.
532. Peterson DA, McNulty NP, Guruge JL, et al. IgA response to symbiotic bacteria as a mediator of gut homeostasis. *Cell Host Microbe* 2007;2:328–339.
533. Geha RS, Jabara HH, Brodeur SR. The regulation of immunoglobulin E class-switch recombination. *Nat Rev Immunol* 2003;3:721–732.
534. Gould HJ, Sutton BJ. IgE in allergy and asthma today. *Nat Rev Immunol* 2008;8:205–217.
535. MacGlashan D Jr. IgE receptor and signal transduction in mast cells and basophils. *Curr Opin Immunol* 2008;20:717–723.
536. Hagan P. IgE and protective immunity to helminth infections. *Parasite Immunol* 1993;15:1–4.
537. Burton OT, Oettgen HC. Beyond immediate hypersensitivity: evolving roles for IgE antibodies in immune homeostasis and allergic diseases. *Immunol Rev* 2011;242:128–143.
538. Kawakami T, Kitaura J. Mast cell survival and activation by IgE in the absence of antigen: a consideration of the biologic mechanisms and relevance. *J Immunol* 2005;175:4167–4173.
539. Gauchat JF, Henchoz S, Mazzei G, et al. Induction of human IgE synthesis in B-cells by mast cells and basophils. *Nature* 1993;365:340–343.
540. Acharya M, Borland G, Edkins AL, et al. CD23/FcepsilonRII: molecular multi-tasking. *Clin Exp Immunol* 2010;162:12–23.
541. Fazilleau N, Mark L, McHeyzer-Williams LJ, et al. Follicular helper T-cells: lineage and location. *Immunity* 2009;30:324–335.
542. Dillon SR, Gross JA, Ansell SM, et al. An APRIL to remember: novel TNF ligands as therapeutic targets. *Nat Rev Drug Discov* 2006;5:235–246.
543. Mackay F, Schneider P. Cracking the BAFF code. *Nat Rev Immunol* 2009;9:491–502.
544. Bernasconi NL, Traggiai E, Lanzavecchia A. Maintenance of serological memory by polyclonal activation of human memory B-cells. *Science* 2002;298:2199–2202.
545. Litinskiy MB, Nardelli B, Hilbert DM, et al. DCs induce CD40-independent immunoglobulin class switching through BLyS and APRIL. *Nat Immunol* 2002;3:822–829.
546. Cerutti A, Puga I, Cols M. Innate control of B-cell responses. *Trends Immunol* 2011;32:202–211.

547. Chorny A, Cerutti A. A gut triumvirate rules homeostasis. *Nat Med* 2011;17:1549–1550.
548. Martin F, Kearney JF. Marginal-zone B-cells. *Nat Rev Immunol* 2002;2:323–335.
549. Griffin DO, Holodick NE, Rothstein TL. Human B1 cells in umbilical cord and adult peripheral blood express the novel phenotype CD20+ CD27+ CD43+ CD70. *J Exp Med* 2011;208:67–80.
550. Pillai S, Cariappa A. The follicular versus marginal zone B lymphocyte cell fate decision. *Nat Rev Immunol* 2009;9:767–777.
551. Cols M, Barra CM, He B, et al. Stromal endothelial cells establish a bidirectional crosstalk with chronic lymphocytic leukemia cells through the TNF-related factors BAFF, APRIL, and CD40L. *J Immunol* 2012;188:6071–6083.
552. He B, Santamaria R, Xu W, et al. The transmembrane activator TACI triggers immunoglobulin class switching by activating B-cells through the adaptor MyD88. *Nat Immunol* 2010;11:836–845.
553. Xu W, He B, Chiu A, et al. Epithelial cells trigger frontline immunoglobulin class switching through a pathway regulated by the inhibitor SLPI. *Nat Immunol* 2007;8:294–303.
554. Macpherson AJ, Gatto D, Sainsbury E, et al. A primitive T-cell-independent mechanism of intestinal mucosal IgA responses to commensal bacteria. *Science* 2000;288:2222–2226.
555. Macpherson AJ, Uhr T. Induction of protective IgA by intestinal dendritic cells carrying commensal bacteria. *Science* 2004;303:1662–1665.
556. Cinamon G, Zachariah MA, Lam OM, et al. Follicular shuttling of marginal zone B-cells facilitates antigen transport. *Nat Immunol* 2008;9:54–62.
557. Song H, Cerny J. Functional heterogeneity of marginal zone B-cells revealed by their ability to generate both early antibody-forming cells and germinal centers with hypermutation and memory in response to a T-dependent antigen. *J Exp Med* 2003;198:1923–1935.
558. Cambier JC, Campbell KS. Membrane immunoglobulin and its accomplices: new lessons from an old receptor. *FASEB J* 1992;6:3207–3217.
559. Kurosaki T, Shinohara H, Baba Y. B-cell signaling and fate decision. *Annu Rev Immunol* 2010;28:21–55.
560. Tamir I, Cambier JC. Antigen receptor signaling: integration of protein tyrosine kinase functions. *Oncogene* 1998;17:1353–1364.
561. Schwartzberg PL. The many faces of Src: multiple functions of a prototypical tyrosine kinase. *Oncogene* 1998;17:1463–1468.
562. Kurosaki T. Molecular mechanisms in B-cell antigen receptor signaling. *Curr Opin Immunol* 1997;9:309–318.
563. DeFranco AL. The complexity of signaling pathways activated by the BCR. *Curr Opin Immunol* 1997;9:296–308.
564. Thome M, Tschopp J. TCR-induced NF-κB activation: a crucial role for Carma1, Bcl10 and MALT1. *Trends Immunol* 2003;24:419–424.
565. Li Q, Verma IM. NF-kappaB regulation in the immune system. *Nat Rev Immunol* 2002;2:725–734.
566. Karin M, Ben-Neriah Y. Phosphorylation meets ubiquitination: the control of NF-[kappa]B activity. *Annu Rev Immunol* 2000;18:621–663.
567. de Gorter DJ, Vos JC, Pals ST, et al. The B-cell antigen receptor controls AP-1 and NFAT activity through Ras-mediated activation of Ral. *J Immunol* 2007;178:1405–1414.
568. Macian F, Lopez-Rodriguez C, Rao A. Partners in transcription: NFAT and AP-1. *Oncogene* 2001;20:2476–2489.
569. Pritchard NR, Smith KG. B-cell inhibitory receptors and autoimmunity. *Immunology* 2003;108:263–273.
570. Tedder TF, Poe JC, Haas KM. CD22: a multifunctional receptor that regulates B lymphocyte survival and signal transduction. *Adv Immunol* 2005;88:1–50.
571. Tedder TF, Tuscano J, Sato S, et al. CD22, a B lymphocyte-specific adhesion molecule that regulates antigen receptor signaling. *Annu Rev Immunol* 1997;15:481–504.
572. Berberich I, Shu GL, Clark EA. Cross-linking CD40 on B-cells rapidly activates nuclear factor-kappa B. *J Immunol* 1994;153:4357–4366.
573. Grammer AC, Lipsky PE. CD40-mediated regulation of immune responses by TRAF-dependent and TRAF-independent signaling mechanisms. *Adv Immunol* 2000;76:61–178.
574. Pullen SS, Miller HG, Everdeen DS, et al. CD40-tumor necrosis factor receptor-associated factor (TRAF) interactions: regulation of CD40 signaling through multiple TRAF binding sites and TRAF hetero-oligomerization. *Biochemistry* 1998;37:11836–11845.
575. Bishop GA, Moore CR, Xie P, et al. TRAF proteins in CD40 signaling. *Adv Exp Med Biol* 2007;597:131–151.
576. Iciek LA, Delphin SA, Stavnezer J. CD40 cross-linking induces Ig epsilon germline transcripts in B-cells via activation of NF-kappaB: synergy with IL-4 induction. *J Immunol* 1997;158:4769–4779.
577. Mackay F, Schneider P, Rennert P, et al. BAFF and APRIL: a tutorial on B-cell survival. *Annu Rev Immunol* 2003;21:231–264.
578. Kawabe T, Naka T, Yoshida K, et al. The immune responses in CD40-deficient mice: impaired immunoglobulin class switching and germinal center formation. *Immunity* 1994;1:167–178.
579. Monroe JG. Tolerance sensitivity of immature-stage B-cells: can developmentally regulated B-cell antigen receptor (BCR) signal transduction play a role? *J Immunol* 1996;156:2657–2660.
580. Cleary AM, Fortune SM, Yellin MJ, et al. Opposing roles of CD95 (Fas/APO-1) and CD40 in the death and rescue of human low density tonsillar B-cells. *J Immunol* 1995;155:3329–3337.
581. Allen RC, Armitage RJ, Conley ME, et al. CD40 ligand gene defects responsible for X-linked hyper-IgM syndrome. *Science* 1993;259:990–993.
582. Ferrari S, Giliani S, Insalaco A, et al. Mutations of CD40 gene cause an autosomal recessive form of immunodeficiency with hyper IgM. *Proc Natl Acad Sci U S A* 2001;98:12614–12619.
583. Korthauer U, Graf D, Mages HW, et al. Defective expression of T-cell CD40 ligand causes X-linked immunodeficiency with hyper-IgM. *Nature* 1993;361:539–541.
584. Schneider P. The role of APRIL and BAFF in lymphocyte activation. *Curr Opin Immunol* 2005;17:282–289.
585. Craxton A, Magaletti D, Ryan EJ, et al. Macrophage- and dendritic cell–dependent regulation of human B-cell proliferation requires the TNF family ligand BAFF. *Blood* 2003;101:4464–4471.

586. Nardelli B, Belvedere O, Roschke V, et al. Synthesis and release of B-lymphocyte stimulator from myeloid cells. *Blood* 2001;97:198–204.
587. Sakurai D, Kanno Y, Hase H, et al. TACI attenuates antibody production costimulated by BAFF-R and CD40. *Eur J Immunol* 2007;37:110–118.
588. Seshasayee D, Valdez P, Yan M, et al. Loss of TACI causes fatal lymphoproliferation and autoimmunity, establishing TACI as an inhibitory BLyS receptor. *Immunity* 2003;18:279–288.
589. Chiu A, Xu W, He B, et al. Hodgkin lymphoma cells express TACI and BCMA receptors and generate survival and proliferation signals in response to BAFF and APRIL. *Blood* 2007;109:729–739.
590. Schiemann B, Gommerman JL, Vora K, et al. An essential role for BAFF in the normal development of B-cells through a BCMA-independent pathway. *Science* 2001;293:2111–2114.
591. Treml LS, Carlesso G, Hoek KL, et al. TLR stimulation modifies BLyS receptor expression in follicular and marginal zone B-cells. *J Immunol* 2007;178: 7531–7539.
592. Castro I, Wright JA, Damdinsuren B, et al. B-cell receptor-mediated sustained c-Rel activation facilitates late transitional B-cell survival through control of B-cell activating factor receptor and NF-kappaB2. *J Immunol* 2009;182: 7729–7737.
593. Rothe M, Pan MG, Henzel WJ, et al. The TNFR2-TRAF signaling complex contains two novel proteins related to baculoviral inhibitor of apoptosis proteins. *Cell* 1995;83:1243–1252.
594. Bossen C, Schneider P. BAFF, APRIL and their receptors: structure, function and signaling. *Semin Immunol* 2006;18:263–275.
595. He B, Chadburn A, Jou E, et al. Lymphoma B-cells evade apoptosis through the TNF family members BAFF/BLyS and APRIL. *J Immunol* 2004;172:3268–3279.
596. Kayagaki N, Yan M, Seshasayee D, et al. BAFF/BLyS receptor 3 binds the B-cell survival factor BAFF ligand through a discrete surface loop and promotes processing of NF-kappaB2. *Immunity* 2002;17:515–524.
597. Armitage RJ, Macduff BM, Spriggs MK, et al. Human B-cell proliferation and Ig secretion induced by recombinant CD40 ligand are modulated by soluble cytokines. *J Immunol* 1993;150:3671–3680.
598. Banchereau J, Rousset F. Human B lymphocytes: phenotype, proliferation, and differentiation. *Adv Immunol* 1992;52:125–262.
599. Shuai K, Liu B. Regulation of JAK-STAT signalling in the immune system. *Nat Rev Immunol* 2003;3:900–911.
600. Attisano L, Wrana JL. Signal transduction by the TGF-beta superfamily. *Science* 2002;296:1646–1647.
601. Cunningham-Rundles C, Ponda PP. Molecular defects in T- and B-cell primary immunodeficiency diseases. *Nat Rev Immunol* 2005;5:880–892.
602. Conley ME, Dobbs AK, Farmer DM, et al. Primary B-cell immunodeficiencies: comparisons and contrasts. *Annu Rev Immunol* 2009;27:199–227.
603. Fischer A, Le Deist F, Hacein-Bey-Abina S, et al. Severe combined immunodeficiency. A model disease for molecular immunology and therapy. *Immunol Rev* 2005; 203:98–109.
604. Notarangelo LD. Primary immunodeficiencies. *J Allergy Clin Immunol* 2010; 125:S182–S194.
605. Chapel H, Lucas M, Lee M, et al. Common variable immunodeficiency disorders: division into distinct clinical phenotypes. *Blood* 2008;112:277–286.
606. Puck JM. Molecular and genetic basis of X-linked immunodeficiency disorders. *J Clin Immunol* 1994;14:81–89.
607. Letterio JJ, Roberts AB. Regulation of immune responses by TGF-beta. *Annu Rev Immunol* 1998;16:137–161.
608. Pestka S, Krause CD, Sarkar D, et al. Interleukin-10 and related cytokines and receptors. *Annu Rev Immunol* 2004;22:929–979.
609. Metzstein MM, Stanfield GM, Horvitz HR. Genetics of programmed cell death in C. elegans: past, present and future. *Trends Genet* 1998;14:410–416.
610. Rathmell JC, Thompson CB. The central effectors of cell death in the immune system. *Annu Rev Immunol* 1999;17:781–828.
611. Hengartner MO. The biochemistry of apoptosis. *Nature* 2000;407:770–776.
612. Kerr JF, Wyllie AH, Currie AR. Apoptosis: a basic biological phenomenon with wide-ranging implications in tissue kinetics. *Br J Cancer* 1972;26:239–257.
613. Kurosaka K, Takahashi M, Watanabe N, et al. Silent cleanup of very early apoptotic cells by macrophages. *J Immunol* 2003;171:4672–4679.
614. Savill J, Fadok V. Corpse clearance defines the meaning of cell death. *Nature* 2000;407:784–788.
615. Earnshaw WC, Martins LM, Kaufmann SH. Mammalian caspases: structure, activation, substrates, and functions during apoptosis. *Annu Rev Biochem* 1999; 68:383–424.
616. Salvesen GS, Dixit VM. Caspases: intracellular signaling by proteolysis. *Cell* 1997;91:443–446.
617. Shi Y. Mechanisms of caspase activation and inhibition during apoptosis. *Mol Cell* 2002;9:459–470.
618. Crawford ED, Wells JA. Caspase substrates and cellular remodeling. *Annu Rev Biochem* 2011;80:1055–1087.
619. Riedl SJ, Shi Y. Molecular mechanisms of caspase regulation during apoptosis. *Nat Rev Mol Cell Biol* 2004;5:897–907.
620. Varfolomeev E, Goncharov T, Maecker H, et al. Cellular inhibitors of apoptosis are global regulators of NF-kappaB and MAPK activation by members of the TNF family of receptors. *Sci Signal* 2012;5:ra22.
621. Bonizzi G, Karin M. The two NF-kappaB activation pathways and their role in innate and adaptive immunity. *Trends Immunol* 2004;25:280–288.
622. Dejardin E, Droin NM, Delhase M, et al. The lymphotoxin-beta receptor induces different patterns of gene expression via two NF-kappaB pathways. *Immunity* 2002;17:525–535.
623. Hayden MS, Ghosh S. Signaling to NF-kappaB. *Genes Dev* 2004;18:2195–2224.
624. Senftleben U, Cao Y, Xiao G, et al. Activation by IKKalpha of a second, evolutionary conserved, NF-kappa B signaling pathway. *Science* 2001;293:1495–1499.
625. Xiao G, Harhaj EW, Sun SC. NF-kappaB-inducing kinase regulates the processing of NF-kappaB2 p100. *Mol Cell* 2001;7:401–409.
626. Bykovskaja SN, Rytenko AN, Rauschenbach MO, et al. Ultrastructural alteration of cytolytic T lymphocytes following their interaction with target cells. II. Morphogenesis of secretory granules and intracellular vacuoles. *Cell Immunol* 1978;40:175–185.
627. Bossi G, Griffiths GM. CTL secretory lysosomes: biogenesis and secretion of a harmful organelle. *Semin Immunol* 2005;17:87–94.
628. Lichtenheld MG, Olsen KJ, Lu P, et al. Structure and function of human perforin. *Nature* 1988;335:448–451.
629. Peters PJ, Borst J, Oorschot V, et al. Cytotoxic T lymphocyte granules are secretory lysosomes, containing both perforin and granzymes. *J Exp Med* 1991;173: 1099–1109.
630. Shi L, Kam CM, Powers JC, et al. Purification of three cytotoxic lymphocyte granule serine proteases that induce apoptosis through distinct substrate and target cell interactions. *J Exp Med* 1992;176:1521–1529.
631. Shi L, Mai S, Israels S, et al. Granzyme B (GraB) autonomously crosses the cell membrane and perforin initiates apoptosis and GraB nuclear localization. *J Exp Med* 1997;185:855–866.
632. Aguilo JI, Anel A, Catalan E, et al. Granzyme B of cytotoxic T-cells induces extra-mitochondrial reactive oxygen species production via caspase-dependent NADPH oxidase activation. *Immunol Cell Biol* 2010;88:545–554.
633. Casey TM, Meade JL, Hewitt EW. Organelle proteomics: identification of the exocytic machinery associated with the natural killer cell secretory lysosome. *Mol Cell Proteomics* 2007;6:767–780.
634. Hirst CE, Buzza MS, Bird CH, et al. The intracellular granzyme B inhibitor, proteinase inhibitor 9, is up-regulated during accessory cell maturation and effector cell degranulation, and its overexpression enhances CTL potency. *J Immunol* 2003;170:805–815.
635. Locksley RM, Killeen N, Lenardo MJ. The TNF and TNF receptor superfamilies: integrating mammalian biology. *Cell* 2001;104:487–501.
636. Hsu H, Xiong J, Goeddel DV. The TNF receptor 1-associated protein TRADD signals cell death and NF-kappa B activation. *Cell* 1995;81:495–504.
637. Ashkenazi A, Dixit VM. Death receptors: signaling and modulation. *Science* 1998;281:1305–1308.
638. Pobezinskaya YL, Kim YS, Choksi S, et al. The function of TRADD in signaling through tumor necrosis factor receptor 1 and TRIF-dependent toll-like receptors. *Nat Immunol* 2008;9:1047–1054.
639. Kelliher MA, Grimm S, Ishida Y, et al. The death domain kinase RIP mediates the TNF-induced NF-kappaB signal. *Immunity* 1998;8:297–303.
640. Carrington PE, Sandu C, Wei Y, et al. The structure of FADD and its mode of interaction with procaspase-8. *Mol Cell* 2006;22:599–610.
641. Chen NJ, Chio II, Lin WJ, et al. Beyond tumor necrosis factor receptor: TRADD signaling in toll-like receptors. *Proc Natl Acad Sci U S A* 2008;105:12429–12434.
642. Devin A, Lin Y, Yamaoka S, et al. The alpha and beta subunits of IkappaB kinase (IKK) mediate TRAF2-dependent IKK recruitment to tumor necrosis factor (TNF) receptor 1 in response to TNF. *Mol Cell Biol* 2001;21:3986–3994.
643. Krammer PH. CD95's deadly mission in the immune system. *Nature* 2000;407: 789–795.
644. Hao Z, Duncan GS, Seagal J, et al. Fas receptor expression in germinal-center B-cells is essential for T and B lymphocyte homeostasis. *Immunity* 2008;29: 615–627.
645. Laytragoon-Lewin N, Duhony E, Bai XF, et al. Downregulation of the CD95 receptor and defect CD40-mediated signal transduction in B-chronic lymphocytic leukemia cells. *Eur J Haematol* 1998;61:266–271.
646. Medema JP, Scaffidi C, Kischkel FC, et al. FLICE is activated by association with the CD95 death-inducing signaling complex (DISC). *EMBO J* 1997;16: 2794–2804.
647. Muzio M, Chinnaiyan AM, Kischkel FC, et al. FLICE, a novel FADD-homologous ICE/CED-3-like protease, is recruited to the CD95 (Fas/APO-1) death–inducing signaling complex. *Cell* 1996;85:817–827.
648. Thome M, Tschopp J. Regulation of lymphocyte proliferation and death by FLIP. *Nat Rev Immunol* 2001;1:50–58.
649. Safa AR, Pollok KE. Targeting the anti-apoptotic protein c-FLIP for cancer therapy. *Cancers (Basel)* 2011;3:1639–1671.
650. Quintavalle C, Incoronato M, Puca L, et al. c-FLIPL enhances anti-apoptotic Akt functions by modulation of Gsk3beta activity. *Cell Death Differ* 2010;17; 1908–1916.
651. Pitti RM, Marsters SA, Ruppert S, et al. Induction of apoptosis by Apo-2 ligand, a new member of the tumor necrosis factor cytokine family. *J Biol Chem* 1996;271:12687–12690.
652. Suliman A, Lam A, Datta R, et al. Intracellular mechanisms of TRAIL: apoptosis through mitochondrial-dependent and -independent pathways. *Oncogene* 2001;20:2122–2133.
653. Sheridan JP, Marsters SA, Pitti RM, et al. Control of TRAIL-induced apoptosis by a family of signaling and decoy receptors. *Science* 1997;277:818–821.
654. Durkop H, Latza U, Hummel M, et al. Molecular cloning and expression of a new member of the nerve growth factor receptor family that is characteristic for Hodgkin's disease. *Cell* 1992;68:421–427.
655. Horie R, Aizawa S, Nagai M, et al. A novel domain in the CD30 cytoplasmic tail mediates NFkappaB activation. *Int Immunol* 1998;10:203–210.
656. Chiarle R, Podda A, Prolla G, et al. CD30 overexpression enhances negative selection in the thymus and mediates programmed cell death via a Bcl-2-sensitive pathway. *J Immunol* 1999;163:194–205.
657. Simhadri VL, Hansen HP, Simhadri VR, et al. A novel role for reciprocal CD30-CD30L signaling in the cross-talk between natural killer and dendritic cells. *Biol Chem* 2012;393:101–106.
658. Estaquier J, Vallette F, Vayssiere JL, et al. The mitochondrial pathways of apoptosis. *Adv Exp Med Biol* 2012;942:157–183.
659. Verhagen AM, Ekert PG, Pakusch M, et al. Identification of DIABLO, a mammalian protein that promotes apoptosis by binding to and antagonizing IAP proteins. *Cell* 2000;102:43–53.
660. Suzuki Y, Imai Y, Nakayama H, et al. A serine protease, HtrA2, is released from the mitochondria and interacts with XIAP, inducing cell death. *Mol Cell* 2001;8:613–621.
661. Shiozaki EN, Chai J, Shi Y. Oligomerization and activation of caspase-9, induced by Apaf-1 CARD. *Proc Natl Acad Sci U S A* 2002;99:4197–4202.
662. Du C, Fang M, Li Y, et al. Smac, a mitochondrial protein that promotes cytochrome c-dependent caspase activation by eliminating IAP inhibition. *Cell* 2000; 102:33–42.
663. Schinzel A, Kaufmann T, Borner C. Bcl-2 family members: integrators of survival and death signals in physiology and pathology [corrected]. *Biochim Biophys Acta* 2004;1644:95–105.
664. Gavathiotis E, Reyna DE, Davis ML, et al. BH3-triggered structural reorganization drives the activation of proapoptotic BAX. *Mol Cell* 2010;40:481–492.

665. Luo X, Budihardjo I, Zou H, et al. Bid, a Bcl2 interacting protein, mediates cytochrome c release from mitochondria in response to activation of cell surface death receptors. *Cell* 1998;94:481–490.

666. Youle RJ, Strasser A. The BCL-2 protein family: opposing activities that mediate cell death. *Nat Rev Mol Cell Biol* 2008;9:47–59.

667. Unkeless JC, Jin J. Inhibitory receptors, ITIM sequences and phosphatases. *Curr Opin Immunol* 1997;9:338–343.

668. Thomas ML. Of ITAMs and ITIMs: turning on and off the B-cell antigen receptor. *J Exp Med* 1995;181:1953–1956.

669. Aman MJ, Lamkin TD, Okada H, et al. The inositol phosphatase SHIP inhibits Akt/PKB activation in B-cells. *J Biol Chem* 1998;273:33922–33928.

670. Pearse RN, Kawabe T, Bolland S, et al. SHIP recruitment attenuates Fc gamma RIIB-induced B-cell apoptosis. *Immunity* 1999;10:753–760.

671. Blair PA, Norena LY, Flores-Borja F, et al. CD19(+)CD24(hi)CD38(hi) B-cells exhibit regulatory capacity in healthy individuals but are functionally impaired in systemic Lupus Erythematosus patients. *Immunity* 2010;32:129–140.

672. Duddy M, Niino M, Adatia F, et al. Distinct effector cytokine profiles of memory and naive human B-cell subsets and implication in multiple sclerosis. *J Immunol* 2007;178:6092–6099.

673. Fillatreau S, Sweenie CH, McGeachy MJ, et al. B-cells regulate autoimmunity by provision of IL-10. *Nat Immunol* 2002;3:944–950.

674. Mauri C, Gray D, Mushtaq N, et al. Prevention of arthritis by interleukin 10–producing B-cells. *J Exp Med* 2003;197:489–501.

675. Mizoguchi A, Mizoguchi E, Takedatsu H, et al. Chronic intestinal inflammatory condition generates IL-10-producing regulatory B cell subset characterized by CD1d upregulation. *Immunity* 2002;16:219–230.

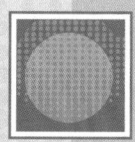

Chapter 3
Immunophenotypic Markers Useful in the Diagnosis and Classification of Hematopoietic and Lymphoid Neoplasms

Kate E. Grimm • Todd S. Barry • Dennis P. O'Malley • Lawrence M. Weiss

Immunohistochemical evaluation of hematologic tissues is a cornerstone of our current diagnostic system. While there are some entities that are defined by clinical, molecular, or genetic findings, in practical terms the combination of morphology and immunophenotype are paramount to the diagnosis, characterization, and classification of hematolymphoid neoplasms.

With this in mind, this chapter has been divided into two distinct sections, each with a different approach to the understanding of immunohistochemical markers. The first segment is meant to function as a stand-alone resource of specific immunohistochemical stains. It is not meant to be an exhaustive list, instead merely a few key stains from each category of antigen followed by a description of the common applications and staining patterns of each stain with instances in which it may be expressed. The subsequent section discusses specific hematolymphoid disorders and their immunohistochemical findings.

When applicable, we refer the reader to other specific chapters in this book that also discuss immunohistochemical analysis in the context of specific disorders. The technical and historical aspects of immunohistochemistry, while interesting, are not within the scope of this chapter. The reader is referred to specialized texts for more information on these details.

 ## APPLICATION OF IMMUNOHISTOCHEMISTRY TO LYMPH NODES

Immunohistochemical studies are useful in the evaluation of lymph nodes for several reasons. First, they are useful in assessing the architecture, important in determining whether the architecture is retained, distorted, partially effaced, or completely effaced. Second, they are useful in determining whether abnormal populations are present, populations that may indicate the presence of lymphoma or another neoplasm. Finally, they are useful in the classification of lymphoma.

 ## LYMPHOID ANTIGENS

B-Cell–Associated Antigens

CD20

CD20 is a nonglycosylated membranous phosphoprotein weighing 35 kDa. It is thought to be involved in B-cell regulation, differentiation, and calcium flux (1–3). L26 is the most commonly used commercial antibody. The staining pattern is membranous.

CD20 is often used as the first-line B-cell lineage–defining antibody (3). It is acquired by late pre-B cells as they mature, and is typically lost as the B cells become plasma cells (3).

The monoclonal antibody against CD20 (i.e., rituximab) has necessitated the use of alternate B-cell lineage–defining markers in patients suspected of relapse (4). CD79a, PAX-5, CD19,

and CD22 are also available for staining B cells in paraffin sections and are useful adjuncts to determine B-cell lineage in patients who have received treatment with rituximab.

Although rare, CD20 expression has been noted on a small subset of nonneoplastic T cells (5). CD20 expression has also been identified in occasional cases of Hodgkin lymphoma, precursor-B acute lymphoblastic leukemia, plasma cell neoplasms, and very rarely in T-cell lymphomas (3,4,6).

PAX-5

PAX-5 (B-cell-specific activator protein) is a nuclear protein belonging to the paired-box-containing (PAX) family of transcription factors (7). PAX-5 is thought to commit B-cell progenitors to the B-cell lineage by suppressing non–B-cell-associated genes and activating B-cell-specific genes (8,9). A broader regulatory role has been described, including regulation of cell adhesion and migration, inducing V-D-J immunoglobulin heavy chain recombination, and facilitating early B-cell receptor signaling to promote development to the mature B-cell stage (9). The staining pattern in B cells is strong and nuclear; Reed-Sternberg cells show a characteristic weak to moderate pattern of nuclear expression (Fig. 3.1).

PAX-5 is used to demonstrate B-cell lineage or to identify Reed-Sternberg cells of classical Hodgkin lymphoma (CHL).

PAX-5 is expressed by nonneoplastic early B-cell precursors as well as mature B cells, and is lost as B cells mature to plasma cells (10). Rare cases of anaplastic large cell lymphoma and lymphomatoid papulosis have been described as expressing PAX-5 (10). Expression also occurs in atypical carcinoids, small cell lung carcinomas, and large cell neuroendocrine carcinomas (11). There is cross-reactivity with the immunohistochemical marker PAX-8.

CD79a

CD79a is associated with the immunoglobulin receptor complex in the B-cell membrane (12). The staining pattern is cytoplasmic.

CD79a is used to demonstrate B-cell lineage. It is the B-cell marker with the broadest sensitivity as it is expressed early in B-cell development, before immunoglobulin heavy chain gene rearrangement, and is only lost in the late plasma cell stage (13).

Although a B-cell lineage antigen, CD79a expression has been rarely reported in cases of T-cell lymphoblastic lymphoma and acute myeloid leukemia (AML) (often in acute promyelocytic leukemia) (14,15).

BCL-6

The BCL-6 gene encodes a 79-kDa zinc finger binding protein that is thought to play a role in B-cell differentiation within the germinal center (16). The staining is nuclear.

BCL-6 is used to identify B cells of germinal center origin, or their neoplastic counterparts. It may also be used in combination

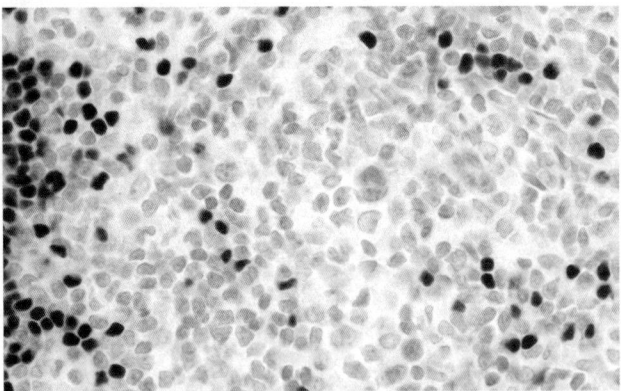

FIGURE 3.1. PAX-5 shows strong nuclear staining of surrounding small B lymphocytes with characteristically weaker nuclear staining of the Reed-Sternberg cells.

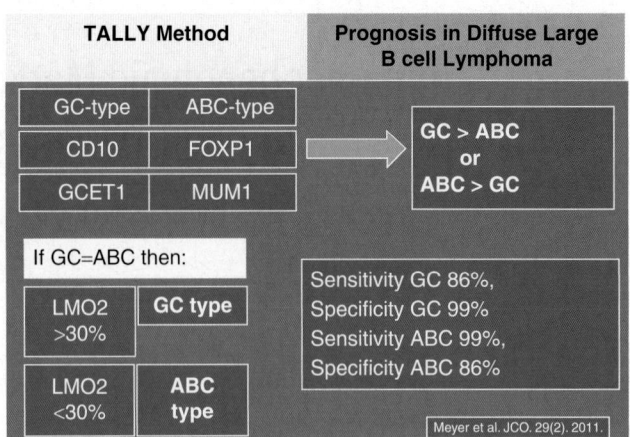

FIGURE 3.3. Immunohistochemical algorithm for assignment into germinal center B-cell or activated B-cell categories. GC type, germinal center-type; ABC type, activated B-cell type. (Adapted from Meyer PN, Fu K, Greiner TC, et al. Hematologic malignancies: immunohistochemical methods for predicting cell of origin and survival in patients with diffuse large B-cell lymphoma treated with rituximab. *JCO* 2011;29(2):200–207, reprinted with permission. Copyright © 2011 American Society of Clinical Oncology. All rights reserved.)

with CD10 and MUM-1 to identify diffuse large B-cell lymphomas (DLBCLs) with a germinal center molecular signature (Fig. 3.2). BCL-6 is also expressed in cells with genetic abnormalities of BCL-6, but expression of BCL-6 protein, as demonstrated through immunohistochemistry, does not correlate well with the presence of a BCL-6 gene rearrangement.

BCL-6 expression is seen in nonneoplastic germinal centers and lymphomas of germinal center origin, such as follicular lymphoma (FL), Burkitt lymphoma, nodular lymphocyte–predominant (LP) Hodgkin lymphoma, or most cases of diffuse large cell lymphoma. Rare cases of BCL-6 expression have been reported in anaplastic large cell lymphoma, and peripheral T-cell lymphoma, particularly those of T-helper phenotype (17,18).

CD10

CD10 (common acute lymphoblastic leukemia antigen—CALLA) is a membrane-bound zinc metalloendopeptidase (24.11-enkephalinase) enzyme thought to play a role in lymphoid development and/or function (19–21). The staining pattern is cytoplasmic.

As with BCL6, CD10 is used to identify B cells of germinal center origin, or their neoplastic counterparts (Fig. 3.2). It may also be used in combination with other stains to identify DLBCLs with a germinal center molecular signature (Fig. 3.3). These germinal center signature lymphomas have been associated with a better prognosis when compared to activated B-cell signature lymphomas (22).

CD10 is expressed on early nonneoplastic lymphoid progenitors and neutrophils in the bone marrow (BM) (19). CD10 is expressed by most acute lymphoblastic leukemias (19).

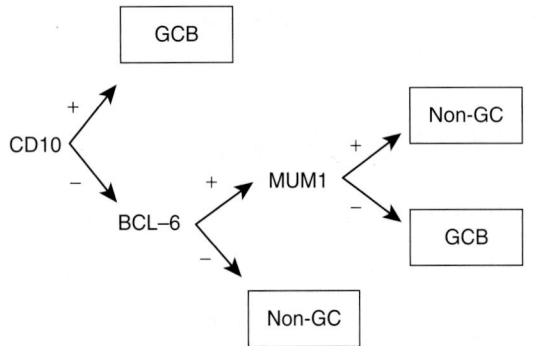

FIGURE 3.2. Immunohistochemical algorithm for assignment into germinal center B-cell or non–germinal center B-cell categories. GCB, germinal center B cell; non-GC, non–germinal center B cell.

GCET1

GCET1 (centrin, SERPINA9) is a serine protease inhibitor (serpin) located on chromosome 14q32, thought to inhibit apoptosis (23). Staining is cytoplasmic (24).

GCET1, LMO2, MUM1, FOXP1, and CD10 are frequently used in combination to identify lymphomas with a germinal center molecular signature that are associated with a better prognosis when compared to activated B-cell signature lymphomas (25,26) (Fig. 3.3).

GCET1 is expressed in a subset of nonneoplastic germinal center B cells and in some, but not all, of the following lymphomas: FL, nodular LP Hodgkin lymphoma, some DLBCLs, T-cell-/histiocyte-rich rich large B-cell lymphoma, and Burkitt lymphoma (23,24).

LMO2

The LIM only 2 domain (rhombotin-like 1; LMO2) is a transcription factor required for hematopoiesis, especially influencing erythroid differentiation and angiogenesis (27). LMO2 is activated by two translocations: t(11;14)p13;q11 or t(7;11)q35;p13, the latter seen predominantly in precursor T acute lymphoblastic leukemia (28). In paraffin sections, LMO2 antibody clone SP51 has been well studied. A cutoff of >30% expressing cells is used by most to define positivity for this marker (27). The staining pattern is nuclear.

LMO2 is most frequently used in combination with other antibodies to identify a subset of DLBCLs with a germinal center molecular signature (27) (Fig. 3.3). An anti-LMO2 drug is being developed (27).

LMO2 is expressed in nonneoplastic cells including germinal center B cells, normal hematopoietic precursors, mantle cells, and splenic marginal zone B cells. LMO2 is expressed in some, but not all, cases of DLBCL, nodular LP Hodgkin lymphoma, CHL, Burkitt lymphoma, FL, precursor B and T acute lymphoblastic lymphoma/leukemia, and rare cases of chronic lymphocytic leukemia/small lymphocytic lymphoma (CLL/SLL) and mantle cell lymphoma (MCL) (27). In addition, LMO2 is expressed in a wide variety of nonhematopoietic tumors (27)

MUM1/IRF4

Multiple myeloma oncogene-1 (MUM1) belongs to the interferon regulatory family (IRF4); it encodes a transcription factor responsible for development in B, T, plasma, dendritic, and myeloid cells (29). Two antibodies are commercially available: Mum-1p (monoclonal) and ICSTAT (polyclonal) (30). The staining pattern is both nuclear and cytoplasmic (31).

MUM1 is often used in combination with other antibodies to identify a subset of DLBCLs with an activated B-cell molecular signature (Figs. 3.2 and 3.3).

Although originally recognized by its up-regulation in multiple myeloma with t(6;14)(p25;q32), MUM1 is not specific for plasmacytic differentiation and in general is thought to parallel CD30 staining (29–31). MUM1 expression is seen in nonneoplastic "activated" T cells, a subset of germinal center B cells, and normal melanocytes (29–31). In lymphomas, MUM1 expression may be seen in some, but not all, cases of lymphoplasmacytic lymphoma (LPL), CLL (particularly highlighting proliferation centers), FL, marginal zone lymphoma, DLBCL, primary mediastinal large B-cell lymphoma, primary effusion lymphoma, Burkitt lymphoma, Hodgkin lymphoma, anaplastic large cell lymphoma, peripheral T-cell lymphoma not otherwise specified, adult T-cell lymphoma/leukemia, and malignant melanoma (29,31).

FOXP1

FOXP1 (Forkhead box protein P1) is a transcription factor that plays a role in early B-cell development (32). The staining pattern is cytoplasmic.

Like GCET and LMO2, FOXP1 is primarily used in combination with other antibodies to identify DLBCLs with an activated B-cell molecular signature (Fig. 3.3) (26,33). FOXP1 is expressed in normal activated B cells, mantle cells, and a subset of nonneoplastic germinal center B cells (33).

OCT2 and BOB.1

OCT2 and its coactivator BOB.1 (OBF1, OCA-B47, Bob-148) are transcription factors of the POU homeo-domain family that bind to the conserved octamer sites in the promoters of the immunoglobulin genes involved in B-cell differentiation and regulation (34,35). The staining pattern is nuclear.

These markers were used to differentiate nodular LP Hodgkin lymphoma from CHL. OCT2 and BOB1 are expressed in the LP ("popcorn cells") of nodular LP Hodgkin lymphoma, and it was originally thought that the Reed-Sternberg cells of CHL were negative for this marker. However, weak expression of OCT2 and BOB.1 in the Reed-Sternberg cells of CHL has been reported in a subset of cases (36,37).

BOB.1 is seen predominantly in precursor and mature B cells (38). Strong consistent expression of OCT2 and BOB.1 is seen in nodular LP Hodgkin lymphoma and in other B-cell non-Hodgkin lymphomas (37). OCT2 and BOB.1 are also expressed in a subset of AMLs, where their expression may have a prognostic relevance (39).

SOX11

SOX11 (Sex-determining region Y-box 11) is a neural transcription factor that maps to chromosome 2p25 and plays a critical role in embryonic neural differentiation and tissue remodeling (40,41). The staining pattern is nuclear.

Expression of SOX11 is highly associated with MCL; however, it may be seen in a subset of hairy cell leukemias (HCLs) (where it is associated with overexpression of cyclin D1), occasional cases of lymphoblastic lymphoma, Burkitt lymphoma, and DLBCL (40–42). Expression of SOX11 cannot be used as a surrogate marker for the molecular rearrangement t(11;14)(q13q32) in non-MCLs (40).

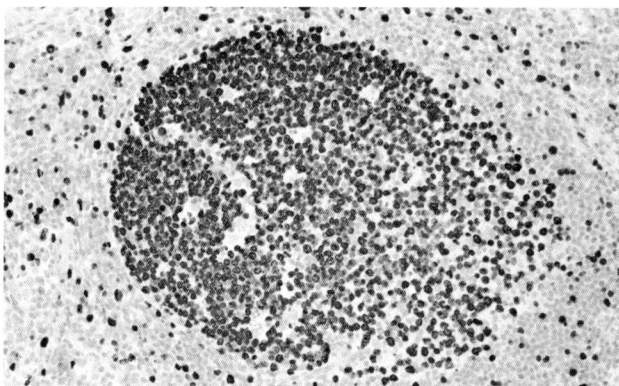

FIGURE 3.4. Ki-67 staining pattern is high in benign reactive secondary germinal centers.

Other Important Markers

Ki67

Ki67 (Mib1) is a nuclear antigen present in all proliferating cells that are in the active part of the cell cycle (i.e., G1, S, G2, and mitosis) and absent in resting cells (i.e., G0 cells) (43,44). The staining pattern is nuclear (44).

Ki67 is used to evaluate the proliferation rate as well as the distribution of proliferating cells (44,45) (Fig. 3.4). In follicular colonization by low-grade lymphoma, an abnormally low proliferation rate in the germinal centers is seen (Fig. 3.5).

CD138

CD138 (syndecan-1) is a 200 kDa member of the transmembrane family of heparin sulfate proteoglycan proteins (46). It is located on chromosome 2p23-p24 and is thought to be a receptor for matrix proteins and a cofactor for growth factors (46,47). The anti-syndecan 1 monoclonal antibody Mi15 is frequently used (46). The staining pattern is membranous (46).

CD138 is most commonly used to demonstrate plasmacytic differentiation, and is seen on both benign plasma cells and their malignant counterparts (plasma cell myeloma).

CD138 expression is seen on nonneoplastic epithelial surfaces and correspondingly has been reported among various types of carcinomas (48). Nonneoplastic early precursor B cells and posttransplant lymphoproliferative disorders also express CD138. Plasmablastic lymphoma, LPL, and a small subset of cases of CLL express CD138 (48). Expression of CD138 on mesenchymal neoplasms and tumors of melanocytic origin have also been reported (48).

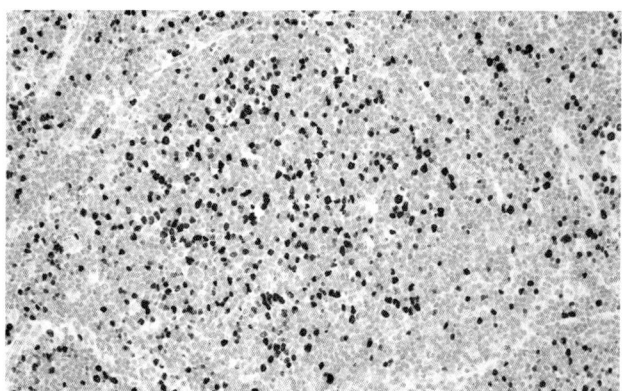

FIGURE 3.5. Ki-67 staining pattern is abnormally low in germinal centers that have been colonized by low-grade lymphoma.

Kappa and Lambda Light Chains

Kappa and lambda light chains are part of the immunoglobulin receptor on the surface and in the cytoplasm of B cells and plasma cells. Both antibodies are polyclonal and are made in rabbits as antibodies to kappa and lambda light chains isolated from the urine of patients with Bence-Jones proteinuria. The antibodies react with free light chains as well as with light chains present in intact immunoglobulin molecules; therefore, background may be high when abundant serum is present in tissue sections. Their cellular staining is membranous or cytoplasmic.

Kappa and lambda are used to demonstrate clonality in paraffin sections. They typically stain best in cells with plasmacytic differentiation but may occasionally work in other B cells. Kappa and lambda *in situ* hybridization is more specific and has the advantage of lower background staining; however, it may be more affected by decalcification and is less preferable in marrow sections.

Heavy Chains

The heavy chain portion of the immunoglobulin receptor is also located on the surface and cytoplasm of B cells and plasma cells in association with the light chains. Small differences in the heavy chain structure dictate the different classes of immunoglobulin. IgM is the first heavy chain produced; through class switching IgD, IgA, IgE, and IgG are made. IgD is usually coexpressed with IgM in naive B cells but can also be seen as IgD-only in centroblasts or memory B cells (49). The staining pattern is membranous or cytoplasmic.

IgM is frequently used in the workup LPL to diagnose Waldenström macroglobulinemia (WM) (50). IgA may be used to identify a distinct subset of extramedullary plasmacytomas with frequent lymph node involvement and a low risk of progression to plasma cell myeloma (51). IgD-positive cases of nodular LP Hodgkin lymphoma identify a subset of cases with distinct clinical features and an interfollicular distribution (49). IgG may be used in the workup for IgG4-related lymphadenopathy, where the IgG to IgG4 plasma cell ratio is helpful for quantification (52).

CD30

CD30 is a membrane-bound phosphorylated glycoprotein weighing 120 kDa that is a member of the tumor necrosis factor receptor superfamily 8 and is thought to be involved in the T-cell–dependent portion of the immune response (53,54). Monoclonal antibodies used in paraffin include Ber-H2, HeFi, HRS-1, HRS-2, HRS-3, M44, M67, and C10 (54). CD30 staining may be membranous or concentrated in the Golgi zone outside the nucleus (paranuclear) (Fig. 3.6).

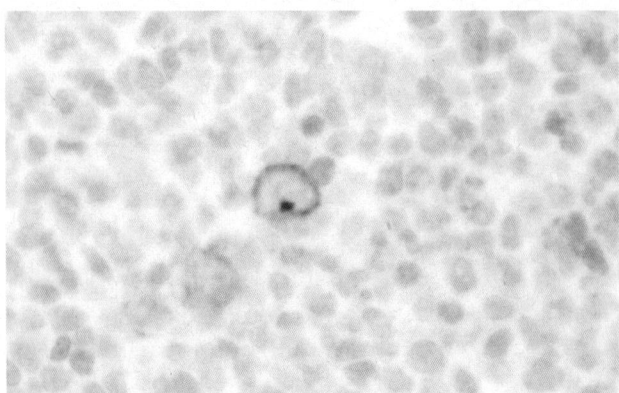

FIGURE 3.6. CD30 showing paranuclear staining in an immunoblast.

CD30 expression may be seen in a multitude of contexts. CD30 is consistently overexpressed in the Reed-Sternberg cells of CHL, lymphomatoid papulosis and anaplastic large cell lymphoma. Brentuximab vedotin is an anti-CD30 chimeric IgG1 monoclonal antibody used to target CD30-positive neoplasms, particularly in the setting of a relapse (53).

CD30 is expressed on normal activated T and B cells, as well as virally transformed B and T cells (Epstein-Barr virus, human T-cell lymphotropic virus-1 or -2, and human immunodeficiency virus [HIV]). Monocytes/macrophages and granulocytes may also constitutively express CD30 (54). In lymph node and tonsil sections a small subset of lymphocytes in the parafollicular areas express CD30 (54). CD30 may be expressed in adult T-cell lymphoma, cutaneous T-cell lymphoma, natural killer (NK) neoplasms, and a subset of B-cell lymphoma (usually DLBCL).

CD15

CD15 (Lewis X/LeuM1/X-hapten) is most frequently used in the workup for CHL. In this context, two potential pitfalls are worth noting: a subset of peripheral T-cell lymphomas may express both CD15 and CD30; large cells and immunoblasts infected by CMV may express CD15 (55). The staining pattern may be membranous, nuclear, or cytoplasmic (56).

CD15 is expressed on nonneoplastic mature neutrophils, some monocytes and histiocytes, and a subset of normal T cells (56). A subset of B-cell lymphomas and cases of AML may also express CD15 (57,58). CD15 expression is also present in adenocarcinomas and normal epithelium (57).

CD45

CD45 (T200 common leukocyte antigen, LCA) is a protein tyrosine phosphatase expressed on hematolymphoid cells (59,60). Although different cell-specific isoforms are produced via alternative splicing, the function of CD45 is the same across all the cells: to regulate growth and division. The staining pattern is membranous or cytoplasmic.

CD45 is often used to confirm the hematologic nature of a poorly differentiated neoplasm, or, in the context of CHL, as a negative finding. CD45 is expressed in both normal and neoplastic B cells, T cells, and myeloid cells.

Cyclin D1

Cyclin D1 (BCL1/PRAD1) is a transcriptional regulator protein involved in the regulation of G1 to the S phase of the cell cycle (61,62). The CCND1 gene is found at chromosome 11q13. The staining is nuclear.

Cyclin D1 is used as the surrogate for the t(11:14)(q13;q32) translocation of MCL (63). In addition, occasional cases of plasma cell myeloma and HCL have been found to express cyclin D1. Focal areas of weak cyclin D1 expression have been described in the proliferation centers of CLL (64). Nonneoplastic lymphoid cells do not express cyclin D1 (61). Overexpression of cyclin D1 is not restricted to hematopoietic malignancies and has been associated with breast carcinoma and non–small cell lung cancer (NSCLC) (62). Scattered nonneoplastic endothelial cells will often express cyclin D1 and can be used as an internal positive control (Fig. 3.7).

C-MYC

C-MYC is one of the most frequently affected genes in cancer; it is overexpressed in hematopoietic, mesenchymal, and epithelial tumors. MYC plays a role in growth control, cell differentiation, and apoptosis. The staining pattern is nuclear and a cutoff of >70% of cells suggests a MYC gene rearrangement according to some authors (65,66).

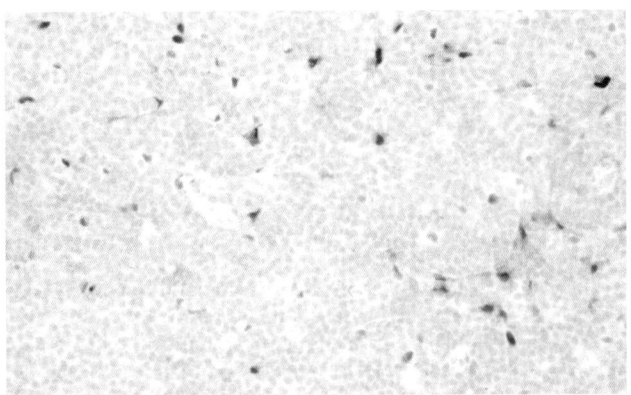

FIGURE 3.7. Cyclin D1–positive internal control staining endothelial cells.

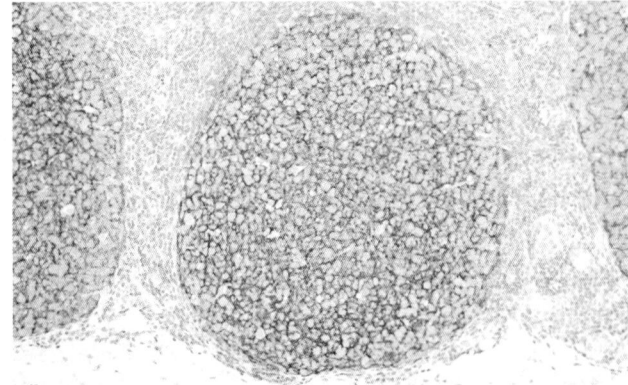

FIGURE 3.9. CD21 highlighting a follicular dendritic cell meshwork in lymph nodes.

C-MYC is used as a screening test for the rearrangement of the MYC gene, seen in Burkitt lymphoma as well as some cases of aggressive DLBCL (65).

BCL2

BCL2 is an antiapoptotic protein that results from the translocation of the BCL2 gene to a position behind the enhancer elements of the Ig heavy chain gene t(14;18)(q32;q21) (67). In addition to inhibiting apoptosis, the resulting BCL2 oncogene may also block chemotherapy-induced cell death (68). Staining is cytoplasmic.

BCL2 expression is typically used to differentiate benign follicular hyperplasia from the neoplastic counterpart follicular lymphoma (FL), as normal germinal center B cells are BCL2-negative (69). Intrafollicular T cells, T and B cells in the interfollicular areas, primary follicles and mantle zone B cells normally express BCL2, while reactive monocytoid B cells are BCL-2-negative (Fig. 3.8). Expression of BCL2 is not limited to lymphomas and is commonly encountered in nonhematopoietic malignancies as well.

CD68, CD163, and Langerin

CD68 is a marker of lysosomes. CD163 is a 130-kDa glycoprotein receptor on macrophages and histiocytes that binds to haptoglobin-hemoglobin complexes (70). With the commercially available clone 10D6, the staining pattern may be cytoplasmic and/or membranous (70).

CD68 and CD163 are used to confirm or quantify histiocytes. Expression is seen on interfollicular macrophages and sinusoidal histiocytes, but not germinal center tingible body macrophages.

Occasional cases of histiocytic sarcoma, littoral cell angioma of the spleen, and acute monoblastic leukemia may express CD68 and CD163 (70). CD68 staining is ubiquitous, with the intensity of staining correlating with the number of lysosomes that a cell possesses. CD163 expression may be seen in cases of atypical fibrous histiocytomas, benign fibrous histiocytomas, atypical fibroxanthomas, and a majority of giant cell tenosynovial tumors, but the staining is seen in the nonneoplastic component (71).

Langerin is a type II transmembrane C-type lectin. It is a highly sensitive and a relatively specific marker of the Birbeck granules of Langerhans cells (72). Langerin is used to confirm or quantify Langerhans cells. The staining pattern is cytoplasmic.

CD21 and CD23

CD21 antibodies recognize the C3d complement receptor, while CD23 antibodies recognized an IgE receptor (73). The staining pattern is membranous and cytoplasmic.

CD21, CD23, and CD35 are often used to identify the follicular dendritic cell meshworks of the lymph node (Fig. 3.9). In addition to the follicular dendritic cell meshworks, subsets of nonneoplastic B cells also express CD21 and CD23, particularly mantle B cells (73).

T-Cell–Associated Antigens

CD3

CD3 is a T-cell antigen composed of four distinct subunits (ε, γ, δ, and ζ) that span the membrane and are associated with the T-cell receptor (TCR) (74,75). The staining pattern is membranous and cytoplasmic.

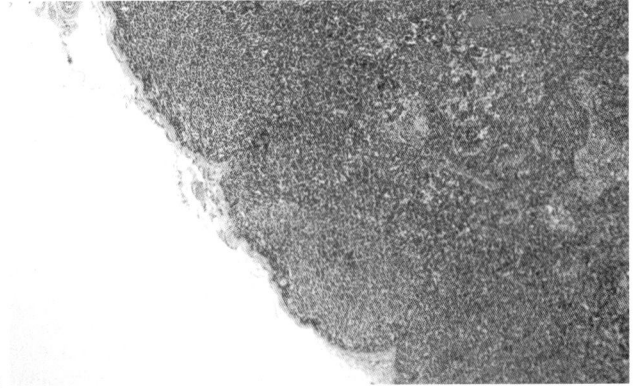

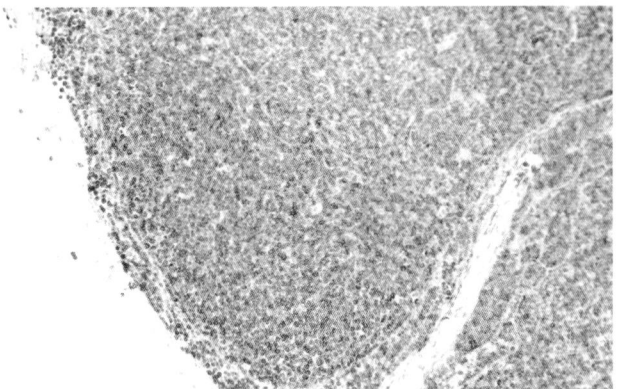

A   **B**

FIGURE 3.8 H&E **(A)** and BCL-2 **(B)**. BCL-2 expression in a primary follicle should not be interpreted as evidence of malignancy.

CD3 is used to identify T cells. It is first found in the cytoplasm of developing T cells as cytoplasmic CD3 (cCD3). As the T cells mature, the CD3 antigen moves to the surface of the cell. Expression on neoplastic cells mirrors this normal development with precursor T-cell neoplasms expressing only the cCD3 antigen and peripheral "mature" T-cell neoplasms expressing surface CD3. NK cells express cytoplasmic, but not membranous, CD3. Although most widely used as a T-cell lineage–specific antigen, CD3 expression (cytoplasmic and membranous) has been reported on B-cell lymphomas, particularly those with expression of Epstein-Barr virus (76).

CD2

CD2 is a 50- to 55-kDa transmembrane glycoprotein thought to play a role in antigen-independent adhesion as well as in T-cell activation (77–79). The staining pattern is cytoplasmic and membranous.

CD2 is used to identify T cells and NK cells (77,80). In T-cell development CD2 expression appears after expression of CD7. CD2 expression is seen on both immature (precursor) T cells and mature (peripheral T cells). Aberrant loss of CD2 expression is seen in T-cell lymphomas. CD2 expression is usually seen in T acute lymphoblastic leukemia and more rarely may be seen on the myeloblasts of AML (81). CD2 expression in mast cells is considered aberrant and supportive of systemic mastocytosis (82).

CD4/CD8

CD4 and CD8 are T-cell antigens that play a role in T-cell recognition and activation by binding to their respective class II and class I major histocompatibility complex (MHC) ligands on a antigen-presenting cells (APCs) (83). CD4 additionally stabilizes the TCR complex; it is also a major target of the human immunodeficiency virus (HIV) (84). The staining pattern for CD4 and CD8 is both cytoplasmic and membranous. Exclusively cytoplasmic CD4 is seen in monocytes and histiocytes.

CD4 and CD8 are used to identify and quantify T cells and to assess their relative proportions. Coexpression of both these markers is seen in early T-cell precursors. As T cells mature they lose one of these antigens to become either CD4 T helper cells or CD8 cytotoxic T cells. CD4 T cells are the predominant population in the T-cell compartment. CD8 T cells are fewer in number in the T-cell compartment of lymph nodes. CD8 additionally highlights the nonneoplastic sinusoids of the spleen.

The majority of T-cell lymphomas express CD4, not CD8, and are thought to be derived from the T-helper lineage. Cytotoxic T-cell lymphomas expressing CD8, not CD4, are a proportionally smaller group of lymphomas. Rarely lymphomas may have aberrant loss of both of these antigens; however, lack of CD4 and CD8 antigens is seen in gamma/delta T cells, and in this context lack of these antigens should not be misinterpreted as aberrant antigen loss.

CD5

CD5 is a 67-kDa type I glycoprotein thought to attenuate signals from the crosslinking of the TCR and its antigen on the MHC of APCs (85,86). The staining pattern is membranous.

CD5 is a T-cell antigen; as such it is often used to identify or quantify T cells. CD5 antibodies may also be used to detect aberrant expression in B cells such as CLL/SLL, MCL or more rarely cases of DLBCL, marginal zone B-cell lymphoma or FL. In addition, expression of CD5 has also been used to distinguish the neoplastic thymocytes of thymic carcinoma from benign thymoma, although this is typically not a reliable discriminator (87).

CD5 is expressed by the majority of peripheral (or mature) T cells; the loss of this marker may be seen as one of the first findings in a developing T-cell lymphoma (86,88). However,

this finding has been reported in reactive populations of T cells as well. In addition, a small nonneoplastic subset of B cells, termed B1a cells, normally express this T-cell marker. B1a lymphocytes are typically identified in the pediatric population, particularly in the tonsils.

CD7

CD7 is a 40-kDa glycoprotein member of the immunoglobulin gene family thought to be involved in signal transduction, proliferation, and adhesion. The CD7 monoclonal antibody CBC.37 shows a membranous staining pattern.

CD7 may be used for T-cell identification or quantification. It is expressed by the majority of peripheral T cells (i.e., mature T cells), NK cells, and precursor T cells (immature T cells).

CD7 is one of the earliest markers in T-cell development (89). Although a T-cell lineage antigen, CD7 expression may be seen in small populations of fetal BM B cells and myeloid precursor cells; however, this is subsequently lost early in differentiation (89). As with CD5, loss of CD7 antigen may be seen in the setting of a T-cell lymphoproliferative process as well as in a benign reactive setting. Loss of CD7 is particularly common in mycosis fungoides (MF) and Sezary syndrome.

Aberrant CD7 expression has been described in the myeloblasts of AML where it has been associated with Fms-like tyrosine kinase-3 internal tandem duplication (FLT3/ITD) mutation, and significantly shorter disease-free/postremission survival (90,91).

CD56/CD57

CD56, or neuronal cell adhesion molecule, is a NK cell marker that is also expressed in the central and peripheral nervous systems (92). The staining of CD56 (monoclonal antibody 123C3) and CD57 are membranous (93).

CD56 and CD57 are frequently used to identify the NK cell lineage; however, they are frequently found expressed in unrelated tissues. Occasionally expression of CD56 is noted in the developing granulocytes of BM, in cases of plasma cell myeloma, and in AML (94).

CD57 is a marker expressed on NK cells as well as other T cells; it is often used in the diagnosis of nodular LP Hodgkin lymphoma to visualize the small T cells ringing the LP cells.

NK cells express CD2, CD7, CD56, and CD57. A proportion express CD8. They are positive for cCD3, but not surface CD3, and do not typically express CD5. The neoplastic counterpart, extranodal NK-/T-cell lymphomas typically express, CD2, cCD3, and CD56 (92,95).

Additional markers for NK cells include killer inhibitory receptors (KIRs). KIR expression is identified using monoclonal antibodies specific for CD94, CD158a, and CD158b (96).

Beta F1

Beta F1 staining identifies the beta portion of the alpha/beta TCR (97). The staining pattern is membranous.

Beta F1 is used to identify and quantify T cells with the alpha/beta TCR, which is normally present in the majority of T cells (i.e., 95%). Similarly, the majority of T-cell lymphomas will express the alpha/beta TCR.

Negativity for beta F1 stain implies that the T cells carry the alternative TCR subunits: gamma/delta. Small subsets of normal gamma/delta T cells are found in the skin, splenic red pulp, mucosal-associated lymphoid tissue, and the medulla of the thymus. Gamma/delta T cells have a distinct immunophenotypic profile, with negativity for CD2, surface CD3, CD4, CD8, and usually CD5. The neoplastic counterparts, hepatosplenic T-cell lymphoma, and cutaneous gamma/delta T-cell lymphoma also express the gamma/delta TCR. However, caution

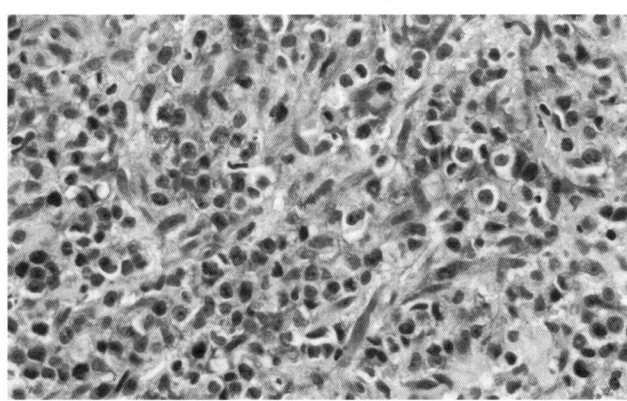 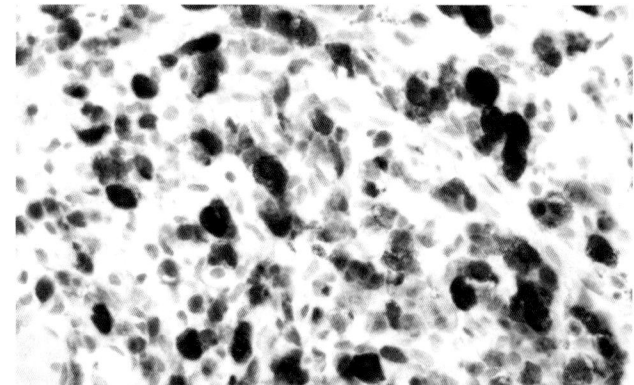

A
B

FIGURE 3.10. H&E (A) and ALK staining (B) in this case of anaplastic large cell lymphoma. When ALK staining is seen in a nuclear and cytoplasmic pattern, as in this case, it is typically associated with the t(2;5) genetic abnormality.

should be used in interpreting this negative staining as evidence of a gamma/delta T-cell derivation as NK cells will also be negative for beta F1; staining with CD56 in this instance will help to identify these cells. Recently, antibodies to the gamma and delta chains have been developed, and may be used as a positive marker of this cell type.

PD1

Programmed death 1 (PD1) is expressed by follicular l center T-helper cells and is thought to play a role in T-cell activation, tolerance, and immune-mediated tissue damage (98,99). The staining pattern is nuclear.

PD1 and other follicular center markers (BCL6, CXCL13, and ICOS) are important to identify a subset of follicular peripheral T-cell lymphoma (F-PTCL) and angioimmunoblastic T-cell lymphoma (AITL) (99). In FL, increasing numbers of PD1 expressing T cells within the neoplastic B-cell follicles have been associated with a better prognosis (99). F-PTCL presenting with Epstein-Barr virus–positive Reed-Sternberg–like cells are a potential mimic of CHL (100).

TIA-1/Granzyme B/Perforin

T-cell intracytoplasmic antigen (TIA-1), granzyme B, and perforin are markers used to identify the cytotoxic CD8-expressing T cells that induce lysis of their targets by using these granule-associated cytotoxic proteins. Expression of TIA-1 can be detected in all cytotoxic cells whereas granzyme B and perforin expression can be detected in high levels only in activated cytotoxic cells (101). The staining pattern is cytoplasmic.

ALK

Anaplastic lymphoma kinase (ALK) is a tyrosine kinase receptor belonging to the insulin receptor superfamily, weighing 220 kDa (102). Staining may be cytoplasmic, nuclear, or membranous; different staining patterns correlate with specific translocations (103) (Fig. 3.10).

Although initially described in anaplastic large cell lymphoma, several other malignancies express ALK either as activated fusion proteins derived from chromosomal rearrangements or as mutationally activated ALK proteins (such as the activating mutations described in neuroblastoma) (104). ALK expression has been reported in cases of B-cell lymphomas, NSCLC, rhabdomyosarcomas, glioblastomas, melanomas, inflammatory myofibroblastic tumors, and esophageal squamous cell carcinomas (104). Crizotinib (PF-02341066), a receptor kinase inhibitor, has been used to treat anaplastic

large cell lymphoma and NSCLC cell lines that harbor ALK translocations (105).

Normal ALK immunohistochemical expression is seen in rare scattered neural cells, endothelial cells, and pericytes in brain of adults (104). ALK was initially described in anaplastic large cell lymphoma where the translocation created a fusion gene from the nucleophosmin gene and the tyrosine kinase receptor gene (ALK). The resulting chimeric gene encoded a constitutively activated tyrosine kinase that is a potent oncogene (103). In addition to the originally described translocation, t(2;5)(p23;q35), at least 15 subsequent ALK fusion proteins have been described (104).

LYMPHOID EVALUATION

Assessment of Immunoarchitecture

Normal lymph nodes are composed of a cortex, paracortical/interfollicular region, and medullary sinuses and cords. Because these nodal components are not always histologically obvious, immunostains can be of great utility in their identification and assessment. The cortex consists of primary and secondary follicles, which normally immunostain with the common B-lineage markers such as CD20, PAX5, and CD79a. Primary follicles generally have a tight network of follicular dendritic cells, which express markers such as CD21 and CD23, and are primarily composed of IgD-positive, CD10-negative, BCL6-negative, and BCL2-positive small B cells that have a low Ki-67 proliferative index (Fig. 3.11). Primary follicle B cells may also be weakly positive for CD21 or CD23. In contrast,

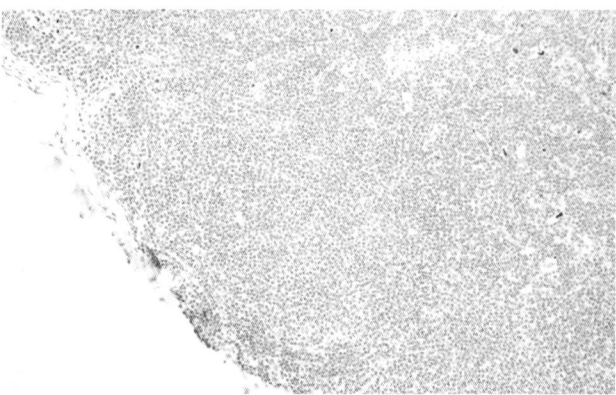

FIGURE 3.11. BCL-6-negative staining pattern in small nonstimulated primary follicles.

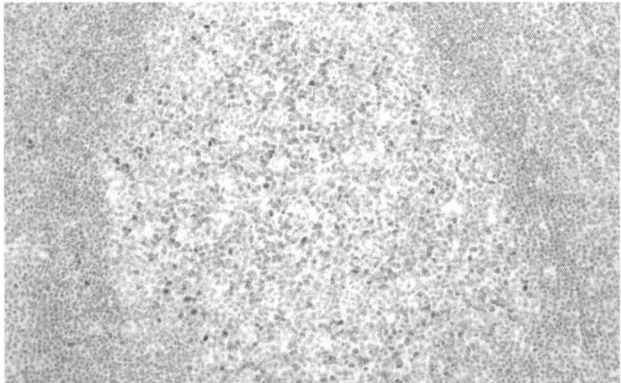

FIGURE 3.12. BCL-6-positive nuclear staining of a stimulated secondary follicle.

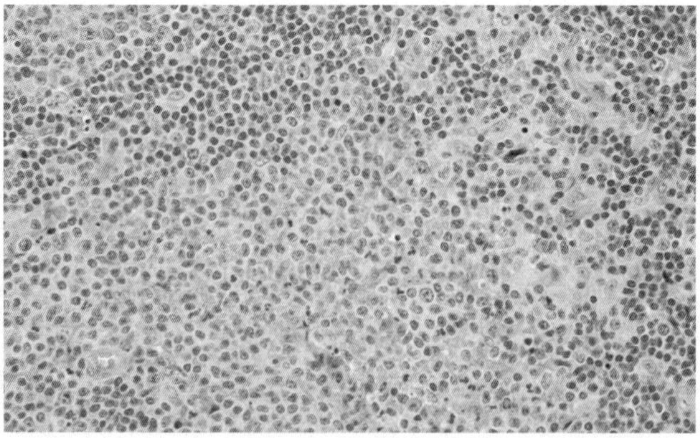

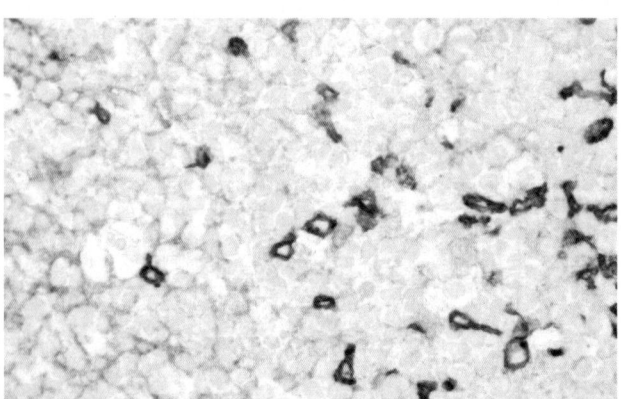

FIGURE 3.13. PD1-positive T helper cells in a benign germinal center.

FIGURE 3.14. Monocytoid B cells with an increased amount of clear cytoplasm are seen admixed with occasional neutrophils; they are BCL-2 negative.

the germinal center cells in secondary follicles usually have a more expanded follicular dendritic cell network, which may show polarization, with CD23 preferentially staining the dendritic cells in the light zone. The germinal center B cells are typically IgG-positive, CD10-positive, BCL6-positive and have a high Ki-67 proliferative index, which often highlights germinal center polarization (Fig. 3.12). Kappa/lambda immunostains can occasionally demonstrate polytypic light chains in reactive germinal centers, which may also have scattered MUM1 or CD138-positive cells, and, in highly reactive cases, occasional CD30-positive cells, usually at the edge of the germinal centers. Germinal centers also contain scattered histiocytes (tingible body macrophages), as well as T-helper cells, which can be stained for PD1, CD57, or T-helper–associated markers (Fig. 3.13). The mantle zone B cells have a similar immunophenotype to the primary follicle, and occasional follicles, seen best in mesenteric lymph nodes, may have a small outer rim of B-lineage and BCL2-positive marginal zone B cells.

In contrast to the follicles, which are predominantly composed of B cells, the interfollicular regions show a marked predominance of T cells that typically show expression of pan-T-cell antigens and BCL2, with sharp demarcation from the follicles. Scattered B cells are present in the interfollicular areas; these are often large cells with immunoblastic features. These B immunoblasts may be CD30-positive, and are often found at the outer edges of the germinal centers. Scattered CD68- and CD163-positive histiocytes and scattered CD138-positive plasma cells are usually evident in the interfollicular areas. The medullary cords may have greater numbers of small B cells and plasma cells. Occasionally, reactive lymph nodes show monocytoid B-cell proliferation, usually present in the subcapsular region or adjacent to trabeculae (Fig. 3.14). In contrast to marginal zone B cells, these cells are typically BCL2 negative.

Lymph nodes involved by lymphoma often have distortion or effacement of the normal lymph node immunoarchitecture. There may be an increase in CD20-, PAX-5-, and CD79a-positive follicles, which may extend throughout the lymph node parenchyma. Expansion in the distribution, size, and complexity of primary follicles into large atypical nodules should raise consideration of nodular LP Hodgkin lymphoma. In these cases, one should examine the margins of the primary follicles carefully for CD20-, PAX-5-, and CD79a-positive large B cells. OCT-2 stains can also be very helpful, as they stain LP cells very strongly, and PD1 and CD57 stains can be useful in demonstrating a ring of positive cells around the large cells (e.g., rosettes). An expansion in the number of small, usual primary follicles can lead to difficulties in its distinction from FL. Although both show BCL2 positivity, FL does not have a predominance of IgD-positive cells and, in contrast to primary follicles, is usually CD10 and BCL6 positive.

The most common difficulty in the evaluation of follicles is the distinction of reactive follicles from FL. CD20, PAX-5, and CD79a can easily demonstrate the increase in the number of follicles that are seen in FL, and can also easily allow assessment of the sizes and shapes of the follicles, with the more regular distribution, and uniformity of size and shape favoring FL. These stains can highlight the interface between the follicles and the interfollicular areas, which is typically sharp in reactive hyperplasia, but occasionally less distinct in FL. The presence of sheets of B cells in the interfollicular areas favors FL, particularly when those cells are CD10- or BCL6-positive. Of course, the most helpful feature in distinguishing reactive follicles from FL is BCL2 staining (69). The cells of FL are BCL2-positive in about 90% of cases, in contrast to the uniform negativity seen in reactive follicles. Consideration must be given to BCL2 positivity of T-helper cells in FL, and comparison to T-lineage stains, such as CD3, may be necessary. In some cases, the BCL2 staining of the FL cells may be weak, and may require high-magnification assessment of the follicles, with special attention to any staining of centroblasts. Cases of BCL2-negative FL are particularly frequent in the higher cytologic grades of FL, particularly grade 3B. In suspected cases of BCL2-negative FL, p53 stains may occasionally show diffuse, strong positivity indicative of lymphoma. The distinction of FL from follicular hyperplasia may be aided by evaluation of proliferation by Ki-67 (44). In FL, the high proliferation of follicular hyperplasia is not seen (Fig. 3.15). The differences between FL, grade 3, and follicular hyperplasia may be more difficult, but

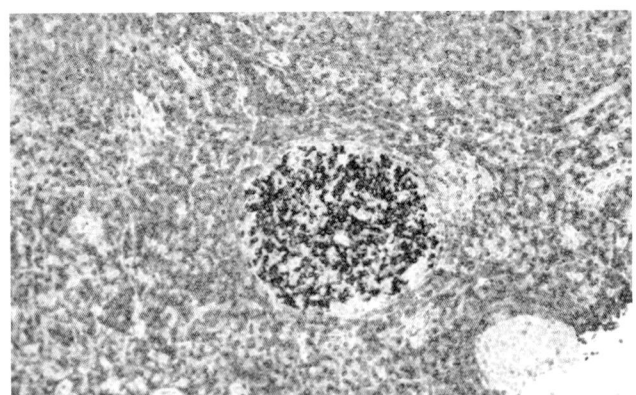

FIGURE 3.15. FL *in situ* with stronger expression of BCL2 as compared with the surrounding mantle cell B cells.

even in these cases, the pattern of proliferation can be quite different. Very rare cases of FL are positive for CD43 or CD5; except in expanding the differential diagnosis, these have no specific impact on diagnosis or prognosis in FL. In addition, immunoglobulin kappa/lambda stains may occasionally show light chain restriction, particularly in cases with predominance of centroblasts.

Occasional cases of FL, particularly cases with only partial involvement, may show only mild distortion of the normal cortex. Thus, close attention to the BCL2 stain may be critical to the diagnosis of FL. This is particularly true of involvement of a lymph node by *in situ* FL. In these cases, the low magnification assessment of the follicles by B-lineage stains shows a normal cortex. However, examination of the BCL2 stain shows increased numbers of BCL2-positive cells in scattered follicles; in addition, the BCL2 staining is often stronger than the adjacent mantle B cells (Fig. 3.15). CD10 staining also often shows an increased staining intensity. Similarly, a normal architecture may be seen in cases of *in situ* MCL. There may even be a normal mantle zone, but cyclin D1/BCL1 stains show scattered positive cells.

Paracortical/interfollicular hyperplasia is characterized by preferential expansion of the interfollicular region of the lymph node. However, it is usually associated with at least some degree of reactive follicular hyperplasia, and often includes a component of reactive B-immunoblastic hyperplasia in the interfollicular region. In diffuse lymphomas, particularly peripheral T-cell lymphomas, the follicles are often diminished in number and "pressed" toward the lymph node capsule. In these situations, B-cell stains may be mandatory to highlight the cortex. Occasionally, hyperplastic follicles may be seen in association with lymphoma, such as those seen in "hyperplastic" cases of AITL. Markers of follicular dendritic cells such as CD21 or CD23 can be very helpful in assessing numbers and sizes of follicles, particularly in small biopsies, cases in which there is both a follicular and diffuse architecture, or cases in which the expansion of the interfollicular regions has "overshadowed" the residual follicles. Dermatopathic lymphadenitis is a specific type of paracortical/interfollicular hyperplasia in which there is a proliferation of interdigitating dendritic cells and Langerhans cells in the interfollicular areas. These cells can be highlighted by S-100 and CD1a stains if necessary. Dermatopathic lymphadenitis never forms mass-forming lesions that distort the adjacent architecture and is not associated with a significant sinusoid component.

Diffuse effacement of architecture usually indicates the presence of lymphoma. But this may be difficult to determine in small specimens such as needle core biopsies of lymph nodes or biopsies of extranodal sites. The presence of diffuse sheets

of B cells is usually indicative of a B-cell lymphoma. However, the presence of diffuse sheets of T cells may be seen in rare B-cell lymphomas (e.g., T-cell-/histiocyte-rich large B-cell lymphoma), T-cell lymphomas, or in CHLs. AITLs commonly have scattered large B cells, which may be EBV-positive, and occasionally, T-cell lymphoma may have atypical cells with the morphologic and often immunohistochemical features of classical Hodgkin cells.

Abnormal Populations of Cells

The first step in assessing the presence of abnormal populations of cells is to determine whether the cells are lymphoid or nonlymphoid. This usually comes into play in the assessment of focal, sinusoidal, or diffuse epithelioid infiltrates or in the assessment of diffuse blastic infiltrates. The differential diagnosis of epithelioid cell infiltrates includes carcinoma, melanoma, sarcoma, lymphoma, and leukemia. Carcinoma can usually be identified by the application of antibodies to keratin. The anticytokeratin antibody OSCAR represents the most sensitive of the broad spectrum cytokeratin antibodies, but has the pitfall in lymph nodes that it also will label a normal dendritic cell meshwork (Fig. 3.16). Pan-cytokeratin cocktails such as AE1/AE3, while not labeling quite as many carcinomas as OSCAR, do not label the dendritic cell network, and thus are often easier to interpret. Melanomas can usually be identified by use of the S-100 protein, Melan A, HMB-45, or SOX-10. However, use of S-100 protein in lymph nodes has the pitfall of also labeling interdigitating dendritic cells, which may be quite numerous in some cases. Sarcoma rarely presents in lymph nodes as an epithelioid tumor, and most cytokeratin and S-100-/SOX-10-negative cases represent malignant lymphoma. Screening markers for lymphoma should usually include CD20, CD3, and CD30, although it must be kept in mind that some plasmablastic lymphomas may lack all these markers. In cases in which all these markers are negative, additional markers such as CD79a (which labels most cases of plasmablastic lymphoma), ALK (which labels all cases ALK-positive B-cell lymphoma), human herpesvirus-8 (which identifies all cases of primary effusion lymphoma), and CD43 (which is a highly sensitive maker of T-cell lymphoma but also stains many cases of leukemia and plasma cell neoplasms) may be necessary. CD138, while a consistent plasma cell marker, is not helpful in the setting of the undifferentiated epithelioid neoplasm, as it stains many cases of carcinoma, including cases that may be cytokeratin-negative. Cases that are only CD43-positive should be stained for additional T-cell markers as well as leukemia markers such as myeloperoxidase, CD34, and CD33.

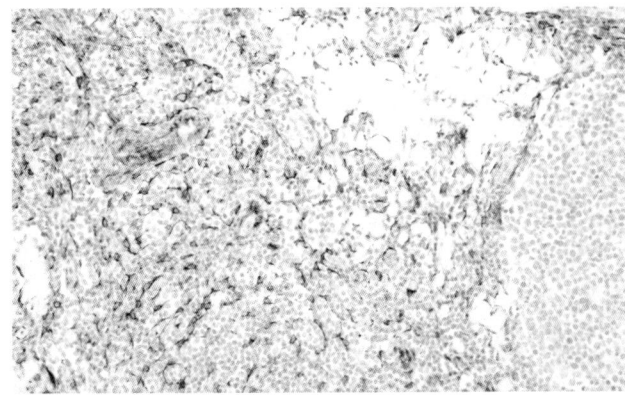

FIGURE 3.16. OSCAR staining in normal dendritic cell meshwork, a potential pitfall in interpretation of this stain in lymph node.

The differential diagnosis of blastic neoplasms includes the entities described above, as well as small round cell neoplasms such as Ewing sarcoma, rhabdomyosarcoma, or neuroblastoma. In evaluating for the possibility of Ewing sarcoma, it must be kept in mind that the most sensitive marker for Ewing sarcoma, CD99, is also commonly expressed on lymphoblastic neoplasms as well as other types of lymphomas. TDT and B- or T-cell lineage markers may be helpful in this regard, as they would be positive in the lymphoblastic lymphomas. Rhabdomyosarcoma can occasionally be present in lymph nodes; muscle markers, including particularly myogenin, will be useful in this setting. Neuroblastoma can be identified by the expression of neural or neuroendocrine markers.

Once a cell is identified as being of B- or T-cell lineage, the identification of aberrant antigen expression is helpful in establishing a diagnosis of lymphoma and may help lead to accurate classification. Aberrant antigen expression would include staining of cells with markers not normal for their lineage, or not seen in their stage of differentiation. An example of this is TDT expression. TDT may be found in occasional BM cells; as scattered cells in the cervical lymph nodes and secondary lymphoid tissues (spleen, tonsil, appendix), particularly in children; or a normal population of cells in thymus or in thymomas. But when a large population of TDT-positive cells is seen outside these contexts, whether of B-cell or T-cell lineage, it is helpful in establishing a diagnosis of lymphoid malignancy (as long as TDT expression in a myeloid leukemia, blastic plasmacytoid dendritic cell tumor, or rare neuroendocrine carcinomas can be excluded), and points to a specific immature classification.

Immunohistologic Criteria for Malignancy in B Cells

The immunohistologic criteria for malignancy in mature B cells include immunoglobulin light chain restriction, BCL2 positivity in B cells with a germinal center cell phenotype or a monocytoid B-cell morphologic appearance, aberrant coexpression of T-cell markers such as CD43 or CD5 on a diffuse B-cell population, and overexpression of certain aberrant or mutant proteins such as cyclin D1/BCL1, ALK, or mutant BRAF protein. However, as discussed below, each of these criteria have certain exceptions and caveats.

Light chain restriction has been the longest used criterion of B-cell malignancy: most reactive conditions have polytypic populations of B cells carrying either kappa or lambda light chains present in a 2:1 ratio, while most lymphomas are composed of cell populations expressing monotypic kappa or lambda light chains. However, light chain staining of B cells can be problematic in paraffin sections and is most reliably detected in cells with plasmacytoid features or reactive germinal center cells. Exceptions to light chain restriction being limited to B-cell lymphomas or plasma cell neoplasms includes HHV-8-infected B cells, which show exclusive lambda light chain usage, even in polyclonal populations (for reasons as yet unknown), and rare light chain–restricted reactive populations in the pediatric population, including some atypical marginal zone B-cell hyperplasia of the tonsil and appendix in children and even some cases of reactive hyperplasia of lymph nodes.

BCL2 positivity in germinal center cells is most often seen in FL but is also be seen in the majority of B-cell lymphomas of all types (Fig. 3.17). Since reactive monocytoid B cells are typically BCL2 negative, BCL2 positivity in a population of monocytoid B cells can be used as evidence to support a diagnosis of marginal zone B-cell lymphoma. However, one must keep in mind that normal marginal zone B cells are BCL2 positive, so this criterion must not be applied to cases of atypical marginal zone B-cell hyperplasia of the spleen or other extranodal marginal zone proliferations (including those in mesenteric lymph nodes).

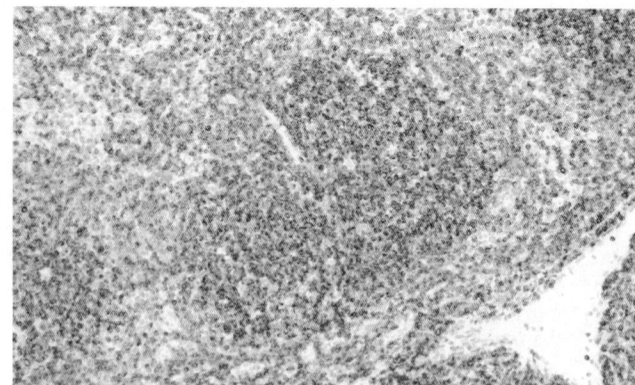

FIGURE 3.17. BCL-2 positivity in the neoplastic follicles of FL.

The coexpression of CD43 or CD5 in a diffuse or follicular B-cell population is often a very useful criterion of B-cell malignancy, particularly in diffuse small B-cell infiltrates. Positivity for either of these markers would be supportive of diagnosis of several B-cell lymphomas including CLL/SLL, MCL, or a nodal or extranodal marginal zone lymphoma (Table 3.1). Often, one can see two intensities of positivity with a population of reactive T cells showing strong expression, and a second population—the B-cell population—with a lower level of expression (Fig. 3.18). In assessing this criterion, it must be kept in mind that there are some small nonneoplastic extranodal populations of B cells that can coexpress CD43, particularly in and around the salivary glands. In addition, individual reactive B immunoblasts may coexpress CD43, and similarly rare mantle cuff B cells coexpress CD5, so it is important to evaluate entire populations of cells rather than individual cells.

The assessment of overexpression of aberrant or mutant proteins in B-lineage populations is perhaps the easiest and surest criterion of B-cell lymphoma, but it is only currently applicable in three situations: expression of cyclin D1/BCL1, ALK, and mutant BRAF. Cyclin D1/BCL1 expression occurs in neoplastic B cells as a result of a t(11;14)(q13;34) translocation and is not seen in normal or reactive B cells. Cyclin D1/BCL1 is strongly expressed in >95% of cases of MCL and shows a cell cycle–dependent variation in staining intensity from cell to cell, allowing easy distinction from artifactual positive staining (Fig. 3.19). Cyclin D1/BCL1 expression may also be seen outside of MCL, in plasma cell neoplasms, prolymphocytic leukemia, and HCL. In t(11;14)-positive plasma cell neoplasms, it should

Table 3.1	IMMUNOHISTOCHEMICAL REACTIVITY OF NEOPLASTIC CELLS OF CHL

- CD45 (<5% +)
- CD30 (98% +)
- CD15 (85% +)
- CD20 (25% + variable)
- CD3 (<5% +)
- MUM-1 (98% +)
- PAX-5 (90% + weak)
- Fascin (90% +)
- EBV LMP-1 (30%–40% +)
- BCL-6 (40% +)
- CD138 (30% +)
- BOB.1, OCT-2, CD79a (15% +)
- EMA (<5% +)
- CD43, Cytotoxic markers (<5% +)
- ALK (0%)

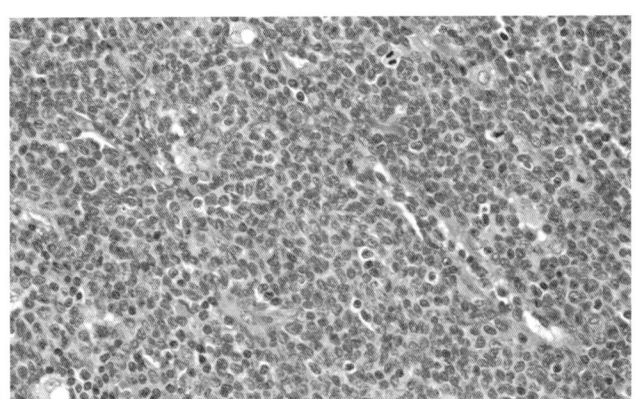 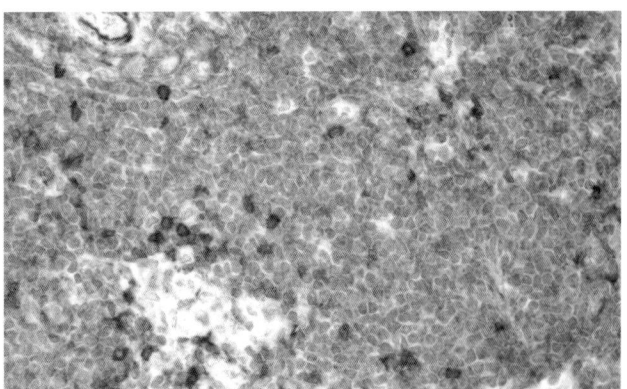

A   B

FIGURE 3.18. H&E (**A**) and CD5 (**B**) showing weak staining in neoplastic B cells, where it is aberrantly coexpressed, and strong staining in the normal T-cell population.

be kept in mind that the positive cells often express CD20 and care should be taken not to mistake this for marrow involvement by MCL. In HCL, BCL1 staining is weak and limited to a subset of the hairy cells (Fig. 3.20). ALK is expressed in a small subset of DLBCL (ALK-positive large B-cell lymphoma), mainly due to a t(2;17)(p23;q23) translocation, leading to fusion of the clathrin (CLTC) gene with the ALK gene and causing constitutive production of a fusion protein detectable with ALK antibodies. HCL shows consistent aberrant expression of the BRAF mutant protein, encoded by the BRAF gene with the V600E gene mutation (discussed subsequently). Mutant BRAF protein is also found in a majority of cases of Langerhans cell histiocytosis and perhaps in other dendritic cell neoplasms as well.

Immunohistologic Criteria of Malignancy in T/NK Cells

It is more difficult to assess malignancy of T cells by immunohistochemical studies. One cannot use the ratio of CD4 to CD8 cells in a similar way to kappa/lambda expression in B cells as the ratio of CD4:CD8 ratio may vary dramatically in reactive conditions (such as HIV infection). The most reliable criterion of malignancy in T cells is the presence of significant cytologic atypia in a diffuse population of T cells (Fig. 3.21). The atypia should not be mild to moderate, as reactive T cells can have a moderate degree of atypia in scattered cells, particularly when there are large numbers of T-cytotoxic cells present.

Another criterion of malignancy is aberrant loss of a pan-T-cell marker or BCL2 in a T-cell population. CD7 loss is common in T-cell neoplasms, and is frequently seen in MF (Fig. 3.22).

CD5, or less frequently CD2 or CD3, may also be lost in T-cell lymphomas. CD3 may lose membrane expression, but may retain cytoplasmic expression. Cytoplasmic expression of CD3 (epsilon chain of CD3) is normally seen in NK-cell populations and NK-cell malignancies. BCL2 is another marker that is frequently lost on neoplastic T cells (40% to 50% of cases). Antigen loss should warrant careful attention and caveats include the loss of CD7 in some reactive T-cell infiltrates, particularly in T-cell infiltrates of the skin. Rarely, BCL2 may be lost by T cells of reactive conditions, such as acute viral infection.

Finally, since alpha/beta T cells make up the overwhelming majority of reactive T-cell infiltrates in lymph nodes and most other extranodal sites (except mucosa), the loss of the TCR-B chain as defined by beta F1 can be used as another criterion of malignancy in most situations, although it is admittedly a rare occurrence, particularly in lymph nodes.

Gain of an "aberrant" marker can be used as another criterion of T-cell malignancy. Most often this will be CD56 and/or EBER in an NK-cell malignancy, but some T-cell lymphomas may also express CD56 or EBER. Rarely, gain of a B-lineage antigen, such as CD20 or even PAX-5, may be seen.

Classical Hodgkin Cell Immunophenotype

The classical Hodgkin cell immunophenotype can be seen as an aberrant immunophenotype consistent with malignancy as it is not seen in normal B- or T-cell populations. The phenotype is summarized in Table 3.1. The Hodgkin cell phenotype is particularly easy to identify when the abnormal large cells coexpress CD30 and CD15 (Figs. 3.23 and 3.24). However,

FIGURE 3.19. Cyclin D1/BCL-1 staining in MCL shows a cell cycle–dependent variation from cell to cell and excludes artifactual positivity.

FIGURE 3.20. BCL-1 showing characteristic weak staining of a subset of cells in HCL.

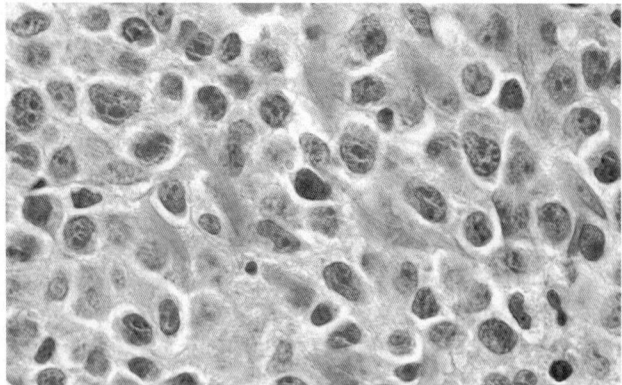

FIGURE 3.21. Significant cytologic atypia in a diffuse population of T cells is an indicator of malignancy.

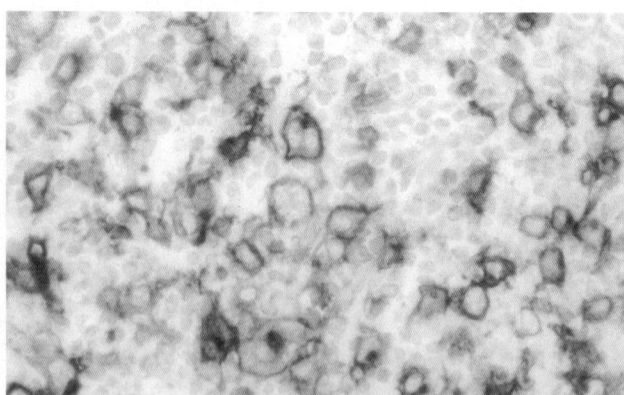

FIGURE 3.23. CD30 showing characteristic staining of a Hodgkin/Reed-Sternberg cell.

one must not mistake the sparse fine dotlike paranuclear staining of cytologically bland histiocytes (Fig. 3.25) or the more coarse granular staining for CD15 on neoplastic T cells (Fig. 3.26). When CD30 is expressed in the absence of CD15, distinction of classical Hodgkin cells from reactive immunoblasts is necessary. Reactive immunoblasts may express many of the other markers of classical Hodgkin cells, including weak expression of PAX-5, but are usually consistently strongly and uniformly CD20-positive. Cases of CHL are CD20 positive in about 20% to 25% of cases and there is usually much less consistent staining of individual abnormal cells with weak and variable staining (Fig. 3.27). Weak to moderate expression of PAX-5 is helpful in distinguishing CHL from peripheral T-cell lymphomas, although a minority of cases of anaplastic large cell lymphoma may show PAX-5 expression. Strong expression of PAX-5 is seen only rarely in CHL, and is more frequently seen in other disorders such as T-cell–/histiocyte-rich large B-cell lymphoma and nodular LP Hodgkin lymphoma. Lack of expression of CD45 can be a very helpful criterion, but the CD45 staining must not be overly strong, or else expression on adjacent cells will be too difficult to distinguish from staining on the large cells. Sometimes, large panels of stains, including CD79a, BOB.1, and OCT-2, are necessary to distinguish classical Hodgkin cells from B-cell lymphoma. Classical Hodgkin cells typically lack strong or uniform expression of most of these pan-B-cell antigens. In approximately 40% of cases, classical Hodgkin cells express evidence of EBV infection, best highlighted by *in situ* staining for EBER. In the appropriate circumstances, this may provide support for a diagnosis of CHL.

Types of Lymphoma

Mature B-Cell Lymphomas

Most B-cell lymphomas express the pan-LCA CD45, as well as the B-lineage markers CD20, PAX-5, and CD79a. Exceptions include the plasmablastic lymphoma, which, by definition, have lost CD45 and/or CD20, and are often also PAX-5-negative. Rituximab-treated B-cell lymphomas also frequently lose CD20, and often also PAX-5, and sometimes CD79a, in recurrences, often necessitating the performance of multiple B-cell markers to demonstrate a B-cell lineage.

Low-Grade B-Cell Lymphomas

The staining profile of most low-grade B-cell lymphomas is summarized in Table 3.2.

Chronic Lymphocytic Leukemia/Small Lymphocytic Lymphoma

CLL/SLL is usually positive for B-lineage markers (unless previously treated with rituximab), as well as coexpresses CD43, CD5, and CD23. MUM-1 is usually positive in the proliferation centers, and Ki-67 can be used in cases in which the proliferation centers are not readily seen. The Ki-67 index is usually low, but can be high in the proliferation centers. A small subset of cases may show weak expression of cyclin D1/BCL1, usually confined to the proliferation centers (Fig. 3.28). A diffusely high Ki-67 index should raise consideration of histologic

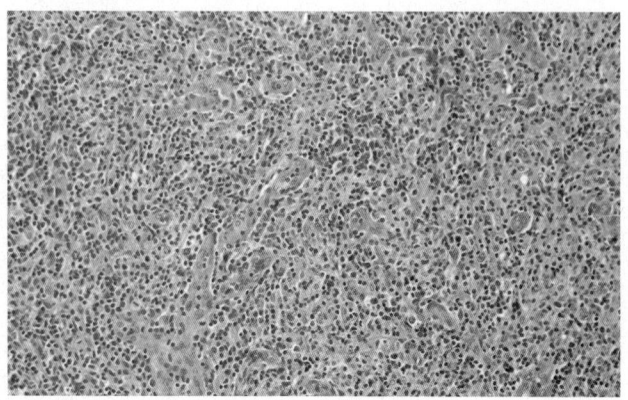

FIGURE 3.22. H&E **(A)** and CD7 **(B)** in T-cell lymphoma. CD7 expression is not seen in the neoplastic T lymphocytes in this case.

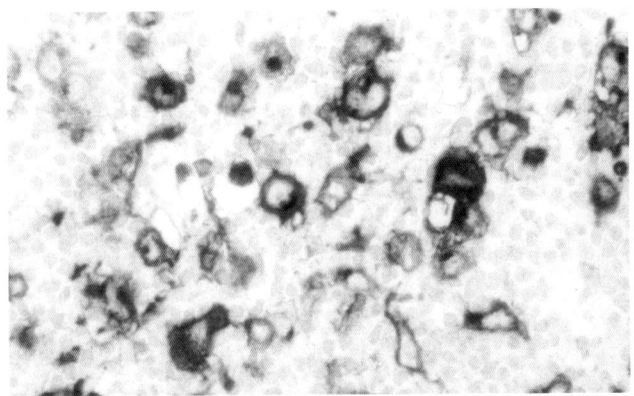

FIGURE 3.24. CD15 showing characteristic staining of a Hodgkin/Reed-Sternberg cell.

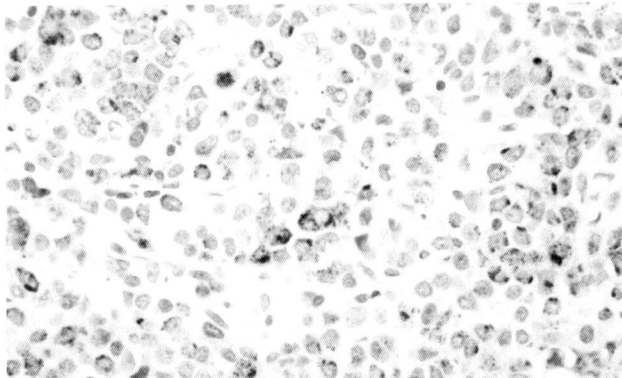

FIGURE 3.26. CD15 showing coarse granular staining of neoplastic T cells; a potential pitfall for Hodgkin/Reed-Sternberg cells.

transformation to a DLBCL, a possibility that should be confirmed through histologic examination. ZAP-70 expression may be used as a paraffin marker to separate the cases into various prognostic groups, as ZAP-70 expression shows a correlation to immunoglobulin heavy chain hypermutation analysis.

Mantle Cell Lymphoma

Like CLL/SLL, MCL usually shows aberrant coexpression of both CD43 and CD5, and it is usually negative for CD23. The most distinctive feature of MCL is the strong, diffuse (but cell cycle dependent) expression of cyclin D1/BCL1, seen in >95% of cases (Fig. 3.29). The strongest expression of cyclin D1/BCL1 tends to be seen in the blastic MCL. It is probably not expressed in all cases, in which the t(11;14) is probably absent and cyclins D2 or D3 are probably of greater pathogenetic significance. Many of the cyclin D1–/BCL1-negative cases are positive for SOX-11 (42). Interestingly, SOX-11 may be negative on indolent cases of cases of MCL. Blastic cases of MCL shows the highest Ki-67 proliferative index although typical cases of MCL may show wide variability in the Ki-67-defined proliferation, and a high Ki-67 index (>30%) is of adverse prognostic significance.

Marginal Zone B-cell Lymphomas

Nodal marginal zone B-cell lymphoma, extranodal marginal zone B-cell lymphoma, and splenic B-cell marginal zone lymphoma are discussed together because, although they are

distinctive lymphomas, they have similar immunophenotypes. All cases express pan-B-cell antigens, are typically BCL2 positive, and have a low proliferation index by Ki-67. All types express myeloid nuclear differentiation antigen (MNDA), and this may be useful in distinguishing them from FLs, although MNDA is also expressed in a subset of other low-grade and even large cell lymphomas. Somewhat <50% of cases coexpress CD43, and only about 5% of cases coexpress CD5. Light chain restriction can be demonstrated by immunohistochemistry in a significant subset of cases, particularly cases of extranodal or nodal marginal zone B-cell lymphomas with plasmacytoid differentiation seen histologically (Fig. 3.29). Extranodal marginal zone B-cell lymphoma may express IgG, IgA, or IgM heavy chain, but not IgD, while splenic marginal zone B-cell lymphoma is IgD-positive, and nodal marginal zone B-cell lymphoma usually expresses IgM, but may express any of the heavy chains.

Lymphoplasmacytic Lymphoma

LPL is distinctive for its consistent expression of immunoglobulins, usually of IgM type. It also commonly shows coexpression of CD43, and may coexpress CD5 and/or CD23 in a minority of cases. CD20 and CD138 stains may sometimes stain separate populations of cells, highlighting lymphoid and plasmacytic cells, respectively. Cells with intermediate features between plasma cells and lymphocytes (e.g., plasmacytoid lymphocytes) may coexpress B-cell markers (CD20, PAX-5) and plasma cell markers (CD138, CD38) in the same cells.

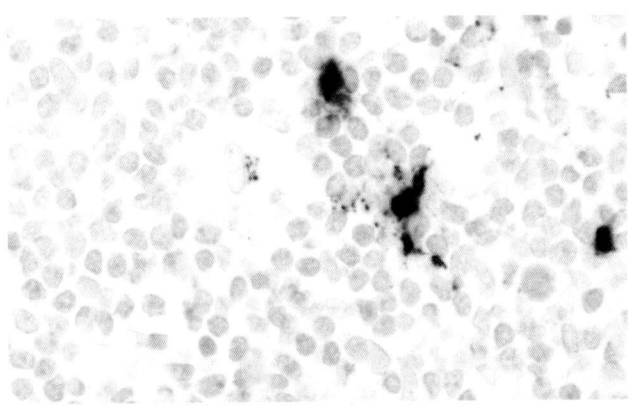

FIGURE 3.25. CD15 showing sparse, fine dotlike paranuclear staining of cytologically bland histiocytes; a potential pitfall for Hodgkin/Reed-Sternberg cells.

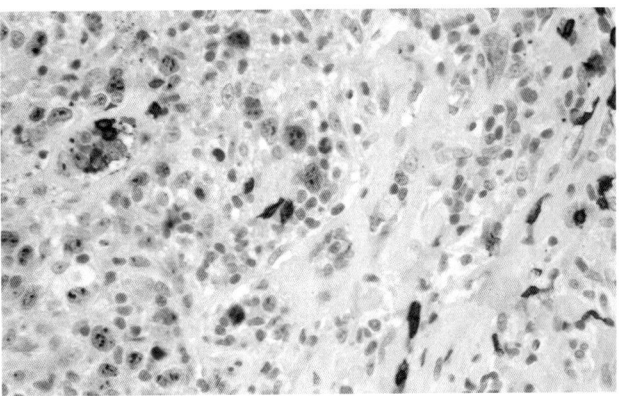

FIGURE 3.27. CD20 staining is seen in a subset of Hodgkin/Reed-Sternberg cells; however, it is usually weak and variable, in contrast to B immunoblasts, which will express strong CD20.

Table 3.2	IMMUNOHISTOCHEMICAL REACTIVITY OF SMALL B-CELL LYMPHOMAS				
	Follicular	SLL/CLL	Marginal	Lym-Plas	Mantle
Ig	90%	98%	98%	98%	98%
Heavy	IgM, G	IgM ± IgD	IgM, D, A	IgM	IgM + IgD
K:L	2:1	2:1	2:1	2:1	1:1
CD20	99%	98%	98%	98%	99%
CD43	2%	98%	50%	60%	80%
CD5	1%	98%	10%	25%	90%
CD10	95%	1%	1%	1%	1%
CD23	15%	90%	5%	10%	5%
Cyclin D1	0%	5%	0%	5%	98%

SLL/CLL, small lymphocytic lymphoma/chronic lymphocytic leukemia; Lym-Plas, lymphoplasmacytic lymphoma; Ig, immunoglobulin; K:L, kappa/lambda light chains.

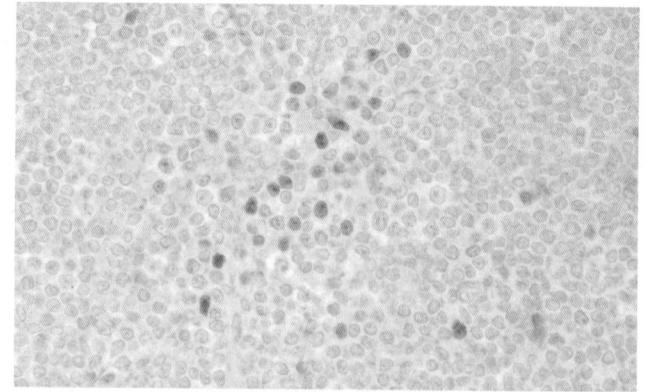

FIGURE 3.28. BCL-1/cyclin-D1 weak staining in a subset of proliferation centers of CLL/SLL.

Follicular Lymphoma

FL usually shows consistent expression of CD10 and BCL6, with the level of CD10 expression often higher than seen in reactive germinal centers. About 90% of FLs show expression of BCL2, with the incidence decreasing with increasing cytologic grade. The staining intensity from case to case may show striking variability, from weak and requiring high-magnification examination, to stronger than the adjacent nonneoplastic mantle cells. The neoplastic cells are usually of IgM or IgG heavy chain, and light chain restriction may be demonstrated by immunohistochemistry in some cases. Cases of higher cytologic grade have a higher Ki-67-defined proliferation, and an elevated Ki-67 index even in the low-grade cases may predict adverse prognosis. Some cases of higher cytologic grade may show strong diffuse expression of p53, and this may predict transformation to DLBCL. The diffuse component of FL often lacks follicular dendritic cells, so that CD21 or CD23 stains may be useful in assessing the architecture of FLs with a possible diffuse component.

Diffuse Large B-Cell Lymphoma

DLBCL encompasses a number of clinicopathologic entities. Most cases express pan-B-cell markers CD20, PAX-5, and CD79a, although the plasmablastic types may lack CD20 and PAX-5 in many cases. Most cases also strongly express the B-cell transcription factors BOB.1 and OCT-2. It has been shown that cases of DLBCL can be separated by gene microarray studies into germinal center versus activated B-cell type, with the activated B-cell type having a worse prognosis (22,25,26). These groups can be reasonably well-separated

by immunohistochemical studies, using either a set of three markers (Hans method; CD10, BCL6, MUM-1) (106) (Fig. 3.2), or, with greater precision, larger sets of antibodies, including the widely used TALLY method (CD10, GCET1, FOXP1, MUM1, LMO2) (107) (Fig. 3.3). Expression of CD5, seen in about 5% of cases, separates out a poor prognosis group, as does uniform strong expression of p53. BCL2 is another adverse prognostic marker, particularly in cases of activated B-cell type or with coexpression of MYC protein (67). A small subset of cases may show expression of cyclin D1/BCL1, usually weak in intensity, and of no significance once the possibility of MCL with a t(11;14) is excluded. Some cases may variably express CD30, which has no specific prognostic significance, but may benefit from anti-CD30 therapies (e.g., Brentuximab). The Ki-67 proliferation index is variable, and, although usually high (>50%), does not correlate well with prognosis.

The different subtypes of DLBCL are sometimes associated with distinctive immunophenotypes. T-cell-/histiocyte-rich large B-cell lymphoma is distinctive because of the large number of antigenically normal CD3-positive T cells of predominantly CD8-positive cytotoxic type and CD68- and CD163-positive histiocytes. The neoplastic B cells are individually dispersed and do not have a distinctive immunophenotype. They express BCL6, CD10, and EMA each in about 50% of cases, and are generally negative for CD5. CD30 may be positive but CD15 is consistently negative. Epstein-Barr virus-positive DLBCL is usually of activated B-cell type, lacking BCL6 and CD10, but expressing MUM-1 and usually also CD30. EBER is consistently positive and EBV-LMP is positive in almost all cases. Lymphomatoid granulomatosis and DLBCL associated with chronic inflammation have a similar phenotype although EBV-LMP is

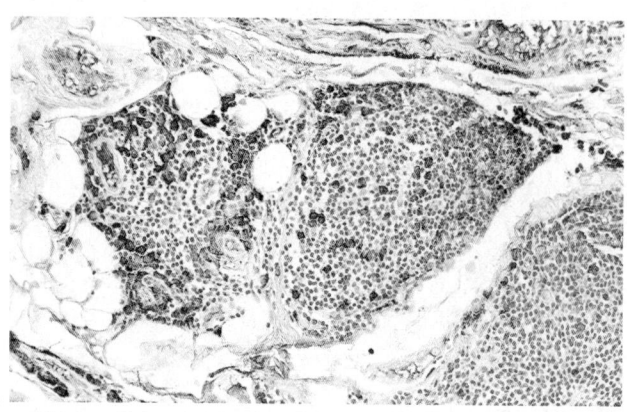 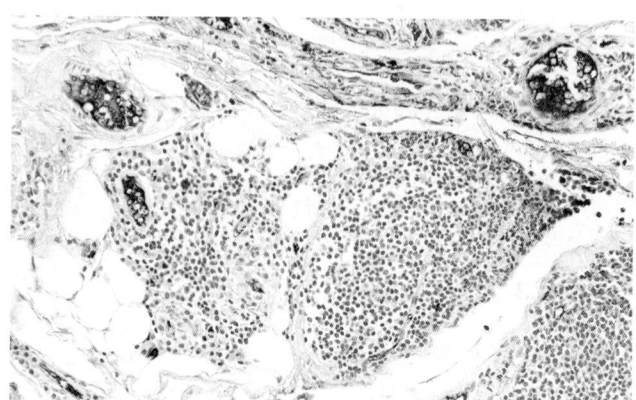

A **B**

FIGURE 3.29. Light chain restriction demonstrated in an extranodal marginal zone B-cell lymphoma showing plasmacytic differentiation (**A**, kappa light chain; **B**, lambda light chain).

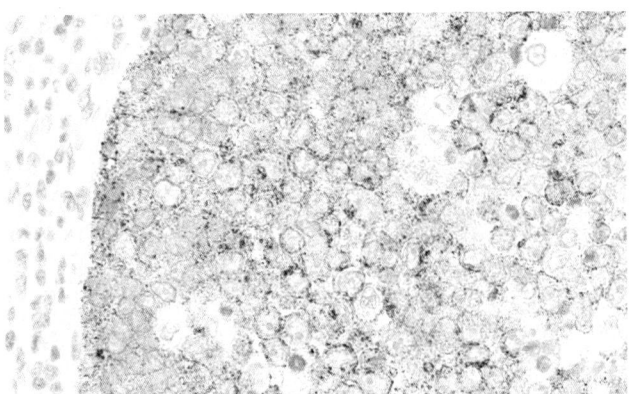

FIGURE 3.30. ALK characteristic granular expression in DLBCL.

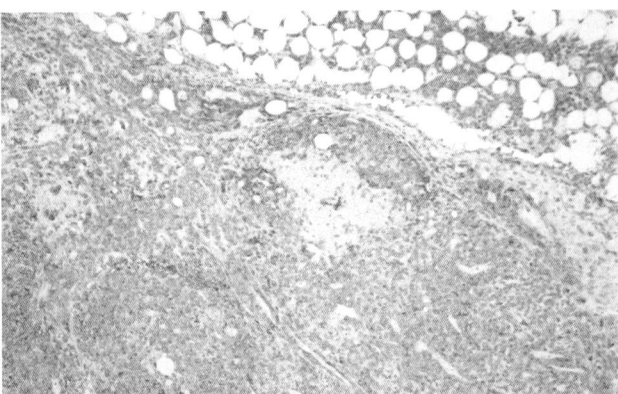

FIGURE 3.31. CD3 staining the neoplastic cells of a peripheral T-cell lymphoma involving the lymph node, showing few residual follicles, with the cortex pressed toward the periphery or adjacent to trabeculae.

usually negative. Primary central nervous system lymphoma and DLBCL, leg type, are also lymphomas of activated B cells, negative for CD10. The leg-type DLBCL characteristically has very strong BCL2 expression, often stronger than the admixed T cells. Primary mediastinal (thymic) large B-cell lymphoma has variable staining for BCL6 and CD10, but characteristically expresses CD23, CD103 (MAL), and CD30.

Plasmablastic lymphoma, ALK-positive large B-cell lymphoma, and HHV8-associated germinotropic lymphoproliferative disorder all have a plasmablastic phenotype, often negative for CD45 and CD20, but positive for MUM-1. ALK-positive large B-cell lymphoma, of course, shows characteristic granular cytoplasmic ALK protein expression (Fig. 3.30), while the HHV-associated germinotropic lymphoproliferative disorder is always HHV-8 LANA protein–positive.

Burkitt Lymphoma and B-Cell Lymphoma, Unclassifiable, with Features Intermediate Between Diffuse Large B-Cell Lymphoma and Burkitt Lymphoma

Burkitt lymphoma has a distinctive germinal center phenotype, with positivity for CD10 and BCL6. CD43 is coexpressed in about 50% of cases, while BCL2 is negative or, at best, weakly positive in rare cases. The Ki-67 proliferation index is usually near 100%. Admixed CD3-positive T cells are infrequent but CD68/163+ macrophages are consistently seen. MUM-1 is positive in about 30% of cases. The intermediate lymphoma has a germinal center–type phenotype that is similar to Burkitt lymphoma but often lacks one or more of the characteristic phenotypes. Most often, there may be strong positivity for BCL2, although negativity for CD10 or BCL6 or a lower Ki-67 proliferation index is sometimes seen.

Mature T-/NK-Cell Lymphomas

Nodal T-/NK-cell lymphomas are predominantly mature T-cell lymphomas of effector T cells that express the alpha/beta TCR of the mature antigen-related immune system, while extranodal T-/NK-cell lymphomas are generally lymphomas of the innate immune system, often either NK-cell type or T-cell gamma/delta type.

Peripheral T-cell Lymphoma, NOS

Peripheral T-cell lymphomas, not otherwise specified, are a mixed group of mature T-cell lymphomas. Involved lymph nodes usually show only a few residual follicles, with the cortex pressed toward the periphery or adjacent to trabeculae (Fig. 3.31). They

are almost always neoplasms of alpha/beta cells, usually (but not always) of CD4$^+$ type, although significant numbers of CD8$^+$ cells are also present. There may be loss of pan-T-cell antigens, most often CD7, CD5, or BCL2. There may be focal positivity for CD30, but it is not the large majority of the neoplastic cells, and it is usually variable rather than consistently strong. There are often admixed large B cells, and rarely there may be cells with the morphologic or phenotypic features of Hodgkin cells, which may or may not express T-cell antigens. Rarely, peripheral T-cell lymphomas may aberrantly coexpress the B-cell marker CD20 (5). The Ki-67 proliferation index is usually high.

Angioimmunoblastic T-Cell Lymphoma

AITL may be regarded as a lymphoma of T-helper cells. This lymphoma also tends to show a compressed rim of B cells toward the nodal periphery. Follicles are usually small, but may have reactive germinal centers in some cases. The atypical cells, in addition to expression of pan-T-cell markers and BCL2, often show expression of BCL6, CD10, and other markers of T-helper cells such as PD-1 or CXCL13. In early cases, the PD-1-positive cells may show a concentration around germinal centers. Follicular dendritic stains such as CD21 and CD23 show expanded networks of follicular dendritic cells outside of the follicles, often with close approximation to the increased high endothelial venules present in this lymphoma (Fig. 3.32). There are often scattered large cells positive for B-lineage antigens, and EBER often shows increased numbers of small and large lymphoid cells; these cells are negative for EBV-LMP.

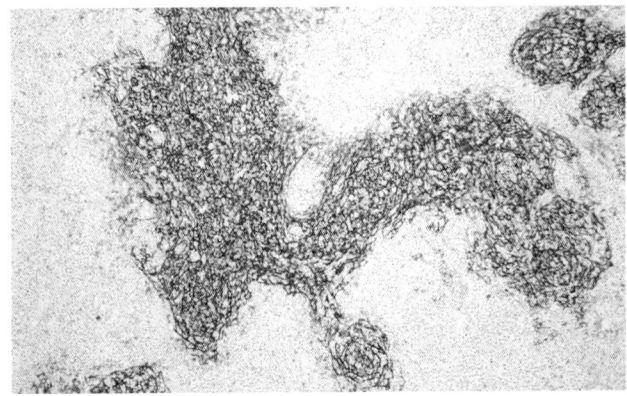

FIGURE 3.32. CD21 in AITL showing expanded networks of follicular dendritic cells outside of the follicles, often with close approximation to the increased high endothelial venules.

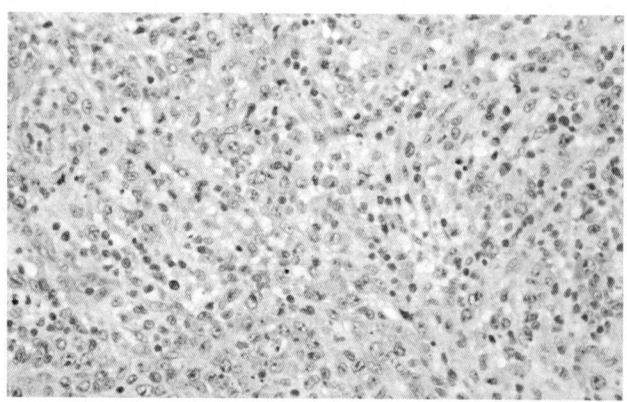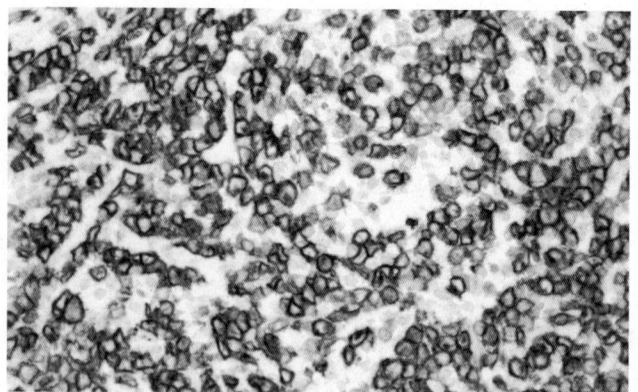

FIGURE 3.33. Anaplastic large cell lymphoma (**A**) and CD30 (**B**) staining the neoplastic T cells of anaplastic large cell lymphoma showing uniform strong expression (usually membranous and paranuclear).

Anaplastic Large Cell Lymphoma, ALK-negative

Anaplastic large cell lymphoma, ALK-negative, is virtually defined as a T-lineage neoplasm with uniform or near-uniform strong expression of CD30 (usually membranous and paranuclear) in the absence of ALK expression (Fig. 3.33). CD45 and CD43 are relatively consistent markers but are still only expressed in about two-thirds of cases. CD4, while nonspecific, and CD2 are also usually expressed, but CD3, CD5, CD7, and BCL2 are only expressed in a minority of cases. Most cases are positive for the cytotoxic markers TIA-1, granzyme B, and perforin. CD25 is also usually expressed, while CD15 is usually negative, or when positive, often shows a coarse granular cytoplasmic staining pattern. On occasion, this neoplasm may aberrantly coexpress a B-lineage marker, including PAX-5, BOB.1, or OCT-2 (10).

Anaplastic Large Cell Lymphoma, ALK positive

Anaplastic large cell lymphoma, ALK-positive, is defined as a T-lineage neoplasm with uniform or near-uniform strong expression of CD30 combined with ALK expression. The ALK staining is usually nuclear and cytoplasmic, but may also be cytoplasmic, or cell membrane, depending on the particularly translocation involving the ALK gene that is present (Fig. 3.34). Like the ALK-negative cases, there is expression of CD45 and CD43 in a majority of cases, although not all. Again, CD4 is usually positive, and CD2 is the pan-T-cell antigen most often expressed. Most cases are also positive for cytotoxic markers.

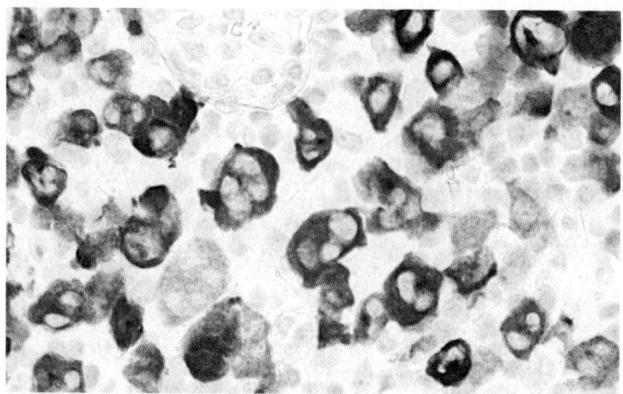

FIGURE 3.34. ALK staining the neoplastic T cells of anaplastic large cell lymphoma; the cytoplasmic staining, without nuclear staining suggests that another translocation, other than the t(2;5), is present in this case.

Extranodal T-Cell Lymphomas

Extranodal NK-/T-cell lymphoma, nasal type, usually expresses CD56, CD2, cCD3, and cytotoxic markers, consistent with NK-cell lineage (Fig. 3.35). A minority of cases may be negative for CD56 and positive for membranous CD3, consistent with a T-cell lineage. Regardless of the phenotype, virtually all cases are EBER-positive, although EBV-LMP is usually negative (Fig. 3.36).

Enteropathy-associated T-cell lymphoma may show two different phenotypes. The type I cases usually show expression of CD3, CD2, and CD7 as well as cytotoxic molecules, while CD5, CD4, CD8, and CD56 are often negative. CD30 may show variable expression. The type II (monomorphic) cases often express CD8 and CD56.

Subcutaneous panniculitic T-cell lymphoma usually shows a mature T-cytotoxic, CD8-expressing phenotype. Cases usually show expression of pan-T-cell antigens and cytotoxic molecules: TIA-1, granzyme B, and perforin.

Cutaneous gamma/delta T-cell lymphoma and most cases of hepatosplenic T-cell lymphoma are neoplasms of gamma/delta T cells rather than alpha/beta T cells. Therefore they are negative for beta-F1, but often positive for markers of gamma/delta T cells such as gamma-F1 or delta-F1. Hepatosplenic T-cell lymphoma often shows expression of TIA-1 but not the other cytotoxic markers.

MF and Sezary syndrome are almost always neoplasms of mature T-helper cells, with consistent loss of CD7. Rare cases of MF are CD8 positive. These CD8-expressing MF cases are not to be confused with the much less common and more aggressive CD8-positive epidermotropic T-cell lymphoma. In contrast to MF, epidermotropic T-cell lymphoma is usually positive for cytotoxic markers and is consistently negative for CD5 and often other pan-T-cell antigens.

Hodgkin Lymphoma

The phenotype of classical Hodgkin cells has already been discussed, and is summarized in Table 3.1. The Hodgkin cells are usually found in a T-cell–rich background, although nodules of B cells may be present in the lymphocyte-rich variant. The classical strongly CD30- and CD15-positive; weakly PAX-5-positive; CD20-, CD3-, and CD45-negative phenotype is seen in only about two-thirds of cases, often necessitating a larger panel to distinguish it from other neoplasms. Addition of CD79a, BOB.1, and OCT-2 is often helpful in the differential diagnosis of CHL from T-cell-/histiocyte-rich large B-cell lymphoma or other B-cell lymphomas, and these markers, with the addition of MUM-1, are useful in distinguishing CHL from nodular LP Hodgkin lymphoma. In young or old patients, the demographic

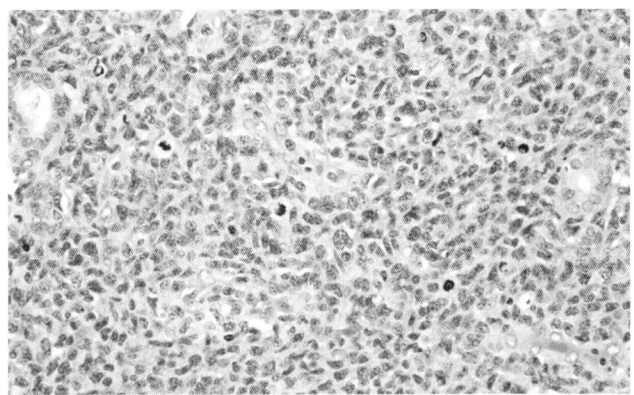 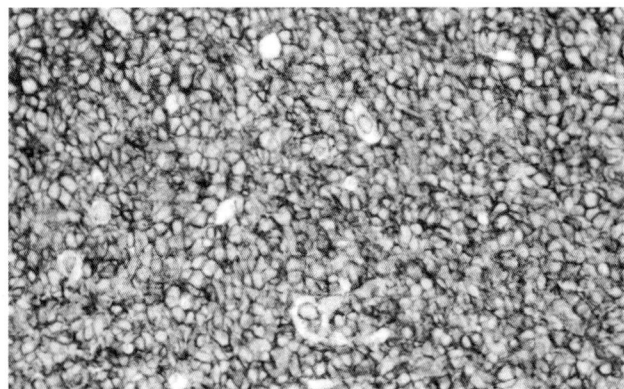

A   **B**

FIGURE 3.35. H&E (**A**) and CD56 (**B**) expression in an extranodal NK-/T-cell lymphoma, nasal type, staining is strong and diffuse.

groups most likely to have EBV-associated CHL, the addition of EBER or EBV-LMP may also be of use. In a small minority of cases, most often seen in the mediastinum, cases may show overlap phenotypic (and morphologic) features between CHL and DLBCL (and primary mediastinal large B-cell lymphoma, in particular). These cases usually show expression of CD45 and/or uniform expression of CD20 and other B-lineage markers in addition to CD30 and CD15. The diagnosis of B-cell lymphoma, unclassified, with features intermediate between DLBCL and CHL is used in the WHO to classify such cases. Anaplastic large cell lymphoma is also a consideration in the immunohistochemical differential diagnosis, sharing consistent strong CD30 expression with CHL. However, it is usually CD15 negative, and when positive usually shows a coarse diffuse granular cytoplasmic staining. Anaplastic large cell lymphoma is usually negative for PAX-5 staining, although staining may be seen for PAX-5, BOB-1, or OCT-2 in about % to 10% of cases (10).

Nodular LP Hodgkin lymphoma shows a distinct phenotype. The LP cells are consistently CD45-postiive and have a B-lineage phenotype, with strong expression of PAX-5 and consistent expression of the B-cell transcription factors BOB.1 and OCT-2. OCT-2 staining is particularly strong, and may be used to highlight the presence of LP cells (Fig. 3.37). They have only weak expression of CD30, are seen in a minority of cases, and are usually negative for CD15. LP cells are usually positive for BCL6, but are often negative for CD10. The LP cells are usually found within, or in the vicinity of, large B-cell nodules with the phenotype of primary follicles or with admixed remnants of germinal centers. EMA staining is seen in about 75% of cases, similar to T-cell-/histiocyte-rich B-cell lymphoma. The LP cells usually express the immunoglobulin-associated J chain, and cases in the pediatric age group are often IgD-positive.

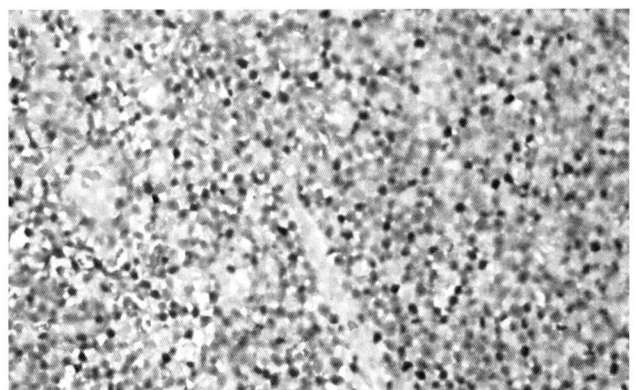

FIGURE 3.36. EBER expression in an extranodal NK-/T-cell lymphoma, nasal type; although rare cases may be negative for CD56, cases with the T-cell immunophenotype will express EBER.

Histiocytic and Dendritic Neoplasms

Histiocytic sarcoma is defined by the expression of two or more relatively specific histiocytic markers, such as CD68 and CD163, in the absence of specific T- or B-lineage markers. Cytoplasmic CD4 expression is seen relatively often, and, without membrane expression, is not considered to be a specific T-lineage marker (Fig. 3.38). CD30 expression, particularly when membranous or paranuclear, is considered to be a specific lymphoid marker, and would rule out a histiocytic neoplasm. The expression of blastic myeloid markers such as CD34 or CD117 would make a myeloid sarcoma showing monocytic differentiation more likely. Rosai-Dorfman disease shows strong expression of S-100 protein along with histiocytic markers. There may be diffuse cytoplasmic staining for CD30, but a paranuclear or membranous pattern of staining is never seen.

Langerhans cell histiocytosis expresses S-100 protein, CD1a, and Langerin. Neoplastic Langerhans cells often carry mutation V600E of BRAF (108), and therefore Langerhans cell histiocytosis is positive for expression of the mutant BRAF protein in a majority of cases; they are also said to be positive for placental alkaline phosphatase in many cases, while normal Langerhans cells are negative.

Indeterminate cell tumor is a neoplasm showing differentiation toward normal indeterminate cells; therefore they have the phenotype of normal indeterminate cell, being S-100 and CD1a positive, but Langerin negative. Similarly, interdigitating cell sarcoma is a neoplasm showing differentiation toward interdigitating cells, with expression of S-100 but absence of CD1a and Langerin. Follicular dendritic cell sarcoma is a tumor showing differentiation toward follicular dendritic cells and therefore expresses one or more of the follicular dendritic cell markers CD21, CD23, CD35, D2-40, or desmoplakin. Often, there is expression of only one or two of these markers in a given case, necessitating performance of multiple stains (or cocktails of antibodies). The extremely rare fibroblastic dendritic cell tumor is probably a neoplasm of the supporting myofibroblastic elements of the lymph node. Thus, it is negative for histiocytic and dendritic cell markers, but often positive for the myofibroblastic marker smooth muscle–specific actin.

Application of Immunohistochemistry to Bone Marrow

Both lymph node and BM biopsy interpretation rely on the clinical context of the patient's age and previous history. However, this is where the similarities end. In lymph node biopsies, location is often a key element in interpretation, while this is usually not a consideration in BM biopsies. In lymph node biopsies, the combination of histology and immunohistochemistry often times

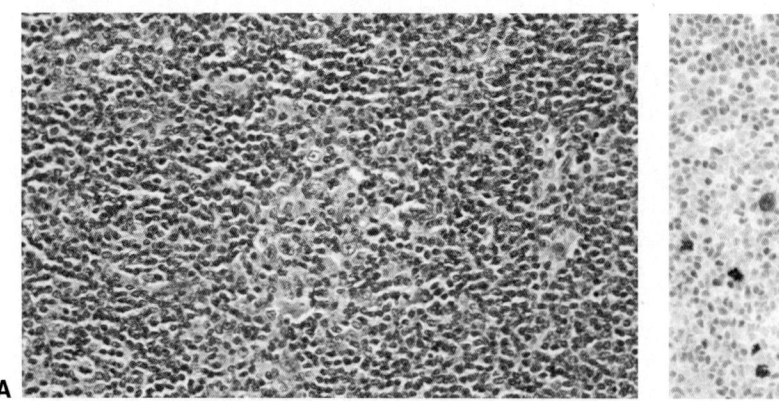 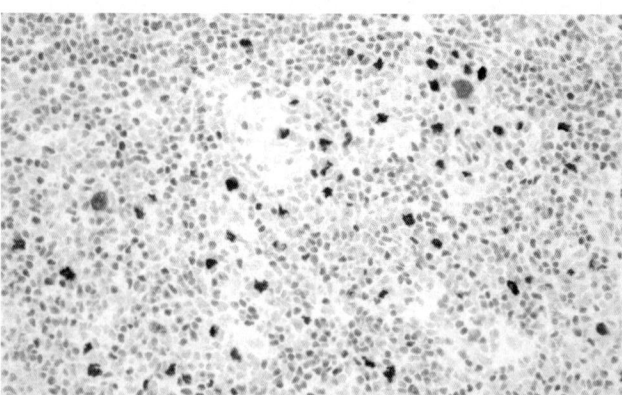

FIGURE 3.37. H&E (**A**) and OCT-2 (**B**) staining in nodular LP Hodgkin lymphoma cells is particularly strong and may be used to highlight the small population of neoplastic cells.

represents the "final word." In contrast, in BM biopsies interpretation is best made in the context of peripheral blood findings and other ancillary studies. These studies may include classical cytogenetics, to look for any clonal genetic abnormality, fluorescent *in situ* hybridization testing, to look for abnormalities associated with myelodysplastic or myeloproliferative syndromes, or flow cytometry, to look for abnormal population of cells. Additionally, unlike lymph node tissue, BM undergoes additional processing for decalcification. It is important to ensure that the immunohistochemical positive and negative controls have been validated on material that has also been subjected to these decalcification solutions. Immunohistochemical evaluation of BM biopsies represents another important tool for interpretation, which in the context of clinical history and ancillary studies will aid in the correct diagnosis and management of patients.

BONE MARROW ANTIGENS

Markers of Blasts

CD34

CD34 is a 115-kDa transmembrane sialomucin encoded on chromosome 1q32.1 (109–112). Most studies evaluating CD34 expression have used the MY 10 or the QBEND/10 monoclonal antibodies; with these the staining is described in blasts as membranous with some cytoplasmic staining.

CD34 is most frequently used to quantify blasts in BM sections where an aspirate was not obtainable (113). CD34 is not restricted to the myeloid lineage; precursor B and T lymphoblasts, hematogones (nonneoplastic early B-cell precursors), and blood vessels also express this marker. In addition, mature megakaryocytes may express CD34 in myelodysplastic syndromes (114).

CD99

CD99 (p30/32mic2) is a cell surface glycoprotein frequently used for peripheral neuroepithelioma and Ewing sarcoma. The monoclonal antibody 013 recognizes a human thymus leukemia antigen and has also been found in immature terminal deoxynucleotidyl transferase (TdT) expressing BM precursors. The staining pattern is cytoplasmic.

As with CD34, CD99 may be used as a marker of immaturity in the BM sections where an aspirate was not obtained. The staining is comparable with TdT; however, it is less sensitive (115).

CD117

CD117 (C-KIT) is a 145-kDa transmembrane tyrosine kinase receptor that is the product of the KIT-gene located on chromosome 4 (4q11-q12) (116,117). The staining pattern in erythroid precursors, abnormal plasma cells, and myeloid blasts is weak and cytoplasmic (Fig. 3.39). The staining pattern in mast cells is strong and cytoplasmic (Fig. 3.40).

CD117 may be helpful in quantifying blasts, abnormal plasma cells, or mast cells in sections. CD117 is not lineage specific and is seen on erythroid precursors, as previously mentioned, and melanocytes as well.

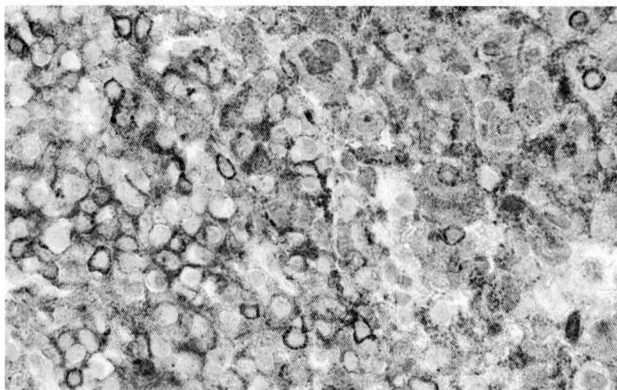 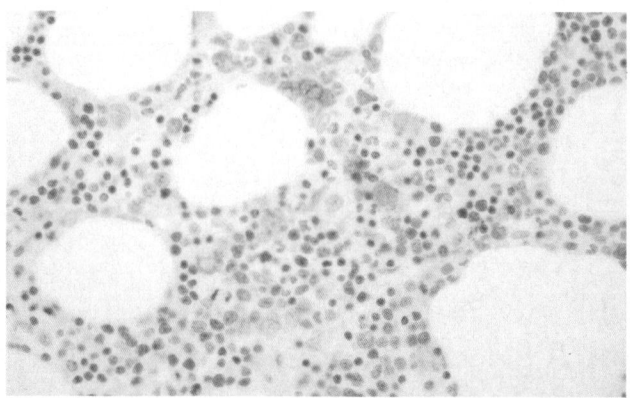

FIGURE 3.38. CD4 staining in a histiocytic sarcoma is cytoplasmic without membrane expression; in this instance it is not considered to be a specific marker of T-cell lineage.

FIGURE 3.39 CD117 staining in erythroid precursors, abnormal plasma cells, and myeloid blasts is weak and cytoplasmic.

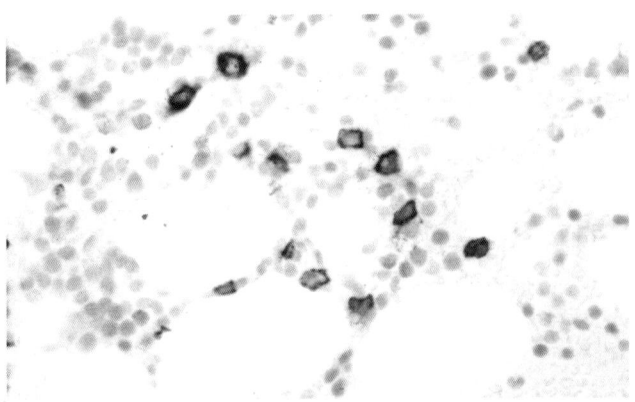

FIGURE 3.40. CD117 staining in mast cells is strong and cytoplasmic.

TdT

TdT is a DNA polymerase that generates antigen receptor diversity by catalyzing the addition of deoxynucleotides to the 3′-hydroxyl terminus of the rearranged immunoglobulin heavy chain and TCR gene segments (118,119). The staining pattern may be nuclear as well as membranous or with paranuclear dotlike positivity (119).

TdT is generally used in marrow sections to identify and quantify blasts when an aspirate was unobtainable. Caution should be used as hematogones (nonneoplastic early B-cell precursors) may also express this marker.

TdT is expressed in the lymphoblasts of acute T or B leukemia/lymphoma, a subset of AMLs and blastic plasmacytoid dendritic cell neoplasm (i.e., hematodermic CD56+/CD4+ neoplasm) (119). Nonhematopoietic malignancies expressing TdT include some pediatric small round blue cell tumors, Merkel cell carcinoma, and small cell lung carcinoma (119).

Granulocytic/Myeloid Antigens

CD33

CD33 (gp67) is a 67-kDa glycosylated transmembrane protein of the sialic acid–binding immunoglobulin-like lectin family that maps to 19q13.1-q13.3 and is thought to play a role in cell adhesion (120). The staining pattern is membranous (120).

CD33 is used to identify cells of myelomonocytic derivation and may be helpful to identify suspected myeloid sarcoma in tissue sections. Anti-CD33-targeted chemotherapy (gemtuzumab ozogamicin, i.e., Mylotarg) is used in cases of AML and acute lymphoblastic leukemia (120).

CD33 is strongly expressed on myeloid precursors including granulocytes, eosinophils, monocytes, macrophages/histiocytes. During maturation granulocytes and eosinophils decrease their expression of CD33 while monocytic or myelomonocytic cells do not (120). CD33 expression is also seen on mast cells and has been reported in one case of plasma cell myeloma (120). No expression of CD33 is reported on lymphocytes, erythroid precursors, megakaryocytes, or normal plasma cells (120). Both myeloid blasts and lymphoblasts may express this marker.

Myeloperoxidase

Myeloperoxidase staining recognizes the primary granules in the cytoplasm of granulocytes, eosinophils, and their precursors (121). The polyclonal antibody staining pattern is cytoplasmic.

Myeloperoxidase is often used as a marker of the myeloid lineage, although cells of monocytic derivation may be only weakly positive or nonreactive to the polyclonal myeloperoxidase antibody. Mast cells, plasma cells, lymphoid cells,

megakaryocytes, and erythroblasts are typically negative for this marker (121).

Lysozyme

The lysozyme antibody is polyclonal and is purified from rabbit antiserum. It is made by reacting the immunoglobulin against urine of patients with monocytic leukemia. The staining pattern is cytoplasmic.

Lysozyme may be used as a granulocytic marker, although myeloperoxidase has higher specificity. The antibody stains granulocytes and granulocyte precursors, as well as monocytes and macrophages/histiocytes.

Megakaryocytic Markers

CD42b

CD42b (gp Ibα) is a glycoprotein that is part of the gpIb-V-IX complex (122,123). The staining pattern is cytoplasmic.

Megakaryocytic markers are used in BM sections to identify blasts with megakaryocytic differentiation, micromegakaryocytes, or to aid in quantification of mature megakaryocytic forms.

CD61

CD61(beta3 integrin) is a membrane-bound glycoprotein that forms a heterodimer with CD41 (alpha IIb) to form the gpIIb/IIIa (CD41/CD61) complex. The staining pattern is cytoplasmic.

CD61, like 42b, is used to identify blasts with megakaryocytic differentiation, micromegakaryocytes, or to aid in quantification of mature megakaryocytes (124).

LAT

LAT (linker for activation of T cells) is a molecule involved in T-cell activation and platelet aggregation (125). The staining pattern is cytoplasmic and may be membranous in occasional cases.

LAT is used to quantify and identify megakaryocytes and megakaryocytic precursors (i.e., blasts with megakaryocytic differentiation). It is expressed at similar strength in both nonneoplastic and neoplastic megakaryocytes and may be better at identifying poorly differentiated megakaryoblasts than other antimegakaryocytic antibodies (125).

Erythroid Markers

CD71

CD71 (transferring receptor-1) mediates the uptake of transferrin-iron complexes and is highly expressed on the surface of erythroid precursors including erythroblasts (126,127). The staining pattern is membranous and cytoplasmic.

CD71 is used to highlight erythroblasts and erythroid precursors with similar staining results to glycophorin A (CD235a) and hemoglobin (127). Mature erythrocytes, lymphocytes, and other marrow elements lack expression of CD71 (127).

Hemoglobin

Hemoglobin is a polyclonal antibody reactive with hemoglobin A and F. The staining pattern is cytoplasmic.

Hemoglobin is primarily used to demonstrate the erythroid nature of the blasts of acute erythroleukemia (formerly AML-M6 of the FAB classification). In addition, hemoglobin may be used to confirm the erythroid nature of the sometimes "worrisome looking" proerythroblasts observed in patients with megaloblastic anemia, myelodysplastic syndromes (MDS), and chemotherapy-induced megaloblastoid changes. Similarly, glycophorin A or C can also be used as a pan-erythroid marker in tissue sections. CD36 is another marker that can be used to identify erythroblasts but is less specific than the others mentioned above.

E-cadherin

E-cadherin is mainly expressed by epithelial cells and was thought to be primarily an adhesion molecule (128). Since its discovery on the developing erythroid cells, a differentiation and signal transduction function has also been proposed (128). The staining pattern is cytoplasmic.

E-cadherin may be used to identify nonneoplastic erythroblasts and normoblasts. Mature erythroid cells do not express this marker. E-cadherin is down-regulated during erythroleukemia on the developing erythroid cells (129).

Other Important Markers

CD25

CD25 recognizes the alpha chain of the interleukin 2 receptor; it is thought to be a marker of activation (130). The staining pattern is cytoplasmic.

CD25 is used predominantly in conjunction with DBA.44 and TRAP in the suspected workup of HCL in the BM. The lack of CD25 on otherwise typical hairy cells may be seen in hairy cell variant cases. CD25 is also expressed at high levels by activated T cells, regulatory T cells, NK cells, and dendritic cells (130).

Strong and diffuse expression of tartrate-resistant acid phosphatase (TRAP) and DBA.44 are highly sensitive markers of HCL. However, they may also be expressed in extranodal marginal zone lymphoma; DBA.44 is typically strongly expressed in cases of splenic red pulp small B-cell lymphoma (131).

T-bet and annexin-1 are also immunohistochemical markers used in the suspected workup of HCL. However, T-bet has not shown sufficient specificity while annexin-1 interpretation is difficult as the myeloid precursors of the BM also express this antigen (132).

With the recent finding that the majority (over 85%) of hairy cell cases contain the BRAF V600E mutation, immunophenotypic findings may be better supported by molecular testing (133).

CD43

CD43 (Leu 22) is a sialomucin expressed on hematopoietic precursors; it is thought to play a role in regulation of hematopoiesis (134). The staining pattern is cytoplasmic.

CD43 may be used as a second-line marker of myeloid lineage; it is expressed on a variety of normal hematopoietic cells including: normal T cells, most marrow-derived cells, and macrophages/histiocytes. Although not typically coexpressed on "resting" mature B cells, CD43 expression is rarely described on B cells actively producing immunoglobulin. CD43 expression is seen in most myeloid cells including myeloblasts and mast cells, immature B cells, lymphoma cells, and rarely metastases of solid neoplasms (135).

CD68

CD68 is a macrophage antigen with three epitopes available: KP-1, PG-M1, and HAM-56. PG-M1 is the most specific, although not very sensitive. The staining pattern is cytoplasmic.

CD68 is used to identify cases of AML with a monocytic component (i.e., formerly AML-M4, M5 especially AML-M5a

subtype, which is negative for myeloperoxidase) (136). CD68 is strongly expressed in marrow macrophages in cases of infection-associated hemophagocytic syndrome, in T-cell lymphoma with associated "histiocytosis," as well as in cases of true malignant histiocytosis (MH) including MH cases associated with mediastinal germ cell tumors. KP-1 is expressed in cases of systemic mastocytosis and Langerhans cell histiocytosis.

CD68 is expressed throughout the monocytic differentiation pathway, usually more intensely in macrophages than in monocytes. Mast cells may also exhibit CD68 (KP-1) positivity, while Langerhans' cells and other dendritic cells are negative.

CD123

CD123 is the alpha chain of the interleukin 3 receptor. The staining pattern is cytoplasmic.

CD123 is used to stain plasmacytoid dendritic cells. It may be used in conjunction with CD2AP, CD56, and BDCA2 for diagnosis of blastic plasmacytoid dendritic cell leukemia (137). In addition, sheets of CD123-expressing plasmacytoid dendritic cells is a relatively specific finding seen in marrows with chronic myelomonocytic leukemia (CMML) (136). Lastly, in BM, CD123 may be used in suspected cases of HCL. In lymph node sections CD123 may be used to highlight the plasmacytoid dendritic cell proliferation seen in Kikuchi-Fujimoto lymphadenopathy and various benign proliferations (138).

CD123 is expressed normally by myeloid precursors, macrophages, dendritic cells, mast cells, basophils, and megakaryocytes. CD123 expression may also be seen on blasts of AML (137).

CD138/Lambda and Kappa Light Chain

CD138, kappa and lambda, antibodies are discussed at greater length under lymphoid antigens (38). They are frequently used together in BM sections to aid in plasma cell quantification and diagnosis of plasma cell disease as well as following therapy. The staining pattern of CD138 is membranous (38). The staining pattern of kappa and lambda are cytoplasmic.

Kappa and lambda are used primarily to look for light chain restriction although nonspecific background staining may make this antibody difficult to interpret. In BM samples kappa and lambda are only capable of recognizing cytoplasmic light chains, not surface ones. As such, they are of little value in the detection of clonal B lymphocytes, which contain surface light chains but no cytoplasmic immunoglobulin.

Kappa and lambda *in situ* hybridization is more sensitive and specific and has the advantage of lower background staining; however, it may be more affected by decalcification and is less preferable in marrow sections because of this.

 ## BONE MARROW EVALUATION

Normal BM consists of a heterogeneous population of cells proceeding along various differentiation pathways. Although most cell types can be easily distinguished on BM aspirate smears and biopsy sections, immunohistochemistry is valuable in identifying specific cell subsets. The evaluation of immunohistochemical stains in BM biopsies is important to the overall evaluation of BM disease. However, because of the frequent concurrent use of flow cytometric analysis in BM samples, immunohistochemical evaluation of BM samples may not always play the primary role such as that seen in lymph node biopsies. Nevertheless, the value of immunohistochemistry in BM pathology cannot be underestimated. In cases where flow samples are not available or in those cases where the marrow aspirates may be nonrepresentative, immunohistochemistry can be the cornerstone of a correct diagnosis.

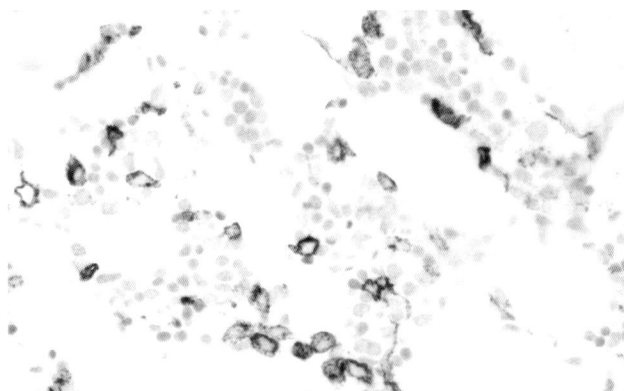

FIGURE 3.41. CD34 staining clusters of blasts in a BM biopsy.

In general, immunohistochemistry in BM is used to approach general categories of disorders including chronic myeloid neoplasms (MDS, myeloproliferative neoplasms [MPNs]), acute leukemias (myeloid, lymphoblastic, other types), lymphoid disorders, plasma cell disorders, and other diseases.

Myelodysplastic Syndrome and Myeloproliferative Neoplasms

The value of BM biopsy in chronic myeloid disorders is generally well established. Immunohistochemistry can be used to increase the diagnostic accuracy of BM biopsy. This is especially important when marrow fibrosis limits the aspirate sample. In cases with limited aspirate smears, BM blasts counts can frequently be reliably evaluated by CD34 staining. CD34 is positive in the blasts of most cases of MDS (139). In any chronic myeloid disorder, including both MDS and MPNs, an increase in CD34-positive blasts at or above 20% is compatible with acute leukemic transformation of the chronic disorder. Additional immunohistochemistry to evaluate type of lineage differentiation (e.g., myeloid versus lymphoid) is necessary as blastic transformations can be of either type. In some circumstances, lineage assignment may be difficult and require several antibodies, as blastic transformations of MPN, specifically chronic myelogenous leukemia (CML), may have aberrant coexpression of lineage antigens, or lineage infidelity.

Blast enumeration by CD117 can be more problematic. In addition to staining blasts in some cases, it can also stain immature erythroid elements and promyelocytes, leading to possible overestimation of blasts. Although not applicable in all cases, aberrant antigen expression in myeloid blast elements (such as TdT or CD7) can also be used as an adjunct to enumerate blasts.

Both an increase in the percentage of CD34-positive cells and a tendency of positive cells to form aggregates have been shown to be a reliable predictor of leukemic transformation and of survival in MDS cases, irrespective of their subtype (Fig. 3.41). Immunostaining for CD34 is especially important in two subsets of patients with MDS: MDS with fibrosis (MDS-f) and MDS with hypocellular marrow (MDS-h). The presence of reticulin fibrosis or fatty changes in the BM of these MDS patients, by causing hemodilution and poorly cellular smears, can make the subclassification very difficult or impossible. The often low cellular yield of the BM aspirate may also be insufficient to obtain adequate cytogenetic analysis, an important diagnostic technique in the assessment of MDS patients.

Myeloproliferative Neoplasms

In general, the category of MPNs do not benefit greatly from immunohistochemistry for their identification or subclassification. Immunohistochemical stains may be used to highlight abnormal distribution of neoplastic marrow elements, including CD42b or CD61 immunostains (among others), to highlight abnormal megakaryocytes (Fig. 3.42).

Systemic Mastocytosis

Systemic mastocytosis is a rare disease characterized by a generalized infiltration of mast cells involving many organs, most notably the BM, spleen, liver, and lymph nodes; cutaneous involvement may or may not be present. An association with malignant hematopoietic disorders has been recognized (140). In the BM, characteristic findings include the presence of clusters of pale cells with oval or reniform nuclei, eosinophilia, and the presence of fibrosis. Immunohistochemical staining for the identification of both normal and neoplastic mast cells is best accomplished by CD117, or the more specific, but less sensitive tryptase (Fig. 3.40). In contrast to normal mast cells, neoplastic mast cells may express CD25 and CD2, although in the case of CD2, distinction from background T lymphocytes may be problematic. CD30 expression in neoplastic mast cells is associated with an especially poor prognosis (141). CD30 positivity is mainly restricted to cases of aggressive systemic mastocytosis, systemic mastocytosis associated with a non–mast cell hematologic malignancy, and mast cell leukemia.

Myelodysplastic/Myeloproliferative Neoplasms

This category of disorders has features that overlap those of both MDS and MPN; its most frequently encountered example is CMML. As in both MDS and MPN, increased blasts may be delineated by CD34 staining. In CMML, the monocytic component may not appear as prominent in the core biopsy as it

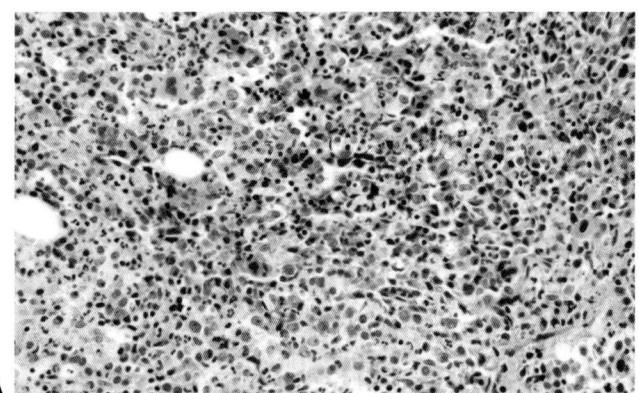

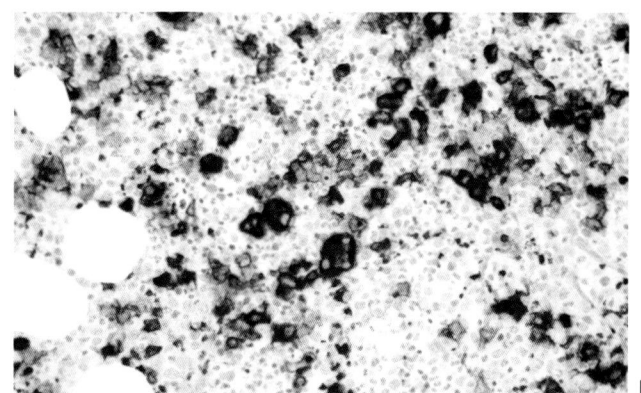

A   B

FIGURE 3.42. H&E (**A**) and CD42b (**B**) staining abnormal megakaryocytes in a BM biopsy of a patient with a MPN.

is in the peripheral blood smear, or in aspirate smears (136). The identification of monocytes in BM biopsy sections can be facilitated by using immunostains for CD14, CD68 (PG-M1), or CD163. As noted earlier in the chapter, these are markers of mature monocytic differentiation, and may not be present in immature or neoplastic monocytes.

Acute Leukemias

Because of significant treatment and prognostic differences, classification of lineage to acute leukemias is of critical importance. As mentioned previously, this is often done by flow cytometry (see Chapter 4). However, certain cases do arise where sample is not available for flow analysis. There are several subtypes, with the most common being AML, and B-lymphoblastic and T-lymphoblastic leukemias.

AMLs are a group of neoplastic proliferations of "blasts" of granulocytic, monocytic, erythroid, or megakaryocytic lineages. Immunohistochemical (or cytochemical) staining for myeloperoxidase is positive in blasts of both neutrophilic and eosinophilic lineages. Cells of monocytic derivation are weakly positive or nonreactive (121). Myeloperoxidase immunostaining is more sensitive than cytochemistry performed on BM aspirates, especially in recognizing minimally and poorly differentiated AML. Lysozyme is less specific, but highly sensitive as a pan-myeloid differentiation antibody.

CD68 is expressed throughout the monocytic differentiation, usually more intensely in macrophages than in monocytes. In BM biopsies, CD68 antibodies are used to identify cases of AML with a monocytic component, the CD68/PG-M1 epitope being preferred for this (136). CD14 and CD163 represent useful markers for identification of monocytic/macrophage lineage. However, each of these antibodies is preferentially expressed in more mature forms of the monocyte lineage, and as such may not be positive in the more immature, abnormal cells of an acute monocytic/monoblastic leukemia.

The abnormal cells of acute erythroleukemia can be identified by the application of several erythroid associated antibodies, including antihemoglobin, antiglycophorin A or C, E-cadherin, or CD71 (127,128). Each of these antibodies has its values, but, in the authors' experience, CD71 has the best combination of sensitivity, specificity, and robust staining for identification of the erythroid lineage. It should also be noted that a simple increase in erythroid cells does not identify acute erythroleukemia and that strict criteria should be applied to make this diagnosis.

Identification of mature megakaryocytes is typically not difficult by morphology. Several immunohistochemical stains that identify the megakaryocytic lineage including factor VIII antigen, CD42b, CD61, CD31, and anti-LAT (linker of activated T cells) are available (123–125). Megakaryocytes are also reactive with antigens typically used for "other" lineages including CD4 and CD79a. All antibodies stain normal megakaryocytes in biopsy sections but only a proportion of cases of acute megakaryoblastic leukemia. Megakaryoblastic leukemia is typically associated with extensive marrow fibrosis, which often precludes the use of aspirates and flow cytometry. Often, a panel of antibodies is necessary to achieve a correct identification. Identification of micromegakaryocytes is useful in confirming acute panmyelosis with myelofibrosis and MDS with fibrosis (MDS-f).

T- and B-Lymphoblastic Leukemias

Acute lymphoblastic leukemia is one of the most common malignancies seen in pediatric patients. Although flow cytometry and cytogenetics retain their dominant role in the evaluation of lymphoblastic leukemias, paraffin immunohistochemistry may provide important adjunct information. TdT, CD34, and CD99 positivity may be used to confirm the immature/blastic nature of leukemic cells. TdT is positive in almost all T- and

most B-lymphoblastic leukemias (118,119). CD79a, CD19, and PAX-5 are positive in almost all B-ALL; CD20 is less frequently positive and can be completely negative in a substantial number of cases. CD10 is positive in the majority of cases of B-lymphoblastic leukemia, and, less frequently (~40%), in T-lymphoblastic leukemia. CD3 is employed, in conjunction with TdT, to identify cases of T-lymphoblastic leukemia. Other T-cell antibodies, including CD2, CD5, CD7, and CD1a, can also be useful in select cases. However, in the setting of a mediastinal mass where the differential diagnosis is between T-lymphoblastic leukemia/lymphoma and a thymoma, the most helpful immunohistochemical stain is likely a cytokeratin and not any of these T-cell markers. This is because the immature T cells of a thymoma will show a similar immunophenotype to that of a T-lymphoblastic leukemia/lymphoma. Islands or strands of cytokeratin-positive epithelial thymic structures in a biopsy of a mediastinal mass will support a diagnosis of thymoma.

Lymphomas in Bone Marrow

Numerous B-cell and T-cell antigens are able to survive fixation and acid decalcification and can be used to confirm the presence of lymphomatous involvement in routinely processed BM biopsy material. Although immunophenotyping of lymphoid malignancies in BM sections can be successfully accomplished, it is always preferable to subtype lymphomas using material from the original involved lymph node or other primarily affected organ. BM should, however, be used to subtype cases of lymphoproliferative disorders that are associated with typical diagnostic findings in this organ (e.g., HCL), or in the rare cases of primary bone lymphomas.

In most cases, one need only determine whether the lymphomatous proliferation in the BM is morphologically compatible with the known subtype of the lymphoma, and quantify its degree of marrow involvement (e.g., in a staging evaluation setting). In this context, immunohistochemistry can be very helpful by allowing an objective comparison of the immunophenotype of the malignant cells in the primary affected organ and in the marrow. This is especially important in cases in which morphology shows discordant cytologic features (e.g., large cell transformation of CLL/SLL). It should be noted that in routinely acid decalcified BM core biopsy, immunoreactivities, background staining and intensity may vary considerably from that displayed by the same antibodies when applied to lymph node or tissue diagnosis. As such, careful selection of antibodies for lymphoma evaluation in BM is necessary.

B-Cell Neoplasms

Chronic Lymphocytic Leukemia/Small Lymphocytic Lymphoma

Morphologically, CLL/SLL often shows lymphoid infiltrates composed of monotonous-looking mature lymphocytes. The infiltrate can be diffuse or multifocal, nodular (but not paratrabecular) or interstitial. The latter, when limited, can be difficult to recognize morphologically. CLL/SLL cells usually show positivity for CD20, CD5, CD23, and often for CD43. CD10 and cyclin D1/BCL1 are negative. Immunohistochemical expression of ZAP-70 has been associated with prognosis; the staining is typically weak as compared to T cells and present in the majority of cells when positive (Fig. 3.43).

Lymphoplasmacytic Lymphoma/Waldenström Macroglobulinemia

LPL is a rare and indolent B-cell lymphoma with proliferations of small lymphocytes, lymphoplasmacytic cells, and plasma cells in varying proportions. In almost all cases, there is BM

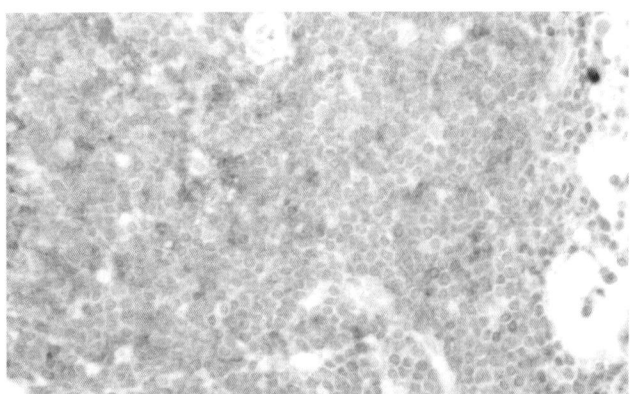

FIGURE 3.43. ZAP-70 expression has been associated with prognosis; the staining is typically weak as compared to T cells and present in the majority of cells when positive.

and peripheral blood involvement, with varying degrees of involvement of spleen and lymph nodes. The morphologic and immunophenotypic distinction of LPL from marginal zone lymphoma (both nodal and extranodal) can be difficult. When associated with a sizable monoclonal protein of IgM type, the preferred diagnosis is WM/LPL.

The immunophenotype of LPL is not distinctive; LPL will express pan B-cell antigens CD19, CD20, CD79a, and PAX-5. BCL2 is positive in almost all cases. There is often expression of IgM by neoplastic lymphoid and plasma cells. Both plasma cells and lymphoplasmacytic cells express plasma cell–associated antigens CD38, VS38c, and CD138, with monoclonal expression of light chains. A minority of cases are positive for CD5 (17% to 43%), with some positive for CD10 (16%) and many positive for CD23 (58%). LPL does not express cyclin D1/BCL1 or BCL6. Most cases of LPL are positive for CD25.

Although not entirely specific, an increase in mast cells has been noted in LPL/WM. Methods to highlight increases in mast cells (including CD117 and/or tryptase staining) could provide diagnostic support in difficult cases.

Mantle Cell Lymphoma

MCL infiltrates the marrow in a pattern similar to that observed in CLL/SLL. Although MCL cells have less regular nuclear outlines than CLL/SLL, these two lymphomas cannot be reliably separated without immunophenotyping. MCL and CLL/SLL are both positive for CD20, CD5, and CD43. However, only MCL expresses cyclin D1/BCL1. In addition, CD23 is negative in the majority of cases of MCL. The blastoid variant of MCL can be difficult to distinguish from lymphoblastic leukemias in BM

biopsies. However, the coexpression of CD5 and CD20 in the former and the lack of staining for TdT and CD99 allows for an objective separation.

Follicular Lymphoma

FL can be distinguished morphologically by its typical multinodular/paratrabecular localization in the BM biopsy. In most cases a mixture of predominantly small cleaved atypical lymphocytes and more rare large noncleaved atypical lymphoid cells is observed. The abnormal lymphocytes are B cells, and when untreated are positive for pan-B-cell antigens including CD20, PAX-5, and CD79a. Loss of CD20 may be seen after therapy with rituximab and other anti-CD20 agents (4). Characterizing the germinal center origin of the FL cells is of benefit in some cases. While there are several antigens associated with germinal center origin, in the authors' experience, HGAL/GCET2 seems to have the most robust staining after decalcification. Still useful, but with potentially misleading false-negative results are CD10 and BCL6. It is not uncommon to find numerous CD3-positive reactive T lymphocytes intermingled with the FL cells. The presence of a "mixed" B- and T-cell infiltrate in these cases may trick the unaware observer into a false-negative interpretation of reactive lymphoid hyperplasia.

Marginal Zone Lymphoma

With the exception of the splenic subtype, marginal zone B-cell lymphoma is only occasionally detected in BM specimens. In cases of splenic marginal zone lymphoma, an intrasinusoidal pattern is frequently seen. It is often only appreciated by immunohistochemical staining for B-cell antigens in the marrow, as the infiltrate may be subtle (Fig. 3.44). Immunophenotypically, marginal zone lymphoma is largely a diagnosis of exclusion. Immunophenotype in marginal zone lymphomas includes expression of pan-B-cell antigens including CD20, PAX-5, and CD19. Generally, SMZL lacks expression of CD5, CD10, CD23, cyclin D1/BCL1, CD43, and CD123. CD103 staining by immunohistochemistry or flow cytometry may be seen in splenic marginal zone lymphoma, and some cases show TRAP expression, but lack expression of DBA.44, in contrast to HCL. Annexin A1 is uniformly negative. Cases with overexpression of p53 may be associated with an aggressive clinical course.

Hairy Cell Leukemia

HCL is a rare, low-grade B-cell lymphoma with prominent involvement of spleen, BM, and peripheral blood. In most circumstances, HCL is identified by flow cytometry of either

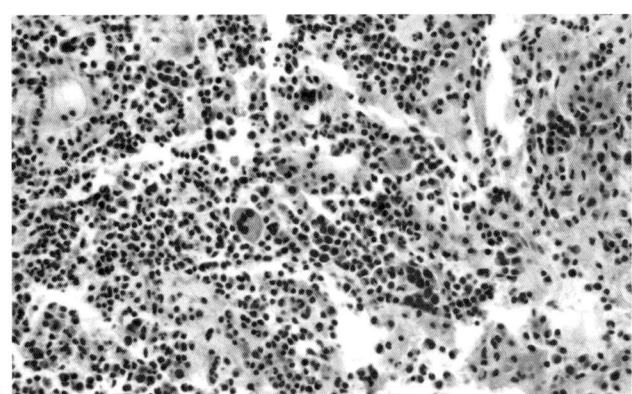
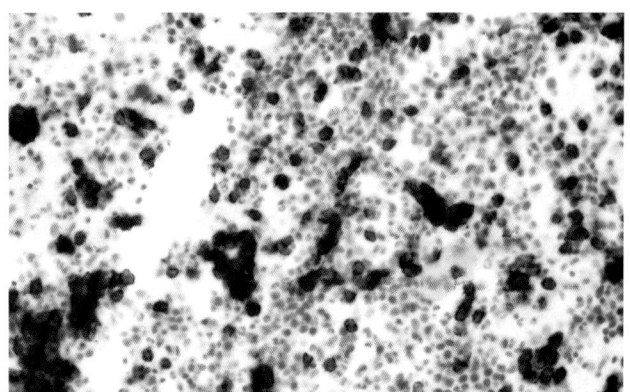

A   B

FIGURE 3.44. H&E (**A**) of Splenic marginal zone lymphoma, an intrasinusoidal pattern is frequently seen. CD20 (**B**) highlights the subtle pattern.

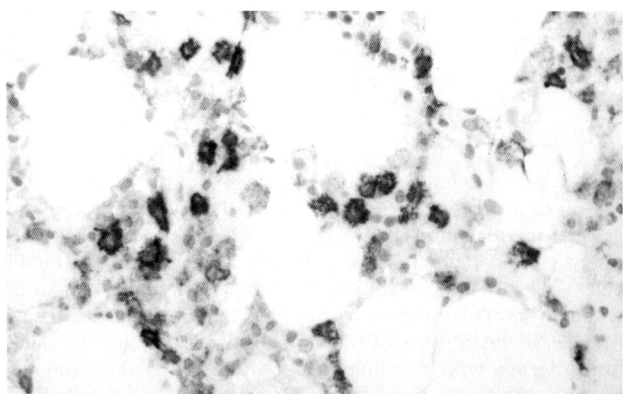

FIGURE 3.45. DBA.44 staining in HCL. This stain can be used to distinguish HCL form other B-cell disorders.

Table 3.3	IMMUNOHISTOCHEMICAL REACTIVITY OF SPLENIC SMALL B-CELL LYMPHOMAS AND HCL			
	SMZL Positive %	SRPL Positive %	HCL-v Positive %	HCL[a] Positive%
CD11c	49%	97% (moderate)	87% (bright)	Pos. (bright)
CD25	8%	Neg.	Neg.	Pos.
CD103	2%	35%	60%	Pos.
CD123	0%	15%	9%	Pos.
CD27	77%	20%	Neg.	Neg.
CD38	23%	3%	Neg.	Neg.
CD76	20% (partial)	90%	Pos. (bright)	Pos. (bright)

IgM/D + G K > L.
IgG + D or IgM/D + G K = L.
IgG alone or in combination K = L.
IgG alone or in combination K = L.
[a]Annexin-A1– and *BRAF* mutation–positive.
SMZL, splenic marginal zone lymphoma; SRPL, splenic red pulp lymphoma; HCL-V, Hairy cell leukemia variant; HCL, Hairy cell leukemia.
Modified from Baseggio L, et al. Relevance of a scoring system including CD11c expression in the identification of splenic diffuse red pulp small B-cell lymphoma (SRPL). *Hematol Oncol* 2011;29:47–51 and Traverse-Glehen A, et al. Splenic marginal zone B-cell lymphoma : a distinct clinicopathological and molecular entity. Recent advances in ontogeny and classification. *Curr Opin Oncol* 2011;23:441–448.

blood or BM samples. The immunophenotype is distinctive, shows expression of pan-B-cell antigens, and includes CD20 and CD19 with restricted light chain expression. HCL also expresses CD103, CD11c, CD22, and CD25. Most cases lack CD5 and CD10 expression, although rare cases of either or both have been reported.

Primary diagnostic immunohistochemical studies of HCL in BM include expression of TRAP and DBA.44 (Fig. 3.45) (131–133). Annexin-1 is positive in almost all cases, but can be difficult to interpret due to extensive staining of normal background elements. Cyclin D1 is positive in a large percentage of cases of HCL, and can be useful in discriminating between HCL and other lymphoma types; it stains less intensely and less uniformly than in cases of MCL (Fig. 3.46). T-bet lacks sensitivity and specificity, but if positive could support a diagnosis of HCL. Neoplastic cells of HCL often carry the V600E mutation of BRAF, and are positive for expression of the mutant BRAF protein in a majority of cases (108). BRAF mutation–specific antibodies will likely find a role in diagnosis of HCL.

Hairy Cell Leukemia-Variant

Hairy cell leukemia-variant (HCL-V) is an exceedingly rare lymphoid neoplasm, with prominent splenic, BM, and peripheral blood involvement. It is more aggressive than conventional HCL, and some cases may be aggressive and refractory to typical treatment. In BM, the abnormal lymphocytes will be intermediate to large in size, with variably prominent nucleoli.

Most cases of HCL-V are identified by flow cytometry of peripheral blood or BM. By immunohistochemical evaluation,

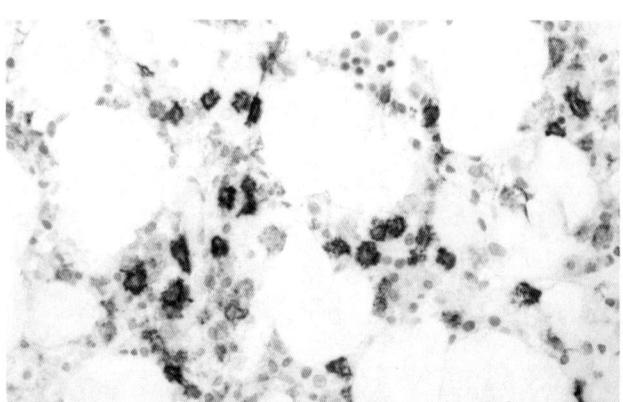

FIGURE 3.46. Cyclin D1 is positive in a large percentage of cases of HCL, and can be useful in discriminating between HCL Nead other lymphoma types; it stains less intensely and less uniformly than in cases of MCL.

HCL-V will be positive for B-cell markers such as CD20, CD19, and PAX-5. They will also express CD11c, CD22, CD103, and DBA.44. In contrast to most cases of conventional HCL, HCL-V will lack expression of cyclin D1, CD123, CD25, TRAP, and annexin-A1. BRAF mutations are typically absent in HCL-V (108). HCL and HCL-V also need to be distinguished from splenic diffuse red pulp small B-cell lymphoma, a provisional entity in the 2008 update of the World Health Organization, which also may express DBA44. In contrast to hairy cell leukemia (HCL), splenic diffuse red pulp lymphoma is negative for CD25, expressing CD11c, CD103, and CD123 (Table 3.3).

Diffuse Large B-Cell Lymphomas

Subclassifying DLBCL in BM sections is impractical and should not be attempted in most cases (Table 3.4). Immunohistochemistry is very useful to confirm the B-cell origin of the neoplastic cells and the degree of involvement in these cases.

DLBCL can be CD20-negative in 15% to 20% of cases, especially after anti-CD20 therapies (4). In these cases, the use of alternate pan-B-cell antigens, such as PAX-5, CD79a, or CD19, is particularly useful in confirming the B-cell derivation of the malignant cells. In cases of B-cell lymphomas in immunodeficient patients, *in situ* identification of EBV infection using EBER probe may be of great benefit.

T-Cell Neoplasms with Prominent Marrow Involvement

Peripheral T-Cell Neoplasms

Although less common than with B-cell lymphomas, involvement of the BM is also seen in cases of T-cell lymphoma. The neoplastic cells in peripheral T-cell lymphoma usually express CD3, CD5, and CD43. CD7 is not uncommonly lost. CD4 is positive in most cases and CD8 expression is less common. CD8-positive T cells are more often seen in marrows with reactive T lymphocytosis such as that seen in patients with viral infections (e.g., EBV) or in cases of infection-associated hemophagocytic syndrome. A gamma/delta derivation (TCR beta-negative using betaF1) is considerably more common than alpha/beta derivation. Peripheral T-cell lymphomas typically lack expression of CD10, BCL6, CXCL13, or PD1 seen in AITL (98,99). CD30 may be positive in a subset of cells; however, if more than 75% are

Table 3.4	IMMUNOHISTOCHEMICAL MARKERS WITH SUBOPTIMAL OR PROBLEMATIC STAINING IN BM	
Antibody	**Usual Reactivity**	**Problems in Marrow Staining**
CD15	Hodgkin lymphoma	Mature granulocytes often express CD15; when staining in marrow there may be numerous positive cells obscuring weak focal staining in Hodgkin lymphoma.
CD10	FL cells; benign follicle center cells	Mature granulocytes often express CD10; when staining in marrow there may be numerous positive cells. FL in marrow may be weak or negative partly due to decalcified sample.
BCL2	Identification of lymphoma cells, usually small B-cell lymphoma	Expressed on most long-lived cells, including granulocytes and erythroid elements, there will be extensive staining in normal marrow elements.
CD43	Coexpressed on several small B-cell lymphomas	Expressed on most elements of myeloid lineage including granulocytes and monocytes and their precursors. Expression in lymphoid cells may be difficult to distinguish from background.
BCL6	Expressed in almost all FLs	Often very weakly expressed in marrow, especially if decalcified. If available, HGAL staining is a robust marker of follicle center origin, which is strongly maintained even in decalcified marrow.
CD68	Expressed in macrophages and monocytes	Extensive nonspecific staining in all cells of myeloid lineage, making interpretation of small populations difficult.
Ki-67	Used to evaluate proliferation rate in lymphomas and other neoplasms	Normal marrow is highly proliferative, so Ki-67 expression will be high. Interpretation in abnormal cells may be difficult from highly proliferative background.
TIA-1	Cytotoxic T cells	Granulocytes, especially neutrophils, strongly express TIA-1, making distinction from cytotoxic T cells difficult.

positive, with strong and uniform expression, a diagnosis of anaplastic large cell lymphoma is more likely.

CD30 is positive in all cases of anaplastic large cell lymphoma involving the marrow. ALK-1 is seen in a subset of cases of anaplastic large cell lymphoma (see above Lymphomas) (103). BM involvement by T-cell lymphomas can occasionally be very subtle and difficult to recognize.

T-Cell Prolymphocytic Leukemia/Lymphoma

T-cell prolymphocytic leukemia/lymphoma is a rare and aggressive T-cell neoplasm. It most often presents as disease of the spleen, peripheral blood, and BM.

T-cell prolymphocytic leukemia/lymphoma is positive for pan-T-cell antigens CD3, CD2, and CD7. It is often negative for CD5. The pattern of CD4/CD8 expression in T-PLL is as follows: 60% CD4 positive/CD8 negative, 25% CD4 positive/CD8 positive, 15% CD4 negative/CD8 positive. T-PLL is almost always positive for TCL1, a protooncogene that acts as an AKT activator. T-PLL is negative for CD1a and TDT, which distinguishes it from T-lymphoblastic leukemia/lymphoma, a frequent differential diagnostic consideration, based on morphology.

Hepatosplenic T-cell Lymphoma

A distinctive T-cell lymphoma, hepatosplenic T-cell lymphoma has a characteristic clinicopathologic presentation. Patients will often have splenic and hepatic involvement, BM is typically involved, but neoplastic cells are only rarely identified circulating in peripheral blood. This lymphoma is associated with a poor prognosis. The lymphoma cells are of T-cell immunophenotype, and in most cases have gamma/delta TCRs, which are normally seen in only 5% of circulating T cells. In typical cases, TCR gamma/delta can be identified, with no staining for TCR gamma/delta (see below). Rare cases will have an alpha/beta immunophenotype; these cases would be positive for TCR beta staining by immunohistochemistry (BetaF1). The lymphoma cells of hepatosplenic T-cell lymphomas also are negative for CD5 and CD4. Hepatosplenic T-cell lymphomas are variably positive for CD8 and CD56, with expression of the cytotoxic T-cell marker TIA-1. They are usually negative for the cytotoxic markers perforin and granzyme B.

T-Cell Large Granular Lymphocytic Leukemia/Lymphoma

T-cell large granular lymphocytic leukemia/lymphoma (T-LGL/L) is a rare disorder that typically involves BM, peripheral blood, and spleen. Patients will often have peripheral blood cytopenias. The proliferation of cells seen are most often intermediate-sized lymphocytes with slightly irregular nuclei, and moderate to large amounts of pale cytoplasm. In most cases, evaluation is by flow cytometry of BM or peripheral blood. By immunophenotypic analysis, the leukemic cells are CD3-positive with expression of CD2, CD8, CD57 (>80%), CD16 (>80%), and TCR alpha/beta. There is frequently abnormal dim or absent expression of CD5 and/or CD7. By immunohistochemical evaluation, these abnormal lymphocytes will express cytotoxic markers TIA1, granzyme B, and perforin. However, these can be especially difficult to interpret in BM, as normal granulocytes will often express these markers. Immunophenotypic variations of T-LGL/L include CD4 expression (very rare), CD4-negative/CD8-negative (very rare), or gamma/delta expression.

Plasma Cell Neoplasms

Plasma cell neoplasms are typically diagnosed by a multiparametric approach that includes clinical, radiologic, and laboratory data. BM aspirate and biopsy is used to assess the number, the distribution pattern, and the degree of cytologic differentiation of the plasma cells. In plasma cell myeloma, the plasma cells usually account for 20% or more of the marrow nucleated cells and frequently appear arranged in cell clusters or large sheets in the BM biopsy (Fig. 3.47).

Several immunohistochemical markers are available for the enumeration of plasma cells in the BM. CD138 is the best antibody to identify and enumerate plasma cells in paraffin-embedded BM biopsies. Virtually all cases of plasma cell myeloma, including plasmablastic and leukemic cases, show strong CD138 immunoreactivity (47,48). Normal plasma cells are also uniformly positive for CD138. Conversely, B-cell lymphomas are almost always negative. In LPL, the plasma cell and plasmacytoid components expresses CD138 while the lymphocytes are negative. Other antigens that may be used to characterize plasma cells are CD79a, CD38, and VS38c. Most plasma cells also express EMA, BCL2, and frequently CD30.

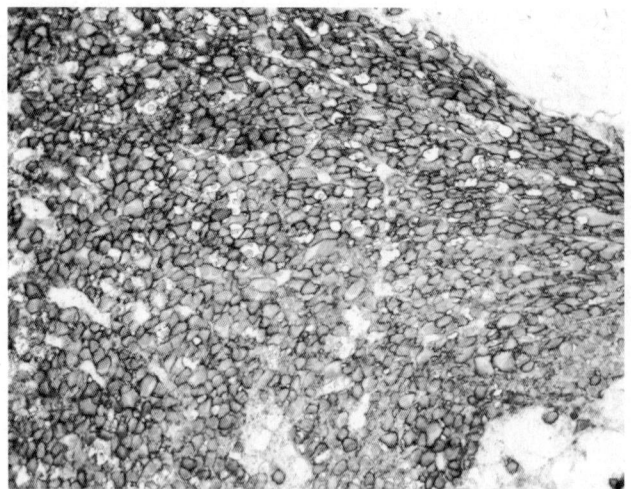

FIGURE 3.47. CD138 staining plasma cell myeloma, the plasma cells usually account for 20% or more of the marrow nucleated cells and frequently appear arranged in cell clusters or large sheets.

In most cases, neoplastic plasma cells do not express pan-B-cell antigens CD20, PAX-5, CD19, or express CD45.

Identification of light chain restriction by kappa and lambda immunostaining is frequently necessary to confirm the presence of a monotypic plasma cell neoplasm. Granted, if there are more than 20% to 30% plasma cells in the marrow, it is quite unlikely to represent a polyclonal pattern and, in the presence of paraproteinemia plus evidence of myeloma-associated organ damage (e.g., lytic bone lesions), the immunohistochemical demonstration of light chain restriction may not be necessary. Immunohistochemical staining for light chains will often have high background staining, and may be difficult to interpret. In situ staining for light chains is not predisposed to background staining due to the presence of paraproteins, but the technique may be somewhat compromised by the decalcification process to which BM biopsies are subjected.

Immunoglobulin heavy chain staining (IgA, IgG, IgM, IgD), which may also be accompanied by a high background staining that makes the interpretation difficult or impossible, is less frequently used. However, heavy chain stains can be useful in cases of heavy chain disease, and rarely to identify IgM staining to support a diagnosis of LPL/WM. IgD can help in identifying BM involvement by splenic marginal zone B-cell lymphoma.

CD56 expression is seen in the majority of cases of PCM (~70%). If CD56 expression is found in small populations of plasma cells, it is a strong indicator of the neoplastic nature of these cells (142). Likewise, CD117 is seen in a subset of neoplastic plasma cells, with moderate cytoplasmic expression (142). This is not seen in normal plasma cells and CD117 would therefore support a diagnosis of neoplastic process.

Cyclin D1/BCL1 expression can be seen in a number of cases of PCM. While most of these cases show evidence of the t(11;14) translocation also seen in MCL, cyclin D1/BCL1 expression in PCM may occasionally be seen in cases without the translocation. A subset of PCM cases with CD20 expression and a small, lymphocyte-like morphology have been identified. Most of these cases will coexpress cyclin D1/BCL1, and should be carefully distinguished from MCL.

Amyloid deposition can be seen in the BM in various types of immunosecretory disorders. Amyloid is usually demonstrated by its characteristic brick-red staining and apple-green birefringence on polarization after staining with Congo red. The distinction between primary (AL) and secondary (AA) amyloidosis is occasionally of benefit. If monotypic plasma cells are identified, then this should represent primary amyloidosis.

Testing for amyloid A and amyloid P proteins may also provide additional information. Amyloid P component is present in all types of amyloid, but is also present in normal elastic tissue and basement membranes. As such, a positive amyloid P is only relevant in the context of a positive Congo red stain. The AA component is present only in secondary amyloidosis and familial Mediterranean type amyloidosis, so immunostains for amyloid A component are positive only in those entities. Cases that are amyloid P–positive/amyloid A–negative include primary amyloidosis, beta2 microglobulin (dialysis-associated) amyloid, and hereditary amyloidosis.

References

1. Riley JK, Sliwkowski MX. CD20: a gene in search of a function. *Semin Oncol* 2000;27:17–24.
2. Shan D, Ledbetter JA, Press OW. Apoptosis of malignant human B cells by ligation of CD20 with monoclonal antibodies. *Blood* 1998;91:1644–1652.
3. Chu PG, Loera S, Huang Q, et al. Lineage determination of CD20- B-Cell neoplasms: an immunohistochemical study. *Am J Clin Pathol* 2006;126:534–544.
4. Plosker GL, Figgitt DP. Rituximab: a review of its use in non-Hodgkin's lymphoma and chronic lymphocytic leukaemia. *Drugs* 2003;63:803–843.
5. Quintanilla-Martinez L, Preffer F, Rubin D, et al. CD20+ T-cell lymphoma. Neoplastic transformation of a normal T-cell subset. *Am J Clin Pathol* 1994;102:483–489.
6. Robillard N, Avet-Loiseau H, Garand R, et al. CD20 is associated with a small mature plasma cell morphology and t(11;14) in multiple myeloma. *Blood* 2003;102:1070–1071.
7. Feldman AL, Dogan A. Diagnostic uses of Pax5 immunohistochemistry. *Adv Anat Pathol* 2007;14:323–334.
8. Medvedovic J, Ebert A, Tagoh H, et al. Pax5: a master regulator of B cell development and leukemogenesis. *Adv Immunol* 2011;111:179–206.
9. Cobaleda C, Schebesta A, Delogu A, et al. Pax5: the guardian of B cell identity and function. *Nat Immunol* 2007;8:463–470.
10. Hagiwara M, Tomita A, Takata K, et al. Primary cutaneous CD30 positive T-cell lymphoproliferative disorders with aberrant expression of PAX5: report of three cases. *Pathol Int* 2012;62:264–270.
11. Song J, Li M, Tretiakova M, et al. Expression patterns of PAX5, c-Met, and paxillin in neuroendocrine tumors of the lung. *Arch Pathol Lab Med* 2010;134:1702–1705.
12. Mason DY, Cordell JL, Brown MH, et al. CD79a: a novel marker for B cell neoplasms in routinely processed tissue samples. *Blood* 1995;86:1453.
13. Chu PG, Arber DA. CD79: a review. *Appl Immunohistochem Mol Morphol* 2001;9:97–106.
14. Li S, Borowitz MJ. CD79a(+) T-cell lymphoblastic lymphoma with coexisting Langerhans cell histiocytosis. *Arch Pathol Lab Med* 2001;125:958–960.
15. Arber DA, Jenkins KA, Slovak ML. CD79 alpha expression in acute myeloid leukemia. High frequency of expression in acute promyelocytic leukemia. *Am J Pathol* 1996;149:1105–1110.
16. Ohno H, Fukuhara S. Significance of rearrangement of the BCL6 gene in B-cell lymphoid neoplasms. *Leuk Lymphoma* 1997;27:53–63.
17. Saglam A, Uner AH. Immunohistochemical expression of Mum-1, Oct-2 and Bcl-6 in systemic anaplastic large cell lymphomas. *Tumori* 2011;97:634–638.
18. Rodríguez-Pinilla SM, Atienza L, Murillo C, et al. Peripheral T-cell lymphoma with follicular T-cell markers. *Am J Surg Pathol* 2008;32:1787–1799.
19. Shipp MA, Vijayaraghavan J, Schmidt EV, et al. Common acute lymphoblastic leukemia antigen (CALLA) is active neutral endopeptidase 24.11 ("enkephalinase"): direct evidence by cDNA transfection analysis. *Proc Natl Acad Sci U S A* 1989;86:297–301.
20. Shipp MA, Stefano GB, Switzer SN, et al. CD10 (CALLA)/neutral endopeptidase 24.11 modulates inflammatory peptide-induced changes in neutrophil morphology, migration, and adhesion proteins and is itself regulated by neutrophil activation. *Blood* 1991;78:1834–1841.
21. Kohn LA, Hao QL, Sasidharan R, et al. Lymphoid priming in human bone marrow begins before expression of CD10 with upregulation of L-selectin. *Nat Immunol* 2012;13:963–971.
22. Choi WW, Weisenburger DD, Greiner TC, et al. A new immunostain algorithm classifies diffuse large B-cell lymphoma into molecular subtypes with high accuracy. *Clin Cancer Res* 2009;15:5494–5502.
23. Montes-Moreno S, Roncador G, Maestre L, et al. Gcet1 (centerin), a highly restricted marker for a subset of germinal center-derived lymphomas. *Blood* 2008;111:351–358.
24. Paterson MA, Hosking PS, Coughlin PB. Expression of the serpin centerin defines a germinal center phenotype in B-cell lymphomas. *Am J Clin Pathol* 2008;130:117–126.
25. Leich E, Hartmann EM, Burek C, et al. Diagnostic and prognostic significance of gene expression profiling in lymphomas. *APMIS* 2007;115:1135–1146.
26. Visco C, Li Y, Xu-Monette ZY, et al. Comprehensive gene expression profiling and immunohistochemical studies support application of immunophenotypic algorithm for molecular subtype classification in diffuse large B-cell lymphoma: a report from the International DLBCL Rituximab-CHOP Consortium Program Study. *Leukemia* 2012;26:2103–2113.
27. Agostinelli C, Paterson JC, Gupta R, et al. Detection of LIM domain only 2 (LMO2) in normal human tissues and haematopoietic and non-haematopoietic tumours using a newly developed rabbit monoclonal antibody. *Histopathology* 2012;61:33–46.
28. Natkunam Y, Zhao S, Mason DY, et al. The oncoprotein LMO2 is expressed in normal germinal-center B cells and in human B-cell lymphomas. *Blood* 2007;109:1636–1642.
29. Natkunam Y, Warnke RA, Montgomery K, et al. Analysis of MUM1/IRF4 protein expression using tissue microarrays and immunohistochemistry. *Mod Pathol* 2001;14:686–694.

30. Gualco G, Weiss LM, Bacchi CE. MUM1/IRF4: A Review. *Appl Immunohistochem Mol Morphol* 2010;18:301–310.
31. Falini B, Fizzotti M, Pucciarini A, et al. A monoclonal antibody (MUM1p) detects expression of the MUM1/IRF4 protein in a subset of germinal center B cells, plasma cells, and activated T cells. *Blood* 2000;95:2084–2092.
32. Hoeller S, Schneider A, Haralambieva E, et al. FOXP1 protein overexpression is associated with inferior outcome in nodal diffuse large B-cell lymphomas with non-germinal centre phenotype, independent of gains and structural aberrations at 3p14.1. *Histopathology* 2010;57:73–80.
33. Yu B, Zhou X, Li B, et al. FOXP1 expression and its clinicopathologic significance in nodal and extranodal diffuse large B-cell lymphoma. *Ann Hematol* 2011;90: 701–708.
34. Sáez AI, Artiga MJ, Sánchez-Beato M, et al. Analysis of octamer-binding transcription factors Oct2 and Oct1 and their coactivator BOB.1/OBF.1 in lymphomas. *Mod Pathol* 2002;15:211–220.
35. Salas M, Eckhardt LA. Critical role for the Oct-2/OCA-B partnership in Ig-secreting cells. *J Immunol* 2003;171:6589–6598.
36. García-Cosío M, Santón A, Martín P, et al. Analysis of transcription factor OCT.1, OCT.2 and BOB.1 expression using tissue arrays in classical Hodgkin's lymphoma. *Mod Pathol* 2004;17:1531–1538.
37. McCune RC, Syrbu SI, Vasef MA. Expression profiling of transcription factors Pax-5, Oct-1, Oct-2, BOB.1, and PU.1 in Hodgkin's and non-Hodgkin's lymphomas: a comparative study using high throughput tissue microarrays. *Mod Pathol* 2006;19: 1010–1018.
38. Matthias P. Lymphoid-specific transcription mediated by the conserved octamer site: who is doing what? *Semin Immunol* 1998;10:155–163.
39. Advani AS, Lim K, Gibson S, et al. OCT-2 expression and OCT-2/BOB.1 co-expression predict prognosis in patients with newly diagnosed acute myeloid leukemia. *Leuk Lymphoma* 2010;51:606–612.
40. Chen YH, Gao J, Fan G, et al. Nuclear expression of sox11 is highly associated with mantle cell lymphoma but is independent of t(11;14)(q13;q32) in non-mantle cell B-cell neoplasms. *Mod Pathol* 2010;23:105–112.
41. Hsiao SC, Cortada IR, Colomo L, et al. SOX11 is useful in differentiating cyclin D1-positive diffuse large B-cell lymphoma from mantle cell lymphoma. *Histopathology* 2012;61:685–693.
42. Xu W, Li JY. SOX11 expression in mantle cell lymphoma. *Leuk Lymphoma* 2010;51:1962–1967.
43. Gerdes J. Ki-67 and other proliferation markers useful for immunohistological diagnostic and prognostic evaluations in human malignancies. *Semin Cancer Biol* 1990;1:199–206.
44. Bryant RJ, Banks PM, O'Malley DP. Ki67 staining pattern as a diagnostic tool in the evaluation of lymphoproliferative disorders. *Br J Histopathol* 2006;48:505–515.
45. Pileri S, Gerdes J, Rivano M, et al. Immunohistochemical determination of growth fractions in human permanent cell lines and lymphoid tumours: a critical comparison of the monoclonal antibodies OKT9 and Ki-67. *Br J Haematol* 1987;65: 271–276.
46. Costes V, Magen V, Legouffe E, et al. The Mi15 monoclonal antibody (anti-syndecan-1) is a reliable marker for quantifying plasma cells in paraffin-embedded bone marrow biopsy specimens. *Hum Pathol* 1999;30:1405–1411.
47. Sebestyén A, Berczi L, Mihalik R, et al. Syndecan-1 (CD138) expression in human non-Hodgkin lymphomas. *Br J Haematol* 1999;104:412–419.
48. O'Connell FP, Pinkus JL, Pinkus GS. CD138 (syndecan-1), a plasma cell marker immunohistochemical profile in hematopoietic and nonhematopoietic neoplasms. *Am J Clin Pathol* 2004;121:254–263.
49. Prakash S, Fountaine T, Raffeld M, et al. IgD positive L&H cells identify a unique subset of nodular lymphocyte predominant Hodgkin lymphoma. *Am J Surg Pathol* 2006;30:585–592.
50. Shaheen SP, Talwalkar SS, Lin P, et al. Waldenström macroglobulinemia: a review of the entity and its differential diagnosis. *Adv Anat Pathol* 2012;19:11–27.
51. Shao H, Xi L, Raffeld M, et al. Nodal and extranodal plasmacytomas expressing immunoglobulin a: an indolent lymphoproliferative disorder with a low risk of clinical progression. *Am J Surg Pathol* 2010;34:1425–1435.
52. Cheuk W, Chan JK. IgG4-related sclerosing disease: a critical appraisal of an evolving clinicopathologic entity. *Adv Anat Pathol* 2010;17:303–332.
53. Gualberto A. Brentuximab Vedotin (SGN-35), an antibody-drug conjugate for the treatment of CD30-positive malignancies. *Expert Opin Investig Drugs* 2012;21:205–216.
54. Gruss H-J, Herrmann F. CD30 ligand, a member of the TNF ligand superfamily, with growth and activation control CD30+ lymphoid and lymphoma cells. *Leuk Lymphoma* 1996;20:397–409.
55. Barry TS, Jaffe ES, Sorbara L, et al. Peripheral T-cell lymphomas expressing CD30 and CD15. *Am J Surg Pathol* 2003;27:1513–1522.
56. Arber DA, Weiss LM. CD15: a review. *Appl Immunohistochem* 1993;1:17–30.
57. Sheibani K, Battifora H, Burke JS, et al. LeuM1 antigen in human neoplasms. An immunohistologic study of 400 cases. *Am J Surg Pathol* 1986;10:227–236.
58. Traweek ST, Arber DA, Rappaport H, et al. Extramedullary myeloid cell tumors: an immunohistochemical and morphologic study of 28 cases. *Am J Surg Pathol* 1993;17:1011–1019.
59. Weiss LM, ArberDA, Chang KL. CD45: a review. *Appl Immunohistochem* 1993;1: 166–181.
60. Trowbridge IS, Thomas ML. CD45: an emerging role as a protein tyrosine phosphatase required for lymphocyte activation and development. *Annu Rev Immunol* 1994;12:85–116.
61. Hasanali Z, Sharma K, Epner E. Flipping the cyclin D1 switch in mantle cell lymphoma. *Best Pract Res Clin Haematol* 2012;25:143–152.
62. Gautschi O, Ratschiller D, Gugger M, et al. Cyclin D1 in non-small cell lung cancer: a key driver of malignant transformation. *Lung Cancer* 2007;55:1–14.
63. Sander B. Mantle cell lymphoma: recent insights into pathogenesis, clinical variability, and new diagnostic markers. *Semin Diagn Pathol* 2011;28:245–255.
64. Gradowski JF, Sargent RL, Craig FE, et al. Chronic lymphocytic leukemia/small lymphocytic lymphoma with cyclin D1 positive proliferation centers do not have CCND1 translocations or gains and lack SOX11 expression. *Am J Clin Pathol* 2012;138:132–139.
65. Green TM, Nielsen O, de Stricker K, et al. High levels of nuclear MYC protein predict the presence of MYC rearrangement in diffuse large B-cell lymphoma. *Am J Surg Pathol* 2012;36:612–619.
66. Hoffman B, Liebermann DA. Apoptotic signaling by c-MYC. *Oncogene* 2008;27:6462–6472.
67. Snuderl M, Kolman OK, Chen YB, et al. B-cell lymphomas with concurrent IGH-BCL2 and MYC rearrangements are aggressive neoplasms with clinical and pathologic features distinct from Burkitt lymphoma and diffuse large B-cell lymphoma. *Am J Surg Pathol* 2010;34:327–340.
68. Kramer MH, Hermans J, Wijburg E, et al. Clinical relevance of BCL2, BCL6, and MYC rearrangements in diffuse large B-cell lymphoma. *Blood* 1998;92:3152–3162.
69. Masir N, Campbell LJ, Goff LK, et al. BCL2 protein expression in follicular lymphomas with t(14;18) chromosomal translocations. *Br J Haematol* 2009;144: 716–725.
70. Lau SK, Chu PG, Weiss LM. CD163: a specific marker of macrophages in paraffin-embedded tissue samples. *Am J Clin Pathol* 2004;122:794–801.
71. Nguyen TT, Schwartz EJ, West RB, et al. Expression of CD163 (hemoglobin scavenger receptor) in normal tissues, lymphomas, carcinomas, and sarcomas is largely restricted to the monocyte/macrophage lineage. *Am J Surg Pathol* 2005;29:617–624.
72. Lau SK, Chu PG, Weiss LM. Immunohistochemical expression of Langerin in Langerhans cell histiocytosis and non-Langerhans cell histiocytic disorders. *Am J Surg Pathol* 2008;32:615–619.
73. Moshkani S, Kuzin II, Adewale F, et al. CD23+ CD21(high) CD1d(high) B cells in inflamed lymph nodes are a locally differentiated population with increased antigen capture and activation potential. *J Immunol* 2012;188:5944–5953.
74. Hawse WF, Champion MM, Joyce MV, et al. Cutting edge: evidence for a dynamically driven T cell signaling mechanism. *J Immunol* 2012;188:5819–5823.
75. Proust R, Bertoglio J, Gesbert F. The Adaptor Protein SAP Directly Associates with CD3ζ Chain and Regulates T cell receptor signaling. *PLoS One* 2012;7:e43200.
76. Oliveira JL, Grogg KL, Macon WR, et al. Clinicopathologic features of b-cell lineage neoplasms with aberrant expression of CD3: a study of 21 cases. *Am J Surg Pathol* 2012;36:1364–1370.
77. Moingeon P, Chang HC, Sayre PH, et al. The structural biology of CD2. *Immunol Rev* 1989;111:111–144.
78. de Vries JE, Yssel H, Spits H. Interplay between the TCR/CD3 complex and CD4 or CD8 in the activation of cytotoxic T lymphocytes. *Immunol Rev* 1989;109:119–141.
79. Bierer BE, Peterson A, Gorga JC, et al. Synergistic T cell activation via the physiological ligands for CD2 and the T cell receptor. *J Exp Med* 1988;168:1145–1156.
80. Choudhuri K, van der Merwe PA. Molecular mechanisms involved in T cell receptor triggering. *Semin Immunol* 2007;19:255–261.
81. Khalidi HS, Medeiros LJ, Chang KL, et al. The immunophenotype of adult acute myeloid leukemia: high frequency of lymphoid antigen expression and comparison of immunophenotpye, French-American-British classification, and karyotypic abnormalities. *Am J Clin Pathol* 1998;109:211–220.
82. Morgado JM, Sánchez-Muñoz L, Teodósio CG, et al. Immunophenotyping in systemic mastocytosis diagnosis: 'CD25 positive' alone is more informative than the 'CD25 and/or CD2' WHO criterion. *Mod Pathol* 2012;25:516–521.
83. Miceli MC, Parnes JR. The roles of CD4 and CD8 in T cell activation. *Semin Immunol* 1991;3:133–141.
84. Killeen N, Davis CB, Chu K, et al. CD4 function in thymocyte differentiation and T cell activation. *Philos Trans R Soc Lond B Biol Sci* 1993;342(1299):25–34.
85. Bamberger M, Santos AM, Gonçalves CM, et al. A new pathway of CD5 glycoprotein-mediated T cell inhibition dependent on inhibitory phosphorylation of Fyn kinase. *J Biol Chem* 2011;286:30324–30336.
86. Sestero CM, McGuire DJ, De Sarno P, et al. CD5-Dependent CK2 Activation Pathway Regulates Threshold for T Cell Anergy. *J Immunol* 2012;189:2918–2930.
87. Hishima T, Fukayama M, Fujisawa M, et al. CD5 expression in thymic carcinoma. *Am J Pathol* 1994;145:268–275.
88. Kawano H, Minagawa K, Wakahashi K, et al. Diminished expression of CD5 and/or CD7 surface antigens as the first clue of diagnosis for monoclonal T lymphocytosis. *Rinsho Ketsueki* 2012;53:785–787.
89. Saati T, Alibaud L, Lamant L, et al. A New Monoclonal Anti-CD7 Antibody Reactive on Paraffin Sections. *Appl Immunohistochem* 2001;9:289–296.
90. Rausei-Mills V, Chang KL, Gaal KK, et al. Aberrant expression of CD7 in myeloblasts is highly associated with de novo acute myeloid leukemias with FLT3/ITD mutation. *Am J Clin Pathol* 2008;129:624–629.
91. Chang H, Yeung J, Brandwein J, et al. CD7 expression predicts poor disease free survival and post-remission survival in patients with acute myeloid leukemia and normal karyotype. *Leuk Res* 2007;31:157–162.
92. Chan JK, Sin VC, Wong KF, et al. Nonnasal lymphoma expressing the natural killer cell marker CD56: a clinicopathologic study of 49 cases of an uncommon aggressive neoplasm. *Blood* 1997;89:4501–4513.
93. Tsang WY, Chan JK, Ng CS, et al. Utility of a paraffin section-reactive CD56 antibody (123C3) for characterization and diagnosis of lymphomas. *Am J Surg Pathol* 1996;20:202–210.
94. Pozdnyakova O, Morgan EA, Li B, et al. Patterns of expression of CD56 and CD117 on neoplastic plasma cells and association with genetically distinct subtypes of plasma cell myeloma. *Leuk Lymphoma* 2012;53:1905–1910.
95. Pongpruttipan T, Sukpanichnant S, Assanasen T, et al. Extranodal NK/T-cell lymphoma, nasal type, includes cases of natural killer cell and αβ, γδ, and αβ/γδ T-cell origin: a comprehensive clinicopathologic and phenotypic study. *Am J Surg Pathol* 2012;36:481–499.
96. Dukers DF, Vermeer MH, Jaspars LH, et al. Expression of killer cell inhibitory receptors is restricted to true NK cell lymphomas and a subset of intestinal enteropathy-type T cell lymphomas with a cytotoxic phenotype. *J Clin Pathol* 2001;54:224–228.
97. Ng CS, Chan JK, Hui PK, et al. Application of a T cell receptor antibody beta F1 for immunophenotypic analysis of malignant lymphomas. *Am J Pathol* 1988; 132:365–371.
98. Saresella M, Rainone V, Al-Daghri NM, et al. The PD-1/PD-L1 pathway in human pathology. *Curr Mol Med* 2012;12:259–267.
99. Gaulard P, de Leval L. Follicular helper T cells: implications in neoplastic hematopathology. *Semin Diagn Pathol* 2011;28:202–213.
100. Moroch J, Copie-Bergman C, de Leval L, et al. Follicular peripheral T-cell lymphoma expands the spectrum of classical Hodgkin lymphoma mimics. *Am J Surg Pathol* 2012;36:1636–1646.
101. Kanavaros P, Boulland ML, Petit B, et al. Expression of cytotoxic proteins in peripheral T-cell and natural killer-cell (NK) lymphomas: association with extranodal site, NK or T gamma delta phenotype, anaplastic morphology and CD30 expression. *Leuk Lymphoma* 2000;38:317–326.

102. Gadgeel SM, Bepler G. Crizotinib: an anaplastic lymphoma kinase inhibitor. *Future Oncol* 2011;7:947–953.
103. Drexler HG, Gignac SM, von Wasielewski R, et al. Pathobiology of NPM-ALK and variant fusion genes in anaplastic large cell lymphoma and other lymphomas. *Leukemia* 2000;14:1533–1559.
104. Ardini E, Magnaghi P, Orsini P, et al. Anaplastic lymphoma kinase: role in specific tumours, and development of small molecule inhibitors for cancer therapy. *Cancer Lett* 2010;299:81–94.
105. Rodig SJ, Shapiro GI. Crizotinib, a small-molecule dual inhibitor of the c-Met and ALK receptor tyrosine kinases. *Curr Opin Investig Drugs* 2010;11: 1477–1490.
106. Hans CP, Weisenburger DD, Greiner TC, et al. Confirmation of the molecular classification of diffuse large B-cell lymphoma by immunohistochemistry using a tissue microarray. *Blood* 2004;103:275–282.
107. Meyer PN, Fu K, Greiner TC, et al. Immunohistochemical methods for predicting cell of origin and survival in patients with diffuse large B-cell lymphoma treated with rituximab. *J Clin Oncol* 2011;29:200–207.
108. Tadmor T, Tiacci E, Falini B, et al. The BRAF-V600E mutation in hematological malignancies: a new player in hairy cell leukemia and Langerhans cell histiocytosis. *Leuk Lymphoma* 2012;53:2339–2340.
109. Tardío JC. CD34-reactive tumors of the skin. An updated review of an ever-growing list of lesions. *J Cutan Pathol* 2009;36:89–102.
110. Drew E, Merzaban JS, Seo W, et al. CD34 and CD43 inhibit mast cell adhesion and are required for optimal mast cell reconstitution. *Immunity* 2005;22: 43–57.
111. Nielsen JS, McNagny KM. CD34 is a key regulator of hematopoietic stem cell trafficking to bone marrow and mast cell progenitor trafficking in the periphery. *Microcirculation* 2009;16:487–496.
112. Lanza F, Healy L, Sutherland DR. Structural and functional features of the CD34 antigen: an update. *J Biol Regul Homeost Agents* 2001;15:1–13.
113. Orazi A. Histopathology in the diagnosis and classification of acute myeloid leukemia, myelodysplastic syndromes, and myelodysplastic/myeloproliferative diseases. *Pathobiology* 2007;74:97–114.
114. Kremer M, Quintanilla-Martínez L, Nährig J, et al. Immunohistochemistry in bone marrow pathology: a useful adjunct for morphologic diagnosis. *Virchows Arch* 2005;447:920–937.
115. Robertson PB, Neiman RS, Worapongpaiboon S, et al. 013 (CD99) positivity in hematologic proliferations correlates with TdT positivity. *Mod Pathol* 1997;10:277–282.
116. Dorfman DM, Bui MM, Tubbs RR, et al. The CD117 immunohistochemistry tissue microarray survey for quality assurance and interlaboratory comparison: a College of American Pathologists Cell Markers Committee Study. *Arch Pathol Lab Med* 2006;130:779–782.
117. Dirnhofer S, Zimpfer A, Went P. The diagnostic and predictive role of kit (CD117). *Ther Umsch* 2006;63:273–278.
118. Chilosi M, Pizzolo G. Review of terminal deoxynucleotidyl transferase. Biologic aspects, methods of detection, and selected diagnostic applications. *Appl Immunohistochem* 1995;3:209–221.
119. Sur M, AlArdati H, Ross C, et al. TdT expression in Merkel cell carcinoma: potential diagnostic pitfall with blastic hematological malignancies and expanded immunohistochemical analysis. *Mod Pathol* 2007;20:1113–1120.
120. Hoyer JD, Grogg KL, Hanson CA, et al. CD33 detection by immunohistochemistry in paraffin-embedded tissues: a new antibody shows excellent specificity and sensitivity for cells of myelomonocytic lineage. *Am J Clin Pathol* 2008;129: 316–323.
121. Pinkus GS, Pinkus JL. Myeloperoxidase: a specific marker for myeloid cells in paraffin sections. *Mod Pathol* 1991;4:733–741.
122. Tomer A. Human marrow megakaryocyte differentiation: multiparameter correlative analysis identifies von Willebrand factor as a sensitive and distinctive marker for early (2N and 4N) megakaryocytes. *Blood* 2004;104:2722–2727.
123. Wickenhauser C, Schmitz B, Baldus SE, et al. Selectins (CD62L, CD62P) and megakaryocytic glycoproteins (CD41a, CD42b) mediate megakaryocyte-fibroblast interactions in human bone marrow. *Leuk Res* 2000;24:1013–1021.
124. Merono A, Lucena C, López A, et al. Immunohistochemical analysis of beta3 integrin (CD61): expression in pig tissues and human tumors. *Histol Histopathol* 2002;17:347–352.
125. Ungari M, Pellegrini W, Borlenghi E, et al. LAT (linker for activation of T cells): a useful marker for megakaryocyte evaluation on bone marrow biopsies. *Pathologica* 2002;94:325–330.
126. Dong HY, Wilkes S, Yang H. CD71 is selectively and ubiquitously expressed at high levels in erythroid precursors of all maturation stages: a comparative immunochemical study with glycophorin A and hemoglobin A. *Am J Surg Pathol* 2011;35:723–732.
127. Marsee DK, Pinkus GS, Yu H. CD71 (transferrin receptor): an effective marker for erythroid precursors in bone marrow biopsy specimens. *Am J Clin Pathol* 2010;134:429–435.
128. Armeanu S, Bühring HJ, Reuss-Borst M, et al. E-cadherin is functionally involved in the maturation of the erythroid lineage. *J Cell Biol* 1995;131:243–249.
129. Armeanu S, Müller CA, Klein G. Involvement of E-cadherin in the Development of Erythroid Cells; Subject Heading. *Hematology* 2000;5:307–316.
130. Driesen J, Popov A, Schultze JL. CD25 as an immune regulatory molecule expressed on myeloid dendritic cells. *Immunobiology* 2008;213:849–858.
131. Dunphy CH. Reaction patterns of TRAP and DBA.44 in hairy cell leukemia, hairy cell variant, and nodal and extranodal marginal zone B-cell lymphomas. *Appl Immunohistochem Mol Morphol* 2008;16:135–139.
132. Sherman MJ, Hanson CA, Hoyer JD. An assessment of the usefulness of immunohistochemical stains in the diagnosis of hairy cell leukemia. *Am J Clin Pathol* 2011;136:390–399.
133. Kreitman RJ. Immunoconjugates and new molecular targets in hairy cell leukemia. *Hematology Am Soc Hematol Educ Program* 2012;2012:660–666.
134. Moore T, Huang S, Terstappen LW, et al. Expression of CD43 on murine and human pluripotent hematopoietic stem cells. *J Immunol* 1994;153:4978–4987.
135. Rupniewska ZM, Roliński J, Bojarska-Junak A. Universal CD43 molecule. *Postepy Hig Med Dosw* 2000;54:619–638.
136. Orazi A, Chiu R, O'Malley DP, et al. Chronic myelomonocytic leukemia: The role of bone marrow biopsy immunohistology. *Mod Pathol* 2006;19:1536–1545.
137. Garnache-Ottou F, Feuillard J, Ferrand C, et al. Extended diagnostic criteria for plasmacytoid dendritic cell leukaemia. *Br J Haematol* 2009;145:624–636.
138. Rollins-Raval MA, Marafioti T, Swerdlow SH, et al. The number and growth pattern of plasmacytoid dendritic cells vary in different types of reactive lymph nodes: an immunohistochemical study. *Hum Pathol* 2012;pii:S0046-817700323-1.
139. Guyotat D, Campos L, Thomas X, et al. Myelodysplastic syndromes: a study of surface markers and in vitro growth patterns. *Am J Hematol* 1990;34:26–31.
140. Wang SA, Hutchinson L, Tang G, et al. Systemic mastocytosis with associated clonal hematological non-mast cell lineage disease: Clinical significance and comparison of chomosomal abnormalities in SM and AHNMD components. *Am J Hematol* 2013;88:219–224.
141. Valent P, Sotlar K, Horny HP. Aberrant expression of CD30 in aggressive systemic mastocytosis and mast cell leukemia: a differential diagnosis to consider in aggressive hematopoietic CD30-positive neoplasms. *Leuk Lymphoma* 2011;52:740–744.
142. Pozdnyakova O, Morgan EA, Li B, et al. Patterns of expression of CD56 and CD117 on neoplastic plasma cells and association with genetically distinct subtypes of plasma cell myeloma. *Leuk Lymphoma* 2012;53:1905–1910.

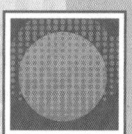

Chapter 4
Flow Cytometry in the Assessment of Hematologic Disorders

Kaaren K. Reichard • Steven H. Kroft

Flow cytometric immunophenotyping plays a central and critical role in the field of hematopathology in the 21st century (1–8). This role largely consists of characterization of myeloid and lymphoid proliferations, assessment for paroxysmal nocturnal hemoglobinuria (PNH), and evaluation of minimal residual disease (MRD). Flow cytometry (FC) is, of course, also a routine tool for evaluation of immunodeficiency syndromes, but discussion of those applications is beyond the scope of this chapter. The powerful ability of FC to rapidly and simultaneously analyze multiple antigens on hematopoietic cells and discriminate normal from abnormal has established FC as a valid and highly useful tool in the diagnosis of neoplasia (9–13). Consequently, flow cytometric immunophenotyping has evolved from being viewed as an "esoteric" ancillary testing modality available in only select centers to a widely used analytic tool.

Few would dispute that multiparametric FC rapidly generates information that is essential for diagnosis, classification, and prognostication of a number of hematologic disorders including acute leukemias and B-cell lymphoproliferative disorders. Newer applications of FC include assessment of tissue specimens for lymphoma; evaluation of prognostic markers in chronic lymphocytic leukemia (CLL) (e.g., ZAP-70 and CD38) and, increasingly, other hematolymphoid neoplasms; and detection of MRD (e.g., CLL, B-lymphoblastic leukemia/lymphoma, and plasma cell myeloma). Additional applications for FC in hematopathology include the assessment of mature T-cell and natural killer (NK)-cell lymphoproliferative disorders and as a component of the evaluation of myelodysplastic and myeloproliferative neoplasms (MPNs). These latter applications are not currently as routinely established in many laboratories, possibly due to lack of consensus on the utility of FC in diagnosing these disorders, variability in interpretative expertise, lack of experience, and lack of standardization of methods and approach across laboratories.

Because of the inherent power of multicolor FC to analyze multiple antigens simultaneously at a single-cell level, clinical laboratories are moving beyond traditional three- and four-color assays and turning to flow cytometers capable of detecting six, eight, or even greater numbers of colors. While such high-color FC is not necessary for traditional FC applications, which typically involve characterization of large and generally homogenous tumor cell populations, higher color FC enables more sophisticated, cutting-edge applications. The power of multiparameter analysis resides in its ability to distinguish populations in a virtual multidimensional FC "space." The more parameters that are assessed, the higher the dimensionality of this virtual space, leading to enhanced power to discriminate immunophenotypically (and biologically) distinct cell populations. What this allows is the robust and reproducible dissection of complex mixtures of cells populations, precise delineation of complex maturation patterns (such as in bone marrow myeloid populations), and detection of small abnormal cell populations in a predominant background of normal cells. The latter is the basis of MRD assessment in hematolymphoid neoplasia, an application that is playing an enlarging role in the monitoring of therapy

in various neoplasms. Multiparameter FC has the ability to accurately and precisely identify and characterize unique, aberrant patterns of expression of multiple antigens, allowing the discrimination of minute neoplastic cell populations against the "noise" of normal cell populations; the sensitivity of this analytic approach improves with the increased dimensionality of the data obtained from high-color FC (14). An additional advantage of high-color FC is that certain lineage-specific panels may now be almost entirely condensed into a single tube, enabling a more precise and complete assessment of the disease in question. For example, initial characterization of a mature B-cell process could be done in eight-color FC with CD19, CD20, CD5, CD10, kappa, lambda, CD23, and an open channel for another desired antibody (e.g., FMC7, CD45, CD103, CD200). Depending on the findings, a subsequent B-cell tube with additional diagnostic (hairy cell leukemia) or prognostic markers (such as for CLL) could be performed: for example, CD19, CD11c, CD22, CD25, and CD103 or CD19, CD5, CD38, CD49d, and ZAP-70, respectively. High-color FC also greatly enhances the evaluation of paucicellular specimens, such as cerebrospinal fluid, fine needle aspirates, and needle core biopsies, as markers needed for a thorough evaluation may be consolidated into fewer tubes (thus requiring fewer cells). Finally, a somewhat banal advantage of high-color FC is that it reduces redundancy of markers across multiple tubes in panels, thus lowering the costs of analysis. The main drawbacks of high-color flow cytometers are the upfront cost of the instruments and the substantially increased technical and interpretative challenges.

Other chapters in this book discuss the application of FC in specific neoplastic hematology topics; so the aim of this chapter is to present a general overview of FC in the practice of hematology. Topics to be covered include general principles of FC, analytical and gating strategies, technical issues and potential pitfalls in interpretation, and a high-level approach to the workup of various hematopathologic neoplastic categories. The text is generously supplemented with illustrative examples of key points. Details regarding the specific immunophenotypic profiles of particular neoplasms and differential diagnostic considerations are left to the other chapters.

 ## INDICATIONS FOR FLOW CYTOMETRY IN HEMATOPATHOLOGY

The number of indications for FC in the evaluation of hematologic abnormalities has grown greatly since its original clinical use to evaluate CD4+ T cells in individuals with human immunodeficiency virus-1 infection/acquired immunodeficiency syndrome (Table 4.1) (2,15,16). In 1995, a group of hematopathology experts convened in Bethesda, MD, and established consensus recommendations on the medical indications for FC, subsequently published in 1997 (16). The consensus group provided detailed recommendations for specimen type and quality, utilization, test ordering, interpretation, specific

Table 4.1	CLINICAL INDICATIONS FOR FC IN THE ASSESSMENT OF HEMATOLOGIC DISORDERS

Clinical and/or laboratory indications strongly suspicious for hematologic neoplasia
- Unexplained cytopenias
- Unexplained elevated monocyte count
- Unexplained elevated lymphocyte count
- Eosinophilia
- Hepatosplenomegaly, lymphadenopathy, extramedullary tissue mass (tissue biopsy)
- Monoclonal protein in serum and/or urine

Pathologic indications
- Lineage assignment in a new acute leukemia
- B-cell lymphoproliferative disorder
- Unexplained plasmacytosis
- Unexplained blasts or abnormal cells
- Amyloidosis
- Therapeutic antibody assessment (e.g., CD20, CD52)
- Prognostic markers in certain neoplasms (e.g., ZAP-70, CD38 in CLL)
- Response to therapy
- Tumor relapse/progression

Indications that are in various stages of integration into clinical practice
- MRD assessment
- Diagnosis of T-cell neoplasia
- Diagnosis and follow-up of plasma cell dyscrasias
- Diagnosis of MPNs
- Diagnosis of MDS

CLL, chronic lymphocytic leukemia; MPN, myeloproliferative neoplasms; MDS, myelodysplastic syndrome.
References: (15–18).

Table 4.2	ADVANTAGES AND DISADVANTAGES OF FC

Advantages
- Rapid results
- Multiparametric (assess multiple [4–10] markers simultaneously on a single-cell basis)
- 0.01% detection sensitivity
- Detect small abnormal populations in a background of normal cells
- Semiquantitative

Disadvantages
- Loss of tissue architecture
- Inability to correlate cytology directly with immunophenotype
- Certain markers not currently available for testing (e.g., infectious agents [Epstein-Barr virus], cyclin D1)
- Potential loss of tumor cells and/or antigens over time

hematologic disease categories, assessment of MRD, and utility in the setting of bone marrow transplantation. These medical indications still apply and are prescient with regard to the potential application of FC in the evaluation of nonacute myeloid disorders and MRD testing.

A second consensus meeting was held in 2006, aimed specifically at identifying clinical and/or laboratory indications (in addition to the already published medical indications) that would support the use of FC in the evaluation for a hematologic malignancy (16). The indications that this group proposed are based on the assumption that that there is a strong suspicion for a hematologic neoplasm and other potential etiologies for the abnormality have been excluded. These clinical indications include unexplained cytopenias, elevated leukocyte counts (excluding neutrophilia), plasmacytosis, monoclonal gammopathy, and tissue mass lesions. Clinical/laboratory findings that were thought to not be an indication for FC included neutrophilia, polyclonal hypergammaglobulinemia, erythrocytosis, thrombocytosis, and basophilia. These clinical conditions either do not typically associate with a hematologic neoplasm or, when associated with a hematologic neoplasm, are not detectable by routine flow cytometric immunophenotyping.

 ## IMMUNOPHENOTYPIC ANALYSIS OF HEMATOLOGIC DISORDERS: FLOW CYTOMETRY VERSUS IMMUNOHISTOCHEMISTRY

FC and immunohistochemistry (IHC) are complementary pathologic techniques with the same ultimate goal—the immunophenotypic characterization of hematopoietic populations. However, important differences exist between these two methodologies that may necessitate the choice of one or both techniques depending on the case type. FC has the advantage

compared to IHC of being rapid (results available within a few hours), highly sensitive, and semiquantitative (Table 4.2). It plays a particularly vital role in situations where solid tissue is not available for immunohistochemical evaluation, particularly in blood, bone marrow aspirate, and body fluid specimens. Perhaps even more important is the ability of FC to simultaneously query multiple antigens on (or in) individual cells, allowing for the distinction and precise characterization of complex mixtures of multiple leukocyte subsets. The main disadvantages of FC include the loss of architectural features, the inability to directly correlate cytologic and immunophenotypic findings, and the requirement for fresh, viable cells. Although FC and IHC are often viewed as alternative methodologies, they actually often provide complementary information. Practice patterns of utilization of these two immunophenotyping methodologies vary widely based on local preferences, but most hematopathologists think that it is necessary to have both available.

SPECIMEN COLLECTION

Essentially any specimen type may be submitted for flow cytometric studies. All specimens should be drawn in a sterile manner following appropriate safety procedures and should never be exposed to a fixative (19). Peripheral blood can be drawn into ethylenediaminetetraacetic acid (EDTA), acid-citrate-dextrose, or sodium heparin anticoagulant. Sodium heparin is the anticoagulant of choice for bone marrow aspirates. If conventional cytogenetic or fluorescence *in situ* hybridization (FISH) studies are anticipated, sodium heparin is the anticoagulant of choice. If a complete blood cell count is to be performed on the peripheral blood, then EDTA is the preferred anticoagulant. Body fluids, including cerebrospinal fluid, should be collected according to standard practice methods. Solid tissue specimens (bone marrow core biopsies, in cases where an adequate aspirate is not obtainable; fine needle aspirations; core needle biopsies; and excisional/incisional biopsies) can be placed in Roswell Park Memorial Institute medium for prompt delivery to the laboratory where disaggregation is subsequently performed.

SAMPLE QUALITY

Specimens should be delivered to the laboratory without delay and without exposure to extremes of temperature to ensure optimal processing and recovery of cells (19). This is of particular importance in cases where the tumor cells have a high proliferative rate and a predilection for rapid cell death. Suboptimal specimens are those that are partially or completely clotted, inadequately bathed in tissue culture medium, exposed to fixative, or exposed to a disproportionately large amount of anticoagulant. Each of these may result in loss of the population of interest, although even suboptimal specimens may often yield informative results. Procurement of an additional sample is advisable, if possible, when a sample is severely compromised.

It is recommended, in general, that most specimens be received and processed within 48 hours of being obtained. Although older specimens can still be analyzed, caution should be exercised when assessing immunophenotypic patterns, as certain antigens are labile and may be falsely negative, nonviable cells may interfere with interpretation, and light scatter properties may be altered. Similarly, the population of interest may no longer be viable, and a disclaimer as to a possible false-negative result should be offered.

Assessment of the proportion of viable cells in an individual sample is useful for knowing the relative degeneration of a submitted specimen. This assessment is most often performed by evaluating staining of nonviable cells. Nonviable cells take up dye (dye inclusion) due to an impaired cell membrane. Commonly available dyes are fluorescent, DNA-binding probes propidium iodide (PI) or 7-amino actinomycin D (7-AAD). It is also worth noting that it is generally possible to exclude nonviable cells in routine analyses based on light scatter properties.

FLOW CYTOMETRY: THE TECHNIQUE

The word "cytometry" derives from the Greek language and translates into the measuring (metry) of a cell/body (cyto). "Flow" cytometry refers to the fact that this measurement occurs when particles flow in a fluid stream. In hematopathology, we are typically accustomed to equating particles to individual cells. However, it is important to note that a variety of other particulate matter can be measured including viruses, DNA fragments, and bacteria.

The technique of FC applied to hematopathology is based on the ability to fluorescently label antibodies that recognize various antigens on the surface, in the nucleus, or in the cytoplasm of cells. A fluorescent dye absorbs light of a certain color and then emits light of a different color of a longer wavelength. After incubation with fluorescently labeled antibody, the emission of fluorescence by a cell after exposure to light of the appropriate wavelength generally indicates the presence of the cognate antigen recognized by the antibody. The ability to simultaneously utilize multiple antibodies to different antigens in a single tube requires that the different fluorochromes emit light at sufficiently distinct wavelengths to be discriminated from one another. If a single laser is used, the number of fluorochromes that excite at the wavelength of the laser and have sufficiently distinct emission spectra is usually limited to three or four. With additional lasers with different wavelengths and the use of tandem fluorochromes (combinations of two fluorochromes in which the light emitted from one fluorochrome is transferred to the second fluorochrome, which then emits at a longer wavelength), one can employ six, eight, or more different antibodies in a single tube. Lasers in common use include gas (argon, helium-neon) and solid state (violet, red diode, green diode, and blue). The excitation and emission wavelengths of commonly used fluorochromes are summarized in Table 4.3.

Cells in suspension are incubated with the fluorescently labeled antibodies and run single file past the laser(s). The point at which the laser beam and the cell flowing through the cytometer meet is often referred to as the interrogation or analysis point. If there are multiple lasers, then there are multiple interrogation points. The fluorescence from each cell passing in front of the laser(s) is collected by photomultiplier tubes (detectors), one detector per fluorochrome. Through a series of filters and

Table 4.3	COMMONLY USED FLUOROCHROMES IN FC AND THEIR MAXIMUM EXCITATION AND EMISSION WAVELENGTHS	
Fluorochrome	Excitation Wavelength (nm)	Emission Wavelength (nm)
BD Horizon V450	404	448
BD Horizon V450	415	500
PerCP	482	678
FITC	494	520
PE	496	578
PE-CY5	496	667
PE-CY7	496	785
PerCP-CY5	482	695
PI	536	617
7-AAD	546	647
Texas Red	589	615
Allophycocyanin (APC)	650	660
APC-CY7	650	785
APC-H7	650	785

BD, Becton Dickinson Biosciences.

mirrors, the light that reaches each detector is restricted to a specific wavelength band. Because the fluorescent light is weak, it is amplified logarithmically by the detectors and displayed on a log scale; the magnitude of amplification is dependent on the voltage supplied to the photomultiplier tube. A logarithmic scale is used to display the FC data because it shows a greater range of positivity, permitting the display of both positive and negative cells in the same dot plot. The fluorescence intensity for each particular fluorochrome is proportional to the amount (if any) of antibody bound to the cell. By extension, this implies that the intensity of fluorescence for each particular fluorochrome is proportional to the number of molecules of a given antigen on or in a cell. However, the precise relationship between fluorescence and antigen density is complex; thus standard FC should be considered semiquantitative.

Additional information regarding physical characteristics of the particles passing in front of the laser is obtained by collecting forward (narrow angle) scattered light and orthogonally scattered light (side scatter). Forward scatter is roughly proportional to cell size, while side scatter is related to cellular complexity (typically cytoplasmic granularity). Since this is scattered incipient laser light (not fluorescence), it is intense and does not require amplification. It is therefore commonly displayed on a linear scale. Note that the axis scales on two-dimensional dot or contour plots are unitless; the numeric designations refer to channel or "bin" numbers employed for the purpose of displaying data in the form of histograms and have no fixed relationship to the actual intensity of fluorescence or scattered laser light. Where a particular event or cluster of events appears in a two-dimensional plot depends on the adjustments of the gains and voltages applied to the scatter detectors and photomultiplier tubes, respectively. These are adjusted to include the events of interest in the window of analysis; such adjustments differ from instrument to instrument, and generally vary over time in a single instrument.

At the end of an acquisition of a single sample, each cell that passed through the cytometer will have a certain number of data points associated with it, depending on the number of parameters queried (e.g., forward scatter, side scatter, fluorescence color[s]). These data points are subsequently stored in a data file in the order that each cell/particle passed through the interrogation point(s). Acquisition of an adequate number of events is essential for accurate analysis. At least 10,000 to 50,000 events per tube should be acquired (19). For the purposes of MRD testing at a detection level of 0.01%, at least 100,000 to 150,000 events should be collected.

ANALYSIS AND GATING STRATEGIES AND INTERNAL CONTROLS

Once all data are acquired and stored, a software program, of which there are several from which to choose, is used to analyze the data. The goal of these analytical tools includes the identification, characterization, and quantification of normal and abnormal cell populations. These programs can typically display the stored data in one of two ways: single-parameter histograms or two-dimensional dot or contour plots. A histogram typically displays fluorescence intensity on the x-axis and the number of events in each fluorescence intensity "bin" on the y-axis. A dot plot displays each event as a single dot in a two-dimensional plot, with the location in the plot determined by the level of fluorescence for that cell with two different antibodies. When data are visualized in this fashion, events with similar levels of expression of the two antigens form visible clusters. Contour plots are similar to dot plots, but instead of dots corresponding to individual events, the density of events in different regions of the plot is conveyed by the distance between adjacent lines, similar to topographical contour maps (i.e., the closer the lines, the more dense are the events in that region of the plot). Two-dimensional dot or contour plots may be displayed for any or all possible combinations of scatter and fluorescence assessed in a given tube.

The identification of a particular population may occur via several analysis strategies. The population may be gated based on light scatter properties (FSC, SSC) and/or a fluorescent marker (e.g., CD45, CD34) (20–23). This approach tends to focus on a predefined position in flow cytometric space, with the assumption that certain populations are expected to occupy that space. Alternatively, the identification of distinct cellular subsets in a sample may be driven by the characteristics of the cellular clusters themselves. These cellular regions can be analyzed from numerous vantage points. This type of analysis is not predicated on any preanalytical presumptions.

Traditional Gating

The traditional approach to analyzing a flow cytometric data file is through a process termed "gating." Gating specifically refers to the selection of a population of interest within the complete data file, with subsequent focused analysis on that particular population. Analysis of all potential subsets within the complete data file is permitted, although the ungated subsets are typically suppressed from view during the focused analysis. If traditional gating analysis is utilized, all ungated data should be initially analyzed in order to determine the best placement of the gate which defines the population of interest (17).

Gates may be set in a variety of ways, although typically they are based on forward (FSC) versus side (SSC) light scatter properties or CD45 versus SSC plots. The various leukocyte populations normally occupy characteristic regions on FSC versus SSC or CD45 versus SSC, such that a "gate" can be drawn around a particular population or region of interest (Fig. 4.1). For example, the CD45/SSC two-dimensional dot plot is widely used to determine the "blast gate" (21). Subsequent displays show all of the events within the preselected gate as various combinations of the antibodies that were tested. Gates can be combined with one another using Boolean logic (AND, OR, NOT) and are also often used sequentially to hone in a particular population or aspect of a population. Back gating is also commonly used when it is unclear on light scatter where a particular gate should be drawn. A region is drawn around the population of interest using a particular fluorescence marker and then visualized on the light scatter dot plot to identify a more accurate region to gate. After gating is complete, based on internal cell populations or isotype

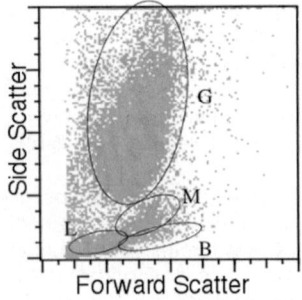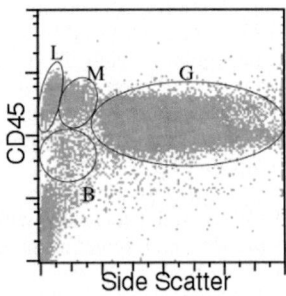

FIGURE 4.1. In traditional gating, regions of either forward scatter/side scatter (FS/SS) or CD45/side scatter (CD45/SS) *dot plots* are selected for analysis based on the characteristic locations of various cell populations. This figure shows typical gates for granulocytes (G), monocytes (M), lymphocytes (L), and blasts (B) in FS/SS (**left**) and CD45/SS (**right**) plots for a normal bone marrow sample.

control tubes, quadrants are assigned to denote positivity or negativity for various antigens on the gated population.

"Gating," as an analytical approach, tends to work best when dealing with quantitatively large and distinct populations of cells. It is generally less optimal for evaluating small populations, subtle immunophenotypic alterations, complex mixtures of multiple populations, a maturational or immunophenotypic spectrum, or MRD.

There are several limitations of the traditional gating strategy. These limitations are not insurmountable, but to overcome them requires a certain degree of expertise and patience. First, not all cell types fall neatly into a region that is identified by a traditional gating strategy. For example, CD45/SSC is a widely utilized dot plot to determine the blast gate based on moderate CD45 expression and moderate side scatter. However, some acute leukemias may show diminished, increased, or even absent expression of CD45 (e.g., B lymphoblastic leukemia/lymphoma is often CD45⁻) or increased side scatter (e.g., acute promyelocytic leukemia). Therefore, if one is using the typical CD45/SSC for gating blasts, the neoplastic population could unintentionally be left out of the typical blast gate analysis and potentially missed. In addition, some acute myeloid leukemias, such as AML with monocytic differentiation, do not show restriction of the blast population to a single "blast gate" but demonstrate a spectrum of maturation into the monocyte and/or granulocyte gates (24). As a consequence, limiting one's gating to the "blast gate" will not allow for the complete characterization of the immunophenotypic profile and full maturational spectrum of the process being evaluated. Second, "gates" are often established from just two parameters (e.g., CD45/SSC), rather than employing the full dimensionality of the multiparametric data to help discriminate populations (e.g., FSC, SCC, CD45, CD34, CD33, and CD19). This introduces some degree of imprecision, as "gates" are not comprised by a single pure population, but rather contain various admixtures of other contaminating cells, depending on the initial gate. For example, the "blast gate" as commonly determined by CD45 and SSC may contain a variety of other cell types in addition to blasts (e.g., basophils, monocytes, granulocytic precursors, hematogones, pronormoblasts) (25) (Fig. 4.2). Thus, immunophenotypic assessment of the blast gate may be imprecise/erroneous, particularly in specimens with a low blast count. Third, if one is using the CD45/SSC dot plot for gating, then CD45 is generally required in every tube to localize the specific population(s) from tube to tube. In some situations, a different antibody may be more useful than CD45 to discriminate a specific population in a particular tube. Fourth, assessing the comparative expression of various antigens relative to each other and to other cell populations can be challenging since all populations are not typically viewed together in the two-dimensional dot plots. Rather than having the analysis strategy determine the

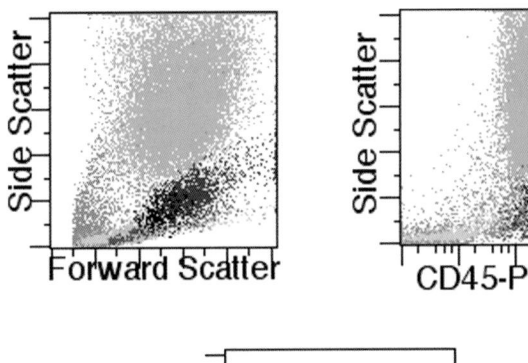

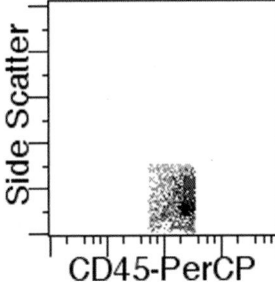

FIGURE 4.2. Locations of normal marrow populations in forward scatter/side scatter and CD45/side scatter plots, and composition of a typical CD45/side scatter "blast gate." The upper left and upper right plots demonstrate an ungated normal marrow containing granulocytes (*green*), monocytes (*dark blue*), lymphocytes (*light blue*), hematogones (*violet*), myeloblasts (*red*), erythroid precursors (*yellow*), and basophils (*black*). A typical CD45/side scatter blast gate of normal marrow contains multiple populations, with blasts typically comprising a minority (~20%) of events in this gate.

populations, particular population(s) should be determined and assessed based on immunophenotypic and scatter attributes. Fifth, using quadrants to assign relative percents of positivity for various antigens on a particular population may not be particularly informative, as it will obscure qualitative immunophenotypic features that may be of interest (e.g., multiple subpopulations, brightness of antigen expression) (17).

Cluster Analysis

"Cluster analysis" is an alternative analysis strategy to traditional "gating." This type of analysis, in contrast to gating, does not presume that certain populations should (or should not) have certain immunophenotypic or light scatter characteristics. Rather, cluster analysis strives to distinguish populations based on whatever features distinguish them in multidimensional flow space. Instead of applying predefined gating approaches, the characteristics of the populations themselves drive the analysis approach. Implicit in this strategy is the assumption that (i) biologically distinct cellular subsets form distinct "clusters" in multidimensional FC space and that (ii) distinct clusters in multidimensional FC space correspond to biologically distinct cellular subsets.

In cluster analysis, all events/populations present in a sample type are viewed as ungated data. Cell aggregates, nonviable cells, and cellular debris are generally removed. In each individual tube, as many of the various cell populations as possible are defined based on cluster formation, antigen expression, and light scatter characteristics. Typically, this is an iterative approach beginning with the two-dimensional dot plot that provides the greatest distinction between populations, and then refining that population through an iterative approach that employs all informative plots in a given tube. Arbitrary colors are assigned to individual populations ("color eventing"), allowing simultaneous visualization of all definable populations in a particular tube. It is evident from this discussion that the success of cluster analysis requires careful selection of antibody combinations/panels (see "Selection of Antibodies and Panels" for more detail), such

that populations of interest can be precisely defined, accurately categorized, and discriminated not only from one another but also from normal hematolymphoid subpopulations, if applicable.

There are several advantages to cluster analysis as the strategy for analyzing cellular populations by FC. First, distinct cellular subsets are readily captured, and a more complete, accurate, and precise immunophenotypic profile is established. These subsets are, by definition, not identified purely by CD45 and scatter characteristics but rather by the combination of antibodies in each tube. Immunophenotypic expression patterns can be determined by comparison with the other background cellular subsets. Second, small clusters of cells are recognized and amenable to complete characterization. For example, a small population of monotypic B cells is more readily identified in a polytypic B-cell background, because a focused assessment on that particular population is the strategy, rather than using an all-encompassing lymphocyte gate that generally contains a variety of cells (e.g., B cells, T cells, and NK cells). Third, by viewing all populations together in each tube, direct immunophenotypic comparisons can be made and subtle immunophenotypic aberrancies or shifts are detected. For example, subtle alterations in the fluorescence intensity of T-cell antigens in a particular T-cell subset can be directly assessed and compared to the background residual normal T cells. This may be the initial clue to the presence of a lymphoproliferative disorder. Fourth, populations with complex maturational patterns (e.g., hematogones, monocytic cells, granulocytic precursors) can be more systematically and precisely characterized. Predefined "gates" do not always contain the complete population of interest; therefore, certain key aspects of the hematologic process (benign or malignant) can be easily overlooked and lead to a misinterpretation. Additionally, by using the actual characteristics of the ungated events to determine distinct cellular subsets, a more complete picture of the relationships of cell populations to one another is revealed.

Controls

Critical for optimal interpretation of FC findings is the ability to reproducibly determine antigen expression (negative or positive) on various cell populations. Isotype controls are one type of control that may be used. An isotype control is an antibody of the same class of immunoglobulin as the specific antibody being tested, conjugated to the same fluorochrome as the antibody of interest, but directed against an irrelevant antigen. Isotype controls are good controls for nonspecific binding and autofluorescence. Internal negative controls are cell populations that do not express the antigen of interest. A negative internal population in a sample is sometimes substituted for an isotype control. However, it is important to recognize that different cell types show different degrees of autofluorescence and nonspecific binding of reagent antibodies (see "Selection of Antibodies and Panels"), and therefore the fluorescence of the population of interest must be compared to that of a similar population of cells (e.g., B cell for T cells, not granulocytes for T cells) (26). Internal positive controls are cell populations that express the antigen of interest. They serve to indicate that the antibody is reacting properly with a predicted normal population (e.g., bright CD33 expression on monocytes), and also may serve as an internal benchmark for assessing the level of antigen expression on other populations. Thus, the expression of markers on normal background cells is useful for assessing aberrant staining patterns of a suspected tumor population.

Selection of Antibodies and Panels

The selection of appropriate antibodies and construction of antibody panels requires a good deal of preparation and validation and is a key component to the success of flow cytometric immunophenotyping. A critical component of the selection process is vetting the interaction of the reagents and the antibody combinations themselves to ensure maximal separation of cellular subsets, discrimination of various populations, and accurately and reproducibly collecting qualitative and semiquantitative data on antigen expression.

Fluorochromes, which are variably conjugated with a number of antibodies, exhibit inherent differences in fluorescence intensity. For example, phycoerythrin (PE) and its tandem fluorochromes are the brightest while fluorescein isothiocyanate (FITC) and peridinin chlorophyll protein (PerCP) are less intense (14). A key consideration is to combine antigens that are more weakly expressed (in a particular cellular subset or disease state) with a brighter fluorochrome (i.e., PE), and a more brightly expressed antigen with a dim fluorochrome (e.g., FITC). Ideally, antibodies should be coupled with appropriate fluorochromes in specific tubes such that all signals can be reliably detected, excessive fluorescence is minimized, and signal to noise ratios are maximized.

Since most antibodies do not recognize antigens that are truly lineage specific, a sufficient breadth of antigens must be tested in order to identify normal and abnormal cell populations. This is becoming easier to accomplish with the use of eight-color or more flow cytometric instruments. An effective combination of these markers allows for the optimal discrimination and characterization of distinct cellular subsets based on antigen specificity for a certain cell lineage, stage of maturation, or aberrant expression.

Antibody panel selection in the evaluation of hematologic disorders can be approached in several ways. A generic, comprehensive panel may be used upfront, with the goal of identifying all possible populations that may be present in a sample. This is probably excessive for the majority of cases, and quite expensive as a routine procedure. Alternatively, a limited triage panel may be used to screen for the presence of an abnormal hematolymphoid cell population, with subsequent reflexing to a targeted panel based on the initial findings (e.g., blast characterization, abnormal mature B- or T-cell population). This approach has the disadvantage of lengthening the turnaround time of the study. An intermediate approach is to design semitargeted panels for various clinical and/or pathologic scenarios. These have sufficient breadth of markers for targeted lineages to cover disorders that are likely in a particular scenario (allowing time-efficient workups), but also contain sufficient markers to detect unexpected findings (which then may trigger additional workup). This approach requires a triage step in which the pathologist evaluates clinical information and, ideally, the morphologic features of a smear, imprint, or cytocentrifuge preparation. Lineage-specific panels efficiently yet confidently determine the lineage of the acute leukemia, B-cell lymphoproliferative disorder, etc. Finally, depending on the projected need, the panels should be sufficient to establish an immunophenotypic "fingerprint" of the neoplastic process in order to facilitate subsequent MRD analysis.

There are several important considerations in the construction of effective antibody panels (18,19,27–29). First, the combined antibodies must be able to adequately separate all cell populations. This requires that antibodies and fluorochromes work effectively in a single tube to allow for accurate separation and assessment of distinct cellular populations. Second, a robust gating strategy should be optimized for all tubes. Although FSC and SSC parameters may provide adequate cellular separation at a screening level, the presence of one or more lineage-associated or lineage-discriminating markers improves the overall gating strategy. Such gating strategies advocate for a "backbone" or "anchor" CD marker(s) as a way to reveal various populations. For example, the insertion of CD19 and CD3 further distinguish B and T lymphocytes from the otherwise "lymphocyte gate" on FSC versus SSC. Additionally, utilization of marker combination(s) that are geared specifically to distinguish and further characterize an individual patient's abnormal cell population is an even more effective analytical tool. For example, if a potentially abnormal

Table 4.4	FC ANTIBODY PANELS USEFUL FOR WORKUP OF AN ABNORMAL POPULATION DETECTED ON A TRIAGE PANEL
Lineage	**Possible Panel**
Mature B cell	CD19, CD20, CD11c, CD22, CD5, CD10, CD23, FMC7, CD25, CD103, kappa and lambda Ig
Mature T cell	CD2, CD3, CD4, CD5, CD7, CD8, alpha-beta, gamma delta, V-beta
T-cell LGL	CD16, CD56, CD57, KIRs, V-beta
NK cell	CD2, CD7, CD8, CD16, CD56, KIRs
Granulocytic	CD13, CD33, CD11b, CD15, CD16
Monocytic	CD36/CD64, CD14, CD4, CD163, CD11b, CD11c
Blasts	CD34, TdT, CD117, CD1a, CD10, CD22, cytoplasmic CD79a, cytoplasmic myeloperoxidase
Erythroid	Hemoglobin A, glycophorin, CD71
Megakaryocytic	CD41, CD42, CD61

LGL, large granular lymphocytic leukemia; KIRs, killer cell immunoglobulin receptors; NK, natural killer

CD3+, CD8+ T-cell population is identified, then subsequent analyses of CD2, CD5, CD7, CD16, C56, and CD57 expression based on CD3 and CD8 gating greatly increases the power of determining the immunophenotypic profile. Finally, such a strategic approach can be deployed for monitoring MRD after therapy.

Many different antibody combinations and consensus panels have been published, but these are generally just lists of CD markers that experts have agreed upon as useful to adequately characterize various hematologic disease categories (18,19,27–29). An effective combination of these markers varies from laboratory to laboratory and is often predicated on personal preference and experience (Table 4.4).

MINIMAL RESIDUAL DISEASE TESTING

Flow cytometric immunophenotyping has emerged as a primary methodology for the detection of MRD in several hematologic malignancies (CLL, mantle cell lymphoma [MCL], plasma cell disorders, and acute leukemia) (30–35). As a rule, the presence of MRD following standard therapy correlates with an increased risk of relapse. In addition to the traditional use of MRD testing as a tool for risk assessment, it is beginning to be used to guide treatment decisions, such as whether an individual should or should not be a candidate for allogeneic stem cell transplantation when a morphologic remission is achieved. Studies of the prognostic impact of MRD typically find that the risk of relapse can be stratified based on the size of the MRD population. Additionally, a lower level cutoff is usually established designating clinically significant MRD. In other words, very low-level MRD detected by highly sensitive methods may not be clinically significant, further emphasizing that MRD assessment needs to be quantitative. Importantly, the precise cutoffs and thresholds established to assess risk vary depending on the type(s) of therapy, extent of disease, timing of MRD assessment following therapy, the pharmacogenomics of the individual, and the genetics of the tumor type (36). Thus, at the present time, MRD analysis is best applied in the context of highly standardized protocols where the majority of those variables may be controlled. It is beyond the scope of this chapter to delve deeply into MRD testing in each of the various disorders, so this section is reserved rather for a general discussion of the application of this technique and a few disease examples.

MRD is defined as the presence of residual tumor cells at sufficiently low levels to be undetectable by routine conventional microscopy. Compared with other techniques that can be used to assess remission status, FC provides the unique combination of high sensitivity (at least 1 tumor cell in 10,000 cells, 0.01%), wide availability, general applicability, and rapid turnaround.

The major barrier to widespread use is interpretative expertise. One of the major criticisms of flow cytometric immunophenotyping in MRD studies is that the interpretation of the data is complex and highly observer dependent. A "nonexpert" who is lacking in significant knowledge of normal or reactive immunophenotypic patterns may miss or overcall MRD.

If FC is to be used to assess MRD, it is very useful to establish a distinctive and aberrant immunophenotypic fingerprint of the tumor cell population at the time of the original diagnosis. This aberrant signature will aid in the identification of any residual tumor cells during follow-up testing and discriminate them from a normal cell population. In the acute leukemia literature, such an aberrant phenotype is referred to as a leukemia-associated immunophenotype (LAIP) and can be detected in essentially 100% of cases of acute lymphoblastic leukemia (ALL) (37–39). Even if a predetermined LAIP is not available, a robust approach to analysis as described below will still allow MRD detection, although a broader panel may be required. Conceptually, the approach to MRD involves identifying a population in a region of multidimensional FC space where no population normally resides.

In order for a method to be useful in the evaluation of MRD, it must achieve adequate analytical sensitivity, be quantitative, and be reproducible. An analytical detection sensitivity of 1 tumor cell in 10,000 cells (10^{-4}) is currently advocated for MRD testing; this is attainable by the majority of FC laboratories. It is generally considered that in order to establish MRD, a cohesive cluster of at least 10 to 20 events must be detected in an abnormal location in a series of dot plots derived from a four-color (six-parameter) tube (40) Therefore, in order to attain a sensitivity of 10^{-4}, at least 100,000 to 200,000 events need to be acquired. Reproducibility of a population across replicate analyses or (preferably) additional tubes with different combination of antibodies greatly enhances the specificity of the MRD determination. In fact, the criterion of reproducibility may allow smaller aberrant clusters (e.g., five events) to constitute definitive evidence of MRD, although this hypothesis has not been tested in a rigorous fashion. It is also arguable that if an LAIP is defined based on a larger number of aberrant antigens in a high-color FC analysis, smaller clusters may be sufficient, since one is effectively shrinking the critical region of multidimensional FC space. Thus, high-color analysis should, in theory, improve both the sensitivity and specificity of MRD analysis.

Appropriate antibody selections and combinations are important for MRD detection. Panels should be designed such that patterns of antigen expression maximally and confidently discriminate abnormal population from the background normal populations. To accomplish this, a fairly broad panel of antigens should probably be tested at diagnosis to establish an LAIP. At follow-up testing, a more limited set of antigens may be tested to target the LAIP seen at diagnosis (37,41–44). Key to panel construction is enabling the analyst to assess the original aberrant immunophenotype, and also allow recognition of immunophenotypic shifts. In B-lymphoblastic leukemia/lymphoma, for example, it has been shown that upward of 70% of cases will show some loss of previous aberrancies and/or gains of new ones (41,43). Although too narrow of an antibody panel may result in a false-negative interpretation, a carefully constructed limited panel may identify most MRD populations (42).

Assessment for the presence/absence of MRD is a powerful prognostic indicator in pediatric B lymphoblastic leukemia (B-LL), both at diagnosis and at transplantation, and has been mainstay of the B-LL evaluation for over a decade (Fig. 4.3) (45–47). Children lacking detectable MRD at the end of induction chemotherapy have an excellent prognosis and are, in general, not in need of treatment intensification or hematopoietic transplantation (48–52). Children with high MRD levels at the end of induction have a worse prognosis and are in need of treatment intensification, alternative therapies, or transplantation (48–52). The persistence of disease is a remarkable predictor of risk of relapse, whether FC or PCR methods are utilized (53). Levels of MRD detection that serve as clinical management and risk stratification endpoints vary between 0.1% and 0.01% depending on the study (48–52). These thresholds can be achieved in most laboratories, although FC may not be as sensitive at levels below 0.01% (54). Persistence of MRD influences clinical decision making and may affect patient management. The timing of MRD measurements, types of specimens (peripheral blood vs. bone marrow) and MRD thresholds vary depending on the research center, but MRD assessment in pediatric B-LL is now standard of care.

In certain subtypes of AML, it has clearly been shown that the molecular demonstration of the absence, persistence, or recurrence of low-level MRD correlates with relapse-free survival (55–58). For example, in AML with t(15;17); *PML-RARA* fusion transcript, persistence of the fusion transcript following consolidation chemotherapy is a powerful predictor of relapse-free survival (59). Using multiparametric FC, a significantly higher rate of relapse was identified in AML patients in morphologic remission who had demonstrable MRD versus MRD-negative individuals (60). In pediatric AML, MRD values have been used both for guiding treatment decisions and for risk assessment (61).

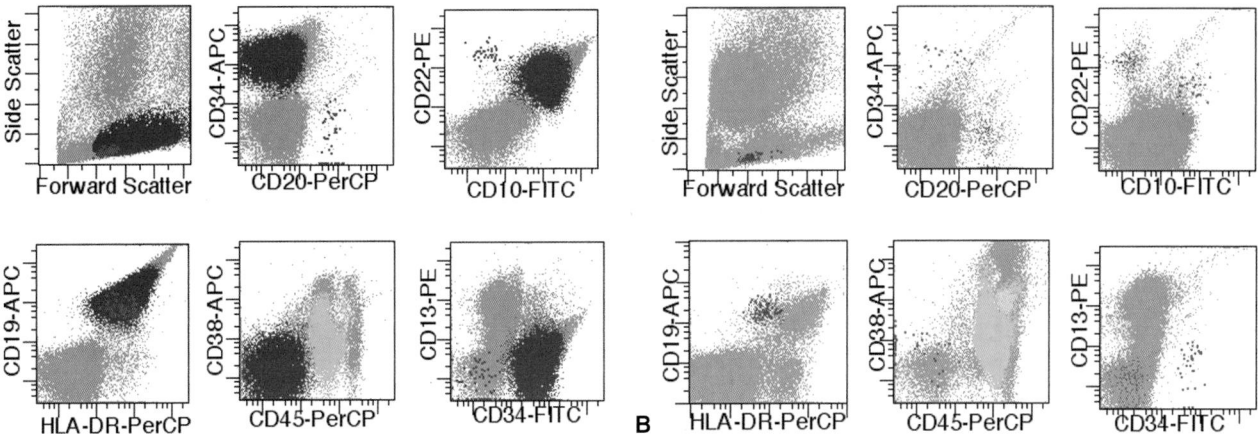

FIGURE 4.3. MRD in B-acute lymphoblastic leukemia/lymphoma. The neoplastic B lymphoblasts (*red*) at diagnosis (**A**) and following therapy at a level of 0.02% (**B**) demonstrate an essentially identical immunophenotype: CD34(+), CD20(–), CD10(bright+), CD22(moderately+), CD19(+), HLA-DR(+), CD38(–), CD45(–), and CD13(partial dim+). Also illustrated are mature B cells (*dark blue*), granulocytes (*green*), and monocytes (*light blue*).

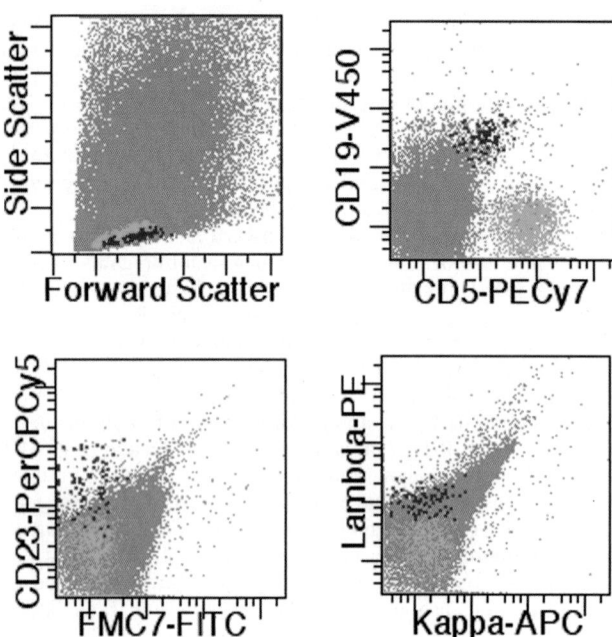

FIGURE 4.4.   MRD in CLL/SLL. In this example, there is a 0.06% population of events (*red*) that have similar light scatter properties as the T cells (*green*) and have a typical CLL/SLL immunophenotype [CD19(+), CD5(+), CD23(+), FMC7(−), and dim surface light chain (lambda)].

Flow cytometric MRD assessment in CLL/small lymphocytic lymphoma (SLL) and MCL is routinely tested as large studies have shown it plays a role in disease management and outcome prediction (Fig. 4.4) (32,34,62–65). In CLL/SLL, one study found that low levels of MRD (<0.01%) were associated with longer progression-free survival and improved overall survival compared to those with higher MRD (34). The MRD level was independently significant when assessed with other known prognostic variables (e.g., deletion *TP53, IGHV* mutational status, beta 2 microglobulin). In MCL, not only is FC more sensitive than morphology (as would be expected), it also correlates with disease presence at another anatomic site or recurrence (62). Furthermore, the detection of MRD may support clinical intervention and/or action (66).

 ## ASSESSMENT OF DNA CONTENT

The DNA content of cells can be determined by measuring the amount of PI staining in individual cells. The DNA staining must be done under fairly standard conditions because the degree of PI fluorescence that is emitted is assumed to be directly proportional to the amount of DNA in that cell. Determining the DNA index (test [tumor] sample/standard DNA fluorescence) is of importance in pediatric B-LL as a DNA index >1.16 and <1.6 generally correlates with a hyperdiploid karyotype and favorable outcome. Obviously, a limitation of the DNA index determination is that the specifics of any genetic gains, losses, or structural abnormalities are not known.

 ## FLOW CYTOMETRY: KEY TECHNICAL AND BIOLOGICAL CONSIDERATIONS

There are numerous technical and biological considerations that influence and impact the routine practice and interpretation of FC. These considerations include improper gating strategies, poor color compensation, doublets/aggregates, nonspecific fluorescence, carryover, atypical immunophenotypes,

and discrepancies between the FC and morphologic findings. Knowledge and expertise are generally necessary to command the optimal performance of this technology.

Color Compensation

One of the main technical problems in the interpretation of multiparameter fluorescence data is the fact that the emission wavelengths of different fluorochromes are not discrete. Rather, the fluorescence emissions from a given fluorochrome form a skewed distribution around a wavelength of maximum intensity with a tail toward longer wavelengths. The emission spectra of commonly used fluorochromes overlap, and there are variable degrees of bleeding of fluorescence from one fluorochrome into the detectors optimized for adjacent fluorochromes at lower and higher wavelengths. This spectral overlap must be accounted for in order to reliably interpret fluorescence data in multiparameter systems, and this correction process is known as "color compensation" (67–70). Briefly, color compensation involves electronically subtracting a portion of the fluorescence of one detector from that of an adjacent detector. The appropriate proportion to electronically subtract is most commonly determined using a series of one-color tubes for each of the fluorochrome/detector pairs using cells or reagent beads that have a high density of antigen-binding sites. The amount of bleeding into adjacent detectors is determined, and the appropriate correction factor is programmed into the instrument settings. Because there are multiple interactions to account for in a multiparameter system, the equation to solve for the appropriate correction factors is complex. While this can be solved manually, modern flow cytometers are equipped with software to accomplish this process automatically. It should be noted that the calculated compensation settings from a series of one-color experiments represent an approximation and do not entirely capture the complexity of the interactions between different fluorochromes; it is safe to say that there is no such thing as a perfectly compensated multicolor instrument (67). It should also be noted that changes in other instrument parameters such as photomultiplier voltage, detector integrity, laser intensity, and laser alignment will affect color compensation. Compensation issues can be minimized through appropriate construction of tubes (pairing brightly expressed antigens with dim fluorochromes and vice versa) and through regular verification of compensation using carefully constructed multicolor verification tubes.

The practical consequence of poor color compensation is the potential for misinterpretation of the positivity or negativity of antigens on populations. If an interaction is undercompensated (not enough fluorescence from one channel subtracted from an adjacent channel), a population may appear to express an antigen when it is actually negative (Fig. 4.5). Conversely, if an interaction is overcompensated (too much fluorescence from one channel subtracted from an adjacent channel), an antigen that is actually dimly expressed may appear negative.

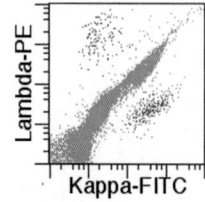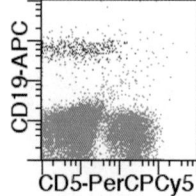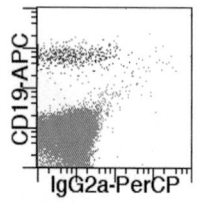

FIGURE 4.5. Poor color compensation. The lambda-expressing subset of this polyclonal B-cell population appears to be CD5(+), whereas the kappa subset is CD5(−). This results from undercompensation of the FL2 (PE) detector on FL3 (PerCP and PerCP-Cy5), whereby the bright CD19-PE fluorescence is bleeding into the adjacent detector. Note that the same phenomenon is observed when an irrelevant mouse antibody is used instead of CD5.

Doublets/Aggregates

Precise characterization of the immunophenotypic characteristics of populations assumes that cells pass in front of the laser singly. However, cells may at times form aggregates that pass through the flow cell as a single "event." In practice, this usually represents aggregates of two cells (doublets) and occasionally three cells (triplets); larger aggregates will usually be off-scale for forward scatter and will not be analyzed. The immunophenotypic features of doublets will essentially be a combination of those of the two cells that are adhering to one another, which may produce confusing immunophenotypic patterns. For example, B-cell/T-cell doublets will appear as large events that coexpress CD19 and CD3, and doublets of B cells may appear to coexpress kappa and lambda. Doublets of the same cell type will show increased levels of fluorescence for all positive antigens. Doublets of lymphocytes and granulocytes or monocytes will possess high side scatter, and thus will not be included in a typical lymphocyte gate, resulting in an underestimation of the number of lymphocytes. In general, lymphocyte doublets with granulocytes and monocytes are assumed to be indiscriminate with respect to different subsets of B cells or T cells. However, we have encountered a scenario in which either kappa- or lambda-expressing B cells preferentially form doublets with granulocytes. Investigation revealed that the dominant light chain type corresponded to the FITC-conjugated reagent antibody in the reaction mixture, whether kappa or lambda (unpublished data). Thus, this binding appears to be mediated through the FITC molecule itself. In such cases, restricting the analysis to the lymphocyte gate will result in skewed light chain ratios in the B cells.

The degree to which doublets are encountered appears dependent on the processing protocol; trial and error may be necessary to reduce the occurrence if it is problematic. In general, doublets are easily recognizable with experience, but occasionally additional investigation with custom antibody sets is necessary to resolve uncertainty.

Nonspecific Fluorescence

Cells that lack antigens reactive with antibodies present in a reaction mixture demonstrate nonzero fluorescence in each of the fluorescence detector bands. This is usually due to one or more of several different phenomena (71). Some degree of autofluorescence is a universal feature of mammalian cells and represents the natural emission of light by intrinsic cellular structures after they absorb light (72). The baseline level of autofluorescence may be easily determined by acquiring processed cell suspension without adding reagent antibody (Fig. 4.6). Nonspecific binding of antibody may occur through various mechanisms. Adsorption of soluble antigen may occur and cause apparently specific reaction with individual antibodies. Most problematic in hematopathology is the nonspecific adsorption of immunoglobulin onto the surface of leukocytes, which may then react with anti-immunoglobulin antibodies. Specific binding of antibody to cells may also occur through a nonidiotype/epitope mechanism: several leukocyte antigens (e.g., CD64 and CD32) represent Fc-gamma receptors that bind the Fc portion of certain subclasses of IgG.

In practice, when the task at hand is to determine whether antigens are or are not expressed on cell populations, it becomes critically important to discriminate specific binding of antibodies to their cognate antigens from nonspecific fluorescence. As previously discussed, a common practice is to employ as controls mixtures of irrelevant mouse antibodies of the same heavy chain isotypes and fluorochromes as reagent antibodies ("isotype controls") (Fig. 4.7). In theory, these will provide an aggregate assessment of the level of nonspecific fluorescence in various cell populations, and in practice they seem to serve this

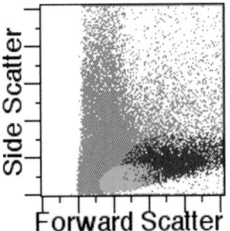
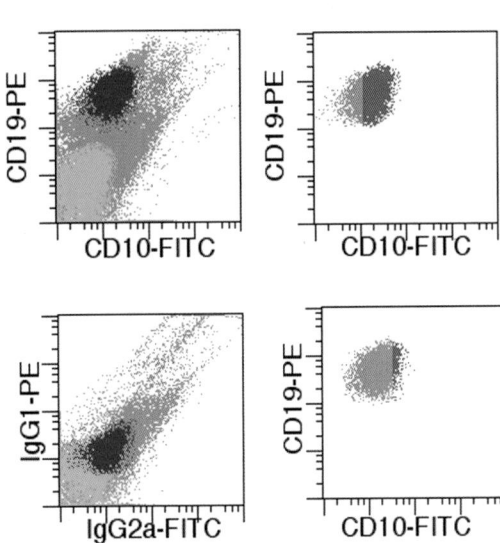

FIGURE 4.6. Increased nonspecific fluorescence in large versus small lymphoid cells. In this example of a diffuse large B-cell lymphoma, the neoplastic B cells (*red*) are larger by forward scatter than the background T cells in the sample (*green*). The neoplastic cells are CD19(+), and appear to be CD10(+), compared to the T cells (**second row**); if the T cells are used as a negative internal control to set a threshold for positivity, 77% of the neoplastic population exceeds the threshold (**middle row, right**). However, it can be seen in the isotypic control tube in the third row of the figure that the neoplastic cells have higher levels of nonspecific fluorescence compared to the small T cells. When the large cell population in the isotypic control tube is used as a negative control, only 7.2% of the population exceeds the threshold (**lower right**), indicating that the lymphoma is actually CD10(−).

purpose in most contexts accurately and reproducibly. Some practitioners forego the use of isotype controls and instead use internal populations that are expected to be negative for various antigens as an internal negative control. This practice ignores the fact that different cell populations have different levels of nonspecific fluorescence. For example, large cells in general

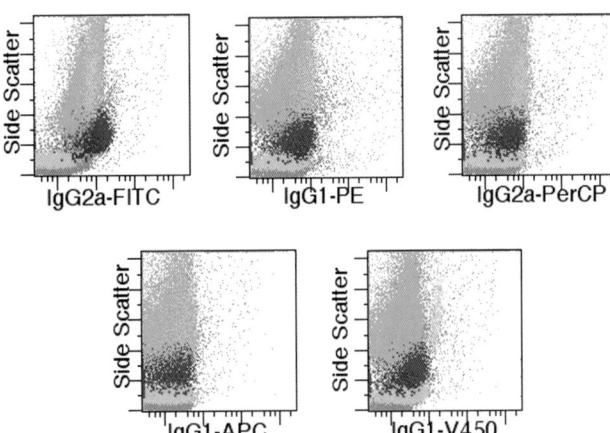

FIGURE 4.7. Nonspecific fluorescence on normal bone marrow populations with several irrelevant mouse antibodies of IgG1 and IgG2a isotypes and several different fluorochromes. *Green*—neutrophilic granulocytes; *yellow*—eosinophils; *blue*—monocytes; *red*—blasts; *cyan*—mature lymphocytes.

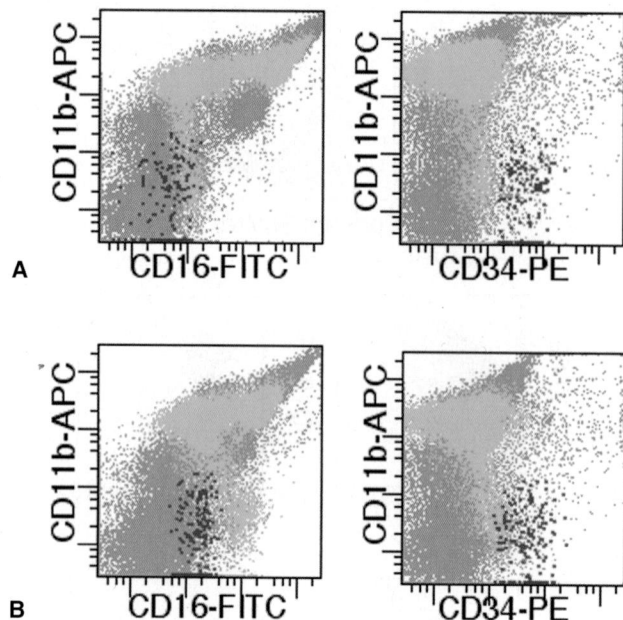

A

B

FIGURE 4.8. Effect of prolonged fixation on autofluorescence. This normal bone marrow sample was stained and fixed on day 0 and then acquired on both day 0 **(A)** and day 3 **(B)** (*green*—granulocytes, *red*—myeloblasts). Both the immature granulocytes [CD11b(−)] and the blasts demonstrate almost a log greater FITC fluorescence on day 3 compared to day 0. Notably, the more mature granulocytes [CD11b(+)] do not exhibit this effect. Note that both the immature granulocytes and myeloblasts are CD16(−) subsets. A similar, but less dramatic effect is evident in the same populations in the PE channel.

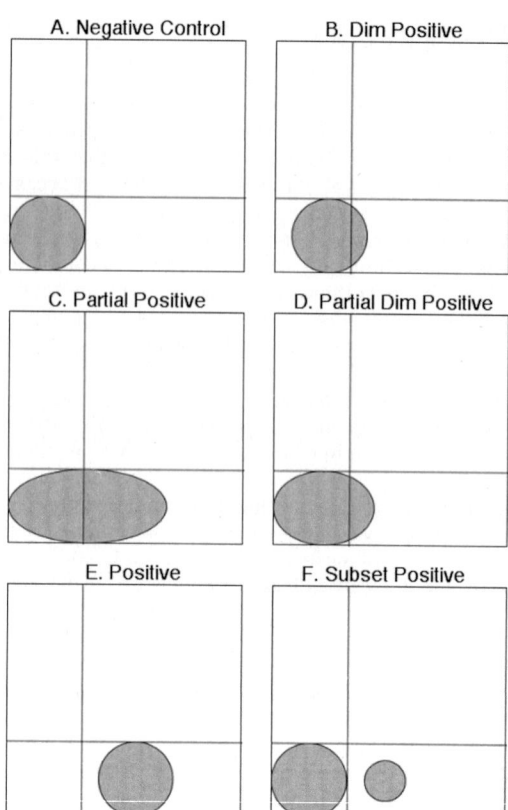

FIGURE 4.9. Examples of qualitative descriptors for antigen expression on populations. This idealized schematic illustrates how the pattern of antigen expression can be described qualitatively. **A:** Negative control. **B:** Compared to the negative control, a dim positive population shows a shift off the baseline without a change in shape, but still substantial overlap with the negative control. This pattern indicates uniform, low-density expression of the antigen on all of the cells in a population; although only a minority of the cells exceeds the threshold, all of the cells in the population express the antigen. The term "dim positive" is also sometimes used to designate an expression level that is lower than that seen in a normal population, even in situations where there is not substantial overlap with the negative control. Consistent usage should be applied to specific situations; additional language may be added to eliminate ambiguity, when necessary. **C,D:** In a partial positive population, the left side of the population remains anchored on the baseline, but the shape of the population becomes elongated, indicating variability of antigen density on the constituent cells of the population. Only a subset exceeds the isotypic threshold. The distinction between partial **(C)** and partial dim **(D)** is somewhat arbitrary; if the right side of the distribution overlaps with the level of fluorescence seen in normal positive cell populations, it can be designated "partial," whereas if it ends short of normal antigen intensity it can be designated "partial dim." **E:** A population is positive when the entire population is shifted and distinct from the negative control. Designation as "positive" or "bright positive" is often made relative to the level of expression seen on normal cells. **F:** Subset positive (**lower right**) is self-explanatory.

have higher levels of background fluorescence than small cells (particularly in the FITC and PE detectors) (Fig. 4.6). Plasma cells are another example of a cell population that often has high levels of nonspecific fluorescence. Furthermore, the level of autofluorescence on a population is not a constant. Dying and dead cells frequently have increased levels of nonspecific fluorescence. We have also found that prolonged exposure to fixative of stained and fixed cells (e.g., over a weekend) significantly increases the nonspecific fluorescence of some populations (e.g., blasts and immature granulocytes) but not others (e.g., lymphocytes and mature granulocytes) (Fig. 4.8). Without the careful use of an isotype control to determine the level of nonspecific fluorescence unique to a particular cell population, errors of interpretation regarding the presence or absence of antigen can and do occur.

The criteria for calling an antigen positive or negative are not clearly defined. A typical approach is to set a negative threshold for the population and antigen of interest based on an isotype control (or, less desirable, an internal population), isolate the population of interest, and determine what percentage of the population events exceed the threshold for that antigen. The precise cutoff employed is arbitrary; 10% and 20% are each commonly employed. It is important to note that the percentage of events exceeding a negative control threshold is not equivalent to the percentage of events positive for an antigen, although this is a common misconception. The actual number of cells in a population expressing an antigen depends on the shape of the distribution and the position of the population relative to a negative control. For example, if an entire population of cells expresses an antigen at low density, the shape of the population will remain the same, but there will be a shift relative to the isotype, resulting in only a minority fraction actually exceeding the isotypic threshold. Therefore, reporting qualitative descriptors of antigen expression on populations (Fig. 4.9) provides more information than listing a percentage of events exceeding an isotypic control (18). Along these same lines,

discrete subpopulations of cells expressing an antigen below the arbitrary 10% or 20% threshold may have biologic relevance, and probably should not be ignored. For example, in the 2008 WHO classification, a distinct myeloid blast population of any size in addition to a lymphoid blast population necessitates a diagnosis of mixed phenotype acute leukemia (73).

It should be noted that isotype controls do not control for reactivity with adsorbed soluble antigens. In the case of light chains, it is useful to include both kappa and lambda in the same tube and display them together. Nonspecific binding of immunoglobulins will result in a coordinate pattern of fluorescence in the kappa and lambda plots (i.e., the events will fall on a diagonal line). Since specific kappa and lambda expression on B cells is mutually exclusive, reactivity for light chains is determined not by distance from the origin in a two-dimensional plot, but by distance from the diagonal. A special case of nonspecific adsorption of immunoglobulin on cells is the scenario of "cytophilic antibodies" in the setting of polyclonal hypergammaglobulinemia. In this situation, there is so much nonspecific

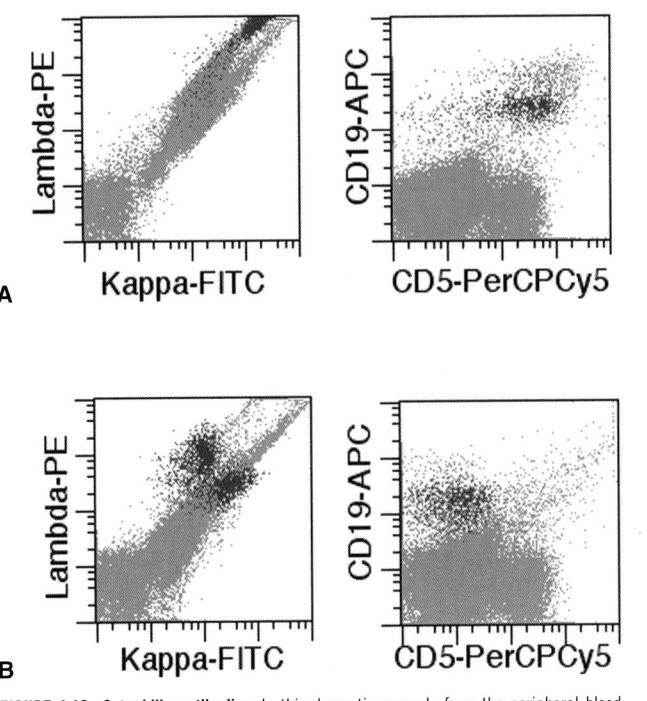

A

B

FIGURE 4.10. Cytophilic antibodies. In this dramatic example from the peripheral blood of a patient with severe polyclonal hypergammaglobulinemia, the B cells appear to brightly coexpress kappa and lambda (**A**). After prewarming at 37°C in phosphate albumin buffer (**B**), enough of the adherent polyclonal immunoglobulin has dissociated to allow discrimination of discrete kappa and lambda clusters. Also notable in this case was the apparent CD5 reactivity in the B cells in the unwarmed samples, which is no longer evident in the warmed sample. This is due to bleeding of the bright PE fluorescence into the PerCPCy5 detector, producing spurious CD5 expression. Under normal circumstances, this would be a minor compensation issue, but it is unmasked by the extremely bright PE fluorescence.

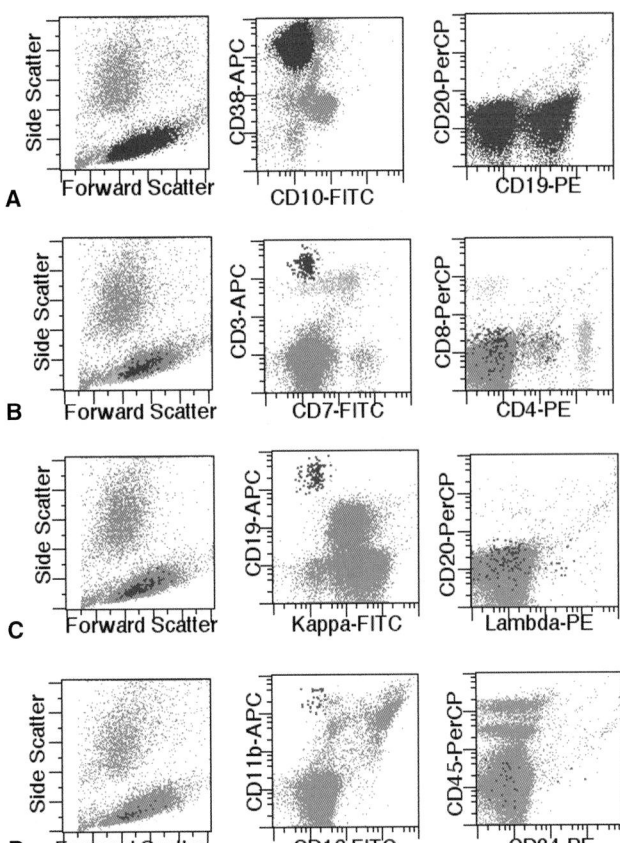

A

B

C

D

FIGURE 4.11. An example of carryover. This peripheral blood specimen contains a plasma cell leukemia population constituting 82% of events (**A**). The following tube (**B**) in the panel contained a 0.53% population of medium-sized cells that appeared to be aberrant T cells that were CD3(bright+), CD7(–), CD4(minor subset+), and CD8(–). The next tube (**C**) contained a 0.41% population of apparently aberrant B cells of medium cell size that were CD19(bright+), CD20(–), kappa(–), and lambda(few+). The last tube in the panel (**D**) contained a 0.11% population of medium-sized cells that were CD11b(bright+), CD16(–), CD45(–) and CD34(predominantly–). The populations in tubes **B–D** all represent carryover of the neoplastic plasma cell population from panel A. The cells in each population still are bound to the antibodies used in panel A, and therefore the populations occupy the same place in the histograms of each subsequent tube.

reactivity for kappa and lambda that the specific reactivity is no longer detectable. This manifests as a B-cell population located in the far upper right corner of a kappa versus lambda plot, with no distinguishable kappa and lambda clusters (Fig. 4.10). In most cases, this can be resolved by prewarming patient cells in a 37°C phosphate albumin buffer for 20 to 45 minutes (74).

Carryover

Occasionally, stained cells from an analysis tube may be adherent to the sample injector of the FC instrument and may dislodge with subsequent sample injections. This carryover can produce very confusing and misleading patterns (Fig. 4.11), since the persistent cells are stained with a different set of antibodies than the operator is expecting in a particular analysis tube. This is particularly challenging when the carryover occurs between two different patient samples. Careful comparison will reveal that these "aberrant" populations due to carryover will reside in the exact position in the fluorescence plots as populations in a prior tube. Some modern analyzers have the ability to flush the sample injector between tubes, essentially eliminating this problem.

Atypical Immunophenotypes

The theoretical basis of the immunophenotypic classification of neoplasia is that a particular tumor expresses a stereotypical pattern of positive and negative antigens. However, malignant cells frequently fail to adhere to textbook definitions, and atypical immunophenotypes are commonly encountered by practitioners who routinely analyze flow cytometric data. For example, CD10 and CD5 expression are fundamental features of the immunophenotypic definitions of follicular lymphoma and MCL, respectively, but a small proportion of cases of either

tumor may lack (or coexpress) these defining markers. Needless to say, this renders the diagnostic process considerably more challenging. It is therefore important in hematologic FC (as in any area of diagnostic pathology) to not rely on a single feature of a tumor for classification purposes, but instead consider the entire morphologic, immunophenotypic, clinical, and possibly genetic picture before rendering a final interpretation. It is also important to recognize that the immunophenotypic signature of a particular neoplasm in a particular patient may vary over time or across different anatomic sites, a factor that complicates follow-up analyses (41,43,75–78).

Discrepancies Between Flow Cytometry and Morphology

The foundation of diagnostic hematopathology remains morphologic analysis. This is particularly true regarding disease definitions that depend on numeric thresholds (e.g., blast or plasma cells as a percentage of marrow cells). Discrepancies between flow cytometric and morphologic counts represent another common pitfall in the analysis of FC. With respect to cell enumeration, FC may be considered truly quantitative only in the context of lymphocyte subset analysis in peripheral blood specimens under carefully controlled conditions. Analysis of bone marrow specimens is subject to several processing variables that are difficult to control, and thus FC cannot be considered an accurate means of quantification of different cell populations. For example, FC specimens generally represent a "second pull" marrow aspirate and are generally contaminated to varying degrees by peripheral blood elements ("hemodilution"). To address this issue, one study proposed the use of a correction factor based on the proportion of granulocytes that are mature based on bright expression of CD16 (79). Such an approach holds promise, but this area requires further investigation. Techniques to lyse erythrocytes also destroy variable numbers of nucleated erythroid cells, altering the marrow differential count. The latter factor can be controlled by using nonerythroid nucleated cells (CD45+) as the denominator of the calculation of cell percentages.

In the case of neoplastic blasts, flow cytometric enumeration may be difficult in situations in which the blasts lack clear-cut markers of immaturity (e.g., CD34, CD117) and/or overlap immunophenotypically with maturing cell populations. Additionally, contamination of the commonly used CD45/side scatter "blast gate" by other cell populations may artifactually inflate the apparent blast percentage (25). Conversely, the entire blast population may not be encompassed in a blast gate, leading to underestimation of blast percentages.

A variety of other preanalytical factors may result in discrepancies between FC and morphology. These include paucicellular specimens with an inadequate number of the cell of interest present for detection, specimens exposed to extreme temperatures or fixative diminishing cell viability and antigen preservation, specimens that are poorly viable, and specimens that contain highly proliferative tumor cells requiring prompt processing. In addition, some neoplasms (e.g., lymphomas and plasma cell myeloma) may show focal (rather than diffuse) tissue involvement, and therefore sampling differences may yield discrepant results between morphology and FC.

FLOW CYTOMETRY: GENERAL APPROACH TO HEMATOLOGIC NEOPLASIA

The identification, diagnosis, and subclassification of hematologic disorders by FC demand baseline recognition of the normal scatter patterns, antigenic profiles, and maturational spectrums of all distinct cellular subsets. Abnormal populations are typically identified and discriminated from normal using a combination of these parameters, and further testing is suggested as necessary (cytogenetics, FISH, PCR, gene sequencing). The final diagnosis of a hematologic neoplasm derives from the integration of clinical, laboratory, morphologic, immunophenotypic, and genetic data and should follow the WHO 2008 classification (1).

A detailed discussion of the immunophenotypic characteristics of each disease category and subtype is beyond the scope of this chapter. However, a general flow cytometric approach to the broad disease categories and their associated immunophenotypic attributes are presented.

Acute Leukemia

FC is indicated in the initial evaluation and workup of acute leukemia. FC determines lineage (myeloid, lymphoid, mixed phenotype, undifferentiated) and certain subtypes (B, T, acute promyelocytic leukemia) that affect disease prognosis, therapy, and posttherapy monitoring. While lineage assignment can be rendered via IHC, there are several significant advantages of FC. First, FC is rapid and can provide an in-depth and extensive immunophenotypic profile within a

few hours. Second, certain immunophenotypic profiles may suggest specific underlying recurrent genetic abnormalities for which a directed rapid genetic assessment could be made. Third, aberrant and cross-lineage antigen expression is readily detected, which may serve as a useful marker for minimal residual monitoring, or to identify the rare cases of mixed phenotype acute leukemias. Finally, quantitative assessment of aberrant weak or strong antigen expression assists in following residual disease.

Using a traditional gating strategy, blasts are usually identified using a CD45 versus side scatter plot given their low side scatter and weak CD45 expression. In such a two-dimensional dot plot, blasts can generally be distinguished from lymphocytes (bright CD45 expression), granulocytes, and precursors (high side scatter) and monocytes (higher side scatter and brighter CD45). However, the so-called "blast gate" is often contaminated with other cell types (e.g., basophils, monocytes, granulocytes, hematogones), such that a pure population of blasts is generally not present, introducing varying degrees of imprecision into the immunophenotypic characterization of the blasts (25) While CD45 is useful for discriminating various populations, neoplasms do not necessarily recapitulate their normal precursors and certain populations may be missed. For example, some B-lymphoblastic leukemia/lymphomas are CD45-. Therefore, regardless of the "gate" selected, a robust and methodical assessment of all events in each case is necessary.

Acute Myeloid Leukemia

AML comprises a heterogeneous group of disorders that are subdivided into four general categories by the WHO; AML with a recurrent genetic abnormality, therapy-related AML, AML with myelodysplasia-related changes, and AML, not otherwise specified (80–83). The blasts in AML may show differentiation along the neutrophilic, monocytic, megakaryocytic, or erythroid lines.

AML is currently defined by the presence of ≥20% blasts/blast equivalents in the bone marrow by morphologic assessment. The exceptions to this definition are the "low blast count" AMLs that may harbor a t(8;21), inv(16), or t(15;17). The finding of any of these recurring genetic abnormalities is diagnostic of AML regardless of blast count.

Flow cytometric immunophenotyping should not serve as a surrogate for the morphologic blast count as the blast percentages may differ due to hemodilution, imprecise gating technique, lysis of red blood cell (RBC) precursors, sampling issues, and loss of blasts during processing. Although FC should not be used as a blast enumeration tool, it is considered the standard-of-care technique to characterize the blast immunophenotypic profile in every new case of acute leukemia. The role of FC in the assessment of a putative new acute leukemia is (i) to determine the presence of blasts/immature cells, (ii) to determine lineage (myeloid, lymphoid), (iii) to establish the immunophenotypic profile, and (iv) to identify unique phenotypic features that suggest a possible genetic correlate (e.g., t(8;21) in AML expressing CD19 and CD56).

The diagnosis of AML by FC typically involves demonstrating cellular immaturity (e.g., CD34, CD117, TdT) coupled with expression of myeloid-associated antigens (e.g., CD13, CD33, and myeloperoxidase) (84). The expression of myeloperoxidase is considered diagnostic of myeloid lineage. It should be mentioned that although CD13 and CD33 are myeloid-associated markers, they are frequently present on lymphoblastic leukemias. Similarly, TdT is typically associated with lymphoblastic leukemias but may be detected in 10% to 20% of AMLs. In addition, aberrant expression of lymphoid-associated markers (e.g., CD2, CD7, CD19) is not uncommon in AML (Fig. 4.12A). Designation of AML as monocytic, erythroid, or megakaryocytic is

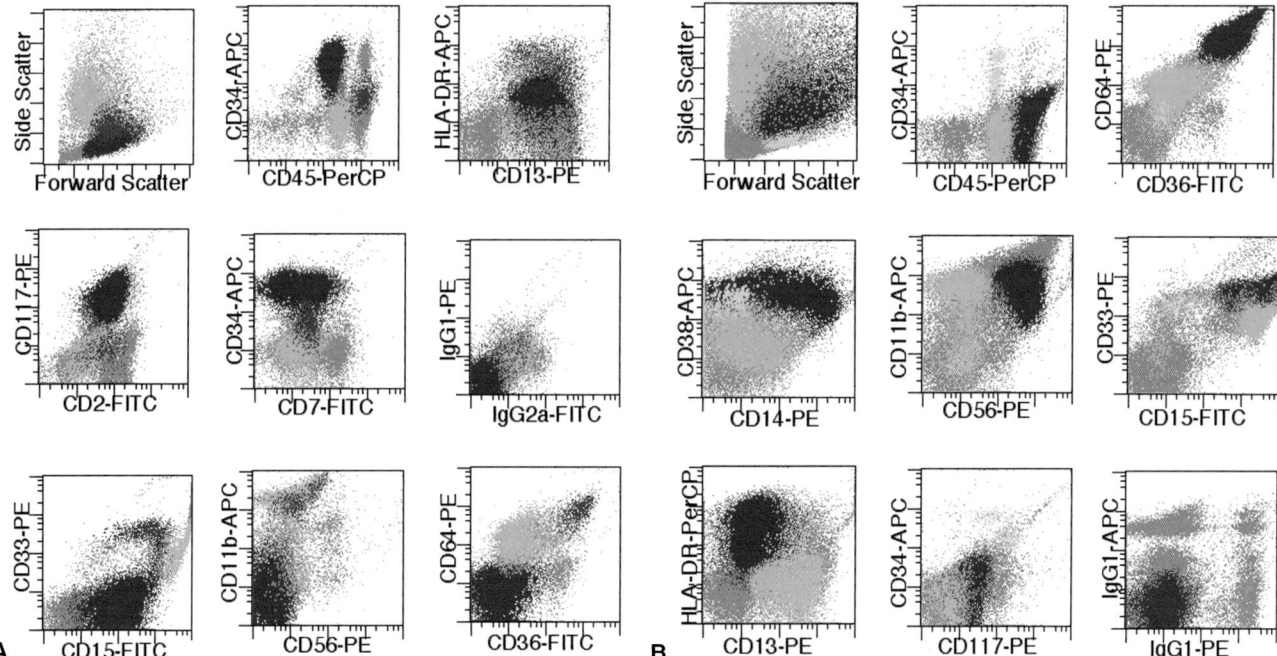

FIGURE 4.12. Two examples of AML at diagnosis. A: In this example of AML, not otherwise specified, there is a large population of blasts (*red*) in the typical low side scatter blast region that express the markers of immaturity CD34 and CD117. The blasts express the myeloid markers CD117, CD13, CD15, and intracytoplasmic myeloperoxidase (not shown). They lack the markers of myelomonocytic differentiation CD36 and CD64, but do asynchronously express CD15, as well showing partial dim expression of CD11b. Other aberrant immunophenotypic findings relative to normal myeloid blasts include expression of the T/NK-associated antigens CD2 and CD7 (compare to isotypic control, **middle right**), predominant lack of CD33, and underexpression of HLA-DR. Maturing granulocytes are illustrated in *green*, monocytes in *blue*. **B:** In this example of acute monoblastic leukemia, the monoblasts (*red*) closely resemble mature monocytes, in that they show light scatter properties approximating normal monocytes; lack the stem cell marker CD34; coexpress CD36, CD64, and CD11b; and show bright expression of CD33 and CD45. However, they show only partial expression of the mature monocyte marker CD14 and show dim C117 expression (compare to the isotypic control, **lower right**). Note that CD15 expression is uniformly bright, whereas on normal monocytes there is variable CD15 expression; this finding is of interest because normal immature monocytes express bright CD15, and then this antigen is down-regulated with maturation. Other aberrant features of this population (compared to normal monocytes) are dim CD13, expression of CD56 (common in monocytic AMLs), and variable HLA-DR. Note also the presence of a minor (1%) population of CD34(+) myeloblasts (*yellow*). These lack evidence of monocytic differentiation, in that they are negative for CD14, CD36, CD64, and CD11b. However, they are aberrant relative to normal myeloid blasts, in that they show a biphasic pattern of both CD34 and CD117 and are abnormally variable for CD33. Maturing granulocytes are shown in *green*.

based on differential antigen expression. Monocytic leukemias may express CD4, CD14, CD11b, CD11c, CD36, CD64, CD68, and/or CD163 (Fig. 4.12B). Importantly, they are often negative for the traditional immature markers CD117 and CD34. Erythroid differentiation is demonstrated by expression of glycophorin A, hemoglobin A, CD36, and bright CD71. CD71 (the transferrin receptor) in and of itself is not specific for erythroid lineage as it may be seen in various AML subtypes and also in other hematopoietic disorders (e.g., lymphoma) and non-hematopoietic neoplasms (various carcinomas). Megakaryocytic differentiation is evidenced by expression of CD41, CD42, and CD61. Care should be taken to exclude the possibility of nonspecific binding of platelets on the blasts or platelet coincidence prior to rendering a diagnosis of acute megakaryoblastic leukemia.

In addition to diagnosing AML, flow cytometric analysis may suggest particular genetic subtypes of AML by virtue of the composite immunophenotypic attributes. For example, AML with t(15;17) (a.k.a. acute promyelocytic leukemia) often shows high side scatter and lacks expression of CD34 and HLA-DR compared with typical blasts. However, this immunophenotypic profile is not specific for APL, and the diagnosis requires correlation with cytology, myeloperoxidase cytochemistry, and/or genetics. Furthermore, a significant minority of APL cases, particularly the hypogranular variant, shows varying degrees of CD34 positivity, potentially leading to the lack of recognition of APL by FC. AML subtypes that may be suggested by their immunophenotypic characteristics are shown in Table 4.5.

Acute Lymphoblastic Leukemia/Lymphoma

ALL is a blastic neoplasm derived from B- or T-cell precursors (B lymphoblastic (a.k.a. precursor B-cell acute lymphoblastic leukemia/lymphoma) and T lymphoblastic (a.k.a. precursor T-cell acute lymphoblastic leukemia/lymphoma) (90–92). Of all pediatric and adult ALL cases, over 80% are of B lineage.

Table 4.5	AML IMMUNOPHENOTYPIC CHARACTERISTICS THAT MAY SUGGEST A PARTICULAR GENETIC CORRELATE	
AML Subtype	**Usual Immunophenotypic Characteristics**	**Comments**
AML with t(15;17)	CD34−, HLA-DR−, CD117+ CD13+, CD33+, high SSC	Substantial minority may show CD34+
AML with t(8;21)	CD34+, CD19+, CD56+, myeloid-associated antigens+	
AML with inv16	CD2+ monocytes, increased eosinophils	
Cytogenetically normal AML with mutated *NPM1* and *FLT3*-ITD wildtype	CD34(−)/weak, CD4+, CD19(+/-), CD56(+/-), HLA-DR(−)	

References: (24,85–89)

B Lymphoblastic Leukemia/Lymphoma

B-LL is defined by the expression of B-lineage–associated antigens on blasts that lack defining features of T-cell or myeloid differentiation. The current WHO 2008 classification definitions for T-, B-, and myeloid lineage are summarized in Table 4.6. A typical immunophenotypic profile for B-LL is CD34+, CD19+, CD22+, CD10+, HLA-DR+, TdT+, surface light chain (–) and dim to negative CD45 (90).

CD19 is not completely specific for B-LL, as it may be seen in a small subset of AMLs, particularly those harboring the genetic abnormality t(8;21)(q22;q22); *RUNX1-RUNX1T1* fusion or cytogenetic variant. CD22 may be detected in virtually all B-LLs and is reportedly rare in AML. CD20 may also be variably detected on B-LL. Kappa and lambda surface light chain expression is negative in the majority of B-LL cases (>95%). However, a small subset of B-LL cases may demonstrate surface light chain expression that may initially lead to confusion and misdiagnosis of a mature B-cell process (Fig. 4.13).

Additional antigens that are not lineage associated but play an important diagnostic role in conjunction with the B-cell markers include CD34, TdT, CD10, and CD45. CD34 and TdT establish an immature phenotype (i.e., blasts), but do not distinguish B-LL from AML or T-lymphoblastic leukemia (T-LL). CD10 (a.k.a. CALLA, common ALL antigen) is expressed in normal B-cell precursors/hematogones as well as B-LL and T-LL.

Aberrant coexpression of the myeloid-associated markers CD13 and CD33 is common in B-LL, and should not lead to confusion in the diagnosis of an otherwise straightforward B-LL. These markers are frequently present in cases showing the genetic abnormalities *BCR-ABL1* and *ETV6-RUNX1* associated with t(9;22)(q34;q11.2) and cryptic t(12;21)(p13;q22), respectively (91).

Certain immunophenotypic profiles have been noted to correlate with particular genetic abnormalities that may be of prognostic significance. For example, B-LL that is CD10(–) and CD15(+) is often associated with the t(4;11)(q21;q23); *AFF1-MLL* fusion (91). Also, while a CD20(–), CD34(–), CD9+ phenotype is associated with the t(1;19)(q23;p13); *PBX1-TCF3* fusion, this is not specific (91).

The main differential diagnostic consideration for B-LL is hematogone hyperplasia. Hematogone is the commonly used term for normal maturing B-cell precursors in the bone marrow. These cells are detectable in the majority of patients with a wide variety of clinical disorders. Recognition of these cells is important for at least three reasons: (i) they are morphologically and (ii) immunophenotypically similar to B lymphoblasts and (iii) they are often increased in postchemotherapy/posttransplantation bone marrows. Although similar immunophenotypically, hematogones and B lymphoblasts are not identical and thus can be distinguished using multiparametric FC.

Hematogones demonstrate a continuous and highly reproducible maturation spectrum, in contrast to B lymphoblasts that show immunophenotypic aberrancies and maturation

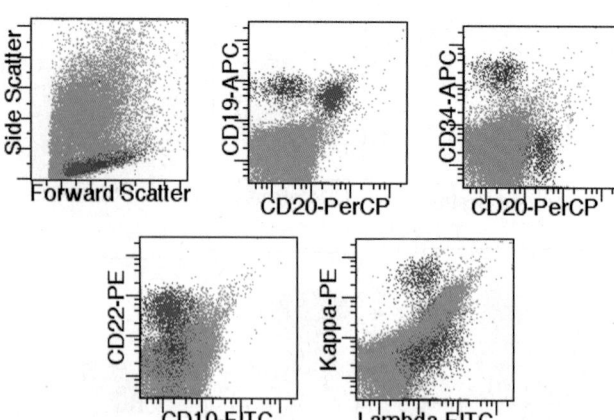

FIGURE 4.13. Surface immunoglobulin-positive B-acute lymphoblastic leukemia/lymphoma (B-ALL). In this example of CD34(+) B-ALL, the neoplastic lymphoblasts (*red*) express weak surface lambda light chain. Mature B cells are also illustrated (*blue*).

arrest (37,41,93–95). The normal maturational pattern of hematogones is shown in Figure 4.14A, and the antigenic pattern is summarized in the figure legend. An antigen combination that is particularly helpful in identifying hematogones and highlighting the maturation pattern is CD45, CD19, CD20, CD10, and CD38. B lymphoblasts deviate from the hematogone maturational pattern in all cases, usually in multiple ways. For example, B lymphoblasts may show uniform expression of CD34 and/or TdT, bright expression of CD10, and/or aberrant myeloid antigen (e.g., CD33) expression (Fig. 4.14B).

A second differential diagnostic challenge is distinguishing the rare case of B-lymphoblastic leukemia/lymphoma with surface light chain (sIg) expression from a mature B-cell lymphoma (96–98). Approximately 5% of B-LL cases are sIg positive, but fortunately the vast majority express CD34 and/or TdT, providing immunophenotypic evidence of immaturity (Fig. 4.13). In addition, most sIg+ B-LL cases show dim or absent CD45 expression. Given that most of the sIg+ B-LL cases express CD10, this raises consideration of Burkitt leukemia/lymphoma, follicular lymphoma, and large B-cell lymphoma. Rarely, one encounters *MLL* gene-rearranged B-LLs that lack both CD34 and TdT; these may also express surface immunoglobulin, but other immunophenotypic features (e.g., lack of CD20, dim CD45) are suggestive of an immature process. Blastoid variants of mature B-cell neoplasms must be excluded in this scenario; the identification of an *MLL* gene rearrangement and lack of mature B-cell lymphoma–associated genetic abnormalities by cytogenetic analysis will confirm a diagnosis of B-LL.

T-Lymphoblastic Leukemia/Lymphoma

T-LL is defined by the expression of T–lineage associated antigens on blasts without otherwise defining features of B-cell or myeloid differentiation (Table 4.6) (92). Expression of CD3 (cytoplasmic and/or surface) is considered lineage specific for T-cell derivation. Given that AMLs frequently express T–cell associated antigens (e.g., CD7, CD2), and that mixed phenotype acute leukemias comprise approximately 5% of all acute leukemias, careful immunophenotypic and cytochemical assessment is required for the best interpretation and subclassification of acute leukemia.

T-LL often presents with a mediastinal mass, and distinction from normal thymus tissue/thymoma can be problematic, particularly in limited tissue specimens. The main difficulty rests in the fact that most thymomas are composed, in part, of a population of immature thymocytes that show variable expression

Table 4.6	WORLD HEALTH ORGANIZATION DEFINITIONS FOR ASSIGNING BLAST LINEAGE (1)	
Lineage	**Definition**
B cell	Strong CD19 expression with ≥1 of strong expression of CD79a, cytoplasmic CD22 or CD10 Weak CD19 expression with ≥2 of strong expression of CD79a, cytoplasmic CD22 or CD10
T cell	Surface or cytoplasmic CD3
Myeloid	Myeloperoxidase or ≥2 NSE, CD11c, CD14, CD36, CD64, lysozyme for monocytic differentiation

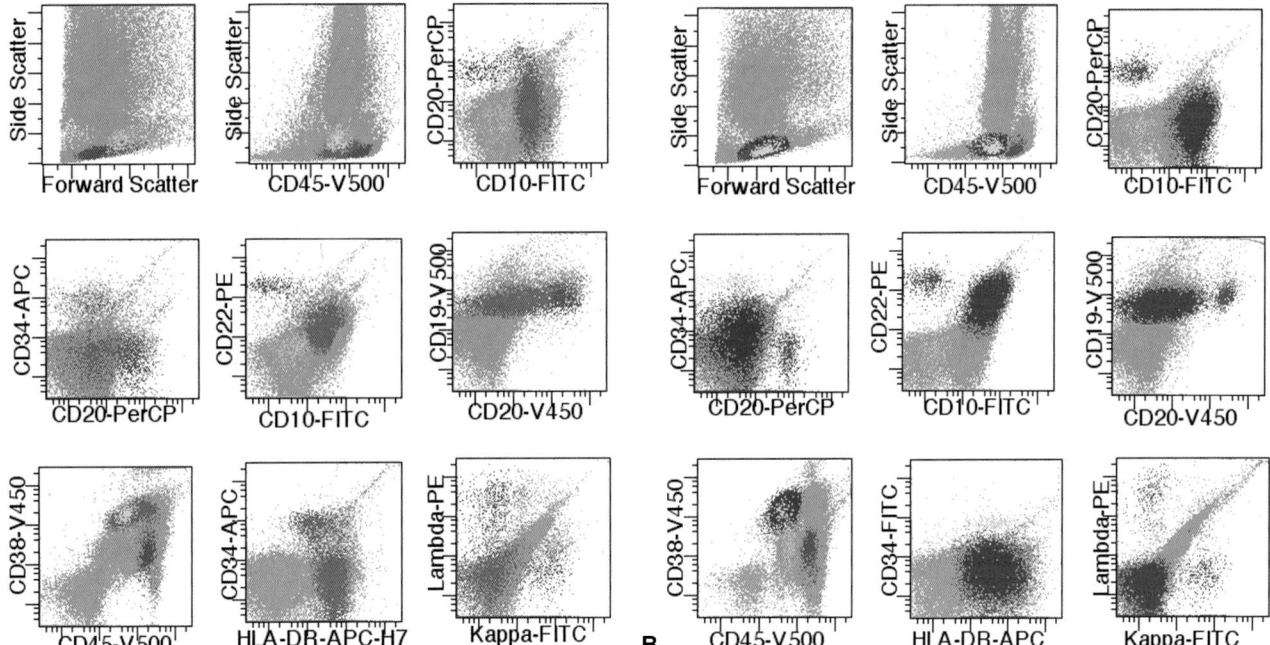

FIGURE 4.14. A: In this example of hematogone hyperplasia, the characteristic and highly reproducible hematogone maturation sequence is observed. The entire hematogone population (*violet*) is CD19(+), CD22(moderately+), CD10(+), and CD38(bright+). They show low side light scatter and variable forward scatter. The earliest hematogones are CD10(bright), CD20(−), CD34(+), CD45(dim), HLA-DR(moderate) and surface immunoglobulin(−). As they mature, CD10 is slightly down-regulated, there is a progressive acquisition of CD20, CD34 expression is lost, CD45 and HLA-DR become brighter, CD38 becomes slightly brighter, and there is limited polyclonal acquisition of surface immunoglobulin. The most mature hematogones express CD20 at a slightly brighter intensity than mature B cells (*blue*) and express CD45 at a similar intensity as mature lymphocytes. Note additionally that CD34 expression is bimodal (rather than exhibiting a continuous progression from positive to negative), and there are no CD34/CD20 coexpressing hematogones. Normal myeloid blasts are also displayed for comparison purposes (*yellow*). **B:** This example of B-acute lymphoblastic leukemia/lymphoma (B-ALL) was analyzed with a similar panel as the hematogones in (A). The neoplastic cells (*red*) resemble hematogones much more closely than most cases of B-ALL, but nevertheless exhibit multiple differences. These differences include brighter-than-normal CD10 and CD22, slightly dim CD19, underexpression of CD20, partial dim expression of CD34 without a discrete CD34(+) subset, and complete lack of surface immunoglobulin. Mature B cells (*blue*) and normal myeloid blasts (*yellow*) are again illustrated for comparison.

of TdT, CD1a, and CD4/CD8 dual expression. However, normal thymocytes, similar to hematogones discussed above, demonstrate a normal and predictable maturational pattern. Thus, T-lymphoblast populations, which deviate from this maturational pattern in all cases, are detected by FC (39,93,99–103).

Assessment of the four antigens CD1a, CD3, CD4, and CD8 is sufficient in most cases to discriminate T-LL from normal immature T cells of the thymus or as part of a thymoma.

The characteristic maturational patterns of normal thymocytes are shown in Figure 4.15A. The earliest thymocytes are

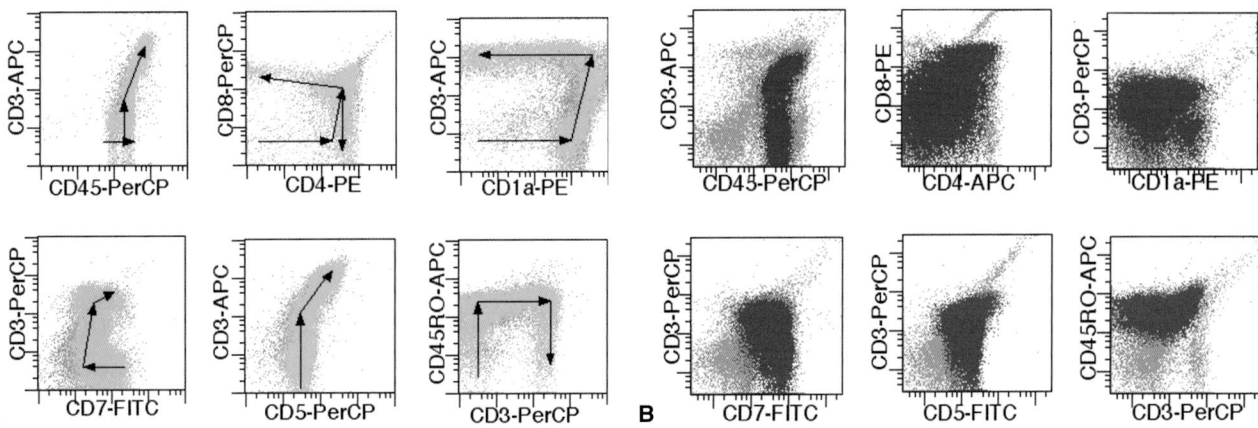

FIGURE 4.15. Thymoma and T-lymphoblastic leukemia/lymphoma. A: Maturing thymocytes in thymomas demonstrate an orderly maturation spectrum, although it is not as rigidly invariant as the maturational sequence seen in hematogones. Maturing thymocytes begin CD1a(−), surface CD3(−), CD5(+), CD7(bright), CD4(−), CD8(−), CD45(dim+), and CD45RO(−). While still CD3(−), they become slightly brighter for CD45, down-regulate CD7 expression, and acquire CD1a, CD4, and CD45RO. This is followed by gain of CD8 expression to become "dual positive cells." They then progressively gain CD3 expression, with up-regulation of CD45 and CD5 toward the end of the acquisition of CD3. Finally, the cells lose CD1a, CD45RO, and either CD4 or CD8, and slightly up-regulate CD7. **B:** This example of T-ALL bears some resemblance to thymocytes, insofar as there is an apparent maturation sequence in the CD3/CD5, CD3/CD7, and CD3/CD45 plots. However, there is a complete lack of any orderly maturation sequence in the CD3/CD1a, CD4/CD8, and CD3/CD45RO plots.

negative for CD4 and CD8, followed by acquisition of CD4, progression to dual CD4 and CD8 positivity, and finally becoming either a CD4 or CD8 positive T-cell (93). CD1a is acquired on thymocytes along with CD4 and remains on CD4/CD8 dual positive cells as surface CD3 becomes expressed. CD1a expression is lost as the T-cells mature to either CD4 or CD8 positive T-cells. CD34 is only expressed in the earliest stage (CD4 and CD8 negative) while CD10 is also seen early and then dissipates. CD2, CD5, and CD7 are essentially expressed throughout the entire maturational sequence. By comparison to normal thymocytes, T-lymphoblasts demonstrate immunophenotypic deviation from the normal maturational pattern (Fig. 4.15B). Myeloid antigen expression is reported to occur in approximately 30% of cases; this finding excludes nonneoplastic thymocytes.

Unlike B-LL, where the detection of certain immunophenotypic profiles may predict an underlying genetic abnormality, no recurring phenotypic-genotypic profiles have been reported to date.

Mature B-Cell Lymphoproliferative Disorders

FC is a critical tool in the immunophenotypic recognition and diagnosis of mature B-cell neoplasms. FC rapidly identifies immunophenotypically aberrant B-cell populations and aids in further subclassification based on differential antigen expression (Table 4.7) (1,2,12). In some circumstances (e.g., CLL/SLL and hairy cell leukemia), the disease definition is almost entirely based on characteristic immunophenotypic features. A detailed discussion of each B-cell entity and immunophenotypic characteristics is provided in its corresponding chapter in this book. In addition to diagnostics, FC also plays an important role in prognosis and/or therapeutics in certain diseases (e.g., CD38 and ZAP-70 expression in CLL, CD52 expression in T-prolymphocytic leukemia) (104–106).

A mature B-cell neoplasm may be distinguished from normal B cells by FC using two main approaches: immunoglobulin light chain restriction/absence and abnormal antigen expression. The traditional approach to identifying B-cell clonality by FC is by assessing the kappa:lambda ratio. Literature values for the normal kappa:lambda ratio are variable, but in general a range of 0.5 to 3.0 is quoted (116–118). Thus, if the ratio in a given case falls within that range, a B-cell clone is presumed to be absent. However, multiparameter FC allows for a more robust approach. Although most B-cell lymphomas are light chain restricted, they also show aberrant expression of other antigens that typically allow their discrimination from normal B cells (1,2). Any normal B-cell marker can be (and often is) expressed at an abnormal level, and lymphoma cells may also show abnormal light scatter properties. If present in a polytypic background, the abnormal B-cell population often forms a separate cluster, distinct from the polytypic B cells or causes abnormal asymmetry of the B-cell cluster in one- or more two-dimensional dot plots. As a consequence, this allows for specific isolation of subpopulations of B cells and demonstration of light chain restriction in such populations. Thus, monoclonal B-cell populations become detectable in a polyclonal B-cell background, regardless of an otherwise overall "normal" B-cell kappa:lambda ratio (Fig. 4.16). Similarly, multiple abnormal B-cell clones may be detected in a polyclonal background (Fig. 4.17). Clearly, recognition of immunophenotypic profiles as "aberrant" requires knowledge of expression patterns in normal B-cell subsets (e.g., hematogones, naïve B-cells, and germinal center cells) and of possible therapeutic effects (e.g., Rituximab) (Fig. 4.18). One important point is that a pure, apparently light chain "restricted" B-cell population without other antigenic aberrancy does not necessarily always correlate with neoplasia/

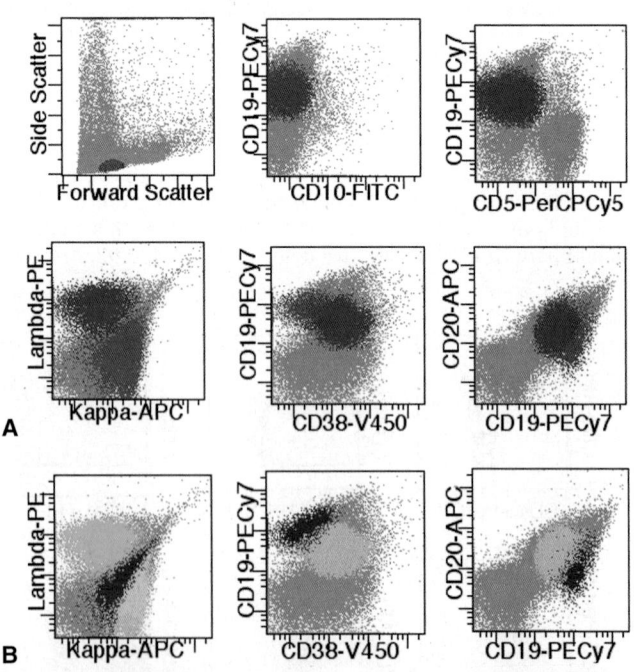

FIGURE 4.16. Small clonal B-cell population in a background of abundant polyclonal B cells. This lacrimal gland mass demonstrates CD5(−)/CD10(−) polyclonal B-cell population with a kappa:lambda ratio of 2.0, within normal limits. However, there is asymmetry in the kappa (*violet*) and lambda (*blue*) clusters in both the CD19/CD38 and CD19/CD20 plots, as well as a hint of a bimodal distribution of the kappa cluster in the kappa/lambda plot **(A)**. After an iterative analysis using maximally informative two-dimensional dot plots, it is evident that there is a dim kappa-restricted B-cell population (*red*) that is bright for CD19 and dim for CD20 **(B)**. The kappa:lambda ratio in the normal B cells (*yellow* and *green*) is 1.7. The clonal B cells represented 4.5% of total events, whereas the background polyclonal population represented 43%. This phenomenon, in which the clonal B cells are outnumbered by polyclonal B cells, is a common finding in extranodal marginal zone lymphomas of mucosa-associated lymphoid tissue.

	IMMUNOPHENOTYPIC FEATURES HELPFUL	
Table 4.7	IN THE SUBCLASSIFICATION OF MATURE B-CELL LYMPHOPROLIFERATIVE DISORDERS	

Antigen Expressed	Typical B-Cell Neoplasm	Comments
CD5	CLL MCL	MCL is CD5(−) in ~5% of cases, Occ. CD5⁺, MZL, LPL, FL
CD10	Follicular lymphoma Burkitt lymphoma Subset of DLBCL	CD10⁺ positive seen in ~10% of HCL, 5% of MCL, 40% of DLBCL
Dim CD19	Common in follicular lymphoma Seems common in BCL, U	
Dim CD20	Common in CLL	Brighter CD20 in CLL tends to correlate with trisomy 12
Bright CD20	Common in follicular and Burkitt lymphomas, HCL	
Dim sIg	Typical of CLL	
Bright sIg	Seen in a variety of tumor subtypes	
Bright CD22	Characteristic of HCL	
Bright CD11c	Characteristic of HCL	
Bright CD38	Uniform feature of Burkitt lymphoma	

Key: CLL, chronic lymphocytic leukemia; MCL, mantle cell lymphoma; DLBCL, diffuse large B-cell lymphoma; BCL, U, B-cell lymphoma, unclassifiable; HCL, hairy cell leukemia.
References: (107–115).

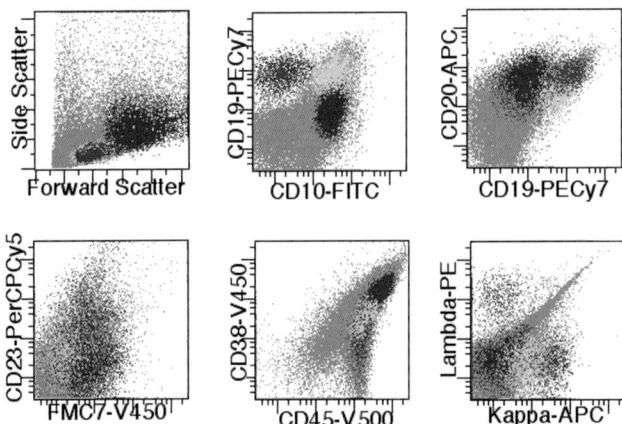

FIGURE 4.17. In this inguinal lymph node from a patient with no prior lymphoma history, there are two distinct CD10(+) clonal B-cell populations. The first population (*yellow*) consists of small cells with CD19 expression similar to normal B cells (*blue*), but with dim CD20, moderate CD38, and dim kappa light chain. The second clonal population (*red*) consists of large cells with distinctly dim CD19, slightly dim CD20, bright CD38, and no surface light chain expression. These findings are strongly suggestive of an aggressive transformation (large cells) of a low-grade follicular lymphoma (small cells). Furthermore, the immunophenotype of the large-cell population (dim CD19, dim CD20, bright CD38, and surface immunoglobulin negative) is predictive of a "double hit" lymphoma (rearrangements of both the *BCL2* and *MYC* genes), a highly aggressive form of non-Hodgkin lymphoma.

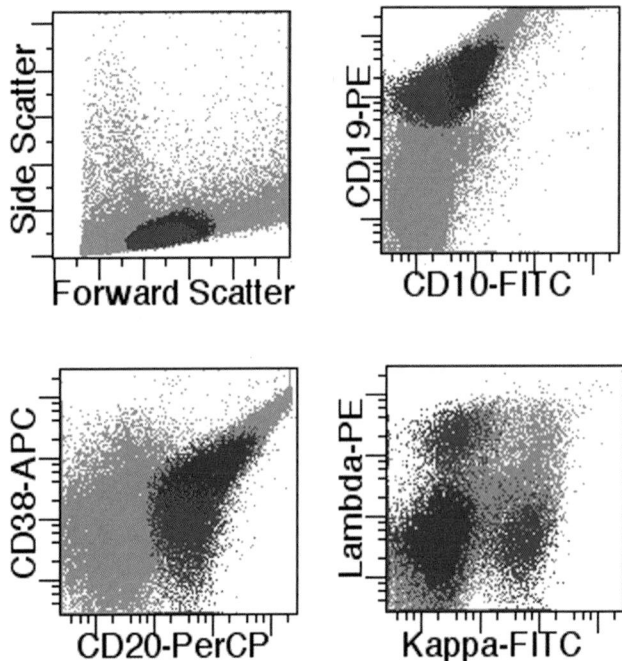

FIGURE 4.19. Surface immunoglobulin-negative lymphoma. This light chain–negative follicular lymphoma (*red*) resembles a normal germinal center population (see Fig. 4.20). However, there is a complete absence of surface light chain staining, in contrast to the limited polytypic staining pattern seen in normal germinal center cells. Additionally, CD20 is slightly dimmer than that seen on normal germinal center cells. Residual polytypic B cells are illustrated in *blue*.

monoclonality (119). Clonal expansion is the normal response of B cells to antigenic stimulation, and therefore clonality in and of itself is not a sufficient criterion to diagnose neoplasia in the lymphoid realm (120). Aberrancy, on the other hand, could be considered a more direct expression of the neoplastic phenotype than clonality.

In this context, B-cell lymphoma may be reliably diagnosed in the absence of surface light chain expression. Although the lack of light chain expression does not "prove" clonality in the traditional sense, it is an abnormal finding, and thus indicative of neoplasia (Fig. 4.19) (121). It has been argued that germinal center cells may normally be surface light chain negative, and that this finding is therefore not specific for neoplastic B cells. While a subset of germinal center B cells does, in fact, lack light chain expression, the entire germinal center population (defined using various combinations of CD10, CD20, and CD38) in fact shows a pattern of partial polytypic antigen expression (Fig. 4.20). CD10(+) B-cell lymphomas that lack surface light chain will almost always show other immunophenotypic aberrancies relative to the characteristic patterns of antigen expression seen on normal germinal center cells (e.g., frequent dim CD19 expression in follicular lymphoma), which will help

confirm the neoplastic nature of a light chain–negative B-cell population. Distinction of surface immunoglobulin-negative, CD10+ B-cell lymphoma from B-lymphoblastic leukemia/lymphoma relies upon other immunophenotypic features of immaturity. It is also important to note that lack of light chain

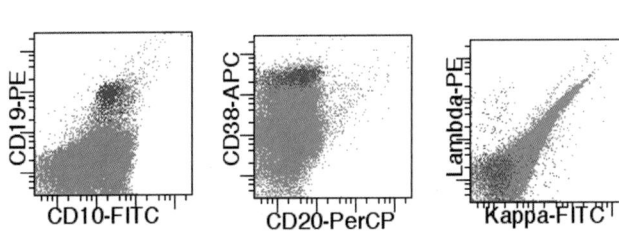

FIGURE 4.18. Rituximab effect on hematogones. A population of CD19(+)/CD10(+)/CD38(bright) hematogones is present, but the population is entirely CD20(−). In addition, there is a complete absence of CD10(−) mature B cells. This pattern is pathognomonic for rituximab effect, and may be evident for several months after the last dose of the drug. Note also there are small numbers of polytypic light chain–expressing hematogones, illustrating that acquisition of surface immunoglobulin on hematogones commences prior to gain of CD20.

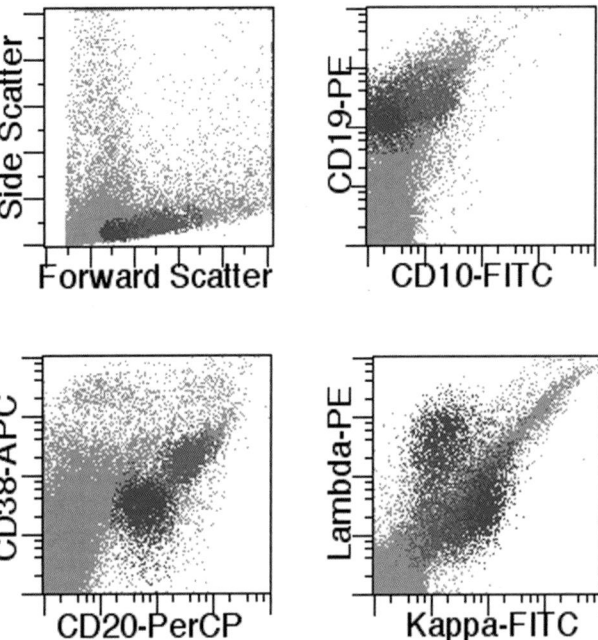

FIGURE 4.20. Follicular hyperplasia. Compared to primary follicle/mantle zone cells (*blue*), germinal center cells (*violet*) are brighter for CD19, CD20, and CD38, in addition to being CD10(+). The germinal center cell population shows partial polytypic light chain expression.

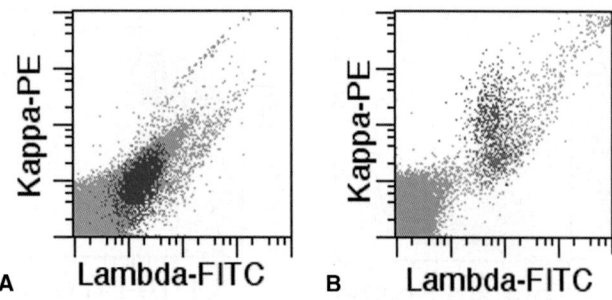

FIGURE 4.21. Artifactual lack of light chain expression in pleural fluid. The B cells in this benign pleural fluid specimen appear to completely lack surface light chain expression **(A)**. A repeat analysis utilizing a 37°C incubation and increased amounts of light chain reagent discriminates kappa and lambda populations **(B)**. This is a common phenomenon in pleural fluid and should not be overinterpreted as lymphoma; the B cells otherwise have normal immunophenotypic features. The cause of this artifact is not known.

expression occasionally represents a technical artifact. Specifically, otherwise normal B cells frequently appear to lack light chain expression in serous body cavity fluids (Fig. 4.21). A 37°C incubation and/or increasing the amount of light chain reagent usually allows demonstration of polytypic light chain expression in this setting (unpublished data). Therefore, lack of light chain expression should be interpreted cautiously in this context. Finally, any individual anti-light chain reagent may fail to react with the monotypic light chain on B-cell lymphoma cells. Use of an alternative light chain reagent (e.g., polyclonal anti-light chain reagents instead of monoclonal, or vice versa) will often allow demonstration of surface light chain restriction (122).

Mature T-Cell and Natural Killer-Cell Lymphoproliferative Disorders

Flow cytometric immunophenotyping is useful in the identification and sometimes in the subclassification of mature T-cell or NK-cell neoplasms, but is typically regarded as a more challenging endeavor than for mature B-cell proliferations. Mature T- and NK-cell neoplasms are generally diagnosed by integrating clinical, morphologic, immunophenotypic, and genetic

(e.g., T-cell receptor gene rearrangement, cytogenetics) data (1) Thus, immunophenotypic results are only one piece of information in the workup and classification of these entities (123–133). In addition, the normal T-cell immune response is complex, with multiple distinct subsets that may differentially expand in different reactive settings. Additionally, expression of individual antigens may be modulated in states of T-cell activation. Therefore, intimate knowledge of the complexity of T- and NK-cell subsets is required for proper interpretation. When a T- or NK-cell neoplasm is identified, FC may also play a role in identifying potential therapeutic targets (e.g., CD52) (134–137). For an in-depth discussion of the diagnostic and immunophenotypic characteristics of specific mature T- and NK-cell lymphoproliferations (see Chapter 38).

The assessment and diagnosis of peripheral T-cell lymphomas by FC has traditionally been hampered by the lack of an immunophenotypic equivalent of kappa and lambda for T cells (although this is no longer the case, as described below). CD4/CD8 ratios may be dramatically skewed in some reactive states, and therefore cannot be relied upon for the purpose of establishing clonality (although prominent skews should serve as a trigger for more in-depth immunophenotypic evaluation of the T cells). However, as in the other settings described earlier in this chapter, immunophenotypic aberrancy can be used as a reliable indicator of neoplasia in most cases of T-cell neoplasia.

Multiparameter FC allows for the direct and simultaneous assessment of multiple antibodies on the T-cell surface, rendering this technique a more robust and sensitive assessment of T-cell antigen aberrancy than IHC. Subtle and gross alterations of antigen expression (gain or loss, weak, or dim) are routinely evaluable by FC. Aberrant global patterns of antigen expression (as opposed to isolated assessment of individual antigens) allow discrimination of abnormal from normal T cells, even when the latter predominate (Fig. 4.22A). As indicated earlier, however, this task is complicated by the complex patterns of T cells in normal and reactive states.

Supplementing the analysis of immunophenotypic aberrancy is the relatively recent availability of antibodies to T-cell V-beta families (133,138–142). The V-beta gene of the T-cell antigen receptor complex codes for 46 genes that are grouped into families based on homology. Antibody kits currently cover 70% of the T-cell V-beta repertoire. Normal and reactive T-cell populations express a mixture of the V-beta

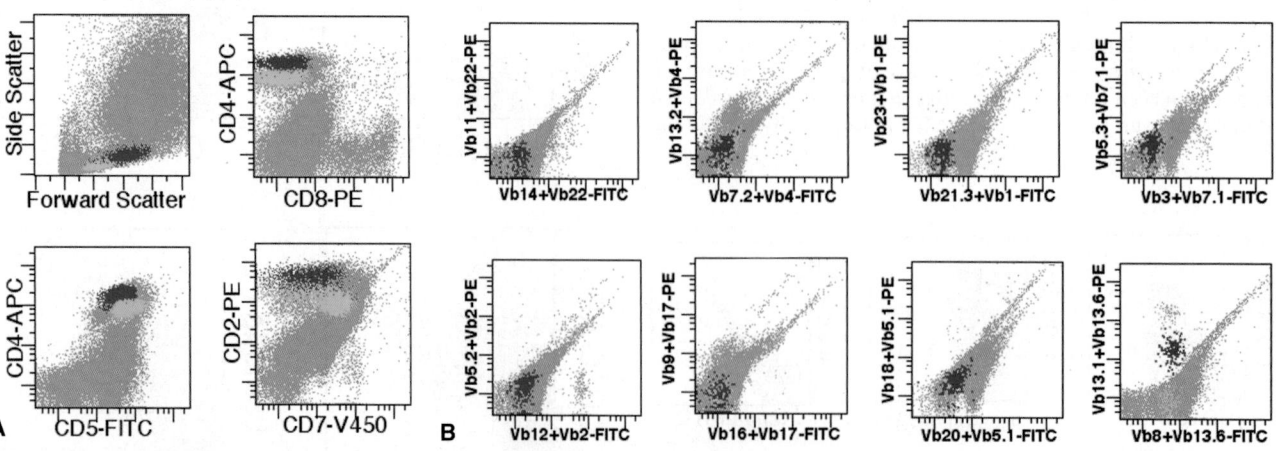

FIGURE 4.22. A: PTCL, not otherwise specified. The lymphoma cells (*red*) are larger in size by forward scatter properties, brighter for CD4, dimmer for CD5, and slightly dimmer for CD7 compared to the normal CD4(+) cells in the sample (*green*). **B:** V-beta analysis of the peripheral blood of the same case illustrated in part A. The V-beta analysis consists of eight tubes, each containing antibodies to three different V-beta families. Antibodies to two of the V-beta families are labeled with either FITC or PE, whereas antibodies to a third V-family are labeled with both FITC and PE. Thus, the upper left quadrant corresponds to positivity for one V-beta family, in the lower right quadrant a second V-beta family, and upper right quadrant the third. In this example, the populations are isolated with additional antibodies in each tube for CD4 and CD5, as illustrated in panel A. The normal CD4(+) T cells (*green*) demonstrate a polytypic pattern of V-beta expression. The lymphoma cells (*red*) are Vb8 restricted, seen in the far lower right dot plot.

family subtypes. When looking at the global V-beta expression on T cells in a sample, abnormal expansions of one family above established normal ranges are indicative of neoplasia. This approach is insensitive and is best suited for support of clonality when the population of interest comprises a sizable proportion of the T cells present. A more robust approach is possible, however, analogous to the refined kappa and lambda assessment described earlier for B cells. Because additional T-cell antibodies may be included in the reaction mixture with the V-beta antibodies (which occupy only the FITC and PE slots in each multicolor tube), immunophenotypically distinct T-cell populations may be isolated and demonstrated to express a single V-beta family, obviating the need to rely on normal ranges established for the entire T-cell repertoire (133). This approach typically follows the detection of an immunophenotypically distinct (aberrant or suspicious) T-cell population by routine analysis, thus triggering a targeted V-beta evaluation (V-beta kits are too expensive and cumbersome to employ routinely). This ability to directly demonstrate clonality in a specific population by immunophenotypic means provides a distinct advantage over gene rearrangement studies by polymerase chain reaction, in which one cannot ascertain which T cells are producing a clonal band in any given case (Fig. 4.22B). Once the V-beta usage of an aberrant population has been determined, V-beta analysis can be useful for MRD monitoring.

NK cells do not express the T-cell receptor and, therefore, there is no utility in assessing for V-beta restriction or T-cell receptor gene rearrangement. Like the case for T cells,

however, neoplastic NK-cell proliferations manifest immunophenotypic aberrancy relative to normal NK cells (Fig. 4.23A). Additionally, analysis of killer cell immunoglobulin receptors (KIRs) and the CD94/NKG2 complex has been recently utilized to support the clonality of NK-cell processes (130,143) (Fig. 4.23B).

Plasma Cell Disorders

Multiparametric flow cytometric immunophenotyping is a useful tool in the identification of clonal/aberrant plasma cells and in the distinction between lymphoplasmacytic and pure plasmacytic neoplasms. Pure plasmacytic neoplasms comprise a heterogeneous group of disorders, ranging from relatively innocuous conditions such as monoclonal gammopathy of uncertain significance (MGUS) to overt malignancies such as plasma cell myeloma. Due to the uniform finding of distinct immunophenotypic aberrancy in plasma cell dyscrasias, FC is a powerful technique for identifying and characterizing abnormal plasma cell populations, even in the presence of polytypic plasma cells.

One limitation of FC in the assessment of plasma cell proliferations is poor recovery of plasma cells. FC on average identifies approximately 70% fewer plasma cells than morphologic differential counts on bone marrow aspirates (144–147). This has been attributed to multiple factors including sampling differences, hemodilution, and loss of plasma cells during processing. It does appear that there is a disproportionate decrement in plasma cells compared to other marrow populations, and it has been postulated that plasma cells are more adherent to the lipid-rich particles in bone marrow aspirate and are therefore less represented in the liquid portion of the marrow that is analyzed by FC (144). Given this limitation, enumeration of plasma cells via FC is inaccurate and generally cannot be used to subclassify plasma cell disorders. Notably, however, a large cooperative group study found that plasma cell percentages by FC were more prognostically relevant than morphologic plasma cell counts (145).

Plasma cells are typically identified by bright expression of bright CD38, with or without the addition of CD138 (Fig. 4.24). Although a wide variety of hematopoietic cells

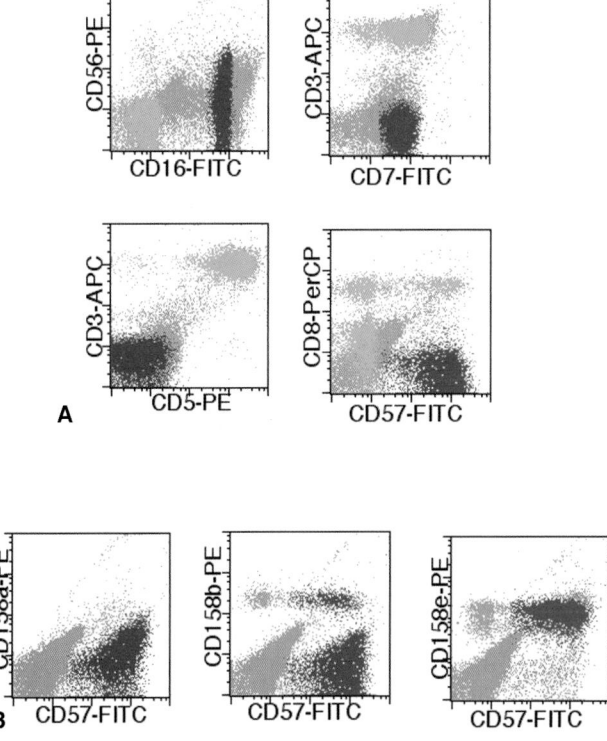

A

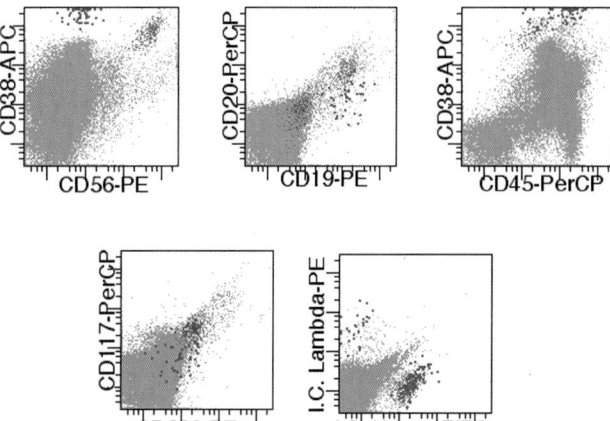

FIGURE 4.23. Chronic lymphoproliferative disorder of NK cells (CLPD-NK). A: In this example of CLPD-NK, the abnormal cells (*red*) share features of normal NK cells, namely expression of CD2 (not shown), CD7, CD16, CD56, and CD57, in the absence of CD3 and CD5. They differ from normal NK cells (not illustrated) in that CD16 is abnormally bright, CD7 is slightly dim (it should be slightly brighter than the upper end of CD7 expression in normal T cells), CD8 is completely absent (normal NK cells show partial dim CD8 expression), and CD56 is only partially expressed. Normal T cells are illustrated in *green*. **B:** KIR analysis of the same case illustrated in part A. Normal NK-cell populations demonstrate a polytypic pattern of expression of CD158a, CD158b, and CD158e. In this case, there is a restricted pattern, in that essentially the entire population expresses CD158e, whereas CD158a and CD158b are minimally expressed.

FIGURE 4.24. Plasma cell myeloma cells and normal plasma cells. In this example, myeloma cells (*red*) and normal plasma cells (*blue*) are present in the same analysis. Normal plasma cells are CD38(bright+), CD19(+), CD20(−), CD45(+), CD117(−), CD200(−), and polytypic with respect to intracellular light chain staining. The myeloma cells in this case are aberrant in that they are CD19(−), CD56(+), CD117(+), CD200(dim+), and intracellular kappa light chain restricted. Also note that the myeloma cells are dimmer for CD38 than the normal plasma cells, although still brighter than other hematolymphoid elements; this is fairly characteristic. CD45 is also slightly dimmer on the myeloma cells than on the normal plasma cells; myeloma cells may express essentially any level of CD45 in any given case. Mature B cells are illustrated in *violet* in this figure.

including hematogones, subsets of T cells, and blasts express CD38, plasma cells are uniquely brighter for CD38. Importantly, abnormal plasma cells may occasionally down-regulate their CD38 expression to levels overlapping other marrow populations, a potential pitfall in analysis. CD138 expression is specific for plasma cells (among hematolymphoid cells), but CD138 assessment may be technically problematic, as it can be affected by clone choice, lysis reagent, and refrigeration (148). Normal plasma cells express CD19 and CD45 and lack CD56 (149). In contrast, the plasma cells in myeloma and other plasma cell dyscrasias lack CD19 in 95% of cases, express CD56 in 75%, and lack CD45 in roughly half of cases. Assessment of these antigens alone will therefore discriminate normal from abnormal plasma cells in the vast majority of cases (Fig. 4.24), and the assessment of additional antigens such as CD20 (aberrantly expressed in 15% to 20% of cases), CD117 (aberrantly expressed in one third of cases), or CD200 (aberrantly expressed in 75% of cases) will likely improve the discriminatory power to essentially 100% (35,150–155). Aberrant antigen expression on plasma cells should be interpreted with caution due to their frequent autofluorescence and nonspecific protein binding (Fig. 4.25). Aberrant antigen expression also may correlate with certain clinical and/or genetic markers (Table 4.8).

FC is able to discriminate normal from abnormal plasma cells based on aberrant antigen expression in the latter, and the presence of residual normal plasma cells in plasma cell dyscrasias has been shown to be prognostically relevant. Specifically, the presence of >5% normal plasma cells (as

Table 4.8 ANTIGEN EXPRESSION IN PLASMA CELL MYELOMA AND POSSIBLE CLINICAL AND/OR GENETIC CORRELATES

Antigen	Comment
CD20	Associated with lymphoid cytology; cyclin D1 protein expression associated with the t(11;14)(q13;q32)
CD23	Associated with t(11;14) (q13;q32) and plasma cell leukemia
CD27	Lack of CD27 expression may correlate with disease progression
CD56	Associated with hyperdiploidy
	Lack of CD56 expression occurs often in leukemic phase; worse prognosis
CD117	Associated with good prognosis and hyperdiploidy
	Lack of CD117 expression associated with nonhyperdiploid genetics enriched for *IGH@* translocations
CD200	Associated with worse event-free survival

References: (153,156–163).

a percentage of total plasma cells) in MGUS or smoldering myeloma portends a much lower rate of disease progression than those patients with <5% polytypic plasma cells. Similarly, in one large study of newly diagnosed plasma cell myeloma patients, those with >5% polytypic plasma cells showed a better overall survival (145).

Nonacute Myeloid Disorders Including Mastocytosis

The general application of FC to diagnose myeloproliferative (MPN), myelodysplastic (MDS), and myelodysplastic/myeloproliferative syndromes is highly complex and, in general, difficult to routinely reproduce in most FC laboratories (164–166). Published data describe abnormalities in both blasts and maturing myeloid elements (11,167,168). Familiarization with what constitutes aberrant maturational patterns/antigen expression requires extensive knowledge of normal expression patterns (11,169). It is currently quite challenging to distill from the published literature truly abnormal versus normal expression patterns. For example, imprecise gating techniques may yield a heterogeneous admixture of blasts and myeloid precursors, rendering determination of antigen expression patterns on pure populations essentially impossible. In addition, alterations in "normal" maturation patterns have been demonstrated in nonneoplastic states (170). Thus, a "left shift" in maturation or robust hematopoietic regeneration in an otherwise nonneoplastic state may alter the typical expected maturation spectrum. Additionally, few studies have employed control groups of nonnormal (but nonneoplastic) bone marrow samples; most use normal bone marrow as the baseline for determining aberrancy. Consequently, the specificity of some abnormalities that have been described in the literature is not clearly established. The sensitivity and specificity of putative aberrancies should be compared not only with conditions of nonclonal cytopenias and stressed bone marrow states but also with age-matched controls. Finally, the patient cohorts in most studies are defined based on traditional morphologic and cytogenetic criteria. The utility of immunophenotyping to detect early or subtle myeloid neoplasia is difficult to document without another available gold standard; cohorts of morphologically borderline cases with lengthy follow-up would be required (171). Consequently, the added value of FC to the diagnostic process in the area of nonacute myeloid disorders is currently not well established.

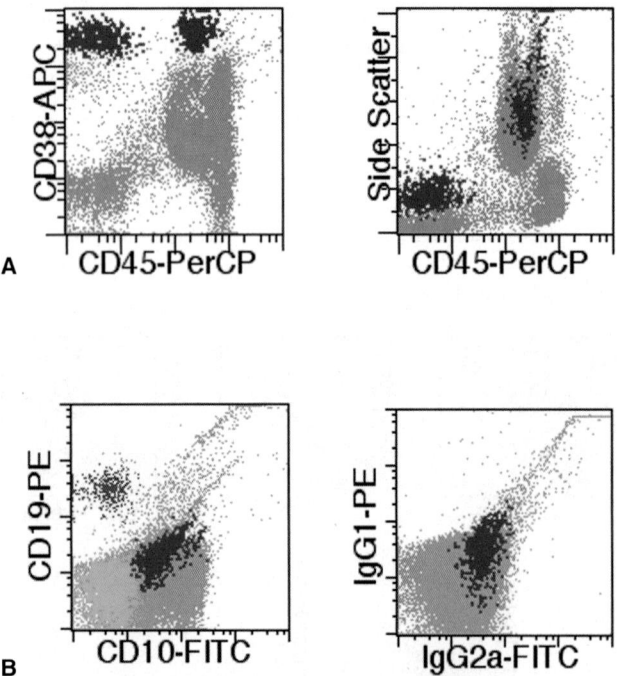

FIGURE 4.25. Interpretive issues in FC of plasma cell myeloma. A: Plasma cell may show prominent adherence to other cell types. In this example, the plasma cell myeloma cells (*red*) appear to show subset CD45 expression. Examination of the CD45/side scatter plot reveals that the CD45(+) subset has distinctly higher side scatter properties than the CD45(−) subset, indicating that this cluster represents plasma cell/granulocyte doublets. The neoplastic plasma cells are, in fact, entirely CD45(−). **B:** Plasma cells characteristically demonstrate high levels of nonspecific fluorescence. In this example, the myeloma cells (*red*) appear to express CD10 and dim CD19. However, the isotype control confirms that the population is negative for both of these antigens. Because myeloma cell populations have variable light scatter and CD45 expression patterns, they are difficult to gate based on forward scatter/side scatter or CD45/side scatter. It is therefore useful to include a CD38 or CD138 in an isotype control tube to precisely delineate the nonspecific fluorescence levels of the plasma cells.

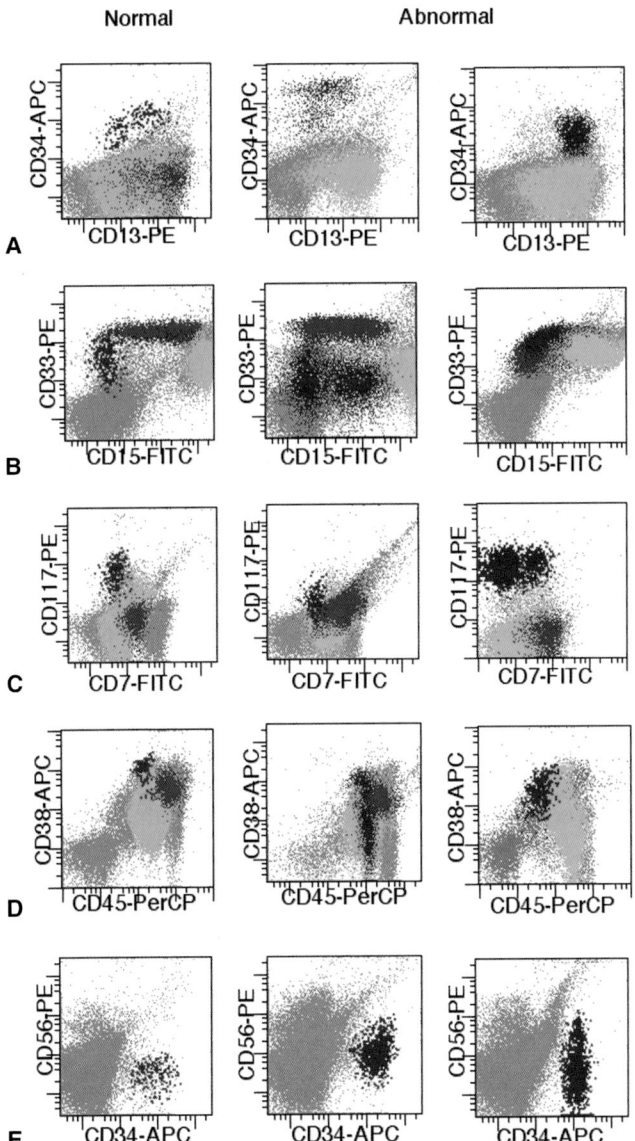

Normal **Abnormal**

FIGURE 4.26. Blast aberrancies in MDS. Blasts—*red*; monocytes—*blue*; granulo-cytes—*green*. **A:** Normal blasts (**left**) show variable CD13, with a biphasic pattern when plotted versus CD34. In the center plot, CD34 expression is predominantly abnormally bright and CD13 is slightly dim. In the right plot, the blasts show uniformly bright CD13 expression. **B:** Normal blasts show moderate CD33 compared to monocytes. They are predominantly CD15−, but a minor population with bright CD33 expression shows variable CD15 expression. The abnormal blasts in the center plot show abnormally variable CD33 and an abnormally large CD15(+) subset that lacks the bright CD33 of the normal CD15(+) blast subset in the left plot. In the right plot, the blasts are abnormally bright for CD33. **C:** The blasts in the center plot show abnormally dim CD117 compared to the normal blasts in the left plot. In the right plot, the blasts show partial CD7 expression. **D:** Normal blasts show predominantly high CD38 and moderate CD45 expression (similar to the bulk of the granulocytes). A small subset is lower for CD38 and slightly brighter for CD45. In the center plot, there is abnormal CD38 variability, with a large CD38(dim) subset. On the right plot, the blasts show abnormally dim CD45 expression. **E:** Normal blasts are CD56(−). The center and right plots show uniform and partial patterns of CD56 expression, respectively.

FC may currently play a more useful role in detecting frank immunophenotypic aberrancy in blasts compared with "normal" precursors. Distinctive immunophenotypic aberrancies that appear to be specific for myeloid neoplasia include expression of CD7, CD36, and/or CD56; decreased expression of/absent CD13, CD33, CD38, and/or CD45; and increased expression of CD34 and CD15 on the blast population (Fig. 4.26) (172). Importantly, when a cohort of nonneoplastic

conditions associated with cytopenias or cytoses is studied, mild nonspecific alterations in antigen expression on blasts may be noted. These include overexpression of CD13, over- or underexpression of CD117, bright HLA-DR, slight overexpression of CD34, and variability of expression of CD33 and CD38 (172). Prior to routine clinical implementation of a grading or scale system to diagnosis myeloid neoplasia by FC, a large-scale assessment of the spectrum of antigenic changes requires external validation.

Myelodysplastic Syndrome

Despite the above caveats, FC is being increasingly used to detect immunophenotypic aberrancies on myeloid progenitors, particularly as a complement in morphologically equivocal cases of possible MDS. Few immunophenotypic abnormalities of myeloid progenitors are individually diagnostic; on the other hand, the presence of multiple immunophenotypic abnormalities appears to have a high predictive value for MDS. While various non-MDS disorders (e.g., growth factor effect, megaloblastic anemia) may show some immunophenotypic alterations, it is the aggregate of multiple abnormalities that points to a diagnosis of MDS. Typical flow cytometric findings in MDS include an abnormal maturation pattern of the maturing myeloid cells (disruption of the CD11b/CD16 and CD13/CD16 curves), diminished side angle light scatter for granulocytes (corresponding to cytoplasmic hypogranularity), abnormal antigen expression on maturing myeloid precursors (e.g., decreased/absent CD13, CD33 on myeloid cells, decreased HLA-DR on monocytes, the presence of lymphoid antigen(s) on a myeloid population, CD56 expression on monocytes and granulocytes), and an aberrant blast population (Figs. 4.26 to 4.28) (172–187).

Despite the ongoing challenges with specificity and the interpretation of flow cytometric analysis in MDS, FC has been proposed as a criterion in the diagnosis of MDS in a consensus statement (188), and therefore standardization is warranted (189). In fact, the WHO 2008 recommends that the presence of three or more immunophenotypic abnormalities in myeloid precursors should be closely evaluated for the development of MDS features in cases without morphologic dysplasia or diagnostic cytogenetic abnormality (1).

A number of flow cytometric scoring systems have been developed for diagnosis of and prognosis in MDS (173,190–193). These systems differ from one another in several ways (number of parameters evaluated, number of cell lineages studied, subpopulations analyzed) but overall show a sensitivity of 75% and specificity of >85% when robust and reproducible parameters are included (189). In terms of a diagnosis of MDS, Chu et al. showed that an FC score >2 was able to reliably discriminate MDS patients from non-MDS patients with cytopenias with a specificity of 100% and sensitivity of 75%. Their three-tiered scoring system ranges from normal/mild (0 to 1 point) to moderate (2 to 3 points) to severe (4 or more points), with points based on detected phenotypic aberrancies. In another multicenter study, it was reported that a majority of low-risk MDS cases could be diagnosed by evaluating four parameters: blast percentage, percent hematogones, aberrant CD45 expression on myeloblasts, and decreased granulocyte side scatter (178,194). Although this type of "diagnostic" testing remains largely restricted to laboratories with expertise in FC, and is very difficult to standardize across laboratories, ongoing effort to standardize and validate this technique is occurring and is likely to result in the integration of flow cytometric analysis in MDS as a distinct data point, along with the other well-known parameters—morphology, blast count, cytopenias, and cytogenetics.

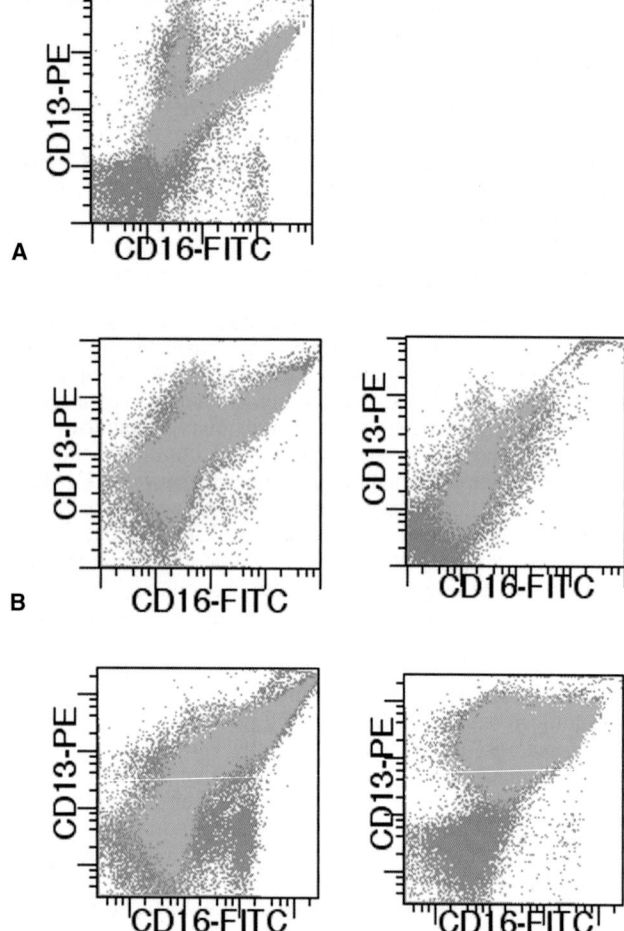

FIGURE 4.27. Normal and abnormal CD13/CD16 granulocyte maturation curves. A: Normal maturing granulocytes begin CD13(bright+)/CD16(−). As they mature, they down-regulate CD13, while remaining CD16(−). Finally, they once again up-regulate CD13 in coordinate fashion with a gain of CD16. **B:** Distorted CD13/CD16 maturation curves are a common finding in MDS.

Several prognostic flow cytometric scoring systems in MDS have also been proposed (190,191). These are fewer in number than the proposed diagnostic systems but suffer from some of the same variabilities. The scoring system of Wells et al. is based on immunophenotypic abnormalities in myeloid precursors, monocytic precursors, and blasts and assigns an overall numerical score that has been validated in subsequent studies (166,190–192). This flow cytometric scoring system correlates

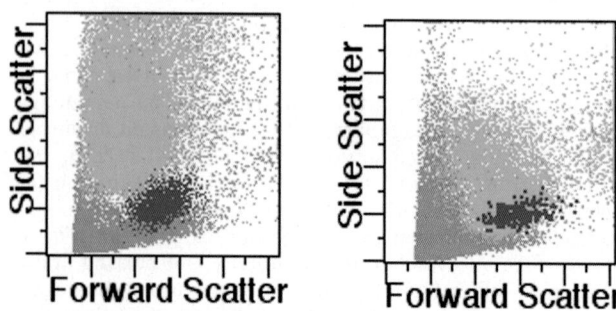

FIGURE 4.28. Diminished side light scatter due to neutrophil hypogranularity in MDS. Normal granulocyte side scatter (**left**) compared to diminished side scatter in a MDS with neutrophil hypogranularity (**right**). Granulocytes are illustrated in *green*; monocytes (*blue*) are included for comparison.

with the International Prognostic Scoring System (IPSS) score (based on cytogenetics, blast percentage, and cytopenias), WHO-adjusted prognostic scoring system, and outcome in MDS after hematopoietic stem cell transplantation (166,190–192). Cases that demonstrated high FC scores were seen preferentially in cases that showed progression to high-grade MDS or AML (166). Chu et al. (190) showed that the FC scoring system may predict overall outcome in patients with MDS and was an independent prognostic parameter after adjusting for IPSS and WPSS.

Mastocytosis

Mastocytosis consists of a heterogeneous group of myeloid disorders characterized by the abnormal proliferation of mast cells in a variety of tissue sites. Systemic mastocytosis is currently classified by the WHO as a MPN (195). Assessment and demonstration of aberrant antigen expression on mast cells is one of the minor criteria that can be used in establishing a diagnosis of systemic mastocytosis. Although mast cells represent a very small fraction of normal bone marrow nucleated cells (<0.5%), they can be accurately and reliably identified by multiparametric flow cytometric techniques, with a detection sensitivity of 1 mast cell per 10,000 nucleated cells. Mast cells are typically identified by bright CD117 expression, light scatter properties, and lack of CD34, CD38, or CD138 expression (196–199). They express CD33 (199,200). The detection of aberrant CD2 and/or CD25 on mast cells qualifies as one of the WHO minor criterion for mastocytosis (Fig. 4.29) (195,201–204). It has recently been proposed that the detection of a distinct CD117+ mast cell population without CD2 or CD25 expression may improve the analytical sensitivity for mastocytosis (205).

Paroxysmal Nocturnal Hemoglobinuria

PNH is an acquired clonal stem cell disorder that is clinically associated with venous thrombosis, intravascular hemolysis, and cytopenias. The primary molecular defect is a mutation

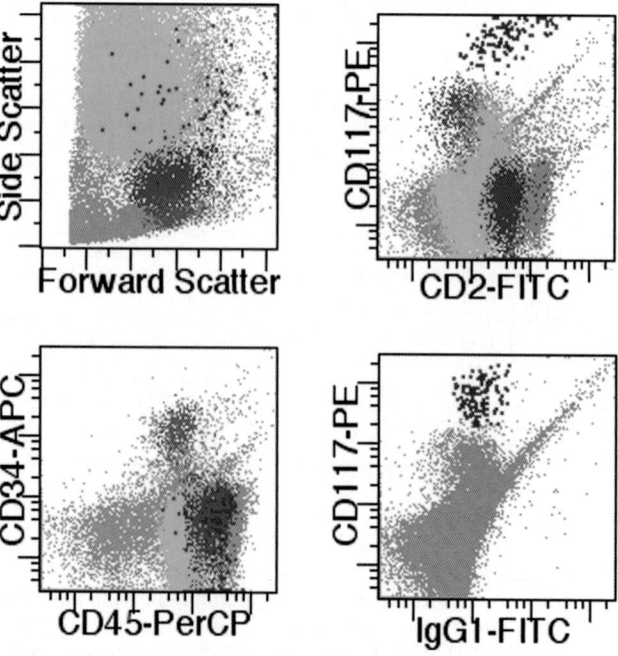

FIGURE 4.29. The mast cells (*red*) are identifiable based on very bright CD117 (brighter than any other myeloid elements). They do not form a distinct cluster by light scatter properties, but instead are scattered among the granulocytes and monocytes in the forward scatter/side scatter plot. In this example, the mast cells show aberrant, partial expression of CD2 relative to the control. (Granulocytes—*green*, monocytes—*blue*, myeloblasts—*violet*.)

in the phosphatidylinositol glycan anchor biosynthesis, class A gene (*PIGA*) located on the X chromosome. This gene is one of multiple genes normally responsible for synthesizing a glycosol phosphatidylinositol (GPI) moiety that anchors various proteins to the cell surface. In PNH, the *PIGA* gene is mutated, resulting in a complete or partial deficiency of the anchored proteins with subsequent enhanced complement-mediated lysis resulting in hemolysis and cytopenias. The *PIGA* gene is located on the X chromosome; therefore, a somatic mutation of only one *PIGA* allele is required to develop PNH since females have inactivation of one X-chromosome in somatic tissues and men only have one X chromosome normally.

More than 20 GPI-linked anchoring proteins are expressed by hematopoietic cells. The progeny of PNH stem cells shows reduced or absent expression of these anchoring proteins, which include CD14, CD16, CD24, CD55, and CD59. RBCs are subclassified into three types based on their GPI-linked anchoring protein expression: Type III cells—complete deficiency,

Type II cells—partially deficient (~90%), relatively resistant to hemolysis, and Type I cells—normal density. Loss of two complement regulatory proteins, CD55 (decay accelerating factor) and CD59 (membrane inhibitor of reactive lysis), are primarily responsible for intravascular hemolysis. Clinical symptoms relate largely to the size of the PNH clone (%).

Flow cytometric analysis of the peripheral blood is considered the gold standard for the identification of PNH clones (8,206–209). Peripheral blood is the preferred specimen type for PNH testing, as cells in earlier stages of maturation often demonstrate variable expression of GPI-linked proteins. Guidelines have been established for both routine (sensitivity 1%) and high sensitivity (sensitivity 0.01%) testing, as well as strategies for identifying rare events (8). Both white blood cells and RBCs are assessed for a deficiency in GPI-linked proteins. The use of FLAER (fluorescein-labeled aerolysin) is advocated for evaluation of granulocytes and monocytes (Fig. 4.30). FLAER directly binds the GPI anchor and best detects small PNH clones. Glycophorin

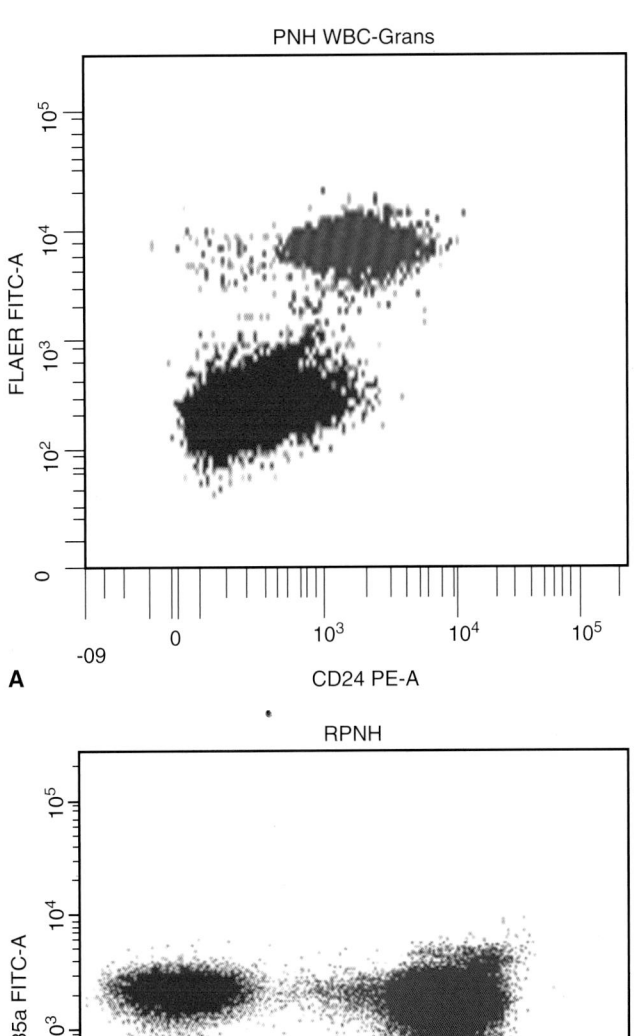

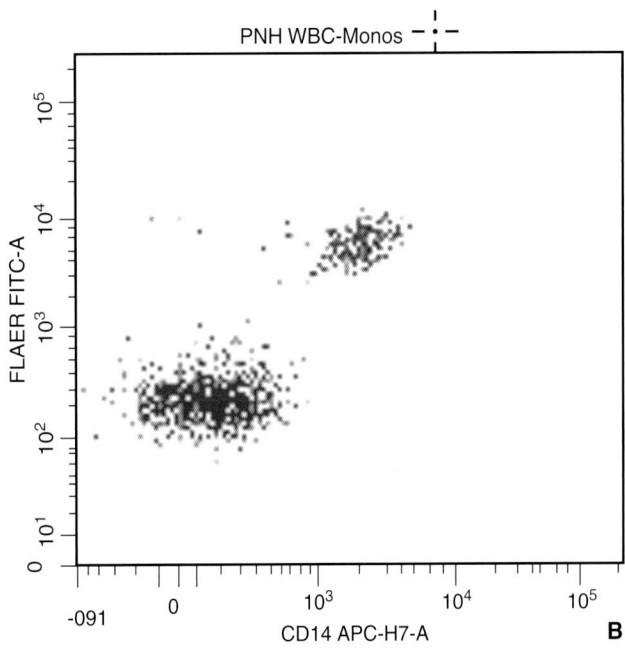

FIGURE 4.30. Detection of a PNH clone in a peripheral blood specimen. A: A distinct cluster of FLAER and CD24⁻ neutrophils is seen (*red* population) compared with the normal residual neutrophils (*green* population) showing preserved expression of FLAER and CD24. **B:** A distinct cluster of FLAER and CD14⁻ monocytes is seen (*red* population) compared with the normal residual monocytes (*maroon* population) showing preserved expression of FLAER and CD14. **C:** A distinct population of RBCs showing loss of CD59 (*red* color) compared to the normal residual RBCs (*blue* color). The percent of the PNH RBC clone is often discrepant (lower) than that detected in the white blood cells due to intravascular hemolysis and/or transfusion.

on RBCs interferes with FLAER binding, preventing its use for analysis of RBCs. For RBC analysis, CD59 is recommended over CD55 as it is more strongly expressed and better detects Type II cells. The erythrocyte PNH clone size is usually underestimated by flow cytometric analysis since PNH+ red cells are rapidly destroyed during hemolysis and diluted by red cell transfusions.

FC may be used to monitor response to therapy in PNH. Assessing the size of the PNH clone may play a role in altering the clinical management of the patient's disease. The monoclonal antibody eculizumab, which targets the C5 component of complement, has shown promising results in reducing transfusion requirements and by nearly eliminating thromboembolic complications (207).

Classical Hodgkin Lymphoma

FC, as is currently performed in the majority of clinical laboratories, is not effective for detecting classical Hodgkin lymphoma cells because of small number of neoplastic cells and rosetting of T cells around the Reed-Sternberg cells. The diagnosis is typically established with the use of IHC on fixed tissue specimens. Recently however, it has been shown that classical Hodgkin cells can be detected via FC using either a nine-color or six-color marker combination (210–212).

CONCLUSION

FC is a powerful tool in the modern-day evaluation of hematologic conditions. Multiple applications for FC exist in this realm, including the detection of abnormal hematolymphoid populations; the diagnosis of acute myeloid and lymphoblastic leukemias, chronic myeloid and lymphoid proliferations, and PNH; the determination of MRD; and disease prognostication (e.g., in CLL). There is ongoing progress in the application of FC in the diagnosis of mature T-cell and NK-cell proliferations and nonacute myeloid disorders. Knowledge of the critical preanalytical, analytical, and postanalytical issues will ensure best practices in FC.

References

1. Swerdlow SH, Campo E., Harris NL, et al., ed. *WHO classification of tumours of haematopoietic and lymphoid tissues*, 3rd ed. Lyon: IARC Press, 2008.
2. Craig FE, Foon KA. Flow cytometric immunophenotyping for hematologic neoplasms. *Blood* 2008;111(8):3941–3967.
3. Calvo KR, McCoy CS, Stetler-Stevenson M. Flow cytometry immunophenotyping of hematolymphoid neoplasia. *Methods Mol Biol* 2011;699:295–316.
4. Stetler-Stevenson M, et al. 2006 Bethesda International Consensus Conference on Flow Cytometric Immunophenotyping of Hematolymphoid Neoplasia. *Cytometry B Clin Cytom* 2007;72(Suppl 1):S3.
5. Martinez A, et al. Routine use of immunophenotype by flow cytometry in tissues with suspected hematological malignancies. *Cytometry B Clin Cytom* 2003;56(1):8–15.
6. Braylan RC. Impact of flow cytometry on the diagnosis and characterization of lymphomas, chronic lymphoproliferative disorders and plasma cell neoplasias. *Cytometry A* 2004;58(1):57–61.
7. Orfao A, et al. Immunophenotyping of acute leukemias and myelodysplastic syndromes. *Cytometry A* 2004;58(1):62–71.
8. Borowitz MJ, et al. Guidelines for the diagnosis and monitoring of paroxysmal nocturnal hemoglobinuria and related disorders by flow cytometry. *Cytometry B Clin Cytom* 2010;78(4):211–230.
9. Wood B. Multicolor immunophenotyping: human immune system hematopoiesis. *Methods Cell Biol* 2004;75:559–576.
10. Loken MR, Wells D, ed. Normal antigen expression in hematopoiesis: basis for interpreting leukemia phenotypes. In: Nicholson J, Stewart C, eds. *Immunophenotyping*. New York: Wiley-Liss, 2000:133–160.
11. Kussick SJ, Wood BL. Using 4-color flow cytometry to identify abnormal myeloid populations. *Arch Pathol Lab Med* 2003;127(9):1140–1147.
12. Stetler-Stevenson M, Braylan RC. Flow cytometric analysis of lymphomas and lymphoproliferative disorders. *Semin Hematol* 2001;38(2):111–123.
13. Weir EG, Borowitz MJ. Flow cytometry in the diagnosis of acute leukemia. *Semin Hematol* 2001;38(2):124–138.
14. Wood B. 9-color and 10-color flow cytometry in the clinical laboratory. *Arch Pathol Lab Med* 2006;130(5):680–690.
15. Davis BH, et al. 2006 Bethesda International Consensus recommendations on the flow cytometric immunophenotypic analysis of hematolymphoid neoplasia: medical indications. *Cytometry B Clin Cytom* 2007;72(Suppl 1):S5–S13.
16. Davis BH, et al. U.S.-Canadian Consensus recommendations on the immunophenotypic analysis of hematologic neoplasia by flow cytometry: medical indications. *Cytometry* 1997;30(5):249–263.
17. Borowitz MJ, et al. U.S.-Canadian Consensus recommendations on the immunophenotypic analysis of hematologic neoplasia by flow cytometry: data analysis and interpretation. *Cytometry* 1997;30(5):236–244.
18. Wood BL, et al. 2006 Bethesda International Consensus recommendations on the immunophenotypic analysis of hematolymphoid neoplasia by flow cytometry: optimal reagents and reporting for the flow cytometric diagnosis of hematopoietic neoplasia. *Cytometry B Clin Cytom* 2007;72(Suppl 1):S14–S22.
19. Stetler-Stevenson MAE, Barnett D, et al. *Clinical flow cytometric analysis of neoplastic hematolymphoid cells. Approved guideline (H43-A2)*. Wayne: Clinical and Laboratory Standards institute, 2007:1–81.
20. Stelzer GT, Shults KE, Loken MR. CD45 gating for routine flow cytometric analysis of human bone marrow specimens. *Ann N Y Acad Sci* 1993;677:265–280.
21. Borowitz MJ, et al. Immunophenotyping of acute leukemia by flow cytometric analysis. Use of CD45 and right-angle light scatter to gate on leukemic blasts in three-color analysis. *Am J Clin Pathol* 1993;100(5):534–540.
22. Sun T, et al. Gating strategy for immunophenotyping of leukemia and lymphoma. *Am J Clin Pathol* 1997;108(2):152–157.
23. Krasinskas AM, et al. The usefulness of CD64, other monocyte-associated antigens, and CD45 gating in the subclassification of acute myeloid leukemias with monocytic differentiation. *Am J Clin Pathol* 1998;110(6):797–805.
24. Xu Y, et al. Immunophenotypic identification of acute myeloid leukemia with monocytic differentiation. *Leukemia* 2006;20(7):1321–1324.
25. Harrington AM, Olteanu H, Kroft SH. A dissection of the CD45/side scatter "blast gate". *Am J Clin Pathol* 2012;137(5):800–804.
26. Stelzer GT, et al. U.S.-Canadian Consensus recommendations on the immunophenotypic analysis of hematologic neoplasia by flow cytometry: standardization and validation of laboratory procedures. *Cytometry* 1997;30(5):214–230.
27. van Dongen JJ, et al. EuroFlow antibody panels for standardized n-dimensional flow cytometric immunophenotyping of normal, reactive and malignant leukocytes. *Leukemia* 2012;26(9):1908–1975.
28. Bene MC, et al. Immunophenotyping of acute leukemia and lymphoproliferative disorders: a consensus proposal of the European LeukemiaNet Work Package 10. *Leukemia* 2011;25(4):567–574.
29. Braylan RC, et al. Optimal number of reagents required to evaluate hematolymphoid neoplasias: results of an international consensus meeting. *Cytometry* 2001;46(1):23–27.
30. Campana D. Minimal residual disease monitoring in childhood acute lymphoblastic leukemia. *Curr Opin Hematol* 2012;19(4):313–318.
31. DiNardo CD, Luger SM. Beyond morphology: minimal residual disease detection in acute myeloid leukemia. *Curr Opin Hematol* 2012;19(2):82–88.
32. Pott C. Minimal residual disease detection in mantle cell lymphoma: technical aspects and clinical relevance. *Semin Hematol* 2011;48(3):172–184.
33. Kern W, et al. The role of multiparameter flow cytometry for disease monitoring in AML. *Best Pract Res Clin Haematol* 2010;23(3):379–390.
34. Bottcher S, et al. Minimal residual disease quantification is an independent predictor of progression-free and overall survival in chronic lymphocytic leukemia: a multivariate analysis from the randomized GCLLSG CLL8 trial. *J Clin Oncol* 2012;30(9):980–988.
35. Gupta R, et al. Flow cytometric immunophenotyping and minimal residual disease analysis in multiple myeloma. *Am J Clin Pathol* 2009;132(5):728–732.
36. Campana D. Minimal residual disease in acute lymphoblastic leukemia. Hematology/the Education Program of the American Society of Hematology. *Am Soc Hematol Educ Prog* 2010;2010:7–12.
37. Seegmiller AC, et al. Characterization of immunophenotypic aberrancies in 200 cases of B acute lymphoblastic leukemia. *Am J Clin Pathol* 2009;132(6):940–949.
38. Olaru D, et al. Multiparametric analysis of normal and postchemotherapy bone marrow: implication for the detection of leukemia-associated immunophenotypes. *Cytometry B Clin Cytom* 2008;74(1):17–24.
39. Fuda F MR, Xu Y, Karandikar N, et al. All cases of precursor T acute lymphoblastic leukemia/lymphoma exhibit multiple immunophenotypic aberrancies [Abstract]. *Mod Pathol* 2006;19:225A.
40. Karandikar NJ, Kroft S, ed. Flow cytometry in the diagnosis of acute leukemias and myelodysplastic/myeloproliferative disorders. In: McCoy J, Keren DF, Carey JL, eds. *Flow cytometry in clinical diagnosis*, 4th ed. Chicago: ASCP Press, 2007:167–214.
41. Borowitz MJ, et al. Comparison of diagnostic and relapse flow cytometry phenotypes in childhood acute lymphoblastic leukemia: implications for residual disease detection: a report from the children's oncology group. *Cytometry B Clin Cytom* 2005;68(1):18–24.
42. Weir EG, et al. A limited antibody panel can distinguish B-precursor acute lymphoblastic leukemia from normal B precursors with four color flow cytometry: implications for residual disease detection. *Leukemia* 1999;13(4):558–567.
43. Chen W, et al. Stability of leukemia-associated immunophenotypes in precursor B-lymphoblastic leukemia/lymphoma: a single institution experience. *Am J Clin Pathol* 2007;127(1):39–46.
44. Sanchez ML, et al. Incidence of phenotypic aberrations in a series of 467 patients with B chronic lymphoproliferative disorders: basis for the design of specific four-color stainings to be used for minimal residual disease investigation. *Leukemia* 2002;16(8):1460–1469.
45. Bruggemann M, Gokbuget N, Kneba M. Acute lymphoblastic leukemia: monitoring minimal residual disease as a therapeutic principle. *Semin Oncol* 2012;39(1):47–57.
46. Dominietto A. Minimal residual disease markers before and after allogeneic hematopoietic stem cell transplantation in acute myeloid leukemia. *Curr Opin Hematol* 2011;18(6):381–387.
47. Szczepanski T. Why and how to quantify minimal residual disease in acute lymphoblastic leukemia? *Leukemia* 2007;21:622–626.
48. van Dongen JJ, et al. Prognostic value of minimal residual disease in acute lymphoblastic leukaemia in childhood. *Lancet* 1998;352(9142):1731–1738.
49. Cave H, et al. Clinical significance of minimal residual disease in childhood acute lymphoblastic leukemia. European Organization for Research and Treatment of Cancer—Childhood Leukemia Cooperative Group. *N Engl J Med* 1998;339(9):591–598.

50. Coustan-Smith E, et al. Immunological detection of minimal residual disease in children with acute lymphoblastic leukaemia. *Lancet* 1998;351(9102):550–554.
51. Nyvold C, et al. Precise quantification of minimal residual disease at day 29 allows identification of children with acute lymphoblastic leukemia and an excellent outcome. *Blood* 2002;99(4):1253–1258.
52. Dworzak MN, et al. Prognostic significance and modalities of flow cytometric minimal residual disease detection in childhood acute lymphoblastic leukemia. *Blood* 2002;99(6):1952–1958.
53. van der Velden V, van Dongen JJ. MRD detection in acute lymphoblastic leukemia patients using Ig/TCR gene rearrangements as targets for real-time quantitative PCR. *Methods Mol Biol* 2009;538:115–150.
54. Denys B, et al. Improved flow cytometric detection of minimal residual disease in childhood acute lymphoblastic leukemia. *Leukemia* 2013;27:635–641.
55. Ravandi F, Jorgensen JL. Monitoring minimal residual disease in acute myeloid leukemia: ready for prime time? *J Natl Compr Canc Netw* 2012;10(8):1029–1036.
56. Freeman SD, Jovanovic JV, Grimwade D. Development of minimal residual disease-directed therapy in acute myeloid leukemia. *Semin Oncol* 2008;35(4): 388–400.
57. San Miguel JF, et al. Immunophenotyping investigation of minimal residual disease is a useful approach for predicting relapse in acute myeloid leukemia patients. *Blood* 1997;90(6):2465–2470.
58. Kern W, Schnittger S. Monitoring of acute myeloid leukemia by flow cytometry. *Curr Oncol Rep* 2003;5(5):405–412.
59. Grimwade D, et al. Prospective minimal residual disease monitoring to predict relapse of acute promyelocytic leukemia and to direct pre-emptive arsenic trioxide therapy. *J Clin Oncol* 2009;27(22):3650–3658.
60. Buccisano F, et al. Cytogenetic and molecular diagnostic characterization combined to postconsolidation minimal residual disease assessment by flow cytometry improves risk stratification in adult acute myeloid leukemia. *Blood* 2010;116(13):2295–2303.
61. Rubnitz JE, et al. Minimal residual disease-directed therapy for childhood acute myeloid leukaemia: results of the AML02 multicentre trial. *Lancet Oncol* 2010;11(6):543–552.
62. Liu W, et al. Usefulness of flow cytometric immunophenotyping for bone marrow staging in patients with mantle cell lymphoma after therapy. *Am J Clin Pathol* 2012;137(4):634–640.
63. Uhrmacher S, Erdfelder F, Kreuzer KA. Flow cytometry and polymerase chain reaction-based analyses of minimal residual disease in chronic lymphocytic leukemia. *Adv Hematol* 2010;2010. pii: 272517. doi: 10.1155/2010/272517. Epub Sep 20, 2010.
64. Varghese AM, Rawstron AC, Hillmen P. Eradicating minimal residual disease in chronic lymphocytic leukemia: should this be the goal of treatment? *Curr Hematol Malig Rep* 2010;5(1):35–44.
65. Bottcher S, et al. Minimal residual disease detection in mantle cell lymphoma: methods and significance of four-color flow cytometry compared to consensus IGH-polymerase chain reaction at initial staging and for follow-up examinations. *Haematologica* 2008;93(4):551–559.
66. Ferrero S, et al. Minimal residual disease detection in lymphoma and multiple myeloma: impact on therapeutic paradigms. *Hematol Oncol* 2011;29(4): 167–176.
67. Roederer M. Spectral compensation for flow cytometry: visualization artifacts, limitations, and caveats. *Cytometry* 2001;45(3):194–205.
68. Tung JW, et al. New approaches to fluorescence compensation and visualization of FACS data. *Clin Immunol* 2004;110(3):277–283.
69. Kalina T, et al. EuroFlow standardization of flow cytometer instrument settings and immunophenotyping protocols. *Leukemia* 2012;26(9):1986–2010.
70. Roederer M. Compensation in flow cytometry. *Curr Protoc Cytom* 2002;1.14.1–1.14.20.
71. Hulspas R, et al. Considerations for the control of background fluorescence in clinical flow cytometry. *Cytometry B Clin Cytom* 2009;76(6):355–364.
72. Shapiro H. *Practical flow cytometry*. Hoboken: John Wiley & Sons, Inc., 2003.
73. Borowitz M, Bene MC, Harris NL, et al. Acute leukemias of ambiguous lineage. In: Swerdlow SH, Campo E, Harris NL, et al., eds. *WHO* classification *of tumours of haematopoietic and lymphoid tissues*. Lyon: IARC Press, 2008:150–155.
74. Fukushima PI, et al. Flow cytometric analysis of kappa and lambda light chain expression in evaluation of specimens for B-cell neoplasia. *Cytometry* 1996;26(4):243–252.
75. Baer MR, et al. High frequency of immunophenotype changes in acute myeloid leukemia at relapse: implications for residual disease detection (Cancer and Leukemia Group B Study 8361). *Blood* 2001;97(11):3574–3580.
76. Langebrake C, et al. Immunophenotypic differences between diagnosis and relapse in childhood AML: Implications for MRD monitoring. *Cytometry B Clin Cytom* 2005;63(1):1–9.
77. van Wering ER, et al. Immunophenotypic changes between diagnosis and relapse in childhood acute lymphoblastic leukemia. *Leukemia* 1995;9(9):1523–1533.
78. Xu Y, et al. Comparison of immunophenotypes of small B-cell neoplasms in primary lymph node and concurrent blood or marrow samples. *Am J Clin Pathol* 2002;118(5):758–764.
79. Loken MR, et al. Normalization of bone marrow aspirates for hemodilution in flow cytometric analyses. *Cytometry B Clin Cytom* 2009;76(1):27–36.
80. Arber D, Vardiman JW, Brunning RD, et al. Acute myeloid leukemia with recurrent genetic abnormalities. In: Swerdlow SH, Campo E, Harris NL, et al., eds. *WHO classification of tumours of haematopoietic and lymphoid tissues*. Lyon: IARC Press, 2008:110–123.
81. Arber D, Porwit A, Brunning RD, et al. Acute myeloid leukemia with myelodysplasia-related changes. In: Swerdlow SH, Campo E, Harris NL, et al., eds. *WHO classification of tumours of haematopoietic and lymphoid tissues*. Lyon: IARC Press, 2008:124–126.
82. Vardiman J, Matutes E, Arber DA, et al. Therapy-related myeloid neoplasms. In: Swerdlow S, Campo E, Harris NL, Jaffe ES, Pileri SA, Stein H, Thiele J, Vardiman JW, eds. *WHO classification of tumours of haematopoietic and lymphoid tissues*. Lyon, France: IARC Press, 2008:127–129.
83. Arber D, Peterson L, Brunning, RD, et al. Acute myeloid leukemia, not otherwise specified. In: Swerdlow S, Campo E, Harris NL, et al., eds. *WHO classification of tumours of haematopoietic and lymphoid tissues*. Lyon, France: IARC Press, 2008.
84. Gorczyca W, et al. Immunophenotypic pattern of myeloid populations by flow cytometry analysis. *Methods Cell Biol* 2011;103:221–266.
85. Dalal BI, et al. Detection of CD34, TdT, CD56, CD2, CD4, and CD14 by flow cytometry is associated with NPM1 and FLT3 mutation status in cytogenetically normal acute myeloid leukemia. *Clin Lymphoma Myeloma Leuk* 2012;12(4):274–279.
86. Dong HY, et al. Flow cytometry rapidly identifies all acute promyelocytic leukemias with high specificity independent of underlying cytogenetic abnormalities. *Am J Clin Pathol* 2011;135(1):76–84.
87. Khalidi HS, et al. The immunophenotype of adult acute myeloid leukemia: high frequency of lymphoid antigen expression and comparison of immunophenotype, French-American-British classification, and karyotypic abnormalities. *Am J Clin Pathol* 1998;109(2):211–220.
88. Khoury H, et al. Acute myelogenous leukemia with t(8;21)—identification of a specific immunophenotype. *Leuk Lymphoma* 2003;44(10):1713–1718.
89. Orfao A, et al. The flow cytometric pattern of CD34, CD15 and CD13 expression in acute myeloblastic leukemia is highly characteristic of the presence of PML-RARalpha gene rearrangements. *Haematologica* 1999;84(5):405–412.
90. Borowitz M, Chan JKC. B lymphoblastic leukemia/lymphoma, not otherwise specified. In: Swerdlow S, Campo E, Harris NL, et al., eds. *WHO classification of tumours of haematopoietic and lymphoid tissues*. Lyon: IARC Press, 2008:168–170.
91. Borowitz M, Chan JKC. B lymphoblastic leukemia/lymphoma with recurrent genetic abnormalities. In: Swerdlow IS, Campo E, Harris NL, et al., eds. *WHO classification of tumours of haematopoietic and lymphoid tissues*. Lyon: IARC Press, 2008:171–175.
92. Borowitz M, Chan JKC. T lymphoblastic leukemia/lymphoma, not otherwise specified. In: Swerdlow S, Campo E, Harris NL, et al., eds. *WHO classification of tumours of haematopoietic and lymphoid tissues*. Lyon: IARC Press, 2008:176–178.
93. Kroft SH. Role of flow cytometry in pediatric hematopathology. *Am J Clin Pathol* 2004;122(Suppl):S19–S32.
94. McKenna RW, Asplund SL, Kroft SH. Immunophenotypic analysis of hematogones (B-lymphocyte precursors) and neoplastic lymphoblasts by 4-color flow cytometry. *Leuk Lymphoma* 2004;45(2):277–285.
95. McKenna RW, et al. Immunophenotypic analysis of hematogones (B-lymphocyte precursors) in 662 consecutive bone marrow specimens by 4-color flow cytometry. *Blood* 2001;98(8):2498–2507.
96. Kansal R, et al. Precursor B lymphoblastic leukemia with surface light chain immunoglobulin restriction: a report of 15 patients. *Am J Clin Pathol* 2004;121(4):512–525.
97. Nelson BP, et al. Surface immunoglobulin positive lymphoblastic leukemia in adults; a genetic spectrum. *Leuk Lymphoma* 2006;47(7):1352–1359.
98. Vasef MA, et al. Surface immunoglobulin light chain-positive acute lymphoblastic leukemia of FAB L1 or L2 type: a report of 6 cases in adults. *Am J Clin Pathol* 1998;110(2):143–149.
99. Gorczyca W, et al. Flow cytometry in the diagnosis of mediastinal tumors with emphasis on differentiating thymocytes from precursor T-lymphoblastic lymphoma/leukemia. *Leuk Lymphoma* 2004;45(3):529–538.
100. Li S, et al. Flow cytometry in the differential diagnosis of lymphocyte-rich thymoma from precursor T-cell acute lymphoblastic leukemia/lymphoblastic lymphoma. *Am J Clin Pathol* 2004;121(2):268–274.
101. Patel JL, et al. The immunophenotype of T-lymphoblastic lymphoma in children and adolescents: a Children's Oncology Group report. *Br J Haematol* 2012;159:454–461.
102. Terstappen LW, Huang S, Picker LJ. Flow cytometric assessment of human T-cell differentiation in thymus and bone marrow. *Blood* 1992;79(3):666–677.
103. Monaghan S, Karandikar NJ. Immunophenotypic differences in T-cell maturation spectrum of thymoma vs. other thymic diseases vs. T-cell lymphoblastic leukemia [Abstract]. *Mod Pathol* 2003;16:245A.
104. Crespo M, et al. ZAP-70 expression as a surrogate for immunoglobulin-variable-region mutations in chronic lymphocytic leukemia. *N Engl J Med* 2003;348(18):1764–1775.
105. Malavasi F, et al. CD38 and chronic lymphocytic leukemia: a decade later. *Blood* 2011;118(13):3470–3478.
106. Matutes E. Novel and emerging drugs for rarer chronic lymphoid leukaemias. *Curr Cancer Drug Targets* 2012;12(5):484–504.
107. Bertram HC, Check IJ, Milano MA. Immunophenotyping large B-cell lymphomas. Flow cytometric pitfalls and pathologic correlation. *Am J Clin Pathol* 2001;116(2):191–203.
108. Harrington AM, et al. The unique immunophenotype of double-hit lymphomas. *Am J Clin Pathol* 2011;135(4):649–650.
109. Jevremovic D, et al. CD5+ B-cell lymphoproliferative disorders: Beyond chronic lymphocytic leukemia and mantle cell lymphoma. *Leuk Res* 2010;34(9): 1235–1238.
110. Kaleem Z, White G, Vollmer RT. Critical analysis and diagnostic usefulness of limited immunophenotyping of B-cell non-Hodgkin lymphomas by flow cytometry. *Am J Clin Pathol* 2001;115(1):136–142.
111. McGowan P, et al. Differentiating between Burkitt lymphoma and CD10+ diffuse large B-cell lymphoma: the role of commonly used flow cytometry cell markers and the application of a multiparameter scoring system. *Am J Clin Pathol* 2012;137(4):665–670.
112. Schniederjan SD, et al. A novel flow cytometric antibody panel for distinguishing Burkitt lymphoma from CD10+ diffuse large B-cell lymphoma. *Am J Clin Pathol* 2010;133(5):718–726.
113. Stetler-Stevenson M, Tembhare PR. Diagnosis of hairy cell leukemia by flow cytometry. *Leuk Lymphoma* 2011;52(Suppl 2):11–13.
114. Venkataraman G, et al. Characteristic CD103 and CD123 expression pattern defines hairy cell leukemia: usefulness of CD123 and CD103 in the diagnosis of mature B-cell lymphoproliferative disorders. *Am J Clin Pathol* 2011;136(4):625–630.
115. Wu D, et al. "Double-Hit" mature B-cell lymphomas show a common immunophenotype by flow cytometry that includes decreased CD20 expression. *Am J Clin Pathol* 2010;134(2):258–265.
116. Chen HI, et al. Restricted kappa/lambda light chain ratio by flow cytometry in germinal center B cells in Hashimoto thyroiditis. *Am J Clin Pathol* 2006;125(1):42–48.
117. Chizuka A, et al. The diagnostic value of kappa/lambda ratios determined by flow cytometric analysis of biopsy specimens in B-cell lymphoma. *Clin Lab Haematol* 2002;24(1):33–36.
118. Reichard KK, McKenna RW, Kroft SH. Comparative analysis of light chain expression in germinal center cells and mantle cells of reactive lymphoid tissues. A four-color flow cytometric study. *Am J Clin Pathol* 2003;119(1):130–136.

119. Kroft SH. Monoclones, monotypes, and neoplasia pitfalls in lymphoma diagnosis. *Am J Clin Pathol* 2004;121(4):457–459.
120. Kussick SJ, et al. Prominent clonal B-cell populations identified by flow cytometry in histologically reactive lymphoid proliferations. *Am J Clin Pathol* 2004;121(4):464–472.
121. Li S, Eshleman JR, Borowitz MJ. Lack of surface immunoglobulin light chain expression by flow cytometric immunophenotyping can help diagnose peripheral B-cell lymphoma. *Am J Clin Pathol* 2002;118(2):229–234.
122. Horna P, et al. Flow cytometric analysis of surface light chain expression patterns in B-cell lymphomas using monoclonal and polyclonal antibodies. *Am J Clin Pathol* 2011;136(6):954–959.
123. Ahmad E, et al. Flow cytometric immunophenotypic profiles of mature gamma delta T-cell malignancies involving peripheral blood and bone marrow. *Cytometry B Clin Cytom* 2005;67(1):6–12.
124. Chen W, et al. Flow cytometric features of angioimmunoblastic T-cell lymphoma. *Cytometry B Clin Cytom* 2006;70(3):142–148.
125. Chen YH, et al. Clinical, morphologic, immunophenotypic, and molecular cytogenetic assessment of CD4-/CD8-gammadelta T-cell large granular lymphocytic leukemia. *Am J Clin Pathol* 2011;136(2):289–299.
126. Hristov AC, Vonderheid EC, Borowitz MJ. Simplified flow cytometric assessment in mycosis fungoides and Sezary syndrome. *Am J Clin Pathol* 2011;136(6): 944–953.
127. Jamal S, et al. Immunophenotypic analysis of peripheral T-cell neoplasms. A multiparameter flow cytometric approach. *Am J Clin Pathol* 2001;116(4):512–526.
128. Jiang NG, et al. Flow cytometric immunophenotyping is of great value to diagnosis of natural killer cell neoplasms involving bone marrow and peripheral blood. *Ann Hematol* 2013;92:89–96.
129. Karube K, et al. Usefulness of flow cytometry for differential diagnosis of precursor and peripheral T-cell and NK-cell lymphomas: analysis of 490 cases. *Pathol Int* 2008;58(2):89–97.
130. Morice WG, et al. Chronic lymphoproliferative disorder of natural killer cells: a distinct entity with subtypes correlating with normal natural killer cell subsets. *Leukemia* 2010;24(4):881–884.
131. Morice WG, et al. A comparison of morphologic features, flow cytometry, TCR-Vbeta analysis, and TCR-PCR in qualitative and quantitative assessment of peripheral blood involvement by Sezary syndrome. *Am J Clin Pathol* 2006;125(3):364–374.
132. Tembhare P, et al. Flow cytometric immunophenotypic assessment of T-cell clonality by vbeta repertoire analysis in fine-needle aspirates and cerebrospinal fluid. *Am J Clin Pathol* 2012;137(2):220–226.
133. Tembhare P, et al. Flow cytometric immunophenotypic assessment of T-cell clonality by Vbeta repertoire analysis: detection of T-cell clonality at diagnosis and monitoring of minimal residual disease following therapy. *Am J Clin Pathol* 2011;135(6):890–900.
134. Geissinger E, et al. CD52 expression in peripheral T-cell lymphomas determined by combined immunophenotyping using tumor cell specific T-cell receptor antibodies. *Leuk Lymphoma* 2009;50(6):1010–1016.
135. Jiang L, et al. Variable CD52 expression in mature T cell and NK cell malignancies: implications for alemtuzumab therapy. *Br J Haematol* 2009;145(2): 173–179.
136. Osuji N, et al. CD52 expression in T-cell large granular lymphocyte leukemia—implications for treatment with alemtuzumab. *Leuk Lymphoma* 2005;46(5): 723–727.
137. Rodig SJ, et al. Heterogeneous CD52 expression among hematologic neoplasms: implications for the use of alemtuzumab (CAMPATH-1H). *Clin Cancer Res* 2006;12(23):7174–7179.
138. Beck RC, et al. Detection of mature T-cell leukemias by flow cytometry using anti-T-cell receptor V beta antibodies. *Am J Clin Pathol* 2003;120(5):785–794.
139. Feng B, et al. TCR-Vbeta flow cytometric analysis of peripheral blood for assessing clonality and disease burden in patients with T cell large granular lymphocyte leukaemia. *J Clin Pathol* 2010;63(2):141–146.
140. Langerak AW, et al. Molecular and flow cytometric analysis of the Vbeta repertoire for clonality assessment in mature TCRalphabeta T-cell proliferations. *Blood* 2001;98(1):165–173.
141. Lima M, et al. Immunophenotypic analysis of the TCR-Vbeta repertoire in 98 persistent expansions of CD3(+)/TCR-alphabeta(+) large granular lymphocytes: utility in assessing clonality and insights into the pathogenesis of the disease. *Am J Pathol* 2001;159(5):1861–1868.
142. Morice WG, et al. Flow cytometric assessment of TCR-Vbeta expression in the evaluation of peripheral blood involvement by T-cell lymphoproliferative disorders: a comparison with conventional T-cell immunophenotyping and molecular genetic techniques. *Am J Clin Pathol* 2004;121(3):373–383.
143. Morice WG, et al. Demonstration of aberrant T-cell and natural killer-cell antigen expression in all cases of granular lymphocytic leukaemia. *Br J Haematol* 2003;120(6):1026–1036.
144. Nadav L, et al. Diverse niches within multiple myeloma bone marrow aspirates affect plasma cell enumeration. *Br J Haematol* 2006;133(5):530–532.
145. Paiva B, et al. Multiparameter flow cytometry quantification of bone marrow plasma cells at diagnosis provides more prognostic information than morphological assessment in myeloma patients. *Haematologica* 2009;94(11):1599–1602.
146. Smock KJ, Perkins SL, Bahler DW. Quantitation of plasma cells in bone marrow aspirates by flow cytometric analysis compared with morphologic assessment. *Arch Pathol Lab Med* 2007;131(6):951–955.
147. Cogbill C, Spears M, Harrington A, et al. Analysis of variables affecting the flow cytometric recovery of plasma cell myeloma in bone marrow aspirates. *Mod Pathol* 2011;224(Suppl 1):291A.
148. Lin, P, et al. Flow cytometric immunophenotypic analysis of 306 cases of multiple myeloma. *Am J Clin Pathol* 2004;121(4):482–488.
149. Liu D, et al. Immunophenotypic heterogeneity of normal plasma cells: comparison with minimal residual plasma cell myeloma. *J Clin Pathol* 2012;65(9): 823–829.
150. Alapat D, et al. Diagnostic usefulness and prognostic impact of CD200 expression in lymphoid malignancies and plasma cell myeloma. *Am J Clin Pathol* 2012;137(1):93–100.
151. Olteanu H, et al. CD200 expression in plasma cell myeloma. *Br J Haematol* 2011;153(3):408–411.
152. Olteanu H, Harrington AM, Kroft SH. Immunophenotypic stability of CD200 expression in plasma cell myeloma. *Am J Clin Pathol* 2012;137(6):1013–1014.
153. Pozdnyakova O, et al. Patterns of expression of CD56 and CD117 on neoplastic plasma cells and association with genetically distinct subtypes of plasma cell myeloma. *Leuk Lymphoma* 2012;53(10):1905–1910.
154. Rawstron AC, et al. Report of the European Myeloma Network on multiparametric flow cytometry in multiple myeloma and related disorders. *Haematologica* 2008;93(3):431–438.
155. Seegmiller AC, et al. Immunophenotypic differentiation between neoplastic plasma cells in mature B-cell lymphoma vs plasma cell myeloma. *Am J Clin Pathol* 2007;127(2):176–181.
156. Bataille R, et al. CD117 (c-kit) is aberrantly expressed in a subset of MGUS and multiple myeloma with unexpectedly good prognosis. *Leuk Res* 2008;32(3):379–382.
157. Buda G, et al. CD23 expression in plasma cell leukaemia. *Br J Haematol* 2010;150(6):724–725.
158. Buonaccorsi JN, et al. Clinicopathologic analysis of the impact of CD23 expression in plasma cell myeloma with t(11;14)(q13;q32). *Ann Diagn Pathol* 2011;15(6):385–388.
159. Heerema-McKenney A, et al. Clinical, immunophenotypic, and genetic characterization of small lymphocyte-like plasma cell myeloma: a potential mimic of mature B-cell lymphoma. *Am J Clin Pathol* 2010;133(2):265–270.
160. Johnsen HE, et al. Improved survival for multiple myeloma in Denmark based on autologous stem cell transplantation and novel drug therapy in collaborative trials: analysis of accrual, prognostic variables, selection bias, and clinical behavior on survival in more than 1200 patients in trials of the Nordic Myeloma Study Group. *Clin Lymphoma Myeloma Leuk* 2010;10(4):290–296.
161. Moreau, P, et al. Lack of CD27 in myeloma delineates different presentation and outcome. *Br J Haematol* 2006;132(2):168–170.
162. Moreaux J, et al. CD200 is a new prognostic factor in multiple myeloma. *Blood* 2006;108(13):4194–4197.
163. Sahara N, Takeshita A. Prognostic significance of surface markers expressed in multiple myeloma: CD56 and other antigens. *Leuk Lymphoma* 2004;45(1):61–65.
164. Porwit A. Role of flow cytometry in diagnostics of myelodysplastic syndromes—beyond the WHO 2008 classification. *Semin Diagn Pathol* 2011;28(4):273–282.
165. Stetler-Stevenson M, Yuan CM. Myelodysplastic syndromes: the role of flow cytometry in diagnosis and prognosis. *Int J Lab Hematol* 2009;31(5):479–483.
166. van de Loosdrecht AA, et al. Rationale for the clinical application of flow cytometry in patients with myelodysplastic syndromes: position paper of an International Consortium and the European LeukemiaNet Working Group. *Leuk Lymphoma* 2013;54(3):472–475.
167. Kussick SJ, et al. Four-color flow cytometry shows strong concordance with bone marrow morphology and cytogenetics in the evaluation for myelodysplasia. *Am J Clin Pathol* 2005;124(2):170–181.
168. Kussick SJ, Wood BL. Four-color flow cytometry identifies virtually all cytogenetically abnormal bone marrow samples in the workup of non-CML myeloproliferative disorders. *Am J Clin Pathol* 2003;120(6):854–865.
169. Ossenkoppele GJ, van de Loosdrecht AA, Schuurhuis GJ. Review of the relevance of aberrant antigen expression by flow cytometry in myeloid neoplasms. *Br J Haematol* 2011;153(4):421–436.
170. Monaghan SA, et al. Altered neutrophil maturation patterns that limit identification of myelodysplastic syndromes. *Cytometry B Clin Cytom* 2012;82(4):217–228.
171. Truong F, et al. The utility of flow cytometric immunophenotyping in cytopenic patients with a non-diagnostic bone marrow: a prospective study. *Leuk Res* 2009;33(8):1039–1046.
172. Harrington A, Olteanu H, Kroft S. The specificity of immunophenotypic alterations in blasts in nonacute myeloid disorders. *Am J Clin Pathol* 2010;134(5): 749–761.
173. Cherian S, et al. Peripheral blood MDS score: a new flow cytometric tool for the diagnosis of myelodysplastic syndromes. *Cytometry B Clin Cytom* 2005;64(1): 9–17.
174. Cherian S, et al. Flow-cytometric analysis of peripheral blood neutrophils: a simple, objective, independent and potentially clinically useful assay to facilitate the diagnosis of myelodysplastic syndromes. *Am J Hematol* 2005;79(3):243–245.
175. Chopra A, et al. Flow cytometry in myelodysplastic syndrome: analysis of diagnostic utility using maturation pattern-based and quantitative approaches. *Ann Hematol* 2012;91(9):1351–1362.
176. Chung JW, et al. A Combination of CD15/CD10, CD64/CD33, CD16/CD13 or CD11b flow cytometric granulocyte panels is sensitive and specific for diagnosis of myelodysplastic syndrome. *Ann Clin Lab Sci* 2012;42(3):271–280.
177. Cutler JA, et al. Phenotypic abnormalities strongly reflect genotype in patients with unexplained cytopenias. *Cytometry B Clin Cytom* 2011;80(3):150–157.
178. Della Porta MG, Lanza F, Del Vecchio L. Flow cytometry immunophenotyping for the evaluation of bone marrow dysplasia. *Cytometry B Clin Cytom* 2011;80(4):201–211.
179. Finn WG, et al. Immunophenotypic signatures of benign and dysplastic granulopoiesis by cytomic profiling. *Cytometry B Clin Cytom* 2011;80(5):282–290.
180. Kern W, et al. Clinical utility of multiparameter flow cytometry in the diagnosis of 1013 patients with suspected myelodysplastic syndrome: correlation to cytomorphology, cytogenetics, and clinical data. *Cancer* 2010;116(19):4549–4563.
181. Malcovati L, et al. Flow cytometry evaluation of erythroid and myeloid dysplasia in patients with myelodysplastic syndrome. *Leukemia* 2005;19(5):776–783.
182. Moon H.W, et al. Immunophenotypic features of granulocytes, monocytes, and blasts in myelodysplastic syndromes. *Korean J Lab Med* 2010;30(2):97–104.
183. Ogata K, et al. Differences in blast immunophenotypes among disease types in myelodysplastic syndromes: a multicenter validation study. *Leuk Res* 2012; 36(10):1229–1236.
184. Stetler-Stevenson M, et al. Diagnostic utility of flow cytometric immunophenotyping in myelodysplastic syndrome. *Blood* 2001;98(4):979–987.
185. Tang G, et al. Multi-color CD34(+) progenitor-focused flow cytometric assay in evaluation of myelodysplastic syndromes in patients with post cancer therapy cytopenia. *Leuk Res* 2012;36(8):974–981.
186. Westers TM, et al. Implementation of flow cytometry in the diagnostic work-up of myelodysplastic syndromes in a multicenter approach: report from the Dutch Working Party on Flow Cytometry in MDS. *Leuk Res* 2012;36(4):422–430.
187. Xu Y, et al. Flow cytometric analysis of monocytes as a tool for distinguishing chronic myelomonocytic leukemia from reactive monocytosis. *Am J Clin Pathol* 2005;124(5):799–806.
188. Valent P, et al. Definitions and standards in the diagnosis and treatment of the myelodysplastic syndromes: Consensus statements and report from a working conference. *Leuk Res* 2007;31(6):727–736.

189. Westers TM, et al. Standardization of flow cytometry in myelodysplastic syndromes: a report from an international consortium and the European LeukemiaNet Working Group. *Leukemia* 2012;26(7):1730–1741.
190. Chu SC, et al. Flow cytometric scoring system as a diagnostic and prognostic tool in myelodysplastic syndromes. *Leuk Res* 2011;35(7):868–873.
191. Scott BL, et al. Validation of a flow cytometric scoring system as a prognostic indicator for posttransplantation outcome in patients with myelodysplastic syndrome. *Blood* 2008;112(7):2681–2686.
192. Wells DA, et al. Myeloid and monocytic dyspoiesis as determined by flow cytometric scoring in myelodysplastic syndrome correlates with the IPSS and with outcome after hematopoietic stem cell transplantation. *Blood* 2003;102(1):394–403.
193. Xu F, et al. Flow cytometric scoring system (FCMSS) assisted diagnosis of myelodysplastic syndromes (MDS) and the biological significance of FCMSS-based immunophenotypes. *Br J Haematol* 2010;149(4):587–597.
194. Della Porta MG, et al. Multicenter validation of a reproducible flow cytometric score for the diagnosis of low-grade myelodysplastic syndromes: results of a European LeukemiaNET study. *Haematologica* 2012;97(8):1209–1217.
195. Horny H, Metcalfe DD, Bennett JM, et al. Mastocytosis. In: Swerdlow S, Campo E, Harris NL, Jaffe ES, Pileri SA, Stein, H, Thiele J, Vardiman JW, eds. *WHO classification of tumours of haematopoietic and lymphoid tissues*. Lyon: IARC Press, 2008:54–63.
196. Escribano L, et al. Immunophenotype of bone marrow mast cells in indolent systemic mast cell disease in adults. *Leuk Lymphoma* 1999;35(3–4):227–235.
197. Escribano L, et al. Immunophenotypic analysis of mast cells in mastocytosis: When and how to do it. Proposals of the Spanish Network on Mastocytosis (REMA). *Cytometry B Clin Cytom* 2004;58(1):1–8.
198. Escribano L, et al. Abnormal expression of CD antigens in mastocytosis. *Int Arch Allergy Immunol* 2002;127(2):127–132.
199. Orfao A, et al. Flow cytometric analysis of mast cells from normal and pathological human bone marrow samples: identification and enumeration. *Am J Pathol* 1996;149(5):1493–1499.
200. Sanchez-Munoz L, et al. Immunophenotypic characterization of bone marrow mast cells in mastocytosis and other mast cell disorders. *Methods Cell Biol* 2011;103:333–359.
201. Escribano L, et al. Utility of flow cytometric analysis of mast cells in the diagnosis and classification of adult mastocytosis. *Leuk Res* 2001;25(7):563–570.
202. Morgado JM, et al. Immunophenotyping in systemic mastocytosis diagnosis: "CD25 positive" alone is more informative than the "CD25 and/or CD2" WHO criterion. *Mod Pathol* 2012;25(4):516–521.
203. Valent P, et al. Standards and standardization in mastocytosis: consensus statements on diagnostics, treatment recommendations and response criteria. *Eur J Clin Invest* 2007;37(6):435–453.
204. Valent P, et al. Diagnostic criteria and classification of mastocytosis: a consensus proposal. *Leuk Res* 2001;25(7):603–625.
205. Pozdnyakova O, et al. High-sensitivity flow cytometric analysis for the evaluation of systemic mastocytosis including the identification of a new flow cytometric criterion for bone marrow involvement. *Am J Clin Pathol* 2012;138(3):416–424.
206. Sutherland DR, Keeney M, Illingworth A. Practical guidelines for the high-sensitivity detection and monitoring of paroxysmal nocturnal hemoglobinuria clones by flow cytometry. *Cytometry B Clin Cytom* 2012;82(4):195–208.
207. Parker CJ. Paroxysmal nocturnal hemoglobinuria. *Curr Opin Hematol* 2012;19(3):141–148.
208. Parker C, et al. Diagnosis and management of paroxysmal nocturnal hemoglobinuria. *Blood* 2005;106(12):3699–3709.
209. Olteanu H, et al. Differential usefulness of various markers in the flow cytometric detection of paroxysmal nocturnal hemoglobinuria in blood and bone marrow. *Am J Clin Pathol* 2006;126(5):781–788.
210. Fromm JR, Thomas A, Wood BL. Flow cytometry can diagnose classical hodgkin lymphoma in lymph nodes with high sensitivity and specificity. *Am J Clin Pathol* 2009;131(3):322–332.
211. Fromm JR, Thomas A, Wood BL. Increased expression of T cell antigens on T cells in classical Hodgkin lymphoma. *Cytometry B Clin Cytom* 2010;78(6):387–388.
212. Fromm JR, Wood BL. Strategies for immunophenotyping and purifying classical Hodgkin lymphoma cells from lymph nodes by flow cytometry and flow cytometric cell sorting. *Methods* 2012;57(3):368–375.

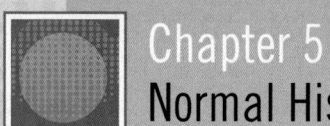

Chapter 5
Normal Histology of the Lymphoid Tissues

J. Han van Krieken

Lymphoid tissue is found all over the body. It occurs in well-organized lymphoid organs, such as the lymph nodes and the spleen, or as extranodal lymphoid tissue as part of the gut, skin, and lung. It may develop in any part of the body under specific conditions.

The lymphoid organs are divided into central and peripheral organs. The bone marrow and the thymus constitute the central lymphoid organs, and the lymph nodes, the spleen, and extranodal lymphoid tissues constitute the peripheral lymphoid organs. The bone marrow is the site of lymphopoiesis. Some lymphocytic precursors develop into B cells, but most become T cells. The generation of a diversity of effector B cells requires a two-step maturation process. The first step occurs in the bone marrow and results in the development of virgin or naive B cells. The second step takes place in the peripheral lymphoid organs, where affinity maturation of the naive B cells takes place on encounter with a specific antigen, resulting in the formation of plasma cells and memory B cells. The generation of mature T cells occurs exclusively in the thymus, where T-cell precursors develop into a variety of mature CD4-positive (CD4⁺) and CD8⁺ T cells through a process of positive and negative selection. T cells do not require further affinity maturation in secondary lymphoid tissues. In contrast to B cells, T cells are activated only in secondary lymphoid organs and start to proliferate on appropriate antigen stimulation.

The architecture of the thymus and of the peripheral lymphoid organs offers the ideal microenvironment for these processes. Knowledge of these structures and the immunophenotype of their cellular components within their natural microanatomic environment has improved significantly by the addition of immunohistochemistry to the morphologic studies on lymphoid tissues. Immunophenotyping allows identification of cell lineage and provides information on the stage of maturation, activation, and differentiation of lymphocytes. Immunohistochemistry has offered the opportunity to identify and distinguish more precisely the nonlymphoid components of the lymphoid tissues as well, including the monocyte-derived antigen-presenting cells and macrophages. The use of antibodies against adhesion molecules expressed by endothelial lining cells and by lymphocytes has led to a better understanding of lymphocyte trafficking and homing.

Molecular techniques performed on tissue fragments and particularly experiments carried out on selected and defined areas, cell clusters, or on single cells dissected from tissue sections, together with *in vitro* experiments, and the development of knockout and transgenic animal's experiments have profoundly changed our understanding of the structure of lymphoid tissues and have resulted in new views and concepts of the functional microanatomy of these tissues as the morphologic substrate of the immune response. This knowledge is essential in the analysis of lymphoid tissues in pathologic conditions, because it is helpful to recognize underlying pathogenic mechanisms.

This chapter discusses the histology and the immunohistology of the thymus, lymph node, and spleen and finally factors governing lymphocyte trafficking. The historical description of the microanatomy of these organs, as reported by classic histology, is presented first. This information is complemented by the results obtained by immunohistochemical analysis. The functional significance of the various compartments identified by morphology is discussed.

The bone marrow, which is the site of lymphopoiesis in postnatal life and represents an additional microenvironment for B-cell maturation, is discussed in Chapter 1. Particular features of extranodal lymphoid tissues are the subject of Chapter 28.

THE THYMUS

The thymus is a lobulated, primary lymphoid organ and has as main function the maturation of T lymphocytes. Its dominant cellular components are epithelial cells and T lymphocytes that mature from the cortex, the peripheral part of the lobules, to the medulla, the central part. The thymus is a completely encapsulated, pyramid-shaped organ located in the anterosuperior mediastinum. It is composed of two lobes that join at their lower poles, which may reach the level of the fourth costal cartilage. The upper poles extend into the neck. The gray color of the thymus during infancy turns yellow with increasing age because of accumulation of fat tissue. Because this fat merely takes the place of normal thymus parenchyma, the organ's shape and volume remain unchanged (1).

Atrophy

In relation to body weight, thymic weight is maximal at birth, and its absolute weight peaks at puberty. Even after excluding age-related differences in the weight of this organ, large interindividual variations exist. These concepts are based on autopsy findings showing a thymus weighing 12 to 15 g at birth and 30 to 40 g at puberty. This prominent increase in absolute mass is followed by a gradual decrease, or "age-related thymic involution," leaving a thymus weighing no more than 10 to 15 g at the age of 60 years. Involution is accompanied by a gradual replacement of the thymic parenchyma by fat tissue until 40 to 50 years of age, after which little changes (1,2). Despite of its notable decrease in size, the thymus never disappears completely, and it remains functionally active even after puberty (1). Nevertheless, the impaired T-cell function that accompanies ageing is attributed to thymic involution resulting in a smaller number of naïve T cells (3). Remnants of the thymus with residual epithelium and cortical thymocytes are preserved, permitting the thymus to act as a site of T-cell differentiation and maturation throughout the entire life (4).

Microscopically, the involution is the result of atrophy of the parenchyma and concomitant accumulation of fat cells (Fig. 5.1A). This gradual decrease of the parenchyma is accompanied by an accentuation of so-called Hassall corpuscles (see Fig. 5.1B). Some of the corpuscles calcify, but others transform into thymic cysts (2). The morphology of the residual epithelial

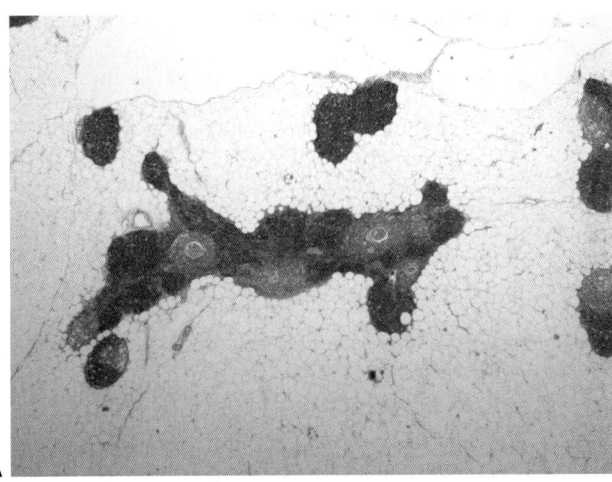
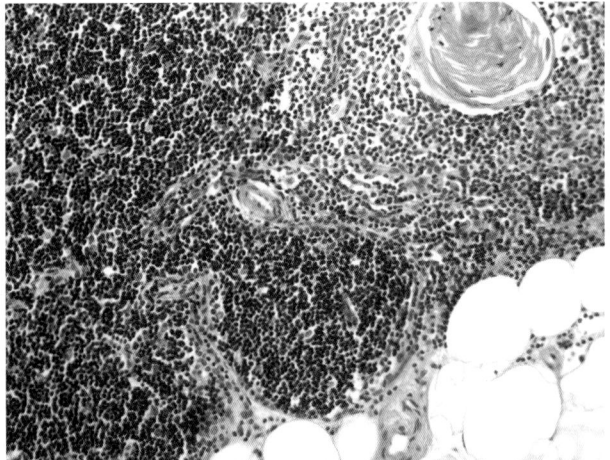

FIGURE 5.1. Hematoxylin and eosin–stained, paraffin-embedded thymic tissue of an adolescent. A: Lobulation of the thymic parenchyma and clear delineation between the dark-stained cortex and the lighter medulla are shown (H&E stain, original magnification: 60× magnification). There is fatty replacement, but the morphology of the thymus tissue is retained. **B:** Detail of the cortex and medulla in which a Hassall corpuscle is present (H&E stain, original magnification: 250× magnification). The cortex contains far more lymphocytes than the medulla. In the medulla, the light-stained large nuclei of the thymic epithelium can be recognized.

cells does not show any significant changes, which probably implies that they remain biologically active. Using immunohistochemistry it became clear that this persistent decrease in the number of epithelial cells and thymocytes is not the only event responsible for age-related thymic involution: there is an even more pronounced decrease in medullary interdigitating dendritic cells (5).

Histology and Immunohistology

Because the fibrous capsule that surrounds the thymus extends into the thymic parenchyma as loose septa, the organ is incompletely subdivided into various lobules measuring 0.5 to 2 mm. These lobules represent the basic structural units of the thymus, which comprises two morphologically distinct areas, a cortex and a medulla (Fig. 5.1). Epithelial cells and T lymphocytes or thymocytes constitute the major components of both regions. The subcapsular area of the cortex is occupied by somewhat larger thymocytes with a blastlike nucleus and a high number of mitotic figures. The distinction between cortex and medulla at the light microscopic level is evident because the amount of lymphocytes in the cortex far outnumbers those in the medulla. In a hematoxylin and eosin (H&E) stain, the medulla appears less intensely stained than the cortex (Fig. 5.1B). The subcapsular and perivascular areas are considered to be a separate compartment of the thymus, referred to as the perivascular space (6).

Thymic Epithelium

The epithelial cells, which especially in the cortex are difficult to recognize by routine light microscopy, are a heterogeneous population of round to spindle-shaped cells. Ultrastructurally, six different subtypes have been identified and described, of which four variants are localized to the cortex and two are confined to the medulla (7). As a whole, epithelial cells provide the appropriate microenvironment for T-cell maturation. However, because the development of T lymphocytes is an extremely complex process, each of the epithelial cell variants exercises its own specific function in the establishment of an effective T-cell compartment.

The epithelial network of the middle and deep cortex consists of cells characterized by their long cytoplasmic processes embracing thymocytes. These cortical epithelial cells represent

the *in vivo* equivalent of thymic nurse cells, a cell population that has been extensively studied *in vitro* (8). The results of these *in vitro* experiments, using cell lines derived from murine thymic nurse cells, suggest that they could be involved in the negative selection process of thymocytes by inducing thymocytic apoptosis (9).

Despite the marked differences in the submicroscopic level appearance of the various epithelial cell types, striking similarities in their morphology, accentuating their common origin, are evident. First, every thymic epithelial cell displays slender cytoplasmic processes, which explains the term *dendritic cell*. These dendrites exhibit well-developed desmosomes at their ends through which the epithelial cells are connected with one another. The whole of thymic epithelial cells creates a firm meshwork throughout the entire parenchyma in which the other cell types are embedded. The epithelial origin of these cells is further confirmed by the presence of a supporting basement membrane. The basal lamina surrounding medullary epithelial cells shows focal gaps, and only cortical epithelial cells lining mesenchymal spaces have a continuous basal membrane to separate them from the neighboring fibrous tissue (1). Immunohistochemistry and electron microscopy of thymic epithelial cells have shown the presence of intermediate and thin filaments within the cytoplasm of these cells. The intermediate filaments, which correspond to tonofilaments, are clustered in thick bundles attached to the desmosomes. They form an extensive filamentous network within the cell body and the cytoplasmic processes of the cortical and the medullary epithelial cells. Bundles of thin actin-like filaments, located immediately underneath the plasma membrane, complete the filamentous cytoskeleton of the epithelial cells. Subcortical epithelial cells typically show an abundance of thin filaments, but this portion of the cytoskeleton is nearly undetectable in medullary epithelial cells (10).

Hassall corpuscles (Fig. 5.1B) are clusters of concentrically arranged epithelial cells located in the medulla, but in addition to their thymic epithelial cell features, they acquire characteristics of squamous epithelium by exhibiting a variable degree of keratinization and staining with antibodies against terminally differentiated epithelium. Their precise function or significance is unresolved. Although interpreted in the past as a terminal phase of a degenerative process, they are considered a dynamic structure that is involved in the intrathymic maturation of T cells (11). The epithelial cells that compose the Hassall corpuscles contain a particularly well-developed framework of tonofilaments (10). These thymic corpuscles do not constitute isolated epithelial islets within the thymic medulla but form, together with the other epithelial components of the inner part of the thymic parenchyma, an uninterrupted epithelial structure.

Subcapsular epithelial cells, a minority of cortical epithelial cells, and almost all medullary epithelial cells can be considered as a functionally distinct group of neuroendocrine cells. These cells strongly express oxytocin, vasopressin, and neurophysin-like peptides (12). These peptides are synthesized within these cells, where the proteins can be demonstrated and the corresponding mRNA is found (13). It has been suggested that, analogous to neurosecretory cells found elsewhere, neuroendocrine cells of the thymus convert neuronal signals into neuropeptide secretion. Accepting this hypothesis, thymic oxytocin and vasopressin, secreted as a result of yet undefined neuronal influences, are expected to exert a direct immunomodulation on T-cell maturation (12).

Antibodies against other substances involved in intercellular signaling—the thymic hormone thymuline, members of the thymosin family, and thymopoietin—immunoreact with a subpopulation of these neuroendocrine cells, particularly subcapsular and medullary epithelial cells (14). These hormones also affect the maturation of T-cell precursors and the expression of T-cell antigens.

The entire cortical epithelium, including the nurse cells, reacts with Mab-MR6, recognizing a component of the interleukin-4 (IL-4) receptor complex. Consequently, these cells may act as an IL-4 reservoir for the surrounding immature cortical thymocytes (15). Antibodies against major histocompatibility complex (MHC) class II molecules (e.g., HLA-DR) stain a fine meshwork of cytoplasmic processes originating from the epithelial cells in the outer cortex that embrace nonreactive thymocytes, arranged singly or in small clusters. Considerable parts of the inner cortex and the medulla are negative for HLA-DR (16).

T Lymphocytes

T lymphocytes (i.e., thymocytes) displaying heterogeneous features corresponding to the various stages of thymocyte maturation predominate in the thymic cortex. The immature lymphoblasts are found in the subcapsular region. Maturation occurs toward the medulla, resulting in medium-sized thymocytes throughout the cortex, and at the corticomedullary junction, mature small lymphocytes are scattered among the epithelial cells in the medulla. This is a complex process involving many transcription factors with the Notch pathway as a key player (17,18).

The most immature thymic T cells (i.e., T-cell precursors) are identified by the expression of TdT, CD34, CD33, CD45RA, and CD38^{low}, typically lacking surface CD2, CD5, CD4, CD8, CD1, and CD3 (15). They express the integrins very late activation (VLA) antigen-4 (VLA-4, $\alpha_4\beta_1$, CD49d/CD29), VLA-5 ($\alpha_5\beta_1$, CD49e/CD29), and PGP-1 (CD44), which potentially mediate homing of the precursors to the thymus (19,20). T-cell receptor (TCR) genes are still in the germline configuration. These multipotent progenitor cells have the capacity to develop into T cells and NK cells (21).

Unlike their predecessors, the earliest committed T-cell progenitors have acquired surface CD1 (Fig. 5.2A), CD2, CD5, CD7, and cytoplasmic CD3, but they are still devoid of surface CD3, CD8, and CD4. These triple-negative thymocytes show an intense proliferative activity (Fig. 5.2B), which depends on IL-7 (22–24) and stem cell factor (25,26). BCL-2, an anti-apoptosis protein, may add to the prolonged cell survival of these early thymocytes (27). During this stage of thymocyte development, the TCR β chain is rearranged. After this pivotal event in T-cell maturation, TCR β is expressed on the cell surface in a complex with gp33 and the pre-TCR α chain. The resultant primitive TCR complex occurs in association with CD3 (28–30). Signaling through this pre-TCR complex is crucial for the next step in the generation of mature T lymphocytes, which comprises three molecular biologic events: the concomitant up-regulation of CD4 and CD8 resulting in double-positive thymocytes, rearrangement of the TCR α locus, and allelic exclusion of the TCR β locus (28–30). As a consequence of this complex event, CD4$^+$CD8$^+$TCR^{low} cortical thymocytes are brought about, representing the first thymic T-cell population to express the definitive TCR $\alpha\beta$ chain (19).

Subsequently, these CD3^{low}, double-positive thymocytes are positively or negatively selected by thymic stromal cells. Many factors, such as the density of the MHC molecules and coreceptors expressed on the auxiliary thymic cells and the nature and concentration of peptides presented on their surface determine the ultimate fate of the T cells subject to this selection process (31–33). However, the level of avidity between TCR and MHC-peptide complexes is the main factor mediating survival signals or deletion by apoptosis. High-affinity binding of the TCR to peptides, derived from autoantigen, superantigens, or both, presented in the context of self-MHC results in clonal deletion

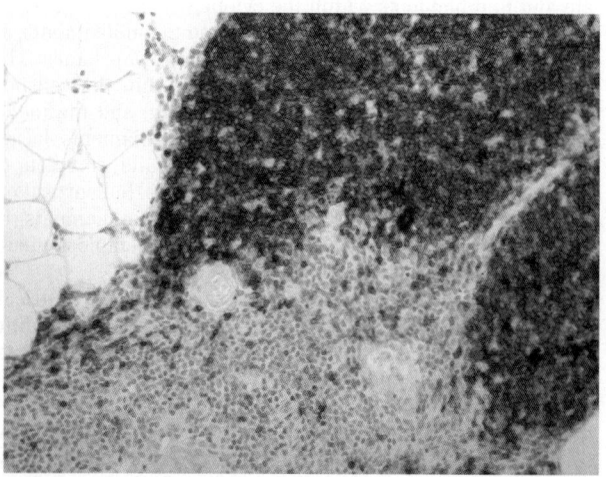
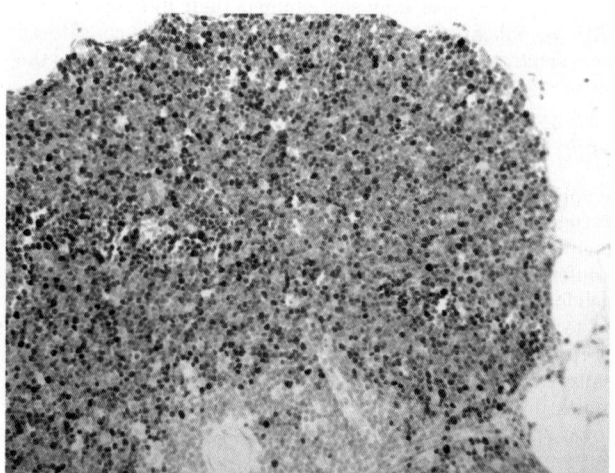

FIGURE 5.2. A: Immunohistochemistry shows expression of CD1a in the cortical thymocytes associated with a high proliferation (**B**, mib1; original magnifications: 250× magnification).

of autoreactive T cells (34,35). In contrast, low or intermediate avidity confers to positive selection, which is indispensable for the final maturation of double-positive thymocytes to CD4 or CD8 single-positive T cells.

Positive selection *in vivo* is mediated predominantly by cortical epithelial cells that express MHC class I or class II molecules (36), whereas *in vitro* experiments suggest that negative selection comes about most efficiently when the antigen is presented by medullary dendritic cells (37). Most thymocytes, unable to pass through the selection process because of defective TCR/MHC interaction, undergo apoptosis. All thymocytes triggered to die, whether apoptosis is a result of negative selection or caused by lack of stimulation, are thoroughly eliminated by the numerous phagocytes in the cortex and medulla, among which are the aforementioned cortical epithelial nurse cells.

B Lymphocytes

The presence of B cells as a consistent component of the human thymus is well established (38–41). There are several subsets of B lymphocytes with distinct B-cell subsets in the perivascular space and in the parenchyma, preferentially in the neighborhood of Hassall corpuscles. This latter subset is morphologically and phenotypically distinct from the B cells composing the B follicle of the lymph node, but they do express most pan-B-cell markers, including CD19, CD20, CD22, CD37, CD72, CD76, and weakly express IgM and IgD (38). An important subset is CD2+ and CD40+, markers that are invariably present on T lymphocytes but only occasionally found on B cells (41). CD2 may mediate the interaction of these B cells with the surrounding thymocytes and epithelial cells through their ligand LFA-3. B and T cells would benefit from this CD2 interaction through the acquisition of improved self-antigen recognition capacity (30,31). Another subpopulation of somewhat larger B cells displaying dendritic cytoplasmic extensions is seen near Hassall corpuscles. These peculiar cells, also designated *asteroid cells*, consistently lack IgD but do express an additional marker, CD23, pointing out their activated status (38).

As a whole, the B cells of the thymic parenchyma belong to the microenvironment of the medulla and do not represent mere passengers derived from the perivascular space, which also comprises a B-lymphocytic population, including B-cell follicles. During fetal development, B lymphocytes initially are restricted to the perivascular compartment, while progressively increasing numbers of these cells are observed within the thymic parenchyma, and it seems likely that thymic medullary B lymphocytes are acquired by migration from the extraparenchymal area. The number of B cells in the thymic medulla is related to the number of individual B lymphocytes and B follicles present in the extraparenchymal compartment, which supports the hypothesis that the intramedullary and extramedullary B-cell compartments do not constitute entirely separate regions but that they are at least subject to similar influences (38).

Based on topographic, morphologic, and immunohistochemical similarities, it has been suggested that intrathymic B cells represent a specific type of marginal zone B cell intrinsic to the thymic parenchyma. Nevertheless, important immunophenotypic differences exist between B lymphocytes of the thymic parenchyma and marginal zone cells as they are observed in the spleen, peripheral lymph, nodes, and mucosa-associated lymphoid tissues (38). This particular subset of B cells awaits further examination to elucidate its precise stage in B-lymphocytic differentiation.

Other Cell Types

Besides thymic epithelial cells and lymphocytes, several other cells have been identified in the thymus. This minor population is composed of various cell types, including macrophages, interdigitating dendritic cells, and myoid cells. Macrophages are mainly found in the cortex, but they also occur in the medulla. As regular phagocytic cells, they are characterized by their α-naphthol esterase and acid phosphatase activity. Being devoid of HLA-DR antigens, these macrophages are not expected to function as genuine antigen-presenting cells. Together with the thymic nurse cells, they eliminate dying thymocytes that have been negatively selected during maturation processes (4).

Interdigitating dendritic cells are exclusively localized in the medulla. These cells stand out by their irregularly shaped and folded nucleus and by their long cytoplasmic processes that embrace the surrounding T cells. Because of this intimate contact and the expression of HLA-DR antigens by interdigitating dendritic cells, investigators have speculated that these cells contribute to the final maturation of medullary T lymphocytes. Although Langerhans cells with characteristic Birbeck granules do occur in the thymus of animals, these cells are consistently lacking in human thymuses (4).

Myoid cells have been identified in adult and fetal thymuses. These cells are unevenly distributed throughout the thymus, with a preferential occurrence in small clusters, predominantly located in the medullary parenchyma. These cells display the ultrastructural features of degenerating striated muscle cells, typically containing myosin and actin filaments in their cytoplasm (10). The presence of acetylcholine receptor–like material (11) has been demonstrated on the surface of thymic myoid cells, a finding that might explain the link between myasthenia gravis and the thymus (38).

Blood vessels and the associated perivascular spaces belong to the extraparenchymal compartment of the thymus. The perivascular space, its macrophages, vascular endothelium, and type 1 thymic epithelium represent the blood-thymus barrier, which was thought to guarantee an antigen-free environment in the thymic cortex, protecting thymocytes from inappropriate stimulation. Nieuwenhuis and associates (42) demonstrated the existence of a transcapsular pathway by which antigens may bypass the thymic-blood barrier. Since these results were published, the functional significance of the blood-thymic barrier was seriously questioned. Nevertheless, cortical thymocytes are undoubtedly efficiently protected against blood-borne antigens, whether this shelter is entirely provided for by the described structures or not. Morphologically, the perivascular space is based on an extensive reticulin meshwork that surrounds the complete vascular system of the thymus. On either side, this specialized region is bordered by a basement membrane, with the one produced by the endothelium on the vascular side and the one lining the type 1 epithelial cells on the other. The overall appearance and the cellular composition of the perivascular area show considerable variation among the two components of the thymic parenchyma. Whereas the medulla generally is poorer in lymphocytes, its wide perivascular spaces contain many of these cells. The cortex is provided with narrow perivascular areas, mostly devoid of lymphocytes.

The vascular network embedded in this fibrous tissue is derived from interlobular arteries, in particular the arterioles at the corticomedullary junction and a capillary network located in the cortex. In the subcapsular area, they unite in an anastomosing arcade that drains in postcapillary venules. The extraparenchymal compartment contains lymphatics and nerves. Whereas afferent lymphatic vessels are consistently absent, efferent ones, arising from the medulla and the corticomedullary junction, run along with arteries and veins. Eventually, they leave the organ also by perforating the capsule, particularly in the clefts formed by the interlobular septa, meanwhile having drained the perivascular spaces (43). The thymus is innervated by autonomic nerves that are derived from the sympathetic chain and the vagal nerve and are mainly restricted to the capsule and its septa. A neural plexus is formed along the corticomedullary junction by closely interwoven sympathetic and vagal fibers. This autonomic innervation is crucial to vasomotor control but probably also serves other purposes (43).

THE LYMPH NODE

Lymph nodes are bean-shaped encapsulated lymphoid organs, generally measuring only a few millimeters in the longest dimension. In a stimulated state they enlarge to reach a size of more than 1 cm. These organs occur throughout the entire body, invariably intercalated in the lymph stream. They are most frequent in the axillary, cervical, and inguinal regions, in the mediastinum, and in the retroperitoneum. They serve innate and specific immunity. Their macrophages ingest the bulk of invading, lymph-borne microorganisms, reducing the load of foreign antigens that is carried along with the lymphatics. Lymphocytes may continuously enter the lymph node parenchyma through the highly specialized postcapillary venules, allowing a recruitment of specific lymphocytes from a large circulating pool. In this way, a system capable of generating an adequate immune response to nearly all lymph-borne antigens is created (44).

Histology and Immunohistology

The lymph node has a fibrous capsule from which septa derive, resulting in an incomplete subdivision of the parenchyma into segments. Several afferent lymphatics reach the lymph node at its convex margin to end into the subcapsular or marginal sinus, which can be regarded as a lymph reservoir (Fig. 5.3). Subsequently, the lymph percolates through the cortical sinuses that communicate with the medullary sinuses and eventually converge to give rise to only one efferent lymph vessel that leaves the lymph node at its hilus. The sinus network does not randomly drain the lymph node. Instead, it constitutes an ingenious irrigation system, relating each afferent lymphatic to a well-defined functional compartment (45).

The sinuses form a labyrinth of wide, irregular spaces that resemble thin-walled blood vessels (46). The sinus lacework is bordered by a discontinuous monolayer of sinus lining cells to which delicate collagen fibers are attached. This supportive fibrous skeleton stretches out in the lumen, preventing the sinus walls from collapsing. Broad intercellular gaps in the sinus lining allow unimpeded contact between the luminal contents and the surrounding tissue. The absence of a basal

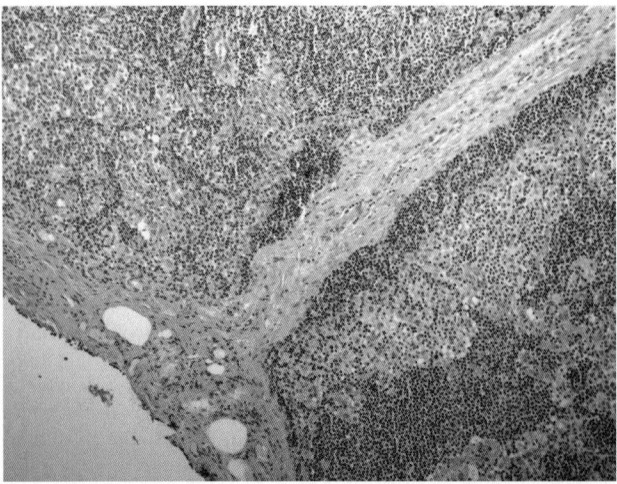

FIGURE 5.3. Lymph node capsule and septum derived from it with entering lymph vessels. The subcapsular sinus is filled with lymphocytes and not well visible (125× magnification).

membrane promotes direct interaction between the circulating lymph and the lymph node parenchyma. In contrast, a basal membrane is found underlying the cellular monolayer, lining the capsular side of the marginal sinus (47).

In normal lymph nodes, sinus lining cells are inconspicuous and can hardly be distinguished from the macrophages and other mononuclear cells abundantly present in the sinus lumen. Sinus lining cells have long dendrites that connect the cell with its neighbors through well-developed desmosomes. Another feature of sinus lining cells is their intimate association with reticulin fibers from the sinus cavity. These components of the fibrous network supporting the sinuses, typically composed of type IV collagen, are engulfed by slender protrusions extending from the cell's body (47,48).

Based on marked morphologic similarities, it has been suggested that the sinus lining cells originate from dendritic cells. However, unlike follicular dendritic cells and interdigitating dendritic cells, they do not display any phagocytic activity. Moreover, they consistently lack S-100 protein and CD1a, molecules frequently present on interdigitating dendritic cells. In contrast, they do react with antibodies directed against the highly restricted antigens Ki-M9 and Ki-M4, which have only been identified on the surface of follicular dendritic cells. The latter finding, together with the demonstration of IL-6 production by sinus lining cells (49), strongly suggests that these cells really function as genuine antigen-binding and -presenting cells (48).

The nodal arteries enter the lymph node through the hilus and give rise to arterioles that follow the fibrous trabeculae. From these small vessels, extensive capillary networks branch off that are connected with postcapillary venules. Most of these highly specialized vessels, also called high endothelial venules because of their unusual morphology, are situated in the paracortex. High endothelial venules, also designated as epithelioid venules, are easily distinguished by their plump, cuboidal to cylindrical endothelial cell lining and typically display a large, round nucleus and abundant cytoplasm. Scanning electron microscopy has shown that the tridimensional structure of these vessels is unique. Extensive portions of the high endothelial venules show a cobblestone surface with lymphocytes located in the crevices separating adjacent endothelial cells. Because of these peculiar features, turbulent blood flow is brought about along the high endothelial venules, which may account for an important improvement of the interactions between circulating lymphocytes and the endothelial surface. These specialized postcapillary vessels play a crucial part in the recruitment of circulating lymphocytes into the lymph node parenchyma, for this process is essentially based on cell-cell interactions between endothelial cells and lymphocytes. Important molecules in this process are nepmucin and autotaxin, both expressed by high endothelial venules (50). The trafficking is steered by several chemokines and chemoattractants (51) with a key role for chemokine receptor 7 (CCR7) (52).

After its passage through the high endothelial venules, the blood is drained by the nodal veins, which leave the node together with the efferent lymphatic. In humans, no communications exist between the sinuses and the vascular system. A detailed description of the microvascular structures supporting the lymphocyte trafficking is beyond the scope of this book (53).

The lymph node parenchyma is subdivided in the cortex, comprised of B-cell follicles, the paracortex, consisting predominantly of T cells, and the medulla, the innermost region (Fig. 5.4). The B follicle is responsible for humoral immunity; the T-cell area accounts for cellular immunity. Immunoglobulin-secreting plasma cells, together with long-lived, antigen-specific memory B cells, are generated in the former area, and in the latter region, antigen-specific T lymphocytes become activated, which results in an impressive clonal expansion of these cells.

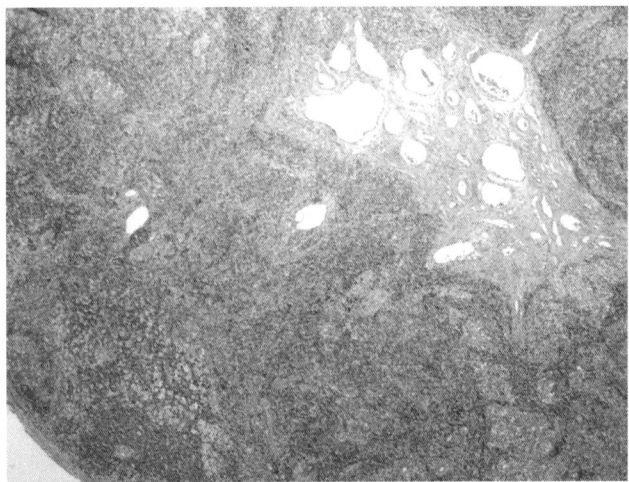

FIGURE 5.4. Hematoxylin and eosin–stained, paraffin-embedded sections of reactive lymph node, both with paracortical hyperplasia and secondary follicles.

The impressive variation in the appearance of a lymph node as a reflection of different pathologic conditions represents adaptation to the specific type of antigen. In follicular hyperplasia, for example, the B-cell follicles increase in size to respond to mainly bacterial antigens, whereas in paracortical hyperplasia the T-cell compartment is enlarged in response to antigens presented by dendritic cells (Fig. 5.5A and B).

The B-Cell Follicle

The B-cell follicle consists of a framework of follicular dendritic cells colonized by B cells, a specific subpopulation of T cells, and tingible body macrophages (Fig. 5.6A and B). In nonstimulated lymphoid tissue, only small, mainly round lymphocytes are embedded in this underlying follicular dendritic cell network. These elementary B follicles are designated as primary B follicles. Secondary B follicles arise as the result of antigenic stimulation and can be distinguished from their unstimulated counterparts by the presence of a well-developed germinal center or follicle center. As a result, the secondary follicle consists of the following compartments: the germinal center, the follicle mantle, and sometimes the marginal zone. In mesenteric lymph nodes, the spleen, and Peyer patches, this

marginal zone is common, but a clear-cut marginal zone is only occasionally demarcated in other lymph nodes (54); in these the marginal zone B cells usually occur as a minor population, inconspicuously intermingled with the small lymphocytes of the outer part of the mantle zone (54,55).

Newly formed germinal centers represent oligoclonal B-cell populations (56–59), because on average each mature germinal center is derived from only one to three B-cell clones. The germinal center reaction reaches its maximum by day 10 to 12 of primary immune responses. Without further antigenic stimulation, germinal centers wane by 21 days after immunization. In the germinal center at least two B-cell types are recognized morphologically: small irregular cells (i.e., centrocytes) and large cells (i.e., centroblasts) (Fig. 5.5B). Centrocytes are identified by an ample amount of clear cytoplasm and an irregular, somewhat elongated nucleus with rather dense nuclear chromatin and inconspicuous nucleoli resulting in a paler staining part of the germinal center. Centroblasts occupy the remaining of the follicle center, which stains considerably more intensely because its large cellular constituents are packed together in a small area. Centroblasts have a small rim of cytoplasm and a round nucleus with less condensed chromatin and several nucleoli located along the nuclear membrane. Germinal centre cells are characterized by the lack of BCL-2. Centroblasts and centrocytes, typically lacking this cytoplasmic protein involved in the protection against apoptosis, are programmed to die, unless they are rescued by high-affinity interaction between their antigen receptor and a given antigen. After apoptosis the cell remnants accumulate in macrophages within the germinal center, the tingible body macrophages, displaying the classic phenotype of macrophages as they express neuron-specific enolase, acid phosphatase, CD11b, CD14, CD68, and HLA-DR (48,60).

Germinal center cells can also be recognized by their expression of the nuclear phosphoprotein BCL-6 (61–63). With its expression strictly confined to the follicle center, at least in nonneoplastic lymphoid tissues, it has been speculated that this transcription factor controls the proliferation and differentiation of B cells within the germinal center (64–66).

Following the differentiation scheme of B lymphocytes, IgD+ B lymphocytes that also express CD38 are the first ones to show the features of a genuine germinal center cell. They are immunoreactive with antibodies directed against CD10, CD71, and FAS. They are highly proliferative as can be demonstrated by the expression of Ki-67. Two subpopulations of these IgD+CD38+ B lymphocytes are recognized. An IgM+ subset, called Bm2',

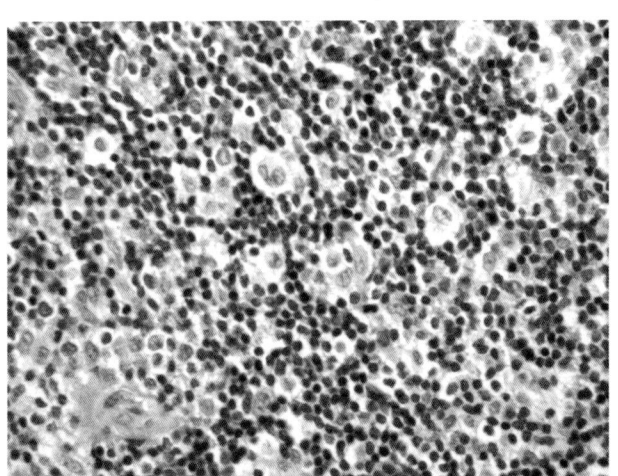

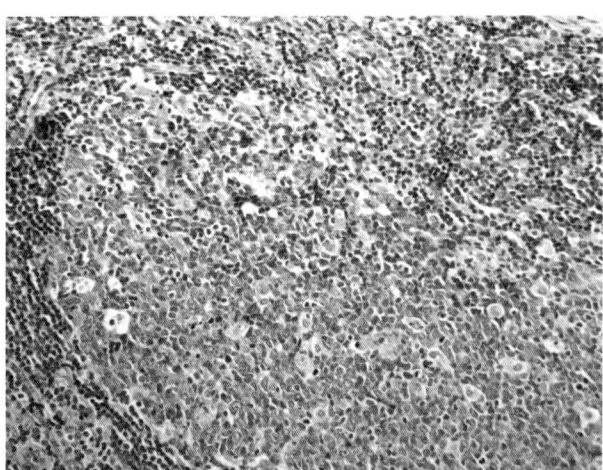

FIGURE 5.5. **A:** A primary T-cell reaction is typically visible by light-appearing interdigitating dendritic cells admixed with T lymphocytes (H&E stain, original magnification: 600× magnification). **B:** B-cell follicle with germinal centre, defining it as a secondary lymphoid follicle, surrounded by the mantle zone. No marginal zone can be identified (H&E stain, original magnification: 125× magnification).

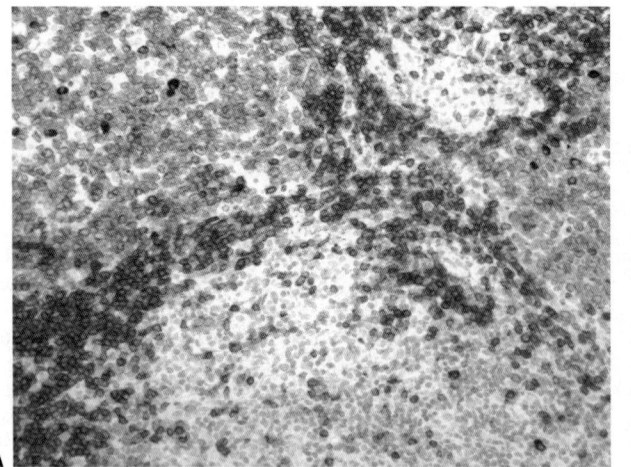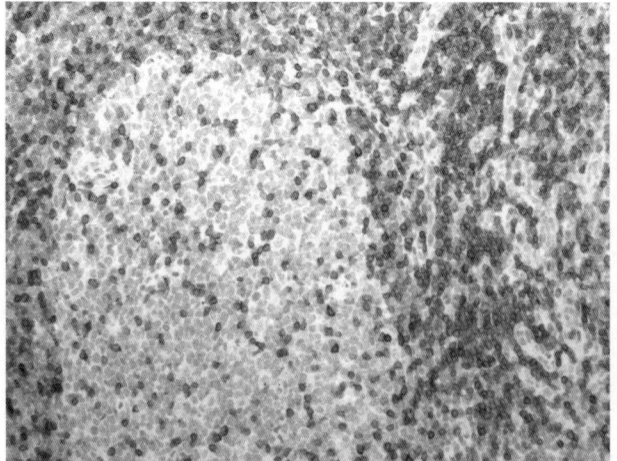

FIGURE 5.6. **A:** Immunohistochemical staining for CD79A of the germinal center of a B follicle of a reactive lymph node (original magnification: 250× magnification). Note the different levels of expression with weak staining by germinal centre cells, strong staining of the mantle B cells and very strong staining of the plasma cells in the germinal center. **B:** Immunohistochemical staining for CD3 showing staining of both paracortical and germinal center T cells.

may correspond to germinal center founder cells, because their immunoglobulin variable genes (V_H) carry few or no mutations. The other IgD⁺CD38⁺ cells, which show no IgM expression, display an extraordinarily high number of somatic mutations in their V_H genes. Most of the IgD⁺CD38⁺ cells with a high number of mutations undergo apoptosis, leaving only a small portion of IgD⁺ germinal center cells provided with low to intermediate numbers of mutations. The latter cells eventually differentiate into mature plasma cells or long-lived memory B cells.

IgD⁻CD38⁺ cells represent the main germinal center cell population, consistently expressing CD10, CD71, and FAS and demonstrating intense proliferative activity, as well. Also these germinal centre cells lack BCL-2 and thus are programmed to die, unless they are selected by an appropriate signal, which can be provided by a specific antigen or by CD40 ligand. The two characteristic properties of these follicle center cells—their impressive mitotic rate and their propensity to undergo apoptosis—should both be conferred by their elevated levels of P53, MYC, BAX, and FAS.

Germinal centers harbor a significant number of CD2⁺, CD3⁺, and CD4⁺-only T cells (Fig. 5.6B). These granular lymphocytes co-express CD57 (67) and are CD45RA⁻ and CD45RO⁺. Although the specific activation marker CD69 can be demonstrated on this particular subset of helper T cells, other surface molecules indicating cellular activation, such as CD25 (IL-2 receptor) and CD71 (transferrin receptor), are consistently absent. This unusual phenotype correlates with the observation that, on activation, these CD57⁺ T cells produce various cytokines but never secrete IL-2, IL-4, interferon-γ, and tumor necrosis factor (67,68). This peculiar T-cell population may reach its activated state through stimulation by antigen-presenting B lymphocytes, because complex bidirectional interactions take place between T lymphocytes on one hand and centroblasts and centrocytes on the other. Various adhesive and costimulatory receptor-counterreceptor systems are involved, particularly CD80/CD86, CD40, LFA-1, and LFA-3 expressed on B cells and CD28, CD40 ligand, CD54, and CD2 on the T-cell surface.

Although the primary follicle and the mantle zone of the secondary follicle are mainly composed of morphologically similar small lymphoid cells, the phenotype and function of these lymphocytes is variable. IgD⁺CD38⁻ B cells found in the follicle mantle are small resting B cells expressing IgM, CD5, CD44, and BCL-2 protein. They correspond to naive B cells as they have not yet undergone somatic mutation. Based on the differential expression of CD23, two subpopulations of these mantle

cells can be distinguished. The CD23⁻ subset, designated as Bm1, probably represents recently generated naive B cells, and the acquisition of this surface marker by the remainder of these B lymphocytes, Bm2, could reflect their selection by a particular ligand.

The marginal zone, when present, is composed predominantly of typical marginal zone B cells, somewhat larger cells with abundant clear cytoplasm, and an irregular bean-shaped nucleus containing vesicular chromatin and an inconspicuous nucleolus. By pure morphology, marginal zone B cells resemble monocytoid cells and centrocytes of the germinal center. They were previously designated immature sinus histiocytes in the lymph node and centrocyte-like cells in Peyer patches of the small intestine. Nevertheless, marginal zone B cells have a distinct phenotype. Studies demonstrating Ki-67 expression in marginal zone cells (69) indicate that, in contrast with the traditional point of view (70), they display proliferative activity. Marginal zone cells express pan-B-cell markers and surface IgM but little or no IgD. They are not reactive with antibodies against surface CD5, CD10, and CD23. Phenotypic features frequently used to accentuate these cells include their alkaline phosphatase positivity and their expression of CD21 and CD25. The unique positioning at the entrance of the antigenic influx considerably facilitates their exposure to and interaction with foreign antigens.

In addition to the characteristic marginal zone cell population, a variable number of different B lymphocytes is observed, among which larger cells with immunoblast-like features and plasma cells expressing cytoplasmic IgM can be recognized. The diversity characterizing the cellular composition of the marginal zone is reflected in the heterogeneity of marginal zone cell lymphomas of the lymph node, the spleen, and extranodal sites (69). Admixed with these peculiar lymphocytic elements, other cells such as macrophages, granulocytes, and ordinary small lymphocytes are also detected (71).

The cells of the follicle lay embedded in a cellular lacework built up by follicular dendritic cells, a unique cell population exclusively found in primary and secondary lymphoid follicles. These cells stand out by their ability to retain antigens integrated in large immune complexes on their surface for a prolonged period (72–74). By routine light microscopy alone, it takes a considerable effort to identify these cells, because only by their nucleus, which displays a very open chromatin pattern in contrast with the rather condensed one observed in the surrounding lymphoid cells, can they be distinguished from the surrounding cells. Nevertheless, immunohistologic and ultrastructural examinations of the B follicle allowed unequivo-cal detection of these peculiar cells and comprehensible descrip-tion of their unique features.

Electron microscopy demonstrates that follicular dendritic cells have one or more large, irregularly shaped nuclei with vesic-ular chromatin and long cytoplasmic dendrites connected by des-mosomes, which together form an intricate network of delicate processes seeded with lymphocytes. Along the slender cellular protrusions, small globular structures or iccosomes, representing immune complex–coated bodies, are observed. By visualizing the immune complexes bound on their surface, phenotyping of fol-licular dendritic cells highlights the network they form.

All follicular dendritic cells express the monocytic marker CD14, the three types of complement receptors—CD35 (CR-1), the long isoform of CD21 (CR-2), and CD11b (CR-3)—and the immunoglobulin Fc receptor CD32 (75,76). Displaying the lat-ter receptors on their plasma membrane, the entire population of follicular dendritic cells is provided with an efficient mecha-nism to trap passing antigen-antibody-C3 (Ag-Ab-C3) com-plexes. A subset of the follicular dendritic cells in the light zone of the germinal center additionally expresses CD23, which is the low-affinity receptor for IgE, and one of the ligands for CD21, allowing them to bind complexes containing CD21 with higher affinity and to interact with IgE.

The T-Cell Area

In contrast to the extensive studies that succeeded in unravel-ing almost the entire microarchitecture of its B-cell counter-part, the architecture of the T-cell area is less well appreciated. Moreover, depending on the stage of the immune response or the particular features of the antigen involved, the morphology of the T-cell area may vary from a well-delineated nodule with dendritic cells at the periphery to a less well-defined aggre-gate composed of a variable number of interdigitating dendritic cells, with or without an admixture of Langerhans cells, and T cells. Demarcation of the T-cell area is subject to consider-able variation, and its precise cellular composition shows even greater fluctuations, depending on the particular features of the antigen involved and on the stage of the immune response.

In contrast with B lymphocytes, T cells cannot be activated by soluble antigen; they require contact of their TCR with anti-genic peptide presented on autologous MHC molecules—MHC class I for CD8+ T cells and MHC class II for CD4+ T cells. At the time of antigen recognition, numerous other cognate interac-tions occur, many of which serve to stabilize the interaction between the antigen-presenting cell and the T lymphocyte.

Immunochemical studies have demonstrated that CD80 and CD86 are expressed in the T-cell area, which har-bors a specific dendritic cell population, the interdigitating den-dritic cells. By means of their numerous cytoplasmic processes, these cells establish a tridimensional network that envelops T lymphocytes and creates a unique microenvironment for T-cell activation and proliferation (77). In contrast with follicular dendritic cells, for which well-developed desmosomes serve as connection between the dendritic protrusions of different cells, the cellular extensions of interdigitating dendritic cells join, as their name indicates, by forming *interdigitations*. These cells have abundant, pale-staining cytoplasm encompassing a large, elongated, bizarre, but very characteristic nucleus. Its outline is provided with several deep clefts and folds, and it contains very delicate chromatin and inconspicuous nucleoli (78). These den-dritic cells derive from bone marrow monocytes and display quite similar light microscopic, ultrastructural, and phenotypic features to Langerhans cells of the epidermis but lack Birbeck granules, a specific, racquet-shaped cell organelle. Langerhans cells are known to migrate to the lymph node. The resultant image of Langerhans cells and interdigitating dendritic cells

occurring side by side in an extended paracortex is particularly prominent in dermatopathic lymphadenitis (79–81) (see Chap-ter 15). Dendritic cells express CD11c leukocyte integrin, the DEC-205 multilectin receptor for antigen presentation, very high levels of MHC class I and MHC class II products, and many accessory molecules such as CD40, CD54, and CD86 (82). More-over, they synthesize high levels of IL-2 (83). The dendritic cells are particularly well equipped to stimulate the growth and acti-vation of a variety of T lymphocytes, including CD8+ cytotoxic T cells and CD4+ helper T cells. Westermann and his group (84) demonstrated that, at least in rats, memory T cells migrate through the T-cell area at a very high rate, and as they continu-ously recirculate, meanwhile surveying the surface of the inter-digitating dendritic cells, they could eventually encounter their specific antigen. Because mature interdigitating dendritic cells and completely differentiated Langerhans cells have acquired the appropriate accessory surface molecules on encounter with their specific antigen presented by the aforementioned cells, selected T lymphocytes undergo activation and eventually pro-liferate intensely. The specific state of the immune response determines which T cells are predominant in the T-cell area.

In conclusion, the T-cell area of the lymph node contains a diverse population of dendritic and T lymphocytes reflecting different stages in their development from immature cells to potent, well-equipped professional antigen-presenting cells and immunologic capable T cells.

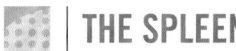 THE SPLEEN

The spleen is an abdominal organ, situated in the left hypo-chondrium beneath the diaphragm. The weight of the spleen varies considerably depending on the age, sex, size, and weight of the individual. In general, a weight of 150 g is considered normal.

Histology and Immunohistology

On its freshly sectioned surface, the two components of the spleen can be distinguished even with the naked eye. Elongated or rounded gray areas, measuring 0.2 to 0.7 cm in diameter and called the white pulp, correspond microscopically to accumula-tions of lymphoid tissue. The reddish, soft mass that they are embedded in, the red pulp, represents the entire vascular laby-rinth that carries the blood along the splenic parenchyma. The red pulp consists of pulp cords and sinuses. The red pulp cords contain the arterial branches that gradually branch into arteri-oles and capillaries; the sinuses form a network that drains into the veins. The spleen functions as an ingenious filter, interca-lated in the bloodstream. Its entire structure is therefore based on the vascular supply provided by the splenic artery. This branch of the truncus celiacus perforates the splenic capsule that completely surrounds the spleen at the hilus to give rise to two smaller vessels, which further subdivide into segmental arteries, each supplying one splenic segment.

The arterial branches, together with their concomitant vein and lymphatics, form a vascular triad embedded in fibrous, mainly collagenous tissue (85). The arteries end up as smaller arterioles, which are no longer accompanied by venules and collagenous fibers but are partially surrounded by a cuff of lymphoid tissue, the T-cell areas. Subsequently, capillaries, oriented perpendicularly to the arterioles, branch off and terminate partially in a specialized vascular structure highly characteristic for the spleen: the sheathed capillaries or periar-teriolar macrophage sheaths.

At this level of the splenic vascularization, the endothelium of the capillaries is replaced by concentrically arranged macro-phages. Blood is forced through these sheathed capillaries and reaches the sinuses through the cordal stroma of the red pulp and after having crossed the basal membrane lining the sinus endothelium. Alternatively, blood can enter the perifollicular zone, a distinct part of the red pulp immediately adjacent to the white pulp that directly gives entrance to the sinuses (86). The sinusoidal channels, covered by a flattened, elongated endothelial lining, form a blind ending system that debouch into the veins, which parallel the arteries (85). As a whole, the sinuses constitute a complex meshwork with many interconnections and bulblike extensions inside the intersinus reticular tissue, which are known as the cords of Billroth. These cords contain reticulum cells, macrophages, and plasma cells, and the predominant population of CD8 positive T cells. Together with the sinus labyrinth, they account for the main mass of the red pulp, representing 75% of the splenic weight.

Most blood cells pass through the perifollicular zone, the region bordering both the follicles and the T-cell areas, that combined form the white pulp. Microanatomic data on this region caused confusion because they resulted from studies on spleens from various species, mainly rodents. In humans it comprises sheathed capillaries; blood-filled, large flattened spaces; terminal sinuses; and scattered B cells, T cells, and macrophages (86). Because the perifollicular zone drains directly into the venous sinuses, most of the splenic blood flow is found bypassing the filtration beds of the red pulp cords.

The white pulp of the spleen is composed of primary and secondary B follicles and the T-cell areas that border or surround arterioles. The follicles are very similar to those in the lymph node, the difference being the more extensive marginal zone. In contrast to other species, there is no marginal zone surrounding the T-cell areas. The T-cell areas differ from the paracortex in the lymph node, since they consist mainly of CD4 positive cells. It is therefore likely that new B-cell follicles arise in the red pulp, probably in the so-called nonfiltering areas. These red pulp cord parts are devoid of sheathed capillaries and contain CD8 positive T cells.

LYMPHOCYTE TRAFFICKING

Lymphocytes not only travel from bone marrow to thymus or lymph nodes for maturation purposes but also circulate to be able to react properly to antigens (87). Specific B and T cells have specific routes for recirculation. For instance, lymphocytes that have matured at a specific extranodal site, that is, the gut, will home to the stomach after recirculation, due to down-regulation of L-selectin and CCR7 and expression $\alpha 4\beta 7$ and CCR9 (88). Many of the factors that determine the recirculation process are known, but the picture is still far from complete. The most important of the molecules are chemokine receptors and adhesion molecules.

T lymphocytes enter the lymph node paracortex from the blood by passing the high endothelial venules to encounter antigen-presenting interdigitating dendritic cells or enter from the lymph vessels through the marginal sinus after activation by antigen in tissues. Crucial factors for transport through the HEV are the chemokines CCL19 and CCL21 that can bind to the chemokine receptor CCR7 and LFA1 on activated peripheral blood T lymphocytes. More recently, the importance of the sphingosine-1-phosphate receptor signaling has been demonstrated to be important as well (88). The process is supported by ICAM1 expression on paracortical stromal cells. B lymphocytes and follicular helper T cells expressing CCR5 and LFA1 are attracted by CXCL13, ICAM1, and VCAM1 on the follicular dendritic cells (89). In the spleen, HEV are lacking, but similar molecules are expressed on parts of the red pulp cord sinuses (90). After encountering antigen-presenting cells in the T-cell area, the T lymphocytes are trapped and activated, resulting in the large expansion of the paracortical area one commonly encounters in reactive lymph nodes.

References

1. Kendall MD, Johnson HR, Singh J. The weight of the human thymus gland at necropsy. *J Anat* 1980;131:483–497.
2. Rosai J, Levine GD. Nonneoplastic conditions of the thymus. In: Rosai J, Levine G, eds. *Tumors of the thymus*, vol 13. Washington, DC: Armed Forces Institute of Pathology, 1976:22–33.
3. Calder AE, Hince MN, Dudakov JA, et al. Thymic involution: where endocrinology meets immunology. *Neuroimmunomodulation* 2011;18:281–289.
4. von Gaudecker B, Muller Hermelink HK. Ontogeny and organization of the stationary non-lymphoid cells in the human thymus. *Cell Tissue Res* 1980;207:287–306.
5. Nakahama M, Mohri N, Mori S, et al. Immunohistochemical and histometrical studies of the human thymus with special emphasis on age-related changes in medullary epithelial and dendritic cells. *Virchows Arch B Cell Pathol Incl Mol Pathol* 1990;58:245–251.
6. Flores KG, Sempowski GD, Haynes BF, et al. Analysis of the human thymic perivascular space during aging. *J Clin Invest* 1999;104:1031–1039.
7. von Gaudecker B. The development of the human thymus microenvironment. *Curr Top Pathol* 1986;75:1–41.
8. Wekerle H, Ketelsen UP, Ernst M. Thymic nurse cells. Lymphoepithelial cell complexes in murine thymuses: morphological and serological characterization. *J Exp Med* 1980;151:925–944.
9. Hiramine C, Nakagawa T, Hojo K. Murine nursing thymic epithelial cell lines capable of inducing thymocyte apoptosis express the self-superantigen Mls-1a. *Cell Immunol* 1995;160:157–162.
10. Drenckhahn D, von Gaudecker B, Muller Hermelink HK, et al. Myosin and actin containing cells in the human postnatal thymus. Ultrastructural and immunohistochemical findings in normal thymus and in myasthenia gravis. *Virchows Arch B Cell Pathol Incl Mol Pathol* 1979;32:33–45.
11. Kao I, Drachman DB. Thymic muscle cells bear acetylcholine receptors: possible relation to myasthenia gravis. *Science* 1977;195:74–75.
12. Moll UM, Lane BL, Robert F, et al. The neuroendocrine thymus. Abundant occurrence of oxytocin-, vasopressin-, and neurophysin-like peptides in epithelial cells. *Histochemistry* 1988;89:385–390.
13. Geenen V, Legros JJ, Franchimont P, et al. The neuroendocrine thymus: coexistence of oxytocin and neurophysin in the human thymus. *Science* 1986;232:508–511.
14. Schmitt D, Monier JC, Dardenne M, et al. Location of FTS (facteur thymique serique) in the thymus of normal and auto-immune mice. *Thymus* 1982;4:221–231.
15. von Gaudecker B. Functional histology of the human thymus. *Anat Embryol (Berl)* 1991;183:1–15.
16. Bhan AK, Reinherz EL, Poppema S, et al. Location of the T-cell and the major histocompatibility complex antigens in the human thymus. *J Exp Med* 1980;152:771–782.
17. Naito T, Tanaka H, Naoe Y, et al. Transcriptional control of T-cell development. *Int Immunol* 2011;23:661–668.
18. Billiard F, Kirshner JR, Tait M, et al. Ongoing Dll4-Notch signaling is required for T-cell homeostasis in the adult thymus. *Eur J Immunol* 2011;41:2207–2216.
19. Spits H, Lanier LL, Phillips JH. Development of human T and natural killer cells. *Blood* 1995;85:2654–2670.
20. Peschon JJ, Morrissey PJ, Grabstein KH, et al. Early lymphocyte expansion is severely impaired in interleukin 7 receptor-deficient mice. *J Exp Med* 1994;180:1955–1960.
21. Conlon PJ, Morrissey PJ, Nordan RP, et al. Murine thymocytes proliferate in direct response to interleukin-7. *Blood* 1989;74:1368–1373.
22. Watson JD, Morrissey PJ, Namen AE, et al. Effect of IL-7 on the growth of fetal thymocytes in culture. *J Immunol* 1989;143:1215–1222.
23. Matsuzaki Y, Gyotoku J, Ogawa M, et al. Characterization of c-kit positive intrathymic stem cells that are restricted to lymphoid differentiation. *J Exp Med* 1993;178:1283–1292.
24. Rodewald HR, Kretzschmar K, Swat W, et al. Intrathymically expressed c-kit ligand (stem cell factor) is a major factor driving expansion of very immature thymocytes in vivo. *Immunity* 1995;3:313–319.
25. Veis DJ, Sentman CL, Bach EA, et al. Expression of the Bcl-2 protein in murine and human thymocytes and in peripheral T lymphocytes. *J Immunol* 1993;151:2546–2554.
26. Raulet DH, Garman RD, Saito H, et al. Developmental regulation of T cell receptor gene expression. *Nature* 1985;314:103–107.
27. Groettrup M, Ungewiss K, Azogui O, et al. A novel disulfide-linked heterodimer on pre-T cells consists of the T cell receptor beta chain and a 33 kd glycoprotein. *Cell* 1993;75:283–294.
28. Saint Ruf C, Ungewiss K, Groettrup M, et al. Analysis and expression of a cloned pre-T cell receptor gene. *Science* 1994;266:1208–1212.
29. Philpott KL, Viney JL, Kay G, et al. Lymphoid development in mice congenitally lacking T cell receptor alpha beta-expressing cells. *Science* 1992;256:1448–1452.
30. Uematsu Y, Ryser S, Dembic Z, et al. In transgenic mice the introduced functional T cell receptor beta gene prevents expression of endogenous beta genes. *Cell* 1988;52:831–841.
31. Crump AL, Grusby MJ, Glimcher LH, et al. Thymocyte development in major histocompatibility complex–deficient mice: evidence for stochastic commitment to the CD4 and CD8 lineages. *Proc Natl Acad Sci U S A* 1993;90:10739–10743.
32. von Boehmer H. Positive selection of lymphocytes. *Cell* 1994;76:219–228.
33. Nossal GJ. Negative selection of lymphocytes. *Cell* 1994;76:229–239.
34. Allen PM. Peptides in positive and negative selection: a delicate balance. *Cell* 1994;76:593–596.
35. Ashton Rickardt PG, Tonegawa S. A differential-avidity model for T cell selection. *Immunol Today* 1994;15:362–366.
36. Anderson G, Owen JJ, Moore NC, et al. Thymic epithelial cells provide unique signals for positive selection of CD4+CD8+ thymocytes in vitro. *J Exp Med* 1994;179:2027–2031.
37. Mazda O, Watanabe Y, Gyotoku J, et al. Requirement of dendritic cells and B cells in the clonal deletion of Mls-reactive T cells in the thymus. *J Exp Med* 1991;173:539–547.
38. Fend F, Nachbaur D, Oberwasserlechner F, et al. Phenotype and topography of human thymic B cells: an immunohistologic study. *Virchows Arch B Cell Pathol Incl Mol Pathol* 1991;60:381–388.
39. Isaacson PG, Norton AJ, Addis BJ. The human thymus contains a novel population of B lymphocytes. *Lancet* 1987;2:1488–1491.

40. Spencer J, Choy M, Hussell T, et al. Properties of human thymic B cells. *Immunology* 1992;75:596–600.
41. Punnonen J, de Vries JE. Characterization of a novel CD2⁺ human thymic B cell subset. *J Immunol* 1993;151:100–110.
42. Nieuwenhuis P, Stet RJ, Wagenaar JP, et al. The transcapsular route: a new way for (self-) antigens to bypass the blood-thymus barrier? *Immunol Today* 1988;9:372–375.
43. Bannister L, Kendall M. Lymphoid cells and tissues: thymus. In: Williams PL, Bannister LH, Berry MM, et al., eds. *Gray's anatomy*, 38th ed. New York: Churchill Livingstone, 1995:1423–1431.
44. Fossum S, Ford WL. The organization of cell populations within lymph nodes: their origin, life history and functional relationships. *Histopathology* 1985;9:469–499.
45. Sainte-Marie G, Peng FS, Belisle, C. Overall architecture and pattern of lymph flow in the r at lymph node. *Am J Anat* 1982;164:275–309.
46. Kurokawa T, Ogata T. A scanning electron microscopic study on the lymphatic microcirculation of the rabbit mesenteric lymph node: a corrosion cast study. *Acta Anat* 1980;107:439–466.
47. Castenholz A. Architecture of the lymph node with regard to its function. In: Grundmann E, Vollmer E, eds. *Reaction patterns of the lymph node*, vol 1. Berlin: Springer-Verlag, 1990:1–32.
48. Wacker HH, Frahm SO, Heidebrecht HJ, et al. Sinus-lining cells of the lymph nodes recognized as a dendritic cell type by the new monoclonal antibody Ki-M9. *Am J Pathol* 1997;151:423–434.
49. Peters J, Krams M, Wacker HH, et al. Detection of rare RNA sequences by single enzyme in situ RT-PCR: high resolution analysis of interleukin-6 mRNA in paraffin sections of lymph nodes. *Am J Pathol* 1996;150:469–476.
50. Umemoto E, Hayasaka H, Bai Z, et al. Novel regulators of lymphocyte trafficking across high endothelial venules. *Crit Rev Immunol* 2011;31:147–169.
51. Kehrl JH, Hwang IY, Park C. Chemoattract receptor signaling and its role in lymphocyte motility and trafficking. *Curr Top Microbiol Immunol* 2009;334:107–127.
52. Förster R, Davalos-Misslitz AC, Rot A. CCR7 and its ligands: balancing immunity and tolerance. *Nat Rev Immunol* 2008;8:362–371.
53. Matsuno K, Ueta H, Shu Z, et al. The microstructure of secondary lymphoid organs that support immune cell trafficking. *Arch Histol Cytol* 2010;73:1–21.
54. van Krieken JH, von Schilling C, Kluin PM, et al. Splenic marginal zone lymphocytes and related cells in the lymph node: a morphologic and immunohistochemical study. *Hum Pathol* 1989;20:320–362.
55. van den Oord JJ, de Wolf Peeters C, Desmet VJ. The marginal zone in the human reactive lymph node. *Am J Clin Pathol* 1986;86:475–479.
56. Liu YJ, Johnson GD, Gordon J, et al. Germinal centers in T cell–dependent antibody responses. *Immunol Today* 1992;13:17–21.
57. Jacob J, Kassir R, Kelsoe G. In situ studies of the primary immune response to (4-hydroxy-3-nitrophenyl)acetyl. I. The architecture and dynamics of responding cell populations. *J Exp Med* 1991;173:1165–1175.
58. Jacob J, Miller C, Kelsoe G. In situ studies of the antigen-driven somatic hypermutation of immunoglobulin genes. *Immunol Cell Biol* 1992;70:145–152.
59. Jacob J, Kelsoe G. In situ studies of the primary immune response to (4-hydroxy-3-nitrophenyl)acetyl. II. A common clonal origin for periarteriolar lymphoid sheath-associated foci and germinal centers. *J Exp Med* 1992;176:679–687.
60. Kroese FGM, Timens W, Niewenhuis P. Germinal center reaction and B lymphocytes: morphology and function. In: Grundmann E, Vollmer E, eds. *Reaction patterns of the lymph node*, vol 1, part 1. Berlin: Springer-Verlag, 1990:116–117.
61. Allman D, Jain A, Dent A, et al. BCL-6 expression during B cell activation. *Blood* 1996;87:5257–5268.
62. Cattoretti G, Chang CC, Cechova K, et al. BCL-6 protein is expressed in germinal-center B cells. *Blood* 1995;86:45–53.
63. Onizuka T, Moriyama M, Yamochi T, et al. BCL-6 gene product, a 92- to 98-kD nuclear phosphoprotein, is highly expressed in germinal center B cells and their neoplastic counterparts. *Blood* 1995;86:28–37.
64. Ye BH, Cattoretti G, Shen Q, et al. The BCL-6 proto-oncogene controls germinal-center formation and Th2-type inflammation. *Nat Genet* 1997;16:161–170.
65. Dent AL, Shaffer AL, Yu X, et al. Control of inflammation, cytokine expression, and germinal center formation by BCL-6. *Science* 1997;276:589–592.
66. Pittaluga S, Ayoubi TA, Wlodarska I, et al. BCL-6 expression in reactive lymphoid tissue and in B cell non-Hodgkin's lymphomas. *J Pathol* 1996;179:145–150.
67. Velardi A, Mingari MC, Moretta L, et al. Functional analysis of cloned germinal center CD4⁺ cells with natural killer cell–related features: divergence from typical T helper cells. *J Immunol* 1986;137:2808–2813.
68. Bowen MB, Butch A, Parvin CA, et al. Germinal center T cells are distinct helper-inducer T cells. *Hum Immunol* 1991;31:67–75.
69. Tierens A, Delabie J, Michiels L, et al. Marginal zone B cells in the human lymph node and spleen show somatic hypermutation and display clonal expansion. *Blood* 1999;93:226–234.
70. Liu YJ, Oldfield S, MacLennan IC. Memory B cells in T cell–dependent antibody responses colonize the splenic marginal zones. *Eur J Immunol* 1988;18:355–362.
71. Kraal G. Cells in the marginal zone of the spleen. *Int Rev Cytol* 1992;132:31–74.
72. Kaplan MH, Coons AH, Deane HW. Localization of antigen in tissue cells. III. Cellular distribution of pneumococcal polysaccharides types II and III in the mouse. *J Exp Med* 1950;91:15–29.
73. Szakal AK, Gieringer RL, Kosco MH, et al. Isolated follicular dendritic cells: cytochemical antigen localization, Nomarski, SEM, and TEM morphology. *J Immunol* 1985;134:1349–1359.
74. Nossal GJ, Abbot A, Mitchell J, et al. Antigens in immunity. XV. Ultrastructural features of antigen capture in primary and secondary lymphoid follicles. *J Exp Med* 1968;127:277–290.
75. Tew JG, Kosco MH, Burton GF, et al. Follicular dendritic cells as accessory cells. *Immunol Rev* 1990;117:185–211.
76. Dijkstra CD, Van den Berg TK. The follicular dendritic cell: possible regulatory roles of associated molecules. *Res Immunol* 1991;142:227–231.
77. Crivellato E, Baldini G, Basa M, et al. The three-dimensional structure of interdigitating cells. *Ital J Anat Embryol* 1993;98:243–258.
78. van der Valk P, Meijer CJ. The histology of reactive lymph nodes. *Am J Surg Pathol* 1987;11:866–882.
79. van den Oord JJ, de Wolf-Peeters C, Desmet VJ, et al. Nodular alteration of the paracortical area. An in situ immunohistochemical analysis of primary, secondary, and tertiary T nodules. *Am J Pathol* 1985;120:55–66.
80. van den Oord JJ, de Wolf Peeters C, de Vos R, et al. The paracortical area in dermatopathic lymphadenitis and other reactive conditions of the lymph node. *Virchows Arch* 1984;45:289–299.
81. Gould E, Porto R, Albores Saavedra J, et al. Dermatopathic lymphadenitis: the spectrum and significance of its morphologic features. *Arch Pathol Lab Med* 1988;112:1145–1150.
82. Inaba K, Pack M, Inaba M, et al. High levels of a major histocompatibility complex II–self peptide complex on dendritic cells from the T cell areas of lymph nodes. *J Exp Med* 1997;186:665–672.
83. Banchereau J, Steinman RM. Dendritic cells and the control of immunity. *Nature* 1998;392:245–252.
84. Westermann J, Geismar U, Sponholz A, et al. CD4⁺ T cells of both the naive and the memory phenotype enter rat lymph nodes and Peyer's patches via high endothelial venules: within the tissue their migratory behavior differs. *Eur J Immunol* 1997;27:3174–3181.
85. van Krieken JH, te Velde J. Normal histology of the human spleen. *Am J Surg Pathol* 1988;12:777–785.
86. Steiniger B, Barth P, Herbst B, et al. The species-specific structure of microanatomical compartments in the human spleen: strongly sialoadhesin-positive macrophages occur in the perifollicular zone, but not in the marginal zone. *Immunology* 1997;92:307–316.
87. Matsuno K, Ueto H, Shu Z, et al. The microstructure of the secondairy lymphoid organs that support immune cell trafficking. *Arch Histol Cytol* 2010;73:1–21.
88. Davis MD, Kehrl JH. The influence of sphingosine-1-phosphate receptor signaling on lymphocyte trafficking. *Immunol Res* 2009;43:187–197.
89. Mora JR, von Adrian UH. T-cell homing specificity and plasticity: new concepts and future challenges. *Trends Immunol* 2006;27:235–243.
90. van Krieken JH, Te Velde J, Kleiverda K, et al. The human spleen; a histological study in splenectomy specimens embedded in methylmethacrylate. *Histopathology* 1985;9:571–585.

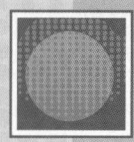

Chapter 6
Antigen Receptor Genes: Structure, Function, and Molecular Analysis in Clinical Applications

Y. Lynn Wang • Ethel Cesarman • Daniel M. Knowles

Antigen receptors, including immunoglobulin (Ig) and T-cell receptors (TCRs), are the primary effector molecules of the adaptive immune system. They are produced by either B cells or T cells and are responsible for antigen recognition. In order to recognize a vast variety of specific antigens, such as bacteria, viruses, and toxins, the genes encoding these molecules undergo rearrangement and somatic hypermutation to generate diversity in antigen receptors, allowing the human body to combat pathogens with billions of effector molecules (1).

In this chapter, we first review the protein structure and function of the antigen receptors. We then describe the major molecular mechanisms that are responsible for generating sequence diversity in the antigen receptor genes, including gene rearrangement, somatic hypermutation, and class switching. A description of the gene structure and the physiologic process of gene rearrangement then follows. In the latter part of the chapter, we focus on clinical applications of such knowledge to the diagnosis and prognosis of lymphoid malignancies.

PROTEIN STRUCTURE OF IMMUNOGLOBULIN AND T-CELL RECEPTORS

Structure of Immunoglobulins

Immunoglobulins are produced by B cells in both secreted and membrane-bound forms. While secreted Igs act as antibodies of adaptive immunity, membrane-bound Ig molecules serve as the antigen-binding part of the B-cell receptor (BCR) complex (2). Immunoglobulin molecules form a basic Y-shaped structure that consists of two paired heavy and light chains (Fig. 6.1A). Both polypeptide chains are divided into constant and variable regions (C and V regions), which are further organized in domain structure. Heavy chains have three to four domains in the C region (C_H1, C_H2, etc.) and one domain in the V region (V_H), while light chains have one domain in the C region (C_L) and the other in the V region (V_L). V regions from both heavy and light chains are highly variable in sequence and form the antigen-binding site. V regions, according to amino acid variability, are further divided into three complementarity-determining regions (CDRs) with highly variable sequences interspersed among three framework regions (FRs) with relatively reduced amino acid variation. The CDRs of the heavy and light chains directly contact antigens in the antigen-binding site (Fig. 6.1B).

The C regions of heavy chains interact with effector cells or molecules such as phagocytes or complements. Each Ig molecule has two antigen-binding sites and is therefore bivalent. Bivalent recognition allows antigen cross-linking and enhances the stability of antigen binding.

According to sequences in the C region of the heavy chains, Igs are divided into five major classes: IgA, IgD, IgE, IgG, and IgM. According to sequences in the C region of the light chains, they are divided into kappa (κ) and lambda (λ) chains. Either type of light chain can be associated with any one of the five classes of the heavy chains, but a given Ig molecule always has two identical heavy chains that are joined to each other by disulfide bonds, paired with two identical light chains that are joined by disulfide bonds to heavy chains (Fig. 6.1A).

The proteolytic enzymes papain and pepsin digest Ig molecules into characteristic fragments with distinct functions (3,4) (Fig. 6.1C). Papain cuts at the N-terminal side of the disulfide bonds. This cut produces two identical antigen-binding fragments (Fab), each with one antigen-binding site, plus a disulfide-linked Fc fragment that binds to effector cells or molecules. Fc imparts functional differences among the five major Ig classes. Meanwhile, protease pepsin cuts at the C-terminal side of the disulfide bonds and generates F(ab') fragments covalently linked together by the disulfide bonds into one $F(ab')_2$ fragment. $F(ab')_2$ is bivalent and retains the capability to cross-link antigens. The C-terminal of the molecule is digested into smaller fragments by the enzyme.

Major Classes of Immunoglobulin

There are no known functional differences between κ and λ light chains. However, heavy chains differ in both structure, especially in the structure of the Fc portions, and physiologic functions. The Igs formed by both the heavy and light chains are thus divided into five major classes (also known as isotypes) according to which heavy chain the Ig contains: IgA, IgD, IgE, IgG, and IgM, with their respective heavy chains α, δ, ε, γ, and μ. Among the five classes, IgG is the most abundant in the plasma. An Ig molecule with a particular antigen specificity can switch from one class to another through a process called class switching (see below). There are five classes of Ig:

IgA is secreted by mucosal lymphoid tissues and is the major mucosal immunoglobulin. It may be present as a monomer or a dimer joined by a joining (J) chain. On the mucosal surface, IgA molecules act mainly as neutralizing antibodies to react with microorganisms that attempt to penetrate the mucosa and prevent their invasion into the body (5–7).

IgD is present in a monomeric form. At the membrane location, it mainly coexists with IgM on the surface of mature naive B cells serving as part of the BCR that initiates B-cell activation. In its circulating form, IgD may also bind to basophils and activate them to produce antimicrobial, opsonizing, inflammatory, and B-cell-stimulating factors to enhance immune surveillance (8,9).

IgE is present in a monomeric form. It is produced at very low levels by plasma cells and can be found in blood and extracellular fluid of bodily tissues. IgE molecules are avidly bound to specific IgE receptors on the surface of mast cells and basophils where they trigger the release of chemical mediators that initiate allergic and inflammatory reactions

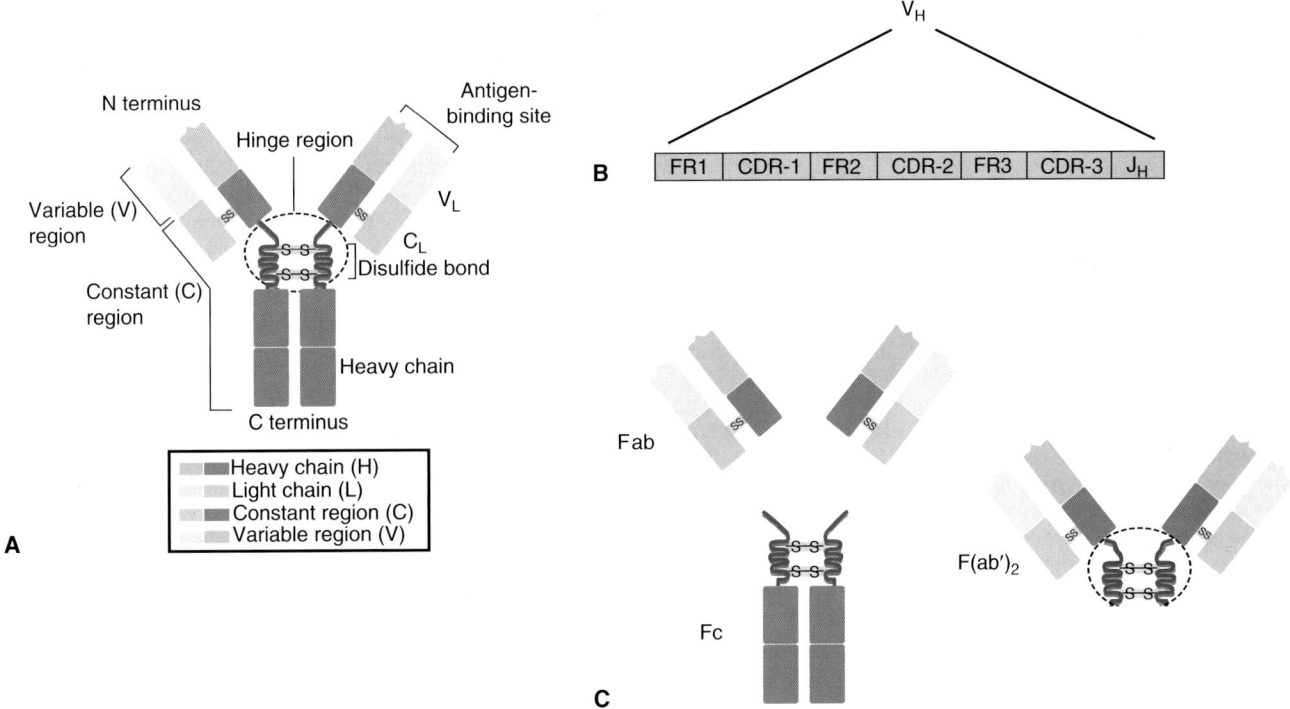

FIGURE 6.1.   A: Schematic diagram of the protein structure of an immunoglobulin molecule. B: Regions of the V$_H$ domain. FR, framework regions; CDR, complementarity-determining regions. **C:** Cleavage of immunoglobulins with papain results in two F(ab´) fragments and one Fc fragment, while cleavage with pepsin yields a bivalent F(ab´)$_2$ fragment, plus several smaller fragments (not shown).

and serve as chemoattractants for other cells. IgE, therefore, is the most important Ig class in allergic reactions and reactions against infecting parasites (10,11).

IgG is always present in a monomeric form. It can be found in blood and extracellular fluid of bodily tissues. IgG is the only Ig that crosses the placenta to provide immune protection to the fetus. It is the major class of immunoglobulins that is produced in large quantities during secondary immune responses. Besides activating the complement system, the Fc portions of IgG molecules bind to Fc receptors on the surface of phagocytes, allowing these cells to destroy infecting microorganisms (12).

IgM can be rapidly produced without class switching, so IgM molecules are the first antibodies made against invading microorganisms during the early phase of the immune response. IgM of pentamers (with 10 antigen-binding sites) are held together by joining (J) chains. Due to this large size, the antibodies penetrate poorly into tissues and stay mostly in blood and lymph to fight against infections. The large pentameric structure of IgM also makes it highly efficient in activating the complement system for infection control (13).

Structure of T-Cell Receptors

The TCR consists of two polypeptide chains: alpha (TCRα) and beta (TCRβ). The heterodimer is held together by disulfide bonds and resembles in structure the Fab fragment of an Ig molecule. Similar to immunoglobulin, both α and β chains are organized in domains of variable regions (V) and constant regions (C) (Fig. 6.2). The V regions of both α and β chains form the antigen recognition site. But unlike immunoglobulin, TCR does not have any structure equivalent to the Fc fragment and thus lacks effector function. TCR is membrane bound with

a transmembrane domain and a short cytoplasmic tail and cannot be secreted like immunoglobulin.

The receptor is monovalent with only one antigen-binding site. Through this antigen-binding site, TCR recognizes antigens presented as peptide sequences in complex with major histocompatibility complex (MHC) on antigen-presenting cells. Helper T cells with co-receptor CD4 recognize cells bearing an MHC-II complex while cytotoxic T cells with co-receptor CD8 recognize cells bearing the MHC-I complex (14–16). Activation of CD4 and CD8 T cells leads to activation of other effector cells of the immune system and the killing of infected cells, respectively. Some T cells can also suppress immune responses and are called regulatory T cells (Tregs); these are FOXP3, CD25, and, most frequently, CD4 positive. A minority

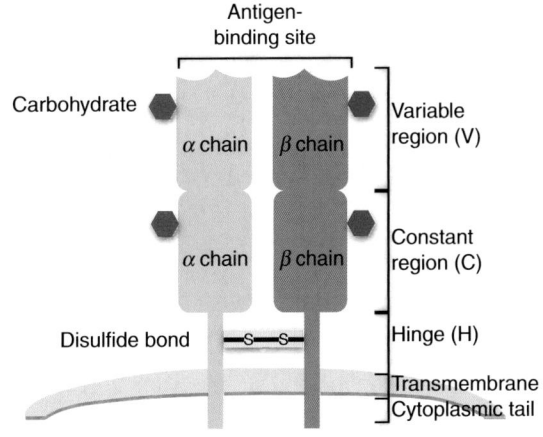

FIGURE 6.2.   Schematic diagram of the protein structure of a TCR molecule.

of TCRs are composed of a heterodimer of γ and δ polypeptide chains. These $\gamma\delta$ TCRs resemble TCR$\alpha\beta$ in structure (17). However, the function of $\gamma\delta$ TCRs and their ligands remain unknown. They may recognize antigens directly and may not require antigen processing or MHC-mediated antigen presentation (18).

 # MOLECULAR MECHANISMS FOR DIVERSITY GENERATION

One of the major functions of the antigen receptors, Ig in B cells and TCR in T cells, is to recognize the antigens that come in all forms, that is, bacteria, viruses, their products, and toxins. Receptors produced by each lymphocyte are unique with a specific antigen-binding site. Billions of antigen-specific lymphocytes exist in any given individual. However, each unique receptor is not encoded by a unique gene. Instead, the genes encoding antigen receptors are organized into gene segments. Three genetic mechanisms are in play to ensure the generation of a vast variety of antigen receptors with diverse amino acid sequences. These include V(D)J gene rearrangement, somatic hypermutation, and class switching of Ig. Gene rearrangement occurs in both B and T cells; however, the latter two processes occur only in B cells and not T cells, and thus they do not affect the TCR gene.

Gene Rearrangements

Gene rearrangement (more details below) is a somatic (as opposed to germ line) process occurring in immature lymphocytes that recombines the gene segments of Ig or TCR to form the V gene sequences that encode the V regions of antigen receptor proteins (19,20) (Fig. 6.3). The fundamental mechanism of gene rearrangement is similar for Ig (both heavy chains and light chains of Ig) and TCR. Diversity results from different combinations of gene segments (combinatorial diversity) as well as insertions or deletions of nucleotides at the joints (junctional diversity). This knowledge has been applied to clinical practice primarily to help determine the clonality of lymphoid lesions (see below).

Somatic Hypermutation

Somatic hypermutation is also a somatic process carried out by coordinated actions of several enzymes that create point mutations in already rearranged V gene sequences (21). An enzyme called activation-induced cytidine deaminase (AID) is expressed in germinal center (GC) B cells and is critical for this process: AID deficiency results in lack of somatic mutation, as well as class switching. The process occurs after B cells are exposed to antigens in conjunction with signals from activated T cells in the GCs (Fig. 6.3) (22). Mutations in the CDRs that result in enhanced antigen binding will be favorably selected, while those that decrease affinity to antigen or

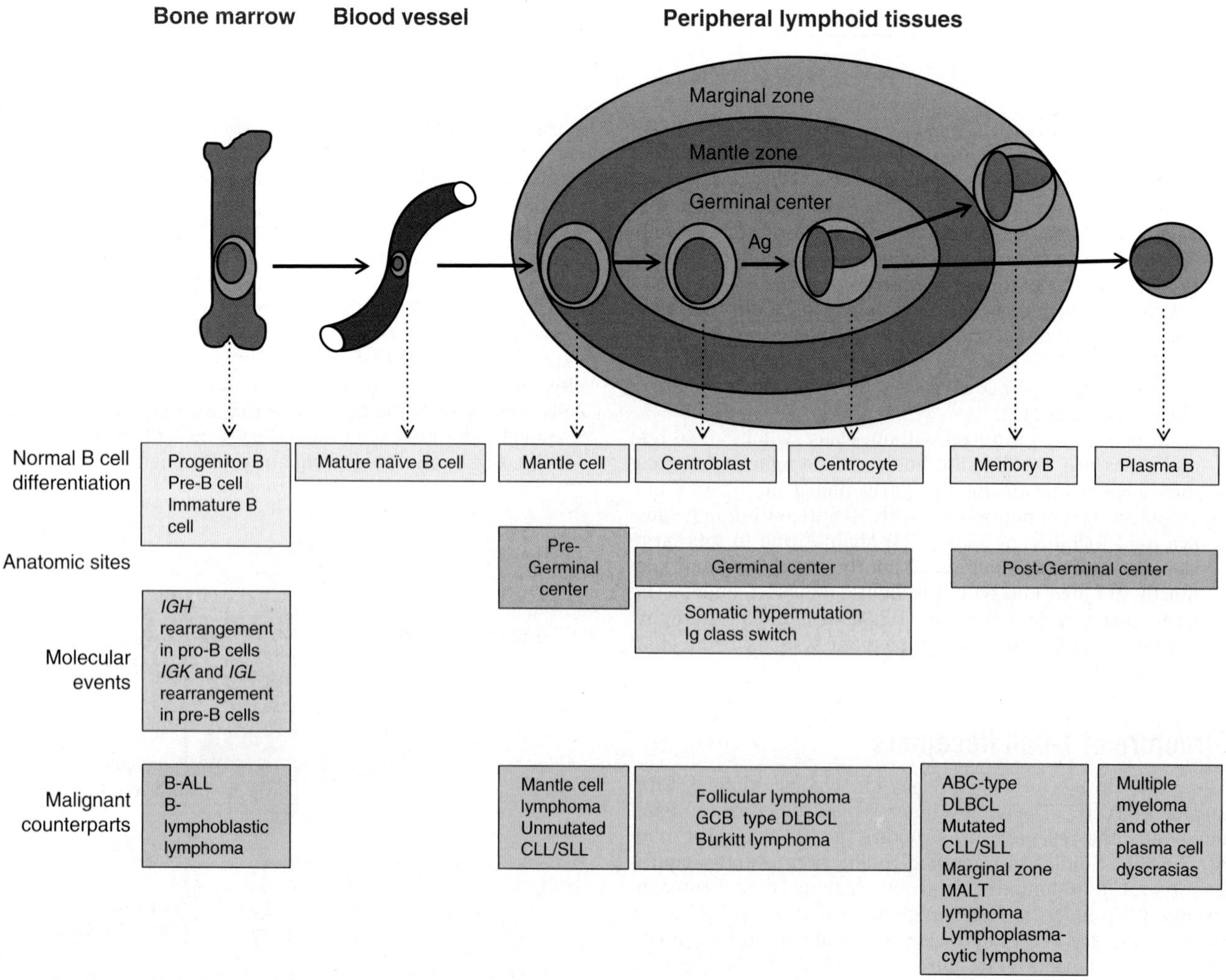

FIGURE 6.3. B-cell development showing sites, concurring molecular events, and malignant counterparts of various B-cell stages.

disrupt the Ig structures will be selected against. In clinical practice, analysis of V gene mutations helps derive prognostic information for patients with chronic lymphocytic leukemia (CLL; see below).

Class Switching of Ig

Class switching is another somatic process that occurs after an antigen encounter (Fig. 6.3). This process allows B cells to switch C regions while maintaining the same V regions to make an Ig of a different class to carry out specific effector functions (23). The initial Ig made by B cells are of either IgM or IgD class and they can subsequently change to IgG, IgA, or IgE through class switching.

In B cells, these three processes occur during distinct stages of B-cell development at different anatomic sites. Figure 6.3 illustrates that *IGH, IGK*, and *IGL* gene rearrangements occur in pro-B or pre-B cells in the bone marrow. Meanwhile, somatic hypermutation and class switching occur in the GCs of lymph nodes. So B-cell lymphomas of GC or post-GC origin, such as follicular lymphoma, have undergone somatic hypermutation that impacts the clonal detection of *IG* rearrangement in these lymphomas (see below).

GERM LINE STRUCTURE OF IG AND TCR GENES

The Ig heavy chain gene locus is located near the telomere of the long arm of chromosome 14 in band 14q32.3 (Fig. 6.4). It spans over an approximately 1.2-Mb region and consists of gene segments of variable (V_H), diversity (D), joining (J_H), and constant (C_H) regions, which are placed in the order of $5'$-V_H-D_H-J_H-C_H-$3'$ (24,25). There are approximately 46 to 52 functional V_H segments that are categorized into 6 or 7 families according to sequence homology (26). The most frequently used families by B-cell malignancies are V_H3, V_H4, and V_H1, that altogether cover 75% to 95% of V_H usage (27–29). Each family has a unique $5'$ flanking region and members of the same family share a consensus nucleotide sequence with 80% or greater homology, while sequences among different families have <70% homology. Within the V gene sequences, there are relatively conserved nucleotide sequences that encode the three FRs (see above) as well as highly variable sequence clusters

that encode the CDRs (see above) of the Ig proteins (Fig. 6.1B). There are about 27 functional D_H segments and 6 functional J_H segments. There are nine functional C_H segments located about 8 kb downstream of the last J_H fragment. Besides functional V, D, and J gene segments, there exist nonfunctional pseudo gene fragments that carry mutations that prevent them from making a functional protein. V_H, D_H, and J_H segments are randomly selected and linked to each other by DNA recombination through a process also known as gene rearrangement, whereas joining of rearranged VDJ to C gene is carried out at the RNA level by RNA splicing. V_H, D_H, and J_H segments jointly encode the V regions of the heavy chain while C_H gene encodes the C region of the Ig protein molecule (see Figs. 6.4 and 6.6).

The human κ light chain locus, *IGK*, is located on chromosome 2p12, occupying about 1.1 Mb of DNA (30–32) (Fig. 6.4). It is composed of 34 to 48 functional V_κ segments, five J_κ segments, and one C_κ gene. The *IGK* gene does not contain any D segments but contains a Kde element lying approximately 24 kb downstream of the C_κ region. Besides, V_κ to J_κ recombination, Kde may rearrange with V_κ to form V_κ-Kde, or rearrange to the intron between J_κ and C_κ to form intron-Kde.

The human λ light chain locus, *IGL*, is located on chromosome 22q11.2, covering about 1.2 Mb of DNA (33,34) (Fig. 6.4). It consists of 29 to 33 functional V_λ segments that are localized 14 kb upstream from 4 to 5 functional J_λ-C_λ clusters. Unlike other *IG* genes, J_λ-C_λ are present as tandem pairs at the *IGL* locus.

There are four TCR gene loci, *TCRA, TCRB, TCRG*, and *TCRD* that encode the TCR α, β, γ and δ chains, respectively. The structure of *TCRA* and *TCRB* genes are much more complex than that of *TCRG* and *TCRD* genes.

TCRA and *TCRD* are located on chromosome 14q11.2 at the same locus, covering approximately 0.9 Mb of DNA (35,36) (Fig. 6.5). It consists of 70 to 80 Vα interspersed with 7 Vδ segments, 5 of these 7 Vδ segments can be shared between the *TCRA* and *TCRD* genes. The V gene segments are spread over >600 kb of DNA and are followed by three Dδ, three to four Jδ, one Cδ, and then one Vδ in reverse orientation. Lying approximately 100 kb downstream are 61 Jα gene segments and 1 Cα approximately 5 kb further downstream from Jα. There are no known D segments for the *TCRA* gene.

The *TCRB* locus is located on chromosome band 7q34, occupying about 700 kb of DNA (37) (Fig. 6.5). It has 52 functional Vβ segments, two D_β segments, 13 J_β segments, and two C regions (31). D_β, J_β, C_β form two tandem clusters in the order of $D_\beta1$-$J_\beta1$-$C_\beta1$ and $D_\beta2$-$J_\beta2$-$C_\beta2$.

Heavy-chain locus, 14q32.3

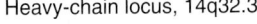

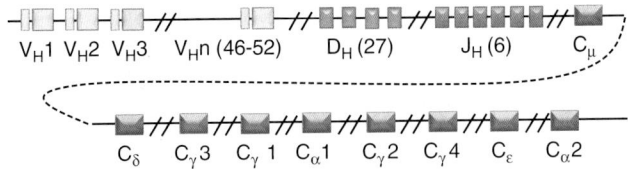

FIGURE 6.4. Germ line structure of *IG* genes.

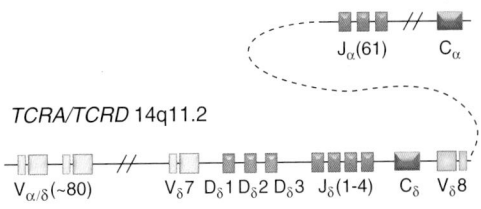

FIGURE 6.5. Germ line structure of *TCR* genes.

The *TCRG* locus is located on chromosome 7p14 spreading over approximately 130 kb of DNA (38,39) (Fig. 6.5). It has 12 to 14 Vγ segments grouped into families, with some families containing a single member. Six of the Vγ segments are functional, and the remainder are pseudogenes that also participate in gene rearrangement, although they do not encode functional γ chains (40,41). There are no known D segments in the *TCRG* locus. The Vγ segments are followed at the 3′ end by five Jγ and two Cγ gene segments. Nucleotide sequences of Cγ1 and Cγ2 share high homology.

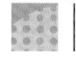 **GENE REARRANGEMENT**

All seven loci encoding the Ig heavy and light (κ, λ) chains and the TCR (α, β, γ, δ) chains undergo somatic DNA rearrangement to form a complete V domain from V, (D), and J segments (D is in parenthesis since some of the genes do not contain D segments) (42,43). C segments of the gene are joined to V(D)J after transcription through RNA splicing (42,44–47). V(D)J gene rearrangement occurs during lymphocyte development, in the bone marrow for *IG* and in the thymus for *TCR*, involving similar genetic mechanisms carried out by the same enzymes. All seven *IG* and *TCR* genes are rearranged in a hierarchical order. Knowledge of this hierarchical order helps us to understand the rearrangement patterns of different *IG* and *TCR* genes in lymphoid malignancies derived from cells at different developmental stages. In the bone marrow, *IGH* is rearranged first in pro-B cells followed by κ light chain rearrangement in pre-B cells (48) (Fig. 6.3). If *IGK* rearrangement fails to generate functional κ light chains, B cells will then initiate the rearrangement of the *IGL* locus. As a consequence, all B cells expressing λ light chains have a rearranged *IGK* locus. In thymus, *TCRD* is rearranged first, followed by *TCRG*, to generate TCR$\gamma\delta$. *TCRB* is then recombined followed by *TCRA* rearrangement to produce TCR$\alpha\beta$. Since *TCRD* is embedded in the *TCRA* locus, *TCRD* gene segments are looped out and deleted when *TCRA* is rearranged. For a specific gene locus, if arrangement of the first allele is not leading to a functional protein product, the B or T cell will proceed to rearrange the second allele (49). So, there may exist up to two rearranged alleles for a single gene in a given B or T cell and its daughter cells (clone).

Figure 6.6 illustrates the step-wise process of gene rearrangement using *IGH* as an example. For genes that

contain D segments, including *IGH*, *TCRB*, and *TCRD*, the recombination machinery, including RAG1 and RAG2 recombinase, randomly selects one D and joins it to a J segment. This event is followed by V to D-J recombination to generate recombinatorial diversity. At each junction, D to J and V to DJ, variable nucleotides are deleted or inserted (including palindromic P nucleotides and non-template encoding N nucleotides) by specialized enzymes to create junctional diversity. For genes that do not contain D, including *IGK*, *IGL*, *TCRA* and *TCRG*, V segments are directly combined with J segments. Again, random nucleotides are inserted at the joints that create a vast array of DNA sequence diversity encoding the antigen contact residues of CDRs of TCR and Ig proteins. Thus, V(D)J recombination plus junctional insertions/deletions are major contributors to the diversity of the antigen receptor repertoire. In the meantime, because of the chance of out-of-frame joining and stop codons generation, nonfunctional rearranged genes are also created as side products.

 MOLECULAR ANALYSIS OF ANTIGEN RECEPTOR GENE REARRANGEMENT IN CLINICAL APPLICATIONS

Clinical Utilities

The V(D)J rearrangement that results in the generation of antigen receptor diversity are not merely of academic interest. They can be applied to answer crucial and practical clinical questions concerning the clonality and lineage of a particular lymphoid lesion (50,51) V(D)J rearrangement is unique for each B or T cell and a particular V(D)J recombination is highly enriched during clonal expansion of a malignant lymphocyte (Fig. 6.7). Thus, identification in the laboratory of any particular V(D)J rearrangement suggests that the lesion is monoclonal and thus is likely to mark a malignant clone. On the contrary, if all V(D)J are more or less equally represented by the population of lymphocytes analyzed, the finding suggests the lesion is polyclonal.

In 10% to 30% of lymphoproliferative lesions, in which histologic examination and immunophenotyping are not

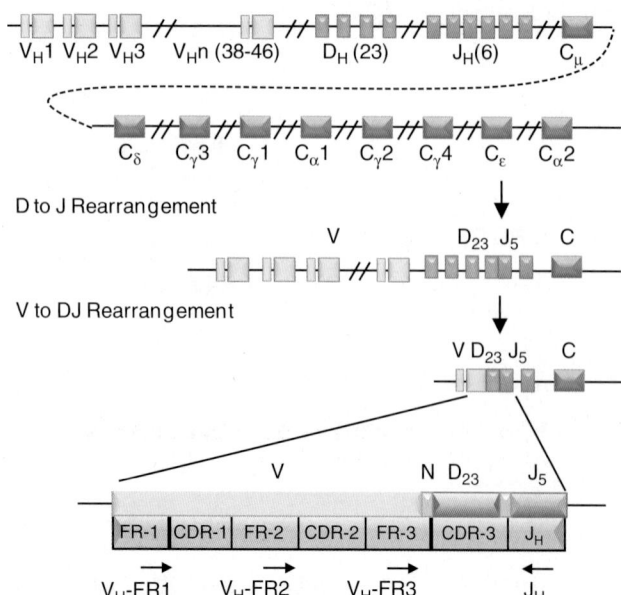

FIGURE 6.6. Gene rearrangement. *IGH* is illustrated here as an example. At the bottom, the *purple bar* depicts the regions of the V$_H$ gene and common primers used for clonality detection.

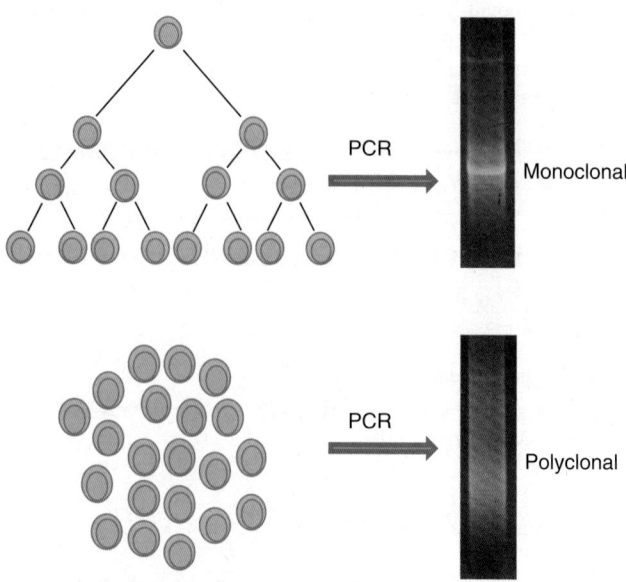

FIGURE 6.7. PCR analysis of clonality. Top: Showing monoclonal cell expansion and the corresponding gel pattern. **Bottom:** Showing polyclonal cell population and the corresponding gel pattern.

definitive, gene rearrangement analysis may be applied to aid in diagnosis to

1. Distinguish malignant from benign lesions (see below for caveats)
2. Distinguish between a B-cell lesion and a T-cell lesion (see below for caveats)
3. Assess whether there is bone marrow involvement by a lymphoid malignancy for staging
4. Determine the pathologic relationship of two tumors from different anatomic sites or between a primary and a secondary tumor present at different times (is the secondary tumor new or recurrent?)

Methods for Analysis

Since the late 1990s, polymerase chain reaction (PCR) has replaced Southern blot analysis as the most often used method to detect V(D)J rearrangement of *IG* and *TCR* due to its ease to perform, speed, analytic sensitivity, feasibility with scant materials, and compatibility with formalin-fixed, paraffin-embedded (FFPE) tissues (52). The principle of PCR reaction is described in detail elsewhere (53). Many types of clinical samples including peripheral blood, aspirated bone marrow, fresh tissues or cells, and FFPE tissues can be used for the analysis. PCR does not work with any tissues fixed with fixatives containing Bouin's or mercury since these fixatives inhibit Taq polymerase, the key enzyme that catalyzes the PCR reaction (54). The major steps of the tests involve (i) DNA extraction, (ii) PCR in a thermocycler, and (iii) gel or capillary electrophoresis to resolve and visualize the PCR products.

High degrees of sequence variations at *IG* and *TCR* loci made it challenging to design PCR primers for the detection of gene rearrangement. Primers containing mismatches to the DNA template may fall off during the reaction and generate false-negative results. Thus, the diagnostic sensitivity of the analysis may be reduced. Normally, a pair of upstream and downstream oligonucleotide primers, each about 20 bases long and complementary to opposite strands of the target sequence, are required for each reaction. The primer pairs are usually placed <400 bp apart to ensure successful amplification from cross-linked FFPE material. Ideally, primers should be precisely complementary to their target sequences, but may bear some mismatches, if the target sequence cannot be predicted precisely (52). Mismatches at the 5′ ends or the middle of the primers may be tolerated, but mismatches at the 3′ ends prevent primer extension by Taq DNA polymerase and significantly affect the efficiency of PCR amplification.

Due to the presence of sequence diversity at *IG* and *TCR* loci, the design of primers with perfect match to the target DNA is impossible. So, the design either targets the consensus sequences of relatively conserved regions, like FRs within the V segments, or targets particular V, D, or J families. Figure 6.6 illustrates the FR regions for the *IGH* locus. Within the V_H gene, there are three FRs called FR1, FR2, and FR3. Upstream PCR primers are normally hybridized to one of these regions and are referred to as FR1, FR2, or FR3 primers. The downstream primers usually target J segments.

Owing to the extensive sequence variations with *IG* and *TCR* genes, the traditional PCR design with one pair of upstream and downstream primers yields frequent false-negative results. To maximize the rate of clonality detection, a large European collaborative group developed standardized BIOMED-2 assays using a multiplex PCR approach that involves multiple pairs of consensus or family primers in a few PCR reactions for each locus of *IG* and *TCR* (55). Figure 6.8 illustrates the concept of multiplex PCR for the *TCRG* locus where each PCR reaction tube contains several upstream and downstream primers. The PCR products can be detected by either gel or capillary electrophoresis as bands or

TCRG tube A:
V_γ If and V_γ 10 primers+ J_γ 1.1/2.1 and J_γ 1.3/2.3

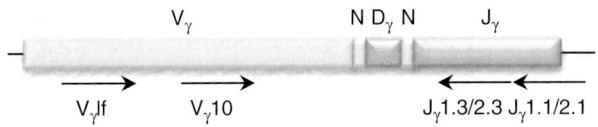

TCRG tube B:
V_γ 9 and V_γ 11 primers+ J_γ 1.1/2.1 and J_γ 1.3/2.3

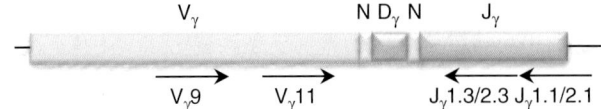

FIGURE 6.8. Multiplex PCR for TCRG locus. The assay consists of two-tube reactions with each tube including more than one pair of PCR primers.

peaks, respectively (Figs. 6.9 and 6.10). The assays, available as commercial prepackaged kits, have been widely used in clinical laboratories since their publication in 2003 (55).

Interpretation and Caveats

Normally, the interpretation of clonality assays is straightforward. Monoclonal gene rearrangement appears as a predominant monoclonal band or as a peak on a background of polyclonal bands or peaks (Figs. 6.9 and 6.10) whereas polyclonal gene rearrangements appear as a ladder of multiple bands or peaks. The absence of bands/peaks suggests amplification failure, which may result for a number of reasons, including the presence of very few lymphoid cells in the specimen (nonlymphoid tissue, cerebrospinal fluid, fine needle aspiration, etc.), the presence of PCR inhibitors in the specimen (from medicines taken by patients, Bouin's, and other fixatives containing heavy metals), or DNA damage caused by overfixation (leading to extensive cross-linking).

Like any other clinical test, clonality by PCR analysis sometimes yields false positives or false negatives due to either technical or biologic issues. In this section of the chapter, we discuss caveats related to the interpretation of PCR results.

False Positives from PCR Contamination

First and foremost, false positives resulting from PCR contamination must be ruled out. Since PCR involves many cycles of DNA target amplification, the technique is extremely sensitive to carry-over contamination. Stringent quality control measures need to be built into the clinical assay to maximize the chance of contamination detection. The assays require minimally three quality controls: monoclonal control, polyclonal control, and H_2O control. If a monoclonal band or peak is observed with what are supposed to be polyclonal or H_2O control samples, contamination has likely occurred. With the aid of these controls, false positives can be easily detected.

Nonspecific Bands

Nonspecific hybridization of primers may occur and may be mistaken as evidence for clonal gene rearrangement. When interpreting PCR results, one should be aware of the sizes of commonly seen nonspecific bands. These normally fall outside the range of legitimate PCR products from V(D)J rearrangement.

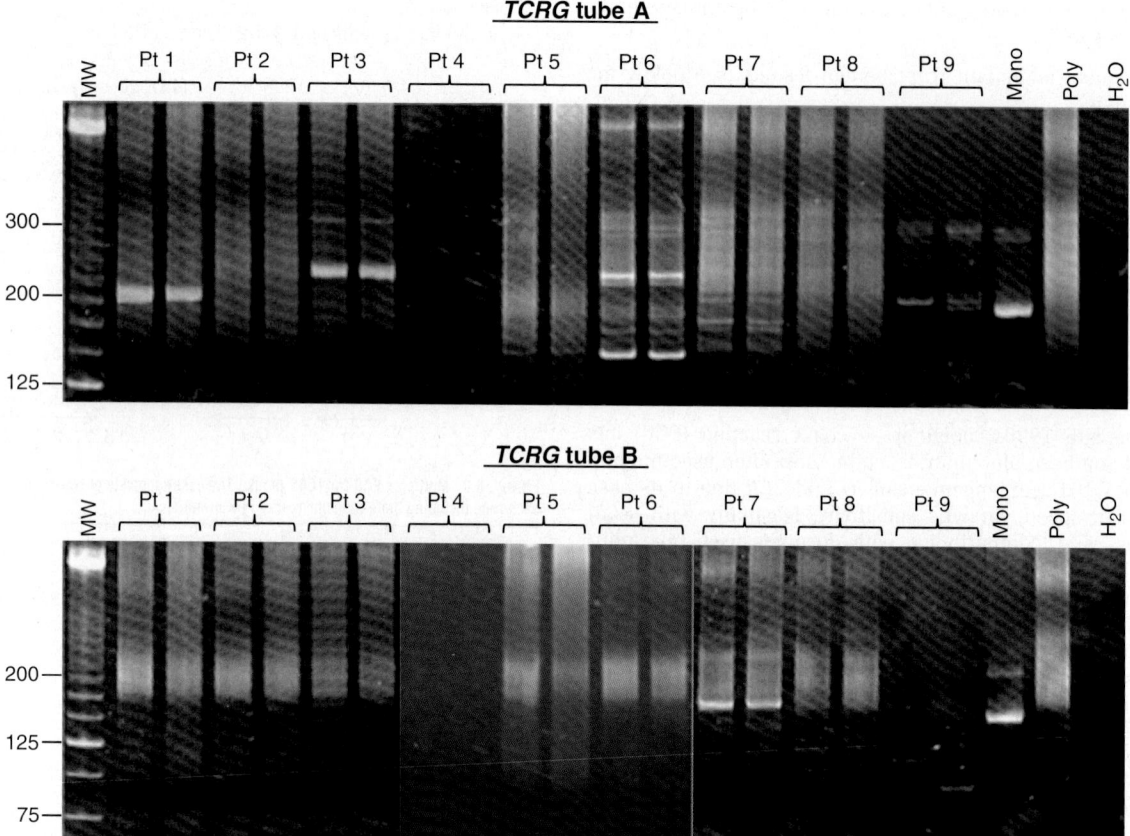

FIGURE 6.9. Gel electrophoretic analysis of *TCRG* gene rearrangement. Each sample is shown in duplicate. Pt, patient. MW, 25 bp DNA molecular weight ladder. Mono, positive control. Poly, negative control. H₂O, water control. Monoclonal gene rearrangements detected in Pt 1, 3, 6, and 7. Polyclonal gene rearrangements detected in Pt 2, 5, and 8. Pt 4's lanes were blank suggesting problem with DNA quality. Pt 9's specimen was of skin origin, and the lesion had a small lymphocytic infiltrate.

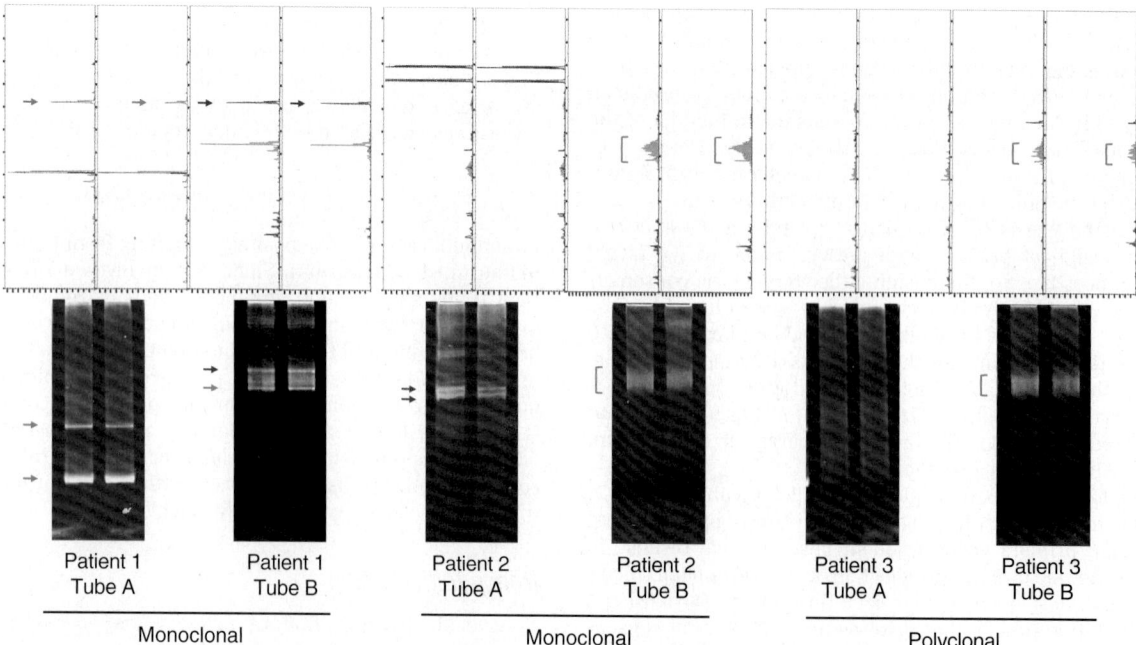

FIGURE 6.10. Gel and capillary electrophoretic analysis of *TCRG* gene rearrangement. Each sample is shown in duplicate. *Arrows* indicate monoclonal gene rearrangements and brackets indicate polyclonal gene rearrangement. Primers are conjugated with either *green* or *blue* fluorochome that target different V and J regions of the *TCRG* locus.

Monoclonality as Tumor Markers

Results of clonality analysis should be interpreted with consideration of other clinical, morphologic, immunophenotypic, and cytogenetic findings. Although monoclonal gene rearrangement is frequently used as a marker for a B- or T-cell neoplasm, it is *not* synonymous with malignancy. *IGH* and *TCR* gene rearrangement has been demonstrated in 3% to 9% of non-neoplastic lymphoid tissue samples from patients with benign pathologic conditions (56,57). Meanwhile, polyclonality is not equivalent to a benign process either. Failure to detect monoclonal gene rearrangement may result from primer hybridization failure caused by extensive sequence variations in the *IG* and *TCR* genes. False-negative findings happen more often in lymphomas of germinal-center or post-GC origins since these tumor cells have undergone somatic hypermutation (Fig. 6.3).

Clonality in Benign Pathologic Conditions

As mentioned above, monoclonality can be found in benign pathologic conditions. When interpreting a monoclonal result, one needs to be aware of the fact that (i) T-cell clones may be found in the peripheral blood of older normal individuals with no apparent pathologic conditions; (ii) in skin, clonal gene rearrangement can be found in lymphomatoid papulosis, a benign cutaneous lesion; (iii) oligoclonality can result from infection due to expansions of several B or T clones that recognize specific epitopes of a particular antigen; (iv) oligoclonality can result from immune suppression where there is a paucity of lymphocytes; and (v) pseudoclonality can be observed in nonlymphoid tissues with a small lymphocytic infiltrate. When specific V(D)J genes from individual lymphocytes are amplified by PCR, the electrophoresis pattern may appear to be monoclonal or oligoclonal. The best way to differentiate these situations from true clonality is to perform duplicate PCR reactions. Benign oligoclonality or pseudoclonality would not reproduce the same rearranged bands/peaks in two independent PCR reactions.

IG and TCR Rearrangement as Lineage Markers

IG and *TCR* rearrangement is frequently used as a linage marker to characterize a lymphoid lesion, *IG*-rearranged tumors are more likely of B-cell origin and *TCR*-rearranged tumors are more likely of T-cell origin. However, exceptions to this rule are not uncommon. Among B-cell malignancies, up to 25% may carry a *TCR* gene rearrangement (58). In immature B-cell malignancies, lineage infidelity is even more frequent: >90% precursor B-acute lymphoblastic leukemias (ALL) may carry *TCR* gene rearrangement (59). Among T-cell malignancies, up to 10% may contain *IG* rearrangement (60). In large studies using PCR methods independent of BIOMED-2 assays, a dual genotype was observed in approximately 10% of B-cell and approximately 10% of T-cell lymphomas (56,61).

Presence of Multiple Rearrangements

Clonality assays complement each other. Besides the monoclonal single band/peak pattern, other monoclonal rearrangement patterns can be observed: (i) same rearrangement detected by multiple primer sets (e.g., by *IGH* FR1, FR2, and FR3 primer sets); (ii) two rearrangements detected on the same allele (e.g., by Vβ-Jβ and Dβ-Jβ primer sets); (iii) biallelic rearrangements detected in the same clonal cell population (two bands/peaks with one set of PCR primers, see Figs. 6.9 and 6.10); (iv) rearrangement detected at more than one locus (e.g., *IGH* and *IGK*); and (v) a malignant process with both *IG* and *TCR* rearrangements detected as mentioned in the previous paragraph. All these patterns may be observed in a clonal lymphoid lesion.

Correlation with Immunophenotyping

Gene rearrangement results cannot be directly correlated with immunophenotyping results. Since B cells rearrange the *IGK* locus before the *IGL* locus, λ-restricted tumor has undergone *IGK* rearrangement already. So an *IGK*-rearranged tumor can be either κ- or λ-restricted. In T cells, the order of gene rearrangements is D-G-B-A. TCRαβ T cells may have rearranged *TCRG* and TCRγδ may also have rearranged *TCRB* in some cases; thus, detection of *TCRB* or *TCRG* monoclonality is not indicative of malignancies of TCRαβ or TCRγδ type.

Presence of a Weak Band/Small Peak

A small clone that comprises <10% of a total cell population may be missed due to the polyclonal background. This limited analytic sensitivity of clonality assays restricts their use in minimal residual disease assessment or assessment of bone marrow involvement. For diagnostic tissues, a weak band/small peak may mean a number of different scenarios: (i) a small clone in the tissue; (ii) inefficient PCR amplification due to suboptimal primer hybridization; and (iii) reactive lymphoproliferations where a particular clone may be preferentially expanded due to a strong antigenic drive. Up to 15% of benign lesions contain a weak band/peak in a polyclonal background. The weak band/small peak is normally seen in one isolated gene rearrangement assays (57).

Presence of Several Rearranged Bands/Peaks

Gene rearrangement analysis may reveal two or three monoclonal bands/peaks for the same locus. This may be the result of several scenarios: (i) The lesion rearranged both alleles. As mentioned above, if V(D)J rearrangement does not generate a functional *IG* or *TCR* gene product, the lymphocyte would initiate the rearrangement of the second allele. This perhaps is the most common scenario when two bands are identified, and should be interpreted accordingly. (ii) The lesion contains two lymphoid clones. The finding of two rearranged band/peaks may support a diagnosis of composite lymphoma. Occasional presence of three or even four bands is also consistent with a composite lymphoma. (iii) Amplification from both an upstream and a downstream J segment. For example, the consensus J$_{\rm H}$ primer may hybridize to both J$_5$ and J$_6$ segments of the *IGH* gene and give rise to two PCR products out of the same VDJ rearrangement. This is possible since all J segments cluster in a relatively small region: J$_{\rm H}$ spans an approximately 2.3-kb region, Jκ an approximately 1.4-kb region, and Jβ an approximately 1.1-kb region (55).

Sensitivities of Clonality Analysis in Major Types of non-Hodgkin Lymphomas

For mature lymphoid malignancies, B-cell tumors are more frequent than T-cell tumors. However, among cases of ALL, 15% to 20% are of T-cell origin, and among cutaneous lymphomas, two-thirds are of T-cell origin. Most lymphomas can be diagnosed based on morphologic and immunophenotypic evaluation. In 10% to 30% cases, molecular studies are instrumental in helping differentiate lesions between malignant and benign, and between B- and T-cell neoplasms (see "Clinical Utilities"). For lymphoid malignancies requiring molecular clonality studies, ideally, all *IG* and *TCR* tests should be carried out to maximize the chance of finding a PCR-detectable clone. However, in reality, this approach increases the labor, time, and patient care cost dramatically, so a step-wise algorithm is more feasible. Among *IG* and *TCR* loci, *TCRA* rearrangement is not routinely analyzed due to its highly complex gene structure. In addition, since it is the last rearranged locus in T cells, virtually

Table 6.1	DIAGNOSTIC SENSITIVITIES OF *IG* CLONALITY ASSAYS IN MAJOR TYPES OF B-CELL NHLS						
	MCL *n* = 54 (%)	CLL/SLL *n* = 56 (%)	FL *n* = 109 (%)	MALT Extranodal *n* = 31 (%)	MZL Nodal *n* = 10 (%)	DLBCL *n* = 109 (%)	Total *n* = 369 (%)
IGH genes							
VDJ cases (%)	54 (100)	56 (100)	92 (84)	26 (84)	10 (100)	86 (79)	324 (88)
DHJH cases (%)	6 (11)	24 (43)	21 (19)	18 (58)	3 (30)	33 (30)	105 (28)
All IGH	54 (100)	56 (100)	94 (86)	29 (94)	10 (100)	93 (95)	336 (91)
IGK genes	54 (100)	56 (100)	92 (84)	26 (84)	8 (80)	87 (80)	232 (88)
IGL genes	24 (44)	17 (30)	23 (21)	9 (29)	3 (30)	30 (28)	106 (29)
Combined IG gene							
VH-JH+IGK	54 (100)	56 (100)	109 (100)	29 (94)	10 (100)	105 (96)	364 (99)
All IGH+IGK	54 (100)	56 (100)	109 (100)	31 (100)	10 (100)	107 (98)	367 (99)
Total IGH+IGK+IGL	54 (100)	56 (100)	109 (100)	31 (100)	10 (100)	107 (98)	367 (99)

MCL, mantle cell lymphoma; CLL, chronic lymphocytic leukemia; SLL, small lymphocytic lymphoma; FL, follicular lymphoma; MALT, mucosa-associated lymphoid tissue; MZL, marginal zone lymphoma; DLBCL, diffuse large B-cell lymphoma.

all T-cell malignancies with rearranged *TCRA* have rearranged *TCRB* and most of them have rearranged *TCRG* locus. Analysis of *TCRB* and *TCRG* normally obviates the need to analyze *TCRA*. *TCRD*, which occupies the same locus as *TCRA*, is deleted when *TCRA* is rearranged.

Overall, BIOMED-2 assays detect clonality in 99% of B-cell non-Hodgkin lymphomas (NHLs) and 94% of T-cell NHLs. Diagnostic sensitivities of each multiplex assay in major types of NHLs are shown in Table 6.1 (B) and Table 6.2 (T). The *IG* rearrangement could be demonstrated in approximately 80% of Hodgkin lymphoma in a small study of 24 cases (62). Regarding these assays, a few points are worth special notice: (i) the *IGK* assay has particular value in lymphomas of GC and post-GC origin, increasing the clonality detection rate in follicular lymphoma by 15% to 30% (58,63–65); (ii) *IGL* clonality appears to add little value; and (iii) *TCRB* and *TCRG* each detects approximately 90% of T-cell malignancies. Together, they detect 94% of all T-cell tumors; (iv) *TCRD* is particularly useful in immature T-cell malignancies and in TCRγδ tumors; and (v) *TCR* clonality assays have the lowest detection rate in anaplastic large cell lymphoma (ALCL); up to 25% of ALCL cases may lack a PCR-detectable clone (58).

For laboratories that intend to perform these tests in the most efficient manner, meaning running the fewest reactions without a significant compromise in diagnostic sensitivity, BIOMED-2 action has developed a testing algorithm that is shown in Figure 6.11. The most useful tests for suspected B-cell malignancies are assays that detect complete *IGH* rearrangement (V$_H$-J$_H$, including FR1, FR2, and FR3) and *IGK* rearrangement. For T-cell tumors, assays that detect complete *TCRG* rearrangement and *TCRB* rearrangement are the most informative and useful. More recently, a large study with more than 300 FFPE tumor specimens showed that *IGH* FR2 plus

IGK generate a >90% detection rate in B-cell malignancies, and *TCRG* test alone detects clonality in approximately 95% of T-cell malignancies (66).

 ## ANALYSIS OF IGHV GENE MUTATION IN CLL PROGNOSIS

While CLL is often an indolent disease with a median survival of more than 10 years, some patients have a more aggressive clinical course (67). The first indication that different subtypes of CLL exist came from morphologic and cytogenetic studies, where in CLL cases with typical morphology the most common karyotypic abnormalities are in 3q14 while those with atypical cytology frequently have a trisomy 12 and a less favorable clinical outcome (68,69). Subsequent studies found that cases with trisomy 12 had a minimal number of somatic mutations in the *IGHV* regions, while cases with 13q14 abnormalities had significant somatic hypermutation (70). This observation was followed by a number of larger studies clearly documenting that unmutated germ line configuration of *IGHV* is an adverse prognostic factor in CLL (71–73). The unmutated cases can be distinguished with variable accuracy by flow cytometry showing CD38 and ZAP-70 positivity (72,74,75). With cutoff values for CD38 and ZAP-70 positivity of 20% to 30%, the concordance between CD38 or ZAP-70 expression and *IGVH* mutation status is around 75%, and between CD38 expression and ZAP-70 expression is also close to 75% (72–78). While one study found that ZAP-70 expression is the best predictor of time to treatment in patients with early disease (79), other studies based on multivariate analysis have found that unmutated *IGVH* is an independent prognostic factor for time to first treatment

Table 6.2	DIAGNOSTIC SENSITIVITIES OF TCR CLONALITY ASSAYS IN MAJOR TYPES OF T-CELL NHLS						
	T-PLL *n* = 33 (%)	T-LGL *n* = 28 (%)	PTCL-NOS *n* = 47 (%)	AILT *n* = 37 (%)	ALCL (ALK+) *n* = 34 (%)	ALCL (ALK−) *n* = 9 (%)	Total *n* = 188 (%)
TCRB PCR	33 (100)	27 (96)	46 (98)	33 (89)	25 (74)	7 (78)	171 (91)
TCRG PCR	31 (94)	27 (96)	97 (94)	97 (92)	90 (71)	99 (89)	80 (89)
TCRD PCR	2 (6)	8 (29)	7 (15)	13 (35)	4 (12)	0 (0)	34 (18)
Total TCR	33 (100)	28 (100)	47 (100)	35 (95)	26 (76)	8 (89)	177 (94)

T-PLL, T-cell prolymphocytic leukemia; T-LGL, T-cell large granular lymphocytic leukemia; PTCL-NOS, peripheral T-cell lymphoma (not otherwise specified); AILT, angioimmunoblastic T-cell lymphoma; ALCL, anaplastic large cell lymphoma.

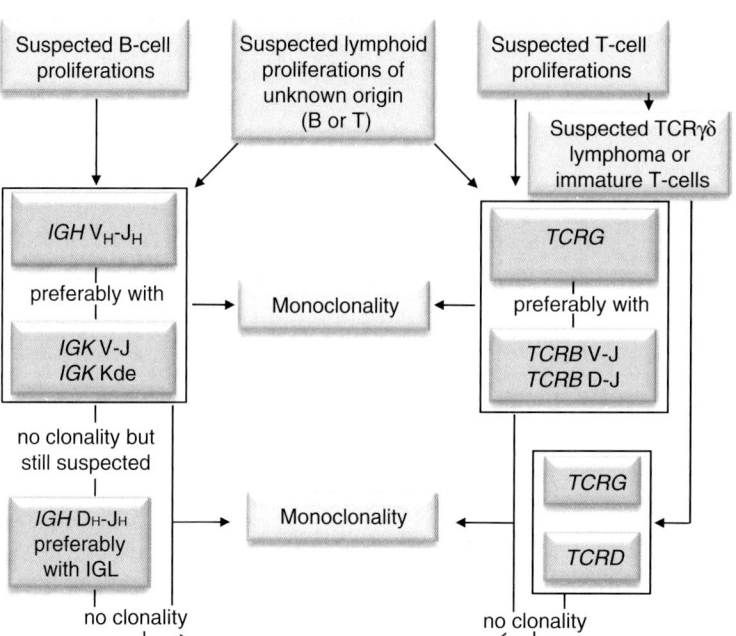

FIGURE 6.11. Testing algorithm in suspected lymphoid lesions.

and overall survival, in addition to other indicators, like 17p deletion, 11q deletion, age, lymphocyte doubling time, white blood cell counts, and lactate dehydrogenase (LDH) (76,80). An overall survival of approximately 12 years has been reported in cases without *IGVH* mutations as opposed to 23 years in patients with mutations (76). Therefore, assessment of mutations in the *IGHV* region has become useful in the clinical care of CLL. In addition, usage of the *VH3-21* gene segment in CLL has been reported to confer a poor prognosis, regardless of the *IGVH* mutation status. So sequence analysis of this region, which also reveals the *VH* segment used, may provide additional prognostic information (79,81).

Various specific methods have been used by clinical laboratories to assess the presence of somatic hypermutation in CLL, thereby providing prognostic information. These essentially rely upon amplification of cDNA or genomic DNA using consensus primers to the CDR and FR regions followed by sequencing. Alignment is then done to public databases, such as the international immunogenetics information (IMGT) (*http://imgt.org*) database of human immunoglobulin sequences with alignment programs like V-QUEST. This type of analysis provides the closest matching germ line *VH* segment and the percentage of sequence identity. If IGHV sequence identity to germ line is ≥98%, the CLL case is considered unmutated, which imparts an inferior prognosis. On the other hand, if the sequence homology is <98%, the case is interpreted as mutated.

More recent studies with careful analysis of the mutation pattern in *IGHV* in larger cohorts of patients with CLL, and a comparison with extensive sequencing of normal B-cell subsets, have shown that while these mutations reflect the classical somatic hypermutation machinery, CLL also has "stereotyped" IGH V sequences, which are more frequent than in normal GC B cells and are therefore "CLL biased." A further subdivision has been proposed into two additional categories for the subset of cases with somatic hypermutation: one with stereotyped and the other with nonstereotyped IGHV sequences, where the latter is twice as common (82,83). However, the prognostic or therapeutic implications of this additional subgrouping are not yet evident.

 | **SUMMARY AND CONCLUSIONS**

The determination of clonality based on immunoglobulin gene rearrangements for the diagnosis of lymphoma in humans was demonstrated to be useful since 10 years after the discovery that these rearrangements occur (84,85). Similar analysis of TCR gene rearrangements followed soon thereafter (86). The first studies involved Southern blotting, which required relatively large amounts of DNA extracted from fresh or frozen tissue. The clinical applications of this methodology to support the pathologic interpretation for the diagnosis of leukemias and lymphomas were the first molecular diagnostic assays, and paved the way for the current molecular pathology laboratories. While the technologies have evolved greatly, with PCR now being the basic diagnostic platform for clonality, the basic principles remain the same. Sequence information has allowed multiplexing to detect the majority of rearrangements, and technical platforms, such as capillary electrophoresis, have allowed shortening of procedure time, and more accurate interpretation. Sequencing has already been brought to the clinical arena for the prognostication of CLL. With evolving high-throughput next-generation sequencing being taken into the diagnostic clinical setting, it may soon be common diagnostic practice to sequence the rearranged immunoglobulin and TCR genes to gather information about clonality, the biologic origin of the specific neoplasm that may have diagnostic and prognostic implication, and to develop patient-specific primers to increase sensitivity and specificity and implementation of quantitative assays for the evaluation of response to therapy and minimal residual disease.

References

1. Hood L, Kronenberg M, Hunkapiller T. T cell antigen receptors and the immunoglobulin supergene family. *Cell* 1985;40:225–259.
2. Kurosaki T. Genetic analysis of B cell antigen receptor signaling. *Ann Rev Immunol* 1999;17:555–592.
3. Van Vunakis H, Langone JJ, eds. *Methods in enzymology.* New York: Academic Press, 1980.
4. Langone JJ, Van Vunakis H, eds. *Methods in enzymology.* Orlando: Academic Press, 1986.

5. Kaetzel CS, Robinson JK, Chintalacharuvu KR, et al. The polymeric immunoglobulin receptor (secretory component) mediates transport of immune complexes across epithelial cells: a local defense function for IgA. *Proc Natl Acad Sci U S A* 1991;88:8796–8800.
6. Macpherson AJ, Slack E. The functional interactions of commensal bacteria with intestinal secretory IgA. *Curr Opin Gastroenterol* 2007;23:673–678.
7. Fagarasan S, Honjo T. Intestinal IgA synthesis: regulation of front-line body defences. *Nat Rev Immunol* 2003;3:63–72.
8. Ohta Y, Flajnik M. IgD, like IgM, is a primordial immunoglobulin class perpetuated in most jawed vertebrates. *Proc Natl Acad Sci U S A* 2006;103:10723–10728.
9. Chen K, Xu W, Wilson M, et al. Immunoglobulin D enhances immune surveillance by activating antimicrobial, proinflammatory and B cell-stimulating programs in basophils. *Nat Immunol* 2009;10:889–898.
10. Winter WE, Hardt NS, Fuhrman S. Immunoglobulin E: importance in parasitic infections and hypersensitivity responses. *Arch Pathol Lab Med* 2000;124: 1382–1385.
11. Gould HJ, Sutton BJ, Beavil AJ, et al. The biology of IGE and the basis of allergic disease. *Ann Rev Immunol* 2003;21:579–628.
12. Indik ZK, Park JG, Hunter S, et al. The molecular dissection of Fc gamma receptor mediated phagocytosis. *Blood* 1995;86:4389–4399.
13. Casali P, Schettino EW. Structure and function of natural antibodies. *Curr Top Microbiol Immunol* 1996;210:167–179.
14. Germain RN. MHC-dependent antigen processing and peptide presentation: providing ligands for T lymphocyte activation. *Cell* 1994;76:287–299.
15. Reinherz EL, Tan K, Tang L, et al. The crystal structure of a T cell receptor in complex with peptide and MHC class II. *Science* 1999;286:1913–1921.
16. Rudolph MG, Stanfield RL, Wilson IA. How TCRs bind MHCs, peptides, and coreceptors. *Ann Rev Immunol* 2006;24:419–466.
17. Allison TJ, Winter CC, Fournie JJ, et al. Structure of a human gammadelta T-cell antigen receptor. *Nature* 2001;411:820–824.
18. Carding SR, Egan PJ. Gammadelta T cells: functional plasticity and heterogeneity. *Nat Rev Immunol* 2002;2:336–345.
19. Schatz DG. V(D)J recombination. *Immunol Rev* 2004;200:5–11.
20. Jung D, Giallourakis C, Mostoslavsky R, et al. Mechanism and control of V(D)J recombination at the immunoglobulin heavy chain locus. *Ann Rev Immunol* 2006;24:541–570.
21. Odegard VH, Schatz DG. Targeting of somatic hypermutation. *Nat Rev Immunol* 2006;6:573–583.
22. Muramatsu M, Kinoshita K, Fagarasan S, et al. Class switch recombination and hypermutation require activation-induced cytidine deaminase (AID), a potential RNA editing enzyme. *Cell* 2000;102:553–563.
23. Chaudhuri J, Basu U, Zarrin A, et al. Evolution of the immunoglobulin heavy chain class switch recombination mechanism. *Adv Immunol* 2007;94:157–214.
24. Ravetch JV, Siebenlist U, Korsmeyer S, et al. Structure of the human immunoglobulin mu locus: characterization of embryonic and rearranged J and D genes. *Cell* 1981;27:583–591.
25. Ichihara Y, Matsuoka H, Kurosawa Y. Organization of human immunoglobulin heavy chain diversity gene loci. *EMBO J* 1988;7:4141–4150.
26. Matsuda F, Ishii K, Bourvagnet P, et al. The complete nucleotide sequence of the human immunoglobulin heavy chain variable region locus. *J Exp Med* 1998;188:2151–2162.
27. Rettig MB, Vescio RA, Cao J, et al. VH gene usage is multiple myeloma: complete absence of the VH4.21 (VH4-34) gene. *Blood* 1996;87:2846–2852.
28. Pritsch O, Troussard X, Magnac C, et al. VH gene usage by family members affected with chronic lymphocytic leukaemia. *Br J Haematol* 1999;107:616–624.
29. Camacho FI, Algara P, Rodriguez A, et al. Molecular heterogeneity in MCL defined by the use of specific VH genes and the frequency of somatic mutations. *Blood* 2003;101:4042–4046.
30. Malcolm S, Barton P, Murphy C, et al. Localization of human immunoglobulin kappa light chain variable region genes to the short arm of chromosome 2 by *in situ* hybridization. *Proc Natl Acad Sci U S A* 1982;79:4957–4961.
31. McBride OW, Hieter PA, Hollis GF, et al. Chromosomal location of human kappa and lambda immunoglobulin light chain constant region genes. *J Exp Med* 1982;155:1480–1490.
32. Zachau HG. The immunoglobulin kappa locus-or-what has been learned from looking closely at one-tenth of a percent of the human genome. *Gene* 1993;135:167–173.
33. Vasicek TJ, Leder P. Structure and expression of the human immunoglobulin lambda genes. *J Exp Med* 1990;172:609–620.
34. Combriato G, Klobeck HG. V lambda and J lambda-C lambda gene segments of the human immunoglobulin lambda light chain locus are separated by 14 kb and rearrange by a deletion mechanism. *Eur J Immunol* 1991;21:1513–1522.
35. Sim GK, Yague J, Nelson J, et al. Primary structure of human T-cell receptor alpha-chain. *Nature* 1984;312:771–775.
36. Chien YH, Iwashima M, Kaplan KB, et al. A new T-cell receptor gene located within the alpha locus and expressed early in T-cell differentiation. *Nature* 1987;327:677–682.
37. Tunnacliffe A, Kefford R, Milstein C, et al. Sequence and evolution of the human T-cell antigen receptor beta-chain genes. *Proc Natl Acad Sci U S A* 1985;82: 5068–5072.
38. Lefranc MP, Chuchana P, Dariavach P, et al. Molecular mapping of the human T cell receptor gamma (TRG) genes and linkage of the variable and constant regions. *Eur J Immunol* 1989;19:989–994.
39. Pfeffer K, Schoel B, Gulle H, et al. Analysis of primary T cell responses to intact and fractionated microbial pathogens. *Curr Top Microbiol and Immunol* 1991;173:173–178.
40. Raulet DH. The structure, function, and molecular genetics of the gamma/delta T cell receptor. *Ann Rev Immunol* 1989;7:175–207.
41. Lefranc MP, Rabbitts TH. The human T-cell receptor gamma (TRG) genes. *Trends Biochem Sci* 1989;14:214–218.
42. Tonegawa S. Somatic generation of antibody diversity. *Nature* 1983;302:575–581.
43. Davis MM, Bjorkman PJ. T-cell antigen receptor genes and T-cell recognition. *Nature* 1988;334:395–402.
44. von Boehmer H, Fehling HJ. Structure and function of the pre-T cell receptor. *Ann Rev Immunol* 1997;15:433–452.
45. Krangel MS, Hernandez-Munain C, Lauzurica P, et al. Developmental regulation of V(D)J recombination at the TCR alpha/delta locus. *Immunol Rev* 1998;165:131–147.
46. Gellert M. A new view of V(D)J recombination. *Genes Cells* 1996;1:269–275.
47. Alt FW, Oltz EM, Young F, et al. VDJ recombination. *Immunol Today* 1992;13:306–314.
48. Perlot T, Alt FW. Cis-regulatory elements and epigenetic changes control genomic rearrangements of the IgH locus. *Adv Immunol* 2008;99:1–32.
49. Waldmann TA. The arrangement of immunoglobulin and T cell receptor genes in human lymphoproliferative disorders. *Adv Immunol* 1987;40:247–321.
50. Diss TC, Pan L. Polymerase chain reaction in the assessment of lymphomas. *Cancer Surv* 1997;30:21–44.
51. Medeiros LJ, Carr J. Overview of the role of molecular methods in the diagnosis of malignant lymphomas. *Arch Pathol Lab Med* 1999;123:1189–1207.
52. Wan JH, Trainor KJ, Brisco MJ, et al. Monoclonality in B cell lymphoma detected in paraffin wax embedded sections using the polymerase chain reaction. *J Clin Pathol* 1990;43:888–890.
53. Saiki RK, Scharf S, Faloona F, et al. Enzymatic amplification of beta-globin genomic sequences and restriction site analysis for diagnosis of sickle cell anemia. *Science* 1985;230:1350–1354.
54. Greer CE, Peterson SL, Kiviat NB, et al. amplification from paraffin-embedded tissues. Effects of fixative and fixation time. *Am J Clin Pathol* 1991;95:117–124.
55. van Dongen JJ, Langerak AW, Bruggemann M, et al. Design and standardization of PCR primers and protocols for detection of clonal immunoglobulin and T-cell receptor gene recombinations in suspect lymphoproliferations: report of the BIOMED-2 Concerted Action BMH4-CT98-3936. *Leukemia* 2003;17:2257–2317.
56. Theriault C, Galoin S, Valmary S, et al. PCR analysis of immunoglobulin heavy chain (IgH) and TcR-gamma chain gene rearrangements in the diagnosis of lymphoproliferative disorders: results of a study of 525 cases. *Mod Pathol* 2000; 13(12):1269–1279.
57. Langerak AW, Molina TJ, Lavender FL, et al. Polymerase chain reaction-based clonality testing in tissue samples with reactive lymphoproliferations: usefulness and pitfalls. A report of the BIOMED-2 Concerted Action BMH4-CT98-3936. *Leukemia* 2007;21:222–229.
58. Evans PA, Pott C, Groenen PJ, et al. Significantly improved PCR-based clonality testing in B-cell malignancies by use of multiple immunoglobulin gene targets. Report of the BIOMED-2 Concerted Action BHM4-CT98-3936. *Leukemia* 2007;21:207–214.
59. Szczepanski T, Beishuizen A, Pongers-Willemse MJ, et al. Cross-lineage T cell receptor gene rearrangements occur in more than ninety percent of childhood precursor-B acute lymphoblastic leukemias: alternative PCR targets for detection of minimal residual disease. *Leukemia* 1999;13:196–205.
60. Bruggemann M, White H, Gaulard P, et al. Powerful strategy for polymerase chain reaction-based clonality assessment in T-cell malignancies Report of the BIOMED-2 Concerted Action BHM4 CT98-3936. *Leukemia* 2007;21:215–221.
61. Vergier B, Dubus P, Kutschmar A, et al. Combined analysis of T cell receptor gamma and immunoglobulin heavy chain gene rearrangements at the single-cell level in lymphomas with dual genotype. *J Pathol* 2002;198:171–180.
62. Hebeda KM, Van Altena MC, Rombout P, et al. PCR clonality detection in Hodgkin lymphoma. *J Hematopathol* 2009;2:34–41.
63. Halldorsdottir AM, Zehnbauer BA, Burack WR. Application of BIOMED-2 clonality assays to formalin-fixed paraffin embedded follicular lymphoma specimens: superior performance of the IGK assays compared to IGH for suboptimal specimens. *Leuk Lymphoma* 2007;48:1338–1343.
64. Berget E, Helgeland L, Molven A, et al. Detection of clonality in follicular lymphoma using formalin-fixed, paraffin-embedded tissue samples and BIOMED-2 immunoglobulin primers. *J Clin Pathol* 2011;64:37–41.
65. Payne K, Wright P, Grant JW, et al. BIOMED-2 PCR assays for IGK gene rearrangements are essential for B-cell clonality analysis in follicular lymphoma. *Br J Haematol* 2011;155:84–92.
66. Liu H, Bench AJ, Bacon CM, et al. A practical strategy for the routine use of BIOMED-2 PCR assays for detection of B- and T-cell clonality in diagnostic haematopathology. *Br J Haematol* 2007;138:31–43.
67. Chiorazzi N, Rai KR, Ferrarini M. Chronic lymphocytic leukemia. *N Engl J Med* 2005;352:804–815.
68. Oscier DG. Cytogenetic and molecular abnormalities in chronic lymphocytic leukaemia. *Blood Rev* 1994;8:88–97.
69. Matutes E, Oscier D, Garcia-Marco J, et al. Trisomy 12 defines a group of CLL with atypical morphology: correlation between cytogenetic, clinical and laboratory features in 544 patients. *Br J Haematol* 1996;92:382–388.
70. Oscier DG, Thompsett A, Zhu D, et al. Differential rates of somatic hypermutation in V(H) genes among subsets of chronic lymphocytic leukemia defined by chromosomal abnormalities. *Blood* 1997;89:4153–4160.
71. Hamblin TJ, Davis Z, Gardiner A, et al. Unmutated Ig V(H) genes are associated with a more aggressive form of chronic lymphocytic leukemia. *Blood* 1999;94:1848–1854.
72. Damle RN, Wasil T, Fais F, et al. Ig V gene mutation status and CD38 expression as novel prognostic indicators in chronic lymphocytic leukemia. *Blood* 1999;94:1840–1847.
73. Hamblin TJ, Orchard JA, Gardiner A, et al. Immunoglobulin V genes and CD38 expression in CLL. *Blood* 2000;95:2455–2457.
74. Rassenti LZ, Huynh L, Toy TL, et al. ZAP-70 compared with immunoglobulin heavy-chain gene mutation status as a predictor of disease progression in chronic lymphocytic leukemia. *N Engl J Med* 2004;351:893–901.
75. Orchard JA, Ibbotson RE, Davis Z, et al. ZAP-70 expression and prognosis in chronic lymphocytic leukaemia. *Lancet* 2004;363:105–111.
76. Pepper C, Majid A, Lin TT, et al. Defining the prognosis of early stage chronic lymphocytic leukaemia patients. *Br J Haematol* 2012;156:499–507.
77. Hamblin TJ, Orchard JA, Ibbotson RE, et al. CD38 expression and immunoglobulin variable region mutations are independent prognostic variables in chronic lymphocytic leukemia, but CD38 expression may vary during the course of the disease. *Blood* 2002;99:1023–1029.
78. Del Principe MI, Del Poeta G, Buccisano F, et al. Clinical significance of ZAP-70 protein expression in B-cell chronic lymphocytic leukemia. *Blood* 2006;108:853–861.
79. Ghia EM, Jain S, Widhopf GF II, et al. Use of IGHV3-21 in chronic lymphocytic leukemia is associated with high-risk disease and reflects antigen-driven, post-germinal center leukemogenic selection. *Blood* 2008;111:5101–5108.
80. Krober A, Seiler T, Benner A, et al. V(H) mutation status, CD38 expression level, genomic aberrations, and survival in chronic lymphocytic leukemia. *Blood* 2002;100:1410–1416.
81. Thorselius M, Krober A, Murray F, et al. Strikingly homologous immunoglobulin gene rearrangements and poor outcome in VH3-21-using chronic lymphocytic leukemia patients independent of geographic origin and mutational status. *Blood* 2006;107:2889–2894.

82. Murray F, Darzentas N, Hadzidimitriou A, et al. Stereotyped patterns of somatic hypermutation in subsets of patients with chronic lymphocytic leukemia: implications for the role of antigen selection in leukemogenesis. *Blood* 2008;111:1524–1533.

83. Agathangelidis A, Darzentas N, Hadzidimitriou A, et al. Stereotyped B-cell receptors in one-third of chronic lymphocytic leukemia: a molecular classification with implications for targeted therapies. *Blood* 2012;119:4467–4475.

84. Eichmann K, Tung AS, Nisonoff A. Linkage and rearrangement of genes encoding mouse immunoglobulin heavy chains. *Nature* 1974;250:509–511.

85. Cleary ML, Chao J, Warnke R, et al. Immunoglobulin gene rearrangement as a diagnostic criterion of B-cell lymphoma. *Proc Natl Acad Sci U S A* 1984;81:593–597.

86. Flug F, Pelicci PG, Bonetti F, et al. T-cell receptor gene rearrangements as markers of lineage and clonality in T-cell neoplasms. *Proc Natl Acad Sci U S A* 1985;82:3460–3464.

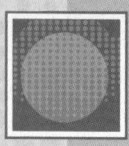

Chapter 7
Protooncogenes and Tumor Suppressor Genes in Hematopoietic Malignancies

Wayne Tam • Laura Pasqualucci

Cancer derives from alterations of the cellular genome (1). The breakthrough in the identification of specific cellular genes involved in carcinogenesis took place nearly three decades ago with the development of recombinant DNA technology (2,3). Eukaryotic genes related to the viral oncogenes carried by acute transforming retroviruses were discovered. At about the same time, biologically active cellular oncogenes were identified by the ability of tumor DNA, but not normal cellular DNA, to induce transformation in gene transfer assays (1,4–9). Viral and cellular oncogenes were later shown to be genetically altered, or "activated," versions of normal cellular genes called *protooncogenes* (1). This finding implicates cellular oncogene activation in the pathogenesis of human cancers.

Malignant cells are often characterized by the loss of specific genetic material. This finding led to the concept and demonstration of the existence of tumor suppressor genes (TSG), the inactivation of which is involved in tumorigenesis (10,11).

Studies of the normal and oncogenic functions of protooncogenes and tumor suppressor genes in hematopoietic neoplasms are critical to the understanding of their pathogenesis. In this chapter, we begin with an introduction of the concept of protooncogenes and tumor suppressor genes, with particular reference to hematopoietic neoplasms. The next section outlines the mechanisms of their activation and inactivation. This is followed by a discussion of the most common protooncogenes and tumor suppressor genes involved in the pathogenesis of hematologic neoplasms of lymphoid and myeloid origin. Emphasis is placed on how these genes become activated or inactivated and on the mechanisms by which alterations of these genes result in transformation of hematopoietic cells. Additional information regarding the specific roles of these genetic alterations can be found in the chapters focusing on specific tumor types.

 ## PROTOONCOGENES

Protooncogenes can be defined as normal cellular genes that possess the potential to contribute to tumorigenesis when their expression or structure is altered, resulting in aberrant function. They represent a heterogeneous family of genes that play a critical role in many cellular processes, including cell proliferation, growth, differentiation, and apoptosis. Some of these genes are involved specifically in subtypes of lymphoid or myeloid neoplasms; others are implicated in a variety of human cancers. The protooncogenes involved in hematopoietic neoplasms can generally be classified as encoding transcription factors and chromatin remodelers, signal transducers, cell death regulators, growth factor receptors, and a recently discovered class of noncoding RNA called microRNAs (miRNAs) (12).

Transcription Factors and Chromatin Remodelers

The class of protooncogenes that produces transcription factors is particularly important in the pathogenesis of hematopoietic neoplasms because they are frequently the targets of chromosomal translocations (13–16). Transcription factors include nuclear proteins with functional domains that mediate specific DNA binding and protein-protein interactions, as well as components of the transcription machinery that interact with other transcription factors but do not contact DNA directly (i.e., coactivators and corepressors). Transcription factors can be classified into different families based on the presence of specific functional domains. On receiving signals from the cytoplasm of the cells conveyed through signal transduction pathways, activation of transcription factors results in an increase (activation) or decrease (repression) of transcription of the target genes. In this way, transcription factors play a pivotal role in regulating cellular processes, including cell proliferation, cell differentiation, and apoptosis. Oncogenic conversion of transcription factors by chromosomal translocations occurs by two mechanisms: deregulated expression due to heterologous regulatory sequences or alteration of function due to fusion with another protein (16). Frequently, these transcription factors mediate expression of multiple target genes through interaction with chromatin remodelers that modify histones through methylation and acetylation. The pattern of histone modification in turn determines the structure of chromatin and gene transcriptional activity (17,18). These chromatin remodelers can be targets of gain-of-function and loss-of-function somatic mutations.

Signal Transducers

Signal transducers are a class of proteins that play central roles in transmitting extracellular signals to their terminal components (i.e., transcription factors within the nucleus) through essential signal transduction pathways. Via this function, they control many important cellular processes, including cell cycle entry and apoptosis (19–21). The signal transducers that are involved in hematologic malignancies include three groups: tyrosine kinases (receptor and nonreceptor type), serine/threonine protein kinases, and guanine nucleotide (GTP)-binding proteins. Tyrosine kinases and serine/threonine kinases are protein kinases that relay signals by phosphorylating intracellular signaling molecules at tyrosine or serine/threonine residues, respectively. Receptor tyrosine kinases include proteins that possess an extracellular ligand-binding domain linked to a membrane-spanning segment and an intracellular effector kinase domain. Binding of the ligand to the extracellular domain results in oligomerization of the receptor and activation of the kinase activity. An example of receptor tyrosine kinase involved in hematopoietic neoplasms is the orphan receptor tyrosine kinase ALK, a target of chromosomal translocation t(2;5) (22,23). Abelson murine leukemia viral oncogene homolog 1 (*ABL1*), activated by chromosomal translocation in chronic myelogenous leukemia (CML), encodes a nonreceptor tyrosine kinase (24,25). ABL1 is present in the nucleus and cytoplasm, where it has distinct cellular functions. Its biologic activity depends on multiple protein-protein interactions, protein-DNA interactions, and its kinase activity (26–28). An example of serine/threonine kinase is breakpoint cluster region protein (BCR), the fusion partner of ABL1 in t(9;22) translocations (29).

Among the GTP-binding proteins, one subclass that is involved in hematopoietic malignancies is *rat* sarcoma (RAS), whose role in cancer has been well established. There are three members of the RAS family: HRAS, KRAS, and NRAS. Mutations in the RAS family occur in about 30% of human cancers, although with heterogeneous frequency among different types (30). RAS is a plasma membrane protein that is active in the GTP-bound state but inactive in the GDP-bound state. Regulation of GTP binding and hydrolysis is mediated by positive and negative regulators (21,31). In general, the conversion of these signal transducers to oncogenes occurs by a variety of structural alterations, the result of which is increased deregulated catalytic activity (20,31,32). Not only can the RAS signaling pathway be abnormally activated due to mutations in the RAS genes themselves, it can also be activated due to alterations in upstream or downstream signaling components (33). For example, GTP-bound RAS can bind to and activate the serine/threonine kinase RAF, which has three closely related members (c-RAF, BRAF, and ARAF), leading to the phosphorylation and activation of downstream targets MEKs (mitogen-activated protein kinases) and ERK (extracellular-regulated kinases). Recently, it has been demonstrated that all cases of hairy cell leukemia harbor a V600E somatic mutation in BRAF that results in constitutive activation of the RAF-MEK-ERK pathway (34), underscoring the important role of aberrant RAS signaling in this leukemia subtype.

Cell Death Regulators

Regulation of programmed cell death, called *apoptosis*, is essential for maintaining homeostasis of the hematopoietic cell population and is mediated by positive and negative regulators. Ineffective apoptosis can lead to disturbances in the homeostasis of hematopoietic cells and consequently to tumorigenesis (35–37). There are two pathways leading to apoptosis, the intrinsic or stress pathway, and the extrinsic or death receptor pathway. The former pathway is activated by stress stimuli such as cell damage, activation of oncogenes, and growth factor deprivation. The death receptor pathway is activated by binding of cell death–inducing ligands, such as Fas ligand, TRAIL, and tumor necrosis factor alpha (TNF-α), to the corresponding factors (38). Both pathways eventually lead to the activation of caspase 3, a proteolytic enzyme that in turn cleaves a series of substrates and orchestrates the death of the cell.

Negative regulators of apoptosis can act as protooncogenes (39). The prototype of an antiapoptotic gene is *BCL2*, the target of the chromosomal translocation t(14;18) in follicular lymphoma. *BCL2* encodes an integral membrane protein localized to the inner mitochondrial membrane, endoplasmic reticulum, and nuclear membranes. It belongs to a family of BCL2–related apoptosis regulators, which include BAX, BAD, BCL-X, and many others (38–40). The BCL2 protein is an integral member of the stress apoptotic pathway and functions through heterodimerization with BAX and BAK and inhibition of their proapoptotic activities. BCL2 itself is inhibited by interaction with the BH3 (BCL2 homology 3)-only BCL2 family members, some of which, for example, BIM and PUMA, can also directly activate BAX/BAK. Deregulation of BCL2 (or similar antiapoptotic factors, such as BCLx) results in abnormal constitutive inhibition of BAX and BAK, which leads to cell survival. Activation of negative regulators of apoptosis is likely to represent an early step in the pathogenesis of hematologic malignancies in which the neoplastic cells are long-lived and nonproliferative, such as in chronic lymphocytic leukemia (CLL) and follicular lymphoma. Acquisition of antiapoptotic lesions can also be an important event in tumor progression of hematopoietic malignancies composed of highly proliferative cells (36).

Growth Factor Receptors

Alterations of growth-factor receptors are found in many human cancers. Typically, growth factor receptors are transmembrane proteins possessing tyrosine kinase activity and an extracellular ligand-binding domain, which, upon activation by the ligand, phosphorylates tyrosine residues in the intracellular domain and initiates signaling transduction cascades. In hematopoietic malignancies, genetic abnormalities affecting growth factor receptors are present mainly in two categories of the WHO classification: myeloid and lymphoid malignancies associated with eosinophilia, and mast cell disease. In the former category, the PDGFRA, PDGFRB, or FGFR1 genes are rearranged due to reciprocal translocations, leading to the generation of fusion proteins composed of partner sequences at the N-terminal portions and receptor sequences at the C-terminal portions. A common theme of these fusion proteins is their constitutive tyrosine kinase activity. However, the mechanisms of activation appear different between fusion proteins formed by PDGFRA rearrangements and those generated by PDGFRB or FGFR1 rearrangements. PDGFRA is typically fused to FIP1L1 because of an interstitial deletion of chromosome 4q12. The resulting gene fusion, FIP1L1-PDGFRA, removes the transmembrane domain of PDGFRA and generates a cytoplasmic protein. Interestingly, the breakpoints found in FIP1L1-PDGFRA typically result in the removal of part of the autoinhibitory juxtamembrane domain, which in turn may lead to constitutive activation of receptor tyrosine kinase activity (41). The partners of PDGFRB and FGFR1 are much more promiscuous (42). These fusion proteins retain the transmembrane domain. Unlike the FIP1L1-PDGFRA fusion protein, constitutive tyrosine kinase activity of the PDGFRB and FGFR1 fusion proteins is likely to result from ligand-independent receptor dimerization mediated by the translocation partner (43).

Mastocytosis is frequently associated with somatic point mutations, predominantly at D816, in KIT (stem cell factor receptor), another tyrosine kinase receptor. This mutation results in ligand-independent, constitutive activation of tyrosine kinase activity (44). Unlike the PDGFRA/B or FGFR-associated fusions, the KIT D816V mutant is not inhibited by imatinib.

MicroRNA Genes

miRNAs are small RNA regulators about 22 nt long that inhibit gene expression by binding to specific sites mostly at the 3′ untranslated region (UTR) of target mRNAs. Binding of miRNAs to these sites in animal cells involves a perfect complementarity between the seed region at the 5′ portion of the miRNA and the 3′ portion of the binding site, and imperfect complementarity in the rest of the sequence. The biological consequence of this specific interaction is the inhibition of the translation of the target mRNAs, often associated with mRNA degradation (45). MiRNAs are derived from precursors that are transcribed from the genome. The primary precursors (pri-miRNA) are processed in the nucleus by Drosha into about 70-bp-long pre-miRNAs that are then exported to the cytoplasm by exportin-5. Pre-miRNAs are then further processed into mature miRNAs by Dicer. More than a thousand human miRNA genes have been identified to date, and each of them is predicted to target multiple genes. MiRNAs play important roles in almost all cellular processes, including cell proliferation, differentiation, apoptosis and development (46,47).

The involvement of miRNAs in cancer development is supported by the observation that miRNAs are frequently located at regions of chromosomal fragile sites and that miRNA expression profiles are broadly altered in cancers (48,49). Because miRNAs are negative regulators of gene expression, changes in the amounts of these RNAs can be tumorigenic if they target mRNAs for either a tumor suppressor or an oncogene.

For example, miRNAs that target tumor suppressor genes function as oncogenes when overexpressed, by reducing the amount of those protective factors. In contrast, miRNAs that target protooncogenes may function as tumor suppressors. Down-regulated expression of these tumor suppressor miRNAs may lead to excessive amounts of the oncogenic protein and promote tumorigenesis (50). Activation of oncogenic miRNAs and inactivation of tumor suppressor miRNAs may result from several genetic and epigenetic alterations. Changes in the copy number of genes encoding miRNAs are often responsible, with amplifications leading to up-regulation of miRNA expression and genomic deletions causing down-regulation of miRNA expression (46). Epigenetic deregulation of the primary transcripts encoding miRNAs, such as abnormal DNA methylation or histone modification, have also been implicated in changing the levels of some miRNAs (51). Finally, miRNA expression may be altered at the processing step (52). For example, the MLL gene that is frequently translocated in acute leukemias can actually direct Drosha to precursor mRNAs of miR-191 and enhance their processing, resulting in increased mature miR-191 levels (53). Although germline sequence variants of miRNA precursors are rather common in cancer cells, mutations that affect the production of normal mature miRNAs are infrequent (54). Thus, further studies are needed to address the role of single point mutations in activating or inactivating oncogenic and tumor suppressor miRNAs.

MECHANISMS OF ONCOGENE ACTIVATION IN HEMATOPOIETIC NEOPLASMS

The type and nature of genetic alterations associated with hematologic malignancies and solid tumors are in part different. Tumors of epithelial origin are associated with general random genomic instability, characterized by marked aneuploidy, nonreciprocal translocations, large deletions, and a significant number of nonclonal alterations. In contrast, the genomes of leukemias and lymphomas are relatively stable during most stages of the disease, with few clonal alterations, including balanced reciprocal translocations, as well as deletions, amplifications, and point mutations (55). Most of these nonrandom chromosomal aberrations are predominantly associated with a specific subtype of hematologic malignancy. The relatively "simple" nature of chromosomal abnormalities in hematologic neoplasms provided ample opportunities for the identification and characterization of the involved protoonocogenes.

Activation by Chromosomal Translocation

One major mechanism by which oncogenes are activated in hematopoietic malignancies is chromosomal translocation. Chromosomal translocations are detected, at variable frequencies, in virtually all types of hematologic malignancies of lymphoid and myeloid lineages. The chromosomal translocations associated with activation of protooncogenes in leukemias and lymphomas represent recurrent, reciprocal, balanced recombination events that involve the exchange of portions of chromosome between two chromosomes without apparent loss of genetic material. These events are clonally represented in the tumor cells and are often predominantly associated with a specific type of leukemia or lymphoma, where they are usually observed in most cases, thus representing the hallmark of the disease. An example is t(14;18), which involves BCL2 and the immunoglobulin heavy chain (IgH) locus in 85% of follicular lymphoma cases. Less frequently, a chromosomal region may be translocated to multiple partner chromosomal sites in different cases of a certain tumor type. Examples of promiscuous

translocations include translocations affecting the MLL gene at chromosomal band 11q23 in acute myeloid leukemia (AML) and acute lymphoblastic leukemia (ALL), and those affecting BCL6 at 3q27 in diffuse large B-cell lymphoma (DLBCL).

Because of the translocation, the affected protooncogene can be altered in either its expression pattern or its structure and function. In the first scenario, the regulatory sequences of a heterologous gene juxtaposed by the translocation in front of the protooncogene may deregulate its pattern or degree of expression, with preservation of the structure of the coding domain (56). This mechanism of activation is consistently seen in most types of B-NHL. Alternatively, chromosomal translocations can result in the juxtaposition of two genes to form a chimeric gene that codes for a fusion protein with novel function. This mechanism is common in acute leukemias but rare in NHLs, except for the t(2;5)(p23;q35) of anaplastic large cell lymphoma (ALCL) and t(11;18)(p21;q21) of extranodal marginal zone B-cell lymphoma of mucosa-associated lymphoid tissues (MALT).

Although the precise mechanisms leading to chromosomal translocations in hematopoietic neoplasms are not completely understood, studies thus far have demonstrated that RAG (recombination activating gene) and AID (activation-induced cytidine deaminase) are the two major enzymes required for these lesions in lymphoid cancers. RAG mediates the site-specific recombination between the variable (V), diversity (D) and joining (J) genes to generate diversity of the immunoglobulin and T-cell receptor. RAG initiates this process by recognizing and binding to specific recombination signal sequences (RSS) composed of heptamers and nonamers separated by 12 or 23 bp spacer regions flanking the V, D, and J genes, and induces nicks followed by hairpin formation (57). The hairpins are resolved and converted to double-strand breaks (DSBs), which are joined using the nonhomologous end joining (NHEJ) machinery, one of the DSB repair pathways in higher eukaryotes. The model for RAG-mediated chromosomal translocation is supported by several observations. First, a significant fraction of translocations involve chromosomal breakpoints within the Ig or TCR loci. Second, in B-cell NHL, breakpoints within the Ig loci are often located precisely within sequences that normally mediate Ig gene rearrangement in B cells. Moreover, N-nucleotides, which are template-independent nucleotide additions generated at the site of VDJ recombination by terminal deoxynucleotidyl transferase (TdT), can be detected at certain breakpoint junctions, suggesting the action of the recombinase. Third, similarity has been shown between the sequences surrounding the breakpoints and recombination targeting motifs, such as the heptamers or nonamers and the bp45 nuclease-binding sequence. It is believed that RAG can misrecognize these cryptic RSS elements in other non-antigen receptor genes and induce nicks that are converted to DSB and then joined erroneously to the antigen receptor genes by the components of the NHEJ pathway. RAG can also recognize single-stranded regions of non-B DNA structures, especially in the context of cytosines, and induce DSBs. This latter mechanism seems to underlie the genesis of the t(14;18) translocation involving the major breakpoint region (MBR) in the 3′ UTR of the BCL2 gene, which was shown to adopt a non-B DNA structure (56,58).

AID is the major enzyme required for both somatic hypermutation and class switch recombination, two DNA remodeling reactions that occur in germinal center (GC) B cells (59). Errors in the repair of DNA breaks induced by AID are believed to be largely responsible for chromosomal translocations occurring in GC-derived lymphoid malignancies, such as Burkitt lymphoma (BL) and DLBCL (60). AID can deaminate cytosines on DNA to form uracil, which results in a G-U mismatch and initiates the base excision repair mechanism. The U base is removed by uracil N-glycosylase, leaving an abasic site which, on replication, can be repaired or result in mutations. Alternatively, the abasic site may be cleaved and converted to a single-strand break by the Mre11/Rad50/Nbs1 (MRN) complex. These single-strand breaks are processed by a low-fidelity polymerase that can lead to mutations. If unrepaired, single-strand breaks in close proximity can act as DSBs, which can serve as physiological intermediates of class switching (when taking place in the heavy chain isotype genes) or as substrates for illegitimate joining and chromosomal translocations. Although the immunoglobulin gene is the major site of action of AID, non-Ig genes have also been shown to be targets of AID-mediated somatic hypermutation in the GC (61–65). The demonstration of AID activity beyond the Ig gene provides a mechanistic explanation for the observation of AID-mediated chromosomal translocations between Ig genes and non-Ig genes. Consistent with this model, a large fraction of DLBCL cases harbor multiple aberrant somatic mutations in the 5′ genomic regions of transcribed genes that also coincide with chromosomal translocations breakpoints (66). Furthermore, it was recently discovered that AID can induce reproducible DNA breaks at a large number of non-Ig loci in activated B cells (ABCs), many of which occur near the regions of translocations (67).

The t(8;14) translocation characteristically seen in BL is a prototypical example of AID-mediated translocation. This hypothesis was first supported by the observation that the breakpoints at the IgH loci in endemic BL are not directly adjacent to the RSS that mediates VDJ recombination, but are located in the J intron or within rearranged VJ genes (i.e., the target region for hypermutation) (60,68). In addition, breakpoints in sporadic BL tend to occur in the Ig switch region. Later it was demonstrated that breaks at the c-myc gene in t(8;14) translocations are also induced by AID (69). Additionally, mice deficient in miR-155, a negative regulator of AID expression, or with a mutated miR-155-binding site in AID, have increased AID activity and increased frequency of t(8;14) (70,71). Although not demonstrated formally in a mouse model, AID is likely to play a role also in the generation of chromosomal translocations at the BCL6 locus, which is targeted by somatic hypermutation in both normal GC cells and DLBCL (see BCL6 section). Importantly, removal of AID was sufficient to prevent the development of mature (GC-experienced) B-cell lymphomas in lymphoma-prone mouse models (72), documenting a direct link between AID activity and lymphomagenesis.

Since RAG and AID have restricted expressions in immature B/T cells and GC-B cells, respectively, these two enzymes may not play a major role in chromosomal translocations associated with other hematopoietic malignancies beyond lymphoid cancers. In addition to receptor loci remodeling processes, other mechanisms can be involved in facilitating chromosomal translocations. DNA DSBs can be generated by exogenous and endogenous sources (e.g., chemicals, oxygen free radicals), which may lead to chromosomal rearrangements. A defect in DNA damage repair mechanisms may be responsible for at least some translocations. For example, based on sequence analysis of reciprocal chromosomal breakpoints, the chromosomal translocation t(4;11), seen in acute leukemias of the B lineage, appears to be initiated by several DNA DSBs on participating chromosomes and subsequent DNA repair by an "error-prone" DNA repair mechanism. Similarly, analysis of the breakpoint junction sequence at TEL (also called ETV6) in t(12;21)(p13;q22) supports the occurrence of staggered DNA DSBs followed by DNA repair (73). Abnormal down-regulation of NHEJ efficiency due to BCL2 overexpression and its interaction with KU proteins may result in chromosomal translocation (74,75). In addition, some chromosomal translocations are mediated by Alu repeats (76). For example, Alu-mediated intrachromosomal recombination was seen in the MLL gene associated with AML (77). The BCR-ABL translocation is also possibly Alu-mediated (78). Finally, palindromic sequences

may also play a role in promoting chromosomal translocations. Examples of translocations that are associated with palindromic sequences are t(11;22)(q23;q11), t(1;22)(p21;q11), t(4;22)(q35;q11), t(17;22)(q11;q11), and t(X;22). These palindromic sequences tend to adopt DNA structures that may be cleaved by DNA nucleases resulting in breakage.

Activation by Aberrant Somatic Hypermutation

A unique mechanism of genetic lesion in mature B-cell malignancies, particularly in DLBCL, is represented by aberrant somatic hypermutation (ASHM) (79). This mechanism appears to be due to an abnormal functioning of the physiologic SHM process that normally operates in GC B cells, as suggested by several observations: first, the mutations are typically distributed within approximately 2 kb from the transcription initiation site, which represents the hypermutable domain in the Ig and BCL6 genes. Second, the mutations target expressed genes, consistent with the requirement of active transcription for SHM. Third, the mutation features are strongly reminiscent of those described for the SHM process, including the significantly high frequency, the predominance of single point mutations with occasional small deletions and duplications, a bias for transitions over transversions, and the preferential targeting of hotspot motifs (59,80).

ASHM targets numerous genes in DLBCL, including well-known protooncogenes such as MYC and PIM1 (66). Depending on the genomic configuration of the target gene, the mutations may affect nontranslated as well as coding regions, potentially altering the response to transcriptional regulators or key protein structural and functional properties (66). This is the case of MYC, where a significant number of events lead to amino acid changes with proven functional consequences in activating its oncogenic potential. Overall, ASHM affects over 50% of DLBCL cases, as well as a few other lymphoma types including, among others, AIDS-associated B-NHL, primary central nervous system lymphomas, posttransplant lymphoproliferative disorders, and Hodgkin lymphoma (81–84). However, a comprehensive characterization of the potentially extensive genetic damage caused by ASHM is still missing.

Activation by Point Mutation

A protooncogene can be converted to an oncogene by a DNA base pair mutation in the coding sequence, causing a change in the amino acid sequence that alters the structure of the protein. Oncogene activation by point mutation is best demonstrated by the RAS family. RAS mutations are found in a variety of human neoplasms at three specific codons: 12, 13, and 61. The genetic mutations result in amino acid substitutions leading to constitutive activation of the signal-transducing function of RAS. NRAS mutations are the most frequent and occur in approximately 10% to 30% of some hematologic malignancies, including AML, ALL, multiple myeloma (MM), and myelodysplastic syndromes, but they are virtually absent in mature B-NHL. RAS mutations result in constitutive activation of RAS, which remains in the GTP-bound state regardless of regulatory signals. This event results in deregulated activity of multiple signal transduction pathways, including the mitogen-activated protein kinase pathway, which leads to abnormal activation of transcription factors and to gene deregulation.

Activation by Gene Amplification

Gene amplification is defined as an excess copy number of a given oncogene, and represents one of the molecular mechanisms by which gene expression can be deregulated. A number of amplifications involving protooncogenes have been characterized in various human cancers. These alterations can be detected at different levels of resolution by conventional cytogenetics, comparative genomic hybridization (CGH), fluorescence *in situ* hybridization (FISH), Southern blot analysis, and most recently developed genome-wide technologies such as single nucleotide polymorphism (SNP) array hybridization. The best-characterized examples of oncogene amplification in human cancers are the amplification of the *MYCN* gene in neuroblastoma, *NEU* gene amplification in breast and ovarian carcinoma, and *ERBB1* gene amplification in glioblastoma (85).

By CGH, the frequency of involvement of gene amplification ranges from 10% to 20% of lymphoma cases overall, with some preference for individual phenotypic subgroups. In primary mediastinal B-cell lymphoma, gains of band 9p24, including the genes encoding for the tyrosine kinase JAK2 and the regulators of immune responses PDL1 and PDL2, are observed in approximately 70% of cases (86,87). *REL* amplification is associated with extranodal presentation. The advent of more sensitive techniques such as array-based CGH and high-density SNP array analysis have demonstrated that oncogene amplification is a much more wide-spread phenomenon than previously thought in lymphomas (88). Nowadays, high-throughput global sequencing may enable more accurate determination of gene copy number and allows precise identification of genes involved in amplification.

COMMONLY INVOLVED ONCOGENES

The list of oncogenes known to be involved in hematologic malignancies is ever expanding. Below, we discuss selections of oncogenes that are more commonly involved in these tumors, highlighting their mechanisms of action and mode of activation. For the sake of discussion, these oncogenes are divided into those that are generated by gene fusions, those that are deregulated by immunoglobulin-associated translocations, and those that are activated primarily by somatic mutations.

Fusion Oncogenes

BCR-ABL

A pathognomonic feature of CML is the juxtaposition of the *BCR* gene on chromosome 22 and the *ABL* gene on chromosome 9 to form the chimeric *BCR-ABL* gene because of the chromosomal translocation t(9;22)(q34;q11). In more than 95% of cases, the translocation can be detected as the Philadelphia (Ph1) chromosome by standard cytogenetic analysis. In the remaining cases, the translocation is masked karyotypically and can only be detected by other more sensitive molecular techniques.

ABL is a tyrosine kinase that is predominantly in the nucleus but is also present in the cytoplasm. It contains tandem SRC homology 3 (SH3), SH2 and the tyrosine kinase (Y-kinase domain) at its N-terminal half portion, as well as SH3-, DNA- and actin-binding domains at the C-terminal portion. The SH3, SH2, and Y-kinase domains can form an auto-inhibitory structure, in which the SH3 and SH2 domains can maintain the tyrosine kinase activity in an off state. ABL transduces signals from cell-surface growth factor and adhesion receptors to regulate cytoskeletal structure (89,90). BCR is a ubiquitously expressed cytoplasmic protein that possesses serine/threonine kinase activity at the N-terminal portion. This region is also capable of interacting with the SH2 domain. In front of this serine/threonine kinase domain is a coiled-coil oligomerization domain at the N-terminus. Following the S/T kinase domain, BCR contains a Dbl/CDC24 guanine-nucleotide exchange factor homology domain, a pleckstrin homology activating domain, and an RAC guanosine-triphosphatase activating protein domain within the C-terminal portion. Depending on the precise breakpoint within the *BCR* gene, fusion proteins of two different molecular masses, 210 kDa (BCR-ABL p210) or 190 kDa (BCR-ABL p190), can be produced (Fig. 7.1). Both p190 and p210 contain the same *ABL*-derived coding sequence, but they differ in the number of *BCR*-derived amino acids. In almost all cases of CML, the breakpoint in the *BCR* gene is grouped in the major breakpoint cluster region (M-BCR). This results in the production of the larger chimeric protein p210. In rare cases of CML, the breakpoint occurs 40 kb upstream of the M-BCR in the *BCR* gene (i.e., minor breakpoint cluster region [m-bcr]). This leads to the production of the smaller chimeric protein p190, which is mainly associated with precursor B-ALL. In both p210 and p190, the coiled-coil oligomerization domain and the serine/threonine kinase domain and SH2 domain of BCR are fused to almost the entire coding domain of ABL (Fig. 7.1).

BCR-ABL is required for the initiation, maintenance and disease progression of CML. BCR-ABL transforms the multipotent self-renewing hematopoietic stem cell, which is capable of proliferating and differentiating into most, if not all, hematopoietic lineages. In fact, BCR-ABL may enhance differentiation of long-term repopulating hematopoietic stem cells and decrease their self-renewal capacity. There seems to be a bias towards differentiation of the granulocytic series and suppression of lymphopoiesis, as production of B and T cells from the neoplastic clone occurs at very low levels. The oncogenic potential of BCR-ABL has been demonstrated using *in vitro* transformation assays and *in vivo* mouse models. Several earlier *in vivo* mouse models using a murine stem cell retroviral vector to transduce the *BCR-ABL* oncogene in hematopoietic stem/progenitor cells resulted with high efficiency in a myeloproliferative disease (MPD) that resembled CML. A transgenic mouse model has been generated that directed conditional, tetracycline-regulated expression of BCR-ABL specifically to hematopoietic stem cells through the use of a mouse stem cell leukemia (SCL) enhancer. This model comes closest to faithfully recapitulating CML, and provides the best available *in vivo* system to study leukemogenic mechanisms of BCR-ABL and to investigate drugs for CML treatment. Mice carrying the *BCR-ABL* transgene expressing p190 develop acute leukemia of the B-cell lineage, analogous to precursor B-ALL in humans. The difference in phenotypes of these transgenic mice demonstrates the difference in biologic activities of the p210 and p190 proteins.

The ABL kinase domain and the BCR sequences have been shown to be essential for the ability of BCR-ABL to cause MPD *in vivo*. The fusion of BCR sequences to ABL increases the latter's tyrosine kinase activity, probably through activation by the BCR N-terminal coiled-coil oligomerization domain and by binding of the BCR N-terminal to the ABL SH-2 domain, which inhibits the negative regulatory activity on tyrosine kinase activity. However, activation of the kinase activity of ABL alone is necessary but not sufficient to induce CML-like disease, and other BCR-ABL domains are also critical in the pathogenesis of CML. The BCR fusion brings new regulatory/catalytic domains to ABL, such as the growth factor receptor–bound protein 2 (GRB2) SH2-binding site. Phosphorylation of tyrosine Y177 at the BCR serine/threonine kinase domain in BCR-ABL generates this high-affinity site and leads to binding of GRB2 to BCR-ABL through its SH2 domain, as well as its binding to SOS and GAB2 through its SH3 site. SOS in turn activates RAS; while phosphorylation of GAB2 by BCR-ABL leads to recruitment of PI3K and SHP2. Activation of these signal transduction pathways is at least partly responsible for the increased cell proliferation and survival seen in CML. Thus, through protein-protein interactions mediated by multiple functional domains, BCR-ABL can bind to and phosphorylate different effectors, activating signal transduction pathways important for regulating many cellular functions including increased proliferation and survival, and altered cell adhesion and migration. Further research is necessary to fully decipher the role played by these pathways and the cellular functions affected by BCR-ABL.

Although it appears that BCL-ABL is sufficient to induce a CML-like myeloproliferative disorder in mice, it remains

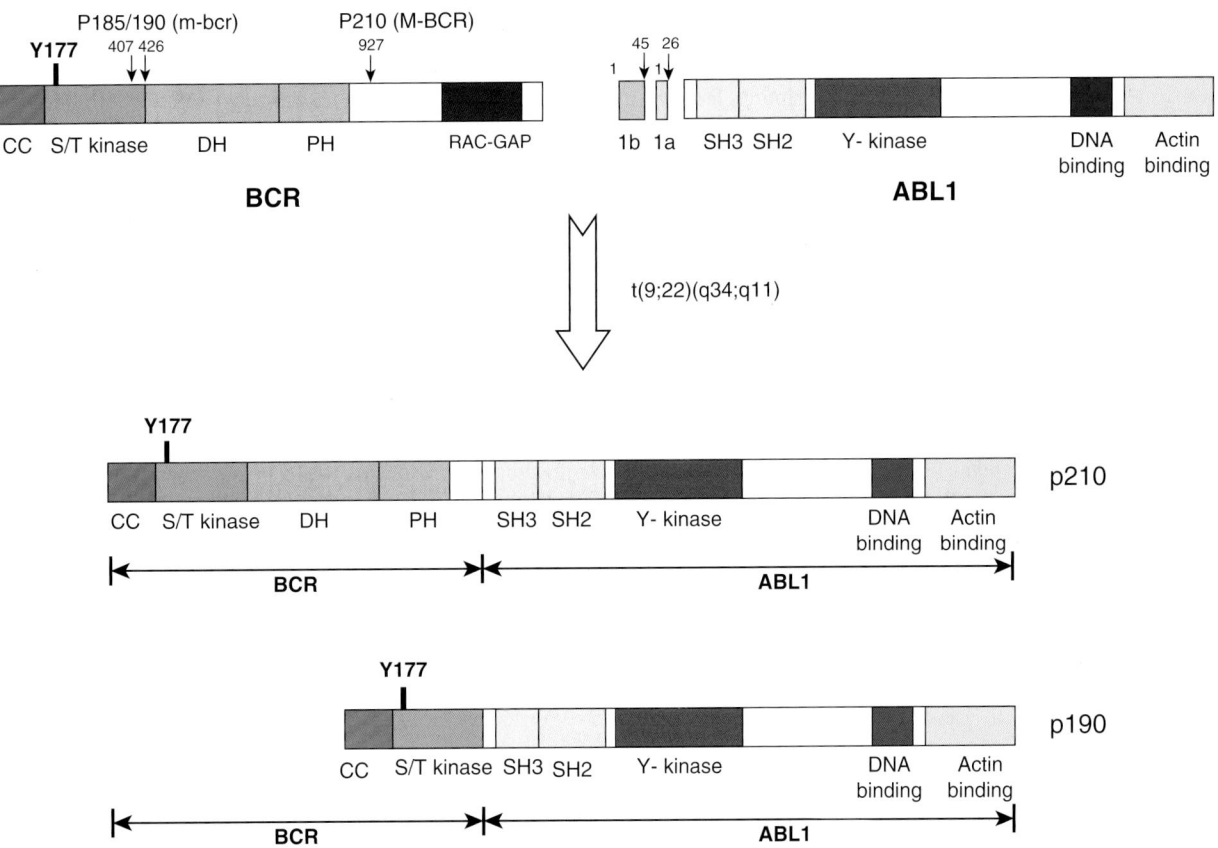

FIGURE 7.1. Schematic representation of the protein fusion between BCR and ABL1 in t(9;22)(q34;q11). The modular organizations of BCR and ABL1 are shown in the **top panel**. CC, coiled-coil oligomerization domain; S/T kinase, serine/threonine kinase domain; DH, Dbl/CDC24 guanine-nucleotide exchange factor homology domain; PH, Pleckstrin homology domain; RAC-GAP, RAC guanosine triphosphatase-activating protein domain; SH3 and SH2, SRC homology 3 and 2, respectively; Y-kinase, tyrosine kinase domain. The SH3, SH2, and Y-kinase domains of ABL1 can form an auto-inhibitory structure, in which the SH3 and SH2 domains act as a clamp to keep the kinase in an "off" state. The C-terminal of ABL1 harbors a DNA-binding and an actin-binding domain. Phosphorylation of the tyrosine at position 177 (Y177) generates a high-affinity SH2-binding site for GRB2 as well as ABL1. ABL1 has two isoforms, types 1a and 1b, generated by alternative splicing of exon 1. *Vertical arrows* indicate the breakpoints where the proteins are fused. The number corresponds to the amino acid number where the breakpoints occur. The point of fusion at the carboxyl terminus of BCR depends on whether the translocation breakpoints are located at the M-BCR or m-bcr. The point of fusion at the amino terminus of ABL1 is located at amino acid 26 of type 1a ABL1, which corresponds to amino acid 45 of type 1b ABL1. BCR-ABL1 p210 produced by t(9;22) involving the M-BCR consists of 927 BCR-derived amino acids fused to ABL1. BCR-ABL1 p185/190 produced by t(9;22) involving the m-bcr consists of 407 or 426 amino acids (depending on the exact location of the breakpoint at m-bcr) fused to ABL1. In both p210 and p185/190, the ABL1-derived sequence is the same and represents the near full-length product (amino acids encoded by *ABL1* exon 1 are not present). Constitutive activation of the ABL1 kinase activity in BCR-ABL1 results from oligomerization mediated by the CC domain, which leads to trans-autophosphorylation of the Y-kinase domain, and the interaction between the SH2-binding domain of BCR (Y177) and the SH2 domain of ABL1.

unclear whether this applies to humans. BCR-ABL fusion can be detected in healthy individuals, but only a subset of them eventually develop CML, suggesting that additional mutations are required for the development of full-blown CML in humans. In addition, CML can progress from an indolent phase to a blast crisis characterized by the accumulation of myeloid or lymphoid blast cells due to a block in cell differentiation. This disease progression is associated with additional genetic alterations beyond BCR-ABL expression. Accumulating evidence shows that mutations in *TP53* are associated with 15% to 20% of blast crises but rarely with the chronic phase. *TP53* mutations in these cases are closely associated with the loss of chromosome 17p, the site of p53, through the formation of isochromosome i(17)q and, less frequently, through unbalanced translocations. The importance of p53 inactivation in the blast crisis is directly demonstrated by a study that shows that *BCR-ABL* (p210) transgenic, *TP53*⁻ heterozygous (p53⁺/⁻) mice develop a short latency blastic crisis preceded by a chronic myeloproliferative phase. The residual *TP53* allele is frequently inactivated in the tumor tissues. Other genetic alterations involved in blast crisis include inactivation of p16. Homozygous deletions of p16 occur in up to 40% to 50% of blast crises of the lymphoid type but are

not present in blast crises of the myeloid type. Another genetic lesion associated with blast crisis is the fusion between the *AML* and *EVI1* genes due to chromosomal translocation t(3;21) (q26;q22), which can be detected in up to 1% of AML cases. This translocation results in the formation of a chimeric oncogenic transcription factor consisting of the *runt* homology domain of AML1 and the zinc finger DNA-binding and acidic trans-activation domains of EVI-1. Other translocations associated with BCR-ABL in CML include AML-ETO in t(8;21)(q22;q22), NUP98-HOXA9 in t(7;11)(p15;p15), and CBFβ-SMMHC in inv 16 (p13;q22) (91). BCR-ABL can cooperate with these oncogenic transcription factors in blocking myeloid differentiation, resulting in transformation of CML from chronic phase to blast phase. This is supported by mouse bone marrow transplant models in which retrovial transduction of both BCR-ABL and AML-ETO or NUP98-HOXA9 in bone marrow cells led to rapid induction of AML that resembled blast crisis of CML (92,93).

PML-RARA

Acute promyelocytic leukemia (APL) is characterized by a malignant proliferation of myeloid cells blocked at the promyelocytic stage of differentiation. It is invariably associated with reciprocal chromosomal translocations involving the gene *(RARA)* for the retinoic acid receptor-α (RARα) on chromosome 17. RARα belongs to the nuclear ligand-activated transcription factor family (94). It contains several functional domains, including a DNA-binding domain, a ligand-binding domain, and a heterodimerization domain with RXRα. In >99% of APL cases, t(15;17)(q22;q21) results in translocation of *RARA* to a gene called promyelocytic leukemia *(PML)* on chromosome 15 (95–97), which encodes a component of a marcomolecular organelle called PML oncogenic domains (or PML nuclear bodies) (98,99). In <1% of cases, *RARA* translocates to *PLZF* on chromosome 11, which codes for a transcription factor. Translocations of *RARA* to *NUMA1* (coding for an essential component for the function of mitotic spindles), *NPM* (coding for a RNA-binding nucleolar phosphoprotein), STAT5b, PRKAR1A, and BCOR are rare (100–104). The result of the translocations is the production of fusion between the same sequence (domains B to F) of RARα, and variable portions of proteins encoded by partner genes (X), creating RARα-X and X-RARα proteins. All these protein products of the partner genes contain dimerization domains at their N-terminal portions. These heterologous dimerization domains promote the formation of chimeric receptor homodimers and, together with the DNA-binding domain of RARα, are critical for the oncogenic activities of the fusion proteins (105).

PML-RARα and the other variants of RARα fusion proteins play crucial roles in the pathogenesis of APL. Transgenic mice carrying *PML-RARA, PLZF-RARA,* or *NPM-RARA* fusion genes develop leukemias ranging from typical APL to CML-like leukemia preceded by a preleukemic phase, indicating that the *X-RARA* fusion genes are necessary but not sufficient for leukemogenicity. The oncogenicity of the fusion protein appears to rely on the interference of retinoic acid (RA)–mediated transactivation in the RARα/RXRα pathway and on disruption of normal function of the RARα partner proteins. Since most of the studies have focused on PML-RARα, it will be the main subject of subsequent discussion.

The PML-RARα proteins, irrespective of the breakpoints, are identical in their RARα-derived sequence and retain the domains for DNA and ligand (RA) binding, as well as the region for heterodimerization with retinoic X-receptor (RXRα). They also contain the homodimerization domain of PML1 (Fig. 7.2). In the absence of RA, RARα is a transcription repressor (106). It binds to DNA as a heterodimer with RXRα, recruits co-repressors and silences target gene expression. On binding to RA, RXR-RARα undergoes conformational change and recruits transcription activation complex, leading to increased gene expression. PML-RARα dimerizes and binds DNA in conjunction with RXRα. However, PML-RARα loses the potential to respond to physiologic amounts of RA and therefore function as

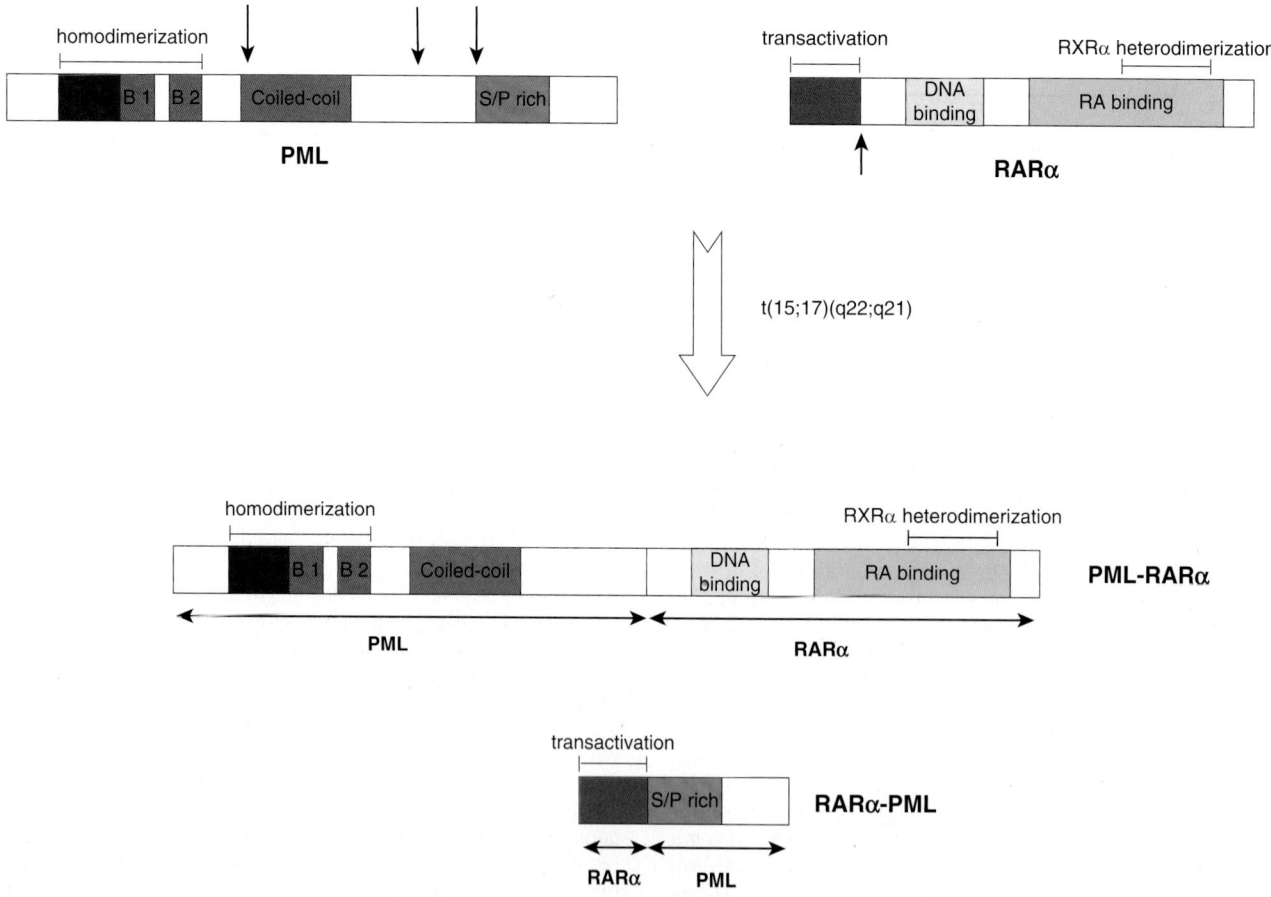

FIGURE 7.2. Schematic representation of the wild-type *RARA, PML,* and their fusion proteins resulting from t(15;17). The modular configurations of RARα and PML with their distinct functional domains are indicated in the **top panel.** RARα contains a transactivation domain and a DNA-binding domain at its N-terminal portion and an RA-binding domain and RXRα dimerization domain at its C-terminal portion. PML contains at its N-terminal part a RING finger-B Box domain, which represents the homodimerization interface for PML. The breakpoints where the proteins are fused are indicated by *vertical arrows.* PML-RARα contains the RING and B-box (with or without the coiled-coil region) of PML fused to almost the entire RARα. Because of the functional domains contributed by the partner proteins, PML-RARα can interfere with the RA-mediated transactivation pathway and the normal function of the wild-type PML. The reciprocal fusion protein RARα-PML consists of the transactivation domain of RARα fused to the C-terminal portion of PML. No definite biochemical functions have been attributed to RARα-PML.

constitutive transcriptional repressors. HDAC appears to play a major role in maintaining the repressed chromatin architecture in PML-RARα binding sites, as an increase in histone H3 acetylation is observed in the majority of PML-RARα binding sites upon all-trans retinoic acid (ATRA) treatment (107). This observation supports the inclusion of HDAC inhibitor as an ancillary treatment regimen for APL.

Apart from altering transcriptional regulation of classical RAR/RXR target genes, PML-RARa affects RAR signaling in APL cells via additional mechanisms. Recently, global analysis of binding sites of PML-RARα using the Chip-seq or chip-on-chip techniques demonstrated that PML-RARα binds to promoter regions of RAR genes themselves, suggesting direct regulation of these genes by PML-RARα. In addition, PML-RARα exhibited a gain of DNA-binding capacity toward genes with more degenerate RAR response element motifs, implying an abnormally extended transcriptional repression repertoire compared to RARα. PML-RARa may also contribute to its oncogenic activity through regulation of the expressions and functions of other transcriptional factors, such as PU.1, GATA-2, and AP-1, through transcription modulation and direct interaction. Furthermore, genes capable of modifying chromatin structure, for example, DNA methyltransferase (DNMT3), histone methyltransferases (JMJD3, JMJD1A, SETB1), and histone deacetylases (HDAC 4 and 9), are putative targets of PML-RARa, suggesting a potential for PML-RARα to alter the epigenome through regulating expressions of these chromatin modifiers (108).

The sensitivity of these corepressor interactions to RA also determines the responsiveness of APL to pharmacologic doses of RA. High-dose RA can induce the differentiation of malignant cells into mature granulocytes resulting in complete, albeit transient, remission in all cases of APL with PML-RARa as well as in ATRA-sensitive genetic variants of APL (NUMA-RARA, NPM1-RARA, FIPILI-RARA). In the cases with PML-RARA, ATRA (and arsenic oxide) mediates degradation of PML-RARA, which results in replacement by RARA/RXR, dissociation of HDAC and recruitment of histone acetyltransferase, leading to transcriptional activation. However, APL associated with translocation between *RARA* and *PLZF* has a worse prognosis and a poor response to RA. Consistent with this, PML-RARα and NPM-RARα transgenic mice develop RA–sensitive leukemia, whereas PLZF-RARα transgenic mice develop RA–resistant leukemia (109–111). Corepressors can be dissociated from the complexes formed by PML-RARα or NPM-RARα by high-dose RA, but PLZF forms corepressor complexes that are insensitive to high-dose RA (110,111). These findings indicate a crucial role for interactions of these fusion proteins with corepressors and transcriptional silencing in APL pathogenesis and resistance to RA in APL.

The X-RARα fusion proteins can also interfere with the normal functions of the partner proteins through heterodimerization with the native partner proteins and inhibit their normal function in a dominant-negative fashion. Among the RARα partner proteins, PML has been the most studied. It contains domains for protein-protein interaction, including the RING finger domain, and it modulates key tumor suppressor pathways including growth suppression, apoptosis and cellular senescence. It is associated with the nuclear matrix and is responsible for the formation of PML nuclear bodies, the presence of which is essential for the growth- and tumor suppressor potential of PML (112,113). PML is a mediator of apoptosis by multiple signals, including FAS, TNF, and interferons. In APL with t(15;17) translocation, expression of PML-RARα leads to disruption of the nuclear bodies (113,114) and resistance of apoptosis in hematopoietic progenitor cells (115) presumably by a dominant-negative manner. This implicates a critical role for disruption of the growth- or tumor-suppressing and apoptosis-inducing function of PML in the pathogenesis of APL.

AML-ETO

The t(8;21)(q22;q22.3) translocation is present in approximately 10% to 15% of AMLs. It is predominantly, but not exclusively, associated with the AML subtype M2 (about 25% of M2 AML) and involves rearrangement of the *AML1* gene on chromosome 21 and the *ETO* gene on chromosome 8 (116,117). AML1 is a widely expressed transcription factor with approximately 70% homology to the *Drosophila* pair-rule gene, called *runt*, at its 5′ portion (118,119). It forms the α subunit of the heterodimeric core-binding factor (CBF). The runt homology protein mediates specific DNA-binding and protein-protein interactions of AML1. The C-terminal end of AML contains a transactivation domain and nuclear-matrix–targeting signal that direct the protein to the appropriate nuclear matrix–associated foci. Based on the analysis of knockout mice, AML is an important regulator for hematopoiesis and regulates many hematopoietic genes (120,121). ETO, originally thought of as a DNA-binding transcription factor (122) was found to be a corepressor for the PLZF protein (123). Its C-terminal end was shown to interact with other corepressors, such as SMRT and N-CoR. Like AML1, it is also associated with the nuclear matrix (124). ETO itself has transforming properties *in vitro* (125).

The t(8;21) translocation fuses the N terminus of AML containing the DNA-binding runt domain to near full-length ETO (116,124,126,127). The C-terminal portion of AML1, which contains the transactivation domain and the nuclear matrix–targeting signal, is not retained in the fusion protein. However, AML1-ETO can bind to DNA and dimerize with the CBPβ subunit. Consequently, this fusion with ETO alters the intranuclear targeting and transcriptional activity of AML1. First, AML1-ETO is misrouted by the ETO component to alternate nuclear matrix–associated foci, leading AML1 away from its native foci that support gene expression (128). Second, the substitution of the C-terminal portion of AML1 by the C-terminal part of ETO generates an aberrant and potent transcriptional repressor because of the ability of ETO to recruit the transcriptional corepressors SMRT and N-CoR (123) and ability to form oligomeric complexes with histone deacetylases (HDAC) and DNA methyltransferases (129,130). While binding of AML1 to its binding site is permissive for transcription, AML1-ETO biding results in histone hypoacetylation and hypermethylation of CpGs in DNA, leading to repressed transcription. AML-ETO therefore can antagonize the normal AML1 activity in a dominant-negative fashion. Both of these mechanisms can result in deregulation of AML effector genes, which is likely to be important for the pathogenesis of AML (120) Transgenic mice with a knockin *AML1-ETO* allele have impaired hematopoiesis similar to AML1-deficient mice, demonstrating the dominant-negative action of AML-ETO (120,131,132). Not only does AML1-ETO inhibit AML1-dependent transcriptional activation, it may also block the activities of other transcriptional factors via protein-protein interactions mediated by the runt domain of AML1. For example, AML1-ETO can bind to and inhibit the transcriptional activation activity of C/EBPα, which also results in a decrease in C/EBPα expression (133). AML1-ETO can inactivate PU.1 (134); it can also interfere with tumor growth factor (TGF)-β signaling by inhibiting SMAD proteins (135).

AML1-ETO most likely contributes to AML by enhancing self renewal and maintenance of hematopoietic stem cells, and interfering with differentiation (136). Elucidation of the exact mechanisms has been facilitated by identification of the target genes and pathways affected by AML1-ETO. Among the genes targeted by AML1-ETO via transcriptional repression or protein-protein interaction, many are factors with potentially important roles in hematopoietic stem cell renewal and differentiation. For example, inactivation of C/EBPα and PU.1 by AML1-ETO can impair granulocytic differentiation (133,134). AML-ETO also represses expression of miR-223, a critical regulator of myelopoiesis, and results in differentiation blockade (137). It also inhibits p14 (ARF) and therefore disrupts p53 signaling, which may have an anti-apoptotic role. Blockade of the TGFβ anti-growth signals through SMAD inhibition may contribute to cell proliferation.

MLL

Chromosomal translocations affecting 11q23 are seen in approximately 5% to 10% of AMLs, about 5% of ALLs and virtually all cases of biphenotypic acute leukemia (138,139). Among the AML cases with 11q23 rearrangements, 50% are M5a, 20% are M4, 10% are M1 or M5b, and 5% are M2 (140,141). These chromosomal translocations are promiscuous, resulting in fusion of the *MLL* gene (also called *ALL1* or *HRX*) on chromosome 11q23 to many alternative (>50) partner genes in different cases (141–144). The breakpoints at 11q23 span a genomic region of 8 kb between exons 5 and 11 of MLL, whereas the breakpoints at the partner genes are more variable (141,143). Based on molecular and cytogenetic data, the crucial chimeric gene is the 5'*MLL*-3'-partner fusion, which is consistently obtained in tumor cells (145).

The *MLL* gene encodes a large, 3969 amino-acid nuclear transcription factor that shares homology with the Drosophila trithorax protein (146). It contains multiple domains, including (i) an N-terminal AT-hook DNA-binding motif of high mobility group proteins; (ii) a transcriptional repression domain with two subdomains, consisting of a DNA methyltransferase homology domain with CxxC zinc finger motif and another domain that recruits histone deacetylase HDAC1 and HDAC2; (iii) a centrally located plant homology domain (PHD) with zinc finger–like motifs that mediate binding of cyclophilin CYP33; (iv) a transactivation domain that recruits the transactivation co-activator CREB-binding protein; and (v) a C-terminal SET domain with homology to trithorax that possesses histone H3K4 methyltransferase activity (147–149). The 11q23 translocations result in the formation of chimeric proteins that retain the N-terminal portion of MLL, including the AT-hook domain, the DNA methyltransferase domain, and the zinc finger–like domain fused to the partner protein (44). The AT-hook domain and the DNA methyltransferase domains are essential for MLL fusion transformation ability (150). Except for MLL-PTD, all MLL fusion proteins lose the H3K4 methyltransferase domain.

More than 50 chimeric genes formed by translocations involving *MLL* have been identified (142,144). The partner genes that fuse to *MLL* are heterogeneous; some of them can be generally classified into the following groups:

1. Nuclear proteins: These are DNA-binding proteins with functions in transcription control and elongation (151). Examples are AF4, AF9, ENL, AF10, and ELL. Fusions with these genes account for >80% of MLL-rearranged leukemias. The three major fusion partner genes in pediatric ALL are AF4 (34%), ENL (24%), and AF9 (18%); in adult ALL, AF4 is found in 90% of cases. The two major fusion partner genes in adult AML are AF9 (32%) and ENL (14%).
2. Cytoplasmic proteins, with coiled-coil oligomerization domains: Examples are EPS15, GAS7, EEN, AF6, and AFX. The oligomerization domains are important for their transformation potential (152,153) MLL fusions with these genes account for >10% of MLL-rearranged leukemias.
3. Cytoplasmic proteins, septin family: Mammalian septins interact with cytoskeletal filaments and are involved in diverse processes such as cell-cycle control, vesicle trafficking and plasma membrane compartmentalization (154). Examples include SEPT2, SEPT5, SEPT6, SEPT9, and SEPT11.
4. Histone acetyltransferases: CBP (CREB-binding protein) (155) and P300 (156). These are nuclear proteins that function in transcription activation.

The leukemogenicity of the fusion proteins was first demonstrated in transgenic mice carrying the fusion gene *MLL-AF9*. These mice developed AML preceded by a nonmalignant myeloproliferation, indicating that *MLL-AF9* is necessary but not sufficient for the development of acute leukemia (157,158). Recent models employ the technique of retroviral gene transfer in which mouse hematopoietic stem cells or human cord blood progenitor cells are transduced with retroviruses expressing the MLL fusion proteins and injected into immunodeficient mice to assess for leukemia development. This approach has been used to demonstrate the leukemogenicity of MLL-GAS7, MLL-ENL, and MLL-AF9 (159–161). The mechanism by which MLL fusion proteins lead to leukemogenesis does not appear to be due simply to the loss of the H3K4 methyltransferase domain but rather to gene activation mediated by the fusion partner, as target gene expressions are increased in most MLL-rearranged acute leukemias. In addition, it has been shown that MLL-ENL fusion protein is a potent transcriptional activator and that the DNA-binding motifs present in the N terminus of MLL and transcriptional transactivation domain of ENL are indispensable for the transforming activity of MLL-ENL (150). This observation supports a model of AML pathogenesis in which the fusion protein induces transformation by deregulating subordinate genes through a gain-of-function mechanism. The MLL fusion partner may mediate gene activation by more than one mechanism (144). These may include (i) transcriptional activation through chromatin remodeling. A transcriptionally active gene may have unique histone marks, for example, histone methylation at H3K4 at the promoter region, H3K36 at the coding region, and H3K79 at both the promoter and coding regions. MLL normally mediates H3K4 methylation. A major group of MLL fusion partners, for example, AF9, AF10, AF4, and ENL, are nuclear factors involved in transcriptional control and elongation, and appear to interact, either directly or indirectly, with the H3K79 methyltransferase DOTIL, which may lead to aberrant activation of transcription of HOXA and other target genes by these MLL fusion proteins by virtue of H3K79 methylation; (ii) intrinsic histone acetyltransferase activity, for example, MLL-p300 and MLL-CBP; (iii) oligomerization of the MLL fusion proteins mediated by the MLL partners may be the major mechanism for gene activation in a subset of MLL fusion proteins, for example, MLL-GAS7 and MLL-AF1P.

Most studies suggest that MLL fusions may reprogram committed progenitors or convert hematopoietic stem cells to leukemic stem cells. Through the aberrant transcriptional activation capacity, MLL fusion proteins may impart stem cell properties, for example, self-renewal and extensive proliferation, in committed progenitors that already lose these properties by activating a set of genes (including the HoxA cluster) that are normally expressed at high levels in hematopoietic stem cells. Alternatively, MLL fusion proteins may transform hematopoietic stem cells themselves by constitutively maintaining their self-renewal capacity.

CBFβ–SMMHC (MYH11)

Inv(16)(p13q22) and its variants, t(16;16)(p13;q22) and del(16)(q22), are detected in 5% to 10% of AMLs. The 16q22 anomaly is present in all M4Eo cases but is rare in other AML subtypes (162,163). The gene involved is the heterodimeric CBF β subunit gene on 16q, which becomes rearranged to the smooth muscle myosin heavy chain gene *(MYH11)* on 16p. This rearrangement generates a CBFβ-SMMHC fusion protein, composed of the first 165 amino acids of CBFβ fused to the C-terminal coiled-coil region of SMMHC (164,165). CBFβ interacts with the DNA-binding AML1 (RUNX1, CBPα) transcription factor and either activate or repress transcription (166). CBFβ-SMMHC contributes to leukemogenesis by dominantly inhibiting functional activities of AML1 (167). This fusion protein is capable of binding to AML1, and recruits co-repressors such as Sin3A and HDAC8 facilitated by multimerization mediated by the coiled-coil myosin tail domain of SMMHC in the fusion protein (168,169). Thus, AML1 is converted to a dedicated transcription repressor, thereby interfering with normal transcriptional regulation by the AML1/CBFβ complex.

CBFβ-MYH11 knock-in mice exhibited a similar phenotype as RUNX1 knock out mice, consistent with a dominant-negative effect of the fusion protein on AML1 (132). These mice have defective hematopoiesis and blockade of hematopoietic differentiation at the stem-cell level (132,162,163). They do not develop acute leukemia spontaneously but are predisposed to AML, implying that CBF11-MYH11 is insufficient for leukogenesis and that additional genetic alterations are required for full transformation (162). Several candidate cooperating genes, for example PLAG1 and PLAG2, have been identified by retroviral insertional mutagenesis in CBFβ-MYH11 transgenic mice (164). They are thought to contribute to leukemogenesis in these mice by promoting proliferation and expanding hematopoietic progenitors (165). The observation that both subunits of CBF (i.e., AML1 [CBFα] and CBFβ) are the targets of chromosomal translocations in AML underscores the importance of the CBF complex in myeloid differentiation.

E2A-PBX1

The t(1:19)(q23;p13) translocation is common in precursor B-ALL, occurring in approximately 25% to 30% of childhood cytoplasmic Ig⁺ precursor B-ALLs and 1% of childhood cytoplasmic Ig⁻ precursor B-ALLs, and is associated with a poor prognosis (170). This translocation juxtaposes a transcription factor *E2A* gene on chromosome 19p13 with a homeobox gene *PBX1* on 1q23, leading to the formation of a fusion gene that encodes a chimeric transcription factor (171,172). The E2A protein is widely expressed in human tissues and contains the transcriptional activation domain at the N-terminal portion and a basic helix-loop-helix DNA-binding site at the C terminus. It is an important regulator in B-lymphocyte development. PBX1 is a homeodomain transcription factor that is ubiquitously expressed except in the B and T lineages, although close members PBX2 and PBX3 are expressed in B cells. It contains the DNA-binding domain and the adjacent HOX-cooperativity domain for interaction with HOX homeodomain proteins. The E2A-PBX1 fusion protein contains the N-terminal transactivation domain of E2A fused to the C-terminal DNA-binding homeodomain and HOX cooperativity motif of PBX1 (171–173).

The E2A-PBX1 fusion transcription factor has been demonstrated to have oncogenic potential by *in vitro* and *in vivo* experiments. E2A-PBX1 causes T-cell lymphomas and myeloid leukemia in mice, transforms fibroblasts, and blocks differentiation of cultured myeloid progenitors (174–177). It was also shown to cause immortalization and inhibit terminal differentiation of pro-T cells (178,179). To date, transformation of B-cell precursors by E2A-PBX1 *in vivo* has yet to be demonstrated. However, the B-cell leukemogenic potential of E2A-PBX1 has been suggested by an experiment in which reduction of E2A-PBX1 by siRNA increases apoptosis in a B-ALL cell line (180). A transgenic mouse model is needed to fully delineate the role of E2A-PBX1 in the pathogenesis of B-ALL.

The oncogenicity of E2A-PBX1 depends on its unique biochemical properties (181). First, the fusion results in the conversion of a DNA-binding nonactivator PBX1 to a constitutive transcriptional activator that can activate transcription through PBX1-binding sites. Normally, the cooperative binding of HOX with PBX family proteins represses the transcription of a subset of HOX/PBX target genes; however, association of HOX with E2A-PBX1 disrupts the normal regulation and aberrantly activates transcription of HOX/PBX target genes. Second, E2A-PBX1 is capable of interacting with HOX but not MEIS/PREP family proteins because of the loss of an MEIS/PREP interacting motif at the N-terminal of PBX1. Thus, while many genes normally downregulated by HOX/PBX will be ectopically activated by E2A-PBX1, E2A-PBX1 fails to activate genes normally regulated by MEIS/PBX. Third, E2A-PBX1 may sequester co-factors that are normally required by E2A homodimers to regulate expression of genes important for cell-cycle control, resulting in inappropriately repressed expression of E2A target genes and uncontrolled cell cycle. Thus, deregulated expression due to E2A-PBX1 of tissue- and developmental-specific genes normally regulated by PBX and E2A proteins in B cells is likely to be primarily responsible for its oncogenicity in B-ALL (182).

Studies on the target genes of E2A-PBX1 have provided additional insights into the mechanism of transformation by E2A-PBX1. Through comparison of genes expressed in B-ALL with or without E2A-PBX1 translocations, several genes have been shown to be up-regulated by E2A-PBX1. These include genes for granulocyte colony-stimulating factor (183); *EB1*, a tyrosine kinase signal transduction gene not normally expressed in B-cell precursors (182); *WNT16*, a member of the *WNT* gene family (184); and the gene for angiogenin-3, a new member of the angiogenin family (185). EB1 and WNT16b mRNA levels are decreased upon siRNA treatment of B-ALL cell lines with E2A-PBX1, supporting that these two genes are indeed targets of E2A-PBX1 (180). These targets may contribute to pathogenesis of B-ALL mediated by E2A-PBX1.

NPM1-ALK

The t(2;5)(p23;q35) chromosomal translocation occurs frequently in ALCL (186). The percentage of cases positive for the t(2;5) translocation, as measured with excellent correlation by cytogenetics, FISH, RT-PCR, or immunohistochemistry using antibodies (p80 and ALK-1) directed against the fusion protein, varies from 25%–30% to approximately 70% (187–190). This spectrum probably reflects the types of ALCL cases examined in the different studies. The t(2;5) translocation is associated with specific clinical characteristics in ALCL. It occurs in a younger patient population and is associated with a better survival rate (191,192).

Molecular characterization of the breakpoint shows that the t(2;5) translocation causes the fusion of two genes, the nucleophosmin *(NPM)* gene, encoding for a nucleolar phosphoprotein on chromosome 5, and the anaplastic lymphoma kinase *(ALK)* gene, encoding for a novel orphan receptor tyrosine kinase on chromosome 2. This creates an 80-kDa fusion protein that contains the amino-terminal portion of NPM joined to the entire cytoplasmic catalytic portion of ALK (22,23). NPM-ALK has transforming ability *in vitro* (193,194). The first demonstration of a direct causative role for NPM-ALK in human lymphoma was provided by a study in which infection of bone marrow cells with a retrovirus expressing NPM-ALK results in a B-cell lymphoma (195). Subsequently, it was shown that targeted expression of NPM-ALK in T cells results in T-cell lymphoma in mice (196,197), which serve as a useful model to study ALK-induced T lymphomagenesis.

Between 10% and 20% of ALK-positive ALCLs express ALK-fusion proteins other than NPM-ALK (198,199). An example is the TRK-fused gene *(TFG)* (200). The ALK breakpoints in these other translocations involving TRK are the same as in the classic t(2;5) translocation, almost invariably located in the intron between exons 16 and 17. Each of these translocations results in the fusion of the 5′ portion of the chromosomal partner to the ALK cytoplasmic tyrosine kinase domain at the 3′ portion. The fusion the of *NPM,* or other partner genes, to *ALK* has two distinct consequences, both of which are important in the oncogenicity of their fusion protein. First, it leads to the ectopic expression of the fusion proteins in T cells, which normally lack ALK (194). Second, a universal theme of these fusion proteins is the constitutive activation of the tyrosine kinase activity of ALK, in almost all cases through induction of spontaneous dimerization mediated by the 5′ fusion partners. Constitutive ALK kinase activity triggers several downstream signal transduction pathways that are interconnected and overlapping. Among the most important ones are the RAS-ERK, JAK-STAT, and PI3K-AKT pathways. Increased proliferation of the lymphoma cells triggered by ALK fusion proteins is primarily mediated by activation of the RAS-ERK pathway, while antiapoptotic mechanisms generated by ALK fusion proteins are due to activation of the other two pathways (199). STAT3 is the key component in the survival mechanism mediated by ALK fusion proteins, and is required for NPM-ALK–mediated lymphomagenesis (201). STAT3 is activated by NPM-ALK directly or through Janus kinase 3 (JAK3), and exerts its anti-apoptotic functions by up-regulating BCL2, BCL-XL, MCL1, C/EBPβ, and survivin. In addition, ALK fusion proteins can modulate cytoskeletal rearrangements and increase cell migration and invasion, through activation of SRC, SHP2, p1130Cas, and RAC1 (202–205). ALK fusion proteins also modulate immunophenotype, for example, CD30 expression by the ERK and STAT3 pathway (206,207) and CD274 by the STAT3 pathway (208,209).

API2-MALT1

Little was known about the molecular genetics of MALT lymphoma until the t(11;18)(q21;q21) translocation was identified as a recurrent genetic lesion, occurring in approximately 50% of low-grade MALT lymphomas with cytogenetic abnormalities (210–213). The t(11;18)(q21;21) is present frequently in *Helicobacter Pylori*-negative gastric MALT and serves as a clinical marker that is associated with nonresponsiveness to *H. Pylori* eradication. This translocation leads to rearrangements of the *API2* (*BIRC3*) gene on chromosome 11 and the *MALT1* gene on chromosome 18, generating abnormal chimeric mRNAs that code for a API2-MALT fusion protein (214–218). BIRC3 is a member of the inhibitors of apoptosis (IAP) protein family, which consist of suppressors of apoptosis that act by inhibiting caspases, the integral components of many cell-death programs. It contains three baculovirus IAP repeats (BIR) at its N-terminal portion and the caspase recruitment domain (CARD) at its C-terminal region. MALT1 is a component of the trimolecular complex of signaling proteins (CARD11, BCL10, and MALT1) that play a key role in antigen receptor-mediated nuclear factor-κB (NF-κB) activation, regulating lymphocyte activation, proliferation, apoptosis, and development (219,220). These signaling components also participate in CD40-dependent activation of B cells. Upon receptor-mediated activation of tyrosine kinases, this signaling complex activates inhibitor of NF-κB kinase (IKK), which phosphorylates IκB, leading to its ubiquitination and degradation, and enabling NF-κB to translocate to the nucleus and regulate gene transcription. MALT1 is a caspase-like protein (paracaspase) with an amino-terminal death domain, two immunoglobulin-(Ig)-like domains, and a carboxyl-terminal caspase-like domain. MALT1 directly interacts with BCL10 through its Ig-like domain (221,222). The physical interaction between MALT1 and BCL10 is crucial for optimal NF-κB activation. Mice lacking MALT1 have impaired BCR- and CD40-induced proliferation, diminished humoral response and T-cell response, and reduced number of marginal zone B cells and peritoneal B1 cells (223,224).

Breakpoints at *API2* occur in an intron that separates the exons coding for the BIR domains and the CARD domain. The API2-MALT1 fusion protein contains the BIR domains of API2 fused to the C-terminal portion of MALT1, which contains the caspase-like domain but not the immunoglobulin C2 domains. The mechanisms of API2-MALT1 in lymphomagenesis are not exactly known; however, it is very likely that the fusion protein bypasses the normal BCL10/MALT1 signaling mechanism.

Oligomerization mediated by the API2 portion in the fusion protein may result in deregulated activation of NF-κB activity (222), which may lead to up-regulation of antiapoptotic genes. In addition, API2-MALT1 may also have anti-apoptotic activity through direct inhibition of caspases and other apoptotic regulators (220,225).

Oncogenes Activated by Ig-associated Translocations

BCL2

The protein product of the *BCL2* gene is a mitochondrial integral membrane protein that acts as a negative regulator of apoptosis. BCL2 belongs to the large BCL2 family proteins that regulate apoptosis. All members in this family contain at least one of four BH (BCL2 homology) domains. Certain members, such as BCL2, BCL-xl, and MCL1, are anti-apoptotic, whilst others are proapoptotic. The proapoptotic group of BH proteins can be further sub-divided into the structurally diverse "BH3" only proteins (e.g., BID, NOXA, PUMA, and BAD) and the multidomain proteins that share BH1 to 4 (e.g., BAX and BAK). Most BCL2 family members contain a C-terminal transmembrane domain that functions to target these proteins to the outer mitochondrial and other intracellular membranes (38). BCL2 is a major regulator of the intrinsic pathway of apoptosis, which is activated by various cytotoxic insults and developmental cues, such as DNA damage, viral infection, and growth factor deprivation. Upon activation of this pathway, BH3-only proapoptotic proteins are induced or post-translationally activated. These active BH-3-only proteins inhibit BCL2 and relieve the latter's inhibition of BAX and BAK, which are critical for inducing permeabilization of the outer mitochondrial membrane and the subsequent release of cytochrome C that leads to APAF1 assembly into apoptosome, caspase 9 activation and finally caspase 3 activation. Abnormal accumulation of BCL2 may override the inhibitory activity of upstream BH-3-only proteins on BCL2 upon activation of the intrinsic pathway, resulting in reduced apoptotic response.

In 80% to 90% of follicular lymphomas, BCL2 is overexpressed due to the t(14;18)(q32;q21) translocation. This translocation juxtaposes the 3′ portion of the *BCL2* gene to the IgH locus (226–230) (Fig. 7.3). Approximately 70% of the breakpoints are in the MBR, joining the *BCL2* 3′ UTR with the J_H segment. The remaining breakpoints are clustered within the minor cluster region (mcr) located 3′ of the MBR (231). Novel t(14;18) breakpoints have been found approximately 800 bp downstream of the MBR in the 3′ UTR of BCL2. The t(14;18) translocation results in overexpression of a normal BCL2 protein, mainly through transcriptional activation by the Ig-regulatory elements. In those follicular lymphomas with t(14;18) breakpoints located at the MBR region, BCL2-Ig fusion mRNAs with J_H and Cμ 3′ end can also be produced. These fusion mRNAs have a posttranscriptional processing advantage, possibly related to RNA splicing or nucleocytoplasmic transport.

In the B-cell compartment, BCL2 appears to be important for the emergence of long-living memory cells by promoting survival of antigen-selected GC cells (232). Deregulation of BCL2 expression can contribute to the pathogenesis of follicular lymphoma by preventing apoptosis of GC cells that are normally destined to die. The role of this mechanism in follicular lymphomagenesis is supported by the studies of transgenic mice with enforced expression of BCL2 in B cells, which develop follicular lymphoproliferative disease composed of long-lived B cells analogous to human follicular lymphoma (233). Like human follicular lymphomas, a fraction of these indolent follicular lymphomas can progress to large cell lymphoma. In mice, this histologic transformation is frequently associated with *MYC* gene rearrangements.

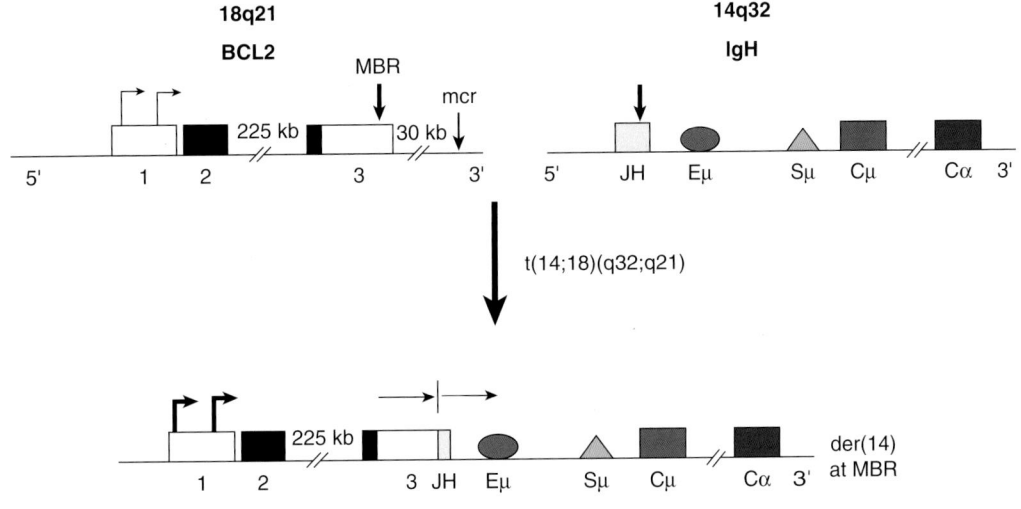

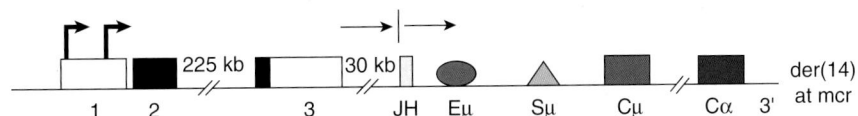

FIGURE 7.3. Schematic representation of t(14;18) translocations involving the _BCL2_ gene. The germline configuration of the human _BCL2_ gene is shown in the **top left panel**. It consists of three exons with a large intron 2. The coding region is indicated in black and the noncoding region in white. The major breakpoint region (MBR) and the minor cluster region (mcr) are indicated by _vertical arrows_. The promoters of _BCL2_ within _BCL2_ exon 1 are marked by _arrows_. MBR is located in the 3′ untranslated region of _BCL2_ and mcr is located approximately 30 kb 3′ of exon 3. The immunoglobulin heavy chain (IgH) locus with the J$_H$ region, the IgH core enhancer (Eμ), the switch recombination region (Sμ), and the constant region (Cμ to Cα) are shown in the **top right panel**. Breakpoints at IgH are located at the J$_H$ region (_vertical arrow_). The t(14;18) translocation results in the juxtaposition of the IgH locus to _BCL2_ in a head to tail fashion, resulting in transcriptional deregulation of _BCL2_ by the IgH-regulatory elements, including Eμ. A translocated _BCL2_ allele at der(14) involving the MBR or the mcr is represented in the **bottom panel**. Transcripts generated from the translocated _BCL2_ allele involving MBR consists of a fusion between the _BCL2_ exon 3 and the JH-Cμ sequence derived from IgH. Normal BCL2 transcripts are generated from the translocated _BCL2_ allele involving mcr. Both types of transcripts give rise to a normal BCL2 protein.

BCL6

The *BCL6* protooncogene was originally identified by virtue of its involvement in recurrent chromosomal translocations affecting the 3q27 region in DLBCL (234–238). *BCL6* encodes a 95-kDa nuclear phosphoprotein belonging to the POZ/zinc finger family of transcriptional repressors (239–241). In the B-cell lineage, expression of BCL6 is specifically restricted to the GC (242,243), where it acts as a transcriptional switch integrating various signals important for GC development, including the control of apoptosis and cell cycle, the sensing and response to DNA damage, the response to T/B cell activation and numerous cytokines/chemokines, and terminal B-cell differentiation (244–253).

Indeed, BCL6 is an essential requirement for the formation of GCs, as documented by the observation that mice deficient for a functional BCL6 protein are not capable of forming these structures and show a complete lack of affinity maturation (254,255). Expression of BCL6 must then be turned off in the late phases of the GC reaction, in order to allow further differentiation into plasma cells and memory B cells (253). At least two signals have been documented to be involved in the down-regulation of BCL6 expression: engagement of the antigen receptor by the antigen (256) and CD40-CD40 ligand interaction (257).

This strictly regulated dynamic is disrupted in tumors carrying rearrangements of the *BCL6* locus, including approximately 35% of DLBCLs as well as a minority (5% to 10%) of follicular

lymphomas (258). A notable feature of BCL6 translocations, which is apparently unique among B-NHLs, is the involvement of various partner chromosomal sites, including IgH (14q23), Igκ (2p12), Igκ (22q11), and at least 20 other chromosomal sites unrelated to the Ig loci; hence the term "promiscuous translocations." The latter include *PIM1*, *RhoH/TTF*, the major histocompatibility complex (MHC) class II transactivator *CIITA*, *OCAB*, *Histone H4*, *IKAROS*, and *HSP89A* among many others (259,260). In all cases, the translocation results in the juxtaposition of heterologous promoters in front of an intact *BCL6* protein-coding sequence leading to its transcriptional deregulation (261,262) (Fig. 7.4). Notably, the common denominator of these heterologous promoters is a broader spectrum of activity throughout B-cell development, including expression in the post-GC differentiation stage. Consequently, the translocation will prevent the normal down-regulation of BCL6 expression that occurs during differentiation into post-GC B cells. By blocking the normal exit of GC B cells and maintaining an environment that is permissive for DNA damage and proliferation while being resistant to apoptosis, BCL6 translocations play a critical role in the pathogenesis of DLBCL, as also confirmed in a mouse model where deregulated expression of BCL6 under the Iμ promoter causes the development of lymphoma in up to 40% of cases (263).

Besides promoter substitution, the *BCL6* gene can also be altered by somatic mutations at its 5′-noncoding region. These mutations largely reflect the derivation from a GC B-cell, where

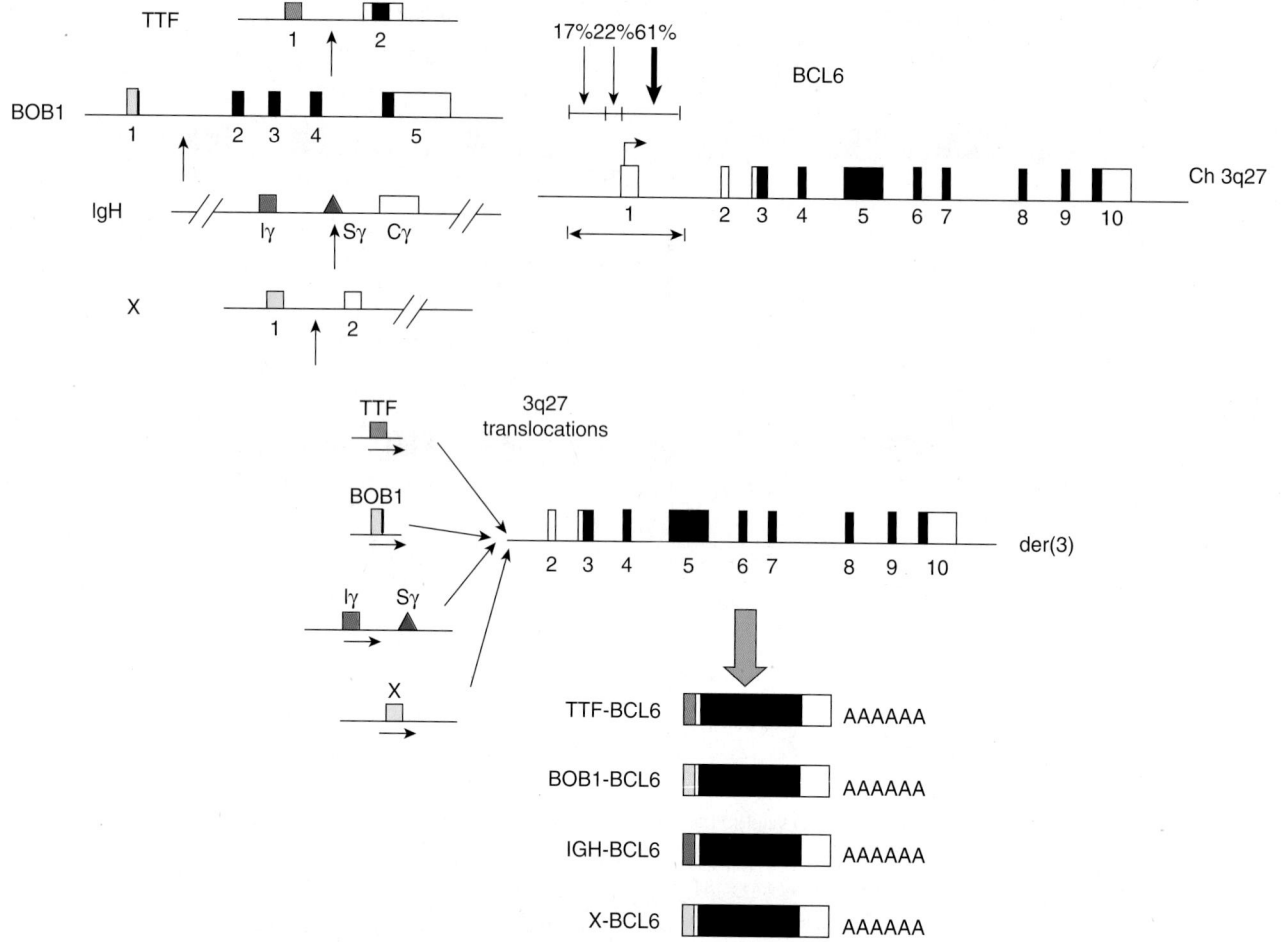

FIGURE 7.4. BCL6 deregulation by promoter substitution in promiscuous translocations affecting 3q27. The **top right panel** is a schematic representation of the human *BCL6* gene, showing the clusters of chromosomal breakpoints with their respective frequency among diffuse large B-cell lymphoma (DLBCL) cases carrying rearranged *BCL6* (*vertical arrows*) and the region targeted by somatic hypermutation (*horizontal double arrows*). The coding and noncoding exons are indicated by filled and empty boxes, respectively. Most breakpoints at *BCL6* are located in intron 1, but they can also occur within exon 1 or 5′ of exon 1. The **top left panel** shows the exon-intron structure of the partner genes (e.g., *TTF*, *BOB1*, IgH, others [X]) involved in 3q27 translocations. Only the 5′ region of partner gene X is schematically represented. The breakpoints at the partner chromosomes are indicated by *arrows*. In the translocations shown here, the promoter and exon 1 of *BCL6* are replaced by the sequences derived from the partner genes. These sequences provide a heterologous promoter to *BCL6*, leading to transcriptional deregulation (i.e., promoter substitution). The **bottom panel** represents the fusion transcripts (i.e., TTF/BCL6, BOB1/BCL6, Iγ/BCL6, and X/BCL6) generated from the translocated alleles. These fusion transcripts contain a heterologous exon spliced to exon 2 of *BCL6*. The entire coding region of *BCL6* is retained, which translates into a normal BCL6 protein.

BCL6 is normally targeted by the physiologic SHM process (61,62,65), and are thus observed in all GC-derived B-NHLs, including DLBCL (73% of cases) (264,265). However, a subset of mutations have been found exclusively in lymphoma, suggesting selection for a pathogenic role. These events include mutations disrupting two BCL6-binding sites within the first noncoding exon of the gene, which abrogate an autoregulatory feedback loop by which BCL6 controls its own expression, and may contribute to tumorigenesis by altering BCL6 basal level transcription (266). Additional mutations in the *BCL6* promoter sequences have been shown to impair the response to IRF4-mediated transcriptional repression, further supporting the role of *BCL6* deregulation in the pathogenesis of DLBCL (257). Finally, an alternative mechanism for deregulation of BCL6 activity may be represented by the recently discovered mutations inactivating the CREBBP and EP300 acetyltransferases (see section on CREBBP and EP300) (267). Acetylation of the BCL6 protein represents an important mechanism for down-regulation of its transrepression activity by preventing the interaction with HDACs (268); thus, inactivation of CREBBP/EP300 may lead to improperly high BCL6 oncogenic activity, favoring malignant transformation.

CCND1

Mantle cell lymphoma (MCL) is characterized cytogenetically by the chromosomal translocation t(11;14)(q13;q32) (269). The 11q13 breakpoints are dispersed over a genomic region of more than 100 kb. However, in approximately 50% of cases, the breakpoints are tightly clustered in the major translocation cluster (MTC) region at the *CCND1 (BCL1)* locus. *CCND1* encodes cyclin D1, a member of the G1 cyclins, which is not normally expressed in lymphocytes. Its expression is related to the cell cycle, and its levels are highest in the G1 phase and lowest in S phase. The t(11;14) translocation results in deregulation of the *CCND1* gene by regulatory elements of the IgH locus. *CCND1* gene overexpression is a highly sensitive and specific marker of MCL. Overexpression of cyclin D1 can be detected in most MCLs and is only rarely present in other benign or malignant lymphoproliferative disorders. Further up-regulation of cyclin D1 mRNA and protein expression may result from truncations of the 3′UTR of cyclin D1 mRNA, which remove mRNA destabilizing elements and binding sites for miR-15/16. These truncated cyclin D1 transcripts are associated with higher tumor proliferation and are predictive of short survival.

Cyclin D1 is important for triggering cells to progress from the G1 to S phase of the cell cycle and for promoting cell proliferation. Its function depends on the formation of a complex with the cyclin-dependent kinases (CDK)-4, which binds to and phosphorylate RB, resulting in the release of E2F transcription factors and G1/S phase transition (270). In addition, cyclin D1/CDK-4 promotes G1 phase transition via a kinase-independent mechanism, sequestering CDK inhibitors such as p27 and p21 and thereby efficiently activating cyclin E/CDK2 complexes. Increased cyclin D1 expression due to genetic alterations in CCND1 will enhance cyclin D1/CDK4 activity and leads to increased cell proliferation. Overexpression of cyclin D1 in the B-cell compartment of transgenic mice leads to B-cell lymphomas in cooperation with MYC, demonstrating the lymphomagenicity of cyclin D1 (271,272). However, despite the established biochemical role of cyclin D1 in cell-cycle control and the increase in cellular proliferation observed on constitutive cyclin D1 expression in murine epithelial tissues (273–275), enforced expression of cyclin D1 alone in the B-cell compartment of transgenic mice does not cause a tumorigenic phenotype, indicating that cyclin D1 overexpression *per se* is not sufficient for lymphoma development. These data suggest that cells possess additional regulatory mechanisms to tightly control cyclin D1 functional activity and limit its neoplastic potential.

In normal cells, after G1 progression to S phase, cyclin D1 is phosphorylated on threonine 286 by GSK3β and exported from the nucleus to the cytoplasm by CRM-1. Here the phosphorylated cyclin D1 is polyubiquitinated by the E3 ligase SKp1-CUL1-F box protein and degraded through the proteasome. This mechanism serves to limit accumulation of nuclear cyclin D1 during S phase. A critical event in cyclin D1-induced lymphomagenesis appears to be the aberrant, constitutive nuclear accumulation of cyclin D1/CDK4 (276,277). Increased nuclear cyclin D1 in S phase enhances its oncogenic potential, as evidenced by a mouse model in which transgenic expression of mutant T286A cyclin D1 leads to the development mature B-cell lymphomas (278). In cancer cells, an aberrant increase in nuclear cyclin D1 during S phase may occur through a T286A point mutation that prevents phosphorylation of cyclin D1 by GSK3β or mutations in the E3 ubiquitin ligase complex that inhibits ubiquitin-dependent degradation. These two mechanisms, however, are only observed in solid tumors and have not been observed in MCL. In the latter, inhibition of GSK3β by activated PI3K/AKT and WNT pathways may be an alternative mechanism for constitutive cyclin D1 accumulation. Active cyclin D1/CDK4 in the nucleus during S phase stabilizes CDT1 and induces re-replication of chromosomal segments, giving rise to increased DSBs and genomic instability. This cyclin D1-induced genomic instability may cooperate with defective DNA damage responses in the pathogenesis of MCL. For example, besides t(11;14), deletion of chromosomal region 11q22-q23 is a frequent chromosomal aberration in MCL. The *ATM* tumor suppressor gene located at this chromosomal site, which is critically involved in the cellular response to DNA damage (see also paragraph ATM below), is inactivated in about 75% of MCL cases by deletion and deleterious point mutations. The tumor suppressor gene *TP53* acts downstream of ATM and plays an important role in DNA damage responses. P53 mutations and deletions have been detected primarily in blastoid MCL cases. Expression of CHK1 and CHK2, two serine-threonine kinases downstream of S-phase checkpoints and involved in DNA damage response, was found to be reduced in cases of MCL with high degree of genomic instability. In addition, deletions or loss of expression of genes encoding for the cell-cycle inhibitors p15, p16, and p21 are associated with aggressive variants of MCL. Deletions and loss of expression of p16 and p21 appear to occur in a subset of aggressive variants of MCL with a wild-type p53, suggesting that these genetic alterations may represent alternate pathways in the pathogenesis of these aggressive variants of MCL.

Cyclin D1 may also have an anti-apoptotic function by sequestering the proapoptotic BAX protein in the cytoplasm and therefore enhancing BCL2 antiapoptotic function. Thus, the oncogenic role of cyclin D1 is not only due to the increased cell proliferation, as induced by deregulation of the cell cycle at the G1/S transition, and initiation of genomic instability, but is also linked to its potential to deregulate apoptosis in B cells.

MYC

The MYC gene encodes a transcription factor that contains an N-terminal transactivation domain and a C-terminal basic helix-loop-helix leucine zipper (bHLHLZ) domain. The MYC protein functions mainly as a transcriptional activator by binding to specific DNA sequences when heterodimerized with a partner protein, called MAX. MAX also heterodimerizes with members of the Mxd (formerly MAD) family, which provides another layer of mechanism to functionally antagonize MYC activity through protein-protein interaction and specific DNA binding. In addition to MAD, MYC can interact with other proteins through the N-terminal transactivation domain, which contains the highly conserved elements known as Myc box I, II, and III, and the C-terminal bHLHLZ domain. These protein-protein interactions can modulate the ability of MYC to interact with the transcriptional machinery, providing additional complexity in the regulation of MYC function. Recently, it was demonstrated that MYC/MAX can activate gene transcription by recruiting histone acetylation complexes through interaction with TRRAP and by recruiting the SWI-SNF chromatin remodeling complex through interaction with INI1 (hSnf5). MYC can also promote transcription elongation through P-TEFb (positive transcriptional elongation factor) and promote mRNA cap methylation. Besides functioning as a transcriptional activator, MYC can also act as a transcriptional repressor by binding to DNA-binding transcriptional activators such as nuclear factor Y (NFY), SP1 and MYC-interacting zinc finger 1 (MYZ1), resulting in displacement of coactivators and recruitment of co-repressors.

MYC is capable of directing numerous important cellular functions through its role as a global transcriptional regulator. MYC-regulated activities are diverse and include cell cycle regulation, differentiation, cell growth, metabolism and protein synthesis, cell adhesion and migration, apoptosis, angiogenesis, DNA damage and chromosomal instability, stem cell self-renewal and/or differentiation, and DNA replication. Using an unbiased genome-wide analysis approach, MYC was shown to occupy more than 15% of gene promoters and to regulate numerous target genes associated with these promoters in BL cell lines. For a comprehensive description of MYC target genes, readers are referred to the database "MYC Cancer gene." (http://www.myc-cancer-gene.org/)

The *MYC* protooncogene is the target of the translocation on 8q24. MYC translocations are consistently found in BLs of all subtypes, and frequently in B-cell lymphomas, unclassifiable, with features intermediate between BL and DLBLC, and a subset of DLBCL. In all affected cases, the translocation involves region 8q24 and one of the immunoglobulin loci on chromosomes 2, 14, or 22 (279–283). Specifically, IGH is present in 80% of the cases. The remaining 20% have t(2;8)(p11;q24) involving the Igκ locus (15%) or t(8;22)(q24;q11) involving the Igκ locus (5%). Because of the chromosomal translocation, *MYC* becomes juxtaposed to the Ig locus. In BL, *MYC* chromosomal translocations are most likely the result of errors occurring during somatic hypermutation in the GC (see Section Oncogene Activation by Chromosomal Translocation). The t(8;14), t(2;8), and t(8;22) translocations are somewhat different in the precise locations of the breakpoints. The t(8;14) breakpoints are located 5′ and centromeric to *MYC,* whereas the breakpoints map 3′ and telomeric to *MYC* in t(2;8) and t(8;22). Within t(8;14), the molecular architecture of the translocation region varies between different subtypes. The endemic form of BL is associated predominantly with breakpoints at an undefined distance (>100 kb) 5′ to the *MYC* locus on chromosome 8 and within or in proximity to the Ig J$_H$ region on chromosome 14. In contrast, the t(8;14) translocation in sporadic and in AIDS-associated BLs involves sequences within or immediately 5′ (<3 kb) to *MYC* on chromosome 8 and sequences within the IgH switch region on chromosome 14 (284–286) (Fig. 7.5).

The common effect of t(8;14), t(2;8), and t(8;22) is that *MYC* becomes transcriptionally deregulated by at least two mechanisms: juxtaposition of heterologous regulatory elements from the Ig loci in front to *MYC* and removal or mutations in the 5′ regulatory region, including exon 1, of *MYC* (287). In all forms of BL, the full-length MYC protein is constitutively expressed. However, about 50% of BL harbor mutations in the N-terminal transactivation domain. These mutations are clustered in several hotspots in the MYC box1 and are also present in the MYC box 2. Those mutations, particularly the one at Thr58, present in MYC Box 1, have been shown to enhance the transcriptional and transforming activity of MYC, possibly by interfering with the physiologic ability of p107, a protein related to RB, to modulate MYC transcriptional activity (288,289). Mutations at

Thr58 were also shown to result in insufficient ubiquitination and decreased proteasome-mediated turnover, leading to accumulation of the MYC protein. Interestingly, mutations in the MYC Box 2 were found to decrease its transforming ability and simultaneously its ability to induce apoptosis without altering its transactivation ability.

The pathogenic role of deregulated MYC in BL has been demonstrated by *in vitro* and *in vivo* experiments. *In vitro*, constitutive expression of MYC in Epstein-Barr virus (EBV)-immortalized human B-cell lines results in their malignant transformation. *In vivo*, mice transgenic for *MYC* driven by the immunoglobulin enhancer develop pre-B and B-cell lymphomas at relatively high frequency. The oncogenicity of MYC in lymphoma is most likely related to deregulation in its global transcriptional regulatory function with consequent abnormal expression of many target genes. Constitutive expression of MYC can lead to multiple tumorigenic consequences that contribute to lymphoma development: (i) it promotes cell-cycle progression and increased cell proliferation; (ii) it enhances cell growth by providing cells with building blocks, increasing cell metabolism and protein synthesis; (iii) it contributes to genomic instability; (iv) it induces angiogenesis; (v) it potentiates the

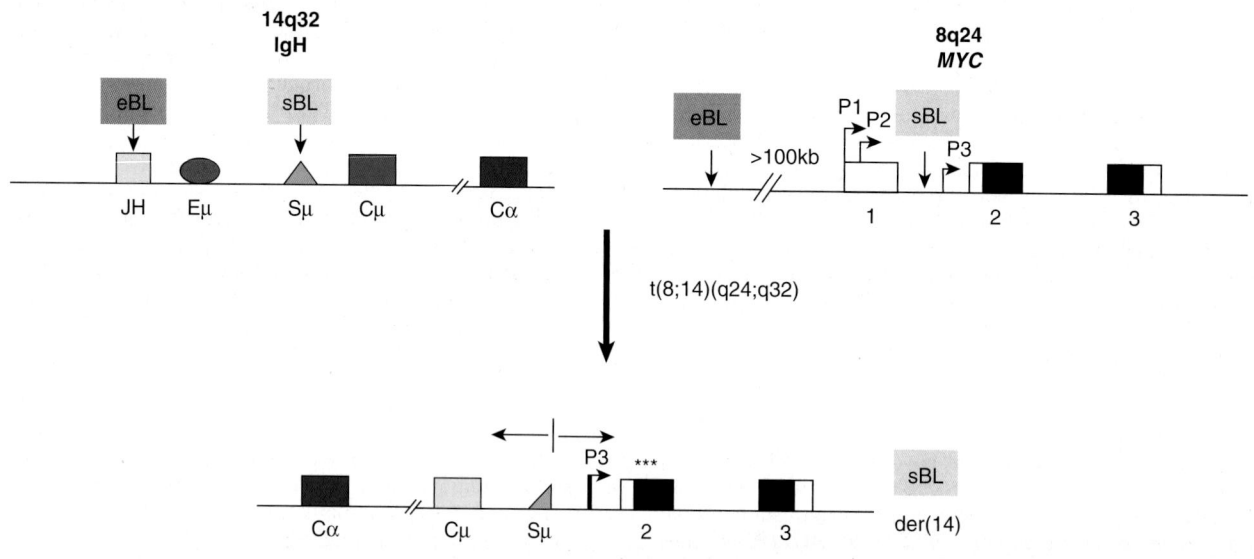

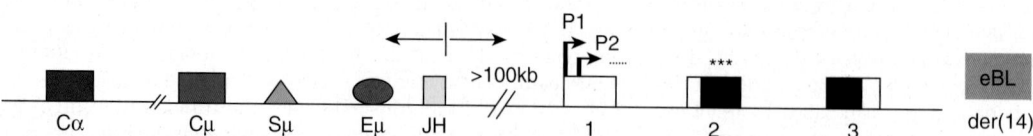

FIGURE 7.5. Schematic diagram of t(8;14) in sporadic and endemic Burkitt lymphomas. The germline configuration of human *MYC* is shown in the **top left panel**. It consists of three exons. The coding region is indicated in *black* and the noncoding region in *white*. The two major promoters of *MYC*, P1, and P2, and the minor intronic promoter P3, are marked by *arrows*. The **top right panel** represents the germline configuration of the immunoglobulin heavy chain (IgH) locus, including the J$_H$ region, the core enhancer (Eμ), the switch recombination region (Sμ), and the constant region (Cμ to Cα). The breakpoint regions in sporadic Burkitt lymphoma (sBL) and endemic Burkitt lymphoma (eBL) are indicated by *vertical arrows*. The configurations of the translocated *MYC* alleles in sBL and eBL are represented in the **bottom panel**. In the case of t(8;14) in sBL, the breakpoints tend to cluster in intron 1 of *MYC* and the Sμ region of IgH. The exon 1, including the major promoters of *MYC*, is deleted. Translocation results in deregulation of *MYC* transcription initiated near the intronic promoter P3 by immunoglobulin regulatory elements. Because the coding domain is structurally intact, a full length MYC protein is generated. In the case of t(8;14) in eBL, the breakpoints are located more than 100 kb 5′ of the first exon of *MYC* and at the J$_H$ region of IgH. As a result of the translocation, *MYC* transcription initiated from P1 and P2 is deregulated by regulatory elements of the IgH locus, including Eμ. Mutations can be detected in the exon 1–intron 1 border (*dots*), where *MYC* transcriptional regulatory sequences are located. As in the case of sBL, a full-length MYC protein is produced. In both types of translocated *MYC* alleles, the coding region in exon 2 frequently harbor point mutations that result in amino acid substitutions at the N-terminal transactivation domain of *MYC* (*asterisks*). These mutations contribute to the oncogenicity of *MYC*.

initiation and maintenance of tumor stem cells, and it may lead to inappropriate DNA replication MYC activation can also lead to cell apoptosis through multiple pathways, the major one being the p14ARF-MDM2-p53 pathway. In this pathway, MYC up-regulates ARF, which in turn activates p53 to regulate a cohort of target genes mediating cell apoptosis. MYC can also induce apoptosis through activation of the proapoptotic BAX protein and indirect up-regulation of the proapoptotic BIM protein (290). Since MYC–potentiated apoptosis can nullify its hyperproliferative effect, abrogation of the former by additional genetic events is essential for full transformation.

MALT1 and BCL10

Besides t(11;18)(q21;q21), which results in the fusion of MALT1 to API2, MALT1 is also frequently involved by translocation t(14;18)(q32;21), which results in juxtaposition of the MALT1 gene to the IgH locus. MALT1 might be overexpressed as a consequence of this translocation, leading to increased NF-κB activation.

Another recurrent but infrequent chromosomal abnormality in MALT lymphoma is t(1;14)(p22;q32). The breakpoint at chromosome 1 is located upstream of the promoter of the BCL10 gene. BCL10, a cellular homologue of the equine herpesvirus-2 E10 gene, contains the CARD domain. Like MALT1, BCL10 acts as a crucial signaling molecule in antigen receptor–induced NF-κB activation (222). Mediated by a CARD-CARD interaction, BCL10 binds to and acts down-stream of CARD11. It also interacts with MALT1 through a short motif down-stream of its CARD domain. Translocation of BCL10 to the Ig locus results in its increased expression, which leads to constitutive NF-κB activation. Abnormal nuclear BCL10 expression has also been reported in cases with API2-MALT1 fusion and BCL10 translocation and may be associated with more advanced or aggressive disease. This abnormal subcellular localization may induce its binding to proteins that do not normally interact with BCL10.

Rather high frequencies of BCL10 mutations were originally reported in MALT lymphomas with the t(1;14) translocations (291,292). These mutations were frameshift mutations producing truncations in or distal to the CARD domain. However, BCL10 mutations have been found at very low frequency in other studies, suggesting that they may not play a significant role in the pathogenesis of MALT lymphomas (293–296).

ONCOGENIC MUTATIONS

In B-NHL, and particularly in DLBCL, oncogenic point mutations have been found in a number of genes that are involved in the activation of the NF-κB transcription complex and of the BCR signaling pathway. Up to 30% of DLBCL cases belonging to the activated B cell like (ABC) subtype (297) display mutations in the MYD88 gene, which encodes for an adaptor molecule mediating signal transduction from the Toll-like-receptor (TLR)/IL1 receptor to both NF-κB and STAT3 (298). The majority of MYD88 mutations target the evolutionarily invariant amino acid residue L265 within the Toll/IL1 receptor (TIR) domain, and have been shown to enhance the ability of MYD88 to interact with two kinases that are critical for downstream signaling activation, namely IRAK1 and IRAK4 (298). An additional 20% of DLBCL patients, also of the ABC subtype, carry activating mutations of the CD79B gene, encoding for the immunoglobulin coreceptor (299). In the majority of cases, the mutations substitute the Tyrosine 158 residue, a phosphorylation site within the ITAM motif, which is required for activation of the BCR signaling pathway (299). The CARD11 gene, encoding for an adaptor molecule in the same pathway which also converges on activation of NF-κB, is mutated in approximately 9% of ABC-DLBCL (300), while less frequent mutations

have been found in genes encoding for other components of the NF-κB signaling cascade, including TRAF2, TRAF5, and the RANK receptor (301). A common consequence shared by the aforementioned mutations is the constitutive activation of the NF-κB signaling pathway, which is a hallmark of ABC-DLBCL (302); however, mutations in CD79B may trigger the activation of other signaling pathways downstream to the BCR, including PI3K, MAPK, and ERK (299), while enforced expression of MYD88 mutated alleles been shown to induce a signature of STAT3 activation (298).

Recent genome-wide sequencing efforts have revealed the presence of recurrent missense mutations affecting the EZH2 gene in 7.2% of follicular lymphoma (FL) and 21.7% of GCB-DLBCL (303). EZH2 encodes for a lysine methyltransferase that forms the catalytic subunit of the Polycomb-Repressive Complex 2 (PRC2) (304–306). The EZH2 protein mediates mono-, di- and tri-methylation of histone H3 on lysine 27 (H3K27), the latter two modifications being generally associated with transcriptional repression. Through this activity, EZH2 plays essential roles in both developmental and differentiation processes, including the maintenance of hematopoietic and progenitor cells (304–306). In the vast majority of affected cases, the mutations target a hotspot residue (Tyrosine 641) and seem to play a gain-of-function role by altering the substrate specificity of the EZH2 protein and by increasing its trimethyltransferase activity on H3K27, as documented by several biochemical studies (307,308). Thus, dysregulation of EZH2 may contribute to lymphoma development by subverting the transcriptional regulation of important cellular programs and by promoting the epigenetic remodeling of the cancer cell.

TUMOR SUPPRESSOR GENES INACTIVATION IN HEMATOPOIETIC NEOPLASMS

The mechanisms by which tumor suppressor genes are inactivated in hematologic malignancies include point mutations, genomic deletions, and promoter hypermethylation. Point mutations are mostly represented by nucleotide substitutions affecting the coding region of the target gene, and resulting in premature stop codons (nonsense mutations) or amino acid changes (missense mutations) that inactivate the protein function. Less frequently, mutations may affect splicing sites or regulatory sequences of the target gene. Small deletions and insertions in the coding region that lead to a shift in the reading frame can also occur. Larger genomic deletions result in removal of the entire gene locus or of large portions of it. Hypermethylation occurs at CpG islands in the gene promoter and can lead to transcriptional silencing in the absence of any structural alterations (309).

In most tumor suppressor genes, both alleles are inactivated by genetic and/or epigenetic mechanisms, usually through gross deletion of one allele and nonsense/missense mutation in the second allele, and less frequently through homozygous deletions or copy number neutral loss of heterozygosity (due to duplication of the mutated allele). Alternatively, promoter hypermethylation can lead to gene inactivation by affecting intact alleles or by silencing the remaining allele when the second allele has been deleted. Although Knudson two hit model of tumor suppressor gene inactivation holds true for many classical TSGs, a number of genes have been identified in which haploinsufficiency, that is, the loss or inactivation of only one allele, can contribute to tumorigenesis due to reduction in gene dosage (310).

A number of chromosomal deletions are specifically associated with hematopoietic malignancies, suggesting the presence of TSGs in these regions. The detailed dissection of these chromosomal abnormalities to delineate the minimal deleted region has been instrumental in the identification of TSG with critical roles in lymphomagenesis. Recently, genome-wide sequencing approaches combined with high-density SNP array analyses have enabled the unbiased identification of recurrent mutations and/or deletions in several novel genes, suggesting a tumor suppressor role. The list of TSGs discussed here is not meant to be exhaustive, but rather to provide an illustration of the spectrum of TSG that can be affected. These TSGs have various functions relevant to the specific contexts of genesis of the different lymphoma subtypes.

ATM (Ataxia Telangiectasia)

The ataxia teleangiectasia mutated (*ATM*) gene is located on chromosomal band 11q22-q23 and encodes a nuclear 370-kDa phosphoprotein with leucine zipper, helix-loop-helix, and PI3-K motifs. It belongs to the PI3K-like protein kinase (PIKK) family consisting of six members, all of which possess a PI3-K domain that harbors the catalytic site. ATM is known to associate with chromosomal regions containing DSBs, and acts as a upstream mediator of multiple kinase signaling cascades that respond to DSBs induced by damaging agents or by normal processes, such as meiotic or V(D)J recombination. These responses involve the activation of cell cycle checkpoints, DNA repair, and apoptosis (81–83,311). Upon DSB, ATM is rapidly autophosphorylated and activated, leading to the phosphorylation of its substrates. More than a dozen substrates have so far been identified for ATM, including p53, CHK2, and BRCA1. A series of ATM-dependent p53 modifications, including direct phosphorylation, indirect phosphorylation through CHK2, and phosphorylation of its inhibitor MDM2, result in activation and stabilization of p53. This leads to increased transcription of p21, the inhibitor of the CDK2-cyclin E complex, thus establishing the G1/S cell-cycle checkpoint. Phosphorylation of CHK2, a checkpoint kinase, activates it to phosphorylate the checkpoint phosphatase CDC25A and marks it for degradation. Since CDC25A dephosphorylates and maintains the activity of CDK1 and CDK2, which drives G2/M and G1/S phase transitions respectively, destruction of CDC25A contributes to the G2/M and G1/S checkpoints. Phosphorylation of other substrates besides p53 and CHK2 by ATM results in activation of multiple cell-cycle checkpoints in response to DSB. ATM may also directly control the DNA repair process through activation of the ABL tyrosine kinase and subsequent phosphorylation of the RAD51 and RAD52 proteins that are major players in the homologous recombination pathway (312,313).

ATM germline mutations are consistently present in patients with ataxia telangiectasia, who have strong predisposition to develop lymphoid malignancies among other phenotypes (314). This suggests that *ATM* can act as a tumor suppressor gene. Consistent with this, ATM-deficient mice develop thymic lymphomas with a relatively short latency (315,316). Biallelic alterations of ATM, including deletion and mutation or biallelic mutations, are present in the majority (about 75%) of MCLs. These mutations are primarily somatic in origin, and distributed across the entire coding region; deleterious mutations are more frequently seen than missense mutations (317–320). ATM alterations are also detected at high frequency (about 40% to 60%) in T-prolymphocytic leukemia (T-PLL), where they show a mode of inactivation typical of classical tumor-suppressor gene, that is, deletion in one allele and mutation in the second allele (321,322). Interestingly, the point mutations seen in T-PLL are primarily missense mutations clustering in the PI3-K region. Biallelic ATM alterations and/or deficient ATM expression are also common (about 25% to 40%) in CLL/small lymphocytic

lymphoma (SLL), and are associated with a poor prognosis (323–326). Mutations ATM alterations are also observed at lower frequency in other lymphomas, including FL, DLBLC, as well as in childhood ALL (320). Thus, ATM alteration is a common event in a wide array of sporadic lymphoproliferative disorders, supporting an important tumor suppressor role in these tumors.

Cyclin-Dependent Kinase Inhibitors

The mammalian cell cycle is regulated by CDKs, a family of serine/threonine protein kinases that are activated at specific points of the cycle by complexing with their activating proteins, the cyclins (327). For example, CDK4 and CDK6 bind to D-type cyclins (cyclin D1, cyclin D2, cyclin D3), and these CDK-cyclin D complexes are essential for G1 entry and progression. The CDK2-cyclin E complex is important for G1/S transition. The activity of CDKs is negatively regulated by a group of cell-cycle inhibitory proteins, called CDK inhibitors, which bind to CDK alone or to the CDK-cyclin complex and regulate CDK activity (327). Two classes of CDK inhibitors, the INK4 family and Cip/Kip family, have been identified. The INK4 family includes p15 (INK4b), p16 (INK4a), and p18 (INK4c), which specifically inactivate G1 CDK (CDK4 and CDK6). The Cip/Kip family includes p21 (Waf1, Cip1), p27 (Cip2), and p57 (Kip2). These proteins inhibit the G1 CDK-cyclin complexes. Deficiency in functions of CDK inhibitor functions results in unbalanced CDK activities and abnormal cell-cycle regulation.

CDK inhibitors are altered at variable frequency in hematopoietic malignancies. The most frequent alterations are inactivation of p15 and p16 because of deletions (usually biallelic) or 5′ CG island promoter methylation (328). Homozygous deletions in p15 and p16 are most frequent in ALL (precursor B and T) but much less frequent in B- and T-cell NHLs, AML, and CML. Methylation of the p15 and p16 genes was detected, respectively, in 64% and 32% of B-cell lymphomas, in 44% and 22% of T-cell lymphomas, and is more frequent in aggressive primary and transformed lymphomas than in indolent lymphomas, suggesting a role in tumor progression (329,330). Point mutations in p15 or p16 are uncommon. p16 alterations frequently co-exist with p14[ARF] aberrations in B-cell lymphomas (330,331), suggesting that simultaneous inactivation of these two regulatory pathways may cooperate to promote B-cell lymphomagenesis. p21 promoter methylation is rare in lymphomas and acute leukemias (226,227,332,333). P27 methylation is also infrequent in acute leukemia (227), but is present in about 25% of lymphomas (228). Loss of p27 not associated with hypermethylation, inactivating mutation, or deletion has been found in a subset of lymphomas, including MCL (228–230).

MicroRNA-15a/MicroRNA-16

Using interphase cytogenetics, the most frequent chromosomal aberrations in CLL/SLL are deletions involving chromosome band 13q14, followed by deletions of the genomic region 11q22.3-q23.1, trisomy 12, and deletions at 17p13 (94,95). Deletion of 13q14.3 is seen in approximately 50% of cases. It is now known that this region harbors two miRNAs, miR-15a and miR-16. MiRNAs are very small noncoding RNAs that function as regulators of gene expression by sequence-specific base-paring with the 3′ UTR of mRNA, and have been implicated as oncogenes and tumor suppressor genes (46). MiRNAs down-regulate target gene expressions by promoting mRNA degradation and by inhibiting protein translation. In 48% of CLL/SLL, miR-15a and miR-16 are down-regulated by hemizygous or homozygous deletion, or other unknown mechanisms (334). In one case, a point mutation in the precursor molecule for miR-16 has been shown to compromise the generation of the mature miR-16. This mutation is associated with a family history of CLL, when the other, normal, allele is deleted (335). Though this classic mechanism of TSG inactivation appears to be rare in the inactivation of miRNAs, it does provide further evidence for a tumor suppressor roles of miR-15a and miR-16. The tumor suppressor role of the miR-15a/miR-16 cluster was demonstrated in a mouse model in which deletion of the region encompassing these genetic elements resulted in an indolent clonal B-cell lymphoproliferative disorder akin to human CLL/SLL (336).

The tumor suppressor activities of miR-15a and miR-16 in CLL are mediated mainly through their ability to target genes that regulate apoptosis and cell cycles (337). These two miRNAs negatively regulate the expression of the antiapoptotic factor BCL2. Thus, down-regulation of miR-15a and miR-16 could result in higher BCL2 protein level and higher anti-apoptotic activity. Additional target genes related to anti-apoptosis, including MCL-1 and PDCD6IP, have also been identified in CLL. MCL-1 belongs to the BCL2 protein family and inhibits apoptosis. PDCD6IP binds to and affects the function of PDCD6, a protein required for apoptosis. Furthermore, miR-15a/miR-16 modulate expression of genes controlling cell-cycle progression. MiR-15a/miR-16 alterations result in increased expressions of these target genes, leading to enhanced cell survival, increased proliferation, and tumor progression.

TP53

The *TP53* tumor suppressor gene is the most frequently mutated gene in human cancers. An extensive review of the structure and function of p53 is beyond the scope of this chapter and can be found elsewhere (338). In brief, p53 is a 393–amino acid sequence-specific transcription factor that has a key role in integrating cellular responses to different types of stress. The ability of p53 to transcriptionally regulate a large group of genes is critical for activation of those responses. However, p53 can also have functions independent of its transcriptional activity. For sample, p53 can function as a proapoptotic BH3 (BCL2-homology domain-3)-only protein and antagonizes antiapoptotic BH proteins (339), which complements the ability of p53 to activate expression of proapoptotic BH3-only proteins such as PUMA. It is proposed that p53 has different responses depending on the stress levels. P53 responds to low or constitutive stress normally encountered during growth and development by promoting cell-cycle arrest and DNA repair. In response to acute stress such as oncogene activation, p53 is switched from promoting survival to induction of apoptosis in order to eliminate the damaged cell. It was originally thought that p53-mediated tumor suppression is dependent on the ability of p53 to respond to DNA damage. However, this notion was challenged by a recent mouse model, which suggested that p53 induction in response to signals that persist beyond DNA damage, for example, activated oncogenes, is the key to tumor suppression (340,341). In contrast, other studies, using precancerous models, support that p53 response to genotoxic stress is responsible for p53-mediated tumor suppression (342,343).

Inactivation of p53 in hematologic neoplasms, as in solid cancers, can occur through point mutation in one allele and deletion of the other allele (344). The impairment of the normal functions of p53 is critical for its effects on tumor progression. Interestingly, unlike many other TSGs that harbor deleterious mutations, about 80% of the mutations in p53 are missense point mutations, mostly clustered in exons 5 to 10 (amino acids 120 to 290), which encode for the DNA-binding domain (344). These mutations result in the disruption of normal p53 function and accumulation of high levels of p53 mutant proteins that have aberrant functions. Some of these mutations can lead to the formation of dominant-negative p53 mutants that act as inhibitory proteins interfering with the normal functions of the wild-type protein, if the normal allele is still retained (345). Others have been suggested to have gain-of-function and even oncogenic activity (346,347). One of the mechanisms by which these p53 mutants exert their oncogenic potential is by binding to, and interfering with the activities of p63 and p73, relatives of p53 (348). Mutant p53 may also acquire novel transcriptional activities that have oncogenic potential (349,350). Furthermore, p53 activity may be compromised by alterations in p14^{ARF}, a protein product generated by an alternative reading frame in the p16/INK4a locus. p14^{ARF} is considered to be an upstream regulator of p53 function. Experimental studies have shown that p14^{ARF} interacts physically with MDM2, thus preventing p53 degradation and promoting p53 stabilization and accumulation (351–354). Loss of p14 function may increase degradation of p53 and result in a defective p53-regulatory pathway.

Alterations of *TP53* are present in different types of hematopoietic neoplasms at variable frequencies. In general, they are less common (10% to 15%) in hematologic malignancies than in solid tumors. *TP53* gene alterations have been found in 20% of CML blast crisis, 15% of AML, 2% of ALL (up to 50% of L3 ALL), 10% of CLL and 40% of Richter transformation, 30% to 40% of adult T-cell leukemia, 5% to 10% of MM, and 30% of high grade B-cell NHLs (rare in low-grade NHL) (355). Genomic deletions and, more rarely, missense mutations in p14^{ARF} have been identified in about 20% of aggressive B-cell lymphomas, where they mainly occur in cases with wild-type p53 (330).

PRDM1/Blimp-1

The *PRDM1/Blimp-1* gene is expressed in two isoforms, PRDM1α and PRDM1β, the former representing the larger functional isoform. The former isoform has a PR domain at the N-terminal portion of the protein, which is related to the SET domain found in many histone methyltransferases (HMTs). However, in contrast to *bona fide* SET-domain proteins, the PR domain of PRDM1 does not possess intrinsic HMT activity. Five C2H2-type zinc fingers, which represent the DNA-binding domain, are present at the C-terminal portion of the protein. PRDM1β lacks the N-terminal 101 amino acids of PRDM1α and has a truncated PR domain. PRDM1β has been shown to be functionally impaired in its transcriptional repression activity. PRDM1 is a transcriptional repressor that binds to specific DNA sequences through its zinc finger domains, and functions as a scaffold for recruiting co-repressors that catalyze histone modifications. PRDM1 has been shown to mediate transcriptional silencing via interactions with the H3 lysine methyltransferase G9a (356), the histone deacetylases HDAC1 and HDAC2 (357), and the H3 lysine demethylase LSD1 (358). PRDM1 can also tether the Groucho family of transcription factors to mediate repression of gene transcription (359).

PRDM1 was originally identified as a novel repressor of human beta-interferon gene expression called PRDI-BF1 (positive regulatory domain I–binding factor 1) (360). Blimp-1 (B-lymphocyte–induced maturation protein), which represents the murine homolog of PRDI-BF1 (361), was later discovered as a protein the enforced expression of which was sufficient to drive plasma cell differentiation of a mouse lymphoma cell line with an ABC phenotype (362). Studies since then have revealed important roles for PRDM1 in differentiation, homeostasis and development of multiple cell types, including B and T cells, natural killer (NK) cells, macrophages, dendritic cells, as well as nonhematopoietic cells. In B cells, PRDM1 is the master regulator of plasma cell differentiation, critical for the generation of immunoglobulin-secreting plasma cells and the maintenance of long-lived plasma cells (363–365). It mediates terminal B-cell differentiation by extinguishing gene programs related to B-cell signaling and proliferation (366), and allowing the induction of XBP1, which in turn coordinates phenotypic changes, including expansion of tendoplasmic reticulum and increased protein synthesis, that define the plasma cell phenotype (367).

Inactivation or down-regulation of PRDM1 appears to be an important event in the pathogenesis of DLBCLs of the ABC/non-GCB subtype. In up to 50% of DLBCLs of this subtype, PRDM1 is inactivated by truncating or missense mutations, biallele gene deletions or transcription repression by a constitutively active, translocated BCL6 (368–370). *PRDM1* mutations are detected in about 24% to 35% of the ABC/non-GCB subtype of DLBCL and have not been identified in GCB-like DLBCL. The types of somatic mutations observed in *PRDM1* include splice site mutations, frameshift insertions/deletions, and less frequently, nonsense and missense mutations. The vast majority of these mutations result in the generation of truncated proteins lacking one or more of the critical domains including the PR, proline-rich region, and zinc fingers. Most of the somatic mutations (about 90%) are associated with inactivation of the second allele by deletion, consistent with biallelic inactivation characteristic of a tumor suppressor gene. Mutations in acute leukemias and solid tumors have not been identified (371). In non-GCB/ABC-like DLBCL without genetic lesions, asynchronous PRDM1 mRNA and protein expressions have been observed, suggesting posttranscriptional down-regulation (370,372). miRNAs have been postulated as a potential mechanism of down-regulation (372).

PRDM1 has been shown to function as a tumor suppressor gene in mouse models (370,373). Mice lacking *Blimp-1* are predisposed to develop lymphoproliferative disorders resembling human ABC-like DLBCL. One of these mouse models also demonstrated a cooperative pathogenic effect between *PRDM1* inactivation and constitutive NF-κB activation (373). These findings suggest that *PRDM1* inactivation contributes to the pathogenesis of ABC-like DLBCL by inhibiting terminal B-cell differentiation induced by constitutive canonical NF-κB activation characteristically present in this lymphoma type.

In addition, PRDM1 is a tumor suppressor gene in aggressive NK cell malignancies (374–376) and is implicated in the etiology of radiation-therapy induced secondary malignancy neoplasms in pediatric patients with classical Hodgkin lymphomas (377).

Retinoblastoma 1 (RB1)

The *RB1* gene was one of the first tumor suppressor genes to be identified, by virtue of its role in hereditary retinoblastoma (378). The RB protein encodes a 107-kDa nuclear phosphoprotein belonging to a family of three proteins that also include p107 and p130. RB is now viewed as a transcription co-factor that can bind to and either potentiate or antagonize activities of more than one hundred transcription factors, thereby regulating transcription of numerous target genes by recruitment of chromatin modifier complexes (379). In addition, RB may serve as a nonchromosome-associated adaptor protein. For example, RB can bind to APC/C (anaphase promoting complex/cyclosome) and SKP2 (S-phase kinase-associated protein 2), promoting the latter's degradation (380,381).

The ability of RB to control expression of a vast array of genes mediates its pleotropic cellular functions, including controlling cell-cycle arrest, inducing differentiation, maintaining genomic stability, and inducing senescence in response to oncogenic stresses. Its binding partners and the functional consequences of interactions with these proteins determine the molecular mechanisms underlying RB functions (379,382). The role of RB as a major cell-cycle inhibitor is largely mediated through its interaction with the E2F transcription factors (383).

RB suppresses the G1/S transition in the cell cycle by binding to E2F and inhibiting E2F-mediated transactivation of a variety of genes involved in initiating DNA synthesis, such as *MYC, MYB,* and *CDC2,* and those for dihydrofolate reductase and thymidine kinase, by recruiting several chromosomal remodeling enzymes (including HDAC and DNMT1) to repress transcription. RB function is regulated by phosphorylation mediated by CDKs, the activity of which is regulated by CDK inhibitors including the INK4 and Cip/Kip families. When hypophosphorylated or dephosphorylated, RB is activated and binds to E2F, thereby inducing cell-cycle arrest; in contrast, phosphorylated RB is inactivated, and cannot bind E2F, thereby promoting entry of cells into S phase. The ability of RB to mediate cell-cycle control is not solely mediated by interactions with E2F; it may also be promoted the interaction of RB with APC/c, which results in stabilization of the CDK inhibitor p27 (380,381). Other cellular functions of RB can be E2F-dependent or mediated by interaction with other protein partners. It was originally believed that the tumor suppressor function of RB is largely due to its ability to control cell cycle arrest, but most likely other cellular functions also contribute. The presence of RB may also inhibit tumorigenesis by inducing differentiation, maintaining genomic stability, and inducing senescence in response to oncogenic stresses. Which function(s) is/are most crucial for tumor suppression is likely to be dependent on the biological context, for example, the cell and tissue type of the tumors.

RB can be inactivated by point mutations, deletions, or binding to transforming viral proteins encoded by SV40, adenovirus, and human papillomavirus. Inactivation of RB can lead to cancer initiation and tumor progression. For initiation of cancer, abrogation of the control of the G1/S checkpoint and subsequent deregulation of cell-cycle control due to RB inactivation may be the key (384,385). However, this may only be crucial under specific conditions, such as tumor initiation from cycling progenitor cells, and may not universally apply to stem cells or differentiated cells. The role of RB inactivation in tumor progression is less clear, and may be related to a decrease in differentiation potential, chromosomal instability, inhibition of cellular senescence, promotion of angiogenesis and increase in metastatic potential (379).

Direct or indirect inactivation of RB can be found in almost all human cancers. In most cancers, RB deletion and mutations result in complete loss or marked reduction in RB expression (386). Although down-regulation of RB expression is frequent in leukemias, *RB1* mutations or deletions are not common among hematopoietic malignancies, except in about 20% of cases of CML in blast crisis (387,388). RB alterations due to deletions are infrequent and mutations are very rare in lymphoid malignancies. In general, loss of RB expression is uncommon in lymphomas, although it has been reported in ALCL (389). In contrast, indirect inactivation through phosphorylation of RB by loss of activity of CDK inhibitors such as p16 is common in lymphomas (390).

TNFAIP3/A20

The *TNFAIP3/A20* gene is located at the tumor suppressor gene locus 6q23, a known target of deletions in aggressive lymphomas (391,392). It was originally identified as a gene rapidly induced after TNF-α stimulation (393) and acts as an ubiquiting-editing enzyme with an essential role in terminating NF-κB activation in response to a variety of cell stimuli, including those that trigger the TNF receptor (TNFR), TLR pathways, CD40 and EBV LMP1 (394–398). The mechanism by which A20 terminates NF-κB signaling downstream of TNFR involves sequential deubiquitination of K-63 chains and ubiquitination of K-48 lysines in the TNF receptor-interacting protein (RIP), which is then targeted for proteasomal degradation (399). A20 also negatively regulates NF-κB activation induced by TLRs by disrupting the E2 ubiquitin enzyme complexes and consequently inhibiting the E3 ligase activities of TRAF6 and TRAF2 (400). The *TNFAIP3/A20* gene is inactivated by mutations and/or deletions in several lymphoma types characterized by the presence of constitutive NF-κB activity, including DLBCL (7% of all cases, and up to 30% of ABC-DLBCL cases) (301,401), marginal zone lymphoma (22%) (402,403), nodular sclerosis Hodgkin lymphoma (25%) (404), primary mediastinal B-cell lymphoma (36%) (404), and EBV-related neoplasms (405). In most of these cases, both alleles are lost due to focal deletions, somatic point mutations or promoter hypermethylation. This biallelic pattern of inactivation suggests that A20 may function as a classic tumor-suppressor gene. However, monoallelic inactivation by deletion or mutation alone has been also observed in these diseases, as well as in a small fraction of NK-cell lymphomas and MCLs (406), suggesting that A20 may contribute to tumorigenesis through reduction of gene dosage. Promoter methylation has been found in DLBCL, MCL and MALT lymphoma with a frequency of 26% to 42% (402,406).

Given its central role in terminating NF-κB responses, the loss or reduction of A20 activity may result in abnormally prolonged NF-κB activation in the presence of external stimulatory signals (397). Indeed, restoration of A20 in A20-deficient cell lines that are dependent on NF-κB results in decreased cell proliferation, increased apoptosis, and decreased tumorigenecity associated with reduced NF-κB activity (301,401).

Mixed-Lineage Leukemia 2 (MLL2)

Over the past 2 years, studies based on genome-wide, high-throughput sequencing analysis have uncovered a new class of mutated genes that had not been previously recognized and appear to play a major role as TSGs in hematologic malignancies. The identified genes include a number of histone lysine modification enzymes, with MLL2 and CREBBP (CREB-binding protein) representing the two most commonly mutated in B-NHL (267,303,407).

MLL2 encodes a highly conserved and ubiquitously expressed HMT that controls gene transcription by modifying the lysine-4 position of Histone 3 (H3K4) and by promoting PolII-dependent activation of target genes (284,285). H3K4 trimethylation represents a conserved mark of transcriptionally active chromatin and is closely associated with early transcribed regions of active genes, where it favors the recruitment of chromatin-remodeling enzymes by opposing the repressive function associated with H3K9 and H3K27 methylation (284). Up to 30% of DLBCLs and 89% of FLs harbor inactivating mutations of *MLL2*, including stop codons, frameshift mutations and splice site mutations that are predicted to generate truncated proteins lacking the C-terminal cluster of enzymatic domains (303,407). Missense mutations were also found in a smaller number of cases, although their functional significance has not been tested. While, in nearly one-third of DLBCL patients, both *MLL2* alleles are disrupted by mutations, consistent with the classical two-hit model for TSGs, the remaining large fraction of cases appear to have lost only one allele, suggesting that *MLL2* haploinsufficiency may have a tumorigenic role (303,407). Notably, monoallelic mutations of *MLL2* represent the causative lesion in Kabuki syndrome, an autosomal congenital disorder characterized by multiple developmental and intellectual abnormalities, documenting that reduction in *MLL2* gene dosage has pathogenic effects (286,408). Although further studies will be required to elucidate the precise role of *MLL2* in lymphomagenesis, the extremely high frequency of DLBCL and FL cases carrying MLL2 mutations suggests a major contribution to the development of these malignancies.

CREBBP and EP300

The *CREBBP* gene and its paralog *EP300* encode for two members of the KAT3 family of acetyltransferases that enhance transcription by acetylating a variety of histone and nonhistone nuclear proteins, also including BCL6 and P53 (409,410). Up to 40% of both DLBCLs and FLs display genomic deletions and/or somatic mutations that disrupt the enzymatic activity of the protein by either completely removing its acetyl transferase (AT) domain (stop codons, frameshift mutations and splice site mutations) or by reducing its affinity for acetyl-CoA (missense mutations in the AT domain) (267). With very few exceptions, these lesions are monoallelic, and the expression of the residual wild type allele is retained, suggesting that CREBBP and EP300 function as haploinsufficient TSGs. This model is strongly supported by the observation that haploinsufficiency of CREBBP and, in a smaller proportion of patients, EP300 plays a causative role in an autosomal congenital disease known as Rubinstein-Taybi syndrome, which is associated with predisposition to the development of tumors including malignant lymphomas (411,412).

SUMMARY AND CONCLUSIONS

Similar to other human cancers, hematopoietic malignancies occur through the activation of protooncogenes and the inactivation of tumor suppressor genes. The genome of hematopoietic neoplasms is characterized by the preponderance of reciprocal balanced chromosomal translocations. The molecular dissection of these alterations has led to the identification of protooncogenes that have been shown to contribute to the pathogenesis of these tumors. Although some of these genes are also involved in solid tumors, many of them are specific to lymphoid or myeloid tumors. Alterations of these genes lead to subversion of the normal cellular processes that control growth, proliferation, apoptosis, and differentiation of the hematopoietic cell, resulting in neoplastic transformation.

From a clinical standpoint, the identification and characterization of protooncogenes and tumor suppressor genes are important in several aspects. First, because many protooncogenes in hematopoietic malignancies are specific to certain subtypes, they can be used as diagnostic adjuncts for routine histopathologic analysis. This is exemplified by the utility of the detection of CCND1 and *BCL2* gene rearrangements in the diagnosis of MCL and follicular lymphoma, respectively. Second, studies of genes involved in leukemias and lymphomas may help refine the classification of hematologic tumors and allow the identification of subsets within each subtype, which may not be possible based on histologic analysis alone. Third, rearrangements and fusions involving protooncogenes provide sensitive and specific parameters for the detection of minimal residual disease, particularly in acute leukemia. Finally, the identification of protooncogenes and tumor suppressor genes involved in hematopoietic malignancies may provide the basis for the development of targeted therapeutic strategies.

References

1. Bishop JM. Molecular themes in oncogenesis. *Cell* 1991;64(2):235–248.
2. Stehelin D, Varmus HE, Vogt PK. DNA related to the transforming gene(s) of avian sarcoma viruses is present in normal avian DNA. *Nature* 1976;260(5547):170–173.
3. Stehelin DD, Guntaka RVR, Bishop JM. Purification of DNA complementary to nucleotide sequences required for neoplastic transformation of fibroblasts by avian sarcoma viruses. *J Mol Biol* 1976;101(3):349–365.
4. Krontiris TGT, Cooper GMG. Transforming activity of human tumor DNAs. *Proc Natl Acad Sci U S A* 1981;78(2):1181–1184.
5. Shih C, Padhy LC, Murray M, et al. Transforming genes of carcinomas and neuroblastomas introduced into mouse fibroblasts. *Nature* 1981;290(5803):261–264.
6. Perucho M, Goldfarb M, Shimizu K, et al. Human-tumor-derived cell lines contain common and different transforming genes. *Cell* 1981;27(3 Pt 2):467–476.

7. Hall A, Marshall CJ, Spurr NK, et al. Identification of transforming gene in two human sarcoma cell lines as a new member of the ras gene family located on chromosome 1. *Nature* 1983;303(5916):396–400.
8. Pulciani S, Santos E, Lauver AV, et al. Oncogenes in human tumor cell lines: molecular cloning of a transforming gene from human bladder carcinoma cells. *Proc Natl Acad Sci U S A* 1982;79(9):2845–2849.
9. Shimizu K, Goldfarb M, Suard Y, et al. Three human transforming genes are related to the viral ras oncogenes. *Proc Natl Acad Sci U S A* 1983;80(8): 2112–2116.
10. Marshall CJ. Tumor suppressor genes. *Cell* 1991;64(2):313–326.
11. Stanbridge E. Human tumor suppressor genes. *Annu Rev Genet* 1990.
12. Croce CM. Oncogenes and cancer. *N Engl J Med* 2008;358(5):502–511.
13. Barr FG. Chromosomal translocations involving paired box transcription factors in human cancer. *Int J Biochem Cell Biol* 1997;29(12):1449–1461.
14. Rabbitts THT. Perspective: chromosomal translocations can affect genes controlling gene expression and differentiation—why are these functions targeted? *J Pathol* 1999;187(1):39–42.
15. Cleary ML. Oncogenic conversion of transcription factors by chromosomal translocations. *Cell* 1991;66(4):619–622.
16. Nichols J, Nimer SD. Transcription factors, translocations, and leukemia. *Blood* 1992;80(12):2953–2963.
17. Strahl BD, Allis CD. The language of covalent histone modifications. *Nature* 2000;403(6765):41–45.
18. Jenuwein T, Allis CD. Translating the histone code. *Science* 2001;293(5532): 1074–1080.
19. Joneson T, Bar-Sagi D. Ras effectors and their role in mitogenesis and oncogenesis. *J Mol Med* 1997;75(8):587–593.
20. Sawyers CL. Signal transduction pathways involved in BCR-ABL transformation. *Baillieres Clin Haematol* 1997;10(2):223–231.
21. Rebollo A, Martínez AC. Ras proteins: recent advances and new functions. *Blood* 1999;94(9):2971–2980.
22. Morris CM, Kirtsein M, Valentine M, et al. Fusion of a kinase gene, Alk, to a nucleolar protein gene, Npm, in non-Hodgkins-lymphoma. *Science* 1994;263(5151):1281–1284.
23. Ladanyi MM. The NPM/ALK gene fusion in the pathogenesis of anaplastic large cell lymphoma. *Cancer Surv* 1997;30:59–75.
24. Warmuth M, Danhauser-Riedl S, Hallek M. Molecular pathogenesis of chronic myeloid leukemia: implications for new therapeutic strategies. *Ann Hematol* 1999;78(2):49–64.
25. Gishizky ML. Molecular mechanisms of Bcr-Abl-induced oncogenesis. *Cytokines Mol Ther* 1996;2(4):251–261.
26. Laneuville P. Abl tyrosine protein kinase. *Semin Immunol* 1995.
27. Shaul YY. C-Abl: activation and nuclear targets. *Cell Death Differ* 2000;7(1):10–16.
28. Wang JYJ. Abl tyrosine kinase in signal transduction and cell-cycle regulation. *Curr Opin Genet Dev* 1993;3(1):35–43.
29. Gotoh A, Broxmeyer HE. The function of BCR/ABL and related proto-oncogenes. *Curr Opin Hematol* 1997;4(1):3–11.
30. BOS J. Ras Oncogenes in human cancer—a review. *Cancer Res* 1989;49(17): 4682–4689.
31. Maruta H, Burgess AW. Regulation of the Ras signalling network. *Bioessays* 1994;16(7):489–496.
32. Cantley LC, Auger KR, Carpenter C, et al. Oncogenes and signal transduction. *Cell* 1991;64(2):281–302.
33. Downward J. Targeting RAS signalling pathways in cancer therapy. *Nat Rev Cancer* 2003;3(1):11–22.
34. Tiacci E, Trifonov V, Schiavoni G, et al. BRAF mutations in hairy-cell leukemia. *N Engl J Med* 2011;364(24):2305–2315.
35. Wickremasinghe RG, Hoffbrand AV. Biochemical and genetic control of apoptosis: relevance to normal hematopoiesis and hematological malignancies. *Blood* 1999;93(11):3587–3600.
36. McKenna SL, Cotter TG. Functional aspects of apoptosis in hematopoiesis and consequences of failure. *Adv Cancer Res* 1997;71:121–164.
37. Yoshida Y, Anzai N, Kawabata H. Apoptosis in normal and neoplastic hematopoiesis. *Crit Rev Oncol Hematol* 1996;24(3):185–211.
38. Youle RJ, Strasser A. The BCL2 protein family: opposing activities that mediate cell death. *Nat Rev Mol Cell Biol* 2008;9(1):47–59.
39. Korsmeyer SJ. BCL2 initiates a new category of oncogenes: regulators of cell death. *Blood* 1992;80(4):879–886.
40. Chao DT, Korsmeyer SJ. BCL2 family: regulators of cell death. *Annu Rev Immunol* 1998;16:395–419.
41. Cools J, Stover EH, Wlodarska I, et al. The FIP1L1-PDGFR[alpha] kinase in hypereosinophilic syndrome and chronic eosinophilic leukemia. *Curr Opin Hematol* 2004;11(1):51.
42. Bain BJ, Fletcher SH. Chronic eosinophilic leukemias and the myeloproliferative variant of the hypereosinophilic syndrome. *Immunol Allergy Clin North Am* 2007;27(3):377–388.
43. Golub TR, Barker GF, Lovett M, et al. Fusion of PDGF receptor beta to a novel ets-like gene, tel, in chronic myelomonocytic leukemia with t(5;12) chromosomal translocation. *Cell* 1994;77(2):307–316.
44. Tefferi A, Pardanani A. Clinical, genetic, and therapeutic insights into systemic mast cell disease. *Curr Opin Hematol* 2004;11(1):58–64.
45. Bartel DP. MicroRNAs: genomics, biogenesis, mechanism, and function. *Cell* 2004;116(2):281–297.
46. Zhang W, Dahlberg JE, Tam W. MicroRNAs in tumorigenesis: a primer. *Am J Pathol* 2007;171(3):728–738.
47. Davidson-Moncada J, Papavasiliou FN, Tam W. MicroRNAs of the immune system: roles in inflammation and cancer. *Ann N Y Acad Sci* 2010;1183:183–194.
48. Calin GA, Sevignani C, Croce CM, et al. Human microRNA genes are frequently located at fragile sites and genomic regions involved in cancers. *Proc Natl Acad Sci U S A* 2004;101(9):2999–3004.
49. Calin GA, Croce CM. MicroRNA signatures in human cancers. *Nat Rev Cancer* 2006;6(11):857–866.
50. Shenouda SK, Alahari SK. MicroRNA function in cancer: oncogene or a tumor suppressor? *Cancer Metastasis Rev* 2009;28(3–4):369–378.
51. Chuang JC, Jones PA. Epigenetics and microRNAs. *Pediatr Res* 2007;61(5 Pt 2): 24R–29R.
52. Zhang L, Huang J, Yang N, et al. MicroRNAs exhibit high frequency genomic alterations in human cancer. *Proc Natl Acad Sci U S A* 2006;103(24):9136–9141.
53. Nakamura T, Canaani E, Croce CM. Oncogenic All1 fusion proteins target Drosha-mediated microRNA processing. *Proc Natl Acad Sci U S A* 2007;104(26): 10980–10985.
54. Diederichs SS, Haber DAD. Sequence variations of microRNAs in human cancer: alterations in predicted secondary structure do not affect processing. *Cancer Res* 2006;66(12):6097–6104.
55. Johansson BB, Mertens FF, Mitelman FF. Primary vs. secondary neoplasia-associated chromosomal abnormalities—balanced rearrangements vs. genomic imbalances? *Genes Chromosomes Cancer* 1996;16(3):155–163.
56. Kuppers R, Dalla-Favera R. Mechanisms of chromosomal translocations in B cell lymphomas. *Oncogene* 2001;20(40):5580–5594.
57. Fugmann S, Lee A, Shockett P, et al. The rag proteins and V(D)J recombination: complexes, ends, and transposition. *Annu Rev Immunol* 2000;18:495–527.
58. Nambiar M, Raghavan SC. How does DNA break during chromosomal translocations? *Nucleic Acids Res* 2011;39(14):5813–5825.
59. Teng G, Papavasiliou FN. Immunoglobulin somatic hypermutation. *Annu Rev Genet* 2007;41(1):107–120.
60. Nussenzweig A, Nussenzweig MC. Origin of chromosomal translocations in lymphoid cancer. *Cell* 2010;141(1):27–38.
61. Pasqualucci L, Migliazza A, Fracchiolla N, et al. BCL-6 mutations in normal germinal center B cells: evidence of somatic hypermutation acting outside Ig loci. *Proc Natl Acad Sci U S A* 1998;95(20):11816–11821.
62. Shen HM, Peters A, Baron B, et al. Mutation of BCL-6 gene in normal B cells by the process of somatic hypermutation of Ig genes. *Science* 1998;280(5370): 1750–1752.
63. Gordon MS, Kanegai CM, Doerr JR, et al. Somatic hypermutation of the B cell receptor genes B29 (Igbeta, CD79b) and mb1 (Igalpha, CD79a). *Proc Natl Acad Sci U S A* 2003;100(7):4126–4131.
64. Tanaka A, Shen HM, Ratnam S, et al. Attracting AID to targets of somatic hypermutation. *J Exp Med* 2010;207(2):405–415.
65. Peng HZ, Du M-Q, Koulis A, et al. Nonimmunoglobulin gene hypermutation in germinal center B cells. *Blood* 1999;93(7):2167–2172.
66. Pasqualucci L, Neumeister P, Goossens T, et al. Hypermutation of multiple proto-oncogenes in B-cell diffuse large-cell lymphomas. *Nature* 2001;412(6844): 341–346.
67. Staszewski O, Baker RE, Ucher AJ, et al. Activation-induced cytidine deaminase induces reproducible DNA breaks at many non-Ig Loci in activated B cells. *Mol Cell* 2011;41(2):232–242.
68. Neri A, Barriga F, Knowles DM, et al. Different regions of the immunoglobulin heavy-chain locus are involved in chromosomal translocations in distinct pathogenetic forms of Burkitt lymphoma. *Proc Natl Acad Sci U S A* 1988;85(8):2748–2752.
69. Robbiani DF, Bothmer A, Callen E, et al. AID is required for the chromosomal breaks in c-myc that lead to c-myc/IgH translocations. *Cell* 2008;135(6): 1028–1038.
70. Teng G, Hakimpour P, Landgraf P, et al. MicroRNA-155 is a negative regulator of activation-induced cytidine deaminase. *Immunity* 2008;28(5):621–629.
71. Dorsett Y, McBride KM, Jankovic M, et al. MicroRNA-155 suppresses activation-induced cytidine deaminase-mediated Myc-Igh translocation. *Immunity* 2008;28(5):630–638.
72. Pasqualucci L, Bhagat G, Jankovic M, et al. AID is required for germinal center-derived lymphomagenesis. *Nat Genet* 2008;40(1):108–112.
73. Romana S, Poirel H, Valle Della V, et al. Molecular analysis of chromosomal breakpoints in three examples of chromosomal translocation involving the TEL gene. *Leukemia* 1999;13(11):1754–1759.
74. Wang Q, Gao F, May WS, et al. BCL2 negatively regulates DNA double-strand-break repair through a nonhomologous end-joining pathway. *Mol Cell* 2008;29(4): 488–498.
75. Kumar TS, Kari V, Choudhary B, et al. Anti-apoptotic protein BCL2 down-regulates DNA end joining in cancer cells. *J Biol Chem* 2010;285(42):32657–32670.
76. Kolomietz E, Meyn MS, Pandita A, et al. The role of Alu repeat clusters as mediators of recurrent chromosomal aberrations in tumors. *Genes Chromosomes Cancer* 2002;35(2):97–112.
77. Hess JL. MLL: a histone methyltransferase disrupted in leukemia. *Trends Mol Med* 2004;10(10):500–507.
78. Jeffs AR, Wells E, Morris CM. Nonrandom distribution of interspersed repeat elements in the BCR and ABL1 genes and its relation to breakpoint cluster regions. *Genes Chromosomes Cancer* 2001;32(2):144–154.
79. Gu X, Shivarov V, Strout MP. The role of activation-induced cytidine deaminase in lymphomagenesis. *Curr Opin Hematol* 2012;19:292–298.
80. Gagyi E, Balogh Z, Bödör C, et al. Somatic hypermutation of IGVH genes and aberrant somatic hypermutation in follicular lymphoma without BCL2 gene rearrangement and expression. *Haematologica* 2008;93(12):1822–1828.
81. Gaidano G, Pasqualucci L, Capello D, et al. Aberrant somatic hypermutation in multiple subtypes of AIDS-associated non-Hodgkin lymphoma. *Blood* 2003;102(5):1833–1841.
82. Cerri M, Capello D, Muti G, et al. Aberrant somatic hypermutation in post-transplant lymphoproliferative disorders. *Br J Haematol* 2004;127(3):362–364.
83. Liso A, Capello D, Marafioti T, et al. Aberrant somatic hypermutation in tumor cells of nodular-lymphocyte-predominant and classic Hodgkin lymphoma. *Blood* 2006;108(3):1013–1020.
84. Montesinos-Rongen M, Van Roost D, Schaller C, et al. Primary diffuse large B-cell lymphomas of the central nervous system are targeted by aberrant somatic hypermutation. *Blood* 2004;103(5):1869–1875.
85. Schwab M. Oncogene amplification in solid tumors. *Semin Cancer Biol* 1999;9(4):319–325.
86. Rui L, Emre NCT, Kruhlak MJ, et al. Cooperative epigenetic modulation by cancer amplicon genes. *Cancer Cell* 2010;18(6):590–605.
87. Green MR, Monti S, Rodig SJ, et al. Integrative analysis reveals selective 9p24.1 amplification, increased PD-1 ligand expression, and further induction via JAK2 in nodular sclerosing Hodgkin lymphoma and primary mediastinal large B-cell lymphoma. *Blood* 2010;116(17):3268–3277.
88. Wessendorf S, Schwaenen C, Kohlhammer H, et al. Hidden gene amplifications in aggressive B-cell non-Hodgkin lymphomas detected by microarray-based comparative genomic hybridization. *Oncogene* 2003;22(9):1425–1429.
89. Hernández SE, Krishnaswami M, Miller AL, et al. How do Abl family kinases regulate cell shape and movement? *Trends Cell Biol* 2004;14(1):36–44.
90. Woodring PJ, Hunter T, Wang JYJ. Regulation of F-actin-dependent processes by the Abl family of tyrosine kinases. *J Cell Sci* 2003;116(Pt 13):2613–2626.

91. Deininger M, Goldman J, Melo J. The molecular biology of chronic myeloid leukemia. *Blood* 2000;96(10):3343–3356.
92. Dash AB, Williams IR, Kutok JL, et al. A murine model of CML blast crisis induced by cooperation between BCR/ABL and NUP98/HOXA9. *Proc Natl Acad Sci U S A* 2002;99(11):7622–7627.
93. Cuenco GM, Ren R. Cooperation of BCR-ABL and AML1/MDS1/EVI1 in blocking myeloid differentiation and rapid induction of an acute myelogenous leukemia. *Oncogene* 2001;20(57):8236–8248.
94. Chambon P. A decade of molecular biology of retinoic acid receptors. *FASEB J* 1996;10(9):940–954.
95. Borrow J, Goddard AD, Sheer D, et al. Molecular analysis of acute promyelocytic leukemia breakpoint cluster region on chromosome 17. *Science* 1990;249(4976):1577–1580.
96. de Thé H, Chomienne C, Lanotte M, et al. The t(15;17) translocation of acute promyelocytic leukaemia fuses the retinoic acid receptor alpha gene to a novel transcribed locus. *Nature* 1990;347(6293):558–561.
97. Alcalay M, Zangrilli D, Fagioli M, et al. Expression pattern of the RAR alpha-PML fusion gene in acute promyelocytic leukemia. *Proc Natl Acad Sci U S A* 1992;89(11):4840–4844.
98. Dyck JA, Maul GG, Miller WH, et al. A novel macromolecular structure is a target of the promyelocyte-retinoic acid receptor oncoprotein. *Cell* 1994;76(2):333–343.
99. Hodges M, Tissot C, Howe K, et al. Structure, organization, and dynamics of promyelocytic leukemia protein nuclear bodies. *Am J Hum Genet* 1998;63(2): 297–304.
100. Redner RL, Rush EA, Faas S, et al. The t(5;17) variant of acute promyelocytic leukemia expresses a nucleophosmin-retinoic acid receptor fusion. *Blood* 1996;87(3):882–886.
101. Wells RA, Catzavelos C, Kamel-Reid S. Fusion of retinoic acid receptor alpha to NuMA, the nuclear mitotic apparatus protein, by a variant translocation in acute promyelocytic leukaemia. *Nat Genet* 1997;17(1):109–113.
102. Catalano A, Dawson MA, Somana K, et al. The PRKAR1A gene is fused to RARA in a new variant acute promyelocytic leukemia. *Blood* 2007;110(12):4073–4076.
103. Arnould C, Philippe C, Bourdon V, et al. The signal transducer and activator of transcription STAT5b gene is a new partner of retinoic acid receptor {alpha} in acute promyelocytic-like leukaemia. *Hum Mol Genet* 1999;8(9):1741–1749.
104. Yamamoto Y, Tsuzuki S, Tsuzuki M, et al. BCOR as a novel fusion partner of retinoic acid receptor alpha in a t(X;17)(p11;q12) variant of acute promyelocytic leukemia. *Blood* 2010;116(20):4274–4283.
105. Lin RJ, Evans RM. Acquisition of oncogenic potential by RAR chimeras in acute promyelocytic leukemia through formation of homodimers. *Mol Cell* 2000;5(5):821–830.
106. Hong SH, David G, Wong CW, et al. SMRT corepressor interacts with PLZF and with the PML-retinoic acid receptor alpha (RARalpha) and PLZF-RARalpha oncoproteins associated with acute promyelocytic leukemia. *Proc Natl Acad Sci U S A* 1997;94(17):9028–9033.
107. Villa R, Pasini D, Gutierrez A, et al. Role of the polycomb repressive complex 2 in acute promyelocytic leukemia. *Cancer Cell* 2007;11(6):513–525.
108. Martens JHA, Brinkman AB, Simmer F, et al. PML-RARalpha/RXR alters the epigenetic landscape in acute promyelocytic leukemia. *Cancer Cell* 2010;17(2): 173–185.
109. He LZ, Merghoub T, Pandolfi PP. In vivo analysis of the molecular pathogenesis of acute promyelocytic leukemia in the mouse and its therapeutic implications. *Oncogene* 1999;18(38):5278–5292.
110. Cheng GX, Zhu XH, Men XQ, et al. Distinct leukemia phenotypes in transgenic mice and different corepressor interactions generated by promyelocytic leukemia variant fusion genes PLZF-RARalpha and NPM-RARalpha. *Proc Natl Acad Sci U S A* 1999;96(11):6318–6323.
111. He LZ, Guidez F, Tribioli C, et al. Distinct interactions of PML-RARalpha and PLZF-RARalpha with co-repressors determine differential responses to RA in APL. *Nat Genet* 1998;18(2):126–135.
112. Mu ZM, Le XF, Glassman AB, et al. The biologic function of PML and its role in acute promyelocytic leukemia. *Leuk Lymphoma* 1996;23(3–4):277–285.
113. Grimwade D, Solomon E. Characterisation of the PML/RAR alpha rearrangement associated with t(15;17) acute promyelocytic leukaemia. *Curr Top Microbiol Immunol* 1997;220:81–112.
114. Seeler JSJ, Dejean AA. The PML nuclear bodies: actors or extras? *Curr Opin Genet Dev* 1999;9(3):362–367.
115. Wang ZG, Ruggero D, Ronchetti S, et al. PML is essential for multiple apoptotic pathways. *Nat Genet* 1998;20(3):266–272.
116. Ohki M. Molecular basis of the t(8;21) translocation in acute myeloid leukaemia. *Semin Cancer Biol* 1993;4(6):369–375.
117. Andrieu V, RadfordWeiss I, Troussard X, et al. Molecular detection of t(8;21)/AML1-ETO in AML M1/M2: Correlation with cytogenetics, morphology and immunophenotype. *Br J Haematol* 1996;92(4):855–865.
118. Lo Coco F, Pisegna S, Diverio D. The AML1 gene: a transcription factor involved in the pathogenesis of myeloid and lymphoid leukemias. *Haematologica* 1997;82(3):364–370.
119. Meyers S, Downing JR, Hiebert SW. Identification of AML-1 and the (8;21) translocation protein (AML-1/ETO) as sequence-specific DNA-binding proteins: the runt homology domain is required for DNA binding and protein-protein interactions. *Mol Cell Biol* 1993;13(10):6336–6345.
120. Okuda T, van Deursen J, Hiebert SW, et al. AML1, the target of multiple chromosomal translocations in human leukemia, is essential for normal fetal liver hematopoiesis. *Cell* 1996;84(2):321–330.
121. Wang Q, Stacy T, Binder M, et al. Disruption of the Cbfa2 gene causes necrosis and hemorrhaging in the central nervous system and blocks definitive hematopoiesis. *Proc Natl Acad Sci U S A* 1996;93(8):3444–3449.
122. Erickson PF, Robinson M, Owens G, et al. The ETO portion of acute myeloid leukemia t(8;21) fusion transcript encodes a highly evolutionarily conserved, putative transcription factor. *Cancer Res* 1994;54(7):1782–1786.
123. Melnick AM, Westendorf JJ, Polinger A, et al. The ETO protein disrupted in t(8;21)-associated acute myeloid leukemia is a corepressor for the promyelocytic leukemia zinc finger protein. *Mol Cell Biol* 2000;20(6):2075–2086.
124. Le XF, Claxton D, Kornblau S, et al. Characterization of the ETO and AML1-ETO proteins involved in 8;21 translocation in acute myelogenous leukemia. *Eur J Haematol* 1998;60(4):217–225.
125. Wang JJ, Wang MM, Liu JMJ. Transformation properties of the ETO gene, fusion partner in t(8:21) leukemias. *Cancer Res* 1997;57(14):2951–2955.
126. Erickson P, Gao J, Chang KS, et al. Identification of breakpoints in t(8;21) acute myelogenous leukemia and isolation of a fusion transcript, AML1/ETO, with similarity to *Drosophila* segmentation gene, runt. *Blood* 1992;80(7):1825–1831.
127. Nucifora G, Rowley J. AML1 and the 8;21 and 3;21 translocations in acute and chronic myeloid leukemia. *Blood* 1995;86(1):1–14.
128. McNeil S, Zeng C, Stein GS. The t(8;21) chromosomal translocation in acute myelogenous leukemia modifies intranuclear targeting of the AML1/CBFalpha2 transcription factor. *Proc Natl Acad Sci U S A* 1999;96(26):14882–14887.
129. Liu Y, Cheney MD, Gaudet JJ, et al. The tetramer structure of the Nervy homology two domain, NHR2, is critical for AML1/ETO's activity. *Cancer Cell* 2006;9(4):249–260.
130. Liu S, Shen T, Huynh L, et al. Interplay of RUNX1/MTG8 and DNA methyltransferase 1 in acute myeloid leukemia. *Cancer Res* 2005;65(4):1277–1284.
131. Yergeau DA, Hetherington CJ, Wang Q, et al. Embryonic lethality and impairment of haematopoiesis in mice heterozygous for an AML1-ETO fusion gene. *Nat Genet* 1997;15(3):303–306.
132. Castilla LH, Wijmenga C, Wang Q, et al. Failure of embryonic hematopoiesis and lethal hemorrhages in mouse embryos heterozygous for a knocked-in leukemia gene CBFB-MYH11. *Cell* 1996;87(4):687–696.
133. Pabst T, Mueller BU, Harakawa N, et al. AML1-ETO downregulates the granulocytic differentiation factor C/EBPalpha in t(8;21) myeloid leukemia. *Nat Med* 2001;7(4):444–451.
134. Vangala R, Heiss-Neumann M, Rangatia J, et al. The myeloid master regulator transcription factor PU.1 is inactivated by AML1-ETO in t(8;21) myeloid leukemia. *Blood* 2003;101(1):270–277.
135. Jakubowiak A, Pouponnot C, Berguido F, et al. Inhibition of the transforming growth factor beta 1 signaling pathway by the AML1/ETO leukemia-associated fusion protein. *J Biol Chem* 2000;275(51):40282–40287.
136. Nimer SD, Moore MAS. Effects of the leukemia-associated AML1-ETO protein on hematopoietic stem and progenitor cells. *Oncogene* 2004;23(24):4249–4254.
137. Fazi F, Racanicchi S, Zardo G, et al. Epigenetic silencing of the myelopoiesis regulator microRNA-223 by the AML1/ETO oncoprotein. *Cancer Cell* 2007;12(5): 457–466.
138. Meyer C, Schneider B, Jakob S, et al. The MLL recombinome of acute leukemias. *Leukemia* 2006;20(5):777–784.
139. De Braekeleer M, Morel F, Le Bris M-J, et al. The MLL gene and translocations involving chromosomal band 11q23 in acute leukemia. *Anti Cancer Res* 2005; 25(3B):1931–1944.
140. Poirel H, Rack K, Delabesse E, et al. Incidence and characterization of MLL gene (11q23) rearrangements in acute myeloid leukemia M1 and M5. *Blood* 1996;87(6):2496–2505.
141. Bernard OA, Berger R. Molecular basis of 11q23 rearrangements in hematopoietic malignant proliferations. *Genes Chromosomes Cancer* 1995;13(2):75–85.
142. Downing JR, Look AT. MLL fusion genes in the 11q23 acute leukemias. *Cancer Treat Res* 1996;84:73–92.
143. Rubnitz JE, Behm FG, Downing JR. 11q23 rearrangements in acute leukemia. *Leukemia* 1996;10(1):74–82.
144. Krivtsov AV, Armstrong SA. MLL translocations, histone modifications and leukaemia stem-cell development. *Nat Rev Cancer* 2007;7(11):823–833.
145. Johansson B, Moorman AV, Secker-Walker LM. Derivative chromosomes of 11q23-translocations in hematologic malignancies. European 11q23 Workshop participants. *Leukemia* 1998;12(5):828–833.
146. Mbangkollo D, Burnett R, McCabe N, et al. The human MLL gene: nucleotide sequence, homology to the Drosophila trx zinc-finger domain, and alternative splicing. *DNA Cell Biol* 1995;14(6):475–483.
147. Broeker PL, Harden A, Rowley JD, et al. The mixed lineage leukemia (MLL) protein involved in 11q23 translocations contains a domain that binds cruciform DNA and scaffold attachment region (SAR) DNA. *Curr Top Microbiol Immunol* 1996;211:259–268.
148. Milne TA, Briggs SD, Brock HW, et al. MLL targets SET domain methyltransferase activity to Hox gene promoters. *Mol Cell* 2002;10(5):1107–1117.
149. Nakamura T, Mori T, Tada S, et al. ALL-1 is a histone methyltransferase that assembles a supercomplex of proteins involved in transcriptional regulation. *Mol Cell* 2002;10(5):1119–1128.
150. Slany RK, Lavau C, Cleary ML. The oncogenic capacity of HRX-ENL requires the transcriptional transactivation activity of ENL and the DNA binding motifs of HRX. *Mol Cell Biol* 1998;18(1):122–129.
151. Slany RK. When epigenetics kills: MLL fusion proteins in leukemia. *Hematol Oncol* 2005;23(1):1–9.
152. So CW, Cleary ML. Common mechanism for oncogenic activation of MLL by forkhead family proteins. *Blood* 2003;101(2):633–639.
153. So CW, Lin M, Ayton PM, et al. Dimerization contributes to oncogenic activation of MLL chimeras in acute leukemias. *Cancer Cell* 2003;4(2):99–110.
154. Hall PA, Russell SEH. The pathobiology of the septin gene family. *J Pathol* 2004;204(4):489–505.
155. Sobulo O, Borrow J, Tomek R, et al. MLL is fused to CBP, a histone acetyltransferase, in therapy-related acute myeloid leukemia with a t(11;16)(q23;p13.3). *Proc Natl Acad Sci U S A* 1997;94(16):8732–8737.
156. Ida K, Kitabayashi I, Taki T, et al. Adenoviral E1A-associated protein p300 is involved in acute myeloid leukemia with t(11;22)(q23;q13). *Blood* 1997;90(12): 4699–4704.
157. Corral J, Lavenir I, Impey H, et al. An Mll-AF9 fusion gene made by homologous recombination causes acute leukemia in chimeric mice: a method to create fusion oncogenes. *Cell* 1996;85(6):853–861.
158. Dobson CL, Warren AJ, Rabbitts TH, et al. The mll-AF9 gene fusion in mice controls myeloproliferation and specifies acute myeloid leukaemogenesis. *EMBO J* 1999;18(13):3564–3574.
159. So CW, Karsunky H, Passegué E, et al. MLL-GAS7 transforms multipotent hematopoietic progenitors and induces mixed lineage leukemias in mice. *Cancer Cell* 2003;3(2):161–171.
160. Zeisig BB, García-Cuéllar MP, Winkler TH, et al. The Oncoprotein MLL–ENL disturbs hematopoietic lineage determination and transforms a biphenotypic lymphoid/myeloid cell. *Oncogene* 2003;22(11):1629–1637.
161. Barabé F, Kennedy JA, Hope KJ, et al. Modeling the initiation and progression of human acute leukemia in mice. *Science* 2007;316(5824):600–604.
162. Castilla LH, Garrett L, Adya N, et al. The fusion gene Cbfb-MYH11 blocks myeloid differentiation and predisposes mice to acute myelomonocytic leukaemia. *Nat Genet* 1999;23(2):144–146.

163. Kundu M, Chen A, Anderson S, et al. Role of Cbfb in hematopoiesis and perturbations resulting from expression of the leukemogenic fusion gene Cbfb-MYH11. *Blood* 2002;100(7):2449–2456.
164. Castilla LH, Perrat P, Martinez NJ, et al. Identification of genes that synergize with Cbfb-MYH11 in the pathogenesis of acute myeloid leukemia. *Proc Natl Acad Sci U S A* 2004;101(14):4924–4929.
165. Landrette SF, Kuo Y-H, Hensen K, et al. Plagl and Plagl2 are oncogenes that induce acute myeloid leukemia in cooperation with Cbfb-MYH11. *Blood* 2005;105(7):2900–2907.
166. Lutterbach B, Hiebert SW. Role of the transcription factor AML-1 in acute leukemia and hematopoietic differentiation. *Gene* 2000;245(2):223–235.
167. Shigesada K, van de Sluis B, Liu P. Mechanism of leukemogenesis by the inv(16) chimeric gene CBFB/PEBP2B-MHY11. *Oncogene* 2004;23(24):4297–4307.
168. Lutterbach B, Hou Y, Durst KL, et al. The inv(16) encodes an acute myeloid leukemia 1 transcriptional corepressor. *Proc Natl Acad Sci U S A* 1999;96(22): 12822–12827.
169. Durst KL, Lutterbach B, Kummalue T, et al. The inv(16) fusion protein associates with corepressors via a smooth muscle myosin heavy-chain domain. *Mol Cell Biol* 2003;23(2):607–619.
170. Troussard X, Rimokh R, Valensi F, et al. Heterogeneity of t(1;19)(q23;p13) acute leukaemias. French Haematological Cytology Group. *Br J Haematol* 1995;89(3):516–526.
171. Nourse J, Mellentin JD, Galili N, et al. Chromosomal translocation t(1;19) results in synthesis of a homeobox fusion mRNA that codes for a potential chimeric transcription factor. *Cell* 1990;60(4):535–545.
172. Kamps MP, Murre C, Sun XH, et al. A new homeobox gene contributes the DNA binding domain of the t(1;19) translocation protein in pre-B ALL. *Cell* 1990;60(4):547–555.
173. Hunger SPS. Chromosomal translocations involving the E2A gene in acute lymphoblastic leukemia: clinical features and molecular pathogenesis. *Blood* 1996;87(4):1211–1224.
174. Kamps MP, Wright DD. Oncoprotein E2A-Pbx1 immortalizes a myeloid progenitor in primary marrow cultures without abrogating its factor-dependence. *Oncogene* 1994;9(11):3159–3166.
175. Kamps MP. E2A-Pbx1 induces growth, blocks differentiation, and interacts with other homeodomain proteins regulating normal differentiation. *Curr Top Microbiol Immunol* 1997;220:25–43.
176. Kamps MP, Baltimore D. E2A-Pbx1, the t(1;19) translocation protein of human pre-B-cell acute lymphocytic leukemia, causes acute myeloid leukemia in mice. *Mol Cell Biol* 1993;13(1):351–357.
177. Dedera D, Waller E, Lebrun D, et al. Chimeric homeobox gene E2a-Pbx1 induces proliferation, apoptosis, and malignant-lymphomas in transgenic mice. *Cell* 1993;74(5):833–843.
178. Sykes D, Kamps M. E2a/Pbx1 induces the rapid proliferation of stem cell factor-dependent murine pro-t cells that cause acute T-lymphoid or myeloid leukemias in mice. *Mol Cell Biol* 2004;24(3):1256–1269.
179. Bourette RP, Grasset M-F, Mouchiroud G. E2a/Pbx1 oncogene inhibits terminal differentiation but not myeloid potential of pro-T cells. *Oncogene* 2007;26(2): 234–247.
180. Casagrande G, Kronnie G, Basso G. The effects of siRNA-mediated inhibition of E2A-PBX1 on EB-1 and Wnt16b expression in the 697 pre-B leukemia cell line. *Haematologica* 2006;91(6):765–771.
181. Aspland SE, Bendall HH, Murre C. The role of E2A-PBX1 in leukemogenesis. *Oncogene* 2001;20(40):5708–5717.
182. Fu X, Kamps MP. E2a-Pbx1 induces aberrant expression of tissue-specific and developmentally regulated genes when expressed in NIH 3T3 fibroblasts. *Mol Cell Biol* 1997;17(3):1503–1512.
183. de Lau WBW, Hurenkamp JJ, van Dijk MA, et al. The gene encoding the granulocyte colony-stimulating factor receptor is a target for deregulation in pre-B ALL by the t(1;19)-specific oncoprotein E2A-Pbx1. *Oncogene* 1998;17(4):503–510.
184. McWhirter J, Neuteboom S, Wancewicz E, et al. Oncogenic homeodomain transcription factor E2A-Pbx1 activates a novel WNT gene in pre-B acute lymphoblastoid leukemia. *Proc Natl Acad Sci U S A* 1999;96(20):11464–11469.
185. Fu X, Roberts WG, Nobile V, et al. MAngiogenin-3, a target gene of oncoprotein E2a-Pbx1, encodes a new angiogenic member of the angiogenin family. *Growth Factors* 1999;17(2):125–137.
186. Kadin ME, Morris SW. The t(2;5) in human lymphomas. *Leuk Lymphoma* 1998;29(3–4):249–256.
187. Lamant L, Meggetto F, Delsol G, et al. High incidence of the t(2;5)(p23;q35) translocation in anaplastic large cell lymphoma and its lack of detection in Hodgkin's disease. Comparison of cytogenetic analysis, reverse transcriptase-polymerase chain reaction, and P-80 immunostaining. *Blood* 1996;87(1):284–291.
188. Cataldo KA, Jalal SM, Law ME, et al. Detection of t(2;5) in anaplastic large cell lymphoma: comparison of immunohistochemical studies, FISH, and RT-PCR in paraffin-embedded tissue. *Am J Surg Pathol* 1999;23(11):1386–1392.
189. Mathew P, Sanger WG, Weisenburger DD, et al. Detection of the t(2;5)(p23;q35) and NPM-ALK fusion in non-Hodgkin's lymphoma by two-color fluorescence in situ hybridization. *Blood* 1997;89(5):1678–1685.
190. Pulford K, Lamant L, Morris SW, et al. Detection of anaplastic lymphoma kinase (ALK) and nucleolar protein nucleophosmin (NPM)-ALK proteins in normal and neoplastic cells with the monoclonal antibody ALK1. *Blood* 1997;89(4):1394–1404.
191. Shiota M, Nakamura S, Ichinohasama R, et al. Anaplastic large cell lymphomas expressing the novel chimeric protein p80NPM/ALK: a distinct clinicopathologic entity. *Blood* 1995;86(5):1954–1960.
192. Shiota M, Mori S. Anaplastic large cell lymphomas expressing the novel chimeric protein p80NPM/ALK: a distinct clinicopathologic entity. *Leukemia* 1997;11(Suppl 3):538–540.
193. Bai RY, Dieter P, Peschel C, et al. Nucleophosmin-anaplastic lymphoma kinase of large-cell anaplastic lymphoma is a constitutively active tyrosine kinase that utilizes phospholipase C-gamma to mediate its mitogenicity. *Mol Cell Biol* 1998;18(12):6951–6961.
194. Bischof D, Pulford K, Morris SW, et al. Role of the nucleophosmin (NPM) portion of the non-Hodgkin's lymphoma-associated NPM-anaplastic lymphoma kinase fusion protein in oncogenesis. *Mol Cell Biol* 1997;17(4):2312–2325.
195. Kuefer MU, Look AT, Pulford K, et al. Retrovirus-mediated gene transfer of NPM-ALK causes lymphoid malignancy in mice. *Blood* 1997;90(8):2901–2910.
196. Chiarle R, Gong JZ, Guasparri I, et al. NPM-ALK transgenic mice spontaneously develop T-cell lymphomas and plasma cell tumors. *Blood* 2003;101(5):1919–1927.
197. Jäger R, Hahne J, Jacob A, et al. Mice transgenic for NPM-ALK develop non-Hodgkin lymphomas. *Anticancer Res* 2005;25(5):3191–3196.
198. Falini B, Pulford K, Pucciarini A, et al. Lymphomas expressing ALK fusion protein(s) other than NPM-ALK. *Blood* 1999;94(10):3509–3515.
199. Chiarle R, Voena C, Ambrogio C, et al. The anaplastic lymphoma kinase in the pathogenesis of cancer. *Nat Rev Cancer* 2008;8(1):11–23.
200. Hernández L, Pinyol M, Hernández S, et al. TRK-fused gene (TFG) is a new partner of ALK in anaplastic large cell lymphoma producing two structurally different TFG-ALK translocations. *Blood* 1999;94(9):3265–3268.
201. Chiarle RR, Simmons WJW, Inghirami GG, et al. Stat3 is required for ALK-mediated lymphomagenesis and provides a possible therapeutic target. *Nat Med* 2005;11(6):623–629.
202. Ambrogio C, Voena C, Manazza AD, et al. P130Cas mediates the transforming properties of the anaplastic lymphoma kinase. *Blood* 2005;106(12):3907–3916.
203. Colomba A, Courilleau D, Ramel D, et al. Activation of Rac1 and the exchange factor Vav3 are involved in NPM-ALK signaling in anaplastic large cell lymphomas. *Oncogene* 2008;27(19):2728–2736.
204. Voena C, Conte C, Ambrogio C, et al. The tyrosine phosphatase Shp2 interacts with NPM-ALK and regulates anaplastic lymphoma cell growth and migration. *Cancer Res* 2007;67(9):4278–4286.
205. Cussac D, Greenland C, Roche S, et al. Nucleophosmin-anaplastic lymphoma kinase of anaplastic large-cell lymphoma recruits, activates, and uses pp60c-src to mediate its mitogenicity. *Blood* 2004;103(4):1464–1471.
206. Watanabe M, Sasaki M, Itoh K, et al. JunB induced by constitutive CD30-extracellular signal-regulated kinase 1/2 mitogen-activated protein kinase signaling activates the CD30 promoter in anaplastic large cell lymphoma and reed-sternberg cells of Hodgkin lymphoma. *Cancer Res* 2005;65(17):7628–7634.
207. Hsu FY-Y, Johnston PB, Burke KA, et al. The expression of CD30 in anaplastic large cell lymphoma is regulated by nucleophosmin-anaplastic lymphoma kinase-mediated JunB level in a cell type-specific manner. *Cancer Res* 2006;66(18):9002–9008.
208. Marzec M, Zhang Q, Goradia A, et al. Oncogenic kinase NPM/ALK induces through STAT3 expression of immunosuppressive protein CD274 (PD-L1, B7-H1). *Proc Natl Acad Sci U S A* 2008;105(52):20852–20857.
209. Niedobitek G, Agathanggelou A, Rowe M, et al. Heterogeneous expression of Epstein-Barr virus latent proteins in endemic Burkitt's lymphoma. *Blood* 1995;86(2):659–665.
210. Bertoni F, Cotter FE, Zucca E. Molecular genetics of extranodal marginal zone (MALT-type) B-cell lymphoma. *Leuk Lymphoma* 1999;35(1):57–68.
211. Horsman D, Gascoyne R, Klasa R, et al. T(11;18)(q21;q21.1): a recurring translocation in lymphomas of mucosa-associated lymphoid tissue (MALT)? *Genes Chromosomes Cancer* 1992;4(2):183–187.
212. Auer IA, Gascoyne RD, Connors JM, et al. T(11;18)(q21;q21) is the most common translocation in MALT lymphomas. *Ann Oncol* 1997;8(10):979–985.
213. Ott GG, Katzenberger TT, Müller-Hermelink HKH, et al. The t(11;18)(q21;q21) chromosome translocation is a frequent and specific aberration in low-grade but not high-grade malignant non-Hodgkin's lymphomas of the mucosa-associated lymphoid tissue (MALT-) type. *Cancer Res* 1997;57(18):3944–3948.
214. Dierlamm J, Baens M, Wlodarska I, et al. The apoptosis inhibitor gene API2 and a novel 18q gene, MLT, are recurrently rearranged in the t(11;18)(q21;q21) associated with mucosa-associated lymphoid tissue lymphomas. *Blood* 1999; 93(11):3601–3609.
215. Morgan J, Yin Y, Borowsky A, et al. Breakpoints of the t(11;18)(q21;q21) in mucosa-associated lymphoid tissue (MALT) lymphoma lie within or near the previously undescribed gene MALT1 in chromosome 18. *Cancer Res* 1999;59(24): 6205–6213.
216. Suzuki H, Motegi M, Akagi T, et al. API1-MALT1-MLT is involved in mucosa-associated lymphoid tissue lymphoma with t(11;18)(q21;q21). *Blood* 1999;94(9): 3270–3271.
217. Akagi T, Motegi M, Tamura A, et al. A novel gene, MALT1 at 18q21, is involved in t(11;18) (q21;q21) found in low-grade B-cell lymphoma of mucosa-associated lymphoid tissue. *Oncogene* 1999;18(42):5785–5794.
218. Akagi T, Tamura A, Motegi M, et al. Molecular cytogenetic delineation of the breakpoint at 18q21.1 in low-grade B-cell lymphoma of mucosa-associated lymphoid tissue. *Genes Chromosomes Cancer* 1999;24(4):315–321.
219. Thome M. CARMA1, BCL-10 and MALT1 in lymphocyte development and activation. *Nat Rev Immunol* 2004;4(5):348–359.
220. Hosokawa Y. Anti-apoptotic action of API2-MALT1 fusion protein involved in t(11;18)(q21;q21) MALT lymphoma. *Apoptosis* 2005;10(1):25–34.
221. Uren AG, O'Rourke K, Aravind LA, et al. Identification of paracaspases and metacaspases: two ancient families of caspase-like proteins, one of which plays a key role in MALT lymphoma. *Mol Cell* 2000;6(4):961–967.
222. Lucas PC, Yonezumi M, Inohara N, et al. Bcl10 and MALT1, independent targets of chromosomal translocation in malt lymphoma, cooperate in a novel NF-kappa B signaling pathway. *J Biol Chem* 2001;276(22):19012–19019.
223. Ruland J, Duncan GS, Wakeham A, et al. Differential requirement for Malt1 in T and B cell antigen receptor signaling. *Immunity* 2003;19(5):749–758.
224. Ruefli-Brasse AA, French DM, Dixit VM. Regulation of NF-kappaB-dependent lymphocyte activation and development by paracaspase. *Science* 2003;302(5650): 1581–1584.
225. Roy N, Deveraux QL, Takahashi R, et al. The c-IAP-1 and c-IAP-2 proteins are direct inhibitors of specific caspases. *EMBO J* 1997;16(23):6914–6925.
226. Toyota M. Methylation profiling in acute myeloid leukemia. *Blood* 2001; 97(9):2823–2829.
227. Chim CS, Wong ASY, Kwong YL. Epigenetic inactivation of the CIP/KIP cell-cycle control pathway in acute leukemias. *Am J Hematol* 2005;80(4):282–287.
228. Nakatsuka S-I, Liu A, Yao M, et al. Methylation of promoter region in p27 gene plays a role in the development of lymphoid malignancies. *Int J Oncol* 2003;22(3):561–568.
229. Quintanilla-Martinez L, Thieblemont C, Fend F, et al. Mantle cell lymphomas lack expression of p27Kip1, a cyclin-dependent kinase inhibitor. *Am J Pathol* 1998; 153(1):175–182.
230. Go JH. Methylation analysis of cyclin-dependent kinase inhibitor genes in primary gastrointestinal lymphomas. *Mod Pathol* 2003;16(8):752–755.
231. Cleary ML, Galili N, Sklar J. Detection of a second t(14;18) breakpoint cluster region in human follicular lymphomas. *J Exp Med* 1986;164(1):315–320.
232. Nunez G, Hockenbery D, McDonnell TJ, et al. BCL2 maintains B cell memory. *Nature* 1991;353(6339):71–73.

233. McDonnell TJ, Deane N, Platt FM, et al. BCL2-immunoglobulin transgenic mice demonstrate extended B cell survival and follicular lymphoproliferation. *Cell* 1989;57(1):79–88.
234. Ye BHB, Lista FF, Coco Lo FF, et al. Alterations of a zinc finger-encoding gene, BCL-6, in diffuse large-cell lymphoma. *Science* 1993;262(5134):747–750.
235. Ye BH, Rao PH, Chaganti RS, et al. Cloning of bcl-6, the locus involved in chromosome translocations affecting band 3q27 in B-cell lymphoma. *Cancer Res* 1993;53(12):2732–2735.
236. Miki T, Kawamata N, Hirosawa S, et al. Gene involved in the 3q27 translocation associated with B-cell lymphoma, BCL5, encodes a Krüppel-like zinc-finger protein. *Blood* 1994;83(1):26–32.
237. Kerckaert JP, Deweindt C, Tilly H, et al. LAZ3, a novel zinc-finger encoding gene, is disrupted by recurring chromosome 3q27 translocations in human lymphomas. *Nat Genet* 1993;5(1):66–70.
238. Baron BW, Nucifora G, McCabe N, et al. Identification of the gene associated with the recurring chromosomal translocations t(3;14)(q27;q32) and t(3;22)(q27;q11) in B-cell lymphomas. *Proc Natl Acad Sci U S A* 1993;90(11):5262–5266.
239. Deweindt C, Albagli O, Bernardin F, et al. The LAZ3/BCL6 oncogene encodes a sequence-specific transcriptional inhibitor: a novel function for the BTB/POZ domain as an autonomous repressing domain. *Cell Growth Differ* 1995;6(12):1495–1503.
240. Seyfert V, Allman D, He Y, et al. Transcriptional repression by the proto-oncogene BCL-6. *Oncogene* 1996;12(11):2331–2342.
241. Chang CC, Ye BH, Chaganti RS, et al. BCL-6, a POZ/zinc-finger protein, is a sequence-specific transcriptional repressor. *Proc Natl Acad Sci U S A* 1996;93(14):6947–6952.
242. Cattoretti G, Chang CC, Cechova K, et al. BCL-6 protein is expressed in germinal-center B cells. *Blood* 1995;86(1):45–53.
243. Allman D, Jain A, Dent A, et al. BCL-6 expression during B-cell activation. *Blood* 1996;87(12):5257–5268.
244. Basso K, Dalla-Favera R. BCL6: master regulator of the germinal center reaction and key oncogene in B cell lymphomagenesis. *Adv Immunol* 2010;105(105):193–210.
245. Saito M, Novak U, Piovan E, et al. BCL6 suppression of BCL2 via Miz1 and its disruption in diffuse large B cell lymphoma. *Proc Natl Acad Sci U S A* 2009;106(27):11294–11299.
246. Parekh S, Polo JM, Shaknovich R, et al. BCL6 programs lymphoma cells for survival and differentiation through distinct biochemical mechanisms. *Blood* 2007;110(6):2067–2074.
247. Basso K, Saito M, Sumazin P, et al. Integrated biochemical and computational approach identifies BCL6 direct target genes controlling multiple pathways in normal germinal center B cells. *Blood* 2010;115(5):975–984.
248. Phan RT, Dalla-Favera R. The BCL6 proto-oncogene suppresses p53 expression in germinal-centre B cells. *Nature* 2004;432(7017):635–639.
249. Ci W, Polo JM, Cerchietti L, et al. The BCL6 transcriptional program features repression of multiple oncogenes in primary B cells and is deregulated in DLBCL. *Blood* 2009;113(22):5536–5548.
250. Ranuncolo SM, Polo JM, Dierov J, et al. Bcl-6 mediates the germinal center B cell phenotype and lymphomagenesis through transcriptional repression of the DNA-damage sensor ATR. *Nat Immunol* 2007;8(7):705–714.
251. Poholek AC, Hansen K, Hernandez SG, et al. In vivo regulation of Bcl6 and T follicular helper cell development. *J Immunol* 2010;185(1):313–326.
252. Tunyaplin C, Shaffer AL, Angelin-Duclos CD, et al. Direct repression of prdm1 by Bcl-6 inhibits plasmacytic differentiation. *J Immunol* 2004;173(2):1158–1165.
253. Shaffer AL, Yu X, He Y, et al. BCL-6 represses genes that function in lymphocyte differentiation, inflammation, and cell cycle control. *Immunity* 2000;13(2):199–212.
254. Ye BH, Cattoretti G, Shen Q, et al. The BCL-6 proto-oncogene controls germinal-centre formation and Th2-type inflammation. *Nat Genet* 1997;16(2):161–170.
255. Dent AL, Shaffer AL, Yu X, et al. Control of inflammation, cytokine expression, and germinal center formation by BCL-6. *Science* 1997;276(5312):589–592.
256. Niu H, Ye BH, Dalla-Favera R. Antigen receptor signaling induces MAP kinase-mediated phosphorylation and degradation of the BCL-6 transcription factor. *Genes Dev* 1998;12(13):1953–1961.
257. Saito M, Gao J, Basso K, et al. A signaling pathway mediating downregulation of BCL6 in germinal center B cells is blocked by BCL6 gene alterations in B cell lymphoma. *Cancer Cell* 2007;12(3):280–292.
258. Lococo F, Ye B, Lista F, et al. Rearrangements of the Bcl6 gene in diffuse large-cell non-Hodgkin's-lymphoma. *Blood* 1994;83(7):1757–1759.
259. Ohno H. Pathogenetic role of BCL6 translocation in B-cell non-Hodgkin's lymphoma. *Histol Histopathol* 2004;19(2):637–650.
260. Yoshida S, Kaneita Y, Aoki Y, et al. Identification of heterologous translocation partner genes fused to the BCL6 gene in diffuse large B-cell lymphomas: 5'-RACE and LA—PCR analyses of biopsy samples. *Oncogene* 1999;18(56):7994–7999.
261. Chen W, Iida S, Louie DC, et al. Heterologous promoters fused to BCL6 by chromosomal translocations affecting band 3q27 cause its deregulated expression during B-cell differentiation. *Blood* 1998;91(2):603–607.
262. Ye BH, Chaganti S, Chang CC, et al. Chromosomal translocations cause deregulated BCL6 expression by promoter substitution in B cell lymphoma. *EMBO J* 1995;14(24):6209–6217.
263. Cattoretti G, Pasqualucci L, Ballon G, et al. Deregulated BCL6 expression recapitulates the pathogenesis of human diffuse large B cell lymphomas in mice. *Cancer Cell* 2005;7(5):445–455.
264. Migliazza A, Martinotti S, Chen W, et al. Frequent somatic hypermutation of the 5' noncoding region of the BCL6 gene in B-cell lymphoma. *Proc Natl Acad Sci U S A* 1995;92(26):12520–12524.
265. Capello D, Vitolo U, Pasqualucci L, et al. Distribution and pattern of BCL-6 mutations throughout the spectrum of B-cell neoplasia. *Blood* 2000;95(2):651–659.
266. Pasqualucci L, Migliazza A, Basso K, et al. Mutations of the BCL6 proto-oncogene disrupt its negative autoregulation in diffuse large B-cell lymphoma. *Blood* 2003;101(8):2914–2923.
267. Pasqualucci L, Dominguez-Sola D, Chiarenza A, et al. Inactivating mutations of acetyltransferase genes in B-cell lymphoma. *Nature* 2011;471(7337):189–195.
268. Bereshchenko OR, Gu W, Dalla-Favera R. Acetylation inactivates the transcriptional repressor BCL6. *Nat Genet* 2002;32(4):606–613.
269. Raffeld M, Jaffe ES. Bcl-1, t(11;14), and mantle cell-derived lymphomas. *Blood* 1991;78(2):259–263.
270. Weinberg RA. The retinoblastoma protein and cell cycle control. *Cell* 1995;81(3):323–330.
271. Bodrug SE, Warner BJ, Bath ML, et al. Cyclin D1 transgene impedes lymphocyte maturation and collaborates in lymphomagenesis with the myc gene. *EMBO J* 1994;13(9):2124–2130.
272. Lovec H, Grzeschiczek A, Kowalski M, et al. Cyclin D1 Bcl-1 Cooperates with Myc Genes in the Generation of B-Cell Lymphoma in Transgenic Mice. *EMBO J* 1994;13(15):3487–3495.
273. Mueller A, Odze R, Jenkins TD, et al. A transgenic mouse model with cyclin D1 overexpression results in cell cycle, epidermal growth factor receptor, and p53 abnormalities. *Cancer Res* 1997;57(24):5542–5549.
274. Robles AI, Larcher F, Whalin RB, et al. Expression of cyclin D1 in epithelial tissues of transgenic mice results in epidermal hyperproliferation and severe thymic hyperplasia. *Proc Natl Acad Sci U S A* 1996;93(15):7634–7638.
275. Wang TC, Cardiff RD, Zukerberg L, et al. Mammary hyperplasia and carcinoma in MMTV-cyclin D1 transgenic mice. *Nature* 1994;369(6482):669–671.
276. Kim JK, Diehl JA. Nuclear cyclin D1: an oncogenic driver in human cancer. *J Cell Physiol* 2009;220(2):292–296.
277. Pérez-Galán P, Dreyling M, Wiestner A. Mantle cell lymphoma: biology, pathogenesis, and the molecular basis of treatment in the genomic era. *Blood* 2011;117(1):26–38.
278. Gladden AB, Woolery R, Aggarwal P, et al. Expression of constitutively nuclear cyclin D1 in murine lymphocytes induces B-cell lymphoma. *Oncogene* 2006;25(7):998–1007.
279. Dalla-Favera R, Bregni M, Erikson J, et al. Human c-myc onc gene is located on the region of chromosome 8 that is translocated in Burkitt lymphoma cells. *Proc Natl Acad Sci U S A* 1982;79(24):7824–7827.
280. Dalla-Favera R, Martinotti S, Gallo R, et al. Translocation and rearrangements of the C-Myc oncogene locus in human undifferentiated B-cell lymphomas. *Science* 1983;219(4587):963–967.
281. Taub R, Kirsch I, Morton C. Translocation of the c-myc gene into the immunoglobulin heavy chain locus in human Burkitt lymphoma and murine plasmacytoma cells. *Proc Natl Acad Sci U S A* 1982;79:7837–7841.
282. Davis M, Malcolm S, Rabbitts TH. Chromosome translocation can occur on either side of the c-myc oncogene in Burkitt lymphoma cells. *Nature* 1984;308(5956):286–288.
283. Hollis GF, Mitchell KF, Battey J, et al. A variant translocation places the λ immunoglobulin genes 3' to the c-myc oncogene in Burkitt's lymphoma. *Nature* 1984;307(5953):752–755.
284. Eissenberg JC, Shilatifard A. Histone H3 lysine 4 (H3K4) methylation in development and differentiation. *Dev Biol* 2010;339(2):240–249.
285. Prasad R, Zhadanov AB, Sedkov Y, et al. Structure and expression pattern of human ALR, a novel gene with strong homology to ALL-1 involved in acute leukemia and to Drosophila trithorax. *Oncogene* 1997;15(5):549–560.
286. Ng SB, Bigham AW, Buckingham KJ, et al. Exome sequencing identifies MLL2 mutations as a cause of Kabuki syndrome. *Nat Genet* 2010;42(9):790–793.
287. Cesarman E, Dalla-Favera R, Bentley D, et al. Mutations in the first exon are associated with altered transcription of c-myc in Burkitt lymphoma. *Science* 1987;238(4831):1272–1275.
288. Hoang A, Lutterbach B, Lewis B, et al. A link between increased transforming activity of lymphoma-derived myc mutant alleles, their defective regulation by P107, and altered phosphorylation of the C-Myc transactivation domain. *Mol Cell Biol* 1995;15(8):4031–4042.
289. Gu W, Bhatia K, Magrath IT, et al. Binding and suppression of the Myc transcriptional activation domain by p107. *Science* 1994;264(5156):251–254.
290. Sakamuro D, Eviner V, Prendergast GC, et al. C-Myc induces apoptosis in epithelial cells by both p53-dependent and p53-independent mechanisms. *Oncogene* 1995;11(11):2411–2418.
291. Willis TG, Jadayel DM, Du M-Q, et al. Bcl10 is involved in t(1;14)(p22;q32) of MALT B cell lymphoma and mutated in multiple tumor types. *Cell* 1999;96(1):35–45.
292. Zhang Q, Siebert R, Yan M, et al. Inactivating mutations and overexpression of BCL10, a caspase recruitment domain-containing gene, in MALT lymphoma with t(1;14)(p22;q32). *Nat Genet* 1999;22(1):63–68.
293. Luminari S, Intini D, Baldini L, et al. BCL10 gene mutations rarely occur in lymphoid malignancies. *Leukemia* 2000;14(5):905–908.
294. Tadokoro J, Nakamura Y, Furusawa S, et al. Low frequency of BCL10 gene mutations in B-cell non-Hodgkin's lymphoma. *Int J Hematol* 2001;73(2):222–225.
295. Fakruddin JM, Chaganti RS, Murty VV. Lack of BCL10 mutations in germ cell tumors and B cell lymphomas. *Cell* 1999;97(6):683–684; discussion 686–688.
296. Maes B. BCL10 mutation does not represent an important pathogenic mechanism in gastric MALT-type lymphoma, and the presence of the API2-MLT fusion is associated with aberrant nuclear BCL10 expression. *Blood* 2002;99(4):1398–1404.
297. Alizadeh AA, Eisen MB, Davis RE, et al. Distinct types of diffuse large B-cell lymphoma identified by gene expression profiling. *Nature* 2000;403(6769):503–511.
298. Ngo VN, Young RM, Schmitz R, et al. Oncogenically active MYD88 mutations in human lymphoma. *Nature* 2011;470(7332):115–119.
299. Davis RE, Ngo VN, Lenz G, et al. Chronic active B-cell-receptor signalling in diffuse large B cell lymphoma. *Nature* 2010;463(7277):88–92.
300. Lenz G, Davis RE, Ngo VN, et al. Oncogenic CARD11 mutations in human diffuse large B cell lymphoma. *Science* 2008;319(5870):1676–1679.
301. Compagno M, Lim WK, Grunn A, et al. Mutations of multiple genes cause deregulation of NF-kappaB in diffuse large B-cell lymphoma. *Nature* 2009;459(7247):717–721.
302. Rui L, Schmitz R, Ceribelli M, et al. Malignant pirates of the immune system. *Nat Immunol* 2011;12(10):933–940.
303. Morin RD, Mendez-Lago M, Mungall AJ, et al. Frequent mutation of histone-modifying genes in non-Hodgkin lymphoma. *Nature* 2011;476(7360):298–303.
304. Cao R, Wang L, Wang H, et al. Role of histone H3 lysine 27 methylation in Polycomb-group silencing. *Science* 2002;298(5595):1039–1043.
305. Czermin B, Melfi R, McCabe D, et al. Drosophila enhancer of Zeste/ESC complexes have a histone H3 methyltransferase activity that marks chromosomal polycomb sites. *Cell* 2002;111(2):185–196.
306. Müller J, Hart CM, Francis NJ, et al. Histone methyltransferase activity of a Drosophila Polycomb group repressor complex. *Cell* 2002;111(2):197–208.
307. Yap DB, Chu J, Berg T, et al. Somatic mutations at EZH2 Y641 act dominantly through a mechanism of selectively altered PRC2 catalytic activity, to increase H3K27 trimethylation. *Blood* 2011;117(8):2451–2459.
308. Sneeringer CJ, Scott MP, Kuntz KW, et al. Coordinated activities of wild-type plus mutant EZH2 drive tumor-associated hypertrimethylation of lysine

27 on histone H3 (H3K27) in human B-cell lymphomas. *Proc Natl Acad Sci* 2010;107(49):20980–20985.

309. Esteller M. CpG island hypermethylation and tumor suppressor genes: a booming present, a brighter future. *Oncogene* 2002;21(35):5427–5440.

310. Santarosa M, Ashworth A. Haploinsufficiency for tumour suppressor genes: when you don't need to go all the way. *Biochim Biophys Acta* 2004;1654(2):105–122.

311. Shiloh Y. ATM and related protein kinases: safeguarding genome integrity. *Nat Rev Cancer* 2003;3(3):155–168.

312. Chen G, Yuan SS, Liu W, et al. Radiation-induced assembly of Rad51 and Rad52 recombination complex requires ATM and c-Abl. *J Biol Chem* 1999;274(18):12748–12752.

313. Shafman T, Khanna KK, Kedar P, et al. Interaction between ATM protein and c-Abl in response to DNA damage. *Nature* 1997;387(6632):520–523.

314. Shiloh Y, Rotman G. Ataxia-telangiectasia and the ATM gene: linking neurode-generation, immunodeficiency, and cancer to cell cycle checkpoints. *J Clin Immunol* 1996;16(5):254–260.

315. Xu Y, Ashley T, Brainerd EE, et al. Targeted disruption of ATM leads to growth retardation, chromosomal fragmentation during meiosis, immune defects, and thymic lymphoma. *Genes Dev* 1996;10(19):2411–2422.

316. Barlow C, Hirotsune S, Paylor R, et al. Atm-deficient mice: a paradigm of ataxia telangiectasia. *Cell* 1996;86(1):159–171.

317. Schaffner C, Idler I, Stilgenbauer S, et al. Mantle cell lymphoma is characterized by inactivation of the ATM gene. *Proc Natl Acad Sci U S A* 2000;97(6):2773–2778.

318. Stilgenbauer S, Schaffner C, Winkler D, et al. The ATM gene in the pathogenesis of mantle-cell lymphoma. *Ann Oncol* 2000;11(Suppl 1):127–130.

319. Stilgenbauer S, Winkler D, Ott G, et al. Molecular characterization of 11q dele-tions points to a pathogenic role of the ATM gene in mantle cell lymphoma. *Blood* 1999;94(9):3262–3264.

320. Gumy-Pause F, Wacker P, Sappino A-P. ATM gene and lymphoid malignancies. *Leukemia* 2004;18(2):238–242.

321. Stilgenbauer S, Schaffner C, Litterst A, et al. Biallelic mutations in the ATM gene in T-prolymphocytic leukemia. *Nat Med* 1997;3(10):1155–1159.

322. Vorechovský I, Luo L, Dyer MJ, et al. Clustering of missense mutations in the ataxia-telangiectasia gene in a sporadic T-cell leukaemia. *Nat Genet* 1997;17(1):96–99.

323. Bullrich FF, Rasio DD, Croce CMC. ATM mutations in B-cell chronic lymphocytic leukemia. *Cancer Res* 1999;59(1):24–27.

324. Starostik P, Manshouri T, O'Brien S, et al. Deficiency of the ATM protein expression defines an aggressive subgroup of B-cell chronic lymphocytic leukemia. *Cancer Res* 1998;58(20):4552–4557.

325. Schaffner C, Stilgenbauer S, Rappold GA, et al. Somatic ATM mutations indicate a pathogenic role of ATM in B-cell chronic lymphocytic leukemia. *Blood* 1999;94(2):748–753.

326. Stankovic T, Weber P, Taylor AM, et al. Inactivation of ataxia telangiectasia mutated gene in B-cell chronic lymphocytic leukaemia. *Lancet* 1999;353(9146):26–29.

327. Vermeulen K, Van Bockstaele DR, Berneman ZN. The cell cycle: a review of regulation, deregulation and therapeutic targets in cancer. *Cell Prolif* 2003;36(3):131–149.

328. Drexler HG. Review of alterations of the cyclin-dependent kinase inhibitor INK4 family genes p15, p16, p18 and p19 in human leukemia-lymphoma cells. *Leukemia* 1998;12(6):845–859.

329. Baur AS, Shaw P, Burri N, et al. Frequent methylation silencing of p15(INK4b) (MTS2) and p16(INK4a) (MTS1) in B-cell and T-cell lymphomas. *Blood* 1999;94(5):1773–1781.

330. Pinyol M, Hernández L, Cazorla M, et al. Deletions and loss of expression of p16INK4a and p21Waf1 genes are associated with aggressive variants of mantle cell lymphomas. *Blood* 1997;89(1):272–280.

331. Nakamura M, Sakaki T, Hashimoto H, et al. Frequent alterations of the p14(ARF) and p16(INK4a) genes in primary central nervous system lymphomas. *Cancer Res* 2001;61(17):6335–6339.

332. Ying J, Srivastava G, Gao Z, et al. Promoter hypermethylation of the cyclin-dependent kinase inhibitor (CDKI) gene p21WAF1/CIP1/SDI1 is rare in various lymphomas and carcinomas. *Blood* 2004;103(2):743–746.

333. Shen L, Kondo Y, Issa J-P, et al. Lack of p21(CIP1) DNA methylation in acute lymphocytic leukemia. *Blood* 2002;100(9):3432–3434.

334. Calin GA, Dumitru CD, Shimizu M, et al. Frequent deletions and down-regulation of micro- RNA genes miR15 and miR16 at 13q14 in chronic lymphocytic leukemia. *Proc Natl Acad Sci U S A* 2002;99(24):15524–15529.

335. Calin GA, Ferracin M, Cimmino A, et al. A MicroRNA signature associated with prognosis and progression in chronic lymphocytic leukemia. *N Engl J Med* 2005;353(17):1793–1801.

336. Klein U, Lia M, Crespo M, et al. The DLEU2/miR-15a/16-1 cluster controls B cell proliferation and its deletion leads to chronic lymphocytic leukemia. *Cancer Cell* 2010;17(1):28–40.

337. Aqeilan RI, Calin GA, Croce CM. MiR-15a and miR-16-1 in cancer: discovery, function and future perspectives. *Cell Death Differ* 2010;17(2):215–220.

338. Vousden KH, Lane DP. P53 in health and disease. *Nat Rev Mol Cell Biol* 2007;8(4):275–283.

339. Yee KS, Vousden KH. Complicating the complexity of p53. *Carcinogenesis* 2005;26(8):1317–1322.

340. Efeyan A, Garcia-Cao I, Herranz D, et al. Tumour biology: Policing of oncogene activity by p53. *Nature* 2006;443(7108):159–159.

341. Christophorou M, Ringshausen I, Finch A, et al. The pathological response to DNA damage does not contribute to p53-mediated tumour suppression. *Nature* 2006;443(7108):214–217.

342. Bartkova J, Ho ejší Z, Koed K, et al. DNA damage response as a candidate anti-cancer barrier in early human tumorigenesis. *Nat Cell Biol* 2005;434(7035):864–870.

343. Gorgoulis VG, Vassiliou L-VF, Karakaidos P, et al. Activation of the DNA dam-age checkpoint and genomic instability in human precancerous lesions. *Nature* 2005;434(7035):907–913.

344. Hollstein M, Sidransky D, Vogelstein B, et al. P53 mutations in human cancers. *Science* 1991;253(5015):49–53.

345. May P, May E. Twenty years of p53 research: structural and functional aspects of the p53 protein. *Oncogene* 1999;18(53):7621–7636.

346. Lang GA, Iwakuma T, Suh Y-A, et al. Gain of function of a p53 hot spot mutation in a mouse model of Li-Fraumeni syndrome. *Cell* 2004;119(6):861–872.

347. Olive KP, Tuveson DA, Ruhe ZC, et al. Mutant p53 gain of function in two mouse models of Li-Fraumeni syndrome. *Cell* 2004;119(6):847–860.

348. Irwin M. Family feud in chemosensitvity—p73 and mutant p53. *Cell Cycle* 2004;3(3):319–323.

349. Sigal A, Rotter V. Oncogenic mutations of the p53 tumor suppressor: the demons of the guardian of the genome. *Cancer Res* 2000;60(24):6788–6793.

350. Kim E, Deppert W. Transcriptional activities of mutant p53: when mutations are more than a loss. *J Cell Biochem* 2004;93(5):878–886.

351. Zhang Y, Xiong Y, Yarbrough WG. ARF promotes MDM2 degradation and stabi-lizes p53: ARF-INK4a locus deletion impairs both the Rb and p53 tumor suppres-sion pathways. *Cell* 1998;92(6):725–734.

352. Honda RR, Yasuda HH. Association of p19(ARF) with Mdm2 inhibits ubiquitin ligase activity of Mdm2 for tumor suppressor p53. *EMBO J* 1999;18(1):22–27.

353. Tao WW, Levine AJA. P19(ARF) stabilizes p53 by blocking nucleo-cytoplasmic shuttling of Mdm2. *Proc Natl Acad Sci U S A* 1999;96(12):6937–6941.

354. Weber JD, Taylor LJ, Roussel MF, et al. Nucleolar Arf sequesters Mdm2 and acti-vates p53. *Nat Cell Biol* 1999;1(1):20–26.

355. Imamura J, Miyoshi I, Koeffler HP. P53 in hematologic malignancies. *Blood* 1994;84(8):2412–2421.

356. Gyory I, Fejer G, Ghosh N, et al. Identification of a functionally impaired positive regulatory domain I binding factor 1 transcription repressor in myeloma cell lines. *J Immunol* 2003;170(6):3125–3133.

357. Yu J, Angelin-Duclos C, Greenwood J, et al. Transcriptional repression by blimp-1 (PRDI-BF1) involves recruitment of histone deacetylase. *Mol Cell Biol* 2000;20(7):2592–2603.

358. Su ST, Ying HY, Chiu YK, et al. Involvement of histone demethylase LSD1 in blimp-1-mediated gene repression during plasma cell differentiation. *Mol Cell Biol* 2009;29(6):1421–1431.

359. Ren B, Chee KJ, Kim TH, et al. PRDI-BF1/Blimp-1 repression is mediated by corepressors of the Groucho family of proteins. *Genes Dev* 1999;13(1):125–137.

360. Keller AD, Maniatis T. Identification and characterization of a novel repressor of beta-interferon gene expression. *Genes Dev* 1991;5(5):868–879.

361. Huang S. Blimp-1 is the murine homolog of the human transcriptional repressor PRDI-BF1. *Cell* 1994;78(1):9.

362. Turner CA, Mack DH, Davis MM. Blimp-1, a novel zinc finger-containing protein that can drive the maturation of B lymphocytes into immunoglobulin-secreting cells. *Cell* 1994;77(2):297–306.

363. Shapiro-Shelef M, Lin K, McHeyzer-Williams L, et al. Blimp-1 is required for the formation of immunoglobulin secreting plasma cells and pre-plasma memory B cells. *Immunity* 2003;19(4):607–620.

364. Shapiro-Shelef M, Lin K-I, Savitsky D, et al. Blimp-1 is required for maintenance of long-lived plasma cells in the bone marrow. *J Exp Med* 2005;202(11):1471–1476.

365. Martins G, Calame K. Regulation and Functions of Blimp-1 in T and B Lympho-cytes. *Annu Rev Immunol* 2008;26(1):133–169.

366. Shaffer AL, Lin K-I, Kuo TC, et al. Blimp-1 orchestrates plasma cell differen-tiation by extinguishing the mature B cell gene expression program. *Immunity* 2002;17(1):51–62.

367. Shaffer AL, Shapiro-Shelef M, Iwakoshi NN, et al. XBP1, downstream of Blimp-1, expands the secretory apparatus and other organelles, and increases protein synthesis in plasma cell differentiation. *Immunity* 2004;21(1):81–93.

368. Tam W, Gomez M, Chadburn A, et al. Mutational analysis of PRDM1 indi-cates a tumor-suppressor role in diffuse large B-cell lymphomas. *Blood* 2006;107(10):4090–4100.

369. Pasqualucci L, Compagno M, Houldsworth J, et al. Inactivation of the PRDM1/BLIMP1 gene in diffuse large B cell lymphoma. *J Exp Med* 2006;203(2):311–317.

370. Mandelbaum J, Bhagat G, Tang H, et al. BLIMP1 Is a tumor suppressor gene frequently disrupted in activated B cell-like diffuse large B cell lymphoma. *Cancer Cell* 2010;18(6):568–579.

371. Hangaishi A, Kurokawa M. Blimp-1 is a tumor suppressor gene in lymphoid malignancies. *Int J Hematol* 2010;91(1):46–53.

372. Nie K, Zhang T, Allawi H, et al. Epigenetic down-regulation of the tumor suppres-sor gene PRDM1/blimp-1 in diffuse large B cell lymphomas a potential role of the microRNA let-7. *Am J Pathol* 2010;177(3):1470–1479.

373. Calado DP, Zhang B, Srinivasan L, et al. Constitutive canonical NF-κB activation cooperates with disruption of BLIMP1 in the pathogenesis of activated B cell-like diffuse large cell lymphoma. *Cancer Cell* 2010;18(6):580–589.

374. Iqbal J, Kucuk C, deLeeuw RJ, et al. Genomic analyses reveal global functional alterations that promote tumor growth and novel tumor suppressor genes in natural killer-cell malignancies. *Leukemia* 2009;23(6):1139–1151.

375. Karube K, Nakagawa M, Tsuzuki S, et al. Identification of FOXO3 and PRDM1 as tumor suppressor gene candidates in NK cell neoplasms by genomic and func-tional analyses. *Blood* 2011;0(2011):201104346.

376. Küçük C, Iqbal J, Hu X, et al. PRDM1 is a tumor suppressor gene in natural killer cell malignancies. *Proc Natl Acad Sci* 2011;108(50):20119–20124.

377. Best T, Li D, Skol AD, et al. Variants at 6q21 implicate PRDM1 in the etiology of therapy-induced second malignancies after Hodgkin's lymphoma. *Nat Med* 2011;17(8):941–943.

378. Weinberg RA. The Rb gene and the negative regulation of cell growth. *Blood* 1989;74(2):529–532.

379. Burkhart DL, Sage J. Cellular mechanisms of tumour suppression by the retino-blastoma gene. *Nat Rev Cancer* 2008;8(9):671–682.

380. Binné UK, Classon MK, Dick FA, et al. Retinoblastoma protein and anaphase-promoting complex physically interact and functionally cooperate during cell-cycle exit. *Nat Cell Biol* 2007;9(2):225–232.

381. Ji P, Jiang H, Rekhtman K, et al. An Rb-Skp2-p27 pathway mediates acute cell cycle inhibition by Rb and is retained in a partial-penetrance Rb mutant. *Mol Cell* 2004;16(1):47–58.

382. Goodrich DW. The retinoblastoma tumor-suppressor gene, the exception that proves the rule. *Oncogene* 2006;25(38):5233–5243.

383. Hatakeyama M, Weinberg RA. The role of RB in cell cycle control. *Prog Cell Cycle Res* 1995;1:9–19.

384. Benedict WF, Xu HJ, Takahashi R. The retinoblastoma gene: its role in human malignancies. *Cancer Invest* 1990;8(5):535–540.

385. Vooijs M, Berns A. Developmental defects and tumor predisposition in Rb mutant mice. *Oncogene* 1999;18(38):5293–5303.

386. Classon MM, Harlow EE. The retinoblastoma tumour suppressor in development and cancer. *Nat Rev Cancer* 2002;2(12):910–917.

387. Zhu YM, Haynes AP, Keith FJ, et al. Abnormalities of retinoblastoma gene expres-sion in hematological malignancies. *Leuk Lymphoma* 1995;18(1–2):61–67.

388. Beck Z, Kiss A, Tóth FD, et al. Alterations of P53 and RB genes and the evolution of the accelerated phase of chronic myeloid leukemia. *Leuk Lymphoma* 2000;38(5–6):587–597.

389. Rassidakis GZ, Lai R, Herling M, et al. Retinoblastoma protein is frequently absent or phosphorylated in anaplastic large-cell lymphoma. *Am J Pathol* 2004;164(6):2259–2267.

390. Leoncini L, Bellan C, De Falco G. Retinoblastoma gene family expression in lymphoid tissues. *Oncogene* 2006;25(38):5309–5314.

391. Offit KK, Parsa NZN, Gaidano GG, et al. 6q deletions define distinct clinico-pathologic subsets of non-Hodgkin's lymphoma. *Blood* 1993;82(7):2157–2162.

392. Gaidano G, Hauptschein RS, Parsa NZ, et al. Deletions involving two distinct regions of 6q in B-cell non-Hodgkin lymphoma. *Blood* 1992;80(7):1781–1787.

393. Dixit VM, Green S, Sarma V, et al. Tumor necrosis factor-alpha induction of novel gene products in human endothelial cells including a macrophage-specific chemotaxin. *J Biol Chem* 1990;265(5):2973–2978.

394. Sarma V, Lin Z, Dixit VM. Activation of the B-cell surface receptor CD40 induces A20, a novel zinc finger protein that inhibits apoptosis. *J Biol Chem* 1995;270(21):12343–12346.

395. Fries KLK, Miller WEW, Raab-Traub NN. The A20 protein interacts with the Epstein-Barr virus latent membrane protein 1 (LMP1) and alters the LMP1/TRAF1/TRADD complex. *Virology* 1999;264(1):159–166.

396. Coornaert B, Carpentier I, Beyaert R. A20: Central Gatekeeper in Inflammation and Immunity. *J Biol Chem* 2008;284(13):8217–8221.

397. Lee EG, Boone DL, Chai S, et al. Failure to regulate TNF-induced NF-kappaB and cell death responses in A20-deficient mice. *Science* 2000;289(5488):2350–2354.

398. Boone DL, Turer EE, Lee EG, et al. The ubiquitin-modifying enzyme A20 is required for termination of Toll-like receptor responses. *Nat Immunol* 2004;5(10):1052–1060.

399. Heyninck K, Beyaert R. A20 inhibits NF-kappaB activation by dual ubiquitin-editing functions. *Trends Biochem Sci* 2005;30(1):1–4.

400. Shembade N, Ma A, Harhaj EW. Inhibition of NF-kappaB signaling by A20 through disruption of ubiquitin enzyme complexes. *Science* 2010;327(5969):1135–1139.

401. Kato M, Sanada M, Kato I, et al. Frequent inactivation of A20 in B-cell lymphomas. *Nature* 2009;459(7247):712–716.

402. Chanudet E, Huang Y, Ichimura K, et al. A20 is targeted by promoter methylation, deletion and inactivating mutation in MALT lymphoma. *Leukemia* 2010;24(2):483–487.

403. Novak U, Rinaldi A, Kwee I, et al. The NF-{kappa}B negative regulator TNFAIP3 (A20) is inactivated by somatic mutations and genomic deletions in marginal zone lymphomas. *Blood* 2009;113(20):4918–4921.

404. Schmitz R, Hansmann M-L, Bohle V, et al. TNFAIP3 (A20) is a tumor suppressor gene in Hodgkin lymphoma and primary mediastinal B cell lymphoma. *J Exp Med* 2009;206(5):981–989.

405. Giulino L, Mathew S, Ballon G, et al. A20 (TNFAIP3) genetic alterations in EBV-associated AIDS-related lymphoma. *Blood* 2011;117(18):4852–4854.

406. Honma K, Tsuzuki S, Nakagawa M, et al. TNFAIP3/A20 functions as a novel tumor suppressor gene in several subtypes of non-Hodgkin lymphomas. *Blood* 2009;114(12):2467–2475.

407. Pasqualucci L, Trifonov V, Fabbri G, et al. Analysis of the coding genome of diffuse large B-cell lymphoma. *Nat Genet* 2011;43(9):830–837.

408. Paulussen ADC, Stegmann APA, Blok MJ, et al. MLL2 mutation spectrum in 45 patients with Kabuki syndrome. *Hum Mutat* 2011;32(2):E2018–E2025.

409. Goodman RH, Smolik S. CBP/p300 in cell growth, transformation, and development. *Genes Dev* 2000;14(13):1553–1577.

410. Kalkhoven E. CBP and p300: HATs for different occasions. *Biochem Pharmacol* 2004;68(6):1145–1155.

411. Petrij F, Giles RH, Dauwerse HG, et al. Rubinstein-Taybi syndrome caused by mutations in the transcriptional co-activator CBP. *Nature* 1995;376(6538):348–351.

412. Roelfsema JH, Peters DJM. Rubinstein-Taybi syndrome: clinical and molecular overview. *Expert Rev Mol Med* 2007;9(23):1–16.

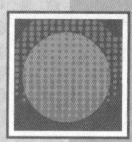

Chapter 8
Application of Molecular Genetics to the Diagnosis and Classification of Hematologic Neoplasms

Christopher David Watt • Michele Renee Roullet • Adam Bagg

 INTRODUCTION

Although once considered an ancillary tool, molecular genetic studies have become an essential component in the evaluation of hematologic neoplasms. In fact, WHO diagnostic criteria for several diseases are based primarily on the presence (or, in some cases, absence) of specific genetic lesions (Table 8.1) (1). Molecular diagnostics provide clinically relevant insights that cannot otherwise be obtained through traditional histomorphologic and immunophenotypic assessment.

Although sometimes interrelated, there are four broad indications for molecular genetic studies in hematologic neoplasms: (a) initial diagnosis and classification, (b) determination of prognosis, (c) directing specific therapy, and (d) posttherapy monitoring. Importantly, molecular diagnostics are not universally indicated; there are neoplasms where these tools are either not needed or not available. In other neoplasms, even though a specific tumor type is associated with a prototypic genetic abnormality (e.g., follicular lymphoma [FL] and t(14;18)(q32;q21) translocation), it is not (always) necessary to detect the translocation to render the diagnosis of FL, and the presence of the translocation in a lymphoma does not definitively indicate that it is an FL. Thus, specific applications, as is discussed in this chapter, vary as a function of the disease, the concomitant genetic lesion, and, most importantly, the particular clinicopathologic scenario. With the advent of more rigorous and robust genomic applications in cancer, this limitation may be changing (2).

Genetic lesions in hematologic neoplasms are primarily evaluated by a combination of approaches including conventional cytogenetics, fluorescence *in situ* hybridization (FISH), and polymerase chain reaction (PCR)-based strategies. Other technologies, including array comparative genomic hybridization (aCGH), single nucleotide polymorphism (SNP) arrays, and next-generation sequencing (NGS) platforms, are emerging in the clinical laboratory; these new technologies are poised to redefine and evolve the field of molecular diagnostics. Gene expression arrays, by contrast, despite having been used for over a decade as tremendous discovery tools, are not (yet) ready for diagnostic prime time. A brief comparison of these techniques, highlighting diagnostic advantages and limitations, is provided in Table 8.2. Importantly, a single unified methodology or platform for the genetic analysis of hematologic neoplasms does not exist; different nucleic acid-based studies complement each other and extend the information provided by other diagnostic modalities including conventional metaphase cytogenetic studies and FISH (e.g., identification of cryptic translocations) (3). A discussion of cytogenetics and FISH can be found elsewhere in this book (see Chapter 9). Here, we focus primarily on the applications of PCR and its related technologies.

When considering the spectrum of genetic phenomena evaluated in hematologic neoplasms, and for the most part neoplasms in general, the majority can be divided into one of four broad categories: (a) gene mutations, (b) altered levels of gene expression including epigenetic alterations, (c)

gene rearrangements, both physiologic (which are typically restricted to lymphoid cells) and pathologic, and (d) numeric genetic abnormalities including gains, losses, and copy number variations (CNVs). Collectively, this conceptual framework forms the backbone of the discussion.

Molecular Genetic Methods

Molecular techniques in the clinical laboratory have evolved over the preceding 30 years, and especially so in the past decade; consequently, it may have become challenging for the "general" or "nonmoleculocentric" hematopathologist to keep pace. Initially Southern blots dominated the landscape; this powerful but technically and logistically demanding method was supplanted by a variety of facile PCR-based methods. The accessibility and versatility of PCR has, in part, lead to its widespread adoption in clinical laboratories. Technologies such as RNA expression profiling, as currently designed, appear unlikely to become standard diagnostic tools. SNP arrays and NGS platforms are experiencing slow rates of universal application in the clinical setting, as compared to PCR, due to not only significant operational costs but also a number of substantial administrative, technical, and interpretive challenges (4–7). However, both, particularly the latter, are poised to become extremely useful tools. These issues notwithstanding, there is one thing in common for past, present, and future technologies: the need for purified nucleic acid.

Nucleic Acid Isolation

The hematologic specimens most frequently evaluated by DNA- and RNA-based molecular genetic studies include peripheral blood, bone marrow, and lymph nodes, but in many circumstances other types of tissue (e.g., skin) and fluid (e.g., cerebrospinal fluid) may be analyzed. A distinct advantage of PCR-based technologies, as compared to conventional cytogenetics, is that they can routinely be performed on any of fresh, frozen, or fixed tissue. This allows specimens that have been processed for routine histology to be evaluated in a retrospective manner; in fact, useable DNA has been isolated from histology blocks archived for 25 years (8).

Peripheral blood and bone marrow aspiration specimens need to be collected in either an ethylenediaminetetraacetic acid (EDTA)- or an acid citrate dextrose–containing tube. Heparin, another commonly used anticoagulant, should be avoided as it is an inhibitor of PCR through its interactions with *Taq* polymerase (9,10). While a heparinized specimen is suitable for conventional cytogenetics and FISH, heparin is not efficiently removed by many nucleic acid isolation methods; extractions utilizing silica columns in conjunction with chaotropic salts may have better success than other organic-based methods (e.g., phenol-chloroform extraction). Occasionally, the only clinical specimen available is in a heparin-containing tube. In these situations, clinical laboratories may attempt nucleic acid isolation, but partial to complete inhibition of amplification would not be unexpected. Care should also be taken with hemolyzed

| Table 8.1 | LIST OF 2008 WHO CATEGORIES WHERE THE PRESENCE OF SPECIFIC MOLECULAR GENETIC ABNORMALITIES PLAYS A CRITICAL DIAGNOSTIC ROLE | |

Hematologic Neoplasm	Molecular Genetic Lesion	Significance of Genetic Lesion[a]
AML		
AML with recurrent translocations	t(8;21)(q22;q22); *RUNX1-RUNX1T1* inv(16)(p13.1q22); *CBFB-MYH11* or t(16;16)(p13.1;q22); *CBFB-MYH11* t(15;17)(q24;q12); *PML-RARA*[b] t(9;11)(q22;q23); *MLLT3-MLL* t(6;9)(q23;q34); *DEK-NUP214* inv(3)(q21q26.2); *RPN-EVI1* or t(3;3)(q21;q26.2); *RPN-EVI1* t(1;22)(p13;q13); *RBM15-MKL1*	Each translocation defines a specific disease entity
AML with gene mutations	Mutated *NPM1*[c] Mutated *CEBPA*[c]	Disease-defining diagnostic criteria
Myeloproliferative Neoplasms		
CML	t(9;22)(q34;q11.2); *BCR-ABL1*	Disease-defining diagnostic criterion
PV	*JAK2* V617F mutation *JAK2* exon 12 mutations	Major diagnostic criterion
PMF	*JAK2* V617F mutation Mutated *MPL*	Major diagnostic criterion
ET	JAK2 V617F mutation Mutated *MPL*	Major diagnostic criterion
Mastocytosis	*KIT* D816V mutation	Minor diagnostic criterion
Myeloid and Lymphoid Neoplasms with Eosinophilia and Abnormalities of PDGFRA, PDGFRB, and FGFR1		
Myeloid and lymphoid neoplasms with *PDGFRA* rearrangement	del(4)(q12); *FIP1L1-PDGFRA* or related translocation involving *PDGFRA*	Disease-defining diagnostic criterion
Myeloid neoplasms with *PDGFRB* rearrangement	t(5;12)(q31~q33;p12); *ETV6-PDGFRB* or related translocation involving *PDGFRB*	Disease-defining diagnostic criterion
Myeloid and lymphoid neoplasms with *FGFR1* rearrangement	t(8;13)(p11;q12); *ZNF198-FGFR1* or related translocation involving *FGFR1*	Disease-defining diagnostic criterion
MDS		
MDS with isolated del(5q)	Isolated del(5q)	Disease-defining diagnostic criteria
B Lymphoblastic Leukemia/Lymphoma		
B-ALL with recurrent genetic abnormalities	t(9;22)(q34;q11.2); *BCR-ABL1* t(v;11q23); *MLL* rearranged (12;21)(p13;q22); *ETV6-RUNX1* t(5;14)(q31;q32); *IL3-IGH@* t(1;19)(q23;p13.3); *TCF3-PBX1* Hyperdiploidy Hypodiploidy	Each abnormality defines a specific disease entity
Mature T-Cell Neoplasms		
Anaplastic large cell lymphoma, ALK positive	t(2;5)(p23;q35); *NPM1-ALK* or related variant with 2p23	Disease-defining diagnostic criterion[d]

[a]In the appropriate clinical and hematologic context.
[b]*PML* was originally assigned to 15q22 but has since been reassigned to 15q24.
[c]These are provisional diagnostic categories.
[d]Immunohistochemical detection of ALK is an alternative (and perhaps more frequently used) diagnostic surrogate.

samples (e.g., freeze-thawed blood sample) as hemoglobin is another potent inhibitor of PCR (11). Fortunately, hemoglobin is readily removed by most contemporary extraction techniques. Both DNA and RNA can be isolated from peripheral blood and bone marrow aspirate specimens; however, the extremely labile nature of RNA dictates that specimens be refrigerated and extracted as quickly as possible. As the more stable molecule, DNA can be successfully recovered from a fresh specimen within 3 days (and in some circumstances up to 7 days) after collection as long as it has been stored at 4°C (12). RNA, on the other hand, is extremely unstable due to the pervasive existence of environmental RNAses. Ideally, RNA extraction should occur within 4 hours of specimen collection (12); as this is not always practical for clinical laboratories, usable RNA can still typically be isolated from samples up to 48 to 72 hours after collection. If nucleic acid extraction is to be delayed for any reason, samples can be stored at –20°C for longer periods of time if erythrocytes are removed before freezing the samples. Finally, a number of specimen collection tubes with RNA stabilization

agents are available commercially. These commercial systems lyse the cells immediately after collection and then stabilize the RNA, using proprietary technology, allowing blood and bone marrow specimens to be stored for days at room temperature before being extracted (13–15).

Body fluids (e.g., cerebrospinal fluid) are not typically collected in a container with an anticoagulant. This may only be problematic if the sample becomes heavily contaminated with blood. DNA and RNA can be obtained from a body fluid sample assuming it is refrigerated and/or extracted in a timely manner (12). Fresh tissue specimens should be submitted promptly for nucleic acid isolation either in a stabilizing transport medium lacking any fixative (e.g., saline or Michel's medium) or snap frozen, usually through embedding in optimal cutting temperature solution, and transported to the laboratory on dry ice.

Paraffin-embedded tissue (PET) may also be suitable for genetic studies. An important consideration is the fixative used in preparing the tissue as this directly impacts the quality and quantity of the recovered DNA and RNA. Neutral buffered

| Table 8.2 | CLINICAL APPLICATIONS OF MOLECULAR DIAGNOSTIC APPROACHES |

Sample Type	Method	Approximate Analytical Sensitivity (%)	Widely Available in Clinical Laboratories					Emerging in Clinical Laboratories		
			Identify Gene Mutations	Evaluate Gene Expression Levels	Profile Antigen Receptor Gene Rearrangements	Detect Balanced Chromosomal Translocations	Identify Numeric Chromosomal Changes[a]	Gene Methylation	CNVs	aUPD
DNA	PCR	<1	Yes	—	Yes	Yes	—	Yes	Limited	—
	Sanger sequencing	20	Yes	—	—	Yes	—	Yes	—	—
	Pyrosequencing	10	Yes	—	—	—	—	Yes	—	—
	NGS sequencing	5	Yes	—	—	—	—	—	Yes	—
	SNP array	20	—	—	—	—	Yes	—	Yes	Yes
	Array CGH	30	—	—	—	—	Yes	—	Yes	—
RNA	RT-PCR	<1	Yes	Yes	—	Yes	—	—	—	—
	Sanger sequencing	20	Yes	—	—	Yes	—	—	—	—
Cells	Karyotype[b]	10	—	—	—	Yes	Yes	—	—	—
	FISH	1	—	—	—	Yes	Yes	—	Limited	—

[a]While conventional karyotyping and FISH are able to distinguish multiple and distinct clones within a patient sample, SNP arrays and array CGH cannot.
[b]Conventional karyotyping requires viable dividing cells whereas FISH (as well as all the other methods noted here) does not. Consequently, FISH can be performed on a wide range of cells and tissues including paraffin-embedded material.

formalin, the most widely used fixative, degrades nucleic acid through a series of chemical reactions including protein and nucleic acid cross-linking. Conventional extraction methods are able to reverse a number of these modifications; however, DNA and RNA isolated from formalin-fixed PET are highly fragmented. While the degree of fragmentation is variable, the average recovered DNA fragment is 300 to 400 bp, which is suitable for most PCR-based assays (16). Larger amplifiable DNA fragments (i.e., >1,000 bp) have been reported (17). RNA, not surprisingly, is often degraded to fragments 200 bp or less in size (18,19). Furthermore, not all methods are suitable and/ or efficient at RNA extraction from PET (18). Thus, RNA-based diagnostics from PET are much less readily available as compared to DNA-based assays. Fixatives containing mercuric chloride, like B-5 and Zenker's fixative, are not appropriate for molecular analysis. Mercuric chloride forms protein complexes, which are resistant to protease digestion and thus prevent the recovery of DNA from fixed tissue (20,21). The acids contained in some fixatives, like the picric acid in Bouin's fixative, are also problematic. The acid degrades DNA and RNA. Not surprisingly, acidic decalcifying solutions such as those used for bone marrow biopsy processing are also contraindicated for genetic studies due to the negative effects on nucleic acid stability (21). In contrast, alcohol-based fixatives (e.g., ethanol or methanol found in many cytology preparations) are excellent for PCR-based studies because they preserve the integrity of the nucleic acid with limited fragmentation (20,21).

Specimen Enrichment

To improve assay sensitivity and specificity, selective cell enrichment can be performed in certain specimen types. In liquid specimens such as peripheral blood, leukocyte "enrichment" can be obtained through either centrifugation, and by analyzing the buffy coat cells, or selective erythrocyte lysis. If more specific enrichment is needed (e.g., CD3+ cellular subset of peripheral blood in the context of post–stem cell transplant chimerism analysis), then antibody-based selection using either coated magnetic beads or fluorescent-activated cell sorting can be employed (22,23). However, not all of these approaches are widely available in clinical laboratories. By contrast, plasma cell enrichment (or identification) using CD138, for example, is essential to evaluating chromosomal abnormalities by FISH in plasma cell neoplasms (PCNs) (24,25).

PET specimens also can be selectively enriched by micro- or macrodissecting the tissue of interest, thereby increasing the relative representation of the lesional cells in the extracted specimen, off of unstained or stained slides (26). While not utilized as commonly in hematopathology as compared to other malignancies, microdissection can prove useful especially when investigating putative composite lymphomas (27).

Identification of Gene Mutations

A wide spectrum of gene mutations have been described in hematologic neoplasms including point mutations, insertions, deletions, and other complex alterations. The detection of gene mutations in the clinical setting is based largely upon a single, highly versatile technique: PCR.

Polymerase Chain Reaction

First developed by Kary Mullis et al. (28) in the 1980s, PCR is based upon a simple principle of thermocycling in the presence of a heat-stable DNA-dependent DNA polymerase. In a typical PCR reaction, a DNA sequence is selected for exponential amplification (Fig. 8.1). The specificity of the amplification is dictated, in large part, through the design of the PCR primers. Primers are manufactured short oligonucleotide sequences complementary to a portion of the target sequence that is used by a DNA polymerase to initiate DNA synthesis in the PCR reaction. The principal components of the PCR reaction are (a) intact double-stranded DNA from the patient sample, (b) PCR primers, (c) a thermostable DNA-dependent DNA polymerase, such as *Taq* polymerase, and (d) deoxynucleotide triphosphates (dNTPs), which serve as substrate for the polymerase. Through repeated cycles of (a) DNA denaturation, (b) PCR primer annealing, and (c) primer extension by the polymerase, the exponential amplification of the target sequence is achieved. While the level of amplification is dependent on the overall efficiency of the reaction, a 35-cycle PCR theoretically amplifies the target sequence more than 10 billion fold (i.e., 2^{35}). To provide a sense of scale, if a single teaspoon of water (1 mL) was amplified to this degree, there would be enough water to fill nearly 14

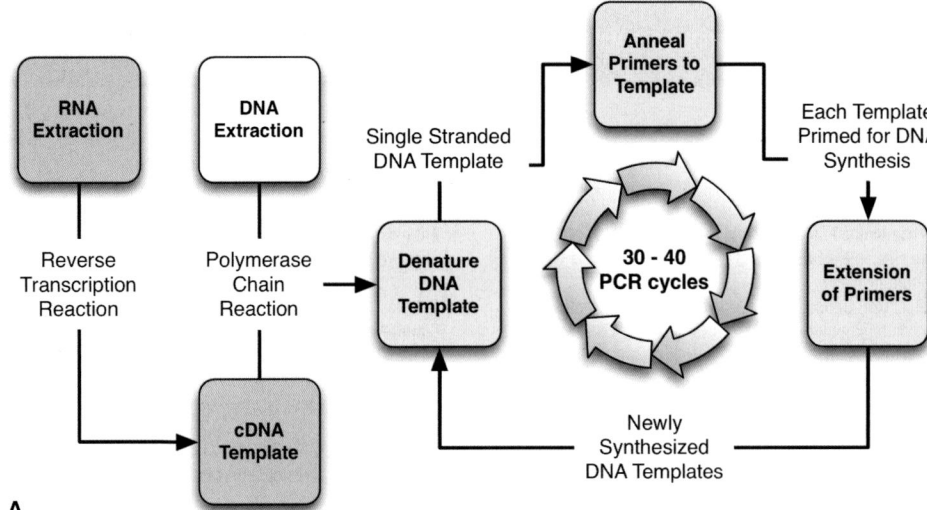

A

FIGURE 8.1. Polymerase chain reaction overview. A: A schematic overview of the steps involved in a PCR amplification beginning with either DNA or RNA extraction and ending with the evaluation of the PCR product. PCR products can be evaluated qualitatively via agarose gel electrophoresis or capillary electrophoresis. Amplified template from a completed PCR reaction can also serve as starting material for additional analytical methods such as Sanger sequencing reactions. B: Each PCR cycle results in the doubling of the starting template material, leading to an exponential accumulation of the targeted segment.

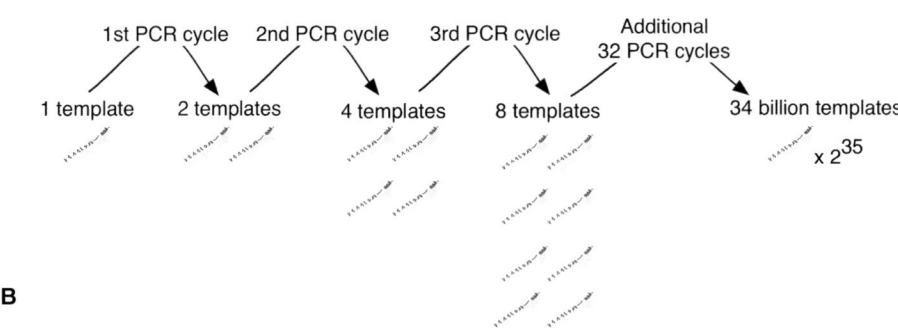

B

Olympic-sized swimming pools. This level of amplification is what gives PCR its tremendous analytical sensitivity. Many PCR assays are capable of detecting the equivalent of one leukemia or lymphoma cell in 100,000 normal cells, thus making PCR an outstanding tool in the monitoring of minimal residual disease.

As the universal adaptor of molecular diagnostics, PCR is not limited to the evaluation of DNA. In addition to interrogating samples for specific genomic lesions, PCR is also the gold standard for measuring RNA transcripts. Reverse-transcription PCR (RT-PCR) mirrors traditional PCR with one minor exception: the starting material is RNA (Fig. 8.1). Using RNA-dependent DNA polymerase (retroviral reverse transcriptase), single-stranded RNA isolated from the patient sample is converted into double-stranded complementary DNA (cDNA). The cDNA, which is more stable than RNA, then serves as the template in the subsequent PCR reaction that produces an exponential amount of DNA from the starting cDNA template.

Several alternative methods to PCR have been developed to amplify the signal from nucleic acid templates. These non-PCR–based approaches include transcription-mediated amplification, ligase chain reaction, loop mediate amplification (29), invader assay (30), branched DNA assay (31), and several others that have been variably implemented in the clinical laboratory; however, most of these methods are not routinely used in the evaluation of hematologic neoplasms.

One of the strengths of PCR is its tremendous versatility, with each PCR variation having its own distinct advantages and applications. For example, allele-specific PCR is a variant used primarily in the detection of point mutations. Primer sequences are specifically designed to interrogate the variant position. By using multiple reactions with allele-specific primers, one can readily distinguish heterozygous and homozygous mutant

sequences from wild-type. This approach has been employed extensively in the evaluation of hematologic disorders including the detection of *JAK2* V617F and *KIT* D816V mutations in myeloproliferative neoplasms (MPNs) (32,33). A thorough and exhaustive description of all PCR variants exceeds what is practical for this discussion; Table 8.3 summarizes the PCR variants used in the evaluation of hematopoietic neoplasms.

A number of molecular diagnostic techniques, including DNA sequencing, are based on the evaluation and/or manipulation of the amplified template from a PCR reaction. When evaluating a clinical specimen for mutations, the direct evaluation of the DNA sequence can be a robust and powerful tool. In the context of hematologic malignancies, and indeed cancer in general, somatically acquired mutations are typically evaluated; on occasion, assessment of constitutional (i.e., inherited) mutations may also be indicated. The principal sequencing approaches include traditional Sanger sequencing and pyrosequencing, with NGS emerging as a potentially superior technology. Each sequencing method has its own inherent strengths and weaknesses (Table 8.4). Given the effort associated with sequencing, a number of laboratories are utilizing high-resolution melt curve analysis as an initial screening tool to enrich for somatic mutations. By leveraging the thermodynamic properties of DNA, high-resolution melt curve analysis can readily detect sequence variants in a simple and cost effective manner (34).

Sanger Sequencing

Developed in the 1970s by Sanger et al. (36), Sanger sequencing is a multistep process based on DNA synthesis with random chain termination events. The technique involves five major steps: (a) PCR amplification of target sequence, (b) PCR template cleanup

Table 8.3	VARIATIONS OF PCR USED IN THE EVALUATION OF HEMATOLOGIC NEOPLASMS			

Common PCR Variants	Template	Typical Application	Example Application
Allele specific PCR	DNA	Identification point mutations and SNPs	Diagnostic assay for *JAK2* V617F mutation
Methlyation-dependent PCR	DNA	Characterizes epigenetic changes by evaluating methylation status of CpG islands	*Hpa*II tiny fragment enrichment by ligation-mediated PCR (HELP) assay for genome-wide DNA methylation profiling
Multiplex PCR	DNA	By combining multiple primer sets in a single reaction, one can efficiently evaluate multiple targets in a single gene simultaneously	Antigen receptor gene rearrangements (e.g., *IGH@* PCR and *TRG@* PCR)
RT-PCR	RNA	Detect RNA transcripts both physiologic and pathologic	Diagnostic assay for t(15;17); *PML-RARA* translocation
Multiplex reverse transcription PCR	RNA	By combining multiple primer sets in a single reaction, one can efficiently evaluate multiple recurrent translocations	Simultaneous detection of recurrent translocations in acute leukemia
Quantitative PCR	DNA	Monitor levels of a specific clonal rearrangement in response to therapy; may require sequencing the specific gene, synthesizing patient-specific primers, and a real-time PCR instrument	Allele-specific quantitative *IGH@* PCR in B-cell ALL (for minimal residual disease)
Quantitative RT-PCR	RNA	Monitor levels of a RNA transcript in response to therapy; requires a real-time PCR instrument	Quantitative t(9;22); *BCR-ABL1* transcript monitoring in CML (for minimal residual disease)

to remove extraneous PCR primers and dNTPs, which serve as substrate for the polymerase, (c) the PCR template is denatured into single strands, (d) the single-stranded DNA serves as a template for DNA synthesis, with the reaction containing fluorescently tagged chain terminating nucleotides, and (e) after multiple rounds of DNA synthesis the DNA fragments are then evaluated via electrophoresis. Sanger was awarded the Nobel Prize in the 1980s for the Sanger sequencing methodology, which has been the workhorse in clinical laboratories as well as in the Human Genome Project (37,38). Although capable of detecting a full spectrum of mutations (e.g., insertion, deletions, point mutations), Sanger sequencing has limited analytical sensitivity as compared to other mutation detection methods. While Sanger sequencing is well suited to diagnostic indications, minimal residual disease detection is better accomplished by other methods.

Pyrosequencing

Pyrosequencing emerged in the late 1990s (39) and is a rapid, flexible, and cost-effective alternative to traditional Sanger sequencing. It differs from the Sanger approach (i.e., sequencing by termination) in that it relies on the release of a pyrophosphate following the incorporation of a dNTP into DNA (i.e., sequencing by synthesis). The technique involves four major steps, the first three of which are quite similar to Sanger sequencing: (a) PCR amplification of the target sequence, (b) PCR template cleanup to remove extraneous PCR primers and dNTPS, (c) the PCR template is denatured into a single strand

and immobilized on beads, and (d) DNA synthesis then occurs in a cyclical manner by the controlled dispensation of a single type of dNTP. Through a series of reactions, an incorporated dNTP results in the generation of light while unincorporated dNTPs are destroyed. The chemistry of pyrosequencing makes it advantageous for mutation analysis over short sequences with high-quality and quantitative sequence information. Hence, pyrosequencing lends itself to the targeted evaluation of clustered mutation "hotspots" (e.g., mutations in *MPL* codon 515).

Next-Generation Sequencing

Alternative high-throughput DNA sequencing methods have been an area of rapid technologic growth. Innovations have lead to improved speed, throughput, and accuracy while reducing the cost per megabase sequenced (6). The first human genome took 15 years to go from conception to completion and required thousands of scientists and cost billions of dollars (40). Over 10 years later, this same level of information can be obtained in days for a fraction of the cost. Although NGS is becoming faster and cheaper every year, there are still barriers for clinical implementation including the high cost of the equipment and reagents, the relatively large batch sizes of each run, and the expense and complexity of analysis and interpretation (2,5,40). A variety of hematologic neoplasms (including acute myeloblastic leukemia, acute lymphoblastic leukemia, chronic lymphocytic leukemia (CLL), mantle cell lymphoma (MCL), FL, diffuse large B-cell leukemia, hairy cell leukemia,

Table 8.4	GENERALIZED COMPARISON OF PRINCIPAL SEQUENCING TECHNOLOGIES		

	Sanger Sequencing	Pyrosequencing	Next-Generation Sequencing[a]
Relative cost[b]	Low	Low	High
Relative assay complexity	Low	Low	High
Allele quantitation	Limited	Yes	Yes
Sequence read length[c]	~600 bp	~60 bp	~100 to 1,000 bp
Sequence output per assay[d]	~0.06 Mb	~0.006 Mb	~10 to 100,000 Mb
Analytical sensitivity[e]	20%	10%	5%

[a]NGS platforms are evolving at a rapid rate, so these generalizations do not apply to all platforms and to all applications of the technology.
[b]Based on a mid 2011 report, the approximate reagent cost for a single NGS run varied, depending on the technology, from $500 to over $20,000 (6). By comparison, the reagent cost for a 96-well Sanger sequencing run was approximately $100.
[c]Approximate length of evaluable sequence from a single sequencing reaction measured in base pairs (bp). NGS generates tremendous data through massive parallel sequencing reactions.
[d]The total amount of sequence data, measured in megabase pairs (Mb), from a single run (6). 1 Mb = 1,000,000 bases.
[e]Analytical sensitivity for NGS varies as a function of the assay design; in specific settings the technology can achieve sensitivities as low as 0.001% (35).

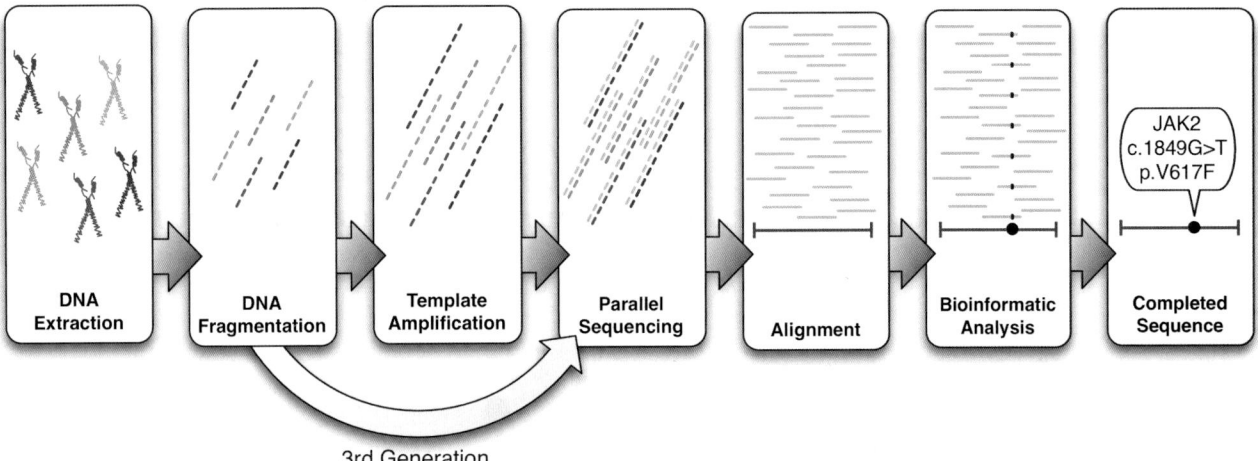

3rd Generation

FIGURE 8.2. Generalized overview of next-generation sequencing. Genomic DNA is isolated and then fragmented. Although not depicted, the fragmented DNA template is typically immobilized on a solid support (e.g., slide or bead) as a means to spatially separate the templates during the massive parallel sequencing step. Most current methods (i.e., "second-generation" NGS technology) utilize a DNA template amplification step. In contrast, emerging "third-generation" NGS technologies are not reliant on template amplification, thus reducing a potential source of error and bias (51). The next step involves a multitude of short sequencing reactions that are carried out in parallel across the entire template. These reactions result in a number of overlapping sequencing reads such that each DNA base position in the template is independently evaluated multiple times. Once the massive parallel sequencing reactions are completed, the individual sequencing reads (*light blue lines*) are aligned to a reference sequence (*dark red line*) using software tools. Using bioinformatic tools, the final sequence is assembled, interpreted, and annotated for sequence variants.

and T-cell malignancies) have been (at the least partially) sequenced in the past 5 years using different variations of this technology, including whole genome, exome, transcriptome, or RNA sequencing (41–47). The data derived therefrom has provided tremendous insights into the pathophysiology of these leukemias and lymphomas, while simultaneously providing new diagnostic and therapeutic information, as well as identifying specific lesions for targeted therapy. The pace at which genomic data is being obtained currently exceeds the rate at which the data can then be applied in the current clinical setting. In fact, much of the cancer genome data originated in cell lines that fail to replicate the tumor heterogeneity revealed by multiregional sequencing in human cancer (48). An international effort is under way to generate annotated genomic data from a large number of cancers (49).

NGS (a term that is neither ideal nor universally accepted; "massively parallel sequencing" might be a preferred term) refers to technology that does not depend on traditional electrophoresis-based Sanger sequencing (i.e., the first generation). A variety of alternative chemistries and technologies are available in NGS (6,50). Broadly, NGS platforms can be divided into second generation (i.e., methods requiring template amplification before sequencing) and more recently third generation (i.e., methods that sequence templates directly without amplification). The common thread for all NGS methods is the massive parallel sequencing of millions of short segments of DNA or RNA (Fig. 8.2). Sophisticated computational tools are required to map and assemble the massive amounts of data generated from a single NGS reaction. Clinical laboratories, as currently configured, lack the bioinformatics infrastructure to generate and annotate an entire human genome (let alone a heterogeneous cancer genome) in a clinically relevant time frame. This has led many institutions to employ NGS in a more limited fashion through targeted exome sequencing where only a subset of exons is sequenced at very high levels of coverage.

Evaluation of Gene Expression Levels

There is a growing list of genes implicated in hematologic malignancies whose coding sequence is completely unaltered; however, their expression is dysregulated. The etiology of the altered expression remains poorly understood but may be a consequence of a mutation or epigenetic alteration in a regulatory element, or an effect of microRNA (miRNA). Altered gene expression may be a contributing factor to neoplastic transformation, or alternatively it may be simply a biomarker of the disease and/or prognosis. Regardless, data are accumulating that certain gene expression levels should be measured as they may have an impact on patient management including risk stratification (52). Routine monitoring of gene expression levels is only at the initial phases of integration of clinical implementation. A primary limitation for implementation is the need to perform these studies on RNA samples that, as previously discussed, are highly unstable. Furthermore, reference ranges will need to be established before gene expression tests can become routine and practical.

Real-Time PCR

PCR, whether using DNA or RNA (i.e., reverse transcription PCR) as the initial template, can be designed to generate binary end-point data: DNA or mRNA transcript present or absent. While this qualitative end-point analysis has important practical uses, PCR truly shines when it is performed on an instrument that can monitor amplicon generation in real time, that is, so-called real-time PCR.

"Real-time" technology allows for highly sensitive and specific amplification of DNA (and RNA) templates. By incorporating standard curves, the data generated from real-time PCR and real-time RT-PCR assays can be quantitative. Employed correctly, quantitative real-time assays can be immensely useful in monitoring disease progression or response to therapy. Examples of DNA-based real-time methods include the measurement of clone-specific antigen receptor gene rearrangements in childhood acute lymphoblastic leukemia, *JAK2* allelic burden in MPNs, and Epstein-Barr virus (EBV) viral loads in lymphoproliferative disorders (53,54). Germane RNA applications include quantitative expression analysis fusion transcripts (e.g., *BCR-ABL1* in chronic myelogenous leukemia [CML]) (55). The basic tenet of real-time PCR and real-time RT-PCR is the measurement of fluorescence during each PCR cycle; three principal fluorescent technologies are employed to achieve this goal

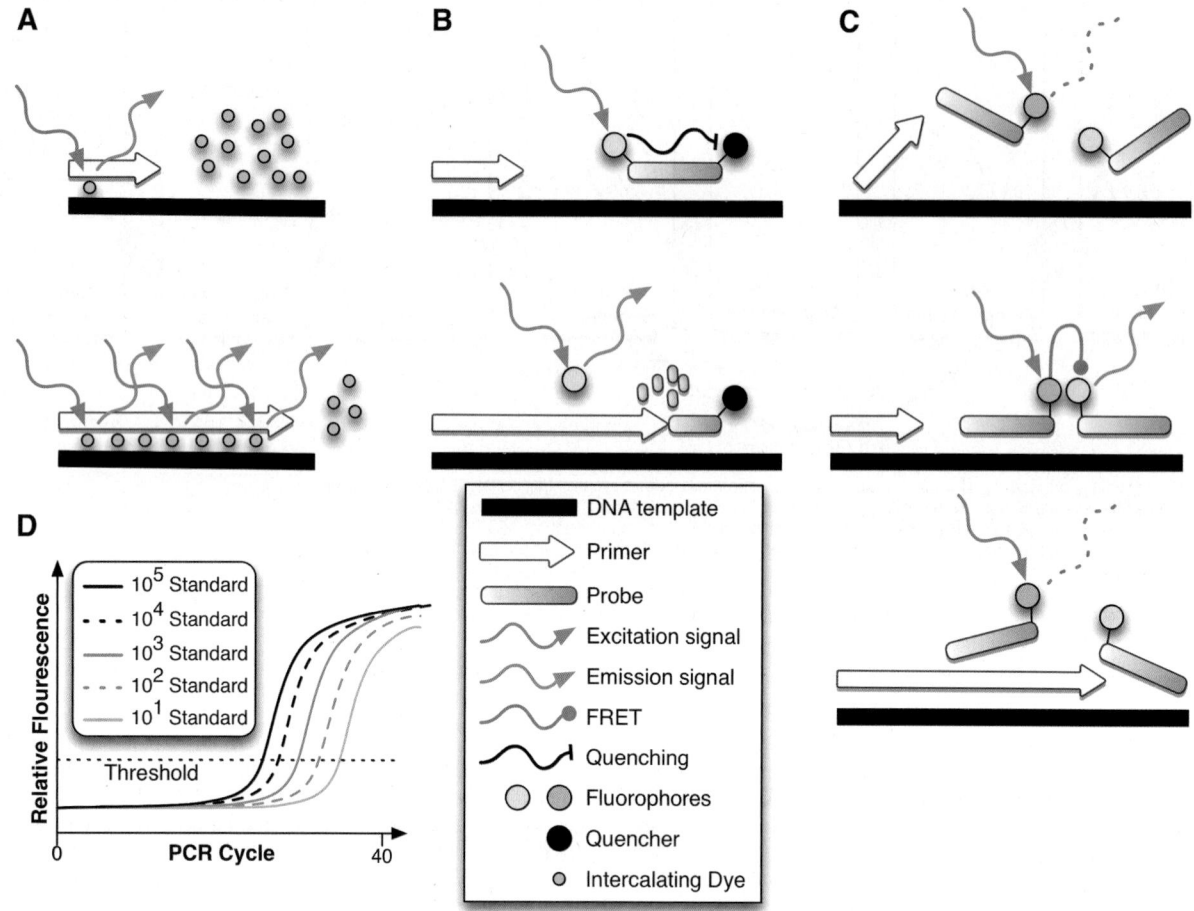

FIGURE 8.3. Principal methodologies of real-time PCR. **A**: Intercalating fluorescent dye (e.g., SYBR green) binds nonspecifically to double-stranded DNA. **B**: Sequence-specific (e.g., Taqman) probe containing a fluorophore and a quencher. **C**: Two-probe system based on FRET. **D**: Real-time PCR curves for a series of 10-fold dilutions. Note the inverse relationship between the amount of starting material and the PCR cycle; the individual reaction exceeds the fluorescence threshold. See text for details.

(Fig. 8.3). The first involves an intercalating fluorescent dye, such as SYBR green, that binds nonspecifically to the double-stranded DNA produced in the PCR reaction. As the amount of PCR product increases, the amount of bound dye increases leading to a proportional rise in the fluorescent signal (Fig. 8.3A). However, intercalating dyes bind to all double-stranded DNA including nonspecific products like dimerized PCR primers. So in this approach, the specificity of intercalating dye fluorescence is often assessed with an end-point melt curve analysis. A melt curve analysis leverages the fact that the temperature of double-stranded DNA dissociation is directly related to the sequence composition of the molecule (i.e., different DNA molecules have different dissociation curves). The two remaining approaches involve the use of fluorescently labeled probes. An advantage of sequence-specific probes is a reduction in background fluorescence as compared to intercalating dyes. Fluorescently labeled probes also have the added advantage of multiplexing (i.e., one can detect and distinguish multiple analytes in a single reaction). One approach uses a (Taqman) probe containing a reporter fluorophore and a quencher; when intact, the quencher prevents fluorescent signal emission. During the primer extension step of PCR, the probe binds to DNA and is subsequently cleaved by the exonuclease activity of *Taq* polymerase. This results in the separation of the reporter fluorophore from the quencher leading to fluorescent signal emission in proportion to the amount of PCR amplicon (Fig. 8.3B). The third general method utilizes two fluorescently labeled probes that anneal to adjacent regions

on the PCR amplicon. When unbound, the appropriate fluorescent signal is not detected from either probe. But when both probes are bound to DNA in close proximity to each other, fluorescent energy transfer (FRET) results in a detectable fluorescent signal emission (Fig. 8.3C). As the PCR reaction progresses, more of the probes are able to participate in FRET leading to an increase in signal generation.

Gene Expression Microarrays

An array refers to an orderly collection of molecules (e.g., capture probes) on a solid support surface such as a nylon membrane or silicon surface. An array can be macroscopic (e.g., a line probe assay) or miniaturized to be microscopic (e.g., SNP microarrays). The advantage of a microarray is the density of the analytes that can be assembled on a single array; potentially hundreds of thousands of unique sequences can be evaluated simultaneously. A gene expression microarray is engineered with thousands of probes that bind fluorescently tagged cDNA. Once the data from the array are captured, appropriate computer software then aids in the analysis of these fluorescent signals, allowing one to evaluate the relative level of expression of each evaluated gene. Global patterns of gene expression can then be assayed and used to classify disease states. Gene expression arrays have not reached the clinical setting. In part this is due to the massive amount of data generated from an array since this requires a robust bioinformatics infrastructure to facilitate interpretation. In addition, validation and quality assurance are challenging given the number of assays that are being performed in parallel.

Characterizing Epigenetic Alterations

Cancer is driven by not only genetic alterations but also epigenetic abnormalities (56,57). Epigenetics refers to changes in gene expression that occur without altering genomic sequence. The most common epigenetic mechanisms are DNA methylation, histone modification, and posttranscriptional gene regulation by miRNAs. Alterations that disturb these epigenetic processes have been documented to contribute to malignancy. A variety of molecular methods are available to detect epigenetic changes, both qualitatively and quantitatively. However, direct clinical applications currently remain limited.

DNA Methylation

DNA methylation plays an important role in transcriptional regulation. Methylation frequently, but not exclusively, involves the cytosine within a CpG dinucleotide sequence. Clusters of CpG sequences form so-called CpG islands. More than half of the CpG islands occur within gene regulatory elements (58). As DNA methylation increases, especially in CpG islands located in promoters, there is a concomitant repression of transcription. Silencing of tumor suppressor genes through hypermethylation appears to be an important mechanism in neoplastic transformation (57). Likewise, genomic hypomethylation contributes to cancer by promoting genomic instability (e.g., chromosomal translocations), favoring (onco)gene activation and disrupting genomic imprinting (57). In addition to primary defects in methylation, this phenomenon may also be dysregulated as a consequence of mutations of genes that encode proteins involved in the DNA methylation pathway (e.g., *DNMT3A*, *TET2*, and *IDH1/2*).

Methylated DNA can be identified by using sodium bisulfite. Treating genomic DNA with this compound converts unmethylated cytosine (C) to uracil (U) but leaves methylated cytosine unaltered. Bisulfite-converted DNA can then be interrogated by a variety of mechanisms including enzymatic digestion, sequencing, and methylation-specific PCR (MSP). MSP is a variation of allele-specific PCR in as much as primers are specifically designed to recognize either methylated or unmethylated DNA. Qualitative or quantitative data can be obtained from sodium bisulfite-based approaches. Another method to evaluate DNA methylation, which is not dependent on sodium bisulfite treatment, is the use of restriction enzymes that are sensitive or insensitive to CpG island methylation (e.g., *Hpa*II and its methylation insensitive isoschizomer *Msp*I). One particularly relevant variant of this approach is called the HELP assay (*Hpa*II tiny fragment enrichment by ligation PCR). Briefly, genomic DNA is digested separately by *Hpa*II and *Msp*I. The resulting DNA fragments are then PCR amplified and hybridized to an array for comparison (59). The *Hpa*II digested fraction is enriched for hypomethylated DNA while the *Msp*I fraction serves as a control. HELP can be used for genome-wide or gene-specific DNA methylation profiling. Applications of MSP and other technologies to assess methylation in hematologic neoplasms are likely to enter into the clinical laboratory in the near future. For example, a 15-gene methylation panel, based on HELP, has been described that predicts overall survival in acute myeloid leukemia (AML) (60).

Histone Modification

Histone modification alters chromatin structure, which can have an important impact on gene expression. Histones are small basic proteins that comprise a portion of chromatin. Post-translational protein modifications such as acetylation, methylation, phosphorylation, ubiquitination, and sumoylation, among others, lead to structural changes in chromatin. These reversible protein modifications are controlled by a variety of enzymes, and ultimately the collection of modifications drive chromatin into one of two configurations: transcriptionally inactive heterochromatin or transcriptionally active euchromatin. As with DNA methylation, histone modification may also be dysregulated as a consequence of gene mutations that encode proteins involved in these pathways (e.g., *EZH2*, *MLL*, and *ASXL1*). As posttranslation events, histone modifications themselves are best evaluated by immunoassays, immunohistochemistry (IHC), or mass spectrometry and thus might be considered outside of the realm of molecular genetics (61–63).

MicroRNAs

miRNAs are endogenous short (~22 bp) noncoding RNA molecules that posttranscriptionally regulate gene expression. MiRNAs target complementary sequences in the untranslated regions of messenger RNA transcripts. These interactions lead to either the degradation of the targeted mRNA or the inhibition of translation. Hundreds of miRNAs have been described, and thousands more have been predicted (64). As miRNAs play a crucial role in numerous biologic processes including the regulation of epigenetic machinery, it is not surprising that they have been implicated in the initiation and progression of cancer (65). In fact, miRNA profiling has been useful in the classification of certain hematologic malignancies (66).

MiRNA expression levels can be gauged by a variety of methods (67,68). Northern blotting, the RNA-based variant of Southern blotting, is one of the most widely used methods. However, like Southern blotting, it is labor intensive and has a limited throughput. Given this, quantitative RT-PCR based methods have been adapted for sensitive and specific detection and quantification of miRNAs. When appropriate, microarray technology can also be employed for high-throughput evaluations of miRNAs.

Detection of Translocations

The most frequent genetic phenomenon that is currently routinely evaluated in hematologic malignancies is pathologic rearrangements, that is, nonrandom recurrent chromosomal translocations. Importantly, translocations are often (but not always) disease specific, so identifying them provides critical diagnostic information. They can be grouped into two broad categories with regard to the consequence of the translocation: (a) quantitative and (b) qualitative. Quantitative translocations are more commonly found in lymphoid malignancies. For example, in FL, the juxtaposition of a contextually transcriptionally active gene (e.g., *IGH@* in a B cell) with a protooncogene (e.g., *BCL2*) results in dysregulated expression of an unaltered wild-type BCL2 protein. These types of translocations arise as a consequence of an error in normal V(D)J antigen receptor gene rearrangement that occurs in the bone marrow or thymus; as well as at the time of somatic hypermutation (SHM) or class switch recombination in the germinal centers (69). Hence, most quantitative translocations often involve antigen receptor genes, and are restricted to lymphoid neoplasms. Qualitative translocations, on the other hand, are more often, but not exclusively, seen in myeloid malignancies. Qualitative translocations result in the creation of a novel gene fusion due to the simultaneous disruption of the coding sequence for both of the genes involved. Examples include the *BCR-ABL1* fusion gene in the t(9;22) translocation of and *NPM1-ALK* fusion in the t(2;5) translocation seen in ALK-positive anaplastic large cell lymphoma (ALCL). It is worth noting that methods for the diagnostic detection of pathologic rearrangements are typically binary (i.e., absent/present), while those for physiologic rearrangements (i.e., antigen receptor gene rearrangements) are designed to assess the heterogeneity (or lack thereof) of the genes.

Table 8.5	**COMPARISON OF METAPHASE CYTOGENETICS, FISH, AND PCR-BASED METHODS IN THE DETECTION OF CHROMOSOMAL ABNORMALITIES**		
	Metaphase Cytogenetics	**FISH**	**PCR-based Methods**
Requires viable dividing cells	Yes	No	No
Typical turnaround time[a]	1–2 wk	1–5 d	1–5 d
Detect cryptic translocations	No	Yes	Yes
Detect rare or variable translocations	Yes	Yes	No[b]
Detect numeric abnormalities	Yes	Yes	No
Analytical sensitivity	5%–10%	1%–5%	0.001%–1%

[a]PCR-based methods and FISH can, in urgent clinical situations, be completed within 1 working day (i.e., 6–8 hours). This shortened turnaround time is exceedingly useful in diseases such as t(15;17); *PML-RARA*-positive AML where a rapid diagnosis can dramatically impact clinical care and outcome. If cells in a submitted sample are sufficiently mitotic with adequate metaphases, results from conventional cytogenetics can be obtained in 1–2 days.

[b]PCR-based methods are only useful in the detection of translocations specifically covered by the primers in the assay. Testing for uncommon or variant translocations not covered by the assay will result in (false)-negative results.

Translocations can be detected by a variety of methods including conventional cytogenetics and FISH (Table 8.5). Translocations can, in many cases, also be detected by PCR or RT-PCR. Translocations with quantitative consequences are typically analyzed by DNA PCR (e.g., *IGH@-BCL2* in the t(14;18) translocation). By contrast, the location of genomic breakpoints in gene fusions tends to be variable across large segments of DNA, making their detection by traditional DNA-based PCR untenable (e.g., *BCR-ABL1* in the t(9;22) translocation). As part of RNA processing, introns are spliced out of immature RNA transcripts leading to the juxtaposition of exons from each gene. By targeting primers to the exons typically involved at the junction of the fusion transcript, RT-PCR becomes the method of choice for detecting these types of recurrent balanced translocations. However, not all recurrent translocations are amenable to RT-PCR analysis.

Southern Blot

The Southern blot, a technique developed in the 1970s by Sir Edwin Mellor Southern (70), was an early tool in the molecular genetic evaluation of hematologic malignancies including chromosomal translocations and antigen receptor gene rearrangements. In a typical Southern blot, the DNA sample was digested by restriction enzymes and then fractionated by gel electrophoresis. The DNA was then physically transferred through "blotting" to a solid support medium (e.g., nitrocellulose) that was subsequently interrogated by a labeled probe. Analysis would then be based on the detected banding patterns. The technique proved to be both time-consuming and laborious for clinical laboratories. Furthermore, because the target DNA sequence is not amplified following extraction, a large amount of high-quality DNA was required for a Southern blot. Consequently, many specimens were not suitable for Southern blot analysis including formalin-fixed paraffin-embedded tissue given the DNA fragmentation. For technical and analytical reasons, Southern blotting has largely been supplanted by PCR and its contemporaries.

Profiling Antigen Receptor Gene Rearrangements

The rearrangement of antigen receptor genes (i.e., *IGH@*, *IGK@*, *IGL@* and *TRG@*, *TRD@*, *TRA@*, *TRB@*) is a defining feature of essentially all lymphocytes other than NK cells. As it is part of normal lymphoid maturation, antigen receptor gene rearrangements are not considered pathologic. Instead, these alterations can serve as an important biomarker, since documenting monoclonality in a lymphoid process can help, when incorporated with pertinent clinical and pathologic findings, distinguish a neoplastic process from a reactive one. Please see Chapter 6 for a detailed discussion.

Identification of Numeric Abnormalities

Beyond numeric abnormalities in whole chromosomes, which are of clear clinical utility but are best evaluated by either conventional cytogenetics or FISH, are a series of subkaryotypic alterations in genomic content: so-called CNVs. CNVs are a common and widespread phenomenon in nonneoplastic cells. Acquired CNVs have also been identified in a variety of hematologic neoplasms and are likely collateral damage from other genetic lesions such as insertions, deletions, and translocations (71). In one study, CNVs were detected in 24% of patients with a normal karyotype AML and 40% with an abnormal karyotype with an average of approximately two CNVs per genome (72). Although CNVs are likely an important mechanism in pathogenesis of hematologic neoplasms, the prognostic and diagnostic utility of CNV discovery has not been definitively demonstrated. Initial work suggests an evaluation of CNVs may be an independent prognostic factor when integrated with age and conventional karyotyping (73). However, assessment of CNVs is currently more useful as a discovery tool than as a clinical tool.

Array CGH

Microarray-based comparative genomic hybridization (aCGH) can identify copy number gains and losses (74). DNA from a patient sample and a reference control sample are each labeled with a different fluorophore. Once labeled, both samples are cohybridized to a DNA microarray containing probes composed of either genomic fragments or oligonucleotides. Fluorescent data are then captured and analyzed for differences in the ratio of signal from each genome. A genomic gain or loss in the patient sample would be indicated by a concomitant increase or decrease in the fluorescence signal across a series of contiguous probes. Depending on the design of the aCGH, this method can detect copy number changes from several thousand base pairs in size to several hundred (75,76). For comparison, conventional cytogenetics has a resolution for chromosomal abnormalities on the order of several million base pairs in size (75).

SNP Arrays

Another application of DNA array technology is the genome-wide evaluation of SNPs, which are DNA sequence variants occurring at single nucleotide positions in the genome and commonly having only two alleles. Briefly, genomic DNA is amplified, labeled, and then hybridized to the SNP array. As SNPs are not evenly distributed throughout the genome, many SNP arrays extend their ability to detect numeric changes by including thousands of CNV probes (74). By analyzing changes in signal intensity and allelic ratios, over contiguous regions of the genome, deletions and amplifications can be detected. However, not all copy number changes detected by SNP arrays are pathologic. CNV databases, which are employed in the analysis of the data, are far from complete (77). To distinguish inherited from neoplastic CNVs, SNP array data should be obtained and analyzed from matched neoplastic and normal tissue, allowing one to readily identify "private" CNVs that are not yet available in the CNV database (77).

Acquired uniparental disomy (aUPD) is a genetic lesion readily detected by SNP arrays but missed by traditional

Table 8.6	REPRESENTATIVE EXAMPLES OF GENE MUTATION NOMENCLATURE IN HEMATOLOGIC NEOPLASMS					
Colloquial Nomenclature	**HGNC Gene Name**	**Reference Sequence**	**HGVS DNA**	**HGVS Protein**	**Standardized Nomenclature**[a]	
BRAF V600E mutation	*BRAF*	NM_004333.4	c.1799T>A	p.V600E	*BRAF* NM_004333.4: c.1799T>A (p.V600E)	
CEBPA N-terminal mutation	*CEBPA*	NM_004364.2	c.247delC	p.Q83fs*77	*CEBPA* NM_004364.2: c.247delC (p.Q83fs*77)	
CEBPA C-terminal mutation	*CEBPA*	NM_004364.2	c.937_939delAAG	p.K313del	*CEBPA* NM_004364.2: c.937_939delAAG (p.K313del)	
JAK2 V617F mutation	*JAK2*	NM_004972.3	c.1849G>T	p.V617F	*JAK2* NM_004972.3: c.1849G>T (p.V617F)	
KIT D816V mutation	*KIT*	NM_000222.2	c.2447A>T	p.D816V	*KIT* NM_000222.2: c.2447A>T (p.D816V)	
NPM1 Type A mutation	*NPM1*	NM_002520.4	c.863_864insTCTG	p.W288fs*12	*NPM1* NM_002520.4: c.863_864insTCTG (p.W288fs*12)	

[a]The HGVS standardized nomenclature consists of three components. The first is the HGNC-approved gene name. The second component is the reference sequence (i.e., the refseq). The National Center for Biotechnology Information (NCBI) hosts a database (www.ncbi.nlm.nih.gov/RefSeq) of nonredundant annotated biomolecules (e.g., protein, RNA and DNA sequences) that serve as the reference standard in molecular genetic testing. In the examples above, the reference sequence from the mature mRNA transcript (NM) is provided. The third and final component is the description of the molecular change using the HGVS system. Examples for a variety of changes at the coding DNA level (c.) and the protein level (p.) are presented. The typical layout is as follows: *Gene name* Reference sequence: Sequence Variation. Variant abbreviations: deletion (del), insertion (ins), frameshift (fs*), nucleotide substitutions (G>T).

cytogenetics and aCGH. Caused by either chromosomal nondisjunction or homologous recombination during cell division, uniparental disomy (UPD) contributes to transformation by leading to copy-neutral loss of heterozygosity of mutated genes such as *JAK2*, *CEBPA*, *WT1*, *RUNX1*, *CBL*, and *FLT3* (78–80). Some *FLT3* mutations, for example, are only prognostically important when there is loss of wild type via UPD. Y371 mutations of *CBL*, which are also associated with UPD, are not pathologic when present in the "heterozygous" states (81). Thus, there is a synergy between certain mutations and UPD that may reflect distinct pathophysiology. Detection of UPD is primarily performed by SNP arrays because of its ability to genotype the SNP. The clinical utility of assessing UPD in hematologic malignancies is uncertain and at this point remains, like CNV, primarily a discovery tool for novel genetic lesions.

Standardized Gene and Mutation Nomenclature

Gene nomenclature is a potential source of confusion in molecular genetic testing. Often, a single gene will have multiple symbols and names. For example, *MLL* has been variably referred to in the literature as *ALL-1*, *CXXC7*, *HRX*, *HTRX-1*, *KMT2A*, *MLL1A*, and *TRX1*. The problem worsens when one considers recurrent translocations; *AML1-ETO*, *AML1-MTG8*, *AML1-CDR*, *CBFA2-ETO*, *CBFA2-CBFA2T1*, and *RUNX1-CBFA2T1* are all references to the *RUNX1–RUNX1T1* gene fusion resulting from the t(8;21)(q22;q22) translocation. In the clinical setting, it is critical that the results of molecular diagnostic testing be communicated in a clear, concise, and unambiguous manner. The Human Genome Organization (HUGO) gene nomenclature committee (HGNC) is an internationally recognized authority charged with the standardization and unification of human gene nomenclature (82); HGNC currently curates a database (www.genenames.org) of over 33,000 unique gene names and symbols. The HGNC has been embraced by contemporary clinical diagnostic criteria, including the 2008 WHO guidelines. In addition, most biomedical databases, including the Catalogue of Somatic Mutations in Cancer (COSMIC, cancer.sanger.ac.uk/cancergenome/projects/cosmic), use the HGNC nomenclature. Equally confusing and ambiguous are gene mutations. For example, V617F and G1849T both have been used in the literature (appropriately) to refer to the same mutation in *JAK2* with the former referencing the change at the amino acid level and the latter at the nucleotide level. Not surprisingly, individuals have inadvertently interpreted this information as two separate but common mutations in JAK2 (e.g., can you test my V617F-negative patient for the G1849T mutation?). Fortunately, a nomenclature system for gene mutations and sequence variations has been developed by the Human Genome Variation Society (HGVS, www.hgvs.org) (83). Representative examples

of gene mutations in hematologic neoplasms are presented in Table 8.6. Although the HGVS system allows for unambiguous communication, which makes it well suited for full clinical reports, the system does not lend itself to verbal communication and as such colloquial mutation nomenclature will continue to be used in written and oral communications.

 ## MYELOID NEOPLASMS

Myeloid neoplasms can be parsed into five variably and broadly distinct categories. These are AML, MPNs, neoplasms with eosinophila, myelodysplastic syndromes (MDS), and mixed myelodysplastic/MPNs. For each broad category, there are distinctive clinical, morphologic, and biologic characteristics (see chapters 41 and 43–45 for detailed discussions of these), and each has its own somewhat distinctive genetic underpinnings. However, some of the targeted genes are not unique to a category, and appear to be mechanistically involved across these categories. Table 8.7 summarizes the enormous genetic complexity evident in these different myeloid neoplasms.

Acute Myeloid Leukemia

AML is, in simplest terms, a clonal expansion of immature myeloid elements (myeloblasts and their morphologic equivalents) emanating from the bone marrow. How this occurs, from a molecular perspective, is rather complex. At a minimum, neoplastic transformation requires two major genetic

Table 8.7	RECURRENT GENETIC LESIONS IN MYELOID NEOPLASMS	
Disease	**Genes with Recurrent Mutations**[a]	**Recurrent Structural Chromosomal Abnormalities**[b]
AML	198	819
MDS	29	147
Myeloproliferative neoplasms (MPN)[c]	23	411
MDS/MPN	21	45
Eosinophilic neoplasms	Rare	39

[a]Recurrent genetic lesions (i.e., events documented in at least two instances) based on available data from COSMIC (84), Mitelman Database of Chromosome Aberrations and Gene Fusions in Cancer (85) and the 2008 WHO classification (1).
[b]Of the recurrent structural chromosomal abnormalities associated with MPN, the majority (i.e., 86) were documented in association with CML; this high number includes numerous variant translocations as well as cases that are undergoing transformation.

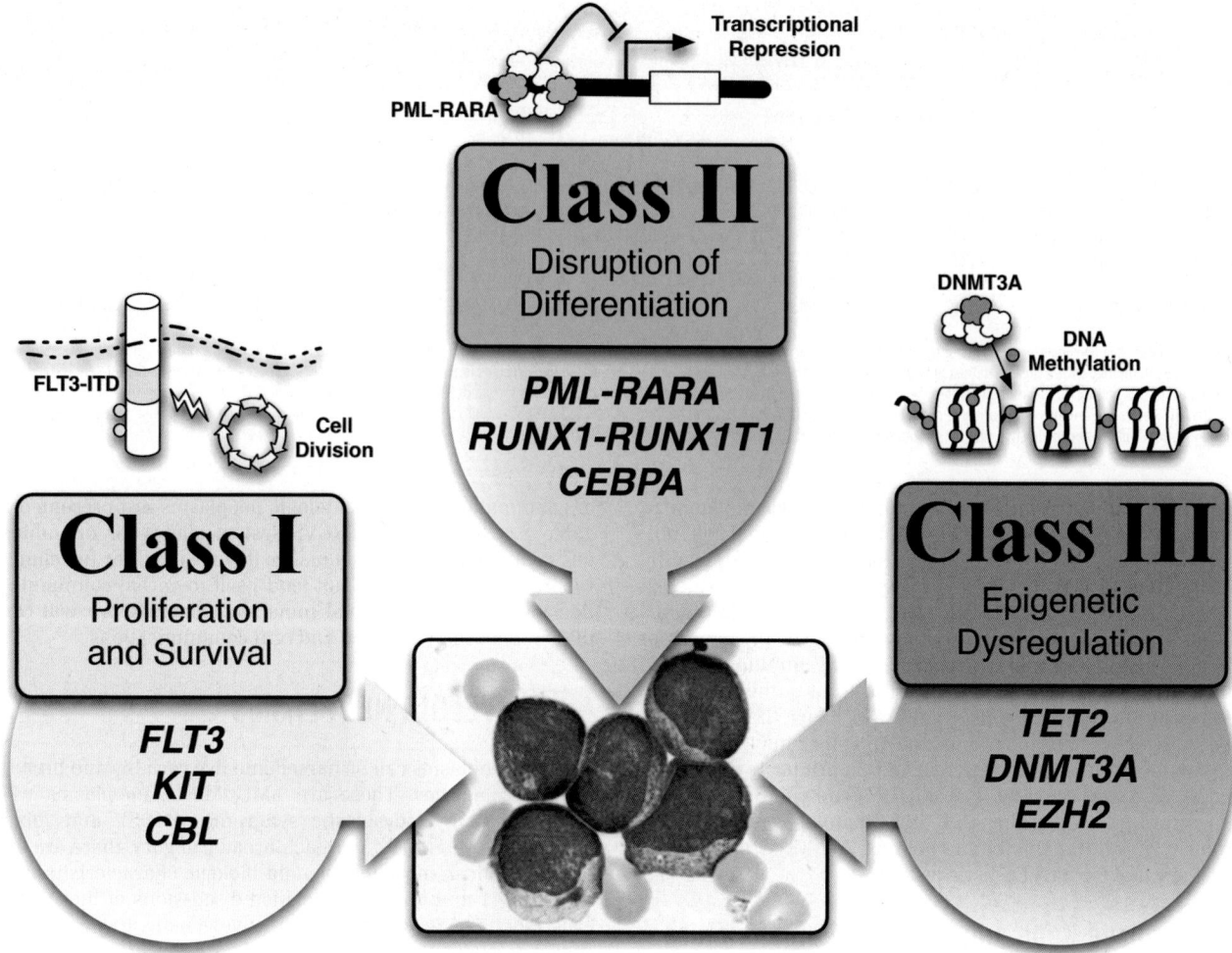

FIGURE 8.4.   Molecular basis of AML. While it remains unclear how many genetic hits are required to induce neoplastic transformation, the current model highlights (at least) three major pathways, which are recurrently disrupted in AML. Some studies have shown the presence of approximately 10 somatic mutations per AML genome, and other targeted pathways (or classes) might include those that affect cellular interactions (with the stroma or other cells), DNA damage repair (such as TP53), and RNA splicing (spliceosome genes).

lesions: a disruption in proliferation or survival (i.e., class I mutations) and a defect in differentiation (i.e., class II mutations). Gene mutations that disrupt signal transduction pathways (e.g., *FLT3* and *KIT* mutations) are categorized as class I mutations. As for archetypal class II mutations, gene fusions (e.g., *PML-RARA* and *RUNX1-RUNX1T1*) clearly impair normal differentiations of hematopoietic stem cells. A third pathway seems to be recurrently disrupted in AML; thus, it has been proposed that those that modify epigenetic mechanisms (such as DNA methylation, histone modifications) be considered class III mutations (Fig. 8.4). While all classes of mutations might be present simultaneously in all AMLs, this model probably oversimplifies the process. In fact, it has become increasingly clear that AML is a tremendously heterogeneous disease and that the diversity truly reveals itself at the molecular level (Fig. 8.5). Although multiple genetic mechanisms (e.g., altered gene expression, epigenetic changes, and copy number alterations) have been implicated in the pathophysiology of the disease, only chromosomal translocations and a small number of gene mutations are currently formally recognized as clinically relevant abnormalities. The inclusion of seven diagnostic recurrent translocations and two provisional diagnostic categories based on gene mutations in the 2008 WHO classification system has promoted the concept that AML is a genetic disease.

Over 800 recurrent chromosomal aberrations have been described in AML (85). Of these structural abnormalities, at least 250 are recurrent translocations. However, the seven recurrent translocations recognized by WHO as distinct entities represent, in aggregate, approximately 25% of all AML cases. Thus, the identification of these seven specific translocations is particularly relevant to clinical diagnosis as well as prognosis.

t(8;21)(q22;q22); RUNX1–RUNXT1

Core binding factor (CBF) is a heterodimeric transcription complex. As CBF is an important regulator of hematopoiesis, it is not surprising that genetic abnormalities that dysregulate CBF lead to a number of myeloid neoplasms including AML. In fact, two of the components of CBF, *RUNX1* and *CBFB*, are common targets of translocations in AML. One of the two major AML translocations involving CBF is t(8;21)(q22;q22), which occurs in approximately 5% to 8% of all AML (1,88) and is associated with a favorable prognosis. While enriched in the previously FAB-designated morphologic category of AML-M2 (myeloblastic with maturation), many cases with this translocation are associated with cytologically characteristic blasts, with numerous and occasionally very large azurophilic granules, as well as single Auer rods. Immunophenotypically, this category of AMLs is noteworthy for the expression of some B-cell–associated

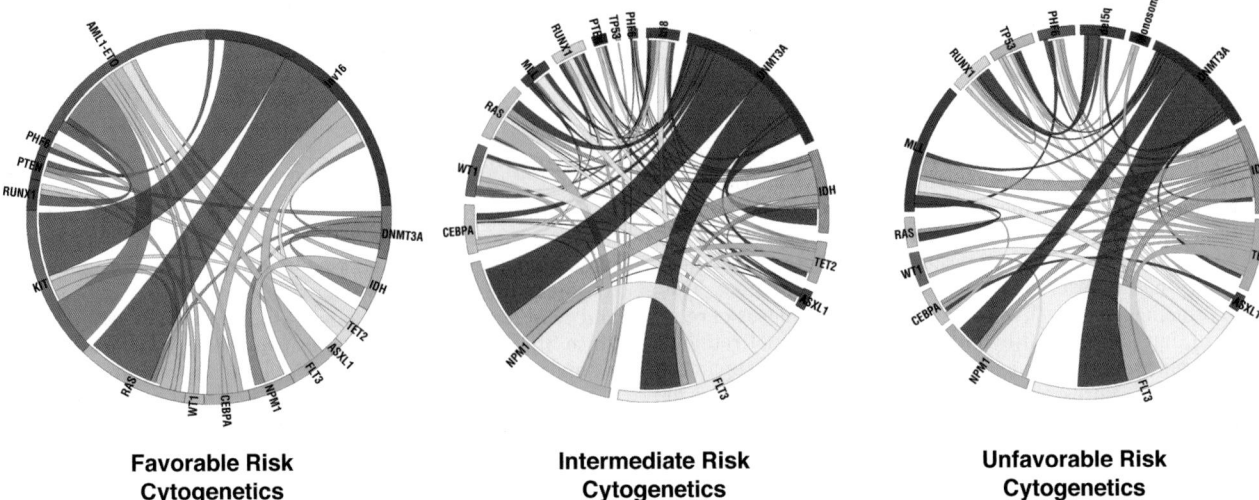

Favorable Risk Cytogenetics   **Intermediate Risk Cytogenetics**   **Unfavorable Risk Cytogenetics**

FIGURE 8.5. Mutational complexity of AML. Circos diagrams demonstrating the relative frequency and co-occurrence of genetic lesions in the three cytogenetically defined risk categories of AML. The length of the colored arc corresponds to the frequency of the genetic lesion. Colored ribbons connect genetic lesions that co-occurred; the width of the ribbon is proportional to the percentage of cases with the paired genetic lesions. Within the favorable risk group, the recurrent chromosomal rearrangements associated with core binding factor (CBF) AML predominate. These CBF AMLs include those with "AML1-ETO," which is equivalent to those with the *RUNX1-RUNX1T1* fusion, and "inv16," which is equivalent to those with the *CBFB-MY11* fusion (see text for details). However, data from t(15;17) AML are not available for comparison in this figure. Approximately 15% of AML with favorable cytogenetics have two or more mutations. In comparison, approximately 24% of unfavorable risk and nearly 70% of intermediate risk AMLs have two or more mutations, highlighting the mutational complexity of these two categories. Mutation patterns are becoming increasingly evident. Note the frequent association between *KIT* mutations and CBF AML as well as *DNMT3A* mutations with *NPM1*, *FLT3*, and *IDH1* mutations. It is also apparent that *IDH1/2* mutations are mutually exclusive with *TET2* and *WT1* mutations. Adapted from Patel JP, Gönen M, Figueroa ME, et al. Prognostic relevance of integrated genetic profiling in acute myeloid leukemia. *N Engl J Med,* 2012;366:1079–1089, with permission (87). Copyright © 2012 Massachusetts Medical Society. MLL, MLL partial tandem duplications; IDH, *IDH1* and *IDH2;* tri8, trisomy 8; del5q, deletion 5q.

antigens, including CD19 and PAX5. *RUNX1* on 21q22 is fused with part of the *RUNX1T1* gene on 8q22. The resulting fusion protein, RUNX1–RUNX1T1, disrupts hematopoiesis by repressing transcription of a number of critical target genes including *MPO, GM-CSF, IL-3,* and the *TRB@* (89). Both RT-PCR and FISH, in addition to metaphase cytogenetics, may be used to detect this translocation. Given that the breakpoints cluster within a single intron for each gene, the t(8;21) translocation can be readily detected by a simple RT-PCR assay. Quantitative RT-PCR studies are also available clinically and may prove useful in monitoring minimal residual disease. Importantly, detectable fusion transcripts have been reported in patients with long-term survival (90,91), indicating that qualitative transcript detection may be of limited clinical utility. Rather, as is true of posttherapy molecular monitoring for minimal residual disease across the spectrum of hematologic malignancies, the kinetics of transcript-level changes appears to be more clinically relevant with rising levels predictive of AML relapse (52).

inv(16)(p13q22) or t(16;16)(p13;q22); CBFB-MYH11

Another recurrent translocation in CBF AML results from either a pericentric inversion of chromosome 16 or a molecularly identical t(16;16) translocation. With a frequency of 5% to 10%, the AML resulting from these structural rearrangements is characteristically associated with abnormal eosinophils (i.e., FAB entity AML M4Eo) (1,88). Although most often associated with M4Eo, this recurrent genetic lesion can be found in other subtypes of AML; conversely, not all M4Eos harbor this genetic fusion. These particular chromosome 16 rearrangements result in the fusion of *CBFB* gene with one of the myosin heavy chain genes, *MYH11.* *CBFB-MYH11* disrupts CBF activity by sequestering the RUNX1 protein in the cytoplasm (92). The fusion protein may also act more directly by repressing transcription (92). Since the inversion can be subtle, it can often be missed by conventional cytogenetic analysis. Curiously, inv(16) AML is commonly associated

with a secondary +22 abnormality. As +22 is a relatively uncommon finding in other AMLs, an apparently isolated +22 in AML should be carefully evaluated for a cryptic inv(16). Even more curious, the presence of a +22 in a young adult with inv(16) AML is associated with a better clinical outcome (93); typically secondary cytogenetic abnormalities are associated with adverse clinical outcomes. Given the diagnostic difficulties associated with cytogenetics, other molecular methods have increased relevance in the diagnosis of *CBFB-MHY11*-associated AML. The breakpoints in *CBFB* occur almost exclusively in intron 5 while the breakpoints in *MYH11* are more varied with seven different exons involved. Consequently, at least 10 different fusion transcripts have been described. Fortunately, one specific rearrangement, designated type A, accounts for approximately 90% of the fusion transcripts. Two other *CBFB-MHY11* transcripts, type D and type E, account for an additional 5% of the rearrangements. Although FISH assays will likely detect a larger fraction of translocations, sensitive and specific RT-PCR assays capable of detecting the most common breakpoints (e.g., type A, D, and E) are readily available in the clinical setting. FISH studies serve a complementary role in the ability to detect all breakpoints. Much like in the case of t(8;21), systematic monitoring of inv(16) transcript levels by quantitative RT-PCR may be useful in predicting relapse in a minimal residual disease setting (94). Finally, mutations in *KIT*, encoding a type III tyrosine kinase, are common in both inv(16) and t(8;21) AML with a reported frequency of 16% to 46% (95,96). While CBF-associated AMLs typically have a favorable prognosis, the presence of an activating *KIT* mutation in exon 8 or 17 is associated, at least in adults, with a worse prognosis in both types of CBF+ AML (95,97).

t(15;17)(q24;q12); PML-RARA

The t(15;17)(q24;q12) translocation is the prototypical molecular abnormality in acute promyelocytic leukemia (APL); it also forms the basis for one of the most compelling genotype-phenotype-targeted therapy correlations in AML. The t(15;17) translocation can frequently be predicted due to the characteristic hypergranular (or hypogranular) morphology, including the quite distinctive nuclear features with shapes resembling cottage loaves. At the genetic level, the translocation fuses the *PML* gene on 15q24 (originally assigned to 15q22, [98]) with the *RARA* gene on 17q12, which encodes a retinoic acid–responsive component of a heterodimeric transcriptional repressor complex. The protein product of *PML* is a ubiquitously expressed nuclear protein with complex functions. The *PML-RARA* gene fusion generates a potent transcriptional repressor that interferes with myeloid differentiation. The fusion protein is no longer sensitive to physiologic doses of retinoic acid, but is degraded by pharmacologic doses of retinoic acid (i.e., all-trans-retinoic acid or ATRA). Therapy disrupts the transcriptional repressor functions of PML-RARA leading to differentiation of the malignant cells (99).

Besides the traditional t(15;17) translocations, at least four alternative translocations have been described. These alternative fusions—t(11;17)(q23;q12); *ZBTB16-RARA*, t(11;17)(q13;q12); *NUMA1-RARA*, t(5;17)(q35;q12); *NPM1-RARA* and t(17;17)(q11.2;q12); *STAT5B-RARA*—were originally grouped together with t(15;17) in the 2001 WHO classification system. However, these alternative translocations are now considered separately in so much as not all of them are sensitive to ATRA treatment. For example, the t(11;17)(q23;q21) translocation results in a *ZBTB16-RARA* fusion that is resistant because *ZBTB16* itself acts as a transcriptional repressor whose function cannot be abrogated by pharmacologic doses of ATRA. Thus, it is clinically necessary to identify patients with rare alternative *RARA* partners; FISH analysis may prove useful in patients suspected of having APL but lacking the t(15;17) gene fusion by RT-PCR. Interestingly, there may be morphologic correlates with the alternative *RARA* translocations. For example, an increased number of Pelger-Huet–like cells has been described in t(11;17) leukemia.

In terms of (15;17) testing, *RARA* breakpoints are primarily in intron 2 while *PML* harbors two major breakpoints in introns 3 and 6. Thus, a simple RT-PCR assay consisting of a single downstream *RARA* primer and two upstream primers for *PML* can detect the majority of *PML-RARA* fusions. Occasionally, breakpoints in *PML* occur in exon 6. These rare variant forms of *PML-RARA* can be missed by an RT-PCR assay targeting the traditional breakpoints.

t(9;11)(p22;q23); MLLT3-MLL

The *MLL* gene on 11q23 is notable for its involvement in at least 121 recurrent translocations with 79 different cloned gene partners (100). *MLL* translocations are not limited to *de novo* AML as 11q23 rearrangements are also seen in therapy-related AML, acute lymphoblastic leukemia, and MDS. How the multitude of MLL translocations promote neoplasia has not been completely resolved, but it likely results from the dysregulation of MLL's histone methyltransferase activity leading to aberrant *HOX* gene expression (101). The t(9;11)(p22;q23) translocation, which occurs more frequently in children than in adults, is the most common 11q23 rearrangement in AML, and is typically accompanied by myelomonocytic morphology. Unlike most of the other *MLL* translocations that are associated with a poor prognosis, the t(9;11)(p22;q23) translocation has an intermediate prognosis, and it appears that this better outcome may be mediated by the overexpression of *BRE* (102). The other exceptional *MLL* translocation, which is actually associated with a favorable prognosis in the pediatric context, is t(1;11)(q21;q23), involving *MLLT11* as a partner. *FLT3* mutations occur less commonly (8%) in t(9;11) as compared to other AMLs; however, *RAS* mutations are frequent (36%) and may be associated with slightly worse clinical outcome (103). Although the breakpoints

in *MLL* cluster in the 8.3-kb region of the gene containing exons 5 to 11, the heterogeneity of fusion partners makes detection of *MLL* rearrangements by PCR assay challenging. FISH and conventional cytogenetics are the preferred methods for detecting *MLL* translocations, including t(9;11)(p22;q23) (104).

t(6;9)(p23;q34); DEK-NUP214

AML with t(6;9)(p23;q34) is a rare form of the disease accounting for at most 1% of all AML cases (1). Frequently associated with basophilia and multilineage dysplasia, the prognosis for this leukemia is generally poor. The translocation involves *DEK* and *NUP214* on chromosomes 6p23 and 9q34, respectively. Since the breakpoints for this translocation cluster within a single intron in each gene, the gene fusion can be readily detected by RT-PCR (105,106). Conventional cytogenetics and FISH are equally useful in the detection of the translocation (107). Of note, *FLT3* ITD mutations are extremely common in t(6;9)(p23;q34) AML with an estimated frequency of 70% to 80% (108,109).

inv(3)(q21q26.2) or t(3;3)(q21;q26.2); RPN1-EVI1

AML with inv(3)(q21q26.3) or t(3;3)(q21;q26.2) is another rare form of leukemia (i.e., ~1% to 2% of all AML) with a poor prognosis (1). Cases often present with distinctive hypolobated megakaryocytes and multilineage dysplasia. In contrast to other recurrent translocations in AML, these chromosome rearrangements do not generate a novel fusion protein (i.e., a qualitative translocation). Rather, these rearrangements result in the overexpression of *EVI1*, a quite complicated transcription factor. *EVI1* has multiple alternative splice variants whose regulation is poorly understood; one notable splice variant results in the (nonpathogenic) fusion of *EVI1* with an adjacent gene on chromosome 3 *MDS1* (110). To better represent the regulatory complexity of this locus, HGNC changed the approved gene symbol for *EVI1* and *MDS1* to *MECOM* (i.e., *MDS1 and EVI1 complex locus*). Despite this somewhat confusing name change, one of the gene products produced by *MECOM* is in fact EVI1. In inv(3) and t(3;3) rearrangements, a regulatory element from *RPN1*, a constitutively expressed protein found in the endoplasmic reticulum, becomes associated with the *EVI1* portion of *MECOM*. The end result is pathologic overexpression of wild-type *EVI1*. Molecular detection by PCR-based methods is not widely available for this rare form of AML. The breakpoints in *RPN1* are quite varied and span an approximately 100 kb region, which makes assay development quite challenging. In comparison, FISH assays are readily available and they appear to be more accurate than conventional karyotyping (111).

t(1;22)(p13;q13); RBM15-MKL1

Presenting almost exclusively in infants and small children, AML with t(1;22)(p13;q13) is a rare disease (i.e., <1% of all AML) notable for its megakaryoblastic features and its tendency to present with a soft tissue mass, potentially mimicking other small blue round cell tumors (1). This recurrent translocation results in a fusion gene that contains almost the entire coding regions of *RBM15* from chromosome 1p13 and *MKL1* from chromosome 22q13 (112). The pathophysiology of the RBM15-MKL1 fusion protein remains poorly understood; however, data suggest that the fusion may disrupt Notch signaling and serum response factor activity (113,114). Clinically, this type of AML is probably associated with a favorable prognosis. While the translocation is readily detected by conventional cytogenetics and FISH, sensitive RT-PCR-based methods are also available and may be helpful in cases with limited numbers of blasts (perhaps secondary to disease-associated myelofibrosis) (115).

Gene Mutations in AML

One of the challenges associated with AML is how to integrate the ever-growing list of genetic lesions into clinical practice. Although nearly 200 recurrent gene mutations have been identified in AML (Table 8.8), only *NPM1*, *CEBPA*, and *FLT3*

have a well-defined role in current clinical practice (the detection of *KIT* mutations is also becoming increasingly important, particularly in CBF AMLs). In fact, AMLs with *NPM1* and *CEBPA* were given provisional diagnostic status in the 2008 WHO classification system; *FLT3* mutations are also important to test for, despite the fact that their presence does not define

Table 8.8	GENE MUTATIONS IN AML					
Gene	**Chromosome Location**	**Mutation Frequency**[a]	**Mutation Location**	**Biologic Function of Protein**	**Mutation Effect**	**Clinical Significance**
NPM1	5q35	~32%	Exon 12	Phosphoprotein with diverse and complex biologic activity; shuttles between nucleus and cytoplasm	Create a nuclear export signal that results in cytoplasmic mislocalization that may lead to dysregulation of the p53 pathway, among others	Favorable
FLT3	13q12	~20%	ITD: Exons 14 and 15 TKD: D835	Component of signal transduction pathway; class III receptor tyrosine kinase	Constitutive activation of signal transduction; increased proliferation, and decreased apoptosis	ITD: Unfavorable TKD: Unclear
CEBPA	19q13	~9%	Varied	Transcriptional regulation; intron-less transcription factor that mediates lineage specification	Diminished transcriptional activity through dominant negative mechanisms	Favorable
TET2	4q24	~17%	Varied	Epigenetic regulation; promotes DNA demethylation by converting methylcytosine to 5-hydroxymethylcytosine	Loss-of-function mutations leading to DNA hypermethylation	Unfavorable
DNMT3A	2p23	~17%	R882	Epigenetic regulation; a DNA methyltransferase thought to function in *de novo* methylation as opposed to maintenance methylation	Effect of loss-of-function mutations are unclear, but alterations in epigenetic regulation are suspected	Unfavorable
NRAS	1p13	~12%	G12, G13 and Q61	Component of signal transduction pathway; member of the *RAS* family of GTPase signaling proteins	Constitutive activation of signal transduction	Unclear
RUNX1	21q22	~11%	Varied	Transcription factor; alpha subunit of the heterodimeric CBF	Dominant negative effect leading to decreased transcription	Unfavorable
TP53	17p13	~11%[b]	Varied	Involved in responses to cellular stresses through regulation of cell cycle, apoptosis, and DNA repair	Mutations lead to loss of tumor suppressor activity	Unfavorable
IDH2	15q26	~9%	R140 and R172	Metabolic function; mitochondrial isoform of isocitrate dehydrogenases that catalyzes the oxidative decarboxylation of isocitrate to 2-oxoglutarate	New enzymatic activity leading to production of a putative oncometabolite (2-hydroxyglutarate) and ultimately DNA hypermethylation	Unclear; possibly favorable (R140)
WT1	11p13	~9%	Exon 7 and 9	Transcriptional regulation; encodes a zinc finger transcription factor	Unclear, but likely loss of function	Unclear
ASXL1	20q11	~9%	Exon 12	Epigenetic regulation; a chromatin-binding protein that interacts with polycomb complex proteins	Unclear, but loss-of-function mechanisms are currently favored over a dominant negative effect	Unfavorable
KIT[c]	4q12	~8%	Exons 8 and 17	Component of signal transduction pathway; class III receptor tyrosine kinase	Constitutive activation of signal transduction	Unfavorable
MLL	11q23	~7%	PTD: Exons 5 to 12	Chromatin remodeling; histone methyltransferase modulates gene expression	Partial tandem duplication leading to disruptions in transcriptional regulation	Unfavorable
IDH1	2q34	~6%	R132	Metabolic function; cytoplasmic isoform of isocitrate dehydrogenases that catalyzes the oxidative decarboxylation of isocitrate to 2-oxoglutarate	New enzymatic activity leading to production of a putative oncometabolite (2-hydroxyglutarate) and ultimately DNA hypermethylation	Unclear; possibly unfavorable
BCORL1	Xq25-q26	~6%	Varied	Transcriptional corepressor, perhaps via association with histone deacetylases and BCL6	Unclear, putative tumor suppressor	Unfavorable
KRAS	12p12	~4%	G12, G13 and Q61	Component of signal transduction pathway; member of the *RAS* family of GTPase signaling proteins	Constitutive activation of signal transduction	Unclear
PHF6	Xq26	~3%	Varied	Potential role in transcriptional regulation and/or chromatin remodeling	Unclear, putative tumor suppressor	Unfavorable
GATA2	3q21	~2%	Exons 4 and 5	Transcriptional regulation; zinc finger transcription factor involved in hematopoiesis	Disruption of DNA-binding activity, with altered transcription of target genes	Favorable
EZH2	7q35-q36	~1%	Varied	Epigenetic regulation; component of the polycomb repressor complex 2 that methylates histones to repress transcription	Effects of loss-of-function mutations are unclear, but alterations in epigenetic regulation are likely	Unclear

ITD, internal tandem duplication; TKD, tyrosine kinase domain; PTD, partial tandem duplication.
[a]Mutation frequency is based primarily on aggregate data for AML provided by COSMIC database (84), which is not without potential limitations and biases.
[b]*TP53* is altered in ~80% of AMLs with a monosomal karyotype.
[c]Enriched in CBF AML (~20% of cases).

an entity, provisional or otherwise. Evaluating for these three mutations (and certainly others in the near future) provides important prognostic and predictive information for AML patients, especially those patients with a normal karyotype who tend to harbor more gene mutations than other cytogenetic categories (87).

NPM1

NPM1 on 5q35 encodes for a functionally diverse protein that actively shuttles between the nucleus and the cytoplasm (116,117). Mutations in NPM1 are quite common in cytogenetically normal AML. They are detected in approximately 50% of adult and 20% of pediatric AMLs with a normal karyotype, but are virtually absent in cases of AML with recurrent translocations (118–122). NPM1 mutations are not, however, restricted to normal karyotype AML. Approximately 15% of NPM1 mutations occur in patients with cytogenetic abnormalities other than the recurrent translocations. Over 50 NPM1 mutations have been described in AML; curiously, they almost entirely consist of small (4 to 11 bp) insertions in exon 12 (123). Each of these insertion mutations creates a frameshift in NPM1 resulting in a novel nuclear export signal that shifts the localization of the protein from the nucleus to the cytoplasm. This mislocalization of NPM1 can potentially be detected at the cellular level by both IHC and flow cytometry (123,124). However, assessment at the genetic level is recommended to confirm the presence of an NPM1 mutation; a variety of DNA- and RNA-based PCR methods are available for NPM1 mutation analysis (125). In patients with cytogenetically normal AML, an isolated NPM1 mutation is associated with a good prognosis. However, 40% of NPM1 mutated patients have a concurrent FLT3-ITD mutation (126). In patients with both mutations, the negative impact of the FLT3-ITD mutation nullifies the positive prognostic effect of an NPM1 mutation. Additionally, it appears that the good prognosis associated with NPM1 mutations may be restricted to those AMLs that harbor coexistent IDH2 mutations (87). Finally, NPM1 mutations appear well-suited for quantitative minimal residual disease detection given the high frequency with which they occur and their stability over time (i.e., the mutation remains detectable at relapse unlike other less stable mutations such as FLT3) (127). In fact, studies suggest quantitative NPM1 monitoring may be predictive of relapse and long-term survival (128,129).

CEBPA

CEBPA, a transcription factor involved in granulocytic differentiation (130,131), is mutated primarily in cytogenetically normal AML with an incidence of approximately 5% to 14% (132). Mutations in CEBPA are diverse; over 200 different genetic lesions have been described in both the N- and C-terminal regions (84). Mutations are thought to diminish normal CEBPA activity through a variety of dominant negative mechanisms. AML with mutated CEBPA is associated with a favorable prognosis; however, the benefit is restricted to those patients where both alleles of CEBPA are mutated (133,134). Interestingly, when both alleles are affected, they tend to harbor different mutations; often one will have an N-terminal lesion and the other allele will have a C-terminal lesion (130). Nearly half of AMLs with a mutated CEBPA carry only one mutant allele; patients with only one mutant allele typically have a prognosis similar to that in patients with a wild-type CEBPA. An exception is that when a concurrent NPM1 mutation is present, a monoallelic CEBPA mutation is a positive modifier on the already favorable NPM1 mutation (135). Data also suggest that promoter hypermethylation may be yet another mechanism to silence CEBPA (136). Promoter hypermethylation appears to correlate with prognosis (137). The diversity of genetic lesions

in CEBPA and its GC- rich sequence makes routine clinical testing challenging (138,138a).

FLT3

FLT3, a type III receptor tyrosine kinase expressed early during hematopoiesis, is frequently mutated in AML. There are two major types of mutations in FLT3. Internal tandem duplications (ITDs) of the juxtamembranous domain are the most common and occur in approximately 23% of cytogenetically normal AMLs. The second type of mutation is a missense mutation, most often in codon 835, that has a frequency of approximately 7% in cytogenetically normal AMLs. Both mutations result in constitutive activation of FLT3 signaling. Clinically, only the FLT3-ITD is clearly associated with adverse clinical outcome. ITD dosage is an important determinant, as prognosis is influenced by the relative amount of the mutant allele (139,140). Loss of heterozygosity due to UPD appears to be an important mechanism contributing to increased allelic burden of mutated FLT3 (139). Mutations in codon 835 are of less clear clinical significance; in fact, evidence suggests this mutation may not be associated with an adverse clinical outcome. However, FLT3 codon 835 (along with other) mutations may have future therapeutic implications as these genetic lesions appear to confer resistance to FLT3 inhibitors (141). A handful of PCR-based methods are available for FLT3 mutation analysis. For FLT3-ITD, PCR amplification followed by capillary electrophoresis is a useful technique in that it allows one to not only size the length of the ITD, but also, in a semiquantitative way, determine the allelic burden of the ITD mutation. ITD length is of uncertain clinical significance. FLT3 mutations may be of limited utility in MRD monitoring, as these mutations are not stable in all instances; however, this is not a major impediment as such changes are seen in only approximately 5% to 10% of cases (142).

Emerging Gene Mutations

An increasing number of recurrent mutations have been identified in AML (Table 8.8); a subset of these mutations appears to have compelling clinical significance. For example, integrated genetic profiling of approximately 20–25 genes (including NPM1, FLT3, CEBPA, IDH1, IDH2, RUNX1, ASXL1, PHF6, TET2, and DNMT3A) appears to better risk-stratify AML patients with intermediate cytogenetics (87,142a,142b). Additional studies will be needed to extend and confirm these studies and it will be equally important to establish clinical approaches that can readily and accurately profile a large panel of gene mutations. It is also becoming clear that the interaction and coexistence of various mutations is likely nonrandom (Fig. 8.5), as evidenced by the observation that certain mutations frequently co-occur (e.g., NPM1 and FLT3) while others are seemingly mutually exclusive (e.g., TET2 and IDH1/2). In addition to these numerous mutational defects, there are a number of genes that when overexpressed in AML appear to have prognostic relevance in AML (Table 8.9). While not currently routinely assayed, they may play a future role in the evaluation of AML.

Myeloproliferative Neoplasms

The MPNs can be considered to be classical or nonclassical. The classical MPNs are CML and its well-defined association with t(9;22)(q34;q11); BCR-ABL1, and the so-called non-CML MPNs (including polycythemia vera [PV], primary myelofibrosis [PMF], and essential thrombocythemia [ET]). The nonclassical MPNs include systemic mastocytosis and eosinophilic neoplasms; some of the latter are assigned to their own category by WHO 2008. As our molecular understanding of MPN has evolved, an increasing number of genetic lesions, many of which involve tyrosine kinases, have been identified that have diagnostic utility (1).

	Table 8.9	**GENES OVEREXPRESSED IN AML**	

Gene	Chromosome Location	Biologic Function of Protein	Clinical Significance
ERG	21q22	Transcriptional regulation; encodes an erythroblast transformation-specific (ETS) transcription factor involved in the regulation of hematopoiesis	Unfavorable
MN1	22q12	Transcriptional regulation; encodes a transcriptional coregulator	Unfavorable
BAALC	8q22	Unclear function	Unfavorable
MIR-3151	8q22	Unclear function, located within *BAALC*, but is prognostically independent	Unfavorable
FOXO3	6q21	Transcriptional regulation; encodes a forkhead transcriptional activator likely involved in the regulation of apoptosis	Unfavorable
EVI1[a]	3q26	Transcriptional regulation; encodes a zinc finger transcription factor	Unfavorable
WT1	4q11-q12	Transcriptional regulation; encodes a zinc finger transcription factor	Unfavorable
OGG1	3p26	DNA repair; participates in mutagenic base excision repair	Unfavorable
SET	9q34	Protein phosphatase 2A inhibitor 2 involved in a variety of cellular processes including chromatin remodeling, transcription, and cell cycle regulation	Unfavorable
GATA2	3q21	Transcriptional regulation; encodes a zinc finger transcription factor	Unfavorable
CDKN1B	12p13.1-p12	Regulation of cell cycle progression; encodes a cyclin-dependent kinase inhibitor	Unfavorable
FLI1	11q24.1-q24.3	Transcriptional regulation; encodes an ETS transcription factor involved in the regulation of hematopoiesis	Unfavorable
MIR-155	21q21	miRNA regulating genes involved in the immune response	Unfavorable
LEF1	4q23-q25	Transcriptional regulation; encodes a transcription factor that participates in the Wnt signaling pathway	Favorable
BRE	2p23	Component of the BRCA1-BARD1 DNA repair complex	Favorable[b]
MIR-212	17p13	miRNA regulating genes involved in the immune response	Favorable

[a]*EVI* is a transcript expressed from *MECOM* gene.
[b]Appears to account for the favorable prognosis of t(9;11); *MLL-MLLT3* AML.

Chronic Myelogenous Leukemia t(9;22); BCR-ABL1 Positive

The initial discovery of the Philadelphia chromosome (the 22q–) by Peter Nowell and David Hungerford in 1960 was subsequently shown by Janet Rowley in 1973 to be due to the balanced t(9;22)(q34;q11) translocation. The identification of the consequently generated BCR-ABL1 tyrosine kinase oncoprotein was followed by the development of remarkably effective targeted inhibitor therapy, with this series of events serving as a paradigm for genetic diagnosis and therapy in hematologic neoplasms. The translocation generates a novel fusion protein containing the 5′ portion of the *BCR* gene from chromosome 22 and the 3′ portion of the *ABL1* gene on chromosome 9. The intronic breakpoint in *ABL1* occurs variably within a 300 kb portion of chromosome 9 centered on the 5′ end of the gene near exon 1a or exon 1b (143). Despite the heterogeneity in the location of the breakpoint, the exons *ABL1* contributes to the fusion transcript is highly consistent. This is in part because exons 1a and 1b are ultimately spliced out of the mature fusion transcript regardless of the breakpoint location; thus, *ABL1* exons 2 through 11 are most often incorporated into the fusion protein. Rarely, exon 2 is also excluded along with exons 1a and 1b, but this does not appear to have any functional significance. In contrast, the breakpoints in *BCR* are more diverse, occurring mostly in three primary clusters. The first is called the major breakpoint cluster region (i.e., M-BCR) and it defines an approximately 6 kb section of the *BCR* gene spanning exons 12 through 16. In CML, two fusion transcripts predominate in M-BCR breakpoints. These fusion transcripts contain the first 13 or 14 exons of *BCR* and the last 10 exons of *ABL1* beginning with exon 2, widely referred to as e13a2 and e14a2, respectively. More historical nomenclature designates the fusion transcripts involving the major breakpoints in *BCR* as b2a2 (i.e., e13a2) and b3a2 (i.e., e14a2). Both transcripts produce a 210 kDa fusion protein. The other two breakpoint clusters are rarely involved in CML. The minor breakpoint cluster region (i.e., m-BCR), which defines a 55 kb region of *BCR* within intron 1, is most often, but not exclusively, associated with B-cell acute

lymphoblastic leukemia. Extremely rare cases of CML that harbor a m-BCR breakpoint tend to be associated with monocytosis. The fusion transcripts resulting from an m-BCR breakpoint are referred to as e1a2 and result in a smaller 190 kD fusion protein. The third and final hotspot is the micro breakpoint cluster region (i.e., μ-BCR) located in the 3′ end of the *BCR* gene. The resulting fusion transcript involves the first 19 exons of *BCR* and is referred to as e19a2. Not surprisingly, the fusion protein from a μ-BCR is larger (230 kDa). Rare cases of CML, typically with a greater proportion of neutrophils, contain the e19a2. Other less common breakpoints have been reported including those that involve intron 6 of *BCR* (143).

A number of methods, such as classic metaphase cytogenetics, FISH, and RT-PCR, are available for the detection of the t(9;22) translocation. However, no single method adequately addresses every patient, and frequently more than one methodology must be employed. Up to 10% of CML patients have cryptic or complex translocations that are not readily detectable by conventional cytogenetics (144). In addition, conventional karyotyping takes several days to complete. Given this, either RT-PCR or FISH may be the preferred diagnostic approach for increased diagnostic sensitivity and turnaround time. Most RT-PCR assays for the *BCR-ABL1* fusion transcript typically target the common CML breakpoints (i.e., e13a2 and e14a2, as well as e1a2). However, more comprehensive RT-PCR assays that detect fusions from all three breakpoint clusters (i.e., including e19) have been described, but they are not widely used (145). FISH is also more rapid than conventional cytogenetics and it has the added benefit of increased diagnostic sensitivity since it can detect rare or variant t(9;22) breakpoints not covered by standard RT-PCR assays. The limitation of FISH is that the precise breakpoint is not defined by this method. The ability to monitor a patient's response to therapy requires knowledge of the breakpoint as it has important implications for minimal residual disease monitoring. Importantly, while either FISH or RT-PCR is required at diagnosis, these modalities do not preclude the need for conventional cytogenetics, which, among others, has value in identifying additional chromosomal abnormalities that neither FISH nor RT-PCR can detect. Hence, all three approaches are considered complementary, although it may not be necessary to do both FISH and RT-PCR at diagnosis.

Response to therapy can be assessed by a variety of parameters (i.e., hematologic, cytogenetic, and molecular). One of the most important milestones, major molecular response (MMR), is defined by a quantitative measurement of *BCR-ABL1* transcripts with a real-time RT-PCR assay, and represents a 3-log reduction from a standardized baseline. More recently, deeper levels of MMR, down to 4.5-log reductions, have been recognized (146,147). Please see Chapter 44 for a complete discussion on the time-dependent clinical significance of minimal residual disease monitoring in CML. Quantitative *BCR-ABL1* RT-PCR assays often detect only major breakpoint fusions (i.e., e13a2 or e14a2). Quantitative assays that also monitor e1a2 transcripts have also been described (148). These assays (whether qualitative, which suffice at diagnosis, or quantitative, which are essential for posttherapeutic monitoring) begin with RNA. As mentioned previously, RNA is very unstable and ideally should be extracted soon after specimen collection. This instability makes quantitative RT-PCR assays for fusion transcripts particularly prone to variability due to differences in RNA quality and quantity. Thus, a control gene must be evaluated in parallel with *BCR-ABL1*; this principle also applies to other quantitative PCR assays. Reporting results as a ratio of fusion transcripts to control gene transcripts allows one to compensate for variability due to specimen integrity (i.e., RNA degradation) as well as variance introduced in the extraction and RT-PCR steps. Selecting an appropriate control gene is not a trivial matter. *ABL1*, *BCR*, or *GUSB* are the most suitable control genes. A potentially important limitation of using *ABL1* as a control gene is that its primers may also detect the *BCR-ABL1* fusion. At very high levels of *BCR-ABL1* (e.g., at diagnosis of CML), this may lead to an inadvertent overestimation of *ABL1* and hence an underestimation of the *BCR-ABL1/ABL1* ratio. However, since quantitation appears to be more important for monitoring at levels several orders of magnitude below the diagnostic range, this limitation is not of major clinical significance.

Another critical issue with regard to quantitative *BCR-ABL1* testing is that there is tremendous variability in how the assay is performed. As there is not yet an FDA-approved assay, each clinical laboratory develops and validates their chosen method and reference values. Consequently, measurements obtained at one laboratory are not directly comparable with those obtained at a separate laboratory (149–151). To try and address this problem, an international effort created standardized reference material, so that any laboratory could report on the international scale (IS), which was established in 2006 to standardized tests measurements across laboratories (152,153). While a WHO international standard has been created, these reagents are in limited supply. Thus, the principal function of the international standard is to facilitate the creation of secondary reference reagents by commercial entities. Clinical laboratories would then employ the secondary reference materials to align their laboratory-developed *BCR-ABL1* test to the IS, through a conversion factor, which is analogous to the INR used in coagulation testing.

CML patients may fail first-generation tyrosine kinase inhibitor (TKI) therapy (i.e., imatinib) or have a suboptimal response, for a number of different reasons, including noncompliance. The major cause of *bona fide* resistance is mutations in the kinase domain of *ABL1* (154), the frequency of which increases with progression from chronic through accelerated and blast phase. Over 100 different mutations have been reported, and not all are created equal. For some, increasing the dose of imatinib suffices. For others, switching to second- and third-generation TKIs (such as nilotinib, dasatinib or bosutinib) is indicated. T315I point mutations are the most recalcitrant, since neither first- nor second-generation TKIs are efficacious in its presence (154,155). Various methods are available to detect kinase domain mutations including sequencing and allele-specific PCR

(154). Allele-specific PCR is highly sensitive, but can only detect a targeted subset of kinase domain mutations. Furthermore, the clinical significance of a very low-level kinase domain mutation (e.g., 0.01%) in the setting of failed therapy is uncertain. Thus, the recommended detection method is (the relatively less sensitive) direct Sanger sequencing of the *BCR-ABL1* transcript (i.e., RNA sequencing) (154). Importantly, the identification of a mutation in the kinase domain does not necessarily explain the clinical finding of TKI resistance. Resistance mechanisms are complex and are not limited to kinase domain mutations. *BCR-ABL1* gene amplification and overexpression along with alterations in drug efflux kinetics also account for resistance.

BCR-ABL1-Negative Myeloproliferative Neoplasms

The classical *BCR-ABL1*-negative MPNs (PV, ET, and PMF) are distinct from CML not only hematologically, but also genetically because these disease entities do not harbor the t(9;22) translocation. Moreover, their diagnosis lacked, until recently, well-defined molecular genetic abnormalities. The discoveries of *JAK2* (and to some degree *MPL*) mutations have had a significant impact on the diagnosis of these MPNs. Other more recently discovered mutations are likely to have a role in diagnosis in the future.

The *JAK2* gene located on chromosome 9p24 encodes for a nonreceptor tyrosine kinase. The prototypical V617F mutation in exon 14 of *JAK2* was first described in 2005; this mutation, which results in constitutive activation of the STAT signal transduction pathway, is present in approximately 95% of PV cases and approximately 50% of ET and PMF. Its identification dramatically simplified the diagnostic process for *BCR-ABL1*-negative MPNs. Importantly, however, this mutation is not specific for individual types of MPN; thus other important diagnostic criteria, including hematologic and histopathologic features, must be integrated to arrive at the correct diagnosis. Furthermore, the absence of a *JAK2* mutation does not preclude a diagnosis of *BCR-ABL1*-negative MPN, since not 100% of cases carry this mutation.

A subset of *JAK2* mutations are "homozygous" due to the presence of segmental aUPD (156,157). This phenomenon occurs primarily in PV (25% to 30%) and only rarely in ET and PMF, and may be associated with a different symptoms and laboratory findings. However, the diagnostic and prognostic significance of *JAK2* V617F allelic burden appears to be minimal (158). A variety of PCR-based methods are available for *JAK2* mutation analysis; most methods differ in their analytical sensitivity. For example, methods based on melt curve analysis may lack the analytical sensitivity to detect all mutation-positive patients (159). A qualitative allelic discrimination method is also available and has an estimated analytical sensitivity of approximately 2%. Quantitative PCR methods may be useful in monitoring response to therapy especially following allogeneic stem cell transplantation (53); while currently available JAK2 inhibitors used, in particular, to treat PMF do ameliorate some clinical features, they do not seem to have a profound impact on reducing the levels of mutant *JAK2* (160).

The majority of patients with *JAK2* V617F-negative PV harbor a mutation in exon 12 of *JAK2* (161–163). Unlike V617F, most of these mutations occur in a heterozygous state in PV and appear to be specific for PV. Hence, a *JAK2* mutation can be detected in virtually 100% of cases of PV. Mutations in *MPL*, which encodes the thrombopoietin receptor, have been described in a small percentage of ET (~3%) and PMF (~10%) cases. The majority of abnormalities are point mutations in exon 10 (e.g., W515L and W515K) (164).

Other genes mutated in *BCR-ABL1*-negative MPNs include *TET2*, *IKZF1*, *NRAS*, *TP53*, *RUNX1*, *LNK*, *SOCS*, *ASXL1*, *IDH1*, *IDH2*, *EZH2*, *DNMT3A*, and *CBL* (Table 8.10). Some are more likely to be seen at the time of more aggressive transformation

| Table 8.10 | GENES MUTATED IN *BCR-ABL1*-NEGATIVE MYELOPROLIFERATIVE NEOPLASMS |

Gene	Chromosome Location	Mutation Frequency			Mutation Location	Mutation Effect
		PV	ET	PMF		
JAK2	9p24	~95%	~50%	~50%	V617F	Constitutively active JAK2 causing uncontrolled gene transcription
		~3%	—	—	Exon 12	
MPL	1q34	—	~3%	~10%	Exon 10	Constitutively active thrombopoietin receptor leading to megakaryocytic proliferation
TET2	4q24	~16%	~5%	~17%	Several exons	DNA hypermethylation causing impaired myelopoiesis
DNMT3A	2p23	~7%	—	~7%	R882	Impaired DNA methyltransferase leading to altered DNA methylation patterns
IDH1/IDH2	2q34/15q26	~2%	~1%	~4%	Exon 4	Increased production of 2-hydroxyglutarate leading to DNA hypermethylation causing impaired myelopoiesis
ASXL1	20q11	—	~3%	~13%	Exon 12	Wild-type ASXL1 is thought to have a role in transcription factor activation and transcription repression
EZH2	7q36	—	~3	~7%	Exons 10, 18, 20	Loss of function of a part of the histone methyltransferase complex
CBL	11q23	Rare	Rare	~6%	Exon 8 and 9	Loss of function of E3 ubiquitin ligase that marks mutant kinases for destruction
LNK	12q24	Rare	Rare	Rare	Exon 2	Loss of negative regulation of JAK2 signaling

Adapted with permission from Schmidt AE, Oh ST, Pathology Consultation on Myeloproliferative Neoplasms. *Am J Clin Pathol* 2012;138:12–19. Ref. (165). Copyright © 2012–2013 American Society for Clinical Pathology and Copyright © 2012–2013 American Journal of Clinical Pathology.

of the underlying MPN. Many of these mutations can occur simultaneously with *JAK2*; however, the diagnostic and prognostic utility of these mutations still needs to be established in MPN, although it is anticipated that they may become diagnostically useful in the future.

Mastocytosis

Mastocytosis is a rare and heterogeneous neoplasm of mast cells. *KIT*, a protooncogene located on human chromosome 4q, codes for a type III receptor tyrosine kinase (i.e., the same family as *FLT3*, *PDGFRA*, and *PDGRFB*), which is critical for the development of multiple cell types including those of hematopoietic lineage. Mutations causing constitutive activation of *KIT* promote cell proliferation and decreased apoptosis. Heterozygous *KIT* D816V mutations in exon 17 are present in approximately 90% of cases of systemic mastocytosis (166). The genetic lesion has clinical significance; the presence of a *KIT* D816V mutation is one of the minor diagnostic criteria in the 2008 WHO classification scheme (1). Other less common (<5%) somatic *KIT* mutations have been identified in adult systemic mastocytosis in exon 17 as well as exons 8, 9, 10, and 11 (166). Importantly, D816V mutations predict resistance to most currently available TKIs whereas some non-D816V mutations (e.g., transmembrane domain mutation F522C and juxtamembrane domain mutation V559G) may be sensitive (167). While detecting the D816V mutation appears to be a rather straightforward endeavor, the reality is that the disease burden (i.e., the percentage of cells harboring the abnormality in the submitted sample) may be relatively low especially from a bone marrow that is characteristically fibrotic. Thus, molecular assays must have sufficient analytical sensitivity to be employed in the clinical setting; otherwise, a false-negative result may be obtained, affecting both diagnosis and therapy. Available methods include allele-specific PCR, RT-PCR with restriction fragment length polymorphism analysis, peptide nucleic acid-mediated PCR, and more recently real-time quantitative PCR (168,169). Measuring *KIT* D816V levels by quantitative PCR may be useful in monitoring treatment response (170).

Neoplasms with Eosinophilia

An abundance of eosinophils can prove to be a diagnostic dilemma; are the eosinophils reactive or neoplastic? Reactive eosinophilia can be seen in a variety of nonneoplastic conditions including allergy and parasitic infections. However, neoplastic processes can also induce a reactive eosinophilia; for example, Hodgkin lymphoma (HL), mastocytosis, and T-cell lymphomas. Once reactive causes have been excluded, neoplastic eosinophilia includes disease entities with well-defined molecular abnormalities (i.e., *PDGFR*- and *FGFR1*-associated neoplasms), those with other evidence of clonality (i.e., chronic eosinophilic leukemia [CEL]), and finally those without documented clonality (i.e., hypereosinophilic syndrome).

Myeloid and Lymphoid Neoplasms with PDGFRA Abnormalities

Platelet derived growth factor receptor alpha (*PDGFRA*) is a member of the type III family of receptor tyrosine kinases. *PDGFRA*-associated neoplasms characteristically have a *FIP1L1*-*PDGFRA* gene fusion, although *PDGFRA* may associate with a number of other partners (e.g., *KIF5B*, *CDK5RAP2*, *STRN*, *ETV6*, and *BCR*) (1). The *FIP1L1-PDGFRA* gene fusion is created not by a chromosomal translocation, but by an 800 kb deletion on 4q12 that also results in the deletion of *CHIC2*, a gene between *FIP1L1* and *PDGFRA*. The breakpoints in *FIP1L1* vary significantly while the breakpoints in *PDGFRA* are very stable; presumably, the disruption of an autoinhibitory domain of *PDGFRA* leads to constitutive activation of the receptor tyrosine kinase. The fusion gene can be detected by either RT-PCR or FISH analysis; the 800 kb deletion at 4q12 is too small to be detected by conventional karyotyping. However, the variability in the breakpoints in *FIP1L1* makes RT-PCR less useful than FISH. FISH analysis often includes a probe to *CHIC2* since it is deleted during the rearrangement. *FIP1L1-PDGFRA* neoplasms are exquisitely sensitive to tyrosine kinase therapy (171). Since *PDGFRA*-associated neoplasms may share clinical and morphologic features with other neoplasms (e.g., those of mast cells) that do not respond to small molecular TKIs, this highlights the utility and importance of molecular genetic testing.

Myeloid Neoplasms with PDGFRB Abnormalities

PDGFRB-associated myeloid neoplasm most often occur in association with the t(5;12)(q31~q33;p12), the *ETV6-PDGRFB* fusion gene; however, 15 other rearrangements with *PDGFRB* at 5q have been described. Fusion partners include *SPECC1*, *RABEP1*, *NDE1*, *TP53BP1*, *KIAA1509*, *NIN*, *GIT2*, *CCDC6*, *HIP1*, *GOLGA4*, *PRKG2*, *PDE4DIP*, *TPM3*, *GPIAP1*, and *WDR48*. Like *PDGFRA*-associated neoplasms, neoplasms with *PDGFRB* lesions are responsive to TKIs. Given the large number of potential partners, FISH-based analysis using a breakapart probe is practical in the clinical setting. However, the common t(5;12) translocation should also be confirmed at the molecular level (using fusion FISH probes or RT-PCR) because not all t(5;12) translocations result in the *ETV6-PDGFRB* fusion gene (1).

Myeloid and Lymphoid Neoplasms with FGFR1 Abnormalities

A very rare disease entity with heterogeneous presentations (including eosinophila, AML, or even acute lymphoblastic leukemia), *FGFR1*-associated neoplasms have one common feature: translocations involving *FGFR1* at 8p11 that result in a constitutively active tyrosine kinase (1). The most common translocation is t(8;13)(p11;q12); *ZNF198-FGFR1*. Other translocations have been described including fusions of *FGFR1* with one of the following genes: *CEP110*, *FGFR1OP1*, *BCR*, *TRIM24*, *MYO18A*, *HERVK*, and *FGFR1OP2*. Diagnosis is dependent on the identification of an *FGFR1* rearrangement, typically accomplished by conventional cytogenetics or FISH at the 8p11 locus. Unlike PDGFR-associated neoplasms, this disease entity is not sensitive to currently available tyrosine receptor kinase inhibitor therapy. However, research suggests that newer TKIs (e.g., PKC412 and AP24534) may be effective in the treatment of *FGFR1*-associated neoplasms (172,173).

Chronic Eosinophilic Leukemia, Not Otherwise Specified

Formally classified as a MPN, CEL is a clonal proliferation of eosinophils, which lacks, by definition, defined genetic features of other neoplasms including *BCR-ABL1* and rearrangements of *PDGFRA*, *PDGFRB*, and *FGFR1*. Although disease-defining genetic lesions are still lacking for CEL, clonality has been demonstrated by the identification of other cytogenetic abnormalities, gene mutations (e.g., *JAK2*), and X chromosome inactivation studies (174,175).

Myelodysplastic Syndromes

Presenting typically with cytopenias of one or more lineage and characteristic dysplastic morphology, the MDS are a somewhat enigmatic collection of heterogeneous diseases. Given the sometimes subtle morphologic features, the detection of recurring cytogenetic changes is a central facet of diagnosis. Most of these abnormalities consist of numeric chromosomal changes, among the more frequent of which are gains and losses such as +8, −5, −5q, and −7. A good-quality metaphase analysis usually suffices for the detection of these (and other) abnormalities; data indicate that FISH analysis is only of value in the context of a suboptimal cytogenetic analysis. However, nearly half of patients with *de novo* MDS present with normal cytogenetics. The International Prognostic Scoring System (IPSS) is one widely used tool that incorporates clinical findings with karyotype to risk-stratify patients (176). In the original report, seven different cytogenetic abnormalities were recognized, and were incorporated into the four different prognostic groups. However, the role of cytogenetics has been expanded, and in the recently updated IPSS-R (revised IPSS), 17 different cytogenetic abnormalities are featured in the now expanded five prognostic groups (177). In addition, data are accumulating on a growing number of mutations and other molecular aberrations in MDS.

A number of loss-of-function gene mutations have been discovered in MDS. *TET2*, a poorly understood gene that appears to function in normal hematopoiesis perhaps through epigenetic regulation, is mutated in approximately 20% of patients and portends a poor prognosis. A handful of other less commonly mutated genes, which include *ASXL1*, *IDH1*, *ETV6*, *EZH2*, *RUNX1*, and *TP53*, have also been found to be independent predictors of poor survival (178). In patients with lower-risk MDS, mutations in *EZH2* seem to predict a worse prognosis (179). While the identification of these genetic lesions has provided insight to the molecular pathogenesis of MDS (e.g., dysregulation of epigenetic mechanisms, impaired DNA damage repair, altered splicing), their role in the diagnosis and risk stratification of MDS needs further investigation. Furthermore, gene mutations do not fully explain the genesis of MDS because some of these mutations are also commonly found in other myeloid malignancies and roughly 20% of MDS cases currently have no known genetic changes.

Alternative splice variants are a common phenomenon in cancer. Until recently, mutations in target genes were thought to be the major drivers of alternative splicing. It now appears that defects specifically in genes encoding proteins in the splicing machinery may underlie this process. For example, mutations in the spliceosome machinery, specifically *SF3B1*, *SRSF2*, *U2AF35*, *U2AF1*, *ZRSR2*, *SF3A*, *SF1*, and *U2AF65*, have been described in MDS, with *SF3B1* mutations being the most common (20% to 45%) (180). *SF3B1* mutations correlate rather impressively with the specific MDS subtype of refractory anemia with ringed sideroblasts (181). Mutations of others, including *SRSF2*, appear to portend a poor prognosis (182). The clinical utility of these abnormalities still needs to be further unraveled, although it is likely that they will have some clinical (diagnostic and prognostic) value. Furthermore, mutations in some of these spliceosome genes are not restricted to MDS, and can be found in other myeloid (such as chronic myelomonocytic leukemia [CMML]) and even lymphoid (e.g., CLL) neoplasms.

The 5q− syndrome is the single genetically defined subtype of MDS, with characteristic hematologic findings (macrocytic anemia, normal or elevated platelet count, monolobated megakaryocytes) and clinical features (more common in women, low likelihood of progression to AML). Importantly, and sometimes confusingly, not all MDS patients with 5q− have the 5q− syndrome, and 5q− is also seen in AML. There appear to be subtle (but not necessarily always absolute) differences in the deleted regions in these two scenarios. In the 5q− syndrome, the commonly deleted region (CDR) is more distal, at 5q32-q33.3 (and designated CDR2), while in the nonsyndromic cases, 5q31. 1-q31.2 (CDR1) is typically deleted. Candidate genes in CDR2 are *RPS14*, encoding a short ribosomal protein and *SPARC*, which encodes osteonectin; candidate genes in CDR1 include *EGR1*, *CTNNA1*, and *CDC25C*.

It is becoming clear that mutations acquired after the initiation of MDS may be clinically relevant especially as it pertains to progression to AML. Mutations associated with disease progression include *FLT3* and *NRAS*; these activation mutations (i.e., class I mutations) likely drive proliferation of the myeloid neoplasm. Additional genetic defects that block differentiation (i.e., class II mutations), such as dysregulated *EVI1* expression, likely contribute to the development of AML.

Myelodysplastic/Myeloproliferative Neoplasms

MDS/MPN are a group of neoplasms with clinical, hematologic, and pathologic features of both MDS and MPN. Only recently has their genetic basis been dissected, albeit incompletely; consequently, there are no formally recognized molecular subtypes of MDS/MPN. Disruption of signal transduction pathways, in particular the *RAS/RAF/MAPK* pathway, is emerging as a common theme in some MDS/MPN. These disruptions may account for the proliferative features of these neoplasms. Data from SNP arrays and array CGH have revealed copy number abnormalities in many cases of MDS/MPN, including microdeletions and microduplications, which would otherwise be missed by routine cytogenetics. More importantly, these studies demonstrated that segmental aUPD occurs quite frequently in MDS/MPN (169) and that this may, in a manner analogous to *JAK2* mutations in MPN and *CEBPA* mutations in AML, contribute to the formation of pathologically significant "homozygous" gene mutations (81).

Juvenile Myelomonocytic Leukemia

An aggressive disease of early childhood, juvenile myelomonocytic leukemia (JMML) is characterized by a clonal expansion of the myeloid cells, especially of the monocytic lineage. The RAS signal transduction pathway has been implicated in the pathogenesis of JMML, manifesting with characteristic *in vitro* hypersensitivity of precursor cells to granulocyte macrophage colony stimulating factor. Somatic mutations have been identified in several components of the RAS signaling pathway; these mutations appear to be mutually exclusive. Activating missense mutations in *PTPN11*, a nonreceptor protein tyrosine phosphatase, occurs with the highest frequency (i.e., ~30%) in JMML (183). Point mutations in codons 12 and 13 of either *NRAS* or *KRAS*, two members of a GTPase signaling family, are the next most common having been identified in approximately 20% of patients (183). Inactivating mutations in *NF1*, a GTPase-activating protein associated with neurofibromatosis type 1, occur in approximately 15% of cases of JMML (183). *CBL*, which encodes an ubiquitin protein ligase not directly linked to RAS signaling, is mutated in 10% to 15% of JMML patients (184). Germ line mutations in these same components have also been implicated in the pathogenesis (183,185–187). Identifying mutations in *NF1*, *NRAS*, *KRAS*, *PTPN11*, and *CBL* support a diagnosis of JMML, although this is not (yet) inculcated into the WHO classification.

Chronic Myelomonocytic Leukemia

Over 90% of cases of CMML carry at least one somatic mutation (188). Genes that are frequently targeted for mutation in CMML are *TET2* (~50%), *ASXL1* (~40%), *SRSF2* (~30% to 45%), *U2AF1* (~15%), and *CBL* (~15%); a variety of less common somatic mutations include those affecting *RAS*, *JAK2*, *EZH2*, *IDH1*, *IDH2*, and *RUNX1* (189). Mutations in CMML are not mutually exclusive; in fact, approximately 40% of patients have two or more mutations (190). Interestingly, spliceosome gene mutations (of which *SRSF2* and *U2AF1* are examples) are frequent events in CMML, but extremely rare in JMML. The diagnostic, prognostic, and therapeutic significance of these genetic lesions is still being defined, but it is likely that the detection of at least a subset of these may become clinically important.

Atypical Chronic Myeloid Leukemia, BCR-ABL1 Negative

The terminology of this entity is unfortunate, since it is quite distinct from CML and hence one of its defining features is the absence of t(9;22);*BCR-ABL1* translocation, to avoid any potential confusion with CML. Patients with atypical chronic myeloid leukemia (aCML) typically present with myeloproliferative findings such as leukocytosis and splenomegaly; however, unlike

---

Table 8.11 | **INHERITED GENETIC PREDISPOSITION TO HEMATOLOGIC NEOPLASMS**

Inherited Disorder	Inherited Genetic Abnormality[a]	Predisposition[b]
Familial mosaic monosomy 7 syndrome	Monosomy 7	AML, MDS
Down syndrome	Trisomy 21	AML, ALL, MDS
Familial AML with mutated *CEBPA*	*CEBPA*	AML
Familial thrombocytopenia with predisposition to acute myelogenous leukemia	*RUNX1*	AML
Familial MDS and AML associated with mutated GATA2	*GATA2*	AML, MDS
Diamond-Blackfan anemia	*RPS19, RPL5, RPL11, RPL35, RPS24, RPS17, RPS7, RPS10, RPS26*	AML, MDS
Dyskeratosis congenita	*DKC1, TERC, TERT, TINF2, NHP2, NOP10, WRAP53*	AML, MDS
Fanconi anemia	*FANCA, FANCB, FANCC, BRCA2, FANCD2, FANCE, FANCF, FANCG, FANCI, BRIP1, FANCL, FANCM, PALB2, RAD51C, SLX4*	AML, MDS
Kostmann syndrome (congenital neutropenia)	*ELANE*	AML, MDS
Shwachman-Diamond syndrome	*SBDS*	AML, MDS
X-Linked neutropenia	*WAS*	AML, MDS
Bloom syndrome	*BLM*	AML, ALL, lymphoma
Li-Fraumeni syndrome	*TP53*	AML, ALL
Noonan syndrome	*PTPN11*	JMML, AML, ALL
LEOPARD syndrome	*PTPN11*	JMML, AML, ALL
Neurofibromatosis 1	*NF1*	JMML
Cardiofaciocutaneous syndrome	*BRAF, MAP2K1, MAP2K2, KRAS*	ALL, lymphoma
Ataxia-telangiectasia syndrome	*ATM*	ALL, lymphoma
X-linked lymphoproliferative disease	*SH2D1A*	Lymphoma
Nijmegen breakage syndrome	*NBN*	Lymphoma
Autoimmune lymphoproliferative syndrome	*FAS, FASLG, CASP10*	Lymphoma
Autosomal dominant hyper IgE syndrome	*STAT3*	Lymphoma
Common variable immune deficiency	*TNFRSF13B, ICOS, CD19*	Lymphoma
Baller-Gerold syndrome	*RECQL4*	Lymphoma
Cartilage-hair hypoplasia	*RMRP*	Lymphoma
Wiskott-Aldrich syndrome	*WAS*	Lymphoma
X-linked hyper IgM syndrome	*CD40LG*	Lymphoma

[a]A list of mutated genes and numeric chromosomal abnormalities associated with the inherited disorders is provided. A spectrum of autosomal dominant (e.g., neurofibromatosis 1), autosomal recessive (e.g., ataxia-telangiectasia syndrome) and X-linked (e.g., X-linked lymphoproliferative disease) inheritance patterns are represented. Additional details about these inherited disorders can be found online at *GeneReviews* (192).
[b]Lymphomas include B-cell lymphomas, T-cell lymphomas, and HL; in general, most are B-cell lymphomas and many are EBV-associated.

CML, dysplasia, particularly of the granulocytic lineage, is very prominent. aCML harbors cytogenetic abnormalities in up to 80% of patients. Mutations in *CSF3R* and *SETBP1* are quite frequent in aCML and are likely to become useful diagnostic assays (191,191a,191b).

Inherited Disorders

A variety of inherited disorders predispose individuals to develop hematologic neoplasms. While a through and exhaustive discussion of these disease processes is beyond the scope of this chapter, Table 8.11 highlights some of the more common diseases.

LYMPHOID NEOPLASMS

As with myeloid neoplasms, molecular studies aid in the diagnosis, classification, prognostication, and tracking of minimal residual diseases in lymphoid neoplasms. In addition to the evaluation of specific acquired genetic abnormalities, another (physiologic) phenomenon conveniently lends itself to analysis in malignancies of lymphocytes. The study of antigen receptor gene rearrangements, of both immunoglobulin and T-cell receptor (TCR) genes, provides invaluable information regarding the clonality of lymphoproliferations that can be utilized for diagnosis and sensitively monitoring disease following therapy. This is discussed in further detail in Chapter 6.

Errors at the time of V(D)J rearrangements, which occur in the bone marrow in B-cells, result in the generation of a number of hallmark translocations, especially in B-cell, but also in T-cell (where such rearrangements occur in the thymus), neoplasms. In B-cells, there are two additional phases in which there are physiologic breaks in the immunoglobulin genes, in particular the heavy chain gene. Here too, at the time of SHM and class switch recombination, there is the potential for rejoining of double-stranded DNA breaks to go awry, resulting in recurrent translocations (Fig. 8.6). While many of these translocations are characteristic of the lymphoma subtypes with which they are associated, in contrast to, for example, CML and APL, in which the translocation is *a sine qua non* for the diagnosis (t(9;22)(q34;q11); *BCR-ABL1* and t(15;17) (q24;q12); *PML-RARA*, respectively), this is not the case with these translocations in lymphoma.

Mature B-Cell Neoplasms

Follicular Lymphoma

The t(14;18)(q32;q21), which results in *BCL2* on chromosome 18 coming under the control of the *IGH@* enhancer on chromosome 14, is seen in 85% to 95% of cases of FL (193). The translocation occurs as an error in the normal physiologic VDJ recombination at the *IGH@* locus in early B-cell development, as alluded to above (194). The consequential overexpression of the BCL2 protein protects the cell from apoptosis, providing a critical (but not sufficient) step in the genesis of this lymphoma.

The t(14;18) is prototypically associated with FL; however, the frequency of the translocation varies with the grade,

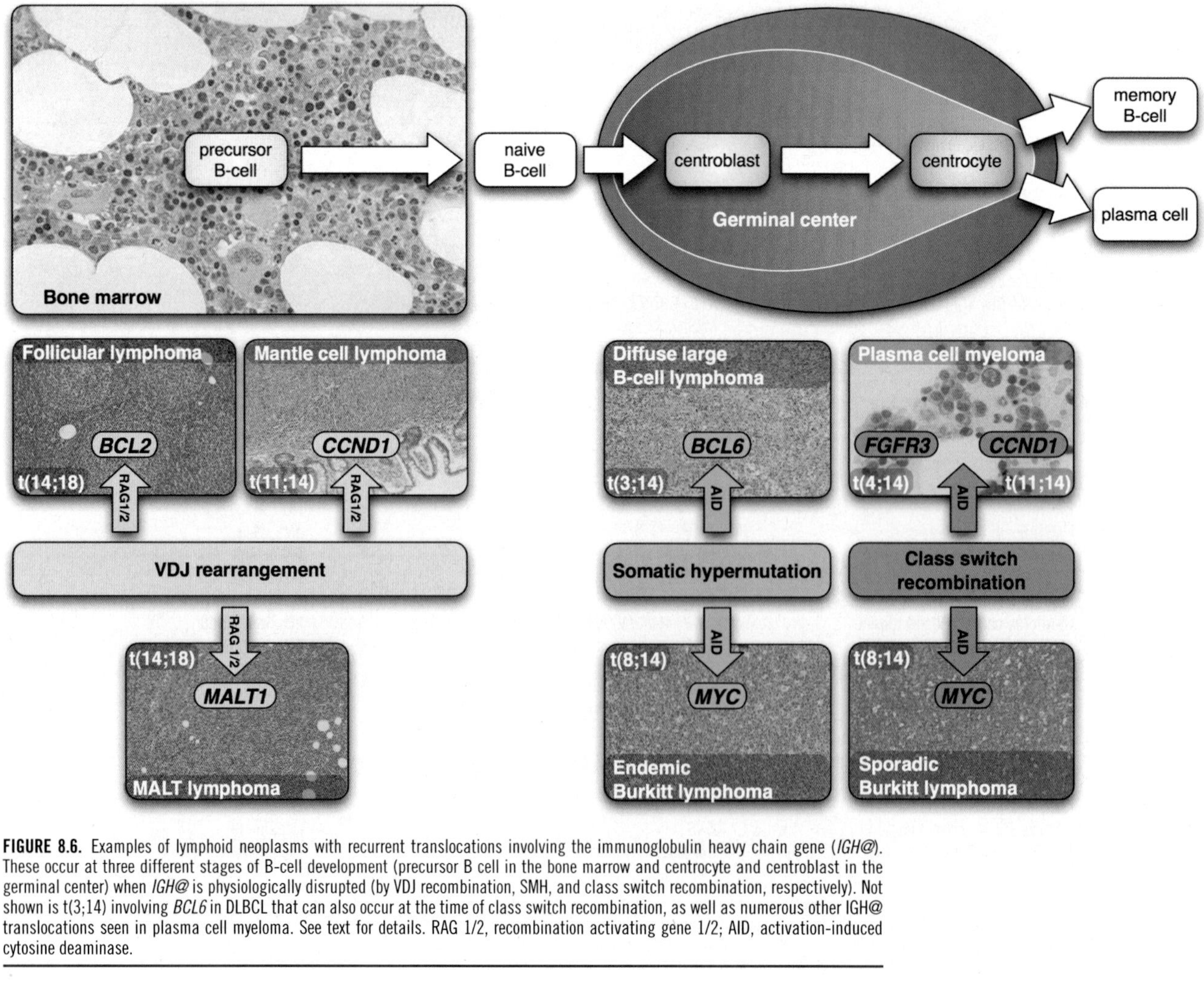

FIGURE 8.6. Examples of lymphoid neoplasms with recurrent translocations involving the immunoglobulin heavy chain gene (*IGH@*). These occur at three different stages of B-cell development (precursor B cell in the bone marrow and centrocyte and centroblast in the germinal center) when *IGH@* is physiologically disrupted (by VDJ recombination, SMH, and class switch recombination, respectively). Not shown is t(3;14) involving *BCL6* in DLBCL that can also occur at the time of class switch recombination, as well as numerous other IGH@ translocations seen in plasma cell myeloma. See text for details. RAG 1/2, recombination activating gene 1/2; AID, activation-induced cytosine deaminase.

location, and patient characteristics, and is the exception rather than the rule in some scenarios. For example, t(14;18) is found in only 10% of grade 3B FL cases, which are more likely to harbor *BCL6* translocations (see below in this section) (195,196). Extranodal FL (in particular cutaneous and testicular forms) and pediatric cases are also less likely to have the translocation (197,198). While primary cutaneous FL is typically t(14;18) negative by PCR, FISH may detect the translocation in up to 40% of cases (199).

Nevertheless, the detection of the t(14;18) by molecular techniques can be very helpful in facilitating the diagnosis of FL when the histology and/or immunophenotype are not definitive. The *BCL2* breakpoints are tightly clustered, allowing for the development of simple PCR assays. Most PCR assays detect the translocation in 75% of cytogenetically detectable cases. The major breakpoint region (mbr), in the nontranslated 3′ region of exon 3 of *BCL2*, is involved in approximately 60% of translocations, while breakpoints of 20 to 30 kb further downstream in the minor cluster region occur in approximately 10% to 15% of cases (200). Translocations involving the intermediate cluster region of *BCL2* are quite common (~15%), and adding primers for this region improves the diagnostic yield. Occasionally the immunoglobulin light chain genes may be the translocation partners (201). Formalin-fixed paraffin embedded tissue (FFPET) is suitable to detect most *IGH@-BCL2* translocations; however, some breakpoints result in PCR products that are very large and may not be detected in FFPET due to the inability to yield adequately sized DNA. FISH is actually diagnostically superior to PCR and can detect almost all rearrangements (202). IG PCR may be useful for PCR-based detection of clonality in cases without the translocation. However, *IGH@* PCR has unacceptably high false-negative rates in FL due to the presence of a high load of ongoing SHM, which may abrogate the ability of primers to anneal. The addition of *IGK@* PCR overcomes much of this problem (203). *BCL2* point mutations may render the protein unrecognizable by the widely used 124 clone, despite the presence of t(14;18) and overexpression of the BCL2 protein, due to an altered epitope. The development of alternative antibodies (E17 and SP66) to a different epitope may be useful to recognize these otherwise "negative" cases in which the protein is not "seen" (204).

Qualitative detection of *IGH@-BCL2* is sufficient for diagnostic purposes; however, measurement of fusion levels by quantitative PCR may yield prognostic information. Levels in the marrow at diagnosis may predict treatment time and long-term outcome (205). The rate of clearance of *IGH@-BCL2* fusions following therapy may be associated with a better outcome, although not all studies demonstrated this finding (205). The t(14;18) can be detected in healthy individuals using highly sensitive nested PCR (206). Importantly, nested PCR is not usually employed in clinical laboratories and hence this phenomenon should not confound diagnostic assays. However, this highlights the notion that the translocation is likely necessary but not sufficient to induce FL. Indeed, FL at presentation typically harbors not only the t(14;18) translocation, but also an average of six additional karyotypically detectable abnormalities, including 1p−, 6q−, +7, +12, and +X (207). *EPHA7* is a target of deletions of 6q; it encodes a tumor suppressor, and is inactivated in approximately 70% of FLs (208).

Translocations other than those involving *BCL2* occur in FL. The second most common target for translocation in FL is *BCL6*, occurring in approximately 5% to 15% of cases overall, and up to approximately 40% in grade 3B FL. A number of different breakpoints occur around this gene in the most common t(3;14) translocation. Another translocation seen in FL is the t(6;14)(p25;q32); *IGH@-IRF4*, which is recurrent, albeit infrequently (<5%), in pediatric FL (209).

A variety of point mutations have been detected in FL, with *MLL2* being targeted most frequently. *TNFRSF14* mutations have been found to be associated with a poor prognosis in some, but not all studies (210,211). *BCL2* mutations are also present and can confound immunohistochemical analysis as alluded to above, although their biologic significance is not yet known (212). *EZH2* codon 641 mutations are recurrent and presumably affect histone methylation (213). *CREBBP* mutations occur in up to approximately 35% of cases and *EP300* mutations occur in approximately 10% of cases of FL (214). The mutations lead to deficient acetylation, by CREBBP and EP300 proteins, of BCL6 and P53, likely contributing to oncogenesis.

Gene expression profiling (GEP) in FL reveals that the composition of the tumor microenvironment, rather than the tumor cells themselves, is prognostically significant, showing two gene expression signatures, designated immune response 1 and 2. Immune response 1 includes transcripts of T-cell genes while immune response 2 contains transcripts from myeloid and monocytic cells. Although somewhat oversimplified, a dominant T-cell–like response is associated with a good prognosis (immune response 1) while a macrophage response is associated with a poor prognosis (immune response 2) (215). Attempts to translate these mRNA profiles into user-friendly IHC assays have not been straightforward. Expression profiling demonstrates that grade 3B FL clusters separately from grade 3A FL and grade 1 to 2 FL, supporting the notion that this form of FL may warrant its own separate classification (216).

aCGH and SNP arrays reveal that minimally evolved cases with a simple karyotype display copy-neutral loss of heterozygosity profiles similar to cytogenetically complex cases (217). It has also been shown that deletion of 1p36 and 6q23 correlate with inferior survival and higher transformation risk (218). Deletion of 1p32 is also associated with a diffuse variant of t(14;18)-negative FL that typically presents with large but localized inguinal disease (219). Germ line SNPs of *FCRIIIA*, which encodes CD16, may alter the efficacy of rituximab in FL via disrupted binding of the Fc portion of this monoclonal antibody to effector cells (220). Prognostically important immune response SNPs (*IL12B, IL1RN, IL2,* and *IL8*) also appear to predict outcome (221). Unlike most small B-cell lymphomas, the genome in FL tends to be hypermethylated (222).

Although the mechanisms underlying large cell transformation of FL are still not fully understood, several genetics factors have been identified as having a role. aCGH shows that dup(1q), dup7, del(6q), and der18 are early events in the evolution of FL. Additional secondary genetic events associated with transformation include translocations involving *MYC*, mutations of *TP53*, and loss of *CDKN2A* and *CDKN2B*. Cases acquiring an *MYC* translocation in combination with the t(14;18) constitute a subset of cases of "double-hit" lymphomas. Transformation may occur from a common subclone or reflect divergent evolution (223).

Mantle Cell Lymphoma

The t(11;14)(q13;q32), involving *IGH@* on chromosome 14 and *CCND1* on chromosome 11, characterizes MCL. As with the t(14;18) in FL, this translocation occurs at the precursor B-cell stage of differentiation in the bone marrow as a result of an error in normal physiologic *IGH@* VDJ recombination. The *CCND1* gene encodes cyclin D1, a cell cycle regulator that has a role at the G1-S phase transition by binding CDK4/6 kinases and phosphorylating RB1. The translocation results in dysregulated *CCND1* expression by the *IGH@* enhancer.

There are several breakpoints around the *CCND1* gene. The most common breakpoints (~30% to 40%) are in the major translocation cluster (MTC) region, located 120 kb centromeric to *CCND1*. The remainder occur at a variety of sites, including MTC2. However, most PCR assays detect the MTC breakpoints only, rendering standard PCR assays suboptimal for diagnostic use. Indeed, FISH for the *CCND1* translocation and IHC for aberrant expression of the cyclin D1 protein both have a higher diagnostic sensitivity than DNA PCR analysis. The *CCND1* gene can be alternatively spliced into cyclin D1a and cyclin D1b isoforms. Shorter cyclin D1a transcripts lacking a 3′UTR predict short survival and high proliferation as they are more stable than the long transcript and correlate with higher cyclin D1 levels; however, the different transcripts are not routinely evaluated in clinical laboratories (224).

Approximately 10% of otherwise classic MCLs do not harbor the translocation or express cyclin D1 (225). Nevertheless, these cases have a gene expression profile and pattern of secondary genetic abnormalities that are indistinguishable from cyclin D1-positive cases (225). Cyclin D2 or D3 may be overexpressed in some of these; although this may be due to *IG@* translocations in a subset of cases, the mechanisms are not always known. Unlike the situation for CCND1 translocations and IHC, CCND2 protein expression is not specific for MCL, and RT-PCR may be superior to IHC for evaluating CCND2 overexpression (226).

The t(11;14) translocation, involving both *CCND1* and *IGH@*, can be seen in a subset of myelomas, albeit with different breakpoints (see section on plasma cell neoplasms). Lymphoid neoplasms other than MCL, such as diffuse large B-cell lymphoma (DLBCL), hairy cell leukemia, and even small lymphocytic lymphoma (SLL)/CLL (particularly in proliferation centers) can express CCND1 by IHC, but these occur in the absence of the hallmark translocation (227–230).

In addition to the hallmark translocation noted above, mutations are also noted in MCL. These include those affecting *NOTCH1* (~12% to 20% of cases) (231). *ATM* and *TP53* mutations are seen in cases with 11q and 17p losses. aCGH demonstrates that MCL contains a higher number of alterations than most other lymphomas, emphasizing their genomic instability (232). Gain of 3q27-q29 and losses of 1p, 6q, and 13q are recurrent, although their significance is not yet fully understood. Both homozygous and monoallelic deletions may occur. Regions with homozygous deletions include 9p21.3, (*CDKN2A*, *CDKN2B*, *MTAP*), 1p33 (*FAF1*, *CDKN2C*), 2q13 (*BCL2L11*), and 2q37 (*SP100*). Recurrent monoallelic deletions affect multiple regions including 17p (*TP53*), 11q (*ATM*), 13q14.2 (*RB1*), and 6q23.3 (*TNFAIP3*).

Since MCL is assumed to arise from a naive, pregerminal center B cell, it might be expected that their *IGH@* genes would be unmutated. However, a subset of cases does indeed show SHM of this gene; as is the case with CLL/SLL, these cases are associated with more indolent behavior and nonnodal presentations (233).

GEP in MCL identifies different prognostically important proliferation signatures (234). While Ki67 can serve as an immunohistochemical surrogate, a 5-gene model (*RAN*, *MYC*, *TNFRSF10B*, *POLE2*, and *SLC29A2*) using quantitative RT-PCR seems superior, although it has yet to be adopted as an assay in diagnostic laboratories (235). GEP has also uncovered different signatures associated with classic and rare indolent forms as well as between nodal and nonnodal MCL (236,237). miRNAs are also dysregulated in MCL. Amplification of chromosome 13q31-q32 leads to overexpression of *MIR17-92*, which negatively impacts the PTEN/AKT pathway, and is associated with chemoresistance and diminished survival (238). Further, a miRNA classifier, which can be performed on FFPET, can serve as a prognosticator in MCL (239).

Marginal Zone Lymphomas

In general, our current understanding of the genetic basis of extranodal marginal zone lymphomas is better than that of nodal or splenic forms. There are four major mutually exclusive translocations that occur in extranodal marginal zone lymphomas (mucosa-associated lymphoid tissue [MALT] lymphomas).

The translocations are t(11;18)(q21;q21), t(14;18)(q32;q21), t(1;14)(p22;q32), and t(3;14)(p14.1;q32).

The most common translocation is t(11;18)(q21;q21), occurring in approximately one-third of cases of MALT lymphoma. The translocation involves *BIRC3* (formerly *API2*) at 11q21 and *MALT1* at 18q21. The result is a BIRC3-MALT fusion protein with antiapoptotic activity and activation of the NF-κB pathway (240). The frequency of this translocation varies with site. Gastric (~25% to 50%) and lung (~50%) MALT lymphomas most commonly harbor t(11;18), which is not seen in the splenic and primary nodal marginal zone lymphomas (241–243). Gastric MALT lymphomas with this translocation may not respond to treatment for *Helicobacter pylori* (244). Multiple breakpoint sites are described for *BIRC3-MALT* generating eight variant fusion transcripts. The fusion protein contains the N terminus of BIRC3 and C terminus of MALT1 with a caspase-like domain. The fusion protein forms homodimers via the BIRC3 portion. The homodimers activate NF-κB and inhibit apoptosis. RT-PCR or FISH can be used to detect the translocation.

The t(14;18)(q32;q21) brings *MALT1* under the transcriptional control of the *IGH@* gene. As is thematic, this translocation is also the result of a mistake in normal physiologic VDJ rearrangements. The t(14;18) occurs in 5% to 10% of cases of MALT lymphoma, typically those in the parotid, liver, and ocular adnexa, while it is rare in the stomach and lung (245). Of note, this translocation is cytogenetically identical to that seen in FL, but is submicroscopically distinct as it involves *MALT1* rather than *BCL2*. The *BCL10* gene on chromosome 1p22 can also be translocated to the *IGH@* locus. The t(1;14)(p22;q32) is found in approximately 2% of MALT lymphomas overall, usually in the lung (up to 10% of cases) and stomach. The translocation results in abnormal nuclear localization of the BCL10 protein, which might provide a useful IHC surrogate (245). Translocations involving *FOXP1* as a consequence of t(3;14) (p14;q32) have been described in MALT lymphomas, especially those of the thyroid, ocular adnexa, and skin (246). The translocation leads to overexpression of the FOXP1 protein, which is involved in B-cell development, although the exact mechanism of how this translocation contributes to lymphomagenesis is unknown (247). FOXP1 protein expression in MALT lymphomas may portend a poor prognosis (248). A less common translocation, t(X;14)(p11;q32), is recurrent in marginal zone lymphomas, which arise in the setting of autoimmune disorders. This translocation leads to up-regulation of *GPR34*, although its role in lymphomagenesis is unknown (249).

SNP arrays have uncovered genetic lesions specific to the different subtypes of marginal zone lymphomas, some which may correlate with prognosis (250). Most recurrent copy number changes in MALT lymphomas are, unlike translocations, site independent although some have a higher frequency at specific sites. These include gains of 6p and 8q, which are more common in the ocular adnexa and gastric locations, respectively (251). FISH studies are useful to demonstrate recurrent trisomies that have been described in marginal zone lymphomas, which include those of chromosomes 3, 12, and 18.

Several recurrent abnormalities have been described in splenic marginal zone lymphomas (SMZL). Deletions of 7q31-q32 occur in up to 30% to 40% of cases and the potential genetic targets include the protection of telomere 1 (*POT1*), sonic hedgehog (*SHH*), and interferon regulatory factor 5 (*IRF5*) genes (252,253). More proximal deletions of the long arm of chromosome 7 at q22 have also been found to be recurrent in a number of studies (254). Mutations and copy number alterations of NF-κB genes are seen in approximately a third of cases of SMZL. The abnormalities involve genes in both the canonical (*TNFAIP3* and *IKBKB*) and noncanonical (*BIRC3*, *TRAF3*, *MAP3K14*) NF-κB pathways (255). The most commonly targeted single gene in SMZL is *NOTCH2*. A spectrum of at least 30 different gain-of-function mutations is concentrated in the

C-terminal PEST domain, and occurs in 20% to 25% of cases (256). These mutations are associated with adverse clinical outcomes, and are likely to prove to be useful diagnostic and therapeutic targets.

Chronic Lymphocytic Leukemia/Small Lymphocytic Lymphoma

Chromosomal abnormalities can be detected in approximately 40% of cases of CLL/SLL by metaphase cytogenetics, although the yield can be increased with the use of mitogens. With FISH, abnormalities can be detected in up to 80% of cases. Unlike FL, MCL, and extranodal MZL, numeric abnormalities, rather than translocations, dominate the genetic landscape of CLL/SLL. The most common, recurrent abnormalities are deletions of 13q14 (~55%), 11q22-q23 (~18%), and 17p13 (7%), and trisomy 12 (~16%).

Chromosome 13q14 deletions, which target (albeit not exclusively) the miRNAs *MIR15A* and *MIR16-1*, have traditionally been associated with a good prognosis, and can now be segregated into two distinct molecular subtypes. Type I deletions are exclusive of *RB1* and type II deletions are inclusive of *RB1*. The larger type II deletions, seen in approximately 20% of cases, are actually associated with short survival (257). Similarly, the number of nuclei containing the deletion may also be relevant with >70% positivity associated with a worse prognosis (258). 17p deletions, resulting in the loss of *TP53*, are associated with a poor prognosis and chemotherapy resistance. 11q22-q23 deletions, affecting *ATM*, also portend a poor prognosis; clinically, there is often impressive adenopathy. Trisomy 12 is associated with atypical morphologic and immunophenotypic features as well as overexpression of *HIP1R*. Many traditional CLL FISH panels are directed at these four abnormalities, but adding probes for del(6q) and *IGH@* translocations may provide additional useful information. *IGH@* translocations can be seen in approximately 7% of cases and they are associated with a worse prognosis (259). Deletions of 6q also occur in approximately 7% of patients and appear to convey an intermediate prognosis (260). Rare *BCL2* translocations, involving the *IGK@* or *IGL@*, may occur in CLL/SLL, involving the 5′ variable cluster region of *BCL2*.

Testing for *TP53* mutations is especially informative in CLL/SLL, as their presence is associated with fludarabine resistance and ultra-high-risk disease (261,262). *TP53* mutations may occur in association with deletion of 17p; however in approximately 4% of cases, the mutation occurs in the absence of a 17p deletion. IHC can detect a majority of cases with *TP53* mutations; however, in some studies, up to 25% of *TP53* mutated cases may be negative by IHC due to the mutation causing a deletion or truncation (263). Hence, genomic evaluation for mutations is preferred. Mutations in a spliceosome gene *SF3B1*, more likely to be encountered in cases with 11q22-q23 deletions, may also be associated with fludarabine resistance, faster disease progression, and poor overall survival (264,265). Similarly, mutations of *BIRC3* and *ATM* may also serve as markers for poor outcome and chemorefractoriness (266). *NOTCH1* mutations also appear to be associated with a dismal prognosis (267). These mutations are enriched in trisomy 12 cases where they impart a poor prognosis in this typically intermediate category (268).

The presence or absence of SHM of the *IGH@* variable region correlates with prognosis in CLL patients, with cases lacking SHM having more aggressive disease. Interestingly, the expression profile of both groups is similar, and is one of memory B-cells (269). ZAP70 is differentially expressed between the mutated (generally ZAP70 negative) and unmutated (usually ZAP70-positive) groups (270). Although analysis of ZAP70 expression, either by flow cytometry or by IHC, was once considered a useful surrogate for the SHM testing, it appears to be an independent marker of (adverse) prognosis.

aCGH demonstrates recurrent abnormalities including gains in 2p25.3 in approximately 30% of cases and gains of 20q13.12 in approximately 20% of cases of CLL (271). Gains of 2p25.3 are associated with ZAP70 expression and unmutated *IGH@* V regions; the gain leads to amplification of *ACP1* and *MYCN*. Methylation assays of ZAP70 may be an alternative way to assess expression. Loss of methylation at a specific single CpG dinucleotide in the *ZAP-70* 5′ regulatory sequence appears highly predictive of a poor prognosis (272). Aberrant methylation of the *CRY1* promoter corresponds with a favorable outcome (273).

CLL may transform into DLBCLs, so-called Richter transformation, in approximately 10% of cases. However, while most (~80%) of these are clonally related, not all are. In additional to being biologically interesting, this is clinically relevant, since those that are clonally related are much more aggressive than those DLBCLs that are *de novo*. Both *NOTCH1* and *SF3B1* mutations in the parent CLL are biomarkers that predict transformation to clonally related DLBCL (274). Interestingly, clonal identity, by comparing *IGH@* rearrangements or using aCGH, does not always indicate linear disease progression (275).

Lymphoplasmacytic Lymphoma

While not specific, deletions of chromosome 6q occur in approximately one-half of cases of lymphoplasmacytic lymphoma (LPL), especially those that are bone marrow based, and not primarily nodal (276). Potentially relevant targets include *PRDM1* and *TNFAIP3*. Trisomy 4 is also a recurrent abnormality in LPL, occurring in 10% to 20% of cases. Like CLL, but in contrast to other small B-cell lymphomas, *IGH@* translocations in LPL are quite rare (<3%). Array CGH demonstrates copy number abnormalities in over 90% of cases of LPL, although these tend to overlap with those seen MZLs (277). *MYD88* L265P mutations are very frequent (~90%) in LPL (278), and testing for these mutations is likely to become diagnostically useful, especially in distinguishing LPL from its mimics, in particular other small B-cell lymphomas with plasmacytic differentiation.

Hairy Cell Leukemia

Before 2011, hairy cell leukemia was not known to be associated with a recurrent genetic abnormality; it is now known that virtually all cases have a mutation in *BRAF*, specifically in exon 15 (V600E) (279,280). These mutations may be detected by simple PCR-based assays or IHC (280,281).

Diffuse Large B-Cell Lymphoma

A variety of recurrent translocations occur in DLBCL, typically involving *IGH@*/14q32. Frequent partners include *BCL6* at 3q27 (~30%), *BCL2* at 18q21 (~25%), and *MYC* at 8q24 (~10%).

BCL6 translocations can involve both immunoglobulin and nonimmunoglobulin gene partners, leading to dysregulated BCL6 protein expression via promoter substitution (282,283). BCL6 is a transcriptional repressor expressed in normal germinal center B-cells, and multiple physiologic gene targets have been identified, including those involved in plasma cell differentiation (e.g., *BLIMP1*) and DNA damage repair (e.g., *TP53*). The oncogenic activity of deregulated BCL6 expression is thus largely due to prevention of differentiation into plasma cells and DNA mutagenesis, respectively (284). PIM1 may cooperate with BCL6 in lymphomagenesis.

Physiologic SHM of the *BCL6* gene occurs as normal B-cells transit the germinal center; this is also seen in other genes that are expressed in this stage of B-cell development. Pathologic mutations of *BCL6* can also be found in various types of lymphomas, including DLBCL, and cluster in the same 5′ regulatory region involved in the translocations (285). These mutations may play a role in lymphomagenesis and tumor progression. Mutations occurring in the binding sites in exon 1 may interfere with negative autoregulation by preventing BCL6 from binding its promoter (286,287). *BCL6* mutations are seen in approximately 15% of DLBCLs; hence, together with translocations (~30%), *BCL6* is targeted in almost one-half of all DLBCLs. *BCL6* is not the only target of aberrant SHM, and this may also affect a variety of genes that may be involved in oncogenesis, including *MYC, PAX5, PIM1, PIM2, SOCS1, BACH2, CIITA,* and *TCL1A* (288).

Initially, the presence of t(14;18)(q32;q21) in DLBCL was thought to reflect evolution from FL. However, it is now accepted that this translocation can also occur in *de novo* DLBCL. *BCL2* translocations occur more frequently in DLBCL with a germinal center phenotype by GEP (see below in this section) (289). Gains of BCL2 can be seen in up to 40% of cases of nongerminal center DLBCL by FISH analysis. Initial studies demonstrated that the overexpression of the BCL2 protein, in the expected absence of t(14;18), was an adverse prognostic factor in the activated B-cell (ABC) group of DLBCL (290). However, these data were generated on patients treated with CHOP without rituximab, and not all studies have confirmed this association, suggesting that the addition of rituximab overcomes this inferior outcome (291). Indeed, with the addition of rituximab, BCL2 expression now seems to have (adverse) prognostic relevance in the germinal center B-cell (GCB) subgroup, and no longer any effect in the ABC subgroup (292). When *BCL2* translocations (and/or *BCL6* translocations) are seen in DLBCL that also have an *MYC* translocation, the lymphomas are considered a "double-hit" lymphoma. This subtype is associated with an especially poor prognosis, making its detection critical (293).

MYC translocations can be seen in DLBCL in the context of (a) *de novo* DLBCL (~10%); (b) plasmablastic lymphomas (~50%); (c) lymphomas that fall into the category of "B-cell lymphoma unclassifiable, with features intermediate between DLBCL and BL" (~40%); and (d) DLBCL arising from an underlying indolent small B-cell lymphoma (~5% to 10%). *De novo* DLBCLs that harbor an *MYC* translocation may not have distinguishing morphologic features, yet still have a poorer prognosis in adults, emphasizing the need for detection of this translocation. Conversely, in pediatric and adolescent cases of nodal DLBCL, the presence of an *MYC* translocation may predict a better prognosis. *MYC* expression can be evaluated in FFPET by a quantitative nuclease protections assay.

Translocations affecting *IRF4* (*MUM1*) have been described in a subset (~5%) of cases of DLBCL (209). The t(6;14)(p25;q32) is cytogenetically cryptic and translocates *IRF4* next to *IGH@*. The translocation in DLBCL correlates with younger age of disease onset and a favorable prognosis.

GEP has yielded abundant information on the diversity of DLBCL, including revealing three quite distinct signatures corresponding to potential cells of origin: GCB-like, ABC-like, and one corresponding to primary mediastinal DLBCL (294). Some of the distinctive genetic (and other) features of these are summarized in Table 8.12. Other GEP analyses have demonstrated subgroups based upon the biology of the lymphoma cells and the host response (HR). These groups are oxidative phosphorylation (Ox Phos), B-cell receptor/proliferation (BCR), and HR (295). A clinically appropriate and applicable diagnostic "lymphochip" has remained elusive, and a multitude of surrogate immunohistochemical algorithms have been proposed. These test for, among others, the expression of CD10, BCL6, MUM1 (IRF4), GCET1, GCET2 (HGAL), FOXP1, BCL2, LMO2, and CD137 (TNFRSF9) (291,296,297). The correlation with GEP of these immunohistochemical algorithms ranges from 80% to 93%; however, standardization and reproducibility issues have shown that this approach may not always be reliable (298). The misclassification rate of IHC may be in the range of 30% to 60% and according to some studies, none of these algorithms may reach the predictive prognostic value of GEP analysis. The expression of SPARC, correlating with a stromal signature associated with extracellular matrix deposition and monocyte/macrophage infiltration (and a good prognosis), and CD31, correlating with microvessel density (and a poor prognosis), has also been evaluated immunohistochemically.

Massively parallel and targeted sequencing in DLBCL reveal mutations in genes encoding protein previously implicated in disease pathogenesis (*MYD88, TP53, CARD11, EZH2, CREBBP, PRDM1, TNFAIP3, CD79B*) as well as those involved in DNA and histone methylation (*MLL2, EZH2, KDM2B*), controlling immune recognition by T cells (*B2M, CD58, TNFSF9, CIITA*), B-cell differentiation (*PAX5, IRF4, ETS1, MEF2B*), and others with heterogeneous functions (*MEF2B, BCL2, BTG1, GNA13,*

Table 8.12	**KEY FEATURES DISTINGUISHING DIFFERENT SUBTYPES OF DLBCL BASED UPON CELL OF ORIGIN**		
	GCB	**ABC**	**PMB**
Cell of origin	Germinal center	Post germinal center	Thymic ("asteroid")
Prognosis	Generally good	Typically bad	Often good
5-y survival	~60%	~30%	~65%
Key proteins/ pathways	CD10, BCL6, SERPIN A9 (GCET1), HGAL (GCET2), LMO2	MUM1 (IRF4)[a], BCL2[b], FOXP1, CCNE, CCND2, SCYA2, MALT1, XBP1, PIM2, NF-κB pathway	REL, MAL, FIG1, TRAF1, TNFAIP2
Key genetic events	t(14;18)/*BCL2* (~40%)	t(3q27)/*BCL6* (~45%)	+9p/*JAK2, PDL1, PDL2, JMJD2C* (~45%)
	m*CREBBP* (~40%)	+18q21-22/*BCL2* (~35%)	m*SOCS1* (~45%)
	m*MLL2* (~30%)	−9p/*CDKN2A* (~30%)	t(16p13)/*CIITA* (~35%)
	m*EZH2* (~20%)	m*BLIMP1* (~30%)	m*STAT6* (~35%)
	amp *MIR17-92* (~15%)	m*MYD88* (~30%)	m*TNFAIP3* (~35%)
	−10q23/*PTEN* (~10%)	−6q21-22/*BLIMP1* (~25%)	+2p/*REL, BCL11A* (~20%)
	t(3;3)/*TBL1XR1-TP63* (~5%)	+19q/*SPIB* (~25%)	
	−1p/*TP73*(~25%)	m*TNFAIP3* (~25%)	
	+2p/*REL* (~15%)	m*CD79B* (~20%)	
	+12q12/*CDK2, CDK4* (~10%)	m*BCL6* (~20%)	
	t(6;14)/*IRF4* (young adults) (~5%)	m*CARD11* (~10%)	
		+3/?*FOXP1* (~10%)	

GCB, germinal center B-cell; ABC, activated B-cell; PMB, primary mediastinal B-cell; m, mutation; amp, amplification.
[a]MUM1/IRF4 is expressed in GCB-DLBCLs that have *IRF4* translocations.
[b]BCL2 is expressed in GCB-DLBCLs that harbor the t(14;18) translocation.

ACTB, P2RY8, PCLO, TNFRSF14) (299,300). Some of these mutations are differentially associated with distinct cell-of-origin subtypes (Table 8.12).

Burkitt Lymphoma

MYC translocations characterize Burkitt lymphoma (BL). The t(8;14)(q24;q32), translocating the oncogene *MYC* (8q24) to *IGH@* (14q32), is found in 80% of cases. Less frequent variant translocations, t(2;8)(p11;q24) and t(8;22)(q24;q11), affect *IGK@* and *IGL@*, respectively. The molecular consequence of all these translocations is the same: overexpression of *MYC. MYC* translocations are not specific for BL, and can also occur in posttransplant lymphoproliferative disorders, plasmablastic lymphoma, DLBCL, so-called borderline lymphomas (see section on B-cell lymphoma, unclassifiable, with features intermediate between DLBCL and BL), and during transformation of indolent lymphomas (301). Furthermore, the notion that 100% of cases of BL harbor an *MYC* translocation had been challenged, in that approximately 5% to 10% may lack a translocation, but still up-regulate MYC expression, albeit via alternative mechanisms, sometimes involving miRNA, specifically down-regulation of *MIR34B* (302). Despite the traditional and long-standing association between MYC and BL, it is well known that *MYC* deregulation alone is insufficient for lymphomagenesis. Indeed, additional mutations occur in BL, which lead to aberrations that synergize with overexpressed MYC. Inactivation of *TP53* is well known to occur in BL, while more recently mutations in *CCND3* (~40%) and in genes encoding participants in the PI3K pathway have been identified (303). The PI3K pathway genes, *TCF3* and *ID3* (which encodes a negative regulator of TCF3), are mutated in approximately 70% of cases of BL.

The *MYC* and *IGH@* breakpoints differ in endemic and sporadic BL. In endemic BL, the 8q24 break occurs up to 300 kb 5′ from the coding region of the *MYC* gene, translocating *MYC* near the J region of *IGH@*. In sporadic BL, a break typically occurs within exon 1 of the *MYC* gene and involves the C region of *IGH@*. These different *IGH@* translocations sites suggest that endemic and sporadic BL are derived from errors in SHM and class switch recombination, respectively. These translocations are not amenable to standard PCR assays and hence FISH breakapart probes are the preferred modality for detecting translocations; dual fusion probes are required to identify specific partners. IHC may have a role in detecting lymphoma cases with increased MYC expression, either from translocations or from alternative mechanisms (304,305).

B-Cell Lymphoma, Unclassifiable, with Features Intermediate Between DLBCL and BL

WHO 2008 created a new category to account for lymphoma cases with features overlapping between DLBCL and BL, "B-cell lymphoma, unclassifiable, with features intermediate between DLBCL and BL" (306). While lymphomas in this category are first considered based upon morphologic and immunophenotypic features, genetic studies (conventional karyotyping and FISH) can be particularly helpful in their documentation (Table 8.13). Although there is some overlap, it is important to appreciate, as currently defined, that not all cases in this category are double-hit lymphomas, as alluded to previously in the section on DLBCLs (307). Similarly, not all double-hit lymphomas fall into this category, as some are better classified as DLBCL.

Hodgkin Lymphoma

Molecular analysis is not required in the routine diagnostic evaluation of HL. Historically, however, molecular studies were essential to prove that Hodgkin and Reed Sternberg cells (as well as lymphocyte-predominant cells) are of B-cell origin in virtually all cases. In addition, recent analyses have unraveled

Table 8.13	GENETIC FEATURES OF BL, B CELL LYMPHOMA UNCLASSIFIABLE WITH FEATURES INTERMEDIATE BETWEEN BL AND DIFFUSE LARGE CELL LYMPHOMA (BCLU), AND DIFFUSE LARGE B CELL LYMPHOMA (DLBCL)		
	BL	**BCLU**	**DLBCL**
MYC rearrangement	Yes[a] (~90%)	Common (~40%)	Rare (~10%)
IG-MYC[b]	Yes	Sometimes	Rare
Non-*IG-MYC*	No	Sometimes	Rare
BCL2 but no *MYC* rearrangement	No	Rare	Sometimes
BCL6 but no *MYC* rearrangement	No	Rare	Sometimes
Double-hit lymphoma[c]	No	Sometimes	Rare
MYC-simple karyotype[d]	Yes	Rare	Rare
MYC-complex karyotype[d]	Rare	Common	Rare

[a]Approximately 5%–10% of otherwise classical BL cases lack a detectable *MYC* rearrangement.
[b]*IG-MYC*, juxtaposition of *MYC* to one of the *IG* loci: *IGH@* at 14q32, *IGK@* at 2p12, or *IGL@* at 22q11. Non-*IG-MYC* tumors contain an *MYC* rearrangement but no juxtaposition to one of the *IG* loci.
[c]Double-hit lymphomas contain an *MYC*/8q24 translocation in combination with a *BCL2*/18q21 (most frequent) and/or *BCL6*/3q27 translocation. The partner of *BCL2*/18q21 is mostly the *IGH@* locus at 14q32.
[d]Simple karyotype: no or only few cytogenetic or aCGH abnormalities other than the *MYC* rearrangement. For aCGH, a lymphoma with six or more abnormalities has been assigned as "*MYC* complex."

an array of molecular genetic abnormalities, particularly in classical HL (Table 8.14). In contrast to the plethora of genetic lesions identified in classical Hodgkin lymphoma (CHL), the molecular pathogenesis of nodular lymphocyte-predominant HL (NLPHL) is less well characterized. An exception is the presence of *BCL6* translocations, which are identified in up to 50% of cases of NLPHL, but not in CHL (308).

Plasma Cell Neoplasms

Of the PCNs, myeloma is the best studied. Interestingly, however, many of the genetic abnormalities seen in myeloma can be found in the others as well, including its indolent precursor monoclonal gammopathy of uncertain significance (MGUS). Molecular studies are not necessary for diagnosis, but they are extremely useful in determining prognosis and, on occasion, directing treatment. Metaphase cytogenetics are of low yield, since plasma cells rarely proliferate *ex vivo*, and FISH has become the gold standard for molecular analysis. While not currently part of the routine diagnostic workup, comparative genomic hybridization can also be useful to detect abnormalities.

There are two main chromosomally abnormal pathogenetic groups, each accounting for approximately half the cases of myeloma: hyperdiploid and nonhyperdiploid cases. Hyperdiploid cases contain multiple trisomies of odd-numbered chromosomes other than 13 and 17 (1, 3, 5, 7, 9, 11, 15, 19, and 21). The remaining nonhyperdiploid cases typically have *IGH@* translocations and they are more frequently associated with deletions of 13q. *IGH@* translocations are not restricted to this group and occur in approximately 10% of hyperdiploid cases (310).

A number of different recurrent *IGH@* partners have been identified. The seven most common, which divide myeloma into three translocation groups, are (a) cyclin Ds: *CCND1* at 11q13 (~15%), *CCND2* at 12p12 (<1%), *CCND3* at 6p21 (~2%); (b) MAFs: *MAF* at 16q23 (~5%), *MAFB* at 20q12 (~2%); (c) *FGFR3/MMSET* at 4p16 (~15%) (311). The *IGH@* translocations in myeloma typically occur as a consequence of errors in class switch recombination or SHM. The light chains may also be involved in translocations, and, interestingly, the lambda locus is more frequently involved than the kappa locus. Plasma cell myeloma can also be classified into eight groups based on patterns of translocations and cyclin expression, since the translocations either directly or indirectly lead to cyclin dysregulation (312).

Table 8.14	GENETIC ABNORMALITIES IN HL				
		Frequency			
Gene	**Chromosome Location**	**CHL**	**NLPHL**	**Genetic Alteration**	**Effect of Genetic Lesion**
ETS1	11q23	~65%	—	Deletion	Decreased transcription factor function
MDM2	12q13-q14	~60%	—	Gain	p53 inactivation
CREL	2p13	~50%	—	Amplification	Activation of NF-κB pathway
BCL6	3q27	—	~50%	Translocation	Disrupted B-cell differentiation
SOCS1	16p13	~45%	—	Mutation	Impaired JAK2 degradation, and hence activation of JAK-STAT signaling
TNFAIP3	6q23-q25	~40%	—	Mutation[a]	Activation of NF-κB pathway
NFKBIA and NFKBIE	14q13 6p21	~30%	—	Mutation	Activation of NF-κB pathway
JAK2	9p24	~30%	—	Amplification or translocation[b]	Activation of JAK-STAT signaling
MAP3K14	17q21-q22	~30%	—	Gain	Activation of NF-κB pathway
TRAF3	14q32	~15%	—	Deletion	Lost of inhibition of CD40 signaling
CIITA	16p13	~15%	—	Translocation	Down-regulation of surface HLA class II expression and overexpression of CD273 and CD274, modulating immunogenicity
FAS	10q24	~10%	—	Mutation	Evasion of apoptosis
EBV	N/A	~40%	—	Presence	A subset of CHL, but not NLPHL, is associated with EBV
IGH@	14q32	"crippling" (~25%), static	Functional, ongoing	SHM	Indicates that the neoplastic cells are B-cells, and of germinal center or postgerminal center origin

[a]TNFAIP3 mutations have a somewhat inverse relationship with EBV infection, in that ~70% of EBV-negative but only ~15% of EBV-positive cases harbor TNFAIP3 mutations.
[b]Translocations involving JAK2, in particular those involving the SEC31A gene, in the t(4;9)(q21;p24), are seen in ~3% of CHLs (309).

The t(11;14)(q13;q32) seen in myeloma differs from that seen in MCL regarding breakpoints in both the IGH@ and CCND1 genes. The 11q13 breakpoints in myeloma are more widely scattered throughout the 11q13 region than in MCL and the IGH@ breakpoint typically involves the switch region. CyclinD1 positivity by IHC typically accompanies the translocation, and is usually associated with a good prognosis; however, this technique does not distinguish between cases with a t(11;14) translocation and those with cyclin D1 up-regulation through other mechanisms (313). Patients with 17p13 deletions have a poor prognosis, although this may be improved with bortezomib-based therapy (314). Deletions of 13q14 are associated with a good prognosis; however, this is only the case when it is detected by conventional metaphase karyotyping, since its detection by FISH is not predictive.

Sequencing studies in myeloma patients identify a number of mutations in genes encoding proteins involved in the NF-κB pathway (BTRC, CARD11, CYLD, IKBIP, IKBKB, MAP3K1, MAP3K14, RIPK4, TLR4, TNFRSF1A, TRAF3), RNA processing and protein homeostasis (DIS3, FAM46C, XBP1, LRRK2), and histone-modifying enzymes (MLL, MLL2, MLL3, UTX, WHSC1, WHSC1L1) (315). RAS mutations occur in approximately 40% of myeloma cases.

Gene expression signatures may predict response to certain therapies (316). Additionally, GEP has demonstrated biologically and clinically relevant signatures that may be amenable to multiplex RT-PCR assays (317). These include differing miRNA signatures (318). GEP in smoldering myeloma may yield information regarding risk for progression by examination of expression of four SNORD genes (SNORD25, SNORD27, SNORD30, and SNORD31) (319). Additionally, GEP has implicated the NF-κB pathway in myeloma and MGUS, with both sets of tumors having a signature showing high expression of NF-κB target genes, perhaps related to some of the mutations

described above (320,321). GEPs that have been proposed for use in clinical trials include those that evaluate a 70 (322) or 92 (323) gene signature.

While many of the classical translocations are acquired early on in PCNs, even at the MGUS stage, increasing copy number changes are seen with progression to smoldering myeloma and overt PCM (324). Changes once thought to be exclusive to PCM, including 11q and 21q gains and 16q and 22q deletions, were also seen in a subset of cases of MGUS. Additional prognostically important copy number alterations in PCM are gains of 1q;CKS1B and losses of 1p;CDKN2C and FAM46C, both of which correlate with a poor outcome (325), and amp(5) (q31), which portends a good prognosis (326). Methylation studies in myeloma reveal global hypomethylation but with focal hypermethylation of CDKN2A, which may be associated with a worse outcome (327). Patients with t(4;14) have particularly enriched gene-specific DNA hypermethylation. MMSET dysregulation leads to changes in histone modification that promote cell survival, cell cycle progression, and DNA repair (328).

Mature (Peripheral) T-cell and NK-Cell Lymphomas and Leukemias

As with mature B-cell lymphomas, molecular studies in T-cell neoplasms can be considered in one of two broad scenarios. One is the use of TCR gene rearrangements, to facilitate the determination of monoclonality (discussed in Chapter 6) as a tool for both diagnosis and tracking minimal residual disease, while the other is the detection of nonrandom acquired genetic lesions that are associated with specific neoplasms. However, in contrast to mature B-cell neoplasms, where numerous specific genetic abnormalities have been recognized, the molecular characterization of T-cell neoplasms is somewhat less well developed, aside from a subset of ALCLs (see below in this section). Nevertheless,

Table 8.15	GENETIC FEATURES OF MATURE (PERIPHERAL) T-CELL AND NK-CELL NEOPLASMS, OTHER THAN ALCL		
T-cell Lymphoma Subtype	**Genetic and Molecular Alterations**	**Frequency**	**Effect of Genetic Lesion**
Peripheral T-cell lymphoma, follicular variant	t(5;9)(q33;q22); *SYK-ITK*	~40%	Overexpression of *SYK* with increased proliferation and prosurvival signaling
Peripheral T-cell lymphoma, NOS	*SYK* activation	~95%	Increased proliferation and prosurvival signaling
	PDGFRA overexpression	~90%	Increased STAT activation
	t(6p25); *IRF4*	~7%	Unclear; *IRF4* mRNA and protein levels are the same in cases with and without the translocation
Angioimmunoblastic T-cell lymphoma	*TET2* mutation	~50%	Inactivation leading to DNA hypermethylation
	IDH2 mutation	~20%–45%	Increased production of 2-hydroxyglutarate leading to DNA hypermethylation
ALK-negative ALCL and primary cutaneous ALCL	t(6;7)(p25;q32); *DUSP22-FRA7H*	~45%	Decreased *DUSP22* expression and up-regulated *MIR29* leading to disrupted T-cell antigen receptor signaling
NK/T cell lymphoma	6q deletion	>50%	Unclear
	PDGFRA overexpression	~100%	Increased STAT activation
	JAK3 mutation	~35%	Constitutive activation leading to impaired STAT signaling
Hepatosplenic T-cell lymphoma	iso7q	~50%–60%	Unclear
	FOS, VAV3, S1PR5 overexpression	~35%	Overexpression resulting in increased TCR signaling
	AIM1 underexpression	~70%	Unclear
Enteropathy-associated T-cell lymphoma	9q gains	~60%	Unclear
T-cell prolymphocytic leukemia	inv(14;14)(q11q32) or t(14;14)(q11;q32.1); *TCRAD@-TCL1* t(X;14)(q28;q11); *TCRAD@-MTCP1*	~50%	Aberrant expression of TCL1 leading to enhanced activation of the AKT pathway
Sézary syndrome	*TCF3* deletion	~70%	Enhanced cell cycle progression
T-cell large granular lymphocytic leukemia	*STAT3* mutations	~30%–40%	Constitutive activation resulting in increased transcription
Chronic NK lymphocytosis	*STAT3* mutations	~30%	Constitutive activation resulting in increased transcription

tremendous insights have been gleaned in other mature T-cell malignancies, and these are summarized in the Table 8.15.

Systemic ALCL is subdivided into two subtypes: ALK positive or ALK negative. Among the ALK-positive cases, t(2;5)(p23;q35) is the most common genetic abnormality, occurring in approximately 70%. The cytoplasmic catalytic portion of the receptor tyrosine kinase *ALK* (2p23) is fused to the amino terminal of nucleophosmin, *NPM1* (5q35). An 80 kD chimeric fusion protein with constitutive tyrosine kinase activity is produced. Other *ALK* partners include *TPM3* at 1q21 (~13%), *ATIC* at 2q35 (1%), *TFG* at 3q21 (<1%), *CLTC* at 17q23 (<1%), and *MSN* at Xq11~q12 (<1%). All variant translocations also result in a chimeric fusion protein with dimerization domains inducing up-regulation of *ALK* (329). The ALK protein is not normally expressed in hematopoietic tissue, and hence IHC can be used to detect ALK that is aberrantly expressed as a consequence of these translocations. The subcellular localization of the ALK protein correlates with the translocation partner. Both nuclear and cytoplasmic staining is seen in cases with t(2;5) while only cytoplasmic (and/or membranous) staining is seen in the others. Although the translocations can be detected by FISH or RT-PCR, IHC is a convenient and reliable diagnostic "surrogate." A three-gene model (*TNFRSF8, BATF3, TMOD1*) is able to distinguish ALK-negative ALCL from peripheral T-cell lymphoma, NOS (330).

ALK dysregulation and expression occurs in a diverse spectrum of neoplasms other than ALCL. A subset of DLBCLs harbors the t(2;17) fusing *ALK* with *CLTC* (331). ALK can also be dysregulated in nonhematopoietic tumors in association with a translocation (inflammatory myofibroblastic tumor and lung cancer) and without (neuroblastoma and glioblastoma) (332).

Acute Lymphoblastic Leukemias

Antigen Receptor Gene Rearrangements in ALL

The major role for evaluating antigen receptor gene rearrangements in ALL is primarily to identify clonal markers that can

subsequently be used for quantitative PCR monitoring of minimal residual disease during or after therapy, since the attainment of defined levels of molecular clearance at certain time points is a powerful prognostic indicator, especially in pediatric ALL. However, such analyses are laborious, since they require the synthesis of patient-specific primers and/or probes. Antigen receptor gene rearrangements seen at diagnosis may not be present at relapse; therefore, following more than one rearrangement is recommended (333). The majority of B-cell ALLs have clonal rearrangements of *IGH@*, or, less frequently, of light chain genes. T-cell ALL almost always shows clonal rearrangements of the TCR beta or gamma chains, and may demonstrate simultaneous rearrangements of *IGH@*. "Cross lineage" rearrangements are frequent. Up to 70% of precursor B-cell ALLs demonstrate monoclonal TCR gene rearrangements (334). It is possible that the use of quantitative PCR for determining remission status may be superseded by approaches using massively parallel sequencing (35).

Recurrent Genetic Abnormalities in ALL

Numerous chromosomal and submicroscopic genetic lesions occur in ALL and many of the former are used for classification (Fig. 8.7).

B-Cell ALL

A number of recurrent translocations have been described in B-cell ALL, which are now inculcated into the current (2008) WHO scheme.

t(9;22)(q34;q11); BCR-ABL1

Best known as the disease-defining abnormality in CML, the t(9;22)(q34;q11) is also the most common translocation seen in adult B-cell ALL, occurring in up to 25% of cases. The translocation has a lower occurrence in pediatric B-cell ALL (1% to 4%).

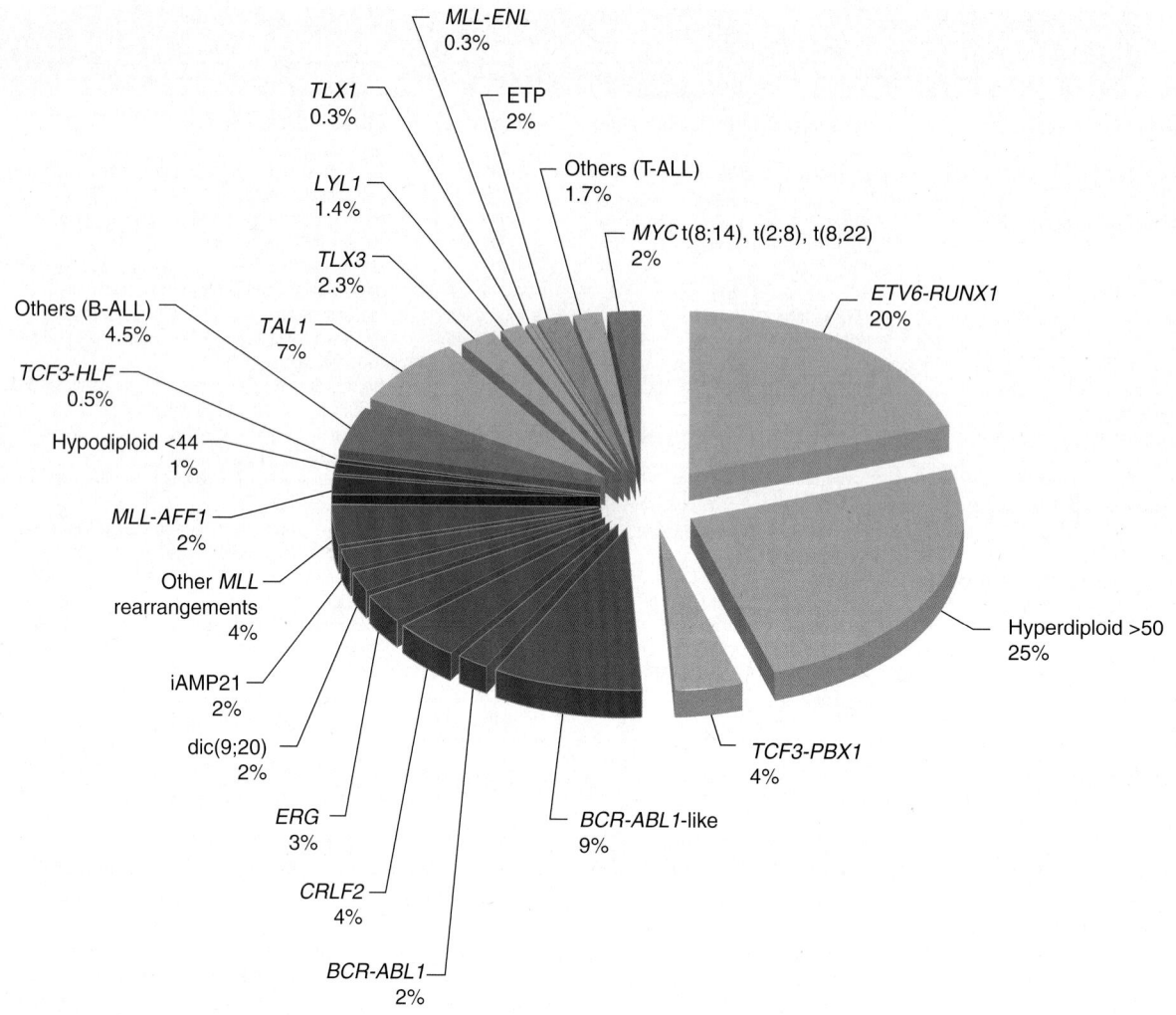

FIGURE 8.7. Examples and estimated frequency of recurrent numerical and structural genetic alterations in childhood B-cell and T-cell ALL. The genetic lesions that are exclusively seen in cases of T-cell ALL are indicated in *gold* and those commonly associated with precursor B-cell ALL in *blue*. The *darker gold* or *blue* colors indicate those subtypes generally associated with poor prognosis, while those in shades of *gray* typically portend a good prognosis. Reproduced with permission from Pui CH, Mullighan CG, Evans WE, et al. Pediatric acute lymphoblastic leukemia: where are we going and how do we get there? *Blood*, 2012;120:1165–1174. Ref. (335). The figure highlights many, but not all, of the recurrent genetic abnormalities in B-cell and T-cell ALL. Please see text and Tables 8.16 and 8.17 for further details on *IKZF1, PAX5, CDKN2A/B, RAS, FLT3, NOTCH1, FBXW7*, among numerous others. For some abnormalities the frequency rates differ between pediatric and adult populations. For example, t(9;22); *BCR-ABL1* is more common in adult B-cell ALL (~25%), while t(12;21); *ETV6-RUNX1* is less common in adults (<5%). B-cell ALL with *MYC* rearrangements likely reflects BL in leukemic phase.

These ALLs are almost exclusively CD10+ precursor B-cell ALLs with frequent coexpression of the myeloid-associated antigens CD13 and CD33. Even with intensified chemotherapy, this translocation is possibly the most important predictor of poor long-term survival (336).

The translocation involves the *ABL1* gene at 9q34 and *BCR* gene at 22q11. As in CML, the breakpoints in the *ABL1* gene typically cluster in intron 1 (after exon 1, termed a1). Occasionally *ABL1* breakpoints may occur in intron 2. Unlike CML, the breakpoints in the *BCR* gene are more variable. The major breakpoint region (M-bcr), located in the introns following exons 13 or 14 (e13 and e14, previously b2 and b3, respectively), is involved in virtually all cases of CML. By contrast, in ALL, the majority of breakpoints occur more 5′ in the intron following exon 1 (e1), the minor breakpoint cluster region (m-bcr). Thus in adults, approximately 60% of breakpoints occur in the m-bcr, while approximately 90% of pediatric cases occur in this region. Hence, two separate RT-PCRs are necessary to detect *BCR-ABL1* transcripts in ALL. These assays utilize two different upstream BCR primers to exon 1 and exon 13. A single *ABL1* primer is sufficient, either to exon 2 (a2) or to exon 3 (a3), with

the latter useful in detecting the rare intron 2 breakpoint. The M-bcr yields a p210 fusion protein while the m-bcr yields a p190 fusion protein.

Either RT-PCR or FISH should be used to document the presence of a *BCR-ABL1* fusion, even if the hallmark cytogenetic translocation is present. This is necessary in order to justify the use of therapy with TKIs and to account for "false-negative" (karyotypically normal) cases, which may occur up to 10% of the time (3).

t(12;21)(p13;q22); ETV6-RUNX1

The cryptic t(12;21)(p13;q22) involving *ETV6* (12p13) and *RUNX1* (21q22) is the most common translocation in pediatric B-cell ALL, occurring in 25% of pediatric cases and <5% of adult cases. Like *BCR-ABL1*+ cases, they tend to have a characteristic CD13+, CD33+, precursor B-cell immunophenotype with bright CD10 expression and absence of CD9. Since the translocation is essentially always cytogenetically cryptic, RT-PCR or FISH is necessary for detection. The translocation results in an in-frame fusion of a portion of *ETV6* with *RUNX1*, both transcription factors needed for normal hematopoiesis. The fusion protein, which is composed of the N-terminal of the non-DNA–binding region of ETV6 and most of RUNX1, acts in a dominant negative manner and interferes with the normal function of RUNX1 by blocking binding to DNA and repressing RUNX1-activated transcription. RT-PCR with primers to exon 5 of *ETV6* and exon 4 of *RUNX1* detect the most common transcripts. The other *ETV6* allele is deleted in many cases with the translocation, suggesting the fusion may function in a recessive manner, requiring the loss of the normal *ETV6* allele (337,338). Both genes in this translocation, namely, *ETV6* and *RUNX1*, are quite promiscuous and can be translocated to a number of different partners in various other hematologic malignancies including AML and MDS (339).

t(1;19)(q23;p13); TCF3-PBX1

The t(1;19)(q23;p13) occurs in approximately 4% to 6% of pediatric and 2% to 3% of adult cases of B-ALL (340). The translocation results in a fusion of the *TCF3* and *PBX1* genes, generating a chimeric oncoprotein. The t(1;19) is associated with a pre-B immunophenotype (Cμ+, CD10+, CD20+, CD34-, TdT-/+). *TCF3* encodes various transcription factors, including the immunoglobulin gene enhancer binding factors E12 and E47, important for B-cell development. *PBX1* encodes a DNA-binding homeodomain protein that is not normally expressed in B-cells. This fusion protein acts as a transcriptional activator and also interferes with transcription factors normally encoded by *TCF3* and *PBX1*. The majority (75%) of translocations are unbalanced, resulting in −19, der(19) t(1;19). An RT-PCR assay using a single pair of primers can detect >90% of t(1;19)-positive cases. The translocation was traditionally associated with an adverse outcome. However, this can be overcome with risk-adapted therapy. Cytogenetic studies can be uninformative in a number of cases, emphasizing the need for molecular genetic studies. A rare variant translocation has been described in children, the t(17;19). This translocation results in a TCF3-HLF fusion protein and it is associated with a poor prognosis (341,342). While this alternative translocation is very rare (~0.1% in children), two molecular subtypes have been described, one associated with disseminated intravascular coagulation and the other with hypercalcemia.

t(v;11q23); MLL Rearranged

Over 100 leukemia-associated translocations involving *MLL* at 11q23 have been described. The translocations of 11q23 seen most frequently in B-cell ALL include t(4;11)(q21;q23), t(11;19)(q23;p13.3), and t(9;11)(p22;q23), which result in a fusion of the 5′ portion of *MLL* to the 3′ portion of *AFF1*, *MLLT1*, and *MLLT3*, respectively (343). Most *MLL* breakpoints occur in a 5′ region between exons 5 and 11. The t(4;11)(q11;q23) is seen in both pediatric and adult patients, but is most common in infantile ALL, where it accounts for 75% of ALLs in this age group. The translocation is associated with a poor prognosis. ALLs with the *AFF1-MLL* fusion overexpress *FLT3*, in the absence of the mutations that are seen in AML, and this confers an even worse prognosis in these cases (344). Since cytogenetics may be negative, RT-PCR or FISH should be considered. RT-PCR analysis with a single exon 8 *MLL* primer and single exon 7 *AFF1* primer may suffice. However, differential breakpoints in different introns and alternative splicing can result in >10 different fusion transcripts, complicating the interpretation of RT-PCR assays. Hence, FISH is preferred for detecting this translocation.

t(5;14); IL3-IGH@

The t(5;14)(q31;q32) occurs in <1% of cases of ALL. The *IL3* gene is translocated to the *IGH@* gene. The resultant *IL3*

overexpression leads to variable degrees of eosinophilia. Standard karyotype analysis or FISH are typically adequate for detection.

Other Genetic Abnormalities in B-Cell ALL

A number of other key genetic abnormalities underlie the pathogenesis of B-cell ALL, in addition to the translocations discussed above (Table 8.16). *IKZF1*, which encodes Ikaros, a zinc finger-containing DNA-binding protein, is frequently targeted. Indeed, microdeletions of *IKZF1* are present in up to 80% of *BCR-ABL1*-positive cases of B-cell ALL, although they are not restricted to this subtype (345). Interestingly, cases with *IKZF1* deletions that are *BCR-ABL1* negative have a gene expression profile similar to *BCR-ABL1*-positive cases, and are referred to as "*BCR-ABL1*-like" or "Ph-like" ALL (346,347). *IKZF1* deletions appear to confer a poor prognosis in children with B-cell ALL, including cases associated with Down syndrome (86,348). The poor prognostic significance may only relate to certain GEP-defined clusters (349). Two multiplex PCR reactions are typically sufficient to detect *IKZF1* deletions, as most involve exon 1 to exon 6 (350). Other microdeletions seen in ALL, both with and without a t(9;22), include those affecting *PAX5* and *CDKN2A/CDKN2B*, each in up to 50% of cases (351). *PAX5* may also be affected by point mutations and translocations (3%). Other genes that encode proteins that are involved in B-cell development, and that are mutated or deleted in B-ALL, include *EBF1*, *RAG1*, *RAG2*, *LEF1*, and *BLINK*.

CRLF2 rearrangements, leading to overexpression of cytokine receptor-like factor 2 (which is measurable by flow cytometry), occur in 5% to 16% of cases of pediatric and adult B-cell ALL. The frequency is even greater in B-cell ALL associated with Down syndrome, where they are seen in >50% of cases (352). This pseudoautosomal gene (located at Xp22.3 and Yp11.3) may be dysregulated by cryptic translocations and deletions, as well as by activating mutations. In the t(X;14)(p22;q32), *CRLF2* rearranges to the *IGH@* enhancer, while in a cryptic interstitial deletion and fusion with another pseudoautosomal gene in the same loci, *CRLF2* rearranges to the *P2RY8* promoter; the former is more common in adults, while the latter is more common in pediatric cases (353). *CRLF2* overexpression is also associated with *JAK2* mutations in up to 50% of cases, particularly in the context of Down syndrome (352); as with IZKF1 alterations noted above, CRLF2 defects are also enriched in "*BCR-ABL1*-like" ALL. Heterozygous mutations of *JAK1*, *JAK2*, and *JAK3* are present in approximately 10% of cases of non-Down syndrome-associated B-ALL, while *BTG1* deletions occur in Down syndrome ALL (354). *LEF1* overexpression may serve as a marker of poor outcome in adult B-ALL (355). Intrachromosomal amplification of chromosome 21 (iAMP21) is seen in a minority (~2%) of cases of pediatric B-cell ALL (356). Three or more copies of the *RUNX1* gene are present. However, amplification of RUNX1 may not be relevant since expression levels are not higher in iAMP cases (357). *RAS* mutations are quite frequent in high-risk B-cell ALL, with mutations of both *NRAS* and *KRAS* each observed in approximately 10% to 15% of cases; mutation of genes encoding participants in the TP53 and RB pathways are also frequently mutated (>50%) in high-risk B-cell ALL (358).

T Lymphoblastic Leukemia/Lymphoma

A variety of recurrent genetic abnormalities have been described in T-cell ALL. An abnormal karyotype can be seen in 50% to 70% of cases (1) and a host of submicroscopic lesions have also been identified (Table 8.17). However, neither karyotypic nor molecular aberrations are currently used in contemporary classification, although their role in the pathogenesis of these neoplasms is clear. Many of the chromosomal alterations

Table 8.16 | MUTATIONS AND OTHER SUBMICROSCOPIC LESIONS IN B-CELL ALL

Gene	Chromosome Location	Frequency	Genetic Alteration	Biologic Function of Protein	Effect of Genetic Lesion	Clinical Significance
IKZF1[a]	7p13	~80% (BCR-ABL1 positive) ~15%–30% (BCR-ABL1 negative)	Mutation or deletion	Transcription factor required for lymphoid development	Decreased transcription results in impaired lymphocyte differentiation	Unfavorable
PAX5	9p13	~30%–40%	Mutation, deletion, or translocation	Transcription factor (B-cell development)	Impaired regulation of early B-cell differentiation	Unclear
CDKN2A/B	9p21	~30%	Deletion	Negative cell cycle regulator	Loss of inhibition of cyclin-dependent kinases, leading to increased cell cycle progression	Unfavorable (especially if BCR-ABL1 positive)
KRAS	12p12	~30% (pediatric)	Mutation at codons 12, 13, and 61	Signal transduction	Constitutive activation of signal transduction	Unfavorable
NRAS	1p13					
FLT3	13q12	Up to ~25% (hyperdiploid cases)	Mostly the same as in AML ITD: Exons 14 and 15 TKD: D835 as well as others	Type III receptor tyrosine kinase	Constitutive activation of signal transduction, increased proliferation and decreased apoptosis	Unclear
CREBBP	16p13	~20% (relapsed cases)	Mutation (almost exclusively in HAT domain for hyperdiploid cases) or deletion	Acetylates histone and nonhistone proteins	Impaired histone acetylation and transcriptional regulation; associated with glucocorticoid resistance	Unfavorable
TP53	17p13	~10%–15% (at relapse)	Mutation (frequently in exon 7 or 8) or deletion	Cell cycle arrest, DNA damage repair, apoptosis	Loss of tumor suppressor activity	Unfavorable
CRLF2[a]	Xp22	~5%–15% >50% in Down syndrome (DS)	Translocations (with IGH@ or P2RY8) or mutations (F232C)	Signal transduction	Constitutive STAT activation with increased proliferation and impaired development	Unfavorable
JAK1[a]	1p21	<5% (JAK1)	Varied including the JAK2 R683 pseudokinase domain mutation	Signal transduction	Constitutive JAK-STAT activation	Unfavorable
JAK2[a]	9p24	~10% (JAK2) ~20%–35% in DS				
RUNX1	21q22	<5%	iAMP21	Transcription factor	DNA amplification including multiple copies of RUNX1; however, may not be accompanied by increased protein	Unfavorable

[a]Alterations in IKZF1, CRLF2 and JAK are enriched in "BCR-ABL1-like" cases (see text for details), and also in B-cell ALL arising in the setting of Down syndrome.

are translocations (~30%), but deletions and duplications also occur. Most commonly, the regulatory region of one of the TCR loci on chromosomes 7, TRB@ (7q35), and TRG@ (7p14-p15) and chromosome 14, TRA@, and TRD@ (both 14q11.2) is juxtaposed to transcription factor genes, resulting in their aberrant expression in developing thymocytes (359,360). Recurrent partners include TLX1 (10q24), TLX3 (5q35), MYC (8q24.1), TAL1 (1p32), LMO1 (11q15), LMO2 (11q13), LYL1 (19p13), and LYK (1p34) (359,361). In addition, gene fusions generating chimeric proteins also occur.

Some recurrent chromosomal abnormalities are cryptic. The submicroscopic nature of these alterations highlights the importance of molecular studies. For example, an interstitial deletion of TAL1 resulting in fusion to the STIL gene occurs in up to 25%. Interestingly, this fusion is mediated by RAG1/2, which typically facilitates physiologic and pathologic V(D)J rearrangements of antigen receptor genes, which are not involved in this genetic event. While the prognostic significance of this translocation is unknown, it may be useful for MRD tracking. A cryptic rearrangement affecting ABL1 gene has also been described. The NUP214-ABL1 fusion with episomal amplification occurs in 6% of cases and the abnormality is associated with responsiveness to tyrosine kinase inhibition, and can be detected by FISH using an ABL1 probe (362).

GEP has been used to classify T-ALL into distinct "molecular-cytogenetic subgroups" that correspond to specific stages of T-cell development. The different groups correlate with genetic rearrangements and overexpression of various transcription factors. These subgroups are HOX11L2, LYL1 plus LMO2, TAL1 plus LMO1 or LMO2, HOX11 and MLL-ENL (363,364). As in B-cell ALL, alterations of CDKN2A and CDKN2B are also common in T-cell ALL and are evident in more than 50% of cases. This occurs via deletion of 9p21 or transcriptional silencing by hypermethylation of 5' CpG islands. FISH, methylation-sensitive PCR, and RT-PCR detect these abnormalities better than conventional cytogenetics (365,366).

Activating mutations in genes involved in normal T-cell development are recurrent events in T-ALL. Mutations in NOTCH1 occur in approximately 55% of cases of T-cell ALL (367,368). These mutations occur in either the extracellular heterodimerization domain or the C-terminal PEST domain. NOTCH1 mutations are usually associated with a favorable prognosis, but this may be modified by the specific treatment protocol (369,370). Examination for both NOTCH1 and FBXW7 mutations appears to be better for risk stratification than evaluating NOTCH1 alone (371). Other genes that may be mutated in T-ALL include CD45, JAK1, and LCK.

Limitations and Rational Use of Molecular Genetic Studies

The practicing hematopathologist is confronted by a daunting, and ever-expanding, array of genetic tests that can be used in the diagnosis, classification, and prognostication of hematologic neoplasms, as well as in the tracking of disease following

Table 8.17   COMMON (≥5%) RECURRENT GENETIC ABNORMALITIES IN T-CELL ALL

Gene	Chromosome Location	Frequency	Genetic Alteration	Biologic Function of Protein	Effect of Genetic Lesion	Clinical Significance
CDKN2A/2B	9p21	~70%	Deletion/hypermethylation	Negative cell cycle regulator	Loss of inhibition of cyclin-dependent kinases, leading to increased cell cycle progression	Unfavorable
NOTCH1	9q34	~55%	Mutation	Membrane receptor needed for normal lymphocyte function	Activation of NOTCH1 pathway resulting in impaired intercellular signaling and development	Favorable (in children); co-occurrence with FBXW7 mutations especially favorable
TAL1	del(1)(p32)	~25%	Deletion resulting in fusion to STIL	Transcription factor for hematopoietic differentiation	Overexpression of TAL1 causing epigenetic dysregulation	Unclear
TLX3-BCL11B	t(5;14)(q35;q32)	~20%	Translocation	Transcription factor	Deregulation of TLX3 with down-regulation of target genes	Unfavorable
FBXW7	4q31	~20%	Mutation	Component of ubiquitin protein ligase that degrades activated NOTCH1	Activation of NOTCH1 pathway	Favorable (in children); co-occurrence with NOTCH1 mutations especially favorable
PHF6	Xq26	~20%	Mutation	Potential role in transcriptional regulation and/or chromatin remodeling	Unclear, putative tumor suppressor	Unfavorable
RUNX1	21q22	~20%	Mutation	Transcription factor	Dominant negative effect leading to decreased transcription	Unfavorable
LEF1	4q23	~20%	Mutation and microdeletion	Component of Wnt signaling pathway	Impaired Wnt signaling	Unclear
JAK1	1p21	~15%	Mutation	Tyrosine kinase	Increased JAK-STAT signaling	Unfavorable
PTEN	10q23	~15%	Mutation	Protein and lipid phosphatase; tumor suppressor	Loss of function, leading to increased cell cycle progression	Unfavorable
TCRAD@-TAL1	t(1;14)(p32;q11)	~15%	Translocation	Transcription factor for hematopoietic differentiation	Overexpression of TAL1 causing epigenetic dysregulation	Favorable
SET-NUP214	del(9)(q34.11q34.13)	~10%	Translocation	Fusion protein may activate members of the HOXA cluster	Elevated expression of HOXA genes	Unclear
IL7R[a]	5p13	~10% (~40% ETP ALL cases)	Mutation	Receptor for IL-7, important for lymphoid differentiation	Gain of function	Unfavorable
BCL11B	14q32	~10%	Mutation	May be involved in TP53 signaling pathway	Impaired differentiation and cell cycle arrest	Unclear
ETV6	12p13	~10%	Mutation	ETS family transcription factor	Loss of function; exact effect unclear	Unclear
MYB	6q22-q23	~10%	Duplication	Transcriptional activator	Increased proliferation	Unclear
ABL1	9q34	~5%	Most often fusion with NUP214 and episomal amplification	Tyrosine kinase	Kinase activation, leading to increased proliferation.	Unclear; sensitive to tyrosine kinase inhibition
PTPN2	18p11	~5%	Deletion	Tyrosine phosphatase	Increased proliferation and cytokine sensitivity	Unclear
FLT3[a]	13q12	~5% (~40% in ETP ALL)	Point mutations and ITDs	Class III receptor tyrosine kinase that regulates hematopoiesis	Constitutive activation of signal transduction, increased proliferation, and decreased apoptosis	Unfavorable

[a]IL7R and FLT3 mutations are enriched in early T-cell precursor (ETP) ALL, but uncommon in other forms of T-cell ALL; conversely, NOTCH1 and FBXW7 mutations are rare in ETP ALL, as compared with the other forms.

therapy. Some tests are a *sine qua non* for specific diagnostic entities (e.g., BCR-ABL1 for CML), while others may be useful but not essential in all cases (e.g., t(14;18) in FL). On occasion, there is more than one test to detect the same lesion, such as metaphase karyotyping, FISH, and PCR. Knowledge of the advantages and limitations of genetic testing, not only when such analysis is indicated, but which specific technology to use and what specimen is required, is essential to ensure the judicious use of molecular studies. Of note, just because a molecular test exists does not mean that it is necessary in all cases; FL (and indeed many others) can be diagnosed quite well without

the need for finding a BCL2-IGH@ fusion (or other disease-associated genetic defect in other lymphomas).

Importantly, molecular genetics findings should not be interpreted in isolation. Despite their excellent sensitivity, specificity, and accuracy, molecular assays are not infallible. This is particularly the case when evaluating antigen receptor gene rearrangements, which have not been a focus of this chapter (see Chapter 6), in that monoclonal rearrangements can be detected in reactive conditions and not all neoplastic lymphoproliferations harbor detectable monoclonal rearrangements (372). Although rare, laboratory errors can occur such as mislabeling a sample, performing the incorrect test, or contaminating a PCR reaction inadvertently with amplicons. Fortunately, good laboratory practices significantly limit these events from occurring in the clinical setting. While the error rate for molecular testing, on the whole, is largely unknown, studies have previously documented a low rate of errors for molecular diagnostics (373).

Perhaps one of the most common issues pertains to specimen selection. For example, submitting a specimen for testing with an inadequate amount of neoplastic cells (i.e., below the analytical sensitivity of the method) where testing may result in a false negative. Also, submitting an improperly handled specimen for an RNA-based assay (e.g., stored at room temperature for an extended period of time) where RNA quality may have degraded enough to alter the analytical performance of the assay. There are obviously other variables, both preanalytic and analytic, which can affect the outcome of a test; however, many are assay and disease specific. Given this, care should be taken to carefully read and integrate any limitations mentioned on the finalized assay report. Molecular diagnostics for hematologic neoplasms are, by and large, laboratory developed tests; consequently, methods and assay performance characteristics for the same molecular analyte can vary widely between laboratories. Thus, results obtained in one laboratory by one PCR method may differ from those obtained in another by an alternative PCR method; similarly, seemingly discordant results are not rare when comparing different technologies (e.g., variant t(15;17) translocation detected by FISH in one laboratory but not detected by RT-PCR in another).

The tremendous sensitivity of PCR can also be problematic. There are numerous reports of healthy individuals with detectable levels of gene translocations including t(8;21), t(9;22), t(14;18), and t(2;5) (374–378). Most of the studies that identified these gene fusions in normal individuals were based on ultrasensitive PCR techniques (e.g., nested RT-PCR, which is not widely used in the clinical laboratory). The ultrasensitivity of molecular diagnostic methods may become problematic in the setting of minimal residual disease; however, assessing the kinetics of low levels of disease is much more relevant than finding an isolated or stable level. Nevertheless, care should be taken to only order molecular tests for minimal residual disease evaluation in which the result will alter clinical care.

Finally, an equally important limitation of molecular analysis is the identification of a genetic lesion of unclear functional or medical significance; often termed variants of unclear significance, these changes can be particularly challenging for the clinician and pathologist alike (379). Hence, it is essential to have molecular genetic data, especially those that are emerging at an explosive pace with NGS, carefully curated by expert molecular hematopathologists so that the end users, the treating clinician and the patient, understand the significance of the findings to that specific neoplasm and that particular patient.

References

1. Swerdlow SH, Campo E, Harris NL, et al., eds. *WHO classification of tumours of haematopoietic and lymphoid tissues*. Lyon: International Agency for Reseach on Cancer, 2008.
2. Taylor BS, Ladanyi M. Clinical cancer genomics: how soon is now? *J Pathol* 2011;223:318–326.
3. King RL, Naghashpour M, Watt CD, et al. A comparative analysis of molecular genetic and conventional cytogenetic detection of diagnostically important translocations in more than 400 cases of acute leukemia, highlighting the frequency of false-negative conventional cytogenetics. *Am J Clin Pathol* 2011;135:921–928.
4. Boguski MS, Arnaout R, Hill C. Customized care 2020: how medical sequencing and network biology will enable personalized medicine. *F1000 Biol Rep* 2009;1:73.
5. Mardis ER. The $1,000 genome, the $100,000 analysis? *Genome Med* 2010;2:84.
6. Glenn TC. Field guide to next-generation DNA sequencers. *Mol Ecol Resour* 2011;11:759–769.
7. Tonellato PJ, Crawford JM, Boguski MS, et al. A National Agenda for the Future of Pathology in Personalized Medicine: Report of the Proceedings of a Meeting at the Banbury Conference Center on Genome-Era Pathology, Precision Diagnostics, and Preemptive Care: A Stakeholder Summit. *Am J Clin Pathol* 2011;135:668–672.
8. Gillio-Tos A, De Marco L, Fiano V, et al. Efficient DNA extraction from 25-year-old paraffin-embedded tissues: study of 365 samples. *Pathology* 2007;39:345–348.
9. Yokota M, Tatsumi N, Nathalang O, et al. Effects of heparin on polymerase chain reaction for blood white cells. *J Clin Lab Anal* 1999;13:133–140.
10. Abu al-Soud W, Radstrom P. Purification and characterization of PCR-inhibitory components in blood cells. *J Clin Microbiol* 2001;39:485–493.
11. Akane A, Matsubara K, Nakamura H, et al. Identification of the heme compound copurified with deoxyribonucleic acid (DNA) from bloodstains, a major inhibitor of polymerase chain reaction (PCR) amplification. *J Forensic Sci* 1994;39:362–372.
12. Rainen L, Arbique JC, Asthana D, et al. *Collection, transport, preparation, and storage of specimens for molecular methods; approved guideline MM13-A*. Wayne: Clinical and Laboratory Standards Institute, 2005.
13. Langebrake C, Günther K, Lauber J, et al. Preanalytical mRNA stabilization of whole bone marrow samples. *Clin Chem* 2007;53:587–593.
14. Günther K, Malentacchi F, Verderio P, et al. Implementation of a proficiency testing for the assessment of the preanalytical phase of blood samples used for RNA based analysis. *Clin Chim Acta* 2012;413:779–786.
15. Prezeau N, Silvy M, Gabert J, et al. Assessment of a new RNA stabilizing reagent (Tempus Blood RNA) for minimal residual disease in onco-hematology using the EAC protocol. *Leuk Res* 2006;30:569–574.
16. Lehmann U, Kreipe H. Real-time PCR analysis of DNA and RNA extracted from formalin-fixed and paraffin-embedded biopsies. *Methods* 2001;25:409–418.
17. Weiss ATA, Delcour NM, Meyer A, et al. Efficient and cost-effective extraction of genomic DNA from formalin-fixed and paraffin-embedded tissues. *Vet Pathol* 2011;48:834–838.
18. Okello JBA, Zurek J, Devault AM, et al. Comparison of methods in the recovery of nucleic acids from archival formalin-fixed paraffin-embedded autopsy tissues. *Anal Biochem* 2010;400:110–117.
19. Castiglione F, Rossi Degl'Innocenti D, Taddei A, et al. Real-time PCR analysis of RNA extracted from formalin-fixed and paraffin-embedded tissues: effects of the fixation on outcome reliability. *Appl Immunohistochem Mol Morphol* 2007;15:338–342.
20. Crisan D, Mattson JC. Retrospective DNA analysis using fixed tissue specimens. *DNA Cell Biol* 1993;12:455–464.
21. Hunt JL. Molecular pathology in anatomic pathology practice: a review of basic principles. *Arch Pathol Lab Med* 2008;132:248–260.
22. Beck O, Seidl C, Lehrnbecher T, et al. Quantification of chimerism within peripheral blood, bone marrow and purified leukocyte subsets: comparison of singleplex and multiplex PCR amplification of short tandem repeat (STR) loci. *Eur J Haematol* 2006;76:237–244.
23. Alison MR, Guppy NJ, Lim SM, et al. Finding cancer stem cells: are aldehyde dehydrogenases fit for purpose? *J Pathol* 2010;222:335–344.
24. Fonseca R, Bergsagel PL, Drach J, et al. International Myeloma Working Group molecular classification of multiple myeloma: spotlight review. *Leukemia* 2009;23:2210–2221.
25. Hartmann L, Biggerstaff JS, Chapman DB, et al. Detection of genomic abnormalities in multiple myeloma: the application of FISH analysis in combination with various plasma cell enrichment techniques. *Am J Clin Pathol* 2011;136:712–720.
26. Morikawa T, Shima K, Kuchiba A, et al. No evidence for interference of H&E staining in DNA testing: usefulness of DNA extraction from H&E-stained archival tissue sections. *Am J Clin Pathol* 2012;138:122–129.
27. Roullet MR, Martinez D, Ma L, et al. Coexisting follicular and mantle cell lymphoma with each having an *in situ* component: A novel, curious, and complex consultation case of coincidental, composite, colonizing lymphoma. *Am J Clin Pathol* 2010;133:584–591.
28. Mullis K, Faloona F, Scharf S, et al. Specific enzymatic amplification of DNA *in vitro*: the polymerase chain reaction. *Cold Spring Harb Symp Quant Biol* 1986;51(Pt 1):263–273.
29. Morlighem J-É, Harbers M, Traeger-Synodinos J, et al. DNA amplification techniques in pharmacogenomics. *Pharmacogenomics* 2011;12:845–860.
30. Olivier M. The Invader® assay for SNP genotyping. *Mutat Res* 2005;573:103–110.
31. Nolte FS. Branched DNA signal amplification for direct quantitation of nucleic acid sequences in clinical specimens. *Adv Clin Chem* 1998;33:201–235.
32. Baxter EJ, Scott LM, Campbell PJ, et al. Acquired mutation of the tyrosine kinase JAK2 in human myeloproliferative disorders. *Lancet* 2005;365:1054–1061.
33. Schumacher JA, Elenitoba-Johnson KSJ, Lim MS. Detection of the c-kit D816V mutation in systemic mastocytosis by allele-specific PCR. *J Clin Pathol* 2008;61:109–114.
34. Vossen RH, Aten E, Roos A, et al. High-resolution melting analysis (HRMA): more than just sequence variant screening. *Hum Mutat* 2009;30:860–866.
35. Wu D, Sherwood A, Fromm JR, et al. High-throughput sequencing detects minimal residual disease in acute T lymphoblastic leukemia. *Sci Transl Med* 2012;4:134ra163.
36. Sanger F, Nicklen S, Coulson AR. DNA sequencing with chain-terminating inhibitors. *Proc Natl Acad Sci U S A* 1977;74:5463–5467.
37. Venter JC, Adams MD, Myers EW, et al. The sequence of the human genome. *Science* 2001;291:1304–1351.
38. Lander ES, Linton LM, Birren B, et al. Initial sequencing and analysis of the human genome. *Nature* 2001;409:860–921.
39. Ronaghi M, Uhlén M, Nyrén P. A sequencing method based on real-time pyrophosphate. *Science* 1998;281:363–365.
40. de Castro DG. Challenges for the implementation of routine molecular diagnostics in cancer care. *Expert Rev Mol Diagn* 2011;11:549–551.
41. Tiacci E, Trifonov V, Schiavoni G, et al. BRAF mutations in hairy-cell leukemia. *N Engl J Med* 2011;364:2305–2315.
42. Ley TJ, Mardis ER, Ding L, et al. DNA sequencing of a cytogenetically normal acute myeloid leukaemia genome. *Nature* 2008;456:66–72.
43. Kridel R, Meissner B, Rogic S, et al. Whole transcriptome sequencing reveals recurrent NOTCH1 mutations in mantle cell lymphoma. *Blood* 2012;119:1963–1971.
44. Zhang J, Ding L, Holmfeldt L, et al. The genetic basis of early T-cell precursor acute lymphoblastic leukaemia. *Nature* 2012;481:157–163.
45. Morin RD, Johnson NA, Severson TM, et al. Somatic mutations altering EZH2 (Tyr641) in follicular and diffuse large B-cell lymphomas of germinal-center origin. *Nat Genet* 2010;42:181–185.
46. Puente XS, Pinyol M, Quesada V, et al. Whole-genome sequencing identifies recurrent mutations in chronic lymphocytic leukaemia. *Nature* 2011;475:101–105.

47. Pasqualucci L, Trifonov V, Fabbri G, et al. Analysis of the coding genome of diffuse large B-cell lymphoma. *Nat Genet* 2011;43:830–837.

48. Gerlinger M, Rowan AJ, Horswell S, et al. Intratumor heterogeneity and branched evolution revealed by multiregion sequencing. *N Engl J Med* 2012;366:883–892.

49. Consortium ICG, Hudson TJ, Anderson W, et al. International network of cancer genome projects. *Nature* 2010;464:993–998.

50. Desai AN, Jere A. Next-generation sequencing: ready for the clinics? *Clin Genet* 2012;81:503–510.

51. Schadt EE, Turner S, Kasarskis A. A window into third-generation sequencing. *Hum Mol Genet* 2010;19:R227–R240.

52. Buccisano F, Maurillo L, Del Principe MI, et al. Prognostic and therapeutic implications of minimal residual disease detection in acute myeloid leukemia. *Blood* 2012;119:332–341.

53. Kröger N, Badbaran A, Holler E, et al. Monitoring of the JAK2–V617F mutation by highly sensitive quantitative real-time PCR after allogeneic stem cell transplantation in patients with myelofibrosis. *Blood* 2007;109:1316–1321.

54. van der Velden VH, Cazzaniga G, Schrauder A, et al. Analysis of minimal residual disease by Ig/TCR gene rearrangements: guidelines for interpretation of real-time quantitative PCR data. *Leukemia* 2007;21:604–611.

55. Cilloni D, Renneville A, Hermitte F, et al. Real-time quantitative polymerase chain reaction detection of minimal residual disease by standardized WT1 assay to enhance risk stratification in acute myeloid leukemia: a European LeukemiaNet study. *J Clin Oncol* 2009;27:5195–5201.

56. Kanwal R, Gupta S. Epigenetic modifications in cancer. *Clin Genet* 2012;81:303–311.

57. Hatziapostolou M, Iliopoulos D. Epigenetic aberrations during oncogenesis. *Cell Mol Life Sci* 2011;68:1681–1702.

58. Wang Y, Leung FCC. An evaluation of new criteria for CpG islands in the human genome as gene markers. *Bioinformatics* 2004;20:1170–1177.

59. Khulan B, Thompson RF, Ye K, et al. Comparative isoschizomer profiling of cytosine methylation: the HELP assay. *Genome Res* 2006;16:1046–1055.

60. Figueroa ME, Lugthart S, Li Y, et al. DNA methylation signatures identify biologically distinct subtypes in acute myeloid leukemia. *Cancer Cell* 2010;17:13–27.

61. Zhang L, Freitas MA, Wickham J, et al. Differential expression of histone post-translational modifications in acute myeloid and chronic lymphocytic leukemia determined by high-pressure liquid chromatography and mass spectrometry. *J Am Soc Mass Spectrom* 2004;15:77–86.

62. Suka N, Suka Y, Carmen AA, et al. Highly specific antibodies determine histone acetylation site usage in yeast heterochromatin and euchromatin. *Mol Cell* 2001;8:473–479.

63. Seligson DB, Horvath S, McBrian MA, et al. Global levels of histone modifications predict prognosis in different cancers. *Am J Pathol* 2009;174:1619–1628.

64. Miranda KC, Huynh T, Tay Y, et al. A pattern-based method for the identification of MicroRNA binding sites and their corresponding heteroduplexes. *Cell* 2006;126:1203–1217.

65. Valeri N, Vannini I, Fanini F, et al. Epigenetics, miRNAs, and human cancer: a new chapter in human gene regulation. *Mamm Genome* 2009;20:573–580.

66. Lu J, Getz G, Miska EA, et al. MicroRNA expression profiles classify human cancers. *Nature* 2005;435:834–838.

67. Cissell KA, Deo SK. Trends in microRNA detection. *Anal Bioanal Chem* 2009;394:1109–1116.

68. Kong W, Zhao J-J, He L, et al. Strategies for profiling microRNA expression. *J Cell Physiol* 2009;218:22–25.

69. Bagg A. B cells behaving badly: a better basis to behold belligerence in B-cell lymphomas. *Hematology Am Soc Hematol Educ Program* 2011;2011:330–335.

70. Southern EM. Detection of specific sequences among DNA fragments separated by gel electrophoresis. *J Mol Biol* 1975;98:503–517.

71. Eklund EA. Genomic analysis of acute myeloid leukemia: potential for new prognostic indicators. *Curr Opin Hematol* 2010;17:75–78.

72. Walter MJ, Payton JE, Ries RE, et al. Acquired copy number alterations in adult acute myeloid leukemia genomes. *Proc Natl Acad Sci U S A* 2009;106:12950–12955.

73. Parkin B, Erba H, Ouillette P, et al. Acquired genomic copy number aberrations and survival in adult acute myelogenous leukemia. *Blood* 2010;116:4958–4967.

74. Choy KW, Setlur SR, Lee C, et al. The impact of human copy number variation on a new era of genetic testing. *BJOG* 2010;117:391–398.

75. Ren H, Francis W, Boys A, et al. BAC-based PCR fragment microarray: high-resolution detection of chromosomal deletion and duplication breakpoints. *Hum Mutat* 2005;25:476–482.

76. Urban AE, Korbel JO, Selzer R, et al. High-resolution mapping of DNA copy alterations in human chromosome 22 using high-density tiling oligonucleotide arrays. *Proc Natl Acad Sci U S A* 2006;103:4534–4539.

77. Heinrichs S, Li C, Look AT. SNP array analysis in hematologic malignancies: avoiding false discoveries. *Blood* 2010;115:4157–4161.

78. Grand FH, Hidalgo-Curtis CE, Ernst T, et al. Frequent CBL mutations associated with 11q acquired uniparental disomy in myeloproliferative neoplasms. *Blood* 2009;113:6182–6192.

79. Fitzgibbon J, Smith L-L, Raghavan M, et al. Association between acquired uniparental disomy and homozygous gene mutation in acute myeloid leukemias. *Cancer Res* 2005;65:9152–9154.

80. Raghavan M, Smith L-L, Lillington DM, et al. Segmental uniparental disomy is a commonly acquired genetic event in relapsed acute myeloid leukemia. *Blood* 2008;112:814–821.

81. Loh ML. Recent advances in the pathogenesis and treatment of juvenile myelomonocytic leukaemia. *Br J Haematol* 2011;152:677–687.

82. Seal RL, Gordon SM, Lush MJ, et al. genenames.org: the HGNC resources in 2011. *Nucleic Acids Res* 2011;39:D514–D519.

83. Ogino S, Gulley ML, den Dunnen JT, et al. Standard mutation nomenclature in molecular diagnostics: practical and educational challenges. *J Mol Diagn* 2007;9:1–6.

84. Forbes SA, Bindal N, Bamford S, et al. COSMIC: mining complete cancer genomes in the Catalogue of Somatic Mutations in Cancer. *Nucleic Acids Res* 2011;39:D945–D950.

85. Mitelman Database of Chromosome Aberrations and Gene Fusions in Cancer (2012). Available at: http://cgap.nci.nih.gov/Chromosomes/Mitelman.

86. Buitenkamp TD, Pieters R, Gallimore NE, et al. Outcome in children with Down's syndrome and acute lymphoblastic leukemia: role of IKZF1 deletions and CRLF2 aberrations. *Leukemia* 2012;26(10):2204–2211.

87. Patel JP, Gönen M, Figueroa ME, et al. Prognostic relevance of integrated genetic profiling in acute myeloid leukemia. *N Engl J Med* 2012;366:1079–1089.

88. Heerema-McKenney A, Arber DA. Acute myeloid leukemia. *Hematol Oncol Clin North Am* 2009;23:633–654.

89. Peterson LF, Zhang D-E. The 8;21 translocation in leukemogenesis. *Oncogene* 2004;23:4255–4262.

90. Jurlander J, Caligiuri MA, Ruutu T, et al. Persistence of the AML1/ETO fusion transcript in patients treated with allogeneic bone marrow transplantation for t(8;21) leukemia. *Blood* 1996;88:2183–2191.

91. Miyamoto T, Weissman IL, Akashi K. AML1/ETO-expressing nonleukemic stem cells in acute myelogenous leukemia with 8;21 chromosomal translocation. *Proc Natl Acad Sci U S A* 2000;97:7521–7526.

92. Shigesada K, van de Sluis B, Liu PP. Mechanism of leukemogenesis by the inv(16) chimeric gene CBFB/PEBP2B-MHY 11. *Oncogene* 2004;23:4297–4307.

93. Grimwade D, Hills RK, Moorman AV, et al. Refinement of cytogenetic classification in acute myeloid leukemia: determination of prognostic significance of rare recurring chromosomal abnormalities among 5876 younger adult patients treated in the United Kingdom Medical Research Council trials. *Blood* 2010;116:354–365.

94. Corbacioglu A, Scholl C, Schlenk RF, et al. Prognostic impact of minimal residual disease in CBFB-MYH11-positive acute myeloid leukemia. *J Clin Oncol* 2010;28:3724–3729.

95. Cairoli R, Beghini A, Grillo G, et al. Prognostic impact of c-KIT mutations in core binding factor leukemias: an Italian retrospective study. *Blood* 2006;107:3463–3468.

96. Paschka P, Marcucci G, Ruppert AS, et al. Adverse prognostic significance of KIT mutations in adult acute myeloid leukemia with inv(16) and t(8;21): a Cancer and Leukemia Group B Study. *J Clin Oncol* 2006;24:3904–3911.

97. Pollard JA, Alonzo TA, Gerbing RB, et al. Prevalence and prognostic significance of KIT mutations in pediatric patients with core binding factor AML enrolled on serial pediatric cooperative trials for de novo AML. *Blood* 2010;115:2372–2379.

98. Stock AD, Dennis TR, Spallone PA. Precise localization by microdissection/reverse ISH and FISH of the t(15;17)(q24;q21.1) chromosomal breakpoints associated with acute promyelocytic leukemia. *Cancer Genet Cytogenet* 2000;119:15–17.

99. Guidez F, Ivins S, Zhu J, et al. Reduced retinoic acid-sensitivities of nuclear receptor corepressor binding to PML- and PLZF-RARalpha underlie molecular pathogenesis and treatment of acute promyelocytic leukemia. *Blood* 1998;91:2634–2642.

100. Meyer C, Hofmann J, Burmeister T, et al. The MLL recombinome of acute leukemias in 2013. *Leukemia* 2013.

101. Dou Y, Hess JL. Mechanisms of transcriptional regulation by MLL and its disruption in acute leukemia. *Int J Hematol* 2008;87:10–18.

102. Noordermeer SM, Monteferrario D, Sanders MA, et al. Improved classification of MLL-AF9-positive acute myeloid leukemia patients based on BRE and EVI1 expression. *Blood* 2012;119:4335–4337.

103. Chandra P, Luthra R, Zuo Z, et al. Acute myeloid leukemia with t(9;11)(p21–22;q23): common properties of dysregulated ras pathway signaling and genomic progression characterize de novo and therapy-related cases. *Am J Clin Pathol* 2010;133:686–693.

104. Keefe JG, Sukov WR, Knudson RA, et al. Development of five dual-color, double-fusion fluorescence in situ hybridization assays for the detection of common MLL translocation partners. *J Mol Diagn* 2010;12:441–452.

105. Soekarman D, von Lindern M, Daenen S, et al. The translocation (6;9) (p23;q34) shows consistent rearrangement of two genes and defines a myeloproliferative disorder with specific clinical features. *Blood* 1992;79:2990–2997.

106. Garçon L, Libura M, Delabesse E, et al. DEK-CAN molecular monitoring of myeloid malignancies could aid therapeutic stratification. *Leukemia* 2005;19:1338–1344.

107. Shearer BM, Knudson RA, Flynn HC, et al. Development of a D-FISH method to detect DEK/CAN fusion resulting from t(6;9)(p23;q34) in patients with acute myelogenous leukemia. *Leukemia* 2004;19:126–131.

108. Oyarzo MP, Lin P, Glassman A, et al. Acute myeloid leukemia with t(6;9)(p23;q34) is associated with dysplasia and a high frequency of flt3 gene mutations. *Am J Clin Pathol* 2004;122:348–358.

109. Slovak ML, Gundacker H, Bloomfield CD, et al. A retrospective study of 69 patients with t(6;9)(p23;q34) AML emphasizes the need for a prospective, multicenter initiative for rare 'poor prognosis' myeloid malignancies. *Leukemia* 2006;20:1295–1297.

110. Nucifora G, Laricchia-Robbio L, Senyuk V. EVI1 and hematopoietic disorders: history and perspectives. *Gene* 2006;368:1–11.

111. Shearer BM, Sukov WR, Flynn HC, et al. Development of a dual-color, double fusion FISH assay to detect RPN1/EVI1 gene fusion associated with inv(3), t(3;3), and ins(3;3) in patients with myelodysplasia and acute myeloid leukemia. *Am J Hematol* 2010;85:569–574.

112. Ma Z, Morris SW, Valentine V, et al. Fusion of two novel genes, RBM15 and MKL1, in the t(1;22)(p13;q13) of acute megakaryoblastic leukemia. *Nat Genet* 2001;28:220–221.

113. Descot A, Rex-Haffner M, Courtois G, et al. OTT-MAL is a deregulated activator of serum response factor-dependent gene expression. *Mol Cell Biol* 2008;28:6171–6181.

114. Mercher T, Raffel GD, Moore SA, et al. The OTT-MAL fusion oncogene activates RBPJ-mediated transcription and induces acute megakaryoblastic leukemia in a knockin mouse model. *J Clin Invest* 2009;119:852–864.

115. Ballerini P, Blaise A, Mercher T, et al. A novel real-time RT-PCR assay for quantification of OTT-MAL fusion transcript reliable for diagnosis of t(1;22) and minimal residual disease (MRD) detection. *Leukemia* 2003;17:1193–1196.

116. Grisendi S, Mecucci C, Falini B, et al. Nucleophosmin and cancer. *Nat Rev Cancer* 2006;6:493–505.

117. Meani N, Alcalay M. Role of nucleophosmin in acute myeloid leukemia. *Expert Rev Anticancer Ther* 2009;9:1283–1294.

118. Falini B, Mecucci C, Tiacci E, et al. Cytoplasmic nucleophosmin in acute myelogenous leukemia with a normal karyotype. *N Engl J Med* 2005;352:254–266.

119. Thiede C, Koch S, Creutzig E, et al. Prevalence and prognostic impact of NPM1 mutations in 1485 adult patients with acute myeloid leukemia (AML). *Blood* 2006;107:4011–4020.

120. Schnittger S, Schoch C, Kern W, et al. Nucleophosmin gene mutations are predictors of favorable prognosis in acute myelogenous leukemia with a normal karyotype. *Blood* 2005;106:3733–3739.

121. Döhner K, Schlenk RF, Habdank M, et al. Mutant nucleophosmin (NPM1) predicts favorable prognosis in younger adults with acute myeloid leukemia and normal cytogenetics: interaction with other gene mutations. *Blood* 2005;106:3740–3746.
122. Boissel N, Renneville A, Biggio V, et al. Prevalence, clinical profile, and prognosis of NPM mutations in AML with normal karyotype. *Blood* 2005;106:3618–3620.
123. Falini B, Sportoletti P, Martelli MP. Acute myeloid leukemia with mutated NPM1: diagnosis, prognosis and therapeutic perspectives. *Curr Opin Oncol* 2009;21:573–581.
124. Gruszka AM, Lavorgna S, Consalvo MI, et al. A monoclonal antibody against mutated nucleophosmin 1 for the molecular diagnosis of acute myeloid leukemias. *Blood* 2010;116:2096–2102.
125. Wertheim G, Bagg A. Nucleophosmin (NPM1) mutations in acute myeloid leukemia: an ongoing (cytoplasmic) tale of dueling mutations and duality of molecular genetic testing methodologies. *J Mol Diagn* 2008;10:198–202.
126. Falini B, Martelli MP, Bolli N, et al. Acute myeloid leukemia with mutated nucleophosmin (NPM1): is it a distinct entity? *Blood* 2011;117:1109–1120.
127. Gorello P, Cazzaniga G, Alberti F, et al. Quantitative assessment of minimal residual disease in acute myeloid leukemia carrying nucleophosmin (NPM1) gene mutations. *Leukemia* 2006;20:1103–1108.
128. Schnittger S, Kern W, Tschulik C, et al. Minimal residual disease levels assessed by NPM1 mutation-specific RQ-PCR provide important prognostic information in AML. *Blood* 2009;114:2220–2231.
129. Krönke J, Schlenk RF, Jensen KO, et al. Monitoring of minimal residual disease in NPM1-mutated acute myeloid leukemia: A study from the German-Austrian acute myeloid leukemia study group. *J Clin Oncol* 2011;29:2709–2716.
130. Lin L-I, Chen C-Y, Lin D-T, et al. Characterization of CEBPA mutations in acute myeloid leukemia: most patients with CEBPA mutations have biallelic mutations and show a distinct immunophenotype of the leukemic cells. *Clin Cancer Res* 2005;11:1372–1379.
131. Pabst T, Mueller BU. Complexity of CEBPA dysregulation in human acute myeloid leukemia. *Clin Cancer Res* 2009;15:5303–5307.
132. Pabst T, Mueller BU, Zhang P, et al. Dominant-negative mutations of CEBPA, encoding CCAAT/enhancer binding protein-alpha (C/EBPalpha), in acute myeloid leukemia. *Nat Genet* 2001;27:263–270.
133. Dufour A, Schneider F, Metzeler KH, et al. Acute myeloid leukemia with biallelic CEBPA gene mutations and normal karyotype represents a distinct genetic entity associated with a favorable clinical outcome. *J Clin Oncol* 2010;28:570–577.
134. Taskesen E, Bullinger L, Corbacioglu A, et al. Prognostic impact, concurrent genetic mutations, and gene expression features of AML with CEBPA mutations in a cohort of 1182 cytogenetically normal AML patients: Further evidence for CEBPA double mutant AML as a distinctive disease entity. *Blood* 2011;117:2469–2475.
135. Dufour A, Schneider F, Hoster E, et al. Monoallelic CEBPA mutations in normal karyotype acute myeloid leukemia: independent favorable prognostic factor within NPM1 mutated patients. *Ann Hematol* 2012;91:1051–1063.
136. Hackanson B, Bennett KL, Brena RM, et al. Epigenetic modification of CCAAT/enhancer binding protein alpha expression in acute myeloid leukemia. *Cancer Res* 2008;68:3142–3151.
137. Figueroa ME, Wouters BJ, Skrabanek L, et al. Genome-wide epigenetic analysis delineates a biologically distinct immature acute leukemia with myeloid/T-lymphoid features. *Blood* 2009;113:2795–2804.
138. Duncavage EJ, Abel HJ, Szankasi P, et al. Targeted next generation sequencing of clinically significant gene mutations and translocations in leukemia. *Mod Pathol* 2012;25:795–804.
138a. Ahn JY, Seo K, Weinberg O, et al. A comparison of two methods for screening CEBPA mutations in patients with acute myeloid leukemia. *J Mol Diagn* 2009;11:319–323.
139. Meshinchi S, Appelbaum FR. Structural and functional alterations of FLT3 in acute myeloid leukemia. *Clin Cancer Res* 2009;15:4263–4269.
140. Thiede C, Steudel C, Mohr B, et al. Analysis of FLT3-activating mutations in 979 patients with acute myelogenous leukemia: association with FAB subtypes and identification of subgroups with poor prognosis. *Blood* 2002;99:4326–4335.
141. Smith CC, Wang Q, Chin CS, et al. Validation of ITD mutations in FLT3 as a therapeutic target in human acute myeloid leukaemia. *Nature* 2012;485:260–263.
142. Warren M, Luthra R, Yin CC, et al. Clinical impact of change of FLT3 mutation status in acute myeloid leukemia patients. *Mod Pathol* 2012;25(10):1405–1412.
142a. Genomic and Epigenomic Landscapes of Adult De Novo Acute Myeloid Leukemia. *N Engl J Med* 2013;368(22):2059–2074.
142b. Wertheim GB, Daber R, Bagg A. Molecular diagnostics of acute myeloid leukemia: it's a (next) generational thing. *J Mol Diagn* 2013;15(1):27–30.
143. Pane F, Intrieri M, Quintarelli C, et al. BCR/ABL genes and leukemic phenotype: from molecular mechanisms to clinical correlations. *Oncogene* 2002;21:8652–8667.
144. Wang YL, Bagg A, Pear W, et al. Chronic myelogenous leukemia: laboratory diagnosis and monitoring. *Genes Chromosomes Cancer* 2001;32:97–111.
145. Chasseriau J, Rivet J, Bilan F, et al. Characterization of the different BCR-ABL transcripts with a single multiplex RT-PCR. *J Mol Diagn* 2004;6:343–347.
146. Branford S, Seymour JF, Grigg A, et al. BCR-ABL messenger RNA levels continue to decline in patients with chronic phase chronic myeloid leukemia treated with imatinib for more than 5 years and approximately half of all first-line treated patients have stable undetectable BCR-ABL using strict sensitivity criteria. *Clin Cancer Res* 2007;13:7080–7085.
147. Ross DM, Branford S, Seymour JF, et al. Patients with chronic myeloid leukemia who maintain a complete molecular response after stopping imatinib treatment have evidence of persistent leukemia by DNA PCR. *Leukemia* 2010;24:1719–1724.
148. Brown JT, Laosinchai-Wolf W, Hedges JB, et al. Establishment of a standardized multiplex assay with the analytical performance required for quantitative measurement of BCR–ABL1 on the international reporting scale. *Blood Cancer J* 2011;1:e13.
149. Branford S, Fletcher L, Cross NCP, et al. Desirable performance characteristics for BCR-ABL measurement on an international reporting scale to allow consistent interpretation of individual patient response and comparison of response rates between clinical trials. *Blood* 2008;112:3330–3338.
150. Branford S, Hughes T. Diagnosis and monitoring of chronic myeloid leukemia by qualitative and quantitative RT-PCR. *Methods Mol Med* 2006;125:69–92.
151. Ou J, Vergilio J-A, Bagg A. Molecular diagnosis and monitoring in the clinical management of patients with chronic myelogenous leukemia treated with tyrosine kinase inhibitors. *Am J Hematol* 2008;83:296–302.
152. Hughes T, Deininger M, Hochhaus A, et al. Monitoring CML patients responding to treatment with tyrosine kinase inhibitors: review and recommendations for harmonizing current methodology for detecting BCR-ABL transcripts and kinase domain mutations and for expressing results. *Blood* 2006;108:28–37.
153. White HE, Matejtschuk P, Rigsby P, et al. Establishment of the first World Health Organization International Genetic Reference Panel for quantitation of BCR-ABL mRNA. *Blood* 2010;116:e111–e117.
154. Jones D, Kamel-Reid S, Bahler D, et al. Laboratory practice guidelines for detecting and reporting BCR-ABL drug resistance mutations in chronic myelogenous leukemia and acute lymphoblastic leukemia: a report of the Association for Molecular Pathology. *J Mol Diagn* 2009;11:4–11.
155. Soverini S, Colarossi S, Gnani A, et al. Contribution of ABL kinase domain mutations to imatinib resistance in different subsets of philadelphia-positive patients: By the GIMEMA working party on chronic myeloid leukemia. *Clin Cancer Res* 2006;12:7374–7379.
156. Levine RL, Wadleigh M, Cools J, et al. Activating mutation in the tyrosine kinase JAK2 in polycythemia vera, essential thrombocythemia, and myeloid metaplasia with myelofibrosis. *Cancer Cell* 2005;7:387–397.
157. Vannucchi AM, Antonioli E, Guglielmelli P, et al. Clinical profile of homozygous JAK2 617V>F mutation in patients with polycythemia vera or essential thrombocythemia. *Blood* 2007;110:840–846.
158. Vannucchi AM, Antonioli E, Guglielmelli P, et al. Clinical correlates of JAK2V617F presence or allele burden in myeloproliferative neoplasms: a critical reappraisal. *Leukemia* 2008;22:1299–1307.
159. Cankovic M, Whiteley L, Hawley RC, et al. Clinical performance of JAK2 V617F mutation detection assays in a molecular diagnostics laboratory: evaluation of screening and quantitation methods. *Am J Clin Pathol* 2009;132:713–721.
160. Verstovsek S, Mesa RA, Gotlib J, et al. A double-blind, placebo-controlled trial of ruxolitinib for myelofibrosis. *N Engl J Med* 2012;366:799–807.
161. Scott LM, Tong W, Levine RL, et al. JAK2 exon 12 mutations in polycythemia vera and idiopathic erythrocytosis. *N Engl J Med* 2007;356:459–468.
162. Pietra D, Li S, Brisci A, et al. Somatic mutations of JAK2 exon 12 in patients with JAK2 (V617F)-negative myeloproliferative disorders. *Blood* 2008;111:1686–1689.
163. Pardanani A, Lasho TL, Finke C, et al. Prevalence and clinicopathologic correlates of JAK2 exon 12 mutations in JAK2V617F-negative polycythemia vera. *Leukemia* 2007;21:1960–1963.
164. Tefferi A. Novel mutations and their functional and clinical relevance in myeloproliferative neoplasms: JAK2, MPL, TET2, ASXL1, CBL, IDH and IKZF1. *Leukemia* 2010;24:1128–1138.
165. Schmidt AE, Oh ST. Pathology consultation on myeloproliferative neoplasms. *Am J Clin Pathol* 2012;138:12–19.
166. Orfao A, Garcia-Montero AC, Sanchez L, et al. Recent advances in the understanding of mastocytosis: the role of KIT mutations. *Br J Haematol* 2007;138:12–30.
167. Tefferi A. Molecular drug targets in myeloproliferative neoplasms: mutant ABL1, JAK2, MPL, KIT, PDGFRA, PDGFRB and FGFR1. *J Cell Mol Med* 2009;13:215–237.
168. Kristensen T, Vestergaard H, Møller MB. Improved detection of the KIT D816V mutation in patients with systemic mastocytosis using a quantitative and highly sensitive real-time qPCR assay. *J Mol Diagn* 2011;13:180–188.
169. Valent P, Akin C, Escribano L, et al. Standards and standardization in mastocytosis: consensus statements on diagnostics, treatment recommendations and response criteria. *Eur J Clin Invest* 2007;37:435–453.
170. Pardanani A, Tefferi A. A critical reappraisal of treatment response criteria in systemic mastocytosis and a proposal for revisions. *Eur J Haematol* 2010;84:371–378.
171. Cools J, DeAngelo DJ, Gotlib J, et al. A tyrosine kinase created by fusion of the PDGFRA and FIP1L1 genes as a therapeutic target of imatinib in idiopathic hypereosinophilic syndrome. *N Engl J Med* 2003;348:1201–1214.
172. Ren M, Qin H, Ren R, et al. Ponatinib suppresses the development ofmyeloid and lymphoid malignancies associated with FGFR1 abnormalities. *Leukemia* 2013;27(1):32–40.
173. Chen J, DeAngelo DJ, Kutok JL, et al. PKC412 inhibits the zinc finger 198–fibroblast growth factor receptor 1 fusion tyrosine kinase and is active in treatment of stem cell myeloproliferative disorder. *Proc Natl Acad Sci U S A* 2004;101:14479–14484.
174. Dunphy CH. Chronic eosinophilic leukemia, not otherwise specified (CEL, NOS). *Curr Cancer Ther Rev* 2012;8:30–34.
175. Dahabreh IJ, Giannouli S, Zoi C, et al. Hypereosinophilic syndrome: another face of janus? *Leuk Res* 2008;32:1483–1485.
176. Greenberg P, Cox C, LeBeau MM, et al. International scoring system for evaluating prognosis in myelodysplastic syndromes. *Blood* 1997;89:2079–2088.
177. Greenberg PL, Tuechler H, Schanz J, et al. Revised International Prognostic Scoring System (IPSS-R) for myelodysplastic syndromes. *Blood* 2012;120(12):2454–2465.
178. Bejar R, Stevenson K, Abdel-Wahab O, et al. Clinical effect of point mutations in myelodysplastic syndromes. *N Engl J Med* 2011;364:2496–2506.
179. Bejar R, Stevenson KE, Caughey BA, et al. Validation of a prognostic model and the impact of mutations in patients with lower-risk myelodysplastic syndromes. *J Clin Oncol* 2012;30(27):3376–3382.
180. Pfeilstöcker M, Stauder R. New developments in MDS. *Memo* 2012:1–4.
181. Papaemmanuil E, Cazzola M, Boultwood J, et al. Somatic SF3B1 mutation in myelodysplasia with ring sideroblasts. *N Engl J Med* 2011;365:1384–1395.
182. Thol F, Kade S, Schlarmann C, et al. Frequency and prognostic impact of mutations in SRSF2, U2AF1, and ZRSR2 in patients with myelodysplastic syndromes. *Blood* 2012;119:3578–3584.
183. Koike K, Matsuda K. Recent advances in the pathogenesis and management of juvenile myelomonocytic leukaemia. *Br J Haematol* 2008;141:567–575.
184. Loh ML, Sakai DS, Flotho C, et al. Mutations in CBL occur frequently in juvenile myelomonocytic leukemia. *Blood* 2009;114:1859–1863.
185. Niemeyer CM, Kang MW, Shin DH, et al. Germline CBL mutations cause developmental abnormalities and predispose to juvenile myelomonocytic leukemia. *Nat Genet* 2010;42:794–800.
186. De Filippi P, Zecca M, Lisini D, et al. Germ-line mutation of the NRAS gene may be responsible for the development of juvenile myelomonocytic leukaemia. *Br J Haematol* 2009;147:706–709.
187. Tartaglia M, Niemeyer CM, Fragale A, et al. Somatic mutations in PTPN11 in juvenile myelomonocytic leukemia, myelodysplastic syndromes and acute myeloid leukemia. *Nat Genet* 2003;34:148–150.
188. Meggendorfer M, Roller A, Haferlach T, et al. SRSF2 mutations in 275 cases with chronic myelomonocytic leukemia (CMML). *Blood* 2012;120(15):3080–3088.

189. Muramatsu H, Makishima H, Maciejewski JP. Chronic myelomonocytic leukemia and atypical chronic myeloid leukemia: novel pathogenetic lesions. *Semin Oncol* 2012;39:67–73.
190. Jankowska AM, Makishima H, Tiu RV, et al. Mutational spectrum analysis of chronic myelomonocytic leukemia includes genes associated with epigenetic regulation: UTX, EZH2, and DNMT3A. *Blood* 2011;118:3932–3941.
191. Tyner JW, Erickson H, Deininger MWN, et al. High-throughput sequencing screen reveals novel, transforming RAS mutations in myeloid leukemia patients. *Blood* 2009;113:1749–1755.
192. Pagon RA, Bird TD, Dolan CR, et al., eds. *GeneReviews*. Seattle: University of Washington, 1993.
193. Huang JZ, Sanger WG, Greiner TC, et al. The t(14;18) defines a unique subset of diffuse large B-cell lymphoma with a germinal center B-cell gene expression profile. *Blood* 2002;99:2285–2290.
194. Raghavan SC, Swanson PC, Wu X, et al. A non-B-DNA structure at the Bcl-2 major breakpoint region is cleaved by the RAG complex. *Nature* 2004;428:88–93.
195. Ott G, Katzenberger T, Lohr A, et al. Cytomorphologic, immunohistochemical, and cytogenetic profiles of follicular lymphoma: 2 types of follicular lymphoma grade 3. *Blood* 2002;99:3806–3812.
196. Bosga-Bouwer AG, van Imhoff GW, Boonstra R, et al. Follicular lymphoma grade 3B includes 3 cytogenetically defined subgroups with primary t(14;18), 3q27, or other translocations: t(14;18) and 3q27 are mutually exclusive. *Blood* 2003;101:1149–1154.
197. Bacon CM, Ye H, Diss TC, et al. Primary follicular lymphoma of the testis and epididymis in adults. *Am J Surg Pathol* 2007;31:1050–1058.
198. Oschlies I, Salaverria I, Mahn F, et al. Pediatric follicular lymphoma—a clinico-pathological study of a population-based series of patients treated within the Non-Hodgkin's Lymphoma—Berlin-Frankfurt-Munster (NHL-BFM) multicenter trials. *Haematologica* 2010;95:253–259.
199. Streubel B, Scheucher B, Valencak J, et al. Molecular cytogenetic evidence of t(14;18)(IGH;BCL2) in a substantial proportion of primary cutaneous follicle center lymphomas. *Am J Surg Pathol* 2006;30:529–536.
200. Buchonnet G, Lenain P, Ruminy P, et al. Characterisation of BCL2-JH rearrangements in follicular lymphoma: PCR detection of 3′ BCL2 breakpoints and evidence of a new cluster. *Leukemia* 2000;14:1563–1569.
201. Weinberg OK, Ai WZ, Mariappan MR, et al. "Minor" BCL2 breakpoints in follicular lymphoma: frequency and correlation with grade and disease presentation in 236 cases. *J Mol Diagn* 2007;9:530–537.
202. Chang CM, Schroeder JC, Huang WY, et al. Non-Hodgkin lymphoma (NHL) subtypes defined by common translocations: utility of fluorescence *in situ* hybridization (FISH) in a case-control study. *Leuk Res* 2010;34:190–195.
203. Payne K, Wright P, Grant JW, et al. BIOMED-2 PCR assays for IGK gene rearrangements are essential for B-cell clonality analysis in follicular lymphoma. *Br J Haematol* 2011;155:84–92.
204. Adam P, Baumann R, Schmidt J, et al. The BCL2 E17 and SP66 antibodies discriminate 2 immunophenotypically and genetically distinct subgroups of conventionally BCL2-"negative" grade 1/2 follicular lymphomas. *Human Pathol* 2013.
205. van Oers MH, Tonnissen E, Van Glabbeke M, et al. BCL-2/IgH polymerase chain reaction status at the end of induction treatment is not predictive for progression-free survival in relapsed/resistant follicular lymphoma: results of a prospective randomized EORTC 20981 phase III intergroup study. *J Clin Oncol* 2010;28:2246–2252.
206. Roulland S, Navarro JM, Grenot P, et al. Follicular lymphoma-like B cells in healthy individuals: a novel intermediate step in early lymphomagenesis. *J Exp Med* 2006;203:2425–2431.
207. Cook JR, Shekhter-Levin S, Swerdlow SH. Utility of routine classical cytogenetic studies in the evaluation of suspected lymphomas: results of 279 consecutive lymph node/extranodal tissue biopsies. *Am J Clin Pathol* 2004;121:826–835.
208. Oricchio E, Nanjangud G, Wolfe AL, et al. The Eph-receptor A7 is a soluble tumor suppressor for follicular lymphoma. *Cell* 2011;147:554–564.
209. Salaverria I, Philipp C, Oschlies I, et al. Translocations activating IRF4 identify a subtype of germinal center-derived B-cell lymphoma affecting predominantly children and young adults. *Blood* 2011;118:139–147.
210. Cheung KJ, Johnson NA, Affleck JG, et al. Acquired TNFRSF14 mutations in follicular lymphoma are associated with worse prognosis. *Cancer Res* 2010;70:9166–9174.
211. Launay E, Pangault C, Bertrand P, et al. High rate of TNFRSF14 gene alterations related to 1p36 region in de novo follicular lymphoma and impact on prognosis. *Leukemia* 2012;26:559–562.
212. Schuetz JM, Johnson NA, Morin RD, et al. BCL2 mutations in diffuse large B-cell lymphoma. *Leukemia* 2012;26:1383–1390.
213. Ryan RJ, Nitta M, Borger D, et al. EZH2 codon 641 mutations are common in BCL2-rearranged germinal center B cell lymphomas. *PLoS One* 2011;6:e28585.
214. Pasqualucci L, Dominguez-Sola D, Chiarenza A, et al. Inactivating mutations of acetyltransferase genes in B-cell lymphoma. *Nature* 2011;471:189–195.
215. Dave SS, Wright G, Tan B, et al. Prediction of survival in follicular lymphoma based on molecular features of tumor-infiltrating immune cells. *N Engl J Med* 2004;351:2159–2169.
216. Piccaluga PP, Califano A, Klein U, et al. Gene expression analysis provides a potential rationale for revising the histological grading of follicular lymphomas. *Haematologica* 2008;93:1033–1038.
217. Cheung KJ, Rogic S, Ben-Neriah S, et al. SNP analysis of minimally evolved t(14;18)(q32;q21)-positive follicular lymphomas reveals a common copy-neutral loss of heterozygosity pattern. *Cytogenet Genome Res* 2011;136:38–43.
218. Cheung KJ, Shah SP, Steidl C, et al. Genome-wide profiling of follicular lymphoma by array comparative genomic hybridization reveals prognostically significant DNA copy number imbalances. *Blood* 2009;113:137–148.
219. Katzenberger T, Kalla J, Leich E, et al. A distinctive subtype of t(14;18)-negative nodal follicular non-Hodgkin lymphoma characterized by a predominantly diffuse growth pattern and deletions in the chromosomal region 1p36. *Blood* 2009;113:1053–1061.
220. Cartron G, Dacheux L, Salles G, et al. Therapeutic activity of humanized anti-CD20 monoclonal antibody and polymorphism in IgG Fc receptor FcgammaRIIIa gene. *Blood* 2002;99:754–758.
221. Cerhan JR, Wang S, Maurer MJ, et al. Prognostic significance of host immune gene polymorphisms in follicular lymphoma survival. *Blood* 2007;109:5439–5446.
222. Choi JH, Li Y, Guo J, et al. Genome-wide DNA methylation maps in follicular lymphoma cells determined by methylation-enriched bisulfite sequencing. *PLoS One* 2010;5:e13020.
223. d'Amore F, Chan E, Iqbal J, et al. Clonal evolution in t(14;18)-positive follicular lymphoma, evidence for multiple common pathways, and frequent parallel clonal evolution. *Clin Cancer Res* 2008;14:7180–7187.
224. Wiestner A, Tehrani M, Chiorazzi M, et al. Point mutations and genomic deletions in CCND1 create stable truncated cyclin D1 mRNAs that are associated with increased proliferation rate and shorter survival. *Blood* 2007;109:4599–4606.
225. Fu K, Weisenburger DD, Greiner TC, et al. Cyclin D1–negative mantle cell lymphoma: a clinicopathologic study based on gene expression profiling. *Blood* 2005;106:4315–4321.
226. Quintanilla-Martinez L, Slotta-Huspenina J, Koch I, et al. Differential diagnosis of cyclin D2+ mantle cell lymphoma based on fluorescence *in situ* hybridization and quantitative real-time-PCR. *Haematologica* 2009;94:1595–1598.
227. O'Malley DP, Vance GH, Orazi A. Chronic lymphocytic leukemia/small lymphocytic lymphoma with trisomy 12 and focal cyclin d1 expression: a potential diagnostic pitfall. *Arch Pathol Lab Med* 2005;129:92–95.
228. Vela-Chavez T, Adam P, Kremer M, et al. Cyclin D1 positive diffuse large B-cell lymphoma is a post-germinal center-type lymphoma without alterations in the CCND1 gene locus. *Leuk Lymphoma* 2011;52:458–466.
229. Sherman MJ, Hanson CA, Hoyer JD. An assessment of the usefulness of immunohistochemical stains in the diagnosis of hairy cell leukemia. *Am J Clin Pathol* 2011;136:390–399.
230. Gradowski JF, Sargent RL, Craig FE, et al. Chronic lymphocytic leukemia/small lymphocytic lymphoma with cyclin D1 positive proliferation centers do not have CCND1 translocations or gains and lack SOX11 expression. *Am J Clin Pathol* 2012;138:132–139.
231. Kridel R, Meissner B, Rogic S, et al. Whole transcriptome sequencing reveals recurrent NOTCH1 mutations in mantle cell lymphoma. *Blood* 2012;119:1963–1971.
232. Bea S, Campo E. Secondary genomic alterations in non-Hodgkin's lymphomas: tumor-specific profiles with impact on clinical behavior. *Haematologica* 2008;93:641–645.
233. Navarro A, Clot G, Royo C, et al. Molecular subsets of mantle cell lymphoma defined by the IGHV mutational status and SOX11 expression have distinct biological and clinical features. *Cancer Res* 2012;72(20):5307–5316.
234. Rosenwald A, Wright G, Wiestner A, et al. The proliferation gene expression signature is a quantitative integrator of oncogenic events that predicts survival in mantle cell lymphoma. *Cancer Cell* 2003;3:185–197.
235. Hartmann E, Fernandez V, Moreno V, et al. Five-gene model to predict survival in mantle-cell lymphoma using frozen or formalin-fixed, paraffin-embedded tissue. *J Clin Oncol* 2008;26:4966–4972.
236. Fernandez V, Salamero O, Espinet B, et al. Genomic and gene expression profiling defines indolent forms of mantle cell lymphoma. *Cancer Res* 2010;70:1408–1418.
237. Del Giudice I, Messina M, Chiaretti S, et al. Behind the scenes of non-nodal MCL: downmodulation of genes involved in actin cytoskeleton organization, cell projection, cell adhesion, tumour invasion, TP53 pathway and mutated status of immunoglobulin heavy chain genes. *Br J Haematol* 2012;156:601–611.
238. Rao E, Jiang C, Ji M, et al. The miRNA-17 approximately 92 cluster mediates chemoresistance and enhances tumor growth in mantle cell lymphoma via PI3K/AKT pathway activation. *Leukemia* 2012;26:1064–1072.
239. Iqbal J, Shen Y, Liu Y, et al. Genome-wide miRNA profiling of mantle cell lymphoma reveals a distinct subgroup with poor prognosis. *Blood* 2012;119:4939–4948.
240. Uren AG, O'Rourke K, Aravind LA, et al. Identification of paracaspases and metacaspases: two ancient families of caspase-like proteins, one of which plays a key role in MALT lymphoma. *Mol Cell* 2000;6:961–967.
241. Streubel B, Simonitsch-Klupp I, Mullauer L, et al. Variable frequencies of MALT lymphoma-associated genetic aberrations in MALT lymphomas of different sites. *Leukemia* 2004;18:1722–1726.
242. Xia H, Nakayama T, Sakuma H, et al. Analysis of API2-MALT1 fusion, trisomies, and immunoglobulin VH genes in pulmonary mucosa-associated lymphoid tissue lymphoma. *Hum Pathol* 2011;42:1297–1304.
243. Remstein ED, James CD, Kurtin PJ. Incidence and subtype specificity of API2-MALT1 fusion translocations in extranodal, nodal, and splenic marginal zone lymphomas. *Am J Pathol* 2000;156:1183–1188.
244. Liu H, Ruskon-Fourmestraux A, Lavergne-Slove A, et al. Resistance of t(11;18) positive gastric mucosa-associated lymphoid tissue lymphoma to *Helicobacter pylori* eradication therapy. *Lancet* 2001;357:39–40.
245. Remstein ED, Dogan A, Einerson RR, et al. The incidence and anatomic site specificity of chromosomal translocations in primary extranodal marginal zone B-cell lymphoma of mucosa-associated lymphoid tissue (MALT lymphoma) in North America. *Am J Surg Pathol* 2006;30:1546–1553.
246. Streubel B, Vinatzer U, Lamprecht A, et al. T(3;14)(p14.1;q32) involving IGH and FOXP1 is a novel recurrent chromosomal aberration in MALT lymphoma. *Leukemia* 2005;19:652–658.
247. Fenton JA, Schuuring E, Barrans SL, et al. t(3;14)(p14;q32) results in aberrant expression of FOXP1 in a case of diffuse large B-cell lymphoma. *Genes Chromosomes Cancer* 2006;45:164–168.
248. Sagaert X, de Paepe P, Libbrecht L, et al. Forkhead box protein P1 expression in mucosa-associated lymphoid tissue lymphomas predicts poor prognosis and transformation to diffuse large B-cell lymphoma. *J Clin Oncol* 2006;24:2490–2497.
249. Baens M, Finalet Ferreiro J, Tousseyn T, et al. t(X;14)(p11.4;q32.33) is recurrent in marginal zone lymphoma and up-regulates GPR34. *Haematologica* 2012;97:184–188.
250. Rinaldi A, Mian M, Chigrinova E, et al. Genome-wide DNA profiling of marginal zone lymphomas identifies subtype-specific lesions with an impact on the clinical outcome. *Blood* 2011;117:1595–1604.
251. Kwee I, Rancoita PM, Rinaldi A, et al. Genomic profiles of MALT lymphomas: variability across anatomical sites. *Haematologica* 2011;96:1064–1066.
252. Vega F, Cho-Vega JH, Lennon PA, et al. Splenic marginal zone lymphomas are characterized by loss of interstitial regions of chromosome 7q, 7q31.32 and 7q36.2 that include the protection of telomere 1 (POT1) and sonic hedgehog (SHH) genes. *Br J Haematol* 2008;142:216–226.
253. Fresquet V, Robles EF, Parker A, et al. High-throughput sequencing analysis of the chromosome 7q32 deletion reveals IRF5 as a potential tumour suppressor in splenic marginal-zone lymphoma. *Br J Haematol* 2012;158:712–726.
254. Robledo C, Garcia JL, Benito R, et al. Molecular characterization of the region 7q22.1 in splenic marginal zone lymphomas. *PLoS One* 2011;6:e24939.
255. Rossi D, Deaglio S, Dominguez-Sola D, et al. Alteration of BIRC3 and multiple other NF-kappaB pathway genes in splenic marginal zone lymphoma. *Blood* 2011;118:4930–4934.

256. Kiel MJ, Velusamy T, Betz BL, et al. Whole-genome sequencing identifies recurrent somatic NOTCH2 mutations in splenic marginal zone lymphoma. *J Exp Med* 2012;209:1553–1565.

257. Ouillette P, Collins R, Shakhan S, et al. The prognostic significance of various 13q14 deletions in chronic lymphocytic leukemia. *Clin Cancer Res* 2011;17:6778–6790.

258. Dal Bo M, Rossi FM, Rossi D, et al. 13q14 deletion size and number of deleted cells both influence prognosis in chronic lymphocytic leukemia. *Genes Chromosomes Cancer* 2011;50:633–643.

259. Cavazzini F, Hernandez JA, Gozzetti A, et al. Chromosome 14q32 translocations involving the immunoglobulin heavy chain locus in chronic lymphocytic leukaemia identify a disease subset with poor prognosis. *Br J Haematol* 2008;142:529–537.

260. Wang DM, Miao KR, Fan L, et al. Intermediate prognosis of 6q deletion in chronic lymphocytic leukemia. *Leuk Lymphoma* 2011;52:230–237.

261. Rossi D, Cerri M, Deambrogi C, et al. The prognostic value of TP53 mutations in chronic lymphocytic leukemia is independent of Del17p13: implications for overall survival and chemorefractoriness. *Clin Cancer Res* 2009;15:995–1004.

262. Zenz T, Eichhorst B, Busch R, et al. TP53 mutation and survival in chronic lymphocytic leukemia. *J Clin Oncol* 2010;28:4473–4479.

263. Marinelli M, Raponi S, Del Giudice I, et al. Is the aberrant expression of p53 by immunocytochemistry a surrogate marker of TP53 mutation and/or deletion in chronic lymphocytic leukemia? *Am J Clin Pathol* 2011;135:173–174.

264. Wang L, Lawrence MS, Wan Y, et al. SF3B1 and other novel cancer genes in chronic lymphocytic leukemia. *N Engl J Med* 2011;365:2497–2506.

265. Rossi D, Bruscaggin A, Spina V, et al. Mutations of the SF3B1 splicing factor in chronic lymphocytic leukemia: association with progression and fludarabine-refractoriness. *Blood* 2011;118:6904–6908.

266. Rossi D, Fangazio M, Rasi S, et al. Disruption of BIRC3 associates with fludarabine chemorefractoriness in TP53 wild-type chronic lymphocytic leukemia. *Blood* 2012;119:2854–2862.

267. Rossi D, Rasi S, Fabbri G, et al. Mutations of NOTCH1 are an independent predictor of survival in chronic lymphocytic leukemia. *Blood* 2012;119:521–529.

268. Del Giudice I, Rossi D, Chiaretti S, et al. NOTCH1 mutations in +12 chronic lymphocytic leukemia (CLL) confer an unfavorable prognosis, induce a distinctive transcriptional profiling and refine the intermediate prognosis of +12 CLL. *Haematologica* 2012;97:437–441.

269. Rosenwald A, Alizadeh AA, Widhopf G, et al. Relation of gene expression phenotype to immunoglobulin mutation genotype in B cell chronic lymphocytic leukemia. *J Exp Med* 2001;194:1639–1647.

270. Crespo M, Bosch F, Villamor N, et al. ZAP-70 expression as a surrogate for immunoglobulin-variable-region mutations in chronic lymphocytic leukemia. *N Engl J Med* 2003;348:1764–1775.

271. Ma D, Chen Z, Patel KP, et al. Array comparative genomic hybridization analysis identifies recurrent gain of chromosome 2p25.3 involving the ACP1 and MYCN genes in chronic lymphocytic leukemia. *Clin Lymphoma Myeloma Leuk* 2011;11 (Suppl 1):S17–S24.

272. Claus R, Lucas DM, Stilgenbauer S, et al. Quantitative DNA methylation analysis identifies a single CpG dinucleotide important for ZAP-70 expression and predictive of prognosis in chronic lymphocytic leukemia. *J Clin Oncol* 2012;30(20):2483–2491.

273. Hanoun M, Eisele L, Suzuki M, et al. Epigenetic silencing of the circadian clock gene CRY1 is associated with an indolent clinical course in chronic lymphocytic leukemia. *PLoS One* 2012;7:e34347.

274. Rossi D, Rasi S, Spina V, et al. Different impact of NOTCH1 and SF3B1 mutations on the risk of chronic lymphocytic leukemia transformation to Richter syndrome. *Br J Haematol* 2012;158:426–429.

275. Liu H, Yan Q, Nuako-Bandoh B, et al. Richter transformation: clonal identity does not indicate a linear disease progression. *Br J Haematol* 2012;157(1):136–139.

276. Cook JR, Aguilera NI, Reshmi S, et al. Deletion 6q is not a characteristic marker of nodal lymphoplasmacytic lymphoma. *Cancer Genet Cytogenet* 2005;162:85–88.

277. Braggio E, Dogan A, Keats JJ, et al. Genomic analysis of marginal zone and lymphoplasmacytic lymphomas identified common and disease-specific abnormalities. *Mod Pathol* 2012;25:651–660.

278. Poulain S, Roumier C, Decambron A, et al. MYD88 L265P mutation in Waldenstrom macroglobulinemia. *Blood* 2013;121:4504–4511.

279. Tiacci E, Trifonov V, Schiavoni G, et al. BRAF mutations in hairy-cell leukemia. *N Engl J Med* 2011;364:2305–2315.

280. Arcaini L, Zibellini S, Boveri E, et al. The BRAF V600E mutation in hairy cell leukemia and other mature B-cell neoplasms. *Blood* 2012;119:188–191.

281. Tiacci E, Schiavoni G, Forconi F, et al. Simple genetic diagnosis of hairy cell leukemia by sensitive detection of the BRAF-V600E mutation. *Blood* 2012;119:192–195.

282. Akasaka H, Akasaka T, Kurata M, et al. Molecular anatomy of BCL6 translocations revealed by long-distance polymerase chain reaction-based assays. *Cancer Res* 2000;60:2335–2341.

283. Ye H, Remstein ED, Bacon CM, et al. Chromosomal translocations involving BCL6 in MALT lymphoma. *Haematologica* 2008;93:145–146.

284. Jardin F, Ruminy P, Bastard C, et al. The BCL6 proto-oncogene: a leading role during germinal center development and lymphomagenesis. *Pathol Biol (Paris)* 2007;55:73–83.

285. Migliazza A, Martinotti S, Chen W, et al. Frequent somatic hypermutation of the 5′ noncoding region of the BCL6 gene in B-cell lymphoma. *Proc Natl Acad Sci U S A* 1995;92:12520–12524.

286. Pasqualucci L, Migliazza A, Basso K, et al. Mutations of the BCL6 proto-oncogene disrupt its negative autoregulation in diffuse large B-cell lymphoma. *Blood* 2003;101:2914–2923.

287. Wang X, Li Z, Naganuma A, et al. Negative autoregulation of BCL-6 is bypassed by genetic alterations in diffuse large B cell lymphomas. *Proc Natl Acad Sci U S A* 2002;99:15018–15023.

288. Jiang Y, Soong TD, Wang L, et al. Genome-wide detection of genes targeted by non-Ig somatic hypermutation in lymphoma. *PLoS One* 2012;7:e40332.

289. Copie-Bergman C, Gaulard P, Leroy K, et al. Immuno-fluorescence *in situ* hybridization index predicts survival in patients with diffuse large B-cell lymphoma treated with R-CHOP: a GELA study. *J Clin Oncol* 2009;27:5573–5579.

290. Iqbal J, Neppalli VT, Wright G, et al. BCL2 expression is a prognostic marker for the activated B-cell-like type of diffuse large B-cell lymphoma. *J Clin Oncol* 2006;24:961–968.

291. Muris JJ, Meijer CJ, Vos W, et al. Immunohistochemical profiling based on Bcl-2, CD10 and MUM1 expression improves risk stratification in patients with primary nodal diffuse large B cell lymphoma. *J Pathol* 2006;208:714–723.

292. Iqbal J, Meyer PN, Smith LM, et al. BCL2 predicts survival in germinal center B-cell-like diffuse large B-cell lymphoma treated with CHOP-like therapy and rituximab. *Clin Cancer Res* 2011;17:7785–7795.

293. Li S, Lin P, Fayad LE, et al. B-cell lymphomas with MYC/8q24 rearrangements and IGH@BCL2/t(14;18)(q32;q21): an aggressive disease with heterogeneous histology, germinal center B-cell immunophenotype and poor outcome. *Mod Pathol* 2012;25:145–156.

294. Rosenwald A, Wright G, Chan WC, et al. The use of molecular profiling to predict survival after chemotherapy for diffuse large-B-cell lymphoma. *N Engl J Med* 2002;346:1937–1947.

295. Monti S, Savage KJ, Kutok JL, et al. Molecular profiling of diffuse large B-cell lymphoma identifies robust subtypes including one characterized by host inflammatory response. *Blood* 2005;105:1851–1861.

296. Choi WW, Weisenburger DD, Greiner TC, et al. A new immunostain algorithm classifies diffuse large B-cell lymphoma into molecular subtypes with high accuracy. *Clin Cancer Res* 2009;15:5494–5502.

297. Meyer PN, Fu K, Greiner TC, et al. Immunohistochemical methods for predicting cell of origin and survival in patients with diffuse large B-cell lymphoma treated with rituximab. *J Clin Oncol* 2011;29:200–207.

298. de Jong D, Xie W, Rosenwald A, et al. Immunohistochemical prognostic markers in diffuse large B-cell lymphoma: validation of tissue microarray as a prerequisite for broad clinical applications (a study from the Lunenburg Lymphoma Biomarker Consortium). *J Clin Pathol* 2009;62:128–138.

299. Pasqualucci L, Trifonov V, Fabbri G, et al. Analysis of the coding genome of diffuse large B-cell lymphoma. *Nat Genet* 2011;43:830–837.

300. Lohr JG, Stojanov P, Lawrence MS, et al. Discovery and prioritization of somatic mutations in diffuse large B-cell lymphoma (DLBCL) by whole-exome sequencing. *Proc Natl Acad Sci U S A* 2012;109:3879–3884.

301. Put N, Van Roosbroeck K, Konings P, et al. Chronic lymphocytic leukemia and prolymphocytic leukemia with MYC translocations: a subgroup with an aggressive disease course. *Ann Hematol* 2012;91:863–873.

302. Leucci E, Cocco M, Onnis A, et al. MYC translocation-negative classical Burkitt lymphoma cases: an alternative pathogenetic mechanism involving miRNA deregulation. *J Pathol* 2008;216:440–450.

303. Schmitz R, Young RM, Ceribelli M, et al. Burkitt lymphoma pathogenesis and therapeutic targets from structural and functional genomics. *Nature* 2012;490(7418):116–120.

304. Green TM, Nielsen O, de Stricker K, et al. High levels of nuclear MYC protein predict the presence of MYC rearrangement in diffuse large B-cell lymphoma. *Am J Surg Pathol* 2012;36:612–619.

305. Kluk MJ, Chapuy B, Sinha P, et al. Immunohistochemical detection of MYC-driven diffuse large b-cell lymphomas. *PLoS One* 2012;7:e33813.

306. Kanungo A, Medeiros LJ, Abruzzo LV, et al. Lymphoid neoplasms associated with concurrent t(14;18) and 8q24/c-MYC translocation generally have a poor prognosis. *Mod Pathol* 2006;19:25–33.

307. Roy DaB, A B-cell lymphoma, unclassifiable, with features intermediate between diffuse large B-cell lymphoma and Burkitt lymphoma. *Pathol Case Rev* 2012;17:84–89.

308. Wlodarska I, Nooyen P, Maes B, et al. Frequent occurrence of BCL6 rearrangements in nodular lymphocyte predominance Hodgkin lymphoma but not in classical Hodgkin lymphoma. *Blood* 2003;101:706–710.

309. Van Roosbroeck K, Cox L, Tousseyn T, et al. JAK2 rearrangements, including the novel SEC31A-JAK2 fusion, are recurrent in classical Hodgkin lymphoma. *Blood* 2011;117:4056–4064.

310. Avet-Loiseau H, Facon T, Grosbois B, et al. Oncogenesis of multiple myeloma: 14q32 and 13q chromosomal abnormalities are not randomly distributed, but correlate with natural history, immunological features, and clinical presentation. *Blood* 2002;99:2185–2191.

311. Chesi M, Bergsagel PL. Many multiple myelomas: making more of the molecular mayhem. *Hematol Am Soc Hematol Educ Prog* 2011;2011:344–353.

312. Bergsagel PL, Kuehl WM. Molecular pathogenesis and a consequent classification of multiple myeloma. *J Clin Oncol* 2005;23:6333–6338.

313. Soverini S, Cavo M, Cellini C, et al. Cyclin D1 overexpression is a favorable prognostic variable for newly diagnosed multiple myeloma patients treated with high-dose chemotherapy and single or double autologous transplantation. *Blood* 2003;102:1588–1594.

314. Neben K, Lokhorst HM, Jauch A, et al. Administration of bortezomib before and after autologous stem cell transplantation improves outcome in multiple myeloma patients with deletion 17p. *Blood* 2011;119:940–948.

315. Chapman MA, Lawrence MS, Keats JJ, et al. Initial genome sequencing and analysis of multiple myeloma. *Nature* 2011;471:467–472.

316. Kumar SK, Uno H, Jacobus SJ, et al. Impact of gene expression profiling-based risk stratification in patients with myeloma receiving initial therapy with lenalidomide and dexamethasone. *Blood* 2011;118:4359–4362.

317. Dickens NJ, Walker BA, Leone PE, et al. Homozygous deletion mapping in myeloma samples identifies genes and an expression signature relevant to pathogenesis and outcome. *Clin Cancer Res* 2010;16:1856–1864.

318. Chi J, Ballabio E, Chen XH, et al. MicroRNA expression in multiple myeloma is associated with genetic subtype, isotype and survival. *Biol Direct* 2011;6:23.

319. Lopez-Corral L, Mateos MV, Corchete LA, et al. Genomic analysis of high risk smoldering multiple myeloma. *Haematologica* 2012;97(9):1439–1443.

320. Annunziata CM, Davis RE, Demchenko Y, et al. Frequent engagement of the classical and alternative NF-kappaB pathways by diverse genetic abnormalities in multiple myeloma. *Cancer Cell* 2007;12:115–130.

321. Keats JJ, Fonseca R, Chesi M, et al. Promiscuous mutations activate the noncanonical NF-kappaB pathway in multiple myeloma. *Cancer Cell* 2007;12:131–144.

322. Shaughnessy JD Jr, Haessler J, van Rhee F, et al. Testing standard and genetic parameters in 220 patients with multiple myeloma with complete data sets: superiority of molecular genetics. *Br J Haematol* 2007;137:530–536.

323. Kuiper R, Broyl A, de Knegt Y, et al. A gene expression signature for high-risk multiple myeloma. *Leukemia* 2012;26(11):2406–2413.

324. Lopez-Corral L, Sarasquete ME, Bea S, et al. SNP-based mapping arrays reveal high genomic complexity in monoclonal gammopathies, from MGUS to myeloma status. *Leukemia* 2012;26(12):2521–2529.

325. Shaughnessy JD Jr, Zhan F, Burington BE, et al. A validated gene expression model of high-risk multiple myeloma is defined by deregulated expression of genes mapping to chromosome 1. *Blood* 2007;109:2276–2284.

326. Avet-Loiseau H, Li C, Magrangeas F, et al. Prognostic significance of copy-number alterations in multiple myeloma. *J Clin Oncol* 2009;27:4585–4590.

327. Walker BA, Wardell CP, Chiecchio L, et al. Aberrant global methylation patterns affect the molecular pathogenesis and prognosis of multiple myeloma. *Blood* 2011;117:553–562.

328. Pei H, Zhang L, Luo K, et al. MMSET regulates histone H4K20 methylation and 53BP1 accumulation at DNA damage sites. *Nature* 2011;470:124–128.

329. Amin HM, Lai R. Pathobiology of ALK+ anaplastic large-cell lymphoma. *Blood* 2007;110:2259–2267.

330. Agnelli L, Mereu E, Pellegrino E, et al. Identification of a 3-gene model as a powerful diagnostic tool for the recognition of ALK-negative anaplastic large-cell lymphoma. *Blood* 2012;120:1274–1281.

331. Chikatsu N, Kojima H, Suzukawa K, et al. ALK+, CD30-, CD20- large B-cell lymphoma containing anaplastic lymphoma kinase (ALK) fused to clathrin heavy chain gene (CLTC). *Mod Pathol* 2003;16:828–832.

332. Li S. Anaplastic lymphoma kinase-positive large B-cell lymphoma: a distinct clinicopathological entity. *Int J Clin Exp Pathol* 2009;2:508–518.

333. Szczepanski T, Willemse MJ, Brinkhof B, et al. Comparative analysis of Ig and TCR gene rearrangements at diagnosis and at relapse of childhood precursor-B-ALL provides improved strategies for selection of stable PCR targets for monitoring of minimal residual disease. *Blood* 2002;99:2315–2323.

334. Bagg A. Malleable immunoglobulin genes and hematopathology—the good, the bad, and the ugly: a paper from the 2007 William Beaumont hospital symposium on molecular pathology. *J Mol Diagn* 2008;10:396–410.

335. Pui CH, Mullighan CG, Evans WE, et al. Pediatric acute lymphoblastic leukemia: where are we going and how do we get there? *Blood* 2012;120:1165–1174.

336. Arico M, Valsecchi MG, Camitta B, et al. Outcome of treatment in children with Philadelphia chromosome-positive acute lymphoblastic leukemia. *N Engl J Med* 2000;342:998–1006.

337. Mullighan CG. Mutations of NOTCH1, FBXW7, and prognosis in T-lineage acute lymphoblastic leukemia. *Haematologica* 2009;94:1338–1340.

338. Hong D, Gupta R, Ancliff P, et al. Initiating and cancer-propagating cells in TEL-AML1-associated childhood leukemia. *Science* 2008;319:336–339.

339. De Braekeleer E, Douet-Guilbert N, Morel F, et al. ETV6 fusion genes in hematological malignancies: a review. *Leuk Res* 2012;36:945–961.

340. Zhou Y, You MJ, Young KH, et al. Advances in the molecular pathobiology of B-lymphoblastic leukemia. *Hum Pathol* 2012;43:1347–1362.

341. Hirose K, Inukai T, Kikuchi J, et al. Aberrant induction of LMO2 by the E2A-HLF chimeric transcription factor and its implication in leukemogenesis of B-precursor ALL with t(17;19). *Blood* 2010;116:962–970.

342. Moorman AV, Ensor HM, Richards SM, et al. Prognostic effect of chromosomal abnormalities in childhood B-cell precursor acute lymphoblastic leukaemia: results from the UK Medical Research Council ALL97/99 randomised trial. *Lancet Oncol* 2010;11:429–438.

343. Meyer C, Kowarz E, Hofmann J, et al. New insights to the MLL recombinome of acute leukemias. *Leukemia* 2009;23:1490–1499.

344. Chillon MC, Gomez-Casares MT, Lopez-Jorge CE, et al. Prognostic significance of FLT3 mutational status and expression levels in MLL-AF4+ and MLL-germline acute lymphoblastic leukemia. *Leukemia* 2012;26(11):2360–2366.

345. Harvey RC, Mullighan CG, Chen IM, et al. Rearrangement of CRLF2 is associated with mutation of JAK kinases, alteration of IKZF1, Hispanic/Latino ethnicity, and a poor outcome in pediatric B-progenitor acute lymphoblastic leukemia. *Blood* 2010;115:5312–5321.

346. Mullighan CG, Su X, Zhang J, et al. Deletion of IKZF1 and prognosis in acute lymphoblastic leukemia. *N Engl J Med* 2009;360:470–480.

347. Den Boer ML, van Slegtenhorst M, De Menezes RX, et al. A subtype of childhood acute lymphoblastic leukaemia with poor treatment outcome: a genome-wide classification study. *Lancet Oncol* 2009;10:125–134.

348. Yang YL, Hung CC, Chen JS, et al. IKZF1 deletions predict a poor prognosis in children with B-cell progenitor acute lymphoblastic leukemia: A multicenter analysis in Taiwan. *Cancer Sci* 2011;102:1874–1881.

349. Harvey RC, Mullighan CG, Wang X, et al. Identification of novel cluster groups in pediatric high-risk B-precursor acute lymphoblastic leukemia with gene expression profiling: correlation with genome-wide DNA copy number alterations, clinical characteristics, and outcome. *Blood* 2010;116:4874–4884.

350. Mullighan CG, Miller CB, Radtke I, et al. BCR-ABL1 lymphoblastic leukaemia is characterized by the deletion of Ikaros. *Nature* 2008;453:110–114.

351. Iacobucci I, Ferrari A, Lonetti A, et al. CDKN2A/B alterations impair prognosis in adult BCR-ABL1–positive acute lymphoblastic leukemia patients. *Clin Cancer Res* 2011;17:7413–7423.

352. Hertzberg L, Vendramini E, Ganmore I, et al. Down syndrome acute lymphoblastic leukaemia, a highly heterogeneous disease in which aberrant expression of CRLF2 is associated with mutated JAK2: a report from the International BFM Study Group. *Blood* 2010;115:1006–1017.

353. Moorman AV. The clinical relevance of chromosomal and genomic abnormalities in B-cell precursor acute lymphoblastic leukaemia. *Blood Rev* 2012;26:123–135.

354. Lundin C, Hjorth L, Behrendtz M, et al. High frequency of BTG1 deletions in acute lymphoblastic leukemia in children with down syndrome. *Genes Chromosomes Cancer* 2012;51:196–206.

355. Kuhnl A, Gokbuget N, Kaiser M, et al. Overexpression of LEF1 predicts unfavorable outcome in adult patients with B-precursor acute lymphoblastic leukemia. *Blood* 2011;118:6362–6367.

356. Harrison CJ, Moorman AV, Barber KE, et al. Interphase molecular cytogenetic screening for chromosomal abnormalities of prognostic significance in childhood acute lymphoblastic leukaemia: a UK Cancer Cytogenetics Group Study. *Br J Haematol* 2005;129:520–530.

357. Strefford JC, van Delft FW, Robinson HM, et al. Complex genomic alterations and gene expression in acute lymphoblastic leukemia with intrachromosomal amplification of chromosome 21. *Proc Natl Acad Sci U S A* 2006;103:8167–8172.

358. Zhang J, Mullighan CG, Harvey RC, et al. Key pathways are frequently mutated in high-risk childhood acute lymphoblastic leukemia: a report from the Children's Oncology Group. *Blood* 2011;118:3080–3087.

359. Graux C, Cools J, Michaux L, et al. Cytogenetics and molecular genetics of T-cell acute lymphoblastic leukemia: from thymocyte to lymphoblast. *Leukemia* 2006;20:1496–1510.

360. Han X, Bueso-Ramos CE. Precursor T-cell acute lymphoblastic leukemia/lymphoblastic lymphoma and acute biphenotypic leukemias. *Am J Clin Pathol* 2007;127:528–544.

361. De Keersmaecker K, Marynen P, Cools J. Genetic insights in the pathogenesis of T-cell acute lymphoblastic leukemia. *Haematologica* 2005;90:1116–1127.

362. Graux C, Stevens-Kroef M, Lafage M, et al. Heterogeneous patterns of amplification of the NUP214-ABL1 fusion gene in T-cell acute lymphoblastic leukemia. *Leukemia* 2009;23:125–133.

363. van Grotel M, Meijerink JP, van Wering ER, et al. Prognostic significance of molecular-cytogenetic abnormalities in pediatric T-ALL is not explained by immunophenotypic differences. *Leukemia* 2008;22:124–131.

364. Meijerink JP, den Boer ML, Pieters R. New genetic abnormalities and treatment response in acute lymphoblastic leukemia. *Semin Hematol* 2009;46:16–23.

365. Usvasalo A, Savola S, Raty R, et al. CDKN2A deletions in acute lymphoblastic leukemia of adolescents and young adults: an array CGH study. *Leuk Res* 2008;32:1228–1235.

366. Kuchinskaya E, Heyman M, Nordgren A, et al. Array-CGH reveals hidden gene dose changes in children with acute lymphoblastic leukaemia and a normal or failed karyotype by G-banding. *Br J Haematol* 2008;140:572–577.

367. Weng AP, Ferrando AA, Lee W, et al. Activating mutations of NOTCH1 in human T cell acute lymphoblastic leukemia. *Science* 2004;306:269–271.

368. Pear WS, Aster JC. T cell acute lymphoblastic leukemia/lymphoma: a human cancer commonly associated with aberrant NOTCH1 signaling. *Curr Opin Hematol* 2004;11:426–433.

369. Breit S, Stanulla M, Flohr T, et al. Activating NOTCH1 mutations predict favorable early treatment response and long-term outcome in childhood precursor T-cell lymphoblastic leukemia. *Blood* 2006;108:1151–1157.

370. Ben Abdelali R, Asnafi V, Leguay T, et al. Pediatric-inspired intensified therapy of adult T-ALL reveals the favorable outcome of NOTCH1/FBXW7 mutations, but not of low ERG/BAALC expression: a GRAALL study. *Blood* 2011;118:5099–5107.

371. Callens C, Baleydier F, Lengline E, et al. Clinical impact of NOTCH1 and/or FBXW7 mutations, FLASH deletion, and TCR status in pediatric T-cell lymphoblastic lymphoma. *J Clin Oncol* 2012;30:1966–1973.

372. Roullet M, Bagg A. The basis and rational use of molecular genetic testing in mature B-cell lymphomas. *Adv Anat Pathol* 2010;17:333–358.

373. Dequeker E, Ramsden S, Grody WW, et al. Quality control in molecular genetic testing. *Nat Rev Genet* 2001;2:717–723.

374. Rowe D, Cotterill SJ, Ross FM, et al. Cytogenetically cryptic AML1–ETO and CBF beta-MYH11 gene rearrangements: incidence in 412 cases of acute myeloid leukaemia. *Br J Haematol* 2000;111:1051–1056.

375. Langabeer SE, Walker H, Rogers JR, et al. Incidence of AML1/ETO fusion transcripts in patients entered into the MRC AML trials. MRC Adult Leukaemia Working Party. *Br J Haematol* 1997;99:925–928.

376. Bose S, Deininger M, Gora-Tybor J, et al. The presence of typical and atypical BCR-ABL fusion genes in leukocytes of normal individuals: biologic significance and implications for the assessment of minimal residual disease. *Blood* 1998;92:3362–3367.

377. Laurent C, Lopez C, Desjobert C, et al. Circulating t(2;5)-positive cells can be detected in cord blood of healthy newborns. *Leukemia* 2012;26:188–190.

378. Schuler F, Hirt C, Dolken G. Chromosomal translocation t(14;18) in healthy individuals. *Semin Cancer Biol* 2003;13:203–209.

379. ten Bosch JR, Grody WW. Keeping up with the next generation: massively parallel sequencing in clinical diagnostics. *J Mol Diagn* 2008;10:484–492.

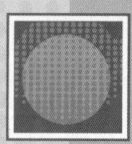

Chapter 9
Role of Cytogenetic Analysis in the Diagnosis and Classification of Hematopoietic Neoplasms

Karen J. Ouyang • Michelle M. Le Beau

The malignant cells in many patients who have leukemia, lymphoma, or another hematologic neoplasm have acquired clonal chromosomal abnormalities. Specific cytogenetic abnormalities are closely, and sometimes uniquely, associated with morphologically and clinically distinct subsets of leukemia or lymphoma (1,2). The detection of a cytogenetic abnormality clearly distinguishes between benign reactive lymphoid or myeloid hyperplasia and a malignant proliferation (1). Moreover, the detection of recurring cytogenetic abnormalities may predict the clinical course, and the likelihood of responding to particular treatments, for example, retinoic acid (RA) in acute promyelocytic leukemia (APL) (3–5). In many cases, the prognostic information derived from cytogenetic analysis is independent of that provided by other clinical features. Patients with favorable prognostic features may be treated with standard regimens, whereas those with less favorable clinical or cytogenetic characteristics may be better treated with more intensive or investigational therapies (3–5). In addition, the disappearance of a chromosomal abnormality, or an abnormal clone, that was present at diagnosis is an important indicator of complete remission following treatment, and its reappearance invariably heralds relapse of the disease. This chapter focuses on the genetics of the leukemias and lymphomas from primarily a cytogenetic perspective.

GENETIC CONSEQUENCES OF CHROMOSOMAL TRANSLOCATIONS

Recurring chromosomal translocations are the hallmark of hematologic malignant diseases. Alterations in the expression of genes that are located at the breakpoints of the chromosomal translocations, or in the properties of the encoded proteins, play an integral role in the process of malignant transformation (6–9). The transforming genes that are involved in chromosomal translocations fall into several functional classes, such as transcription factors, tyrosine protein kinases, cell surface receptors, growth factors, and regulators of apoptosis. Genes encoding proteins that regulate transcription are the most commonly involved. Transcription factors are proteins that recognize and bind to target sequences in the regulatory elements of genes or to other DNA-binding proteins, often in a tissue-specific fashion. They play critical roles in differentiation and development, as well as in maintaining the function of differentiated cells (7–9).

There are two general mechanisms by which chromosomal translocations result in altered gene function. The first is deregulation of gene expression. This mechanism is characteristic of the translocations in lymphoid neoplasms that involve the immunoglobulin genes in B-lineage tumors and the T-cell receptor (TCR) genes in T-lineage tumors (8,9). These rearrangements result in inappropriate expression of an onco-gene (overexpression or aberrant expression in a tissue that does not normally express the gene), with no alteration in its protein structure. The second mechanism is the expression of a novel fusion protein, resulting from the juxtaposition of coding sequences from two genes that are normally located on different chromosomes (6,8,9). Such chimeric genes/proteins are "tumor specific" in that the fusion gene does not exist in nonmalignant cells; the detection of such a fusion gene or protein can be important in the diagnosis or in the detection of residual disease or early relapse. They may also be appropriate targets for tumor-specific therapies, for example, the chimeric BCR-ABL1 protein resulting from the t(9;22) in chronic myelogenous leukemia (CML).

METHODS

Cytogenetic abnormalities may be detected by conventional cytogenetic analysis of metaphase cells, fluorescence *in situ* hybridization (FISH) analysis, reverse transcription-polymerase chain reaction (RT-PCR), or microarray-based genomic copy number analysis (Fig. 9.1).

Conventional Cytogenetic Analysis

Conventional cytogenetic analysis is technically complex but allows for the examination of the entire tumor genome. This is particularly important for the evaluation of hematologic malignancies that have a complex karyotype with multiple genetic abnormalities. In leukemia, the specimen is usually obtained by bone marrow (BM) aspiration (1 to 5 mL of marrow is aspirated aseptically into a syringe coated with preservative-free sodium heparin and transferred to a sterile 15-mL centrifuge tube containing 5 mL of RPMI 1640 culture medium, and 100 units sodium heparin) and is cultured for 24 to 72 hours. When a BM aspirate cannot be obtained, a BM biopsy (bone core specimen) can often be processed successfully. Alternatively, for patients who have a white blood cell (WBC) count higher than 10,000/μL with more than 10% immature myeloid or lymphoid cells, a sample of peripheral blood (PB) drawn aseptically into a syringe coated with preservative-free heparin can be cultured. The karyotype of the dividing cells is similar to that obtained from the BM. Mitogens are not added routinely to PB cultures in acute leukemia, because stimulation of division of normal lymphocytes may interfere with the analysis of spontaneously dividing malignant cells. An involved lymph node or tumor mass specimen or malignant effusion may be processed similarly for the analysis of lymphomas.

Cytogenetic studies are feasible only for specimens that contain viable dividing cells. For this reason, it is critical that the specimen be transported to the laboratory without delay. Overnight shipment of specimens frequently results in loss of cell viability, and most laboratories experience a high proportion of inadequate analyses using such specimens. For optimally handled specimens, approximately 95% of all cases should be adequate for cytogenetic analysis.

A. Metaphase Cytogenetic Analysis

B. Fluorescence *In Situ* Hybridization

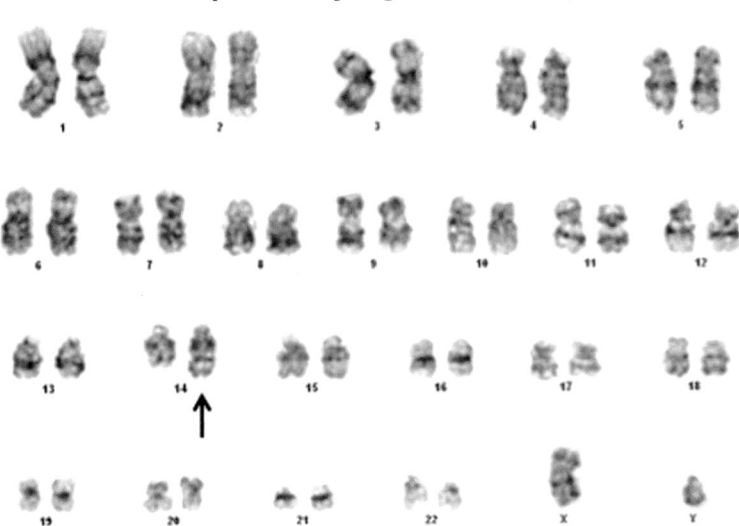

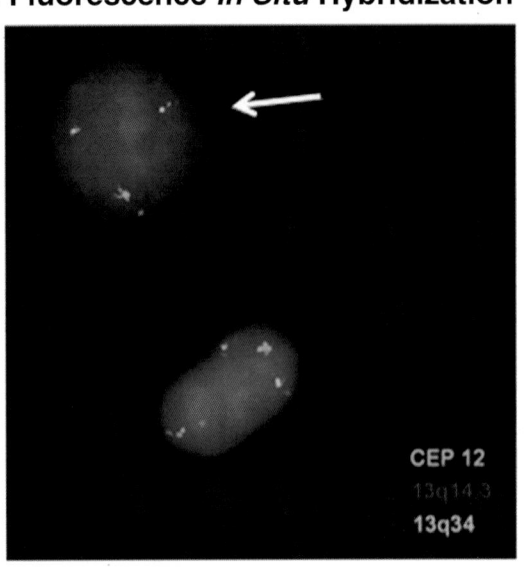

C. Chromosomal SNP Microarray

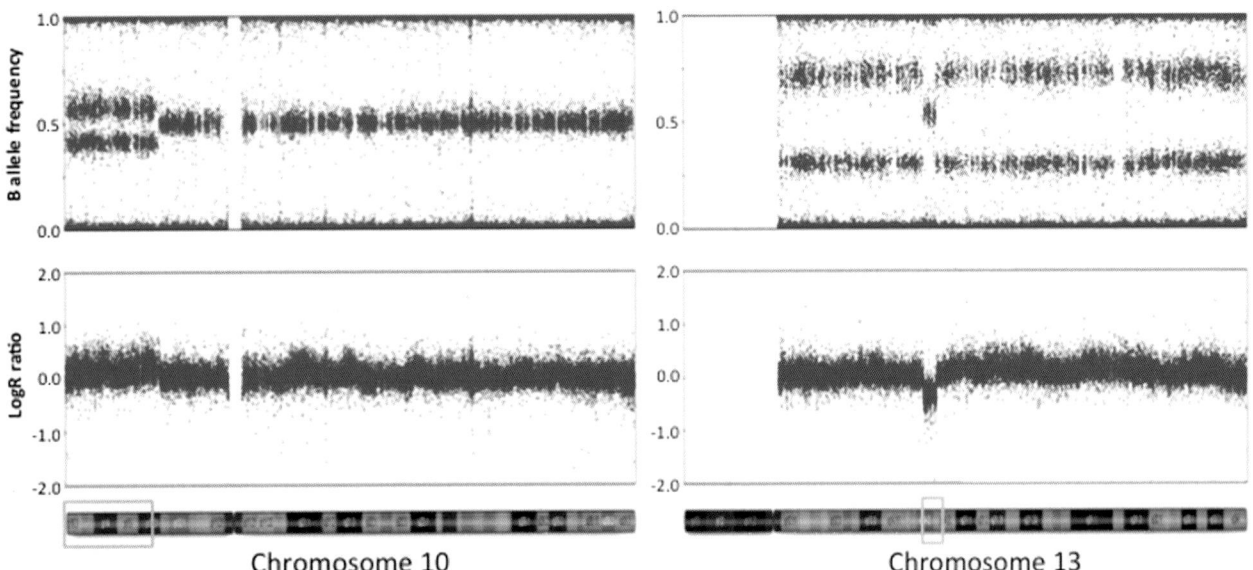

FIGURE 9.1. **Genetic analysis of a BM sample from a patient with CLL using conventional cytogenetic, FISH, and SNP microarray analysis demonstrates the utility and complementarity of each testing methodology in providing a comprehensive analysis of the molecular features. A:** Metaphase cytogenetic analysis revealed a chromosomally abnormal clone, characterized by a structurally rearranged chromosome 14 (*black arrow*) (46,XY,add(14)(q32)[6]/46,XY[14]). **B:** FISH analysis using a panel of probes for CLL revealed a homozygous deletion of sequences from 13q14.3 (see *white arrowed* interphase nucleus) not visible by conventional metaphase analysis in approximately 50% of the cells analyzed. Interphase nuclei were hybridized with the tricolor probe set (CEP12 SpectrumGreen; LSI D13S319 SpectrumOrange; LSI 13q34 SpectrumAqua Probe, Abbott Molecular Diagnostics). **C:** SNP microarray analysis is shown with the LogR ratio diagram (signal intensity) on the bottom and the B-allele frequency (genotype information) diagram directly above. The shifting in intensity values of the LogR ratio combined with the different track patterns in the B-allele frequency diagram provide powerful data for copy number analysis, for example, a normal pattern is visualized as a LogR ratio value of 0, and a pattern of B-allele frequency values at 1.0, 0.5, and 0. There are also additional properties of identifying copy-neutral loss of heterozygosity (CN-LOH) and indicating mosaic mixtures of normal and malignant cells. **Bottom left panel:** An increase in the LogR ratio combined with a splitting of the middle track in the B-allele frequency diagram indicates a duplication of material from 10p (*orange box*) in a proportion of the cells, and likely accounts for the additional material identified on chromosome 14 in the karyotype described above. **Bottom right panel:** The observation of splitting of the middle B-allele frequency track throughout the whole chromosome 13 (besides the deleted region at 13q14.3), without a concurrent rise in the LogR ratio, indicates whole chromosome CN-LOH in a proportion of the cells. A clearly visible decrease in the logR ratio at 13q14.3 (*green box*) combined with the shift in B-allele frequency pattern at that region indicates a homozygous deletion of this region in a proportion of the cells, consistent with the results of FISH analysis. Additionally, these results suggest that the homozygous deletion of 13q14.3 arose from a deletion event involving a single chromosome 13 homolog, followed by gain of the deleted homolog, and loss of the normal chromosome 13 homolog, or by a somatic recombination event near the centromere of chromosome 13. (SNP microarray, Illumina Human Omni1-Quad.)

Fluorescence *In Situ* Hybridization

In FISH analysis, probes are labeled with fluorochromes and hybridized to either metaphase chromosomes or interphase nuclei. This technique is a rapid and sensitive means of detecting recurring numerical and structural abnormalities. FISH is dependent upon the ability of single-stranded DNA to anneal to complementary sequences in the nuclear DNA of interphase cells or the DNA of metaphase chromosomes that are affixed to a glass microscope slide (10). FISH can also be accomplished with BM or PB smears, freshly prepared touch preparations, cytospin slides, or formalin-fixed, paraffin-embedded tissue. Commercially available probes are typically several hundred kilobase bacterial artificial chromosome (BAC) clones, directly labeled with fluorochrome. The use of dual- and triple-pass filters enables the detection of two to three probes simultaneously. In general, there are three types of probes that are used to detect chromosomal abnormalities by FISH. Centromere-specific probes, unique to the repetitive sequences that flank the centromere of each human chromosome, have been used to identify monosomy, trisomy, and other aneuploidies in both leukemias and solid tumors. Locus-specific probes, such as the *BCR* and *ABL1* probes, are usually BAC clones flanking or spanning the relevant gene, labeled in a single color or in two colors (dual-color probes). This type of probe is very useful in detecting structural aberrations, such as translocations or inversions, as well as deletions or gain of gene copy number. Chromosome-specific libraries, which paint the entire chromosome, chromosome arm, or specific chromosomal bands, are particularly useful in identifying marker chromosomes (rearranged chromosomes of unidentified origin) or structural rearrangements, but are rarely used in clinical assays.

The high sensitivity and specificity, rapid turnaround time, capacity to analyze large numbers of cells, and ability to obtain adequate data from samples with a low mitotic index or terminally differentiated cells are the main advantages of FISH. This method is most useful when the analysis is targeted toward those abnormalities that are known to be associated with a particular disease, for example, the *BCR-ABL1* fusion in CML. However, additional abnormalities or multiple clones will not be detected by this method alone. Thus, in the clinical setting, FISH analysis may be used to assess the presence of a recurring abnormality rapidly for therapeutic decisions. Complete cytogenetic analysis should be performed at the time of diagnosis, recurrence, or progression to identify the chromosomal abnormalities in the malignant cells of a particular patient. Thereafter, FISH with the appropriate probes can be used to detect residual disease or early relapse, and to assess the efficacy of therapeutic regimens (10,11). FISH probes are available for the detection of all of the common recurring chromosomal abnormalities in hematologic malignant diseases, including chromosome gains or losses, deletions, and translocations.

As mentioned above, FISH may be utilized to detect and monitor response to therapy, residual disease, and relapse. This requires the establishment of a reference range and cutoff value for a positive result for each probe and assay used to distinguish a low percentage of cells with an abnormal signal pattern from background. The most practical method to determine a cutoff value is to calculate the upper limit of the occurrence of an abnormal signal pattern in normal cells (12). For example, if the cutoff value for a positive test result for trisomy 8 (observed as three distinct fluorescent signals within the boundary of a nucleus) is 2%, the observation of five cells with the abnormal signal pattern out of 200 total cells scored (2.5%) would be considered positive for trisomy 8. However, it is important to note that borderline-positive and borderline-negative results should be interpreted cautiously and in the context of other clinical and laboratory findings.

Although monitoring of residual disease by FISH has been incorporated into the assessment of response in specific diseases such as CML (13), there are few studies that have evaluated the prognostic value of interphase FISH after therapy or in the posttransplant period for hematologic malignancies (14). Furthermore, the sensitivity of FISH probes varies substantially depending on the probe configuration, that is, centromere-specific, dual-color dual-fusion, or break-apart probes, and the cutoff values for a positive result range from 1.5% to 6%, placing practical limits on the applicability of FISH for the detection of minimal residual disease (MRD). Clinical trials and large-scale studies are needed to address the clinical utility of FISH and various other techniques, as well as standardized approaches to allow for reproducibility between laboratories.

Microarray Analysis

Emerging technologies that are starting to play a major role in the diagnosis and management of hematologic disorders include microarray-based genomic copy number analysis and high-resolution genome-wide genotyping using single nucleotide polymorphisms (SNPs) (15,16). This technology facilitates genome-wide association studies for the identification of disease susceptibility loci, as well as the identification of acquired abnormalities, such as genetic imbalances, including cryptic deletions and duplications. SNP arrays can also detect loss of heterozygosity (LOH) that occurs without concurrent changes in the gene copy number, (referred to as copy-neutral LOH [CN-LOH]), which can be attributed to somatic mitotic recombination or acquired uniparental disomy. Several studies have validated the utility of this technology as a diagnostic tool, as well as a discovery tool in research (17). For example, genomic analysis of clonal origins of relapsed acute lymphoblastic leukemia (ALL) revealed that genomic abnormalities contributing to ALL relapse were present prior to treatment, and were selected for during initial treatment, perhaps pointing to new targets for therapeutic intervention (18).

CHROMOSOME NOMENCLATURE

Chromosomal terminology is summarized in Table 9.1, and abnormalities are described according to the International System for Human Cytogenetic Nomenclature (19). To describe the chromosomal complement, the total chromosome number is listed first, followed by the sex chromosome complement, and numerical and structural abnormalities in ascending order. The observation of at least two cells with the same structural rearrangement, for example, translocations, deletions or inversions, or gain of the same chromosome, or three cells each showing loss of the same chromosome, is considered evidence for the presence of an abnormal clone. However, one cell with a normal karyotype is sufficient to define a normal cell line. Patients whose cells show no alteration or nonclonal (single cell) abnormalities are considered to be normal. An exception to this is a single cell characterized by a recurring structural abnormality. In such instances, it is likely that this represents the karyotype of the malignant cells in that particular patient. Following treatment, the detection of a single cell with the clonal abnormalities noted prior to therapy is considered evidence for residual or recurrent disease.

Cytogenetic studies have enabled routine assessment of the clonal composition of malignant cell populations. Cells that have the same chromosome abnormality are considered clonally related, since it is statistically improbable that the same alteration occurs repeatedly and independently in different cells. Unlike some solid tumors, the cytogenetic heterogeneity of hematologic malignancies is relatively low. The presence of

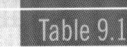

Table 9.1	GLOSSARY OF CYTOGENETIC TERMINOLOGY

Aneuploidy—An abnormal chromosome number due to either gain or loss of chromosomes.

Banded chromosomes—Chromosomes with alternating dark and light segments due to special stains or pretreatment with enzymes before staining. Each chromosome pair has a unique pattern of bands.

Breakpoint—A specific site on a chromosome containing a DNA break that is involved in a structural rearrangement, such as a translocation or deletion.

Centromere—The chromosome constriction that is the site of the spindle fiber attachment. The position of the centromere determines whether chromosomes are *metacentric* (X-shaped, e.g., chromosomes 1–3, 6–12, X, 16, 19, 20) or *acrocentric* (inverted V-shaped, e.g., chromosomes 13–15, 21, 22, Y). During mitosis, the duplicate copies of the DNA in each chromosome (chromatids) are separated by shortening of the spindle fibers attached to opposite sides of the dividing cell.

Clone—In the cytogenetic sense, this is defined as two cells with the same additional or structurally rearranged chromosome, or three cells with loss of the same chromosome.

Deletion—A segment of a chromosome is missing as the result of two breaks and loss of the intervening piece (interstitial deletion). Molecular studies of many recurring deletions have shown that, in each case, the deletions were interstitial, rather than terminal (single break with loss of the terminal segment).

Diploid—Normal chromosome number and composition of chromosomes.

FISH—A molecular-cytogenetic technique based on the visualization of fluorescently labeled DNA probes hybridized to complementary DNA sequences from metaphase or interphase cells, used to detect numerical and structural abnormalities. A short nomenclature description is used to describe the results of *in situ* hybridization. For interphase FISH, the abbreviation "nuc ish" is followed immediately by the locus designation in parentheses (or multiple loci separated by a comma), a multiplication signal, and the number of signals observed. The number of cells scored is placed in brackets. For example, normal results for the *BCR-ABL1* probe are described as "nuc ish(ABL1, BCR) x2[400]." A case with the t(9;22) resulting in the *BCR-ABL1* fusion analyzed using a dual-color, dual-fusion probe would be described as "nuc ish(ABL1x3),(BCRx3),(ABL1 con BCRx2)[400]."

Haploid—Only one-half the normal complement, that is, 23 chromosomes.

Hyperdiploid—Additional chromosomes; therefore, the modal number is 47 or greater.

Hypodiploid—Loss of chromosomes with a modal number of 45 or less.

Inversion—Two breaks occur in the same chromosome with rotation of the intervening segment. If both breaks are on the same side of the centromere, it is called a paracentric inversion. If they are on opposite sides, it is called a pericentric inversion.

Isochromosome—A chromosome that consists of identical copies of one chromosome arm with loss of the other arm. Thus, an isochromosome for the long arm of chromosome 17 [i(17)(q10)] contains two copies of the long arm (separated by the centromere) with loss of the short arm of the chromosome.

Karyotype—Arrangement of chromosomes from a particular cell according to an internationally established system such that the largest chromosomes are first and the smallest ones are last. A normal female karyotype is described as 46,XX and a normal male karyotype is described as 46,XY. An *idiogram* is an idealized representation (diagram) of the chromosomes.

Pseudodiploid—A diploid number of chromosomes accompanied by structural abnormalities.

Recurring abnormality—A numerical or structural abnormality noted in multiple patients who have a similar neoplasm. Such abnormalities are characteristic or diagnostic of distinct subtypes of leukemia and lymphoma that have unique morphologic and/or immunophenotypic features. Recurring abnormalities represent genetic mutations that are involved in the pathogenesis of the corresponding diseases; many recurring abnormalities have prognostic significance.

Translocation—A break in at least two chromosomes with exchange of material. In a reciprocal translocation, there is no obvious loss of chromosomal material. Translocations are indicated by t; the chromosomes involved are noted in the first set of brackets and the breakpoints in the second set of brackets. The Ph translocation is t(9;22)(q34;q11.2).

Nomenclature symbols:

p—Short arm

q—Long arm

+—If before the chromosome, indicates a gain of a whole chromosome (e.g., +8)

−—If before the chromosome, indicates a loss of a whole chromosome (e.g., −7) and if after the chromosome indicates loss of part of the chromosome (e.g., 5q−, loss of part of the long arm of chromosome 5)

?—Indicates uncertainty about the identity of the chromosome or band listed just after the "?"

t—Translocation

del—Deletion

inv—Inversion

i—Isochromosome

mar—Marker chromosome

r—Ring chromosome

Modified from Rowley JD. Chromosome abnormalities in human cancer. In: De Vita VT, Hellman S, Rosenberg S, eds. *Practice and principles of oncology*, 3rd ed. Philadelphia: J.P. Lippincott, 1991.

cytogenetically unrelated clones, though rare, is observed occasionally in pretreatment and posttreatment samples, for example, approximately 2% in acute myeloid leukemia (AML) and 5% in myelodysplastic syndrome (MDS) (20). Clones emerging after therapy may persist for extensive periods of time, without further evidence of disease, as exemplified by the emergence of newly detected clones with a del(20q) or +8 [without the t(9;22)] in CML following treatment with tyrosine kinase inhibitors (TKIs) (21,22). However, a concern when assessing clonality based on "conventional cytogenetic analysis" is that aberrations or mutations below the resolution detectable by cytogenetic analyses are not recognized. It is therefore possible that unifying, submicroscopic alterations, such as microdeletions, cryptic translocations, and point mutations, exist in malignant cell populations with seemingly unrelated chromosome abnormalities.

The utility of new technologies, such as multiplex FISH, genomic arrays, and next-generation sequencing, has increased our ability to detect genomic aberrations, and to address questions regarding the origin, clonality, and evolution of cancers, including acute leukemias, multiple myeloma (MM), and others (23–29). Recent studies have revealed several patterns of clonality in hematologic malignant diseases. In AML arising from MDS, a sequential linear path of clonal evolution has been described (29). In contrast, in ALL and MM, tumor cell evolution more closely mimics a darwinian-like branching hierarchy dynamic, leading to a more complex clonal architecture with substantial clonal diversity and coexistence of wider genetic heterogeneity. Furthermore, the relative proportion of coexisting subclones may alternate over time based on therapeutic- and/or microenvironment-dependent selective pressures. These findings have potential implications in the approach to therapy. Cases in which significant clonal heterogeneity is detected at diagnosis may benefit more from cocktail-based combination therapies instead of single-agent sequential therapies to eradicate not only major clones but also minor clones that may prevail at relapse.

MYELOPROLIFERATIVE NEOPLASMS

In the most recent edition of the World Health Organization (WHO) classification, the previous entity, myeloproliferative disorders, was renamed myeloproliferative neoplasms (MPNs), reflecting an increasing understanding of the molecular and genetic basis of these diseases (1,30). As the distinguished hematologist Dr. William Dameshek predicted in 1951, the MPNs are characterized by uncontrolled clonal proliferation of stem cell–like myeloid progenitor cells. Clonal expansion of erythroid, megakaryocytic, or myeloid cells results from constitutively activated tyrosine kinases (TKs) that are components of the signal transduction pathway regulating the growth and differentiation of normal myeloid cells (30,31).

Chronic Myelogenous Leukemia

CML is a particularly important subtype of leukemia, because the first consistent chromosomal abnormality in a malignant disease was noted in this disease (32). This abnormality, the Philadelphia or "Ph" chromosome, was first described in 1960 by Nowell and Hungerford (33) as a deletion of part of the long arm of a G group chromosome, and later with the use of fluorescence banding techniques as a deletion of chromosome 22. The nature of the chromosomal aberration was clarified in 1973, when Rowley (34) reported that the Ph chromosome resulted from a reciprocal translocation involving chromosomes 9 (break at band q34) and 22 (break at band q11.2). The t(9;22) also represents the first rearrangement shown to result in a fusion protein (Table 9.2) (35,36).

Approximately 92% of CML cases have the conventional t(9;22) (1). Other cases have variant translocations (~8%) that involve additional chromosomes besides chromosomes 9 and 22. In a three-way variant translocation, material from chromosome 9 translocates to chromosome 22, material from 22q translocates to a third chromosome, and material from the third chromosome translocates to 9q (37). In conventional and variant rearrangements, the *ABL1* oncogene on 9q34 is relocated adjacent to the *BCR* gene on 22q11.2 producing the *BCR-ABL1* fusion gene (35). Rare patients have a cryptic rearrangement involving 9q34 and 22q11.2 that cannot be identified by conventional metaphase analysis (38). However, the *BCR-ABL1* fusion gene is present and can be detected by molecular techniques, such as FISH and RT-PCR (37,38).

The breakpoints in the *ABL1* gene on chromosome 9 span a large region of more than 200 kb, upstream of exon 2. In contrast, breakpoints in the *BCR* gene on chromosome 22 usually cluster in a small 5.8-kb region between exons 12 and 16 called the major breakpoint cluster region (M-bcr) (39). The *ABL1* coding sequences are translocated to chromosome 22 and fused in-frame with the *BCR* gene. A novel chimeric 8.5 kb mRNA transcript is produced and translated into the chimeric p210 kilodalton protein, which has persistent and increased TK activity. Recognizing alternative breakpoints in the *BCR* gene of a *BCR-ABL1* translocation is important because these lead to distinct phenotypes and diseases (40,41). Patients who produce a larger fusion protein (p230), resulting from *BCR* breakpoints that span exons 17 to 20, may demonstrate neutrophilic maturation and conspicuous thrombocytosis. Breakpoints spanning exons 1 to 2 (minor breakpoint cluster region, m-bcr) give rise to a smaller fusion protein (p190) that is most frequently associated with Ph-positive ALL (40,41). Rare cases

of CML that express the p190 protein present with increased numbers of monocytes.

The ABL1 protein is a nuclear protein that is regulated by the retinoblastoma protein, RB1. The aberrant BCR-ABL1 protein localizes to the cytoplasmic surface of the cell membrane via the BCR moiety, has constitutive TK activity, and acquires a novel function in transmitting growth-regulatory signals from cell surface receptors to the nucleus through the RAS signal transduction pathway (41,42). BCR-ABL1 promotes abnormal cell proliferation and inhibits apoptosis in hematopoietic cells (42). Evidence that *BCR-ABL1* is transforming was provided by *in vivo* studies in mice showing that expression of BCR-ABL1 in hematopoietic cells leads to leukemia (43).

Knowledge of the molecular pathogenesis of BCR-ABL1-mediated CML prompted the rational design of inhibitors targeted specifically to the aberrant TK activity of the BCR-ABL1 fusion protein. Imatinib inhibits BCR-ABL1 TK activity by competing with ATP for binding to the ABL1 kinase domain, thereby effectively hindering aberrant downstream signaling and reversing oncogenic effects. Clinical use of imatinib since 1998 has dramatically changed the prognosis and natural history of CML. The estimated 7- to 10-year overall survival is 80% to 85%, and 90% to 93% if non–CML-related deaths are excluded (44,45). However, approximately 6% of CML cases in chronic phase and up to 80% to 90% of cases in the advanced phases fail to respond to imatinib treatment (46,47). Second-generation TKIs, such as dasatinib, nilotinib, and ponatinib, were specifically engineered to inhibit the kinase activity in leukemia cells that have acquired mutations in the BCR-ABL1 kinase domain that hinder or decrease the binding of imatinib, and are proving to have even higher efficacy than imatinib first-line therapy (48–50).

The development of novel therapeutics in CML has expanded the use of cytogenetic analysis for monitoring of therapeutic response. Complete cytogenetic response, defined as 0% Ph-positive cells in at least 20 analyzable metaphase cells, has consistently been associated with improved survival following treatment, including imatinib therapy. Although other monitoring techniques, such as FISH, quantitative PCR, and mutation analysis, have been incorporated into various protocols to supplement disease evaluation, achieving a complete cytogenetic response remains the gold standard of TKI therapy in CML (51).

In the era of TKIs, progression to the accelerated and acute phase of CML is uncommon. Although the exact mechanisms of disease progression in CML are still largely unknown, cytogenetic evolution remains the most consistent indicator of progression to advanced disease (52). Eighty percent of patients in blast crisis exhibit additional chromosomal changes. The most common changes, a gain of chromosomes 8, 19, a second Ph (by gain of the first), or i(17q), frequently occur in combination to produce modal chromosome numbers of 47 through 50. Taken together, these changes occur in 70% of cases with secondary abnormalities. Less common abnormalities occurring in about 15% of cases with additional changes include −7, −17, +17, +21, −Y, and the t(3;21)(q26.2;q22) creating the *RUNX1-MDS1/MECOM* fusion. Rarely, one of the recurring abnormalities in AML can be seen with the t(9;22), such as an inv(16) in myelomonocytic blast crisis (52,53).

BCR-ABL1–Negative MPNs

The unifying theme for the group of *BCR-ABL1*–negative MPNs was the discovery of acquired *JAK2* mutations (54–57). However, JAK2 mutations have also been reported in rare cases of *BCR-ABL1*–positive CML (58) and MDS (59–61). The most common mutation, $JAK2^{V617F}$, results in a constitutively active TK that aberrantly drives a cascade of signaling pathways to promote transformation and proliferation of progenitor cells. The discovery of *JAK2* mutations in MPNs has led to the

Table 9.2	RECURRING CHROMOSOME ABNORMALITIES IN MALIGNANT MYELOID DISEASES

Disease[a]	Chromosome Abnormality	Frequency	Involved Genes[b]		Consequence
MPN CML	t(9;22)(q34;q11.2)	~99%[c]	ABL1	BCR	Fusion protein—Altered cytokine signaling pathways, genomic instability
CML blast phase	t(9;22) with +8, i(17q), +19, or +der(22)t(9;22)	~70%			
PV	+8 +9 del(20q) del(13q) partial trisomy 1q	20% (all abnormalities combined)			
MF	+8 +9 −7/del(7q) del(5q)/t(5q) del(20q) del(13q) partial trisomy 1q	30% (all abnormalities combined)			
AML	t(8;21)(q22;q22)	10%	RUNX1T1/ETO	RUNX1/AML1	Fusion protein—Altered transcriptional regulation
	t(15;17)(q24.1;q21.1)	9%	PML	RARA	Fusion protein—Altered transcriptional regulation
	inv(16)(p13.1q22) or t(16;16)(p13.1;q22)	5%	MYH11	CBFB	Fusion protein—Altered transcriptional regulation
	t(9;11)(p22;q23) t(10;11)(p12;q23) t(11;17)(q23;q25) t(11;19)(q23;p13.3) t(11;19)(q23;p13.1) t(6;11)(q27;q23) Other t(11q23) del(11)(q23)	5%–8% for all t(11q23)	MLLT3/AF9 MLLT10/AF10 MLL MLL MLL MLLT4/AF6 MLL	MLL MLL MLLT6/AF17 MLLT1/ENL ELL MLL	MLL histone methyltransferase fusion proteins—Altered chromatin structure and transcriptional regulation
	+8	8%			
	+11	1%–2%	MLL		ITD
	−7 or del(7q)	14%			
	del(5q)/t(5q)	12%			
	t(6;9)(p23;q34)	1%	DEK	NUP214/CAN	
	inv(3)(q21q26.2) or t(3;3)	2%	RPN1	MECOM/EVI1	
	del(20q)	5%			
	t(12p) or del(12p)	2%			
Therapy-related MN	−7 or del(7q)	45%			
	del(5q)/t(5q)	40%			
	der(1;7)(q10;p10)	2%			
	dic(5;17)(q11.1-13;p11.1-13)	5%		TP53	Loss of function—DNA damage response
	t(9;11)(p22;q23)/t(11q23)	3%	MLLT3/AF9	MLL	MLL histone methyltransferase fusion proteins—Altered chromatin structure and transcriptional regulation
	t(11;16)(q23;p13.3)	2% (t-MDS)	MLL	CREBBP	
	t(21q22)	2%	RUNX1/AML1		Fusion protein—Altered transcriptional regulation
	t(3;21)(q26.2;q22)	3%	RPL22L1	RUNX1	
MDS (Unbalanced)	+8	10%			
	−7/del(7q)[d]	12%			
	del(5q)/t(5q)[d]	15%			
	del(20q)	5%–8%			
	−Y	5%			
	i(17q)/t(17p)[d]	3%–5%	TP53		Loss of function, DNA damage response
	−13/del(13q)[d]	3%			
	del(11q)[d]	3%			
	del(12p)/t(12p)[d]	3%			
	del(9q)[d]	1%–2%			
	idic(X)(q13)[d]	1%–2%			
(Balanced)	t(1;3)(p36.3;q21.2)[d]	1%	MMEL1	RPN1	Deregulation of MMEL1—Transcriptional activation?
	t(2;11)(p21;q23)/t(11q23)[d]	1%		MLL	MLL fusion protein—Altered transcriptional regulation
	inv(3)(q21q26.2)/t(3;3)[d]	1%	RPN1	MECOM/EVI1	Altered transcriptional regulation by MECOM
	t(6;9)(p23;q34)[d]	1%	DEK	NUP214	Fusion protein—Nuclear pore protein
CMML	t(5;12)(q33.1;p13)	~2%	PDGFRB	ETV6/TEL	Fusion protein—Altered signaling pathways

[a]AML, acute myeloid leukemia; CML, chronic myelogenous leukemia; CMML, chronic myelomonocytic leukemia; MDS, myelodysplastic syndrome; MPN, myeloproliferative neoplasm.
[b]Genes are listed in order of citation in the karyotype, for example, for CML, ABL1 is at 9q34 and BCR at 22q11.2.
[c]Rare patients with CML have an insertion of ABL1 adjacent to BCR in a normal appearing chromosome 22.
[d]Cytogenetic abnormalities considered in the WHO 2008 Classification as presumptive evidence of MDS in patients with persistent cytopenias(s), but with no dysplasia or increased blasts.

identification of aberrations in additional genes involved in TK signaling, for example, *MPL, CBL, LNK*, epigenetic regulation, for example, *TET2, ASXL1, EZH2*, and promotion of oncogenic pathways, for example, *IDH1, IDH2*, that are relevant to disease pathogenesis (62). Conventional chemotherapy regimens have not been effective in these diseases. Targeted therapies, such as JAK2 inhibitors, are currently being evaluated in clinical trials (63).

Polycythemia Vera

The *JAK2*^{V617F} mutation is found in more than 95% of patients with polycythemia vera (PV) (54–57), and more than 80% of the remaining cases have a different *JAK2* mutation in exon 12 (64). Although *JAK2* mutations are not unique to PV, and are observed in other MPNs, it has become an important indicator for the diagnosis of PV and a critical factor for ruling out reactive causes included in the differential diagnosis (62,65). Cytogenetic abnormalities are relatively uncommon in PV at diagnosis (~11%), but occur at a higher frequency in those individuals who have been treated with cytotoxic agents, or who have progressed to acute leukemia. Although no specific cytogenetic abnormalities are associated with PV, recurring abnormalities include +8, +9, del(20q), del(13q), del(9p), and dup(1q) (66–68). Interestingly, a number of patients with PV show gains of both chromosomes 8 and 9, which may be unique to PV (67).

The presence of cytogenetic abnormalities at diagnosis does not necessarily predict a short survival or the development of leukemia. An evolutionary change in the karyotype during the disease course, however, may be an ominous sign. Approximately 20% of PV cases progress to MDS or AML, and nearly all of these cases have cytogenetic abnormalities (66,68), which overlap with those noted in the polycythemic phase. Loss of chromosome 7 is seen in 20% of leukemic-phase PV, but is almost never present in the polycythemic phase. Rearrangements of chromosome 5, particularly del(5q), are the most frequent changes noted in advanced disease (66,68,69).

Primary Myelofibrosis

JAK2 mutations are seen in 50% of primary myelofibrosis (PMF) cases (54,55,57), and mutations in the gene encoding the thrombopoietin receptor, *MPL*, are observed in 5% of cases (70). Cytogenetic abnormalities occur in 30% of cases (69,71). An abnormal karyotype at presentation is indicative of an adverse prognosis (71,72). As in PV, the most common recurring abnormalities are +8, +9, del(20q), and abnormalities of 1q. A del(13q) leading to loss of q12-q22 and der(6)t(1;6)(q21-q23;p21.3), although not diagnostic, may be strongly suggestive of PMF. Cases of PMF that progress to AML may have a del(5q) or −7/del(7q) (71,73).

Essential Thrombocythemia

Essential thrombocythemia (ET) is an indolent disease characterized by long intervals of unremarkable symptoms peppered with sudden life-threatening episodes of thromboembolism and hemorrhage (1). *JAK2* mutations are seen in 40% to 50% of ET cases (54–57), whereas *MPL* mutations account for a mere 1% of cases (70). Although these mutations are not specific to ET, and can be seen in PV and PMF as well, the identification of these genetic defects is helpful in ruling out reactive thrombocytosis. Because of the rare occurrence of cytogenetic abnormalities in ET at diagnosis (<5%), there are no well-defined recurrent abnormalities. Those abnormalities that have been reported, such as +8, 9q abnormalities, and del(20q), are not unique to ET, and some observers have suggested that such cases actually represent MPNs other than ET (74).

MYELOID AND LYMPHOID NEOPLASMS WITH EOSINOPHILIA AND ABNORMALITIES OF *PDGFRA, PDGFRB,* OR *FGFR1*

The 2008 WHO classification introduced a new category constituting three rare specific disease groups of myeloid and lymphoid neoplasms associated with rearrangements of *PDGFRA, PDGFRB,* or *FGFR1*. These disorders typically present as a MPN, although they can also manifest as a lymphoid neoplasm. Eosinophilia is frequently observed and is characteristic in these cases, but is not a requirement for classification. The unifying feature is the presence of rearrangements in genes that encode components of receptor protein TKs (*PDGFRA, PDGFRB,* or *FGFR1*). The main importance of recognizing these disorders is the sensitivity of the disease to TKIs that can significantly impact outcomes (1,75).

Myeloid and Lymphoid Neoplasms with *PDGFRA* Rearrangements

Cases with *PDGFRA* rearrangements are rare, and usually present as chronic eosinophilic leukemia (CEL) with prominent involvement of the mast cell lineage and, less commonly, as AML or T-lymphoblastic lymphoma, both accompanied by eosinophilia (1,76). There is a male predominance of 17-fold (1). The majority of cases in this subtype present with a normal karyotype, but have the *FIP1L1-PDGFRA* fusion gene as a result of a cryptic deletion at 4q12 (77). This cryptic event can be detected by FISH analysis probing for the presence or absence of *CHIC2* (located between *FIP1L1* and *PDGFRA*) that is deleted in the process of forming the fusion gene, or by RT-PCR. Although very rare, variant rearrangements of *PDGFRA* with other partner genes, such as *BCR* at 22q11.2, *KIF5B* at 10p11.2, *CDK5RAP2* at 9q33, *STRN* at 2p24, and *ETV6* at 12p13, have been reported (78). Additional cytogenetic abnormalities may be observed with disease progression. Because morphologic and metaphase cytogenetic analysis may be inconclusive in these cases, the detection of the *FIP1L1-PDGFRA* fusion gene is especially important in reaching a definitive diagnosis (76), as this disease is highly responsive to TKI therapy. Resistance to TKIs, refractory disease, or progression to AML can occur with the acquisition of specific mutations of *PDGFRA*, such as T674I or D842V. The long-term prognosis for this rare disease is unknown.

Myeloid and Lymphoid Neoplasms with *PDGFRB* Rearrangements

The features of patients with *PDGFRB* rearrangements are pathologically and genetically variable. These diseases are frequently categorized as chronic myelomonocytic leukemia (CMML) but have also been characterized as other disease types, such as atypical CML and juvenile myelomonocytic leukemia (JMML) (usually with eosinophilia) (1). The most common cytogenetic abnormality is the t(5;12)(q33.1;p13) that results in an *ETV6-PDGFRB* fusion (79,80). However, more than 20 distinct fusion gene partners of *PDGFRB* have been described, illustrating the genetic heterogeneity of this subtype. The t(5;12)/*ETV6-PDGFRB* and other variant translocations of *PDGFRB* lead to a constitutively activated TK that consequently sensitizes malignant cells to TKIs (75,81). Prior to the development of TKIs, the median survival of patients was <2 years. Several recent studies based on a small series of patients have reported median survival times of more than 5 years (82,83).

Myeloid and Lymphoid Neoplasms with *FGFR1* Rearrangements

Neoplasms with rearrangements involving *FGFR1* at 8p11.2 are quite heterogeneous and are thought to be derived from a pluripotent hematopoietic stem cell (HSC). Patients often present with CEL, AML, or T-lymphoblastic leukemia and, less frequently, with B-lymphoblastic leukemia/lymphoma. Transformation to AML can occur in patients initially presenting with CEL. This neoplasm affects patients of all ages, with a slight male predominance (1,75). The most common cytogenetic abnormalities include the t(8;13)(p11.2;q12)/*ZNF198-FGFR1*, t(8;9)(p11.2;q33)/*CEP110-FGFR1*, or t(6;8)(q27;p11.2)/*FGFR1OP1-FGFR1*; however, other fusion partner genes have also been reported (1,84). Interestingly, specific translocations correlate with distinct clinicopathologic features. Patients with the t(8;13) are more likely to present with lymphoblastic lymphoma (85), whereas patients with a *BCR-FGFR1* fusion resulting from the t(8;22)(p11.2;q11.2) may have basophilia (86), and cases with the t(6;8) have been associated with PV. The prognosis of this subgroup of neoplasms is poor. Although *FGFR1* encodes a TK, patients with this disease do not respond to the current TKI therapies. The search for other inhibitors that may provide more effective targeted treatment is in progress (87–89).

MYELODYSPLASTIC SYNDROME/ MYELOPROLIFERATIVE NEOPLASM

The MDS/MPNs are clonal myeloid malignancies that display features of both MDS with cellular dysplasia and complications related to ineffective hematopoiesis, and MPN with cytosis and organ infiltration. Patients may present with clinical, laboratory, or morphologic findings anywhere along the continuum between these two myeloid diseases (1). Currently, the proliferative component of most cases of MDS/MPN appears to be related to aberrations in the *RAS/MAPK* signaling pathways (90,91). The MDS/MPN categories of the 2008 WHO classification include CMML, atypical (*BCR-ABL1*–negative) chronic myeloid leukemia (aCML), JMML, and unclassifiable MDS/MPN.

Chronic Myelomonocytic Leukemia

CMML is characterized by persistent monocytosis in the PB, absence of the *BCR-ABL1* fusion, fewer than 20% blasts in the PB and BM, and dysplasia involving one or more myeloid lineages. There is a male predominance of 2:1, and the median age of diagnosis is 65 to 75 years (1,92). CMML cases displaying eosinophilia with *PDGFRA* or *PDGFRB* rearrangements should not be categorized as MDS/MPN, but instead classified in the new category of myeloid and lymphoid neoplasms with eosinophilia and abnormalities of *PDGFRA*, *PDGFR*, or *FGFR1* (1).

Clonal cytogenetic abnormalities are present in 20% to 40% of CMML cases, with +8, –7/del(7q), 12p abnormalities, and complex karyotypes being the most common (69,93); however, none are specific to CMML. Recurrent copy number abnormalities (most commonly at 7q22.1, 4q24, and 11q23.1) and CN-LOH (frequently observed at 1p, 4q, 7q, and 11q) were identified in approximately 50% of CMML cases by microarray analysis (94,95).

Mutations in the *RAS* gene family are observed in 10% to 40% of CMML (96,97). The *JAK2*[V617F] mutation is found in 8% to 10% of patients with CMML, typically in those patients with clinical and pathologic features of the myeloproliferative type of the disease, suggesting a potential role for *JAK2* mutation status in refining the classification of CMML (98). Recent studies have also identified recurrent mutations in other genes, including *CBL*, *RUNX1*, *ASXL1*, *NPM1*, *TET2*, *IDH1*, *IDH2*, and *EZH2*. Although an increasing number of genetic aberrations are being characterized in CMML, the prognostic impact of these lesions remains to be defined (92).

Atypical Chronic Myeloid Leukemia, BCR-ABL1–Negative

aCML is a very rare leukemic disorder characterized by neutrophilic leukocytosis with dysgranulopoiesis and circulating immature granulocytes in the PB, and is generally associated with a poor outcome (90). Approximately 15% to 40% of patients with aCML evolve to AML, and the remainder succumb to BM failure. Cytogenetic abnormalities have been reported in up to 80%; the most common abnormalities are +8 and del(20q), although abnormalities of chromosomes 12, 13, 14, 17, and 19 have been observed as well (99). Karyotypic evolution is associated with leukemic progression. Approximately 30% of aCML cases are associated with acquired mutations of *NRAS* or *KRAS* (100), and recurring mutations have also been identified in *TET2*, *CBL*, *EZH*, and *SETBP1* (91,95,101,102).

Juvenile Myelomonocytic Leukemia

JMML is a rare aggressive myeloid malignancy of childhood characterized by abnormal proliferation of the granulocytic and monocytic lineages, often presenting with anemia and thrombocytopenia. The hallmark and an important diagnostic indicator of JMML is hypersensitivity of myeloid progenitors to granulocyte-monocyte colony–stimulating factor *in vitro*. Approximately 75% of JMML is diagnosed in children <3 years of age with a male predominance of 2:1, and 10% of cases occur in children with neurofibromatosis type I (NF1) (1,103).

Cytogenetic abnormalities are seen in approximately 35% of JMML; –7/del(7q) is most frequent accounting for 25%. In patients presenting with both JMML and NF1, acquired uniparental isodisomy of regions on 17q resulting in duplication of the mutant *NF1* allele were identified in the malignant cells (104,105). The loss of *NF1* function is associated with RAS hyperactivity, since NF1 negatively regulates RAS function (106). Similar studies have also identified CN-LOH regions on 11q that result in homozygosity for *CBL* mutations (95,107,108), which is associated with a high rate of spontaneous resolution of disease (109–111).

Mutations in numerous genes have been identified in JMML, and converge on the RAS/MAPK pathway. The most frequently observed mutations occur in *NF1*, *NRAS*, *KRAS*, *PTPN11*, and *CBL*, indicating that aberrant signal transduction of RAS-dependent pathways plays a critical role in the pathogenesis of this disease (103).

MYELODYSPLASTIC SYNDROMES

The MDSs are a group of heterogeneous clonal HSC diseases characterized by cytopenias, morphologic dysplasia, ineffective hematopoiesis, and increased propensity to develop AML (1). The current classification of MDS is mainly based on blast count and morphologic findings; however, the presence of specific abnormalities, for example, del(5q), –7/del(7q), in the context of refractory cytopenia without morphologic evidence of dysplasia is considered presumptive evidence for MDS (1). The frequency of chromosomal abnormalities in MDS correlates with the severity of disease. Clonal abnormalities can be detected in 40% to 100% of primary MDS at diagnosis (Table 9.2), and the proportion varies with the risk of transformation to AML (112–114). Only 10% to 25% of low-grade MDS cases, refractory cytopenias with unilineage dysplasia (RCUD)

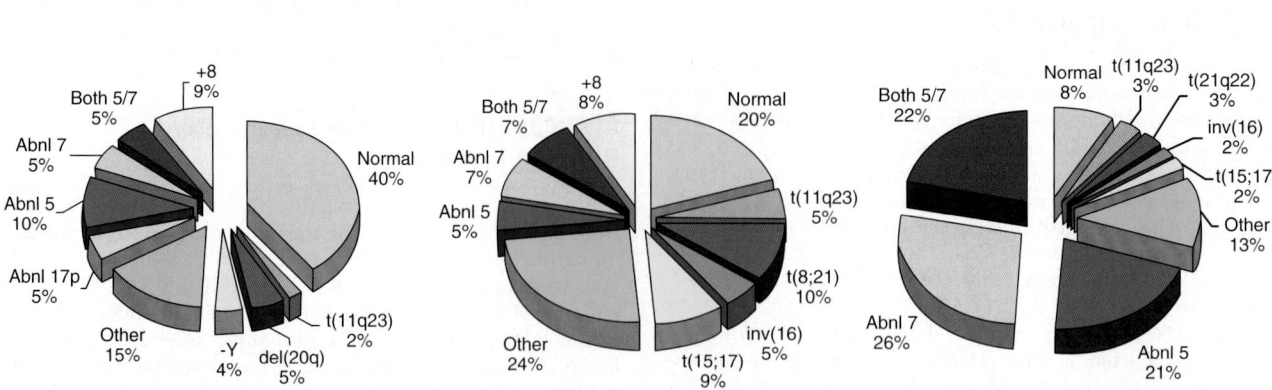

FIGURE 9.2. Frequency of recurring chromosomal abnormalities in primary MDS, AML *de novo*, and t-MN.

and refractory anemia with ring sideroblasts (RARS), have clonal abnormalities, whereas 50% to 70% of the high-grade cases, refractory cytopenia with multilineage dysplasia (RCMD) and refractory anemia with excess blasts (RAEB), present with abnormal karyotypes (1).

Most recurring cytogenetic abnormalities found in MDS are unbalanced, often presenting as loss of a whole chromosome, deletion of part of a chromosome, or an unbalanced translocation. The most common abnormalities are +8, del(5q), −7/del(7q), and del(20q) (Fig. 9.2). Of note, the recurrent balanced translocations, such as t(15;17) and t(8;21), that are closely associated with distinct morphologic subsets in *de novo* AML are rarely seen in MDS (112). The WHO classification identified several clonal cytogenetic abnormalities in MDS that are not definitive evidence for this disorder in the absence of morphologic criteria, for example, +8, −Y, or del(20q).

Although morphologic classification systems are valuable as benchmarks for the diagnosis of MDS (115), they have been less useful for the determination of prognosis, prompting the development of prognostic scoring systems. The International Prognostic Scoring System (IPSS), described in 1977, incorporated diagnostic karyotype, BM blast percentage, and number of cytopenias as critical prognostic factors, and is the most widely used and validated prognostic scoring system for MDS (116). Limitations of the IPSS are (a) the study was validated in previously untreated patients with *de novo* MDS, which limits the ability to use this tool to predict outcomes in patients with MDS treated using contemporary therapies and approaches; (b) the severity of cytopenias is not taken into account; and (c) a limited number of cytogenetic abnormalities were included in the stratification of risk groups. These limitations have led to the development of other scoring systems, as well as the recent release of a revised IPSS (IPSS-R) (114,117). For example, the WHO Prognostic Scoring System incorporated WHO subtype, transfusion dependency, and IPSS cytogenetic risk groups to provide a dynamic prognostic scoring system that has the advantage of being applicable throughout the course of the disease (117,118).

The newly released IPSS-R evaluated a much larger international database of MDS patients ascertained from multiple institutions (114). Although diagnostic karyotype, BM blast percentage, and cytopenias remain the basis of the new system, major refinements have been made to improve the precision of prognostic stratification. The most important changes are the integration of additional cytogenetic abnormalities (16 vs. 6 in the IPSS) into the scoring system, the definition of five (very good, good, intermediate, poor, and very poor) rather than three distinct cytogenetic subgroups, expansion of the ranges of marrow blast percentages, and incorporation of the severity of cytopenias. Other factors that were analyzed in the IPSS-R

model, such as patient age, performance status, serum ferritin, and lactate dehydrogenase, were found to influence survival, but not transformation to AML. Overall, the new IPSS-R stratifies patients into five rather than four prognostic categories, and many patients who were previously placed within the intermediate-1 and -2 categories were more accurately separated using the five IPSS-R categories (114).

Major advances in the classification of cytogenetic risk groups in the IPSS-R were made by integrating more abnormalities as well as stratifying based on the number of abnormalities, creating new subgroups within the heterogeneous category of complex karyotypes. The IPSS-R incorporated those abnormalities considered in the original IPSS [normal karyotype, −Y, del(5q), −7/del(7q), del(20q), and complex karyotype], as well as additional abnormalities [inv(3)/t(3q)/del(3q), +8, del(11q), del(12p), i(17q), +19, and +21] (Table 9.2) (114).

Deletions of Chromosome 5

Loss of genetic material from the long arm of chromosome 5 is the most common cytogenetic abnormality (15% to 20%) observed in primary MDS cases, and is also observed in approximately 40% of therapy-related MDS associated with previous exposure to high-dose alkylating agent chemotherapy (119–121). The presence of 5q deletions in the context of a complex karyotype predicts a poor prognosis with rapid progression to leukemia, resistance to treatment, and shorter overall survival. Conversely, MDS with an isolated del(5q) constitutes a distinct clinical syndrome, originally named "the 5q− syndrome" (122), that is associated with the most favorable outcome of any MDS subtype (113,114). MDS with an isolated del(5q) is characterized by macrocytic anemia, splenomegaly, normal to elevated platelet counts, and hypolobated megakaryocytes in the BM, and occurs predominantly in older women (1). Notably, *JAK2* mutations have been identified in rare cases of MDS with an isolated del(5q) (59–61). The clinical and pathologic features of this small subset of patients are not yet clear; thus, it is most appropriate at present to classify these cases as MDS with an isolated del(5q) instead of as a MDS/MPN, and to indicate the presence of the *JAK2* mutation in the diagnosis (123).

The breakpoints of the del(5q) and hence the deleted regions are variable in nature; however, most patients have larger deletions that encompass approximately 70 Mb. An analysis of the breakpoints and deleted regions of 5q in MDS or AML has resulted in the identification of two distinct commonly deleted regions (CDRs). The proximal region located at band 5q31.2 is associated with t-MDS and the more aggressive forms of MDS and AML; molecular analysis of this CDR is described later in the therapy-related myeloid neoplasms (t-MN) section (124,125).

The distal region at 5q33.1 is associated with MDS with an isolated del(5q) (126). Despite careful molecular analyses, including sequencing of these regions of interest on 5q in MDS or AML samples, no pathogenetic mutations were found on the remaining alleles on the intact chromosome 5 homolog (119,126–128). Moreover, even though acquired CN-LOH is commonly observed in MDS cases, this phenomenon has not been seen on 5q (127). Together, these findings support the hypothesis that haploinsufficiency for one or more genes on 5q is involved in the pathogenesis of this disease, rather than the biallelic inactivation of a tumor suppressor gene (TSG) (129).

RPS14, a gene involved in ribosomal function, was initially identified as a critical gene in the development of MDS with an isolated del(5q) through a functional RNA interference screen of genes in the 5q33.1 region (130). Knockdown of *RPS14* altered the differentiation of cells and recapitulated the erythroid phenotype of this disease. Further studies have shown that down-regulation of *Rps14* in mouse hematopoietic progenitor cells blocks differentiation and increases apoptosis of erythroid cells in a TP53-dependent manner (131). Interestingly, Diamond-Blackfan anemia (DBA), which presents with the same severe macrocytic anemia as MDS with an isolated del(5q), is also caused by haploinsufficiency of other ribosomal proteins (132). Recent studies have revealed that haploinsufficiency for microRNAs, *miR-145* and *miR-146a*, encoded by sequences near the *RPS14* gene cooperate with *RPS14*. The Toll-interleukin-1 receptor domain–containing adaptor protein and *FLI1* are targets of these miRNAs. Haploinsufficiency of miR-145 may account for several features of MDS with an isolated del(5q), including megakaryocytic dysplasia; however, neither *RPS14* nor miR-145 haploinsufficiency is predicted to confer clonal dominance (133,134).

Loss of Chromosome 7 and del(7q)

The presence of monosomy 7 or deletions of the long arm of chromosome 7 is associated with a poor prognosis (93,113), and is observed in isolation or as part of a complex karyotype in approximately 10% of patients with MDS; the frequency increases to 55% in t-MDS (135). In contrast to MDS with an isolated del(5q), "monosomy 7 syndrome" is associated with a poor prognosis and occurs primarily in young children, with 80% of patients being male (136,137). The prognostic significance of a del(7q) versus loss of the whole chromosome (–7) has been controversial, which may reflect the complexity of the karyotype. The IPSS-R found that del(7q) as the sole abnormality was associated with an "intermediate prognosis" (median survival, 2.7 years), whereas –7 as the sole abnormality was associated with a "poor prognosis" (median survival, 1.5 years). However, either abnormality in the context of a double abnormality or three abnormalities was classified as a "poor prognostic subgroup," and as a "very poor prognostic subgroup" when there were more than three abnormalities (114). Molecular analysis of the –7/del(7q) is described in the t-MN section.

Gain of Chromosome 8

A gain of chromosome 8 is observed in approximately 10% of patients, and occurs in all MDS subgroups; trisomy 8 is currently categorized as intermediate risk (93,113,114,138). Patients with an isolated +8 respond well to immunosuppressive therapy (139). However, determining the significance of the gain of chromosome 8 in MDS is complicated in that +8 is often associated with other recurring abnormalities in different prognostic groups, such as abnormalities of chromosomes 5 and 7. An isolated +8 may also be seen in an independent clone, unrelated to the primary clone, in up to 5% of MDS cases. Hematopoietic cells with trisomy 8 express higher levels of antiapoptotic genes, which may contribute to the development of malignant disease.

Loss of the Y Chromosome

Loss of the Y chromosome as a sole abnormality in MDS confers a favorable prognosis (113,114). The clinicopathologic significance is unclear, since –Y is also found in aging healthy men without hematologic disease (140,141). Empirically, the presence of –Y in >75% of BM cells accurately predicts malignant disease.

20q Deletions

A deletion of the long arm of chromosome 20 is seen in approximately 5% of MDS and 7% of t-MDS patients (112,142). Although the presence of del(20q) as the sole abnormality confers a favorable prognosis, the presence of del(20q) in the context of a complex karyotype is considered a poor prognostic indicator (113,114). A CDR containing 19 genes has been identified on 20q; however, the relationship of those genes to the pathogenesis of myeloid neoplasms is not yet clear (143,144).

Rare Recurring Translocations

Recurrent rearrangements involving 3q26.2, such as the inv(3)(q21q26.2) and t(3;21)(q26.2;q22), have been identified in rare cases of MDS and are associated with a poor prognosis (93,113,114). These abnormalities may occur as a sole anomaly, but are often associated with the presence of –7/del(7q) and, less frequently, del(5q). Breakpoints typically involve the *EVI1/MECOM* gene and rearrangements usually lead to overexpression of *EVI1/MECOM*. Overexpression of *EVI1/MECOM* is associated with a poor outcome even in the absence of abnormalities of 3q26.2 (145,146).

Translocations involving the *MLL* (*KMT2A*) gene on 11q23 are noted in 3% to 5% of patients with t-MDS and rarely in primary MDS, and confer a poor prognosis (147–150). The MLL protein is a histone methyltransferase that confers the H3K4me3 mark on histones of target gene promoters and regulates gene transcription. The most common translocations in t-MDS are the t(9;11)(p22;q23) and t(11;16)(q23;p13.3) (151).

Complex Karyotypes

Complex karyotypes are defined by the presence of three or more chromosomal abnormalities. Complex karyotypes are observed in approximately 20% of patients with primary MDS, and in as many as 90% of patients with t-MDS, and are associated with a poor prognosis (112–114). In primary MDS, patients with complex karyotypes with >3 abnormalities (overall survival median of 5.7 months) had a significantly poorer outcome than those with exactly three abnormalities (median of 15.6 months). Abnormalities involving chromosome 5 are present in most cases with complex karyotypes (113).

Molecular Mutations

In addition to the cytogenetic abnormalities discussed above, there is overwhelming evidence that gene mutations play an important role in the pathogenesis and progression of MDS. The involved genes fall into several main classes, namely, genes regulating the DNA damage response, genes encoding hematopoietic transcription factors or proteins that regulate cytokine signaling pathways, proteins that regulate chromatin structure, and proteins regulating mRNA splicing. An increase in the frequency of molecular mutations from low-risk to high-risk MDS or AML evolving from MDS emphasizes the role of these mutations in disease progression (152). The integration of the mutation profile into diagnostic classification and prognostic scoring systems will further stratify MDS into subsets with more consistent clinical phenotypes and prognosis.

INHERITED BONE MARROW FAILURE SYNDROMES ASSOCIATED WITH MYELOID MALIGNANCIES

Inherited BM failure syndromes are rare disorders generally characterized by failure of the BM to produce sufficient blood cells as well as an elevated risk of developing cancer. Great strides have been made in identifying genetic lesions underlying these disorders, making it possible to confirm or exclude a clinical diagnosis in many cases (153,154).

Fanconi anemia (FA) is the most frequent inherited cause of BM failure with a strong predisposition to developing hematologic malignancies, specifically MDS and AML. FA cells display a hallmark feature of increased chromosomal breakage upon exposure to cross-linking agents, such as mitomycin C, suggesting a defect in repair of cross-linked DNA. Indeed, mutations in at least 15 different genes (named *FANC* genes), including *BRCA2*, involved in the repair of interstrand cross-linked DNA during replication have been identified in FA patients (155). It is thought that the background of deficient hematopoiesis coupled with continuous genomic instability in FA cells exerts a strong selective pressure toward clonal evolution resulting in the development of malignancies.

Approximately 40% to 50% of FA patients develop MDS/AML by the age of 50 (156), and specific patterns of acquired chromosomal abnormalities have been identified, including add(1q), add(3q), −7/del(7q), and del(11q) (157–159). Additionally, cryptic alterations involving *RUNX1* on chromosome 21 are observed in about 20% of FA patients with MDS (159). Although −7/del(7q) and *RUNX1* abnormalities are common in non-FA cases of MDS/AML, add(1q) and add(3q), abnormalities appear to be specific to FA. The presence of an isolated add(1q) abnormality has been routinely observed in cells of FA patients before the development of dysplasia and may persist for years without progression to MDS or AML (159).

Shwachman-Diamond syndrome (SDS) is an autosomal recessive disorder characterized by hematologic features of neutropenia and an increased predisposition to leukemia. More than 90% of individuals with SDS carry biallelic mutations of the *SBDS* gene (located at 7q11.23) involved in ribosome biogenesis, and approximately 30% to 40% go on to develop MDS/AML by the age of 30 years (153). Chromosome 7 abnormalities and 20q deletions are common in SDS patients with MDS/AML. Although i(7q) is frequently observed in BM cells from patients with SDS, it is surprisingly not present in the AML cells, suggesting that this abnormality does not contribute to leukemic transformation (160).

Severe congenital neutropenia (SCN) is characterized by low neutrophil count and the arrest of myeloid precursors at the promyelocyte stage of differentiation. Approximately 30% of individuals with SCN carry heterozygous mutations of the *ELANE* gene (located at 19p13.3). Mutations in *HAX1* and *WAS* have also been identified (153). The development of MDS/AML in SCN patients is often preceded by clonal expansion of cells with mutations in the *CSF3R* (G-CSFR) gene, making the presence of *CSF3R* mutations highly predictive of leukemic transformation (161). Additional aberrations including −7/del(7q) as well as mutations in *RUNX1*, *NRAS*, *KRAS*, and *KIT* have also been observed in SCN patients with MDS/AML (162).

Other inherited BM failure syndromes include dyskeratosis congenita, shown to be caused by mutations in genes associated with telomere function (163), and DBA, in which mutations in nine different ribosomal protein genes currently account for approximately 50% of DBA cases (153).

ACUTE MYELOID LEUKEMIA

AML is a clinically, morphologically, and genetically heterogeneous disease resulting from the aberrant clonal expansion of myeloid blasts involving one or more lineages that have altered hematopoietic properties of proliferation, differentiation, and self-renewal (1). Clonal cytogenetic abnormalities are detected in 50% to 80% of cases (Table 9.2; Fig. 9.2). The most recent WHO classification system recognizes the impact of genetic alterations in defining biologically distinct subsets of AML, and has thus categorized a majority of AMLs according to the presence of recurrent genetic abnormalities: t(8;21)(q22;q22)/*RUNX1-RUNX1T1(AML1-ETO)*, inv(16)(p13.1q22) or t(16;16)(p13.1;q22)/*CBFB-MYH11*, t(15;17)(q24.1;q21.1)/*PML-RARA*, t(9;11)(p22;q23)/*MLLT3-MLL*, t(6;9)(p23;q34)/*DEK-NUP214*, inv(3)(q21q26.2) or t(3;3)(q21;q26.2)/*RPN1-EVI1 (RPN1-MECOM)*, and t(1;22)(p13;q13)/*RBM15-MKL1* (1,4,164). Although the diagnosis of AML is based on a percentage of blast cells exceeding 20%, a diagnosis of AML can be made regardless of blast cell count if there is an associated t(8;21), inv(16), t(16;16), or t(15;17). It is not yet clear if cases with the t(9;11), t(6;9), inv(3), t(3;3), or t(1;22) should be classified as AML when the blast cell count does not reach the 20% threshold (1,164). The MDS-related chromosomal alterations commonly observed in AML, such as −7/del(7q) and del(5q), are encompassed by a separate category "AML with myelodysplasia-related changes" (1).

In addition to playing a role in classification, the cytogenetic pattern is also the most powerful independent prognostic factor in AML, and is the basis for the current stratification of patients with respect to complete remission rate, risk of relapse, and treatment options. The various cytogenetic abnormalities are typically categorized into favorable, intermediate (standard), or adverse risk groups. Risk stratification and therapeutic strategies are being further refined based on age at diagnosis and the presence of additional genetic aberrations (3,4).

In recent years, a major advance in the leukemia field has been the explosion of recurrent gene mutations identified in AML (3,17), providing significant insight into the regulation of normal hematopoiesis and the critical mechanisms and pathways that promote leukemogenesis. Molecular profiling has revealed that the genetic profile in AML is not only heterogeneous, but complex. For example, the subgroup of AML with a normal karyotype (20% to 50% of newly diagnosed AML) is genetically heterogeneous, and mutations in *FLT3* and *NPM1* are common in this group. Moreover, multiple aberrations cooperate in a multistep process to give rise to leukemogenesis, including a combination of genetic aberrations that impair myeloid differentiation, promote proliferation, and enhance survival of the neoplastic clone (165).

Although mutations in a number of genes, such as *FLT3*, *NPM1*, *CEBPA*, *KIT*, *IDH1*, *IDH2*, *WT1*, *RUNX1*, *MLL*, and others, have been detected in AML, only the mutation status of *NPM1*, *CEBPA*, and *FLT3* has been shown to date to have independent prognostic significance, and has been integrated into clinical practice to inform diagnosis, risk assessment, and the selection of therapy (3,17). Indeed, one of the most significant changes in the current WHO classification is the inclusion of "AML with *NPM1* mutations" and "AML with *CEPBA* mutations" as provisionary subtypes within the "AML with recurrent genetic abnormalities" category (1). Although *FLT3* mutations are not considered an independent provisional subtype due to the presence of these mutations in several different entities, *FLT3* mutation status is, nonetheless, an important prognostic factor, and should be tested in cytogenetically normal, if not all, cases of AML (1).

Acute Myeloid Leukemia with Recurrent Genetic Abnormalities

AML with t(8;21)(q22;q22)/RUNX1-RUNX1T1(AML1-ETO)

The t(8;21)(q22;q22)/*RUNX1-RUNX1T1(AML1-ETO)* is observed in approximately 5% of AML cases, occurring predominantly in younger patients, and is associated with a favorable prognosis (4,166–168). AML cases with t(8;21) usually show maturation in the neutrophil lineage, an increase in eosinophil precursors, and the presence of Auer rods. There is an increased incidence of extramedullary disease associated with this abnormality (1). Approximately 70% of AML cases with t(8;21) display additional chromosomal abnormalities, such as del(9q), –Y, or –X, which do not adversely impact outcome (4,167,168).

At the molecular level, the t(8;21) is important because it involves an essential transcription factor pathway in hematopoiesis. In the t(8;21), the *RUNX1* gene on 21q22 is fused to the *RUNX1T1* gene on 8q22, and results in a RUNX1-RUNX1T1 chimeric protein. The RUNX1 protein (also known as core binding factor α, CBFA2) heterodimerizes with another protein, CBFB, to form a transcription factor. The *CBFB* gene is located at 16q22 at the breakpoint of the inv(16)/t(16;16). The RUNX1/CBFB transcription factor complex regulates gene expression by binding directly to an enhancer core motif that is present in the regulatory regions of a number of genes that are critical to hematopoietic stem and progenitor cell development as well as myeloid cell differentiation. The RUNX1-RUNX1T1 fusion protein functions by interfering with normal activation of gene expression by the RUNX1/CBFB transcription factor complex. Moreover, RUNX1-RUNX1T1 has gained a new function within the cell and is capable of activating expression of the *MDM2* gene, resulting in suppression of the TP53 pathway. Transformation by *RUNX1-RUNX1T1* likely results from altered transcriptional regulation of normal RUNX1 target genes, combined with the activation of new target genes that prevent programmed cell death or cause aberrant proliferation (169,170).

Mutations in *KIT*, a gene that encodes the receptor for stem cell factor, are found in 20% to 25% of t(8;21)-associated AML cases, and have been associated with an inferior outcome in several studies (171,172). Patients with *KIT* mutations have higher WBC counts and an increased prevalence of extramedullary disease. Clinical trials assessing the efficacy of KIT inhibitors are under way. Furthermore, *KRAS* and *NRAS* mutations have been observed in up to 30% of pediatric AML with the t(8;21) or inv(16)/t(16;16) (173).

AML with inv(16)(p13.1q22) or t(16;16)(p13.1;q22)/CBFB-MYH11

AML with the inv(16)(p13.1q22) or t(16;16)(p13.1;q22)/*CBFB-MYH11*, is characterized by a distinct abnormal eosinophil component, and monocytic and granulocytic differentiation (1,168,174), and accounts for 5% to 8% of all AML. These rearrangements are associated with a good prognosis (167,168). The inv(16)/t(16;16) is a subtle abnormality that may be overlooked by conventional cytogenetic analysis; thus, some laboratories incorporate FISH or RT-PCR methods to detect the *CBFB-MYH11* fusion at diagnosis. A distinct pattern of additional cytogenetic abnormalities is seen in approximately 40% of AML cases with the inv(16)/t(16;16), the most common being +8, +22, +21, and del(7q). Although +8 is often observed in isolation or with an assortment of primary aberrations, +22 is almost never detected with other abnormalities in AML and is quite specific to the inv(16)/t(16;16), and predicts a better outcome (4,167,175). Similar to AML with the t(8;21), mutations in the *KIT* gene have been found in 30% of inv(16)/t(16;16) AML, and are associated with a poor prognosis (171,172).

The inversion breakpoint at 16q22 occurs within the *CBFB* gene, which encodes one subunit of the heterodimeric RUNX1/CBFB transcription factor, whereas the breakpoint at 16p13.1 disrupts the *MYH11* gene that encodes a smooth muscle myosin heavy chain. The resulting chimeric protein consists of the 5′ region of *CBFB*, including the domain that heterodimerizes with *RUNX1*, fused to the 3′ portion of *MYH11* containing a repeated α helical structure involved in myosin filament interactions that may cause multimerization of the fusion protein. Although the precise mechanism by which the CBFB-MYH11 fusion protein mediates leukemogenesis is not yet clear, several models have been proposed: multimeric CBFB-MYH11 aberrantly activates RUNX1; CBFB-MYH11 sequesters RUNX1 preventing its access to DNA-binding sites; and CBFB-MYH11 interferes with the normal function of RUNX1 through steric hindrance (169,174,176).

AML with the inv(16)/t(16;16) has a number of similarities to AML with the t(8;21), and they are jointly referred to as core-binding factor (CBF) AML (169,170,174). At the molecular level, both involve the genes encoding the CBF, a heterodimeric transcription factor that is required for hematopoiesis. Second, they both have distinctive morphologic phenotypes. Third, they both have a good overall prognosis. Fourth, they both frequently have mutations in the *KIT* gene.

Acute Promyelocytic Leukemia with t(15;17)(q24.1;q21.1)/PML-RARA

APL, including the microgranular variant, is characterized by the t(15;17)(q24.1;q21.1)/*PML-RARA* and a predominance of abnormal promyelocytes in the BM and PB, and accounts for 5% to 8% of all AML (177,178). Establishing an accurate diagnosis of APL with the typical t(15;17) is important, because this disease is sensitive to therapy with all trans-retinoic acid (ATRA) (179), whereas other cases of AML, and some of the APL-like disorders associated with variant *RARA* translocations, do not respond to this treatment (180). APL cases treated with the appropriate ATRA and anthracycline regimen have a more favorable prognosis than any other cytogenetic subtype (4). Additional cytogenetic abnormalities are observed in 40% of cases, with +8 being the most common, and have no impact on the prognosis of APL patients (181). Furthermore, approximately 34% to 45% of APL cases have *FLT3* mutations, with internal tandem duplications (ITDs) being the most common. Cases with *FLT3*-ITD mutations have a higher WBC count, microgranular blast cell morphology, and involvement of a specific breakpoint on PML (bcr3); however, the prognostic significance is not yet clear (182,183).

The t(15;17) breakpoint at 17q21.1 occurs within the first intron of the α retinoic acid receptor gene (*RARA*) in most patients, whereas the break at 15q24.1 occurs within the *PML* gene. The RARA protein is a member of a superfamily of nuclear hormone receptors. These proteins have a ligand-binding domain that mediates binding to steroid hormones, including RA, a DNA-binding domain that mediates binding to regulatory elements of target genes, and a dimerization domain that permits heterodimerization with retinoid X receptors (RXRs), a second class of nuclear retinoid receptors. The RA-receptor complex acts as a transcription factor to induce gene expression, and thereby regulates cellular differentiation of myeloid progenitors. The t(15;17) results in a fusion *PML-RARA* gene that contains most of the *PML* coding sequences, and the DNA-binding and ligand-binding domains of the *RARA* gene. The PML RING finger protein is a critical component of the RA pathway, and its absence results in failure of myeloid precursor cells to undergo terminal differentiation. Through its ability to heterodimerize with PML and RXR, the PML-RARA fusion protein is thought to interfere with PML and RAR/RXR RA pathways, acting as a double-dominant negative oncogenic protein (177,178,184).

A small proportion of patients have morphologic features resembling APL and are characterized by variant translocations involving *RARA* (185,186). These variant *RARA* rearrangements include the t(5;17)(q35;q21.1) with the *NPM1* gene, the t(11;17)(q23;q21.1) with *ZBTB16/PLZF*, the t(11;17)(q13;q21.1) with *NUMA1*, the t(4;17)(q12;q21.1) with *FIP1L1*, and the t(X;17)(p11;q21.1) with *BCOR*, as well as 17q alterations involving the *PRKAR1A* and *STAT5B* genes (185–191). Sensitivity to ATRA treatment has been demonstrated in patients with *RARA* translocations involving *PML* (15q22), *NPM1* (5q35), *NUMA1* (11q13), and *FIP1L1* (4q12) (180). However, leukemias with *ZBTB16-RARA* and *STAT5B-RARA* fusions are resistant to ATRA (187,191). Using the most recent WHO classification criteria, cases with variant translocations are diagnosed as "AML with a variant *RARA* translocation."

AML with the t(9;11)(p22;q23)/MLLT3-MLL

Over 100 different rearrangements involving the *MLL* gene at 11q23 have been identified (192). In contrast to the previous framework of encompassing all 11q23 abnormalities in a single category, the t(9;11)(p22;q23)/*MLLT3-MLL* is now considered a distinct entity in AML. This rearrangement is the most common *MLL* translocation in AML, accounting for 2% of adult and 9% to 12% of pediatric patients, and is associated with monocytic features and an intermediate prognosis that is better than AML with other 11q23 rearrangements (4,193,194). Additional cytogenetic abnormalities may be observed, with +8 being the most common, but do not appear to affect outcome (193,195). Other common *MLL* translocations in AML include the t(6;11)(q27;q23) involving *MLLT4(AF6)* and the t(11;19)(q23;p13.3) involving ENL. Although these *MLL* rearrangements occur predominantly in AML, they are also observed rarely in ALL (192,196).

MLL is a DNA-binding protein that methylates histone H3 lysine 4 (H3K4), and positively regulates gene expression by binding to open chromatin structures at the active promoter regions of various genes, including multiple *HOX* genes, that are important in hematopoietic and lymphoid cell development (197,198). The MLL protein contains one potential DNA-binding motif (AT-hooks), a transcriptional activation domain (SET domain) in the COOH-terminus, and a repression domain in the N-terminal portion. Translocations of *MLL* result in the formation of a chimeric gene on the derivative 11 chromosome through juxtaposition of the 5′ region of *MLL* and the 3′ region of the partner gene. The AT hook DNA-binding motif and repression domain of MLL are retained in the fusion protein, but the strong activation domain is lost, leading to the absence of the H3K4 methyltransferase activity (199). A key feature of MLL fusion proteins is their ability to efficiently transform hematopoietic cells into leukemia stem cells. In addition to the contribution of altered *MLL* function to leukemogenesis, the partner gene also appears to be important (197,198). Consistent with this hypothesis is the observation that AML occurs in chimeric mice containing an *MLLT3-MLL* fusion gene from a t(9;11), but not in mice with a disrupted *MLL* gene (200). At least four subgroups of *MLL* partner genes with various putative functions have been identified. Fusions with nuclear DNA-binding proteins account for most MLL rearrangements. Additional partner subgroups include cytoplasmic proteins with coiled-coil oligomerization domains, histone acetyltransferases, and several others; however, only a few key MLL rearrangements have been extensively characterized (201).

AML with the t(6;9)(p23;q34)/DEK-NUP214

The t(6;9)(p23;q34)/*DEK-NUP214* is observed in approximately 1% of AML cases, often as the sole cytogenetic abnormality, and is associated with a poor prognosis (4,195,202). This subtype of AML typically presents with marked basophilia, pancytopenia, and multilineage dysplasia (203). *FLT3* ITD mutations are extremely common in AML with the t(6;9), occurring in 69% of pediatric and 78% of adult patients, and may contribute to the adverse outcome associated with this subtype (204). The t(6;9) forms an aberrant fusion protein through juxtaposition of the *NUP214(CAN)* gene on 9q34 to the 3′ end of the *DEK* gene on 6p23 (203). *NUP214* encodes a component of the nuclear pore complex that permits proper transfer of mRNA and proteins across the nuclear membrane. The resulting NUP214-DEK nucleoporin fusion protein alters nuclear transport, and also acts as an aberrant transcription factor (205).

AML with the inv(3)(q21q26.2) or t(3;3)(q21;q26.2)/RPN1-MECOM(RPN1-EVI1)

AML with the inv(3)(q21q26.2) or t(3;3)(q21;q26.2)/*RPN1-MECOM (RPN1-EVI1)* accounts for 1% to 2% of all AML, and is characterized by thrombocytosis, increased atypical megakaryocytes in the BM (206), and a poor prognosis (4,207). Additional cytogenetic abnormalities are frequent, with monosomy 7 occurring in approximately 50% of cases, followed by 5q deletions and complex karyotypes (207). The *MECOM (EVI1)* gene, located at 3q26.2, is aberrantly expressed due to chromosomal rearrangements 5′ of the gene in the t(3;3) or 3′ of the gene in the inv(3) via juxtaposition of the gene with enhancer elements of the *RPN1* ribophorin gene located at 3q21 (208,209). MECOM is a transcription factor that contains a seven-zinc-finger domain at the N-terminal end, a three-finger domain in the central portion, and an acidic domain distal to the second group of zinc fingers. Depending on its binding partners, MECOM can act as a transcriptional activator to promote the proliferation of HSCs or as a transcriptional repressor inhibiting erythroid differentiation. Aberrant *MECOM* expression results in increased proliferation and impaired differentiation (208,209). Abnormal expression of *MECOM* has also been detected in AML patients with a normal karyotype, and is associated with a poor outcome, suggesting that inappropriate activation of this gene occurs through alternative mechanisms (210).

AML with the t(1;22)(p13;q13)/RBM15-MKL1

AML with the t(1;22)(p13;q13)/*RBM15-MKL1* is a rare entity (<1% of AML), and is characterized by an abundance of megakaryoblasts, presenting mainly in young children and infants, especially in the first 6 months of life. Notably, the t(1;22) is not seen in AML arising in children with Down syndrome (DS) (211,212). The prognosis of AML with the t(1;22) is not clear; however, recent studies have found that these patients respond well to intensive AML chemotherapy (213). The t(1;22) results in juxtaposition of *RBM15* at 1p13, a gene encoding a RNA-binding protein, with *MKL1* (22q13), a gene encoding a DNA-binding protein involved in chromatin organization. The function of the RBM15-MKL1 fusion protein is poorly understood, but may involve modulation of chromatin organization, HOX-mediated differentiation, or extracellular signaling pathways (212,214).

AML with Mutated NPM1 (Provisional WHO Entity)

NPM1 mutations, predominantly in exon 12, are observed in approximately 30% of *de novo* AML and up to 50% of cytogenetically normal AML. The prevalence increases with age (215,216). AML with mutated *NPM1* is characterized by aberrant cytoplasmic expression of NPM1 and prominent myelomonocytic or monocytic features (215,216). Mutations in *NPM1* are usually associated with a normal karyotype and tend to be mutually exclusive with other cytogenetic abnormalities in the "AML with recurrent genetic abnormalities" category, and with *CEBPA* mutations (217). However, approximately 40% of *NPM1*-mutated AML cases also have *FLT3* mutations (215). AML with *NPM1* mutations without concurrent *FLT3* ITD mutations has a good prognosis, comparable to CBF AML (218).

AML with Mutated CEBPA (Provisional WHO Entity)

CEBPA mutations are observed in 6% to 15% of *de novo* AML and 15% to 18% of cytogenetically normal AML. Two types of *CEBPA* mutations—truncating mutations in the N-terminus and insertions or deletions near the C-terminus—have been identified in AML. Approximately 60% of *CEBPA*-mutated AML cases present as compound heterozygous mutations, with a C-terminal mutation on one allele and an N-terminal mutation on the other (219–221). Interestingly, only biallelic mutations of *CEBPA* confer a favorable outcome. The prognosis for AML with a single *CEBPA* mutation is similar to AML with wild-type *CEBPA* (222,223).

Acute Myeloid Leukemia with Myelodysplasia-Related Changes

AML cases arising from a previous MDS, characterized by a MDS-related cytogenetic alteration in the absence of "recurrent genetic abnormalities," or displaying multilineage dysplasia may be designated in the category of "AML with myelodysplasia-related changes," representing 25% to 35% of all AML. This subtype occurs predominantly in elderly patients, and has a poor prognosis (1,224). Cytogenetic abnormalities observed in this category of AML are similar to those found in MDS, with −7/del(7q), del(5q), and complex karyotypes being the most common (112,225). Occupational or environmental exposure to mutagens, benzene exposure, and smoking have been associated with −7/del(7q), del(5q), and complex karyotypes. Although trisomy 8, del(20q), and −Y are also common in MDS, these abnormalities are not disease-specific, and by themselves are insufficient to categorize a case as AML with myelodysplasia-related changes (1). Chromosomal translocations are generally rare in this category of AML, with most translocations involving chromosome bands 5q31-q34. The t(3;5)(q25;q35) that generates the *NPM1-MLF1* fusion is associated with a younger age at presentation compared to other abnormalities in this disease group (226). Although *NPM1* and *FLT3* mutations have been detected in cases of AML with myelodysplasia-related changes, the presence of MDS-related cytogenetic abnormalities takes diagnostic precedence over detection of *NPM1* and *CEBPA* gene mutations with respect to classification (1).

AML with myelodysplasia-related changes is generally associated with an adverse outcome, in which high-risk cytogenetic abnormalities are the most significant prognostic indicators (224). A recent study distinguished a subset of AML cases with a "monosomal karyotype" that is associated with a particularly poor prognosis (227). A "monosomal karyotype" is defined as having loss of an autosomal chromosome combined with either another autosomal chromosome loss or at least one structural abnormality. Overall this classification is overly simplistic, and does not take into account the specificity of the various abnormalities; this group largely comprises cases with an adverse karyotype based on standard classification schemes, for example, −7/del(7q), del(5q), and complex karyotypes.

THERAPY-RELATED MYELOID NEOPLASMS

t-MN are a late complication of cytotoxic therapy (radiation and/or chemotherapy) used in the treatment of both malignant and nonmalignant diseases (135,228–230). These neoplasms are thought to be the direct consequence of mutational events induced by the prior therapy. Although long-term survivors of Hodgkin disease were among the first patients reported to develop t-MN, this complication is now increasingly observed in those patients who are treated for solid tumors, for example, in breast cancer patients treated with a topoisomerase II inhibitor, such as mitoxantrone. t-MN arises in most cases from a multipotential HSC or, less commonly, in a lineage-committed progenitor cell. Survival times of t-MN patients are typically short, because this disorder is less responsive to current forms of therapy than is AML *de novo* (135,228,229,231).

Several distinct cytogenetic and clinical subtypes of t-MN are recognized that are closely associated with the nature of the preceding treatment (Table 9.2). Patients who develop t-MN following alkylating agent therapy (~75% of cases) typically show a latency of 3 to 7 years from alkylating agent exposure (median 5 years), insidious disease onset with an antecedent MDS with peripheral cytopenias, and a poor prognosis (median survival, <8 months) (135,229). This subset of t-MN is typically associated with MDS-related cytogenetic abnormalities, that is, loss, deletion, or rearrangement of chromosomes 5 and/or 7, and complex karyotypes with a predominance of the loss of genetic material. Typically, all three hematopoietic cell lineages (erythroid, myeloid, and megakaryocytic) are involved in the dysplastic process (trilineage dysplasia), suggesting that the disease arises in a multipotent hematopoietic stem or progenitor cell (HSPC). Mild to marked reticulin fibrosis may be present, Auer rods are rarely seen, and myeloperoxidase and nonspecific esterase activity are often only weakly expressed (1). In contrast, patients who develop t-MN following treatment with drugs targeting topoisomerase II are younger, have a shorter latency period (2 to 3 years), and present with AML. Balanced translocations involving *MLL* at 11q23, *RUNX1* at 21q22, *CBFB* at 16q22, or *PML* (15q24.1) and *RARA* (17q21.1) are common in this subgroup, suggesting that these cytogenetic subsets of t-MN arise in a lineage-committed progenitor cell (135,228,232).

t-MN represents an important model for cancer. The incidence of t-MN is rising, as a result of the increasing number of cancer survivors at risk of developing this disorder and the changes in therapeutic trends. Secondly, t-MN provides a unique opportunity to examine the effects of mutagens on carcinogenesis in humans, as well as the role of genetic susceptibility to cancer (228,233). Finally, the mechanisms of leukemogenesis that are uncovered in t-MN will likely apply to those subtypes of AML *de novo* that share the same cytogenetic abnormalities, for example, AML *de novo* with abnormalities of chromosome 5 or 7.

The frequency of recurring abnormalities in t-MN is contrasted to that of AML *de novo* in Figure 9.2. In the University of Chicago series of 386 consecutive patients with t-MN, 349 (90.4%) had a clonal chromosomal abnormality, including 259 (67%) with a clonal abnormality leading to loss, deletion, or rearrangements of chromosomes 5 and/or 7 (referred to as del(5q)/t(5q) and −7/del(7q) herein) (135) (Le Beau MM and Larson RA, *unpublished data*). Overall, 164 patients (42%) had abnormalities of chromosome 5, and 180 (47%) had abnormalities of chromosome 7. A del(5q) was the most common structural abnormality. Complex karyotypes were associated with abnormalities of chromosome 5, rather than chromosome 7. Recurring abnormalities observed at a high frequency (>20%) in patients with del(5q) included +8, and loss of 13q, 16q, 17p (40% of cases), chromosome 18, and 20q, which frequently occurred in the same clone. Other recurring abnormalities were noted in 62 (16%) patients. Recurring translocations were most common, particularly translocations involving the *MLL* gene at 11q23 (4%), the t(8;21)/inv(16) involving the CBF genes, *RUNX1* at 21q22 and *CBFB* at 16q22, (3%), the t(15;17) involving the *PML-RARA* fusion (2%), and +8 (2.5%). Similar results have been reported in other series, with the caveat that newer series ascertained in the past decade show an increase in the percentage of cases with balanced recurring translocations, and a decrease in abnormalities in chromosomes 5 and 7, reflecting therapeutic trends (231).

Molecular Analysis of the del(5q)

Several groups of investigators have defined a CDR on the long arm of chromosome 5, band 5q31.2, predicted to contain a myeloid TSG that is involved in the pathogenesis of the more aggressive forms of MDS and AML (119,125,234). A second, distal CDR of 1.5 Mb within 5q33.1 has been identified in MDS with an isolated del(5q), and was described earlier (126). Despite intense efforts, the identification of TSGs on chromosomes 5 has been challenging, because the deletions of 5q are typically large, and encompass both of these regions. Molecular analysis of the 19 candidate genes within the CDR of 5q31.2 and 44 genes in the 5q33.1 CDR did not reveal inactivating mutations in the remaining alleles, nor was there evidence of transcriptional silencing (126–128). Moreover, CN-LOH is not seen on 5q in MDS or AML. These observations are compatible with a haploinsufficiency model in which loss of one allele of the relevant gene(s) on 5q perturbs cell fate, rather than the biallelic inactivation of a TSG (129). A number of genes and several miRNAs located on 5q, including *RPS14* (130), miRNA-145 (133,134), *EGR1* (235), *APC* (236), *CTNNA1*, *HSPA9*, and *DIAPH1* (234), have been implicated in the development of myeloid disorders due to a gene dosage effect. Key genes on 5q are reviewed below; the role of *RPS14* and miR-145 are described in the section on MDS. Together, these studies support a haploinsufficiency model, in which *loss of a single allele of more than one gene on 5q* acts in concert to alter hematopoiesis, promote self-renewal of HSPCs, induce apoptosis of hematopoietic cells, and disrupt differentiation.

APC. APC is a multifunctional tumor suppressor involved in the pathogenesis of colorectal cancer via regulation of the WNT signaling cascade. The *APC* gene is located at 5q22.2, and is deleted in >95% of patients with a del(5q) (234). Conditional inactivation of a single allele of *Apc* in mice leads to the development of severe macrocytic anemia, a block in erythropoiesis at the early stages of differentiation (proerythroblasts), and an expansion of the short-term and long-term HSCs (236). *Apc* heterozygous myeloid progenitor cells display an increased frequency of apoptosis, and decreased *in vitro* colony-forming capacity, recapitulating several characteristic features of myeloid neoplasms with a del(5q).

EGR1. The early growth response 1 gene (*EGR1*) encodes a member of the WT-1 family of zinc finger transcription factors, and mediates the cellular response to growth factors, mitogens, and stress stimuli. *EGR1* was identified as a TSG in several human tumors, including breast and non–small cell lung cancer. EGR1 is a direct transcriptional regulator of many known TSGs, for example, *TP53, CDKN1A, TGFB1,* and *PTEN. Egr1*-null mice show spontaneous mobilization of HSPCs into the periphery, identifying Egr1 as a transcriptional regulator of stem cell migration (237). In addition, Egr1, and its family member, Egr2, play a pivotal role at a later stage of hematopoiesis, specifically in lineage determination at the level of the granulocyte-monocyte progenitor (GMP), that is, in regulating differentiation into monocytes versus granulocytes. Loss of a single allele of *Egr1* cooperates with mutations induced by an alkylating agent in the development of malignant myeloid diseases in mice, indicating that *Egr1* is a haploinsufficient myeloid suppressor gene (235).

Molecular Analysis of Loss or Deletion of Chromosome 7

A –7/del(7q) is observed in approximately 50% of patients with t-MN (135,231). An emerging paradigm is that the loss of genetic material on 7q cooperates with other mutations that cause deregulated signaling of the RAS pathway in the development of these myeloid neoplasms. Activating mutations in the *NRAS* and *KRAS* genes, inactivating mutations in negative regulators of RAS proteins, such as NF1, or activating mutations in positive regulators of RAS proteins, such as the PTPN11/SHP2 phosphatase, as well as *RUNX1* mutations and methylation silencing of the *CDKN2B* (*p15^{INK4B}*) gene are associated with –7/del(7q) (232,238–240).

To date, three CDRs have been identified on 7q; however, the molecular mechanisms underlying the development of MDS and AML with del(7q) remain poorly understood. We previously identified two distinct CDRs, a 2.52 Mb CDR within 7q22 spanning the interval containing *LRRC17* and *SRPK2*, and a second, less frequent, region in q32-q33 (241). Each of the candidate genes within the CDR at 7q22 has been evaluated for mutations; however, no inactivating mutations have been identified in the remaining allele. Although mice with a conditional heterozygous deletion of this region displayed a defect in the survival of HSPCs, they have normal hematopoiesis, and do not develop malignant disease, suggesting that this region does not contain a haploinsufficient myeloid TSG, or that mutations in cooperating genes are required (242). Recently, Dohner et al. reported the analysis of a large series of patients with abnormalities of 7q using FISH. Whereas most patients had large deletions, they identified an approximately 2 Mb deleted segment in proximal q22 that overlaps with the proximal portion of the CDR we defined, but extends more proximally, and includes the *CUX1 (CUTL1), RASA4, EPO,* and *FBXL13* genes in 7q22.1 (243). This region was confirmed and refined to a 1 Mb interval in 7q22.1 spanning *TRIM56* to *CUX1* (244). As in the del(5q), the observation of reduced expression of the genes within the deleted interval and the lack of mutations in the remaining alleles suggest a haploinsufficiency model. Recent studies using transcriptome sequencing have identified the *CUX1* gene as a haploinsufficient myeloid suppressor gene at 7q22. *CUX1* encodes a lineage-determining transcription factor that regulates HSCs (245). Although the recent discovery that recurrent mutations in *EZH2*, which encodes a histone methyltransferase, located on 7q36.1 in MDS and AML may shed light on disease pathogenesis (101,246), it is unlikely to account for the phenotype associated with chromosome 7 abnormalities, since myeloid neoplasms with *EZH2* mutations do not typically coexist with –7/del(7q) abnormalities, and the del(7q) does not always result in loss of one *EZH2* allele (101,246).

In conclusion, t-MN remains one of the most adverse complications of successful therapy for a variety of malignant and nonmalignant conditions. Researchers are beginning to elucidate the factors, including genetic susceptibility, that place individual patients at risk, which are critical for individualizing therapy directed at minimizing the development of this disease. Recently, an elegant study revealed that genetic programs associated with t-MN are perturbed in hematopoietic progenitor cells long before disease onset in lymphoma patients following autologous HSC transplantation, and may identify patients at risk for this complication (247). Moreover, characterizing the genetic pathways that give rise to t-MN will lead to a greater understanding of the molecular features of the disease and, ultimately, may lead to more effective therapies.

MYELOID PROLIFERATIONS RELATED TO DOWN SYNDROME

One of the best-known examples of a genetic syndrome predisposing to leukemia is constitutional trisomy 21, otherwise known as Down syndrome. Not only do individuals with DS display a markedly elevated risk of developing both ALL and AML, young children under the age of 4 demonstrate a striking

500-fold increased incidence of developing acute megakaryo-blastic leukemia (AMKL). AMKL is characterized by a sub-stantial increase of megakaryoblasts and reticulin deposition in the BM. Megakaryoblasts are positive for platelet peroxi-dase activity, negative for myeloperoxidase, and positive for CD33, CD117, CD36, glycophorin A, CD41, and CD42 (248). There are significant cytogenetic differences between DS and non-DS acute leukemias. Although the t(1;22) discussed in a previous section is associated with AMKL in children without DS, it is absent in cases of children with DS. Furthermore, the recurrent translocations associated with AML are rarely seen in DS-AML. Instead, other cytogenetic abnormalities, such as dup(1q), del(6q), del(7p), dup(7q), +8, +11, +19, and +21, are frequently observed (249).

Interestingly, 10% of infants with DS present with a tran-sient myeloproliferative disorder (TMD), characterized by an accumulation of clonal immature megakaryoblasts in the fetal liver and PB. The majority of cases resolve spontane-ously within a few months. However, after a latency period of 1 to 3 years, approximately 20% to 30% go on to develop AMKL (248). Most notably, acquisition of mutations in the *GATA1* gene, resulting in a truncated GATA1 protein, has been observed in nearly all TMD and DS-AMKL cases (250). *GATA1* mutations have been identified in TMD patient sam-ples as early as at 21 weeks of gestation (251). In contrast, *GATA1* mutations are not seen in non-DS AMKL cases (250). *GATA1*, located on the X chromosome, encodes a transcrip-tion factor involved in regulating development of the erythroid and megakaryocytic lineages. The clonal nature of AMKL and its evolution from TMD have been demonstrated by the pres-ence of identical *GATA1* mutation clones during TMD and then later at onset of AMKL, and the disappearance of the clone at remission (252). Because of the unique clinical, morphologic, and molecular features associated with DS-related myeloid neoplasms, the most recent WHO classification has recognized "myeloid proliferations related to Down syndrome" as a dis-tinct entity under the category of "Acute myeloid leukemia and related precursor neoplasms" (123).

The natural history of leukemogenesis in individuals with DS points to trisomy 21 as one of the most identifiable risk fac-tors for the development of acute leukemia. Thus, identifying the gene(s) on chromosome 21 that contribute to DS-related malignancies will provide a broader understanding of leuke-mogenesis. A critical region of 8.35 Mb has been identified by genetic mapping studies in rare individuals with segmental tri-somies of chromosome 21 (253). A candidate gene within this interval is the *DYRK1A* gene at 21q22.13. Increased expres-sion of the DYRK1A kinase suppresses the "nuclear factor of activated T cells" pathway (thought to be cancer promoting when activated), but promotes development of AMKL (254). It is believed that the combination of a *GATA1* mutation and aberrant expression of *ERG* and *DYRK1A*, among other genes on chromosome 21, promotes TMD (254). Evolution of TMD to AMKL likely requires the acquisition of additional mutations in genes such as *MPL* and *JAK2*, which are associated with aber-rant megakaryopoiesis in the MPNs. This finding sheds light on the observation that individuals with DS have an increased risk of leukemia in childhood, but a decreased risk of solid tumors in adulthood.

PRECURSOR LYMPHOID NEOPLASMS

ALL is the most common leukemia in children, and is char-acterized by an uncontrolled clonal expansion of malignant immature lymphoid cells in the BM. ALL is broadly classi-fied as B-lineage or T-lineage ALL (1). The lymphoblasts in B-ALL are usually positive for the immunophenotypic markers

CD19, cytoplasmic CD79a, and cytoplasmic CD22, which are indicative of a B lineage. The patterns of additional nuclear, cytoplasmic, and cell surface antigens are used to distinguish the degree of differentiation of the lymphoblasts that can have distinct clinical and genetic correlates (1). T-ALL is a high-risk neoplasm of lymphoblasts committed to the T lineage, that is, classified based on the expression of specific immunopheno-typic markers (1). The most useful prognostic indicators in ALL are age, WBC count, cytogenetic pattern, immunophenotype, central nervous system (CNS) status, and MRD after initial therapy (255). It is important to emphasize that recurring cyto-genetic abnormalities distinguish B-ALL and T-ALL, and are associated with distinct outcomes, since the majority of ALL patients have clonal abnormalities (Table 9.3; Fig. 9.3). There are also notable differences in the frequency and outcome of various cytogenetic abnormalities between children and adults (256–258).

The Children's Oncology Group (COG) has sought to develop a consensus classification strategy for treatment of pediatric ALL (255). The current clinical trial for newly diagnosed ALL (COG AALL08B1) stratifies patients with B-ALL into four risk groups (low risk, average risk, high risk, and very high risk) based on age and presenting leukocyte count, initial CNS status, genetic abnormalities, day 8 PB MRD, and day 29 BM morpho-logic response and MRD. Favorable cytogenetic abnormalities include the presence of either hyperdiploidy with trisomies of chromosomes 4 and 10 (double trisomy) or the *ETV6-RUNX1* fusion. Unfavorable cytogenetic abnormalities include hypo-diploidy (<44 chromosomes), an *MLL* rearrangement, and intrachromosomal amplification of chromosome 21 (iAMP21). Other unfavorable characteristics are CNS involvement (CNS3) at diagnosis, induction failure, and age >13 years. The pres-ence of any of these unfavorable cytogenetic abnormalities or characteristics is sufficient to classify a patient as very high risk, regardless of other presenting features. The presence of the *BCR-ABL1* fusion (Ph⁺ ALL) is considered very high risk, and these patients are treated on a separate clinical trial.

B-ALL with Recurrent Genetic Abnormalities

This subgroup of ALL is characterized by recurrent genetic abnormalities that are associated with distinct clinical or phenotypic properties, as well as important prognostic impli-cations. The different categories are biologically distinct and are generally mutually exclusive of each other (1). A signifi-cant breakthrough in the understanding of ALL has been the discovery of not only structural rearrangements, but also an abundance of deletions, amplifications, and point mutations in genes that play a role in the development of ALL (259). SNP array analyses identified copy number changes in several genes involved in B-cell development and differentiation, including *PAX5*, *TCF3*, *EBF1*, *LEF1*, and *IZKF1*, or cell cycle progression, such as *CDKN2A*, *CDKN1B*, and *RB1* (260–262). DNA sequence analysis of a large cohort of childhood ALL cases resulted in the identification of *NRAS*, *KRAS*, *PAX5*, and *JAK2* as the most frequently mutated genes (263). Together, these results have determined that genes in at least four cancer signaling path-ways are involved in a majority of ALL cases: B-cell develop-ment and differentiation, RAS signaling, JAK/STAT signaling, and the TP53/RB1 tumor suppressor pathway. Integration of these newly discovered abnormalities into clinical practice will be an important focus.

ALL with the t(9;22)

The t(9;22)(q34;q11.2)/*BCR-ABL1* is the most commonly observed cytogenetic abnormality in adults with ALL (11% to 29%) (264,265), but is less common in children (2% to 5%) (255).

Table 9.3	CYTOGENETIC-IMMUNOPHENOTYPIC CORRELATIONS IN MALIGNANT LYMPHOID DISEASES

Disease[a]	Chromosome Abnormality	Frequency[b]	Involved Genes[c]		Consequence
ALL					
Precursor B	t(12;21)(p13;q22)	25%	ETV6/TEL	RUNX1/AML1	Fusion protein—TF
	t(9;22)(q34;q11.2)	10%[d]	ABL1	BCR	Fusion protein—Altered cytokine signaling pathways
	t(4;11)(q21;q23)	5%	AFF14	MLL	Fusion protein—TF
	t(17;19)(q22;p13.3)	1%	HLF	TCF3 (E2A)	Fusion protein—TF
	t(11;19)(q23;p13.3)	1%	MLL	MLLT1/ENL	Fusion protein—TF
Pre-B	t(1;19)(q23;p13.3)	6% (30%)	PBX1	TCF3 (E2A)	Fusion protein—TF
B (SIg+)	t(8;14)(q24.2;q32)	5% (95%)	MYC	IGH	Deregulated expression—TF
	t(2;8)(p12;q24.2)	<1% (1%)	IGK	MYC	Deregulated expression—TF
	t(8;22)(q24.2;q11.2)	<1% (4%)	MYC	IGL	Deregulated expression—TF
Other	Hyperdiploidy (50–60)	10%			
	del(12p),t(12p)	10%			
T	t(11;14)(p15;q11.2)	1%	LMO1	TRA	Deregulated expression—TF
	t(11;14)(p13;q11.2)	3%	LMO2	TRA	Deregulated expression—TF
	t(8;14)(q24.2;q11.2)	<1%	MYC	TRA	Deregulated expression—TF
	inv(14)(q11.2q32)	<1%	TRA	TCL1A	Deregulated expression—TF
	t(10;14)(q24;q11.2)	3%	TLX1	TRA	Deregulated expression—TF
	t(1;14)(p32;q11.2)	1%	TALI	TRD	Deregulated expression—TF
	t(7;9)(q34;q34)		TRB	NOTCH1	Deregulated expression—TF
	t(7;19)(q34;p13.2)	2%	TRB	LYL1	
	del(9p),t(9p)	<1% <1% (10%)	CDKN2A, CDKN2B		TSG—cell cycle regulation
NHL					
B-cell NHL					
Burkitt	t(8;14)(q24.2;q32)	95%	MYC	IGH	Deregulated expression—TF
	t(2;8)(p12;q24.2)	1%	IGK	MYC	Deregulated expression—TF
	t(8;22)(q24.2;q11.2)	4%	MYC	IGL	Deregulated expression—TF
Follicular SNCL	t(14;18)(q32;q21.3)	80%	IGH	BCL2	Deregulated expression—Antiapoptosis protein
DLBCL		20%			
DLBCL	t(3;22)(q27;q11.2)	45% for all	BCL6	IGL	Deregulated expression—TF
	t(3;14)(q27;q32)	t(3q27)	BCL6	IGH	Deregulated expression—TF
MCL	t(11;14)(q13;q32)	~100%	CCND1	IGH	Deregulated expression—TF
LPL	t(9;14)(p13;q32)		PAX5	IGH	Deregulated expression—TF
SLL	t(14;19)(q32;q13.3)		IGH	BCL3	Deregulated expression—TF
MALT	t(11;18)(q21;q21.3)	40%–50%	BIRC3/API2	MALT1	Fusion Protein—Increased NF-κB activation
	t(1;14)(p22;q32)	10%	BCL10	IGH	Deregulated expression—Increased NF-κB activation
	t(14;18)(q32;q21.3)	10%–20%	IGH	MALT1	Deregulated expression—Increased NF-κB activation
	t(3;14)(p13;q32)	10%	FOXP1	IGH	Deregulated expression—TF
	t(X;14)(p12;q32)	Rare	GPR34	IGH	Deregulated expression—G protein–coupled receptor
PCMZL	t(14;18)(q32;q21.3)	Rare	IGH	MALT1	Deregulated expression—Increased NFκB activation
PCFCL	t(14;18)(q32;q21.3)	40%	IGH	BCL2	Deregulated expression—Antiapoptosis protein
T-cell NHL					
ALK+ ALCL	t(2;5)(p23;q35.1)	75%	ALK	NPM1	Deregulated expression—TK
ALK− ALCL	t(6;7)(p25.3;q32.3)	10%–15%	IRF4, DUSP22		Deregulated expression of TF (IRF4) and phosphatase (DUSP22)
Nasal/NK cell	i(1q), i(7q), i(17q)				
Hepatosplenic	i(7q)	>95%			
Peripheral	t(5;9)(q33;q22)	15%	ITK	SYK	Constitutively active TK (SYK)
CLL					
B	t(11;14)(q13;q32)	10%	CCND1	IGH	Deregulated expression—Cell cycle regulation
	t(14;19)(q32;q13.2)	5%	IGH	BCL3	Deregulated expression—Increased NF-κB activation
	t(2;14)(p16;q32)	5%	BCL11A	IGH	
	t(14q32)	15%	IGH		
	del(13q)	30%			
	+12	25%			

Table 9.3	CYTOGENETIC-IMMUNOPHENOTYPIC CORRELATIONS IN MALIGNANT LYMPHOID DISEASES (Continued)				
Disease[a]	Chromosome Abnormality	Frequency[b]	Involved Genes[c]		Consequence
T	t(8;14)(q24.2;q11.2)	5%	MYC	TRA	Deregulated expression—TF
	inv(14)(q11.2q32)	5%	TRA/TRD	IGH	Deregulated expression
	inv(14)(q11.2q32)	5%	TRA/TRD	TCL1A	Deregulated expression—TF
MM					
B	−13/del(13q)	40%			
	t(4;14)(p16;q32)	15%	WHSC1/FGFR3	IGH	Deregulated expression—Growth factor receptor
			MMSET	IGH	Deregulated chromatin modification and gene expression—Histone methyltransferase
	t(14;16)(q32;q23)	5%	IGH	MAF	Deregulated expression—TF
	t(6;14)(p21;q32)	4%	CCND3	IGH	Deregulated expression—Cell cycle regulation
	t(11;14)(q13;q32)	15%	CCND1	IGH	Deregulated expression—Cell cycle regulation
	t(14q32)	50%	IGH		
	del(17p)/t(17p)	30%	TP53		Loss of function—DNA damage response
	Gain of 1q				
	Hyperdiploidy: +3, +5, +7, +9, +11	20%			
Adult T-cell Leukemia/Lymphoma					
	t(14;14)(q11.2;q32)		TRA	IGH	Deregulated expression
	inv(14)(q11.2q32)		TRA/TRD	IGH	Deregulated expression
	+3				

[a]SIg, surface immunoglobulin; DLBCL, diffuse large B-cell lymphoma; MCL, mantle cell lymphoma; LPL, lymphoplasmacytoid lymphoma; SLL, small lymphocytic lymphoma; MALT, mucosa-associated lymphoid tumor; PCMZL, primary cutaneous marginal zone lymphoma; PCFCL, primary cutaneous follicular center lymphoma; ALCL, anaplastic large cell lymphoma; CTCL, cutaneous T-cell lymphoma.
[b]The percentage refers to the frequency within the disease overall. The number in the parentheses refers to the frequency within the morphologic or immunologic subtype of the disease.
[c]Genes are listed in order of citation in karyotype, for example, for precursor B ALL, ETV6/TEL is at 12p13 and RUNX1/AML1 is at 21q22.
[d]By cytogenetic analysis, the frequency in children is about 5%, and in adults is about 25%; using molecular probes, this frequency is 30% in adults overall, and 50% in adults over 60 years of age.

The presence of the t(9;22) is associated with a poor outcome in both adult and pediatric patients, and is usually a strong indicator for consideration of allogeneic stem cell transplantation (266,267). Recently, the incorporation of TKIs into the therapeutic regimen has improved event-free survival rates and outcomes after BM transplantation. Further follow-up is required to determine whether these results will translate into increased overall survival (268). Although relapse due to the development of resistance to TKI therapy is a major concern, new-generation TKIs, such as ponatinib, are being employed to address these issues.

Molecular studies of Ph⁺ ALL have revealed two distinct subgroups (269,270). Approximately 30% to 50% of adult patients, but very few childhood ALL patients with the t(9;22), have the p210 fusion protein that is identical to that seen in CML. Many of these patients have persistent metaphase cells with the t(9;22) after chemotherapy-induced hematologic remissions. They also have the t(9;22) in myeloid cells and in myeloid colonies grown *in vitro*, suggesting that they represent cases of CML presenting in lymphoid blast crisis after an unrecognized chronic phase. The majority of children and about half of adults who have ALL with the t(9;22) produce

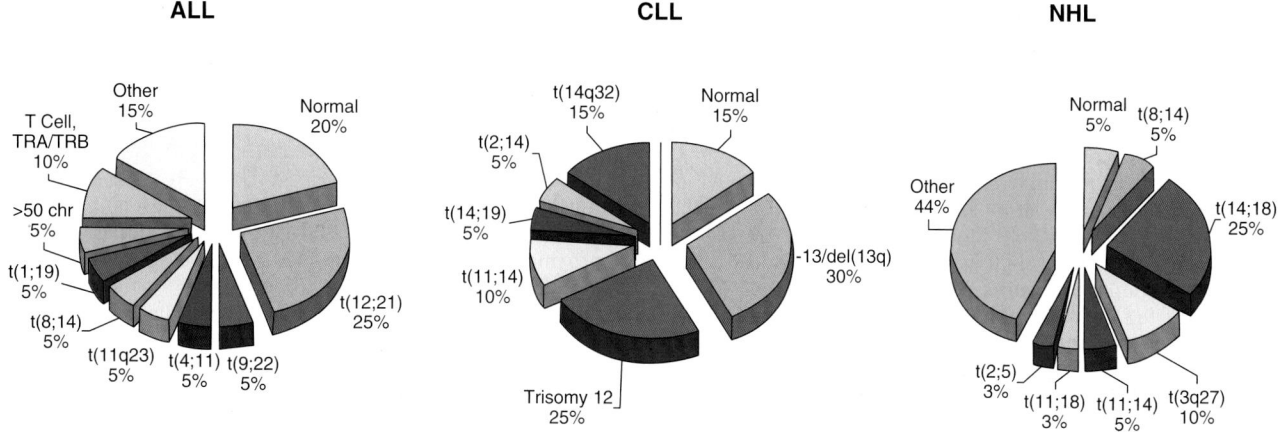

FIGURE 9.3. Frequency of recurring chromosomal abnormalities in ALL, CLL, and NHL.

the smaller p190 fusion protein resulting from an alternative breakpoint (m-bcr) (269,271). Most of these patients lack the additional cytogenetic abnormalities typical of CML blast crisis, do not have the t(9;22) in myeloid cells and colonies, and become Ph⁻ in hematologic remission. These observations suggest that the t(9;22) occurred in a cell that is more restricted in its differentiation potential, perhaps a committed B-lymphoid progenitor. Both the p210 and p190 BCR-ABL1 fusion proteins are involved in constitutive signaling via the RAS pathway of signal transduction and promote leukemogenesis (43,272). No significant clinical differences have been associated with these two fusion gene products.

Approximately 70% of ALL patients have abnormalities in addition to the t(9;22), a frequency that is substantially higher than that observed in chronic-phase CML. The most common secondary changes include gain of an extra Ph chromosome [der(22)t(9;22)(q34;q11.2)], –7 or loss of 7p, and abnormalities involving 9p, +8, +21, and +X (264). Although pediatric and adult Ph⁺ ALL patients with secondary abnormalities of chromosome 7 or 9p have been shown to have a poorer outcome as compared to those with other secondary changes in the pre-TKI era, it is not yet clear if the presence of secondary abnormalities influences prognosis in patients treated with TKIs.

Recent molecular studies have identified a subset of high-risk B-ALL patients who are BCR-ABL1 negative, but exhibit a gene expression signature similar to patients with BCR-ABL1–positive ALL (273). A high proportion of these BCR-ABL1–like leukemias were shown to have deletions or mutations in IKZF1 (located at 7p12.2), which encodes a lymphoid transcription factor (274). Subsequent studies have revealed that aberrations in IKZF1 are observed in about 30% of high-risk B-ALL, and in more than 80% of BCR-ABL1–positive ALL, and are associated with a very poor prognosis (273–275). A subset of patients with IKZF1 deletions were also found to have mutations in the genes encoding JAK kinases, suggesting potential candidates for targeted therapy (276).

Approximately 5% to 10% of all ALL patients, and up to 50% of patients with BCR-ABL1–like ALL, have rearrangements that deregulate expression of CRLF2 (277–279). Notably, CRLF2 abnormalities are more common in children with DS (277). CRLF2 is located on the pseudoautosomal regions of the sex chromosomes and encodes a cytokine receptor. Cryptic translocations, t(X;14)(p22;q32) or t(Y;14)(p11.2;q32), leading to IGH-CRLF2 fusions, deletions within the pseudoautosomal regions giving rise to a P2RY8-CRLF2 fusion, and mutations within CRLF2 itself all lead to the overexpression of CRLF2 (277–279). CRLF2 abnormalities are also strongly correlated with the presence of IKZF1 deletions and JAK2 mutations (280), and have been associated with an adverse outcome (280–282).

ALL with 11q23 (*MLL*) Rearrangements

Chromosomal rearrangements involving the MLL gene on 11q23 are observed in 5% to 7% of ALL patients, and are associated with a poor prognosis (283,284). The frequency of MLL rearrangements is strikingly high in infants with ALL (60% to 80%), but drops sharply in older children (2% to 4%) and in adults (4% to 9%) (264,283). More than 100 MLL translocation partners have been identified (192,285). The most common translocation, observed in 50% of MLL-rearranged ALLs, is the t(4;11)(q21;q23) resulting in a MLL-AFF1(AF4) fusion gene. The presence of the t(4;11) has a particularly dismal outcome in infants <3 months of age and in patients with a poor early response to prednisone (256,286,287). The t(11;19) (q23;p13.3)/MLL-MLLT1(ENL) is the second most frequently observed; however, this rearrangement is not limited to ALL in that about 50% of cases have AML (288). Less frequent translocations include the t(9;11)(p22;q23)/MLL-MLLT3(AF9),

t(10;11) (p12;q23)/MLL-MLLT10(AF10), t(6;11)(q27;q23)/MLL-MLLT4(AF6), and others.

ALL in infants is particularly intriguing because although the incidence is low, the prevalence of MLL rearrangements is as high as 80% (289,290). Evidence that the genetic events causing MLL-rearranged infant ALL occur *in utero* includes the early onset of infant ALL, concordance of leukemia in monozygotic twins, and detection of MLL-AFF1(AF4) fusion sequences in neonatal blood spots from infants diagnosed with ALL (291,292). Recent genome-wide association studies in pediatric leukemia cases have identified specific SNPs in IKZF1 (7p12.2), ARID5B (10q21.2), and CEBPE (14q11.2) that are associated with risk for developing infant ALL (293–295). Replication of these results in independent data sets is warranted, but may be challenging due to the rarity of infant ALL.

MLL encodes a histone methyltransferase involved in the global regulation of gene transcription (201), and MLL-rearranged ALLs display unique gene expression profiles that are distinct from other cytogenetic subsets of ALL (296). Subsequent genome-wide methylation studies have shown that ALLs with the t(4;11) or t(11;19) are characterized by aberrant DNA hypermethylation, suggesting that MLL-rearranged ALLs may be responsive to treatment with demethylating agents (297).

Constitutively activated FLT3 and overexpression of FLT3, frequently seen in cases of AML, have also been observed in MLL-rearranged ALL. These cases respond to FLT3 inhibitors, and clinical trials exploring the efficacy of FLT3 inhibitors in treating MLL-rearranged ALL are currently in progress (298).

ALL with the t(1;19)

The t(1;19)(q23;p13.3)/TCF3(E2A)-PBX1 is observed in approximately 1% to 3% of adult and 5% of childhood ALL (299–302). The t(1;19) occurs in the form of either a reciprocal translocation or an unbalanced translocation characterized by two normal chromosome 1 homologs, and one normal chromosome 19 homolog and a rearranged der(19)t(1;19). The adverse outcome previously noted in children with the t(1;19) in the context of antimetabolite-based therapy has been greatly improved with the use of more aggressive multiagent therapies (303,304). A recent study, however, found that the t(1;19) is associated with a higher risk of CNS relapse (300). The outcome of adult patients with the t(1;19) is controversial.

The t(1;19) involves the TCF3(E2A) gene at 19p13.3, which encodes two transcription factors (E12 and E47) that bind to enhancer elements in the IGK gene, as well as the regulatory elements of other genes. The breakpoint on 1q occurs within PBX1, a homeobox (HOX) gene. HOX genes encode DNA-binding transcription factors that regulate developmental processes. The t(1;19) forms a TCF3(E2A)-PBX1 fusion protein that becomes a potent transcriptional activator driving aberrant expression of a multitude of genes (299,305).

ALL with the t(12;21)

The t(12;21)(p13;q22)/ETV6-RUNX1(TEL-AML1) is a cryptic translocation detectable by FISH or RT-PCR, and is seen in approximately 25% of children with ALL, but almost never in adults (306,307). The t(12;21) fuses the ETV6 gene at 12p13 with the RUNX1 gene at 21q22, resulting in the production of a fusion protein that inhibits activation of genes by the normal RUNX1 protein, alters differentiation, and enhances self-renewal of hematopoietic progenitor cells (308–310). The presence of the t(12;21) is associated with a good prognosis (311). Although there is a higher frequency of late relapses in patients with the t(12;21), these patients tend to have a better outcome than other relapsed patients (312,313). Nearly 75% of

ALL patients with the t(12;21) have additional abnormalities, the most common being deletions of 12p with loss of the second copy of *ETV6*, +21, and gain of an extra der(21)t(12;21). The prognostic significance of these additional abnormalities is not yet clear (314).

The application of FISH for the routine detection of the *ETV6-RUNX1* fusion in ALL patients led to the observation of an intrachromosomal amplification of chromosome 21 (iAMP21). Most cases were negative for the *ETV6-RUNX1* fusion, but instead showed multiple copies of the *RUNX1* signal clustered on the long arm of chromosome 21. The iAMP21 abnormality is observed in approximately 2% of children and 0.5% of adults with ALL, and is associated with a poor prognosis (315,316). The outcome of patients with iAMP21 is impacted by the treatment protocol; thus, reliable detection is important to guide therapy.

ALL with Hypodiploidy

Hypodiploidy, defined as having fewer than 46 chromosomes per cell, is associated with a poor outcome. A lower chromosome number is associated with a progressively worse outcome. The majority of hypodiploid ALLs have 45 chromosomes, and have a significantly better outcome than patients who have fewer than 45 chromosomes. Patients who have low hypodiploidy (31 to 39 chromosomes) do poorly, and those with near-haploidy (24 to 29 chromosomes) have the worst outcome (317,318).

ALL with High Hyperdiploidy

High hyperdiploidy, characterized by the presence of 51 to 65 chromosomes per cell, is seen in 25% to 30% of children, but only 2% to 10% of adults with ALL (264,319). The most commonly gained chromosomes include chromosomes 4, 6, 10, 14, 17, 18, 21, and the X chromosome (320). The overall prognosis of patients with high hyperdiploidy is very good (319,321), and patients with trisomies of chromosomes 4, 10, and 17 have a particularly favorable outcome (322,323). Structural rearrangements occur in up to 50% of high hyperdiploid ALL cases. The most common abnormalities, consisting of duplication and gain of 1q, del(6q), and i(17q), do not appear to significantly influence prognosis (324). However, patients with recurrent translocations, such as the t(9;22) and *MLL* rearrangements, should be risk-classified based on the prognostic significance of the translocation, rather than high hyperdiploidy (325).

Rare cases of hyperdiploid ALL have been shown to arise from the doubling of a hypodiploid clone, for example, a hypodiploid clone of 29 chromosomes undergoes polyploidization resulting in a clone with 58 chromosomes. These patients have a poor outcome that is similar to those with hypodiploidy. True hyperdiploidy can be distinguished from the doubling of a hypodiploid clone by examining the pattern of chromosome gains and losses (317).

Burkitt Leukemia

Based on the French-American-British classification criteria, leukemias that express surface immunoglobulin (Ig) (L3 morphology) and have a *MYC* translocation, t(8;14) or variant, identical to that seen in Burkitt lymphoma (BL), known as mature B-cell or Burkitt leukemia, were previously included as a subtype of ALL. However, the current WHO classification considers BL and Burkitt leukemia to be different manifestations of the same disease; thus, Burkitt leukemia is classified as a variant form of BL (1). Patients with this specific rare form of leukemia should be treated according to protocols for BL (326).

T-Cell Acute Lymphoblastic Leukemia/Lymphoma

T-cell acute lymphoblastic leukemia (T-ALL) represents 15% of childhood and 25% of adult ALL cases (264,327,328). T-ALL often presents with more unfavorable clinical features than B-ALL, such as an older age at diagnosis, high WBC count, bulky adenopathy, large mediastinal masses and pleural effusions, and CNS infiltration (1,301,327). T-ALL patients are at a higher risk for induction failure, early relapse, and isolated CNS relapse. The presence of MRD after initial therapy is associated with a poor prognosis. Although 50% to 70% of patients present with an abnormal karyotype (329), cytogenetic results are not currently incorporated into the decision of risk group classification and the selection of treatment (1).

Cytogenetic abnormalities in T-ALL usually involve rearrangement of one of the TCR loci—the alpha and delta loci (14q11.2), the beta locus (7q34), or the gamma locus (7p14)—with an assortment of partner genes. The consequence of these translocations is dysregulated transcription of the partner gene due to juxtaposition of the gene with TCR regulatory elements (329). A majority of these partner genes encode transcription factors involved in the regulation of genes that are important for T-cell differentiation and development. Several partner genes, *TAL1*, *TAL2*, *LYL1*, and *OLIG2*, are members of the basic helix-loop-helix family of transcription factors. *TAL1* is overexpressed in 20% to 30% of childhood T-ALL; a small percentage (3%) is due to the t(1;14)(p32;q11.2), and the remainder are due to a cryptic interstitial deletion resulting in the fusion of *TAL1* with the nearby *STIL(SIL)* gene (329,330). Up-regulation of *TAL2* as a result of the t(7;9)(q34;q32), *LYL1* from the t(7;19) (q34;p13.2), and *OLIG2* from the t(14;21)(q11.2;q22) occur less commonly (331). Although rearrangements of *TAL1* are the most frequent abnormalities observed in childhood T-ALL, rearrangements of this gene are rarely seen in adult T-ALL.

Other partner genes encode members of the highly conserved homeobox (HOX) family of transcription factors (332,333). The t(10;14)(q24;q11.2) results in overexpression of *TLX1(HOX11)*, and is observed in 7% of childhood and 30% of adult T-ALL, making it the most frequent abnormality in adult T-ALL (334). The cryptic t(5;14)(q35;q32.1), resulting in the fusion of *TLX3(HOX11L2)* with *BCL11B*, is seen in 20% of childhood and 10% to 15% of adult T-ALL (335). The inv(7) (p15q34) and t(7;7)(p15;q34) leads to dysregulated expression of multiple *HOXA* genes by bringing TCR regulatory elements close to the *HOXA* gene cluster (336). Translocations involving cysteine-rich LIM domain–only genes, *LMO1* in the t(11;14) (p15;q11.2) and *LMO2* in the t(11;14)(p13;q11.2), are also recurring in T-ALL (329).

Interestingly, aberrant expression of *TAL1*, *LYL1*, *TLX1*, and *TLX3* has been shown to be mutually exclusive. These findings correlate with specific gene expression signatures that correspond to stages of thymocyte development: $LYL1^+$ represents the pro-T stage, $TLX1^+$ the early cortical stage, and $TAL1^+$ the late cortical thymocyte stage (331). Together, these results suggest that there are nonoverlapping, pathogenetically distinct subgroups that may facilitate better stratification of outcome and treatment for T-ALL in the future.

A subset of abnormalities in T-ALL do not involve the *TCR* genes. The t(10;11)(p12;q14) results in the PICALM-MLLT10 (CALM-AF10) oncogenic fusion protein, and occurs in approximately 10% of patients with T-ALL (337). Rearrangements of the *MLL* gene, the most common being the t(11;19)(q23;p13.3)/ *MLL-ENL*, are seen in 8% of T-ALL cases. Neither translocation is specific to T-ALL, and also occurs in AML or B-ALL, respectively (329). Infrequent rearrangements involving the *ABL1* TK gene have also been detected in T-ALL. The *NUP214-ABL1* fusion is of particular interest because it is specific to T-ALL (6%), and occurs through the formation of episomes resulting in the fusion of the nearby *ABL1* and *NUP214* genes on 9q34, followed by cryptic extrachromosomal amplifications of the fusion segment (338,339). The NUP214-ABL1 fusion protein has constitutive ABL1 TK activity, and the disease responds to TKIs (340).

Mutations in *NOTCH1* and *FBXW7* (encoding a negative regulator of NOTCH1) are seen in approximately 50% and 30% of T-ALL cases, respectively, and represent the most common alterations in T-ALL (341–343). The development of anti-NOTCH1–targeted therapies is an active area of research. Recurrent mutations in T-ALL have also been found in *PHF6*, *PTPN2*, *NRAS*, *FLT3*, *LMO2*, *JAK1*, *WT1*, and *LEF1* (344,345). Furthermore, genome-wide profiling of DNA copy number in T-ALLs has identified del(9p) abnormalities that result in loss of the *CDKN2A* TSG, deletions of *RB1*, amplification of the *MYB* oncogene, and deletions of *PTEN* (260,346,347).

MATURE LYMPHOID NEOPLASMS

The presence of cytogenetic abnormalities in lymphomas, especially non-Hodgkin lymphomas (NHLs), has played an important role in the classification of these neoplasms (Table 9.3) (348,349). This is evident in the most recent WHO classification that broadly groups lymphomas by cell type, such as mature B-cell, T-cell, and NK killer cell, and then further defines the categories using a combination of genetic, clinical, morphologic, and immunophenotypic features (1). Although the correlation of cytogenetic abnormalities with specific disease categories can be equivocal, several recurring translocations are highly associated with distinct subtypes of lymphoma, including the t(14;18) in follicular lymphoma (FL), t(8;14) in BL, t(11;18) in MALT lymphoma, t(3;14) in diffuse large B-cell lymphoma (DLBCL), t(11;14) in mantle cell lymphoma (MCL), and t(2;5) in anaplastic large cell lymphoma (1,348) (Fig. 9.3). The *IGH* gene at 14q32 is frequently involved in translocations in B-cell neoplasms, whereas the majority of T-cell lymphomas are characterized by rearrangements involving TCR genes at 14q11.2, 7q34, and 7p14.

The integration of conventional cytogenetic analysis, FISH techniques, and gene expression profiling with emerging technologies, such as genomic array profiling and next-generation sequencing, promises to provide a better understanding of the pathogenesis of lymphoid malignancies that is expected to impact diagnosis, prognosis, and treatment (Fig. 9.1).

CLL/SLL

Chronic lymphocytic leukemia/small lymphocytic lymphoma (CLL/SLL) is an indolent lymphoproliferative neoplasm characterized by progressive lymphocytosis due to clonal accumulation of monomorphic, small round, CD5+/CD23+ B lymphocytes in the blood, BM, spleen, and lymph nodes, and is often observed in older individuals with an incidence that increases exponentially after the age of 50 (1). SLL refers to the pathologically identical, but nonleukemic form of CLL. Though rare in Eastern countries, CLL is the most common leukemia of adults in Western countries, accounting for approximately 7% of NHLs (350). Variability in the prevalence of CLL between different populations may be attributed to the strong genetic predisposition. In fact, CLL has the highest genetic predisposition of all hematologic malignancies. Between 5% and 10% of patients with CLL have a family history presenting with more than two affected individuals, and first-degree relatives of CLL patients are at an increased risk (two- to sevenfold) of developing CLL (351).

Cytogenetic abnormalities are detected in 80% of CLL cases, and are mainly characterized by genomic imbalances. The most common abnormalities are deletions of 13q14.3 (55%),

11q22-q23 (18%), 17p13 (7%), and trisomy 12 (16%). Other recurrent abnormalities that are seen less frequently include del(6q), +3, +8, +18, and translocations involving the *IGH* gene at 14q32 (352–354) (Fig. 9.3).

del(13q)

The presence of an isolated del(13q) in CLL is associated with a good outcome. The CDR (13q14.2) does not contain the nearby *RB1* gene (354); however, recent chromosomal microarray studies have identified a subset of CLL patients with larger deletions inclusive of *RB1* (355,356). Two microRNA genes, *miR-16-1* and *miR-15a*, that negatively regulate *BCL2* have been identified as candidate genes within the deletion, suggesting a potential role in the pathogenesis of CLL (357,358). Interestingly, mice with genetically engineered deletions of the entire band 13q14.2 developed CLL more frequently and presented with a more aggressive clinical course than mice that had deletions of only the miR sequences, raising the possibility that loss of additional genes in this region contributes to the pathogenesis of CLL (359).

del(11q)

CLL patients with the del(11q) are characterized by a younger age of onset, bulky lymphadenopathy, and a poor prognosis. A consequence of the del(11q) is loss of *ATM*, a TSG involved in the DNA damage response pathway (360). Deletions and mutations that lead to inactivation of the *ATM* gene are usually somatic, but have also been found to be constitutional, suggesting a predisposition of heterozygous *ATM* mutation carriers to develop CLL (361). However, the majority of patients with the del(11q) do not show a disruption of the remaining *ATM* allele, implicating haploinsufficiency as the pathogenic mechanism.

Trisomy 12

Trisomy 12 is frequently associated with increased numbers of atypical lymphoplasmacytic and cleaved cells, and strong surface immunoglobulin and FMC7 expression, and is an intermediate prognostic factor. The mechanism of pathogenesis is thought to be a gene dosage effect of one or more candidate oncogenes on chromosome 12; however, the involved gene(s) has yet to be identified (352).

del(17p)

The presence of the del(17p) confers the poorest prognosis in CLL. The critical mechanism is loss of *TP53*, encoding the tumor suppressor protein, TP53, that is essential in mediating apoptosis or cell cycle arrest after DNA damage (352,353). Patients with monoallelic deletions of 17p usually harbor inactivating point mutations on the remaining *TP53* allele that result in complete loss of TP53 function and a block in the DNA damage response pathway (362). CLL patients with inactivated TP53 respond poorly to purine nucleoside analogues and alkylating agent–based treatments, most likely due to the requirement of TP53-dependent pathways to induce cell death (363,364). This has led to the development of ongoing clinical trials of non-TP53–dependent agents in the treatment of CLL with del(17p) (365,366).

Other Molecular Abnormalities in CLL

Antigen-stimulated B cells enter and form germinal centers in lymphoid follicles, then undergo random somatic mutations in the variable regions of the immunoglobulin gene (*IGHV*) to alter antibody-antigen affinity as a process of affinity maturation. Only B cells with a high antigen-binding affinity will survive and differentiate further. Approximately 50% to 60% of CLL cases show somatic hypermutation of the *IGHV* gene, which is correlated with specific cytogenetic abnormalities (367). CLLs with deletions of 13q, associated with a good prognosis, have a high frequency of mutations, whereas leukemias with deletions of 11q and 17p, characterized by a poor prognosis, have a significantly lower rate. *IGHV* mutation status is an independent prognostic factor; CLL patients with mutated *IGHV* have a better outcome than those with unmutated *IGHV* (368,369).

To identify potential surrogate markers that correlate with *IGHV* mutation status, gene expression profiles were compared between *IGHV* mutated and unmutated CLL cases (370,371). The *ZAP70* gene, which encodes a TK protein involved in transmitting signals from the TCR to downstream pathways, emerged as the top candidate since aberrant expression of *ZAP70* is associated with unmutated *IGHV* CLL in over 80% of cases (372). Flow cytometric assays of *ZAP70* are utilized as a surrogate test for *IGHV* mutation status in CLL (372).

Recently, studies of CLL using next-generation sequencing technologies have identified recurrent mutations in *NOTCH1*, *XPO1*, *MYD88*, *KLHL6*, *POT1*, *CHD2*, *LRP1B*, and *SF3B1*, with mounting evidence that specific mutations are associated with the mutated or unmutated states of *IGHV* (373,374). *NOTCH1* mutated CLL cases have been shown to overexpress *NOTCH1* pathway genes, which predicts a poor outcome (375). Mutations in the *SF3B1* gene, which encodes a spliceosome subunit, were found to be overrepresented in fludarabine-refractory CLL cases compared to a diagnostic cohort, implicating an alternative therapeutic target in cases refractory to routine chemotherapy. SF3B1 inhibitors are currently under preclinical development as anticancer agents.

MALT Lymphoma

MALT lymphoma is an indolent disease characterized by the infiltration of a mixture of morphologically heterogeneous small B cells, including marginal zone cells, cells resembling monocytoid cells, small lymphocytes, and scattered immunoblasts and centroblast-like cells, into extranodal lymphoid tissue (1,376). The gastrointestinal tract, particularly the stomach, is the most common site of MALT lymphoma. The onset of MALT lymphoma is often preceded by chronic inflammation due to infection, autoimmunity, or other unknown stimuli. In particular, infection by the bacteria *Helicobacter pylori* is present in a high proportion of cases. The correlation of distinct cytogenetic abnormalities with specific anatomic site presentations of MALT lymphoma illustrates the potential effect of environmental factors on lymphomagenesis (377).

MALT lymphomas represent 7% to 8% of all B-cell lymphomas. The most common cytogenetic abnormalities are t(11;18) (q21;q21.3)/*BIRC3(API2)-MALT1* (15%), t(14;18)(q32;q21.3)/*IGH-MALT1* (11%), and t(1;14)(p22;q32)/*IGH-BCL10* (2%) (378–382). Trisomy 3 and 18, and partial gains of 3q, 9q, and 18q are also recurrently observed in MALT lymphoma (383).

The t(11;18) is specific to MALT lymphomas, and is the most frequent translocation associated with this disease, occurring predominantly in gastric and pulmonary cases, often as the sole abnormality (378,379). MALT lymphoma with aneuploidy, particularly trisomy 3 and 18, has been shown to be negatively correlated with the presence of the t(11;18) (384). The second most frequent abnormality in MALT lymphoma, the t(14;18)/*IGH-MALT1*, occurs mainly in ocular adnexal and liver tumors (382,385). Although the t(14;18) resulting in either the *IGH-MALT1* fusion or the *IGH-BCL2* fusion (to be detailed in another section) are cytogenetically indistinguishable, they are molecularly and pathologically distinct. Distinguishing between these rearrangements can be accomplished by targeted FISH

analysis. A smaller proportion of MALT lymphomas, usually at gastric and pulmonary sites, have the t(1;14) or more rarely a variant t(1;2)(p22;p12) involving the *IGK* locus, and have strong aberrant nuclear BCL10 immunostaining (381,386,387).

The genes targeted by these translocations, *MALT1* and *BCL10*, induce lymphomagenesis by their common involvement in the NF-κB pathway (380,388,389), a central pathway regulating the expression of genes important in lymphocyte proliferation and survival (390). Constitutive activation of NF-κB occurs via the expression of the *BIRC3(API2)-MALT1* fusion protein as a result of the t(11;18) or overexpression of *MALT1* or *BCL10* as a result of juxtaposition with the *IGH* enhancer following the t(14;18) or t(1;14), respectively (388,389).

Another recurrent rearrangement, the t(3;14)(p14.1;q32)/*IGH-FOXP1*, is most commonly seen in gastric lymphomas, and results in the overexpression of *FOXP1* due to juxtaposition of the gene with *IGH* regulatory elements (391). Although the translocation is rare, overexpression of *FOXP1* is common in MALT lymphomas (392,393). FOXP1 regulates genes involved in VDJ recombination, and is essential for B-cell development (394); however, the role of FOXP1 in lymphomagenesis is largely unknown. Notably, the t(3;14) has also been identified in DLBCLs.

Follicular Lymphoma

FL accounts for 20% of all lymphomas, and is characterized by a follicular growth pattern of germinal center B cells (GCB), typically centrocytes and centroblasts/large transformed cells, and the presence of chromosomal translocations involving the *BCL2* gene at 18q21.3, most commonly the t(14;18)(q32;q21.3)/*IGH-BCL2* (1,395,396). In the current WHO classification, FL can be categorized into grades 1 to 3 based on the number of blasts and the presence or absence of centrocytes (1). A higher grade correlates with disease progression and a worse prognosis. Importantly, progression of FL to an aggressive lymphoma, usually diffuse large cell lymphoma, occurs in 25% to 30% of patients and is associated with a poor outcome (1).

Approximately 70% to 90% of FL cases have the t(14;18), resulting in constitutive expression of *BCL2* by juxtaposition of the *BCL2* gene to *IGH* regulatory elements (397). Variant translocations, t(2;18)(p12;q21.3) and t(18;22)(q21.3;q11.2), involving the *IGK* and *IGL* genes, respectively, are observed less commonly (398). The t(14;18) is characteristic of, but not unique to, FL and is also observed in 30% of DLBCLs and occasionally in CLL. Notably, the t(14;18) is extremely rare in pediatric FL (399). As mentioned previously, it is important to distinguish the t(14;18) involving *BCL2* described here and the t(14;18) involving *MALT1* in MALT lymphoma.

The molecular analysis of *BCL2* led to the discovery of a new class of oncogenes, which instead of promoting proliferation, contribute to development of a neoplastic state by preventing programmed cell death. The *BCL2* gene encodes a mitochondrial membrane protein that functions to increase cell survival (400). Aberrant expression of BCL2 as a consequence of the t(14;18) and other variants is the initiating event in the pathogenesis of FL. Transgenic mice containing an *Ig-Bcl2* minigene develop polyclonal follicular hyperplasia and, after a long latency, some develop high-grade lymphomas, many of which possess translocations involving *Myc* (401). Furthermore, the *IGH-BCL2* fusion can be detected in tonsil and PB lymphocytes of normal individuals (402). These findings suggest that BCL2 overexpression is not transforming *per se*, but cooperates with other transforming events. In this regard, it has been proposed that FL cells expressing BCL2 are unable to undergo apoptosis during affinity maturation and class switching in the germinal centers and, thus, are more likely to accumulate secondary chromosomal alterations during the subsequent somatic hypermutation process (403,404).

Secondary chromosomal alterations, in addition to the t(14;18), are found in 90% of FL and include gains of 1q, 2p, 6p, 7, 8, 12q, 18q, and the X chromosome, as well as deletions of 1p, 6q, 10q, 13q, and 17p (405). The number of additional alterations has been shown to increase with histologic grade and transformation (406–409). Acquisition of secondary or tertiary abnormalities involving 17p (*TP53*), 9p21 (*CDKN2A*), or 8q24.2 (*MYC*) is associated with disease progression and a poor prognosis (410–413).

Although only a small proportion of FL cases lack the t(14;18), the majority of these cases are identified as grade 3 FL (414,415). Furthermore, t(14;18)-negative cases are associated with a higher incidence of abnormalities involving the *BCL6* gene at 3q27 (416,417). BCL6 is a transcriptional regulator involved in germinal center formation and is deregulated by juxtaposition with the *IGH* gene or other partner genes (418,419).

Mantle Cell Lymphoma

MCL represents 3% to 10% of all NHLs with a 2:1 male predominance, and is characterized by a monomorphic lymphoid cell proliferation with a diffuse, mantle zone growth pattern and chromosomal translocations involving the *CCND1* gene at 11q13. MCL displays an aggressive clinical course with a median survival of only 3 to 4 years (1,349,420).

The t(11;14)(q13;q32)/*IGH-CCND1*, which results in overexpression of CCND1 by juxtaposition of the *CCND1* gene to the *IGH* locus, is present in almost all cases of MCL. Rare variant translocations of *CCND1* with the *IGK* and *IGL* genes have also been observed. CCND1 is a member of the conserved cyclin family of proteins and acts to regulate the cell cycle during G1 progression and G1/S transition. CCND1, together with activated cyclin dependent kinase 4 (CDK4), phosphorylates and inactivates RB1, releasing E2F from the complex; E2F is a transcription factor that regulates the expression of genes required for cell division (349,421). Deregulated expression of *CCND1* is thought to overcome the cell cycle–suppressive effect of RB1 and other factors, leading to the development of MCL (422,423).

A small proportion of MCL cases are CCND1 negative and do not have the t(11;14) or variant rearrangements but, interestingly, display a gene expression signature that is indistinguishable from CCND1-positive MCL. These cases have been shown to overexpress *CCND2* or *CCND3* (424,425). Chromosomal rearrangements, t(12;14)(p13;q32)/*IGH-CCND2* and t(2;12)(p12;p13)/*IGK-CCND2*, that juxtapose *CCND2* with *IGH* or *IGK*, respectively, may account for CCND2 overexpression in some cases (426).

The ability of aberrant CCND1 to induce lymphomagenesis appears to depend on cooperation with other oncogenes, since mice ectopically expressing *CCND1* do not develop lymphoma (427). In addition to the t(11;14), a significant proportion of MCL cases also have recurrent secondary chromosomal aberrations including gains of 3q, 7p, and 8q, and losses of 1p, 6q, 9p, 11q, 13q, and 17p (428–431). Trisomy 12 is observed in 25% of cases, and the occurrence of tetraploid clones is associated with a nontypical pleomorphic and blastoid morphology. Abnormalities involving the *MYC* gene at 8q24.2 are occasionally observed in MCL, and are associated with an aggressive clinical course (432). *BCL6* (3q27) rearrangements are also detected rarely in MCL (433). Gains of 3q, deletions of 9q, trisomy 12, and complex karyotypes are associated with an adverse outcome (428,434).

Molecular studies have identified additional genetic aberrations in genes involved in the DNA damage response and cell cycle regulation. Approximately 40% to 75% of MCL cases have inactivating mutations or deletions of the *ATM* gene located at 11q22.3 (435,436). MCLs that are highly proliferative (high mitotic rate) are associated with an adverse outcome, and often have *TP53* mutations, homozygous deletions of the gene encoding the CDK inhibitors, *CDKN2A* and *CDKN2C*, amplification and overexpression of the *BMI1* polycomb and *CDK4* genes, and microdeletions of the *RB1* gene (437).

Diffuse Large B-Cell Lymphoma

DLBCL is a morphologically, biologically, and clinically heterogeneous disease that accounts for 30% to 40% of all NHLs, making it the most prevalent type of lymphoma in Western countries. DLBCL usually arises *de novo*, but may also present as the result of progression (or transformation) from a less aggressive lymphoma, particularly FL. DLBCL is cytogenetically heterogeneous in that several recurrent lymphoma-associated rearrangements are observed, although none are limited to DLBCL. The most common abnormalities include the t(3;14)(q27;q32) involving *BCL6*, the t(14;18)(q21.3;q32) involving *BCL2*, and the t(8;14)(q24.2;q32) involving *MYC* (1,438,439).

Abnormalities of *BCL6* tend to be indiscriminating, and can be found in a wide range of lymphomas. The t(3;14)(q27;q32), observed in 30% of DLBCL cases, is the most frequent abnormality; however, variant translocations involving *IGK*, t(2;3)(p12;q27), and *IGL*, t(3;22)(q27;q11.2), are also detected and result in deregulated expression of *BCL6* (419,439–441). BCL6 is a potent transcriptional repressor; a role in germinal center formation is suggested by topographic restriction of *BCL6* expression in germinal centers of normal human lymphoid tissue, and the fact that mice with targeted disruptions of *Bcl6* are incapable of forming germinal centers (442).

The t(14;18)(q21.3;q32)/*IGH-BCL2* accounts for 20% to 30% of DLBCL cases, but is more common in FL (443). Similarly, translocations involving the *MYC* gene at 8q24.2 are generally considered the hallmark of BL, but are also observed in approximately 10% of DLBCL cases. The presence of *MYC* rearrangements in DLBCL is associated with a complex karyotype and a poor prognosis (443,444). Approximately 20% of cases with a *MYC* rearrangement also have a concurrent *IGH-BCL2* translocation, *BCL6* rearrangement, or both. These so-called double-hit lymphomas usually have a high proliferative status associated with a dismal outcome, and are better categorized as "B-cell lymphomas, unclassified with features intermediate between DLBCL and Burkitt lymphoma" (445).

DLBCL is a heterogeneous disease and gene expression profiling studies have thus far identified three distinct expression signatures (446–448). The first group has the profile of GCB-like, the second has the profile of activated peripheral B cells (ABC-like), and the third group, termed primary mediastinal B-cell lymphoma, seems to originate from a rare B-cell population that resides in the thymus. Patients with a GCB profile of DLBCL have a significantly better clinical outcome than those with the ABC profile (446–449). Furthermore, the GCB and ABC subgroups are associated with the presence of different chromosomal alterations. The GCB group displays frequent gains of 12q12, and cases with *BCL2* abnormalities are almost exclusively the GCB type. The ABC group frequently contains gains of 3q, 18q, and losses of 6q (450,451).

Burkitt Lymphoma

BL is a highly aggressive B-cell lymphoma with an extremely short doubling time, and can be further categorized into three clinical variants, endemic BL, sporadic BL, and immunodeficiency-associated BL, based on differences in clinical presentation, biology, and morphology (1,452,453). The t(8;14)(q24.2;q32), a hallmark of BL, has played an important role in the history of cancer cytogenetics as it was the first chromosomal rearrangement to be characterized in lymphoid neoplasms (454). In 1972, Manolov and Manolova (455) identified a consistent abnormality (14q+) in the cells of primary BLs and in cultured cell lines. Several years later, Zech et al. (453) suggested that the rearrangement was a reciprocal translocation involving chromosomes 8 and 14, t(8;14)(q24.2;q32). As additional Burkitt tumors were examined, it became apparent that at least two other related translocations occur, the t(2;8) (p12;q24.2) and t(8;22)(q24.2;q11.2). All three translocations involve chromosome band 8q24.2, and result in deregulation (constitutive expression) of the *MYC* oncogene through juxtaposition with the enhancer elements of the immunoglobulin loci (453,455). Specifically, the t(8;14) involves a break within the *IGH* locus at 14q32 and a break 5′ or within *MYC* at 8q24.2, and positions the *MYC* coding exons adjacent to *IGH* sequences in a "head to head" orientation. The various breakpoints in the translocation correlate roughly with the forms of BL: endemic BLs usually have breakpoints upstream of *MYC*, whereas sporadic or immunodeficiency-associated BLs usually contain breakpoints within *MYC* (456). *MYC* encodes a transcription factor that plays a role in a number of cellular processes, including proliferation and apoptosis (457,458).

The t(8;14) or variant translocations present as the sole abnormality in 40% of BL cases; the remaining 60% of cases have secondary chromosomal alterations associated with disease progression, the most common being a partial gain of 1q, and trisomy of chromosome 7 and 8. Interestingly, these secondary abnormalities tend to be mutually exclusive in BL progression. Other recurrent abnormalities include loss of 6q, 17p, and 13q (454). It is important to note that recurring translocations involving other oncogenes, for example, *BCL2* (18q21.3), *BCL6* (3q27), and *CCND1* (11q13), are not observed in BL. Molecular studies have identified additional genetic and epigenetic alterations in BL involving *CDKN2A*, *TP53*, *TP73*, *BAX*, *RBL2*, and *BCL6* that may function to promote cell growth and/or inhibit apoptosis (459).

T-Cell Lymphomas

T-cell and NK-cell lymphomas constitute a group of rare and often clinically aggressive diseases, accounting for 15% of all lymphomas. The 18 subtypes of T- and NK-cell neoplasms recognized by the WHO classification can be broadly categorized based on their presentation as predominantly disseminated, extranodal or cutaneous, or nodal diseases. There is significant overlap in morphologic and immunophenotypic features between the different entities, and accurate diagnosis remains a challenge. T- and NK-cell lymphomas can have rearrangements involving the TCR loci, including the TCR α chain and δ chain genes (*TRA*, *TRD*) at 14q11.2 or, less often, one of two regions of chromosome 7 (7q34 and 7p14) to which the TCR β chain (*TRB*) and γ chain (*TRG*) genes are localized, respectively. The involved gene on the partner chromosome may encode a transcription factor, whose expression is deregulated or activated as a result of the rearrangement. Few recurrent genetic alterations have been identified in T- and NK-cell lymphomas, and the molecular pathogenesis in general remains poorly understood. ALK-positive anaplastic large cell lymphoma (ALCL) is currently the sole T- and NK-cell lymphoma subtype in the WHO classification that is defined on a genetic basis (1,460,461).

Anaplastic Large Cell Lymphoma, ALK Positive

ALCL, ALK positive, is a T-cell lymphoma that consists of large lymphoid cells with abundant cytoplasm and pleomorphic nuclei, and is characterized by ALK expression, usually the consequence of *ALK* translocations, and expression of CD30. ALK-positive ALCL is observed in approximately 3% of adult lymphomas, and 10% to 20% of childhood lymphomas, and has a good prognosis compared to ALK-negative ALCL (462).

The most common translocation involving *ALK* at 2p23 is the t(2;5)(p23;q35)/*ALK-NPM1* resulting in the aberrant fusion of the *ALK* gene with the *NPM1* gene on 5q35. *ALK* encodes a TK receptor that is not expressed in normal lymphoid cells. The resultant chimeric fusion protein consists of the 5′ portion of NPM1 fused to the ALK TK domain at the 3′ end, which induces constitutive activation of the ALK TK (463,464). Variant *ALK* translocations involving other partner genes have been observed, such as *TPM3* (1q21), *ATIC* (2q35), *TFG* (3q12), *CLTC* (17q23), *MSN* (Xq11-q12), *TPM4* (19p13.1), *MYH9* (22q13.1), and RNF213 (17q25); however, there is no difference in prognosis (460,461). Genomic profiling studies have identified frequent secondary genetic alterations in ALK-positive ALCL, including gains of chromosome 7, 17p, and 17q, and losses of 4, 11q, and 13q (465).

ALK rearrangements and overexpression are not unique to ALCL, and have also been identified in other cancers, such as non–small cell lung cancer and squamous cell carcinoma (466). A rare aggressive form of ALK-positive, CD30-negative DLBCL has been reported and is associated with a very dismal outcome (467). Several small molecule ALK inhibitors currently in early-phase clinical trials may provide a targeted therapy for ALK-positive ALCL in the future (468).

MULTIPLE MYELOMA

MM (also known as plasma cell myeloma) is a proliferation of malignant monoclonal plasma cells in the BM, and accounts for 13% of all hematologic malignancies. MM is clinically heterogeneous, with a median survival of 3 to 4 years (range 6 months to >10 years) (1,469–471). In the past decade, several subtypes of the disease have been defined at the genetic and molecular level, which are associated with clinicopathologic features and outcomes (472–474). Several recurring cytogenetic and genetic abnormalities have been identified that provide information on the biology, pathogenesis, clinical course, and prognosis of MM (Table 9.3). As a result of the low mitotic index in MM, FISH has become an essential analytical tool in detecting recurring abnormalities (475,476).

To understand the genetic and molecular events underlying MM initiation and progression, it is important to touch upon the development of plasma cells. Initially, immature B cells that leave the BM and encounter antigens migrate to germinal centers. It is here that cells engineer functional and highly specific antibodies by undergoing processes that include somatic hypermutation and class switch recombination. The cells, called plasmablasts at this point, then migrate back to the BM to become long-lived antibody-producing plasma cells (477). Errors in somatic hypermutation and class switch recombination may facilitate genomic instability causing hyperdiploidy and aberrant *IGH* rearrangements, bringing oncogenes under the control of strong immunoglobulin promoters and enhancers. The consequences are the deregulation of tightly coordinated genes, pathways, and networks leading to malignant transformation (477–479).

For plasma cells to thrive in the BM, interaction with the surrounding BM niche microenvironment is critical. Progression of MM to increasingly aggressive disease, such as extramedullary myeloma and plasma cell leukemia, usually requires the ability of clonal cells to proliferate at sites outside of the BM. Most likely, a combination of genetic evolution in both the malignant MM cells and the BM microenvironment contribute to progression (473). Furthermore, MM is almost always preceded by an asymptomatic condition called monoclonal gammopathy of unknown significance (MGUS). The clinical course of MGUS is usually stable and progresses at a rate of just 1% per year to symptomatic disease. The cytogenetic abnormalities observed in MGUS are similar to those found in MM; however, clonal abnormalities are less common (480,481).

Hyperdiploid versus Nonhyperdiploid

Empirically, MM can be broadly divided into two categories: hyperdiploid MM associated with the gain of odd-numbered chromosomes 3, 5, 7, 9, 11, 15, 19, and 21 and nonhyperdiploid MM (482). The hyperdiploid category has a low prevalence of *IGH* translocations, whereas the nonhyperdiploid group is highly enriched for *IGH* translocations (483). Patients with hyperdiploid MM are generally older in age and trend toward a more favorable outcome (472).

t(11;14)(q13;q32)/*IGH-CCND1*

The t(11;14) resulting in the up-regulation of cyclin D1 (*CCND1*) is observed in approximately 15% of all MM cases (476), and is associated with CD20 expression, lymphoplasmacytic morphology, gamma-light chain usage, and a neutral to slightly favorable prognosis using current treatment regimens (484,485). Recently, gene expression profiling studies have identified distinct subsets of t(11;14) with significantly different outcomes, potentially explaining the overall neutral prognosis associated with the t(11;14) (486). It is worth noting, however, that increased expression of cyclin D genes (*CCND1*, *CCND2*, *CCND3*) is found in virtually all MM malignancies, regardless of the presence of the t(11;14) (487).

t(4;14)(p16;q32)

The t(4;14) is associated with a poor clinical response and survival, and is observed in 15% of MM cases (476,488,489). Translocation of the *IGH* locus (14q32) with 4p16 containing adjacent genes (*FGFR3* and *WHSC1-MMSET*) results in the production of two fusion products, 5′*FGFR3*-3′*IGH* on the der(14) and 5′*IGH*-3′*WHSC1* on the der(4) (490). *FGFR3* encodes a receptor TK that is involved in embryonic development, tissue homeostasis, and metabolism. Aberrant overexpression of *FGFR3* is thought to play a role in the oncogenic transformation seen in MM (491), making it an attractive candidate for targeted therapy. Indeed, TKIs specific to FGFR3 have been developed and are currently in clinical trials (492,493). WHSC1 (MMSET) is a histone methyltransferase whose overexpression in MM is associated with changes in chromatin methylation and gene expression. Loss of *WHSC1* expression alters adhesion properties, suppresses growth, and induces apoptosis (494). Although 25% of MM cases with the t(4;14) lack *FGFR3* expression (often coinciding with loss of the der(14)), *WHSC1* is consistently overexpressed (495), identifying WHSC1 as a potential therapeutic target. The development of WHSC1 inhibitors is currently under way.

t(14;16)(q32;q23)/*IGH-MAF*

The t(14;16) is observed in approximately 5% of MM cases, and is associated with a poor prognosis (488,496). This translocation arises from aberrant rearrangement of *IGH* with the *MAF* gene. It is interesting to note that while *MAF* translocations occur in only 5% of cases, almost 50% of myelomas overexpress *MAF* (496). Overexpression of *MAF* has been associated with increased expression of *CCND2* among a large number of other genes that enhance myeloma cell proliferation and adhesion to the BM microenvironment (496). The t(14;20)(q32;q12) involving *MAFB* occurs at a lower frequency (2%) (497), and is correlated with increased *CCND2* expression and a poor outcome.

Chromosome 13 Loss or Deletion

Loss or partial deletion of chromosome 13 is found in approximately 30% to 50% of MM cases by FISH analysis and, less commonly, by conventional cytogenetic analysis. Among these cases, 85% represent monosomy 13, and 15% represent an interstitial deletion of 13q (476,498). Despite observations of prognostic significance of these abnormalities, studies have shown that this is likely due to tight association with other high-risk genetic features (499,500). Notably, 90% of cases with the t(4;14) have chromosome 13 deletions, implicated in clonal expansion in MM (498,501).

Deletion of 17p13

One of the most important cytogenetic factors for prognosis in MM is deletion of 17p13, which results in the loss of the TSG, *TP53*. Deletions of 17p occur in approximately 8% of MM cases at presentation with increasing frequency at later stages of the disease (476,488). Prognosis is dismal with overall shorter survival, more aggressive disease, and higher prevalence of extramedullary disease; the latter is likely to be the consequence of dysfunctional TP53 (502,503). Although MM and MGUS share many of the same abnormalities, deletion of 17p13 is rarely found in MGUS, and is likely to be a later event associated with disease progression.

Chromosome 1 Abnormalities

Chromosome 1 abnormalities are prevalent in MM (476), frequently resulting in both gain of 1q and loss of 1p (504,505), and are associated with a shorter survival (504,506,507). Furthermore, gene expression profiling studies that identified a high-risk disease signature noted a significant enrichment of genes located on chromosome 1 (500,508). For this reason, it is now recommended that a comprehensive FISH testing panel for MM include detection of chromosome 1 abnormalities, particularly using probes for 1q.

Other recurrent genetic abnormalities observed in MM include translocations involving *MYC*, that is, the t(8;14) (q24.2;q32), mutations in genes that lead to the activation of the NF-κB pathway (509), *KRAS* and *NRAS* mutations (510), deletions of the short arm of chromosome 12 (506), and epigenetic and miRNA-related changes that could alter regulation of critical genes (511,512).

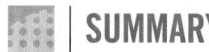 ## SUMMARY

Cytogenetic analysis provides pathologists and clinicians with a powerful tool for the diagnosis and classification of hematologic malignant diseases. The detection of an acquired somatic mutation establishes the diagnosis of a neoplastic disorder, and excludes a reactive hyperplasia or morphologic changes caused by toxic injury or vitamin deficiency. Given an equivocal pathologic diagnosis, the detection of a clonal chromosomal abnormality in a BM specimen or in lymph node tissue provides sufficient justification to institute cytotoxic treatment with radiation therapy or chemotherapy.

Specific cytogenetic abnormalities identify homogeneous subsets of various malignant diseases and enable clinicians to predict their clinical course and their likelihood of responding to particular treatments. In many cases, the prognostic information derived from cytogenetic analysis is independent of that provided by other clinical features. Patients with favorable prognostic features benefit from standard therapies with well-known spectra of toxicities, whereas those with less favorable clinical or cytogenetic characteristics may be better treated with more intensive or investigational therapies. Pretreatment cytogenetic analysis can be useful in choosing between postremission therapies that differ widely in cost, acute and chronic morbidity, and effectiveness. The disappearance of a chromosomal abnormality present at diagnosis is an important indicator of disease remission after treatment, and its reappearance invariably heralds relapse of the disease.

The delineation of recurring chromosomal abnormalities has had an important impact on molecular studies of human tumors. Recurring chromosomal abnormalities represent genetic mutations that are involved in the process of malignant transformation often representing the initiating event. The application of new, rapidly advancing technologies is facilitating the discovery of novel cancer-related genes, and providing insights into the processes that regulate normal cell growth and differentiation as well as malignant transformation.

References

1. Swerdlow SH, Campo C, Harris NL, et al. *WHO classification of tumours of haematopoietic and lymphoid tissues*, 4th ed. Lyon: IARC, 2008.
2. Heim S, Mitelman F. *Cancer cytogenetics: chromosomal and molecular genetic abberations of tumor cells*. Hoboken: Wiley, 2011.
3. Marcucci G, Haferlach T, Dohner H. Molecular genetics of adult acute myeloid leukemia: prognostic and therapeutic implications. *J Clin Oncol* 2011;29(5): 475–486.
4. Grimwade D, Hills RK, Moorman AV, et al. Refinement of cytogenetic classification in acute myeloid leukemia: determination of prognostic significance of rare recurring chromosomal abnormalities among 5876 younger adult patients treated in the United Kingdom Medical Research Council trials. *Blood* 2010;116(3): 354–365.
5. Harrison CJ. Cytogenetics of paediatric and adolescent acute lymphoblastic leukaemia. *Br J Haematol* 2009;144(2):147–156.
6. Greaves MF, Wiemels J. Origins of chromosome translocations in childhood leukaemia. *Nat Rev Cancer* 2003;3(9):639–649.
7. Rosenbauer F, Tenen DG. Transcription factors in myeloid development: balancing differentiation with transformation. *Nat Rev Immunol* 2007;7(2):105–117.
8. Dyer MJ. The pathogenetic role of oncogenes deregulated by chromosomal translocation in B-cell malignancies. *Int J Hematol* 2003;77(4):315–320.
9. Falini B, Mason DY. Proteins encoded by genes involved in chromosomal alterations in lymphoma and leukemia: clinical value of their detection by immunocytochemistry. *Blood* 2002;99(2):409–426.
10. Gozzetti A, Le Beau MM. Fluorescence in situ hybridization: uses and limitations. *Semin Hematol* 2000;37(4):320–333.
11. Buno I, Moreno-Lopez E, Diez-Martin JL. Sequential fluorescence in situ hybridization for the quantification of minimal residual disease in recipient cells after sex-mismatched allogeneic stem cell transplantation. *Br J Haematol* 2002;118(2):349.
12. Mascarello JT, Hirsch B, Kearney HM, et al. Section E9 of the American College of Medical Genetics technical standards and guidelines: fluorescence in situ hybridization. *Gen Med* 2011;13(7):667–675.
13. Baccarani M, Cortes J, Pane F, et al. Chronic myeloid leukemia: an update of concepts and management recommendations of European LeukemiaNet. *J Clin Oncol* 2009;27(35):6041–6051.
14. Bacher U, Kern W, Schoch C, et al. Evaluation of complete disease remission in acute myeloid leukemia: a prospective study based on cytomorphology, interphase fluorescence in situ hybridization, and immunophenotyping during follow-up in patients with acute myeloid leukemia. *Cancer* 2006;106(4):839–847.
15. Maciejewski JP, Mufti GJ. Whole genome scanning as a cytogenetic tool in hematologic malignancies. *Blood* 2008;112(4):965–974.
16. Mullighan CG, Downing JR. Genome-wide profiling of genetic alterations in acute lymphoblastic leukemia: recent insights and future directions. *Leukemia* 2009;23(7):1209–1218.
17. Godley LA, Cunningham J, Dolan ME, et al. An integrated genomic approach to the assessment and treatment of acute myeloid leukemia. *Semin Oncol* 2011;38(2):215–224.
18. Mullighan CG, Phillips LA, Su X, et al. Genomic analysis of the clonal origins of relapsed acute lymphoblastic leukemia. *Science* 2008;322(5906):1377–1380.
19. Shaffer LG, McGowan-Jordan J, Schmid M. *ISCN (2013): An International System for Human Cytogenetic Nomenclature*. Basel: S. Karger, 2013.
20. Han JY, Theil KS, Hoeltge G. Frequencies and characterization of cytogenetically unrelated clones in various hematologic malignancies: seven years of experiences in a single institution. *Cancer Genet Cytogenet* 2006;164(2):128–132.
21. Sun J, Yin CC, Cui W, et al. Chromosome 20q deletion: a recurrent cytogenetic abnormality in patients with chronic myelogenous leukemia in remission. *Am J Clin Pathol* 2011;135(3):391–397.
22. Bacher U, Hochhaus A, Berger U, et al. Clonal aberrations in Philadelphia chromosome negative hematopoiesis in patients with chronic myeloid leukemia treated with imatinib or interferon alpha. *Leukemia* 2005;19(3):460–463.
23. Anderson K, Lutz C, van Delft FW, et al. Genetic variegation of clonal architecture and propagating cells in leukaemia. *Nature* 2011;469(7330):356–361.
24. Ding L, Ley TJ, Larson DE, et al. Clonal evolution in relapsed acute myeloid leukaemia revealed by whole-genome sequencing. *Nature* 2012;481(7382): 506–510.
25. Egan JB, Shi CX, Tembe W, et al. Whole-genome sequencing of multiple myeloma from diagnosis to plasma cell leukemia reveals genomic initiating events, evolution, and clonal tides. *Blood* 2012;120(5):1060–1066.
26. Keats JJ, Chesi M, Egan JB, et al. Clonal competition with alternating dominance in multiple myeloma. *Blood* 2012;120(5):1067–1076.
27. Notta F, Mullighan CG, Wang JC, et al. Evolution of human BCR-ABL1 lymphoblastic leukaemia-initiating cells. *Nature* 2011;469(7330):362–367.
28. Walker BA, Wardell CP, Melchor L, et al. Intraclonal heterogeneity and distinct molecular mechanisms characterize the development of t(4;14) and t(11;14) myeloma. *Blood* 2012;120(5):1077–1086.
29. Walter MJ, Shen D, Ding L, et al. Clonal architecture of secondary acute myeloid leukemia. *N Engl J Med* 2012;366(12):1090–1098.
30. Anastasi J. The myeloproliferative neoplasms: insights into molecular pathogenesis and changes in WHO classification and criteria for diagnosis. *Hematol Oncol Clin North Am* 2009;23(4):693–708.
31. Tefferi A, Vardiman JW. Classification and diagnosis of myeloproliferative neoplasms: the 2008 World Health Organization criteria and point-of-care diagnostic algorithms. *Leukemia* 2008;22(1):14–22.
32. Zhang Y, Rowley JD. Chronic myeloid leukemia: current perspectives. *Clin Lab Med* 2011;31(4):687–698.
33. Nowell PC, Hungerford DA. Chromosome studies on normal and leukemic human leukocytes. *J Natl Cancer Inst* 1960;25:85–109.
34. Rowley JD. Letter: a new consistent chromosomal abnormality in chronic myelogenous leukaemia identified by quinacrine fluorescence and Giemsa staining. *Nature* 1973;243(5405):290–293.
35. Shtivelman E, Lifshitz B, Gale RP, et al. Fused transcript of abl and bcr genes in chronic myelogenous leukaemia. *Nature* 1985;315(6020):550–554.
36. Bartram CR, de Klein A, Hagemeijer A, et al. Translocation of c-ab1 oncogene correlates with the presence of a Philadelphia chromosome in chronic myelocytic leukaemia. *Nature* 1983;306(5940):277–280.
37. Marzocchi G, Castagnetti F, Luatti S, et al. Variant Philadelphia translocations: molecular-cytogenetic characterization and prognostic influence on frontline imatinib therapy, a GIMEMA Working Party on CML analysis. *Blood* 2011;117(25):6793–6800.
38. Ganesan TS, Rassool F, Guo AP, et al. Rearrangement of the bcr gene in Philadelphia chromosome-negative chronic myeloid leukemia. *Blood* 1986;68(4): 957–960.
39. Groffen J, Stephenson JR, Heisterkamp N, et al. Philadelphia chromosomal breakpoints are clustered within a limited region, bcr, on chromosome 22. *Cell* 1984;36(1):93–99.
40. Melo JV, Barnes DJ. Chronic myeloid leukaemia as a model of disease evolution in human cancer. *Nat Rev Cancer* 2007;7(6):441–453.
41. Quintas-Cardama A, Cortes J. Molecular biology of bcr-abl1-positive chronic myeloid leukemia. *Blood* 2009;113(8):1619–1630.
42. Sawyers CL, McLaughlin J, Witte ON. Genetic requirement for Ras in the transformation of fibroblasts and hematopoietic cells by the Bcr-Abl oncogene. *J Exp Med* 1995;181(1):307–313.
43. Daley GQ, Van Etten RA, Baltimore D. Induction of chronic myelogenous leukemia in mice by the P210bcr/abl gene of the Philadelphia chromosome. *Science* 1990;247(4944):824–830.
44. Druker BJ, Guilhot F, O'Brien SG, et al. Five-year follow-up of patients receiving imatinib for chronic myeloid leukemia. *N Engl J Med* 2006;355(23):2408–2417.
45. Hughes TP, Hochhaus A, Branford S, et al. Long-term prognostic significance of early molecular response to imatinib in newly diagnosed chronic myeloid leukemia: an analysis from the International Randomized Study of Interferon and STI571 (IRIS). *Blood* 2010;116(19):3758–3765.
46. Kantarjian HM, Talpaz M, Giles F, et al. New insights into the pathophysiology of chronic myeloid leukemia and imatinib resistance. *Ann Intern Med* 2006;145(12):913–923.
47. Hochhaus A, O'Brien SG, Guilhot F, et al. Six-year follow-up of patients receiving imatinib for the first-line treatment of chronic myeloid leukemia. *Leukemia* 2009;23(6):1054–1061.
48. Weisberg E, Manley PW, Cowan-Jacob SW, et al. Second generation inhibitors of BCR-ABL for the treatment of imatinib-resistant chronic myeloid leukaemia. *Nat Rev Cancer* 2007;7(5):345–356.
49. Talpaz M, Shah NP, Kantarjian H, et al. Dasatinib in imatinib-resistant Philadelphia chromosome-positive leukemias. *N Engl J Med* 2006;354(24):2531–2541.
50. Kantarjian H, Giles F, Wunderle L, et al. Nilotinib in imatinib-resistant CML and Philadelphia chromosome-positive ALL. *N Engl J Med* 2006;354(24):2542–2551.
51. Kantarjian H, Cortes J. Considerations in the management of patients with Philadelphia chromosome-positive chronic myeloid leukemia receiving tyrosine kinase inhibitor therapy. *J Clin Oncol* 2011;29(12):1512–1516.
52. Luatti S, Castagnetti F, Marzocchi G, et al. Additional chromosomal abnormalities in Philadelphia-positive clone: adverse prognostic influence on frontline imatinib therapy: a GIMEMA Working Party on CML analysis. *Blood* 2012;120(4): 761–767.
53. Rowley JD, Testa JR. Chromosome abnormalities in malignant hematologic diseases. *Adv Cancer Res* 1982;36:103–148.
54. Kralovics R, Passamonti F, Buser AS, et al. A gain-of-function mutation of JAK2 in myeloproliferative disorders. *N Engl J Med* 2005;352(17):1779–1790.
55. Baxter EJ, Scott LM, Campbell PJ, et al. Acquired mutation of the tyrosine kinase JAK2 in human myeloproliferative disorders. *Lancet* 2005;365(9464):1054–1061.
56. James C, Ugo V, Le Couedic JP, et al. A unique clonal JAK2 mutation leading to constitutive signalling causes polycythaemia vera. *Nature* 2005;434(7037):1144–1148.
57. Levine RL, Wadleigh M, Cools J, et al. Activating mutation in the tyrosine kinase JAK2 in polycythemia vera, essential thrombocythemia, and myeloid metaplasia with myelofibrosis. *Cancer Cell* 2005;7(4):387–397.
58. Kramer A, Reiter A, Kruth J, et al. JAK2-V617F mutation in a patient with Philadelphia-chromosome-positive chronic myeloid leukaemia. *Lancet Oncol* 2007;8(7):658–660.
59. Chen CY, Lin LI, Tang JL, et al. Acquisition of JAK2, PTPN11, and RAS mutations during disease progression in primary myelodysplastic syndrome. *Leukemia* 2006;20(6):1155–1158.
60. Ingram W, Lea NC, Cervera J, et al. The JAK2 V617F mutation identifies a subgroup of MDS patients with isolated deletion 5q and a proliferative bone marrow. *Leukemia* 2006;20(7):1319–1321.
61. Sokol L, Caceres G, Rocha K, et al. JAK2(V617F) mutation in myelodysplastic syndrome (MDS) with del(5q) arises in genetically discordant clones. *Leuk Res* 2010;34(6):821–823.
62. Tefferi A, Vainchenker W. Myeloproliferative neoplasms: molecular pathophysiology, essential clinical understanding, and treatment strategies. *J Clin Oncol* 2011;29(5):573–582.
63. Passamonti F, Maffioli M, Caramazza D. New generation small-molecule inhibitors in myeloproliferative neoplasms. *Curr Opin Hematol* 2012;19(2):117–123.
64. Scott LM, Tong W, Levine RL, et al. JAK2 exon 12 mutations in polycythemia vera and idiopathic erythrocytosis. *N Engl J Med* 2007;356(5):459–468.
65. Tefferi A, Skoda R, Vardiman JW. Myeloproliferative neoplasms: contemporary diagnosis using histology and genetics. *Nat Rev Clin Oncol* 2009;6(11):627–637.

66. Andrieux JL, Demory JL. Karyotype and molecular cytogenetic studies in polycythemia vera. *Curr Hematol Rep* 2005;4(3):224–229.
67. Westwood NB, Gruszka-Westwood AM, Pearson CE, et al. The incidences of trisomy 8, trisomy 9 and D20S108 deletion in polycythaemia vera: an analysis of blood granulocytes using interphase fluorescence in situ hybridization. *Br J Haematol* 2000;110(4):839–846.
68. Gangat N, Strand J, Lasho TL, et al. Cytogenetic studies at diagnosis in polycythemia vera: clinical and JAK2V617F allele burden correlates. *Eur J Haematol* 2008;80(3):197–200.
69. Bacher U, Haferlach T, Kern W, et al. Conventional cytogenetics of myeloproliferative diseases other than CML contribute valid information. *Ann Hematol* 2005;84(4):250–257.
70. Pardanani AD, Levine RL, Lasho T, et al. MPL515 mutations in myeloproliferative and other myeloid disorders: a study of 1182 patients. *Blood* 2006;108(10):3472–3476.
71. Hussein K, Van Dyke DL, Tefferi A. Conventional cytogenetics in myelofibrosis: literature review and discussion. *Eur J Haematol* 2009;82(5):329–338.
72. Dingli D, Schwager SM, Mesa RA, et al. Presence of unfavorable cytogenetic abnormalities is the strongest predictor of poor survival in secondary myelofibrosis. *Cancer* 2006;106(9):1985–1989.
73. Santana-Davila R, Tefferi A, Holtan SG, et al. Primary myelofibrosis is the most frequent myeloproliferative neoplasm associated with del(5q): clinicopathologic comparison of del(5q)-positive and -negative cases. *Leuk Res* 2008;32(12):1927–1930.
74. Gangat N, Tefferi A, Thanarajasingam G, et al. Cytogenetic abnormalities in essential thrombocythemia: prevalence and prognostic significance. *Eur J Haematol* 2009;83(1):17–21.
75. Bain BJ. Myeloid and lymphoid neoplasms with eosinophilia and abnormalities of PDGFRA, PDGFRB or FGFR1. *Haematologica* 2010;95(5):696–698.
76. Metzgeroth G, Walz C, Score J, et al. Recurrent finding of the FIP1L1-PDGFRA fusion gene in eosinophilia-associated acute myeloid leukemia and lymphoblastic T-cell lymphoma. *Leukemia* 2007;21(6):1183–1188.
77. Cools J, DeAngelo DJ, Gotlib J, et al. A tyrosine kinase created by fusion of the PDGFRA and FIP1L1 genes as a therapeutic target of imatinib in idiopathic hypereosinophilic syndrome. *N Engl J Med* 2003;348(13):1201–1214.
78. Curtis CE, Grand FH, Musto P, et al. Two novel imatinib-responsive PDGFRA fusion genes in chronic eosinophilic leukaemia. *Br J Haematol* 2007;138(1):77–81.
79. Golub TR, Barker GF, Lovett M, et al. Fusion of PDGF receptor beta to a novel ets-like gene, tel, in chronic myelomonocytic leukemia with t(5;12) chromosomal translocation. *Cell* 1994;77(2):307–316.
80. Keene P, Mendelow B, Pinto MR, et al. Abnormalities of chromosome 12p13 and malignant proliferation of eosinophils: a nonrandom association. *Br J Haematol* 1987;67(1):25–31.
81. Bain BJ, Fletcher SH. Chronic eosinophilic leukemias and the myeloproliferative variant of the hypereosinophilic syndrome. *Immunol Allergy Clin North Am* 2007;27(3):377–388.
82. David M, Cross NC, Burgstaller S, et al. Durable responses to imatinib in patients with PDGFRB fusion gene-positive and BCR-ABL-negative chronic myeloproliferative disorders. *Blood* 2007;109(1):61–64.
83. Arefi M, Garcia JL, Penarrubia MJ, et al. Incidence and clinical characteristics of myeloproliferative neoplasms displaying a PDGFRB rearrangement. *Eur J Haematol* 2012;89(1):37–41.
84. Soler G, Nusbaum S, Varet B, et al. LRRFIP1, a new FGFR1 partner gene associated with 8p11 myeloproliferative syndrome. *Leukemia* 2009;23(7):1359–1361.
85. Macdonald D, Reiter A, Cross NC. The 8p11 myeloproliferative syndrome: a distinct clinical entity caused by constitutive activation of FGFR1. *Acta Haematol* 2002;107(2):101–107.
86. Roumiantsev S, Krause DS, Neumann CA, et al. Distinct stem cell myeloproliferative/T lymphoma syndromes induced by ZNF198-FGFR1 and BCR-FGFR1 fusion genes from 8p11 translocations. *Cancer Cell* 2004;5(3):287–298.
87. Ren M, Qin H, Ren R, et al. Ponatinib suppresses the development of myeloid and lymphoid malignancies associated with FGFR1 abnormalities. *Leukemia* 2013;27(1):32–40. doi: 10.1038/leu.2012.188.
88. Chase A, Bryant C, Score J, et al. Ponatinib as targeted therapy for FGFR1 fusions associated with the 8p11 myeloproliferative syndrome. *Haematologica* 2013;(98)1:103–106.
89. Guagnano V, Kauffmann A, Wohrle S, et al. FGFR genetic alterations predict for sensitivity to NVP-BGJ398,a selective pan-FGFR inhibitor. *Cancer Discov* 2012;2(12):1118–1133.
90. Vardiman J, Hyjek E. World health organization classification, evaluation, and genetics of the myeloproliferative neoplasm variants. *Hematology Am Soc Hematol Educ Program* 2011;2011:250–256.
91. Cazzola M, Malcovati L, Invernizzi R. Myelodysplastic/myeloproliferative neoplasms. *Hematology Am Soc Hematol Educ Program* 2011;2011:264–272.
92. Parikh SA, Tefferi A. Chronic myelomonocytic leukemia: 2012 update on diagnosis, risk stratification, and management. *Am J Hematol* 2012;87(6):610–619.
93. Haase D, Germing U, Schanz J, et al. New insights into the prognostic impact of the karyotype in MDS and correlation with subtypes: evidence from a core dataset of 2124 patients. *Blood* 2007;110(13):4385–4395.
94. Jankowska AM, Makishima H, Tiu RV, et al. Mutational spectrum analysis of chronic myelomonocytic leukemia includes genes associated with epigenetic regulation: UTX, EZH2, and DNMT3A. *Blood* 2011;118(14):3932–3941.
95. Grand FH, Hidalgo-Curtis CE, Ernst T, et al. Frequent CBL mutations associated with 11q acquired uniparental disomy in myeloproliferative neoplasms. *Blood* 2009;113(24):6182–6192.
96. Bacher U, Haferlach T, Kern W, et al. A comparative study of molecular mutations in 381 patients with myelodysplastic syndrome and in 4130 patients with acute myeloid leukemia. *Haematologica* 2007;92(6):744–752.
97. Ricci C, Fermo E, Corti S, et al. RAS mutations contribute to evolution of chronic myelomonocytic leukemia to the proliferative variant. *Clin Cancer Res* 2010;16(8):2246–2256.
98. Pich A, Riera L, Sismondi F, et al. JAK2V617F activating mutation is associated with the myeloproliferative type of chronic myelomonocytic leukaemia. *J Clin Pathol* 2009;62(9):798–801.
99. Breccia M, Biondo F, Latagliata R, et al. Identification of risk factors in atypical chronic myeloid leukemia. *Haematologica* 2006;91(11):1566–1568.
100. Vardiman JW. Myelodysplastic/myeloproliferative diseases. *Cancer Treat Res* 2004;121:13–43.
101. Ernst T, Chase AJ, Score J, et al. Inactivating mutations of the histone methyltransferase gene EZH2 in myeloid disorders. *Nat Genet* 2010;42(8):722–726.
102. Reiter A, Invernizzi R, Cross NC, et al. Molecular basis of myelodysplastic/myeloproliferative neoplasms. *Haematologica* 2009;94(12):1634–1638.
103. Loh ML. Recent advances in the pathogenesis and treatment of juvenile myelomonocytic leukaemia. *Br J Haematol* 2011;152(6):677–687.
104. Flotho C, Steinemann D, Mullighan CG, et al. Genome-wide single-nucleotide polymorphism analysis in juvenile myelomonocytic leukemia identifies uniparental disomy surrounding the NF1 locus in cases associated with neurofibromatosis but not in cases with mutant RAS or PTPN11. *Oncogene* 2007;26(39):5816–5821.
105. Stephens K, Weaver M, Leppig KA, et al. Interstitial uniparental isodisomy at clustered breakpoint intervals is a frequent mechanism of NF1 inactivation in myeloid malignancies. *Blood* 2006;108(5):1684–1689.
106. Shannon KM, O'Connell P, Martin GA, et al. Loss of the normal NF1 allele from the bone marrow of children with type 1 neurofibromatosis and malignant myeloid disorders. *N Engl J Med* 1994;330(9):597–601.
107. Dunbar AJ, Gondek LP, O'Keefe CL, et al. 250K single nucleotide polymorphism array karyotyping identifies acquired uniparental disomy and homozygous mutations, including novel missense substitutions of c-Cbl, in myeloid malignancies. *Cancer Res* 2008;68(24):10349–10357.
108. Sanada M, Suzuki T, Shih LY, et al. Gain-of-function of mutated C-CBL tumour suppressor in myeloid neoplasms. *Nature* 2009;460(7257):904–908.
109. Matsuda K, Taira C, Sakashita K, et al. Long-term survival after nonintensive chemotherapy in some juvenile myelomonocytic leukemia patients with CBL mutations, and the possible presence of healthy persons with the mutations. *Blood* 2010;115(26):5429–5431.
110. Niemeyer CM, Kang MW, Shin DH, et al. Germline CBL mutations cause developmental abnormalities and predispose to juvenile myelomonocytic leukemia. *Nat Genet* 2010;42(9):794–800.
111. Perez B, Mechinaud F, Galambrun C, et al. Germline mutations of the CBL gene define a new genetic syndrome with predisposition to juvenile myelomonocytic leukaemia. *J Med Genet* 2010;47(10):686–691.
112. Olney HJ, Le Beau MM. Evaluation of recurring cytogenetic abnormalities in the treatment of myelodysplastic syndromes. *Leuk Res* 2007;31(4):427–434.
113. Schanz J, Tuchler H, Sole F, et al. New comprehensive cytogenetic scoring system for primary myelodysplastic syndromes (MDS) and oligoblastic acute myeloid leukemia after MDS derived from an international database merge. *J Clin Oncol* 2012;30(8):820–829.
114. Greenberg PL, Tuechler H, Schanz J, et al. Revised International Prognostic Scoring System for myelodysplastic syndromes. *Blood* 2012;120(12):2454–2465.
115. Vardiman J. The classification of MDS: From FAB to WHO and beyond. *Leuk Res* 2012;36(12):1453–1458. doi: 10.1016/j.leukres.2012.08.008.
116. Greenberg P, Cox C, Le Beau MM, et al. International scoring system for evaluating prognosis in myelodysplastic syndromes. *Blood* 1997;89(6):2079–2088.
117. Malcovati L, Germing U, Kuendgen A, et al. Time-dependent prognostic scoring system for predicting survival and leukemic evolution in myelodysplastic syndromes. *J Clin Oncol* 2007;25(23):3503–3510.
118. Alessandrino EP, Della Porta MG, Bacigalupo A, et al. WHO classification and WPSS predict posttransplantation outcome in patients with myelodysplastic syndrome: a study from the Gruppo Italiano Trapianto di Midollo Osseo (GITMO). *Blood* 2008;112(3):895–902.
119. Lai F, Godley LA, Joslin J, et al. Transcript map and comparative analysis of the 1.5-Mb commonly deleted segment of human 5q31 in malignant myeloid diseases with a del(5q). *Genomics* 2001;71(2):235–245.
120. Godley LA, Larson R. The syndrome of therapy-related myelodysplasia and myeloid leukemia. In: Bennett JM, ed. *The myelodysplastic syndromes: pathobiology and clinical management.* New York: Marcel Dekker Inc. 2002:136–176.
121. West RR, Stafford DA, White AD, et al. Cytogenetic abnormalities in the myelodysplastic syndromes and occupational or environmental exposure. *Blood* 2000;95(6):2093–2097.
122. Boultwood J, Lewis S, Wainscoat JS. The 5q- syndrome. *Blood* 1994;84(10):3253–3260.
123. Swerdlow SH, Campo E, Harris NL, et al., eds. *WHO classification of tumours of haematopoietic and lymphoid tissues,* 4th ed. Lyon: IARC Press, 2008.
124. Fairman J, Chumakov I, Chinault AC, et al. Physical mapping of the minimal region of loss in 5q- chromosome. *Proc Natl Acad Sci U S A* 1995;92(16):7406–7410.
125. Zhao N, Stoffel A, Wang PW, et al. Molecular delineation of the smallest commonly deleted region of chromosome 5 in malignant myeloid diseases to 1-1.5 Mb and preparation of a PAC-based physical map. *Proc Natl Acad Sci U S A* 1997;94(13):6948–6953.
126. Boultwood J, Fidler C, Strickson AJ, et al. Narrowing and genomic annotation of the commonly deleted region of the 5q- syndrome. *Blood* 2002;99(12):4638–4641.
127. Jerez A, Gondek LP, Jankowska AM, et al. Topography, clinical, and genomic correlates of 5q myeloid malignancies revisited. *J Clin Oncol* 2012;30(12):1343–1349.
128. Graubert TA, Payton MA, Shao J, et al. Integrated genomic analysis implicates haploinsufficiency of multiple chromosome 5q31.2 genes in de novo myelodysplastic syndromes pathogenesis. *PLoS One* 2009;4(2):e4583.
129. Shannon KM, Le Beau MM. Cancer: hay in a haystack. *Nature* 2008;451(7176):252–253.
130. Ebert BL, Pretz J, Bosco J, et al. Identification of RPS14 as a 5q- syndrome gene by RNA interference screen. *Nature* 2008;451(7176):335–339.
131. Barlow JL, Drynan LF, Hewett DR, et al. A p53-dependent mechanism underlies macrocytic anemia in a mouse model of human 5q- syndrome. *Nat Med* 2010;16(1):59–66.
132. Narla A, Ebert BL. Ribosomopathies: human disorders of ribosome dysfunction. *Blood* 2010;115(16):3196–3205.
133. Starczynowski DT, Kuchenbauer F, Argiropoulos B, et al. Identification of miR-145 and miR-146a as mediators of the 5q- syndrome phenotype. *Nat Med* 2010;16(1):49–58.
134. Kumar MS, Narla A, Nomami A, et al. Coordinate loss of a microRNA and protein coding gene cooperate in the pathogenesis of 5q- Syndrome. *Blood* 2011;118:4666–4673.

135. Smith SM, Le Beau MM, Huo D, et al. Clinical-cytogenetic associations in 306 patients with therapy-related myelodysplasia and myeloid leukemia: the University of Chicago series. *Blood* 2003;102(1):43–52.
136. Heerema NA, Nachman JB, Sather HN, et al. Deletion of 7p or monosomy 7 in pediatric acute lymphoblastic leukemia is an adverse prognostic factor: a report from the Children's Cancer Group. *Leukemia* 2004;18(5):939–947.
137. Luna-Fineman S, Shannon KM, Lange BJ. Childhood monosomy 7: epidemiology, biology, and mechanistic implications. *Blood* 1995;85(8):1985–1999.
138. Paulsson K, Sall T, Fioretos T, et al. The incidence of trisomy 8 as a sole chromosomal aberration in myeloid malignancies varies in relation to gender, age, prior iatrogenic genotoxic exposure, and morphology. *Cancer Genet Cytogenet* 2001;130(2):160–165.
139. Sloand EM, Wu CO, Greenberg P, et al. Factors affecting response and survival in patients with myelodysplasia treated with immunosuppressive therapy. *J Clin Oncol* 2008;26(15):2505–2511.
140. Wiktor A, Rybicki BA, Piao ZS, et al. Clinical significance of Y chromosome loss in hematologic disease. *Genes Chromosomes Cancer* 2000;27(1):11–16.
141. Pierre RV, Hoagland HC. Age-associated aneuploidy: loss of Y chromosome from human bone marrow cells with aging. *Cancer* 1972;30(4):889–894.
142. Hasle H. Myelodysplastic and myeloproliferative disorders in children. *Curr Opin Pediatr* 2007;19(1):1–8.
143. Bench AJ, Nacheva EP, Hood TL, et al. Chromosome 20 deletions in myeloid malignancies: reduction of the common deleted region, generation of a PAC/BAC contig and identification of candidate genes. UK Cancer Cytogenetics Group (UKCCG). *Oncogene* 2000;19(34):3902–3913.
144. Wang PW, Eisenbart JD, Espinosa R III, et al. Refinement of the smallest commonly deleted segment of chromosome 20 in malignant myeloid diseases and development of a PAC-based physical and transcription map. *Genomics* 2000;67(1):28–39.
145. Lugthart S, van Drunen E, van Norden Y, et al. High EVI1 levels predict adverse outcome in acute myeloid leukemia: prevalence of EVI1 overexpression and chromosome 3q26 abnormalities underestimated. *Blood* 2008;111(8):4329–4337.
146. Groschel S, Lugthart S, Schlenk RF, et al. High EVI1 expression predicts outcome in younger adult patients with acute myeloid leukemia and is associated with distinct cytogenetic abnormalities. *J Clin Oncol* 2010;28(12):2101–2107.
147. Bain BJ, Moorman AV, Johansson B, et al. Myelodysplastic syndromes associated with 11q23 abnormalities. European 11q23 Workshop participants. *Leukemia* 1998;12(5):834–839.
148. Secker-Walker LM. General report on the European Union Concerted Action Workshop on 11q23, London, UK, May 1997. *Leukemia* 1998;12(5):776–778.
149. Bloomfield CD, Archer KJ, Mrozek K, et al. 11q23 balanced chromosome aberrations in treatment-related myelodysplastic syndromes and acute leukemia: report from an international workshop. *Genes Chromosomes Cancer* 2002;33(4):362–378.
150. Rowley JD, Olney HJ. International workshop on the relationship of prior therapy to balanced chromosome aberrations in therapy-related myelodysplastic syndromes and acute leukemia: overview report. *Genes Chromosomes Cancer* 2002;33(4):331–345.
151. Rowley JD, Reshmi S, Sobulo O, et al. All patients with the T(11;16)(q23;p13.3) that involves MLL and CBP have treatment-related hematologic disorders. *Blood* 1997;90(2):535–541.
152. Bejar R, Levine R, Ebert BL. Unraveling the molecular pathophysiology of myelodysplastic syndromes. *J Clin Oncol* 2011;29(5):504–515.
153. Parikh S, Bessler M. Recent insights into inherited bone marrow failure syndromes. *Curr Opin Pediatr* 2012;24(1):23–32.
154. Shimamura A, Alter BP. Pathophysiology and management of inherited bone marrow failure syndromes. *Blood Rev* 2010;24(3):101–122.
155. Kee Y, D'Andrea AD. Molecular pathogenesis and clinical management of Fanconi anemia. *J Clin Invest* 2012;122(11):3799–3806.
156. Alter BP, Giri N, Savage SA, et al. Malignancies and survival patterns in the National Cancer Institute inherited bone marrow failure syndromes cohort study. *Br J Haematol* 2010;150(2):179–188.
157. Cioc AM, Wagner JE, MacMillan ML, et al. Diagnosis of myelodysplastic syndrome among a cohort of 119 patients with Fanconi anemia: morphologic and cytogenetic characteristics. *Am J Clin Pathol* 2010;133(1):92–100.
158. Mehta PA, Harris RE, Davies SM, et al. Numerical chromosomal changes and risk of development of myelodysplastic syndrome—acute myeloid leukemia in patients with Fanconi anemia. *Cancer Genet Cytogenet* 2010;203(2):180–186.
159. Quentin S, Cuccuini W, Ceccaldi R, et al. Myelodysplasia and leukemia of Fanconi anemia are associated with a specific pattern of genomic abnormalities that includes cryptic RUNX1/AML1 lesions. *Blood* 2011;117(15):e161–e170.
160. Minelli A, Maserati E, Nicolis E, et al. The isochromosome i(7)(q10) carrying c.258+2t>c mutation of the SBDS gene does not promote development of myeloid malignancies in patients with Shwachman syndrome. *Leukemia* 2009;23(4): 708–711.
161. Germeshausen M, Ballmaier M, Welte K. Incidence of CSF3R mutations in severe congenital neutropenia and relevance for leukemogenesis: results of a long-term survey. *Blood* 2007;109(1):93–99.
162. Link DC, Kunter G, Kasai Y, et al. Distinct patterns of mutations occurring in de novo AML versus AML arising in the setting of severe congenital neutropenia. *Blood* 2007;110(5):1648–1655.
163. Dokal I, Vulliamy T, Mason P, et al. Clinical utility gene card for: dyskeratosis congenita. *Eur J Hum Genet* 2011;19(11).
164. Grimwade D, Mrozek K. Diagnostic and prognostic value of cytogenetics in acute myeloid leukemia. *Hematol Oncol Clin North Am* 2011;25(6):1135–1161, vii.
165. Kelly LM, Gilliland DG. Genetics of myeloid leukemias. *Annu Rev Genomics Hum Genet* 2002;3:179–198.
166. Rowley JD. Identification of a translocation with quinacrine fluorescence in a patient with acute leukemia. *Ann Genet* 1973;16(2):109–112.
167. Schlenk RF, Benner A, Krauter J, et al. Individual patient data-based meta-analysis of patients aged 16 to 60 years with core binding factor acute myeloid leukemia: a survey of the German Acute Myeloid Leukemia Intergroup. *J Clin Oncol* 2004;22(18):3741–3750.
168. Appelbaum FR, Kopecky KJ, Tallman MS, et al. The clinical spectrum of adult acute myeloid leukaemia associated with core binding factor translocations. *Br J Haematol* 2006;135(2):165–173.
169. Goyama S, Mulloy JC. Molecular pathogenesis of core binding factor leukemia: current knowledge and future prospects. *Int J Hematol* 2011;94(2):126–133.
170. Martens JH, Stunnenberg HG. The molecular signature of oncofusion proteins in acute myeloid leukemia. *FEBS Lett* 2010;584(12):2662–2669.
171. Paschka P, Marcucci G, Ruppert AS, et al. Adverse prognostic significance of KIT mutations in adult acute myeloid leukemia with inv(16) and t(8;21): a Cancer and Leukemia Group B study. *J Clin Oncol* 2006;24(24):3904–3911.
172. Cairoli R, Beghini A, Grillo G, et al. Prognostic impact of c-KIT mutations in core binding factor leukemias: an Italian retrospective study. *Blood* 2006;107(9):3463–3468.
173. Goemans BF, Zwaan CM, Miller M, et al. Mutations in KIT and RAS are frequent events in pediatric core-binding factor acute myeloid leukemia. *Leukemia* 2005;19(9):1536–1542.
174. Speck NA, Gilliland DG. Core-binding factors in haematopoiesis and leukaemia. *Nat Rev Cancer* 2002;2(7):502–513.
175. Marcucci G, Mrozek K, Ruppert AS, et al. Prognostic factors and outcome of core binding factor acute myeloid leukemia patients with t(8;21) differ from those of patients with inv(16): a Cancer and Leukemia Group B study. *J Clin Oncol* 2005;23(24):5705–5717.
176. Liu P, Tarle SA, Hajra A, et al. Fusion between transcription factor CBF beta/PEBP2 beta and a myosin heavy chain in acute myeloid leukemia. *Science* 1993;261(5124):1041–1044.
177. de The H, Chomienne C, Lanotte M, et al. The t(15;17) translocation of acute promyelocytic leukaemia fuses the retinoic acid receptor alpha gene to a novel transcribed locus. *Nature* 1990;347(6293):558–561.
178. Borrow J, Goddard AD, Sheer D, et al. Molecular analysis of acute promyelocytic leukemia breakpoint cluster region on chromosome 17. *Science* 1990;249 (4976):1577–1580.
179. Castaigne S, Chomienne C, Daniel MT, et al. All-trans retinoic acid as a differentiation therapy for acute promyelocytic leukemia. I. Clinical results. *Blood* 1990;76(9):1704–1709.
180. Grimwade D, Mistry AR, Solomon E, et al. Acute promyelocytic leukemia: a paradigm for differentiation therapy. *Cancer Treat Res* 2010;145:219–235.
181. Cervera J, Montesinos P, Hernandez-Rivas JM, et al. Additional chromosome abnormalities in patients with acute promyelocytic leukemia treated with all-trans retinoic acid and chemotherapy. *Haematologica* 2010;95(3):424–431.
182. Callens C, Chevret S, Cayuela JM, et al. Prognostic implication of FLT3 and Ras gene mutations in patients with acute promyelocytic leukemia (APL): a retrospective study from the European APL group. *Leukemia* 2005;19(7):1153–1160.
183. Kuchenbauer F, Schoch C, Kern W, et al. Impact of FLT3 mutations and promyelocytic leukaemia-breakpoint on clinical characteristics and prognosis in acute promyelocytic leukaemia. *Br J Haematol* 2005;130(2):196–202.
184. Brown NJ, Ramalho M, Pedersen EW, et al. PML nuclear bodies in the pathogenesis of acute promyelocytic leukemia: active players or innocent bystanders? *Front Biosci* 2009;14:1684–1707.
185. Grimwade D, Biondi A, Mozziconacci MJ, et al. Characterization of acute promyelocytic leukemia cases lacking the classic t(15;17): results of the European Working Party. Groupe Francais de Cytogenetique Hematologique, Groupe de Francais d'Hematologie Cellulaire, UK Cancer Cytogenetics Group and BIOMED 1 European Community-Concerted Action "Molecular Cytogenetic Diagnosis in Haematological Malignancies". *Blood* 2000;96(4):1297–1308.
186. Zelent A, Guidez F, Melnick A, et al. Translocations of the RARalpha gene in acute promyelocytic leukemia. *Oncogene* 2001;20(49):7186–7203.
187. Arnould C, Philippe C, Bourdon V, et al. The signal transducer and activator of transcription STAT5b gene is a new partner of retinoic acid receptor alpha in acute promyelocytic-like leukaemia. *Hum Mol Genet* 1999;8(9):1741–1749.
188. Catalano A, Dawson MA, Somana K, et al. The PRKAR1A gene is fused to RARA in a new variant acute promyelocytic leukemia. *Blood* 2007;110(12): 4073–4076.
189. Kondo T, Mori A, Darmanin S, et al. The seventh pathogenic fusion gene FIP1L1-RARA was isolated from a t(4;17)-positive acute promyelocytic leukemia. *Haematologica* 2008;93(9):1414–1416.
190. Yamamoto Y, Tsuzuki S, Tsuzuki M, et al. BCOR as a novel fusion partner of retinoic acid receptor alpha in a t(X;17)(p11;q12) variant of acute promyelocytic leukemia. *Blood* 2010;116(20):4274–4283.
191. Dong S, Tweardy DJ. Interactions of STAT5b-RARalpha, a novel acute promyelocytic leukemia fusion protein, with retinoic acid receptor and STAT3 signaling pathways. *Blood* 2002;99(8):2637–2646.
192. Meyer C, Kowarz E, Hofmann J, et al. New insights to the MLL recombinome of acute leukemias. *Leukemia* 2009;23(8):1490–1499.
193. Mrozek K, Heinonen K, Lawrence D, et al. Adult patients with de novo acute myeloid leukemia and t(9; 11)(p22; q23) have a superior outcome to patients with other translocations involving band 11q23: a cancer and leukemia group B study. *Blood* 1997;90(11):4532–4538.
194. Rubnitz JE, Raimondi SC, Tong X, et al. Favorable impact of the t(9;11) in childhood acute myeloid leukemia. *J Clin Oncol* 2002;20(9):2302–2309.
195. Byrd JC, Mrozek K, Dodge RK, et al. Pretreatment cytogenetic abnormalities are predictive of induction success, cumulative incidence of relapse, and overall survival in adult patients with de novo acute myeloid leukemia: results from Cancer and Leukemia Group B (CALGB 8461). *Blood* 2002;100(13):4325–4336.
196. Shih LY, Liang DC, Fu JF, et al. Characterization of fusion partner genes in 114 patients with de novo acute myeloid leukemia and MLL rearrangement. *Leukemia* 2006;20(2):218–223.
197. Ayton PM, Cleary ML. Molecular mechanisms of leukemogenesis mediated by MLL fusion proteins. *Oncogene* 2001;20(40):5695–5707.
198. Smith ML, Hills RK, Grimwade D. Independent prognostic variables in acute myeloid leukaemia. *Blood Rev* 2011;25(1):39–51.
199. Zeleznik-Le NJ, Harden AM, Rowley JD. 11q23 translocations split the "AT-hook" cruciform DNA-binding region and the transcriptional repression domain from the activation domain of the mixed-lineage leukemia (MLL) gene. *Proc Natl Acad Sci U S A* 1994;91(22):10610–10614.
200. Corral J, Lavenir I, Impey H, et al. An Mll-AF9 fusion gene made by homologous recombination causes acute leukemia in chimeric mice: a method to create fusion oncogenes. *Cell* 1996;85(6):853–861.
201. Krivtsov AV, Armstrong SA. MLL translocations, histone modifications and leukaemia stem-cell development. *Nat Rev Cancer* 2007;7(11):823–833.
202. Slovak ML, Gundacker H, Bloomfield CD, et al. A retrospective study of 69 patients with t(6;9)(p23;q34) AML emphasizes the need for a prospective, multicenter initiative for rare 'poor prognosis' myeloid malignancies. *Leukemia* 2006;20(7):1295–1297.
203. Soekarman D, von Lindern M, Daenen S, et al. The translocation (6;9) (p23;q34) shows consistent rearrangement of two genes and defines a myeloproliferative disorder with specific clinical features. *Blood* 1992;79(11):2990–2997.

204. Oyarzo MP, Lin P, Glassman A, et al. Acute myeloid leukemia with t(6;9)(p23;q34) is associated with dysplasia and a high frequency of flt3 gene mutations. *Am J Clin Pathol* 2004;122(3):348–358.
205. Kohler A, Hurt E. Gene regulation by nucleoporins and links to cancer. *Mol Cell* 2010;38(1):6–15.
206. Bitter MA, Neilly ME, Le Beau MM, et al. Rearrangements of chromosome 3 involving bands 3q21 and 3q26 are associated with normal or elevated platelet counts in acute nonlymphocytic leukemia. *Blood* 1985;66(6):1362–1370.
207. Lugthart S, Groschel S, Beverloo HB, et al. Clinical, molecular, and prognostic significance of WHO type inv(3)(q21q26.2)/t(3;3)(q21;q26.2) and various other 3q abnormalities in acute myeloid leukemia. *J Clin Oncol* 2010;28(24):3890–3898.
208. Goyama S, Kurokawa M. Evi-1 as a critical regulator of leukemic cells. *Int J Hematol* 2010;91(5):753–757.
209. Nucifora G, Laricchia-Robbio L, Senyuk V. EVI1 and hematopoietic disorders: history and perspectives. *Gene* 2006;368:1–11.
210. Russell M, List A, Greenberg P, et al. Expression of EVI1 in myelodysplastic syndromes and other hematologic malignancies without 3q26 translocations. *Blood* 1994;84(4):1243–1248.
211. Ma Z, Morris SW, Valentine V, et al. Fusion of two novel genes, RBM15 and MKL1, in the t(1;22)(p13;q13) of acute megakaryoblastic leukemia. *Nat Genet* 2001;28(3):220–221.
212. Mercher T, Coniat MB, Monni R, et al. Involvement of a human gene related to the *Drosophila* spen gene in the recurrent t(1;22) translocation of acute megakaryocytic leukemia. *Proc Natl Acad Sci U S A* 2001;98(10):5776–5779.
213. Duchayne E, Fenneteau O, Pages MP, et al. Acute megakaryoblastic leukaemia: a national clinical and biological study of 53 adult and childhood cases by the Groupe Francais d'Hematologie Cellulaire (GFHC). *Leuk Lymphoma* 2003;44 (1):49–58.
214. Cheng EC, Luo Q, Bruscia EM, et al. Role for MKL1 in megakaryocytic maturation. *Blood* 2009;113(12):2826–2834.
215. Falini B, Mecucci C, Tiacci E, et al. Cytoplasmic nucleophosmin in acute myelogenous leukemia with a normal karyotype. *N Engl J Med* 2005;352(3):254–266.
216. Falini B, Nicoletti I, Martelli MF, et al. Acute myeloid leukemia carrying cytoplasmic/mutated nucleophosmin (NPMc+ AML): biologic and clinical features. *Blood* 2007;109(3):874–885.
217. Falini B, Mecucci C, Saglio G, et al. NPM1 mutations and cytoplasmic nucleophosmin are mutually exclusive of recurrent genetic abnormalities: a comparative analysis of 2562 patients with acute myeloid leukemia. *Haematologica* 2008;93(3):439–442.
218. Verhaak RG, Goudswaard CS, van Putten W, et al. Mutations in nucleophosmin (NPM1) in acute myeloid leukemia (AML): association with other gene abnormalities and previously established gene expression signatures and their favorable prognostic significance. *Blood* 2005;106(12):3747–3754.
219. Pabst T, Mueller BU, Zhang P, et al. Dominant-negative mutations of CEBPA, encoding CCAAT/enhancer binding protein-alpha (C/EBPalpha), in acute myeloid leukemia. *Nat Genet* 2001;27(3):263–270.
220. Pabst T, Eyholzer M, Fos J, et al. Heterogeneity within AML with CEBPA mutations; only CEBPA double mutations, but not single CEBPA mutations are associated with favourable prognosis. *Br J Cancer* 2009;100(8):1343–1346.
221. Koschmieder S, Halmos B, Levantini E, et al. Dysregulation of the C/EBPalpha differentiation pathway in human cancer. *J Clin Oncol* 2009;27(4):619–628.
222. Wouters BJ, Lowenberg B, Erpelinck-Verschueren CA, et al. Double CEBPA mutations, but not single CEBPA mutations, define a subgroup of acute myeloid leukemia with a distinctive gene expression profile that is uniquely associated with a favorable outcome. *Blood* 2009;113(13):3088–3091.
223. Dufour A, Schneider F, Metzeler KH, et al. Acute myeloid leukemia with biallelic CEBPA gene mutations and normal karyotype represents a distinct genetic entity associated with a favorable clinical outcome. *J Clin Oncol* 2010;28(4):570–577.
224. Arber DA, Stein AS, Carter NH, et al. Prognostic impact of acute myeloid leukemia classification. Importance of detection of recurring cytogenetic abnormalities and multilineage dysplasia on survival. *Am J Clin Pathol* 2003;119(5):672–680.
225. Ebert BL. Genetic deletions in AML and MDS. *Best Pract Res Clin Haematol* 2010;23(4):457–461.
226. Arber DA, Chang KL, Lyda MH, et al. Detection of NPM/MLF1 fusion in t(3;5)-positive acute myeloid leukemia and myelodysplasia. *Hum Pathol* 2003;34(8): 809–813.
227. Haferlach C, Alpermann T, Schnittger S, et al. Prognostic value of monosomal karyotype in comparison to complex aberrant karyotype in acute myeloid leukemia: a study on 824 cases with aberrant karyotype. *Blood* 2012;119(9):2122–2125.
228. Allan JM, Travis LB. Mechanisms of therapy-related carcinogenesis. *Nat Rev Cancer* 2005;5(12):943–955.
229. Godley LA, Larson RA. Therapy-related myeloid leukemia. *Semin Oncol* 2008;35(4):418–429.
230. Vardiman JW, Thiele J, Arber DA, et al. The 2008 revision of the World Health Organization (WHO) classification of myeloid neoplasms and acute leukemia: rationale and important changes. *Blood* 2009;114(5):937–951.
231. Schoch C, Kern W, Schnittger S, et al. Karyotype is an independent prognostic parameter in therapy-related acute myeloid leukemia (t-AML): an analysis of 93 patients with t-AML in comparison to 1091 patients with de novo AML. *Leukemia* 2004;18(1):120–125.
232. Pedersen-Bjergaard J, Andersen MK, Andersen MT, et al. Genetics of therapy-related myelodysplasia and acute myeloid leukemia. *Leukemia* 2008;22(2):240–248.
233. Knight JA, Skol AD, Shinde A, et al. Genome-wide association study to identify novel loci associated with therapy-related myeloid leukemia susceptibility. *Blood* 2009;113(22):5575–5582.
234. Stoddart A, McNerney ME, Bartom E, et al. Genetic pathways leading to therapy-related myeloid neoplasms. *Mediterr J Hematol Infect Dis* 2011;3(1):e2011019.
235. Joslin JM, Fernald AA, Tennant TR, et al. Haploinsufficiency of EGR1, a candidate gene in the del(5q), leads to the development of myeloid disorders. *Blood* 2007;110(2):719–726.
236. Wang J, Fernald AA, Anastasi J, et al. Haploinsufficiency of Apc leads to ineffective hematopoiesis. *Blood* 2010;115(17):3481–3488.
237. Min IM, Pietramaggiori G, Kim FF, et al. The transcription factor EGR1 controls both the proliferation and localization of hematopoietic stem cells. *Cell Stem Cell* 2008;10:380–391.
238. Christiansen DH, Andersen MK, Pedersen-Bjergaard J. Methylation of p15INK4B is common, is associated with deletion of genes on chromosome arm 7q and predicts a poor prognosis in therapy-related myelodysplasia and acute myeloid leukemia. *Leukemia* 2003;17(9):1813–1819.
239. Loh ML, Vattikuti S, Schubbert S, et al. Mutations in PTPN11 implicate the SHP-2 phosphatase in leukemogenesis. *Blood* 2004;103(6):2325–2331.
240. Side LE, Curtiss NP, Teel K, et al. RAS, FLT3, and TP53 mutations in therapy-related myeloid malignancies with abnormalities of chromosomes 5 and 7. *Genes Chromosomes Cancer* 2004;39(3):217–223.
241. Le Beau MM, Espinosa R III, Davis EM, et al. Cytogenetic and molecular delineation of a region of chromosome 7 commonly deleted in malignant myeloid diseases. *Blood* 1996;88(6):1930–1935.
242. Wong JC, Zhang Y, Lieuw KH, et al. Use of chromosome engineering to model a segmental deletion of chromosome band 7q22 found in myeloid malignancies. *Blood* 2010;115(22):4524–4532.
243. Dohner K, Habdank M, Rucker FG, et al. Molecular characterization of distinct hot spot regions on chromosome 7q in myeloid leukemias. *Blood* 2006;108: Abstract 2349.
244. Jerez A, Sugimoto Y, Makishima H, et al. Loss of heterozygosity in 7q myeloid disorders: clinical associations and genomic pathogenesis. *Blood* 2012;119(25):6109–6117.
245. McNerney ME, Brown CD, Wang X, et al. CUX1 is a haploinsufficient tumor suppressor gene on chromosome 7 frequently inactivated in acute myeloid leukemia. *Blood* 2013:121(6):975–983.
246. Nikoloski G, Langemeijer SM, Kuiper RP, et al. Somatic mutations of the histone methyltransferase gene EZH2 in myelodysplastic syndromes. *Nat Genet* 2010;42(8):665–667.
247. Li L, Li M, Sun C, et al. Altered hematopoietic cell gene expression precedes development of therapy-related myelodysplasia/acute myeloid leukemia and identifies patients at risk. *Cancer Cell* 2011;20(5):591–605.
248. Khan I, Malinge S, Crispino J. Myeloid leukemia in Down syndrome. *Crit Rev Oncog* 2011;16(1–2):25–36.
249. Forestier E, Izraeli S, Beverloo B, et al. Cytogenetic features of acute lymphoblastic and myeloid leukemias in pediatric patients with Down syndrome: an iBFM-SG study. *Blood* 2008;111(3):1575–1583.
250. Wechsler J, Greene M, McDevitt MA, et al. Acquired mutations in GATA1 in the megakaryoblastic leukemia of Down syndrome. *Nat Genet* 2002;32(1):148–152.
251. Groet J, McElwaine S, Spinelli M, et al. Acquired mutations in GATA1 in neonates with Down's syndrome with transient myeloid disorder. *Lancet* 2003;361(9369):1617–1620.
252. Hitzler JK, Cheung J, Li Y, et al. GATA1 mutations in transient leukemia and acute megakaryoblastic leukemia of Down syndrome. *Blood* 2003;101(11):4301–4304.
253. Korbel JO, Tirosh-Wagner T, Urban AE, et al. The genetic architecture of Down syndrome phenotypes revealed by high-resolution analysis of human segmental trisomies. *Proc Natl Acad Sci U S A* 2009;106(29):12031–12036.
254. Malinge S, Bliss-Moreau M, Kirsammer G, et al. Increased dosage of the chromosome 21 ortholog Dyrk1a promotes megakaryoblastic leukemia in a murine model of Down syndrome. *J Clin Invest* 2012;122(3):948–962.
255. Schultz KR, Pullen DJ, Sather HN, et al. Risk- and response-based classification of childhood B-precursor acute lymphoblastic leukemia: a combined analysis of prognostic markers from the Pediatric Oncology Group (POG) and Children's Cancer Group (CCG). *Blood* 2007;109(3):926–935.
256. Moorman AV, Ensor HM, Richards SM, et al. Prognostic effect of chromosomal abnormalities in childhood B-cell precursor acute lymphoblastic leukaemia: results from the UK Medical Research Council ALL97/99 randomised trial. *Lancet Oncol* 2010;11(5):429–438.
257. Harrison CJ. Acute lymphoblastic leukemia. *Clin Lab Med* 2011;31(4):631–647, ix.
258. Mrozek K, Harper DP, Aplan PD. Cytogenetics and molecular genetics of acute lymphoblastic leukemia. *Hematol Oncol Clin North Am* 2009;23(5):991–1010, v.
259. Iacobucci I, Papayannidis C, Lonetti A, et al. Cytogenetic and molecular predictors of outcome in acute lymphocytic leukemia: recent developments. *Curr Hematol Malig Rep* 2012;7(2):133–143.
260. Mullighan CG, Goorha S, Radtke I, et al. Genome-wide analysis of genetic alterations in acute lymphoblastic leukaemia. *Nature* 2007;446(7137):758–764.
261. Kawamata N, Ogawa S, Zimmermann M, et al. Molecular allelokaryotyping of pediatric acute lymphoblastic leukemias by high-resolution single nucleotide polymorphism oligonucleotide genomic microarray. *Blood* 2008;111(2): 776–784.
262. Kuiper RP, Schoenmakers EF, van Reijmersdal SV, et al. High-resolution genomic profiling of childhood ALL reveals novel recurrent genetic lesions affecting pathways involved in lymphocyte differentiation and cell cycle progression. *Leukemia* 2007;21(6):1258–1266.
263. Zhang J, Mullighan CG, Harvey RC, et al. Key pathways are frequently mutated in high-risk childhood acute lymphoblastic leukemia: a report from the Children's Oncology Group. *Blood* 2011;118(11):3080–3087.
264. Moorman AV, Harrison CJ, Buck GA, et al. Karyotype is an independent prognostic factor in adult acute lymphoblastic leukemia (ALL): analysis of cytogenetic data from patients treated on the Medical Research Council (MRC) UKALLXII/Eastern Cooperative Oncology Group (ECOG) 2993 trial. *Blood* 2007;109(8):3189–3197.
265. Pullarkat V, Slovak ML, Kopecky KJ, et al. Impact of cytogenetics on the outcome of adult acute lymphoblastic leukemia: results of Southwest Oncology Group 9400 study. *Blood* 2008;111(5):2563–2572.
266. Pui CH, Evans WE. Treatment of acute lymphoblastic leukemia. *N Engl J Med* 2006;354(2):166–178.
267. Stock W. Advances in the treatment of Philadelphia chromosome-positive acute lymphoblastic leukemia. *Clin Adv Hematol Oncol* 2008;6(7):487–488.
268. Schultz KR, Bowman WP, Aledo A, et al. Improved early event-free survival with imatinib in Philadelphia chromosome-positive acute lymphoblastic leukemia: a children's oncology group study. *J Clin Oncol* 2009;27(31):5175–5181.
269. Hermans A, Heisterkamp N, von Linden M, et al. Unique fusion of bcr and c-abl genes in Philadelphia chromosome positive acute lymphoblastic leukemia. *Cell* 1987;51(1):33–40.
270. Anastasi J, Feng J, Dickstein JI, et al. Lineage involvement by BCR/ABL in Ph⁺ lymphoblastic leukemias: chronic myelogenous leukemia presenting in lymphoid blast vs Ph⁺ acute lymphoblastic leukemia. *Leukemia* 1996;10(5):795–802.
271. Fainstein E, Marcelle C, Rosner A, et al. A new fused transcript in Philadelphia chromosome positive acute lymphocytic leukaemia. *Nature* 1987;330(6146): 386–388.
272. van Etten RA. Disease progression in a murine model of bcr/abl leukemogenesis. *Leuk Lymphoma* 1993;11(Suppl 1):239–242.

273. Den Boer ML, van Slegtenhorst M, De Menezes RX, et al. A subtype of childhood acute lymphoblastic leukaemia with poor treatment outcome: a genome-wide classification study. *Lancet Oncol* 2009;10(2):125–134.
274. Mullighan CG, Su X, Zhang J, et al. Deletion of IKZF1 and prognosis in acute lymphoblastic leukemia. *N Engl J Med* 2009;360(5):470–480.
275. Harvey RC, Mullighan CG, Wang X, et al. Identification of novel cluster groups in pediatric high-risk B-precursor acute lymphoblastic leukemia with gene expression profiling: correlation with genome-wide DNA copy number alterations, clinical characteristics, and outcome. *Blood* 2010;116(23):4874–4884.
276. Mullighan CG, Zhang J, Harvey RC, et al. JAK mutations in high-risk childhood acute lymphoblastic leukemia. *Proc Natl Acad Sci U S A* 2009;106(23): 9414–9418.
277. Mullighan CG, Collins-Underwood JR, Phillips LA, et al. Rearrangement of CRLF2 in B-progenitor- and Down syndrome-associated acute lymphoblastic leukemia. *Nat Genet* 2009;41(11):1243–1246.
278. Russell LJ, Capasso M, Vater I, et al. Deregulated expression of cytokine receptor gene, CRLF2, is involved in lymphoid transformation in B-cell precursor acute lymphoblastic leukemia. *Blood* 2009;114(13):2688–2698.
279. Yoda A, Yoda Y, Chiaretti S, et al. Functional screening identifies CRLF2 in precursor B-cell acute lymphoblastic leukemia. *Proc Natl Acad Sci U S A* 2010;107(1):252–257.
280. Harvey RC, Mullighan CG, Chen IM, et al. Rearrangement of CRLF2 is associated with mutation of JAK kinases, alteration of IKZF1, Hispanic/Latino ethnicity, and a poor outcome in pediatric B-progenitor acute lymphoblastic leukemia. *Blood* 2010;115(26):5312–5321.
281. Cario G, Zimmermann M, Romey R, et al. Presence of the P2RY8-CRLF2 rearrangement is associated with a poor prognosis in non-high-risk precursor B-cell acute lymphoblastic leukemia in children treated according to the ALL-BFM 2000 protocol. *Blood* 2010;115(26):5393–5397.
282. Ensor HM, Schwab C, Russell LJ, et al. Demographic, clinical, and outcome features of children with acute lymphoblastic leukemia and CRLF2 deregulation: results from the MRC ALL97 clinical trial. *Blood* 2011;117(7):2129–2136.
283. Pui CH, Chessells JM, Camitta B, et al. Clinical heterogeneity in childhood acute lymphoblastic leukemia with 11q23 rearrangements. *Leukemia* 2003;17(4): 700–706.
284. Harrison CJ, Moorman AV, Barber KE, et al. Interphase molecular cytogenetic screening for chromosomal abnormalities of prognostic significance in childhood acute lymphoblastic leukaemia: a UK Cancer Cytogenetics Group Study. *Br J Haematol* 2005;129(4):520–530.
285. Meyer C, Schneider B, Jakob S, et al. The MLL recombinome of acute leukemias. *Leukemia* 2006;20(5):777–784.
286. Hilden JM, Dinndorf PA, Meerbaum SO, et al. Analysis of prognostic factors of acute lymphoblastic leukemia in infants: report on CCG 1953 from the Children's Oncology Group. *Blood* 2006;108(2):441–451.
287. Pieters R, Schrappe M, De Lorenzo P, et al. A treatment protocol for infants younger than 1 year with acute lymphoblastic leukaemia (Interfant-99): an observational study and a multicentre randomised trial. *Lancet* 2007;370(9583): 240–250.
288. Rubnitz JE, Behm FG, Curcio-Brint AM, et al. Molecular analysis of t(11;19) breakpoints in childhood acute leukemias. *Blood* 1996;87(11):4804–4808.
289. Pieters R. Infant acute lymphoblastic leukemia: lessons learned and future directions. *Curr Hematol Malig Rep* 2009;4(3):167–174.
290. Bueno C, Montes R, Catalina P, et al. Insights into the cellular origin and etiology of the infant pro-B acute lymphoblastic leukemia with MLL-AF4 rearrangement. *Leukemia* 2011;25(3):400–410.
291. Greaves MF, Maia AT, Wiemels JL, et al. Leukemia in twins: lessons in natural history. *Blood* 2003;102(7):2321–2333.
292. Gale KB, Ford AM, Repp R, et al. Backtracking leukemia to birth: identification of clonotypic gene fusion sequences in neonatal blood spots. *Proc Natl Acad Sci U S A* 1997;94(25):13950–13954.
293. Papaemmanuil E, Hosking FJ, Vijayakrishnan J, et al. Loci on 7p12.2, 10q21.2 and 14q11.2 are associated with risk of childhood acute lymphoblastic leukemia. *Nat Genet* 2009;41(9):1006–1010.
294. Trevino LR, Shimasaki N, Yang W, et al. Germline genetic variation in an organic anion transporter polypeptide associated with methotrexate pharmacokinetics and clinical effects. *J Clin Oncol* 2009;27(35):5972–5978.
295. Ross JA, Linabery AM, Blommer CN, et al. Genetic variants modify susceptibility to leukemia in infants: a Children's Oncology Group report. *Pediatr Blood Cancer* 2013;60(1):31–34.
296. Yeoh EJ, Ross ME, Shurtleff SA, et al. Classification, subtype discovery, and prediction of outcome in pediatric acute lymphoblastic leukemia by gene expression profiling. *Cancer Cell* 2002;1(2):133–143.
297. Stumpel DJ, Schneider P, van Roon EH, et al. Specific promoter methylation identifies different subgroups of MLL-rearranged infant acute lymphoblastic leukemia, influences clinical outcome, and provides therapeutic options. *Blood* 2009;114(27):5490–5498.
298. Chillon MC, Gomez-Casares MT, Lopez-Jorge CE, et al. Prognostic significance of FLT3 mutational status and expression levels in MLL-AF4+ and MLL-germline acute lymphoblastic leukemia. *Leukemia* 2012;26(11):2360–2366.
299. Hunger SP. Chromosomal translocations involving the E2A gene in acute lymphoblastic leukemia: clinical features and molecular pathogenesis. *Blood* 1996;87(4):1211–1224.
300. Jeha S, Pei D, Raimondi SC, et al. Increased risk for CNS relapse in pre-B cell leukemia with the t(1;19)/TCF3-PBX1. *Leukemia* 2009;23(8):1406–1409.
301. Uckun FM, Sensel MG, Sun L, et al. Biology and treatment of childhood T-lineage acute lymphoblastic leukemia. *Blood* 1998;91(3):735–746.
302. Garg R, Kantarjian H, Thomas D, et al. Adults with acute lymphoblastic leukemia and translocation (1;19) abnormality have a favorable outcome with hyperfractionated cyclophosphamide, vincristine, doxorubicin, and dexamethasone alternating with methotrexate and high-dose cytarabine chemotherapy. *Cancer* 2009;115(10):2147–2154.
303. Crist WM, Carroll AJ, Shuster JJ, et al. Poor prognosis of children with pre-B acute lymphoblastic leukemia is associated with the t(1;19)(q23;p13): a Pediatric Oncology Group study. *Blood* 1990;76(1):117–122.
304. Uckun FM, Sensel MG, Sather HN, et al. Clinical significance of translocation t(1;19) in childhood acute lymphoblastic leukemia in the context of contemporary therapies: a report from the Children's Cancer Group. *J Clin Oncol* 1998;16(2):527–535.
305. Kamps MP. E2A-Pbx1 induces growth, blocks differentiation, and interacts with other homeodomain proteins regulating normal differentiation. *Curr Top Microbiol Immunol* 1997;220:25–43.
306. Romana SP, Poirel H, Leconiat M, et al. High frequency of t(12;21) in childhood B-lineage acute lymphoblastic leukemia. *Blood* 1995;86(11):4263–4269.
307. Shurtleff SA, Buijs A, Behm FG, et al. TEL/AML1 fusion resulting from a cryptic t(12;21) is the most common genetic lesion in pediatric ALL and defines a subgroup of patients with an excellent prognosis. *Leukemia* 1995;9(12):1985–1989.
308. Golub TR, Barker GF, Bohlander SK, et al. Fusion of the TEL gene on 12p13 to the AML1 gene on 21q22 in acute lymphoblastic leukemia. *Proc Natl Acad Sci U S A* 1995;92(11):4917–4921.
309. Lopez RG, Carron C, Oury C, et al. TEL is a sequence-specific transcriptional repressor. *J Biol Chem* 1999;274(42):30132–30138.
310. Stegmaier K, Pendse S, Barker GF, et al. Frequent loss of heterozygosity at the TEL gene locus in acute lymphoblastic leukemia of childhood. *Blood* 1995;86(1): 38–44.
311. Rubnitz JE, Wichlan D, Devidas M, et al. Prospective analysis of TEL gene rearrangements in childhood acute lymphoblastic leukemia: a Children's Oncology Group study. *J Clin Oncol* 2008;26(13):2186–2191.
312. Forestier E, Heyman M, Andersen MK, et al. Outcome of ETV6/RUNX1-positive childhood acute lymphoblastic leukaemia in the NOPHO-ALL-1992 protocol: frequent late relapses but good overall survival. *Br J Haematol* 2008;140(6): 665–672.
313. Loh ML, Goldwasser MA, Silverman LB, et al. Prospective analysis of TEL/AML1-positive patients treated on Dana-Farber Cancer Institute Consortium Protocol 95-01. *Blood* 2006;107(11):4508–4513.
314. Stams WA, Beverloo HB, den Boer ML, et al. Incidence of additional genetic changes in the TEL and AML1 genes in DCOG and COALL-treated t(12;21)-positive pediatric ALL, and their relation with drug sensitivity and clinical outcome. *Leukemia* 2006;20(3):410–416.
315. Moorman AV, Richards SM, Robinson HM, et al. Prognosis of children with acute lymphoblastic leukemia (ALL) and intrachromosomal amplification of chromosome 21 (iAMP21). *Blood* 2007;109(6):2327–2330.
316. Attarbaschi A, Mann G, Panzer-Grumayer R, et al. Minimal residual disease values discriminate between low and high relapse risk in children with B-cell precursor acute lymphoblastic leukemia and an intrachromosomal amplification of chromosome 21: the Austrian and German acute lymphoblastic leukemia Berlin-Frankfurt-Munster (ALL-BFM) trials. *J Clin Oncol* 2008;26(18):3046–3050.
317. Nachman JB, Heerema NA, Sather H, et al. Outcome of treatment in children with hypodiploid acute lymphoblastic leukemia. *Blood* 2007;110(4):1112–1115.
318. Harrison CJ, Moorman AV, Broadfield ZJ, et al. Three distinct subgroups of hypodiploidy in acute lymphoblastic leukaemia. *Br J Haematol* 2004;125(5):552–559.
319. Paulsson K, Johansson B. High hyperdiploid childhood acute lymphoblastic leukemia. *Genes Chromosomes Cancer* 2009;48(8):637–660.
320. Heerema NA, Raimondi SC, Anderson JR, et al. Specific extra chromosomes occur in a modal number dependent pattern in pediatric acute lymphoblastic leukemia. *Genes Chromosomes Cancer* 2007;46(7):684–693.
321. Arico M, Valsecchi MG, Rizzari C, et al. Long-term results of the AIEOP-ALL-95 Trial for Childhood Acute Lymphoblastic Leukemia: insight on the prognostic value of DNA index in the framework of Berlin-Frankfurt-Muenster based chemotherapy. *J Clin Oncol* 2008;26(2):283–289.
322. Sutcliffe MJ, Shuster JJ, Sather HN, et al. High concordance from independent studies by the Children's Cancer Group (CCG) and Pediatric Oncology Group (POG) associating favorable prognosis with combined trisomies 4, 10, and 17 in children with NCI Standard-Risk B-precursor Acute Lymphoblastic Leukemia: a Children's Oncology Group (COG) initiative. *Leukemia* 2005;19(5):734–740.
323. Harris MB, Shuster JJ, Carroll A, et al. Trisomy of leukemic cell chromosomes 4 and 10 identifies children with B-progenitor cell acute lymphoblastic leukemia with a very low risk of treatment failure: a Pediatric Oncology Group study. *Blood* 1992;79(12):3316–3324.
324. Raimondi SC, Pui CH, Hancock ML, et al. Heterogeneity of hyperdiploid (51-67) childhood acute lymphoblastic leukemia. *Leukemia* 1996;10(2):213–224.
325. Heerema NA, Harbott J, Galimberti S, et al. Secondary cytogenetic aberrations in childhood Philadelphia chromosome positive acute lymphoblastic leukemia are nonrandom and may be associated with outcome. *Leukemia* 2004;18(4):693–702.
326. Meinhardt A, Burkhardt B, Zimmermann M, et al. Phase II window study on rituximab in newly diagnosed pediatric mature B-cell non-Hodgkin's lymphoma and Burkitt leukemia. *J Clin Oncol* 2010;28(19):3115–3121.
327. Heerema NA, Sather HN, Sensel MG, et al. Frequency and clinical significance of cytogenetic abnormalities in pediatric T-lineage acute lymphoblastic leukemia: a report from the Children's Cancer Group. *J Clin Oncol* 1998;16(4):1270–1278.
328. Mancini M, Scappaticci D, Cimino G, et al. A comprehensive genetic classification of adult acute lymphoblastic leukemia (ALL): analysis of the GIMEMA 0496 protocol. *Blood* 2005;105(9):3434–3441.
329. Graux C, Cools J, Michaux L, et al. Cytogenetics and molecular genetics of T-cell acute lymphoblastic leukemia: from thymocyte to lymphoblast. *Leukemia* 2006;20(9):1496–1510.
330. Carroll AJ, Crist WM, Link MP, et al. The t(1;14)(p34;q11) is nonrandom and restricted to T-cell acute lymphoblastic leukemia: a Pediatric Oncology Group study. *Blood* 1990;76(6):1220–1224.
331. Ferrando AA, Neuberg DS, Staunton J, et al. Gene expression signatures define novel oncogenic pathways in T cell acute lymphoblastic leukemia. *Cancer Cell* 2002;1(1):75–87.
332. Soulier J, Clappier E, Cayuela JM, et al. HOXA genes are included in genetic and biologic networks defining human acute T-cell leukemia (T-ALL). *Blood* 2005;106(1):274–286.
333. van Oostveen J, Bijl J, Raaphorst F, et al. The role of homeobox genes in normal hematopoiesis and hematological malignancies. *Leukemia* 1999;13(11):1675–1690.
334. Kees UR, Heerema NA, Kumar R, et al. Expression of HOX11 in childhood T-lineage acute lymphoblastic leukaemia can occur in the absence of cytogenetic aberration at 10q24: a study from the Children's Cancer Group (CCG). *Leukemia* 2003;17(5):887–893.
335. Bernard OA, Busson-LeConiat M, Ballerini P, et al. A new recurrent and specific cryptic translocation, t(5;14)(q35;q32), is associated with expression of the Hox11L2 gene in T acute lymphoblastic leukemia. *Leukemia* 2001;15(10): 1495–1504.

336. Speleman F, Cauwelier B, Dastugue N, et al. A new recurrent inversion, inv(7)(p15q34), leads to transcriptional activation of HOXA10 and HOXA11 in a subset of T-cell acute lymphoblastic leukemias. *Leukemia* 2005;19(3):358–366.
337. Asnafi V, Radford-Weiss I, Dastugue N, et al. CALM-AF10 is a common fusion transcript in T-ALL and is specific to the TCRgammadelta lineage. *Blood* 2003;102(3):1000–1006.
338. Barber KE, Martineau M, Harewood L, et al. Amplification of the ABL gene in T-cell acute lymphoblastic leukemia. *Leukemia* 2004;18(6):1153–1156.
339. Graux C, Cools J, Melotte C, et al. Fusion of NUP214 to ABL1 on amplified episomes in T-cell acute lymphoblastic leukemia. *Nat Genet* 2004;36(10):1084–1089.
340. Quintas-Cardama A, Tong W, Manshouri T, et al. Activity of tyrosine kinase inhibitors against human NUP214-ABL1-positive T cell malignancies. *Leukemia* 2008;22(6):1117–1124.
341. Weng AP, Ferrando AA, Lee W, et al. Activating mutations of NOTCH1 in human T cell acute lymphoblastic leukemia. *Science* 2004;306(5694):269–271.
342. Baldus CD, Thibaut J, Goekbuget N, et al. Prognostic implications of NOTCH1 and FBXW7 mutations in adult acute T-lymphoblastic leukemia. *Haematologica* 2009;94(10):1383–1390.
343. O'Neil J, Grim J, Strack P, et al. FBW7 mutations in leukemic cells mediate NOTCH pathway activation and resistance to gamma-secretase inhibitors. *J Exp Med* 2007;204(8):1813–1824.
344. Zhang J, Ding L, Holmfeldt L, et al. The genetic basis of early T-cell precursor acute lymphoblastic leukaemia. *Nature* 2012;481(7380):157–163.
345. Van Vlierberghe P, Palomero T, Khiabanian H, et al. PHF6 mutations in T-cell acute lymphoblastic leukemia. *Nat Genet* 2010;42(4):338–342.
346. Lahortiga I, De Keersmaecker K, Van Vlierberghe P, et al. Duplication of the MYB oncogene in T cell acute lymphoblastic leukemia. *Nat Genet* 2007;39(5):593–595.
347. Palomero T, Sulis ML, Cortina M, et al. Mutational loss of PTEN induces resistance to NOTCH1 inhibition in T-cell leukemia. *Nat Med* 2007;13(10):1203–1210.
348. Dave BJ, Nelson M, Sanger WG. Lymphoma cytogenetics. *Clin Lab Med* 2011;31(4):725–761.
349. Nogai H, Dorken B, Lenz G. Pathogenesis of non-Hodgkin's lymphoma. *J Clin Oncol* 2011;29(14):1803–1811.
350. Chiorazzi N, Rai KR, Ferrarini M. Chronic lymphocytic leukemia. *N Engl J Med* 2005;352(8):804–815.
351. Goldin LR, Bjorkholm M, Kristinsson SY, et al. Elevated risk of chronic lymphocytic leukemia and other indolent non-Hodgkin's lymphomas among relatives of patients with chronic lymphocytic leukemia. *Haematologica* 2009;94(5):647–653.
352. Van Bockstaele F, Verhasselt B, Philippe J. Prognostic markers in chronic lymphocytic leukemia: a comprehensive review. *Blood Rev* 2009;23(1):25–47.
353. Dohner H, Stilgenbauer S, Benner A, et al. Genomic aberrations and survival in chronic lymphocytic leukemia. *N Engl J Med* 2000;343(26):1910–1916.
354. Haferlach C, Dicker F, Schnittger S, et al. Comprehensive genetic characterization of CLL: a study on 506 cases analysed with chromosome banding analysis, interphase FISH, IgV(H) status and immunophenotyping. *Leukemia* 2007;21(12):2442–2451.
355. Dal Bo M, Rossi FM, Rossi D, et al. 13q14 deletion size and number of deleted cells both influence prognosis in chronic lymphocytic leukemia. *Genes Chromosomes Cancer* 2011;50(8):633–643.
356. Ouillette P, Fossum S, Parkin B, et al. Aggressive chronic lymphocytic leukemia with elevated genomic complexity is associated with multiple gene defects in the response to DNA double-strand breaks. *Clin Cancer Res* 2010;16(3):835–847.
357. Calin GA, Dumitru CD, Shimizu M, et al. Frequent deletions and down-regulation of micro- RNA genes miR15 and miR16 at 13q14 in chronic lymphocytic leukemia. *Proc Natl Acad Sci U S A* 2002;99(24):15524–15529.
358. Cimmino A, Calin GA, Fabbri M, et al. miR-15 and miR-16 induce apoptosis by targeting BCL2. *Proc Natl Acad Sci U S A* 2005;102(39):13944–13949.
359. Klein U, Lia M, Crespo M, et al. The DLEU2/miR-15a/16-1 cluster controls B cell proliferation and its deletion leads to chronic lymphocytic leukemia. *Cancer Cell* 2010;17(1):28–40.
360. Austen B, Skowronska A, Baker C, et al. Mutation status of the residual ATM allele is an important determinant of the cellular response to chemotherapy and survival in patients with chronic lymphocytic leukemia containing an 11q deletion. *J Clin Oncol* 2007;25(34):5448–5457.
361. Skowronska A, Austen B, Powell JE, et al. ATM germline heterozygosity does not play a role in chronic lymphocytic leukemia initiation but influences rapid disease progression through loss of the remaining ATM allele. *Haematologica* 2012;97(1):142–146.
362. Zenz T, Krober A, Scherer K, et al. Monoallelic TP53 inactivation is associated with poor prognosis in chronic lymphocytic leukemia: results from a detailed genetic characterization with long-term follow-up. *Blood* 2008;112(8):3322–3329.
363. Rosenwald A, Chuang EY, Davis RE, et al. Fludarabine treatment of patients with chronic lymphocytic leukemia induces a p53-dependent gene expression response. *Blood* 2004;104(5):1428–1434.
364. Turgut B, Vural O, Pala FS, et al. 17p Deletion is associated with resistance of B-cell chronic lymphocytic leukemia cells to in vitro fludarabine-induced apoptosis. *Leuk Lymphoma* 2007;48(2):311–320.
365. Hillmen P, Skotnicki AB, Robak T, et al. Alemtuzumab compared with chlorambucil as first-line therapy for chronic lymphocytic leukemia. *J Clin Oncol* 2007;25(35):5616–5623.
366. Zenz T, Habe S, Denzel T, et al. Detailed analysis of p53 pathway defects in fludarabine-refractory chronic lymphocytic leukemia (CLL): dissecting the contribution of 17p deletion, TP53 mutation, p53-p21 dysfunction, and miR34a in a prospective clinical trial. *Blood* 2009;114(13):2589–2597.
367. Krober A, Seiler T, Benner A, et al. V(H) mutation status, CD38 expression level, genomic aberrations, and survival in chronic lymphocytic leukemia. *Blood* 2002;100(4):1410–1416.
368. Oscier DG, Gardiner AC, Mould SJ, et al. Multivariate analysis of prognostic factors in CLL: clinical stage, IGVH gene mutational status, and loss or mutation of the p53 gene are independent prognostic factors. *Blood* 2002;100(4):1177–1184.
369. Vasconcelos Y, Davi F, Levy V, et al. Binet's staging system and VH genes are independent but complementary prognostic indicators in chronic lymphocytic leukemia. *J Clin Oncol* 2003;21(21):3928–3932.
370. Haslinger C, Schweifer N, Stilgenbauer S, et al. Microarray gene expression profiling of B-cell chronic lymphocytic leukemia subgroups defined by genomic aberrations and VH mutation status. *J Clin Oncol* 2004;22(19):3937–3949.
371. Vasconcelos Y, De Vos J, Vallat L, et al. Gene expression profiling of chronic lymphocytic leukemia can discriminate cases with stable disease and mutated Ig genes from those with progressive disease and unmutated Ig genes. *Leukemia* 2005;19(11):2002–2005.
372. Crespo M, Bosch F, Villamor N, et al. ZAP-70 expression as a surrogate for immunoglobulin-variable-region mutations in chronic lymphocytic leukemia. *N Engl J Med* 2003;348(18):1764–1775.
373. Puente XS, Pinyol M, Quesada V, et al. Whole-genome sequencing identifies recurrent mutations in chronic lymphocytic leukaemia. *Nature* 2011;475(7354):101–105.
374. Wang L, Lawrence MS, Wan Y, et al. SF3B1 and other novel cancer genes in chronic lymphocytic leukemia. *N Engl J Med* 2011;365(26):2497–2506.
375. Fabbri G, Rasi S, Rossi D, et al. Analysis of the chronic lymphocytic leukemia coding genome: role of NOTCH1 mutational activation. *J Exp Med* 2011;208(7):1389–1401.
376. Isaacson PG, Du MQ. MALT lymphoma: from morphology to molecules. *Nat Rev Cancer* 2004;4(8):644–653.
377. Remstein ED, Dogan A, Einerson RR, et al. The incidence and anatomic site specificity of chromosomal translocations in primary extranodal marginal zone B-cell lymphoma of mucosa-associated lymphoid tissue (MALT lymphoma) in North America. *Am J Surg Pathol* 2006;30(12):1546–1553.
378. Akagi T, Motegi M, Tamura A, et al. A novel gene, MALT1 at 18q21, is involved in t(11;18) (q21;q21) found in low-grade B-cell lymphoma of mucosa-associated lymphoid tissue. *Oncogene* 1999;18(42):5785–5794.
379. Horsman D, Gascoyne R, Klasa R, et al. t(11;18)(q21;q21.1): a recurring translocation in lymphomas of mucosa-associated lymphoid tissue (MALT)? *Genes Chromosomes Cancer* 1992;4(2):183–187.
380. Sagaert X, De Wolf-Peeters C, Noels H, et al. The pathogenesis of MALT lymphomas: where do we stand? *Leukemia* 2007;21(3):389–396.
381. Willis TG, Jadayel DM, Du MQ, et al. Bcl10 is involved in t(1;14)(p22;q32) of MALT B cell lymphoma and mutated in multiple tumor types. *Cell* 1999;96(1):35–45.
382. Ye H, Gong L, Liu H, et al. MALT lymphoma with t(14;18)(q32;q21)/IGH-MALT1 is characterized by strong cytoplasmic MALT1 and BCL10 expression. *J Pathol* 2005;205(3):293–301.
383. Zhou Y, Ye H, Martin-Subero JI, et al. Distinct comparative genomic hybridization profiles in gastric mucosa-associated lymphoid tissue lymphomas with and without t(11;18)(q21;q21). *Br J Haematol* 2006;133(1):35–42.
384. Remstein ED, Kurtin PJ, James CD, et al. Mucosa-associated lymphoid tissue lymphomas with t(11;18)(q21;q21) and mucosa-associated lymphoid tissue lymphomas with aneuploidy develop along different pathogenetic pathways. *Am J Pathol* 2002;161(1):63–71.
385. Streubel B, Simonitsch-Klupp I, Mullauer L, et al. Variable frequencies of MALT lymphoma-associated genetic aberrations in MALT lymphomas of different sites. *Leukemia* 2004;18(10):1722–1726.
386. Zhang Q, Siebert R, Yan M, et al. Inactivating mutations and overexpression of BCL10, a caspase recruitment domain-containing gene, in MALT lymphoma with t(1;14)(p22;q32). *Nat Genet* 1999;22(1):63–68.
387. Chuang SS, Liu H, Martin-Subero JI, et al. Pulmonary mucosa-associated lymphoid tissue lymphoma with strong nuclear B-cell CLL/lymphoma 10 (BCL10) expression and novel translocation t(1;2)(p22;p12)/immunoglobulin kappa chain-BCL10. *J Clin Pathol* 2007;60(6):727–728.
388. Ruland J, Duncan GS, Elia A, et al. Bcl10 is a positive regulator of antigen receptor-induced activation of NF-kappaB and neural tube closure. *Cell* 2001;104(1):33–42.
389. Lucas PC, Yonezumi M, Inohara N, et al. Bcl10 and MALT1, independent targets of chromosomal translocation in malt lymphoma, cooperate in a novel NF-kappa B signaling pathway. *J Biol Chem* 2001;276(22):19012–19019.
390. Hayden MS, Ghosh S. Signaling to NF-kappaB. *Genes Dev* 2004;18(18):2195–2224.
391. Streubel B, Vinatzer U, Lamprecht A, et al. T(3;14)(p14.1;q32) involving IGH and FOXP1 is a novel recurrent chromosomal aberration in MALT lymphoma. *Leukemia* 2005;19(4):652–658.
392. Sagaert X, de Paepe P, Libbrecht L, et al. Forkhead box protein P1 expression in mucosa-associated lymphoid tissue lymphomas predicts poor prognosis and transformation to diffuse large B-cell lymphoma. *J Clin Oncol* 2006;24(16):2490–2497.
393. Goatly A, Bacon CM, Nakamura S, et al. FOXP1 abnormalities in lymphoma: translocation breakpoint mapping reveals insights into deregulated transcriptional control. *Mod Pathol* 2008;21(7):902–911.
394. Hu H, Wang B, Borde M, et al. Foxp1 is an essential transcriptional regulator of B cell development. *Nat Immunol* 2006;7(8):819–826.
395. Leich E, Ott G, Rosenwald A. Pathology, pathogenesis and molecular genetics of follicular NHL. *Best Pract Res Clin Haematol* 2011;24(2):95–109.
396. Anderson JR, Armitage JO, Weisenburger DD. Epidemiology of the non-Hodgkin's lymphomas: distributions of the major subtypes differ by geographic locations. Non-Hodgkin's Lymphoma Classification Project. *Ann Oncol* 1998;9(7):717–720.
397. Tsujimoto Y, Finger LR, Yunis J, et al. Cloning of the chromosome breakpoint of neoplastic B cells with the t(14;18) chromosome translocation. *Science* 1984;226(4678):1097–1099.
398. Johansson B, Mertens F, Mitelman F. Cytogenetic evolution patterns in non-Hodgkin's lymphoma. *Blood* 1995;86(10):3905–3914.
399. Swerdlow SH. Pediatric follicular lymphomas, marginal zone lymphomas, and marginal zone hyperplasia. *Am J Clin Pathol* 2004;122(Suppl):S98–S109.
400. Zinkel S, Gross A, Yang E. BCL2 family in DNA damage and cell cycle control. *Cell Death Differ* 2006;13(8):1351–1359.
401. McDonnell TJ, Korsmeyer SJ. Progression from lymphoid hyperplasia to high-grade malignant lymphoma in mice transgenic for the t(14; 18). *Nature* 1991;349(6306):254–256.
402. Summers KE, Goff LK, Wilson AG, et al. Frequency of the Bcl-2/IgH rearrangement in normal individuals: implications for the monitoring of disease in patients with follicular lymphoma. *J Clin Oncol* 2001;19(2):420–424.
403. Bende RJ, Smit LA, van Noesel CJ. Molecular pathways in follicular lymphoma. *Leukemia* 2007;21(1):18–29.
404. Pasqualucci L, Bhagat G, Jankovic M, et al. AID is required for germinal center-derived lymphomagenesis. *Nat Genet* 2008;40(1):108–112.
405. Hoglund M, Sehn L, Connors JM, et al. Identification of cytogenetic subgroups and karyotypic pathways of clonal evolution in follicular lymphomas. *Genes Chromosomes Cancer* 2004;39(3):195–204.

406. Aamot HV, Torlakovic EE, Eide MB, et al. Non-Hodgkin lymphoma with t(14;18): clonal evolution patterns and cytogenetic-pathologic-clinical correlations. *J Cancer Res Clin Oncol* 2007;133(7):455–470.

407. Cheung KJ, Shah SP, Steidl C, et al. Genome-wide profiling of follicular lymphoma by array comparative genomic hybridization reveals prognostically significant DNA copy number imbalances. *Blood* 2009;113(1):137–148.

408. O'Shea D, O'Riain C, Gupta M, et al. Regions of acquired uniparental disomy at diagnosis of follicular lymphoma are associated with both overall survival and risk of transformation. *Blood* 2009;113(10):2298–2301.

409. O'Shea D, O'Riain C, Taylor C, et al. The presence of TP53 mutation at diagnosis of follicular lymphoma identifies a high-risk group of patients with shortened time to disease progression and poorer overall survival. *Blood* 2008;112(8):3126–3129.

410. Davies AJ, Rosenwald A, Wright G, et al. Transformation of follicular lymphoma to diffuse large B-cell lymphoma proceeds by distinct oncogenic mechanisms. *Br J Haematol* 2007;136(2):286–293.

411. Elenitoba-Johnson KS, Gascoyne RD, Lim MS, et al. Homozygous deletions at chromosome 9p21 involving p16 and p15 are associated with histologic progression in follicle center lymphoma. *Blood* 1998;91(12):4677–4685.

412. Lossos IS, Alizadeh AA, Diehn M, et al. Transformation of follicular lymphoma to diffuse large-cell lymphoma: alternative patterns with increased or decreased expression of c-myc and its regulated genes. *Proc Natl Acad Sci U S A* 2002;99(13):8886–8891.

413. Pinyol M, Cobo F, Bea S, et al. p16(INK4a) gene inactivation by deletions, mutations, and hypermethylation is associated with transformed and aggressive variants of non-Hodgkin's lymphomas. *Blood* 1998;91(8):2977–2984.

414. Horsman DE, Okamoto I, Ludkovski O, et al. Follicular lymphoma lacking the t(14;18)(q32;q21): identification of two disease subtypes. *Br J Haematol* 2003; 120(3):424–433.

415. Ott G, Katzenberger T, Lohr A, et al. Cytomorphologic, immunohistochemical, and cytogenetic profiles of follicular lymphoma: 2 types of follicular lymphoma grade 3. *Blood* 2002;99(10):3806–3812.

416. Guo Y, Karube K, Kawano R, et al. Bcl2-negative follicular lymphomas frequently have Bcl6 translocation and/or Bcl6 or p53 expression. *Pathol Int* 2007;57(3):148–152.

417. Jardin F, Gaulard P, Buchonnet G, et al. Follicular lymphoma without t(14;18) and with BCL-6 rearrangement: a lymphoma subtype with distinct pathological, molecular and clinical characteristics. *Leukemia* 2002;16(11):2309–2317.

418. Jardin F, Ruminy P, Bastard C, et al. The BCL6 proto-oncogene: a leading role during germinal center development and lymphomagenesis. *Pathol Biol (Paris)* 2007;55(1):73–83.

419. Ye BH, Rao PH, Chaganti RS, et al. Cloning of bcl-6, the locus involved in chromosome translocations affecting band 3q27 in B-cell lymphoma. *Cancer Res* 1993;53(12):2732–2735.

420. Parry-Jones N, Matutes E, Morilla R, et al. Cytogenetic abnormalities additional to t(11;14) correlate with clinical features in leukaemic presentation of mantle cell lymphoma, and may influence prognosis: a study of 60 cases by FISH. *Br J Haematol* 2007;137(2):117–124.

421. Sherr CJ, McCormick F. The RB and p53 pathways in cancer. *Cancer Cell* 2002; 2(2):103–112.

422. Perez-Galan P, Dreyling M, Wiestner A. Mantle cell lymphoma: biology, pathogenesis, and the molecular basis of treatment in the genomic era. *Blood* 2011;117(1):26–38.

423. Quintanilla-Martinez L, Davies-Hill T, Fend F, et al. Sequestration of p27Kip1 protein by cyclin D1 in typical and blastic variants of mantle cell lymphoma (MCL): implications for pathogenesis. *Blood* 2003;101(8):3181–3187.

424. Fu K, Weisenburger DD, Greiner TC, et al. Cyclin D1-negative mantle cell lymphoma: a clinicopathologic study based on gene expression profiling. *Blood* 2005;106(13):4315–4321.

425. Rosenwald A, Wright G, Wiestner A, et al. The proliferation gene expression signature is a quantitative integrator of oncogenic events that predicts survival in mantle cell lymphoma. *Cancer Cell* 2003;3(2):185–197.

426. Gesk S, Klapper W, Martin-Subero JI, et al. A chromosomal translocation in cyclin D1-negative/cyclin D2-positive mantle cell lymphoma fuses the CCND2 gene to the IGK locus. *Blood* 2006;108(3):1109–1110.

427. Bodrug SE, Warner BJ, Bath ML, et al. Cyclin D1 transgene impedes lymphocyte maturation and collaborates in lymphomagenesis with the myc gene. *EMBO J* 1994;13(9):2124–2130.

428. Salaverria I, Zettl A, Bea S, et al. Specific secondary genetic alterations in mantle cell lymphoma provide prognostic information independent of the gene expression-based proliferation signature. *J Clin Oncol* 2007;25(10):1216–1222.

429. Rubio-Moscardo F, Climent J, Siebert R, et al. Mantle-cell lymphoma genotypes identified with CGH to BAC microarrays define a leukemic subgroup of disease and predict patient outcome. *Blood* 2005;105(11):4445–4454.

430. Bea S, Campo E. Secondary genomic alterations in non-Hodgkin's lymphomas: tumor-specific profiles with impact on clinical behavior. *Haematologica* 2008;93(5):641–645.

431. Vater I, Wagner F, Kreuz M, et al. GeneChip analyses point to novel pathogenetic mechanisms in mantle cell lymphoma. *Br J Haematol* 2009;144(3):317–331.

432. Vaishampayan UN, Mohamed AN, Dugan MC, et al. Blastic mantle cell lymphoma associated with Burkitt-type translocation and hypodiploidy. *Br J Haematol* 2001;115(1):66–68.

433. Camacho FI, Garcia JF, Cigudosa JC, et al. Aberrant Bcl6 protein expression in mantle cell lymphoma. *Am J Surg Pathol* 2004;28(8):1051–1056.

434. Sander S, Bullinger L, Leupolt E, et al. Genomic aberrations in mantle cell lymphoma detected by interphase fluorescence in situ hybridization. Incidence and clinicopathological correlations. *Haematologica* 2008;93(5):680–687.

435. Schaffner C, Idler I, Stilgenbauer S, et al. Mantle cell lymphoma is characterized by inactivation of the ATM gene. *Proc Natl Acad Sci U S A* 2000;97(6):2773–2778.

436. Camacho E, Hernandez L, Hernandez S, et al. ATM gene inactivation in mantle cell lymphoma mainly occurs by truncating mutations and missense mutations involving the phosphatidylinositol-3 kinase domain and is associated with increasing numbers of chromosomal imbalances. *Blood* 2002;99(1):238–244.

437. Jares P, Colomer D, Campo E. Genetic and molecular pathogenesis of mantle cell lymphoma: perspectives for new targeted therapeutics. *Nat Rev Cancer* 2007;7(10):750–762.

438. Armitage JO, Weisenburger DD. New approach to classifying non-Hodgkin's lymphomas: clinical features of the major histologic subtypes. Non-Hodgkin's Lymphoma Classification Project. *J Clin Oncol* 1998;16(8):2780–2795.

439. Lenz G, Nagel I, Siebert R, et al. Aberrant immunoglobulin class switch recombination and switch translocations in activated B cell-like diffuse large B cell lymphoma. *J Exp Med* 2007;204(3):633–643.

440. Offit K, Lo Coco F, Louie DC, et al. Rearrangement of the bcl-6 gene as a prognostic marker in diffuse large-cell lymphoma. *N Engl J Med* 1994;331(2):74–80.

441. Bastard C, Deweindt C, Kerckaert JP, et al. LAZ3 rearrangements in non-Hodgkin's lymphoma: correlation with histology, immunophenotype, karyotype, and clinical outcome in 217 patients. *Blood* 1994;83(9):2423–2427.

442. Dent AL, Shaffer AL, Yu X, et al. Control of inflammation, cytokine expression, and germinal center formation by BCL-6. *Science* 1997;276(5312):589–592.

443. Hummel M, Bentink S, Berger H, et al. A biologic definition of Burkitt's lymphoma from transcriptional and genomic profiling. *N Engl J Med* 2006;354(23):2419–2430.

444. Dave SS, Fu K, Wright GW, et al. Molecular diagnosis of Burkitt's lymphoma. *N Engl J Med* 2006;354(23):2431–2442.

445. Aukema SM, Siebert R, Schuuring E, et al. Double-hit B-cell lymphomas. *Blood* 2011;117(8):2319–2331.

446. Alizadeh AA, Eisen MB, Davis RE, et al. Distinct types of diffuse large B-cell lymphoma identified by gene expression profiling. *Nature* 2000;403(6769):503–511.

447. Rosenwald A, Wright G, Leroy K, et al. Molecular diagnosis of primary mediastinal B cell lymphoma identifies a clinically favorable subgroup of diffuse large B cell lymphoma related to Hodgkin lymphoma. *J Exp Med* 2003;198(6):851–862.

448. Savage KJ, Monti S, Kutok JL, et al. The molecular signature of mediastinal large B-cell lymphoma differs from that of other diffuse large B-cell lymphomas and shares features with classical Hodgkin lymphoma. *Blood* 2003;102(12):3871–3879.

449. Rosenwald A, Wright G, Chan WC, et al. The use of molecular profiling to predict survival after chemotherapy for diffuse large-B-cell lymphoma. *N Engl J Med* 2002;346(25):1937–1947.

450. Bea S, Zettl A, Wright G, et al. Diffuse large B-cell lymphoma subgroups have distinct genetic profiles that influence tumor biology and improve gene-expression-based survival prediction. *Blood* 2005;106(9):3183–3190.

451. De Paepe P, Achten R, Verhoef G, et al. Large cleaved and immunoblastic lymphoma may represent two distinct clinicopathologic entities within the group of diffuse large B-cell lymphomas. *J Clin Oncol* 2005;23(28):7060–7068.

452. Jaffe ES, Pittaluga S. Aggressive B-cell lymphomas: a review of new and old entities in the WHO classification. *Hematology Am Soc Hematol Educ Program* 2011;2011:506–514.

453. Zech L, Haglund U, Nilsson K, et al. Characteristic chromosomal abnormalities in biopsies and lymphoid-cell lines from patients with Burkitt and non-Burkitt lymphomas. *Int J Cancer* 1976;17(1):47–56.

454. Boerma EG, Siebert R, Kluin PM, et al. Translocations involving 8q24 in Burkitt lymphoma and other malignant lymphomas: a historical review of cytogenetics in the light of todays knowledge. *Leukemia* 2009;23(2):225–234.

455. Manolov G, Manolova Y. Marker band in one chromosome 14 from Burkitt lymphomas. *Nature* 1972;237(5349):33–34.

456. Bellan C, Lazzi S, Hummel M, et al. Immunoglobulin gene analysis reveals 2 distinct cells of origin for EBV-positive and EBV-negative Burkitt lymphomas. *Blood* 2005;106(3):1031–1036.

457. Klapproth K, Wirth T. Advances in the understanding of MYC-induced lymphomagenesis. *Br J Haematol* 2010;149(4):484–497.

458. Adams JM, Harris AW, Pinkert CA, et al. The c-myc oncogene driven by immunoglobulin enhancers induces lymphoid malignancy in transgenic mice. *Nature* 1985;318(6046):533–538.

459. Sanchez-Beato M, Saez AI, Navas IC, et al. Overall survival in aggressive B-cell lymphomas is dependent on the accumulation of alterations in p53, p16, and p27. *Am J Pathol* 2001;159(1):205–213.

460. Vose J, Armitage J, Weisenburger D. International peripheral T-cell and natural killer/T-cell lymphoma study: pathology findings and clinical outcomes. *J Clin Oncol* 2008;26(25):4124–4130.

461. de Leval L, Gaulard P. Tricky and terrible T-cell tumors: these are thrilling times for testing: molecular pathology of peripheral T-cell lymphomas. *Hematology Am Soc Hematol Educ Program* 2011;2011:336–343.

462. Kinney MC, Higgins RA, Medina EA. Anaplastic large cell lymphoma: twenty-five years of discovery. *Arch Pathol Lab Med* 2011;135(1):19–43.

463. Morris SW, Kirstein MN, Valentine MB, et al. Fusion of a kinase gene, ALK, to a nucleolar protein gene, NPM, in non-Hodgkin's lymphoma. *Science* 1994; 263(5151):1281–1284.

464. Mason DY, Bastard C, Rimokh R, et al. CD30-positive large cell lymphomas ('Ki-1 lymphoma') are associated with a chromosomal translocation involving 5q35. *Br J Haematol* 1990;74(2):161–168.

465. Salaverria I, Bea S, Lopez-Guillermo A, et al. Genomic profiling reveals different genetic aberrations in systemic ALK-positive and ALK-negative anaplastic large cell lymphomas. *Br J Haematol* 2008;140(5):516–526.

466. Chiarle R, Voena C, Ambrogio C, et al. The anaplastic lymphoma kinase in the pathogenesis of cancer. *Nat Rev Cancer* 2008;8(1):11–23.

467. Laurent C, Do C, Gascoyne RD, et al. Anaplastic lymphoma kinase-positive diffuse large B-cell lymphoma: a rare clinicopathologic entity with poor prognosis. *J Clin Oncol* 2009;27(25):4211–4216.

468. Webb TR, Slavish J, George RE, et al. Anaplastic lymphoma kinase: role in cancer pathogenesis and small-molecule inhibitor development for therapy. *Expert Rev Anticancer Ther* 2009;9(3):331–356.

469. Greipp PR, San Miguel J, Durie BG, et al. International staging system for multiple myeloma. *J Clin Oncol* 2005;23(15):3412–3420.

470. Kyle RA, Remstein ED, Therneau TM, et al. Clinical course and prognosis of smoldering (asymptomatic) multiple myeloma. *N Engl J Med* 2007;356(25):2582–2590.

471. Sirohi B, Powles R. Epidemiology and outcomes research for MGUS, myeloma and amyloidosis. *Eur J Cancer* 2006;42(11):1671–1683.

472. Fonseca R, Bergsagel PL, Drach J, et al. International Myeloma Working Group molecular classification of multiple myeloma: spotlight review. *Leukemia* 2009;23(12):2210–2221.

473. Morgan GJ, Walker BA, Davies FE. The genetic architecture of multiple myeloma. *Nat Rev Cancer* 2012;12(5):335–348.

474. Slovak ML. Multiple myeloma: current perspectives. *Clin Lab Med* 2011;31(4):699–724, x.

475. Dewald GW, Therneau T, Larson D, et al. Relationship of patient survival and chromosome anomalies detected in metaphase and/or interphase cells at diagnosis of myeloma. *Blood* 2005;106(10):3553–3558.

476. Avet-Loiseau H, Attal M, Moreau P, et al. Genetic abnormalities and survival in multiple myeloma: the experience of the Intergroupe Francophone du Myelome. *Blood* 2007;109(8):3489–3495.

477. Gonzalez D, van der Burg M, Garcia-Sanz R, et al. Immunoglobulin gene rearrangements and the pathogenesis of multiple myeloma. *Blood* 2007;110(9):3112–3121.

478. Hakim O, Resch W, Yamane A, et al. DNA damage defines sites of recurrent chromosomal translocations in B lymphocytes. *Nature* 2012;484(7392):69–74.

479. Bergsagel PL, Kuehl WM. Critical roles for immunoglobulin translocations and cyclin D dysregulation in multiple myeloma. *Immunol Rev* 2003;194:96–104.

480. Landgren O, Kyle RA, Pfeiffer RM, et al. Monoclonal gammopathy of undetermined significance (MGUS) consistently precedes multiple myeloma: a prospective study. *Blood* 2009;113(22):5412–5417.

481. Weiss BM, Abadie J, Verma P, et al. A monoclonal gammopathy precedes multiple myeloma in most patients. *Blood* 2009;113(22):5418–5422.

482. Chng WJ, Van Wier SA, Ahmann GJ, et al. A validated FISH trisomy index demonstrates the hyperdiploid and nonhyperdiploid dichotomy in MGUS. *Blood* 2005;106(6):2156–2161.

483. Fonseca R, Debes-Marun CS, Picken EB, et al. The recurrent IgH translocations are highly associated with nonhyperdiploid variant multiple myeloma. *Blood* 2003;102(7):2562–2567.

484. Garand R, Avet-Loiseau H, Accard F, et al. t(11;14) and t(4;14) translocations correlated with mature lymphoplasmacytoid and immature morphology, respectively, in multiple myeloma. *Leukemia* 2003;17(10):2032–2035.

485. Hoyer JD, Hanson CA, Fonseca R, et al. The (11;14)(q13;q32) translocation in multiple myeloma. A morphologic and immunohistochemical study. *Am J Clin Pathol* 2000;113(6):831–837.

486. Broyl A, Hose D, Lokhorst H, et al. Gene expression profiling for molecular classification of multiple myeloma in newly diagnosed patients. *Blood* 2010;116(14):2543–2553.

487. Bergsagel PL, Kuehl WM, Zhan F, et al. Cyclin D dysregulation: an early and unifying pathogenic event in multiple myeloma. *Blood* 2005;106(1):296–303.

488. Fonseca R, Blood E, Rue M, et al. Clinical and biologic implications of recurrent genomic aberrations in myeloma. *Blood* 2003;101(11):4569–4575.

489. Karlin L, Soulier J, Chandesris O, et al. Clinical and biological features of t(4;14) multiple myeloma: a prospective study. *Leuk Lymphoma* 2011;52(2):238–246.

490. Chesi M, Nardini E, Lim RS, et al. The t(4;14) translocation in myeloma dysregulates both FGFR3 and a novel gene, MMSET, resulting in IgH/MMSET hybrid transcripts. *Blood* 1998;92(9):3025–3034.

491. Chesi M, Nardini E, Brents LA, et al. Frequent translocation t(4;14)(p16.3;q32.3) in multiple myeloma is associated with increased expression and activating mutations of fibroblast growth factor receptor 3. *Nat Genet* 1997;16(3):260–264.

492. Trudel S, Ely S, Farooqi Y, et al. Inhibition of fibroblast growth factor receptor 3 induces differentiation and apoptosis in t(4;14) myeloma. *Blood* 2004;103(9):3521–3528.

493. Trudel S, Li ZH, Wei E, et al. CHIR-258, a novel, multitargeted tyrosine kinase inhibitor for the potential treatment of t(4;14) multiple myeloma. *Blood* 2005;105(7):2941–2948.

494. Marango J, Shimoyama M, Nishio H, et al. The MMSET protein is a histone methyltransferase with characteristics of a transcriptional corepressor. *Blood* 2008;111(6):3145–3154.

495. Martinez-Garcia E, Popovic R, Min DJ, et al. The MMSET histone methyl transferase switches global histone methylation and alters gene expression in t(4;14) multiple myeloma cells. *Blood* 2011;117(1):211–220.

496. Hurt EM, Wiestner A, Rosenwald A, et al. Overexpression of c-maf is a frequent oncogenic event in multiple myeloma that promotes proliferation and pathological interactions with bone marrow stroma. *Cancer Cell* 2004;5(2):191–199.

497. Ross FM, Chiecchio L, Dagrada G, et al. The t(14;20) is a poor prognostic factor in myeloma but is associated with long-term stable disease in monoclonal gammopathies of undetermined significance. *Haematologica* 2010;95(7):1221–1225.

498. Avet-Louseau H, Daviet A, Sauner S, et al. Chromosome 13 abnormalities in multiple myeloma are mostly monosomy 13. *Br J Haematol* 2000;111(4):1116–1117.

499. Chng WJ, Santana-Davila R, Van Wier SA, et al. Prognostic factors for hyperdiploid-myeloma: effects of chromosome 13 deletions and IgH translocations. *Leukemia* 2006;20(5):807–813.

500. Walker BA, Leone PE, Chiecchio L, et al. A compendium of myeloma-associated chromosomal copy number abnormalities and their prognostic value. *Blood* 2010;116(15):e56–e65.

501. Fonseca R, Harrington D, Oken MM, et al. Biological and prognostic significance of interphase fluorescence in situ hybridization detection of chromosome 13 abnormalities (delta13) in multiple myeloma: an eastern cooperative oncology group study. *Cancer Res* 2002;62(3):715–720.

502. Tiedemann RE, Gonzalez-Paz N, Kyle RA, et al. Genetic aberrations and survival in plasma cell leukemia. *Leukemia* 2008;22(5):1044–1052.

503. Xiong W, Wu X, Starnes S, et al. An analysis of the clinical and biologic significance of TP53 loss and the identification of potential novel transcriptional targets of TP53 in multiple myeloma. *Blood* 2008;112(10):4235–4246.

504. Debes-Marun CS, Dewald GW, Bryant S, et al. Chromosome abnormalities clustering and its implications for pathogenesis and prognosis in myeloma. *Leukemia* 2003;17(2):427–436.

505. Carrasco DR, Tonon G, Huang Y, et al. High-resolution genomic profiles define distinct clinico-pathogenetic subgroups of multiple myeloma patients. *Cancer Cell* 2006;9(4):313–325.

506. Avet-Loiseau H, Li C, Magrangeas F, et al. Prognostic significance of copy-number alterations in multiple myeloma. *J Clin Oncol* 2009;27(27):4585–4590.

507. Hanamura I, Stewart JP, Huang Y, et al. Frequent gain of chromosome band 1q21 in plasma-cell dyscrasias detected by fluorescence in situ hybridization: incidence increases from MGUS to relapsed myeloma and is related to prognosis and disease progression following tandem stem-cell transplantation. *Blood* 2006;108(5):1724–1732.

508. Shaughnessy JD Jr, Zhan F, Burington BE, et al. A validated gene expression model of high-risk multiple myeloma is defined by deregulated expression of genes mapping to chromosome 1. *Blood* 2007;109(6):2276–2284.

509. Annunziata CM, Davis RE, Demchenko Y, et al. Frequent engagement of the classical and alternative NF-kappaB pathways by diverse genetic abnormalities in multiple myeloma. *Cancer Cell* 2007;12(2):115–130.

510. Chng WJ, Gonzalez-Paz N, Price-Troska T, et al. Clinical and biological significance of RAS mutations in multiple myeloma. *Leukemia* 2008;22(12):2280–2284.

511. Pichiorri F, Suh SS, Ladetto M, et al. MicroRNAs regulate critical genes associated with multiple myeloma pathogenesis. *Proc Natl Acad Sci U S A* 2008;105(35):12885–12890.

512. Walker BA, Wardell CP, Chiecchio L, et al. Aberrant global methylation patterns affect the molecular pathogenesis and prognosis of multiple myeloma. *Blood* 2011;117(2):553–562.

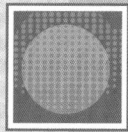

Chapter 10
Organization and Operation of a Hematopathology Laboratory

Wayne Tam • Angela R. Murray • Attilio Orazi • Daniel M. Knowles

Multiple diagnostic dilemmas are commonly encountered in the routine diagnosis and classification of hematopoietic neoplasms. Examples include the differential diagnosis of non-Hodgkin lymphoma versus undifferentiated carcinoma, lymphoid hyperplasia versus non-Hodgkin lymphoma in lymphatic and in extralymphatic tissues, Hodgkin lymphoma versus non-Hodgkin lymphoma, acute leukemias of lymphoid versus myeloid origin, and chronic leukemias of B-cell versus T-cell origin. The application of solely morphologic criteria in these situations is fraught with difficulties. The purely cytomorphologic detection of minimal neoplastic disease, such as partial involvement of lymph nodes by non-Hodgkin lymphoma and the presence of small numbers of lymphoma/leukemia cells in peripheral blood, bone marrow, effusions, and cerebrospinal fluid (CSF), is often difficult. Morphologic criteria are frequently incapable of correctly forecasting the lineage of diffuse aggressive hematologic neoplasms (1–5).

Immunophenotypic analysis is capable of determining the polyclonal or monoclonal B-cell or T-cell nature of a lymphoid proliferation, thereby often distinguishing benign from malignant lymphoid proliferations; determining the lineage, subset, and approximate stage of differentiation of neoplastic hematopoietic cells; and detecting minimal neoplastic disease (6–11). Immunogenotypic analysis, the evaluation of clonal rearrangements of the antigen recognition molecules of B and T cells (immunoglobulin and T-cell receptors, respectively), is capable of determining the lineage and clonality of B- and T-cell proliferations at the molecular level (12–22) and of detecting clonal B- and T-cell populations that escape detection by morphologic examination and immunophenotypic analysis (23–28). Immunogenotypic analysis may help when immunophenotypic analysis is incapable of resolving a diagnostic dilemma. Immunophenotypic analysis and immunogenotypic analysis have become invaluable adjuncts to morphology in the differential diagnosis and classification of hematopoietic neoplasms.

For this reason, physicians providing care to patients who have hematopoietic neoplasms require access to a hematopathology laboratory capable of performing these studies on all solid tissue and fluid pathologic specimens. Unfortunately, some clinical pathologists accustomed to handling high-volume clinical testing with sophisticated automated instrumentation prefer performing cytofluorometric analysis of isolated cells in suspension and fail to correlate their results with the histopathology of the specimens from which the cells were isolated. Many anatomic pathologists accustomed to evaluating tissue sections prefer performing immunohistochemical staining of tissue sections and ignore "wet" hematologic samples. Even worse, many of these individuals extol the virtues of their approach and ignore and remain biased against the other approach, refusing to recognize the advantages as well as the disadvantages of both methodologies. Too few "full-service" hematopathology laboratories exist; many large institutions remain in need of a hematopathologist capable of establishing and operating such a facility.

The hematopathology laboratory, whose organization and operation is described here, is now based at the New York Weill-Cornell campus of New York-Presbyterian Hospital and is currently directed by Dr. Attilio Orazi and managed by Ms. Angela Murray. This laboratory was initially established at the Columbia-Presbyterian Medical Center by Dr. Daniel M. Knowles in 1978. Initially, immunofluorescent analysis of isolated cells in suspension was routinely performed on all specimens because it was believed at that time that this was the best all-around approach for handling the greatest number and variety of pathologic specimens. Since then, the assays performed in the hematopathology laboratory have been continually improved as each new significant technologic advance (i.e., monoclonal antibodies, flow cytometry, immunohistochemistry, antigen retrieval, automated immunohistochemistry, Southern blotting, and polymerase chain reaction [PCR]) has been incorporated into the laboratory, which has been continuously reorganized to accommodate the changes. The result today is a full-service hematopathology laboratory capable of routinely performing the entire array of immunophenotypic, immunogenotypic, and molecular biologic analyses currently available on a large number of solid and fluid pathologic specimens. In this chapter, the organization and daily operation of this laboratory, including the handling and processing of pathologic specimens, reagent maintenance, and our approach to immunophenotypic evaluation and diagnosis, are described. An appendix provides the recipes for performing many of the laboratory's procedures. Many other excellent hematopathology laboratories offering alternative but equally reliable approaches exist, but the intent of this chapter is to provide an overview of the daily routine operation of one laboratory.

LABORATORY ORGANIZATION AND DAILY OPERATION

Immunophenotypic analysis can be performed on virtually any pathologic specimen, including all solid tissues, peripheral blood, aspirated bone marrow, pleural and abdominal effusions, and CSF. A hematopathology laboratory should be capable of effectively analyzing all these different types of samples on any given day. This can be readily accomplished if the laboratory establishes appropriate guidelines for the correct handling and processing of each of these different types of pathologic specimens; is capable of performing cytofluorometric analysis of isolated cells in suspension and immunohistochemical analysis of paraffin tissue sections, frozen sections, and cytospin preparations; is cognizant of the utility and reactivity of the many monoclonal antibodies currently available for cell suspensions and histologic sections and the immunophenotypic profiles of the various hematopoietic neoplasms; is capable of performing antigen receptor gene rearrangement analysis and other molecular genetic assays as an adjunct to immunophenotypic analysis; and tailors the methodologic approach of the analysis to the individual requirements of each pathologic specimen and the specific diagnostic problem requiring resolution. Under these circumstances, the only factors limiting the successful outcome of immunophenotypic analysis are adequacy of sample size, technical difficulties inherent in the various phenotyping techniques, and the limits of immunophenotypic criteria applied to the diagnosis and classification of hematopoietic neoplasms. However, the large volume and diverse nature of the specimens submitted to the hematopathology laboratory and the labor-intensive nature of the assays performed on them dictate that each specimen be handled rapidly and efficiently and that all assays be performed expeditiously but accurately. We have adopted a specific operational approach to the immunophenotypic analysis of pathologic specimens, which is described later. Based on this correlative clinical, morphologic, and immunophenotypic approach, a definitive diagnosis can be made in most cases within 48 hours.

HANDLING AND PROCESSING OF PATHOLOGIC SPECIMENS

Accessioning Specimens and Tracking Data

All specimens submitted to the laboratory for diagnostic leukemia/lymphoma evaluation are accompanied by a New York-Presbyterian Hospital requisition form or paperwork submitted by the referring hospital or physician. Each specimen is logged in the accession book as well as electronically, and assigned a laboratory identification number. Upon accessioning in the Laboratory Information System (LIS), bar code labels are generated for the requisition forms and specimen containers. This procedure is put in place for Material Specimen Tracking and Matching, a specimen management system that ensures that all specimens received are properly identified. The bar codes are scanned at this point to record the appropriate location at which the specimen will be processed. A laboratory data sheet is generated by the LIS, printed, and stapled to the front of the submitted requisition or paperwork so that all the information and paperwork concerning each specimen are grouped together and are available when needed. The laboratory data sheet that includes the patient's name and location, age, sex, hospital number, physician's name and location, referring institution, a summary of the pertinent clinical information, the hematopathology laboratory number, date, time of arrival, and the nature of the specimen is attached to the requisition, and the paperwork remains in the laboratory during the entire workup of the specimen. Notations concerning specimen handling are continuously added to the front sheet during the processing of the specimen. Such information includes viability, cell counts, processing times, and initials of laboratory technologists for work performed. Ongoing laboratory findings can also be added to the front sheet if necessary. In this way, the front sheet becomes a complete summary of the case when the evaluation process is completed, at which time a final hematopathology laboratory report is generated. After a final report is generated, all the information concerning each specimen is stored in the mainframe computer. The specimen data archives are retrievable by patient name, laboratory identification number, patient history number, ICD9 diagnosis code, or SNOMED diagnosis code.

Specimen Collection

All peripheral venous blood and aspirated bone marrow samples submitted for the diagnosis and classification of leukemia/lymphoma must be anticoagulated with either EDTA or sodium heparin to prevent clotting. In general, peripheral blood samples are drawn and submitted in either EDTA lavender tubes or sodium-heparinized green-top tubes, and bone marrow samples are drawn and submitted in a sterile syringe prerinsed with and containing a small residual amount (<1 mL) of sodium heparin or in a sodium-heparinized green-top tube. Overanticoagulation with unnecessarily large volumes of heparin can alter the results of immunophenotypic analysis.

The quantity of peripheral blood necessary to perform immunophenotypic analysis depends on the patient's white blood cell (WBC) count, the proportion of lymphocytes or other mononuclear cells whose analysis is desired, and the number and type of assays to be performed. Approximately 1×10^7 mononuclear cells can be isolated by red blood cell lysis from every 10 mL of peripheral blood obtained from an individual with a normal WBC count. This represents a sufficient number of mononuclear cells for examination with >30 monoclonal antibodies using multicolor flow cytometry (1×10^6 cells per tube). Very large numbers of mononuclear cells, more than adequate for extensive immunophenotypic analysis, can be obtained when a similar amount of peripheral blood is taken from a leukemic patient with a high leukocyte count. In these instances, all cells in excess of that needed for immunodiagnosis are cryopreserved for future studies.

In general, 1 to 3 mL of aspirated bone marrow yields sufficient numbers of cells, usually between 10 and 20×10^6, to permit adequate cytofluorometric analysis. Attempts to aspirate large amounts of bone marrow frequently result in peripheral blood contamination of the bone marrow sample by normal peripheral blood B and T cells. Introducing this artifact may make the immunophenotypic identification and analysis of neoplastic cells from the bone marrow considerably more difficult.

Ideally, the physician desiring immunophenotypic analysis of an effusion should submit a fresh specimen obtained from a recent-onset effusion. Chronic, long-standing effusions may lack sufficient numbers of viable cells for analysis. The physician should submit the entire effusion to the hematopathology laboratory in a sterile container, anticoagulated with heparin and without fixatives, minus the relatively small portions necessary for the microbiology and cytopathology laboratories, so that the maximum number of viable cells can be isolated for immunophenotypic analysis.

Unfortunately, in our experience, this ideal situation is not always achieved. In some instances, physicians fail to heparinize the collection container, which can result in fibrin clots or large blood clots if the effusion is bloody. These clots interfere significantly with cell isolation. Because cells become entrapped within these clots, the number of cells available for analysis is reduced and the sample may be rendered nonrepresentative. However, because most effusions represent an excellent physiologic medium and support cell viability very well, immunophenotypic analysis can be performed on most of these specimens, even if they have not been submitted under ideal conditions.

Immunophenotypic analysis can be performed on CSF samples; the limiting factor is the number of cells necessary to perform the analyses required to resolve the particular diagnostic problem. In our experience, CSF samples containing fewer than 50 cells/mm³ are often inadequate for diagnostic immunophenotypic analysis. The physician should submit the largest volume of CSF that can be safely obtained from the patient in a sterile collection tube without fixative. Heparinization is unnecessary.

Peripheral blood, aspirated bone marrow, and effusions contain single cells in suspension that continue to be bathed in their natural physiologic environment even after removal from the body. In contrast, lymph nodes and other solid tissues generally contain tightly packed clusters and sheets of cells, sometimes surrounded by dense connective tissue, whose nutrient support is wholly dependent on continuous and appropriate vascular perfusion. Removal from the body results in the interruption of blood flow to these cells, alters their physiologic environment, and consequently places their viability at risk almost immediately. All lymph node and other solid tissue specimens must be handled carefully and expeditiously to maximize cell viability and antigen preservation.

The entire lymph node or other solid tissue biopsy specimen should be submitted in sterile RPMI 1640 (preferable) or sterile physiologic saline (if more accessible to the surgeon) in a sterile container immediately after its removal from the patient, transported immediately to the laboratory and be evaluated, handled, and processed without delay on arrival in the laboratory. One factor that unavoidably delays appropriate processing is a request for intraoperative frozen section consultation. Cell viability can decrease rapidly and markedly if the solid tissue is allowed to dry out on a laboratory counter top at room temperature for even 10 minutes. The entire biopsy, or representative portions in the case of large resection specimens, should be floated in tissue culture media or saline during the intraoperative consultation to maximize cell viability.

In general, the typical excisional lymph node biopsy specimen is sufficient in size to permit the preparation of histologic sections, the generation of a cell suspension for cytofluorometric analysis and possibly tumor banking, cytogenetic analysis, and the cryopreservation of tissue blocks for tumor banking. A representative cell suspension totaling about 5×10^7 cells can be prepared from a 0.5 to 0.7 cm^2 piece of lymphoid cell–rich tissue devoid of necrosis and fibrous connective tissue. In the case of smaller biopsy specimens, which are more frequently encountered nowadays with the increasing popularity of needle core biopsies, representative portions are taken first for histology, and without compromising diagnostic evaluation, cryopreservation, and cell suspension in that order of priority if sufficient material remains. Cell suspensions are not usually prepared from densely fibrotic or extensively necrotic tissues because this is usually unsuccessful or the resultant cell suspensions are nonrepresentative.

Specimen Transport

Rapid specimen transport and processing are recommended because this maximizes cell viability and antigen preservation. CSF samples should always be transported immediately because these specimens usually contain very few cells and their analysis is often crucial for diagnosis. In general, peripheral blood, aspirated bone marrow, and effusion specimens should be delivered to the laboratory within 3 hours of being obtained from the patient. However, we and others (29) have found that the mononuclear cells present in most unseparated whole peripheral blood, aspirated bone marrow, and effusion samples, with the possible exception of CD4 T cells, remain viable, without antigen loss, for 24 hours or longer after collection. These specimens should be maintained at room temperature during unavoidable delays in processing. Even specimens obtained in the late evening after the laboratory is closed should be stored overnight at room temperature until they can be processed the next day.

All solid tissue specimens, especially resection specimens too large to be floated in tissue culture media or saline, should be delivered to the laboratory immediately after removal from the patient because cell viability is most difficult to maintain in these specimens. Tissue specimens procured from within the medical center that are delivered promptly to the laboratory and processed immediately on their arrival may be maintained at room temperature. Tissue specimens procured from outside the medical center or that must be in transit for 2 hours or more should be kept cool on ice but not allowed to freeze. This

is especially important on hot summer days, when cell viability may be severely compromised by the excessive heat. However, maintaining tissue samples on ice does not ensure cell viability and antigen preservation if the cells are not also floated in sterile tissue culture media or physiologic saline.

Handling Cell Suspensions

All specimens arriving in the laboratory for diagnostic evaluation of hematopoietic malignancies are examined and handled in a sterile, laminar flow tissue culture hood (Sterilgard Hood, Baker Instrument Co., Baker, ME). Specimen containers are never opened to room air and are never casually examined on a laboratory bench top. All physicians and laboratory personnel handling specimens wear gloves and take appropriate safety precautions. Moreover, all manipulations, including cell isolation, cryopreservation, and thawing of cells, are performed under sterile conditions in a sterile laminar flow tissue culture hood. This approach provides maximum protection to the entire laboratory staff and permits the preparation of sterile cell suspensions useful for a variety of research programs.

All peripheral blood and bone marrow aspirate samples submitted for immunophenotypic analysis are subjected to ammonium chloride bulk lysis to remove contaminating red blood cells (see Appendix 10.1). In the case of solid tissues, we require that the surgeon submit the entire tissue specimen to the laboratory intact in sterile tissue culture media RPMI 1640 (Lonza BioWhittaker, Watersville, MD) or physiologic saline. The only exceptions are cases submitted in consultation from outside institutions. In these instances, we prefer that the local referring pathologist divide the specimen, submit a representative portion of the biopsy fresh and unfixed in RPMI 1640 to the laboratory, process the remainder for histopathology in his or her own laboratory, and send us representative recut histologic slides to review and keep in our files. In our institution, a pathologist examines all gross specimens immediately on their arrival in the laboratory and, after examination of a Diff-Quick (modified Wright-Giemsa)–stained touch preparation (see Appendix 10.2), determines those portions that are suitable for routine histopathology, cell suspension preparation, and snap-freezing. These samples are always handled expeditiously to maximize cell viability and antigen preservation. If a cell suspension is prepared, cell viability and the degree of contamination by erythrocytes, dead cells, and debris are assessed immediately, and a decision to Ficoll or not is made depending on tumor cell viability and degree of red cell contamination (see below).

Examination of a touch preparation of a solid tissue specimen is important for several reasons. The touch preparation gives the pathologist insight into the type of lesion he or she is dealing with, which influences how the tissue should be handled. For example, if a lymph node touch prep shows a mixed cell population containing many eosinophils and large binucleated cells with prominent nucleoli suggestive of Reed-Sternberg cells, the pathologist may choose to freeze tissue blocks and submit tissue for routine histology and not prepare a cell suspension because cytofluorometric analysis is not useful in arriving at a diagnosis of Hodgkin lymphoma. Alternatively, the pathologist may identify metastatic carcinoma, obviating the need to prepare a cell suspension. A touch preparation may suggest that the tissue is largely fibrotic, and it is likely that only a small number of cells will be obtained if an attempt is made to prepare a cell suspension. The touch preparation also gives the pathologist a general idea of the viability of the cells within the specimen. If most cells in the touch prep are not viable, it is often more useful to save the specimen as frozen tissue blocks that can be used for DNA studies rather than place the dying cells in suspension only to lose them during Ficoll separation.

That portion of a lymph node or other tissue specimen used to prepare a cell suspension is placed in a Falcon #1029 Petri dish and covered with a small volume of RPMI 1640 containing 1% penicillin and 1% streptomycin. The cells are isolated from the tissue by a combination of cutting, teasing, and scraping manipulations. However, before placing the entire specimen into suspension, a small number of cells are isolated and their viability checked by Trypan blue dye exclusion (see Appendix 10.4). If the viability is poor (<50%), it is often preferable to preserve the remainder of the specimen as frozen tissue blocks. If the viability is >50%, the tissue is cut into small pieces that are more workable; this also ensures maximum perfusion by the tissue culture media. Each piece is held at the bottom of the Petri dish by a sterile forceps held in one hand and alternately sliced and scraped with a sterile scalpel blade held in the other hand. The maximum number of cells is drawn out of the tissue in the shortest period of time when only a small amount of fluid is maintained around the piece of tissue being teased apart. The media becomes progressively cloudier as cells are scraped out of the tissue and into the fluid. Every few minutes, the cloudy cell-rich supernatant is drawn off with a Pasteur pipette and collected into a Falcon #2070 50-mL tube and a comparable volume of fresh media is added to the Petri dish. This process is continued until all the tissue pieces have been chopped, the fluid is clear, and only white fibrous connective tissue fragments remain. These tissue fragments are then ground to a white fibrous pulp using the flat rubber bottom of a plunger removed from a 60 mL syringe to ensure that the maximum number of cells is collected. In our experience, this approach results in higher cell yields, better viability, and more representative cell suspensions than the commonly used approach of forcing tissue through a nylon mesh.

The 50-mL tube is capped and shaken, the tissue debris is allowed to settle toward the bottom for about 30 to 60 seconds, and the cell-rich supernatant is then drawn off with a Pasteur pipette and placed in another 50-mL tube; the debris remaining at the bottom of the tube is discarded. The cells are examined and counted in a hemocytometer, and their viability is assessed by Trypan blue dye exclusion (see Appendix 10.3). Cell suspensions of <80% viability or containing erythrocytes and cellular debris require Ficoll-Hypaque density gradient centrifugation (see Appendix 10.4). The cells should be suspended to a final concentration of 5 to 10×10^6 cells/mL before adding Ficoll to produce optimum post-Ficoll mononuclear cell layers and maximum cell recovery. Cell suspensions not requiring Ficoll separation are stored overnight, as described in the last paragraph of this section.

Bloody effusion specimens are treated like peripheral blood samples. They are diluted 1:2 to 1:4 with PBS and then placed over Ficoll-Hypaque. Nonbloody effusion specimens are handled like cell suspensions prepared from lymph nodes. The cells are examined and counted on a hemocytometer, and their viability is assessed by Trypan blue dye exclusion. Cell suspensions of <80% viability or containing erythrocytes and cellular debris are suspended to a concentration of 5 to 10×10^6 cells/mL and placed over Ficoll-Hypaque. Cell suspensions not requiring Ficoll-Hypaque separation are stored overnight.

CSF samples are transferred to a sterile 15-mL Falcon #2097 conical tube and pelleted in a ThermoScientific Sorval Legend RT Plus centrifuge at 1,000 rpm for 8 minutes at room temperature. The supernatant is discarded, and the cells are resuspended in a small volume (0.5 to 1.0 mL) of RPMI 1640 and counted. In our experience, these samples never require Ficoll separation and nearly always contain too few cells to do so anyway.

The mononuclear cells isolated and collected from each specimen are counted, their viability is reassessed, and they are resuspended in sterile RPMI 1640 containing 10% heat-inactivated fetal or newborn calf serum (Gibo Laboratories),

1% penicillin, and 1% streptomycin (overnight solution). Diff-Quik (modified Wright-Giemsa)–stained cytocentrifuge slides (cytospins) of each cell suspension are prepared (see Appendix 10.2) to evaluate the morphologic features of the cells and determine the approximate percentage of neoplastic cells in the sample before cytofluorometric analysis. These slides also provide a permanent morphologic record of the cell suspension prepared from each specimen. The resuspended cells are then stored in overnight solution at 4°C. In our experience, viable mononuclear cell suspensions stored in this manner are nearly always as viable the next day and even over the weekend in most cases. The principal exceptions are some high-grade lymphomas, especially Burkitt lymphoma, immunoblastic lymphomas, and plasmacytomas or multiple myeloma. The viability of the cell suspensions prepared from these neoplasms often continues to decrease, even after the harvesting of only viable cells by Ficoll-Hypaque. When possible, these neoplastic cells are analyzed the same day that the specimens are obtained from the patient. The next morning, a technician counts and reassesses the viability of the multiple cell suspensions collected the previous day. After aliquoting the appropriate quantity of cells for cytofluorometric analysis, the residual cells are cryopreserved in liquid nitrogen at −170°C. The proper handling of cell suspensions for cytofluorometric analysis and immunohistochemical analysis of cytospins are discussed in Chapters 5 and 38, respectively.

Handling Frozen and Paraffin-Embedded Tissues

A representative portion of every tissue specimen submitted to the laboratory is snap-frozen and cryopreserved except for exceedingly small biopsies that are entirely submitted for histopathology. In the past, these frozen tissues were preserved both for tumor banking and immunohistochemistry. Nowadays, however, immunohistochemical analysis on frozen tissue is rarely performed because of the availability of a vast array of antibodies that are capable of detecting antigens on paraffin-embedded, formalin-fixed tissue. Thus, frozen tissues are procured mainly for the purpose of tumor banking (see section Banking Cryopreserved Cells and Tissues for Future Studies for detailed procedure). On the rare occasions when immunohistochemical staining is required, the cryopreserved tissue block is removed from the freezer and mounted in a cryostat, and a sufficient number of 4- to 6-μm thick serial sections are prepared. The sections are air dried at room temperature for 1 hour to overnight, depending on when the immunostaining is to be performed, fixed in room temperature acetone for 10 minutes, and then air dried for 5 minutes (see Appendix 10.5). One or two of the sections are stained with Diff-Quik (see Appendix 10.3) to review the morphology of the lesion being analyzed and to help determine the immunostaining panel. The remaining sections are then placed in 0.05% Tween-Tris buffered saline for 5 minutes after which they are loaded onto the Tech Mate 500 Automated Immunostaining System (Ventana, Tuscon, AZ).

Two factors that are critical in achieving optimal frozen tissue sections for immunohistochemical staining are rapidity in handling and processing tissue specimens once they are removed from the patient and the speed of the actual freezing process. The first factor is important for preserving cell surface antigens and reducing diffusion artifact during immunostaining. The second factor is important for preventing ice crystal formation, which results in suboptimal tissue sections that often cannot be interpreted accurately after immunostaining. These and other considerations in handling frozen tissue are discussed in Chapter 4.

Nowadays, immunohistochemistry is routinely done on paraffin-embedded tissues. Paraffin tissue sections are baked overnight in a 56°C oven and are deparaffinized by four serial 5-minute washes in xylene the following morning. The sections are then serially immersed for 5 minutes each in 100% ethanol and 95% ethanol and placed into 0.45% H_2O_2 in methanol (3 mL of 30% H_2O_2 in 200 mL of methanol) for 20 minutes. The sections are then transferred into room temperature distilled water to await antigen retrieval. Tissues that have been fixed in Bouin solution must be debouinized before immunostaining to remove the yellow background color, which may interfere with interpretation. This is accomplished by placing the paraffin tissue sections in a freshly prepared supersaturated solution of lithium carbonate in 70% ethanol for 30 to 60 seconds between the 100% and 95% ethanol steps in the hydration procedure. Tissues fixed in B5 have pigment that must be removed, because it may interfere with interpretation. Before counterstaining, the B5-fixed tissues are immersed in 100 mL of H_2O containing 1 g of iodine and 2 g of potassium iodide for 5 minutes, after which the sections are placed in 0.2% sodium thiosulfate for 8 minutes to remove the pigment (see Appendix 10.5). Because the type of fixative and the duration of fixation affect antigen detection, the fixation used for each specimen (i.e., formalin, Bouin, B5) is always recorded and the monoclonal antibody used to detect a particular antigen is used at the titer appropriate for the particular fixative and detection system employed (see Chapters 4 and 30). Visualization of specific antigens in paraffin tissue sections frequently requires antigen retrieval. The antigen retrieval techniques used in our laboratory include proteolytic digestion with trypsin or protease and special heating procedures involving microwave or pressure cooker techniques. After these preparatory steps, the paraffin tissue sections are loaded onto the TechMate 500 Automated Immunostaining System (Ventana, Tucson, AZ).

Banking Cryopreserved Cells and Tissues for Future Studies

All excess cells isolated from pathologic specimens, including liquid specimens and solid tissues, submitted to the laboratory for immunophenotypic analysis are cryopreserved in a viable state in fetal calf serum and dimethyl sulfoxide and are stored in liquid nitrogen at –170°C (see Appendix 10.6). The laboratory has continuously stored vials of cryopreserved cells in this manner on a daily basis since 1978. Approximately 23,000 vials of lymphoma and leukemia cells have been accumulated since then. These include about 5,000 lymphoid neoplasms encompassing a wide spectrum of indolent and aggressive lymphomas in immunocompetent and immunocompromised patients and about 1,500 myeloid neoplasms including acute leukemias, chronic myeloproliferative neoplasms, and myelodysplastic syndrome. These cells may be stored indefinitely and thawed in the distant future (see Appendix 10.7) to perform additional studies.

Similarly, all excess snap-frozen tissue blocks have been collected and stored since 1982 in –85°C freezers. These frozen tissue blocks are derived from about 5,400 cases, which are predominantly lymphoid neoplasms. A freshly prepared mixture of isopentane and dry ice is used to snap-freeze each tissue specimen. In general, a minimum of one, usually two, but sometimes as many as 10 tissue blocks ranging in size from 0.1 cm³ to 1.0 × 1.0 × 0.3 cm are taken from each pathologic specimen and snap-frozen. Round 2.2-cm cork disks (Superior Technologies, Pittsburgh, PA) are covered with OCT-embedding compound (Tissue-Tek, Naperville, IL). The tissue block is firmly placed in the middle of the OCT-covered disc and covered with additional OCT. The specimen is then held in the isopentane-dry ice mixture with forceps for about 1 to 2 minutes or until thoroughly frozen. The frozen blocks belonging to each

specimen are placed in a zip-lock bag inscribed in indelible ink with the laboratory identification number of the specimen, the tissue type, the number of frozen blocks, and the date. The bag is stored in a –80°C freezer until needed. Recently, this procedure for storing tissue blocks has been slightly modified to facilitate tumor banking. Tissues are frozen on the cork discs with the aid of a plastic cryogenic mold to help create a more uniform configuration. Once the specimen is adequately frozen, the tissue is removed from the mold and transferred to a plastic cassette labeled with the identification number. Cassettes are then stored in cryogenic boxes in –80°C freezers. Recently, we have also begun collecting and banking peripheral blood specimens from patients with lymphomas.

All these materials constitute the core of the hematologic malignancy biobank (HMB). The HMB is supported by a modern, sophisticated, home-brewed software that permits efficient entry and retrieval of a variety of specimen-related data, including demographic information; specimen source; WHO-based diagnosis; specimen procurement information (e.g., date and time of procurement, number of frozen vials and blocks, storage location, etc.); and ancillary immunophenotypic, cytogenetic, and molecular data. It has the capacity to be linked with a parallel clinical database, enabling complete integration of clinical and pathologic information.

These cryopreserved cells and tissues in the HMB have formed the basis for the clinical and basic science research programs of the hematopathology laboratory. They also provide valuable clinically annotated materials for researchers outside the department in collaborative research projects. In the past, cryopreserved cells and tissues have frequently been employed to prepare, screen, and characterize new monoclonal antibodies (30–35) or to further characterize existing monoclonal antibodies (36,37). They have also been frequently employed in immunophenotypic analyses of interesting and unusual hematopoietic neoplasms (38–46) and in large clinicopathologic studies (3,47–55). *In vitro* functional studies have even been successfully performed on lymphoma/leukemia cells cryopreserved in this manner for as long as 10 years (56). High-quality DNA and RNA can be extracted from these cryopreserved cells and tissues for use in a variety of molecular biologic assays. This has enabled the laboratory to perform or participate in numerous original molecular genetic investigations of hematopoietic neoplasia (3,15,17,18,23,24,27,57–108), including studies aimed at detecting Epstein-Barr virus (EBV), human T-cell lymphotropic virus type 1, and other viruses in hematopoietic neoplasms (109–111). Cryopreserved cells and tissues from this laboratory were used in the initial discovery and characterization of the Kaposi sarcoma–associated herpesvirus (112), its presence in a subset of acquired immunodeficiency syndrome–related lymphomas (113), and the subsequent characterization of these lymphomas as a distinct clinicopathologic entity (114). Materials from the bank have also been used to identify genetic alterations critical for lymphomagenesis (106). Frozen materials represent the ideal source for genome-wide discovery using next-generation sequencing and can be utilized for postdiscovery validation studies using standard techniques such as reverse-transcriptase PCR for gene expression analysis, quantitative PCR and FISH for assessing chromosomal rearrangements or gene copy number, and Sanger sequencing for somatic mutations. In addition, peripheral blood from lymphoma patients is a source of materials for germline sequence determination and experimental investigation on circulating tumor cells and nucleic acids, which can serve as potential biomarkers. Together with matching paraffin blocks that permit generation of tissue microarray and immunohistochemical studies, the HMB represents a critical resource for comprehensive analysis of alterations in hematologic malignancies.

ESTABLISHING AND MAINTAINING LABORATORY STANDARDS

Handling Monoclonal Antibodies and Other Reagents

The efficient daily operation of the laboratory requires the establishment and maintenance of a large inventory of commercially available and privately generated monoclonal antibodies, heteroantisera, and other reagents. The laboratory supervisor oversees the maintenance of this inventory, including the replacement of exhausted reagents. As each monoclonal antibody or other reagent is received in the laboratory, its source, identifying lot number, date of receipt, expiration date, storage requirements, date in use, and amount used per test are recorded in a reagent inventory log book. Each new shipment is parallel tested for parity with the most recently used lot. The quality control date is noted on the vial and recorded.

All monoclonal antibodies are stored under the appropriate conditions (usually 4°C) to ensure their reliability and to maximize their shelf life. Before routine use, an aliquot is removed from storage and titered on the appropriate cells or tissue to determine the ideal working dilution of that particular "lot" of antibody for daily use, which is recorded in the reagent inventory log in the computer. The optimal working dilution of each antibody differs in flow cytometry and in frozen and paraffin tissue section immunohistochemistry. The optimal working dilutions of monoclonal antibodies that detect paraffin-resistant antigens vary with the fixative (e.g., formalin, Bouin solution) and with the sensitivity of the detection system used. Each antibody reagent must be titered on the appropriate cells or tissue in each detection system in which it is to be employed.

Quality Control in the Laboratory

Rigorous quality control must be employed in handling and processing specimens, establishing and maintaining reagent panels, and performing cytofluorometric and immunohistochemical analysis of pathologic specimens. Processing normal tissues in conjunction with pathologic specimens in an analogous manner contributes significantly to monitoring the consistency and quality of the laboratory. This approach may also be used to establish the normal values of the laboratory and is an important source of material for positive and negative controls. Fresh tonsils are an excellent source of "normal tissue" for preparing formalin-fixed, paraffin-embedded tissue blocks and cryopreserved tissue blocks for use as positive and negative controls.

All labeled monoclonal antibodies and heteroantisera must be carefully evaluated continuously to ensure their specificity and sensitivity. All reagents should be titered on the appropriate benign or neoplastic cells or tissues that encompass the range of strong positivity to virtual negativity. The proper dilution is the one giving the highest acceptable level of brightness in conjunction with the lowest background. Retitering with additional, more appropriate serial dilutions may be necessary to arrive at the optimal working dilution.

The flow cytometer must be properly aligned, appropriately calibrated, and its settings optimally adjusted daily to consistently perform accurate cytofluorometric analysis. Isotype-matched, murine monoclonal antibodies with irrelevant specificity (e.g., IgG1, IgG2a) are used to establish the background noise level and the zero point of the analysis. Immunostaining for CD45 and CD14 indicates the purity of the analysis gate based on cellular composition with respect to lymphocytes and monocytes. The laboratory participates in the College of American Pathologists proficiency testing program as well as the New York State proficiency testing program (New York State Department of Health, Albany, NY). Quality control procedures in flow cytometry are discussed in more detail in Chapter 5.

Positive and negative controls must be routinely employed in immunohistochemical staining as well. For example, immunostaining of paraffin tissue sections of a diffuse large cell lymphoma with monoclonal antibodies for CD20 and CD43 should be accompanied by parallel immunostaining of paraffin sections of a normal tonsil. Immunostaining of paraffin tissue sections of a suspected case of Hodgkin lymphoma with monoclonal antibodies for CD30 and CD15 should be accompanied by parallel immunostaining of paraffin sections of a known case of Hodgkin lymphoma expressing those antigens. The diagnostic case slides should be evaluated in light of the results obtained with the known positive control slides. If, for example, the Reed-Sternberg cells in the known positive control sections are CD30⁻ or only very weakly positive, CD30⁻ diagnostic case slides are probably invalid, and the immunostaining should be repeated. Negative controls should include sections stained with isotype-matched, irrelevant murine monoclonal antibodies followed by the appropriate labeled secondary antibody and sections stained only with the labeled secondary antibody. Quality control procedures in immunohistochemical staining are discussed in Chapter 4.

APPROACH TO IMMUNOPHENOTYPIC ANALYSIS OF LYMPHOMA AND LEUKEMIA

General Comments

Laboratories approach immunophenotypic analysis differently, often depending on the philosophical biases and the methodologic preferences of the director. Unfortunately, some of the approaches that are commonly chosen fail to achieve a precise immunodiagnosis or do so only after a needless expenditure of time, effort, and money because they are not targeted to the specific diagnostic problem.

The limited screening approach most often results in a failure to achieve a precise immunodiagnosis and, worse, sometimes results in an incorrect diagnosis. In this case, the pathologist tends to screen all cell suspensions and paraffin tissue sections with the same limited panel of monoclonal antibody reagents. This panel may include, for example, anti-B-cell antibody B1 (CD20), anti-T-cell antibody Leu-4 (CD3), anti-monocyte antibody Leu-M3 (CD14), anti-T-cell subset antibodies Leu-3a (CD4) and Leu2a (CD8), and antibodies recognizing κ and λ light chains and an anti-TdT antibody in the case of acute leukemia. The use of this limited panel of antibodies is far from sufficient for diagnostic evaluations in modern-day clinical practice in modern-day hematopathology. This approach fails to consider the special immunophenotypic profiles of the many different entities recognized in the current WHO classification, the precise immunodiagnosis of which can only be made by employing additional monoclonal antibodies (115).

In contrast, the "shot-gun" approach nearly always arrives at a correct immunodiagnosis but at a price. In this case, the pathologist routinely employs a large panel of monoclonal antibodies that detect a wide array of B-cell, T-cell, monocyte-macrophage, myeloid, leukemia-associated, and other antigens to arrive at the correct immunodiagnosis. The price of this approach is an unnecessary expenditure of time, effort, and money.

The other reasons investigators sometimes have difficulty achieving a correct immunodiagnosis are failure to recognize the pitfalls and disadvantages inherent in each immunophenotypic approach; failure or inability to employ an alternative approach when the initial approach fails; and failure to correlate the immunophenotypic results with the clinical information and careful examination of the histopathologic sections. For example, some pathologists exclusively perform flow cytometric analysis of cells in suspension and report their results without correlating their findings with the histopathology. Pitfalls exist in the cytofluorometric analysis of cell suspensions, however. For example, the poor viability of some cell suspensions may result in preferential loss of the neoplastic cells accompanied by selective enrichment of the residual benign T cells. For some cases, the content of the neoplastic cells in the tumor may be low, for example, in Hodgkin lymphoma and T-cell/histiocyte-rich large B-cell lymphoma. In these instances, the pathologist may report the immunophenotypic profile of the normal and not the neoplastic cells, resulting in misdiagnosis. Review of the viability data and the histopathologic sections should alert the pathologist to the discrepant results and the obvious reason for them. The pathologist should reanalyze this case by immunohistochemical staining of paraffin tissue sections. Unfortunately, the failure of some laboratories to recognize and rectify such problems has led some hematopathologists to question the validity of performing cytofluorometric analysis of lymph nodes and other tissue specimens.

However, pathologists who exclusively analyze lymph nodes by frozen section immunohistochemistry sometimes may be unable, for example, to detect partial nodal involvement by a B-cell lymphoma or identify a T-cell–rich B-cell lymphoma. In these instances, preferential gated cytofluorometric analysis of the different constituent cell populations comprising a lymph node or other tissue specimen may detect a monoclonal B-cell population that evades detection in tissue sections.

We believe that a laboratory requires four attributes to routinely perform immunophenotypic analyses of pathologic specimens reliably and reproducibly:

1. Knowledge of the distribution of reactivity of the numerous available monoclonal antibody reagents with benign and malignant hematopoietic cells in cell suspensions and frozen and paraffin tissue sections (Table 10.1) (see Chapter 3)
2. Knowledge of the immunophenotypic profiles of the principal hematopoietic neoplasms (Tables 10.2 through 10.5)
3. Knowledge of the different methodologic approaches to immunophenotypic analysis and an appreciation of the advantages, disadvantages, and pitfalls intrinsic to each (see Chapter 3)
4. The ability to implement the appropriate combination of immunophenotypic methodology and monoclonal antibodies and other reagents to resolve the diagnostic dilemma posed by each individual case

Our Approach

Immunophenotypic analyses of all peripheral blood, bone marrow aspiration, and effusion specimens, as well as all solid tissue specimens, obtained fresh and adequate in size to prepare a representative viable cell suspension are performed by immunofluorescent staining of the cells in suspension followed by cytofluorometric analysis of the immunostained cells. In the past, single-color analysis was performed using unlabeled primary murine monoclonal antibodies followed by affinity-purified, solid-phase human immunoglobulin-absorbed, fluorescein isothiocyanate–conjugated F(ab')$_2$ fragments of sheep anti-mouse immunoglobulin (ICN

Biomedicals, Costa Mesa, CA). Total surface immunoglobulin and the individual immunoglobulin heavy- and light-chain classes are detected with fluoroscein-labeled F(ab')$_2$ fragments of goat anti-human immunoglobulin (BioSource International, Camarillo, CA). Nowadays, the laboratory employs multicolor flow cytometry to analyze coexpression of multiple antigens by the same cell population using labeled antibodies. This is helpful in diagnosing hematologic malignancies with expression of markers of multiple lineages, for example, acute mixed lineage (biphenotypic) leukemias, precisely delineating aberrant gain or loss of antigens, and detecting abnormal intensities in antigen expressions on hematopoietic cells. Multicolor flow cytometry is also useful when only limited numbers of cells are available for analysis, because multiple antigens can be detected using the number of cells normally assayed for one antigen (11). Cell suspension analysis of tissue specimens is also advantageous because it permits nearly all the specimens arriving each day to be batched and analyzed using the same methodology. This allows all the analyses to be performed rapidly in the least labor-intensive and the most time-efficient and cost-effective manner. The technical aspects of cytofluorometric analysis are discussed in detail in Chapter 5.

Immunohistochemical staining of paraffin-embedded tissue sections is performed on solid tissue specimens in which a representative viable cell suspension cannot be prepared for technical reasons or because only fixed tissue is available and when the results of cell suspension analysis are equivocal or do not correlate with the histopathologic sections. One of the major advantages of immunohistochemical staining of paraffin tissue sections is architectural preservation, which permits precise topographic localization of the positively stained cells and their cytomorphologic evaluation. Immunohistochemical staining of paraffin tissue sections requires a separate panel of reagents capable of detecting antigens that are resistant to formalin fixation and paraffin embedding. However, the new antigen retrieval techniques allow a wide range of antigens to be detected in routinely fixed and paraffin-embedded tissues, including many antigens that traditionally have been considered identifiable only in frozen tissue sections.

In most cases, paraffin tissue sections are immunostained by an ABC immunoperoxidase technique (see Appendix 10.5) because this method is both highly sensitive and rapid. One technician can easily perform two or more immunostaining "runs" of 120 slides each day using the Leica Bond III Automated Immunostaining System. Because the pseudoperoxidase activity of erythrocytes and the myeloperoxidase activity of neutrophils and other myeloid cells can make interpretation of immunoperoxidase-stained sections difficult, endogenous peroxidase activity is blocked in paraffin tissue sections before immunoperoxidase staining. The use of a negative control for the identification of endogenous peroxidase activity on frozen sections or the APAAP technique (see Appendix 10.5) on cytospin preparations is preferred.

Our approach to the immunophenotypic analysis of the acute leukemias and non-Hodgkin lymphomas is broadly outlined below.

Acute Leukemia

In most cases, the diagnosis of acute leukemia has already been made or is strongly suspected clinically. In these instances, samples of involved peripheral blood or aspirated bone marrow are usually submitted to determine the immunophenotypic profile and thereby the nature of the leukemic cells. Often, most cells isolated from these specimens are malignant, and only a small number of residual benign cells are present, making analysis of these cases relatively straightforward.

Table 10.1	PRINCIPAL ANTIGENS ANALYZED AND MONOCLONAL ANTIBODIES EMPLOYED IN IMMUNOPHENOTYPIC ANALYSIS

General Category	Antigen	Principal Monoclonal Antibodies for Flow Cytometry and Paraffin Sections Immunohistochemistry	Antigen Recognized (kd)	Principal Pattern of Reactivity	Comments
Hematopoietic	CD45	2D1, HI30, PD7/26/16 and 2B11 (P)	gp180-220,	Pan-hematopoietic cell	Leukocyte common antigen (LCA)
T lineage	CD1a	BL6, DCGM4, HI149, O10, SK9, MTB1 (P)	gp49	Cortical thymocytes, Langerhans cells	
	CD2	39C1.5, 6F10.3, L303.1, RPA-2.10, 1, S5.2, SFCI3Pt2H9, AB75 (P)	gp50	Pan-T lymphocyte, natural killer (NK) cells	Sheep erythrocyte (E) rosette receptor
	CD3	HIT3, SK7, UCHT1, SP7 (P)	gp/p 26, 20, 20, 16, 28	Pan-T lymphocyte, NK cells	CD3 complex of 5 chains; most antibodies detect ε chain; cytoplasmic but not surface expression detected in NK cells
	CD4	13B8.2, BL4, RPA-T4, SFC12T4D11, SK3, 4B12 (P)	gp59	Cortical thymocytes, helper/inducer T cells, monocytes-macrophages	MHC class II receptor, HIV receptor
	CD5	BL1a, L17F12, SFCI24T6G12, UCHT2, 4C7 (P)	gp67	Pan-T lymphocyte, B-lymphocyte subset	
	CD7	3A1E-12H7, 8H8.1, Leu9, 3A1, OKT16, WT1, LP15 (P)	gp40	Pan-T lymphocyte, NK cells	Earliest appearing T-lymphocyte antigen
	CD8	B9.11, SFCI21Thy2D3, HIT8a, RPA-T8, SK1, C8/144B (P)	gp32	Cortical thymocytes, suppressor/cytotoxic T cells, NK cell subset	MHC class I receptor
	CD43	DFT1, Leu22 (L60) (P), MT1 (P)	gp95–135	Stem cells, erythroblasts, megakaryocytes, myeloid cells, macrophages, pan T-cells, all mature WBCs except resting B cells	Sialophorin, leukosialin
	CD45RO	UCHL-1 (P), A6 (P), OPD4 (P)	gp180	T-cell subset, granulocytes, monocytes-macrophages	LCA isoform without A, B or C exons
	TCR $\alpha\beta$	T10B9.1A-31, WT31, 8A3 (P)	gp47–49, 40	T lymphocytes expressing $\alpha\beta$ T-cell receptor	
	TCR $\gamma\delta$	B1, 11F2, 5A6.E9	gp40, 43	T lymphocytes expressing $\gamma\delta$ T-cell receptor	<5% normal T cells
	ZAP70	1E7.2, 17A/P-ZAP70, J34-602, 2F32 (P)	ZAP70	T cells, NK cells	70 kd, Syk family protein kinase, associated with the CD3/TCR complex zeta chain; also expressed in some CLL cells; correlates with IgVh somatic hypermutation. Used as a prognostic marker in CLL
B lineage	CD19	4G7, 89B, HIB19, J3-119, SJ25C1, BT51E (P)	gp95	Pan-B lymphocyte	Earliest appearing B-lymphocyte antigen
	CD20	2H7, B9E9, H1, H299, L27, L26 (P)	p33	Pan-B lymphocyte	Appears after CD19 and CD22 in B-cell ontogeny
	CD21	1048, B-ly4, BL13, 2G9 (P)	gp145	Mature B-lymphocyte subset, follicular dendritic cells	C3d/EBV receptor (CR2)
	CD22	HD239, HIB22, S-HCL-1, SJ10.1H11, FPC1 (P)	gp130/140	Pan-B lymphocyte	Appears early in B-cell ontogeny, after CD19
	CD45RA	2H4LDH11LDB9, ALB11, DBB42, 4KB5 (P)	gp205–220	Pan-B lymphocyte, NK cells	LCA isoforms containing exon A
	CD79a	HM47 (P), JCB117 (P)	gp33	Pan-B lymphocyte, plasma cells	Surface Ig receptor complex, expressed throughout B-cell differentiation, from early immature B cells to plasma cells
	PAX5	24/PAX5 (P), SP34 (P)	PAX5/ B-cell lineage specific activator protein (BSAP)	Pan-B lymphocyte	42 kDa, paired box (PAX) family of transcription factors, also known as BSAP; not expressed in normal plasma cells
	OCT2	C-20 (Pt)	OCT2	Pan-B lymphocyte	58 kDa, Octamer transcription factor-2 (OCT2), belongs to the POU family of transcription factors; specifically binds to the octamer motif to activate transcription of immunoglobulingene and other genes; weakly expressed to absent in Hodgkin/Reed Sternberg cells
	NA	Immunoglobulin (Ig) $\mu, \delta, \gamma, \alpha, \kappa, \lambda$		B lymphocytes	Precursor B cells contain cytoplasmic μ, mature B cells express surface Ig, plasma cells contain cytoplasmic Ig
	CD138	1D4, DL101, MI15, B-A38 (P)	Syndecan-1	Plasma cells	Not expressed in mature B cells; strong expression in epithelial cells.

Table 10.1	PRINCIPAL ANTIGENS ANALYZED AND MONOCLONAL ANTIBODIES EMPLOYED IN IMMUNOPHENOTYPIC ANALYSIS *(Continued)*				
Myeloid/monocytic lineages	CD11b	94, Bear1, D12, ICRF44	gp165	Monocytes-macrophages, granulocytes, NK cells	iC3b receptor (CR3)
	CD11c	B-Ly6, BU15, LeuM5 (S-HCL3), 5D11 (P)	gp150	Granulocytes, monocytes-macrophages, NK cells, activated T and B cells	Hairy cell leukemia-associated
	CD13	36, Immu103.44, L138, SJ1D1, WM15, 38C12 (P)	gp130–150	Myeloid cells, monocytes-macrophages	Aminopeptidase N, coronavirus receptor
	CD14	116, 322A-1, MφP9, M5E2, RMO52, 7 (P)	gp55	Monocytes-macrophages, granulocytes	Expressed in mature monocytes; not expressed in immature monocytes
	CD15	80H5, CSLEX1, HI98, MMA, W6D3, LeuM1 (P), MMA (P)	X-hapten, Lewis antigen	Granulocytes, eosinophils, activated T cells, monocytes-macro-phages, Langerhans cells	Expressed by Reed-Sternberg cells of Hodgkin lymphoma
	CD33	906, P67.6, WM53, D3HL60, PWS44 (P)	gp67	Immature myeloid cells, granulocytes, monocytes-macrophages	Function unknown
	CD36	FA6.152, CB38	gp88	Megakaryocytes, platelets, monocytes, endothelial cells, very early erythroid precursors	Platelet GPIV, receptor for extracellular matrix proteins such as collagen and thrombospondin
	CD41	69, P2, SZ22, MWReg30, PBM 6.4, 5B12	gp120/23	Megakaryocytes, platelets	Platelet glycoprotein GPIIb (integrin αIIb chain) forms complex with GPIIIa (CD61)
	CD42b	HIP1, SZ2, MM2/174 (P)	gp135	Megakaryocytes, platelets	Platelet glycoprotein Ib alpha chain that is disulfide bonded to CD42c (GPIb beta) to form 170 kDa heterodimer GPIb which is noncovalently complexed with CD42a and CD42d to form the CD42 complex, the receptor for von Willebrand factor
	CD61	1/integrin beta 3 chain, RUU-PL7F12, SZ21, 2f2 (P)	gp105	Megakaryocytes, platelets	Platelet glycoprotein GPIIIa (integrin β3 subunit), noncovalently bound to GPIIb (CD41) to form the GPIIb-GPIIIa complex on platelets and megakaryocytes; also expressed on endothelial cells, macrophages, osteoblasts, fibroblasts, and smooth muscle; complex with CD51 (integrin αV) to form the vitronectin receptor
	CD64	10.1	gp75	Monocytes-macrophages, subset of dendritic cells	High-affinity receptor for IgG (FcγRI); also expressed in granulocytes when they are activated with IFN-γ
	CD68	KP-1 (P), PG-M1 (P)	gp110	Monocytes-macrophages, granulocytes, mast cells	PG-M1 is more restricted toward CD68 expression in monocytes-macrophages
	CD71	2/transferrin, L01.1, M-A712, YDJ1.2.2, H68.4 (P)	gp95	Erythroid precursors, activated B and T cells, macrophages	Transferrin receptor, present as dimers. Expression in mature erythrocytes is minimal, therefore facilitating evaluation of erythroid precursors in bone marrow biopsy
	Glycophorin A (CD235a)	GA-R2, 11E48-7-6, KC16, JC159 (P)	Sialoglycoprotein	Erythroid precursors excluding BFU-E and CFU-E, mature erythrocytes	M, N blood group antigens
	MPO	1B10, 5B8, 59A5 (P)	p140	Granulocytes, monocytes (low density)	Lyzosomal enzyme
Natural killer	CD16	B73.1, 3G8, 2H7 (P)	gp50–80	NK cells, granulocytes, macrophages	FcγRIII
	CD56	B159, CD218, My31, N901, CD564 (P), 1b6 (P)	gp180	NK cells, T-cell subset	Neural cell adhesion molecule
	CD57	HNK-1, NC1, NK-1, Leu7 (HNK-1) (P)	gp110	NK cell subset, T-cell subset	Expressed by various carcinomas (e.g., small cell lung carcinoma), associated with myelin-associated glycoprotein; function unknown
Proliferation associated	Ki-67	35/Ki-67, B56, MIB-1 (P)	NR	Proliferating cells	Nuclear proliferation antigen
Activation associated	CD23	9P25, EBVCS-5, HD50, M-L233, 1B12 (P)	gp45	Follicle mantle B cells, activated B cells, follicular dendritic cells, monocytes, platelets	FcεRII
	CD25	1HT44H3, 2A3, 33B3.1, B1.49.9, M-A251, 4C9 (P)	gp55	Activated T cells, B cells and monocytes	Interleukin-2 receptor

(continued)

| Table 10.1 | PRINCIPAL ANTIGENS ANALYZED AND MONOCLONAL ANTIBODIES EMPLOYED IN IMMUNOPHENOTYPIC ANALYSIS *(Continued)* |

General Category	Antigen	Principal Monoclonal Antibodies for Flow Cytometry and Paraffin Sections Immunohistochemistry	Antigen Recognized (kd)	Principal Pattern of Reactivity	Comments
	CD30	BerH8, Ber-H83, E59.126, HRS4, KDR-1, Ber-H2 (P)	gp105–120	Activated B and T cells	Member of the tumor necrosis factor receptor superfamily; interacts with CD153 (CD30 ligand), consistently expressed by Hodgkin/Reed-Sternberg cells of Hodgkin lymphoma and anaplastic large cell lymphoma
	CD38	HB7, LS198-4-3, T16, SPC32 (P)	gp46	Immature B lymphocytes, thymocytes, activated Tcells, plasma cells, NK cells, myeloblasts and erythroblasts	
	HLA-DR	46-6, BB.12.2, Immu-357, TU36, Tu39, TAL.1B5 (P)	gp29, 34	B lymphocytes, monocytes-macrophages, activated T cells and immature cells of many lineages	
Precursor	CD34	581,8G12, QBend/10 (P)	gp110	Myeloid, lymphoid and stromal progenitor cells, vascular endothelial cells	Earliest stem cell antigen
	CD117	95C3, 104D2, YB5.B8	p145	Myeloblasts, early erythroid precursors, mast cells	Stem cell factor receptor
	TdT	E17-1519, HT1 + HT4 + HT8 + HT9, SEN28(P)	p60	Precursor B and T cells	Intranuclear DNA polymerase involved in the formation of nucleotide (N) regions
Oncogene and tumor suppressor gene products	BCL-2	124 (P)	p24–26	Medullary thymocytes, T and nongerminal center B cells	Useful in distinguishing follicular lymphoma (BCL2 positive in most cases) and follicular hyperplasia (BCL2 negative)
	BCL-6	PG-B6p (P)	p87	Germinal center B cells, subset of T cells and macrophages	Expression of BCL6 is deregulated in DLBCL by *BCL6* gene rearrangement and somatic hypermutation
	Cyclin D1	DCS-6 (P), SP4 (P)	p36	Absent in normal lymphoid cells	Aberrantly expressed in vast majority of mantle cell lymphomas as a result of BCL1/CCND1 gene rearrangement in t(11;14); can also be aberrantly expressed in hairy cell leukemia and plasma cell neoplasm; one of the D-type cyclins involved in cell cycle control
	p53	AM240-10M (P), D01 (P), D07 (P), 1801 (P)	p53	Absent in normal lymphoid tissue	p53 protein overexpression and gene mutations do not necessarily correlate
	IRF4/MUM1	MUM1p (P)	p52	Subset of germinal center cells (committed to plasmacytic differentiation), subset of activated T cells, plasma cells	Interferon regulatory factor 4. Originally identified as a IgH translocation partner in a *MU*ltiple *M*yeloma cell line with (6;14) (p25;q32). Also expressed in melanocytes. Variable expression in B- and T-cell lymphomas. Positive in vast majority of plasma cell neoplasms. Consistently expressed in Hodgkin/Reed-Sternberg cells in classical Hodgkin lymphomas
	PRDM1/ Blimp-1	3H2E8 (P)	p88	Subset of germinal center cells (committed to plasmacytic differentiation), subset of activated T cells, plasma cells	Tumor suppressor gene in DLBCL. Deleted and mutated in DLBCL of the non–germinal center B-cell type. Considered a master regulator of plasma cell differentiation. Expressed in B-cell lymphomas with plasmablastic/plasmacytic differentiation and consistently expressed in plasma cell neoplasms
Other	CD10	J5, BA-3, CALLA	gp100	Precursor B cells, mature B-cell subset, granulocytes	Neutral endopeptidase

gp, Glycoprotein; p, protein; kDa, kilodaltons; P, paraffin.
Compiled from references (6,7,9,10,29,116–173), personal observations.

Table 10.2 IMMUNOPHENOTYPIC PROFILES OF SUBCATEGORIES OF ALL AND LYMPHOBLASTIC LYMPHOMA

Category		Common Immunophenotypic Profile	Comments
B ALL/LBL, NOS			~80%, ALLs, ~20% of LBLs; variable CD34, CD13 and CD33 expression
	Precursor B-ALL/Pro-B-ALL	TdT(+), HLA-DR(+), CD19(+), cCD22(+), cCD79a(+), CD10(−), CD20(−)	~10% of B-ALL/LBLs
	Common type	TdT(+), HLA-DR(+), CD19(+), cCD22(+), cCD79a(+), CD10(+), CD20(−/+)	~70% of B-ALL/LBLs
	Pre-B cell	TdT(+), HLA-DR(+), CD19(+), CD10(+), CD20(+), cytoplasmic μ(+)	~20% of B-ALL/LBLs
B ALL/LBL with recurrent genetic abnormalities			
	t(9;22)(q34;q11.2), BCR-ABL1	TdT(+), CD34(±), HLA-DR(+), CD19(+), cCD22(+), cCD79a(+), CD10(+), CD20(−/+), CD13(±), CD33(±), CD25(±)	CD13 and CD33 expression is frequent (~40%–60%). High association with CD25 expression
	t(v;11q23), MLL rearranged	TdT(+), CD34(+), HLA-DR(+), CD19(+), cCD22(+), cCD79a(+), CD10(−), CD20(−), CD15(±), CD13(-), CD33(−)	Frequent CD15 expression; precursor B phenotype
	t(12;21)(p13;q22); TEL-AML1	TdT(+), CD34(+), HLA-DR(+), CD19(+), cCD22(+), cCD79a(+), CD10(+), CD20(−), CD13(±), CD33(±)	Frequent CD13 and CD33 expressions
	Hyperdiploidy	TdT(+), CD34(+), HLA-DR(+), CD19(+), cCD22(+), cCD79a(+), CD10(+), CD20(−), CD13(−), CD33(−)	
	t(1;19)(q23;p13.3); E2A-PBX1	TdT(+), CD34(-), HLA-DR(+), CD19(+), cCD22(+), cCD79a(+), CD10(+), CD20(±), cytoplasmic μ(±)	Most have pre-B-cell phenotype
Precursor T cell			~20% of ALLs; ~80% of LBLs CD79a positive in 10% of cases, CD13 and CD33 positive in 16%–32% of cases, CD117 occasionally positive
	Pro-T (prothymocyte)	TdT(+), CD34(±), HLA-DR(±), CD7(+), CD2(−), CD5(−), CD1a(−), cCD3(+), sCD3(−), CD4(−), CD8(−)	~70% of T-ALLs and ~30% of T-LBLs express prothymocyte and immature thymocyte phenotypes
	Pre-T (immature/early thymocyte)	TdT(+), CD34(±), HLA-DR(±), CD7(+), CD2(+), CD5(+), CD1a(−), cCD3(+), sCD3(−), CD4(−), CD8(−)	
	Cortical T (common thymocyte)	TdT(+), CD34(−), HLA-DR(−), CD7(+), CD2(+), CD5(+), CD1a(+), cCD3(+), sCD3(−), CD4(+), CD8(+)	~30% of T-ALLs and ~70% of T-LBLs express common and mature thymocyte phenotypes
	Mature (medullary) thymocyte	TdT(+), CD34(−), HLA-DR(−), CD7(+), CD2(+), CD5(+), CD1a(−), cCD3(+), sCD3(+), CD4(+) or CD8(+)	~1% of T-ALLs

ALL, acute lymphoblastic leukemia; LBL, lymphoblastic lymphoma; cCD3, cytoplasmic CD3; sCD3, surface CD3; cCD22, cytoplasmic CD22; cCD79a, cytoplasmic CD79a.
Compiled from references (6,7,9,10,29,174–177) and personal observations.

If a sufficient number of cells is available, acute leukemias are analyzed in cell suspension with a comprehensive antibody panel that not only permit their subclassification as B-cell acute lymphoblastic leukemia (ALL), T-cell ALL, acute myeloid leukemia (AML), or acute mixed lineage (biphenotypic) leukemia but also provides a detailed phenotypic profile. This panel can be performed as an initial screen (Table 10.6) followed by additional immunophenotypic analyses depending on the initial results (Table 10.7). If an insufficient number of cells are present, select markers that include the more lineage-specific antigens (e.g., CD19, cCD3, MPO, etc.) should be used to allow general categorization of acute leukemia. Clinical information and morphologic examination of smears and Diff-Quik–stained cytospin preparations are helpful in narrowing the differential diagnosis and selecting a condensed panel when materials are limited. For example, a 12-year-old boy presenting with a large mediastinal mass and a WBC count of 75,000/mm³ probably has T-cell ALL. In this case, if cells for flow cytometry are in short supply, essential markers will include TdT and cCD3, and preferably more T-cell markers should be included, in addition to MPO (for evaluation of a T/myeloid biphenotypic acute leukemia), CD19, and CD10 (for evaluation of T/B-bilineage acute leukemia). A carefully planned immunophenotypic analysis based on review of all of the available information and material is always strongly recommended.

Occasionally, a patient has a near normal peripheral blood WBC count and differential count and a bone marrow packed with leukemic cells but that cannot be aspirated. In these cases, immunophenotypic analysis can be performed on paraffin tissue sections prepared from a bone marrow biopsy core. The hematopoietic cell antigens that are most helpful in the diagnosis of acute leukemia in routinely processed paraffin tissue sections overlap to some extent with the antigens evaluated by flow cytometry. Some antigens, for example, CD19, CD13, and CD33, which could only be assessed before by flow cytometry, can now be evaluated by immunohistochemistry on paraffin sections because of the availability of new commercially available antibodies. For the evaluation of B-cell lineage in acute leukemia on paraffin tissue sections, PAX5, though not 100% specific, is useful. CD68, CD163, and lysozyme can be used to assess granulocytic/monocytic lineage (see Chapters 4 and 38).

In some instances, other types of pathologic specimens (e.g., cutaneous punch biopsies, testicular and liver needle biopsies, effusions, CSF) are submitted for identification and analysis of leukemic cells. The same leukemia antibody panels may be employed in these situations. However, it is sometimes more

Table 10.3	IMMUNOPHENOTYPIC PROFILES OF SUBCATEGORIES OF AML

Category		FAB Classification	Common Immunophenotypic Profile
AML with recurrent genetic abnormalities			
	AML with t(8;21)(q22;q22), *RUNX1-RUNX1T1 (AML1/ETO)*	M2	CD34(+), CD117(+), HLA-DR(+), CD13(+, bright), CD33(−) or CD33(+, dim), MPO (+, bright), CD11b(−), CD15(+), CD14(−), TdT(±), CD19 (+, dim), CD56(±), CD2(−), CD7(−)
	AML with inv16(p13.1q22) or t(16;16)(p13.1;q22), *CBFB-MYH11*	M4(Eo)	CD34(+), CD117(+), HLA-DR(+), CD13(+), CD33(+), MPO(+), CD11b(+), CD15(+), CD14(+), TdT(−), CD19(−), CD56(−), CD4(+), CD2(±), CD7(−)
	AML with t(15;17)(q22;q12), *PML-RARA*	M3	CD34(−), CD117(±), HLA-DR(−), CD13(+), CD33(+, bright homogeneous), MPO(+), CD11b(−), CD15(−), CD14(−), TdT(−), CD19(−), CD56(±), CD2(±), CD7(−)
	AML with 11q23 abnormalities, *MLL* rearrangement	M4/5	CD34(±), CD117(±), HLA-DR(+), CD13(−), CD33(+), MPO(±), CD11b(+), CD15(+), CD14(+), TdT (−), CD19(−), CD56(±), CD4(+), CD2(−), CD7(−), NG2(+)
AML, NOS			
	AML with minimal differentiation	M0	CD34(+), CD117(+), HLA-DR(+), CD13(+), CD33(±), CD11b(−), CD15(−), CD14(−), CD64(−), MPO(−), TdT(±), CD7(±)
	AML without maturation	M1	CD34(±), CD117(±), HLA-DR(±), CD13(+), CD33(+), CD11b(±), CD15(−), CD14(−), CD64(−), MPO(+), CD7(±)
	AML with maturation	M2	CD34(±), CD117(±), HLA-DR(±), CD13(+), CD33(+), CD11b(±), CD15(±), CD14(−), CD64(−), MPO(+), CD7(±)
	AML myelomonocytic leukemia	M4	CD34(±), CD117(±), HLA-DR(+), CD13(+), CD33(+), MPO(+), CD11b(+), CD15(+), CD14(+), CD36(+), CD64(+), TdT(−), CD4(+), CD2(±), CD7(−)
	AML monoblastic/monocytic leukemia	M5	CD34(±), CD117(±), HLA-DR(+), CD13(+), CD33(+), MPO(±), CD11b(+), CD15(+), CD14(+), CD36(+), CD64(+), TdT(−), CD4(+), CD7(±), CD56(±)
	Acute erythroblastic leukemia	M6	CD34(−), CD117(−), HLA-DR(−), MPO(−), Glycophorin A(±)
	Acute megakaryoblastic leukemia	M7	CD34(−), CD117(−), HLA-DR(−), MPO(−), CD41(+), CD61(+)

FAB, French-American-British classification (178).
Compiled from references (7,9,29,118,177,179) and personal observations.

difficult to analyze these specimens because of the small size of the tissue biopsy, the limited numbers of cells that can be harvested from the specimen, and the presence of many residual normal cells. In these instances, it is important to employ the immunodiagnostic reagents in order of diagnostic priority, such as CD34, CD117, and TdT before κ or λ. If flow cytometry is employed, it is important to preferentially gate the neoplastic cells, thereby eliminating the normal cells from analysis and avoiding confusion in determining the immunophenotype of the leukemic cells.

Table 10.4	IMMUNOPHENOTYPIC PROFILES OF PRINCIPAL CATEGORIES OF MATURE B-CELL LYMPHOMA AND LYMPHOID LEUKEMIA

Category	Common Immunophenotypic Profile
Small lymphocytic lymphoma/chronic lymphocytic leukemia	CD19(+), CD20(+, weak), CD22(+, weak), HLA-DR(+), surface Ig(+, weak), CD5(+), CD23(+), CD10(−), FMC7(−)
B-cell prolymphocytic leukemia	CD19(+), CD20(+), CD22(+), HLA-DR(+), surface Ig(+), CD5(−), CD23(v), CD10(−), FMC7(+), CD11c(±), CD25(±)
Mantle cell lymphoma	CD19(+), CD20(+), CD22(+), HLA-DR(+), surface Ig(+), CD5(+), CD10(−), CD23(− or weak), cyclin D1(+), SOX11(+)
Lymphoplasmacytic lymphoma	CD19(+), CD20(+), CD22(±), HLA-DR(+), surface and cytoplasmic Ig(+, predominantly M, sometimes G, rarely A), CD5(−), CD10(−), CD23(−), CD138(+ in plasma cells)
Follicular lymphoma	CD19(+), CD20(+), CD22(+), HLA-DR(+), surface Ig(±), CD5(−), CD10(±), CD23(v)
Marginal zone lymphoma (nodal and MALT-type)	CD19(+), CD20(+), CD22(+), HLA-DR(+), surface Ig(+, usually M, less often G/A), CD5(−, + in small subset), CD10(−), CD23(−), CD11c(v)
Splenic marginal zone lymphoma	CD19(+), CD20(+), CD22(+), HLA-DR(+), surface Ig(+, MD), CD5(−, + in small subset), CD10(−), CD23(v), CD11c(v)
Hairy cell leukemia	CD19(+), CD20(+), CD22(+), HLA-DR(+), surface Ig(+, G), CD11c(+), CD25(+), CD103(+), CD5(−), CD10(−), CD23(−), TRAP(+), DBA.44(+), Annexin A1, cyclin D1(+, weak)
Diffuse large B-cell lymphoma, NOS	CD19(+), CD20(+), CD22(+), HLA-DR(+), surface Ig(±), BCL6(v), CD10(v), MUM1(−), CD138(±)
Primary mediastinal large B-cell lymphoma	CD19(+), CD20(+), CD22(+), HLA-DR(+), surface Ig(±), BCL6(v), CD10(v), MUM1(±), CD30(±), CD23(±)
Burkitt lymphoma	CD19(+), CD20(+), CD22(+), HLA-DR(+), surface Ig(+, M), BCL6(+), CD10(+), MUM1(v)
Plasmablastic lymphoma	CD19(−), CD20(−), CD22(−), HLA-DR(−), CD138(+), surface Ig(−), cytoplasmic Ig (±), BCL6(−), MUM1(+), EBER (EBV)(±)
Plasmacytoma; multiple myeloma	CD19(−), CD20(−), CD22(−), HLA-DR(−), CD10(±), CD138(+), cytoplasmic Ig(+), surface Ig(−), CD56(±)

Ig, immunoglobulin; v, variable.
Compiled from references (6,7,9,10,29,160,164,180–193) and personal observations.

Table 10.5 IMMUNOPHENOTYPIC PROFILES OF PRINCIPAL CATEGORIES OF POSTTHYMIC T-CELL NON-HODGKIN LYMPHOMA AND LYMPHOID LEUKEMIA

Category	Common Immunophenotypic Profile[a]	Comments
Mycosis fungoides; Sezary syndrome	CD2(+), CD3(+), CD5(+), CD7(±), CD4(+), CD8(−), TCRαβ(+)	Two-thirds of cases show partial or complete loss of CD7, occasionally CD4(−)CD8(+), rarely CD4(+)CD8(+) or CD4(−)CD8(−) CD30 can be expressed in larger cells
T-cell prolymphocytic leukemia	CD2(+), CD3(+), CD5(+), CD7(+), CD4(±), CD8(±), TCRαβ(+), TCL1(+)	CD4(+)CD8(−) (~60%), CD4(+)CD8(+) (25%), CD4(−)CD8(+)(15%) Membrane CD3 is negative in 20% of cases
T-cell large granular lymphocytic leukemia	CD2(+), CD3(+), CD5(+), CD7(+), CD4(−), CD8(+), CD16(±), CD56(±), CD57(+), TCRαβ(+), TIA1(+), Granzyme B(+)	Rare variants: TCRαβ and CD4(+)CD8(−) or CD4(+)CD8(+) or CD4(−)CD8(−) TCRγδ and CD4(±)CD8(±) CD5 expression tends to be weak
Adult T-cell leukemia/lymphoma	CD2(+), CD3(+), CD5(+), CD7(−), CD4(+), CD8(−), CD25(+), TCRαβ(+)	CD30 can be expressed in the larger cells
Angioimmunoblastic T-cell lymphoma	CD2(+), CD3(+), CD5(+), CD7(+), CD4(+), CD8(−), CD10(±), BCL6(±), CXCL13(+), PD1(+)	Neoplastic T cells are believed to derive from the follicular helper T-cell subset (TFH) Expanded CD21-positive follicular dendritic cell meshworks EBV-positive B cells/B-cell proliferation (detectable by EBER and/or LMP)
Anaplastic large cell lymphoma	CD30(+), CD15(−), CD2(±), CD3(±), CD5(±), CD7(±), CD4(±), CD8(−), EMA(±), CD43 (±), CD25(±), TIA-1(±), Granzyme B (±), clusterin (±), ALK (±)	Clusterin is expressed in all cases of systemic ALCL but not in primary cutaneous ALCL
Peripheral T-cell lymphoma, NOS	CD2/CD3/CD5 and/or CD7 (±), CD4(±), CD8(±), TCRαβ(±), CD30(±), CD56(±), BCL6(±), CD10(±), CXCL13(±), PD1(±), TIA1(±), Granzyme B(±)	PTCL, NOS usually lacks TFH phenotype (CD10+, BCL6+, CXCL13+, PD1+), but ~25% of them may express at least two TFH markers. Follicular variant of PTCL, NOS express the TFH phenotype CD30 is variably expressed, often in occasional tumor cells

[a]Postthymic T-cell neoplasms are uniformly CD1a and TdT negative.
Compiled from references (6–10,29,174,194–214) and personal observations.

Table 10.6 MAJOR MONOCLONAL ANTIBODIES EMPLOYED IN THE IMMUNOPHENOTYPIC ANALYSIS OF ACUTE LEUKEMIA AND THEIR REACTIVITY WITH NEOPLASTIC CELLS

Antigen	Monoclonal Antibody	Reactivity with Neoplastic Cells		
		B cells	T cells	Myeloid Cells
TdT	6	~100% B-ALL/LBL, absent from mature B-NHLs/LLs	~100% precursor T-ALL/LBL; absent from postthymic T-NHLs/LLs	~20% AMLs
HLA-DR	L243	~100% B-ALL/LBL ~100% mature B-NHLs/LLs	~5% T-ALL/LBL ~50% postthymic T-NHLs/LLs	~75% AMLs
CD10	HI10a	~70% B-ALL/LBL, variable among B-NHLs/LLs	~20% T-ALL/LBL Absent from postthymic T-NHLs/LLs in the vast majority of cases	Absent
CD19	4G7	~95% B-ALL/LBL ~95% mature B-NHLs/LLs	Absent	~5% AMLs
CD20	L27	~50% B-ALL/LBL ~95% mature B-NHLs/LLs	Absent	Absent
CD7	4H9	Absent	~100% T-ALL/LBL ~60% postthymic T-NHLs/LLs	~20% AMLs
CD5	L17F12	Variable among mature B-NHLs/LLs Absent in B-ALL/LBL	~90% T-ALL/LBL ~60% postthymic T-NHLs/LLs	Absent
CD2	S5.2	Absent	~60% T-ALL/LBL	~3% AMLs
cCD3		Absent (except in B/T biphenotypic leukemia)	100% T-ALL/LBL ~100% postthymic T-NHLs/LLs	Absent (except T/myeloid biphenotypic leukemia)
CD13	L138	Absent	~20% T-ALL/LBL	~80% AMLs
CD33	P67.6	Absent	~7% T-ALL/LBL	~80% AMLs
MPO	CLB-MPO-1	Absent (except in B/myeloid biphenotypic leukemia)	Absent (except in B/myeloid biphenotypic leukemia)	~75% AMLs
CD34	8G12	~80% B-ALL/LBL	~40% precursor T-ALL/LBL	~60% AMLs
CD117	104D2	Absent	Absent	~50% AMLs

TdT, terminal deoxynucleotidyl transferase; ALL, acute lymphoblastic leukemia; LBL, lymphoblastic lymphoma; AML, acute myeloid leukemia; NHL, non-Hodgkin lymphoma; LL, lymphoid leukemia.
Compiled from references (6–10,29,174–177,179,194,215–219) and personal observations.

| Table 10.7 | DIAGNOSTIC IMPLICATIONS AND EXPANDED IMMUNOPHENOTYPIC PROFILES PERFORMED BASED ON THE RESULTS OF THE LEUKEMIA SCREEN |

Results of Leukemia Screen	Diagnostic Implications	Expanded Immunophenotypic Profiles
TdT(+), HLA-DR(+), CD19(+), CD20(±), CD10(±), others (−)	Precursor B-cell ALL; chronic myelogenous leukemia in lymphoid blast crisis	
TdT(+), CD7(+), CD5(±), CD2(±), cCD3, CD10(±), others (−)	Precursor T-cell ALL	CD1a, CD3, CD4, CD8,
CD34(+), CD117(±), HLA-DR(±), TdT(−), CD13 and/or CD33(+), MPO(±), others (−)	AML; chronic myelogenous leukemia in myeloid blast crisis	CD11b, CD11c, CD14, CD15, CD36, CD64, CD41, CD71
TdT(−), CD34(−), CD2, CD7 and/or CD5(+), cCD3(+), HLA-DR(±), others (−)	Postthymic T-cell leukemia/lymphoma	CD3, CD4, CD8, CD25
TdT(−), CD19(+), CD20(+), HLA-DR(+), CD10(±), others (−)	Mature B-cell leukemia/lymphoma	Surface immunoglobulin μ, δ, γ, α, κ, λ; others as necessary or desired for precise classification
CD34(+), CD117(±), TdT(+), CD19(+), CD20(±), CD13 and/or CD33(+), HLA-DR(+), CD10(±), MPO(±), others (−)	Acute B/myeloid mixed-lineage (biphenotypic) leukemia	CD79a, cytoplasmic CD22; if MPO negative, CD11c, CD14, CD64, lysozyme
CD34(+), CD117(±), TdT(+), CD7, CD2, and/or CD5(+), cCD3(+), CD13 and/or CD33(+), MPO(±), others (−)	Acute T/myeloid mixed-lineage (biphenotypic) leukemia	CD1a, CD3, CD4, CD8; if MPO negative, CD11c, CD14, CD64, lysozyme

Compiled from references (6,7,9,10,29,174,179,194) and personal observations.

B-Cell and T-Cell Non-Hodgkin Lymphomas and Chronic Leukemias

Cell suspensions prepared from pathologic specimens are analyzed using an algorithm (Fig. 10.1) composed of an initial antibody panel catered toward a classification of lymphoid proliferations as polyclonal or monoclonal B cell or T cell, followed by additional immunophenotypic analysis of the cell suspensions and/or other studies (on the cell suspensions or paraffin sections) aimed at further classifying the nature of

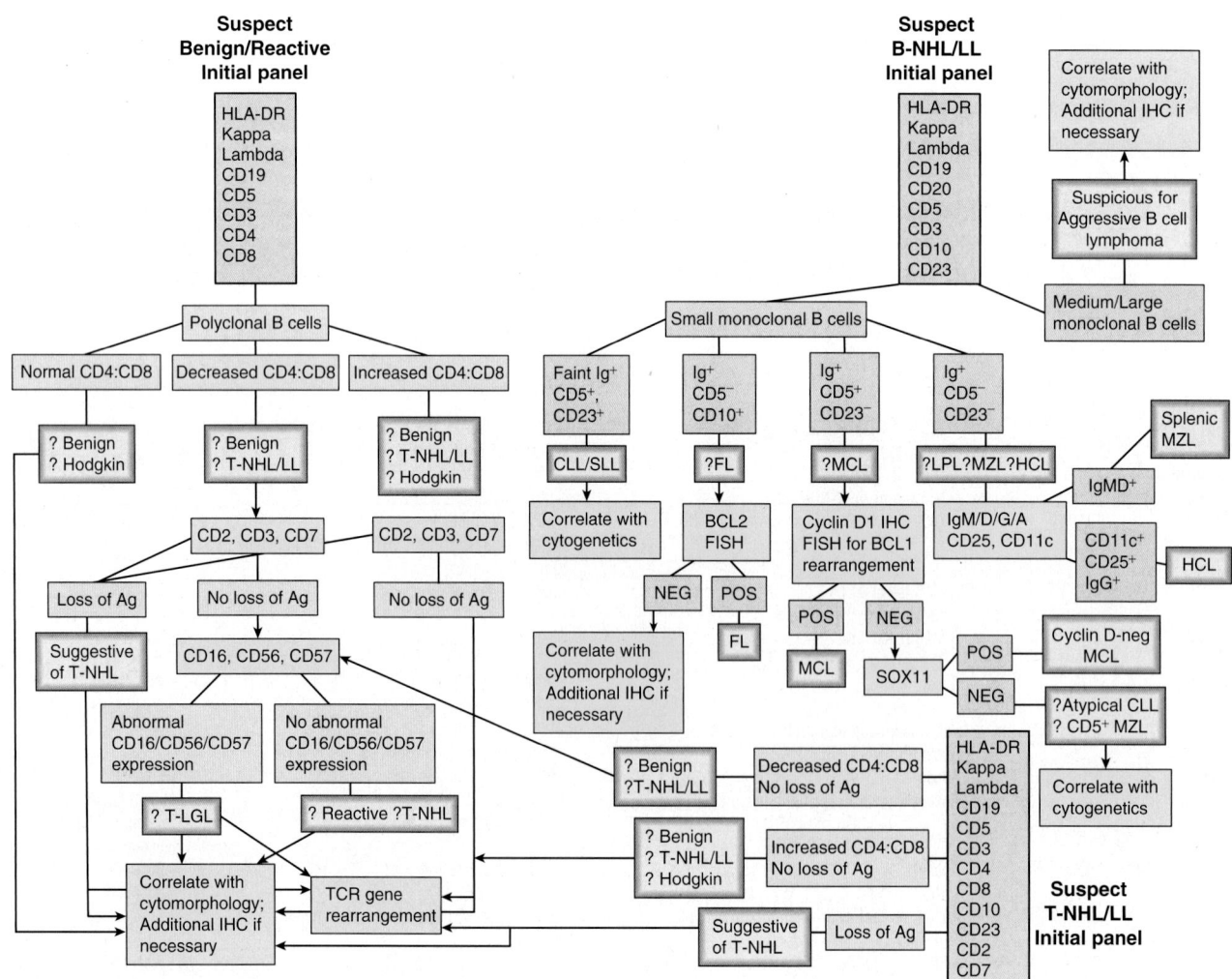

FIGURE 10.1. An algorithm employed in the immunophenotypic analysis of mature B- and T-cell non-Hodgkin lymphoma (NHL) and lymphoid leukemia (LL) starting from flow cytometric analysis of cell suspensions. An initial panel (*blue*) is used based on results of evaluation of cytospin morphology and clinical data. Depending on the diagnostic implications (*gray*), an expanded immunophenotypic profiling is used, with correlations with cytomorphology, immunohistochemistry, and cytogenetics, if necessary (*yellow*).

the process based on the results of the initial screen. Careful consideration of the clinical information and morphologic examination of touch imprints and Diff-Quik–stained cytospin preparations nearly always helps narrowing the differential diagnosis significantly. A single-step definitive immunophenotypic analysis is possible in most cases if these factors are carefully evaluated before analysis. The immunodiagnostic reagents should always be used in order of diagnostic priority when the number of cells or the amount of tissue is severely limited. For example, if a B-cell lymphoma/leukemia is strongly suspected, immunostaining for κ and λ light chains, a pan-B-cell antigen (CD19, CD20, or CD22), and a pan-T-cell antigen (CD3) should be performed in that order. Preferential gated analysis should be performed in the case of flow cytometry.

In the case of lymph nodes and other solid tissue specimens, the results of cell suspension analysis are always correlated immediately with the histopathologic sections (Fig. 10.1). Additional cell suspension studies are performed if it is believed that they will contribute to the further understanding of the case or if the results of morphologic examination and immunophenotypic analysis fail to correlate with one another or are equivocal. Immunostaining of paraffin tissue sections may be performed, depending on the specific diagnostic problem. If the results of all these additional studies are still nondiagnostic, it may be necessary to perform antigen receptor gene rearrangement analysis and possibly other molecular genetic studies on DNA extracted from the residual cells or cryopreserved tissue block.

Role of Antigen Receptor Gene Rearrangement Analysis

This laboratory has contributed significantly to the general understanding of the role of antigen receptor gene rearrangement analysis in the diagnosis and classification of hematopoietic neoplasia (3,15,17,18,23,24,27,46,57–59,61–64,67,89,90,174). Nonetheless, most hematopoietic neoplasms encountered in daily practice can be accurately diagnosed and classified on the basis of morphologic examination and immunophenotypic analysis alone. The routine application of this technology to lymphoma and leukemia samples is therefore unnecessary. This laboratory therefore reserves the performance of antigen receptor gene rearrangement analysis for diagnostic dilemmas unresolvable by morphologic and immunophenotypic analysis and those occasional situations where such analyses may provide additional useful information.

For example, some follicular lymphomas lack surface immunoglobulin (6,7,9), precluding the determination of B-cell clonality by light chain restriction. Follicular and diffuse B-cell lymphomas sometimes only partially involve lymphatic and extralymphatic tissues or are surrounded by a significant inflammatory response. In these instances, it may be impossible to demonstrate a monotypic surface immunoglobulin-positive cell population and thereby confirm the morphologic diagnosis of B-cell lymphoma. The demonstration of clonal immunoglobulin heavy and light chain gene rearrangements can be very helpful in confirming the diagnosis of B-cell lymphoma in all these situations. Small B-cell populations in small biopsies, for example in gastric biopsies, can occasionally be difficult to interpret based on morphologic and immunophenotypic analyses as to whether they represent a reactive or neoplastic process. This can be particularly challenging when the infiltrate is minimal as seen in cases where the patients are treated for gastric MALT lymphoma and the question is whether there is residual disease. For these cases, immunoglobulin gene rearrangement will be extremely helpful to determine B-cell clonality.

Unlike B cells, for which monotypic surface immunoglobulin can be used to infer clonality, no phenotypic markers of T-cell clonality exist. Thus, even with the benefit of immunophenotypic analysis, it is sometimes difficult to make a definitive diagnosis of peripheral T-cell lymphoma. Mature T-cell lymphomas frequently contain many reactive T cells, which may lead to difficult interpretations or ambiguous results by morphologic or immunophenotypic evaluations. Diagnosis of a subset of T-cell lymphomas, for example, Lennert lymphoma (lymphoepithelioid variant of peripheral T-cell lymphoma, not otherwise specified), can be challenging because of the potential masking by the prominent granulomatous proliferation and the absence of significant cytologic atypia and immunophenotypic aberrations in the T cells. Distinguishing between a reactive T-cell large granular lymphocytic population and a T-cell large granular lymphocytic leukemia can be problematic by morphology and immunophenotype alone, especially when the T cells do not show aberrant loss of T-cell antigens. The demonstration of clonal T-cell receptor gene rearrangements is extremely helpful in confirming the morphologic diagnosis of T-cell lymphoma and leukemia in these instances.

However, employing antigen receptor gene rearrangement analysis in the diagnosis of hematopoietic neoplasia is not without complication. First, clonal immunoglobulin and T-cell receptor gene rearrangements are not entirely lineage specific. Approximately 10% of B- and T-cell leukemias/lymphomas are bigenotypic (57), and rare T-cell malignancies have been reported to display clonal light chain gene rearrangements (220,221). Some AMLs exhibit clonal immunoglobulin and T-cell receptor gene rearrangements (61). Second, the demonstration of clonality does not necessarily indicate malignancy. Clonal immunoglobulin gene rearrangements have been demonstrated in hyperplastic lymph nodes from human immunodeficiency virus (HIV)-infected patients (23), in extranodal lymphoid hyperplasias (24,27,28), in the benign lymphoepithelial lesions of Sjögren syndrome (25,27), and in systemic Castleman disease (26). Clonal T-cell receptor gene rearrangements have been demonstrated in lymphomatoid papulosis (222,223) and in a variety of cutaneous lymphoproliferative disorders (174). Considerable caution should be exercised in interpreting the results of antigen receptor gene rearrangement analysis. This is discussed in Chapter 9.

ANALYSIS AND INTERPRETATION OF IMMUNOPHENOTYPIC DATA

The accurate morphologic evaluation of hematopoietic neoplasms ranges from easy to difficult, depending on the knowledge, expertise, and experience of the pathologist. The same holds true for the accurate immunophenotypic evaluation of hematopoietic neoplasms. Ideally, the person analyzing, interpreting, and reporting the results of immunophenotypic analysis should have knowledge of the clinical characteristics and be expert in the morphologic evaluation of hematopoietic neoplasia, as well as have considerable experience in performing immunophenotypic analysis and analyzing and interpreting the results. If such a person is not available to perform these diagnostic studies, two or more individuals possessing these skills in combination should coordinate the diagnostic activities.

In the late afternoon in our laboratory, the entire physician staff reviews the results of all cytofluorometric and immunohistochemical studies in conjunction with the clinical information, morphologic review of the histopathologic sections, and any other available information for difficult cases, and renders a definitive diagnosis or requests additional studies in each case under study. The correlative morphologic examination and immunophenotypic analysis of each specimen is usually completed within 48 hours, unless extensive additional studies are necessary.

The two most important factors to be considered in the analysis and interpretation of immunophenotypic data are the clinical characteristics of the patient and the results of morphologic evaluation of the pathologic specimen. Immunophenotypic data should always be interpreted in light of, and never reported without considering, this information. Failure to do so may result in erroneous conclusions with grave consequences for the patient.

In general, it is best to approach each case systematically, taking all the available information into consideration and asking yourself the critical questions as you proceed. First, the clinical characteristics of the patient and the results of other pertinent laboratory tests that have been performed should be reviewed. Based on this information, what is the most likely diagnosis? What are the other diagnostic possibilities? Second, the morphology of the histopathologic sections, peripheral blood, bone marrow smears, and other pathologic material should be carefully evaluated. Is a hematopoietic neoplasm present? If so, can it be definitively diagnosed and classified? If diagnosis and classification are not possible, what is the diagnostic dilemma—benign versus malignant, Hodgkin lymphoma versus non-Hodgkin lymphoma, B cell versus T cell, or lymphoid versus myeloid? Third, the Diff-Quik–stained cytocentrifuge slides prepared from the cell suspension or the Diff-Quik–stained frozen tissue sections should be reviewed. Are the cells or tissue present in these slide preparations the same as those in the histopathologic sections? In other words, are these preparations representative? What is the proportion of neoplastic cells or tissue in these preparations? Fourth, the immunophenotypic results should be reviewed. Do these results correlate with the histopathologic interpretation? If a hematopoietic neoplasm is present, does the immunophenotypic profile clearly indicate its lineage and classification? If the results do not correlate with the morphologic interpretation, why not? Is this because of technical problems encountered during immunophenotypic analysis? Is the initial morphologic interpretation incorrect? What additional studies can be performed to resolve this discrepancy? If the morphologic evaluation of the pathologic specimen did not lead to a definitive diagnosis, do the results of the immunophenotypic analysis resolve the diagnostic dilemma? Will the performance of additional studies provide additional important diagnostic or prognostic information? Does the final morphologic and immunophenotypic diagnosis in this case correlate with the clinical scenario? If so, a definitive diagnosis is rendered.

SUMMARY AND CONCLUSIONS

Multiple diagnostic dilemmas are commonly encountered in the routine diagnosis and classification of hematopoietic neoplasms. Immunophenotypic analysis is a useful adjunct to histopathology and can be of considerable assistance in resolving many of these diagnostic dilemmas. Immunophenotypic analysis can be performed on virtually any pathologic specimen using flow cytometric cell suspension or paraffin tissue section immunohistochemistry. Each of these methodologic approaches has distinct advantages and disadvantages. Utmost attention must be paid to all steps of the life history of the specimens. They need to be handled properly during transportation and upon arrival within the laboratory. It is

essential that tissue specimens are triaged in such a way as to ensure proper diagnosis but at the same time, that materials be procured for tumor banking. The cell suspensions have to be prepared with maximum viability and suitability for flow cytometric assessment. Tissues have to be fixed and processed adequately to allow proper morphologic evaluation and immunohistochemical analysis. Quality control is essential to maintain the functionality of reagents and equipment. Moreover, immunophenotypic analysis should be tailored to the nature of the pathologic specimen and individualized according to the particular diagnostic problem. Results of immunophenotypic analysis should always be correlated with the clinical findings and histopathologic examination of the pathologic specimen under analysis. In addition, the modern hematopathology laboratory, being a central source of neoplastic and non-neoplastic hematopoietic tissues in multiple forms (cell suspensions and tissue blocks), should be an integral contributor to tumor banking and an essential resource for translational research.

APPENDICES

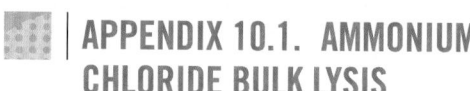

APPENDIX 10.1. AMMONIUM CHLORIDE BULK LYSIS

All samples should be processed under sterile conditions using aseptic techniques and reagents in a Sterilgard laminar flow hood (Baker Co., Sanford, ME).

1. Prepare working lysis solution by mixing 100 mL of Pharm Lyse (BD Biosciences) with 900 mL of distilled water. Working solution can be stored at room temperature.
2. Pour the bone marrow aspirate or peripheral blood samples into a 15- or 50-mL Falcon tube.
3. Add about 10 to 15 mL PBS. Rinse syringe or vacutainer with PBS and add to tube.
4. Spin for 5 minutes at 20,000 rpm.
5. Aspirate the supernatant. Add 10 mL of lysing agent for each milliliter of packed bone marrow or peripheral blood.
6. Vortex and incubate at room temperature for 10 minutes.
7. Spin for 5 minutes at 2,000 rpm. A white cell pellet should be seen at the bottom of the tube. Decant the supernatant and wash once.
8. Resuspend the cells in overnight solution and count the cells using a hemocytometer. Adjust the cell concentration to 5×10^6 cells/mL.

APPENDIX 10.2. DIFF-QUIK (MODIFIED WRIGHT-GIEMSA) STAIN OF CYTOCENTRIFUGE SLIDE PREPARATIONS, TOUCH PREPARATIONS, AND FROZEN TISSUE SECTIONS

Diff-Quik stain is a modification of Wright stain (Dade Diagnostics of P.R., Inc., Aguada, Puerto Rico).

1. Prepare cytocentrifuge slides, touch preparations, and frozen tissue sections.
2. Dip the slide in fixative solution five times, 1 second each time. Allow the excess to drain off.
3. Dip the slide in solution I five times, 1 second each time. Allow the excess to drain off.

4. Dip the slide in solution II five times, 1 second each time. Allow the excess to drain off.
5. Rinse the slide with distilled or deionized water.
6. Allow the slide to dry, dip in xylene, coverslip with Permount, and examine with a light microscope.

The intensity of staining can be changed by increasing or decreasing the number of dips in solutions I and II, but do not go below three dips of one full second each time.

APPENDIX 10.3. MANUAL CELL COUNTING AND VIABILITY ASSESSMENT

1. Clean a hemocytometer with alcohol before use.
2. Place a clean coverslip over the counting chamber of the hemocytometer.
3. Combine a 50 μL representative aliquot of the cell suspension with 50 μL of 0.4% Trypan blue dye (Gibco, Grand Island, NY) and allow to sit for 30 to 60 seconds.
4. Load one side of the hemocytometer with about 50 μL of a representative aliquot of the cell suspension (do not overfill).
5. Load the other side of the hemocytometer with about 50 μL of the cell suspension treated with Trypan blue dye (do not overfill).
6. Allow the cells to settle on the hemocytometer for 30 to 60 seconds before counting.
7. Place the loaded hemocytometer on the light microscope stage, focus on the counting chamber filled with non–Trypan blue dye-treated cells with the 10× objective, and then focus with the 40× objective.
8. Count all the leukocytes (excluding any contaminant erythrocytes) present in one row of five squares comprising one 4 × 4 grid. Multiply this number by 5 to obtain the total field count and then by 10^4 to obtain the cell count per milliliter.
9. Focus the 40× objective on the other side of the counting chamber containing the cells treated with Trypan blue dye. The clear cells are viable while the blue cells are dead. Count a total of 200 consecutive cells (clear and blue) and calculate the viability as follows: live (clear) cells/total of live (clear) and dead (blue) cells × 100 = percent (%) viability.
10. The number of viable cells per milliliter is calculated by multiplying the cell count/mL by the percent viability.

APPENDIX 10.4. FICOLL-HYPAQUE DENSITY GRADIENT CENTRIFUGATION

All samples should be processed under sterile conditions using aseptic techniques and reagents in a Sterilgard laminar flow hood (Baker Co., Sanford, ME).

1. Place 15 mL of room temperature Ficoll-Hypaque (Pharmacia, Piscataway, NJ) into a Falcon #2070 screw-cap 50-mL tube.
2. Hold the 50-mL tube at a 45-degree angle, and slowly but steadily overlay the Ficoll-Hypaque with up to 30 mL of the appropriately diluted sample using a 10- or 25-mL disposable serologic pipette.
3. Recap the tube and centrifuge at 1,900 rpm (400 g) in a Sorvall RC3B centrifuge for 30 minutes at room temperature without applying a brake.
4. After centrifugation, using a Pasteur pipette or a disposable transfer pipette, carefully remove the supernatant to within 1 cm above the mononuclear cell layer and discard.

5. Carefully remove the mononuclear cell layer with a Pasteur pipette and transfer the cells to a Falcon #2070 50-mL tube. Up to 30 mL of cell-rich fluid may be combined into each 50-mL tube. Be careful not to place the Pasteur pipette too far below the mononuclear cell layer because this draws in Ficoll and neutrophils.
6. Fill the tubes containing the harvested cells to 50 mL with PBS.
7. Discard the original tubes containing residual Ficoll and pellets composed of erythrocytes, dead cells, and debris.
8. Centrifuge the 50-mL tubes at 1,900 rpm in a Sorvall RC3B centrifuge for 10 minutes at room temperature. The brake may now be applied.
9. Decant the supernatant from each of the tubes, resuspend the cells in small volumes of PBS, combine the cells from each tube into one 50-mL tube, and fill the tube with PBS.
10. Centrifuge the cells at 1,100 rpm in a Sorvall RC3B centrifuge for 10 minutes at room temperature.
11. Decant the supernatant and resuspend the cells in RPMI 1640 containing 10% heat-inactivated fetal calf serum, 1% penicillin, and 1% streptomycin (overnight media).
12. Count the cells, assess their viability by Trypan blue dye exclusion (see Appendix 10.4), prepare Diff-Quik–stained cytocentrifuge slides for morphologic examination (see Appendix 10.3), and adjust the final concentration to 5 × 10^6 cells/mL.

In the case of smaller sample volumes, Falcon #2097 tubes may be filled with 4 mL of Ficoll-Hypaque and overlaid with 8 mL of sample. The second wash (step 10) may be eliminated to reduce cell loss if the cell pellet is observed to be very small after the first wash (step 8).

APPENDIX 10.5. IMMUNOHISTO-CHEMICAL STAINING OF PARAFFIN TISSUE SECTIONS

All immunohistochemical staining is performed using the Leica Bond III Automated Immunohistochemical System (Leica Biosystems, Germany).

Preparation of Paraffin Tissue Sections for Immunostaining

1. Cut paraffin tissue sections 4 μm thick and place onto Leica Gap Plus slides (Leica Biosystems, Germany).
2. Place the slides in a rack and bake in a 60°C oven for 35 minutes.
3. Remove the slides from the oven. The slides are ready to be placed in the fully automated BOND system for immunostaining or for manual staining, if necessary (see below).

Immunostaining of Paraffin Tissue Sections (Manual Procedure)

1. Deparaffinize the slides by placing them in a tub of xylene for 15 minutes. Then serially dunk slides 20 times in 100% ethanol, 20 times in 70% alcohol containing approximately 0.75 g of LiCO$_3$ and 20 times in 95% alcohol.
2. Place the slides in a mixture of 3 mL of 30% H_2O_2 in 200 mL of methanol for 10 minutes. Then transfer the slides into room-temperature distilled H_2O until antigen retrieval is performed. A variety of antigen retrieval methods are used depending on the antibody being employed. These include heating methods (i.e., microwave and pressure cooker techniques) and enzymatic digestion methods (i.e., trypsin and protease treatments).

3. After the antigen retrieval process is completed, cool off by running tap water.
4. Rinse in water three times.
5. Quench endogenous peroxidase in Dako Dual Endogenous Enzyme Block (Dako, Cat# S2003) for 5 minutes.
6. Apply 200 μL per slide of primary antibody and incubate in humidified incubation chamber for 40 minutes.
7. Rinse with PBS.
8. Apply 200 μL per slide of appropriate secondary antibody and incubate in humidified incubation chamber for 30 minutes.
9. Make DAB solution while secondary antibody is incubating.
10. Rinse with ITBS.
11. Place 200 μL of freshly prepared DAB solution for 15 minutes in humidified incubation chamber.
12. Rinse slides with tap water.
13. Counterstain with hematoxylin for 2 minutes.
14. Rinse with tap water.
15. Place in ammonia-water for 1 minutes.
16. Rinse with tap water.
17. Place in 95% alcohol for 2 minutes.
18. Dehydrate in 100% alcohol for 2 minutes. Repeat.
19. Mount in Cytoseal XYL (Richard-Allan Scientific, Cat# 8312-4)

TBS is 10 L of distilled H_2O, 80 g of NaCl, 6.05 g of Tris (hydroxymethyl) aminomethane (Sigma, St. Louis, MO). Adjust the pH to 7.4 with 40 mL of 1 N HCl.

 ## APPENDIX 10.6. CELL CRYOPRESERVATION USING METHANOL FREEZING METHOD

Freezing Solution

1. Slowly add (drop by drop) one volume of dimethyl sulfoxide (DMSO) to nine volumes of heat-inactivated fetal bovine serum (FBS). For example, add 5 mL of DMSO to 45 mL of FBS.
2. Filter the solution through a 0.22-μm syringe or bottle transfer system and then transfer the filtered solution to a Falcon #2070 screw-cap 50-mL tube. This freezing solution can be used fresh or stored at –20°C for up to 2 weeks for later use.

Freezing Procedure

1. Determine the total number of cells to be cryopreserved; this determines the total number of vials and the cell concentration per vial. The best cell viability is achieved when the number of cells per vial lies in the range of 20 to 50 × 10^6 cells.
2. Write the patient's name, freeze number, specimen, and number of cells on each 1.8-mL cryotube (Nunc #368632).
3. Prepare fresh freezing solution, or thaw previously prepared freezing solution in a 37°C water bath. Determine the total number of vials to be cryopreserved and the total volume of freezing solution needed; 1.5 mL of freezing solution is required for each vial to be frozen. Place the freezing solution on ice until ready to use.
4. Pellet the cells by centrifugation at 1,500 rpm in a Sorvall RT 6000 centrifuge for 10 minutes at 4°C and decant the supernatant.
5. Remove the caps from the vials carefully under sterile conditions and place them into a sterile Petri dish screw side down.
6. With a serologic pipette, add the calculated volume of cold freezing solution to the pellet. Resuspend the cells well.

Carefully distribute the suspended cells among the vials (1.5 mL per vial) using a serologic pipette and place immediately on ice. Recap the vials and transfer quickly to a Styrofoam container. Cover with another Styrofoam container and tape in place to create a protected environment. Store at –80°C for 24 hours and then transfer to a liquid nitrogen storage tank (–170°C). Note the location of the vials in the cell cryopreservation log.

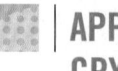 ## APPENDIX 10.7. RECONSTITUTING CRYOPRESERVED CELLS

Thawing media consists of RPMI 1640 and 20% fetal calf serum.

1. Place 30 mL of thawing media in a Falcon #2070 screw-cap 50-mL tube labeled with the patient's name.
2. Remove a vial of cryopreserved cells from the liquid nitrogen storage tank and thaw quickly by immersion in a 37°C water bath.
3. After the vial of cells is thawed, carefully open the vial under sterile conditions. Using a sterile transfer pipette, carefully add 100 to 200 μL of thawing media and gently resuspend the cells.
4. Transfer 0.5 mL of suspended cells to the Falcon tube containing the thawing media. Repeat this procedure until all the cells in the vial have been transferred to the Falcon tube.
5. Centrifuge the cells at 600 rpm in a Sorvall RT6000 centrifuge for 10 minutes at 4°C.
6. Decant the supernatant, and resuspend the cells in thawing media to a final concentration of 5 × 10^6 cells/mL.
7. Assess the viability of the cells by Trypan blue dye exclusion (see Appendix 10.3).

References

1. Jaffe ES, Strauchen JA, Berard CW. Predictability of immunologic phenotype by morphologic criteria in diffuse aggressive non-Hodgkin's lymphomas. *Am J Clin Pathol* 1982;77:46–49.
2. Wood GS, Burke JS, Horning S, et al. The immunologic and clinicopathologic heterogeneity of cutaneous lymphomas other than mycosis fungoides. *Blood* 1983; 62:464–472.
3. Knowles DM, Dodson LG, Burke JS, et al. SIg⁻ E⁻ ("null cell") non-Hodgkin's lymphomas: multiparametric determination of their B- or T-cell lineage. *Am J Pathol* 1985;120:356–370.
4. Chan LC, Pegram SM, Greaves MF. Contribution of immunophenotype to the classification and differential diagnosis of acute leukaemia. *Lancet* 1985;1:475–479.
5. Krause JR, Penchansky L, Contis L, et al. Flow cytometry in the diagnosis of acute leukemia. *Am J Clin Pathol* 1988;89:341–346.
6. Knowles DM. Lymphoid cell markers: their distribution and usefulness in the immunophenotypic analysis of lymphoid neoplasms. *Am J Surg Pathol* 1985; 9(Suppl):85–108.
7. Foon KA, Todd RF. Immunologic classification of leukemia and lymphoma. *Blood* 1986;68:1–31.
8. Picker LJ, Weiss LM, Medeiros JL, et al. Immunophenotypic criteria for the diagnosis of non-Hodgkin's lymphoma. *Am J Pathol* 1987;128:181–201.
9. Freedman AS, Nadler LM. Cell surface markers in hematologic malignancies. *Semin Oncol* 1987;14:193–212.
10. Deegan MJ. Membrane antigen analysis in the diagnosis of lymphoid leukemias and lymphomas. *Arch Pathol Lab Med* 1989;113:606–618.
11. Craig FE, Foon KA. Flow cytometric immunophenotyping for hematologic neoplasms. *Blood* 2008;111(8):3941–3967.
12. Korsmeyer SJ, Arnold A, Bakhshi A, et al. Immunoglobulin gene rearrangement and cell surface antigen expression in acute lymphocytic leukemias of T-cell and B-cell precursor origins. *J Clin Invest* 1983;71:301–313.
13. Arnold A, Cossman J, Bakhski A, et al. Immunoglobulin gene rearrangements as unique clonal markers in human lymphoid neoplasms. *N Engl J Med* 1983; 309:1593–1599.
14. Cleary ML, Chao J, Warnke R, et al. Immunoglobulin gene rearrangement as a diagnostic criterion of B-cell lymphoma. *Proc Natl Acad Sci U S A* 1984;81: 593–597.
15. Flug F, Pelicci PG, Bonetti F, et al. T cell receptor gene rearrangements as markers of lineage and clonality in T cell neoplasms. *Proc Natl Acad Sci U S A* 1985; 82:3460–3464.
16. Waldmann TA, Davis MM, Bongiovanni KF, et al. Rearrangements of gene for the antigen receptor on T cells as markers of lineage and clonality in human lymphoid neoplasms. *N Engl J Med* 1985;313:776–783.
17. Rambaldi A, Pelicci PG, Allavena P, et al. T cell receptor β chain gene rearrangements in lymphoproliferative disorders of large granular lymphocytes/natural killer cells. *J Exp Med* 1985;162:2156–2162.

18. Knowles DM, Neri A, Pelicci PG, et al. Immunoglobulin and T cell receptor beta chain gene rearrangement analysis of Hodgkin's disease: implications for lineage determination and differential diagnosis. *Proc Natl Acad Sci U S A* 1986; 83:7942–7946.
19. Bruggemann M, White H, Gaulard P, et al. Powerful strategy for polymerase chain reaction-based clonality assessment in T-cell malignancies report of the BIOMED-2 Concerted Action BHM4 CT98-3936. *Leukemia* 2007;21(2):215–221.
20. Evans PA, Pott C, Groenen PJ, et al. Significantly improved PCR-based clonality testing in B-cell malignancies by use of multiple immunoglobulin gene targets. Report of the BIOMED-2 Concerted Action BHM4-CT98-3936. *Leukemia* 2007; 21(2):207–214.
21. Langerak AW, Molina TJ, Lavender FL, et al. Polymerase chain reaction-based clonality testing in tissue samples with reactive lymphoproliferations: usefulness and pitfalls. A report of the BIOMED-2 Concerted Action BMH4-CT98-3936. *Leukemia* 2007;21(2):222–229.
22. van Krieken JH, Langerak AW, Macintyre EA, et al. Improved reliability of lymphoma diagnostics via PCR-based clonality testing: report of the BIOMED-2 Concerted Action BHM4-CT98-3936. *Leukemia* 2007;21(2):201–206.
23. Pelicci PG, Knowles DM, Arlin Z, et al. Multiple monoclonal B cell expansions and c-myc oncogene rearrangements in acquired immune deficiency syndrome-related lymphoproliferative disorders: implications for lymphomagenesis. *J Exp Med* 1986;164:2049–2060.
24. Neri A, Jakobiec FA, Pelicci PG, et al. Immunoglobulin and T cell receptor β chain gene rearrangement analysis of ocular adnexal lymphoid neoplasms: clinical and biologic implications. *Blood* 1987;70:1519–1529.
25. Fishleder A, Tubbs R, Hessie B, et al. Uniform detection of immunoglobulin gene rearrangement in benign lymphoepithelial lesions. *N Engl J Med* 1987;316: 1118–1121.
26. Hanson CA, Frizzera G, Patton DF, et al. Clonal rearrangement of immunoglobulin and T-cell receptor genes in systemic Castleman's disease: association with Epstein-Barr virus. *Am J Pathol* 1988;131:84–91.
27. Knowles DM, Athan E, Ubriaco A, et al. Extranodal noncutaneous lymphoid hyperplasias represent a continuous spectrum of B-cell neoplasia: demonstration by molecular genetic analysis. *Blood* 1989;73:1635–1645.
28. Wood GS, Ngan BY, Tung R, et al. Clonal rearrangements of immunoglobulin genes and progression to B cell lymphoma in cutaneous lymphoid hyperplasia. *Am J Pathol* 1989;135:13–19.
29. Foucar K, Chen IM, Crago S. Organization and operation of a flow cytometric immunophenotyping laboratory. *Semin Diagn Pathol* 1989;6:13–36.
30. Knowles DM, Tolidjian B, Marboe CC, et al. A new human B lymphocyte surface antigen (BL2) detectable by a hybridoma monoclonal antibody: distribution on benign and malignant lymphoid cells. *Blood* 1983;62:191–198.
31. Knowles DM, Tolidjian B, Marboe CC, et al. Distribution of antigens defined by OKB monoclonal antibodies on benign and malignant lymphoid cells and non-lymphoid tissues. *Blood* 1984;63:886–896.
32. Wang CY, Azzo W, Al-Katib A, et al. Preparation and characterization of monoclonal antibodies recognizing three distinct differentiation antigens (BL1, BL2, BL3) on human B lymphocytes. *J Immunol* 1984;133:684–691.
33. Peng R, Al-Katib A, Knowles DM, et al. Preparation and characterization of monoclonal antibodies recognizing two distinct differentiation antigens (Pro-Im1, Pro-Im2) on early hematopoietic cells. *Blood* 1984;64:1169–1178.
34. Knowles DM, Tolidjian B, Marboe CC, et al. Monoclonal anti-human monocyte antibodies OKM1 and OKM5 possess distinctive tissue distributions including differential reactivity with vascular endothelium. *J Immunol* 1984;132:2170–2173.
35. Posnett DN, Marboe CC, Knowles DM, et al. A membrane antigen (HC1) selectively present on hairy cell leukemia cells, endothelial cells and epidermal basal cells. *J Immunol* 1984;132:2700–2702.
36. Knowles DM, Halper JP, Azzo W, et al. The expression and distribution of Leu1 on benign and malignant human lymphoid cells: correlation with conventional cell markers and with monoclonal antibody OKT1. *Cancer* 1983;52:1369–1377.
37. Chadburn A, Inghirami G, Knowles DM. Hairy cell leukemia-associated antigen LeuM5 (CD11c) is preferentially expressed by benign activated and neoplastic CD8 T cells. *Am J Pathol* 1990;136:29–37.
38. Friedman SM, Thompson G, Halper JP, et al. OT-CLL: a human chronic lymphocytic leukemia that produces IL2 in high titer. *J Immunol* 1982;128:935–940.
39. Bonetti F, Knowles DM, Chilosi M, et al. A distinctive cutaneous malignant neoplasm expressing the Langerhans cell phenotype: synchronous occurrence with B-chronic lymphocytic leukemia. *Cancer* 1985;55:2417–2425.
40. Wieczorek R, Greco MA, McCarthy K, et al. Familial erythrophagocytic lymphohistiocytosis: immunophenotypic, immunohistochemical and ultrastructural demonstration of its relationship to sinus histiocytes. *Hum Pathol* 1986;17: 55–63.
41. Wieczorek R, Suhrland M, Ramsay D, et al. LeuM1 antigen expression in advanced (tumor) stage mycosis fungoides. *Am J Clin Pathol* 1986;86:25–32.
42. Bonetti F, Chilosi M, Menestrina F, et al. Immunohistological analysis of Rosai-Dorfman histiocytosis: a disease of S-100$^+$ CD1$^-$ histiocytes. *Virchows Arch A* 1987;411:129–135.
43. Franchino C, Reich C, Distenfeld A, et al. A clinicopathologically distinctive primary splenic histiocytic neoplasm: demonstration of its histiocytic derivation by immunophenotypic and molecular genetic analysis. *Am J Surg Pathol* 1988;12: 398–404.
44. Thomas FP, Vallejos U, Foitl DR, et al. B-cell small lymphocytic lymphoma and chronic lymphocytic leukemia with peripheral neuropathy; two cases with neuropathological findings and lymphocyte marker analysis. *Acta Neuropathol* 1990;80:198–203.
45. Wisniewski T, Sisti M, Inghirami G, et al. Intracerebral solitary plasmacytoma. *Neurosurgery* 1990;27:826–829.
46. Gold JE, Louis-Charles A, Ghali V, et al. T-cell chronic lymphocytic leukemia with unusual morphologic, phenotypic, and karyotypic features in association with light-chain amyloidosis. *Cancer* 1992;70:86–93.
47. Knowles DM, Halper JP. Human T cell malignancies: correlative clinical, histopathologic, immunologic and cytochemical analysis of 23 cases. *Am J Pathol* 1982;106: 197–203.
48. Wieczorek R, Burke JS, Knowles DM. Leu M1 antigen expression in T cell neoplasia. *Am J Pathol* 1985;121:374–380.
49. Flug F, Dodson L, Wolff J, et al. B lymphocyte associated differentiation antigen expression by "non-B, non-T" acute lymphoblastic leukemia. *Leuk Res* 1985;9: 1051–1058.
50. McNally L, Jakobiec FA, Knowles DM. Clinical, morphologic, immunophenotypic and molecular genetic analysis of bilateral ocular adnexal lymphoid neoplasms: clinical and biological implications. *Am J Ophthalmol* 1987;103:555–568.
51. Inghirami G, Wieczorek R, Zhu BY, et al. Differential expression of LFA-1 molecules in non-Hodgkin's lymphoma and lymphoid leukemia. *Blood* 1988; 72:1431–1434.
52. Knowles DM, Chamulak G, Subar M, et al. Clinicopathologic, immunophenotypic and molecular genetic analysis of AIDS-associated lymphoid neoplasia: clinical and biological implications. *Pathol Ann* 1988;23:33–67.
53. Knowles DM, Chamulak GA, Subar M, et al. Lymphoid neoplasia associated with AIDS: the New York University Medical Center experience with 105 cases (1981–1986). *Ann Intern Med* 1988;108:744–753.
54. Knowles DM, Jakobiec FA, McNally L, et al. Lymphoid hyperplasia and malignant lymphoma occurring in the ocular adnexa (orbit, conjunctiva, and eyelids): a prospective multiparametric analysis of 108 cases during 1977–1987. *Hum Pathol* 1990;21:959–973.
55. Inghirami G, Lederman S, Yellin MJ, et al. Phenotypic and functional characterization of T-BAM (CD40 ligand) positive T cell non-Hodgkin's lymphomas. *Blood* 1994;84:866–872.
56. Yang C, Lu P, Lee FY, et al. Tyrosine kinase inhibition in diffuse large B-cell lymphoma: molecular basis for antitumor activity and drug resistance of dasatinib. *Leukemia* 2008;22(9):1755–1766.
57. Pelicci PG, Knowles DM, Dalla-Favera R. Lymphoid tumors displaying rearrangements of both immunoglobulin and T-cell receptor genes. *J Exp Med* 1985;162:1015–1024.
58. Foa R, Migone N, Lauria F, et al. Analysis of T-cell receptor gene rearrangements demonstrates the monoclonal nature of T-cell chronic lymphoproliferative disorders. *Blood* 1986;67:247–250.
59. Knowles DM, Pelicci PG, Dalla-Favera R. T-cell receptor beta chain gene rearrangements: genetic markers of T cell lineage and clonality. *Hum Pathol* 1986; 17:546–551.
60. Pelicci PG, Knowles DM, Magrath I, et al. Chromosomal breakpoints and structural alterations of the c-myc locus differ in endemic and sporadic forms of Burkitt lymphoma. *Proc Natl Acad Sci U S A* 1986;83:2984–2988.
61. Seremetis SV, Pelicci PG, Tabilio A, et al. High frequency of clonal immunoglobulin or T-cell receptor gene rearrangements in the subset of acute myelogenous leukemia expressing terminal deoxynucleotidyl transferase. *J Exp Med* 1987;165: 1703–1712.
62. Pelicci P, Allavena P, Alessandro R, et al. T-cell receptor (α, β, γ) gene rearrangements and expression distinguish large granular lymphocyte/natural killer cells. *Blood* 1987;70:1500–1508.
63. Subar M, Pelicci PG, Neri A, et al. T-gamma gene rearrangements: different patterns in T- and B-cell neoplasms. *Leukemia* 1988;2:19–26.
64. Neri A, Knowles DM, Magrath IT, et al. Different regions of the immunoglobulin heavy chain locus are involved in chromosomal translocations in endemic and sporadic forms of Burkitt lymphoma. *Proc Natl Acad Sci U S A* 1988;85: 2748–2752.
65. Subar M, Neri A, Inghirami G, et al. Frequent c-myc oncogene activation and infrequent presence of Epstein-Barr virus genome in AIDS-associated lymphoma. *Blood* 1988;7:667–671.
66. Neri A, Knowles DM, McCormick F, et al. Analysis of RAS oncogene in human lymphoid malignancies. *Proc Natl Acad Sci U S A* 1988;85:9268–9272.
67. Knowles DM, Inghirami G, Ubriaco A, et al. Molecular genetic analysis of three AIDS-associated neoplasms of uncertain lineage demonstrates their B-cell derivation and the possible pathogenetic role of the Epstein-Barr virus. *Blood* 1989; 73:792–799.
68. Logtenberg T, Schutte MEM, Inghirami G, et al. Immunoglobulin V_H gene expression in human B cell lines and tumors: biased V_H gene expression in chronic lymphocytic leukemia. *Int Immunol* 1989;1:362–366.
69. Neri A, Barriga F, Inghirami G, et al. Epstein-Barr virus infection precedes clonal expansion in Burkitt's and AIDS-associated lymphoma. *Blood* 1991;77: 1092–1095.
70. Athan E, Foitl DR, Knowles DM. Bcl-1 gene rearrangement: frequency and clinical significance among B cell chronic lymphocytic leukemias and non-Hodgkin's lymphomas. *Am J Pathol* 1991;138:591–597.
71. Gaidano G, Ballerini P, Gong JZ, et al. P53 mutations in human lymphoid malignancies: association with Burkitt's lymphoma and chronic lymphocytic leukemia. *Proc Natl Acad Sci U S A* 1991;88:5413–5417.
72. Berman JE, Nickerson KG, Pollock RR, et al. V_H gene usage in humans: biased usage of the V_H6 gene in immature B lymphoid cells. *Eur J Immunol* 1991;21: 1311–1314.
73. Athan E, Chadburn A, Knowles DM. The bcl-2 gene translocation is undetectable in Hodgkin's disease by Southern blot hybridization and polymerase chain reaction. *Am J Pathol* 1992;141:193–201.
74. Gaidano G, Hauptschein RS, Parsar NZ, et al. Deletions involving two distinct regions of 6q in B-cell non-Hodgkin lymphoma. *Blood* 1992;80:1781–1787.
75. Cesarman E, Chadburn A, Inghirami G, et al. Structural and functional analysis of oncogenes and tumor suppressor genes in adult T-cell leukemia/lymphoma (ATLL) reveals frequent p53 mutations. *Blood* 1992;80:3205–3216.
76. Gaidano G, Parsa NZ, Tassi V, et al. In vitro establishment of AIDS-related lymphoma cell lines: phenotypic characterization, oncogene and tumor suppressor gene lesions, an heterogeneity in Epstein-Barr virus infection. *Leukemia* 1993;7: 1621–1629.
77. Cesarman E, Inghirami G, Chadburn A, et al. High levels of p53 protein expression do not correlate with p53 gene mutations in anaplastic large cell lymphoma. *Am J Pathol* 1993;143:1–12.
78. Ballerini P, Gaidano G, Gong JZ, et al. Multiple genetic lesions in AIDS-related non-Hodgkin lymphoma. *Blood* 1993;81:166–176.
79. Ye BH, Lista F, LoCoco F, et al. Alterations of a zinc-finger encoding gene, BCL-6, in diffuse large cell lymphoma. *Science* 1993;262:747–750.
80. Corradini P, Ladetto M, Voena C, et al. Mutational activation of N- and K-ras oncogenes in plasma cell dyscrasias. *Blood* 1993;81:2708–2714.
81. Cesarman E, Liu YF, Knowles DM. The MDM2 oncogene is rarely amplified in human lymphoid tumors and does not correlate with p53 gene expression [Letter]. *Int J Cancer* 1994;56:457–458.
82. Matsushima AY, Cesarman E, Chadburn A, et al. Post-thymic T cell lymphomas frequently overexpress p53 protein but infrequently exhibit p53 gene mutations. *Am J Pathol* 1994;144:573–584.

83. Gaidano G, Lo Coco F, Ye BH, et al. Rearrangements of the BCL-6 gene in AIDS-associated non-Hodgkin's lymphoma: association with diffuse large-cell subtype. *Blood* 1994;84:397–402.
84. Matolcsy A, Inghirami G, Knowles DM. Molecular genetic demonstration of the diverse evolution of Richter's syndrome (chronic lymphocytic leukemia and subsequent large cell lymphoma). *Blood* 1994;83:1363–1372.
85. Lo Coco F, Ye BH, Lista F, et al. Rearrangements of the BCL6 gene in diffuse large-cell non Hodgkin's lymphoma. *Blood* 1994;83:1757–1759.
86. Riboldi P, Gaidano G, Schettino EW, et al. Two AIDS-associated Burkitt's lymphomas produce specific anti-i IgM cold agglutinins utilizing somatically mutated V_H4-21 segments. *Blood* 1994;83:2952–2961.
87. Inghirami G, Macri L, Cesarman E, et al. Molecular characterization of CD30 positive anaplastic large cell lymphoma: high frequency of c-myc proto-oncogene activation. *Blood* 1994;83:3581–3590.
88. Corradini P, Inghirami G, Astolfi M, et al. Inactivation of tumor suppressor genes, p53 and RB1, in plasma cell dyscrasias. *Leukemia* 1994;8:758–767.
89. Knowles DM, Cesarman E, Chadburn A, et al. Correlative morphologic and molecular genetic analysis demonstrates three distinct categories of post-transplantation lymphoproliferative disorders. *Blood* 1995;85:552–565.
90. Chadburn A, Cesarman E, Liu YF, et al. Molecular genetic analysis demonstrates that multiple post-transplantation lymphoproliferative disorders occurring in one anatomic site in a single patient represent distinct primary lymphoid neoplasms. *Cancer* 1995;75:2747–2756.
91. Matolcsy A, Chadburn A, Knowles DM. De novo CD5 positive and Richter's syndrome associated diffuse large B cell lymphomas are genotypically distinct. *Am J Pathol* 1995;147:207–216.
92. Chadburn A, Suciu-Foca N, Cesarman E, et al. Post-transplantation lymphoproliferative disorders (PT-LPDs) arising in solid organ transplant recipients are usually of recipient origin. *Am J Pathol* 1995;174:1862–1870.
93. Matolcsy A, Casali P, Knowles DM. Different clonal origin of B cell populations of chronic lymphocytic leukemia and large cell lymphoma in Richter's syndrome. *Ann N Y Acad Sci* 1995;764:496–503.
94. Migliazza A, Martinotti S, Chen W, et al. Frequent somatic hypermutation of the 5′ non-coding region of the BCL6 gene in B cell lymphoma. *Proc Natl Acad Sci U S A* 1995;92:12520–12524.
95. Tsang P, Cesarman E, Chadburn A, et al. Molecular characterization of primary mediastinal B cell lymphoma. *Am J Pathol* 1996;148:2017–2025.
96. Gamberi B, Gaidano G, Parsa N, et al. Microsatellite instability is rare in B-cell non-Hodgkin's lymphomas. *Blood* 1997;89:975–979.
97. Matolcsy A, Casali P, Liu Y, et al. Molecular characterization of IgA- and/or IgG-switched chronic lymphocytic leukemia B cells. *Blood* 1997;89:1732–1739.
98. Matolcsy A, Warnke RA, Knowles DM. Somatic mutations of the translocated bcl-2 gene are associated with morphologic transformation of follicular lymphoma to diffuse large cell lymphoma. *Ann Oncol* 1997;8(Suppl 2):119–122.
99. Horenstein MG, Nador RG, Chadburn A, et al. Epstein-Barr virus latent gene expression in primary effusion lymphomas containing Kaposi's sarcoma-associated herpesvirus/human herpesvirus-8. *Blood* 1997;90:1186–1191.
100. Scheinfeld AG, Nador RG, Cesarman E, et al. Epstein-Barr virus latent membrane protein-1 oncogene deletion in post-transplantation lymphoproliferative disorders. *Am J Pathol* 1997;151:805–812.
101. Chiu A, Pan L, Li Z, et al. DNA polymerase mu gene expression in B-cell non-Hodgkin's lymphomas: an analysis utilizing in situ hybridization. *Am J Pathol* 2002;161(4):1349–1355.
102. Li Z, Pan L, Cesarman E, et al. Alterations of mRNA splicing in primary effusion lymphomas. *Leuk Lymphoma* 2003;44(5):833–840.
103. Nador RG, Chadburn A, Gundappa G, et al. Human immunodeficiency virus (HIV)-associated polymorphic lymphoproliferative disorders. *Am J Surg Pathol* 2003;27(3):293–302.
104. Chadburn A, Hyjek E, Mathew S, et al. KSHV-positive solid lymphomas represent an extra-cavitary variant of primary effusion lymphoma. *Am J Surg Pathol* 2004; 28(11):1401–1416.
105. Fan W, Bubman D, Chadburn A, et al. Distinct subsets of primary effusion lymphoma can be identified based on their cellular gene expression profile and viral association. *J Virol* 2005;79(2):1244–1251.
106. Tam W, Gomez M, Chadburn A, et al. Mutational analysis of PRDM1 indicates a tumor-suppressor role in diffuse large B-cell lymphomas. *Blood* 2006; 107(10):4090–4100.
107. Czuchlewski DR, Csernus B, Bubman D, et al. Expression of the follicular lymphoma variant translocation 1 gene in diffuse large B-cell lymphoma correlates with subtype and clinical outcome. *Am J Clin Pathol* 2008;130(6):957–962.
108. Nie K, Zhang T, Allawi H, et al. Epigenetic down-regulation of the tumor suppressor gene PRDM1/Blimp-1 in diffuse large b cell lymphomas a potential role of the microRNA Let-7. *Am J Pathol* 2010;177(3):1470–1479.
109. Inghirami G, Chilosi M, Knowles DM. Western thymomas lack Epstein-Barr virus by Southern blotting analysis and by polymerase chain reaction. *Am J Pathol* 1990; 136:1429–1436.
110. Chadburn A, Athan E, Wieczorek R, et al. Detection and characterization of HTLV-I associated T cell neoplasms in an HTLV-I non-endemic region by polymerase chain reaction. *Blood* 1991;77:2419–2430.
111. Frank D, Cesarman E, Liu YF, et al. Post-transplantation lymphoproliferative disorders frequently contain type A and not type B Epstein-Barr virus. *Blood* 1995; 85:1396–1403.
112. Chang Y, Cesarman E, Pessin MS, et al. Kaposi's sarcoma-associated DNA sequences of nonhuman origin: evidence for a new human herpes virus. *Science* 1994;266:1865–1869.
113. Cesarman E, Chang Y, Moore PS, et al. Kaposi's sarcoma-associated herpesvirus-like DNA sequences in AIDS-related body-cavity based lymphomas. *N Engl J Med* 1995;332:1186–1191.
114. Nador RG, Cesarman E, Chadburn A, et al. Primary effusion lymphoma: a distinct clinicopathologic entity associated with the Kaposi's sarcoma-associated herpesvirus. *Blood* 1996;88:645–656.
115. Swerdlow SH, Campo E, Harris NL, et al., eds. *WHO classification of tumors of haematopoietic and lymphoid tissues*. Lyon: IARC, 2008.
116. Gahmberg CG, Jokinen M, Andersson LC. Expression of the major sialoglycoprotein (glycophorin) on erythroid cells in human bone marrow. *Blood* 1978; 52:379–387.
117. Robinson J, Sieff C, Delia D, et al. Expression of cell-surface HLA-DR, HLA-ABC and glycophorin during erythroid differentiation. *Nature* 1981;289:68–71.
118. Greaves MF, Sieff C, Edwards PAW. Monoclonal antiglycophorin as a probe for erythroleukemias. *Blood* 1983;61:645–651.
119. Warnke RA, Gatter KC, Falini B, et al. Diagnosis of human lymphoma with monoclonal antileukocyte antibodies. *N Engl J Med* 1983;309:1275–1281.
120. Civin CI, Strauss IC, Brovall C, et al. Antigenic analysis of hematopoiesis. III. A hematopoietic progenitor cell surface antigen defined by a monoclonal antibody raised against KG la cells. *J Immunol* 1984;133:157–165.
121. Pinkus GS, Thomas P, Said J. Leu M1—a marker for Reed-Sternberg cells in Hodgkin's disease. *Am J Pathol* 1985;119:244–252.
122. Sheibani K, Battifora H, Burke JS, et al. Leu-M1 antigen in human neoplasms: an immunohistologic study of 400 cases. *Am J Surg Pathol* 1986;10:227–236.
123. Banks L, Matlashewski G, Crawford L. Isolation of human p53-specific monoclonal antibodies and their use in the studies of human p53 expression. *Eur J Biochem* 1986;159:529–534.
124. Andrews RG, Singer JW, Bernstein ID. Monoclonal antibody 12-8 recognizes a 115-kd molecule present on both unipotent and multipotent hematopoietic colony-forming cells. *Blood* 1986;67:842–845.
125. Norton AJ, Ramsay AD, Smith SA, et al. Monoclonal antibody (UCHL1) that recognizes normal and neoplastic T cells in routinely fixed tissues. *J Clin Pathol* 1986; 39:399–405.
126. Brenner MB, McLean J, Scheft H, et al. Characterization and expression of the human $\alpha\beta$ T cell receptor using a framework monoclonal antibody. *Immunology* 1987;138:1502–1509.
127. Linder J, Ye Y, Harrington DS, et al. Monoclonal antibodies marking T lymphocytes in paraffin-embedded tissue. *Am J Pathol* 1987;127:1–8.
128. Cartun RW, Coles FB, Pastuszak WT. Utilization of monoclonal antibody L26 in the identification and confirmation of B-cell lymphomas: a sensitive and specific marker applicable to formalin and B5-fixed, paraffin-embedded tissues. *Am J Pathol* 1987;129:415–421.
129. Dobson CM, Myskow MW, Krajewski AS, et al. Immunohistochemical staining of non-Hodgkin's lymphoma in paraffin sections using the MB1 and MT1 monoclonal antibodies. *J Pathol* 1987;153:203–212.
130. Hall PA, Lindeman R, Butler MG, et al. Demonstration of lymphoid antigens in decalcified bone marrow trephines. *J Clin Pathol* 1987;40:870–873.
131. Norton AJ, Isaacson PG. Monoclonal antibodies (MT1, MT2, MB1, MB2, MB3) reactive with leukocyte subsets in paraffin embedded tissue sections. *Am J Pathol* 1987; 127:418–429.
132. Schwarting R, Gerdes J, Stein H. Ber H-2: a new monoclonal antibody of the Ki-1 family for the detection of Hodgkin's disease in formaldehyde fixed tissue. In: McMichael AJ, Beverley PCL, Cobbold S, et al., eds. *Leucocyte typing, III. White cell differentiation antigens.* Oxford: Oxford University Press, 1987:574–575.
133. Band H, Hochstenbach F, McLean J, et al. Immunochemical proof that a novel rearranging gene encodes the T cell receptor δ subunit. *Science* 1987;238: 682–684.
134. Chittal SM, Caveriviere P, Schwarting R, et al. Monoclonal antibodies in the diagnosis of Hodgkin's disease: the search for a rational panel. *Am J Surg Pathol* 1988; 12:9–21.
135. Pinkus GS, Said JW. Hodgkin's disease, lymphocyte predominance type, nodular. Further evidence for a B cell derivation: L & H variants of Reed-Sternberg cells express L26, a pan B cell marker. *Am J Pathol* 1988;133:211–217.
136. Pallesen G, Hamilton-Dutoit SJ. Ki-1 (CD30) antigen is regularly expressed by tumor cells of embryonal carcinoma. *Am J Pathol* 1988;133:446–450.
137. Ng CS, Chan JKC, Hui PK, et al. Monoclonal antibodies reactive with normal and neoplastic T cells in paraffin sections. *Hum Pathol* 1988;19:295–303.
138. Wieczorek R, Buck D, Bindl J, et al. Monoclonal antibody Leu-22 (L60) permits the demonstration of some neoplastic T cells in routinely fixed and paraffin-embedded tissue sections. *Hum Pathol* 1988;19:1434–1443.
139. Mason DY, Krissansen GW, Davey FR, et al. Antisera against epitopes resistant to denaturation on T3 (CD3) antigen can detect reactive and neoplastic T cells in paraffin embedded tissue biopsy specimens. *J Clin Pathol* 1988;41:121–127.
140. Borst J, van Dongen JJM, Bolhuis RLH, et al. Distinct molecular forms of human T cell receptor γ/δ detected on viable T cells by a monoclonal antibody. *J Exp Med* 1988;167:1625–1644.
141. Pulford K, Rigney E, Jones M, et al. KP1 (CD68)—a new monoclonal antibody detecting a monocyte/macrophage associated antigen in routinely processed tissue sections. *J Clin Pathol* 1989;42:414–421.
142. Mason DY, Cordell J, Brown M, et al. Detection of T cells in paraffin wax embedded tissue using antibodies against a peptide sequence from the CD3 antigen. *J Clin Pathol* 1989;42:1194–1200.
143. Ngan BY, Picker LJ, Medeiros J, et al. Immunophenotypic diagnosis of non-Hodgkin's lymphoma in paraffin sections: co-expression of L60 (Leu-22) and L26 antigens correlates with malignant histologic findings. *Am J Clin Pathol* 1989; 91:579–583.
144. Clark JR, Williams ME, Swerdlow SH. Detection of B- and T-cells in paraffin-embedded tissue sections: diagnostic utility of commercially obtained 4KB5 and UCHL-1. *Am J Clin Pathol* 1990;93:58–69.
145. Fina L, Molgaard HV, Robertson D, et al. Expression of the CD34 gene in vascular endothelial cells. *Blood* 1990;75:2417–2426.
146. Pezzella F, Tse AGD, Cordell JL, et al. Expression of the bcl-2 oncogene protein is not specific for the 14;18 chromosomal translocation. *Am J Pathol* 1990; 137:225–232.
147. Hockenbery D, Nunez G, Milliman C, et al. Bcl-2 is an inner mitochondrial membrane protein that blocks programmed cell death. *Nature* 1990;348:334–336.
148. Zutter M, Hockenbery D, Silverman GA, et al. Immunolocalization of the Bcl-2 protein within hematopoietic neoplasms. *Blood* 1991;78:1062–1068.
149. van Noesel CJM, van Lier RAW, Cordell JL, et al. The membrane IgM-associated heterodimer on human B cells is a newly defined B cell antigen that contains the protein product of the mb-1 gene. *J Immunol* 1991;146:3881–3888.
150. Simmons PJ, Torok-Storb B. CD34 expression by stromal precursors in normal human adult bone marrow. *Blood* 1991;78:2848–2853.
151. Vojtesck B, Bartek J, Midgley CA, et al. An immunohistochemical analysis of the human nuclear phosphoprotein p53: new monoclonal antibodies and epitope mapping using recombinant p53. *J Immunol Methods* 1992;151;237–244.
152. Chadburn A, Husain S, Knowles DM. Monoclonal antibody OPD4 detects neoplastic T cells but does not distinguish between CD4 and CD8 neoplastic T cells in paraffin tissue sections. *Hum Pathol* 1992;23:940–947.
153. Cattoretti G, Pileri S, Parravicini C, et al. Antigen unmasking on formalin-fixed paraffin-embedded tissue sections. *J Pathol* 1993;171:83–98.

154. Falini B, Flenghi L, Pileri S, et al. PG-M1: a new monoclonal antibody directed against a fixative-resistant epitope on the macrophage-restricted form of the CD68 molecule. *Am J Pathol* 1993;142:1359–1372.
155. Jiang W, Zhang YJ, Kahn SM, et al. Altered expression of the cyclin D1 and retinoblastoma genes in human esophageal cancer. *Proc Natl Acad Sci U S A* 1993;90:9026–9030.
156. Cesarman E, Inghirami G, Chadburn A, et al. High levels of p53 expression do not correlate with p53 gene mutations in anaplastic large cell lymphoma. *Am J Pathol* 1993;43:845–846.
157. Matsushima AY, Cesarman E, Chadburn A, et al. Post-thymic T cell lymphomas frequently overexpress p53 protein but infrequently exhibit p53 gene mutations. *Am J Pathol* 1994;144:573–584.
158. Bartkova J, Lukas J, Strauss M, et al. Cell cycle-related variation and tissue-restricted expression of human cyclin D1 protein. *J Pathol* 1994;172:237–245.
159. Yang WI, Zukerberg LR, Motokura T, et al. Cyclin D1 (Bcl-1, PRAD1) protein expression in low-grade B-cell lymphomas and reactive hyperplasia. *Am J Pathol* 1994;145:86–96.
160. Cuevas EC, Bateman AC, Wilkins BS, et al. Microwave antigen retrieval in immunocytochemistry: a study of 80 antibodies. *J Clin Pathol* 1994;47:448–452.
161. Norton AJ, Jordan S, Yeomans P. Brief, high-temperature heat denaturation (pressure cooking): a simple and effective method of antigen retrieval for routinely processed tissues. *J Pathol* 1994;173:371–379.
162. Pezzella F, Gatter K. What is the value of bcl-2 protein detection for histopathologists? *Histopathology* 1995;26:89–93.
163. Zukerberg LR, Yang WI, Arnold A, et al. Cyclin D1 expression in non-Hodgkin's lymphomas. *Am J Clin Pathol* 1995;103:756–760.
164. Mason DY, Cordell JL, Brown MH, et al. CD79a: a novel marker for B-cell neoplasms in routinely processed tissue samples. *Blood* 1995;86:1453–1459.
165. Shi SR, Gu J, Kalra KL, et al. Antigen retrieval technique: a novel approach to immunohistochemistry on routinely processed tissue sections. *Cell Vision* 1995; 2:7–22.
166. Schlossman SF, Boumsell L, Gilks W, et al., eds. *Leukocyte typing, V: white cell differentiation antigens.* New York: Oxford University Press, 1995.
167. Tsang WYW, Chan JKC, Pau MY. Utility of a paraffin section-reactive CD56 antibody (123C3) for characterization and diagnosis of lymphomas. *Am J Surg Pathol* 1996;20:202–210.
168. Bonsing BA, Corver WE, Gorsira MCB, et al. Specificity of seven monoclonal antibodies against p53 evaluated with Western blotting, immunohistochemistry, confocal laser scanning microscopy, and flow cytometry. *Cytometry* 1997;28:11–24.
169. Wang H, Kadlecek TA, Au-Yeung BB, et al. ZAP-70: an essential kinase in T-cell signaling. *Cold Spring Harb Perspect Biol* 2010;2(5):a002279.
170. Cobaleda C, Schebesta A, Delogu A, et al. Pax5: the guardian of B cell identity and function. *Nat Immunol* 2007;8(5):463–470.
171. Browne P, Petrosyan K, Hernandez A, et al. The B-cell transcription factors BSAP, Oct-2, and BOB.1 and the pan-B-cell markers CD20, CD22, and CD79a are useful in the differential diagnosis of classic Hodgkin lymphoma. *Am J Clin Pathol* 2003;120(5):767–777.
172. Gualco G, Weiss LM, Bacchi CE. MUM1/IRF4: a review. *Appl Immunohistochem Mol Morphol* 2010;18(4):301–310.
173. Tam W. PRDM1 (PR domain containing 1, with ZNF domain). *Atlas Genet Cytogenet Oncol Haematol* 2012;16(2):135–140.
174. Knowles DM. Immunophenotypic and antigen receptor gene rearrangement analysis in T cell neoplasia. *Am J Pathol* 1989;134:761–785.
175. Thalhammer-Scherrer R, Mitterbauer G, Simonitsch I, et al. The immunophenotype of 325 adult acute leukemias: relationship to morphologic and molecular classification and proposal for a minimal screening program highly predictive for lineage discrimination. *Am J Clin Pathol* 2002;117(3):380–389.
176. Han X, Bueso-Ramos CE. Precursor T-cell acute lymphoblastic leukemia/lymphoblastic lymphoma and acute biphenotypic leukemias. *Am J Clin Pathol* 2007; 127(4):528–544.
177. Hrusak O, Porwit-MacDonald A. Antigen expression patterns reflecting genotype of acute leukemias. *Leukemia* 2002;16(7):1233–1258.
178. Bennett JM, Catovsky D, Daniel MT, et al. Proposals for the classification of the acute leukemias: French-American-British (FAB) co-operative Group. *Br J Haematol* 1976;33:451–458.
179. Griffin JD. The use of monoclonal antibodies in the characterization of myeloid leukemias. *Hematol Pathol* 1987;1:81–91.
180. Zukerberg LR, Medeiros LJ, Ferry JA, et al. Diffuse low-grade B-cell lymphomas: four clinically distinct subtypes defined by a combination of morphologic and immunophenotypic features. *Am J Clin Pathol* 1993;100:373–385.
181. Dorfman DM, Pinkus GS. Distinction between small lymphocytic and mantle cell lymphoma by immunoreactivity for CD23. *Mod Pathol* 1994;7:326–331.
182. Matutes E, Owusu-Ankomah K, Morilla R, et al. The immunological profile of B-cell disorders and proposal of a scoring system for the diagnosis of CLL. *Leukemia* 1994;8:1640–1650.
183. Kroft SH, Finn WG, Peterson LC. The pathology of the chronic lymphoid leukaemias. *Blood Rev* 1995;9(4):234–250.
184. Dungarwalla M, Matutes E, Dearden CE. Prolymphocytic leukaemia of B- and T-cell subtype: a state-of-the-art paper. *Eur J Haematol* 2008;80(6):469–476.
185. Campo E, Raffeld M, Jaffe ES. Mantle-cell lymphoma. *Semin Hematol* 1999;36(2): 115–127.
186. Mozos A, Royo C, Hartmann E, et al. SOX11 expression is highly specific for mantle cell lymphoma and identifies the cyclin D1-negative subtype. *Haematologica* 2009;94(11):1555–1562.
187. San Miguel JF, Vidriales MB, Ocio E, et al. Immunophenotypic analysis of Waldenstrom's macroglobulinemia. *Semin Oncol* 2003;30(2):187–195.
188. Matutes E. Immunophenotyping and differential diagnosis of hairy cell leukemia. *Hematol Oncol Clin North Am* 2006;20(5):1051–1063.
189. Nathwani BN, Drachenberg MR, Hernandez AM. Primary nodal marginal zone lymphomas of splenic and MALT type. *Am J Surg Pathol* 2000;24(2):317–319.
190. Gaulard P, Harris NL, Pileri SA, et al. Primary mediastinal (thymic) large B-cell lymphoma. In: Swerdlow SH, Campo E, Harris NL, et al., eds. *WHO classification of tumors of haematopoietic and lymphoid tissues.* Lyon: IARC, 2008:250–251.
191. Berglund M, Thunberg U, Amini RM, et al. Evaluation of immunophenotype in diffuse large B-cell lymphoma and its impact on prognosis. *Mod Pathol* 2005;18(8): 1113–1120.
192. de Leval L, Harris NL. Variability in immunophenotype in diffuse large B-cell lymphoma and its clinical relevance. *Histopathology* 2003;43(6):509–528.
193. Montes-Moreno S, Gonzalez-Medina A-R, Rodriguez-Pinilla S-M, et al. Aggressive large B-cell lymphoma with plasma cell differentiation: immunohistochemical characterization of plasmablastic lymphoma and diffuse large B-cell lymphoma with partial plasmablastic phenotype. *Haematologica* 2010;95(8):1342–1349.
194. Knowles DM. The human T-cell leukemias: clinical, cytomorphologic, immunophenotypic, and genotypic characteristics. *Hum Pathol* 1986;17:14–33.
195. Kelemen K, White CR, Gatter K, et al. Immunophenotypic correlation between skin biopsy and peripheral blood findings in mycosis fungoides. *Am J Clin Pathol* 2010; 134(5):739–748.
196. Wood GS, Abel EA, Hoppe RT, et al. Leu-8 and Leu-9 antigen phenotypes: immunologic criteria for the distinction of mycosis fungoides from cutaneous inflammation. *J Am Acad Dermatol* 1986;14(6):1006–1013.
197. Matutes E, Brito-Babapulle V, Swansbury J, et al. Clinical and laboratory features of 78 cases of T-prolymphocytic leukemia. *Blood* 1991;78(12):3269–3274.
198. Herling M, Khoury JD, Washington LT, et al. A systematic approach to diagnosis of mature T-cell leukemias reveals heterogeneity among WHO categories. *Blood* 2004; 104(2):328–335.
199. Chan WC, Link S, Mawle A, et al. Heterogeneity of large granular lymphocyte proliferations: delineation of two major subtypes. *Blood* 1986;68(5):1142–1153.
200. Richards SJ, Short M, Scott CS. Clonal CD3 + CD8 + large granular lymphocyte (LGL)/NK-associated (NKa) expansions: primary malignancies or secondary reactive phenomena? *Leuk Lymphoma* 1995;17(3-4):303–311.
201. Morice WG, Kurtin PJ, Tefferi A, et al. Distinct bone marrow findings in T-cell granular lymphocytic leukemia revealed by paraffin section immunoperoxidase stains for CD8, TIA-1, and granzyme B. *Blood* 2002;99(1):268–274.
202. Waldmann TA, White JD, Goldman CK, et al. The interleukin-2 receptor: a target for monoclonal antibody treatment of human T-cell lymphotrophic virus I-induced adult T-cell leukemia. *Blood* 1993;82(6):1701–1712.
203. Ohtsuka E, Kikuchi H, Nasu M, et al. Clinicopathological features of adult T-cell leukemia with CD30 antigen expression. *Leuk Lymphoma* 1994;15(3-4):303–310.
204. Attygalle A, Al-Jehani R, Diss TC, et al. Neoplastic T cells in angioimmunoblastic T-cell lymphoma express CD10. *Blood* 2002;99(2):627–633.
205. Dogan A, Attygalle AD, Kyriakou C. Angioimmunoblastic T-cell lymphoma. *Br J Haematol* 2003;121(5):681–691.
206. Dunleavy K, Wilson WH, Jaffe ES. Angioimmunoblastic T cell lymphoma: pathobiological insights and clinical implications. *Curr Opin Hematol* 2007;14(4):348–353.
207. Stein H, Foss HD, Durkop H, et al. CD30(+) anaplastic large cell lymphoma: a review of its histopathologic, genetic, and clinical features. *Blood* 2000;96(12):3681–3695.
208. Delsol G, Al Saati T, Gatter KC, et al. Coexpression of epithelial membrane antigen (EMA), Ki-1, and interleukin-2 receptor by anaplastic large cell lymphomas. Diagnostic value in so-called malignant histiocytosis. *Am J Pathol* 1988;130(1):59–70.
209. Foss HD, Anagnostopoulos I, Araujo I, et al. Anaplastic large-cell lymphomas of T-cell and null-cell phenotype express cytotoxic molecules. *Blood* 1996;88(10): 4005–4011.
210. Wellmann A, Thieblemont C, Pittaluga S, et al. Detection of differentially expressed genes in lymphomas using cDNA arrays: identification of clusterin as a new diagnostic marker for anaplastic large-cell lymphomas. *Blood* 2000;96(2):398–404.
211. Rodriguez-Pinilla SM, Atienza L, Murillo C, et al. Peripheral T-cell lymphoma with follicular T-cell markers. *Am J Surg Pathol* 2008;32(12):1787–1799.
212. Went P, Agostinelli C, Gallamini A, et al. Marker expression in peripheral T-cell lymphoma: a proposed clinical-pathologic prognostic score. *J Clin Oncol* 2006;24(16): 2472–2479.
213. Jones D, Fletcher CD, Pulford K, et al. The T-cell activation markers CD30 and OX40/CD134 are expressed in nonoverlapping subsets of peripheral T-cell lymphoma. *Blood* 1999;93(10):3487–3493.
214. Asano N, Suzuki R, Kagami Y, et al. Clinicopathologic and prognostic significance of cytotoxic molecule expression in nodal peripheral T-cell lymphoma, unspecified. *Am J Surg Pathol* 2005;29(10):1284–1293.
215. Borowitz MJ, Shuster JJ, Civin CI, et al. Prognostic significance of CD34 expression in childhood B-precursor acute lymphocytic leukemia: a Pediatric Oncology Group study. *J Clin Oncol* 1990;8:1389–1398.
216. Pui CH, Hancock ML, Head DR, et al. Clinical significance of CD34 expression in childhood acute lymphoblastic leukemia. *Blood* 1993;82:889–894.
217. Thomas X, Archimbaud E, Charrin C, et al. CD34 expression is associated with major adverse prognostic factors in adult acute lymphoblastic leukemia. *Leukemia* 1995;9:249–253.
218. Sperling C, Buchner T, Creutzig U, et al. Clinical, morphologic, cytogenetic and prognostic implications of CD34 expression in childhood and adult de novo AML. *Leuk Lymphoma* 1994;17:417–426.
219. Borowitz MJ, Bene M-C, Harris NL, et al. Acute leukemias of ambiguous lineage. In: Swerdlow SH, Campo E, Harris NL, et al., eds. *WHO classification of tumors of haematopoietic and lymphoid tissues.* Lyon: IARC, 2008:150–155.
220. Ha-Kawa K, Hara J, Keiko Y, et al. Kappa-chain gene rearrangement in an apparent T-lineage lymphoma. *J Clin Invest* 1986;78:1439–1442.
221. Sheibani K, Wu A, Ben-Ezra J, et al. Rearrangement of κ-chain and T-cell receptor β-chain genes in malignant lymphomas of "T-cell" phenotype. *Am J Pathol* 1987; 129:201–206.
222. Weiss LM, Wood GS, Trela M, et al. Clonal T-cell population in lymphomatoid papulosis: evidence of a lymphoproliferative origin for a clinically benign disease. *N Engl J Med* 1986;315:475–479.
223. Kadin ME, Vonderheid ED, Sako D, et al. Clonal composition of T cells in lymphomatoid papulosis. *Am J Pathol* 1987;126:13–17.

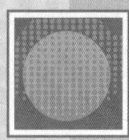

Chapter 11
Technical Factors in the Preparation and Evaluation of Lymph Node Biopsies

Sonam Prakash • Peter M. Banks

The most underrepresented aspect of hematopathology in publications is that of specimen preparation. This belies the subject's importance, because high-quality conventional paraffin section preparations are the essential starting point for accurate diagnosis (1).

The pathologist's charge has grown considerably over the past several decades as ancillary studies of diagnostic importance have become a part of established practice, requiring special tissue allocations. It is sobering to realize that in modern practice the failure to allocate biopsied tissue appropriately could represent a greater failure than an erroneous interpretation of the disease process itself. Although the latter error can often be corrected by consultative review, the former may oblige the patient to an additional surgical procedure. The task is made all the more difficult by current trends toward ever smaller biopsy samples.

Pathologists should regularly reevaluate and update the quality of their stock-in-trade, the conventional paraffin tissue section products of their laboratory, as well as their practices in tissue allocation of lymph node and related tissue biopsy specimens.

 ## CONVENTIONAL PARAFFIN TISSUE SECTIONS

The importance of consistently high-quality paraffin tissue sections to the hematopathologist cannot be exaggerated. Conventional microscopy remains the gold standard and starting point for our understanding of lymphoid proliferations. It is always a top priority, at least in initial samplings, that representative tissue blocks be submitted for conventional paraffin processing. The quality of the paraffin used for conventional processing has improved greatly with the addition of plastic polymers, which enhance its physical characteristics for sectioning. The commercial availability of almost innumerable useful antibodies that can be used with immunohistochemistry (IHC) to identify antigens in paraffin preparations makes high-quality sections all the more valuable. More recently, *in situ* hybridization assays have become available for the demonstration of RNA and DNA sequences, and these depend likewise on the same high-quality paraffin sections.

Because of the long sequence involved in the production of paraffin tissue sections, potential shortcomings are many and diverse. The critical reviews of slide preparations by the pathologist and technologist allow recognition of telltale deficiencies specific to particular steps in processing (2) (Table 11.1). A chronology of routine processing with reference to morphologic artifacts follows; it can be used as a guide for troubleshooting.

Specimen Delivery

Even when the laboratory receives biopsy specimens directly from the operating rooms, irreversible drying artifacts can be introduced if transport is in dry towels or surgical sponges.

The surface tissue is desiccated, resulting in dehydrational denaturation of cellular proteins, commonly recognizable as a dark edge in hematoxylin and eosin (H&E)–stained sections (Fig. 11.1). This can be a serious problem with small samples, such as needle biopsies, especially if delivered on gauze pads in which the delicate tissue adheres to the dry interstices and may be damaged in an attempt to remove it or even be effectively inextricable. To avoid such catastrophes, the investigator should instruct surgeons and nurse circulators to submit all specimens on paper or fine-mesh synthetic pads moistened with sterile saline. Transport and short-term storage within sealed jars containing saline or tissue culture media are also satisfactory, and cooling the specimen to 4°C delays autolysis, a problem related to the metabolic activity of the sampled process. For morphologic purposes, storage at 4°C for up to 24 hours is usually satisfactory, and the preservation of immunoreactivity for most markers and nucleic acids is surprisingly durable (3–5).

Tissue Blocking

Representation of the biopsy specimen in paraffin tissue sections should never be jeopardized, and in fashioning tissue blocks, the pathologist frames the image of the sampling as it ultimately will appear on the microscope stage. A large, sweeping cut through the long axis of a small lymph node ensures assessment of nodal architecture. The block should be no more than 3 mm thick to allow adequate diffusion of liquids during fixation and processing. Today's thin-profile tissue cassettes, serving doubly as labels for storage as well, require an especially thin block to allow circulation of fluid within the interior space. If too thick a block is submitted, the result is a paraffin-embedded block that is soft in the center (Fig. 11.2). Adequate sections simply cannot be made from such a preparation, because the central portion retracts from the microtome knife, and in the paraffin ribbons, these areas crack and disintegrate on contact with the water bath (Fig. 11.3) (blocking procedures are discussed further under "Allocation of Tissue Specimens").

Fixation

Fixatives are substances that denature cellular and extracellular tissue constituents to preserve them and render them suitable for treatments such as dehydration, infiltration by a supporting medium, and staining. There is no one fixative that is best for all purposes, and the examiner must select a fixative that best suits the potential study needs of the case.

The most universal fixative in hospital pathology is 10% formalin (3.7% aqueous formaldehyde solution). This fixative is relatively safe, is inexpensive, rapidly diffuses into tissues, and is not an environmental disposal problem. For a number of reasons, a slightly alkaline buffer is added. This not only retards the formation of formene pigment, a black, insoluble polymeric product of formaldehyde, but also guarantees uniform reaction times for IHC and *in situ* methods. Aldehyde fixatives, such as formalin solution, act chemically by producing

Table 11.1	COMMON ERRORS IN ROUTINE TISSUE PROCESSING AND THEIR CONSEQUENCES	

Step	Error	Result
Delivery	Specimen on dry towel	"Edge" artifact due to desiccation of surface tissue (Fig. 11.1)
Blocking	Tissue blocks too thick	"Soft" central core of block that fragments in sections (Figs. 11.2 and 11.3)
Fixation	Inadequate time for fixation	Uniform fragmentation of sections
Dehydration	Aqueous contamination of alcohols or inadequate time in alcohols in processor	Sections show small, irregular cracks with faint staining, blurred nuclear chromatin
Clearing	Excessive time in xylenes; alcohol contaminating xylenes with poor paraffin infiltration	Tissue hard and brittle; sections compressed and wrinkled; do not ribbon
Infiltration	Paraffin too hot	Cellular shrinkage and retraction; collagen basophilic
Embedding	Delay in embedding after removal from paraffin bath	Air spaces around tissue, poor connection to surrounding paraffin disrupts sections
Sectioning	Improper knife angle; defective knife edge	"Venetian blind" shutter effect lines across sections
Floating section	Inadequate attention to teasing sections flat on water bath	Folds and/or tears in sections (Fig. 11.4)
Drying	Oven temperature set too high	Nuclear "bubbling" in large, delicate nuclei
Staining	Inadequate rinse after eosin stain	Sections have overall red hue; even nucleoli in immunoblasts are eosinophilic

Data from Beard C, Nabers K, Bowling MC, et al. Achieving technical excellence in lymph node specimens: an update. *Lab Med* 1985;16:468–475.

methylene or longer carbon chain bridges between sterically apposed amino groups of proteins. This is a very delicate quality of fixation, ideal, for example, for ultrastructural studies, as with glutaraldehyde. However, for the purposes of paraffin section cytomorphology, this type of fixation predisposes to the common nuclear bubbling artifact. Large nuclei with dispersed chromatin are disrupted by sectioning. At the moment of deparaffinization, if physical rigidity is insufficient, there is coalescence into strands of chromatin with clearing of chromatin.

A variety of fixatives have been used in the past, either instead of formalin or after initial formalin fixation, to avoid nuclear bubbling artifact. These are all protein-precipitating agents that produce physically rigid denaturation of nucleoproteins. Some of these are acids, which denature proteins by taking them away from their isoelectric points (e.g., acetic acid and picric acid in Bouin solution). Others are metallic cationic solutions, which form large, insoluble coordination complexes with the organic groups that extend out from the amino acid chains of proteins (i.e., mercuric chloride and zinc chloride solutions). Many fixatives consist of a mixture of formaldehyde solution with a protein precipitating agent (e.g., zinc chloride or zinc sulfate) (6).

Protein-precipitating agents afford sharper nuclear detail in H&E sections and they enhance immunoreactivity. Surprisingly,

the cytomorphologic and immunoreactive limitations of formalin fixation can be improved by "runback" procedures in which paraffin-embedded tissue is sequenced back to aqueous solution and then refixed in a protein precipitant. The refixed block is then forward processed in standard sequence to paraffin (7). Zinc-formalin also offers the advantage of being suitable for DNA *in situ* and amplification studies (8,9).

Alcohol mixtures are good for immunopreservation and genetic probe analysis (10). However, conventional H&E histology is often suboptimal, with cellular shrinkage and drying artifact in small biopsy specimens.

While zinc-formalin is ideal for most purposes, the zinc may result in some interference with polymerase chain reaction DNA assays (11). Therefore, in most laboratories, to serve the most diverse possibilities for ancillary studies, neutral buffered formalin remains the fixative of choice.

Automated Processing

Automated sequence processing is carried out in laboratories using a variety of commercially available processors. Some models offer the option of rapid sequencing, with heat and vacuum applied to accelerate diffusion and reactivity of the reagents. Minimal time required for adequate fixation, dehydration, clearing, and paraffin infiltration depends on the

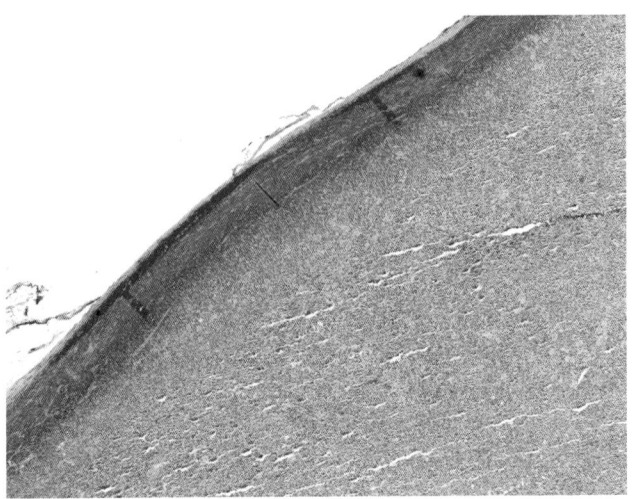

FIGURE 11.1. "Edge" artifact in a lymph node biopsy (paraffin section) is introduced by delivery of the specimen in a surgical towel, with resulting irreversible denaturation of proteins by drying (H&E stain, original magnification: 2×).

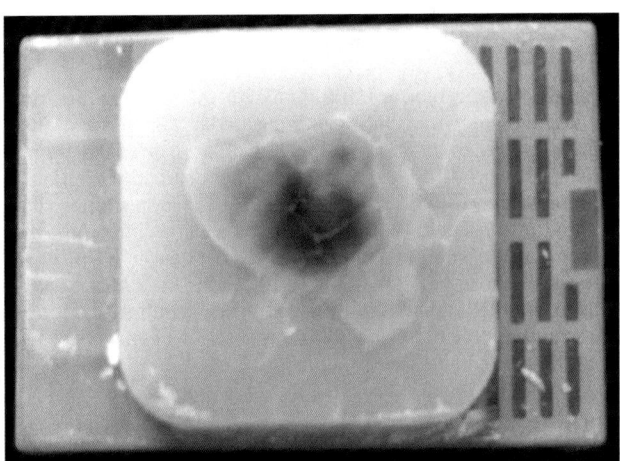

FIGURE 11.2. A poorly processed block inadequately infiltrated by paraffin, resulting in a soft central region that retracts from the cutting surface. This most commonly results from blocks that are too thick.

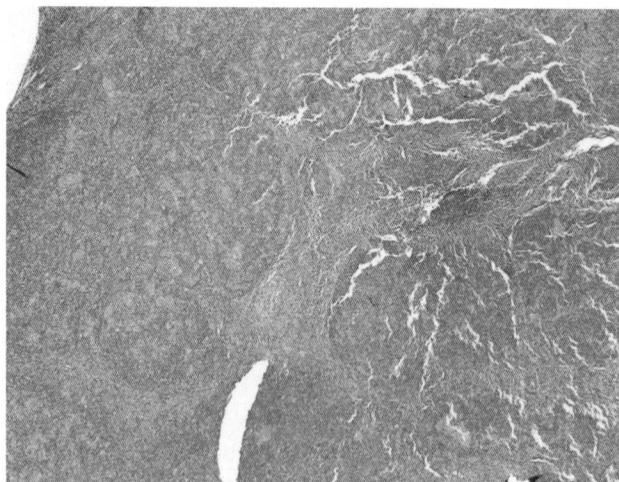

FIGURE 11.3. Section resulting from poorly processed tissue block due to inadequate fixation displays fragmentation (H&E stain, original magnification: 10×).

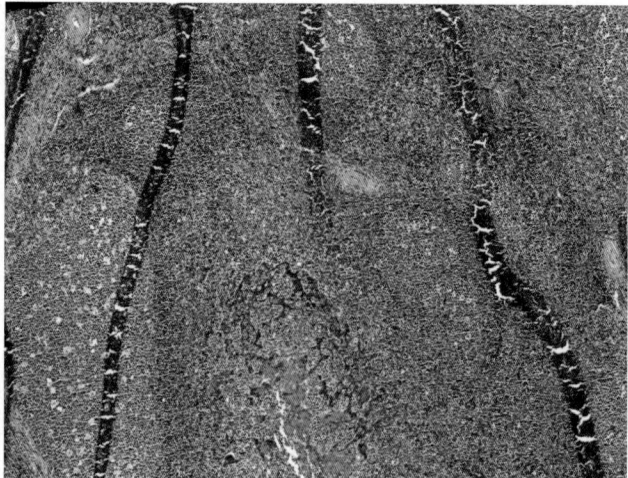

FIGURE 11.4. Poor sectioning technique renders architectural interpretation difficult. Notice the folds in this example (H&E stain, original magnification: 4×).

size and quality of the specimens; a very thin block of porous tissue such as lung is adequately processed much more rapidly than a thick block of an impervious tissue such as muscle. Fixation and subsequent processing of bloody tissues such as spleen can be enhanced by initially agitating thin cut blocks in a jar of buffered formalin. In general, perfectly satisfactory processing can be carried out with an overnight schedule (total of 12 hours), as long as the tissue blocks are <3 mm thick. At least 6 hours of fixation should be allowed (4).

It is important to replace the fluids in the processor regularly, and this can be done in part with a "forward shift" of identical reagent sequence; yesterday's second 95% ethanol becomes today's first 95% ethanol bath. The alcohol sequence used for dehydration should be graded, starting with 70% or 80% ethanol, and absolute ethanol should not be used for more than a total time of 2 hours. Initial exposure to concentrated alcohol or prolonged time in absolute alcohol can produce a "burned" effect, in which sections show contracted nuclei and a pale gray refractile hematoxylin tint with excessive eosin staining.

The temperature of the melted paraffin should be checked periodically. Excessive heat (>70°C) leads to "cooking", with thermal denaturation of proteins with shrunken cells and collagen that stains more hematoxyphilic than is normally seen. For the purpose of preserving antigens for immunostaining, it is best to maintain the paraffin temperature below 62°C.

Embedding

Processed tissue blocks infiltrated with melted paraffin must be aligned in position for sectioning under the cassette base, a process known as *embedding*. This often overlooked hands-on step is crucial because, if tissue is not correctly oriented in relation to the cutting surface, the plane of section cannot allow optimal microscopic interpretation of tissue architecture, and much of the tissue block is wasted in an attempt to cut down into the block adequately. For lymph nodes, it is best to carefully orient the largest, flattest tissue surface against the bottom of the embedding mold so that minimal tissue need be cut away to reach a complete sectioning face.

Sectioning

The most difficult and most laborious step in the production of high-quality slides is sectioning. Pathologists should regularly review slides with histotechnologists to maintain optimal sectioning technique. Sloppy sectioning results in tears and folds

in the tissue ribbon, precluding low-magnification assessment of lymphoid architecture (Fig. 11.4). Such problems are related to poor cutting techniques and to mounting (i.e., when the section ribbons are teased out smoothly on the surface of the water bath). Proper temperature and the addition to the water bath of proteins, detergents, or both augment section mounting, because they reduce electrostatic tension along the interface, resulting in adherence of the sections to the glass more perfectly.

Because many hematolymphoid cells are relatively small in diameter, thin sections (3 or 4 μm) are needed for cytomorphologic assessment (Fig. 11.5). However, the thinner the sections, the more difficult is the task of producing large, undisrupted preparations free of imperfections. It is particularly important that microtome knives be sharp and even -edged (Fig. 11.6). Nowadays, in most laboratories, disposable blade systems are used to encourage frequent switching to a new, perfect edge. To avoid "shuttering" or the "Venetian blind" effect, the knife cutting angle must be maintained sufficiently acute to the sectioning surface.

Proper sectioning can be carried out only if the tissue block has been adequately fixed and processed (Fig. 11.7). Minor shortcomings can sometimes be remedied with trick methods, such as smearing glycerol on the cutting surface when tissue has been excessively dehydrated in alcohols or applying an ice cube to the block face when insufficient fixation has led to a soft tissue core.

Section Drying

Wet mounted sections are annealed to the underlying glass slides by oven drying. The temperature should not exceed 55°C to avoid the production of disruptions in the chromatin of large, delicate vesicular nuclei (nuclear "bubbling" artifact). With excessive heat, the supportive paraffin medium becomes so soft that water vapor penetrates through the section selectively at points of least physical resistance. Usually 2 hours at 45°C is adequate for drying, depending on ambient humidity. In some laboratories, commercial grade heater blowers are used to accelerate the process.

Staining

Thorough deparaffinization in xylenes or some similar hydrophobic solvent is necessary before the sections can be gradually hydrated in graded alcohols, making regular rotation and replacement of the xylenes mandatory. In general, the progressive

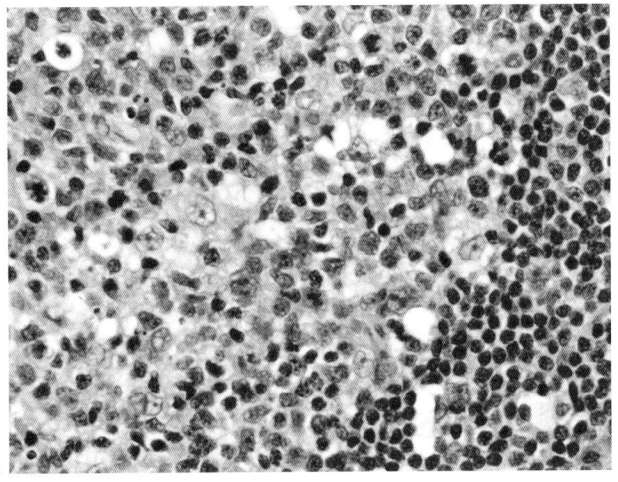 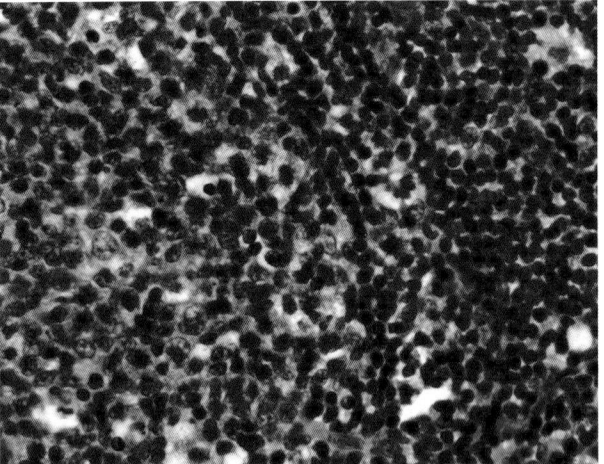

FIGURE 11.5. The importance of preparing adequately thin paraffin sections for cytomorphologic evaluation is demonstrated in this comparison of thick and thin sections from the same paraffin block in a case of follicular hyperplasia. **A:** This sample was sectioned at 3 μm, enabling recognition of centroblasts, centrocytes, and mantle zones (H&E stain, original magnification: 40×). **B:** This sample was sectioned at 6 μm, resulting in obscuration of even large cells by superimposition of cell nuclei (H&E stain, original magnification: 40×).

type of hematoxylin solution (Mayer, Schmitt) is superior to the regressive type (Harris) because the variability from slide to slide with the extra decolorization step is not a problem. Progressive hematoxylins do not form precipitates requiring daily filtration, as do the regressive types.

The balance between H&E is important for distinguishing cell types in hematopathology and not merely an arbitrary or subjective matter of esthetic preference. For example, the nucleoli of large transformed follicle center cells and of reactive immunoblasts should be hematoxyphilic and not eosinophilic, while those in Reed-Sternberg cells should be eosinophilic. To avoid overstaining with eosin, the technologist should thoroughly rinse the slides in 95% alcohol before dehydrating, clearing, and coverslipping. Automated staining systems are widely used today, but the settings must be monitored closely to assure balanced staining.

Coverslipping

Although shortcomings in coverslipping are usually not serious and can be repaired, they are nonetheless inconvenient and can obscure sections. Mounting medium should not be

diluted by too much xylene remaining on slides, because this leads to air bubbles forming underneath the coverslip. This is a particularly big issue with automated coverslipping, since the temptation is to use a medium too dilute. Even very old slides can be recoverslipped as long as the investigator is patient enough to allow release of the old coverslip by soaking in xylene or alternative solutions. When this method fails, the slide can be pressed against a hot plate for a few seconds. Such heat usually quickly releases the coverslip. Then the preparation can be rinsed in xylene or alternative solutions and coverslipped afresh.

Strict adherence to all these recommended procedural guidelines results in production of high-quality H&E paraffin tissue sections. Such preparations provide large, intact tissue architecture and fine cytologic detail for microscopic evaluation (Fig. 11.7).

ALLOCATION OF TISSUE SPECIMENS

Intraoperative Interpretations

There is a common fallacy among pathologists and surgeons that intraoperative microscopic interpretations should not be attempted on lymph nodes biopsied for suspected lymphoma. Although it is true that accurate diagnosis and classification of lymphoma should not be attempted by this means, such on-the-spot interpretations are beneficial for confirmation of adequate sampling and for selection of tissue allocations. It is far better to inform the surgeon during surgery that the sampling is inadequate for diagnosis than to do so 1 or 2 days postoperatively! Imprints or scrape smear preparations can be used in place of frozen tissue sections for intraoperative microscopy.

The pathologist should communicate fully with the managing physician and surgeon before the biopsy to render the best possible interpretation of the intraoperative frozen section or cytology preparation. If there is evidence of inflammation (e.g., suppuration or granuloma formation, especially in a patient with signs or symptoms of infection), fresh sterile tissue should be sent for microbial cultures.

Pathologists should recognize their role as stewards of the sampled tissue. They are responsible for its proper handling and division for appropriate special studies. It is essential that the strengths and weaknesses of the various available ancillary studies be understood in order that tissue allocations and

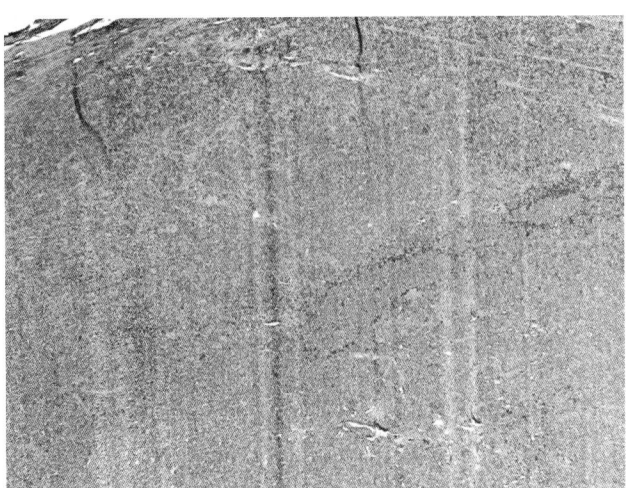

FIGURE 11.6. Lines from an irregular microtome blade produce poor-quality section with folds due to poor sectioning technique (H&E stain, original magnification: 4×). Such materials are difficult for the pathologist to interpret.

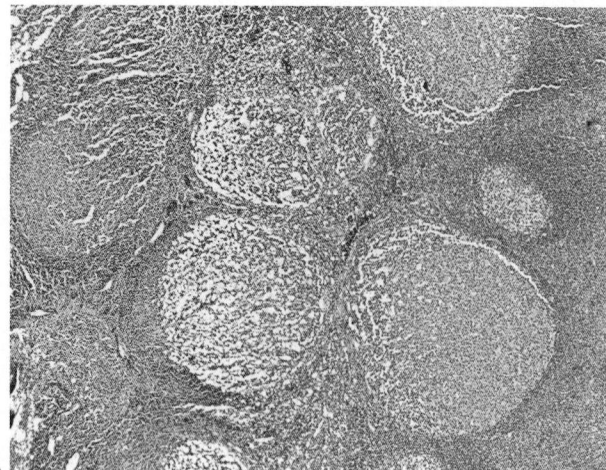
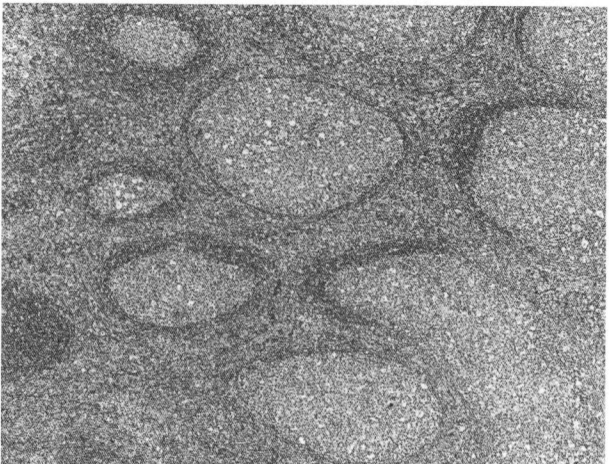

FIGURE 11.7. Comparison of sections from poorly fixed and well-fixed tissue blocks. A: Poorly fixed tissue resulting in disrupted sections. **B:** A properly fixed and processed block correctly sectioned allows evaluation of architecture under low magnification (H&E stain, original magnification: 4×).

the subsequent studies are selected appropriately, in a manner that most directly affords a definitive diagnosis and is least wasteful. In most instances involving a possible diagnosis of lymphoma, tissue will be allocated for flow cytometric and cytogenetic studies whenever adequate tissue is available. Flow cytometric immunophenotypic studies are especially valuable for determining clonality when the touch imprints demonstrate predominantly small lymphoid cells.

Blocking for Conventional Processing

Selection and production of the portion of tissue to be submitted for conventional processing is critical. Optimal plane of section and representation of the pathologic process must be obtained. It is usually best to stabilize the lymph node on a dry, rough-surfaced base, such as a paper towel. A large scalpel or sharp knife is then used to cut away the encapsulated deep aspect of the specimen. The fresh-cut deep surface of the upper portion is then quickly stabilized on another dry surface, and with a decisive slice parallel to and about 2 to 3 mm away from the paper towel, a large, thin block is produced. Imprints can then be produced from any of the freshly cut tissue surfaces. It is best to use pieces of node with adherent capsule for purposes other than conventional processing. These are not suitable for paraffin blocks because the capsule serves as a barrier to fluid diffusion.

Immediately after division of the specimen, the portions are immersed in one sort of fluid or another, according to the type of allocation, to avoid drying artifact. Although ideally the pathologist could submit some tissue sampling for all possible ancillary studies (12), in practice this may not be feasible, especially with small specimens. Based on the combination of preoperative clinical differential diagnosis and intraoperative cytomorphologic interpretation, tissue is allocated according to priority of anticipated importance of the respective ancillary studies that can derive from these.

Imprints and Smears

Monolayers of cells can be obtained by direct touch preparations of lymph nodes, offering preparations similar to those of fine needle aspiration cytology or cytocentrifuge methods for detailed single-cell analysis (Fig. 11.8). The allocation is simple, inexpensive, and effectively consumes no tissue. It should not be attempted on very small specimens that may suffer cellular crush artifact from such maneuvers. Densely sclerotic processes

do not yield intact cells. When attempts to produce cellular imprints are unsuccessful, it is unlikely that flow cytometry will be successfully carried out.

Imprint slides should be labeled ahead of time, usually six to eight, depending on the needs of the individual case. Anchoring one end of the slide face down against the cutting surface (i.e., towel) adjacent to a fresh-cut specimen surface, the slide is gently levered down into contact with the tissue surface and then pulled away, avoiding any sideways shearing motion. The first two preparations, carrying the thickest layer of cells, are immediately placed in a Coplin jar containing formalin or 95% alcohol solution; the remaining imprints are allowed to air dry. Alternatively, cells can be extruded from the fresh-cut surface by gently scraping with the edge of a slide. The wet cellular material is then quickly smeared over the surface of another slide and fixed or air dried. Such preparations can be stained immediately for intraoperative cytomorphologic interpretation. Compared with frozen tissue section methods, imprints can be produced faster, can conserve sampled tissue, and can be produced from bony tissues.

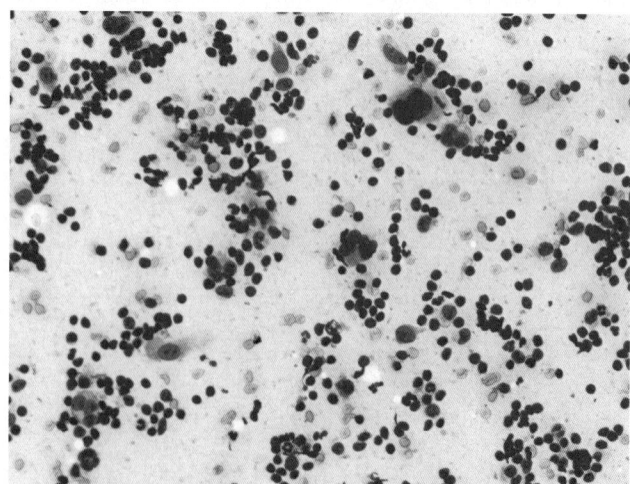

FIGURE 11.8. Diff-Quik–stained alcohol-fixed imprint preparations from a lymph node involved by classical Hodgkin lymphoma. Note the large bilobated and polylobated atypical nuclei in a polymorphous inflammatory background (original magnification: 20×). Such preparations are useful for immediate intraoperative evaluation as to adequacy of the sample and likely ancillary studies needed.

To avoid infectious disease contamination problems, all imprint preparations can be fixed; those initially air dried can be placed in a 50:50 mixture of acetone and methanol for 1 minute. This retains immunoreactivity and cytochemical properties and can be especially useful for fluorescence *in situ* hybridization studies, if needed. Solutions of 95% ethanol are almost as effective for preservation of antigens.

Wet-fixed imprints can be stained with H&E for cytomorphology equivalent to that in H&E-stained paraffin tissue sections, with clear nuclear detail provided. Air-dried preparations show less cellular shrinkage than those wet fixed, and Romanovsky-type stains, such as Wright-Giemsa or Diff-Quik, can be used to achieve cytoplasmic staining, as is favored in hematology (Fig. 11.8). Cytochemical (13) and immunocytochemical (14) preparations of imprints are typically of outstanding clarity, in contrast to corresponding frozen tissue section preparations.

Fixation of air-dried imprints should be in accord with the type of study to be done. Thoroughly dried preparations stored at 20°C retain most antigens for about 1 week; however, maintaining air-dried imprints at −70°C allows immunocytochemical analysis months or even years later. It is necessary to store such imprints in sealed five-slide plastic containers so that warming to 20°C can be done without direct exposure to ambient air, because this results in wet, runny-appearing preparations. Anhydrous acetone is generally the gentlest fixative; however, brief (1 minute) fixation in a 50:50 mixture of absolute methanol and anhydrous acetone at 20°C is superior for diminished nonspecific background staining. Enzyme cytochemical studies often require formol-acetone fixation (15).

Frozen Tissue

Tissue representative of the pathologic process should be frozen away whenever possible because this represents an insurance policy for some of the most powerful ancillary studies in hematopathology. Even mRNA is preserved in such preparations for studies such as gene expression array analysis (16).

The faster tissue is frozen, the more intact the cellular structures. Although ideally supercooled liquids such as liquid nitrogen or isopentane are used, for practical diagnostic purposes, the rapid freeze chuck accessory in a cryotome is perfectly suitable. However, it is imperative that the block of tissue for freezing be thin (<2 mm). When intraoperative frozen tissue sections are to be rendered, the tissue should be rapidly frozen and stored afterward for the potential ancillary studies mentioned. The production of "frozen section control" paraffin blocks is seldom useful diagnostically anyway. Because most cryotomes feature automatic defrost cycles, it is necessary to transfer the frozen block to a −70°C freezer for safekeeping. If long-term storage is a possibility, covering the tissue with a hyperviscous mounting medium such as OCT is necessary to prevent desiccation.

Fresh Tissue Allocations

No morphologist can surrender fresh tissue to other laboratories without some apprehension regarding its disappearance. However, some such studies are definitely indicated in many cases. A common situation is flow cytometry for immunophenotyping (17). Compared with frozen or paraffin tissue section IHC, the method is complementary. It is very rapid, safely handles infectious tissues, and is particularly sensitive for the detection of surface antigens, many of which can be compared simultaneously with multiple channel analysis. However, the method is less convenient than IHC because it must be carried out on fresh samples. Maintaining samples in tissue culture medium

for up to 48 hours at 4°C allows delay in performing such studies until at least the initial H&E-stained paraffin sections can be interpreted. Small compartments of cells, especially large, cohesive tumor cells, may not be detectable or even survive into the suspension to be analyzed. Some degree of reassurance can be given to the anxious morphologist by using a small portion of the cell suspension to produce cytocentrifuge slides, stained ones for cytomorphologic correlation and unstained ones for potential immunocytochemical studies. The most fastidious allocation requirements are those for microbial culture or cytogenetics, because sterile fresh tissue is needed. A sealed sterile container should then preferably be sent from the operating or procedural room directly to the appropriate laboratories without contamination in the pathology gross room, where it is easy to envision a microbial veneer covering all surfaces.

Conventional Special Stains

Stains that have been available for many decades as adjuncts to H&E in paraffin tissue sections are sometimes very informative, extremely fast, convenient, and low cost, but today they are often overlooked. Giemsa staining of sections was recommended by Professor Karl Lennert, one of the pioneers of modern lymphoma classification, as a primary stain for paraffin sections in the interpretation of lymphoid tissues because of its differential cytoplasmic tinctorial qualities, which are superior to those of H&E (18). However, careful alcoholic differentiation is necessary with microscopic monitoring of stain balance to obtain an optimal stain; a bad Giemsa stain is definitely worse than a good H&E stain. Conventional histochemical methods such as periodic acid–Schiff, mucicarmine, and reticulin silver impregnation should not be forgotten in hematopathology. A useful enzyme cytochemical marker, chloroacetate esterase, is preserved in paraffin sections. This is a practical means to detect myeloid (granulocytic) and mast cells in conventional preparations (2,13).

It is a mark of mastery to employ simple, rapid methods rather than more sophisticated and expensive ones to solve a diagnostic problem. Special stains for microorganisms are an important and necessary everyday tool for modern hematopathology. Spontaneous and acquired immunodeficiencies can result in the presence of opportunistic infectious agents without an inflammatory response recognizable in H&E sections alone. Stains such as acid-fast and silver methods for fungi, *Pneumocystis*, and even catscratch bacilli are required on a regular basis.

SUMMARY AND CONCLUSIONS

Technical factors in the preparation of lymph node specimens are of critical importance for accurate interpretation. The pathologist should work with the laboratory's technologists to constantly monitor the quality of conventional paraffin section slides, troubleshooting avoidable problems.

Intraoperative interpretation is appropriate for cases of suspected lymphoproliferative disease. This ensures adequacy of sampling and can be used to determine appropriate allocation of tissue for ancillary studies. Such interpretations can be based on frozen tissue sections, imprints, or both. For initial biopsy specimens, top priority in allocation must always be given to adequate representation in conventionally processed paraffin section material. Imprints are usually a no-risk method of preparation suitable for diverse special staining purposes. A frozen tissue block, stored after intraoperative frozen section interpretation, serves as an insurance policy for powerful ancillary studies, including frozen tissue section IHC and genetic probe analysis.

ACKNOWLEDGMENTS

Linda Streckfus and Faye Blakeney assisted in the production of the first edition manuscript. Coranelle Shelton provided valuable technical consultation. Lilian Antonio and Edy Daniel assisted in preparing slides and blocks to demonstrate artifacts from technical issues.

References

1. Banks PM, Long JC, Howard CA. Preparation of lymph node biopsy specimens. *Hum Pathol* 1979;10:617–621.
2. Berard C, Nabers K, Bowling MC, et al. Achieving technical excellence in lymph node specimens: an update. *Lab Med* 1985;16:468–475.
3. Pelstring RJ, Allred DC, Esther RJ, et al. Differential antigen preservation during tissue autolysis. *Hum Pathol* 1991;22:237–241.
4. Gown AM. Current issues in ER and HER2 testing by IHC in breast cancer [Review]. *Mod Pathol* 2008;21(Suppl 2):S8–S15.
5. Moatamed NA, Nanjangud G, Pucci R, et al. Effect of ischemic time, fixation time, and fixative type on HER2/neu immunohistochemical and fluorescence in situ hybridization results in breast cancer. *Am J Clin Pathol* 2011;136:754–761.
6. Herman GE, Chlipala E, Bochenski G, et al. Zinc formalin fixative for automated tissue processing. *J Histotechnol* 1988;11:85–89.
7. Abbondanzo SL, Allred DC, Lampkin S, et al. Enhancement of immunoreactivity among lymphoid malignant neoplasms in paraffin-embedded tissues by refixation in zinc sulfate formalin. *Arch Pathol Lab Med* 1991;115:31–33.
8. Babic A, Loftin IR, Stanislaw S, et al. The impact of pre-analytical processing on staining quality for H&E, dual hapten, dual color in situ hybridization and fluorescent in situ hybridization assays. *Methods* 2010;52:287–300.
9. Wester K, Asplund A, Bäckvall H, et al. Zinc-based fixative improves preservation of genomic DNA and proteins in histoprocessing of human tissues. *Lab Invest* 2003;83:889–899.
10. Smith LJ, Braylan RC, Nutkis JE, et al. Extraction of cellular DNA from human cells and tissues fixed in ethanol. *Anal Biochem* 1987;160:135–138.
11. Ahrens K, Braylan R, Almasri N, et al. IgH PCR of zinc formalin-fixed, paraffin-embedded non-lymphomatous gastric samples produces artifactual "clonal" bands not observed in paired tissues unexposed to zinc formalin. *J Mol Diagn* 2002;4:159–163.
12. Collins RD. Lymph node examination. What is an adequate workup? *Arch Pathol Lab Med* 1985;109:796–799.
13. Sun T, Li CY, Yam LT, eds. *Atlas of cytochemistry and immunocytochemistry of hematologic neoplasms*. Chicago: American Society of Clinical Pathologists Press, 1985:22–33.
14. Banks PM, Caron BL, Morgan TW. Use of imprints for monoclonal antibody studies: suitability of air-dried preparations from lymphoid tissues with an immunohistochemical method. *Am J Clin Pathol* 1983;79:438–442.
15. Witzig TE, Banks PM, Stenson MJ, et al. Rapid immunotyping of B cell non-Hodgkin's lymphomas by flow cytometry: a comparison with the standard frozen section methods. *Am J Clin Pathol* 1990;94:280–286.
16. Bea S, Zettl A, Wright G, et al. Lymphoma/leukemia molecular profiling project. Diffuse large B-cell lymphoma subgroups have distinct genetic profiles that influence tumor biology and improve gene-expression-based survival prediction. *Blood* 2005;106:3183–3190.
17. Craig FE, Foon KA. Flow cytometric immunophenotyping for hematologic neoplasms [Review]. *Blood* 2008;111:3941–3967.
18. Lennert K, ed. *Histopathology of non-Hodgkin's lymphomas (based on the Kiel classification)*. New York: Springer-Verlag, 1981:119.

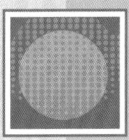

Chapter 12

The Role of Fine Needle Aspiration Biopsy in the Diagnosis and Management of Hematopoietic Neoplasms

Rana S. Hoda

 | FINE NEEDLE ASPIRATION

Introduction

Fine needle aspiration (FNA) is a well-established minimally invasive technique for the cytologic evaluation of suspicious mass lesions involving lymph nodes and other organs. The 2008 WHO classification of tumors of hematopoietic and lymphoid tissues utilizes a multiparametric approach based on cytomorphologic, immunophenotypic, and cytogenetic features to classify these tumors (1). This approach can be applied to FNA cytologic specimens (2–8), of both nodal and extranodal sites. About 25% to 40% of lymphoid neoplasms arise outside of the lymph node system, and dissemination of nodal neoplasms may occur to almost any anatomical site, presenting as an extranodal mass (8). FNA in conjunction with flow cytometry (FCM) has been shown to be useful for the diagnosis and subclassification of lymphoma (2–4,8–10).

The use of FNA for in the initial workup of patients with hematolymphoid neoplasms, particularly for patients who present with lymphadenopathy, remains underutilized (Table 12.1). Lymphoma constitutes approximately 10% of cases diagnosed by FNA (2,7,9–11).

Indications of FNA of Lymph Nodes

The utility of FNA in lymphadenopathy varies with the clinical situation (Table 12.2). The majority of cases of lymphadenopathy are benign or reactive, and FNA can be particularly advantageous in the diagnosis and appropriate management thereof (12).

Accuracy of Reporting FNA of Lymph Nodes

Diagnostic accuracy of FNA for high-grade non-Hodgkin lymphoma (NHL) and Hodgkin lymphoma (HL) (with the exception of lymphocytic predominant variant) is high (70% to 90%) (2,13). However, FNA has significant limitations in the assessment of low-grade B-cell lymphomas with a relatively low diagnostic accuracy (67%), inherent to the loss of architecture (14). False-negative rate of FNA for lymphoid lesions ranges from 5% to 15%, with low-grade lymphomas accounting for a significant percentage of the false-negative or indeterminate cases (14,15). The major strength of FNA in the workup of hematopoietic and lymphoid lesions is its high specificity (85% to 100%) even in extranodal sites. The diagnostic sensitivity of FNA in the initial workup of hematolymphoid lesions is enhanced when it is used in conjunction with FCM and/or needle core biopsy (16). A close interaction between cytopathologists and hematopathologists to coordinate the morphologic and immunophenotypic data is also required (7,8).

Cytologic Preparations for FNA Specimens

Aspirated material for evaluation of hematolymphoid lesions is first processed as direct smears, both air-dried and alcohol-fixed smears (Fig. 12.1). Air-dried smears are stained with a Romanowsky method. In this respect, Diff-Quik (DQ) stain, which provides better assessment of background and cytoplasmic features, is preferred. Alcohol-fixed smears are best stained with Papanicolaou (Pap) stain, which is useful for assessing nuclear features. Hematoxylin and eosin (H&E) stain can also be used for fixed smears. Residual material is rinsed for preparation of liquid-based preparations (LBPs), such as ThinPrep (TP [Hologic Inc., Bedford, MA]) or SurePath (SP [BD Diagnostics, Burlington, NC]), or for the preparation of cell block (17). LBPs are preferably not used as the sole preparation type for FNA of suspected lymphoma because of artifactual aggregation and clumping of lymphoid cells (Fig. 12.2), but are best suited for immunocytochemistry (ICC) and molecular analyses.

FNA Technique and Triage

Superficial FNA, by palpation only, is usually performed using thin needles, generally 22 to 27 gauge, and most often 1 to 1.5 inch in length attached to a 5 or 10 mL disposable

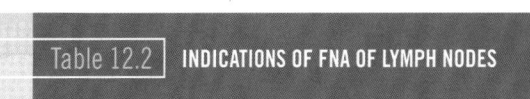 Table 12.1	REASONS FOR UNDERUTILIZATION OF FNA FOR HEMATOLYMPHOID LESIONS

- Relative ease of excisional biopsy
- Ignorance of terminologies and classification
- Limited experience
- Limited availability of cytopathologists
- Nonavailability of ancillary tests
- Lack of histologic architecture
- Morphologic difficulty in distinguishing reactive and low-grade lymphomas

Table 12.2	INDICATIONS OF FNA OF LYMPH NODES

- Distinguish between benign and neoplastic lesions
- Diagnosis of infection and to obtain material for bacterial or fungal cultures
- Confirmation of suspected metastases
- Diagnosis of hematolymphoid lesions and to obtain ancillary studies
- Document disease extent, relapse, progression, or transformation of hematolymphoid neoplasm
- Monitor effects of therapy in hematolymphoid neoplasms

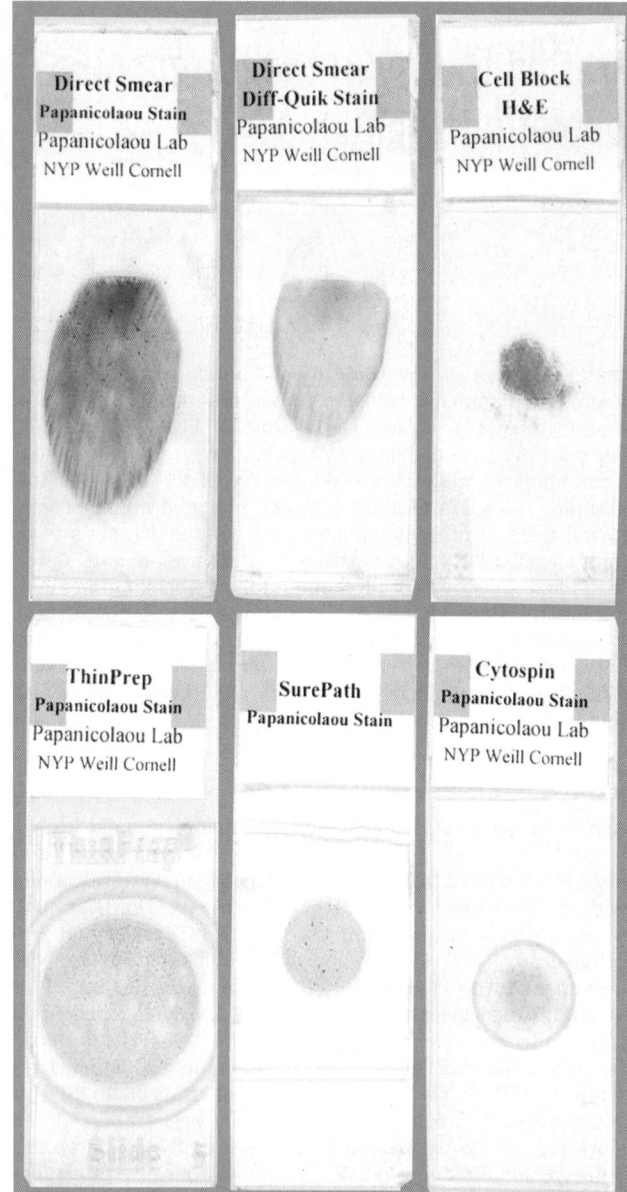

FIGURE 12.1. Gross appearance of various types of cytologic preparations. (Top row from left to right) Diff-Quik (DQ)-stained direct smear (DS), Papanicolaou (Pap)-stained DS, hematoxylin and eosin (H&E)-stained cell block section; **(bottom row from left to right)** ThinPrep (TP [20 mm diameter circle]), SurePath (SP [13 mm diameter circle]), and cytospin (CS [12 mm diameter circle]).

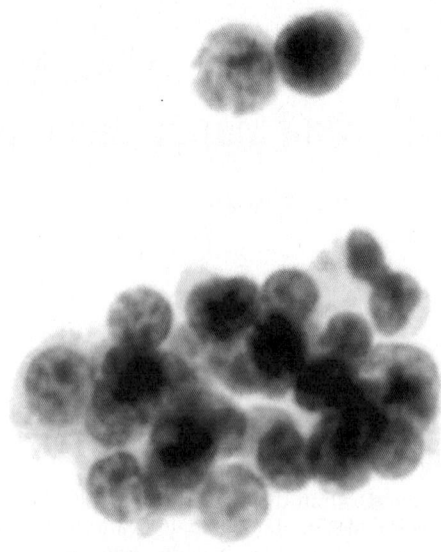

FIGURE 12.2. Both liquid-based techniques, TP and SP, produce artificial aggregations of lymphocytes that may be mistaken for epithelial cells (Pap stain, TP ×60 objective).

plastic syringe that may be placed on a Cameco aspiration gun. Shorter gauge needles or "butterfly" needles may be used for superficial subcutaneous lesions (18).

High-resolution ultrasound (US) technology is considered the "gold standard" for evaluation of superficially located targets. Pathologists are currently being trained and certified by the College of American Pathologists (CAP) in performing US-guided FNA (19). Image guidance enables anatomic localization of the target and its relationship to adjacent tissues. Specific features of the target including its size and shape can be visualized.

Suspected lymphomas of deep-seated organs are sampled by the help of radiologic techniques including computed tomography (CT) or endoscopic ultrasound (EUS) techniques. Transthoracic and transabdominal FNA are generally performed by radiologists with CT guidance using a 21- and 22-gauge Chiba needle (20,21). EUS-FNA is considered the procedure of choice for tissue sampling of abdominal and mediastinal nodes that may be difficult to reach by percutaneous CT guidance. EUS-FNA combined with FCM has a reported accuracy of 70% to 90% in the diagnosis of intrathoracic and intra-abdominal lymphoma (14,22,23). EUS also has the ability to obtain biopsy for histologic evaluation (14,23).

A cytologist should assess on-site adequacy at the time of FNA by the air-dried DQ-stained smears and perform proper specimen triage (24,25). When a hematolymphoid lesion is suspected, residual and additional specimen is rinsed in either a phosphate-buffered saline solution or RPMI (Roswell Park Memorial Institute) cell media for FCM. When an inflammatory/infectious etiology is suspected, microbiology studies can be obtained. Tables 12.3 to 12.5 outline the advantages and limitations of FNA.

Strategies of FNA Interpretation

Strategies for the evaluation of FNA of lymph nodes are outlined in Figure 12.3. Interpretive problems may result from improper FNA technique, faulty smearing technique, or lesional characteristics: (i) improper FNA technique fails to yield smears that are sufficiently cellular; (ii) faulty smearing

Table 12.3	ADVANTAGES OF SUPERFICIAL FNA

- Simple, easy, safe, rapid
- Cost-effective
- Noninvasive
- Preserves native lymph node architecture
- Ability to sample multiple lymph nodes
- Can be combined with FCM
- Fresh and pure tumor cells obtained for molecular tests
- Easily repeated allowing serial (pretherapy and posttherapy) sampling
- Complications are rare

Table 12.4	ADVANTAGES OF RADIOLOGICALLY GUIDED FNA

- Small or deep-seated targets can be sampled
- Nature of target (solid or cystic) can be assessed
- Reduced number of nondiagnostic biopsies, after on-site cytologic assessment of adequacy
- Follow-up of benign tumors for growth or change at defined intervals with US
- No ionizing radiation exposure with US
- Inability to subclassify lymphoma
- Loss of important architectural patterns
- Inability to reliably distinguish RHL from low-grade lymphomas
- Inability to reliably distinguish between various types of low-grade lymphoma
- False-negative results due to
  - Sampling error with inadequate sampling due to
    - Poor biopsy technique
    - Peripheral blood contamination
    - Marked nodal fibrosis
    - Partial involvement of lymph node by tumor
    - Extensive necrosis or inflammation
  - Interpretive errors
    - Faulty smearing techniques
    - Paucity of diagnostic cells such as Reed-Sternberg cells
- Rare, post-FNA changes in lymph nodes that may occur and interfere with histologic assessment
  - Total infarction
  - Hemorrhage
  - Granulation tissue

Table 12.5	LIMITATIONS OF FNAB

- Inability to subclassify lymphoma
- Loss of important architectural patterns
- Inability to reliably distinguish RHL from low-grade lymphomas
- Inability to reliably distinguish between various types of low-grade lymphoma
- False-negative results due to
  - Sampling error with inadequate sampling due to[a]
    - Poor biopsy technique
    - Peripheral blood contamination
    - Marked nodal fibrosis
    - Partial involvement of lymph node by tumor
    - Extensive necrosis or inflammation
  - Interpretive errors
    - Faulty smearing techniques
    - Paucity of diagnostic cells such as Reed-Sternberg cells
- Rare, post-FNA changes in lymph nodes that may occur and interfere with histologic assessment
  - Total infarction
  - Hemorrhage
  - Granulation tissue

[a]Three or more passes with sampling from different parts of the lesion or lymph node will reduce sampling error. Sampling error may be reduced with the use of US guidance.

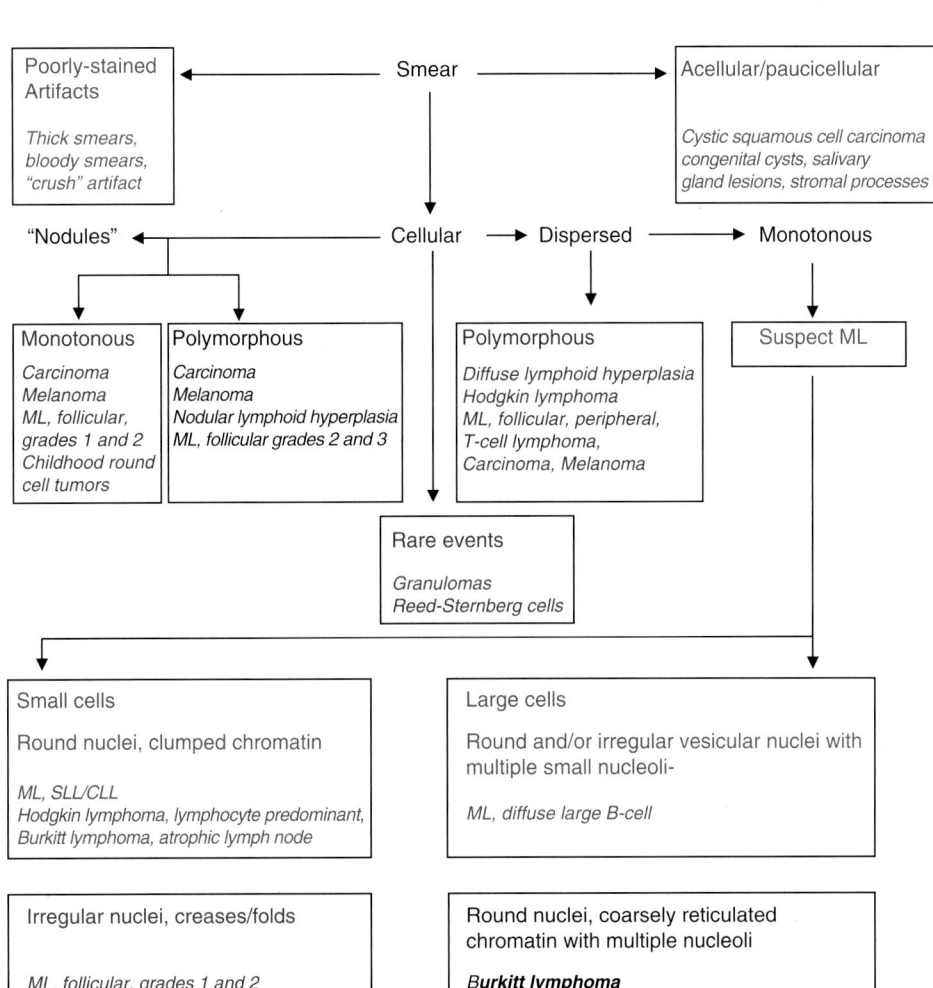

FIGURE 12.3. Strategies of FNA interpretation.

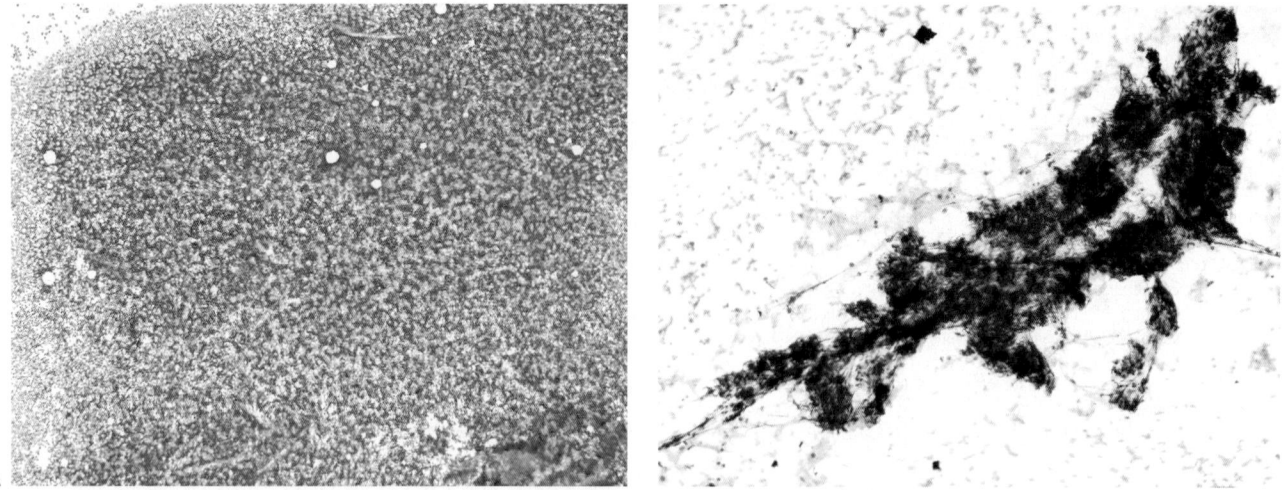

FIGURE 12.4. Technical issues with lymph node aspirate preparation. A: A smear preparation with unevenly distributed cellular material that is too concentrated for proper staining. **B:** Excessive pressure during smear preparation showing "crush" artifact (**A** and **B**, DQ stain, DS ×20 objective).

technique can result in concentration of the cellular material, resulting in poorly stained smears (Fig. 12.4A) or excessive pressure during smear preparation may result in "crush" artifact (Fig. 12.4B); or (iii) lesional characteristics—centrally necrotic masses are best sampled at the periphery or it may result in adequate sampling. Some lymphoid neoplasms are associated with marked sclerosis, such as nodular sclerosing Hodgkin lymphoma (NSCHL), and may yield paucicellular samples (26,27).

Histologic evaluation of hematolymphoid processes is based on interpretation of architectural and cellular patterns that provide important clues in interpretation. Adopting the histopathologic approach to cytologic evaluation of lymph nodes enables the cytopathologist to discern vague architectural patterns on scanning magnification. Small cellular aggregates or dispersed cells pattern can be identified (Fig. 12.5A and B). Lymph nodes that display cellular patterns of an admixture of small, medium-sized, and large lymphocytes (polymorphous population) in addition to tingible body macrophages and histiocytes are usually associated with benign or reactive conditions (Fig. 12.6A–C).

In contrast, a monotonous or monomorphous cell population generally implies a malignant condition (Fig. 12.7A–C). Several exceptions to this rule exist including HL and lymphoma with a high content of epithelioid histiocytes that may show polymorphous cells (Fig. 12.7D). Monotony in a lymph node aspirate also does not always indicate lymphoma. Carcinomas may appear discohesive and monotonous (Fig. 12.8). Examination of cytologic features at high magnification allows further separation into monomorphous and polymorphous lymphoid cell populations (Fig. 12.9A and B).

Proliferative and apoptotic indices may also be used on FNA samples for subclassification and histologic grading of B-cell NHL (28,29). An increase in the mean Ki-67 proliferation index has been reported with tumor aggressiveness. The Ki-67 median percentages of 15% for indolent lymphomas and 50% for aggressive lymphomas have been reported that show good correlation with histologic samples (Fig. 12.9C) (28). Apoptotic index may be incorporated with other cytomorphologic criteria. An apoptotic index of more than 3.5% may indicate a high-grade lymphoma (Fig. 12.9D) (29).

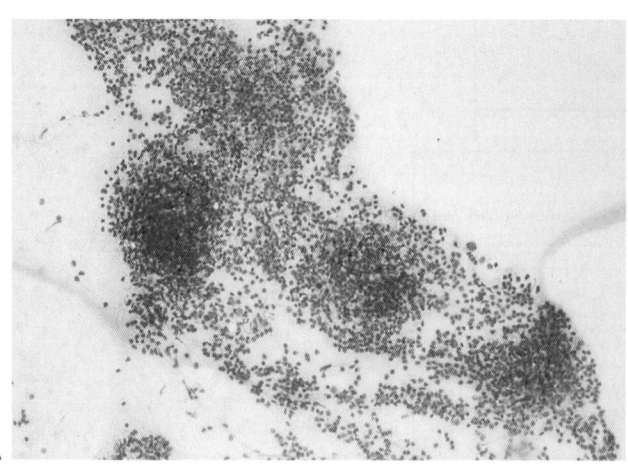

FIGURE 12.5. Architectural patterns on scanning magnification on cytologic smears. A: Small nodular aggregates indicating lymphoid follicles in reactive follicular hyperplasia. **B:** A dispersed cell pattern from a reactive lymph node (**A** and **B**, DQ stain, DS ×20 objective).

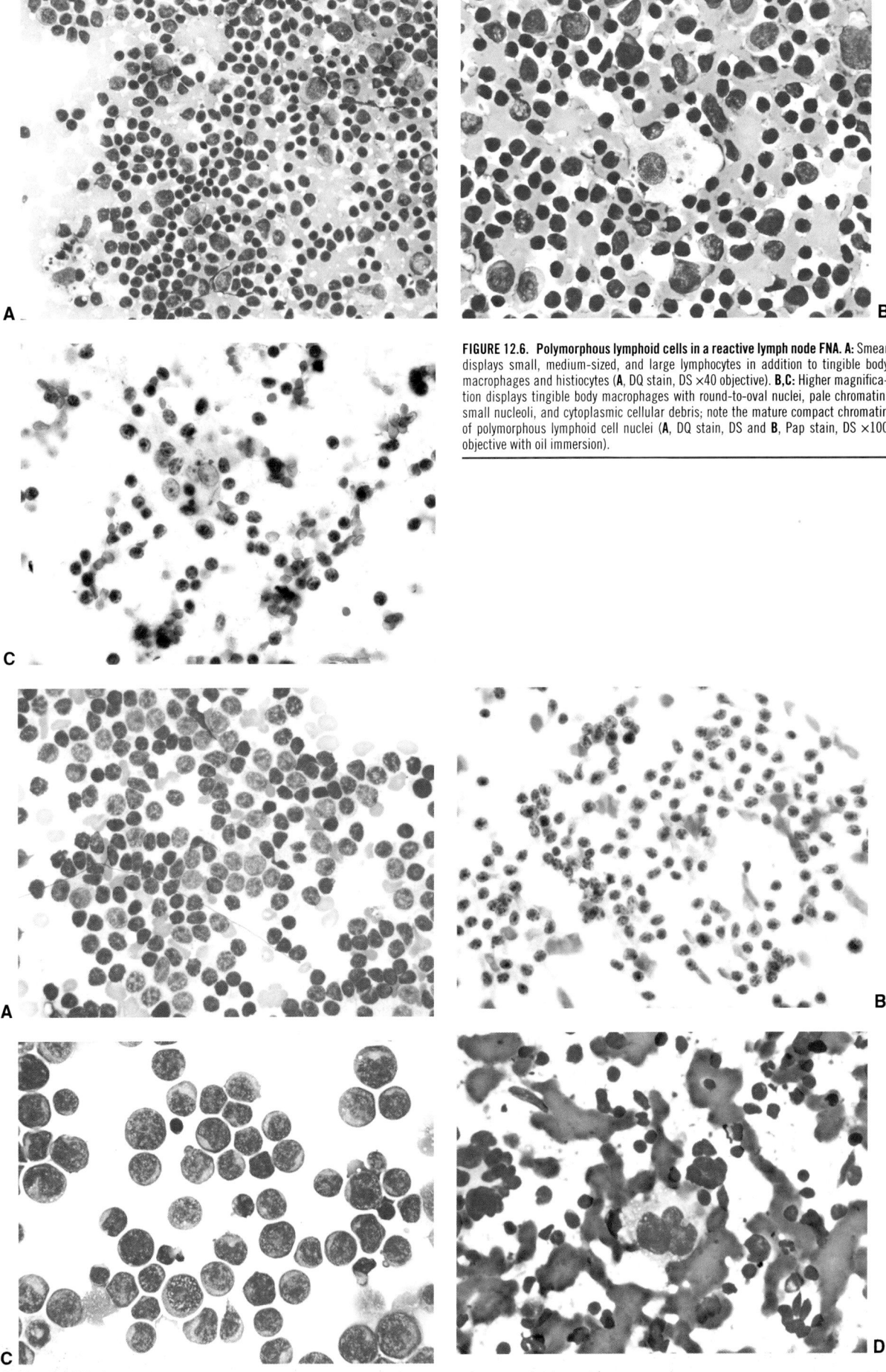

FIGURE 12.6. Polymorphous lymphoid cells in a reactive lymph node FNA. A: Smear displays small, medium-sized, and large lymphocytes in addition to tingible body macrophages and histiocytes (**A**, DQ stain, DS ×40 objective). **B,C:** Higher magnification displays tingible body macrophages with round-to-oval nuclei, pale chromatin, small nucleoli, and cytoplasmic cellular debris; note the mature compact chromatin of polymorphous lymphoid cell nuclei (**A**, DQ stain, DS and **B**, Pap stain, DS ×100 objective with oil immersion).

FIGURE 12.7. Nature of lymphoid cells in lymphoma. A,B: Smear from CLL depicts a monotonous small cell population that generally implies malignancy. Compare the size of neoplastic lymphoid cells with red blood cells (RBCs [**A**, DQ stain, DS and **B**, Pap stain, DS ×60 objective]). **C:** Smear from a case of DLBCL displaying monotonous population of large neoplastic lymphoid cells. Compare the nuclear size with scattered benign lymphoid cells (DQ stain, DS ×100 objective with oil immersion). **D:** HL and lymphoma with a high content of epithelioid histiocytes that may show polymorphous cells (DQ stain, DS ×60 objective).

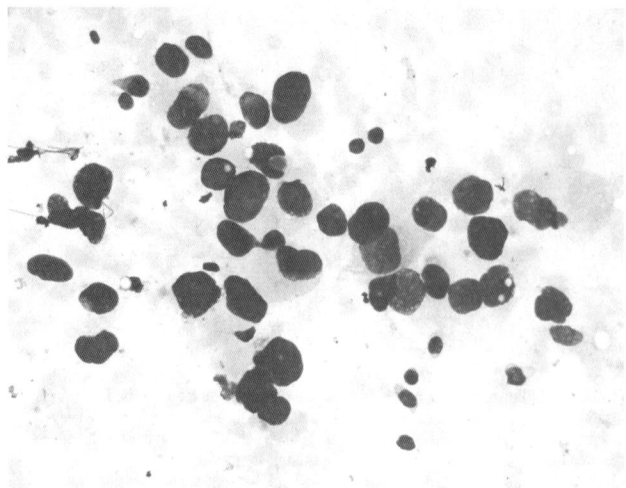

FIGURE 12.8. Occasionally, carcinomas may appear discohesive and monotonous. In this case of metastatic urothelial carcinoma in lung, the smear shows monomorphic epithelial cells. Clinical history, review of urothelial carcinoma histology, and a cercariform cell (11 o'clock position) provide a helpful clue to the primary malignancy (DQ stain, DS ×60 objective).

ANCILLARY METHODS FOR DIAGNOSIS OF HEMATOPOIETIC AND LYMPHOID LESIONS

The success of FNA in the diagnosis of hematolymphoid lesions relies on adopting a multidisciplinary approach, that is, analyzing cytomorphology, ICC, and FCM (2–8,27,30–35). Molecular studies further enhance diagnostic sensitivity and specificity of FNA (36).

Immunochemistry

The application of ICC has enhanced the ability to diagnose and classify lymphomas. ICC can be successfully applied to FNA specimens. ICC is preferable in those cases where FCM has a high false-negative rate such as large cell lymphomas, HL, and metastases (37,38). An abbreviated antibody panel including leukocyte common antigen (CD45), cytokeratin (AE1/AE3), and S-100 protein can be applied initially. In suspected hematolymphoid lesions, an expanded battery of monoclonal antibodies can be employed including CD20, CD79a, and PAX5 (markers for B-cell lymphoma) (Figs. 12.9C and 12.10A and B). The presence of

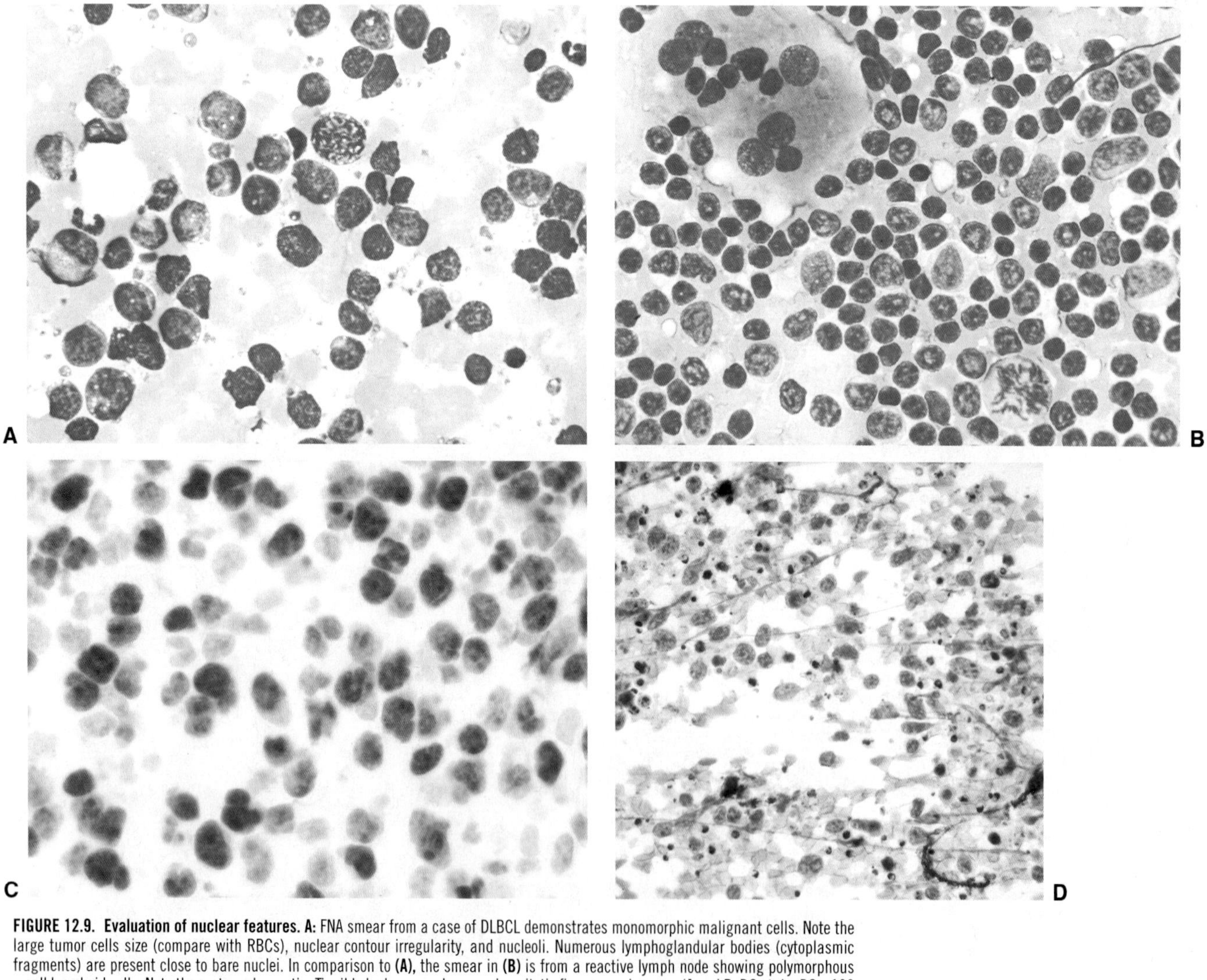

FIGURE 12.9. Evaluation of nuclear features. A: FNA smear from a case of DLBCL demonstrates monomorphic malignant cells. Note the large tumor cells size (compare with RBCs), nuclear contour irregularity, and nucleoli. Numerous lymphoglandular bodies (cytoplasmic fragments) are present close to bare nuclei. In comparison to **(A)**, the smear in **(B)** is from a reactive lymph node showing polymorphous small lymphoid cells. Note the mature chromatin. Tingible body macrophage and a mitotic figure are also seen (**A** and **B**, DQ stain, DS ×100 objective with oil immersion). **C:** Cells from a case of DLBCL showing a Ki-67 index of 100% (DS ×60 objective). **D:** Increased apoptosis from a case of a high-grade lymphoma (Pap stain, DS ×60 objective).

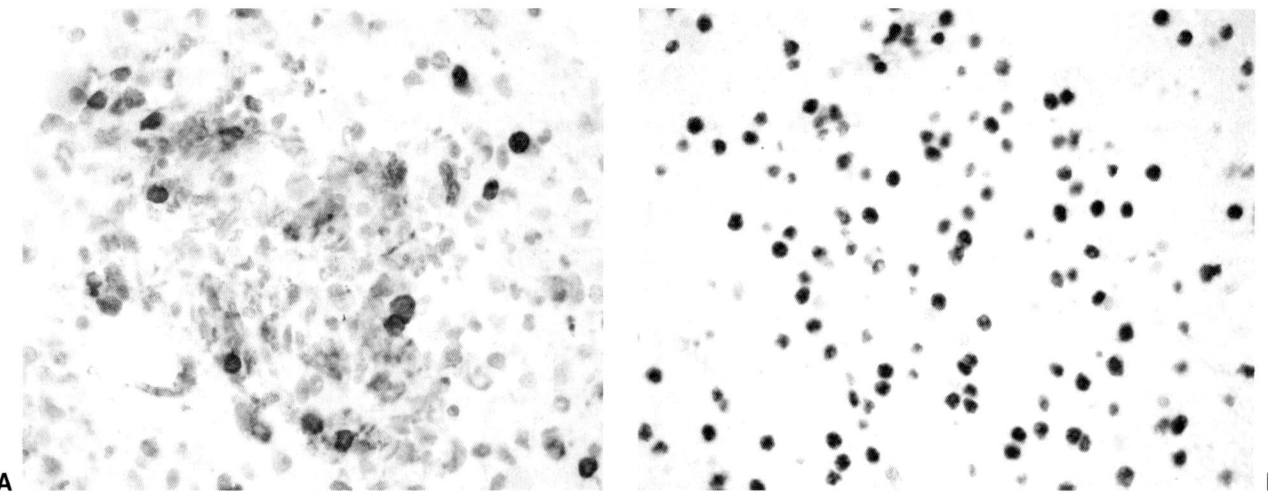

FIGURE 12.10. Immunocytochemistry. A: Cytoplasmic positivity for CD45 in a case of DLBCL. **B:** Strong nuclear positivity for Pax5 in a case of CLL/SLL (DS ×60 objective).

light-chain restriction may be the most useful criterion for determining B-cell malignancy and can be applied to limited cytology sample or in cell block sections of adequate sample (31). Evaluation of antigen loss, crucial to the immunologic diagnosis of peripheral T-cell lymphoma (PTCL), may be more difficult to perform in FNA smears than in frozen sections, because assessment of antigen expression within specific regions of the lymph node is not possible. In cytology, ICC can be performed on additional LBP including TP or SP, cytospins, or cell block sections (37).

The advantages of ICC over FCM are the requirement of a small sample, preservation of cellular morphology, use in cases of large cell lymphomas where FCM may be falsely negative, and ability to assess staining pattern and intensity of staining. The disadvantage of ICC is that evaluation of double antigen expression (e.g., CD5/CD23 or CD10/BCL2) is not possible.

Flow Cytometry

Immunophenotyping by FCM in the diagnosis of lymphoma is performed for the detection of clonality, which distinguishes lymphoma from reactive lymphoid hyperplasia (RLH). The utility of FNA in conjunction with FCM for definitive diagnosis of NHL is well documented (2,4,7,9,13,30,39–42). Several studies of FNA and FCM have used the REAL/WHO classification system for diagnosis and subclassification of NHL. Meda et al. (2) evaluated 290 aspirates from 275 patients. A definitive diagnosis of NHL was made in 76.7% on the basis of FNA and FCM, which resulted in a sensitivity of 95% and specificity of 85%. Dong et al. (4) diagnosed 67% of primary and recurrent lymphomas using FNA combined with FCM. In another reported series, all 74 cases of lymphoma on FNA were correctly diagnosed (9). In this study, correct classification was more accurate in 53 cases that were also subjected to concurrent FCM (84% vs. 33%). These studies indicate the importance of using FNA

Table 12.6	**FALSE-NEGATIVE FLOW CYTOMETRY**

- Sampling error
- Partial involvement of lymph node by disease
- Insufficient number of neoplastic cells
- Few viable cells
- Peripheral blood contamination
- Large cell lymphoma
- Primary T-cell lymphoma

in conjunction with FCM for diagnosis and subclassification of lymphoma.

FCM is sensitive, provides quantitative results, and can detect a small abnormal cell population in a reactive background. FCM has the advantages of multiparametric analysis and objective interpretation. The panel of antibodies utilized in FCM depends on the amount of FNA material provided. The use of an FCM panel comprising of B- and T-cell counts, kappa and lambda, CD4/CD8 ratio, and proliferation index is effective in detection of NHL subtypes and distinguishing them from RLH. The ability to distinguish between monotypic and polytypic lymphoid cell population is considered a major advantage of FCM.

The overall accuracy for diagnosis and subclassification of B-cell lymphomas by FCM performed on FNA samples is reported to be 88.4% with a sensitivity of 86% and specificity of 93% (39). Similar concordance (88%) has been reported for FCM performed from excised tissue and subsequent histopathologic diagnoses (2,4,9,10). The sensitivity of FCM for T-cell NHL is poor and reported to be 36.4% (39).

FCM may be false negative in large cell NHL and HL. However, the cellular abnormalities in these lesions are easily appreciated on FNA smears and should prompt additional diagnostic studies. FCM may be misinterpreted as polyclonal due to a small fraction of tumor compared to a prominent component of benign/reactive lymphocytes such as in T-cell lymphomas. When cellularity is limited because of fibrosis, extensive necrosis, or cellular damage, FCM results may be inconclusive (Table 12.6) (2,40).

Molecular Analyses

Molecular analyses in the diagnosis of lymphoma are performed for the detection of genetic abnormalities such as translocations, deletions or aneuploidy, and gene rearrangement. Sufficient DNA and RNA may be obtained from FNA-derived material for analysis by polymerase chain reaction (PCR), or fluorescence *in situ* hybridization (FISH) and nucleic acid microarrays/gene profiling techniques. For molecular analyses, specimen can be directly collected into RNA-preserving or extracting solutions or in PreservCyt solution (cell collection and preservation medium for TP [Hologic Inc., Bedford, MA]) that retains both cytologic features and RNA for assessment (36,43,44). These techniques can also be applied to archival cytologic material (TP, alcohol-fixed or formalin-fixed, paraffin-embedded). The results are comparable to those in excision biopsies (36). DNA obtained from FNA samples may be analyzed by PCR for the presence of specific chromosomal translocations, viral genomes, activated or amplified oncogenes, and gene rearrangements. For example, detection of t(14;18) (q32;q21) on PCR may provide evidence of a follicular lymphoma (FL) and t(11;14)(q13;q32) evidence for mantle cell lymphoma (MCL) (36,43). In addition, PCR studies on cytology specimens may be used to determine viral load in patients infected with HIV. The pattern of gene rearrangements obtained on analysis of DNA from FNA cytology specimens is comparable to that obtained on excised lymph nodes (30). In an appropriate sample, interphase FISH can exploit intact interphase nuclei and detect structural and numerical chromosomal abnormalities (36,43). DNA microarrays can rapidly provide information on many genes at the mRNA level. It has been possible to use amplified RNA from small FNA samples for gene expression profiling in combination with morphology and immunophenotyping for subtyping of diffuse large B-cell lymphoma (DLBCL). The amount of RNA recovered from FNA has been shown to be comparable to that from a core biopsy (36,41).

NON-HODGKIN LYMPHOMA

Cytologic subclassification of NHL, particularly of small mature B-cell lymphomas, is controversial and underutilized (2,7,9–11). However, FNA in combination with ancillary tests including ICC, FCM, and/or molecular analyses can be used in the evaluation of NHL (2,4,7,9,13,27,30,36–44). Ninety percent of NHLs are B-cell type, with more than half representing either DLBCL or FL. Some lymphomas have characteristic cytologic appearances, and it may be possible in these cases to render a diagnosis of lymphoma based on cytomorphology alone, at least in general terms. On FNA of most NHL, a monotonous lymphoid cell population with uniform nuclear size and chromatin is evident (Figs. 12.7A–C and 12.9A). Once the monotony

FIGURE 12.11. An algorithmic approach to evaluating FNA of lymph nodes.

of the lymphoid population is appreciated, the initial subclassification into small and large lymphoid cells requires the comparison of the suspect neoplastic lymphoid cells to typical small mature lymphocytes, red blood cells, plasma cells (PCs), or histiocytes (Figs. 12.7A–C and 12.9A). Nuclei of histiocytes can be used as an internal reference to assess the relative size of the lymphoid cells and separate them into small- and large cell types (Figs. 12.6B, C and 12.9B). Careful evaluation of nuclear features including contour, chromatin pattern, and nucleolus aids in further subclassifying lymphoid cells on cytology (Figs. 12.6B, C, 12.7C, and 12.9A and B) (26,27).

DIAGNOSTIC CATEGORIES OF FNA FOR HEMATOPOIETIC LESIONS

Cytologic diagnostic categories for FNA of hematopoietic and lymphoid neoplasms include "atypical lymphoproliferative lesion," "atypical lymphoid infiltrate," "suspicious for lymphoma," "malignant lymphoma," or "B-cell lymphoma" (the latter, if immunophenotyping has been performed) (7,25). Figure 12.11 outlines an algorithmic approach to evaluating FNA of lymph nodes for appropriate diagnostic categorization.

B-Cell Neoplasms

Lymphoblastic Lymphoma

Lymphoblastic lymphoma (LBL) is of either precursor B- or T-cell differentiation (Table 12.7). It is discussed in the T-Cell and Natural Killer-Cell Lymphoma section.

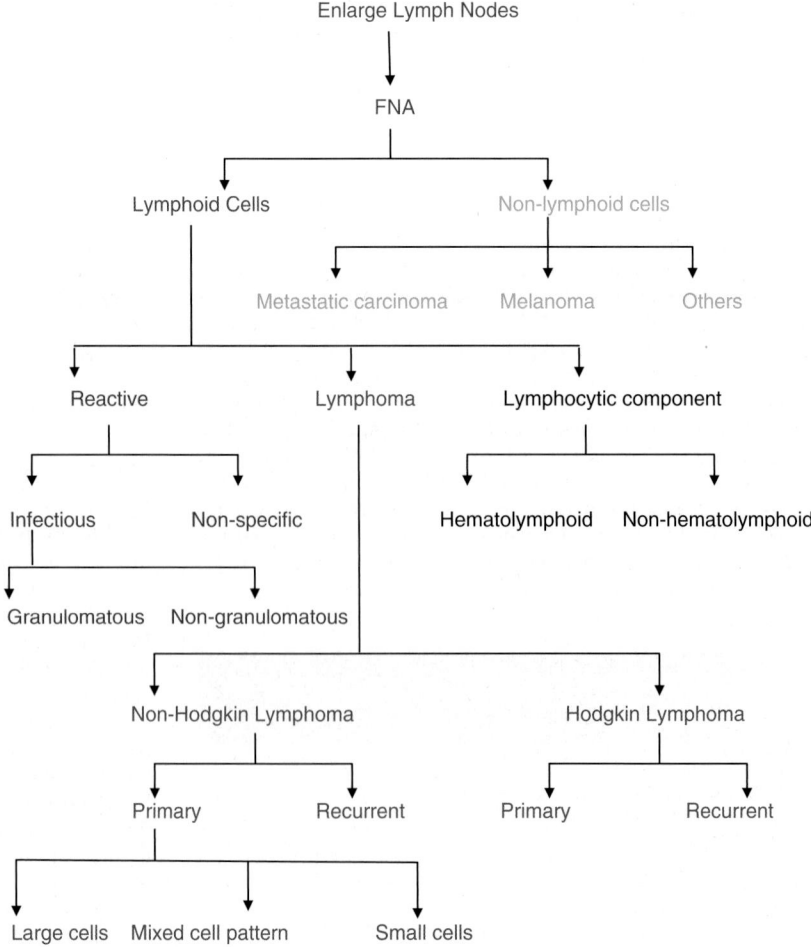

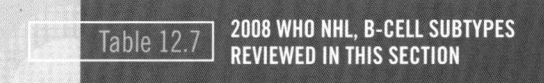

Table 12.7	2008 WHO NHL, B-CELL SUBTYPES REVIEWED IN THIS SECTION

- Precursor B-cell lymphoblastic lymphoma
- Mature B-cell neoplasms
  - *SLL*
    - CLL/SLL
    - LPL
    - Plasmacytoma
    - Extranodal MZL of MALTtype
    - N-MZL
    - FL
    - MCL
  - *Aggressive B-cell lymphomas*
    - DLBCL, not otherwise specified
    - PBL
    - BL

Mature B-cell Neoplasms

Chronic Lymphocytic Leukemia/ Small Lymphocytic Lymphoma

Key Cytologic Features
- Monomorphic small lymphocytes
- Regular round nuclei, clumped chromatin, small to inconspicuous nucleoli
- Scant cytoplasm
- Promyelocytes and paraimmunoblasts

Clinical Features. Chronic lymphocytic leukemia/small lymphocytic lymphoma (CLL/SLL) is a B-cell neoplasm that constitutes about 5% of all NHLs. SLL is regarded as a tissue manifestation of B-cell CLL and often involves lymph nodes. It predominantly occurs in older adults and is more common in men. Patients are usually asymptomatic, but anemia, hepatosplenomegaly, and generalized lymphadenopathy may be present. Patients also have peripheral blood and bone marrow involvement at the time of presentation. Although CLL/SLL is an indolent lymphoma, approximately 5% of cases can transform to a higher-grade lymphoma clinically referred to as Richter syndrome or transformation. FNA can be used to evaluate patients with a history of CLL/SLL who are subsequently clinically suspected of having the Richter syndrome (45).

Cytology. In CLL/SLL, a predominantly dispersed cell pattern of homogenous population of small lymphocytes that are the same size or slightly larger than a small, mature lymphocyte is evident on smears. The nuclei are round and regular or slightly irregular, with clumped chromatin, small to inconspicuous nucleoli, and scant pale to slightly basophilic cytoplasm (Fig. 12.12A and B). Occasionally, larger lymphocytes representing prolymphocytes and paraimmunoblasts are noted (Fig. 12.12C). These cells have centrally placed smooth nuclei and abundant pale cytoplasm. The prolymphocytes display single and central nucleoli while the paraimmunoblasts contain either multiple, peripherally located nucleoli or a single prominent nucleolus. Mitoses are rare and tingible body macrophages or lymphohistiocytic aggregates are not seen.

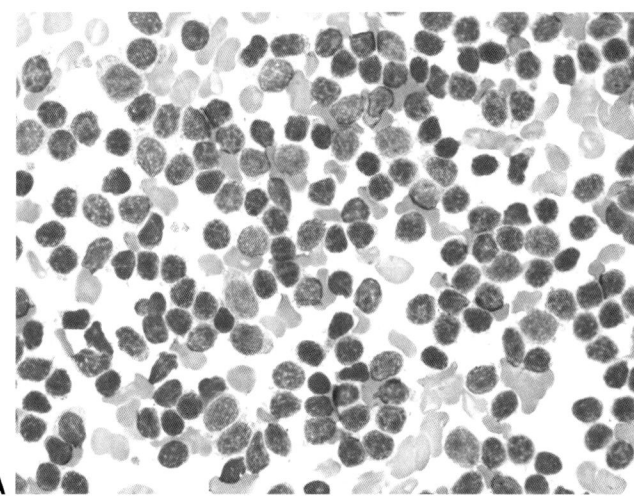

A

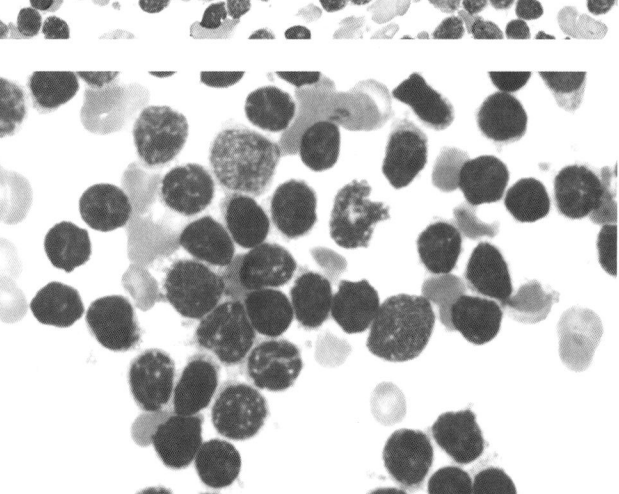

C

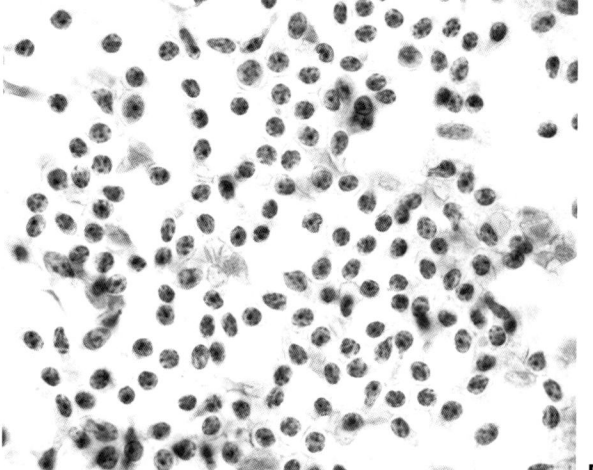

B

FIGURE 12.12. Chronic lymphocytic leukemia/small lymphocytic lymphoma. A,B: Homogenous population of small lymphocytes (slightly larger than RBCs) is evident on smears (**A**, DQ stain, DS and **B**, Pap stain, DS ×60 objective). **C:** Nuclei are round and slightly irregular with coarse clumped chromatin, small-to-inconspicuous nucleoli, and scant basophilic cytoplasm (**C**, DQ stain DS ×100 objective with oil immersion).

Tingible (stainable) bodies are the phagocytosed apoptotic cells and cell debris in the macrophage cytoplasm. In cases of Richter syndrome, there are large numbers of blastic cells with round nuclei with vesicular chromatin and prominent nucleoli and scant basophilic cytoplasm (2,15).

Phenotype. Positive for CD5, CD23, and Pax5 (Fig. 12.10B) and negative for CD10, FMC-7, and CD79b. CD20 and surface immunoglobulin (sIg), light-chain expression are typically dim. The proliferation index is usually low (<10%) with proliferation marker Ki-67. A proliferation index of >30% may indicate transformation (42). A newer marker LEF-1 is positive in approximately 100% of CLL/SLL (46). A subset of DLBCL and grade 3 FL are also positive for LEF-1 (46).

Cytogenetics. Deletion 13q14 (50%), deletion 11q (20%), and trisomy 12 (10% to 15%). 17p deletion is associated with disease progression and increased risk of death and is treated differently (47).

Differential Diagnosis. Reactive lymphadenitis and other mature SLLs and large cell lymphomas when there is Richter transformation.

Lymphoplasmacytic Lymphoma

Key Cytologic Features
- Small lymphocytes
- Plasmacytoid lymphocytes
- Mature PCs with Dutcher and Russell bodies
- Mast cells
- Epithelioid histiocytes

Clinical Features. Lymphoplasmacytic lymphoma (LPL) is an uncommon low-grade B-cell malignancy comprising <2% of all NHL. The disease affects older men. LPL usually presents with bone marrow involvement, splenomegaly, and generalized lymphadenopathy. The clinical course is generally indolent, but transformation to large cell lymphoma occurs in 5% to 10% of cases (48).

Cytology. Smears depict a mixed population of small lymphocytes (similar to CLL/SLL) and plasmacytoid lymphocytes. The latter have eccentric nuclei with coarse chromatin and inconspicuous nucleoli. The chromatin, however, is lymphocyte-like and does not demonstrate the "cartwheel" pattern as seen in PCs. Cytoplasm is moderate and basophilic with occasional paranuclear "hof" (large Golgi zone) (Fig. 12.13). Mature PCs containing Russell bodies (cytoplasmic globular eosinophilic immunoglobulin inclusions) and Dutcher bodies (intranuclear immunoglobulin inclusions) are also seen. Occasional multinucleated cells may be present. Mitoses are rare. Increased mast cells and epithelioid histiocytes may be seen (15,49,50).

Phenotype. Positive for CD20, Ig light chains, and IgM and usually positive for BCL2 and negative for CD5 (usually), CD10, CD23, Cyclin D1, and BCL6. Lymphoplasmacytoid cells are positive for CD38, and mature PCs are positive for CD38 and CD138.

Cytogenetics. Lacks a distinct molecular genetic hallmark. Deletion of 6q21-q23, a nonspecific finding, is the most common aberration reported in 40% to 70% of patients (50).

Differential Diagnosis. Distinguishing the LPL from other small cell lymphomas, especially marginal zone lymphoma (MZL) with plasmacytic differentiation, may be problematic. PC neoplasms are also in the differential (50).

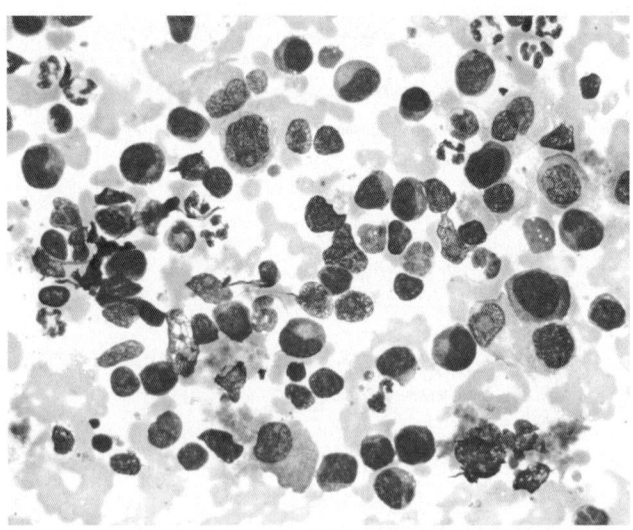

FIGURE 12.13. Lymphoplasmacytic lymphoma. Small lymphocytes (similar to CLL/SLL) and plasmacytoid lymphocytes. The latter has eccentric nuclei, lymphocyte-like coarse chromatin, and inconspicuous nucleoli. Cytoplasm shows occasional paranuclear "hof" (DQ stain, DS ×60 objective).

Plasmacytoma

Key Cytologic Features
- Mature and immature PCs
  - Eccentric nuclei, "cartwheel" chromatin
  - Basophilic cytoplasm, perinuclear "hof"
  - Some binucleated cells
- Dutcher bodies and Russell bodies
- Mitosis
- Amyloid
- Blastic morphology in plasmablastic form
- Anaplastic morphology in anaplastic form

Clinical Features. PC neoplasms encompass clonal PC proliferations with a wide range of clinical manifestations and behavior. In most cases, PC neoplasms are associated with the production of a monoclonal immunoglobulin, or M protein which is detectable in the serum and urine. PC neoplasms constitute approximately 15% of all hematopoietic neoplasms and are rare before the age of 40. Plasmacytoma is a neoplasm of mature and immature PCs that presents as a discrete tumor mass. They can be multiple osteolytic tumors (multiple myeloma [MM]) or solitary. Solitary or extramedullary plasmacytomas (EMPs) are rare, constituting approximately 3% to 5% of all plasma cell neoplasms (PCN) and have no associated bone marrow or systemic disease. EMP can occur in any organ; however, approximately 90% are found in the head and neck region involving the upper aerodigestive tract. EMP may also present as a metastatic deposit from another soft tissue plasmacytoma or as a consequence of MM. Primary plasmacytoma of lymph nodes is uncommon, and metastasis should be excluded before making this diagnosis (51,52).

Cytology. Smears are dominated by PCs, with varying degrees of maturity. These cells are arranged singly and in sheets and clusters. The mature PCs show monomorphic round and eccentric nuclei with condensed "cartwheel" chromatin and indistinct nucleoli. Cytoplasm is abundant and basophilic and shows a perinuclear "hof." Binucleated cells are usually present (Fig. 12.14A and B). The plasmablastic form has a more blastic morphology with enlarged nuclei and bi- or multinucleation, open chromatin structure, prominent nucleoli, higher N:C ratio, and bare nuclei. Anaplastic plasmacytomas may

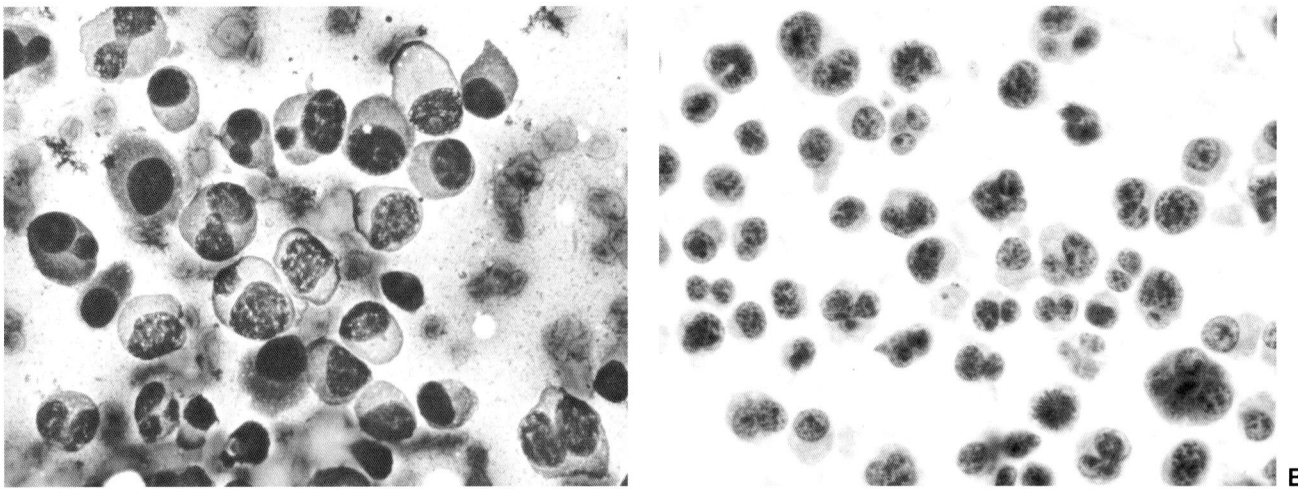

FIGURE 12.14. Plasmacytoma. A,B: PCs with varying degrees of maturity. Mature PCs show condensed "cartwheel" chromatin. Occasional binucleated forms are seen. Note the crisp nuclear features in the Pap-stained smear (**A**, DQ stain, DS and **B**, Pap stain, DS ×100 objective with oil immersion).

show considerable pleomorphism and need to be differentiated from DLBCL. Tumor cells may contain Dutcher bodies and Russell bodies. Mitotic rate is high in the pleomorphic types. Extracellular eosinophilic material representing amyloid may be seen in some cases and will show apple-green birefringence with Congo red stain on polarizing light microscopy (51,52).

Phenotype. PCs lose many of the surface markers of mature B cells and are frequently negative for CD45 and CD20, but usually express CD79a, CD38, and CD138. The tumor cells synthesize Ig, most commonly of IgA and IgG isotype and show light-chain restriction.

Cytogenetics. Translocations involving Ig genes. Many involve the switch region of the immunoglobulin heavy chain gene, consistent with the expression of IgA or IgG. The t(11;14)(q13;q32) occurs in 25% to 30% of myelomas, leading to overexpression of cyclin D1.

Differential Diagnosis. MZL and LPL, both of which may have evidence of plasmacytic differentiation, should be considered in the differential diagnosis of PCN. Ancillary tests usually help with this differential. Reactive plasmacytosis is composed of a polymorphous collection of PCs and other inflammatory cells.

Marginal Zone B-Cell Lymphoma

Key Cytologic Features
- Nodal MZL (N-MZL) and extranodal MZL of mucosa-associated lymphoid tissue (MALT lymphoma) are cytologically similar
- Heterogeneous lymphoid cells
  - Monocytoid B cells
  - Small-to-intermediate centrocyte-like cells
- Plasmacytoid cells (especially in MALT lymphoma)
- Occasional immunoblasts
- Few PCs
- Occasional tingible body macrophages and lymphohistiocytic aggregates
- Rare mitoses

Clinical Features. MZL is a low-grade indolent B-cell lymphoma that is derived from monocytoid B cells. It is divided into two types, extranodal MZL (MALT lymphoma) and N-MZL. Both

types are morphologically and immunophenotypically similar. N-MZL is rare and has no extranodal or splenic disease.

MALT lymphoma constitutes 7% to 8% of all B-cell lymphomas and is more common in older women, but may also occur in children. Up to half involve the gastrointestinal tract, with stomach being the most frequent site. However, other sites, not usually thought of as mucosa associated, can also be involved including salivary glands, thyroid, lung, breast, and urinary bladder. Most MALT lymphomas are associated with a predisposing infectious or autoimmune condition, such as *Helicobacter pylori*–associated chronic gastritis, Hashimoto thyroiditis, and Sjögren Syndrome (50).

Cytology. Smears show a dispersed cell pattern comprising of various proportions of lymphocytes with monocytoid B cells and small-to-intermediate cells with centrocyte-like morphology. The monocytoid B cells are medium-sized lymphoid cells with round, reniform, or indented nuclei, with condensed chromatin and small indistinct nucleoli. Cytoplasm may be scant to abundant, and pale staining or clear. Small- to intermediate-sized lymphoid cells contain slightly irregular nuclei and small nucleoli and are thus centrocyte-like (Fig. 12.15A and B). Plasmacytoid cells, scattered immunoblasts, and monoclonal PCs are also seen. The latter are most common in the MALT type. Lymphohistiocytic aggregates are common, while tingible body macrophages may be seen in some cases. Mitoses are rare. MZLs can transform to DLBCL in about 10% of the cases (53–55).

Phenotype. Positive for CD19, CD20, CD79a (Fig. 12.15C), and bcl-2 and negative for CD5, CD10, CD23, BCL6, and cyclin D1. A subset is also positive for IgD (53).

Cytogenetics. t(11;18) is seen in up to one third of low-grade extranodal MZL and trisomy 3 has been described in both nodal and extranodal MZL (50).

Differential Diagnosis. Reactive lymphocyte proliferation and other small B-cell lymphomas should be considered in the differential diagnosis. Cytomorphology, specific phenotypic, and genetic features, such as absence of coexpression of CD19/CD5, seen in SLL/CLL and MCL, cyclin D1 expression in MCL, CD10 expression in FL, and the characteristic t(14;18) translocation involving the BCL2 locus in FL and the t(11;14) translocation in MCL may be helpful in this regard (53).

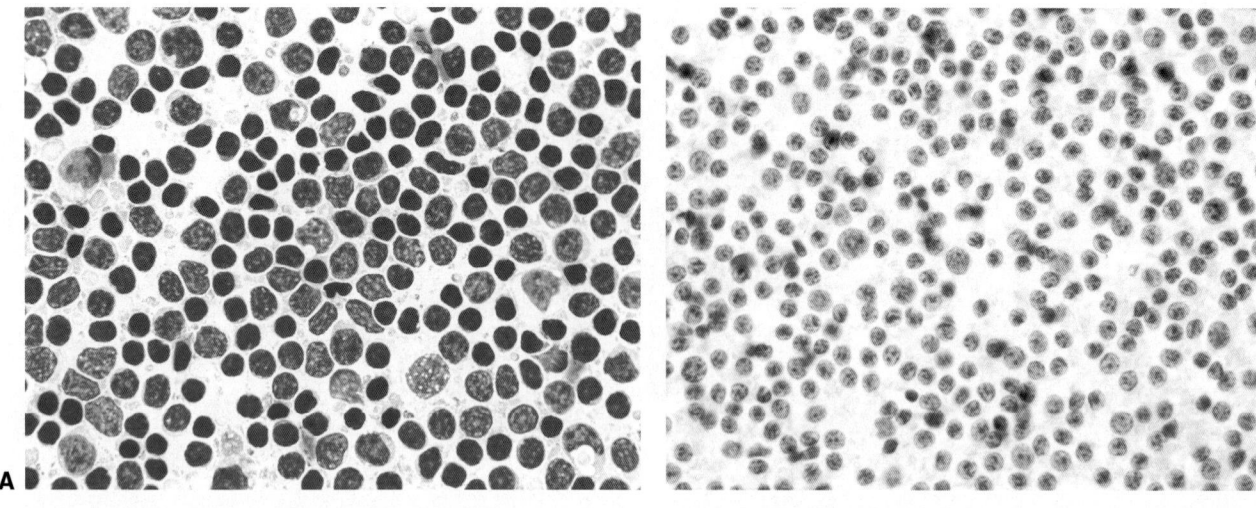

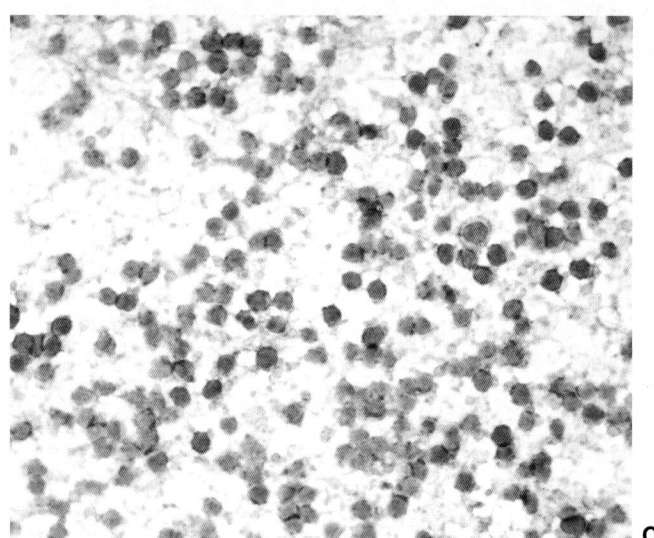

FIGURE 12.15. Nodal marginal zone lymphoma. A,B: Dispersed cell pattern comprising various proportions of lymphocytes with monocytoid B cells and small-to-intermediate cells with centrocyte-like morphology (**A**, DQ stain, DS ×100 objective with oil immersion and **B**, Pap stain, DS ×60 objective); **C:** Positive immunostain for CD20 (DS ×60 objective).

Follicular Lymphoma

Key Cytologic Features

- Polymorphous lymphoid cells with centrocytes and centroblasts
- Lymphoid cell aggregates in one third of cases
- Centrocytes (cleaved cells) predominate
- Approximately 10% centroblasts (large transformed noncleaved cells)
- Lymphoglandular bodies (cytoplasmic fragments of lymphocytes)
- Reactive T lymphocytes
- Increasing number of centroblasts with increasing grade
- Increased mitoses with increasing grade

Clinical Features. FL is a B-cell neoplasm of follicular center cell origin, comprising of two cell types found in normal germinal centers, centrocytes (cleaved cells), and centroblasts (large transformed noncleaved cells). It is a common form of NHL in adults and accounts for about 20% to 40% of cases. Median age at presentation is 55 years with equal sex incidence. The vast majority of cases present with advanced disseminated disease with spleen, bone marrow, and lymph node involvement (33,56,57). Transformation to an aggressive large B-cell lymphoma may occur in 25% to 30% and is associated with rapid progression (34,58).

The WHO recommends a three-tier grading system (grades 1 to 3) for FLs based on the absolute number of centroblasts per high-power microscopic field (hpf) in 10 neoplastic follicles on histology (34). Grades 1 and 2 FLs, often combined together, are indolent tumors and may not be treated, whereas grade 3 FLs are aggressive but potentially curable with chemotherapy. Since FL may also have a diffuse growth pattern both The WHO 2008 and REAL classifications also recommend that the degree of follicle formation (predominantly follicular, follicular, diffuse, and predominantly diffuse) should also be reported. Grade 1 has an average of <6, grade 2, 6 to 15, and grade 3 >15 centroblasts/hpf counted in 10 neoplastic follicles. This method of grading system has prognostic implications (34).

Cytology. On FNA smears, a loose follicular pattern or dense lymphoid aggregates suggest follicle formation in these lymphomas (Fig. 12.16A). Lymphoid cells are polymorphous and consist of two cell types, the centrocytes and centroblasts (Fig. 12.16B). The predominant cells are centrocytes. These are small- to intermediate-sized lymphocytes (slightly larger than benign lymphocytes) with cleaved nuclei with deep folds in the membrane, occasionally imparting a bilobed appearance. Chromatin is coarsely clumped and nucleoli are inconspicuous. Cytoplasm is scant and pale or lightly basophilic with poorly defined borders (Fig. 12.16C and D). The centroblasts, constituting about 10% of the cells, are large noncleaved lymphocytes (twice the size of benign lymphocytes), with round-to-oval nuclei, with occasional indentation. Chromatin is reticular and nucleoli may be single and central or multiple and peripheral. Cytoplasm is scant and dense basophilic or amphophilic. The nuclear membrane

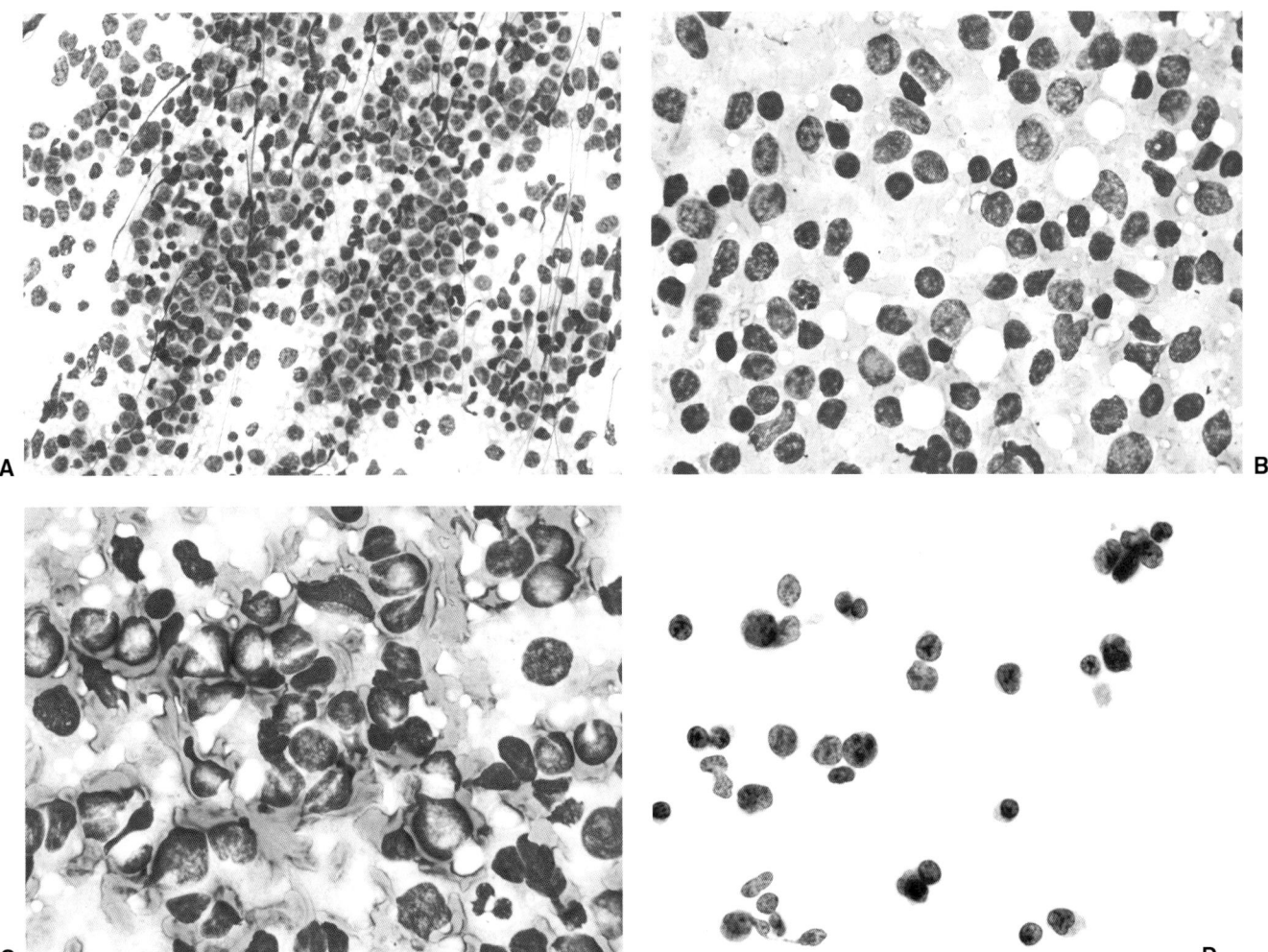

FIGURE 12.16. Follicular lymphoma. A: Loose clusters of small lymphoid cells indicating follicle formation (DQ stain, DS ×40 objective). **B:** Lymphoid cells are polymorphous with predominant centrocytes with occasional centroblasts (**B**, DQ stain, DS ×100 objective with oil immersion). **C,D:** Centrocytes are angulated or cleaved small lymphoid cells with deep nuclear folds (**C**, DQ stain. DS and **D**, Pap stain, TP ×100 objective with oil immersion).

abnormalities are similar to those identified in histologic sections of small cleaved cell lymphoma, both follicular and diffuse. Small mature reactive T lymphocytes are also seen. Numerous lymphoglandular bodies (clumped cytoplasmic fragments) are present. There are few or no mitoses in low-grade FL (56,57,59).

The relative lack of architecture in FNA remains a limitation in grading FL. Cytologic grading may be performed after a morphologic and immunophenotypic diagnosis of FL (57). Methods include counting centroblasts only in clusters resembling follicular structures and evaluating the proliferation index by Ki-67 and DNA image analysis (60) or counting centroblasts, either in 300 lymphoid cells or per 10 hpf in TP slides (61). Grading can also be performed on cell blocks, which may better preserve follicular architecture (57). When the large cells/hpf approach 20% to 50%, the cases may be classified as grade II (mixed small cleaved and large cells) and when the large cells constitute more than 50% of the cells/hpf, the cases may be classified as grade III (variable mixture of large noncleaved cells, large cleaved cells, and occasional immunoblasts) (2,57,58,60).

Phenotype. Positive for CD19, CD20, CD79a, CD10, and Bcl-6. Approximately 85% are positive for Bcl-2. CD5, CD23, and CD43 are negative.

Cytogenetics. t(14;18)(q32;q21) occurs in 95% of FL (62,63).

Differential Diagnosis. RLH and MCL should be considered in the differential diagnosis of FL grades 1 and 2. Low-grade FL may be indistinguishable morphologically from normal or reactive lymph nodes because of a mixed pattern of small and large lymphocytes. This distinction between reactive hyperplasia and low-grade FL poses a serious obstacle to the use of FNA in the diagnosis of malignant lymphoma. FL must also be differentiated from other small or mixed small lymphomas including MCL. Morphologically, FL tends to be less monotonous and contains a mixture of small and large cleaved and large noncleaved cells, whereas MCL is composed of predominantly small irregular cells. The tumor cells of MCL are characteristically CD5 and cyclin D1 positive. FL-3 needs to be distinguished from DLBCL (62).

Mantle Cell Lymphoma

Key Cytologic Features

- Monotonous small- to medium-sized lymphoid cells
- Irregular (centrocyte-like) nuclei
- Epithelioid histiocytes
- Lymphoid cell aggregates
- Rare plasmacytoid lymphocytes
- Rare tingible body macrophages
- Mitoses

- Blastoid variant has intermediate to large cells—resemble lymphoblasts
- Pleomorphic type has large cells—resemble centroblasts

Clinical Features. MCL is an aggressive B-cell lymphoma that is uncommon, constituting approximately 5% to 10% of all NHLs. These tumors mostly occur in older men. MCL is usually widespread at presentation, with generalized lymphadenopathy, hepatosplenomegaly, multiple lymphomatous polyposis within the gastrointestinal tract, and bone marrow involvement. Transformation to an aggressive blastoid variant is frequent (33,34).

Cytology. Smears demonstrate a monotonous population of small- to medium-sized lymphoid cells, slightly larger than normal lymphocytes. Nuclei resemble centrocytes and are oval and irregular containing dispersed mature chromatin and inconspicuous nucleoli. Cytoplasm is scant and mildly basophilic (Fig. 12.17A and B). The cell proliferation is homogeneous, without the presence of larger cells with prominent nucleoli. Epithelioid histiocytes with large oval nuclei and abundant eosinophilic cytoplasm are commonly present. Lymphoid cell aggregates are seen in one third of the cases. Plasmacytoid lymphocytes and tingible body macrophages are rare. Mitoses may be identified (53,64).

In the blastoid variant of MCL, the cells resemble lymphoblasts and are medium to large with irregular nuclei containing finely granular chromatin and multiple irregular nucleoli. The mitotic and apoptotic rate is high (Fig. 12.17C and D). Terminal deoxynucleotidyl transferase (TdT) is negative (65). The pleomorphic type has large cells which resemble centroblasts.

Phenotype. Positive for pan B-cell antigens CD19, CD20, and PAX5. MCL is also positive for CD79a, CD5, and FMC7 and negative for CD10, BCL6, and CD23. The tumor cells express monotypic sIg, with lambda light-chain restriction being more common. Almost all show nuclear positivity for cyclin D1 that provides a specific marker for MCL (66). SOX11, a transcription factor for CNS development, is positive in >95% of MCL. It is also found in Burkitt lymphoma (BL) and LBL and some grade 3 FL. SOX11 is not found in other small B-cell lymphomas (67).

Cytogenetics. MCL are characterized by t(11;14)(q13;q32) resulting in BCL1 gene rearrangement with characteristic overexpression of cyclin D1 in >95% of cases (47). In B-cell NHL, cyclin D1 overexpression is limited to MCL and provides a useful marker for this tumor (66).

Differential Diagnosis. Includes other small cell lymphomas such as CLL/SLL, low-grade FL, and MZL. This differential is important since MCL has a relatively worse prognosis. Immunophenotyping may be critical in this differential. CLL/SLL is CD23 positive and FL is CD10 and BCL6 positive. Difficulty in diagnosing MCL can result from aberrant phenotypes. Positivity

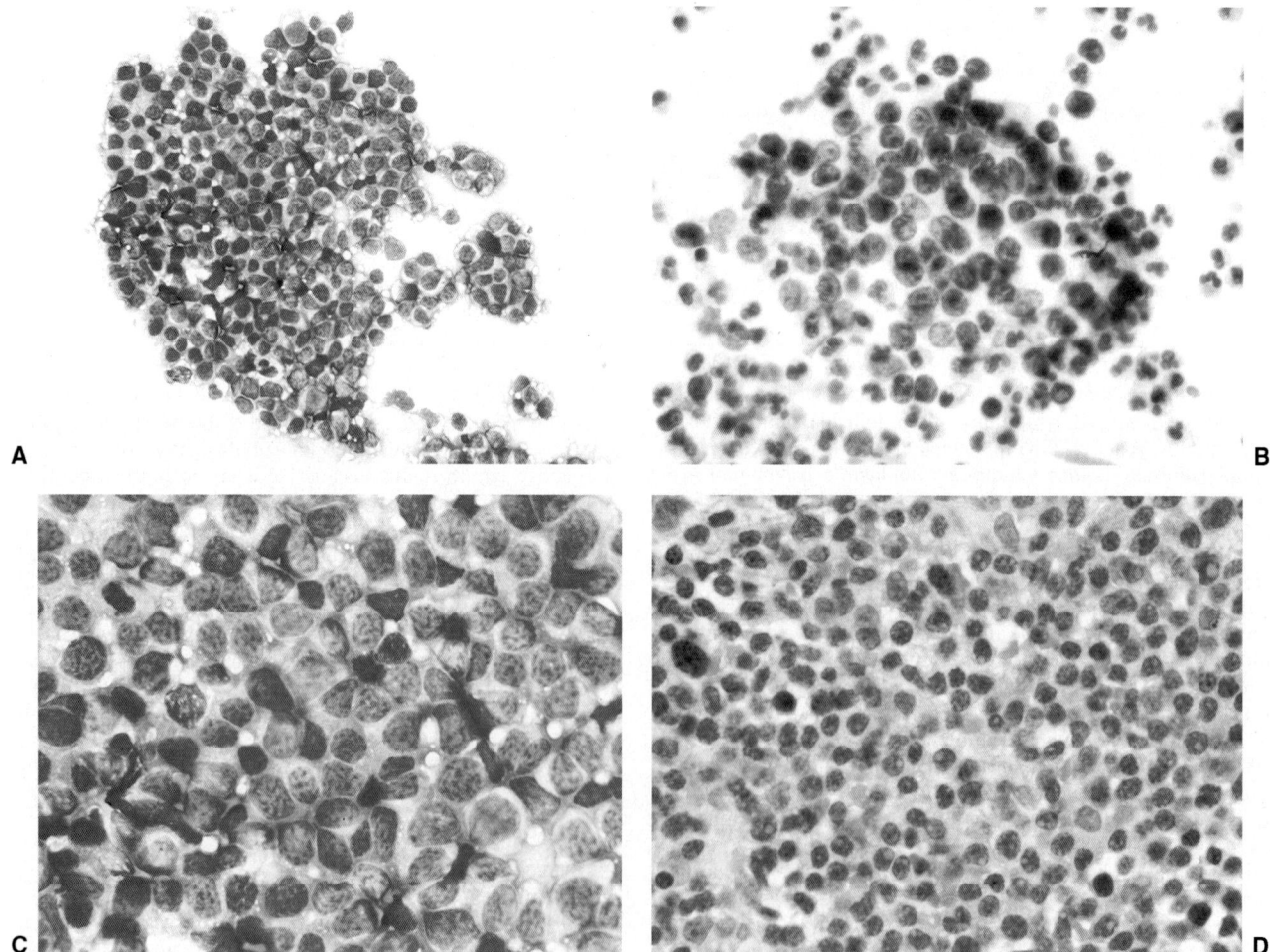

FIGURE 12.17. Mantle cell lymphoma. A,B: Homogeneous population of small to medium-sized lymphoid cells with oval and irregular nuclei, dispersed mature chromatin, inconspicuous nucleoli, and scant and mildly basophilic cytoplasm (**A**, DQ stain, DS and **B**, Pap stain, DS ×60 objective). **C,D:** Blastoid variant with lymphoblast-like cells showing open coarsely granular chromatin (**C**, DQ stain, DS and **D**, H&E-stained cell block ×100 objective with oil immersion).

for SOX11 may be helpful in the rare cases of CD5-negative/equivocal or negative cyclin D1 MCL and CD5-positive MZL (67).

Diffuse Large B-Cell Lymphoma, Not Otherwise Specified

Key Cytologic Features
- Monotonous population of large cells
- Several morphologic subtypes
  - Centroblastic
  - Immunoblastic
  - T cell rich
  - Anaplastic
- Epithelioid histiocytes and tingible body macrophages
- Necrosis, mitoses
- Artifacts of smearing

Clinical Features. DLBCL is characterized by a variety of morphologic and clinical characteristics, suggesting an underlying pathogenetic heterogeneity. DLBCL is a common subtype of aggressive but potentially curable NHL that constitutes approximately 30% of adult lymphomas. It can occur at any age including childhood. Primary extranodal disease may be present. Lymph nodes are also frequently involved. Most cases of DCLBL arise *de novo*, while some cases represent transformation of a pre-existing low-grade lymphoma. DLBCL may also occur in patients with immunodeficiencies such as AIDS or may represent a post-transplant lymphoproliferative disorder (59,68).

Cytology. DLBCL has a variable morphology. Smears of DLBCL show a dispersed pattern of monotonous cells (Fig. 12.9A). Usually, the smears are moderately cellular and recognizable as abnormal due to the presence of large atypical. Morphology may vary with the specific subtype—centroblastic, immunoblastic, or anaplastic. The centroblastic type is most common. It shows a preponderance of cells with medium-to-large cells with round-to-oval nuclei with distinct smooth or irregular contours, vesicular chromatin, and multiple prominent nucleoli, often peripheral. Cytoplasm is scant basophilic and may show vacuoles (Fig. 12.18A and B). There may be admixed immunoblasts. The immunoblastic type is composed predominantly of immunoblasts (>90%). Immunoblasts are larger than centroblasts, have smooth round or oval nuclei, and single central prominent nucleoli, a characteristic feature of this subtype. Cytoplasm is abundant pale or clear to intensely basophilic and may displace the nucleus eccentrically, imparting a plasmacytoid appearance (Fig. 12.18C and E). Cells of this type are seen in a large proportion of centroblastic lymphomas. Anaplastic type shows large, occasionally multinucleated pleomorphic cells (Fig. 12.18F and G). In the T-cell–rich type, small mature T cells dominate the smears with a variable

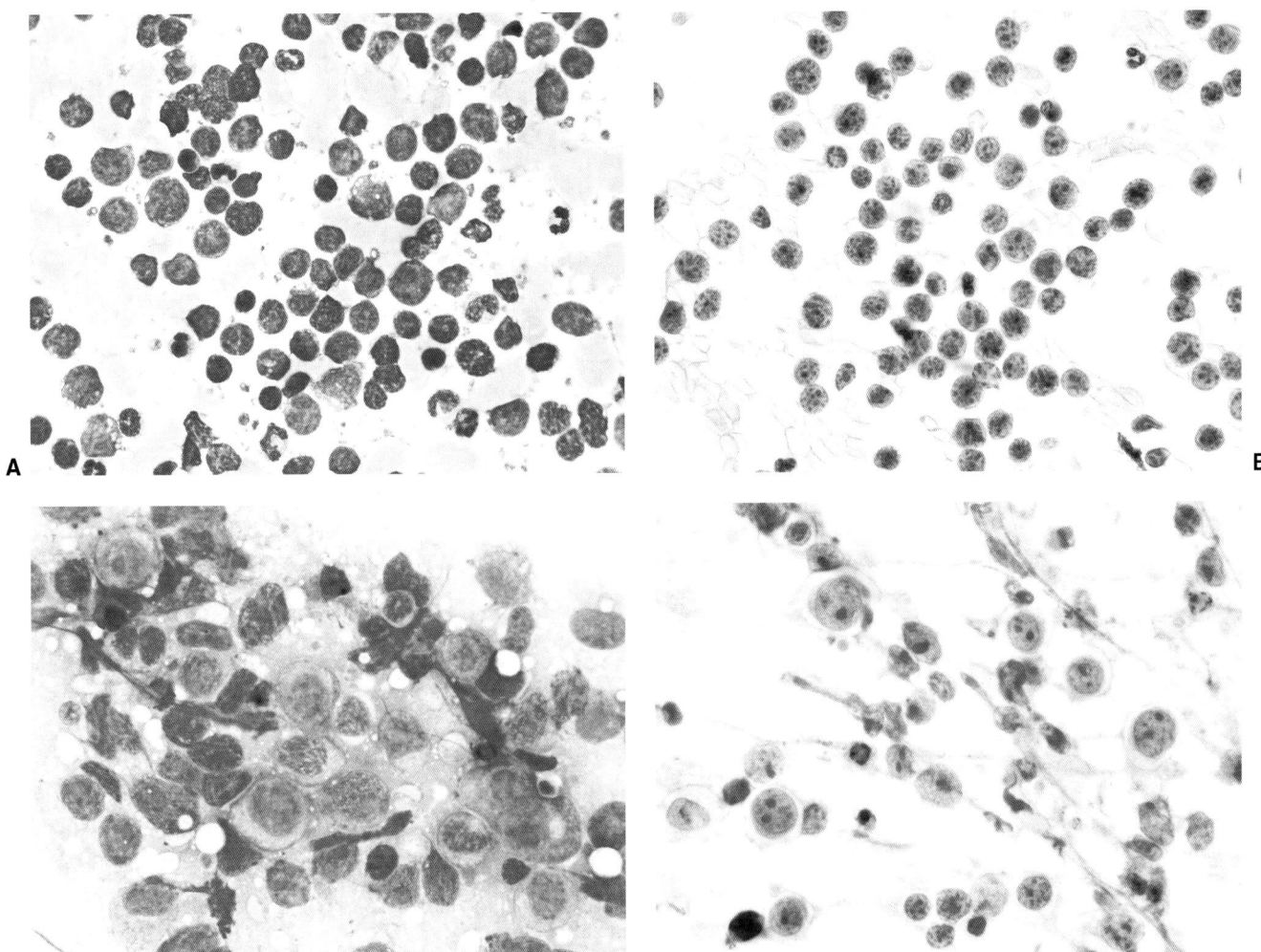

FIGURE 12.18. Diffuse large B-cell lymphoma. A,B: Centroblastic type morphology with medium-to-large cells tumor cells, round-to-oval nuclei with smooth or irregular contours, and basophilic cytoplasm with small vacuoles. Nucleoli are more obvious in the Pap-stained DS (**A**, DQ stain, DS and **B**, Pap stain, DS ×100 objective with oil immersion).

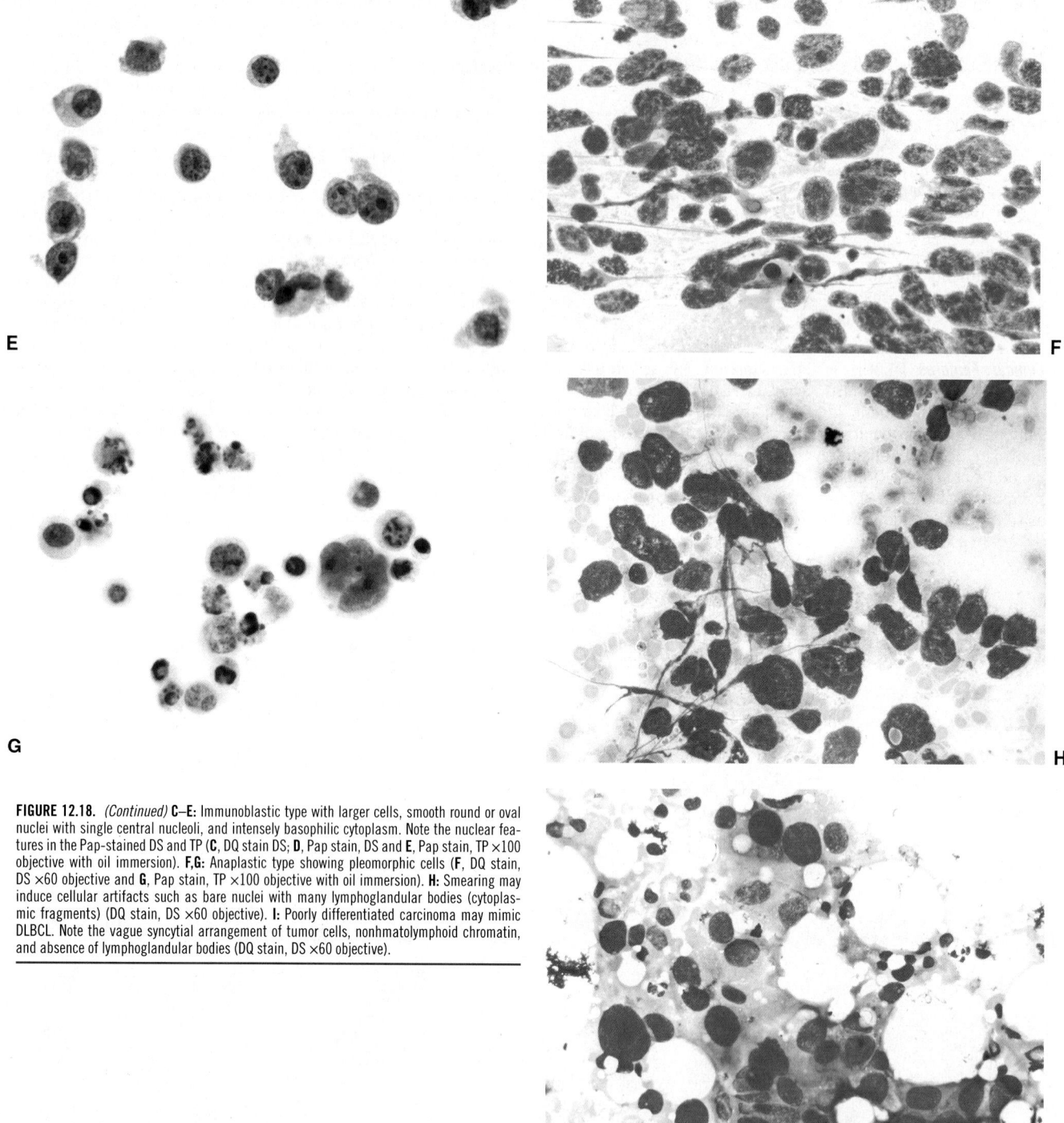

FIGURE 12.18. *(Continued)* **C–E:** Immunoblastic type with larger cells, smooth round or oval nuclei with single central nucleoli, and intensely basophilic cytoplasm. Note the nuclear features in the Pap-stained DS and TP (**C**, DQ stain DS; **D**, Pap stain, DS and **E**, Pap stain, TP ×100 objective with oil immersion). **F,G:** Anaplastic type showing pleomorphic cells (**F**, DQ stain, DS ×60 objective and **G**, Pap stain, TP ×100 objective with oil immersion). **H:** Smearing may induce cellular artifacts such as bare nuclei with many lymphoglandular bodies (cytoplasmic fragments) (DQ stain, DS ×60 objective). **I:** Poorly differentiated carcinoma may mimic DLBCL. Note the vague syncytial arrangement of tumor cells, nonhmatolymphoid chromatin, and absence of lymphoglandular bodies (DQ stain, DS ×60 objective).

admixture of histiocytes. Large tumor cells are scattered and constitute <10% of all cells. All subtypes show variable numbers of epithelioid histiocytes and tingible body macrophages. Cells of DLBCL are fragile. Smearing may induce artifacts such as loss of cytoplasm, which appears as lymphoglandular bodies, and resultant distorted bare nuclei (Fig. 12.18H). Poorly differentiated carcinoma (PDCa) cells may mimic DLBCL (Fig. 12.18I).

Phenotype. Cells of DLBCL express CD45 and B-cell markers CD20 and CD79a. Most DLBCL also express surface or cytoplasmic Ig. The anaplastic variant expresses CD30. DLBCL of centroblastic morphology frequently express CD10, indicating a follicular center cell derivation. Expression for BCL6 may also be seen. Large cell lymphomas have a false-negative or nondiagnostic rate of approximately 27% by FCM analyses. Possible causes of such a high rate include small sample size, necrosis, or cell fragility (7,69,70).

Cytogenetics. Frequent molecular characteristics are 3q27 break involving BCL6 gene in 30%, BCL2 t(14;18) in 25%, and MYC rearrangement in 10%. The latter may make it difficult to distinguish DLBCL from Burkitt (34). Clonal rearrangement of Ig heavy- and light-chain genes is also seen.

Differential Diagnosis. Tumor cells in the T-cell–rich subtype and the anaplastic subtypes of DLBCL may resemble RS cells. Other entities that should be considered in the differential diagnoses include FL-3, blastoid variant of MCL, BL, and PDCa (Fig. 12.18I). Immunophenotyping will aid in the differential (33,70,71).

Primary Mediastinal (Thymic) Large B-Cell Lymphoma

Key Cytologic Features
- Monotonous large neoplastic cells
- Enlarged irregular nuclei, granular chromatin, nucleoli
- Pale blue cytoplasm with distinct outer border
- High N:C
- Lymphoglandular bodies
- Mitoses

Clinical Features. Primary mediastinal large B-cell lymphoma (PMBL), a unique subtype of DLBCL, is rare. It arises in the thymus, the cell of origin is most likely the CD19+/CD21– thymic B cell normally found clustering around Hassall corpuscles. The disease usually affects young women and displays a unique combination of clinical, histologic, immunologic, and cytogenetic features. Patients commonly present with a rapidly enlarging mass in the mediastinum that infiltrates surrounding structures and causes compression symptom including superior vena cava syndrome. It often involves the lungs and may eventually metastasize to other organs. Bone marrow involvement is uncommon at diagnosis. FNA is usually part of the initial workup of the patient.

Cytology. Smears show a monotonous population of atypical lymphocytes, with predominance of large cells. The nuclei are enlarged (>5 times the size of a normal lymphocyte), irregular, cleaved or noncleaved, and lobulated, with coarsely granular chromatin and occasional prominent nucleoli. Cytoplasm is pale blue, scant to moderate in amount, and forms a narrow pale-to-clear rim with a distinct cell border. Nuclear-to-cytoplasmic ratio is high. Lymphoglandular bodies and mitoses are present (72). FNA of primary DLBCL of the mediastinum may show low cellularity due to sclerosis (69,72).

Phenotype. Distinct phenotype includes weak and non-homogenous positivity for CD30 in 80% and CD23 positivity in 70% of cases. Expression of surface and cytoplasmic Ig is often absent as is CD21 expression. BCL6 mutations and BCL2 gene rearrangement are lacking.

Differential Diagnosis. Includes mediastinal involvement with peripheral DLBCL, HL, anaplastic large cell lymphoma (ALCL), thymoma, and carcinoma. PMBL can be distinguished from these entities by ICC, FCM, and molecular features.

Plasmablastic Lymphoma

Key Cytologic Features
- Large tumor cells
- Round, eccentrically located nuclei, nucleoli
- Occasional bi- or multinucleated cells
- Basophilic or clear cytoplasm with distinct borders

Clinical Features. Plasmablastic lymphoma (PBL) is an uncommon aggressive Epstein-Barr virus (EBV)–associated lymphoma of the oral cavity, which is usually but not always associated with HIV. Primary PBL may also occur at other extraoral sites, predominantly in the gastrointestinal tract and lung (73). Rarely, PBL may also occur in HIV-negative immunodeficient and immunocompetent individuals. Such cases are more common in lymph nodes.

Cytology. Smears show singly dispersed, highly atypical large-to-intermediate, round-to-oval tumor cells. Nuclei are round and eccentrically located with prominent nucleoli (plasmablastic differentiation). The cytoplasm is scant to moderate in amount, densely basophilic with occasional fine vacuoles and distinct cell borders (Fig. 12.19A). Some cells are binucleated or multinucleated (Fig. 12.19B). Plasmacytoid morphology is more evident on air-dried DQ-stained slides (58,73,74).

Phenotype. Plasmablastic differentiation is confirmed by diffuse and strong positivity for PC markers CD38, CD138, MUM1, and PRDM1/Blimp-1. Lymphocytic and B-cell marker CD79a is positive (50% to 85%), while others including CD45 and CD20 and PAX5 are negative. EBER is positive and EBV LMP1 (Latency Pattern 1) is negative. The proliferation index with Ki-67 immunochemistry approaches 100% (35).

Cytogenetics. Clonal Ig kappa light-chain gene rearrangement (73).

Differential Diagnosis. Plasmablastic myeloma must be distinguished from PBL because of the different clinical management pathways. Typically, the presence of serum paraprotein and/or lytic bone lesions in older patients favors MM. However, widely disseminated bone disease and monoclonal serum Ig have been described in PBL and could lead to major confusion with MM. Although PBL and MM have nearly identical

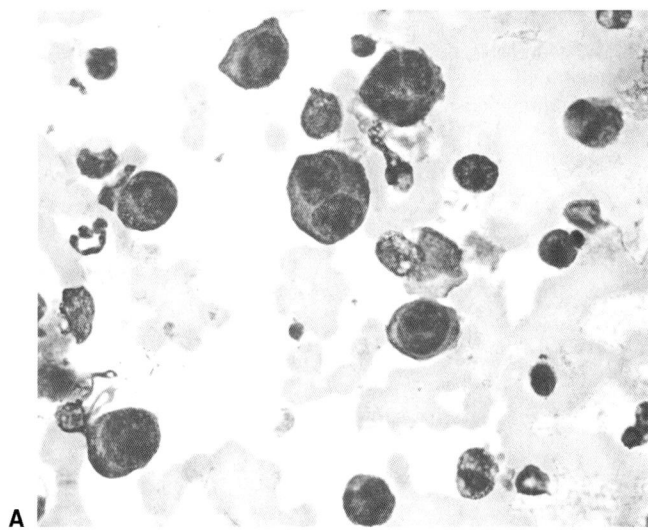

A

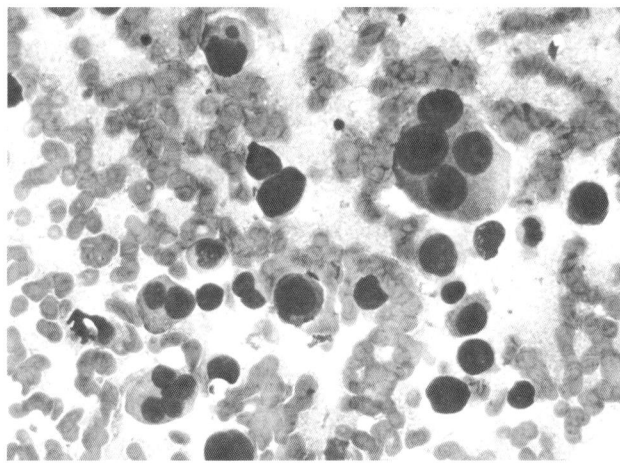

B

FIGURE 12.19. Plasmablastic lymphoma. A,B: Singly dispersed atypical tumor cells with plasmablastic differentiation; some cells are bi- or multinucleated (**A**, DQ stain, DS ×100 objective with oil immersion and **B**, DQ stain, DS ×60 objective).

immunophenotypic profiles, CD56 positivity, occasionally cyclin D1 positivity, and a relatively lower Ki-67 can help identify secondary extramedullary plasmablastic MM (58).

Burkitt Lymphoma

Key Features
- Monomorphic medium-sized tumor cells
- Round nuclei, clumped chromatin, small nucleoli
- Deeply basophilic cytoplasm with small clear vacuoles
- Tingible body macrophages in a "starry sky" pattern
- Mitoses and apoptosis

Clinical Features. BL is an aggressive mature B-cell lymphoma that may occur in extranodal sites. There are three major subtypes of BL—endemic, sporadic, and immunodeficiency associated. These subtypes of BL have similar morphology but differ clinically and biologically. Endemic BL occurs in equatorial Africa in areas of endemic malaria, strongly associated with the EBV (95%) (75). It commonly occurs in children, 4 to 7 years old, and affects mandible, gonads, and kidney. It is the most common childhood malignancy in Africa. Sporadic BL is the most common NHL in children and young adults in the developed countries. It commonly presents as an intra-abdominal tumor. Lymphoid tissue of Waldeyer ring may also be involved. Immunodeficiency-associated BL is often associated with HIV infection and may present with nodal and extranodal disease with bone marrow involvement. BL is a fast-growing bulky disease. All types have a high risk of CNS, ovary, breast, and kidney involvement. The EBV genome is present in the neoplastic cells in all cases of endemic BL. EBV is detected in approximately 33% of sporadic and immunodeficiency-associated BL (75).

Cytology. Smears show a largely monomorphic population of medium-to-large tumor cells. These cells bear round and uniform nuclei with occasional clefts or indentations, clumped chromatin, multiple small central nucleoli, and moderate amount of deeply basophilic and vacuolated cytoplasm (Fig. 12.20A). Similar cytoplasmic vacuoles can be seen in DLBCL (Fig. 12.18A). Numerous tingible body macrophages impart a "starry sky" pattern (Fig. 12.20B and C). Mitotic rate is brisk. Background looks "dirty" due to individual cell necrosis (apoptosis) (76). Some cases of BL may show tumor cells with plasmacytoid features, particularly in immunodeficiency-associated BL, or nuclear pleomorphism with more prominent nucleoli.

Phenotype. Tumor cells express light-chain restriction and germinal center phenotype expressing CD10 and BCL6. Proliferation index is high with nearly 100% positivity with Ki-67. Cells are negative for CD5, CD23, TdT, and bcl-2.

Cytogenetics. t(8:14) in 90%. EBV genome can be demonstrated in all endemic BL and approximately 30% to 40% of other subtypes.

Differential Diagnosis. Includes DLBCL and childhood small round blue cell tumors. These can be distinguished by immunostains and cytogenetic findings (77).

T-Cell and Natural Killer–Cell Lymphoma

T-cell lymphomas, which are more common in Asia, are a heterogeneous group of lymphomas with diverse morphology. In the United States, they are much less common than B-cell lymphomas and constitute about 10% to 20% of all NHL. T-cell lymphomas are derived from post-thymic or mature T cells at different

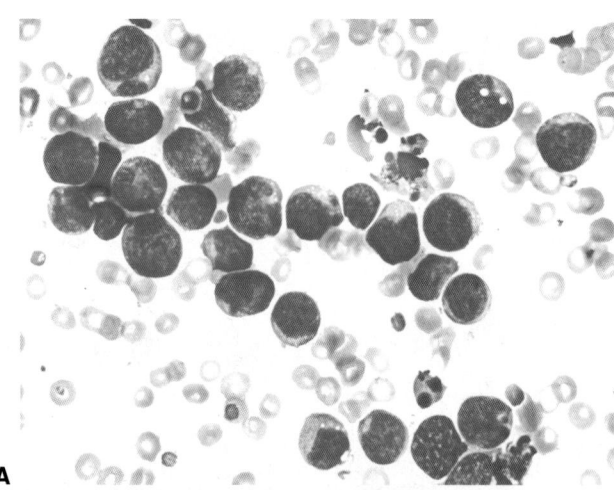

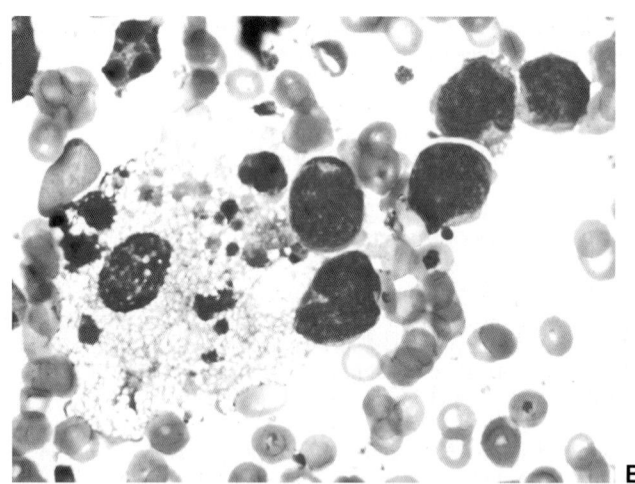

FIGURE 12.20. Burkitt lymphoma. A: Monomorphic medium-to-large tumor cells with round nuclei with occasional clefts and clumped chromatin. Note the small clear lipid-containing cytoplasmic vacuoles (DQ stain, DS ×100 objective with oil immersion). **B,C:** Tingible body macrophages impart a "starry sky" pattern (**B**, DQ stain DS ×100 objective with oil immersion and **C**, Pap stain, TP ×60 objective).

stages of differentiation and are divided into two broad categories in the WHO classification—precursor T-cell LBL and mature T-cell and natural killer-cell lymphomas. T-cell lymphomas have a poorer prognosis and response to treatment compared to B-cell lymphomas. The section will cover only those entities that may be encountered on FNA including precursor T-cell LBL/leukemia, PTCL (unspecified and angioimmunoblastic), and ALCL.

Precursor B- and T-Cell Lymphoblastic Lymphoma/Leukemia (B- and T-LBL)

Key Cytologic Features in B- and T-LBL
- Small- or intermediate-sized blasts
- Round or highly convoluted nuclei, distinct nucleoli, delicate blastlike chromatin
- Scant-to-moderate amount of nongranular cytoplasm with frequent protrusions
- Tingible body macrophages
- Numerous mitoses

Clinical Features. Precursor T-cell LBL/leukemia are composed of precursor B or T cells and involve the bone marrow and peripheral blood occasionally accompanied by primary nodal or extranodal site involvement. The neoplasm is rare. It occurs in all age groups, but has a relatively high incidence in children and young adults. B-LBL is most common in children and may present with skin nodules, bone lesions, and lymphadenopathy. T-LBL most frequently presents as symptomatic mediastinal mass with pleural and pericardial effusions and subdiaphragmatic lymphadenopathy. Both have coexistent leukemic involvement (78).

Cytology. Smears contain small or intermediate-sized blasts with round-to-convoluted nuclei with delicate blastlike chromatin, distinct nucleoli, and scant-to-moderate weakly basophilic nongranular cytoplasm (Fig. 12.21). Numerous mitoses are present. Tingible body macrophages may be present (79).

Phenotype. Lymphoblasts in both B- and T-LBL are positive for TdT. The T-LBL is positive for T-cell antigens CD2, CD3, CD5, CD7, and CD1a and the B-LBL is positive for B-cell antigens CD19, CD79a, and PAX5.

Cytogenetics. B-LBL show clonal but unmutated rearrangements of Ig genes, two thirds show clonal Ig heavy-chain

rearrangements. T-LBL almost always has T-cell receptor gene rearrangements.

Differential Diagnoses. Include BL and blastoid variant of MCL. However, T-LBL is distinguished from B-cell lymphomas due to absent B-cell markers and positivity for CD7 and other T-cell markers.

Peripheral T-Cell Lymphoma Unspecified (PTCL, NOS), Including Angioimmunoblastic T-Cell Lymphoma

Key Cytologic Features
- Small, intermediate and large lymphocytes
- Irregular nuclei, nucleoli
- Pale-staining cytoplasm
- Epithelioid histiocytes, PCs, and eosinophils
- Mitoses
- Reed-Sternberg (RS)–like cells

Clinical Features. PTCL is rare and constitutes <10% of all NHL in the Western countries. It is primarily a disease of adults with no sex predilection. Clinically, PTCL is a more aggressive form of NHL. It is a heterogeneous group of tumors with variable clinical presentation, morphologic appearance, and prognosis. Patients commonly present with pruritus, lymphadenopathy, and extranodal disease (80,81).

Cytology. PTCL most commonly shows a polymorphous pattern with variable admixture of small, intermediate, and large neoplastic cells. Percentage of large cells may range from 20% to 90%. Smears in PTCL appear to be monomorphous when one cell type predominates. The nuclei vary considerably in size and exhibit significant membrane irregularities with protrusions and indentations. Nucleoli may be present. Cytoplasm is scant to moderate in amount, pale to basophilic, and has well-defined borders (Fig. 12.22). Mitoses are numerous. Epithelioid histiocytes, eosinophils, and PCs may be seen. Occasionally, scattered large cells with vesicular nuclei and prominent nucleoli, resembling RS-like cells, may be observed (80,81).

Phenotype. Neoplastic cells express T-cell phenotype including CD2, CD3, CD4, CD5, CD7, CD8, CD43 and CD45RO and are

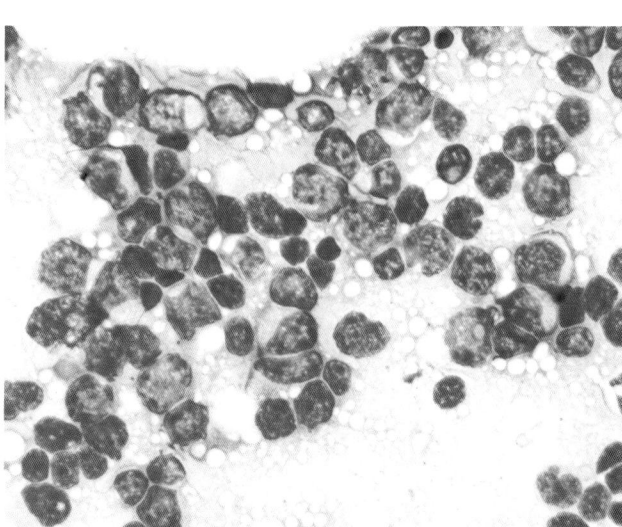

FIGURE 12.21. Precursor T-cell LBL displays intermediate-sized blasts with nuclear irregularities (DQ stain, DS ×100 objective with oil immersion).

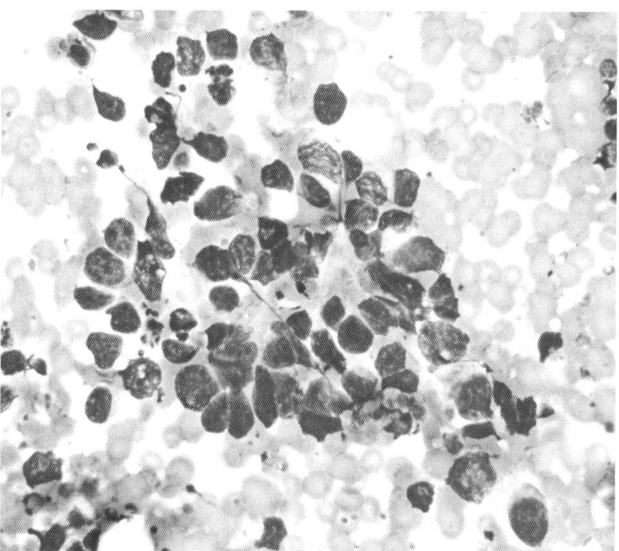

FIGURE 12.22. PTCL shows large neoplastic cells with variably-sized nuclei with membrane irregularities and scant cytoplasm (DQ stain, DS ×60 objective).

negative for B-cell antigens. The RS-like cells may have similar phenotype to RS-cells in HL with CD20, CD30 and occasionally CD15 positivity.

Cytogenetics. Clonal rearrangement of T-cell receptor genes is seen.

Differential Diagnoses. Includes reactive hyperplasia, HL, ALCL and DLBCL. A combination of cytomorphologic criteria, immunophenotyping and molecular analyses are useful to distinguish PTCL from these entities.

Anaplastic Large Cell Lymphoma

Key Cytologic Features
- Three variants: common, small cell and lymphohistiocytic types
- "Hallmark" cells: large with irregular horseshoe-shaped nuclei, prominent nucleoli,
- "Doughnut" cells: multiple nuclei arranged in a "wreath-like" pattern
- RS-like cells
- Histiocytes
- PCs
- Erythrophagocytosis
- Necrosis and inflammation
- Mitoses and apoptosis

Clinical Features. Ki-1 (CD30)-positive ALCL is a rare T-cell lymphoma. ALCL can have diverse clinical, histologic and cytologic presentation. It is divided into morphologically indistinct but clinically distinct ALK-positive (ALK⁺) ALCL and ALK-negative (ALK⁻) ALCL according to the presence or absence of ALK protein. ALK⁺ ALCL is more common in children and young men. It involves both lymph nodes and extranodal sites (skin, bone, soft tissue, lungs, liver). ALK⁻ ALCL tends to occur in older patients with a lower male to female ratio and exhibits immunophenotypic heterogeneity. Response to treatment and prognosis of ALK⁺ ALCL patients is comparatively better than in ALK⁻ ALCL and other PTCL (82,83).

Cytology. ALCL shows a broad morphologic spectrum which makes it difficult to make a definitive diagnosis on FNA (82). The three distinct morphologic variants are the common large cell and the less common lymphohistiocytic and small cell patterns. The "hallmark" cells, so-called because they constitute a hallmark of ALCL, are seen in all variants. These are large pleomorphic cells with eccentric lobulated (horseshoe-shaped or kidney-shaped) nuclei, finely granular chromatin, multiple basophilic nucleoli and abundant basophilic or clear cytoplasm. Usually a prominent perinuclear clear "hof," corresponding to the Golgi region is evident (Fig. 12.23A) (83). The other notable cells are the "doughnut cells" which are multinucleated giant cells, with nuclei arranged in a wreathlike pattern close to the cytoplasmic border (Fig. 12.23B). RS-like cells are also present. Background shows reactive lymphocytes, histiocytes, and PCs (Fig. 12.23C). Erythrophagocytosis can occasionally be seen. Necrosis, mitoses, and apoptosis are frequent. The small cell variant shows medium-sized neoplastic cells with clear

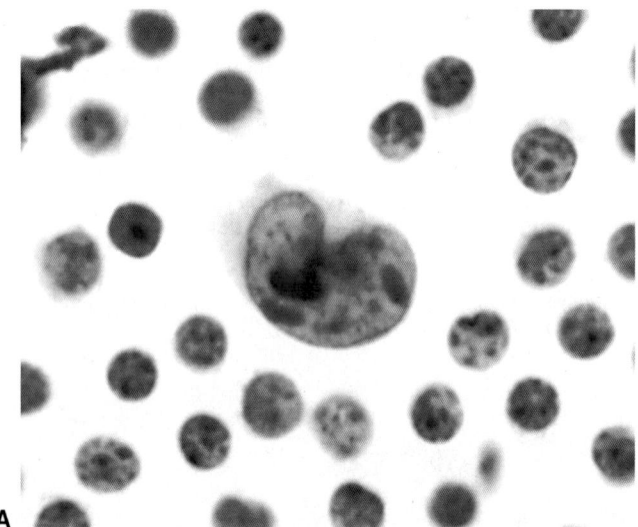

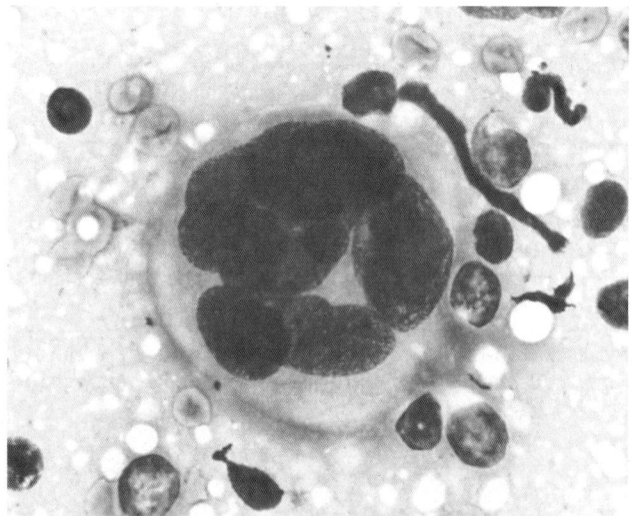

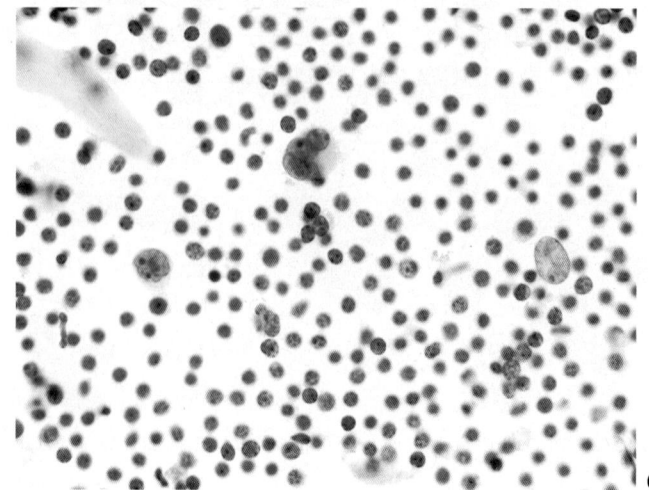

FIGURE 12.23. Anaplastic large cell lymphoma. A: "Hallmark" cell with eccentric lobulated, horseshoe-shaped, or kidney-shaped nucleus (Pap stain, DS ×100 objective with oil immersion). **B:** "Doughnut" cell with nuclei arranged in a wreathlike pattern (DQ stain, DS ×100 objective with oil immersion). **C:** Background shows reactive lymphocytes. Compare the size of the neoplastic cells with the benign lymphoid cells (Pap stain, DS ×60 objective).

cytoplasm and distinct cell membranes. Nuclei are irregular with clumped chromatin resembling the horseshoe-shaped nuclei of the classical "hallmark" cells. The lymphohistiocytic variant contains similar small cells admixed with abundant pale histiocytes (82).

Immunocytochemistry. Positive for ALK, CD30, EMA, CD45, and one or more T-cell markers including CD2 and CD5.

Cytogenetics. T-cell receptor gene rearrangements, t(2;5) translocation in >80% of ALK$^+$ ALCL cases.

Differential Diagnosis. Includes other large cell lymphomas, anaplastic carcinoma, melanoma and HL. These tumors can be distinguished based on morphology and ICC. Caution should be exercised in interpreting positive EMA stain in a specimen with carcinoma-like features as EMA is also a characteristic marker for ALCL. ALCL and HL have overlapping morphologic and ICC features. Careful evaluation of the latter two features and clinical presentation would be helpful (84).

HODGKIN LYMPHOMA

WHO 2008 Classification of Hodgkin Lymphoma

- Classical HL
  - Nodular sclerosis classical HL
  - Mixed cellularity classical HL
  - Lymphocyte-rich classical HL
  - Lymphocyte-depleted classical HL
- Nodular lymphocytic predominant HL

HL is a relatively uncommon form of lymphoma (~10% to 20%). The two distinct groups are the classical (CHL) and the nodular lymphocytic predominant Hodgkin lymphoma (NLPHL) types. These two groups differ in their epidemiology, clinical features, phenotype, genetics, and association with EBV but share RS cells and its variants. CHL includes four subtypes: nodular sclerosis (NSCHL), mixed cellularity (MCCHL), lymphocyte rich (LRCHL) and lymphocyte depleted (LDCHL) (85).

The role of FNA as a sole diagnostic modality in HL is controversial; however, FNA can be reliably used in the diagnosis of recurrent HL. A cytologic diagnosis of HL is dependent on the recognition of RS cells. Diagnostic RS cells may or may not be easy to identify on FNA, depending on the histopathologic type of HL. On FNA, the diagnostic accuracy of HL, not otherwise specified, is >90%, but the accuracy of subtyping the disease is lesser (86,87). However, accurate subtyping, as per WHO 2008, is not considered crucial for management purposes. Rarely, RS cells are seen in the absence of HL (88). FNA of HL may be false-negative due to sampling error or fibrosis. When the findings on FNA do not correlate with the clinical and radiologic impression, repeat FNA or histologic biopsy should be performed (89,90).

Key Cytologic Features

- Classical HL
  - NSCHL may show low cellularity due to fibrosis
  - Characteristic cells are classic RS cells or its variants (Hodgkin cells)
  - Background of inflammatory cells in NSCHL and MCCHL
- Nodular lymphocytic predominant HL
  - Characteristic cell are LP or "popcorn" cells
  - Background shows small and large lymphocytes
  - Histiocytes and PCs

Classical HL
Clinical Features. Classical HL accounts for >95% of all HL and shows a bimodal age distribution—younger and older age groups with a male to female ratio of 2:1. Cervical lymph nodes are the commonest site of presentation followed by mediastinal, axillary, and inguinal lymph nodes. The spleen is involved in a minority of cases. Other extranodal sites are uncommon except in late stages. EBV infection is seen in 40% of CHL, with the highest incidence in patients with AIDS.

NSCHL is the commonest subtype accounting for 70% of cases, primarily affects young people, and shows a female predominance. The mediastinum is involved in the majority of cases and more than one half of patients present with stage II disease (86,87).

MCCHL constitutes about 20% of cases, while LRCHL and LDCHL types are rare; the former constitute <5% of all CHL and the latter <5% in the Western countries. MCCHL and LDCHL have overlapping epidemiologic, clinical, and biologic features; both are more common in developing countries, are most commonly associated with HIV infection, and commonly involve peripheral lymph nodes and bone marrow. MCCHL shows a bimodal age distribution while LDCHL is more common in the elderly. These three subtypes of CHL show a male predominance (85).

Cytology. The smears often show low cellularity in NSCHL due to sclerosis. Small- to medium-sized lymphoid cells, eosinophils, and other inflammatory cells with scattered, RS cells or their mononuclear cell variants, the Hodgkin (H) cells, are present (Fig. 12.24A and B). Classic RS cells are large, three to four times the size of small lymphocytes and are binucleate or have a bilobed nucleus with prominent eosinophilic nucleoli (often occupying 25% of the nuclear diameter), giving the cells an "owl-eyed" appearance. Cytoplasm is moderate and basophilic (Fig. 12.24C–E). The RS variant, Hodgkin cell, has a large nucleus, distinct nucleolus, and abundant pale-blue cytoplasm (Fig. 12.24F). The nuclei may be irregular and polylobated. If diagnostic RS cells are identified in the appropriate polymorphous, dispersed population, the diagnosis of HL may be rendered (Fig. 12.24A). In MCCHL, H/RS cells are seen in a background of small- to medium-sized lymphoid cells, some centroblasts, eosinophils, PCs, neutrophils, and epithelioid histiocytes with occasionally granulomas. In some cases of MCCHL, granulomatous inflammation may dominate the smear and obscure the diagnostic cells. Smears of LRCHL show H/RS cells in a background showing a spectrum of lymphoid cells without eosinophils or histiocytes. In LDCHL, H/RS cells dominate the smear (35).

Immunocytochemistry. CD15 and CD30 are positive (Fig. 12.24G and H) and EMA, CD45, and usually CD20 are negative. Positivity for EBV will be seen in EBV-associated cases.

Differential Diagnosis. Difficulties encountered in the diagnosis of HL are attributable to overlapping features of RS cells and a variety of benign and malignant cells. These RS cell mimics or RS-like cells may be seen in large cell NHL (ALCL, T-cell–rich B-cell lymphoma, PTCL), carcinoma (breast, gastric, and nasopharyngeal), melanoma, sarcoma, germ cell tumor, infectious mononucleosis (IM), and RLH (86,87).

ALCL and PTCL sometimes show large cells with large nuclei and prominent nucleoli that resemble RS cells. Nuclei in ALCL show prominent nuclear contour irregularities and cells are negative for CD15. p63 protein may be used as a potential tool in the differential diagnosis between ALCL and CHL. p63 is frequently expressed in a subset of ALCL cases while HL has shown to be negative (89). Gene rearrangement studies can be used to distinguish RS cells from T-cell lymphomas (90). The occasional bizarre cells of nasopharyngeal carcinoma (NPC) may mimic RS cells. Melanoma occasionally shows large, atypical cells that may mimic RS cells. MCCHL may be mistaken for RLH if diagnostic RS cells are sparse or not noticed (12).

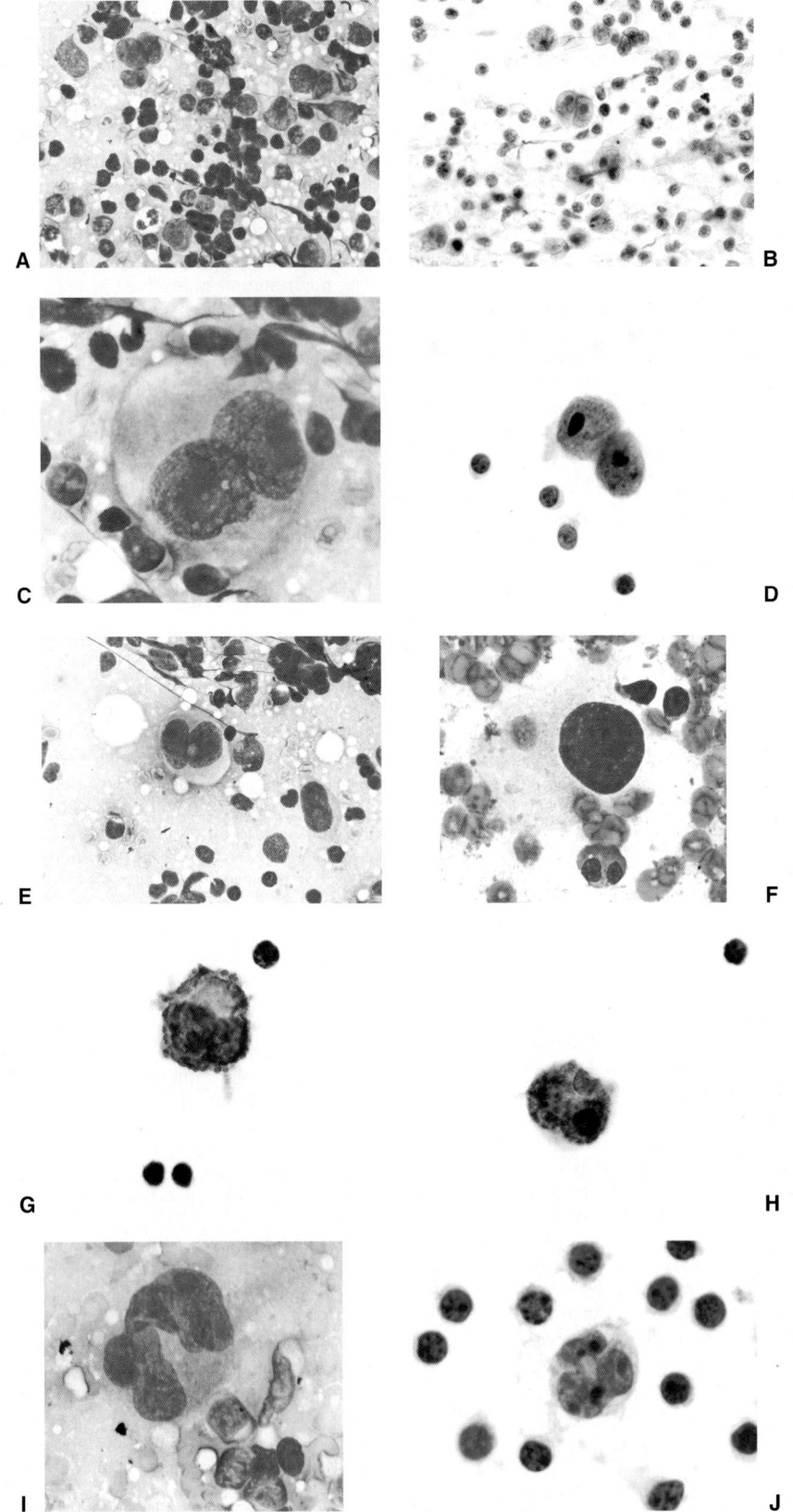

FIGURE 12.24. Hodgkin lymphoma. *Classical (CHL)* in **(A,B)** shows a mixture of small and large lymphoid cells with scattered Reed-Sternberg (RS) cells (**A**, DQ stain, DS and **B**, Pap stain, DS ×60 objective). **C,D:** Diagnostic RS cells, also known as "owl-eyed" cell with "mirror image" nuclei (**C**, DQ stain, DS and **D**, Pap stain, DS ×100 objective with oil immersion). **E:** Classic binucleated RS cell in an inflammatory background (DQ stain, DS ×100 objective with oil immersion). **F:** Mononuclear variant of RS cell (Hodgkin cell). Note the eosinophil and benign lymphoid cells (DQ stain, DS ×100 objective with oil immersion). **G,H:** Positive ICC for CD15 and CD30 (**G** and **H**, TP ×100 objective with oil immersion). *NLPHL in* **(I,J)** shows LP (popcorn) cell with multilobed nucleus and prominent nucleoli (**I**, DQ stain, DS and **J**, Pap stain, DS ×100 objective with oil immersion).

Nodular Lymphocytic Predominant HL

Clinical Features. NLPHL is rare accounting for <5% of all HL. It differs from CHL in its clinical, epidemiologic, pathologic, immunophenotype, and genetic features. It has a male predominance and peaks in the fourth decade. The majority of patients present with lymphadenopathy in the cervical, axillary, or inguinal regions. NLPHL is rarely associated with EBV. It is has a good prognosis even though recurrence is common (91).

Cytology. The LP cells are sparse and may be difficult to find on FNA smears. The nuclei are folded or multilobated with fine chromatin and distinct nucleoli (Fig. 12.24I and J). Classical RS cells are not seen in NLPHL. The background shows small and large lymphocytes. Histiocytes, singly or in clusters, and PCs may be seen. Eosinophils and neutrophils are not present (91).

Immunocytochemistry. The neoplastic cells of NLPHL are B cells and express CD45, CD20, CD79a, and BCL6. They are also positive for B-cell transcription factors PAX5, OCT2, and BOB-1 and negative for CD30 and CD15.

Genetics. Monoclonal rearrangements of the Ig genes.

Differential Diagnosis. Includes CHL and T-cell–rich B-cell lymphoma (TCRBCL). CHL shows positivity for CD30 and CD15. NLPHL is morphologically and immunophenotypically similar to TCRBCL, and the differential diagnosis between the two is controversial and a difficult task (97). Other entities such as PTCL may need molecular studies to distinguish from NLPHL (33).

HISTIOCYTIC AND DENDRITIC CELL NEOPLASMS

Dendritic cells are antigen-presenting cells. Their main function is to process antigen material and present it on the surface to other cells of the immune system. Dendritic cells include Langerhans cells (on the skin), interdigitating dendritic cells (IDDCs) (in the lymph node), and follicular dendritic cells (FDCs) (in lymph node follicle). Neoplasms of dendritic cells are rare. Langerhans cell histiocytosis (LCH) usually affects children between 1 and 15 years old and is traditionally divided into three groups: unifocal, multifocal unisystem, and multifocal multisystem. The key to diagnosing LCH is the identification of the characteristic nuclear features of Langerhans cells,

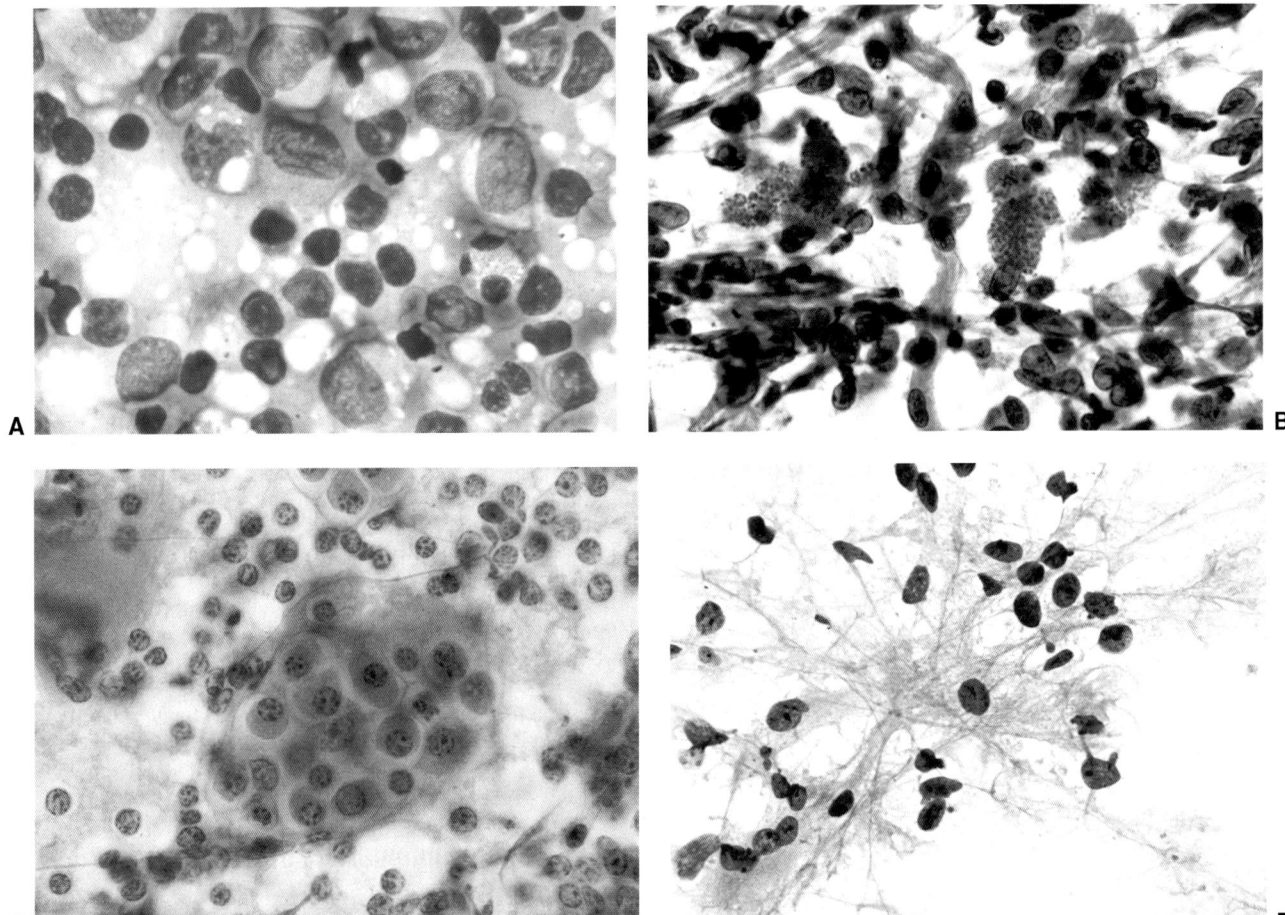

FIGURE 12.25. A: Smear from a case of Langerhans histiocytosis showing large neoplastic cells with elongated grooved nuclei, prominent nucleoli, and light blue cytoplasm. Note the eosinophils in the background (DQ stain, DS ×100 objective with oil immersion). *Courtesy of Stephan Papmbuccian, MD, Department of Pathology, University of Minnesota Medical Center, Minneapolis, MN.* **B:** Dermatopathic lymphadenitis shows histiocytes containing melanin pigment, Langerhans cells, and scattered lymphocytes (Pap stain, DS ×60 objective). **C:** Rosai-Dorfman disease shows a histiocyte with engulfed PCs (Pap stain, DS ×60 objective). *Both* **(B,C)** *courtesy of Ricardo Bardales, MD, Department of Pathology, Mercy General Hospital, Sacramento, CA.* **D:** FDC sarcoma shows spiderweb-like network of thin, radiating, multipolar processes interconnecting single tumor cells (Ultrafast stain, DS ×60 objective). *Courtesy of Grace Yang, MD, Department of Pathology & Laboratory Medicine, Weill Cornell Medical Center, New York, NY.*

which usually are admixed with numerous eosinophils. Langerhans cell nuclei have a folded, indented, or grooved appearance, generally with a fine chromatin pattern, inconspicuous nucleoli, and a thin nuclear membrane (Fig. 12.25A). Dermatopathic lymph nodes may contain numerous Langerhans cells and eosinophils; therefore, dermatopathic lymphadenitis is in the cytologic differential diagnosis (Fig. 12.25B). FNA in sinus histiocytosis with massive lymphadenopathy (Rosai-Dorfman disease) shows large histiocyte-like cells with abundant pale, eosinophilic cytoplasm containing well-preserved lymphocytes and occasional PCs and granulocytes. The diagnosis can be supported by the demonstration of S-100 protein in the large cells (Fig. 12.25C) (92).

IDDCs sarcoma predominantly occurs in adults. Morphologically, IDDCs have a folded nucleus, in contrast to FDC sarcoma, which appear to have an elongated nucleus. On electron microscopy, IDDCs have long and fine cytoplasmic extensions that intermingle with similar cells. In contrast to FDCs, they lack desmosomes, and in contrast to Langerhans cells they lack Birbeck granules. Immunostains for S-100 and CD1a are positive.

FDC sarcoma also predominantly occurs in adults. On FNA, the smears are cellular and show cells in syncytial fragments in addition to a prominent single-cell population. The nuclei are round to oval and moderately pleomorphic with vesicular chromatin, small nucleoli, occasional grooves, and pseudoinclusions. Cytoplasm is abundant, eosinophilic, and shows spiderweb-like network of thin, radiating, multipolar processes interconnecting single tumor cells (Fig. 12.25D). Delicate cytoplasmic strands are also seen in the small syncytial fragments, sprinkled with small lymphocytes. Positive immunostaining for CD21, CD23, and CD35 confirms the diagnosis (93).

Benign Conditions that Mimic Lymphoma

Reactive Lymphoid Hyperplasia

Key Cytologic Features
- Dispersed polymorphous lymphoid cells
- Predominantly small mature lymphocytes, centrocytes, and centroblasts
- Immunoblasts
- PCs, eosinophils, neutrophils
- Tingible body macrophages,
- Lymphohistiocytic aggregates
- Mitoses

Clinical Features. Nonspecific RLH is usually of unknown cause and frequently affects children and young adults. It is the most common cause of lymphadenopathy in children and largely attributed to the repeated antigenic stimulation encountered in early life. In adults, RLH is less common. The enlarged lymph nodes in RLH are usually < 3cm, soft, small, oval, mobile, and single or multiple. RLH commonly involves the cervical, axillary, or inguinal lymph nodes. The lymphadenopathy may last up to a few weeks to months. In the clinical setting of persistent or increasing lymphadenopathy, FNA may be warranted to exclude lymphoma.

Cytology. FNA smears show a polymorphous population dominated by small mature lymphocytes. The latter have round nuclei and condensed dark chromatin. Other cells include transformed lymphocytes including centrocytes, centroblasts, and immunoblasts, scattered histiocytes including tingible body macrophages, which are specialized histiocytes predominantly found in germinal centers and PCs (Figs. 12.6A–C, 12.9B, and 12.26). Lymphohistiocytic aggregates and mitoses are also present (12,38).

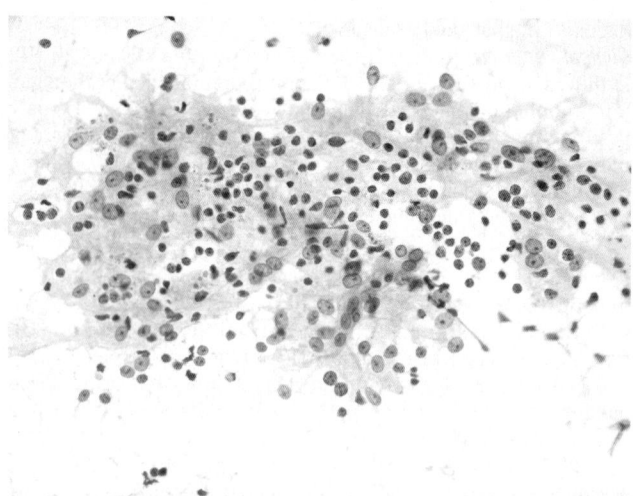

FIGURE 12.26. RHL shows a lymphohistiocytic aggregate comprising of small and large lymphoid cells and tingible body macrophages. The latter are present both within and at the periphery of the aggregate (Pap stain, DS ×60 objective). Figures 12.5A–C and 12.8B depict other characteristics of a reactive lymph node.

Immunophenotype. Positive for pan-B-cell markers including CD19, CD20, CD22, CD79a, and PAX5 with no light-chain restriction nor any cytogenetic abnormalities, as well as pan-T-cell markers including CD3, CD2, and CD5.

Cytogenetics. Absence of t(14;18) is helpful in distinguishing reactive from neoplastic proliferations.

Differential Diagnosis. In some lymphoid malignancies, a heterogeneous lymphoid pattern may be seen. These include low-grade FL, MZL, HL, and PTCL. These malignant entities can be distinguished from RLH by FCM and molecular analyses and by finding large atypical cells with CD15 and CD30 positivity in HL (12,38).

Granulomatous Processes

Some infectious processes may incite a granulomatous response; however, clusters of epithelioid histiocytes, multinucleated giant cells, or a "sarcoid-like reaction" can be seen in some malignant conditions affecting the lymph node. These conditions include HL and NHL and metastatic tumors (94,95).

Histiocytes typically seen in granulomas have elongated or curved nuclei with fine, evenly dispersed chromatin, small nucleoli, and moderate amount of finely vacuolated cytoplasm. Multinucleated histiocytic giant cells are commonly encountered (see specific types of granulomas in the Infectious Granulomatous Condition section below).

When granulomatous inflammation is diagnosed on FNA, special stains for organisms, including acid-fast bacillus (AFB) and Grocott methenamine silver stains, should be obtained. Microbiology culture studies should be performed when possible.

Infectious Granulomatous Condition

Tuberculous Lymphadenitis

Key Cytologic Features
- Caseating granulomas
  - Histiocytes, reactive lymphocytes, central caseous necrosis
- Langhans giant cells
- Background of neutrophils and necrosis
- Intracellular and extracellular "negative" images of bacilli on DQ stain in atypical mycobacteria (MAC) cases

In TB, the most common finding, seen in about 50% of cases, is the presence of epithelioid clusters with or without Langhans giant cells (large cells with nuclei arranged in a horseshoe-shaped pattern in the cell periphery) with necrosis (Fig. 12.27A and B); necrosis is absent in about one third of cases. FNA shows a sensitivity of about 75% in the detection of tuberculous lymphadenitis (94). AFBs may be identified by AFB special stain (Fig. 12.27C). In AIDS patient, MAC appear as intracellular and extracellular "negative images" in air-dried DQ-stained smears.

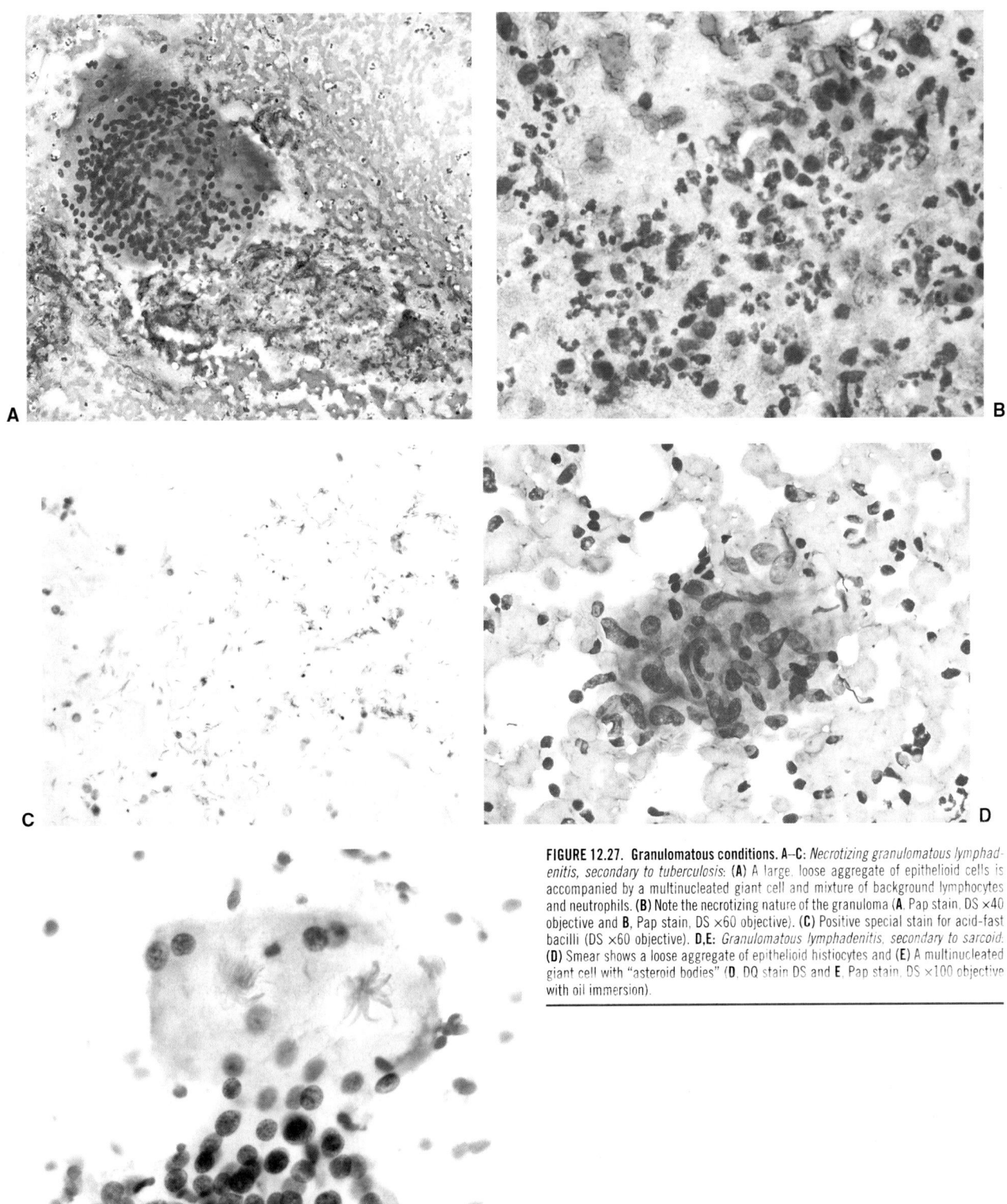

FIGURE 12.27. **Granulomatous conditions. A–C:** *Necrotizing granulomatous lymphadenitis, secondary to tuberculosis:* (**A**) A large, loose aggregate of epithelioid cells is accompanied by a multinucleated giant cell and mixture of background lymphocytes and neutrophils. (**B**) Note the necrotizing nature of the granuloma (**A**, Pap stain, DS ×40 objective and **B**, Pap stain, DS ×60 objective). (**C**) Positive special stain for acid-fast bacilli (DS ×60 objective). **D,E:** *Granulomatous lymphadenitis, secondary to sarcoid:* (**D**) Smear shows a loose aggregate of epithelioid histiocytes and (**E**) A multinucleated giant cell with "asteroid bodies" (**D**, DQ stain DS and **E**, Pap stain, DS ×100 objective with oil immersion).

Noninfectious Granulomatous Condition

Sarcoidosis

Key Cytologic Features
- Noncaseating granulomas
  - Epithelioid histiocytes, reactive lymphoid cells
  - Multinucleated giant cells
  - Cytoplasmic asteroid bodies or Schaumann bodies in sarcoid
- No necrosis

Sarcoidosis is a systemic disease of unknown cause characterized by noncaseating granulomas. The disease predominantly affects adult and middle-aged African American women. Although any organ can be affected, sarcoidosis frequently involves mediastinal lymph nodes and lungs. Cytologically, the main findings are well-formed noncaseating granulomas comprising of epithelioid histiocytes, multinucleated giant cells, and lymphocytes without necrosis (Fig. 12.27D). Asteroid bodies (star-shaped intracytoplasmic cytoskeletal elements) (Fig. 12.27E) and Schaumann bodies (calcium oxalate crystals) may be observed. Sarcoidosis is a diagnosis of exclusion; a foreign-body giant cell reaction, an infectious etiology, or a malignancy need to be excluded. Cytologic findings should be correlated with clinical and imaging features (95).

Infectious Mononucleosis

Key Cytologic Features
- Polymorphous lymphocytes
- Immunoblasts
- Plasmacytoid lymphocytes
- Tingible body macrophages
- Occasional PCs
- Mitosis and apoptosis

IM is an acute self-limited disease caused by EBV. It is usually seen in adolescents and young adults. In the acute infection, the virus replicates in the perifollicular B cells, simulating a vigorous humoral and cellular immune response. Typically, patients present with fever, pharyngitis, and cervical lymphadenopathy (75).

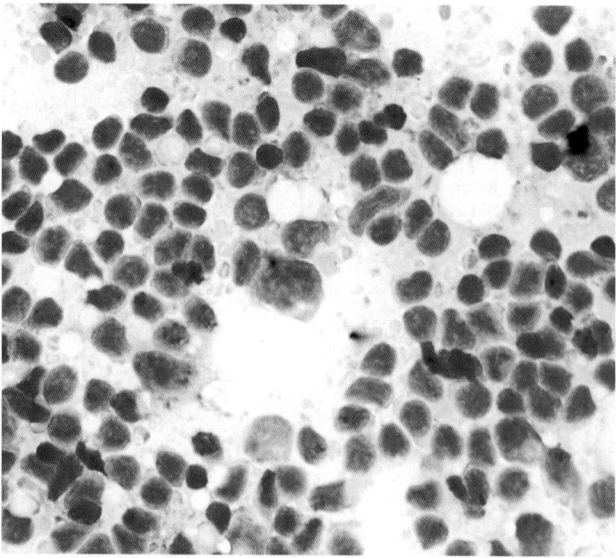

FIGURE 12.28. Infectious mononucleosis. Smear shows immunoblasts, reactive lymphocytes, and rare PCs (DQ stain DS ×100 objective with oil immersion).

Cytologically, IM displays large and small lymphocytes and large numbers of immunoblastic cells than are usually seen in a reactive lymph node. Immunoblasts are large cells with a large nucleus and nucleolus and basophilic cytoplasm (Fig. 12.28). Occasionally binucleated immunoblasts resembling RS cells are seen, a feature more commonly noted in the tonsils. Plasmacytoid lymphocytes, tingible body macrophages, and PCs are also seen. Mitosis and apoptosis are evident. In FNA smears, a polymorphic immunoblastic proliferation is suggestive of IM (Fig. 12.18A). ICC shows that these are of both B- and T-lymphocyte phenotype. Serologic studies confirm the diagnosis.

Primary and Metastatic Neoplasms

Primary and metastatic neoplasms including carcinomas, melanomas, germ cell tumors and sarcomas can mimic lymphoma (38,96).

Poorly Differentiated Carcinoma

Key Cytologic Features
- Loosely cohesive cell clusters and single cells
- Cell crowding
- High-grade nuclei
- Less or no cytoplasmic differentiation

Metastatic carcinoma represents about 50% of cases in FNA of lymph nodes. Well- to moderately differentiated carcinoma usually shows cohesive cell clusters with community cell borders (Fig. 12.29A) and can easily be recognized as being of epithelial origin on FNA. In adenocarcinomas, cytoplasmic differentiation such as mucinous vacuoles may be present. In squamous cell carcinomas, keratinized cytoplasm is usually seen. PDCa predominantly exhibit dispersed single cells or loosely cohesive cell clusters and may mimic lymphoma. Differential diagnosis of PDCa includes DLBCL (Fig. 12.29B). A history of a previous carcinoma is usually present. Epithelial markers including cytokeratin in conjunction with tumor-specific markers, such as thyroid-transcription factor (TTF-1) for lung and thyroid, PSMA for prostatic, and CDX2 for gastrointestinal adenocarcinomas, can be applied to various types of cytology preparations. Artifactual aggregation of cells in lymphoma may simulate carcinoma (Fig. 12.29C). Small cell carcinoma may also be mistaken for lymphomas (Fig. 12.30). Careful evaluation for the classic nuclear features of molding, "salt and pepper" chromatin with crush artifact, and ICC positivity for endocrine markers including chromogranin, synaptophysin, and CD56 help to distinguish it from lymphoma (97).

FNA smears of metastatic NPC show neoplastic single cells and clusters in a reactive lymphoid background (mixed pattern). Most single neoplastic cells present as large, pleomorphic bare nuclei. Metastatic NPC and HL may have a similar reactive lymphoid background, with eosinophils, PCs, and sometimes epithelioid-cell granulomas, and can be distinguished by ICC (98).

Melanoma

Melanoma demonstrates monomorphous mono- or binucleated cells in a dispersed cell pattern. Nuclei are large and round with smooth chromatin and prominent nucleoli. Cytoplasm is scanty and may contain melanin pigment (Fig. 12.31). The large binucleated melanoma cells with prominent nucleoli may mimic RS cells or cells of ALCL. Immunoreactivity for S-100 protein, HMB-45, and Melan A is characteristic.

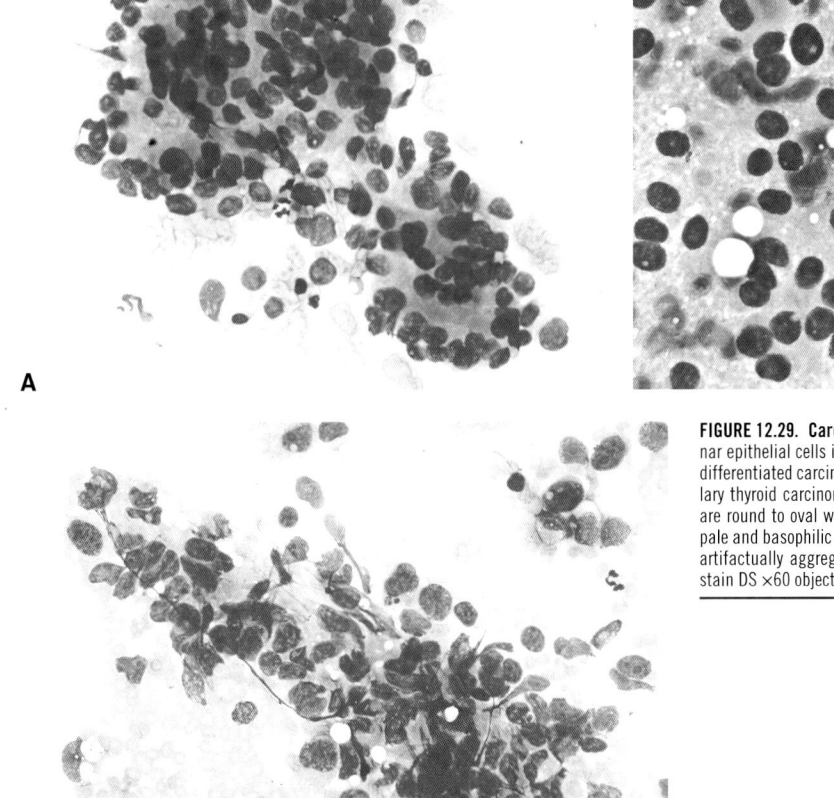

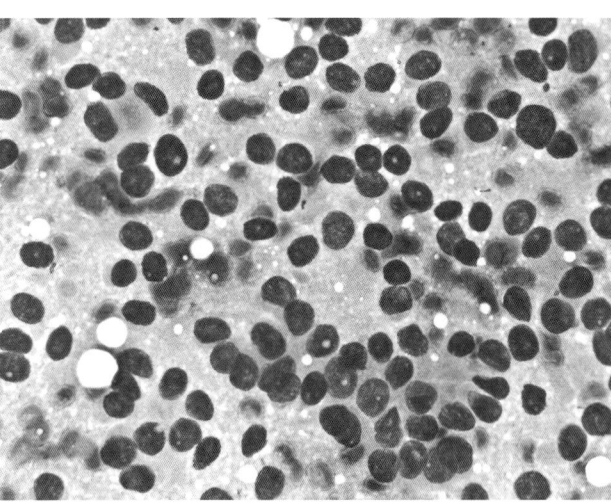

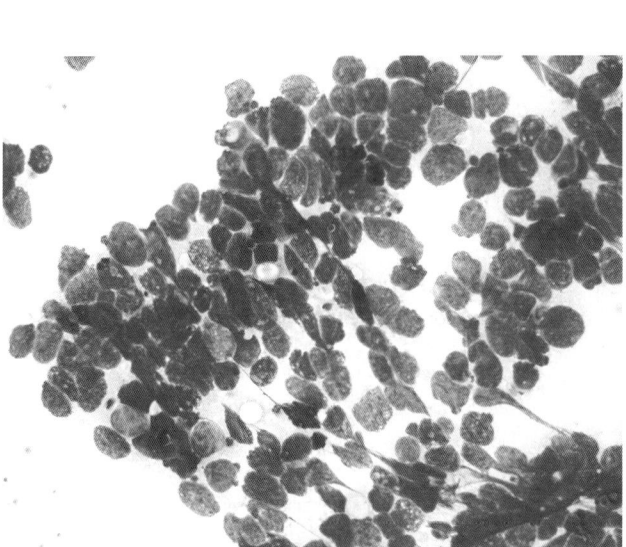

FIGURE 12.29. Carcinoma. A: Well-differentiated carcinoma of lung depicting colum-nar epithelial cells in a glandular architecture (DQ stain, DS ×60 objective). **B:** Poorly differentiated carcinoma may mimic DLBCL. In this case of poorly differentiated papil-lary thyroid carcinoma, cells are arranged in a vague follicular arrangement. Nuclei are round to oval with occasional intranuclear inclusions and grooves. Cytoplasm is pale and basophilic (Pap stain, DS ×60 objective). **C:** Cells of large cell lymphoma may artifactually aggregate and may need ICC for confirmation of lymphoid nature (DQ stain DS ×60 objective).

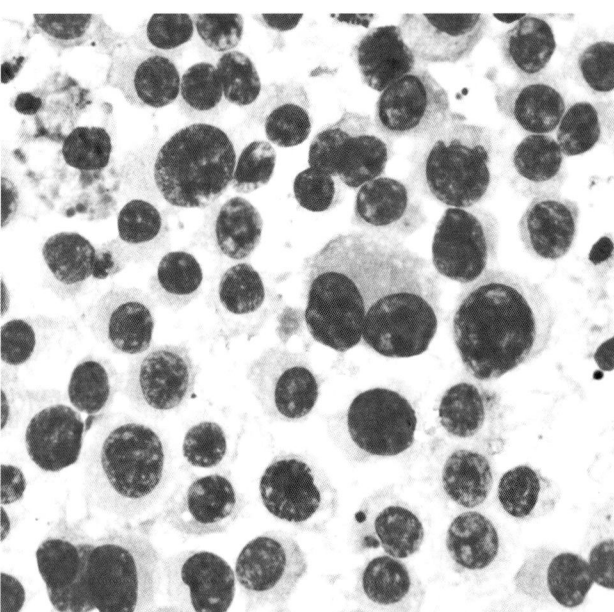

FIGURE 12.30. Metastatic small cell undifferentiated carcinoma of the lung. Aggregate of cohesive tumor cells with nuclear molding, fine to coarse, evenly dispersed chromatin, and scant to absent cytoplasm is easily identified. Note occasional nuclear elongation indicating crush artifact and apoptotic bodies (DQ stain DS ×60).

FIGURE 12.31. Metastatic melanoma showing dispersed neoplastic cells with eccentri-cally placed nuclei, prominent nucleoli, and granular blue-to-purple staining cytoplasm. Bi- and multinucleation and intranuclear cytoplasmic inclusions were also noted (DQ stain DS ×100 oil immersion).

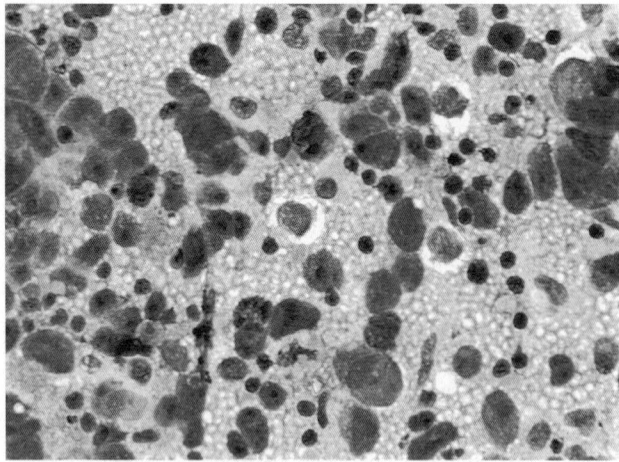

FIGURE 12.32. FNA of seminoma shows the characteristic "tigroid background" and monomorphic tumor cells with hyperchromatic round-to-oval nuclei and prominent nucleoli and lymphocytes (DQ stain DS ×100 oil immersion). Courtesy of Grace Yang, MD, Department of Pathology & Laboratory Medicine, Weill Cornell Medical Center, New York, NY.

Small Round Blue Cell Tumors

A group of undifferentiated malignancies known as the small round blue-cell tumors include neuroblastoma, Ewing family of tumors consisting of Ewing sarcoma and primitive neuroectodermal tumors, rhabdomyosarcoma, and lymphoblastic leukemia. These tumors share cytomorphologic similarities that can make them indistinguishable from each other and from lymphomas.

On FNA, neuroblastoma, Ewing sarcoma, and rhabdomyosarcoma frequently form small cellular aggregates in addition to discohesive cells. Other specific architectural features may be evident such as pseudorosettes in Ewing sarcoma and neuroblastoma and neurophil-like material in neuroblastoma. Rhabdomyosarcoma nuclei tend to be round with a vesicular chromatin pattern, occasionally with prominent nucleoli and relatively abundant cytoplasm. Ewing sarcoma tends to have spherical to ellipsoid nuclei with faintly stippled chromatin and small nucleoli.

ICC and cytogenetic studies can facilitate the distinction between lymphoma and other types of small round blue-cell tumors. Thus, for example, a panel composed of CD99 and TdT, lymphocytic markers (LCA, CD20, CD3), and vimentin appears to be sensitive and specific for distinguishing Ewing sarcoma from LBL (99). Ewing sarcoma also shows cytogenetic abnormality of t(11;22) in the majority of cases and t(21;22) in a small number of cases. Immunoreactivity for CD56 and chromogranin are effective in detecting neuroblastoma cells, and desmin and myogenin are useful in rhabdomyosarcoma.

Seminoma

Dispersed monomorphic cells with thick nuclear membranes, prominent nucleoli, and vacuolated cytoplasm with a lymphocytic component are characteristic for seminoma and may simulate lymphoma. The "tigroid background" of seminoma, produced by strands of cytoplasm and proteinaceous material, provides a helpful clue on DQ stain (Fig. 12.32).

Immunoreactivity for nuclear OCT4, membranous c-kit, and new marker SALL4 and 12p abnormality by FISH are seen in seminoma (100).

References

1. Swerdlow SH, Campo E, Harris NL, et al., eds. *World Health Organization classification of tumors of the hematopoietic and lymphoid tissues.* Lyon: IARC Press, 2008.

2. Meda BA, Buss DH, Woodruff RD, et al. Diagnosis and subclassification of primary and recurrent lymphoma. The usefulness and limitations of combined fine-needle aspiration cytomorphology and flowcytometry. *Am J Clin Pathol* 2000;113:688–699.

3. Wakely PE Jr. Fine-needle aspiration cytopathology in diagnosis and classification of malignant lymphoma: accurate and reliable? *Diagn Cytopathol* 2000;22:120–125.

4. Dong HY, Harris NL, Preffer FI, et al. Fine-needle aspiration biopsy in the diagnosis and classification of primary and recurrent lymphoma: a retrospective analysis of the utility of cytomorphology and flow cytometry. *Mod Pathol* 2001;14:472–481.

5. Landgren O, Porwit MacDonald A, et al. A prospective comparison of fine-needle aspiration cytology and histopathology in the diagnosis and classification of lymphomas. *Hematol J* 2004;5:69–76.

6. Katz RL. Modern approach to lymphoma diagnosis by fine-needle aspiration: restoring respect to a valuable procedure. *Cancer* 2005;105:429–431.

7. Wakely PE Jr. The diagnosis of non-Hodgkin lymphoma using fine-needle aspiration cytopathology: a work in progress. *Cancer Cytopathol* 2010;118:238–243.

8. Orucevic A, Reddy VB, Selvaggi SM, et al. Fine-needle aspiration of extranodal and extramedullary hematopoietic malignancies. *Diagn Cytopathol* 2000;23:318–321.

9. Mourad WA, Tulbah A, Shoukri M, et al. Primary diagnosis and REAL/WHO classification of non-Hodgkin's lymphoma by fine-needle aspiration: cytomorphologic and immunophenotypic approach. *Diagn Cytopathol* 2003;28:191–195.

10. Sigstad E, Dong HP, Davidson B, et al. The role of flow cytometric immunophenotyping in improving the diagnostic accuracy in referred fine-needle aspiration specimens. *Diagn Cytopathol* 2004;31:159–163.

11. Hehn ST, Grogan TM, Miller TP. Utility of fine-needle aspiration as a diagnostic technique in lymphoma. *J Clin Oncol* 2004;22:3046–3052.

12. Monaco SE, Khalbuss WE, Pantanowitz L. Benign non-infectious causes of lymphadenopathy: a review of cytomorphology and differential diagnosis. *Diagn Cytopathol* 2012;40(10):925–938.

13. Bangerter M, Brudler O, Heinrich B, et al. Fine needle aspiration cytology and flow cytometry in the diagnosis and subclassification of non-Hodgkin's lymphoma based on the World Health Organization classification. *Acta Cytol* 2007;51:390–398.

14. Ribeiro A, Pereira D, Escalón MP, et al. EUS-guided biopsy for the diagnosis and classification of lymphoma. *Gastrointest Endosc* 2010;71:851–855.

15. Chhieng DC, Cohen JM, Cangiarella JF. Cytology and immunophenotyping of low- and intermediate-grade non-Hodgkin's lymphomas with a predominant small-cell component: a study of 56 cases. *Diagn Cytopathol* 2001;24:90–97.

16. Amador-Ortiz C, Chen L, Hassan A, et al. Combined core needle biopsy and fine-needle aspiration with ancillary studies correlate highly with traditional techniques in the diagnosis of nodal-based lymphoma. *Am J Clin Pathol* 2011;135:516–524.

17. Hoda RS. Non-gynecologic cytology on liquid-based preparations: a morphologic review of facts and artifacts. *Diagn Cytopathol* 2007;35:621–634.

18. Ljung BM. Techniques of fine needle aspiration, smear preparation and principles of interpretation. In: Koss G, Melamed MR, eds. *Koss' diagnostic cytology and its histopathologic bases,* 5th ed. Philadelphia: Lippincott Williams & Wilkins, 2006:1056–1581.

19. Lieu D. Value of cytopathologist-performed ultrasound-guided fine needle aspiration as a screening test for ultrasound-guided core-needle biopsy in nonpalpable breast masses. *Diagn Cytopathol* 2009;37:262–269.

20. Gong JZ, Snyder MJ, Lagoo AS, et al. Diagnostic impact of core-needle biopsy on fine-needle aspiration of non-Hodgkin lymphoma. *Diagn Cytopathol* 2004;31:23–30.

21. Assaad MW, Pantanowitz L, Otis CN. Diagnostic accuracy of image-guided percutaneous fine needle aspiration biopsy of the mediastinum. *Diagn Cytopathol* 2007;35:705–709.

22. Ko HM, da Cunha Santos G, Darling G, et al. Diagnosis and subclassification of lymphomas and non-neoplastic lesions involving mediastinal lymph nodes using endobronchial ultrasound-guided transbronchial needle aspiration. *Diagn Cytopathol.* Published online 2011 May 31. PubMed PMID: 21630485.

23. Marshall CB, Jacob B, Patel S, et al. The utility of endobronchial ultrasound-guided transbronchial needle aspiration biopsy in the diagnosis of mediastinal lymphoproliferative disorders. *Cancer Cytopathol* 2011;119:118–126.

24. Griffin AC, Schwartz LE, Baloch ZW. Utility of on-site evaluation of endobronchial ultrasound-guided transbronchial needle aspiration specimens. *Cytojournal* 2011;8:20.

25. Florentine BD, Staymates B, Rabadi M, et al. Cancer Committee of the Henry Mayo Newhall Memorial Hospital. The reliability of fine-needle aspiration biopsy as the initial diagnostic procedure for palpable masses: a 4-year experience of 730 patients from a community hospital-based outpatient aspiration biopsy clinic. *Cancer* 2006;107:406–416.

26. Punia RS, Dhingra N, Chopra R, et al. Lymph node infarction and its association with lymphoma: a short series and literature review. *N Z Med J* 2009;122:40–44.

27. Caraway NP. Strategies to diagnose lymphoproliferative disorders by fine-needle aspiration by using ancillary studies. *Cancer* 2005;105:432–442.

28. Ali AE, Morgen EK, Geddie WR, et al. Classifying B-cell non-Hodgkin lymphoma by using MIB-1 proliferative index in fine-needle aspirates. *Cancer Cytopathol* 2010;118:166–172.

29. Symmans WF, Cangiarella JF, Symmans PJ, et al. Apoptotic index from fine needle aspiration cytology as a criterion to predict histologic grade of non-Hodgkin's lymphoma. *Acta Cytol* 2000;44:194–204.

30. Dey P. Role of ancillary techniques in diagnosing and subclassifying non-Hodgkin's lymphomas on fine needle aspiration cytology. *Cytopathology* 2006;17:275–287.

31. Weiss LM, Loera S, Bacchi CE. Immunoglobulin light chain immunohistochemistry revisited, with emphasis on reactive follicular hyperplasia versus follicular lymphoma. *Appl Immunohistochem Mol Morphol* 2010;18:199–205.

32. Theodossiou C, Schwarzenberger P. Non-Hodgkin's lymphomas. *Clin Obstet Gynecol* 2002;45:820–829.

33. Pambuccian SE, Bardales RH. *Lymph node cytopathology. Essentials in cytopathology.* New York: Springer, 2011.

34. Wright DH, Leong A S-Y, Addis BJ. *Diagnostic lymph node pathology,* 2nd ed. Canada: Hodder Arnold Publishers, 2011.

35. Skooj L, Tani E. *FNA cytology in the diagnosis of lymphoma*. Basel, Switzerland: Karger, 2009.
36. Kocjan G. Best Practice No 185. Cytological and molecular diagnosis of lymphoma. *J Clin Pathol* 2005;58:561–567.
37. Rossi ED, Larghi A, Verna EC, et al. Endoscopic ultrasound-guided fine-needle aspiration with liquid-based cytologic preparation in the diagnosis of primary pancreatic lymphoma. *Pancreas* 2010;39:1299–1302.
38. Gupta RK, Naran S, Lallu S, et al. The diagnostic value of fine needle aspiration cytology (FNAC) in the assessment of palpable supraclavicular lymph nodes: a study of 218 cases. *Cytopathology* 2003;14:201–207.
39. Savage EC, Vanderheyden AD, Bell AM, et al. Independent diagnostic accuracy of flow cytometry obtained from fine-needle aspirates: a 10-year experience with 451 cases. *Am J Clin Pathol* 2011;135:304–309.
40. Zeppa P, Vigliar E, Cozzolino I, et al. Fine needle aspiration cytology and flow cytometry immunophenotyping of non-Hodgkin lymphoma: can we do better? *Cytopathology* 2010;21:300–310.
41. Barrena S, Almeida J, Del Carmen García-Macias M, et al. Flow cytometry immunophenotyping of fine-needle aspiration specimens: utility in the diagnosis and classification of non-Hodgkin lymphomas. *Histopathology* 2011;58:906–918.
42. Schmid S, Tinguely M, Cione P, et al. Flow cytometry as an accurate tool to complement fine needle aspiration cytology in the diagnosis of low grade malignant lymphomas. *Cytopathology* 2011;22:397–406.
43. Zhang S, Abreo F, Lowery-Nordberg M, et al. The role of fluorescence in situ hybridization and polymerase chain reaction in the diagnosis and classification of lymphoproliferative disorders on fine-needle aspiration. *Cancer Cytopathol* 2010;118:105–112.
44. Goy A, Stewart J, Barkoh BA, et al. The feasibility of gene expression profiling generated in fine-needle aspiration specimens from patients with follicular lymphoma and diffuse large B-cell lymphoma. *Cancer* 2006;108:10–20.
45. Reading CF, Schlette EJ, Stewart JM, et al. Fine-needle aspiration biopsy findings in patients with small lymphocytic lymphoma transformed to Hodgkin lymphoma. *Am J Clin Pathol* 2007;128:571–578.
46. Tandon B, Peterson L, Gao J, et al. Nuclear overexpression of lymphoid-enhancer-binding factor 1 identifies chronic lymphocytic leukemia/small lymphocytic lymphoma in small B-cell lymphomas. *Mod Pathol* 2011;24:1433–1443.
47. Caraway NP, Thomas E, Khanna A, et al. Chromosomal abnormalities detected by multicolor fluorescence in situ hybridization in fine-needle aspirates from patients with small lymphocytic lymphoma are useful for predicting survival. *Cancer* 2008;114:315–322.
48. Lin P, Medeiros LJ. Lymphoplasmacytic lymphoma/waldenstrom macroglobulinemia: an evolving concept. *Adv Anat Pathol* 2005;12:246–255.
49. Vitolo U, Ferreri AJ, Montoto S. Lymphoplasmacytic lymphoma-Waldenstrom's macroglobulinemia. *Crit Rev Oncol Hematol* 2008;67:172–185.
50. Berger F, Traverse-Glehen A, Felman P, et al. Clinicopathologic features of Waldenstrom's macroglobulinemia and marginal zone lymphoma: are they distinct or the same entity? *Clin Lymphoma* 2005;5:220–224.
51. Goel G, Rai S, Naik R, et al. Cytodiagnosis of extramedullary plasmacytomas. *Acta Cytol* 2010;54:255–258.
52. Sarin H, Manucha V, Verma K. Extramedullary plasmacytoma, a report of five cases diagnosed by FNAC. *Cytopathology* 2009;20:328–231.
53. Murphy BA, Meda BA, Buss DH, et al. Marginal zone and mantle cell lymphomas: assessment of cytomorphology in subtyping small B-cell lymphomas. *Diagn Cytopathol* 2003;28:126–130.
54. Kaba S, Tokoro Y, Washiya K, et al. Cytology of pulmonary marginal zone B-cell lymphoma of MALT type: lessons learned for intra-operative diagnosis. *Cytopathology* 2011;22:346–349.
55. Crapanzano JP, Lin O. Cytologic findings of marginal zone lymphoma. *Cancer* 2003;99:301–309.
56. Saikia UN, Dey P, Saikia B, et al. Fine-needle aspiration biopsy in diagnosis of follicular lymphoma: cytomorphologic and immunohistochemical analysis. *Diagn Cytopathol* 2002;26:251–256.
57. Young NA. Grading follicular lymphoma on fine-needle aspiration specimens—a practical approach. *Cancer* 2006;108:1–9.
58. Ouansafi I, He B, Fraser C, et al. Transformation of follicular lymphoma to plasmablastic lymphoma with c-myc gene rearrangement. *Am J Clin Pathol* 2010;134:972–981.
59. Cibas ES, Ducatman BS. *Cytology: diagnostic principals and clinical correlates*, 3rd ed. Philadelphia: Elsevier Health Sciences, 2009.
60. Sun W, Caraway NP, Zhang HZ, et al. Grading follicular lymphoma on fine needle aspiration specimens. Comparison with proliferative index by DNA image analysis and Ki-67 labeling index. *Acta Cytol* 2004;48:119–126.
61. Brandao GD, Rose R, McKenzie S, et al. Grading follicular lymphomas in fine-needle aspiration biopsies: the role of ThinPrep slides and flowcytometry. *Cancer* 2006;108:319–323.
62. da Cunha Santos G, Ko HM, Geddie WR, et al. Targeted use of fluorescence in situ hybridization (FISH) in cytospin preparations: results of 298 fine needle aspirates of B-cell non-Hodgkin lymphoma. *Cancer Cytopathol* 2010;118:250–258.
63. Richmond J, Bryant R, Trotman W, et al. FISH detection of t(14;18) in follicular lymphoma on Papanicolaou-stained archival cytology slides. *Cancer* 2006;108:198–204.
64. Bangerter M, Brudler O, Heinrich B, et al. Fine needle aspiration cytology and flow cytometry in the diagnosis and subclassification of non-Hodgkin's lymphoma based on the World Health Organization classification. *Acta Cytol* 2007;51: 390–398.
65. Parrens M, Belaud-Rotureau MA, Fitoussi O, et al. Blastoid and common variants of mantle cell lymphoma exhibit distinct immunophenotypic and interphase FISH features. *Histopathology* 2006;48:353–362.
66. Athanasiou E, Kotoula V, Hytiroglou P, et al. In situ hybridization and reverse transcription-polymerase chain reaction for cyclin D1 mRNA in the diagnosis of mantle cell lymphoma in paraffin-embedded tissues. *Mod Pathol* 2001;14: 62–71.
67. Zeng W, Fu K, Quintanilla-Fend L, et al. Cyclin D1-negative blastoid mantle cell lymphoma identified by SOX11 expression. *Am J Surg Pathol* 2012;36:214–219.
68. de Leval L, Hasserjian RP. Diffuse large B-cell lymphomas and burkitt lymphoma. *Hematol Oncol Clin North Am* 2009;23:791–827.
69. Verstovsek G, Chakraborty S, Ramzy I, et al. Large B-cell lymphomas: fine-needle aspiration plays an important role in initial diagnosis of cases which are falsely negative by flow cytometry. *Diagn Cytopathol* 2002;27:282–285.
70. Desouki MM, Post GR, Cherry D, et al. PAX-5: a valuable immunohistochemical marker in the differential diagnosis of lymphoid neoplasms. *Clin Med Res* 2010;8:84–88.
71. Daneshbod Y, Omidvari S, Daneshbod K, et al. Diffuse large B cell lymphoma of thyroid as a masquerader of anaplastic carcinoma of thyroid diagnosed by FNA: a case report. *Cytojournal* 2006;3:23.
72. Hoda RS, Picklesimer L, Green KM, et al. Fine-needle aspiration of a primary mediastinal large B-cell lymphoma: a case report with cytologic, histologic, and flow cytometric considerations. *Diagn Cytopathol* 2005;32:370–337
73. Rafaniello Raviele P, Pruneri G, et al. Plasmablastic lymphoma: a review. *Oral Dis* 2009;15:38–45.
74. Reid-Nicholson M, Kavuri S, Ustun C, et al. Plasmablastic lymphoma: cytologic findings in 5 cases with unusual presentation. *Cancer* 2008;114(5):333–341.
75. Rezk SA, Weiss LM. Epstein-Barr virus-associated lymphoproliferative disorders [Review]. *Hum Pathol* 2007;38:1293–304.
76. Troxell ML, Bangs CD, Cherry AM, et al. Cytologic diagnosis of Burkitt lymphoma. *Cancer* 2005;105:310–318.
77. Bellan C, Stefano L, Giulia de F, et al. Burkitt lymphoma versus diffuse large B-cell lymphoma: a practical approach. *Hematol Oncol* 2009;27:182–185.
78. Mann G, Attarbaschi A, Steiner M, et al. Austrian Berlin-Frankfurt-Münster (BFM) group. Early and reliable diagnosis of non-Hodgkin lymphoma in childhood and adolescence: contribution of cytomorphology and flow cytometric immunophenotyping. *Pediatr Hematol Oncol* 2006;23:167–176.
79. Wakely P Jr, Frable WJ, Kneisl JS. Soft tissue aspiration cytopathology of malignant lymphoma and leukemia. *Cancer* 2001;93:35–39.
80. Yao JL, Cangiarella JF, Cohen JM, et al. Fine-needle aspiration biopsy of peripheral T-cell lymphomas. A cytologic and immunophenotypic study of 33 cases. *Cancer* 2001;93:151–159.
81. Mathur S, Verm K. Peripheral T-cell lymphoma not otherwise specified vs. Hodgkin's lymphoma on fine needle aspiration cytology. *Acta Cytol* 2005;49:373–377.
82. Das P, Iyer VK, Mathur SR, et al. Anaplastic large cell lymphoma: a critical evaluation of cytomorphological features in seven cases. *Cytopathology* 2010;21: 251–258.
83. McEvoy JR, Cady FM, Hoda RS. "Wreath cell" in recurrent anaplastic large cell lymphoma. *Diagn Cytopathol* 2006;34:112–113.
84. Buxton D, Bacchi CE, Gualco G, et al. Frequent expression of CD99 in anaplastic large cell lymphoma: a clinicopathologic and immunohistochemical study of 160 cases. *Am J Clin Pathol* 2009;131:574–579.
85. Eberle FC, Mani H, Jaffe ES. Histopathology of Hodgkin's lymphoma. *Cancer J* 2009;15:129–137.
86. Das DK, Francis IM, Sharma PN, et al. Hodgkin's lymphoma: diagnostic difficulties in fine-needle aspiration cytology. *Diagn Cytopathol* 2009;37:564–573.
87. Jiménez-Heffernan JA, Vicandi B, López-Ferrer P, et al. Value of fine needle aspiration cytology in the initial diagnosis of Hodgkin's disease. Analysis of 188 cases with an emphasis on diagnostic pitfalls. *Acta Cytol* 2001;45:300–306.
88. Iacobuzio-Donahue CA, Clark DP, Ali SZ. Reed-Sternberg-like cells in lymph node aspirates in the absence of Hodgkin's disease: pathologic significance and differential diagnosis. *Diagn Cytopathol* 2002;27:335–339.
89. Gualco G, Weiss LM, Bacchi CE. Expression of p63 in anaplastic large cell lymphoma but not in classical Hodgkin's lymphoma. *Hum Pathol* 2008;39: 1505–1510.
90. Mourad WA, al Nazer M, Tulbah A. Cytomorphologic differentiation of Hodgkin's lymphoma and Ki-1+ anaplastic large cell lymphoma in fine needle aspirates. *Acta Cytol* 2003;47:744–748.
91. Subhawong AP, Ali SZ, Tatsas AD. Nodular lymphocyte-predominant Hodgkin lymphoma: cytopathologic correlates on fine-needle aspiration. *Cancer Cytopathol* 2012;120(4):254–260.
92. Kumar PV, Mousavi A, Karimi M, et al. Fine needle aspiration of Langerhans cell histiocytosis of the lymph nodes. A report of six cases. *Acta Cytol* 2002;46:753–756.
93. Yang GC, Wang J, Yee HT. Interwoven dendritic processes of follicular dendritic cell sarcoma demonstrated on ultrafast papanicolaou-stained smears: a case report. *Acta Cytol* 2006;50:534–538.
94. Mittal P, Handa U, Mohan H, et al. Comparative evaluation of fine needle aspiration cytology, culture, and PCR in diagnosis of tuberculous lymphadenitis. *Diagn Cytopathol* 2011;39:822–826.
95. Mehrotra R, Dhingra V. Cytological diagnosis of sarcoidosis revisited: a state of the art review. *Diagn Cytopathol* 2011;39:541–548.
96. Anderson GG, Weiss LM. Determining tissue of origin for metastatic cancers: meta-analysis and literature review of immunohistochemistry performance. *Appl Immunohistochem Mol Morphol* 2010;18:3–8. Review.
97. De Las Casas LE, Gokden M, Mukunyadzi P, et al. A morphologic and statistical comparative study of small-cell carcinoma and non-Hodgkin's lymphoma in fine-needle aspiration biopsy material from lymph nodes. *Diagn Cytopathol* 2004;31:229–234.
98. Kollur SM, El Hag IA. Fine-needle aspiration cytology of metastatic nasopharyngeal carcinoma in cervical lymph nodes: comparison with metastatic squamous-cell carcinoma, and Hodgkin's and non-Hodgkin's lymphoma. *Diagn Cytopathol* 2003;28:18–22.
99. Lucas DR, Bentley G, Dan ME, et al. Ewing sarcoma vs lymphoblastic lymphoma. A comparative immunohistochemical study. *Am J Clin Pathol* 2001;115:11–17.
100. Iwamoto N, Ishida M, Yoshida K, et al. Mediastinal seminoma: a case report with special emphasis on sall4 as a new immunocytochemical marker. *Diagn Cytopathol*. Published online 2012 Feb 1. Pubmed PMID: 22298374.

OVERVIEW

Lymph nodes are composed of multiple interrelated functional compartments. Although the following histologic appearances are described separately, they are often seen in combination. Instead of separate categories, they are better thought of as predominant patterns.

Maturation of the follicular dendritic cell meshwork is thought to be a first step in the development of the primary follicle and subsequent secondary follicle formation. Follicular dendritic cells produce the chemokine CXCL13 (B-cell–attracting chemokine) that interacts with a highly expressed receptor on naive B cells, CXCR5, recruiting B cells to the primary follicle (1). B cells and T cells are segregated into their respective compartments within the lymph node by following fluctuations in chemokine concentration gradients (1). Germinal center (GC) formation is typically the result of a T-cell–dependent B-cell response to an antigen. B cells in T-cell zones interact with specific T cells that have already been primed to a specific antigen; B cells then can differentiate into antibody-forming cells or GCs that give rise to plasma cells and memory B cells (1). The exact signals that bias this response are still unclear.

Antigen stimulation triggers transformation from the primary follicle (Fig. 13.1) to the secondary follicle (Fig. 13.2), followed by eventual termination of the GC reaction via GC dissolution (progressive transformation, regression, or fragmentation) (Fig. 13.3) (2). Primary follicles are small nodular collections of unstimulated small B cells in a follicular dendritic meshwork. Primary follicles express a distinct immunophenotype with up-regulation of BCL-2 protein and in contrast to secondary follicles do not express CD10 or BCL-6. Similarly, the naive follicular dendritic cell meshworks of the primary follicle do not express CD21 or CD23, markers that are expressed strongly in the follicular dendritic cell meshworks of the secondary follicle (3). Secondary follicles are composed of a GC surrounded circumferentially by a mantle zone. The GC contains small B lymphocytes (centrocytes and centroblasts), some small T helper lymphocytes, follicular dendritic cells, and tingible body macrophages. There are two functional microenvironments of the GC that typically show a distinctive polarization due to the direction of antigen presentation: a dark zone (facing the medulla) and a light zone (facing the capsule) (2). B cells of the dark zone, centroblasts, proliferate and undergo somatic hypermutation. B cells of the light zone, centrocytes, are selected for their affinity to antigen and nonaffinity (or tolerance) to self. The centrocytes of the light zone are the centroblasts from the dark zone that have exited the cell cycle and become long-lived plasma cells and memory B cells. Centrocytes with self-reactivity or low-affinity antibodies undergo apoptosis, resulting in much of the cellular debris seen inside tingible body macrophages. In contrast to the immunophenotype of primary follicles,

secondary follicles have down-regulation of BCL-2 protein and express the follicle center markers CD10 and BCL-6. The surrounding mantle zone is composed of small unstimulated B cells that had previously made up the primary follicle. Both immunoglobulin M (IgM) and immunoglobulin D (IgD) are expressed on the B cells of the mantle zone. An additional concentric layer of small marginal zone B cells may be seen surrounding the mantle zone, primarily in mesenteric lymph nodes and spleen. B cells that make up the marginal zone express IgM and do not express IgD. Rarely this third layer may be expanded in reactive conditions.

Follicular Hyperplasia

Follicular hyperplasia (FH) (Fig. 13.4) refers to an increase in secondary follicles per unit area. Follicles are often increased in size (e.g., hypertrophy) as well (Fig. 13.5). Histologically, a spectrum of variably sized and shaped secondary follicles is seen. Classically, they retain their polarization, distinct mantle zones, and tingible body macrophages in the GCs. These findings support a reactive proliferation over a neoplastic process. Typically, in follicular hyperplasia, overall lymph node architecture is retained, sinuses are patent, there is no capsular fibrosis, and extracapsular extension is minimal or absent. Benign, reactive proliferations may show a temporal sequence of primary follicles, follicular hyperplasia, and areas of GC breakdown. Rarely, a marginal zone pattern may be seen in combination with follicular hyperplasia (4).

The differential diagnosis of follicular hyperplasia is broad and encompasses neoplastic, infectious, and autoimmune etiologies. Often no specific etiologic agent is identified; however, some classic associations are rheumatoid arthritis (RA), human immunodeficiency virus (HIV)-related lymphadenopathy, syphilis, and plasma cell subtype of Castleman disease. BCL-2 expression is often used to differentiate neoplastic from reactive follicles. Neoplastic follicles of follicular lymphoma express BCL-2 protein in the majority of cases (>75%), while reactive secondary follicles do not show up-regulation of this protein. An important caveat to use of this immunohistochemical staining is that high-grade follicular lymphoma (follicular lymphoma grade 3) may not show expression of BCL-2; consequently this stain cannot exclude a neoplastic proliferation. Focal staining of BCL-2 in secondary follicles has been referred to as "follicular lymphoma *in situ*" and is thought to be a precursor lesion to frank follicular lymphoma (see Chapter 22) (Table 13.1) (5). BCL-2 staining also highlights the intrafollicular T-helper cells, which can be highly variable in number. Comparison of the BCL-2 stain with a CD3 stain, to assess the number of T cells within the follicle, is recommended.

Rarely, follicular hyperplasia may show clonal B-cell populations by flow cytometric evaluation. These clonal populations may coexpress the follicle center marker CD10, and have been found to be in excess of 20% of cells analyzed (6).

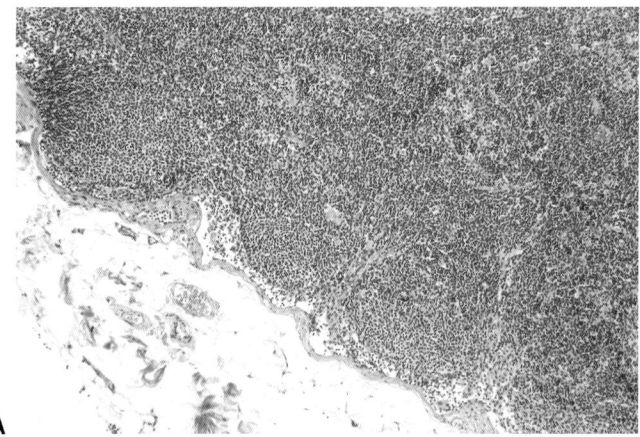

A

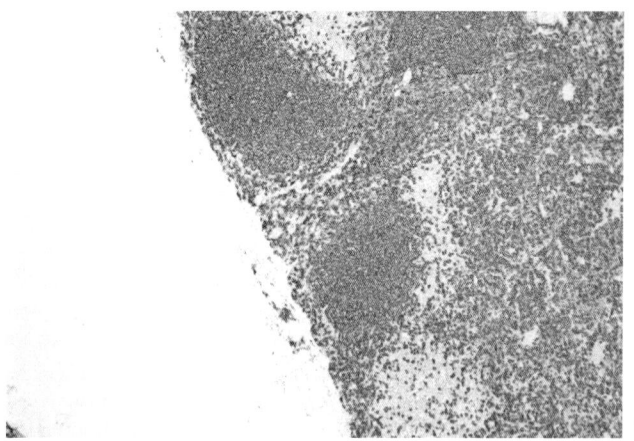

B

FIGURE 13.1. Primary follicle composed of small unstimulated B lymphocytes, BCL-2 positive. Nodular aggregates of lymphoid cells at the periphery of the lymph node. These nodules are uniform in appearance and composed of *small dark blue*, "mantle-type" lymphocytes **(A)**. This is a primary follicle that is composed of mostly naive, CD20-positive B cells **(B)**, which are positive for bcl-2 **(C)**.

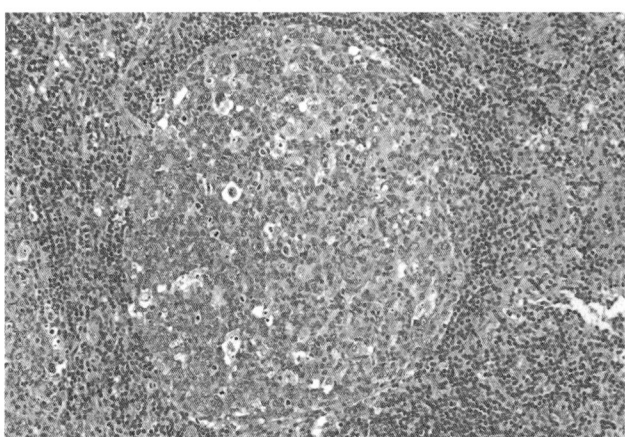

C

Similarly, evaluation of follicular hyperplasia by molecular studies for immunoglobulin gene rearrangements by PCR may occasionally lead to aberrant clonal results (7). In these cases, it should be noted that this is a possibility and if there are compelling morphologic and immunophenotypic evidence of a benign process, then these ancillary studies should be taken in the overall context and not overinterpreted.

Follicular hyperplasia is thought to be an immunologic response to an allergenic challenge. In children and young adults, follicular hyperplasia is easily explained as exposure to a new antigen and the resulting mounting of a humoral immune response. In older adults, more clinical correlation may be needed, as FH in this age group has been associated with concurrent or subsequent diagnosis of non-Hodgkin lymphoma (8,9). Additionally, follicular hyperplasia has been associated with IgG4-related lymphadenopathy in older adults (see Chapter 14).

Mantle Zone/Primary Follicle Hyperplasia

Mantle zone hyperplasia, or primary follicle hyperplasia, is a proliferation of naive B cells of the mantle zone, and is a rare occurrence. This term is used to describe both the expansion or

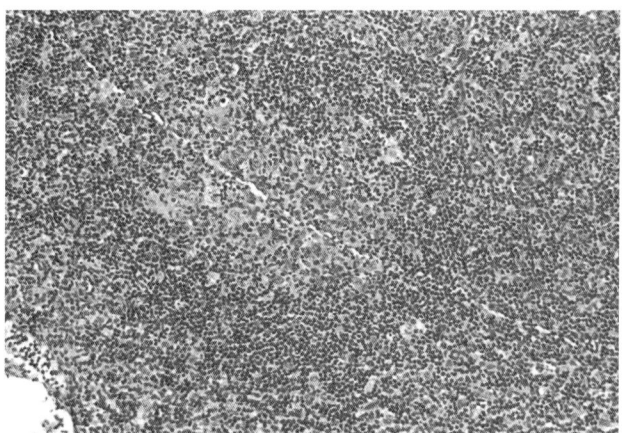

FIGURE 13.2. Secondary follicle composed of a GC showing a light **(right)** and dark **(left)** zone, polarization, with tingible body macrophages, follicular dendritic cells, surrounded by a mantle cell zone of small lymphocytes.

FIGURE 13.3. GC dissolution. Small follicle in center has lost sharp borders distinguishing mantle from GC. The GC cells are still present, but other features of reactive GCs (polarization, tingible body macrophages) are not seen.

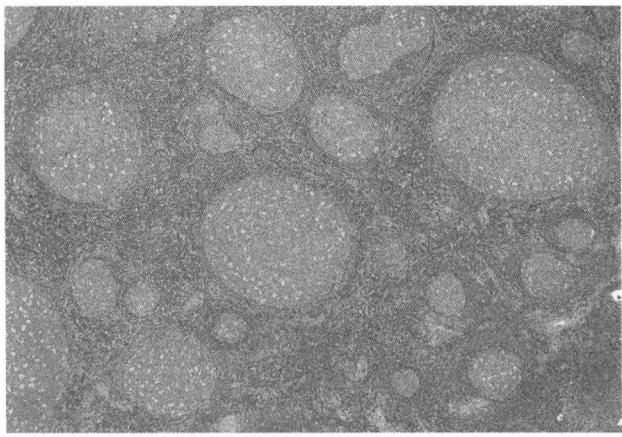

FIGURE 13.4. Follicular hyperplasia. There is an increase in the number of follicles per unit area, the definition of follicular hyperplasia.

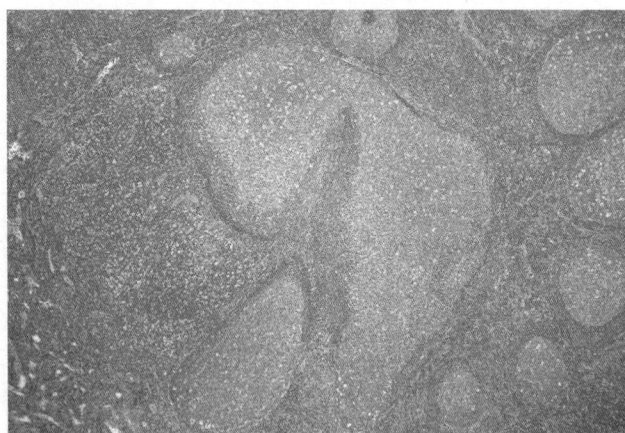

FIGURE 13.5. Hypertrophy, or an increase in size, of follicles that usually accompanies a follicular hyperplasia, an increase in number. In this case, there is fusion of follicular structures forming a large dumbbell-shaped follicle.

thickening of the mantle cell zone (Fig. 13.6) and an increase in the number of primary follicles per unit area.

The cells of the mantle zone are small in size with round nuclear contours, inconspicuous nucleoli, mature chromatin, and a scant amount of cytoplasm. Rarely a moderate amount of pale cytoplasm may be seen, giving the appearance of a monocytoid or marginal zone B cell (10). Mantle zone hyperplasia is thought to represent the earliest phase of a reactive GC reaction. It may be seen in association with progressive transformation of germinal centers (PTGCs) and hyaline vascular Castleman disease (HV-CD). The differential diagnosis includes low-grade lymphomas such as mantle cell lymphoma (MCL) or small lymphocytic lymphoma (SLL). MCL expresses cyclin D1 (BCL-1) and SLL expresses CD43, and in contrast benign mantle cells do not express these markers. However, the benign mantle cells express BCL-2 protein, and in cases with PTGCs this is a potential pitfall in the diagnosis of floral variant of follicular lymphoma.

Marginal Zone/Monocytoid B-Cell Hyperplasia

The marginal zone refers to a third outer layer of the secondary follicle, or a proliferation of monocytoid B cells in interfollicular areas (Fig. 13.7). The normal marginal zone is seen only in spleen, mesenteric lymph nodes, or mucosal sites. When marginal zone hyperplasia is present, it may be seen in any site. The ontogeny of the marginal zone has not been completely explained. This compartment is a mixture of immature B cells, memory B cells, naive recirculating B cells, and B1 cells (1). The relationship between marginal zone hyperplasia and monocytoid B-cell hyperplasia is not clear, and these processes may be somehow related.

The cells of the marginal zone are small to medium sized with mature chromatin, rounded to indented nuclei, inconspicuous nucleoli, and a moderate amount of pale to clear cytoplasm. Neutrophils almost always accompany the cells of monocytoid B-cell hyperplasia. Atypia and mitotic figures are not characteristic. Included in the differential diagnosis of marginal zone hyperplasia are lymphomas such as nodal marginal zone lymphoma, follicular lymphoma with marginal zone differentiation, SLL, MCL, and peripheral T-cell lymphoma (11). Viral infections (Cytomegalovirus [CMV], Epstein-Barr virus [EBV], and HIV), toxoplasmosis, cat scratch disease (CSD), and lymphogranuloma venereum are specific infectious manifestations associated with marginal zone or monocytoid B-cell hyperplasia. Normal marginal zone B cells (infrequently seen in lymph nodes) are typically BCL-2 positive, but reactive monocytoid hyperplasia is BCL-2 negative (11,12). Higher levels of IgM as well as high levels of CD21 and low levels of CD23 are seen in this population (1). Differentiation from neoplastic proliferations may be difficult by morphology. Immunohistochemical stains and/or evaluation for a clonal population using molecular gene rearrangement studies may be necessary.

Immunoblastic Hyperplasia

Immunoblastic hyperplasia is most commonly seen as a nonspecific response. It is characterized by an increase in large activated lymphocytes (immunoblasts) in interfollicular zones (Fig. 13.8). The immunoblasts are accompanied by a heterogeneous population with varying numbers of small lymphocytes, eosinophils, plasma cells, histiocytes, and interdigitating reticulum cells, imparting a mottled appearance at low magnification.

Table 13.1 COMPARISON OF IMMUNOHISTOCHEMICAL STAINING: PRIMARY FOLLICLE, FOLLICULAR HYPERPLASIA, FOLLICULAR LYMPHOMA *IN SITU*, AND FOLLICULAR LYMPHOMA

Immunohistochemical Stain	Primary Follicle	Follicular Hyperplasia	Follicular Lymphoma *In Situ*	Follicular Lymphoma
BCL-2	+	–	+	+ in about 75%
CD20	+	+	+	+
BCL-6/CD10	–	+	+	+
CD21/CD23	+ in follicular dendritic networks	+ in follicular dendritic networks	+ in follicular dendritic networks	+ in follicular dendritic networks
Ki-67	Low	High	Focal low	Low

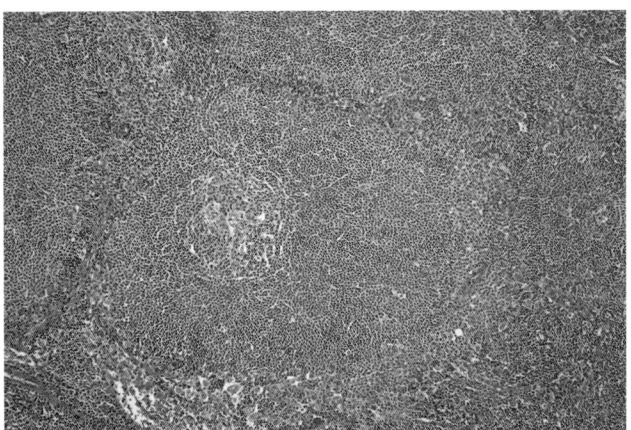

FIGURE 13.6. Expanded mantle cell zone in mantle zone hyperplasia.

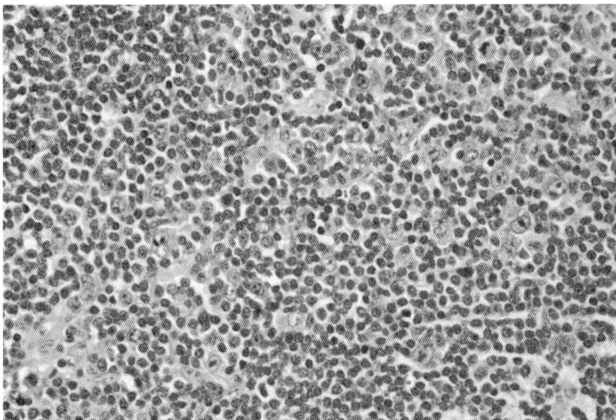

FIGURE 13.8. Expanded immunoblasts in an interfollicular expansion/immunoblastic hyperplasia. Increased immunoblasts are seen in the interfollicular areas. These have some prominent nucleoli and moderate amounts of blue cytoplasmic.

Immunoblastic hyperplasia is a common finding in viral infections, including EBV (discussed later in Herpesviridae section). Other identified causes include postvaccinal and drug-related lymphadenopathy (particularly Dilantin) (13). The differential diagnosis includes diffuse large B-cell lymphoma, early nodal involvement by Hodgkin lymphoma, nodal marginal zone lymphoma, lymphoplasmacytic lymphoma, anaplastic large cell lymphoma, peripheral T-cell lymphoma, and plasmacytoma as these all show preferential distribution in the interfollicular zones.

Immunohistochemical staining shows that the immunoblasts are a mixture of B and T cells. The B immunoblasts may show down-regulation of CD20 as well as expression of CD30 (a marker of activation). CD15 staining is negative in these immunoblasts; however, focal weak staining in histiocytes may be seen, making a diagnosis of classical Hodgkin lymphoma a common pitfall. Immunoblasts show expression of CD45 while Hodgkin cells are negative for this marker. Additionally, B immunoblasts show strong nuclear expression of Pax-5, while Hodgkin cells have a characteristic decreased intensity of expression for this marker.

Germinal Center Breakdown

PTGCs are thought to be one of multiple pathways of GC breakdown (2,14). PTGC results in a markedly expanded nodule, roughly three to five times the size of a typical reactive follicle (Fig. 13.9). The nodule is composed of small mantle zone B cells that have infiltrated the GC and markedly expanded the follicular dendritic cell meshwork. Occasionally, epithelioid histiocytes may be seen in a concentric ring surrounding the nodule, a finding described as perifollicular granulomas.

The differential diagnosis of PTGC includes nodular lymphocyte predominant Hodgkin lymphoma (NLPHL) (see Chapter 15), follicular colonization by low-grade B-cell lymphomas, such as mantle cell or marginal zone lymphoma, as well as the floral variant of follicular lymphoma. In PTGC, T cells are seen clustering around GC remnants; however, this phenomenon is not seen in follicular colonization by low-grade lymphoma (2). PTGC may be seen in a number of different contexts. In the context of follicular hyperplasia one or more areas of PTGC may be seen in 10% to 15% of enlarged lymph nodes (14,15). PTGC may also occur as a predominant pattern, often called florid PTGC. This finding is often seen in the pediatric or young adult age group. In these cases it is most often reported as solitary painless lymphadenopathy in males with the cervical region most commonly affected followed by the inguinal and axillary regions (16). Persistent or recurrent PTGC is often reported in the pediatric age group (2). The presence of PTGC is associated with Hodgkin lymphoma, especially NLPHL; however, it is not considered a premalignant condition (15,17).

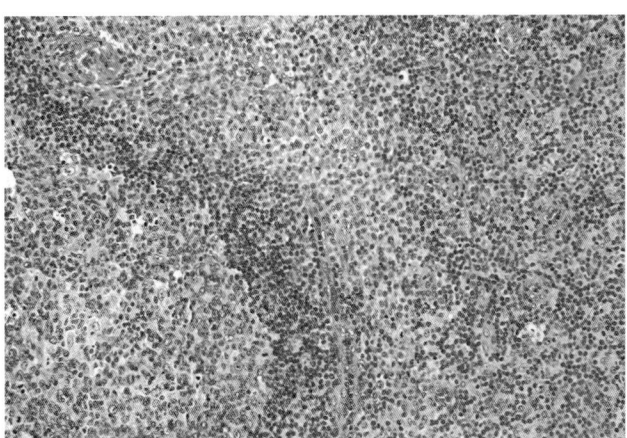

FIGURE 13.7. Marginal zone hyperplasia. The marginal zone (**center**) is usually found adjacent to the mantle zone, and composed of lymphocytes with round to slightly irregular nuclei and moderate amounts of pale cytoplasm.

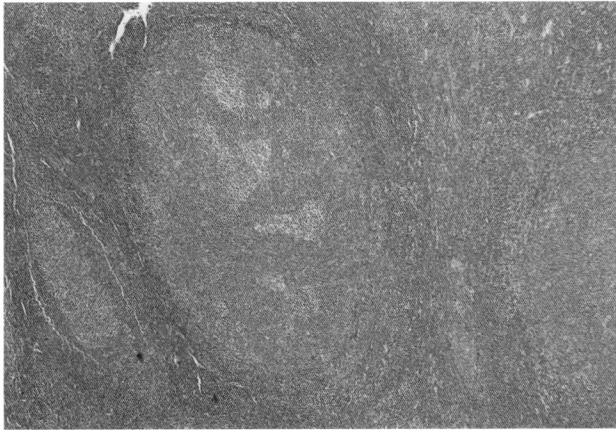

FIGURE 13.9. Progressive transformation of germinal centers (PTGCs). PTGCs are very large nodules composed of mostly *dark blue*, small lymphocytes. In the central regions there are some larger, more pale cells (GC cells).

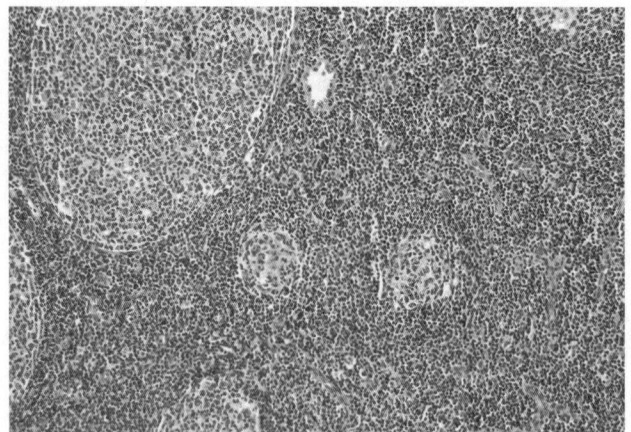

FIGURE 13.10. Regression of GCs. A large GC (**upper left**) is compared to two regressed follicles in the more central area. There are small mantle zones and reduced numbers of GC cells.

In contrast to PTGC, regression of GCs ends in small atrophic follicles. Regression of GCs is often seen in the context of a follicular hyperplasia. Stromal cells of the follicles are prominent, lymphocytes and tingible body macrophages are depleted, and often the mantle zone is preserved (Fig. 13.10). Similar changes can be seen in patients with connective tissue disease or in patients who have received nodal radiation or systemic immunosuppressive chemotherapy (2). Regressed follicles may appear similar to the small atrophic follicles of HV-CD (see Chapter 14); however, they lack the large atypical follicular dendritic cells seen in HV-CD. The number of regressed GCs with prominent hyalinization increases with increasing age (18).

Sinus Histiocytosis

Sinus histiocytosis is an exaggeration of normal lymph node compartment and is part of a functional immunologic response. In sinus histiocytosis, the normally compact and inapparent lymph node sinuses are distended by a prominent population of histiocytes (Fig. 13.11). The histiocytes are of uniform size with oval-shaped, bland-appearing nuclei and a copious amount of clear or pale cytoplasm. Rare cases with a signet ring cell appearance of the histiocytes have been reported (19). Sinus histiocytosis may show phagocytosis (with cellular debris); however, emperipolesis (retention of intact cells such as lymphocytes) is not seen, an important distinction from Rosai-Dorfman disease.

Most cases of sinus histiocytosis do not have a specific etiology. This pattern may be seen in lymph nodes draining tumors. As such, it is important to exclude metastatic tumor (bland appearing carcinoma or melanoma). If the tumor has a mucinous component an expanded population of sinus histiocytes containing mucin (muciphages) may be seen. Additionally, a primarily sinusoidal pattern is classically associated with anaplastic large cell lymphoma. Sinus histiocytosis may also be present as part of hemophagocytic lymphohistiocytosis (HLH)/ hemophagocytic syndrome (discussed later in Hemophagocytic lymphohistiocytic syndrome).

Paracortical Hyperplasia

In paracortical hyperplasia the paracortex (the region between the B-cell follicles and the medulla) is expanded by immunoblasts, small T lymphocytes, histiocytes, and occasional collections of plasmacytoid dendritic cells. The heterogeneous population combined with histiocytes and immunoblasts imparts a mottled appearance at low power (Fig. 13.12). The histologic appearance is similar to dermatopathic lymphadenitis (see below in Dermatopathic lymphadenitis section); however, phagocytized melanin or pigment is not apparent. Most cases of paracortical hyperplasia do not have a specific etiology. Classically, a hyperplasia of the paracortical region is associated with a viral lymphadenitis as well as postvaccinal lymphadenopathy.

Dermatopathic Lymphadenitis

Dermatopathic lymphadenitis is a paracortical proliferation originally described in lymph nodes draining chronically inflamed skin (20–22). Generally, dermatopathic lymphadenitis is a benign condition that can be diagnosed histologically without the clinical history of dermatitis (23). It is classically described in axillary lymph nodes, but may occasionally be seen in the head and neck region and throughout the body (23).

Lymph nodes with dermatopathic lymphadenitis show irregular areas in the cortex or the paracortex composed of increased numbers of interdigitating reticulum cells, Langerhans cells, and histiocytes imparting a mottled appearance on low power. The histologic findings are identical to paracortical hyperplasia with the addition of dermatopathic pigment. The histiocytes have a bland-appearing nucleus and copious amounts of pale cytoplasm containing phagocytized melanin (or occasionally hemosiderin) (Fig. 13.13). Increased numbers of plasma cells, eosinophils, and occasional neutrophils

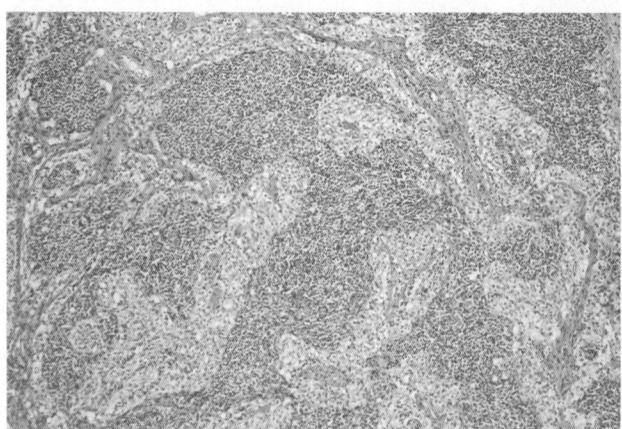

FIGURE 13.11. Histiocytes distend the normally compact lymph node sinuses in sinus histiocytosis.

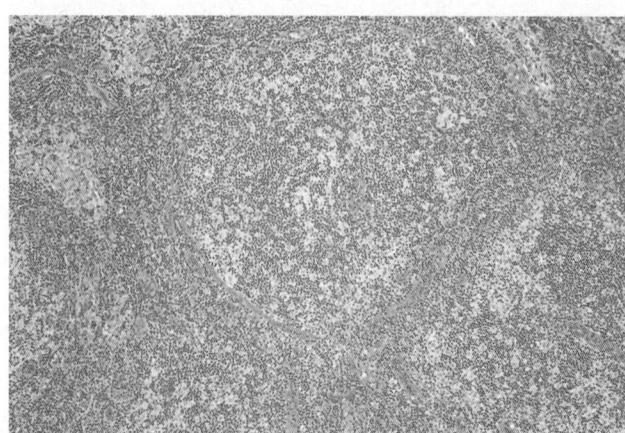

FIGURE 13.12. Paracortical hyperplasia imparts a mottled appearance on low power, may be seen in either a nodular or a diffuse pattern.

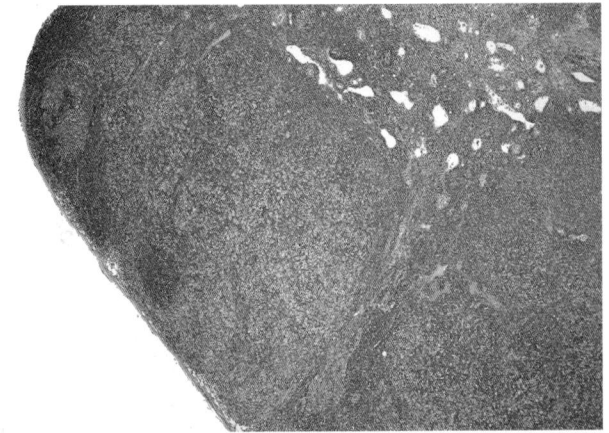

A

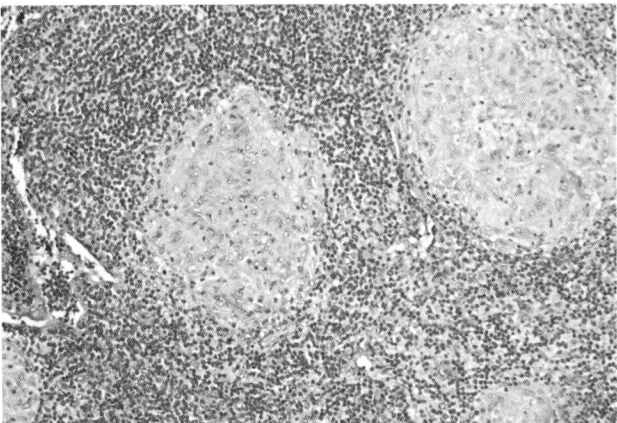

FIGURE 13.14. Granuloma. Several epithelioid granulomas within the interfollicular areas and follicles. The epithelioid histiocytes have bland nuclei and voluminous pale, *pink* cytoplasm.

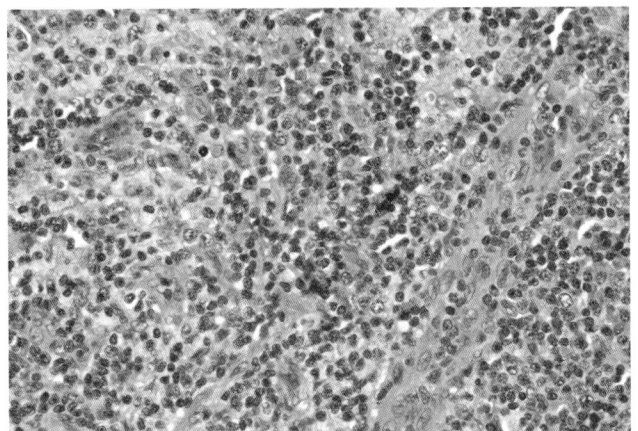

B

FIGURE 13.13. Dermatopathic lymphadenitis appears histologically similar to paracortical hyperplasia (**A**); however, the histiocytes contain phagocytized melanin (**B**—high magnification).

may also be seen admixed in the paracortex and medulla. Immunohistochemical staining shows that interdigitating reticulum cells are S-100 positive and negative for CD1a and Langerin. However, CD1a⁺ and Langerin may also be present in florid cases. Although the histologic appearance is characteristic, a potential pitfall is early involvement by cutaneous T-cell lymphoma (such as mycosis fungoides) (23). Molecular testing for the presence of T-cell antigen receptor gene rearrangements may be necessary to make this distinction.

Granulomas

An innate immune response, granuloma formation is the morphologic manifestation of a delayed hypersensitivity reaction. The histology of granulomas is diverse: it may be as vague as loose collections of macrophages or as clearly defined as well-formed epithelioid macrophages in tight, nodular collections. In all instances, the macrophages that make up the granulomas have oval or elongated nuclei with copious amounts of pink cytoplasm (Fig. 13.14). Activated macrophages of the granuloma are frequently accompanied by other inflammatory cells including neutrophils, lymphocytes, and plasma cells. Often macrophages may coalesce into multinucleated giant cells. The cytoplasm may contain polarizable material or microorganisms.

Inciting agents may be foreign material, tumors, infectious agents (notably fungi or mycobacteria), or the granulomas may be part of an autoimmune response. Special stains for acid-fast bacilli, fungi, and bacteria may help to identify infectious causes of granuloma formation. Of note, both Hodgkin and non-Hodgkin lymphoma as well as other epithelial malignancies may be associated with granulomatous inflammation, so the background cellularity should be assessed for atypical cells.

Infectious Agents Overview

The histologic changes seen in lymph node biopsies may not be indicative of the underlying infectious etiology. In general and with many exceptions, bacterial infections evoke a neutrophilic infiltrate with or without granulomatous inflammation; viral infections may cause a paracortical hyperplasia or immunoblastic reaction, and fungal and mycobacterial infections may cause granulomatous inflammation with or without necrosis (24).

Herpesviridae

Eight herpes viruses infect humans: herpes simplex virus (HSV)-1 and HSV-2, CMV, varicella zoster virus (VZV), EBV, and human herpesvirus (HHV) 6, 7, and 8 (also called Kaposi sarcoma-associated herpesvirus—KSHV) (25). Although they all share a common viral structure and replication cycle, differences in cell tropism contribute to the diverse clinical manifestations of infection (25). All have an asymptomatic latent infection in immune-competent hosts. Once an infection is established, it persists through chronic and latent stages and is shed throughout the lifetime of an individual with few or no symptoms of illness (26). T-cell–mediated immunity keeps the virus latent in infected cells. When T-cell immunity is lost, in immune-compromised hosts, reactivation of the virus may occur (26). In immune-compromised individuals severe, potentially fatal infections can be seen.

Many of the herpes virus family members evoke a similar histologic appearance; therefore, they will be described together. One of the most prominent findings is an interfollicular expansion of immunoblasts that may partially efface lymph node architecture (see "Immunoblastic Hyperplasia"). Monocytoid B-cell collections may also be seen in the interfollicular areas. Paracortical areas may show an increase in plasma cells, eosinophils, and vascular elements. Focal areas of necrosis may be seen with any of the Herpesviridae and are often prominent with HSV-1 and HSV-2. Follicular dendritic cell meshworks are enlarged, with variable degrees of follicular hyperplasia. Proliferating lymphocytes are accompanied by histiocytes that engulf nuclear debris (e.g., tingible body macrophages). There may be extracapsular extension of lymphoid tissue, and sinuses may appear effaced or compacted, mimicking lymphoma. Sinus histiocytosis may also be present. The immunoblastic proliferation may be marked, with sheets of immunoblasts (mostly T cells) resembling large cell lymphoma, or nodular expansions in the paracortex (Fig. 13.15). Occasional immunoblasts may have a Reed-Sternberg—like appearance (Fig. 13.16). Eosinophilic, large viral intranuclear inclusions may be seen, usually at the

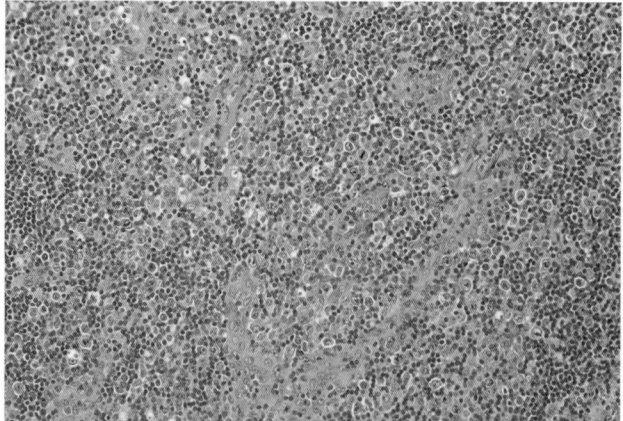

FIGURE 13.15. Sheets of immunoblasts in the paracortex resembling large cell lymphoma.

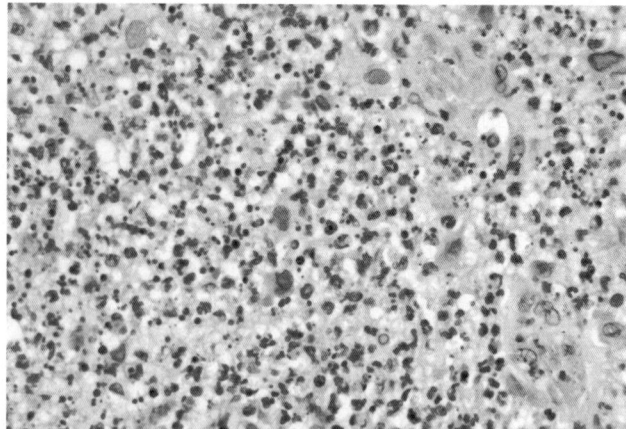

FIGURE 13.17. Herpesviridae intranuclear inclusion. Note the nuclear clearing and smudged appearance. This indicated the presence of viral particles, pushing the normal chromatin to the periphery.

periphery of necrotic areas or in the medulla at the corticomedullary junction. The intranuclear inclusions often show a surrounding area of clearing, described as a "halo" (Fig. 13.17). In addition to the intranuclear viral inclusions seen in all the members of the Herpesviridae family members, CMV may also show basophilic cytoplasmic viral inclusions. HHV-8 associated lymph node changes include florid follicular hyperplasia with increased numbers of plasma cells, including atypical forms, plasmablasts in interfollicular areas, and an increased vascular proliferation. HHV-8 is often seen in association with HIV infection and concurrent EBV infection. Some cases may show a combination of histologic features from these viruses (Table 13.2).

Immunohistochemical staining highlights a mixture of CD20-expressing B immunoblasts and CD3-expressing T immunoblasts, differentiating it from a large cell lymphoma. Reed-Sternberg-like cells (immunoblasts) do not express CD15, although they may express CD30. The Reed-Sternberg-like cells are enlarged immunoblasts, and will be surrounded by other immunoblasts with more typical morphology. The differential diagnosis of herpes virus family includes angioimmunoblastic T-cell lymphoma as well as other infections including entities with necrosis, such as tuberculosis or CSD. These should have granulomas in addition to necrosis. The necrosis accompanying Kikuchi lymphadenitis lacks neutrophils (see Chapter 14). Lupus lymphadenitis may have a similar histology, but frequently has hematoxylin bodies, as well as a more prominent plasmacytic infiltrate. The differential diagnosis of HHV-8 includes the entities outlined

above, as well as plasma cell neoplasms. Immunohistochemical staining for specific viral entities (HHV-8, HSV, CMV, EBV) may provide definitive diagnosis; however, clinical and serologic studies are often necessary to support a specific diagnosis.

HSV is an alpha-herpesvirus with two main serotypes HSV-1 and HSV-2. HSV-1 is usually acquired in childhood and when symptomatic usually forms an orolabial lesion; however, it can also affect the genitalia (27). HSV-2 is usually acquired via sexual contact and is more frequently associated with genital lesions, although it may also produce orolabial lesions as well (27). HSV lymphadenitis is rare; it may present as generalized or localized lymphadenopathy with disseminated HSV infection and a concomitant rash. Lymph nodes most commonly affected are those draining skin or organ lesions. A peripheral blood lymphocytosis is not associated with HSV1 or HSV2 infection.

CMV is a beta-herpesvirus. Primary infection is often subclinical, although the virus has been reported to cause an infectious mononucleosis-type presentation in rare cases (28). Reactivation of CMV and acute illness are seen in immunecompromised patients (29,30). Lymph node involvement in disseminated CMV infection is one of the acquired immune deficiency syndrome (AIDS)-defining illnesses. Lymph nodes draining the site of involvement are most frequently involved. In the peripheral blood a lymphocytosis with atypical lymphocytes may be present. CMV has not been shown to be oncogenic; however, it has been associated with CD4+ T-cell large granular lymphocyte expansions (28).

VZV is an alpha-herpesvirus. Primary mucocutaneous infection manifests as varicella (chickenpox) in childhood. After initial infection, the virus enters a latent phase and if reactivated later in life presents as herpes zoster (shingles) (31). Varicella herpes zoster lymphadenitis may be seen in the cervical supraclavicular and axillary regions. In the peripheral blood, a lymphocytosis and viremia may be present (32).

HHV-6 is a beta-herpesvirus. It is frequently seen in infants and children as a sixth disease (or roseola infantum) presenting with fever and a rash. HHV-6 is increasingly recognized as an opportunistic pathogen in adults. HHV-6 has been found in rare cases of malignant lymphomas and leukemias; however, a causal relationship has not been substantiated. In rare cases of benign reactive lymphadenopathies in immune-competent patients, HHV-6 has been demonstrated (33). Additionally, in some cases of Rosai-Dorfman disease late viral antigens of HHV-6 have been seen in the histiocytes and follicular dendritic cells (28). Although much research has been devoted to discovering associations between HHV-6 and neoplastic proliferations, no clear causal relationship has been established (34).

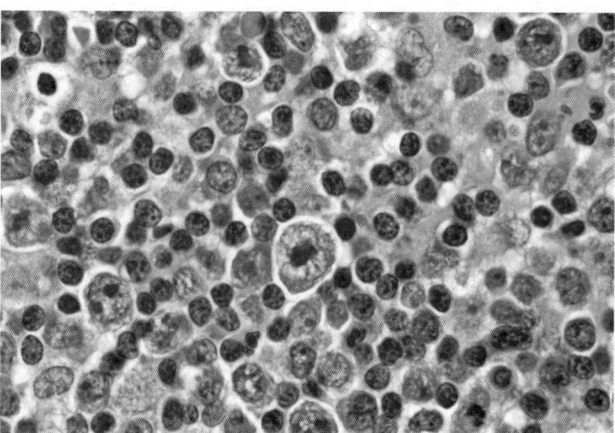

FIGURE 13.16. Immunoblast with a Reed-Sternberg–like appearance. Individual immunoblasts may appear similar to the mononuclear variant of Hodgkin cells (pictures) or more rarely, bi- or multinucleated Reed-Sternberg cells.

	Table 13.2	HERPESVIRIDAE		
Virus	**Type**	**Inclusions**	**Prominent Histologic Features**	**Other**
CMV	Beta	Eosinophilic nuclear and basophilic cytoplasmic	Marginal zone hyperplasia	Seen in immune-compromised patients
EBV	Gamma	None	Sheet-like expansion of immunoblasts in the interfollicular areas	Infectious mononucleosis seen in immune-competent young adults
HSV1/HSV2	Alpha	Eosinophilic nuclear	Necrosis	Seen in immune-compromised. Often seen in association with lymphomas such as CLL/SLL and MCL
VZV	Alpha	Eosinophilic nuclear (rare)	Sheet-like expansion of immunoblasts in the interfollicular areas	Seen in young patients as chicken pox/older patients as shingles. Lymphadenopathy relatively rare.
HHV-8	Gamma	Eosinophilic nuclear	Interfollicular plasma cell proliferations and increased vascular proliferation	Seen in plasma cell Castleman disease, primary effusion lymphoma and HHV8+ diffuse large B-cell lymphoma; seen commonly in HIV/AIDS
HHV-6/HHV-7	Beta	Eosinophilic nuclear or cytoplasmic	Sheet-like expansion of immunoblasts in the interfollicular areas	Seen in immunocompromised patients

CLL/SLL, chronic lymphocytic leukemia/small lymphocytic lymphoma.

HHV-8 is a Rhadinovirus, a member of the gamma group of HHV (with Epstein-Barr). Alternate names include Kaposivirus and KSHV (35). HHV-8 is found in both HIV-positive and HIV-negative plasma cell Castleman disease, multicentric Castleman disease–associated plasmablastic lymphoma, primary effusion lymphoma, and Kaposi sarcoma (KS) (28,36). In the setting of HIV virus, HHV-8 drives systemic inflammation complementing HIV virus infection and producing multicentric plasma cell Castleman disease (36). HHV-8 is the causal agent of KS and has also been linked to the development of body cavity–based lymphomas (such as primary effusion lymphoma) that are often coinfected with EBV (36).

EBV is a gamma-herpesvirus that establishes a lifelong infection. Most infections are asymptomatic, however, when exposure is delayed until young adulthood or adulthood, primary infection can be associated with the clinical syndrome of infectious mononucleosis (37). In immune-suppressed patients who have undergone a bone marrow transplant or a solid organ transplant, EBV primary infection or reactivation may result in posttransplant lymphoproliferative disease (see Chapter 25).

Human Immunodeficiency Virus/Acquired Immune Deficiency Syndrome

HIV is a member of the lentivirus subfamily of the retroviruses (38). After a clinically silent interval, HIV infection leads to depletion of CD4+ T cells and subsequent clinical development of AIDS (39). Clinical symptomatic AIDS manifests as dementia, diarrhea/wasting disease, and hematologic deficiencies (38). The most frequent nodal sites of AIDS-related lymphadenopathy include cervical, axillary, and inguinal lymph nodes (40).

Classic histologic findings associated with AIDS-related lymphadenopathy are described in three temporal stages. The first stage is that of florid follicular hyperplasia. The follicles are characteristically large with irregular shapes and often without surrounding mantle cell zones, a finding referred to as "naked germinal centers" (Fig. 13.18). The hyperplasia is so striking as to mimic follicular lymphoma. Prominent tingible body macrophages in the expanded follicles are a typical feature. In this proliferative phase, follicular lysis and intrafollicular hemorrhage are often seen. The interfollicular areas may be expanded by increased plasma cells, immunoblasts, macrophages, and neutrophils. Giant cells including Warthin-Finkeldey-like multinucleated giant cells may be seen. Proliferating small blood vessels in GCs and interfollicular areas mimicking Castleman disease may be apparent. Areas of monocytoid B-cell hyperplasia may be in the interfollicular areas. The late stage of AIDS-related lymphadenopathy shows marked depletion of lymphocytes, with the organization of follicles and paracortex lost. Only residual stromal and vascular elements remain (Fig. 13.19). It is in this later "burned-out" stage that opportunistic infections and associated neoplastic proliferations are more likely to be encountered. Between the early phase and the late phase, a "mixed" histologic picture including elements of both stages is described.

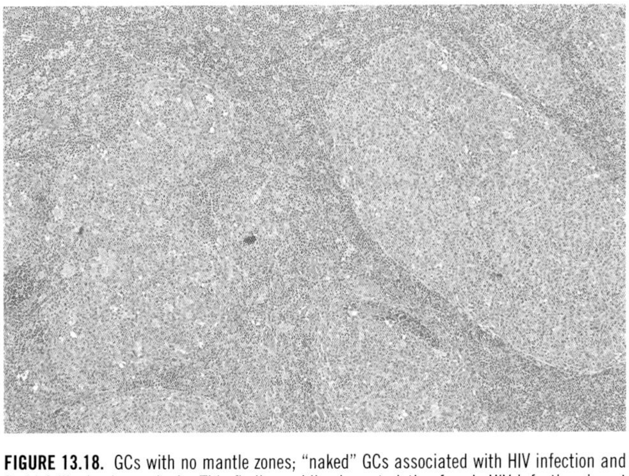

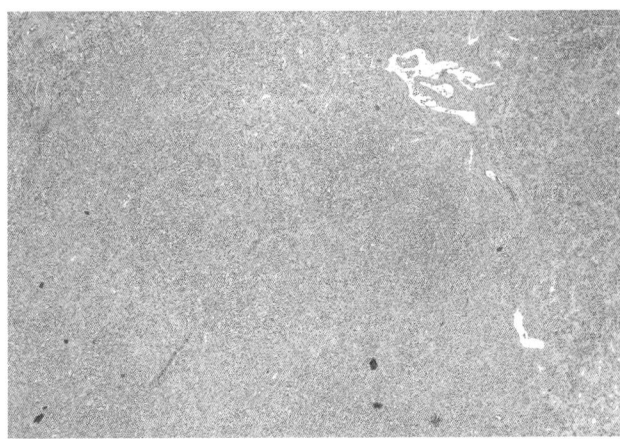

FIGURE 13.18. GCs with no mantle zones; "naked" GCs associated with HIV infection and florid follicular hyperplasia. This finding, while characteristic of early HIV infection, is not pathognomonic.

FIGURE 13.19. The late stage of HIV-related lymphadenopathy showing depletion of the lymphocytes and only residual stromal and vascular elements remaining.

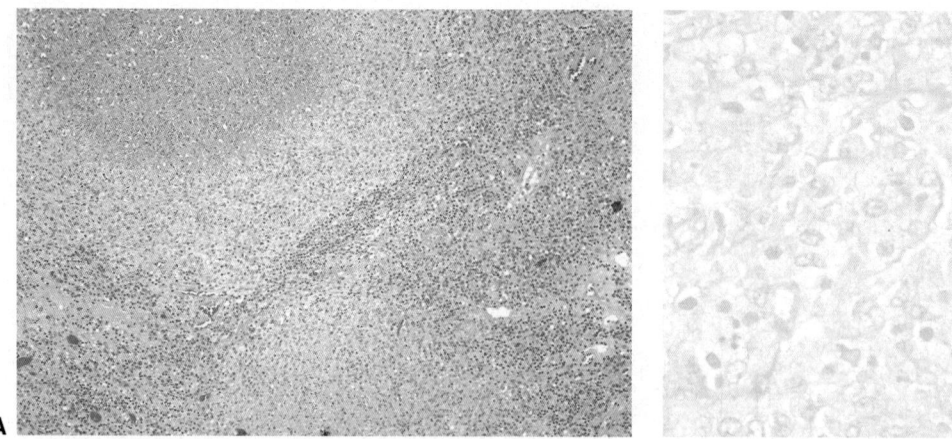
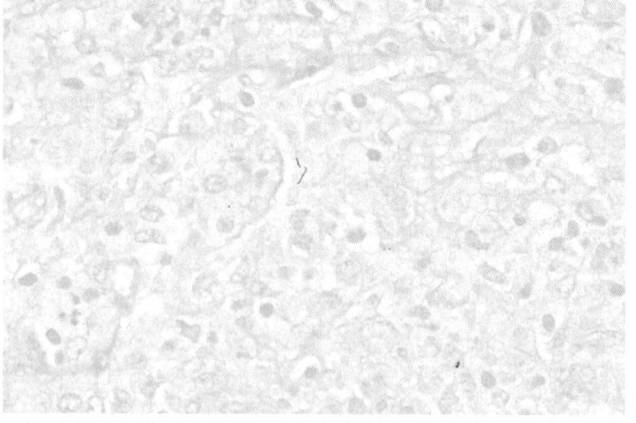

FIGURE 13.20. Epithelioid granulomas in mycobacterium infection. In this example of *M. tuberculosis* infection, the granulomas have areas of central, fragmented necrosis (e.g., caseation) (**A**). An AFB stain shows rare, rod-shaped organisms (**B**).

In addition to the histologic changes associated with this viral infection, histologic changes associated with immune suppression may be seen in HIV/AIDS patients. These findings include necrotizing granulomas from tuberculosis and the nontuberculosis mycobacteria, extensive necrosis, sarcoid-like nonnecrotizing granulomas, foamy macrophage or pseudo-Gaucher cell response, and inflammatory pseudotumor-like changes (41). No one histologic finding seen in lymphadenopathy is diagnostic of HIV-related lymphadenopathy; the histologic findings reflect the immune status in the overall progression of this immune destructive disease. A constellation of histologic and clinical findings is necessary for diagnosis (42).

The development of highly active antiretroviral therapy (HAART) is thought to have slowed the spread of HIV and significantly decreased mortality. Treatment with HAART has been shown to reverse the burnt-out histology associated with the later stages of AIDS-related lymphadenopathy, but does not affect the "early" proliferative histology.

Bacterial

Bacterial infections only rarely have specific histologic findings in lymph nodes. In most cases, there are general responses to bacterial infection typical of other sites with infiltration by granulocytes, necrosis, and abscess formation. Only a small number of bacterial infections have fairly distinctive findings in lymph node that necessitate further description. These fall into two general categories: mycobacterial and nonmycobacterial infections in lymph nodes.

Mycobacterial infections in lymph nodes are uncommon, and are more typical of systemic infection rather than localized disease (43,44). However, mycobacterial infection can be prominent in lymph nodes or other extranodal lymphoid sites, and present as a primary site for biopsy and diagnosis. As in other sites, lymph node involvement by *Mycobacterium tuberculosis* is characterized by the presence of epithelioid granulomas (Fig. 13.20). In most circumstances, these granulomas have central necrosis or caseation. Granulomas are often surrounded by generalized reactive changes of lymphoid tissue, including follicular or interfollicular hyperplasias. Immunoblasts may also be increased. Organisms are most often identified by acid fast bacillus (AFB) stains of various types, but immunohistochemical staining for tuberculosis is also available. In addition, PCR studies to confirm tuberculosis are available and it is prudent to confirm a diagnosis of *M. tuberculosis* infection with appropriate microbiologic testing.

Less commonly, other mycobacterial infections may be seen in lymph nodes and lymphoid tissues (43). *Mycobacterium avium-intracellulare* is most often seen as an opportunistic infection in patients with advanced HIV/AIDS (45). When involved, there are proliferations of plump histiocytes that have a granular cytoplasm (Fig. 13.21). These may form nodules/granulomas or be more diffuse in distribution. *M. avium-intracellulare* is positive for PAS, in contrast to *M. tuberculosis*, as well as AFB stains.

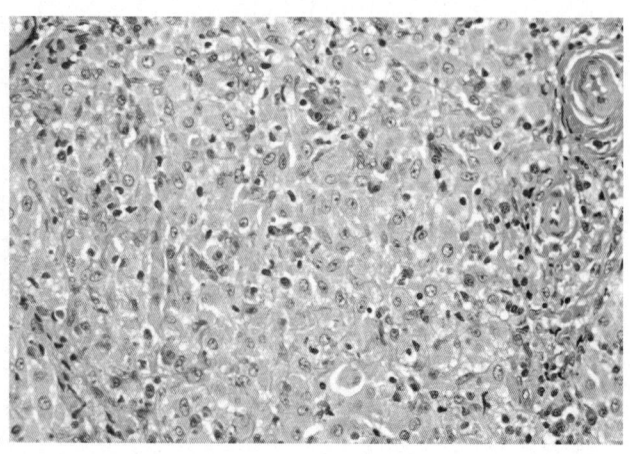
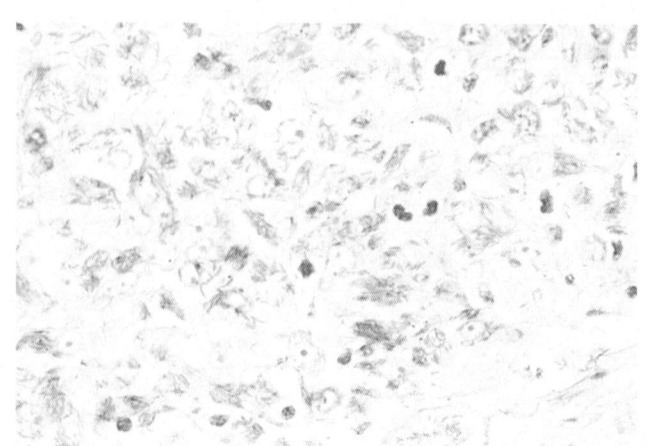

FIGURE 13.21. Plump histiocytes with a granular cytoplasm in *M. avium-intracellulare* infection (**A**). In contrast to *M. tuberculosis*, *M. avium-intracellulare* has numerous organisms staining for AFB in most cases (**B**).

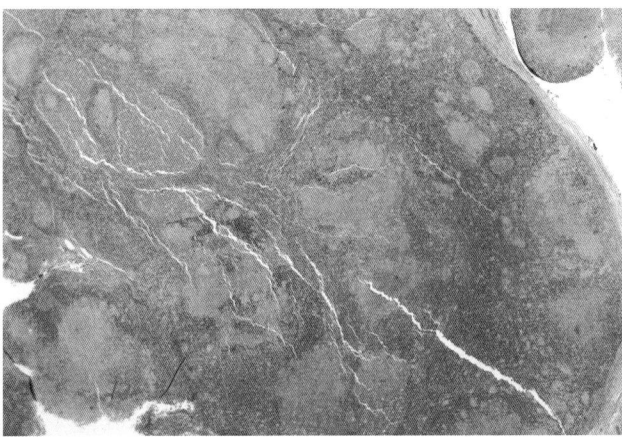

FIGURE 13.22. Necrotizing granulomatous lymphadenitis of catscratch lymphadenitis. Low magnification of lymph node with multiple necrotizing granulomas. Some of these are stellate in shape, a finding typical of catscratch lymphadenitis.

This pattern of staining is not entirely specific for *M. avium-intracellulare*, but usually suffices for histologic identification. If exact speciation is necessary, then PCR methods or other microbiologic studies such as cultures should be performed. Atypical mycobacteria of various types may be seen rarely in lymph nodes (45). They are most often associated with granuloma formation but can only be fully characterized by microbiologic studies.

Nonmycobacterial infections of lymph node with distinctive findings are uncommon. Perhaps most frequently seen is the typical presentation of infection by *Bartonella henselae*, known as CSD. As the name implies, the causative organism, *B. henselae*, is often introduced by a bite or scratch from a cat, and this history may be elicited in exceptional cases. Also, given the site of inoculation, unilateral nodes draining the extremities (antecubital, axillary, inguinal) are most commonly affected. The typical morphologic findings of CSD are those of necrotizing granulomatous lymphadenitis (Figs. 13.22 and 13.23). In the most developed stages, prominent areas of necrosis with central abscess formation are found. The granuloma may have irregular shapes including a stellate appearance. Rare multinucleated giant cells, as well as proliferations of plasmacytoid dendritic cells, may be seen (46). *Bartonella henselae* organisms are not apparent by hematoxylin and eosin (H&E) staining but may be found using Warthin-Starry or tissue Gram stains; they appear as individual or clusters of small, pleomorphic bacteria. An immunohistochemical stain for *B. henselae* is available, and is more specific and more sensitive

than silver stains. However, in at least 20% of cases, the immunohistochemical stain are negative. As such, if indicated for patient management or to confirm a diagnosis, serologic or PCR studies for *B. henselae* can be performed. It should be noted that some other infections, notably tularemia (*Francisella tularensis*) and lymphogranuloma venereum (infection by *Chlamydia trachomatis* serovar L1-L3), may also cause necrotizing lymphadenitis, and cannot be easily distinguished from CSD by morphology alone (47). Antibiotic therapy is curative in CSD.

Syphilis infection in lymph node, also called luetic lymphadenitis, has distinctive features (48). The infection is caused by *Treponema pallidum*, and lymphadenopathy is not an uncommon finding. The morphologic features are not distinctive individually, but as a group can be quite suggestive of the diagnosis. The most characteristic combination of findings is fibrous thickening of the lymph node capsule, follicular hyperplasia, small granulomas, and a polyclonal plasmacytosis (Fig. 13.24). Plasma cells may be seen within the capsule material, in interfollicular areas, and within follicles themselves. Less commonly, there are areas with more extensive fibrosis, increased vascular elements, and a lymphocytic vasculitis. In rare cases, the degree of fibrosis in the lymph node may be so extensive as to mimic inflammatory pseudotumor (IPT) (49). Organisms are not apparent on H&E stains, but may be found on careful examination using Warthin-Starry (or other silver stains). However, immunohistochemical stains for *T. pallidum* or spirochetes reveal numerous organisms. While uncommon, it is prudent to evaluate lymph nodes with an IPT-like pattern with stains for syphilis. Conversely, in cases where the morphologic findings are suspicious for syphilis but the staining does not show organisms, it may be appropriate to suggest serologic studies.

Whipple disease is caused by infection by *Tropheryma whipplei* bacteria. It presents as a relapsing multiorgan illness, with prominent gastrointestinal abnormalities such as malabsorption. Lymphadenitis occurrences are fairly frequent, and may be a site of primary biopsy. Lymph nodes that are affected are enlarged with aggregates and clusters of pale or pink histiocytes (Fig. 13.25). These histiocytes may be associated with or surround large empty vacuoles within the lymph nodes. In some cases more typical granulomatous reactions may be seen. Individual epithelioid histiocytes have voluminous pink granular cytoplasm. In rare cases, gray-blue granular material can be seen as well. Organisms are positive for PAS and are frequently quite numerous within the histiocytes. They do not stain for AFB, in contrast to mycobacteria, such as *M. avium-intracellulare*. Immunohistochemical stains for *T. whipplei* are available, as are PCR studies for confirmation of the organism (50–52). Therapy for Whipple disease is typically antibiotics that may

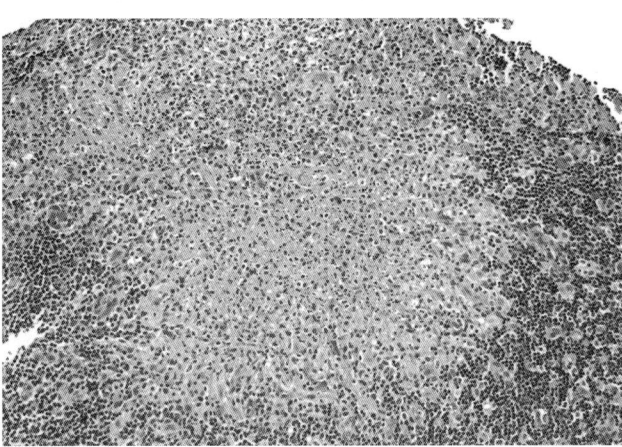

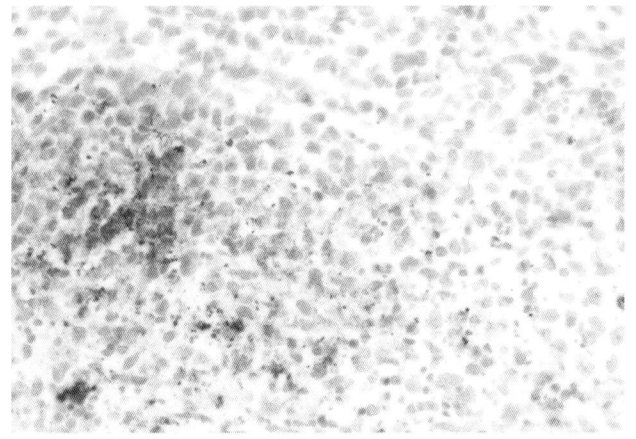

A   **B**

FIGURE 13.23. Necrotizing granulomatous lymphadenitis of cat scratch lymphadenitis. Central portions of the granulomas show necrotic debris and neutrophils **(A)**. An immunohistochemical stain for the cat scratch organism (*B. henselae*) is positive in this case (organisms stain *red*; **B**).

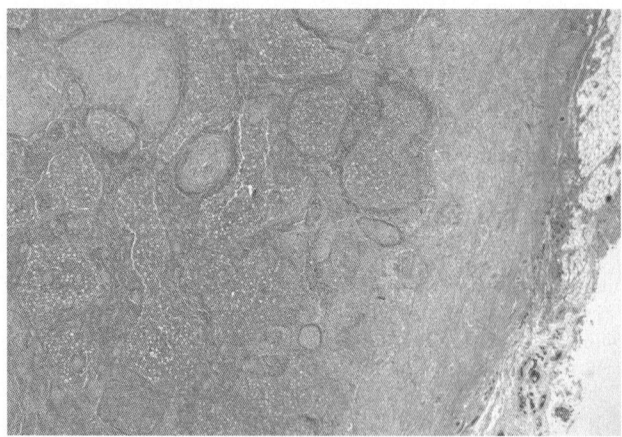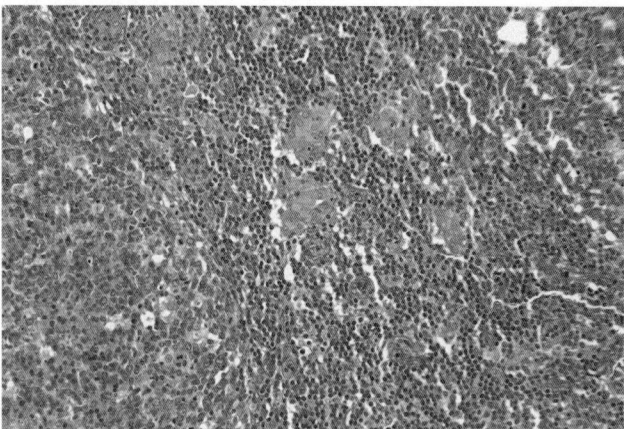

FIGURE 13.24. Histologic findings associated with syphilis lymphadenitis. Fibrous thickening of the lymph node capsule, follicular hyperplasia, small granulomas, and polyclonal plasmacytosis are seen **(A,B)**.

be necessary for 12 to 18 months for complete resolution of the disorder.

Fungal Lymphadenitis

Systemic infections by fungi are relatively uncommon. As such, fungal lymphadenitis is also rare. Only occasionally is lymph node the initial site of diagnosis. Further, fungal lymphadenitis is most commonly seen in patients who are immune-compromised. Only a limited number of more common fungal infections in the lymph node will be addressed.

Cryptococcus infection in the lymph node is quite uncommon, and most cases have been described in patients with HIV/AIDS (53–55). This is most often as a part of a systemic infection. The affected lymph nodes show varying degrees of noncaseating granulomatous inflammation (Fig. 13.26). Many epithelioid histiocytes, occasional multinucleated histiocytes, and a polymorphous lymphoplasmacytic infiltrate are present. Yeast forms are monomorphic and round; when present budding is single and narrow based. The organisms are quite difficult to see with standard H&E staining. Careful examination of sections stained for mucin show organisms with a thick mucopolysaccharide capsule. Confirmation of the organisms should be performed by microbiologic culture and immunohistochemical or PCR tests.

Histoplasma infection in the lymph node may occur in both immune-competent and immune-compromised hosts. *Histoplasma capsulatum* is a dimorphic fungus, endemic in the

Ohio and Mississippi river valleys. Yeast forms may be identified inside macrophages in affected lymph nodes (Fig. 13.27). The sinuses and medulla are involved initially, but large areas of granulomatous inflammation can replace much of the node. Yeast forms in macrophages are highlighted by PAS and GMS stains. However, as with other fungi, confirmation by culture, immunohistochemistry, or PCR studies is recommended.

Coccidioidomycosis is endemic in the Western United States and Mexico; infection may also be seen in Central and South America. While primary infection is typically pulmonary, lymph node involvement may be seen in exceptional cases (56). The incidence is significantly increased in certain racial groups as well as in immune-compromised patients (57). Lymph nodes have necrotizing granulomas. They are formed from epithelioid histiocytes with occasional giant cells. Roughly spherical organisms, termed sporangia, are present that can be large in size (up to 40 µm) with a thick wall. Often they are filled with small round endospores, which spread when the sporangium ruptures. As with other fungi, PAS and GMS stains are positive. Confirmation of coccidioidomycosis should be performed by ancillary methods to ensure species and optimize therapy.

Pneumocystis jiroveci (formerly *Pneumocystis carinii*) has undergone reclassification as a fungus, after previously being classified as a protozoan, as a result of DNA sequence studies (58). It is seen in significantly immune-compromised hosts. Exposure is most commonly pulmonary and this is the most frequent site of infection and diagnosis. Lymph node involvement is rare, and typically part of widespread systemic disease.

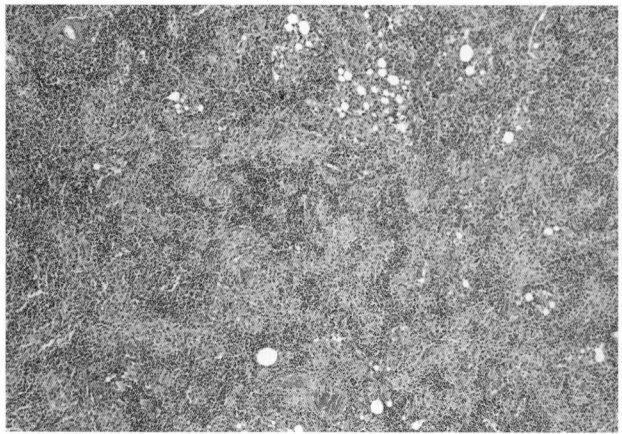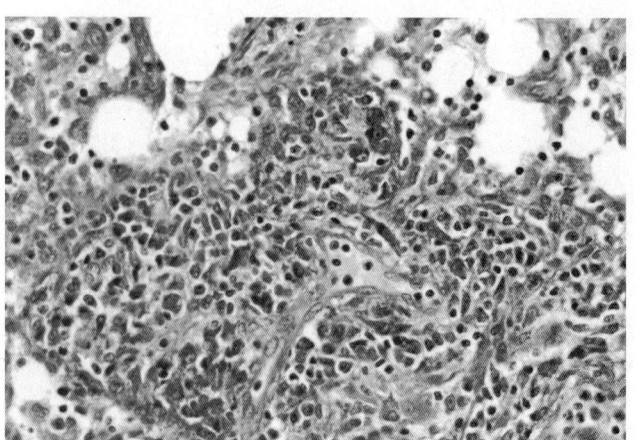

FIGURE 13.25. Clusters of pale histiocytes containing organisms in Whipple disease **(A)**, which are positive for PAS staining **(B)**.

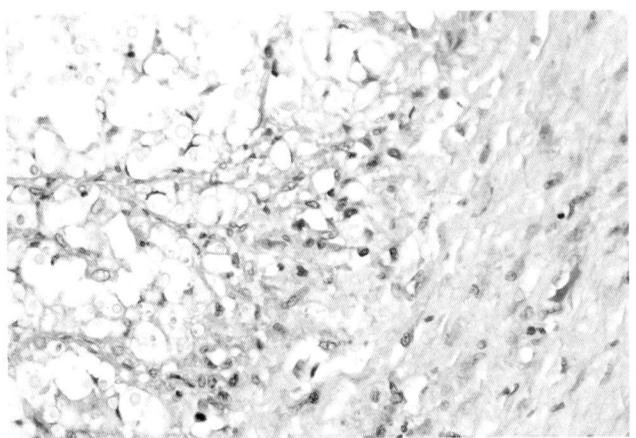

FIGURE 13.26. *Cryptococcus* lymphadenitis. A thickened lymph node capsule (**right**) and numerous organisms with thick clear capsules.

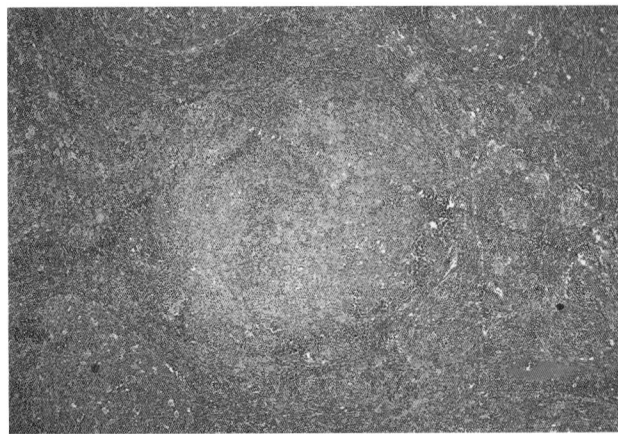

FIGURE 13.28. Follicular hyperplasia and monocytoid B-cell hyperplasia associated with *Toxoplasma* infection.

Involvement in lymph nodes may show areas of necrosis. Minimal inflammation is present. Most characteristic, *P. jiroveci* is associated with a pink frothy material. This fibrinous exudate contains the *P. jiroveci* organisms that can be highlighted by special stains. When evaluated using a GMS stain, the organisms appear as spheres, or more commonly as "crushed ping pong balls." An immunohistochemical stain can confirm the diagnosis. Also, organisms can be identified by culture or PCR studies. Therapy requires specific antibiotics, and most AIDS patients take prophylactic trimethoprim-sulfamethoxazole, which greatly reduces *P. jiroveci* infections.

Protozoal/Parasitic Infections

Toxoplasma gondii is a protozoal infection that has a characteristic appearance in lymph node. While exact incidences are difficult to calculate, it is a relatively common cause of lymphadenopathy with an identifiable benign etiology (59–62). Exposure is most commonly from cat feces. Lymph nodes are enlarged and show hyperplastic features. The three hallmark findings of toxoplasmic lymphadenitis are (i) follicular hyperplasia, (ii) increases in marginal zone/monocytoid B cells, and (iii) epithelioid microgranulomas (Figs. 13.28 and 13.29). Follicular hyperplasia is of usual type with typical benign features. Increases in marginal zone or monocytoid B cells are seen commonly in paracortical regions. These B cells are typically small with round mature nuclei and increased amounts of pale cytoplasm, imparting a monocytoid appearance. These

cells almost always have some rare accompanying neutrophils admixed. Finally, there are variable numbers of microgranulomas formed from small clusters of epithelioid histiocytes. While these can occur in any location in the lymph node, they are most characteristic when seen impinging on GCs. Organisms are almost never seen, although in some severe cases with immune-compromised patients, cyst forms can be identified (63).

The histologic findings with an appropriate clinical context can be strongly supportive of a diagnosis. Infection is typically self-limited and does not require specific treatment. If necessary, diagnosis confirmation can be obtained by serologic or PCR studies (64). Immunohistochemical staining for the cysts of *Toxoplasma* typically used in extranodal tissues throughout the body, as in the brain, are typically negative in the lymph nodes.

Systemic and Autoimmune

The etiology and pathophysiology of many of these entities have not been thoroughly explained yet. Many are thought to be caused by immune system dysfunction, possibly driven by derangements of regulatory T/B cells with aberrant cytokine production to explain the associated clinical and histologic findings. In general, they are largely systemic diseases with abnormal histologic findings in the lymph node; their diagnosis is better made on clinical grounds in the full context of the patient's presentation. Histology in the lymph node may be

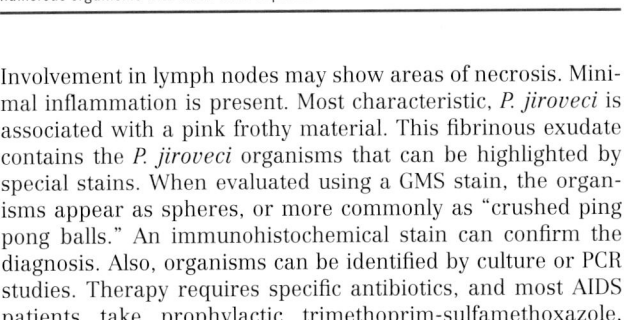

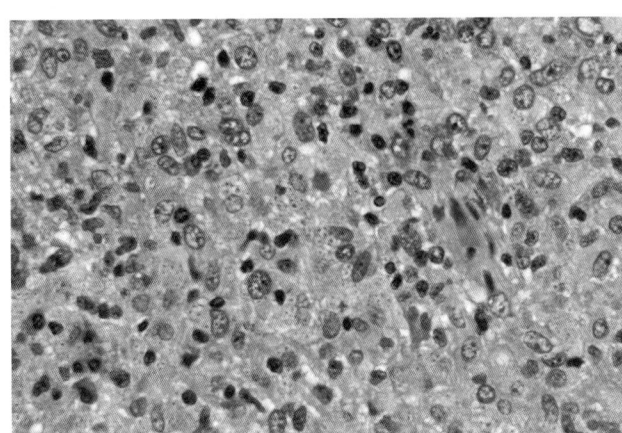

FIGURE 13.27. Intracellular yeast forms of *H. capsulatum*.

FIGURE 13.29. Epithelioid microgranulomas associated with *Toxoplasma* infection.

suggestive of these diseases but is not sufficiently distinctive for a diagnosis independent of clinical findings.

Rheumatoid Arthritis

RA is a chronic systemic autoimmune disease. While the most crippling effects are usually seen in joints, the results of chronic inflammation are seen throughout the body. Women are three times more likely to be affected with onset between 40 and 50 years old. Clinical presentation includes a lymphadenopathy that is usually localized and not generalized (65). Fever, anemia, weight loss, and hypergammaglobulinemia are associated with rheumatoid lymphadenopathy. The incidence of lymphadenopathy in patients with RA may be as high as 82% (65). Men are more likely to have lymphadenopathy than women (65). Lymphadenopathy may occur in any site; however, an association has been seen in enlarged lymph nodes draining affected joints (65).

Histology of lymphadenopathy associated with RA shows a florid follicular hyperplasia, with an expanded interfollicular plasma cell population in cluster or sheets (intrafollicular plasma cells may also be seen) (Fig. 13.30). The differential diagnosis includes follicular lymphoma, plasma cell Castleman disease, IgG4-related lymphadenopathy, or infectious etiologies. Immunohistochemical staining for BCL-2 protein may help exclude follicular lymphoma. The absence of HHV-8 staining may exclude plasma cell Castleman disease in many cases. The lack of increased IgG4 plasma cells exclude IgG4-related lymphadenopathy. Exclusion of infectious etiologies, demonstration of polyclonal plasma cells, and clinical results of serologic studies may help to diagnose RA-related lymphadenopathy.

Patients with RA have a two- to threefold risk of development of lymphoma when compared with the general population (66,67). It is unclear if the increased risk is attributable to an underlying pathophysiology of RA, one of the multiple medications used to treat RA, or a combination of both. Treatment of RA is usually a combination of disease-modifying agents (DMARDs), biologic agents, and anti-inflammatory agents. Rituximab therapy has also been shown to be helpful in a subset of patients (68).

Systemic Lupus Erythematosus

SLE is an aberrant autoimmune reaction that can involve any part of the body and subsequently has a variable presentation (69). In the United States, an increased prevalence is seen in patients of Hispanic, Asian, and African decent (69). Women are far more often affected than men (69,70). Patients with

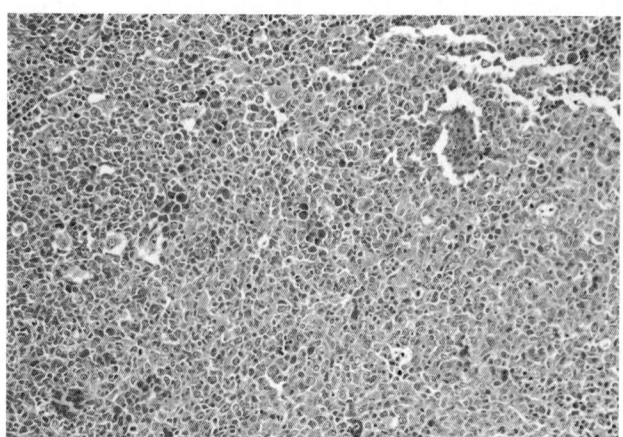

FIGURE 13.30. Expanded plasma cell interfollicular infiltrate seen in RA-associated lymphadenopathy. In this case, many intracytoplasmic immunoglobulin inclusions (Russell bodies, Mott cells) are seen.

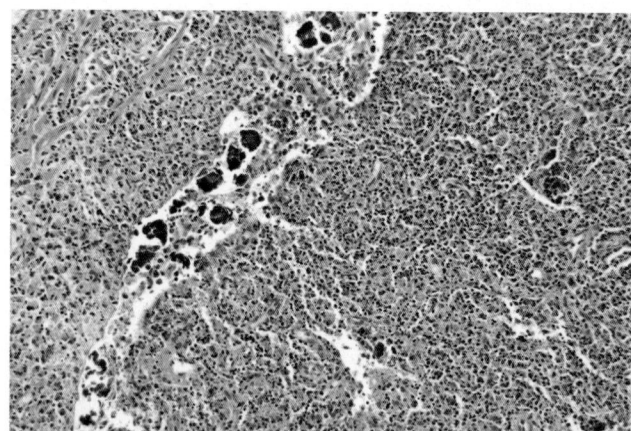

FIGURE 13.31. Prominent hematoxylin body formation seen with SLE-associated lymphadenopathy.

SLE produce antibodies to ubiquitous self-antigens (usually intranuclear antigens such as double-stranded DNA). Clinical symptoms are diverse and include skin rash (malar or discoid), photosensitivity, oral ulcers, arthritis, serositis (pleuritis or pericarditis), glomerulonephritis (renal failure), neurologic symptoms (including seizures), hemolytic anemia, leukopenia, and thrombocytopenia (70). Immune complexes, autoantibodies, autoreactive lymphocytes, dendritic cells, and locally increased cytokines are all involved in clinical manifestations (70).

Histologic changes in the lymph node associated with SLE include necrosis, with formation of hematoxylin bodies, and a prominent follicular hyperplasia (Fig. 13.31). Scattered macrophages, immunoblasts, and plasma cells are seen in the interfollicular areas. The increase in interfollicular polyclonal plasma cells may be seen in combination with a vascular proliferation (71). The differential diagnosis of SLE includes other entities with a predominantly necrotic histologic picture, including Kikuchi lymphadenitis. In contrast to Kikuchi lymphadenitis, SLE necrosis contains neutrophils and hematoxylin bodies. Bacterial infections, such as CSD, often show prominent necrosis containing neutrophils. Viral etiologies, such as infectious mononucleosis, should also be excluded. Treatment of SLE has been largely dependent on corticosteroids.

Sarcoidosis

Sarcoidosis is a systemic disease in which noncaseating granulomas are found throughout the body. The most common sites of involvement are the lungs, lymph nodes, skin, eyes, and central nervous system (72). It is estimated that one-third of patients have palpable peripheral lymph nodes (72). Systemic symptoms may be present including fatigue, weight loss, dyspnea, cough, and fever (72). Sarcoidosis is more common in women than in men and in African Americans than in Caucasians (72).

The histologic hallmarks of sarcoidosis-associated lymphadenopathy are multiple well-formed noncaseating granulomas. Circumscribed granulomas are formed by epithelioid macrophages with bland nuclei and copious amounts of pale cytoplasm, which may contain Schaumann bodies or asteroid bodies (Fig. 13.32). Small T lymphocytes are often seen within the granuloma. These lymphocytes are thought to be involved in the formation of the granulomas. Multinucleated giant cells may be found throughout the lymph nodes. The differential diagnosis includes infectious etiologies, lymphomas (Hodgkin lymphoma), carcinoma, or Langerhans cell histiocytosis. Hodgkin lymphoma may present with a prominent granulomatous reaction; CD30 and other immunohistochemical staining may be necessary to exclude occult Hodgkin cells. Special stains for acid-fast bacilli

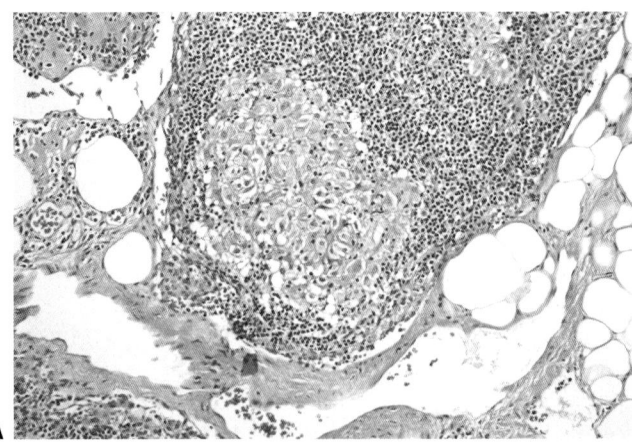 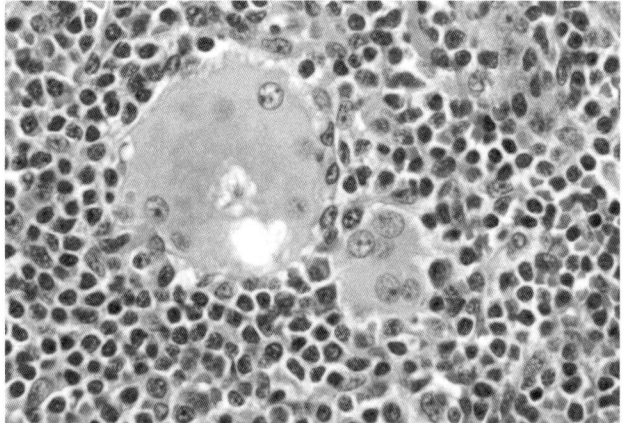

FIGURE 13.32. Epithelioid granulomas of sarcoidosis in the lymph node (**A**) and an asteroid body seen within one histiocyte (**B**).

and fungi are required to exclude infectious organisms. Polarization may be necessary to exclude granulomas due to foreign material. Treatment is corticosteroids with immunosuppressive agents used in refractory cases.

Kawasaki Disease

Kawasaki disease is a clinical syndrome presenting predominantly in children with enlarged lymph nodes, systemic symptoms, and a potentially life-threatening vasculitis. There is a slight male predominance, with a median age of 2 years (73). Children of Asian/Pacific Islander descent have a higher incidence of Kawasaki disease as compared with other ethnicities (73).

Associated histologic changes seen in the lymph node include prominent necrosis and microthrombi of small vessels. The necrosis may be geographic or in confluent sheets. Swollen endothelial cells are seen in areas adjacent to the necrosis. In contrast to Kikuchi disease, the necrosis contains neutrophils.

The self-limiting nature of the majority of the cases combined with the observed seasonality suggests an infectious agent, although no associations have yet been documented, in combination with a genetic susceptibility. Diagnosis and prompt treatment are essential as one of the most feared clinical outcomes is myocardial ischemia due to cardiac vascular compromise. Intravenous immunoglobulin therapy is the mainstay of treatment.

Hemophagocytic Lymphohistiocytic Syndrome

HLH is a potentially life-threatening syndrome of excessive inflammatory response associated with defects in the perforin-dependent cytotoxic pathway (74–76). The loss of perforin function results in increased levels of proinflammatory cytokines producing organ dysfunction (with the liver being the most commonly affected organ) (74). Hemophagocytosis may not be seen in all patients at the onset; it is considered neither sensitive nor specific for this disease (74,76). HLH presents in both children and adults and exists in a sporadic (secondary) form as well as an inherited (primary) form. Although commonly thought of as a disease of children, the primary form may occur at any age and has been documented as late as 70 years of age by genetic testing (74). The secondary form may be in association with: infections (EBV being most common), rheumatologic disorders (macrophage activation syndrome), metabolic diseases, and malignancies (74). Malignancy-associated HLH is associated with peripheral T-cell lymphoma, natural killer (NK)/T-cell leukemia, EBV-positive NK/T-cell lymphoma, EBV-negative B-cell lymphomas, acute monoblastic leukemia, and acute lymphoblastic leukemia.

Lymph node sections show a prominent population of histiocytes expanding the sinuses. The histiocytes have a bland-appearing nucleus and copious amounts of pale cytoplasm containing engulfed red blood cells, lymphocytes, granulocytes, or platelets. Capsular involvement and extracapsular extension are often seen. The differential diagnosis includes histiocytic neoplasms, monocytoid B-cell lymphoma, and nonhematopoietic entities such as carcinoma or amelanotic melanoma.

Histologic findings alone are not used for diagnosis. Soluble CD25 (sCD25), also known as the alpha chain of the IL-2 receptor or (sIL-2), and soluble CD163 (sCD163) are used for diagnosis and follow-up (74,76). Screening for problems in degranulation via flow cytometry using CD107a and perforin protein are used as a surrogate testing for esoteric genetic testing (74). Treatment with chemotherapy and stem cell transplant are used.

Foreign Materials and Chemicals

Because of their function filtering lymph fluid, lymph nodes may occasionally have deposition of foreign materials. Items such as tattoo pigment are frequently seen, and usually do not elicit a significant host response (77) (Fig. 13.33). In other circumstances, foreign materials may be associated with significant response such as the talc granulomas seen in the lymph nodes of intravenous drug abusers. A selection of significant foreign materials and inclusions is discussed below.

Proteinaceous lymphadenopathy is caused by the deposition of amorphous protein within the lymph node (78,79). This

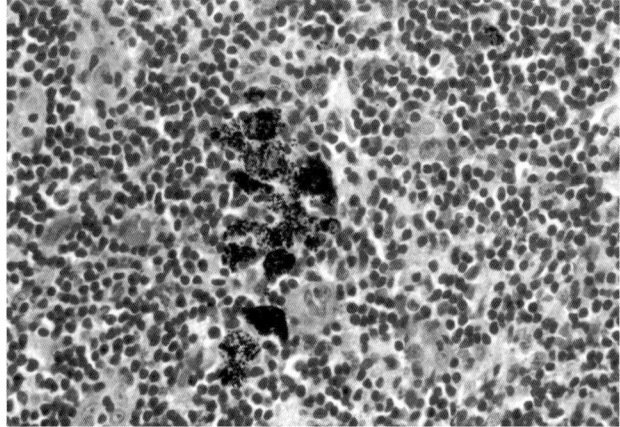

FIGURE 13.33. Tattoo pigment in lymph node. Careful inspection reveals black pigment (*ink*) and in this case, some rare green pigment as well. Typically, there is no granulomatous or histiocytic response to tattoo pigment deposition.

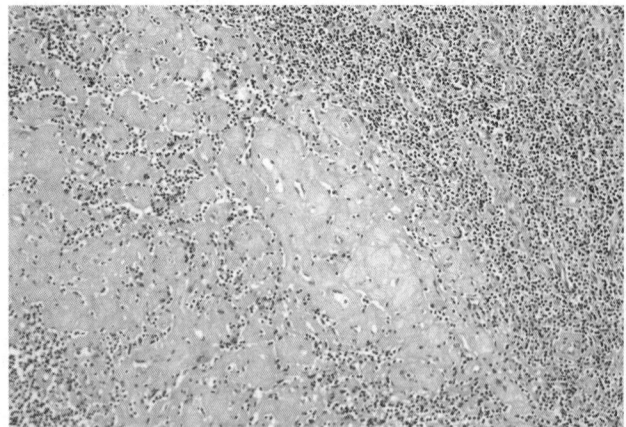

FIGURE 13.34. Hypocellular pink material of proteinaceous lymphadenopathy.

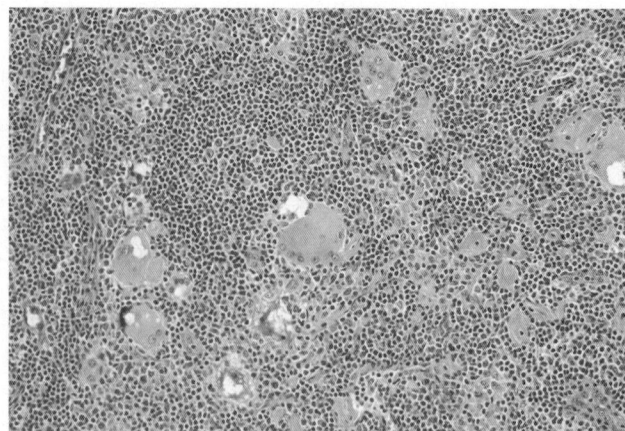

FIGURE 13.36. Gold in colloidal or crystalline form in lymph nodes for treatment of autoimmune disorders. The gold is associated with formation of foreign body giant cells and small granulomas. Subtle crystalline structures are present within some of the clear spaces, representing crystalline forms of the injectable gold.

material is typically hypocellular, pink with a dense hyaline appearance. In contrast to amyloid, it is not positive for Congo red staining (Fig. 13.34). In many cases, it is deposition of a nonamyloid immunoglobulin material. It may or may not be associated with monoclonal B-cell disorders, such as plasma cell or lymphoplasmacytic neoplasms.

Silicone deposition is most often a result of leakage from silicone breast implants. It is found most frequently in axillary lymph nodes (80,81). The silicone may evoke a granulomatous response (Fig. 13.35). Histiocytes, with frequent cytoplasmic vacuoles, and giant cells are seen. Most of these are clear, but occasionally, there may be evidence of vaguely crystalline material within. The granulomas are composed of typical components including histiocytes, plasma cells, and small lymphocytes. The remaining lymph node may show generalized reactive changes including follicular hyperplasia, paracortical hyperplasia, and sinus histiocytosis.

Although currently rare, lymphangiogram was formerly a frequently used diagnostic procedure (77). A radiopaque agent was injected in small lymphatics, (usually between the toes) and the agent traveled through the lymphatic system being deposited in lymph nodes. Scans would show filling defects, which suggested involvement of nodes by disease. In many cases, the radiopaque dyes used would induce significant changes in the lymph nodes. Beside an overall hyperplasia, there were prominent granulomatous reactions with deposition of the oily dye material. On histologic exam, this would leave large empty holes, imparting a "Swiss cheese" appearance to the nodes.

Rarely, metal debris associated with joint replacement can be seen within lymph nodes (82,83). Most often, these are seen in inguinal nodes draining the region of a hip replacement, although other sites can also be seen. The debris is most often within macrophages. The metallic debris may appear black or gray in color, with an irregular or even crystalline shape. Associated reaction with granulomas, lymphoid hyperplasia, and prominent sinus histiocytosis may also be seen.

Although extremely rare, gold in colloidal or crystalline forms is used as a therapy for disorders, including some autoimmune disorders such as RA (77) (Fig. 13.36). The gold may accumulate in lymph nodes. It will often evoke a granulomatous response, and be entrapped within vacuoles of histiocytes and giant cells. Rarely it may be associated with lymph node necrosis (84–86). There may be formation of small or intermediate-sized granulomas. These are most often seen adjacent to sinuses in interfollicular areas of the lymph node.

Vascular Abnormalities and Cellular Inclusions

Infarction in lymph node can present significant diagnostic challenges (Fig. 13.37). While a number of cases may be attributed to benign or reactive causes, the possibility of infarction of a lymphoma or other neoplastic disorder can be difficult to exclude entirely (84–88). In these cases, several studies

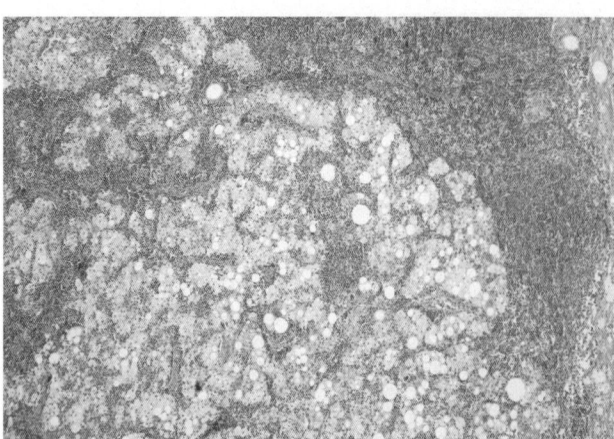

FIGURE 13.35. Silicone produces a granulomatous response in lymph nodes. It is most often deposited in axillary lymph nodes of women with silicone breast implants that have leaked material into soft tissue.

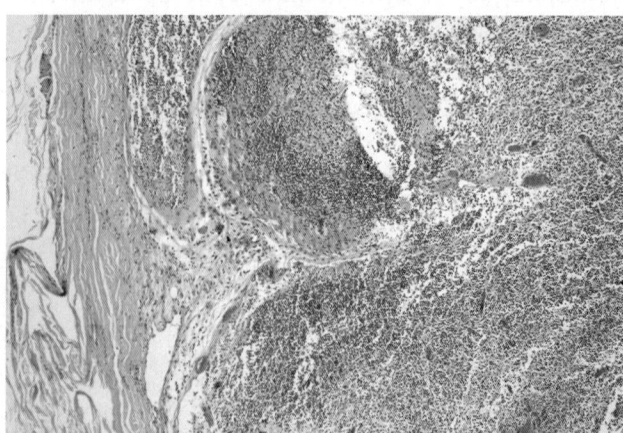

FIGURE 13.37. Infarcted lymph node. An example of a partially infarcted lymph node. Approximately half of the cells are necrotic with half retaining definition of their nuclei. There is some hint of residual nodal structures. In complete infarction, there are few viable cells and a loss of architectural features.

have addressed the use of immunohistochemical staining in infarcted cells. Immunoreactivity for different antigens is variably affected by tissue infarction. In some cases of infarcted tissue, PCR studies for B- and/or T-cell clonality have been informative (89). In all cases, it is important to do appropriate studies to exclude a malignant diagnosis and if not, to obtain additional viable tissue for diagnosis.

Vascular transformation of sinuses (VTS) is a rare benign change in lymph nodes (90–92). Most often, this change has been associated with occlusion, either mechanically or in upstream areas by masses or sometimes tumors. It is proposed that as a result of increased pressure to the outflow of lymph, there is a subsequent proliferation of vascular elements of the lymph node. Sometimes, this process may be so dramatic as to replace much of the parenchyma of the lymph node by vascular elements. In most cases the histologic appearance of VTS is of small-caliber, thin-walled anastomosing vessels in the lymph node (Fig. 13.38). They may arise from the sinuses of the node or the hilum. These small vessels have little intervening stroma. The individual endothelial cells are bland, with no significant atypia. VTS is primarily concerning because it can be a morphologic mimic of KS in the lymph node, or less commonly, a benign vascular neoplasm, such as hemangioma. VTS is positive for endothelial markers including Factor VIII antigen and CD31. Recent reports suggest that VTS is positive for D2-D40, suggesting a proliferation of lymphatic endothelial elements (93). In contrast to KS, VTS will not have any evidence of HHV-8 infection.

Epithelial cell inclusions in lymph nodes are uncommon but can be a vexing diagnostic problem. They have been reported in almost all body regions, and the types of inclusions are typically embryologically related to the tissue drained by the particular lymph node group (Fig. 13.39). In all cases, the histologic appearance of the glands is characterized by a benign cytology of (usually) simple glands. These are preferentially located within or adjacent to the lymph node capsule. When located within the parenchyma of the node, they are more often near fibrous trabeculae extending from the capsule. In contrast to most cases of metastatic disease, benign inclusions typically lack a desmoplastic stromal response.

Small inclusions of thyroid and parathyroid glands have been identified in cervical lymph nodes (94). Lymph nodes in the regions of salivary glands may have small glandular elements within the node. Likewise, benign breast tissue has been reported in predominantly axillary lymph nodes. These may be problematic, especially in evaluating sentinel lymph nodes for minimal involvement by breast cancer (95). Apocrine- or squamous-lined inclusions may also be rarely seen in axillary

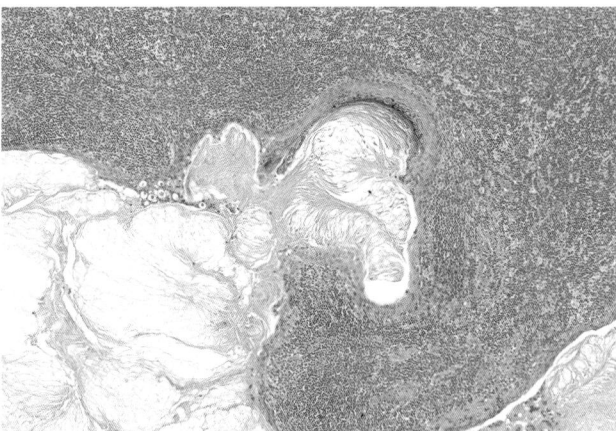

FIGURE 13.39. Epithelial cell inclusions in the lymph node. An example of an epithelial cystic structure within a lymph node. The cystic structure is filled with keratinaceous debris. A granular layer can be seen in the epithelial lining.

lymph nodes. Inclusions have also been noted in perirenal lymph nodes from kidney resections. While most commonly seen in resections for pediatric renal tumors, such as Wilms tumor (96), they can also be seen in adult lymph nodes (77). Unlike other circumstances, in perirenal lymph nodes, glandular elements may also be accompanied by depositions of Tamm-Horsfall protein (97). Mullerian inclusions in lymph nodes may be somewhat more problematic

Similar to the circumstances described above, nevus cell inclusions can be seen in lymph nodes throughout the body. While often cytologically bland, they can be quite problematic when evaluating sentinel lymph node biopsies for melanoma. In most circumstances, the inclusions are small, cytologically bland, and located adjacent to or within the node capsule. However, because of the gravity of possible metastatic melanoma, care must be taken to exclude a melanoma diagnosis. Immunohistochemical evaluation may be of benefit, with some differential features allowing reasonable distinction of nevus from melanoma. In nevus, proliferation by Ki67 should be low to negative. Nevus cells should not express WT-1 or HMB-45, in contrast to melanoma. Both are typically strongly positive for S-100 protein. Capsular inclusions of amorphous material have been described as a benign phenomenon. This is thought to represent elastotic material passively transported form the skin (98).

References

1. Vinuesa CG, Cook MC. The molecular basis of lymphoid architecture and B cell responses: implications for immunodeficiency and immunopathology. *Curr Mol Med* 2001;1:689–725.
2. Jones D. Dismantling the germinal center: comparing the processes of transformation, regression, and fragmentation of the lymphoid follicle. *Adv Anat Pathol* 2002;9:129–138.
3. Bagdi E, Krenacs L, Krenacs T, et al. Follicular dendritic cells in reactive and neoplastic lymphoid tissues: a reevaluation of staining patterns of CD21, CD23, and CD35 antibodies in paraffin sections after wet heat-induced epitope retrieval. *Appl Immunohistochem Mol Morphol* 2001;9:117–124.
4. Kojima M, Nakumura S, Motoori T, et al. Follicular hyperplasia presenting with marginal zone pattern in a reactive lymph node lesion. *APMIS* 2002;110:325–331.
5. Cong P, Raffeld M, Teruya-Feldstein J, et al. *In situ* localization of follicular lymphoma: description and analysis by laser capture microdissection. *Blood* 2002;99:3376–3382.
6. Kussick SJ, Kalnoski M, Braziel RM, et al. Prominent clonal B-cell populations identified by flow cytometry in histologically reactive lymphoid proliferations. *Am J Clin Pathol* 2004;121:464–472.
7. Nam-Cha SH, San-Millán B, Mollejo M, et al. Light-chain-restricted germinal centers in reactive lymphadenitis: report of eight cases. *Histopathology* 2008;52:436–444.
8. Osborne BM, Butler JJ. Clinical implications of nodal reactive follicular hyperplasia in the elderly patient with enlarged lymph nodes. *Mod Pathol* 1991;4:24–30.
9. Kojima M, Nakumura S, Itoh H, et al. Clinical implication of florid reactive follicular hyperplasia in Japanese patients 60 years or older: a study of 46 cases. *J Surg Pathol* 2005;13:175–180.
10. Hunt JP, Chan JA, Samoszuk M, et al. Hyperplasia of mantle/marginal zone B cells with clear cytoplasm in peripheral lymph nodes: a clinicopathologic study of 35 cases. *Am J Clin Pathol* 2001;116:550–559.

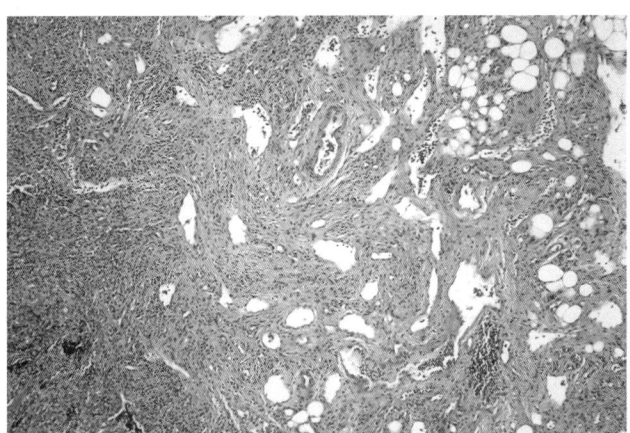

FIGURE 13.38. Thin-walled anastomosing vessels with little intervening stroma, seen in VTS of lymph node.

11. Kojima M, Nakamura S, Motoori T, et al. Follicular hyperplasia presenting with a marginal zone pattern in a reactive lymph node lesion. *APMIS* 2002;110: 325–331.

12. Lai R, Arber DA, Chang KL, et al. Frequency of bcl-2 expression in non-Hodgkin lymphoma: a study of 778 cases with comparison of marginal zone lymphoma and monocytoid B-cell hyperplasia. *Mod Pathol* 1998;11:864–869.

13. Abbondazo SL, Irey NS, Frizzera G. Dilantin-associated Lymphadenopathy: spectrum of histopathologic patterns. *Am J Surg Pathol* 1995;19:675–686.

14. Chang C, Osipov V, Wheaton S, et al. Follicular hyperplasia, follicular lysis, and progressive transformation of germinal centers: a sequential spectrum of morphologic evolution in lymphoid hyperplasia. *Am J Clin Pathol* 2003;120:322–326.

15. Hicks J, Flaitz C. Progressive transformation of germinal centers: review of histopathologic and clinical features. *Int J Pediatr Otorhinolaryngol* 2002;65: 195–202.

16. Kojima M, Nakamura S, Motoori T, et al. Progressive transformation of germinal centers: a clinicopathological study of 42 Japanese patients. *Int J Surg Pathol* 2003;11:101–107.

17. Poppema S. Lymphocyte-predominance Hodgkin's disease. *Semin Diagn Pathol* 1992;9:257–264.

18. Taniguchi I, Murakami G, Sato A, et al. Lymph node hyalinization in elderly Japanese. *Histol Histopathol* 2003;18:1169–1180.

19. Gould E, Perez J, Albores-Saavedra J, et al. Signet ring cell sinus histiocytosis: a previously unrecognized histologic condition mimicking metastatic adenocarcinoma in lymph nodes. *Am J Clin Pathol* 1989;92:509–512.

20. van der Oord JJ, de Wolf-Peeters C, de Vos R, et al. The paracortical area in dermatopathic lymphadenitis and other reactive conditions of the lymph node. *Virchows Arch B Cell Pathol Incl Mol Pathol* 1984;45:289–299.

21. Merad M, Ginhoux F, Collin M. Origin, homeostasis and function of Langerhans cells and other langerin-expressing dendritic cells. *Nat Rev Immunol* 2008;8: 935–947.

22. Geissmann F, Dieu-Nosjean MC, Dezutter C, et al. Accumulation of immature Langerhans cells in human lymph nodes draining chronically inflamed skin. *J Exp Med* 2002;196:417–430.

23. Winter LK, Spiegel JH, King T. Dermatopathic lymphadenitis of the head and neck. *J Cutan Pathol* 2007;34:195–197.

24. Segal G, Perkins SL, Kjeldsberg CR. Benign lymphadenopathies in children and adolescents. *Semin Diagn Pathol* 1995;12:288–302.

25. van Lint AL, Knipe DM. Herpesviridae. In: Schaechter M, ed. *Encyclopedia of microbiology*, 3rd ed. Elsevier: Oxford, UK, 2009:376–390.

26. Goodrum F, Caviness K, Zagallo P. Human Cytomegalovirus persistence. *Cell Microbiol* 2012;14(5):644–655.

27. Looker KJ, Garnett GP. A systematic review of the epidemiology and interaction of herpes simplex virus types 1 and 2. *Sex Transm Infect* 2005;81:103–107.

28. Quadrelli C, Barozzi P, Riva G, et al. β-HHVs and HHV-8 in lymphoproliferative disorders. *Mediterr J Hematol Infect Dis* 2011;3:e2011043.

29. Boeckh M, Geballe AP. Cytomegalovirus: pathogen, paradigm, and puzzle. *J Clin Invest* 2011;121:1673–1680.

30. Britt W. Manifestations of human cytomegalovirus infection: proposed mechanisms of acute and chronic disease. *Curr Top Microbiol Immunol* 2008;325:417–470.

31. Santos RA, Padilla JA, Hatfield C, et al. Antigenic variation of varicella zoster virus Fc receptor gE: loss of a major B cell epitope in the ectodomain. *Virology* 1998;249:21–31.

32. Abendroth A, Arvin AM. Immune evasion as a pathogenic mechanism of varicella zoster virus. *Semin Immunol* 2001;13:27–39.

33. Maric I, Bryant R, Abu-Asab M, et al. Human herpesvirus-6-associated acute lymphadenitis in immunocompetent adults. *Mod Pathol* 2004;17:1427–1433.

34. Ogata M. Human herpesvirus 6 in hematological malignancies. *J Clin Exp Hematop* 2009;49:57–67.

35. Gantt S, Casper C. Human herpesvirus 8-associated neoplasms: the roles of viral replication and antiviral treatment. *Curr Opin Infect Dis* 2011;24:295–301.

36. Schulte KM, Talat N. Castleman's disease: a two compartment model of HHV8 infection. *Nat Rev Clin Oncol* 2010;7:533–543.

37. Pietersma F, Piriou E, van Baarle D. Immune survelience of EBV-infected B cells and the development of non-Hodgkin lymphomas in immunocompromised patients. *Leuk Lymphoma* 2008;49:1028–1041.

38. Greene WC. The molecular biology of human immunodeficiency virus type 1 infection. *N Engl J Med* 1991;324:308–317.

39. Cicala C, Arthos J, Fauci AS. HIV-1 envelope, integrins and co-receptor use in mucosal transmission of HIV. *J Transl Med* 2011;9(Suppl 1):S2.

40. Vanhems P, Toma E. Recognizing primary HIV-1 infection. *Infect Med* 1999; 16:104–108.

41. Wannakrairot P, Leong TY, Leong AS. The morphological spectrum of lymphadenopathy in HIV infected patients. *Pathology* 2007;39:223–227.

42. Stanley MW, Frizzera G. Diagnosis specificity of histologic features in lymph node biopsy specimens from patients at risk for the acquired immunodeficiency syndrome. *Hum Pathol* 1983;17:1231–1239.

43. Chao SS, Loh KS, Tan KK, et al. Tuberculous and nontuberculous cervical lymphadenitis: a clinical review. *Otolaryngol Head Neck Surg* 2002;126:176–179.

44. Ramanathan VD, Jawahar MS, Paramasivan CN, et al. A histological spectrum of host responses in tuberculous lymphadenitis. *Indian J Med Res* 1999;109: 212–220.

45. Kraus M, Benharroch D, Kaplan D, et al. Mycobacterial cervical lymphadenitis: the histological features of non-tuberculous mycobacterial infection. *Histopathology* 1999;35:534–538.

46. Kojima M, Morita Y, Shimizu K, et al. Plasmacytoid monocytes in cat scratch disease with special reference to the histological diversity of suppurative lesions. *Pathol Res Pract* 2006;202:17–22.

47. Sutinen S, Syrjala H. Histopathology of human lymph node tularemia caused by *Francisella tularensis* var palaearctica. *Arch Pathol Lab Med* 1986;110:42–46.

48. Farhi DC, Wells SJ, Siegel RJ. Syphilitic lymphadenopathy: histology and human immunodeficiency virus status. *Am J Clin Pathol* 1999;112:330–334.

49. Facchetti F, Incardona P, Lonardi S, et al. Nodal inflammatory pseudotumor caused by luetic infection. *Am J Surg Pathol* 2009;33:447–453.

50. Alkan S, Beals TF, Schnitzer B. Primary diagnosis of Whipple disease manifesting as lymphadenopathy: use of polymerase chain reaction for detection of *Tropheryma whippelii*. *Am J Clin Pathol* 2001;116:898–904.

51. Baisden BL, Lepidi H, Raoult D, et al. Diagnosis of Whipple disease by immunohistochemical analysis: a sensitive and specific method for the detection of *Tropheryma whipplei* (the Whipple bacillus) in paraffin-embedded tissue. *Am J Clin Pathol* 2002;118:742–748.

52. Gras E, Matias-Guiu X, Garcia A, et al. PCR analysis in the pathological diagnosis of Whipple's disease: emphasis on extraintestinal involvement or atypical morphological features. *J Pathol* 1999;188:318–321.

53. Mohanty SK, Vaiphei K, Dutta U, et al. Granulomatous cryptococcal lymphadenitis in immunocompetent individuals: report of two cases. *Histopathology* 2003;42:96–97.

54. Fish DG, Ampel NM, Galgiani JN, et al. Coccidioidomycosis during human immunodeficiency virus infection: a review of 77 patients. *Medicine (Baltimore)* 1990;69:384–391.

55. Khan ZU, Al-Anezi AA, Chandy R, et al. Disseminated cryptococcosis in an AIDS patient caused by a canavanine-resistant strain of *Cryptococcus neoformans* var. grubii. *J Med Microbiol* 2003;52:271–275.

56. Robinson MJ, Fogel R. Granulomatous lymphadenitis caused by *Coccidioides immitis*. *J Am Osteopath Assoc* 1994;94:578–572.

57. Hector RF, Rutherford GW, Tsang CA, et al. The public health impact of coccidioidomycosis in Arizona and California. *Int J Environ Res Public Health* 2011;8:1150–1173.

58. Sritangratanakul S, Nuchprayoon S, Nuchprayoon I. Pneumocystis pneumonia: an update. *J Med Assoc Thai* 2004;87(Suppl 2):S309–S317.

59. Dorfman RF, Remington JS. Value of lymph node biopsy in the diagnosis of acute acquired toxoplasmosis. *N Engl J Med* 1973;289:878–881.

60. Eapen M, Mathew CF, Aravindan KP. Evidence based criteria for the histopathological diagnosis of toxoplasmic lymphadenopathy. *J Clin Pathol* 2005;58: 1143–1146.

61. Jayaram N, Ramaprasad AV, Chethan M, et al. Toxoplasma lymphadenitis: analysis of cytologic and histopathologic criteria and correlation with serologic tests. *Acta Cytol* 1997;41:653–658.

62. McCabe RE, Brooks RG, Dorfman RF, et al. Clinical spectrum in 107 cases of toxoplasmic lymphadenopathy. *Rev Infect Dis* 1987;9:754–774.

63. Aisner SC, Aisner J, Moravec C, et al. Acquired toxoplasmic lymphadenitis with demonstration of the cyst form. *Am J Clin Pathol* 1983;79:125–127.

64. Lin MH, Kuo TT. Specificity of the histopathological triad for the diagnosis of toxoplasmic lymphadenitis: polymerase chain reaction study. *Pathol Int* 2001;51:619–623.

65. Robertson MD, Hart FD, White WF, et al. Rheumatoid lymphadenopathy. *Ann Rheum Dis* 1968;27:253–260.

66. Kaiser R. Incidence of lymphoma in patients with rheumatoid arthritis: a systematic review of the literature. *Clin Lymphoma Myeloma* 2008;8:87–89.

67. Baecklund E, Askling J, Rosenquist R, et al. Rheumatoid arthritis and malignant lymphomas. *Curr Opin Rheumatol* 2004;16:254–261.

68. Sellam J, Rouanet S, Hendel-Chavez H, et al. Blood memory B cells are disturbed and predict the response to rituximab in patients with rheumatoid arthritis. *Arthritis Rheum* 2011;63:3692–3701.

69. Tsokos GC. Systemic lupus erythematosus. *N Engl J Med* 2011;365:2110–2121.

70. Crispín JC, Liossis SN, Kis-Toth K, et al. Pathogenesis of human systemic lupus erythematosus: recent advances. *Trends Mol Med* 2010;16:47–57.

71. Kojima M, Nakamura S, Morishita Y, et al. Reactive follicular hyperplasia in the lymph node lesions from systemic lupus erythematosus patients: a clinicopathological and immunohistochemical study of 21 cases. *Pathology International* 2000;50:304–312.

72. Sekhri V, Sanal S, DeLorenzo LJ, et al. Cardiac sarcoidosis: a comprehensive review. *Arch Med Sci* 2011;7:546–554.

73. Holman RC, Belay ED, Christensen K, et al. Hospitalizations for Kawasaki syndrome among children in the United States, 1997–2007. *Pediatr Infect Dis J* 2010;29:483–488.

74. Weitzman S. Approach to hemophagocytic syndromes. *Am Soc Hematol Educ Program* 2011;2011:178–183.

75. Risma K, Jordan MB. Hemophagocytic lymphohistiocytosis: updates and evolving concepts. *Curr Opin Pediatr* 2012;24:9–15.

76. Jordan MB, Allen CE, Weitzman S, et al. How I treat hemophagocytic lymphohistiocytosis. *Blood* 2011;118:4041–4052.

77. O'Malley DP, George TI, Orazi A, et al. Foreign bodies and chemicals. In: *Atlas of non-tumor pathology: benign and reactive conditions of lymph node and spleen*. Washington, DC: American Registry of Pathology, 2009.

78. al Rikabi AC, Naddaf HO, al Balla SR, et al. Proteinaceous lymphadenopathy in a patient with known rheumatoid arthritis—case report and review of the literature. *Br J Rheumatol* 1995;34:1087–1089.

79. Michaeli J, Niesvizky R, Siegel D, et al. Proteinaceous (angiocentric sclerosing) lymphadenopathy: a polyclonal systemic, nonamyloid deposition disorder. *Blood* 1995;86:1159–1162.

80. Katzin WE, Centeno JA, Feng LJ, et al. Pathology of lymph nodes from patients with breast implants: a histologic and spectroscopic evaluation. *Am J Surg Pathol* 2005;29:506–511.

81. van Diest PJ, Beekman WH, Hage JJ. Pathology of silicone leakage from breast implants. *J Clin Pathol* 1998;51:493–497.

82. Forest M, Carlioz A, Vacher Lavenu MC, et al. Histological patterns of bone and articular tissues after orthopaedic reconstructive surgery (artificial joint implants). *Pathol Res Pract* 1991;187:963–977.

83. Gray MH, Talbert ML, Talbert WM, et al. Changes seen in lymph nodes draining the sites of large joint prostheses. *Am J Surg Pathol* 1989;13:1050–1056.

84. Roberts C, Batstongbn PJ, Goodlad JR. Lymphadenopathy and lymph node infarction as a result of gold injections. *J Clin Pathol* 2001;54:562–564.

85. Kojima M, Nakamura S, Yamane Y, et al. Antigen preservation in infarcted nodal B-cell lymphoma, with special reference to follicular center cell markers. *Int J Surg Pathol* 2004;12:251–255.

86. Nasuti JF, Gupta PK, Baloch ZW. Clinical implications and immunohistochemical staining in the evaluation of lymph node infarction after fine-needle aspiration. *Diagn Cytopathol* 2001;25:104–107.

87. Strauchen JA, Miller LK. Lymph node infarction: an immunohistochemical study of 11 cases. *Arch Pathol Lab Med* 2003;127:60–63.

88. Vega F, Lozano MD, Alcalde J, Pardo-Mindan FJ. Utility of immunophenotypic and immunogenotypic analysis in the study of necrotic lymph nodes. *Virchows Arch* 1999;434:245–248.

89. Laszewski MJ, Belding PJ, Feddersen RM, et al. Clonal immunoglobulin gene rearrangement in the infarcted lymph node syndrome. *Am J Clin Pathol* 1991;96:116–120.

90. Chan JKC, Warnke RA, Dorfman R. Vascular transformation of sinuses in lymph nodes: a study of its morphological spectrum and distinction from Kaposi's sarcoma. *Am J Surg Pathol* 1991;15:732–743.
91. Chan JK, Frizzera G, Fletcher CD, et al. Primary vascular tumors of lymph nodes other than Kaposi's sarcoma: analysis of 39 cases and delineation of two new entities. *Am J Surg Pathol* 1992;16:335–350.
92. Ide F, Shimoyama T, Horie N. Vascular transformation of sinuses in bilateral cervical lymph nodes. *Head Neck* 1999;21:366–369.
93. Fukunaga M. Expression of D2-40 in lymphatic endothelium of normal tissues and in vascular tumours. *Histopathology* 2005;46:396–402.
94. Veras E, Sturgis EM, Luna MA. Heterotopic parathyroid inclusion in a cervical lymph node. *Head Neck* 2007;29:1160–1163.

95. Norton LE, Komenaka IK, Emerson RE, et al. Benign glandular inclusions a rare cause of a false positive sentinel node. *J Surg Oncol* 2007;95:593–596.
96. Weeks DA, Beckwith JB, Mierau GW. Benign nodal lesions mimicking metastases from pediatric renal neoplasms: a report of the National Wilms' Tumor Study Pathology Center. *Hum Pathol* 1990;21:1239–1244.
97. Zanetti G. Epithelial inclusions and Tamm-Horsfall protein in paranephric lymph nodes: a light microscopy and immunocytochemical study. *Virchows Arch A Pathol Anat Histopathol* 1986;408:593–601.
98. Pulitzer MP, Gerami P, Busam K. Solar elastotic material in dermal lymphatics and lymph nodes. *Am J Surg Pathol* 2010;34:1492–1497.

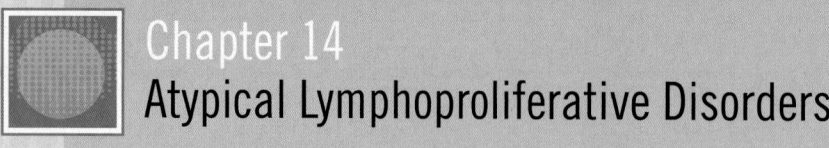

Chapter 14
Atypical Lymphoproliferative Disorders

Dennis P. O'Malley • Kate E. Grimm

 ## INTRODUCTION

This chapter addresses some causes of lymphadenopathy that either are obscure or fall in a gray zone between truly reactive or infectious processes and neoplastic processes. Individually, these cases can present as striking and impressive causes of adenopathy and/or symptoms, which raise concern for lymphoma clinically. They also present a set of unique problems with histologic examination and with mimicry of other, more serious problems in some circumstances.

The general topic of atypical lymphoid hyperplasia (ALH) is covered, including circumstances for use of this terminology and potential diagnostic approaches to address this somewhat vexing circumstance. The specific entities of Castleman disease (CD), Kikuchi-Fujimoto disease (KFD), Kimura disease, and Rosai-Dorfman disease (RDD) are also addressed. Unusual lymphadenopathies associated with medications are covered. A relatively newly described entity, IgG4-related lymphadenopathy (IgG4-RL), is addressed, including its relationship with a broader category of IgG4-related sclerosing disease (IgG4-RSD). Finally, the difficult topics of inflammatory pseudotumor of lymph node (IPT-LN) and the immunodeficiency disorder, autoimmune lymphoproliferative syndrome (ALPS), are discussed.

Atypical Lymphoid Hyperplasia

ALH is not a specific diagnosis. Rather, it describes a circumstance where the exact nature of a lymphoid proliferation cannot be determined in the current circumstance (Table 14.1). ALH should not be diagnosed without a specific discussion of the reason(s) for atypicality, as well as a proposed resolution to clarify the diagnosis (1). In many ways, while an unclear diagnosis, it is an actionable diagnosis, because inherent to the diagnosis are suggestions or explanations of the next steps for patient evaluation.

An ALH diagnosis can be based on a variety of features, but can mostly be described in terms of atypical findings of architecture, cytology, or immunohistochemistry (1). Three histologic circumstances generally account for the majority of ALH diagnoses: the presence of one or more atypical follicles or follicular structures (Fig. 14.1), the presence of increased immunoblasts beyond what is expected in a normal reactive condition (Fig. 14.2), and finally the presence of any individual large atypical cells that could mimic a Hodgkin or Reed-Sternberg cell (Fig. 14.3). Other proliferations that disrupt normal lymph node architecture, expansions of unusual compartments (such as mantle or marginal zones), or interfollicular proliferation of polymorphous cells could also be considered, albeit less commonly. In each case, the differential diagnosis and appropriate further evaluation are slightly different, and the reader is referred to the appropriate chapters for specific diagnostic features.

As mentioned above, each diagnosis of ALH should be accompanied by an explanation or suggestions of additional diagnostic steps. In some circumstances, it is appropriate to further evaluate the submitted tissue by additional ancillary studies. In cases that are suspicious for B-cell lymphoma, polymerase chain reaction (PCR) studies for B-cell clonality may be adequate to resolve a diagnosis of ALH (2). In the appropriate circumstance, a positive PCR study for B-cell clonality in ALH would confirm a diagnosis of a B-cell lymphoma. Likewise, if IgH/BCL2 fluorescence *in situ* hybridization (FISH) studies were performed in a case of ALH and were positive, this would likely provide support for a diagnosis of follicular lymphoma. In cases of possible T-cell lymphoma, PCR studies for T-cell clonality may provide useful ancillary information. In cases of possible Hodgkin lymphoma, if an exhaustive immunohistochemical evaluation has been performed, and the diagnosis cannot be resolved, then either additional biopsy materials or careful clinical follow-up with subsequent biopsies may be appropriate. As in all circumstances, overall clinical context, histologic findings, and molecular or other ancillary studies need to be correlated. In many circumstances, the appropriate course for an ALH diagnosis may be careful clinical follow-up or, in cases of samples limited in size or quality, repeat biopsy. In any case, ALH as a specific diagnosis should not be used frequently; in each case, an attempt should be made to provide a more definitive diagnosis.

Castleman Disease

CD encompasses two main subtypes described together, but with marked histologic and clinical differences. Clinical presentation is divided into unicentric and multicentric subtypes. Histologically, CD is divided into hyaline-vascular subtype and plasma cell subtype. The histologic classification is favored by pathologists, who may not be aware of the extent of disease involvement at the time of diagnosis. The two different classification schemes are often combined, as hyaline vascular Castleman disease (HV-CD) frequently is unicentric in presentation and plasma cell Castleman disease (PC-CD) is often multicentric in presentation. In the time since its first description by Benjamin Castleman in 1957, CD has been expanded to include different histologic subtypes and different clinical presentations and has consequently become an even more complex diagnostic group (Fig. 14.4) (3).

Hyaline Vascular Castleman Disease

HV-CD presents as a mass or solitary enlarged lymph node, with few or no systemic symptoms (Table 14.2) (4–6). Early series reported presentation in the mediastinal or thoracic lymph nodes as the most common sites of involvement; subsequent series have found cervical, axillary, and abdominal locations to be equally as common (7). However, a diverse number of lymph node locations and organs have been reported (8). Involved lymph nodes are frequently large, ranging in size from

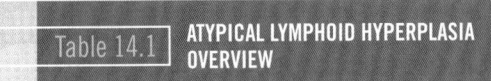

Table 14.1	ATYPICAL LYMPHOID HYPERPLASIA OVERVIEW

Lymph node histology
Atypical follicles or follicular structures, the presence of increased immunoblasts or individual large atypical cells

1 to 25 cm (median 6 to 7 cm) (7) (Fig. 14.5) giving rise to one of this entity's previous names: giant lymph node hyperplasia. Angiofollicular lymph node hyperplasia, angiomatous lymphoid hamartoma, and follicular lymphoreticuloma are all previous names used to describe this disease. HV-CD has a median age at presentation in the third and fourth decades with no clear gender predilection (3–5,7). Pediatric cases are well documented (9).

Lymph node sections show a distinctive histologic appearance at low power, with an overall increase of small atrophic follicles. In contrast to a reactive or normal follicle center, the follicular centers of HV-CD have diminished numbers of germinal center B cells and are composed mostly of residual follicular dendritic cells (Fig. 14.6). Dysplastic or atypical-appearing dendritic cells may be found in the follicle centers or in the interfollicular areas (Fig. 14.7). These cells are large and may be multinucleated with small nucleoli, or a smudged appearance. Pink hyalinized material may often be seen in the atrophic follicle centers. The mantle zone is characteristically expanded. Small, mature-appearing lymphocytes of the mantle zone are seen in single-file concentric rings around the atrophic follicles, imparting an "onion skin" appearance. A single ring of mantle cells may be seen surrounding multiple small follicles. Radially penetrating, hyalinized vessels combined with the "onion skinning" is what has been described as the lollipop appearance (Fig. 14.8). Interfollicular areas often show an increase in hyalinized vasculature. Plasma cells may be mildly increased in number in the interfollicular areas, as well as present in the follicle centers themselves. Increased paracortical plasmacytosis, if pronounced, may overlap with the histologic findings of PC-CD.

The multinucleated dysplastic follicular dendritic cells may superficially resemble Hodgkin cells; however, they express CD21 or CD35 (follicular dendritic cell markers) and do not express CD30 or Pax-5. Immunohistochemical stains may be helpful to exclude minimal involvement by Hodgkin lymphoma.

The etiology and exact prevalence of HV-CD are still unknown, although many different disease associations have

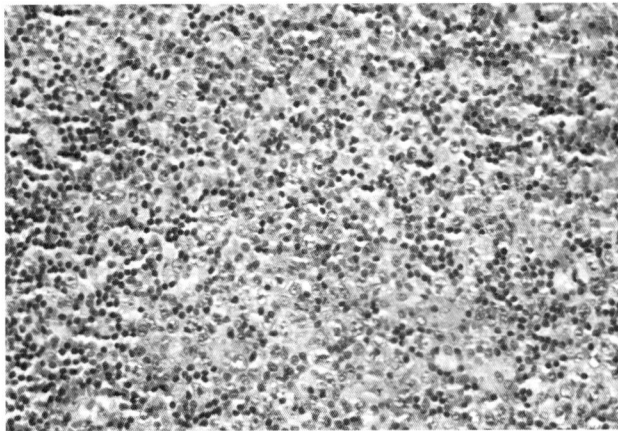

FIGURE 14.2. "ALH" with an increase in interstitial immunoblasts. The combination of morphologic and immunophenotypic findings should be correlated, but in equivocal cases, additional studies, such as PCR, may be necessary.

been reported and may be clues to the underlying pathology. Etiologically, some authors have proposed that HV-CD represents a neoplasm of follicular dendritic cells (10–12). In this context, the histologic findings of HV-CD represent a reaction to the neoplastic proliferation of dendritic cells in the same manner that the neoplastic cells of classical Hodgkin lymphoma produce a heterogeneous histologic response. Clonal cytogenetic abnormalities of the follicular dendritic cells of HV-CD have been described (13), and the association between HV-CD and dendritic cell sarcomas has been well documented (5,14–17). In addition to the association with dendritic cell sarcoma, nonneoplastic entities including paraneoplastic pemphigus and thrombotic thrombocytopenic purpura have also been associated with HV-CD (7). Other authors have proposed that the hyaline-vascular and plasma cell subtypes are a lymphoproliferative reaction to an unknown viral stimulus with the different subtypes representing different points in time (4). In this context, PC-CD represents the early presentation and HV-CD represents the later, scarred end stage.

The prognosis of HV-CD is excellent. Excision is considered curative (7,18,19).

Plasma Cell Castleman Disease

PC-CD frequently presents as regional lymphadenopathy with systemic symptoms such as fever, night sweats, and malaise

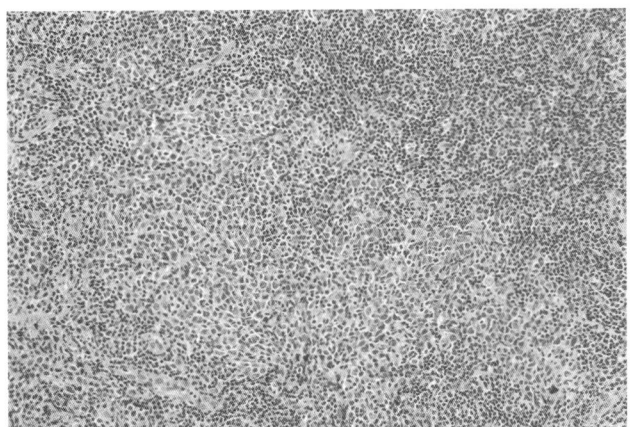

FIGURE 14.1. An example of "ALH" with an abnormal follicle. In this case, the follicle shows some features of a benign follicle (polymorphous cellularity), but other atypical features such as a lack of polarization and a well-formed mantle zone. Further studies (immunohistochemistry, flow cytometry, FISH, PCR) would be appropriate to evaluate the specimen.

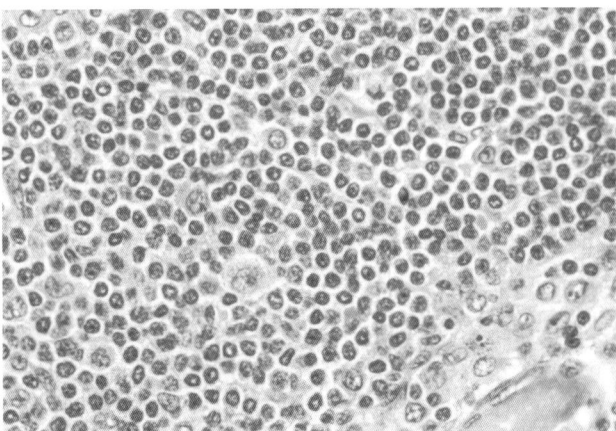

FIGURE 14.3. "ALH" with a large cell suggesting a diagnosis of classical Hodgkin lymphoma. In cases such as this, the lack of an appropriate immunophenotype for classical Hodgkin lymphoma (e.g., CD15+, CD30+, PAX-5 weak+) would make the diagnosis challenging.

FIGURE 14.4. Schematic overview of CD.

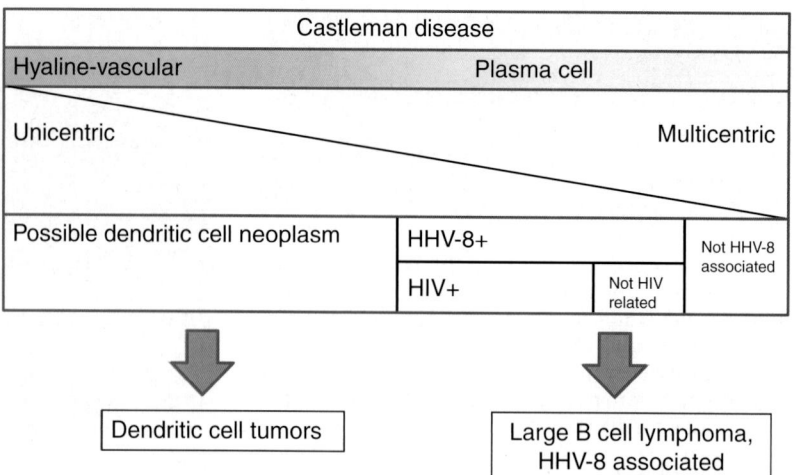

(Table 14.3). Laboratory findings may include elevated serum interleukin 6 (IL-6), elevated lactate dehydrogenase (LDH), cytopenias (most commonly thrombocytopenia or anemia), an elevated C-reactive protein (CRP), or renal insufficiency. On physical exam, hepatosplenomegaly may be identified (5–7,20). PC-CD, like HV-CD, has a broad age range with no clear gender predilection. Given the historical classifications, studies have differed slightly in their reported age ranges. The "unicentric plasma cell variant" is reported in a slightly younger group, with a median age of 30. The "multicentric plasma cell variant" is reported in the fifth and sixth decades (5,7). However, both age distribution and even gender predilection may be skewed as a subset of patients with "multicentric CD" have concomitant infection with human immunodeficiency virus (HIV) and human herpes virus type 8 (HHV-8).

The histologic findings in PC-CD are nonspecific and may be seen in a variety of other settings, making this a diagnosis of exclusion. The overall architecture of the lymph node is typically not effaced; the sinuses are patent and may be dilated. The histologic hallmarks of PC-CD are expanded interfollicular zones with paracortical plasmacytosis, often with plasmacytoid immunoblasts (Fig. 14.9). Paracortical areas often show hypervascularity (Fig. 14.10). The accompanying follicular hyperplasia includes a spectrum of appearances including large hypertrophic follicles to small atrophic follicles (as seen in the hyaline-vascular subtype). Comparable histology may be seen in lymph nodes adjacent to both hematopoietic and nonhematopoietic malignancies. Lymph nodes in patients with HIV infection, autoimmune diseases (such as rheumatoid arthritis [RA]), or reactive lymphadenopathies associated with immunodeficiency may have a similar appearance (5,21,22). Additionally, strikingly similar histologic changes may be seen in syphilitic (luetic) lymphadenitis (8).

Immunohistochemical studies show most cases have a polytypic plasmacytosis; however, a subset of cases may have a lambda monoclonal population, often in a polytypic background. Frank light chain restriction should be carefully evaluated in the overall context and is suggestive of HHV-8 infection, although a neoplastic proliferation such as a plasma cell dyscrasia, a lymphoma with prominent plasmacytic differentiation

(lymphoplasmacytic lymphoma or marginal zone lymphoma), or an IgA plasmacytoma should be excluded (see Chapter 37). Immunohistochemical staining for HHV-8 is often positive, as a subset of PC-CD cases are associated with this viral infection (5) (Fig. 14.11). Cases that are HHV-8 positive are associated with more aggressive clinical disease. The plasma cells may show monotypic lambda light chain restriction in up to one half of cases; however, these cases are not associated with more aggressive disease. In addition, immunohistochemical staining for IgG4 should be performed to exclude IgG4-RL.

HHV-8 is a gamma-herpesvirus, closely related to the Epstein-Barr virus (EBV), (7) and is also found in Kaposi sarcoma and primary effusion lymphoma (23–25). The role of HHV-8 infection in PC-CD is still being explored. Recent reports have focused on the increased production of IL-6 (23,26,27). HHV-8 produces a viral analog of IL-6 (vIL-6), which has 50% homology with the human IL-6 (hIL-6) gene (7). vIL-6 stimulates the normal intrinsic hIL-6 janus kinase-mediated activation of the signal transducers and activators of transcription (Jak-STAT) pathways through the cytokine receptor glycoprotein 130. However, since it is not an intrinsic signal it is not subject to normal negative regulatory feedback mechanisms (5,23,28). In the context of CD, IL-6 is thought to induce B-cell proliferation and differentiation, mediate the inflammatory clinical symptoms, and induce angiogenesis via VEGF production (28).

Although HHV-8 is not identified in all cases of PC-CD, when present it is almost universally in association with HIV

Table 14.2	HYALINE-VASCULAR CASTLEMAN OVERVIEW

Younger patients with single enlarged lymph node, usually thoracic in location
Asymptomatic
Lymph node histology: Atrophic follicles, onion skinning and lollipop formation, interfollicular vascular hyperplasia, dysplastic dendritic cells

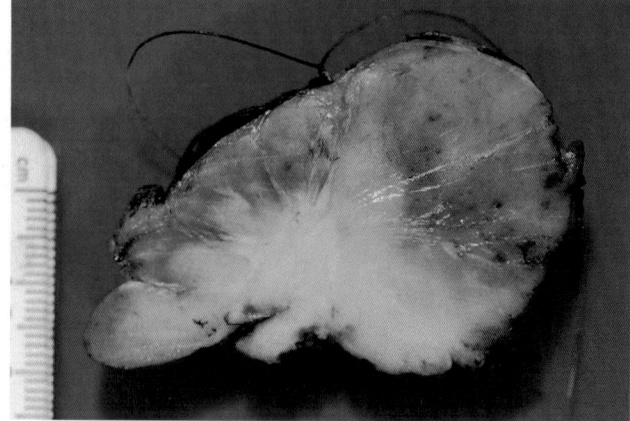

FIGURE 14.5. Gross image of lymph node with diffuse involvement by hyaline-vascular CD. The lymph node is mostly replaced by a diffuse proliferation of stromal and vascular elements (*yellow tan*) while residual lymphoid tissue has a faint *brown* appearance.

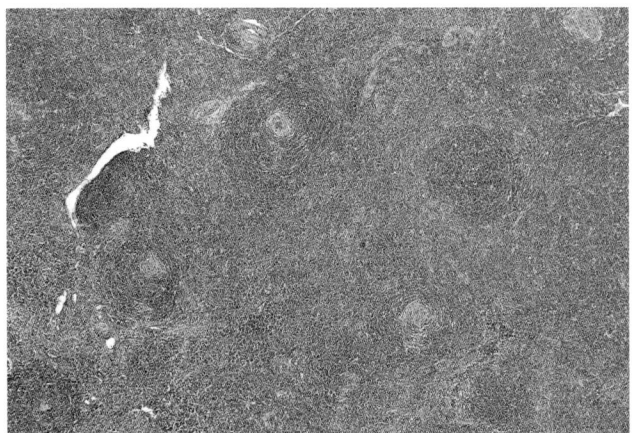

FIGURE 14.6. Low-magnification image of hyaline-vascular CD. The follicular structures seen are quite small in size due to regression of the central portions of follicles. There are increased numbers of mantle-type lymphocytes imparting a *deep blue* appearance at low magnification. Some hyalinized vessels are also seen.

infection (5). HHV-8 infection is viewed as the primary etiology of PC-CD in HIV-positive patients (29). These cases are more frequently multicentric in presentation and are associated with a poor prognosis, with survival times measured in months (5,30). In addition, they are also at higher risk for non-Hodgkin lymphomas. Large B-cell lymphoma arising in HHV-8-associated multicentric CD (HHV-8–positive plasmablastic lymphoma) has been described as a rare but specific entity (31). The neoplastic cells of this lymphoma arise from naive IgM-producing plasma cells without immunoglobulin hypermutation (5,31).

PC-CD (both multicentric and unicentric presentations) is associated with POEMS syndrome (polyneuropathy, organomegaly, endocrinopathy, M protein, and skin changes) in a small percentage of cases (5,7,32). HHV-8 is detected in POEMS patients with multicentric PC-CD almost five times more often than in patients with POEMS disease without multicentric CD (75% vs. 13% in a study of 22 patients) (33). Kaposi sarcoma is also often associated with PC-CD, as would be expected considering HHV-8 infection (7,23).

Treatment and prognosis is different depending on clinical presentation (multicentric vs. unicentric), HHV-8 infections, or HIV infection. Unicentric PC-CD, an uncommon presentation, is reportedly cured by excision alone. Multicentric PC-CD requires systemic therapy (5,7,18,19). Removal of the affected lymph nodes is associated with clinical improvement and a decrease

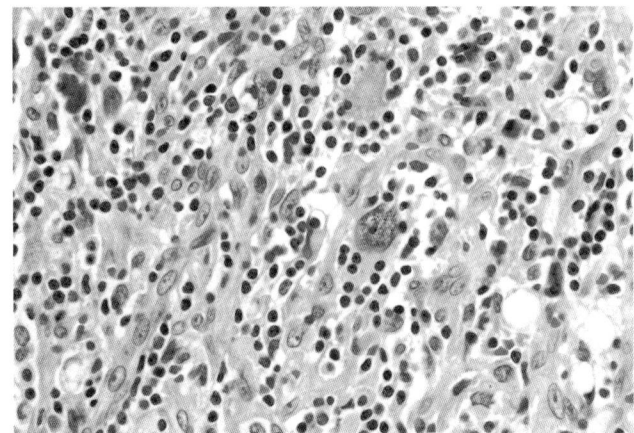

FIGURE 14.7. High magnification of an enlarged, hyperchromatic dendritic cell seen in interfollicular areas in hyaline-vascular CD. In some cases of hyaline-vascular CD, these dendritic cells have proven to be clonal.

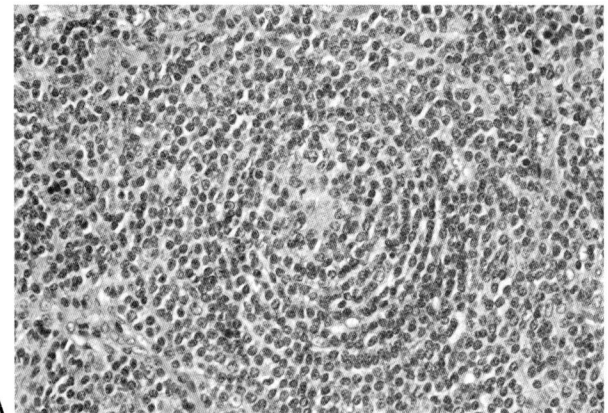

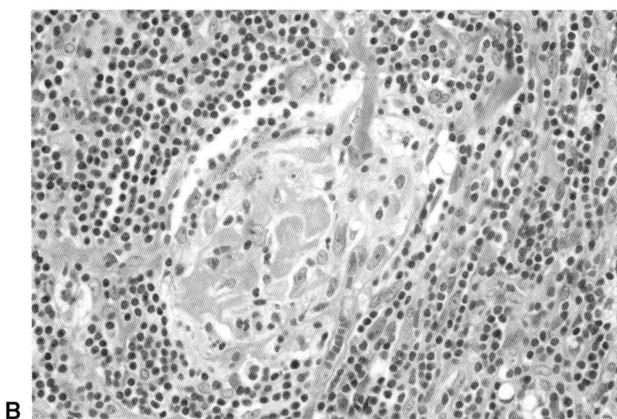

FIGURE 14.8. One typical feature of hyaline-vascular Castleman is the presence of small regressed follicles with a laminated appearance to the mantle zone lymphocytes imparting an "onion-skin" appearance **(A)**. High-magnification microscopic image of hyaline-vascular CD. Note the hyalinized vessel penetrating the small, atrophic follicle structure. These vessels may impart the appearance of a "lollipop" when seen in conjunction with the laminated, onion-skin appearance of surround mantle-type lymphocytes **(B)**.

in IL-6 levels (34). Numerous treatment interventions have been documented for multicentric PC-CD. Cytoreductive therapy has shown documented remissions lasting from 1 to 10 years; however, the HHV-8 status of the patients was not known in these patients (7,18,35). Immune modulators (steroids, interferon alpha, all-trans retinoic acid, and thalidomide), monoclonal antibodies (including anti-IL-6 and rituximab), and antiviral therapy (ganciclovir, foscarnet, and cidofovir for patients with documented HHV-8–positive PC-CD) have all been used in small reports with varying degrees of success (7).

Kikuchi-Fujimoto Disease

KFD is a rare cause of necrotizing lymphadenitis. Its importance in recognition cannot be underestimated, as it can be frequently misinterpreted as lymphoma.

Table 14.3	PLASMA CELL CASTLEMAN OVERVIEW

Older patient with regional lymphadenopathy/multicentric involvement
Fever, POEMS, HHV-8 association, increased levels of IL-6, association with HIV infection
Lymph node histology: Hyperplastic enlarged germinal centers, interfollicular sheets of plasma cells, may show lambda light chain monotypia

at\!

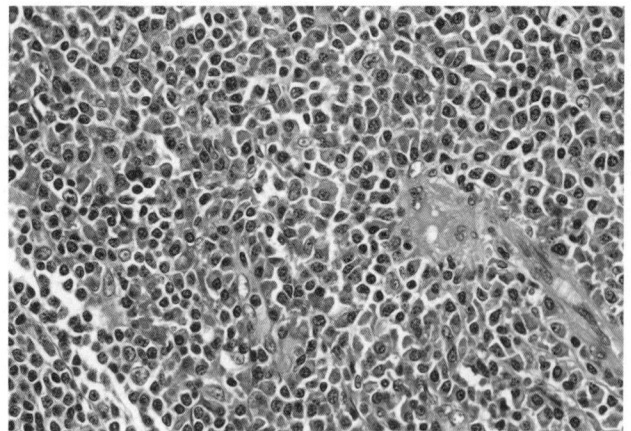

FIGURE 14.9. Interfollicular plasma cells of PC-CD. Some atypical forms are seen including occasional cells with numerous cytoplasmic immunoglobulin inclusions (Mott cells), binucleated forms, and some with enlarged, plasmablastic morphology.

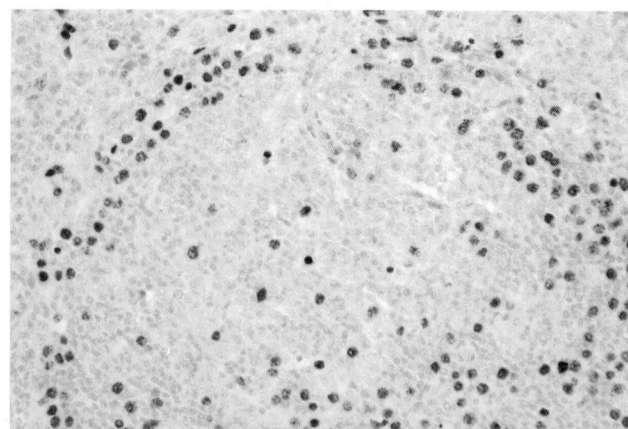

FIGURE 14.11. Immunohistochemical staining for HHV-8 in a case of PC-CD associated with HIV infection.

KFD presents in a young adult age range with a mean age of 21 years (36–38). The male-to-female ratio is 1:1 despite early reports that had showed a female predominance (36,39) (Table 14.4). KFD presents most often as cervical lymphadenopathy (posterior cervical triangle) and may be accompanied by low-grade fever, night sweats, or upper respiratory symptoms (36,37). Enlarged lymph nodes may be tender and range in size from 0.5 to 4 cm (36). Ancillary lab testing is usually normal but may show anemia, increased LDH, increased liver function tests, elevated sedimentation rate, elevated CRP, mild leukopenia, or leukocytosis or circulating atypical lymphocytes (36,37). Extranodal involvement is uncommon; however, skin lesions associated with KFD are well described in the literature. The face and upper body are the most common sites of skin involvement, which may be in the form of erythematous papules, plaques, indurated lesions, or ulcers (37).

KFD can have a range of histologic appearances, based on the stage of disease. There are considered to be three stages, corresponding to early, middle, and late disease, also referred to as proliferative, necrotizing, and xanthogranulomatous stages.

Proliferative Stage

The proliferative stage will often have clusters of plasmacytoid dendritic cells (PDCs), transformed lymphocytes, and histiocytes, but true necrosis is minimal or absent (Fig. 14.12).

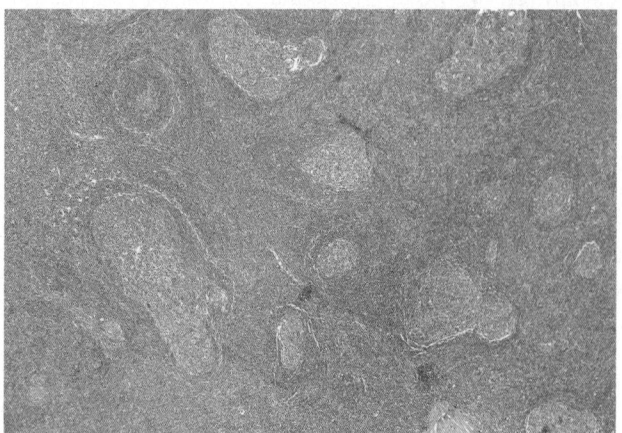

FIGURE 14.10. Low-magnification image of lymph node involved by PC-CD. In this case, there are reactive, hyperplastic follicles present with expanded interfollicular areas. The expanded interfollicular areas contain increased numbers of plasma cells.

Careful examination reveals individual cells or small fragments from rare individual cell necrosis. At low magnification, these areas seem more pale, pink, and less cellular than normal nodal areas. PDCs tend to cluster into small nodules, which may mimic germinal centers, and have a characteristic immunophenotype. They express myeloperoxidase, lysozyme, CD68, CD4, CD43, and CD123. The latter marker is one of the most specific and sensitive for PDCs.

Necrotizing Stage

The lymph node capsule is typically not thickened (although this may occur in the later stages). Extracapsular extension of lymphoid tissue may be seen, contributing to the mimicry of a lymphomatous process. Sinuses may be patent, but will likely be inconspicuous. Depending on the degree of involvement, there may be partial retention of normal nodal architecture, with reactive germinal centers and unremarkable interfollicular areas. The most prominent finding will be areas of necrosis (Fig. 14.13). These will vary in size, and can be found in interfollicular or paracortical areas. Within the central necrotic core, there is cellular debris (karyorrhexis) and fragments of apoptotic cells. Importantly, within this central core, neutrophils are not found. Also, no evidence of organisms or viral inclusions is seen. Surrounding these areas of necrosis are increased numbers of histiocytes, large transformed lymphocytes, and a cell type that is fairly characteristic of KFD, the PDC (Fig. 14.14). The immunoblasts are almost always large transformed T cells with a cytotoxic T-cell immunophenotype (CD8+), although rare B immunoblasts can also be seen.

Xanthogranulomatous Stage

In the late stage, lymphoid tissue is mostly replaced by foamy histiocytes and granulomatous material (Fig. 14.15). There is an overall increase of fibrosis and hypocellularity of the affected

Table 14.4	KIKUCHI-FUJIMOTO DISEASE OVERVIEW

Young adult patients with cervical lymphadenopathy
Fever upper respiratory symptoms or cutaneous lesions
Lymph node histology: Partially preserved lymph node architecture with patchy necrosis, apoptosis, nuclear debris, histiocytes, PDCs, CD8+ T cells, absence of neutrophils and eosinophils

FIGURE 14.12. **A low-magnification image of an early phase of KFD.** In this case, there is a *pale* area with increased histiocytes, PDCs, and transformed lymphocytes. However, the necrosis typical of later stages of KFD is not seen.

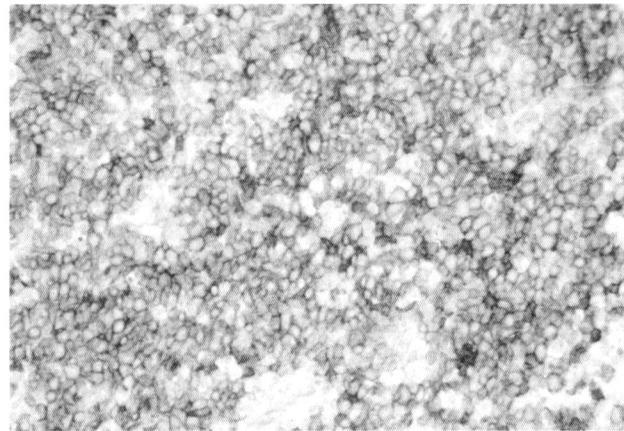

FIGURE 14.14. **Immunohistochemical staining for CD123 in KFD.** Increases in PDCs are typical in KFD, and while PDC are positive for many markers, CD123 is among the most sensitive and specific.

areas. PDCs are still present, but areas of necrosis are obscured by the histiocytic proliferation. This stage may be more likely confused with infectious or sclerosing etiologies, compared to other stages.

The differential diagnosis of the early and middle stages of KFD includes large cell lymphomas, acute lupus lymphadenitis, Hodgkin lymphoma, and other causes of necrotizing lymphadenitis (40,41). Acute lupus lymphadenitis and KFD may be morphologically "identical." One difference that is notable is that there can be hematoxylin bodies (degenerated cells with homogenized nuclear debris) seen in lupus lymphadenitis, although this may not be present or prominent in many cases. Also, acute lupus can have neutrophils and plasma cells associated with the necrosis, but not in all cases. Capsular inflammation and vasculitis may be seen in lupus but are not common in KFD. In these cases, serologic studies to exclude autoantibodies are critical. Because of the remarkable similarities between the histologic findings of acute lupus lymphadenitis and KFD, there have been continual attempts to declare all cases of KFD as a *forme fruste* (incomplete form) of systemic lupus (Fig. 14.16). It should be noted that all cases of KFD probably should be screened for autoimmune disease, and cases that are positive for lupus autoantibodies should be diagnosed as such. This only emphasizes the histologic similarities between KFD and acute lupus lymphadenitis.

Other necrotizing lymphadenopathies to consider include herpes simplex lymphadenitis (viral inclusions are present), tuberculosis and other atypical mycobacterial infections (use of

acid-fast bacillus [AFB] and Fite stains will exclude), and other infections including cat scratch disease, toxoplasmosis, bacterial, fungal, and viral infections. Acute EBV infection can rarely mimic KFD. If significant EBV positivity is identified (EBER or EBV-LMP) then a diagnosis of KFD should not be rendered. In general, viral lymphadenitis shows less prominent histiocytic infiltrate, more neutrophils, and more plasma cells (37).

To exclude large B-cell lymphoma, immunohistochemical stains should be used. The lack of a significant population of CD20-positive large B cells will help exclude this diagnosis. Also, a lack of light chain–restricted B cells by flow cytometry or a negative PCR study for B-cell clonality would help to exclude B-cell lymphoma. T-cell lymphoma is more difficult to exclude, as T-cell receptor gene rearrangements may be positive in this nonneoplastic setting. Flow cytometry may show increased numbers of CD8+ cells in KFD, which may help to exclude a T-cell lymphoproliferative process as most are CD4+ with aberrant antigen expression or antigen loss. The scattered CD30-positive immunoblasts seen in KFD do not coexpress CD15, in contrast to Hodgkin cells. Likewise, an increase in eosinophils and plasma cells is often seen in classical Hodgkin lymphoma, but rarely in KFD.

KFD was originally described in Japan independently by Drs. Kikuchi (42) and Fujimoto (43). The etiology is not currently known; however, there have been many studies attempting to identify an underlying infectious agent. Some nonviral etiologies including *Yersinia enterocolitica* and toxoplasma have been suggested. Many studies have tested for the presence of a wide

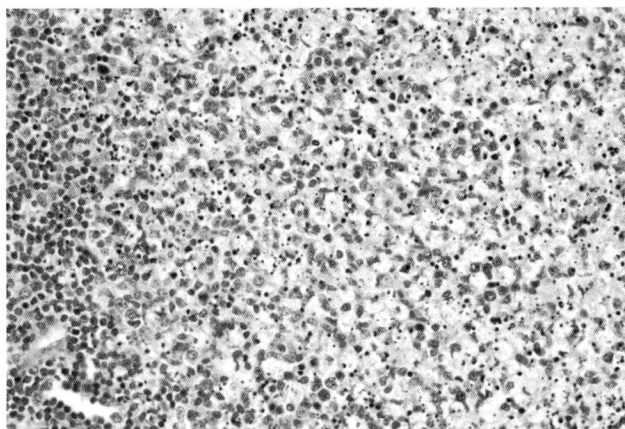

FIGURE 14.13. **High magnification of the necrotic phase of KFD.** Karyorrhectic debris is seen within the cytoplasm of histiocytes, in a background rich with lymphocytes and PDCs. Note that despite the necrosis, there are no neutrophils.

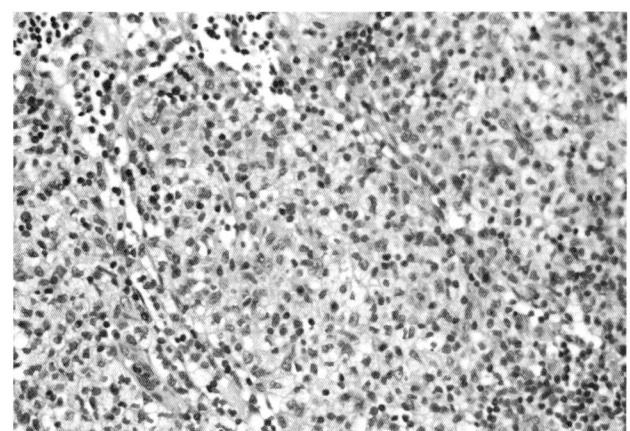

FIGURE 14.15. Late stage of KFD with foamy histiocytes and a more granulomatous appearance.

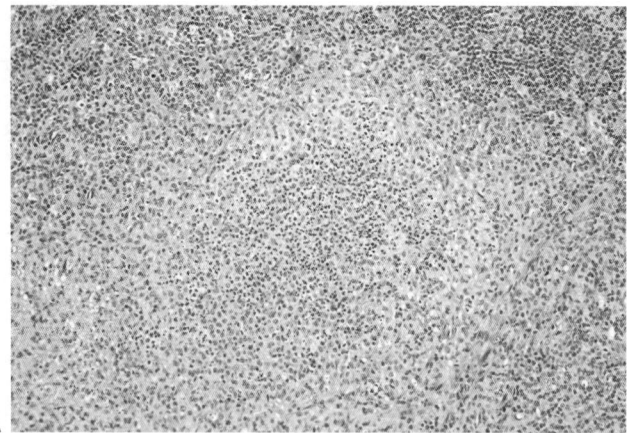 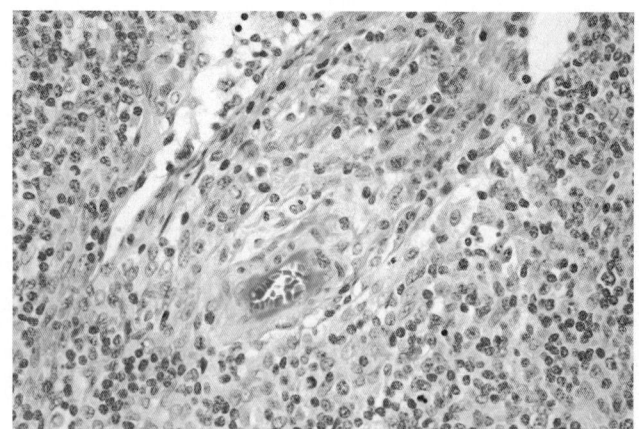

A   B

FIGURE 14.16. Histologic appearance of lupus lymphadenitis. Intermediate magnification of acute lupus lymphadenitis with necrotic areas rich in neutrophils **(A)**. A high-magnification image of acute lupus lymphadenitis shows prominent vasculitis within the lymph node **(B)**.

variety of viruses, including EBV, HHV-6, HHV-8, HIV, hepatitis B, human T-lymphotrophic virus type 1, parvovirus B19, paramyxovirus, and parainfluenza virus (44–47). Studies have not confirmed a specific virus as causative. No specific genetic basis has been identified in KFD, although a higher prevalence among Japanese and other Asiatic people have been reported (36). One hypothesis proposes that KFD may represent an overactive T-cell response to certain antigens in genetically susceptible individuals.

KFD is typically a self-limited disease with complete resolution in 3 to 4 months (37). Rare cases have been associated with recurrences (36). Treatment is usually limited to management of symptoms. In cases with severe symptomatology or in recurrent cases, steroids are sometimes used (37).

Kimura Disease

Kimura disease is a rare cause of lymphadenopathy associated with increased eosinophils. Cases commonly present as subcutaneous nodules in the head and neck, often in salivary glands and regional lymph nodes (48,49). Kimura disease is more prevalent in Asia, although it can be seen in Western countries as well (48). Young to middle-aged adults are most often affected, with a mean age of 32 years and a male-to-female ratio of 6:1 (48,49). Common clinical findings include peripheral blood eosinophilia and elevated serum IgE (49). Systemic symptoms such as fever or weight loss are rare. Nephrotic syndrome is seen in 12% to 16% of patients with Kimura disease (50,51). Renal disease may develop concurrently or before diagnosis of Kimura disease. The clinical course of Kimura disease is often chronic with periods of waxing and waning. There may be long-term recurrences (48,49,52).

In extranodal tissues, lymphoid infiltrate is often prominent with the formation of follicles and follicular hyperplasia. In lymph nodes, the nodal architecture is generally preserved (Table 14.5). Interfollicular areas often have an increase in vascular elements, including plump high-endothelial venules. Eosinophils are increased; they may be seen in interfollicular

areas or within follicles. Frequently clusters and aggregates of eosinophils, or eosinophilic microabscesses, are seen (Fig. 14.17). In addition to these findings, there are scattered multinucleated dendritic cells seen. These have the features of Warthin-Finkeldey cells, similar to those classically seen in measles infections (Fig. 14.18). These multinucleated cells are found both within the germinal centers and in interfollicular areas. Other histologic findings that are frequently seen include vascularization of germinal centers and proteinaceous deposition within germinal centers and fibrosis (Fig. 14.19). In some cases, necrosis of germinal centers is seen. Rarely, progressive transformation of germinal centers (PTGCs) may be seen in association with Kimura disease.

There is a broad differential of disorders with eosinophilic proliferations in lymphoid tissue. It is critical to exclude other diseases with eosinophilia including allergic responses, infections (human T-cell lymphoma/leukemia-virus 1, parasitic), Churg-Strauss disease, Wiskott-Aldrich syndrome, dermatopathic lymphadenitis, and medication reactions. Other differential diagnostic considerations include Hodgkin lymphoma, T-cell lymphomas (including angioimmunoblastic T-cell lymphoma), Langerhans cell histiocytosis, CD, systemic mastocytosis, and myeloid and lymphoid neoplasms with eosinophilia and abnormalities of PDGFRA, PDGFRB, and FGFR1. "Angiolymphoid hyperplasia with eosinophilia" was originally confused with

Table 14.5	**KIMURA DISEASE OVERVIEW**

Young adult patient, typically male, with lymphadenopathy in the neck or preauricular areas +/− subcutaneous nodules, involvement of salivary gland or kidney
Peripheral blood: eosinophilia/increased levels of IgE
Lymph node histology: Follicular hyperplasia, increased eosinophils including eosinophilic microabscesses and infiltration into follicle centers, multinucleated dendritic cells

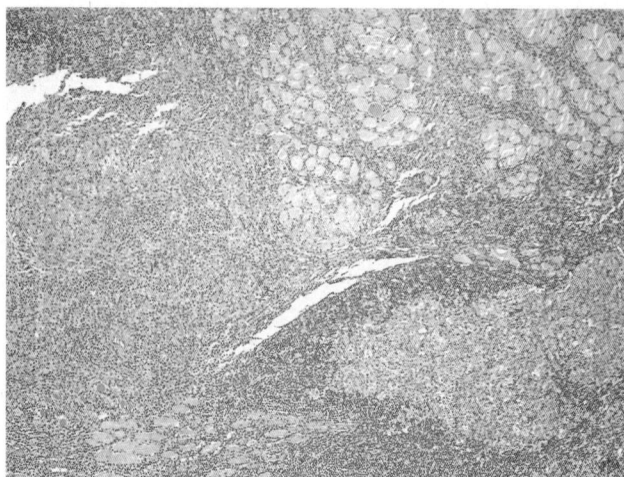

FIGURE 14.17. A low-magnification image of Kimura disease with hyperplastic follicles **(lower right)** and markedly increased eosinophils. This case shows infiltration of skeletal muscle.

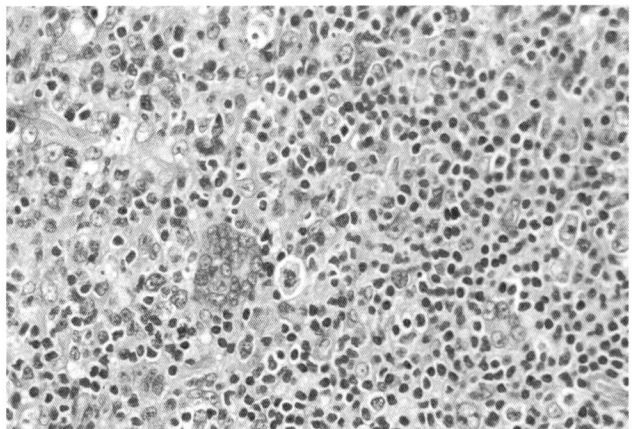

FIGURE 14.18. High magnification of Kimura disease showing a characteristic polykaryotic cell. These likely represent dendritic cells or histiocytes, and their appearance has fueled theories suggesting a viral etiology for Kimura disease.

Kimura disease (53). It presents in similar sites and has lymphoid cells in association with eosinophils; however, it was ultimately recognized as an *epithelioid hemangioma with eosinophilia*, as evidenced by staining with vascular markers (54).

Kimura disease was originally described in China by Kim (55) as "eosinophilic hyperplastic granuloma" in 1937. The eponym derives from a later description by Kimura (56) from Japan in 1948. Historically, there has been a great deal of confusion associated with this disease due to a broad range of names used to describe it.

The etiology and exact prevalence of Kimura disease is unknown. It can be seen in the context of hypereosinophilic syndrome (57).

Multiple therapeutic options have been attempted. Some studies suggest that localized radiotherapy (20 to 45 Gy) is more effective than other treatment modalities (58). Local excision of affected tissues and steroid therapy are commonly used, with some effect. Case reports and small studies suggest effectiveness of many other treatment options including cyclosporine and low-dose imatinib (49,59). At present, no single therapy has proven to be completely effective.

Rosai-Dorfman Disease (Sinus Histiocytosis with Massive Lymphadenopathy)

RDD, also known as sinus histiocytosis with massive lymphadenopathy, is defined as a proliferation of atypical histiocytes

Table 14.6	ROSAI-DORFMAN DISEASE OVERVIEW

Children and young adults, long-standing massive cervical lymphadenopathy
Fever, polyclonal hypergammaglobulinemia
Lymph node histology: Dilated sinuses, large, pale histiocytes with emperipolesis (S100+)

that accumulate in tissues or lymph nodes causing masses or lymphadenopathy (Table 14.6). Although it is a benign disease, individual cases may have significant morbidity due to local damage of critical tissues.

The most common clinical presentation is painless, bilateral massive enlargement of neck lymph nodes (8). The median age of presentation is 20 years, with a slightly higher prevalence in males and those of African descent (8). Patients may present with fever and weight loss; associated laboratory findings include leukocytosis, elevated ESR, and hypergammaglobulinemia (60). Rarely, patients exhibit positive rheumatoid factor or antinuclear antibodies. Extranodal presentations occur in 25% to 40% of cases (61). Extranodal sites that are most commonly affected are skin, upper respiratory tract, soft tissue, orbit, bone, salivary gland, central nervous system, breast, and pancreas (62). Presentation in the bone marrow has also been reported (63).

In affected nodes, the sinuses are typically expanded by large abnormal histiocytes. However, histiocytic cells within the parenchyma of the node in sheets and clusters are not unusual. Nodal architecture is effaced by the histiocytic proliferation and other typical, reactive features are also usually present. The histiocytes of RDD are characteristic. They have intermediate-to-large round nuclei; open, vesicular chromatin; and distinct, but relatively small nucleoli (Fig. 14.20). They have ample amounts of pale or clear cytoplasm. One of the most characteristic findings is the presence of emperipolesis (Fig. 14.21) or the presence of intact inflammatory cells within the cytoplasm of these histiocytes. Any cell type can be seen, although most commonly, these are small lymphocytes, plasma cells, and red blood cells. Eosinophils are not usually seen. RDD histiocytes are positive for S100 protein (Fig. 14.22). This is typically strong and both cytoplasmic and nuclear in distribution. RDD histiocytes also express typical histiocyte-related antigens, lysozyme, CD4, fascin, CD11c, CD14, CD33, and CD68. CD30 is positive in some cases. These cells lack CD1a and langerin expression, in contrast to Langerhans cell histiocytosis. Molecular studies up to this point have shown the histiocytes to be polyclonal via HUMARA assays (63).

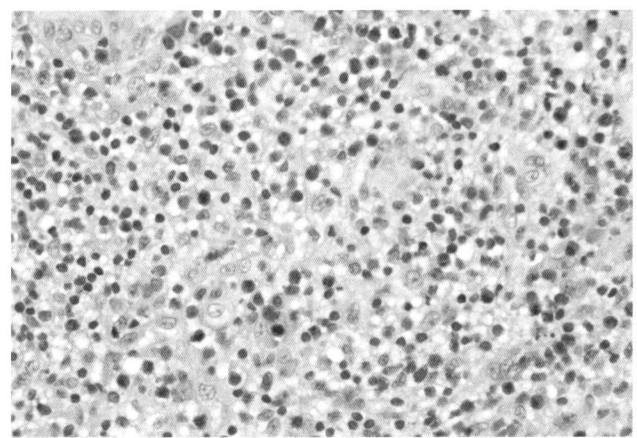

FIGURE 14.19. Intermediate magnification of Kimura disease showing an increase in mature eosinophils. In this case, there is an increase in background histiocytes.

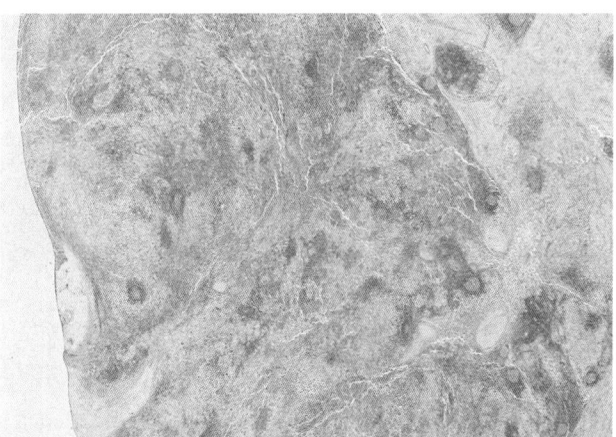

FIGURE 14.20. A low-magnification image of a lymph node with RDD. The sinuses are massively expanded by pale histiocytes. These abnormal histiocytes displace normal lymphoid structures.

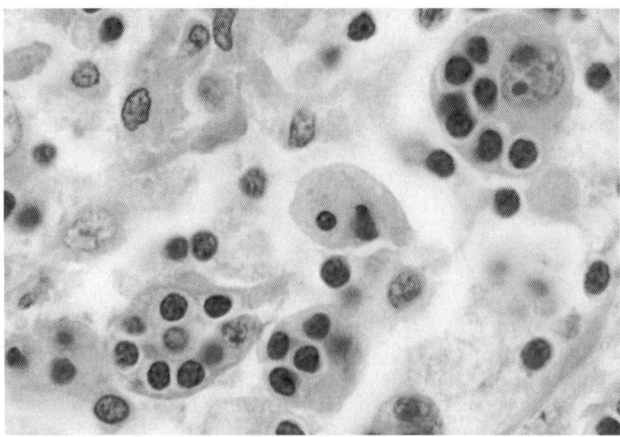

FIGURE 14.21. The characteristic histiocytes of RDD have large round to oval nuclei with dispersed chromatin. They have voluminous pale cytoplasm, and often have ingested, intact cells, known as emperipolesis.

The histologic differential diagnosis of RDD includes sinus histiocytosis of "usual type," sinus histiocytosis induced by joint replacement (metal fragments or debris), hemophagocytic syndrome, Langerhans cell histiocytosis, leprosy, storage diseases, as well as metastatic melanoma or other metastatic malignancies. It should be noted that RDD has been associated with several hematopoietic neoplasms (60). In light of this, in cases with RDD, careful examination of the remaining tissue is required to exclude concurrent pathologies. Flow cytometry does not play a specific role in the diagnosis of RDD, but may be useful to exclude concurrent hematolymphoid disorders.

RDD was originally described in the literature by Rosai and Dorfman in 1969 (64,65). Their original series combined with subsequent publications defined all of the essential features of RDD (66). Since its initial description no specific etiologic agent has been identified in RDD. In a subset of cases, studies have shown positivity for HHV-6 and more recently polyomavirus (67,68). RDD has been reported concurrently and following Hodgkin and non-Hodgkin lymphomas (including acute lymphoblastic leukemia). In addition to the hematopoietic neoplasms, RDD has also been associated with other diseases such as ALPS-type 1 cases and concurrent Langerhans cell histiocytosis (69,70). There are some cases of familial RDD, or perhaps more precisely a disease that has features of RDD in association with a variety of other

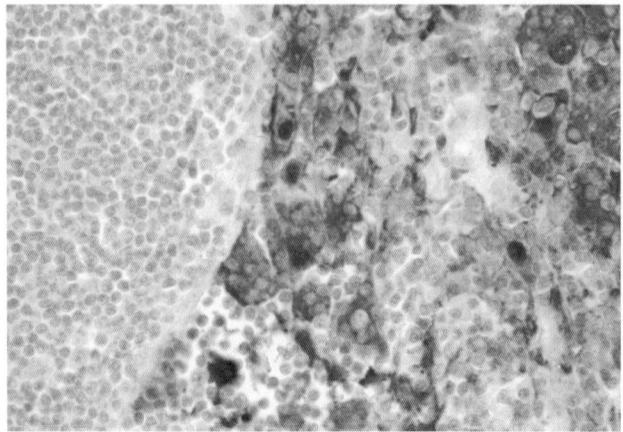

FIGURE 14.22. Strong staining for S-100 protein in the cytoplasm of the histiocytes of RDD. Careful inspection may reveal intracytoplasmic cells (e.g., emperipolesis) that do not stain for S-100.

manifestations of a broader genetic disorder. Recent studies have associated these cases with mutations in *SLC29A3* hENT3 (chromosome 10q22.1) (sodium-dependent nucleotide transporter) (71,72).

RDD is typically associated with an indolent clinical course. It usually lasts 3 to 9 months with spontaneous remission. A small subset of cases have recurrences and pursue an aggressive clinical course (73,74). Surgical excision or localized radiotherapy may be used in cases where vital organ functions are compromised. Although there are anecdotal cases of responses to chemotherapy or other biologic agents (cytokines, etc.), there are no clear data to support a single, specific therapy.

IgG4-Related Lymphadenopathy

IgG4-related sclerosing disease is the name given to a recently described systemic disorder that presents as mass-forming lesions in soft tissues (often exocrine glands). A characteristic triad of lymphoplasmacytic infiltrate, fibrosis, and phlebitis is diagnostic in extranodal locations. Plasma cells are polyclonal and predominantly of the IgG4 subtype. Reported sites of involvement and disease associations are diverse including central nervous system (pituitary gland, pachymeningitis), lacrimal gland, parotid gland, submandibular gland (Mikulicz disease), sclerosing sialadenitis (Kuttner tumor), thyroid gland, pulmonary lesions, breast, liver, retroperitoneum (idiopathic retroperitoneal fibrosis, inflammatory aortic aneurysm), pancreas (type 1 autoimmune pancreatitis, sclerosing cholangitis), kidney, skin, and lymph node (75). *IgG4-related lymphadenopathy* shows increased numbers of IgG4 plasma cells; however, in contrast to other sites, fibrosis is rarely present and phlebitis is not seen. IgG4-RL may precede, coexist with, or follow extranodal manifestations of disease.

The clinical presentation varies widely, depending on affected sites. Lymphadenopathy may be seen alone or in combination with an elevated sedimentation rate and/or autoantibodies including antinuclear antibodies or rheumatoid factor (Table 14.7) (75). Symptoms such as fever and night sweats have not been reported in IgG4-RL. Radiologic evidence of a mass and surrounding lymphadenopathy may mimic carcinoma with metastatic disease in regional lymph nodes. In one study, 80% of patients presenting with IgG4-RSD in the pancreas also showed enlarged regional lymph nodes IgG4-RL (76).

Laboratory findings seen in a many patients may include increased serum levels of IgG, IgG4, or IgE. Serum IgG4 levels are considered elevated at >135 mg/dL. Serum elevations are thought to coincide with disease activity and the number of involved sites. Patients who have been diagnosed with IgG4-RSD by fulfilling histologic criteria may not have elevated IgG4 serum levels, and elevated IgG4 serum levels may be seen in other conditions, such as atopic dermatitis pemphigus and parasitic diseases (75). In initial reports of IgG4-RSD a male predominance and advanced age are described in this patient population (77). In lymph nodes with increased numbers of IgG4 plasma cells this male predominance was not observed (78).

Multiple histologic patterns are described in association with IgG4-RL. Increased IgG4 plasma cells are the common finding among the various histologies, making diagnosis of this

Table 14.7	IGG4-RELATED LYMPHADENOPATHY OVERVIEW

Middle-aged to older adult, with mass-forming lesions +/− lymphadenopathy
Lymph node histology: Increased polyclonal plasma cells or plasma cells infiltrate into follicle centers, PTGC, IPT-like changes, PC-CD-like changes

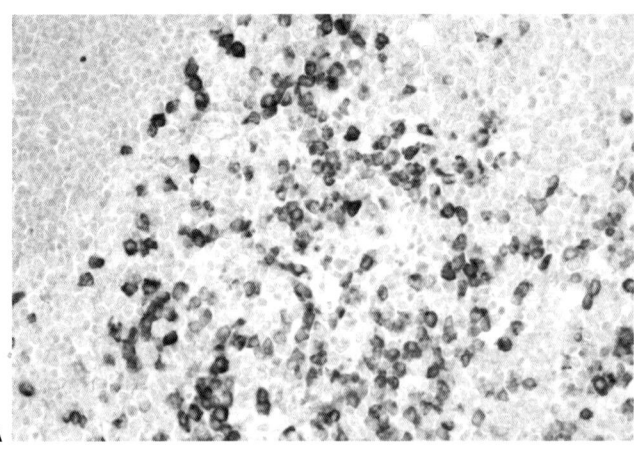
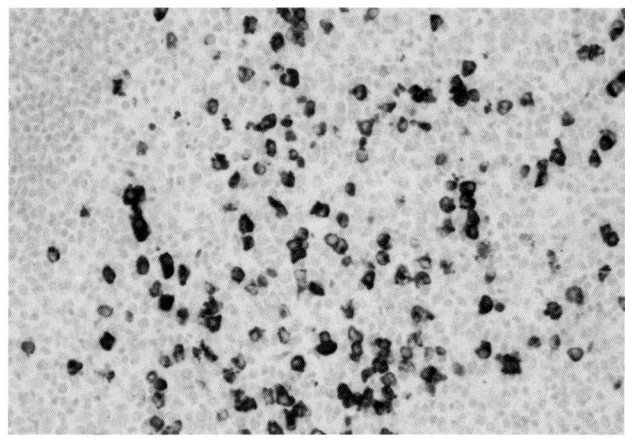

A   **B**

FIGURE 14.23. Stains for IgG **(A)** and IgG4 **(B)** in a case of IgG4-RL. In normal lymph nodes, there are almost no IgG4-positive plasma cells. In IgG4-RL, IgG4-positive plasma cells are present in increased numbers (often clusters of 50 or more) with an IgG4/IgG ratio of >40%.

entity largely dependent on suspicion and subsequent immuno-histochemical findings (Fig. 14.23). On hematoxylin and eosin sections, plasma cell increases range from mild to marked. Their distribution may be interfollicular and/or within the follicle centers. Mild increases in eosinophils are also seen in many cases. Additional findings include follicular hyperplasia, interfollicular expansion (expanded by scattered immunoblasts and/or vascular proliferation), PTGCs, or a nodal inflammatory pseudotumor (IPT)–like appearance (Fig. 14.24) (75,79). Proposed histologic criteria in lymph node include all of the following: a morphology compatible with those outlined above, an increase in plasma cells, and an increased number of IgG4 cells measured in absolute number, >50 per high-power field, as well as by a percentage of IgG4-positive/IgG-positive cells >40% (75). Plasma cells should be evaluated in areas of the highest density of positive cells, averaged over three high-power fields (75). Patchy or an uneven distribution of IgG4 plasma cells may be seen, making negative IgG4 staining on a needle core biopsy insufficient to exclude IgG4-RL lymphadenopathy.

The differential diagnosis of IgG4-RL is wide, encompassing reactive, infectious, immunologic, and neoplastic etiologies. A predominantly fibrotic pattern in lymph node, described as IPT-like, is differentiated from a true IPT by the lack of IgG4 plasma cells (80). When plasma cell increases are marked and predominantly interfollicular in distribution, PC-CD must be excluded. Increased levels of serum IL-6 and a clinical presentation including fever

and expression of HHV-8 in tissue support a diagnosis of PCCD and have not been reported in IgG4-RL (81). The presence of a light chain–restricted B-cell or plasma cell population excludes a diagnosis of IgG4-RL. Lymphomas associated with IgG4 production have been reported (82–84). The relationship between IgG4-positive benign disorders and the subsequent development of IgG4-positive lymphomas has not been thoroughly evaluated at this point. Increased numbers of IgG4 plasma cells may be seen in a variety of unrelated settings including occasional cases of RA, RDD, syphilis infections, perforating collagenosis, autoimmune atrophic gastritis, and sclerosing variant of mucoepidermoid carcinoma of salivary gland (75,85).

The etiology and prevalence of IgG4-RSD or IgG4-RL are not known. The role of the IgG4 plasma cells in the mechanism underlying this disease remains unclear and may represent a biomarker of underlying pathophysiology (86). Recognition of IgG4-RSD and IgG4-RL is of significant importance, as adverse clinical outcomes resulting from underdiagnosing may include loss of function of exocrine glands, local destruction from mass lesions, aortic dissection, and exposure to unnecessary surgical interventions. IgG4-RSD has been shown to be exquisitely responsive to steroids as well as rituximab, (75,77,87). Prompt diagnosis and treatment will prevent significant patient morbidity (75,87–89).

Inflammatory Pseudotumor

IPT-LN are lesions with partial or complete effacement of lymph node architecture by proliferations of spindle cells with a mixed inflammatory infiltrate. The majority of these lesions have a benign clinical course.

The clinical presentations reported include lymphadenopathy and systemic symptoms such as fever, fatigue, and night sweats (Table 14.8). Lymph nodes may be enlarged up to 3 cm or greater. Similar lesions have been previously referred to as plasma cell granulomas in other anatomic sites, including lung and bronchus, skin, and the gastrointestinal tract. Rarely, cases

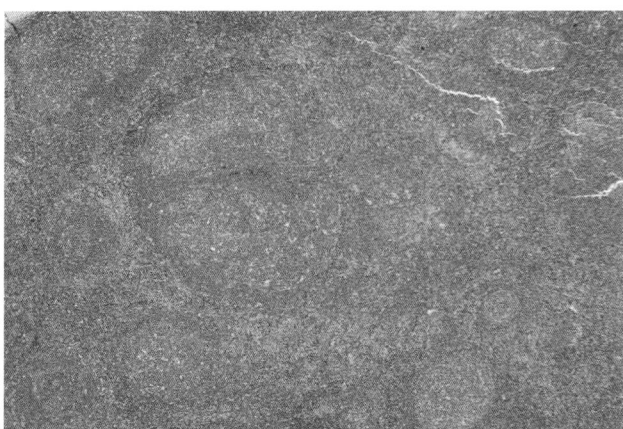

FIGURE 14.24. Low-magnification image of IgG4-RL. In this case, there is the combination of follicular hyperplasia and progressively transformed germinal centers. These cases will often have increased numbers of plasma cells within follicles and in interfollicular areas.

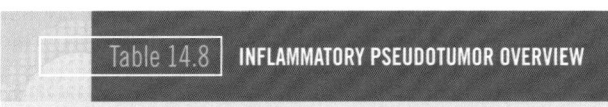

Table 14.8	INFLAMMATORY PSEUDOTUMOR OVERVIEW

Lymphadenopathy and systemic symptoms
Lymph node histology: Hyperplastic stromal elements including spindle cells and histiocytes with varying degrees of sclerosis, marked vascularity, and mixed inflammatory cell infiltrate

A

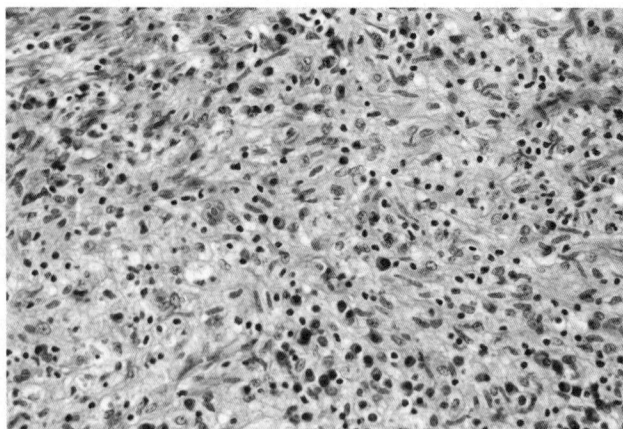
B

FIGURE 14.25. Spindled cells of IPT-LN. Low magnification of IPT **(A)** replacing much of the lymph node with a proliferation of bland spindle cells with infiltration by acute and chronic inflammatory elements **(B)**.

have presented with multiple sites of involvement or disseminated disease (90,91). IPT-LN may occur at any age with no clear gender predilection.

Histologically, IPT-LN demonstrate hyperplastic stromal elements including spindle cells and histiocytes with varying degrees of sclerosis (Fig. 14.25). There is marked vascularity and a mixed inflammatory cell infiltrate, including numerous plasma cells. Necrosis and infarction are rare (92,93). The characteristic spindle cells are reactive with vimentin, and variably reactive for CD68 and/or smooth-muscle actin, supporting a fibroblastic/myofibroblastic origin. Immunohistochemical staining of the inflammatory cells shows a mixture of B and T cells, and rare CD30-positive transformed lymphocytes.

The differential diagnosis of IPT-LN includes both benign and malignant lesions. Some of the more common entities that show similar histologic features include follicular lymphoma with sclerosis (93), CD (94), medication-related lymphadenopathy (95), Langerhans cell histiocytosis, dendritic cell neoplasms, peripheral T-cell lymphoma, and Hodgkin lymphoma. Other entities such as syphilitic (luetic) lymphadenitis (96), Kaposi sarcoma, intranodal hemorrhagic spindle cell tumor with amianthoid fibers or palisaded myofibroblastoma, amyloidosis, and proteinaceous lymphadenopathy are also in the differential diagnosis of IPT-LN (8). The expression of ALK-1 by immunohistochemistry is not seen in IPT-LN and would indicate an alternate diagnosis, such as inflammatory myofibroblastic tumor. Cases should be evaluated for IgG4 expression by plasma cells. If there are significant numbers of IgG4-positive plasma cells or if there are focal increases with a high IgG4/IgG ratio, then this should be considered as part of the spectrum of IgG4-related disease. When prominent follicular hyperplasia is present, the possibility of syphilis infection should be considered (96). IPT-LN should lack evidence of active infection, and stains for microorganisms, such as AFB, GMS, and PAS, may be warranted to exclude infectious etiologies. However, evidence of EBV infection may be present in IPT-LN when evaluated by EBER *in situ* stains (97), although the EBV is not in the spindled cells in IPT-LN.

IPT-LN was first reported by Perrone et al. (98) in seven patients in 1988. Some studies suggest that "true" IPT-LN may represent an evolving, dynamic process with different histologic features depending on its stage of evolution.

In virtually all cases of IPT-LN, resection is typically curative. In cases with associated clinical symptomatology, these may resolve after complete resection of the lesion. If cases have increases in IgG4-positive plasma cells, then treatments for IgG4-related disease, such as steroid or rituximab, may be of benefit.

Autoimmune Lymphoproliferative Syndrome

ALPS is a genetically heterogeneous syndrome resulting from defective apoptosis of activated lymphocytes. Clinically ALPS presents in early childhood and is characterized by nonmalignant lymphoproliferation, lymphadenopathy, and/or splenomegaly, an increase in double-negative CD4-CD8 T cells, hypergammaglobulinemia, and autoimmune abnormalities (99,100).

Patients present at a median age of 9 months (ranging from 2 months to 5 years) with marked lymphadenopathy and/or splenomegaly that frequently distorts normal anatomical landmarks (Table 14.9) (101). The male-to-female ratio is 1.8:1 (102). Associated autoimmune phenomenon include hemolytic anemia, idiopathic thrombocytopenic purpura (ITP), urticarial rash, and neutropenia. Glomerulonephritis and Guillan-Barre–like presentations have rarely been reported as well (101,102). Opportunistic infections or increased susceptibility to infection has not been reported (101,103).

Overall lymph node architecture remains intact (101,104). Florid follicular hyperplasia with marked paracortical expansion may be accompanied by PTGCs or rarely follicular involution (Fig. 14.26) (101,104). The interfollicular areas are expanded by T cells of the alpha/beta receptor CD4-CD8 double-negative phenotype expressing CD57 (104). Paracortical plasmacytosis is also present (104). Ki-67 shows prominent proliferative activity in the paracortex (104). Focal areas of lymph node may show features of RDD (103).

A lymphocytosis may be seen in the peripheral blood. Flow cytometry shows the characteristic CD4-CD8- double-negative T cells (101,104). CD3+ T cells are often within normal limits, but CD4+ cells are relatively decreased leading to an inverted CD4:CD8 ratio or a 1:1 ratio (104). In addition, a CD20+ polyclonal B lymphocytosis may be present, often with coexpression of CD5 (104).

The differential diagnosis of ALPS includes peripheral T-cell lymphoma not otherwise specified (103,104). Viral

Table 14.9	ALPS OVERVIEW

Child or young adult with extensive lymphadenopathy and/or splenomegaly
Autoimmune phenomenon, hypergammaglobulinemia, no increased opportunistic infections
Peripheral blood: Double-negative CD4 and CD8 T cells, CD5-expressing B cells
Lymph node histology: Follicular hyperplasia, paracortical expansion by double-negative CD4- CD8 T cells, PTGCs

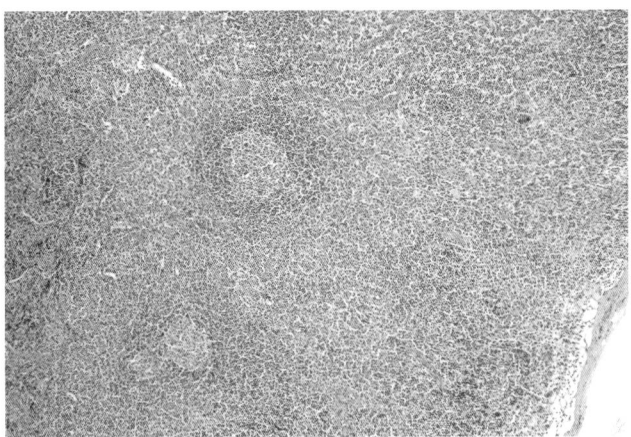

FIGURE 14.26. Low magnification of lymph nodes from ALPS. Follicles are present with expanded and atypical-appearing interfollicular zones.

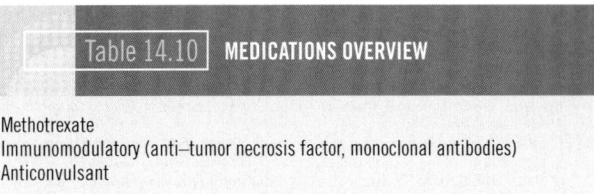

Table 14.10	MEDICATIONS OVERVIEW

Methotrexate
Immunomodulatory (anti–tumor necrosis factor, monoclonal antibodies)
Anticonvulsant

lymphadenitis may show similar histologic changes; however, histiocytes containing apoptotic debris are conspicuously absent in ALPS (101).

Also called Canale-Smith syndrome, ALPS was first described by Canale and Smith in 1967 as a benign lymphoproliferative disease and autoimmune cytopenia (99,102). Diagnostic criteria used to identify cases of ALPS include a characteristic triad of chronic accumulation of nonmalignant lymphoid cells, increased α/β^+ double-negative T cells, and defective *in vitro* receptor-mediated lymphocyte apoptosis (102). Defective lymphocyte apoptosis is thought to be due to genetic mutations of the underlying apoptotic pathway, all of which have not been defined yet. The best characterized abnormality is the binding of FAS to the FAS ligand (FAS-L) to trigger apoptosis (105). The genetic and molecular basis of ALPS was identified in 1995 by demonstrating the mutation of TNFRSF6 (formerly called APT1) gene encoding a surface receptor, FAS (CD95/Apo1) in patients with lymphocyte apoptotic defects (99,106). Subsequent identification of other (non-FAS) defects in ALPS patients led to the current classification system based on genetic defects. ALPS-0 patients are homozygous and ALPS-Ia patients are heterozygous for inherited mutations of the FAS gene. ALPS-Ib patients have mutations in the FAS-L. ALPS-IIa and IIb patients have mutations in the CASPASE-10 and CASPASE-8. ALPS-III patients have unknown genetic mutation but clinically display mild ALPS. ALPS-IV patients have *NRAS* mutations. ALPS-Im patients have somatic mosaic FAS mutations (99).

Treatment of ALPS is largely symptomatic, with associated severe autoimmune phenomenon (such as hemolytic anemia or ITP) being treated by systemic corticosteroid therapy (99).

Atypical Lymphoid Proliferations Associated with Medications and Therapies

Medication and treatment effects can be a challenging area of diagnosis in lymph node pathology. In many cases, without adequate history, some cases may be diagnosed as lymphomas, or often as ALHs (see **Atypical Lymphoid Hyperplasia section**). In any case, the effects of several medications may have a profound impact on the histology of lymph nodes leading to some significant histopathologic findings (Table 14.10).

It should be noted that many of the medications that have prominent effects on lymph nodes are those used in treating autoimmune and inflammatory conditions. In these circumstances, it is often difficult to distinguish specific medication effects from those of concomitant therapies or the underlying disease (107). This is especially problematic when considering RA, systemic lupus, and therapy with methotrexate.

Methotrexate-associated lymphoid proliferations can range from "typical" hyperplasias to frank lymphoma (108). These proliferations are most often associated with long-term and low-dose therapy, with a median treatment time of 3 years (107). Most challenging are ALH and the distinctions from underlying changes seen in the primary disorders, such as RA. In most circumstances, the proliferations seen with methotrexate are polymorphous and expand the interfollicular zones of lymph nodes. There may be increases in immunoblasts and in certain cases, Hodgkin-like cells are seen. Thus, mimicry of T-cell lymphomas, diffuse large B-cell lymphoma, and both classical and nodular lymphocyte-predominant Hodgkin lymphoma can be seen. Approximately 40% of these proliferations are EBV positive (107). In these circumstances, PCR studies for B- and T-cell clonality may be supportive of a diagnosis of an overt lymphoproliferative disorder. The clinical behavior of methotrexate-associated lymphoproliferative disorders is unpredictable. However, it may also be prudent to exercise caution in diagnosing these cases; if possible, attempts should be made to withdraw the drug to evaluate for possible improvement or resolution of the lymphoid proliferation, especially if the proliferations are EBV associated (107,109).

A comparable range of lymphoid proliferations has been identified with immunomodulatory agents, including the group of anti-tumor necrosis factor monoclonal antibodies used to treat autoimmune disorders (110). In these cases a broad variety of benign, atypical, and frankly malignant lymphoid proliferations have been noted. Approximately one half of cases have associated EBV infections. Further, in addition to B-cell proliferations, some T-cell lymphomas and atypical T-cell proliferations have been noted. As in other circumstances, sorting the effects of the immunomodulatory agents from disease effects as well as previous therapies (such as methotrexate) can be challenging. In each circumstance, careful correlation of medication history, disease course, and overall histologic, molecular, and genetic findings is recommended.

Anticonvulsant medications, including phenytoin, ethosuximide, carbamazepine, and mesantoin, have been associated with lymphadenopathy (111). Some cases of outright lymphoma have been reported. However, the majority of cases are associated with reactive lymphadenopathies. These medications most often induce changes of germinal center hyperplasia with increased immunoblasts, increased immunoblasts with germinal center atrophy, or other atypical lymphoid proliferations. PCR and flow cytometric studies will be polyclonal in reactive cases (112). As in other disorders associated with medications, correlation with medication history, evaluation after drug withdrawal, and prudent use of immunohistochemical and molecular studies will most often guide appropriate diagnosis and management.

References

1. Bagg A. Malleable immunoglobulin genes and hematopathology—the good, the bad, and the ugly: a paper from the 2007 William Beaumont hospital symposium on molecular pathology. *J Mol Diagn* 2008;10:396–410.
2. Good DJ, Gascoyne RD. Atypical lymphoid hyperplasia mimicking lymphoma. *Hematol Oncol Clin North Am* 2009;23:729–745.
3. Castleman B, Iverson L, Menendez VP. Localized mediastinal lymph node hyperplasia resembling thymoma. *Cancer* 1956;9:822–830.

4. Keller AR, Hochholzer L, Castleman B. Hyaline-vascular and plasma cell types of giant lymph node hyperplasia of the mediastinum and other locations. *Cancer* 1972;29:670–683.
5. Cronin DMP, Warnke RA. Castleman disease an update on classification and the spectrum of associated lesions. *Adv Anat Pathol* 2009;16:236–246.
6. Frizzera G. Castleman's disease and related disorders. *Semin Diagn Pathol* 1988;5:346–364.
7. Casper C. The etiology and management of Castleman disease at 50 years: translating pathophysiology to patient care. *Br J Haematol* 2005;129:3–17.
8. O'Malley DP, George TI, Orazi A, et al. *Atlas of nontumor pathology first series Fascicle 7. Benign and reactive conditions of lymph node and spleen*. Washington, DC: ARP press, 2009.
9. Smir BN, Greiner TC, Weisenberger DD. Multicentric angiofollicular lymph node hyperplasia in children: a clinicopathologic study of eight patients. *Mod Pathol* 1996;9:1135–1142.
10. Pauwels P, Dal Cin P, Vlasveld LT, et al. A chromosomal abnormality in hyaline vascular Castleman disease: evidence for clonal proliferation of dysplastic stromal cells. *Am J Surg Pathol* 2000;24:882–888.
11. Hsi ED. *Castleman disease. Hematopathology.* Philadelphia: Churchill Livingstone Elsevier, 2007:150–155.
12. Cokelaere K, Debiec-Rychter M, De Wolfe-Peeters C, et al. Hyaline vascular Castleman's disease with HMGIC rearrangement in follicular dendritic cells: molecular evidence of mesenchymal tumorigenesis. *Am J Surg Pathol* 2002;26:662–669.
13. Chen WC, Jones D, Ho CL, et al. Cytogenetic abnormalities in hyaline vascular Castleman disease: report of two cases with reappraisal of histogenesis. *Cancer Genet Cytogenet* 2006;164:110–117.
14. Chan JK, Tsang WY, Ng CS. Follicular dendritic cell tumor and vascular neoplasm complicating hyaline vascular Castleman's disease. *Am J Surg Pathol* 1994;18:517–525.
15. Lin O, Frizzera G. Angiomyoid and follicular dendritic cell proliferative lesions in Castleman's disease of hyaline-vascular type: a study of 10 cases. *Am J Surg Pathol* 1997;21:1295–1306.
16. Chan AC, Chan KW, Chan JK, et al. Development of follicular dendritic cell sarcoma in hyaline-vascular Castleman's disease of the nasopharynx: tracing its evolution by sequential biopsies. *Histopathology* 2001;38:510–518.
17. Kazakov DV, Morrison C, Plaza JA, et al. Sarcoma arising in hyaline-vascular Castleman disease of skin and subcutis. *Am J Dermatopathol* 2005;27:327–332.
18. Bowne WB, Lewis JJ, Filippa DA, et al. The management of unicentric and multicentric Castleman disease: a report of 16 cases and a review of the literature. *Cancer* 1999;85:706–717.
19. Herrada J, Cabanillas F, Rice L, et al. The clinical behavior of localized and multicentric Castleman disease. *Ann Intern Med* 1998;128:657–662.
20. Menke DM, Camoriano JK, Banks PM. Angiofollicular lymph node hyperplasia: a comparison of unicentric, multicentric, hyaline vascular, and plasma cell types of disease by morphometric and clinical analysis. *Mod Pathol* 1992;5:525–530.
21. McClain KL, Natkunam Y, Swerdlow SH. Atypical cellular disorders. *Hematology Am Soc Hematol Educ Program* 2004;1:283–296.
22. McCarty MJ, Vukelja SJ, Banks PM, et al. Angiofollicular lymph node hyperplasia (Castleman disease). *Cancer Treat Rev* 1995;21:291–310.
23. Waterston A, Bower M. Fifty years of multicentric Castleman's disease. *Acta Oncol* 2004;43:698–704.
24. Chang Y, Cesarman E, Pessin MS, et al. Identification of herpesvirus-like DNA sequences in AIDS-associated Kaposi's sarcoma. *Science* 1994;266:1865–1869.
25. Moore PS, Chang Y. Detection of herpesvirus-like DNA sequences in Kaposi sarcoma lesions from persons with and without HIV infection. *New Engl J Med* 1995;332:1181–1185.
26. Van Kooten C, Resnik I, Aarden L, et al. Effect of Il-4 and Il-6 on the proliferation and differentiation of B-chronic lymphocytic leukemia cells. *Leukemia* 1993;7:618–624.
27. Foss HD, Araujo I, Demel G, et al. Expression of vascular endothelial growth factor in lymphomas and Castleman's disease. *J Pathol* 1997;183:44–50.
28. Schulte KM, Talat N. Castleman's disease—a two compartment model of HHV-8 infection. *Nat Rev Clin Oncol* 2010;7:533–543.
29. van Rhee F, Stone K, Szmania S, et al. Castleman disease in the 21st century: an update on diagnosis assessment and therapy. *Clin Adv Hematol Oncol* 2010;8:486–498.
30. Peterson BA, Frizzera G. Multicentric Castleman's disease. *Semin Oncol* 1993;20:636–647.
31. Jaffe ES, Harris NL, Stein H, et al., eds. *Pathology and genetics of tumours of haematopoietic and lymphoid tissues. World Health Organization classification of tumours.* Lyon (France): IARC Press, 2001.
32. Dispenzieri A, Kyle RA, Lacy MQ, et al. POEMS syndrome: definitions and long-term outcome. *Blood* 2003;101:2496–2506.
33. Bélec L, Mohamed AS, Authier FJ, et al. Human herpesvirus 8 infection in patients with POEMS syndrome-associated multicentric Castleman disease. *Blood* 1999;93:3643–3653.
34. Leger-Ravet MB, et al. Interleukin-6 gene expression in Castleman's disease. *Blood* 1991;78:2923–2930.
35. Chronowski GM, Ha CS, Wilder RB, et al. Treatment of unicentric and multicentric Castleman disease and the role of radiotherapy. *Cancer* 2001;92:670–676.
36. Bosch X, Guilabert A, Miquel R, et al. Enigmatic Kikuchi-Fujimoto disease: a comprehensive review. *Am J Clin Pathol* 2004;122:141–152.
37. Hutchinson CB, Wang E. Kikuchi-Fujimoto disease. *Arch Pathol Lab Med* 2010;134:289–293.
38. Lin HC, Su CY, Huang CC, et al. Kikuchi's disease: a review and analysis of 61 cases. *Otolaryngol Head Neck Surg* 2003;128:650–653.
39. Kuo T. Kikuchi's disease (histiocytic necrotizing lymphadenitis): a clinicopathologic study of 79 cases with an analysis of histologic subtypes, immunohistology, and DNA ploidy. *Am J Surg Pathol* 1995;19:798–809.
40. Kucukardali Y, Solmazgul E, Kunter E, et al. Kikuchi-Fujimoto disease: analysis of 244 cases. *Clin Rheumatol* 2007;26:50–54.
41. Tsang WY, Chan JK, Ng CS. Kikuchi's lymphadenitis. A morphologic analysis of 75 cases with special reference to unusual features. *Am J Surg Pathol* 1994;18:219–231.
42. Kikuchi M. Lymphadenitis showing focal reticulum cell hyperplasia with nuclear debris and phagocytosis. *Nippon Ketsueki Gakkai Zasshi* 1972;35:378–380.
43. Fujimoto Y, Kozima Y, Hamaguchi K. Cervical necrotizing lymphadenitis: a new clinicopathological agent. *Naika* 1972;20:920–927.
44. Hudnall SD. Kikuchi-Fujimoto disease. Is Epstein-Barr virus the culprit? *Am J Clin Pathol* 2000;113:761–764.
45. Hudnall SD, Chen T, Amr S, et al. Detection of human herpesvirus DNA in Kikuchi-Fujimoto disease and reactive lymphoid hyperplasia. *Int J Clin Exp Pathol* 2008;1:362–368.
46. Cho MS, Choi HJ, Park HK, et al. Questionable role of human herpesviruses in the pathogenesis of Kikuchi disease. *Arch Pathol Lab Med* 2007;131:604–609.
47. George TI, Jones CD, Zehnder JL, et al. Lack of human herpesvirus 8 and Epstein-Barr virus in Kikuchi's histiocytic necrotizing lymphadenitis. *Hum Pathol* 2003;34:130–135.
48. Chen H, Thompson LD, Aguilera NS, et al. Kimura disease: a clinicopathologic study of 21 cases. *Am J Surg Pathol* 2004;28:505–513.
49. Iwai H, Nakae K, Ikeda K, et al. Kimura disease: diagnosis and prognostic factors. *Otolaryngol Head Neck Surg* 2007;137:306–311.
50. Abuel-Haija M, Hurford MT. Kimura disease. *Arch Pathol Lab Med* 2007;131:650–651.
51. Sun Q-F, Xu D-Z, Pan S-H. Kimura disease: review of the literature. *Intern Med J* 2008;38:668–674.
52. Hong C, Thompson LDR, Ives-Aguilera NS, et al. Kimura Disease. A clinicopathologic study of 21 cases. *Am J Surg Pathol* 2004;28:505–513.
53. Suster S. Nodal angiolymphoid hyperplasia with eosinophilia. *Am J Clin Pathol* 1987;88:236–239.
54. Chan JK, Hui PK, Ng CS, et al. Epithelioid hemangioma (angiolymphoid hyperplasia with eosinophilia) and Kimura's disease in Chinese. *Histopathology* 1989;15:557–574.
55. Kim HT, Szeto C. Eosinophilic hyperplastic lymphogranuloma, comparison with Mikulicz's disease. *Chin Med J* 1937;23:699–700.
56. Kimura T, Yoshimura S, Ishikawa E. On the unusual granulation combined with hyperplastic changes of lymphatic tissue. *Trans Soc Pathol Jpn* 1948;37:179–180.
57. Roufosse FE, Goldman M, Cogan E. Hypereosinophilic syndromes. *Orphanet J Rare Dis* 2007;2:37.
58. Chang AR, Kim K, Kim HJ, et al. Outcomes in Kimura's disease after radiotherapy or non radiotherapeutic treatment modalities. *Int J Radiat Oncol Biol Phys* 2006;65:1233–1239.
59. Sato S, Kawashima H, Kuboshima S, et al. Combined treatment of steroids and cyclosporine in Kimura disease. *Pediatrics* 2006;118:921–923.
60. Lu D, Estalilla OC, Manning JT, et al. Sinus histiocytosis with massive lymphadenopathy and malignant lymphoma involving the same lymph node: a report of four cases and review of the literature. *Mod Pathol* 2000;13:414–419.
61. Foucar E, Rosai J, Dorfman RF. Sinus histiocytosis with massive lymphadenopathy (Rosai-Dorfman disease: review of the entity. *Sem in Diagn Pathol* 1990;7:19–73.
62. Huang Q, Chang KL, Weiss LM. Extranodal Rosai-Dorfman disease involving the bone marrow: a case report. *Am J Surg Pathol* 2006;30:1189–1192.
63. Paulli M, Bergamaschi G, Tonon L, et al. Evidence for a polyclonal nature of the cell infiltrate in sinus histiocytosis with massive lymphadenopathy (Rosai-Dorfman disease). *Br J Haematol* 1995;91:415–418.
64. Dorfman RF. The true story behind Rosai-Dorfman disease. *Adler Mus Bull* 2008;34:13–17.
65. Rosai J, Dorfman RF. Sinus histiocytosis with massive lymphadenopathy: a newly recognized benign clinicopathologic entity. *Arch Pathol* 1969;87:63–70.
66. Rosai J, Dorfman RF. Sinus histiocytosis with massive lymphadenopathy: a pseudolymphomatous benign disorder. Analysis of 34 cases. *Cancer* 1972;30:1174–1188.
67. Levine PH, Jahan N, Murari P, et al. Detection of human herpesvirus 6 in tissues involved by sinus histiocytosis with massive lymphadenopathy (Rosai-Dorfman disease). *J Infect Dis* 1992;166:291–295.
68. Al-Daraji W, Anandan A, Klassen-Fischer M, et al. Soft tissue Rosai-Dorfman disease: 29 new lesions in 18 patients, with detection of polyoma virus antigen in 3 abdominal cases. *Ann Diagn Pathol* 2010;14:309–316.
69. O'Malley DP, Duong A, Barry T, et al. Co-occurrence of Langerhans cell histiocytosis and Rosai-Dorfman disease: possible relationship of two histiocytic disorders in rare cases. *Mod Pathol* 2010;23:1616–1623.
70. Venkataraman G, McLain KL, Pittauluga S, et al. Development of disseminated histiocytic sarcoma in a patient with autoimmune lymphoproliferative syndrome and associated Rosai-Dorfman disease. *Am J Surg Pathol* 2010;34:589–594.
71. Morgan NV, Morris MR, Cangul H, et al. Mutations in SLC29A3, encoding an equilibrative nucleoside transporter ENT3, cause a familial histiocytosis syndrome (Faisalabad Histiocytosis) and familial Rosai-Dorfman disease. *PLoS Genet* 2010;6(2):e1000833.
72. Kang N, Jun A, Bhutia Y, et al. Human equilibrative nucleoside transporter-3 (hENT3) spectrum disorders mutations impair nucleoside transport, protein localization, and stability. *J Biol Chem* 2010;285:28343–28352.
73. de Silva D, Joshi N. Rosai-Dorfman disease recurrence with bilateral orbital masses following immunosuppressant therapy. *Orbit* 2005;24:51–53.
74. Wang F, Qiao G, Lou X, et al. Intracranial recurrences of Rosai-Dorfman disease in the sellar region: two illustrative cases. *Acta Neurochir (Wien)* 2011;153:859–867.
75. Cheuk W, Chan JKC. IgG4-related sclerosing disease a critical appraisal of an evolving clinicopathologic entity. *Adv Anat Pathol* 2010;17:303–332.
76. Hamano H, Arakura N, Muraki T, et al. Prevalence and distribution of extrapancreatic lesions complicating autoimmune pancreatitis. *J Gastroenterol* 2006;41:1197–1205.
77. Sato Y, Notohara K, Kojima M, et al. IgG4-related disease: historical overview and pathology of hematological disorders. *Pathol Int* 2010;60:247–258.
78. Grimm KE, Barry TS, Chizhevsky V, et al. Histopathological findings in 29 lymph node biopsies with increased IgG4 plasma cells. *Mod Pathol* 2012;25(3):480–491.
79. Cheuk W, Yuen HK, Chu SYY, et al. Lymphadenopathy of IgG4-related sclerosing disease. *Am J Surg Pathol* 2008;32:671–681.
80. Saab ST, Hornick JL, Fletcher CD, et al. IgG4 plasma cells in inflammatory myofibroblastic tumor: inflammatory marker or pathogenic link? *Mod Pathol* 2011;24:606–612.
81. Sato Y, Kojima M, Takata K, et al. Systemic IgG4-related lymphadenopathy: a clinical and pathologic comparison to multicentric Castleman's disease. *Mod Pathol* 2009;22:589–599.
82. Cheuk W, Yuen HK, Chan AC, et al. Ocular adnexal lymphoma associated with IgG4+ chronic sclerosing dacryoadenitis: a previously undescribed complication of IgG4-related sclerosing disease. *Am J Surg Pathol* 2008;32:1159–1167.

83. Sato Y, Takata K, Ichimura K, et al. IgG4-producing marginal zone B-cell lymphoma. *Int J Hematol* 2008;88:428–433.
84. Venkataraman G, Rizzo KA, Chavez JJ, et al. Marginal zone lymphomas involving the meningeal dura: possible link to IgG4-related diseases. *Mod Pathol* 2011;24:355–366.
85. Strehl JD, Hartman A, Agaimy A. Numerous IgG4-positive plasma cells are ubiquitous in diverse localized non-specific chronic inflammatory conditions and need to be distinguished from IgG4-related systemic disorders. *J Clin Pathol* 2011;64:237–243.
86. Nirula A, Glaser SM, Kalled SL, et al. What is IgG4? A review of the biology of a unique immunoglobulin subtype. *Curr Opin Rheumatol* 2011;23:119–124.
87. Lim EJ, Bhathal PS, Tagkalidis PP, et al. Catching a chameleon: IgG4-related systemic disease. *Med J Aust* 2010;193:418–420.
88. Khosroshahi A, Bloch DB, Deshpande V, et al. Rituximab therapy leads to a rapid decline of serum IgG4 levels and prompt clinical improvement in IgG4-related systemic disease. *Arthritis Rheum* 2010;62:1755–1762.
89. Chari ST, Smyrk TC, Levy MJ, et al. Diagnosis of autoimmune pancreatitis: the Mayo Clinic experience. *Clin Gastroenterol Hepatol* 2006;4:1010–1016.
90. Kemper CA, Davis RE, Deresinski SC, et al. Inflammatory pseudotumor of intraabdominal lymph nodes manifesting as recurrent fever of unknown origin: a case report. *Am J Med* 1991;90:519–523.
91. Miras-Parra FJ, Parra-Ruiz J, Gómez-Morales M, et al. Inflammatory pseudotumor of lymph nodes with focal infiltration in liver and spleen. *Dig Dis Sci* 2003;48:2003–2004.
92. Davis RE, Warnke RA, Dorfman RF. Inflammatory pseudotumor of lymph nodes. Additional observations and evidence for an inflammatory etiology. *Am J Surg Pathol* 1991;15:744–756.
93. Kojima M, Matsumoto M, Miyazawa Y, et al. Follicular lymphoma with prominent sclerosis ("sclerosing variant of follicular lymphoma") exhibiting a mesenteric bulky mass resembling inflammatory pseudotumor. Report of three cases. *Pathol Oncol Res* 2007;13:74–77.
94. Frizzera G. Castleman's disease and related disorders. *Semin Diagn Pathol* 1988;5:346–364.
95. Abbondazo SL, Irey NS, Frizzera G. Dilantin-associated lymphadenopathy. Spectrum of histopathologic patterns. *Am J Surg Pathol* 1995;19:675–686.
96. Facchetti F, Incardona P, Lonardi S, et al. Nodal inflammatory pseudotumor caused by luetic infection. *Am J Surg Pathol* 2009;33:447–453.
97. Arber DA, Kamel OW, van de Rijn M, et al. Frequent presence of the Epstein-Barr virus in inflammatory pseudotumor. *Hum Pathol* 1995;26:1093–1098.
98. Perrone T, De Wolf-Peeters C, Frizzera G. Inflammatory pseudotumor of lymph nodes. A distinctive pattern of nodal reaction. *Am J Surg Pathol* 1988;12:351–361.
99. Magerus-Chatinet A, Stolzenberg MC, Loffredo MS, et al. Fas-L, IL-10, and double-negative CD4-CD8-TCR a/b+ T cells are reliable markers of autoimmune lymphoproliferative syndrome (ALPS) associated with FAS loss of function. *Blood* 2009;113:3027–3030.
100. Sneller MC, Dale JL, Straus SE. Autoimmune lymphoproliferative syndrome. *Curr Opin Rheumatol* 2003;15:417–421.
101. Sneller MC, Wang J, Dale JK, et al. Clinical, immunologic, and genetic features of an autoimmune lymphoproliferative syndrome associated with abnormal lymphocyte apoptosis. *Blood* 1997;89:1341–1348.
102. Bleesing JJH, Brown MR, Straus SE, et al. Immunophenotypic profiles in families with autoimmune lymphoproliferative syndrome. *Blood* 2001;98:2466–2473.
103. Chan JKC, Kwang YL. Common misdiagnosis in lymphomas and avoidance strategies. *Lancet Oncol* 2010;11:579–588.
104. Lim MS, Straus SE, Dale JK, et al. Pathological findings in human autoimmune lymphoproliferative syndrome. *Am J Pathol* 1998;153:1541–1550.
105. Aspinall AI, Pinto A, Auer IA, et al. Identification of new Fas mutations in a patient with autoimmune lymphoproliferative syndrome (ALPS) and eosinophilia. *Blood Cells Mol Dis* 1999;25:227–238.
106. Fleisher TA, Straus SE, Bleesing JJ. A genetic disorder of lymphocyte apoptosis involving the FAS pathway: the autoimmune lymphoproliferative syndrome. *Curr Allergy Asthma Rep* 2001;1:534–540.
107. Bagg A. Therapy-associated lymphoid proliferations. *Adv Anat Pathol* 2011;18:199–205.
108. Rizzi R, Curci P, Delia M, et al. Spontaneous remission of "methotrexate-associated lymphoproliferative disorders" after discontinuation of immunosuppressive treatment for autoimmune disease. Review of the literature. *Med Oncol* 2009;26:1–9.
109. Salloum E, Cooper DL, Howe G, et al. Spontaneous regression of lymphoproliferative disorders in patients treated with methotrexate for rheumatoid arthritis and other rheumatic diseases. *J Clin Oncol* 1996;14:1943–1949.
110. Hasserjian RP, Chen S, Perkins SL, et al. Immunomodulator agent-related lymphoproliferative disorders. *Mod Pathol* 2009;22:1532–1540.
111. Abbondazo SL, Irey NS, Frizzera G. Dilantin-associated lymphadenopathy. Spectrum of histopathologic patterns. *Am J Surg Pathol* 1995;19:675–686.
112. Chevrel G, Berger F, Miossec P, et al. Hodgkin's disease and B cell lymphoproliferation in rheumatoid arthritis patients treated with methotrexate: a kinetic study of lymph node changes. *Arthritis Rheum* 1999;42:1773–1776.

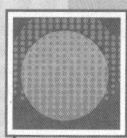

Chapter 15
Hodgkin Lymphoma: Histopathology and Differential Diagnosis

Jerome S. Burke

In 1832, Thomas Hodgkin (1) described seven patients with an unusual lymphoma of lymph nodes that became known by his name more than 30 years later (2). The latter half of the 19th century also saw the first descriptions of the characteristic giant cell of Hodgkin lymphoma, but it is Sternberg and Reed who are recognized as having provided the first detailed descriptions and illustrations of the giant cells and the other histopathologic characteristics that define Hodgkin lymphoma (3). During the period in which Sternberg and Reed defined the pathologic aspects of Hodgkin lymphoma, and until very recently, the precise nature of the disorder was controversial, but today, the malignant nature of Hodgkin lymphoma is established. The past 50 years have witnessed remarkable achievements in the understanding of the clinical patterns of Hodgkin lymphoma both at the onset of the disorder and during progression, in the development of new diagnostic techniques for accurate staging, in the illumination of the pathologic characteristics, and in the establishment of successful therapeutic protocols (4,5). Despite the current relative stability of the understanding of Hodgkin lymphoma in terms of overall pathologic characteristics and therapy, especially viewed in contrast with the non-Hodgkin lymphomas, Hodgkin lymphoma remains a subject of intense investigation. The sustained interest in Hodgkin lymphoma results not only from the continuous refinement in the pathologic criteria and therapeutic regimens but also because of the greater understanding of the molecular and biologic aspects of the lymphoma as exemplified by the establishment of the germinal center B-cell derivation of the neoplastic cells in both the classical and lymphocyte predominant (LP) forms, as well as the significance of the microenvironment (6–9).

This chapter concentrates on the current histopathologic concepts and characteristics of Hodgkin lymphoma, including the differential diagnosis, and emphasizes the salient clinicopathologic correlations at the time of initial biopsy, staging, and relapse. The immunobiology and pathogenesis of Hodgkin lymphoma, as well as the origin of the Reed-Sternberg cell, are not stressed, because these subjects are discussed in Chapter 16. Nor is any attempt made to recapitulate all details concerning the history, epidemiology, clinical characteristics, and therapeutic aspects of Hodgkin lymphoma, which are described in both texts and superb reviews (5,10–15).

HISTOPATHOLOGIC CLASSIFICATION AND DEFINITION

Almost 50 years have elapsed since Lukes and Butler (16,17) proposed their histopathologic classification of Hodgkin lymphoma. This classification was based on the predominant histologic features seen in pretherapy lymph node biopsies and was an attempt to further the earlier concepts of Jackson and Parker (18) in the identification of histologic groups of Hodgkin lymphoma that were prognostically significant. Lukes and

Butler introduced the concept of nodular sclerosis and identified a nodular variant of the former paragranuloma group of Jackson and Parker, resulting in a classification containing six categories (Table 15.1). The histopathologic categories in the Lukes and Butler classification reflect the significance of lymphocytic proliferation, the inverse relationship between the number of lymphocytes and that of Reed-Sternberg cells, and the presence of two distinctly different types of connective tissue proliferation found in nodular sclerosis and diffuse fibrosis (16,17).

The original Lukes and Butler classification persists as the foundation for the modern classification of Hodgkin lymphoma, despite the popular simplification of the six categories of Lukes and Butler to four groups at the Rye Conference, and the addition of a lymphocyte-rich classical form in the Revised European-American Lymphoma (REAL) and World Health Organization (WHO) classifications (19–23). In both the REAL classification and current WHO scheme, the categories of nodular sclerosis, mixed cellularity, and lymphocytic depletion are combined under the designation *classical Hodgkin lymphoma (cHL)*, in order to underscore the tight bond among these histologic types, and their distinction from the nodular lymphocyte predominant (NLP) form (20–23). The WHO classification also emphasizes that LP Hodgkin lymphoma is essentially nodular and provides the option of dividing nodular sclerosis into two grades based mainly on European data showing that cases of nodular sclerosis with significant nuclear pleomorphism or lymphocyte depletion or increased eosinophils (grade II or high grade) are associated with a poorer prognosis, particularly in patients with intermediate- and advanced-stage disease (23–26); however, grading is restricted for investigational purposes and is not routinely required. The lymphocyte-depleted subtype is retained in the WHO classification, but this category includes cases that provisionally were denoted in the REAL classification as *anaplastic large cell lymphoma* (ALCL) *Hodgkin-like* (20,21). In fact, ALCL Hodgkin-like is rare accounting for <3% of genuine ALCL cases (27). Most cases so classified are examples of *anaplastic large cell lymphoma–like classical Hodgkin lymphoma* of either lymphocyte-depleted or nodular sclerosis with lymphocyte depletion (grade II) type (21,23). The WHO classification also alters the idiom *Hodgkin disease* to *Hodgkin lymphoma* in order to lend credence to the fact that this disorder is actually neoplastic (23).

Notwithstanding these new proposals, the pathologist should continue to be familiar with the criteria and terminology of the original Lukes and Butler classification. The original classification provides specific criteria and descriptive histologic categories that aid in the pathologic diagnosis and in the differentiation from benign and malignant conditions that may simulate Hodgkin lymphoma (28–30). Although modern therapy has reduced the differences in prognosis and survival traditionally found among the histologic groups of Hodgkin lymphoma, pathologic classification of Hodgkin lymphoma

Table 15.1	COMPARISON OF HISTOLOGIC CLASSIFICATIONS OF HODGKIN LYMPHOMA		
Lukes and Butler	**Rye**	**REAL**	**WHO (Hodgkin lymphoma)**
Lymphocytic and Histiocytic Nodular Diffuse	Lymphocyte predominance	Lymphocyte predominance	Nodular lymphocyte predominant
		Lymphocyte-rich classical	Lymphocyte-rich classical
Nodular sclerosis	Nodular sclerosis	Nodular sclerosis	Nodular sclerosis
Mixed cellularity	Mixed cellularity	Mixed cellularity	Mixed cellularity
Diffuse fibrosis	Lymphocytic depletion	Lymphocytic depletion	Lymphocyte-depleted
Reticular			

REAL, Revised European-American Lymphoma; WHO, World Health Organization.

remains important, because the various histologic groups correlate with specific clinical parameters including geographic patterns of disease as well as prognosis (31,32).

The definition of Hodgkin lymphoma that unifies the different histologic types is the *identification of diagnostic Reed-Sternberg cells in the appropriate cellular environment*. Both parts of this definition are essential. The diagnostic Reed-Sternberg cell is a large cell that may be lobated, binucleated, or multinucleated and contains homogeneous, acidophilic, inclusion-like nucleoli that are approximately one-quarter of the size of the nucleus (17,28) (Fig. 15.1); the cytoplasm is usually abundant and amphophilic. Variants of Reed-Sternberg cells that aid in the diagnosis include a mononuclear variant, the folded and lobated ("popcorn") cell of the NLP type that currently is referred to as a LP cell, and the lacunar cell of nodular sclerosis (23,28) (Fig. 15.2). Because cells similar to Reed-Sternberg cells and its variants are found in conditions other than Hodgkin lymphoma, including infectious mononucleosis and non-Hodgkin lymphomas, the identification of only a Reed-Sternberg cell is insufficient for an absolute diagnosis of Hodgkin lymphoma (33,34). Reed-Sternberg cells must be viewed in the context of one of the described histologic types of Hodgkin lymphoma. The cellular background is usually heterogeneous in Hodgkin lymphoma, particularly in the nodular sclerosis and mixed cellularity types. In these classical types of Hodgkin lymphoma, the heterogeneous cell population includes diverse mixtures of small lymphocytes devoid of significant nuclear membrane irregularities, plasma cells, large lymphoid cells, histiocytes, and varying mixtures of inflammatory cells including eosinophils and polymorphonuclear leukocytes, with or without necrosis (Fig. 15.3). Parenthetically, the presence of increased eosinophils

correlates with a poor prognosis in nodular sclerosis but not in mixed cellularity (35), whereas increased numbers of macrophages that express CD68 and/or CD163 are associated with an adverse prognosis in cHL, a discovery that has been validated by computer image analysis of the CD68 and CD163 immunohistochemical stains (36,37). The definition of an *appropriate* cellular environment, however, is somewhat vague, because this environment is mutable, and similar heterogeneous cell populations including Reed-Sternberg–like cells may be observed in a variety of non-Hodgkin lymphomas, especially peripheral T-cell lymphomas (PTCLs), T-cell/histiocyte-rich large B-cell lymphomas (THRLBCLs), and ALCL (27,38–42).

A modern definition of Hodgkin lymphoma, therefore, requires expansion, with the incorporation of immunologic criteria in order to differentiate cHL and the Reed-Sternberg cell from those non-Hodgkin lymphomas that histologically simulate, and can be indistinguishable from, Hodgkin lymphoma. This differentiation includes cases of B-cell lymphoma, unclassifiable, with features intermediate between those of diffuse large B-cell lymphoma (DLBCL) and cHL (gray zone lymphoma), in addition to PTCL, THRLBCL, and ALCL (23,38–46). Although a variety of antibodies are expressed in classical Hodgkin cells, the most commonly employed and relevant are CD15 and CD30, as well as PAX5, fascin, CD3, CD20, and CD45 (Fig. 15.4, Table 15.2). In selected cases, the B-cell transcription factors Oct2 and BOB.1 also are expedient (47). For patients with cHL of nodular sclerosis and mixed cellularity types, moreover, the immunophenotype appears to have a direct impact on clinical prognosis (48). In contrast to patients with a classic CD15-, CD30-positive immunophenotype, patients who lack CD15 have a significantly worse freedom from treatment failure and survival (48); CD20, antiapoptotic factor bcl-2, CD279 or programmed death 1 (PD-1), and MAL expression by Hodgkin cells also are reported to be independent adverse predictive factors in cHL (49–52). Among patients 50 years or older, Epstein-Barr virus (EBV) positivity is associated with a significantly poorer prognosis (53), and low levels of tumor-infiltrating regulatory T cells (FOXP3) and high-expression cytotoxic T/NK cells expressing granzyme B and/or TIA-1 equally tally with poor overall survival (54).

EPIDEMIOLOGY, GENERAL CLINICAL CHARACTERISTICS INCLUDING PATTERNS OF DISSEMINATION, STAGING, AND THERAPY

Hodgkin lymphoma has a characteristic bimodal age curve with one peak in early adult life (15 to 34 years) and a second increase in incidence at 55 years of age or older (55). Employing surveillance, epidemiology, and end results (SEER) data, in the

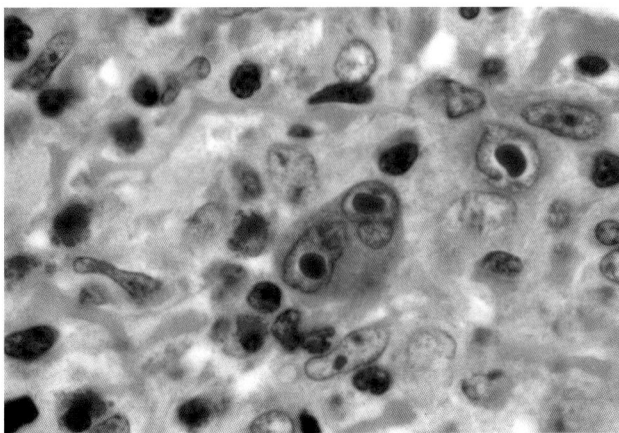

FIGURE 15.1. Classic binucleated Reed-Sternberg cell with characteristic large acidophilic, mirror-image nucleoli. A mononuclear variant also is present (hematoxylin and eosin stain, original magnification: 1,500× magnification).

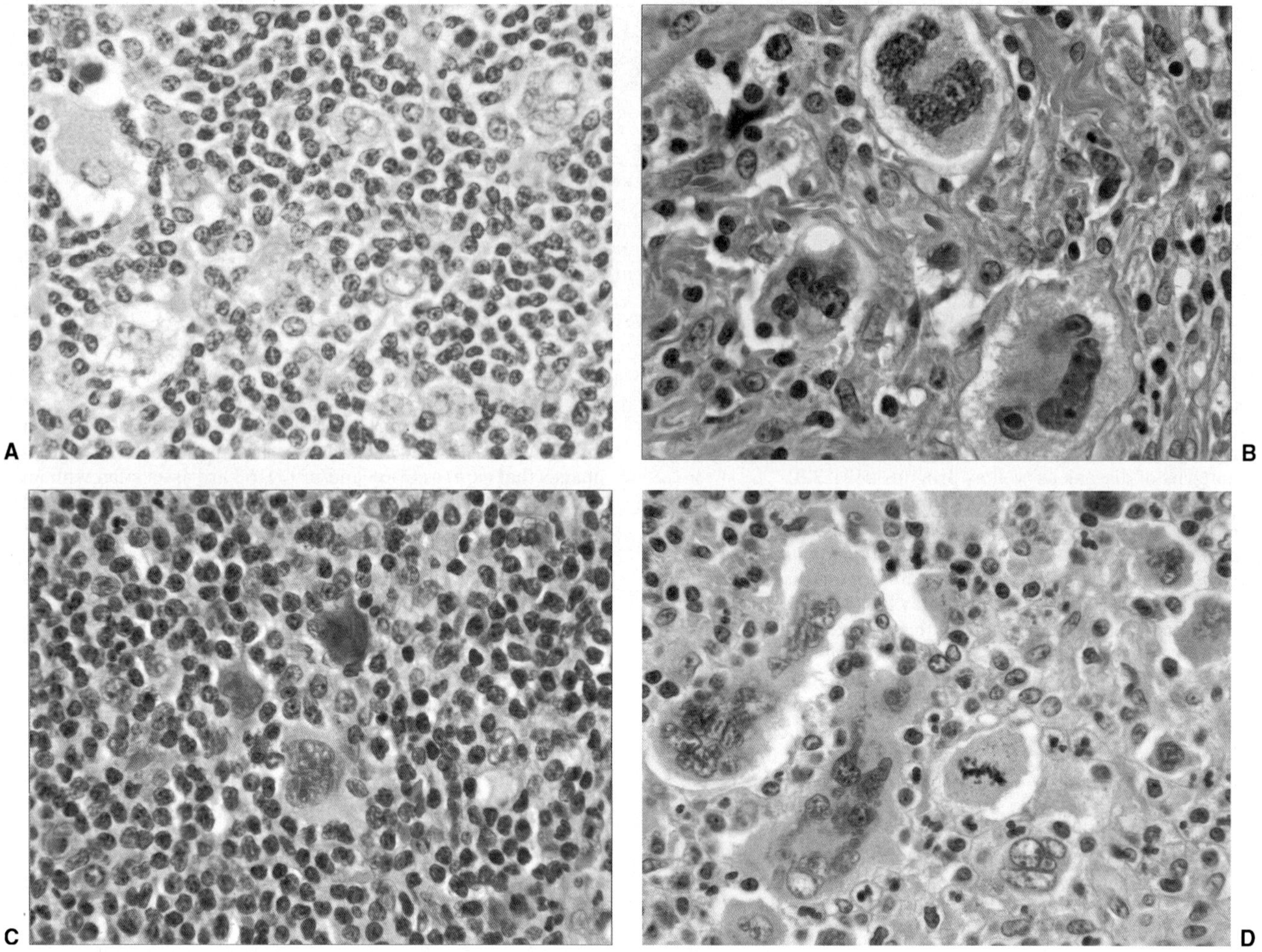

FIGURE 15.2. Variants of Reed-Sternberg cells. A: Folded and lobated ("popcorn") LP cells are typical of NLP Hodgkin lymphoma (hematoxylin and eosin stain, original magnification: 600× magnification). **B:** Hyperlobated lacunar cells are another variant characteristically found in nodular sclerosis (hematoxylin and eosin stain, original magnification: 600× magnification). **C:** Degenerating Reed-Sternberg cells are common in cHL and usually referred to as "mummified" cells (hematoxylin and eosin stain, original magnification: 600× magnification). **D:** In grade II or high-grade nodular sclerosis, the lacunar cells are often pleomorphic and atypical and may be confused with another neoplasm (hematoxylin and eosin stain, original magnification: 600× magnification).

United States from 2004 to 2008 the median age at diagnosis was 38 years with 31.5% of cases diagnosed between the ages of 20 and 34 years (56). The age-adjusted incidence rate during this period was 2.8 cases per 100,000 men and women per year (56), and in 2012, it was estimated that 9,060 patients would be diagnosed with Hodgkin lymphoma in the United States (57). Curiously, the incidence trend of Hodgkin lymphoma from 1975 to 2008 is declining (56). Part of the falling incidence of Hodgkin lymphoma in older patients likely is related to earlier overdiagnosis of lymphocyte-depleted Hodgkin lymphoma and underdiagnosis of non-Hodgkin lymphomas (55).

In the United States, Hodgkin lymphoma accounts for 10% to 15% of malignant lymphomas and ranks fourth following DLBCL, chronic lymphocytic leukemia/small lymphocytic lymphoma (CLL/SLL), and follicular lymphoma (FL) (58). In Europe, Hodgkin lymphoma supersedes FL in incidence (59). The epidemiologic pattern of Hodgkin lymphoma differs according to the socioeconomic level of a region; for example, in Third World countries and in referral medical centers serving populations at lower socioeconomic levels in the United States, there is an increased incidence of symptomatic, advanced lymphoma, often in children, with a higher rate of the mixed cellularity and even lymphocyte-depleted types (60). In developing countries, this

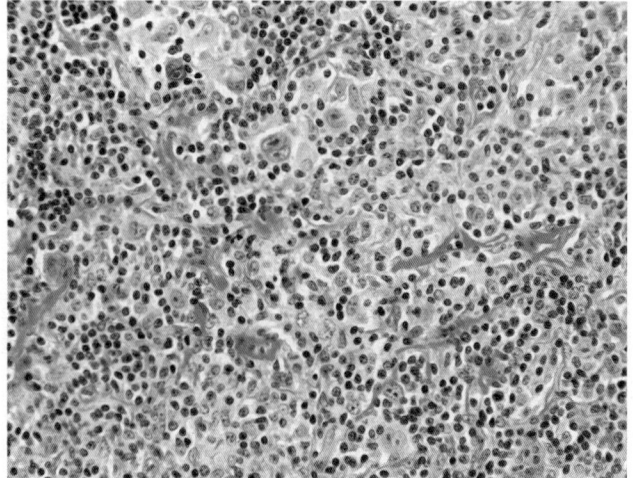

FIGURE 15.3. A heterogeneous cell population is characteristic of most types of Hodgkin lymphoma and includes varying numbers of small lymphocytes, plasma cells, histiocytes, eosinophils, and polymorphonuclear leukocytes as well as Reed-Sternberg cells (hematoxylin and eosin stain, original magnification: 300× magnification).

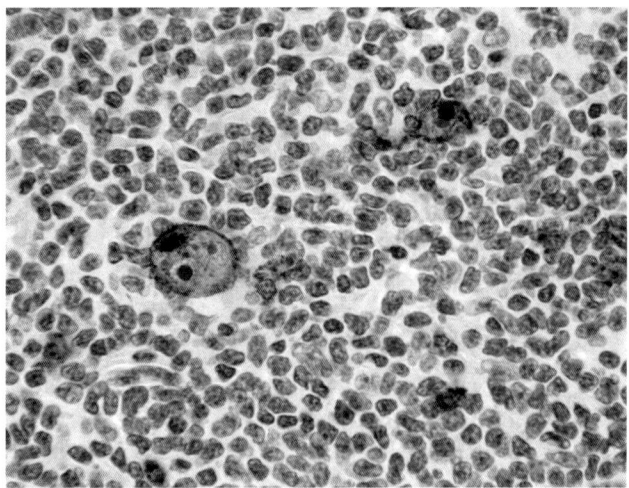

FIGURE 15.4. Positive reactivity for CD15 is characteristic, but not pathognomonic, of the Reed-Sternberg cells in cHL. Reactivity is both membranous and in the paranuclear area corresponding to the Golgi zone (immunoperoxidase stain, original magnification: 600× magnification).

pattern appears to be changing and is likely related to continuing economic development with subsequent modifications of environmental factors including EBV infection (61,62). In contrast, patients from relatively affluent areas are usually young adults and present with asymptomatic, low-stage lymphoma and nodular sclerosis histology. The risk of Hodgkin lymphoma is increased significantly by 10-fold among patients with AIDS (63). The incidence of Hodgkin lymphoma is especially high in regions with populations at increased risk for HIV infection (55), and the natural history and biologic features of Hodgkin lymphoma associated with HIV typically are altered, with an increased incidence of advanced-stage lymphoma, involvement of extranodal sites at presentation, increased proportions of the mixed cellularity and lymphocyte-depleted histologic types, a high frequency of EBV infection in the Reed-Sternberg cells, and a more aggressive clinical course compared with Hodgkin lymphoma in the general population (55,63,64). In the

Table 15.2	HISTOPATHOLOGIC AND IMMUNOLOGIC DEFINITION OF cHL

Histopathologic criterion: Diagnostic Reed-Sternberg cells in the appropriate cellular environment
Immunologic Criteria:

Reed-Sternberg Cells	
CD15	+
CD30	+
PAX5	+
Fascin	+
Vimentin	+
CD200	+
MUM1	+
EBV	+/−
CD45	−
CD20	−/+
CD3	−
Oct2/BOB.1	−/+
Grb2	−
EMA	−
ALK	−
Surrounding cells: T cells, predominantly CD4⁺, TIA-1⁺	

Grb2, growth factor receptor-bound protein 2; EMA, epithelial membrane antigen; ALK, anaplastic lymphoma kinase.

current combination antiretroviral therapy period, a paradoxical increase in cHL has developed, specifically nodular sclerosis, which occurs at higher CD4 counts with less aggressive disease and better survival (63–65) (see Chapter 25).

Constitutional symptoms, age, and histopathologic type classically are the most important factors influencing the clinical evaluation of Hodgkin lymphoma (10). Patients with night sweats, fever, or significant weight loss are more likely to have an accelerated pace of lymphoma and more widespread dissemination. Patients older than 60 years of age also are reported to have more advanced lymphoma compared with children and young adults (66). At one extreme, LP histology typically is associated with an overall indolent course; at the other, lymphocyte-depleted Hodgkin lymphoma is associated with constitutional symptoms, wide dissemination, and historically a rapidly fatal course (10,32,67–70). Nodular sclerosis and mixed cellularity Hodgkin lymphoma tend to have intermediate rates of evolution. In general, modern therapy is diminishing the differences in survival rates and the prognoses of the histopathologic types of Hodgkin lymphoma (10,12,70).

Many of the accomplishments in the treatment of Hodgkin lymphoma in the past 50 years are directly attributable to the development of superior diagnostic methods to quantitate the extent of lymphoma. The advent of bipedal lymphangiography, staging laparotomy with splenectomy and selective biopsies, computed tomography (CT), positron emission tomography (PET), and PET combined with fluorodeoxyglucose F¹⁸ (FDG-PET) has allowed critical assessment of the spleen and retroperitoneal lymph nodes and accurate staging of patients (5,10,12,15). Lymphangiography led to the observation that the spread of Hodgkin lymphoma is nonrandom and that there is an orderly progression of lymphoma, with dissemination to contiguous lymph node groups including the spleen (10,71). *Contiguity* refers to the existence of direct connections between pairs of lymph node chains by way of lymphatic channels that do not have to pass through, and be filtered by, intervening lymph nodes or other lymphatic tissue barriers (10,71). As a result, paraaortic or celiac lymph node involvement is associated with a high probability of splenic involvement, and splenic involvement commonly is followed by involvement of the liver and bone marrow. In the chest, the sequence of spread appears to be from the mediastinal to the hilar lymph nodes and then to the pulmonary parenchyma. Vascular invasion and hematogeneous dissemination of Hodgkin lymphoma are less clear. Vascular invasion appears more common in patients with lymphocyte-depleted but also may occur in lymph nodes and spleens from patients with nodular sclerosis and mixed cellularity Hodgkin lymphoma (72–74). These studies demonstrate an association between vascular invasion and extranodal involvement; however, a review of the original lymph node biopsies from 11 patients who had localized Hodgkin lymphoma, and who later developed extranodal dissemination, failed to identify vascular invasion (75).

Staging laparotomy with splenectomy and selective biopsies also greatly contributed to the understanding of the patterns of Hodgkin lymphoma (76,77). This procedure was employed not only to define the extent of Hodgkin lymphoma but also to select patients primarily for radiation therapy. Staging laparotomy has become obsolete because of the increased diagnostic accuracy of combined PET-CT and FDG-PET scans in identifying involvement of abdominal lymph nodes in Hodgkin lymphoma, and the widespread employment of multiagent chemotherapy for most clinical settings, including patients with large mediastinal masses as well as patients with nonbulky early-stage lymphoma (5,12–15).

The development of more accurate diagnostic techniques for determining the extent and pattern of Hodgkin lymphoma at presentation resulted in the adoption of the Ann Arbor staging

Table 15.3	ANN ARBOR STAGING CLASSIFICATION OF HODGKIN LYMPHOMA
Stage I	Involvement of a single lymph node region (I) or a single extralymphatic organ or site (I_E)
Stage II	Involvement of two or more lymph node regions on the same side of the diaphragm (II) or localized involvement of a single associated extralymphatic organ or site and its regional lymph node(s), with or without involvement of other lymph node regions on the same side of the diaphragm (II_E)
Stage III	Involvement of lymph node regions on both sides of the diaphragm (III), which may also be accompanied by localized involvement of an associated extralymphatic organ or site (III_E), by involvement of the spleen (III_S) or by both (III_{E+S})
Stage IV	Disseminated (multifocal) involvement of one or more extralymphatic organs with or without associated lymph node involvement, or isolated extralymphatic organ involvement with distant (nonregional) nodal involvement

A, No systemic symptoms present; B, Unexplained fevers >38°C; drenching night sweats; or weight loss >10% of body weight (within 6 months prior to diagnosis).

classification in 1971 (78); this system persists as the basis for the current staging classification of Hodgkin lymphoma (13–15) (Table 15.3). The Ann Arbor scheme divides Hodgkin lymphoma into four stages depending on the extent of nodal or extranodal lymphoma: *E* denotes extranodal lymphoma by direct extension from lymph nodes and is distinguished from stage IV disseminated extranodal Hodgkin lymphoma. The absence (*A*) or presence (*B*) of specific clinical symptoms is affixed to each stage (13). The *Cotswolds modification* was introduced to revise the Ann Arbor system by adding CT results, modifying the criteria for clinical involvement of the spleen and liver to include evidence of focal defects on two imaging techniques, designating bulky lymphoma (>10 cm) with *X*, and introducing a new category of response to therapy, unconfirmed or uncertain complete remission—*CR(u)*—in order to accommodate the difficulty of persistent radiologic abnormalities of uncertain significance (5,14,79).

It is beyond the scope of this chapter to provide a detailed account of the remarkable progress in the therapy of Hodgkin lymphoma. Highlights include the development of the linear accelerator and the standardization of the mantle, inverted Y, and total nodal lymphoid fields for radiotherapy; the use of combination chemotherapy regimens such as doxorubicin, bleomycin, vinblastine, and dacarbazine (ABVD); mechlorethamine, doxorubicin, vinblastine, vincristine, bleomycin, and prednisone (Stanford V); and, more recently, escalated-dose bleomycin, etoposide, doxorubicin, cyclophosphamide, vincristine, procarbazine, and prednisone (BEACOPP) for patients with advanced lymphoma; and the strategy of employing combined modality therapy (5,11–15). For example, the overall 5-year relative survival of Hodgkin lymphoma for 2001 to 2007 from 17 SEER geographic areas was 83.9% (56). Over the past 25 years, the increased survival was particularly pronounced for patients aged 45 to 59 years and 60 years and older (66); however, an age gradient persists for patients more than 60 years of age who have a 10-year relative survival of 44.9% in contrast to 92.7% for patients aged 15 to 24 years. Therapy continues to be refined, with protocols designed to determine the chemotherapy regimen that is the least toxic or most successful including the use of rituximab, an anti-CD20 antibody, the best treatment options for patients with both early- and advanced-stage lymphoma, and the most effective salvage treatment for progressive disease encompassing high-dose chemotherapy stem-cell rescue for patients who experience relapses (5,11–15). There also is a concerted effort to reduce many of the late complications of therapy, such as thyroid, cardiovascular, and

pulmonary dysfunction induced by radiation therapy; gonadal dysfunction as a result of chemotherapy; and secondary malignancies, specifically acute myeloid leukemias, non-Hodgkin lymphomas, and solid tumors (13,14). Although the risk of adverse therapeutic sequelae may be reduced with modern treatment regimens, secondary malignancies remain a significant cause of death developing more than 10 years after completion of Hodgkin lymphoma therapy. Carcinomas of lung and breast are the most common secondary solid malignancies, but the largest relative risk (20-fold) is for mesothelioma (80). Thirty-year cumulative risks of solid cancers for men and women diagnosed at 30 years were 18% and 26%, respectively, in comparison with 7% and 9%, respectively, in the general population (80). For pediatric patients, the risk also is high with excess mortality from secondary malignancies and cardiovascular disease persisting more than 20 years in Hodgkin lymphoma survivors and, therefore, necessitating lifelong observation (81).

PATHOLOGIC FEATURES, CLINICOPATHOLOGIC CORRELATIONS, AND DIFFERENTIAL DIAGNOSIS

Nodular Lymphocyte-Predominant Hodgkin Lymphoma

The NLP type comprises approximately 5% of cases of Hodgkin lymphoma (13,68). Despite its relative rarity, NLP has generated considerable interest since the demonstration that this form of Hodgkin lymphoma has not only unique morphologic features but also clinical, immunophenotypic, and molecular characteristics that differ from those of cHL (5–8,10,13–15,22,45,67,68,82,83). Although the LP category traditionally included both the nodular and diffuse lymphocytic and histiocytic (L&H) types noted by Lukes and Butler, the existence of a pure diffuse form is rare (16,17,19,22). For example, a report from the European Task Force on Lymphoma indicated that only 7 of 219 cases (3%) of LP Hodgkin lymphoma fulfilled the criteria for the diffuse type (84). For practical purposes, LP Hodgkin lymphoma is considered virtually synonymous with the nodular type (21,22) (Fig. 15.5). The majority of diffuse cases in the earlier studies, including those by Lukes and Butler, likely would be incorporated into the nodular type today, because the

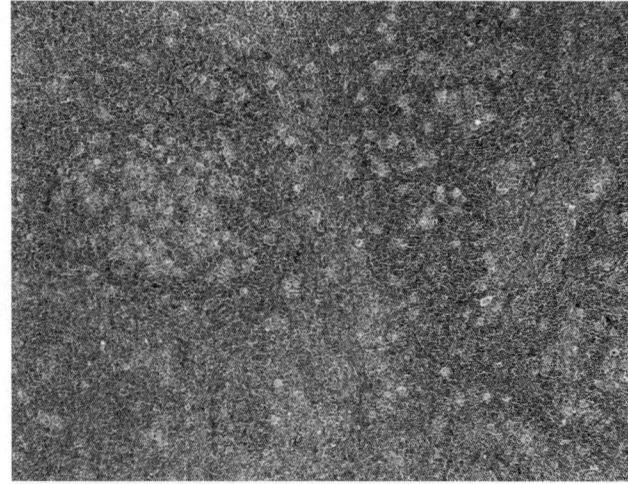

FIGURE 15.5. In NLP Hodgkin lymphoma, the nodules vary in size and frequently are poorly defined (hematoxylin and eosin stain, original magnification: 60× magnification).

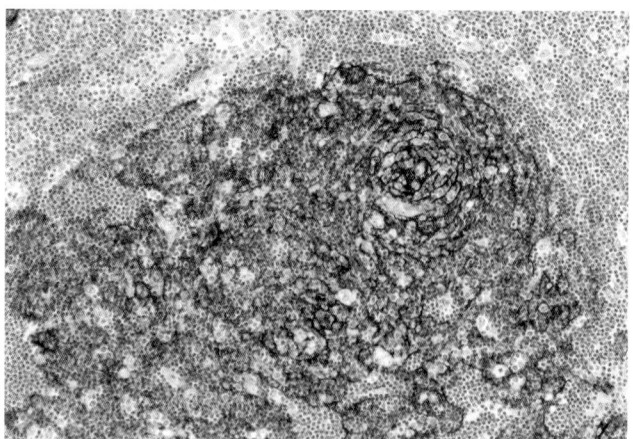

FIGURE 15.6. A stain for CD21 highlights the large spherical follicular dendritic cell meshwork in NLP Hodgkin lymphoma. A similar dendritic cell pattern is found in progressive transformation of germinal centers (immunoperoxidase stain, original magnification: 150× magnification).

presence of a solitary nodule is sufficient for the diagnosis of NLP Hodgkin lymphoma and a focal nodular architecture may be subtle, masked in thick sections, and sometimes evident only with a reticulin stain or the demonstration of a follicular dendritic cell meshwork by immunohistochemistry (22,28,85) (Fig. 15.6). Other cases of so-called diffuse LP Hodgkin lymphoma conceivably are examples of lymphocyte-rich cHL or THRLBCL (20,40,41,45).

NLP Hodgkin lymphoma is composed of a diverse mixture of small lymphocytes with round nuclear contours and reactive histiocytes (Fig. 15.7). The histiocytes may be single or clustered, suggesting epithelioid or sarcoid granulomas (16,22,28). The nodal architecture almost always is effaced, and although small residual germinal centers occasionally may be discovered in the neoplastic nodules, germinal centers, if present, usually are confined to a subcapsular position; the capsule is characteristically intact, and there usually is no capsular thickening, but foci of intranodal fibrosis are reported in up to 20% of cases (28,86,87). Eosinophils, plasma cells, and necrosis are rare. The nodules are variable in size and often poorly defined, with vague borders that may be accentuated by the use of a reticulin stain or by immunohistochemistry employing CD21 to illustrate an expanded follicular dendritic cell meshwork

(22,45,84,85). The nodules often exhibit increased numbers of small lymphocytes and only a few histiocytes; any diffuse areas more likely contain a predominance of histiocytes and smaller numbers of lymphocytes. It should be realized that the pattern of nodularity and immunoarchitecture in this form of Hodgkin lymphoma is variable. In addition to the classic pattern of nodules dominated by CD20⁺ B cells, other B-cell patterns encompass a serpiginous or interconnecting pattern of nodules, nodules with significant numbers of extranodular LP cells, a T-cell–rich nodular form, and two diffuse patterns including one with a T-cell–rich background imitating THRLBCL and another with B cells dominating the diffuse cellular milieu (87).

The most pathognomonic characteristic of NLP Hodgkin lymphoma is the proliferation of so-called LP variants (formerly L&H cells) of Reed-Sternberg cells, which represent up to 10% of the cell population (17,28). These cells have a polyploid shape with abundant pale-staining cytoplasm and large folded, twisted, or even lobated or multilobated "popcorn-like" nuclei with lacy chromatin, thin nuclear membranes, and small nucleoli (17,22) (Fig. 15.8). The LP cells frequently concentrate in the center of the nodules but are not cohesive (16). Most significantly, Reed-Sternberg cells, including mononuclear variants, usually are uncommon and difficult to identify, as they comprise only a small proportion of the neoplastic cells and may not be present in NLP Hodgkin lymphoma (82,84). The paucity of classic Reed-Sternberg cells is as important for the classification of NLP Hodgkin lymphoma as is the surfeit of lymphocytes. If classic Reed-Sternberg cells can be identified readily, then the classification of NLP Hodgkin lymphoma probably is incorrect and the correct classification is more likely lymphocyte-rich cHL or mixed cellularity Hodgkin lymphoma (20,28). Historically, a diagnostic Reed-Sternberg cell was mandatory for the diagnosis of Hodgkin lymphoma, but currently diagnostic classic Reed-Sternberg cells are not required and they are no longer essential for the diagnosis in cases that otherwise have the characteristic morphologic and immunophenotypic features of the NLP form of Hodgkin lymphoma (82,86).

NLP Hodgkin lymphoma expresses immunophenotypic characteristics that are distinct from the classical types of Hodgkin lymphoma (21,22,45,82–84,88). As is detailed in Chapter 16, the LP cells in NLP Hodgkin lymphoma consistently express B-cell-lineage–restricted antigens, such as CD20. They also express CD45 (leukocyte common antigen) and frequently epithelial membrane antigen (EMA). Approximately 25% of cases express IgD and such cases more often involve the interfollicular region in a setting with a surfeit of T cells (89). Despite the B-cell phenotype, immunoglobulin light chain restriction usually is not demonstrable by standard immunohistochemical methods but may be shown by *in situ* hybridization for light chain messenger RNA (mRNA) (90); this is in contrast to cHL, in which such RNA is not detectable in Reed-Sternberg cells (91). The B-cell transcription factor Oct2 and its coactivators, BOB. 1/OBF.1, are coexpressed in NLP Hodgkin lymphoma as opposed to almost no expression in the classical forms (47).

Of most pragmatic and diagnostic significance and unlike cHL, the LP cells of NLP Hodgkin lymphoma rarely express CD15 and CD30; only approximately 7% of NLP Hodgkin cases express either CD15 or CD30 (88,92), but the expression of both CD15 and CD30 in the same case clearly indicates classical and not the NLP type. Similarly, vimentin, fascin, and CD200 are not expressed by LP cells (45,46,93). As stated above, employing CD21, NLP Hodgkin lymphoma exhibits large, spherical follicular dendritic cell meshworks that are either absent or ill-defined and small in the alleged diffuse variety (84,85). With the correct morphologic features, the presence of even one CD21⁺ meshwork is sufficient for the diagnosis (22). At least 50% of the small lymphocytes in the nodular areas are B cells. The T cells present may be positive for both CD4 and CD8 (94) and are phenotypically parallel

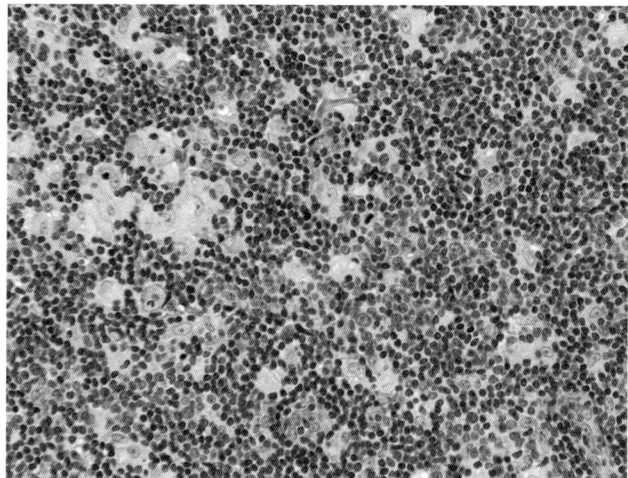

FIGURE 15.7. In addition to LP cells, the cell population in NLP Hodgkin lymphoma mainly is composed of a mixture of small lymphocytes and reactive histiocytes, including epithelioid histiocytes (hematoxylin and eosin stain, original magnification: 300× magnification).

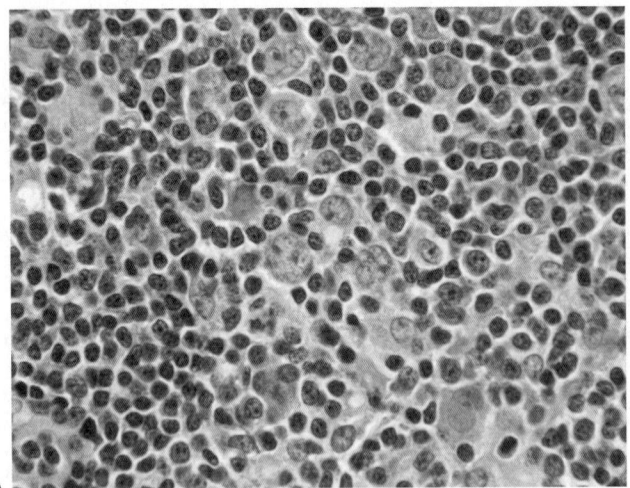

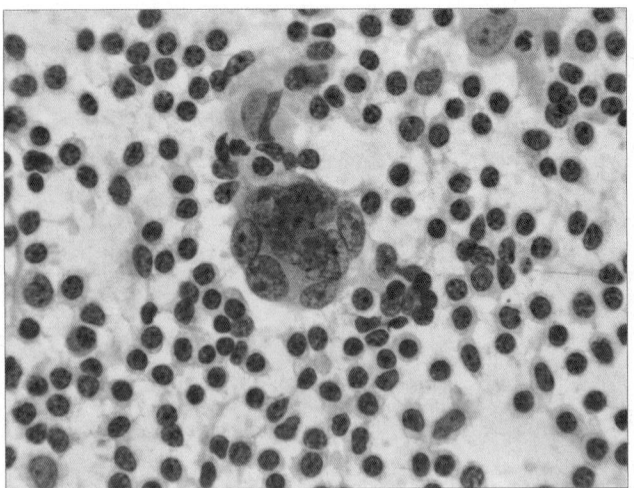

A

B

FIGURE 15.8. A: The LP cell variants of Reed-Sternberg cells typically have a polyploid shape with folded, twisted, and often lobated nuclei with small nucleoli. Note the absence of classic Reed-Sternberg cells (hematoxylin and eosin stain, original magnification: 600× magnification). **B:** A touch imprint exhibits the characteristic multilobated "popcorn-type" nucleus of an LP cell (hematoxylin and eosin stain, original magnification: 600× magnification).

to intrafollicular T cells in that they frequently express CD57 with bcl-6 coexpression and form rosettes around LP cells (22,84,88); the CD57+ rosetting pattern can be a diagnostic aid in differentiating NLP Hodgkin lymphoma from THRLBCL (95). CD279 or PD-1, a newer follicular T-cell antigen, was initially reported to be even more accurate than CD57 in this differential diagnosis (96) (Fig. 15.9); in contrast to PD-1 rosettes in NLP Hodgkin lymphoma, THRLBCL cases allegedly lack the rosettes. If ambiguous cases between the two lymphomas display PD-1 rosettes, the implication is that such cases are, in fact, examples of NLP Hodgkin lymphoma (96). The proposal to employ PD-1 in this context, however, has come into question. In a Stanford study, THRLBCL cases expressed PD-1 in 33% to 40% of cases (97).

The discovery that NLP Hodgkin lymphoma is composed of B cells correlates with the proposal that this form of Hodgkin lymphoma is a germinal-center–derived lymphoma (6,22) and that an identifiable early-phase–designated *intrafollicular neoplasia* may exist, parallel to FL *in situ* (98). The diagnosis of intrafollicular neoplasia is predicated on the recognition of CD20+, bcl-6+ LP cells surrounded by PD-1+ T-cell rosettes in

CD21+, or CD23+ altered follicles with encircling IgD+ B cells. This hypothesis coincides with earlier suggestions that NLP Hodgkin lymphoma is related to a form of reactive hyperplasia found in 3.5% to 10% of lymph nodes with chronic nonspecific lymphadenitis and referred to as *progressive transformation of germinal centers* (PTGC) (99,100). This is a condition in which the follicles become enlarged as a result of the infiltration by small B lymphocytes, leading to distortion of the germinal centers and sometimes completely masking them (99) (Fig. 15.10). The small lymphocytes of PTGC exhibit the immunologic characteristics of mantle zone lymphocytes, and it has been suggested that they represent early, transient stages in the transformation of primary into secondary lymphoid follicles (100,101). There is a remarkable similarity between the patterns of PTGC and NLP Hodgkin lymphoma; however, LP cells are absent in PTGC (102). Moreover, the lymph node usually is not replaced totally in PTGC, and there is associated, frequently florid reactive follicular hyperplasia. This is in contrast to NLP Hodgkin lymphoma, in which the architecture generally is effaced completely, and any residual germinal centers are compressed and usually confined to

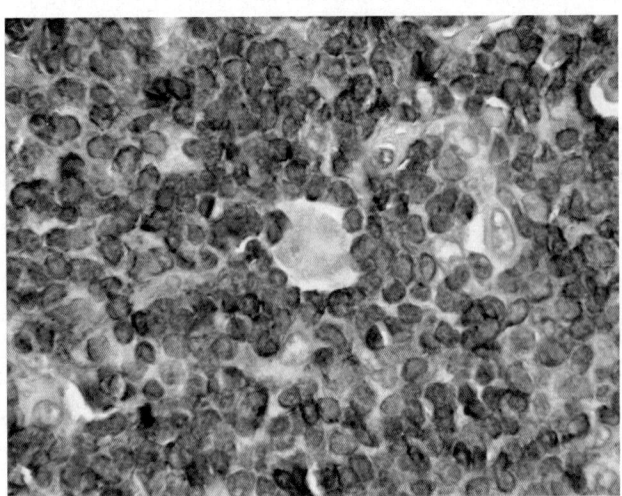

FIGURE 15.9. In NLP Hodgkin lymphoma, PD-1+ follicular T-helper cells characteristically form rosettes around LP cells (immunoperoxidase stain, original magnification: 600× magnification).

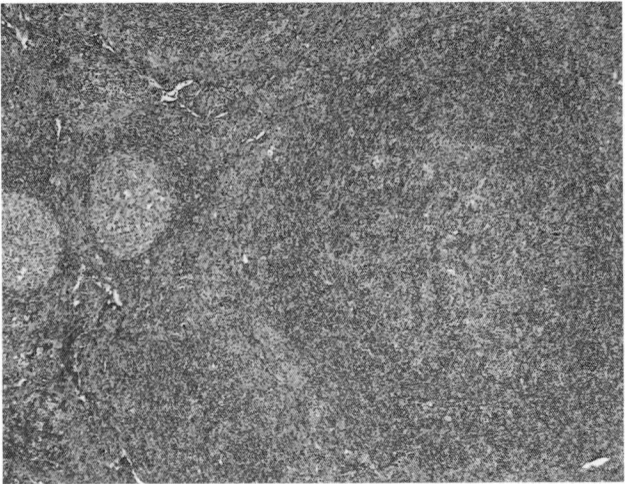

FIGURE 15.10. A large progressively transformed germinal center is seen in association with smaller reactive follicles. PTGC resembles NLP Hodgkin lymphoma, but in LP reactive follicles are uncommon or generally limited to the subcapsular region of the lymph node (hematoxylin and eosin stain, original magnification: 60× magnification).

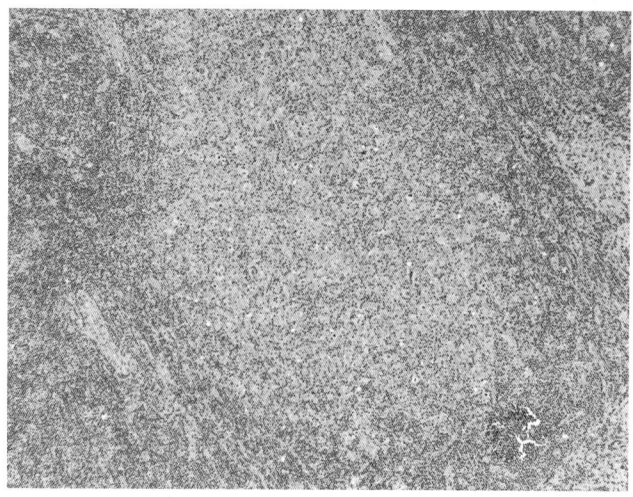
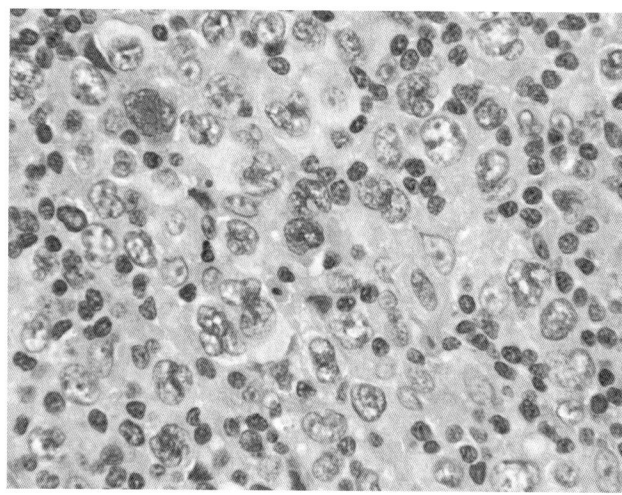

FIGURE 15.11. **A:** Pale-staining clusters of LP cells in the LP-cell–rich or syncytial variant of NLP Hodgkin lymphoma (hematoxylin and eosin stain, original magnification: 60× magnification). **B:** The aggregates of LP cells may be mistaken for large cell lymphoma, but the LP-cell–rich cases do not have clonal immunoglobulin heavy chain rearrangements employing standard techniques (hematoxylin and eosin stain, original magnification: 600× magnification).

the subcapsular region (16,28,86). Nonetheless, the histologic similarity between PTGC and NLP Hodgkin lymphoma, coupled with the discovery of an association between the two conditions in some cases, led to the proposal that PTGC represents a prelymphomatous disorder (99). In one study, 18% of 171 cases of NLP Hodgkin lymphoma coexisted with PTGC in the same lymph node (103); two additional patients had PTGC in lymph node biopsies prior to developing NLP Hodgkin lymphoma, and three patients with histologically proven Hodgkin lymphoma were found on subsequent lymph node biopsy to have PTGC. The association between these two disorders, however, is tenuous. Independent studies have shown that in most cases PTGC arises in patients, especially pediatric patients and young adults, who have not had and will not develop Hodgkin lymphoma (100,102,104); a minority of patients who have associated PTGC and Hodgkin lymphoma develop classical mixed cellularity and nodular sclerosis as well as the NLP type (100).

Most patients who have LP Hodgkin lymphoma are men in the fourth decade of life and present with localized, persistent lymph node enlargement (10,13,14,16). They usually have clinical stage I or IIA lymphoma with few risk factors, rare involvement of the mediastinum, and relatively indolent clinical courses with a superior prognosis compared to patients with cHL (10,13,14,22,68,105); only a minority of patients have advanced lymphoma including bone marrow involvement (106), and some may present in extranodal sites (107,108). Despite a propensity for relapse, patients with NLP Hodgkin lymphoma still pursue an indolent course, with only a few deaths resulting from Hodgkin lymphoma (67); the majority of patients who experience relapse have histologic persistence of their NLP Hodgkin lymphoma (109). Although late but salvageable relapses are associated with NLP Hodgkin lymphoma, patients respond to therapy that is standard for classical forms of Hodgkin lymphoma and survive these relapses better than or equal to patients with such forms (68,84,105). For example, in a large study of 8,298 Hodgkin lymphoma patients of whom 394 had the NLP type, the overall survival for LP and cHL patients was 96% and 92%, respectively (P = 0.0166) (68). The current strategy is to seek less intensive treatment protocols for patients with NLP Hodgkin lymphoma, including the use of rituximab and a "wait and watch" approach in pediatric patients, as a means of reducing treatment toxicities (13,14,68,105,110,111).

Earlier reports indicate that relapse in the LP type of Hodgkin lymphoma can be associated with histologic progression toward morphologically more classic forms (16,112). Moreover, rare cases of composite and synchronous NLP and cHL have been reported, including a case in which the LP and classical Hodgkin cells were clonally identical (113,114). Rather than cHL, 3% to 14% of patients with NLP Hodgkin lymphoma relapse or evolve to DLBCL, coexisting in the same biopsy specimen or distant from the presenting site (115–120). The large B cells may be multilobated and similar to LP cells or resemble centroblasts or immunoblasts or even be T-cell/histiocyte–rich (117,118). In some patients, in whom the condition was termed *L&H cell–rich* (LP-cell–rich), the large cells appear to arise from clustering and aggregation of the LP cells but do not fulfill criteria for frank DLBCL (116,121) (Fig. 15.11). The LP-cell–rich cases likely are similar, if not identical, to the clustered *T-cell/histiocyte–rich* or *syncytial* form of NLP Hodgkin lymphoma that were described subsequently (122,123). Clinically, patients with this variant form of NLP Hodgkin lymphoma present at a higher stage and with B symptoms similar to THRLBCL, but have an excellent survival as in the usual form of NLP Hodgkin lymphoma (122). From a biologic perspective, the LP-cell–rich cases do not exhibit clonal immunoglobulin heavy chain gene rearrangements (IgHGRs) by standard polymerase chain reaction (PCR) analysis, to add to the thesis that such cases are merely NLP Hodgkin lymphoma with increased numbers of LP cells (121). In contrast, cases of unequivocal DLBCL arising in patients with NLP Hodgkin lymphoma are clonal with IgHGR by standard PCR or *in situ* hybridization for light chain mRNA (121,124,125). Despite evident clonality in the large cell component, a clonal link between the DLBCL and the preceding NLP type of Hodgkin lymphoma usually is not detectable or is found only in a small minority of cases (121,124); however, a direct clonal link between the NLP and large B-cell lymphoma constituents is demonstrable by the analysis of single LP cells isolated from sections by micromanipulation (126). Despite advanced-stage disease, patients with transformed DLBCL associated with NLP Hodgkin lymphoma generally differ clinically from the usual cases of *de novo* DLBCL. In most reports, patients with DLBCL arising from NLP Hodgkin lymphoma exhibit a relatively favorable clinical course rather than the typically aggressive course of many *de novo* DLBCL (116,117,119). Other reports, however, describe no significant difference in survival between patients with DLBCL arising in NLP Hodgkin lymphoma patients and age- and sex-matched patients with *de novo* DLBCL (118). Curiously, rare cases of concurrent or subsequent LP Hodgkin lymphomas and molecularly confirmed PTCL are described, but the pathogenetic relationship between the synchronous LP Hodgkin lymphoma and PTCL is enigmatic (127,128). Caution is required in the diagnosis of PTCL associated with NLP Hodgkin lymphoma. Rare cases of NLP Hodgkin lymphoma exhibit cytologic atypia among the background T cells to simulate PTCL or a composite lymphoma (129). Despite characteristic B-cell nodular areas of LP Hodgkin lymphoma, in these unusual cases sheets of atypical T cells surround follicles to imitate the T-zone pattern of PTCL or atypical T cells form large clusters at the periphery of the B-cell nodules. Unlike PTCL, the atypical T lymphocytes show no loss of pan T-cell antigens or anomalous T-cell antigen expression, molecular studies do not reveal T-cell clonality, and, of most significance, the overall survival is as in patients with NLP Hodgkin lymphoma without atypical-appearing T cells (129).

The differential diagnosis of LP Hodgkin lymphoma usually depends on whether the pattern is classic nodular or the uncommon nodular with predominately diffuse areas type (87). For the classic nodular variety, the main differential diagnosis concerns PTGC and the nodular variant of lymphocyte-rich cHL. The distinction from PTGC is related directly to both pattern and cytologic characteristics. In NLP Hodgkin lymphoma, the nodules are poorly defined, closely approximated, and coalescent and blend into diffuse areas. Reactive follicles usually are not present or small or are limited to the periphery of the node (16,28,87,89). In PTGC, the nodules are sharply circumscribed, discrete, and set amid a score of reactive follicles (102). Cytologically, the conditions have many small lymphocytes and variable numbers of epithelioid histiocytes, but in NLP Hodgkin lymphoma LP cells are appreciated readily, whereas in PTGC LP cells are absent and there are only scattered follicle center cells. Immunohistochemical stains are of marginal utility in distinguishing NLP Hodgkin lymphoma from PTGC (130). Both conditions contain CD21+ follicular dendritic cell meshworks. B and T cells are found in the nodules of NLP Hodgkin lymphoma and PTGC, but there are distributional differences. In NLP Hodgkin lymphoma, B cells are dispersed irregularly with a mottled pattern, whereas in PTGC B cells form well-circumscribed confluent nodules. T cells in NLP Hodgkin lymphoma aggregate and surround LP cells; in contrast, T cells in PTGC are scattered but may form rings around transformed lymphocytes (130). One distinct immunophenotypic difference is the presence of CD57 and PD-1 rosettes around LP cells in NLP Hodgkin lymphoma; CD57 or PD-1 rosettes are not found in PTGC. Reactivity for EMA also is seen in NLP Hodgkin lymphoma, but not in PTGC.

The differential diagnosis of the uncommon variant of LP Hodgkin lymphoma with a predominately diffuse pattern mainly concerns classical types of Hodgkin lymphoma, particularly lymphocyte-rich cHL, in which the differential diagnosis is discussed in the next section, and THRLBCL (87). In THRLBCL, the lymph node architecture is effaced by a proliferation of small, mainly round lymphocytes (Fig. 15.12) and varying numbers of histiocytes. The histiocytes may obscure atypical large cells, including cells resembling LP cells and even classic Reed-Sternberg–type cells. As in LP Hodgkin lymphoma, patients generally are male and in their 40s. The patients with THRLBCL, however, mainly have advanced lymphoma, stage III or IV, with frequent splenomegaly, liver, and bone marrow involvement (40,131–133). Patients with THRLBCL do not respond to standard Hodgkin lymphoma protocols and have aggressive disease with a prognosis equivalent to the more typical form of DLBCL (133,134). Immunophenotypic analysis may not absolutely separate LP Hodgkin lymphoma from THRLBCL because of considerable immunohistochemical overlap between these entities, especially NLP Hodgkin lymphoma with extensive diffuse areas (41,45,122)

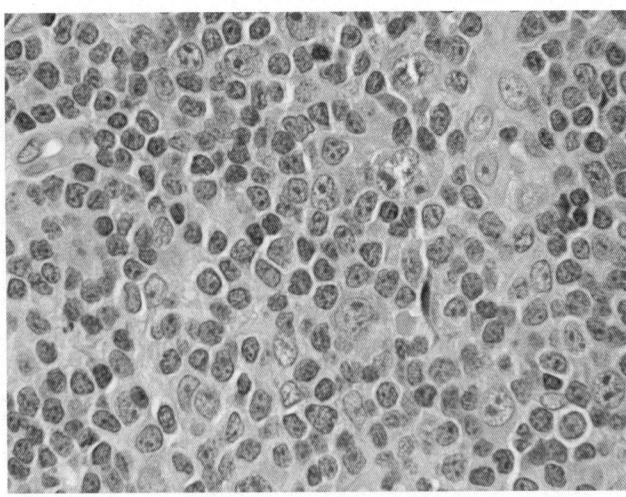

FIGURE 15.12. The cellular constituents of THRLBCL are confused easily with those of NLP and lymphocyte-rich cHL. Immunophenotypic analysis is mandatory to accurately differentiate these entities (hematoxylin and eosin stain, 600× magnification).

(Table 15.4). Although clonal IgHGR are detectable in cases of THRLBCL, important differences between both entities are found in the background cell population (40,45,122). For example, follicular dendritic cell meshworks expressing CD21 are found in LP Hodgkin lymphoma, whereas they are absent in THRLBCL (40,122,131). In NLP Hodgkin lymphoma, the small lymphocytes include many B cells, as well as T cells; the T cells are usually CD57+ and PD-1+, form rosettes, but do not express TIA-1 (95,96,122). The background lymphocytes in THRLBCL are virtually exclusively CD3+ T cells of CD8 class that are TIA-1+ (40,122). Although most cases lack CD57 and PD-1 rosetting activity, as noted earlier, up to 40% of THRLBCL exhibit positivity for PD-1 so that the discovery of T rosettes in equivocal cases does not necessarily equate with a diagnosis of NLP Hodgkin lymphoma (97). The overlapping morphologic and immunophenotypic features, as well as reports of concurrent or subsequent THRLBCL and NLP Hodgkin lymphoma, suggest a histogenetic relationship between at least a subgroup of the two disorders (41,122). In most cases, however, the identification of even a single nodule with the features of LP Hodgkin lymphoma is sufficient to exclude THRBCL (22), whereas the diagnosis of THRBCL should be limited to cases where the neoplastic large B cells are set in the background of T cells and histiocytes without small B cells (122) (see Chapter 23). For the variant cases of

Table 15.4	IMMUNOHISTOCHEMICAL PANEL COMPARING NLP HODGKIN LYMPHOMA AND THRLBCL	
	NLP	**THRLBCL**
CD45	+	+
CD20	+	+
CD15	–/+ (~7%+)	–
CD30	–/+ (~7%+)	–
Oct2/BOB.1	+	+
EMA	+/–	–/+
CD3 background	–/+	+
CD8 background	–	+
CD20 background	+/–	–
CD21 background	+	–
TIA-1 background	–	–/+
CD57/PD-1 background	+	–

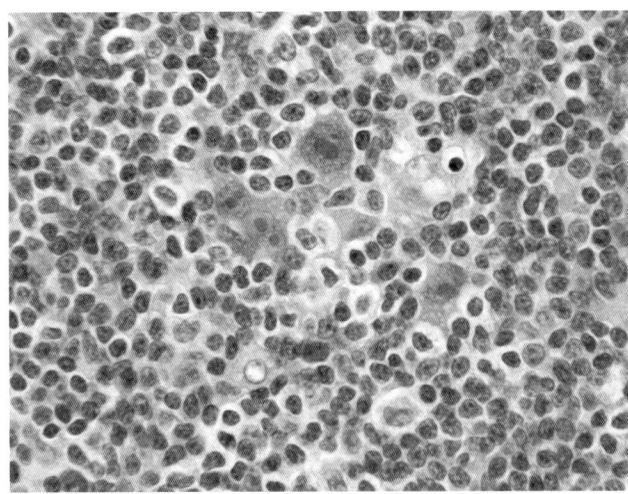

FIGURE 15.13. A classic Reed-Sternberg cell and variants can be identified in lymphocyte-rich classical, as opposed to the virtual absence of such cells in NLP Hodgkin lymphoma (hematoxylin and eosin stain, original magnification: 600× magnification).

NLP Hodgkin lymphoma that recur and exhibit a predominately diffuse architecture dominated by T cells to simulate THRBCL, the designation of *NLP Hodgkin lymphoma, THRBCL-like* is advised (22,83,87).

Lymphocyte-Rich Classical Hodgkin Lymphoma

Lymphocyte-rich cHL is a subtype that originally was proposed as a provisional entity by the proponents of the REAL classification and now has been incorporated into the WHO classification (20,23). According to the original definition, lymphocyte-rich cHL is "a diffuse tumor with relatively infrequent Reed-Sternberg cells, which are of the classic type, rather than the variants seen in nodular lymphocyte predominance; some lacunar cells may be present, in a background of lymphocytes, with infrequent eosinophils or plasma cells. There is morphologic overlap with diffuse lymphocyte predominance, the cellular phase of nodular sclerosis, and mixed cellularity. In contrast to diffuse lymphocyte predominance, the Reed-Sternberg cells have the morphology and immunophenotype of classic Reed-Sternberg cells" (20) (Fig. 15.13). A nodular or follicular variant also occurs and, in fact, forms the majority of

cases (84,135,136) (Fig. 15.14). In a seminal study, 80 (70%) of 115 cases of lymphocyte-rich cHL were nodular (84). In nodular lymphocyte-rich cHL, the nodules are composed of IgM+, IgD+ mantle zone lymphocytes with a loose CD21+ follicular dendritic cell meshwork. The nodules usually exhibit eccentrically located, atrophic-appearing germinal centers containing a condensed follicular dendritic cell meshwork. Diagnostic classic and lacunar variants of Reed-Sternberg cells are scattered and usually found at the periphery of the mantle zone nodules (135,136). The Reed-Sternberg cells in both the diffuse and nodular forms of lymphocyte-rich cHL variably express the cHL-associated antigens CD15 and CD30, as well as fascin, and almost a third of nodular cases are CD20+ (20,46,84,135–137). The lymphocytes in the less common diffuse cases are predominately T cells. Like NLP Hodgkin lymphoma, cases of lymphocyte-rich cHL may form CD57+ and PD-1+ T-cell rosettes (138). Marker analysis discloses that lymphocyte-rich cHL displays features intermediate between those of NLP and cHL. As well as exhibiting a follicular T-cell microenvironment with PD-1 expression, cases of lymphocyte-rich cHL express B-cell transcription factors such as Oct2 and BOB.1. Alternatively and comparable to cHL, nuclear factor kappa B (NF-κB) markers, for example, TRAF1, p50, and MUM1, are present in lymphocyte-rich cHL. The immunophenotype and microenvironment in lymphocyte-rich cHL imply that the Hodgkin cells originate from the outer zone of the germinal center (138).

The immunophenotype is essential for the diagnosis of lymphocyte-rich cHL and, despite an overlap, its distinction from LP Hodgkin lymphoma. For example, in an immunohistochemical analysis from the German Hodgkin Study Group, 104 morphologically confirmed cases of LP Hodgkin lymphoma were compared with 104 cHL cases that originally had been classified as LP and subsequently revised by a panel of pathologists (139). In 25 (24%) of 104 cases, immunohistochemistry altered the morphologic diagnosis of LP Hodgkin lymphoma by the panel to cHL, and 13 (12%) of 104 cases originally regarded by the panel as cHL showed an LP phenotype. The study from the European Task Force on Lymphoma also demonstrated the value of employing immunohistochemical criteria to aid in the classification of LP and lymphocyte-rich cHL (84). Of 388 initial cases that morphologically were interpreted as LP Hodgkin lymphoma, only 219 (56.5%) cases were classified as LP Hodgkin lymphoma following histologic review coupled with immunohistochemical studies. Lymphocyte-rich cHL constituted 115 (29.5%) cases and, as mentioned above, 80 (70%) of the

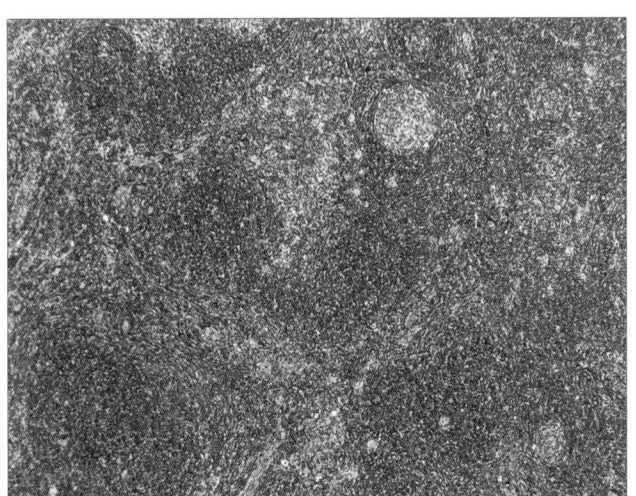

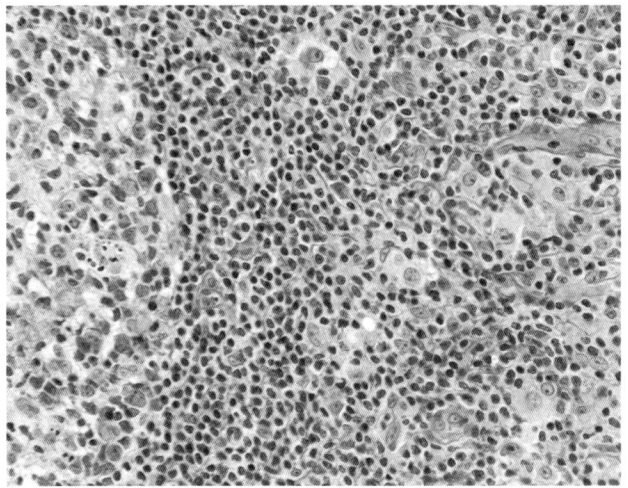

FIGURE 15.14. A: The nodular variant of lymphocyte-rich cHL is a result of expanded mantle zones with frequent eccentrically located germinal centers (hematoxylin and eosin stain, original magnification: 60× magnification). **B:** Reed-Sternberg cell variants are at the periphery of the nodule adjacent to a germinal center on the **left** (hematoxylin and eosin stain, original magnification: 300× magnification).

lymphocyte-rich classical cases were the nodular type. The remaining cases in the study were a mixture of other forms of cHL, non-Hodgkin lymphomas, and reactive lesions or were considered as technically inadequate (84).

The clinical features of lymphocyte-rich cHL have been clarified and compared with LP Hodgkin lymphoma (105,140). In one review of 2,715 patients with Hodgkin lymphoma with follow-up information, 100 (4%) were classified as lymphocyte-rich classical type and 115 (5%) as LP (140). Like patients with NLP Hodgkin lymphoma, patients who have lymphocyte-rich cHL are predominantly male and have early-stage lymphoma and few risk factors; however, the patients who have lymphocyte-rich cHL tend to be older (105,140). Survival and failure-free survival rates are similar for both groups and comparable to those for stage-matched patients with other forms of cHL (nodular sclerosis and mixed cellularity). The clinical data, particularly the mode of presentation, suggest that lymphocyte-rich cHL is more closely related to LP Hodgkin lymphoma, in spite of its distinct immunophenotype, and likely corresponds to an early stage in the spectrum of cHL (105,140,141).

The differential diagnosis of lymphocyte-rich cHL includes not only LP Hodgkin lymphoma but also THRLBCL. This is

particularly relevant to the diffuse form of lymphocyte-rich cHL since THRLBCL usually is associated with a diffuse small lymphocytic milieu that mimics lymphocyte-rich cHL (40,84,131,132). The identification of classic Reed-Sternberg cells and variants that express CD15 and/or CD30 with no or only weak CD20 reactivity and CD45 negativity usually distinguishes the diffuse lymphocyte-rich classical cases from THRLBCL, but rare cases may fall into the category of gray zone lymphoma (132).

In addition to THRLBCL, the diffuse form of lymphocyte-rich cHL must be distinguished from CLL/SLL and related lymphoproliferative disorders, such as lymphoplasmacytic lymphoma (LPL). The differential diagnosis is especially pertinent in cases of CLL/SLL and LPL containing epithelioid histiocytes and even blasts with Reed-Sternberg-cell–like features (142–145). One morphologic aid is the fact that capsular invasion is common in CLL/SLL but usually does not occur in Hodgkin lymphoma. Studies to determine clonality are important in differentiating between these two conditions, as well as determining whether any Reed-Sternberg–like cells express CD15 or CD30. Compounding the diagnostic difficulty, rare cases of CLL/SLL and LPL may coexist with genuine Hodgkin lymphoma, including cases of NLP Hodgkin lymphoma (146–150); in most instances, Hodgkin lymphoma develops after an initial diagnosis of

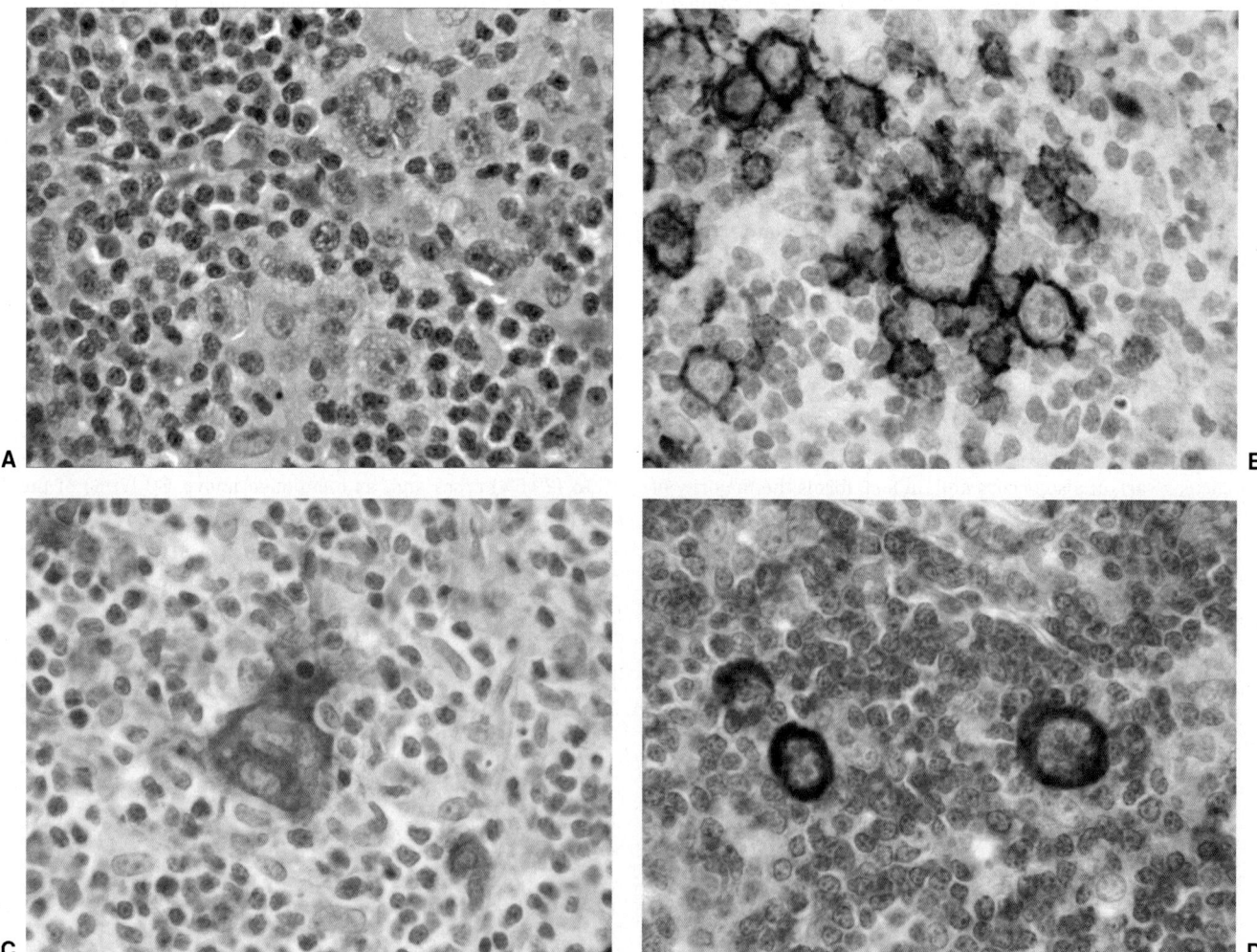

FIGURE 15.15. A: Lymph node biopsy from patient with CLL/SLL contains Reed-Sternberg cells compatible with Richter transformation (hematoxylin and eosin stain, original magnification: 600× magnification). **B:** As in CLL/SLL, the Reed-Sternberg cells express CD20, as well as CD5 (not shown) (immunoperoxidase stain, original magnification: 600× magnification). **C:** Typical of Hodgkin lymphoma, the Reed-Sternberg cells express CD30, in addition to other Hodgkin lymphoma markers, including CD15, fascin, and PAX5 (not shown) (immunoperoxidase stain, original magnification: 600× magnification). **D:** EBV, in this case LMP, also is positive in the Reed-Sternberg cells of Hodgkin-type Richter transformation of CLL/SLL (immunoperoxidase stain, original magnification: 600× magnification).

CLL/SLL or LPL, like Richter syndrome, and frequently is of the nodular sclerosis or mixed cellularity type. In a series of 4,121 patients with CLL/SLL, 18 (0.4%) patients developed Hodgkin lymphoma (149). Composite CLL/SLL and Hodgkin lymphoma, however, may occur at presentation, and in these cases the classic Reed-Sternberg cells or LP cells have their usual immunophenotypic characteristics of Hodgkin lymphoma, in contrast to the clonal B-cell immunophenotype of the surrounding neoplastic small lymphocytes (147,148). In other cases, the Reed-Sternberg cells may be intimately intermingled with the cells of CLL/SLL and, whereas the Hodgkin cells express Hodgkin-associated antigens such as CD15 and CD30, they also may express CD20 (Fig. 15.15). The typical Reed-Sternberg cells in such cases contain EBV-encoded RNA, but the surrounding CLL/SLL cells do not have EBV (151). Employing microdissection and PCR on isolated single neoplastic cells, a clonal relationship may be discovered between the cells of CLL/SLL and the Reed-Sternberg cells in some cases of Hodgkin-type Richter syndrome, but in other cases the CLL/SLL and Hodgkin cells are clonally distinct (152–155) (see Chapter 18). Among current patients with Hodgkin-type Richter transformation, many were treated with fludarabine, which may play a causative role in the onset of the syndrome (154,156). The prognosis of Hodgkin-type Richter syndrome is inferior to *de novo* Hodgkin lymphoma with a median failure-free survival of 0.4 years and median overall survival of 0.8 years (149).

Because of the nodular pattern in some cases, lymphocyte-rich cHL may be mistaken for FL. In FL, the follicles typically are small, uniform, and sharply demarcated in contrast to the macronodules seen in lymphocyte-rich cHL; the lymphocytes in FL are centrocytes and centroblasts, in contrast to the usual round nuclear contours of the benign mantle cells found in nodular-lymphocyte–rich cHL (135,136). Reed-Sternberg–like cells, however, occasionally can be observed in FL (34). The Reed-Sternberg–like cells usually are in the center of the neoplastic follicles, in which case they probably represent transformed follicle center cells (Fig. 15.16), but occasionally they are located in the interfollicular regions or even are associated with epithelioid histiocytes (145,157). In addition to histologic features, these cases are differentiated from nodular-lymphocyte-rich cHL by immunologic studies that demonstrate reactivity of the Reed-Sternberg–like cells with antibodies directed against B-cell antigens found in FL and, although CD30 may be expressed, CD15 is not; in this setting, microdissection and PCR discloses that the Reed-Sternberg–like cells are clonally related to the centrocytes and centroblasts of

the FL (145,157) (see Chapter 22). Rarely, the follicular variant of PTCL may mimic cHL, such as the nodular lymphocyte-rich type, due to the presence of B cells with Reed-Sternberg-like features that express CD15 and CD30 (157a,157b); the Reed-Sternberg-like cells may express EBV. The correct diagnosis is established by the recognition of atypical CD3+ T cells that express follicular helper T-cell antigens, such as BCL-6, PD-1 and CXCL13.

Nodular Sclerosis Classical Hodgkin Lymphoma

Nodular sclerosis is the most common type of Hodgkin lymphoma, comprising more than 60% of cases in the United States and Europe (23,140,158). This type of Hodgkin lymphoma equally affects females as well as males and is most prevalent between the ages of 15 and 34 years (5,23,31,58). Nodular sclerosis tends to involve the lower cervical and supraclavicular lymph nodes, with mediastinal lymphadenopathy discovered in 80% of patients and bulky disease in 40% (5,16); the majority of patients have stage II lymphoma at presentation and have an excellent prognosis (5,23,140).

The diagnosis of nodular sclerosis can be suspected at the time of gross examination by the delineation of distinct nodules defined by retracted gray-white interconnecting bands on the cut surface of a lymph node (16) (Fig. 15.17). This histologic type of cHL is characterized by orderly bands of interconnecting collagenous connective tissue that partially or entirely subdivide abnormal lymphoid tissue into isolated cellular nodules (16,17) (Fig. 15.18). The degree of collagen and the character of the cellular proliferation vary widely even within the same specimen. The connective tissue bands are identified as collagen by their birefringent character as seen under polarized light (Fig. 15.19). In some cases, the entire lymph node undergoes spontaneous sclerosis. At the opposite extreme, the process may be predominantly cellular and the formation of collagen bands and isolation of nodules limited to only a small portion of the specimen (16). Minimal alteration usually is related to focal thickening of the lymph node capsule, from which a collagen band extends into the cortex to at least partially encircle a nodule (23,28,30) (Fig. 15.20). The collagen found in nodular sclerosis likely reflects specific cytokine activity, such as interleukin-13, in comparison to other forms of cHL, specifically mixed cellularity (159). When gene expression profiling is used, cases of nodular sclerosis exhibit a significantly higher expression of genes involved

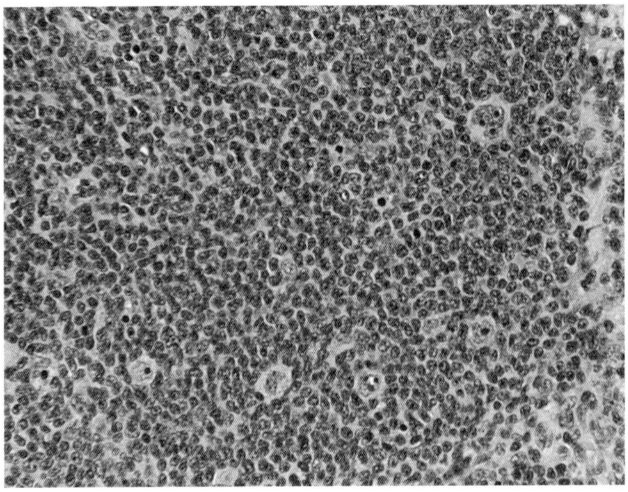

FIGURE 15.16. A giant cell indistinguishable from a Reed-Sternberg cell is found in the center of a FL, grade 1 type. In this context, the Reed-Sternberg–like cell is interpreted as a transformed follicle center B cell (hematoxylin and eosin stain, original magnification: 300× magnification).

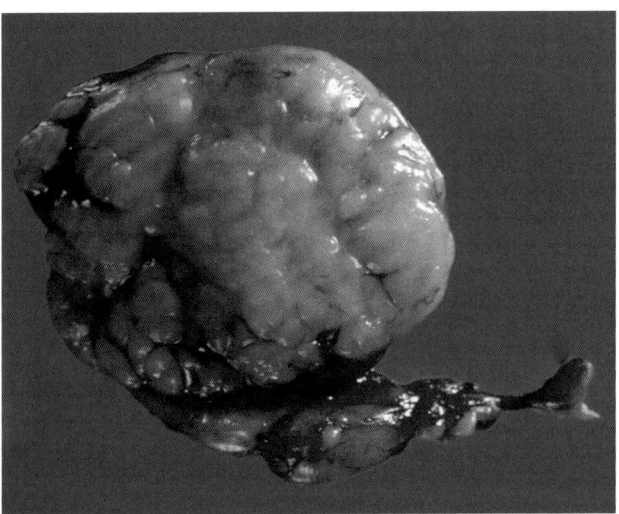

FIGURE 15.17. The distinct nodules on the cut surface of this lymph node strongly suggest the nodular sclerosis type of Hodgkin lymphoma.

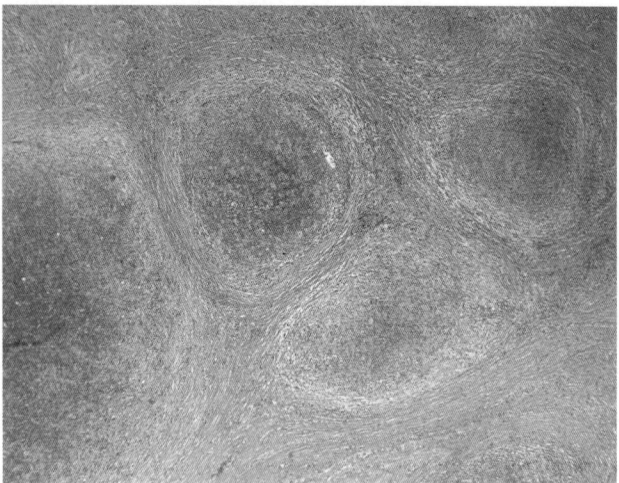

FIGURE 15.18. In typical nodular sclerosis, bands of fibrous connective tissue subdivide the lymph node into a series of nodules (hematoxylin and eosin stain, original magnification: 30× magnification).

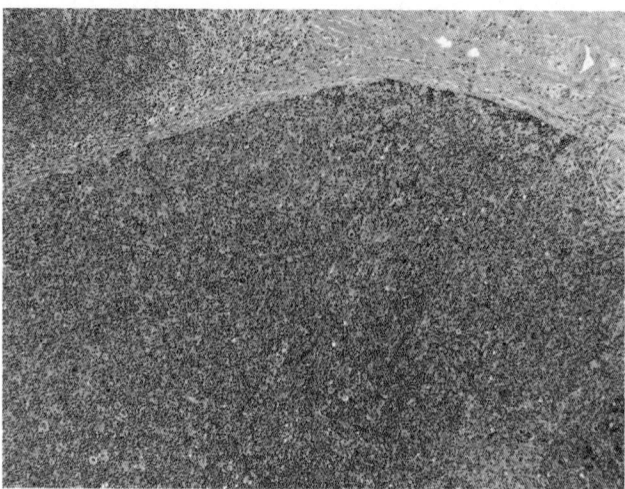

FIGURE 15.20. In minimal nodular sclerosis, the capsule is thickened with formation of an early collagen band extending into the cortex. Lacunar cells are barely evident at this magnification. This pattern has been termed by some the *cellular phase* of nodular sclerosis (hematoxylin and eosin stain, original magnification: 60× magnification).

in extracellular matrix remodeling and deposition similar to wound healing (160). The nodular-sclerosis–related genes are mainly expressed by macrophages and fibroblasts. Macrophages and Reed-Sternberg cells also express connective tissue growth factor protein to correlate with the degree of fibrosis (161). The type of fibrosis also appears as a significant factor in survival. By separately tabulating the amount of collagen or acellular sclerosis from the number of visible, plump, spindled fibroblasts, patients with increased numbers of fibroblasts have a shorter duration of relapse-free survival (158). Some cases with the "fibroblastic variant" of nodular sclerosis may have a spindle and storiform pattern reminiscent of a pleomorphic sarcoma (Fig. 15.21).

The cellular proliferation within the abnormal lymphoid nodules is highly variable, but the distinctive feature is the presence of the lacunar variants of Reed-Sternberg cells. These cells occur in clusters and are characterized by abundant and water-clear to slightly eosinophilic cytoplasm with sharply defined cellular borders situated in a lacuna-like space (16,17) (Fig. 15.22); the lacuna-like spaces are artifacts of formalin fixation and are less prominent in tissues fixed in a mercury-type fixative, such as B5. Moreover, with the use

of modern vacuum tissue processors, the lacuna-type spaces also appear less conspicuous. The nuclei of the lacunar cells usually are hyperlobated, with delicate nuclear chromatin, and contain small nucleoli. Paradoxically, classic diagnostic Reed-Sternberg cells may be difficult to identify in nodular sclerosis despite the presence of numerous lacunar variants (86). The cellular constituents associated with lacunar cells and Reed-Sternberg cells are variable. They may be predominantly lymphocytic or exhibit a mixed composition, with the addition of mature granulocytes and numerous eosinophils as well as increased small blood vessels. Eosinophilic abscesses and areas of central necrosis may occur (158) (Fig. 15.23). Necrosis often is associated with a predominance of Reed-Sternberg cells, which form cohesive clusters and sheets (17). The Reed-Sternberg cells frequently appear degenerated and shrunken to impart a "mummified" appearance; these cells sometimes are referred to as "zombie" cells. In some cases, the areas of necrosis may be accompanied by foamy macrophages, which may mask Hodgkin lymphoma and lead to a misdiagnosis of a lipid storage disease or even sinus histiocytosis with massive lymphadenopathy (158,162) (Fig. 15.24).

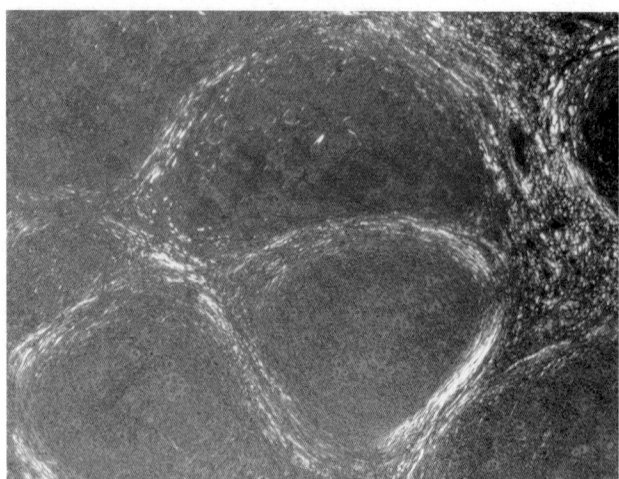

FIGURE 15.19. The bands of fibrous connective tissue in nodular sclerosis appear characteristically birefringent in examination under polarized light (hematoxylin and eosin stain, original magnification: 60× magnification).

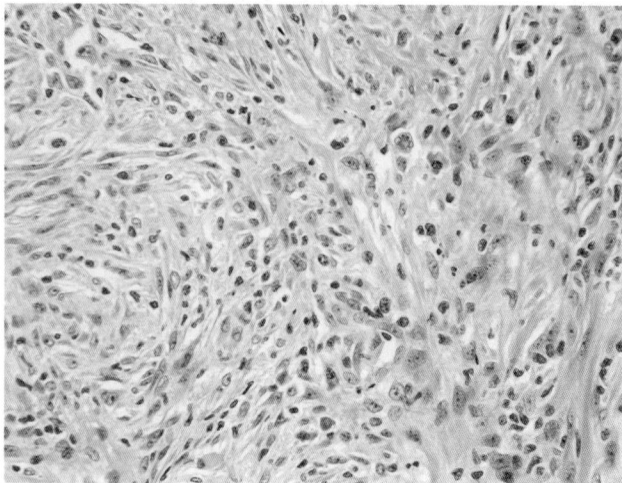

FIGURE 15.21. The "fibroblastic variant" of nodular sclerosis is associated with a shorter duration of relapse-free survival and may be confused with a pleomorphic sarcoma (hematoxylin and eosin stain, original magnification: 300× magnification).

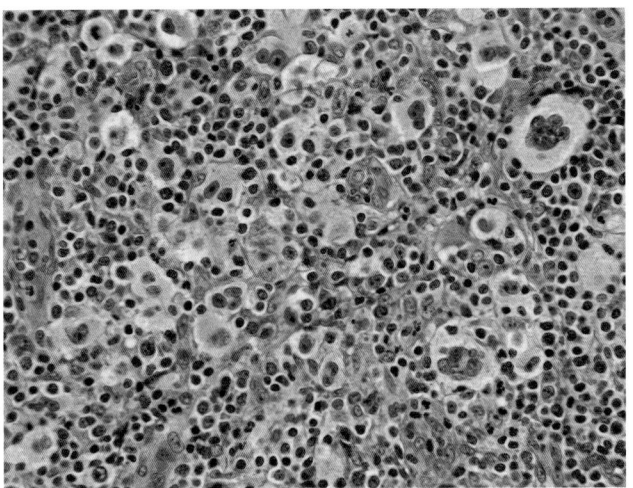

FIGURE 15.22. Clusters of lacunar cells are characteristic of the lymphoid islands in nodular sclerosis. The nuclei frequently are hyperlobated, and the nucleoli generally are smaller than those seen in classic Reed-Sternberg cells (hematoxylin and eosin stain, original magnification: 300× magnification).

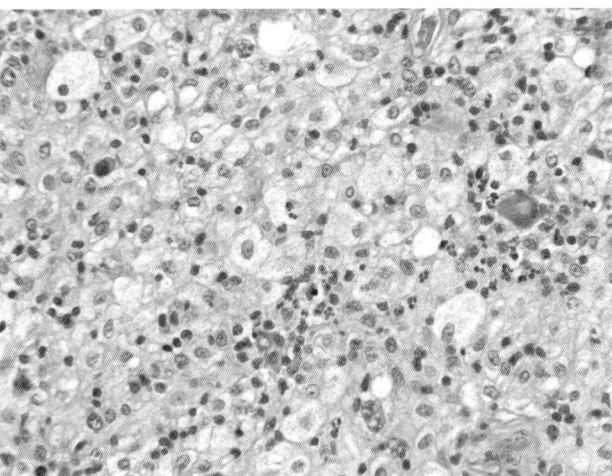

FIGURE 15.24. In nodular sclerosis, areas of necrosis and degeneration may occur associated with a proliferation of foamy macrophages. The macrophages may obscure the diagnosis of Hodgkin lymphoma (hematoxylin and eosin stain, original magnification: 300× magnification).

The presence of both lacunar cells and collagen bands, usually in association with a thickened capsule, is required for an absolute diagnosis of nodular sclerosis, and the diagnosis is more reproducible if both criteria are used (23,28). The finding of lacunar cells without fibrous septa raises the question of the so-called cellular phase of nodular sclerosis (28). Definitions of nodular sclerosis vary from one requiring only the identification of cellular nodules containing clusters of lacunar cells but without demonstrable fibrosis to another in which there must be at least a single band of collagen extending from a thickened capsule in association with the characteristic cellular proliferation containing lacunar cells (16,17,112,163,164). Lukes (28) acknowledged that occasional cases may exhibit a true cellular phase without collagen bands, but in order to achieve diagnostic consistency, these cases should be classified with the mixed cellularity type. This proposal was supported by a study in which cases that were categorized as nodular sclerosis, cellular phase exhibited clinical features and an overall survival that was more like

patients with mixed cellularity Hodgkin lymphoma than those with nodular sclerosis (158).

The classification of nodular sclerosis takes precedence over other histologic types that appear to be present in the same section, even if the area of nodular sclerosis is small (164). Lymph node involvement by nodular sclerosis may exhibit wide architectural variations to encompass even focal involvement (28). Focal involvement of the lymph node by Hodgkin lymphoma is observed with the mixed cellularity as well as nodular sclerosis types. Focal involvement by Hodgkin lymphoma, also referred to as *interfollicular Hodgkin lymphoma*, usually is characterized by an essentially preserved lymph node architecture associated with reactive follicular hyperplasia (28,165,166) (Fig. 15.25). However, the interfollicular region exhibits vague expansion as a result of a heterogeneous proliferation of small lymphocytes, plasma cells, eosinophils, epithelioid histiocytes, and diagnostic Reed-Sternberg cells that frequently are difficult to identify (28,165,166). Cases may be mistaken for benign reactive

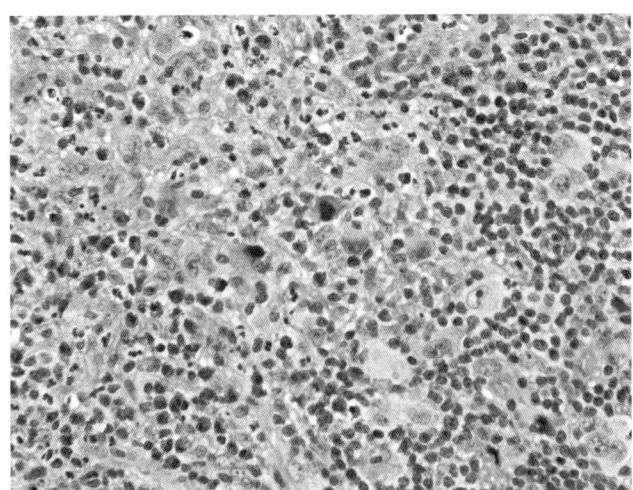

FIGURE 15.23. Eosinophils form an abscess-like lesion in nodular sclerosis. Increased eosinophils are regarded as a negative prognostic factor in nodular sclerosis, specifically in intermediate and advanced-stage disease. Note the degenerating Reed-Sternberg cell that is commonly referred to as a "mummified" or "zombie" cell (hematoxylin and eosin stain, original magnification: 300× magnification).

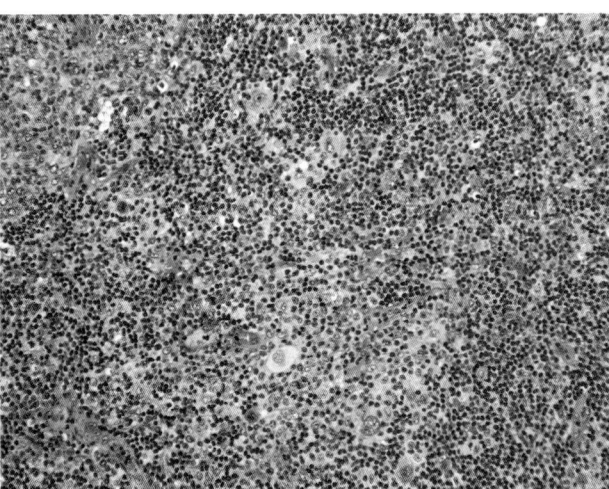

FIGURE 15.25. Adjacent to a germinal center in the **upper left**, the interfollicular region is expanded because of focal involvement by Hodgkin lymphoma (hematoxylin and eosin stain, original magnification: 150× magnification).

follicular hyperplasia, including toxoplasmic lymphadenitis, especially if interfollicular epithelioid histiocytes are prominent. Focal Hodgkin lymphoma also has been reported to occur in monocytoid B-cell clusters within lymph nodes, and monocytoid B cells have been described at the periphery of the nodules of nodular sclerosis (167,168). Because focal involvement of the lymph node by Hodgkin lymphoma is of limited size, accurate classification according to the WHO classification is not possible, but often deeper sections or a second biopsy specimen reveal nodular sclerosis or mixed cellularity (28,166). The pattern of focal or interfollicular cHL has no bearing on prognosis (158).

Because the cellular composition of nodular sclerosis is so variable, several investigators have attempted to determine whether subdividing nodular sclerosis according to the predominant histologic type has any prognostic significance. The results are inconsistent. Studies, mainly in Europe, demonstrated a relationship between the histopathologic composition in nodular sclerosis and both survival and relapse rates (24,25,169,170). Cases of nodular sclerosis were classified as grade I or II. For grade II, more than 25% of the cellular nodules were required to contain areas of pleomorphic lymphocyte depletion or numerous bizarre and anaplastic-appearing lacunar cells without lymphocyte depletion (Fig. 15.26), or 80% or more of the cellular nodules had to have a fibrohistiocytic variant of lymphocytic depletion (24); grade I included all other types of nodular sclerosis, comprising approximately 73% to 83% of cases. These studies concluded that nodular sclerosis with extensive areas of lymphocytic depletion or pleomorphic lacunar cells is associated with a statistically significant poor response to initial therapy, an increased relapse rate, and a decreased survival rate compared with other forms of nodular sclerosis (24,25,169,170). In contrast, most American studies conclude that grading of either advanced- or limited-stage nodular sclerosis, including uniformly staged and treated patients, has no predictive clinical value (171–173). Stemming from an analysis that demonstrated that tissue eosinophilia in nodular sclerosis correlated with poor prognosis (35), a new system for grading nodular sclerosis was proposed based on the criteria of eosinophilia, lymphocyte depletion, and atypia of the Hodgkin/Reed-Sternberg cells (26). This grading system was applied to 965 uniformly staged patients with nodular sclerosis enrolled in a multicenter trial and found no differences in clinical outcome between low- and

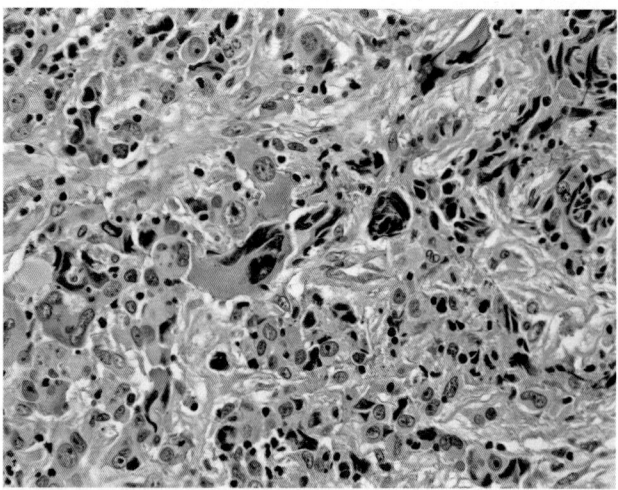

FIGURE 15.26. Cases of nodular sclerosis may have areas of lymphocyte depletion containing bizarre and pleomorphic lacunar cells. In some studies, these cases have been associated with a worse prognosis (hematoxylin and eosin stain, original magnification: 300× magnification).

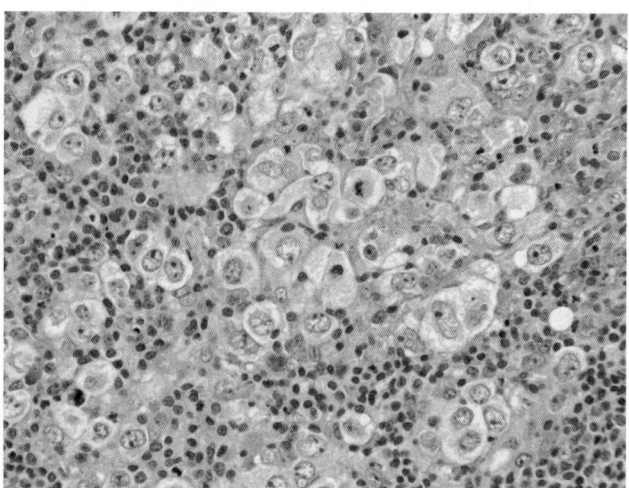

FIGURE 15.27. Sheets or clusters of lacunar cells and mononuclear Reed-Sternberg–type cells characterize the syncytial variant of nodular sclerosis. Especially in core biopsy specimens, these cases often are misdiagnosed as large cell lymphoma, metastatic carcinoma, or malignant melanoma (hematoxylin and eosin stain, original magnification: 300× magnification).

high-grade nodular sclerosis among patients with early-stage Hodgkin lymphoma; however, in intermediate and advanced stages, significant differences in prognosis were revealed between the histologic grades (26). Despite the controversy and the complex variability in results on the grading of nodular sclerosis, pathologists have the option to grade nodular sclerosis, or at least acknowledge the more pleomorphic grade II or high-grade type if present, so that additional data can be accumulated and clinicians can have the grading results to possibly employ as another parameter in guiding treatment and for research protocols (23).

Cases of nodular sclerosis that are composed predominantly of clusters and sheets of pleomorphic lacunar cells and mononuclear Reed-Sternberg cells also have been termed the *syncytial variant* (86,174) (Fig. 15.27). The atypical-appearing lacunar cells and mononuclear Reed-Sternberg cells often concentrate around areas of necrosis; because they form cohesive aggregates with only a few lymphocytes, such cases frequently are misdiagnosed as large cell lymphoma, metastatic carcinoma, seminoma, or melanoma (86,174). The syncytial variant of nodular sclerosis is diagnosed by recognizing the lacunar-like spaces associated with the proliferating cells, the discovery of more typical areas of nodular sclerosis in other parts of the biopsy specimen, and the employment of immunologic studies to verify the Reed-Sternberg nature of the large cells and exclude other malignancies.

The pattern of classic nodular sclerosis with broad, birefringent collagen bands outlining lymphoid nodules may be mimicked by a number of disorders. Similar patterns are observed in some cases of reactive lymphadenitis, carcinomatous metastases, sarcomas, and large cell lymphomas with sclerosis. Reactive lymphadenitis with an infectious etiology frequently leads to thickening of the fibrous capsule and intranodal fibrosis. Although occasionally double-nucleated immunoblasts may resemble Reed-Sternberg cells, lacunar cells and true Reed-Sternberg cells are absent in these reactive lesions. Metastases, such as metastatic lymphoepithelial carcinoma of nasopharyngeal origin, may evoke a desmoplastic response and form islands in lymphoid tissue (Fig. 15.28); however, the metastatic lesions are distinguished from nodular sclerosis, including the syncytial variant, through identification of cohesive aggregates of malignant epithelial cells and the use of immunohistochemical stains employing a panel of antibodies directed against cytokeratin, CD45, CD15, and CD30 (174–176). Occasionally, the

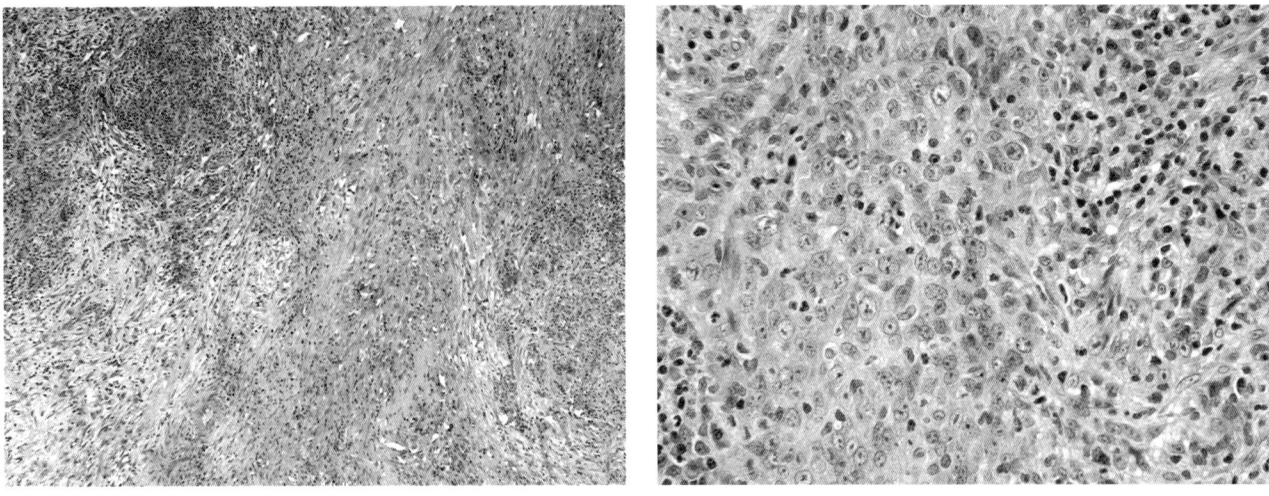

FIGURE 15.28. A: The pattern of nodular sclerosis is mimicked by metastatic lymphoepithelial carcinoma of nasopharynx (hematoxylin and eosin stain, original magnification: 60× magnification). **B:** The metastatic lymphoepithelial carcinoma forms syncytial groups of neoplastic cells but, in contrast to nodular sclerosis, the neoplastic cells are cohesive and do not express Hodgkin lymphoma–associated antigens; however, they express cytokeratin to verify the diagnosis of a metastasis (hematoxylin and eosin stain, original magnification: 300× magnification).

giant and atypical cells in various sarcomas and mesenchymal tumors, notably those with inflammatory and lymphocytic infiltrates, may resemble Reed-Sternberg cells and be confused with Hodgkin lymphoma (177,178). Complicating matters, a storiform pattern may be present in the fibroblastic variant of nodular sclerosis (158). A sarcoma is distinguished from Hodgkin lymphoma by the absence of true lacunar cells in the sarcoma, coupled with the use of appropriate immunohistochemical or molecular studies.

Lacunar and Reed-Sternberg–like cells cause special difficulty in distinguishing nodular sclerosis from primary mediastinal large B-cell lymphoma (PMBL); this difficulty is compounded in small needle biopsy specimens (Fig. 15.29). In PMBL, the large cells often have clear cytoplasm and simulate lacunar cells, and they also may exhibit considerable nuclear pleomorphism and resemble classic Reed-Sternberg cells (179–181). Despite this difficulty, in large cell lymphoma the sclerosis tends to compartmentalize small groups of lymphoma cells rather than produce true lymphoid islands (179). Immunologic studies almost always substantiate the non-Hodgkin nature of PMBL

by demonstrating a B-cell lineage and, with sufficient tissue, PMBL are found to express the transcription factors Oct2, BOB.1, and PU.1 in contrast to nodular sclerosing Hodgkin lymphoma (181). With needle core biopsy specimens, however, appropriate caution is required in the interpretation of immunophenotypic studies because, like nodular sclerosis, PMBL often expresses CD30, although the staining pattern is more sporadic than in Hodgkin lymphoma (182). In fact, considerable immunophenotypic overlap exists between these entities so that the distinction may not always be blatant (Table 15.5). Prediction for Hodgkin lymphoma reportedly includes reactivity for CD15, cyclin E, and EBV-latent membrane protein (LMP), whereas PMBL is predicted chiefly by expression of B-cell antigens, especially CD79a in addition to CD20, BOB.1, and CD23, as well as p63 and growth-factor-receptor–bound protein 2 (183,184). Although demonstration of B-cell clonality by PCR traditionally has indicated B-cell non-Hodgkin lymphoma, current advanced PCR techniques are sufficiently sensitive in cases of cHL to also identify B-cell clonality without the use of microdissection (185); consequently, the discovery of a B-cell clone

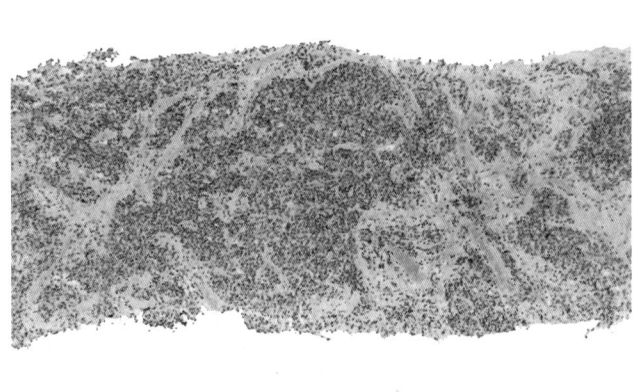

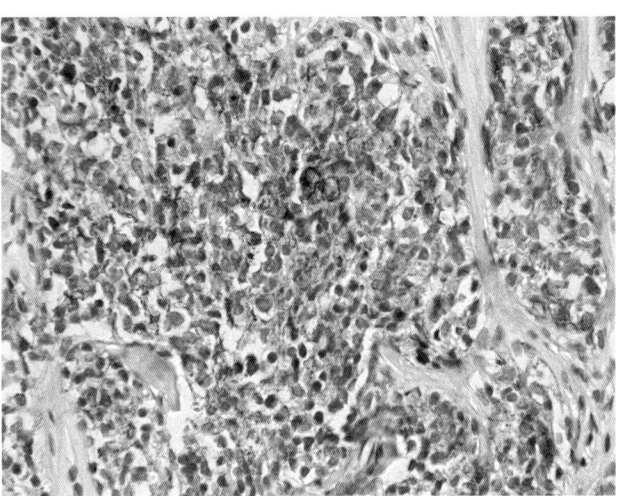

Figure 15.29. A: PMBL can occasionally simulate the pattern of nodular sclerosis in a core biopsy specimen (hematoxylin and eosin stain, original magnification: 60× magnification). **B:** Like cHL, the neoplastic large cells in PMBL commonly express CD30 (immunoperoxidase stain, original magnification: 300× magnification).

Table 15.5	IMMUNOHISTOCHEMICAL PANEL TO DISTINGUISH cHL, MAINLY NODULAR SCLEROSIS, FROM PMBL	
	cHL	**PMBL**
CD15	+/−	−
CD30	+	+/−
CD45	−	+
Cyclin E	+	−
CD20, CD79a	−/+	+
PAX5	+	+
Oct2/BOB.1	−/+	+
CD200	+	+
TNFAIP2	+	+
EBV	+/−	−
CD23	−	+/−
p63	−	+
Grb2	−/+	+
MAL	−/+	+

TNFAIP2, tumor necrosis factor-α-inducible protein-2; Grb2, growth factor receptor-bound protein 2.

is not beneficial in distinguishing cHL from non-Hodgkin lymphoma, including PMBL. In this vein, gene expression profiling demonstrates that PMBL cases, as opposed to other forms of DLBCL, share a common gene expression signature with cHL, thereby adding additional evidence that both PMBL and nodular sclerosis are related tumors (186,187); both tumors also aberrantly express the dendritic cell marker, tumor-necrosis-factor-α-inducible protein-2 (TNFAIP2), whereas TNFAIP2 is rarely expressed in DLBCL, not otherwise specified (188) (see Chapters 16 and 23).

It is not surprising, therefore, that rare cases exhibit an intermediate or transitional appearance and immunophenotype rendering them unclassifiable as to either DLBCL or cHL. In the WHO lymphoma classification such cases are referred to as *B-cell lymphoma, unclassifiable, with features intermediate between diffuse large B-cell lymphoma and cHL*, also known as *gray zone lymphoma* (43,44,189). The differential diagnosis of most of these unclassifiable cases is with nodular sclerosis and PMBL. Some mediastinal gray zone lymphoma cases histologically resemble nodular sclerosis with fibrous bands, but also with sheets of pleomorphic large cells, a weakened inflammatory environment, deficiency of CD15 reactivity, and robust CD20 expression (44,190,191). Other cases exhibit the morphology of PMBL, but equally contain admixed Hodgkin and lacunar cells, absent or weak CD20 reactivity, and variable positivity for CD15, CD30, and CD45 (44,191,192). B-cell transcription factor expression in the gray zone cases parallels PMBL; most cases exhibit features in keeping with activation of the NF-κB pathway, and cyclin E and p63 are similarly expressed in both groups of gray zone cases (44,190–192). Genetic alterations involving 2p and 9p are found in gray zone lymphomas to mirror those described in cHL and PMBL (191). MAL reactivity is also common in gray zone lymphoma (44). MAL, a gene that is overexpressed in PMBL, is not completely restricted to PMBL (193); approximately 20% of cHL cases are MAL+ and such expression correlates with nodular sclerosis, especially the grade II variety (52). Patients with Hodgkin lymphoma who express MAL have an adverse clinical outcome, providing support for the connection between cHL and PMBL. The clinical course of the gray zone cases usually is aggressive and the ideal therapeutic management remains unsettled (43).

The unclassifiable category between DLBCL and cHL does not include composite, synchronous, or metachronous (sequential) cases of both neoplasms (194). Patients with composite lymphomas, in which Hodgkin lymphoma and non-Hodgkin

lymphoma (excluding CLL/SLL) coexist in the same anatomic site, are uncommon, but well described (44,191,195). Although any type of non-Hodgkin lymphoma, such as mantle cell lymphoma or marginal zone lymphoma, can occur (196,197), the most common combination is nodular sclerosis and PMBL. Unlike the unclassifiable cases in which Reed-Sternberg–like or true Reed-Sternberg cells are admixed intimately with non-Hodgkin lymphoma, in true composite lymphoma with both Hodgkin lymphoma and a non-Hodgkin lymphoma, such as PMBL, there generally is some demarcation between the different histologic types with only a minor transitional area (44,189,191,195). In some respects, the pattern is analogous to that seen in the cases of NLP Hodgkin lymphoma associated with DLBCL (116–121,124–126); however, in composite lymphomas in which the Hodgkin lymphoma component has a nodular sclerosis appearance, the Reed-Sternberg cells reflect an immunophenotype that is typical of the classical form (44,191,195). This is in contrast to the B-cell phenotype of the PMBL component. In some examples of composite lymphoma, the Hodgkin and non-Hodgkin components are clonally related (198). In addition to composite lymphoma, clonally related nodular sclerosis and PMBL may develop in a synchronous or metachronous fashion (44,191). The most common sequence is nodular sclerosis followed by PMBL, generally after a short interval. Alternatively, metachronous Hodgkin lymphoma, most frequently nodular sclerosis, occasionally may develop in patients with PMBL and other B-cell non-Hodgkin lymphomas, such as FL (44,191,199). Patients with non-Hodgkin lymphomas are at an almost threefold risk of developing subsequent Hodgkin lymphoma (200). cHL also has been described in association with T-cell lymphomas, including cases arising in patients with mycosis fungoides and cutaneous CD30+ T-cell lymphoproliferative disorders (201–203). In this setting, the diagnosis of Hodgkin lymphoma has been based on histologic criteria and usually supplemented by immunohistochemistry demonstrating CD15 and CD30 expression on the putative Reed-Sternberg cells. However, substantial histologic and immunohistologic commonality exists between cHL and cutaneous CD30+ T-cell lymphoproliferative disorders, including expression of both CD15 and CD30 in some T-cell lymphomas (38). In fact, almost all cases of alleged cHL affiliated with mycosis fungoides and cutaneous CD30+ T-cell lymphoproliferative disorders are T-cell lymphomas that simulate Hodgkin lymphoma with Hodgkin-like cells that express CD15 and CD30 (204). Unlike Hodgkin lymphoma, the cells mimicking Reed-Sternberg cells often have multiple nucleoli that are smaller than in genuine Hodgkin cells, are more variable in size with frequent mitotic figures, cluster or form sheets with frequent sinusoidal invasion, exhibit a T-cell phenotype and genotype, and fail to express B-cell marker PAX5 (204).

Mixed Cellularity Classical Hodgkin Lymphoma

The mixed cellularity type of cHL follows the nodular sclerosis type in frequency comprising 27% of cases (140). It is slightly more common in males and often is associated with systemic symptoms. Approximately 70% of cases are EBV-associated with an incidence of 100% in many developing regions (23,62,205). Mixed cellularity occurs in all clinical stages and traditionally has a prognosis intermediate between those of the NLP and lymphocyte-depleted types (10,16,158).

Histologically, mixed cellularity Hodgkin lymphoma also occupies an intermediate position between the lymphocyte-rich and depleted groups (16,17,28). The mixed cellularity type is a repository for cases that do not fit into the other types in the original Lukes and Butler classification (16,17,28,86). It usually is characterized by a heterogeneous cell population composed of variable numbers of small lymphocytes with either no or minimal nuclear membrane irregularities, plasma cells,

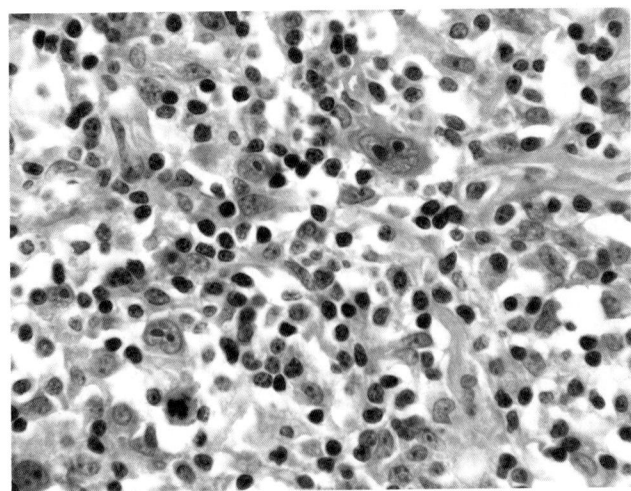

FIGURE 15.30. Mixed cellularity Hodgkin lymphoma typically is composed of a polymorphous cell population with fluctuating numbers of small lymphocytes, plasma cells, eosinophils, neutrophils, histiocytes, and diagnostic Reed-Sternberg cells (hematoxylin and eosin stain, original magnification: 600× magnification).

neutrophils, and eosinophils (Fig. 15.30). Of interest, tissue eosinophilia has no significant effect on survival in patients with mixed cellularity as opposed to patients with nodular sclerosis in whom increased eosinophils are deemed an adverse prognostic factor (26,35). As well as eosinophils, in mixed cellularity there generally are also a variable number of reactive histiocytes, which often form small clusters (Fig. 15.31), and an inconsistent degree of disorderly fibrosis without collagen formation. Necrosis also may be present, but this is usually not overly conspicuous. Typically, Reed-Sternberg cells can be detected easily (16,17). As a reflection of the heterogeneous inflammatory-type background in mixed cellularity, this form of Hodgkin lymphoma expresses genes related to inflammation in contrast to the expression of genes involved in extracellular matrix remodeling found in nodular sclerosis (160). The nodal architecture often is effaced completely in mixed cellularity Hodgkin lymphoma, but focal or interfollicular involvement occasionally occurs (16,17,30,86,165,166).

Because mixed cellularity occupies a central position in the spectrum from lymphocyte-rich classical to lymphocyte-depleted, there is considerable overlap. For example, cases where typical diagnostic Reed-Sternberg cells can be identified with minimal search are classified as the lymphocyte-rich classical or mixed cellularity type depending on whether a surfeit of lymphocytes are present or whether the background cell population comprises plasma cells, eosinophils, and other inflammatory-type cells. Also, cases containing numerous variants of Reed-Sternberg cells but few absolutely diagnostic Reed-Sternberg cells with characteristic large nucleoli are not included in the reticular form of lymphocyte-depleted Hodgkin lymphoma but qualify for the mixed cellularity group (28). The mixed cellularity group also comprises cases with lacunar cells in which there is an absence of sclerosis (86,158).

The differential diagnosis of mixed cellularity Hodgkin lymphoma is broad, encompassing cases with a heterogeneous cell population. This includes viruses and non-Hodgkin lymphomas, specifically angioimmunoblastic T-cell lymphoma (AILT) and PTCL of the mixed medium and large cell type, embracing those with epithelioid histiocytes (lymphoepithelioid cell or Lennert lymphoma). Virus-induced lymphadenopathies frequently lead to a proliferation of immunoblasts, and the binucleated forms may resemble Reed-Sternberg cells, such as in infectious mononucleosis (33,34). These lesions are distinguished morphologically from Hodgkin lymphoma by the recognition of immunoblasts with their characteristic strongly amphophilic and pyroninophilic cytoplasm; the immunoblasts almost always display a mottled pattern if seen on low-power microscopy and PD-1 commonly is expressed (206). AILT also contains immunoblasts and expresses PD-1 (207), but lacks a mottled pattern. In AILT, there is marked arborizing vascularity, deposition of periodic-acid-Schiff–positive interstitial material, and a clinical history that differs from Hodgkin lymphoma (208). Frequently, EBV-infected B cells are present in AILT, and such cells can mimic Reed-Sternberg cells. Unlike mixed cellularity Hodgkin lymphoma, AILT is a form of T-cell lymphoma derived from follicular T-helper cells, which is verifiable by immunologic, cytogenetic, and molecular studies (207–209) (see Chapter 26).

Other types of PTCL, such as those with a mixed cellular composition, including the Lennert variant, also may be difficult to distinguish objectively from cHL (38,39,144,210,211). In Lennert lymphoma, for example, the architectural characteristics and cellular composition often are identical to the

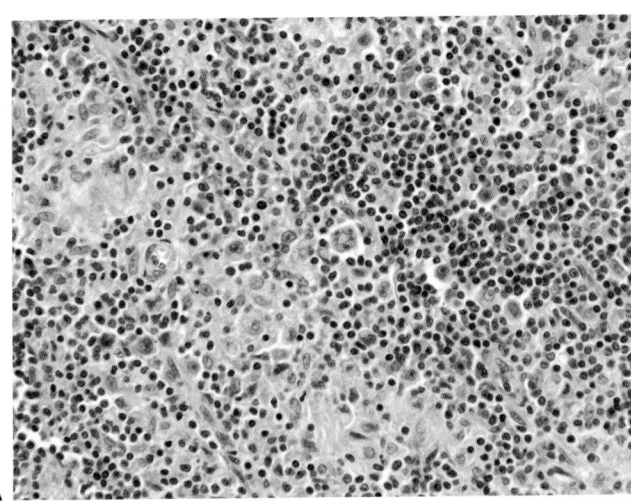

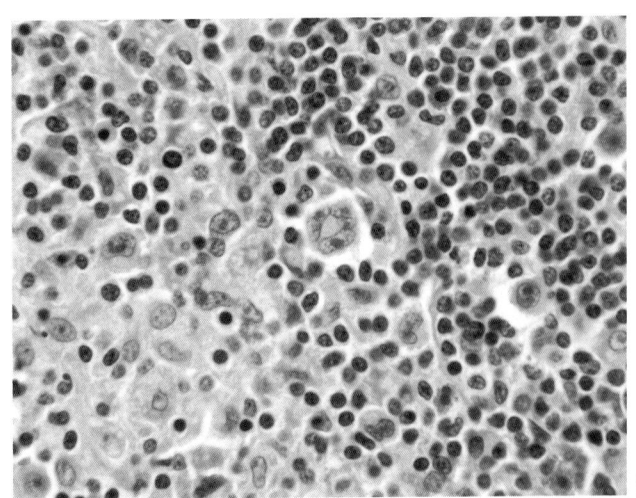

FIGURE 15.31. A: Some cases of mixed cellularity Hodgkin lymphoma contain numerous clusters of epithelioid histiocytes and have a pattern indistinguishable from a PTCL of Lennert type (hematoxylin and eosin stain, original magnification: 300× magnification). **B:** Unlike Lennert lymphoma, mixed cellularity Hodgkin lymphoma has readily identifiable Reed-Sternberg cells and variants. Note that the small lymphocytes are not atypical (hematoxylin and eosin stain, original magnification: 600× magnification).

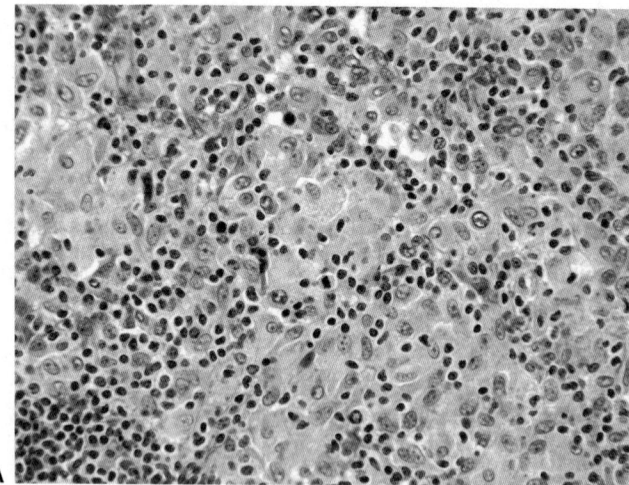 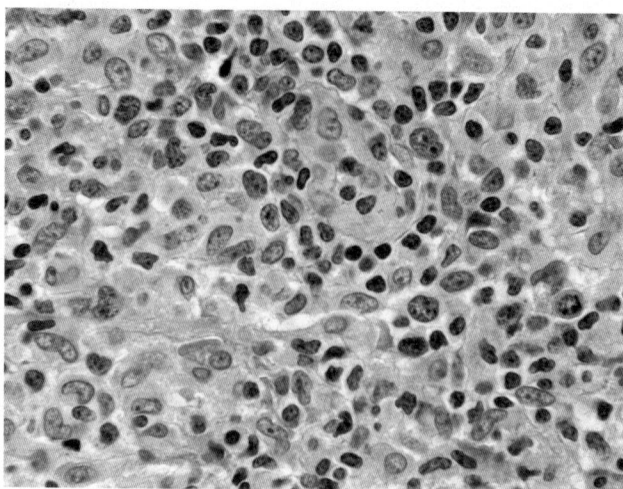

FIGURE 15.32. A: Clusters of epithelioid histiocytes characterize the lymphoepithelioid variant (Lennert lymphoma) of PTCL to evoke a differential diagnosis that encompasses THRLBCL as well as mixed cellularity Hodgkin lymphoma (hematoxylin and eosin stain, original magnification: 300× magnification). **B:** The small and medium-sized lymphocytes in this case of PTCL have irregular nuclear contours. Compare with Figure 15.31. The small and large lymphocytes, including the double-nucleated cell, expressed T-cell lineage–associated antigens and a clonal T-cell gene rearrangement was demonstrable (hematoxylin and eosin stain, original magnification: 600× magnification).

mixed cellularity type, with many epithelioid histiocytes, but in contrast to the small, generally round lymphocytes found in Hodgkin lymphoma, the lymphocytes in Lennert lymphoma are atypical with nuclear membrane irregularities (Fig. 15.32). Other histologic features that distinguish the Lennert form of PTCL from Hodgkin lymphoma are capsular invasion and a lack of sufficient numbers of diagnostic Reed-Sternberg cells. Fortunately, Lennert lymphoma is rare and in one series constituted only 8% of 340 cases of PTCL, not otherwise specified (212). In a review of 97 registry cases of lymphomas with a high content of epithelioid histiocytes, 8 cases (8%) were interpreted as Lennert lymphoma with the remaining cases representing additional forms of PTCL (41%), B-cell lymphomas (26%) such as THRLBCL, Hodgkin lymphoma (22%), and others (3%) (144). In many cases the histologic differences are subtle, and morphologic differentiation of mixed cellularity cHL from PTCL or even THRLBCL may not be objectively reliable (38–41). Immunohistologic studies are almost mandatory for diagnostic verification, with the qualification that a panel of antibodies must be employed because of the observation that the CD15 antigen often is expressed in the pleomorphic large cells, including the Reed-Sternberg–like cells, of PTCL, as well as in the diagnostic Reed-Sternberg cells of Hodgkin lymphoma (38,45,213). To add to the diagnostic difficulty, PTCL cases may simultaneously express CD15 and also CD30, as well as histologically mimic cHL (38). In contrast to Hodgkin lymphoma in which Hodgkin cells are unrelated to the background lymphocytes, in the CD15+, CD30+ PTCL cases the Reed-Sternberg–like cells and the background T cells express T-cell–associated markers, exhibit loss of T-cell–associated antigens and reveal T-cell receptor gene rearrangements by PCR (38). The coexpression of CD15 and CD30 in some cases of PTCL emphasizes that this immunophenotype is not absolute for cHL and the necessity of employing a comprehensive immunohistochemical panel augmented by molecular analysis (38,204) (see Chapter 26).

Lymphocyte-Depleted Classical Hodgkin Lymphoma

Lymphocyte-depleted is the least common form of Hodgkin lymphoma, found in <1% of cases (70,140). It is the Hodgkin lymphoma type causing the most contention, which is reflected by the recent history as to whether lymphocyte-depleted should be a category of ALCL (21,23). Two recent reports, however, verified the existence of the lymphocyte-depleted subtype and stressed that these cases express Hodgkin-associated antigens encompassing CD15, CD30, fascin, and PAX5, as well as EBV (214,215). Lymphocyte-depleted is retained in the WHO classification and includes cases that formerly were considered Hodgkin-like ALCL but that currently are reinterpreted as ALCL-like Hodgkin lymphoma (20,21,23,27,42). The latter is an aggressive form of Hodgkin lymphoma that also may embrace cases of nodular sclerosis, of grade II or the syncytial variant, and cases of lymphocyte-depleted Hodgkin lymphoma.

Lymphocyte-depleted traditionally comprises the diffuse fibrosis and reticular types of Lukes and Butler (16,17). The diffuse fibrosis type is characterized by a disordered proliferation of nonbirefringent connective tissue of noncollagenous type (Fig. 15.33). The fibrous connective tissue often is fibrillar, loosely cellular, and random in distribution (16,17). It occasionally has a fibroblastic appearance or resembles amorphous proteinaceous material. In addition to the connective tissue, this type of Hodgkin lymphoma overall is depleted of cells, particularly of lymphocytes, but rare cellular areas may be observed, with increased numbers of Reed-Sternberg cells. The reticular type of lymphocyte-depleted Hodgkin lymphoma is characterized by two essential patterns. One pattern may resemble mixed cellularity Hodgkin lymphoma, but with a predominance of Reed-Sternberg cells. In the other pattern, there also are increased numbers of Reed-Sternberg cells, but these appear pleomorphic and almost sarcomatous (16,17). The presence of Reed-Sternberg cells in almost every high-power microscopic field is the main characteristic of the reticular type of lymphocyte-depleted Hodgkin lymphoma (28) (Fig. 15.34). In some biopsy specimens, areas with diffuse fibrosis and reticular patterns may coexist (17).

Lymphocyte-depleted Hodgkin lymphoma generally occurs in elderly patients with constitutional symptoms and stage III or IV lymphoma at the time of diagnosis (10,69,70). Historically, the lymphocyte-depleted type of Hodgkin lymphoma has been the most aggressive, with the shortest median length of survival (10,17,31,70). In one early study, lymphocyte-depleted appeared to define a syndrome in which the patients were older (median age, 51 years) and presented with fevers, wasting, and hepatic dysfunction (69); peripheral lymphadenopathy was uncommon, but there was extensive subdiaphragmatic lymphoma, with

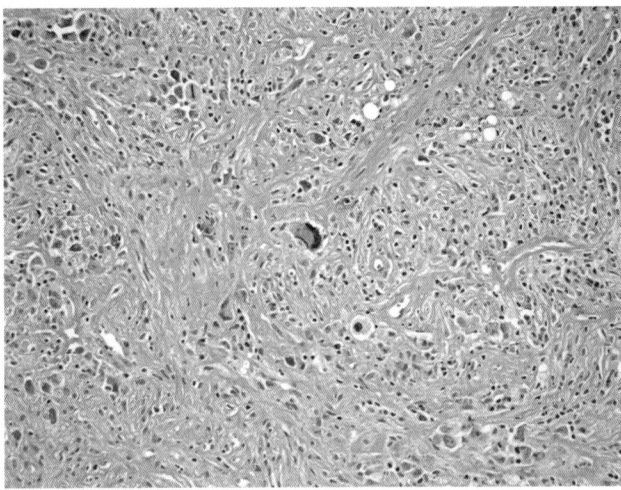
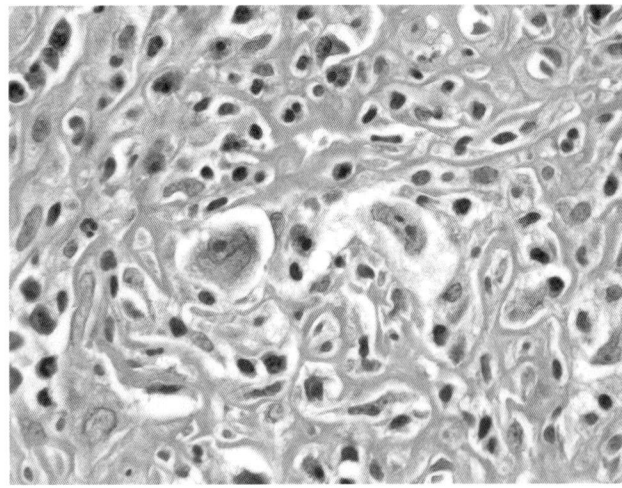

A

B

FIGURE 15.33. **A:** The diffuse fibrosis type of lymphocyte-depleted Hodgkin lymphoma typically has broad areas of amorphous nonbirefringent connective tissue of noncollagenous type (hematoxylin and eosin stain, original magnification: 150× magnification). **B:** In addition to a paucity of lymphocytes, Reed-Sternberg cells also may be difficult to identify (hematoxylin and eosin stain, original magnification: 600× magnification).

involvement of liver, spleen, retroperitoneal lymph nodes, and bone marrow. Yet another series, describing 25 patients with lymphocyte-depleted Hodgkin lymphoma, concluded that some patients conform to the syndrome described, including constitutional symptoms, subdiaphragmatic lymphoma, frequent marrow involvement, and advanced-stage lymphoma, but others had clinical symptoms paralleling those found in other patients with Hodgkin lymphoma, including mixed cellularity type (216). A recent study of 84 patients with lymphocyte-depleted Hodgkin lymphoma, gleaned from four different generations of clinical trials, compared the lymphocyte-depleted patients to patients with other histologic types of Hodgkin lymphoma (70). Parallel to the earlier series, in the more recent review the lymphocyte-depleted patients had a higher incidence of unfavorable characteristics, for example, advanced stage, B symptoms, large mediastinal masses, extranodal disease, involvement of three or more lymph node groups, and a higher International Prognostic Score, as well as a greater rate of bone marrow and liver involvement. They also exhibited a lower progression-free survival and overall survival at 5 years; however, the patients with lymphocyte-depleted Hodgkin lymphoma who received therapy

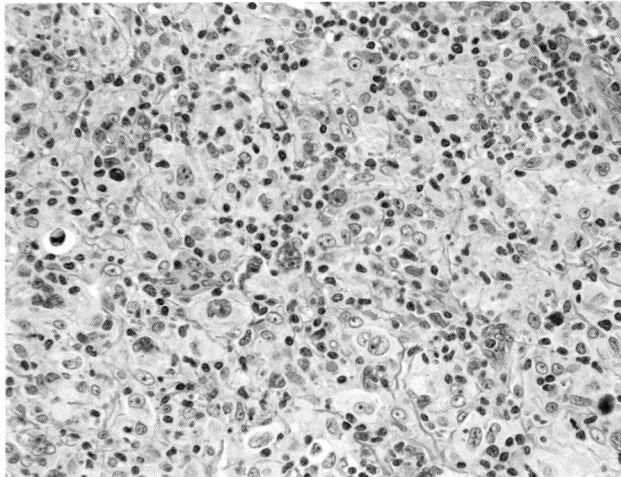

FIGURE 15.34. In the reticular type of lymphocyte-depleted, Reed-Sternberg cells are evident in virtually every high-power microscopic field (hematoxylin and eosin stain, original magnification: 300× magnification).

with intensified-dose BEACOPP had comparable outcomes to patients with other forms of Hodgkin lymphoma (70).

The differential diagnosis of lymphocyte-depleted Hodgkin lymphoma includes, in addition to ALCL, other forms of Hodgkin lymphoma, particularly nodular sclerosis grade II together with the syncytial variant, and the mixed cellularity type with increased numbers of mononuclear cells rather than true diagnostic Reed-Sternberg cells (27,28,42,174). In fact, most historical cases of the lymphocyte-depleted type of Hodgkin lymphoma do not represent that entity. In one histologic review of 39 cases considered originally to reflect the lymphocyte-depleted form, only 9 (23%) were regarded as morphologically acceptable for that entity (217); the remaining cases were examples of nodular sclerosis with lymphocytic depletion (grade II) and probably included the syncytial variant, other forms of Hodgkin lymphoma, and non-Hodgkin large cell lymphomas. Other studies combining both morphologic and immunologic assessment confirmed that a variety of large cell malignant neoplasms, including metastatic carcinomas as well as other varieties of Hodgkin lymphoma and non-Hodgkin lymphomas, may be confused with lymphocyte-depleted (86,214,215).

The most difficult cases to differentiate from lymphocyte-depleted Hodgkin lymphoma are those of ALCL (Fig. 15.35), because there may be a continuous spectrum between these disorders with clinical, morphologic, and immunologic overlap to echo the unclassifiable or gray zone cases between cHL and DLBCL. Cases of common ALCL tend to have sinusoidal and perivascular patterns of infiltration by sheets of pleomorphic, cohesive large cells with eccentric, frequently horseshoe-shaped nuclei with small nucleoli associated with active mitotic figures (42,218). This morphologic appearance, however, is inconsistent, and there may be morphologic ambiguity, with cells indistinguishable from Reed-Sternberg cells, together with an inflammatory background, fibrous bands, and a thickened capsule (20,21,27,42,218). An immunohistochemical panel is paramount in attempting to resolve such cryptic cases, and although generally successful, a panel may not always settle the ambiguity (Table 15.6). For example, cases of lymphocyte-depleted Hodgkin lymphoma tend to be CD15+, PAX5+, CD45−, T cell−, EMA−, and, most significantly, anaplastic lymphoma kinase (ALK) negative; the opposite usually is found in ALCL (27,42,219). Nonetheless, CD15 expression is lacking in approximately 25% of cHL cases and cases of ALCL may exhibit a null cell immunophenotype and/or be ALK− (42,48,219). For the ALK− cases, EBV determination is

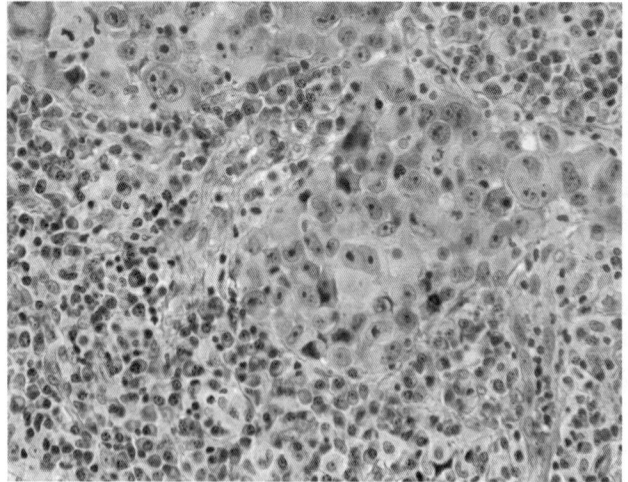

FIGURE 15.35. Like ALCL, pleomorphic large cells, including some Reed-Sternberg–like cells, infiltrate a peripheral lymph node sinus. Although the large cells were CD30⁺, they also were CD15⁺ and CD45⁻. Moreover, T-cell antigens were not expressed, ALK was negative, and no T-cell gene rearrangements were manifest. As in this case, ALCL can be difficult to separate from lymphocyte-depleted Hodgkin lymphoma (hematoxylin and eosin stain, original magnification: 300× magnification).

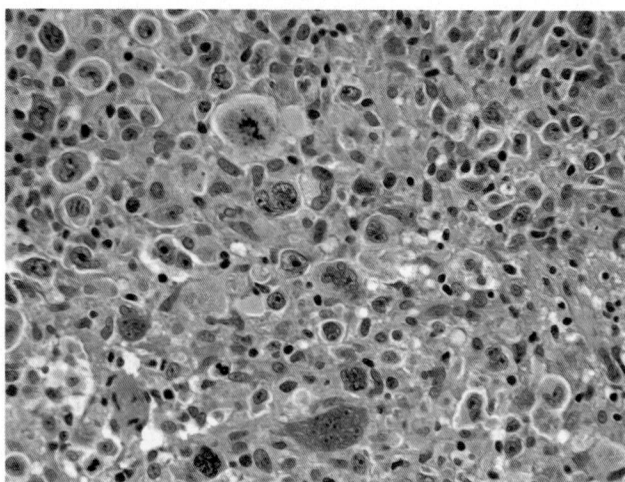

FIGURE 15.36. EBV⁺ DLBCL of the elderly can be morphologically indistinguishable from lymphocyte-depleted Hodgkin lymphoma (hematoxylin and eosin stain, original magnification: 300× magnification).

useful since ALCL is reliably EBV⁻, but PAX5 and CD43 are recommended as the most valuable markers in distinguishing between cHL, such as the lymphocyte-depleted form, and ALK⁻ ALCL (220); however, aberrant PAX5 expression has been documented in rare cases of ALCL and may be associated with extra copies of the *PAX5* gene (221). For such unusual cases, an expanded panel is required employing other markers that are positive for ALCL, such as clusterin, p63, and CD99 (222–224). For example, p63 expression is absent in Hodgkin lymphoma, but is reported in a significant minority of cases of ALK⁺ and ALK⁻ cases of ALCL, including the rare CD45⁻, ALK⁻, null cell subtype (223). In the differential diagnosis between ALCL and classical lymphocyte-depleted Hodgkin lymphoma, the continuous development of a reliable immunohistochemical library coupled with awareness of the morphologic nuances and the use of molecular genetics has significantly reduced the number of the intriguing borderline, unclassifiable, or gray zone cases.

In addition to ALCL, EBV⁺ DLCBL of the elderly is another lymphoma that may be confused with EBV⁺ cHL encompassing the lymphocyte-depleted form (189) (Fig. 15.36). Although uncommon in the West, EBV⁺ DLCBL of the elderly comprises up to 10% of DLBCL cases in Asia (225). In a study from Japan,

patients with EBV⁺ DLBCL of the elderly tended to have a more aggressive clinical course than patients with EBV⁺ cHL, with a higher age of onset, lower male predominance, and a higher rate of involvement of extranodal sites including the skin, gastrointestinal tract, and lung (226). Histologically, cases of EBV⁺ DLBCL of the elderly contain a polymorphous cell population with prominent reactive component and numerous large lymphocytes, as well as Hodgkin and Reed-Sternberg–like cells. As opposed to cHL, the cases of EBV⁺ DLCBL of the elderly exhibit more geographic necrosis, and greater increase in cytotoxic T cells among background lymphocytes; both EBV⁺ DLBCL of the elderly cases and age-matched cases of EBV⁺ Hodgkin lymphoma express CD30, but the DLBCL cases demonstrate an absence of CD15 expression, more consistent expression of B-cell markers, including CD79a as well as CD20 with strong reactivity for PAX5, in addition to the transcription factors Oct2 and BOB.1 (225,226). Despite these diagnostic parameters, as in ALCL, some examples may bridge features of both EBV⁺ DLBCL of the elderly and EBV⁺ cHL, such as lymphocyte-depleted, and are either synchronous cases or unclassifiable/gray zone lymphoma (189,227).

PATHOLOGY OF STAGING

Pathologic staging for Hodgkin lymphoma is currently restricted to bone marrow and is especially appropriate for patients with advanced clinical disease (228). The criteria for involvement of bone marrow, as well as liver and spleen, remain those proposed at the Ann Arbor conference of 1971 (164). Because the amount of tissue available for histological examination in bone marrow biopsy and liver biopsy specimens is relatively small, classic Reed-Sternberg cells may not be discovered. Multiple sections should be obtained to search for the cells; if none are found, however, proof of involvement of these sites is not as rigorous as that required for an initial diagnosis of Hodgkin lymphoma. A mononuclear cell with a single large nucleolus found in a cellular environment appropriate for Hodgkin lymphoma suffices for an absolute diagnosis. In the bone marrow, foci of fibrosis should lead to serial sectioning in the search for diagnostic Reed-Sternberg cells or the mononuclear variants (164,229) (Fig. 15.37). Bone marrow involvement by cHL is found in 4% to 10% of patients, with the greatest risk to patients with the mixed cellularity and lymphocyte-depleted types (69,163,229). Immunohistochemical confirmation is advised, but antigenic

Table 15.6	IMMUNOHISTOCHEMICAL PANEL TO DISTINGUISH cHL, SUCH AS LYMPHOCYTE-DEPLETED, FROM ALCL	
	cHL	**ALCL**
CD15	+/−	−
CD30	+	+
CD45	−	+/−
CD3, 4, 5, 43, 45RO	−	+/−
PAX5	+	−
EMA	−	+/−
Clusterin	−	+
Fascin	+	+/−
EBV	+/−	−
ALK	−	+/−
p63	−	−/+
CD99	−	+/−
TIA-1	−/+	+/−

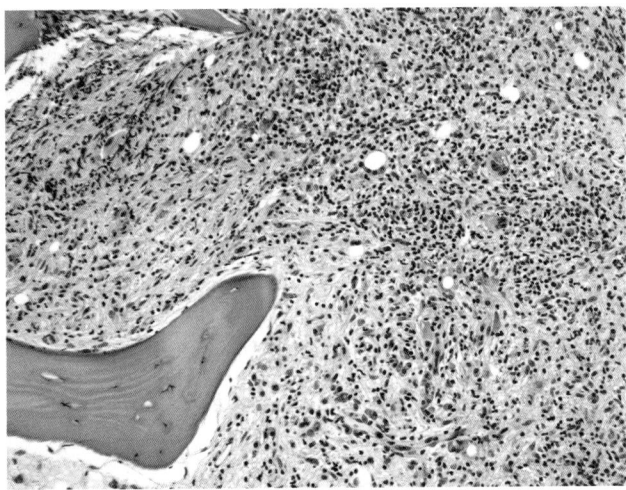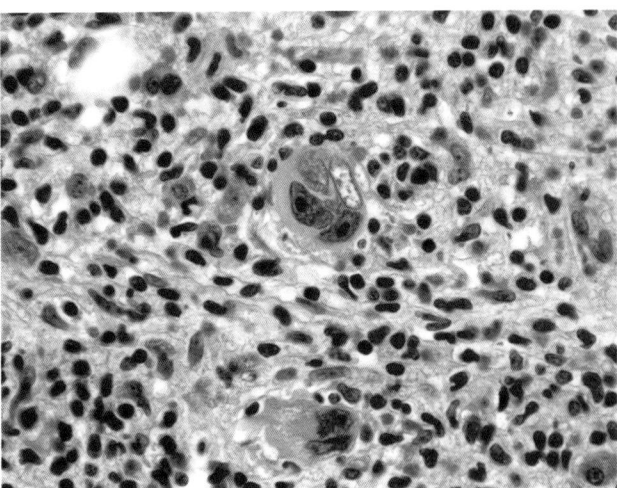

FIGURE 15.37. A: Fibrosis often is a morphologic clue that the bone marrow may contain Hodgkin lymphoma (hematoxylin and eosin stain, original magnification: 150× magnification). **B:** A diagnostic Reed-Sternberg cell corroborates the diagnosis, but a mononuclear variant of a Reed-Sternberg cell in an area of fibrosis would be sufficient for a diagnosis of Hodgkin lymphoma in the bone marrow in a patient with established Hodgkin lymphoma (hematoxylin and eosin stain, original magnification: 600× magnification).

degradation may develop as a result of decalcification (229) so that morphologic features remain the standard for diagnosis. The uninvolved bone marrow frequently exhibits a variety of nonspecific reactions including stromal edema, hypocellularity, myeloid hyperplasia, and benign lymphoid nodules (229,230). For patients with NLP Hodgkin lymphoma, the bone marrow rarely may be involved and such cases exhibit large B cells associated with a prominent T cell and histiocytic background (106); these patients have a reduced prognosis and could well be examples of THRLBCL. In the liver, lymphocytic infiltrates in the portal areas frequently are observed, but these have no definite relationship to Hodgkin lymphoma (28). Patients with hepatic involvement by Hodgkin lymphoma are much more likely to have histological evidence of large portal infiltrates, with a predominance of atypical lymphocytes, and also may exhibit changes of acute cholangitis and portal edema (231).

Pathologic documentation of Hodgkin lymphoma in spleen is currently uncommon in contrast to the era of staging laparotomy. Splenic involvement by Hodgkin lymphoma was discovered in 39% of patients at staging laparotomy, but the weight of the spleen had no bearing on predicting involvement (163). Typically, Hodgkin lymphoma in spleen forms multiple, single or coalescent, white, discrete nodules scattered throughout the parenchyma in a miliary-type distribution (232) (Fig. 15.38) (see Chapter 50). Many spleens with Hodgkin lymphoma,

however, manifest tumor involvement by only a solitary nodule measuring from 1 to 3 mm in diameter (163). Unless the spleen is sectioned meticulously and examined at 2- to 3-mm intervals, these isolated small nodules may be overlooked (232). Solitary splenic nodules often are limited to the T zones of the spleen in the periarteriolar lymphoid sheaths or periphery of the marginal zones (Fig. 15.39). The cytologic criteria for the diagnosis of Hodgkin lymphoma in the spleen are identical to those employed in lymph nodes. All histologic types of lymphoma may be found in the spleen and may be so designated (28); however, in many cases the distinction between nodular sclerosis and mixed cellularity Hodgkin lymphoma is not possible, but subclassification is not mandatory and is not a crucial factor in therapy (10). There may be confusion in the diagnosis of Hodgkin lymphoma in the spleen because of the presence of clusters of histiocytes forming epithelioid or sarcoid-like granulomas (233). Granulomas are observed in up to 9% of cases of Hodgkin lymphoma and may even form visible nodules on the splenic cut surface. The discovery of granulomas in the spleen or other organs does not indicate involvement of these organs by Hodgkin lymphoma.

EXTRANODAL HODGKIN LYMPHOMA

With the exception of patients with AIDS (55,63), primary-stage IE extranodal Hodgkin lymphoma is very rare. In extranodal sites, an initial diagnosis of Hodgkin lymphoma should be viewed with skepticism, because most cases likely represent other conditions with Reed-Sternberg–like cells, such as PTCL, ALCL, EBV+ DLBCL of the elderly, metastatic carcinoma, and metastatic melanoma or are a result of contiguous or retrograde lymphatic spread from another site containing Hodgkin lymphoma. To unequivocally establish a diagnosis of extranodal Hodgkin lymphoma, the diagnostic requisites are the same as in lymph nodes, and immunologic verification must be sought (28).

The lung is among the most common extralymphatic site for Hodgkin lymphoma apart from the liver, but even in the lung Hodgkin lymphoma is rare. Most cases of pulmonary Hodgkin lymphoma are of the nodular sclerosis type and are a result of contiguous spread from the mediastinum (28,234) (Fig. 15.40). The criteria for the diagnosis of primary pulmonary Hodgkin lymphoma are restriction of the lymphoma to the lung with

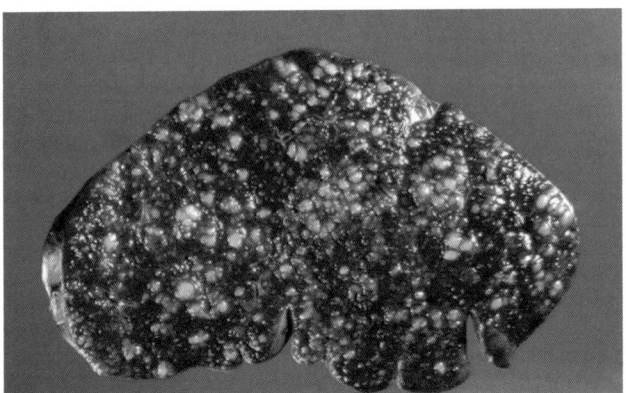

FIGURE 15.38. Multiple, random, pale tumor nodules are characteristic of Hodgkin lymphoma in the spleen.

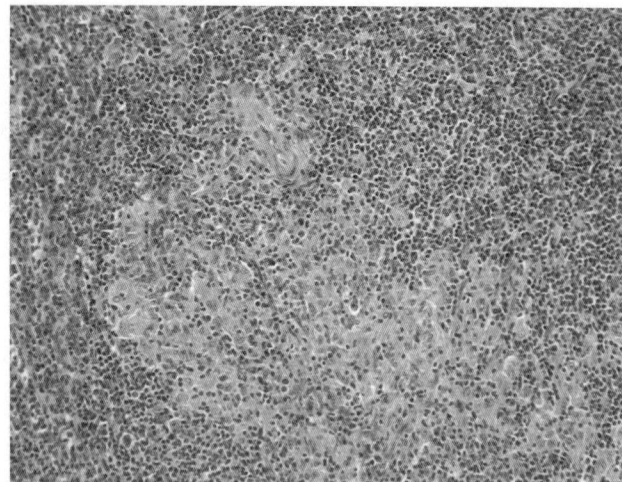
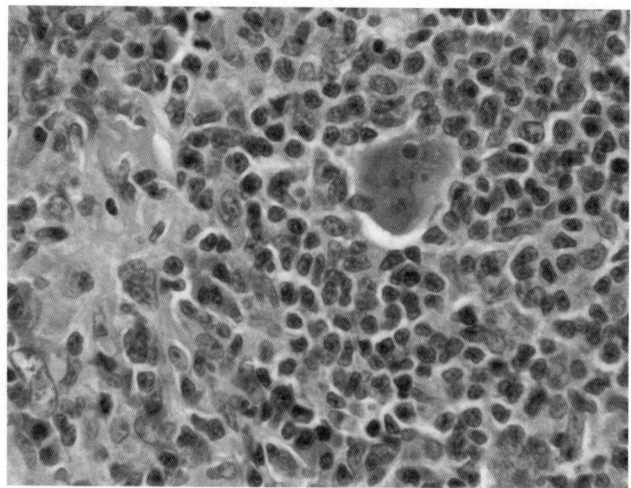

A   B

FIGURE 15.39. A: Hodgkin lymphoma in the spleen usually concentrates in the T zones, such as the periarteriolar lymphoid sheaths (hematoxylin and eosin stain, original magnification: 150× magnification). **B:** A Reed-Sternberg cell is found adjacent to epithelioid histiocytes. Epithelioid histiocytes may form sarcoid-type granulomas in the spleen but are not an indication of Hodgkin lymphoma unless an appropriate Reed-Sternberg cell is identified (hematoxylin and eosin stain, original magnification: 600× magnification).

minimal or no hilar lymph node involvement, exclusion of lymphoma at distant sites, and documentation of the typical histologic features of Hodgkin lymphoma (235). Hodgkin lymphoma of the lung occurs more frequently in women and radiologically appears as a solitary nodule or multinodular lymphoma, occasionally with cavitation (235). As well as forming a solid, nodular tumor mass, Hodgkin lymphoma in the lung may exhibit a peribronchial-perivascular distributional pattern and/or involve the pleura (236). All cases must be differentiated from Wegener granulomatosis and non-Hodgkin lymphomas that simulate Hodgkin lymphoma.

Primary extranodal Hodgkin lymphoma in other sites is similarly rare, with many descriptions limited to single anecdotal case reports and with only the contemporary cases validated by appropriate immunohistochemical studies. For example, in one classic series of 2,185 patients with Hodgkin lymphoma, none had intracranial lymphoma at presentation, and only 12 patients (0.5%) later developed documented intracranial lymphoma (237). A report from an international collaborative group discovered only 16 patients with Hodgkin lymphoma

of the central nervous system (CNS) (238). Eight patients presented with Hodgkin lymphoma of the CNS of whom two had disease limited to the CNS, whereas eight other patients developed CNS involvement at relapse. Most patients had Hodgkin lymphoma in brain parenchyma, others in dura/meninges, and a few patients exhibited multifocal disease. All patients were classified as cHL, either not otherwise specified [7], nodular sclerosis type [7], or mixed cellularity type [2] (238). Although uncommon, extradural Hodgkin lymphoma leading to spinal cord compression is a well-recognized clinical presentation of Hodgkin lymphoma (10,239). Patients with Hodgkin lymphoma in the spinal epidural space usually are discovered to have advanced disease.

An incidence of 0.5% also has been cited for cutaneous involvement of Hodgkin lymphoma (240). Skin involvement in Hodgkin lymphoma generally manifests in the formation of small papules and nodules, as a result of retrograde lymphatic spread of regionally involved lymph nodes. The majority of patients with cutaneous Hodgkin lymphoma have a rapid clinical course, and skin involvement is regarded as a symptom of stage IV lymphoma (240). Bona fide cases of primary cutaneous Hodgkin lymphoma are exceedingly rare and may not even exist. Most reports of primary cutaneous Hodgkin lymphoma likely represent cases of primary cutaneous CD30+ T-cell lymphoproliferative disorders with Reed-Sternberg–like cells (204,240) (Fig. 15.41) or are an example of EBV+ mucocutaneous ulcer, a condition associated with different forms of immunosuppression (241). In EBV+ mucocutaneous ulcer, skin involvement manifests by sharply circumscribed ulcers containing a polymorphous cell population with atypical large B cells that display frequent Reed-Sternberg–like features. In addition to EBV positivity, the B cells are CD30+ and also may coexpress CD15 to add to the confusion with Hodgkin lymphoma (241). Unlike cHL, the Reed-Sternberg–like cells in EBV+ mucocutaneous ulcer usually express CD45 and Oct2. The morphologic and immunophenotypic differences between EBV+ mucocutaneous ulcer and cHL are subtle, but the knowledge that primary extranodal Hodgkin lymphoma of skin is so rare should allow one to be constantly dubious of cutaneous Hodgkin lymphoma and to broaden consideration for another pathologic entity. Further caution also is required in the diagnosis of primary cutaneous Hodgkin lymphoma because of the risk of unnecessary therapy, as patients with EBV+ mucocutaneous ulcer tend to regress spontaneously with no treatment (241), like patients with lymphomatoid papulosis.

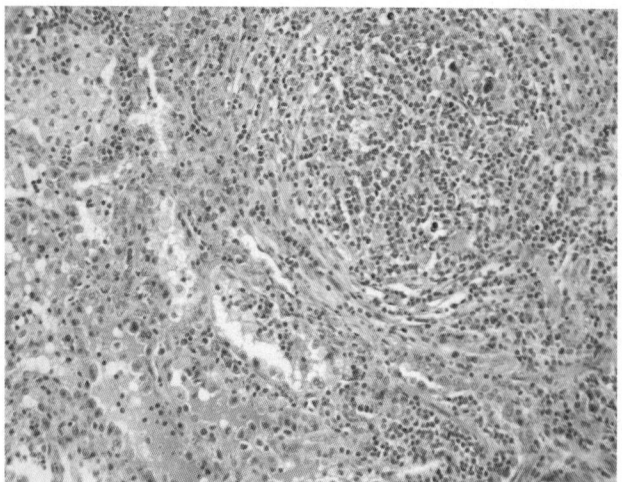

FIGURE 15.40. Hodgkin lymphoma in the lung usually is of the nodular sclerosis type and often is a consequence of contiguous spread from the mediastinum (hematoxylin and eosin stain, original magnification: 150× magnification).

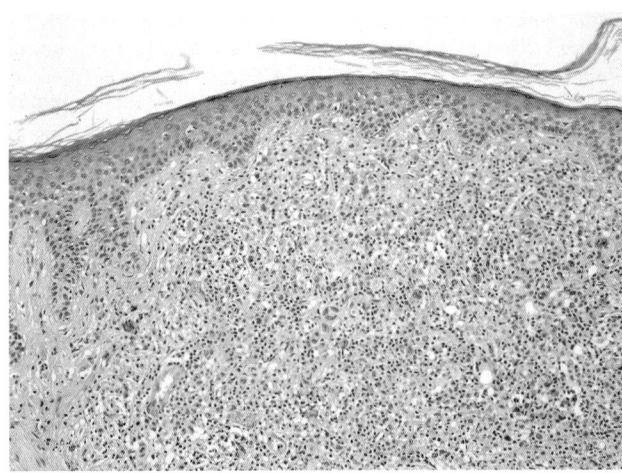
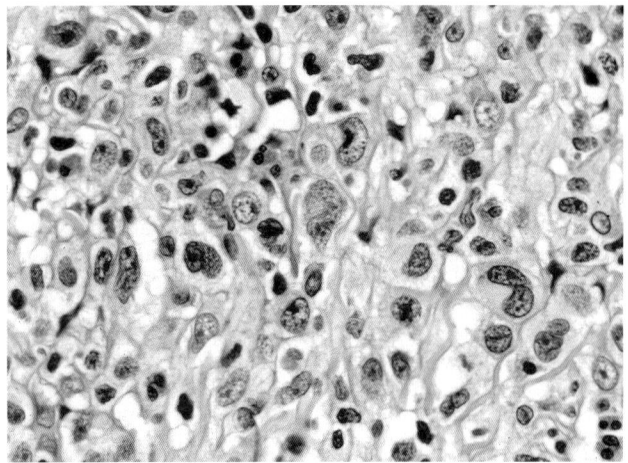

FIGURE 15.41. A: This cutaneous lesion contains a polymorphous dermal infiltrate including Reed-Sternberg–like cells (hematoxylin and eosin stain, original magnification: 150× magnification). **B:** Detail of the dermal lymphocytes encompassing double-nucleated forms with Reed-Sternberg–like features. Clinical and immunophenotypic studies indicated that the lesion was a primary cutaneous CD30+ lymphoproliferative disorder (hematoxylin and eosin stain, original magnification: 900× magnification).

Like the skin, breast involvement by Hodgkin lymphoma also is uncommon. In one large series, only six cases of Hodgkin lymphoma of the breast were encountered over a 22-year period (242). All six were of the nodular sclerosis type. No case was interpreted to be primary in the breast; all were considered likely to have resulted from Hodgkin lymphoma in the intramammary or internal mammary lymph nodes or direct mediastinal extension into the breast and chest wall (242). Chest wall invasion by Hodgkin lymphoma is a significant adverse prognostic factor (234).

The gastrointestinal tract is rarely involved by Hodgkin lymphoma, and most of the earlier described cases of primary gastrointestinal Hodgkin lymphoma likely were non-Hodgkin lymphomas of various aggressive types. Identical to other alleged cases of primary extranodal Hodgkin lymphoma, the morphologic diagnosis of gastrointestinal Hodgkin lymphoma requires rigorous immunologic and clinical confirmation. For example, cases of intestinal Hodgkin lymphoma arising in a setting of inflammatory bowel or diverticular disease are described with the characteristic immunophenotype of Hodgkin lymphoma, and are EBV+ associated with immunodeficiency (243). In retrospect, these cases likely are examples of EBV+ mucocutaneous ulcer affecting the gastrointestinal tract (241) (Fig. 15.42). A similar case of an EBV+ lymphoid infiltrate simulating Hodgkin lymphoma with eventual regression in the anorectal area is described, but in an immunocompetent patient (244). On the other hand, genuine rare cases of primary gastrointestinal Hodgkin lymphoma likely exist and can originate in any part of the tract (245–247).

Waldeyer ring is another uncommon site for Hodgkin lymphoma (10). Moreover, many cases purported in the past to be Hodgkin lymphoma in Waldeyer ring likely represent non-Hodgkin lymphoma of the Lennert type (248). More recent reports using large patient data bases, however, describe 38 cases of Waldeyer ring Hodgkin lymphoma of predominantly mixed cellularity, nodular sclerosis, and lymphocyte-rich classical types (249,250); immunohistochemical studies verified the diagnoses. EBV was detected in Reed-Sternberg cells in 67% of the cases studied in both series; this high

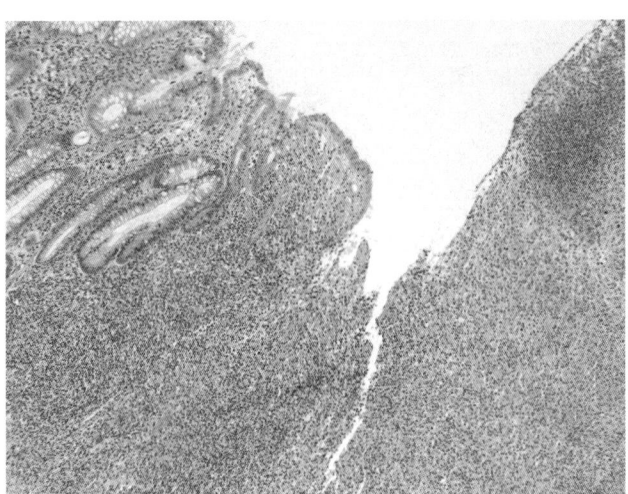
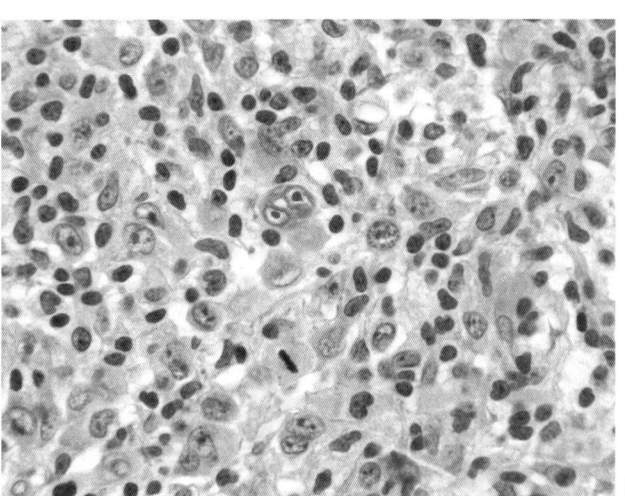

FIGURE 15.42. A: An ulcerated mass in the sigmoid colon of an elderly patient exhibits a dense polymorphous lymphocytic infiltrate (hematoxylin and eosin stain, original magnification: 60× magnification). **B:** The colonic infiltrate includes cells indistinguishable from Reed-Sternberg cells. Moreover, the lesional cells expressed Hodgkin lymphoma–associated antigens CD15 and CD30 and were CD20+ and EBV+. Although originally thought to be Hodgkin lymphoma, the case is likely an example of EBV+ mucocutaneous ulcer (hematoxylin and eosin stain, original magnification: 600× magnification).

incidence was felt to reflect the fact that Waldeyer ring is a reservoir for EBV (249,250).

Hodgkin lymphoma also may present rarely as a primary solitary or multifocal bone tumor (251,252). In a review from the Mayo Clinic, 25 patients with osseous Hodgkin lymphoma were identified over a 70-year span (252); 17 patients initially presented with bone tumors, and the remainder had recurrent Hodgkin lymphoma involving bone. Bone pain was the main symptom, and most lesions were in the axial and proximal appendicular skeleton. Radiologic features included osteoblastic, osteolytic, and osteosclerotic patterns. Most patients subsequently were discovered to have nonosseous, particularly nodal Hodgkin lymphoma (252). In bone, Hodgkin lymphoma usually infiltrates between bony trabeculae and may be associated with reactive new bone formation. Although Reed-Sternberg cells were identified in all cases, and there was immunophenotypic verification, necrosis also was seen that led to an occasional misdiagnosis of acute osteomyelitis (252). Most patients with primary Hodgkin lymphoma of bone do well with modern therapy (251,252).

The thyroid is a very rare site for presentation of Hodgkin lymphoma (253). When present, the patients may provide histories of chronic thyroiditis. They frequently have a cold nodule or a diffusely enlarged gland. Most cases are of the classical nodular sclerosis type involving females, but fibrosis may result in diagnostic difficulty (253). Patients usually respond to Hodgkin therapy.

PATHOLOGY OF RELAPSE

Notwithstanding the phenomenal success of modern therapy for Hodgkin lymphoma, 10% to 30% of patients subsequently relapse (11,254). The timing of relapse is relevant because early relapse from complete remission portends more aggressive or refractory disease as opposed to late relapse usually developing 12 to 18 months after complete remission (255). The probability of being refractory to complete remission increases with advanced disease and relapse equally increases with advanced disease, such as the presence of systemic symptoms and bulky mediastinal lymphoma. Most patients experience relapse in lymph nodes, but relapse also may occur in extranodal sites; for example, almost half of patients with Hodgkin lymphoma at autopsy are shown to have extranodal involvement, particularly in the liver and lung although any extranodal site may be involved (256,257).

Autopsy studies of patients with Hodgkin lymphoma reflect the effects of modern therapy and provide considerable data on relapse and persistent lymphoma. Autopsy of patients who died of Hodgkin lymphoma before the current era of therapy often disclosed widespread Hodgkin lymphoma (10,16). Persistent Hodgkin lymphoma also was found in a small group of asymptomatic long-term survivors who died from apparently unrelated causes (256). Patients who die after treatment for Hodgkin lymphoma in the modern era often have a reduction in the extent of lymphoma, and one-third of patients have no evidence of residual Hodgkin lymphoma (256,257); the latter patients often die of complications of therapy. In fact, adults and children who are treated for Hodgkin lymphoma are at increased risk of dying of causes unrelated to progressive Hodgkin lymphoma compared with population-based statistics and despite successful therapy (11,14,80,81). The main causes of death include second malignancies and cardiovascular disease.

A change in cell type of Hodgkin lymphoma at clinical relapse is well recognized and usually interpreted as histologic progression to a more aggressive form of Hodgkin lymphoma (16,112). Only cases of the nodular sclerosis type exhibit a high degree of persistence in sequential biopsies, although some studies indicate that NLP Hodgkin lymphoma also is characterized by histologic persistence (109,112). The immunophenotype of classic Reed-Sternberg cells also is relatively constant in sequential biopsy specimens of Hodgkin lymphoma. In one study, 82% of cases exhibited immunophenotypic stability, as opposed to a previous report of only 19% consistency in patients with Hodgkin lymphoma undergoing biopsies at different times (258,259). The latter study preceded the use of routine antigen-retrieval techniques in immunohistochemistry.

Although a comprehensive study of the pathologic aspects of relapse of Hodgkin lymphoma after modern therapy has not materialized for more than 30 years, studies in the early 1980s reported that the histologic appearance depends on whether relapse occurs in an untreated or previously treated site (260,261). The vast majority of patients (89%) experiencing a relapse maintain the histologic appearance in biopsy specimens from an untreated site (260). An increase in epithelioid cell granulomatous reactions is observed among those patients who have an interval before relapse >1 year. Histologic persistence is far less common in patients who develop relapse in treated sites. Almost half of these patients exhibit some alteration from their original histology and 20% are unclassifiable because of an unusual appearance, with loss of lymphocytes and increased numbers of pleomorphic cells, including bizarre Reed-Sternberg cells (261) (Fig. 15.43). These findings are identical to those described at autopsy (256,257). Curiously, the histologic appearance or subclassification at relapse does not necessarily portend a poor prognosis (261).

It is important to stress that the development of a mass in a patient after treatment for Hodgkin lymphoma may not indicate recurrent lymphoma. Large, bulky masses in the mediastinum or retroperitoneum may represent masses of fibrosis, with or without other degenerative changes, probably as a consequence of therapy (254,262,263). Patients with Hodgkin lymphoma also are susceptible to infections such as toxoplasmosis after therapy and can develop lymphadenopathy, which may simulate clinical recurrence. In order to document clinical relapse of Hodgkin lymphoma, diagnostic rebiopsy is recommended, particularly for patients with late relapse or if an alternative diagnosis is favored (13,254).

As mentioned previously, patients treated for Hodgkin lymphoma are prone to develop secondary malignancies including not only solid tumors but also acute myeloid leukemia and non-Hodgkin lymphoma (13,14,80,81). Patients who have

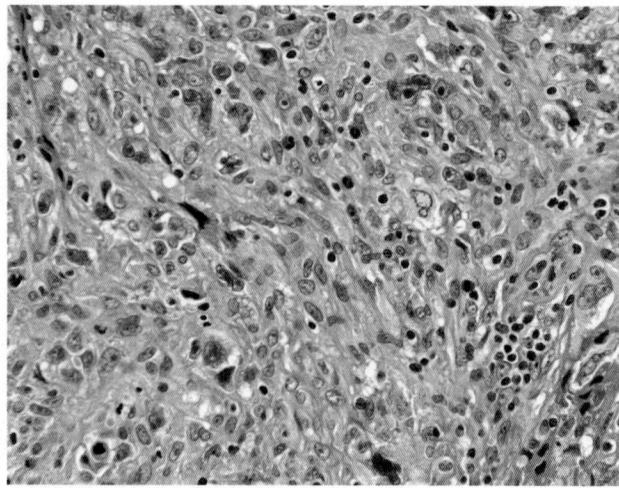

FIGURE 15.43. Recurrent cHL in a treated site often is unclassifiable as to exact type. This case in the mediastinum resembles lymphocyte-depleted Hodgkin lymphoma, but lacks sufficient numbers of diagnostic Reed-Sternberg cells for that entity. The original diagnosis was nodular sclerosis (hematoxylin and eosin stain, original magnification: 300× magnification).

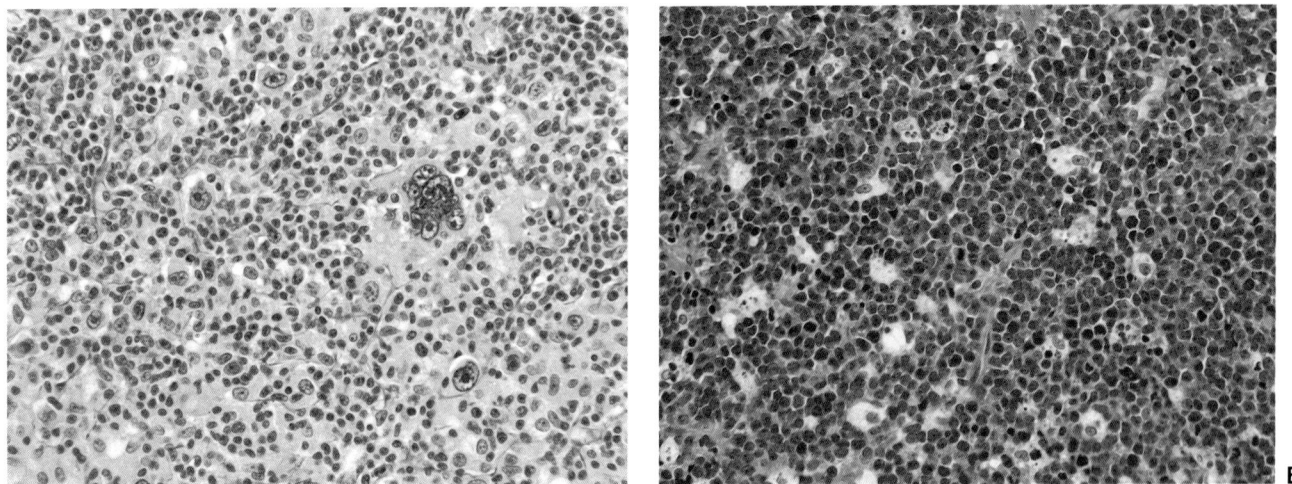

FIGURE 15.44. A: Initial diagnostic biopsy of mixed cellularity Hodgkin lymphoma (hematoxylin and eosin stain, original magnification: 300× magnification). **B:** Burkitt lymphoma presenting as an abdominal mass several years after the original diagnosis and combined-modality therapy (hematoxylin and eosin stain, original magnification: 300× magnification).

Hodgkin lymphoma and later develop non-Hodgkin lymphoma develop these secondary tumors late, usually after 6 years or more, although the risk may be less with current treatment regimens compared to those used in the preceding decade (14). Patients with secondary non-Hodgkin lymphoma frequently have abdominal presentations, including involvement of the gastrointestinal tract, and mainly have DLBCL or Burkitt lymphoma (264,265) (Fig. 15.44). According to one case report, an aggressive B-cell non-Hodgkin lymphoma was not related clonally to the preceding treated Hodgkin lymphoma (266). Rare cases of PTCL have been reported after therapy for Hodgkin lymphoma (267). The etiology of the B-cell aggressive lymphomas that arise in patients treated for Hodgkin lymphoma may be a consequence of either an immunosuppressive or a mutagenic effect of combined-modality therapy or may develop secondary to Hodgkin lymphoma–associated defective immunity (264,265,268). The onset of B-cell lymphoma after Hodgkin therapy does not appear to be related to EBV infection (268).

SUMMARY AND CONCLUSIONS

The advances in the understanding of Hodgkin lymphoma in the past 50 years have been multidisciplinary. Clinical progress sprang from the development of new diagnostic techniques including lymphangiography, staging laparotomy, PET-CT, and more recently FDG-PET that led to the elucidation of the general orderly and contiguous pattern of dissemination of Hodgkin lymphoma. The employment of more accurate diagnostic methods also resulted in the worldwide acceptance of the Ann Arbor system for staging the extent of disease. The ability to stage Hodgkin lymphoma accurately culminated in the development of new therapeutic regimens with innovative modes of radiation therapy and the evolution of chemotherapy, combined-modality therapy, and bone marrow transplantation. Consequently, 80% or more of patients who develop Hodgkin lymphoma are cured at major centers in all parts of the world.

During this same era, the pathologic contributions to the understanding of Hodgkin lymphoma have been equally dynamic. The now historic clinicopathologic studies of Lukes and Butler resulted in a pathologic classification system, including the subsequent Rye modification, that has proven its relevance and reproducibility. Although the classification scheme

of Lukes and Butler provides the base for the pathologic understanding of Hodgkin lymphoma, their concepts have undergone considerable redefinition and refinement and have been superseded by the modifications offered in the WHO classification. NLP Hodgkin lymphoma is a distinct entity differing from other types of Hodgkin lymphoma in that the LP variants of Reed-Sternberg cells, as well as most of the surrounding small lymphocytes, react with antibodies directed against CD45 and, significantly, express B-cell-lineage–restricted antigens but rarely the Hodgkin lymphoma–associated antigens CD15 and CD30. Approximately 3% to 14% of patients with NLP Hodgkin lymphoma evolve to DLBCL but, like most patients with NLP without transformation, the patients with DLBCL also tend to have localized clinical lymphoma and, in most reports, exhibit a high rate of long-term survival.

Lymphocyte-rich cHL is the new category of Hodgkin lymphoma formalized in the REAL and WHO classifications. The majority of cases have a nodular or follicle-like architecture, and some cases of lymphocyte-rich cHL could be placed in either the cellular phase of nodular sclerosis or mixed cellularity groups. Unlike NLP, the lymphocyte-rich form has identifiable classic Reed-Sternberg cells with a classic immunophenotypic profile (CD15+CD30+CD20−CD45−). The immunophenotype is significant, and an immunophenotypic panel is mandatory to absolutely differentiate lymphocyte-rich cHL from NLP and THRLBCL. Lymphocyte-rich cHL shares many clinical, pathologic, and immunophenotypic traits with NLP Hodgkin lymphoma, for example, the manner of presentation and the formation of PD-1+ rosettes; however, like patients with other types of cHL, patients with lymphocyte-rich cHL are similar with respect to the patterns of relapse and the expression NF-κB markers. Because of the overlapping features with both NLP and cHL, lymphocyte-rich cHL probably relates to an early stage in the continuum of cHL.

Classical nodular sclerosis is the most accurately diagnosed type of Hodgkin lymphoma, but there are histologic variants that may lead to a diagnostic conundrum. The two essential criteria for diagnosis of this type are sclerotic bands and clusters of the lacunar variants of Reed-Sternberg cells. Variants of nodular sclerosis include a fibroblastic type in which the fibroblasts almost mimic the appearance of a sarcoma; this variant is associated with a shorter-duration relapse-free survival. Another variant is a pleomorphic grade II type of Hodgkin lymphoma that may encompass the syncytial variant. These cases are mistaken easily for metastatic carcinoma or large cell lymphoma, and it appears that the high-grade cases of nodular sclerosis with a combination of anaplastic lacunar cells, significant areas of lymphocyte depletion, and/or increased eosinophils are associated with a worse prognosis compared with the more common grade I type of nodular sclerosis in patients with intermediate- or advanced-stage disease. The differential diagnosis of nodular sclerosis is broad and is most difficult with respect to PMBL, particularly in light of the fact that gene expression profiling has demonstrated that these two entities are closely related. Although usually separable, a small number of cases exhibit intermediate morphologic and immunophenotypic features rendering such cases as unclassifiable or gray zone lymphomas.

Mixed cellularity cHL has a highly variable morphologic appearance, because the classification essentially is a repository for cases that do not fit into the other types of Hodgkin lymphoma. Our understanding of the subtleties of the morphology of the mixed cellularity type essentially derives from expansion of the differential diagnosis to refine the broad histologic criteria for this type of Hodgkin lymphoma. The differential diagnosis of mixed cellularity Hodgkin lymphoma includes virus-induced florid reactive hyperplasia, AILT, and other PTCLs including cases with epithelioid histiocytes (Lennert lymphoma). Mixed cellularity Hodgkin lymphoma also may be confused with THRLBCL. In all cases, morphologic criteria have been expounded, but an absolute diagnosis is dependent on verification by immunologic means. In addition, both the mixed cellularity and nodular sclerosis types may affect only a portion of a lymph node; such cases have been designated as focal or interfollicular Hodgkin lymphoma.

Lymphocyte-depleted is the least common type of Hodgkin lymphoma and, with the advances in both immunology and molecular genetics, the number of cases being filed in pathology archives under this type is being reduced further. Many historical cases identified as lymphocyte-depleted were in fact the syncytial or high-grade variants of nodular sclerosis, other types of Hodgkin lymphoma, and non-Hodgkin lymphomas of large cell type, most notably ALCL and probably also EBV⁺ DLBCL of the elderly. Both morphologic reappraisal and immunophenotypic analysis are mandatory in the contemplation of any diagnosis of lymphocyte-depleted Hodgkin lymphoma.

The pathology of Hodgkin lymphoma at staging by laparotomy essentially has not changed, probably because of the almost universal abandonment of this diagnostic procedure. The pathologic criteria for involvement of bone marrow, as well as spleen and liver, and at pathologic staging remain those proposed at the Ann Arbor conference in 1971. The most significant proposal of the criteria for establishing Hodgkin lymphoma at staging is that a mononuclear cell with a single large nucleolus is acceptable for diagnosis in a small biopsy specimen from bone marrow in patients with histologically established Hodgkin lymphoma. Extranodal Hodgkin lymphoma is rare, except in patients with AIDS, and should be regarded with initial disbelief. Genuine cases of extranodal Hodgkin lymphoma can arise in a variety of sites such as the lung, gastrointestinal tract, Waldeyer ring, bone, and thyroid, but other conditions that mimic Hodgkin lymphoma need to be excluded, for example, EBV⁺ mucocutaneous ulcer.

Studies of Hodgkin lymphoma at relapse indicate that almost all patients exhibit persistence of the original histologic appearance if relapse occurs in an untreated site. If relapse develops in a treated site, the morphologic appearance becomes more pleomorphic and more difficult to classify, and the histology resembles that seen in Hodgkin lymphoma at autopsy. Intriguingly, there is no correlation of pleomorphism with prognosis. Patients who relapse also may develop an aggressive non-Hodgkin lymphoma of B-cell type that seems related to combined-modality therapy.

References

1. Hodgkin T. On some morbid appearances of the absorbent glands and spleen. *Med Chir Trans* 1832;17:68–114.
2. Wilks S. Cases of enlargement of the lymphatic glands and spleen (or, Hodgkin's disease), with remarks. *Guys Hosp Rep* 1865;11:56–67.
3. Rather LJ. Who discovered the pathognomonic giant cell of Hodgkin's disease? *Bull N Y Acad Med* 1972;48:943–950.
4. Diehl V. Hodgkin's disease–from pathology specimen to cure. *N Engl J Med* 2007;357:1968–1971.
5. Hoppe RT, Mauch PM, Armitage JO, et al., eds. *Hodgkin lymphoma*, 2nd ed. Philadelphia: Lippincott Williams & Wilkins, 2007.
6. Marafioti T, Hummel M, Foss HD, et al. Hodgkin and Reed-Sternberg cells represent an expansion of a single clone originating from a germinal center B-cell with functional immunoglobulin gene rearrangements but defective immunoglobulin transcription. *Blood* 2000;95:1443–1450.
7. Re D, Thomas RK, Behringer K, et al. From Hodgkin disease to Hodgkin lymphoma: biologic insights and therapeutic potential. *Blood* 2005;105:4553–4560.
8. Küppers R. The biology of Hodgkin's lymphoma. *Nat Rev Cancer* 2009;9:15–27.
9. Steidl C, Connors JM, Gascoyne RD. Molecular pathogenesis of Hodgkin lymphoma: increasing evidence of the importance of the microenvironment. *J Clin Oncol* 2011;29:1812–1826.
10. Kaplan HS. *Hodgkin's disease*, 2nd ed. Cambridge: Harvard University Press, 1980.
11. Connors JM. State-of-the-art therapeutics: Hodgkin's lymphoma. *J Clin Oncol* 2005;23:6400–6408.
12. Ansell SM, Armitage JO. Management of Hodgkin lymphoma. *Mayo Clin Proc* 2006;81:419–426.
13. Hoppe RT, Advani RH, Ai WZ, et al. NCCN clinical practice guidelines in oncology: Hodgkin lymphoma 2012 v.2. www.nccn.org; 2012.
14. Hoppe RT, Advani RH, Ai WZ, et al. Hodgkin lymphoma. *J Natl Compr Canc Netw* 2011;9:1020–1058.
15. Eichenauer DA, Engert A, Dreyling M. Hodgkin's lymphoma: ESMO clinical practice guidelines for diagnosis, treatment and follow-up. *Ann Oncol* 2011;22(Suppl 6):vi55–vi58.
16. Lukes RJ, Butler JJ. The pathology and nomenclature of Hodgkin's disease. *Cancer Res* 1966;26:1063–1081.
17. Lukes RJ, Butler JJ, Hicks EB. Natural history of Hodgkin's disease as related to its pathologic picture. *Cancer* 1966;19:317–344.
18. Jackson H Jr, Parker F Jr. *Hodgkin's disease and allied disorders.* New York: Oxford University Press, 1947.
19. Lukes RJ, Craver LF, Hall TC, et al. Report of the nomenclature committee. *Cancer Res* 1966;26:1311.
20. Harris NL, Jaffe ES, Stein H, et al. A revised European-American classification of lymphoid neoplasms: a proposal from the International Lymphoma Study Group. *Blood* 1994;84:1361–1392.
21. Harris NL. Hodgkin's disease: classification and differential diagnosis. *Mod Pathol* 1999;12:159–176.
22. Poppema S, Delsol G, Pileri SA, et al. Nodular lymphocyte predominant Hodgkin lymphoma. In: Swerdlow SH, Campo E, Harris NL, et al., eds. *WHO classification of tumours of haemotopoietic and lymphoid tissues*, 4th ed. Lyon: IARC Press, 2008:323–325.
23. Stein H, Delsol G, Pileri SA, et al. Classical Hodgkin lymphoma. In: Swerdlow SH, Campo E, Harris NL, et al., eds. *WHO classification of tumours of haemotopoietic and lymphoid tissues*, 4th ed. Lyon: IARC Press, 2008:326–334.
24. MacLennan KA, Bennett MH, Tu A, et al. Relationship of histopathologic features to survival and relapse in nodular sclerosing Hodgkin's disease: a study of 1659 patients. *Cancer* 1989;64:1686–1693.
25. Wijlhuizen TJ, Vrints LW, Jairam R, et al. Grades of nodular sclerosis (NSI-NSII) in Hodgkin's disease: are they of independent prognostic value? *Cancer* 1989;63:1150–1153.
26. von Wasielewski S, Franklin J, Fischer R, et al. Nodular sclerosing Hodgkin disease: new grading predicts prognosis in intermediate and advanced stages. *Blood* 2003;101:4063–4069.
27. Vassallo J, Lamant L, Brugieres L, et al. ALK-positive anaplastic large cell lymphoma mimicking nodular sclerosis Hodgkin's lymphoma: a report of 10 cases. *Am J Surg Pathol* 2006;30:223–229.
28. Lukes RJ. Criteria for involvement of lymph node, bone marrow, spleen, and liver in Hodgkin's disease. *Cancer Res* 1971;31:1755–1767.
29. Eberle FC, Mani H, Jaffe ES. Histopathology of Hodgkin lymphoma. *Cancer J* 2009;15:129–137.
30. Schnitzer B. Hodgkin lymphoma. *Hematol Oncol Clin North Am* 2009;23:747–768.
31. Butler JJ. Relationship of histological findings to survival in Hodgkin's disease. *Cancer Res* 1971;31:1770–1775.
32. Allemani C, Sant M, De Angelis R, et al. Hodgkin disease survival in Europe and the U.S.: prognostic significance of morphologic groups. *Cancer* 2006;107:352–360.
33. Tindle BH, Parker JW, Lukes RJ. "Reed-Sternberg cells" in infectious mononucleosis? *Am J Clin Pathol* 1972;58:607–617.
34. Strum SB, Park JK, Rappaport H. Observation of cells resembling Sternberg-Reed cells in conditions other than Hodgkin's disease. *Cancer* 1970;26:176–190.
35. von Wasielewski R, Seth S, Franklin J, et al. Tissue eosinophilia correlates strongly with poor prognosis in nodular sclerosing Hodgkin's disease, allowing for known prognostic factors. *Blood* 2000;95:1207–1213.
36. Steidl C, Lee T, Shah SP, et al. Tumor-associated macrophages and survival in classic Hodgkin lymphoma. *N Engl J Med* 2010;363:875–885.
37. Tan KL, Scott DW, Hog F, et al. Tumor-associated macrophages predict inferior outcomes in classic Hodgkin lymphoma: a correlative study from the E2496 Intergroup trial. *Blood* 2012;120:3280–3287.
38. Barry TS, Jaffe ES, Sorbara L, et al. Peripheral T-cell lymphomas expressing CD30 and CD15. *Am J Surg Pathol* 2003;27:1513–1522.
39. Vose J, Armitage J, Weisenburger D. International peripheral T-cell and natural killer/T-cell lymphoma study: pathology findings and clinical outcomes. *J Clin Oncol* 2008;26:4124–4130.
40. Fraga M, García-Rivero A, Sánchez-Verde L, et al. T-cell/histiocyte-rich large B-cell lymphoma is a disseminated aggressive neoplasm: differential diagnosis from Hodgkin's lymphoma. *Histopathology* 2002;41:216–229.
41. Pittaluga S, Jaffe ES. T-cell/histiocyte-rich large B-cell lymphoma. *Haematologica* 2010;95:352–356.

42. Stein H, Foss HD, Dürkop H, et al. CD30+ anaplastic large cell lymphoma: a review of its histopathologic, genetic, and clinical features. *Blood* 2000;96:3681–3695.
43. Jaffe ES, Stein H, Swerdlow SH, et al. B-cell lymphoma, unclassifiable, with features intermediate between diffuse large B-cell lymphoma and classical Hodgkin lymphoma. In: Swerdlow SH, Campo E, Harris NL, et al., eds. *WHO classification of tumours of haemotopoietic and lymphoid tissues*, 4th ed. Lyon: IARC Press, 2008:267–268.
44. Traverse-Glehen A, Pittaluga S, Gaulard P, et al. Mediastinal gray zone lymphoma: the missing link between classic Hodgkin's lymphoma and mediastinal large B-cell lymphoma. *Am J Surg Pathol* 2005;29:1411–1421.
45. Rüdiger T, Ott G, Ott MM, et al. Differential diagnosis between classic Hodgkin's lymphoma, T-cell-rich B-cell lymphoma, and paragranuloma by paraffin immunohistochemistry. *Am J Surg Pathol* 1998;22:1184–1191.
46. Bakshi NA, Finn WG, Schnitzer B, et al. Fascin expression in diffuse large B cell lymphoma, anaplastic large cell lymphoma, and classical Hodgkin lymphoma. *Arch Pathol Lab Med* 2007;131:742–747.
47. Stein H, Marafioti T, Foss HD, et al. Down-regulation of BOB.1/OBF.1 and Oct2 in classical Hodgkin disease but not in lymphocyte predominant Hodgkin disease correlates with immunoglobulin transcription. *Blood* 2001;97:496–501.
48. von Wasielewski R, Mengel M, Fischer R, et al. Classic Hodgkin's disease: clinical impact of the immunophenotype. *Am J Pathol* 1997;151:1123–1130.
49. Portlock CS, Donnelly GB, Qin J, et al. Adverse prognostic significance of CD20 positive Reed-Sternberg cells in classical Hodgkin's disease. *Br J Haematol* 2004;125:701–708.
50. Sup SJ, Alemañy CA, Pohlman B, et al. Expression of bcl-2 in classical Hodgkin's lymphoma: an independent predictor of poor outcome. *J Clin Oncol* 2005;23:3773–3779.
51. Muenst S, Hoeller S, Dirnhofer S, et al. Increased programmed death-1+ tumor-infiltrating lymphocytes in classical Hodgkin lymphoma substantiate reduced overall survival. *Hum Pathol* 2009;40:1715–1722.
52. Hsi E, Sup SJ, Alemany C, et al. MAL is expressed in a subset of Hodgkin lymphoma and identifies a population of patients with poor prognosis. *Am J Clin Pathol* 2006;125:776–782.
53. Diepstra A, van Imhoff GW, Schaapveld M, et al. Latent Epstein-Barr virus infection of tumor cells in classical Hodgkin lymphoma predicts adverse outcome in older adult patients. *J Clin Oncol* 2009;27:3815–3821.
54. Koreishi AF, Saenz AJ, Persky DO, et al. The role of cytoxic regulatory T cells in relapsed/refractory Hodgkin lymphoma. *Appl Immunohistochem Mol Morphol* 2010;18:206–211.
55. Medeiros LJ, Greiner TC. Hodgkin's disease. *Cancer* 1995;75:357–369.
56. Surveillance Epidemiology and End Results (SEER) Program Howlander N, Noone AM, Krapcho M, et al., eds. *SEER Cancer Statistics Review 1975–2008*. Bethesda: National Cancer Institute, based on November 2010 SEER data submission, posted to the SEER web site (www.seer.cancer.gov), 2011.
57. Siegel R, Naishadham D, Jemal A. Cancer statistics, 2012. *CA Cancer J Clin* 2012;62:10–29.
58. Morton LM, Wang SS, Devesa SS, et al. Lymphoma incidence patterns by WHO subtype in the Unites States, 1992–2001. *Blood* 2006;107:265–276.
59. Sant M, Allemani C, Tereanu C, et al. Incidence of hematologic malignancies in Europe by morphologic subtype: results of the HAEMCARE project. *Blood* 2010;116:3724–3734.
60. Hu E, Hufford S, Lukes R, et al. Third-world Hodgkin's disease at Los Angeles County-University of Southern California Medical Center. *J Clin Oncol* 1988;6:1285–1292.
61. Macfarlane GJ, Evstifeeva T, Boyle P, et al. International patterns in the occurrence of Hodgkin's disease in children and young adult males. *Int J Cancer* 1995;61:165–169.
62. Cader FZ, Kearns P, Young L, et al. The contribution of the Epstein-Barr virus to the pathogenesis of childhood lymphomas. *Cancer Treat Rev* 2010;36:348–353.
63. Biggar RJ, Jaffe ES, Goedert JJ, et al. Hodgkin lymphoma and immunodeficiency in persons with HIV/AIDS. *Blood* 2006;108:3786–3791.
64. Glaser SL, Clarke CA, Gulley ML, et al. Population-based patterns of human immunodeficiency virus-related Hodgkin lymphoma in the greater San Francisco Bay area, 1988–1998. *Cancer* 2003;98:300–309.
65. Dunleavy K, Wilson WH. How I treat HIV-associated lymphoma. *Blood* 2012;119:3245–3255.
66. Brenner H, Gondos A, Pulte D. Ongoing improvement in long-term survival of patients with Hodgkin disease at all ages and recent catch-up of older patients. *Blood* 2008;111:2977–2983.
67. Regula DP Jr, Hoppe RT, Weiss LM. Nodular and diffuse types of lymphocyte predominance Hodgkin's disease. *N Engl J Med* 1988;318:214–219.
68. Nogová L, Reineke T, Brillant C, et al. Lymphocyte-predominant and classical Hodgkin's lymphoma: a comprehensive analysis from the German Hodgkin Study Group. *J Clin Oncol* 2008;26:434–439.
69. Neiman RS, Rosen PJ, Lukes RJ. Lymphocyte-depletion Hodgkin's disease: a clinicopathological entity. *N Engl J Med* 1973;288:751–754.
70. Klimm B, Franklin J, Stein H, et al. Lymphocyte-depleted classical Hodgkin's lymphoma: a comprehensive analysis from the German Hodgkin Study Group. *J Clin Oncol* 2011;29:3914–3920.
71. Rosenberg SA, Kaplan HS. Evidence for an orderly progression in the spread of Hodgkin's disease. *Cancer Res* 1966;26:1225–1231.
72. Naeim F, Waisman J, Coulson WF. Hodgkin's disease: the significance of vascular invasion. *Cancer* 1974;34:655–662.
73. Strum SB, Hutchison GB, Park JK, et al. Further observations on the biologic significance of vascular invasion in Hodgkin's disease. *Cancer* 1971;27:1–6.
74. Strum SB, Allen LW, Rappaport H. Vascular invasion in Hodgkin's disease: its relationship to involvement of the spleen and other extranodal sites. *Cancer* 1971;28:1329–1334.
75. Lamoureux KB, Jaffe ES, Berard CW, et al. Lack of identifiable vascular invasion in patients with extranodal dissemination of Hodgkin's disease. *Cancer* 1973;31:824–825.
76. Glatstein E, Guernsey JM, Rosenberg SA, et al. The value of laparotomy and splenectomy in the staging of Hodgkin's disease. *Cancer* 1969;24:709–718.
77. Gamble JF, Fuller LM, Martin RG, et al. Influence of staging celiotomy in localized presentations of Hodgkin's disease. *Cancer* 1975;35:817–825.
78. Carbone PP, Kaplan HS, Musshoff K, et al. Report of the committee on Hodgkin's disease staging classification. *Cancer Res* 1971;31:1860–1861.
79. Lister TA, Crowther D, Sutcliffe SB, et al. Report of a committee convened to discuss the evaluation and staging of patients with Hodgkin's disease: Cotswolds meeting. *J Clin Oncol* 1989;7:1630–1636.
80. Hodgson DC, Gilbert ES, Dores GM, et al. Long-term solid cancer risk among 5-year survivors of Hodgkin's lymphoma. *J Clin Oncol* 2007;25:1489–1497.
81. Castellino SM, Geiger AM, Mertens AC, et al. Morbidity and mortality in long-term survivors of Hodgkin lymphoma: a report from the Childhood Cancer Survivor Study. *Blood* 2011;117:1806–1816.
82. Mason DY, Banks PM, Chan J, et al. Nodular lymphocyte predominance Hodgkin's disease: a distinct clinicopathological entity. *Am J Surg Pathol* 1994;18:526–530.
83. Smith LB. Nodular lymphocyte predominant Hodgkin lymphoma: diagnostic pearls and pitfalls. *Arch Pathol Lab Med* 2010;134:1434–1439.
84. Anagnostopoulos I, Hansmann ML, Franssila K, et al. European Task Force project on lymphocyte predominance Hodgkin's disease: histologic and immunohistologic analysis of submitted cases reveals 2 types of Hodgkin's disease with a nodular growth pattern and abundant lymphocytes. *Blood* 2000;96:1889–1899.
85. Hansmann ML, Stein H, Dallenbach F, et al. Diffuse lymphocyte-predominant Hodgkin's disease (diffuse paragranuloma): a variant of the B-cell-derived nodular type. *Am J Pathol* 1991;138:29–36.
86. Butler JJ. The histologic diagnosis of Hodgkin's disease. *Semin Diagn Pathol* 1992;9:252–256.
87. Fan Z, Natkunam Y, Bair E, et al. Characterization of variant patterns of nodular lymphocyte predominant Hodgkin lymphoma with immunohistologic and clinical correlation. *Am J Surg Pathol* 2003;27:1346–1356.
88. Uherova P, Valdez R, Ross CW, et al. Nodular lymphocyte predominant Hodgkin lymphoma: an immunophenotypic reappraisal based on a single-institution experience. *Am J Clin Pathol* 2003;119:192–198.
89. Prakash S, Fountaine T, Raffeld M, et al. IgD positive L&H cells identify a unique subset of nodular lymphocyte predominant Hodgkin lymphoma. *Am J Surg Pathol* 2006;30:585–592.
90. Stoler MH, Nichols GE, Symbula M, et al. Lymphocyte predominance Hodgkin's disease: evidence for a κ light chain-restricted monotypic B-cell neoplasm. *Am J Pathol* 1995;146:812–818.
91. von Wasielewski R, Wilkens L, Nolte M, et al. Light-chain mRNA in lymphocyte-predominant and mixed-cellularity Hodgkin's disease. *Mod Pathol* 1996;9:334–338.
92. Venkataraman G, Raffeld M, Pittaluga S, et al. CD15-expressing nodular lymphocyte predominant Hodgkin lymphoma [Letter]. *Histopathology* 2011;58:803–805.
93. Dorfman DM, Shahsafaei A. CD200 (OX-2 membrane glycoprotein) expression in B-cell derived neoplasms. *Am J Clin Pathol* 2010;134:726–733.
94. Rahemtullah A, Harris NL, Dorn ME, et al. Beyond the lymphocyte predominant cell: CD4+CD8+ T-cells in nodular lymphocyte predominant Hodgkin lymphoma. *Leuk Lymphoma* 2008;49:1870–1878.
95. Kamel OW, Gelb AB, Shibuya RB, et al. Leu 7 (CD57) reactivity distinguishes nodular lymphocyte predominance Hodgkin's disease from nodular sclerosing Hodgkin's disease, T-cell-rich B-cell lymphoma and follicular lymphoma. *Am J Pathol* 1993;142:541–546.
96. Nam-Cha SH, Roncador G, Sanchez-Verde L, et al. PD-1, a follicular T-cell marker useful for recognizing nodular lymphocyte-predominant Hodgkin lymphoma. *Am J Surg Pathol* 2008;32:1252–1257.
97. Churchill HRO, Roncador G, Warnke RA, et al. Programmed death 1 expression in variant immunoarchitectural patterns of nodular lymphocyte predominant Hodgkin lymphoma: comparison with CD57 and lymphomas in the differential diagnosis. *Hum Pathol* 2010;41:1726–1734.
98. Carbone A, Gloghini A. "Intrafollicular neoplasia" of nodular lymphocyte predominant Hodgkin lymphoma: description of a hypothetic early stage of the disease. *Hum Pathol* 2012;43:619–628.
99. Poppema S, Kaiserling E, Lennert K. Hodgkin's disease with lymphocytic predominance, nodular type (nodular paragranuloma) and progressively transformed germinal centres–a cytohistological study. *Histopathology* 1979;3:295–308.
100. Hansmann ML, Fellbaum C, Hui PK, et al. Progressive transformation of germinal centers with and without association to Hodgkin's disease. *Am J Clin Pathol* 1990;93:219–226.
101. Van den Oord JJ, de Wolf-Peeters C, Desmet VJ. Immunohistochemical analysis of progressively transformed follicular centers. *Am J Clin Pathol* 1985;83:560–564.
102. Osborne BM, Butler JJ. Clinical implications of progressive transformation of germinal centers. *Am J Surg Pathol* 1984;8:725–733.
103. Burns BF, Colby TV, Dorfman RF. Differential diagnostic features of nodular L&H Hodgkin's disease, including progressive transformation of germinal centers. *Am J Surg Pathol* 1984;8:253–261.
104. Ferry JA, Zukerberg LR, Harris NL. Florid progressive transformation of germinal centers: a syndrome affecting young men, without early progression to nodular lymphocyte predominance Hodgkin's disease. *Am J Surg Pathol* 1992;16:252–258.
105. Diehl V, Sextro M, Franklin J, et al. Clinical presentation, course, and prognostic factors in lymphocyte-predominant Hodgkin's disease and lymphocyte-rich classic Hodgkin's disease: report from the European Task Force on Lymphoma project on lymphocyte-predominant Hodgkin lymphoma. *J Clin Oncol* 1999;17:776–783.
106. Khoury JD, Jones D, Yared MA, et al. Bone marrow involvement in patients with nodular lymphocyte predominant Hodgkin lymphoma. *Am J Surg Pathol* 2004;28:489–495.
107. Chang KL, Kamel OW, Arber DA, et al. Pathologic features of nodular lymphocyte predominance Hodgkin's disease in extranodal sites. *Am J Surg Pathol* 1995;19:1313–1324.
108. Siebert JD, Stuckey JH, Kurtin PJ, et al. Extranodal lymphocyte predominance Hodgkin's disease: clinical and pathologic features. *Am J Clin Pathol* 1995;103:485–491.
109. Regula DP Jr, Weiss LM, Warnke RA, et al. Lymphocyte predominance Hodgkin's disease: a reappraisal based upon histological and immunophenotypical findings in relapsing cases. *Histopathology* 1987;11:1107–1120.
110. Eichenauer DA, Fuchs M, Pluetschow A, et al. Phase 2 study of rituximab in newly diagnosed stage IA nodular lymphocyte-predominant Hodgkin lymphoma: a report from the German Hodgkin Study Group. *Blood* 2011;118:4363–4365.
111. Pellegrino MJ, Terrier-Lacombe MJ, Oberlin O, et al. Lymphocyte-predominant Hodgkin's lymphoma in children: therapeutic abstention after initial lymph node resection–a study of the French Society of Pediatric Oncology. *J Clin Oncol* 2003;21:2948–2952.
112. Strum SB, Rappaport H. Interrelations of the histologic types of Hodgkin's disease. *Arch Pathol* 1971;91:127–134.

113. Gelb AB, Dorfman RF, Warnke RA. Coexistence of nodular lymphocyte predominance Hodgkin's disease and Hodgkin's disease of the usual type. *Am J Surg Pathol* 1993;17:364–374.
114. Song JY, Eberle FC, Xi L, et al. Coexisting and clonally identical classic Hodgkin lymphoma and nodular lymphocyte predominant Hodgkin lymphoma. *Am J Surg Pathol* 2011;35;767–772.
115. Miettinen M, Franssila KO, Saxen E. Hodgkin's disease, lymphocytic predominance nodular: increased risk for subsequent non-Hodgkin lymphomas. *Cancer* 1983;51:2293–2300.
116. Sundeen JT, Cossman J, Jaffe ES. Lymphocyte predominant Hodgkin's disease nodular subtype with coexistent "large cell lymphoma": histological progression or composite malignancy? *Am J Surg Pathol* 1988;12:599–606.
117. Hansmann ML, Stein H, Fellbaum C, et al. Nodular paragranuloma can transform into high-grade malignant lymphoma of B type. *Hum Pathol* 1989;20: 1169–1175.
118. Huang JZ, Weisenburger DD, Vose JM, et al. Diffuse large B-cell lymphoma arising in nodular lymphocyte predominant Hodgkin lymphoma. A report of 21 cases from the Nebraska Lymphoma Study Group. *Leuk Lymphoma* 2003;44:1903–1910.
119. Al-Mansour M, Connors JM, Gascoyne RD, et al. Transformation to aggressive lymphoma in nodular lymphocyte-predominant Hodgkin's lymphoma. *J Clin Oncol* 2010;28:793–799.
120. Cotta CV, Coleman JF, Li S, et al. Nodular lymphocyte predominant Hodgkin lymphoma and diffuse large B-cell lymphoma: a study of six cases concurrently involving the same site. *Histopathology* 2011;59:1194–1203.
121. Greiner TC, Gascoyne RD, Anderson ME, et al. Nodular lymphocyte-predominant Hodgkin's disease associated with large-cell lymphoma: analysis of Ig gene rearrangements by V-J polymerase chain reaction. *Blood* 1996;88:657–666.
122. Boudová L, Torlakovic E, Delabie J, et al. Nodular lymphocyte-predominant Hodgkin lymphoma with nodules resembling T-cell/histiocyte-rich B-cell lymphoma: differential diagnosis between nodular lymphocyte-predominant Hodgkin lymphoma and T-cell/histiocyte rich B-cell lymphoma. *Blood* 2003;102: 3753–3758.
123. Drakos E, Rassidakis GZ, Leventaki V, et al. Nodular lymphocyte predominant Hodgkin lymphoma with clusters of LP cells, acute inflammation, and fibrosis; a syncytial variant. *Am J Surg Pathol* 2009;33:1725–1731.
124. Wickert RS, Weisenburger DD, Tierens A, et al. Clonal relationship between lymphocytic predominance Hodgkin's disease and concurrent or subsequent large-cell lymphoma of B lineage. *Blood* 1995;86:2312–2320.
125. Hell K, Hansmann ML, Pringle JH, et al. Combination of Hodgkin's disease and diffuse large cell lymphoma: an in situ hybridization study for immunoglobulin light chain messenger RNA. *Histopathology* 1995;27:491–499.
126. Ohno T, Huang JZ, Wu G, et al. The tumor cells in nodular lymphocyte-predominant Hodgkin disease are clonally related to the large cell lymphoma occurring in the same individual: direct demonstration by single cell analysis. *Am J Clin Pathol* 2001;116:506–511.
127. Delabie J, Greiner TC, Chan WC, et al. Concurrent lymphocyte predominance Hodgkin's disease and T-cell lymphoma: a report of three cases. *Am J Surg Pathol* 1996;20:355–362.
128. Arevalo A, Caponetti GC, Hu Q, et al. Cytotoxic peripheral T cell lymphoma arising in a patient with nodular lymphocyte predominant Hodgkin lymphoma: a case report. *J Hematop* 2010;3:23–28.
129. Sohani AR, Jaffe ES, Harris NL, et al. Nodular lymphocyte-predominant Hodgkin lymphoma with atypical T cells: a morphologic variant mimicking peripheral T-cell lymphoma. *Am J Surg Pathol* 2011;35:1666–1678.
130. Nguyen PL, Ferry JA, Harris NL. Progressive transformation of germinal centers and nodular lymphocyte predominance Hodgkin's disease: a comparative immunohistochemical study. *Am J Surg Pathol* 1999;23:27–33.
131. Achten R, Verhoef G, Vanuytsel L, et al. Histiocyte-rich, T-cell-rich B-cell lymphoma: a distinct diffuse large B-cell lymphoma subtype showing characteristic morphologic and immunophenotypic features. *Histopathology* 2002;40:31–45.
132. Lim MS, Beaty M, Sorbara L, et al. T-cell/histiocyte-rich large B-cell lymphoma: a heterogeneous entity with derivation from germinal center B cells. *Am J Surg Pathol* 2002;26:1458–1466.
133. Ripp JA, Loiue DC, Chan W, et al. T-cell rich B-cell lymphoma: clinical distinctiveness and response to treatment in 45 patients. *Leuk Lymphoma* 2002;43:1573–1580.
134. Bouabdallah R, Mounier N, Guettier C, et al. T-cell/histiocyte-rich large B-cell lymphomas and classical diffuse large B-cell lymphomas have similar outcome after chemotherapy: a matched-control analysis. *J Clin Oncol* 2003;21: 1271–1277.
135. Ashton-Key M, Thorpe PA, Allen JP, et al. Follicular Hodgkin's disease. *Am J Surg Pathol* 1995;19:1294–1299.
136. Kansal R, Singleton TP, Ross CW, et al. Follicular Hodgkin lymphoma: a histopathologic study. *Am J Clin Pathol* 2002;117:29–35.
137. Bhargava P, Pantanowitz L, Pinkus GS, et al. Utility of fascin and JunB in distinguishing nodular lymphocyte predominant from classical lymphocyte-rich Hodgkin lymphoma. *Appl Immunohistochem Mol Morphol* 2010;18:16–23.
138. Nam-Cha SH, Montes-Moreno S, Salcedo MT, et al. Lymphocyte-rich classical Hodgkin lymphoma: distinctive tumor and microenvironment markers. *Mod Pathol* 2009;22:1006–1015.
139. von Wasielewski R, Werner M, Fischer R, et al. Lymphocyte-predominant Hodgkin lymphoma: an immunohistochemical analysis of 208 reviewed Hodgkin's disease cases from the German Hodgkin Study Group. *Am J Pathol* 1997;150:793–803.
140. Shimabukuro-Vornhagan A, Haverkamp H, Engert A, et al. Lymphocyte-rich classical Hodgkin's lymphoma: clinical presentation and treatment outcome in 100 patients treated within German Hodgkin's Study Group trials. *J Clin Oncol* 2005;23:5739–5745.
141. de Jong D, Bosq J, MacLennan KA, et al. Lymphocyte-rich classical Hodgkin lymphoma (LRCHL): clinico-pathological characteristics and outcome of a rare entity. *Ann Oncol* 2006;17:141–145.
142. Patsouris E, Noel H, Lennert K. Lymphoplasmacytic/lymphoplasmacytoid immunocytoma with a high content of epithelioid cells: histologic and immunohistochemical findings. *Am J Surg Pathol* 1990;14:660–670.
143. Sargent RL, Cook JR, Aguilera NI, et al. Fluorescence immunophenotypic and interphase cytogenetic characterization of nodal lymphoplasmacytic lymphoma. *Am J Surg Pathol* 2008;32:1643–1653.
144. Hartmann S, Agostinelli C, Klapper W, et al. Revising the historical collection of epithelioid cell-rich lymphomas of the Kiel Lymph Node Registry: what is Lennert's lymphoma nowadays? *Histopathology* 2011;59:1173–1182.
145. Shin SS, Ben-Ezra J, Burke JS, et al. Reed-Sternberg-like cells in low-grade lymphomas are transformed neoplastic cells of B-cell lineage. *Am J Clin Pathol* 1993;99:658–662.
146. Brecher M, Banks PM. Hodgkin's disease variant of Richter's syndrome: report of eight cases. *Am J Clin Pathol* 1990;93:333–339.
147. Williams J, Schned A, Cotelingam JD, et al. Chronic lymphocytic leukemia with coexistent Hodgkin's disease: implications for the origin of the Reed-Sternberg cell. *Am J Surg Pathol* 1991;15:33–42.
148. Weisenberg E, Anastasi J, Adeyanju M, et al. Hodgkin's disease associated with chronic lymphocytic leukemia: eight additional cases, including two of the nodular lymphocyte predominant type. *Am J Clin Pathol* 1995;103:479–484.
149. Tsimberidou AM, O'Brien S, Kantarjian HM, et al. Hodgkin transformation of chronic lymphocytic leukemia: the M. D. Anderson Cancer Center experience. *Cancer* 2006;107:1294–1302.
150. Rosales CM, Lin P, Mansoor A, et al. Lymphoplasmacytic lymphoma/Waldenström macroglobulinemia associated with Hodgkin disease: a report of two cases. *Am J Clin Pathol* 2001;116:34–40.
151. Momose H, Jaffe ES, Shin SS, et al. Chronic lymphocytic leukemia/small lymphocytic lymphoma with Reed-Sternberg-like cells and possible transformation to Hodgkin's disease: mediation by Epstein-Barr virus. *Am J Surg Pathol* 1992;16:859–867.
152. Ohno T, Smir BN, Weisenburger DD, et al. Origin of the Hodgkin/Reed-Sternberg cells in chronic lymphocytic leukemia with "Hodgkin transformation." *Blood* 1998;91:1757–1761.
153. Kanzler H, Küppers R, Helmes S, et al. Hodgkin and Reed-Sternberg–like cells in B-cell chronic lymphocytic leukemia represent the outgrowth of single germinal-center B-cell–derived clones: potential precursors of Hodgkin and Reed-Sternberg cells in Hodgkin's disease. *Blood* 2000;96:1023–1031.
154. de Leval L, Vivario M, De Prijck B, et al. Distinct clonal origin in two cases of Hodgkin's lymphoma variant of Richter's syndrome associated with EBV infection. *Am J Surg Pathol* 2004;28:679–686.
155. Mao Z, Quintanilla-Martinez L, Raffeld M, et al. IgVH mutational status and clonality analysis of Richter's transformation: diffuse large B-cell lymphoma and Hodgkin lymphoma in association with B-cell chronic lymphocytic leukemia (B-CLL) represent 2 different pathways of disease evolution. *Am J Surg Pathol* 2007;31:1605–1614.
156. Fong D, Spizzo G, Gastl G, Tzankov A. Hodgkin's disease variant of Richter's syndrome in chronic lymphocytic leukaemia patients previously treated with fludarabine. *Br J Haematol* 2005;129:199–205.
157. Bayerl MG, Bentley G, Bellan C, et al. Lacunar and Reed-Sternberg-like cells in follicular lymphomas are clonally related to the centrocytic and centroblastic cells as demonstrated by laser capture microdissection. *Am J Clin Pathol* 2004;122:858–864.
157a. Moroch J, Copie-Bergman C, de Leval L, et al. Follicular peripheral T-cell lymphoma expands the spectrum of classical Hodgkin lymphoma mimics. *Am J Surg Pathol* 2012;36:1636–1646.
157b. Nicolae A, Pittaluga S, Venkataraman G, et al. Peripheral T-cell lymphomas of follicular T-helper cell derivation with Hodgkin/Reed-Sternberg cells of B-cell lineage: both EBV-positive and EBV-negative variants exist. *Am J Surg Pathol* 2013;37:816–826.
158. Colby TV, Hoppe RT, Warnke RA. Hodgkin's disease: a clinicopathologic study of 659 cases. *Cancer* 1982;49:1848–1858.
159. Ohshima K, Akaiwa M, Umeshita R, et al. Interleukin-13 and interleukin-13 receptor in Hodgkin's disease: possible autocrine mechanism and involvement in fibrosis. *Histopathology* 2001;38:368–375.
160. Birgersdotter A, Baumforth KRN, Porwit A, et al. Inflammation and tissue repair markers distinguish the nodular sclerosis and mixed cellularity subtypes of classical Hodgkin's lymphoma. *Br J Cancer* 2009;101:1393–1401.
161. Birgersdotter A, Baumforth KRN, Wei W, et al. Connective tissue growth factor is expressed in malignant cells of Hodgkin lymphoma but not in other mature B-cell lymphomas. *Am J Clin Pathol* 2010;133:271–280.
162. Variakojis D, Strum SB, Rappaport H. The foamy macrophages in Hodgkin's disease. *Arch Pathol* 1972;93:453–456.
163. Kadin ME, Glatstein E, Dorfman RF. Clinicopathologic studies of 117 untreated patients subjected to laparotomy for the staging of Hodgkin's disease. *Cancer* 1971;27:1277–1294.
164. Rappaport H, Berard CW, Butler JJ, et al. Report of the committee on histopathological criteria contributing to staging of Hodgkin's disease. *Cancer Res* 1971;31:1864–1865.
165. Strum SB, Rappaport H. Significance of focal involvement of lymph nodes for the diagnosis and staging of Hodgkin's disease. *Cancer* 1970;25:1314–1319.
166. Doggett RS, Colby TV, Dorfman RF. Interfollicular Hodgkin's disease. *Am J Surg Pathol* 1983;7:145–149.
167. Mohrmann RL, Nathwani BN, Brynes RK, et al. Hodgkin's disease occurring in monocytoid B-cell clusters. *Am J Clin Pathol* 1991;95:802–808.
168. Ohsawa M, Kanno H, Naka N, et al. Occurrence of monocytoid B-lymphocytes in Hodgkin's disease. *Mod Pathol* 1994;7:540–543.
169. Haybittle JL, Hayhoe FGJ, Easterling MJ, et al. Review of British National Lymphoma Investigation studies of Hodgkin's disease and development of prognostic index. *Lancet* 1985;1:967–972.
170. Ferry JA, Linggood RM, Convery KM, et al. Hodgkin's disease, nodular sclerosis type: implications of histologic subclassification. *Cancer* 1993;71:457–463.
171. Masih AS, Weisenburger DD, Vose JM, et al. Histologic grade does not predict prognosis in optimally treated, advanced-stage nodular sclerosing Hodgkin's disease. *Cancer* 1992;69:228–232.
172. d'Amore ESG, Lee CKK, Aeppli DM, et al. Lack of prognostic value of histopathologic parameters in Hodgkin's disease, nodular sclerosis type: a study of 123 patients with limited stage lymphoma who had undergone laparotomy and were treated with radiation therapy. *Arch Pathol Lab Med* 1992;116:856–861.
173. Hess JL, Bodis S, Pinkus G, et al. Histopathologic grading of nodular sclerosis Hodgkin's disease: lack of prognostic significance in 254 surgically staged patients. *Cancer* 1994;74:708–714.
174. Strickler JG, Michie SA, Warnke RA, et al. The "syncytial variant" of nodular sclerosing Hodgkin's disease. *Am J Surg Pathol* 1986;10:470–477.
175. Bacchi CE, Dorfman RF, Hoppe RT, et al. Metastatic carcinoma in lymph nodes simulating "syncytial variant" of nodular sclerosing Hodgkin's disease. *Am J Clin Pathol* 1991;96:589–593.
176. Zarate-Osorno A, Jaffe ES, Medeiros LJ. Metastatic nasopharyngeal carcinoma initially presenting as cervical lymphadenopathy: a report of two cases that resembled Hodgkin's disease. *Arch Pathol Lab Med* 1992;116:862–865.

177. Khalidi HS, Singleton TP, Weiss SW. Inflammatory malignant fibrous histiocytoma: distinction from Hodgkin's disease and non-Hodgkin lymphoma by a panel of leukocyte markers. *Mod Pathol* 1997;10:438–442.
178. Montgomery EA, Devaney KO, Giordano TJ, et al. Inflammatory myxohyaline tumor of distal extremities with virocyte or Reed-Sternberg-like cells: a distinctive lesion with features simulating inflammatory conditions, Hodgkin's disease, and various sarcomas. *Mod Pathol* 1998;11:384–391.
179. Cazals-Hatem D, Lepage E, Brice P, et al. Primary mediastinal large B-cell lymphoma: a clinicopathologic study of 141 cases compared with 916 nonmediastinal large B-cell lymphomas, a GELA ("Groupe d'Etude des Lymphomes de l'Adulte") study. *Am J Surg Pathol* 1996;20:877–888.
180. Paulli M, Sträter J, Gianelli U, et al. Mediastinal B-cell lymphoma: a study of its histomorphologic spectrum based on 109 cases. *Hum Pathol* 1999;30:178–187.
181. Pileri SA, Gaidano G, Zinzani PL, et al. Primary mediastinal B-cell lymphoma: high frequency of bcl-6 mutations and consistent expression of the transcription factors OCT-2, BOB.1 and PU.1in the absence of immunoglobulins. *Am J Pathol* 2003;162:243–253.
182. Higgins JP, Warnke RA. CD30 expression is common in mediastinal large B-cell lymphoma. *Am J Clin Pathol* 1999;112:241–247.
183. Hoeller S, Zihler D, Zlobec I, et al. BOB.1, CD79a and cyclin E are the most appropriate markers to discriminate classical Hodgkin lymphoma from primary mediastinal large B-cell lymphoma. *Histopathology* 2010;56:217–228.
184. Miles RR, Mankey CC, Seiler CE, et al. Expression of Grb2 distinguishes classical Hodgkin lymphomas from primary mediastinal B-cell lymphomas and other diffuse large B-cell lymphomas. *Hum Pathol* 2009;40:1731–1737.
185. Tapia G, Sanz C, Mate JL, et al. Improved clonality detection in Hodgkin lymphoma using the BIOMED-2-based heavy and kappa chain assay: a paraffin-embedded tissue study. *Histopathology* 2012;60:768–773.
186. Rosenwald A, Wright G, Leroy K, et al. Molecular diagnosis of primary mediastinal B cell lymphoma identifies a clinically favorable subgroup of diffuse large B cell lymphoma related to Hodgkin lymphoma. *J Exp Med* 2003;198:851–862.
187. Savage KJ, Monti S, Kutok JL, et al. The molecular signature of mediastinal large B-cell lymphoma differs from that of other diffuse large B-cell lymphomas and shares features with classical Hodgkin lymphoma. *Blood* 2003;102:3871–3879.
188. Kondratiev S, Duraisamy S, Unitt CL, et al. Aberrant expression of the dendritic cell marker TNFAIP2 by the malignant cells of Hodgkin lymphoma and primary mediastinal large B-cell lymphoma distinguishes these tumor types from morphologically and phenotypically similar lymphomas. *Am J Surg Pathol* 2011;35:1531–1539.
189. Quintanilla-Martinez L, de Jong D, de Mascarel A, et al. Gray zones around diffuse large B cell lymphoma. Conclusions based on the workshop of the XIV meeting of the European Association for Hematopathology and the Society of Hematopathology in Bordeaux, France. *J Hematopathol* 2009;2:211–236.
190. García JF, Mollejo M, Fraga M, et al. Large B-cell lymphoma with Hodgkin's features. *Histopathology* 2005;47:101–110.
191. Eberle FC, Salaverria I, Steidl C, et al. Gray zone lymphoma: chromosomal aberrations with immunophenotypic and clinical correlations. *Mod Pathol* 2011;24:1586–1597.
192. Gualco G, Natkunam Y, Bacchi CE. The spectrum of B-cell lymphoma, unclassifiable, with features intermediate between diffuse large B-cell lymphoma and classical Hodgkin lymphoma: a description of 10 cases. *Mod Pathol* 2012;25:661–674.
193. Copie-Bergman C, Plonquet A, Alonso MA, et al. MAL expression in lymphoid cells: further evidence for MAL as a distinct molecular marker of primary mediastinal large B-cell lymphomas. *Mod Pathol* 2002;15:1172–1180.
194. Campo E, Swerdlow SH, Harris NL, et al. The 2008 WHO classification of lymphoid neoplasms and beyond: evolving concepts and practical applications. *Blood* 2011;117:5019–5032.
195. Gonzalez CL, Medeiros LJ, Jaffe ES. Composite lymphoma: a clinicopathologic analysis of nine patients with Hodgkin's disease and B-cell non-Hodgkin lymphoma. *Am J Clin Pathol* 1991;96:81–89.
196. Caleo A, Sánchez-Aguilera A, Rodríguez S, et al. Composite Hodgkin lymphoma and mantle cell lymphoma: two clonally unrelated tumors. *Am J Surg Pathol* 2003;27:1577–1580.
197. Zettl A, Rüdiger T, Marx A, et al. Composite marginal zone B-cell lymphoma and classical Hodgkin's lymphoma: a clinicopathological study of 12 cases. *Histopathology* 2005;46:217–228.
198. Huang Q, Wilczynski SP, Chang KL, et al. Composite recurrent Hodgkin lymphoma and diffuse large B-cell lymphoma: one clone, two faces. *Am J Clin Pathol* 2006;126:222–229.
199. Zarate-Osorno A, Medeiros LJ, Kingma DW, et al. Hodgkin's disease following non-Hodgkin lymphoma: a clinicopathologic and immunophenotypic study of nine cases. *Am J Surg Pathol* 1993;17:123–132.
200. Travis LB, Gonzalez CL, Hankey BF, et al. Hodgkin's disease following non-Hodgkin lymphoma. *Cancer* 1992;69:2337–2342.
201. Chan WC, Griem ML, Grozea PN, et al. Mycosis fungoides and Hodgkin's disease occurring in the same patient: report of three cases. *Cancer* 1979;44:1408–1413.
202. Davis TH, Morton CC, Miller-Cassman R, et al. Hodgkin's disease, lymphomatoid papulosis, and cutaneous T-cell lymphoma derived from a common T-cell clone. *N Engl J Med* 1992;326:1115–1122.
203. Brown JR, Weng AP, Freedman AS. Hodgkin disease associated with T-cell non-Hodgkin lymphomas: case reports and review of the literature. *Am J Clin Pathol* 2004;121:701–708.
204. Eberle FC, Song JY, Xi L, et al. Nodal involvement by cutaneous CD30-positive T-cell lymphoma mimicking classical Hodgkin lymphoma. *Am J Surg Pathol* 2012;36:716–725.
205. Glaser SL, Lin RJ, Stewart SL, et al. Epstein-Barr virus-associated Hodgkin's disease: epidemiologic characteristics in international data. *Int J Cancer* 1997;70:375–382.
206. Krishnan C, Warnke RA, Arber DA, et al. PD-1 expression in T-cell lymphomas and reactive lymphoid entities: potential overlap in staining patterns between lymphoma and viral lymphadenitis. *Am J Surg Pathol* 2010;34:178–189.
207. Yu H, Shahsafaei A, Dorfman DM. Germinal-center T-helper-cell markers PD-1 and CXCL13 are both expressed by neoplastic cells in angioimmunoblastic T-cell lymphoma. *Am J Clin Pathol* 2009;131:33–41.
208. Dogan A, Attygalle AD, Kyriakou C. Angioimmunoblastic T-cell lymphoma. *Br J Haematol* 2003;121:681–691.
209. de Leval L, Rickman DS, Thielen C, et al. The gene expression profile of nodal peripheral T-cell lymphoma demonstrates a molecular link between angioimmunoblastic T-cell lymphoma (AITL) and follicular helper T (T_{FH}) cells. *Blood* 2007;109:4952–4963.
210. Patsouris E, Noel H, Lennert K. Histological and immunohistological findings in lymphoepithelioid cell lymphoma (Lennert's lymphoma). *Am J Surg Pathol* 1988;12:341–350.
211. Patsouris E, Noel H, Lennert K. Cytohistologic and immunohistochemical findings in Hodgkin's disease, mixed cellularity type, with a high content of epithelioid cells. *Am J Surg Pathol* 1989;13:1014–1022.
212. Weisenburger DD, Savage KJ, Harris NL, et al. Peripheral T-cell lymphoma, not otherwise specified: a report of 340 cases from the International Peripheral T-cell Lymphoma Project. *Blood* 2011;117:3402–3408.
213. Sheibani K, Battifora H, Burke JS, et al. Leu-M1 antigen in human neoplasms: an immunohistologic study of 400 cases. *Am J Surg Pathol* 1986;10:227–236.
214. Benharroch D, Levy A, Gopas J, et al. Lymphocyte-depleted classic Hodgkin lymphoma–a neglected entity? *Virchows Arch* 2008;453:611–616.
215. Slack GW, Ferry JA, Hasserjian RP, et al. Lymphocyte depleted Hodgkin lymphoma: an evaluation with immunophenotyping and genetic analysis. *Leuk Lymphoma* 2009;50:937–94.
216. Greer JP, Kinney MC, Cousar JB, et al. Lymphocyte-depleted Hodgkin's disease: clinicopathologic review of 25 patients. *Am J Med* 1986;81:208–214.
217. Kant JA, Hubbard SM, Longo DL, et al. The pathologic and clinical heterogeneity of lymphocyte-depleted Hodgkin's disease. *J Clin Oncol* 1986;4:284–294.
218. Benharroch D, Meguerian-Bedoyan Z, Lamant L, et al. ALK-positive lymphoma: a single disease with a broad spectrum of morphology. *Blood* 1998;91:2076–2084.
219. Inghirami G, Pileri SA. European T-cell lymphoma study group. Anaplastic large-cell lymphoma. *Semin Diagn Pathol* 2011;28:190–201.
220. Stein H, Johrens K, Anagnostopoulos I. Non-mediastinal grey zone lymphomas and report from the workshop. *Eur J Haematol* 2005;75(Suppl 66):42–44.
221. Feldman AL, Law ME, Inwards DJ, et al. PAX5-positive T-cell anaplastic large cell lymphomas associated with extra copies of the *PAX5* gene locus. *Mod Pathol* 2010;23:593–602.
222. Nascimento AF, Pinkus JL, Pinkus GS. Clusterin, a marker for anaplastic large cell lymphoma immunohistochemical profile in hematopoietic and nonhematopoietic malignant neoplasms. *Am J Clin Pathol* 2004;121:709–717.
223. Gualco G, Weiss LM, Bacchi CE. Expression of p63 in anaplastic large cell lymphoma but not in classical Hodgkin's lymphoma. *Hum Pathol* 2008;39:1505–1510.
224 Buxton D, Bacchi CE, Gualco G, et al. Frequent expression of CD99 in anaplastic large cell lymphoma: a clinicopathologic and immunohistochemical study of 160 cases. *Am J Clin Pathol* 2009;131:574–579.
225. Adam P, Bonzheim I, Fend F, et al. Epstein-Barr-positive diffuse large B-cell lymphomas of the elderly. *Adv Anat Pathol* 2011;18:349–355.
226. Asano N, Yamamoto K, Tamaru JI, et al. Age-related Epstein-Barr virus (EBV)–associated B-cell lymphoproliferative disorders: comparison with EBV-positive classic Hodgkin lymphoma in elderly patients. *Blood* 2009;113:2629–2636.
227. Hwang YY, Leung AYH, Lau WH, et al. Synchronous Epstein-Barr virus-positive diffuse large B-cell lymphoma of the elderly and Epstein-Barr virus-positive classical Hodgkin lymphoma [Letter]. *Histopathology* 2011;59:352–355.
228. Howell SJ, Grey M, Chang J, et al. The value of bone marrow examination in the staging of Hodgkin's lymphoma: a review of 955 cases seen in a regional cancer centre. *Br J Haematol* 2002;119:408–411.
229. Zhang QY, Foucar K. Bone marrow involvement by Hodgkin and non-Hodgkin lymphoma. *Hematol Oncol Clin North Am* 2009;23:873–902.
230. Te Velde J, Den Ottolander GJ, Spaander PJ, et al. The bone marrow in Hodgkin's disease: the non-involved marrow. *Histopathology* 1978;2:31–46.
231. Dich NH, Goodman ZD, Klein MA. Hepatic involvement in Hodgkin's disease: clues to histologic diagnosis. *Cancer* 1989;64:2121–2126.
232. Burke JS. The spleen. In: Mills SE, Carter D, Greenson JK, et al., eds. *Sternberg's diagnostic surgical pathology*, 5th ed. Philadelphia: Lippincott Williams & Wilkins, 2010:745–771.
233. Sacks EL, Donaldson SS, Gordon J, et al. Epithelioid granulomas associated with Hodgkin lymphoma: clinical correlations in 55 previously untreated patients. *Cancer* 1978;41:562–567.
234. Hodgson DC, Tsang RW, Pintillie M, et al. Impact of chest wall and lung invasion on outcome of stage I–II Hodgkin's lymphoma after combined modality therapy. *Int J Radiat Oncol Biol Phys* 2003;57:1374–1381.
235. Yousem SA, Weiss LM, Colby TV. Primary pulmonary Hodgkin's disease: a clinicopathologic study of 15 cases. *Cancer* 1986;57:1217–1224.
236. Costa MBG, Siqueira SAC, Saldiva PHN, et al. Histologic patterns of lung infiltration of B-cell, T-cell, and Hodgkin lymphomas. *Am J Clin Pathol* 2004;121:718–726.
237. Sapozink MD, Kaplan HS. Intracranial Hodgkin's disease: a report of 12 cases and review of the literature. *Cancer* 1983;52:1301–1307.
238. Gerstner ER, Abrey LE, Schiff D, et al. CNS Hodgkin lymphoma. *Blood* 2008;112:1658–1661.
239. Gupta V, Srivastava A, Bhatia B. Hodgkin disease with spinal cord compression. *J Pediatr Hematol Oncol* 2009;31:771–773.
240. Smith JL Jr, Butler JJ. Skin involvement in Hodgkin's disease. *Cancer* 1980;45:354–361.
241. Dojcinov SD, Venkataraman G, Raffeld M, et al. EBV positive mucocutaneous ulcer—a study of 26 cases associated with various sources of immunosuppression. *Am J Surg Pathol* 2010;34;405–417.
242. Meis JM, Butler JJ, Osborne BM. Hodgkin's disease involving the breast and chest wall. *Cancer* 1986;57:1859–1865.
243. Kumar S, Fend F, Quintanilla-Martinez L, et al. Epstein-Barr virus–positive primary gastrointestinal Hodgkin's disease: association with inflammatory bowel disease and immunosuppression. *Am J Surg Pathol* 2000;24:66–73.
244. Vasiliu V, Suarez F, Canioni D, et al. Anorectal Epstein-Barr virus infection mimicking Hodgkin lymphoma in an immunocompetent man. *Am J Surg Pathol* 2010;34:1715–1719.
245. Perez MT, Cabello-Inchausti B, Castellano-Sanchez A, et al. Primary gastroesophageal-ileal Hodgkin lymphoma: a case report and review of the literature. *Arch Pathol Lab Med* 2002;126:1534–1537.
246. Venizelos I, Tamiolakis D, Bolioti S, et al. Primary gastric Hodgkin's lymphoma: a case report and review of the literature. *Leuk Lymphoma* 2005;46:147–150.
247. da Costa AA, Flora AC, Stroher M, et al. Primary Hodgkin lymphoma of the rectum: an unusual presentation. *J Clin Oncol* 2011;29:e268–e270.
248. Todd GB, Michaels L. Hodgkin's disease involving Waldeyer's lymphoid ring. *Cancer* 1974;34:1769–1778.

249. Kapadia SB, Roman LN, Kingma DW, et al. Hodgkin's disease of Waldeyer's ring: clinical and histoimmunophenotypic findings and association with Epstein-Barr virus in 16 cases. *Am J Surg Pathol* 1995;19:1431–1439.
250. Quiñones-Avila Mdel P, Gonzalez-Longoria AA, Admirand JH, et al. Hodgkin lymphoma involving Waldeyer ring: a clinicopathologic study of 22 cases. *Am J Clin Pathol* 2005;123:651–656.
251. Ozdemirli M, Mankin HJ, Aisenberg AC, et al. Hodgkin's disease a presenting as a solitary bone tumor: a report of four cases and review of the literature. *Cancer* 1996;77:79–88.
252. Ostrowski ML, Inwards CY, Strickler JG, et al. Osseous Hodgkin's disease. *Cancer* 1999;85:1166–1178.
253. Wang, SA, Rahemtullah A, Faquin WC, et al. Hodgkin's lymphoma of the thyroid: a clinicopathologic study of five cases and review of the literature. *Mod Pathol* 2005;18:1577–1584.
254. Kuruvilla J, Keating A, Crump M. How I treat relapsed and refractory Hodgkin lymphoma. *Blood* 2011;117:4208–4217.
255. Canellos GP. Relapsed and refractory Hodgkin's lymphoma: new avenues? *Hematol Oncol Clin N Am* 2007;21:929–941.
256. Colby TW, Hoppe RT, Warnke RA. Hodgkin's disease at autopsy: 1972–1977. *Cancer* 1981;47:1852–1862.
257. Grogan TM, Berard CW, Steinhorn SC, et al. Changing patterns of Hodgkin's disease at autopsy: a 25-year experience at the National Cancer Institute, 1953–1978. *Cancer Treat Rep* 1982;66:653–665.
258. Vasef MA, Alsabeh R, Medeiros LJ, et al. Immunophenotype of Reed-Sternberg and Hodgkin cells in sequential biopsy specimens of Hodgkin's disease: a paraffin-section immunohistochemical study using the heat-induced epitope retrieval method. *Am J Clin Pathol* 1997;108:54–59.
259. Chu WS, Abbondanzo SL, Frizzera G. Inconsistency of the immunophenotype of Reed-Sternberg cells in simultaneous and consecutive specimens from the same patients: a paraffin section evaluation in 56 patients. *Am J Pathol* 1992;141:11–17.
260. Colby TV, Warnke RA. The histology of the initial relapse of Hodgkin's disease. *Cancer* 1980;45:289–292.
261. Dolginow D, Colby TV. Recurrent Hodgkin's disease in treated sites. *Cancer* 1981;48:1124–1126.
262. Chao N, Levine J, Horning SJ. Retroperitoneal fibrosis following treatment for Hodgkin's disease. *J Clin Oncol* 1987;5:231–232.
263. Chen JL, Osborne BM, Butler JJ. Residual fibrous masses in treated Hodgkin's disease. *Cancer* 1987;60:407–413.
264. Krikorian JG, Burke JS, Rosenberg SA, et al. Occurrence of non-Hodgkin lymphoma after therapy for Hodgkin's disease. *N Engl J Med* 1979;300:452–458.
265. Zarate-Orsorno A, Medeiros LJ, Longo DL, et al. Non-Hodgkin lymphomas arising in patients successfully treated for Hodgkin's disease: a clinical, histologic, and immunophenotypic study of 14 cases. *Am J Surg Pathol* 1992;16:885–895.
266. Ohno T, Trenn G, Wu G, et al. The clonal relationship between nodular sclerosis Hodgkin's disease with a clonal Reed-Sternberg cell population and a subsequent B-cell small noncleaved cell lymphoma. *Mod Pathol* 1998;11:485–490.
267. Gaulier A, Teillet F, Davi F, et al. Pleomorphic medium-sized T-cell lymphoma following Hodgkin's disease (nodular sclerosis type). *Arch Pathol Lab Med* 1997;121:411–416.
268. Kingma DW, Medeiros LJ, Barletta J, et al. Epstein-Barr virus is infrequently identified in non-Hodgkin lymphomas associated with Hodgkin's disease. *Am J Surg Pathol* 1994;18:48–61.

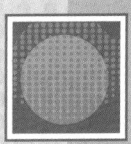

Chapter 16
Hodgkin Lymphoma: Cell of Origin, Immunobiology, and Pathogenesis

Ralf Küppers • Sylvia Hartmann • Martin-Leo Hansmann

 ## INTRODUCTION AND MORPHOLOGY

Hodgkin lymphoma (HL) is a heterogeneous lymphoid malignancy usually characterized by enlarged lymph nodes. During progression, involvement of nonlymphoid organs may be seen. The diagnosis is done by hematopathologists using histologic sections, with no need for additional molecular investigations in most cases. The tumor cells, the Hodgkin and Reed-Sternberg (HRS) cells, show a broad cytologic spectrum ranging from small to medium-sized mononuclear blast cells with slightly irregular nuclei (the Hodgkin cells) to large multinucleated cells, the so-called Reed-Sternberg (RS) cells, which are a hallmark for the diagnosis. Without immunostains, RS cells are much easier to recognize than the smaller Hodgkin cells (Fig. 16.1). The tumor cells in HL are a minority in the tumor tissue (<1% of cells), and their occurrence alone is not enough to establish the diagnosis of HL. The typical histologic background, in addition to HRS cells, is needed for the classification of a malignant lymphoma in the category of classical HL, which consists of four different subtypes (1). These subtypes are called nodular sclerosis, mixed cellularity, lymphocyte-rich classical, and lymphocyte depleted (Table 16.1). Typical for all these subtypes is the large number of small lymphocytes, which are mainly T helper (TH) cells, as well as varying numbers of macrophages, eosinophils, and a few plasma cells (Fig. 16.1). The cellular composition of the HL infiltrate can show similarities with a granulomatous process. For this reason, for many years, there was a controversial discussion as to whether HL is an infectious or inflammatory process and not a malignant tumor. As in inflammations, fibroblasts can produce collagen, which can form broad bands surrounding lymphoma infiltrates in HL, characteristic for nodular sclerosis HL (1). This histologic pattern, in which at least one nodule is surrounded by collagen, has HRS cells with special features showing a broad pale cytoplasm and a retraction of the cytoplasm due to an embedding artifact (Fig. 16.2). These HRS cells are called lacunar cells and are characteristic of nodular sclerosis HL, which account for about 80% of cases of this disease (see Chapter 15).

In contrast to classical HL, a small group of about 5% of all cases is categorized as nodular lymphocyte predominant HL (NLPHL), which shows special morphologic, immunohistochemical, and clinical features (Fig. 16.3), which justifies categorizing these cases separately (Table 16.1). In NLPHL, the tumor cells were previously called lymphocytic and histiocytic cells, but have recently been renamed lymphocyte predominant (LP) cells (1). NLPHL usually occurs in male patients of 20 to 40 years of age, is often confined to one localization, and usually has an excellent prognosis even without any therapy (see Chapter 15).

Although the classification of types and subtypes in HL is without any doubt useful, it became more and more evident that gray zones exist between the HL categories and between HL subtypes and particular types of non-Hodgkin lymphoma (NHL). The question arose as to whether these gray zones

exist because of biologic overlaps or because of insufficiency in diagnostic procedures. Based on the fact that HRS cells of classical HL and LP cells of NLPHL are germinal center (GC) B-cell–derived cells, it is not amazing that HL can show overlaps with other GC B-cell–derived lymphomas, such as diffuse large B-cell lymphoma, follicular lymphoma, and others, in particular as these lymphomas may also share some transforming events. However, these gray zone constellations or real combinations of HL and NHL are rare events. Best known are gray zone lymphomas of the mediastinum with features of nodular sclerosis and diffuse large B-cell lymphoma, as well as NLPHL and the T-cell–rich B-cell lymphoma or T-cell–rich B-cell lymphoma-like tumors. Especially, the latter case of gray zone category is often a difficult problem for diagnosis and therapy decisions, which could not be clarified up to now even using global gene expression strategies (2) (see Chapters 15 and 23). The current state of our understanding of the immunohistochemical and molecular findings of tumor cells and the background infiltrate in the composition and behavior of different HL types, including their morphologic appearance and immunohistochemical properties, is discussed.

 ## IMMUNOPHENOTYPE AND DIFFERENTIAL DIAGNOSIS

HRS cells express various markers related to myeloid, dendritic, or T-cells, such as CD30, CD15, fascin, CD23, CD4, perforin, TIA1, or granzyme B (Table 16.2; Fig. 16.2). Whereas most B-cell markers such as CD20, CD79a, and CD19, as well as the common leukocyte antigen CD45, are usually not expressed or only in a subset of HRS cells, a typically weak expression of PAX5 can be always demonstrated in these cells (3,4) (Fig. 16.2) and is the most reliable marker in the differential diagnosis with ALK-negative anaplastic large cell lymphoma or a secondary nodal manifestation of a cutaneous CD30+ lymphoproliferative disease, which can also mimic HL. In rare classical HL expressing B-cell markers, there is a considerable overlap with diffuse large B-cell lymphoma and particularly with primary mediastinal B-cell lymphoma (1). The reactive infiltrate in classical HL is usually composed of CD3+/CD4+ T-cells and epithelioid cells as well as eosinophils. Whereas IgD+ mantle zone B-cells and CD21+ or CD23+ follicular dendritic cells are usually present only in low numbers at the margins of the infiltrate in classical HL, the LP cells of NLPHL are frequently found in between mantle zone cells and follicular dendritic cells. PD-1+ and CD57+ T-cells rosetting around the tumor cells, which can also be present in the lymphocyte-rich subtype of classical HL, are much more common in NLPHL (5). In rare cases of NLPHL, T-cell rosettes can also be MUM1 positive, whereas MUM1 expression in the LP cells is usually much weaker than in HRS cells of classical HL. In contrast to classical HL, LP cells generally show expression of B-cell markers as well as B-cell–related transcription factors, such as OCT2, BOB.1, and PU.1, as well

Table 16.1	HISTOLOGIC CHARACTERISTICS OF THE DIFFERENT HL SUBTYPES

Histologic Subtype	Histologic Characteristics
NLPHL	• LP cells show lobulated nuclei, express B-cell markers, and are found in most cases in large nodules of small B-cells and dendritic cells • T-cell rosetting is frequently found
Lymphocyte-rich subtype of classical HL	• HRS cells are frequently found in small B-cell nodules that can surround regressive GCs • T-cell rosetting is frequently found • Eosinophils may be present
Nodular sclerosing subtype of classical HL	• At least one nodule is surrounded by fibrous collagen tissue • HRS cells are frequently arranged around regressive naive follicles or necroses and can be numerous • Typical lacunar cells
Mixed cellularity subtype of classical HL	• Slightly nodular or diffuse, often interfollicular patchy infiltrate rich in epitheloid cells and eosinophils containing single HRS cells
Lymphocyte-depleted subtype of classical HL	• HRS cells lying in diffuse fibrosis or predominance of HRS cells concurrent with strong depletion of reactive inflammatory infiltrate

as the GC B-cell markers CD75 and BCL6. LP cells also show an active immunoglobulin transcription machinery, detected by expression of J chain and frequently kappa light chains (Table 16.2; Fig. 16.3) (6,7). Expression of these markers in the tumor cells strongly argues for the diagnosis of NLPHL in the differential diagnosis of lymphocyte-rich subtype of classical HL. In some cases of NLPHL, the intensity of the B-cell markers expressed in the LP cells can be reduced (2,8), which can make it difficult to identify LP cells in the tissue section. The LP cells are never Epstein-Barr virus (EBV) infected, whereas EBV infection of HRS cells can be demonstrated in 30% to 40% of classical HL, particularly in mixed cellularity and lymphocyte-depleted subtypes as well as human immunodeficiency virus–associated HL.

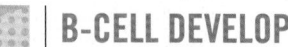

B-CELL DEVELOPMENT

Before discussing the cellular derivation of HRS and LP cells, it is useful to consider central aspects of normal B-cell development and differentiation. B-cells are generated from hematopoietic stem cells in the bone marrow in a multistep differentiation process (9). This process is classified according to the structure of the immunoglobulin (Ig) genes, in line with the key role of the B-cell antigen receptor (BCR) for B-cell survival and function. Hematopoietic stem cells give rise among other descendents to common lymphoid progenitors, the precursors of B- and T-lineage cells. The first step in B-cell development from these common lymphoid progenitors is the generation of pro-B-cells, which perform somatic rearrangements of the D_H and J_H gene segments of the variable (V) region of Ig heavy chains (9). In the next step, rearrangements of V_H gene segments to $D_H J_H$ joints are made, and cells carrying productive $V_H D_H J_H$ gene rearrangements allowing expression of an Ig heavy chain have reached the stage of pre-B-cells. As there are about 50 functional V_H, 27 D_H, and 6 J_H gene segments in the IgH locus, many different combinations are possible. Enormous additional diversity is generated at the joining sites of the gene segments, because at the ends of the rearranging segments nucleotides can be removed, and additional, nongermline–encoded N nucleotides are often added. This generates a practically limitless diversity of heavy chain rearrangements, which hence can be used as clonal markers for B-cells. Because of the randomness of nucleotide loss and addition, the correct reading frame of the V_H region gene is often lost in the rearrangement process. B-cell precursors can perform IgH gene rearrangements on both heavy chain alleles, increasing the chance that a functional heavy chain is generated.

Heavy chain rearrangements are followed by rearrangements of V and J gene segments at the kappa light chain locus (there are no D segments in the light chain loci). If no functional $V_\kappa J_\kappa$ region genes are generated on one of the two Igκ alleles, $V_\lambda J_\lambda$ rearrangements are performed at the Igλ loci. B-cell precursors that do not generate functional heavy and light chain rearrangements will undergo apoptosis. Once a B-cell expresses a heavy and light chain as a surface IgM receptor, the cells are selected against (strong) autoreactivity and then differentiate

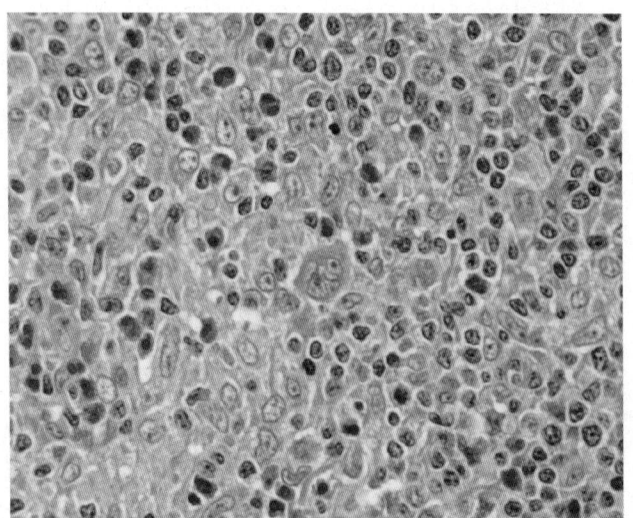

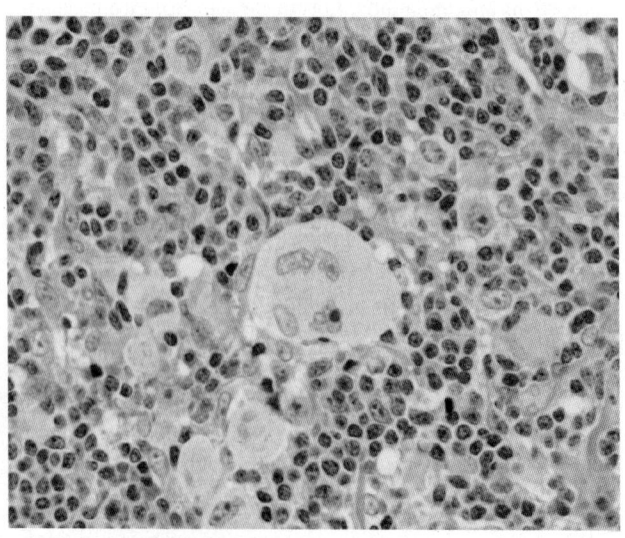

FIGURE 16.1. Histologic picture of classical HL. A: In the middle of the picture is a typical HRS cell showing a multilobulated nucleus with three large nucleoli and abundant cytoplasm. In addition, lymphocytes, histiocytes, epitheloid cells, and numerous eosinophilic granulocytes are seen. Classical HL mixed type, hematoxylin and eosin staining. **B:** Several large lacunar cells with irregularly shaped nuclei, large nucleoli, and extremely abundant pale cytoplasm. Many lymphocytes, several histiocytes, and single as well as eosinophilic granulocytes arranged in small clusters are seen. Classical HL, nodular sclerosis type, hematoxylin and eosin staining.

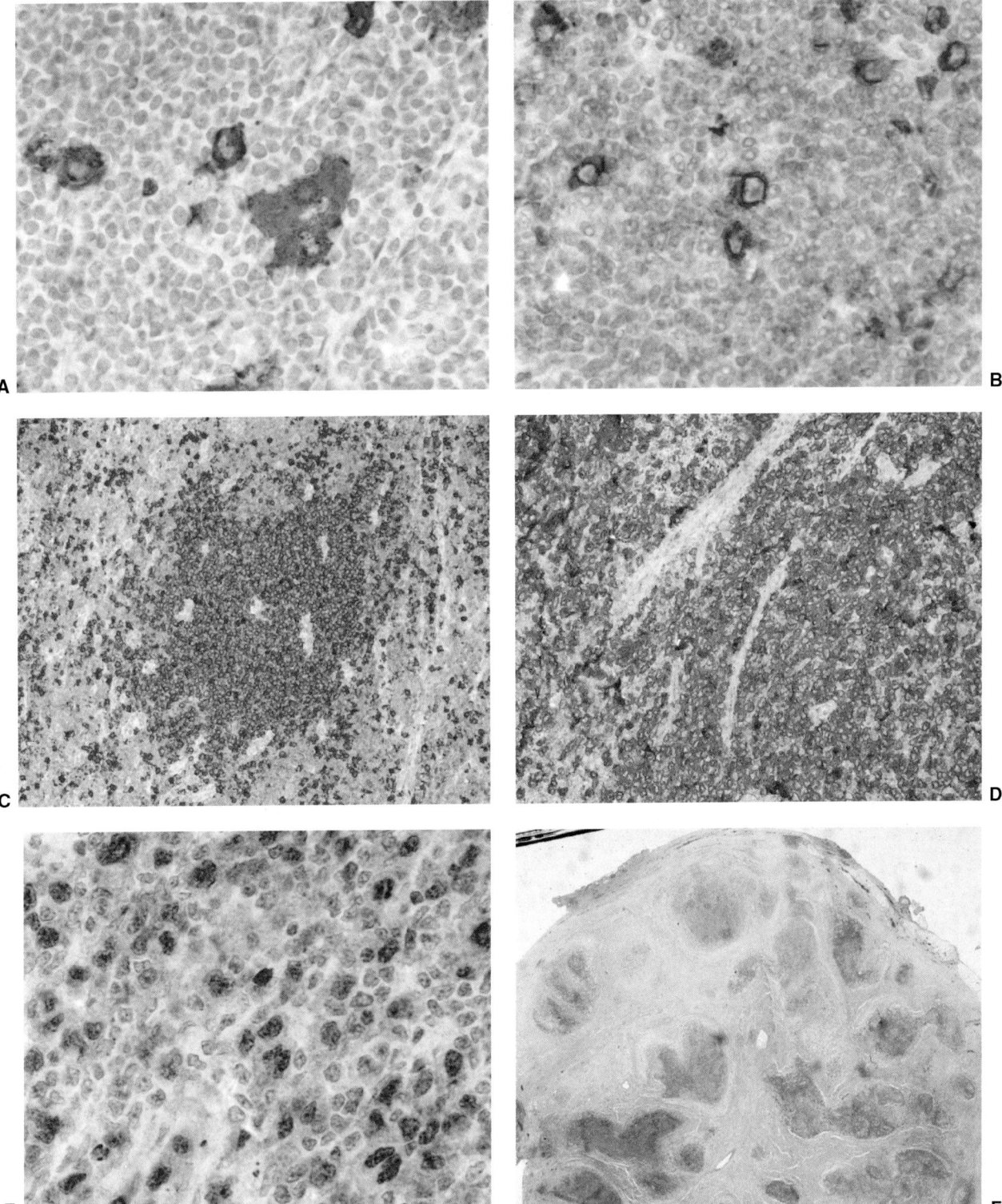

FIGURE 16.2. Immunohistochemical features of classical HL. A: Several large HRS cells are positively immunostained for CD15. The immunostaining is mainly seen in the cytoplasm and has a granular distribution. Classical HL nodular sclerosis type. **B:** Hodgkin cells with large nucleoli are visualized with anti-CD30 antibody staining in a case of classical HL lymphocyte-rich type, alkaline phosphatase immunoreaction. **C:** A nodular infiltrate of small B-cells in a case of classical HL lymphocyte-rich type is shown. Alkaline phosphatase immunoreaction, CD20. **D:** Large clusters of blasts as well as Hodgkin cells strongly immunostained for CD30. Classical HL lymphocyte-depleted type. Immunoalkaline phosphatase reaction. **E:** This picture shows a case of classical HL lymphocyte-depleted type immunostained for PAX5. The immunoreaction is mainly localized in the nuclei of the large HRS cells, which form clusters. In between the tumor cells, there are only few lymphocytes and histiocytes. Lymphocyte-depleted HL, alkaline phosphatase immunoreaction. **F:** The lymph node shows large nodules composed of lymphoid cells surrounded by broad bands of collagen fibers. This is the typical picture of classical HL of nodular sclerosis type showing a destroyed lymph node structure, hematoxylin and eosin.

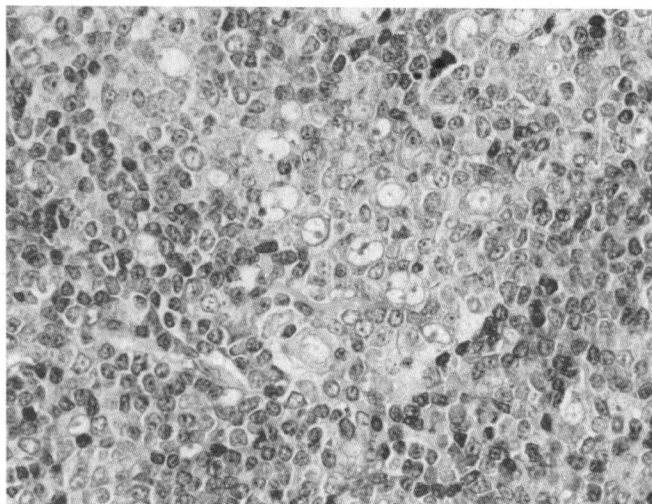

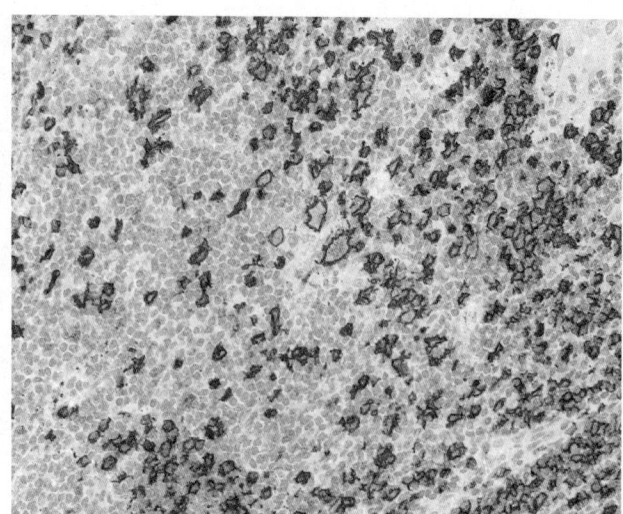

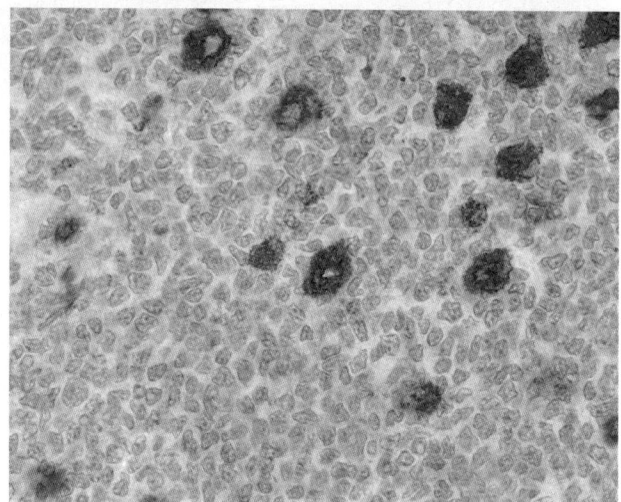

FIGURE 16.3. Histologic and immunohistochemical features of NLPHL. A: In the middle of the picture are several LP cells with lobulated nuclei and medium-sized to occasionally large nucleoli. Most cells are small lymphocytes, NLPHL, Giemsa staining. **B:** Part of a nodular infiltrate showing B-cell immunostaining (CD20) with a few LP cells in the middle of the picture and clusters of small B lymphocytes. NLPHL, immunoalkaline phosphatase reaction. **C:** This picture shows several LP cells immunostained for J chain. NLPHL, immunoalkaline phosphatase reaction.

Table 16.2	IMMUNOPHENOTYPE OF THE TUMOR CELLS OF CLASSICAL HL AND NLPHL	
	HRS Cells	**LP Cells**
CD30	+	– (+)
CD15	+/–	– (+)
CD20	– (+)	+
CD79a	–	+
CD19	–	–/+
CD23	+/–[a]	– (+)
PAX5	Weakly	+
CD45	–	+
BCL6	–	+
CD75	–	+
MUM1	+	Weakly
IgD	–	+/–
Oct2	–	+
BOB.1	–	+
P63	–	+
EMA	–	+
EBER/LMP1	+/–	–

[a]CD23 positivity is particularly observed in the nodular sclerosing subtype of classical HL.
+, positive; –, negative; +/–, positive in a large fraction of cases; –/+, positive in a minor fraction of cases; – (+), partly positive in a subset of tumor cells in some cases.

into mature, naive B-cells, which coexpress the BCR as IgM and IgD molecules, and which are released into the periphery (9) (see Chapter 6).

If a mature B-cell is activated by binding of foreign antigens to the BCR, and if T-cell help is available, a T-dependent immune response is initiated. This happens in secondary lymphoid organs, such as lymph nodes. Antigen-activated B-cells enter B-cell follicles and establish particular histologic structures, the GC. In the GC, the B-cells undergo rapid proliferation and activate the process of somatic hypermutation, through which the V region genes of the Ig heavy and light chains are molecularly modified (Fig. 16.4) (10). As the somatic hypermutation process is largely random, most mutations will be unfavorable, for example when they cause a reduction of the affinity of the BCR to the antigen. They can also impair BCR expression at all, for example, when mutations generate stop codons or when deletions or insertions destroy the correct reading frame. GC B-cells with such disadvantageous mutations are efficiently eliminated by apoptosis (11). Only the few GC B-cells that acquire affinity-increasing replacement mutations will be positively selected and undergo further rounds of proliferation, mutation, and selection (Fig. 16.4). For the selection process, the interaction of GC B-cells with follicular TH cells and follicular dendritic cells plays a central role. Many GC B-cells undergo a further Ig gene

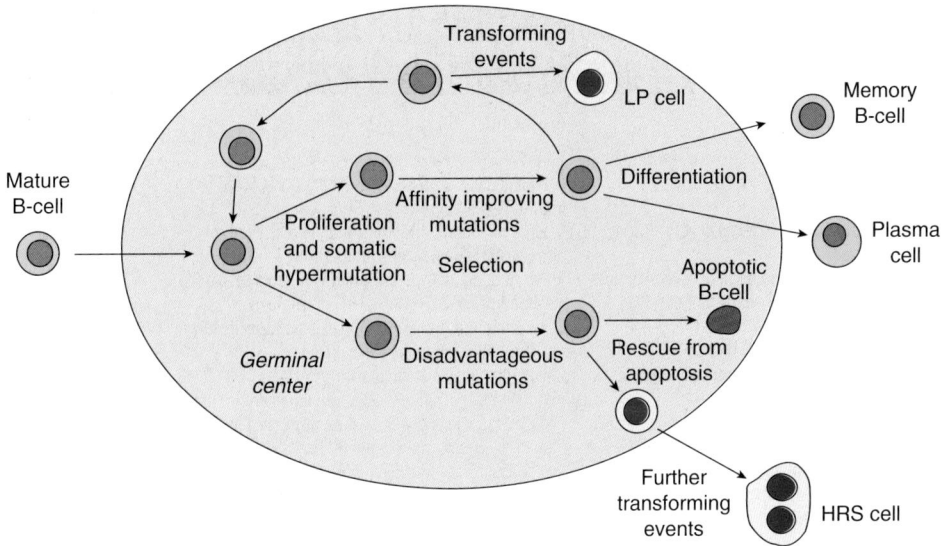

FIGURE 16.4. The GC reaction and a scenario for the origin of HRS and LP cells. Antigen-activated mature B-cells after initial stimulation by TH cells enter B-cell follicles and establish GC. In the GC, the B-cells undergo massive proliferation and activate the process of somatic hypermutation, which introduces point mutations and some deletions or duplications into the rearranged Ig V genes. Most mutations are disadvantageous for the cells and cause their apoptotic death as the default program. Only those GC B-cells acquiring affinity-increasing mutations are positively selected and survive. GC B-cells usually undergo multiple rounds of proliferation, mutation, and selection before they finally differentiate into either memory B-cells or plasma cells and exit the GC. LP cells are likely derived from mutating and positively selected GC B-cells. HRS cells likely originate from GC B-cells that acquired disadvantageous mutations and normally would have undergone apoptosis. (Adapted from Küppers R, Rajewsky K. The origin of Hodgkin and Reed/Sternberg cells in Hodgkin disease. *Annu Rev Immunol* 1998;16:471–493.)

remodeling process, that is, class switch recombination. In this process, the genes for the originally expressed IgM and IgD constant region genes are deleted, and one of the IgH constant region genes located further 3′ in the IgH locus (four IgG, two IgA, and one IgE genes are available for this) is expressed. Positively selected GC B-cells expressing a high-affinity BCR finally differentiate into either long-lived plasma cells or memory B-cells and exit the GC (see Chapter 2).

POSTULATED NORMAL COUNTERPART

As HRS cells show an unusual morphology and coexpress markers of various types of hematopoietic cells, the cellular origin of these cells remained unclear for a long time. An origin from dendritic cells, B-cells, T-cells, myeloid cells, and fibroblasts was postulated. A few cell lines that were established from HL biopsy samples were of B-cell, T-cell, or nonlymphoid origin, so that their analysis did not clarify the issue (12). Moreover, it was unclear whether the initially established cell lines indeed derived from the HRS cells in the patient. Other studies searched for Ig or T-cell receptor gene rearrangements as molecular markers for B- and T-lineage cells, respectively, by Southern blot or polymerase chain reaction (PCR) analyses of whole-tissue DNA. Clonal Ig gene rearrangements were obtained from some of the cases (13). However, because of the rarity of HRS cells in the tissue, it remained unclear as to whether the rearrangements stemmed from the HRS cells, and whether the lack of an amplificate in PCR-negative cases was due to the rarity of these cells.

The issue of a potential B-cell origin of HRS cells was clarified when we established a method to isolate single HRS cells from frozen tissue sections by hydraulic micromanipulation and to analyze these cells for rearranged Ig heavy and light chain genes by single-cell PCR (10,14). This analysis revealed a B-cell origin of HRS cells (14,15). Several other studies using similar approaches initially did not come to the same result, reporting either polyclonal or mixed polyclonal and monoclonal populations of B-cell–derived HRS cells, or an absence of Ig

gene rearrangements in these cells (16–18). However, numerous follow-up studies verified that HRS cells represent monoclonal populations of B-cell–derived tumor cells in nearly all cases (19–23).

In nearly all instances, the rearranged Ig V genes amplified from HRS cells carry a high load of somatic mutations (15,19–23). This demonstrates that the tumor cells derive from mature B-cells that are undergoing or have undergone a GC reaction (Table 16.1). Intraclonal diversity is not or to only a very minor extent observed, showing that the process of somatic hypermutation is silenced in these cells. There are rare cases of HL in which the HRS cells carry unmutated Ig V genes (24,25). However, also these cases may derive from GC B-cells, because GC founder cells acquire the propensity to undergo apoptosis even before they acquire somatic mutations (26).

A surprising finding of our studies was that in about 25% of cases of classical HL, the HRS cells carry clearly destructive V gene mutations, such as nonsense mutations and frameshift-causing deletions, in originally functional V gene rearrangements (15,19). As discussed above, such crippling mutations normally cause the immediate death of the cells through apoptosis. Thus, it is highly likely that the GC B-cells that acquired the destructive mutations already carried or acquired some transforming event(s) that prevented their apoptosis. On this ground, we argued that HRS cells are derived from (preapoptotic) GC B-cells, as critical steps in the malignant transformation process occurred at the GC B-cell stage of differentiation (Fig. 16.4) (15,27). As many disadvantageous mutations cannot be easily identified by evaluating the V gene sequences (e.g., replacement mutations that cause a reduction of the affinity of the BCR to the cognate antigen), we speculated that HRS cells as a rule derive from preapoptotic GC B-cells (15,27).

The GC B-cell origin of HRS cells is further supported by additional genetic features of these cells (Table 16.3). HL cell lines and presumably also primary HRS cells show class-switch recombination, which is as also a V gene recombination and somatic hypermutation B-cell–specific process (28,29). HRS cells also frequently show aberrant somatic hypermutation

Table 16.3	GENETIC ARGUMENTS FOR A B-CELL ORIGIN OF HRS CELLS IN CLASSICAL HL	
Feature	**Argument**	**References**
Clonal Ig heavy and light chain gene rearrangements in HRS cells of nearly all classical HL	V_H and V_L gene rearrangements take place only in B-lineage cells, and presence of both is specific for mature B-cells	(14,15,19,21,22)
Somatic mutations in Ig V genes of HRS cells of nearly all HL	Process of somatic hypermutation is restricted to antigen-activated B-cells proliferating in GC	(14,15,19,21,22)
Aberrant somatic hypermutation of several protooncogenes in HRS cells of nearly half of HL	Aberrant somatic hypermutation is highly specific for several types of GC B-cell–derived lymphomas	(30)
Class switch recombination in most HL cell lines and presumably also primary HRS cells	Class switch recombination takes place specifically in antigen-activated mature B-cells	(28,29)
Clonally related composite lymphomas of a classical HL and a B-cell NHL	Clonal relationship of composite lymphomas with V gene mutation pattern suggesting a derivation of the clones from distinct members of a GC B-cell clone demonstrates the B-cell origin of the HRS cells in these cases	(31–35)
Ig loci-associated chromosomal translocations in HRS cells of about 20% of classical HL	Ig loci-associated translocations take place only in B-cells as side products of Ig gene-remodeling processes	(29)

of several protooncogenes, which is specifically happening in several types of GC B-cell–derived lymphomas (30).

Although the structure of the *IG* loci in HRS cells clearly points to a derivation of HRS cells from (preapoptotic) GC B-cells, it may well be that there is an even more specific precursor of these cells. For example, in most cases, nodular sclerosis HL has a primary presentation in the mediastinum, and it has been discussed that this subtype of HL may derive from an unusual population of B-cells present in the thymus (36,37). Moreover, as HRS cells consistently express the CD30 marker, and as rare CD30+ large normal B-cells are found outside as well as inside the GC in reactive lymph nodes (38), it is an intriguing question as to whether HRS cells show a specific relationship with these cells. Finally, when assigning a B-cell lymphoma to a specific B-cell subset as the cell of origin, it needs to be considered that lymphoma development is a multistep process. The HRS cell precursors may well have already carried some genetic lesions when they entered the GC reaction (e.g., *IG* loci-associated translocations that happened as mistakes of V gene recombination in B-cell precursors in the bone marrow [39]). Moreover, some final transforming events may happen after the HRS cells left the GC microenvironment. What we want to argue is that decisive steps in HL development occur in GC B-cells.

The observations that two presumed HL cell lines are of T-cell origin (HDLM2 and L540) and that some cases of classical HL show expression of several cytotoxic and T-cell antigens by the HRS cells prompted the analysis of such cases for a potential T-cell derivation. Indeed, in a fraction of cases studied, clonal T-cell receptor gene rearrangements were amplified from the HRS cells, and these cases lacked Ig gene rearrangements (40,41). Thus, a few cases diagnosed as typical classical HL are derived from T-cells. It is a matter of debate whether such cases should be called classical HL or considered as a rare form of T-cell lymphoma with features resembling HL. Notably, in gene expression studies, the T-cell–derived HL line HDLM2 was more similar to B-cell–derived HL cell lines than to cell lines of the T-cell lymphoma anaplastic large cell lymphoma, arguing for a close relationship of B-cell– and T-cell–derived classical HL (42). It should also be mentioned that most of the cases of classical HL with T-cell marker expression are B-cell derived, showing that this marker expression does not specify T-cell HL cases. Overall, it seems that <2% of cases diagnosed as classical HL originate from T-cells (40).

For NLPHL, the cellular origin of the LP cells from B-cells was presumed based on numerous phenotypic and histologic features. LP cells express many B-cell markers, including CD20, CD79, surface Ig, and PAX5 (43). They do not show an

expression of many non-B-cell genes, as HRS cells do. Moreover, LP cells express key markers of GC B-cells, such as BCL6, centerin, HGAL, and activation-induced cytidine deaminase, the master regulator of somatic hypermutation and class-switch recombination (43). As they also grow in follicular structures resembling GC in association with follicular dendritic cell networks and follicular TH cells, all these features point to a close relationship to, and hence origin from, GC B-cells. The first genetic proof for a GC B-cell origin of LP cells was the demonstration of clonal and somatically mutated Ig V genes in isolated LP cells in a study by our group (14). This finding was later verified by three additional studies that showed clonal Ig gene rearrangements in LP cells (44–46). The Ig V genes were consistently mutated, but crippling mutations were not found (44,45,47). About half of the cases showed intraclonal diversity of the Ig V genes, demonstrating active somatic hypermutation during clonal expansion of the tumor clone (44,45,48). Thus, all these features taken together show that LP cells represent transformed GC B-cells that retain key features of their cells of origin upon malignant transformation (Fig. 16.4).

THE RELATIONSHIP OF HODGKIN TO RS CELLS AND PUTATIVE HRS STEM CELLS

Based on the frequent aneuploidy of HRS cells, the multinuclearity of the RS cells, and the "mixed" phenotype of the HRS cells, it was discussed that the HRS cell clone as such or the RS cells may be generated through cell fusions (49). However, a detailed molecular analysis of *IG* or *TCR* loci in B-cell– or T-cell–derived HRS cells, respectively, strongly argued against a role for cell fusion in the generation of the HRS cell clone (50). Studies with HL cell lines also argued against fusion of Hodgkin cells as the source for the multinucleated RS cells (51). Indeed, there is now comprehensive evidence that Hodgkin cells give rise to RS cells through a process resembling endomitosis, that is, nuclear division without cell division (52,53). RS cells have little proliferative capacity, so that the population of HRS cells is maintained by proliferation of mononuclear Hodgkin cells, which produce more Hodgkin cells and also RS cells (53).

A related issue concerned the question whether the typical CD30+ HRS cells represent the whole tumor cell clone, or whether additional clone members can be found among CD30- cells (54). A cytogenetic analysis initially pointed to the existence of CD30- cells with the same genetic lesions as the HRS cells (55). However, as single numerical chromosomal abnormalities, which were studied in that work, are not stringent clonal markers, this study could not unequivocally resolve that issue. Moreover, in a study of EBV⁺ HL, where all tumor clone members should be EBV infected, because of the clonal EBV infection pattern of HRS cells (56), the molecular *IG* gene analysis of CD30⁺ HRS cells and small CD30⁻ EBV-infected B-cells revealed that HRS clone members do not exist among the CD30⁻ EBV⁺ B-cells, or are at least very rare (57). A recent publication reported the existence of HRS cell clone members among CD20⁺BCR⁺ and CD30⁻ peripheral blood B-cells in several HL patients (58). However, the validity of this finding was questioned based on technical aspects (59). In addition, an older highly sensitive PCR study for HRS clone members in peripheral blood did not detect cells with HRS cell–specific *IG* gene rearrangements in the patients analyzed (23).

Side population cells are cells that extrude the Hoechst dye 33342, usually because of expression of ABC transporters, and hence appear negative for the stain in flow cytometric analyses with the dye (60). Side population cells among tumor cells are usually resistant to numerous chemotherapeutic drugs, as the ABC transporters also expel drugs from the cells, and there is an interesting link between side population cells and cancer stem cells, although these are not identical, but at most overlapping populations in several types of cancers (60). Two recent studies described the identification of rare side population cells (about 0.5% of HRS cells) also in HL cell lines (61,62). The side population cells were found among mononuclear Hodgkin cells and had a CD30⁺CD20⁻ phenotype. Importantly, these cells showed increased chemoresistance and could efficiently reestablish HRS cell populations in subcloning experiments (61,62).

These features might indicate that side population cells represent stem cell–like cells for the HRS cell clones. However, side population cells were not seen in all HL cell lines (61,62), arguing against an essential and general role of these cells for HRS cells. In addition, although side population cells were also detected in HL lymph node suspensions, it remains to be determined whether these cells belong to the HRS cell clones.

LOST B-CELL PHENOTYPE OF HRS CELLS

Among all B-cell lymphomas, classical HL is unique in the extent to which the tumor B-cells have lost the phenotype of their cells of origin (63). The down-regulation of B-cell–typical genes not only affects a number of immunohistochemical markers but is a genome-wide phenomenon (3,64). As the loss of the gene expression program of their cells of origin is such a specific and consistent feature of HRS cells, it is likely a central aspect of HL pathogenesis. It is therefore important to clarify the mechanisms that cause this "reprogramming" of HRS cells. The initiating events for this process are still unclear, but several factors are known that contribute to the down-regulation of B-cell–typical genes (Fig. 16.5). First, HRS cells posses low or undetectable expression of the important B-cell transcription factors OCT2, BOB1, EBF1, and PU.1 (65–67). This is most likely a reason why many target genes of these factors are not expressed in HRS cells. Second, E2A, another central B-cell transcription factor, is found in HRS cells, but its activity is inhibited by ID2 and ABF1 (68,69). ID2 is normally expressed by natural killer (NK) cells

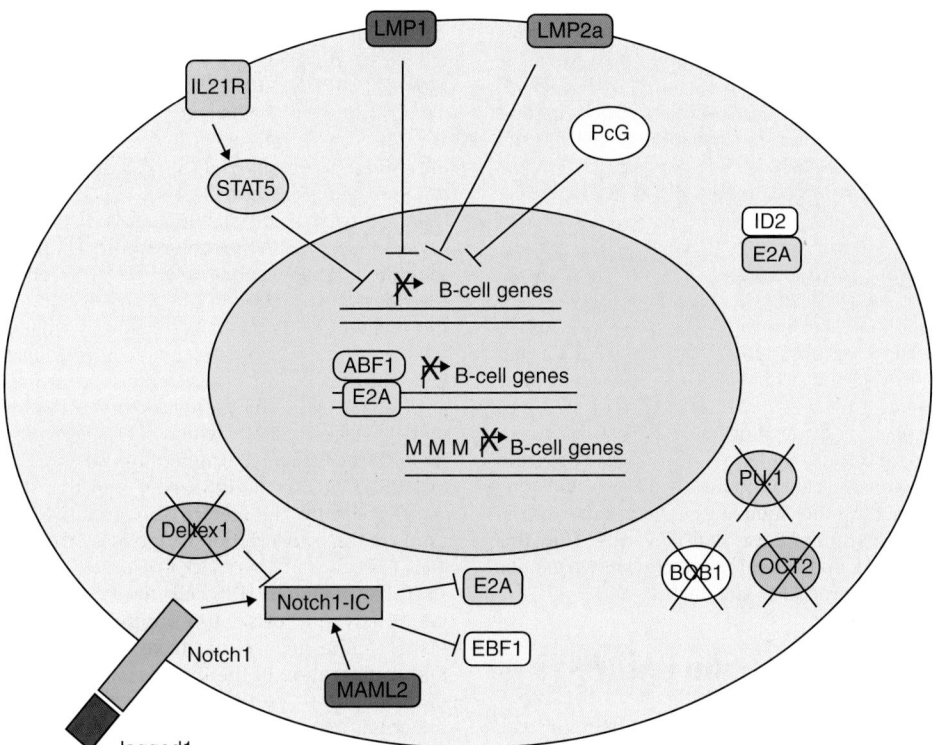

FIGURE 16.5. Factors contributing to the lost B-cell phenotype of HRS cells. The down-regulation of the B-cell gene expression program in HRS cells is mediated by multiple factors. The transcription factors OCT2, BOB1, and PU.1 are down-regulated in HRS cells. The transcription factor E2A is still expressed, but its activity is inhibited. ID2 retains E2A in the cytoplasm. E2A bound by ABF1 can still bind to DNA but is unable to activate its target genes. B-cell gene expression is also inhibited by active STAT5, by polycomb group (PcG) repressive factors, and by the EBV-encoded genes LMP1 and LMP2a. The T-cell transcription factor NOTCH1 and its coactivator MAML2 show aberrant expression in HRS cells. It is activated through its ligand JAGGED1, which is expressed on cells in the HL microenvironment. Moreover, the NOTCH inhibitor DELTEX is down-regulated in HRS cells. Active NOTCH1 inhibits the B-cell transcription factors E2A and ABF1. Many B-cell genes are also silenced through epigenetic mechanisms, such as methylation of CpG sites (denoted as "M") in their regulatory elements. (Adapted from Küppers R. The biology of Hodgkin lymphoma. *Nat Rev Cancer* 2009;9:15–27.)

and promotes the generation of NK cells from lymphoid precursors by inhibiting B-cell master regulators, such as E2A. The physiologic role of ABF1 is not well understood; its expression is induced in activated B-cells. Third, HRS cells express active NOTCH1, which is a master regulator of T-cell development and which inhibits B-cell development (70,71). Also Mastermind-like 2 (MAML2), an important cofactor for NOTCH1 activity, shows elevated expression in HRS cells (72). Fourth, HRS cells express constitutively active STAT5a and b, and *in vitro* studies have shown that enforced expression of active STAT5 in B-cell lines induces a phenotype resembling HRS cells, including the downregulation of a number of B-cell genes (73). Fifth, in EBV+ cases of classical HL, the EBV-encoded latent membrane proteins 1 and 2a (LMP1 and LMP2a, respectively) also contribute to a reduced expression of B-cell genes (74,75). Sixth, HRS cells coexpress multiple members of the polycomb repressive complexes 1 and 2, and these factors function in hematopoietic stem cells and lymphoid precursors by dampening B-cell gene expression and enabling the coexpression of markers of various hematopoietic cell types (76,77). Seventh, the silencing of many B-cell genes is also stabilized by epigenetic mechanisms, as many B-cell–specific genes show a hypermethylation of CpG sites in their regulatory regions (78–80).

Curiously, PAX5, which is considered to be the master commitment and maintenance factor for B-cell identity, is still expressed in HRS cells, albeit at a low level. It is not well understood why PAX5 does not drive the B-cell program in HRS cells. Perhaps, factors like NOTCH1 inhibit PAX5 activity (70).

Although the vast majority of B-cell–typical genes are downregulated in HRS cells, among the genes that are usually still expressed, one finds CD40, CD80, and CD86. These are genes that play an important role in the interaction of mature B-cells with TH cells. As HRS cells are usually directly surrounded by CD4+ T-cells, one may speculate that this interaction is of critical importance for HRS cells. However, in about 40% of cases, HRS cells have down-regulated the expression of MHC class II (81,82), so that a cognate interaction between HRS cells and T-cells via MHC class II and the T-cell receptor is at least not generally involved in the HRS cell–T-cell interaction.

LP cells of NLPHL have largely retained the gene expression program of the GC B-cells from which they are derived, as discussed above. However, by global gene expression profiling, we observed a moderate down-regulation of numerous B-cell–typical genes in these cells as well (2).

Could there be a pathophysiologic role for the consistent downregulation of the B-cell program in HRS cells? Considering that HRS cells appear to derive from crippled GC B-cells that normally would undergo apoptosis, we speculated that a loss of the B-cell phenotype may represent a strategy of the HRS precursor cells to escape the selectional force to undergo the apoptosis program (15,27). By losing their B-cell identity, the GC B-cells with disadvantageous mutations lose the signaling pathways that would execute the apoptosis program of these "failed" B-cells. How this reprogramming is initiated, and whether as-yet-unknown genetic lesions are involved in this process is still unclear.

 DEREGULATED SIGNALING PATHWAYS

Usually cells receive transient signals to promote their survival, to induce differentiation processes, or to regulate their proliferation. In tumor cells, signaling pathways are often deregulated, causing sustained proliferation of the tumor cells and preventing their apoptosis. In HRS cells, a large number of signaling pathways and transcription factors show deregulated and sometimes aberrant activation. We already discussed the aberrant activity of NOTCH1 signaling, and of the ID2 transcription factor, as well as deregulated activity of STAT5 and of polycomb repressor family complexes in these cells.

HRS cells also show constitutive activation of the NF-κB signaling pathway (83). The NF-κB family consists of five members (p50, p52, p65, Rel, and RelB), which function as homo- or heterodimers. A canonical and a noncanonical NF-κB pathway is distinguished. In the canonical pathway, upstream signals activate the IκB complex that induces the degradation of the main NF-κB inhibitor IκBα. IκBα usually binds to NF-κB dimers and prevents their translocation into the nucleus. Hence, when IκBα is degraded, NF-κB is released and can activate the transcription of multiple genes, including numerous antiapoptotic genes and genes promoting cell proliferation. In the noncanonical pathway, the kinase NIK induces processing of inactive p105 to p50, which then as a heterodimer with RelB functions as an active transcription factor. In HRS cells, both NF-κB pathways are active (83). This activation is partly mediated through signals in the microenvironment, for example stimulation of CD30, CD40, RANK, and BCMA on HRS cells through their respective ligands on cells in the vicinity of HRS cells (43). Also viral genes and genetic lesions play an important role in NF-κB activation. Constitutive NF-κB activity is essential for the survival of HRS cells, as its inhibition in HL cell lines is toxic for the cells (83).

The main signaling pathway for cytokines is the JAK/STAT pathway. Upon binding of cytokines to their receptors, JAK kinases bound to these receptors become active and phosphorylate STAT factors. Phosphorylated homo- or heterodimers of STAT factors are active, translocate into the nucleus, and function as transcription factors. Various cytokines presumably contribute to activating JAK/STAT signaling in HRS cells, including IL-13 and IL-21 (73,84). The main active STAT factors in HRS cells are STAT3, STAT5, and STAT6 (73,84–86).

Receptor tyrosine kinases are a family of receptors with multiple functions in the regulation of cell growth and differentiation. In HRS cells, several of these receptors are expressed, which are not usually seen in normal B-cells, including DDR2, PDGFR2, EPHB1, RON, TRKA, and TRKB (87). Expression of each of these molecules was found in 30% to 70% of classical HL. The most pronounced expression was seen in EBV– cases of nodular sclerosis HL (88). For at least some of the receptor tyrosine kinases, there is evidence that they are activated by auto- or paracrine mechanisms in HRS cells (87). CSF1R is a myeloid cell-specific receptor tyrosine kinase that was recently identified as being expressed in HRS cells, too (89). Notably, the aberrant expression of CSF1R in HRS cells is mediated by the reactivation of a long terminal repeat sequence located upstream of the *CSF1R* gene, so that *CSF1R* is transcribed in HRS cells from a long terminal repeat promoter (89).

Further signaling pathways that show deregulated activity in HRS cells, and for which there is evidence that the activity of these pathways promote the survival and/or proliferation of HRS cells, are the PI3K/AKT and the MAPK/ERK pathways (90–93). Lastly, the factors JUN and JUNB, which are components of the transcription factor AP1, are overexpressed in HRS cells (94).

Taken together, HRS cells are characterized by the deregulated activation of a large number of signaling pathways and transcription factors that have essential roles for the survival and proliferation of the tumor cells. The constitutive activation of these pathways and factors is mediated by multiple factors, including autocrine stimulation, interaction with other cells in the microenvironment, genetic lesions, epigenetic alterations, and viral products.

HL CELL LINES

In vitro growing cell lines are important tools for the molecular analysis and for functional studies of tumor cells. Numerous attempts have been made to establish cell lines from HRS or

Table 16.4 | FEATURES OF HL CELL LINES

Cell Line	HL Subtype	Cell Type	EBV	Mutated Oncogenes or Tumor Suppressor Genes	Remarks
L428	Classical	B-cell	−	NFKBIA, NFKBIE, SOCS1, TP53	
L540	Classical	T-cell	−		
L591	Classical	B-cell	+		EBV gene expression pattern distinct from EBV⁺ primary HRS cells
L1236	Classical	B-cell	−	TNFAIP3, CD95, SOCS1, TP53, t(4:18)(q27;q24) involving PDE5A and ZHX2	Only line with proven derivation from HRS cells
KMH2	Classical	B-cell	−	NFKBIA, TNFAIP3, CYLD, CTIIA (translocation)	
HDLM2	Classical	T-cell	−	TNFAIP3, SOCS1, TP53, UTX, TNFSF7, TNFSF9	
SUP-HD1	Classical	B-cell	−	TNFAIP3, PTPN2	
U-HO1	Classical	B-cell	−	TNFAIP3, TRAF3	
DEV	NLPHL	B-cell	−	SOCS1, BCL6 (translocation)	

LP cells, but only a few lines have been obtained. The main reason for the difficulties in establishing HRS cell lines is most likely the dependency of HRS and LP cells from survival signals in their microenvironment. In support of this, HRS cells are very rarely found in the peripheral blood, and primary HRS cells do not survive in immunodeficient mice (95). Indeed, all existing HL cell lines have been established from patients with advanced stages of HL and from extranodal biopsy material—peripheral blood, bone marrow, or pleural effusions—indicating that only HRS cells that already had lost the dependency on the lymph node microenvironment in the patient—perhaps due to acquisition of additional transforming events—can survive in vitro. Only nine cell lines are currently used in the field: L428, L540, L591, L1236, KMH2, HDLM2, SUP-HD1, DEV, and U-HO1 (12,96,97) (Table 16.4). L1236 is the only cell line for which the derivation from the HRS cells of the respective patient was molecularly proven (21). L591 is the only EBV⁺ HL line (12). However, the EBV gene expression pattern of L591 is not typical for primary HRS cells, which needs to be taken into consideration when using this line (98). L540 and HDLM2 are T-cell derived, whereas all other lines have a B-cell origin. DEV is the only line obtained from a case of NLPHL (99,100). Originally, cell line CO was described as a HL cell line, too, but it turned out to be a cell culture contamination (101). HD-MYZ was for a long time also considered as an HRS cell line. However, this line differs phenotypically significantly from the primary HRS cells of the patient from whom it was established (102). More importantly, HD-MYZ is not of B- or T-cell but likely myeloid origin (103). As HRS cells are derived from B- or T-cells, this strongly argues against an HRS cell origin of HD-MYZ, so that the line should no longer be used as a model for HRS cells.

When using HL cell lines, one needs to consider that these lines are adapted to grow in suspension without the normal HL microenvironment. Nevertheless, these lines are very valuable, because many key features, deregulated signaling pathways, and genetic lesions of HRS cells were initially found in HL cell lines and later also confirmed in primary HRS cells.

CYTOGENETICS

For many years, cytogenetic analysis of HL was hampered by the low tumor cell content in the infiltrate and the polyploidy of the tumor cells (104). By the development of comparative genomic hybridization (CGH) of microdissected HRS cells, several loci of recurrent copy number aberrations could

be identified, including gains of 2p (54%), 9p, 12q, 16p, 17p, 17q, and 20q as well as losses of 13q (105,106). Overexpression of REL and JAK2 proteins, located in 2p and 9p, respectively, was demonstrated (105,107). Recent studies showed that the frequent gain on 9p24 not only involved JAK2 but at least three additional genes with pathogenetic relevance in HL, that is, the PD-1 ligands PD-L1 and PD-L2 and the histone demethylase JMJD2C (108,109). These as well as additional genomic aberrations were confirmed by array CGH of microdissected HRS cells. Gains involved 2p12-16, 5q15-23, 6p22, 8q13, 8q24, 9p21-24, 9q34, 12q13-14, 17q12, 19p13, 19q13, and 20q11, losses involved Xp21, 6q23-24, and 13q22 (110). Genomic regions with gains included several genes known to be constitutively overexpressed in classical HL, such as NOTCH1, STAT6, and JUNB. In a larger CGH array study of microdissected HRS cells of 53 patients, enriched for those with treatment failure, gains were found on 2p15-16.1, 9p21.1, 9p24.1-24.3, 17q21.31-32, 20q13.11-13.12, and 20q13.2, and the most frequent losses were located on 6q23.2, 11q22.3, and 13q14.3-21.1 (111). In this study, a gain of 16p12.1-13.3 in the HRS cells was significantly correlated with treatment failure, and the overexpression of multidrug resistance gene ABCC1, located in this genomic region, was shown in HL cell line KMH2.

Recurrent translocations involving the IG loci and protooncogenes are a hallmark of many B-cell NHLs (112). Indications for IG loci-associated translocations were also seen in HRS cells in about 20% of classical HL (29). In a few instances, the translocation partners were identified as BCL1, BCL2, BCL3, MYC, and REL, but for most cases, the translocation partners are not known (29,39,113). Notably, in B-cell NHL, the translocations usually function through the dysregulated expression of the protooncogenes, driven by the strongly active IG loci regulatory elements. However, as HRS cells have largely silenced the IG loci, it is unclear to which extent the translocated protooncogenes are still expressed in HRS cells (39). Perhaps these genes were important for HL pathogenesis during early stages of lymphoma development, when the HRS precursor cells still had a B-cell phenotype, but became less important in the established HRS cell clone upon acquisition of further transforming events. One may also speculate that perhaps in some cases these translocations involve tumor suppressor genes that are inactivated through the translocation.

There are only a few cytogenetic studies of NLPHL. Microdissected LP cells were characterized by CGH, and distinct recurrent copy number aberrations were observed on 1p12-22, 1q21-31, 2q24-31, 3p13-21, 3q12-13, 4q12-25, 5q23, 6p,

6q12-24, 8q21, 11q12-22, 12q12, 12q14-15, Xp, and Xq23-26 (gains) and 6p, 8p, 10p, 11q, 16p, and 17p (losses) (114). Whereas the identification of target genes located in these genomic regions was difficult, translocations to the *BCL6* gene locus were detected in LP cells in over 40% of cases (115,116). Therefore, also from a cytogenetic point of view, classical HL and NLPHL show remarkably different mechanisms of oncogenesis.

ONCOGENE AND TUMOR SUPPRESSOR GENE MUTATIONS

The identification of somatic mutations in oncogenes and tumor suppressor genes that are involved in the pathogenesis of HL has been very much hampered by the rarity of the HRS cells in the tumor. Often, candidate genes were first analyzed in HL cell lines, and if mutations were found, the genes were then analyzed in microdissected HRS cells.

As constitutive activity of the NF-κB transcription factor is a consistent finding in HRS cells, members of this transcription factor family and several regulators of its activity have been studied. Genomic gains involving the NF-κB factor REL were found in about 40% of cases, as already mentioned in Cytogenetics section (106,117). These gains are likely of functional relevance, because they are correlated with strong immunostaining for the REL protein (107). Gains are also frequent for the *NIK* gene (111,118). Inactivating mutations in *NFKBIA*, the gene encoding IκBα, are present in 10% to 20% of classical HL (119–122). One study also reported mutations in the *NFKBIE* gene, encoding IκBε, another negative regulator of NF-κB, in a few cases (123). The gene *TNFAIP3* encodes the dual ubiquitinase and deubiquitinase A20, which inhibits NF-κB signaling upstream of the IKK complex in the canonical pathway. Mutations in this gene were found in several HL cell lines and in HRS cells of about 40% of classical HL (124,125). *TNFAIP3* mutations were mostly found in EBV⁻ HL (70% of EBV⁻ HL with *TNFAIP3* mutations), suggesting that EBV infection and A20 inactivation are complementary transforming events in classical HL (125). As reconstitution of A20 in A20-deficient HL cell lines caused reduced NF-κB activity and cell survival, *TNFAIP3* functions as a tumor suppressor gene in HRS cells (125). In rare instances, mutations were also found in *CYLD* and *TRAF3*, two further inhibitors of NF-κB activity, and some HL carry translocations of the *BCL3* gene, which can positively regulate NF-κB function (118,126,127).

In several HL cell lines, mutations in more than one of the NF-κB pathway genes mentioned above were found (Table 16.2). This indicates that often a genetic lesion in one of the regulators of the NF-κB pathway is not sufficient for the HRS cells, and that a concerted distortion of this pathway is required to obtain the strong and constitutive activation of this transcription factor family. Notably, although LP cells of NLPHL also show strong NF-κB activity (2), the mechanisms for NF-κB activation in LP cells seem to be different from those observed in HRS cells, because no inactivating mutations in *NFKBIA* or *TNFAIP3* were found in LP cells (100), and there is also no indication for *REL* gains in these cells.

Recurrent genetic lesions were also found in members of the JAK/STAT signaling pathway. *JAK2* frequently shows genomic gains and in rare instances is involved in chromosomal translocations (105,128). About 40% of cases of HL carry mono- or biallelic inactivating mutations in the gene *SOCS1*, encoding a negative regulator of STAT signaling (129).

Numerous other genes that were studied for mutations in HRS cells were either found to be mutated only in rare instances or not at all (reviewed in Ref. [43]). Mutations in *CD95*, a receptor of the TNFR family that usually promotes apoptosis upon activation, were detected in only 3 of 39 cases (43). No mutations were found in other factors of CD95 signaling, that is, *FADD*, caspase 8, and caspase 10 (130). For *TP53*, a main regulator of apoptosis and the most frequently mutated tumor suppressor gene in human cancers, mutations were found only in rare primary cases, but in three HL cell lines (131,132). As the mutations in the cell lines were not restricted to the typically mutated exons of the gene and included larger deletions, it may well be that the previous analyses of primary HRS cells for mutations within exons 5 to 9 underestimate the true frequency of *TP53* alterations in HRS cells.

Little is known about the genetic lesions in LP cells. *BCL6* translocations involving the *IG* loci or other partner genes are frequently found (115,116,133). LP cells also frequently carry *SOCS1* mutations, suggesting an important role of deregulated STAT signaling in the LP cells (134).

ROLE OF EPSTEIN-BARR VIRUS IN HL

EBV is a member of the γ herpes virus family that infects about 90% of the human population worldwide. After primary infection, which is usually asymptomatic when it occurs in children, a lifelong persistent infection is established. The reservoir of the virus is B-cells, and in healthy virus carriers, the frequency of EBV genome harboring B-cells is usually about $1/10^5$ to $1/10^6$. However, the virus is not always a harmless passenger, and it is associated with several malignancies, including Burkitt lymphoma and nasopharyngeal carcinoma. In 1989, EBV was detected in HRS cells for the first time (56). In EBV⁺ cases of HL, with very rare exceptions, all HRS cells carry the virus and the infection pattern is clonal (56), showing that EBV infection is an early and clonal event in HRS cells. In classical HL patients in the Western world, about 30% to 40% of the cases show EBV infection of the HRS cells. In childhood HL in Central America, the frequency is even higher, reaching up to 90% of cases. EBV is not found in the LP cells of NLPHL.

In EBV⁺ HRS cells, the virus shows a latency form that is called latency II. This is defined by expression of the EBV-encoded genes EBV nuclear antigen 1 (*EBNA1*), *LMP1*, and *LMP2a*. In addition, several non–protein-coding EBV RNAs are produced. EBNA1 is essential for the replication of the episomal EBV genome in proliferating cells. Whether EBNA1 also has a direct pathogenetic role in the lymphoma cells is still debated. LMP1 has a cytoplasmic domain that resembles an activated CD40 receptor (135,136). Hence, LMP1 causes constitutive NF-κB activity. LMP2a has a cytoplasmic domain that resembles the key signaling module of the BCR (137). As LMP2a recruits components of the BCR signaling machinery to itself and hence away from the BCR, it was suggested that LMP2a dampens BCR signaling. However, LMP2a itself causes a constitutive low-level activity of the BCR signaling machinery and thereby may provide a (tonic) survival signal for the LMP2a-expressing B-cells (138). Importantly, CD40 and BCR signaling are the two main survival signals of GC B-cells in the selection for high-affinity BCR in the GC reaction (11). Thus, by mimicking activation of these receptors, EBV may be able to rescue crippled GC B-cells from apoptosis. This is supported by studies that showed that BCR-deficient GC B-cells can be immortalized by EBV *in vitro* (139,140). LMP2a has a central role in this process (141). That EBV has an essential role in particular for those cases of HL in which somatic Ig gene mutations prevent the expression of a BCR at all is suggested from the observation that all classical HL with such mutations analyzed so far are EBV⁺ (142). The role of LMP2a as a replacement for the BCR may be less relevant in the established HRS cell clones, because HRS cells have down-regulated most of the BCR signaling machinery, so that it is unlikely that LMP2a can still function in this way.

In general, it remains unclear at which stage of development of an EBV⁺ HL the infection with the virus occurred, for example, whether an already EBV-infected B-cell was driven into a GC reaction, or whether EBV infection occurred later, within the GC. However, we described one example for the latter scenario. In a composite lymphoma of a classical HL and a mantle cell lymphoma, only a subclone of the HRS cells was EBV infected, and this subclone had a slightly different Ig V gene mutation pattern than the EBV⁻ HRS cells, indicating that in this case, EBV infection happened in an HRS cell precursor mutating in the GC (31).

The finding of EBV in a fraction of classical HL prompted numerous studies to search for other viruses in HRS cells. However, no indication was found for an infection of HRS cells with polyomaviruses or herpes viruses other than EBV (143). It was initially reported that HRS cells are infected by measles virus in a fraction of cases (144). However, this finding could not be validated (145). Recently, the infection of an HL cell line with Torque teno (TT) virus was reported, but it remains currently unclear whether infection occurred in culture and whether primary HRS cells also carry the virus (146). Finally, an infection of HRS cells with human herpes virus 6 was also recently reported (147), but further studies are needed to validate this finding, which was based only on immunohistochemistry for a viral protein and not on detection of viral genomes in isolated HRS cells.

COMPOSITE LYMPHOMAS

Composite lymphomas are rare combinations of an HL and an NHL. The NHL in these combinations is diverse, including follicular lymphomas, diffuse large B-cell lymphomas, mantle cell lymphomas, and even T-cell lymphomas. In the strict definition, they occur concurrently in the patient, either at the same site or in different locations. There are, however, also cases where an HL and an NHL develop at different time points in a patient. By molecular analysis, it was shown that in some cases of composite lymphoma the two lymphomas are unrelated to each other, representing the chance occurrence of two malignancies in one patient (148). Interestingly, however, in most concurrently occurring composite lymphomas, molecular studies of rearranged Ig genes (or T-cell receptor genes when the NHL was a T-cell lymphoma) revealed that the two lymphomas shared a common ancestor (25,32–34). In most of the related B-cell lymphomas, a striking pattern of Ig V gene mutations was found: The HRS cells and the B-cell NHL cells had not only shared somatic mutations but also mutations that were found only in one or the other of the two lymphomas. Such a mutation pattern strongly supports a scenario in which the two lymphomas develop from a common precursor, a mutating GC B-cell, and that two separate descendents of this cell (recognized by the additional separate mutations) developed to the two distinct lymphomas (32). Thus, the two lymphomas do not represent the transformation of one lymphoma into the other, but the parallel evolution from a common ancestor. The close relationship of HRS cell clones in several composite lymphomas with typical GC-derived B-cell lymphomas and the indication for a GC B-cell as the common precursor is a strong further argument for the derivation of HRS cells from GC B-cells (see above and Table 16.3).

In two instances where classical HL was combined with T-cell malignancies, molecular analysis of the tumor cells revealed that they carried clonally related T-cell receptor gene rearrangements and that hence the HRS cells are also T-cell derived (149,150). Thus, these cases further support that there are rare cases diagnosed as classical HL with a T-cell derivation.

Composite lymphomas are also excellent models to study the multistep transformation process in lymphomagenesis. It is highly likely that in clonally related composite lymphomas, the common precursors already carried some transforming event(s), and that additional events were acquired during the GC reaction in separate clone members of the premalignant GC B-cell clone, causing the development of two distinct lymphomas from a common cell of origin. In combinations of HL with a follicular lymphoma or a mantle cell lymphoma, we observed that the clonally related lymphomas in the first instance shared the typical t(14;18) IgH-*BCL2* translocation for follicular lymphomas, and in the latter instance the typical t(11;14) IgH-*BCL1* translocation of mantle cell lymphomas (39). Thus, these are examples of shared genetic lesions that were present already in the common precursor of the composite lymphomas. In a combination of HL with a diffuse large B-cell lymphoma, a somatic *TP53* mutation was found only in the B-cell NHL, hence representing a distinct genetic lesion that contributed only to the pathogenesis of the diffuse large B-cell lymphoma, but not of the HL (39).

MICROENVIRONMENTAL INTERACTIONS

As HRS cells with very rare exceptions remain a small subpopulation of cells in the affected lymph nodes, although they are malignant tumor cells, it is likely that the microenvironment plays an essential role in the pathophysiology of the disease. The cellular infiltrate in many aspects resembles an inflammatory response, as it consists of CD4⁺ and CD8⁺ T-cells, B-cells, neutrophils, eosinophils, mast cells, macrophages, plasma cells, and other cell types. There is comprehensive evidence that HRS cells orchestrate this infiltrate by producing multiple chemokines and cytokines. For example, HRS cells produce high levels of the chemokine CCL17 and thereby attract TH2 and regulatory T (Treg) cells (151). HRS cells also secrete CCL5, which attracts mast cells and eosinophils (151). Eosinophils are additionally attracted through production of IL-5 and CCL28 by HRS cells (151).

The cells attracted by the HRS cells into the microenvironment of the lymphoma presumably promote the survival and proliferation of the HRS cells in various ways. For example, mast cells and eosinophils express CD30L and may thus stimulate CD30 signaling in the CD30⁺ HRS cells, thereby contributing to NF-κB activity of the latter cells. Neutrophils express the BCMA ligand APRIL and may thereby stimulate the BCMA-expressing HRS cells (152).

CD4⁺ T-cells usually represent the largest cell population in classical HL tissues. The CD4⁺ T-cell population in classical HL is composed of TH2 TH and Treg cells (153,154). The helper function of T-cells for HRS cells includes secretion of IL-13, which stimulates the IL-13R-positive HRS cells, and cellular interaction between CD40L on T-cells and CD40 on HRS cells. The observation that HRS cells have down-regulated nearly all B-cell–typical genes but still express genes important for interaction with TH cells (CD40, CD54, CD80, CD86) indeed indicates an important role of the interaction between HRS cells and CD4⁺ T-cells for HL pathogenesis.

A large fraction of the CD4⁺ T-cells in HL tissues are Treg cells (153,154). The main role of these cells may be to rescue HRS cells from an attack by cytotoxic T-cells or NK cells. Secretion of IL-10 by the Treg cells is one of the main factors in this regard. HRS cells themselves produce further factors that contribute to an immunosuppressive milieu, including IL-10, TGFβ, galectin 1, prostaglandin E2, PD1L, and CD95 (64).

SUMMARY AND CONCLUSIONS

Molecular analysis of isolated tumor cells has established that not only LP cells of NLPHL but also HRS cells of classical HL derive from mature B-cells. These are most likely antigen-selected GC B-cells in the case of NLPHL and "crippled" GC B-cells in case of classical HL. Some lymphomas currently diagnosed as typical classical HL have a T-cell origin. Classical HL is unique among B-cell lymphomas in the extent to which the tumor cells have lost the phenotype and gene expression pattern of their cells of origin. This loss of the B-cell phenotype may be related to the presumed origin of HRS cells from preapoptotic GC B-cells, may be a strategy of the HRS cell precursors to escape from the pressure to undergo apoptosis as "failed B-cells," and hence may be a central pathogenetic event.

The pattern of genetic lesions identified so far in HRS cells is quite diverse, in all instances affecting only a fraction of cases. However, the detection of multiple lesions in members and regulators of the NF-κB and JAK/STAT pathway points to an important role of the deregulation of these pathways in the development of HL. HRS cells show deregulated activation of multiple other signaling pathways and transcription factors, but to what extent this is also mediated through gene mutations is not known. Certainly, multiple microenvironmental interactions, which are another hallmark of HL pathogenesis, are also involved in the "hyperactivated" state of HRS cells.

References

1. Swerdlow SH, Campo E, Harris NL, et al. *Classification of tumours of haematopoietic and lymphoid tissues.* Lyon: IARC Press, 2008:323–325.
2. Brune V, Tiacci E, Pfeil I, et al. Origin and pathogenesis of nodular lymphocyte-predominant Hodgkin lymphoma as revealed by global gene expression analysis. *J Exp Med* 2008;205:2251–2268.
3. Schwering I, Bräuninger A, Klein U, et al. Loss of the B-lineage-specific gene expression program in Hodgkin and Reed-Sternberg cells of Hodgkin lymphoma. *Blood* 2003;101:1505–1512.
4. Foss HD, Reusch R, Demel G, et al. Frequent expression of the B-cell-specific activator protein in Reed-Sternberg cells of classical Hodgkin's disease provides further evidence for its B-cell origin. *Blood* 1999;94:3108–3113.
5. Nam-Cha SH, Roncador G, Sanchez-Verde L, et al. PD-1, a follicular T-cell marker useful for recognizing nodular lymphocyte-predominant Hodgkin lymphoma. *Am J Surg Pathol* 2008;32:1252–1257.
6. Schmid C, Sargent C, Isaacson PG. L and H cells of nodular lymphocyte predominant Hodgkin's disease show immunoglobulin light-chain restriction. *Am J Pathol* 1991;139:1281–1289.
7. Steimle-Grauer SA, Tinguely M, Seada L, et al. Expression patterns of transcription factors in progressively transformed germinal centers and Hodgkin lymphoma. *Virchows Arch* 2003;442:284–293.
8. Tedoldi S, Mottok A, Ying J, et al. Selective loss of B-cell phenotype in lymphocyte predominant Hodgkin lymphoma. *J Pathol* 2007;213:429–440.
9. Rajewsky K. Clonal selection and learning in the antibody system. *Nature* 1996;381:751–758.
10. Küppers R, Zhao M, Hansmann ML, et al. Tracing B cell development in human germinal centres by molecular analysis of single cells picked from histological sections. *EMBO J* 1993;12:4955–4967.
11. Liu YJ, Joshua DE, Williams GT, et al. Mechanism of antigen-driven selection in germinal centres. *Nature* 1989;342:929–931.
12. Drexler HG. Recent results on the biology of Hodgkin and Reed-Sternberg cells. II. Continuous cell lines. *Leuk Lymphoma* 1993;9:1–25.
13. Tamaru J, Hummel M, Zemlin M, et al. Hodgkin's disease with a B-cell phenotype often shows a VDJ rearrangement and somatic mutations in the VH genes. *Blood* 1994;84:708–715.
14. Küppers R, Rajewsky K, Zhao M, et al. Hodgkin disease: Hodgkin and Reed-Sternberg cells picked from histological sections show clonal immunoglobulin gene rearrangements and appear to be derived from B cells at various stages of development. *Proc Natl Acad Sci U S A* 1994;91:10962–10966.
15. Kanzler H, Küppers R, Hansmann ML, et al. Hodgkin and Reed-Sternberg cells in Hodgkin's disease represent the outgrowth of a dominant tumor clone derived from (crippled) germinal center B cells. *J Exp Med* 1996;184:1495–1505.
16. Delabie J, Tierens A, Gavriil T, et al. Phenotype, genotype and clonality of Reed-Sternberg cells in nodular sclerosis Hodgkin's disease: results of a single-cell study. *Br J Haematol* 1996;94:198–205.
17. Roth J, Daus H, Trümper L, et al. Detection of immunoglobulin heavy-chain gene rearrangement at the single-cell level in malignant lymphomas: no rearrangement is found in Hodgkin and Reed-Sternberg cells. *Int J Cancer* 1994;57:799–804.
18. Hummel M, Ziemann K, Lammert H, et al. Hodgkin's disease with monoclonal and polyclonal populations of Reed-Sternberg cells. *N Engl J Med* 1995;333:901–906.
19. Bräuninger A, Wacker HH, Rajewsky K, et al. Typing the histogenetic origin of the tumor cells of lymphocyte-rich classical Hodgkin's lymphoma in relation to tumor cells of classical and lymphocyte-predominance Hodgkin's lymphoma. *Cancer Res* 2003;63:1644–1651.
20. Irsch J, Nitsch S, Hansmann ML, et al. Isolation of viable Hodgkin and Reed-Sternberg cells from Hodgkin disease tissues. *Proc Natl Acad Sci U S A* 1998;95:10117–10122.
21. Kanzler H, Hansmann ML, Kapp U, et al. Molecular single cell analysis demonstrates the derivation of a peripheral blood-derived cell line (L1236) from the Hodgkin/Reed-Sternberg cells of a Hodgkin's lymphoma patient. *Blood* 1996;87:3429–3436.
22. Marafioti T, Hummel M, Foss H-D, et al. Hodgkin and Reed-Sternberg cells represent an expansion of a single clone originating from a germinal center B-cell with functional immunoglobulin gene rearrangements but defective immunoglobulin transcription. *Blood* 2000;95:1443–1450.
23. Vockerodt M, Soares M, Kanzler H, et al. Detection of clonal Hodgkin and Reed-Sternberg cells with identical somatically mutated and rearranged VH genes in different biopsies in relapsed Hodgkin's disease. *Blood* 1998;92:2899–2907.
24. Müschen M, Küppers R, Spieker T, et al. Molecular single-cell analysis of Hodgkin- and Reed-Sternberg cells harboring unmutated immunoglobulin variable region genes. *Lab Invest* 2001;81:289–295.
25. Rosenquist R, Roos G, Erlanson M, et al. Clonally related splenic marginal zone lymphoma and Hodgkin lymphoma with unmutated V gene rearrangements and a 15-yr time gap between diagnoses. *Eur J Haematol* 2004;73:210–214.
26. Lebecque S, de Bouteiller O, Arpin C, et al. Germinal center founder cells display propensity for apoptosis before onset of somatic mutation. *J Exp Med* 1997;185:563–571.
27. Küppers R, Rajewsky K. The origin of Hodgkin and Reed/Sternberg cells in Hodgkin's disease. *Annu Rev Immunol* 1998;16:471–493.
28. Irsch J, Wolf J, Tesch H, et al. Class switch recombination was specifically targeted to immunoglobulin (Ig)G4 or IgA in Hodgkin's disease-derived cell lines. *Br J Haematol* 2001;113:785–793.
29. Martin-Subero JI, Klapper W, Sotnikova A, et al. Chromosomal breakpoints affecting immunoglobulin loci are recurrent in Hodgkin and Reed-Sternberg cells of classical Hodgkin lymphoma. *Cancer Res* 2006;66:10332–10338.
30. Liso A, Capello D, Marafioti T, et al. Aberrant somatic hypermutation in tumor cells of nodular-lymphocyte-predominant and classic Hodgkin lymphoma. *Blood* 2006;108:1013–1020.
31. Tinguely M, Rosenquist R, Sundstrom C, et al. Analysis of a clonally related mantle cell and Hodgkin lymphoma indicates Epstein-Barr virus infection of a Hodgkin/Reed-Sternberg cell precursor in a germinal center. *Am J Surg Pathol* 2003;27:1483–1488.
32. Bräuninger A, Hansmann ML, Strickler JG, et al. Identification of common germinal-center B-cell precursors in two patients with both Hodgkin's disease and Non-Hodgkin's lymphoma. *N Engl J Med* 1999;340:1239–1247.
33. Küppers R, Sousa AB, Baur AS, et al. Common germinal-center B-cell origin of the malignant cells in two composite lymphomas, involving classical Hodgkin's disease and either follicular lymphoma or B-CLL. *Mol Med* 2001;7:285–292.
34. Marafioti T, Hummel M, Anagnostopoulos I, et al. Classical Hodgkin's disease and follicular lymphoma originating from the same germinal center B cell. *J Clin Oncol* 1999;17:3804–3809.
35. Rosenquist R, Menestrina F, Lestani M, et al. Indications for peripheral light-chain revision and somatic hypermutation without a functional B-cell receptor in precursors of a composite diffuse large B-cell and Hodgkin's lymphoma. *Lab Invest* 2004;84:253–262.
36. Isaacson PG, Norton AJ, Addis BJ. The human thymus contains a novel population of B lymphocytes. *Lancet* 1987;2:1488–1491.
37. Rosenwald A, Wright G, Leroy K, et al. Molecular diagnosis of primary mediastinal B cell lymphoma identifies a clinically favorable subgroup of diffuse large B cell lymphoma related to Hodgkin lymphoma. *J Exp Med* 2003;198:851–862.
38. Brown P, Marafioti T, Kusec R, et al. The FOXP1 transcription factor is expressed in the majority of follicular lymphomas but is rarely expressed in classical and lymphocyte predominant Hodgkin's lymphoma. *J Mol Histol* 2005;36:249–256.
39. Schmitz R, Renné C, Rosenquist R, et al. Insight into the multistep transformation process of lymphomas: IgH-associated translocations and tumor suppressor gene mutations in clonally related composite Hodgkin's and non-Hodgkin's lymphomas. *Leukemia* 2005;19:1452–1458.
40. Müschen M, Rajewsky K, Bräuninger A, et al. Rare occurrence of classical Hodgkin's disease as a T cell lymphoma. *J Exp Med* 2000;191:387–394.
41. Seitz V, Hummel M, Marafioti T, et al. Detection of clonal T-cell receptor gamma-chain gene rearrangements in Reed-Sternberg cells of classic Hodgkin disease. *Blood* 2000;95:3020–3024.
42. Willenbrock K, Küppers R, Renne C, et al. Common features and differences in the transcriptome of large cell anaplastic lymphoma and classical Hodgkin's lymphoma. *Haematologica* 2006;91:596–604.
43. Schmitz R, Stanelle J, Hansmann M-L, et al. Pathogenesis of classical and lymphocyte-predominant Hodgkin lymphoma. *Annu Rev Pathol* 2009;4:151–174.
44. Braeuninger A, Küppers R, Strickler JG, et al. Hodgkin and Reed-Sternberg cells in lymphocyte predominant Hodgkin disease represent clonal populations of germinal center-derived tumor B cells. *Proc Natl Acad Sci USA* 1997;94:9337–9342.
45. Marafioti T, Hummel M, Anagnostopoulos I, et al. Origin of nodular lymphocyte-predominant Hodgkin's disease from a clonal expansion of highly mutated germinal-center B cells. *N Engl J Med* 1997;337:453–458.
46. Ohno T, Stribley JA, Wu G, et al. Clonality in nodular lymphocyte-predominant Hodgkin's disease. *N Engl J Med* 1997;337:459–465.
47. Küppers R, Rajewsky K, Braeuninger A, et al. L&H cells in lymphocyte-predominant Hodgkin's disease (Letter to the Editor). *N Engl J Med* 1998;338:763–764.
48. Klein U, Goossens T, Fischer M, et al. Somatic hypermutation in normal and transformed human B cells. *Immunol Rev* 1998;162:261–280.
49. Michels KB. The origins of Hodgkin's disease. *Eur J Cancer Prev* 1995;4:379–388.
50. Küppers R, Bräuninger A, Müschen M, et al. Evidence that Hodgkin and Reed-Sternberg cells in Hodgkin disease do not represent cell fusions. *Blood* 2001;97:818–821.
51. Re D, Benenson E, Beyer M, et al. Cell fusion is not involved in the generation of giant cells in the Hodgkin-Reed Sternberg cell line L1236. *Am J Hematol* 2001;67:6–9.
52. Newcom SR, Kadin ME, Phillips C. L-428 Reed-Sternberg cells and mononuclear Hodgkin's cells arise from a single cloned mononuclear cell. *Int J Cell Cloning* 1988;6:417–431.
53. Ikeda J, Mamat S, Tian T, et al. Tumorigenic potential of mononucleated small cells of Hodgkin lymphoma cell lines. *Am J Pathol* 2010;177:3081–3088.
54. Küppers R, Engert A, Hansmann M-L. Hodgkin lymphoma. *J Clin Invest* 2012;122:3439–3447.
55. Jansen MP, Hopman AH, Bot FJ, et al. Morphologically normal, CD30⁻ B-lymphocytes with chromosome aberrations in classical Hodgkin's disease: the progenitor cell of the malignant clone? *J Pathol* 1999;189:527–532.
56. Weiss LM, Movahed LA, Warnke RA, et al. Detection of Epstein-Barr viral genomes in Reed-Sternberg cells of Hodgkin's disease. *N Engl J Med* 1989;320:502–506.

57. Spieker T, Kurth J, Küppers R, et al. Molecular single-cell analysis of the clonal relationship of small Epstein-Barr virus-infected cells and Epstein-Barr virus-harboring Hodgkin and Reed/Sternberg cells in Hodgkin disease. *Blood* 2000;96:3133–3138.
58. Jones RJ, Gocke CD, Kasamon YL, et al. Circulating clonotypic B cells in classic Hodgkin lymphoma. *Blood* 2009;113:5920–5926.
59. Küppers R. Clonogenic B cells in classic Hodgkin lymphoma. *Blood* 2009; 114:3970–3971.
60. Wu C, Alman BA. Side population cells in human cancers. *Cancer Lett* 2008; 268:1–9.
61. Nakashima M, Ishii Y, Watanabe M, et al. The side population, as a precursor of Hodgkin and Reed-Sternberg cells and a target for nuclear factor-kappaB inhibitors in Hodgkin's lymphoma. *Cancer Sci* 2010;101:2490–2496.
62. Shafer JA, Cruz CR, Leen AM, et al. Antigen-specific cytotoxic T lymphocytes can target chemoresistant side-population tumor cells in Hodgkin lymphoma. *Leuk Lymphoma* 2010;51:870–880.
63. Küppers R. Mechanisms of B-cell lymphoma pathogenesis. *Nat Rev Cancer* 2005;5:251–262.
64. Küppers R. The biology of Hodgkin's lymphoma. *Nat Rev Cancer* 2009;9:15–27.
65. Re D, Müschen M, Ahmadi T, et al. Oct-2 and Bob-1 deficiency in Hodgkin and Reed Sternberg cells. *Cancer Res* 2001;61:2080–2084.
66. Stein H, Marafioti T, Foss HD, et al. Down-regulation of BOB.1/OBF.1 and Oct2 in classical Hodgkin disease but not in lymphocyte predominant Hodgkin disease correlates with immunoglobulin transcription. *Blood* 2001;97:496–501.
67. Torlakovic E, Tierens A, Dang HD, et al. The transcription factor PU.1, necessary for B-cell development is expressed in lymphocyte predominance, but not classical Hodgkin's disease. *Am J Pathol* 2001;159:1807–1814.
68. Mathas S, Janz M, Hummel F, et al. Intrinsic inhibition of transcription factor E2A by HLH proteins ABF-1 and Id2 mediates reprogramming of neoplastic B cells in Hodgkin lymphoma. *Nature Immunol* 2006;7:207–215.
69. Renné C, Martin-Subero JI, Eickernjager M, et al. Aberrant expression of ID2, a suppressor of B-cell-specific gene expression, in Hodgkin's lymphoma. *Am J Pathol* 2006;169:655–664.
70. Jundt F, Acikgoz O, Kwon SH, et al. Aberrant expression of Notch1 interferes with the B-lymphoid phenotype of neoplastic B cells in classical Hodgkin lymphoma. *Leukemia* 2008;22:1587–1594.
71. Jundt F, Anagnostopoulos I, Förster R, et al. Activated Notch 1 signaling promotes tumor cell proliferation and survival in Hodgkin and anaplastic large cell lymphoma. *Blood* 2001;99:3398–3403.
72. Köchert K, Ullrich K, Kreher S, et al. High-level expression of Mastermind-like 2 contributes to aberrant activation of the NOTCH signaling pathway in human lymphomas. *Oncogene* 2011;30:1831–1840.
73. Scheeren FA, Diehl SA, Smit LA, et al. IL-21 is expressed in Hodgkin lymphoma and activates STAT5; evidence that activated STAT5 is required for Hodgkin lymphomagenesis. *Blood* 2008;111:4706–4715.
74. Portis T, Dyck P, Longnecker R. Epstein-Barr virus (EBV) LMP2A induces alterations in gene transcription similar to those observed in Reed-Sternberg cells of Hodgkin lymphoma. *Blood* 2003;102:4166–4178.
75. Vockerodt M, Morgan SL, Kuo M, et al. The Epstein-Barr virus oncoprotein, latent membrane protein-1, reprograms germinal centre B cells towards a Hodgkin's Reed-Sternberg-like phenotype. *J Pathol* 2008;216:83–92.
76. Hu M, Krause D, Greaves M, et al. Multilineage gene expression precedes commitment in the hemopoietic system. *Genes Dev* 1997;11:774–785.
77. Miyamoto T, Iwasaki H, Reizis B, et al. Myeloid or lymphoid promiscuity as a critical step in hematopoietic lineage commitment. *Dev Cell* 2002;3:137–147.
78. Ammerpohl O, Haake A, Pellissery S, et al. Array-based DNA methylation analysis in classical Hodgkin lymphoma reveals new insights into the mechanisms underlying silencing of B cell-specific genes. *Leukemia* 2012;26:185–188.
79. Doerr JR, Malone CS, Fike FM, et al. Patterned CpG methylation of silenced B cell gene promoters in classical Hodgkin lymphoma-derived and primary effusion lymphoma cell lines. *J Mol Biol* 2005;350:631–640.
80. Ushmorov A, Leithäuser F, Sakk O, et al. Epigenetic processes play a major role in B-cell-specific gene silencing in classical Hodgkin lymphoma. *Blood* 2005;107:2493–2500.
81. Steidl C, Shah SP, Woolcock BW, et al. MHC class II transactivator CIITA is a recurrent gene fusion partner in lymphoid cancers. *Nature* 2011;471:377–381.
82. Diepstra A, van Imhoff GW, Karim-Kos HE, et al. HLA class II expression by Hodgkin Reed-Sternberg cells is an independent prognostic factor in classical Hodgkin's lymphoma. *J Clin Oncol* 2007;25:3101–3108.
83. Bargou RC, Emmerich F, Krappmann D, et al. Constitutive nuclear factor-kappaB-RelA activation is required for proliferation and survival of Hodgkin's disease tumor cells. *J Clin Invest* 1997;100:2961–2969.
84. Kapp U, Yeh WC, Patterson B, et al. Interleukin 13 is secreted by and stimulates the growth of Hodgkin and Reed-Sternberg cells. *J Exp Med* 1999;189:1939–1946.
85. Baus D, Nonnenmacher F, Jankowski S, et al. STAT6 and STAT1 are essential antagonistic regulators of cell survival in classical Hodgkin lymphoma cell line. *Leukemia* 2009;23:1885–1893.
86. Kube D, Holtick U, Vockerodt M, et al. STAT3 is constitutively activated in Hodgkin cell lines. *Blood* 2001;98:762–770.
87. Renné C, Willenbrock K, Küppers R, et al. Autocrine and paracrine activated receptor tyrosine kinases in classical Hodgkin lymphoma. *Blood* 2005;105:4051–4059.
88. Renné C, Hinsch N, Willenbrock K, et al. The aberrant coexpression of several receptor tyrosine kinases is largely restricted to EBV-negative cases of classical Hodgkin's lymphoma. *Int J Cancer* 2007;120:2504–2509.
89. Lamprecht B, Walter K, Kreher S, et al. Derepression of an endogenous long terminal repeat activates the CSF1R proto-oncogene in human lymphoma. *Nat Med* 2010;16:571–579.
90. Dutton A, Reynolds GM, Dawson CW, et al. Constitutive activation of phosphatidylinositide 3 kinase contributes to the survival of Hodgkin's lymphoma cells through a mechanism involving Akt kinase and mTOR. *J Pathol* 2005;205:498–506.
91. Georgakis GV, Li Y, Rassidakis GZ, et al. Inhibition of the phosphatidylinositol-3 kinase/Akt promotes G1 cell cycle arrest and apoptosis in Hodgkin lymphoma. *Br J Haematol* 2006;132:503–511.
92. Nagel S, Burek C, Venturini L, et al. Comprehensive analysis of homeobox genes in Hodgkin lymphoma cell lines identifies dysregulated expression of HOXB9 mediated via ERK5 signaling and BMI1. *Blood* 2007;109:3015–3023.
93. Zheng B, Fiumara P, Li YV, et al. MEK/ERK pathway is aberrantly active in Hodgkin disease: a signaling pathway shared by CD30, CD40, and RANK that regulates cell proliferation and survival. *Blood* 2003;102:1019–1027.
94. Mathas S, Hinz M, Anagnostopoulos I, et al. Aberrantly expressed c-Jun and JunB are a hallmark of Hodgkin lymphoma cells, stimulate proliferation and synergize with NF-kappa B. *EMBO J* 2002;21:4104–4113.
95. Kapp U, Wolf J, Hummel M, et al. Hodgkin's lymphoma-derived tissue serially transplanted into severe combined immunodeficient mice. *Blood* 1993;82:1247–1256.
96. Wolf J, Kapp U, Bohlen H, et al. Peripheral blood mononuclear cells of a patient with advanced Hodgkin's lymphoma give rise to permanently growing Hodgkin-Reed Sternberg cells. *Blood* 1996;87:3418–3428.
97. Mader A, Brüderlein S, Wegener S, et al. U-HO1, a new cell line derived from a primary refractory classical Hodgkin lymphoma. *Cytogenet Genome Res* 2007;119:204–210.
98. Vockerodt M, Belge G, Kube D, et al. An unbalanced translocation involving chromosome 14 is the probable cause for loss of potentially functional rearranged immunoglobulin heavy chain genes in the Epstein-Barr virus-positive Hodgkin's lymphoma-derived cell line L591. *Br J Haematol* 2002;119:640–646.
99. Maggio EM, Van Den Berg A, Visser L, et al. Common and differential chemokine expression patterns in RS cells of NLP, EBV positive and negative classical Hodgkin lymphomas. *Int J Cancer* 2002;99:665–672.
100. Schumacher MA, Schmitz R, Brune V, et al. Mutations in the genes coding for the NF-kappaB regulating factors IkappaBalpha and A20 are uncommon in nodular lymphocyte-predominant Hodgkin's lymphoma. *Haematologica* 2010;95: 153–157.
101. Drexler HG, Dirks WG, MacLeod RA. False human hematopoietic cell lines: cross-contaminations and misinterpretations. *Leukemia* 1999;13:1601–1607.
102. Stein H, Diehl V, Marafioti T, et al. The nature of Reed-Sternberg cells, lymphocytic and histiocytic cells and their molecular biology in Hodgkin's disease. In: Armitage JO, Diehl JO, Hoppe RT, Weiss LM, eds. *Hodgkin's disease*. Philadelphia: Lippincott Williams & Wilkins, 1999:121–137.
103. Bargou RC, Mapara MY, Zugck C, et al. Characterization of a novel Hodgkin cell line, HD-MyZ, with myelomonocytic features mimicking Hodgkin's disease in severe combined immunodeficient mice. *J Exp Med* 1993;177:1257–1268.
104. Weber-Matthiesen K, Deerberg J, Poetsch M, et al. Numerical chromosome aberrations are present within the CD30+ Hodgkin and Reed-Sternberg cells in 100% of analyzed cases of Hodgkin's disease. *Blood* 1995;86:1464–1468.
105. Joos S, Küpper M, Ohl S, et al. Genomic imbalances including amplification of the tyrosine kinase gene JAK2 in CD30+ Hodgkin cells. *Cancer Res* 2000;60: 549–552.
106. Joos S, Menz CK, Wrobel G, et al. Classical Hodgkin lymphoma is characterized by recurrent copy number gains of the short arm of chromosome 2. *Blood* 2002;99:1381–1387.
107. Barth TF, Martin-Subero JI, Joos S, et al. Gains of 2p involving the REL locus correlate with nuclear c-Rel protein accumulation in neoplastic cells of classical Hodgkin lymphoma. *Blood* 2003;101:3681–3686.
108. Green MR, Monti S, Rodig SJ, et al. Integrative analysis reveals selective 9p24.1 amplification, increased PD-1 ligand expression, and further induction via JAK2 in nodular sclerosing Hodgkin lymphoma and primary mediastinal large B-cell lymphoma. *Blood* 2010;116:3268–3277.
109. Rui L, Emre NC, Kruhlak MJ, et al. Cooperative epigenetic modulation by cancer amplicon genes. *Cancer Cell* 2010;18:590–605.
110. Hartmann S, Martin-Subero JI, Gesk S, et al. Detection of genomic imbalances in microdissected Hodgkin and Reed-Sternberg cells of classical Hodgkin's lymphoma by array-based comparative genomic hybridization. *Haematologica* 2008;93:1318–1326.
111. Steidl C, Telenius A, Shah SP, et al. Genome-wide copy number analysis of Hodgkin Reed-Sternberg cells identifies recurrent imbalances with correlations to treatment outcome. *Blood* 2010;116:418–427.
112. Küppers R, Dalla-Favera R. Mechanisms of chromosomal translocations in B cell lymphomas. *Oncogene* 2001;20:5580–5594.
113. Szymanowska N, Klapper W, Gesk S, et al. BCL2 and BCL3 are recurrent translocation partners of the IGH locus. *Cancer Genet Cytogenet* 2008;186:110–114.
114. Franke S, Wlodarska I, Maes B, et al. Lymphocyte predominance Hodgkin disease is characterized by recurrent genomic imbalances. *Blood* 2001;97: 1845–1853.
115. Renné C, Martin-Subero JI, Hansmann ML, et al. Molecular cytogenetic analyses of immunoglobulin loci in nodular lymphocyte predominant Hodgkin's lymphoma reveal a recurrent IGH-BCL6 juxtaposition. *J Mol Diagn* 2005;7:352–356.
116. Wlodarska I, Nooyen P, Maes B, et al. Frequent occurrence of BCL6 rearrangements in nodular lymphocyte predominance Hodgkin lymphoma but not in classical Hodgkin lymphoma. *Blood* 2003;101:706–710.
117. Martin-Subero JI, Gesk S, Harder L, et al. Recurrent involvement of the REL and BCL11A loci in classical Hodgkin lymphoma. *Blood* 2002;99:1474–1477.
118. Otto C, Giefing M, Massow A, et al. Genetic lesions of the TRAF3 and MAP3K14 genes in classical Hodgkin lymphoma. *Br J Haematol* 2012;157:702–708.
119. Cabannes E, Khan G, Aillet F, et al. Mutations in the IκBα gene in Hodgkin's disease suggest a tumour suppressor role for IκBα. *Oncogene* 1999;18:3063–3070.
120. Emmerich F, Meiser M, Hummel M, et al. Overexpression of I kappa B alpha without inhibition of NF-kappaB activity and mutations in the I kappa B alpha gene in Reed-Sternberg cells. *Blood* 1999;94:3129–3134.
121. Jungnickel B, Staratschek-Jox A, Bräuninger A, et al. Clonal deleterious mutations in the iκBα gene in the malignant cells in Hodgkin's disease. *J Exp Med* 2000;191:395–401.
122. Lake A, Shield LA, Cordano P, et al. Mutations of NFKBIA, encoding IkappaBalpha, are a recurrent finding in classical Hodgkin lymphoma but are not a unifying feature of non-EBV-associated cases. *Int J Cancer* 2009;125:1334–1342.
123. Emmerich F, Theurich S, Hummel M, et al. Inactivating I kappa B epsilon mutations in Hodgkin/Reed-Sternberg cells. *J Pathol* 2003;201:413–420.
124. Kato M, Sanada M, Kato I, et al. Frequent inactivation of A20 in B-cell lymphomas. *Nature* 2009;459:712–716.
125. Schmitz R, Hansmann ML, Bohle V, et al. TNFAIP3 (A20) is a tumor suppressor gene in Hodgkin lymphoma and primary mediastinal B cell lymphoma. *J Exp Med* 2009;206:981–989.
126. Martin-Subero JI, Wlodarska I, Bastard C, et al. Chromosomal rearrangements involving the BCL3 locus are recurrent in classical Hodgkin and peripheral T-cell lymphoma. *Blood* 2006;108:401–402.

127. Schmidt A, Schmitz R, Giefing M, et al. Rare occurrence of biallelic CYLD gene mutations in classical Hodgkin lymphoma. *Genes Chromosomes Cancer* 2010;49:803–809.
128. Van Roosbroeck K, Cox L, Tousseyn T, et al. JAK2 rearrangements, including the novel SEC31A-JAK2 fusion, are recurrent in classical Hodgkin lymphoma. *Blood* 2011;117:4056–4064.
129. Weniger MA, Melzner I, Menz CK, et al. Mutations of the tumor suppressor gene SOCS-1 in classical Hodgkin lymphoma are frequent and associated with nuclear phospho-STAT5 accumulation. *Oncogene* 2006;25:2679–2684.
130. Thomas RK, Schmitz R, Harttrampf AC, et al. Apoptosis-resistant phenotype of classical Hodgkin's lymphoma is not mediated by somatic mutations within genes encoding members of the death-inducing signaling complex (DISC). *Leukemia* 2005;19:1079–1082.
131. Feuerborn A, Moritz C, Von Bonin F, et al. Dysfunctional p53 deletion mutants in cell lines derived from Hodgkin's lymphoma. *Leuk Lymphoma* 2006;47:1932–1940.
132. Maggio EM, Stekelenburg E, Van den Berg A, et al. TP53 gene mutations in Hodgkin lymphoma are infrequent and not associated with absence of Epstein-Barr virus. *Int J Cancer* 2001;94:60–66.
133. Wlodarska I, Stul M, De Wolf-Peeters C, et al. Heterogeneity of BCL6 rearrangements in nodular lymphocyte predominant Hodgkin's lymphoma. *Haematologica* 2004;89:965–972.
134. Mottok A, Renné C, Willenbrock K, et al. Somatic hypermutation of SOCS1 in lymphocyte-predominant Hodgkin lymphoma is accompanied by high JAK2 expression and activation of STAT6. *Blood* 2007;110:3387–3390.
135. Kilger E, Kieser A, Baumann M, et al. Epstein-Barr virus-mediated B-cell proliferation is dependent upon latent membrane protein 1, which simulates an activated CD40 receptor. *EMBO J* 1998;17:1700–1709.
136. Gires O, Zimber-Strobl U, Gonnella R, et al. Latent membrane protein 1 of Epstein-Barr virus mimics a constitutively active receptor molecule. *EMBO J* 1997;16:6131–6140.
137. Alber G, Kim KM, Weiser P, et al. Molecular mimicry of the antigen receptor signalling motif by transmembrane proteins of the Epstein-Barr virus and the bovine leukemia virus. *Curr Biol* 1993;3:333–339.
138. Caldwell RG, Wilson JB, Anderson SJ, et al. Epstein-Barr virus LMP2A drives B cell development and survival in the absence of normal B cell receptor signals. *Immunity* 1998;9:405–411.
139. Chaganti S, Bell AI, Begue-Pastor N, et al. Epstein-Barr virus infection in vitro can resue germinal centre B cells with inactivated immunoglobulin genes. *Blood* 2005;106:4249–4252.
140. Bechtel D, Kurth J, Unkel C, et al. Transformation of BCR-deficient germinal-center B cells by EBV supports a major role of the virus in the pathogenesis of Hodgkin and posttransplantation lymphomas. *Blood* 2005;106:4345–4350.
141. Mancao C, Hammerschmidt W. Epstein-Barr virus latent membrane protein 2A is a B-cell receptor mimic and essential for B-cell survival. *Blood* 2007;110:3715–3721.
142. Bräuninger A, Schmitz R, Bechtel D, et al. Molecular biology of Hodgkin and Reed/Sternberg cells in Hodgkin's lymphoma. *Int J Cancer* 2006;118:1853–1861.
143. Jarrett R. The role of viruses in the pathogenesis of Hodgkin lymphoma. In: Engert A, Horning SJ, eds. *Hodgkin lymphoma*. Berlin: Springer-Verlag, 2011:21–32.
144. Benharroch D, Shemer-Avni Y, Myint YY, et al. Measles virus: evidence of an association with Hodgkin's disease. *Br J Cancer* 2004;91:572–579.
145. Maggio E, Benharroch D, Gopas J, et al. Absence of measles virus genome and transcripts in Hodgkin-Reed/Sternberg cells of a cohort of Hodgkin lymphoma patients. *Int J Cancer* 2007;121:448–453.
146. zur Hausen H, de Villiers EM. Virus target cell conditioning model to explain some epidemiologic characteristics of childhood leukemias and lymphomas. *Int J Cancer* 2005;115:1–5.
147. Lacroix A, Collot-Teixeira S, Mardivirin L, et al. Involvement of human herpesvirus-6 variant B in classic Hodgkin's lymphoma via DR7 oncoprotein. *Clin Cancer Res* 2010;16:4711–4721.
148. Caleo A, Sanchez-Aguilera A, Rodriguez S, et al. Composite Hodgkin lymphoma and mantle cell lymphoma: two clonally unrelated tumors. *Am J Surg Pathol* 2003;27:1577–1580.
149. Davis TH, Morton CC, Miller-Cassman R, et al. Hodgkin's disease, lymphomatoid papulosis, and cutaneous T-cell lymphoma derived from a common T-cell clone. *N Engl J Med* 1992;326:1115–1122.
150. Willenbrock K, Ichinohasama R, Kadin ME, et al. T-cell variant of classical Hodgkin's lymphoma with nodal and cutaneous manifestations demonstrated by single-cell polymerase chain reaction. *Lab Invest* 2002;82:1103–1109.
151. Ma Y, van den Berg A, Atayar C, et al. Cytokines, cytokine receptors, and chemokines in Hodgkin lymphoma. In: Hoppe RT, Mauch PM, Armitage JO, Diehl V, Weiss LM, eds. *Hodgkin lymphoma*. Lippincott Wiliams & Wilkins, Philadelphia, 2007:87–98.
152. Chiu A, Xu W, He B, et al. Hodgkin lymphoma cells express TACI and BCMA receptors and generate survival and proliferation signals in response to BAFF and APRIL. *Blood* 2007;109:729–739.
153. Gandhi MK, Lambley E, Duraiswamy J, et al. Expression of LAG-3 by tumor-infiltrating lymphocytes is coincident with the suppression of latent membrane antigen-specific CD8+ T-cell function in Hodgkin lymphoma patients. *Blood* 2006;108:2280–2289.
154. Marshall NA, Christie LE, Munro LR, et al. Immunosuppressive regulatory T cells are abundant in the reactive lymphocytes of Hodgkin lymphoma. *Blood* 2004;103:1755–1762.

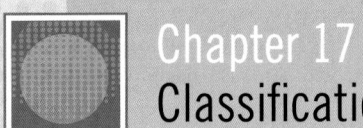

Chapter 17
Classification of Non-Hodgkin Lymphomas

Lawrence M. Weiss • Karen L. Chang

PRINCIPLES OF LYMPHOMA CLASSIFICATION

Many years ago, Henry Rappaport proposed criteria for a sound classification of lymphoma: that a successful classification should be clinically useful, reproducible, easy to teach, and easy to learn. These days, one might add that it should be scientifically accurate and cost-effective, but there is little else to quibble with Rappaport's simple but profound statement. A rational classification of non-Hodgkin lymphomas has been slow in the making, with many false starts and blind alleys, but much progress has been seen in recent years. We are now at the point of a rational classification that is agreed upon by almost all hematopathologists and which only needs minor updating from time to time (1,2).

The original classifications of lymphomas depended exclusively upon histologic analysis, necessary since even rudimentary knowledge of immunology and molecular biology was unknown at the time they were devised (3). Some later classifications tried to encompass an increasing knowledge of immunology, attempting to distinguish B- from T-lineage neoplasms and recognizing the phenomenon of lymphocyte transformation (3–5), but failed due to either an insufficient knowledge base or lack of appropriate diagnostic tools at the time the classifications were proposed to recognize specific lymphoma types. The ultimate expression of these principles was the Working Formulation of Non-Hodgkin Lymphoma for Clinical Usage, published in 1982 (Table 17.1) (6–8). While craftily proposed as a way to "translate" between the different classifications used at the time, it itself became a major classification of non-Hodgkin lymphoma, recognizing 10 major morphologic categories organized into three major prognostic groups. Useful clinically for many years, it ultimately failed as a classification scheme because it was not scientifically accurate. It became increasingly clear that morphologic schemes that did not address immunology or molecular biology in a comprehensive way could not capture many true lymphoma entities. Contemporaneously, diagnostic tools such as immunohistochemistry, flow cytometry, monoclonal antibodies, and molecular studies (most notably Southern blotting and polymerase chain reaction analyses) were becoming available, and these have enabled the diagnostic pathologist to apply the newly discovered knowledge to individual cases.

The first major lymphoma classification to truly address lymphoma biology in a comprehensive way was the Revised European American Lymphoma (REAL) classification (Table 17.2) (9). The overarching principle of this classification separated lymphoma types by cell lineage and degree of maturation. On the other hand, recognizing the limitations of the current state of knowledge in defining different lymphoma types based solely on biology, the classification utilized a multiparameter approach including clinical presentation and other clinical features, morphologic assessment, immunophenotype, molecular features, and virology. Thus, it was realized that extranodal localization was the key to recognizing a new biologic entity of extranodal marginal zone lymphoma of mucosa-associated lymphoid tissue (MALT). Similarly, mediastinal localization was key to the recognition of primary mediastinal (thymic) large B-cell lymphoma. The result was a list of various lymphomas, sorted by B versus T/natural killer (NK) and precursor versus mature neoplasms.

The principles established by the REAL classification were further developed in the 2001 World Health Organization (WHO) classification of lymphomas (strictly speaking, the third edition) (1). Significant enhancements included not only incorporation of our increasing knowledge of the biology of lymphocytes and malignant lymphomas but the admirable inclusion of a large representation of expert hematopathologists from around the world and the formal input from clinical advisory committees, constituting worldwide experts on lymphoma treatment. This emphasis on universality was reflected by the inclusion of lymphoma entities not commonly seen in Western populations, but identified in other populations. The grounding of the WHO classification in two large hematopathology societies (Society for Hematopathology and European Association of Hematopathology) has provided an anchor for future modifications, as exemplified by the 2008 update of this classification (fourth edition) (2). The 2008 WHO classification is the classification primarily used in this book, reflecting its near-universal acceptance by hematopathologists and surgical pathologists around the world.

It is widely acknowledged that the current 2008 WHO classification is the most scientifically accurate classification of lymphoma yet devised, but what of Rappaport's other three criteria, as well as the added criterion of cost-effectiveness? Surprisingly, there have been no major studies reporting on the reproducibility of the WHO classification. However, a major study of the REAL classification involving over 1,400 cases demonstrated that both diagnostic accuracy and reproducibility of the diagnosis was about 85% (10). Is the classification easy to teach and easy to learn? These are questions for which it is difficult to design a study to answer. The anecdotal experience of most hematopathologists would suggest that the WHO classification is teachable and learnable. Nonetheless, the multiparameter approach requires a highly knowledgeable pathologist with ready access to immunophenotyping in most cases and more advanced technology in some cases to accurately apply the classification. It also requires a clinician who is knowledgeable about the classification, to understand the full implications of the diagnosis. Rightfully or wrongfully, the new classification requires more specialization on the part of both the pathologist and the clinician to apply and interpret the classification most successfully, as well as good communication between the two. Finally, is the classification cost-effective? Again, this is a question that is not easy to answer via scientific studies. In some cases, a sophisticated (read: expensive) workup is necessary to establish the proper diagnosis. However, one must

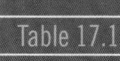

Table 17.1 WORKING FORMULATION

Low Grade
- Malignant lymphoma, small lymphocytic (chronic lymphocytic leukemia)
- Malignant lymphoma, follicular, predominantly small cleaved cell
- Malignant lymphoma, follicular, mixed (small cleaved and large cell)

Intermediate Grade
- Malignant lymphoma, follicular, predominantly large cell
- Malignant lymphoma, diffuse, small cleaved cell
- Malignant lymphoma, diffuse, mixed small and large cell
- Malignant lymphoma, diffuse, large cell

High Grade
- Malignant lymphoma, large cell, immunoblastic
- Malignant lymphoma, lymphoblastic
- Malignant lymphoma, small noncleaved cells (Burkitt lymphoma)

Adapted from National Cancer Institute sponsored study of classifications of non-Hodgkin's lymphomas: summary and description of a working formulation for clinical usage. The Non-Hodgkin's Lymphoma Pathologic Classification Project. *Cancer* 1982;49:2112–2135, with permission from John Wiley and Sons, Inc.

also consider the economic consequences of misdiagnosis in this age of specific disease-directed therapies. One may argue, however costly a pathology workup may be, its cost pales in comparison to either the costs of the complex radiologic studies necessary to diagnose and stage lymphoma patient or the costs of therapy. It is far preferable to spend precious resources

Table 17.2 REVISED EUROPEAN-AMERICAN LYMPHOMA (REAL) CLASSIFICATION

B-Cell Neoplasms
I. Precursor B-cell neoplasm: precursor B-acute lymphoblastic leukemia/lymphoblastic lymphoma (B-ALL, LBL)
II. Peripheral B-cell neoplasms
   A. B-cell chronic lymphocytic leukemia/small lymphocytic lymphoma
   B. B-cell prolymphocytic leukemia
   C. Lymphoplasmacytic lymphoma/immunocytoma
   D. Mantle cell lymphoma
   E. Follicular lymphoma
   F. Extranodal marginal zone B-cell lymphoma of MALT type
   G. Nodal marginal zone B-cell lymphoma (+/− monocytoid B-cells)
   H. Splenic marginal zone lymphoma (+/− villous lymphocytes)
   I. Hairy cell leukemia
   J. Plasmacytoma/plasma cell myeloma
   K. Diffuse large B-cell lymphoma
      Primary mediastinal B-cell lymphoma
      Primary effusion lymphoma
   L. Burkitt lymphoma

T-Cell and Putative NK-Cell Neoplasms
I. Precursor T-cell neoplasm: precursor T-acute lymphoblastic leukemia/lymphoblastic lymphoma (T-ALL, LBL)
II. Peripheral T-cell and NK-cell neoplasms
   A. T-cell chronic lymphocytic leukemia/prolymphocytic leukemia
   B. T-cell granular lymphocytic leukemia
   C. Mycosis fungoides/Sezary syndrome
   D. Peripheral T-cell lymphoma, not otherwise characterized
   E. Hepatosplenic gamma/delta T-cell lymphoma
   F. Subcutaneous panniculitis-like T-cell lymphoma
   G. Angioimmunoblastic T-cell lymphoma
   H. Extranodal T/NK-cell lymphoma, nasal type
   I. Enteropathy-type intestinal T-cell lymphoma
   J. Adult T-cell lymphoma/leukemia (HTLV-1+)
   K. Anaplastic large cell lymphoma, primary systemic type
   L. Anaplastic large cell lymphoma, primary cutaneous type
   M. Aggressive NK-cell leukemia Hodgkin lymphoma

Adapted from Harris NL, Jaffe ES, Stein H, et al. A revised European-American classification of lymphoid neoplasms: a proposal from the International Lymphoma Study Group. *Blood* 1994; 84:1361–1392, with permission from the American Society of Hematology (ASH).

directed against the correct diagnosis than an incorrect diagnosis that may not have a hope of responding to the selected course of treatment (e.g., rituxan in a peripheral T-cell lymphoma).

GENERAL BASIS OF LYMPHOMA DIAGNOSIS

In general, the non-Hodgkin lymphomas tend to recapitulate a specific stage of B-, T-, and NK-cell development. In a perfect world, one would like to identify that specific stage and arrange the lymphomas in an orderly progression of lymphocyte differentiation. Unfortunately, we still do not know the "cell type of origin" for many categories of lymphoma. In fact, some lymphomas seem to defy that characterization (e.g., hairy cell lymphoma), while other lymphomas of markedly different biology and behavior seem to share a similar developmental stage (e.g., follicular lymphoma and Burkitt lymphoma). Thus, there are obviously other biologic factors that are of greater importance in terms of classification.

Optimally, one would like to identify a single biologic feature or a simple constellation of features that would identify a specific lymphoma type with clinical significance. This is possible in a number of situations. In some cases, for example chronic lymphocytic leukemia/small lymphocytic lymphoma showing proliferation centers or follicular lymphoma showing obvious follicular architecture throughout the lesion, histologic assessment may be sufficient for a confident diagnosis. However, more often than not, proper classification also requires the performance of immunophenotyping studies, using either immunohistochemistry or flow cytometry, occasionally supplemented by molecular or virologic studies. Immunophenotyping studies are invaluable in determining the lineage and differentiation stage of a lymphoid proliferation (particularly immature vs. mature, but also germinal center vs. activated B cell vs. plasmablastic, etc.) and can in many circumstances by itself be useful in establishing a specific diagnosis. Again, using the example of chronic lymphocytic leukemia/small lymphocytic lymphoma, the identification of an aberrant CD20+, CD5+, CD43+, and CD23+ population of cells is characteristic of this neoplasm, and therefore very helpful in establishing the diagnosis. On the other hand, the identification of single antigens rarely is sufficient to establish a specific diagnosis. For example, ALK expression, the hallmark of anaplastic large cell lymphoma, ALK+, may also be found in rare ALK+ large B-cell lymphomas (11) and cyclin D1 expression, the hallmark of mantle cell lymphoma, may also be found in a subset of cases of plasma cell myeloma (12). An example of a pathognomonic molecular feature that alone can establish a specific diagnosis would be the identification of specific translocations in specific variants of B-lymphoblastic leukemia/lymphoma. Nonetheless, in most cases, this is not possible. While many molecular findings are characteristic of specific lymphoma types, they are usually not pathognomonic. Thus, translocations involving the MYC gene are characteristic of Burkitt lymphoma but may be also seen in a subset of cases of diffuse large B-cell lymphoma (DLBCL) (13). Similarly, t(14;18) is characteristic of most cases of follicular lymphoma but may also be seen in a subset of cases of DLBCL and may even be seen in the peripheral blood of a significant proportion of older individuals without malignant lymphoma (14). Similarly, virologic studies may be helpful in establishing a specific lymphoma type. The identification of monoclonally integrated human T-cell leukemia/lymphoma virus 1 (HTLV-1) may be used to definitively establish the diagnosis of adult T-cell leukemia/lymphoma (15). Yet again, other than this example, virologic studies are not pathognomonic of a specific lymphoma type. For example, while the presence of human herpesvirus 8 (HHV-8) is universal in primary effusion lymphoma, it also may be seen in large B-cell lymphoma arising in HHV-8–associated Castleman disease (16). In some still poorly studied and rare lymphoma types, particularly T or NK neoplasms, one must depend heavily on clinical features, since the pathologic and biologic features are not distinctive enough, or at least not well characterized enough, to provide a definitive diagnosis in some or even a majority of cases without the clinical features. Therefore, one usually must depend on a multiparameter approach, which will vary depending upon the specific differential diagnosis.

Even when a diagnosis of specific type of malignant lymphoma may be confidently rendered, the diagnosis alone may not be sufficient for clinical use. For example, it is usually relatively easy to establish a diagnosis of chronic lymphocytic leukemia/small lymphocytic lymphoma on histologic and immunophenotypic features, but additional prognostic pathologic data are often required. This may include additional phenotyping studies (e.g., ZAP-70 and CD38) (17), molecular studies (e.g., somatic mutation in the IGH@ variable region genes) (18), or cytogenetic studies (e.g., identification of specific translocations or numerical abnormalities) (19). The performance of additional studies will depend on the specific lymphoma type. Finally, clinicians will supplement these data with clinical data such as the International Prognostic Index to provide the most accurate prognostic information to the patient and to design the most appropriate treatment plan (20,21).

WHO CLASSIFICATION

The most recent WHO classification of non-Hodgkin lymphoma divides lymphomas into precursor neoplasms, mature B-cell neoplasms, and mature T- and NK-cell neoplasms. This section concentrates on some salient or controversial points of classification for each of the entities below.

Precursor Neoplasms

Within the category of precursor neoplasms, there is subdivision into B-lymphoblastic leukemia/lymphoma, NOS or with recurrent genetic abnormalities, and T-lymphoblastic leukemia/lymphoma. There is no formal cutoff between leukemia and lymphoma, although many clinical protocols still regard >25% bone marrow blasts as leukemia. Contrary to the criteria in acute myeloid leukemia, there is no lower limit for the percentage of blasts required for the diagnosis of precursor B or T neoplasms, although it is stated that "the diagnosis should be avoided when there are fewer than 20% blasts" (1). While many prior classifications included Burkitt leukemia within the definition of B-lymphoblastic leukemia/lymphoma (L3), the former disease is now excluded and considered part of the spectrum of Burkitt lymphoma. Similarly, the morphologic designations L1 and L2 of the previous French-American-British (FAB) classification are discarded, since there is no clinical or biologic significance to these distinctions. The specific recurrent genetic abnormalities to be distinguished from B-lymphoblastic leukemia/lymphoma, not otherwise specified, include both translocations (BCR-ABL1, MLL, TEL-AML1, IL3-IGH, and E2A-PBX1) and alterations in chromosome number (hyperdiploidy, hypodiploidy). In general, these specific abnormalities were chosen because they defined a discrete group of patients and were associated with distinctive clinical, phenotypic, or biologic findings, and particularly if there was prognostic significance to the grouping. In contrast, all cases of T-lymphoblastic leukemia/lymphoma are considered together in one category, because specific recurrent genetic abnormalities within this neoplasm have not yet been found to have strikingly distinctive characteristics (Table 17.3).

Table 17.3	2008 WHO CLASSIFICATION OF PRECURSOR LYMPHOID NEOPLASMS

- B-lymphoblastic leukemia/lymphoma, not otherwise specified
- B-lymphoblastic leukemia/lymphoma with recurrent genetic abnormalities
  - B-lymphoblastic leukemia/lymphoma with t(9;22) (q34;q11.2); BCR/ABL
  - B-lymphoblastic leukemia/lymphoma with t(v;11q23); MLL rearranged
  - B-lymphoblastic leukemia/lymphoma with t(12;21)(p13;q22); TEL/AML1 (ETV6-RUNX1)
  - B-lymphoblastic leukemia/lymphoma with hyperdiploidy
  - B-lymphoblastic leukemia/lymphoma with hypodiploidy (hypodiploid ALL)
  - B-lymphoblastic leukemia/lymphoma with t(5;14)(q31;q32)(IL3-IGH)
  - B-lymphoblastic leukemia/lymphoma with t(1;19)(Q23;P13.3); (E2A-PBX1; TCF3/PBX1)
- T-lymphoblastic leukemia/lymphoma

Adapted from Swerdlow SH, Campo E, Harris NL, et al. *WHO Classification of Tumours of Haematopoietic and Lymphoid Tissues.* Lyon: International Agency for Research on Cancer, 2008, with permission.

Mature B-Cell Neoplasms

Mature B-cell neoplasms constitute about two dozen separate categories, with several of the categories containing additional entities. For example, in the category of DLBCL, NOS, there are the four subentities of DLBCL, although it is not entirely clear why these are placed here and not regarded as separate categories, as was the case for other variants of DLBCL, such as DLBCL associated with chronic inflammation (Table 17.4).

Chronic Lymphocytic Leukemia/Small Lymphocytic Lymphoma

Chronic lymphocytic leukemia/small lymphocytic lymphoma constitute the first category within mature B-cell neoplasms. There is no formal distinction between leukemia and lymphoma; however, it is noted that one group of investigators requires lymphadenopathy, absence of cytopenias due to marrow infiltration, and $<5 \times 10^9$/L B cells with the characteristic phenotype in the peripheral blood for the diagnosis of small lymphocytic lymphoma (22). In fact, in the absence of extramedullary tissue involvement, a diagnosis of chronic lymphocytic leukemia cannot be made unless there are $>5 \times 10^9$/L B cells with the characteristic phenotype in the peripheral blood. Cases in which there are $<5 \times 10^9$/L monoclonal or oligoclonal B cells in the peripheral blood have been designated monoclonal B-cell lymphocytosis, the clinical significance of which is still yet not clear (23,24). Cases of transformation of chronic lymphocytic leukemia/small lymphocytic lymphoma to B-cell prolymphocytic leukemia, diffuse large cell lymphoma, or Hodgkin lymphoma are not given a separate category within the WHO classification.

B-Cell Prolymphocytic Leukemia

B-cell prolymphocytic leukemia is defined as having >55% B prolymphocytes in the peripheral blood (2). It must be distinguished from cases of prolymphocytic transformation of chronic lymphocytic leukemia, a task that may be quite difficult if not impossible without knowledge of the prior clinical course. Cases that otherwise resemble B-cell prolymphocytic leukemia but carrying a t(11;14) are also excluded from the definition, although many of these cases behave better than typical cases of mantle cell lymphoma (25). Even with these restrictions, B-cell prolymphocytic leukemia still appears to be a heterogeneous entity, which may undergo refinement as the field advances.

Table 17.4	2008 WHO CLASSIFICATION OF LYMPHOID NEOPLASMS: MATURE B-CELL NEOPLASMS

Chronic lymphocytic leukemia/small lymphocytic lymphoma
- B-cell prolymphocytic leukemia
- Splenic marginal zone B-cell lymphoma
- Hairy cell leukemia
- Splenic lymphoma/leukemia, unclassifiable
  - Splenic diffuse red pulp small B-cell lymphoma
  - Hairy cell leukemia-variant
- Lymphoplasmacytic lymphoma
  - Waldenstrom macroglobulinemia
- Heavy chain diseases
  - Gamma heavy chain disease
  - Mu heavy chain disease
  - Alpha heavy chain disease
- Plasma cell neoplasms
  - Monoclonal gammopathy of unknown significance
  - Plasma cell myeloma
  - Solitary plasmacytoma of bone
  - Extraosseous plasmacytoma
  - Monoclonal immunoglobulin deposition diseases
- Extranodal marginal zone lymphoma of MALT
- Nodal marginal zone lymphoma
- Follicular lymphoma
- Primary cutaneous follicle center lymphoma
- Mantle cell lymphoma
- Diffuse large B-cell lymphoma (DLBCL), NOS
  - T-cell/histiocytes-rich large B-cell lymphoma
  - Primary DLBCL of the CNS
  - Primary cutaneous DLBCL, leg type
  - EBV+ DLBCL of the elderly
- DLBCL associated with chronic inflammation
- Lymphomatoid granulomatosis
- Primary mediastinal (thymic) large B-cell lymphoma
- Intravascular large B-cell lymphoma
- ALK+ large B-cell lymphoma
- Plasmablastic lymphoma
- Large B-cell lymphoma arising in HHV8-associated multicentric Castleman disease
- Primary effusion lymphoma
- Burkitt lymphoma
- B-cell lymphoma, unclassifiable, with features intermediate between DLBCL and Burkitt lymphoma
- B-cell lymphoma, unclassifiable, with features intermediate between DLBCL and classical Hodgkin lymphoma

Adapted from Swerdlow SH, Campo E, Harris NL, et al. *WHO Classification of Tumours of Haematopoietic and Lymphoid Tissues.* Lyon: International Agency for Research on Cancer, 2008, with permission.

Splenic B-Cell Lymphomas

The WHO classification recognizes several categories of lymphoma primarily occurring in the spleen (2). Splenic marginal zone lymphoma is a distinctive neoplasm that probably accounts for many cases previously regarded as CD5⁻ chronic lymphocytic leukemia or splenic lymphoma with circulating villous lymphocytes (26). It shows a characteristic appearance in the spleen, with a central zone or rim of small lymphocytes around a germinal center merging with a peripheral zone of slightly larger cells, with effacement of the mantle zone (Fig. 17.1) (27). Although the red pulp is commonly involved, it rarely shows a predominantly red pulp pattern of involvement (28). The classification of splenic lymphomas with predominantly red pulp involvement such as hairy cell leukemia and two provisional variants is still problematic. Hairy cell leukemia is a clinically, pathologically, and molecularly distinctive neoplasm that is important to recognize due to the availability of specific and effective treatment (29). In addition, the WHO classification recognizes two provisional entities within the greater category of splenic B-cell lymphoma/leukemia, unclassifiable:

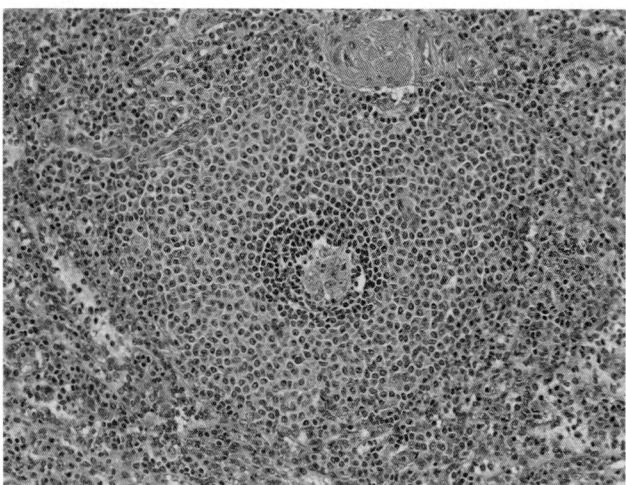

FIGURE 17.1. Splenic marginal zone B-cell lymphoma. There is an atrophic germinal center surrounded by a rim of smaller cells and a much larger peripheral zone of marginal zone B cells. Both the rim of small cells (which is not a normal mantle zone) and the larger peripheral zone represent part of the neoplastic process.

splenic diffuse red pulp small B-cell lymphoma and hairy cell leukemia-variant (2). Splenic diffuse red pulp small B-cell lymphoma, as its name suggests, is defined by its diffuse pattern of involvement of the red pulp by small lymphocytes, in which other clearly defined entities have been excluded (Fig. 17.2) (27). There is probably some degree of overlap with hairy cell leukemia-variant, which is defined by resembling classic hairy cell leukemia, but exhibiting variant "cytohematologic" features (30,31). In my opinion, this is an inappropriate designation, as there are many cytologic, cytochemical, or immunophenotypic differences with hairy cell leukemia, and probably represents a neoplasm biologically distinctive from classic hairy cell leukemia, and patients with hairy cell leukemia variant do not respond to the treatments so effective in hairy cell leukemia. Obviously, the area of non–hairy cell but primarily splenic red pulp lymphomas needs additional study.

Lymphoplasmacytic Lymphoma

B-cell lymphomas with plasmacytic differentiation have been problematic in lymphoma classification. Plasmacytic

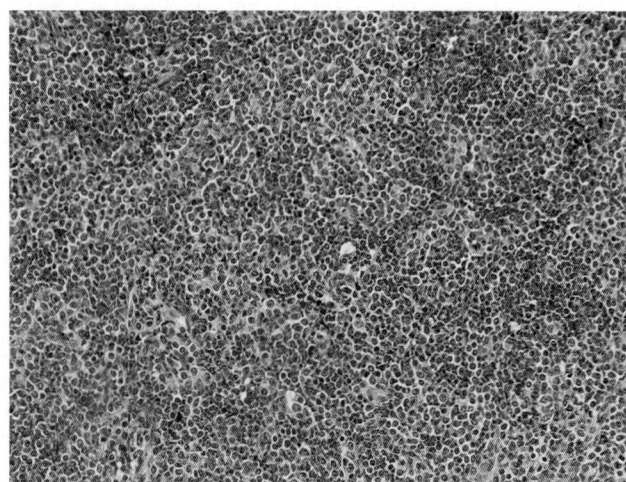

FIGURE 17.2. Splenic red pulp B-cell lymphoma. All other known types of lymphoma, including splenic marginal zone B-cell lymphoma with prominent red pulp involvement, must be ruled out.

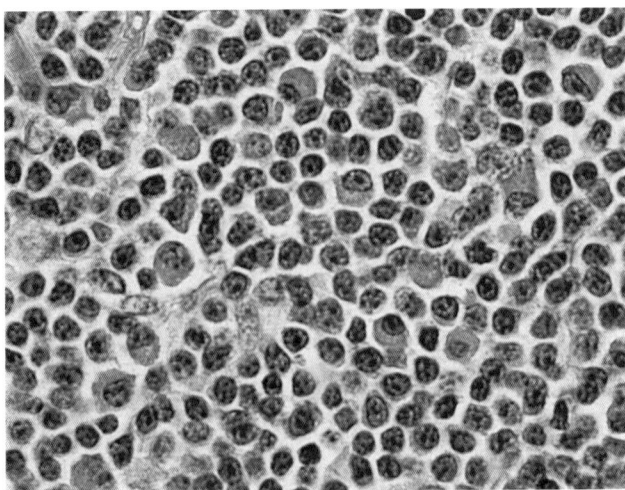

FIGURE 17.3. Lymphoplasmacytic lymphoma. There is a complete spectrum of cells from mature B lymphocytes to plasma cells, mixed haphazardly.

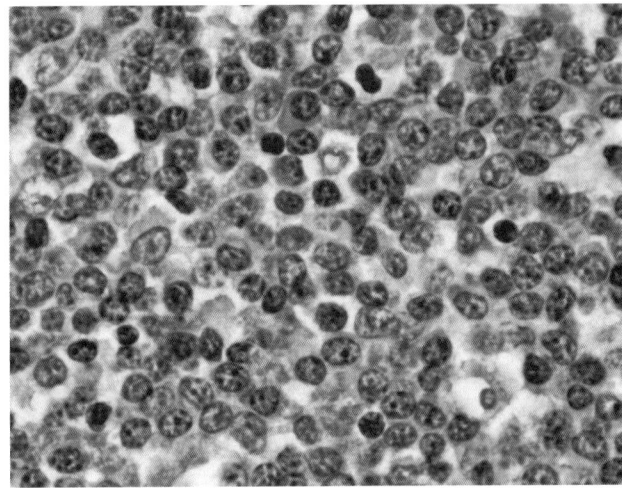

FIGURE 17.5. Gamma heavy chain disease. The histologic appearance is identical to lymphoplasmacytic lymphoma. Laboratory data are crucial to the correct diagnosis.

differentiation may be a defining feature of some neoplasms, but may also be a characteristic of other well-defined lymphoma types. For example, plasmacytic differentiation may be seen in nodal or extranodal marginal zone B-cell lymphoma, chronic lymphocytic leukemia/small lymphocytic lymphoma, or DLBCL, but is a defining feature of lymphoplasmacytic lymphoma and the plasma cell neoplasms.

Lymphoplasmacytic lymphoma is defined as a neoplasm of small B-lymphocytes, plasmacytoid lymphocytes, and plasma cells in which other specific diagnoses have been excluded (Fig. 17.3) (2). It includes the clinicopathologic entity Waldenstrom macroglobulinemia, which clearly represents a distinctive neoplasm (32). It probably also includes cases of gamma heavy chain disease, with which it shares very similar histologic changes (33). Once those two entities are removed, the category of lymphoplasmacytic lymphoma becomes more nebulous and difficult to distinguish from cases of nodal marginal zone lymphoma with plasmacytic differentiation or, less commonly, other lymphomas showing plasmacytic differentiation. Cases of nodal marginal zone lymphoma with plasmacytic differentiation can often be recognized by architectural dichotomization between the lymphoid and lymphoplasmacytoid areas (Fig. 17.4), in distinction to lymphoplasmacytic lymphoma, in which the plasmacytoid and nonplasmacytoid areas are intermixed. If lymphoplasmacytic lymphoma exists as a true lymphoma distinct from Waldenstrom macroglobulinemia and gamma heavy chain disease, it is quite rare.

Heavy Chain Diseases

Heavy chain diseases are rare neoplasms that produce monoclonal heavy chains without light chains (34). As stated in the previous paragraph, gamma heavy chain disease typically shows histologic overlap with lymphoplasmacytic lymphoma (Fig. 17.5) (35). Alpha heavy chain disease, previously known as immunoproliferative small intestinal disease, is regarded to be a distinctive variant of extranodal marginal zone lymphoma of MALT of the intestinal tract, mainly the small intestine and regional mesenteric lymph nodes (36). Mu heavy chain disease is extremely rare and has a resemblance to chronic lymphocytic leukemia, often with the addition of vacuolated plasma cells in the bone marrow (37).

Plasma Cell Neoplasms

Plasma cell neoplasms comprise monoclonal gammopathy of undetermined significance (MGUS); plasma cell myeloma and its three variants, namely, asymptomatic (smoldering) myeloma, nonsecretory myeloma, and plasma cell leukemia; solitary plasmacytoma of bone; extraosseous (extramedullary) plasmacytoma; and the immunoglobulin deposition diseases (primary amyloidosis and systemic light- and heavy chain deposition diseases; and osteosclerotic myeloma [POEMS syndrome]) (2). The function of the pathologist is to determine whether there is a monoclonal proliferation of plasma cells, and the specific classification is made based on a correlation of clinical, pathologic, and radiologic features. MGUS is defined as the presence of <30 g/L M protein in the serum and <10% clonal plasma cells in the absence of both end-organ damage and any neoplasm known to produce an M protein (38). It is distinguished from asymptomatic (smoldering) myeloma by the presence of either >30 g/L M protein or >10% plasma cells, again in the absence of end-organ damage (39). In nonsecretory myeloma, there is an absence of an M protein, although in up to two-thirds of cases, elevated or abnormal serum free light chains may be present (40). Plasma cell leukemia is an aggressive variant in which the number of clonal plasma cells in the peripheral blood is >2 × 10⁹/L or >20% of the white blood cells (41). Solitary plasmacytoma of bone is a single

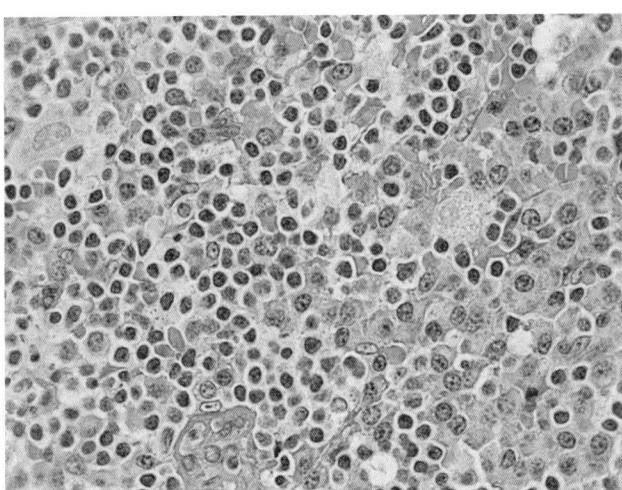

FIGURE 17.4. Nodal marginal zone B-cell lymphoma, with prominent plasmacytoid differentiation. Note the architectural segregation of the plasma cell component.

Table 17.5	**PLASMA CELL NEOPLASMS**

- Monoclonal gammopathy of unknown significance
- Plasma cell myeloma
  - Asymptomatic (smoldering) myeloma
  - Nonsecretory myeloma
  - Plasma cell leukemia
- Solitary plasmacytoma of bone
- Extraosseous plasmacytoma
- Monoclonal immunoglobulin deposition diseases
  - Primary amyloidosis
  - Systemic light and heavy chain deposition diseases
  - Osteosclerotic myeloma (POEMS syndrome)

Adapted from Swerdlow SH, Campo E, Harris NL, et al. *WHO Classification of Tumours of Haematopoietic and Lymphoid Tissues.* Lyon: International Agency for Research on Cancer, 2008, with permission.

localized osseous lesion consisting of clonal plasma cells without evidence of systemic involvement, including the absence of clonal plasma cells in random bone marrow specimens (42). Extraosseous plasmacytoma are identical lesions found in extraosseous sites (43). They are distinguished from the more common extranodal marginal zone B-cell lymphomas with extensive plasmacytoid differentiation by the complete absence of a lymphoid component in the former; conversely, the presence of any lymphoid component, no matter how small (and often recognizable by CD20 stains), would warrant the latter diagnosis (44) (Table 17.5).

Monoclonal immunoglobulin deposition diseases are characterized by deposition of immunoglobulin by clonal plasma cells or lymphoplasmacytic cells, leading to compromised organ function (45). In primary amyloidosis, there is formation of amyloid (46), while in monoclonal light and heavy chain deposition disease, the deposited immunoglobulin fragments do not form amyloid (45,47). Osteosclerotic myeloma is a plasma cell neoplasm that is characterized by peculiar paratrabecular fibrotic and osteosclerotic changes of the bone with embedded clonal plasma cells (48). It is usually (but not always) associated with the POEMS syndrome of polyneuropathy, organomegaly, endocrinopathy, monoclonal gammopathy, and skin changes.

Marginal Zone Lymphomas

Extranodal marginal zone lymphoma of MALT is a family of related extranodal lymphomas that are most commonly found, but not exclusively seen, in mucosal locations (49,50). As the name implies, they are thought to derive from B-cells of the marginal zone of follicles, possibly due to persistent antigen stimulation, which may vary at different sites of the body (51). They show similar morphologic appearance, immunophenotype, and molecular genetic findings at the various sites, although the incidence of the various cytogenetic abnormalities may vary from site to site (Fig. 17.4). Nodal marginal zone lymphoma is considered to be a distinct category of lymphoma, and patients with lymph node involvement by a marginal zone lymphoma are considered to have extranodal marginal zone lymphoma if there is a previous or concurrent (or subsequent) extranodal marginal zone lymphoma or even a history of an autoimmune disorder such as Sjögren syndrome (52). The absence of the characteristic translocations found in extranodal marginal zone lymphoma and not in nodal marginal zone lymphoma is a key piece of evidence suggesting that the two types of lymphomas are distinct neoplasms. In addition, it appears that pediatric nodal marginal zone lymphomas may be a distinct neoplasm from adult cases (53). While the immunophenotypic findings are identical, histologically there is often a close intermingling of the neoplastic cells with progressively

transformed germinal centers, and clinically the cases are usually relatively asymptomatic, present at low stage, and have an excellent outcome, as compared to adult cases.

Follicular Lymphoma

Follicular lymphoma is probably the one lymphoma category that has stayed the most stable as the numerous classifications of lymphoma have evolved throughout the last century. Nonetheless, there have been a number of refinements in recent years. For many years, pathologists have been asked to separate follicular lymphomas into three cytologic grades based on the proportions of small and large cells in the follicles (predominantly small cleaved, 1; mixed small and large cells, 2; and predominantly large cell, 3). Due to the irreproducibility of distinguishing between the first two categories, as well as its lack of clinical significance, they have been combined into a category of 1/2 (2). One must still distinguish these cases from grade 3 cases with >15 centroblasts (large, noncleaved cells) per hpf; moreover, one must distinguish grade 3A, with scattered centrocytes (small, cleaved cells), from grade 3B, composed of solid sheets of centroblasts (Fig. 17.6). In addition, one must report the architectural pattern, ranging from follicular (>75% follicular), follicular and diffuse (25% to 75% follicular), focally follicular (<25% follicular), and diffuse. Thus one can make the seemingly paradoxical diagnosis of a diffuse follicular lymphoma, although one must ensure that the sampling is adequate, and that the cells have the immunophenotypic or molecular (e.g., t(14;18)) findings indicative of a follicular center cell lymphoma. In addition, there are several variants of follicular lymphoma now recognized. Similar to pediatric nodal marginal zone lymphoma, a pediatric variant of follicular lymphoma is now recognized (54). These latter patients usually present in low stage; a high proportion of cases are bcl-2⁻ and grade 3 and have an excellent prognosis. Primary intestinal follicular lymphoma is a rare variant of follicular lymphoma that has a particular predilection for the second portion of the duodenum (55). Although it has similar biologic features to nodal follicular lymphoma, it has been separated out because of its usual low stage at presentation and excellent prognosis (even without treatment). Finally, similar to the relationship of monoclonal B-cell lymphocytosis to chronic lymphocytic leukemia, a lesion of intrafollicular neoplasia/"*in situ*" follicular lymphoma has been recognized, in which isolated neoplastic follicles are seen in the context of a normal or reactive lymph nodes (56). It is usually identified by a bcl-2 stain, which often

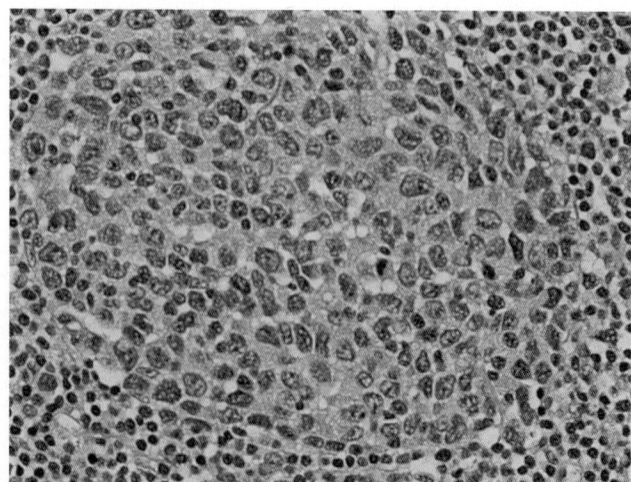

FIGURE 17.6. Follicular lymphoma, grade 3B. A pure population of centroblasts is seen, without scattered small or large cleaved cells.

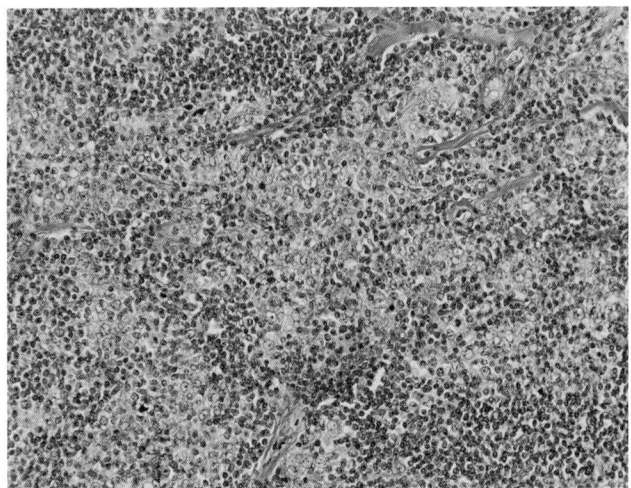

FIGURE 17.7. **Primary cutaneous follicular center lymphoma.** While this lymphoma of the dermis did not form discrete follicles, the phenotype of the large cells was that of follicular center B cells.

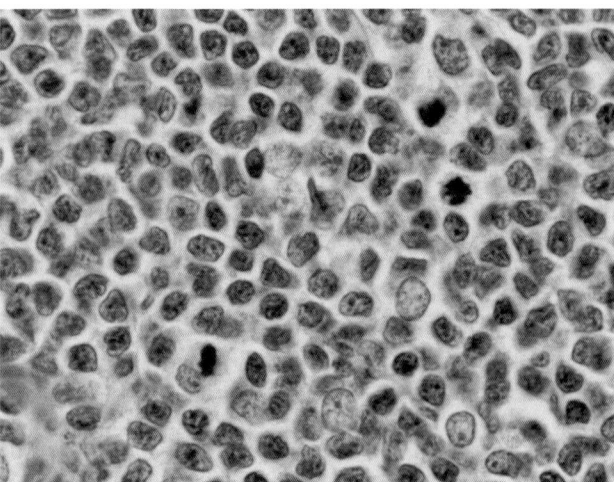

FIGURE 17.8. **Blastic mantle cell lymphoma.** The cells have a finer chromatin pattern than cases of typical mantle cell lymphoma. Note the high mitotic rate.

shows a stronger level of bcl-2 staining than in the adjacent normal B-lymphocyte mantle cells. Once further investigation has ruled out the possibility of concurrent systemic lymphoma, these patients may be followed without treatment.

While adult follicular lymphoma has remained a relatively homogeneous entity for classification purposes, one can speculate that it may be subdivided into the future. There is increasing evidence that t(14;18) and bcl-2 cases may be a different biologic subtype of follicular lymphoma than the much more frequent t(14;18) and bcl-2 positive cases (57,58). This may partially account for why grade 3 cases, and particularly grade 3B cases, behave worse than other cases, because these cases are most likely to be t(14;18) and bcl-2 negative.

Primary Cutaneous Follicle Center Lymphoma

Primary cutaneous follicle center lymphoma is a distinct lymphoma category separate from follicular lymphoma. It contains lymphomas that would previously have been called primary follicular lymphoma of the skin (due to the presence of a follicular pattern) as well as lymphomas primary in the skin showing the morphology of diffuse large cell lymphomas but having a germinal center cell phenotype (Fig. 17.7). Interestingly, the majority of cases of primary cutaneous follicle center lymphoma fail to express bcl-2 or carry the t(14;18) but carry a high frequency of abnormalities of 3q27, including *BCL6* rearrangements, suggesting that this category may have a different pathogenesis than typical follicular lymphoma involving lymph nodes and other sites.

Mantle Cell Lymphoma

Mantle cell lymphoma is a distinctive B-cell neoplasm characterized by overexpression of cyclin D1 (and if not cyclin D1, then either cyclin D2 or D3) (59). However, it is not a completely homogenous neoplasm, morphologically or genetically. Rare cases are characterized by limited involvement of the inner mantle zone or an attenuated mantle ("*in situ*" mantle cell lymphoma) (60). More commonly, cases may show a mantle zone pattern (limitation to an expanded mantle), a "follicular" growth pattern (obliteration of the follicle along with involvement of the mantle), or a diffuse pattern with effacement of nodal architecture. Cytologically, there is variation as well, as both blastoid and pleomorphic aggressive variants are recognized, probably representing genetic progression of classical mantle cell lymphoma (Fig. 17.8) (61).

Diffuse Large Cell B-Cell Lymphoma

DLBCL is a large category of non-Hodgkin lymphoma, both epidemiologically and in terms of classification. DLBCL constitutes about one-quarter to one-third of all non-Hodgkin lymphomas in Western countries. The 2008 WHO classification recognizes diffuse large cell lymphoma, not otherwise specified; four distinct DLBCL subtypes; eight other lymphomas of large B-cells; as well as two categories of large cell lymphoma borderline with other types of lymphoma (2). Unfortunately, the vast majority of large B-cell lymphomas still fall within the category of "not otherwise specified." In addition, the WHO criteria for what constitutes a subtype of DLBCL versus other lymphoma of large B-cells are not given and appear to be somewhat arbitrary.

Diffuse Large B-Cell Lymphoma, NOS

DLBCL, not otherwise specified, contains morphologic variants as well as both molecular and immunohistochemical subgroups. The morphologic variants include the centroblastic variant, the immunoblastic variant, and the anaplastic variant. The centroblastic variant represents the overwhelmingly most common variant, particularly because diagnosis of the immunoblastic variant requires that >90% of the neoplastic cells have the morphologic features of immunoblasts (2). The morphologic variants provide no significant prognostic or biologic data, and their importance lies more in framing the differential diagnosis rather than imparting information to clinicians. Gene expression profiling, on the other hand, has provided a basis for the separation of cases into germinal center B-cell like versus activated B-cell like (62). This subgrouping does have biologic significance, as different genetic abnormalities are associated with each group of cases, and cases of the germinal center B-cell–like group have a significantly better clinical outcome than those of the activated B-cell–like group, at least in the era of conventional chemotherapy. While gene expression profiling is not ready for routine clinical use, surrogate markers for each group have been identified by immunohistochemical studies. Various combinations of antibodies have been proposed that may provide a similar separation of cases into germinal center B-cell like and activated B-cell like, with similar if not identical prognostic significance as the gene expression profiling studies (63). It is likely that future classifications of non-Hodgkin lymphoma will include the distinction between germinal center cell–like and activated

B-cell–like cases as a major discriminant in subclassifying cases of DLBCL.

The four subtypes of DLBCL include T-cell/histiocyte-rich large B-cell lymphoma, primary DLBCL of the central nervous system, primary cutaneous DLBCL, leg type, and Epstein-Barr virus (EBV) positive DLBCL of the elderly.

T-Cell/Histiocyte-Rich Large B-Cell Lymphoma

T-cell/histiocyte-rich large B-cell lymphoma represents the largest of the four subtypes of DLBCL. Minimum criteria in terms of either numbers of large B cells or numbers of T cells or histiocytes for its diagnosis are not given in the 2008 WHO classification (2). It is not clear whether cases without significant numbers of histiocytes belong in this category (64). In addition, the relationship of T-cell/histiocyte-rich large B-cell lymphoma and histologically virtually identical neoplasms in patients with a previous history of nodular lymphocyte predominance Hodgkin lymphoma is also not yet clear (65). Nonetheless, however as it is currently defined, T-cell/histiocyte-rich large B-cell lymphoma appears to define a distinctive aggressive subtype of lymphoma.

Primary Diffuse Large B-Cell Lymphoma of the Central Nervous System

Primary DLBCL of the central nervous system is defined to exclusively include primary lymphomas of intracerebral and intraocular sites arising in nonimmunosuppressed patients. Specifically excluded are those lymphomas of the dura, intravascular large cell lymphoma (even when the central nervous system is the only known site of disease), any secondary manifestations from primary lymphoma elsewhere in the body, and any lymphomas arising in the setting of immunosuppression, for example, lymphomas of the brain arising in patients with acquired immunodeficiency syndrome (2). As defined, this lymphoma is a non-EBV-associated lymphoma of activated B-cell–like type with distinctive patterns of spread (mostly to other sites within the central nervous system and infrequently to bone marrow or other common sites of secondary lymphoma involvement) (66,67).

Primary Cutaneous Diffuse Large Cell Lymphoma, Leg Type

Primary cutaneous diffuse large cell lymphoma, leg type is defined as a lymphoma composed almost exclusively of centroblasts and immunoblasts of activated B-cell–like phenotype; this lymphoma occurs mostly on the lower extremities (68). The name is perhaps somewhat unfortunate, leaving the pathologist open to ridicule in the minority of cases that do not occur on the legs, and should perhaps be more appropriately named primary cutaneous diffuse large cell lymphoma, activated B-cell like (69). Nonetheless, it seems important to distinguish these cases from primary cutaneous follicle center lymphoma, as the latter lymphoma behaves in a much more indolent fashion than the former (67).

Epstein-Barr Virus–Positive Diffuse Large Cell Lymphoma of the Elderly

EBV-positive DLBCL of the elderly is defined as an EBV-associated DLBCL in an elderly patient without a history of immunodeficiency (70). Epidemiologically, these cases occur in increasing incidence with increasing age, hence the name (71). Arbitrarily, the age cutoff has been set at >50 years, although there is no biologic age cutoff. These cases are significantly more common in Asian than Western countries. Rare cases

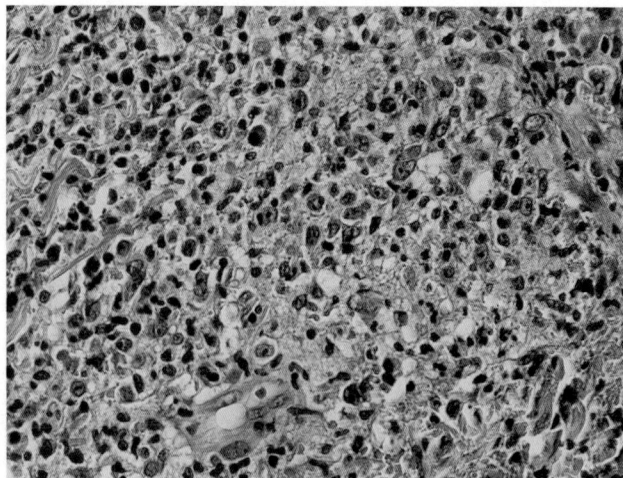

FIGURE 17.9. Epstein-Barr virus–positive diffuse large cell lymphoma of the elderly. Note the polymorphous morphology and the areas of necrosis at the periphery.

have been noted in younger seemingly immunocompetent individuals. For this reason, renaming this entity as DLBCL, EBV associated, should be considered, with the description that these cases are much more common in the elderly. In any event, this lymphoma variant is worthy of recognition, as these cases have somewhat distinctive clinical, morphologic, and prognostic features (Fig. 17.9). They tend to occur in extranodal sites, usually have foci of necrosis, and often have a polymorphic infiltrate that may include Hodgkin-like cells.

Diffuse Large B-Cell Lymphoma Associated with Chronic Inflammation

DLBCL associated with chronic inflammation is a rare lymphoma occurring in the specific setting of very long-standing chronic inflammation, often decades long (72). It is another EBV-associated lymphoma and is generally a lymphoma of activated B-cell–like phenotype (73). While its morphologic features are not distinguishable from DLBCL, not otherwise specified, its distinctive clinical setting probably merits recognition as a separate entity. Nonetheless, it is not clear why it is considered as one of the "lymphomas of large B-cells" as opposed to a subtype within the larger category of DLBCL, such as is the case with EBV-positive DLBCL of the elderly.

Lymphomatoid Granulomatosis

Lymphomatoid granulomatosis, despite the retention of the name suggesting an inflammatory disorder, is now considered to be a variant of B-cell lymphoma, given the recognition that the lesional cells are clonal, EBV-positive large B-cells, admixed with reactive T-cells (Fig. 17.10) (74). It is now also recognized that most of the patients with lymphomatoid granulomatosis have a history of either overt (e.g., history of a primary immunodeficiency) or subtle immunodeficiency (e.g., decreased immune function noted on careful analysis) (75). There is a morphologic grading system within the diagnosis, ranging from grade 1 to 3, depending upon the number of neoplastic cells (76).

Primary Mediastinal Large (Thymic) B-Cell Lymphoma

Primary mediastinal large (thymic) B-cell lymphoma is by far the most frequent of the specific variants of large B-cell lymphoma. Gene expression microarray studies have shown that this neoplasm is biologically distinct from either germinal

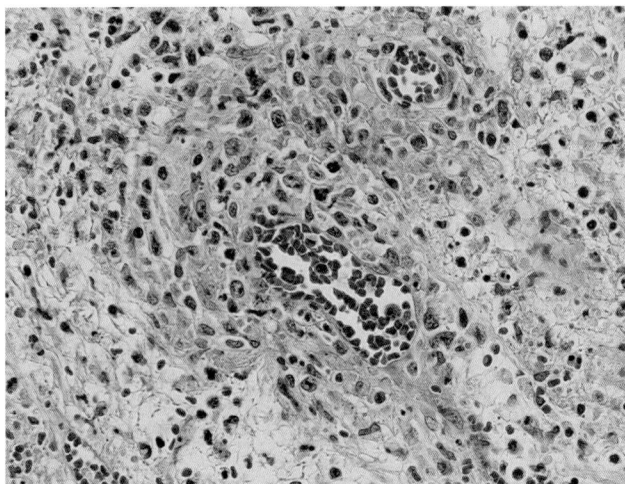

FIGURE 17.10. **Lymphomatoid granulomatosis**. This lung biopsy showed widespread areas of necrosis with perivascular collections of large cells, which were EBV⁺ B cells.

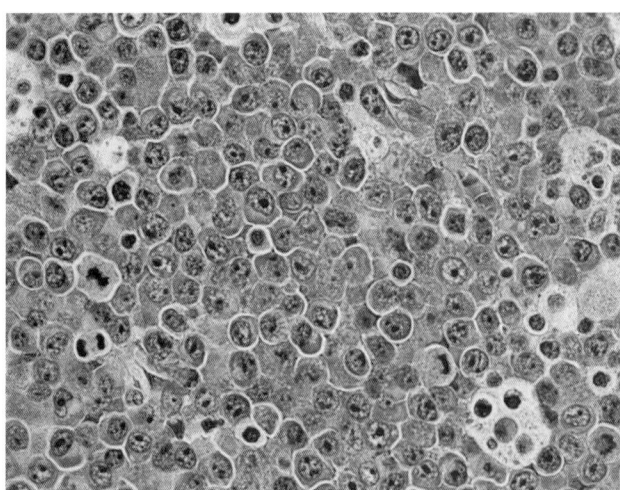

FIGURE 17.12. **Plasmablastic lymphoma**. This anal lesion had the morphologic features of immunoblasts combined with the phenotype of plasma cells.

center B-cell–like and activated B-cell–like large cell lymphomas and actually shares many biologic similarities with classical Hodgkin lymphoma (77). There are also some differences in morphology (e.g., compartmentalization of medium-sized to large cells with abundant pale cytoplasm) and immunophenotype (e.g., lack of immunoglobulin and presence of CD30, MUM1, and CD23) from DLBCL, not otherwise specified (Fig. 17.11) (78,79). Nonetheless, on a routine basis, its most distinctive feature is still its location, and it is difficult to distinguish this lymphoma from a DLBCL, not otherwise specified, that just happened to occur in a mediastinal lymph node. Similarly, it may be difficult to distinguish this lymphoma from a borderline lymphoma intermediate with classical Hodgkin lymphoma.

Intravascular Large B-Cell Lymphoma

Intravascular large B-cell lymphoma is an extremely rare variant of large cell lymphoma with an unusual predilection for the lumina of the smallest vessels. Two clinicopathologic forms are recognized, one more common in Asian patients (systemic symptoms), while the other more common in Western patients (specific organ-related symptoms) (80). This suggests that

biologically it may represent at least two different neoplasms. Nonetheless, its morphologic appearance is quite distinctive and easy to differentiate from other malignant lymphomas.

Plasmablastic Lymphoma

Plasmablastic lymphoma is a malignant lymphoma with the morphologic appearance of immunoblasts but an immunophenotype more consistent with plasma cells (Fig. 17.12) (81). Many patients have a history of immunodeficiency, most often due to HIV infection, iatrogenic immunosuppression, or even age related. In contrast to ALK⁺ large B-cell lymphoma, plasmablastic lymphoma has an association with EBV in about two-thirds of cases, is usually CD30⁺, is most often IgG expressing, and is associated with translocations involving the *MYC* gene in about 50% of cases (82,83).

ALK⁺ Large B-Cell Lymphoma

ALK⁺ large B-cell lymphoma is defined by ALK expression within a B-lineage lymphoma (84). It shows a morphologic overlap with other lymphomas showing immunoblastic or plasmablastic differentiation (Fig. 17.13). In addition, it also shows

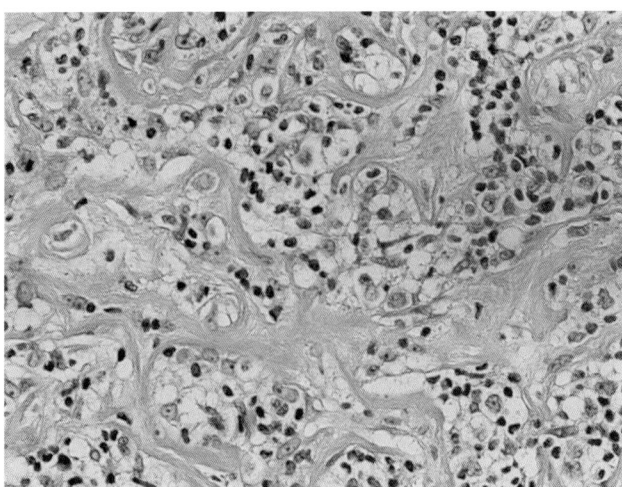

FIGURE 17.11. **Primary mediastinal large (thymic) B-cell lymphoma**. This case was recognizable by the site of biopsy and by the characteristic compartmentalizing sclerosis.

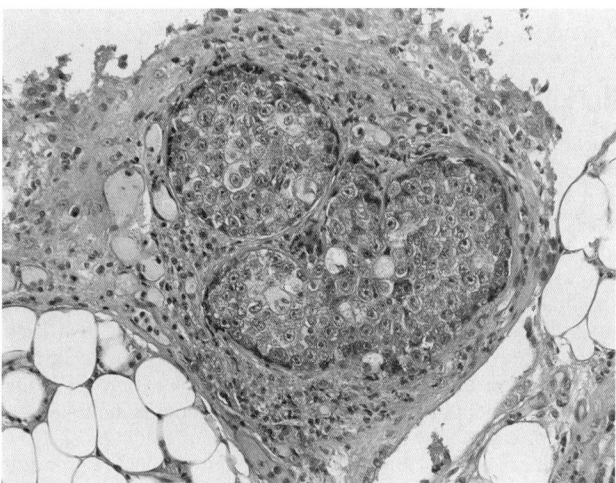

FIGURE 17.13. **ALK⁺ large B-cell lymphoma**. Carcinoma was originally suspected, due to the sinusoidal distribution of the neoplasm. The individual neoplastic cells have the morphologic features of immunoblasts.

many phenotypic similarities with plasmablastic lymphoma, with frequent expression of epithelial membrane antigen, the plasma cell markers CD138 and VS38, and cytoplasmic immunoglobulin (but most often IgA, instead IgG), as well as frequent negativity for CD45 and the B-lineage markers CD20 and CD79a. In contrast to many plasmablastic lymphomas, which show an association with human immunodeficiency virus-1 (HIV-1) infection or other immunodeficiency states, ALK+ large B-cell lymphoma appears to be a lymphoma of immunocompetent children and adults (11). Nonetheless, one may make the case that ALK+ large B-cell lymphoma represents a subtype of plasmablastic lymphoma.

Large B-Cell Lymphoma Arising in HHV-8 Associated Multicentric Castleman Disease

Large B-cell lymphoma arising in HHV-8–associated multicentric Castleman disease may be viewed as another variant of plasmablastic lymphoma associated with a unique clinicopathologic setting (85). Arising as a plasma cell proliferation in the setting of the plasmablastic variant of HHV-8–associated multicentric Castleman disease, the lymphoma progresses from single cells to clusters to sheets of atypical plasmablasts to eventually completely obliterate the nodal or splenic architecture and to involve other organs. The cells have the morphologic features of plasmablasts and have an immunophenotype suggestive of plasmablastic differentiation, with CD20 and CD38 variably positive, CD79-, and IgM+ with consistent lambda light chain restriction; however, CD138 is negative. Interestingly, this neoplasm is invariably HHV-8+ and EBV-, a characteristic finding only shared with a minority of cases of primary effusion lymphoma.

Primary Effusion Lymphoma

Primary effusion lymphoma is yet another lymphoma category with morphologic and immunophenotypic features that may closely resemble plasmablastic lymphoma. The morphologic features are plasmablastic to highly anaplastic, and although the cells usually express CD45 and CD30, they are usually negative for pan-B-cell markers and express the plasma cells markers CD138, CD38, VS38, and epithelial membrane antigen (86). However, in contrast to other plasmablastic lymphomas, surface or cytoplasmic immunoglobulin is absent. Similar to large B-cell lymphoma arising in HHV-8–associated multicentric Castleman disease, the neoplastic cells are HHV-8 positive, but they are also EBV+ in a majority of cases.

Burkitt Lymphoma

Burkitt lymphoma is a very distinctive B-cell lymphoma that occurs in three clinicopathologic settings: endemic, sporadic, and immunodeficiency associated (87–89). It now includes cases with dominant bone marrow involvement, which used to be considered L3 acute B-lymphoblastic leukemia (90). The majority of cases are easy to diagnose, due to their characteristic clinical setting, morphologic appearance (starry-sky on low magnification; homogeneous medium-sized cells with a high mitotic rate on high magnification); germinal center immunophenotype; and characteristic MYC translocation involving an immunoglobulin heavy or light chain gene. Nonetheless, a subset of cases may be notoriously difficult to diagnose (91). In these cases, the clinical setting is often atypical (e.g., adult rather than children); the phenotype may be atypical (e.g., bcl-2 expression); and the MYC translocation may be absent, juxtaposed to a nonimmunoglobulin gene site, or associated with additional cytogenetic abnormalities.

B-Cell Lymphoma, Unclassifiable, with Features Intermediate Between Diffuse Large B-Cell Lymphoma and Burkitt Lymphoma

The category B-cell lymphoma, unclassifiable, with features intermediate between DLBCL and Burkitt lymphoma, has been created for entities that appear to show overlap between DLBCL of germinal center B-cell-like type and Burkitt lymphoma (2). This category probably represents a subset of the cases that used to be classified as Burkitt-like lymphoma or small, noncleaved lymphoma, non-Burkitt type. Unfortunately, the criteria used for this category will vary from case to case. It is clear that this diagnosis should not be used for a case of DLBCL in which only the proliferative rate is very high or for which a MYC translocation can be identified, as these features alone are still within the spectrum of DLBCL (13). Acceptable features for this category might include a moderately or strongly positive bcl-2 stain in an otherwise typical case of Burkitt lymphoma or a characteristic germinal center immunophenotype in a case that is morphologically suggestive of but still atypical for Burkitt lymphoma, or a case morphologically resembling Burkitt lymphoma but a complex karyotype is seen or one including a BCL2 translocation in addition to a MYC translocation (Fig. 17.14) (92,93). These latter cases ("double-hit" lymphoma) may represent transformation of follicular lymphoma, whether present in the clinical history or clinically occult, and consideration should be given in the future to separating these cases out as a separate, highly aggressive lymphoma category (92).

B-Cell Lymphoma, Unclassifiable, with Features Intermediate Between Diffuse Large B-Cell Lymphoma and Classical Hodgkin Lymphoma

The final category of mature B-cell lymphoma recognized in the 2008 WHO is B-cell lymphoma, unclassifiable, with features intermediate between DLBCL and classical Hodgkin lymphoma (2). Similar to the other unclassifiable category described above, this lymphoma entity is most easily defined by what it is not rather than by reproducible criteria that may be applied in every case. The cases on the one hand do not have clearly defined features of DLBCL, usually primary

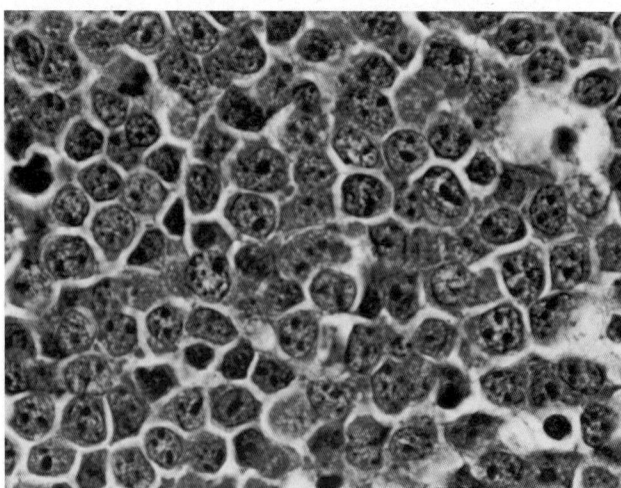

FIGURE 17.14. B-cell lymphoma, unclassifiable, with features intermediate between diffuse large B-cell lymphoma and Burkitt lymphoma. This case had a typical low magnification appearance for Burkitt lymphoma, but has more vesicular cytoplasm, fewer nucleoli, and more prominent nucleoli than usual. This case had translocations of both the MYC and BCL2 genes.

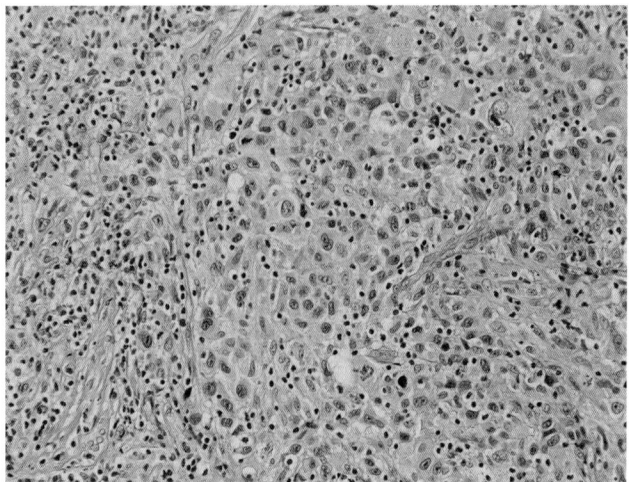

FIGURE 17.15. B-cell lymphoma, unclassifiable, with features intermediate between diffuse large B-cell lymphoma and classical Hodgkin lymphoma. This mediastinal case had fibrous bands suggestive of nodular sclerosis, but featured sheets of large cells in the nodules, with some of the large cells having features of Hodgkin cells. This case was CD30⁺, CD15⁺, CD20⁺, and CD45⁺.

Table 17.6	2008 WHO CLASSIFICATION OF MATURE T-CELL NEOPLASMS

- T-cell prolymphocytic leukemia
- T-cell large granular lymphocytic leukemia
- Aggressive NK-cell leukemia
- EBV⁺ T-cell lymphoproliferative disorders of childhood
  - Systemic EBV⁺ T-cell lymphoproliferative disease
  - Hydroa vacciniforme–like lymphoma
- Adult T-cell leukemia/lymphoma
- Extranodal NK/T-cell lymphoma, nasal type
- Enteropathy-associated T-cell lymphoma
- Hepatosplenic T-cell lymphoma
- Subcutaneous panniculitis-like T-cell lymphoma
- Mycosis fungoides/Sezary syndrome
- Primary cutaneous anaplastic large cell lymphoma/lymphomatoid papulosis
- Primary cutaneous gamma-delta T-cell lymphoma
- Primary cutaneous aggressive epidermotropic CD8⁺ cytotoxic T-cell lymphoma *(provisional)*
- Primary cutaneous small/medium CD4⁺ T-cell lymphoma *(provisional)*
- Angioimmunoblastic T-cell lymphoma
- Peripheral T-cell lymphoma, not otherwise specified
- Anaplastic large cell lymphoma, ALK⁺
- Anaplastic large cell lymphoma, ALK⁻

Adapted from Swerdlow SH, Campo E, Harris NL, et al. *WHO Classification of Tumours of Haematopoietic and Lymphoid Tissues.* Lyon: International Agency for Research on Cancer, 2008, with permission.

mediastinal (thymic) large B-cell lymphoma, and on the other hand lack clearly defined features of classical Hodgkin lymphoma (Fig. 17.15) (94,95). In some cases, the lymphoma presents with one area or site with a histologic appearance resembling one of these neoplasms and another area or site (including recurrence) with a histologic appearance resembling the other neoplasm. The immunophenotype is confusing, usually showing overlapping features of both neoplasms, often with CD45, CD20, CD30, and CD15 positivity. Support for a true biologic entity includes the overlap in gene expression microarray studies between primary mediastinal (thymic) large B-cell lymphoma and classical Hodgkin lymphoma. However, additional studies, particularly karyotypic and molecular genetic studies, are warranted before confident conclusions can be drawn. Unfortunately, such testing is difficult to perform in these rare neoplasms.

Mature T- and NK-Cell Lymphomas

Mature T- and NK-cell lymphomas constitute about 18 different entities (Table 17.6) (2). While the classification of mature B-cell neoplasms depends heavily on morphologic appearance, these features are much less important in the classification of mature T- and NK-cell neoplasms. First, all mature T-cell lymphomas show diffuse architecture, and there is no equivalent to the follicles of follicular lymphoma or the pseudoproliferation centers of chronic lymphocytic leukemia. Second, many different mature T- and NK-cell lymphomas share a similar wide range in cytologic appearance and host infiltrate. In addition, immunophenotype is much less important for classifying mature T- and NK-cell lymphomas than mature B-cell lymphomas. There is significant overlap between T- versus NK-cell phenotype and clinicopathologic entities. For example, there are no significant differences in clinical behavior between T-cell versus NK-cell phenotype extranodal NK/T-cell lymphoma, nasal type. In addition, aberrant T-cell phenotypes, particularly loss of pan-T-cell markers or bcl-2, are common in a wide variety of categories of T-cell lymphoma. Furthermore, T-cell and NK-cell lymphomas are much less common than B-cell lymphomas, the former entities constitute <10% of all cases of malignant lymphoma, and thus, a lot less is known about their karyotypes and molecular genetics (10). Furthermore, many of the mature T-cell lymphomas occur in distinctive extranodal sites, and their varying clinical presentations

have been the greatest help in sorting out the various mature T- and NK-cell lymphomas. Therefore, classification is generally based on a constellation of clinical, histologic, phenotypic, genotypic, and viral findings.

A helpful conceptual framework for understanding of T and NK cells and their corresponding characteristics is knowledge of the innate versus adaptive immune system. The innate immune system is the more primitive of the two and responds to antigens in a nonspecific nonmajor histocompatibility complex (MHC)–restricted way, obviating the need for antigen-presenting cells. CD3⁺ and CD56⁺ alpha-beta T-cells, gamma-delta T-cells, and NK cells contribute to the innate system, which is primarily located in extranodal organs, as a first line of defense. The adaptive immune system is the more ontologically developed mechanism of defense and responds to antigen presented by antigen-presenting cells in a specific and MHC-restricted way, leading to the development of immunologic memory. Both CD4⁺ (helper) and CD8⁺ (cytotoxic/suppressor) alpha-beta T-cells contribute to the adaptive immune system, which operates primarily in the lymph nodes. Therefore, it is not surprising that neoplasms of the innate immune system (including neoplasms of CD56⁺ alpha-beta T cells, gamma-delta T-cells, and NK cells) tend to occur in younger patients and at extranodal sites, while neoplasms of the adaptive system tend to occur in lymph nodes of adults (96).

T-Cell Prolymphocytic Leukemia

T-cell prolymphocytic leukemia is a distinctive leukemic T-cell proliferation, usually characterized by the presence of medium-sized T lymphocytes with variably shaped nuclei and a visible nucleolus in the peripheral blood and a relatively mature T-cell phenotype (97). In about one-quarter of cases, the cells are small and may lack nucleoli. This is considered to be a small cell variant of T-cell prolymphocytic leukemia rather than T-cell chronic lymphocytic leukemia, a disease that is no longer considered to exist. Molecular genetic studies have shown that both the common and the small cell variant share similar cytogenetic abnormalities, particularly involving the T-cell receptor alpha gene (98).

T-Cell Large Granular Lymphocytic Leukemia

T-cell large granular lymphocytic leukemia is problematic in lymphoma classification, as it has been definitively shown to be a clonal disorder (as shown by T-cell receptor gamma chain gene studies), yet it often has a nonprogressive course (99). The minimum criteria for the diagnosis include a >6-month increase in the number of peripheral blood T-large granular lymphocytes, because similar but reactive clonal or oligoclonal populations may be seen transiently following allogeneic bone marrow transplantation or in association with low-grade B-cell lymphomas (2,100). Cytogenetic abnormalities have been noted in only a minority of cases. Survival greater than a decade is the norm, and death due to disease is rare. Thus, the question still remains whether most proliferations of even >6-month duration truly represent a neoplastic process.

Chronic Lymphoproliferative Disorders of NK Cells

As the plural name implies, there is uncertainty as to whether chronic lymphoproliferative disorders of NK cells represent a homogeneous category. While having an immunophenotype of NK cells rather than the mature T-cell phenotype of T-cell large granular lymphocytic leukemia, it nonetheless shares many features with the latter disorder. The minimum criteria for the diagnosis of chronic lymphoproliferative disorders of NK cells also include a >6-month increase in peripheral blood NK cells, since similar but clearly reactive populations may be seen in a variety of other diseases (101,102). Although analysis of the antigen receptor genes for clonality does not apply to NK-cell neoplasms since NK cells do not rearrange either their immunoglobulin or T-cell receptor genes, studies of X-chromosome inactivation are consistent with a clonal process (103). However, cytogenetic abnormalities have only been noted in a minority of cases, and prolonged survival is typically seen. Thus, similar to T-cell large granular lymphocytic leukemia, the question still remains whether most cases of these disorders represent a true neoplastic process, or only gain neoplastic potential when subsequent cytogenetic abnormalities occur.

Aggressive NK-Cell Leukemia

Aggressive NK-cell leukemia is a distinctive aggressive neoplasm of NK cells (104). Some investigators have suggested that it may represent a leukemic variant of extranodal NK/T-cell lymphoma, nasal type, since it shares many features with the latter neoplasm, including a predilection for Asian patients, almost constant association with EBV, and a very similar immunophenotype. Nonetheless, cytogenetic studies have shown significant differences between the two neoplasms, and aggressive NK-cell leukemia clearly represents a more aggressive neoplasm clinically (105). Other investigators have noted similarities between aggressive NK-cell leukemia and EBV⁺ T-cell lymphoproliferative disorders of childhood, as some patients have a history of EBV-associated chronic infectious mononucleosis (similar to systemic EBV⁺ T-cell lymphoproliferative disease of childhood), while other patients have a history of hypersensitivity to mosquito bites (similar to hydroa vacciniforme–like lymphoma) (106).

EBV⁺ T-Cell Lymphoproliferative Disorders of Childhood

The EBV⁺ T-cell lymphoproliferative disorders of childhood include two separate rare neoplasms that occur in childhood, have a marked increased incidence in Asians, and in which EBV plays a significant role in the pathogenesis. Systemic EBV⁺

T-cell lymphoproliferative disease of childhood is a fulminant systemic disorder arising either subsequent to primary or chronic Epstein-Barr infection (107,108). Although the proliferating EBV⁺ T cells lack significant cytologic atypia and no recurrent cytogenetic abnormalities have been reported, they have monoclonal rearrangements of the T-cell receptor genes. Hydroa vacciniforme-like lymphoma is usually an indolent disorder (at least initially) based in the skin, associated with sensitivity to insect bites and sun exposure (109). Again, most cases occur in childhood or adolescence. Most cases have monoclonal rearrangements of the T-cell receptor genes, although a minority of cases are of NK lineage and lack rearrangements of the antigen receptor genes.

Adult T-Cell Leukemia/Lymphoma

Adult T-cell leukemia/lymphoma is a unique mature T-cell lymphoma invariably associated with monoclonal integration of HTLV-1 into the neoplastic cells (110). Several clinical subtypes are recognized, including acute, chronic smoldering, and lymphomatous (111). A wide range of organ involvement may be seen, spanning from involvement of peripheral blood, to involvement of skin and other extranodal organs, and lymph nodes and spleen (112). Most patients have systemic disease at presentation. The appearance in involved lymph nodes may simulate a wide variety of mature T-cell lymphomas, and the neoplastic cells have the phenotype of mature T-cells, usually with strong CD25 expression (Fig. 17.16).

Extranodal NK/T-cell Lymphoma, Nasal Type

Extranodal NK/T-cell lymphoma, nasal type, is a distinctive mature T-cell lymphoma with an angiocentric and angiodestructive pattern infiltrate, a variable cytologic appearance, and a strong predilection for nasal involvement (Fig. 17.17). Most common in Asians, there is a very strong association with EBV in all populations studied (113,114). The epidemiologic features, association with EBV, and common NK-cell phenotype are all similarities shared with aggressive NK-cell leukemia, an entity with which some investigators believe this neoplasm may have a relationship. Extranodal NK/T-cell lymphoma, nasal type, is easiest to recognize when it occurs in the nose or nasal sinuses, but may be identified outside of this location by its association with Epstein-Barr infection and its most common phenotype: CD2, CD56, cytotoxic marker and cytoplasmic CD3⁺, and surface CD3⁻ immunophenotype (115).

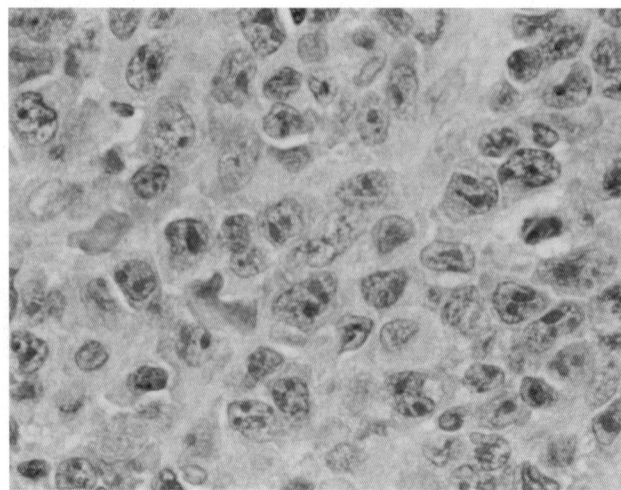

FIGURE 17.16. Adult T-cell leukemia/lymphoma. This case features highly pleomorphic cells.

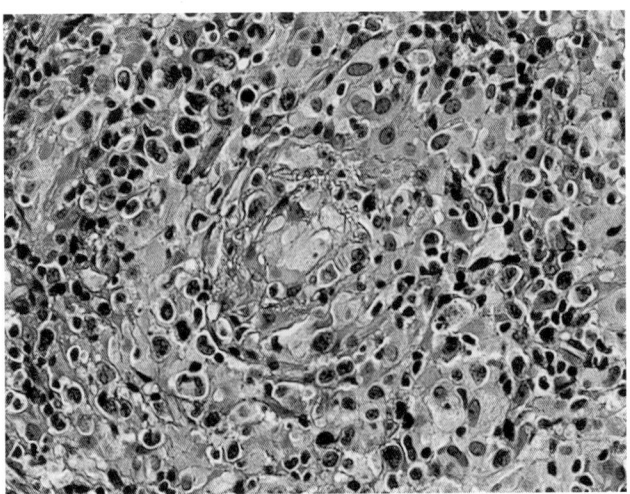

FIGURE 17.17. Extranodal NK/T-cell lymphoma, nasal type. A pleomorphic infiltrate is seen centered around blood vessels.

The NK/T designation stems from the fact that a minority of cases may show a T-cell phenotype (and have monoclonal rearrangements of the T-cell receptor genes), but are otherwise indistinguishable from the NK-phenotype cases (116).

Enteropathy-Associated T-Cell Lymphoma

Enteropathy-associated T-cell lymphoma is an intestinal lymphoma probably derived from intraepithelial T and NK lymphocytes, associated with inflammatory changes of the adjacent intestinal mucosa (Fig. 17.18). While an uncommon lymphoma category as presently defined, it may in fact represent at least two distinct types of lymphomas. In the common variant, constituting about 80% of the patients (at least in Europe), there is a strong association with adult- or childhood-onset celiac disease, with or without ulceration (117). The cytologic features are variable, and most cases show a CD3+, CD7+, CD5−, CD4−, and CD8− phenotype. In the variant described as type II or the monomorphic intestinal T-cell lymphoma, which constitutes about 20% of the patients in Europe (but possibly higher in the United States and Asia), there is no association with celiac disease, although there are still atrophic and inflammatory changes in the adjacent mucosa, with striking intraepithelial

lymphocytosis (118). As the name implies, the cytologic features are monomorphic, with medium-sized cells showing round nuclei and a rim of moderate pale cytoplasm, and the cells are CD8+ and CD56+ (in contrast to the common type). Nonetheless, both types share various cytogenetic abnormalities, although the incidence of each particular alternation various between the two types (118). Both types must be distinguished from other types of T-cell lymphomas involving the intestine; these latter cases have their own distinctive features and should not have inflammatory changes in the adjacent intestinal mucosa.

Hepatosplenic T-Cell Lymphoma

Hepatosplenic T-cell lymphoma is a distinctive clinicopathologic entity, and only one of two lymphoma types predominantly derived from cytotoxic T-cells of gamma-delta lineage (the other is primary cutaneous gamma-delta lymphoma) (119,120). The cells are monotonous, with medium-sized nuclei, but the neoplasm is most recognizable by the pattern of organ involvement (liver, spleen, and bone marrow), as well as the pattern within involved organs—predominantly sinusoidal (Fig. 17.19). As mentioned above, most cases are of gamma-delta phenotype, although a minority of cases may be of alpha-beta type (121); interestingly, these cases seem to be otherwise indistinguishable from the gamma-delta cases. Most cases have expression of TIA-1 but not granzyme A or perforin, indicating a nonactivated cytotoxic phenotype. A unifying feature is the presence of abnormalities 7q in nearly all cases, usually manifested by isochromosome 7q or less commonly a ring chromosome (122).

Subcutaneous Panniculitis-Like T-Cell Lymphoma

Subcutaneous panniculitis-like T-cell lymphoma is a cytotoxic T-cell lymphoma that has a marked predilection for the subcutaneous adipose tissue (Fig. 17.20) (123,124). In the past, some cases of primary cutaneous gamma-delta lymphoma were probably mixed in with this entity, but presently cases of gamma-delta phenotype are excluded from the definition, as the latter more aggressive cases often show involvement of the epidermis and dermis, in contrast to the near exclusive involvement of the subcutaneous tissue in this entity. As defined, cases have a mature alpha-beta phenotype and are usually CD8+, with expression of cytotoxic molecules. The clinical course is usually indolent, unless a hemophagocytic syndrome supervenes.

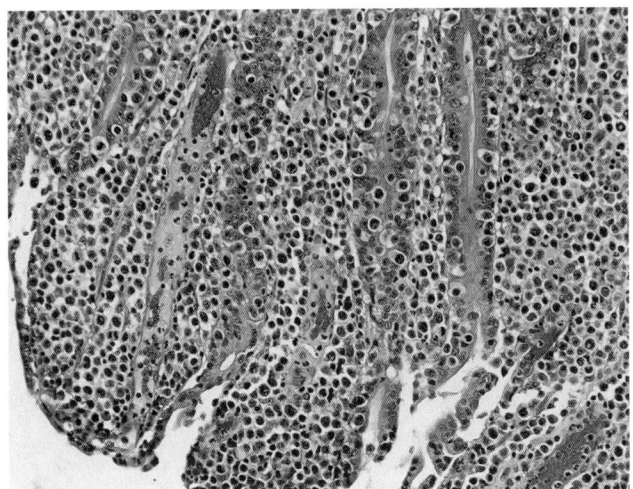

FIGURE 17.18. Enteropathy-associated T-cell lymphoma. Notice the involvement of the intestinal mucosa.

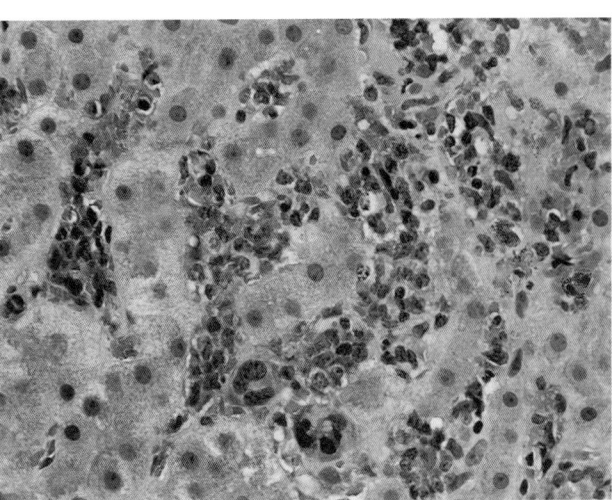

FIGURE 17.19. Hepatosplenic T-cell lymphoma. A atypical lymphoid infiltrate is present in the hepatic sinusoids.

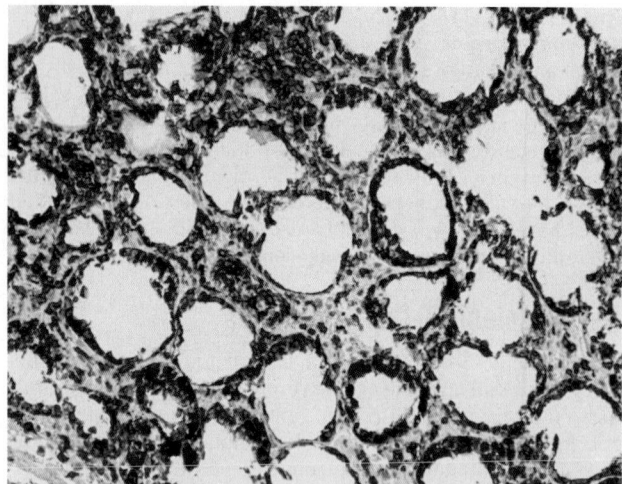

FIGURE 17.20. Subcutaneous panniculitis-like T-cell lymphoma. This CD8 stain shows characteristic ringing of the atypical cells around individual adipocytes.

Mycosis Fungoides

Mycosis fungoides is an epidermotropic lymphoma of helper T lymphocytes that progresses from skin patches to plaques to tumors, with eventual involvement of regional lymph nodes and systemic organs. Sezary syndrome is specifically excluded from the definition and is discussed in the next paragraph. While uncommon, mycosis fungoides is the most common primary skin lymphoma (68). The cytologic features are characteristic, with small to medium-sized cells with highly convoluted or cerebriform nuclei. These cells accumulate first at the lowest level of the epidermis, eventually forming clusters of cells (Pautrier abscesses) and infiltrating the dermis (Fig. 17.21) (125). Common variants of mycosis recognized by the 2008 WHO classification include folliculotropic MF, in which the atypical cells show preferential involvement of hair follicles (126), often associated with follicular mucinosis; Pagetoid reticulosis (Woringer-Kolopp disease) in which there is a nearly exclusive intraepidermal infiltrate without significant dermal involvement over a large patch or plaque (127); and granulomatous slack skin disease, a rare but very distinctive variant in which there are large folds of lax skin containing a granulomatous infiltrate admixed with the neoplastic cells (128).

Sezary Syndrome

Sezary syndrome shares many similarities with mycosis fungoides, including a similar cell of origin, an epidermotropic helper T lymphocyte, and a similar histology in the skin. The syndrome is characterized by a triad of erythroderma, generalized lymphadenopathy, and the presence of a clonal cerebriform T-cell proliferation in the skin, lymph nodes, and peripheral blood. By definition, there is an absolute Sezary cell count of at least 1×10^3/L, and CD4/CD8 ratio of >10:1, or loss of at least one specific pan-T-cell antigens in the peripheral blood (2). It is now thought that Sezary syndrome differs from mycosis fungoides in its presentation because it is a neoplasm of central memory T-cells expressing CCR7, L-selectin, and CD27, while mycosis fungoides is a neoplasm of skin-resident effector memory T-cells, expressing CCR4 and CLA (14).

Primary Cutaneous CD30+ T-Cell Lymphoproliferative Disorders

The primary cutaneous CD30+ T-cell lymphoproliferative disorders are a family of related neoplasms, ranging from primary cutaneous anaplastic large cell lymphoma on the one hand to lymphomatoid papulosis on the other. Primary cutaneous anaplastic large cell lymphoma comprises sheets of lymphoid cells in the dermis with large anaplastic nuclei and relatively abundant cytoplasm that strongly express (Fig. 17.22) CD30 (129). By definition, cases of transformation of mycosis fungoides or spread from a systemic anaplastic large cell lymphoma are excluded. Most of these cases have an indolent course, often with at least partial regression, although relapse in the skin is relatively common. There is a translocation involving chromosome 6p25, in at least a subset of these cases. Lymphomatoid papulosis is more histologically variable and usually contains only scattered (type A) or clusters to sheets of large CD30+ cells (type C), although occasionally it may have an appearance and phenotype simulating mycosis fungoides (type B) (and may in fact be more closely related to mycosis fungoides) (129). Clinically, it has an excellent prognosis, although recurrences may still occur. Borderline cases are composed primarily of lesions in which there is no clear correlation between the clinical and histologic characteristics. Both primary cutaneous anaplastic large cell lymphoma and lymphomatoid papulosis contain monoclonal T-cell receptor gene rearrangements in the majority of cases, which does not correlate with clinical aggressiveness (130,131). However, the translocations involving 6q25 are

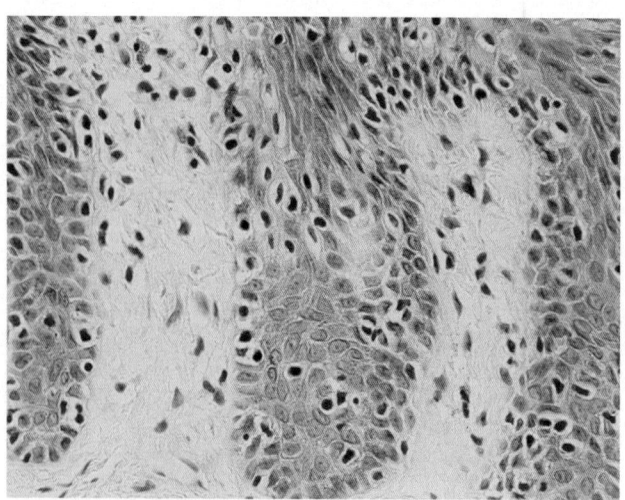

FIGURE 17.21. Mycosis fungoides. Although Pautrier abscesses were not present, there are numerous atypical lymphoid cells within the basal layer of the epidermis.

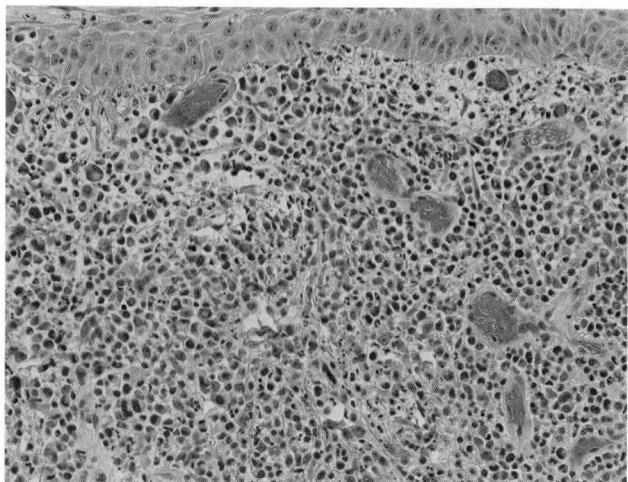

FIGURE 17.22. Cutaneous anaplastic large cell lymphoma. The atypical cells were all CD30+. Despite the worrisome histologic features, an indolent course is seen in most patients.

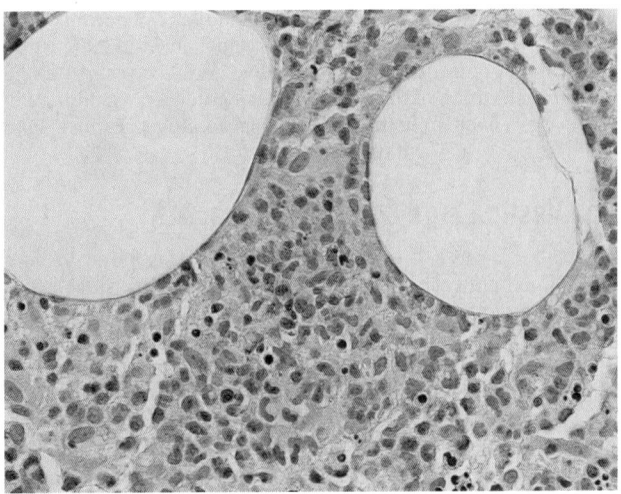

FIGURE 17.23. **Primary cutaneous gamma-delta T-cell lymphoma.** Extensive infiltrate, from the epidermis to the subcutaneous tissue, is usually seen.

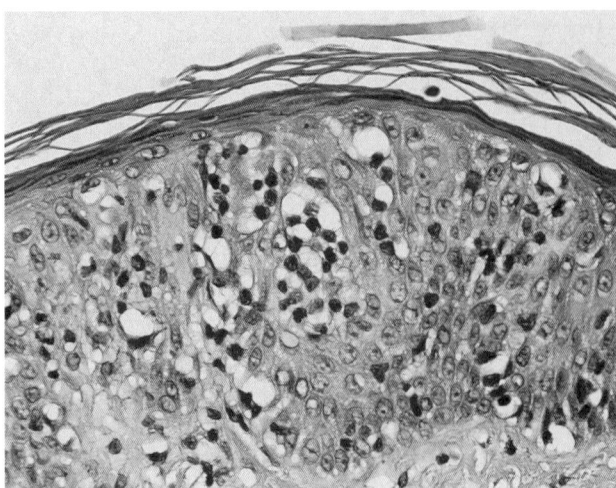

FIGURE 17.24. **Primary cutaneous CD8⁺ aggressive epidermotropic cytotoxic T-cell lymphoma.** The epidermotropism and cytologic atypia are often easier to appreciate than cases of mycosis fungoides.

only found in cutaneous anaplastic large cell lymphoma (seen in about 20% of cases) (132).

Primary Cutaneous Gamma-Delta T-Cell Lymphoma

Besides hepatosplenic T-cell lymphoma, primary cutaneous gamma-delta T-cell lymphoma is the only other lymphoma composed of gamma-delta T cells (124,133). As defined, this entity includes cases that at one time were considered to be gamma-delta variants of subcutaneous panniculitis-like T-cell lymphoma. As defined, it includes cases in which the primary localization of skin involvement may be epidermotropic, dermal, or subcutaneous; quite often, multiple regions are involved in a single case (Fig. 17.23). In addition to gamma-delta expression, the neoplastic cells are consistently positive for CD56, often positive for CD7, and occasionally positive for CD8.

The recognition of this entity raises the issue of how rare gamma-delta T-cell lymphoma not primary in the liver, spleen, or skin should be classified (134). Presumably, this will be addressed in a future WHO classification as more of these cases are recognized and studied.

Primary Cutaneous CD8⁺ Aggressive Epidermotropic Cytotoxic T-Cell Lymphoma

This is a rare lymphoma that is only a provisional category in the 2008 WHO classification. These cases have an exquisitely epidermotropic localization, even more pronounced than seen in mycosis fungoides (Fig. 17.24) (135). While some cases of mycosis fungoides may have a CD8⁺ rather than CD4⁺ T-cell phenotype, they are distinguished from primary cutaneous CD8⁺ aggressive epidermotropic cytotoxic T-cell lymphoma by the clinical features and indolent course more typical of mycosis fungoides, rather than the obviously aggressive presentation and clinical course seen in this neoplasm.

Primary Cutaneous CD4⁺ Small/Medium T-Cell Lymphoma

Primary cutaneous CD4⁺ small/medium T-cell lymphoma is also only a provisional entity in the 2008 WHO classification. It consists of a relatively homogeneous population of medium-sized but pleomorphic cells within the dermis, without being

associated with the epidermotropism of mycosis fungoides (Fig. 17.25) (136). The cells are T cells expressing CD4, but often have aberrant loss of pan-T-cell antigens. These cases may be important to recognize as a separate category of lymphoma because of their allegedly good prognosis (137).

Angioimmunoblastic T-Cell Lymphoma

Angioimmunoblastic T-cell lymphoma is a mature T-cell lymphoma with a distinctive morphologic appearance and immunophenotype. It occurs primarily in lymph nodes and is actually the most common T-cell lymphoma to involve the lymph nodes. There is frequent involvement of other organs. Its morphologic appearance includes a neoplastic infiltrate of small to medium-sized lymphoid cells clustered around an intense proliferation of high endothelial venules, starting in the perifollicular regions around reactive follicles and progressing to complete involvement of the paracortex with regression of the follicles (Fig. 17.26) (138,139). The immunophenotype is that of a CD4⁺ follicular helper T-cell, usually expressing CD10, bcl-6, and PD-1, and often associated with

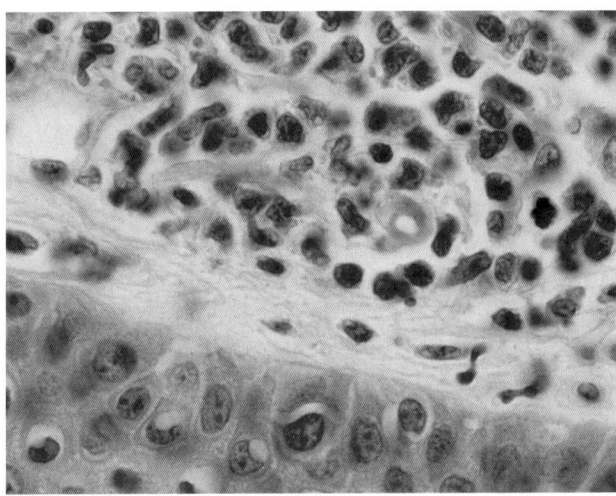

FIGURE 17.25. **Primary cutaneous CD4⁺ small/medium T-cell lymphoma.** Note the absence of epidermotropism. The cells are homogeneous from one to another, but show atypical nuclear features.

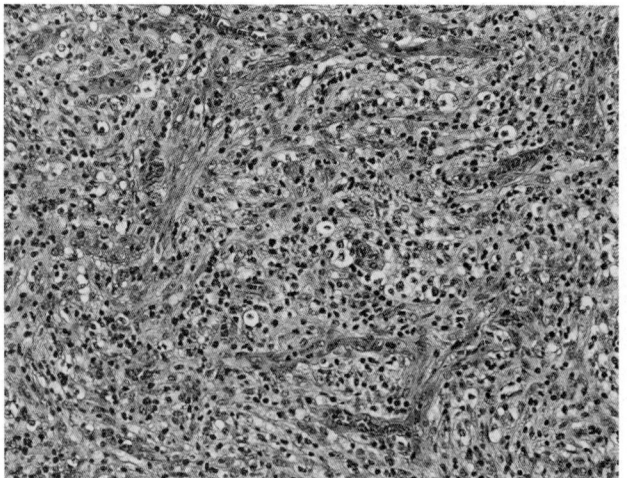

FIGURE 17.26. **Angioimmunoblastic T-cell lymphoma.** There is intense vascularity, with a cell poor infiltrate that includes clusters of large cells, particularly around high-endothelial venules.

expansion of the CD21+ follicular dendritic cell network enveloping the high endothelial venules (140,141). A consistent feature of angioimmunoblastic T-cell lymphoma is a proliferation of B immunoblasts, often expressing EBER, and occasionally giving rise to the detection of clonal immunoglobulin genes in addition to the consistent detection of monoclonal T-cell receptor gene rearrangements (142). The distinctive immunophenotype and consistent proliferation of EBER+ B immunoblasts are most helpful in distinguishing this lymphoma from other peripheral T-cell lymphomas.

Anaplastic Large Cell Lymphoma, ALK+

Anaplastic large cell lymphoma, ALK+, is a very distinctive lymphoma type defined as a T-cell lineage lymphoma with strong, consistent expression of CD30 and ALK, the latter finding reflecting the presence of a chromosomal translocation involving the ALK gene (143). While the histologic appearance may vary, there is usually a population of large lymphoid cells with abundant cytoplasm and eccentric, horseshoe-shaped nuclei referred to as hallmark cells (Fig. 17.27). This neoplasm is to be distinguished from anaplastic large cell lymphoma, ALK−, because both are of T lineage, have strong, consistent

expression of CD30, and may have a similar appearance in a subset of cases. It must also be distinguished from ALK+ large B-cell lymphoma. Although both have ALK expression along with translocation of the ALK gene, the latter is by definition of B lineage. This lymphoma category has a better prognosis than other peripheral T-cell lymphomas.

Anaplastic Large Cell Lymphoma, ALK−

Anaplastic large cell lymphoma, ALK−, is considered to be a provisional entity in the 2008 WHO classification, since it has not been definitively demonstrated in multiple studies that there are clear differences in clinical presentation, prognosis, or cytogenetic or molecular findings from peripheral T-cell lymphoma, not otherwise specified. However, there are some data to suggest that there are differences from the latter disorder (144). It is defined as a non–skin-based mature T-lineage lymphoma that has an anaplastic histologic appearance, with consistent and strong expression of CD30 on all or nearly all of the neoplastic cells and lacks ALK protein expression and translocation of the ALK gene (Fig. 17.28). Thus, it is distinguished from its ALK+ counterpart by the lack of ALK expression or translocation, from anaplastic B-cell lymphomas by its T-lineage, from primary cutaneous anaplastic large cell lymphoma by its predominant localization outside the skin, and from other peripheral T-cell lymphomas by its anaplastic cytologic appearance and strong and consistent CD30 expression in all or nearly all the neoplastic cells.

Peripheral T-Cell Lymphoma, Not Otherwise Specified

As its name implies, peripheral T-cell lymphoma, not otherwise specified, is defined by what it is not—it is a mature T-cell lymphoma without characteristics that would warrant classification as another specific type of T-cell lymphoma. Although most commonly occurring in lymph nodes, it may occur in any organ, particularly the skin, gastrointestinal tract, liver and spleen, and bone marrow (145). Within this category, several morphologic variants have been recognized. The lymphoepithelioid variant (Lennert lymphoma) is characterized by numerous epithelioid histiocytes, singly and in small clusters, which may be so numerous to partially obscure the neoplastic infiltrate (146). This variant must be distinguished from cases of angioimmunoblastic T-cell lymphoma, which may also have large numbers of epithelioid histiocytes. The follicular variant

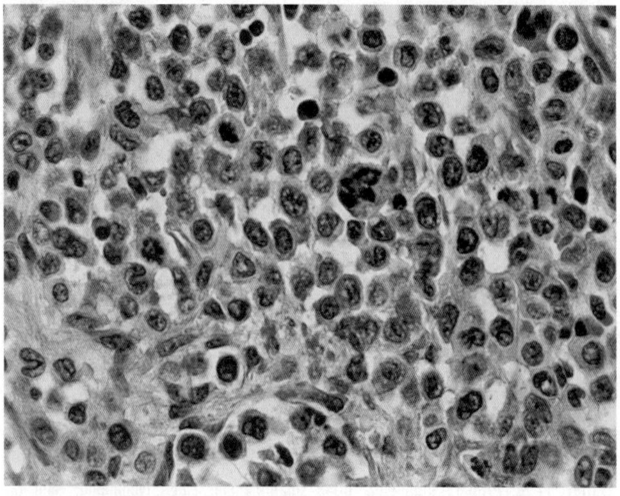

FIGURE 17.27. **Anaplastic large cell lymphoma, ALK+.** The neoplastic cells have large nuclei, with occasional horseshoe forms.

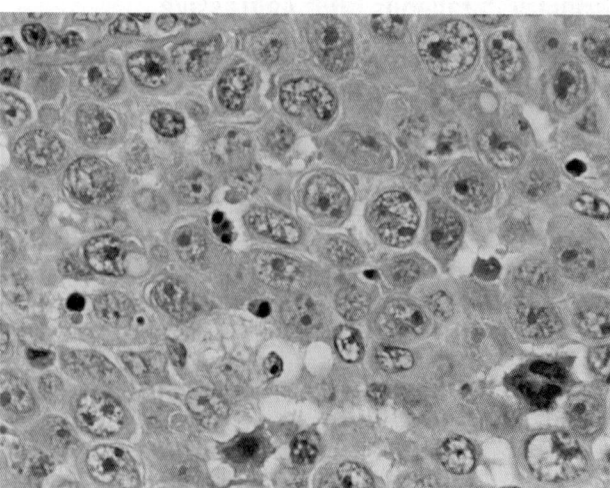

FIGURE 17.28. **Anaplastic large cell lymphoma, ALK−.** The cells are highly pleomorphic. The differential diagnosis would include carcinoma and melanoma.

is characterized by aggregates of atypical T cells within or surrounding follicles, which are often expanded (147). It shares a CD4+ follicular helper T-cell phenotype with angioimmunoblastic T-cell lymphoma and may represent an early form of that neoplasm, although it has a distinctive translocation, t(5;9), in at least a subset of cases (148). The T-zone variant shows an exclusive perifollicular/paracortical pattern of involvement, with retained follicles (149). To date, there is no convincing evidence that this variant represents a distinct clinicopathologic entity rather than just a characteristic histologic appearance, and it must be distinguished from an early variant of angioimmunoblastic lymphadenopathy.

CRITIQUE OF 2008 WHO CLASSIFICATION AND FUTURE DIRECTIONS

The 2008 WHO classification is the best attempt yet at a scientifically accurate classification that is also useful for patient care. Its greatest shortcoming is not intrinsic to the classification itself but rather due to the biology of malignant lymphoma: it appears that there truly are a large number of biologically distinct types of malignant lymphoma. Thus, while scientifically accurate to separate of all of these entities, it may make the design of clinical trials of the rare entities impractical, as it may require the cooperation of numerous institutions and years of enrollment to conduct meaningful studies for many of the rarer lymphoma types. Thus, it may be helpful in the future attempt to group some of these entities into intermediate hierarchies in order to overcome this problem. For example, plasmablastic lymphoma, ALK+ large B-cell lymphoma, large B-cell lymphoma arising in HHV-8–associated multicentric Castleman disease, and primary effusion lymphoma, while clearly representing distinct clinicopathologic entities, might be grouped together under a common designation, since these neoplasms, while representing distinct lymphoma types, share many common characteristics.

Finally, science and technology keep marching forward. Gene expression microarray studies, comparative genomic hybridization, particularly array-based comparative genomic hybridization, and epigenetic studies continue to add new information to the field, and high-throughput sequencing and proteomic studies are just beginning to add their contribution. While it is still unlikely that these technologies will be available in the near future for direct clinical use for the classification of individual tumor specimens, these studies are adding information every week that allows us to better understand the biology of these neoplasms and provide a more scientifically accurate classification. It is likely that these studies will be applied to currently difficult areas, such as B-prolymphocytic leukemia, splenic red pulp lymphomas, the two unclassifiable B-cell lymphomas intermediate between DLBCL and either Burkitt's lymphoma or classical Hodgkin lymphoma, chronic lymphoproliferative disorders of NK cells, and particularly the area of peripheral T-cell lymphoma, not otherwise specified, in an attempt to provide a more rational basis for classification. In addition, these studies may give us the knowledge to enable the design of surrogate markers using more practical technologies (such as immunohistochemistry) and help apply this newly gained knowledge to routine lymphoma classification of our daily cases.

References

1. Jaffe E, Harris N, Stein H, et al. *Pathology and genetics of tumours of haematopoietic and lymphoid tissues.* Lyon: IARC Press, 2001.
2. Swerdlow SH, Campo E, Harris NL, et al. *WHO classification of tumours of haematopoietic and lymphoid tissues.* Lyon: International Agency for Research on Cancer, 2008.
3. Lukes RJ, Collins RD. Immunologic characterization of human malignant lymphomas. *Cancer* 1974;34:1488–1503.
4. Lennert K, Mohri N, Stein H, et al. The histopathology of malignant lymphoma. *Br J Haematol* 1975;31(Suppl):193–203.
5. Stansfeld AG, Diebold J, Kapanci Y, et al. Updated Kiel classification for lymphomas (letter). *Lancet* 1988;1:292–293.
6. National Cancer Institute sponsored study of classifications of non-Hodgkin's lymphomas: summary and description of a working formulation for clinical usage. The Non-Hodgkin's Lymphoma Pathologic Classification Project. *Cancer* 1982;49:2112–2135.
7. Committee NCIn-HsCPW. Classification of non-Hodgkin's lymphomas. Reproducibility of major classification systems. *Cancer* 1985;55:91–95.
8. Simon R, Durrleman S, Hoppe RT, et al. The Non-Hodgkin Lymphoma Pathologic Classification Project. Long-term follow-up of 1153 patients with non-Hodgkin lymphomas. *Ann Intern Med* 1988;109:939–945.
9. Harris NL, Jaffe ES, Stein H, et al. A revised European-American classification of lymphoid neoplasms: a proposal from the International Lymphoma Study Group. *Blood* 1994;84:1361–1392.
10. A clinical evaluation of the International Lymphoma Study Group classification of non-Hodgkin's lymphoma. The Non-Hodgkin's Lymphoma Classification Project. *Blood* 1997;89:3909–3918.
11. Reichard KK, McKenna RW, Kroft SH. ALK-positive diffuse large B-cell lymphoma: report of four cases and review of the literature. *Mod Pathol* 2007;20:310–319.
12. Sawyer JR, Waldron JA, Jagannath S, et al. Cytogenetic findings in 200 patients with multiple myeloma. *Cancer Genet Cytogenet* 1995;82:41–49.
13. Yunis JJ, Mayer MG, Amesen MA. bcl-2 and other genomic alterations in the prognosis of large-cell lymphoma. *N Engl J Med* 1989;320:1047–1054.
14. Schmitt C, Balogh B, Grundt A, et al. The bcl-2/IgH rearrangement in a population of 204 healthy individuals: occurrence, age and gender distribution, breakpoints, and detection method validity. *Leuk Res* 2006;30:745–750.
15. Tsukasaki K, Tsushima H, Yamamura M, et al. Integration patterns of HTLV-1 provirus in relation to the clinical course of ATL: frequent clonal change at crisis from indolent disease. *Blood* 1997;89:948–956.
16. Dupin N, Fisher C, Kellam P, et al. Distribution of human herpesvirus-8 latently infected cells in Kaposi's sarcoma, multicentric Castleman's disease, and primary effusion lymphoma. *Proc Natl Acad Sci U S A* 1999;96:4546–4551.
17. Ghia P, Guida G, Stella S, et al. The pattern of CD38 expression defines a distinct subset of chronic lymphocytic leukemia (CLL) patients at risk of disease progression. *Blood* 2003;101:1262–1269.
18. Hamblin TJ, Davis Z, Gardiner A, et al. Unmutated Ig V(H) genes are associated with a more aggressive form of chronic lymphocytic leukemia. *Blood* 1999;94:1848–1854.
19. Dohner H, Stilgenbauer S, Benner A, et al. Genomic aberrations and survival in chronic lymphocytic leukemia. *N Engl J Med* 2000;343:1910–1916.
20. A predictive model for aggressive non-Hodgkin's lymphoma. The International Non-Hodgkin's Lymphoma Prognostic Factors Project. *N Engl J Med* 1993;329:987–994.
21. Sehn LH, Berry B, Chhanabhai M, et al. The revised International Prognostic Index (R-IPI) is a better predictor of outcome than the standard IPI for patients with diffuse large B-cell lymphoma treated with R-CHOP. *Blood* 2007;109:1857–1861.
22. Hallek M, Cheson BD, Catovsky D, et al. Guidelines for the diagnosis and treatment of chronic lymphocytic leukemia: a report from the International Workshop on Chronic Lymphocytic Leukemia updating the National Cancer Institute-Working Group 1996 guidelines. *Blood* 2008;111:5446–5456.
23. Marti GE, Rawstron AC, Ghia P, et al. Diagnostic criteria for monoclonal B-cell lymphocytosis. *Br J Haematol* 2005;130:325–332.
24. Rawstron AC, Green MJ, Kuzmicki A, et al. Monoclonal B lymphocytes with the characteristics of "indolent" chronic lymphocytic leukemia are present in 3.5% of adults with normal blood counts. *Blood* 2002;100:635–639.
25. Orchard J, Garand R, Davis Z, et al. A subset of t(11;14) lymphoma with mantle cell features displays mutated IgVH genes and includes patients with good prognosis, nonnodal disease. *Blood* 2003;101:4975–4981.
26. Isaacson PG, Matutes E, Burke M, et al. The histopathology of splenic lymphoma with villous lymphocytes. *Blood* 1994;84:3828–3834.
27. Mollejo J, Men'rguez J, Lloret E, et al. Splenic marginal zone lymphoma: a distinctive type of low-grade B-cell lymphoma—a clinicopathological study of 13 cases. *Am J Surg Pathol* 1995;19:1146–1157.
28. Mollejo M, Algara P, Mateo M, et al. Splenic small B-cell lymphoma with predominant red pulp involvement: a diffuse variant of splenic marginal zone lymphoma? *Histopathology* 2002;40:22–30.
29. Basso K, Liso A, Tiacci E, et al. Gene expression profiling of hairy cell leukemia reveals a phenotype related to memory B cells with altered expression of chemokine and adhesion receptors. *J Exp Med* 2004;199:59–68.
30. Matutes E, Wotherspoon A, Catovsky D. The variant form of hairy-cell leukaemia. *Best Pract Res Clin Haematol* 2003;16:41–56.
31. Saikia T, Advani S, Dasgupta A, et al. Characterisation of blast cells during blastic phase of chronic myeloid leukaemia by immunophenotyping–experience in 60 patients. *Leuk Res* 1988;12:499–506.
32. Owen R, Treon S, Al-Katib A, et al. Clinicopathological definition of Waldenstrom's macroglobulinemia: consensus panel recommendations from the Second International Workshop on Waldenstrom's Macroglobulinemia. *Semin Oncol* 2003;30:110–115.
33. Munoz L, Nomdedeu JF, Villamor N, et al. Acute myeloid leukemia with MLL rearrangements: clinicobiological features, prognostic impact and value of flow cytometry in the detection of residual leukemic cells. *Leukemia* 2003;17:76–82.
34. Fermand JP, Brouet JC. Heavy-chain diseases. *Hematol Oncol Clin North Am* 1999;13:1281–9124.
35. Munshi NC, Digumarthy S, Rahemtullah A. Case records of the Massachusetts General Hospital. Case 13-2008. A 46-year-old man with rheumatoid arthritis and lymphadenopathy. *N Engl J Med* 2008;358:1838–1848.
36. Price SK. Immunoproliferative small intestinal disease: a study of 13 cases with alpha heavy-chain disease. *Histopathology* 1990;17:7–17.
37. Ballard HS, Hamilton LM, Marcus AJ, et al. A new variant of heavy-chain disease (mu-chain disease). *N Engl J Med* 1970;282:1060–1062.
38. Kyle RA, Therneau TM, Rajkumar SV, et al. Prevalence of monoclonal gammopathy of undetermined significance. *N Engl J Med* 2006;354:1362–1369.
39. Kyle RA, Greipp PR. Smoldering multiple myeloma. *N Engl J Med* 1980;302:1347–1349.

40. Kyle RA, Gertz MA, Witzig TE, et al. Review of 1027 patients with newly diagnosed multiple myeloma. *Mayo Clin Proc* 2003;78:21–33.
41. Criteria for the classification of monoclonal gammopathies, multiple myeloma and related disorders: a report of the International Myeloma Working Group. *Br J Haematol* 2003;121:749–757.
42. Soutar R, Lucraft H, Jackson G, et al. Guidelines on the diagnosis and management of solitary plasmacytoma of bone and solitary extramedullary plasmacytoma. *Br J Haematol* 2004;124:717–726.
43. Dimopoulos MA, Kiamouris C, Moulopoulos LA. Solitary plasmacytoma of bone and extramedullary plasmacytoma. *Hematol Oncol Clin North Am* 1999;13:1249–1257.
44. Hussong JW, Perkins SL, Schnitzer B, et al. Extramedullary plasmacytoma. A form of marginal zone cell lymphoma? *Am J Clin Pathol* 1999;111:111–116.
45. Buxbaum J. Mechanisms of disease: monoclonal immunoglobulin deposition. Amyloidosis, light chain deposition disease, and light and heavy chain deposition disease. *Hematol Oncol Clin North Am* 1992;6:323–346.
46. Kyle RA, Gertz MA. Primary systemic amyloidosis: clinical and laboratory features in 474 cases. *Semin Hematol* 1995;32:45–59.
47. Herzenberg AM, Lien J, Magil AB. Monoclonal heavy chain (immunoglobulin G3) deposition disease: report of a case. *Am J Kidney Dis* 1996;28:128–131.
48. Miralles GD, O'Fallon JR, Talley NJ. Plasma-cell dyscrasia with polyneuropathy. The spectrum of POEMS syndrome. *N Engl J Med* 1992;327:1919–1923.
49. Isaacson PG, Spencer J. Malignant lymphoma of mucosa-associated lymphoid tissue. *Histopathology* 1987;11:445–462.
50. Isaacson PG, Wotherspoon AC, Diss T, et al. Follicular colonization in B cell lymphoma of mucosa associated lymphoid tissue. *Am J Surg Pathol* 1991;15:819–828.
51. Isaacson PG. Gastrointestinal lymphoma. *Hum Pathol* 1994;25:1020–1029.
52. Arcaini L, Paulli M, Burcheri S, et al. Primary nodal marginal zone B-cell lymphoma: clinical features and prognostic assessment of a rare disease. *Br J Haematol* 2007;136:301–304.
53. Taddesse-Heath L, Pittaluga S, Sorbara L, et al. Marginal zone B-cell lymphoma in children and young adults. *Am J Surg Pathol* 2003;27:522–531.
54. Agrawal R, Wang J. Pediatric follicular lymphoma: a rare clinicopathologic entity. *Arch Pathol Lab Med* 2009;133:142–146.
55. Sato Y, Ichimura K, Tanaka T, et al. Duodenal follicular lymphomas share common characteristics with mucosa-associated lymphoid tissue lymphomas. *J Clin Pathol* 2008;61:377–381.
56. Cong P, Raffeld M, Teruya-Feldstein J, et al. In situ localization of follicular lymphoma: description and analysis by laser capture microdissection. *Blood* 2002;99:3376–3382.
57. Katzenberger T, Ott G, Klein T, et al. Cytogenetic alterations affecting BCL6 are predominantly found in follicular lymphomas grade 3B with a diffuse large B-cell component. *Am J Pathol* 2004;165:481–490.
58. Ott G, Katzenberger T, Lohr A, et al. Cytomorphologic, immunohistochemical, and cytogenetic profiles of follicular lymphoma: 2 types of follicular lymphoma grade 3. *Blood* 2002;99:3806–3812.
59. Fu K, Weisenburger DD, Greiner TC, et al. Cyclin D1-negative mantle cell lymphoma: a clinicopathologic study based on gene expression profiling. *Blood* 2005;106:4315–4321.
60. Richard P, Vassallo J, Valmary S, et al. "In situ-like" mantle cell lymphoma: a report of two cases. *J Clin Pathol* 2006;59:995–996.
61. Lardelli P, Bookman MA, Sundeen J, et al. Lymphocytic lymphoma of intermediate differentiation. Morphologic and immunophenotypic spectrum and clinical correlations. *Am J Surg Pathol* 1990;14:752–763.
62. Alizadeh AA, Eisen MB, Davis RE, et al. Distinct types of diffuse large B-cell lymphoma identified by gene expression profiling. *Nature* 2000;403:503–511.
63. Choi WW, Weisenburger DD, Greiner TC, et al. A new immunostain algorithm classifies diffuse large B-cell lymphoma into molecular subtypes with high accuracy. *Clin Cancer Res* 2009;15:5494–5502.
64. Greer JP, Macon WR, Lamar RE, et al. T-cell-rich B-cell lymphomas: diagnosis and response to therapy of 44 patients. *J Clin Oncol* 1995;13:1742–1750.
65. Boudova L, Torlakovic E, Delabie J, et al. Nodular lymphocyte-predominant Hodgkin lymphoma with nodules resembling T-cell/histiocyte-rich B-cell lymphoma: differential diagnosis between nodular lymphocyte-predominant Hodgkin lymphoma and T-cell/histiocyte-rich B-cell lymphoma. *Blood* 2003;102:3753–3758.
66. Camilleri-Broet S, Criniere E, Broet P, et al. A uniform activated B-cell-like immunophenotype might explain the poor prognosis of primary central nervous system lymphomas: analysis of 83 cases. *Blood* 2006;107:190–196.
67. Liu YJ. IPC: professional type 1 interferon-producing cells and plasmacytoid dendritic cell precursors. *Annu Rev Immunol* 2005;23:275–306.
68. Willemze R, Jaffe ES, Burg G, et al. WHO-EORTC classification for cutaneous lymphomas. *Blood* 2005;105:3768–3785.
69. Senff NJ, Hoefnagel JJ, Jansen PM, et al. Reclassification of 300 primary cutaneous B-Cell lymphomas according to the new WHO-EORTC classification for cutaneous lymphomas: comparison with previous classifications and identification of prognostic markers. *J Clin Oncol* 2007;25:1581–1587.
70. Oyama T, Ichimura K, Suzuki R, et al. Senile EBV + B-cell lymphoproliferative disorders: a clinicopathologic study of 22 patients. *Am J Surg Pathol* 2003;27:16–26.
71. Oyama T, Yamamoto K, Asano N, et al. Age-related EBV-associated B-cell lymphoproliferative disorders constitute a distinct clinicopathologic group: a study of 96 patients. *Clin Cancer Res* 2007;13:5124–5132.
72. Iuchi K, Aozasa K, Yamamoto S, et al. Non-Hodgkin's lymphoma of the pleural cavity developing from long-standing pyothorax. Summary of clinical and pathological findings in thirty-seven cases. *Jpn J Clin Oncol* 1989;19:249–257.
73. Petitjean B, Jardin F, Joly B, et al. Pyothorax-associated lymphoma: a peculiar clinicopathologic entity derived from B cells at late stage of differentiation and with occasional aberrant dual B- and T-cell phenotype. *Am J Surg Pathol* 2002;26:724–732.
74. Guinee D Jr, Jaffe E, Kingma D, et al. Pulmonary lymphomatoid granulomatosis. Evidence for a proliferation of Epstein-Barr virus infected B-lymphocytes with a prominent T-cell component and vasculitis. *Am J Surg Pathol* 1994;18:753–764.
75. Haque AK, Myers JL, Hudnall SD, et al. Pulmonary lymphomatoid granulomatosis in acquired immunodeficiency syndrome: lesions with Epstein-Barr virus infection. *Mod Pathol* 1998;11:347–356.
76. Lipford EH, Margolich JB, Longo DL, et al. Angiocentric immunoproliferative lesions: a clinicopathologic spectrum of post-thymic T cell proliferations. *Blood* 1988;72:1674–1681.
77. Rosenwald A, Wright G, Leroy K, et al. Molecular diagnosis of primary mediastinal B cell lymphoma identifies a clinically favorable subgroup of diffuse large B cell lymphoma related to Hodgkin lymphoma. *J Exp Med* 2003;198:851–862.
78. Calaminici M, Piper K, Lee AM, et al. CD23 expression in mediastinal large B-cell lymphomas. *Histopathology* 2004;45:619–624.
79. Pileri SA, Gaidano G, Zinzani PL, et al. Primary mediastinal B-cell lymphoma: high frequency of BCL-6 mutations and consistent expression of the transcription factors OCT-2, BOB.1, and PU.1 in the absence of immunoglobulins. *Am J Pathol* 2003;162:243–253.
80. Ferreri AJ, Dognini GP, Campo E, et al. Variations in clinical presentation, frequency of hemophagocytosis and clinical behavior of intravascular lymphoma diagnosed in different geographical regions. *Haematologica* 2007;92:486–492.
81. Delecluse HJ, Anagnostopoulos I, Dallenbach F, et al. Plasmablastic lymphomas of the oral cavity: a new entity associated with the human immunodeficiency virus infection. *Blood* 1997;89:1413–1420.
82. Dong HY, Scadden DT, de LL, et al. Plasmablastic lymphoma in HIV-positive patients: an aggressive Epstein-Barr virus-associated extramedullary plasmacytic neoplasm. *Am J Surg Pathol* 2005;29:1633–1641.
83. Valera A, Balague O, Colomo L, et al. IG/MYC rearrangements are the main cytogenetic alteration in plasmablastic lymphomas. *Am J Surg Pathol* 2010;34:1686–1694.
84. Gascoyne RD, Lamant L, Martin-Subero JI, et al. ALK-positive diffuse large B-cell lymphoma is associated with Clathrin-ALK rearrangements: report of 6 cases. *Blood* 2003;102:2568–2573.
85. Dupin N, Diss TL, Kellam P, et al. HHV-8 is associated with a plasmablastic variant of Castleman disease that is linked to HHV-8-positive plasmablastic lymphoma. *Blood* 2000;95:1406–1412.
86. Nador RG, Cesarman E, Chadburn A, et al. Primary effusion lymphoma: a distinct clinicopathologic entity associated with the Kaposi's sarcoma-associated herpes virus. *Blood* 1996;88:645–656.
87. Facer CA, Playfair JH. Malaria, Epstein-Barr virus, and the genesis of lymphomas. *Adv Cancer Res* 1989;53:33–72.
88. Magrath IT, Sariban E. Clinical features of Burkitt's lymphoma in the USA. *IARC Sci Publ* 1985:119–127.
89. Raphael M, Gentilhomme O, Tulliez M, et al. Histopathologic features of high-grade non-Hodgkin's lymphomas in acquired immunodeficiency syndrome. *Arch Pathol Lab Med* 1991;115:15–20.
90. Soussain C, Patte C, Ostronoff M, et al. Small noncleaved cell lymphoma and leukemia in adults. A retrospective study of 65 adults treated with the LMB pediatric protocols. *Blood* 1995;85:664–674.
91. Seegmiller AC, Garcia R, Huang R, et al. Simple karyotype and bcl-6 expression predict a diagnosis of Burkitt lymphoma and better survival in IG-MYC rearranged high-grade B-cell lymphomas. *Mod Pathol* 2010;23:909–920.
92. Le GS, Talmant P, Touzeau C, et al. The clinical presentation and prognosis of diffuse large B-cell lymphoma with t(14;18) and 8q24/c-MYC rearrangement. *Haematologica* 2007;92:1335–1342.
93. Hummel M, Bentink S, Berger H, et al. A biologic definition of Burkitt's lymphoma from transcriptional and genomic profiling. *N Engl J Med* 2006;354:2419–2430.
94. Gallagher CJ, Gregory WM, Jones AE, et al. Follicular lymphoma: prognostic factors for response and survival. *J Clin Oncol* 1986;4:1470–1480.
95. Traverse-Glehen A, Pittaluga S, Gaulard P, et al. Mediastinal gray zone lymphoma: the missing link between classic Hodgkin's lymphoma and mediastinal large B-cell lymphoma. *Am J Surg Pathol* 2005;29:1411–1421.
96. Jaffe ES. Pathobiology of peripheral T-cell lymphomas. *Hematol Am Soc Hematol Educ Program* 2006:317–322.
97. Matutes E, Brito-Babapulle V, Swansbury J, et al. Clinical and laboratory features of 78 cases of T-prolymphocytic leukemia. *Blood* 1991;78:3269–3274.
98. Maljaei SH, Brito-Babapulle V, Hiorns LR, et al. Abnormalities of chromosomes 8, 11, 14, and X in T-prolymphocytic leukemia studied by fluorescence in situ hybridization. *Cancer Genet Cytogenet* 1998;103:110–116.
99. Lamy T, Loughran TP Jr. Current concepts: large granular lymphocyte leukemia. *Blood Rev* 1999;13:230–240.
100. French LE, Alcindor T, Shapiro M, et al. Identification of amplified clonal T cell populations in the blood of patients with chronic graft-versus-host disease: positive correlation with response to photopheresis. *Bone Marrow Transplant* 2002;30:509–515.
101. Rabbani GR, Phyliky RL, Tefferi A. A long-term study of patients with chronic natural killer cell lymphocytosis. *Br J Haematol* 1999;106:960–966.
102. Lima M, Almeida J, Montero AG, et al. Clinicobiological, immunophenotypic, and molecular characteristics of monoclonal CD56-/+dim chronic natural killer cell large granular lymphocytosis. *Am J Pathol* 2004;165:1117–1127.
103. Kelly A, Richards SJ, Sivakumaran M, et al. Clonality of CD3 negative large granular lymphocyte proliferations determined by PCR based X-inactivation studies. *J Clin Pathol* 1994;47:399–404.
104. Ruskova A, Thula R, Chan G. AGGRESSIVE natural killer-cell leukemia: report of five cases and review of the literature. *Leuk Lymphoma* 2004;45:2427–2438.
105. Nakashima Y, Tagawa H, Suzuki R, et al. Genome-wide array-based comparative genomic hybridization of natural killer cell lymphoma/leukemia: different genomic alteration patterns of aggressive NK-cell leukemia and extranodal Nk/T-cell lymphoma, nasal type. *Genes Chromosomes Cancer* 2005;44:247–255.
106. Ishihara S, Okada S, Wakiguchi H, et al. Clonal lymphoproliferation following chronic active Epstein-Barr virus infection and hypersensitivity to mosquito bites. *Am J Hematol* 1997;54:276–281.
107. Quintanilla-Martinez L, Kumar S, Fend F, et al. Fulminant EBV(+) T-cell lymphoproliferative disorder following acute/chronic EBV infection: a distinct clinicopathologic syndrome. *Blood* 2000;96:443–451.
108. Kimura H, Hoshino Y, Kanegane H, et al. Clinical and virologic characteristics of chronic active Epstein-Barr virus infection. *Blood* 2001;98:280–286.
109. Barrionuevo C, Anderson VM, Zevallos-Giampietri E, et al. Hydroa-like cutaneous T-cell lymphoma: a clinicopathologic and molecular genetic study of 16 pediatric cases from Peru. *Appl Immunohistochem Mol Morphol* 2002;10:7–14.
110. Yamaguchi K. Human T-lymphotropic virus type I in Japan. *Lancet* 1994;343:213–216.
111. Shimoyama M. Diagnostic criteria and classification of clinical subtypes of adult T-cell leukaemia-lymphoma. A report from the Lymphoma Study Group (1984-87). *BrJ Haematol* 1991;79:428–437.
112. Ohshima K. Pathological features of diseases associated with human T-cell leukemia virus type I. *Cancer Sci* 2007;98:772–778.

113. Arber DA, Weiss LM, Albujar PF, et al. Nasal lymphomas in Peru: high incidence of T-cell immunophenotype and Epstein-Barr virus infection. *Am J Surg Pathol* 1993;17:392–399.
114. Kanavaros P, Lescs MC, Briere J, et al. Nasal T-cell lymphoma: a clinicopathologic entity associated with peculiar phenotype and with Epstein-Barr virus. *Blood* 1993;81:2688–2695.
115. Chim CS, Ma ES, Loong F, et al. Diagnostic cues for natural killer cell lymphoma: primary nodal presentation and the role of in situ hybridisation for Epstein-Barr virus encoded early small RNA in detecting occult bone marrow involvement. *J Clin Pathol* 2005;58:443–445.
116. Ng SB, Lai KW, Murugaya S, et al. Nasal-type extranodal natural killer/T-cell lymphomas: a clinicopathologic and genotypic study of 42 cases in Singapore. *Mod Pathol* 2004;17:1097–1107.
117. Wright D. Enteropathy associated T cell lymphoma. *Cancer Surv* 1997;30:249–261.
118. Deleeuw RJ, Zettl A, Klinker E, et al. Whole-genome analysis and HLA genotyping of enteropathy-type T-cell lymphoma reveals 2 distinct lymphoma subtypes. *Gastroenterology* 2007;132:1902–1911.
119. Cooke CB, Krenacs L, Stetler-Stevenson M, et al. Hepatosplenic T-cell lymphoma: a distinct clinicopathologic entity of cytotoxic gamma delta T-cell origin. *Blood* 1996;88:4265–4274.
120. Belhadj K, Reyes F, Farcet JP, et al. Hepatosplenic gammadelta T-cell lymphoma is a rare clinicopathologic entity with poor outcome: report on a series of 21 patients. *Blood* 2003;102:4261–4269.
121. Suarez F, Wlodarska I, Rigal-Huguet F, et al. Hepatosplenic alphabeta T-cell lymphoma: an unusual case with clinical, histologic, and cytogenetic features of gammadelta hepatosplenic T-cell lymphoma. *Am J Surg Pathol* 2000;24:1027–1032.
122. Wlodarska I, Martin-Garcia N, Achten R, et al. Fluorescence in situ hybridization study of chromosome 7 aberrations in hepatosplenic T-cell lymphoma: isochromosome 7q as a common abnormality accumulating in forms with features of cytologic progression. *Genes Chromosomes Cancer* 2002;33:243–251.
123. Kumar S, Krenacs L, Medeiros J, et al. Subcutaneous panniculitic T-cell lymphoma is a tumor of cytotoxic T-lymphocytes. *Hum Pathol* 1998;29:397–403.
124. Willemze R, Jansen PM, Cerroni L, et al. Subcutaneous panniculitis-like T-cell lymphoma: definition, classification, and prognostic factors: an EORTC Cutaneous Lymphoma Group Study of 83 cases. *Blood* 2008;2:838–845.
125. Massone C, Kodama K, Kerl H, et al. Histopathologic features of early (patch) lesions of mycosis fungoides: a morphologic study on 745 biopsy specimens from 427 patients. *Am J Surg Pathol* 2005;29:550–560.
126. van DR, Scheffer E, Willemze R. Follicular mycosis fungoides, a distinct disease entity with or without associated follicular mucinosis: a clinicopathologic and follow-up study of 51 patients. *Arch Dermatol* 2002;138:191–198.
127. Haghighi B, Smoller BR, LeBoit PE, et al. Pagetoid reticulosis (Woringer-Kolopp disease): an immunophenotypic, molecular, and clinicopathologic study. *Mod Pathol* 2000;13:502–510.
128. van Haselen CW, Toonstra J, van der Putte SJ, et al. Granulomatous slack skin. Report of three patients with an updated review of the literature. *Dermatology* 1998;196:382–391.
129. Bekkenk MW, Geelen FA, van Voorst Vader PC, et al. Primary and secondary cutaneous CD30(+) lymphoproliferative disorders: a report from the Dutch Cutaneous Lymphoma Group on the long-term follow-up data of 219 patients and guidelines for diagnosis and treatment. *Blood* 2000;95:3653–3661.
130. Weiss LM, Wood GS, Trela MJ, et al. Clonal T cell populations in lymphomatoid papulosis. Evidence for a lymphoproliferative etiology in a clinically benign disease. *N Engl J Med* 1986;315:475–479.

131. Kadin ME. Pathobiology of CD30+ cutaneous T-cell lymphomas. *J Cutan Pathol* 2006;33(Suppl 1):10–17.
132. Wada DA, Law ME, Hsi ED, et al. Specificity of IRF4 translocations for primary cutaneous anaplastic large cell lymphoma: a multicenter study of 204 skin biopsies. *Mod Pathol* 2011;24:596–605.
133. Toro JR. Gamma-delta T-Cell phenotype is associated with significantly decreased survival in cutaneous T-cell lymphoma. *Blood* 2003:3407–3412.
134. De Wolf-Peeters C, Achten R. gammadelta T-cell lymphomas: a homogeneous entity? *Histopathology* 2000;36:294–305.
135. Berti E, Tomasini D, Vermeer MH, et al. Primary cutaneous CD8-positive epidermotropic cytotoxic T cell lymphomas. A distinct clinicopathological entity with an aggressive clinical behavior. *Am J Pathol* 1999;155:483–492.
136. Bekkenk MW, Vermeer MH, Jansen PM, et al. Peripheral T-cell lymphomas unspecified presenting in the skin: analysis of prognostic factors in a group of 82 patients. *Blood* 2003;102:2213–2219.
137. Garcia-Herrera A, Colomo L, Camos M, et al. Primary cutaneous small/medium CD4+ T-cell lymphomas: a heterogeneous group of tumors with different clinicopathologic features and outcome. *J Clin Oncol* 2008;26:3364–3371.
138. Ottaviani G, Bueso-Ramos CE, Seilstad K, et al. The role of the perifollicular sinus in determining the complex immunoarchitecture of angioimmunoblastic T-cell lymphoma. *Am J Surg Pathol* 2004;28:1632–1640.
139. Ree HJ, Kadin ME, Kikuchi M, et al. Angioimmunoblastic lymphoma (AILD-type T-cell lymphoma) with hyperplastic germinal centers. *Am J Surg Pathol* 1998;22:643–655.
140. Dorfman DM, Brown JA, Shahsafaei A, et al. Programmed death-1 (PD-1) is a marker of germinal center-associated T cells and angioimmunoblastic T-cell lymphoma. *Am J Surg Pathol* 2006;30:802–810.
141. de LL, Rickman DS, Thielen C, et al. The gene expression profile of nodal peripheral T-cell lymphoma demonstrates a molecular link between angioimmunoblastic T-cell lymphoma (AITL) and follicular helper T (TFH) cells. *Blood* 2007;109:4952–4963.
142. Weiss LM, Jaffe ES, Liu X, et al. Detection and localization of Epstein-Barr viral genomes in angioimmunoblastic lymphadenopathy and angioimmunoblastic lymphadenopathy-like lymphomas. *Blood* 1992;79:1789–1795.
143. Benharroch D, Meguerian-Bedoyan Z, Lamant L, et al. ALK-positive lymphoma: a single disease with a broad spectrum of morphology. *Blood* 1998;91:2076–2084.
144. Savage KJ, Harris NL, Vose JM, et al. ALK- anaplastic large-cell lymphoma is clinically and immunophenotypically different from both ALK+ ALCL and peripheral T-cell lymphoma, not otherwise specified: report from the International Peripheral T-Cell Lymphoma Project. *Blood* 2008;111:5496–5504.
145. Rizvi MA, Evens AM, Tallman MS, et al. T-cell non-Hodgkin lymphoma. *Blood* 2006;107:1255–1264.
146. Suchi T, Lennert K, Tu LY, et al. Histopathology and immunohistochemistry of peripheral T cell lymphomas: a proposal for their classification. *J Clin Pathol* 1987;40:995–1015.
147. Rahemtullah A, Reichard KK, Preffer FI, et al. A double-positive CD4+CD8+ T-cell population is commonly found in nodular lymphocyte predominant Hodgkin lymphoma. *Am J Clin Pathol* 2006;126:805–814.
148. Streubel B, Vinatzer U, Willheim M, et al. Novel t(5;9)(q33;q22) fuses ITK to SYK in unspecified peripheral T-cell lymphoma. *Leukemia* 2006;20:313–318.
149. Warnke RA, Jones D, Hsi ED. Morphologic and immunophenotypic variants of nodal T-cell lymphomas and T-cell lymphoma mimics. *Am J Clin Pathol* 2007;127:511–527.

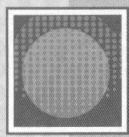

Chapter 18

Chronic Lymphocytic Leukemia/Small Lymphocytic Lymphoma and B-Cell Prolymphocytic Leukemia

David Czuchlewski • Kathryn Foucar

Chronic lymphoid neoplasms that generate a predominant leukemic blood and bone marrow picture encompass a broad spectrum of disorders with distinct clinical, morphologic, and immunophenotypic features. Chronic lymphocytic leukemia (CLL) is by far the most common of these chronic leukemias (Table 18.1). Perhaps because of its relatively high prevalence, CLL has received close attention from primary and translational researchers. These investigations have yielded landmark insights into the pathogenesis of CLL and hastened the arrival of ancillary studies that establish prognostic expectations for individual patients with CLL. In this chapter, we focus on CLL and its tissue-based manifestation, small lymphocytic lymphoma (SLL). In addition, we discuss an entirely separate neoplastic entity, B-cell prolymphocytic leukemia (B-PLL), and touch upon the evolving concept of monoclonal B lymphocytosis (MBL). Together, these diseases present a complex challenge to the diagnostician in that they demand integration of clinical features, morphology, immunophenotypic findings, and molecular data for optimal subclassification, therapeutic decision making, and prognostic assessment. In this sense, the diagnostic approach to these cases reflects the modern, multimodal philosophy championed by successive editions of the World Health Organization (WHO) Classification of Tumours of Haematopoietic and Lymphoid Tissues (1,2).

CHRONIC LYMPHOCYTIC LEUKEMIA/ SMALL LYMPHOCYTIC LYMPHOMA

Diagnostic Criteria/Definitions

CLL/SLL is a clonal proliferation of small, mature B cells that typically possess conspicuously condensed chromatin, round nuclear contours, and scant cytoplasm. Admixed with this predominant population may be slightly larger B cells with nucleoli ("prolymphocytes"), or even larger B cells with very prominent nucleoli ("paraimmunoblasts"); all these cell types are part of the clonal population (7). Prolymphocytes may be observed circulating in the peripheral blood in CLL/SLL, while in nodal disease the prolymphocytes and paraimmunoblasts are concentrated in collections known as proliferation centers. The neoplastic cells usually express CD5 and CD23, in addition to showing other characteristic immunophenotypic features.

The relative anatomic distribution of the malignant cells serves to distinguish CLL from SLL. Cases with lymphadenopathy and/or splenomegaly that also lack significant numbers of circulating B cells ($<5 \times 10^9$/L) are considered to be SLL (7,8). Involvement of lymph nodes, other organs, soft tissue, and bone marrow may be seen in *both* CLL and SLL; thus, the key distinction is the extent of peripheral blood involvement. There is clearly a degree of clinical and biologic overlap between CLL and SLL that is not entirely captured in these definitions. For example, if highly sensitive techniques are utilized, some minimal degree of blood involvement is the rule rather

than the exception even in patients with apparent pure SLL (9). CLL and SLL are united at the molecular level as well, in that both share the same common cytogenetic abnormalities and certain molecular changes (9–11). Finally, there is clinical overlap between CLL and SLL, with up to 35% of the latter evolving toward a leukemic picture over the course of their disease (9). Thus, CLL and SLL are best considered to be different appearances of *one* entity—much as steam and ice are different phases of the atomic entity H_2O. The combination of CLL and SLL into the overall diagnostic category "CLL/SLL" in the WHO classification highlights this continuum between tissue-based and leukemic disease (7,12). For the sake of readability, in this chapter we generally refer to "chronic lymphocytic leukemia/ small lymphocytic lymphoma" simply as CLL, reserving specific mentions of SLL and CLL/SLL for those instances in which the precise sites of involvement are of special importance.

A second key definitional distinction is between CLL and the recently recognized MBL (13,14). In population-based screening, a percentage (~3% to 4%) of healthy, older adults can be shown to harbor small monoclonal B-cell populations circulating in their peripheral blood (15). Indeed, if unusually sensitive analysis is employed, even higher incidence of MBL can be documented, especially in elderly patients (16–19). Many, though not all, of these clones show an immunophenotype reminiscent of CLL, and similar genetic abnormalities (especially deletion of 13q) are seen in both CLL and MBL (14,15,20); but because these small populations do not cause the B-cell count to exceed 5×10^9/L, they are *not* instances of CLL, and are usually instead designated as MBL. Interestingly, some cases of MBL will eventually progress to outright CLL (~1% per year) (14,21), and retrospective analysis reveals that the vast majority of CLL patients can be shown to have met criteria for MBL some time before their CLL diagnosis (22). Thus, MBL is a precursor lesion to CLL—a situation analogous to the relationship between monoclonal gammopathy of undetermined significance and plasma cell myeloma.

In practice, given the immunophenotypic overlap with many cases of MBL, a firm diagnosis of CLL/SLL should be made only when the absolute count of monoclonal B cells is $>5 \times 10^9$/L; *or*, failing that, a diagnosis of CLL/SLL can be entertained if extramedullary tissue involvement,* cytopenias, and/or disease-related symptoms are present (7,8,23). Conversely, a diagnosis of MBL should be rendered if the B-cell count is $<5 \times 10^9$/L, *and* there is no evidence of lymphadenopathy, organomegaly, cytopenias, disease-related symptoms, autoimmune syndromes, infectious

---

*While the 5×10^9/L threshold for a diagnosis of CLL is usually thought to be relevant only in the *absence* of extramedullary tissue involvement, recent data has called this absolute distinction into question. Certain patients meeting peripheral blood criteria for MBL but also showing incidental or minimal nodal involvement followed an indolent course if imaging showed lymphadenopathy <1.5 cm in maximum diameter and/ or the nodes lacked proliferation centers. The term "tissue involvement by CLL/SLL-like cells of uncertain significance" has been suggested for such cases, but this has not been endorsed by consensus committees and has not entered routine clinical practice (19).

Table 18.1	INCIDENCE OF CHRONIC LYMPHOID LEUKEMIAS
Type	**Frequency (%)**
CLL/SLL	>80
Hairy cell leukemia	10
B-PLL	<5
Peripheralized lymphomas	<5
All T-cell leukemias	<5

Adapted from references (3–6).

Table 18.2	CLL INCIDENCE AND MORTALITY BY AGE	
Age Group	**% of Total CLL Cases Diagnosed in Given Age Group**	**% of Total CLL-Attributable Deaths in Given Age Group**
<20	0.1	0.0
20–34	0.2	0.1
35–44	1.5	0.5
45–54	8.8	3.0
55–64	20.3	10.6
65–74	26.6	20.9
75–84	28.9	35.3
85+	13.6	29.6

Adapted from reference (36).

disease, or findings meeting criteria for diagnosis of any other lymphoma (7,8,13,23). Some degree of bone marrow involvement does not necessarily exclude a diagnosis of MBL (23).

It should be noted that the WHO 2008 Classification requires "$\geq 5 \times 10^9$ *monoclonal* lymphocytes with a CLL phenotype" for a diagnosis of CLL in the absence of extramedullary tissue involvement, cytopenias, and/or symptoms (emphasis added) (7,23). Recent European Society for Medical Oncology clinical practice guidelines likewise call for $\geq 5{,}000$ monoclonal B lymphocytes per microliter (24). The most recent IWCLL guidelines for diagnosis of CLL specify "the presence of at least 5×10^9/L B lymphocytes" in the peripheral blood and note that the "clonality of the circulating B lymphocytes needs to be confirmed by flow cytometry" (8). However, the established definition of MBL cites absolute, not monoclonal, "B-lymphocyte count $>5 \times 10^9$/L" as an exclusionary criterion (13). In practice, the absolute B-cell count and monoclonal B-cell count are often quite close. Indeed, in cases with an absolute B-cell count $>4 \times 10^9$/L, very few circulating normal B cells typically remain (25,26), suggesting that absolute B-cell count is probably a reasonable surrogate for monoclonal B-cell count in patients near the 5×10^9/L threshold.

Although the distinction between MBL and CLL may belie a true biologic continuum, it nevertheless has practical clinical relevance; comparisons between MBL and low-stage CLL show that the latter diagnosis carries comparatively higher risk and a less favorable prognosis (17,27). Even so, it has been observed that there is a difference between so-called low count and high count MBL, with the former less likely to progress (14,28,29). In addition, alternative cutoff values for the absolute B-cell count may in fact better categorize patients according to clinically relevant parameters such as overall survival or requirement for treatment (26,30).

Epidemiology and Incidence

CLL is the most common leukemia of adults in the West, with an incidence of up to 50 cases per 100,000 persons older than 80 years of age (31–33). Almost 15,000 cases are currently diagnosed every year in the United States, with a mean age at diagnosis of around 72 years (34–36). Individuals born at the time of this book's publication stand a 0.5% risk of being diagnosed with CLL at some point during their lifetime (36). Both incidence and disease-related mortality are concentrated in patients past the fifth decade of life (Table 18.2) (31,32,34, 36–39). Despite its rarity, well-characterized case reports of CLL in young adults and children have been published (40–44). Men are diagnosed with CLL more often than women, with a male-to-female ratio of approximately 1:4 to 2:1 (36,45). Increased risk of CLL has been demonstrated in farmers, rubber manufacturing and asbestos workers, and persons exposed to benzene (31–33,46). Unlike many other types of leukemia, CLL is not linked to prior radiation exposure (33). Familial aggregation of CLL has been well described, indicating that inherited polymorphisms or mutations can predispose to the development of the disease.

In contrast to the high prevalence observed in the West, CLL is much less common in some other parts of the world, notably Japan and China (47,48). Careful epidemiologic investigations have attempted to disentangle the contributions of genetics and environment to this discrepancy. The incidence of CLL in Asian Americans (both those who emigrate from Asia and their descendants born in the United States) remains below that of the general U.S. population, indicating that inherent genetic susceptibility plays an important role (49,50). However, Asian individuals born in the United States have an increased risk of developing CLL when compared to those who immigrate to the United States from Asia, and the risk seems to correlate with the degree of acculturation—suggesting that some slight degree of environmental effect may also be contributory (51). Differences in CLL incidence and disease course have also been observed in other races and ethnicities (52–54).

Clinical Features

Given the relatively indolent behavior observed in many cases of CLL, it is common for CLL to be discovered incidentally in an essentially asymptomatic older patient upon routine complete blood count and peripheral blood smear analysis. However, in other patients, clinical manifestations are apparent and include weakness, night sweats, weight loss, and bleeding. Although generally mild, lymphadenopathy and splenomegaly are evident in most patients. Peripheral blood abnormalities range from isolated leukocytosis to lymphocytosis with severe cytopenias. The white blood cell count varies widely, and although absolute lymphocyte counts usually are lower than 100×10^9/L, about 5% of patients who have CLL have hyperleukocytosis exceeding 500×10^9/L, which may be associated with hyperviscosity or leukostasis (3,32,39,55,56). About one-half of CLL patients are mildly anemic at presentation, whereas anemia and mild thrombocytopenia are simultaneously demonstrated in one-fourth of patients (32,55). Cytopenias arise in the setting of CLL through several possible mechanisms, especially splenic enlargement and progressive bone marrow replacement by the neoplastic infiltrate. In addition, during their disease course up to a quarter of CLL patients develop autoimmune phenomena, most of which feature elements of the peripheral blood as target cells (57,58). Coombs-positive hemolytic anemia is seen in between 2% and 10% of cases, and immune thrombocytopenia occurs about 2% of the time (58,59). These autoimmune findings may be attributable in part to aberrant antigen presentation by the malignant B cells and/or impaired function of regulatory T cells (58).

Although it is uncommon, red cell aplasia in the setting of CLL is well described and can occur at any time during the disease course (39,55,60–64). This is generally thought to be immune mediated, and treatment with immunomodulatory agents is often successful in this setting (61,62,65–70). The specific mechanism may involve an autoantibody directed against erythropoietin or red blood cell precursors, though abnormal activity of cytotoxic T cells has also been implicated (60,71–75). In addition, infection with parvovirus B19 is recognized as causative in rare cases of CLL-associated red cell aplasia (76,77). Careful pathologic assessment of red blood cell precursors as a proportion of the residual hematopoietic marrow is essential in differentiating red cell aplasia from autoimmune hemolytic anemia and marrow infiltration as causes for anemia in patients with CLL.

Most patients with CLL show prominent abnormalities of circulating gamma globulin fractions, most often in the form of hypogammaglobulinemia and/or monoclonal gammopathy. These abnormalities can be shown to precede the diagnosis of CLL by up to a decade (78). Hypogammaglobulinemia is seen in up to half of all CLL patients and is associated with increased risk of infection (79–81). At the other extreme, almost 50% of CLL patients have a monoclonal gammopathy. The amount of monoclonal immunoglobulin usually is low and may require highly sensitive techniques for detection (82). Of note, the M protein produced by the neoplastic cells is not typically responsible for the autoimmune features discussed above; rather, the autoreactive antibodies are typically polyclonal in nature and appear to reflect the more global disarray of the immune system in the setting of CLL (58).

Pathologic Features

Peripheral Blood

Although a monotonous lymphocyte population generally predominates, the morphologic spectrum of CLL is fairly broad, overlapping with various reactive disorders and with other B-cell lymphoproliferative disorders (3,4,32,37,39,55). In typical cases of CLL, the blood contains a relatively homogeneous lymphocyte population characterized by cells with a high nuclear-to-cytoplasmic ratio, scant to moderate nongranular cytoplasm, and round nuclei with highly condensed chromatin and inconspicuous nucleoli (Fig. 18.1). The exaggerated chromatin clumping results in a characteristic "blocky" separation of chromatin and parachromatin.

Admixed with these mature-appearing lymphocytes may be prolymphocytes, which generally account for <10% of the lymphocyte population (4,37,39). Prolymphocytes are distinguished from prototypic CLL cells by their greater amounts of cytoplasm, less condensed chromatin, and prominent central nucleoli. Cases with increased prolymphocytes (>10% but <55%) were originally described as "CLL/PLL," a term that has not been incorporated into the WHO classification. However, these cases are associated with specific cytogenetic

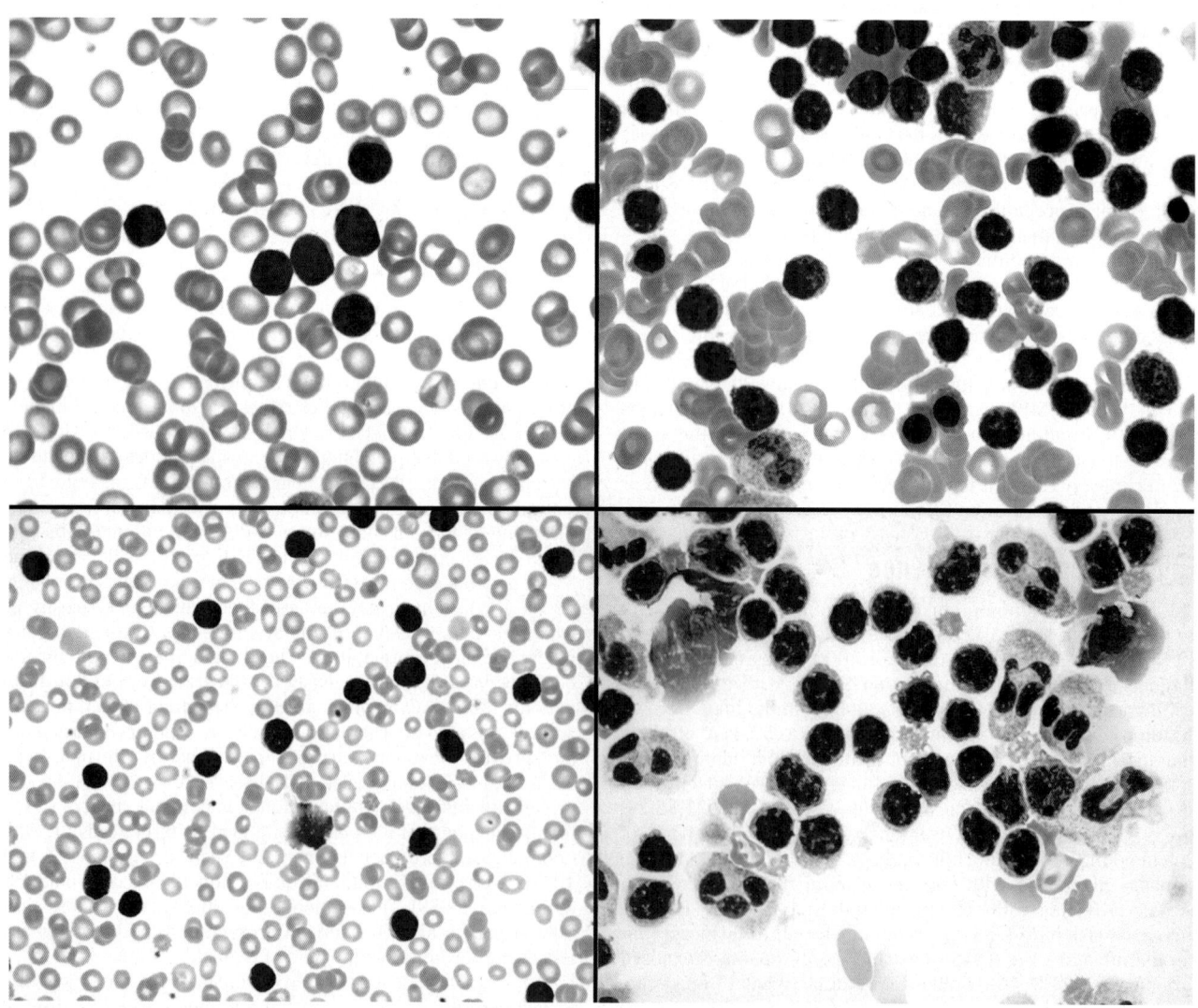

FIGURE 18.1. Typical CLL cells shown in several common preparations: peripheral blood (**lower left**), albumin preparation (**upper left**), bone marrow aspirate smear (**upper right**), and cytospin preparation (**lower right**). Note the cellular monotony, relatively small cell size, condensed chromatin, scant cytoplasm, and round nuclear contours. The peripheral blood smear on the lower left also shows a smudge cell.

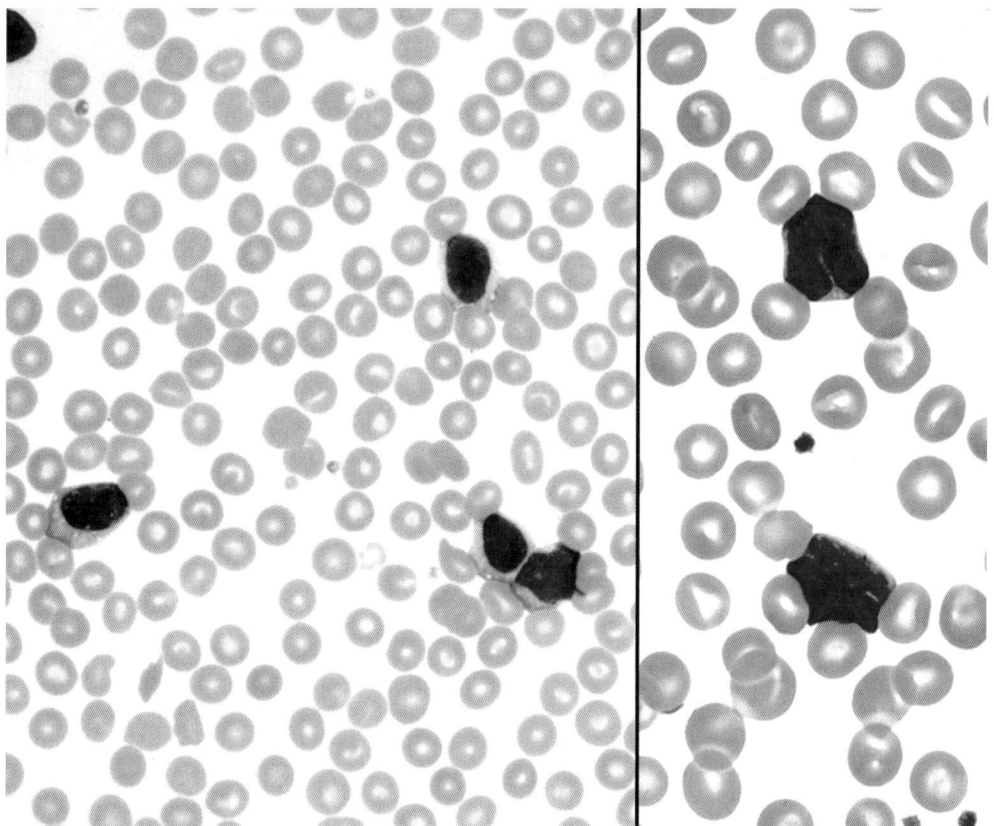

FIGURE 18.2. Two examples of morphologically atypical CLL. The cells in the case on the left have increased cytoplasm, while the case on the right is characterized by conspicuously cleaved nuclear contours. These features are significant departures from typical CLL morphology.

abnormalities (83,84). The absolute number of prolymphocytes in such cases also seems to hold prognostic significance, with cases showing prolymphocytes in excess of 15×10^9/L associated with poor outcome (85,86).

The nuclear irregularity described in some cases of CLL typically occurs in only a minority of lymphocytes and is characterized by prominent nuclear clefting and notching (4,37,39). However, in some cases, the lymphocyte population is substantially more heterogeneous with fair numbers of clefted lymphocytes, or larger cells with more cytoplasm, prominent nucleoli, or plasmacytoid features; these cases are sometimes described as "atypical CLL" (87,88) (Fig. 18.2). Associations of atypical CLL include the presence of trisomy 12, immunophenotypic aberrancy, and worse outcome (88–90). In about 5% to 10% of cases of CLL, cytoplasmic inclusions, such as rod-like bodies, crystals, and vacuoles, are identified (91). These inclusions generally are derived from immunoglobulin and, when present, are found in a variable percentage of the CLL cells (91,92). "Smudge cells" (*aka* "Gumprecht shadows") are common in CLL and are produced when the neoplastic cells are mechanically disrupted during the preparation of the blood smear (Fig. 18.1). The addition of albumin to the specimen can stabilize the cells and prevent this phenomenon (93); in our experience, the condensed chromatin typically associated with CLL is less obvious in such a preparation (Fig. 18.1). The percentage of smudge cells may have prognostic implications (94,95). In addition to evaluating the morphology and absolute lymphocyte count, assessment of normal hematopoietic elements is essential in CLL patients; abnormalities in number and/or morphology of these "bystander" cells may point to autoimmune cytopenias or marrow infiltration by malignant cells and are also crucial in the clinical staging of the disease.

Bone Marrow

Because peripheral blood involvement is a defining feature of CLL, bone marrow examination is generally not required to establish the diagnosis. Aspirate smears typically reveal a mature lymphocytosis that exceeds 30% of the differential cell count (8) (Fig. 18.1). These cells are similar to those present in the blood, although foci of transformed cells may rarely be evident (39). Mast cells may be increased, and plasma cells are often decreased.

The patterns of bone marrow infiltration in biopsy sections are helpful in distinguishing CLL infiltrates from benign lymphoid aggregates and in offering prognostic information (Table 18.3) (3,4,37,55,96–99). Benign lymphoid nodules are generally well circumscribed, are nonparatrabecular, and surround a blood vessel (3,100–102). In contrast, the infiltrates of CLL may be nodular (i.e., focal), interstitial, or diffuse, and various combinations of these patterns have been described

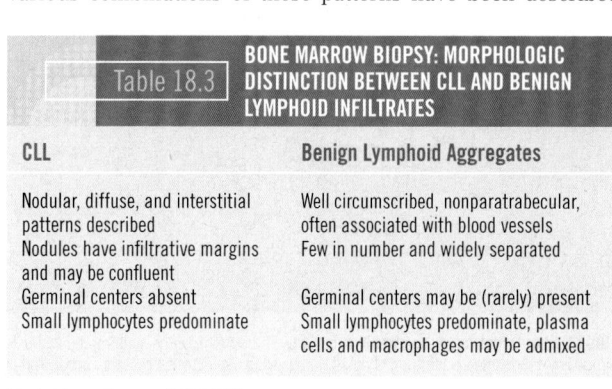

Table 18.3	BONE MARROW BIOPSY: MORPHOLOGIC DISTINCTION BETWEEN CLL AND BENIGN LYMPHOID INFILTRATES	
CLL		**Benign Lymphoid Aggregates**
Nodular, diffuse, and interstitial patterns described		Well circumscribed, nonparatrabecular, often associated with blood vessels
Nodules have infiltrative margins and may be confluent		Few in number and widely separated
Germinal centers absent		Germinal centers may be (rarely) present
Small lymphocytes predominate		Small lymphocytes predominate, plasma cells and macrophages may be admixed

Adapted from references (4,100–103).

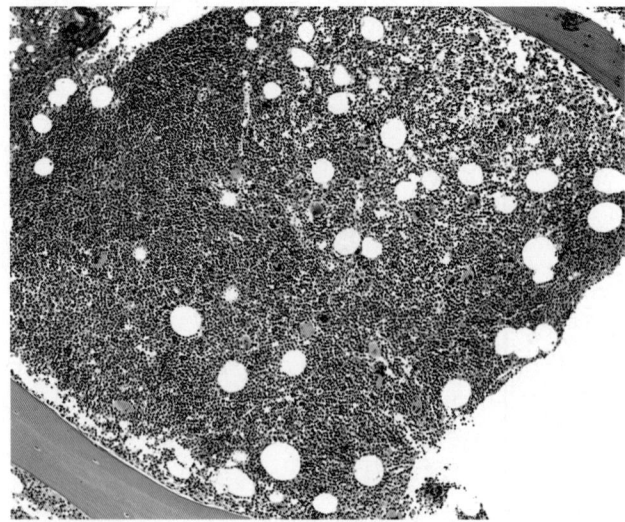

FIGURE 18.3. Diffuse bone marrow infiltration by CLL. This pattern of infiltration is tied to adverse prognosis in CLL.

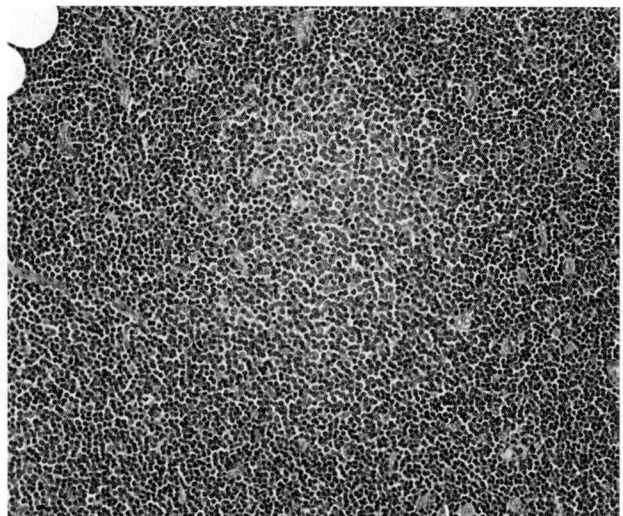

FIGURE 18.5. Proliferation centers in CLL contain significant numbers of prolymphocytes and paraimmunoblasts.

(3,39,55,98). Nodular infiltrates are characterized by dense, localized aggregations of CLL cells that are nonparatrabecular, have infiltrative margins, and may be confluent. In contrast, interstitial infiltrates of CLL cells are admixed with fat cells and hematopoietic elements, whereas bone marrow architecture is completely effaced in the packed diffuse infiltrates (Fig. 18.3). It has been observed that diffuse bone marrow infiltration in CLL is associated with worse prognosis (89,96–98).

Other Sites

Although CLL/SLL infiltrates have been identified in numerous organ systems, lymph nodes and spleen are the most commonly evaluated extramedullary sites (32,37,55,104,105). The lymph nodes generally exhibit diffuse architectural effacement by a monotonous infiltrate of small lymphocytes with round nuclear contours, inconspicuous nucleoli, and scant cytoplasm (Fig. 18.4). Proliferation centers that consist of intermediate-sized cells with more cytoplasm and more readily apparent mitotic activity are frequently present (Figs. 18.4 and 18.5).

These larger cells are thought to constitute the proliferative component of the neoplasm (106,107). Occasionally, the intermediate-sized cells are admixed diffusely with the small lymphocytes of CLL/SLL (104). Different lymph node histology has been described in patients with atypical CLL/SLL (105). In these cases the proliferation foci are larger, more distinct, and contain large transformed cells. Greater nuclear irregularity of the small lymphocytes may be evident. Although infiltration by small lymphocytes is the most common morphologic pattern at presentation, nodal morphology may change during the course of CLL/SLL, and the lymph node may be the initial site of transformation of CLL/SLL to large cell lymphoma (Fig. 18.6).

Splenomegaly caused by leukemic infiltration is a common clinical finding in CLL/SLL (55,108–111). Although the leukemic cells infiltrate the white and red pulp, white pulp disease usually dominates, creating a miliary nodular pattern grossly. The larger cells tend to be concentrated in the white pulp and form proliferation foci like those seen in lymph nodes. These cells express proliferation markers such as Ki-67, whereas "resting" B cells are concentrated in the red pulp cords (111). Spleens from CLL/SLL patients may also demonstrate trabecular, subendothelial, and prominent sinus involvement (108).

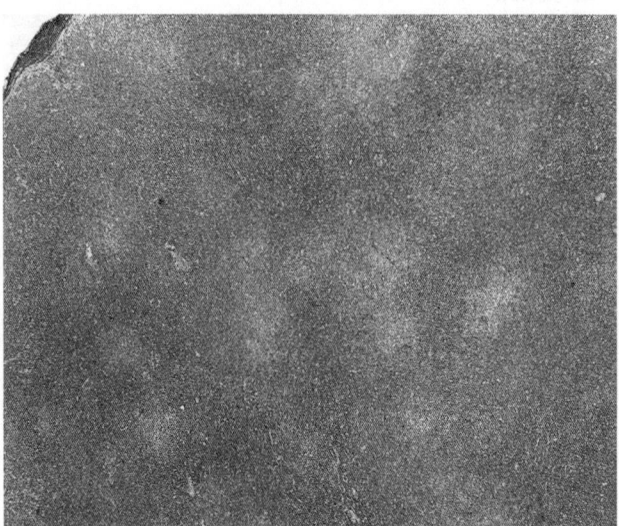

FIGURE 18.4. Lymph node involvement by CLL. The normal lymph node architecture is effaced by a monotonous infiltrate of small lymphocytes. Proliferation centers appear at this low-power magnification as ill-defined pale areas.

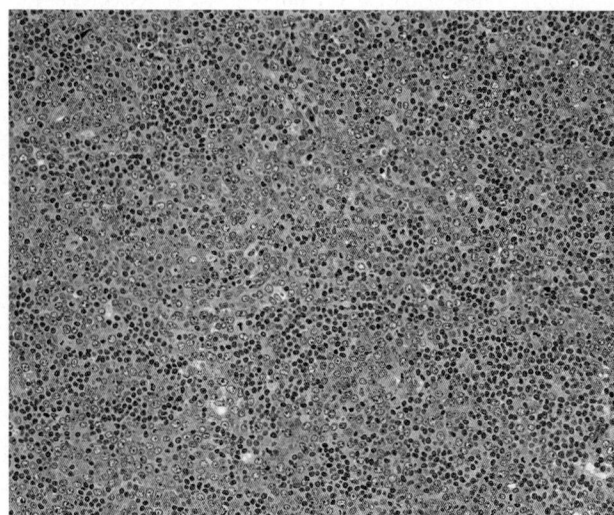

FIGURE 18.6. Lymph node showing Richter transformation of CLL to DLBCL.

Table 18.4	EXTRAMEDULLARY ORGAN INVOLVEMENT IN CLL/SLL		
Site	**Usual Pattern of Infiltration**	**Comments**	**References**
Lymph node	Diffuse; proliferation foci present	May see variation in morphology with disease progression, duration, and in cases of atypical CLL	(37,55,104,105,118)
Spleen	May see white pulp–predominant or red pulp–predominant patterns, but infiltration of both sites generally present	Splenomegaly in majority of patients, usually mild	(55,108–111)
Liver	Usually portal tract involvement predominates; may be associated with fibrosis	Liver involvement common; may be associated with cholestatic jaundice or other liver function abnormalities	(55,110)
Skin	Dermal infiltrates	Clinical spectrum including localized or generalized papules, plaques, nodules, or large tumor masses; incidental involvement of the skin may be noted in the vicinity of unrelated cutaneous pathology	(55,112–117)
Lung	Variable	Generally involves hilar nodes with resulting bronchial compression or lymphatic obstruction causing effusions	(55)
Gastrointestinal tract	Mucosal infiltrates described in stomach, small bowel, and large bowel	May cause malabsorption (small bowel infiltrates)	(55,119)
Bone	Variable	Diffuse demineralization (<5% patients); rare patient develops osteolytic lesions with hypercalcemia	(55)
Central nervous system	Variable	<2% of patients develop CNS symptoms that range from meningeal signs to tumor masses (usually associated with transformation to large cell lymphoma)	(55,120–124)
Heart, adrenal, kidney	Diffuse infiltrates of small lymphocytes	Usually subclinical but may be associated with fibrosis	(110)

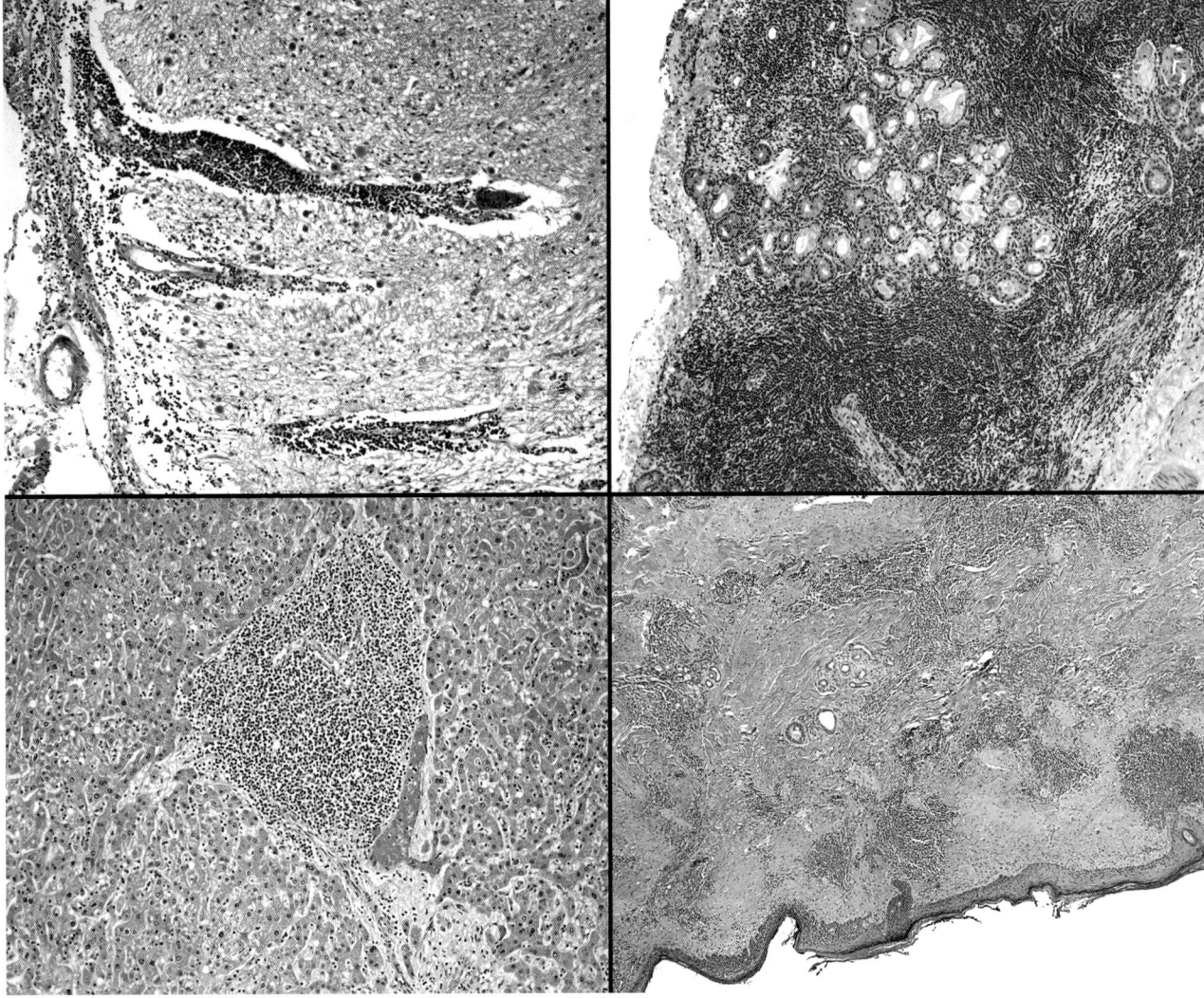

FIGURE 18.7. Unusual sites of involvement by CLL include brain (**upper left**), ethmoid sinus (**upper right**), liver (**lower left**), and skin (**lower right**).

Table 18.4 details the patterns of CLL/SLL infiltration in other sites, including liver, skin, lung, gastrointestinal tract, bone, central nervous system, heart, adrenal, and kidney (Fig. 18.7). In all of these sites, CLL/SLL infiltrates may be associated with fibrosis (110). Dermal infiltration by CLL/SLL is not uncommonly noted in the vicinity of unrelated cutaneous lesions (112–117). Hepatic involvement is also well described, but clinically significant infiltrates of other soft tissue sites are only infrequently encountered in clinical practice. Autopsy studies, however, have documented a wide extent of anatomic disease distribution.

Immunophenotype

By applying a battery of monoclonal antibodies, a spectrum of immunophenotypic characteristics has been delineated that generally can be used to distinguish CLL from other B-lymphoproliferative disorders (3,4,32,37,39,55,125–128). The comprehensive surface antigenic profile of prototypic CLL entails expression of weak monotypic immunoglobulin, CD19, CD23, CD5, and weak or absent CD20, CD22, FMC7, and CD11c; CD10 is not expressed (Table 18.5) (3,37,55,125,126,128). The use of both monoclonal and polyclonal antibodies for the detection of surface light chain can assist in documenting light chain restriction in CLL (129). *Bona fide* CD5-negative cases of CLL are rare (130,131). By using this broad antigenic fingerprint of the leukemic clone, CLL can usually be distinguished from other mature B-cell neoplasms such as peripheralizing mantle cell lymphoma, follicular lymphoma, splenic marginal zone lymphoma (SMZL), hairy cell leukemia, and B-PLL. Indeed, an immunophenotypic scoring system has been proposed as a diagnostic aide (126,132). Significant deviation from the classic CLL immunophenotype is associated with inferior prognosis (133). In addition, CD38 and ZAP-70 can be detected by flow cytometric analysis and figure prominently in establishing prognostic expectations in a given case of CLL; they will be discussed in more detail below. CD8 expression by the CLL cells is a very rare phenomenon (1%), but when present is associated with more aggressive disease (134). A novel application of flow cytometric analysis in CLL is the detection of minimal residual disease in patients who have been treated with modern chemoimmunotherapy regimens (135–137). Nuclear staining for p53 by immunohistochemistry may to some degree mirror the presence of *TP53* mutations, but is generally considered inadequate for clinical detection of this important mutation (138–140).

Because flow cytometric analysis is highly sensitive, small (<5 × 10⁹/L) clonal populations of cells with a CLL-type immunophenotype may be identified. Even if alternative B-cell lymphomas are excluded, such populations may represent *either* CLL/SLL *or* monoclonal B lymphocytosis, as described above. Therefore, the diagnostician should exercise great caution in the interpretation of isolated flow cytometric data in this setting, and careful clinical and morphologic correlation must be undertaken to ascertain the true significance of low-level clones.

Prognostic Factors

The overall 5-year relative survival for CLL patients in the United States between the years 2001 and 2007 was 78% (36),

but there is a wide range of possible clinical behavior in CLL. Indeed, roughly a third of patients diagnosed with CLL experience nonprogressive disease with little associated morbidity. However, the remainder of patients will show progression of disease, with a subset experiencing a markedly more aggressive clinical course. A critical task has been to identify clinical or laboratory features that discriminate between indolent and aggressive disease. In fact, the search for such markers has led to almost an "embarrassment of riches": a huge and ever-expanding catalogue of biomarkers tied to disease behavior and prognosis. A list of these is provided in Table 18.6. Here we concentrate on the features most commonly used in practice to establish prognostic expectations, and conclude with a discussion of the problem of discordance between these parameters.

Clinical Stage

As in all neoplasms, the purpose of staging CLL patients is to segregate them into good-, intermediate-, and poor-risk categories. Although several researchers have proposed classification systems that attempt to stratify CLL patients, the two most commonly used systems in clinical medicine are those proposed by Rai and Binet (34,39,55,202–206). Rai et al. proposed a five-stage classification system for CLL, based on the extent of anatomic involvement of lymphoid organs and the presence or absence of anemia and thrombocytopenia (Table 18.7). Although the clinical relevance of the Rai staging system for CLL is well established, several groups recommended a combination of the stages to establish low-risk (stage 0), intermediate-risk (stages I and II), and high-risk (stages III and IV) categories (207). Median survival times have been determined for patients categorized by the Rai staging system (204,205). Subsequent studies have confirmed that survival correlates with the Rai stage, though in modern case series the median survival for patients with high-stage disease is significantly longer than originally described by Rai (208); these differences are a measure of the relative success of current therapeutic regimens (201).

Binet et al. proposed a simplified staging system, designating stages A, B, and C (Table 18.8) (203,206). In this staging system, lymphoid areas relevant to classification include three lymph node groups (cervical, axillary, and inguinal) plus the spleen and liver. Patients are categorized according to the number of these lymphoid areas that are enlarged and the degree of anemia or thrombocytopenia. The clinical relevance of the Binet classification system has also been established in clinical trials. As with the Rai staging system, modern case series show a significant improvement in median survival compared to the original description by Binet, particularly for patients with stage C disease (206,208).

Because both classification systems are successful in segregating patients into broad prognostic groups, the International Workshop on CLL recommended that patients be staged using a combined Rai-Binet classification system, as follows: A(0), A(I), A(II), B(I), B(II), C(III), and C(IV); however, the complexity of this combined staging system has been emphasized by subsequent investigators, and it has not been widely used (209).

Although the Rai and Binet classification systems segregate groups of patients into general survival groups, they have

	SIg	CD19	CD20	CD22	CD79a	CD5	CD23	FMC7	CD10	CD11c	CD25	CD103	Cyclin D1
CLL	W	+	W	W	W	+	+	–	–	W	–	–	–
B-PLL	+	+	+	+	+	V	–	+	–	V	V	–	–

Table 18.5 TYPICAL IMMUNOPHENOTYPIC FEATURES OF CLL AND B-PLL

Adapted from references (141,142).

Table 18.6 | A SAMPLING OF ESTABLISHED AND PROPOSED PROGNOSTIC MARKERS IN CLL

Clinical
Stage
Lymphocyte doubling time
Pattern of bone marrow involvement
Age
Gender
Percent smudge cells (94,95)
Circulating prolymphocytes
Minimal residual disease status (136,137)
Treatment response
Duration of response
Performance status
Absolute lymphocyte count
High white blood cell count (143)
Number of nodal groups involved
Atypical morphology (88)

Molecular
IGHV@ mutation status
Interphase FISH
Karyotype
TP53 mutation (144–148)
IGHV@ V region usage
Stereotyped B-cell receptor
IRF4 mutation (149)
MDM2 SNP
BCL2 polymorphism
BCL6 mutation
Telomere length (150)
Nucleolar morphology
NOTCH1 mutations (151–154)
SF3B1 mutation (155,156)
LDOC1 expression (157)
Overall complexity by array comparative genomic hybridization (158)
TOSO overexpression (159)
LRP4 SNP (160)
PDE7B expression (161)
Abnormal methylation patterns (162,163)
Gene expression signatures (164–166)
FCRL2 expression (167)
HLA-G expression (168–170)
HLA-DOA expression (171)
LPL expression (172)
LPL/ADAM29 expression ratio (173)
MicroRNA signature (174)
SKI and *SLAMF1* gene signature (175)
BCL2L12 expression (176)
SET oncoprotein expression (177)
CLLU1 expression (178)

Cytokine/Soluble Molecule
Beta-2 microglobulin
VEGF
bFGF
IL6
IL8
Thrombospondin-1
Plasma thrombopoietin
ICAM-1
NKG2D ligands
Soluble CD23
Soluble CD27
Free light chains (179)
Angiopoietin-2
Circulating Ki-67
Lipoprotein lipase
Serum thymidine kinase
TNF-alpha
Cytokine expression "clusters" (180)
APRIL (181,182)
Monoclonal paraprotein (183)
CCL3 (MIP-1α) (184)
BAFF (182,185)
CD52 and CD20 levels (186)

Cell Based
CD38
ZAP-70
CD49d
CD26
CD69 (187)
FCRL2 (188)
P27
Immature laminin receptor expression (189)
Cytoplasmic nucleophosmin (190)
Atypical immunophenotype (133)

Miscellaneous
Bone marrow vessel density
Direct antiglobulin test
relA DNA binding
Circulating endothelial cells
Vitamin D deficiency (191,192)
PD-1 positive follicular helper T cells in the microenvironment (193)
Number of regulatory T cells (194,195)
Relative numbers of CD4 and CD8 T cells (196)
Dipeptidyl peptidase 2 apoptosis assay (197)
Proliferative response to CpG-ODN (mitogen) stimulation (198)
T/leukemic lymphocyte ratio (143)
CD8(+)PD-1(+) replicative senescence phenotype (199)
In vitro response to CD40 ligation (200)

Modified from reference (201).

Table 18.7 | RAI STAGING SYSTEM FOR CLL

Risk group	Stage	Criteria	Median Survival (mo), Original Description by Rai	Median Survival (mo), Modern Case Series
Low	0	Lymphocytosis only (>15 × 10⁹/L)	>150	138
Intermediate	I	Lymphocytosis plus lymphadenopathy	101	132
	II	Lymphocytosis with hepatomegaly or splenomegaly	71	93.6
High	III	Lymphocytosis with anemia (hemoglobin <11 g/dL)	19	63.6
	IV	Lymphocytosis with thrombocytopenia (<100 × 10⁹/L)	19	84

Adapted from references (8,205,208).

Table 18.8	BINET STAGING SYSTEM FOR CLL		
Stage	Criteria	Median Survival (y), Original Description by Binet	Median Survival (y), Modern Case Series
A	No anemia, no thrombocytopenia, involvement of fewer than three lymphoid areas[a]	Not different from age- and sex-matched unaffected population	11.5
B	No anemia, no thrombocytopenia, involvement of three or more lymphoid areas[a]	7	8.6
C	Anemia (<10 g/dL) or thrombocytopenia (<100 × 10⁹/L)	2	7.0

[a]Cervical, axillary, inguinal node groups, spleen, and liver constitute the "lymphoid areas."
Adapted from references (8,206,208).

some significant shortcomings. Especially for the early stages (Rai 0 or Binet A), the clinical staging systems do not fully capture the heterogeneity of disease (201). The ability to identify which early-stage patients are at risk for disease progression facilitates patient counseling and influences the selection of intervals for clinical follow-up (210). The fact that the majority of CLL patients fall into early clinical stages at diagnosis only heightens the need for additional biomarkers that can refine prognostic expectations.

IGHV@ Mutational Status

The specific nucleotide sequence within the *IGH@* region constitutes a key prognostic variable in that it reveals the presence or absence of somatic hypermutation in the variable region of the rearranged immunoglobulin heavy chain locus (*IGHV@*). Somatic hypermutation is a physiologic process, usually occurring within the germinal center, in which B cells acquire random changes to nucleotides in regions encoding the immunoglobulin components (211). By chance, in some cells these changes permit production of an immunoglobulin molecule that will bind antigen with increased affinity, thus enhancing the immune response. Cases of CLL may be sorted into favorable and unfavorable groups based on the presence and absence, respectively, of such somatic hypermutation (212–214). The laboratory analysis involves sequencing the variable region of the heavy chain locus and comparing the result to known germline configurations of the various V regions. A significant divergence (by general consensus, >2% of nucleotides different) from the closest germline V-region sequence is the hallmark of "mutated CLL" (M-CLL), while a sequence with greater homology to the germline is considered "unmutated CLL" (U-CLL). The detection of unmutated *IGHV@* predicts a greater likelihood of early progression, treatment requirement, and shorter survival (215–217); M-CLL, on the other hand, is associated with more indolent behavior and better outcome. The median survival of patients with M-CLL is 25 years, as compared to 8 years for those with U-CLL (213). CLL patients are almost equally divided between these groups, with a slight preponderance of mutated cases (89). There is also some data to suggest that M-CLL with a very low burden of somatic hypermutation (between 2% and 3% divergence from germline) may follow an intermediate prognostic course (218). With modern chemoimmunotherapy regimens the achievement of complete remission is comparable between U-CLL and M-CLL, while the duration of the remission is significantly shorter in U-CLL (219).

An additional molecular parameter of prognostic significance emerges almost as a by-product of the analysis described above. In comparing the sequence from a clonal population to the known library of human V-region sequences, it is easy to determine which of the various V regions was selected by the B

cell for incorporation into its coding immunoglobulin sequence at the time of initial VDJ recombination. The usage of V regions in CLL clones is not random, as CLL cases tend to utilize specific V regions (as will be discussed further below). Clinically, use of V(H)3-21 is associated with adverse prognosis regardless of mutational status (220–222). If this V region is identified in the course of somatic hypermutation analysis for a given patient, most laboratories will note or report the finding. Similarly, use of V(H)3-23 by M-CLL predicts shorter time to treatment than would be typical of a case with somatic hypermutation (223). In a further application of this type of analysis, the specific sequence of nucleotides that encode the complementarity-determining region-3 (CDR3) of the immunoglobulin molecule may also permit greater refinement of prognostic expectations, though the clinical application of such "stereotypy" remains a work in progress (224–226).

CD38

CD38 is a cell surface transmembrane glycoprotein present on a number of hematopoietic cell types and associated with cellular activation. Functionally, it is an "ectoenzyme," meaning that the extracellular portion of the molecule catalyzes a reaction, in this case involving cyclic adenosine diphosphate ribose (227). Expression of CD38 appears to facilitate antiapoptotic signaling and microenvironmental interactions (228,229). Normal B cells express CD38 in a highly regulated manner. It is present on progenitor cells, germinal center cells, and plasma cells. It is also expressed in some cases of CLL, a finding associated with an adverse prognosis (212,214,230–232). Flow cytometric detection of CD38 is easily accomplished at the time of the original immunophenotypic diagnosis, and therefore CD38 expression is one of the most commonly assessed prognostic factors in CLL. Because CLL cells often show a spectrum of CD38 expression (rather than discrete, uniform positivity or negativity), a quantitative threshold of expression must be established to discriminate between CD38-positive and CD38-negative cases. While historically there has been some controversy as to the proper set point for this threshold (230,233,234), many laboratories consider a case of CLL to be CD38 positive when >30% of the monoclonal cells express this antigen. There are several important caveats in assessing CD38 expression in CLL. First, there is potential variability in CD38 expression between anatomic sites (235). Even in a single patient, CLL cells from the peripheral blood and lymph node may show slightly different levels of CD38 expression. Second, there is some temporal variability, with expression levels sometimes changing over time within a given patient (214). Third, CD38 expression is discordant with the *IGHV@* mutational status in up to one-third of cases (236–238). Consequently, CD38 expression may be a relatively less robust prognostic indicator than some of the other available biomarkers (237,239).

ZAP-70

Zeta associated protein-70 (ZAP-70), a tyrosine kinase necessary for T-cell receptor signaling, is not normally expressed in B cells. Gene expression studies identified ZAP-70 expression in some cases of CLL, and it was soon recognized that there was good correlation between ZAP-70 expression and the mutational status of the IGHV@ region (ZAP-70-positive cases tend to be unmutated) (240,241). Thus, ZAP-70 became an attractive surrogate marker for mutational status and poor prognosis, especially in the recent past when IGHV@ mutational analysis was less frequently available as a clinical assay (242). Unfortunately, ZAP-70 expression has historically proven difficult to assess in the clinical laboratory (243). Both flow cytometric analysis and immunohistochemistry have been utilized (244). Despite recent data suggesting that reproducible and standardized ZAP-70 analysis is indeed achievable in the clinical laboratory (245,246), the optimal method of analysis remains a point of discussion (247–253). There is discordance between ZAP-70 status and IGHV@ mutation status in between 5% and 20% of cases studied for both markers (141), some of which may be attributable to the presence of other independent high-risk genetic lesions (221). Interestingly, while IGHV@ mutational analysis is now increasingly available as a standard and widely performed assay, some studies indicate that ZAP-70 expression retains independent prognostic significance even when IGHV@ mutational status is known (239). ZAP-70 expression is also intriguing in relation to the pathobiology of CLL, as it appears to enhance B-cell receptor signaling, thus tying disease behavior to the functional activity of this signaling pathway (254–256).

Cytogenetic Findings

Cytogenetic analysis is often performed in cases of CLL to assess for the presence of recurrent cytogenetic abnormalities associated with specific clinical behavior and prognosis (Fig. 18.8). These abnormalities are neither sensitive nor specific for a diagnosis of CLL, as they are frequently absent in *bona fide* cases of CLL and may also occur in a wide array of other neoplasms, including other low-grade chronic B-cell leukemias and lymphomas. Historically, CLL has been difficult to analyze in the cytogenetic laboratory because the malignant cells have a low spontaneous rate of *in vitro* cellular replication, a feature that hinders cell culture and conventional karyotyping (257). The use of B-cell mitogens, which stimulate B cells and induce

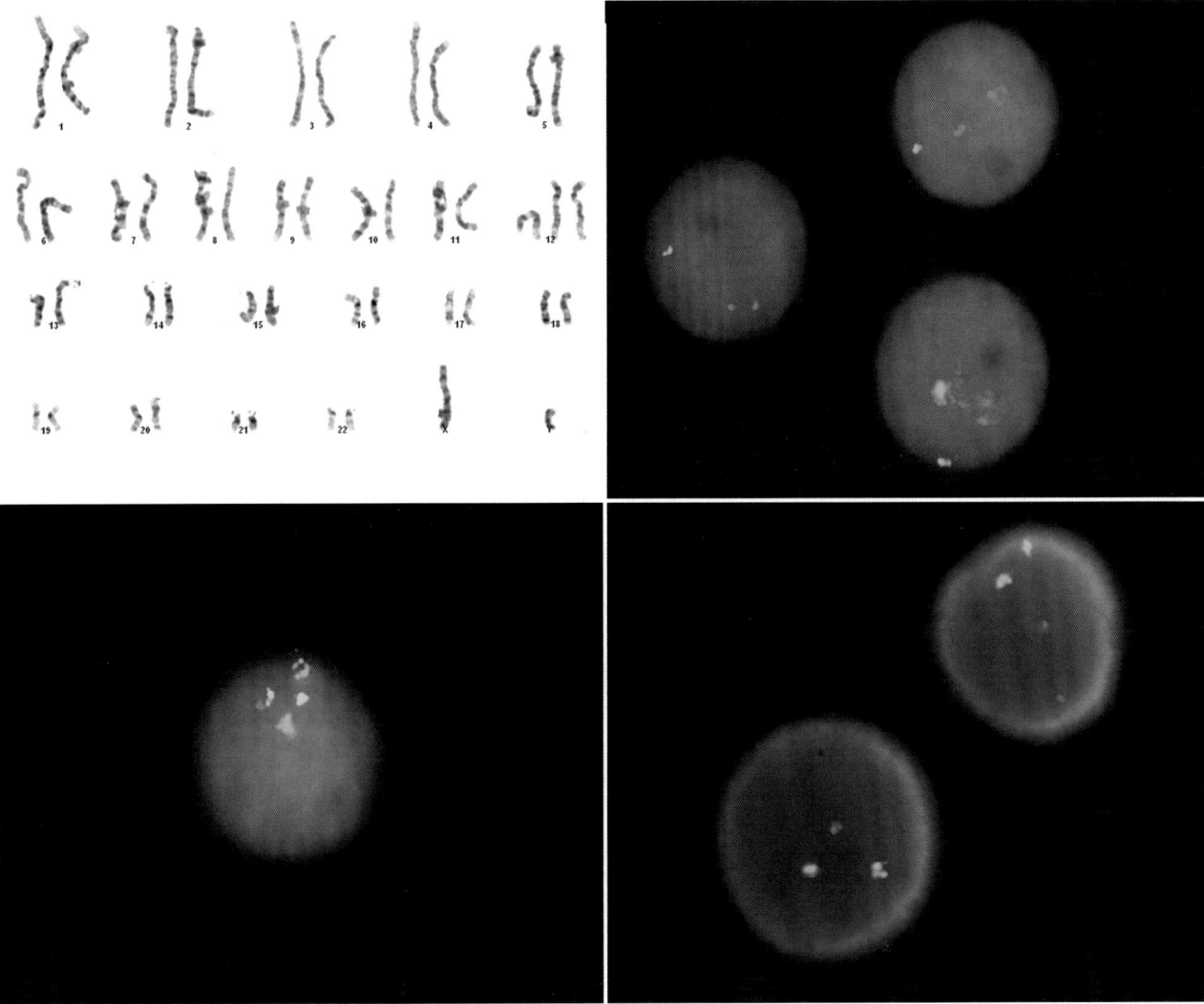

FIGURE 18.8. Cytogenetic analysis of CLL can reveal several recurrent abnormalities of prognostic significance. The karyotype in the upper left panel shows trisomy 12. Interphase FISH analysis reveals deletion of 11q22.3 (**upper right**, *green probe*), 13q14.3 (**lower left**, *red probe*), and 17p13.1 (**lower right**, *red probe*).

Table 18.9	CYTOGENETIC FEATURES OF CLL COMMONLY ASSESSED VIA FISH ANALYSIS

Cytogenetic Abnormality	Approximate Incidence in CLL	Comment
13q14 deletion	>50%	As sole abnormality, associated with good-risk disease; recent data suggest that biallelic 13q deletions may behave similarly
11q22-23 deletion	~20%	Higher risk disease, though better than 17p13 deletion
Trisomy 12	~20%	Associated with atypical morphology and/or immunophenotype; intermediate risk disease; *NOTCH1* mutations are relatively common in this group and appear to adversely impact survival
17p13 deletion	<10%	Very high-risk disease

Adapted from references (152,262,267–270).

cellular proliferation, has facilitated the conventional cytogenetic analysis of CLL (258,259). Indeed, conventional banding performed in this fashion is capable of finding clonal abnormalities is up to 83% of cases of CLL, and can identify the presence of complex karyotypes and translocations, which may influence prognosis (260,261). Nevertheless, clinical assessment for cytogenetic abnormalities in CLL is often accomplished by fluorescence *in situ* hybridization (FISH), which permits cost-effective detection of small deletions. The specific regions that are typically investigated in cases of CLL include 13q14, 11q22-23, and 17p13; a probe directed to chromosome 12 is also employed to detect trisomy of this chromosome. The established prognostic associations of these findings are summarized in Table 18.9 (262). Importantly, changing therapeutic paradigms continue to modify the prognostic expectations associated with these cytogenetic abnormalities; for example, in patients with relatively poor prognostic del(11q), the regimen of fludarabine, cyclophosphamide, and rituximab results in progression-free survival more similar to that expected in cases with normal cytogenetics (24,263,264). However, the del(11q) retains some poor prognostic weight, because these patients remain at higher risk for relapse and have inferior overall survival (265). Other relatively common recurrent cytogenetic abnormalities in CLL are summarized in Table 18.10; in addition, even rarer recurrent karyotypic abnormalities have been reported (266).

Novel array-based karyotyping methods have also been applied to cases of CLL. These techniques (array comparative genomic hybridization and single nucleotide polymorphism arrays) are capable of detecting the recurrent abnormalities as well as additional small deletions, duplications, and other changes throughout the genome of the malignant cells

(158,273–280). These more sensitive methods are also adept at documenting clonal evolution, a phenomenon that has been linked (at least at the karyotypic level) to disease progression (280–283). Array-based analysis is quite well suited to CLL, a disease characterized by frequent copy number gains and losses as well as lackluster growth in culture. At present, the clinical applications of array-based analysis in assessment of CLL continue to evolve (276,284).

Integration of Multiple Prognostic Indicators

The sheer number of reported biomarkers that bear on prognosis in CLL (Table 18.6) creates potential confusion. How many markers should be studied in a given case? Are some more valuable than others? And what should be done when there is discordance between the results of different tests (e.g., CD38 expression indicates more aggressive disease but the *IGHV@* region is hypermutated)?

Among the best ways to judge the relative strength of prognostic predictors is through studies of large cohorts in which multivariable analysis can be used to achieve direct relative comparison of the variables. One such study found that both ZAP-70 and *IGHV@* are independent prognostic variables, with ZAP-70 attaining a slight edge in predictive power (239). CD38 expression was not as strongly linked to outcome. Based on this study, it was proposed that CLL could be efficiently risk-stratified by ZAP-70 and *IGHV@* status, with ZAP-70–positive patients considered high risk regardless of mutation status, and ZAP-70–negative cases segregated into low and intermediate risk by mutated and unmutated *IGHV@* status, respectively (210,239). Similarly, in another multivariable analysis, CD38

Table 18.10	ADDITIONAL CYTOGENETIC FEATURES OF CLL

Cytogenetic Abnormality	Approximate Incidence in CLL	Comment
6q deletion	3%–9%	Linked to unmutated *IGHV@*, atypical morphology, high white blood cell count, bulky lymphadenopathy, marked splenomegaly, and shorter interval to therapy
Abnormalities of 3q27/*BCL6*	~3%	Translocations involving BCL6 include t(3;4) with *RHOH*, t(3;6) with *H1F1*, t(3;11) with *OBF1*, and t(3;13) with *LCP1*. Trisomy 3q27 is also rarely observed.
MYC translocation	Rare	Associated with disease acceleration/prolymphocytoid transformation
t(14;19)(q32;q13) IGH@-BCL3	~1%	Associated with younger age, atypical morphology, atypical immunophenotype reminiscent of mantle cell lymphoma, unmutated *IGHV@*, rapid disease progression, and poor prognosis
t(2;14) BCL11A-IGH@	Rare	Associated with younger age (including children), atypical morphology, unmutated *IGHV@*, aggressive disease
Other 14q32 *IGH@* translocations	<10%	Regardless of translocation partner, associated with unmutated *IGHV@* and poor prognosis
Complex karyotype	10%–40%	Associated with aggressive disease course
Karyotypic evolution	>25% (over 5 y of follow-up)	Independent predictor of adverse prognosis, especially if high-risk cytogenetic abnormalities are acquired; may be more common in cases with unmutated *IGHV@*

Adapted from references (84,210,216,257,269,271,272).

expression was not identified as an independent prognostic factor (285). Instead, Krober et al. proposed a combined cytogenetic/molecular classification, in which cases with del(17p) are high risk; cases with del(11q) and/or unmutated *IGHV@* are intermediate risk; and cases with mutated *IGHV@* [in the absence of del(17p) or del(11q)] are low risk (210,285). In contrast, however, another multivariable analysis found that *IGHV@* and CD38 have independent prognostic value at diagnosis (286). Yet another multivariable analysis advocated the use of serum thymidine kinase, lymphocytosis, β_2-microglobulin, and CD38 expression (287); another imputed essentially equivalent prognostic weights to CD38, *IGHV@* status, and ZAP-70 expression (288); another stressed the prognostic significance of lymphadenopathy in early stage CLL (289); and still another endorsed *IGHV@* and 17p deletion, but not CD38 or ZAP-70 (290). The very existence of discordance between *IGHV@*, CD38, and/or ZAP-70 has been noted to alter prognostic expectations (242,291–293). Clearly, further work is necessary if these disparate biomarkers are to be integrated into a simple and coherent system for prognostic assessment.

An alternative strategy for assessing risk in CLL patients has been the creation of nomograms. Wierda and colleagues created a nomogram for prognostic expectations based on six clinical and laboratory parameters that are comparatively routine and widely available: age, β_2-microglobulin, absolute lymphocyte count, sex, Rai stage, and number of involved lymph node groups (208). This model has been validated using additional data sets (294,295). However, competing nomograms and indices (which take into account various combinations of age, sex, Binet staging, beta-2 microglobulin, *IGHV@* mutation status, serum VEGF and lipoprotein lipase, and 17p deletion) have also been proposed (290,296,297). Subsequently, Wierda et al. created yet another nomogram (298) that calculates individualized 2- and 4-year expected time to first treatment based on a combination of both traditional and esoteric (FISH, *IGHV@*) variables. These types of statistical approaches, applied to large and well-characterized data sets, seem to offer some hope for clarity in an otherwise complex area.

Pathogenesis

Investigation of the cellular and molecular underpinnings of CLL has been an exceptionally fertile area of basic and translational research. Here we will describe five broad areas of inquiry and technical findings, and then conclude with general observations about our current understanding of CLL pathogenesis.

Cell of Origin

Because lymphoma cells often recapitulate stages of normal B-cell development, the physiologic counterpart of the CLL cell has long been sought in an effort to better understand the nature of the transformative events driving lymphomagenesis. Historically, the counterpart of the CLL cell was thought to be the naive B cell. This theory was complicated by the discovery that roughly half of CLL cases bear the imprint of somatic hypermutation, implying that these cases had undergone exposure to antigen and were therefore not "naive" at all. Still more recently, it has been demonstrated that, in fact, all CLL clones (whether unmutated or mutated) show tell-tale characteristics of prior antigen exposure. This contention is supported by gene expression profiling studies in which both mutated and unmutated cases show gene expression signatures similar to those of marginal zone or memory B cells (299,300). Current dogma holds that CLL is exclusively a disease of memory-type B cells that have experienced antigen either in the germinal center or, alternatively, in a T-cell-independent manner, perhaps in the marginal zone. More specific "cells of origin" have been also been proposed. Normal human marginal zone cells

show some features reminiscent of CLL, including expression of CD27, but the lack of CD5 expression in typical marginal zone B cells argues against this site as harboring a discrete cell of origin (301). Some CLL cases show stereotyped B-cell receptors (discussed further in the next section) and/or produce polyreactive "natural" antibodies—characteristics held in common with a normal constituent of the murine immune system, the CD5-positive B-1 cell. While the B-1 cell presents a very attractive candidate for the CLL cell of origin, such a hypothesis is complicated—if not entirely refuted—by the fact that a human counterpart of the B-1 cell has never been conclusively demonstrated (301). Some have suggested that CLL may represent the neoplastic counterpart of a normal human CD5-positive peripheral blood B lymphocyte usually present in very low numbers (34,135,302). Normal B cells with an immunophenotypic pattern similar to CLL also have been identified in mantle zones of lymph node, tonsil, and blood, whereas abundant CD5-positive B cells are present in fetal lymph node, spleen, and blood (34,302,303). However, these normal CD5-positive B cells do not produce antibodies with the same characteristics as those produced by CLL cells (301). Alternatively, the expression of CD5 could be induced in B cells by activation with certain antigens (302). A recent proposal even suggests that CLL-associated transforming events occur at the level of the hematopoietic stem cell (304,305). Thus, at present, the exact cell of origin in CLL remains elusive and controversial.

Biased V-Region Usage and Stereotypical Immunoglobulin Structure

Individual B cells have two opportunities to generate unique and specific immunoglobulin proteins (which, when expressed on the cell surface with other proteins, also constitute the B-cell receptor, or BCR). First, VDJ recombination early in B-cell development juxtaposes different segments of the immunoglobulin loci, much like a card dealer blindly selecting cards from a deck. Second, somatic hypermutation changes nucleotides in order to create immunoglobulins with increased affinity for antigen. Both of these processes operate based on random chance and generate the broadly diverse contingent of normal B cells necessary for proper immune function. If CLL clones were to arise without bias from this background, the selected V, D, and J regions and somatic hypermutation-induced changes would be expected to reflect this diversity. In fact, CLL clones show a more restricted pattern of these changes. Mutated cases, for example, preferentially utilize a subset of V regions, including VH4-34, while unmutated cases are much more likely to use VH1-69 and VH4-39 (306). These observations have led to the proposal that the specific configuration of the BCR is important in the pathogenesis of CLL (307). Indeed, so consistent are the changes that several clusters of CLL have been described, each characterized by specific combinations of heavy or light chain VDJ regions and/or specific matching amino acid sequences in the complementarity determining region 3 (CDR3) of the immunoglobulin molecule. Such "stereotyped" BCRs are detected in 20% to 30% of CLL cases (301,308), and about 1% of cases display virtually identical immunoglobulin molecules (309).

Because each BCR recognizes a specific antigen or subset of antigens, the biased distribution in CLL immediately leads one to ask: *to what do these nonrandom CLL BCRs bind?* Both self and foreign molecules have been proposed as sources of antigen recognized by the CLL BCR. Some of the stereotyped clusters have been investigated for the specificity of their immunoglobulin, revealing reactivity with ubiquitous cellular constituents including nonmuscle myosin heavy chain IIA, calreticulin, and vimentin, possibly reflecting epitopes displayed during apoptosis or on stromal cells (310–313). Similarly, some CLL BCRs share a propensity to bind superantigens such as

Staphylococcus aureus protein A and the cytomegalovirus phosphoprotein pUL32 (314,315). The binding of such antigens or superantigens may be crucial in the development of CLL clones and/or modulation of their clinical behavior (316). Indeed, the "strength" of BCR signaling, as judged by the expression of downstream target genes, appears to correlate with disease aggressiveness, and the intracellular response to BCR stimulation differs for U-CLL and M-CLL (106,317–319). Thus, although CLL cells usually express only low levels of surface immunoglobulin, signaling through the BCR may be among the most critical factors influencing biologic behavior and disease progression (319,320).

Genetic Changes Associated with Familial CLL

Genetic predisposition to the development of CLL is the strongest among all the hematologic neoplasms. Large cohort studies place CLL in the company of solid tumors with known heritable risk such as breast and colon cancer (7,321). Supporting the contention that inherited genetic factors influence the development of CLL, familial aggregation of CLL has been well documented (46,48,322,323). Members of these families show predisposition to CLL that is non-Mendelian in nature (i.e., not overtly dominant or recessive). Similarly, up to 15% of relatives in affected families have MBL, an incidence in excess of the occurrence in the general population (20,324,325). Even in cases of apparently sporadic CLL, first-degree relatives of newly diagnosed patients have up to an 8.5-fold increase in their own risk of such a diagnosis, consistent with inherited susceptibility (326–330). Similarly, up to 10% of newly diagnosed patients have a family history of CLL (45). While early attempts at linkage analysis were largely disappointing, more recent genome-wide association studies have uncovered several loci putatively associated with increased risk of CLL (331–333). The relative risk associated with each locus is modest, on the order of one to twofold. However, the risk appears to be additive and the polymorphisms are relatively common. Among the 2% of individuals carrying a very high burden of these variant alleles, the relative risk of CLL is increased approximately eightfold compared to the general population (48). Some loci have been verified in subsequent, independent case-control studies or further genome-wide association studies, providing additional evidence for their relevance (333–335). A few of the genes near the implicated polymorphisms have a "logical" connection to lymphomagenesis (e.g., *IRF4*, which encodes MUM-1, is intimately involved in control of B-cell development) (336). Interestingly, a small fraction (~2%) of sporadic CLL cases carry acquired mutations of *IRF4*, thus linking familial risk and some cases of sporadic disease through the same genetic lesion (149). Similarly, linkage studies have identified a susceptibility locus as 2q21, which harbors the gene encoding the CXCR4 chemokine receptor thought to be critical in proproliferative interactions between CLL cells and their microenvironment (45,337,338). The role of the other implicated loci in disease pathogenesis remains to be more fully explored (339). Very intriguingly, inherited abnormalities that alter patterns of DNA methylation may be responsible for the disease risk in some CLL families (340,341), suggesting that susceptibility may be modulated at the epigenetic level as well.

Somatic Genetic Drivers, Including Those in Minimally Deleted Regions of CLL-Associated Recurring Cytogenetic Abnormalities

When a recurrent chromosomal deletion is associated with a specific phenotype, either in the neoplastic or in the constitutional setting, the minimal region that is deleted in all affected patients is likely to hold genes or regulatory regions important in disease pathogenesis. In CLL, the recurrent deletions of 13q14, 11q22-23, and 17p13 provide such an opportunity for investigation.

The 13q14 deletion, the most common cytogenetic abnormality in CLL, is identified by FISH in 40% to 60% of cases (257). The presence of the *RB1* tumor suppressor gene in the vicinity initially prompted suggestions that loss of *RB1* could be important in the development of CLL. However, while *RB1* is indeed deleted in many cases with the del(13q), in fact the minimally deleted region held in common by all patients lies slightly telomeric to *RB1* at band 13q14.3 (342). In addition, even in cases with deletion of one copy of *RB1*, disruption of the remaining *RB1* allele by mutation or methylation is rare. These observations cast some doubt on a central role for *RB1* in the pathogenesis of CLL. Investigation of several other genes in the region, however, failed to identify a promising candidate until sequences encoding two microRNAs—miR-15a and miR-16-1—were identified (343). As with all microRNAs, these small molecules bind specific mRNA transcripts and modulate their translation into protein (344). Among the targets of miR-15a and miR-16-1 are *BCL2* transcripts; thus, the deletion of the microRNAs at 13q14 is believed to de-repress BCL2 translation and foster antiapoptotic effects via increased BCL2 protein levels (345–348). As attractive as this hypothesis might be, there are at least two lines of evidence to suggest that there is more to the story of the 13q14 deletion. First, mouse models have been created in which the animals carry deletion of either the minimally deleted region or the microRNA cluster only; while both types of mice develop a lymphoproliferative disease resembling CLL, those with the slightly larger deletion have a more aggressive disease (349,350). Second, fine mapping studies have demonstrated heterogeneity in the size of deletions at 13q14, with larger losses (including those extending to the *RB1* locus) associated with more aggressive disease (351–355). The gene *DLEU7* in the minimally deleted region has drawn attention as a possible cooperating tumor suppressor involved in regulation of NF-κB (345,356). It has been suggested that the relatively good prognosis associated with the 13q14 deletion applies equally to cases with monoallelic and biallelic loss (267,357).

The recurrent deletion at 11q22.3-q23.1 encompasses the tumor suppressor *ATM*, which participates in DNA damage detection and cell cycle control (257). Because *ATM* mutations are associated with lymphoma (358), loss of the gene may be pathogenic in CLL. Indeed, *ATM* mutations are found in 12% of patients with CLL overall and are associated with an adverse prognosis (359). Moreover, CLL cells with the 11q deletion show impaired responses to DNA damaging events, as would be expected based on the known function of the ATM protein (360). The remaining *ATM* allele in patients with 11q22.3-q23.1 deletion is mutated 36% of the time (361). In addition, cases with *ATM* mutations in the absence of 11q deletion may share prognostic and biologic features with the deleted cases (362). Interestingly, *ATM* falls outside of the deleted region in very rare cases (277), and attention has also been given to other possible tumor suppressors in the area, including *NPAT*, *CUL5*, *PPP2R1B*, and miR-34b/miR-34c (363,364).

Deletion of the *TP53* tumor suppressor gene clearly underlies the recurrent 17p13 deletion. Up to 90% of patients with 17p13 deletion show mutation of the remaining *TP53* allele, leading to a complete breakdown of this signaling pathway critical for DNA damage repair and cell cycle control (365). As a consequence, 17p13 deletion and *TP53* mutations are linked to genomic instability, refractory disease unresponsive to standard fludarabine-based treatment, and extremely poor prognosis (144,366). A subset of cases with *TP53* mutation in the absence of deletion also shares this adverse prognosis (144–147). miR-34a has been identified as a prime downstream effector that is reliably disturbed in CLL cases with *TP53* abnormalities (367–370).

The contributions of genes involved in other CLL-associated cytogenetic abnormalities is less clear. For example, trisomy for the entirety of chromosome 12 could implicate any of a large number of genes, though detailed analysis seems to have identified a "hot spot" around 12q13-q21 as particularly important (371,372).

In addition, genetic drivers of CLL may be suggested by other approaches, including some at the forefront of molecular technology. Massively parallel next-generation sequencing has recently documented *SF3B1* mutations in 15% of CLL patients (155,156,373); this gene, which encodes a component of the spliceosome, was not previously suspected to be relevant to CLL (374). Other recurrent mutations identified in this manner include *NOTCH1, XPO1, MYD88,* and *KLHL6* (375). SNP array analysis has detected a recurrent gain of 3.5 Mb that includes the *BCL11A* oncogene (376); because *BCL11A* is also involved in the recurrent t(2;14)(p13;q32) seen in rare cases of CLL (377), it may be a promising focus of future research. Finally, mouse models demonstrating that forced expression of *TCL1* leads to an aggressive CLL-like disease (378) have uncovered a possible role for this oncogene in the pathogenesis of some cases of CLL (345,379–381). Integration of these molecular-level observations with clinical information, prognostic variables, and the relevant immunobiology remains largely in its infancy.

The Microenvironment and CLL

With antigen stimulation via the BCR important in the pathogenesis of CLL, interactions between the B cell and its immediate surroundings serve to sustain and propagate the B-cell clone (106,313,382,383). Indeed, the requirement for such interactions is highlighted by the propensity of CLL cells to undergo apoptosis when removed from their natural microenvironment(s) (384). In the lymph node, CLL/SLL cells are associated with CD14-positive cells known as nurselike cells (NLCs); in the bone marrow, mesenchymal stromal cells serve a similar function (45,385,386). These cell types secrete a number of cytokines that enhance B-cell viability (386), including CXCL12. This cytokine binds its receptor CXCR4 on the CLL cells, activating intracellular signaling pathways that promote cellular proliferation. Blockade of this interaction has been shown to inhibit the survival of the neoplastic cells (383,387). Other important microenvironmental interactions include the secretion of B-cell activating factor (BAFF) and a proliferation-inducing ligand (APRIL) by the NLCs, and the stimulatory engagement between CD40 on the B cells and CD40L on neighboring helper T cells (45,388). The variable infiltration of the tumor microenvironment by PD-1–positive follicular helper T cells appears to be an important event, and may hold independent prognostic significance (193). It appears that the proliferation centers are the sites of most active microenvironmental stimulation and consequent neoplastic proliferation (106,107,389).

Summary of Pathogenesis

Our understanding of CLL has evolved significantly in recent years. No longer is the disease thought to represent a single uniform process characterized by the indolent accumulation of senescent B cells that are essentially identical between patients. Rather, there are important functional differences between cases of CLL. Indeed, it would appear from the diversity of V-region characteristics and the differing, but recurrent, cytogenetic abnormalities that there is more than one way for a B-cell clone to "become" CLL. Despite the complexity of the transforming events, we can make some general synoptic observations about the pathogenesis of CLL, as presently understood:

- *CLL clones may show either the presence or the absence of somatic hypermutation.* These disease subsets are

biologically distinct, and likely reflect differences in the preceding process of lymphomagenesis.
- *There is a familial contribution to the disease in some cases.* The existence of familial aggregation of both CLL and associated MBL hints at a multistep model of disease development.
- *MBL is a precursor lesion to CLL.* "Low-count" MBL may be oligoclonal and infrequently progress to CLL, while "high-count" cases are more likely to progress (28,29,390).
- *The specific configuration of the B-cell receptor and the immunoglobulin molecule is important in the development and clinical course of CLL.* The existence of V-region bias and stereotyped BCR confirm the importance of antigen stimulation.
- *Cytogenetic deletions and alterations in microRNA networks appear to be central in the development of CLL.* Although molecular pathways continue to be elaborated and debated, many of the somatic genetic lesions in CLL affect tumor suppressors and/or microRNA expression. Some investigators have even proposed a kind of "unified theory" in which feedback interactions between *TP53* and the microRNA clusters at 11q and 13q explain the recurrent nature of genetic abnormalities at these locations (364).
- *The microenvironment assists in the propagation and maintenance of the clonal population.* Interaction with T cells and supporting cells appears to take place within lymph node proliferation centers and the bone marrow.

Treatment

Because of the highly variable clinical course of CLL, determining optimal therapy and the appropriate time to initiate therapy are major problems. The dilemma is only heightened by a recent trend in which patients are increasingly diagnosed with low-stage disease (391). Currently, treatment for CLL is initiated only once the patient develops clinically "progressive or symptomatic ... active" disease, defined as progressive marrow failure, massive/progressive/symptomatic splenomegaly or lymphadenopathy, progressive lymphocytosis (increase of 50% in 2 months or lymphocyte doubling time <6 months), refractory autoimmune manifestations, and/or constitutional symptoms (8). In other words, it is *not* standard of care to initiate early treatment—even in patients found to have high-risk prognostic features based on interphase FISH, ZAP-70, CD38, and/or *IGHV@* mutation status. Several trials have failed to demonstrate improved outcome with early treatment (392–395). However, these older studies used chlorambucil (now superseded by more effective agents) and included many patients with indolent disease (201). Thus, the possible benefit of early treatment using modern protocols in high-risk (but low-stage) patients remains very much an open question. A large trial designed to explore this approach failed to accrue sufficient numbers of patients. More recently, a multicenter trial sponsored by the German CLL Study Group has completed accrual, but data were not available at the time of this writing.

Once it is determined that treatment is indicated for an individual patient with CLL, the pharmacologic armamentarium is comparatively large. Options include fludarabine, chlorambucil, cyclophosphamide, rituximab, alemtuzumab, bendamustine, ofatumumab, and lenalidomide. A number of landmark studies have established some preferred combinations (268). In brief, fludarabine plus cyclophosphamide (FC) is superior in many respects to single agent fludarabine (396–398); fludarabine plus rituximab (FR) is superior to single agent fludarabine (399); and fludarabine plus cyclophosphamide plus rituximab (FCR) is superior to FC (366,400–402). (Insufficient data exist pitting FCR against FR.) In practice, FCR is now a standard first-line therapy in patients without significant comorbidity (24,201,265,268,403). This strategy of "chemoimmunotherapy" has fundamentally shifted the goal of treatment in CLL toward complete remission, eradication of minimal residual disease, and improved survival (137,404–406). However, one noteworthy complication of fludarabine-based regimens is the development of subsequent therapy-related myeloid neoplasm, at an incidence of between 4% and 8% (407,408). Stem cell transplantation is an option for some CLL patients, including those with unmutated *IGHV@* in combination with high-risk interphase cytogenetics, and younger patients with poor response to therapy or early relapse (24,409,410). A wide array of alternative agents, targeted inhibitors, and drug combinations remain under investigation in clinical trials, and treatment recommendations are expected to continue to evolve over time (268,319,383,388,411,412). In particular, the optimal therapy for elderly and/or less physically fit patients remains to be established (413–415). The significance of standard prognostic tests may also differ when applied to elderly patients (416).

Although FISH abnormalities currently play no role in determining the *timing* of treatment initiation, certain findings do have significant impact on the *selection* of treatment regimen. The deletion of 11q is a poor prognostic marker, but FCR therapy brings these patients closer to standard-risk CLL in terms of treatment response (24,263,264,417). However, del(11q) remains adverse in the sense that these patients remain at higher risk of relapse and show an inferior overall survival (265,268). Patients with del(17p) are particularly refractory to purine nucleoside analogues, and for this reason are commonly treated with alemtuzumab, an anti-CD52 monoclonal antibody that appears to work in a non–p53-dependent manner (24,265,418–422). However, alemtuzumab appears to be less effective in patients with bulky lymphadenopathy, and in general the duration of response to alemtuzumab in patients with del(17p) is suboptimal (201). While patients with del(17p) are often considered for allogeneic hematopoietic stem cell transplantation or clinical trials (409), some data indicate that patients with *de novo* del(17p) at diagnosis may constitute a more heterogeneous group (423), and other genetic lesions (such as mutations or deletions affecting *BIRC3*) also contribute to fludarabine refractoriness (424). Nevertheless, because FISH abnormalities are so important in treatment selection, and because the neoplastic clone may acquire cytogenetic abnormalities over time, it has been recommended that the FISH prognostic panel be repeated at the time of treatment initiation, even if previously performed in a patient at the time of original diagnosis (404). In addition, up to 5% of patients harbor *TP53* mutation even in the absence of a 17p deletion, yet follow a similar adverse clinical course (144,145,147). Thus, recent consensus recommendations call for molecular analysis for *TP53* mutations at the time of treatment selection (146,147).

In addition to targeting the neoplastic CLL clone, it may also be necessary to treat secondary complications. Autoimmune hemolytic anemia is often addressed with corticosteroids, though other options include immunosuppressive agents such as cyclosporine or even splenectomy in refractory cases (58). CLL patients are at significantly increased risk of infection, and intravenous immunoglobulin may reduce this risk in patients with severe hypogammaglobulinemia, though this approach is not recommended on a routine basis and does not seem to impact overall survival (24,425–427). The relative frequency of specific causes of death in the setting of CLL, with cytopenias and immune dysfunction as key determinants, is detailed in Table 18.11.

Morphologic Transformation

CLL can undergo morphologic changes during the course of the disease. The most common transformation of CLL is prolymphocytoid transformation, which occurs in about 15% of all CLL patients (3,31,32,85,428–433). Exact definitions vary, but generally there is a notable and sustained increase in the proportion of prolymphocytes, exceeding 10% of the total lymphoid cells (430). Clinically there is progressive increase in absolute lymphocyte count and refractoriness to treatment. The lymphocytes in the blood tend to be more heterogeneous than those seen in *de novo* PLL, and they may retain the immunophenotypic characteristics of the earlier CLL or demonstrate brighter surface immunoglobulin, as well as variable CD5 and FMC7 positivity. Prolymphocytoid transformation is linked to the acquisition of additional genetic abnormalities (434). After prolymphocytoid transformation has occurred, the median survival is generally about 1 year.

The next most frequent type of transformation is Richter syndrome, which occurs in 3% to 10% of patients and is characterized by the abrupt onset of fever, weight loss, increasing organomegaly, and rising serum lactate dehydrogenase (3,31,435–452). Because rapidly enlarging tumor masses typically develop, positron emission tomography/computed tomography imaging is particularly useful in evaluating suspicious cases (453). The transformation is typically detected in lymph node specimens, though other anatomic locations are also possible (Table 18.12). Biopsy of these tumor masses reveals distinct areas that fulfill criteria for large cell lymphoma. In most cases (>80%), the large cells show centroblastic features, with the remainder immunoblastic (454). The tumor cells may also show some degree of pleomorphism and can include multinucleated cells with prominent nucleoli that resemble Reed-Sternberg cells. The diffuse large B-cell lymphoma (DLBCL) component is immunophenotypically compatible with an activated B-cell profile in 80% of cases (454,455). Many molecular or immunologic studies confirm a clonal relationship between the large cell lymphoma and the underlying CLL (437,443,445,447,448,452). The genetic lesions that accompany this progression are heterogeneous, though chromosomal gains, deletions, and translocations bearing on *MYC* and *TP53* function are recurrent (456). However, some cases of Richter syndrome represent secondary neoplasms that have arisen in a background of CLL-associated immunosuppression (450,457).

Table 18.11	MORTALITY IN CLL PATIENTS	
Cause of Death	**Percentage of All Causes of Death in Patients with CLL**	
"Active" CLL	37	
Infection	16	
Autoimmune hemolytic anemia	1	
Cardiac	3	
Second malignancy	16	
Unrelated to CLL/unknown	~27	

Adapted from reference (208).

Table 18.12	ANATOMIC LOCATIONS OF RICHTER TRANSFORMATION	
Location	**Total Richter Transformation**	
Lymph node	59%	
GI tract	14%	
Bone marrow	12%	
Tonsil	8%	
Skin	5%	
Liver	2%	
Ocular, CNS, nasal, bronchial	Rare	

Adapted from references (454,467).

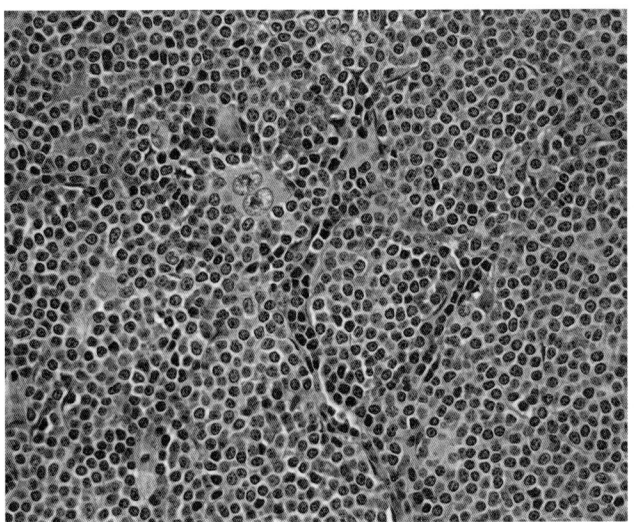

FIGURE 18.9. Rare cases of CLL can harbor admixed large cells reminiscent of Reed-Sternberg cells. A diagnosis of transformation to Hodgkin lymphoma should only be made if there is a cellular milieu appropriate for such a diagnosis.

Chemotherapy, particularly with fludarabine, has also been implicated as an iatrogenic cause of immunodeficiency-associated secondary lymphoproliferative disorders in CLL (458–460). EBV is detected in the large cells in about 16% of all cases of Richter syndrome and has been hypothesized to play an especially notable role in postfludarabine cases (460,461). There are some interesting correlations between the type of Richter transformation and the underlying characteristics of the CLL clone. Transformations in which the large cell component is clonally related to the CLL clone generally take place in U-CLL, while clonally unrelated large cell lymphomas are more likely to arise in M-CLL (454,462). Immunophenotypic differences from the preceding CLL (e.g., loss of CD5 or CD23 expression) may be seen in both clonally related and unrelated cases (454). Certain biologic characteristics—including *CD38* and *LRP4* polymorphisms, CD38 expression, the absence of 13q14 deletion, use of IGHV4-39, certain stereotyped B-cell receptors, *NOTCH1* mutation, and lymph node size—appear to predict greater likelihood of Richter transformation (151,160,225,455,463–465). The clinical course of Richter syndrome is that of a rapidly progressive, high-grade neoplasm with generally short median survivals. Prognosis for individual patients with Richter transformation is affected by performance status, LDH, platelet count, tumor size, and number of prior therapies (466). Richter transformation is typically treated in a manner similar to other high-grade lymphomas (268,455).

Rare cases (<1%) show progression to classical Hodgkin lymphoma (442,468). This phenomenon must be distinguished histologically from cases of CLL that show admixed background Reed-Sternberg–like cells (Fig. 18.9); the diagnosis of transformation to outright Hodgkin lymphoma requires that the Reed-Sternberg cells be present in a milieu appropriate for the diagnosis of classical Hodgkin lymphoma (7). It should be noted that CLL may also be a participant in a so-called composite lymphoma, some rare cases of which constitute a combination of CLL and Hodgkin lymphoma.

Other types of transformation in CLL are less frequent (Table 18.13). Of particular note among these rare cases is paraimmunoblastic transformation—a diffuse, usually nodal, proliferation of the paraimmunoblasts (with some admixed prolymphocytes) that are otherwise limited to proliferation centers in typical CLL (469,470).

Differential Diagnosis

When all causes of blood and bone marrow lymphocytoses are considered, the differential diagnosis of CLL is extensive. The difficulty in distinguishing CLL from reactive lymphocytoses and other lymphoproliferative disorders varies considerably from case to case. Often, a morphologic review of the blood smear is all that is required, whereas sophisticated immunologic and even molecular techniques may be necessary for successful diagnosis. In general, reactive lymphocytoses in blood exhibit morphologic heterogeneity, have a predominance of T cells, and are associated with a specific underlying cause, such as infection or drug treatment. A rare and unusual mimic of CLL is a poorly understood entity of "persistent polyclonal B-cell lymphocytosis," in which polyclonal, expanded populations of small B lymphocytes persist in the peripheral blood. This phenomenon is seen mostly in middle-aged women who are smokers, and is associated with a specific HLA genotype (484,485). While the polyclonal nature of these processes is easily established via flow cytometric analysis of kappa and lambda light chain expression, the diagnostician should bear in mind that rare cases of CLL consist of two separate clones (486,487). If, in these "biclonal" or "bitypic" cases, one clone expresses kappa and the other lambda, then the light chain histogram could be interpreted as polyclonal. Clues to the presence of a biclonal CLL include atypically "tight" populations as assessed on the histograms, as well as immunophenotypic abnormalities, including CD5 coexpression by B cells.

Table 18.13	TYPES OF TRANSFORMATION OF CLL	
Transformation Type	**Incidence (% of Total Cases of CLL)**	**Features**
Prolymphocytoid transformation	15	Increasing percentage of prolymphocytes; progressive cytopenias, lymphadenopathy, splenomegaly, refractoriness to therapy
Richter syndrome	3–10	Large cell transformation; etiologically and morphologically heterogeneous
Blastic transformation	<1	Rare lymphoblastic leukemia clonally related to underlying CLL (myeloid cases are somewhat more common and may be secondary to therapy)
Plasmacytoid transformation	<1	Plasma cell myeloma, plasmacytoma, and plasmablastic leukemia described; rare cases clonally related to underlying CLL
Paraimmunoblastic variant of SLL	<1	Diffuse nodal proliferation of paraimmunoblasts; may be analogous to prolymphocytoid transformation that is node based
Histiocytic/dendritic cell sarcoma	<1%	Rare case reports, including some in which clonal relationship with CLL cells (i.e., transdifferentiation) was documented

Adapted from references (469–483).

Lymphoid aggregates in the bone marrow present another possible differential diagnostic dilemma. Although benign lymphoid aggregates are common in the bone marrow, especially in the elderly, increased lymphoid aggregates are also found in young patients who have collagen vascular diseases. Benign lymphoid aggregates consist predominantly of T cells, and the B cells present are polyclonal. The morphologic distinction between benign lymphoid aggregates and CLL is detailed in Table 18.3.

Once reactive processes are excluded, CLL must be distinguished from other B-cell lymphoproliferative disorders, lymphomas, and leukemias, including MBL, B-PLL, mantle cell lymphoma, hairy cell leukemia, and splenic lymphomas. Various morphologic and immunologic findings can be used to distinguish these disorders from B-CLL. The numerical and clinical features that define the borderland between MBL and CLL were discussed earlier. A diagnosis of B-PLL requires at least 55% circulating prolymphocytes, and is excluded in cases of CLL with increased prolymphocytes/prolymphocytoid transformation. Mantle cell lymphoma shows aberrant coexpression of CD5 and therefore deserves special mention in the differential diagnosis of CLL (488). Mantle cell lymphoma tends to lack most or all of the immunophenotypic features classically associated with CLL (e.g., dim surface immunoglobulin, dim CD20, absence of FMC7, coexpression of CD23). However, some cases of *bona fide* CLL also demonstrate deviation from the classic CLL-associated immunophenotype. In these cases, FISH for evidence of the t(11;14)(q13;q32) and/or paraffin immunohistochemistry for cyclin D1 overexpression should be performed—keeping in mind the important caveat that rare cases of mantle cell lymphoma may show negative results with these techniques (118,489).

B-CELL PROLYMPHOCYTIC LEUKEMIA

Diagnostic Criteria/Definitions

The clinical and pathologic features of B-PLL, originally described in 1974 by Galton and coworkers, have been well delineated (490). B-PLL is characterized by splenomegaly, marked monoclonal B-cell lymphocytosis, an absence of significant lymphadenopathy, and >55% circulating prolymphocytes (491,492). Interestingly, the morphologic prolymphocytes that characterize B-PLL may also be present among the malignant clone in cases of CLL, and patients with CLL may acquire increased prolymphocytes as a feature of disease progression or transformation. Nevertheless, B-PLL is a strictly defined entity that *excludes* such cases of CLL, and as such B-PLL is characterized by distinct clinical, immunophenotypic, and prognostic features that differ from CLL and justify its designation as an independent diagnostic entity. B-PLL shows a gene expression signature that is different from CLL, supporting the contention that it is biologically dissimilar (492). Indeed, although there has been historical controversy over the definitional borderlands of B-PLL, the WHO 2008 clearly recognizes B-PLL as a well-defined, distinctive neoplasm (491). While older descriptions of B-PLL included cases with the t(11;14)(q13;q32), these are now considered to be cases of peripheralized/splenomegalic mantle cell lymphoma rather than B-PLL (491–493). Strictly defined in this manner, B-PLL is very rare, accounting for only approximately 1% of lymphocytic leukemias and standing in sharp contrast to the highly prevalent entities (CLL, MBL) discussed elsewhere in this chapter.

Pathologic Features

Peripheral Blood

The prolymphocyte has distinct morphologic features, including moderate to abundant pale blue agranular cytoplasm and a round nucleus with moderately condensed chromatin

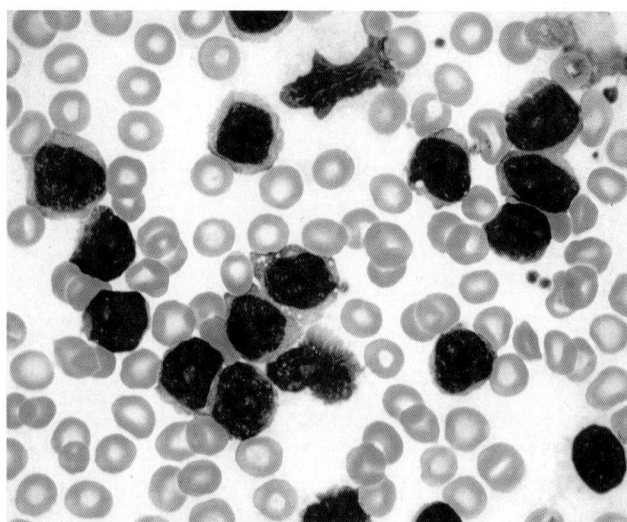

FIGURE 18.10. Peripheral blood smear from a patient with B-PLL shows the characteristic prolymphocytes. Note the prominent central nucleoli.

that contains a large, prominent central vesicular nucleolus (Fig. 18.10). Although the nuclear morphology of prolymphocytes shows some variation, the chromatin generally is less condensed than that of typical CLL but not as finely dispersed as that seen in lymphoblasts (3–5,37,39,55,86,490,494–498). The marked leukocytosis present at diagnosis in at least three-fourths of patients who have B-PLL is characterized by absolute lymphocyte counts that exceed 100×10^9/L. There is also evidence of substantial bone marrow failure in that thrombocytopenia, anemia, and neutropenia are common at presentation.

Bone Marrow

B-PLL patients who present with a marked lymphocytosis generally exhibit extensive and diffuse infiltration of the bone marrow (4,39,495). In some patients with less advanced disease, however, a mixed nodular and diffuse pattern is identified (3,37,39). On histologic sections, the distinct nucleoli, intermediate cell size, and moderate amounts of cytoplasm are readily apparent.

Other Organs

Massive splenic involvement by B-PLL is a characteristic feature of this disease. Because of prominent white pulp involvement, a miliary nodular pattern can be appreciated grossly. Microscopic examination reveals extensive infiltration of both white pulp and red pulp. The larger cells tend to be concentrated in the white pulp, often forming an inverse pseudofollicular pattern with a central collection of small lymphocytes surrounded by a broad cuff of pale prolymphocytes (39,109). Even though lymphadenopathy is not generally a prominent feature of B-PLL, diffuse or vaguely nodular replacement of nodal architecture by neoplastic prolymphocytes with prominent nucleoli can be identified (494,496,497). Within the liver, a sinusoidal pattern of infiltration can be appreciated, especially in patients who show high numbers of circulating prolymphocytes. Rare cases of cutaneous and central nervous system infiltration by B-PLL have been recorded, although these are not major sites of disease involvement (499,500).

Immunophenotype

In contrast to CLL, the surface immunoglobulin expressed in B-PLL is brightly intense, and bright CD22 and FMC7 expression are evident. CD5 is present in less than one-third of

B-PLL cases, while CD23 is expressed even less frequently (Table 18.5) (142,491). Expression of CD38 is heterogeneous and does not correlate with either *IGHV@* somatic hypermutation status or prognosis (142). Most cases of B-PLL are positive for ZAP-70, though expression of this antigen does not track with *IGHV@* somatic hypermutation status; counterintuitively, ZAP-70 expression in B-PLL may correlate with improved outcome (142).

Cytogenetic and Molecular Features

Most cases of B-PLL show deletions and/or mutations of *TP53*. While this recurring abnormality is not specific for a diagnosis of B-PLL, the consistency of the finding (50% to 75% of cases of B-PLL) has led to the suggestion that the aggressive clinical course in B-PLL may be tied to genetic lesions at this locus (142,491,501). However, the presence of del(17p) does not independently predict poor outcome in B-PLL (142), and it is often present in the setting of a complex karyotype (502). Deletions of 11q23 and 13q14 are also common in B-PLL (as they are in CLL) underscoring the fact that cytogenetic results alone cannot establish a diagnosis of *de novo* B-PLL (503). Translocation of *MYC* has been reported in several cases of B-PLL (271,504–508), a finding that is particularly interesting given that overexpression of *MYC* is characteristic of B-PLL (492). *MYC* translocations have also been associated with prolymphocytoid transformation of CLL, again highlighting that molecular findings must be integrated with clinical and morphologic data for most appropriate interpretation (84). Given the historical association of the t(11;14)(q13;q32) with the category of B-PLL, it is worth reiterating that cases with this translocation are now considered to be mantle cell lymphomas rather than instances of B-PLL (491–493).

B-PLL is about evenly divided between cases showing *IGHV@* somatic hypermutation and cases lacking this finding (142). In contrast to CLL, *IGVH@* mutation status does not correlate with CD38 or ZAP-70 expression and does not seem to predict outcome (142). B-PLL cases exclusively utilize VH3 and VH4 family gene segments, with V3–23, V4–59, and V4–34 the most common (142,509). In this, B-PLL differs from CLL and other B-cell neoplasms, again suggesting a unique underlying biology.

Differential Diagnosis

The main differential diagnostic considerations are neoplastic processes that show circulating prolymphocytes or morphologically similar cells. Such cells are characteristic of T-cell prolymphocytic leukemia (T-PLL), as its name implies, and T-PLL shares with B-PLL additional features including a propensity for high white blood cell counts and splenomegaly. However, T-PLL differs clinically from B-PLL in its association with prominent lymphadenopathy. In the end, the distinction from B-PLL is rather simple on immunophenotypic grounds, as T-PLL shows a mature T-cell phenotype.

Circulating prolymphocytes or similar cells may be present in a number of B-cell neoplasms, including CLL, mantle cell lymphoma, SMZL, and the hairy cell leukemia variant (HCL-v; i.e., splenic B-cell lymphoma/leukemia, unclassifiable according to the WHO 2008). As detailed above, cases of CLL with increased prolymphocytes or frank prolymphocytoid transformation should not be classified as B-PLL, which is by definition a *de novo* entity. Most cases of CLL with increased prolymphocytes are recognizable by a background population of small cells with more typical CLL morphology. Circulating mantle cell lymphoma may adopt a prolymphocytic appearance, and conventional cytogenetic or FISH analysis for the t(11;14)(q13;q32) and/or immunohistochemistry for cyclin D1 expression should be employed liberally when a diagnosis of B-PLL is considered.

Indeed, in our practice we would hesitate to make a definitive diagnosis of B-PLL without first exploring the possibility of mantle cell lymphoma in this manner. Prolymphocytes may constitute a proportion of the circulating neoplastic cells in SMZL, though in this setting they are usually accompanied by lymphocytes with villous polar projections and lymphocytes with plasmacytoid features. The prototypic patterns of bone marrow infiltration also differ between B-PLL and SMZL, with a diffuse interstitial infiltrate more common in B-PLL and SMZL associated with nodular and intrasinusoidal involvement. The neoplastic cells in HCL-v can show hybrid morphology between B-PLL and classic hairy cell leukemia, with prominent nucleoli and cytoplasmic projections of variable prominence. HCL-v also resembles B-PLL clinically, in that both are characterized by marked splenomegaly and high white blood cell counts. HCL-v is usually positive for CD103, whereas CD103 is only rarely detected in B-PLL (142,510). In addition, the pattern of splenic infiltration is distinctly different, with exclusive red pulp involvement in HCL-v and a mixed red pulp/white pulp pattern in B-PLL (141).

Treatment and Survival

Most patients with B-PLL have advanced-stage disease and follow a corresponding steady downhill course, with median survivals in the range of 2 or 3 years (142,494). Some investigators have identified B-PLL patients who follow a more indolent course (511). A contemporary study using stringent WHO-endorsed criteria confirmed the overall poor prognosis for patients with B-PLL, showing a median overall survival of 35 months. Interestingly, however, even this study documented a few patients with unexpectedly long survival (142). While traditionally B-PLL has responded poorly to therapies utilized in the treatment of CLL, successes have been reported with multiagent strategies, immunotherapy, and/or fludarabine-based regimens (511–516).

▦ | SUMMARY AND CONCLUSIONS

The past several decades have seen substantial improvements in our understanding of CLL and B-PLL. Particularly in the case of CLL, this has enabled real-world progress in diagnosis, prognostic prediction, and treatment. Given the high prevalence of CLL and the substantial foundation of knowledge already established, large numbers of researchers will undoubtedly continue to focus on CLL and discover new insights. Of particular interest will be the refinement and integration of prognostic markers and their possible application to treatment decisions. For the diagnostic pathologist in the foreseeable future, CLL will likely retain its status as an entity that is equally common and complex.

References

1. Swerdlow SH, Campo E, Harris NL, et al., eds. *WHO classification of tumours of haematopoietic and lymphoid tissues*. Lyon: International Agency for Research on Cancer, 2008.
2. Jaffe ES, Harris NL, Stein H, et al., eds. *Pathology and genetics of tumours of haematopoietic and lymphoid tissues*. Lyon: International Agency for Research on Cancer Press, 2001.
3. Foucar K. Chronic lymphoproliferative disorders. In: Foucar K, ed. *Bone marrow pathology*. Chicago: ASCP Press, 1995:275–314.
4. Foucar K. Chronic lymphoid leukemias and lymphoproliferative disorders. *Mod Pathol* 1999;12:141–150.
5. Bennett JM, Catovsky D, Daniel MT, et al. Proposals for the classification of chronic (mature) B and T lymphoid leukaemias. French-American-British (FAB) Cooperative Group. *J Clin Pathol* 1989;42:567–584.
6. Greaves MF, Gross CE, Ferrarini M. Lymphoproliferative disorders. In: Zucker-Franklin D, Greaves MF, Grossi CE, eds. *Atlas of blood cells: function and pathology*, vol 2. Philadelphia: Lea & Febiger, 1988:445–548.
7. Muller-Hermelink H, Montserrat E, Catovsky D, et al. Chronic lymphocytic leukaemia/small lymphocytic lymphoma. In: Swerdlow SH, Campo E, Harris NL,

et al., eds. *WHO classification of tumours of haematopoietic and lymphoid tissues.* Lyon: International Agency for Research on Cancer, 2008:180–182.

8. Hallek M, Cheson BD, Catovsky D, et al. Guidelines for the diagnosis and treatment of chronic lymphocytic leukemia: a report from the International Workshop on Chronic Lymphocytic Leukemia updating the National Cancer Institute-Working Group 1996 guidelines. *Blood* 2008;111:5446–5456.

9. Ben-Ezra J. Small lymphocytic lymphoma. In: Knowles DM, ed. *Neoplastic hematopathology*, 2nd ed. Philadelphia: Lippincott Williams & Wilkins, 2001:773–787.

10. Levine EG, Arthur DC, Frizzera G, et al. There are differences in cytogenetic abnormalities among histologic subtypes of the non-Hodgkin's lymphomas. *Blood* 1985;66:1414–1422.

11. Correlation of chromosome abnormalities with histologic and immunologic characteristics in non-Hodgkin's lymphoma and adult T cell leukemia-lymphoma. Fifth International Workshop on Chromosomes in Leukemia-Lymphoma. *Blood* 1987;70:1554–1564.

12. Muller-Hermelink H, Montserrat E, Catovsky D, et al. Chronic lymphocytic leukaemia/small lymphocytic lymphoma. In: Jaffe ES, Harris NL, Stein H, et al., eds. *Tumours of haematopoietic and lymphoid tissues.* Lyon: IARC Press, 2001:127–130.

13. Marti GE, Rawstron AC, Ghia P, et al. Diagnostic criteria for monoclonal B-cell lymphocytosis. *Br J Haematol* 2005;130:325–332.

14. Rawstron AC, Bennett FL, O'Connor SJ, et al. Monoclonal B-cell lymphocytosis and chronic lymphocytic leukemia. *N Engl J Med* 2008;359:575–583.

15. Rawstron AC, Green MJ, Kuzmicki A, et al. Monoclonal B lymphocytes with the characteristics of "indolent" chronic lymphocytic leukemia are present in 3.5% of adults with normal blood counts. *Blood* 2002;100:635–639.

16. Dagklis A, Fazi C, Sala C, et al. The immunoglobulin gene repertoire of low-count chronic lymphocytic leukemia (CLL)-like monoclonal B lymphocytosis is different from CLL: diagnostic implications for clinical monitoring. *Blood* 2009;114:26–32.

17. Shanafelt TD, Ghia P, Lanasa MC, et al. Monoclonal B-cell lymphocytosis (MBL): biology, natural history and clinical management. *Leukemia* 2010;24:512–520.

18. Nieto WG, Almeida J, Romero A, et al. Increased frequency (12%) of circulating chronic lymphocytic leukemia-like B-cell clones in healthy subjects using a highly sensitive multicolor flow cytometry approach. *Blood* 2009;114:33–37.

19. Almeida J, Nieto WG, Teodosio C, et al. CLL-like B-lymphocytes are systematically present at very low numbers in peripheral blood of healthy adults. *Leukemia* 2011;25:718–722.

20. Lanasa MC, Allgood SD, Slager SL, et al. Immunophenotypic and gene expression analysis of monoclonal B-cell lymphocytosis shows biologic characteristics associated with good prognosis CLL. *Leukemia* 2011;25:1459–1466.

21. Rawstron AC, Hillmen P. Clinical and diagnostic implications of monoclonal B-cell lymphocytosis. *Best Pract Res Clin Haematol* 2010;23:61–69.

22. Landgren O, Albitar M, Ma W, et al. B-cell clones as early markers for chronic lymphocytic leukemia. *N Engl J Med* 2009;360:659–667.

23. Gibson SE, Swerdlow SH, Ferry JA, et al. Reassessment of small lymphocytic lymphoma in the era of monoclonal B-cell lymphocytosis. *Haematologica* 2011;96:1144–1152.

24. Eichhorst B, Dreyling M, Robak T, et al. Chronic lymphocytic leukemia: ESMO Clinical Practice Guidelines for diagnosis, treatment and follow-up. *Ann Oncol* 2011;22(Suppl 6):50–54.

25. Mulligan CS, Thomas ME, Mulligan SP. Monoclonal B-cell lymphocytosis and chronic lymphocytic leukemia. *N Engl J Med* 2008;359:2065–2066; author reply 2066.

26. Shanafelt TD, Kay NE, Jenkins G, et al. B-cell count and survival: differentiating chronic lymphocytic leukemia from monoclonal B-cell lymphocytosis based on clinical outcome. *Blood* 2009;113:4188–4196.

27. Rossi D, Sozzi E, Puma A, et al. The prognosis of clinical monoclonal B cell lymphocytosis differs from prognosis of Rai 0 chronic lymphocytic leukaemia and is recapitulated by biological risk factors. *Br J Haematol* 2009;146:64–75.

28. Lanasa MC, Allgood SD, Volkheimer AD, et al. Single-cell analysis reveals oligoclonality among 'low-count' monoclonal B-cell lymphocytosis. *Leukemia* 2010;24:133–140.

29. Fazi C, Scarfo L, Pecciarini L, et al. General population low-count CLL-like MBL persists over time without clinical progression, although carrying the same cytogenetic abnormalities of CLL. *Blood* 2011;118:6618–6625.

30. Molica S, Mauro FR, Giannarelli D, et al. Differentiating chronic lymphocytic leukemia from monoclonal B-lymphocytosis according to clinical outcome: on behalf of the GIMEMA chronic lymphoproliferative diseases working group. *Haematologica* 2011;96:277–283.

31. O'Brien S, del Giglio A, Keating M. Advances in the biology and treatment of B-cell chronic lymphocytic leukemia. *Blood* 1995;85:307–318.

32. Keating MJ. Chronic lymphocytic leukemia. In: Henderson ES, Lister TA, Greaves MF, eds. *Leukemia*, 6th ed. Philadelphia: W.B. Saunders, 1996:554–586.

33. Linet MS, Blattner WA. The epidemiology of chronic lymphocytic leukemia. In: Polliack A, Catovsky D, eds. *Chronic lymphocytic leukemia*. New York: Harwood Academic Publishers, 1988:11–32.

34. Rozman C, Montserrat E. Chronic lymphocytic leukemia. *N Engl J Med* 1995;333:1052–1057.

35. Horner MJ, Ries LAG, Krapcho M, et al. *SEER cancer statistics review, 1975–2006*: National Cancer Institute, 2009. Available at: http://seer.cancer.gov/csr/1975_2006/. Accessed November 23, 2011.

36. Howlander N, Noon AM, Krapcho M, et al. *SEER cancer statistics review, 1975–2008*. Bethesda: National Cancer Institute, 2011.

37. Kroft SH, Finn WG, Peterson LC. The pathology of the chronic lymphoid leukaemias. *Blood Rev* 1995;9:234–250.

38. Brittinger G, Hellriegel KP, Hiddemann W. Chronic lymphocytic leukemia and hairy-cell leukemia-diagnosis and treatment: results of a consensus meeting of the German CLL Co-operative Group. *Leukemia* 1997;11(Suppl 2):S1–S3.

39. Brunning RD, McKenna RW. Small lymphocytic leukemias and related disorders. In: Brunning RD, McKenna RW, eds. *Tumors of the bone marrow*. Washington: Armed Forces Institute of Pathology, 1993:255–322.

40. Sonnier JA, Buchanan GR, Howard-Peebles PN, et al. Chromosomal translocation involving the immunoglobulin kappa-chain and heavy-chain loci in a child with chronic lymphocytic leukemia. *N Engl J Med* 1983;309:590–594.

41. Yoffe G, Howard-Peebles PN, Smith RG, et al. Childhood chronic lymphocytic leukemia with (2;14) translocation. *J Pediatr* 1990;116:114–117.

42. Fell HP, Smith RG, Tucker PW. Molecular analysis of the t(2;14) translocation of childhood chronic lymphocytic leukemia. *Science* 1986;232:491–494.

43. Spier CM, Kjeldsberg CR, Head DR, et al. Chronic lymphocytic leukemia in young adults. *Am J Clin Pathol* 1985;84:675–678.

44. De Rossi G, Mandelli F, Covelli A, et al. Chronic lymphocytic leukemia (CLL) in younger adults: a retrospective study of 133 cases. *Hematol Oncol* 1989;7:127–137.

45. Lanasa MC. Novel insights into the biology of CLL. *Hematol Am Soc Hematol Educ Prog* 2010;2010:70–76.

46. Fernhout F, Dinkelaar RB, Hagemeijer A, et al. Four aged siblings with B cell chronic lymphocytic leukemia. *Leukemia* 1997;11:2060–2065.

47. Chan LC, Lam CK, Yeung TC, et al. The spectrum of chronic lymphoproliferative disorders in Hong Kong. A prospective study. *Leukemia* 1997;11:1964–1972.

48. Crowther-Swanepoel D, Houlston RS. Genetic variation and risk of chronic lymphocytic leukaemia. *Semin Cancer Biol* 2010;20:363–369.

49. Gale RP, Cozen W, Goodman MT, et al. Decreased chronic lymphocytic leukemia incidence in Asians in Los Angeles County. *Leuk Res* 2000;24:665–669.

50. Haenszel W, Kurihara M. Studies of Japanese migrants. I. Mortality from cancer and other diseases among Japanese in the United States. *J Natl Cancer Inst* 1968;40:43–68.

51. Clarke CA, Glaser SL, Gomez SL, et al. Lymphoid malignancies in U.S. Asians: incidence rate differences by birthplace and acculturation. *Cancer Epidemiol Biomarkers Prev* 2011;20:1064–1077.

52. Marquez ME, Deglesne PA, Lopez JL, et al. Unexpectedly high frequency of European parentage in Venezuelan patients with chronic lymphocytic leukemia. *Leuk Lymphoma* 2012;53:235–241.

53. Shenoy PJ, Malik N, Sinha R, et al. Racial differences in the presentation and outcomes of chronic lymphocytic leukemia and variants in the United States. *Clin Lymphoma Myeloma Leuk* 2011;11:498–506.

54. Ruiz-Arguelles GJ, Velazquez BM, Apreza-Molina MG, et al. Chronic lymphocytic leukemia is infrequent in Mexican mestizos. *Int J Hematol* 1999;69:253–255.

55. Jandl JH. Chronic lymphatic leukemia. In: Jandl JH, ed. *Blood—textbook of hematology*. Boston: Little Brown, 1996:991–1018.

56. Baer MR, Stein RS, Dessypris EN. Chronic lymphocytic leukemia with hyperleukocytosis. The hyperviscosity syndrome. *Cancer* 1985;56:2865–2869.

57. Zent CS, Kay NE. Autoimmune complications in chronic lymphocytic leukaemia (CLL). *Best Pract Res Clin Haematol* 2010;23:47–59.

58. Dearden C. Disease-specific complications of chronic lymphocytic leukemia. *Hematol Am Soc Hematol Educ Prog* 2008;2008:450–456.

59. Zent CS, Ding W, Reinalda MS, et al. Autoimmune cytopenia in chronic lymphocytic leukemia/small lymphocytic lymphoma: changes in clinical presentation and prognosis. *Leuk Lymphoma* 2009;50:1261–1268.

60. Yamada O, Yun-Hua W, Motoji T, et al. Clonal T-cell proliferation causing pure red cell aplasia in chronic B-cell lymphocytic leukaemia: successful treatment with cyclosporine following in vitro abrogation of erythroid colony-suppressing activity. *Br J Haematol* 1998;101:335–337.

61. Radosevich CA, Gordon LI, Weil SC, et al. Complete resolution of pure red cell aplasia in a patient with chronic lymphocytic leukemia following antithymocyte globulin therapy. *JAMA* 1988;259:723–725.

62. Chikkappa G, Pasquale D, Phillips PG, et al. Cyclosporin-A for the treatment of pure red cell aplasia in a patient with chronic lymphocytic leukemia. *Am J Hematol* 1987;26:179–189.

63. Vashi P, Patel B, Musson P, et al. Corticosteroid-responsive pure red cell aplasia in chronic lymphatic leukemia. *Am J Hematol* 1987;26:279–284.

64. D'Arena G, Cascavilla N. Chronic lymphocytic leukemia-associated pure red cell aplasia. *Int J Immunopathol Pharmacol* 2009;22:279–286.

65. D'Arena G, Vigliotti ML, Dell'Olio M, et al. Rituximab to treat chronic lymphoproliferative disorder-associated pure red cell aplasia. *Eur J Haematol* 2009;82:235–239.

66. Cesana C, Carlo-Stella C, Mangoni L, et al. Response to cyclosporin A and recombinant human erythropoietin in a case of B cell chronic lymphocytic leukemia and pure red cell aplasia. *Leukemia* 1996;10:1400–1401.

67. Sivakumaran M, Bhavnani M. Cyclosporin therapy for pure red cell aplasia in patients with chronic lymphocytic leukemia. *Am J Hematol* 1994;45:192.

68. Chikkappa G, Pasquale D, Zarrabi MH, et al. Cyclosporine and prednisone therapy for pure red cell aplasia in patients with chronic lymphocytic leukemia. *Am J Hematol* 1992;41:5–12.

69. Christen R, Morant R, Fehr J. Cyclosporin-A therapy of pure red cell aplasia in a patient with B-cell chronic lymphocytic leukemia. *Eur J Haematol* 1989;42:303–307.

70. Reid IS. Reversal of pure red cell aplasia by cyclosporin-A in a patient with chronic lymphocytic leukemia. *J Ark Med Soc* 1988;85:253–254.

71. Diehl LF, Ketchum LH. Autoimmune disease and chronic lymphocytic leukemia:autoimmune hemolytic anemia, pure red cell aplasia, and autoimmune thrombocytopenia. *Semin Oncol* 1998;25:80–97.

72. Estrov Z, Berrebi A, Kusminsky G, et al. Circulating mononuclear cells from pure red cell aplasia of chronic lymphocytic leukemia suppress in vitro erythropoiesis. *Acta Haematol* 1989;81:213–216.

73. Kay NE, Oken MM, Ascensao J, et al. Lymphocytotoxic T lymphocytes in a patient with B-chronic lymphocytic leukemia and pure red cell aplasia. *Leuk Res* 1985;9:1189–1194.

74. Mangan KF, Chikkappa G, Farley PC. T gamma (T gamma) cells suppress growth of erythroid colony-forming units in vitro in the pure red cell aplasia of B-cell chronic lymphocytic leukemia. *J Clin Invest* 1982;70:1148–1156.

75. Mangan KF, Chikkappa G, Scharfman WB, et al. Evidence for reduced erythroid burst (BFUE) promoting function of T lymphocytes in the pure red cell aplasia of chronic lymphocytic leukemia. *Exp Hematol* 1981;9:489–498.

76. Itala M, Kotilainen P, Nikkari S, et al. Pure red cell aplasia caused by B19 parvovirus infection after autologous blood stem cell transplantation in a patient with chronic lymphocytic leukemia. *Leukemia* 1997;11:171.

77. Sharma P, Singh T, Mishra D, et al. Parvovirus B-19 induced acute pure red cell aplasia in patients with chronic lymphocytic leukemia and neurofibromatosis type-1. *Hematology* 2006;11:257–259.

78. Tsai HT, Caporaso NE, Kyle RA, et al. Evidence of serum immunoglobulin abnormalities up to 9.8 years before diagnosis of chronic lymphocytic leukemia: a prospective study. *Blood* 2009;114:4928–4932.

79. Barton JC, Ratard RC. Vibrio vulnificus bacteremia associated with chronic lymphocytic leukemia, hypogammaglobulinemia, and hepatic cirrhosis: relation to host and exposure factors in 252 V. vulnificus infections reported in Louisiana. *Am J Med Sci* 2006;332:216–220.

80. Freeland HS, Scott PP. Recurrent pulmonary infections in patients with chronic lymphocytic leukemia and hypogammaglobulinemia. *South Med J* 1986;79:1366–1369.
81. Morrison VA. Infectious complications in patients with chronic lymphocytic leukemia: pathogenesis, spectrum of infection, and approaches to prophylaxis. *Clin Lymphoma Myeloma* 2009;9:365–370.
82. Deegan MJ, Abraham JP, Sawdyk M, et al. High incidence of monoclonal proteins in the serum and urine of chronic lymphocytic leukemia patients. *Blood* 1984;64:1207–1211.
83. Bacher U, Kern W, Schoch C, et al. Discrimination of chronic lymphocytic leukemia (CLL) and CLL/PL by cytomorphology can clearly be correlated to specific genetic markers as investigated by interphase fluorescence in situ hybridization (FISH). *Ann Hematol* 2004;83:349–355.
84. Huh YO, Lin KI, Vega F, et al. MYC translocation in chronic lymphocytic leukaemia is associated with increased prolymphocytes and a poor prognosis. *Br J Haematol* 2008;142:36–44.
85. Melo JV, Catovsky D, Galton DA. Chronic lymphocytic leukemia and prolymphocytic leukemia: a clinicopathological reappraisal. *Blood Cells* 1987;12:339–353.
86. Melo JV, Catovsky D, Gregory WM, et al. The relationship between chronic lymphocytic leukaemia and prolymphocytic leukaemia. IV. Analysis of survival and prognostic features. *Br J Haematol* 1987;65:23–29.
87. Criel A, Verhoef G, Vlietinck R, et al. Further characterization of morphologically defined typical and atypical CLL: a clinical, immunophenotypic, cytogenetic and prognostic study on 390 cases. *Br J Haematol* 1997;97:383–391.
88. Oscier DG, Matutes E, Copplestone A, et al. Atypical lymphocyte morphology: an adverse prognostic factor for disease progression in stage A CLL independent of trisomy 12. *Br J Haematol* 1997;98:934–939.
89. Hsi ED. Pathologic and molecular genetic features of chronic lymphocytic leukemia. *Semin Oncol* 2012;39:74–79.
90. Frater JL, McCarron KF, Hammel JP, et al. Typical and atypical chronic lymphocytic leukemia differ clinically and immunophenotypically. *Am J Clin Pathol* 2001;116:655–664.
91. Peters O, Thielemans C, Steenssens L, et al. Intracellular inclusion bodies in 14 patients with B cell lymphoproliferative disorders. *J Clin Pathol* 1984;37:45–50.
92. Ralfkiaer E, Hou-Jensen K, Geisler C, et al. Cytoplasmic inclusions in lymphocytes of chronic lymphocytic leukaemia. A report of 10 cases. *Virchows Arch A Pathol Anat Histol* 1982;395:227–236.
93. *Reference leukocyte (WBC) differential count (proportional) and evaluation of instrumental methods; approved standard*, 2nd ed. Wayne: Clinical and Laboratory Standards Institute, 2007.
94. Nowakowski GS, Hoyer JD, Shanafelt TD, et al. Percentage of smudge cells on routine blood smear predicts survival in chronic lymphocytic leukemia. *J Clin Oncol* 2009;27:1844–1849.
95. Nowakowski GS, Hoyer JD, Shanafelt TD, et al. Using smudge cells on routine blood smears to predict clinical outcome in chronic lymphocytic leukemia: a universally available prognostic test. *Mayo Clin Proc* 2007;82:449–453.
96. Rozman C, Montserrat E, Rodriguez-Fernandez JM, et al. Bone marrow histologic pattern—the best single prognostic parameter in chronic lymphocytic leukemia: a multivariate survival analysis of 329 cases. *Blood* 1984;64:642–648.
97. Pangalis GA, Roussou PA, Kittas C, et al. B-chronic lymphocytic leukemia. Prognostic implication of bone marrow histology in 120 patients experience from a single hematology unit. *Cancer* 1987;59:767–771.
98. Montserrat E, Villamor N, Reverter JC, et al. Bone marrow assessment in B-cell chronic lymphocytic leukaemia: aspirate or biopsy? A comparative study in 258 patients. *Br J Haematol* 1996;93:111–116.
99. Bartl R, Frisch B, Burkhardt R, et al. Assessment of marrow trephine in relation to staging in chronic lymphocytic leukaemia. *Br J Haematol* 1982;51:1–15.
100. Faulkner-Jones BE, Howie AJ, Boughton BJ, et al. Lymphoid aggregates in bone marrow: study of eventual outcome. *J Clin Pathol* 1988;41:768–775.
101. Rywlin AM, Ortega RS, Dominguez CJ. Lymphoid nodules of bone marrow: normal and abnormal. *Blood* 1974;43:389–400.
102. Navone R, Valpreda M, Pich A. Lymphoid nodules and nodular lymphoid hyperplasia in bone marrow biopsies. *Acta Haematol* 1985;74:19–22.
103. Foucar K. Reactive lymphoid proliferations in blood and bone marrow. In: Foucar K, ed. *Bone marrow pathology*, 1st ed. Chicago: ASCP Press, 1995:255–274.
104. Dick FR, Maca RD. The lymph node in chronic lymphocytic leukemia. *Cancer* 1978;41:283–292.
105. Bonato M, Pittaluga S, Tierens A, et al. Lymph node histology in typical and atypical chronic lymphocytic leukemia. *Am J Surg Pathol* 1998;22:49–56.
106. Herishanu Y, Perez-Galan P, Liu D, et al. The lymph node microenvironment promotes B-cell receptor signaling, NF-kappaB activation, and tumor proliferation in chronic lymphocytic leukemia. *Blood* 2011;117:563–574.
107. Ponzoni M, Doglioni C, Caligaris-Cappio F. Chronic lymphocytic leukemia: the pathologist's view of lymph node microenvironment. *Semin Diagn Pathol* 2011;28:161–166.
108. Edelman M, Evans L, Zee S, et al. Splenic micro-anatomical localization of small lymphocytic lymphoma/chronic lymphocytic leukemia using a novel combined silver nitrate and immunoperoxidase technique. *Am J Surg Pathol* 1997;21:445–452.
109. Lampert IA, Thompson I. The spleen in chronic lymphocytic leukemia and related disorders. In: Polliack A, Catovsky D, eds. *Chronic lymphocytic leukemia*. New York: Harwood Academic Publishers, 1988:193–208.
110. Schwartz JB, Shamsuddin AM. The effects of leukemic infiltrates in various organs in chronic lymphocytic leukemia. *Hum Pathol* 1981;12:432–440.
111. Lampert IA, Hegde U, Van Noorden S. The splenic white pulp in chronic lymphocytic leukaemia: a microenvironment associated with CR2 (CD21) expression, cell transformation and proliferation. *Leuk Lymphoma* 1990;1:319–326.
112. Ziemer M, Bornkessel A, Hahnfeld S, et al. 'Specific' cutaneous infiltrate of B-cell chronic lymphocytic leukemia at the site of a florid herpes simplex infection. *J Cutan Pathol* 2005;32:581–584.
113. Kakagia D, Tamiolakis D, Lambropoulou M, et al. Systemic B-cell chronic lymphocytic leukemia first presenting as a cutaneous infiltrate arising at the site of a herpes simplex scar. *Minerva Stomatol* 2005;54:161–163.
114. Cerroni L, Zenahlik P, Kerl H. Specific cutaneous infiltrates of B-cell chronic lymphocytic leukemia arising at the site of herpes zoster and herpes simplex scars. *Cancer* 1995;76:26–31.
115. Pujol RM, Matias-Guiu X, Planaguma M, et al. Chronic lymphocytic leukemia and cutaneous granulomas at sites of herpes zoster scars. *Int J Dermatol* 1990;29:652–654.
116. Wilson ML, Elston DM, Tyler WB, et al. Dense lymphocytic infiltrates associated with non-melanoma skin cancer in patients with chronic lymphocytic leukemia. *Dermatol Online J* 2010;16:4.
117. Robak E, Robak T. Skin lesions in chronic lymphocytic leukemia. *Leuk Lymphoma* 2007;48:855–865.
118. Swerdlow SH, Campo E, Seto M, et al. Mantle cell lymphoma. In: Swerdlow SH, Campo E, Harris NL, et al., eds. *WHO classification of tumours of haematopoietic and lymphoid tissues*. Lyon: International Agency for Research on Cancer, 2008:229–232.
119. Kuse R, Lueb H. Gastrointestinal involvement in patients with chronic lymphocytic leukemia. *Leukemia* 1997;11(Suppl 2):S50–S51.
120. O'Neill BP, Habermann TM, Banks PM, et al. Primary central nervous system lymphoma as a variant of Richter's syndrome in two patients with chronic lymphocytic leukemia. *Cancer* 1989;64:1296–1300.
121. Miller K, Budke H, Orazi A. Leukemic meningitis complicating early stage chronic lymphocytic leukemia. *Arch Pathol Lab Med* 1997;121:524–527.
122. Garicochea B, Cliquet MG, Melo N, et al. Leptomeningeal involvement in chronic lymphocytic leukemia identified by polymerase chain reaction in stored slides: a case report. *Mod Pathol* 1997;10:500–503.
123. Moazzam AA, Drappatz J, Kim RY, et al. Chronic lymphocytic leukemia with central nervous system involvement: report of two cases with a comprehensive literature review. *J Neurooncol* 2012;106:185–200.
124. Tonino SH, Rijssenbeek AL, Oud ME, et al. Intracerebral infiltration as the unique cause of the clinical presentation of chronic lymphocytic leukemia/small lymphocytic leukemia. *J Clin Oncol* 2011;29:e837–e839.
125. Foon KA, Gale RP, Todd RF III. Recent advances in the immunologic classification of leukemia. *Semin Hematol* 1986;23:257–283.
126. Moreau EJ, Matutes E, A'Hern RP, et al. Improvement of the chronic lymphocytic leukemia scoring system with the monoclonal antibody SN8 (CD79b). *Am J Clin Pathol* 1997;108:378–382.
127. Davis BH, Foucar K, Szczarkowski W, et al. U.S.-Canadian Consensus recommendations on the immunophenotypic analysis of hematologic neoplasia by flow cytometry: medical indications. *Cytometry* 1997;30:249–263.
128. Hamblin TJ, Oscier DG. Chronic lymphocytic leukaemia: the nature of the leukaemic cell. *Blood Rev* 1997;11:119–128.
129. Horna P, Olteanu H, Kroft SH, et al. Flow cytometric analysis of surface light chain expression patterns in B-cell lymphomas using monoclonal and polyclonal antibodies. *Am J Clin Pathol* 2011;136:954–959.
130. Huang JC, Finn WG, Goolsby CL, et al. CD5- small B-cell leukemias are rarely classifiable as chronic lymphocytic leukemia. *Am J Clin Pathol* 1999;111:123–130.
131. Shapiro JL, Miller ML, Pohlman B, et al. CD5- B-cell lymphoproliferative disorders presenting in blood and bone marrow. A clinicopathologic study of 40 patients. *Am J Clin Pathol* 1999;111:477–487.
132. Matutes E, Owusu-Ankomah K, Morilla R, et al. The immunological profile of B-cell disorders and proposal of a scoring system for the diagnosis of CLL. *Leukemia* 1994;8:1640–1645.
133. Cro L, Ferrario A, Lionetti M, et al. The clinical and biological features of a series of immunophenotypic variant of B-CLL. *Eur J Haematol* 2010;85:120–129.
134. Kern W, Bacher U, Haferlach C, et al. Frequency and prognostic impact of the aberrant CD8 expression in 5,523 patients with chronic lymphocytic leukemia. *Cytometry B Clin Cytom* 2011;82:145–150.
135. Durrieu F, Genevieve F, Arnoulet C, et al. Normal levels of peripheral CD19(+) CD5(+) CLL-like cells: toward a defined threshold for CLL follow-up—a GEIL-GOELAMS study. *Cytometry B Clin Cytom* 2011;80:346–353.
136. Rawstron AC, Kennedy B, Evans PA, et al. Quantitation of minimal disease levels in chronic lymphocytic leukemia using a sensitive flow cytometric assay improves the prediction of outcome and can be used to optimize therapy. *Blood* 2001;98:29–35.
137. Rawstron AC, Villamor N, Ritgen M, et al. International standardized approach for flow cytometric residual disease monitoring in chronic lymphocytic leukaemia. *Leukemia* 2007;21:956–964.
138. Chang H, Jiang AM, Qi CX. Aberrant nuclear p53 expression predicts hemizygous 17p (TP53) deletion in chronic lymphocytic leukemia. *Am J Clin Pathol* 2010;133:70–74.
139. Marinelli M, Raponi S, Del Giudice I, et al. Is the aberrant expression of p53 by immunocytochemistry a surrogate marker of TP53 mutation and/or deletion in chronic lymphocytic leukemia? *Am J Clin Pathol* 2011;135:173–174.
140. Schlette EJ, Admirand J, Wierda W, et al. p53 expression by immunohistochemistry is an important determinant of survival in patients with chronic lymphocytic leukemia receiving frontline chemo-immunotherapy. *Leuk Lymphoma* 2009;50:1597–1605.
141. Viswanatha DS, Montgomery KD, Foucar K. Mature B-cell neoplasms: chronic lymphocytic leukemia-small lymphocytic lymphoma, B-cell prolymphocytic leukemia, and lymphoplasmacytic lymphoma. In: Jaffe ES, Harris NL, Vardiman JW, et al., eds. *Hematopathology*. Philadelphia: W.B. Saunders, 2011:221–246.
142. Del Giudice I, Davis Z, Matutes E, et al. IgVH genes mutation and usage, ZAP-70 and CD38 expression provide new insights on B-cell prolymphocytic leukemia (B-PLL). *Leukemia* 2006;20:1231–1237.
143. Del Giudice I, Mauro FR, De Propris MS, et al. White blood cell count at diagnosis and immunoglobulin variable region gene mutations are independent predictors of treatment-free survival in young patients with stage A chronic lymphocytic leukemia. *Haematologica* 2011;96:626–630.
144. Stilgenbauer S, Zenz T. Understanding and managing ultra high-risk chronic lymphocytic leukemia. *Hematol Am Soc Hematol Educ Prog* 2010;2010:481–488.
145. Rossi D, Cerri M, Deambrogi C, et al. The prognostic value of TP53 mutations in chronic lymphocytic leukemia is independent of Del17p13: implications for overall survival and chemorefractoriness. *Clin Cancer Res* 2009;15:995–1004.
146. Pospisilova S, Gonzalez D, Malcikova J, et al. ERIC recommendations on TP53 mutation analysis in chronic lymphocytic leukemia. *Leukemia* 2012;26(7):1458–1461.
147. Gonzalez D, Martinez P, Wade R, et al. Mutational status of the TP53 gene as a predictor of response and survival in patients with chronic lymphocytic leukemia: results from the LRF CLL4 trial. *J Clin Oncol* 2011;29:2223–2229.
148. Trbusek M, Smardova J, Malcikova J, et al. Missense mutations located in structural p53 DNA-binding motifs are associated with extremely poor survival in chronic lymphocytic leukemia. *J Clin Oncol* 2011;29:2703–2708.
149. Havelange V, Pekarsky Y, Nakamura T, et al. IRF4 mutations in chronic lymphocytic leukemia. *Blood* 2011;118:2827–2829.

150. Rampazzo E, Bonaldi L, Trentin L, et al. Telomere length and telomerase levels delineate subgroups of B-cell chronic lymphocytic leukemia with different biological characteristics and clinical outcomes. *Haematologica* 2012;97:56–63.
151. Rossi D, Rasi S, Fabbri G, et al. Mutations of NOTCH1 are an independent predictor of survival in chronic lymphocytic leukemia. *Blood* 2012;119:521–529.
152. Del Giudice I, Rossi D, Chiaretti S, et al. NOTCH1 mutations in +12 chronic lymphocytic leukemia (CLL) confer an unfavorable prognosis, induce a distinctive transcriptional profiling and refine the intermediate prognosis of +12 CLL. *Haematologica* 2011;97:437–441.
153. Sportoletti P, Baldoni S, Cavalli L, et al. NOTCH1 PEST domain mutation is an adverse prognostic factor in B-CLL. *Br J Haematol* 2010;151:404–406.
154. Di Ianni M, Baldoni S, Rosati E, et al. A new genetic lesion in B-CLL: a NOTCH1 PEST domain mutation. *Br J Haematol* 2009;146:689–691.
155. Rossi D, Bruscaggin A, Spina V, et al. Mutations of the SF3B1 splicing factor in chronic lymphocytic leukemia: association with progression and fludarabine-refractoriness. *Blood* 2011;118(26):6904–6908.
156. Quesada V, Conde L, Villamor N, et al. Exome sequencing identifies recurrent mutations of the splicing factor SF3B1 gene in chronic lymphocytic leukemia. *Nat Genet* 2012;44:47–52.
157. Duzkale H, Schweighofer CD, Coombes KR, et al. LDOC1 mRNA is differentially expressed in chronic lymphocytic leukemia and predicts overall survival in untreated patients. *Blood* 2011;117:4076–4084.
158. Kay NE, Eckel-Passow JE, Braggio E, et al. Progressive but previously untreated CLL patients with greater array CGH complexity exhibit a less durable response to chemoimmunotherapy. *Cancer Genet Cytogenet* 2010;203:161–168.
159. Yi S, Yu Z, Zhou K, et al. TOSO is overexpressed and correlated with disease progression in Chinese patients with chronic lymphocytic leukemia. *Leuk Lymphoma* 2011;52:72–78.
160. Rasi S, Spina V, Bruscaggin A, et al. A variant of the LRP4 gene affects the risk of chronic lymphocytic leukaemia transformation to Richter syndrome. *Br J Haematol* 2011;152:284–294.
161. Zhang L, Murray F, Rassenti LZ, et al. Cyclic nucleotide phosphodiesterase 7B mRNA: an unfavorable characteristic in chronic lymphocytic leukemia. *Int J Cancer* 2011;129:1162–1169.
162. Irving L, Mainou-Fowler T, Parker A, et al. Methylation markers identify high risk patients in IGHV mutated chronic lymphocytic leukemia. *Epigenetics* 2011; 6:300–306.
163. Fabris S, Bollati V, Agnelli L, et al. Biological and clinical relevance of quantitative global methylation of repetitive DNA sequences in chronic lymphocytic leukemia. *Epigenetics* 2011;6:188–194.
164. Rodriguez A, Villuendas R, Yanez L, et al. Molecular heterogeneity in chronic lymphocytic leukemia is dependent on BCR signaling: clinical correlation. *Leukemia* 2007;21:1984–1991.
165. Stamatopoulos B, Meuleman N, De Bruyn C, et al. A molecular score by quantitative PCR as a new prognostic tool at diagnosis for chronic lymphocytic leukemia patients. *PLoS One* 2010;5:e12780.
166. Herold T, Jurinovic V, Metzeler KH, et al. An eight-gene expression signature for the prediction of survival and time to treatment in chronic lymphocytic leukemia. *Leukemia* 2011;25:1639–1645.
167. Nuckel H, Collins CH, Frey UH, et al. FCRL2 mRNA expression is inversely associated with clinical progression in chronic lymphocytic leukemia. *Eur J Haematol* 2009;83:541–549.
168. Erikci AA, Karagoz B, Ozyurt M, et al. HLA-G expression in B chronic lymphocytic leukemia: a new prognostic marker? *Hematology* 2009;14:101–105.
169. Rebmann V, Nuckel H, Duhrsen U, et al. HLA-G in B-chronic lymphocytic leukaemia: clinical relevance and functional implications. *Semin Cancer Biol* 2007;17:430–435.
170. Nuckel H, Rebmann V, Durig J, et al. HLA-G expression is associated with an unfavorable outcome and immunodeficiency in chronic lymphocytic leukemia. *Blood* 2005;105:1694–1698.
171. Souwer Y, Chamuleau ME, van de Loosdrecht AA, et al. Detection of aberrant transcription of major histocompatibility complex class II antigen presentation genes in chronic lymphocytic leukaemia identifies HLA-DOA mRNA as a prognostic factor for survival. *Br J Haematol* 2009;145:334–343.
172. van't Veer MB, Brooijmans AM, Langerak AW, et al. The predictive value of lipoprotein lipase for survival in chronic lymphocytic leukemia. *Haematologica* 2006;91:56–63.
173. Maloum K, Settegrana C, Chapiro E, et al. IGHV gene mutational status and LPL/ADAM29 gene expression as clinical outcome predictors in CLL patients in remission following treatment with oral fludarabine plus cyclophosphamide. *Ann Hematol* 2009;88:1215–1221.
174. Calin GA, Ferracin M, Cimmino A, et al. A MicroRNA signature associated with prognosis and progression in chronic lymphocytic leukemia. *N Engl J Med* 2005;353:1793–1801.
175. Schweighofer CD, Coombes KR, Barron LL, et al. A two-gene signature, SKI and SLAMF1, predicts time-to-treatment in previously untreated patients with chronic lymphocytic leukemia. *PLoS One* 2011;6:e28277.
176. Papageorgiou SG, Kontos CK, Pappa V, et al. The novel member of the BCL2 gene family, BCL2L12, is substantially elevated in chronic lymphocytic leukemia patients, supporting its value as a significant biomarker. *Oncologist* 2011;16: 1280–1291.
177. Christensen DJ, Chen Y, Oddo J, et al. SET oncoprotein overexpression in B-cell chronic lymphocytic leukemia and non-Hodgkin lymphoma: a predictor of aggressive disease and a new treatment target. *Blood* 2011;118:4150–4158.
178. Buhl AM, Jurlander J, Geisler CH, et al. CLLU1 expression levels predict time to initiation of therapy and overall survival in chronic lymphocytic leukemia. *Eur J Haematol* 2006;76:455–464.
179. Morabito F, De Filippi R, Laurenti L, et al. The cumulative amount of serum-free light chain is a strong prognosticator in chronic lymphocytic leukemia. *Blood* 2011;118:6353–6361.
180. Yan XJ, Dozmorov I, Li W, et al. Identification of outcome-correlated cytokine clusters in chronic lymphocytic leukemia. *Blood* 2011;118:5201–5210.
181. Tecchio C, Nichele I, Mosna F, et al. A proliferation-inducing ligand (APRIL) serum levels predict time to first treatment in patients affected by B-cell chronic lymphocytic leukemia. *Eur J Haematol* 2011;87:228–234.
182. Ferrer G, Hodgson K, Pereira A, et al. Combined analysis of levels of serum B-cell activating factor and a proliferation-inducing ligand as predictor of disease progression in patients with chronic lymphocytic leukemia. *Leuk Lymphoma* 2011;52:2064–2068.
183. Xu W, Wang YH, Fan L, et al. Prognostic significance of serum immunoglobulin paraprotein in patients with chronic lymphocytic leukemia. *Leuk Res* 2011;35: 1060–1065.
184. Sivina M, Hartmann E, Kipps TJ, et al. CCL3 (MIP-1alpha) plasma levels and the risk for disease progression in chronic lymphocytic leukemia. *Blood* 2011;117: 1662–1669.
185. Molica S, Digiesi G, Battaglia C, et al. Baff serum level predicts time to first treatment in early chronic lymphocytic leukemia. *Eur J Haematol* 2010;85:314–320.
186. Alatrash G, Albitar M, O'Brien S, et al. Circulating CD52 and CD20 levels at end of treatment predict for progression and survival in patients with chronic lymphocytic leukaemia treated with fludarabine, cyclophosphamide and rituximab (FCR). *Br J Haematol* 2010;148:386–393.
187. Del Poeta G, Del Principe MI, Zucchetto A, et al. CD69 is independently prognostic in chronic lymphocytic leukemia: a comprehensive clinical and biological profiling study. *Haematologica* 2012;97:279–287.
188. Li FJ, Ding S, Pan J, et al. FCRL2 expression predicts IGHV mutation status and clinical progression in chronic lymphocytic leukemia. *Blood* 2008;112:179–187.
189. Friedrichs B, Siegel S, Reimer R, et al. High expression of the immature laminin receptor protein correlates with mutated IGVH status and predicts a favorable prognosis in chronic lymphocytic leukemia. *Leuk Res* 2011;35:721–729.
190. Rees-Unwin KS, Faragher R, Unwin RD, et al. Ribosome-associated nucleophosmin 1: increased expression and shuttling activity distinguishes prognostic subtypes in chronic lymphocytic leukaemia. *Br J Haematol* 2010;148:534–543.
191. Molica S, Digiesi G, Antenucci A, et al. Vitamin D insufficiency predicts time to first treatment (TFT) in early chronic lymphocytic leukemia (CLL). *Leuk Res* 2011;36(4):443–447.
192. Shanafelt TD, Drake MT, Maurer MJ, et al. Vitamin D insufficiency and prognosis in chronic lymphocytic leukemia. *Blood* 2011;117:1492–1498.
193. Richendollar BG, Pohlman B, Elson P, et al. Follicular programmed death 1-positive lymphocytes in the tumor microenvironment are an independent prognostic factor in follicular lymphoma. *Hum Pathol* 2011;42:552–557.
194. D'Arena G, Laurenti L, Minervini MM, et al. Regulatory T-cell number is increased in chronic lymphocytic leukemia patients and correlates with progressive disease. *Leuk Res* 2011;35:363–368.
195. Weiss L, Melchardt T, Egle A, et al. Regulatory T cells predict the time to initial treatment in early stage chronic lymphocytic leukemia. *Cancer* 2011;117:2163–2169.
196. Gonzalez-Rodriguez AP, Contesti J, Huergo-Zapico L, et al. Prognostic significance of CD8 and CD4 T cells in chronic lymphocytic leukemia. *Leuk Lymphoma* 2010;51:1829–1836.
197. Danilov AV, Danilova OV, Brown JR, et al. Dipeptidyl peptidase 2 apoptosis assay determines the B-cell activation stage and predicts prognosis in chronic lymphocytic leukemia. *Exp Hematol* 2010;38:1167–1177.
198. Tarnani M, Laurenti L, Longo PG, et al. The proliferative response to CpG-ODN stimulation predicts PFS, TTT and OS in patients with chronic lymphocytic leukemia. *Leuk Res* 2010;34:1189–1194.
199. Nunes C, Wong R, Mason M, et al. Expansion of a CD8+PD-1+ replicative senescence phenotype in early stage CLL patients is associated with inverted CD4:CD8 ratios and disease progression. *Clin Cancer Res* 2012;18:678–687.
200. Scielzo C, Apollonio B, Scarfo L, et al. The functional in vitro response to CD40 ligation reflects a different clinical outcome in patients with chronic lymphocytic leukemia. *Leukemia* 2011;25:1760–1767.
201. Furman RR. Prognostic markers and stratification of chronic lymphocytic leukemia. *Hematol Am Soc Hematol Educ Prog* 2010;2010:77–81.
202. Rai KR. The different staging systems proposed in chronic lymphocytic leukemia. In: Polliack A, Catovsky D, eds. *Chronic lymphocytic leukemia*. New York: Harwood Academic Publishers, 1988:105–110.
203. Binet JL. Clinical classifications and treatment of chronic lymphocytic leukemia: the experience of the French Cooperative Group trials. In: Polliack A, Catovsky D, eds. *Chronic lymphocytic leukemia*. New York: Harwood Academic Publishers, 1988:123–140.
204. Montserrat E, Rozman C. Prognostic factors in chronic lymphocytic leukemia. In: Polliack A, Catovsky D, eds. *Chronic lymphocytic leukemia*. New York: Harwood Academic Publishers, 1988:111–122.
205. Rai KR, Sawitsky A, Cronkite EP, et al. Clinical staging of chronic lymphocytic leukemia. *Blood* 1975;46:219–234.
206. Binet JL, Auquier A, Dighiero G, et al. A new prognostic classification of chronic lymphocytic leukemia derived from a multivariate survival analysis. *Cancer* 1981;48:198–206.
207. Rai KR, Han T. Prognostic factors and clinical staging in chronic lymphocytic leukemia. *Hematol Oncol Clin North Am* 1990;4:447–456.
208. Wierda WG, O'Brien S, Wang X, et al. Prognostic nomogram and index for overall survival in previously untreated patients with chronic lymphocytic leukemia. *Blood* 2007;109:4679–4685.
209. Cheson BD, Bennett JM, Grever M, et al. National Cancer Institute-sponsored Working Group guidelines for chronic lymphocytic leukemia: revised guidelines for diagnosis and treatment. *Blood* 1996;87:4990–4997.
210. Shanafelt TD. Predicting clinical outcome in CLL: how and why. *Hematol Am Soc Hematol Educ Prog* 2009:421–429.
211. Teng G, Papavasiliou FN. Immunoglobulin somatic hypermutation. *Annu Rev Genet* 2007;41:107–120.
212. Damle RN, Wasil T, Fais F, et al. Ig V gene mutation status and CD38 expression as novel prognostic indicators in chronic lymphocytic leukemia. *Blood* 1999;94:1840–1847.
213. Hamblin TJ, Davis Z, Gardiner A, et al. Unmutated Ig V(H) genes are associated with a more aggressive form of chronic lymphocytic leukemia. *Blood* 1999;94: 1848–1854.
214. Hamblin TJ, Orchard JA, Ibbotson RE, et al. CD38 expression and immunoglobulin variable region mutations are independent prognostic variables in chronic lymphocytic leukemia, but CD38 expression may vary during the course of the disease. *Blood* 2002;99:1023–1029.
215. Smit LA, van Maldegem F, Langerak AW, et al. Antigen receptors and somatic hypermutation in B-cell chronic lymphocytic leukemia with Richter's transformation. *Haematologica* 2006;91:903–911.
216. Stilgenbauer S, Sander S, Bullinger L, et al. Clonal evolution in chronic lymphocytic leukemia:acquisition of high-risk genomic aberrations associated with unmutated VH, resistance to therapy, and short survival. *Haematologica* 2007;92:1242–1245.
217. Byrd JC, Gribben JG, Peterson BL, et al. Select high-risk genetic features predict earlier progression following chemoimmunotherapy with fludarabine and

rituximab in chronic lymphocytic leukemia: justification for risk-adapted therapy. *J Clin Oncol* 2006;24:437–443.
218. Hamblin TJ, Davis ZA, Oscier DG. Determination of how many immunoglobulin variable region heavy chain mutations are allowable in unmutated chronic lymphocytic leukaemia—long-term follow up of patients with different percentages of mutations. *Br J Haematol* 2008;140:320–323.
219. Lin KI, Tam CS, Keating MJ, et al. Relevance of the immunoglobulin VH somatic mutation status in patients with chronic lymphocytic leukemia treated with fludarabine, cyclophosphamide, and rituximab (FCR) or related chemoimmunotherapy regimens. *Blood* 2009;113:3168–3171.
220. Thorselius M, Krober A, Murray F, et al. Strikingly homologous immunoglobulin gene rearrangements and poor outcome in VH3-21-using chronic lymphocytic leukemia patients independent of geographic origin and mutational status. *Blood* 2006;107:2889–2894.
221. Krober A, Bloehdorn J, Hafner S, et al. Additional genetic high-risk features such as 11q deletion, 17p deletion, and V3-21 usage characterize discordance of ZAP-70 and VH mutation status in chronic lymphocytic leukemia. *J Clin Oncol* 2006;24:969–975.
222. Falt S, Merup M, Tobin G, et al. Distinctive gene expression pattern in VH3-21 utilizing B-cell chronic lymphocytic leukemia. *Blood* 2005;106:681–689.
223. Bomben R, Dal-Bo M, Benedetti D, et al. Expression of mutated IGHV3-23 genes in chronic lymphocytic leukemia identifies a disease subset with peculiar clinical and biological features. *Clin Cancer Res* 2010;16:620–628.
224. Maura F, Cutrona G, Fabris S, et al. Relevance of stereotyped B-cell receptors in the context of the molecular, cytogenetic and clinical features of chronic lymphocytic leukemia. *PLoS One* 2011;6:e24313.
225. Rossi D, Spina V, Cerri M, et al. Stereotyped B-cell receptor is an independent risk factor of chronic lymphocytic leukemia transformation to Richter syndrome. *Clin Cancer Res* 2009;15:4415–4422.
226. Bomben R, Dal Bo M, Capello D, et al. Molecular and clinical features of chronic lymphocytic leukaemia with stereotyped B cell receptors: results from an Italian multicentre study. *Br J Haematol* 2009;144:492–506.
227. Hamblin T. CD38: What is it there for? *Blood* 2003;102:1939–1940.
228. Malavasi F, Deaglio S, Damle R, et al. CD38 and chronic lymphocytic leukemia: a decade later. *Blood* 2011;118:3470–3478.
229. Lund FE, Yu N, Kim KM, et al. Signaling through CD38 augments B cell antigen receptor (BCR) responses and is dependent on BCR expression. *J Immunol* 1996;157:1455–1467.
230. Ghia P, Guida G, Stella S, et al. The pattern of CD38 expression defines a distinct subset of chronic lymphocytic leukemia (CLL) patients at risk of disease progression. *Blood* 2003;101:1262–1269.
231. Ibrahim S, Keating M, Do KA, et al. CD38 expression as an important prognostic factor in B-cell chronic lymphocytic leukemia. *Blood* 2001;98:181–186.
232. Durig J, Naschar M, Schmucker U, et al. CD38 expression is an important prognostic marker in chronic lymphocytic leukaemia. *Leukemia* 2002;16:30–35.
233. Gentile M, Mauro FR, Calabrese E, et al. The prognostic value of CD38 expression in chronic lymphocytic leukaemia patients studied prospectively at diagnosis: a single institute experience. *Br J Haematol* 2005;130:549–557.
234. Domingo-Domenech E, Domingo-Claros A, Gonzalez-Barca E, et al. CD38 expression in B-chronic lymphocytic leukemia: association with clinical presentation and outcome in 155 patients. *Haematologica* 2002;87:1021–1027.
235. Patten PE, Buggins AG, Richards J, et al. CD38 expression in chronic lymphocytic leukemia is regulated by the tumor microenvironment. *Blood* 2008;111:5173–5181.
236. Hamblin TJ, Orchard JA, Gardiner A, et al. Immunoglobulin V genes and CD38 expression in CLL. *Blood* 2000;95:2455–2457.
237. Thunberg U, Johnson A, Roos G, et al. CD38 expression is a poor predictor for VH gene mutational status and prognosis in chronic lymphocytic leukemia. *Blood* 2001;97:1892–1894.
238. Matrai Z, Lin K, Dennis M, et al. CD38 expression and Ig VH gene mutation in B-cell chronic lymphocytic leukemia. *Blood* 2001;97:1902–1903.
239. Rassenti LZ, Jain S, Keating MJ, et al. Relative value of ZAP-70, CD38, and immunoglobulin mutation status in predicting aggressive disease in chronic lymphocytic leukemia. *Blood* 2008;112:1923–1930.
240. Crespo M, Bosch F, Villamor N, et al. ZAP-70 expression as a surrogate for immunoglobulin-variable-region mutations in chronic lymphocytic leukemia. *N Engl J Med* 2003;348:1764–1775.
241. Wiestner A, Rosenwald A, Barry TS, et al. ZAP-70 expression identifies a chronic lymphocytic leukemia subtype with unmutated immunoglobulin genes, inferior clinical outcome, and distinct gene expression profile. *Blood* 2003;101:4944–4951.
242. Del Principe MI, Del Poeta G, Buccisano F, et al. Clinical significance of ZAP-70 protein expression in B-cell chronic lymphocytic leukemia. *Blood* 2006;108:853–861.
243. Chen YH, Peterson LC, Dittmann D, et al. Comparative analysis of flow cytometric techniques in assessment of ZAP-70 expression in relation to IgVH mutational status in chronic lymphocytic leukemia. *Am J Clin Pathol* 2007;127:182–191.
244. Admirand JH, Knoblock RJ, Coombes KR, et al. Immunohistochemical detection of ZAP70 in chronic lymphocytic leukemia predicts immunoglobulin heavy chain gene mutation status and time to progression. *Mod Pathol* 2010;23:1518–1523.
245. Hassanein NM, Perkinson KR, Alcancia F, et al. A single tube, four-color flow cytometry assay for evaluation of ZAP-70 and CD38 expression in chronic lymphocytic leukemia. *Am J Clin Pathol* 2010;133:708–717.
246. Gachard N, Salviat A, Boutet C, et al. Multicenter study of ZAP-70 expression in patients with B-cell chronic lymphocytic leukemia using an optimized flow cytometry method. *Haematologica* 2008;93: 215–223.
247. Smolej L, Vroblova V, Motyckova M, et al. Quantification of ZAP-70 expression in chronic lymphocytic leukemia:T/B-cell ratio of mean fluorescence intensity provides stronger prognostic value than percentage of positive cells. *Neoplasma* 2011;58:140–145.
248. Rossi FM, Del Principe MI, Rossi D, et al. Prognostic impact of ZAP-70 expression in chronic lymphocytic leukemia: mean fluorescence intensity T/B ratio versus percentage of positive cells. *J Transl Med* 2010;8:23.
249. Wang YH, Fan L, Xu W, et al. Detection methods of ZAP-70 in chronic lymphocytic leukemia. *Clin Exp Med* 2011;12(2):69–77.
250. Degheidy HA, Venzon DJ, Farooqui MZ, et al. Combined normal donor and CLL: Single tube ZAP-70 analysis. *Cytometry B Clin Cytom* 2011;82(2):67–77.
251. Degheidy HA, Venzon DJ, Farooqui MZ, et al. Improved ZAP-70 assay using two clones, multiple methods of analysis and clinical correlation. *Cytometry B Clin Cytom* 2011;85:309–317.
252. Degheidy HA, Venzon DJ, Farooqui MZ, et al. Methodological comparison of two anti-ZAP-70 antibodies. *Cytometry B Clin Cytom* 2011;80:300–308.
253. Preobrazhensky SN, Szankasi P, Bahler DW. Improved flow cytometric detection of ZAP-70 in chronic lymphocytic leukemia using experimentally optimized isotypic control antibodies. *Cytometry B Clin Cytom* 2011;82;78–84.
254. Kipps TJ. The B-cell receptor and ZAP-70 in chronic lymphocytic leukemia. *Best Pract Res Clin Haematol* 2007;20:415–424.
255. Gobessi S, Laurenti L, Longo PG, et al. ZAP-70 enhances B-cell-receptor signaling despite absent or inefficient tyrosine kinase activation in chronic lymphocytic leukemia and lymphoma B cells. *Blood* 2007;109:2032–2039.
256. Chen L, Widhopf G, Huynh L, et al. Expression of ZAP-70 is associated with increased B-cell receptor signaling in chronic lymphocytic leukemia. *Blood* 2002; 100:4609–4614.
257. Hoehn D, Medeiros LJ, Konoplev S. Molecular pathology of chronic lymphocytic leukemia. In: Crisan D, ed. *Hematopathology, genomic mechanisms of neoplastic diseases*. New York: Humana Press, 2010:255–291.
258. Heerema NA, Byrd JC, Dal Cin PS, et al. Stimulation of chronic lymphocytic leukemia cells with CpG oligodeoxynucleotide gives consistent karyotypic results among laboratories: a CLL Research Consortium (CRC) Study. *Cancer Genet Cytogenet* 2010;203:134–140.
259. Muthusamy N, Breidenbach H, Andritsos L, et al. Enhanced detection of chromosomal abnormalities in chronic lymphocytic leukemia by conventional cytogenetics using CpG oligonucleotide in combination with pokeweed mitogen and phorbol myristate acetate. *Cancer Genet* 2011;204:77–83.
260. Haferlach C, Dicker F, Schnittger S, et al. Comprehensive genetic characterization of CLL: a study on 506 cases analysed with chromosome banding analysis, interphase FISH, IgV(H) status and immunophenotyping. *Leukemia* 2007;21:2442–2451.
261. Dicker F, Schnittger S, Haferlach T, et al. Immunostimulatory oligonucleotide-induced metaphase cytogenetics detect chromosomal aberrations in 80% of CLL patients: a study of 132 CLL cases with correlation to FISH, IgVH status, and CD38 expression. *Blood* 2006;108:3152–3160.
262. Dohner H, Stilgenbauer S, Benner A, et al. Genomic aberrations and survival in chronic lymphocytic leukemia. *N Engl J Med* 2000;343:1910–1916.
263. Mougalian SS, O'Brien S. Adverse prognostic features in chronic lymphocytic leukemia. *Oncology (Williston Park)* 2011;25:692–696, 699.
264. Grever MR, Lucas DM, Dewald GW, et al. Comprehensive assessment of genetic and molecular features predicting outcome in patients with chronic lymphocytic leukemia: results from the US Intergroup Phase III Trial E2997. *J Clin Oncol* 2007;25:799–804.
265. Hillmen P. Using the biology of chronic lymphocytic leukemia to choose treatment. *Hematol Am Soc Hematol Educ Prog* 2011;2011:104–109.
266. Cavazzini F, Cuneo A, de Angeli C, et al. Abnormalities of chromosomes 1p34–36, 4p16, 4q35, 9q11–32 and +7 represent novel recurrent cytogenetic rearrangements in chronic lymphocytic leukemia. *Leuk Lymphoma* 2004;45:1197–1203.
267. Van Dyke DL, Shanafelt TD, Call TG, et al. A comprehensive evaluation of the prognostic significance of 13q deletions in patients with B-chronic lymphocytic leukaemia. *Br J Haematol* 2010;148:544–550.
268. Gribben JG, O'Brien S. Update on therapy of chronic lymphocytic leukemia. *J Clin Oncol* 2011;29:544–550.
269. Foucar K. Mature B- and T-cell lymphoproliferative neoplasms. In: Foucar K, ed. *Bone marrow pathology*, 3rd ed. Chicago: ASCP Press, 2010:475–521.
270. Balatti V, Bottoni A, Palamarchuk A, et al. NOTCH1 mutations in CLL associated with trisomy 12. *Blood* 2012;119:329–331.
271. Put N, Van Roosbroeck K, Konings P, et al. Chronic lymphocytic leukemia and prolymphocytic leukemia with MYC translocations: a subgroup with an aggressive disease course. *Ann Hematol* 2011;91(6):863–873.
272. Huh YO, Schweighofer CD, Ketterling RP, et al. Chronic lymphocytic leukemia with t(14;19)(q32;q13) is characterized by atypical morphologic and immunophenotypic features and distinctive genetic features. *Am J Clin Pathol* 2011;135: 686–696.
273. Kolquist KA, Schultz RA, Slovak ML, et al. Evaluation of chronic lymphocytic leukemia by oligonucleotide-based microarray analysis uncovers novel aberrations not detected by FISH or cytogenetic analysis. *Mol Cytogenet* 2011;4:25.
274. O'Malley DP, Giudice C, Chang AS, et al. Comparison of array comparative genomic hybridization (aCGH) to FISH and cytogenetics in prognostic evaluation of chronic lymphocytic leukemia. *Int J Lab Hematol* 2011;33:238–244.
275. Hagenkord JM, Monzon FA, Kash SF, et al. Array-based karyotyping for prognostic assessment in chronic lymphocytic leukemia: performance comparison of Affymetrix 10K2.0, 250K Nsp, and SNP6.0 arrays. *J Mol Diagn* 2010;12:184–196.
276. Gunn SR. The vanguard has arrived in the clinical laboratory: array-based karyotyping for prognostic markers in chronic lymphocytic leukemia. *J Mol Diagn* 2010;12:144–146.
277. Gunn SR, Hibbard MK, Ismail SH, et al. Atypical 11q deletions identified by array CGH may be missed by FISH panels for prognostic markers in chronic lymphocytic leukemia. *Leukemia* 2009;23:1011–1017.
278. Gunn SR, Mohammed MS, Gorre ME, et al. Whole-genome scanning by array comparative genomic hybridization as a clinical tool for risk assessment in chronic lymphocytic leukemia. *J Mol Diagn* 2008;10:442–451.
279. Rodriguez AE, Robledo C, Garcia JL, et al. Identification of a novel recurrent gain on 20q13 in chronic lymphocytic leukemia by array CGH and gene expression profiling. *Ann Oncol* 2012;23:2138–2146.
280. Gunnarsson R, Mansouri L, Isaksson A, et al. Array-based genomic screening at diagnosis and during follow-up in chronic lymphocytic leukemia. *Haematologica* 2011;96:1161–1169.
281. Zhang L, Znoyko I, Costa LJ, et al. Clonal diversity analysis using SNP microarray: a new prognostic tool for chronic lymphocytic leukemia. *Cancer Genet* 2011;204:654–665.
282. Knight SJ, Yau C, Clifford R, et al. Quantification of subclonal distributions of recurrent genomic aberrations in paired pre-treatment and relapse samples from patients with B-cell chronic lymphocytic leukemia. *Leukemia* 2012;26: 1564–1575.
283. Braggio E, Kay NE, Vanwier S, et al. Longitudinal genome wide analysis of patients with chronic lymphocytic leukemia reveals complex evolution of clonal architecture at disease progression and at the time of relapse. *Leukemia* 2012;26:1698–1701.
284. Rinaldi A, Mian M, Kwee I, et al. Genome-wide DNA profiling better defines the prognosis of chronic lymphocytic leukaemia. *Br J Haematol* 2011;154:590–599.

285. Krober A, Seiler T, Benner A, et al. V(H) mutation status, CD38 expression level, genomic aberrations, and survival in chronic lymphocytic leukemia. *Blood* 2002;100:1410–1416.
286. Pepper C, Majid A, Lin TT, et al. Defining the prognosis of early stage chronic lymphocytic leukaemia patients. *Br J Haematol* 2011;156:499–507.
287. Letestu R, Levy V, Eclache V, et al. Prognosis of Binet stage A chronic lymphocytic leukemia patients:the strength of routine parameters. *Blood* 2010;116:4588–4590.
288. Morabito F, Cutrona G, Gentile M, et al. Definition of progression risk based on combinations of cellular and molecular markers in patients with Binet stage A chronic lymphocytic leukaemia. *Br J Haematol* 2009;146:44–53.
289. Oliveira AC, de la Banda E, Domingo-Domenech E, et al. Prospective study of clinical and biological prognostic factors at diagnosis in patients with early stage B-cell chronic lymphocytic leukemia. *Leuk Lymphoma* 2011;52:429–435.
290. Bulian P, Rossi D, Forconi F, et al. IGHV gene mutational status and 17p deletion are independent molecular predictors in a comprehensive clinical-biological prognostic model for overall survival prediction in chronic lymphocytic leukemia. *J Transl Med* 2012;10:18.
291. Morilla A, Gonzalez de Castro D, Del Giudice I, et al. Combinations of ZAP-70, CD38 and IGHV mutational status as predictors of time to first treatment in CLL. *Leuk Lymphoma* 2008;49:2108–2115.
292. Gladstone DE, Swinnen L, Kasamon Y, et al. Importance of immunoglobulin heavy chain variable region mutational status in del(13q) chronic lymphocytic leukemia. *Leuk Lymphoma* 2011;52:1873–1881.
293. Gladstone DE, Blackford A, Cho E, et al. The importance of IGHV mutational status in del(11q) and del(17p) chronic lymphocytic leukemia. *Clin Lymphoma Myeloma Leuk* 2012;12:132–137.
294. Shanafelt TD, Jenkins G, Call TG, et al. Validation of a new prognostic index for patients with chronic lymphocytic leukemia. *Cancer* 2009;115:363–372.
295. Molica S, Mauro FR, Callea V, et al. The utility of a prognostic index for predicting time to first treatment in early chronic lymphocytic leukemia: the GIMEMA experience. *Haematologica* 2010;95:464–469.
296. Bulian P, Tarnani M, Rossi D, et al. Multicentre validation of a prognostic index for overall survival in chronic lymphocytic leukaemia. *Hematol Oncol* 2011;29:91–99.
297. Antic D, Mihaljevic B, Cokic V, et al. Patients with early stage chronic lymphocytic leukemia: new risk stratification based on molecular profiling. *Leuk Lymphoma* 2011;52:1394–1397.
298. Wierda WG, O'Brien S, Wang X, et al. Multivariable model for time to first treatment in patients with chronic lymphocytic leukemia. *J Clin Oncol* 2011;29:4088–4095.
299. Klein U, Tu Y, Stolovitzky GA, et al. Gene expression profiling of B cell chronic lymphocytic leukemia reveals a homogeneous phenotype related to memory B cells. *J Exp Med* 2001;194:1625–1638.
300. Rosenwald A, Alizadeh AA, Widhopf G, et al. Relation of gene expression phenotype to immunoglobulin mutation genotype in B cell chronic lymphocytic leukemia. *J Exp Med* 2001;194:1639–1647.
301. Chiorazzi N, Ferrarini M. Cellular origin(s) of chronic lymphocytic leukemia: cautionary notes and additional considerations and possibilities. *Blood* 2011;117:1781–1791.
302. Freedman AS, Nadler LM. The relationship of chronic lymphocytic leukemia to normal activated B cells. *Leuk Lymphoma* 1990;1:293–300.
303. Caligaris-Cappio F, Riva M, Tesio L, et al. Human normal CD5+ B lymphocytes can be induced to differentiate to CD5- B lymphocytes with germinal center cell features. *Blood* 1989;73:1259–1263.
304. Kikushige Y, Ishikawa F, Miyamoto T, et al. Self-renewing hematopoietic stem cell is the primary target in pathogenesis of human chronic lymphocytic leukemia. *Cancer Cell* 2011;20:246–259.
305. Alizadeh AA, Majeti R. Surprise! HSC are aberrant in chronic lymphocytic leukemia. *Cancer Cell* 2011;20:135–136.
306. Szankasi P, Bahler DW. Clinical laboratory analysis of immunoglobulin heavy chain variable region genes for chronic lymphocytic leukemia prognosis. *J Mol Diagn* 2010;12:244–249.
307. Murray F, Darzentas N, Hadzidimitriou A, et al. Stereotyped patterns of somatic hypermutation in subsets of patients with chronic lymphocytic leukemia: implications for the role of antigen selection in leukemogenesis. *Blood* 2008;111:1524–1533.
308. Stamatopoulos K, Belessi C, Moreno C, et al. Over 20% of patients with chronic lymphocytic leukemia carry stereotyped receptors: pathogenetic implications and clinical correlations. *Blood* 2007;109:259–270.
309. Widhopf GF II, Rassenti LZ, Toy TL, et al. Chronic lymphocytic leukemia B cells of more than 1% of patients express virtually identical immunoglobulins. *Blood* 2004;104:2499–2504.
310. Chu CC, Catera R, Hatzi K, et al. Chronic lymphocytic leukemia antibodies with a common stereotypic rearrangement recognize nonmuscle myosin heavy chain IIA. *Blood* 2008;112:5122–5129.
311. Chu CC, Catera R, Zhang L, et al. Many chronic lymphocytic leukemia antibodies recognize apoptotic cells with exposed nonmuscle myosin heavy chain IIA: implications for patient outcome and cell of origin. *Blood* 2010;115:3907–3915.
312. Catera R, Silverman GJ, Hatzi K, et al. Chronic lymphocytic leukemia cells recognize conserved epitopes associated with apoptosis and oxidation. *Mol Med* 2008;14:665–674.
313. Binder M, Lechenne B, Ummanni R, et al. Stereotypical chronic lymphocytic leukemia B-cell receptors recognize survival promoting antigens on stromal cells. *PLoS One* 2010;5:e15992.
314. Dal-Bo M, Del Giudice I, Bomben R, et al. B-cell receptor, clinical course and prognosis in chronic lymphocytic leukaemia: the growing saga of the IGHV3 subgroup gene usage. *Br J Haematol* 2011;153:3–14.
315. Steininger C, Widhopf GF II, Ghia EM, et al. Recombinant antibodies encoded by IGHV1–69 react with pUL32, a phosphoprotein of cytomegalovirus and B-cell superantigen. *Blood* 2012;119:2293–2301.
316. Lanemo Myhrinder A, Hellqvist E, Sidorova E, et al. A new perspective: molecular motifs on oxidized LDL, apoptotic cells, and bacteria are targets for chronic lymphocytic leukemia antibodies. *Blood* 2008;111:3838–3848.
317. Petlickovski A, Laurenti L, Li X, et al. Sustained signaling through the B-cell receptor induces Mcl-1 and promotes survival of chronic lymphocytic leukemia B cells. *Blood* 2005;105:4820–4827.
318. Coscia M, Pantaleoni F, Riganti C, et al. IGHV unmutated CLL B cells are more prone to spontaneous apoptosis and subject to environmental prosurvival signals than mutated CLL B cells. *Leukemia* 2011;25:828–837.
319. Stevenson FK, Krysov S, Davies AJ, et al. B-cell receptor signaling in chronic lymphocytic leukemia. *Blood* 2011;118:4313–4320.
320. Packham G, Stevenson F. The role of the B-cell receptor in the pathogenesis of chronic lymphocytic leukaemia. *Semin Cancer Biol* 2010;20:391–399.
321. Kerber RA, O'Brien E. A cohort study of cancer risk in relation to family histories of cancer in the Utah population database. *Cancer* 2005;103:1906–1915.
322. Neuland CY, Blattner WA, Mann DL, et al. Familial chronic lymphocytic leukemia. *J Natl Cancer Inst* 1983;71:1143–1150.
323. Conley CL, Misiti J, Laster AJ. Genetic factors predisposing to chronic lymphocytic leukemia and to autoimmune disease. *Medicine (Baltimore)* 1980;59:323–334.
324. Marti GE, Carter P, Abbasi F, et al. B-cell monoclonal lymphocytosis and B-cell abnormalities in the setting of familial B-cell chronic lymphocytic leukemia. *Cytometry B Clin Cytom* 2003;52:1–12.
325. Rawstron AC, Yuille MR, Fuller J, et al. Inherited predisposition to CLL is detectable as subclinical monoclonal B-lymphocyte expansion. *Blood* 2002;100:2289–2290.
326. Cartwright RA, Bernard SM, Bird CC, et al. Chronic lymphocytic leukaemia: case control epidemiological study in Yorkshire. *Br J Cancer* 1987;56:79–82.
327. Linet MS, Van Natta ML, Brookmeyer R, et al. Familial cancer history and chronic lymphocytic leukemia. A case-control study. *Am J Epidemiol* 1989;130:655–664.
328. Goldin LR, Pfeiffer RM, Li X, et al. Familial risk of lymphoproliferative tumors in families of patients with chronic lymphocytic leukemia: results from the Swedish Family-Cancer Database. *Blood* 2004;104:1850–1854.
329. Pottern LM, Linet M, Blair A, et al. Familial cancers associated with subtypes of leukemia and non-Hodgkin's lymphoma. *Leuk Res* 1991;15:305–314.
330. Goldin LR, Bjorkholm M, Kristinsson SY, et al. Elevated risk of chronic lymphocytic leukemia and other indolent non-Hodgkin's lymphomas among relatives of patients with chronic lymphocytic leukemia. *Haematologica* 2009;94:647–653.
331. Di Bernardo MC, Crowther-Swanepoel D, Broderick P, et al. A genome-wide association study identifies six susceptibility loci for chronic lymphocytic leukemia. *Nat Genet* 2008;40:1204–1210.
332. Crowther-Swanepoel D, Broderick P, Di Bernardo MC, et al. Common variants at 2q37.3, 8q24.21, 15q21.3 and 16q24.1 influence chronic lymphocytic leukemia risk. *Nat Genet* 2010;42:132–136.
333. Slager SL, Rabe KG, Achenbach SJ, et al. Genome-wide association study identifies a novel susceptibility locus at 6p21.3 among familial CLL. *Blood* 2011;117:1911–1916.
334. Slager SL, Goldin LR, Strom SS, et al. Genetic susceptibility variants for chronic lymphocytic leukemia. *Cancer Epidemiol Biomarkers Prev* 2010;19:1098–1102.
335. Crowther-Swanepoel D, Mansouri M, Enjuanes A, et al. Verification that common variation at 2q37.1, 6p25.3, 11q24.1, 15q23, and 19q13.32 influences chronic lymphocytic leukaemia risk. *Br J Haematol* 2010;150:473–479.
336. Gualco G, Weiss LM, Bacchi CE. MUM1/IRF4: a review. *Appl Immunohistochem Mol Morphol* 2010;18:301–310.
337. Crowther-Swanepoel D, Qureshi M, Dyer MJ, et al. Genetic variation in CXCR4 and risk of chronic lymphocytic leukemia. *Blood* 2009;114:4843–4846.
338. Sellick GS, Goldin LR, Wild RW, et al. A high-density SNP genome-wide linkage search of 206 families identifies susceptibility loci for chronic lymphocytic leukemia. *Blood* 2007;110:3326–3333.
339. Skowronska A, Austen B, Powell JE, et al. ATM germline heterozygosity does not play a role in chronic lymphocytic leukemia initiation but influences rapid disease progression through loss of the remaining ATM allele. *Haematologica* 2012;97:142–146.
340. Raval A, Tanner SM, Byrd JC, et al. Downregulation of death-associated protein kinase 1 (DAPK1) in chronic lymphocytic leukemia. *Cell* 2007;129:879–890.
341. Martin-Guerrero I, Enjuanes A, Richter J, et al. A putative "hepitype" in the ATM gene associated with chronic lymphocytic leukemia risk. *Genes Chromosomes Cancer* 2011;50:887–895.
342. Bouyge-Moreau I, Rondeau G, Avet-Loiseau H, et al. Construction of a 780-kb PAC, BAC, and cosmid contig encompassing the minimal critical deletion involved in B cell chronic lymphocytic leukemia at 13q14.3. *Genomics* 1997;46:183–190.
343. Calin GA, Dumitru CD, Shimizu M, et al. Frequent deletions and down-regulation of micro- RNA genes miR15 and miR16 at 13q14 in chronic lymphocytic leukemia. *Proc Natl Acad Sci U S A* 2002;99:15524–15529.
344. Lee SK, Calin GA. Non-coding RNAs and cancer: new paradigms in oncology. *Discov Med* 2011;11:245–254.
345. Pekarsky Y, Zanesi N, Croce CM. Molecular basis of CLL. *Semin Cancer Biol* 2010;20:370–376.
346. Cimmino A, Calin GA, Fabbri M, et al. miR-15 and miR-16 induce apoptosis by targeting BCL2. *Proc Natl Acad Sci U S A* 2005;102:13944–13949.
347. Calin GA, Cimmino A, Fabbri M, et al. MiR-15a and miR-16–1 cluster functions in human leukemia. *Proc Natl Acad Sci U S A* 2008;105:5166–5171.
348. Raveche ES, Salerno E, Scaglione BJ, et al. Abnormal microRNA-16 locus with synteny to human 13q14 linked to CLL in NZB mice. *Blood* 2007;109:5079–5086.
349. Klein U, Lia M, Crespo M, et al. The DLEU2/miR-15a/16–1 cluster controls B cell proliferation and its deletion leads to chronic lymphocytic leukemia. *Cancer Cell* 2010;17:28–40.
350. Lia M, Carette A, Tang H, et al. Functional dissection of the chromosome 13q14 tumor suppressor locus using transgenic mouse lines. *Blood* 2011;119:2981–2990.
351. Mian M, Rinaldi A, Mensah AA, et al. Del(13q14.3) length matters: an integrated analysis of genomic, fluorescence *in situ* hybridization and clinical data in 169 chronic lymphocytic leukaemia patients with 13q deletion alone or a normal karyotype. *Hematol Oncol* 2011;30(1):46–49.
352. Dal Bo M, Rossi FM, Rossi D, et al. 13q14 deletion size and number of deleted cells both influence prognosis in chronic lymphocytic leukemia. *Genes Chromosomes Cancer* 2011;50:633–643.
353. Ouillette P, Erba H, Kujawski L, et al. Integrated genomic profiling of chronic lymphocytic leukemia identifies subtypes of deletion 13q14. *Cancer Res* 2008;68:1012–1021.
354. Parker H, Rose-Zerilli MJ, Parker A, et al. 13q deletion anatomy and disease progression in patients with chronic lymphocytic leukemia. *Leukemia* 2011;25:489–497.
355. Ouillette P, Collins R, Shakhan S, et al. The prognostic significance of various 13q14 deletions in chronic lymphocytic leukemia. *Clin Cancer Res* 2011;17:6778–6790.
356. Palamarchuk A, Efanov A, Nazaryan N, et al. 13q14 deletions in CLL involve cooperating tumor suppressors. *Blood* 2010;115:3916–3922.
357. Garg R, Wierda W, Ferrajoli A, et al. The prognostic difference of monoallelic versus biallelic deletion of 13q in chronic lymphocytic leukemia. *Cancer* 2011;118(14):3531–3537.

358. Gumy-Pause F, Wacker P, Sappino AP. ATM gene and lymphoid malignancies. *Leukemia* 2004;18:238–242.
359. Austen B, Powell JE, Alvi A, et al. Mutations in the ATM gene lead to impaired overall and treatment-free survival that is independent of IGVH mutation status in patients with B-CLL. *Blood* 2005;106:3175–3182.
360. Stankovic T, Stewart GS, Fegan C, et al. Ataxia telangiectasia mutated-deficient B-cell chronic lymphocytic leukemia occurs in pregerminal center cells and results in defective damage response and unrepaired chromosome damage. *Blood* 2002;99:300–309.
361. Austen B, Skowronska A, Baker C, et al. Mutation status of the residual ATM allele is an important determinant of the cellular response to chemotherapy and survival in patients with chronic lymphocytic leukemia containing an 11q deletion. *J Clin Oncol* 2007;25:5448–5457.
362. Guarini A, Marinelli M, Tavolaro S, et al. ATM gene alterations in chronic lymphocytic leukemia patients induce a distinct gene expression profile and predict disease progression. *Haematologica* 2012;97:47–55.
363. Kalla C, Scheuermann MO, Kube I, et al. Analysis of 11q22-q23 deletion target genes in B-cell chronic lymphocytic leukaemia: evidence for a pathogenic role of NPAT, CUL5, and PPP2R1B. *Eur J Cancer* 2007;43:1328–1335.
364. Fabbri M, Bottoni A, Shimizu M, et al. Association of a microRNA/TP53 feedback circuitry with pathogenesis and outcome of B-cell chronic lymphocytic leukemia. *JAMA* 2011;305:59–67.
365. Zenz T, Mertens D, Dohner H, et al. Importance of genetics in chronic lymphocytic leukemia. *Blood Rev* 2011;25:131–137.
366. Hallek M, Fischer K, Fingerle-Rowson G, et al. Addition of rituximab to fludarabine and cyclophosphamide in patients with chronic lymphocytic leukaemia: a randomised, open-label, phase 3 trial. *Lancet* 2010;376:1164–1174.
367. Mraz M, Pospisilova S, Malinova K, et al. MicroRNAs in chronic lymphocytic leukemia pathogenesis and disease subtypes. *Leuk Lymphoma* 2009;50:506–509.
368. Merkel O, Asslaber D, Pinon JD, et al. Interdependent regulation of p53 and miR-34a in chronic lymphocytic leukemia. *Cell Cycle* 2010;9:2764–2768.
369. Zenz T, Mohr J, Eldering E, et al. miR-34a as part of the resistance network in chronic lymphocytic leukemia. *Blood* 2009;113:3801–3808.
370. Zenz T, Habe S, Denzel T, et al. Detailed analysis of p53 pathway defects in fludarabine-refractory chronic lymphocytic leukemia (CLL): dissecting the contribution of 17p deletion, TP53 mutation, p53-p21 dysfunction, and miR34a in a prospective clinical trial. *Blood* 2009;114:2589–2597.
371. Merup M, Juliusson G, Wu X, et al. Amplification of multiple regions of chromosome 12, including 12q13–15, in chronic lymphocytic leukaemia. *Eur J Haematol* 1997;58:174–180.
372. O'Connor SJ, Su'ut L, Morgan GJ, et al. The relationship between typical and atypical B-cell chronic lymphocytic leukemia. A comparative genomic hybridization-based study. *Am J Clin Pathol* 2000;114:448–458.
373. Wang L, Lawrence MS, Wan Y, et al. SF3B1 and other novel cancer genes in chronic lymphocytic leukemia. *N Engl J Med* 2011;365:2497–2506.
374. Villanueva MT. Genetics: splicing the pieces of the chronic lymphocytic leukemia puzzle. *Nat Rev Clin Oncol* 2011;9:66.
375. Puente XS, Pinyol M, Quesada V, et al. Whole-genome sequencing identifies recurrent mutations in chronic lymphocytic leukaemia. *Nature* 2011;475:101–105.
376. Pfeifer D, Pantic M, Skatulla I, et al. Genome-wide analysis of DNA copy number changes and LOH in CLL using high-density SNP arrays. *Blood* 2007;109:1202–1210.
377. Yin CC, Lin KI, Ketterling RP, et al. Chronic lymphocytic leukemia with t(2;14)(p16;q32) involves the BCL11A and IgH genes and is associated with atypical morphologic features and unmutated IgVH genes. *Am J Clin Pathol* 2009;131:663–670.
378. Bichi R, Shinton SA, Martin ES, et al. Human chronic lymphocytic leukemia modeled in mouse by targeted TCL1 expression. *Proc Natl Acad Sci U S A* 2002;99:6955–6960.
379. Pekarsky Y, Santanam U, Cimmino A, et al. Tcl1 expression in chronic lymphocytic leukemia is regulated by miR-29 and miR-181. *Cancer Res* 2006;66:11590–11593.
380. Palamarchuk A, Yan PS, Zanesi N, et al. Tcl1 protein functions as an inhibitor of *de novo* DNA methylation in B-cell chronic lymphocytic leukemia (CLL). *Proc Natl Acad Sci U S A* 2012.
381. Pekarsky Y, Palamarchuk A, Maximov V, et al. Tcl1 functions as a transcriptional regulator and is directly involved in the pathogenesis of CLL. *Proc Natl Acad Sci U S A* 2008;105:19643–19648.
382. Ghia P, Chiorazzi N, Stamatopoulos K. Microenvironmental influences in chronic lymphocytic leukaemia: the role of antigen stimulation. *J Intern Med* 2008;264:549–562.
383. Burger JA. Nurture versus nature: the microenvironment in chronic lymphocytic leukemia. *Hematol Am Soc Hematol Educ Prog* 2011;2011:96–103.
384. Munk Pedersen I, Reed J. Microenvironmental interactions and survival of CLL B-cells. *Leuk Lymphoma* 2004;45:2365–2372.
385. Ferretti E, Bertolotto M, Deaglio S, et al. A novel role of the CX3CR1/CX3CL1 system in the cross-talk between chronic lymphocytic leukemia cells and tumor microenvironment. *Leukemia* 2011;25:1268–1277.
386. Ysebaert L, Fournie JJ. Genomic and phenotypic characterization of nurse-like cells that promote drug resistance in chronic lymphocytic leukemia. *Leuk Lymphoma* 2011;52:1404–1406.
387. Burger M, Hartmann T, Krome M, et al. Small peptide inhibitors of the CXCR4 chemokine receptor (CD184) antagonize the activation, migration, and antiapoptotic responses of CXCL12 in chronic lymphocytic leukemia B cells. *Blood* 2005;106:1824–1830.
388. Hayden RE, Pratt G, Roberts C, et al. Treatment of chronic lymphocytic leukemia requires targeting of the protective lymph node environment with novel therapeutic approaches. *Leuk Lymphoma* 2011;53(4):537–549.
389. Balogh Z, Reiniger L, Rajnai H, et al. High rate of neoplastic cells with genetic abnormalities in proliferation centers of chronic lymphocytic leukemia. *Leuk Lymphoma* 2011;52:1080–1084.
390. Rawstron AC, Shanafelt T, Lanasa MC, et al. Different biology and clinical outcome according to the absolute numbers of clonal B-cells in monoclonal B-cell lymphocytosis (MBL). *Cytometry B Clin Cytom* 2010;78 Suppl 1:S19–S23.
391. Molica S, Levato D. What is changing in the natural history of chronic lymphocytic leukemia? *Haematologica* 2001;86:8–12.
392. Dighiero G, Maloum K, Desablens B, et al. Chlorambucil in indolent chronic lymphocytic leukemia. French Cooperative Group on Chronic Lymphocytic Leukemia. *N Engl J Med* 1998;338:1506–1514.
393. Shustik C, Mick R, Silver R, et al. Treatment of early chronic lymphocytic leukemia: intermittent chlorambucil versus observation. *Hematol Oncol* 1988;6:7–12.
394. Effects of chlorambucil and therapeutic decision in initial forms of chronic lymphocytic leukemia (stage A): results of a randomized clinical trial on 612 patients. The French Cooperative Group on Chronic Lymphocytic Leukemia. *Blood* 1990;75:1414–1421.
395. Chemotherapeutic options in chronic lymphocytic leukemia: a meta-analysis of the randomized trials. CLL Trialists' Collaborative Group. *J Natl Cancer Inst* 1999;91:861–868.
396. Eichhorst BF, Busch R, Hopfinger G, et al. Fludarabine plus cyclophosphamide versus fludarabine alone in first-line therapy of younger patients with chronic lymphocytic leukemia. *Blood* 2006;107:885–891.
397. Flinn IW, Neuberg DS, Grever MR, et al. Phase III trial of fludarabine plus cyclophosphamide compared with fludarabine for patients with previously untreated chronic lymphocytic leukemia: US Intergroup Trial E2997. *J Clin Oncol* 2007;25:793–798.
398. Catovsky D, Richards S, Matutes E, et al. Assessment of fludarabine plus cyclophosphamide for patients with chronic lymphocytic leukaemia (the LRF CLL4 Trial): a randomised controlled trial. *Lancet* 2007;370:230–239.
399. Byrd JC, Rai K, Peterson BL, et al. Addition of rituximab to fludarabine may prolong progression-free survival and overall survival in patients with previously untreated chronic lymphocytic leukemia: an updated retrospective comparative analysis of CALGB 9712 and CALGB 9011. *Blood* 2005;105:49–53.
400. Tam CS, O'Brien S, Wierda W, et al. Long-term results of the fludarabine, cyclophosphamide, and rituximab regimen as initial therapy of chronic lymphocytic leukemia. *Blood* 2008;112:975–980.
401. Keating MJ, O'Brien S, Albitar M, et al. Early results of a chemoimmunotherapy regimen of fludarabine, cyclophosphamide, and rituximab as initial therapy for chronic lymphocytic leukemia. *J Clin Oncol* 2005;23:4079–4088.
402. Wierda W, O'Brien S, Wen S, et al. Chemoimmunotherapy with fludarabine, cyclophosphamide, and rituximab for relapsed and refractory chronic lymphocytic leukemia. *J Clin Oncol* 2005;23:4070–4078.
403. Molica S. Progress in the treatment of chronic lymphocytic leukemia: results of the German CLL8 trial. *Expert Rev Anticancer Ther* 2011;11:1333–1340.
404. Gribben JG. Are prognostic factors in CLL overrated? *Oncology (Williston Park)* 2011;25:703–706.
405. Uhrmacher S, Erdfelder F, Kreuzer KA. Flow cytometry and polymerase chain reaction-based analyses of minimal residual disease in chronic lymphocytic leukemia. *Adv Hematol* 2010;2010.
406. Varghese AM, Rawstron AC, Hillmen P. Eradicating minimal residual disease in chronic lymphocytic leukemia: should this be the goal of treatment? *Curr Hematol Malig Rep* 2010;5:35–44.
407. Zhou Y, Tang G, Medeiros LJ, et al. Therapy-related myeloid neoplasms following fludarabine, cyclophosphamide, and rituximab (FCR) treatment in patients with chronic lymphocytic leukemia/small lymphocytic lymphoma. *Mod Pathol* 2012;25:237–245.
408. Smith MR, Neuberg D, Flinn IW, et al. Incidence of therapy-related myeloid neoplasia after initial therapy for chronic lymphocytic leukemia with fludarabine-cyclophosphamide versus fludarabine: long-term follow-up of US Intergroup Study E2997. *Blood* 2011;118:3525–3527.
409. Dreger P, Corradini P, Kimby E, et al. Indications for allogeneic stem cell transplantation in chronic lymphocytic leukemia: the EBMT transplant consensus. *Leukemia* 2007;21:12–17.
410. Gladstone DE, Fuchs E. Hematopoietic stem cell transplantation for chronic lymphocytic leukemia. *Curr Opin Oncol* 2012;24(2):176–181.
411. Hillmen P. Targeted therapy for chronic lymphocytic leukemia: a glimpse into the future. *J Clin Oncol* 2011;30(5):469–470.
412. Roberts AW, Seymour JF, Brown JR, et al. Substantial susceptibility of chronic lymphocytic leukemia to BCL2 inhibition: results of a phase I study of navitoclax in patients with relapsed or refractory disease. *J Clin Oncol* 2011;30(5):488–496.
413. Tadmor T, Polliack A. Optimal management of older patients with chronic lymphocytic leukemia: some facts and principles guiding therapeutic choices. *Blood Rev* 2012;26:15–23.
414. Del Giudice I, Mauro FR, Foa R. Chronic lymphocytic leukemia in less fit patients: "slow-go". *Leuk Lymphoma* 2011;52:2207–2216.
415. Badoux XC, Keating MJ, Wen S, et al. Lenalidomide as initial therapy of elderly patients with chronic lymphocytic leukemia. *Blood* 2011;118:3489–3498.
416. Shanafelt TD, Rabe KG, Kay NE, et al. Age at diagnosis and the utility of prognostic testing in patients with chronic lymphocytic leukemia. *Cancer* 2010;116:4777–4787.
417. Tsimberidou AM, Tam C, Abruzzo LV, et al. Chemoimmunotherapy may overcome the adverse prognostic significance of 11q deletion in previously untreated patients with chronic lymphocytic leukemia. *Cancer* 2009;115:373–380.
418. Stilgenbauer S, Dohner H. Campath-1H-induced complete remission of chronic lymphocytic leukemia despite p53 gene mutation and resistance to chemotherapy. *N Engl J Med* 2002;347:452–453.
419. Lozanski G, Heerema NA, Flinn IW, et al. Alemtuzumab is an effective therapy for chronic lymphocytic leukemia with p53 mutations and deletions. *Blood* 2004;103:3278–3281.
420. Hillmen P, Skotnicki AB, Robak T, et al. Alemtuzumab compared with chlorambucil as first-line therapy for chronic lymphocytic leukemia. *J Clin Oncol* 2007;25:5616–5623.
421. Keating MJ, Flinn I, Jain V, et al. Therapeutic role of alemtuzumab (Campath-1H) in patients who have failed fludarabine: results of a large international study. *Blood* 2002;99:3554–3561.
422. Parikh SA, Keating MJ, O'Brien S, et al. Frontline chemoimmunotherapy with fludarabine, cyclophosphamide, alemtuzumab, and rituximab for high-risk chronic lymphocytic leukemia. *Blood* 2011;118:2062–2068.
423. Tam CS, Shanafelt TD, Wierda WG, et al. *De novo* deletion 17p13.1 chronic lymphocytic leukemia shows significant clinical heterogeneity: the M. D. Anderson and Mayo Clinic experience. *Blood* 2009;114:957–964.
424. Rossi D, Fangazio M, Rasi S, et al. Disruption of BIRC3 associates with fludarabine chemorefractoriness in TP53 wild type chronic lymphocytic leukemia. *Blood* 2012;119(12):2854–2862.
425. Griffiths H, Brennan V, Lea J, et al. Crossover study of immunoglobulin replacement therapy in patients with low-grade B-cell tumors. *Blood* 1989;73:366–368.
426. Raanani P, Gafter-Gvili A, Paul M, et al. Immunoglobulin prophylaxis in chronic lymphocytic leukemia and multiple myeloma: systematic review and meta-analysis. *Leuk Lymphoma* 2009;50:764–772.

427. Intravenous immunoglobulin for the prevention of infection in chronic lymphocytic leukemia. A randomized, controlled clinical trial. Cooperative Group for the Study of Immunoglobulin in Chronic Lymphocytic Leukemia. *N Engl J Med* 1988; 319:902–907.
428. Ghani AM, Krause JR, Brody JP. Prolymphocytic transformation of chronic lymphocytic leukemia. A report of three cases and review of the literature. *Cancer* 1986;57:75–80.
429. Kjeldsberg CR, Marty J. Prolymphocytic transformation of chronic lymphocytic leukemia. *Cancer* 1981;48:2447–2457.
430. Economopoulos T, Fotopoulos S, Hatzioannou J, et al. 'Prolymphocytoid' cells in chronic lymphocytic leukaemia and their prognostic significance. *Scand J Haematol* 1982;28:238–242.
431. Enno A, Catovsky D, O'Brien M, et al. 'Prolymphocytoid' transformation of chronic lymphocytic leukaemia. *Br J Haematol* 1979;41:9–18.
432. Roberts JD, Tindle BH, MacPherson BR. Prolymphocytic transformation of chronic lymphocytic leukemia: a case report of lengthy survival after intensive chemotherapy. *Am J Hematol* 1989;31:131–132.
433. Scott CS, Stark AN, Head C, et al. Diagnostic features and survival in typical and prolymphocytoid variants of chronic lymphocytic leukemia. *Hematol Oncol* 1989;7:175–179.
434. Reiniger L, Bodor C, Bognar A, et al. Richter's and prolymphocytic transformation of chronic lymphocytic leukemia are associated with high mRNA expression of activation-induced cytidine deaminase and aberrant somatic hypermutation. *Leukemia* 2006;20:1089–1095.
435. Giardino AA, O'Regan K, Jagannathan JP, et al. Richter's transformation of chronic lymphocytic leukemia. *J Clin Oncol* 2011;29:e274–e276.
436. Flandrin G. Richter's syndrome. In: Polliack A, Catovsky D, eds. *Chronic lymphocytic leukemia.* New York: Harwood Academic Publishers, 1988:209–218.
437. Bertoli LF, Kubagawa H, Borzillo GV, et al. Analysis with antiidiotype antibody of a patient with chronic lymphocytic leukemia and a large cell lymphoma (Richter's syndrome). *Blood* 1987;70:45–50.
438. Bayliss KM, Kueck BD, Hanson CA, et al. Richter's syndrome presenting as primary central nervous system lymphoma. Transformation of an identical clone. *Am J Clin Pathol* 1990;93:117–123.
439. Richter MN. Generalized reticular cell sarcoma of lymph nodes associated with lymphatic leukemia. *Am J Pathol* 1928;4:285–292 287.
440. Foucar K, Rydell RE. Richter's syndrome in chronic lymphocytic leukemia. *Cancer* 1980;46:118–134.
441. Strauchen JA, May MM, Crown J. Large cell transformation of subclinical small lymphocytic leukemia/lymphoma: a variant of Richter's syndrome. *Hematol Oncol* 1987;5:167–174.
442. Brecher M, Banks PM. Hodgkin's disease variant of Richter's syndrome. Report of eight cases. *Am J Clin Pathol* 1990;93:333–339.
443. Michiels JJ, van Dongen JJ, Hagemeijer A, et al. Richter's syndrome with identical immunoglobulin gene rearrangements in the chronic lymphocytic leukemia and the supervening non-Hodgkin lymphoma. *Leukemia* 1989;3:819–824.
444. Lane PK, Townsend RM, Beckstead JH, et al. Central nervous system involvement in a patient with chronic lymphocytic leukemia and non-Hodgkin's lymphoma (Richter's syndrome), with concordant cell surface immunoglobulin isotypic and immunophenotypic markers. *Am J Clin Pathol* 1988;89:254–259.
445. Cherepakhin V, Baird SM, Meisenholder GW, et al. Common clonal origin of chronic lymphocytic leukemia and high-grade lymphoma of Richter's syndrome. *Blood* 1993;82:3141–3147.
446. Momose H, Jaffe ES, Shin SS, et al. Chronic lymphocytic leukemia/small lymphocytic lymphoma with Reed-Sternberg-like cells and possible transformation to Hodgkin's disease. Mediation by Epstein-Barr virus. *Am J Surg Pathol* 1992; 16:859–867.
447. Nakamine H, Masih AS, Sanger WG, et al. Richter's syndrome with different immunoglobulin light chain types. Molecular and cytogenetic features indicate a common clonal origin. *Am J Clin Pathol* 1992;97:656–663.
448. Miyamura K, Osada H, Yamauchi T, et al. Single clonal origin of neoplastic B-cells with different immunoglobulin light chains in a patient with Richter's syndrome. *Cancer* 1990;66:140–144.
449. Sun T, Susin M, Desner M, et al. The clonal origin of two cell populations in Richter's syndrome. *Hum Pathol* 1990;21:722–728.
450. Matolcsy A, Inghirami G, Knowles DM. Molecular genetic demonstration of the diverse evolution of Richter's syndrome (chronic lymphocytic leukemia and subsequent large cell lymphoma). *Blood* 1994;83:1363–1372.
451. Fayad L, Robertson LE, O'Brien S, et al. Hodgkin's disease variant of Richter's syndrome: experience at a single institution. *Leuk Lymphoma* 1996;23:333–337.
452. Ohno T, Smir BN, Weisenburger DD, et al. Origin of the Hodgkin/Reed-Sternberg cells in chronic lymphocytic leukemia with "Hodgkin's transformation". *Blood* 1998;91:1757–1761.
453. Bruzzi JF, Macapinlac H, Tsimberidou AM, et al. Detection of Richter's transformation of chronic lymphocytic leukemia by PET/CT. *J Nucl Med* 2006;47: 1267–1273.
454. Mao Z, Quintanilla-Martinez L, Raffeld M, et al. IgVH mutational status and clonality analysis of Richter's transformation: diffuse large B-cell lymphoma and Hodgkin lymphoma in association with B-cell chronic lymphocytic leukemia (B-CLL) represent 2 different pathways of disease evolution. *Am J Surg Pathol* 2007;31:1605–1614.
455. Molica S. A systematic review on Richter syndrome: what is the published evidence? *Leuk Lymphoma* 2010;51:415–421.
456. Scandurra M, Rossi D, Deambrogi C, et al. Genomic profiling of Richter's syndrome: recurrent lesions and differences with *de novo* diffuse large B-cell lymphomas. *Hematol Oncol* 2010;28:62–67.
457. van Dongen JJ, Hooijkaas H, Michiels JJ, et al. Richter's syndrome with different immunoglobulin light chains and different heavy chain gene rearrangements. *Blood* 1984;64:571–575.
458. Foo WC, Huang Q, Sebastian S, et al. Concurrent classical Hodgkin lymphoma and plasmablastic lymphoma in a patient with chronic lymphocytic leukemia/ small lymphocytic lymphoma treated with fludarabine: a dimorphic presentation of iatrogenic immunodeficiency-associated lymphoproliferative disorder with evidence suggestive of multiclonal transformability of B cells by Epstein-Barr virus. *Hum Pathol* 2010;41:1802–1808.
459. Abruzzo LV, Rosales CM, Medeiros LJ, et al. Epstein-Barr virus-positive B-cell lymphoproliferative disorders arising in immunodeficient patients previously treated with fludarabine for low-grade B-cell neoplasms. *Am J Surg Pathol* 2002;26:630–636.
460. Thornton PD, Bellas C, Santon A, et al. Richter's transformation of chronic lymphocytic leukemia. The possible role of fludarabine and the Epstein-Barr virus in its pathogenesis. *Leuk Res* 2005;29:389–395.
461. Ansell SM, Li CY, Lloyd RV, et al. Epstein-Barr virus infection in Richter's transformation. *Am J Hematol* 1999;60:99–104.
462. Timar B, Fulop Z, Csernus B, et al. Relationship between the mutational status of VH genes and pathogenesis of diffuse large B-cell lymphoma in Richter's syndrome. *Leukemia* 2004;18:326–330.
463. Fangazio M, De Paoli L, Rossi D, et al. Predictive markers and driving factors behind Richter syndrome development. *Expert Rev Anticancer Ther* 2011;11: 433–442.
464. Rossi D, Cerri M, Capello D, et al. Biological and clinical risk factors of chronic lymphocytic leukaemia transformation to Richter syndrome. *Br J Haematol* 2008; 142:202–215.
465. Fabbri G, Rasi S, Rossi D, et al. Analysis of the chronic lymphocytic leukemia coding genome: role of NOTCH1 mutational activation. *J Exp Med* 2011;208:1389–1401.
466. Rossi D, Gaidano G. Richter syndrome: molecular insights and clinical perspectives. *Hematol Oncol* 2009;27:1–10.
467. Omoti CE, Omoti AE. Richter syndrome: a review of clinical, ocular, neurological and other manifestations. *Br J Haematol* 2008;142:709–716.
468. Bockorny B, Codreanu I, Dasanu CA. Hodgkin lymphoma as Richter transformation in chronic lymphocytic leukaemia: a retrospective analysis of world literature. *Br J Haematol* 2012;156:50–66.
469. Pugh WC, Manning JT, Butler JJ. Paraimmunoblastic variant of small lymphocytic lymphoma/leukemia. *Am J Surg Pathol* 1988;12:907–917.
470. Chuang SS, Liao YL, Liou CP, et al. Chronic lymphocytic leukemia with paraimmunoblastic transformation—with comparative genomic hybridization and review of the literature. *Pathol Res Pract* 2010;206:276–281.
471. Stano-Kozubik K, Malcikova J, Tichy B, et al. Inactivation of p53 and amplification of MYCN gene in a terminal lymphoblastic relapse in a chronic lymphocytic leukemia patient. *Cancer Genet Cytogenet* 2009;189:53–58.
472. Torelli UL, Torelli GM, Emilia G, et al. Simultaneously increased expression of the c-myc and mu chain genes in the acute blastic transformation of a chronic lymphocytic leukaemia. *Br J Haematol* 1987;65:165–170.
473. Zarrabi MH, Grunwald HW, Rosner F. Chronic lymphocytic leukemia terminating in acute leukemia. *Arch Intern Med* 1977;137:1059–1054.
474. Laurent G, Gourdin MF, Flandrin G, et al. Acute blast crisis in a patient with chronic lymphocytic leukemia. Immunoperoxidase study. *Acta Haematol* 1981;65:60–66.
475. Frenkel EP, Ligler FS, Graham MS, et al. Acute lymphocytic leukemic transformation of chronic lymphocytic leukemia: substantiation by flow cytometry. *Am J Hematol* 1981;10:391–398.
476. Januszewicz E, Cooper IA, Pilkington G, et al. Blastic transformation of chronic lymphocytic leukemia. *Am J Hematol* 1983;15:399–402.
477. Asou N, Osato M, Horikawa K, et al. Burkitt's type acute lymphoblastic transformation associated with t(8;14) in a case of B cell chronic lymphocytic leukemia. *Leukemia* 1997;11:1986–1988.
478. Fermand JP, James JM, Herait P, et al. Associated chronic lymphocytic leukemia and multiple myeloma: origin from a single clone. *Blood* 1985;66:291–293.
479. Brouet JC, Fermand JP, Laurent G, et al. The association of chronic lymphocytic leukaemia and multiple myeloma: a study of eleven patients. *Br J Haematol* 1985;59:55–66.
480. Saltman DL, Ross JA, Banks RE, et al. Molecular evidence for a single clonal origin in biphenotypic concomitant chronic lymphocytic leukemia and multiple myeloma. *Blood* 1989;74:2062–2065.
481. Aktan M, Akkaya A, Dogan O, et al. Chronic lymphocytic leukemia and multiple myeloma in the same patient: case report. *Leuk Lymphoma* 2003;44:1421–1424.
482. Fraser CR, Wang W, Gomez M, et al. Transformation of chronic lymphocytic leukemia/small lymphocytic lymphoma to interdigitating dendritic cell sarcoma: evidence for transdifferentiation of the lymphoma clone. *Am J Clin Pathol* 2009;132:928–939.
483. Shao H, Xi L, Raffeld M, et al. Clonally related histiocytic/dendritic cell sarcoma and chronic lymphocytic leukemia/small lymphocytic lymphoma: a study of seven cases. *Mod Pathol* 2011;24:1421–1432.
484. Troussard X, Cornet E, Lesesve JF, et al. Polyclonal B-cell lymphocytosis with binucleated lymphocytes (PPBL). *Onco Targets Ther* 2008;1:59–66.
485. Delage R, Jacques L, Massinga-Loembe M, et al. Persistent polyclonal B-cell lymphocytosis: further evidence for a genetic disorder associated with B-cell abnormalities. *Br J Haematol* 2001;114:666–670.
486. Hsi ED, Hoeltge G, Tubbs RR. Biclonal chronic lymphocytic leukemia. *Am J Clin Pathol* 2000;113:798–804.
487. Xu D. Dual surface immunoglobulin light-chain expression in B-cell lymphoproliferative disorders. *Arch Pathol Lab Med* 2006;130:853–856.
488. Ho AK, Hill S, Preobrazhensky SN, et al. Small B-cell neoplasms with typical mantle cell lymphoma immunophenotypes often include chronic lymphocytic leukemias. *Am J Clin Pathol* 2009;131:27–32.
489. Mozos A, Royo C, Hartmann E, et al. SOX11 expression is highly specific for mantle cell lymphoma and identifies the cyclin D1-negative subtype. *Haematologica* 2009;94:1555–1562.
490. Galton DA, Goldman JM, Wiltshaw E, et al. Prolymphocytic leukaemia. *Br J Haematol* 1974;27:7–23.
491. Campo E, Catovsky D, Montserrat E, et al. B-cell prolymphocytic leukemia. In: Swerdlow SH, Campo E, Harris NL, et al., eds. *WHO classification of tumours of haematopoietic and lymphoid tissues.* Lyon: International Agency for Research on Cancer, 2008:183–184.
492. Del Giudice I, Osuji N, Dexter T, et al. B-cell prolymphocytic leukemia and chronic lymphocytic leukemia have distinctive gene expression signatures. *Leukemia* 2009;23:2160–2167.
493. Ruchlemer R, Parry-Jones N, Brito-Babapulle V, et al. B-prolymphocytic leukaemia with t(11;14) revisited: a splenomegalic form of mantle cell lymphoma evolving with leukaemia. *Br J Haematol* 2004;125:330–336.
494. Stone RM. Prolymphocytic leukemia. *Hematol Oncol Clin North Am* 1990;4:457–471.
495. Catovsky D. Prolymphocytic and hairy cell leukemia. In: Henderson ES, Lister TA, eds. *Leukemia*, 5th ed. Philadelphia: W.B. Saunders, 1990:639–660.
496. Owens MR, Strauchen JA, Rowe JM, et al. Prolymphocytic leukemia: histologic findings in atypical cases. *Hematol Oncol* 1984;2:249–257.
497. Pallesen G, Madsen M, Pedersen BB. B-prolymphocytic leukaemia—a mantle zone lymphoma? *Scand J Haematol* 1979;22:407–416.

498. Jandl JH. Prolymphocytic and hairy cell leukemias. In: Jandl JH, ed. *Blood: textbook of hematology*. Boston: Little Brown, 1996:1019–1039.

499. Logan RA, Smith NP. Cutaneous presentation of prolymphocytic leukaemia. *Br J Dermatol* 1988;118:553–558.

500. Pamuk GE, Puyan FO, Unlu E, et al. The first case of *de novo* B-cell prolymphocytic leukemia with central nervous system involvement: description of an unreported complication. *Leuk Res* 2009;33:864–867.

501. Lens D, De Schouwer PJ, Hamoudi RA, et al. p53 abnormalities in B-cell prolymphocytic leukemia. *Blood* 1997;89:2015–2023.

502. Schlette E, Bueso-Ramos C, Giles F, et al. Mature B-cell leukemias with more than 55% prolymphocytes. A heterogeneous group that includes an unusual variant of mantle cell lymphoma. *Am J Clin Pathol* 2001;115:571–581.

503. Lens D, Matutes E, Catovsky D, et al. Frequent deletions at 11q23 and 13q14 in B cell prolymphocytic leukemia (B-PLL). *Leukemia* 2000;14:427–430.

504. Lens D, Coignet LJ, Brito-Babapulle V, et al. B cell prolymphocytic leukaemia (B-PLL) with complex karyotype and concurrent abnormalities of the p53 and c-MYC gene. *Leukemia* 1999;13:873–876.

505. Brennscheidt U, Eick D, Kunzmann R, et al. Burkitt-like mutations in the c-myc gene locus in prolymphocytic leukemia. *Leukemia* 1994;8:897–902.

506. Merchant S, Schlette E, Sanger W, et al. Mature B-cell leukemias with more than 55% prolymphocytes: report of 2 cases with Burkitt lymphoma-type chromosomal translocations involving c-myc. *Arch Pathol Lab Med* 2003;127:305–309.

507. Kuriakose P, Perveen N, Maeda K, et al. Translocation (8;14)(q24;q32) as the sole cytogenetic abnormality in B-cell prolymphocytic leukemia. *Cancer Genet Cytogenet* 2004;150:156–158.

508. Crisostomo RH, Fernandez JA, Caceres W. Complex karyotype including chromosomal translocation (8;14) (q24;q32) in one case with B-cell prolymphocytic leukemia. *Leuk Res* 2007;31:699–701.

509. Davi F, Maloum K, Michel A, et al. High frequency of somatic mutations in the VH genes expressed in prolymphocytic leukemia. *Blood* 1996;88:3953–3961.

510. Dong HY, Weisberger J, Liu Z, et al. Immunophenotypic analysis of CD103+ B-lymphoproliferative disorders: hairy cell leukemia and its mimics. *Am J Clin Pathol* 2009;131:586–595.

511. Shvidel L, Shtalrid M, Bassous L, et al. B-cell prolymphocytic leukemia: a survey of 35 patients emphasizing heterogeneity, prognostic factors and evidence for a group with an indolent course. *Leuk Lymphoma* 1999;33:169–179.

512. Chow KU, Kim SZ, von Neuhoff N, et al. Clinical efficacy of immunochemotherapy with fludarabine, epirubicin and rituximab in the treatment for chronic lymphocytic leukaemia and prolymphocytic leukaemia. *Eur J Haematol* 2011;87:426–433.

513. Telek B, Batar P, Rejto L, et al. [Successful treatment of B-cell prolymphocytic leukemia (B-PLL) with FCR-Lite (fludarabine, cyclophosphamide, rituximab) protocol]. *Orv Hetil* 2010;151:1261–1263.

514. Tempescul A, Feuerbach J, Ianotto JC, et al. A combination therapy with fludarabine, mitoxantrone and rituximab induces complete immunophenotypical remission in B-cell prolymphocytic leukaemia. *Ann Hematol* 2009;88:85–88.

515. Kantarjian HM, Childs C, O'Brien S, et al. Efficacy of fludarabine, a new adenine nucleoside analogue, in patients with prolymphocytic leukemia and the prolymphocytoid variant of chronic lymphocytic leukemia. *Am J Med* 1991;90:223–228.

516. Mourad YA, Taher A, Chehal A, et al. Successful treatment of B-cell prolymphocytic leukemia with monoclonal anti-CD20 antibody. *Ann Hematol* 2004;83:319–321.

Chapter 19
Lymphoplasmacytic Lymphoma

Michiel van den Brand • J. Han van Krieken

Lymphoplasmacytic lymphoma (LPL) is a relatively rare mature B-cell lymphoma that typically involves the bone marrow, consisting of cells ranging from lymphocytes to plasma cells. It is frequently associated with a monoclonal IgM gammopathy, allowing a diagnosis of Waldenström macroglobulinemia (WM). LPL is frequently diagnosed by exclusion, because no positive marker exists. The differential diagnosis with marginal zone lymphoma can be particularly difficult, if not impossible.

DEFINITION AND HISTORICAL BACKGROUND

Earlier classification systems classified LPL as "lymphoplasmacytoid (immunocytic)" (Kiel classification, 1974) (1), "lymphoplasmacytic/cytoid (LP immunocytoma)" (Updated Kiel classification, 1988) (2), and "lymphoplasmacytoid lymphoma" (Revised European American Lymphoma Classification, 1994) (3).

In the current 2008 World Health Organization (WHO) classification, LPL is defined as a neoplasm that consists of a spectrum of cells ranging from small B lymphocytes to plasmacytoid lymphocytes and plasma cells. It usually involves the bone marrow and sometimes lymph nodes and spleen. Importantly, other lymphoid neoplasms that may show plasmacytic differentiation need to be excluded (4). In its current definition, LPL is no longer regarded as synonymous to WM. This is in contrast with the former WHO classification, which grouped LPL/WM as a single entity (5).

WM, first described in 1944, is currently considered a clinicopathologic entity that requires the presence of LPL in the bone marrow and an IgM monoclonal gammopathy of any concentration (6,7). According to the clinicopathologic definition, established at a consensus panel meeting in 2002, patients with IgA- and IgG-secreting LPLs are not considered to have WM (7). No minimum level of monoclonal IgM is needed for a diagnosis of WM. However, in addition to monoclonal IgM, a diagnosis of WM does require bone marrow infiltration by LPL. It is recognized that other lymphomas can secrete IgM and cause a WM-like syndrome, but these patients do not have WM according to current definitions.

Because the definitions of LPL and WM have changed significantly over time and because different authors have used different definitions, the overview presented in this chapter unavoidably covers a somewhat heterogeneous population.

EPIDEMIOLOGY

LPL accounts for approximately 2% of all hematologic malignancies, with a reported incidence of 3.4 to 7.3 for males and 1.7 to 4.2 for females per 1 million years at risk (8–11). Its incidence increases with age, with a median age around 70 years at diagnosis (12–15). However, patients in their twenties and teens have been reported (15–17). A racial predilection for whites has been recognized, as opposed to multiple myeloma (MM), which occurs more frequently in African Americans (9,10). Men are affected with a slightly higher frequency, with a male:female ratio varying between 1.16:1 and 2.5:1 in larger studies (9–15,17–21).

Clustering of LPL in families has been reported (22–24). Also, larger studies show that first-degree relatives of LPL patients have an increased risk of both LPL and other non-Hodgkin lymphomas, with a familial predisposition in up to 20% of patients (17,25). Although the causes of this familial clustering remain to be elucidated, some studies have shown familial cases to associate with autoimmune disease, infections, and exposure to farming, pesticides, wood dust, and organic solvents (22,26,27).

Patients with a history of autoimmune conditions or infections are at increased risk of developing LPL (28,29). Reported autoimmune conditions associated with LPL include Sjögren syndrome, systemic sclerosis, autoimmune hemolytic anemia, immune thrombocytopenic purpura, polymyalgia rheumatica, giant cell arteritis, and Crohn disease. A large variety of infectious and chronic inflammatory disorders have been reported in association with LPL. The association between LPL and hepatitis C virus has been reported in some studies (30,31), but not in others (32,33), possibly related to geographical differences.

CLINICAL FEATURES

The presenting clinical features of LPL show great variation (7,12–16,18–20,34–36). Approximately one-third of patients are asymptomatic at diagnosis. Symptoms can be a result of bone marrow infiltration or an effect of antibody production. The typical LPL patient presents with complaints of weakness and fatigue due to anemia, which is present in about two-thirds of patients. In addition to displacement of the normal bone marrow, anemia can be caused by hemolysis, chemotherapy, and dilution of the blood due to high IgM levels that cause an increased oncotic pressure. In addition, the production of hepcidin by lymphoma cells, which causes decreased intestinal absorption of iron and iron sequestration in monocytes and macrophages, could contribute to the anemia (37). B-symptoms are reported in 16% to –77% of patients. About 10% to 20% have thrombocytopenia, and 5% to 10% of patients have neutropenia; 7% to 18% of patients have lymphocytosis. Lymphadenopathy, splenomegaly, and hepatomegaly are present in 15% to 40%, 12% to 43%, and 9% to 24% of patients, respectively.

Most patients with LPL have monoclonal antibodies in the peripheral blood (paraproteins), usually of the IgM isotype. Although paraproteins tend to be higher in LPL in comparison with other B-cell lymphomas, the overlap in paraprotein levels limits its use in differential diagnosis. At present, the diagnosis of WM is based on the presence of bone marrow infiltration rather than paraprotein levels (7).

If a patient presents with a lymphoma and IgM paraproteinemia, one study showed a chance of 60% of a final diagnosis of LPL (38). Other diagnoses included chronic lymphocytic leukemia (CLL) (20%), marginal zone lymphoma (7%), follicular lymphoma (5%), mantle cell lymphoma (3%), and diffuse large B-cell lymphoma (2%). In this particular study, all patients with a diagnosis other than LPL had an IgM lower than 3 g/L. However, another study by Owen et al. (39) did show IgM levels above 3 g/L in patients with other lymphoma types.

The antibodies produced by the malignant cells can cause symptoms in different ways. Hyperviscosity is present in roughly one-fifth of patients, although its prevalence varies strongly between studies. Symptoms of hyperviscosity include visual disturbances, skin and mucosal bleeding, and neurologic symptoms (40). Congestive heart failure and other cardiovascular manifestations do occur, but infrequently. Funduscopic examination shows venous engorgement with retinal hemorrhage and microaneurysms in a later stage.

A small subset of patients (2% to 3%) has amyloidosis (12,18). Autoantibody activity is present in 13% of patients (18). Peripheral neuropathy is a relatively frequent autoimmune phenomenon, with a prevalence of 7% to 17% (12,18,41). About half of WM patients show axon loss with electrodiagnostic studies, as compared to only 19% of controls (42). More rare presentations of autoimmunity include acquired von Willebrand disease, myasthenia gravis, and acquired C1 esterase deficiency. In addition, thrombocytopenia and cryoglobulins can be a result of autoantibodies instead of bone marrow infiltration and paraproteins, respectively.

Slightly more than half of LPL patients have an increased β_2-microglobulin, which is of prognostic value. Lactate dehydrogenase (LDH) is increased in 10% to 18% of patients, and has also been proposed to be of diagnostic value (16).

Involvement of other organs is rare, with skin, gut, lung, and kidney involvement in 3% to 4% of patients (19). Central nervous system manifestations of LPL, known as the Bing-Neel syndrome, are rare. They can be due to direct infiltration of LPL cells or to IgM deposition (43,44).

MORPHOLOGY

In studies predating the current WHO classification, the diagnosis of LPL showed very poor reproducibility (45). Although a recent report showed better agreement (46), LPL remains a lymphoma type that can be difficult to diagnose accurately. This is mostly due to the lack of a specific immunohistochemical or genetic marker that characterizes this entity, making it a diagnosis of exclusion.

General Morphology

LPL usually involves the bone marrow. Lymph nodes and the spleen are less commonly involved. As its name implies, LPL displays a morphology ranging from small lymphocytes to plasmacytoid cells to cells that have a mature plasma cell morphology. In addition, rare blasts can be encountered. The extent of plasma cell differentiation varies strongly between cases (18). In rare cases, cells with mature plasma cell morphology are the predominant cell type, requiring immunophenotypic studies to allow differentiation from plasma cell myeloma (PCM) (41). Although one study attributed prognostic value to cellular morphology, this difference in prognosis was most likely due to differences in marrow infiltration (18,47). Remstein et al. (36) have reported rare cases of LPL with hairy cell–like, signet ring cell, and monocytoid morphology.

Peripheral Blood

Lymphocytosis is present in a small subset of patients. Circulating plasmacytoid cells and plasma cells can be observed (Fig. 19.1A). Rouleaux formation of red blood cells due to high IgM levels is frequently observed.

Bone Marrow

The extent of bone marrow infiltration varies; most studies report a median percentage of lymphoid cells in the bone marrow of around 30% (Fig. 19.1B) (13,41,48). Unlike in MM, no lower limit for bone marrow infiltration has been defined (7). The growth pattern is variable and can be diffuse, nodular, interstitial, and paratrabecular (Figs. 19.2 through 19.4). Frequently, a mixed pattern of infiltration is observed. Of note, paratrabecular growth can be predominant or even the sole growth pattern.

The extent of plasma cell differentiation as well as the distribution of plasma cells varies. Plasma cells can either be intermingled with the lymphoid cells or form discrete aggregates (41). These aggregates can be separated from

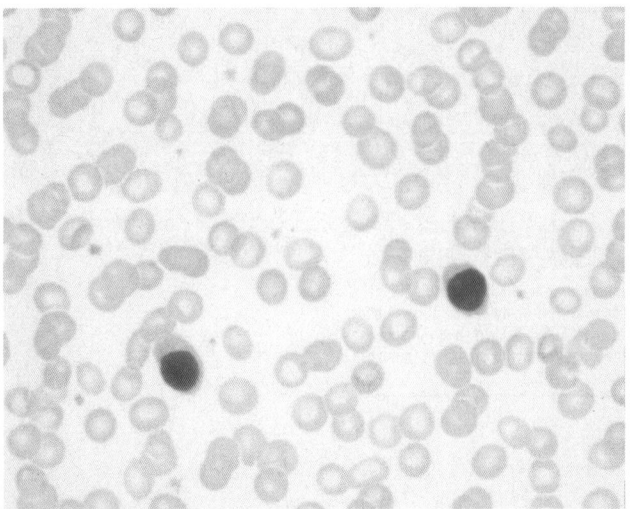
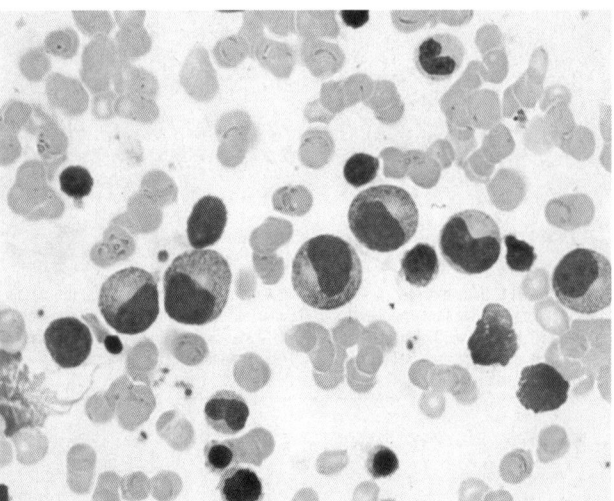

A

B

FIGURE 19.1. Peripheral blood and bone marrow cytology. A: Peripheral blood showing frequent lymphoplasmacytoid cells with some rouleaux formation of erythrocytes. **B:** Bone marrow aspirate showing increased numbers of lymphoplasmacytoid cells among haematopoietic elements. (Courtesy of Dr. MacKenzie, Radboud University Medical Center, Nijmegen, the Netherlands.)

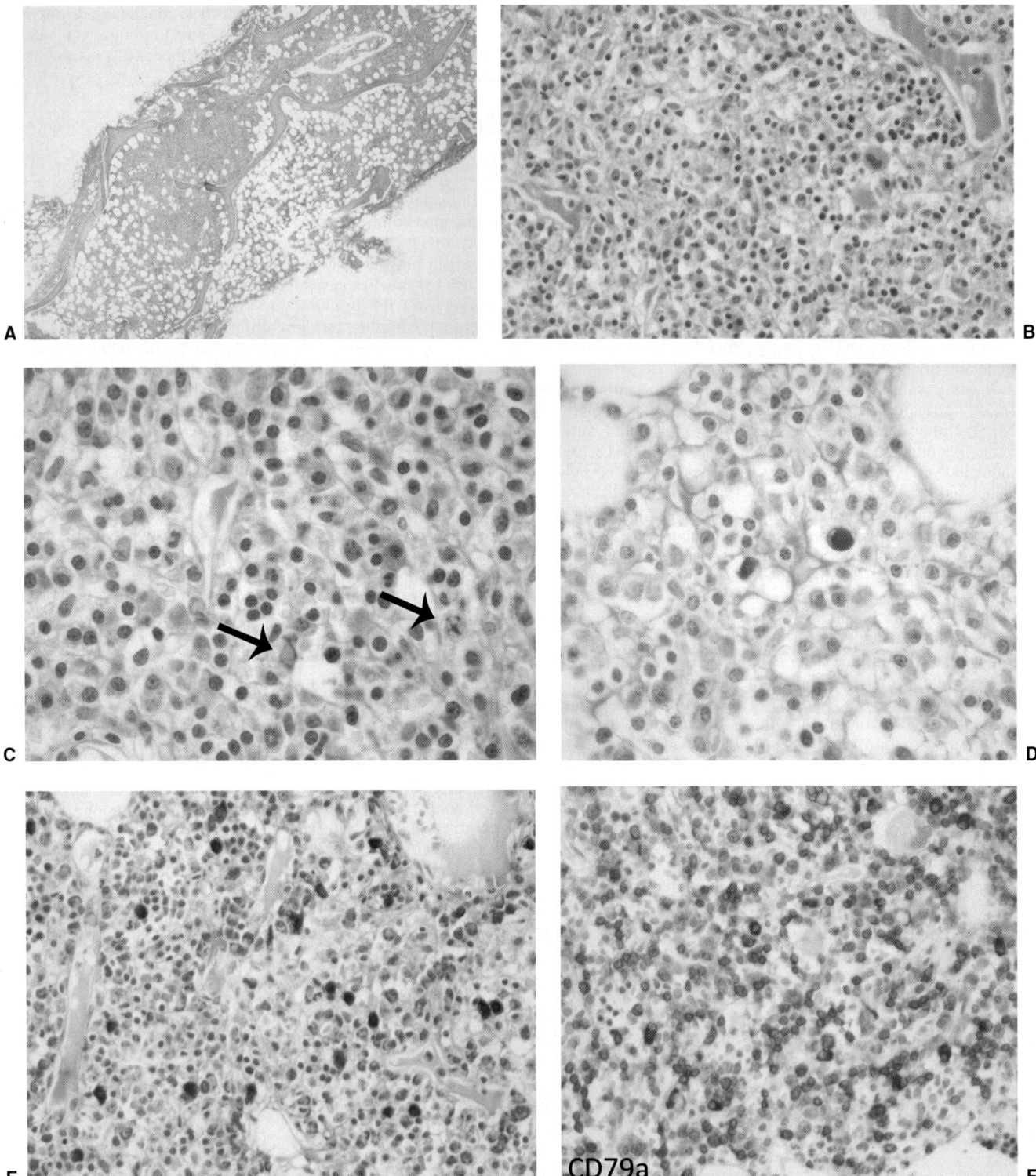

FIGURE 19.2. LPL, bone marrow. A: Overview, showing nodular and interstitial infiltration of the bone marrow. H&E 12.5×. **B:** LPL cells with morphology varying from lymphocytes to plasma cells. H&E 200×. **C:** Detail showing a Dutcher body (**left arrow**) and a Russell body (**right arrow**). H&E 400×. **D:** Periodic acid Schiff (PAS) staining, highlighting immunoglobulin inclusions. 400×. **E:** Giemsa stain, showing an increased number of mast cells. 200×. **F:** CD79a immunohistochemistry, showing a heterogeneous pattern with stronger staining in the plasma cell component. 200×

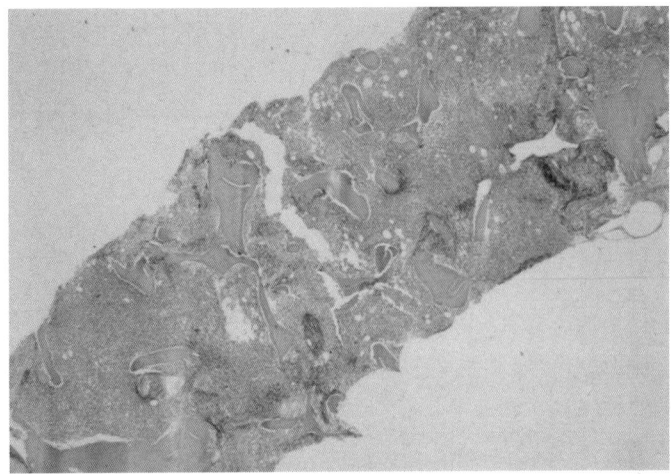

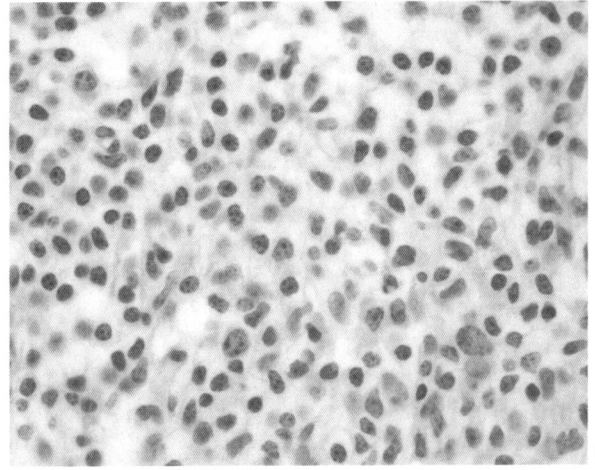

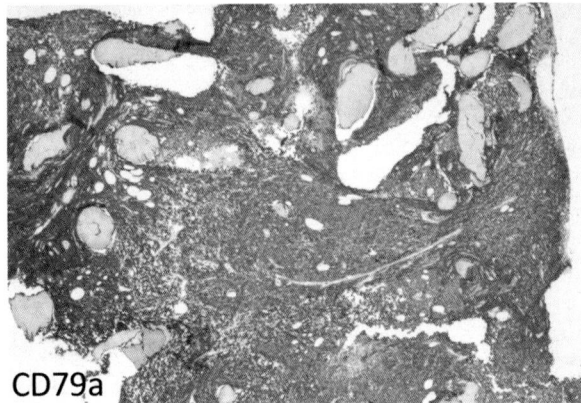

FIGURE 19.3. Bone marrow, diffuse pattern. A: Overview, showing bone marrow with maximal cellularity. H&E 12.5×. **B:** Detail, showing LPL cells with no residual hematopoiesis. H&E 400×. **C:** CD79a immunohistochemistry accentuating the diffuse infiltration. 25×.

the lymphoid component and can be the sole plasmacytoid component. Dutcher bodies or Russell bodies are found in the majority of cases (Fig. 19.2C and D). An increased number of mast cells is observed in one-third to one-fifth of cases (Fig. 19.2E). These mast cells appear to stimulate tumor growth via CD154, a marker that is present on tumor-derived mast cells, but not on bone marrow mast cells of healthy individuals (49). Increased reticulin staining is a frequent phenomenon, present in 67% to 89% of cases, with usually only mild increases in reticulin fibers (18,34). Germinal center

formation, necrosis, and granulomas are not specific features of LPL (48). Finally, one should be aware of possible amyloid deposits.

Lymph Nodes

Whereas LPL can be diagnosed in the bone marrow with fair precision, its diagnosis in lymph nodes is more problematic. In its classical form, a lymph node affected by LPL shows an architecture that is at least partially retained with intact

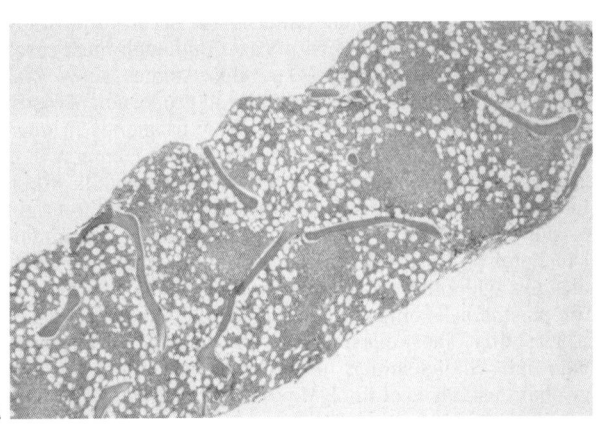

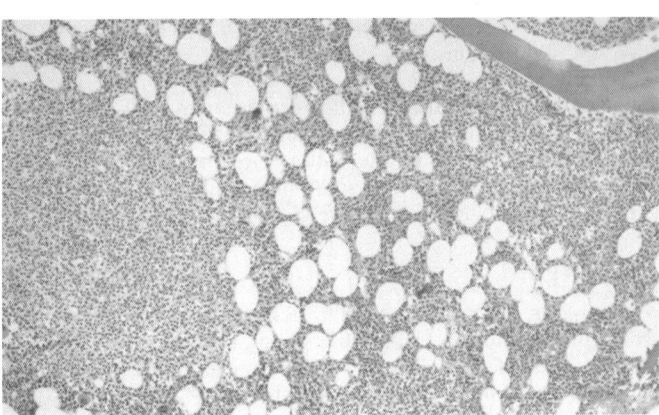

FIGURE 19.4. LPL, bone marrow, nodular pattern. A,B: Low power, showing nodular infiltrates with intervening fat tissue and hematopoiesis. H&E 12,5× (**A**) and 50× (**B**).

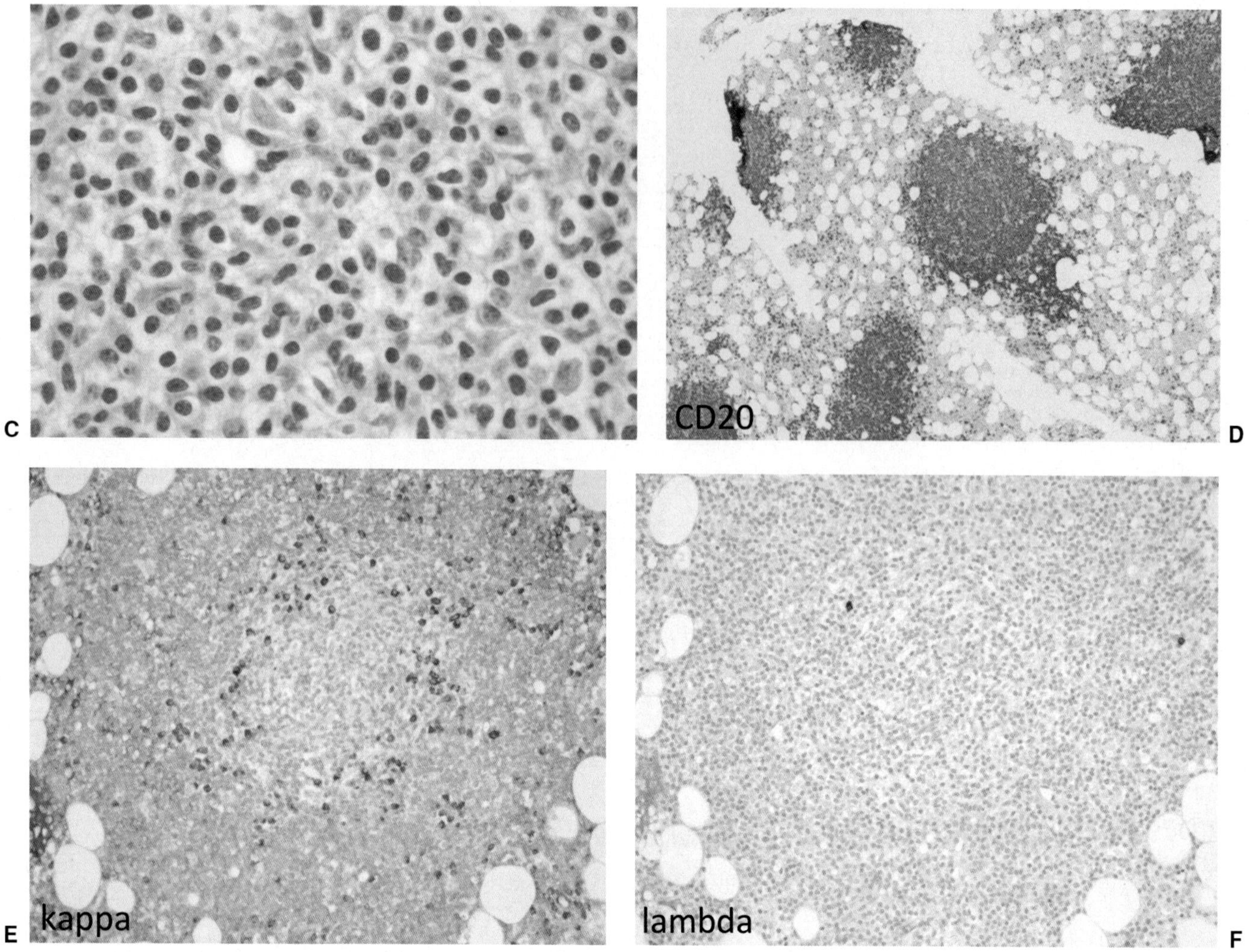

C

CD20   D

E kappa   lambda F

FIGURE 19.4. *(Continued)* **C:** Detail of a tumor nodule, showing lymphoplasmacytoid morphology. H&E 400×. **D:** CD20 immunohistochemistry, accentuating the nodular pattern of infiltration. 25×. **E:** Kappa immunohistochemistry, showing kappa light chain restriction of LPL cells with stronger staining of tumor cells with plasma cell differentiation at the periphery of the nodule. 100×. **F:** Lambda immunohistochemistry of the same nodule, showing only rare positive cells. 100×.

sinuses that are often dilated and contain periodic acid Schiff (PAS)-positive material (Fig. 19.5A and B) (46,50,51). Hemosiderin deposition near vessels or sinuses is frequently present. Follicles are generally small, and the neoplastic cells are rather monotonous. However, other patterns that show a more pronounced or complete effacement of the architecture do occur. Sometimes a vaguely nodular pattern is present. Other possible features include numerous reactive germinal centers and the presence of epithelioid granulomas (52). Dutcher bodies and Russell bodies are frequently observed. Also, amyloid deposition and crystal-storing histiocytosis have been reported (53). The latter consists of numerous macrophages that have cytoplasmic eosinophilic deposits that consist of immunoglobulins in crystal form.

Other Organs

In the spleen, the pattern of infiltration can involve both the white and red pulp, both in a diffuse and in a nodular manner (Fig. 19.5C–F) (53). The cellular morphology corresponds to that in the bone marrow and lymph nodes, with lymphocytes, plasmacytoid cells, plasma cells, and scattered blasts. The other most commonly affected organs are skin, lung, and the gastrointestinal tract (53,54).

IMMUNOPHENOTYPE

The typical LPL case has a mature monoclonal B-cell phenotype with expression of CD19, CD20, CD22, CD79a, and PAX5 and lacks expression of CD5, CD10, and CD23 (18,35,36,38,41). However, atypical expression patterns do occur. One study reported CD5 expression in 43% of cases, although most cases showed only partial staining (41). Other studies show CD5 expression in a smaller, but not insignificant proportion of cases. CD23 expression is also reported relatively frequently in most studies. Coexpression of CD5 and CD23 is less common. For the distinction from CLL/small lymphocytic lymphoma (SLL), the heterogeneous expression of CD5 and CD23 and the bright expression of CD20 in LPL are important features. With immunohistochemistry, CD20 staining can be weak, requiring additional stains with other pan B-cell markers like CD79a or PAX5.

The plasma cell component can be highlighted with CD138 or CD38 stains. These plasma cells show restricted immunoglobulin light chains similar to the lymphoid component. The heavy chain usually is of the IgM type, less frequently IgG, and even more rarely IgA.

Expression of CD10 is infrequent, being present in 0% to 10% of cases (18,35,36,41). Cyclin D1 is negative (36).

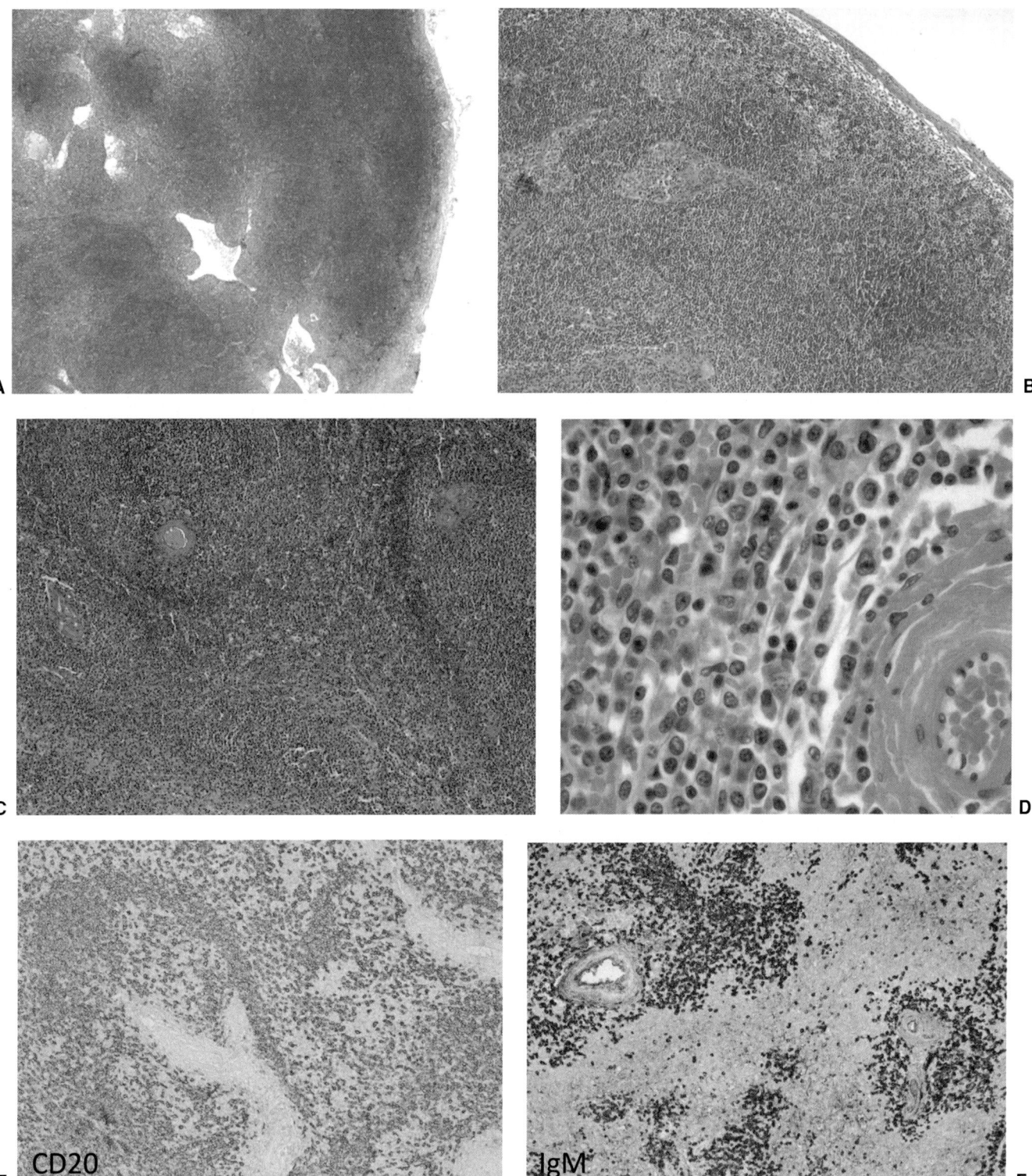

FIGURE 19.5. LPL, lymph node (A and B) and spleen (C–F). A,B: Lymph node infiltrated by LPL, showing the classical pattern with sparing of sinuses and sinusoidal dilatation. H&E 12.5× (**A**) and 50× (**B**). **C,D:** Spleen involved by LPL, showing mainly white pulp infiltration with less pronounced infiltration of the red pulp. H&E 50× (**C**) and 400× (**D**). **E:** CD20 immunohistochemistry confirms the infiltration of the white pulp and red pulp by B cells. 50×. **F:** IgM immunohistochemistry displaying IgM heavy chain expression of the neoplastic cells.

CYTOGENETICS AND MOLECULAR CHARACTERISTICS

No specific cytogenetic abnormalities have been reported in LPL thus far. With conventional cytogenetic techniques, abnormal karyotypes are observed in approximately one-third of patients (55,56). The most frequently observed structural chromosomal abnormality is a deletion of 6q, which is present in more than half of patients in some studies using highly sensitive fluorescence *in situ* hybridization approaches. However, the incidence of del6q varies strongly between studies (55–64). Two studies that specifically looked at nodal LPL, showed no 6q deletions (51,65). Some studies have reported recurrent gains of chromosome 4 (61,66), monosomy/deletion of chromosome 8 (55,56,59), monosomy 18 (56), trisomy 5 (55), and del 20q (67).

In the 2001 WHO classification, t(9;14)(p13;q32) was reported as characteristic of LPL/WM, following a study by Offit et al. (68) who reported the presence of this translocation in SLL with plasmacytoid features. This translocation was shown to involve the *PAX5* gene, a B-cell-specific transcription factor (69). However, after subsequent studies that showed no *PAX5* translocations in LPL, we have to conclude that it is not a specific feature of LPL (55,70,71).

Translocations involving the immunoglobulin heavy chain locus have been reported incidentally, but are certainly not a specific feature of LPL (51). Moreover, because LPL is a diagnosis of exclusion, one could imagine that such cases actually represent other types of B-cell lymphomas. Also, translocations involving *MALT1* have been reported in WM (66,72). However, under the current definitions, these cases are probably better regarded as IgM-secreting marginal zone lymphomas that cause a "WM-like" clinical syndrome.

Gene expression profiling studies show a specific gene expression signature in WM, which allowed separation from CLL and MM (73,74). The expression pattern in WM was reported to be more similar to CLL than MM. Another study, in which the B-lymphocyte and plasma cell component were separately analyzed, showed clustering of the B-lymphocyte component with CLL and clustering of the plasma cell component with MM (74). Both studies showed upregulation of interleukin-6.

A proteomics study showed dysregulation of numerous proteins, including members of the Ras and Rho family, histone deacetylases (HDACs), and the heat shock protein 90 (HSP90). HDAC and HSP90 inhibitors caused growth inhibition and apoptosis in WM cell lines, suggesting that these proteins can be a therapeutic target. Also, a microRNA expression profiling study showed changes in expression of microRNAs that regulate histone acetylation (75,76). Also, the HDAC inhibitor panobinostat showed activity against WM cells *in vitro* (76). Finally, antitumor activity of panobinostat has been reported in a phase II trial (77).

Multiple pathways that are known to have a role in oncogenesis show dysregulation in WM. The PI3K/Akt/mTOR pathway is constitutively activated in WM and inhibition of this pathway by means of the inhibitor perifosine causes reduced tumor growth *in vivo* and *in vitro* (78). In addition, 37 WM patients were treated with perifosine in a phase II clinical trial in which 35% of patients achieved at least a minimal response (79). Also, mTOR inhibitors have shown efficacy in a preclinical study, and in a phase II trial in patients with relapsed or refractory WM (80,81).

The PI3K/Akt/mTOR pathway indirectly activates the NF-κB pathway (82). One immunohistochemical study showed NF-κB activation in WM, whereas another study did not (83,84). Leleu et al. (85) showed increased levels of NF-κB in WM cells and also showed growth inhibition of WM cells treated with the proteasome inhibitor bortezomib, which inhibits NF-κB. Accordingly, bortezomib treatment has shown efficacy in WM, both in relapsed patients and as a primary treatment (86–90).

POSTULATED NORMAL COUNTERPART

LPL has been shown to be a clonal proliferation of B cells that have undergone rearrangement of immunoglobulin light and heavy chains (91). The plasma cells are part of the malignant clone. The presence of multiple clones has been reported (92–94). Most cases show extensive somatic mutations, corresponding with antigen-exposed B cells (95,96). However, statistical analysis of the specific mutations showed no evidence of antigen-driven selection in a significant proportion of cases, suggesting that part of LPL cases might be derived from B cells that have undergone somatic hypermutation by means other than the germinal center (97). Although ongoing somatic hypermutation has been reported, most cases show intraclonal homogeneity (91,94,98,99). The fact that somatic hypermutation has ceased in most cases suggests that LPL has a memory B-cell origin. However, CD27 expression, which correlates with memory B-cell status, is absent in most cases (91,100). Possibly, LPL cells could be derived from a CD27-negative population of memory B cells (101).

For WM, studies have shown that class switch recombination is impaired, although the class switch machinery appears intact (102). However, this statement cannot be extrapolated to LPL, which can also have IgG or IgA heavy chains.

CLINICAL COURSE AND PROGNOSTIC ASSESSMENT

LPL is an incurable disease with a clinical course that is generally indolent, but highly variable. This is reflected in the possible treatment strategies, varying from no therapy in asymptomatic patients to aggressive treatment in symptomatic patients. Patients with asymptomatic WM, also known as smouldering or indolent WM, are best left untreated, considering the fact that progression to symptomatic disease occurs in only 3% to 12% of patients per year (103–106).

For patients with symptomatic WM, treatment is indicated. A large number of different effective therapeutic regimens have been reported. The choice of treatment should take patient factors into account including age, comorbidities, severity of symptoms, and whether the patient is a transplantation candidate. Possible first-line therapeutic approaches include rituximab, alkylators (e.g., cyclophosphamide, melphalan, chlorambucil), purine nucleoside analogs (fludarabine, cladribine), doxorubicin, vincristin, thalidomide, and steroids (prednisone, dexamethasone) (107–111). The Mayo Clinic has published treatment guidelines (Mayo Stratification of Macroglobulinemia and Risk-Adapted Therapy—mSMART; available online at www.mSMART.org) in which symptomatic patients are treated with either rituximab alone or rituximab in combination with dexamethasone and cyclophosphamide, depending on the severity of symptoms (110).

Patients with hyperviscosity are treated with plasmapheresis for short-term viscosity decrease with concomitant start of chemotherapy for a long-term effect. Rituximab treatment can cause an IgM flare; a transient increase in serum IgM that may require plasmapheresis (112).

Treatment options for relapses include a repeat of the first-line therapy or another first-line treatment regimen. Other options include bone marrow transplantation or treatment with more recently developed agents, including those discussed under "genetics and molecular findings." Alemtuzumab, an

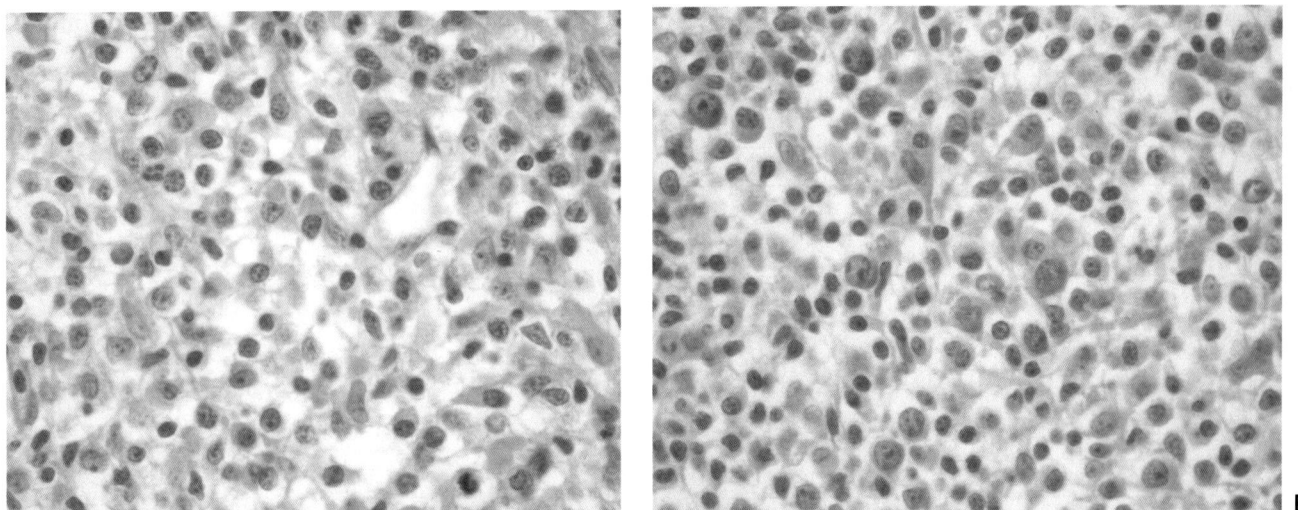

FIGURE 19.6. LPL, bone marrow, with local increase of centroblasts. A: Bone marrow showing infiltration by LPL with low-grade morphology among preexistent hematopoiesis. H&E 400×. **B:** Same case as in (**A**), showing another part of the bone marrow with more frequent centroblasts. Although transformation in LPL is not defined precisely, this could be indicative of a more aggressive disease course. H&E 400×.

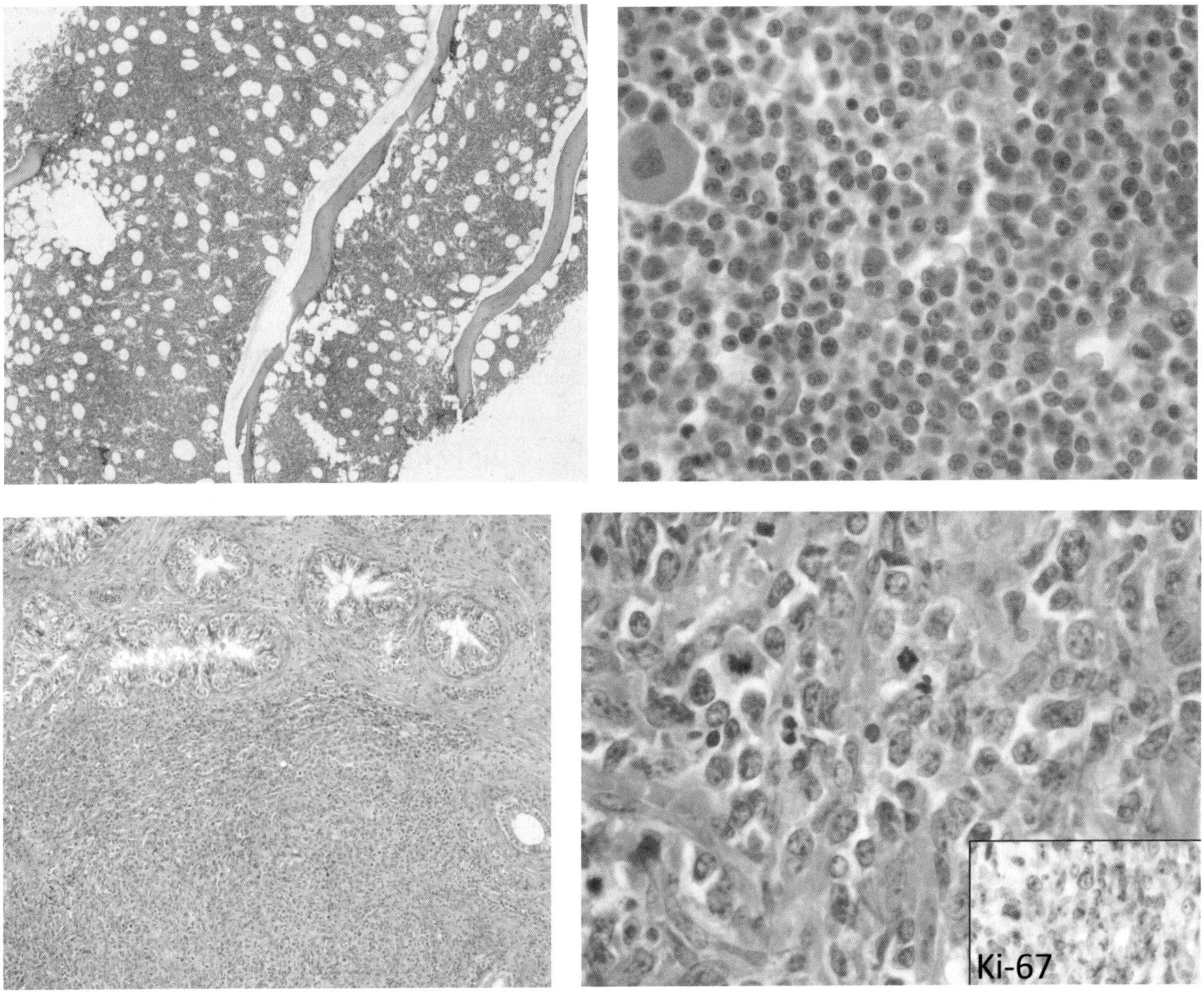

FIGURE 19.7. LPL, transformation. A,B: Bone marrow, showing interstitial infiltration by LPL with low-grade morphology. H&E 25× (**A**) and 400× (**B**). **C:** Orchidectomy specimen of the same patient, showing infiltration by lymphoma among preexistent ducts. H&E 50×. **D:** High-power view, showing diffuse aggregates of large blasts with numerous mitoses. Ki-67 immunohistochemistry (**inset**) confirms the high proliferative activity. H&E 400×.

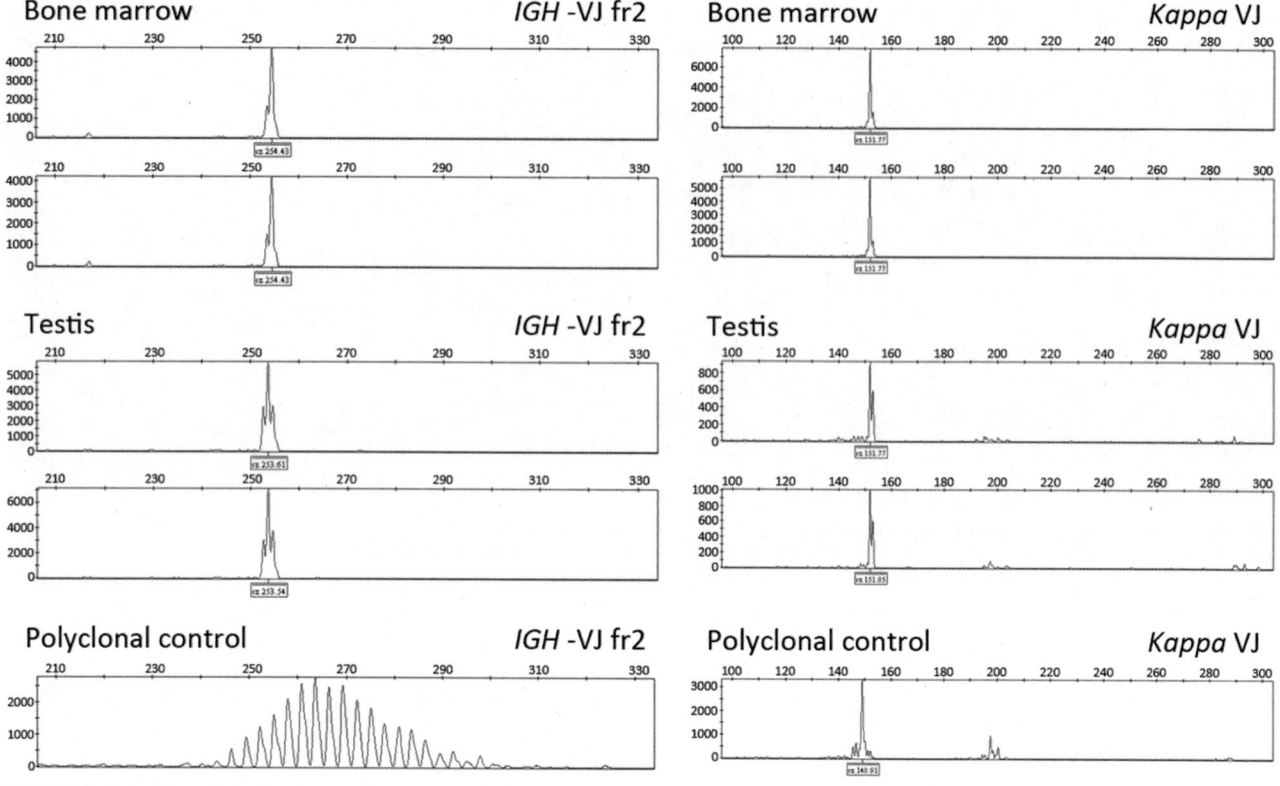

FIGURE 19.8. Ig clonality analysis. GeneScan clonality patterns, in duplicate, from DNA specimens obtained from bone marrow (**top**) and testis (**middle**) of the same patient as in Figure 19.7, using primers targeting the immunoglobulin heavy chain (*IGH*) V_H-J_H region framework 2 and *IGK*-VJ, according to Euroclonality/ BIOMED-2. Clonality analysis shows clonal *IGH* and *IGK* products of identical sizes in bone marrow and testis, confirming that the high-grade lymphoma in the testis is indeed a transformation of the low-grade lymphoma in the bone marrow. Polyclonal controls are displayed in the **bottom** panels. (Courtesy of Dr. Groenen, Radboud University Medical Center, Nijmegen, the Netherlands.)

anti-CD52 monoclonal antibody that targets both LP cells and mast cells, is another agent that is active against LPL, but also displays frequent toxicity (113).

Median overall survival is 5 to 8 years (7,13,36,114,115). Numerous studies have sought factors that determine prognosis. Adverse prognostic factors identified with multivariate analysis include age, cytopenias, increased β_2-microglobulin, increased LDH, weight loss, cryoglobulinemia, low serum albumin, and M-protein levels (12–15,19,21,103,114). In 2009, a prognostic scoring system for WM was proposed and validated, in which five adverse covariates were identified: (i) age >65 years, (ii) hemoglobin ≤11.5 g/dL, (iii) platelet count ≤100 × 10⁹/L, (iv) β_2-microglobulin >3 mg/L, and (v) serum monoclonal protein concentration >7.0 g/dL (114). This scoring system, the International Prognostic Scoring System for Waldenström Macroglobulinemia, was validated by another study that showed additional prognostic value of elevated serum LDH (defined as LDH >250 IU/L) (16).

Transformation to a high-grade lymphoma (analogous to Richter syndrome in CLL) can occur in LPL, with an incidence of 6.2% and a median time to development of 5 years in a large study (116). Treatment with nucleoside analogs appears to increase the risk of transformation (116,117). Interestingly, the blood of patients treated with nucleoside analogs less frequently contains clonal expansions of specific cytotoxic T cells that are associated with a good prognosis, possibly due to antitumor activity (118). The histology of the transformed component is usually that of a diffuse large B-cell lymphoma that can consist of either centroblasts or immunoblasts, with frequent mitoses and a high proliferative index as shown by Ki-67 immunohistochemistry (Figs. 19.6 through 19.8) (119). In addition, LPL has been rarely reported in association with

Hodgkin lymphoma (116,120). Positivity for Epstein-Barr varies between reports, being negative in most cases currently documented (119–122).

DIFFERENTIAL DIAGNOSIS

Monoclonal Gammopathy of Uncertain Significance

Patients with monoclonal gammopathy of uncertain significance (MGUS) have a serum M protein of <30 g/L without significant bone marrow infiltration (<10% clonal plasma cells) and without lytic bone lesions or myeloma-related end-organ damage (123). Fifteen to twenty percent of MGUS patients have an IgM paraprotein. Instead of an increased risk of MM, like in patients with IgG and IgA MGUS, patients with IgM MGUS have a strongly increased risk of LPL/WM. A study by Kyle et al. (124) reported a relative risk of 262 compared to the general population, with a risk of progression to lymphoma or a related disorder of 14% in 10 years. In addition to LPL/WM, IgM MGUS patients can progress to CLL, other non-Hodgkin lymphomas, and amyloidosis. Progression to MM is seen only very rarely (124,125).

Nodal Marginal Zone Lymphoma

Differentiating LPL from nodal marginal zone lymphoma (NMZL) can be problematic, especially in lymph nodes. This is due to the frequent plasmacytic differentiation in NMZL and because both NMZL and LPL lack specific immunohistochemical or genetic markers. Morphologically, the presence of monocytoid lymphoid cells with abundant pale cytoplasm favors NMZL. In the bone marrow, the presence of lymphoid follicles favors NMZL. Especially for diagnoses on lymph nodes, it might be best to employ three diagnostic categories (46,126). The first category includes those cases that show the classical morphology of LPL, as described above under "morphology." The second category includes cases that can be confidently diagnosed as NMZL, with a marginal zone growth pattern and disruption and colonization of preexistent follicles with disruption of dendritic cell meshworks. The third category contains those cases in which no reliable differentiation can be made, which can be termed "small B-cell lymphoma with plasmacytic differentiation." Features favoring LPL are a preserved architecture and a more monotonous cellular morphology. Although there is a high need for better criteria to distinguish LPL from NMZL, from a clinical point of view this distinction might not be that important, since treatment is based on IgM levels and symptoms rather than a diagnosis of LPL or NMZL (127).

Splenic Marginal Zone Lymphoma

Like NMZL, splenic marginal zone lymphoma (SMZL) also frequently shows plasmacytic differentiation and may be difficult to distinguish from LPL. Clinically, SMZL patients show more extensive splenomegaly. On bone marrow biopsy, SMZL is characterized by sinusoidal infiltration and more frequently shows a nodular pattern in comparison with LPL. Other helpful features are the increased presence of mast cells and more extensive CD138 positivity in LPL (128,129). Cytogenetic studies can be helpful if they show a loss of chromosome 7q31-q32, which is present in up to 40% of SMZLs (130). In the peripheral blood, villous lymphocytes are typical of SMZL.

Extranodal Marginal Zone Lymphoma of Mucosa-Associated Lymphoid Tissue Lymphoma

Mucosa-associated lymphoid tissue (MALT) lymphomas have a specific tissue distribution with rare bone marrow involvement (±15%) (131,132). Therefore, on clinical grounds, LPL or MALT lymphoma can be favored. However, MALT lymphomas do sometimes involve the bone marrow and LPL can have its primary presentation at an extranodal site, resulting in rare cases in which differentiation is difficult or impossible. Histological discrimination between LPL and MALT lymphoma includes features described under NMZL. In addition, cytogenetic studies can show specific translocations in MALT lymphoma, with frequencies depending on the primary site of involvement (133,134).

Plasma Cell Myeloma

PCM is usually easily distinguished from LPL. However, cases of LPL with predominant or exclusive plasmacytoid morphology and PCM with lymphoid morphology can cause difficulties. A LPL with predominant plasmacytoid morphology can usually be distinguished from PCM by the absence of lytic bone lesions and hypercalcemia, expression of CD19, and lack of CD56 expression (135). Aggregates consisting solely of monoclonal plasma cells can remain in the bone marrow of treated LPL patients (136,137). In these cases, adequate clinical information is essential. Finally, some PCM cases show lymphoid morphology, associated with CD20 and cyclin D1 expression and translocations involving the cyclin D1 gene. These can be distinguished from LPL based on clinical features and immunoglobulin heavy chain isotype. Also, cyclin D1 expression and translocations involving the cyclin D1 gene are not features of LPL.

Chronic Lymphocytic Leukemia/Small Lymphocytic Lymphoma

Rare cases of LPL express both CD5 and CD23, causing possible confusion with CLL/SLL. However, this staining is heterogeneous in comparison with CLL/SLL. Also, CD20 expression is brighter in LPL. Morphologically, LPL does not show proliferation centers, has more pronounced plasma cell differentiation, and has increased intratumoral mast cells.

References

1. Gerard-Marchant R, Hamlin I, Lennert K, et al. Classification of non-Hodgkin's lymphoma. *Lancet* 1974;304(7877):406–408.
2. Stansfeld AG, Diebold J, Noel H, et al. Updated Kiel classification for lymphomas. *Lancet* 1988;1(8580):292–293.
3. Harris NL, Jaffe ES, Stein H, et al. A revised European-American classification of lymphoid neoplasms: a proposal from the International Lymphoma Study Group. *Blood* 1994;84(5):1361–1392.
4. Swerdlow SH, Berger F, Pileri SA, et al. Lymphoplasmacytic lymphoma. In: Swerdlow SH, Campo E, Harris NL, et al., eds. *WHO classification of tumors of hematopoietic and lymphoid tissues.* Lyon: IARC, 2008:194–195.
5. Berger F, Müller-Hermelink HK, Isaacson PG, et al. Lymphoplasmacytic lymphoma/Waldenström macroglobulinemia. In: Jaffe ES, Harris NL, Stein H, et al., eds. *Tumors of haematopoietic and lymphoid tissues.* Lyon: IARC, 2001:132–134.
6. Waldenström J. Incipient myelomatosis or "essential" hyperglobulinemia with fibrogenopenia—a new syndrome? *Acta Med Scand* 1944;117:216–247.
7. Owen RG, Treon SP, Al-Katib A, et al. Clinicopathological definition of Waldenström's macroglobulinemia: consensus panel recommendations from the Second International Workshop on Waldenström's Macroglobulinemia. *Semin Oncol* 2003; 30(2):110–115.
8. Dimopoulos MA, Alexanian R. Waldenstrom's macroglobulinemia. *Blood* 1994; 83(6):1452–1459.
9. Herrinton LJ, Weiss NS. Incidence of Waldenstrom's macroglobulinemia. *Blood* 1993;82(10):3148–3150.
10. Groves FD, Travis LB, Devesa SS, et al. Waldenstrom's macroglobulinemia: incidence patterns in the United States, 1988–1994. *Cancer* 1998;82(6):1078–1081.
11. Phekoo KJ, Jack RH, Davies E, et al. The incidence and survival of Waldenstrom's macroglobulinaemia in South East England. *Leuk Res* 2008;32(1):55–59.
12. Dimopoulos MA, Hamilos G, Zervas K, et al. Survival and prognostic factors after initiation of treatment in Waldenstrom's macroglobulinemia. *Ann Oncol* 2003;14(8):1299–1305.
13. Morel P, Monconduit M, Jacomy D, et al. Prognostic factors in Waldenström macroglobulinemia: a report on 232 patients with the description of a new scoring system and its validation on 253 other patients. *Blood* 2000;96(3):852–858.
14. Facon T, Brouillard M, Duhamel A, et al. Prognostic factors in Waldenstrom's macroglobulinemia: a report of 167 cases. *J Clin Oncol* 1993;11(8):1553–1558.
15. Merlini G, Baldini L, Broglia C, et al. Prognostic factors in symptomatic Waldenstrom's macroglobulinemia. *Semin Oncol* 2003;30(2):211–215.
16. Kastritis E, Kyrtsonis MC, Hadjiharissi E, et al. Validation of the International Prognostic Scoring System (IPSS) for Waldenstrom's macroglobulinemia (WM) and the importance of serum lactate dehydrogenase (LDH). *Leuk Res* 2010;34(10):1340–1343.
17. Kristinsson SY, Bjorkholm M, Goldin LR, et al. Risk of lymphoproliferative disorders among first-degree relatives of lymphoplasmacytic lymphoma/Waldenstrom macroglobulinemia patients: a population-based study in Sweden. *Blood* 2008;112(8):3052–3056.
18. Owen RG, Barrans SL, Richards SJ, et al. Waldenstrom macroglobulinemia. Development of diagnostic criteria and identification of prognostic factors. *Am J Clin Pathol* 2001;116(3):420–428.
19. Garcia-Sanz R, Montoto S, Torrequebrada A, et al. Waldenstrom macroglobulinaemia: presenting features and outcome in a series with 217 cases. *Br J Haematol* 2001;115(3):575–582.
20. Dhodapkar MV, Jacobson JL, Gertz MA, et al. Prognostic factors and response to fludarabine therapy in patients with Waldenstrom macroglobulinemia: results of United States intergroup trialSouthwest Oncology Group S9003). *Blood* 2001; 98(1):41–48.
21. Gobbi PG, Bettini R, Montecucco C, et al. Study of prognosis in Waldenstrom's macroglobulinemia: a proposal for a simple binary classification with clinical and investigational utility. *Blood* 1994;83(10):2939–2945.
22. Blattner WA, Garber JE, Mann DL, et al. Waldenstrom's macroglobulinemia and autoimmune disease in a family. *Ann Intern Med* 1980;93(6):830–832.
23. Renier G, Ifrah N, Chevailler A, et al. Four brothers with Waldenstrom's macroglobulinemia. *Cancer* 1989;64(7):1554–1559.
24. Massari R, Fine JM, Metais R. Waldenstrom's macroglobulinaemia observed in two brothers. *Nature* 1962;196:176–178.
25. Treon SP, Hunter ZR, Aggarwal A, et al. Characterization of familial Waldenstrom's macroglobulinemia. *Ann Oncol* 2006;17(3):488–494.
26. Royer RH, Koshiol J, Giambarresi TR, et al. Differential characteristics of Waldenstrom macroglobulinemia according to patterns of familial aggregation. *Blood* 2010;115(22):4464–4471.
27. Linet MS, Humphrey RL, Mehl ES, et al. A case-control and family study of Waldenstrom's macroglobulinemia. *Leukemia* 1993;7(9):1363–1369.
28. Kristinsson SY, Koshiol J, Bjorkholm M, et al. Immune-related and inflammatory conditions and risk of lymphoplasmacytic lymphoma or Waldenstrom macroglobulinemia. *J Natl Cancer Inst* 2010;102(8):557–567.
29. Koshiol J, Gridley G, Engels EA, et al. Chronic immune stimulation and subsequent Waldenstrom macroglobulinemia. *Arch Intern Med* 2008;168(17): 1903–1909.

30. Mele A, Pulsoni A, Bianco E, et al. Hepatitis C virus and B-cell non-Hodgkin lymphomas: an Italian multicenter case-control study. *Blood* 2003;102(3):996–999.

31. Nieters A, Kallinowski B, Brennan P, et al. Hepatitis C and risk of lymphoma: results of the European multicenter case-control study EPILYMPH. *Gastroenterology* 2006;131(6):1879–1886.

32. Leleu X, O'Connor K, Ho AW, et al. Hepatitis C viral infection is not associated with Waldenstrom's macroglobulinemia. *Am J Hematol* 2007;82(1):83–84.

33. Veneri D, Aqel H, Franchini M, et al. Prevalence of hepatitis C virus infection in IgM-type monoclonal gammopathy of uncertain significance and Waldenstrom macroglobulinemia. *Am J Hematol* 2004;77(4):421.

34. Andriko JA, Aguilera NS, Chu WS, et al. Waldenstrom's macroglobulinemia: a clinicopathologic study of 22 cases. *Cancer* 1997;80(10):1926–1935.

35. San Miguel JF, Vidriales MB, Ocio E, et al. Immunophenotypic analysis of Waldenstrom's macroglobulinemia. *Semin Oncol* 2003;30(2):187–195.

36. Remstein ED, Hanson CA, Kyle RA, et al. Despite apparent morphologic and immunophenotypic heterogeneity, Waldenstrom's macroglobulinemia is consistently composed of cells along a morphologic continuum of small lymphocytes, plasmacytoid lymphocytes, and plasma cells. *Semin Oncol* 2003;30(2):182–186.

37. Ciccarelli BT, Patterson CJ, Hunter ZR, et al. Hepcidin is produced by lymphoplasmacytic cells and is associated with anemia in Waldenstrom's macroglobulinemia. *Clin Lymphoma Myeloma Leuk* 2011;11(1):160–163.

38. Lin P, Hao S, Handy BC, et al. Lymphoid neoplasms associated with IgM paraprotein: a study of 382 patients. *Am J Clin Pathol* 2005;123(2):200–205.

39. Owen RG, Parapia LA, Higginson J, et al. Clinicopathological correlates of IgM paraproteinemias. *Clin Lymphoma* 2000;1(1):39–43.

40. Stone MJ. Waldenstrom's macroglobulinemia: hyperviscosity syndrome and cryoglobulinemia. *Clin Lymphoma Myeloma* 2009;9(1):97–99.

41. Morice WG, Chen D, Kurtin PJ, et al. Novel immunophenotypic features of marrow lymphoplasmacytic lymphoma and correlation with Waldenstrom's macroglobulinemia. *Mod Pathol* 2009;22(6):807–816.

42. Levine T, Pestronk A, Florence J, et al. Peripheral neuropathies in Waldenstrom's macroglobulinaemia. *J Neurol Neurosurg Psychiatry* 2006;77(2):224–228.

43. Ly KI, Fintelmann F, Forghani R, et al. Novel diagnostic approaches in Bing-Neel syndrome. *Clin Lymphoma Myeloma Leuk* 2011;11(1):180–183.

44. Malkani RG, Tallman M, Gottardi-Littell N, et al. Bing-Neel syndrome: an illustrative case and a comprehensive review of the published literature. *J Neurooncol* 2010;96(3):301–312.

45. A clinical evaluation of the International Lymphoma Study Group classification of non-Hodgkin's lymphoma. The Non-Hodgkin's Lymphoma Classification Project. *Blood* 1997;89(11):3909–3918.

46. Lin P, Molina TJ, Cook JR, et al. Lymphoplasmacytic lymphoma and other nonmarginal zone lymphomas with plasmacytic differentiation. *Am J Clin Pathol* 2011;136(2):195–210.

47. Bartl R, Frisch B, Mahl G, et al. Bone marrow histology in Waldenstrom's macroglobulinaemia. Clinical relevance of subtype recognition. *Scand J Haematol* 1983;31(4):359–375.

48. Arber DA, George TI. Bone marrow biopsy involvement by non-Hodgkin's lymphoma: frequency of lymphoma types, patterns, blood involvement, and discordance with other sites in 450 specimens. *Am J Surg Pathol* 2005;29(12):1549–1557.

49. Tournilhac O, Santos DD, Xu L, et al. Mast cells in Waldenstrom's macroglobulinemia support lymphoplasmacytic cell growth through CD154/CD40 signaling. *Ann Oncol* 2006;17(8):1275–1282.

50. Harrison CV. The morphology of the lymph node in the macroglobulinaemia of Waldenstrom. *J Clin Pathol* 1972;25(1):12–16.

51. Sargent RL, Cook JR, Aguilera NI, et al. Fluorescence immunophenotypic and interphase cytogenetic characterization of nodal lymphoplasmacytic lymphoma. *Am J Surg Pathol* 2008;32(11):1643–1653.

52. Andriko JA, Swerdlow SH, Aguilera NI, et al. Is lymphoplasmacytic lymphoma/immunocytoma a distinct entity? A clinicopathologic study of 20 cases. *Am J Surg Pathol* 2001;25(6):742–751.

53. Lin P, Bueso-Ramos C, Wilson CS, et al. Waldenstrom macroglobulinemia involving extramedullary sites: morphologic and immunophenotypic findings in 44 patients. *Am J Surg Pathol* 2003;27(8):1104–1113.

54. Fadil A, Taylor DE. The lung and Waldenstrom's macroglobulinemia. *South Med J* 1998;91(7):681–685.

55. Mansoor A, Medeiros LJ, Weber DM, et al. Cytogenetic findings in lymphoplasmacytic lymphoma/Waldenstrom macroglobulinemia. Chromosomal abnormalities are associated with the polymorphous subtype and an aggressive clinical course. *Am J Clin Pathol* 2001;116(4):543–549.

56. Ocio EM, Schop RF, Gonzalez B, et al. 6q deletion in Waldenstrom macroglobulinemia is associated with features of adverse prognosis. *Br J Haematol* 2007;136(1):80–86.

57. Buckley PG, Walsh SH, Laurell A, et al. Genome-wide microarray-based comparative genomic hybridization analysis of lymphoplasmacytic lymphomas reveals heterogeneous aberrations. *Leuk Lymphoma* 2009;50(9):1528–1534.

58. Chang H, Qi X, Xu W, et al. Analysis of 6q deletion in Waldenstrom macroglobulinemia. *Eur J Haematol* 2007;79(3):244–247.

59. Schop RF, Kuehl WM, Van Wier SA, et al. Waldenstrom macroglobulinemia neoplastic cells lack immunoglobulin heavy chain locus translocations but have frequent 6q deletions. *Blood* 2002;100(8):2996–3001.

60. Schop RF, Van Wier SA, Xu R, et al. 6q deletion discriminates Waldenstrom macroglobulinemia from IgM monoclonal gammopathy of undetermined significance. *Cancer Genet Cytogenet* 2006;169(2):150–153.

61. Braggio E, Keats JJ, Leleu X, et al. Identification of copy number abnormalities and inactivating mutations in two negative regulators of nuclear factor-kappaB signaling pathways in Waldenstrom's macroglobulinemia. *Cancer Res* 2009;69(8):3579–3588.

62. Poulain S, Roumier C, Cheok M, et al. Genome wide SNP analysis reveals frequent cryptic clonal chromosomal aberrations including uniparental disomy (UPD) in waldenstrom's macroglobulinemia. *Blood* 2009;114:1512 (abstract 3932).

63. Bang SM, Seo JW, Park KU, et al. Molecular cytogenetic analysis of Korean patients with Waldenstrom macroglobulinemia. *Cancer Genet Cytogenet* 2010; 197(2):117–121.

64. Poulain S, Braggio E, Roumier C, et al. High-throughput genomic analysis in Waldenstrom's macroglobulinemia. *Clin Lymphoma Myeloma Leuk* 2011;11(1):106–108.

65. Cook JR, Aguilera NI, Reshmi S, et al. Deletion 6q is not a characteristic marker of nodal lymphoplasmacytic lymphoma. *Cancer Genet Cytogenet* 2005;162(1):85–88.

66. Terre C, Nguyen-Khac F, Barin C, et al. Trisomy 4, a new chromosomal abnormality in Waldenstrom's macroglobulinemia: a study of 39 cases. *Leukemia* 2006;20(9):1634–1636.

67. Kitahara T, Umezu T, Ando K, et al. Non-random chromosomal deletion clustering at 20q in Waldenstrom macroglobulinemia. *Hematology* 2011;16(3):139–142.

68. Offit K, Parsa NZ, Filippa D, et al. t(9;14)(p13;q32) denotes a subset of low-grade non-Hodgkin's lymphoma with plasmacytoid differentiation. *Blood* 1992;80(10):2594–2599.

69. Iida S, Rao PH, Nallasivam P, et al. The t(9;14)(p13;q32) chromosomal translocation associated with lymphoplasmacytoid lymphoma involves the PAX-5 gene. *Blood* 1996;88(11):4110–4117.

70. Cook JR, Aguilera NI, Reshmi-Skarja S, et al. Lack of PAX5 rearrangements in lymphoplasmacytic lymphomas: reassessing the reported association with t(9;14). *Hum Pathol* 2004;35(4):447–454.

71. George TI, Wrede JE, Bangs CD, et al. Low-grade B-cell lymphomas with plasmacytic differentiation lack PAX5 gene rearrangements. *J Mol Diagn* 2005;7(3):346–351.

72. Hirase N, Yufu Y, Abe Y, et al. Primary macroglobulinemia with t(11;18)(q21;q21). *Cancer Genet Cytogenet* 2000;117(2):113–117.

73. Chng WJ, Schop RF, Price-Troska T, et al. Gene-expression profiling of Waldenstrom macroglobulinemia reveals a phenotype more similar to chronic lymphocytic leukemia than multiple myeloma. *Blood* 2006;108(8):2755–2763.

74. Gutierrez NC, Ocio EM, de Las RJ, et al. Gene expression profiling of B lymphocytes and plasma cells from Waldenstrom's macroglobulinemia: comparison with expression patterns of the same cell counterparts from chronic lymphocytic leukemia, multiple myeloma and normal individuals. *Leukemia* 2007;21(3):541–549.

75. Roccaro AM, Sacco A, Chen C, et al. microRNA expression in the biology, prognosis, and therapy of Waldenstrom macroglobulinemia. *Blood* 2009;113(18):4391–4402.

76. Roccaro AM, Sacco A, Jia X, et al. microRNA-dependent modulation of histone acetylation in Waldenstrom macroglobulinemia. *Blood* 2010;116(9):1506–1514.

77. Issa GC, Ghobrial IM, Roccaro AM. Novel agents in Waldenstrom macroglobulinemia. *Clin Investig (Lond)* 2011;1(6):815–824.

78. Leleu X, Jia X, Runnels J, et al. The Akt pathway regulates survival and homing in Waldenstrom macroglobulinemia. *Blood* 2007;110(13):4417–4426.

79. Ghobrial IM, Roccaro A, Hong F, et al. Clinical and translational studies of a phase II trial of the novel oral Akt inhibitor perifosine in relapsed or relapsed/refractory Waldenstrom's macroglobulinemia. *Clin Cancer Res* 2010;16(3):1033–1041.

80. Roccaro AM, Sacco A, Husu EN, et al. Dual targeting of the PI3K/Akt/mTOR pathway as an antitumor strategy in Waldenstrom macroglobulinemia. *Blood* 2010;115(3):559–569.

81. Ghobrial IM, Gertz M, Laplant B, et al. Phase II trial of the oral mammalian target of rapamycin inhibitor everolimus in relapsed or refractory Waldenstrom macroglobulinemia. *J Clin Oncol* 2010;28(8):1408–1414.

82. Romashkova JA, Makarov SS. NF-kappaB is a target of AKT in anti-apoptotic PDGF signalling. *Nature* 1999;401(6748):86–90.

83. Merzianu M, Jiang L, Lin P, et al. Nuclear BCL-10 expression is common in lymphoplasmacytic lymphoma/Waldenstrom macroglobulinemia and does not correlate with p65 NF-kappaB activation. *Mod Pathol* 2006;19(7):891–898.

84. Leitch D, Barrans SL, Jack AS, et al. Dysregulation of apoptosis in Waldenstrom's macroglobulinemia does not involve nuclear factor kappa B activation. *Semin Oncol* 2003;30(2):161–164.

85. Leleu X, Eeckhoute J, Jia X, et al. Targeting NF-kappaB in Waldenstrom macroglobulinemia. *Blood* 2008;111(10):5068–5077.

86. Dimopoulos MA, Anagnostopoulos A, Kyrtsonis MC, et al. Treatment of relapsed or refractory Waldenstrom's macroglobulinemia with bortezomib. *Haematologica* 2005;90(12):1655–1658.

87. Chen CI, Kouroukis CT, White D, et al. Bortezomib is active in patients with untreated or relapsed Waldenstrom's macroglobulinemia: a phase II study of the National Cancer Institute of Canada Clinical Trials Group. *J Clin Oncol* 2007;25(12):1570–1575.

88. Treon SP, Hunter ZR, Matous J, et al. Multicenter clinical trial of bortezomib in relapsed/refractory Waldenstrom's macroglobulinemia: results of WMCTG Trial 03-248. *Clin Cancer Res* 2007;13(11):3320–3325.

89. Treon SP, Ioakimidis L, Soumerai JD, et al. Primary therapy of Waldenstrom macroglobulinemia with bortezomib, dexamethasone, and rituximab: WMCTG clinical trial 05-180. *J Clin Oncol* 2009;27(23):3830–3835.

90. Ghobrial IM, Hong F, Padmanabhan S, et al. Phase II trial of weekly bortezomib in combination with rituximab in relapsed or relapsed and refractory Waldenstrom macroglobulinemia. *J Clin Oncol* 2010;28(8):1422–1428.

91. Kriangkum J, Taylor BJ, Treon SP, et al. Clonotypic IgM V/D/J sequence analysis in Waldenstrom macroglobulinemia suggests an unusual B-cell origin and an expansion of polyclonal B cells in peripheral blood. *Blood* 2004;104(7):2134–2142.

92. Kriangkum J, Taylor BJ, Treon SP, et al. Molecular characterization of Waldenstrom's macroglobulinemia reveals frequent occurrence of two B-cell clones having distinct IgH VDJ sequences. *Clin Cancer Res* 2007;13(7):2005–2013.

93. Schulz R, David D, Farkas DH, et al. Molecular analysis in a patient with Waldenstrom's macroglobulinemia reveals a rare case of biclonality. *Mol Diagn* 1996;1(3):159–166.

94. Ciric B, VanKeulen V, Rodriguez M, et al. Clonal evolution in Waldenstrom macroglobulinemia highlights functional role of B-cell receptor. *Blood* 2001;97(1):321–323.

95. Aoki H, Takishita M, Kosaka M, et al. Frequent somatic mutations in D and/or JH segments of Ig gene in Waldenstrom's macroglobulinemia and chronic lymphocytic leukemia (CLL) with Richter's syndrome but not in common CLL. *Blood* 1995;85(7):1913–1919.

96. Wagner SD, Martinelli V, Luzzatto L. Similar patterns of V kappa gene usage but different degrees of somatic mutation in hairy cell leukemia, prolymphocytic leukemia, Waldenstrom's macroglobulinemia, and myeloma. *Blood* 1994;83(12):3647–3653.

97. Kriangkum J, Taylor BJ, Reiman T, Belch AR, Pilarski LM. Origins of Waldenstrom's macroglobulinemia: does it arise from an unusual B-cell precursor? *Clin Lymphoma* 2005;5(4):217–219.

98. Sahota SS, Forconi F, Ottensmeier CH, et al. Origins of the malignant clone in typical Waldenstrom's macroglobulinemia. *Semin Oncol* 2003;30(2):136–141.

99. Sahota SS, Forconi F, Ottensmeier CH, et al. Typical Waldenstrom macroglobulinemia is derived from a B-cell arrested after cessation of somatic mutation but prior to isotype switch events. *Blood* 2002;100(4):1505–1507.

100. Klein U, Rajewsky K, Kuppers R. Human immunoglobulin (Ig)M+IgD+ peripheral blood B cells expressing the CD27 cell surface antigen carry somatically mutated variable region genes: CD27 as a general marker for somatically mutated (memory) B cells. *J Exp Med* 1998;188(9):1679–1689.

101. Stone MJ, Pascual V. Pathophysiology of Waldenstrom's macroglobulinemia. *Haematologica* 2010;95(3):359–364.

102. Kriangkum J, Taylor BJ, Strachan E, et al. Impaired class switch recombination (CSR) in Waldenstrom macroglobulinemia (WM) despite apparently normal CSR machinery. *Blood* 2006;107(7):2920–2927.

103. Dhodapkar MV, Hoering A, Gertz MA, et al. Long-term survival in Waldenstrom macroglobulinemia: 10-year follow-up of Southwest Oncology Group-directed intergroup trial S9003. *Blood* 2009;113(4):793–796.

104. Kyle RA, Benson J, Larson D, et al. IgM monoclonal gammopathy of undetermined significance and smoldering Waldenstrom's macroglobulinemia. *Clin Lymphoma Myeloma* 2009;9(1):17–18.

105. Kyle RA, Dispenzieri A, Kumar S, et al. IgM monoclonal gammopathy of undetermined significance (MGUS) and smoldering Waldenstrom's macroglobulinemia (SWM). *Clin Lymphoma Myeloma Leuk* 2011;11(1):74–76.

106. Baldini L, Goldaniga M, Guffanti A, et al. Immunoglobulin M monoclonal gammopathies of undetermined significance and indolent Waldenstrom's macroglobulinemia recognize the same determinants of evolution into symptomatic lymphoid disorders: proposal for a common prognostic scoring system. *J Clin Oncol* 2005;23(21):4662–4668.

107. Gertz MA, Anagnostopoulos A, Anderson K, et al. Treatment recommendations in Waldenstrom's macroglobulinemia: consensus panel recommendations from the Second International Workshop on Waldenstrom's macroglobulinemia. *Semin Oncol* 2003;30(2):121–126.

108. Treon SP, Gertz MA, Dimopoulos M, et al. Update on treatment recommendations from the Third International Workshop on Waldenstrom's macroglobulinemia. *Blood* 2006;107(9):3442–3446.

109. Dimopoulos MA, Gertz MA, Kastritis E, et al. Update on treatment recommendations from the Fourth International Workshop on Waldenstrom's Macroglobulinemia. *J Clin Oncol* 2009;27(1):120–126.

110. Ansell SM, Kyle RA, Reeder CB, et al. Diagnosis and management of Waldenstrom macroglobulinemia: Mayo stratification of macroglobulinemia and risk-adapted therapy (mSMART) guidelines. *Mayo Clin Proc* 2010;85(9):824–833.

111. Gertz MA. Waldenstrom macroglobulinemia: 2011 update on diagnosis, risk stratification, and management. *Am J Hematol* 2011;86(5):411–416.

112. Ghobrial IM, Fonseca R, Greipp PR, et al. Initial immunoglobulin M "flare" after rituximab therapy in patients diagnosed with Waldenstrom macroglobulinemia: an Eastern Cooperative Oncology Group Study. *Cancer* 2004;101(11):2593–2598.

113. Treon SP, Soumerai JD, Hunter ZR, et al. Long-term follow-up of symptomatic patients with lymphoplasmacytic lymphoma/Waldenstrom macroglobulinemia treated with the anti-CD52 monoclonal antibody alemtuzumab. *Blood* 2011;118(2):276–281.

114. Morel P, Duhamel A, Gobbi P, et al. International prognostic scoring system for Waldenstrom macroglobulinemia. *Blood* 2009;113(18):4163–4170.

115. Kastritis E, Kyrtsonis MC, Hatjiharissi E, et al. No significant improvement in the outcome of patients with Waldenstrom's macroglobulinemia treated over the last 25 years. *Am J Hematol* 2011;86(6):479–483.

116. Leleu X, Soumerai J, Roccaro A, et al. Increased incidence of transformation and myelodysplasia/acute leukemia in patients with Waldenstrom macroglobulinemia treated with nucleoside analogs. *J Clin Oncol* 2009;27(2):250–255.

117. Ling S, Joshua DE, Gibson J, et al. Transformation and progression of Waldenstrom's macroglobulinemia following cladribine therapy in two cases: natural evolution or iatrogenic causation? *Am J Hematol* 2006;81(2):110–114.

118. Li J, Sze DM, Brown RD, et al. Clonal expansions of cytotoxic T cells exist in the blood of patients with Waldenstrom macroglobulinemia but exhibit anergic properties and are eliminated by nucleoside analogue therapy. *Blood* 2010;115(17):3580–3588.

119. Lin P, Mansoor A, Bueso-Ramos C, et al. Diffuse large B-cell lymphoma occurring in patients with lymphoplasmacytic lymphoma/Waldenstrom macroglobulinemia. Clinicopathologic features of 12 cases. *Am J Clin Pathol* 2003;120(2):246–253.

120. Rosales CM, Lin P, Mansoor A, et al. Lymphoplasmacytic lymphoma/Waldenstrom macroglobulinemia associated with Hodgkin disease. A report of two cases. *Am J Clin Pathol* 2001;116(1):34–40.

121. Owen RG, Bynoe AG, Varghese A, et al. Heterogeneity of histological transformation events in Waldenstrom's macroglobulinemia (WM) and related disorders. *Clin Lymphoma Myeloma Leuk* 2011;11(1):176–179.

122. Varghese AM, Sayala H, Evans PA, et al. Development of EBV-associated diffuse large B-cell lymphoma in Waldenstrom macroglobulinemia and mantle cell lymphoma. *Leuk Lymphoma* 2008;49(8):1618–1619.

123. Criteria for the classification of monoclonal gammopathies, multiple myeloma and related disorders: a report of the International Myeloma Working Group. *Br J Haematol* 2003;121(5):749–757.

124. Kyle RA, Therneau TM, Rajkumar SV, et al. Long-term follow-up of IgM monoclonal gammopathy of undetermined significance. *Blood* 2003;102(10):3759–3764.

125. Morra E, Cesana C, Klersy C, et al. Predictive variables for malignant transformation in 452 patients with asymptomatic IgM monoclonal gammopathy. *Semin Oncol* 2003;30(2):172–177.

126. Molina TJ, Lin P, Swerdlow SH, et al. Marginal zone lymphomas with plasmacytic differentiation and related disorders. *Am J Clin Pathol* 2011;136(2):211–225.

127. Shaheen SP, Talwalkar SS, Lin P, et al. Waldenstrom macroglobulinemia: a review of the entity and its differential diagnosis. *Adv Anat Pathol* 2011;18(1):11–27.

128. Arcaini L, Varettoni M, Boveri E, et al. Distinctive clinical and histological features of Waldenstrom's macroglobulinemia and splenic marginal zone lymphoma. *Clin Lymphoma Myeloma Leuk* 2011;11(1):103–105.

129. Kyrtsonis MC, Levidou G, Korkolopoulou P, et al. CD138 expression helps distinguishing Waldenstrom's macroglobulinemia (WM) from splenic marginal zone lymphoma (SMZL). *Clin Lymphoma Myeloma Leuk* 2011;11(1):99–102.

130. Mateo M, Mollejo M, Villuendas R, et al. 7q31–32 allelic loss is a frequent finding in splenic marginal zone lymphoma. *Am J Pathol* 1999;154(5):1583–1589.

131. Montalban C, Castrillo JM, Abraira V, et al. Gastric B-cell mucosa-associated lymphoid tissue (MALT) lymphoma. Clinicopathological study and evaluation of the prognostic factors in 143 patients. *Ann Oncol* 1995;6(4):355–362.

132. Thieblemont C, Berger F, Dumontet C, et al. Mucosa-associated lymphoid tissue lymphoma is a disseminated disease in one third of 158 patients analyzed. *Blood* 2000;95(3):802–806.

133. Remstein ED, Dogan A, Einerson RR, et al. The incidence and anatomic site specificity of chromosomal translocations in primary extranodal marginal zone B-cell lymphoma of mucosa-associated lymphoid tissue (MALT lymphoma) in North America. *Am J Surg Pathol* 2006;30(12):1546–1553.

134. Streubel B, Simonitsch-Klupp I, Mullauer L, et al. Variable frequencies of MALT lymphoma-associated genetic aberrations in MALT lymphomas of different sites. *Leukemia* 2004;18(10):1722–1726.

135. Seegmiller AC, Xu Y, McKenna RW, et al. Immunophenotypic differentiation between neoplastic plasma cells in mature B-cell lymphoma vs. plasma cell myeloma. *Am J Clin Pathol* 2007;127(2):176–181.

136. Goteri G, Olivieri A, Ranaldi R, et al. Bone marrow histopathological and molecular changes of small B-cell lymphomas after rituximab therapy: comparison with clinical response and patient's outcome. *Int J Immunopathol Pharmacol* 2006;19(2):421–431.

137. Varghese AM, Rawstron AC, Ashcroft AJ, et al. Assessment of bone marrow response in Waldenstrom's macroglobulinemia. *Clin Lymphoma Myeloma* 2009;9(1):53–55.

Chapter 20
Mantle Cell Lymphoma

James R. Cook • Steven H. Swerdlow

Mantle cell lymphoma (MCL) has been recognized as a distinct entity for almost four decades, and it acquired its current name about two decades later. Although originally defined solely based on its morphologic appearance and included among the other cytologically low-grade lymphomas in the Kiel classification, it has long been recognized as an aggressive but generally incurable neoplasm. However, with better ancillary tools to help define MCL, it is now known to have a much broader morphologic and clinical spectrum than when originally described. In addition, it has served as a model in terms of understanding B-cell lymphomagenesis and progression (1,2).

 ## DEFINITION AND HISTORICAL BACKGROUND

MCL is defined in the 2008 WHO classification as "a B-cell neoplasm generally composed of monomorphic small to medium-sized lymphoid cells with irregular nuclear contours and a *CCND1* translocation. Neoplastic transformed cells (centroblasts), paraimmunoblasts, and proliferation centers are absent" (3). A small proportion of MCLs are also known to be cyclin D1 and *CCND1* translocation negative (4). Reflecting its wide morphologic and clinical spectrum, several variants of MCL are recognized. There are two clinically relevant aggressive variants recognized in the WHO classification, namely, blastoid and pleomorphic MCL. Small cell and marginal zone–like morphologic variants are also recognized with the former considered to be distinctive by some. Although not graded, it is considered very important to assess the proliferative fraction in MCL based on mitotic count or Ki-67 staining. Finally, there is current interest in recognizing two more clinically indolent variants. The first is defined by the presence of peripheral blood, marrow, and sometimes splenic involvement but without peripheral adenopathy (5) and the other is *in situ* mantle cell lymphoma (ISMCL) (6).

MCL was first described with the name "diffuse germinocytoma" by K. Lennert in 1973 and included in the 1974 Kiel classification as centrocytic lymphoma (7). It was thought to be derived from pure centrocytes, rather than a combination of centrocytes and centroblasts, which characterized other germinal center–derived neoplasms. The first manuscript describing "centrocytic lymphoma" in detail was published in 1980 (8). The criteria for MCL variably overlapped what was also being diagnosed at the time as "malignant lymphoma, lymphocytic, intermediate grade of differentiation" or "intermediate lymphocytic lymphoma"; however, many accepted the presence of proliferation centers or transformed cells/centroblasts in these entities while others suggested excluding those cases (9). A subset of MCL (as well as some other types of B-cell lymphomas that had a mantle zone growth pattern) was also diagnosed as "mantle zone lymphoma." Lennert had also recognized that MCL had a mantle zone growth pattern in newly infiltrated lymph nodes. In 1992, the International Lymphoma Study Group proposed the current term of MCL and noted that "Lennert's ... characterization of centrocytic lymphoma remains one of the best descriptions of the morphology of this lymphoma, although we would add that residual, nonneoplastic germinal centers are frequently seen" (10). By this time, it was recognized that MCL was not a germinal center–derived lymphoma and that it was strongly associated with translocations of what subsequently turned out to be the cyclin D1 (*CCND1*) gene (previously known as *BCL1* or *PRAD1*) usually with the *IgH* gene (11). Documentation of cyclin D1 expression followed, which, together with the demonstration of *CCND1* translocations by molecular or cytogenetic techniques, allowed for greater and more definitive recognition of the full spectrum of MCL. Additional criteria were reviewed and agreed upon at the first workshop of the European Task Force on Lymphoma held in Annecy, France, in February 1994 (12). Since then, the spectrum of MCL has continued to expand even further. In addition, numerous studies have continued to expand the "complex landscape" of genetic and epigenetic alterations present in MCL (2).

 ## EPIDEMIOLOGY

MCL represents approximately 2% to 6% of all non-Hodgkin lymphomas (3,13,14) with a reported incidence of 0.55/100,000 in the United States and a similar rate of 0.45/100,000 in Europe (15,16). The median age at first diagnosis is 68 years, and diagnosis under the age of 50 is uncommon (14–16). There is a significant male predominance (M:F ratio 2–2.5:1) (14–16). Analysis of data from the United States shows evidence of racial differences, with the incidence in Caucasians reported to be approximately twice that in African Americans or other races (16). Several studies have demonstrated skewed immunoglobulin variable gene segment usage (17–22), suggesting that antigen selection contributes to lymphomagenesis, but a definitive link to underlying infectious agents or autoimmune diseases has not been identified (14,16).

 ## CLINICAL FEATURES

Following recognition of MCL as a distinct entity, numerous studies clarified the typical clinical features at presentation (Table 20.1) (11,12,23–37). The majority of patients present with generalized adenopathy, splenomegaly, bone marrow involvement, and high-stage disease (Ann Arbor stage III–IV). Overt leukemic involvement, identified by peripheral blood lymphocytosis, is present in approximately 25% of cases, but using more sensitive flow cytometric studies, peripheral blood involvement is identified in >90% of patients (38).

Extranodal involvement is common, usually in the presence of widespread lymphadenopathy. A distinctive form of extranodal presentation with disease predominantly limited to the gastrointestinal tract is known as multiple lymphomatous polyposis (MLP) (39–43). In MLP, the MCL forms innumerable polypoid

Table 20.1	CLINICAL FEATURES AT PRESENTATION
Generalized adenopathy	90%
Splenomegaly	55%
Hepatomegaly	35%
Bone marrow infiltration	75%
Peripheral blood lymphocytosis	25%
Overt gastrointestinal involvement	15%
Waldeyer's ring involvement	10%
Ann Arbor stage III–IV	90%
B symptoms	35%
Bulky disease	30%
Poor performance status	20%
Elevated LDH	40%
Elevated β_2-microglobulin	50%

Adapted from Zucca E, Stein H, Coiffier B. European Lymphoma Task Force (ELTF): report of the workshop on mantle cell lymphoma (MCL). *Ann Oncol* 1994;5(6):507–511, with permission.

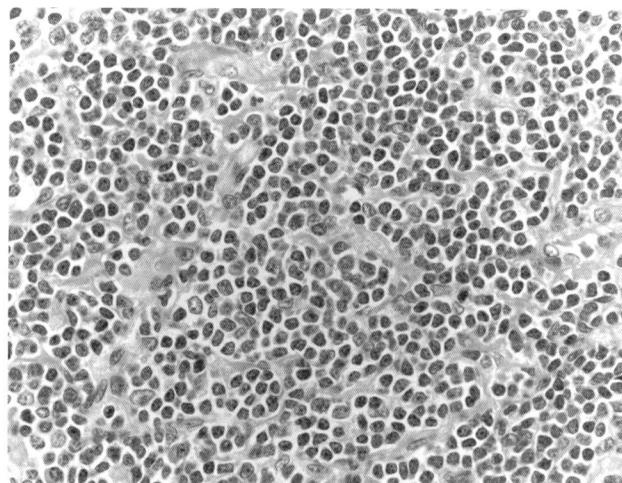

FIGURE 20.1. Typical histologic features of classic MCL. The cells are small to intermediate in size with angulated nuclear contours and indistinct nucleoli.

lesions throughout the small and large intestine. Patients with MLP frequently present with abdominal pain, weight loss, diarrhea, and iron deficiency anemia. The preferential localization within the gastrointestinal tract appears to be mediated in many MLP cases by expression of the $\alpha 4\beta 7$ integrin, which facilitates homing to the gastrointestinal tract (44). Intestinal involvement, however, is not limited to patients with MLP. Endoscopy studies have shown that intestinal involvement is present in >80% of MCL patients overall, even in the absence of altered mucosa on endoscopy (45). While MLP is highly associated with MCL, it should be noted that this type of presentation may also be seen in follicular lymphoma and MALT lymphomas (46–50).

Central nervous system (CNS) involvement, although rare at initial diagnosis, has been reported at time of relapse in 4% to 25% of patients (51,52). The risk of CNS involvement is reportedly increased in patients with blastoid morphology and a high proliferation index as determined by Ki-67 immunohistochemistry (IHC).

MORPHOLOGY

Lymph Nodes

In the classic form of the disease, the neoplastic cells are small to intermediate in size with irregular, angulated nuclear contours, scant cytoplasm, and relatively clumped chromatin with indistinct nucleoli (Fig. 20.1) (3,53,54). Large transformed cells are rare to absent. Three main histologic growth patterns are recognized in lymph nodes: diffuse, nodular, and mantle zone (Fig. 20.2), with many cases showing a mixture of the diffuse and nodular patterns (11,27,53,55). In the diffuse pattern, which is the most common, the nodal architecture is effaced by a diffuse proliferation of small neoplastic cells, often admixed with epithelioid-appearing histiocytes and with hyalinized vessels. In the nodular growth pattern, the neoplastic cells form large, often somewhat vague nodules that may become confluent. Lastly, the mantle zone pattern, which is the least common (<2% of cases) (53,55), shows residual hyperplastic germinal centers surrounded by widened neoplastic mantle zones. The mantle zone pattern must be distinguished from so-called ISMCL as described in the *In Situ* Mantle Cell Lymphoma section.

Peripheral Blood

In peripheral blood smears, the neoplastic cells are usually small to intermediate in size with irregular to clefted nuclear contours, mature chromatin, and sometimes distinct nucleoli (Fig. 20.3). There is cytologic overlap with the findings in chronic

lymphocytic leukemia (CLL), especially CLL with trisomy 12, which is associated with atypical cytology (56–59). Uncommonly, cases may present with a predominance of prolymphocyte-like cells. While such cases were frequently diagnosed as prolymphocytic leukemia (PLL) with t(11;14)(q13;q32) in the past, today these are generally accepted as MCL (3,60).

Spleen

In MCL with splenic involvement (Fig. 20.4), gross and microscopic examination of the spleen shows diffuse enlargement with prominent expanded white pulp nodules (61–63). Gross macronodules are not present. Residual germinal centers may be seen in the white pulp nodules, and there may be red pulp involvement. The periphery of the nodules may show more abundant cytoplasm, creating a differential diagnosis that includes splenic marginal zone lymphoma (64,65).

Gastrointestinal Tract

In MLP, there are numerous polypoid masses throughout the small and large bowel (39–43). Histologically, these lesions are composed of large aggregates of neoplastic cells infiltrating through the mucosa. Occasionally, reactive germinal centers may be identified. Destructive lymphoepithelial lesions, characteristic of extranodal MALT lymphomas, are not present, although intraepithelial neoplastic cells may be identified. Gastrointestinal involvement is also frequently seen in patients with typical nodal MCL where solitary tumoral masses or ulcerated lesions composed of tumor cells may occur. Endoscopic biopsy may also show patchy involvement by MCL even in areas of unremarkable mucosa (45,66).

Cytologic Variants

Several cytologic variants have been described in MCL. Two aggressive variants, the blastoid and pleomorphic types, are associated with an adverse prognosis and are therefore important to recognize in routine practice (3,23,53,55,67). Other variants have also been described, whose identification is not required but that are important to recognize because of their varied differential diagnoses.

Blastoid Variant

In blastoid MCL, the cells are small to intermediate in size with finely dispersed chromatin (Fig. 20.5A). Tingible body

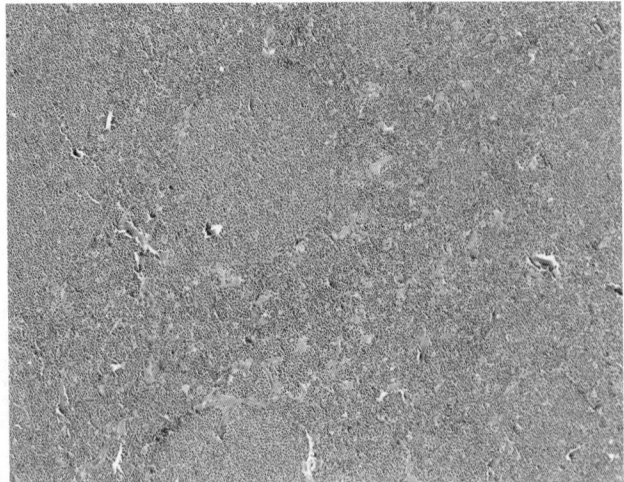

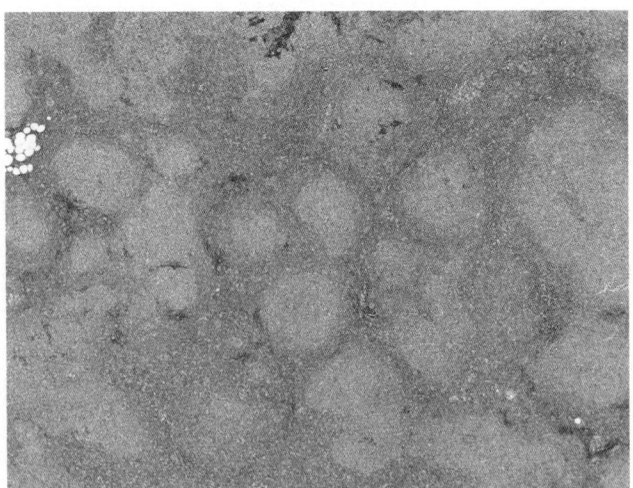

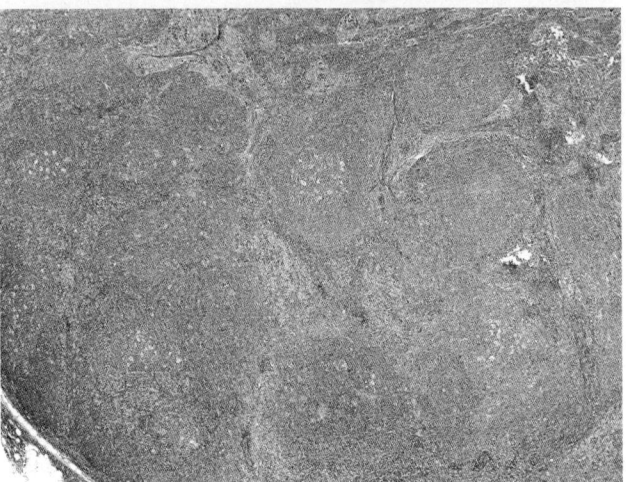

FIGURE 20.2. Growth patterns of MCL: predominantly diffuse with occasional vague nodules (**A**), markedly nodular (**B**), and mantle zone (**C**).

macrophages may be present, creating a "starry sky" pattern. This variant frequently displays prominent mitotic figures (>2 to 3/hpf). The differential diagnosis in blastoid MCL includes lymphoblastic lymphoma. Blastoid MCL in the peripheral blood may create a differential diagnosis that includes PLL or other aggressive B-cell lymphomas.

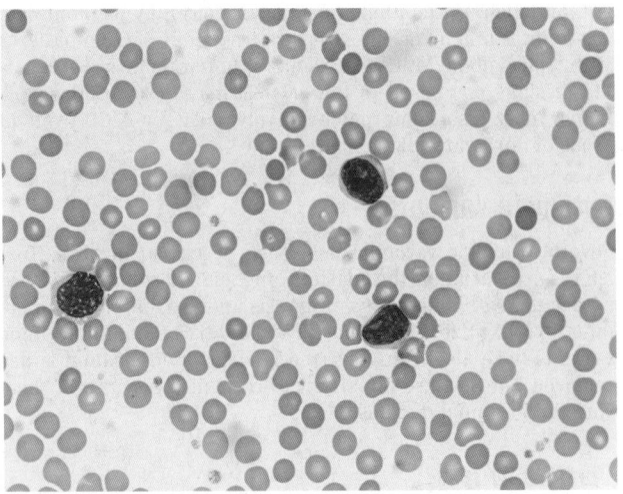

FIGURE 20.3. MCL in the peripheral blood. The neoplastic cells are small to intermediate in size with round to irregular nuclei, sometimes with small nucleoli.

Pleomorphic Variant

In the pleomorphic type, the cells are intermediate to large with round to irregular nuclear contours, vesicular chromatin, and often nucleoli (Fig. 20.5B). Morphologically, such cases may closely resemble diffuse large B-cell lymphoma (DLBCL). Some MCL cases may display a mixture of classic and pleomorphic cytologic features.

Other Cytologic Variants

In the small cell variant, which is reported to represent <10% of MCL, the neoplastic cells are small with round nuclear contours, scant cytoplasm, and condensed chromatin, resembling the cells of CLL/small lymphocytic lymphoma (SLL) (55,68). A minority of cases may show more abundant pale cytoplasm, resembling the monocytoid or marginal zone–type cells of a marginal zone lymphoma (11,69). Plasmacytic differentiation, although only rarely described in MCL (70,71), may also occur and leads to a differential diagnosis that includes marginal zone lymphoma, lymphoplasmacytic lymphoma, or a potentially unrelated plasma cell neoplasm.

In Situ Mantle Cell Lymphoma

As with the *IGH/BCL2* translocation, the presence of very low levels of *IGH/CCND1* fusion transcripts can also be detected in a small subset of apparently healthy controls (72). What is believed to often be the tissue equivalent of this phenomenon,

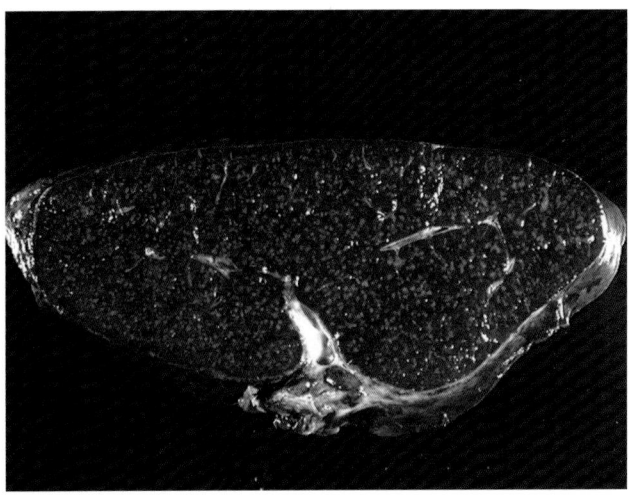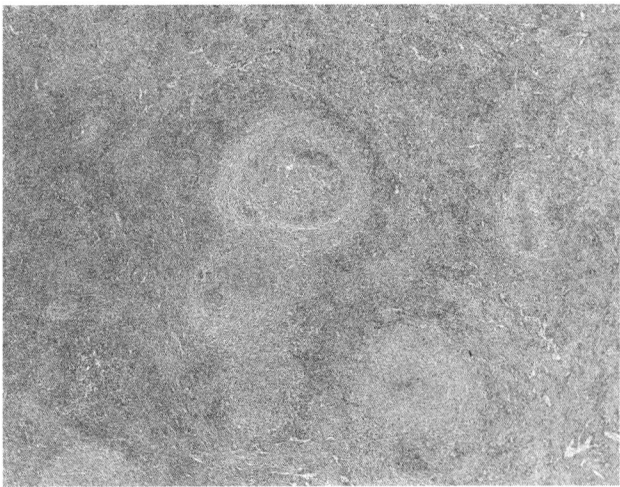

FIGURE 20.4. Splenic involvement by MCL. A: Gross examination reveals prominent white pulp nodules without a focal mass lesion. **B:** Histologically, the neoplastic cells are found in the white pulp nodules with variable amounts of red pulp infiltration.

commonly known as *in situ* mantle cell lymphoma (ISMCL), is seen in occasional lymph node biopsies with completely preserved lymph node architecture, but with focal germinal centers surrounded by mantle zones containing CD5 variably positive, cyclin D1–positive B cells (Fig. 20.6) (6,73,74). In contrast to cases of overt MCL with a mantle zone growth pattern, cases of ISMCL usually do not have widened mantle zones. If the mantle zones are widened, the cyclin D1–positive cells are only a subset of the cells present within the mantles. Because of the minimal morphologic changes in such cases, this phenomenon is almost always detected only incidentally after cyclin D1 IHC. Interestingly, cases of ISMCL have recently been reported to lack SOX11 expression more frequently than classic MCL (73,75). This finding has suggested that cases of ISMCL may contain *IGH/CCND1* as a "single hit" abnormality, but lack additional abnormalities including SOX11 dysregulation, required for progression to overt lymphoma. One group, however, has reported SOX11 negativity to be associated with more aggressive disease (76), highlighting the need for additional studies to clarify the clinical significance of this subset of patients. These cases of aggressive SOX11-negative MCL often have strong p53 expression (76). Retrospective studies of patients with overt MCL have reported that lymph nodes sampled prior to the diagnosis of overt MCL

may contain ISMCL, although the incidence of this finding is currently controversial (77a,77b). This finding suggests that ISMCL may precede most, if not all, cases of overt MCL. Nevertheless, out of concern that at least some of these cases do not represent a true malignancy, the term "MCL-like B cells of uncertain significance" has recently been proposed for these lesions (78).

PHENOTYPE

Most cases of MCL may be confidently diagnosed on the basis of morphology and characteristic phenotypic findings (Fig. 20.7). MCL is typically positive for B-cell antigens (CD19, CD20, CD22, CD79a) with intermediate to bright surface immunoglobulin light chain expression. Lambda light chains are found more frequently than kappa (3,11,53,79). The immunoglobulin heavy chain is IgM in the vast majority of cases, usually with coexpression of IgD. Characteristically, MCL shows coexpression of CD5 and FMC7 (a CD20 epitope) and absence of CD23. Importantly, this prototypic phenotype is not completely specific for MCL and is also seen in a minority of cases of CLL (80). Similarly, MCL not uncommonly lacks this prototypic phenotype. Absence of CD5 expression has been reported in 5%

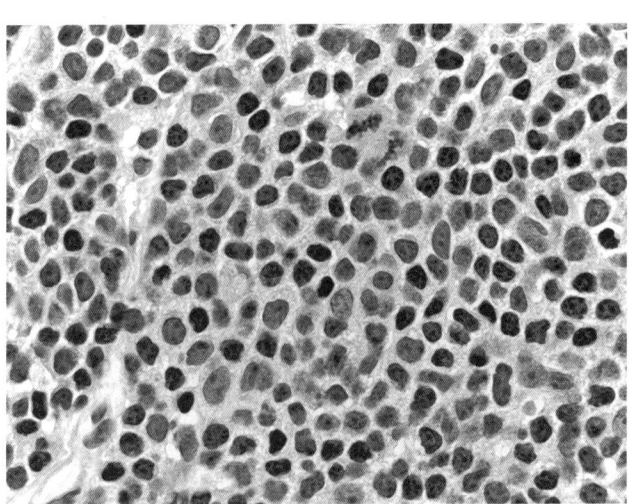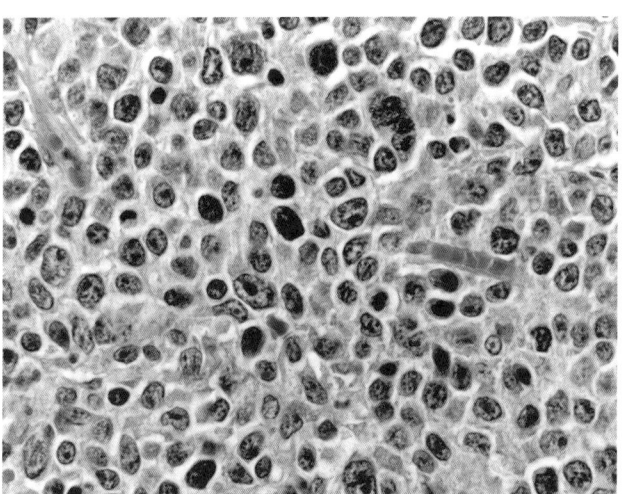

FIGURE 20.5. Cytologic variants of MCL. In the blastoid type (**A**), the cells display finely dispersed chromatin and frequent mitotic figures. The pleomorphic type (**B**) shows larger cells with vesicular chromatin and distinct nucleoli.

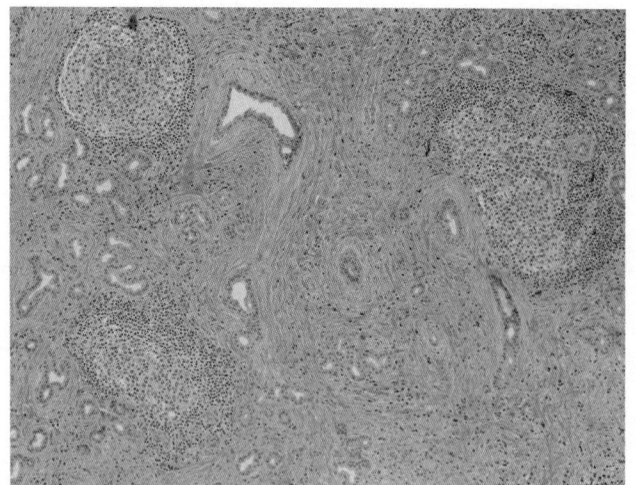

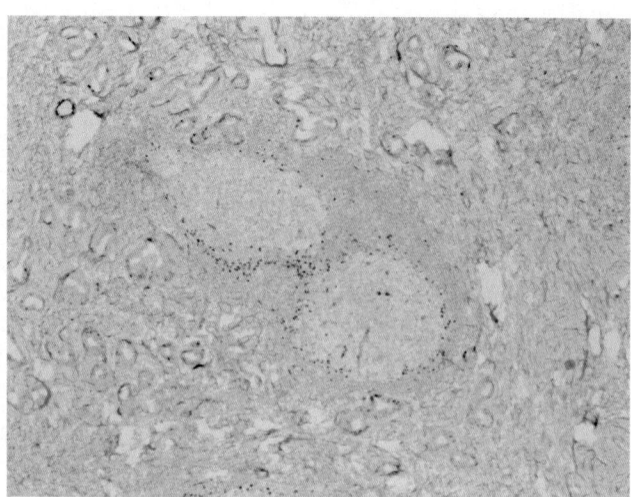

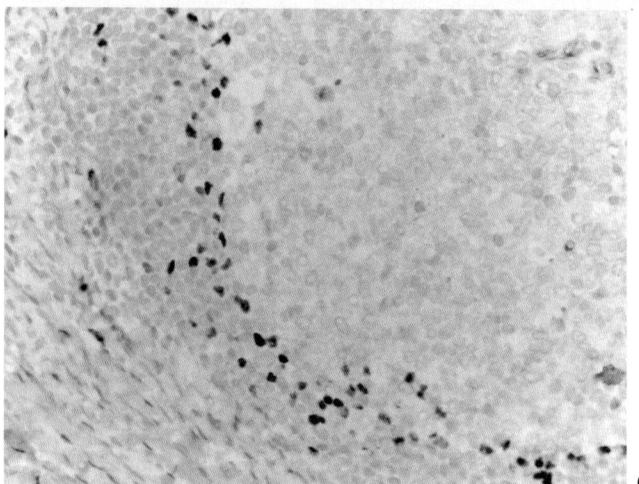

FIGURE 20.6. *In situ* **mantle cell lymphoma (ISMCL).** This lacrimal gland contains a sclerotic chronic inflammatory infiltrate with scattered hyperplastic germinal centers (**A**, H&E). A cyclin D1 immunostain shows thin rims of cyclin D1–positive B cells surrounding the germinal centers (**B**). The cyclin D1–positive cells are largely confined to the innermost layers of the mantle zone (**C**).

to 17% of MCL (81–83). Aberrant expression of the germinal center–associated marker BCL6, often in the setting of *BCL6* gene abnormalities, has been described in approximately 10% of cases, while CD10 is reported only rarely, usually only by a minority of the neoplastic cells (82,84,85). IRF4/MUM1 expression is seen in approximately one-third of cases (85). CD23 expression is found in one quarter of cases, and may be associated with a more favorable prognosis (82,86).

The vast majority of cases (>95%) are positive for cyclin D1 by IHC with rabbit monoclonal antibodies to cyclin D1, introduced almost a decade ago, showing positivity in a greater proportion of neoplastic cells than earlier mouse monoclonal antibodies and having less nonspecific cytoplasmic staining (87,88). Although in the past cyclin D1 expression by IHC or translocations by fluorescence *in situ* hybridization (FISH) were considered to be defining features of MCL, more recently the existence of cyclin D1–negative cases has become widely accepted (4,89–92).

A newer marker useful in the differential diagnosis of MCL is SOX11, a transcription factor that is important for embryonic development of the nervous system (75). SOX11 staining has been reported in 93% to 95% of MCL cases and is positive in cyclin D1–negative MCL, including blastoid forms (75,89,90). It also may be helpful when cyclin D1 staining is suboptimal or otherwise difficult to interpret. SOX11 expression, however, is not unique to MCL and may also be seen in lymphoblastic lymphoma, Burkitt lymphoma, hairy cell leukemia, and T-cell PLL (89). SOX11 also seems to be absent in a subset of cases of ISMCL and in some patients with leukemic disease and a remarkably indolent clinical course (described below). Diminished p27

expression in classical MCL has also been reported to be of help in distinguishing MCL from other small B-cell neoplasms where p27 is usually strongly expressed (93–95).

CYTOGENETIC AND MOLECULAR ABNORMALITIES

Cyclin D1 Translocation

The cytogenetic hallmark of MCL is the t(11;14)(q13;q32) *IGH/CCND1* translocation, which places the *CCND1* gene under the control of the *IGH* locus enhancer element (Fig. 20.8). This translocation is identified in >95% of cases (96–98). Variant translocations involving *CCND1* and either the *IGK* or *IGL* loci have rarely been reported (99). *CCND1* translocations can be identified by metaphase cytogenetics, FISH or PCR techniques although the yield with PCR (or even Southern blot) studies is much lower than with cytogenetic studies (100). FISH studies utilizing a *CCND1* break-apart strategy are also particularly valuable as these may also detect the rare *CCND1* translocations other than the *IGH/CCND1*. The presence of a *CCND1* translocation results in expression of the cyclin D1 protein, which is not normally expressed in lymphocytes.

Two cyclin D1 mRNA transcripts are produced in MCL through alternative splicing. The first, full-length transcript contains exons 1 to 5 and a 3′ untranslated region that includes an AUUUA sequence that leads to decreased mRNA stability.

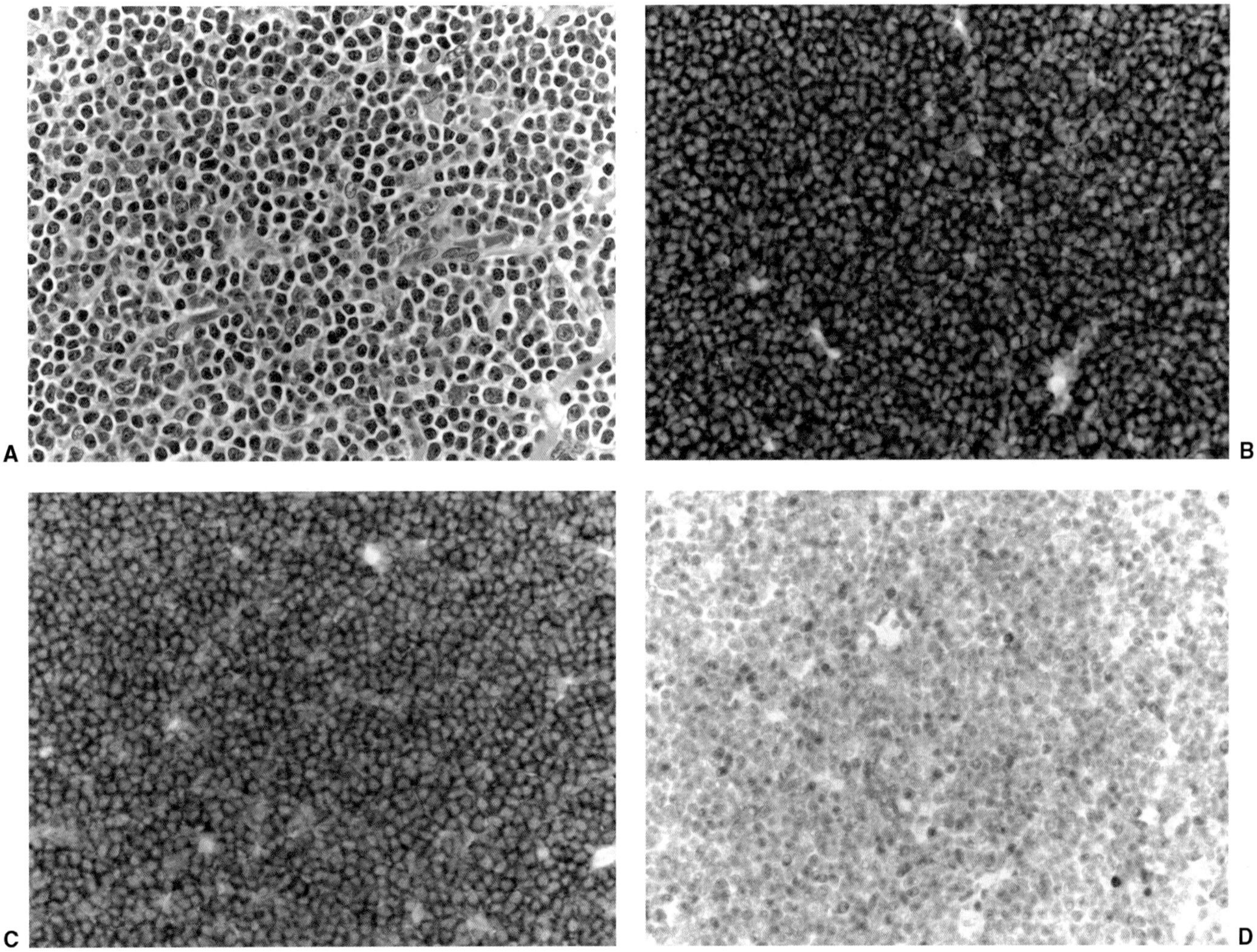

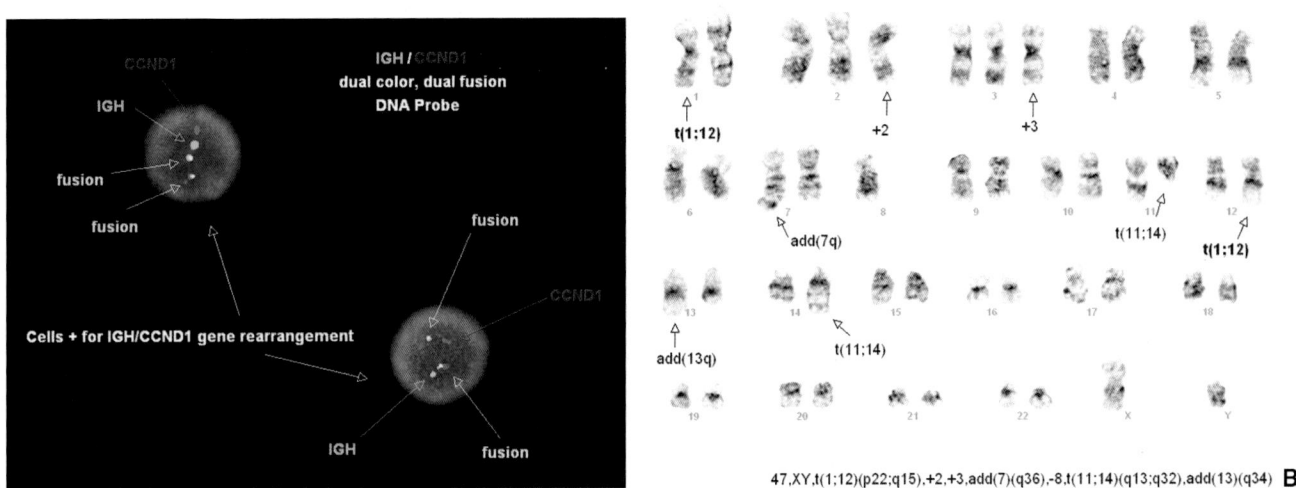

FIGURE 20.7. Immunohistochemical profile of MCL. This typical case (**A**) displays positive staining for CD20 (**B**), CD5 (**C**), and cyclin D1 (**D**).

47,XY,t(1;12)(p22;q15),+2,+3,add(7)(q36),-8,t(11;14)(q13;q32),add(13)(q34) **B**

FIGURE 20.8. Detection of the IGH/CCND1 translocation in MCL. A: Interphase FISH analysis using a dual-color, dual-fusion probe. **B:** Metaphase cytogenetic analysis revealing a complex karyotype including t(11;14)(q13;q32). (Courtesy Maureen Sherer and Susanne M. Gollin, Pittsburgh Cytogenetics Laboratory at Magee-Womens Hospital of the University of Pittsburgh Medical Center.)

FIGURE 20.9. The role of cyclin D1 in cell cycle regulation. Cyclin D1 associates with the cyclin-dependent kinases CDK4 and CDK6, resulting in phosphorylation of the retinoblastoma protein (RB1), which allows the E2F transcription factor to promote the transition from the G1 to the S phase. Cyclin D1/CDK activity is inhibited by p16-INK4a. Loss of p16-INK4a activity, which occurs with deletions of the *CDKN2A* locus at 9p21.3, enhances cyclin D1 function. Cyclin D1/CDK complexes also associate with p27, removing p27-mediated inhibition of cyclin E/CDK2 activity and further promoting cell cycle progression.

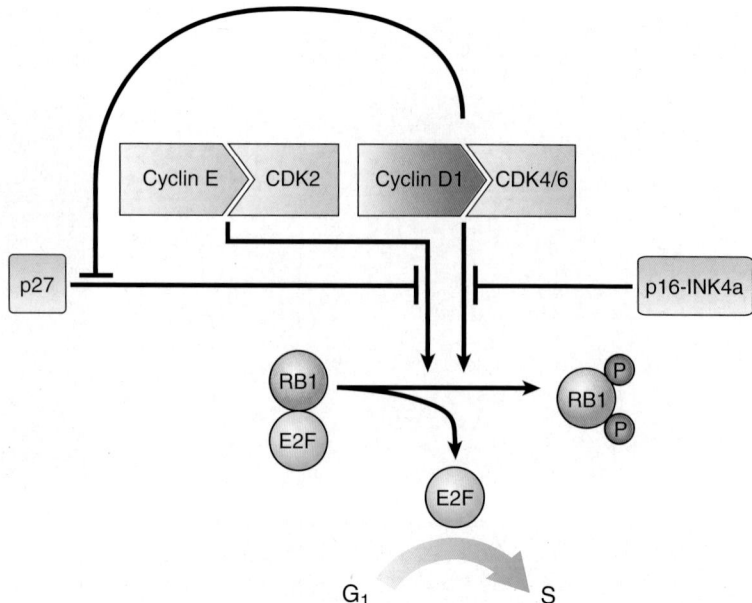

The second transcript, termed cyclin D1b, is shortened, containing exons 1 to 4 with a portion of intron 4, and lacking exon 5 and 3′ UTR (101–105). This truncated isoform is associated with longer half-life and increased nuclear protein accumulation. Both isoforms are oncogenic and are found in varying proportions in MCL. Cases of MCL with increased levels of the truncated isoform are associated with blastoid cytology, increased cyclin D1 protein expression, increased proliferative fraction, and more aggressive behavior (104,106).

Cyclin D1 protein plays a critical role in cell cycle control (Fig. 20.9). Specifically, cyclin D1 interacts with CDK4/6 kinases to promote inactivation of the retinoblastoma 1 protein (RB1) by phosphorylation (94,96,97,107). The formation of pRB1 leads to dissociation of the E2F transcription factor, promoting progression from the G1 to the S phase. This pathway may be further enhanced by additional abnormalities in MCL, such as loss of the CDKN2A locus on chromosome 9p. Increased cyclin D1 also promotes cell cycle progression through binding and sequestering p27. Decreased availability of p27 protein allows cyclin E/CDK2 complexes to also enhance phosphorylation of RB and cell cycle progression.

Cyclin D1–Negative MCL

Although the nature of reported MCL without cyclin D1 expression or a *CCND1* translocation were initially viewed with some skepticism (91,96,108), the existence of cyclin D1–negative MCL has been confirmed on the basis of gene expression profiling studies that show a gene signature identical to that in typical MCL, but lacking *CCND1* dysregulation (4,109). Follow-up studies have confirmed the existence of cases of MCL that show morphologic and phenotypic findings identical to that observed in MCL, except for the absence of cyclin D1 staining (Fig. 20.10) (89,92,110,111a).

In these rare cases of MCL lacking cyclin D1 expression, there is consistent expression of cyclin D2 and/or D3 protein. Approximately half of cyclin D1 negative MCL have been reported to contain *CCND2* translocations, while only rare cases of *CCND3* translocations have been described (4,92,111b). Assessment of cyclin D2 or D3 protein is difficult in routine practice because many commercially available antibodies do not completely discriminate between the various D type cyclins, and because cyclin D2 and D3 are each found in other types of B-cell lymphomas as well (112). Recent studies have indicated

that cyclin D1–negative MCL, like typical MCL, are positive for SOX11 (75,89). While formal criteria for the diagnosis of cyclin D1–negative MCL have not yet been established, this diagnosis should currently be reserved for cases showing typical histologic features, expression of CD5 and SOX11, and lack of cyclin D1 staining and *CCND1* translocations by FISH.

Other Cytogenetic and Molecular Abnormalities

Multiple lines of evidence indicate that the *IGH/CCND1* translocation alone is not sufficient for lymphomagenesis. In transgenic mouse models of the *IGH/CCND1* translocation, spontaneous lymphomas do not develop, and the lymphomas that are induced in these model systems invariably contain abnormalities in other molecular pathways that lead to transformation, such as *MYC* (113–115). In humans, screening studies have identified very low levels of *IGH/CCND1* fusion transcripts in approximately 7% of asymptomatic adults (72). This "preclinical" clonal population is stable over time, and does not develop into overt lymphoma in most patients. In keeping with this concept of *IGH/CCND1* as necessary but not sufficient for the development of MCL, secondary abnormalities are found in the majority of cases of MCL. Cases of MCL with an unusually indolent clinical course, however, have been reported to frequently show simple karyotypes with an isolated t(11;14)(q13;q32) (116,117).

Using traditional metaphase cytogenetics, only one-third of cases yield a simple karyotype with an apparently isolated, balanced t(11;14)(q13;q32) (118,119). The remaining two-thirds of cases show additional abnormalities. Overall, the median number of karyotypic abnormalities observed in MCL is approximately four. An even greater incidence of complex karyotypes, and a greater median number of abnormalities is observed in cases with blastoid cytology with tetraploidy, a feature most frequently seen in the pleomorphic variant (120). In recent years, studies using comparative genomic hybridization (CGH) and single nucleotide polymorphism (SNP) arrays have further delineated the common secondary abnormalities seen in MCL (Table 20.2) (2,121–124). Using SNP arrays, acquired uniparental disomy (aUPD) also occurs in 27% to 61% of cases, and predominantly affects regions that also show copy number loss. Among the recurrent gains and losses, gains of chromosome 3q and losses of 17p have been shown to be associated with poor outcome in multivariate analysis (2,121,122,125).

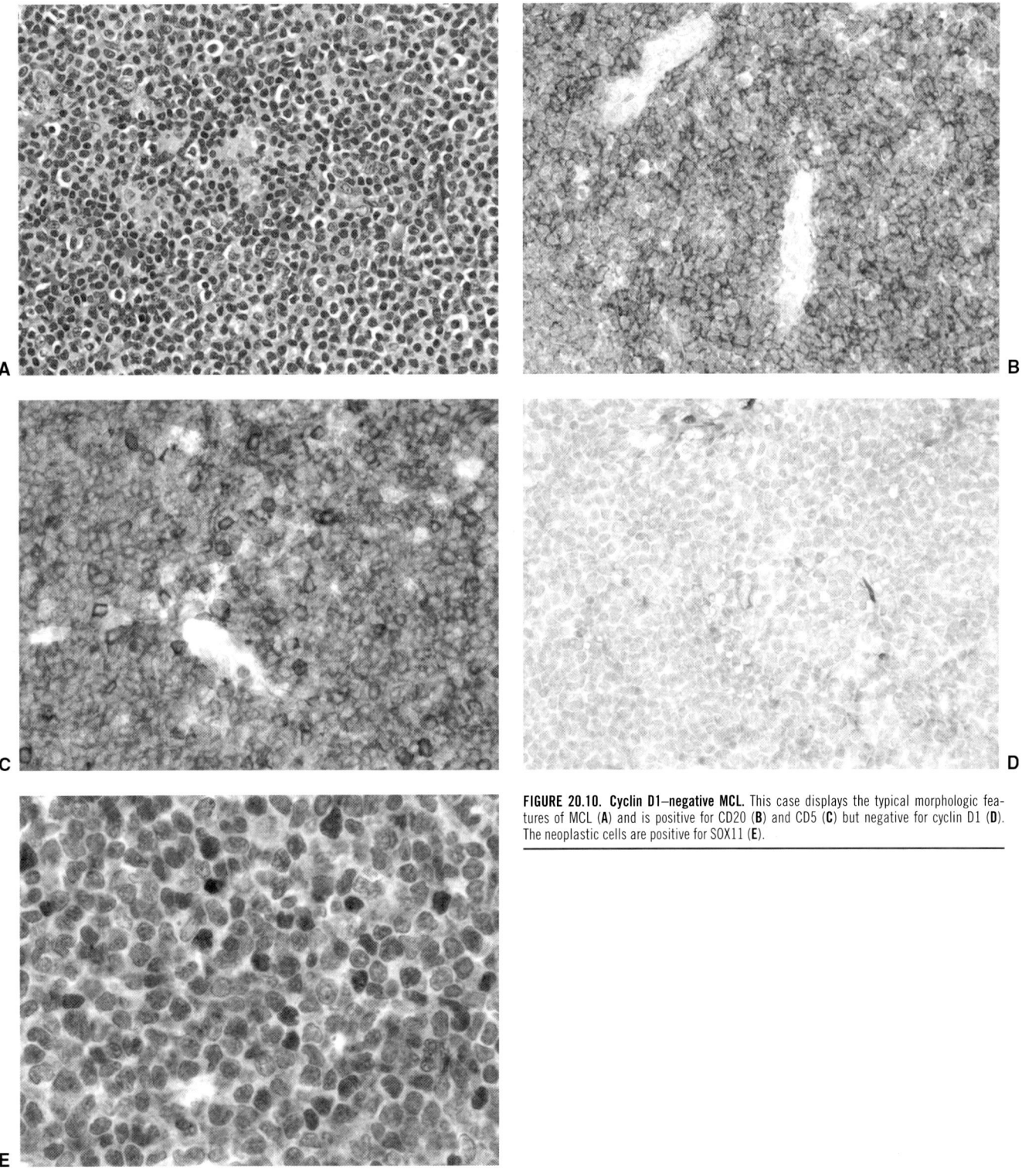

FIGURE 20.10. Cyclin D1–negative MCL. This case displays the typical morphologic features of MCL (**A**) and is positive for CD20 (**B**) and CD5 (**C**) but negative for cyclin D1 (**D**). The neoplastic cells are positive for SOX11 (**E**).

One secondary abnormality, deletion of the *CDKN2A* locus on chromosome 9p21.3, has been extensively characterized (1,96,108). This locus encodes both p16^{INK4a} and ARF. The ability of cyclin D1/CDK4 or cyclin D1/CDK6 complexes to phosphorylate RB is normally inhibited by p16^{INK4a}. Decreased p16^{INK4a} expression leads to loss of such inhibition and increased cyclin D1/CDK activity. ARF normally functions to stabilize p53 by blocking degradation by MDM2. Loss of ARF therefore leads to loss of p53 function. Increased MDM2 protein expression has also been reported in MCL, which similarly leads to decreased p53 activity (131,132). The basis of MDM2 dysregulation in

MCL, however, remains unclear as amplification of the MDM2 locus does not appear to occur.

Several types of alterations of the *TP53* locus at chromosome 17p13 may occur in MCL. Mutations in *TP53* have been reported in approximately 20% of cases of MCL and have been associated with a poor outcome (106,133,134). Cases with mutated *TP53* may also show a deletion of the normal 17p13 locus, resulting in decreased p53 function. However, the presence of *TP53* mutations and deletions of 17p13 are not necessarily concurrent. Some cases show deletions of 17p13 without *TP53* mutations, and some cases show mutant *TP53*

Table 20.2	RECURRENT SECONDARY MOLECULAR CYTOGENETIC ABNORMALITIES REPORTED IN >10% OF MCL BY METAPHASE KARYOTYPING, CGH ARRAY, OR SNP ARRAY	
Region	**Alteration**	**Putative Gene**
1p21-p31	Loss, UPD	
2q13	Loss	BCL2L11
3q21-qter	Gain	
4p12-p13	Gain	
6q23-q27	Loss	TNFAIP3
7p21-p22	Gain	
8p21-ter	Loss	
8q21-qter	Gain	MYC
9p21-p22	Loss, UPD	CDKN2A, ARF1
9q22	Gain	
9q21-qter	Loss	
10p11-p12	Gain	
10p14-p15	Loss	
11q13.3	Gain	CCND1
11q22-q23	Loss, UPD	ATM
12q13	Gain	CDK4
13q14-q34	Loss	
17p13-pter	Loss, UPD	TP53
18q11-q23	Loss	BCL2
22q11-q12	Loss	

Refs. 2,22,96,118,119,121–130.

with retention of two 17p13 loci. Some studies have reported that loss of the 17p region is associated with a poor outcome (119,126,127). Other studies, however, have reported that deletions of 17p are not associated with differences in prognosis while the detection of a TP53 mutation by sequencing studies is associated with poor outcome (2,135).

Abnormalities leading to impaired DNA repair are also frequent in MCL. Mutations in the ataxia-telangiectasia-mutated (ATM) gene, which usually are associated with deletion of the other ATM allele on chromosome 11q23, are reported in 40% to 75% of MCL (133,136–138). ATM is a serine/threonine kinase that normally plays a vital role in the repair of double-stranded DNA breaks. Loss of ATM function is thought to lead to genomic instability and progressive accumulation of secondary chromosomal abnormalities. Similarly, decreased function of CHK2 and CHK1, which are kinases downstream of the ATM pathway, have also been identified in MCL secondary to mutations, deletion, or decreased protein expression (139).

High-level amplifications of specific loci have been identified in 36% of MCL (2,121–123). Amplification of 18q21, identified in 10% to 20% of cases, includes the BCL2 locus, leading to increased levels of BCL2 expression. Amplification of the CCND1 locus has been identified in 14% of cases, and is associated with high levels of cyclin D1 mRNA expression (121,124). Interestingly, this amplification generally involves the translocated CCND1 locus, leading to complex rearrangements which may be detected by metaphase karyotyping or FISH.

A recent whole transcriptome sequencing study has identified the presence of NOTCH1 mutations in 12% of MCL (140). The NOTCH1 gene encodes a transmembrane protein that functions as a ligand-activated transcription factor. Activating mutations in NOTCH1 appear to increase proliferation, and are associated with poor prognosis in MCL.

 ## POSTULATED NORMAL COUNTERPART

Based largely upon the growth pattern of ISMCL and its immunophenotype, the neoplastic cells in MCL are believed to be most closely related to the CD5+ B cells of the inner mantle zone. It has also been suggested that because of their typically

more intense CD5 expression, they may be more closely related to fetal type CD5+ B cells (141), although the fetal cells do not localize to mantle zones and, with current immunohistochemical stains, CD5 expression can be seen in normal mantle zone B cells and sometimes even in paraffin-embedded tissue sections. While usually representing naive B cells, a significant minority of MCL have mutated immunoglobulin genes; however, the full implication of this finding is unknown since immunoglobulin gene somatic mutation may occur outside of germinal centers.

CLINICAL COURSE AND PROGNOSTIC ASSESSMENT

Patients with MCL are generally considered to have an overall median survival of 3 to 5 years (3). It has been reported that patients with advanced stage MCL have shown an improvement in overall survival over the last several decades. A German study reports a median survival of only 2.7 years for the time period 1975 to 1986 but a 4.8-year median survival for the time period 1996 to 2004 (142). An American study based on SEER data reported no significant increase in overall survival for patients with MCL for the periods 1992 to 1999, 2000 to 2003, and 2004 to 2007; however, the median survival for patients with advanced stage disease showed a significant increase from 32 to 38 months (143). The median survival for those with localized disease showed a nonsignificant increase from 56 to 65 months. Although some newer regimens raise hope for better survivals, MCL remains a very aggressive neoplasm. It is important to recognize the very different expectations for patients with the two types of "indolent" MCL. Patients who lack peripheral adenopathy and have peripheral blood, bone marrow, and sometimes splenic involvement have a median survival of 79 months (versus 30 months for those with nodal disease) (5). Patients with ISMCL are reported to pursue a very indolent course often without progression over many years, sometimes without any therapy (6). However, there may be persistent disease and progression to overt MCL can occur.

Prognostic Indicators

Clinical risk factors have been identified that are associated with prognosis in MCL. The International Prognostic Index (IPI), published in 1993, was designed to assess prognosis in diffuse large B-cell lymphomas (144). Following recognition of MCL as a distinct entity, many studies attempted to employ the IPI to assess prognosis in MCL with generally disappointing results (23,25,34,36,37,55,145–150). For this reason, an MCL-specific clinical prognostic index (the Mantle Cell International Prognostic Index, or MIPI) was designed. The MIPI uses age, Eastern Cooperative Oncology Group (ECOG) performance status, lactate dehydrogenase (LDH) level, and white blood cell (WBC) count, each of which are of independent prognostic significance in MCL as continuous variables to assess prognosis. A simplified MIPI, easily computed at the bedside, was also developed that shows a high correlation with the calculated MIPI (Table 20.3). The MIPI has subsequently been validated by several independent groups (151–156), and is now widely used in routine practice.

Several pathologic findings have also been associated with prognosis in MCL. Blastoid cytology, gains of chromosome 3q, and loss of chromosome 17p have each been associated with a poor prognosis (2,121,122,125). The diffuse growth pattern has been reported to be associated with a worse survival compared to patients with nodular architecture (55). Perhaps most importantly, it is clear that the proliferative rate in MCL is a key prognostic factor. The proliferative rate was initially

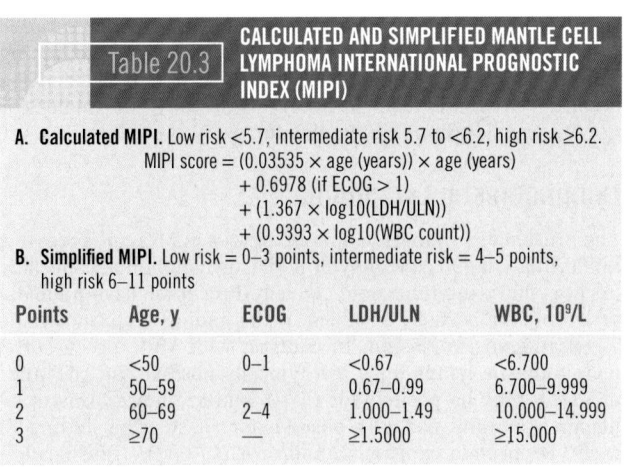

	CALCULATED AND SIMPLIFIED MANTLE CELL LYMPHOMA INTERNATIONAL PROGNOSTIC INDEX (MIPI)
Table 20.3	

A. Calculated MIPI. Low risk <5.7, intermediate risk 5.7 to <6.2, high risk ≥6.2.

$$\text{MIPI score} = (0.03535 \times \text{age (years)}) \times \text{age (years)}$$
$$+ 0.6978 \text{ (if ECOG > 1)}$$
$$+ (1.367 \times \log10(\text{LDH/ULN}))$$
$$+ (0.9393 \times \log10(\text{WBC count}))$$

B. Simplified MIPI. Low risk = 0–3 points, intermediate risk = 4–5 points, high risk 6–11 points

Points	Age, y	ECOG	LDH/ULN	WBC, 10⁹/L
0	<50	0–1	<0.67	<6.700
1	50–59	—	0.67–0.99	6.700–9.999
2	60–69	2–4	1.000–1.49	10.000–14.999
3	≥70	—	≥1.5000	≥15.000

Abbreviations: LDH, lactate dehydrogenase; ULN, laboratory upper limit of normal for LDH; WBC, white blood cell; ECOG, Eastern Cooperative Oncology Group performance status.

studied using mitotic counts, which showed that cases with >1 to 2 mitosis/hpf are associated with poor prognosis (23,25,53). Later studies emphasized the use of Ki-67 to stratify patients. Studies have employed various cutoffs from 10% to 40% positive nuclei, but an increased Ki-67 rate is clearly associated with poor outcome (53,55,157–159). Some investigators have proposed incorporating the Ki-67 index into a "biologic" MIPI for routine prognostic assessment (152). More recently, gene expression profiling studies have identified a "proliferation signature" that is associated with poor outcome (109,160).

THERAPEUTIC STRATEGIES

Conventional Immunochemotherapy and Bone Marrow Transplantation

Frontline treatment of MCL remains a difficult challenge for clinicians, as MCL is characterized by both aggressive behavior and little apparent success for long-term cure with currently available chemotherapy regimens (161,162). Immunochemotherapy protocols used for many DLBCL (e.g., rituximab, cyclophosphamide, doxorubicin, vincristine, and prednisone; R-CHOP) are frequently used in current community practice, especially for elderly patients. These result in a high overall response rate (>95%), but poor complete response rate and a disappointing progression-free survival of about 16 months (163–166). The use of intensive chemotherapy regimens with highly active drugs such as cytarabine (Ara-C) ("HyperCVAD") and autologous stem cell rescue has been shown to lead to improved survival compared to conventional immunochemotherapy, but essentially all patients still eventually relapse with this approach (167–174). Other intensive chemotherapy regimens also using high-dose cytarabine (e.g., rituximab, hyperfractionated cyclophosphamide, vincristine, doxorubicin, dexamethasone, high dose Ara-C, and high-dose methotrexate; R-HCVAD-AM) have been reported to improve survival without the need for autologous stem cell transplant (175,176). In light of concern for late relapses, however, it remains unclear whether autologous stem cell rescue may safely be omitted from such regimens (162).

Relapsed MCL generally shows poor response rates to salvage chemotherapy regimens, and there currently is no consensus on standard therapy. Newer agents showing high activity in the relapsed setting include bortezomib (177,178) or

the mammalian target of rapamycin (mTOR) kinase inhibitor, temsirolimus (179,180). Other options include bendamustine, immunomodulatory agents such as lenalidomide, or allogenic stem cell transplant (181,182).

Watch and Wait

In light of the aggressive behavior of most MCL, current treatment strategies have generally emphasized the need for immediate therapy. Nevertheless, some studies have suggested that in asymptomatic patients, therapy can be safely deferred until symptoms develop with a median time to treatment of about 1 year (183–185). Patients with one of the indolent types of MCL may be particularly well suited for a watch-and-wait approach. However, definitive identification of such cases remains challenging, and further studies are required to more precisely delineate which patients may be safely monitored without immediate therapy.

DIFFERENTIAL DIAGNOSIS

In routine practice, MCL must be distinguished from reactive lymphoid hyperplasia and from other B-cell non-Hodgkin lymphomas that may show overlapping histologic features. In most cases, this is readily accomplished using routine histology and a panel of immunohistochemical stains (Table 20.4). FISH or other cytogenetic studies are not necessary in most circumstances, but can be helpful in confirming the presence of an *IGH/CCND1* translocation in challenging cases.

Reactive Hyperplasia

While the great majority of cases of MCL demonstrate architectural effacement, MCL with a mantle zone growth pattern, especially when only partially involving the node, or ISMCL may be mistaken for reactive lymphoid hyperplasia (53,73,78). In mantle zone pattern MCL, mantles are conspicuously widened by CD5-positive, cyclin D1–positive B cells, often with some infiltration of the interfollicular areas. It should be noted that dim CD5 expression may also be seen in benign mantle zones in some cases, and this finding alone should not prompt a diagnosis of malignancy. ISMCL by definition displays a preserved architecture, and only small rims of cyclin D1–positive cells within the mantle zone region that do not fill or expand the mantle zones. These cases therefore will likely go undetected in the absence of cyclin D1 IHC.

	CHARACTERISTIC PHENOTYPIC AND GENOTYPIC MARKERS OF SMALL B-CELL NEOPLASMS
Table 20.4	

Marker	FL	CLL/SLL	MCL	NMZL	LPL
CD5	−	+	+	−	−
CD10	+	−	−	−	−
BCL6	+	−	−	−	−
CD23	+/−	+	−	−/+	−/+
LMO2	+	−	−	−	−
HGAL	+	−	−	−	−
GCET1	+	−	−	−	−
SOX11	−	−	+	−	−
LEF-1	−/+	+	−	−	−
IGH/BCL2	+/−	Rare	−	−	−
IGH/CCND1	−	−	+	−	−
t(*BCL6*)	−/+	−	Rare	Rare	−

Note that there are exceptions to these findings in a small percentage of cases, as discussed in the text.

Chronic Lymphocytic Leukemia/Small Lymphocytic Lymphoma

Many cases of MCL, especially those with a diffuse growth pattern, create a differential diagnosis with CLL/SLL. The neoplastic cells of MCL generally have more irregular or angulated nuclear contours with slightly more dispersed chromatin, compared to the usually round nuclei with condensed chromatin of CLL/SLL. However, there is substantial cytologic overlap between the two entities. Cases of CLL/SLL with trisomy 12, in particular, frequently show atypical cytologic features that may resemble MCL (186–188) and the small cell variant of MCL by definition resembles the cytology of CLL/SLL. Proliferation centers are not seen in MCL, and are one of the most helpful histologic features in this differential; however, MCL may have paler foci with large cells that can mimic proliferation centers (69). Similarly, mitotic figures are frequently seen in MCL, but are unusual in CLL/SLL outside of the proliferation centers. In most cases, this differential diagnosis is resolved with immunophenotypic studies. Extensive cyclin D1 staining is not expected in CLL/SLL although weak and variable staining with cyclin D1 may occasionally be seen in the proliferation centers of up to about 20% to 30% of CLL/SLL (189–191). SOX11 expression is seen in >90% of cases of MCL, including cyclin D1–negative cases, but is absent in CLL/SLL (75,89,90,191). In contrast, LEF-1 staining is observed in >95% of cases of CLL/SLL and is absent in MCL (192).

Follicular Lymphoma

The angulated nuclei of MCL often resemble the centrocytes of follicular lymphoma, a finding that led to the original diagnostic term of centrocytic lymphoma, and infrequent cases of MCL can have a very follicular growth pattern (3,53). Careful examination in such cases of MCL, however, will show a more monotonous proliferation without significant numbers of centroblasts and also may identify focal residual germinal centers surrounded by neoplastic cells, facilitating the correct diagnosis. IHC for CD10 and BCL6, or newer germinal center markers such as LMO2, GCET1, and HGAL (193–195), readily resolves this differential diagnosis in most cases; however, expression of CD10 and BCL6 has been reported in occasional cases, especially in the blastoid variant (82,84,85).

Other Small B-cell Lymphomas

Because the neoplastic cells in MCL sometimes have abundant pale cytoplasm, and can grow around reactive germinal centers, they may mimic a marginal zone lymphoma. Distinction is based on the marginal zone lymphomas being negative for cyclin D1 and SOX11. It should be remembered that MZL can be CD5 positive and MCL can be CD5 negative. In bone marrow biopsies, the differential diagnosis may include hairy cell leukemia, particularly since HCL may be cyclin D1 and SOX11 positive. Other immunophenotypic studies can be used to make a confident diagnosis of HCL such as CD103, CD123, or annexin A1 expression. *CCND1* translocations are rarely if ever found in HCL (196).

Diffuse Large B-cell Lymphoma

In the pleomorphic variant of MCL, the malignant cells may resemble the transformed cells of centroblastic, immunoblastic, or even anaplastic diffuse large B-cell lymphomas. Such cases are easily misdiagnosed as diffuse large B-cell lymphoma unless IHC for cyclin D1 or molecular or cytogenetic studies for the *IGH/CCND1* translocation are performed. For this reason, routine staining of presumptive DLBCL for cyclin D1 may be useful. It should be noted that DLBCL, often of nongerminal center type, may occasionally display weak and variable expression of cyclin D1 in a subset of nuclei, and this finding should not prompt a diagnosis of MCL (197–199). When the cyclin D1 IHC is equivocal, SOX11 IHC and FISH studies for *CCND1* translocations can be helpful.

Lymphoblastic Lymphoma

The presence of numerous mitotic figures in MCL may create a differential diagnosis with lymphoblastic lymphoma, especially in cases that exhibit blastoid cytology. Precursor T lymphoblastic lymphoma is easily excluded by the finding of characteristic T-cell antigen expression. In contrast with MCL, precursor B lymphoblastic lymphomas are typically positive for TdT and/or CD34, may be positive for CD10, and are more likely to be negative or only partially positive for CD20. The finding of cyclin D1 protein expression and/or *IGH/CCND1* translocation by FISH confirms the diagnosis of MCL.

 ## SUMMARY AND CONCLUSIONS

Over the last four decades since its original description and more than two decades since its documented association with *CCND1*("*BCL1*") translocations, much has been learned about MCL. At the same time, MCL has taught us, and continues to teach us, much about lymphomagenesis, including the stepwise but varied pathways to neoplasms of increasing clinical aggressiveness, the importance of cell cycle machinery and its control, and the importance of chromosomal instability. MCL has gone from being a largely morphologically identified rather homogeneous entity to one diagnosed with the aid of a multiparameter approach, which has a broad clinical spectrum from very indolent to extremely aggressive. Unfortunately, many patients have at least a moderately aggressive neoplasm, with little, if any, chance for a cure. In spite of some improvement in survival for those with advanced disease, there is a pressing need for improved therapeutic modalities. Whether measured by mitotic counts, Ki-67 immunohistochemical staining or gene expression profiling, the proliferative activity in MCL remains an extremely important prognostic indicator that must be reported by pathologists. We continue to learn about the biologic and clinical importance of a variety of secondary molecular genetic and epigenetic events documented by classical and high-throughput molecular cytogenetic technologies, and most recently from genomic sequencing studies.

References

1. Navarro A, et al. Molecular pathogenesis of mantle cell lymphoma: new perspectives and challenges with clinical implications. *Semin Hematol* 2011;48(3):155–165.
2. Royo C, et al. The complex landscape of genetic alterations in mantle cell lymphoma. *Semin Cancer Biol* 2011;21(5):322–334.
3. Swerdlow SH, et al. Mantle cell lymphoma. In: Swerdlow SH, et al., eds. *WHO classification of tumours of haematopoietic and lymphoid tissues*. Lyon: IARC Press, 2008:229–232.
4. Fu K, et al. Cyclin D1-negative mantle cell lymphoma: a clinicopathologic study based on gene expression profiling. *Blood* 2005;106(13):4315–4321.
5. Orchard J, et al. A subset of t(11;14) lymphoma with mantle cell features displays mutated IgVH genes and includes patients with good prognosis, nonnodal disease. *Blood* 2003;101(12):4975–4981.
6. Carvajal-Cuenca A, et al. In situ mantle cell lymphoma: clinical implications of an incidental finding with indolent clinical behavior. *Haematologica* 2012;97(2):270–278.
7. Gerard-Marchant R, et al. Classification of non-Hodgkin Lymphomas. *Lancet* 1974;304:406–408.
8. Tolksdorf G, Stein H, Lennert K. Morphological and immunological definition of a malignant lymphoma derived from germinal-centre cells with cleaved nuclei (centrocytes). *Br J Cancer* 1980;41(2):168–182.
9. Lardelli P, et al. Lymphocytic lymphoma of intermediate differentiation. Morphologic and immunophenotypic spectrum and clinical correlations. *Am J Surg Pathol* 1990;14(8):752–763.
10. Banks PM, et al. Mantle cell lymphoma. A proposal for unification of morphologic, immunologic, and molecular data. *Am J Surg Pathol* 1992;16(7):637–640.

11. Swerdlow SH Williams ME. From centrocytic to mantle cell lymphoma: a clinicopathologic and molecular review of 3 decades. *Hum Pathol* 2002;33(1):7–20.
12. Zucca E, Stein H, Coiffier B, European Lymphoma Task Force (ELTF): Report of the workshop on Mantle Cell Lymphoma (MCL). *Ann Oncol* 1994;5(6):507–511.
13. A clinical evaluation of the International Lymphoma Study Group classification of non-Hodgkin's lymphoma. The Non-Hodgkin's Lymphoma Classification Project. *Blood* 1997;89(11):3909–3918.
14. Smedby KE, Hjalgrim H. Epidemiology and etiology of mantle cell lymphoma and other non-Hodgkin lymphoma subtypes. *Semin Cancer Biol* 2011;21(5):293–298.
15. Sant M, et al. Incidence of hematologic malignancies in Europe by morphologic subtype: results of the HAEMACARE project. *Blood* 2010;116(19):3724–3734.
16. Zhou Y, et al. Incidence trends of mantle cell lymphoma in the United States between 1992 and 2004. *Cancer* 2008;113(4):791–798.
17. Agathangelidis A, et al. Unlocking the secrets of immunoglobulin receptors in mantle cell lymphoma: implications for the origin and selection of the malignant cells. *Semin Cancer Biol* 2011;21(5):299–307.
18. Camacho FI, et al. Molecular heterogeneity in MCL defined by the use of specific VH genes and the frequency of somatic mutations. *Blood* 2003;101(10):4042–4046.
19. Garcia-Munoz R, et al. Autoimmunity and lymphoma: is mantle cell lymphoma a mistake of the receptor editing mechanism? *Leuk Res* 2009;33(11):1437–1439.
20. Hadzidimitriou A, et al. Is there a role for antigen selection in mantle cell lymphoma? Immunogenetic support from a series of 807 cases. *Blood* 2011;118(11):3088–3095.
21. Schraders M, et al. Hypermutation in mantle cell lymphoma does not indicate a clinical or biological subentity. *Mod Pathol* 2009;22(3):416–425.
22. Thelander EF, Rosenquist R. Molecular genetic characterization reveals new subsets of mantle cell lymphoma. *Leuk Lymphoma* 2008;49(6):1042–1049.
23. Argatoff LH, et al. Mantle cell lymphoma: a clinicopathologic study of 80 cases. *Blood* 1997;89(6):2067–2078.
24. Berger F, et al. Nonfollicular small B-cell lymphomas: a heterogeneous group of patients with distinct clinical features and outcome. *Blood* 1994;83(10):2829–2835.
25. Bosch F, et al. Mantle cell lymphoma: presenting features, response to therapy, and prognostic factors. *Cancer* 1998;82(3):567–575.
26. Fisher RI, et al. A clinical analysis of two indolent lymphoma entities: mantle cell lymphoma and marginal zone lymphoma (including the mucosa-associated lymphoid tissue and monocytoid B-cell subcategories): a Southwest Oncology Group study. *Blood* 1995;85(4):1075–1082.
27. Majlis A, et al. Mantle cell lymphoma: correlation of clinical outcome and biologic features with three histologic variants. *J Clin Oncol* 1997;15(4):1664–1671.
28. Norton AJ, et al. Mantle cell lymphoma: natural history defined in a serially biopsied population over a 20-year period. *Ann Oncol* 1995;6(3):249–256.
29. Pittaluga S, et al. Prognostic significance of bone marrow trephine and peripheral blood smears in 55 patients with mantle cell lymphoma. *Leuk Lymphoma* 1996;21(1–2):115–125.
30. Pittaluga S, et al. Mantle cell lymphoma: a clinicopathological study of 55 cases. *Histopathology* 1995;26(1):17–24.
31. Swerdlow SH, et al. Centrocytic lymphoma: a distinct clinicopathologic and immunologic entity. A multiparameter study of 18 cases at diagnosis and relapse. *Am J Pathol* 1983;113(2):181–197.
32. Teodorovic I, et al. Efficacy of four different regimens in 64 mantle-cell lymphoma cases: clinicopathologic comparison with 498 other non-Hodgkin's lymphoma subtypes. European Organization for the Research and Treatment of Cancer Lymphoma Cooperative Group. *J Clin Oncol* 1995;13(11):2819–2826.
33. Vandenberghe E, et al. The clinical outcome of 65 cases of mantle cell lymphoma initially treated with non-intensive therapy by the British National Lymphoma Investigation Group. *Br J Haematol* 1997;99(4):842–847.
34. Velders GA, et al. Mantle-cell lymphoma: a population-based clinical study. *J Clin Oncol* 1996;14(4):1269–1274.
35. Weisenburger DD, Armitage JO. Mantle cell lymphoma—an entity comes of age. *Blood* 1996;87(11):4483–4494.
36. Weisenburger DD, et al. Mantle cell lymphoma. A clinicopathologic study of 68 cases from the Nebraska Lymphoma Study Group. *Am J Hematol* 2000;64(3):190–196.
37. Samaha H, et al. Mantle cell lymphoma: a retrospective study of 121 cases. *Leukemia* 1998;12(8):1281–1287.
38. Ferrer A, et al. Leukemic involvement is a common feature in mantle cell lymphoma. *Cancer* 2007;109(12):2473–2480.
39. Burke JS. Lymphoproliferative disorders of the gastrointestinal tract: a review and pragmatic guide to diagnosis. *Arch Pathol Lab Med* 2011;135(10):1283–1297.
40. Hashimoto Y, et al. Multiple lymphomatous polyposis of the gastrointestinal tract is a heterogenous group that includes mantle cell lymphoma and follicular lymphoma: analysis of somatic mutation of immunoglobulin heavy chain gene variable region. *Human Pathol* 1999;30(5):581–587.
41. Kodama T, et al. Lymphomatous polyposis of the gastrointestinal tract, including mantle cell lymphoma, follicular lymphoma and mucosa-associated lymphoid tissue lymphoma. *Histopathology* 2005;47(5):467–478.
42. Moynihan MJ, et al. Lymphomatous polyposis. A neoplasm of either follicular mantle or germinal center cell origin. *Am J Surg Pathol* 1996;20(4):442–452.
43. Ruskone-Fourmestraux A, et al. Multiple lymphomatous polyposis of the gastrointestinal tract: prospective clinicopathologic study of 31 cases. Groupe D'etude des Lymphomes Digestifs. *Gastroenterology* 1997;112(1):7–16.
44. Geissmann F, et al. Homing receptor alpha4beta7 integrin expression predicts digestive tract involvement in mantle cell lymphoma. *Am J Pathol* 1998;153(6):1701–1705.
45. Romaguera JE, et al. Frequency of gastrointestinal involvement and its clinical significance in mantle cell lymphoma. *Cancer* 2003;97(3):586–591.
46. Misdraji J, et al. Primary follicular lymphoma of the gastrointestinal tract. *Am J Surg Pathol* 2011;35(9):1255–1263.
47. Schmatz AI, et al. Primary follicular lymphoma of the duodenum is a distinct mucosal/submucosal variant of follicular lymphoma: a retrospective study of 63 cases. *J Clin Oncol* 2011;29(11):1445–1451.
48. Shia J, et al. Primary follicular lymphoma of the gastrointestinal tract: a clinical and pathologic study of 26 cases. *Am J Surg Pathol* 2002;26(2):216–224.
49. Takata K, et al. Primary gastrointestinal follicular lymphoma involving the duodenal second portion is a distinct entity: a multicenter, retrospective analysis in Japan. *Cancer Sci* 2011;102(8):1532–1536.
50. Yoshino T, et al. Increased incidence of follicular lymphoma in the duodenum. *Am J Surg Pathol* 2000;24(5):688–693.
51. Ferrer A, et al. Central nervous system involvement in mantle cell lymphoma. *Ann Oncol* 2008;19(1):135–141.
52. Gill S, et al. Mantle cell lymphoma with central nervous system involvement: frequency and clinical features. *Br J Haematol* 2009;147(1):83–88.
53. Klapper W. Histopathology of mantle cell lymphoma. *Semin Hematol* 2011;48(3):148–154.
54. Kurtin PJ. Indolent lymphomas of mature B lymphocytes. *Hematol Oncol Clin North Am* 2009;23(4):769–790.
55. Tiemann M, et al. Histopathology, cell proliferation indices and clinical outcome in 304 patients with mantle cell lymphoma (MCL): a clinicopathological study from the European MCL Network. *Br J Haematol* 2005;131(1):29–38.
56. Criel A, Michaux L, De Wolf-Peeters C. The concept of typical and atypical chronic lymphocytic leukaemia. *Leuk Lymphoma* 1999;33(1–2):33–45.
57. Criel A, et al. Further characterization of morphologically defined typical and atypical CLL: a clinical, immunophenotypic, cytogenetic and prognostic study on 390 cases. *Br J Haematol* 1997;97(2):383–391.
58. Criel A, et al. Trisomy 12 is uncommon in typical chronic lymphocytic leukaemias. *Br J Haematol* 1994;87(3):523–528.
59. Que TH, et al. Trisomy 12 in chronic lymphocytic leukemia detected by fluorescence in situ hybridization: analysis by stage, immunophenotype, and morphology. *Blood* 1993;82(2):571–575.
60. Ruchlemer R, et al. B-prolymphocytic leukaemia with t(11;14) revisited: a splenomegalic form of mantle cell lymphoma evolving with leukaemia. *Br J Haematol* 2004;125(3):330–336.
61. Angelopoulou MK, et al. The splenic form of mantle cell lymphoma. *Eur J Haematol* 2002;68(1):12–21.
62. Kansal R, et al. Histopathologic features of splenic small B-cell lymphomas. A study of 42 cases with a definitive diagnosis by the World Health Organization classification. *Am J Clin Pathol* 2003;120(3):335–347.
63. Pittaluga S, et al. "Small" B-cell non-Hodgkin's lymphomas with splenomegaly at presentation are either mantle cell lymphoma or marginal zone cell lymphoma. A study based on histology, cytology, immunohistochemistry, and cytogenetic analysis. *Am J Surg Pathol* 1996;20(2):211–223.
64. Piris MA, et al. A marginal zone pattern may be found in different varieties of non-Hodgkin's lymphoma: the morphology and immunohistology of splenic involvement by B-cell lymphomas simulating splenic marginal zone lymphoma. *Histopathology* 1998;33(3):230–239.
65. Cook JR, Splenic B-cell lymphomas/leukemia. *Surg Pathol Clin* 2010;3:933–954.
66. Salar A, et al. Gastrointestinal involvement in mantle cell lymphoma: a prospective clinic, endoscopic, and pathologic study. *Am J Surg Pathol* 2006;30(10):1274–1280.
67. Bernard M, et al. Blastic variant of mantle cell lymphoma: a rare but highly aggressive subtype. *Leukemia* 2001;15(11):1785–1791.
68. Kimura Y, et al. Small cell variant of mantle cell lymphoma is an indolent lymphoma characterized by bone marrow involvement, splenomegaly, and a low Ki-67 index. *Cancer Sci* 2011;102(9):1734–1741.
69. Swerdlow SH, et al. The morphologic spectrum of non-Hodgkin's lymphomas with BCL1/cyclin D1 gene rearrangements. *Am J Surg Pathol* 1996;20(5):627–640.
70. Visco C, et al. Molecular characteristics of mantle cell lymphoma presenting with clonal plasma cell component. *Am J Surg Pathol* 2011;35(2):177–189.
71. Young KH, et al. Mantle cell lymphoma with plasma cell differentiation. *Am J Surg Pathol* 2006;30(8):954–961.
72. Lecluse Y, et al. t(11;14)-positive clones can persist over a long period of time in the peripheral blood of healthy individuals. *Leukemia* 2009;23(6):1190–1193.
73. Carbone A, Santoro A. How I treat: diagnosing and managing "in situ" lymphoma. *Blood* 2011;117(15):3954–3960.
74. Nodit L, et al. Indolent mantle cell lymphoma with nodal involvement and mutated immunoglobulin heavy chain genes. *Hum Pathol* 2003;34(10):1030–1034.
75. Xu W, Li J-Y. SOX11 expression in mantle cell lymphoma. *Leuk Lymphoma* 2010;51(11):1962–1967.
76. Nygren L, Baumgartner Wennerholm S, Klimkowska M, et al. Prognostic role of SOX11 in a population-based cohort of mantle cell lymphoma. Blood 2012;119(18):4215–4223.
77a. Racke F, et al. Evidence of long latency periods prior to development of mantle cell lymphoma. *Blood* 2010;116(21):147–147.
77b. Adam P, Schiefer AI, Prill S, et al. Incidence of preclinical manifestations of mantle cell lymphoma and mantle cell lymphoma in situ in reactive lymphoid tissues. *Mod Pathol* 2012;25(12):1629–1636.
78. Campo E, et al. The 2008 WHO classification of lymphoid neoplasms and beyond: evolving concepts and practical applications. *Blood* 2011;117(19):5019–5032.
79. Campo E, Raffeld M, Jaffe ES. Mantle-cell lymphoma. *Semin Hematol* 1999;36(2): 115–127.
80. Ho AK, et al. Small B-cell neoplasms with typical mantle cell lymphoma immunophenotypes often include chronic lymphocytic leukemias. *Am J Clin Pathol* 2009;131(1):27–32.
81. Liu Z, et al. CD5- mantle cell lymphoma. *Am J Clin Pathol* 2002;118(2):216–224.
82. Gao J, et al. Immunophenotypic variations in mantle cell lymphoma. *Am J Clin Pathol* 2009;132(5):699–706.
83. Matutes E, et al. The leukemic presentation of mantle-cell lymphoma: disease features and prognostic factors in 58 patients. *Leuk Lymphoma* 2004;45(10):2007–2015.
84. Camacho FI, et al. Aberrant Bcl6 protein expression in mantle cell lymphoma. The American journal of surgical pathology, 2004;28(8):1051–1056.
85. Gualco G, et al. BCL6, MUM1, and CD10 expression in mantle cell lymphoma. *Appl Immunohistochem Mol Morphol* 2010;18(2):103–108.
86. Kelemen K, et al. CD23+ mantle cell lymphoma: a clinical pathologic entity associated with superior outcome compared with CD23- disease. *Am J Clin Pathol* 2008;130(2):166–177.
87. Cheuk W, et al. Consistent immunostaining for cyclin D1 can be achieved on a routine basis using a newly available rabbit monoclonal antibody. *Am J Surg Pathol* 2004;28(6):801–807.
88. Pruneri G, et al. SP4, a novel anti-cyclin D1 rabbit monoclonal antibody, is a highly sensitive probe for identifying mantle cell lymphomas bearing the t(11;14)(q13;q32) translocation. *Appl Immunohistochem Mol Morphol* 2005;13(4):318–322.
89. Mozos A, et al. SOX11 expression is highly specific for mantle cell lymphoma and identifies the cyclin D1-negative subtype. *Haematologica* 2009;94(11):1555–1562.
90. Zeng W, et al. Cyclin D1-negative Blastoid Mantle Cell Lymphoma Identified by SOX11 Expression. *Am J Surg Pathol* 2012;36(2):214–219.

91. Yatabe Y, et al. Significance of cyclin D1 overexpression for the diagnosis of mantle cell lymphoma: a clinicopathologic comparison of cyclin D1-positive MCL and cyclin D1-negative MCL-like B-cell lymphoma. *Blood* 2000;95(7):2253–2261.
92. Wlodarska I, et al. Translocations targeting CCND2, CCND3, and MYCN do occur in t(11;14)-negative mantle cell lymphomas. *Blood* 2008;111(12):5683–5690.
93. Izban KF, et al. Multiparameter immunohistochemical analysis of the cell cycle proteins cyclin D1, Ki-67, p21WAF1, p27KIP1, and p53 in mantle cell lymphoma. *Arch Pathol Lab Med* 2000;124(10):1457–1462.
94. Quintanilla-Martinez L, et al. Sequestration of p27Kip1 protein by cyclin D1 in typical and blastic variants of mantle cell lymphoma (MCL): implications for pathogenesis. *Blood* 2003;101(8):3181–3187.
95. Quintanilla-Martinez L, et al. Mantle cell lymphomas lack expression of p27Kip1, a cyclin-dependent kinase inhibitor. *Am J Pathol* 1998;153(1):175–182.
96. Jares P, Colomer D, Campo E. Genetic and molecular pathogenesis of mantle cell lymphoma: perspectives for new targeted therapeutics. *Nat Rev Cancer* 2007;7(10):750–762.
97. Perez-Galan P, Dreyling M, Wiestner A. Mantle cell lymphoma: biology, pathogenesis, and the molecular basis of treatment in the genomic era. *Blood* 2011;117(1):26–38.
98. Williams ME, et al. Mantle cell lymphoma: report of the 2010 Mantle Cell Lymphoma Consortium Workshop. *Leuk Lymphoma* 2011;52(1):24–33.
99. Komatsu H, et al. A variant chromosome translocation at 11q13 identifying PRAD1/cyclin D1 as the BCL-1 gene. *Blood* 1994;84(4):1226–1231.
100. Cook JR. Paraffin section interphase fluorescence in situ hybridization in the diagnosis and classification of non-hodgkin lymphomas. *Diagn Mol Pathol* 2004;13(4):197–206.
101. Betticher DC, et al. Alternate splicing produces a novel cyclin D1 transcript. *Oncogene* 1995;11(5):1005–1011.
102. Knudsen KE, et al. Cyclin D1: polymorphism, aberrant splicing and cancer risk. *Oncogene* 2006;25(11):1620–1628.
103. Lu F, Gladden AB, Diehl JA. An alternatively spliced cyclin D1 isoform, cyclin D1b, is a nuclear oncogene. *Cancer Res* 2003;63(21):7056–7061.
104. Shakir R, Ngo N, Naresh KN. Correlation of cyclin D1 transcript levels, transcript type and protein expression with proliferation and histology among mantle cell lymphoma. *J Clin Pathol* 2008;61(8):920–927.
105. Solomon DA, et al. Cyclin D1 splice variants. Differential effects on localization, RB phosphorylation, and cellular transformation. *J Biol Chem* 2003;278(32):30339–30347.
106. Slotta-Huspenina J, et al. The impact of cyclin D1 mRNA isoforms, morphology and p53 in mantle cell lymphoma: p53 alterations and blastoid morphology are strong predictors of a high proliferation index. *Haematologica* 2012;97(9):1422–1430.
107. Kim JK, Diehl JA. Nuclear cyclin D1: an oncogenic driver in human cancer. *J Cell Physiol* 2009;220(2):292–296.
108. Obrador-Hevia A, et al. Molecular biology of mantle cell lymphoma: from profiling studies to new therapeutic strategies. *Blood Rev* 2009;23(5):205–216.
109. Rosenwald A, et al. The proliferation gene expression signature is a quantitative integrator of oncogenic events that predicts survival in mantle cell lymphoma. *Cancer Cell* 2003;3(2):185–197.
110. Chen YH, et al. Nuclear expression of sox11 is highly associated with mantle cell lymphoma but is independent of t(11;14)(q13;q32) in non-mantle cell B-cell neoplasms. *Mod Pathol* 2010;23(1):105–112.
111a. Hunt KE, Reichard KK, Wilson CS. Mantle cell lymphoma lacking the t(11;14) translocation: a case report and brief review of the literature. *J Clin Pathol* 2008;61(7):869–870.
111b. Salaverria I, Royo C, Carvajal-Cuenca A, et al. CCND2 rearrangements are the most frequent genetic events in cyclin D1 negative mantle cell lymphoma. *Blood* 2013;121(8):1394–1402.
112. Metcalf RA, et al. Characterization of D-cyclin proteins in hematolymphoid neoplasms: lack of specificity of cyclin-D2 and D3 expression in lymphoma subtypes. *Mod Pathol* 2010;23(3):420–433.
113. Bodrug SE, et al. Cyclin D1 transgene impedes lymphocyte maturation and collaborates in lymphomagenesis with the myc gene. *EMBO J* 1994;13(9):2124–2130.
114. Lovec H, et al. Cyclin D1/bcl-1 cooperates with myc genes in the generation of B-cell lymphoma in transgenic mice. *EMBO J* 1994;13(15):3487–3495.
115. Smith MR, et al. Murine model for mantle cell lymphoma. *Leukemia* 2006;20(5):891–3.
116. Fernandez V, et al. Genomic and gene expression profiling defines indolent forms of mantle cell lymphoma. *Cancer Res* 2010;70(4):1408–1418.
117. Ondrejka SL, et al. Indolent mantle cell leukemia: a clinicopathological variant characterized by isolated lymphocytosis, interstitial bone marrow involvement, kappa light chain restriction, and good prognosis. *Haematologica* 2011;96(8):1121–1127.
118. Au WY, et al. Cytogenetic analysis in mantle cell lymphoma: a review of 214 cases. *Leuk Lymphoma* 2002;43(4):783–791.
119. Espinet B, et al. Incidence and prognostic impact of secondary cytogenetic aberrations in a series of 145 patients with mantle cell lymphoma. *Genes Chromosomes Cancer* 2010;49(5):439–451.
120. Ott G, et al. Blastoid variants of mantle cell lymphoma: frequent bcl-1 rearrangements at the major translocation cluster region and tetraploid chromosome clones. *Blood* 1997;89(4):1421–1429.
121. Bea S, et al. Uniparental disomies, homozygous deletions, amplifications, and target genes in mantle cell lymphoma revealed by integrative high-resolution whole-genome profiling. *Blood* 2009;113(13):3059–3069.
122. Flordal Thelander E, et al. Detailed assessment of copy number alterations revealing homozygous deletions in 1p and 13q in mantle cell lymphoma. *Leuk Res* 2007;31(9):1219–1230.
123. Salaverria I, et al. Specific secondary genetic alterations in mantle cell lymphoma provide prognostic information independent of the gene expression-based proliferation signature. *J Clin Oncol* 2007;25(10):1216–1222.
124. Kawamata N, et al. Identified hidden genomic changes in mantle cell lymphoma using high-resolution single nucleotide polymorphism genomic array. Exp Hematol, 2009;37(8):937–946.
125. Vater I, et al. GeneChip analyses point to novel pathogenetic mechanisms in mantle cell lymphoma. *Br J Haematol* 2009;144(3):317–331.
126. Allen JE, et al. Identification of novel regions of amplification and deletion within mantle cell lymphoma DNA by comparative genomic hybridization. *Br J Haematol* 2002;116(2):291–298.
127. Rubio-Moscardo F, et al. Mantle-cell lymphoma genotypes identified with CGH to BAC microarrays define a leukemic subgroup of disease and predict patient outcome. *Blood* 2005;105(11):4445–4454.
128. de Leeuw RJ, et al. Comprehensive whole genome array CGH profiling of mantle cell lymphoma model genomes. Hum Mol Genet, 2004;13(17):1827–1837.
129. Jarosova M, et al. High incidence of unbalanced chromosomal changes in mantle cell lymphoma detected by comparative genomic hybridization. *Leuk Lymphoma* 2004;45(9):1835–1846.
130. Kohlhammer H, et al. Genomic DNA-chip hybridization in t(11;14)-positive mantle cell lymphomas shows a high frequency of aberrations and allows a refined characterization of consensus regions. *Blood* 2004;104(3):795–801.
131. Hartmann E, et al. Increased MDM2 expression is associated with inferior survival in mantle-cell lymphoma, but not related to the MDM2 SNP309. *Haematologica* 2007;92(4):574–575.
132. Hernandez L, et al. CDK4 and MDM2 gene alterations mainly occur in highly proliferative and aggressive mantle cell lymphomas with wild-type INK4a/ARF locus. *Cancer Res* 2005;65(6):2199–2206.
133. Greiner TC, et al. Mutation and genomic deletion status of ataxia telangiectasia mutated (ATM) and p53 confer specific gene expression profiles in mantle cell lymphoma. *Proc Natl Acad Sci U S A* 2006;103(7):2352–2357.
134. Stefancikova L, et al. Loss of the p53 tumor suppressor activity is associated with negative prognosis of mantle cell lymphoma. *Int J Oncol* 2010;36(3):699–706.
135. Halldorsdottir AM, et al. Impact of TP53 mutation and 17p deletion in mantle cell lymphoma. *Leukemia* 2011;25(12):1904–1908.
136. Camacho E, et al. ATM gene inactivation in mantle cell lymphoma mainly occurs by truncating mutations and missense mutations involving the phosphatidylinositol-3 kinase domain and is associated with increasing numbers of chromosomal imbalances. *Blood* 2002;99(1):238–244.
137. Schaffner C, et al. Mantle cell lymphoma is characterized by inactivation of the ATM gene. *Proc Natl Acad Sci U S A* 2000;97(6):2773–2778.
138. Stilgenbauer S, et al. The ATM gene in the pathogenesis of mantle-cell lymphoma. Ann Oncol 2000;11(Suppl 1):127–130.
139. Fernandez V, et al. Pathogenesis of mantle-cell lymphoma: all oncogenic roads lead to dysregulation of cell cycle and DNA damage response pathways. *J Clin Oncol* 2005;23(26):6364–6369.
140. Kridel R, et al. Whole transcriptome sequencing reveals recurrent NOTCH1 mutations in mantle cell lymphoma. *Blood* 2012;119(9):1963–1971.
141. Su W, Yeong KF, Spencer J. Immunohistochemical analysis of human CD5 positive B cells: mantle cells and mantle cell lymphoma are not equivalent in terms of CD5 expression. *J Clin Pathol* 2000;53(5):395–397.
142. Herrmann A, et al. Improvement of overall survival in advanced stage mantle cell lymphoma. *J Clin Oncol* 2009;27(4):511–518.
143. Chandran R, et al. Survival trends in mantle cell lymphoma in the United States over 16 years 1992–2007. *Leuk Lymphoma* 2012;53(8):1488–1493.
144. A predictive model for aggressive non-Hodgkin's lymphoma. The International Non-Hodgkin's Lymphoma Prognostic Factors Project. *N Engl J Med* 1993;329(14):987–994.
145. Andersen NS, et al. A Danish population-based analysis of 105 mantle cell lymphoma patients: incidences, clinical features, response, survival and prognostic factors. *Eur J Cancer* 2002;38(3):401–408.
146. Decaudin D, et al. Mantle cell lymphomas: characteristics, natural history and prognostic factors of 45 cases. *Leuk Lymphoma* 1997;26(5–6):539–550.
147. Oinonen R, et al. Mantle cell lymphoma: clinical features, treatment and prognosis of 94 patients. *Eur J Cancer* 1998;34(3):329–336.
148. Raty R, et al. Ki-67 expression level, histological subtype, and the International Prognostic Index as outcome predictors in mantle cell lymphoma. *Eur J Haematol* 2002;69(1):11–20.
149. Schrader C, et al. Topoisomerase IIalpha expression in mantle cell lymphoma: a marker of cell proliferation and a prognostic factor for clinical outcome. *Leukemia* 2004;18(7):1200–1206.
150. Zucca E, et al. Patterns of survival in mantle cell lymphoma. *Ann Oncol* 1995;6(3):257–262.
151. Chiappella A, et al. Retrospective analysis of 206 mantle cell lymphoma patients at diagnosis: Mantle Cell International Prognostic Index (MIPI) is a good predictor of death event in patients treated either with rituximab-chemotherapy or rituximab-high-dose-chemotherapy. *Blood* 2010;116(21):744–745.
152. Geisler CH, et al. The Mantle Cell Lymphoma International Prognostic Index (MIPI) is superior to the International Prognostic Index (IPI) in predicting survival following intensive first-line immunochemotherapy and autologous stem cell transplantation (ASCT). *Blood* 2010;115(8):1530–1533.
153. Hoster E, et al. Confirmation of the Mantle Cell Lymphoma International Prognostic Index (MIPI) in an independent prospective patient cohort. *Blood* 2009;114(22):64–64.
154. Romaguera JE, et al. Ten-year follow-up after intense chemoimmunotherapy with Rituximab-HyperCVAD alternating with Rituximab-high dose methotrexate/cytarabine (R-MA) and without stem cell transplantation in patients with untreated aggressive mantle cell lymphoma. *Br J Haematol* 2010;150(2):200–208.
155. Salek D, et al. Mantle cell lymphoma international prognostic score is valid and confirmed in unselected cohort of patients treated in rituximab era. *Blood* 2008;112(11):1283–1283.
156. van de Schans SAM, et al. Validation, revision and extension of the Mantle Cell Lymphoma International Prognostic Index in a population-based setting. *Haematologica* 2010;95(9):1503–1509.
157. Determann O, et al. Ki-67 predicts outcome in advanced-stage mantle cell lymphoma patients treated with anti-CD20 immunochemotherapy: results from randomized trials of the European MCL Network and the German Low Grade Lymphoma Study Group. *Blood* 2008;111(4):2385–2387.
158. Katzenberger T, et al. The Ki67 proliferation index is a quantitative indicator of clinical risk in mantle cell lymphoma. *Blood* 2006;107(8):3407.
159. Klapper W, et al. Ki-67 as a prognostic marker in mantle cell lymphoma-consensus guidelines of the pathology panel of the European MCL Network. *J Hematop* 2009;2(2):103–111.

160. Martinez N, et al. The molecular signature of mantle cell lymphoma reveals multiple signals favoring cell survival. *Cancer Res* 2003;63(23):8226–8232.
161. Brody J, Advani R. Treatment of mantle cell lymphoma: current approach and future directions. *Crit Rev Oncol Hematol* 2006;58(3):257–265.
162. Harel S, et al. Treatment of younger patients with mantle cell lymphoma. *Semin Hematol* 2011;48(3):194–207.
163. Dreyling M, Hiddemann W. Current treatment standards and emerging strategies in mantle cell lymphoma. *Hematology Am Soc Hematol Educ Program* 2009:542–551.
164. Ghielmini M, Zucca E. How I treat mantle cell lymphoma. *Blood* 2009;114(8):1469–1476.
165. Kluin-Nelemans HC, Doorduijn JK. Treatment of elderly patients with mantle cell lymphoma. *Semin Hematol* 2011;48(3):208–213.
166. Howard OM, et al. Rituximab and CHOP induction therapy for newly diagnosed mantle-cell lymphoma: molecular complete responses are not predictive of progression-free survival. *J Clin Oncol* 2002;20(5):1288–1294.
167. Dreyling M, et al. Early consolidation by myeloablative radiochemotherapy followed by autologous stem cell transplantation in first remission significantly prolongs progression-free survival in mantle cell lymphoma: results of a prospective randomized trial of the European MCL Network. *Blood* 2005;105(7):2677–2684.
168. Lefrere F, et al. Sequential chemotherapy regimens followed by high-dose therapy with stem cell transplantation in mantle cell lymphoma: an update of a prospective study. *Haematologica* 2004;89(10):1275–1276.
169. Magni M, et al. High-dose sequential chemotherapy and in vivo rituximab-purged stem cell autografting in mantle cell lymphoma: a 10-year update of the R-HDS regimen. *Bone Marrow Transplant* 2009;43(6):509–511.
170. van't Veer MB, et al. High-dose Ara-C and beam with autograft rescue in R-CHOP responsive mantle cell lymphoma patients. *Br J Haematol* 2009;144(4):524–530.
171. Vandenberghe E, et al. Outcome of autologous transplantation for mantle cell lymphoma: a study by the European Blood and Bone Marrow Transplant and Autologous Blood and Marrow Transplant Registries. *Br J Haematol* 2003;120(5):793–800.
172. Nabhan C, et al. Hematopoietic SCT for mantle cell lymphoma: is it the standard of care? *Bone Marrow Transplant* 2010;45(9):1379–1387.
173. Damon LE, et al. Immunochemotherapy and autologous stem-cell transplantation for untreated patients with mantle-cell lymphoma: CALGB 59909. *J Clin Oncol* 2009;27(36):6101–6108.
174. Geisler CH, et al. Long-term progression-free survival of mantle cell lymphoma after intensive front-line immunochemotherapy with in vivo-purged stem cell rescue: a nonrandomized phase 2 multicenter study by the Nordic Lymphoma Group. *Blood* 2008;112(7):2687–2693.
175. Merli F, et al. Rituximab plus HyperCVAD alternating with high dose cytarabine and methotrexate for the initial treatment of patients with mantle cell lymphoma, a multicentre trial from Gruppo Italiano Studio Linfomi. *Br J Haematol* 2012;156(3):346–353.
176. Romaguera JE, et al. High rate of durable remissions after treatment of newly diagnosed aggressive mantle-cell lymphoma with rituximab plus hyper-CVAD alternating with rituximab plus high-dose methotrexate and cytarabine. *J Clin Oncol* 2005;23(28):7013–7023.
177. Fisher RI, et al. Multicenter phase II study of bortezomib in patients with relapsed or refractory mantle cell lymphoma. *J Clin Oncol* 2006;24(30):4867–4874.
178. Goy A, et al. Bortezomib in patients with relapsed or refractory mantle cell lymphoma: updated time-to-event analyses of the multicenter phase 2 PINNACLE study. *Ann Oncol* 2009;20(3):520–525.
179. Ansell SM, et al. Low-dose, single-agent temsirolimus for relapsed mantle cell lymphoma: a phase 2 trial in the North Central Cancer Treatment Group. *Cancer* 2008;113(3):508–514.
180. Witzig TE, et al. Phase II trial of single-agent temsirolimus (CCI-779) for relapsed mantle cell lymphoma. *J Clin Oncol* 2005;23(23):5347–5356.
181. Cortelazzo S, et al. Mantle cell lymphoma. *Crit Rev Oncol Hematol* 2012;82(1):78–101.
182. Diefenbach CS, O'Connor OA. Mantle cell lymphoma in relapse: the role of emerging new drugs. *Curr Opin Oncol* 2010;22(5):419–423.
183. Eve HE, et al. Time to treatment does not influence overall survival in newly diagnosed mantle-cell lymphoma. *J Clin Oncol* 2009;27(32):e189–e190; author reply e191.
184. Martin P, et al. Outcome of deferred initial therapy in mantle-cell lymphoma. *J Clin Oncol* 2009;27(8):1209–1213.
185. Martin P, Leonard J. Is there a role for "watch and wait" in patients with mantle cell lymphoma? *Semin Hematol* 2011;48(3):189–193.
186. Ciccone M, et al. Proliferation centers in chronic lymphocytic leukemia: correlation with cytogenetic and clinicobiological features in consecutive patients analyzed on tissue microarrays. *Leukemia* 2012;26(3):499–508.
187. Frater JL, et al. Typical and atypical chronic lymphocytic leukemia differ clinically and immunophenotypically. *Am J Clin Pathol* 2001;116(5):655–664.
188. Matutes E, et al. Trisomy 12 defines a group of CLL with atypical morphology: correlation between cytogenetic, clinical and laboratory features in 544 patients. *Br J Haematol* 1996;92(2):382–388.
189. Choi WW, et al. Chronic lymphocytic leukemia/small lymphocytic lymphoma with focal D-type cyclin expression in proliferation centers: a report of four cases. *Leuk Res* 2010;34(8):e219–e220.
190. O'Malley DP, Vance GH, Orazi A. Chronic lymphocytic leukemia/small lymphocytic lymphoma with trisomy 12 and focal cyclin d1 expression: a potential diagnostic pitfall. *Arch Pathol Lab Med* 2005;129(1):92–95.
191. Gradowski JF, et al. Chronic lymphocytic leukemia/small lymphocytic lymphoma with Cyclin D1 positive proliferation centers do not have CCND1 translocations or gains and lack SOX11 expression. *Am J Clin Pathol* 2012;138(1):132–139.
192. Tandon B, et al. Nuclear overexpression of lymphoid-enhancer-binding factor 1 identifies chronic lymphocytic leukemia/small lymphocytic lymphoma in small B-cell lymphomas. *Mod Pathol* 2011;24(11):1433–1443.
193. Goteri G, et al. Comparison of germinal center markers CD10, BCL6 and human germinal center-associated lymphoma (HGAL) in follicular lymphomas. *Diagn Pathol* 2011;6(1):97.
194. Montes-Moreno S, et al. Gcet1 (centerin), a highly restricted marker for a subset of germinal center-derived lymphomas. *Blood* 2008;111(1):351–358.
195. Natkunam Y, et al. Expression of the human germinal center-associated lymphoma (HGAL) protein, a new marker of germinal center B-cell derivation. *Blood* 2005;105(10):3979–3986.
196. Chen D, et al. A case of hairy cell leukemia with CCND1-IGH@ translocation: indolent non-nodal mantle cell lymphoma revisited. *Am J Surg Pathol* 2011;35(7):1080–1084.
197. Rodriguez-Justo M, et al. Cyclin D1-positive diffuse large B-cell lymphoma. *Histopathology* 2008;52(7):900–903.
198. Teruya-Feldstein J, Gopalan A, Moskowitz CH. CD5 negative, Cyclin D1-positive diffuse large B-cell lymphoma (DLBCL) presenting as ruptured spleen. *Appl Immunohistochem Mol Morphol* 2009;17(3):255–258.
199. Vela-Chavez T, et al. Cyclin D1 positive diffuse large B-cell lymphoma is a post-germinal center-type lymphoma without alterations in the CCND1 gene locus. *Leuk Lymphoma* 2011;52(3):458–466.

Chapter 21

Nodal Marginal Zone B-Cell Lymphoma

Alexandra Traverse-Glehen • Françoise Berger

 ## HISTORICAL BACKGROUND

Nodal marginal zone lymphoma (NMZL) is classified in the group of marginal zone lymphomas (MZLs), first separated from corresponding extranodal or mucosa-associated lymphoid tissue (MALT) lymphomas, in particular in the works of Isaacson (1,2), and subsequently from their primary splenic form. NMZL corresponds to the entity described in the 1980s by the American authors Sheibani and Cousar under the name of monocytoid B-cell lymphoma (MBCL) (3) and parafollicular lymphoma (4), respectively. The initial descriptions and the terms used to designate these neoplasms emphasized frequent architectural (parafollicular) or cytologic (monocytoid) features of the tumors. Historical background resumed in Table 21.1.

Monocytoid B Cells

These cells were described for the first time by Lennert (5) in 1959 and Stansfeld (6) in 1961 in toxoplasmic lymphadenitis and in early-stage Hodgkin lymphoma. They are small to medium in size with abundant pale cytoplasm, and their nuclei and cytoplasm have a superficial resemblance to those of peripheral blood monocytes. The nucleus is central, round, or slightly irregular, with moderately clumped chromatin and inconspicuous nucleoli (7). These morphologic similarities and the subsequent demonstration of B-cell phenotype led to the designation of their name. They are mostly located in parafollicular or parasinusoidal areas and in perivascular spaces, with a predilection around the marginal sinus, or, more rarely, the medullary sinus, sometimes with marginal topography. They form noncohesive sheets distinct from the epithelioid histiocytes in toxoplasmic lymph node, resulting in its initial designation as "immature sinus histiocytosis." Phenotypically, they are B lymphocytes expressing IgM or IgG, without expression of CD5 or CD23. These cells are also observed in other reactive processes or other diseases (e.g., autoimmune diseases, Epstein-Barr virus, hepatitis C or human immunodeficiency infection, and T-cell lymphoma) (8,9). The biologic significance of this particular subpopulation is not well understood. The close association of these cells with reactive follicular hyperplasia suggests they may represent a transient B-cell differentiation stage, related to follicular activation (7,10). A relationship between these cells and lymphocytes of the marginal zone has been suggested based on the topographic distribution and similar morphologic and phenotypic characteristics (11).

Marginal Zone

The marginal zone is a microanatomic site, the most external area of the follicle, outside the mantle cell corona. This is well developed in reactive spleen, Peyer patches, and mesenteric lymph nodes but less evident in other lymph node sites (12–14). It is a heterogeneous compartment of B cells, with some T cells and macrophages associated with it. The composition of the marginal zone is not clearly elucidated, but seems to include different types of memory B lymphocytes and cells involved in a T-cell–independent immune response to poorly immunogenic antigens, such as polysaccharide (15–20).

MALT Lymphomas

In 1983, more than 20 years after the description of monocytoid B cells, Isaacson and Wright introduced the term lymphoma of the mucosa-associated lymphoid tissue or MALT (1) to define primary gastric small B-cell lymphoma. Gradually, the definition of MALT lymphoma extended to other locations, to include extranodal low-grade lymphomas derived from lymphoid tissue acquired in an infectious and/or autoimmune context. For example, the lung, salivary glands, and thyroid have MALT similar to that of the gastrointestinal tract, allowing definition of the group of MALT lymphomas.

Monocytoid B-Cell Lymphoma/NMZL

The first case of lymphoma constituted by monocytoid B cells was described in 1985 in a paper from the Collins team. On clinical, morphologic, and immunologic grounds, this lymphoma presented the characteristics of a small B-cell lymphoma (21). The cytologic features resembled hairy cell leukemia, with some differences, in particular the massive infiltration of node. A short time later, in 1986, Sheibani introduced the term MBCL to describe this entity (3), by presenting three cases of lymphomas in which lymphoma cells had an appearance similar to reactive monocytoid B cells. These atypical monocytoid cells were medium in size, with clearly limited moderately abundant cytoplasm. The nucleus was oval, sometimes reniform, with compact chromatin and an indiscernible nucleolus. Electron microscopic studies showed similarities between reactive monocytoid B cells and the tumor cells.

Between 1985 and 1990, 56 cases of MBCL were published (4,22,23). These cases were of both nodal and extranodal location. At this time, the discussions focused essentially on the differential diagnosis with hairy cell leukemia, because of the clear cytoplasm. However, the nodal location, the absence of blood and bone marrow (BM) invasion, the absence of splenomegaly, and the phenotypic differences seemed to allow distinguishing this lymphoma. Both entities are considered very differently today, with hairy cell leukemia having clearly been recognized as a unique B-cell neoplasm.

In 1988, Piris suggested the origin of the MBCL in the marginal zone (11), in view of the frequent marginal zone topography, expression of IgM, and a phenotype distinct from the other nodal B-cell populations (11). In the 1990s, several series reported frequent extranodal location or splenomegaly and an association with follicular lymphoma (24–28). The existence of NMZL was discussed for a long time as a different entity or representing the nodal counterpart of splenic marginal zone (MZ),

Table 21.1	HISTORY AND CHARACTERIZATION OF NMZL
1959 Lennert (5); 1961 Stansfeld (6)	*"Immature sinus histiocytosis" and monocytoid B cells*
1983 Isaacson (1), 1984 Isaacson (31)	*MALT lymphoma*
1984 Sheibani et al. (10); 1984 Stein (32); 1984 de Almeida (33)	*Benign monocytoid B cells*
	Relationship between marginal zone and immature sinus histiocyte
1986 Van den Oord et al. (12); 1984 Cousar et al. (21), 1986 Sheibani (3) and 1988 Sheibani (34); 1987 Ng and Chan (22)	*MBCL and parafollicular B-cell lymphoma*
1987 Isaacson (35)	*Extranodal location of MALT*
1988 Piris et al. (11)	*Relationship between MBCL and marginal zone*
1990 Cogliatti et al. (27)	*Relationship with MALT*
1990 Lennert (29)	*Lennert classification*
1991 Nizze (36); 1992 Ortiz-Hidalgo and Wright (77)	*Association between MBCL and FL*
1991 Ngan et al. (23); 1996 Hammer (37)	*SMZL cases*
1992 Nathwani et al. (24)	*MBCL series*
1994 Harris (38)	*REAL classification SMZL: provisional entity*
1994 Isaacson (39); 1994 Mollejo (40); 1996 Dierlamm et al. (60); 1997 De Wolf-Peeters (41); 1996 Isaacson (42)	*MZL of different sites share similar cytogenetic and morphologic features*
1997 NHL Classification Project-Armitage (43)	*Clinical evlauation of International Lymphoma Study Group Classification*
1999 Campo et al. (46);2000 Berger et al. (44)	*NMZL series*
2001–2008	*WHO classification*
2003 Camacho et al. (47)-2004 Arcaini et al. (46)-2006 Traverse-Glehen et al. (49)-2005 Petit et al. (51)-2006 Oh et al. (52)-2007 Arcaini et al. (50)-2007 Kojima et al. (53)-Salama et al. (55) 2009-Naresh 2008 (59)	*NMZL series*

clearly described in 1992 (29), or MALT lymphomas. It was included in the REAL classification in 1994 as a provisional entity. It shares with MALT lymphoma and splenic marginal zone lymphoma (SMZL) several morphologic, immunophenotypic, and cytogenetic characteristics. However, differences were revealed that demonstrated it to be a different entity; in recognition of this, NMZL was admitted as a distinct lymphoma by the 2001 WHO.

In contrast to MALT lymphoma, well-characterized and extensively studied at both the clinical and molecular levels, NMZL remains poorly understood. This chapter reviews the pathologic and clinical characteristics of NMZL and the differential diagnosis with other lymphomas that may occasionally adopt a marginal zone pattern. Discrepancies remain, however, concerning the morphologic, biologic, and clinical characteristics of this disease, as well as the therapeutic recommendations. In addition, the recent update of the 2008 WHO Lymphoma Classification (30) has included a pediatric variant of NMZL, with some distinctive clinical and morphologic features.

NODAL MARGINAL ZONE LYMPHOMA

Frequency and Epidemiology

Among other lymphomas, NMZL is rare, representing between 1.5% and 1.8% of the cases analyzed within an international study (43) and a single-center series (44). Two-thirds of the cases of the Southwest Oncology Group study were described as "composite lymphomas" with concomitant follicular lymphoma, and may include follicular lymphomas with marginal zone differentiation (45). Other series probably include cases corresponding to nodal spread of extranodal MZL or cases disseminated at diagnosis, with peripheral lymph nodes associated with extranodal or splenic involvement. Association with hepatitis C virus (HCV) infection has been reported in the Italian (46) and Spanish series (47) but appears rather rare in other settings.

Clinical Presentation

Given the recent identification of NMZL, few reports present detailed patient clinical and outcome data, with a relatively small numbers of patients (26,44,46–53). The median age is 50 to 64 years (range 29 to 87), with a differing sex ratio in several series. The lymphoma is localized in peripheral lymph nodes, mostly cervical, and inguinal, with frequent involvement of other thoracic or abdominal nodes. The clinical stage at diagnosis is variable according to series, but the majority of patients usually present with advanced clinical stage III or IV. Only two series reported patients with stage I and II (47,53). BM involvement is observed between 19% and 62% of cases, and peripheral blood involvement is very rare. Presence of B symptoms is infrequent. Elevated β_2-microglobulin is found in one-third of the patients. An M component is infrequently detected (10%). A few cases are reported to be associated with HCV (HCV seroprevalence was reported in 24% in a series from Italy, in 20% from Spain, and in 5% from Korea). Cryoglobulins may be present when associated with HCV infection. In contrast to the other MZL entities, a history of autoimmune disease is lacking in most patients with NMZL, although autoimmune hemolytic anemia has been reported in a subset of patients. Nodal involvement of other MZL is strictly excluded for diagnosis. Therefore, a careful clinical assessment is important when evaluating these cases.

Morphology

Architecture

The lymph nodes in NMZL may show different patterns of involvement (44,47,49,54,55): marginal zone–like/perifollicular (Fig. 21.1A), "inverse follicular" (Fig. 21.1B), interfollicular (Fig. 21.1C and D), nodular (Fig. 21.1E), follicular colonization of reactive follicles (less frequent than in MALT lymphomas), or diffuse (Fig. 21.1F). A combination of different patterns in a single case is a common finding. The morphologic evolution of the disease often starts with a perifollicular pattern

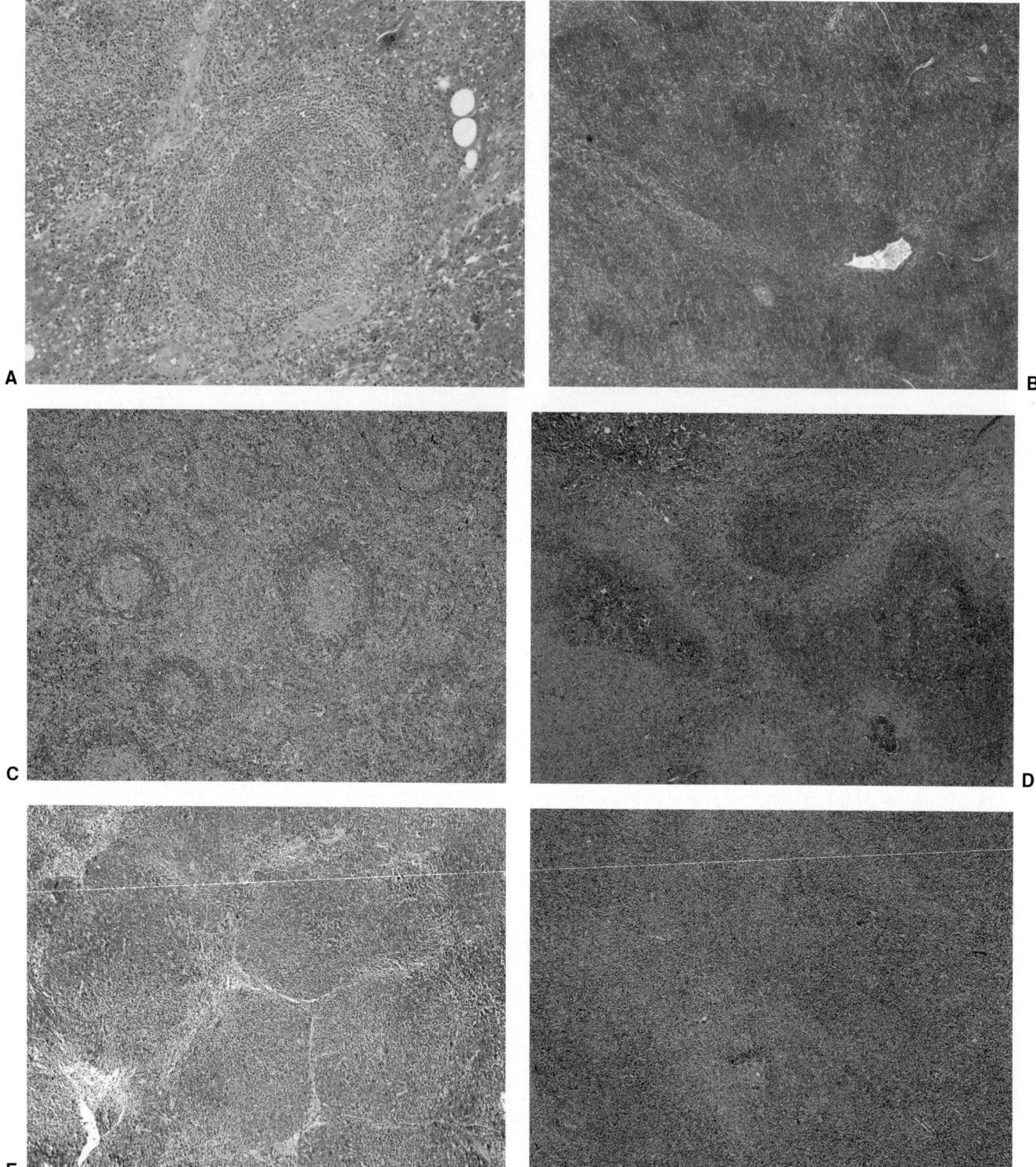

FIGURE 21.1. Nodal marginal zone lymphoma. Architectural patterns (hematoxylin-eosin-safran stain, original magnification: 20×).
A: Perifollicular or marginal zone–like pattern, **(B)** "inverse follicular" (with dark center and clear corona), **(C,D)** interfollicular, **(E)** nodular, or **(F)** diffuse.

by enlargement of the MZ, followed by an expansion into the interfollicular areas and follicular colonization, with formation of large nodules. In this situation, the mantle cuff may be preserved. In advanced cases, the lymph node architecture is effaced, with resulting diffuse architecture. Residual atrophic follicles, rarely hyperplasic, are usually seen.

Few data about BM histology are available (49,56). A nodular and interstitial pattern has been most often reported. A sinusoidal localization, more typical of SMZL, is also frequently described in NMZL. As in SMZL, histology seems to be more sensitive than flow cytometry in detecting BM infiltration (57).

Cytology

NMZL are cytologically heterogeneous (47,49,55,58). Several cell types can be encountered in varying proportions (Fig. 21.2): small cells with irregular nuclei, clumped chromatin, and clear cytoplasm; cells resembling small lymphocytes, small cells

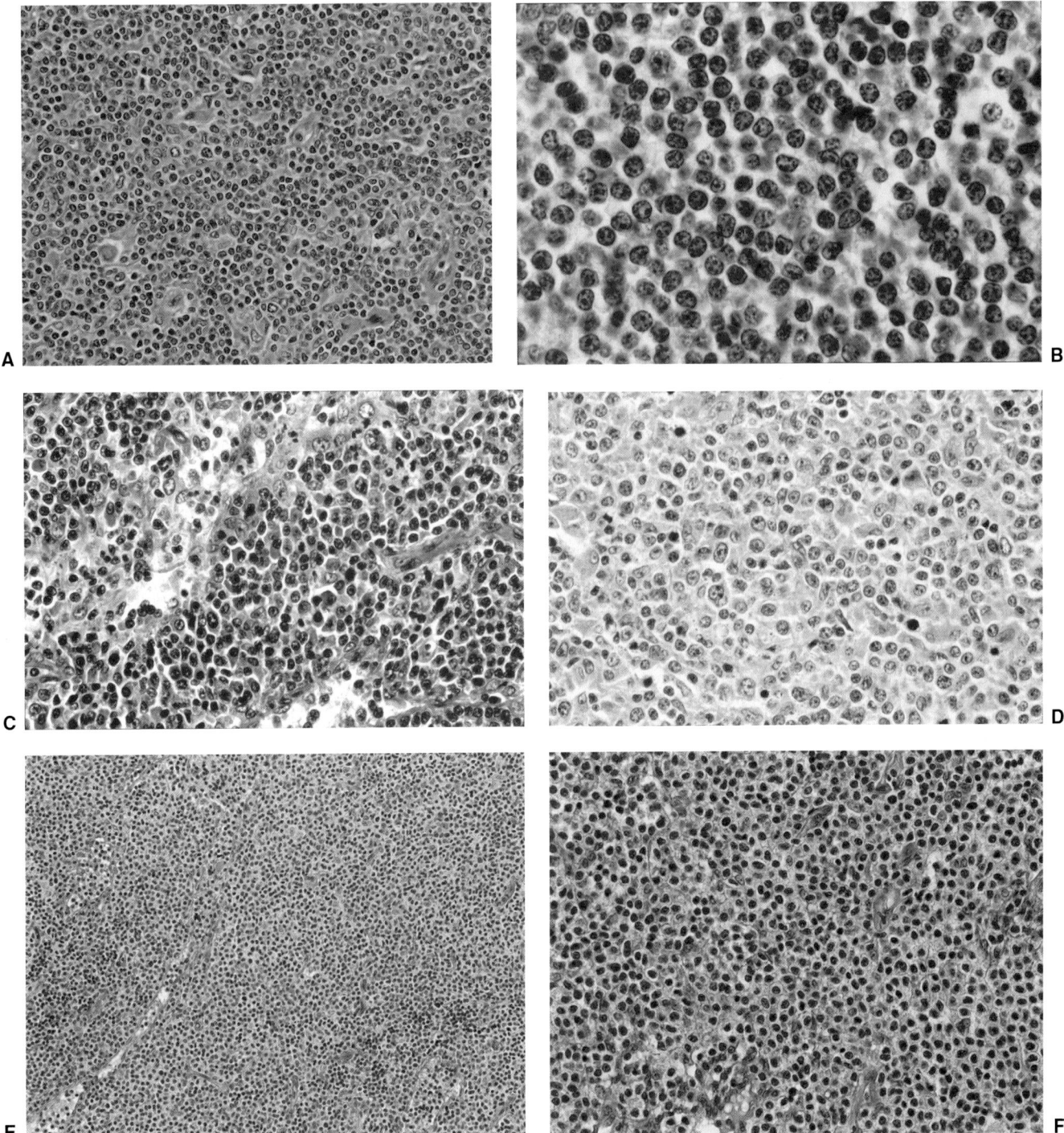

FIGURE 21.2. Nodal marginal zone lymphoma. Cytologic features: **A:** At low power: small cells mixed with large cells. **B:** At high power: small cells with round nucleus and clumped chromatin; **(C)** plasmacytic differentiation predominant around the sinus area. **D:** Large amount of large cells with abundant cytoplasm, admixed with few neoplastic small cells. **E,F:** Neoplastic cells resembling monocytoid cells, with abundant clear cytoplasm (hematoxylin-eosin-safran stain, original magnification: 200× and 400×).

with a plasmacytoid differentiation; plasma cells; and a variable content of medium to large cells that are centroblast- or immunoblast-like. Follicular dendritic cells, usually arranged in a nodular meshwork or restricted to the perifollicular areas (marginal zone pattern), are always present. "Monocytoid" B cells, with more abundant and clear cytoplasm, are not usually predominant, and pure MBCLs are less frequent than cases with plasmacytoid or plasmacytic differentiation (49). Monotypic plasmacytoid or plasmacytic differentiation is reported in almost 30% of cases. Unlike MALT lymphoma and SMZL, the proportion of large cells is often relatively high (more than 20%), and the mitotic index is also frequently elevated. This questions the classification of NMZL as a low-grade lymphoma. The large component is usually sparse, but in some cases may be more abundant; however, it is always admixed with a small B-cell component, without sheets of large cells, and sometimes colonizing the follicle (and may sometimes represent residual germinal center cells). These cases should not be considered as *de novo* diffuse large B-cell lymphoma if they retain the morphology previously described in NMZL. NMZL with a purely small cell component is rarely seen at diagnosis, probably because biopsies are more often performed in symptomatic patients and those with advanced stage disease, suggesting a very indolent progression at the beginning. This high content of large cells and mitoses may explain the more aggressive clinical course reported in some series. However, the number of large cells does not seem to influence the outcome of patients that have been treated with intensive polychemotherapy (49). Scattered neutrophils, eosinophils, and epithelioid histiocytes can be observed occasionally.

Immunophenotype

The phenotype, usually identical to extranodal MZL, is an important diagnostic feature that can help to distinguish these cases from other small B-cell lymphomas: typically, the lymphoma cells are sIgM$^{+/-}$D/G$^+$ cIg$^{+/-}$ CD19$^+$ CD20$^+$ CD79a$^+$ Oct2$^+$ Pax5$^+$ CD5$^-$ CD10$^-$ CD23$^-$ BCL2$^+$ cyclinD1$^-$. Some cases have been reported with expression of CD5 and CD23, each occurring in about 5% to 10% of cases. CD43 is reported in up to 50% of cases. The expression of IgD has been reported by Campo (58), who described "splenic type" and "MALT type" of NMZL (Table 21.2). The splenic type (in absence of splenic involvement) shows a nodular pattern with IgD positivity. In contrast, the "MALT type" shows a perivascular/perisinusoidal and parafollicular pattern, without expression of IgD. However, this subtyping is still debatable, and IgD expression has not been confirmed in a recent series including 51 cases (55). Plasmacytic differentiation is usually associated with the expression

of CD38, CD138, and MUM1 (47). In the largest series, the CD138 expression reflected an increase in plasma cell numbers in about half of the cases (24/51) (55). In cases with follicle colonization (Fig. 21.3), the benign reactive follicle center cells express CD10 and Bcl-6 and are negative for Bcl-2 and MUM1 (49,59). In contrast, the colonizing MZL cells express Bcl-2 and often MUM1 and are negative for CD10 and Bcl-6. Partially colonized follicles showed a "moth-eaten" appearance on CD10, Bcl-2, Bcl-6, and MUM1 immunohistochemistry. Ki67 expression is much higher among the residual benign/reactive follicle center cells as compared to the lymphoma cells in most cases (59).

Cytogenetic and Molecular Features

Cytogenetics may help in recognizing the lymphoma mainly by ruling out other small B-cell lymphomas, but it is difficult to establish a characteristic cytogenetic profile for NMZL (28,49,60,61). Clonal aberrations are found in the majority of cases and the karyotype is most frequently complex. Recurrent clonal abnormalities also found in the other types of MZL, such as trisomy 3, trisomy 18, trisomy 7, trisomy 12, or del6q, may contribute to the diagnosis. The presence of trisomy 12 may possibly be more frequent than in MALT lymphoma or SMZL. The translocations characteristic of MALT or the 7q deletion recurrent in SMZL have not been reported in NMZL. Rare cases (<10%) of TP53 gene heterozygous deletions detected by fluorescence in situ hybridization (FISH) have been reported.

Genomic DNA copy number analysis (50) and gene expression studies (63) demonstrate the absence of major specific lesions in NMZL, but underline the lack of the SMZL-related 7q losses and a profile more similar to MALT lymphomas. Inactivation of the A20 gene (localized in 6q23) by either somatic mutation or deletion has been described in 33% of NMZL (3/9 cases), representing a common genetic aberration across all MZL subtypes, which may contribute to lymphomagenesis, by inducing constitutive NF-κB activation (62,63).

The variable immunoglobulin heavy chain (IGHV) gene mutational status has been investigated in limited series (47,64–68). The majority of cases (87%) contain somatic mutations of the IGHV genes, with a biased usage of IGHV4-34 or IGHV1-69 in cases associated with HCV infection, and evidence of antigen selection in most cases, but without ongoing mutations. VH1-69-encoded antibodies have been shown to be specific for the viral antigen E2. No outcome difference was described between mutated and not mutated cases.

Differential Diagnosis

Differential diagnosis can be difficult with other small B-cell lymphomas, which sometimes have a MZ pattern or contain monocytoid B cells. The diagnosis of NMZL implies the exclusion of lymph node involvement by extranodal or splenic marginal zone B-cell lymphoma. Extensive plasma cell differentiation in MZL may suggest the diagnosis of lymphoplasmacytic lymphoma (LPL). Another rare but difficult differential diagnosis is with angioimmunoblastic T-cell lymphoma (AITL).

Benign Versus Malignant Proliferation

The distinction of lymphoma from reactive conditions, including T-zone hyperplasia, marginal zone expansion, or monocytoid B-cell proliferation, is sometimes problematic. Morphologically, confluent areas of monocytoid cells, presence of cytologic atypias, transformed cells, and mitotic activity suggest lymphoma, rather than a reactive process. BCL2 expression has been reported as negative in reactive monocytoid B cells, whereas it is frequently positive in marginal zone hyperplasia and MZL. Immunoglobulin light-chain restriction

Table 21.2	MALT TYPE AND SPLENIC TYPE OF NMZL	
Features	**MALT Type**	**Splenic Type**
Residual germinal centers	Prominent	Indistinct, regressed
Mantle zones	Prominent	Generally absent
Cytoplasmic membranes	Usually prominent	Indistinct
Monocytoid B cells	Often prominent	Absent
Admixed neutrophils	Common	Absent
Blast cells	May be present	May be present
Plasmacytoid features	May be present	May be present
IgD	Negative	Weakly positive
BCL-2 protein	Positive	Positive
Intrafollicular T cells	Not increased	Increased

From Campo E, Miquel R, Krenacs L, et al. Primary nodal marginal zone lymphomas of splenic and MALT type. *Am J Surg Pathol* 1999;23:59–68.

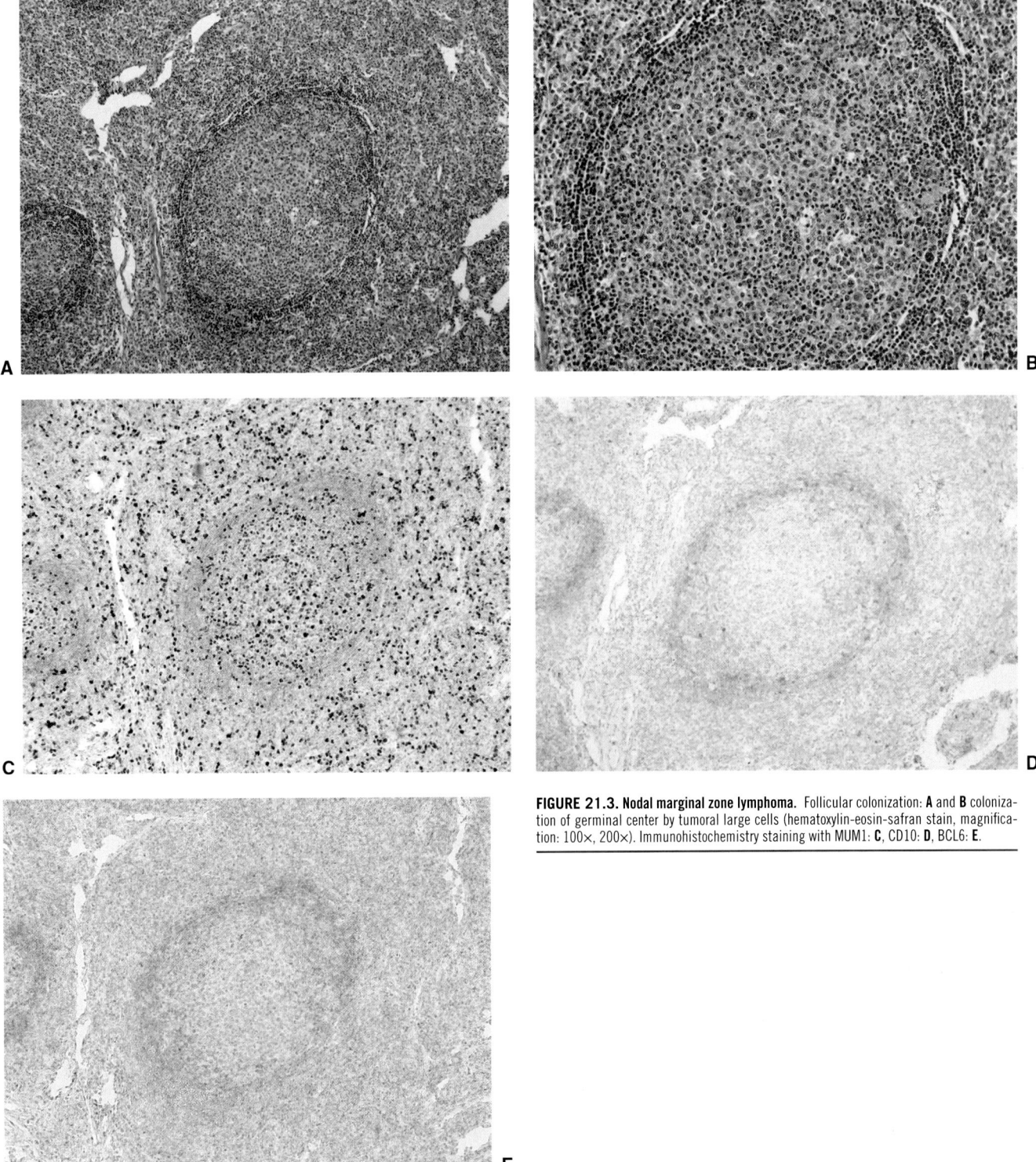

FIGURE 21.3. Nodal marginal zone lymphoma. Follicular colonization: **A** and **B** colonization of germinal center by tumoral large cells (hematoxylin-eosin-safran stain, magnification: 100×, 200×). Immunohistochemistry staining with MUM1: **C**, CD10: **D**, BCL6: **E**.

by flow cytometry or immunohistochemistry, and above all, monoclonality by molecular techniques may be useful in the differential diagnosis.

Monocytoid Differentiation and Marginal Zone Pattern in Other Lymphomas

Several types of B-cell lymphoma may occasionally display a monocytoid appearance with abundant clear cytoplasm and/ or marginal growth pattern that may lead to misdiagnosis as

MZL. Those features can be observed in chronic lymphocytic leukemia/small lymphoid lymphoma (CLL/SLL), as well as mantle cell lymphoma (MCL) and FL. These features, initially considered as composite lymphomas, have been demonstrated as a morphologic variant of the underlying lymphomas and not a different entity, with related clone and similar cytogenetic abnormalities. The diagnosis of MCL or CLL, sometimes challenging in peripheral blood, can be eliminated easily by specific phenotype and characteristic chromosomal abnormalities. However, the differential diagnosis between follicular

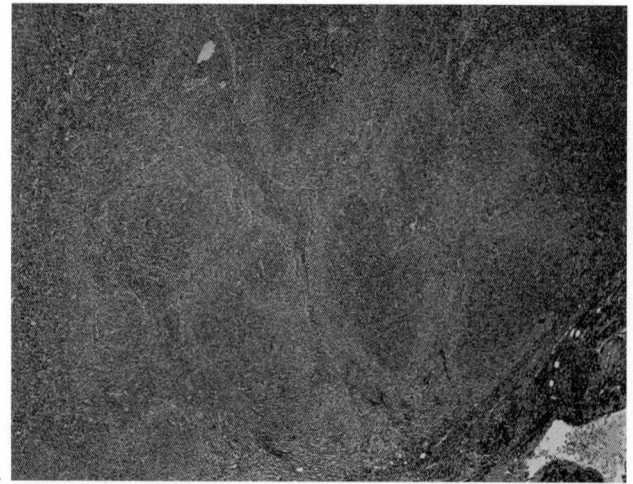

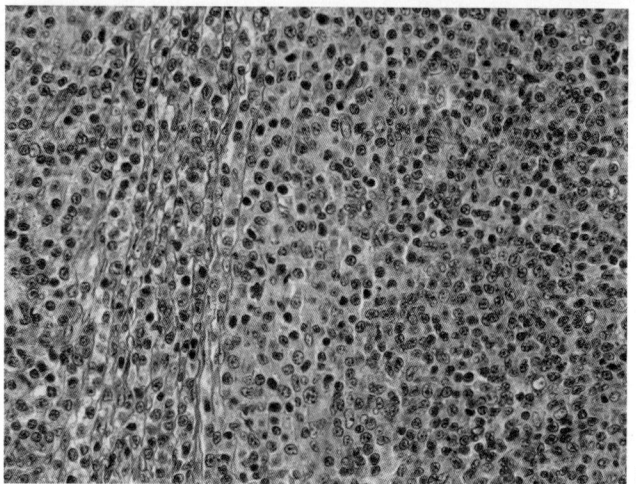

FIGURE 21.4. Follicular lymphoma with a marginal zone pattern. A,B: An inverse follicular pattern is seen, with a dark center and a pale rim (hematoxylin-eosin-safran stain, original magnification: 100×, 200×). **C:** Neoplastic cells at the periphery of the follicle contain more abundant cytoplasm. The transition in cytologic appearance is gradual (hematoxylin-eosin-safran stain, original magnification: 400×).

lymphoma with marginal zone differentiation and NMZL with follicular colonization is more difficult (Figs. 21.3 and 21.4). In many follicles from NMZL cases, the colonization is often partial, and follicles also contain a reactive germinal center component. Immunophenotypic features are helpful to clarify these cases. Germinal center–associated markers that highlight follicular lymphoma cells are typically absent in NMZL. Aberrant expression of CD10 has been reported in only one case (59). A subset of follicular lymphoma may lack some germinal center–associated markers, which could make the differential diagnosis particularly difficult (55). It seems that, for those challenging cases, additional germinal center markers (BCL6, HGAL, and LMO2) show more sensitivity and specificity for follicular lymphoma cells. Follicular lymphomas that do not express CD10, as most cases of high-grade 3B, express MUM1, lack BCL2 gene translocation but present BCL6 gene abnormalities. Cytogenetics studies (BCL2 and/or BCL6 rearrangement by FISH) is then of great interest for the diagnosis. In a gene expression profiling study (69), a set of markers is differentially expressed in NMZL compared with FL, including myeloid cell nuclear differentiation antigen (MNDA), a nuclear protein expressed by myeloid cells and a subset of B cells. MNDA is expressed in normal tissue by a subset of the MZ B cells and especially expressed by the three lymphoma entities derived from the MZ, but are rarely observed in FL, a characteristic that is of potential value in distinguishing between NMZL and FL. One study suggests that FL with monocytoid differentiation may behave more aggressively than conventional FL (70).

Lymphoplasmacytic Lymphoma

The differential diagnosis with LPL is also challenging with overlapping features between those two entities. LPL is considered in the 2008 WHO classification (30) as a lymphoma occurring in adults in the second part of their life, involving BM and, less frequently (15% to 30%), lymph nodes, spleen, liver, and sometimes peripheral blood. It is often associated with an IgM paraprotein. Waldenström macroglobulinemia (WM) is defined as LPL with BM involvement and an IgM monoclonal gammopathy. In lymph nodes, the normal architecture is usually preserved, with dilated sinuses and sometimes atrophic residual germinal centers. Increased mast cells and hemosiderin are frequent. Other features are, however, possible and several aspects are shared with NMZL: diffuse or vaguely nodular pattern, plasmacytic differentiation, absence of specific phenotype, trisomy 3, and an association with hepatitis C, although data concerning LPL are limited and controversial. Immunoglobulin heavy chain variable gene (IGHV) analysis are reported in few cases (in total 46 NMZL (47,64–68) and 64 LPL (71–75) and seems to be distinct between NMZL and LPL but more studies are needed to confirm this feature. Using a comparative genomic hybridization approach, the majority of the recurrent chromosome abnormalities identified in WM is shared with MZL, including deletions of 6q23 and 13q14 and gains of 3q13-q28, 6p, and 18q. However, trisomy 4 seems to be recurrent in WM, as well as gains of 4q and 8q, but have not been described as being common abnormalities in MZL. The search for a MyD88 mutation could be of interest in the differential diagnosis since only 1/5 (20%) NMZL tested has been found to be mutated versus 46/51 (90%) of LPL/Waldenström cases (76). This recent finding needs to be confirmed in other and larger cohorts of patients.

Transformation to Diffuse Large B-Cell Lymphoma

As the component of large cells is often high, many NMZL cases are perhaps considered among the diffuse large B-cell lymphomas, and the clinical significance of the content of large cells is not well established. In some studies, the presence of large cells has been associated with plasmacytoid differentiation (25). Transformation to diffuse large B-cell lymphoma has been described occurring 10 to 76 months after the original diagnosis of low-grade tumor (54,77,78) and is in some studies associated with short survival (51,79).

Castleman Disease

Cases with prominent atrophic germinal centers and hyaline vascular penetration may closely resemble hyaline vascular Castleman disease (HV-CD), leading to misdiagnosis (80). In contrast with HV-CD, B-cell lymphomas with HV-CD-like features are more likely to manifest clinically with systemic symptoms or generalized lymphadenopathy. Careful histopathologic examination, supported by immunohistochemical studies, flow cytometric immunophenotyping, and judicious use of cytogenetic and molecular analyses, allows identification of the masked neoplastic process.

Angioimmunoblastic T-Cell lymphoma

In a subset of cases, the differential diagnosis with AITL may be difficult, in particular in cases with diffuse or predominant interfollicular infiltration with numerous plasma cells, eosinophils, sparse immunoblastic large B cells, and abundant T cells. The histology in those cases may favor AITL, but the immunophenotype is not typical, with the absence of a T-helper marker (CD10, BCL6) or EBV-positive cells by *in situ* hybridization. The demonstration of monoclonality of the B cells by PCR and cytogenetic analysis are important for a definitive diagnosis.

Treatment and Outcome

There is no standardized treatment for this disease. Patients with truly localized disease may be considered for localized radiation therapy, with a good local tumor control. Treatment may be delayed in patients with a low tumor burden, or sometimes single-agent chemotherapy or immunotherapy may be given. In patients with more aggressive features, a standard immunochemotherapy regimen may be proposed, but a substantial proportion of patients do not achieve a complete response. A more dose-intensive strategy, eventually including autologous BM transplantation, is sometimes applied to younger patients, with a high mitotic rate and adverse clinical prognostic factors. Radiation therapy may also be considered as a palliative treatment in some cases, using low doses of radiation (46). However, none of these approaches has been prospectively tested. Therefore, no specific therapeutic approach is recommended at this time, and the clinician may decide optimal therapy based upon the specific morphologic and clinical characteristics of each patient. Monoclonal antibodies directed against the CD20 antigen appear to have some efficacy in this setting (15).

The outcome of NMZL patients is very heterogeneous. Complete response to first-line treatment is observed in 50% to 60% of the cases. In the International Lymphoma Study Group, 5-year failure-free survival and overall survival (OS) were only 28% and 56%, respectively. Most studies have reported 5-year

OS in the range of 55% to 75%, with better outcomes in more recent series, possibly reflecting the increased use of rituximab. This trend toward a poor prognosis was also found for patients with a low or intermediate International Prognostic Index score, although the use of this index in NMZL is clearly exploratory. The 5-year OS is somewhat lower than that seen for follicular lymphoma and CLL, two of the most common low-grade B-cell neoplasms. Time to progression seems to be short, only 1.3 years, but median OS is close to 5 years, indicating that this disease may remain indolent for several years (49). A poor performance status at diagnosis was identified as a clinical parameter significantly influencing the outcome (52,53). The FLIPI score also identified one-third of patients with a significantly shorter survival (50). Of note, a higher proportion of large cells in the diagnostic lymph node was not associated with a different outcome (49). Patients achieving a complete response to first-line treatment may also have a better prognosis. At the time of relapse, nodal sites are usually predominantly involved by disease, although splenic or extranodal site involvement may be encountered, reminiscent of clinical features of the other MZL subtypes. However, histologic progression toward diffuse large-cell lymphomas appears to occur quite frequently and there is no evidence of plateau on survival curves to suggest that this disease is currently curable.

There are limited data concerning other prognostic markers in NMZL. In one study (47), loss of survivin and caspase-3 was associated with shorter failure-free survival, whereas a shorter OS was associated with increased age (more than 60 years) and overexpression of cyclin E. In another study, patients lacking expression of MUM1 or expressing Ki67 in <5% of tumor cells had a better prognosis (51).

PEDIATRIC NODAL MARGINAL ZONE LYMPHOMA

Pediatric NMZL is described as a separate variant of NMZL in the 2008 WHO classification (30). It has a distinctive morphology and clinical presentation and stands out as an indolent disease, with a remarkably better overall prognosis as compared to classic NMZL. The median age of presentation is 16 years with a striking male predominance (sex ratio 20:1). In affected lymph nodes, the lymphoma cells have a predominantly interfollicular distribution, with marked expansion of the MZL. The cell component is similar to the classic form, but with few large cells. A characteristic feature is follicular expansion with features of progressive transformation of germinal centers ("floral variant of NMZL"). Follicular colonization is also observed. Most of the cases present with isolated nodal site of stage I disease and do well with a conservative approach, following simple excision of the nodal mass. A few similar cases have been reported in adults and it seems that the recognition is important to avoid unnecessary overtreatment of this indolent form. The differential diagnosis is especially with atypical marginal zone hyperplasia. Pediatric NMZL involves clonal rearrangement of the IG genes and numerical genetic aberrations similar to those observed in adults. Therefore, it is difficult to understand the pathophysiology of these cases.

CONCLUSION

It is likely that NMZL is underrecognized in routine practice, and remains a diagnostic and therapeutic dilemma. The morphologic and phenotypic description of NMZL is still incomplete in the literature. Cases that are truly borderline—for example, very similar to or perhaps overlapping with other types of lymphomas—appear to exist, and sorting through the differential diagnosis on the basis of morphology and phenotype may still sometimes be tenuous. Clinical and biologic studies of NMZL are hampered by the lack of specific diagnostic markers and the low reproducibility of this diagnosis. Furthermore, descriptions of NMZLs repeatedly raise the question of the genuine existence of LPLs, and the literature is not clear yet on this matter. Overall, there is a strong need for a better individualization of these lymphomas and for an understanding of the mechanisms involved in their pathogenesis. Genomic and proteomic approaches are needed that can identify candidate markers specific to the diagnosis.

References

1. Isaacson P, Wright DH. Malignant lymphoma of mucosa-associated lymphoid tissue. A distinctive type of B-cell lymphoma. *Cancer* 1983;52:1410–1416.
2. Isaacson PG, Du MQ. MALT lymphoma: from morphology to molecules. *Nat Rev Cancer* 2004;4:644–653.
3. Sheibani K, Sohn CC, Burke JS, et al. Monocytoid B-cell lymphoma. A novel B-cell neoplasm. *Am J Pathol* 1986;124:310–318.
4. Cousar JB, McGinn DL, Glick AD, et al. Report of an unusual lymphoma arising from parafollicular B-lymphocytes (PBLs) or so-called "monocytoid" lymphocytes. *Am J Clin Pathol* 1987;87:121–128.
5. Lennert KFA. Diagnose and Atiologie der Piringer'sschen Lymphaneditis. *Ver Dtsch Ges Pathol* 1959;42:203–208.
6. Stansfeld AG. The histological diagnosis of toxoplasmic lymphadenitis. *J Clin Pathol* 1961;14:565–573.
7. Plank L, Hansmann ML, Fischer R. The cytological spectrum of the monocytoid B-cell reaction: recognition of its large cell type. *Histopathology* 1993;23: 425–431.
8. Mohrmann RL, Nathwani BN, Brynes RK, et al. Hodgkin's disease occurring in monocytoid B-cell clusters. *Am J Clin Pathol* 1991;95:802–808.
9. Plank L, Hansmann ML, Fischer R. Monocytoid B-cell reaction associated with peripheral T-cell lymphomas. *Pathol Res Pract* 1995;191:1152–1158.
10. Sheibani K, Fritz RM, Winberg CD, et al. "Monocytoid" cells in reactive follicular hyperplasia with and without multifocal histiocytic reactions: an immunohistochemical study of 21 cases including suspected cases of toxoplasmic lymphadenitis. *Am J Clin Pathol* 1984;81:453–458.
11. Piris MA, Rivas C, Morente M, et al. Monocytoid B-cell lymphoma, a tumour related to the marginal zone. *Histopathology* 1988;12:383–392.
12. van den Oord JJ, de Wolf-Peeters C, Desmet VJ. The marginal zone in the human reactive lymph node. *Am J Clin Pathol* 1986;86:475–479.
13. van Krieken JH, von Schilling C, Kluin PM, et al. Splenic marginal zone lymphocytes and related cells in the lymph node: a morphologic and immunohistochemical study. *Hum Pathol* 1989;20:320–325.
14. Dono M, Zupo S, Colombo M, et al. The human marginal zone B cell. *Ann N Y Acad Sci* 2003;987:117–124.
15. Weller S, Reynaud CA, Weill JC. Splenic marginal zone B cells in humans: where do they mutate their Ig receptor? *Eur J Immunol* 2005;35:2789–2792.
16. Weller S, Braun MC, Tan BK, et al. Human blood IgM "memory" B cells are circulating splenic marginal zone B cells harboring a prediversified immunoglobulin repertoire. *Blood* 2004;104:3647–3654.
17. Martin F, Kearney JF. B-cell subsets and the mature preimmune repertoire. Marginal zone and B1 B cells as part of a "natural immune memory". *Immunol Rev* 2000;175:70–79.
18. Martin F, Oliver AM, Kearney JF. Marginal zone and B1 B cells unite in the early response against T-independent blood-borne particulate antigens. *Immunity* 2001;14:617–629.
19. Kraal G. Cells in the marginal zone of the spleen. *Int Rev Cytol* 1992;132:31–74.
20. Weill JC, Weller S, Reynaud CA. A bird's eye view on human B cells. *Semin Immunol* 2004;16:277–281.
21. Cousar JB, Glick AD, York JC, et al. Peripheral blood and bone marrow involvement by non-Hodgkin's lymphoma: morphological, immunological and cytochemical features. *Prog Clin Pathol* 1984;9:173–196.
22. Ng CS, Chan JK. Monocytoid B-cell lymphoma. *Hum Pathol* 1987;18:1069–1071.
23. Ngan BY, Warnke RA, Wilson M, et al. Monocytoid B-cell lymphoma: a study of 36 cases. *Hum Pathol* 1991;22:409–421.
24. Nathwani BN, Mohrmann RL, Brynes RK, et al. Monocytoid B-cell lymphomas: an assessment of diagnostic criteria and a perspective on histogenesis. *Hum Pathol* 1992;23:1061–1071.
25. Davis GG, York JC, Glick AD, et al. Plasmacytic differentiation in parafollicular (monocytoid) B-cell lymphoma. A study of 12 cases. *Am J Surg Pathol* 1992;16:1066–1074.
26. Nathwani BN, Anderson JR, Armitage JO, et al. Marginal zone B-cell lymphoma: a clinical comparison of nodal and mucosa-associated lymphoid tissue types. Non-Hodgkin's Lymphoma Classification Project. *J Clin Oncol* 1999;17: 2486–2492.
27. Cogliatti SB, Lennert K, Hansmann ML, et al. Monocytoid B cell lymphoma: clinical and prognostic features of 21 patients. *J Clin Pathol* 1990;43:619–625.
28. Banerjee SS, Harris M, Eyden BP, et al. Monocytoid B cell lymphoma. *J Clin Pathol* 1991;44:39–44.
29. Lennert KFA. *Histopathologie der non Hodgkin's lymphoma (rach der aktuaPirienton Kiel-klassification)*. Berlin: Springer Verlag, 1990.
30. Swerdlow SH. *WHO classification of tumours of haematopoietic and lymphoid tissues*. Lyon: IARC Press, 2008.
31. Isaacson PJ, Wright DH. Extranodal malignant lymphoma arising from mucosa-associated lymphoid tissue. *Cancer* 1984;53(11):2515–2524.
32. Stein H, Lennert K, Mason DY, et al. Immature sinus histiocytes: Their identification as a novel B cell population. *Am J Pathol* 1984;117:44–52.
33. de Almeida C, Harris NL, Bhan AK. Characterization of immature sinus histiocytes (monocytoid cells) in reactive lymph nodes by use of monoclonal antibodies. *Hum Pathol* 1984;15(4):330–335.
34. Sheibani K, Burke JS, Swartz WG, et al. Monocytoid B-cell lymphoma. Clinicopathologic study of 21 cases of a unique type of low-grade lymphoma. *Cancer* 1988;62(8):1531–1538.
35. Isaacson PG, Spencer J. Malignant lymphoma of mucosa-associated lymphoid tissue. *Histopathology* 1987;11:445–462.
36. Nizze H, Cogliatti SB, von Schilling C, et al. Monocytoid B-cell lymphoma: morphological variants and relationship to low-grade B-cell lymphoma of the mucosa-associated lymphoid tissue. *Histopathology* 1991;18:403–414.
37. Hammer RD, Glick AD, Greer JP, et al. Splenic marginal zone lymphoma: A distinct B-cell neoplasm. *Am J Surg Pathol* 1996;20:115–132.
38. Harris NL, Jaffe ES, Stein H, et al. A revised European-American classification of lymphoid neoplasms: a proposal from the International Lymphoma Study Group. *Blood* 1994;84(5):1361–1392.
39. Isaacson PG, Matutes E, Burke M, et al. The histopathology of splenic lymphoma with villous lymphocytes. *Blood* 1994;84(11):3828–3834.
40. Mollejo M, Menárguez J, Cristóbal E, et al. Monocytoid B-cells: A comparative clinical pathological study of their distribution in different types of low-grade lymphomas. *Am J Surg pathol* 1994;18(11):1131–1139.
41. de Wolf-Peeters C, Pittaluga S, Dierlamm J, et al. Marginal zone B-cell lymphomas including mucosa-associated lymphoid tissue type lymphoma (MALT), monocytoid B-cell lymphoma and splenic marginal zone cell lymphoma and their relation to the reactive marginal zone. *Leuk Lymphoma* 1997;26:467–478.
42. Isaacson PG. Splenic marginal zone lymphoma. *Blood* 1996;88:751–752.
43. A clinical evaluation of the International Lymphoma Study Group classification of non-Hodgkin's lymphoma. The Non-Hodgkin's Lymphoma Classification Project. *Blood* 1997;89:3909–3918.
44. Berger F, Felman P, Thieblemont C, et al. Non-MALT marginal zone B-cell lymphomas: a description of clinical presentation and outcome in 124 patients. *Blood* 2000;95:1950–1956.
45. Fisher RI, Dahlberg S, Nathwani BN, et al. A clinical analysis of two indolent lymphoma entities: mantle cell lymphoma and marginal zone lymphoma (including the mucosa-associated lymphoid tissue and monocytoid B-cell subcategories): a Southwest Oncology Group study. *Blood* 1995;85:1075–1082.
46. Arcaini L, Paulli M, Boveri E, et al. Splenic and nodal marginal zone lymphomas are indolent disorders at high hepatitis C virus seroprevalence with distinct presenting features but similar morphologic and phenotypic profiles. *Cancer* 2004;100:107–115.
47. Camacho FI, Algara P, Mollejo M, et al. Nodal marginal zone lymphoma: a heterogeneous tumor: a comprehensive analysis of a series of 27 cases. *Am J Surg Pathol* 2003;27:762–771.
48. Armitage JO, Weisenburger DD. New approach to classifying non-Hodgkin's lymphomas: clinical features of the major histologic subtypes. Non-Hodgkin's Lymphoma Classification Project. *J Clin Oncol* 1998;16:2780–2795.
49. Traverse-Glehen A, Felman P, Callet-Bauchu E, et al. A clinicopathological study of nodal marginal zone B-cell lymphoma. A report on 21 cases. *Histopathology* 2006;48:162–173.
50. Arcaini L, Paulli M, Burcheri S, et al. Primary nodal marginal zone B-cell lymphoma: clinical features and prognostic assessment of a rare disease. *Br J Haematol* 2007;136:301–304.
51. Petit B, Chaury MP, Le Clorennec C, et al. Indolent lymphoplasmacytic and marginal zone B-cell lymphomas: absence of both IRF4 and Ki67 expression identifies a better prognosis subgroup. *Haematologica* 2005;90:200–206.
52. Oh SY, Ryoo BY, Kim WS, et al. Nodal marginal zone B-cell lymphoma: analysis of 36 cases. Clinical presentation and treatment outcomes of nodal marginal zone B-cell lymphoma. *Ann Hematol* 2006;85:781–786.
53. Kojima M, Inagaki H, Motoori T, et al. Clinical implications of nodal marginal zone B-cell lymphoma among Japanese: study of 65 cases. *Cancer Sci* 2007;98: 44–49.
54. Nathwani BN, Drachenberg MR, Hernandez AM, et al. Nodal monocytoid B-cell lymphoma (nodal marginal-zone B-cell lymphoma). *Semin Hematol* 1999;36: 128–138.
55. Salama ME, Lossos IS, Warnke RA, et al. Immunoarchitectural patterns in nodal marginal zone B-cell lymphoma: a study of 51 cases. *Am J Clin Pathol* 2009;132:39–49.
56. Boveri E, Arcaini L, Merli M, et al. Bone marrow histology in marginal zone B-cell lymphomas: correlation with clinical parameters and flow cytometry in 120 patients. *Ann Oncol* 2009;20:129–136.
57. Traverse-Glehen A, Baseggio L, Salles G, et al. Splenic marginal zone B-cell lymphoma: a distinct clinicopathological and molecular entity. Recent advances in ontogeny and classification. *Curr Opin Oncol* 2011;23:441–448.
58. Campo E, Miquel R, Krenacs L, et al. Primary nodal marginal zone lymphomas of splenic and MALT type. *Am J Surg Pathol* 1999;23:59–68.
59. Naresh KN. Nodal marginal zone B-cell lymphoma with prominent follicular colonization—difficulties in diagnosis: a study of 15 cases. *Histopathology* 2008;52:331–339.
60. Dierlamm J, Pittaluga S, Wlodarska I, et al. Marginal zone B-cell lymphomas of different sites share similar cytogenetic and morphologic features. *Blood* 1996;87:299–307.
61. Slovak ML, Weiss LM, Nathwani BN, et al. Cytogenetic studies of composite lymphomas: monocytoid B-cell lymphoma and other B-cell non-Hodgkin's lymphomas. *Hum Pathol* 1993;24:1086–1094.
62. Rinaldi A, Mian M, Chigrinova E, et al. Genome-wide DNA profiling of marginal zone lymphomas identifies subtype-specific lesions with an impact on the clinical outcome. *Blood* 2011;117:1595–1604.
63. Novak U, Basso K, Pasqualucci L, et al. Genomic analysis of non-splenic marginal zone lymphomas (MZL) indicates similarities between nodal and extranodal MZL and supports their derivation from memory B-cells. *Br J Haematol* 2011;155:362–365.
64. Traverse-Glehen A, Davi F, Ben Simon E, et al. Analysis of VH genes in marginal zone lymphoma reveals marked heterogeneity between splenic and nodal tumors and suggests the existence of clonal selection. *Haematologica* 2005;90:470–478.
65. Tierens A, Delabie J, Pittaluga S, et al. Mutation analysis of the rearranged immunoglobulin heavy chain genes of marginal zone cell lymphomas indicates an origin from different marginal zone B lymphocyte subsets. *Blood* 1998;91: 2381–2386.
66. Conconi A, Bertoni F, Pedrinis E, et al. Nodal marginal zone B-cell lymphomas may arise from different subsets of marginal zone B lymphocytes. *Blood* 2001;98:781–786.

67. Kuppers R, Hajadi M, Plank L, et al. Molecular Ig gene analysis reveals that monocytoid B cell lymphoma is a malignancy of mature B cells carrying somatically mutated V region genes and suggests that rearrangement of the kappa-deleting element (resulting in deletion of the Ig kappa enhancers) abolishes somatic hypermutation in the human. *Eur J Immunol* 1996;26:1794–1800.

68. Miranda RN, Cousar JB, Hammer RD, et al. Somatic mutation analysis of IgH variable regions reveals that tumor cells of most parafollicular (monocytoid) B-cell lymphoma, splenic marginal zone B-cell lymphoma, and some hairy cell leukemia are composed of memory B lymphocytes. *Hum Pathol* 1999;30:306–312.

69. Novak U, Rinaldi A, Kwee I, et al. The NF-{kappa}B negative regulator TNFAIP3 (A20) is inactivated by somatic mutations and genomic deletions in marginal zone lymphomas. *Blood* 2009;113:4918–4921.

70. Nathwani BN, Anderson JR, Armitage JO, et al. Clinical significance of follicular lymphoma with monocytoid B cells. Non-Hodgkin's Lymphoma Classification Project. *Hum Pathol* 1999;30:263–268.

71. Aoki H, Takishita M, Kosaka M, et al. Frequent somatic mutations in D and/or JH segments of Ig gene in Waldenström's macroglobulinemia and chronic lymphocytic leukemia (CLL) with Richter's syndrome but not in common CLL. *Blood* 1995;85:1913–1919.

72. Sahota SS, Forconi F, Ottensmeier CH, et al. Typical Waldenström macroglobulinemia is derived from a B-cell arrested after cessation of somatic mutation but prior to isotype switch events. *Blood* 2002;100:1505–1507.

73. Kriangkum J, Taylor BJ, Reiman T, et al. Origins of Waldenström's macroglobulinemia: does it arise from an unusual B-cell precursor? *Clin Lymphoma* 2005;5:217–219.

74. Rollett RA, Wilkinson EJ, Gonzalez D, et al. Immunoglobulin heavy chain sequence analysis in Waldenström's macroglobulinemia and immunoglobulin M monoclonal gammopathy of undetermined significance. *Clin Lymphoma Myeloma* 2006;7:70–72.

75. Parrens M, Gachard N, Petit B, et al. Splenic marginal zone lymphomas and lymphoplasmacytic lymphomas originate from B-cell compartments with two different antigen-exposure histories. *Leukemia* 2008;22:1621–1624.

76. Xu L. A somatic variant of MYD88 (L265P) revealed by whole genome sequencing differentiates lymphoplasmacytic lymphoma from marginal zone lymphomas. In: Blood (ed.) ASH Annual Meeting, Edition San Diego Convention Center: Blood 2011.

77. Ortiz-Hidalgo C, Wright DH. The morphological spectrum of monocytoid B-cell lymphoma and its relationship to lymphomas of mucosa-associated lymphoid tissue. *Histopathology* 1992;21:555–561.

78. Kojima M, Tsukamoto N, Miyazawa Y, et al. Nodal marginal zone B-cell lymphoma associated with Sjögren's syndrome: a report of three cases. *Leuk Lymphoma* 2007;48:1222–1224.

79. Kaur P. Nodal marginal zone lymphoma with increased large cells: myth versus entity. *Arch Pathol Lab Med* 2011;135:964–966.

80. Siddiqi IN, Brynes RK, Wang E. B-cell lymphoma with hyaline vascular Castleman disease-like features: a clinicopathologic study. *Am J Clin Pathol* 2011;135:901–914.

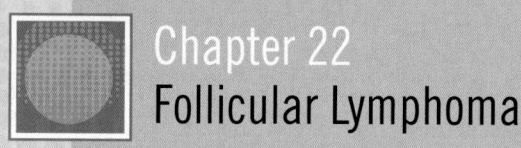

Chapter 22
Follicular Lymphoma

Grant Nybakken • Roger Warnke • Yasodha Natkunam

DEFINITION AND HISTORY OF FOLLICULAR LYMPHOMA

The 2008 edition of the World Health Organization (WHO) classification defines follicular lymphoma (FL) as a neoplasm of germinal center–derived B cells that exhibits at least a partially follicular growth pattern (1). Neoplastic follicles are composed of a variable mixture of centroblasts and centrocytes, and this cellular composition forms the basis of the WHO grading system. Although the nodular growth pattern is a key diagnostic feature, centrocyte-predominant diffuse areas can be present or even form the entirety of the lesion. Primary cutaneous presentations are considered separately as primary cutaneous follicle center lymphoma.

The diagnostic features of FL have evolved from the initial recognition of follicle-like structures in lymphoma by Ghon and Roman (2) in 1916. Separately, Brill et al. (3) and Symmers (4) noted an expansion of giant follicular hyperplasia involving the lymph nodes and spleen, but sparing the peripheral blood. Although initially favoring a benign process, the neoplastic nature and potential for progression of "Brill-Symmers disease" ultimately became clear.

Gall et al. (5) described the first large cohort and delineated the distinction from other types of lymphoma, noting the widespread nodal and splenic involvement with sparing of extranodal sites. Furthermore, they demonstrated the relative indolence (79% 2-year survival vs. 56% 2-year survival in other forms of lymphoma), a lack of constitutional symptoms, and a high rate of involvement of retroperitoneal nodes. A four-stage grading system was proposed that resembles that used in the current classification (1).

Hicks et al. (6) confirmed and furthered the description, but also focused on the cellular composition in contrast to the follicular architecture. They proposed that FL forms a nodular, more indolent version of diffuse lymphomas with the same cellular composition (centrocytic and centroblastic), while also acknowledging the tendency of nodular lymphomas to progress to diffuse lymphoma. They also recognized the cellular composition as a reliable feature in separating lymphoma from reactive follicular hyperplasia.

The Kiel (7), Lukes and Collins (8), and Working formulation (9) classification systems separated the diagnosis from other lymphomas; however, the definition continued to be based upon the cellular composition rather than architectural features.

The Revised European American Lymphoma Classification (10) built upon this work and defined a distinct diagnosis called follicle center lymphoma, an entity consisting of a mixture of centrocytes and centroblasts exhibiting at least a partially follicular growth pattern. Furthermore, they recognized the relative composition of centrocytes and centroblasts to be prognostically important. The WHO, in its 2001 (11) and 2008 (1) editions, retained this disease definition, under the rubric FL. Although a provisional diffuse form of these lymphomas

was previously entertained, it is currently considered a rare (if controversial) type of FL.

The clinical, morphologic, immunophenotypic, and genetic spectrum of FL is described in detail below.

CLINICAL FEATURES

FL is common, accounting for 22% of all non-Hodgkin lymphomas worldwide (12) and 35% in the United States, with approximately 15,000 new cases diagnosed each year (13). It has considerable geographic variability with higher rates in the United States and Western Europe and lower rates in Eastern Europe and Asia. Ethnicity also impacts prevalence as Caucasians have an incidence of around 3 in 100,000 and African Americans have an incidence a third of that (14). It is predominantly a disease of adults with a median age at diagnosis in the sixth decade and infrequent occurrences before the age of 20. The male:female ratio is roughly 1:1 for adult FL, but pediatric FL primarily afflicts males (15).

Patients typically present with mass lesions, either disseminated (12) or, less commonly, localized tumors that may be peripheral (cervical, axillary) or central (retroperitoneal, thoracic). These masses are most commonly nodal (14), but extranodal and hematogenous (spleen, bone marrow, peripheral blood) involvement is also frequent. In fact, bone marrow involvement is seen in around 70% of patients at diagnosis in staging biopsies (12). Interestingly, primary presentation at extranodal sites, in particular skin and gastrointestinal tract, can portend a distinctly better prognosis from more classical nodal FL, as is discussed below. Aside from symptoms related to mass effect, FL is typically asymptomatic. The presence of B symptoms, such as fever and weight loss, is frequently associated with progression of disease.

Although FL is generally an indolent disease, various factors influence survival. A five-part clinical index known as the Follicular Lymphoma International Prognostic Index (FLIPI (16)) has been developed to stratify risk in affected patients. This index has been further refined in FLIPI2 (17), which modifies the FLIPI by substituting β_2-microglobulin levels instead of lactose dehydrogenase and the longest diameter of the involved lymph node instead of number of nodal areas; however, FLIPI2 is not in widespread use as yet. The FLIPI divides patients into low-, intermediate-, and high-risk groups with respective 5-year survivals of 91%, 78%, and 52% and 10-year survivals of 71%, 51%, and 36%. New treatments have markedly improved the prognosis for FL, with 5-year survival increasing from 64% to 95% over the past 30 years (18). Equally as important, failure-free survival has improved from 29% to 60%, demonstrating the success of new frontline treatments, most notably the anti-CD20 monoclonal antibody therapy, rituximab.

Although FL itself is indolent, transformation of FL is followed by an aggressive disease course (19). Transformation occurs in 3% of cases per year over the first 15 years of observation, and cases most commonly transform to diffuse large

B-cell lymphoma (20–22). Minor subsets, however, transform to even more aggressive lymphomas such as blastic FL and those with Burkitt lymphoma–like features. Histologically defined progression of FL is associated with a short life expectancy, with a median survival of 1.7 years (25% 5-year survival) (20). This shortened survival period was closely matched by a survival of 1.8 years when progression was defined clinically and without histologic confirmation. Although progression is not immediate, it appears to be the natural course of the disease when left untreated. In an autopsy study performed before current therapies, 70% of patients with a previous diagnosis of FL had progressed. Only 6% had evidence of residual nodular FL (23).

The indolence of FL both belies and explains the difficulty in clinical management of patients with this lymphoma subtype. Conventional therapeutics can slow but not cure the disease, and this is largely a consequence of a low proliferative rate. Low stage, which manifests with localized disease, is frequently treated with radiation therapy, although watchful waiting can also be employed. Among a selected group of low-stage patients, a median survival of 19 years was observed, despite 67% of patients receiving no treatment for at least 7 years (24). Stage III and IV disease is much more common at diagnosis. Even at high stage, asymptomatic disease does not require immediate treatment. In recent decades, rituximab has been employed successfully in FL, resulting in increased survival rates and longer times to retreatment (25).

REACTIVE GERMINAL CENTERS

An understanding of the composition, architecture, and function of the reactive germinal center provides a foundation for understanding the diagnosis, grading, and treatment of FL. The germinal center is the site of B-cell maturation in primary and secondary immune responses. Following the initial encounter with antigen in the parafollicular areas, naive IgD⁺/IgM⁺ B cells migrate to the B-cell follicles. Once in the B-cell follicles, they proliferate, expanding the follicular dendritic cell meshwork and creating a germinal center. This rapid growth pushes aside the naive B cells in the primary follicle, forming a mantle zone around the germinal center (26). The antigen-induced cells transform to large (3 to 4× a normal lymphocyte) centroblasts with round to oval nuclei, vesicular chromatin with peripheral condensation, one to three marginated basophilic nucleoli, and scant amounts of basophilic cytoplasm. These cells are polarized in the germinal center to form a "dark zone" generally distal to the antigenic source (subcapsular sinus in lymph nodes and the crypts in tonsil) (Fig. 22.1). The germinal center B cells divide rapidly (cell cycle time of 6 to 12 hours) and have a distinct immunophenotype with decreased sIg and increased CD10 and BCL-6 expression. BCL6 proves to be a critical regulator of germinal center development (27) and down-regulates multiple effectors, including repression of BCL2 (28), BLIMP1

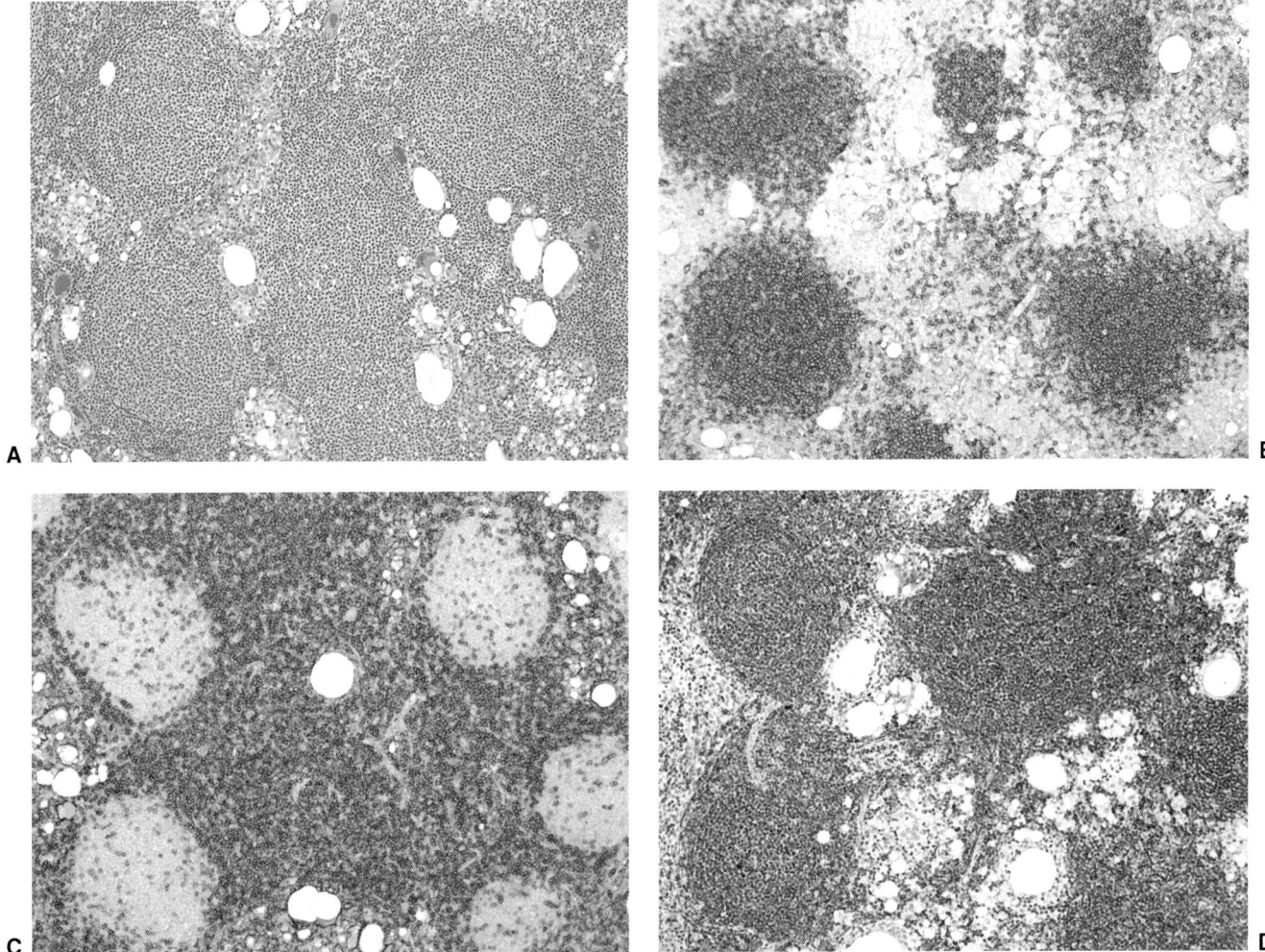

FIGURE 22.1. Reactive lymph nodes. Primary lymphoid follicles characterized by nodules of small lymphoid cells, mature chromatin, and scant cytoplasm (**A**), with a normal immunoarchitecture highlighted by CD20 (**B**), CD3 (**C**), and BCL2 (**D**) expression.

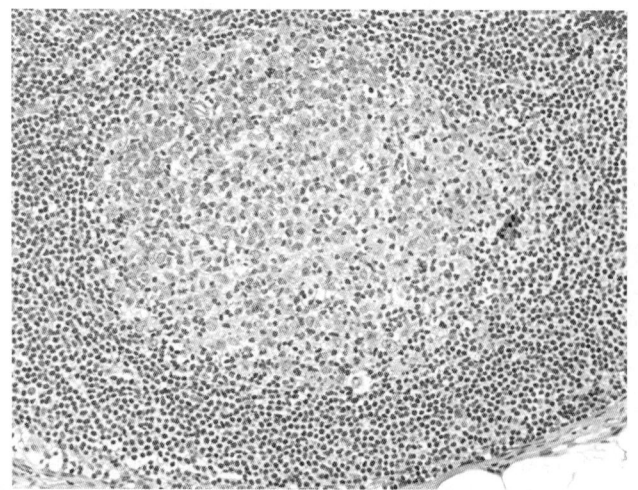

E

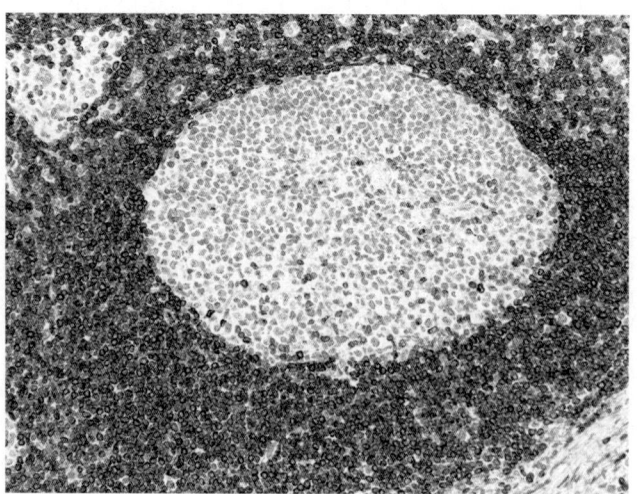

F

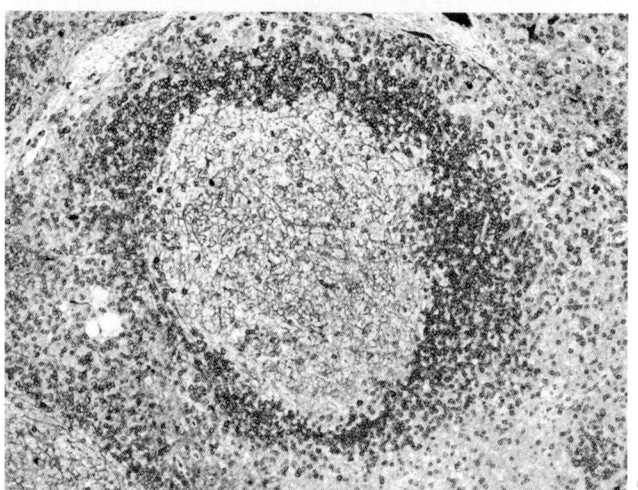

G

FIGURE 22.1. *(Continued)* Secondary lymphoid follicle characterized by a germinal center composed of a heterogeneous population of centrocytes, centroblasts, dendritic cells, and tingible body macrophages **(E)**. A normal immunoarchitecture is highlighted by lack of expression of BCL2 protein within germinal center B cells although expression is present in scattered T cells as well as mantle zone B cells **(F)**. An immunostain for IgM highlights immune complexes within follicles as well as mantle zone cells although the germinal center cells lack staining **(G)**.

(29), p53 (30), ATR (31), and BCR/CD40 signaling mediators (31). Decreased BCL2 leaves the cells vulnerable to apoptosis, while reduced p53 and ATR simultaneously inure the cells to somatic mutations. BLIMP1 suppression prevents maturation toward plasma cells, and BCR/CD40 alterations modulate survival signals from the BCR and CD40 receptors. Somatic hypermutation begins to create diversity in antibody affinity and class switching occurs, potentially generating IgG, IgA, or IgE antibodies. Somatic hypermutation is not limited to the immunoglobulin genes as variability is noted in the promoter region of both *BCL2* and *BCL6*. The cells also mature, becoming centrocytes, medium-sized cells with angular nuclei, even chromatin, inconspicuous nucleoli, and scant pale cytoplasm.

The centrocytes polarize to the "pale zone" of the germinal center, which is rich in follicular dendritic cells; they also express sIg. The decreased expression of BCL2 and increased expression of Fas (a proapoptotic receptor), due to its role in cell death homeostasis, leave the cells acutely vulnerable to apoptosis, allowing for selection of antibody clones with higher affinity. Tingible body macrophages clear the cellular debris formed by the massive apoptosis, creating a "starry-sky" pattern to the germinal center. The follicular dendritic cells generate the appropriate microenvironment through secretion of chemokines and cytokines and present antigen along their dendritic processes. B cells process and present the antigen to germinal center T cells that coexpress CD4, CD57, CXCR5, CXCL-13, and PD-1. T-cell activation and expression of CD40 ligand allows costimulatory signaling through CD40 expressed on B cells, preventing cell death from apoptosis. The cellular

and signaling milieu then prompts migration to the marginal zone and maturation toward effector functions, including plasma cells and memory B cells, with loss of germinal center markers, including CD10 and BCL-6 and reexpression of BCL2.

MORPHOLOGY

Histologically, FL is characterized by effacement of the nodal architecture by a proliferation of follicle center B cells. Not surprisingly, these atypical proliferations often display a follicular growth pattern; however, an intermixed diffuse pattern is common. The follicles can vary markedly in size from case to case with some resembling small germinal centers and others forming serpiginous structures resembling the geographic formations of florid follicular hyperplasia. The recapitulation of the normal germinal center is incomplete, however, as these nodules are often closely packed and have partial or absent mantle zones. An invasive growth pattern is common with frequent infiltration beyond the capsule into surrounding soft tissues (Fig. 22.2).

The cellular composition of reactive and neoplastic follicles is different. Unlike many malignancies, which consist of monotonous cellular proliferations, FL is composed of a mixed cellular milieu. Two follicular B-cell populations are typically seen: centrocytes and centroblasts. Centrocytes are elongate or angulated cells with inconspicuous nucleoli whereas centroblasts are large cells with vesicular chromatin and one to three peripherally placed small nucleoli. The distinct distribution pattern of these cells is a criterion for malignancy. In reactive

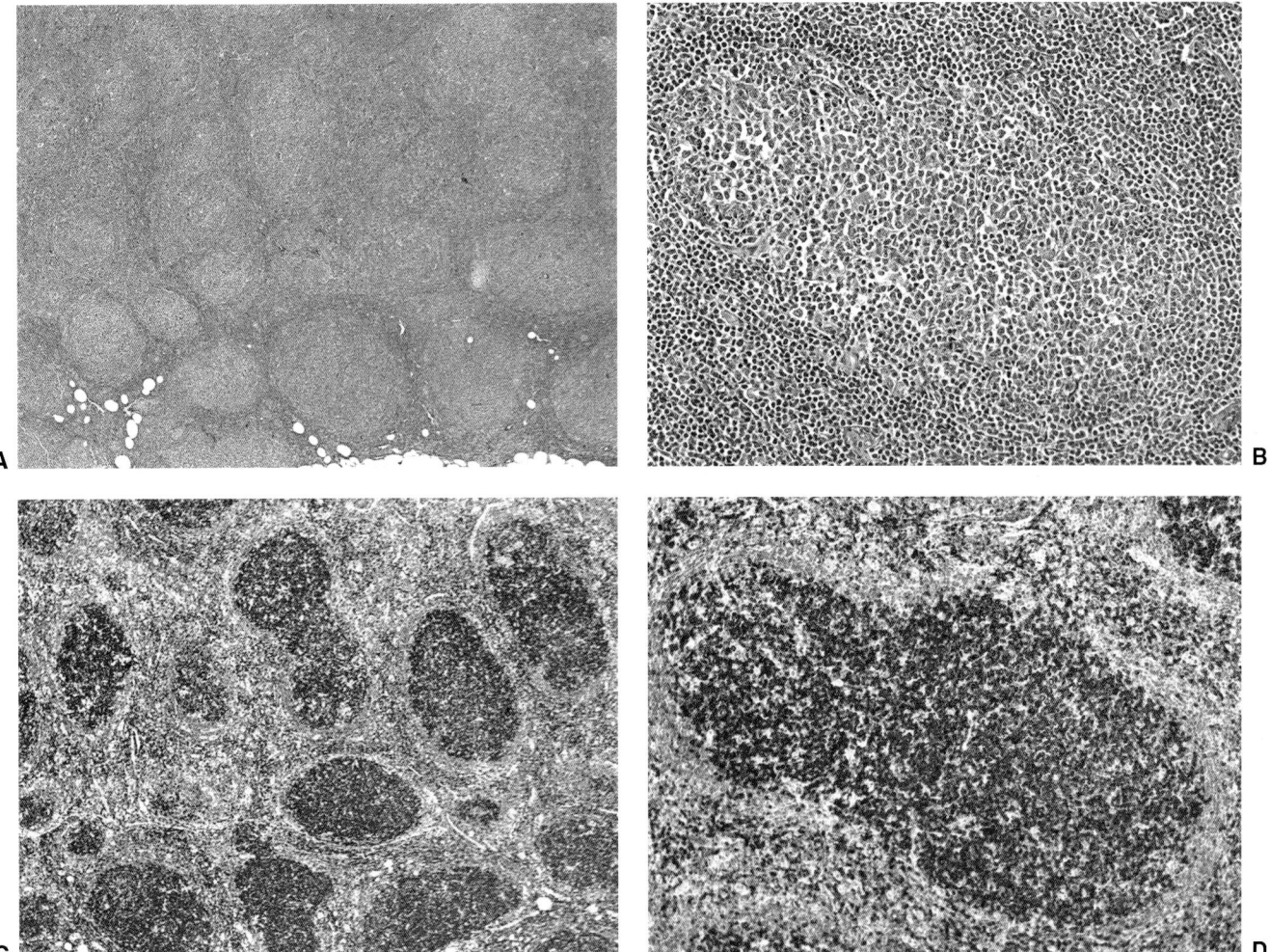

FIGURE 22.2. Follicular lymphoma. FL is characterized by effacement of immunoarchitecture by overcrowded follicles that lack polarization, mantle zones, and a heterogeneous cellular composition within follicles **(A,B)**; immunohistologic stains show expression of BCL2 protein within neoplastic follicles **(C,D)**.

nodes, they are commonly distributed in a gradient, providing a polarized appearance to the germinal center. The germinal center is typically spotted with tingible body macrophages, consistent with the tremendously high turnover associated with the normal functions of the germinal center including clonal expansion, antigen selection, and affinity maturation. In contrast, FL consists of a mixture of centrocytes and centroblasts that frequently lack both polarization and tingible body macrophages.

Many cellular elements of the physiologic germinal center encompass the microenvironment of the follicular B cells. Some, if not all, FLs are thought to remain antigen driven (32,33). Therefore it is not surprising that follicular dendritic cells, with their capacity for antigen presentation, are retained within the neoplastic follicles. However, they typically lack Ig in the form of immune complexes as seen in germinal centers. In fact, they typically form an entire network surrounding the follicular cells, a useful feature during immunophenotypic characterization. Furthermore, follicular T-helper cells also remain in the germinal center. As noted previously, in low-grade lesions, with low proliferative and apoptotic indices, tingible body macrophages are characteristically absent and provide an important diagnostic feature in distinguishing FL from reactive follicular hyperplasia.

The interfollicular regions are frequently inconspicuous, but are occasionally increased in size and can resemble diffuse areas. Unlike a reactive lymph node, the cellular composition is more monotonous and often contains neoplastic centrocytes scattered amongst small T cells with condensed chromatin. Immunoblasts and plasma cells are generally lacking in most cases, which further aides in the separation from reactive follicular hyperplasia. Vessels in the interfollicular regions often demonstrate vascular invasion by individual neoplastic lymphocytes with infiltration of the smooth muscle wall.

Sclerosis is common in the interfollicular and diffuse areas at the periphery of masses of FL. This may complicate diagnosis by either disguising the nodular growth pattern or through low-power mimicry of nodular sclerosis Hodgkin lymphoma, but may be helpful in the separation from reactive hyperplasias.

Apart from the classic features of FL, there are also a number of well-described morphologic variants. These variants generally do not have independent prognostic significance, but recognizing these variants is critical for differentiation from other entities and for appropriate grading.

The marginal zone variant is the most common of the morphologic variants, found in around 9% of FLs (34). Although similar in morphology to conventional FL, the follicles are surrounded by apparent marginal zones. These cells are medium sized with clear cytoplasm, which imparts a monocytoid appearance to the follicular B cells. This feature may provide the impression of a coincident marginal zone lymphoma; in fact, this entity was originally described as a composite lymphoma. Studies have since indicated a common clonal origin for both cell groups, and this entity is now considered a variant of FL (35,36). These monocytoid cells display a germinal center immunophenotype and express CD10 and BCL6. In addition to the t(14;18) translocation, a number of these cases have been found to have trisomy 3, a common alteration in marginal zone lymphoma, which suggests a potential mechanism behind the morphologic marginal zone differentiation (34) (Fig. 22.3A and B).

A plasmacytoid variant has been described as well (37,38). Despite resembling FL at low power, at high power, the follicular or interfollicular cells are plasmacytoid with eccentric nuclei, abundant cytoplasm, and a perinuclear hof. These cells, however, also retain a germinal center immunophenotype and cytogenetic profile (39). There are clinical implications as well; patients with plasmacytoid differentiation can demonstrate a paraproteinemia (40). Therefore, positive staining for plasma cell markers, such as CD38, CD138, and IRF4/MUM1, should not be misinterpreted as a marginal zone lymphoma with plasmacytic differentiation or a plasma cell neoplasm (Fig. 22.3C–E).

The floral variant of FL demonstrates a prominent mantle zone surrounding ragged follicles (41–43). Two patterns have

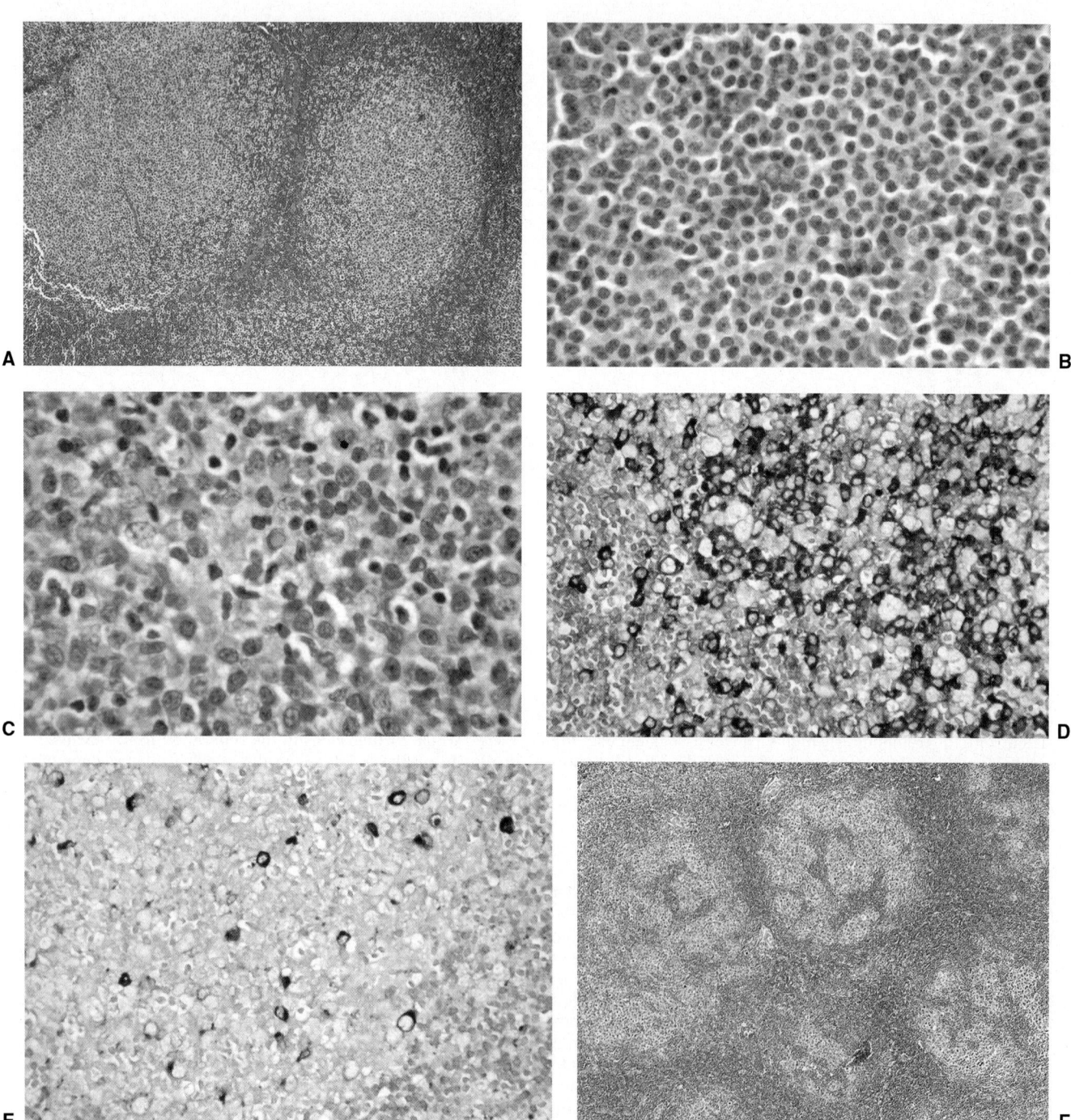

FIGURE 22.3. Variant morphology of FL. FL shows several variant morphologic features including marginal zone differentiation with monocytoid appearance of follicular cells (**A,B**); plasmacytoid features (**C**); positive staining for kappa light chains (**D**): and lack of staining for lambda light chains (**E**). Floral variant with serrated or unusual follicle structures (**F**);

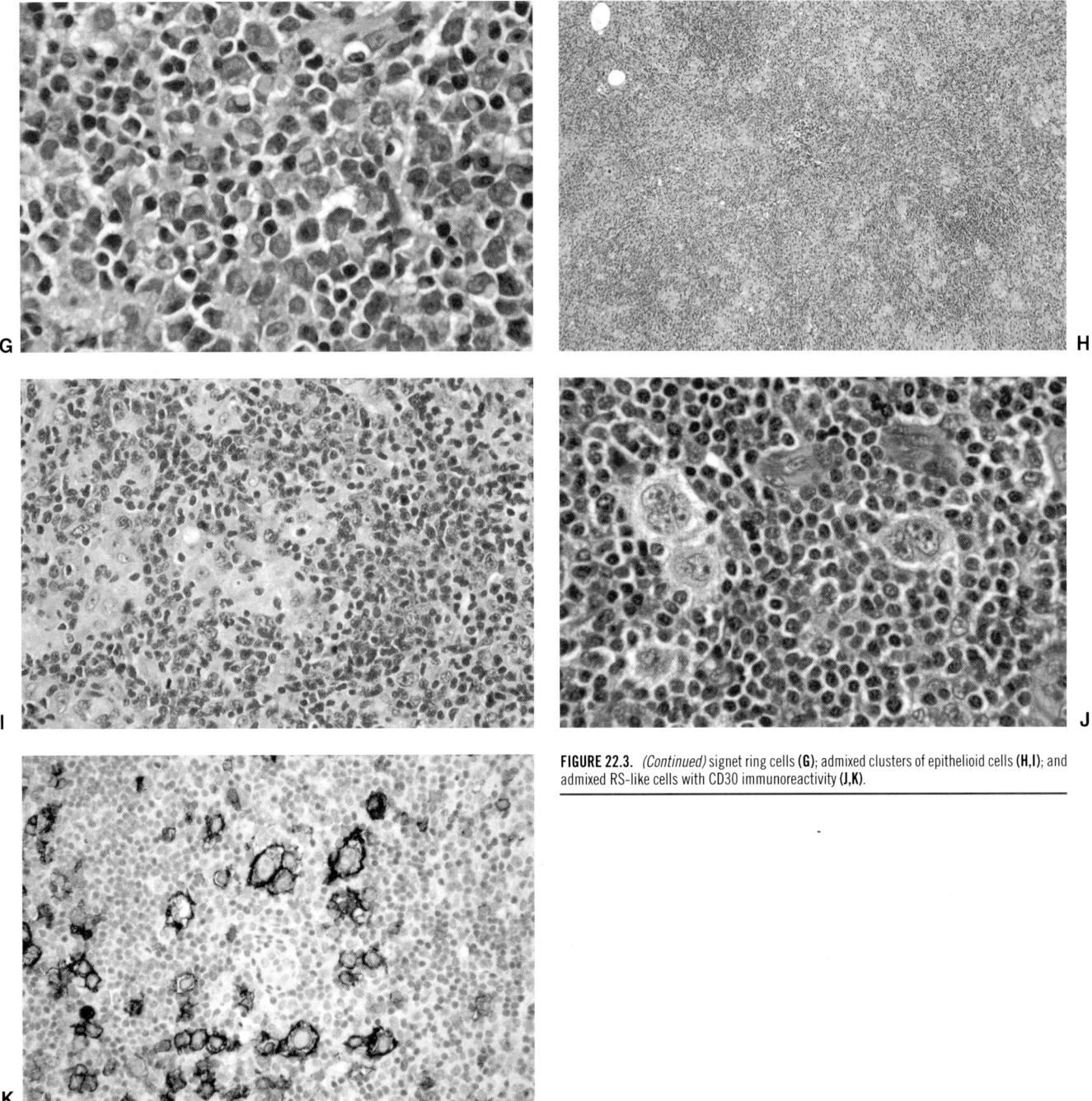

FIGURE 22.3. *(Continued)* signet ring cells (**G**); admixed clusters of epithelioid cells (**H,I**); and admixed RS-like cells with CD30 immunoreactivity (**J,K**).

been described: one in which the mantle zone pushes into large germinal centers creating a scalloped, flower-like appearance and another with near-complete disruption of the germinal centers by mantle zone lymphocytes (41). The first appearance mimics a progressively transformed germinal center, while the second may resemble nodular lymphocyte-predominant Hodgkin lymphoma. Compounding this histologic quandary is the expanded follicular dendritic network highlighted by CD21 immunohistochemistry. The B cells retain the traditional immunophenotype, and express CD10 and BCL2 within follicles but lack CD5, CD43, and cyclin D1. Furthermore, they have monotypic light chains and demonstrate clonal immunoglobulin gene rearrangements (42) (Fig. 22.3F).

A signet ring variant of FL is characterized by centrocytes containing large cytoplasmic inclusions that indent the nucleus. Three different types of inclusions have been described, each with different ultrastructural appearances: round eosinophilic periodic acid-Schiff after diastase (PASD)-positive inclusions associated with IgM accumulation in dense granular vesicle-filled cisternae of rough endoplasmic reticulum; round, clear, PASD-negative inclusions associated with IgG accumulation; and an electron-lucent vacuole with a smooth membrane. Finally, there are ill-defined PASD-negative cytoplasmic forms that are not heavy chain specific, but demonstrate non–membrane delimited granular-fibrillar and crystalline cytoplasmic material (44) (Fig. 22.3G).

The epithelioid variant of FL typically shows admixed clusters of pale-staining epithelioid cells. These epithelioid cell clusters can be so numerous as to complicate recognition of a follicular pattern as well as grading (Fig. 22.3H and I).

FL also has been demonstrated to have Reed-Sternberg (RS)–like cells. Unlike cases of composite lymphoma, the RS-like cells are found within the neoplastic follicles and surrounding areas generally lack the background of mixed inflammatory infiltrates. Laser-capture microdissection followed by molecular analysis has shown that these RS-like cells are clonally related to the surrounding FL B cells (45). Immunophenotypically, these RS-like cells typically express CD30 and other germinal center B-cell markers, but lack expression of CD15 (Fig. 22.3J and K).

GRADING AND REPORTING FOLLICULAR LYMPHOMA

Grading of FL is a controversial issue. The debate covers not only the appropriate method for determining the grade, but also the significance of the grades once they have been determined. In general, however, the prognosis of FL worsens with greater proportions of centroblasts. Although the intraobserver variability is acceptable, the interobserver variability is high, leading to the proposal of multiple methods for grade determination. The optimal method for grading FL, and the clinical significance of the grades in the modern therapeutic era, remains unclear. Regardless, adequate sampling of lymph nodes is required for optimal assessment of pattern, cytologic content and detail for accurate classification.

The 2008 edition of the WHO classification proposes the most commonly used method (Berard method), counting or estimating the number of centroblasts within neoplastic follicles with cutoffs for grades 1, 2, and 3 established (somewhat arbitrarily) at 0 to 5, 6 to 15, >15 centroblasts/high-power fields (hpf), respectively. Grades 1 and 2 are considered to represent low-grade and grade 3, high-grade FL. Grade 3 is divided further into those with increased centroblasts admixed with centrocytes (grade 3A) or sheets of centroblasts without any centrocytes (grade 3B). The average number of centroblasts over at least 10 hpf is then applied to determine the grade. This

technique is fraught with technical issues, including appropriate standardization of the counted field (0.159 mm² hpf), with appropriate adjustments required for any given microscope and a particular set of objective lenses and eyepieces. Furthermore, the thickness of the histologic section could provide variable numbers of cells and, if not optimally prepared, further hamper this estimate. Since the evaluation is based on an ordinal, rather than percentage count, this estimate could lead to skewing of results.

Others have recommended modifying these criteria, such that grade 3 is applied to instances with >50% of the cells centroblasts. The use of a percentage obviates the requirement for standardization of the hpf, and simplifies the analysis. With this method, the distinction between 3A and 3B remains, with the presence of remnant centrocytes mandating a diagnosis of 3A. Some studies have demonstrated this method to have greater interobserver variability than the Berard method (46,47). Others have noted that the Berard method results in skewing toward grade 3, with some finding 60% of cases to have >15 centroblasts/hpf (48).

The proliferative fraction is also correlated with the grade of the lymphoma. The proliferative fraction of low-grade FLs is generally under 20%, while that of grade 3 FLs is typically over 40%. As a consequence, Ki-67 proliferative fraction is used by some as a method for determining grade. The prognostic value of this method remains uncertain. Some studies have demonstrated the centroblast method to be superior (48,49). Others have demonstrated decreased survival in histologically low-grade FL with increased proliferation (50), although the numbers of reported cases are small and the findings have not been validated in larger cohorts of patients or in prospective studies. The WHO currently regards Ki-67 as an auxiliary to the Berard method.

The clinical utility of the grades has evolved since their initial proposal. The original three-level grading system has recently

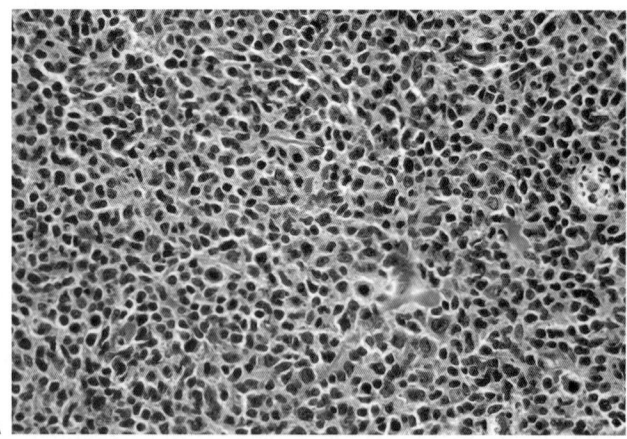

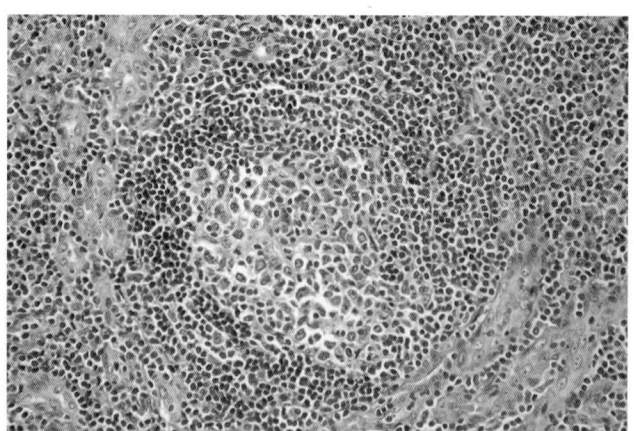

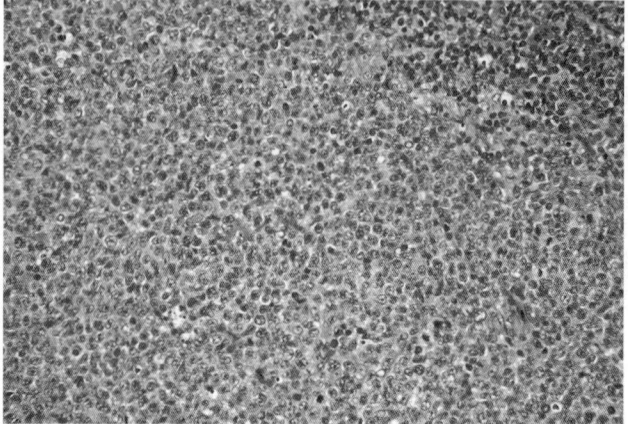

FIGURE 22.4. Grading of FL. The current 2008 WHO classification places FL into three grades based on the relative composition of centrocytes and centroblasts within neoplastic follicles: grade 1 to 2 is classified as low grade (**A**); grade 3 is further divided into 3A, which is characterized by the predominance of large cells with admixed centrocytes (**B**), and 3B, which shows sheets of large cells without admixed centrocytes (**C**).

been simplified. As there is no clinical distinction either prognostically or therapeutically between grades 1 and 2, they have been consolidated into a single grade 1 to 2 or "low grade." Grade 3, as mentioned above, remains divided into two categories: 3A and 3B (Fig. 22.4A–C). The largest study yet (51) found no utility in separating grades 1 to 2 and grade 3A, postulating that the only critical distinction is in separating grade 3B from all other grades of FL; however, other smaller studies, have differed (52,53). Grades 1 to 3A were found to be indolent and incurable, whereas 3B was associated with an aggressive clinical course and higher mortality, which with appropriate therapy was curable (51). Similarly, recent gene expression profiling studies have demonstrated a consistent gene expression signature for grades 1 to 3A, but an overlapping although discrete pattern for grade 3B. Comparison with diffuse large B-cell lymphoma, however, demonstrated a clear distinction, suggesting that although grade 3B is divergent from lower-grade FL, it should continue to be classified separately from diffuse large B-cell lymphoma (54).

PATTERN

The growth patterns of FL are divided into four categories according to the 2008 WHO classification: follicular (>75% follicular), follicular and diffuse (25% to 75% follicular), focally follicular (<25% follicular), and diffuse (0% follicular). Diffuse areas are defined as areas that lack morphologic or immunophenotypic evidence of a follicular growth pattern, but maintain a cellular composition similar to that of neoplastic follicles. It is recommended that the proportion of follicular growth as well as the presence and proportion of diffuse areas be noted in the pathology report. The presence of neoplastic follicular cells in the interfollicular areas does not constitute a diffuse component, and in some cases, separating diffuse areas from the interfollicular component can be difficult and subjective. There is some disagreement about the existence of a true diffuse FL and some believe it may simply represent incomplete sampling. In fact, on biopsies, it is recommended that the potential for sampling error should be noted in the pathology reports in such cases. An excisional biopsy should be recommended for better characterization and grading when this occurs. Regardless, a diffuse pattern FL may be diagnosed in the appropriate setting, with a mixture of centrocytes and centroblasts lacking associated follicular dendritic cells, with an appropriate immunophenotype (BCL2+ with expression of germinal center B-cell markers) and/or the presence of a t(14;18) BCL2-IGH translocation.

The clinical import of these categories is of debate in cases of low-grade FL (55–57). In tumors with sheets of centroblastic cells or other large follicle center cells, however, the clinical significance is clear, as they are associated with inferior survival (58). These should no longer be classified as FL, and rather mandate a separate diagnosis of diffuse large B-cell lymphoma.

Although partial node involvement can be seen, complete effacement of the node is the rule rather than the exception in FL. Infrequently, when partial nodal involvement is seen in conjunction with reactive germinal centers, this pattern should be noted in the diagnostic report. The neoplastic follicles may either be intermixed with reactive follicles or congregate to separate portions of the lymph node. In instances with intermixed reactive follicles, care must be taken to differentiate partial involvement of FL from "in situ FL" (discussed later in Follicular Lymphoma In Situ section).

Studies have demonstrated that partial involvement is associated with good prognosis and low-stage disease. Following excision of the involved node, a significant fraction of patients may lack overt involvement elsewhere and fail to develop further disease even upon longitudinal follow-up (59,60).

EXTRANODAL FOLLICULAR LYMPHOMA

Spleen

Splenic involvement by FL is common and in many respects resembles that seen in lymph nodes. The neoplastic follicles expand the white pulp with a nodular infiltrate. Although nodular involvement of the red pulp is seen, diffuse involvement is decidedly less common. At low power, it may resemble marginal zone lymphoma and should prompt immunophenotypic assessment. Since BCL2 is often positive in splenic marginal zone lymphoma, assessment for germinal center markers such as CD10, human germinal center-associated lymphoma (HGAL), and BCL6 or fluorescence in situ hybridization (FISH) studies for t(14;18) is warranted to separate FL involving the spleen from splenic marginal zone lymphoma (Fig. 22.5A).

Bone Marrow

Bone marrow involvement by FL is quite common as 70% to 80% of patients present with stage III or IV disease. The characteristic appearance is that of circumscribed lymphoid aggregates that are closely associated with the bony trabeculae, so-called paratrabecular lymphoid aggregates, seen in 86% of FLs (61). These extended aggregates often closely conform to the bone in direct apposition, providing a characteristic low-power appearance. True paratrabecular aggregates, especially extensive ones, are suspicious for lymphomatous involvement, especially FL (90% of cases with pure paratrabecular patterns) (61). FL less commonly demonstrates nodular or diffuse patterns. Interstitial patterns are infrequent, but have been described (Fig. 22.5B).

Treatment, in particular treatment with rituximab, can complicate morphologic interpretation of bone marrow biopsies. Posttreatment marrows frequently demonstrate lymphoid infiltrates that are suggestive of lymphoma by hematoxylin-eosin (H&E). Immunohistochemical stains and flow cytometry, however, demonstrate that a majority of these cases lack involvement by lymphoma.

Flow cytometry is frequently used to aid in the determination of marrow involvement during staging or at follow-up. Overall concordance between histology and flow cytometry is around 80% to 90% for non-Hodgkin lymphoma (62). FL, however, generally has lower rates of agreement (around 10% lower), due primarily to histologic involvement in the context of negative flow cytometry. This is thought to be due to lymphoid aggregate-associated reticulin fibrosis preventing aspiration of the lymphocytes (62). The less frequent finding of positive flow cytometry with negative histology is generally considered to be secondary to sampling artifact.

The cellular composition of marrow involvement characteristically is small cells with a centrocytic appearance. Centroblasts and other large cells are infrequently encountered, even in grade 3 FL. Discordance is seen in 39% of FLs with rates approaching 60% at grade 3 (61). As a result, grading of FL should be restricted to adequate extramedullary biopsies.

Peripheral Blood

Morphologically detectable peripheral blood involvement occurs in about 18% of patients (61). Immunophenotypically or molecularly detectable involvement is much more frequent (63,64). The lymphoid cells are typically small with cleaved nuclei and condensed chromatin, resembling centrocytes. These findings, however, are nonspecific and require architectural and immunophenotypic correlation to differentiate from other low-grade B-cell lymphomas (Fig. 22.5C).

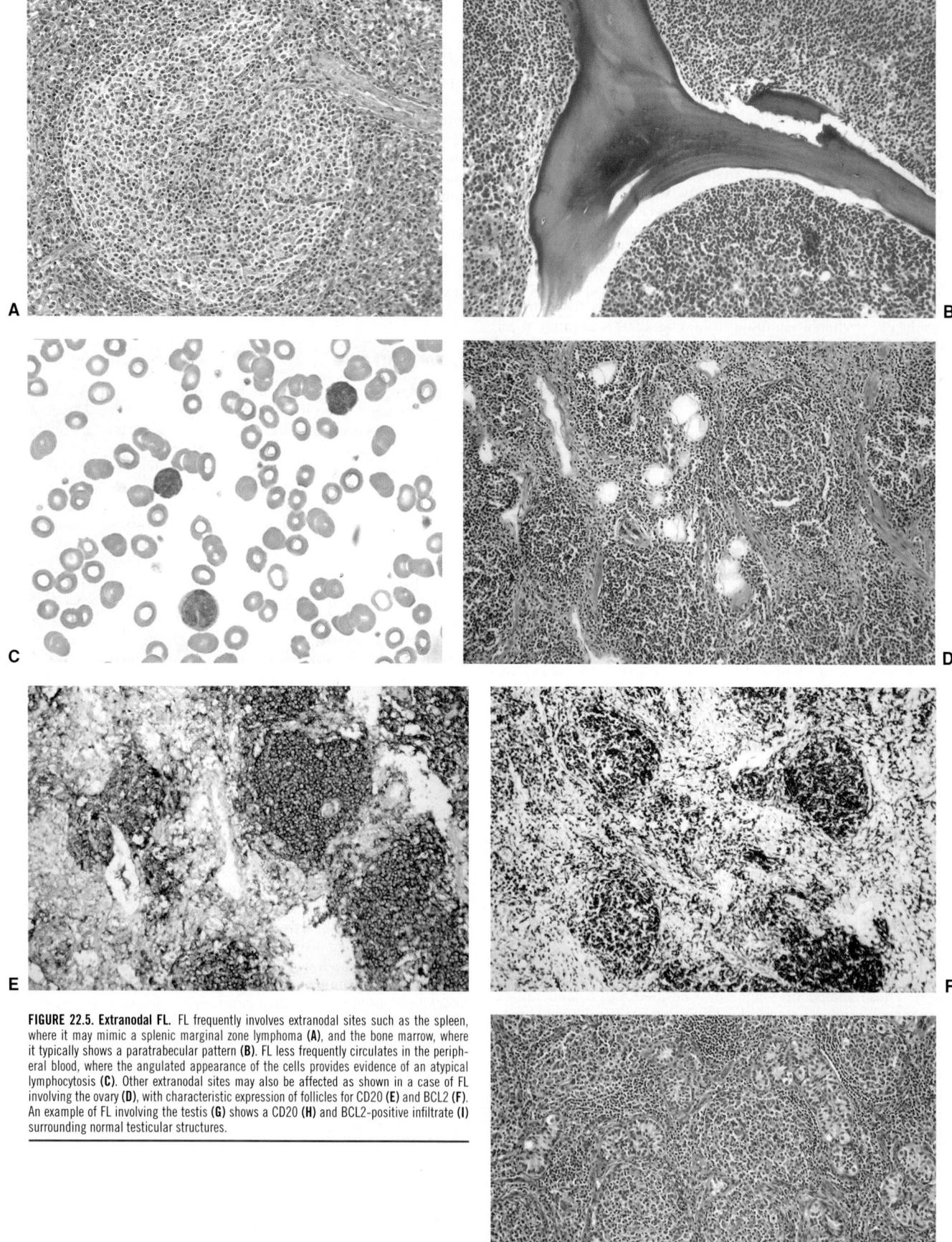

FIGURE 22.5. Extranodal FL. FL frequently involves extranodal sites such as the spleen, where it may mimic a splenic marginal zone lymphoma (**A**), and the bone marrow, where it typically shows a paratrabecular pattern (**B**). FL less frequently circulates in the peripheral blood, where the angulated appearance of the cells provides evidence of an atypical lymphocytosis (**C**). Other extranodal sites may also be affected as shown in a case of FL involving the ovary (**D**), with characteristic expression of follicles for CD20 (**E**) and BCL2 (**F**). An example of FL involving the testis (**G**) shows a CD20 (**H**) and BCL2-positive infiltrate (**I**) surrounding normal testicular structures.

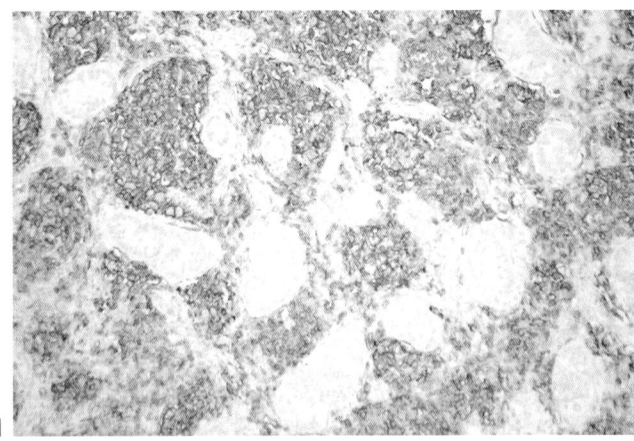

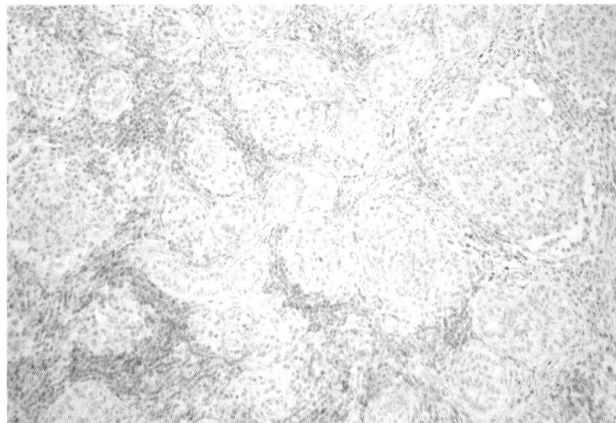

H

I

FIGURE 22.5. *(Continued).*

Other Extranodal Sites

FL may also involve other extranodal sites including the liver, gastrointestinal tract, and gonads. The criteria for diagnosis are similar to those involving the lymph node, although the site may influence differential diagnostic considerations.

 ## IMMUNOPHENOTYPE

FL has an immunophenotype that closely resembles that of normal germinal center B cells. The neoplastic cells express pan-B antigens, including CD19, CD20, CD22, CD79a, and PAX5. They also express markers specific for germinal center B cells, including CD10 (70% to 90%), BCL6 (80% to 90%), HGAL (>95%), and LMO2 (90%) (65–67). Staining for these markers is typically stronger in neoplastic follicles than in reactive ones (Fig. 22.6).

BCL2 is one of the most useful diagnostic markers, particularly in low-grade FL. It serves as a surrogate marker for the IGH-BCL2 translocation seen in the majority of FL cases. BCL2 positivity is seen in roughly 80% of cases, although that number is dependent on grade: 90% of grade 1 to 2 FLs are positive for BCL2, while only 50% to 75% of grade 3 FLs are positive (68,69). The lack of staining in FL may sometimes be due to mutations within BCL2 epitopes, preventing antibody binding (70). BCL2 positivity is aberrant in germinal center B cells and is essentially diagnostic of FL in the appropriate setting. There are a few caveats to interpretation of BCL2 in a germinal center: in marginal zone lymphoma, the neoplastic B cells that colonize the germinal center are BCL2 positive, therefore careful correlation with the pattern of a corresponding germinal center marker or a follicular dendritic cell marker such as CD21 may be required. Additionally, follicular T cells are also BCL2 positive and may be increased in reactive settings.

FL, like most low-grade lymphomas, is generally IgM positive with a subset of cells showing costaining for IgD. There is, however, a significant minority of cases that stain for IgG, indicating that the cells have progressed further in the germinal center reaction and engaged in class switch recombination. IgA is only rarely expressed in FLs; however, one study has demonstrated that a majority of primary intestinal FLs are IgA positive, which may reflect their tissue origin (71).

Other immunostains such as CD5, CD23, and CD43 that are used in the diagnosis of B cell lymphomas are generally negative, although one or more of these can show positivity in a subset of cases. CD23 stains around 30% of FLs and is enriched in low-grade lymphoma and in inguinal presentations (72,73).

CD43 is typically negative in FL, although rare cases have been reported to be positive (74).

In the bone marrow, immunohistologic staining is much less consistent, with CD10 and HGAL being the most effective markers, but only staining 50% and 60% of cases, respectively (66). Other markers of germinal center B cells were positive <20% of the time. Although they can be helpful when positive, germinal center markers are frequently absent or weakly expressed, which makes the classification of paratrabecular lymphoid aggregates difficult.

Flow cytometry is frequently very helpful to diagnose FL. A population of light chain–restricted CD10$^+$ B cells raises concern for this diagnosis, with a differential diagnosis that includes other germinal center–derived lymphomas, including Burkitt lymphoma and diffuse large B-cell lymphoma. Caution is warranted, however, as light chain restriction (or absence) has been reported in follicular hyperplasia and other reactive conditions and correlation with histology is recommended (75,76). Small biopsies also pose challenges, as only 70% of FL diagnoses rendered on small biopsies were found accurate following resection. The most frequent discrepancies resulted from errors in grading, missing an adjacent diffuse large B-cell lymphoma and misdiagnosis of reactive lymphoid hyperplasia (77).

The germinal center milieu also provides useful diagnostic markers for clarifying architecture. Stains directed at follicular dendritic cell networks such as CD21, CD23, CD35, and D2-40 can differentiate grade 3B FL from diffuse large B-cell lymphoma, by highlighting a subtle follicular architecture that may not be easily appreciated on H&E-stained sections. Additionally, in cases with apparently diffuse architecture, these stains are useful to demonstrate areas with follicular architecture that may constitute a lower-grade component, which often has implications for therapy and prognosis. Furthermore, they can be useful in the separation from marginal zone lymphoma colonizing follicles by delineating the boundaries of the disrupted dendritic meshworks.

Gene expression profiling studies have implicated the microenvironment and host response cells as important factors in the pathogenesis and prognosis of FL. As a result, studies have attempted to take advantage of immunohistochemistry to develop prognostic markers. As yet, the results for follicular helper T cells, regulatory T cells, and macrophages have been mixed and have not yielded a uniform predictor amenable for clinical use. These differences may reflect different methodologies used in the studies, and, consequently, further studies are needed to validate initial observations and determine their clinical utility (78).

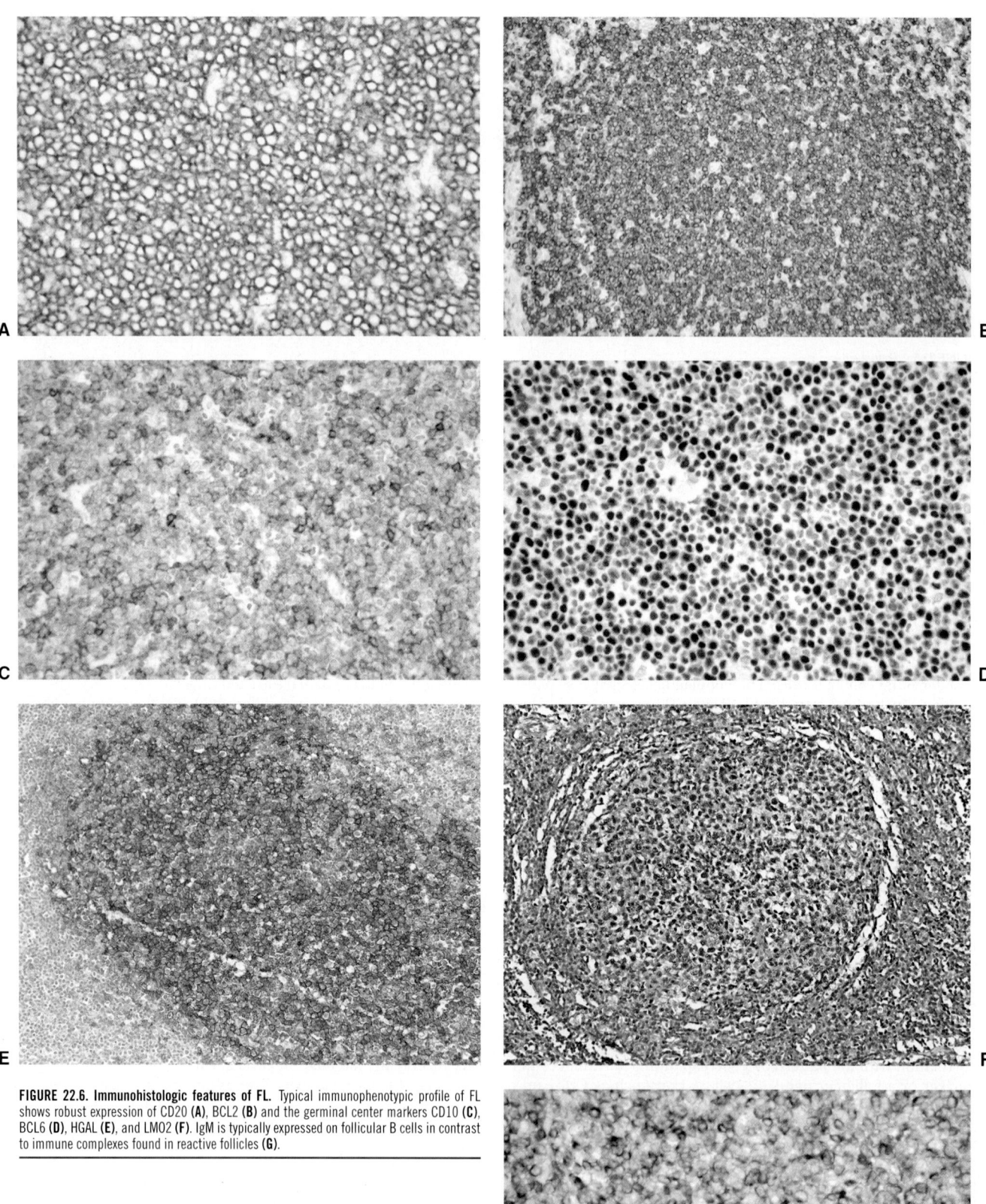

FIGURE 22.6. Immunohistologic features of FL. Typical immunophenotypic profile of FL shows robust expression of CD20 (**A**), BCL2 (**B**) and the germinal center markers CD10 (**C**), BCL6 (**D**), HGAL (**E**), and LMO2 (**F**). IgM is typically expressed on follicular B cells in contrast to immune complexes found in reactive follicles (**G**).

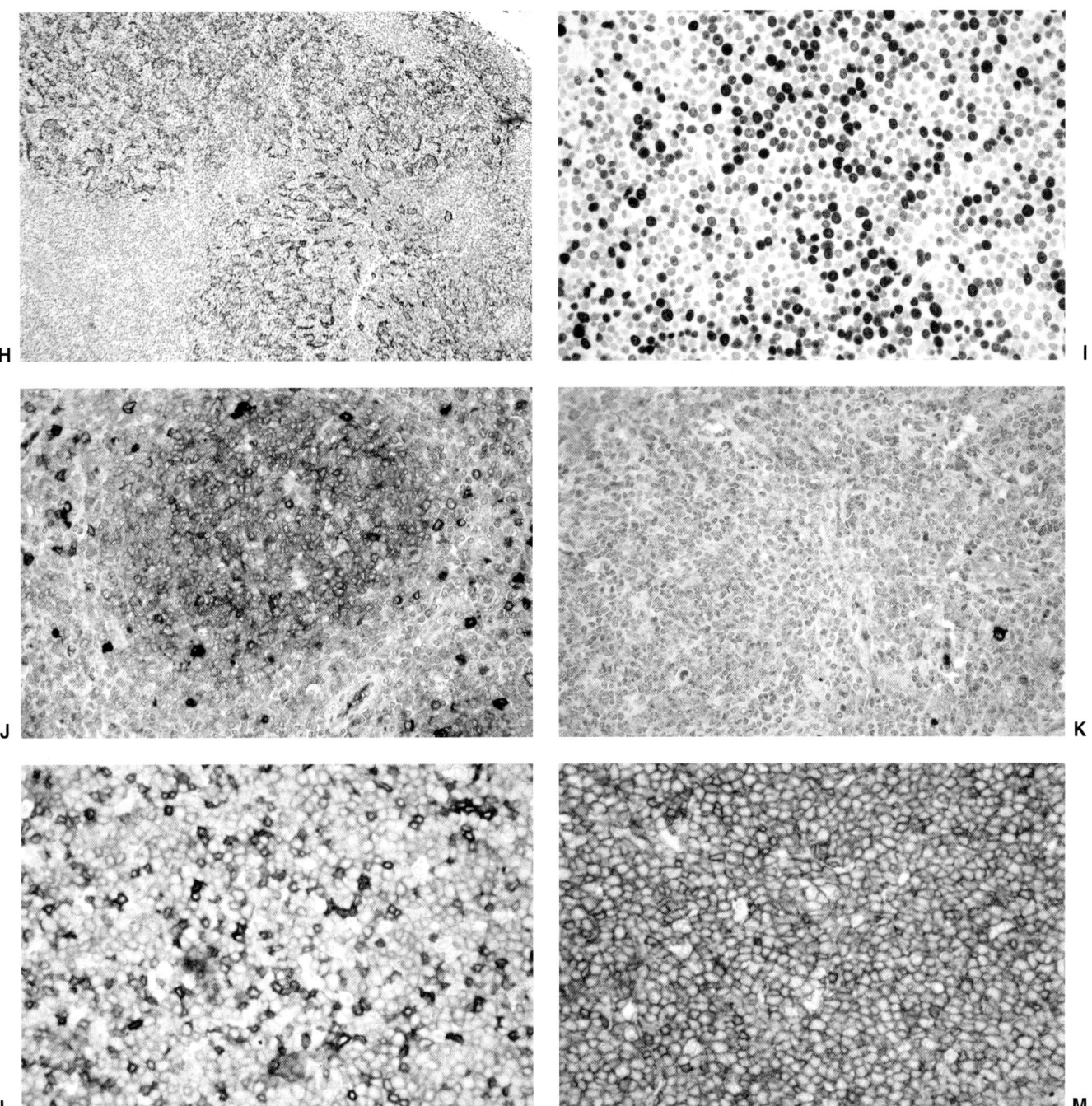

FIGURE 22.6. *(Continued)* Follicular dendritic cell meshworks are highlighted by CD21 (**H**). Ki-67 shows a proliferation index that is well below the threshold of that seen in reactive germinal centers (**I**). Kappa and lambda light chain stains show a restricted pattern of expression indicative of a clonal neoplastic proliferation (**J,K**). In rare cases, aberrant coexpression of CD5 (**L**) and CD43 (**M**) may be present.

FOLLICULAR LYMPHOMA VARIANTS

Variants of FL that are recognized in the WHO 2008 classification scheme include pediatric, primary intestinal, primary cutaneous, other extranodal, and *in situ* FL.

Pediatric Follicular Lymphoma

FL is generally a disease of older adults, but a discrete subset of cases occurs in children and young adults, and manifests distinct clinical and diagnostic features (15). Patients with pediatric FL are younger and have a marked male predominance. Nodal involvement of the head and neck and extranodal involvement of Waldeyer ring and testis are the most common distributions. In contrast to adult FL, disease is typically localized and of low stage (79). A good prognosis is characteristic and progression is infrequent; in fact, patients generally display no evidence of disease following surgery and conservative therapy is suggested (80). Liu et al. (15) have recently recommended classifying nodal and testicular pediatric FL as a monoclonal B-cell proliferation of undetermined significance (Fig. 22.7).

As in adult FL, the histologic pattern involves closely packed follicles. Unlike adult FL, where grade 1 to 2 lesions predominate, grade 3A lesions are the most frequent, and tingible body macrophages are a frequent feature. Nodal and extranodal

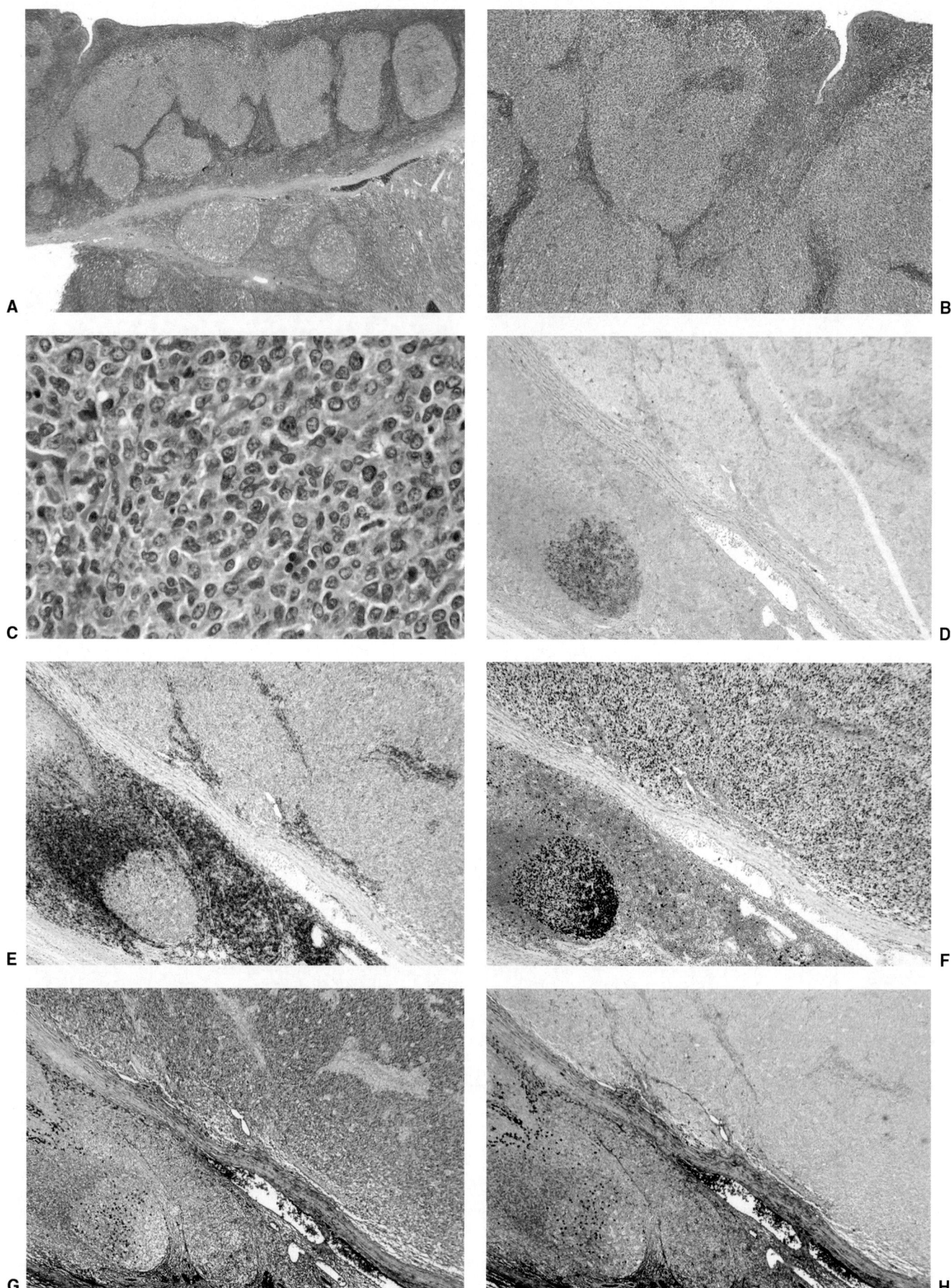

FIGURE 22.7. Pediatric FL. Tonsil tissue shows involvement by FL with large somewhat serpiginous and poorly defined follicles and a predominance of large cells, some with blastoid morphology (**A–C**). The neoplastic follicles lack expression of CD10 (**D**) and BCL2 (**E**). Ki67 shows a moderate growth fraction (**F**). Kappa and lambda light chain stains show a kappa light chain restriction in the neoplastic follicles (**G,H**).

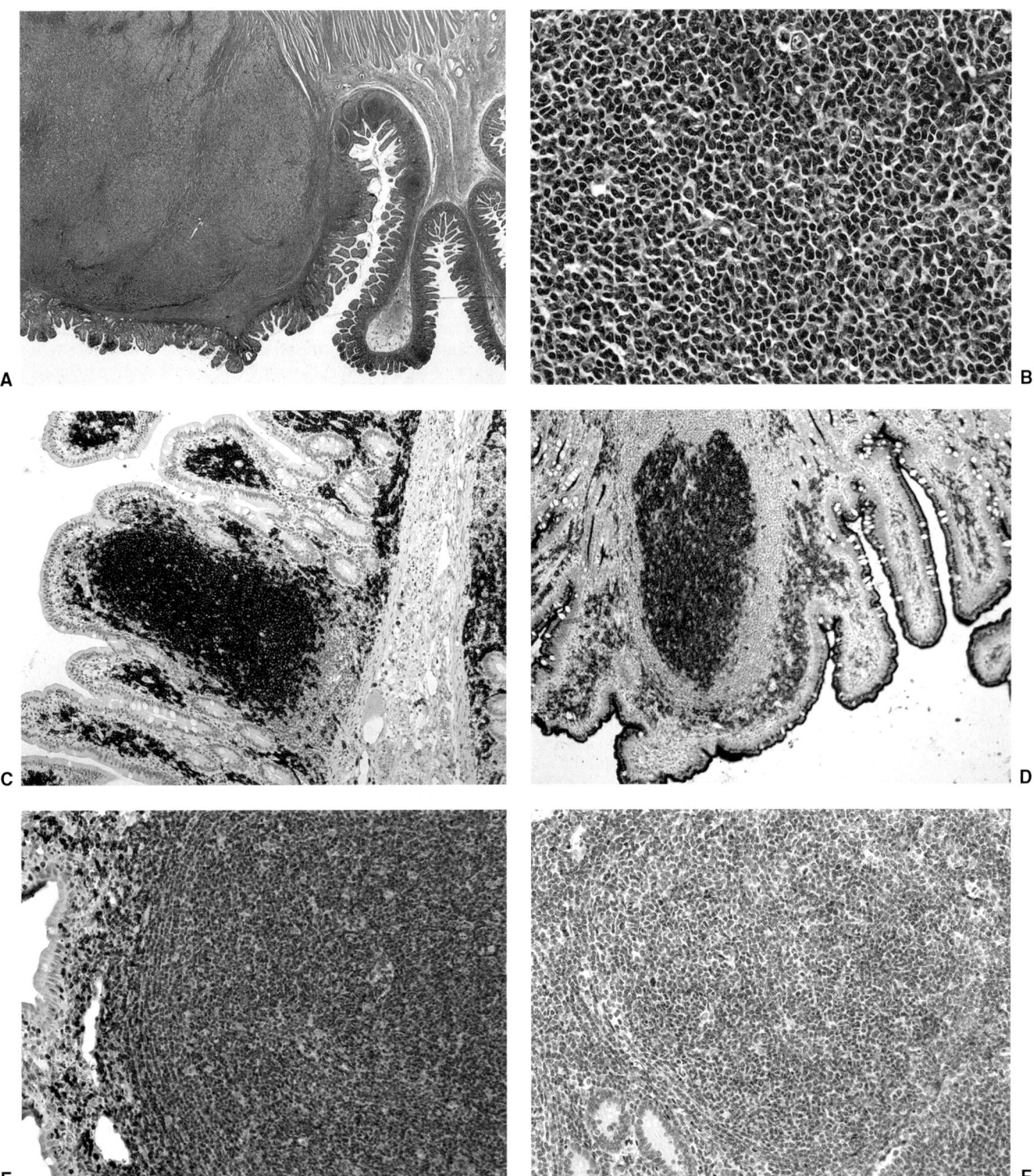

FIGURE 22.8. Primary intestinal FL.   An example of primary intestinal FL occurring in the small intestine shows nodules of neoplastic cells with angulated cytologic features **(A,B)**. Immunohistologic stains for CD20 **(C)**, CD10 **(D)**, and BCL2 **(E)** highlight a typical immunoprofile of FL, whereas BCL6 **(F)** is negative.

disease also differ morphologically and immunophenotypically. Nodal disease has large poorly defined follicles, often with serpiginous topography, whereas tonsilar disease often has blastoid cells of intermediate size instead of centroblasts, and is typically associated with tingible body macrophages. They also have BCL2 and MUM1 expression in the follicles, a finding lost in nodal pediatric FL. Testicular disease has small, nonpolarized follicles percolating amongst seminiferous tubules.

The cytogenetic and immunophenotypic features are also distinct. Nearly all cases have rearranged immunoglobulin genes. The t(14;18) is generally absent in nodal and testicular disease, but is present in a significant number of tonsilar cases. The tonsilar cases also had IRF4 rearrangements, providing a correlate for the observed MUM1 staining and suggesting a potential for a more aggressive course for tonsilar cases (15). BCL6 rearrangements were not found (15).

Primary Intestinal Follicular Lymphoma

Primary intestinal FL is a distinct extranodal presentation of FL (81). It histologically, immunophenotypically and genetically resembles nodal FL, but presents in and is generally localized to the intestinal tract. The duodenum followed by other locations in the small intestine are the most common locations and can have an endoscopic appearance similar to that of lymphomatoid polyposis. They are generally grade 1 to 2, and do not grow in size when observed over time. In keeping with the role of IgA in mucosal immunity, primary intestinal FL typically expresses IgA, which suggests a role for antigen-mediated signaling in its pathogenesis (71). Interestingly, these have a generally good prognosis, and in fact, resection in many cases is curative with additional therapy needed only in a subset of cases (81) (Fig. 22.8).

Follicular Lymphoma *In Situ*

B-cell lymphomas, once thought to arise following a crucial genetic event, are increasingly recognized to have precursor lesions. The diagnosis and management of these precursors pose significant challenges as criteria for diagnosis, appropriate terminology for early lesions, and assessment of clinical implications for patients with *in situ* lesions or partial involvement by lymphomas derived from small B cells are still poorly understood (Table 22.1).

Several reports have now documented the existence of *in situ* FL or intrafollicular neoplasia, where select follicles that express strong BCL2 and CD10 proteins are observed in an otherwise architecturally and immunophenotypically normal lymph node (82–84). These BCL2 and CD10 brightly positive cells may occupy one or a few follicles within the node, be widely scattered throughout the node, or partially involve otherwise normal secondary follicles. Typically, the affected follicles show a predominance of centrocytes and are sharply demarcated from the surrounding mantle cuffs without an interfollicular component. Interestingly, *in situ* FL has been documented in patients with synchronous or metachronous FL as well as in patients who do not have any evidence of overt FL even after several years of clinical follow-up. Using a combination of microdissection techniques and PCR, a clonal relationship between the *in situ* and overt components of FL has been established in patients who demonstrate both lesions (82,83). Clonality assessments on partially replaced follicles have further shown that an oligoclonal pattern similar to what is observed in a normal germinal center is represented in the affected follicles (84). This finding suggests that preexisting normal germinal centers are colonized by BCL2-positive atypical B cells that represent early involvement by FL. However, in patients without evidence of overt FL, whether the intrafollicular lesion represents an early form of FL or a preneoplastic condition is up for debate. The association of *in situ* FL with lymphoproliferative disorders other than FL (82,83) suggests that these early lesions may represent an underlying preneoplastic condition, and that

additional genetic alterations dictate whether and what type of lymphoproliferative disorder subsequently develops in the affected individual (Fig. 22.9).

The phenomenon of *in situ* FL is thought to be the tissue counterpart of t(14;18)-bearing circulating B cells described in a subset of healthy individuals, where at least in some patients, it may represent an early lesion of FL (85–87). *In situ* FL, even if multifocal or recurrent, does not represent clinical progression. The clinical implications of this *in situ* or early phenomenon, however, are not fully understood, particularly in patients who show no other evidence of FL. Given that the relationship of *in situ* FL to overt FL is unclear, the name of "*in situ* involvement by FL-like B cells of uncertain clinical significance," has been suggested. Although long, this terminology most aptly captures the current knowledge that these atypical cells resemble FL cells, but may not represent a neoplastic proliferation. Regarding clinical management, it is generally recommended that patients with early lesions undergo complete clinical staging, including a bone marrow biopsy. Unless overt FL is found at another site that warrants therapeutic intervention, patients should be followed without treatment. Only atypical follicular hyperplasia should elicit an immunophenotypic workup, including a stain for BCL2 and CD10; screening all reactive lymph nodes to find early lesions is not clinically necessary or cost-effective. Additional investigations are awaited to fully understand the extent of the clinical implications and the insight these early lesions are likely to furnish with regard to lymphomagenesis.

Primary Cutaneous Follicle Center Lymphoma

This entity appears to be a genetically and clinically distinct lesion from nodal and other extranodal FLs and is not covered in this chapter.

Other Extranodal Follicular Lymphoma

Extranodal FL has the characteristic histologic appearance of nodal FL. It also shares the t(14;18) translocation and immunophenotype, suggesting a similar pathogenesis. Interestingly, these are frequently restricted to their sites of presentation with infrequent systemic involvements. Furthermore, as is seen with primary intestinal FL, these generally have a better prognosis than nodal disease (88).

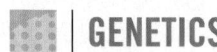 **GENETICS**

Cytogenetics

The cytogenetics of FL prominently feature the t(14;18) translocation. Found in approximately 90% of FLs, this translocation juxtaposes the BCL2 gene downstream of the IGH promoter leading to BCL2 overexpression (89,90). Three dominant breakpoint regions have been described in FL, the major breakpoint region (MBR), minor cluster region (mcr),

Table 22.1	COMPARISON OF *IN SITU* AND PARTIAL INVOLVEMENT BY FOLLICULAR LYMPHOMA	
Attribute	*In Situ* FL	Partial Involvement by FL
Lymph node architecture	Intact	Distorted
Involved follicles	Normal size; widely scattered	Expanded; mixture of reactive and neoplastic follicles
Boundary of affected follicles	Sharply demarcated from mantle cuffs	Diffuse or blurred edges
Cell milieu	Predominance of centrocytes	Mixture of centrocytes and centroblasts; FL of all grades
Immunophenotype	Strong expression of BCL2 and CD10	Variable expression of BCL2 and CD10

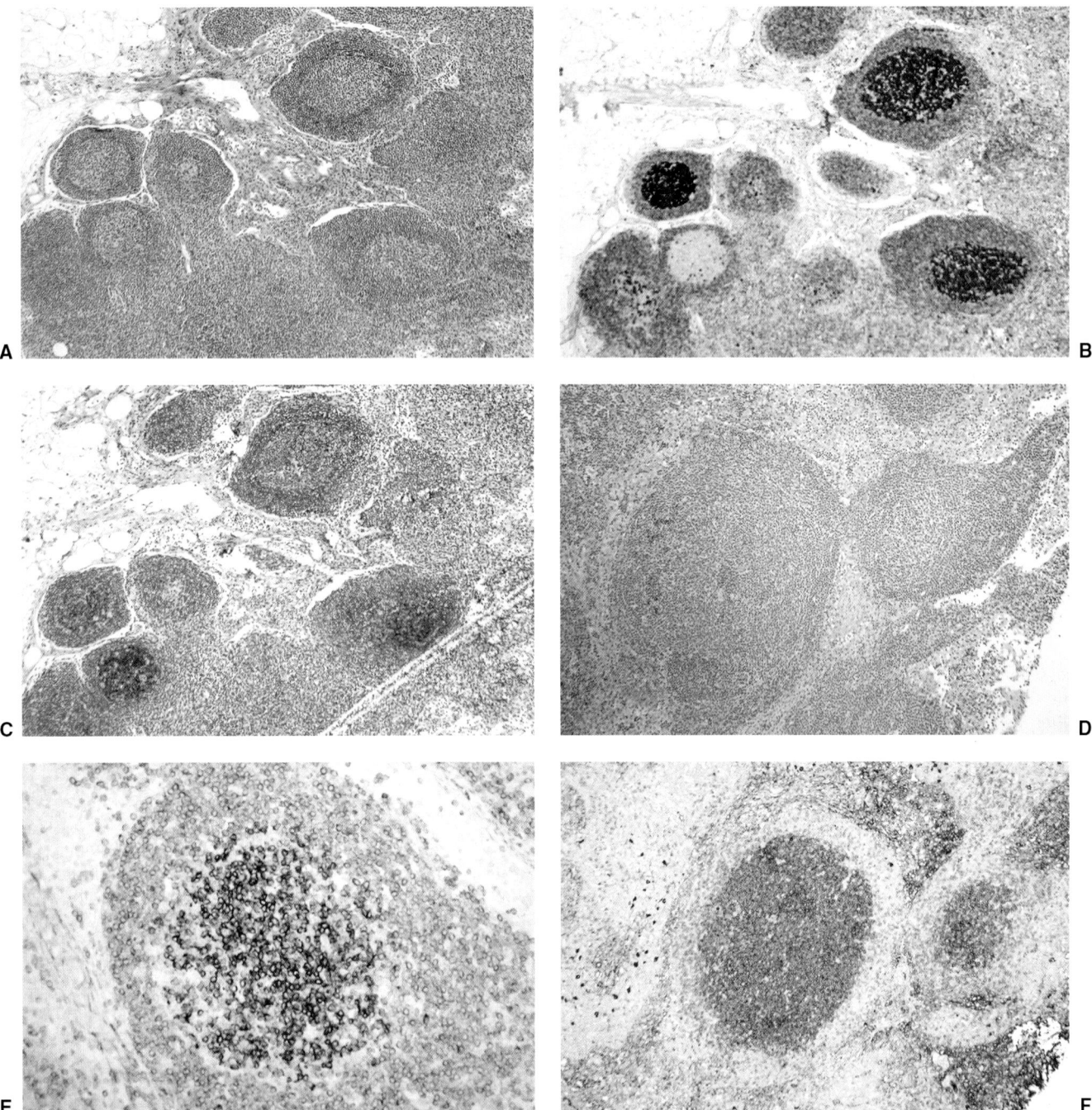

FIGURE 22.9. Follicular lymphoma *in situ*. FL *in situ* is characterized by occasional dispersed follicles in an otherwise unenlarged lymph node (**A**), within which brightly positive BCL2 (**B**) and CD10 (**C**) staining is present. The involved follicles are sharply demarcated from the mantle cuffs and are not associated with an interfollicular component as shown in the higher magnification images (**D–F**).

and the intermediate cluster region (icr), although a number of other breakpoints have also been identified. Infrequently, alternative BCL2 translocations involving either the kappa or lambda light chains on chromosome 2 (91) or 22 (92), respectively, have been described. These translocations are thought to occur in the bone marrow, predating arrival in the lymph node. Although the t(14;18) is the most common cause of BCL2 overexpression, gene amplification has also been observed in higher-grade disease, demonstrating the critical role of BCL2 in the pathogenesis of FL (93).

A number of methods have been used to detect the translocation, including Southern blot, conventional cytogenetics, FISH, and PCR. FISH and PCR are currently the most frequently used methods as the fresh tissue required for Southern blot and conventional cytogenetics is not always available for clinical samples. PCR testing is hampered by the multiple rearrangement hotspots, but by testing the three dominant breakpoints (MBR, mcr, and icr) the sensitivity has improved (94). FISH, however, remains the most sensitive method for detecting a BCL2-IGH rearrangement, identifying them in 96% of low-grade FLs (95).

Sensitive nested PCR studies can detect the t(14;18) translocation in the peripheral blood of people without evidence of disease. The frequency increases with age; however, there is no clear increased risk for development of FL (96). These translocations are thought to occur in the bone marrow and are found in a variety of cells, including memory B cells, suggesting that they can still traverse the germinal center (97). As a result, the presence of this translocation should not be equated with FL in particular or B-cell lymphoma in general. The characteristic morphologic and immunophenotypic features are necessary for the diagnosis.

Although the t(14;18) is commonly found, it is rarely the only cytogenetic abnormality. About 90% of FLs also have other abnormalities including most commonly +X, +7, +12, +18, +der(18), del(6q,10q,17p), dup(1q,12q), der(1p/q) (89,98,99), as determined by conventional karyotype. Chromosomal abnormalities tend to accumulate with higher grade, but do not necessarily correlate with progression. Certain cytogenetic abnormalities have been associated with adverse prognosis, including 1p21-p22, 6q23-q27, 17p, a coincident c-myc translocation, or ≥6 breaks (99,100). Translocations involving BCL6 and/or 3q27 are also found in 5% to 15% of cases and are correlated with grade 3 disease and t(14;18)-negative FLs (101,102).

Initial studies with array comparative genomic hybridization found similar results to those found by karyotype (103). They have also emphasized the prognostic significance of 1p36 and 6q (103). More recent methodologies, more sensitive to small changes, and coupled with single nucleotide polymorphism (SNP) analysis, have furthered the analysis. Copy-neutral loss of heterozygosity is frequently found and often affects large chromosomal regions (median size >26 Mb), such as entire chromosomal arms. These often overlap with deleted regions detected by conventional cytogenetics, emphasizing their importance. In fact, 52% of cases are altered at 1p and 44% of cases at 6p, a frequency beginning to rival that of t(14;18) (104,105). Additionally, SNP arrays have demonstrated frequent involvement of single genes that are not found in the commonly deleted regions. These genes frequently encode cancer-related proteins, such as CDKN2A and CDKN2B.

Gene expression profiling studies have probed FL and demonstrated a high percentage of cells expressing genes associated with their germinal center origin, like BCL6 and LMO2 (106). Interestingly, when determining prognostic groups, the expression patterns clustered with gene expression profiles of non-B cells. The good prognosis group (immune response 1) tended to have upregulated genes from T cells and macrophages. In contrast, the poor prognosis group (immune response 2) was associated with gene signatures of macrophages and dendritic cells (106).

Detection of Clonality

As with nearly all mature B-cell lymphomas, FL has clonally rearranged immunoglobulin heavy and light chains. The detection of these rearrangements through generally sensitive methods, like PCR, was lower than expected, historically. Due to the germinal center origin of the cells, they are undergoing continuous somatic hypermutation and these mutations affect the binding sites of primers, reducing the ability to detect clones (107). Unlike in chronic lymphocytic leukemia, however, these mutations are not of prognostic import.

Newer sets of primers have been more successful at detecting rearrangements. The BIOMED-2 primers were designed to help these issues and increase the sensitivity by testing two IGH framework regions and the IGK locus. Older testing methods had positive rates of around 70% (108,109), but the addition of kappa primer improves the sensitivity to around 90% to 95% (108,110). The improvement seen with kappa primer is due to lower rates of somatic hypermutation in the light chains than in the heavy chain loci (107).

Molecular Alterations

Sequencing has clarified specific genes that are essential in developing or preventing the genesis of FL (Table 22.2). Not surprisingly, BCL2 often plays a dominant role. Further mutations are frequently found in BCL2 (96%), immunoglobulin heavy and light chains (79%) (111), EPHA7 (72%) (112), BCL6 (47%) (113,114), TNFRSF14 (18% to 46%) (115,116), CREBBP (33%) (117,118), EP300 (9%) (117,118), EZH2 (7%) (119), TNFAIP3 (2% to 26%) (112,120,121), and TP53 (<5%). These analyses have provided novel and interesting clues to the pathogenesis of FL. A number of them occur through somatic hypermutation (BCL2, BCL6, immunoglobulin heavy and light chains). Interestingly, the immunoglobulin mutations frequently result in the creation of N-linked glycosylation sites that are postulated to bind lectins in the FL microenvironment (111,122). Some of these mutations may explain the

| Table 22.2 | MOLECULAR ALTERATIONS IN FOLLICULAR LYMPHOMA |

Gene	Full Name	Locus	Function	Mutation Rate (%)
BCL2	B-cell CLL/lymphoma 2	18q21.3	Inhibits caspases blocking apoptosis	96
IGH/IGK/IGL	Immunoglobulin heavy and light chains	14q32.33; 2p12; 22q11.2	Antibody subunits	79
EPHA7	EPH receptor A7	6q16.1	Receptor tyrosine kinase	72
BCL6	B-cell CLL/lymphoma 6	3q27	Transcriptional repressor	47
TNFRSF14	Tumor necrosis factor receptor super-family, member 14	1p36.32	BTLA receptor, TNFSF14 receptor	18–46
CREBBP	cAMP-responsive binding protein	16p13.3	Histone acetylase, activates ALX1 with EP300	33
EP300	E1A binding protein p300	22q13.2	Histone acetyltransferase, HIF1A activator	9
EZH2	Enhancer of zeste homolog 2	7q35-q36	Histone methylase	7
TNFAIP3/A20	Tumor necrosis factor, alpha-induced protein 3	6q23	Ubiquitin editing enzyme	2–26
TP53	Tumor protein 53	17p13.1	Tumor suppressor	<5
MLL2	Myeloid/lymphoid leukemia 2	12q13.12	Histone methyltransferase	89
MEF2B	Myocyte enhancer factor 2B	19q13.11	Transcriptional activator	13

mechanism behind chromosomal losses in FL pathogenesis. TNFRSF14, a member of the TNF receptor superfamily, is found on 1p36 and frequently has truncating mutations. TNFAIP3/A20 and EPHA7 both frequently show mutations and are contained on 6q. MLL2, an H3K4-specific methyltransferase, was found to have inactivating mutations in 89% of FLs, suggesting a critical role for histone modification in pathogenesis (118). MEF2B (118) and EZH2, also involved in histone modification, were frequent targets as well. These rates were higher than those found in DLBCL of germinal center origin, suggesting a role in pathogenesis, rather than progression. Mutations found in DLBCL of germinal center origin, but not FL, include BTG1, CD58, CD70, and STAT3, suggesting a potential role in higher-grade disease. Further studies will be necessary to clarify the role of these molecules in the pathogenesis of FL and its progression toward diffuse large B-cell lymphoma (118).

DIFFERENTIAL DIAGNOSIS

Reactive Follicular Hyperplasia

Reactive follicular hyperplasia is often in the differential diagnosis of FL as they have a similar nodular appearance (Table 22.3). In needle biopsies or other specimens with limited material or comparative architecture, this can be a particularly difficult distinction. A combination of morphologic, immunophenotypic, and molecular findings, however, can reliably distinguish the entities.

Scrupulous adherence to the morphologic criteria for diagnosis of FL can generally allow differentiation from follicular hyperplasia. Unlike reactive follicles, which have populations of centroblasts and centrocytes polarized to opposite ends of the germinal center, FL generally comprises an even distribution of centrocyte-predominant cells. Localization is often a key feature with centrocytes escaping from germinal centers into interfollicular areas and invasion into the extracapsular adipose tissue. Follicles are generally closely packed and frequently lack mantle zones. Tingible body macrophages in the germinal centers can be helpful to suggest a reactive process

in low-grade FL; however, higher-grade lesions and some lower-grade FLs can have a "starry sky" appearance. These features are even more compelling when coupled with lymph nodes with a diffuse effacement. More subtle features to look for include intralymph node fibrosis and permeation of vascular walls by centrocytes.

Immunohistochemical stains can help solidify a diagnosis in borderline cases. The expression of BCL2 in a follicle center B cell is diagnostic of FL. The follicle center nature of the B cell can be determined through morphology or through coexpression with germinal center B-cell markers (CD10, BCL6, HGAL, etc.). Furthermore, germinal center B-cell markers can help demonstrate extrafollicular spread of centrocytes, which is specific for FL. Ki-67, which typically highlights >90% of cells in a reactive germinal center, can be helpful as it stains a lower percentage in most FLs.

Flow cytometry can also be helpful in conjunction with histology. Light chain restriction is highly specific for lymphoma, and coexpression of a germinal center B-cell marker is consistent with FL. Reactive conditions have been demonstrated to develop monotypic germinal center B cells, and therefore, rendering a FL diagnosis without histologic correlation must be approached with caution, particularly in children.

Marginal Zone Lymphoma

Marginal zone lymphoma can commonly be confused with FL due to the frequent maintenance of reactive germinal centers in the effaced node. Furthermore, the reactive germinal centers can be colonized by marginal zone lymphocytes, giving them an atypical appearance. Adding to the potential confusion, marginal zone cells can be angulated and have an appearance similar to that of centrocytes. The growth pattern, however, yields some clues. FL is dominated by closely packed follicles, whereas marginal zone lymphoma generally has more widely spaced follicles, as the neoplastic cells expand the interfollicular areas and colonize preexisting follicles. The cells of marginal zone lymphoma are also often monocytoid with more abundant cytoplasm and appear to be spaced apart on histologic section. Immunohistochemical stains can be helpful, but should be used with caution as there is no characteristic

Table 22.3	DIFFERENTIAL DIAGNOSIS OF FOLLICULAR LYMPHOMA				
Diagnosis	Cell Types	Architecture in Lymph Node	Architecture/Pattern in Bone Marrow	Immunophenotype	Cytogenetics/Molecular
Follicular lymphoma	Small cleaved cells to large pleomorphic cells	Close packed, nonpolarized follicles ± diffuse areas	Paratrabecular lymphoid aggregates	CD5− CD10+ CCND1− BCL2+ BCL6+	t(14;18) IGH-BCL2
Reactive follicular hyperplasia	Centrocytes, centroblasts	Polarized follicles, noneffaced node	Nonparatrabecular lymphoid aggregates	CD5− CD10+ CCND1− BCL2− BCL6+	None
SLL	Small round to cleaved cells, prolymphocytes, paraimmunoblasts	Proliferation centers within a diffuse pattern	Paratrabecular, nonparatrabecular, interstitial and/or mixed	CD5+ CD10− CCND1− BCL2+ BCL6−	Trisomy 12; del(13q); del(11q); del(6q)
Marginal zone lymphoma	Range from small round cells to plasmacytoid cells to plasma cells, monocytoid B cells	Colonized germinal centers, interfollicular, and diffuse patterns	Nodular, paratrabecular and/or interstitial	CD5− CD10− CCND1− BCL2+ BCL6−	t (11;18); Trisomy 3; t(1;14)
Mantle cell lymphoma	Variable small to medium size and variable shape, with somewhat open chromatin	Diffuse, vaguely nodular, and mantle zone patterns	Diffuse	CD5+ CD10− CCND1+ BCL2+ BCL6−	t(11;14)
Lymphoplasmacytic lymphoma	Range from small round cells to plasmacytoid cells to plasma cells	Diffuse	Diffuse	CD5− CD10− CCND1− BCL2+ BCL6−	None; L265P hotspot mutation in MYD88

immunophenotype ascribed to marginal zone lymphoma. The absence of CD5 and CD10 can be helpful to distinguish marginal zone lymphoma from FL, especially by flow cytometry. Furthermore, the follicular dendritic networks in FL are typically compact, whereas in marginal zone lymphoma they are often disrupted as the follicle is colonized by marginal zone cells. These neoplastic marginal zone cells will also show a different immunophenotype from germinal center B cells, allowing their separation from FL in most cases. Finally, the BCL2-IGH translocation is found in FL, but not in marginal zone lymphoma. The separation of BCL2-IGH-negative FL from marginal zone lymphoma can be challenging. Newer immunohistologic markers, such as myeloid nuclear differentiating antigen that recognizes marginal zone B cells but not follicular B cells, are useful in conjunction with germinal center B-cell markers in separating marginal zone and FL in borderline cases (Fig. 22.10A).

Mantle Cell Lymphoma

Mantle cell lymphoma, although typically consisting of a diffuse sheet of cells, can occasionally show a nodular pattern (mantle zone pattern) that may resemble FL. The cellular composition is usually monotonous and small to medium sized, although the exceptions of pleomorphic and blastic variants should be noted. FL is characterized by a mixture of neoplastic and normal cells, including follicular T cells and follicular dendritic cells. Mantle cell lymphoma is usually monotonous and devoid of intervening populations of cells. Once again, the immunophenotype of mantle cell lymphoma is characteristic. Mantle cell lymphoma, like SLL, expresses CD5 and lacks CD10; in addition, the expression of cyclin D1 in nodal small B cells is highly sensitive and specific for mantle cell lymphoma. Finally, the BCL2-IGH translocation is found in FL, but not in mantle cell lymphoma, which contains a CCND1-IGH translocation (Fig. 22.10B).

Small Lymphocytic Lymphoma

Small lymphocytic lymphoma (SLL) is typified by a vaguely nodular pattern created by the proliferation centers, which could be confused with serpiginous or poorly formed germinal centers or neoplastic follicles. The cellular composition is usually distinct as is the immunophenotype. SLL generally has a background of small round lymphocytes with condensed chromatin. Proliferation centers feature an admixture of slightly larger cells with nucleoli. The cells are rarely angulated or cleaved and typically show a spectrum of morphologies, rather than the bimodal appearance of centrocytes and centroblasts. SLL typically expresses CD5 and lacks CD10, while FL is generally the opposite. Finally, the BCL2-IGH translocation is found in FL, but not in SLL (Fig. 22.10C).

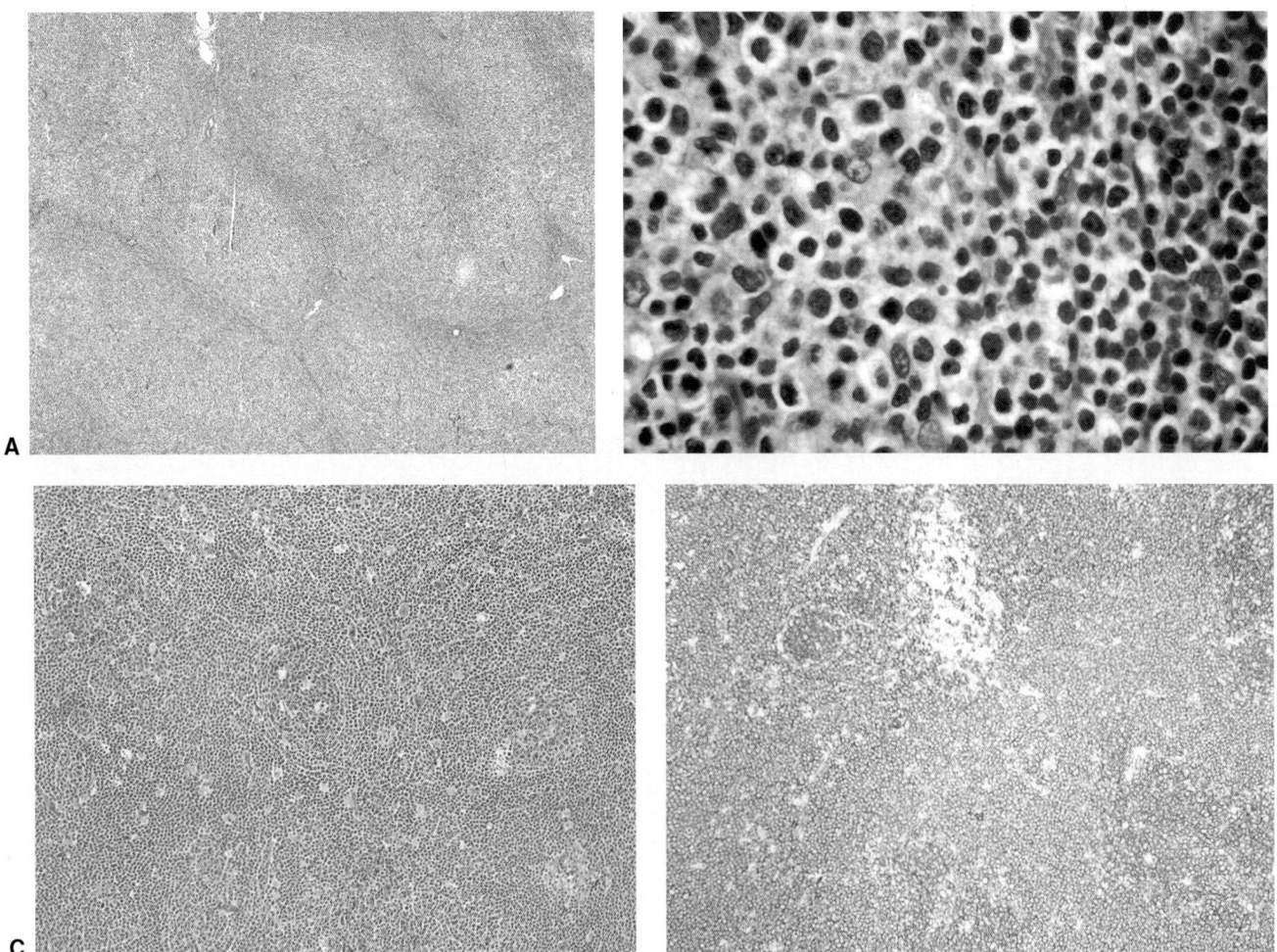

FIGURE 22.10. Differential diagnosis of FL. An example of marginal zone lymphoma shows a nodular growth pattern with colonization of follicles (**A**), by an atypical infiltrate of small lymphoid cells with monocytoid appearance (**B**). An example of mantle cell lymphoma shows a nodular growth pattern and a monotonous small to medium-sized lymphoid infiltrate that spares germinal centers (**C**); the atypical infiltrate is defined by expression of CD20 (**D**),

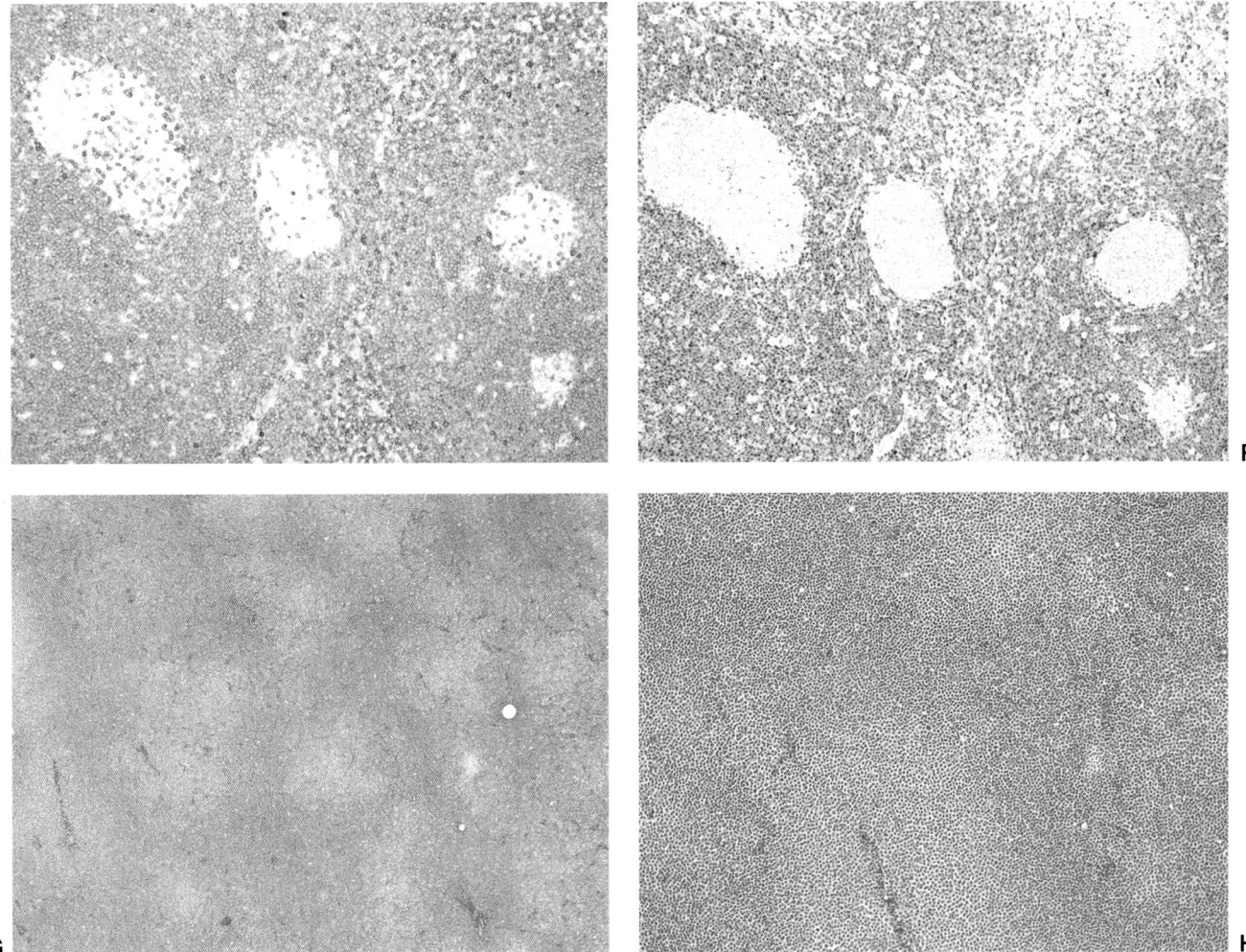

FIGURE 22.10 *(Continued)* CD5 (**E**), and BCL1 (**F**). An example of SLL/chronic lymphocytic leukemia shows a vaguely nodular growth pattern imparted by the presence of proliferation centers (**G**) and monotonous sheets of small lymphoid cells (**H**).

References

1. Swerdlow SH; International Agency for Research on Cancer, World Health Organization, Louis A. Duhring Fund. *WHO classification of tumours of haematopoietic and lymphoid tissues.* Lyon: International Agency for Research on Cancer, 2008.
2. Ghon A, Roman B. Uber das Lymphosarkom. *J Frankfurt Zischr f Path* 1916; 19:1–138.
3. Brill NE, Baehr G, Rosenthal N. Generalized giant lymph follicle hyperplasia of lymph nodes and spleen. *JAMA* 1925;84:668–671.
4. Symmers D. Follicular lymphadenopathy with splenomegaly. A newly recognized disease of the lymphatic system. *Arch Pathol Lab Med* 1927;3:816–820.
5. Gall EA, Morrison HR, Scott AT. The follicular type of malignant lymphoma: a survey of 63 cases. *Ann Intern Med* 1941;14:2073–2090.
6. Hicks EB, Rappaport H, Winter WJ. Follicular lymphoma: a re-evaluation of its position in the scheme of malignant lymphoma, based on a survey of 253 cases. *Cancer* 1956;9:792–821.
7. Lennert K. *Malignant lymphomas other than Hodgkin's disease.* New York: Springer-Verlag, 1978.
8. Lukes RJ, Collins RD. Immunologic characterization of human malignant lymphomas. *Cancer* 1974;34(Suppl):1488–1503.
9. The Non-Hodgkin's Lymphoma Pathologic Classification Project. National Cancer Institute sponsored study of classifications of non-Hodgkin's lymphomas: summary and description of a working formulation for clinical usage. *Cancer* 1982;49:2112–2135.
10. Harris NL, et al. A revised European-American classification of lymphoid neoplasms: a proposal from the International Lymphoma Study Group. *Blood* 1994;84: 1361–1392.
11. Jaffe ES; International Agency for Research on Cancer. *Pathology and genetics of tumours of haematopoietic and lymphoid tissues.* Lyon: IARC Press, 2000.
12. The Non-Hodgkin's Lymphoma Classification Project. A clinical evaluation of the International Lymphoma Study Group classification of non-Hodgkin's lymphoma. *Blood* 1997;89:3909–3918.
13. Siegel R, Naishadham D, Jemal A. Cancer statistics, 2012. *CA Cancer J Clin* 2012; 62:10–29.
14. Groves FD, Linet MS, Travis LB, et al. Cancer surveillance series: non-Hodgkin's lymphoma incidence by histologic subtype in the United States from 1978 through 1995. *J Natl Cancer Inst* 2000;92:1240–1251.
15. Liu Q, et al. Follicular lymphomas in children and young adults: a comparison of the pediatric variant with usual follicular lymphoma. *Am J Surg Pathol* 2013;37(3):333–343.
16. Solal-Celigny P, et al. Follicular lymphoma international prognostic index. *Blood* 2004;104:1258–1265.
17. Federico M, et al. Follicular lymphoma international prognostic index 2: a new prognostic index for follicular lymphoma developed by the international follicular lymphoma prognostic factor project. *J Clin Oncol* 2009;27:4555–4562.
18. Liu Q, et al. Improvement of overall and failure-free survival in stage IV follicular lymphoma: 25 years of treatment experience at The University of Texas M.D. Anderson Cancer Center. *J Clin Oncol* 2006;24:1582–1589.
19. Wong E, Dickinson M. Transformation in follicular lymphoma: biology, prognosis, and therapeutic options. *Curr Oncol Rep* 2012;14:424–432.
20. Al-Tourah AJ, et al. Population-based analysis of incidence and outcome of transformed non-Hodgkin's lymphoma. *J Clin Oncol* 2008;26:5165–5169.
21. Bastion Y, et al. Incidence, predictive factors, and outcome of lymphoma transformation in follicular lymphoma patients. *J Clin Oncol* 1997;15:1587–1594.
22. Conconi A, et al. Incidence, risk factors and outcome of histological transformation in follicular lymphoma. *Br J Haematol* 2012;157:188–196.
23. Garvin AJ, et al. An autopsy study of histologic progression in non-Hodgkin's lymphomas. 192 cases from the National Cancer Institute. *Cancer* 1983;52: 393–398.
24. Advani R, Rosenberg SA, Horning SJ. Stage I and II follicular non-Hodgkin's lymphoma: long-term follow-up of no initial therapy. *J Clin Oncol* 2004;22: 1454–1459.
25. Freedman A. Follicular lymphoma: 2012 update on diagnosis and management. *Am J Hematol* 2012;87:988–995.
26. Victora GD, Nussenzweig MC. Germinal centers. *Annu Rev Immunol* 2012;30: 429–457.
27. Dent AL, Shaffer AL, Yu X, et al. Control of inflammation, cytokine expression, and germinal center formation by BCL-6. *Science* 1997;276:589–592.
28. Saito M, et al. BCL6 suppression of BCL2 via Miz1 and its disruption in diffuse large B cell lymphoma. *Proc Natl Acad Sci U S A* 2009;106:11294–11299.

29. Shaffer AL, et al. BCL-6 represses genes that function in lymphocyte differentiation, inflammation, and cell cycle control. *Immunity* 2000;13:199–212.

30. Phan RT, Dalla-Favera R. The BCL6 proto-oncogene suppresses p53 expression in germinal-centre B cells. *Nature* 2004;432:635–639.

31. Ranuncolo SM, et al. Bcl-6 mediates the germinal center B cell phenotype and lymphomagenesis through transcriptional repression of the DNA-damage sensor ATR. *Nat Immunol* 2007;8:705–714.

32. Zelenetz AD, Chen TT, Levy R. Clonal expansion in follicular lymphoma occurs subsequent to antigenic selection. *J Exp Med* 1992;176:1137–1148.

33. Bahler DW, Zelenetz AD, Chen TT, et al. Antigen selection in human lymphomagenesis. *Cancer Res* 1992;52:5547s–5551s.

34. Goodlad JR, Batstone PJ, Hamilton D, et al. Follicular lymphoma with marginal zone differentiation: cytogenetic findings in support of a high-risk variant of follicular lymphoma. *Histopathology* 2003;42:292–298.

35. Abou-Elella A, et al. Lymphomas with follicular and monocytoid B-cell components. Evidence for a common clonal origin from follicle center cells. *Am J Clin Pathol* 2000;114:516–522.

36. Yegappan S, Schnitzer B, Hsi ED. Follicular lymphoma with marginal zone differentiation: microdissection demonstrates the t(14;18) in both the follicular and marginal zone components. *Mod Pathol* 2001;14:191–196.

37. Keith TA, Cousar JB, Glick AD, et al. Plasmacytic differentiation in follicular center cell (FCC) lymphomas. *Am J Clin Pathol* 1985;84:283–290.

38. Schmid U, Karow J, Lennert K. Follicular malignant non-Hodgkin's lymphoma with pronounced plasmacytic differentiation: a plasmacytoma-like lymphoma. *Virchows Arch A Pathol Anat Histopathol* 1985;405:473–481.

39. Gradowski JF, et al. Follicular lymphomas with plasmacytic differentiation include two subtypes. *Mod Pathol* 2010;23:71–79.

40. Vago JF, Hurtubise PE, Redden-Borowski MM, et al. Follicular center-cell lymphoma with plasmacytic differentiation, monoclonal paraprotein, and peripheral blood involvement. Recapitulation of normal B-cell development. *Am J Surg Pathol* 1985;9:764–770.

41. Kojima M, et al. Histological variety of floral variant of follicular lymphoma. *APMIS* 2006;114:626–632.

42. Goates JJ, Kamel OW, LeBrun DP, et al. Floral variant of follicular lymphoma. Immunological and molecular studies support a neoplastic process. *Am J Surg Pathol* 1994;18:37–47.

43. Osborne BM, Butler JJ. Follicular lymphoma mimicking progressive transformation of germinal centers. *Am J Clin Pathol* 1987;88:264–269.

44. Navas-Palacios JJ, Valdes MD, Lahuerta-Palacios JJ. Signet-ring cell lymphoma. Ultrastructural and immunohistochemical features of three varieties. *Cancer* 1983;52:1613–1623.

45. Bayerl MG, et al. Lacunar and Reed-Sternberg-like cells in follicular lymphomas are clonally related to the centrocytic and centroblastic cells as demonstrated by laser capture microdissection. *Am J Clin Pathol* 2004;122:858–864.

46. Nathwani BN, et al. What should be the morphologic criteria for the subdivision of follicular lymphomas? *Blood* 1986;68:837–845.

47. Metter GE, et al. Morphological subclassification of follicular lymphoma: variability of diagnoses among hematopathologists, a collaborative study between the Repository Center and Pathology Panel for Lymphoma Clinical Studies. *J Clin Oncol* 1985;3:25–38.

48. Martin AR, et al. Prognostic value of cellular proliferation and histologic grade in follicular lymphoma. *Blood* 1995;85:3671–3678.

49. Ellison DJ, et al. Mitotic counts in follicular lymphomas. *Hum Pathol* 1987;18:502–505.

50. Wang SA, et al. Low histologic grade follicular lymphoma with high proliferation index: morphologic and clinical features. *Am J Surg Pathol* 2005;29:1490–1496.

51. Wahlin BE, et al. Clinical significance of the WHO grades of follicular lymphoma in a population-based cohort of 505 patients with long follow-up times. *Br J Haematol* 2012;156:225–233.

52. Hsi ED, et al. A clinicopathologic evaluation of follicular lymphoma grade 3A versus grade 3B reveals no survival differences. *Arch Pathol Lab Med* 2004;128:863–868.

53. Shustik J, et al. Follicular non-Hodgkin lymphoma grades 3A and 3B have a similar outcome and appear incurable with anthracycline-based therapy. *Ann Oncol* 2011;22:1164–1169.

54. Piccaluga PP, et al. Gene expression analysis provides a potential rationale for revising the histological grading of follicular lymphomas. *Haematologica* 2008;93:1033–1038.

55. Bhagavathi S, et al. Does a diffuse growth pattern predict for survival in patients with low-grade follicular lymphoma? *Leuk Lymphoma* 2009;50:900–903.

56. Warnke RA, Kim H, Fuks Z, et al. The coexistence of nodular and diffuse patterns in nodular non-Hodgkin's lymphomas: significance and clinicopathologic correlation. *Cancer* 1977;40:1229–1233.

57. Ezdinli EZ, Costello WG, Kucuk O, et al. Effect of the degree of nodularity on the survival of patients with nodular lymphomas. *J Clin Oncol* 1987;5:413–418.

58. Hans CP, et al. A significant diffuse component predicts for inferior survival in grade 3 follicular lymphoma, but cytologic subtypes do not predict survival. *Blood* 2003;101:2363–2367.

59. Jegalian AG, et al. Follicular lymphoma in situ: clinical implications and comparisons with partial involvement by follicular lymphoma. *Blood* 2011;118:2976–2984.

60. Adam P, et al. Presence of preserved reactive germinal centers in follicular lymphoma is a strong histopathologic indicator of limited disease stage. *Am J Surg Pathol* 2005;29:1661–1664.

61. Arber DA, George TI. Bone marrow biopsy involvement by non-Hodgkin's lymphoma: frequency of lymphoma types, patterns, blood involvement, and discordance with other sites in 450 specimens. *Am J Surg Pathol* 2005;29:1549–1557.

62. Merli M, et al. Assessment of bone marrow involvement in non-Hodgkin's lymphomas: comparison between histology and flow cytometry. *Eur J Haematol* 2010;85:405–415.

63. Ault KA. Detection of small numbers of monoclonal B lymphocytes in the blood of patients with lymphoma. *N Engl J Med* 1979;300:1401–1415.

64. Gribben JG, et al. All advanced stage non-Hodgkin's lymphomas with a polymerase chain reaction amplifiable breakpoint of bcl-2 have residual cells containing the bcl-2 rearrangement at evaluation and after treatment. *Blood* 1991;78:3275–3280.

65. Goteri G, et al. Comparison of germinal center markers CD10, BCL6 and human germinal center-associated lymphoma (HGAL) in follicular lymphomas. *Diagn Pathol* 2011;6:97.

66. Younes SF, et al. The efficacy of HGAL and LMO2 in the separation of lymphomas derived from small B cells in nodal and extranodal sites, including the bone marrow. *Am J Clin Pathol* 2011;135:697–708.

67. Younes SF, et al. Immunoarchitectural patterns in follicular lymphoma: efficacy of HGAL and LMO2 in the detection of the interfollicular and diffuse components. *Am J Surg Pathol* 2010;34:1266–1276.

68. Lai R, Arber DA, Chang KL, et al. Frequency of bcl-2 expression in non-Hodgkin's lymphoma: a study of 778 cases with comparison of marginal zone lymphoma and monocytoid B-cell hyperplasia. *Mod Pathol* 1998;11:864–869.

69. Nguyen PL, Zukerberg LR, Benedict WF, et al. Immunohistochemical detection of p53, bcl-2, and retinoblastoma proteins in follicular lymphoma. *Am J Clin Pathol* 1996;105:538–543.

70. Masir N, et al. BCL2 protein expression in follicular lymphomas with t(14;18) chromosomal translocations. *Br J Haematol* 2009;144:716–725.

71. Bende RJ, et al. Primary follicular lymphoma of the small intestine: alpha4beta7 expression and immunoglobulin configuration suggest an origin from local antigen-experienced B cells. *Am J Pathol* 2003;162:105–113.

72. Thorns C. et al. Significant high expression of CD23 in follicular lymphoma of the inguinal region. *Histopathology* 2007;50:716–719.

73. Olteanu H, et al. CD23 expression in follicular lymphoma: clinicopathologic correlations. *Am J Clin Pathol* 2011;135:46–53.

74. Lai R, Weiss LM, Chang KL, et al. Frequency of CD43 expression in non-Hodgkin lymphoma. A survey of 742 cases and further characterization of rare CD43+ follicular lymphomas. *Am J Clin Pathol* 1999;111:488–494.

75. Nam-Cha SH, et al. Light-chain-restricted germinal centres in reactive lymphadenitis: report of eight cases. *Histopathology* 2008;52:436–444.

76. Zhao XF, et al. Expanded populations of surface membrane immunoglobulin light chain-negative B cells in lymph nodes are not always indicative of B-cell lymphoma. *Am J Clin Pathol* 2005;124:143–150.

77. Farmer PL, Bailey DJ, Burns BF, et al. The reliability of lymphoma diagnosis in small tissue samples is heavily influenced by lymphoma subtype. *Am J Clin Pathol* 2007;128:474–480.

78. Solal-Celigny P, Cahu X, Cartron G. Follicular lymphoma prognostic factors in the modern era: what is clinically meaningful? *Int J Hematol* 2010;92:246–254.

79. Lorsbach RB, et al. Clinicopathologic analysis of follicular lymphoma occurring in children. *Blood* 2002;99, 1959–1964.

80. Atra A, et al. Conservative management of follicular non-Hodgkin's lymphoma in childhood. *Br J Haematol* 1998;103:220–223.

81. Schmatz AI, et al. Primary follicular lymphoma of the duodenum is a distinct mucosal/submucosal variant of follicular lymphoma: a retrospective study of 63 cases. *J Clin Oncol* 2011;29:1445–1451.

82. Cong P, et al. In situ localization of follicular lymphoma: description and analysis by laser capture microdissection. *Blood* 2002;99:3376–3382.

83. Montes-Moreno S, et al. Intrafollicular neoplasia/in situ follicular lymphoma: review of a series of 13 cases. *Histopathology* 2010;56:658–662.

84. Su W, Spencer J, Wotherspoon AC. Relative distribution of tumour cells and reactive cells in follicular lymphoma. *J Pathol* 2001;193:498–504.

85. Agopian J, et al. Agricultural pesticide exposure and the molecular connection to lymphomagenesis. *J Exp Med* 2009;206:1473–1483.

86. Roulland S, et al. Early steps of follicular lymphoma pathogenesis. *Adv Immunol* 2011;111:1–46.

87. Roulland S, et al. Follicular lymphoma-like B cells in healthy individuals: a novel intermediate step in early lymphomagenesis. *J Exp Med* 2006;203:2425–2431.

88. Fernandez de Larrea C, et al. Initial features and outcome of cutaneous and non-cutaneous primary extranodal follicular lymphoma. *Br J Haematol* 2011;153:334–340.

89. Cook JR, Shekhter-Levin S, Swerdlow SH. Utility of routine classical cytogenetic studies in the evaluation of suspected lymphomas: results of 279 consecutive lymph node/extranodal tissue biopsies. *Am J Clin Pathol* 2004;121:826–835.

90. Horsman DE, Gascoyne RD, Coupland RW, et al. Comparison of cytogenetic analysis, southern analysis, and polymerase chain reaction for the detection of t(14;18) in follicular lymphoma. *Am J Clin Pathol* 1995;103:472–478.

91. Bentley G, Palutke M, Mohamed AN. Variant t(14;18) in malignant lymphoma: a report of seven cases. *Cancer Genet Cytogenet* 2005;157:12–17.

92. Lin P, et al. Translocation (18;22)(q21;q11) in B-cell lymphomas: a report of 4 cases and review of the literature. *Hum Pathol* 2008;39:1664–1672.

93. Guo Y, et al. Low-grade follicular lymphoma with t(14;18) presents a homogeneous disease entity otherwise the rest comprises minor groups of heterogeneous disease entities with Bcl2 amplification, Bcl6 translocation or other gene aberrances. *Leukemia* 2005;19:1058–1063.

94. Weinberg OK, et al. "Minor" BCL2 breakpoints in follicular lymphoma: frequency and correlation with grade and disease presentation in 236 cases. *J Mol Diagn* 2007;9:530–537.

95. Espinet B, et al. FISH is better than BIOMED-2 PCR to detect IgH/BCL2 translocation in follicular lymphoma at diagnosis using paraffin-embedded tissue sections. *Leuk Res* 2008;32:737–742.

96. Schuler F, et al. Prevalence and frequency of circulating t(14;18)-MBR translocation carrying cells in healthy individuals. *Int J Cancer* 2009;124:958–963.

97. Hirt C, Dolken G, Janz S, et al. Distribution of t(14;18)-positive, putative lymphoma precursor cells among B-cell subsets in healthy individuals. *Br J Haematol* 2007;138:349–353.

98. Horsman DE, Connors JM, Pantzar T, et al. Analysis of secondary chromosomal alterations in 165 cases of follicular lymphoma with t(14;18). *Genes Chromosomes Cancer* 2001;30:375–382.

99. Chaganti RS, Nanjangud G, Schmidt H, et al. Recurring chromosomal abnormalities in non-Hodgkin's lymphoma: biologic and clinical significance. *Semin Hematol* 2000;37:396–411.

100. Tilly H, et al. Prognostic value of chromosomal abnormalities in follicular lymphoma. *Blood* 1994;84:1043–1049.

101. Gu K, et al. t(14;18)-negative follicular lymphomas are associated with a high frequency of BCL6 rearrangement at the alternative breakpoint region. *Mod Pathol* 2009;22:1251–1257.

102. Horn H, et al. Follicular lymphoma grade 3B is a distinct neoplasm according to cytogenetic and immunohistochemical profiles. *Haematologica* 2011;96:1327–1334.

103. Cheung KJ, et al. Genome-wide profiling of follicular lymphoma by array comparative genomic hybridization reveals prognostically significant DNA copy number imbalances. *Blood* 2009;113:137–148.

104. Fitzgibbon J, et al. Genome-wide detection of recurring sites of uniparental disomy in follicular and transformed follicular lymphoma. *Leukemia* 2007;21:1514–1520.

105. Ross CW, Ouillette PD, Saddler CM, et al. Comprehensive analysis of copy number and allele status identifies multiple chromosome defects underlying follicular lymphoma pathogenesis. *Clin Cancer Res* 2007;13:4777–4785.

106. Dave SS, et al. Prediction of survival in follicular lymphoma based on molecular features of tumor-infiltrating immune cells. *N Engl J Med* 2004;351:2159–2169.

107. Payne K, et al. BIOMED-2 PCR assays for IGK gene rearrangements are essential for B-cell clonality analysis in follicular lymphoma. *Br J Haematol* 2011;155:84–92.

108. Gong JZ, et al. Detection of immunoglobulin kappa light chain rearrangements by polymerase chain reaction. An improved method for detecting clonal B-cell lymphoproliferative disorders. *Am J Pathol* 1999;155:355–363.

109. Amara K, et al. PCR-based clonality analysis of B-cell lymphomas in paraffin-embedded tissues: diagnostic value of immunoglobulin kappa and lambda light chain gene rearrangement investigation. *Pathol Res Pract* 2006;202:425–431.

110. Kaeffer B, et al. Histocompatible miniature pig (d/d haplotype): generation of hybridomas secreting A or M monoclonal antibody. *Hybridoma* 1991;10:731–744.

111. Zhu D, et al. Acquisition of potential N-glycosylation sites in the immunoglobulin variable region by somatic mutation is a distinctive feature of follicular lymphoma. *Blood* 2002;99:2562–2568.

112. Oricchio E, et al. The Eph-receptor A7 is a soluble tumor suppressor for follicular lymphoma. *Cell* 2011;147:554–564.

113. Jardin F, Sahota SS. Targeted somatic mutation of the BCL6 proto-oncogene and its impact on lymphomagenesis. *Hematology* 2005;10:115–129.

114. Migliazza A, et al. Frequent somatic hypermutation of the 5′ noncoding region of the BCL6 gene in B-cell lymphoma. *Proc Natl Acad Sci U S A* 1995;92:12520–12524.

115. Launay E, et al. High rate of TNFRSF14 gene alterations related to 1p36 region in de novo follicular lymphoma and impact on prognosis. *Leukemia* 2012;26:559–562.

116. Cheung KJ, et al. Acquired TNFRSF14 mutations in follicular lymphoma are associated with worse prognosis. *Cancer Res* 2010;70:9166–9174.

117. Pasqualucci L, et al. Inactivating mutations of acetyltransferase genes in B-cell lymphoma. *Nature* 2011;471:189–195.

118. Morin RD, et al. Frequent mutation of histone-modifying genes in non-Hodgkin lymphoma. *Nature* 2011;476:298–303.

119. Morin RD, et al. Somatic mutations altering EZH2 (Tyr641) in follicular and diffuse large B-cell lymphomas of germinal-center origin. *Nat Genet* 2010;42:181–185.

120. Honma K, et al. TNFAIP3/A20 functions as a novel tumor suppressor gene in several subtypes of non-Hodgkin lymphomas. *Blood* 2009;114:2467–2475.

121. Kato M, et al. Frequent inactivation of A20 in B-cell lymphomas. *Nature* 2009;459:712–716.

122. Coelho V, et al. Glycosylation of surface Ig creates a functional bridge between human follicular lymphoma and microenvironmental lectins. *Proc Natl Acad Sci U S A* 2010;107:18587–18592.

Chapter 23
Diffuse Large B-Cell Lymphoma

Ken H. Young • L. Jeffrey Medeiros • Wing C. Chan

This chapter provides a comprehensive review of diffuse large B-cell lymphoma (DLBCL), the most common type of non-Hodgkin lymphoma (NHL) worldwide. DLBCL is a clinically aggressive disease with a 5-year overall survival rate of approximately 50% to 60% with currently used chemotherapy regimens. One roadblock to better therapy has been a limited understanding of DLBCL, reflected in its current definition. It has become increasingly clear, however, that DLBCL is highly heterogeneous, with variable clinical, pathologic, and biologic features (1).

In previous attempts to describe DLBCL, including the Kiel classification and the Working Formulation, centroblastic and immunoblastic lymphomas were accepted as two major DLBCL types (2,3). Due to low reproducibility in distinguishing between centroblastic and immunoblastic lymphomas, the Revised European American Lymphoma classification and the 2001 World Health Organization (WHO) classification defined DLBCL as a single entity (4,5). In recognition of the weaknesses used in the previous classification approaches, the 2008 WHO classification has proposed several clinicopathologic subtypes, distinct subgroups, and distinct disease entities based on clinicopathologic, immunophenotypic, and molecular features (Table 23.1; Fig. 23.1). This classification was a step forward and is reasonably reproducible. Nevertheless, recent efforts have begun to identify unique abnormalities in specific molecular pathways that are potential targets of novel therapy. Knowledge of those targets likely supports to the development of novel targeted therapies that will be tailored to individual patients, leading to improved outcome. The abnormalities will also likely be incorporated into future classification system as they will identify additional subtypes of DLBCL.

 ## DEFINITION

DLBCL is defined as a mature B-cell neoplasm with a diffuse pattern of infiltration that is composed of neoplastic cells with nuclei equal to or greater than the size of a benign histiocyte nucleus (1–5). Cases that do not fall into defined subtypes are classified as DLBCL, not otherwise specified (NOS).

 ## EPIDEMIOLOGY AND ETIOLOGY

DLBCL accounts for 30% to 40% of all NHLs. No significant difference is observed regarding the incidence of lymphoma among different ethnic and racial populations. In some countries, such as Eastern Europe and Asia, the relative frequency of DLBCL is slightly higher than in North America (6,7). This may be a function of a truly higher incidence, but also is likely related to a lower frequency of low-grade B-cell lymphomas in these countries.

The median age of patients is 64 years. The disease can impact any age, but is more common in older adults. There is a mild male predominance with a male-to-female ratio of 1.2:1 (6,7).

The etiology of DLBCL is unknown for most patients although a subset of patients can have known underlying risk factors, including immunodeficiency, chronic inflammatory diseases, autoimmune disorders, or a history of treatment with certain medications. Some cases of DLBCL arise in individuals with congenital or acquired immunodeficiency. Acquired immunodeficiency is seen in patients with human immunodeficiency virus (HIV) infection or iatrogenic scenario following organ transplantation, methotrexate, and other immunosuppressive therapies for patients with autoimmune disorders. Epstein-Barr virus (EBV) and human herpesvirus 8 (HHV8) appear to play an important role in the immunodeficiency setting (see Chapter 25).

It has been reported that chronic inflammation or irritation is associated with increased risk of DLBCL, including postmastectomy or postimplant lymphedema, chronic inflammation in skin, previous surgery and metallic implants, longstanding rheumatoid arthritis, systemic lupus erythromatosis, and pyothorax. The 2008 WHO classification defines some of these lesions as distinct entities, including DLBCL associated with chronic inflammation, pyothorax-associated DLBCL, and methotrexate-related lymphoproliferative disease.

EBV infection is present in several DLBCL subtypes, particularly plasmablastic lymphoma (PBL), primary effusion lymphoma (PEL), DLBCL arising in the setting of immunodeficiency, autoimmune disorders treated with immunosuppressive medications, chronic inflammation (e.g., pyothorax-associated), lymphomatoid granulomatosis (LYG), and DLBCL in the setting of angioimmunoblastic T-cell lymphoma. In EBV⁺ DLBCL of the elderly, EBV is an essential part of the definition. Immune function is believed to be compromised as part of the aging process in patients with EBV⁺ DLBCL (6–9).

Most cases of DLBCL, 80% to 90%, arise *de novo*, but some cases are transformed from low-grade B-cell lymphomas, such as chronic lymphocytic leukemia/small lymphocytic lymphoma (CLL/SLL), follicular lymphoma (FL), marginal zone lymphoma (MZL), lymphoplasmacytic lymphoma, and nodular lymphocyte–predominant Hodgkin lymphoma (NLPHL).

 ## CLINICAL FEATURES

Approximately 60% to 70% of DLBCL patients present with enlarged lymph nodes or a mass lesion. Some patients initially develop DLBCL at extranodal sites, but 60% to 70% patients have extranodal involvement during the course of disease (8,10). The most common extranodal sites include the gastrointestinal tract, skin, central nervous system (CNS), mediastinum, and bone. Several unique anatomic locations, particularly the skin, CNS, retroperitoneum, and testis, show distinctive clinicopathologic and biologic features as well as unique genetic aberrations. The 2008 WHO classification defines some of these tumors as distinct entities, including primary cutaneous DLBCL, leg type; primary DLBCL of the CNS; and intravascular large B-cell lymphoma.

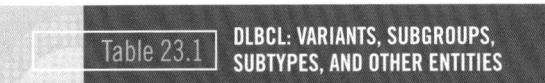

| Table 23.1 | DLBCL: VARIANTS, SUBGROUPS, SUBTYPES, AND OTHER ENTITIES |

DLBCL, NOS
Common morphologic variants
    Centroblastic
    Immunoblastic
    Anaplastic
Rare morphologic variants
    Myxoid
    Spindle
    Fibrillary matrix
    Signet ring cell morphology
    Alveolar
    Rosette formation
    Increased eosinophils
    Microvillous morphology
    Admixed crystal-storing histiocytosis
    Intrasinusoidal
Molecular subgroups
    GCB-like
    ABC-like
Immunohistochemical subgroups
    CD5-positive *de novo* DLBCL
    GCB-like
    Non–germinal center B-cell–like

DLBCL, Subtypes
T-cell-/histiocyte-rich large B-cell lymphoma
Primary DLBCL of the CNS (see Chapters 25 and 33)
Primary cutaneous DLBCL, leg type
EBV-positive DLBCL of the elderly

DLBCL, Other Distinct Entities
Primary mediastinal (thymic) large B-cell lymphoma
Intravascular large B-cell lymphoma
DLBCL associated with chronic inflammation
Lymphomatoid granulomatosis (see Chapters 28, 31, and 33)
ALK-positive large B-cell lymphoma
Plasmablastic lymphoma
Large B-cell lymphoma arising in HHV8-associated MCD (see Chapter 25)
PEL
CD30-positive *de novo* large B-cell lymphoma (not listed in the WHO classification)

Borderline Cases
B-cell lymphoma, unclassifiable, with features intermediate between DLBCL and Burkitt lymphoma (see Chapter 24)
B-cell lymphoma, unclassifiable, with features intermediate between DLBCL and classical Hodgkin lymphoma

ALK, anaplastic lymphoma kinase; DLBCL, diffuse large B-cell lymphoma; EBV, Epstein-Barr virus; HHV8, human herpesvirus 8; WHO, World Health Organization.
From Swerdlow SH, Campo E, Harris NL, et al., eds. *WHO classification of tumours of haematopoietic and lymphoid tissues.* Lyon: IARC, 2008.

Approximately 50% to 60% of patients with DLBCL present with stage I to II disease, 30% to 40% have B symptoms, and 15% to 20% patients have bone marrow involvement. The bone marrow can be involved by DLBCL (concordant histology) or low-grade B-cell lymphoma, most often FL (discordant histology). The latter group appears to have a better overall survival (10,11).

MORPHOLOGY

In most lymph node biopsy specimens, there is complete or subtotal effacement of the architecture by an infiltrate of lymphoid cells in a diffuse pattern (1–6). Extension into perinodal tissues is common (Fig. 23.2). In some cases, the lymphoma cells may exhibit a vaguely nodular pattern, often attributable to compartmentalization by residual structures or sclerosis (Fig. 23.3). In rare cases, the cells may preferentially involve sinusoids (Fig. 23.3), often focally, mimicking metastatic carcinoma. A "starry sky" pattern manifested by scattered

histiocytes with phagocytosed cell debris can be seen in highly proliferative cases of DLBCL (Fig. 23.4). Coagulative necrosis can be seen and may be extensive or the only evidence of disease in a biopsy specimen (Fig. 23.5). Sclerosis can be seen, particularly in extranodal biopsy specimens obtained from the mediastinum and retroperitoneum (Fig. 23.5). Involved lymph nodes can show simultaneous evidence of low-grade lymphoma, such as FL and CLL/SLL, and more rarely Hodgkin lymphoma (Fig. 23.6).

Cytologically, DLBCL is composed of predominantly large lymphoid cells. The most common cytologic variant resembles centroblasts (large noncleaved cells); less common variants resemble immunoblasts or are anaplastic (1–6). Often a case of DLBCL shows a mixture of cell types. Centroblasts demonstrate round or oval nuclei, vesicular chromatin, one to three nucleoli apposed to the nuclear membrane, and a small amount of amphophilic cytoplasm (Fig. 23.7). Centroblasts can have multilobated, angulated, or cleaved nuclei (Figs. 23.7 and 23.8). Immunoblasts exhibit round or oval nuclei and vesicular chromatin, and usually each cell has a single, central, and prominent nucleolus, with a moderate amount of basophilic cytoplasm (Fig. 23.9). Immunoblasts can have plasmacytoid features, with an eccentrically located nucleus and a paranuclear hof. Anaplastic DLBCL cells have multinucleated or multilobated, folded, bizarre or polygonal nuclei, vesicular or dense chromatin, one or more prominent eosinophilic nucleoli, and abundant amphophilic cytoplasm (Fig. 23.10).

The immunoblastic variant of DLBCL can be confidently recognized when most of the lymphoma cells are immunoblasts (1–6). It is accepted that the immunoblastic DLBCL variant is rendered when >90% of the lymphoma cells are immunoblasts, whereas those with <90% immunoblasts are defined as the centroblastic variant (large noncleaved cell). However, in some scenarios, it may be difficult to discern whether a lymphoma cell represents a centroblast or an immunoblast, and many DLBCL cells demonstrate an admixed feature of both cell types. The anaplastic DLBCL variant is composed mostly of anaplastic cells and commonly shows a cohesive or sinusoidal growth pattern (Fig. 23.10). Rare DLBCL cases show plasmacytic differentiation, in which lymphoma cells are admixed with variable numbers of plasma cells and plasmablasts. Such cases are commonly associated with EBV infection (Fig. 23.11A). A small subset of DLBCL cases exhibits blastic cytologic features (Fig. 23.11B).

Some morphologic variants tend to be associated with molecular subtypes defined by gene expression profiling (GEP) and/or genomic studies. Typical centroblastic variants commonly demonstrate the germinal center B-cell (GCB)-DLBCL phenotype, whereas immunoblastic or anaplastic variants often exhibit the activated B-cell (ABC)-DLBCL phenotype.

In some cases of DLBCL, reactive cells admixed with the lymphoma cells can be numerous, including small T cells, histiocytes, and less commonly plasma cells, neutrophils, or eosinophils. Increased histiocytes or small clusters of epithelioid histiocytes can mimic the lymphoepithelioid variant of peripheral T-cell lymphoma (PTCL) (so-called Lennert lymphoma). Sheets of large cells can be seen at the late stage (Fig. 23.11C). Some rare morphologic variants of DLBCL, summarized in Table 23.2, include cases associated with spindle cell or signet ring cell features, myxoid or fibrillary stroma, rosettes, crystal-storing histiocytes, alveolar morphology, microvillous features, and an intrasinusoidal distribution (Fig. 23.11D–H).

At extranodal locations, DLBCL typically forms a mass lesion and is often associated with destruction of normal tissue and loss of function, such as seminiferous tubules in the testis (Fig. 23.12). Some cases of extranodal DLBCL can be shown to arise from an extranodal marginal zone B-cell lymphoma of mucosa-associated lymphoid tissue (MALT lymphoma), and both DLBCL and MALT lymphoma can coexist in a biopsy

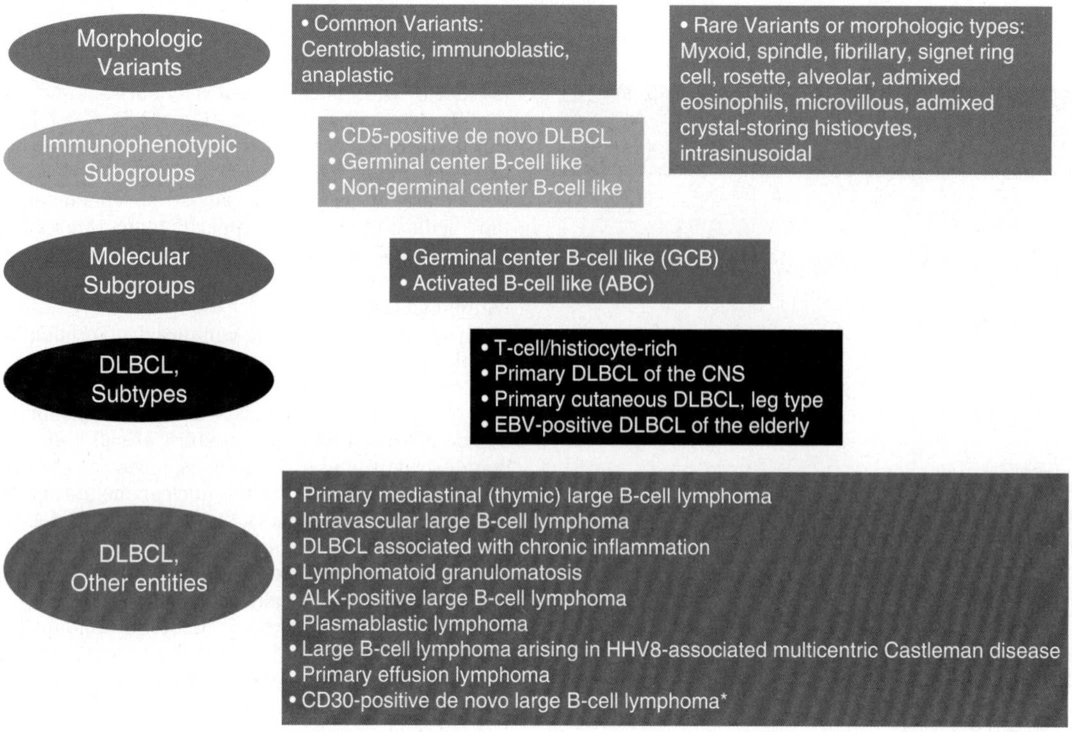

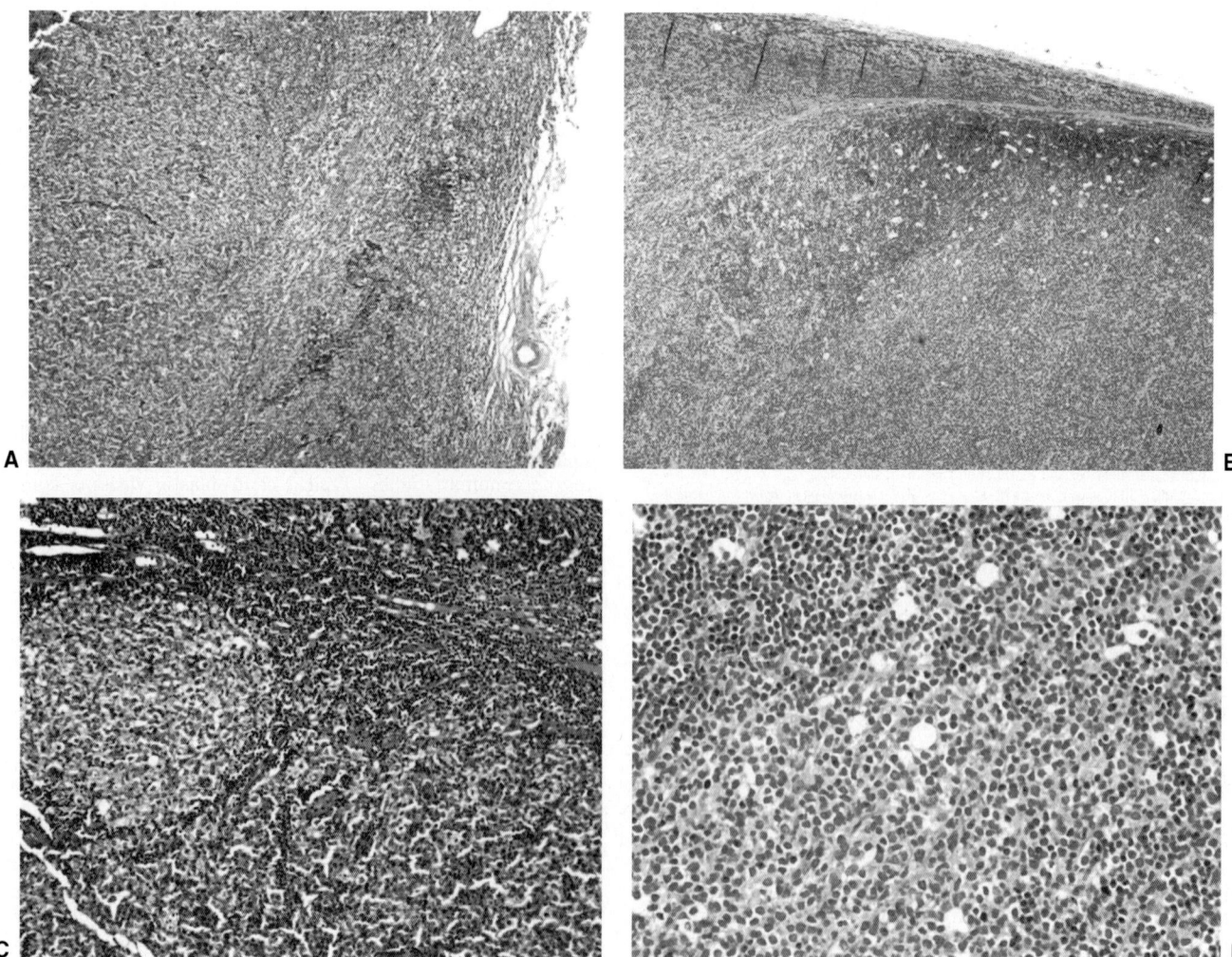

FIGURE 23.1. DLBCL: variants, subgroups, subtypes, and other entities.

Morphologic Variants
- Common Variants: Centroblastic, immunoblastic, anaplastic
- Rare Variants or morphologic types: Myxoid, spindle, fibrillary, signet ring cell, rosette, alveolar, admixed eosinophils, microvillous, admixed crystal-storing histiocytes, intrasinusoidal

Immunophenotypic Subgroups
- CD5-positive de novo DLBCL
- Germinal center B-cell like
- Non-germinal center B-cell like

Molecular Subgroups
- Germinal center B-cell like (GCB)
- Activated B-cell like (ABC)

DLBCL, Subtypes
- T-cell/histiocyte-rich
- Primary DLBCL of the CNS
- Primary cutaneous DLBCL, leg type
- EBV-positive DLBCL of the elderly

DLBCL, Other entities
- Primary mediastinal (thymic) large B-cell lymphoma
- Intravascular large B-cell lymphoma
- DLBCL associated with chronic inflammation
- Lymphomatoid granulomatosis
- ALK-positive large B-cell lymphoma
- Plasmablastic lymphoma
- Large B-cell lymphoma arising in HHV8-associated multicentric Castleman disease
- Primary effusion lymphoma
- CD30-positive de novo large B-cell lymphoma*

FIGURE 23.2. Nodal DLBCL. A: The lymph node architecture is effaced by a diffuse neoplastic lymphoid infiltrate, with extension into the surrounding soft tissue. **B–D:** The lymph node is partially effaced by a neoplastic lymphoid infiltrate. Some residual normal lymph node tissue is seen (upper field). **C:** The lymphoma cells form nodules that demonstrate a clear interface with the surrounding microenvironment. **D:** In this example, the lymphoma selectively involves the interfollicular zone, mimicking reactive lymphoid hyperplasia. Features supportive of a diagnosis of lymphoma include a monotonous population of interfollicular large lymphoid cells.

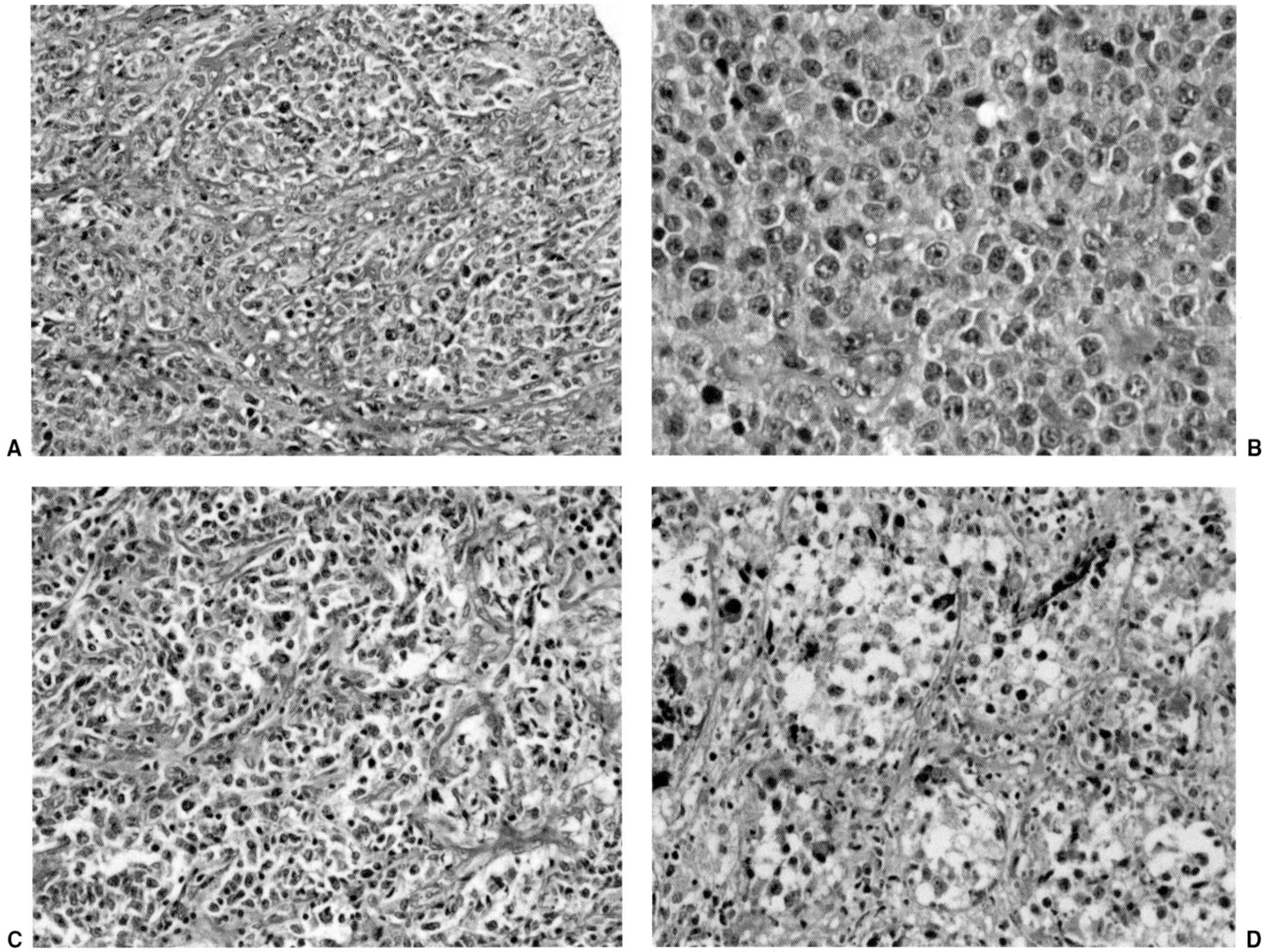

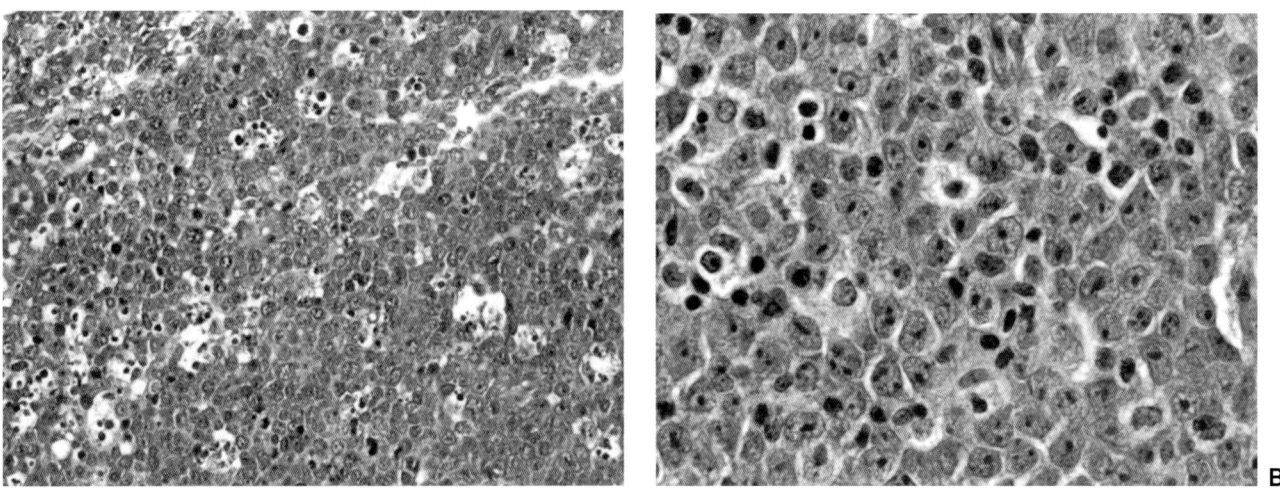

FIGURE 23.3. Nodal DLBCL. A: The lymphoma cells can exhibit a nodular pattern with a clear demarcation from the surrounding microenvironment, mimicking metastatic carcinoma. **B:** Most DLBCL cases are composed of noncohesive neoplastic lymphoid cells with a diffuse pattern. **C:** The lymphoma cells form an alveolar pattern defined by the fibrovascular stroma, mimicking the architecture of rhabdomyosarcoma because of the alveolar architecture. **D:** The lymphoma cells form an intrasinusoidal infiltrative pattern, mimicking metastatic carcinoma.

FIGURE 23.4. A high-grade B-cell lymphoma, unclassifiable with features between DLBCL and Burkitt lymphoma. A–C: The lymphoma is mainly composed of intermediate- and large-sized cells, but the lesion does not fulfill the current diagnostic criteria for Burkitt lymphoma. The lymphoma cells are those of centroblasts and immunoblasts.

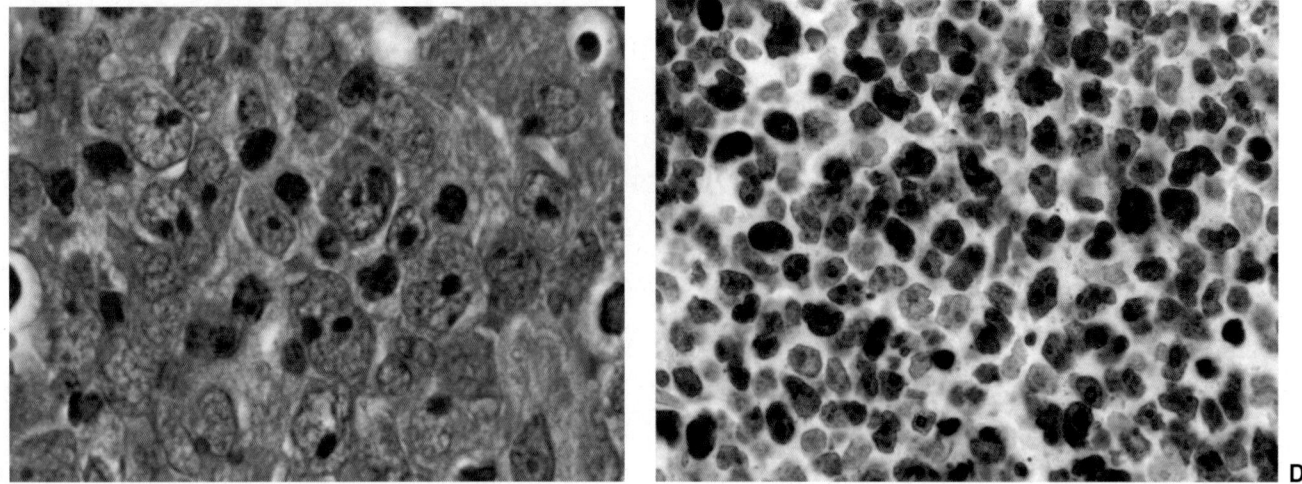

FIGURE 23.4. *(Continued)* **D:** The neoplastic cells in this case had a CD45⁺, CD20⁺, Pax-5⁺, CD10⁺, Bcl-2⁻, MUM-1⁻, Bcl-6⁺ immunophenotype, and show a high index of 80% to 90% by Ki-67 staining (shown).

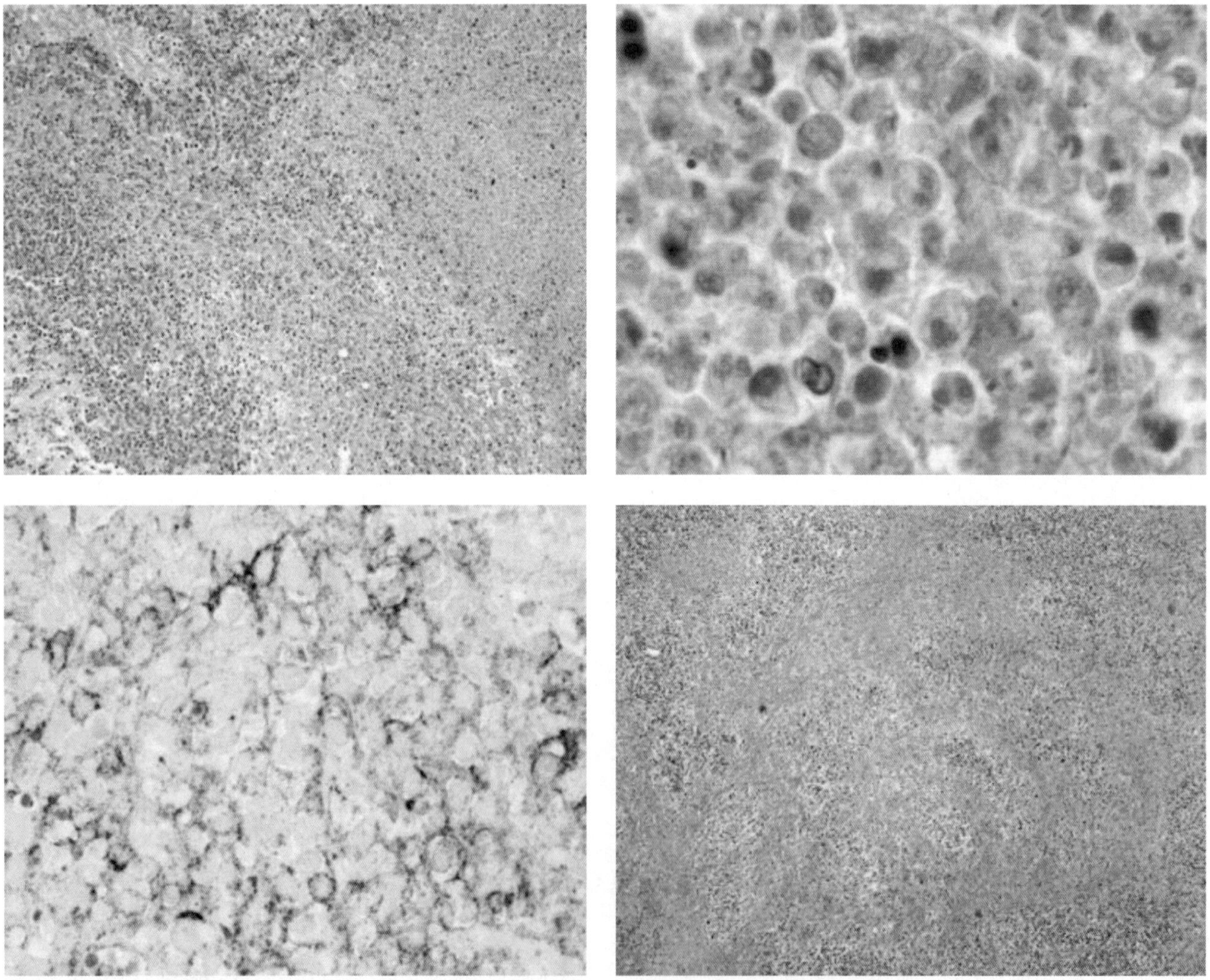

FIGURE 23.5. Diffuse large B-cell lymphoma. A,B: Geographic coagulative necrosis is commonly seen. **C:** These necrotic lymphoma cells are confirmed by a CD20⁺ immunophenotype. Immunostaining for CD20 may be nonspecific in necrotic specimens, so viable cells must be shown to stain to ascertain that the staining is specific. **D,E:** DLBCL with fibrosis. Geographic fibrotic bands delineate the tumor into variable and irregular aggregates. Lymphoma cells entrapped in the fibrotic areas often exhibit retracted or clear cytoplasm with crush artifact.

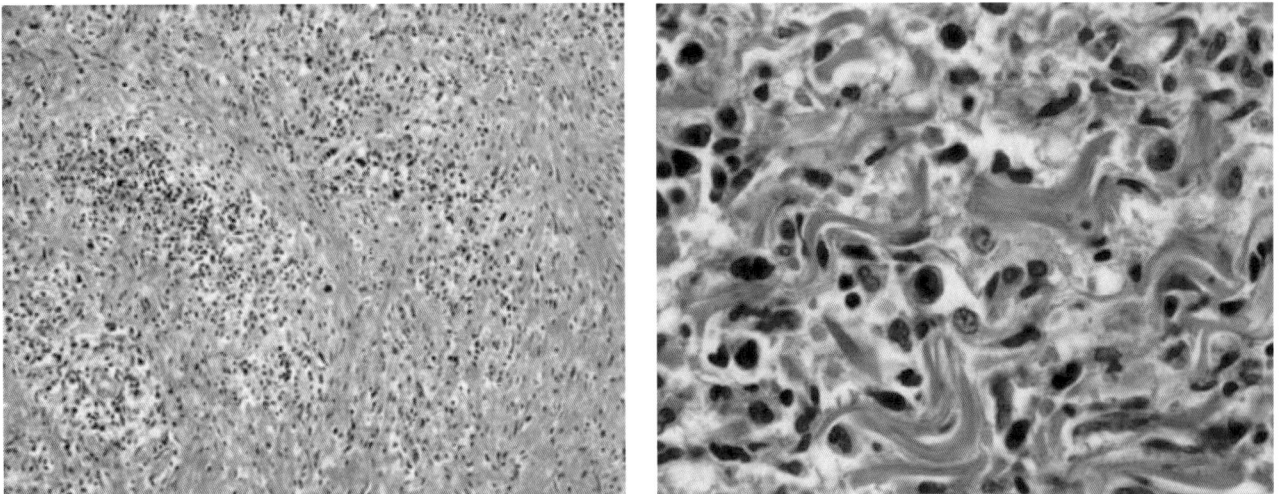

FIGURE 23.5. *(Continued)* **F:** Thin and refined fibrotic bands commonly entrap the lymphoma cells individually and in small aggregates.

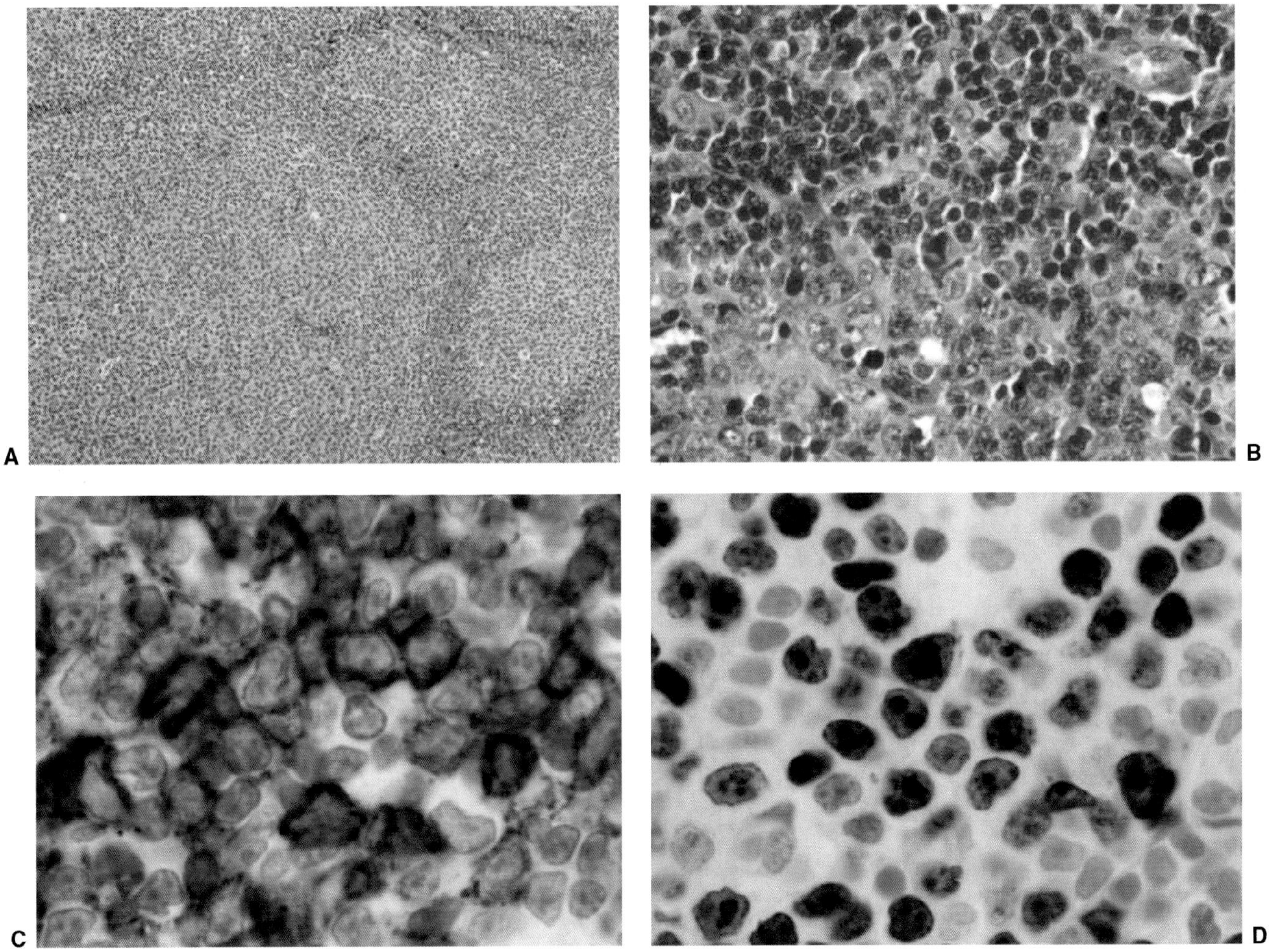

FIGURE 23.6. DLBCL transformed from FL and CLL. A: A large nodule composed of sheets of large lymphoma cells with adjacent coexisting FL components, consisting of small centrocytes and large centroblasts; these cells were clonal with a CD20⁺, CD10⁺, Bcl-2⁺, Bcl-6⁺ immunophenotype. **B:** A DLBCL transformed from preexisting CLL (Richter syndrome). The lower field shows diffuse sheets of large lymphoma cells. The upper field shows the preexisting CLL, consisting of monotonous small lymphoid cells. **C,D:** The neoplastic cells were clonal with a CD20⁺, CD5⁺, CD23⁺ (**C**), CD10⁻ immunophenotype and show a high index of Ki-67 positivity (**D**).

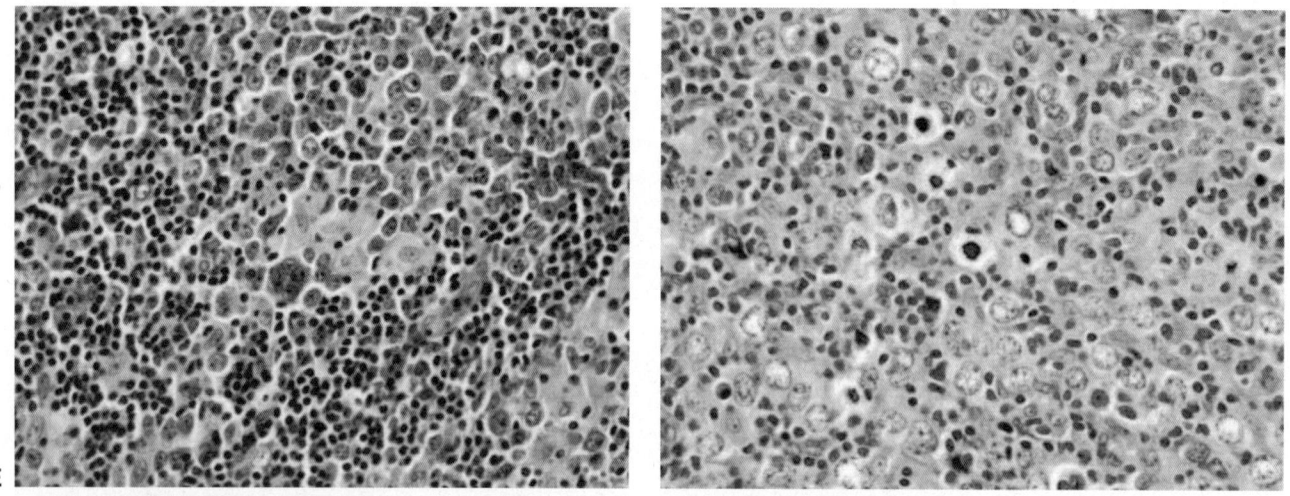

E

F

FIGURE 23.6. *(Continued)* **E:** DLBCL transformed from NLPHL: coexisting NLPHL components, consisting of scattered large LP type cells; these cells show a CD45+, CD20+, CD15−, CD30−, Pax-5+, Bcl6+ immunophenotype. **F:** A DLBCL transformed from NLPHL. These transformed neoplastic cells had a CD45+, CD20+, CD15−, CD30−, PAX-5+, Bcl-6+ immunophenotype. (Courtesy of Dr. Dennis O'Malley, MD, Clarient Reference Laboratory, Aliso Viejo, CA.)

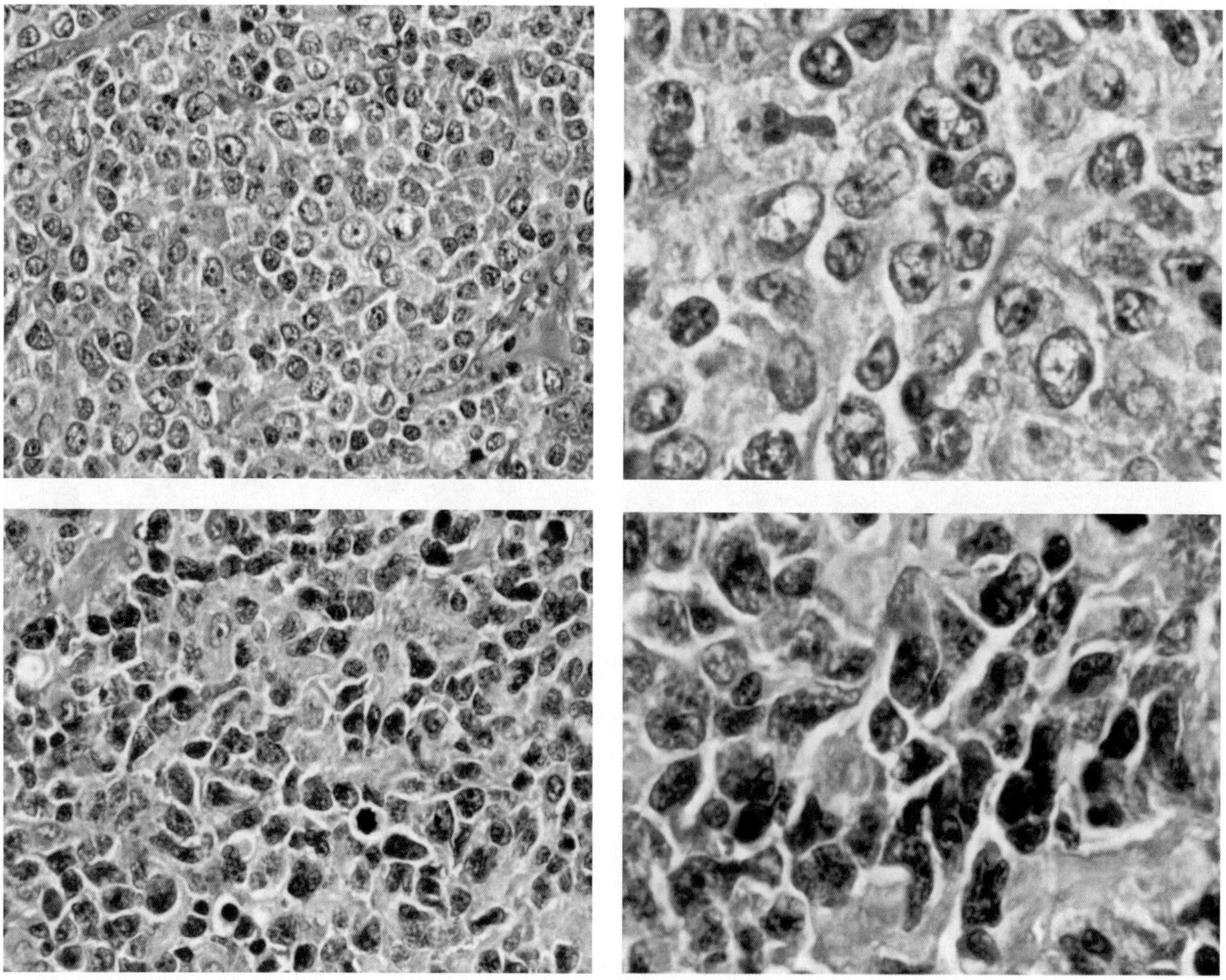

A

B

C

D

FIGURE 23.7. DLBCL, centroblastic subtype. A,B: The centroblasts have round or oval nuclei, finely vesicular chromatin, one to two small nucleoli adjacent to the nuclear membrane, and a thin rim of cytoplasm. **C,D:** The large lymphoma cells show angulated, triangular, or cleaved nuclei. The small nucleoli are obscured by the dense chromatin.

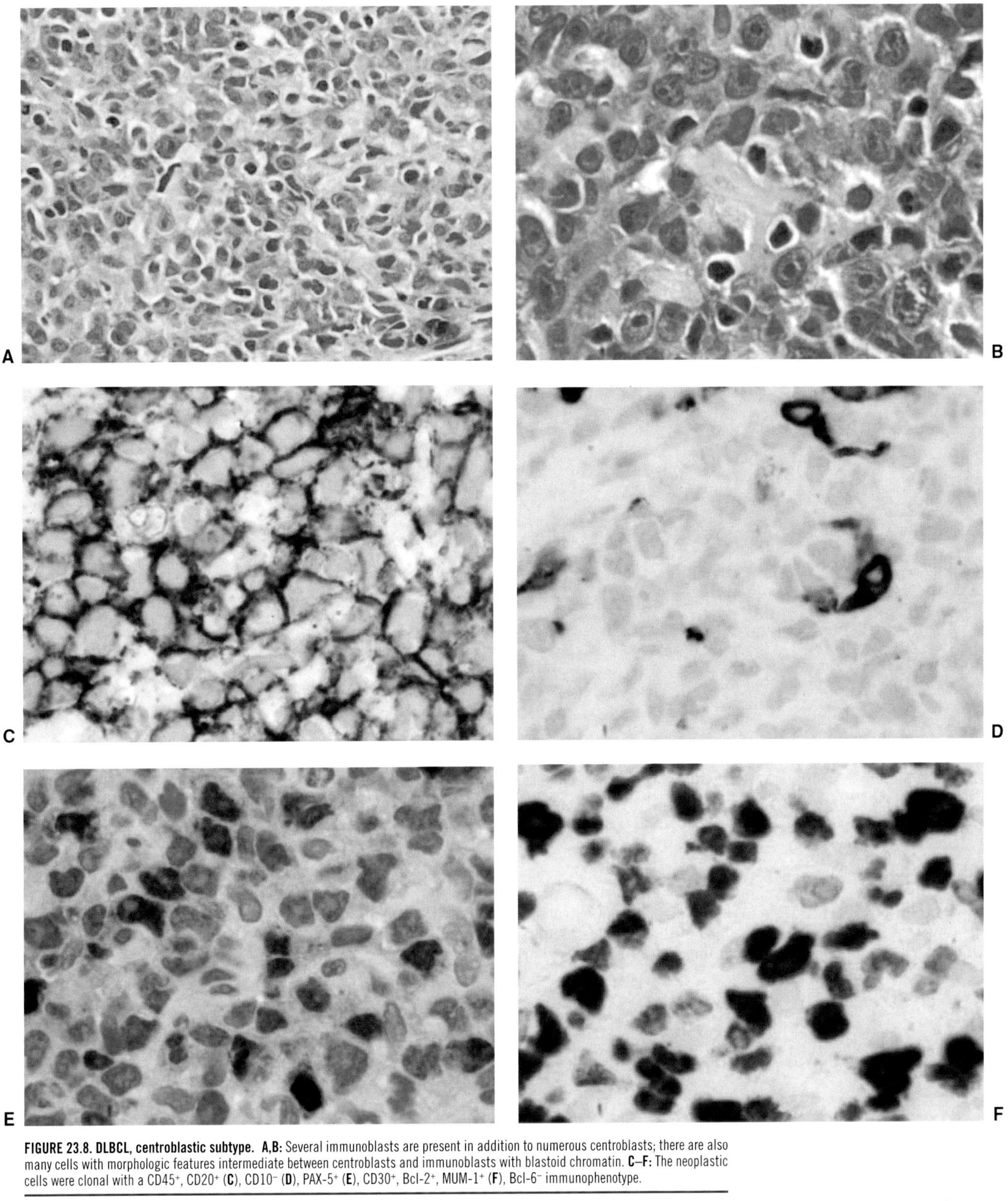

FIGURE 23.8. DLBCL, centroblastic subtype. **A,B:** Several immunoblasts are present in addition to numerous centroblasts; there are also many cells with morphologic features intermediate between centroblasts and immunoblasts with blastoid chromatin. **C–F:** The neoplastic cells were clonal with a CD45⁺, CD20⁺ (**C**), CD10⁻ (**D**), PAX-5⁺ (**E**), CD30⁺, Bcl-2⁺, MUM-1⁺ (**F**), Bcl-6⁻ immunophenotype.

specimen. Typically, the low-grade component infiltrates the epithelium and demonstrates lymphoepithelial lesions.

DLBCL can develop in extranodal locations, and they can have distinct clinical and pathologic features that require different clinical management. The 2008 WHO classification defines several entities, such as primary cutaneous DLBCL, leg type; primary DLBCL of the CNS; and intravascular large cell lymphoma. Each of them is discussed in this chapter.

 POSTULATED NORMAL COUNTERPART

Using GEP, DLBCL patients can be divided into distinctive subgroups (12,13). In the study by the Leukemia Lymphoma Molecular Profiling Project, DLBCL is divided into subgroups reflecting different stages of B-cell differentiation: germinal center B-cell–like (GCB)-DLBCL and activated B-cell–like

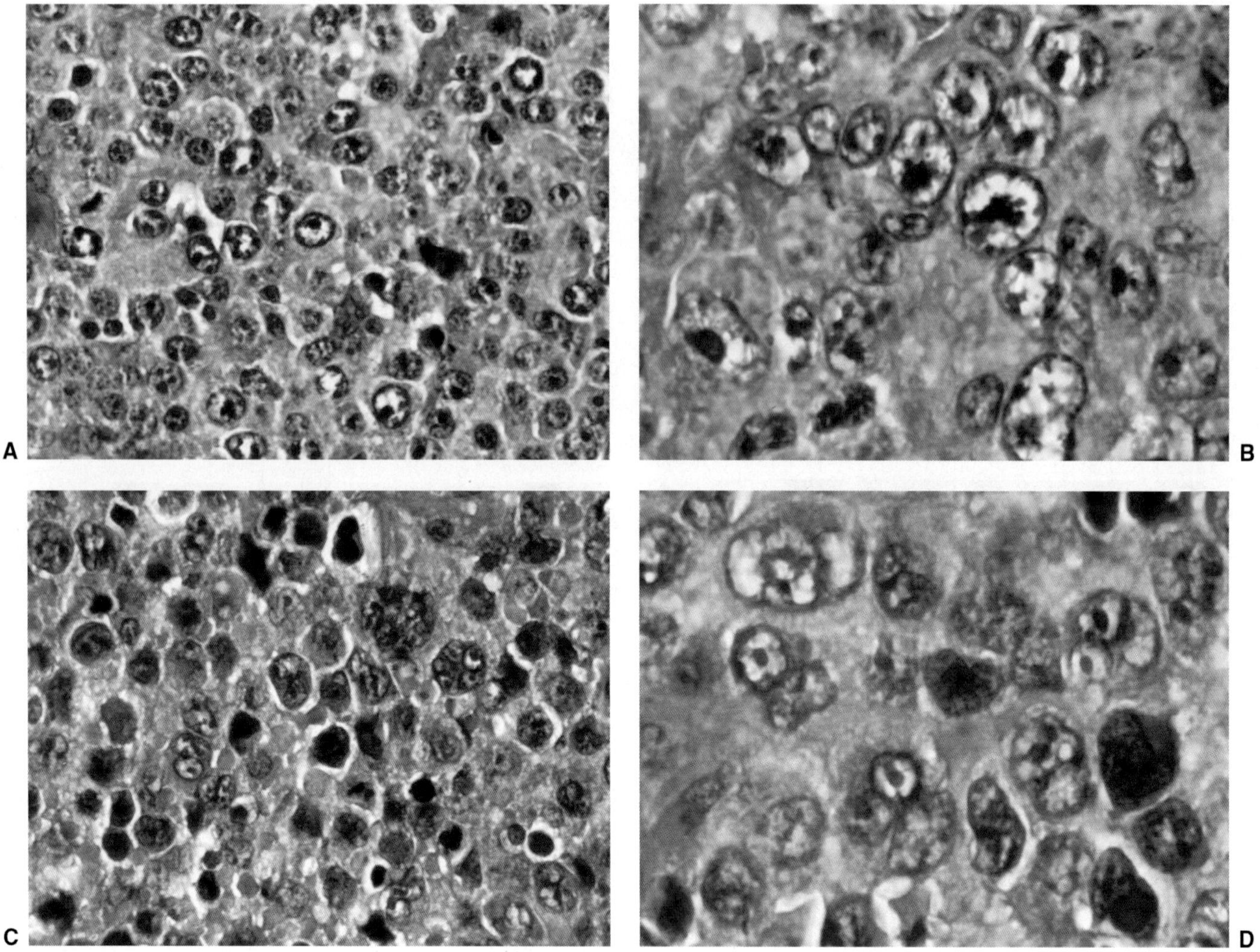

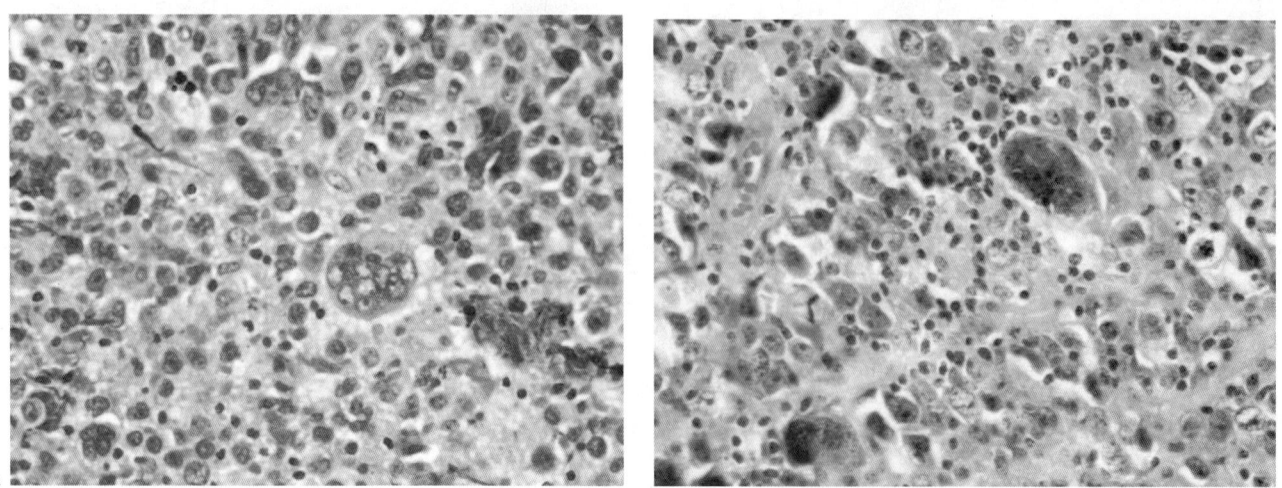

FIGURE 23.9. DLBCL, immunoblastic subtype. A,B: Nearly all the large lymphoma cells show round or oval nuclei, coarsely vesicular chromatin, prominent central nucleoli, and a broad rim of amphophilic cytoplasm. **C,D:** Another case shows occasional multilobated nuclei with prominent central nucleoli and active apoptosis.

(ABC)-DLBCL that express genes associated with GCB or genes induced during *in vitro* activation of peripheral blood B cells, respectively (Fig. 23.13). GCB-DLBCL patients demonstrate a phenotype of B cells in the dark zones of the GC, the stage in which B cells undergo somatic mutations in the variable region of the *Ig* gene. ABC-DLBCL cases do not have ongoing mutations and are possibly derived from a late–GC (light zone) or post–GC stage plasmablasts (Fig. 23.14). Using GEP signatures, a small subset of cases cannot be classified into either subgroup (12,13).

FIGURE 23.10. DLBCL, anaplastic subtype. The lymphoma cells are very large, with multilobulated (**A**), irregularly folded nuclei (**B**),

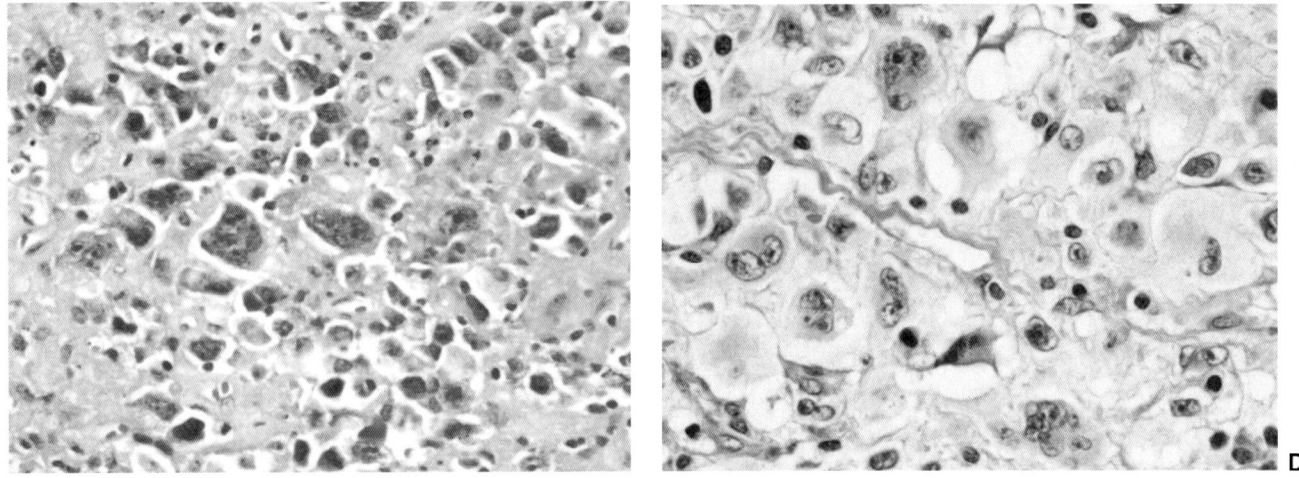

FIGURE 23.10. *(Continued)* abundant cytoplasm **(C)**, or indented **(D)**, resembling those seen in T-/null cell ALCL or Hodgkin lymphoma cells. (Courtesy of Dr. Dennis O'Malley, MD, Clarient Reference Laboratory, Aliso Viejo, CA.)

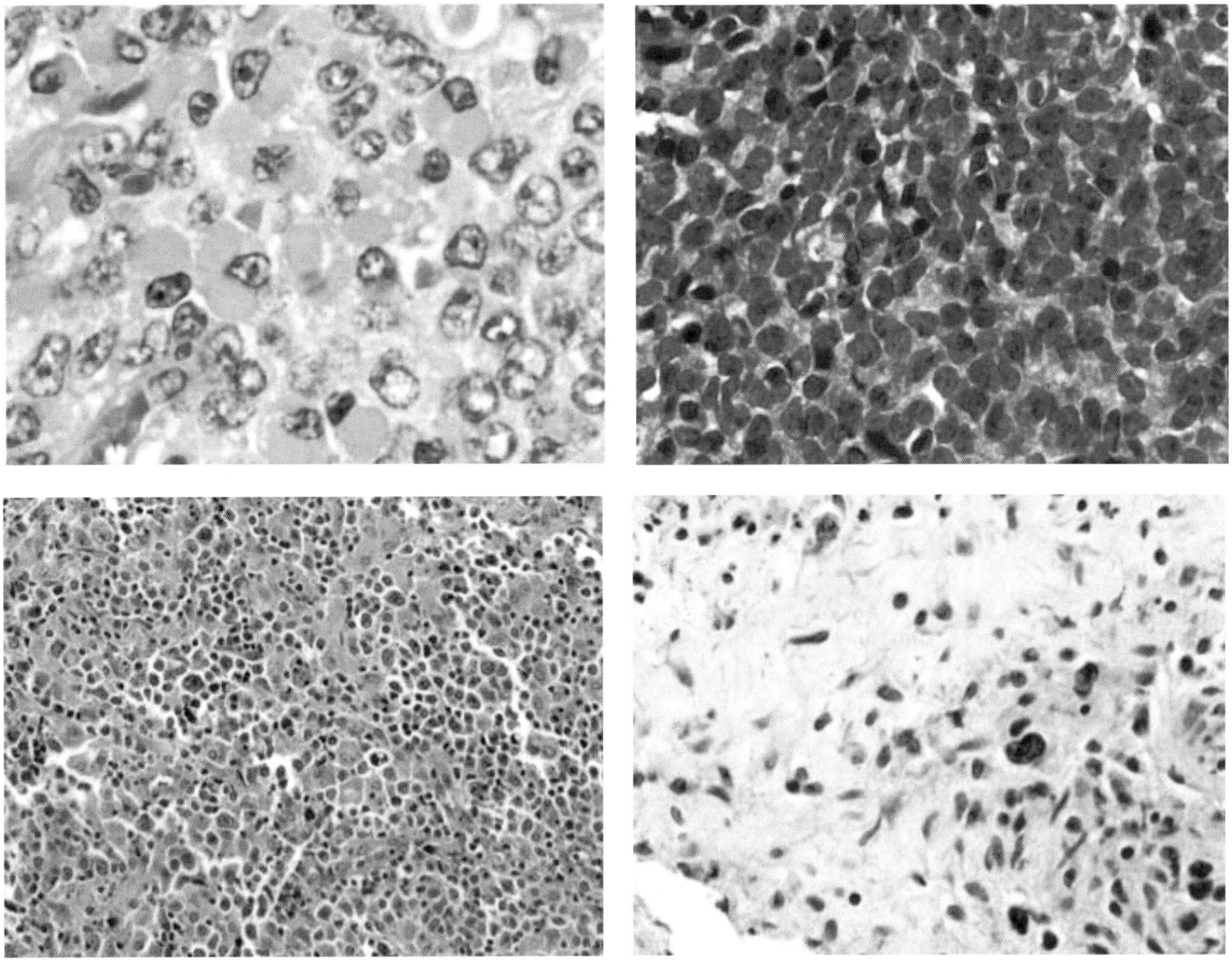

FIGURE 23.11. DLBCL, unusual morphologic features. A: DLBCL with plasma cell differentiation. The lymphoma is composed of large-sized centroblasts admixed with plasmablasts and atypical plasma cells. This feature is similar to that seen in the polymorphic type of PTLD. **B:** DLBCL with blastoid features. A diffuse lymphoid infiltrate is composed of large lymphoma cells with blastoid chromatin. **C:** DLBCL, T-cell-/histiocytic-rich with many interspersed small T cells and scattered and small aggregates of histiocytes. Clusters of epithelioid histiocytes forming granulomata, reminiscent of Lennert lymphoepithelioid T-cell lymphoma, can be seen. **D:** DLBCL with abundant myxoid stroma, mimicking extraskeletal myxoid chondrosarcoma or myxofibrosarcoma.

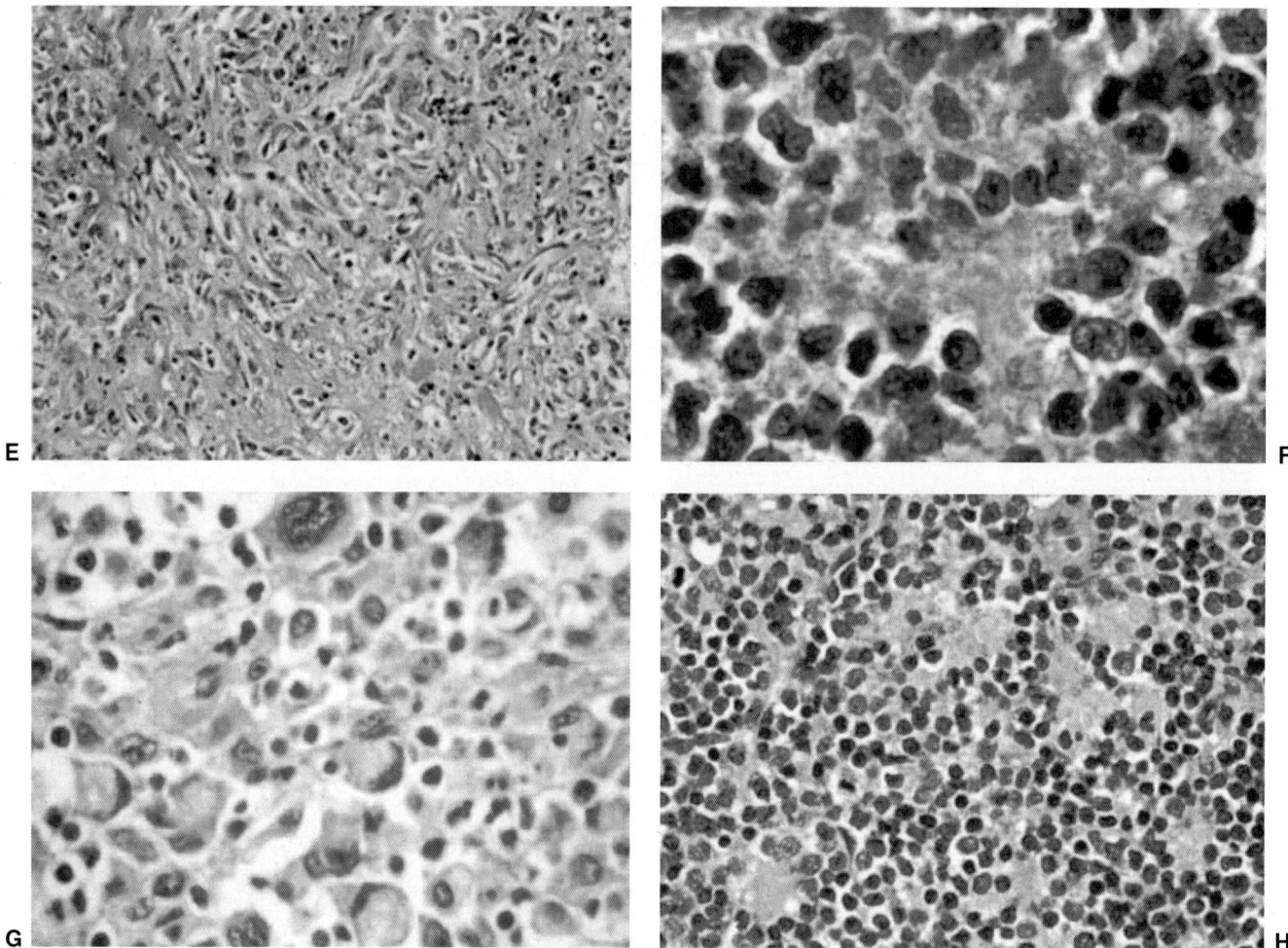

FIGURE 23.11. *(Continued)* **E:** DLBCL with spindle morphology. The large lymphoma cells show elongated and spindle nuclei, dense chromatin, indistinct nucleoli, and a broad rim of cytoplasm. **F:** DLBCL with fibrillary matrix. The large lymphoma cells are associated with abundant eosinophilic fibrillary matrix. The matrix is actually formed by cell membrane materials from the lymphoma cells, as demonstrated by positive CD20 immunostaining. **G:** DLBCL with signet ring cell features. The large lymphoma cells have eccentric nuclei, dense chromatin, indistinct nucleoli, and abundant eosinophilic cytoplasm. (Courtesy of Dr. Dennis O'Malley, MD, Clarient Reference Laboratory, Aliso Viejo, CA.) **H:** DLBCL with rosette formation. The large lymphoma cells are associated with rosette structures. The rosette matrix is actually formed by cell membrane materials from the lymphoma cells, and is positive for CD20.

IMMUNOPHENOTYPE

Almost all cases of DLBCL express pan–B-cell markers with variable intensity, including CD19, CD20, CD22, CD79a, and PAX-5. These tumors also express B-cell transcription factors, such as Oct-2, BOB.1, and PU.1. Surface or cytoplasmic immunoglobulin (Ig) heavy chains (IgM > IgG > IgA > IgD) and light chains and CD45/LCA are commonly expressed. T-cell markers, including CD2, CD3, CD4, CD7, CD8, and T-cell receptors (TCRs), are typically negative, but rare cases express CD2 or CD3 (14). CD5 is expressed in approximately 8% to 10% of DLBCL cases. CD5+ DLBCL can exhibit centroblastic or immunoblastic morphology, and most are of ABC subtype. In patients with DLBCL treated with rituximab (anti-CD20) or anti-CD22 antibodies in recurrent disease, CD20 or CD22 can be negative, perhaps due to therapy effect or more likely clonal evolution (15).

CD10 is expressed in 30% to 40% of DLBCL, with uniform intensity, particularly in the GCB type (16). CD10 expression significantly correlates with t(14;18)(q32;q21), another distinctive feature of GCB-DLBCL. Bcl-2 is expressed in 60% of cases. Bcl-2 expression correlates with t(14;18) and 18q21-q22 amplification, which are distinct features of GCB and ABC DLBCL,

respectively (17,18). Bcl-6 is expressed in approximately 70% of DLBCLs (16,19).

CD5 is expressed in approximately 8% to 10% of cases. CD5+ DLBCL can exhibit centroblastic or immunoblastic morphology, as well as in GCB or ABC molecular subtype. Some DLBCLs are positive for post-GC or plasma cell–associated markers, including CD38, CD138 (syndecan), FOXP-1, and IRF4/MUM-1. CD138 expression is typically seen in cases with plasmacytic differentiation (20). A small subset of cases expresses the activation marker CD30. CD30 expression is commonly heterogeneous and present in a variable percentage of the lymphoma cells. CD30+ DLBCLs can have centroblastic, immunoblastic, or anaplastic morphology, as well as a GCB or ABC molecular profile. Anaplastic cases can be characterized by uniform and strong CD30 expression. EBV+ DLBCLs are frequently associated with CD30 positivity (60% to 70% cases) and this feature should lead to examination for morphologic features suggestive of EBV infection. Ki-67 shows a high proliferation index, frequently ranging from 30% to 80%, although some aggressive cases of DLBCL can have an index of 95% to 100% (21,22).

MYC protein overexpression is seen in 25% to 40% of DLBCLs, and is expressed in both the GCB and ABC subtypes with similar frequency, suggesting that Myc involves a biologic pathway or mechanism independent of cell of origin. In contrast,

Table 23.2	RARE MORPHOLOGIC VARIANTS OF DLBCL AND DIFFERENTIAL DIAGNOSIS		
Rare Morphologic Variant	**Pathologic and Histologic Finding**	**Differential Diagnosis Entity**	**Studies to Support Other Entities**
Myxoid stroma	Individual or small groups of lymphoma cells present in myxoid stroma	Several types of sarcomas with myxoid stroma: • Myxoid chondrosarcoma • Myxofibrosarcoma	• CD68, CD99, desmin, S-100, muscle actin (HHF-35) • t(9;22)(q22;q12) or variant t(9;17) (q22;q11)
Spindle cell	Lymphoma cells have a spindle-shaped morphology, commonly seen in soft tissue and skin	• Various types of spindle cell sarcomas • Spindle cell carcinoma • Desmoplastic neoplasms	• CD99, desmin, S-100, muscle actin (HHF-35), SMA • Cytokeratin • t(11;22)(p13;q12)-WT1-EWS fusion
Signet ring cell morphology	Lymphoma cells have cytoplasmic vacuoles or inclusions, which may be due to abnormal immunoglobulin accumulation or aberrant membrane recycling	• Signet ring cell carcinoma • Liposarcoma	• Cytokeratin, S-100, muscle actin (HHF-35), SMA • t(12;16) or variant t(12;22)
Fibrillary matrix or rosette formation	• Lymphoma cells associated with fibrillary matrix and rosette formation • The fibrillary material results from interdigitating cytoplasmic processes, composed of cell membrane materials, and shows strong staining for CD10 and CD20	• Neuroblastoma • Primitive neuroectodermal tumor	• PGP9.5, Synaptopysin, CD99, S-100, neurofilament, NSE • EWS chimeric fusion transcript • N-myc (1p) amplification
Admixed crystal-storing histiocytes	Lymphoma cells admixed with histiocytes with abnormal crystallized immunoglobulin	• Rhabdomyoma	PTAH stain
Alveolar morphology	Lymphoma cells are arranged in an alveolar pattern and delineated by alveolar fibrovascular septa	• Rhabdomyosarcoma, alveolar type	• t(2;13)(q35;q14) - Pax3-FKHR fusion • Variant t(1;13)(p36;q14) and Pax7-FKHR fusion
Increased eosinophil	Lymphoma cells admixed with numerous eosinophils	• Hodgkin lymphoma • Peripheral T-cell lymphoma	Pan–T-/B-cell markers, CD15, CD30, CD45, Pax-5, EBER, Oct-2, BOB.1
Microvillous DLBCL	Several microvillous projections on ultrastructural examination	• Anaplastic large cell lymphoma • ALK⁺ DLBCL • Metastatic carcinoma • Metastatic melanoma	• ALCL (CD20⁻, CD3⁻/⁺, EMA⁻/⁺, ALK⁺/⁻) • ALK⁺ DLBCL (CD30⁻, ALK⁺) • Metastatic carcinoma (cytokeratin⁺) • Metastatic melanoma (S-100⁺, melanin⁺)
Sinusoidal CD30-positive DLBCL	Lymphoma cells are confined within the sinuses, CD20⁺, CD30⁺, EMA⁻/⁺, ALK⁻	• Anaplastic large cell lymphoma • ALK⁺ DLBCL • Metastatic carcinoma • Metastatic melanoma	• ALCL (CD20⁻, CD3⁺/⁻, EMA⁺/⁻, ALK⁺/⁻) • Microvillous DLBCL (CD30⁻) • ALK⁺ DLBCL (CD30⁻, ALK⁺) • Metastatic carcinoma (cytokeratin⁺) • Metastatic melanoma (S-100⁺, melanin⁺)

ALK, anaplastic lymphoma kinase-1; BOB.1, POU class 2 associating factor *1* (a ubiquitous protein associates with the POU domain of octamer proteins Oct-1 and Oct-2 and alters their recognition specificity); EBER, EBV-encoded RNA; EMA, epithelial membrane antigen; EWS, Ewing sarcoma; FKHR, Forkhead (*Drosophila*) homolog 1 (rhabdomyosarcoma) (13q14.1); OCT-2, POU class 3 homeobox 2 (both ubiquitous and lymphoid-specific POU transcription factors, members of the NF-κB/Rel family); Pax, Paired box gene; SMA, smooth muscle actin.

the *MYC* translocation is only present in 25% of patients with Myc protein overexpression and only in GCB subtype. Given its broad roles in the regulation of cell-cycle progression, metabolism, protein synthesis, stem-cell renewal, apoptotic signaling, p53, and NF-κB pathways, Myc protein expression in DLBCL

may represent a final integrator of all or most of the oncogenic mechanisms that underlie the GCB/ABC classification.

Viral infection has been implicated in a subset of DLB-CLs, and EBV (EBER, Epstein-Barr virus–encoded RNA) is expressed in 3% to 4% of immunocompetent patients with

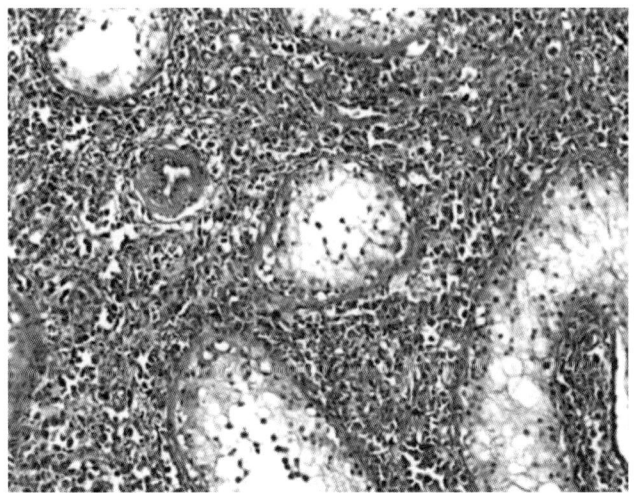

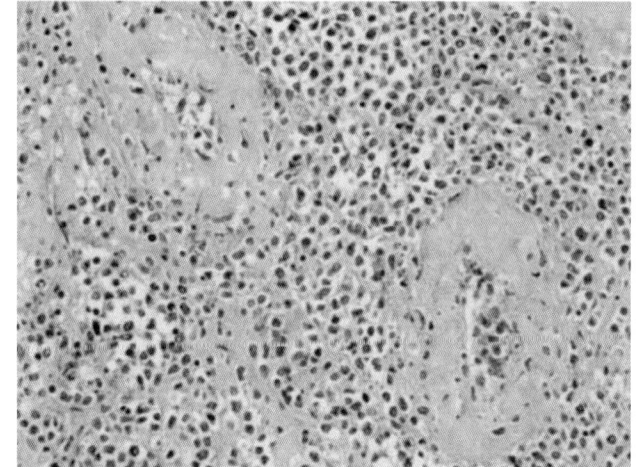

FIGURE 23.12. Extranodal DLBCL. A,B: An interstitial infiltrative pattern in the testis stroma with preserved (**A**) and fibrotic testicular seminiferous tubules (**B**).

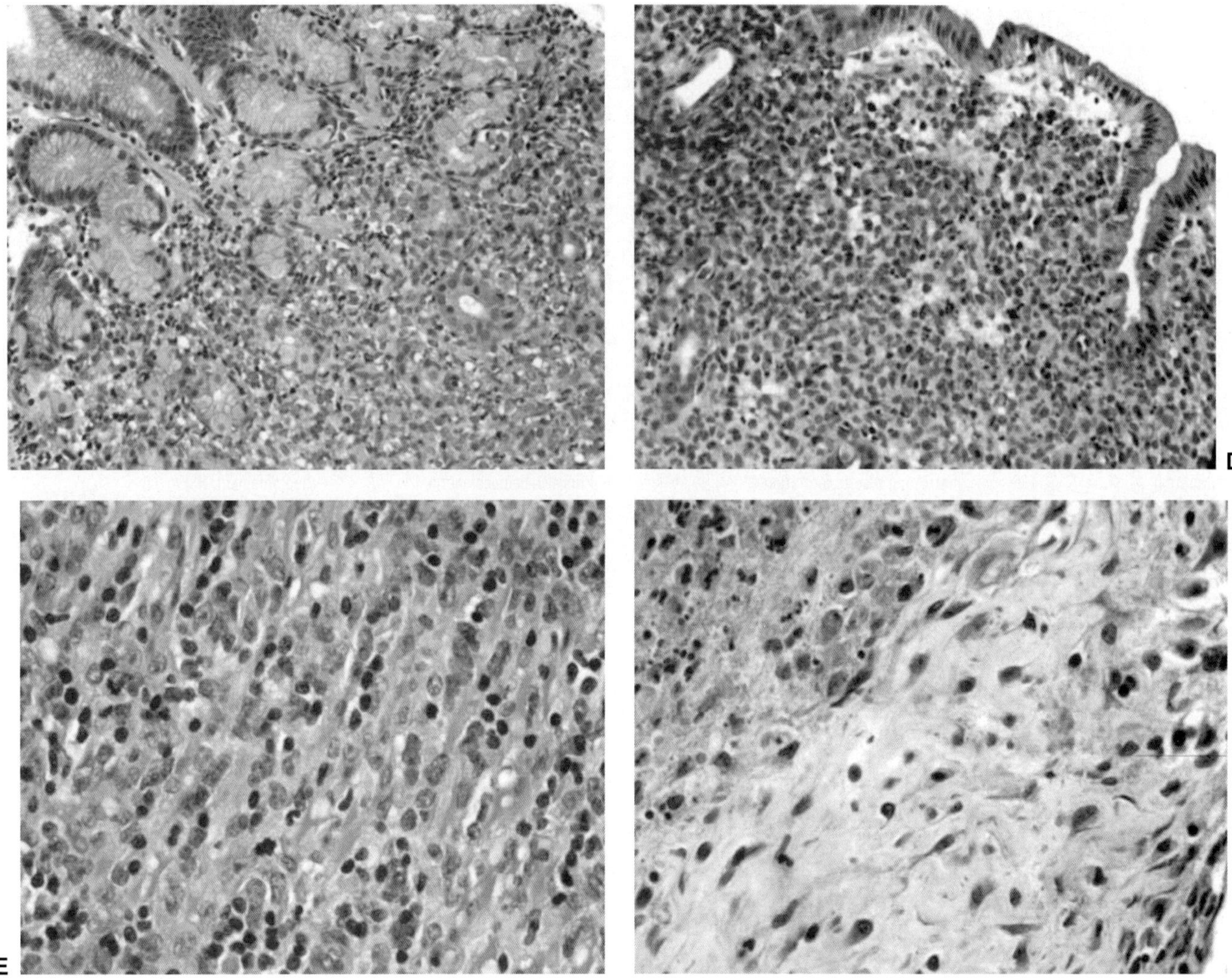

C

D

E

F

FIGURE 23.12. *(Continued)* **C:** An interstitial infiltrative pattern is shown in gastric mucosa. **D:** An interstitial infiltrative pattern is shown in colonic mucosa. **E:** The interstitial infiltrative pattern in the fibrous soft tissue and the tumor cells forms a single-file pattern of infiltration intervening by fibrovascular septa. **F:** The neoplastic lymphoid cells are present in a background of myxoid stroma.

DLBCL, particularly in extranodal DLBCL cases, and usually in elderly patients. A substantial proportion of EBV⁺ cases are of ABC molecular subtype, and significantly correlate with Bcl-2 expression and NF-κB activation. The tumor cells commonly show immunoblastic or plasmablastic features. In immunocompromised patients, the frequency of EBV infection is much higher and approximates 60% to 70% of cases (see Chapters 24 and 25).

Association with hepatitis C is seen in 10% of immunocompetent DLBCL patients, but the frequency is much higher in

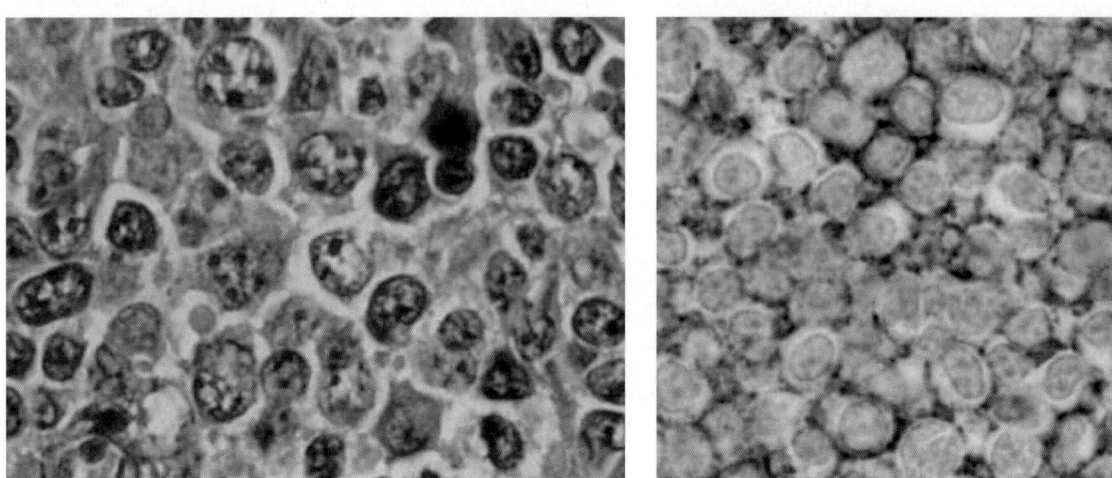

A

B

FIGURE 23.13. Immunohistochemistry of DLBCL. A–F: Germinal center B-cell–like (GCB) molecular subtype. **A:** The lymphoma cells exhibit typical centroblastic morphology. **B:** Strong staining for CD10.

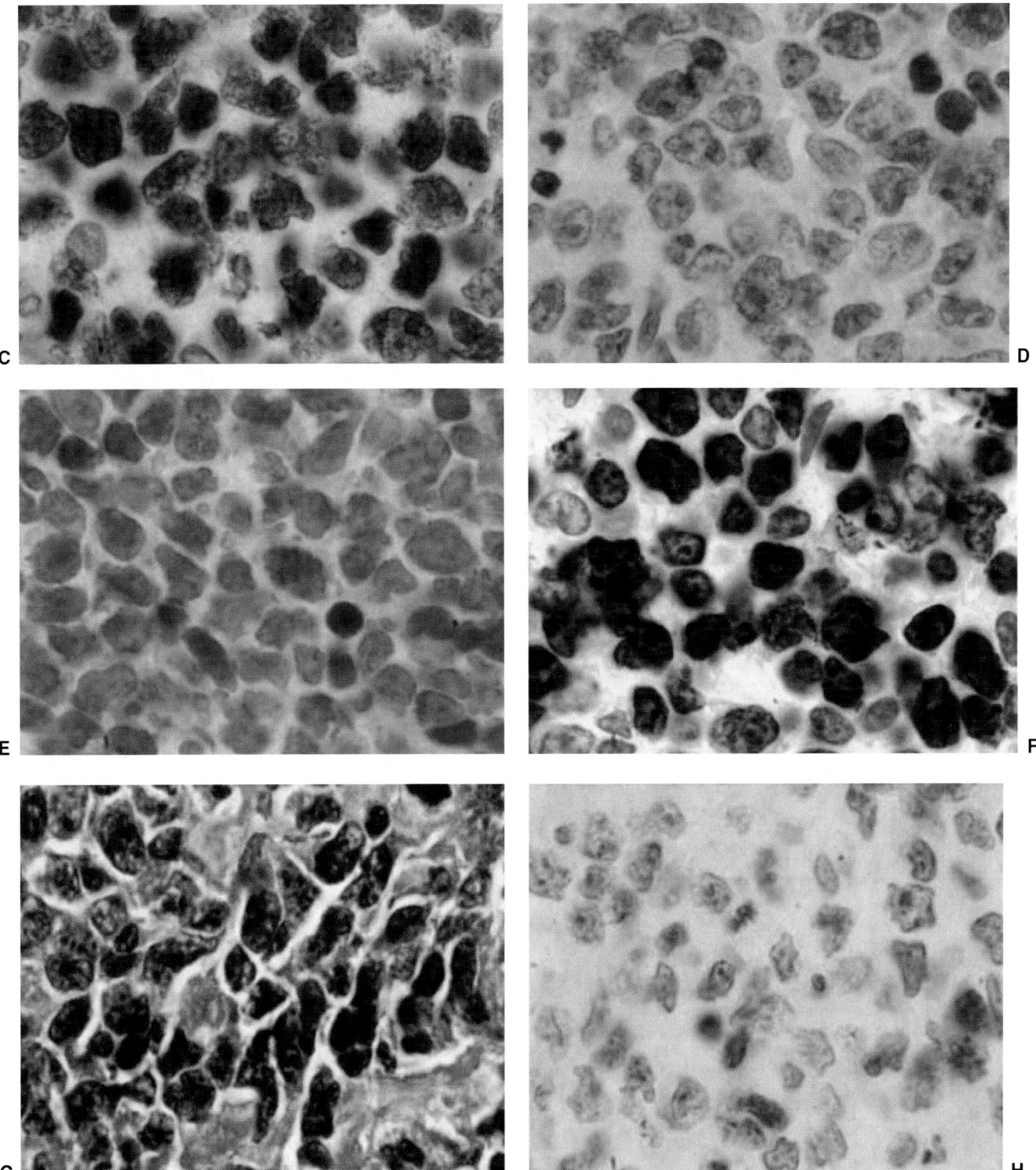

FIGURE 23.13. *(Continued)* **C:** Strong staining for Bcl-6. **D,E:** The lymphoma cells are not immunoreactive for MUM-1 and FOXP-1. **F:** The neoplastic cells show a high Ki-67 index of 70% to 80%. **G–L:** ABC-like or non-GCB molecular subtype. **G:** The lymphoma cells show cleaved or anaplastic morphology and strong cell membrane staining for CD20 (not shown). **H,I:** The lymphoma cells are not immunoreactive for CD10 **(H)** and Bcl-6 **(I)**, but the scattered reactive small T lymphocytes are highlighted by the immunostains.

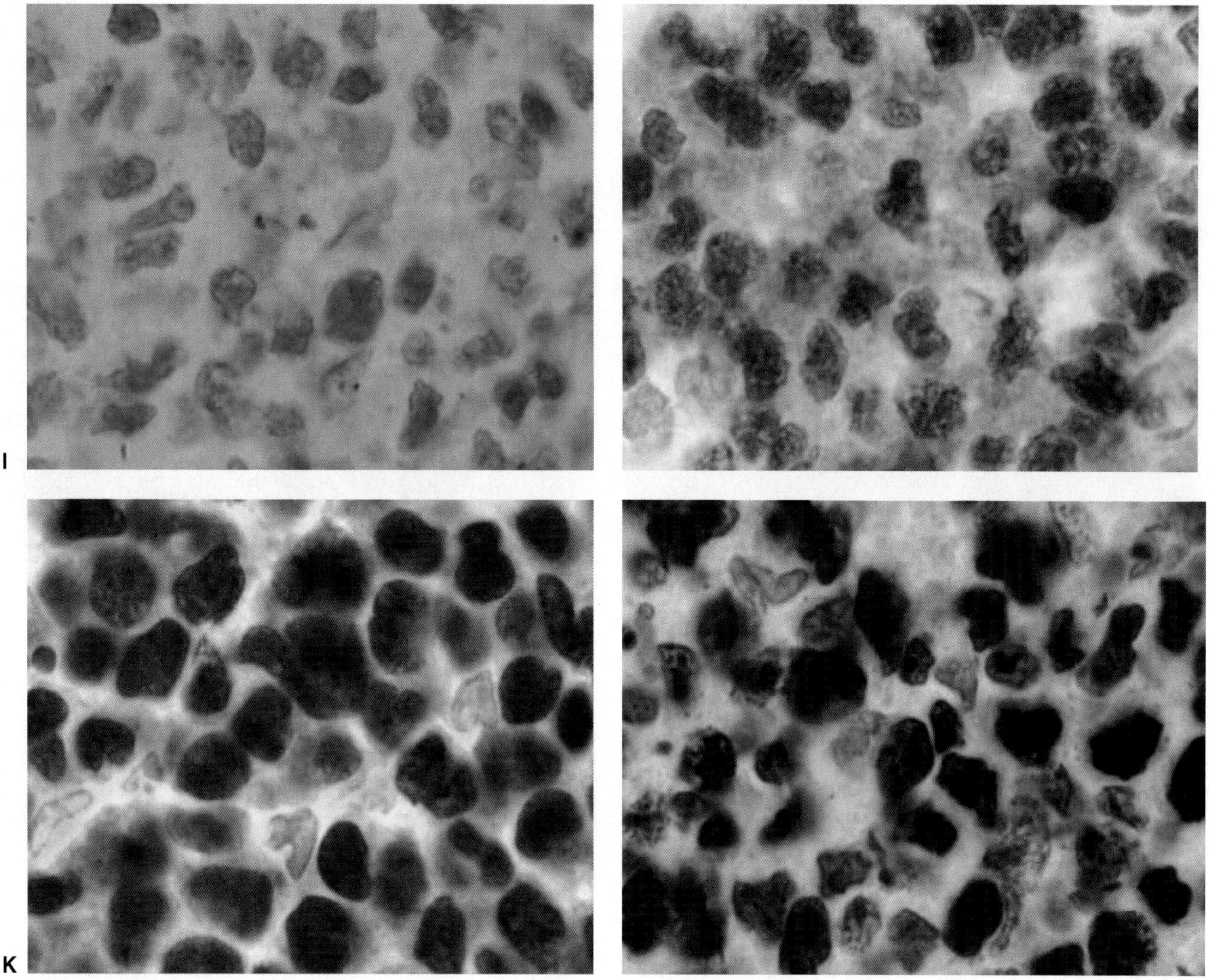

FIGURE 23.13. *(Continued)* **J,K:** In this case, most lymphoma cells show nuclear staining for MUM-1 **(J)** and FOXP-1 **(K)**. **L:** The neoplastic cells show a high proliferation index of 80% to 90% by Ki-67 expression.

some European countries, suggesting that there are geographical differences. Hepatitis B virus (HBV) infection impacts about 350 million people with the highest rates seen in Asia and Africa. An association between HBV infection and NHL has been reported with conflicting results. Epidemiologic studies suggest a positive association between HBV infection and DLBCL, FL, and MZL, but no association with CLL/SLL and T-cell lymphomas. Fulminant hepatitis caused by HBV has emerged as a serious clinical problem due to reactivation of HBV infection in some DLBCL patients. Molecular mechanisms responsible for lymphomagenesis in chronic HBV patients remain to be investigated.

Several immunophenotyping algorithms have been developed to distinguish GCB and non-GCB cases of DLBCL. The Hans algorithm is the most frequently used and was established using CHOP-treated cases, but has approximately 80% correlation with GEP-defined subtypes. More recently reported algorithms, such as Choi, Visco/Young, and Tally methods, show a higher concordance with GEP results (23–26) (Fig. 23.15; Table 23.3).

To simulate the GEP signature, a biologic prognostic model based on immunohistochemistry that incorporates the cell of origin and surrogates for the stromal-1 and stromal-2 signatures is proposed. The results are highly predictive of overall survival and event-free survival, and could be used with the

International Prognostic Index (IPI) to stratify patients for novel or risk-adapted therapies (27).

COMPARATIVE GENOMIC HYBRIDIZATION

In general, conventional cytogenetic studies have not been performed on lymphomas with the same frequency as they have been on acute leukemias. As a result, other cytogenetic approaches that can be applied to routinely processed tissue have been used, such as comparative genomic hybridization (CGH), fluorescence *in situ* hybridization (FISH), and spectral karyotyping (SKY) to obtain genetic information (28). These studies have found frequent gains involving chromosomes 1q, 2p, 3, 6p, 7, 8q, 9q, 11, 12, 13p, 16p, 18, 22q, and X; and losses in chromosomes 1p, 6q, 8p, and X (29). SKY has discovered new breakpoints and new translocations, such as t(3;14)(q21;q32), t(1;13)(p32;q14), t(1;7) (q21;q22), and t(6;8)(q11;q11) in DLBCL cases (30).

GCB-DLBCL shows frequent gains of 12q12, whereas ABC-DLBCL shows frequent trisomy 3, gains of 3q and 18q21-q22, and losses of 6q21-q22. CGH analysis has shown that gains involving chromosomal region 3p11-p12 are associated with a poor prognosis (31,32). In contrast, deletion of the *INK4α/ARF*

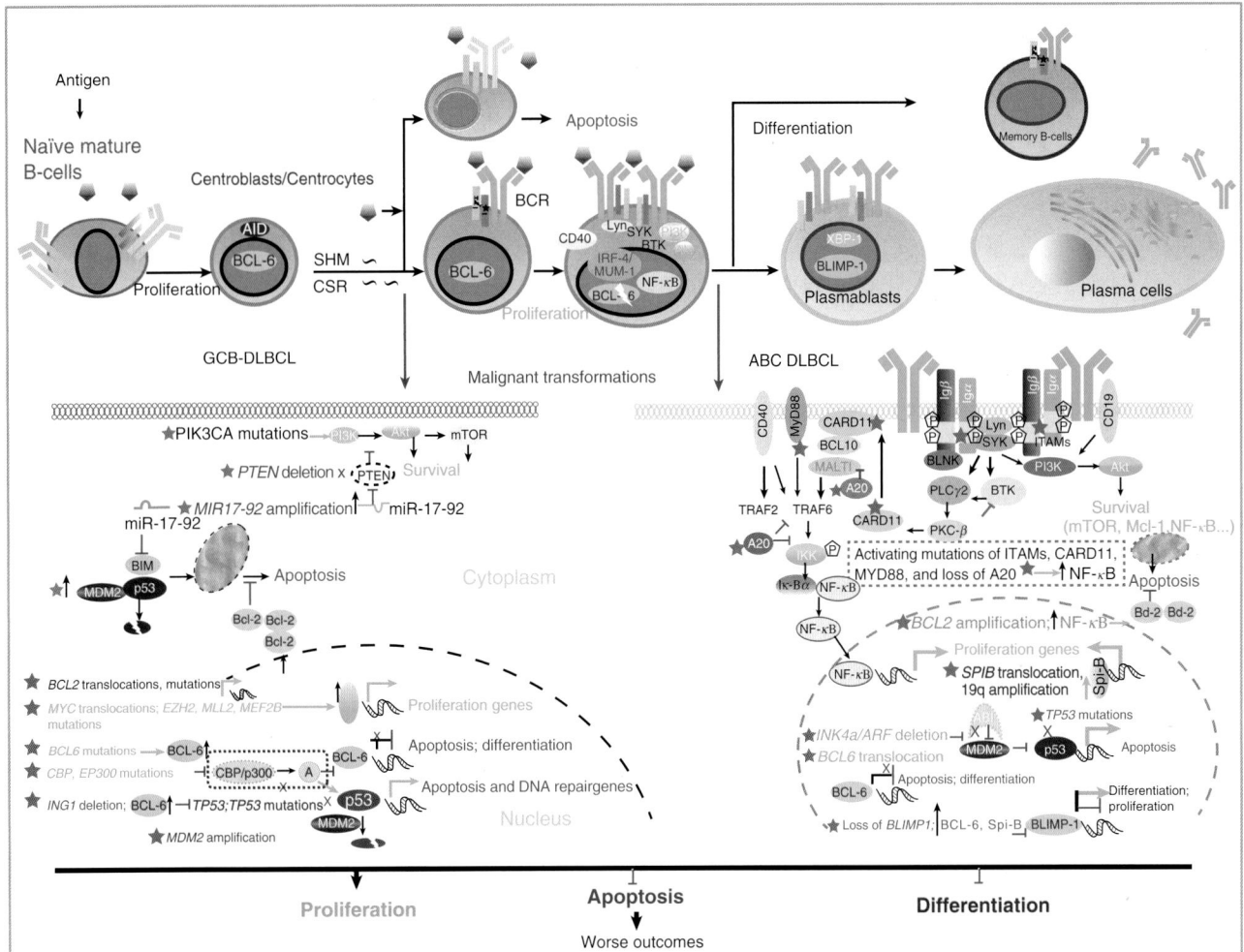

FIGURE 23.14. Molecular mechanisms of DLBCL pathogenesis. Illustration of various molecular pathways (indicated by *red stars*) involved in GCB-DLBCL and ABC-DLBCL that arise from different stages of B-cell development from centroblasts to plasma cells (during and after germinal center reaction). The positive and negative consequences of these genomic lesions are indicated by *green arrows* and red signs, respectively. AID/AICDA, activation-induced cytidine deaminase; BCL-6, B-cell lymphoma 6 protein; SHM, somatic hypermutation; CSR, class switch recombination; BCR, B-cell antigen receptor; SYK, spleen tyrosine kinase; BLNK, protein B-cell linker protein; ITAMs, immunoreceptor tyrosine–based activation motifs; BLIMP-1/PRDM-1, PR domain zinc finger protein 1.

tumor suppressor locus and trisomy 3 seem to occur almost exclusively in ABC-DLBCL and are associated with inferior outcome within this subtype. *FOXP1* is a potential oncogene in ABC-DLBCL that is up-regulated by trisomy 3 and is focally amplified.

In one study, CGH analysis showed 20 recurrent genetic lesions that impacted the clinical course of DLBCL patients. Loss of genomic material at 8p23.1 had the strongest impact on prognosis and was associated with additional aberrations, such as 17p– and 15q–. Unsupervised clustering identified five DLBCL clusters with distinct genetic profiles, clinical characteristics, and outcomes (33).

SPIB, which encodes an ETS family transcription factor on chromosome 19, was highly up-regulated and detected in 26% of ABC-DLBCLs, but in only 3% of GCB DLBCL and primary mediastinal large B-cell lymphoma (PMBCL). Inhibition of *SPIB* by RNA interference was toxic to ABC-DLBCL cell lines, suggesting that *SPIB* is an oncogene important to the pathogenesis of ABC-DLBCL (34).

Gains affecting chromosome 7 are common in DLBCL, especially in the GCB subgroup. Several miRNAs, including mir-96, mir-182, mir-589, and mir-25, are significantly up-regulated in 7q+ DLBCL. Amplification of the oncogenic mir-17-92 microRNA cluster and deletion of the tumor suppressor *PTEN* are recurrent in GCB-DLBCL, and are not present in ABC-DLBCL.

Deletions at 13q14.3 occur in 13% of DLBCLs and might contribute to DLBCL pathogenesis by two mechanisms: deregulating cell-cycle control mainly due to *RB1* loss and contributing to immune escape, as a result of FAS downregulation (35).

In PMLBCL, a unique profile of chromosomal abnormalities is found, including frequent gains of chromosomes 2p, 9p, 7q, 9q, 12q, Xq, and loss of chromosome 1p. Gains in 9p include *JAK2, PDL1, PDL2,* and *SMARCA2* genes, whereas gains in 2p are associated with amplification of the *REL* protooncogene. Rearrangements of *CIITA* gene at chromosome 16p13 have been found in 38% of PMLBCLs; this abnormality results in down-regulation of human leukocyte antigen (HLA) class II expression and reduced tumor cell immunogenicity.

MOLECULAR CHARACTERISTICS

In DLBCL, the immunoglobulin heavy (*IgH*) and light chain genes (*IgK* and *IgL*) are rearranged. In most cases, the immunoglobulin genes have hypermutated variable regions, evidence of passing through the germinal center. Some cases may show ongoing somatic mutations (1–5,36). The TCR genes are usually in the germline configuration.

A. Visco/Young algorithm (four markers)

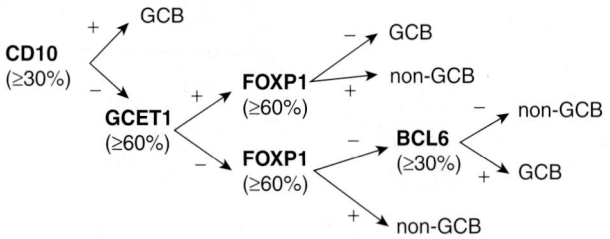

B. Visco/Young algorithm (three markers)

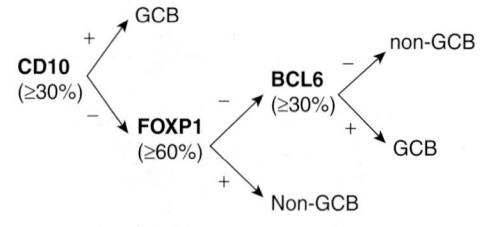

C. Hans algorithm (three markers)

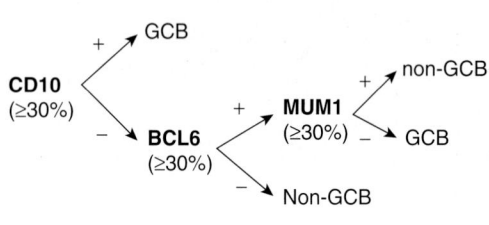

D. Choi algorithm (five markers)

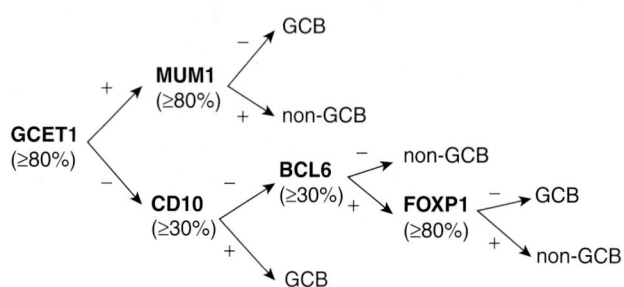

E. Muris algorithm (three markers)

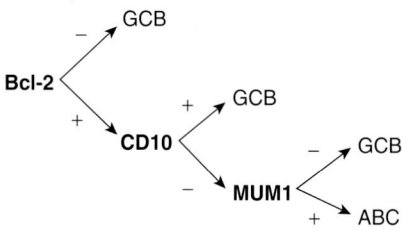

F. Tally algorithm (five markers)

GCB	ABC
CD10	MUM1
GCET1	FOXP1

→ **GCB > ABC** or **ABC > GCB**

If GCB = ABC

LMO2 > 30% → **GCB**
LMO2 < 30% → **ABC**

FIGURE 23.15. Molecular classification of DLBCL by immunophenotyping algorithms (A–F).

t(14;18)(q32;q21), resulting in *BCL2* rearrangement, is a genetic hallmark of FL, and also is present in 20% to 25% of DLBCLs (37). These cases arise *de novo*, may transform from FL, or have a coexisting occult or clinical history of former FL. The t(14;18)(q32;q21) is found in approximately 30% of GCB-DLBCL. The t(14;18) or Bcl-2 expression may predict significantly poorer survival in patients with GCB-DLBCL treated with R-CHOP. *BCL2* translocation correlates with *REL* amplification, which is also characteristically seen in the GCB subgroup (38–40). Additional

genetic alterations, such as *TP53* mutation, *MYC* and *BCL6* aberrations, as well as epigenetic abnormalities, are secondary events required for GCB-DLBCL development (Fig. 23.14). The t(14;18)(q32;q21) is found in <5% of ABC-DLBCsL. *BCL2* gene amplification occurs in 20% of ABC-DLBCLs.

The *BCL6* gene plays an important role in *de novo* DLBCL pathogenesis. *BCL6* (3q27) rearrangement has been reported in 30% to 40% of DLBCLs (41,42). The translocation partner can be *IgH*, in the form of t(3;14)(q27;q32), but many other

Table 23.3 MOLECULAR CLASSIFICATION OF DLBCL BY GEP AND IMMUNOPHENOTYPING ALGORITHMS—CONCORDANCE BETWEEN GEP ANALYSIS AND EACH OF THE IMMUNOPHENOTYPING ALGORITHMS

Algorithms	GEP Classification	Concordance (%)	Sensitivity (%)	Specificity (%)	PPV (%)	NPV (%)	EFS-HR	OS-HR
Visco-Young	GCB = 231	92.6	93	92	93	92	1.9	1.8
	ABC = 200		92	93	92	93		
Hans	GCB = 87	86	82	90	90	82	2.5	2.2
	ABC = 82		90	82	82	90		
Choi	GCB = 87	87	85	89	89	85	2.5	2.4
	ABC = 82		89	85	85	89		
Muris	GCB = 85	77	99	54	69	98	3.4	3.2
	ABC = 82		54	99	98	69		
Tally	GCB = 87	93	86	99	99	87	2.5	2.2
	ABC = 83		99	86	87	99		
Nyman	GCB = 87	81	67	95	94	73	1.7	1.6
	ABC = 83		95	67	73	94		

partners may be involved. *BCL6* somatic mutations have been reported in 30% to 70% of DLBCLs and are independent of *BCL6* gene rearrangement. However, the frequency of *BCL6* somatic mutations, similar to *TP53* mutations, is highly variable among different ethnic populations, suggesting that *BCL6* mutations may play different roles in DLBCL pathogenesis (43–45).

Bcl-6 protein is a master regulator of the GCB cell program and is considered a unique marker for B cells at the GC stage of differentiation. However, in DLBCL, Bcl-6 is also often expressed in the post–GC stage of differentiation. Therefore, it is a less specific marker for GCB-DLBCL. *In vitro* and animal model studies have demonstrated that aberrant Bcl-6 protein expression in B cells associated with *BCL6* translocation can give rise to DLBCL, probably through inhibition of B-cell differentiation and repression of other important genes such as *TP53* (43–45).

MYC (8q24) rearrangement, a genetic hallmark of Burkitt lymphoma, is found in approximately 5% to 8% of DLBCL cases overall, and is more common in highly proliferative DLBCL

(46,47). *MYC* rearrangement is often a part of complex cytogenetic aberrations and likely represents a secondary abnormality. The translocation partner can be one of the immunoglobulin genes or a nonimmunoglobulin gene (48) (Fig. 23.16).

TP53 dysfunction is common in many types of lymphoma. In DLBCL, *TP53* mutations are found in approximately 20% and deletion of *TP53* in 8% of cases. By comparison, p53 protein expression is observed in approximately 40% of DLBCL. No direct correlation is observed between the protein expression and genetic aberrations (49). *TP53* dysfunction plays a critical role in GCB-DLBCL pathogenesis and is often present in association with high-grade transformation from an underlying low-grade lymphoma. The prognostic effect of *TP53* mutation is more prominent in patients with mutations in the DNA-binding domains (50–53), specially those mutations in the loop-sheet-helix and L3 motifs in the DNA-binding domain that are thought to be the most critical. In contrast, *TP53* deletion and loss of heterozygosity does not confer worse survival.

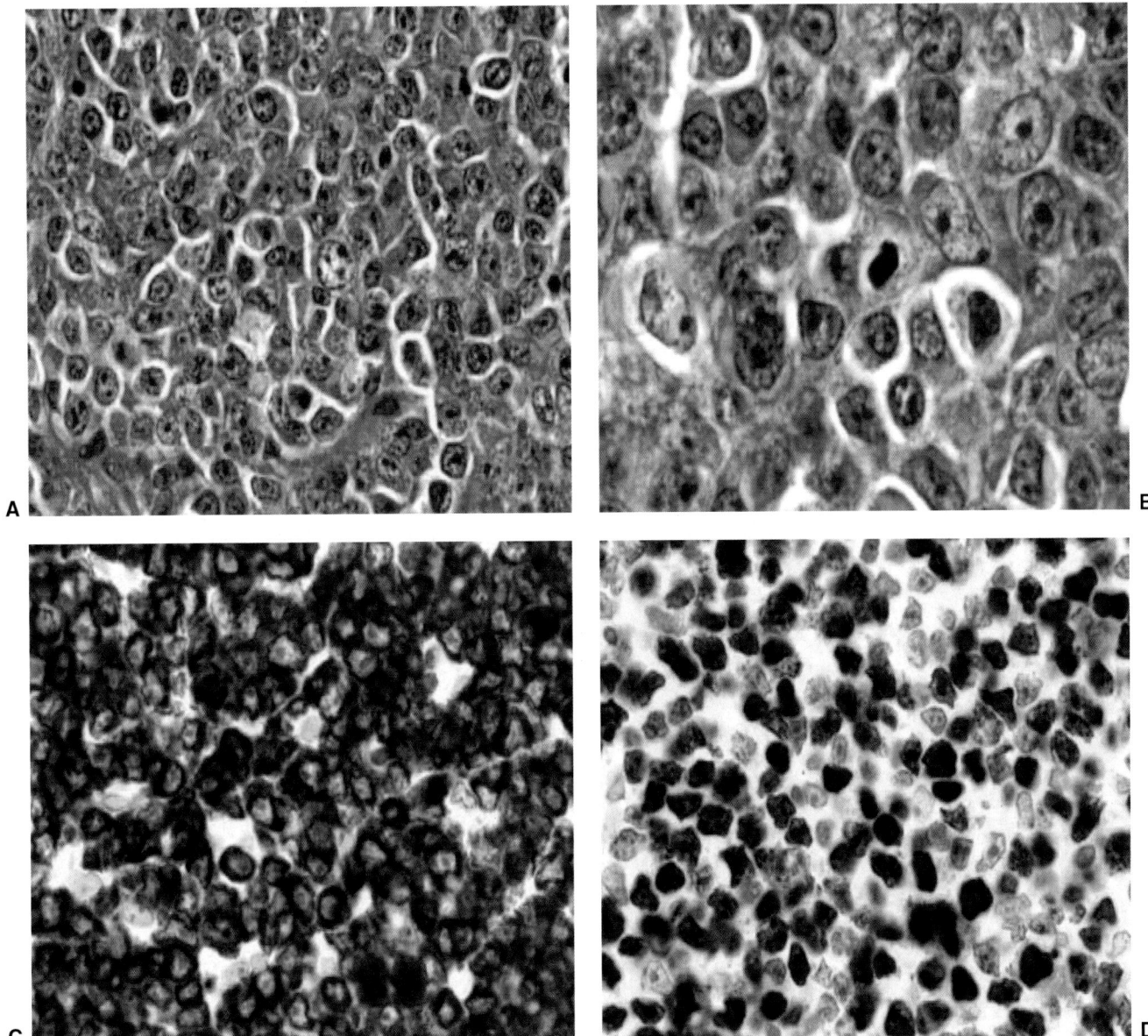

FIGURE 23.16. DLBCL, *MYC* and *BCL2* double-hit. A–D: The lymphoma cells in this case were associated with a typical MYC translocation t(8;14). The neoplastic cells were clonal with a CD45+, CD20+, PAX-5+, CD10+, and Bcl-2+ (**C**), MUM-1−, Bcl-6+ immunophenotype, and a high proliferation index of 70% to 80% by Ki-67 expression (**D**).

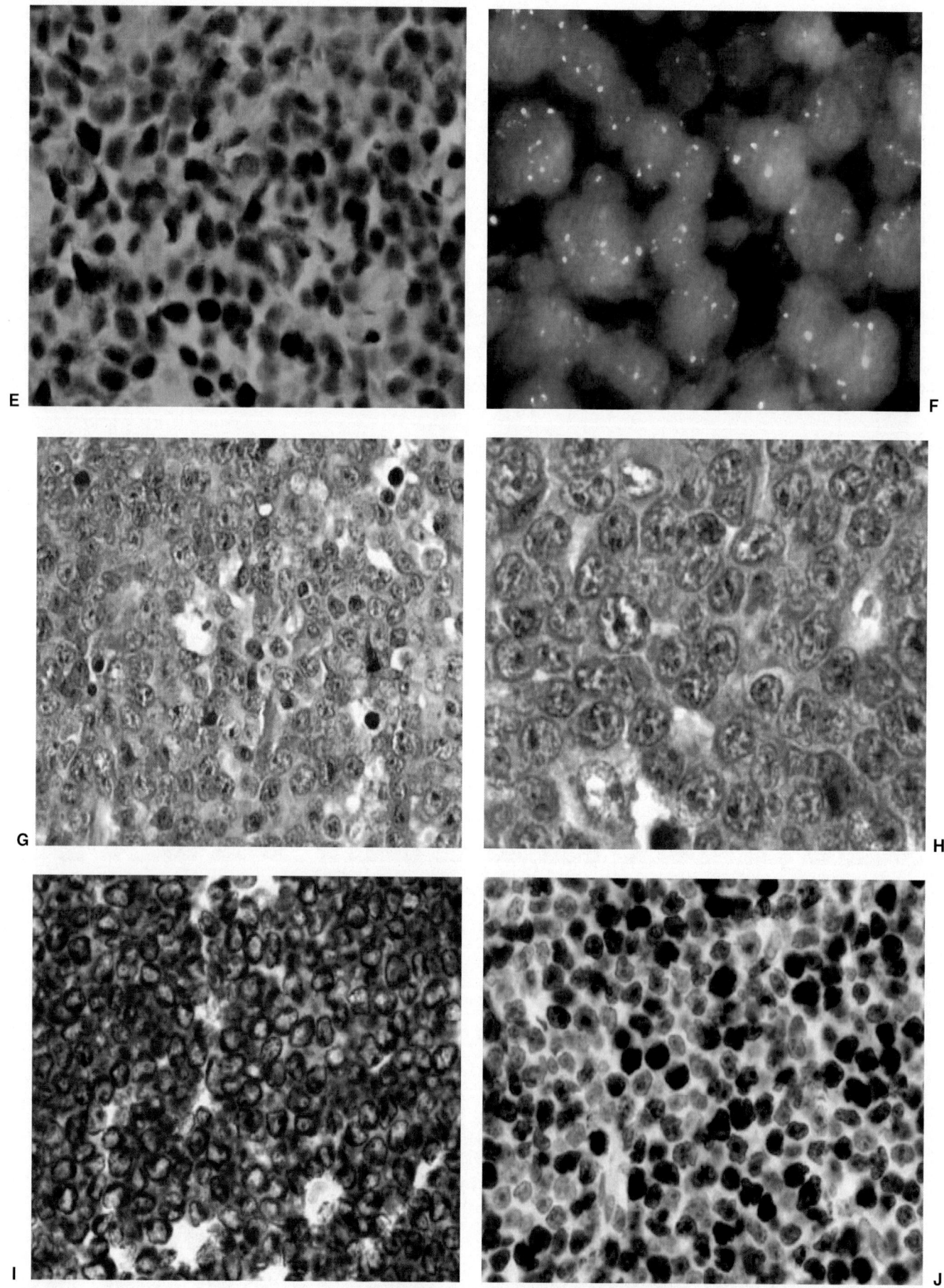

FIGURE 23.16. *(Continued)* **E,F:** The lymphoma cells show 100% positivity for Myc **(E)** by immunostain, and *MYC* translocation t(8;14). **G–J,** The lymphoma cells in this case were associated with alternative *MYC* translocation t(8;22). The neoplastic cells showed a CD45+, CD20+, Pax-5+, CD10+, and Bcl-2+ **(G)**, MUM-1−, Bcl-6+ immunophenotype, and a high proliferation index of 70% to 80% by Ki-67 expression **(H).**

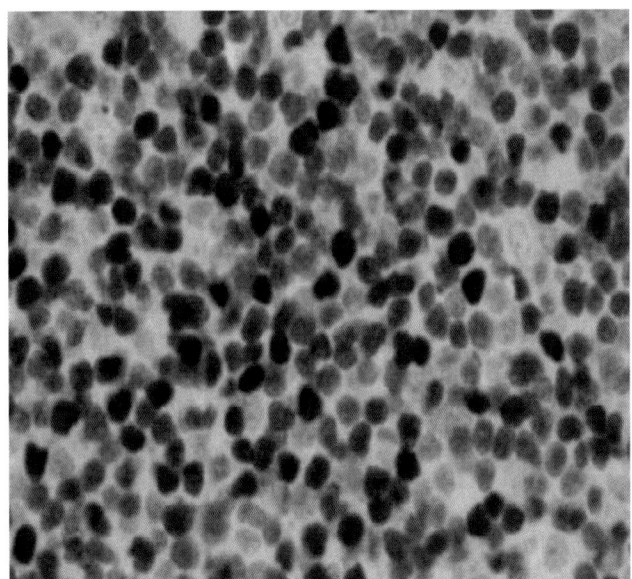
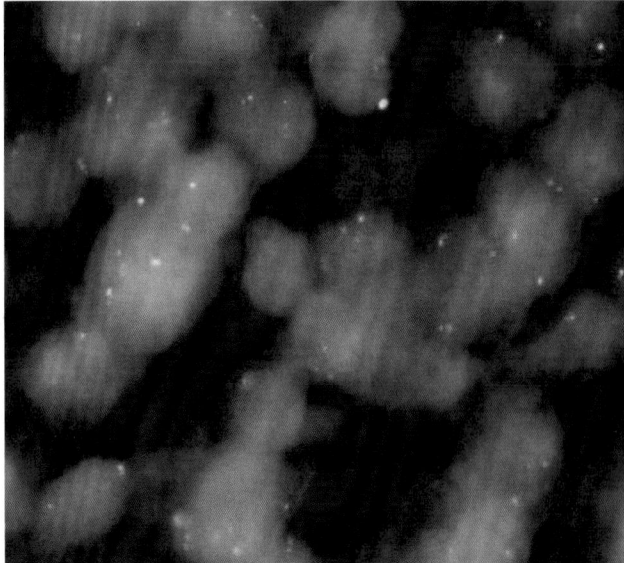

K

L

FIGURE 23.16. *(Continued)* **K,L:** The lymphoma cells show 95% positivity for Myc by immunostain **(K)**, and alternative *MYC* translocation by FISH **(L)**. t(8;22).

Recently, whole genome sequencing analysis of DLBCL has shown a number of recurrent gene mutations that involve a variety of cellular pathways (54). The pattern of gene mutations differs in the GCB and ABC subgroups. In GCB-DLBCL, many genes that regulate histone modification, such as *EZH2, MLL2,* and *MEF2B,* are mutated (55,56). *CREBBP/EP300* may also cause protein acetylation in addition to histone acetylation. *BCL2* and *MYC* translocations are predominantly seen in GCB-DLBCL. Hypermutations of some protooncogenes, including *PIM1, MYC, RhoH/TTF (ARHH),* and *PAX5,* have also been reported in DLBCL although with low frequency, and their presence may be associated with genomic instability. In ABC-DLBCL, specific mutations, such as *CARD11, CD79B, TNFAIP3 (A20),* and *MYD88,* are present in 10%, 20%, 25%, and 30% of cases, respectively, and result in activation of the NF-κB signaling pathway and dysfunction of the B-cell receptor (BCR) pathway. No mutations are identified in the BTK gene. Other signaling pathways, such as PI3K and MAPK pathways, may also be deregulated by *CARD11* and *CD79B* mutations, similar to Janus kinase 2 (JAK2)–signal transducers and activators of transcription (STAT) pathway regulation by *MYD88* mutations (7,55,56).

The JAK-STAT pathway plays an important role in hematologic malignancies. JAKs are important components of the receptor-mediated signal transduction of growth factors, hormones, and cytokines in association with a phosphorylated JAK as a binding ligand for STAT. In turn, STAT becomes phosphorylated, dimerizes, and subsequently migrates to the nucleus to induce transcription of target genes. *STAT* is regulated by protein inhibitors of activated STAT (PIAS), phosphotyrosine phosphatases, and suppressors of cytokine signaling (SOCS). *STAT3* and particularly *STAT5* are the preferred downstream targets of phosphorylated JAK2. Both *STAT3* and *STAT5* have been shown to be of functional importance in lymphomas. Constitutive STAT3 activation is an important prognostic factor in ABC-DLBCL. The JAK2-STAT pathways seem to be of particular oncogenic significance in PMBCL, as they are targeted by multiple genetic aberrations (JAK2 locus gains, point mutations, and deletions of SOCS1).

Mutations and translocations of the *JAK2* gene, mapped at 9p24, lead to constitutive activation of Jak2 and its downstream targets, including *STAT5* and *STAT6* (57). Mutations of *JAK2, STAT3, STAT5,* and *STAT6* are only seen in 1% to 3% of

DLBCL patients (58,59). However, the dysfunctional JAK-STAT pathway has been seen in a significant proportion of DLBCLs as manifested by the higher-level expression of the JAK/STAT pathway–related serum cytokines (i.e., IL-6, IL-10, epidermal growth factor, and IL-2) (60).

EZH2, CREBBP/EP300, PI3K, CD79a, and *PRDM1* are involved in DLBCL pathogenesis. *PRDM1,* a direct target of *BCL6,* is inactivated due to truncating mutations and/or biallelic 6q21-q22 deletions in 30% and 25% of ABC-DLBCL cases, resulting in disruption of terminal B-cell differentiation. In PMLBCL, rearrangements of the *CIITA* gene result in downregulation of HLA class II expression. Mutations of *STAT6* are seen in nearly 30% of PMBCLs in the DNA-binding domains, and this distribution of mutations correlates with *CIITA* gene rearrangements (61). Mutations of *SOCS1* are seen in 45% of PMLBCLs (62,63). The results suggest that the *STAT6* mutations and *CIITA* gene rearrangement represent a genetic signature of PMBCL, whereas they are rarely present in conventional DLBCL. Genetic and molecular features are compared among GCB-DLBCL, ABC-DLBCL, and PMLBCL in Table 23.4.

The tumor microenvironment is also thought to play an important role in the pathogenesis of DLBCL. Based on GEP analysis, a favorable stromal-1 signature is identified that reflects extracellular matrix deposition and infiltration of the lymphoma by macrophages. By contrast, an adverse stromal-2 signature is associated with a high blood vessel density or high vascular marker expression (64). Increased granzyme B-positive T cells, increased expression of integrin family members, decreased CD8+ T cells, decreased FOXP3-positive regulatory T cells, macrophage with CD68 or CD163 expression, and loss of HLA-DR or major histocompatibility complex (MHC) are associated with a poor outcome (65–68).

Some DLBCLs are transformed from a low-grade lymphoma: these constitute approximately 10% to 20% of DLBCLs (Fig. 23.6). Most DLBCLs that transform from FL harbor *BCL2* rearrangement t(14;18)(q32;q21) with strong Bcl-2 protein expression. High cyclin D3 expression, with t(6;14)(p21;q32), has been found to be present in transformation of MALT lymphoma into DLBCL (69). Other genetic alterations, such as *TP53* mutation, del p14/16, *MYC,* or *BCL6* aberrations, as well as mir-17-92 gain/amplification, have been reported to play critical roles during DLBCL transformation or progression (70).

Table 23.4	GENETIC, MOLECULAR AND CLINICAL FEATURES IN DLBCL: GCB, ABC, AND PMLBCL		
Features	**GCB**	**ABC**	**PMLBCL**
Frequency	~50%	~45%	~5%
Disease features	Late relapse	Early relapse	Mediastinal, ~35 y women
5-year survival	~60%	30%–40%	~70%
Centroblastic/immunoblastic	20/1	2/1	20/1
IgH mutation and SHM	Ongoing	No	No
Oncogenic activation	BCL2 translocation	NF-κB activation	NF-κB activation
Translocations	• BCL2, 35%–45% • MYC, 15%	• BCL6 (3q27), 24%–35%	• CIITA (MHC2TA), 38%
Amplifications	• MDM2, 45% • CDK2, CDK4(12q12), 20% • c-Rel (2p), 15% • mir 17–92, 12%–15%	• BCL2 (18q21-22), 30%–35% • FOXP1 (3q) gain, 26% • Trisomy 3, 26% • SPIB (19q), 25% • 9p gain, 6% • 12q12, 5%	• JMJD2C, 45% • JAK2 (9p) gain, 35% • c-Rel (2p), BCL11A, 20% • 3q gain, 5% • 12q12, 5%
Deletions	• PTEN (10q23), 10%–15% • ING1, 10% • IRF4, 5%	• TNFAIP3 (A20), 30% • PRDM1 (BLIMP1, 6q21-22), 25% • CDKN2A (INK4A/ARF, 9p), 20%–30%	No
Mutations	• BCL6, 75% • BCL2, 40% • CREBBP/EP300, 39% • MLL2, 30% • TP53, 21% • EZH2, 20% • MEF2B, 9% • PI3K, 8%	• MYD88, 30% • PRDM1 (BLIMP1), 30% • TNFAIP3, 25% • TP53, 24% • CD79B, 20% • BCL6, 20% • CARD11, 10%	• SOCS1, 45% • STAT6, 20%
Unique protein biomarkers	CD10, GCET1, GCET2, BCL6, LMO2	MUM1/IRF4, Bcl-2, FOXP1, MALT1, XBP1, CCND2, CCNE	REL, MAL, TRAF1, FIG1

PMLBCL, primary mediastinal large B-cell lymphoma; A20 (TNFAIP3), tumor necrosis factor, alpha-induced protein 3; BCL2, B-cell CLL/lymphoma 2; BCL6, B-cell CLL/lymphoma 6; CARD11, caspase recruitment domain family, member 11; CDK2 and CDK4, cyclin-dependent kinase 2 and 4; CDKN2A/ARF/p16, cyclin-dependent kinase inhibitor 2A (melanoma, p16, inhibits CDK4); CREBBP/EP300, CREB binding protein; c-Rel, v-*rel* reticuloendotheliosis viral oncogene homolog (avian); EZH2, enhancer of zeste homolog 2 (*Drosophila*); FOXP1, forkhead box P1; GCET1 and GCET2, germinal center expressed transcript 1 and 2; JAK2, Janus kinase 2; ING1, inhibitor of growth family, member; IRF4, interferon regulatory factor 4; LMO2, LIM domain only 2 (rhombotin-like 1); MAL, *mal*, T-cell differentiation protein; MDM2, *Mdm2* p53 binding protein homolog; MEF2B, myocyte enhancer factor 2B; mir 17–92, microRNA 17–92; MLL2, myeloid/lymphoid or mixed-lineage leukemia 2; MUM1, melanoma-associated antigen (mutated); Myc, myelocytomatosis viral oncogene homolog; PI3K, phosphoinositide-3-kinase; PRDM1/BLIMP1, PR domain containing 1, with ZNF domain; PTEN, phosphatase and tensin homolog; SOCS1, suppressor of cytokine signaling 1; SPIB, Spi-B transcription factor (Spi-1/PU.1 related); TP53, tumor protein p53; TRAF1, TNF receptor-associated factor 1.

CLINICAL COURSE AND PROGNOSTIC ASSESSMENT

Although complete remission can be achieved in approximately 60% of patients, many patients relapse, or are refractory to current treatment regimens, reflecting variable underlying molecular, pathologic, and genetic abnormalities. The most common and major adverse prognostic factors reported in DLBCL are summarized in Figure 23.17.

Clinical

The IPI is a system based on five clinical and laboratory parameters that is helpful for predicting clinical outcome (71). A high IPI score, 4 to 5, is associated with poor survival. The 5-year overall survival in DLBCL patients with a high IPI score is 26%, compared with 73% in the low IPI (score 0 to 1), and 47% in intermediate IPI (score 2 to 3) groups. In patients >60 years old, an age-adjusted IPI is calculated from three unfavorable variables, including poor performance status, advanced Ann Arbor stage, and high serum lactate dehydrogenase (LDH). In the era of R-CHOP chemotherapy, a revised IPI score has been shown to provide a better prediction of outcome (72). However, as helpful as the IPI is, it remains an indirect assessment and a surrogate for the biologic features of DLBCL.

Morphologic

Several studies have shown that patients with immunoblastic, anaplastic, or plasmablastic variants of DLBCL demonstrate a worse outcome in comparison to patients with typical centroblastic DLBCL, but the results are not consistent among these studies (4,73).

Patients with DLBCL can have bone marrow involvement by DLBCL (concordant histology) or low-grade B-cell lymphoma (discordant histology). The latter group has a survival similar to patients without bone marrow disease (74). Concordant bone marrow infiltration is associated with higher serum LDH, a lower remission rate, and a higher progression rate.

Immunohistochemical

Many older studies conducted in the era of CHOP therapy showed that expression of Bcl-2 and CD44 predicted poorer survival. The lack of expression of the GC markers, CD10 and Bcl-6, also showed a similar poor survival tendency. These findings have been validated in the era of R-CHOP therapy in several studies showing that Bcl-2 protein expression and lack of CD10 or Bcl-6 expression are associated with poorer overall survival (16,23,75). Recent studies show that expression of LMO2 and GCET2 (HGAL) are associated with better survival. In contrast, expression of post-GC markers, including IRF4/MUM-1 and FOXP-1, are poor prognostic factors (23,76).

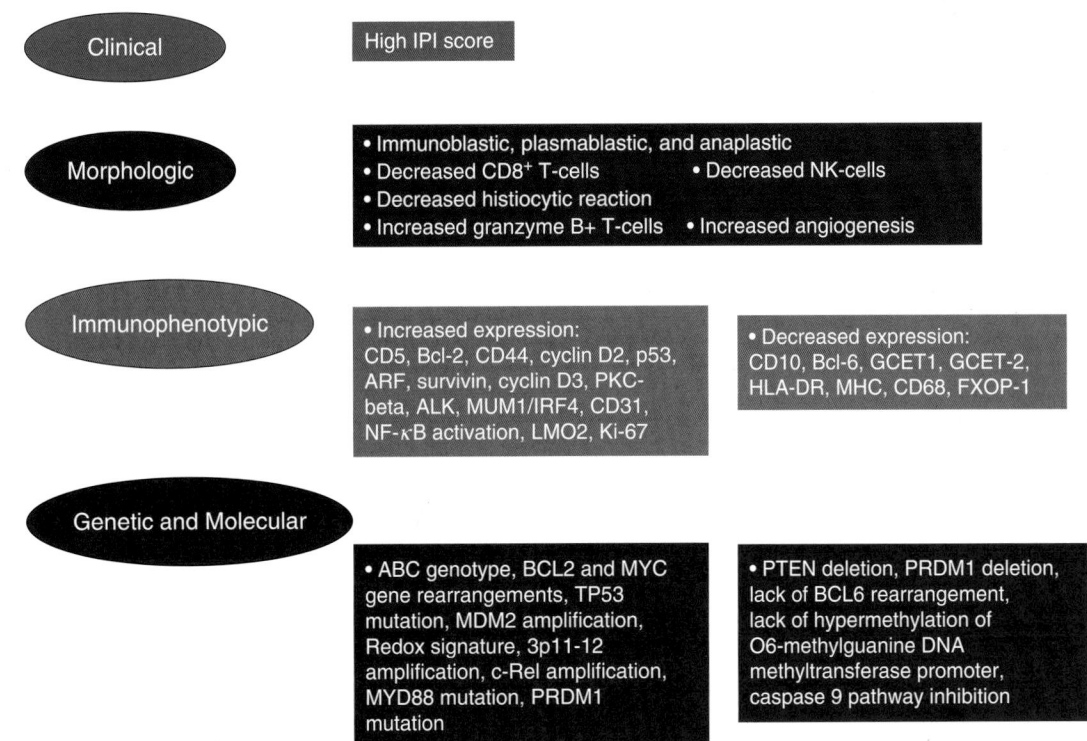

FIGURE 23.17. Adverse prognostic features in patients with DLBCL.

The prognostic significance of the proliferation index, most often assessed by Ki-67 immunohistochemical analysis, is inconsistent in the literature. Some groups reported that a high proliferation index, 60% to 80%, is associated with a worse prognosis, whereas other studies showed opposite results (21,77–79). CD5 expression in DLBCL has been associated with more aggressive disease and poorer survival. Expression of EBV has been seen in a small subset of DLBCL, usually the immunoblastic variant, and may be associated with a poorer outcome.

Expression of B-cell signaling and oncogenic pathway components, such as protein kinase C-β, anaplastic lymphoma kinase (ALK), survivin, caspase 9 inhibition profile, and PIM1, are associated with a worse clinical outcome. The isotype of the BCR expressed by the tumor cells correlates with the molecular subtype and survival. Many GCB-DLBCL cases express a secondary isotype of IgG or IgA, whereas ABC-DLBCL cases express a primary isotype of IgM. A worse outcome and shorter overall survival are found in DLBCL patients with IgM expression, suggesting that the isotype of the BCR is a reliable indicator for the GCB and ABC subtype classification, and that the conservation of IgM is required for ABC-DLBCL lymphomagenesis (80–82).

Expression of cell-cycle regulators, such as cyclin D2 and cyclin D3, has been correlated with a worse prognosis. Activation of NF-κB pathway components, such as p50, p52, p65, and Rel-B, are frequently seen in ABC-DLBCL and are associated with a worse prognosis (83–86).

The JAK-STAT pathway is important in lymphomagenesis and a dysfunctional JAK-STAT pathway has been seen in a significant proportion of DLBCLs. Expression of Jak2, Stat3 and Stat5 has been correlated with a worse prognosis in ABC-DLBCL patients despite rarity of activation mutations in the STAT family genes (60,61).

Expression of p53 protein has been reported to predict for poorer survival, but results are inconsistent. Our recent study reported that immunohistochemical analysis showing >50% cells expressing p53 protein is a useful surrogate and can stratify patients with significantly different prognoses. MDM2 expression does not predict an adverse clinical outcome in DLBCL patients with wild-type p53, but predicts for significantly poorer survival in patients with mutated p53, suggesting that concurrent evaluation of MDM2 and p53 expression is essential to assess their prognostic significance in DLBCL patients. *MDM2* amplification and *MDM2* SNP309 polymorphism do not correlate with survival. Expression of *ARF (P14)* is associated with a more aggressive clinical course, particularly in patients with genetic defects in *TP53, CDKN2A*, and *CDKN1B*, likely representing dysfunction of the cell-cycle regulatory pathways (87).

Coexpression of Myc/Bcl-2 predicts inferior survival and occurs more frequently in ABC-DLBCL patients treated with R-CHOP (88–90). Patients with ABC and GCB-DLBCL without Myc/Bcl-2 coexpression have a similar prognosis. Similarly, ABC-DLBCL and GCB-DLBCL patients with Myc/Bcl-2 coexpression have a similar prognosis. Consistent with the notion that the prognostic difference between the two subtypes was attributable to MYC$^+$/BCL2$^+$ cases, DLBCL patients with Myc/Bcl-2 coexpression demonstrate a signature of marked downregulation of genes encoding proteins involving extracellular matrix deposition/remodeling and cell adhesion, as well as upregulation of proliferation-associated genes. Myc/Bcl-2 coexpression is associated with high-risk gene signatures in DLBCL and an aggressive clinical course and contributes to the overall inferior prognosis of patients with ABC-DLBCL.

Molecular

The GCB group is associated with a better 5-year overall survival than the ABC group (73% vs. 40%) in patients treated with R-CHOP (12,13). Other studies, in an attempt to simplify GEP analysis, have shown that the expression profile of 17 selected genes and subsequently 6 genes (*LMO2, BCL6, FN1, CCND2, SCYA3, BCL2*) can predict survival in CHOP-treated patients (39,91). A recent study proposes a two-gene model, based on LMO2 expressed by tumor cells and TNFRSF9 expressed by cells in the immune microenvironment, that predicts overall survival in DLBCL patients. A poor clinical outcome is also seen in patients exhibiting combined decrease in antioxidant defense enzyme expression and increase in thioredoxin system function (the redox signature score) (92,93).

In the CHOP era, *BCL2* rearrangement was reported to have no prognostic significance in most studies, but may have correlated with shorter disease-free survival or poor response to therapy. A recent study demonstrates that t(14;18), or Bcl-2 expression, is an independent predictor of poorer prognosis in patients with GCB-DLBCL. The GEP of the GCB cases with *BCL2* rearrangement reveals specific activation of NF-κB pathway subunits that are silent in the t(14;18)-negative GCB-DLBCL subgroup (94,95).

BCL6 rearrangement has been reported to have no prognostic significance in most but not all studies. However, patients with higher *BCL6* mRNA or protein expression had a significantly better overall survival (96,97). *BCL6* mutations were detected in 61% of DLBCL cases, with a significantly higher frequency in the GCB (70%) than in the ABC subgroup (44%). The presence of *BCL6* mutations was a significant predictor of favorable survival in DLBCL and in the ABC subgroup, but was of marginal significance in the GCB subgroup (98,99).

TP53 mutation predicts for a poorer outcome in DLBCL. Mutation of *TP53* is associated with a complete remission rate at 27% versus 76% for patients with wild-type *TP53* (49–52). Presence of *MYC* aberrations detectable by break-apart probe, *IGH/MYC* double-fusion probe, and combined break-apart and *IGH/MYC* double-fusion probes was associated with poorer clinical outcome compared to germline cases. The prognostic effect of *MYC* aberration applies primarily to GCB cases. The presence of concurrent *BCL2*, but not BCL6 aberrations, was prognostically additive to the adverse impact of *MYC* (38,46,47).

Several studies have shown that microRNA dysfunction contributes to the pathogenesis of DLBCL (100). Oncogenic mir-155 was found to target the bone morphogenetic protein-responsive transcriptional factor *SMAD5, SHIP1*, and other transcriptional regulatory genes, and its overexpression rendered DLBCL lines resistant to the treatment. mir-155 copy number is found to be 10- to 30-fold higher in DLBCL cells than in normal circulating B cells, and significantly higher levels of mir-155 are present in ABC-DLBCL than in GCB-DLBCL. Recent analysis of global microRNA expression signatures has shown that the microRNA expression signature supports GCB-DLBCL and ABC-DLBCL classification (101). However, expression of the oncogenic mir-155 has played no role on overall or event-free survival of DLBCL patients (102).

Integrated analysis of methylation and gene expression showed a core tumor necrosis factor-α signaling pathway as a principal differentially expressed gene network. Sixteen genes overlapped between the GCB versus ABC methylation and expression signatures, and encoded important proteins such as IKZF1. This concise gene set was an accurate predictor of GCB and ABC subtypes, and could serve as a useful biomarker for GCB- and ABC-DLBCL phenotypes (103).

Hypermethylation of the promoter of the DNA repair gene O⁶-methylguanine DNA methyltransferase, a major mechanism of resistance to alkylating drugs, is associated with a favorable prognosis (104). Loss of promoter methylation of *PRDM1β* was more frequently detected and might be linked to lymphoma progression (105). *p16(INK4a)* methylation has been associated with advanced disease stage and higher IPI, but the role of *p16(INK4a)* promoter methylation as a negative prognostic factor remains to be validated in DLBCL (106).

TREATMENT AND SURVIVAL

DLBCL is a clinically aggressive disease with rapid patient demise if not treated (1–6). Historically, DLBCL patients have been treated with standard CHOP chemotherapy (cyclophosphamide,

doxorubicin, vincristine, and prednisone), followed by radiotherapy in some patients who have a large tumor mass or in specific anatomic locations, such as skin, testis, and brain. Since 2001, rituximab (chimeric CD20 antibody) combined with CHOP has significantly improved overall and progression-free survival. The addition of rituximab particularly benefits older DLBCL patients and some GCB-DLBCL patients with Bcl-2 overexpression, but is less effective in DLBCL patients with *TP53* mutation, *BCL2* or *MYC* translocations, *Rel* gene amplification, and NF-κB activation (12,38,50–52,107,108).

Complete remission can be achieved in approximately 60% of patients, but nearly half of these patients will eventually develop recurrent disease with complex genetic abnormalities. The likelihood of recurrence largely relies on the complexity of the genetic aberrations in the original tumor. Thirty to forty percent of DLBCL patients may fail to achieve complete remission or only attain partial remission, and these patients usually die from the disease within 2 years. The 10-year overall, progression-free, event-free, and disease-free survival rates are 44%, 37%, 34%, and 64%, respectively. Several modified regimens by optimizing the dosing schedule and integrating new drugs, such as lenalidomide, carfilzomib, temsirolimus, histone deacetylase inhibitor, phosphatidylinositol-3-kinase inhibitor, and ibrutinib, have improved patient outcome, particularly in ABC-DLBCL patients (75,109).

DIFFERENTIAL DIAGNOSIS

The diagnosis in most cases of DLBCL is straightforward, and entities in the differential diagnosis can be excluded by ancillary studies. Several common diseases that show overlapping morphologic features with DLBCL are summarized in Table 23.5. A few of these entities are briefly discussed here.

Burkitt lymphoma is a diffuse lymphoma composed of intermediate-sized cells that can have a starry sky pattern and abundant mitotic figures and apoptosis, thereby mimicking high-grade DLBCL (110). In Burkitt lymphoma, the cells are more monotonous with moderate highly basophilic vacuolated cytoplasm, stippled chromatin, clear cytoplasmic borders, and multiple small nucleoli. The Ki-67 index approximates 100% with the typical immunophenotype of CD10⁺, Bcl-2⁻, and Bcl-6⁺ (Fig. 23.18A). *MYC* rearrangement, a characteristic feature of Burkitt lymphoma, is uncommon in DLBCL (5% to 8%). In addition, the karyotype is usually simple in Burkitt lymphoma and more complex in DLBCL (46,110). The WHO defines borderline cases that are difficult to classify as "B-cell lymphoma, unclassifiable, with features intermediate between DLBCL and Burkitt lymphoma" (111) (see Chapter 24).

Mantle cell lymphoma (MCL), pleomorphic variant, contains large pleomorphic cells with irregular nuclei that can mimic DLBCL (112) (Fig. 23.18B). Usually focal evidence of classical MCL is also present, and CD5 and cyclin D1 are positive. Rare cases of DLBCL, approximately 2%, have been reported to be cyclin D1–positive, in association with extra copies of *CCND1*, but are negative for t(11;14) (112–115).

Anaplastic plasmacytoma can mimic DLBCL as this neoplasm has a diffuse pattern and is composed of large cells. The cells in plasmacytoma often have plasmacytoid features with eccentric nuclei, prominent central nucleoli, and an immunophenotype of plasma cells: cytoplasmic immunoglobulin⁺, CD38⁺, CD138⁺, CD20⁻, and CD45⁻.

Classical Hodgkin lymphoma (CHL), including lymphocyte-depleted and nodular sclerosis syncytial variant types, can show morphologic features simulating DLBCL (Fig. 23.18C). The presence of inflammatory cells, including eosinophils in the background, favors CHL. CHL generally has many bizarre RS variants with strong CD30⁺ and often also CD15⁺. Syncytial variant nodular sclerosis Hodgkin lymphoma usually shows

Table 23.5	DIFFERENTIAL DIAGNOSIS OF DLBCL			
Differential Diagnosis	**Pathologic and Histologic Findings to Support DLBCL Diagnosis**	**Accessory Studies to Support DLBCL Diagnosis**	**Pathologic and Histologic Findings to Support the Other Disease**	**Accessory Studies to Support the Other Disease**
Mantle cell lymphoma, pleomorphic variant	• Nucleoli usually prominent • Chromatin pattern is commonly vesicular, or coarsely dispersed	CD5+, 10% Cyclin D1+, ~2%	• Indistinct nucleoli, some cases may have small prominent nucleoli • Dispersed chromatin • Scanty cytoplasm • Eosinophilic epitheloid histiocytes • Hyalinized small vessels • Classic MCL areas are present	CD5+ Cyclin D1+
Paraimmunoblastic variant of CLL	Lymphoma cells are usually larger and heterogeneous	CD5+, ~10% CD10+, ~40% BCL2+, ~60% Ki-67+, 30%–90% (rare cases may reach ~100%)	• Paraimmunoblasts are medium-sized cells, and smaller than DLBCL • Background prolymphocytes and small lymphocytes are prominent	CD5+, ~95% CD23+, ~95%
Diffuse FL, blastoid type	• Nucleoli usually prominent • Chromatin pattern is commonly vesicular, or coarsely dispersed	CD10+, ~80% BCL2+, ~70% Ki-67+, 40%–90% (rare cases may reach ~100%)	• Follicular pattern • Indistinct nucleoli • Blastoid chromatin	CD21 or CD23+, ~95%, shows the dendritic network
Myeloid sarcoma	Cytoplasm of DLBCL cells is commonly amphophilic or basophilic rather than eosinophilic	CD20+, myeloperoxidase−	• Neoplastic myeloid cells are predominantly medium-sized and show blastic or dispersed chromatin feature • Cytoplasm often eosinophilic • Eosinophilic granules may be present • May have admixed differentiating myeloid cells	CD20−, myeloperoxidase+
Histiocytic sarcoma	Cytoplasm of DLBCL cells is commonly amphophilic or basophilic rather than eosinophilic	CD20+, CD68−, CD163−	Sarcoma cells are larger and more heterogeneous with abundant eosinophilic cytoplasm	CD20−, CD68+, CD163+
Classical Hodgkin lymphoma: syncytial variant of nodular sclerosis and lymphocyte-depleted variants	Lymphoma cells usually form large aggregates and clusters with relative uniform morphology	CD20+, monotypic immunoglobulin light chain+, CD30−/+, CD15−, Oct-2+, BOB.1+ EBV+ in ~4% immunocompetent *de novo* cases	Background inflammatory cells, eosinophils, plasma cells, and histiocytes are present	CD30+, CD15+/−, CD20− or heterogeneously CD20+ Oct-2−, BOB.1− EBV+, ~35%–40% cases
Extramedullary hematopoietic tumor	Lymphoma cells usually form large aggregates and clusters with relative uniform morphology	CD20+, myeloperoxidase−	• Large cells are merely megakaryocytes and not neoplastic cells • Heterogeneous composition of other normoblasts and differentiating myeloid cells	CD20−, myeloperoxidase+
Burkitt lymphoma	• Large- and medium-sized, often exhibit more nuclear variation and greater amount of cytoplasm • "Starry sky" pattern is uncommon and distribution is random • More common in elder adults	CD10+, ~40% Bcl-2+, ~60% Ki-67+, 30%–90% (rare cases may reach ~100%) *MYC* gene rearrangement, ~8% *BCL2* gene rearrangement, ~40% *BCL6* gene rearrangement, ~30%	• "Starry sky" pattern is typical • Lymphoma cells are medium-sized, monotonous • More common in children and young adults	CD10+, ~98% BCL2−, ~90% Ki-67+, ~100% *MYC* gene rearranged *BCL2* and *BCL6* genes not rearranged
Peripheral T-cell lymphoma	Lymphoma cells usually form large aggregates and clusters with amphophilic or basophilic cytoplasm	CD20+, CD3−	Admixture of large- and medium-sized cells with greater amount of clear or eosinophilic cytoplasm	CD3+, CD20−, CD30+, ALK+/− for ALCL
NK-cell lymphoma	• Lymphoma cells usually form large aggregates and clusters with amphophilic or basophilic cytoplasm • More common in elder adults	CD20+, CD3−, CD16−, CD56−, CD57−	• Particular anatomic location • More common in young adults	CD16+, CD56+, CD57+
Anaplastic plasmacytoma	Lymphoma cells usually form large aggregates and clusters with amphophilic or basophilic cytoplasm	CD20+	• Admixed small plasma cells frequently present • Possible former history of multiple myeloma	CD20−, CD38+, CD56+/−, CD117+/−, CD138+
Diffuse FL with blastoid morphology	• Lymphoma cells usually form large aggregates and clusters with amphophilic or basophilic cytoplasm • Chromatin pattern is commonly vesicular, or coarsely dispersed	CD10+, ~40% Bcl-2+, ~60% Ki-67+, 30%–90% (rare cases may reach ~100%)	• Admixed small lymphoid cells frequently present • Possible former history of low-grade FL	CD10+, ~80% BCL2+, ~80% Ki-67+, 30%–50%

(Continued)

Table 23.5	DIFFERENTIAL DIAGNOSIS OF DLBCL *(Continued)*			
Differential Diagnosis	**Pathologic and Histologic Findings to Support DLBCL Diagnosis**	**Accessory Studies to Support DLBCL Diagnosis**	**Pathologic and Histologic Findings to Support the Other Disease**	**Accessory Studies to Support the Other Disease**
Nonhematolymphoid malignancies (metastatic melanoma or carcinoma, thymic carcinoma, and mediastinal seminoma)	• Usually noncohesive • Cytoplasm often amphophilic to basophilic • Prominent nuclear lobation or indentation	CD45+, CD20+	• Usually cohesive growth (melanoma usually noncohesive) • Cytoplasm often eosinophilic	CD45−, expression of cell-origin-specific biomarkers (e.g., cytokeratin in carcinoma, S-100 protein and HMB45 in melanoma, CD117 in seminoma)
Infectious mononucleosis	• Large cells often appear monotonous, without maturation toward plasma cells • Large cells commonly exhibit atypia, including basophilic cytoplasms, irregular nuclear contours, vesicular chromatin • Prominent and continuous necrosis • More common in elder adults	• Large cells usually show uniformly strong membrane staining for CD20 • May show monotypic immunoglobulin light-chain expression	• Partial preservation of normal lymphoid tissue architecture • Polymorphic cellular composition: spectrum of cellular differentiation from immunoblasts to plasma cells • Large cells do not show overt nuclear atypia • Large lymphoid cells show polytypic immunoglobulin light chain expression • Geographic necrosis • More common in children and young adults	• Large cells are composed of admixture of CD20+ B and CD3+ T immunoblasts • CD20+ cells often show variable staining intensity due to presence of cells in different stages of maturation • EBV+ or LMP+
Kikuchi lymphadenitis	• Large cells often appear monotonous, without maturation toward plasma cells • Large cells commonly exhibit atypia, including basophilic cytoplasms, irregular nuclear contours, vesicular chromatin • Prominent and continuous necrosis • More common in elder adults	CD20+	• Painful lymphadenopathy, but often lymph node is small • Patchy karyorrhectic foci with scattered crescentic histiocytes • Infiltrate consists of CD68+ histiocytes and plasmacytoid dendritic cells, as well as CD8+ • T cells, but very few CD20+ B cells and CD4+ T cells • No neutrophils	• S-100+, myeloperoxidase+, • Large cells are composed of both CD20+ B and CD3+ T immunoblasts

BCL2, B-cell CLL/lymphoma 2; BCL6, B-cell CLL/lymphoma 6; BOB.1, POU class 2 associating factor *1* (a ubiquitous protein, associates with the POU domain of octamer proteins Oct-1 and Oct-2 and alters their recognition specificity); EBER, EBV-encoded RNA; OCT-2, POU class 3 homeobox 2 (both ubiquitous and lymphoid-specific POU transcription factors, members of the NF-κB/Rel family); LMP-1, EBV-associated latent membrane protein 1; Myc, myelocytomatosis viral oncogene homolog.

prominent central coagulative necrosis. Uniform strong CD20 and CD79a staining supports the diagnosis of DLBCL, whereas negative or variably positive CD20 staining and the presence of EBV favors CHL. B-cell transcription factors Oct-2 and BOB.1 are very helpful as they are often negative in CHL, but are strongly positive in DLBCL. PAX-5 is usually weakly expressed in CHL, but is strongly positive in DLBCL (116,117).

PTCL and anaplastic large cell lymphoma (ALCL) can be composed of large neoplastic lymphoid cells that can morphologically mimic DLBCL. These neoplasms express T-cell antigens, and ALCL is strongly and uniformly positive for CD30 (Fig. 23.18D). Natural killer (NK)–cell lymphomas can be composed of medium-sized or large neoplastic lymphoid cells and morphologically mimic DLBCL. NK-cell lymphomas often arise

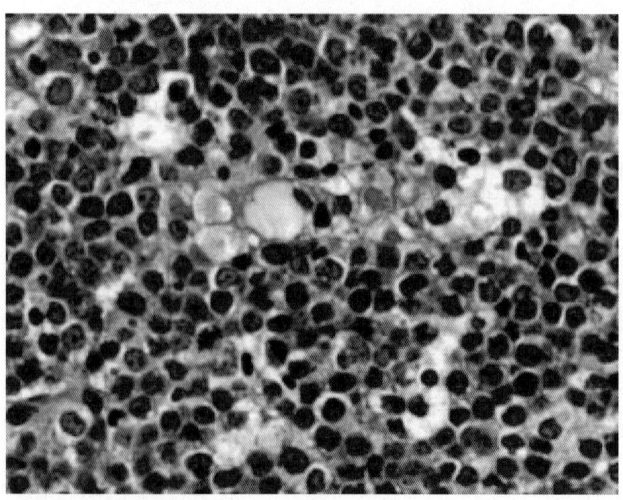

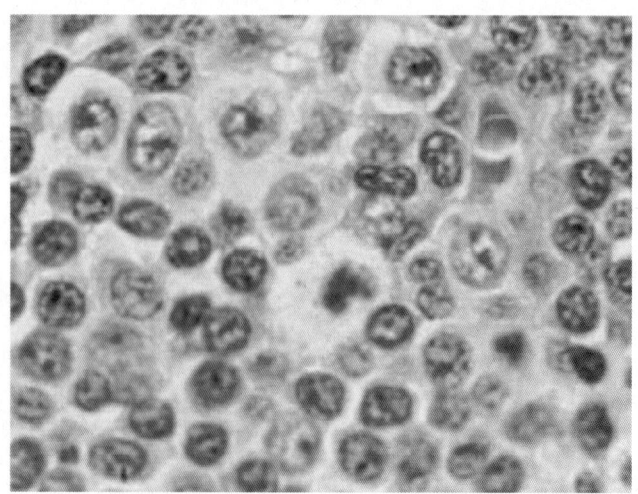

FIGURE 23.18. Differential diagnosis of DLBCL. A: Burkitt lymphoma. The lymphoma cells show monotonous cell size and nuclear features. The neoplastic cells are clonal with a CD45+, CD20+, Pax-5+, CD10+, Bcl-2−, MUM-1−, Bcl-6+ immunophenotype, and a high proliferation index of 100% by Ki-67 expression. **B:** Pleomorphic and blastoid MCL. The lymphoma cells are medium sized and immunoreactive for CD20 and show a high proliferation index. Staining for cyclin D1 is essential for the differential diagnosis.

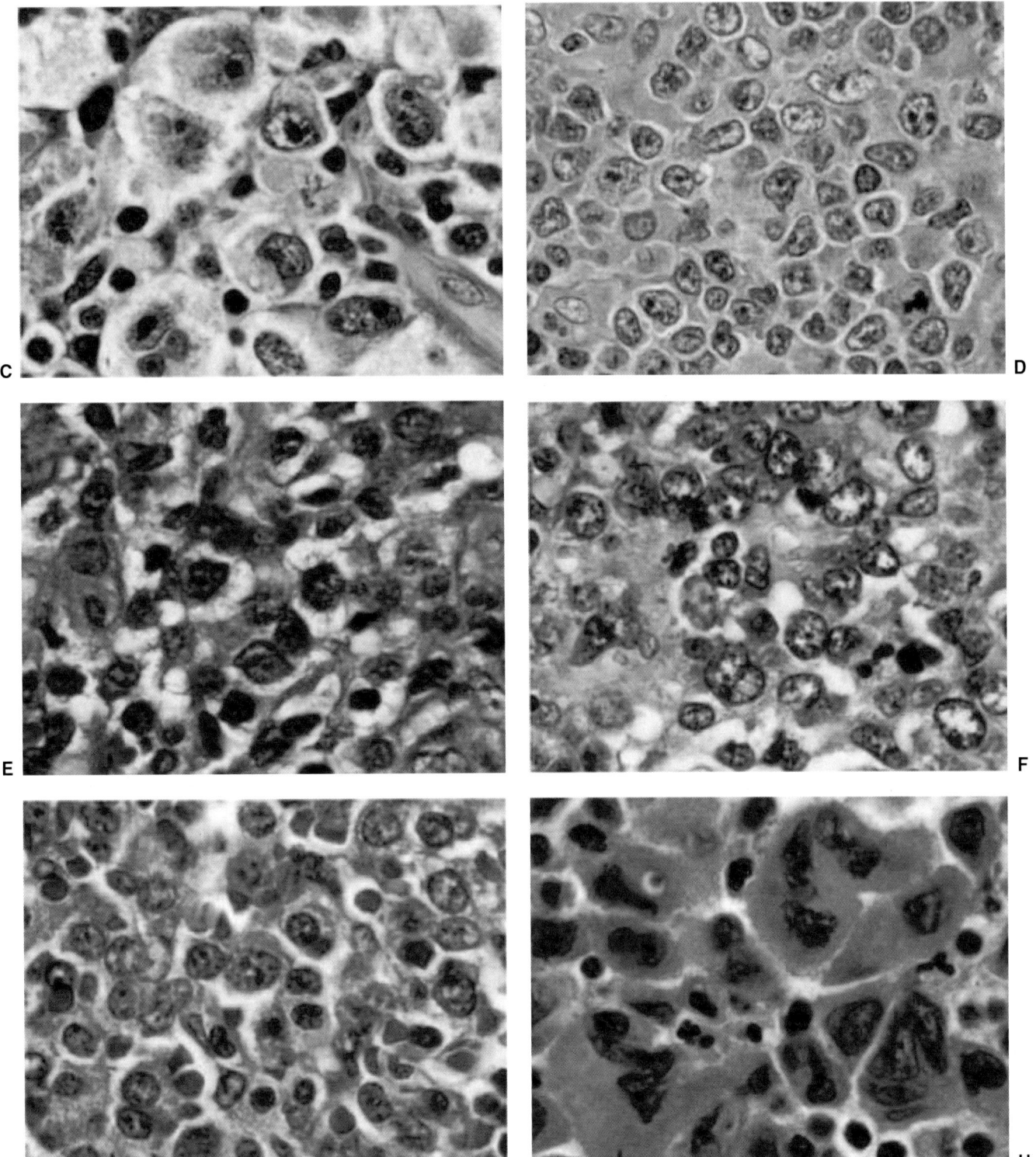

FIGURE 23.18. *(Continued)* **C:** Classical Hodgkin lymphoma. Findings to support the diagnosis include the presence of mixed inflammatory cellular background, unique Hodgkin cell morphology and immunophenotype. **D:** Peripheral T-cell lymphoma. The lymphoma cells may have "centroblastic" features in a background of clusters of epithelioid histiocytes, Lennert lymphoepithelioid pattern. The lymphoma cells are medium sized and show clear cytoplasm with patchy distribution in the lymph node. **E:** Nasal NK-/T-cell lymphoma. The lymphoma cells can form large aggregates with clear cytoplasm, extending into the superimposed squamous epithelial cells. In this case, the lymphoma cells are large sized, and possess eosinophilic cytoplasms and two to three small prominent nucleoli. **F:** Myeloid sarcoma. The myeloid blasts show morphologic similarities to diffuse B-cell lymphoma. Findings to support the diagnosis include the presence of intermingled eosinophilic myelocytes and the eosinophilic cytoplasm with granules. Myeloperoxidase and nonspecific esterase stains highlight specific lineage of differentiating myeloid and monocytic cells. **G:** Chronic myelogenous leukemia and chronic myelomonocytic leukemia involving the lymph node. The differentiating myeloid and monocytic cells show morphologic similarities to diffuse B-cell lymphoma. Findings to support the diagnosis include the presence of eosinophilic myelomonocytic cells, the eosinophilic cytoplasm with granules, and other hematopoietic cells. **H:** Histiocytic sarcoma. Findings to support the diagnosis include the irregular nuclear features, eosinophilic cytoplasm, and inflammatory background. S-100 and CD68 stains confirm the cell origin.

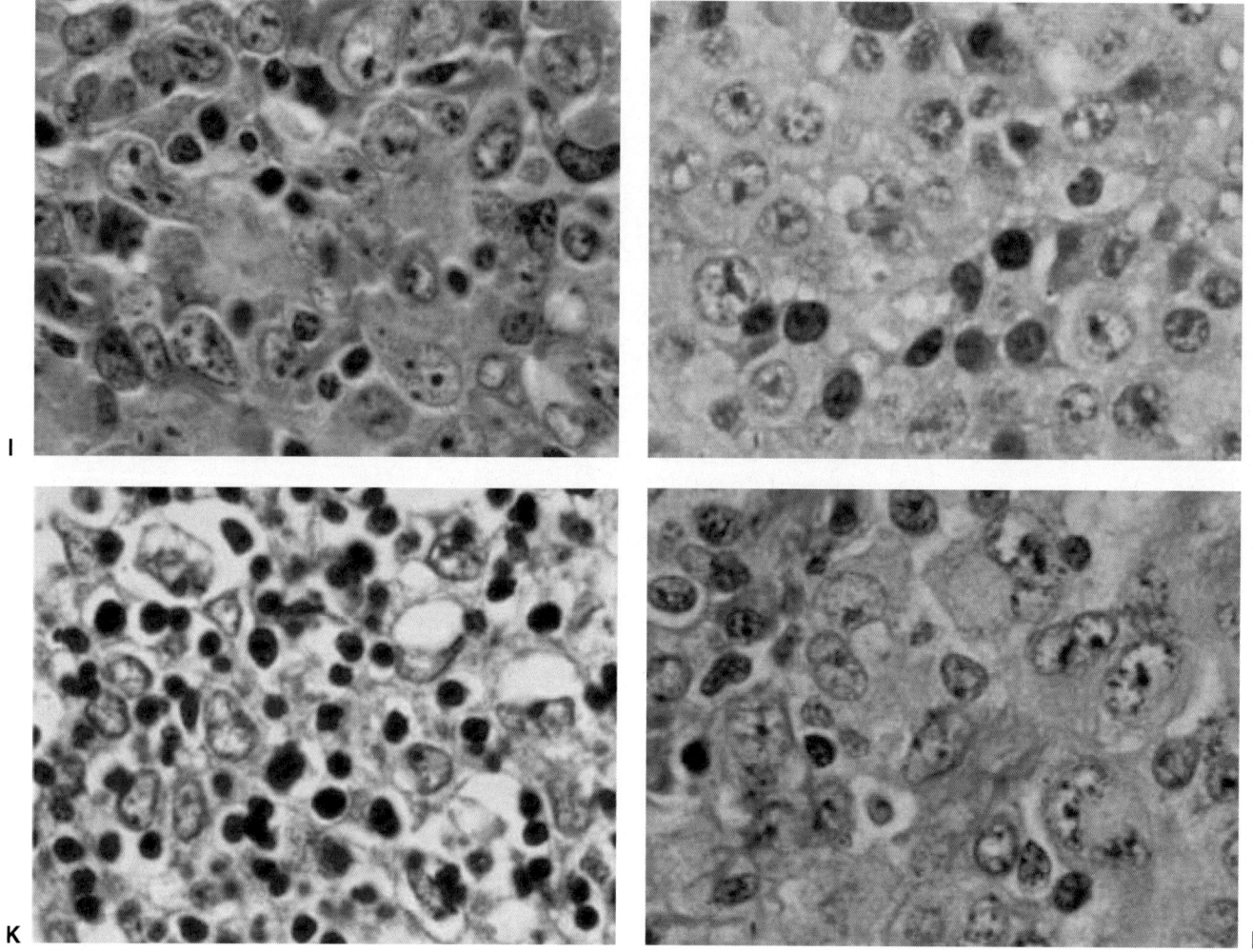

FIGURE 23.18. *(Continued)* **I:** Anaplastic large cell lymphoma. **J:** Anaplastic plasmacytoma. **K:** Thymic carcinoma. **L:** Metastatic melanoma. Valuable information to support the diagnosis includes pertinent clinical history, anatomic location, the presence of surrounding accessory cells, and phenotype.

in distinctive anatomic locations (e.g., nasal and paranasal), express NK-cell markers (CD16 and CD56), and are commonly EBV positive (Fig. 23.18E).

Myeloid sarcoma has a diffuse pattern and is composed of large cells with thin nuclear membranes, blastoid chromatin, small nucleoli, and in some cases the cells have eosinophilic cytoplasmic granules (Fig. 23.18F). The diagnosis can be supported by immunostaining for myeloperoxidase, lysozyme, butyrate esterase, CD34, CD43, and CD117. Patients with myeloid sarcoma may present with *de novo* disease or have a history or simultaneous evidence of a myeloid neoplasm, such as myelodysplastic syndrome or myeloproliferative neoplasm (Fig. 23.18G).

Histiocytic sarcoma is composed of neoplastic histiocytes that are of similar size but have more abundant cytoplasm than the DLBCL cells. Background neutrophils and eosinophils are common (Fig. 23.18H). The neoplastic cells express histiocyte-associated markers, such as CD68 and CD163, and lack expression of pan–B-cell and pan–T-cell markers.

Extramedullary hematopoiesis involving lymph nodes can mimic DLBCL due to the presence of immature erythroid and myeloid precursors. Identification of megakaryocytes and admixed normoblasts and the absence of B-cell markers will point to the correct diagnosis.

Large cell neoplasms of nonhematopoietic lineage are composed of large cells in a diffuse pattern and can mimic DLBCL (Fig. 23.18I–L). The cells in nonhematopoietic tumors tend

to be highly cohesive, and neutrophilic necrosis is common, unlike DLBCL. Other histologic features that support DLBCL include amphophilic or basophilic cytoplasm, vesicular chromatin, marked irregular nuclear contours, a noncohesive growth pattern, sparing of adipocytes when the neoplasm infiltrates adipose tissue, and background small lymphocytes. In nonhematologic tumors, CD45/LCA is consistently negative, and these neoplasms express keratin, S100 protein, or other markers that point to the correct lineage (118).

It is also important to distinguish DLBCL from reactive conditions. In infectious mononucleosis, a lymph node or tonsil specimen can be partially effaced with numerous immunoblasts, resembling DLBCL. Necrosis is very common, and Reed-Sternberg–like cells can be seen (119,120) (Fig. 23.19). The infiltrate is generally more heterogeneous with a range of plasmacytoid cells and plasma cells. CD20 is commonly expressed with variable intensity among the cells reflecting various stages of maturation of immunoblasts to plasma cells (CD20 is negative in plasmablasts and plasma cells) (121). Many EBV+ or LMP1+ cells are present (Fig. 23.19) and EBV serologic studies will support the diagnosis, and provide information regarding the timing of EBV infection (early vs. late).

Other reactive conditions also can have many immunoblasts (e.g., cytomegalovirus infection, drug reactions, and postvaccination response). Unlike DLBCL, these large cells usually do not show significant atypical nuclear features. By

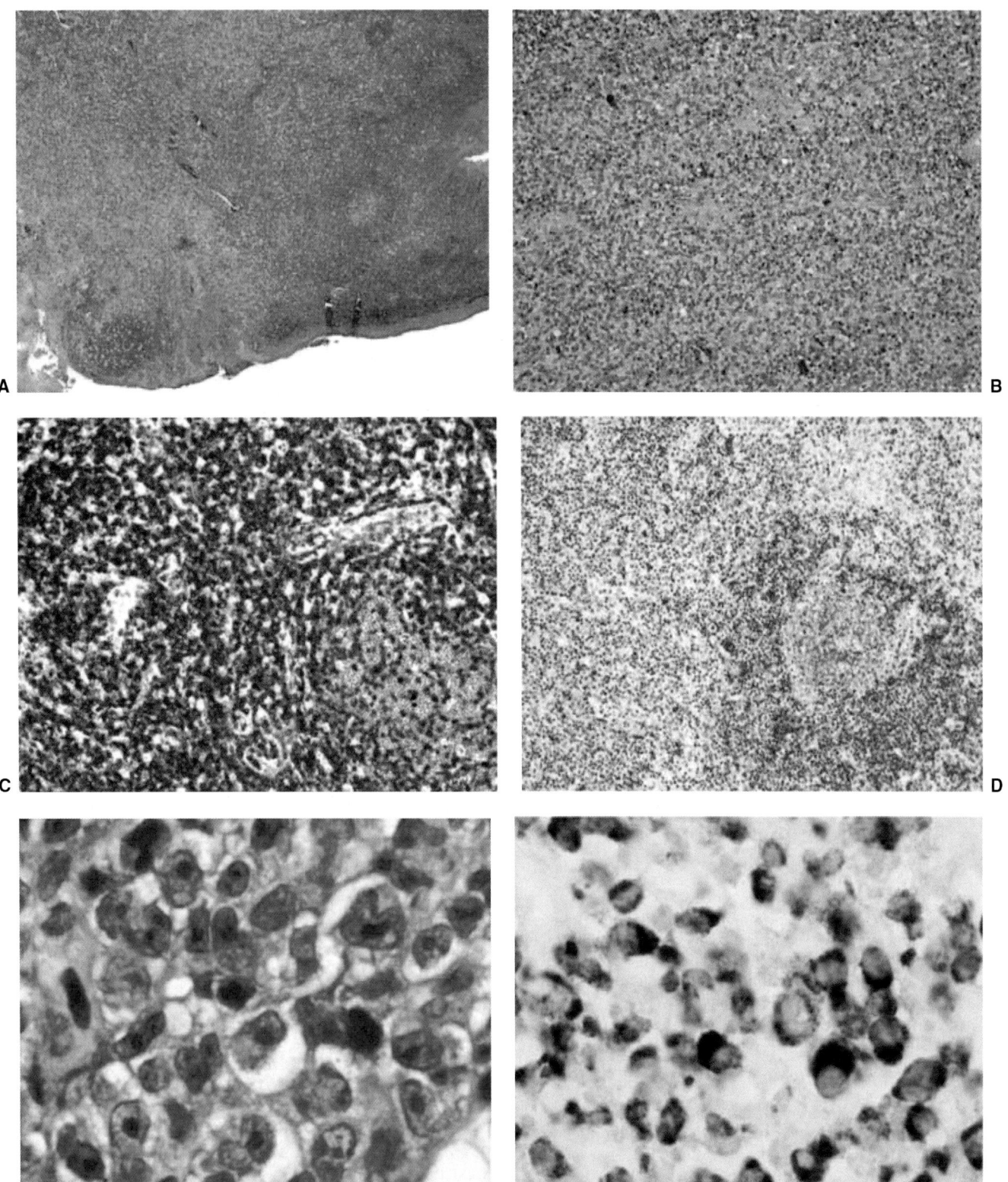

FIGURE 23.19. Infectious mononucleosis. A: A subtotal effacement of lymphoid tissue by large lymphoid cells, in association with multifocal necrosis, raising the consideration of diffuse large cell lymphoma. In mild cases, the large cells do not exhibit prominent atypia and show a transition into recognizable plasmablasts and plasma cells. **B:** The tonsil is commonly involved and exhibits ulceration and multifocal necrosis. **C:** There are often many CD3⁺ cells, including some large T immunoblasts. The valuable clue to the correct diagnosis of infectious mononucleosis is partial preservation of the normal lymphoid tissue architecture, such as the sinuses and lymphoid follicles. **D:** CD20⁺ B cells are often present in preserved lymphoid structure, and the intensity of staining of the large cells is often heterogeneous, indicating that some large cells are plasmablasts (weak or negative for CD20). **E:** In severe cases, a prominent population of large cells is present with round nuclei, vesicular chromatin, prominent nucleoli, and a rich rim of cytoplasm. **F:** Bcl-2 immunostain is negative in the large B-cells, but highlights the T-cells.

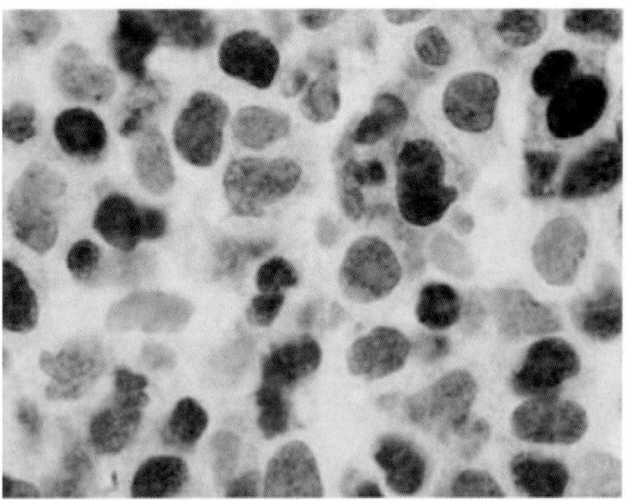

G

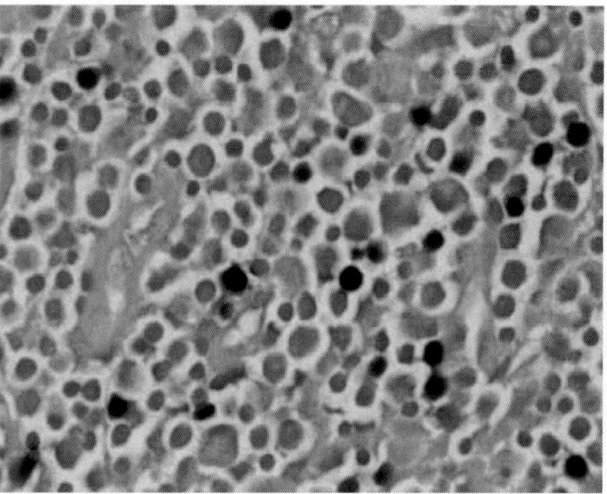

H

FIGURE 23.19. *(Continued)* **G:** The large cells are composed of an admixture of CD3⁺ and CD20⁺ immunoblasts, but they are positive by MUM-1 stain. **H:** A proportion of large cells show nuclear staining for EBER by *in situ* hybridization.

immunohistochemistry, the immunoblasts are composed of a mixture of polytypic B cells and immunophenotypically normal T cells. Kikuchi-Fujimoto lymphadenitis shows patchy and geographical areas of necrosis associated with many histiocytes and large immunoblasts. Karyorrhectic fragments are prominent within these foci and areas; however, neutrophils are not seen. In its earliest phase, when histiocytes and plasmacytoid dendritic cells predominate, the lesion can morphologically mimic DLBCL. The proliferating cells in Kikuchi-Fujimoto lymphadenitis are composed of cytotoxic CD8⁺ T cells, histiocytes (CD68⁺ and myeloperoxidase⁺), and plasmacytoid dendritic cells (CD68⁺, CD123⁺, and myeloperoxidase⁻), with very few CD20⁺ B cells. Some histiocytes have characteristic crescentic or C-shaped nuclei as a result of phagocytosis that compresses the nuclei (122,123).

MORPHOLOGIC SUBTYPES AND DISTINCT ENTITIES

The WHO classification defines four DLBCL subtypes and eight distinct clinicopathologic entities. The major clinical, morphologic, molecular, and immunophenotypic features of these subtypes and entities are summarized and their differential diagnoses are presented in Table 23.6.

T-Cell/Histiocyte-Rich Large B-Cell Lymphoma
Definition

T-cell/histiocyte-rich large B-cell lymphoma (THRLBCL) is a type of DLBCL associated with a prominent component of CD8⁺ reactive T cells and variably admixed histiocytes. The neoplastic large B cells typically represent <10% of all cells in the neoplasm (124–126). THRLBCL is recognized by the 2008 WHO as a distinct clinicopathologic subtype. LYG shows some overlapping morphologic features with THRLBCL but harbors its unique biologic behaviors to be justified as a separate distinct entity.

Epidemiology

The median age of patients with THRLBCL is in the sixth to seventh decades, but young adults also can be affected. The male-to-female ratio is 1.7 to 1.

Etiology

The etiology is unknown. The prominent T-cell infiltration in these tumors may be related to interleukin-4 released by the lymphoma cells, basophils, and helper T cells. The cytotoxic CD8⁺ T cells may be responsible for the tumor cell apoptosis. THRLBCL can show some morphologic similarities to NLPHL, and a subset of THRLBCL cases probably arises from NLPHL. Cases that have a prior history of NLPHL but resemble typical THRLBCL are considered as a separate subset, although they may be morphologically indistinguishable from other THRLBCL. EBV is rarely positive in THRLBCL (127).

Clinical Features

THRLBCL occurs predominantly in lymph nodes, but extranodal sites, such as bone marrow, liver, and spleen, are often involved (128). Patients with THRLBCL often present with advanced-stage disease (~67% in stage III–IV), and bone marrow involvement is common (32% to 62%, vs. 16% in conventional DLBCL). Splenomegaly is seen in approximately 25% patients.

THRLBCL is relatively aggressive, with a 3-year overall survival of 46%. The poor outcome is attributable to the advanced stage of disease at presentation. However, THRLBCL and conventional DLBCL, when matched for IPI, demonstrate similar outcomes after treatment (124). A primary cutaneous form of THRLBCL has been shown to have a much better outcome (124,129). The differential diagnosis of THRLBCL is summarized in Table 23.7.

Histologic Findings

Lymph nodes usually show effacement of architecture by a mixed population of cells in a diffuse pattern. The large neoplastic cells usually constitute <10% of the entire cellular population, and are scattered individually in a background of small lymphocytes and histiocytes. No aggregates or sheets of neoplastic cells are noted, but in some cases these large cells do loosely cluster giving rise to a vaguely nodular pattern.

The large cells can resemble centroblasts or immunoblasts, or have anaplastic features. A subset of neoplastic cells also can be highly pleomorphic with irregularly folded nuclei and can resemble LP or Reed-Sternberg cells (as seen in Hodgkin lymphomas) (Fig. 23.20). The background T lymphocytes are small and can show mildly irregular nuclear contours. In addition, a

(Continued)

Table 23.6 COMPARISON OF MORPHOLOGIC TYPES OF DLBCL

Subtypes	Clinical Features	Morphologic Features	Immunophenotypic Features	Molecular Findings	Prognosis and Treatment	Differential Diagnosis
Conventional DLBCL	• Most common type of NHL • Median age: 64 • Male predominance, 1.4 to 1 • 70% nodal vs. 30% extranodal • 55% stage I–II, 35% III–IV • Complete remission, 60% • 5-year OS, 55% • EBV, 3.8%	• Diffuse pattern • Large- to medium-sized cells • Can be associated with low-grade NHL • Three common morphologic types (centroblastic; immunoblastic, and anaplastic) • Can have several unusual growth patterns	• Pan–B-cell markers+ (CD19, CD20, CD22, CD79am Pax-5) • Ig κ or λ clonal • CD5+, ~10% • CD10−, ~40% • CD30+, ~10% • Bcl-2−, ~60% • Bcl-6+, ~60% • MUM1+, ~40% • FOXP1+, ~30% • NF-κB+, ~60% • Ki-67+, ~50%	• Clonal IgH • Germline TCR • BCL2 rearranged, ~20% • BCL6 rearranged, ~30% • MYC rearranged, ~8% • BCL2 mutation, ~40% • BCL6 mutation, ~70% • TP53 mutation, ~20%	• IPI stratify clinical outcomes • Rituximab with anthracycline-containing regimens • GCB and ABC molecular subtypes benefit from different regimens	• Pleomorphic MCL • Myeloid sarcoma • PTCL and ALCL • NK-cell lymphoma • Lymphoblastic lymphoma • Histiocytic sarcoma • Syncytial Hodgkin lymphoma • Infectious mononucleosis
T-cell/histiocytic large B-cell lymphoma	• 60–70-year-old • Male predominance, 1.7 • 60% nodal vs. 40% extranodal • 33% stage I–II, 67% III–IV • Complete remission in 50% cases • 3-year OS in 46% • EBV in rare cases • Splenomegaly, 25%	• Diffusely scattered large cells • Variable morphologic types (centroblastic, immunoblastic, or Hodgkin-like) • Background activated CD8 TIA+ small T cells, plasma cells, eosinophils, or histiocytes	• Pan–B-cell markers+ • CD5− • CD10− • CD15− • CD30−/− • Bcl-2−, ~40% • Bcl-6+, ~60% • Oct-2+ • BOB.1+ • EMA+, 30% • Background CD3/CD8/TIA1/lysozyme+ T-cells	• Clonal IgH • Germline TCR • EBV− • BCL2 rearranged, ~25%	• Most patients are ABC molecular subtype • May benefit from BTK inhibitor and NF-κB inhibitor regimens	• Reactive florid hyperplasia, PTGC • CHL, lymphocyte-rich type • Nodular lymphocyte–predominant classical Hodgkin lymphoma • Lymphomatoid granulomatosis
Primary DLBCL of the CNS	• Most common type of primary CNS NHL • Median age: 60 • Male predominance • Supratentorial location, 60% • Present with mental status changes, neurologic defect, and headache • EBV− in immunocompetent cases	• Perivascular aggregates of diffuse large cells • Centroblastic or immunoblastic morphology • Age, performance status, LDH serum level are important prognostic variables	• Pan–B-cell markers+ • CD5− • CD10+, 10% • CD15− • CD30+, 10% • Bcl-2+, 60% • Bcl-6+, 70% • MUM1+, 90%	• Clonal IgH • Germline TCR • No BCL2 and MYC rearrangement • BCL6 rearranged, ~35% • Mutation of TP53, BCL6, PIM1, Pax-5 genes • CSF protein concentration and deep lesions are the main prognostic variables	• High-dose methotrexate + high-dose cytarabine combinations followed or not by whole brain irradiation is the first-line treatment. • Rituximab and high-dose chemo supported by ASCT are experimental	• Burkitt lymphoma • Vasculitis • Neuroepithelial tumors • Metastatic lesions • Multiple sclerosis • Gliomas • Toxoplasmosis • Sarcoidosis • Progressive multifocal leukoencephalopathy
Primary cutaneous DLBCL, leg type	• Elderly women • Female predominance, 3.5 • Enlarging mass in lower extremities, 85% • Complete remission, 60% cases • 5-year OS, 50% • EBV-negative	• Diffuse aggregates of large cells • Absence of stromal response • Centroblastic or immunoblastic morphology	• Pan–B-cell markers+ • CD5− • CD10− • CD30+, 20% • Bcl-2+, 100% • Bcl-6+, 90% • MUM1+, 100%	• Clonal IgH • Germline TCR • BCL2 and MALT1 rearrangement, 67% • BCL6 rearranged, ~80% • MYC rearranged, ~30% • CDKN2A and CDKN2B deletion, 67%	• Rituximab with anthracycline-containing regimens • GCB and ABC molecular subtypes benefit from different regimens	• Primary cutaneous follicle center lymphoma • Systemic DLBCL with secondary skin involvement
EBV-positive DLBCL of the elderly	• Median: 71 y (range: 50–92) • Male predominance, 1.4 • 50% stage I–II, 50% III–IV • Variable clinical course • Median survival, 2 y	• Extranodal, 70% cases • Polymorphic infiltrate • Centroblastic, immunoblastic, or intrasinusoidal type • Hodgkin-like cells	• Pan–B-cell markers+ • CD5+, 20% • CD10−, 28% • CD30+, 40% • Bcl-2−, 58% • Bcl-6+, 44% • MUM1+, 80% • FOXP1+, 20% • Blimp1+, 80% • EBER+ and LMP+, 95%	• Clonal IgH • Germline TCR • No BCL2, BCL6, and MYC rearrangements • No TP53 mutation and deletion	• Rituximab with anthracycline-containing regimens • Benefit from specific EBV viral, BTK inhibitor and NF-κB inhibitor regimens	• Plasmablastic lymphoma • Sinusoidal DLBCL • PTLD

Table 23.6 COMPARISON OF MORPHOLOGIC TYPES OF DLBCL (Continued)

Subtypes	Clinical Features	Morphologic Features	Immunophenotypic Features	Molecular Findings	Prognosis and Treatment	Differential Diagnosis
CD5-positive *de novo* DLBCL	• Median: 70 y (range: 55–92) • Female predominance, 1.2 • 40% stage I–II, 60% III–IV • Complete remission in 40% cases • 5-year OS in 34% • EBV negative	• Extranodal, more common than nodal • Similar to typical DLBCL • Centroblastic, immunoblastic, or intrasinusoidal type	• Pan–B-cell markers+ • CD5+ • CD10−/+ • CD29+ • CD30−/+ • Bcl-2+ • Bcl-6+ • MUM1+ • FOXP1+	• Clonal IgH • Germline TCR • No BCL2 and MYC rearrangements	• Rituximab with anthracycline-containing regimens • May benefit from NF-κB inhibitor regimens	• Pleomorphic MCL • Paraimmunoblastic CLL
Primary mediastinal (thymic) large B-cell lymphoma	• Median: 35 y (range: 25–45) • Female predominance, 2/1 • 66% stage I–II, 34% III–IV • Complete remission in 80% cases • 5-year OS in 75% • EBV-negative	• Mediastinal mass • Alveolar fibrosis • Large- to medium-sized cells • Centroblastic, polylobated, or Hodgkin-like cells • Clear cytoplasm	• Pan–B-cell markers+ • CD10+, ~25% • CD15− • CD21− • CD23, ~70% • CD30+, ~80% • Bcl-2+, ~70% • Bcl-6+, ~60% • MUM1+, ~75% • Oct-2/BOB.1/PU.1+ • MAL+, ~70% • c-Rel, TRAF CD54 and CD95+, ~70% • CD57/TIA1− • MHC− • EMA− • EBV−	• Rearranged immunoglobulin IgH genes • Germline TCR genes • BCL6 mutation, ~70% • 9p gain, ~35% • 2p c-Rel amplification, ~50% • 3q, ~5% • 12q12, ~5% • SOCS1 mutation, ~45% • TP53 and ARF mutation, ~5% • No BCL2 and BCL6 gene rearrangements	• Rituximab with anthracycline-containing regimens • May benefit from BTK inhibitor and NF-κB inhibitor regimen	• CHL, nodular sclerosis type • Mediastinal gray zone lymphoma • ALCL • Seminoma • Thymic carcinoma • Neuroendocrine tumor
Intravascular large B-cell lymphoma	• Median age: 71 (13–85) • Male predominance, 1.1 • Skin and CNS most common • 70% stage I–II, 30% III–IV • Complete remission in 30% cases • 5-year OS, ~30% • Aggressive course • EBV-negative	• Small- to medium-sized vessels • Large centroblastic and immunoblastic cells • Intrasinusoidal pattern in liver, bone marrow, and spleen	• Pan–B-cell markers+ • CD5+, 38% • CD10+, 13% • CD15− • CD21− • CD23− • CD29− • CD30+, 30% • CD54− • Bcl-2+, 20% • Bcl-6+, 22% • MUM1+, 90% • EMA−	• Rearranged immunoglobulin IgH genes • Germline TCR genes • No BCL2 and MYC rearrangements	• Rituximab with anthracycline-containing regimens • No appropriate therapy established	• Acute myeloid leukemia with circulating blasts • Acute lymphoblastic leukemia with circulating blasts • Intravascular T- or NK-cell lymphoma • Inflammatory vasculitis
Lymphomatoid granulomatosis	• Median age of 37 (range: 24–76) • Lung, 90% • Skin, liver, and CNS, 10% • Variable clinical course • EBV-positive	• Mass lesion • Necrosis present in higher-grade lesions • Large EBV+ immunoblastic or Hodgkin-like cells • Polymorphic background infiltrate of small lymphocytes, plasma cells, histiocytes • Angiocentric and angiodestructive	• Cyclin D1− • Pan–B-cell markers+ • CD5− • CD10− • CD15− • CD30+, 30% • Bcl-2−, 60% • Bcl-6+, 30% • EBER+; • Grade I: <5/HPF • Grade II: 5–20/HPF • Grade III: >50/HPF	• Rearranged immunoglobulin IgH genes • Germline TCR genes • Clonal EBV viral genome • No recurrent abnormality identified	• Single or multiagent regimens • Immunomodulatory therapy	• Classical Hodgkin lymphoma • Thymic tumor • Metastatic carcinoma

Entity	Clinical features	Morphology	Immunophenotype	Genetics	Treatment	Differential diagnosis
ALK-positive large B-cell lymphoma	• Median age 36 (9–70) • Male predominance, 3/1 • Median survival, 11 mo • Aggressive course • EBV−	• Diffuse aggregates of large cells • Few reactive small lymphocytes • Immunoblastic and plasmablastic nuclei with prominent nucleoli	• CD20+ focal, 3% • CD79a+, 16% • CD4+, 64% • CD5− • CD7+, 40% • CD10− • CD30+ focal, 6% • CD38+ 100% • CD138+, 100% • EMA+/−, 100% • Bcl-6−/+ • MUM1+, 80% • BLIMP1+, 80%	• Rearranged immunoglobulin IgH genes • Germline TCR genes • t(2;19)(p23;q23) • t(2;5)(p23;35) • 3′-ALK cryptic insertion on 4q22-24	• Aggressive rituximab with anthracycline-containing regimens • No appropriate therapy established	• ALK− ALCL • Plasmablastic lymphoma • Sinusoidal DLBCL
Plasmablastic lymphoma	• Median age: 50 • Male predominance • 30% stage I–II, 70% III–IV • Median survival, few months • Aggressive course • EBV+ 70% • HHV8 (KSHV)−	• Oral cavity, most common • Diffuse aggregates of large cells • Minimal reactive small lymphocytes • Immunoblastic and plasmablastic nuclei with prominent nucleoli	• IgA, most common • Pan–B-cell markers− • CD5− • CD10− • CD30+/− • CD38+ • CD56− • CD138+ • EMA+/− • Bcl-6−/+ • MUM1+ • BLIMP1+	• Rearranged immunoglobulin IgH genes • Germline TCR genes • EBV+, ~70% • LMP, ~5% • No recurrent abnormality identified	• Aggressive rituximab with anthracycline-containing regimens • No appropriate therapy established	• DLBCL • Anaplastic plasmacytoma • Burkitt lymphoma
Primary effusion lymphoma	• Median age: 82 (HIV+ cases: 43) • Male predominance • Median survival, few months • Aggressive course • EBV+ • HHV8 (KSHV)+	• Body cavity, most common in pleural • Aggregates of large cells • Anaplastic and immunoblastic and with prominent polymorphism	• IgG, most common • Ki-67, 90%–100% • Pan–B-cell markers− • CD5− • CD10− • CD30+ • CD38+ • CD71+ • CD138+ • EMA+ • Bcl-6− • MUM1+ • BLIMP1+	• Rearranged immunoglobulin IgH genes • Germline TCR genes • No BCL2, BCL6, Myc rearrangements • No TP53 mutation • No RAS mutation • BCL6 mutation, ~70%	• Aggressive rituximab with anthracycline-containing regimens • No appropriate therapy established	• Metastatic carcinoma • Metastatic melanoma • Pneumonia • DLBCL with high proliferation index
High-grade B-cell lymphoma, borderline case, unclassifiable	• 60–70 • Male predominance • Complete remission, ~20% • 5-year OS, ~20% • Aggressive course • Underlying immunodeficiency • EBV+ 10% cases	• Extranodal, common • Diffuse aggregates of large cells • Minimal stromal response • Centroblastic or immunoblastic morphology	• IgG, most common • Pan–B-cell markers+ • CD5− • CD10+/− • CD30+/− • Bcl-2+/− • Bcl-6−/+ • MUM1+ • FOXP1−/+ • EBV+	• Clonal IgH • Germline TCR • Rare BCL2 rearrangement, ~5% • Rare BCL6 rearrangement, ~5% • Rare MYC sole karyotype • Common MYC complex karyotype, ~40% • Common BCL2/MYC double hit, ~20%	• Aggressive rituximab with anthracycline-containing regimens • No appropriate therapy established	• Burkitt lymphoma • DLBCL with high proliferation index

ALCL, anaplastic large cell lymphoma; ALK, anaplastic lymphoma kinase-1; ARF/CDKN2A, cyclin-dependent kinase inhibitor 2A (melanoma, p16, inhibits CDK4); ASCT, allogeneic stem-cell transplantation; BCL2, B-cell CLL/lymphoma 2; BCL6, B-cell CLL/lymphoma 6; BOB.1, POU class 2 associating factor 1 (a ubiquitous protein, associates with the POU domain of octamer proteins Oct-1 and Oct-2 and alters their recognition specificity); CDKN2A/ARF/p16, cyclin-dependent kinase inhibitor 2A (melanoma, p16, inhibits CDK4); c-Rel, v-rel reticuloendotheliosis viral oncogene homolog (avian); EBER, EBV-encoded RNA; EMA, epithelial membrane antigen; FOXP1, forkhead box P1; GCET1 and GCET2, germinal center expressed transcript 1 and 2; IgH, immunoglobulin heavy chain; LMP-1, EBV-associated latent membrane protein 1; MAL, T-cell differentiation protein; MALT1, mucosa-associated lymphoid tissue lymphoma translocation gene 1; MHC, major histocompatibility complex; MUM1, melanoma-associated antigen (mutated); OCT-2, POU class 3 homeobox 2 (both ubiquitous and lymphoid-specific POU transcription factors, members of the NF-κB/Rel family); Pax-5, Paired box gene 5; PIM1, pim-1 oncogene; PRDM1/BLIMP1, PR domain containing 1, with ZNF domain; PTCL, peripheral T-cell lymphoma; PTLD, posttransplant lymphoproliferative disorder; TCR, T-cell receptor; TIA-1, cytotoxic granule–associated RNA binding protein; TP53, tumor protein p53.

	Table 23.7 DIFFERENTIAL DIAGNOSIS OF THRLBCL			
Pathologic Features	**T-Cell-/Histiocyte-Rich Large B-cell Lymphoma**	**Anaplastic Large Cell Lymphoma, ALK⁻**	**Classical Hodgkin Lymphoma**	**Nodular Lymphocyte–Predominant CHL**
Age (median, year-old)	• 60–70 (64-year-old) • Male predominance at 1.7	• 40–65 (52-year-old) • Male predominance at 1.5	• 15–35 and 50–65, bimodal • Predominantly male predominance	• 30–50 (42-year-old) • Predominantly male predominance
Cell origin	Germinal center B cells	Activated mature cytotoxic T cells	Mature B cells at the germinal center stage of differentiation	GCB at the centroblastic stage of differentiation
Disease features	Late relapse	Early relapse	• Indolent, rare relapse • Higher incidence in white Caucasians	Indolent, frequent relapse, but remain responsive to therapy
IgH mutation and SHM	• Rearranged immunoglobulin IgH genes • Germline TCR genes	• Rearranged TCR genes • Germline immunoglobulin gene	• Rearranged immunoglobulin IgH genes • High load of SHMs • No ongoing mutation • Germline TCR genes	• Rearranged immunoglobulin IgH genes • High load of SHMs, 80% • No ongoing mutation • Germline TCR genes • BCL6 translocation, 50%
Anatomic location	Both nodal and extranodal Nodal is more common	Both nodal and extranodal Extranodal is more common	Predominantly involve the lymph node	Predominantly involve the lymph node
Stage, III–IV	67%	70%–80%	40%	5%–25%
Morphology of neoplastic cells	Variable morphologic types, commonly with immunoblastic and anaplastic variants	• Solid, cohesive sheets of tumor cells • Anaplastic nuclei with irregular foldings • Intrasinusoidal pattern • Hallmark cells	Reed-Sternberg cells and mononuclear variants	L&H cells with popcorn-like nuclei, commonly present within the small B-cell nodules
Background microenvironment	Background-activated CD8/TIA⁺ small T cells, plasma cells, eosinophils, or histiocytes	Atypical lymphocytes that show a spectrum of small- to large-sized cells	Admixture of inflammatory cells with small lymphocytes, granulocytes, plasma cells, and histiocytes	Predominance of small B lymphocytes within the nodules and small T lymphocytes between the nodules
Immunophenotype	• CD45⁻ • CD20⁺ • CD8⁺ • CD15⁻ • CD21⁻ • CD30⁻/⁺ • CD57/TIA-1⁻/⁺ • EMA⁻/⁺ • Oct-2/BOB.1⁺ • Vimentin⁻ • J-Chain⁻/⁺	• CD45⁺ • CD20⁻ • CD8⁻ (CD2, CD3, CD4, CD5⁺/⁻) • CD5⁺/⁻ • CD15⁻ • CD21⁻ • CD30⁺ • CD57/TIA-1⁺/⁻ • EMA⁺/⁻ • Oct-2/BOB.1⁻ • Clusterin⁺ • ALK-1⁺/⁻ • Vimentin⁻ • J-chain⁻	• CD45⁻ • CD20⁻/⁺ • CD8⁻ • CD15⁺ • CD21⁻ • CD30⁺ • CD57/TIA-1⁻/⁺ • EMA⁻ • Oct-2/BOB.1⁻/⁺ • Vimentin⁺ • J-chain⁻	• CD45⁺ • CD20⁺ • CD8⁻ • CD15⁻ • CD21⁺ • CD30⁻/⁺ • CD57/TIA-1⁺ • EMA⁺ • Oct-2/BOB.1⁺ • Vimentin⁻ • J-chain⁺/⁻
EBV association	Rare, ~3%	Negative (or very rare)	Common, ~40%	Negative (or very rare)
5-year survival	30% (3-year survival at 46%)	32%	90% (10-year survival at 85%)	90% (10-year survival at 80%)

ALCL, anaplastic large cell lymphoma; ALK, anaplastic lymphoma kinase-1; BCL2, B-cell CLL/lymphoma 2; BCL6, B-cell CLL/lymphoma 6; BOB.1, POU class 2 associating factor *1* (a ubiquitous protein, associates with the POU domain of octamer proteins Oct-1 and Oct-2 and alters their recognition specificity); CDKN2A/ARF/p16, cyclin-dependent kinase inhibitor 2A (melanoma, p16, inhibits CDK4); EBER, EBV-encoded RNA; EMA, epithelial membrane antigen; FOXP1, forkhead box P1; IgH, immunoglobulin heavy chain; LMP-1, EBV-associated latent membrane protein 1; MUM1, melanoma-associated antigen (mutated); OCT-2, POU class 3 homeobox *2* (both ubiquitous and lymphoid-specific POU transcription factors, members of the NF-κB/Rel family); PRDM1/BLIMP1, PR domain containing 1, with ZNF domain; TCR, T-cell receptor; TIA-1, cytotoxic granule–associated RNA binding protein.

variable number of histiocytes or delicate fibrosis can be present. In some cases, clusters of epithelioid histiocytes are present, resembling granulomatous lesions. Plasma cells can be present and are usually few. Granulocytes are typically absent.

Extranodal sites, including involved bone marrow, can show similar histologic features. Splenic THRLBCL commonly exhibits a micronodular pattern composed of scattered large neoplastic cells in a background of small lymphocytes, but lacks follicular dendritic cell meshworks.

Immunophenotypic Features

The large neoplastic cells are positive for pan–B-cell markers, and immunoglobulin light chain restriction can be demonstrated in some cases. CD5, CD10, CD15, and CD30 are usually negative (128). In some cases, the neoplastic cells can

express CD30, usually with variable intensity of staining. Bcl-2 is expressed in 40% of cases, and Bcl-6 in 60% of cases. Epithelial membrane antigen (EMA) expression is variably positive in 30% of cases.

The small cells in the background are mainly composed of CD3⁺ and CD8⁺ cytotoxic T cells (Fig. 23.20E). Small reactive B cells are rare. There are no rosettes of CD57⁺/PD-1⁺ T cells surrounding the large neoplastic cells.

Genetic Findings

THRLBCL has rearranged immunoglobulin *Ig* and germline *TCR* genes. Based on studies on microdissected tumor cells, hypermutated *IgV$_H$* gene and ongoing somatic mutations are present, suggesting antigen selection (130,131). *BCL2* rearrangement is present with a frequency similar to other types of

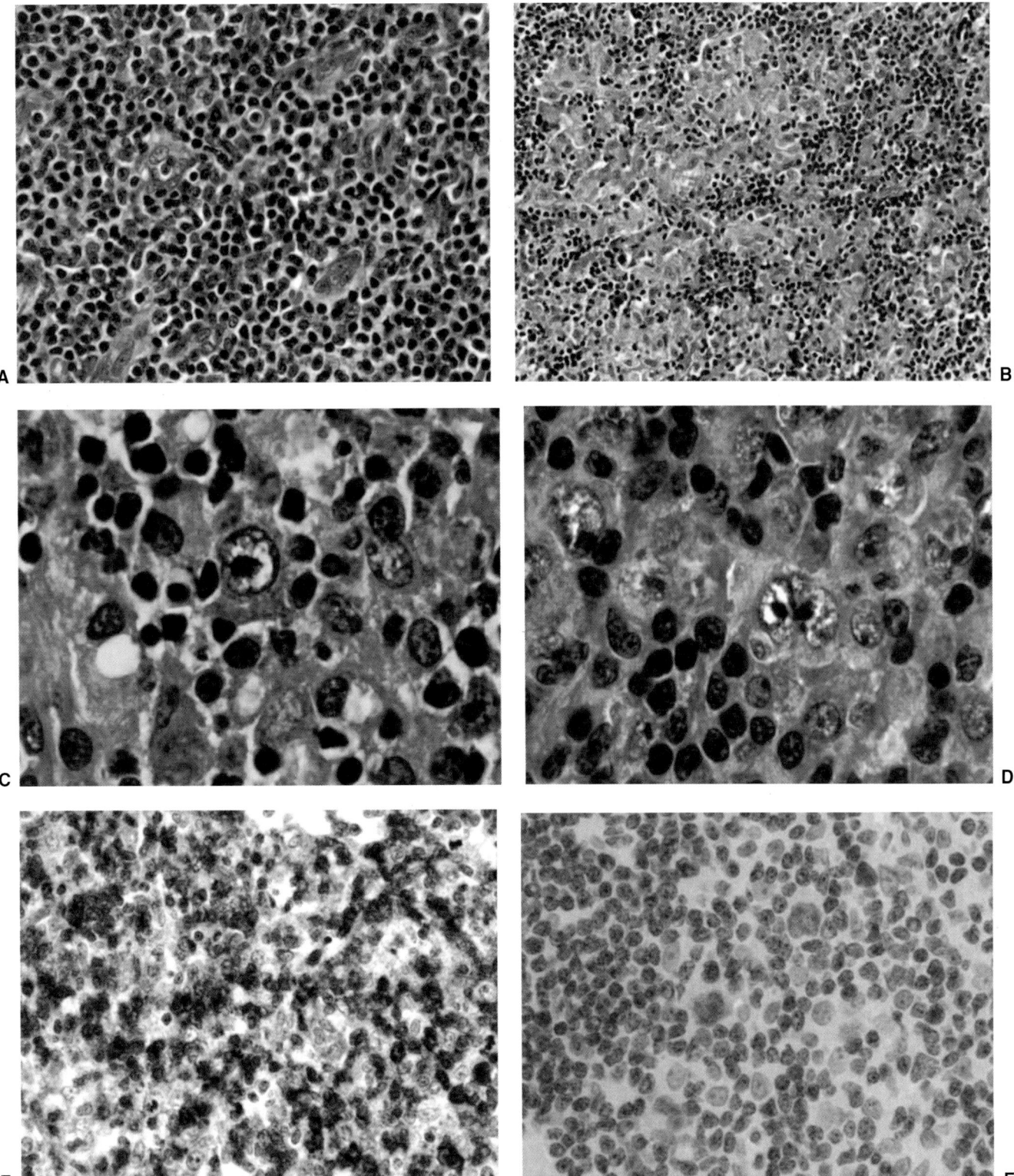

FIGURE 23.20. T-cell/histiocyte-rich large B-cell lymphoma. A: Large lymphoid cells are scattered singly among small lymphocytes, or admixed within small aggregates of histiocytes. **B:** This example is rich in large clusters of epithelioid histiocytes in the lymph node, resembling Lennert lymphoepithelioid T-cell lymphoma. **C,D:** Large cells occur in a background of activated small lymphoid cells, some of which resemble Reed-Sternberg cells **(C)** and anaplastic cells **(D)**. **E:** Numerous small CD3+ T lymphocytes are present in the lesion. **F:** Pax-5 immunostain highlights scattered large B cells.

DLBCL. Array CGH performed on microdissected tumor cells demonstrated several aberrations involving the 4q and 19p chromosomal regions. Most THRLBCL cases are more closely related to GCB-DLBCL than to ABC-DLBCL. GEP has identified a subset of DLBCL cases with features of a host immune response manifested by increased expression of T-/NK-cell receptor and activation pathway components, complement cascade members, macrophage/dendritic cell markers, and inflammatory mediators (132). These cases likely correspond to THRLBCL.

Postulated Cell of Origin

The presence of ongoing somatic mutations, hypermutated immunoglobulin gene, and BCL2 rearrangement supports a GC stage of cell origin, at least in some cases. Similar cytogenetic features between THRLBCL and NLPHL suggest that there are biologic similarities between these two entities.

Differential Diagnosis

Differential diagnosis includes reactive florid hyperplasia, progressive transformation of germinal centers (PTGC), lymphocyte-rich CHL, NLPHL, and LYG. The differential diagnoses in these major categories are summarized in Table 23.7.

In some THRLBCL cases, the large neoplastic cells may overlap with immunoblasts in reactive lymphoid hyperplasia. However, in reactive lymphoid hyperplasia, the large immunoblasts are commonly distributed in small aggregates, and a spectrum of large lymphoid cells from immunoblasts to plasmablasts or plasma cells can be appreciated. By immunostains, CD20 intensity is variable due to different differentiation stages of B cells, and these B cells are polyclonal by immunoglobulin light chain expression. In addition, mild atypia, including irregular nuclear contours, can sometimes be seen in some THRLBCL cases.

CHL, lymphocyte-rich and mixed cellularity types, shows similarities to THRLBCL, but Reed-Sternberg cells or its variants are negative for pan–B-cell markers or show variable staining intensity. They are almost always positive for CD30 and sometimes for CD15. EBV is often positive.

Typical NLPHL can be distinguished from THRLBCL due to the presence of B-cell nodules. In some NLPHL cases with an extensive diffuse component, the cells in the diffuse areas are mostly T cells, which may focally mimic THRLBCL in morphology. However, these T cells usually are negative for cytotoxic T-cell markers. Clinically, NLPHL occurs in younger patients (30 to 50 years), and most patients (80% to 95%) present with early-stage disease (I–II) with a much better overall survival.

PTCL, mixed cell type, should be considered in the differential diagnosis because of many activated CD8+ T cells in the THRLBCL. However, in PTCL, cytologic atypia is more profound, and the atypia is present in all the lymphoid cells of various sizes. The lymphoid cells are composed of a spectrum of cells without clear distinction of large cells as seen in THRLBCL. By immunostains or flow cytometry, the large atypical cells in PTCL express pan–T-cell antigens.

Angioimmunoblastic T-cell lymphoma, which can have a reactive or clonal population of large B cells, can be difficult to distinguish from THRLBCL. Careful evaluation and demonstration of clonal CD10+/CD20+ large B cells and coexisting atypical medium- to large-sized T cells are supportive of such a diagnosis. EBV is commonly positive in AITL, and clonality studies for immunoglobulin and TCR gene rearrangement analyses can be helpful to confirm the diagnostic impression.

LYG has similar features of scattered large atypical B cells in a background of reactive T-cells and histiocytes, but it always presents in specific extranodal sites (lung, brain, and skin), associated with geographic necrosis, and positivity EBV.

Primary DLBCL of the Central Nervous System
Definition

Primary DLBCL of the CNS is defined as a diffuse lymphoma of large B cells that is strictly confined within the CNS. Patients with immunodeficiency are excluded from this category of disease.

Epidemiology

Immunocompromised Patients—Patients with acquired and congenital immunodeficiencies are at increased risk for the development of primary lymphomas in the CNS. The most common cause is AIDS in North America (see Chapter 25). The congenital immunodeficiency associated with the CNS lymphoma is commonly seen in pediatric patients with severe combined immunodeficiency and the Wiskott-Aldrich syndrome. Iatrogenic immunodeficiency, as a result of immunosuppression medication related to solid organ transplantation, also predisposes to the development of EBV+ posttransplant lymphoproliferative disorder (PTLD) in the CNS.

Primary CNS lymphoma is rare, representing <5% of all brain tumors and <1% of all NHL. The median patient age is 60 years. There is a slight male predominance (a male-to-female ratio of 3:2). EBV infection is not involved and the etiology is unknown.

In AIDS patients, primary CNS lymphoma constitutes approximately 20% to 30% of AIDS-related NHL and is a major cause of death. In comparison with the general population, the incidence of CNS lymphoma is 3,600-fold higher in the AIDS population. AIDS-related lymphomas are discussed in detail in Chapter 25.

Clinical Features

The median age is 60 years at diagnosis for immunocompetent patients and 31 years for AIDS patients. A slight male predominance is the case for the immunocompetent population, whereas almost all immunocompromised patients are male AIDS patients.

Primary DLBCL of the CNS in AIDS patients is frequently associated with advanced stages of HIV infection, severe immune dysfunction, and markedly decreased peripheral CD4+ cells. Patients commonly present with systemic AIDS-associated diseases, including various infections (such as cytomegalovirus, *Pneumocystis carinii*, toxoplasmosis, HIV encephalitis), Kaposi sarcoma, and progressive multifocal leukoencephalopathy. In immunocompetent patients, DLBCL is commonly located supratentorially, whereas in AIDS patients, multifocal involvement is typical. The leptomeninges are involved in 5% of cases, whereas intraocular involvement is seen in 20% of cases.

Patients present with neurologic abnormalities. Poor prognostic indicators include B symptoms, high serum LDH level, low performance score, high IPI score, and increased cerebral spinal fluid protein level.

Histologic Findings

The lymphoma is composed of sheets of large neoplastic cells with features of centroblasts or immunoblasts, exhibiting a characteristic perivascular pattern of infiltration. Multiple perivascular concentrically arranged clusters of the tumor cells are separated by brain parenchyma (Fig. 23.21). In AIDS patients, due to multifocal and extensive infiltration by large sheets of lymphoma cells, an angiocentric or perivascular pattern may not be apparent. The tumor cells are admixed with reactive small lymphocytes, macrophages, microglial cells, and astrocytes.

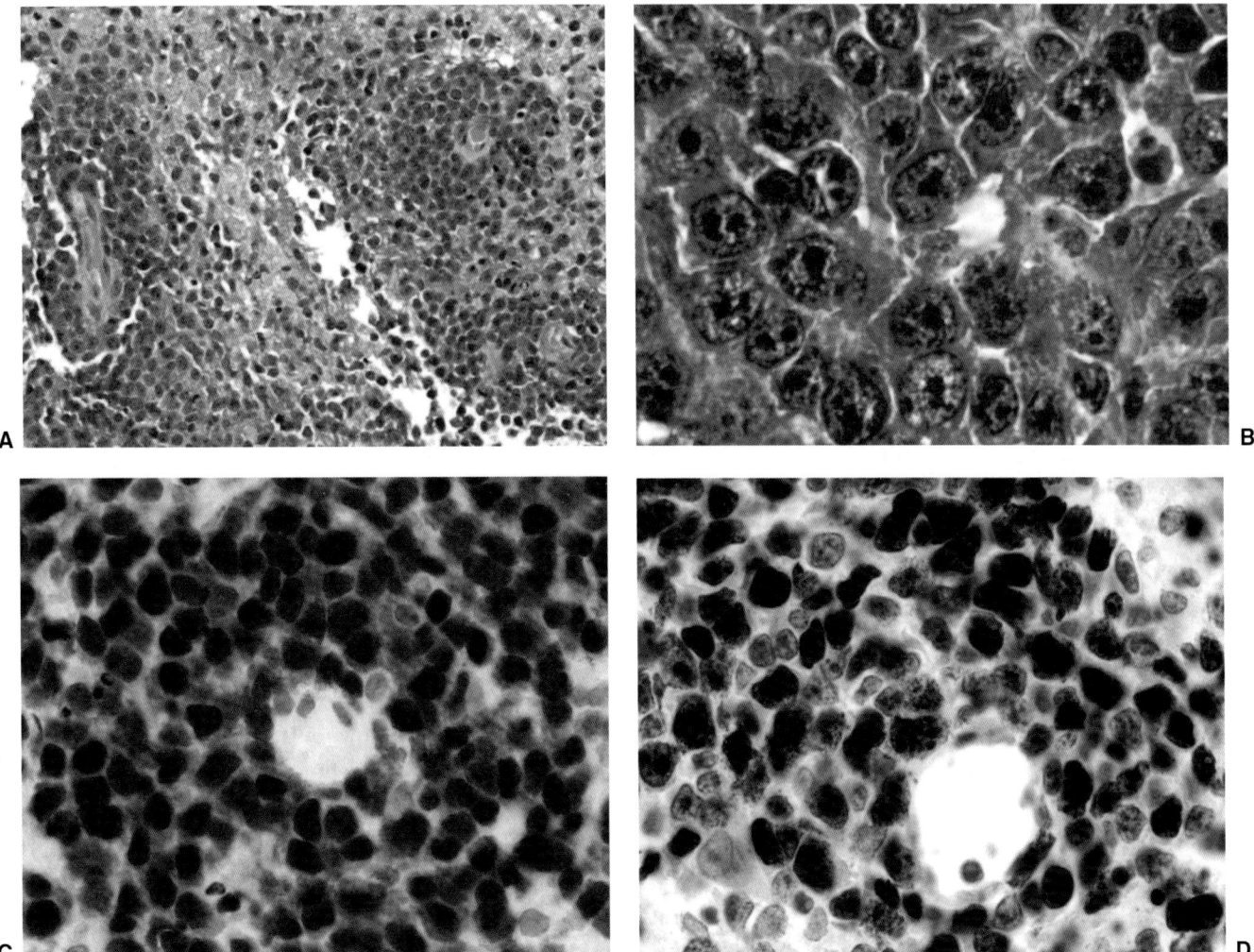

FIGURE 23.21. Primary large B-cell lymphoma of the CNS. A: The large lymphoma cells show the typical perivascular distribution pattern. **B:** This example shows large lymphoma cells admixed with brain parenchyma and form small aggregates. The large lymphoma cells exhibit a typical centroblastic or immunoblastic morphology. The neoplastic cells are CD45+, CD20+, PAX-5+, CD10−, Bcl-2+, MUM-1+ **(C)**, Bcl-6− immunophenotype, and a high proliferation index of 80% to 90% by Ki-67 expression **(D)**.

Immunophenotypic Features

The lymphoma cells express pan–B-cell markers and have a high proliferation index. In immunocompetent patients, EBV is negative. The neoplastic cells frequently express Bcl-2, Bcl-6, MUM1/IRF4, and FOXP1, whereas CD10 expression is seen in only a small subset of cases (Fig. 23.21). Activation biomarkers and adhesion molecules are often expressed, including CD23, CD30, CD38, CD39, CD70, CD18 (LFA1 complex), CD54 (ICAM-1), and CD58 (LFA3) (133). EBV is usually negative in immunocompetent patients.

Genetic Findings

All cases of CNS DLBCL have immunoglobulin *Ig* gene rearrangements and germline *TCR* genes. Hypermutated *IgV$_H$* genes and ongoing somatic mutations are found in 13% to 18% of cases (134). *IgV$_H$* usage is commonly restricted to the *IgV$_H$ 4/34* gene, suggesting that antigenic stimuli direct the *Ig* repertoire and impact the development of CNS lymphoma. Intraclonal diversity of the rearranged *IgH* gene sequences is observed in most cases. Although the pattern of somatic mutation and intraclonal variation suggests that some of the cases

may be derived from GC B cells (134), GEP shows that most CNS DLBCLs have ABC-DLBCL phenotypes.

In immunocompetent patients, *BCL2* rearrangement is present with a frequency similar to conventional DLBCL. Many cases are defined as ABC-DLBCL subtype by GEP. Due to multiple lesions, clonality analysis has shown that these lesions are derived from the same B-cell clone, suggesting that lymphoma cells arise from the same B-cell clone and secondarily disseminate within the CNS. The intriguing finding is that nearly no rearrangements for *BCL2* and *MYC* have been identified in CNS DLBCLs.

Mutations of the 5′ noncoding regions of *BCL6* are found in 42% to 59% of CNS DLBCL, whereas no mutations are found in the regulatory regions of *MYC* (134). Along with *IgV$_H$* gene results, these data suggest that a fraction of cases are derived from GC B cells that subsequently localize to the CNS. However, the frequency of *BCL6* mutations is not different from ABC-DLCBL. *BCL6* gene rearrangements are present in 30% to 40% cases. Array CGH has shown 6q deletion in 47% of cases and gains at chromosome loci 12q, 22q, and 18q21, the latter involving amplification of the *BCL2* and *MALT1* genes in 63% of cases. Small deletions are seen at chromosome 6p21.3 (HLA loci) responsible for the loss of HLA class I and II expression (135).

In immunocompromised patients, nearly all AIDS-related cases are positive for latent EBV infection, while EBV is absent from lymphoma in immunocompetent patients. LMP-1 is expressed in approximately 50% to 60% of the cases and induces Bcl-2 and p53 protein overexpression and BCL6 suppression. LMP-1 also induces EBNA-2 expression, which activates several EBV viral genes, and expression of a variety of adhesion molecules. Some AIDS-related DLBCL cases are found to be positive for ZEBRA-protein expression, a replication activator driving a transition of latent EBV infection to a lytic viral cycle. The presence of HHV8 and its biologic effects in AIDS-related cases remains unclear. More cases need to be analyzed to validate the results by using better *in situ* hybridization and immunohistochemical approaches.

Postulated Cell of Origin

ABC of late GC origin. Due to the paucity of the cases studied, it is important that more cases be analyzed to validate the results on the cell of origin, whether EBV infection has reprogrammed the gene expression phenotype, and whether AIDS-related and AIDS-unrelated primary CNS lymphomas occur via different biologic mechanisms.

Differential Diagnosis

Differential diagnosis includes Burkitt lymphoma, vasculitis, neuroepithelial tumors, metastatic lesions, multiple sclerosis, gliomas, toxoplasmosis, sarcoidosis, and progressive multifocal leukoencephalopathy. A comparison among these entities is given in Table 23.5.

Primary Cutaneous DLBCL, Leg Type

Definition

Primary cutaneous large B-cell lymphomas (PCLBCL) constitute approximately 20% to 25% of all primary cutaneous lymphomas. Based on anatomic location and clinical presentation, the European Organization for Research and Treatment of Cancer classification proposes two large subgroups: primary cutaneous follicle center cell lymphoma (PCFCL) and primary cutaneous DLBCL, leg type.

Primary cutaneous DLBCL, leg type, is confined to the cutaneous region, and composed exclusively of large transformed B cells. It is a subtype of DLBCL recognized by the 2008 WHO as a distinct clinico-pathologic entity.

Epidemiology

PCLBCL, leg type, constitutes approximately 4% of all primary cutaneous lymphomas and 20% to 25% of PCLBCLs. The disease particularly affects elderly patients, frequently relapses, and has a 5-year survival of approximately 50% (136,137).

PCFCL is more common than primary cutaneous DLBCL, leg type. It often shows nodules or masses on skin areas of the head or trunk. These subgroup patients have an excellent prognosis, with a 5-year survival of 95%.

Clinical Features

PCLBCL, leg type, typically presents with nodules or masses on one or both of the lower legs. Although the neoplasm is named leg type based on its most common site or involvement, this tumor also can arise at other skin sites and can frequently disseminate to extracutaneous sites.

Histologic Findings

PCLBCL, leg type, has a diffuse pattern and is composed of large, monotonous cells. The cells exhibit features of centroblasts

or immunoblasts and many cells are round (Fig. 23.22). The tumors usually involve the deep dermis but can extend more deeply or into the superficial dermis, but a Grenz zone is usually present and there is no epidermotropism.

Immunophenotypic Features

PCLBCL, leg type, has a B-cell immunophenotype with expression of CD20 and absence of T-cell–specific antigens. The neoplastic cells frequently express Bcl-6, MUM1/IRF4, and FOXP1 (Fig. 23.22), and nearly all cases express Bcl-2. CD10 is usually negative, but can be positive in a small subset of cases.

Genetic Findings

Most cases of PCLBCL, leg type, have an ABC-DLBCL phenotype. Translocations involving *MYC* or *BCL6* are frequently seen and reported in 45% and 38% PCLBCL, leg type, cases, respectively. The t(14;18) translocation is not present. Array CGH and FISH have identified amplification of the 18q21.31-q33 region, including the *BCL2* and *MALT1* genes, in approximately 67% of the PCLBCL, leg type, cases. Deletion of 9p21.3, containing *CDKN2A* and *CDKN2B*, was identified in two-thirds of cases.

Postulated Cell of Origin

Peripheral B cells of post-GC origin.

Differential Diagnosis

Differential diagnosis includes PCFCL and systemic DLBCL with skin involvement. PCFCL shows similarities to PCLBCL, leg type, but PCFCL is composed of a heterogeneous population of small- to large-sized cells. The lymphoma cells are often negative for Bcl-2 and frequently positive for CD10. Genetic aberrations of *MYC* and *BCL6* translocations are much higher in PCLBCL, leg type, patients.

EBV⁺ Diffuse Large B-Cell Lymphoma of the Elderly

Definition

EBV⁺ DLBCL of the elderly, also known as senile EBV-associated B-cell lymphoproliferative disorder, is defined as an EBV-driven monoclonal B-cell neoplasm occurring in patients older than 50 years without any identifiable immunodeficiency or prior lymphoma (8,138). The neoplasm is believed to result from immunologic deterioration related to the aging process. Rarely, similar tumors can occur in younger patients, but the possibility of an unrecognized underlying immunodeficiency must be excluded. Other well-defined EBV-driven monoclonal B-cell proliferative disorders, including LYG, PEL, PBL, and DLBCL associated with chronic inflammation, are excluded from this category (Fig. 23.23).

Epidemiology and Etiology

EBV⁺ DLBCL of the elderly is most frequently reported in Asian countries and is uncommon in the United States and European countries. In Asia, EBV⁺ DLBCL of the elderly represents 8% to 10% of all cases of DLBCL in patients without immunodeficiency (139–141). In our own experience with DLBCL cases from the United States and Western Europe, the frequency of this entity is about 3% to 4%.

Clinical Features

The median age of affected patients is 71 years with a male-to-female ratio of 1.4 to 1. Extranodal involvement is common, in

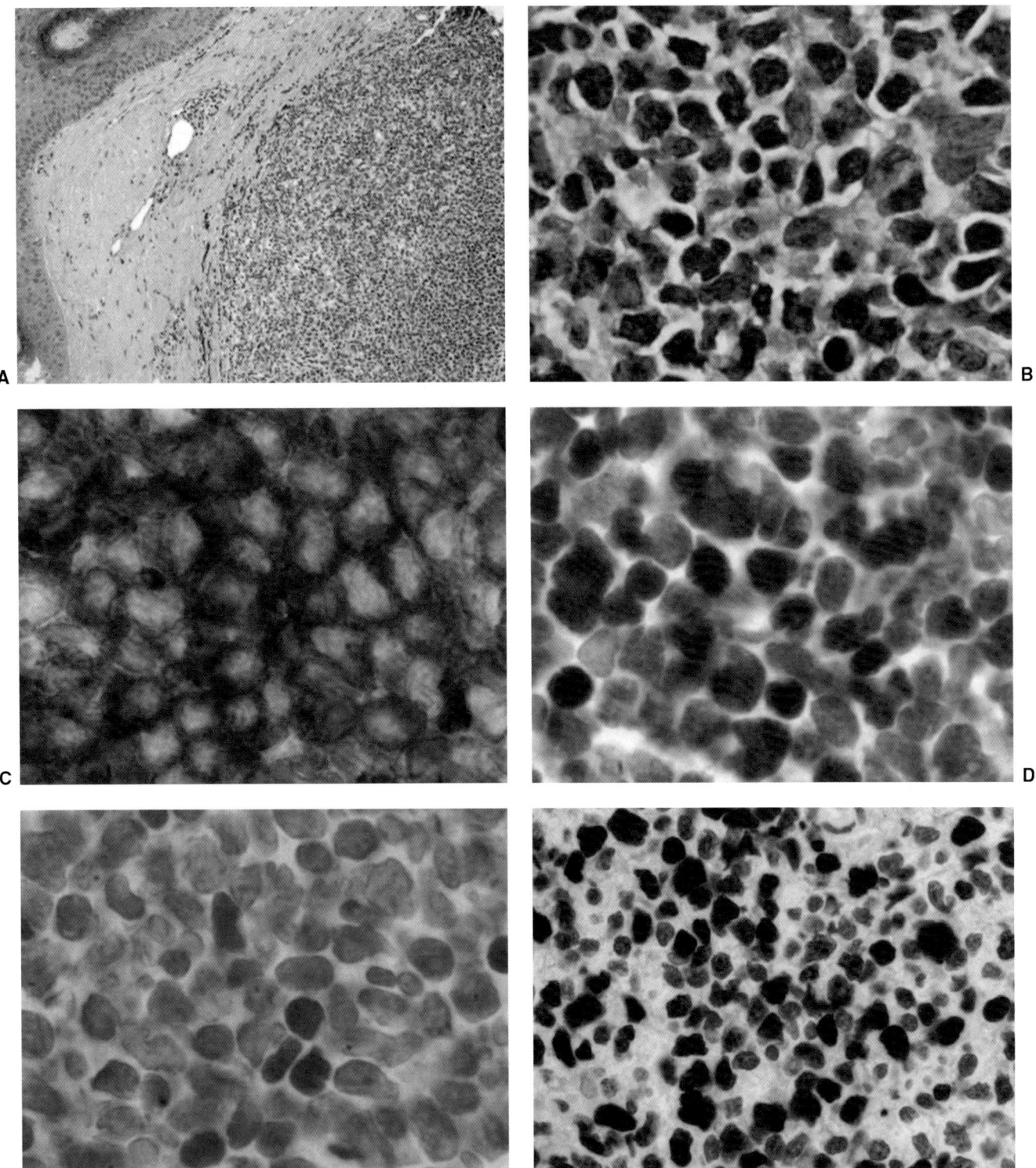

FIGURE 23.22. Primary cutaneous DLBCL, leg type. In this example, (**A**), the large lymphoma cells form a nodular lesion in the deep dermis. **B:** Large lymphoma cells show cleaved nuclear features. The neoplastic cells are CD45+, CD20+, PAX-5+, CD10+ (**C**), Bcl-2+, Bcl-6+ (**D**), MUM-1− (**E**) immunophenotype, and a high proliferation index of 60% by Ki-67 expression (**F**).

approximately 70% of patients, and the most common sites are the skin, lungs, tonsils, and the gastrointestinal tract. Primary nodal disease is seen in 30% the patients. Clinical outcome is poor, with a median survival of 2 years and an overall 5-year survival of approximately 25%. An unfavorable prognosis is associated with B symptoms, high-stage disease, and advanced

age (7,108,110). Most of these studies are reported from Japan, Hong Kong, and Latin America.

Reliable clinical studies are limited in North America. The frequency of this subtype ranges from 3% up to 7% with an even distribution among age groups in the United States. There is a trend toward higher percentage of stage III/IV disease (85%

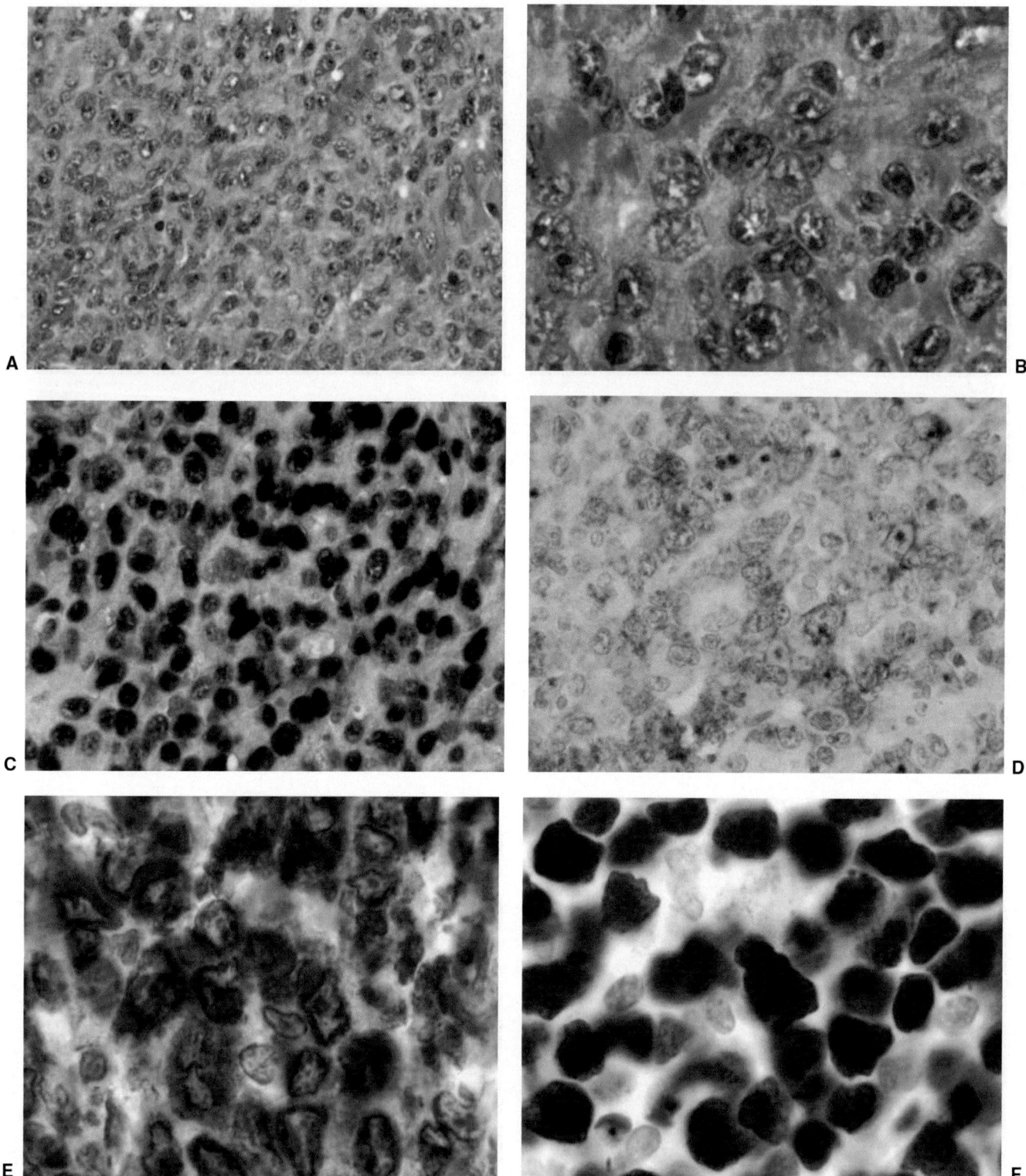

FIGURE 23.23. EBV⁺ DLBCL of the elderly and immunohistochemical features. A: The large lymphoma cells show a diffuse infiltrative pattern in the lymph node. **B:** Large lymphoma cells are composed of admixed centroblasts and immunoblasts with cleaved nuclei. **C,D:** The lymphoma cells are positive for EBER and CD30. The neoplastic cells show a CD45⁺, CD20⁺, PAX-5⁺, Bcl-2⁺ **(E)**, MUM-1⁺, CD10⁻, Bcl-6⁻, FOXP-1⁺, Blimp-1⁺ immunophenotype, and a high proliferation index of 80% to 90% by Ki-67 expression **(F)**.

vs. 57%), and BM involvement (46% vs. 16%), but the disease is not associated with preferential extranodal presentation and further identifiable differences in presenting clinical characteristics. Substantial unique clinical characteristics at presentation for those Caucasian patients with EBV⁺ DLBCL of the elderly are not identified.

The outcomes, including overall survival, progression-free survival, and event-free survival for EBV⁺ DLBCL patients over 50 years old, are no worse than for EBV⁻ counterparts. Similar results are also observed in the EBV⁺ DLBCL patients under the age of 50 years in comparison with EBV⁻ counterparts.

Given the apparent regional and geographical differences in reports of EBV+ DLBCL of the elderly, future clinical series will need to establish a more precise definition or determine more distinctive features to justify adoption of EBV+ DLBCL of the elderly as a full entity in the WHO classification.

Histologic Findings

Extranodal involvement is seen in 70% of the cases, including skin, the gastrointestinal tract, and lung. Primary nodal disease is seen in 30% of the cases. Lymph nodes or extranodal tissues demonstrate a diffuse lymphoid infiltrate. The infiltrate includes numerous large cells with the morphology of centroblasts, immunoblasts, large pleomorphic cells, or Reed-Sternberg–like cells. Coagulative necrosis can be present.

Morphologic features can be variable among the cases in regard to the microenvironment reactions. Monomorphic and polymorphic variants have been described. Nearly 50% of cases are monomorphic and are composed of predominant large lymphoma cells with sparse admixed reactive lymphocytes and frequent mitoses (Fig. 23.23). The polymorphic cases are characterized by many admixed reactive cells, including small reactive T lymphocytes, plasma cells, histiocytes, and epithelioid histiocytes. No clinical significance has been attached to these morphologic variants (8,140).

Immunophenotypic Features

The lymphoma cells usually express pan–B-cell markers, but cases with immunoblastic or plasmablastic features can show variable CD20 expression or be CD20-negative. IRF4/MUM1 is usually positive and CD30 expression is common with variable intensity. EBER is consistently positive in most lymphoma cells. Some cases can show positive EBER staining in a small subset of lymphoma cells. Correlation with EBV-related viral protein expression is required to confirm the EBV status. The EBV-related viral proteins, including LMP1, EBNA1, EBNA2, and ZEBRA, are expressed in 94%, 10%, 28%, and 5% of cases, respectively (8,119). CD10, CD15, and Bcl-6 are usually negative.

Genetic Findings

EBV+ DLBCL of the elderly carries monoclonal immunoglobulin *Ig* gene rearrangements and germline *TCR* genes. Hypermutated *IgV_H* genes are usually present. GEP has shown an ABC-DLBCL phenotype in approximately 80% to 90% of cases, with the remainder having a GCB-DLBCL phenotype (141).

BCL2 and *MYC* translocations are typically absent, but *BCL2* gene amplification has been found in a small subset of the cases. *TP53* mutation is uncommon. Mutations of the 5′ noncoding regions of *BCL6* and *BCL6* gene rearrangement were found in 45% and 30% of cases, respectively.

Clinical Course

The clinical outcome is variable, but overall the outcome is poor in Asian patients, with a median survival of 2 years and an overall 5-year survival of approximately 25%. The addition of rituximab may slightly improve overall response rate, but does not improve the 5-year survival. Reliable results of clinical outcome are lacking from the Western countries.

Postulated Cell of Origin

EBV-transformed mature B cells

Differential Diagnosis

Differential diagnosis includes PBL, conventional DLBCL with intrasinusoidal involvement, and EBV+ PTLD. The presence of Reed-Sternberg–like cells and admixed reactive cellular components may lead to confusion with CHL. EBV+ DLBCL of the elderly more commonly involves extranodal sites; geographic necrosis is more frequent; CD20 is positive, and CD15 is consistently negative.

De Novo CD5+ Diffuse Large B-Cell Lymphoma

Definition

De novo CD5+ DLBCL is a subset of DLBCL with CD5 expression. There is some debate as to whether these neoplasms represent a distinct clinicopathologic entity or an immunophenotypic subgroup, and this category is not specifically teased out from DLBCL NOS in the current WHO classification. However, patients with CD5+ DLBCL appear to have some unique clinicopathologic and genetic features.

Epidemiology

Approximately 8% to 10% of all cases of *de novo* DLBCL are positive for CD5 in Japan. The disease occurs in individuals 55 to 92 year old (median, 70 years), with a male-to-female ratio of 1.2 (142).

Clinical Features

De novo CD5+ DLBCL is associated with an aggressive clinical course (142). A substantial proportion of patients present with a high IPI score, B symptoms, advanced stage, and extranodal involvement. Extranodal involvement is detected in approximately 70% of the cases, with common sites including the bone marrow, skin, soft tissue, and gastrointestinal tract. Primary nodal disease is seen in 30% to 40% patients.

Histologic Findings

Extranodal involvement is common and is seen in approximately 70% of the patients, including bone marrow, skin, soft tissue, and gastrointestinal tract. Primary nodal disease is seen in 30% to 40% of the cases.

Morphologically, *de novo* CD5+ DLBCL overlaps with conventional DLBCL (Fig. 23.24). The neoplastic cells can resemble centroblasts, immunoblasts, or multilobated cells. Four morphologic subtypes—common monomorphic, giant cell–rich, polymorphic, and immunoblastic—have been proposed (142). Some tumors have an intrasinusoidal growth pattern.

Immunophenotype

The lymphoma cells express pan–B-cell markers. MUM-1/IRF and Myc are highly expressed in 70% of cases.

Bcl-2 and Bcl-6 are expressed in 65% and 75% of cases, respectively. CD10 is expressed in approximately 20% of cases. The phenotype of CD5+ DLBCL differs from CLL or MCL, as CD5+ DLBCL is usually CD23- and cyclin D1–negative.

Genetic Findings

De novo CD5+ DLBCL have monoclonal immunoglobulin *Ig* gene rearrangements and germline *TCR* genes. Hypermutated *IgV_H* genes and ongoing somatic mutations are present, but exhibit a lower frequency compared with CD5-negative DLBCL (143,144). GEP shows a GCB-DLBCL and ABC-DLBCL phenotype in approximately 20% and 80% of cases, respectively. Several adhesion molecules, including CD29 (β_1-integrin), are overexpressed by the lymphoma cells, whereas CD36 is overexpressed in vascular structures. A relatively specific GEP signature–associated CD5+ DLBCL has been reported (145–147).

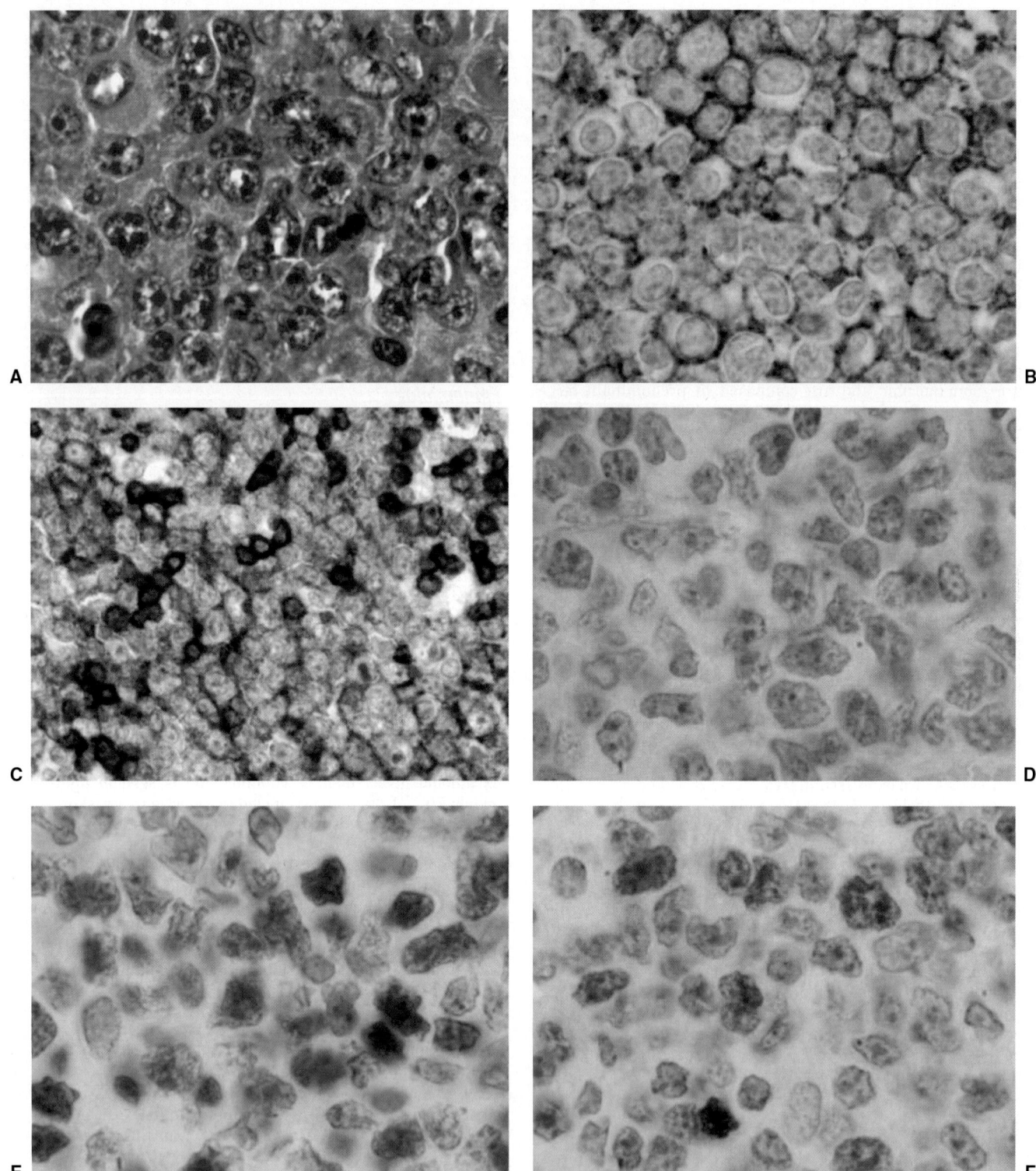

FIGURE 23.24. *De novo* CD5⁺ DLBCL, ABC immunophenotype. A: The lymphoma cells are composed predominantly of immunoblasts admixed with occasional centroblasts. The neoplastic cells are CD45⁺, CD20⁺ **(B)**, PAX-5⁺, CD5⁺ **(C)**, CD10⁻ **(D)**, Bcl-6⁺ **(E)**, FOXP-1⁺, MUM-1⁺, Bcl-2⁺ immunophenotype, and proliferation index of 30% to 40% by Ki-67 expression **(F)**.

BCL2 translocations are very uncommon, whereas *BCL2* gene amplification is present in 20% cases. *BCL6* translocations and amplifications are seen in 30% and 40% cases, respectively. *MYC* translocations are rare or absent. *TP53* mutation is uncommon and found in approximately 3% of cases. Mutations of the 5′ non-coding regions of *BCL6* and *BCL6* gene rearrangement have been shown in approximately 40% and 30% of cases, respectively.

Cytogenetics and CGH studies have shown a high frequency of aberrant gains involving the 8p21 and 11q13 regions; gains of 10p14-p15, 19q13, 11q21-q24, and 16p; and losses of 1q43-q44 and 8p23. This CGH profile seems to be characteristic of CD5⁺ DLBCL compared with the CD5⁻ DLBCL group (148). *De novo* CD5⁺ DLBCL cases are genotypically different from those CD5⁺ DLBCL transformed from CLL/SLL (149).

Clinical Course

Patients with *de novo* CD5+ DLBCL have a worse survival than other DLBCL patients. The 5-year survival rates of CD5+ DLBCL versus CD5- DLBCL are reported to be 34% and 50%, respectively. *De novo* CD5+ DLBCL has a tendency to recur in the CNS (142).

Multivariate analysis has shown that CD5 expression is not an independent prognostic factor, but is an immunophenotypic marker predictive of an aggressive clinical course. However, this category appears to be heterogeneous as a subset of *de novo* CD5+ DLBCL cases with common (monomorphic) histologic features is associated with a better survival (142). Better and reliable studies are required for improving our knowledge of CD5+ DLBCL in North American and European patients.

Postulated Cell of Origin

The presence of somatic hypermutation (SHM) of IgV_H, a low rate of ongoing SHMs, and lack of CD10 expression suggest a post-GC B-cell origin. However, a small subset of cases (15% to 20%) has been found to have a nonmutated immunoglobulin gene, suggesting pre-GC B-cell differentiation. Approximately 80% of cases are classified immunophenotypically as non-GCB DLBCLs according to the immunohistochemical algorithm.

Differential Diagnosis

The differential diagnosis includes the pleomorphic variant of MCL, which is composed of predominantly medium-sized and occasional large pleomorphic cells. Typical morphologic features of MCL are usually present focally with scant cytoplasm, inconspicuous nucleoli, and positive cyclin D1.

The paraimmunoblastic variant of CLL can resemble *de novo* CD5+ DLBCL. It is composed of small neoplastic lymphocytes and many large paraimmunoblasts. Proliferation centers and admixed prolymphocytes are present.

For CLL-transformed DLBCL (Richter syndrome), a former history of CLL, concurrent CLL infiltrate, and CD5+/CD23+ immunophenotype are supportive of the diagnosis.

Primary Mediastinal (Thymic) Large B-Cell Lymphoma

Definition

Primary mediastinal (thymic) large B-cell lymphoma (PMBCL) is thought to arise from B cells normally present in the thymic medulla (150–155). The lymphoma cells are confined to the anterior mediastinum at diagnosis and initial presentation.

Epidemiology and Etiology

PMBCL accounts for 2% to 4% of NHL and is predominantly seen in young adults (median, 35 years). The male-to-female ratio is 1:2. No etiologic factors have been identified (150–155).

Clinical Features

Patients initially present with an anterior mediastinal mass that can compress surrounding organs, resulting in superior vena cava obstruction, dyspnea, or chest discomfort. Rarely, patients may be clinically asymptomatic, but a mediastinal mass is identified by radiographic examination for other reasons. The tumor can infiltrate the chest wall, sternum, pericardium, pleura, and lung.

Most patients present with stage I or II disease that is often bulky (66%). At the time of initial presentation, it is difficult to establish the diagnosis of PMBCL when patients have disseminated disease using currently available criteria. Serum LDH level is frequently elevated, whereas serum β_2-microglobulin level is usually normal or only slightly elevated (156,157).

Histologic Findings

The lymphoma has a diffuse pattern and is composed of medium- to large-sized cells with a variable background of fibrosis. The lymphoma cells can exhibit centroblastic, immunoblastic, or anaplastic features and some neoplasms have Reed-Sternberg–like cells. The cytoplasm is usually moderate to abundant, either pale or clear (Fig. 23.25). Sometimes, the lymphoma cells can involve the large thoracic vessels.

Sclerosis is a common finding, ranging from delicate, thin collagen fibers delineating the lymphoma cells into small aggregates (compartmentalization) to a well-organized "waterfall cascade," broad septa of dense collagen, or extensive fibrous tissue. Remnants of thymic epithelium can be identified and can show atrophic, hyperplastic, or cystic change (157,158). The presence of thymic remnants is helpful for distinguishing PMBCL from DLBCL NOS involving mediastinal lymph nodes.

Immunophenotypic Features

The neoplastic cells express pan–B-cell markers and the immunoglobulin transactivating factors Oct-2, BOB.1, and PU.1, but most cases are negative for surface or cytoplasmic immunoglobulin. The mechanism responsible for the immunoglobulin-negative immunophenotype remains unclear. Messenger RNA transcripts of switched immunoglobulin heavy chain are present in PMBCL (159,160).

PMBCL is positive for CD23 in 70% of cases, as in asteroid B cells normally found in the medulla of the thymus. The lymphoma cells commonly express CD30 (70% to 86%), usually with variable intensity from cell to cell. MAL is expressed in 70% of cases and is uncommon in other types of lymphoma involving the mediastinum, except for a subset of nodular sclerosis CHL cases (161). The cells of PMLBCL are commonly positive for Bcl-2 (70%), Bcl-6 (55% to 100%), MUM1/IRF4 (75%), and c-Rel (70%). CD10 is positive in approximately 25% of cases. The lymphoma cells are negative for CD15, CD57, EMA, EBER, and variable defects in the expression of MHC molecules. Loss of the MHC class II gene is a poor prognostic indicator (162,163). Rare PMBCLs are positive for beta-HCG expression (164).

MAL is expressed in 70% of cases, but is extremely uncommon in other types of lymphoma in the mediastinum or DLBCL arising in other anatomic locations. Therefore, it can be used as a specific marker for this entity. Expression of MAL has been reported in several nodular sclerosis CHL cases.

Genetic Findings

PMBCL shows monoclonal immunoglobulin *Ig* gene rearrangements and germline *TCR* genes. There is a high load of somatic mutations in the immunoglobulin IgV_H variable regions, but no ongoing mutations are present.

PMBCL shows a unique mutational profile (165,166). Mutations of *SOCS1* are seen in 45% of PMBCL cases. Rearrangements of *CIITA* gene have been found in 38% of cases and result in decreased HLA class II expression. *BCL6* rearrangement is uncommon and may occur in 6% to 10% cases, whereas *BCL6* mutation is highly variable and seen in 10% to 70% of cases. Rearrangements of *MYC* or point mutations in *CDKN2A* and *TP53* genes have been detected in occasional cases (157,159). No *BCL1* and *BCL2* rearrangements are identified. *STAT6* mutations are seen in 20% of cases and correlate with *CIITA* gene fusion.

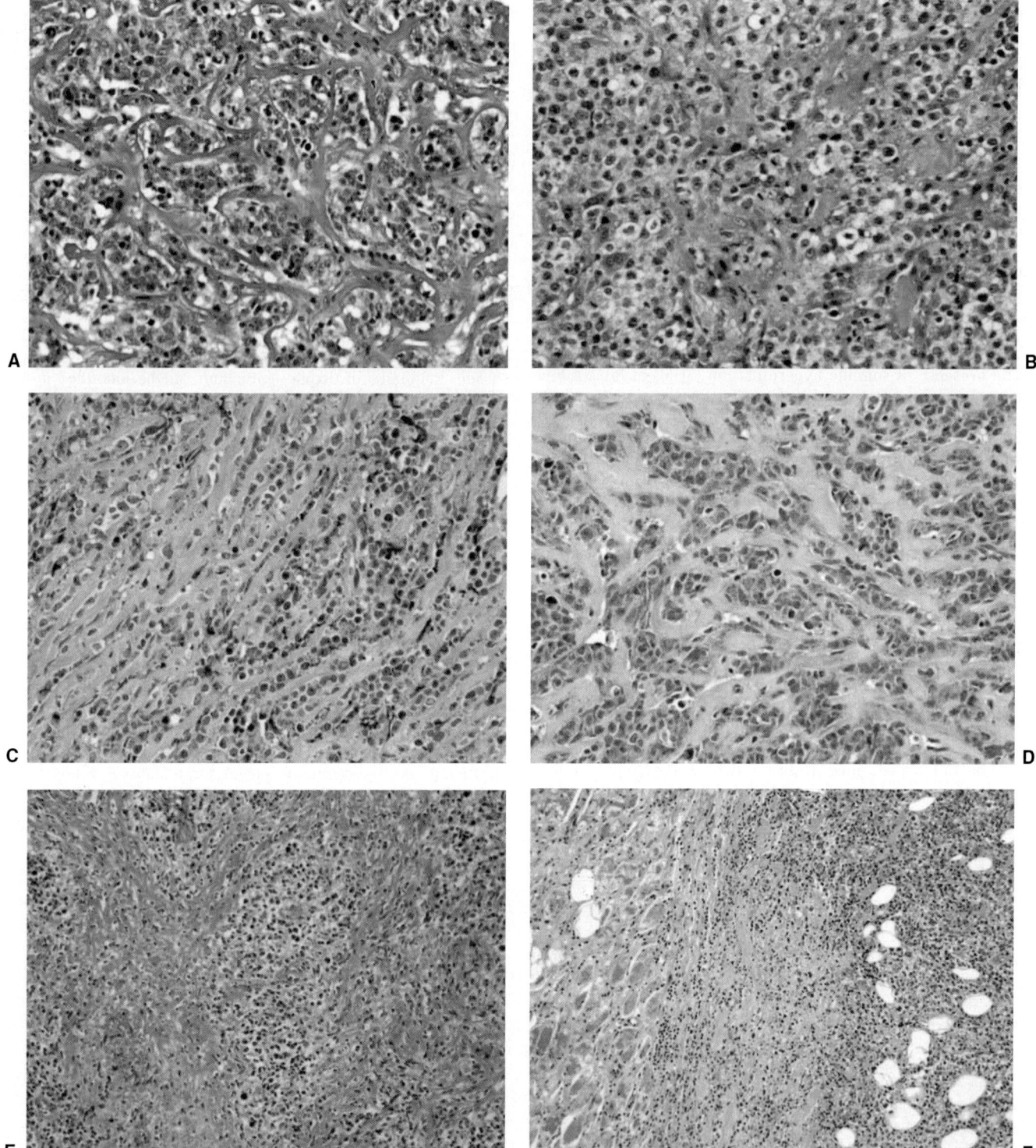

FIGURE 23.25. Primary mediastinal large B-cell lymphoma, patterns of sclerosis. A: Delicate collagen fibrils delineate the lymphoma cells into small aggregates. B: Thinner patchy sclerotic bands demarcate the tumor into packets. C,D: Linear and traversed sclerotic bands separate the tumor into a single file pattern and small aggregates. E: Broad sclerotic bands traverse the tumor to form large lymphoid nodules. F: The lymphoma cells extend into the surrounding fibrovascular and muscular tissue.

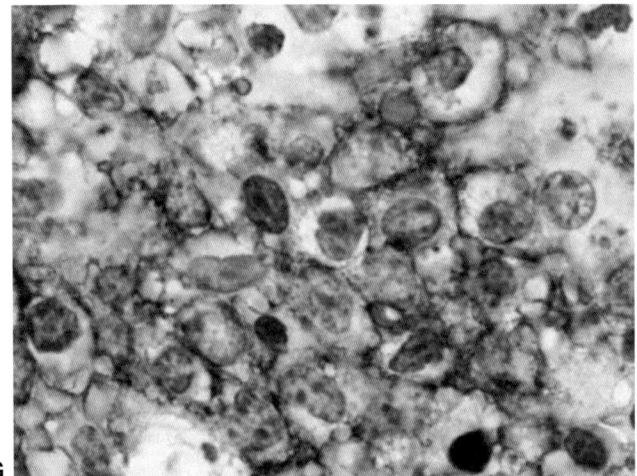

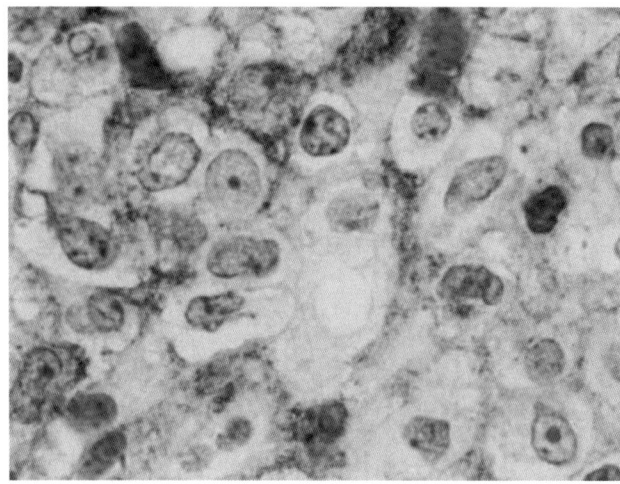

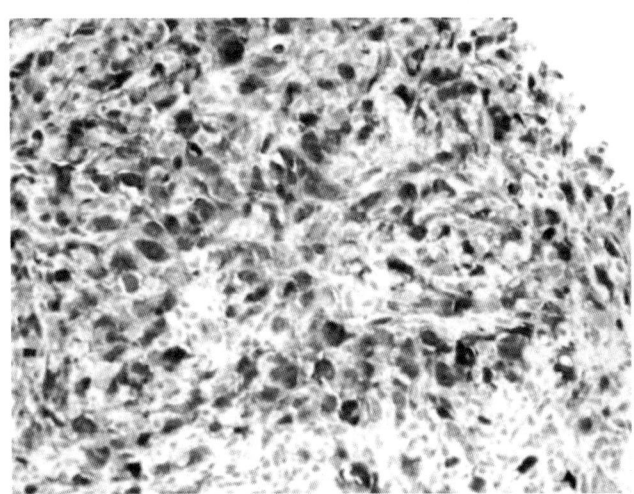

FIGURE 23.25. *(Continued)* In this example, the neoplastic cells are CD45+, CD20+ **(G)**, CD30+ **(H)**, PAX-5+, CD10−, Bcl-6+, FOXP-1−, MUM-1−, Bob.1+ **(I)**, Oct-2+, CD23+ immunophenotype.

CGH and array CGH analyses have shown gains of chromosomal regions 2p15, 7q, 9p24, 9q, 12q, Xp11.4-p21, and Xq24-q26 and losses of the 1p locus. The most frequently observed gain identified on chromosome 9p may involve the *JAK2, JMJD2C, PDL1, PDL2*, and *SMARCA2* genes. Activation of interleukin-4-induced gene 1 (*FIG1*) and *STAT6* has been observed in many cases (167).

Some cases of PMLBCL show a high level of amplifications at chromosome 2p involving the *c-REL* protooncogene and *BCL11A*. Nuclear accumulation of REL protein is common. Combined nuclear REL and cytoplasmic TRAF1 expression is a reflection of activation of the NF-κB signaling pathway, a feature commonly seen in PMBCL and less commonly seen in other types of DLBCL (168,169).

GEP has shown that PMLBCL has a distinct GEP that can distinguish it from DLBCL NOS involving mediastinal lymph nodes and presenting as a mass (167,170). The GEP profile of PMLBCL shares approximately one-third of its genes with the profile derived from many CHL cell lines. In addition, PMLBCL and CHL also share a high frequency of chromosome 9p and 2p abnormalities.

Clinical Course

PMLBCL patients are treated with rituximab plus anthracycline-containing chemotherapy, with or without radiotherapy. Approximately 50% to 80% of patients achieve complete remission. Recent studies have revealed better clinical outcomes compared with historical controls; the improved survival may be attributable to the use of more aggressive chemotherapy regimens, radiotherapy, and rituximab (157,171,172).

Poor prognostic indicators for patients with PMLBCL include pleural or pericardial effusion, nonmediastinal sites of extranodal involvement, B symptoms, advanced stage, high serum LDH level, low performance score, and high IPI score. PMBCL cases demonstrate a typical molecular signature by GEP analysis and it is associated with better clinical outcomes than both the GCB-DLBCL and ABC-DLBCL. A small subset of PMLBCLs relapse or disseminate. Dissemination tends to involve extranodal sites, including the kidney, CNS, adrenal glands, liver, pancreas, gastrointestinal tract, and ovaries.

Postulated Cell of Origin

It is believed that the majority of PMLBCL cases arise from thymic medullary asteroid B cells (154).

A low frequency or lack of *BCL2, BCL6*, and *MYC* rearrangements (0%, 5%, and 0%, compared with 30%, 35%, and 8%, in DLBCL) has been found, supporting PMBCL to be a distinct entity, unrelated to GC differentiation. Some cases show frequent Bcl-6 expression, *BCL6* mutation, and occasional CD10 expression. Although a high load of somatic mutations are seen in the immunoglobulin genes, no ongoing mutation is identified, supporting the post-GC stage of differentiation in PMBCL.

Differential Diagnosis

The most important entities in the differential diagnosis include nodular sclerosis CHL and mediastinal gray zone lymphoma (173–175) (Table 23.8).

Table 23.8	DIFFERENTIAL DIAGNOSIS OF PRIMARY MEDIASTINAL LARGE B-CELL LYMPHOMA

Pathologic Features	Primary Mediastinal Large B-Cell Lymphoma	Anaplastic Large Cell Lymphoma, ALK⁻	Classical Hodgkin Lymphoma	Germ Cell Tumor	Thymic Carcinoma
Age (median, year-old)	• 25–45 (35-years-old) • Female predominance at 2/1	• 40–65 (52-years-old) • Male predominance at 1.5	• 15–35 and 50–65, bimodal • Slight female predominance	• 15–35 • Exclusively in male (except teratoma)	• 50–60 (50-years-old) • Slight male predominance
Cell origin	Thymic medullary B cells	Activated mature cytotoxic T cells	Mature B cells at the germinal center stage of differentiation	Germ cell	Thymic epithelium
Disease features	Late relapse	Early relapse • Stage is the important prognostic factor	Indolent, rare relapse	• Relative aggressive • Stage is the most important prognostic factor	• Aggressive, rapid growth, early recurrence and metastasis
IgH mutation and SHM and other genetic features	• Rearranged Ig genes • Germline TCR genes • Gains of 9p • 2p amplification (c-Rel)	• Rearranged TCR genes • Germline immunoglobulin gene	• Rearranged Ig genes • High load of SHMs • No ongoing mutation • Germline TCR genes	• Germline Ig genes and TCR genes • Isochromosome 12p	Germline Ig genes and TCR genes
Anatomic location	Thymic lymphoid tissue	Both nodal and extranodal Extranodal is more common	Predominantly involve the lymph node	Mediastinal thymus	Mediastinal thymus
Stage, III–IV	34%	70%–80%	40%	30%–40%	33%
Morphology of neoplastic cells	Medium-sized, clear cytoplasm, defined by delicate alveolar fibrovascular septa into nodular aggregates	• Solid, cohesive sheets of tumor cells • Anaplastic nuclei with irregular foldings • Intrasinusoidal pattern • Hallmark cells	Reed-Sternberg cells and mononuclear variants	Aggregates of medium-sized cohesive cells with blastoid chromatin	Scattered or clusters of large cells admixed with small lymphocytes
Background microenvironment	Variable fibrotic reaction and scattered reactive small T cells	Atypical lymphocytes that show a spectrum of small- to large-sized cells	Admixture of inflammatory cells with small lymphocytes, granulocytes, plasma cells, and histiocytes	Predominance of small lymphocytes	Predominance of small mature T lymphocytes
Immunophenotype	• CD45⁺ • CD20⁺ • CD3⁻ • CD15⁻ • CD21⁻ • CD30⁺/⁻ • CD57/TIA-1⁻ • EMA⁻ • Oct-2/BOB.1/PU.1⁺ • Vimentin⁻ • J-chain⁺ • MAL⁺ • CD23⁺ • CD117⁻ • MHC⁻ • Cytokeratin⁻	• CD45⁺ • CD20⁻ • CD8⁻ (CD3, CD4, CD5⁺/⁻) • CD15⁻ • CD21⁻ • CD30⁺ • CD57/TIA-1⁺/⁻ • EMA⁺/⁻ • Oct-2/BOB.1⁻ • Clusterin⁺ • ALK-1⁺/⁻ • Vimentin⁻ • J-Chain⁻ • CD11⁻ • Cytokeratin⁻	• CD45⁻ • CD20⁻/⁺ • CD3⁻ • CD15⁺ • CD21⁻ • CD30⁺ • CD57/TIA-1⁻/⁺ • EMA⁻ • Oct-2/BOB.1⁻/⁺ • Vimentin⁺ • J-chain⁻ • CD117⁻ • Cytokeratin⁻	• CD45⁻ • CD20⁻ • CD3⁻ • CD15⁻ • CD21⁻ • CD30⁻ • CD57/TIA-1⁻ • EMA⁺ • Oct-2/BOB.1⁻ • Vimentin⁻ • J-chain⁻ • PAP⁺ • OCT ¾⁺ • Glycogen⁺ • CD117⁺ • Cytokeratin⁻/⁺ focal • HCG/AFP⁺	• CD45⁻ • CD20⁻/⁺ • CD3⁻ • CD15⁻ • CD21⁻ • CD30⁻ • CD57/Leu-7⁺, variable • EMA⁺ • Oct-2/BOB.1⁻ • Vimentin⁻ • J-chain⁻ • CD117⁻ • Cytokeratin⁺ • CD5⁺, ~70% • Ki67⁺, variable • Neuroendocrine⁺, ~60%
EBV association	Negative or very rare	Negative or very rare	Common, ~40%	Negative	Negative (except lymphoepithelioma-like type, EBV⁺ in 50%)
5-year survival	60%–70%	32%	90% (10-year survival at 85%)	• 85% (seminoma) • 20%–50% (non-seminoma)	• 18% (low stage) • 83% (high stage)

ALCL, anaplastic large cell lymphoma; ALK, anaplastic lymphoma kinase-1; BCL2, B-cell CLL/lymphoma 2; BCL6, B-cell CLL/lymphoma 6; BOB.1, POU class 2 associating factor *1* (a ubiquitous protein, associates with the POU domain of octamer proteins Oct-1 and Oct-2 and alters their recognition specificity); CDKN2A/ARF/p16, cyclin-dependent kinase inhibitor 2A (melanoma, p16, inhibits CDK4); c-Rel, v-*rel* reticuloendotheliosis viral oncogene homolog (avian); EBER, EBV-encoded RNA; EMA, epithelial membrane antigen; FOXP1, forkhead box P1; HCG/AFP, human chorionic gonadotropin/alpha-fetoprotein; IgH, immunoglobulin heavy chain; LMP-1, EBV-associated latent membrane protein 1; MAL, *mal*, T-cell differentiation protein; MUM1, melanoma-associated antigen (mutated); OCT-2, POU class 3 homeobox *2* (both ubiquitous and lymphoid-specific POU transcription factors, members of the NF-κB/Rel family); PRDM1/BLIMP1, PR domain containing 1, with ZNF domain; TCR, T-cell receptor; TIA-1, cytotoxic granule–associated RNA binding protein.

Similarities between PMLBCL and nodular sclerosis CHL include young patient age, anterior mediastinal mass, large cells with variable CD30 expression, and background sclerosis. Nodular sclerosis CHL always demonstrates a variable inflammatory background composed of small lymphocytes, granulocytes, plasma cells, and histiocytes. The Hodgkin cells are uniformly positive for CD30 and at least focally positive for CD15, but are negative for CD45. B-cell markers, such as CD20 and CD79a, may be expressed in Reed-Sternberg cells, but the expression is usually variable in intensity and only partial, in contrast to uniform and strong CD20 and CD79a expression by PMLBCL cells. Reed-Sternberg cells dimly express PAX-5 and are negative or focally weakly positive for Oct-2, BOB.1, and PU.1, whereas PMBCL cells consistently express these B-cell transcription factors. EBV⁺ supports nodular sclerosis CHL over PMBCL (159).

Cases of composite PMBCL and nodular sclerosis CHL have been reported. Clonality studies have demonstrated that the two neoplastic lymphoid components arise from the same precursor in some cases, partially explaining the similarities in the gene expression profiles of each of these two entities (167,170).

The current WHO classification recognizes a provisional category of B-cell lymphoma, unclassifiable, with features intermediate between DLBCL and CHL (155). These cases are also known as gray zone lymphoma or mediastinal gray zone lymphoma as the mediastinum is the most common site. The designation mediastinal gray zone lymphoma includes neoplasms with overlapping histologic features and/or immunophenotypes: cases resembling PMBCL morphologically, but with CD15 or EBV expression; and cases that show the morphology of nodular sclerosis CHL, but have uniform expression of CD20 or other B-cell markers, and lack of CD15 expression (176,177) (see Chapters 15 and 16). Molecular studies of gray zone lymphomas have shown chromosomal aberrations and a methylation profile intermediate between PMLBCL and CHL (177,178).

Clinically, patients with mediastinal gray zone lymphoma show a more aggressive course than typical PMLBCL or CHL although this point is some what controversial (175,176,178). There are also patients who develop sequential PMBCL followed by CHL or *vice versa*. Although not officially part of the gray zone lymphoma definition, many investigators have grouped cases of composite PMBCL and CHL with mediastinal gray zone lymphomas.

Intravascular Large B-Cell Lymphoma

Definition

Intravascular large B-cell lymphoma (IVLBCL), also known as intravascular lymphomatosis or angiotropic lymphoma, is a rare subtype of DLBCL. The lymphoma cells are located predominantly or exclusively within the lumina of small- to medium-sized blood vessels, with rare neoplastic cells circulating in the peripheral blood. Vascular endothelial cells were suspected as the tumor cell origin and the term malignant angioendotheliomatosis was used in the past. It is known now that it is a high-grade B-cell lymphoma arising from peripheral mature B cells (179,180).

Epidemiology and Etiology

IVLBCL is rare and commonly seen in older patients with a range of 13 to 85 years of age (median age 71). In Asians, IVLBCL is often associated with hemophagocytic syndrome resulting in poor outcome. The etiology is unknown. Confinement of the lymphoma cells within blood vessel lumina may be due to the absence of several adhesion molecules on the lymphocyte surface, such as CD29 (β_1-integrin) and CD54 (ICAM-1), which are essential for transvascular migration of white blood cells (181).

Clinical Features

IVLBCL can involve any organ or tissue, but is commonly seen in the CNS, skin, kidneys, lungs, adrenal glands, liver, and bone marrow (179,181–184). Patients do not present with leukemic phase, but rare large cells can be identified at the feathered edge of a peripheral blood smear, and large cells in the blood are commonly detected by flow cytometry. Patients can present with fever, nonspecific neurologic symptoms, skin lesions, or organ dysfunction. The neurologic symptoms are caused by multiple small infarcts due to vascular occlusion by neoplastic cell thrombi. Patients may develop neurologic syndromes, including multifocal cerebrovascular events, spinal cord and root lesions, subacute encephalopathy, and peripheral or cranial

neuropathy. Skin symptoms, commonly seen on the trunk and extremities, are also nonspecific, such as nodular, subcutaneous, firm plaques, with focal hemorrhage or ulceration. Overlying telangiectasia may be present. Patients presenting with disease confined within the skin, a cutaneous variant, have a better survival (183,184).

Some uncommon presentations can be seen in IVLBCL, which often make establishing the diagnosis challenging. Patients can present with interstitial lung disease, pulmonary vasculopathy, adrenal insufficiency, renal nephritic syndrome with minimal change disease, thrombotic microangiopathy, and an epididymal or testicular mass. IVLBCL may be diagnosed by biopsy procedures in those involved organs, including kidney, testicular, bone marrow, nerve and muscle biopsy, but often the morphologic findings are subtle and unexpected and therefore can be missed until autopsy.

IVLBCL can coexist with a patient's other medical illnesses, including autoimmune diseases, acquired immunodeficiency syndrome, hemangioma, lymphangioma, renal cell carcinoma, angiolipoma, and Kaposi sarcoma. Bone marrow involvement is uncommon, and peripheral blood involvement is rare. However, polymerase chain reaction (PCR) methods can identify clonal immunoglobulin gene rearrangement in morphologically negative bone marrow aspirate, suggesting that subtle or minimal involvement is present in the peripheral blood and bone marrow.

Several studies from Japan reported an Asian variant of IVLBCL that is commonly associated with a hemophagocytic syndrome. A few cases reported in Western countries have shown Asian or Caribbean ethnic background. Patients with the Asian variant are elderly and clinically symptomatic with fever, hepatosplenomegaly, anemia, thrombocytopenia, bone marrow involvement, and disseminated intravascular coagulation. Patients usually lack lymphadenopathy, mass lesions, neurologic abnormalities, and skin lesions. No association with EBV and human T-lymphotropic virus-1 has been identified.

Histologic Findings

Large lymphoid cells are found within the lumina of small- to medium-sized blood vessels or sinusoids of liver, spleen, and bone marrow (Fig. 23.26). The neoplastic cells usually have centroblastic or immunoblastic features. These cells can individually circulate in the blood stream; form cohesive aggregates admixed within organized fibrin thrombi and cause vascular occlusion; migrate on the endothelial surface of blood vessels mimicking angiosarcoma; or coexist with underlying endothelial hyperplasia (Fig. 23.26). The vascular occlusion can result in tissue infarction and hemorrhage (158,161). Rare extravascular cells may be identified in some cases by the CD20 stain.

The lymphoma cells can infiltrate tissue focally or can be subtle, especially in the liver, spleen, and bone marrow. Diagnosis often requires immunohistochemical studies to highlight the lymphoma cells. In some patients, extravascular involvement, usually in the abdomen or retroperitoneum, is also present.

Immunophenotypic Features

The lymphoma cells express CD45 and pan–B-cell markers. A small subset of cases expresses CD5, CD10, or Bcl-6 (10% to 38%). CD5 expression is seen in some patients, but is not associated with distinctive clinical features or a worse clinical course (185,186). Factor VIII–related antigen expression has been reported, but this may be explained by passive absorption of antigen by the tumor cells. Rare cases with prostatic acid phosphatase and myeloperoxidase have been reported. Rare IVLBCL cases are EBV-positive (187). The Asian variant of IVLBCL associated with hemophagocytic syndrome shows a similar immunophenotype.

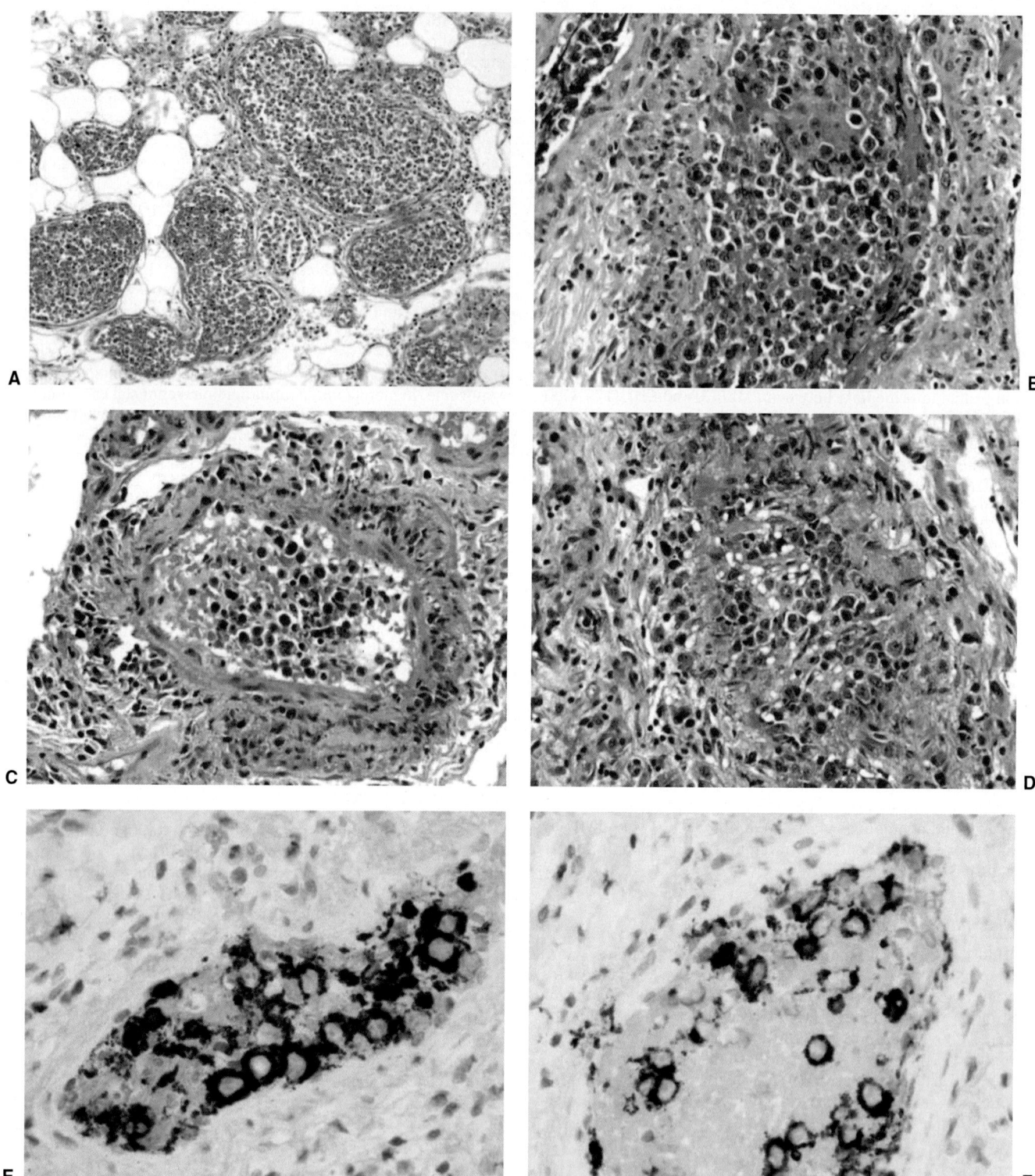

FIGURE 23.26. IVLBCL, the morphologic spectrum. A: The lymphoma cells are present within variably sized capillaries. **B–D:** Lymphoma cells are confined within medium-sized blood vessels of the lung, with complete or partial occlusion (**B,C**), and palisading along the luminal side of the blood vessel with an angiosarcoma-like appearance (**D**). **E,F:** The neoplastic cells within the blood vessels are positive by CD20 immunostain.

Genetic Findings

IVLBCL shows *Ig* gene rearrangements and germline *TCR* genes. Rare cases have *BCL2* gene translocations and may arise from FL. Cytogenetic studies show abnormalities involving chromosomal loci 8p21, 19q13, 14q32, and chromosome 18. A rare case with t(14;19)(q32;q13), probably involving BCL3, has been reported.

Clinical Course

Recent studies demonstrate an increased complete remission rate and prolonged survival in patients treated with aggressive chemotherapy (179,182,188). The addition of rituximab has significantly improved the clinical outcome in both Western and Asian patients. However, diagnostic difficulty or delayed diagnosis precludes early treatment in many patients. The Asian variant with hemophagocytic syndrome is particularly aggressive, with a median survival of only 7 months (189,190). Patients with the rare cutaneous variant, with lesions confined to skin, have a better clinical course and outcome (182,188).

Postulated Cell of Origin

IVLBCL derives from transformed peripheral B cells, with most of the cases showing a ABC-DLBCL immunophenotype.

Differential Diagnosis

The differential diagnosis includes acute leukemia, carcinomatosis, and inflammatory vasculitis.

Leukemic blasts demonstrate fine chromatin, cytoplasmic granules, and prominent nucleoli. The blasts express myeloperoxidase or terminal deoxynucleotidyl transferase (TdT). IVLBCL is persistently negative for TdT. Clusters of carcinoma cells may be seen in the vascular lumina in carcinomatosis patients. The tumor cells are generally cohesive, and they are cytokeratin positive and CD45-.

Inflammatory vasculitis or vascular structures can be involved by lymphocytes in areas adjacent to inflammatory lesions, such as acute appendicitis and pneumonitis. The clinical context is helpful and these lymphoid cells may be smaller than IVLBCL cells.

Diffuse Large B-Cell Lymphoma Associated with Chronic Inflammation

Definition

DLBCL associated with chronic inflammation arises in the setting of a long-standing, persistent chronic inflammation and is associated with EBV infection. Pyothorax-associated lymphoma (PAL) represents the prototype of this type of DLBCL and has been mostly reported from Japan.

Pyothorax-Associated Lymphoma

Epidemiology and Etiology

PAL is a pleural-based, mass-forming, EBV-associated DLBCL that develops from patients with long-standing pyothorax due to artificial pneumothorax, previously used as a treatment for pulmonary tuberculosis, or in patients with tuberculous pleuritis. Artificial pneumothorax for pulmonary tuberculosis was mostly used in Japan and hence PAL has been mostly reported in Japanese patients, with rare cases in Western countries. Patients develop PAL after a long interval with pyothorax, with a median age of 70 years and a male-to-female ratio of 12.3:1 (191).

EBV infection plays a role in the pathogenesis of PAL. EBV in PAL cases shows a type III latency pattern, with expression of LMP1 and EBNA-2 (192). It is believed that EBV-infected B cells proliferate in a locally immunodeficient environment as a result of chronic pyothorax, and eventually undergo malignant transformation. No association with HHV8 has been shown in PAL (193).

Clinical Features

Patients have a long history of chronic pyothorax, with a mean of 10 years, and may develop chest pain, cough, dyspnea, or a mass within the thoracic system. The median interval between the occurrence of pyothorax and the onset of PAL is 37 years (range, 20 to 64 years). Radiographic studies show pleura- or lung-based masses, and the ribs may be involved. The outcome is poor, with a 5-year survival of 20% to 35%. For patients who achieve complete remission, a 5-year survival of 50% has been reported (191,193).

Histologic Findings

PAL is composed of a diffuse infiltrate of large lymphoid cells that are morphologically similar to conventional DLBCL, with either centroblastic or immunoblastic features (Fig. 23.27). These neoplasms also can exhibit plasmacytoid features.

Immunophenotypic Features

The lymphoma cells express CD45, pan–B-cell markers, IRF4/MUM1, and CD138, and are negative for CD10 and Bcl-6. These data suggest a post-GC stage of differentiation (Fig. 23.27). Rare cases aberrantly express T-cell markers, such as CD2, CD3, and CD4.

Genetic Findings

Cases of PAL carry monoclonal *Ig* gene rearrangements and germline *TCR* genes. The *IgV$_H$* genes are mutated but do not show evidence of ongoing mutations. *TP53* mutations occur in approximately 70% of cases and most commonly are identified at dipyrimidine sites. *MYC* amplification is found in approximately 80% cases. Interferon-inducible 27 (IFI27) has been found to be one of the most differentially expressed genes in a gene expression profile study (194).

Differential Diagnosis

The differential diagnosis includes PEL, anaplastic plasmacytoma, and metastatic nonhematolymphoid malignancies.

PEL occurs in HIV-infected patients (see Chapter 25). HHV8 is commonly associated with EBV. In contrast to PAL, PEL cells are usually suspended in the effusion fluid rather than form solid tumor masses. The neoplastic cells are often larger and exhibit profound pleomorphic or immunoblastic morphology. PEL demonstrates a plasmablastic immunophenotype and is commonly negative for pan–B-cell markers, but it expresses CD30, CD38, and CD138. The EBV latency pattern is restricted, with prominent expression of EBNA1, but low level of LMP1 and LMP2A expression.

Plasmacytoma arising from ribs or vertebrae may involve the pleura and lung. Anaplastic plasmacytoma can mimic PAL; however, plasmacytoma patients usually have a myeloma history, presence of smaller plasma cells, and a distinct immunophenotype of CD20-, CD38+, CD138+, and IRF4/MUM-1+.

Metastatic nonhematolymphoid malignancies (e.g., carcinoma, sarcoma, malignant mesothelioma) may show a diffuse growth of large cells, mimicking PAL, but they are negative for CD45 and express their corresponding tissue origin–specific markers.

Other Lymphomas Grouped in the Category of DLBCL Associated with Chronic Inflammation

Other chronic inflammatory conditions can predispose to DLBCL, including chronic osteomyelitis, chronic skin ulcers, prosthetic heart valves, Dacron vascular grafts, surgical mesh implants, and pseudocysts (195,196). The interval between the onset of chronic inflammation and malignant lymphoma in these patients is usually more than 10 years and EBV is involved in the pathogenesis, as in PAL. It therefore has been suggested that these cases represent another form of DLBCL associated with chronic inflammation. However, given that some of these cases are incidentally detected, small neoplasms without associated evidence of chronic inflammation in the pathologic tissues examined, the inclusion of these cases in the category of DLBCL with chronic inflammation is somewhat controversial.

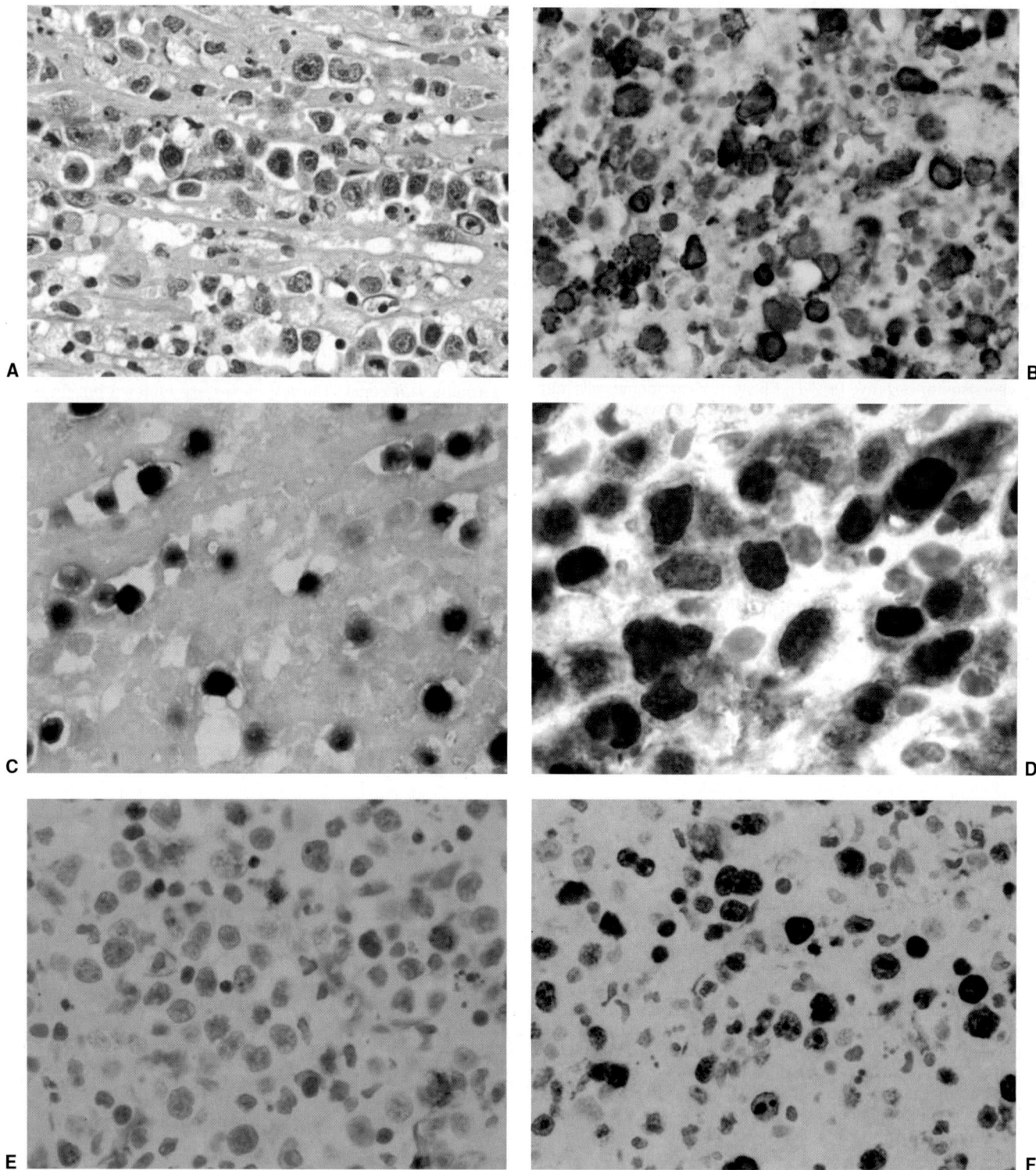

FIGURE 23.27. DLBCL associated with chronic inflammation, PAL. A: The large lymphoma cells are transversed by fibrin and sclerotic stromal components into a linear distribution pattern. **B,C:** The lymphoma cells are positive for CD20 **(B)** and nuclear staining for EBER by *in situ* hybridization **(C)**. In this example, the neoplastic cells are CD45+, CD20+, MUM-1+ **(D)**, PAX-5+, Bcl-6− **(E)**, CD10− immunophenotype and a proliferation index of 80% to 90% by Ki-67 expression **(F)**.

Patients with DLBCL associated with chronic inflammatory conditions may present with symptoms of local pain or a mass lesion, or the tumor is detected incidentally during a surgical procedure for an unrelated medical issue. The morphologic and immunophenotypic features of these tumors are similar to conventional DLBCL except that EBV is commonly positive. These neoplasms carry clonal *Ig* gene rearrangements.

Lymphomatoid Granulomatosis
Definition

LYG is defined as an angiocentric and angiodestructive B-cell lymphoproliferative neoplasm that typically involves the lungs (197), but has also been reported at several other sites, including skin, kidney, liver, and CNS. The pathologic findings are characterized by a histologic triad: a polymorphic lymphoid infiltrate composed of prominent reactive small T lymphocytes, plasma cells, and variable EBV-positive large B cells; angiitis characterized by transmural infiltration of the vascular walls by mononuclear cells; and granulomatosis, which refers to the necrosis occurring within lymphoid nodules rather than true granuloma formation. The histologic grade and clinical aggressiveness correlate with the proportion of EBV-positive large B cells (197).

LYG was first described as a distinct clinicopathologic entity by Liebow et al. in 1972 (198). Katzenstein and Peiper demonstrated EBV positivity by PCR in most cases of LYG, proposing that EBV infection may play an important role in the LYG pathogenesis (199). Subsequently, it was shown that EBV is present in a monoclonal form in LYG and the large lymphoid cells harboring EBV-encoded EBER transcripts express a B-cell phenotype and demonstrate clonal immunoglobulin gene rearrangements in many cases, indicating that LYG represents an EBV-driven B-cell lymphoproliferative neoplasm in a T-cell-rich background (197,200). The proliferation index of B cells in grade 3 LYG is similar to that seen in the conventional DLBCL, indicating that grade 3 LYG is a distinct morphologic variant of DLBCL.

Epidemiology

LYG occurs in adults with a median age of 57 years (range, 24 to 76 years) and a male-to-female ratio of 2:1 (197,198). The presence of lung disease is important for establishing the diagnosis of LYG. However, other extranodal sites can also be involved; these include the skin, liver, kidneys, and brain.

Clinical Features

Symptoms at presentation include cough, hemoptysis, dyspnea, and chest pain. The lungs are involved, with unilateral or more often bilateral nodules or consolidation, mainly involving the lower lobes. The prognosis for LYG is poor, and no optimal therapy has been well established.

Histologic Findings

A histologic triad occurs in LYG: a polymorphic lymphoid infiltrate composed of prominent reactive small T lymphocytes, plasma cells, and variable EBV+ large B cells; angiitis characterized by transmural infiltration of the vascular walls by mononuclear cells; and granulomatosis, which refers to a histiocyte-rich infiltrate and necrosis rather than true granuloma formation. The histologic grade and clinical aggressiveness of LYG correlate with the proportion of EBV-positive large B cells (197,200).

In the lungs, a nodular lymphoid infiltrate with evidence of angiocentricity and angiodestruction is found. Necrosis is present in nearly all cases. The infiltrate consists predominantly of small- to medium-sized reactive lymphocytes. These small lymphocytes can show mild nuclear irregularities. Numerous reactive histiocytes are present and plasma cells are common, but granulocytes are rare. In this background, scattered medium- to large-sized atypical lymphoid cells are present. Most of these large atypical cells exhibit vesicular nuclei, coarsely clumped chromatin, and prominent nucleoli. These large lymphoid cells can exhibit centroblastic or immunoblastic features, and

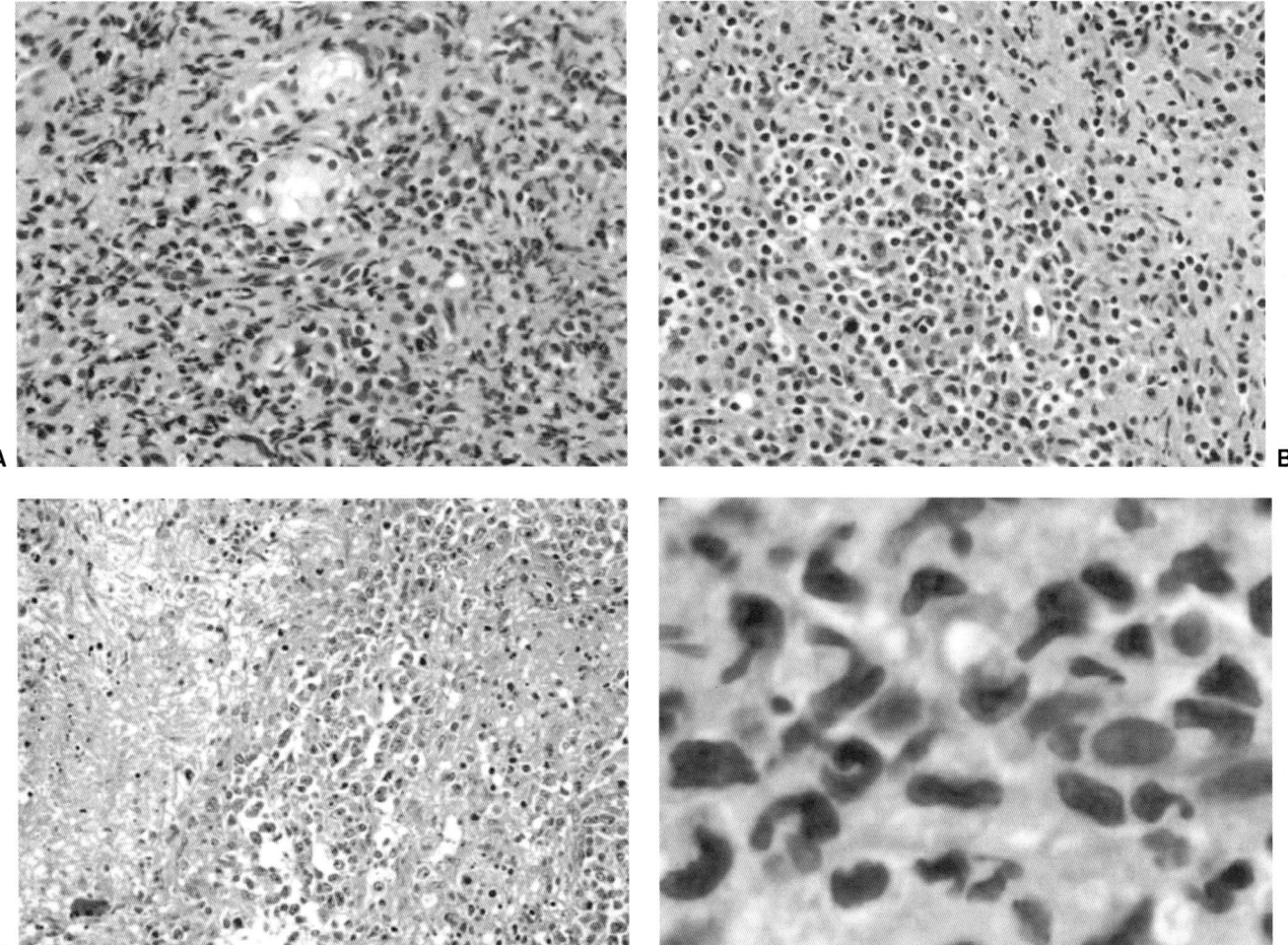

FIGURE 23.28. Diffuse large B-cell lymphoma, lymphomatoid granulomatosis, grade 1 (A,D), grade 2 (B,E), and grade 3 (C,F). The infiltrate is composed mainly of small lymphocytes and histiocytes without significant atypia. The lumen of the infiltrated blood vessel is visible (**A,D**).

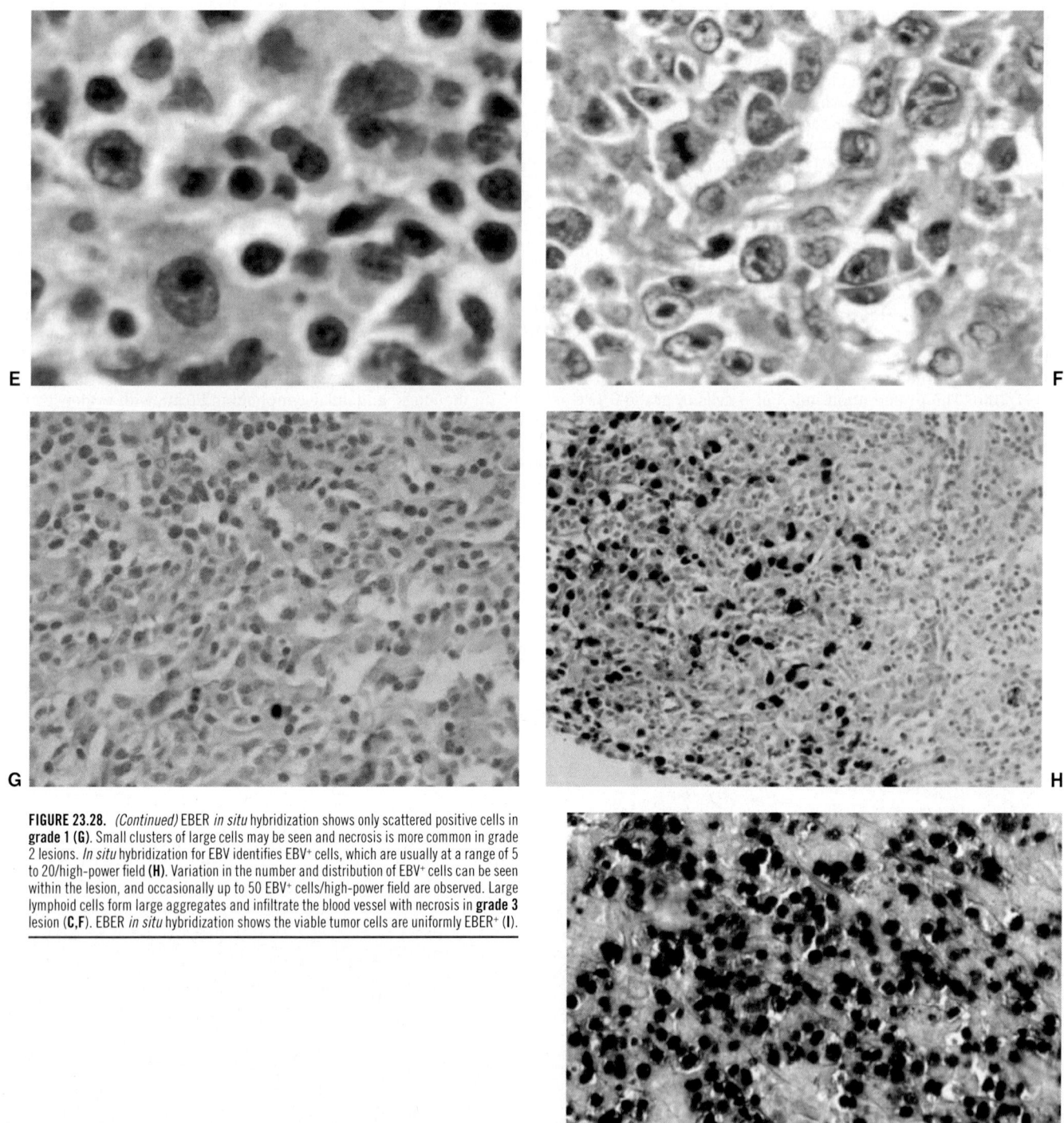

FIGURE 23.28. *(Continued)* EBER *in situ* hybridization shows only scattered positive cells in **grade 1 (G)**. Small clusters of large cells may be seen and necrosis is more common in grade 2 lesions. *In situ* hybridization for EBV identifies EBV+ cells, which are usually at a range of 5 to 20/high-power field **(H)**. Variation in the number and distribution of EBV+ cells can be seen within the lesion, and occasionally up to 50 EBV+ cells/high-power field are observed. Large lymphoid cells form large aggregates and infiltrate the blood vessel with necrosis in **grade 3** lesion **(C,F)**. EBER *in situ* hybridization shows the viable tumor cells are uniformly EBER+ **(I)**.

occasional Reed-Sternberg–like cells can be seen (Fig. 23.28). Vasculitis results from lymphoid infiltration and is often associated with fibrinoid necrosis of the vascular walls. Well-defined granulomas are not present.

The percentage of large cells relative to the background lymphocytes determines the disease aggressiveness and pathologic grading. Grade 1 LYG is defined as a polymorphic infiltrate with no overt cytologic atypia. Large cells are rare or absent, and necrosis is focal. Grade 2 LYG is defined as increased large cells in a polymorphous background. Small clusters of large cells can be present. Necrotic foci are commonly seen. Grade 3 LYG shows large aggregates of large lymphoid cells that infiltrate blood vessels with extensive necrosis (Fig. 23.28).

Immunohistologic Features

The large atypical cells in LYG are B cells, positive for pan-B-cell antigens and EBV, and negative for T-cell antigens including CD5, CD10, and CD15 (197). CD30 is often expressed. Bcl-2 and Bcl-6 expression are seen in 60% and 30% of the cases, respectively. Monotypic cytoplasmic immunoglobulin light chain restriction can be shown in rare cases. The reactive small lymphocytes are T cells, which also participate in the vascular lesions.

Genetic Findings

Most of LYG with sufficient large B cells (e.g., grades 2 and 3) have monoclonal *IgH* gene rearrangements and germline TCR genes. EBV is present in a monoclonal form (197).

Clinical Course

Grade 1 to 2 LYG is associated with a variable clinical outcome (197). Rare patients can demonstrate spontaneous remission without treatment. Interferon-alpha therapy has been used in grade 1 to 2 LYG patients and can achieve complete remission in 60% of pulmonary LYG patients and 90% of CNS LYG patients (201). Nearly 20% of LYG patients on interferon may progress to grade 3 LYG. Patients with grade 3 LYG often show an aggressive course with poor survival (median survival, <2 years), worse than in patients with conventional DLBCL.

Postulated Cell of Origin

EBV transformed mature B cells.

Differential Diagnosis

Pulmonary LYG shares several histologic similarities with EBV-associated lymphoproliferative disorders (EBV-LPD) developing in immunosuppressed individuals. Both diseases can show a similar pattern in pathology, and both lesions are composed of a polymorphous infiltrate, various large atypical cells, and necrotic foci. Both diseases can transform into an overt DLBCL. The B cells can harbor EBV and EBV-LPD can have vascular involvement. EBV-LPD consists predominantly of large B cells without prominent background T cells, and commonly involve the gastrointestinal tract, and head and neck. Cutaneous involvement is uncommon in EBV-LPD.

ALK⁺ Diffuse Large B-Cell Lymphoma

Definition

ALK⁺ DLBCL is defined as a distinct entity of DLBCL with cytoplasmic ALK expression. It was first reported by Delsol et al. in 1997. The ALK⁺ DLBCL represents a distinct clinicopathologic entity with unique clinical, pathologic, and genetic features.

Clinical Features

ALK⁺ DLBCL occurs in young adults with a median age of 36 years (202). Approximately 30% of patients are children with a male-to-female ratio of 3:1. Patients often present with advanced-stage disease and have an aggressive clinical course. Despite rigorous chemotherapy most patients have a poor outcome with a median survival of 11 months for high-stage patients (202,203).

Histologic Findings

The lymphoma cells typically have immunoblastic or plasmablastic features (Fig. 23.29). Intrasinusoidal infiltration is common. The lymphoma cells can appear cohesive mimicking metastatic carcinoma.

Immunophenotypic Features

The lymphoma cells have a distinctive immunophenotype, positive for ALK and usually positive for EMA, CD138, CD45 (~70%), and cytoplasmic Ig (IgA most often) (204,205). Expression of ALK is cytoplasmic or less often nuclear and cytoplasmic. ALK has a granular pattern, in contrast to nuclear staining in ALCL. IRF4/MUM1, Myc, Blimp-1 and phosphorylated STAT3 is usually positive and a subset of cases is positive for CD4 (~65%), CD57 (~40%), and CD79a. ALK⁺ DLBCL is negative for CD10, CD15, CD20, CD30, EBV, and Bcl-6 (206). Rare cases are reported to express cytokeratin.

Genetic Findings

Most cases carry the t(2;17)(p23;q23), which leads to fusion of the clathrin (*CLTC*) gene with the *ALK* gene, resulting in ALK expression that is cytoplasmic and granular. Rare cases demonstrate t(2;5)(p23;q35) (NPM-ALK) translocation, and in these cases ALK expression is both nuclear and cytoplasmic (207,208). MYC gene is not rearranged (206).

Differential Diagnosis

Differential diagnosis includes ALK⁺ ALCL (of T/null cell phenotype), PBL, and conventional DLBCL with intrasinusoidal growth pattern.

Plasmablastic Lymphoma
Definition

PBL is composed of neoplastic cells with morphologic and immunophenotypic features of plasmablasts in a diffuse pattern (209). Other types of lymphoma with plasmablastic features that are excluded from this category include PEL, ALK⁺ DLBCL, DLBCL arising from HHV8⁺ multicentric Castleman disease (MCD), and HHV8⁺ germinotropic lymphoproliferative disorder. Although the WHO classification considers PBL as a subtype of DLBCL, the immunophenotype and poor survival are very different from DLBCL, NOS.

Clinical Features

PBL mainly develops in patients with immunodeficiency, most commonly associated with HIV infection. PBL can also arise in patients with iatrogenic immunosuppression, including organ transplant recipients and patients with autoimmune diseases taking immunosuppressive medications. However, a subset of PBL patients do not have known evidence of immunodeficiency. PBL has a predilection to develop in the oral cavity, but other locations can also be involved, including the nasal cavity, gastrointestinal tract, anus, skin, bone, soft tissue, lung, and lymph nodes (209,210).

Patients with PBL have a median age of 50 years (range, 40 to 55 years), and show a male predominance. A substantial proportion of patients present with high IPI score, B symptoms, advanced stage, and poor prognosis. Approximately 75% of patients die of disease, with a median survival of 7 months (209,210).

Histologic Findings

PBL shows a diffuse infiltrate of large plasmablasts with eccentric nuclei, prominent central nucleoli, paranuclear hofs, and abundant basophilic cytoplasm (209–211) (Fig. 23.30). Admixed plasma cells are sometimes seen. Coagulative necrosis may be present in some cases. Mitotic activity and apoptotic bodies are frequent. A "starry sky" pattern is common. Intermixed reactive cells are usually sparse.

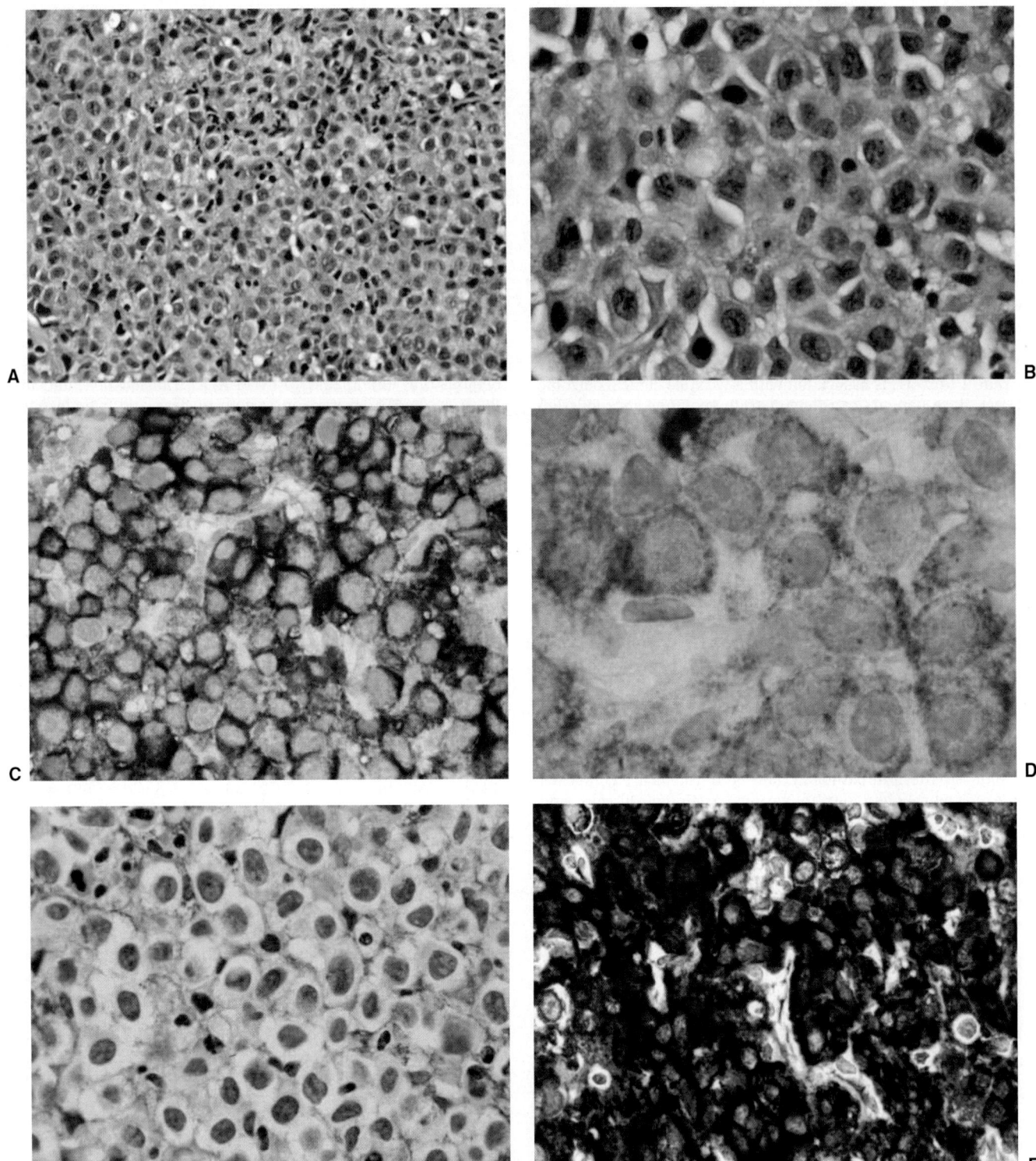

FIGURE 23.29. ALK⁺ large B-cell lymphoma. A,B: The lymphoma cells show a diffuse infiltrative pattern and are large with vesicular or dense chromatin, inclusion-like nucleoli, and voluminous pale cytoplasm. **C:** The lymphoma cells are positive for CD20. **D:** They show granular cytoplasmic immunostaining for the ALK protein. **E,F:** The lymphoma cells are negative for IgM (**E**), and IgG, and positive for IgA (**F**) and EMA stains.

Immunohistologic Features

The immunophenotype of PBL is similar to that of plasma cells, being positive for CD38, CD138, and IRF4/MUM1, and negative for CD10, CD20, CD45, CD56, Bcl-6, and PAX-5. A subset of cases is positive for CD79a, cytoplasmic Ig, and EMA. A high proliferation index in the range of 80% to over 95% is common.

EBER is positive in 60% to 75% of cases and in virtually all HIV⁺ patients. No evidence of HHV8 is identified (212,213). Surface MHC type II protein expression is negative, and aberrant cytoplasmic expression can be seen in some cases. Most cases of AIDS-related PBL have an immunophenotype and tumor suppressor gene expression profile identical to plasmablastic plasma cell myeloma, and different from DLBCL.

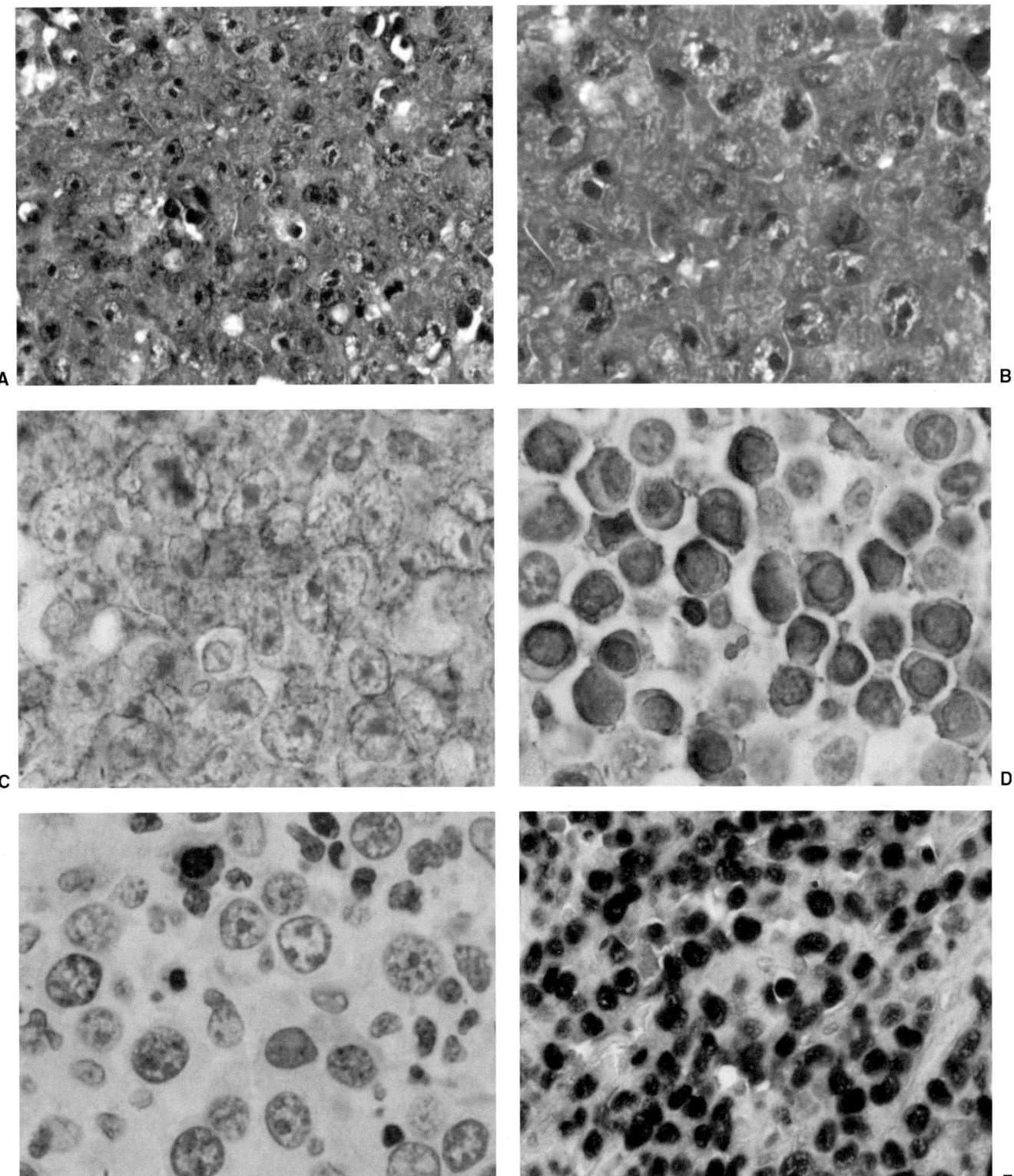

FIGURE 23.30. Plasmablastic lymphoma. A,B: PBL in lymph node. The lymphoma cells exhibit prominent nucleoli and abundant plasmacytoid cytoplasm. The neoplastic cells remain at the stage of plasmablasts, without maturation. **C:** The lymphoma cells are positive for CD138, but lack immunoreactivity for CD20. **D,E:** The lymphoma cells show monotypic cytoplasmic immunostaining for kappa light chains (**D**) and are negative for the lambda light chains (**E**). **F:** The lymphoma cells are positive for nuclear staining for EBER by *in situ* hybridization.

Genetic Findings

PBL carry monoclonal *IgH* gene rearrangements and have germline *TCR* genes. The IgV_H genes can be mutated or unmutated (209). *MYC* rearrangements are a common cytogenetic aberration in about half of cases. The lymphoma cells show a similar prevalence of subhyperdiploid and nonhyperdiploid karyotypes, as observed in plasma cell myeloma cases. Array CGH has shown that the most frequent segmental gains (>40%) include loci at 1p36.11-1p36.33, 1p34.1-1p36.13, 1q21.1-1q23.1, 7q11.2-7q11.23, 11q12-11q13.2, and 22q12.2-22q13.3. This pattern correlates with segmental gains occurring in high frequency in conventional DLBCL cases. GEP has shown an ABC-DLBCL phenotype in most cases assessed.

Postulated Cell of Origin

Plasmablasts, which represent blastic proliferative B cells that have switched their phenotype to the plasma cell program.

Differential Diagnosis

Differential diagnosis of PBL includes anaplastic/plasmablastic plasmacytoma or myeloma, Burkitt lymphoma, immunoblastic variant of DLBCL NOS, and other tumors with plasmablastic morphology. Comparison among these major entities is summarized in Table 23.9.

Anaplastic plasmacytoma shares similar histology and immunophenotype with PBL. In some scenarios, a definitive differential may be difficult to render. A descriptive diagnosis such as "plasmablastic neoplasm, indeterminate between PBL and anaplastic plasmacytoma" may be given. Clinical and laboratory studies, including serum paraprotein SPEP and bone marrow evaluation, may help resolve the diagnostic difficulty. The clinical information, such as immunodeficiency history, oral involvement, absence of bone marrow involvement, along with high proliferation index and EBV positivity, favor the diagnosis of PBL over anaplastic plasmacytoma. In some plasmacytoma cases, CD56 or CD117 may be aberrantly expressed in plasma cells; in such situations, it may support the diagnosis.

The "starry sky" pattern and the high proliferation index should include Burkitt lymphoma as a differential. The Burkitt lymphoma cells are medium-sized, monotonous, lack plasmacytic differentiation, and are uniformly CD45, CD20, and Bcl-6 positive and CD38 and CD138 negative.

Highly proliferative DLBCL cells usually show amphophilic or eosinophilic, instead of prominent basophilic, cytoplasm and are uniformly positive for CD45 and CD20. Overall, the proliferation index is lower in DLBCL than in PBL.

DLBCL arising in HHV8-associated MCD is often seen in HIV-positive patients, which has been named as PBL in the literature in the past. However, this is a distinct entity of DLBCL and different from extranodal PBL. This lymphoma occurs predominantly in lymph nodes or spleen, and has a history of HHV8-associated disease, but is negative for EBV. The lymphoma cells show variable CD20 expression, and are positive for IgM and lambda light chains, with unmutated immunoglobulin variable region genes.

Table 23.9	DIFFERENTIAL DIAGNOSIS OF PBL		
Pathologic Features	**Conventional DLBCL**	**Plasmablastic Lymphoma**	**Extraosseous Plasmacytoma**
Age (median, year-old)	• Median age 64-years-old • Slight male predominance, 1.4	• Median age 50-years-old • Striking male predominance	• Median age 55-years-old • Male predominance, 2.0
Cell origin	Germinal center or postgerminal B cells	Plasmablasts	Plasma cells
Disease features	Late relapse	• Early relapse • Aggressive clinical course	Indolent, 85% cases
IgH mutation and SHM	• Rearranged immunoglobulin IgH genes • Germline TCR genes	• Rearranged immunoglobulin IgH genes • Germline TCR genes	• Rearranged immunoglobulin IgH genes • Germline TCR genes
Anatomic location	• Both nodal and extranodal • Nodal is more common	• Both nodal and extranodal • Extranodal is more common	Predominantly involve the upper respiratory tract, can be other organs (gastrointestinal, CNS, bladder, thyroid, breast, testis, parotid, and skin)
Stage, III–IV	35%	70%–80%	<5%
Morphology of neoplastic cells	Variable morphology, commonly with centroblastic and immunoblastic variants	Immunoblastic and plasmablastic nuclei with prominent nucleoli	Atypical plasma cells, mostly medium sized, but show a spectrum of small- to large-sized at different differentiating stages
Background microenvironment	Variable reactive small lymphocytes	Few reactive small lymphocytes	Few reactive small lymphocytes
Immunophenotype	• CD45+ • CD20+ • CD5− • CD10+/− • CD30−/+ • CD38− • CD56− • CD117− • CD138− • EMA− • Bcl-6+/− • MUM1−/+ • BLIMP1−/+ • IgM, IgG	• CD45− • CD20−/+ • CD5−/+ • CD10− • CD30+/− • CD38+ • CD56− • CD117− • CD138+ • EMA+/− • Bcl-6−/+ • MUM1+ • BLIMP1+ • IgG	• CD45− • CD20−/+ • CD5− • CD10− • CD30− • CD38+ • CD56−/+ • CD117−/+ • CD138+ • EMA+/− • Bcl-6− • MUM1+ • BLIMP1+ • IgG, IgA, IgM, IgD
EBV association	Rare, ~4%	Common, ~70%	Common, ~7%
5-year survival	55%	Median survival in few months	80%–90%

BCL2, B-cell CLL/lymphoma 2; BCL6, B-cell CLL/lymphoma 6; EBER, EBV-encoded RNA; EMA, epithelial membrane antigen; FOXP1, forkhead box P1; IgH, immunoglobulin heavy chain; MUM1, melanoma-associated antigen (mutated); PRDM1/BLIMP1, PR domain containing 1, with ZNF domain; TCR, T-cell receptor.

Large B-Cell Lymphoma Arising in HHV8-Associated Multicentric Castleman Disease

Definition and Clinical Features

DLBCL arising in HHV8-associated MCD is rare. These cases of DLBCL are consistently HHV8 positive and EBV negative.

These tumors occur almost exclusively in immunocompromised HIV⁺ adults. The disease most often involves lymph nodes or spleen, but can disseminate to other organs. Patients usually present with immunodeficiency, lymphadenopathy, splenomegaly and may develop Kaposi sarcoma. Patients respond poorly to conventional chemotherapy or radiotherapy (214,215). The addition of rituximab is a step forward in therapy.

Histologic and Immunophenotypic Findings

In early lesions, lymph node or splenic architecture is largely preserved, but germinal centers of follicles are expanded due to partial replacement by large clusters of cells that can resemble plasmablasts or immunoblasts. In more fully developed lesions, the entire lymph node can be replaced. The neoplastic large cells express IgM, monotypic lambda, CD38, CD138, and IRF4/MUM-1, with variable B-cell marker expression, and can be positive for CD10, Bcl-2, and Bcl-6. Clonal immunoglobulin lambda light chain expression can be seen in some cases. The neoplastic cells are always positive for HHV8, but EBV is usually negative (214). Morphologic features of HHV8⁺ plasma cell variant of Castleman disease are also typically present (214) (Fig. 23.31).

Genetic Findings

PCR analysis of the *Ig* genes shows an oligoclonal or polyclonal pattern in some cases, but the *Ig* genes are monoclonal in advanced disease. The *TCR* genes are germline (214,216).

Differential Diagnosis

The differential diagnosis includes HHV8⁺/EBV⁺ germinotropic lymphoproliferative disorder. However, these patients are immunocompetent adults and HIV-negative. Morphologic features of Castleman disease are typically lacking. The plasmablasts are negative for pan–B-cell markers, Bcl-2, CD10, and Bcl-6, but positive for CD38, CD138, and IRF4/MUM-1. Clonal immunoglobulin light chain expression can be seen in some cases. The neoplastic cells harbor both HHV8 and EBV.

FL may mimic the HHV8-associated lymphoproliferative disorder due to the presence of large centroblasts in the follicles. FL is immunoreactive for CD20 and Bcl-6, and lacks both HHV8 and EBV.

Primary Effusion Lymphoma

Definition

PEL is a rare type of DLBCL that presents as a lymphomatous effusion in body cavities. A tissue-based variant also occurs. PEL usually occurs in immunocompromised patients and HHV8 is detected in all cases (see Chapter 25).

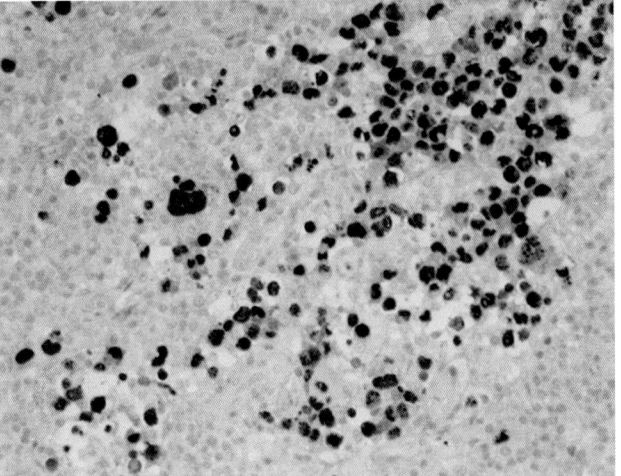
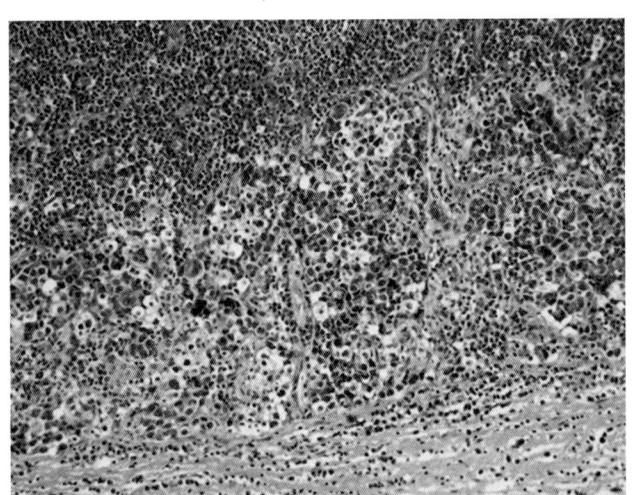
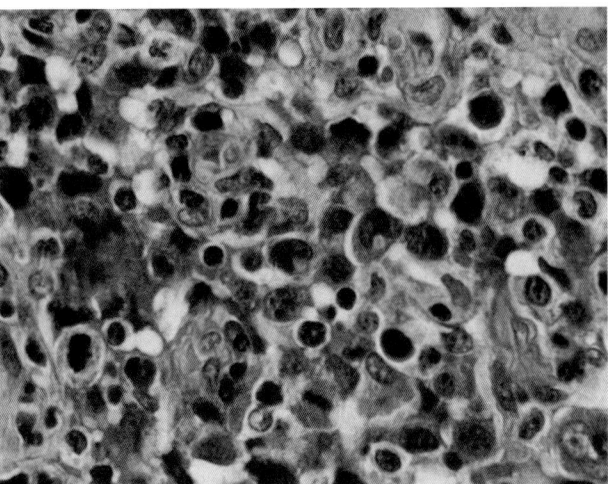

FIGURE 23.31. DLBCL arising from HHV8-associated MCD. **A:** The lymph node shows reactive follicles with large germinal centers populated by large lymphoma cells in the periphery. **B:** The lymphoma cells have round or multilobated nuclei with pleomorphic nuclei. **C:** The HHV8 stain is positive in a few large lymphoma cells. **D:** Clusters of large lymphoma cells, in which several hallmark tumor cells are seen.

Clinical Features

Many patients present with a high IPI score and B symptoms. PEL typically presents initially as serous lymphomatous effusions in the serous body cavities, such as pleural, pericardial, and peritoneal cavities, without contiguous solid tumor masses. The lymphoma cells usually remain confined to the body cavity of origin and only rarely spread to local lymph nodes or distant locations. PEL usually arises in HIV+ patients with severe immunodeficiency, but can be seen in non-HIV patients. The median age of presentation is approximately 40 years in HIV+ patients (216,217). Non-HIV patients with PEL tend to be older and are more common in HHV8-endemic regions.

Rare HIV patients develop HHV8+ lymphomas that involve solid organs, without evidence of effusion (218). Extranodal sites involved include the skin, lung, gastrointestinal tract, CNS, and lymph nodes. This extracavitary or solid variant of PEL can be the sole presentation, or precede or follow a typical case of PEL. The extracavitary solid variants of PEL show similar morphology, immunophenotype, genotype, and HHV8 infection as seen in typical PEL cases.

Histologic Findings

The neoplastic cells exhibit cytologic features that are often intermediate between plasmablasts and immunoblasts (216,217). The lymphoma cells demonstrate moderate to abundant basophilic cytoplasm and have perinuclear hofs. The nuclei may have round or irregular nuclear contours, and one to three large prominent nucleoli (Fig. 23.32).

Immunophenotypic Features

The lymphoma cells express CD45 and antigens related to the post-GC stages of B-cell differentiation, such as CD30, CD38, CD71, CD138, and EMA, and are negative for surface/cytoplasmic immunoglobulin, pan–B-cell markers, and Bcl-6 (217,218).

HHV8-associated latent nuclear antigen-1 (LANA-1) appears to be a robust marker for the immunohistochemical diagnosis of PEL, and HHV8-associated Kaposi sarcoma and MCD. LANA-1 is encoded by viral ORF73, composed of a 1,162–amino acid protein with no sequence similarity to any EBV latent nuclear antigens. Therefore, immunohistochemical staining for LANA-1 is valuable to support the diagnosis.

Genetic Features

PELs have monoclonal *IgH* gene rearrangements. *TCR* gene rearrangement has been reported in some cases. Hypermutated IgV_H genes are present, but ongoing somatic mutations are not seen. The pattern of somatic mutation and the immunophenotype suggest a post-GC cell, and possibly a plasma cell origin (216).

Infection by HHV8 is the hallmark of PEL, and plays a critical role in PEL pathogenesis. Infection is characterized by a high viral load, approximating 60 to 100 copies of HHV8 per lymphoma cell. The virus displays a marked restriction of viral gene expression consistent with latent infection in most PEL cells (216,217,219,220). HHV8 harbors more than 10 genes with structural and functional similarities to *BCL-2*, interleukin-6, cyclin D, and interleukin-8 receptor genes. These HHV8 genes are constitutively expressed in PEL cells, contributing to PEL development (221–223). However, HHV8 infection alone is not sufficient for lymphoma development and other genetic alterations are required for malignant transformation. One such "genetic" factor may arise from EBV.

EBV infection has been detected in nearly all PEL cases. Analysis of EBV latent gene expression has revealed expression of EBNA-1 and LMP2A viral proteins in PEL cells (216,217). LMP-1 mRNA can be detected in some cases at a low level, but protein expression is not identified by immunohistochemistry. It is unclear if EBV is essential to lymphomagenesis. PEL cells lack genetic alterations that are seen in conventional and other types of DLBCL. They lack *BCL6*, *BCL2*, and *MYC* rearrangements. No *RAS* and *TP53* gene mutations are found in PEL cases. Mutations in the 5′ noncoding regions of the *BCL6* gene have been found in most cases (224).

Array CGH analysis has identified frequent gains of chromosome loci 1q21-41, 4q28.3-35, 7q, 8q, 11, 12, 17q, 19p, and 20q, and losses of 4q, 11q25, and 14q32. Recurrent amplification was focally seen on chromosomes 7, 8, and 12. High-resolution chromosome-specific tile-path array CGH identified selectin-P ligand and coronin-1C as targets of a cryptic amplification at 12q24.11.

GEP analysis of PEL cell lines has demonstrated a distinctive plasmablastic gene expression profile with overexpression of genes involved in inflammation, adhesion, and invasion, and different from HHV8-negative B-cell lymphomas (221). Up-regulated KSHV-encoded latent protein vFLIP K13 has been shown to enhance expression of a number of NF-κB-responsive genes, including REL-B and NFKB-2, involved in cytokine signaling, cell death, adhesion, inflammation, and immune response.

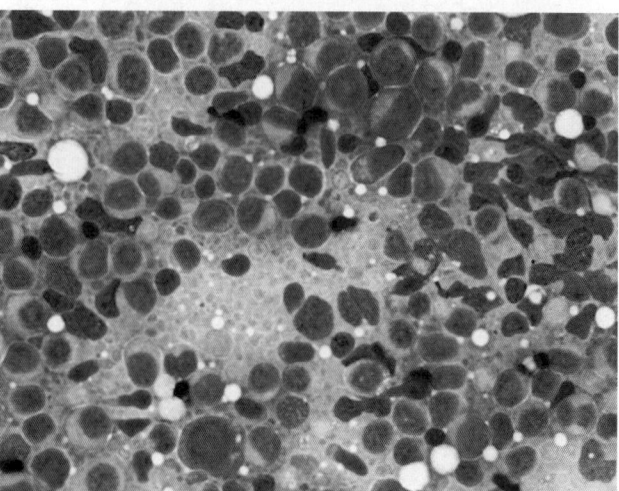

A

B

FIGURE 23.32. Primary effusion lymphoma. A: The lymphoma cells exhibit marked pleomorphism with prominent nucleoli and abundant plasmacytoid cytoplasm. The neoplastic cells remain at the stage of plasmablast differentiation. The lymphoma cells are positive for EBER. **B:** The lymphoma cells seem more uniform in the histologic sections than in the cytospin preparations. (Courtesy of Professor Yun Gong, MD, Department of Cytopathology, The University of Texas MD Anderson Cancer Center, Houston, TX.)

De Novo CD30⁺ Diffuse Large B-cell Lymphoma

Definition

De novo CD30⁺ DLBCL is characterized by uniform and strong CD30 expression (225–229). A newly FDA-approved drug, brentuximab vedotin, has significantly improved clinical outcome for CHL and ALCL patients who demonstrate uniform CD30 expression, and has been shown to be helpful for treating patients with *de novo* CD30⁺ DLBCL (230). Although this category is not recognized in the WHO classification, recent data suggest that *de novo* CD30⁺ DLBCL represents a clinicopathologic and genetic entity (229–232). Brentuximab vedotin treatment, as a single agent, is able to reach a 36% overall response rate in *de novo* CD30⁺ DLBCL patients. A substantial proportion of EBV⁺ DLBCL of the elderly and PBL expresses CD30, and these are not included in this category.

Epidemiology and Etiology

Approximately 15% of all *de novo* DLBCLs are positive for CD30. The disease occurs in individuals with an age range of 12 to 92 years (median, 64 years). There is a male-to-female ratio of 1.4:1 (229).

Clinical Features

De novo CD30⁺ DLBCLs mostly involve lymph nodes and are associated with better clinical course. A substantial subset of

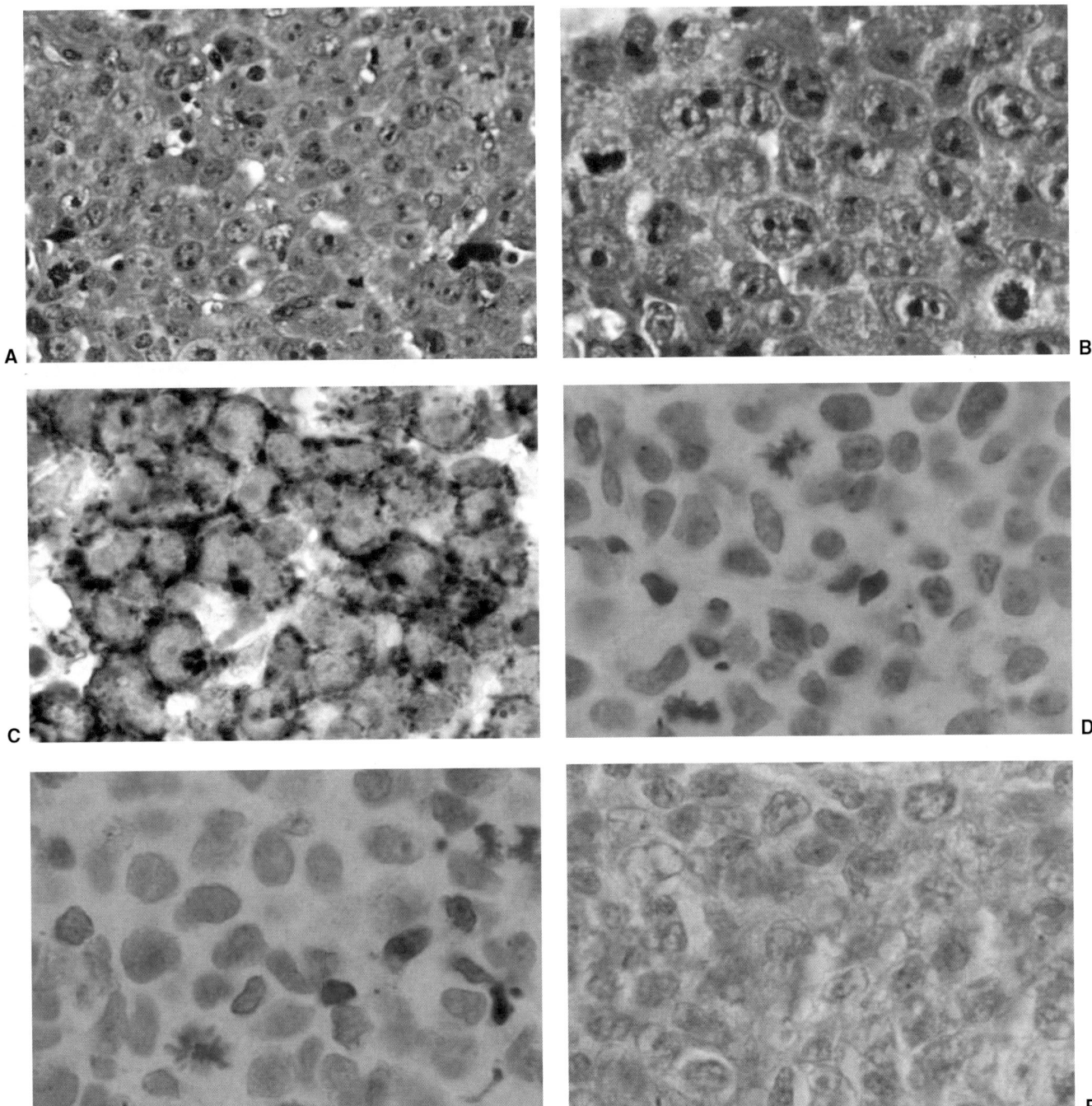

FIGURE 23.33. *De novo* **CD30⁺ DLBCL. A,B:** The lymphoma is composed of admixed centroblasts and immunoblasts. It cannot be distinguished from conventional DLBCL. **C:** The lymphoma cells are positive for CD30. **D–F:** The lymphoma cells are negative for CD10 (**D**), Bcl-6 (**E**), and EBER (**F**) by *in situ* hybridization.

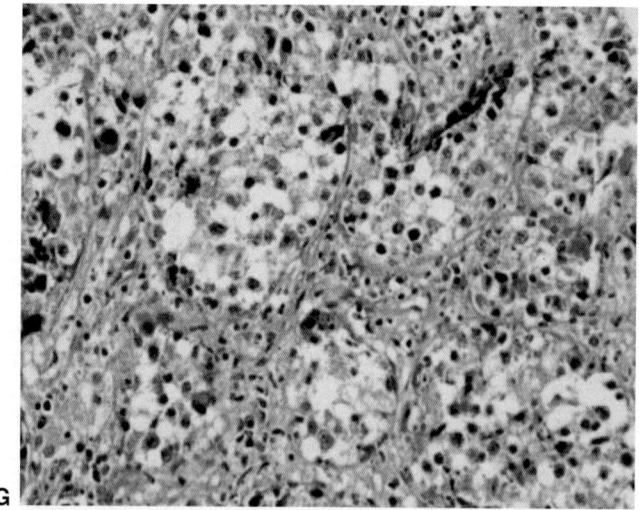

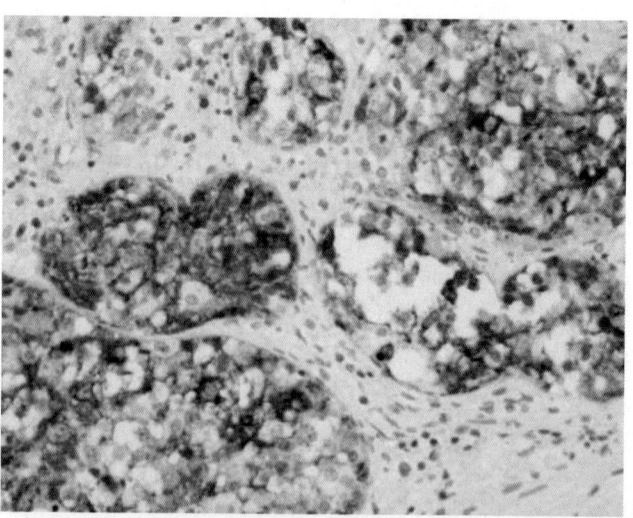

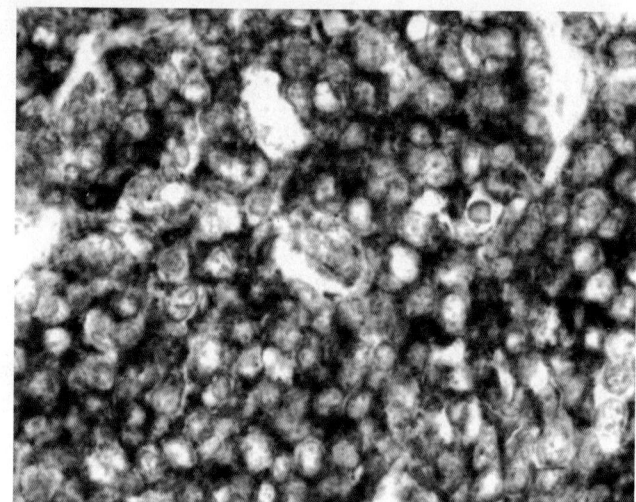

FIGURE 23.33. *(Continued)* **G:** In this CD30⁺ *de novo* DLBCL case, the lymphoma cells are confined to the sinuses of the lymph node. **H,I:** The lymphoma cells are positive for CD20 (**H**) and CD30 (**I**).

patients presents with good performance score and lower IPI. Nearly 52% of patients demonstrate advanced clinical stage and an elevated serum LDH level. However, there is no significant difference between patients with CD30⁺ and CD30⁻ DLBCL with respect to age, clinical stage, extranodal involvement, IPI risk, and GCB/ABC distribution.

Histologic Findings

Lymph node involvement occurs in approximately 90% of patients. Extranodal involvement can affect skin, soft tissue, gastrointestinal tract, testis, and CNS. Morphologically, *de novo* CD30⁺ DLBCL shows centroblastic features in approximately two-thirds of cases. One-third of cases have anaplastic morphology and rarely these tumors are immunoblastic (228,229) (Fig. 23.33). Rare cases have an intravascular or intrasinusoidal growth pattern.

Immunophenotype

The lymphoma cells express CD30 and pan–B-cell markers. CD30 is expressed in a membranous and Golgi pattern, identical to that of CHL and ALCL. Bcl-2 and Bcl-6 are expressed in 56% and 78% of cases, respectively. CD10 is expressed in 30% of the cases. MUM-1 expression is relatively common and seen in 61% of cases. The immunophenotype differs from ALCL and CHL, as the lymphoma cells are negative for T-cell antigens and CD15.

Genetic Findings

The lymphoma cells have monoclonal *Ig* gene rearrangements and germline *TCR* genes. Hypermutated *IgV*$_H$ genes and ongoing somatic mutations are present, and occur at a higher frequency compared with CD30-negative DLBCL. *BCL2* translocations are seen in 18% of cases. *BCL2* gene amplification is relatively uncommon (5%) compared to CD30⁻ DLBCL cases (17%). Mutations of the 5′ noncoding regions of *BCL6* and *BCL6* gene rearrangement are found in 43% and 38% of cases, respectively.

GEP has shown a GCB-DLBCL or ABC-DLBCL phenotype in 52% and 48% of cases, respectively. GEP studies have shown down-regulation of *MYC* and up-regulation of *FAS* and other death receptors/ligands expression (229). Multiple genes encoding proteins negatively regulating the NF-κB pathway and lymphocyte survival have been identified. The up-regulated genes include *I-κBα TNFAIP3, TRAF1, DUSP4,* and *SOCS1.* The down-regulated genes include *IgH μ, NF-ATc1,* and *PKCβ. IgH μ* chain, which encodes a component of BCR required for lymphocyte survival and is absent in other lymphomas, is also down-regulated in *de novo* CD30⁺ DLBCL. *DUSP4* encodes a protein inhibiting MAPK pathways and *SOCS1* inhibits STAT signaling. The inhibition of these pathways may render lymphoma cells susceptible to chemotherapy-induced apoptosis.

Like PMBCL, *de novo* CD30⁺ DLBCLs show up-regulation of genes related to the cytokine and TNFR pathways (including IL-13R, FAS, TRAF1, TNFAIP3, and TNFRAIP6) and down-regulation of genes in the BCR pathway (including IgM, IgL@, PKC-beta, NF-ATc1, and FOXP1). However, they obviously demonstrate different cytokine profiles as only 1 (IL-13Rα1) of 21 differentially expressed genes presents in both. Second, PMBCL shows down-regulated but *de novo* CD30⁺. DLBCL shows up-regulated MHC genes. Although both lymphomas show an incomplete B-cell program, PMBCL appears to lose more B-cell differentiation biomarkers. These markers, down-regulated in PMBCL but not in the CD30⁺ DLBCL, include CD22, BLK, SAB, BLNK, and AKT-1, as well as SPIB and IKAROS. In addition, many costimulatory molecules (such as CD80, CD86, MAL, and SLAM) that are up-regulated in PMBCL are not up-regulated in CD30⁺ DLBCL.

Rosenwald et al. used a 46-gene signature to distinguish PMBCL from other DLBCLs, including 35 genes highly expressed in PMBCL and 11 highly expressed in DLBCL. Of these 46 differentially expressed genes, only 6 were identified in *de novo* CD30⁺ DLBCL GEP studies, including 5 (CD30, FAS, TRAF1, SAMSN1, and FNBP1) up-regulated and 1 (TCL1A) down-regulated in CD30⁺ DLBCL (167,170,229).

STAT6 mutation is present in nearly 30% of PMBCLs, but is rarely seen in *de novo* CD30⁺ DLBCL. The presence of *STAT6* mutation did not correlate with Stat6 protein expression and CD30 protein expression. The *STAT6* mutation showed no impact on survival in PMBCL patients, and it represents a genetic signature for PMBCL patients, but not for *de novo* CD30⁺ DLBCL. Genomic *CIITA* breaks or fusions are highly recurrent in PMBCL (38%) and CHL (15%), but uncommon in CD30⁺ DLBCL. As functional consequences of *CIITA* breaks, the surface HLA class II expression is down-regulated and CD274/PDL1 and CD273/PDL2 are up-regulated. GEP analysis of *de novo* CD30⁺ DLBCL did not reveal the up-regulation of CD274/PDL1 and CD273/PDL2 or the down-regulation of surface HLA class II expression. It is likely that *de novo* CD30⁺ DLBCL patients harbor the normal *CIITA* loci. These results are consistent with the notion that the gene signature of CD30⁺ DLBCL is far closer to that of CD30⁻ DLBCL rather than to PMBCL (231).

TP53 point mutations are found in 23% of cases, but no *MYC* translocations are identified. The absence of *MYC* and lower frequency of *BCL2* aberrations might contribute to its favorable prognosis.

Clinical Course

Patients with *de novo* CD30⁺ DLBCL have a superior survival to patients with conventional DLBCL when treated with R-CHOP therapy. The 5-year survival rates of CD30⁺ DLBCL versus CD30⁻ DLBCL are reported at 77% and 58%, respectively (229). Multivariate analysis has shown that CD30 expression is an independent prognostic factor for better survival and is independent of the IPI score. In light of the favorable prognosis of *de novo* CD30⁺ DLBCL, the different gene expression signatures and the availability of a targeted therapeutic agent (brentuximab vedotin), it is probably appropriate to consider CD30⁺ DLBCL as a provisional entity (232,233).

SUMMARY AND CONCLUSIONS

The current WHO classification system for DLBCL, based on clinical features, morphology, immunophenotype, and genetic information, was an important step in recognizing the heterogeneous nature of DLBCL. Nevertheless, this was only an early step in our efforts to better understand and characterize this disease.

Molecular analyses including GEP and whole genomic sequencing studies of DLBCL have shown activation of oncogenic pathways in different tumors, some of which are associated with the presence of translocations, somatic mutations, and epigenetic changes in specific genes, including *BCL2, BCL6, MYC, TP53, MDM2, MDM4, ARF*, that are critical in determining lymphomagenesis and progression. This knowledge has provided value in predicting treatment response, recurrence, disease progression, and survival. The results of these studies have benefited DLBCL classification and have provided some evidence of differentiation stage and cell of origin (234,235).

GEP was another useful step. Using microarrays to quantitatively analyze the expression of the entire human functional genome, we have shown preferential gene expression in particular types of lymphoid cells with suspected roles that facilitated lymphoma classification and supported immunology and cancer translational research. Analysis of *de novo* DLBCL revealed major groups of cases with the most popular system devised by the LLMPP being GCB-DLBCL, ABC-DLBCL, and PMLBCL. GCB-DLBCL expresses genes that define a GC B-cell signature. In contrast, ABC-DLBCL expresses such genes at low or undetectable levels, but exhibits the signature of activated peripheral blood B cells. Correlation with histology has revealed that the gene expression subgroups defined with this approach did not show a clear relationship to the morphologic subtypes of DLBCL. The investigators also tested a possible correlation of the gene expression patterns with the clinical characteristics of the patients. It became evident that GCB-like and ABC-like DLBCL were associated with statistically significant differences in overall survival and event-free survival; 76% of the GCB-like DLBCL patients were still alive after 5 years, although this was the case for only 30% of the ABC-like DLBCL patients. The molecular subtype-oriented treatment regimens and ongoing clinical trials, such as ibrutinib, histone deacetylase inhibitor, and phosphatidylinositol-3-kinase inhibitor or their combinations, have been providing a hope to these patients by rendering personalized treatment regimens.

The apparent next step in better understanding DLBCL biology will be whole genome sequencing studies (236). Although the two DLBCL subgroups identified by GEP have clinical value, it is unclear which of the genes that distinguish GCB-like from ABC-like DLBCL are the most important. Whole genome sequencing will identify additional driver mutations and help to decipher functional consequences of these abnormalities (55,237). This knowledge will likely strengthen observations made by previously used methods, and provide results that will identify genes that can be targeted by specific therapies, that is, true personalized cancer therapy. These data will also be critical to advance our understanding of the biology of DLBCL and are likely to improve, perhaps radically, future classification schemes for DLBCL.

 ## ACKNOWLEDGMENTS

We thank our colleagues at various academic centers for their assistance with aspects of this chapter, especially Drs. Carlo Visco, Roberto N. Miranda, Shimin Hu, Chi Young Ok, Cesar Moran, Jeanne Meis, Alexander Tzankov, and Michael B. Møller. We appreciate the sharing of several rare cases by Drs. Dennis O'Malley, Yun Gong, and Roger Warnke. We also thank Dr. Ann Sutton, Ph.D., from the Department of Scientific Publications at MD Anderson Cancer Center for editing this chapter. K.H.Y is supported by The University of Texas MD Anderson Cancer Center Institutional R & D Fund, an Institutional Research Grant Award, an MD Anderson Lymphoma Specialized Programs of Research Excellence (SPORE) Research Development Program Award, an MD Anderson Myeloma SPORE Research Development Program Award, MD Anderson Collaborative Research Funds with High-Throughput Molecular Diagnostics and Roche Molecular Systems, National Cancer Institute and National Institutes of Health grants (R01CA138688, 1RC1CA146299, P50CA136411 and P50CA142509), and MD Anderson Cancer Center Support Grant CA016672.

References

1. Stein H, Warnke RA, Chan WC, et al. Diffuse large B-cell lymphoma, not otherwise specified. In: Swerdlow SH, Campo E, Harris NL, et al., eds. *WHO classification of tumours of haematopoietic and lymphoid tissues*, 4th ed. Lyon: IARC, 2008:233–237.
2. Lennert K, Feller AC. *High grade malignant lymphoma of B-cell type. Histopathology of non-Hodgkin's lymphoma*, 2nd ed. Berlin: Springer-Verlag, 1990.
3. The Non-Hodgkin's Lymphoma Pathologic Classification Project Writing Committee. National Cancer Institute sponsored study of classifications of non-Hodgkin's lymphomas: summary and description of a working formulation for clinical usage. The Non-Hodgkin's Lymphoma Pathologic Classification Project. *Cancer* 1982;49:2112–2135.
4. Harris NL, Jaffe ES, Stein H, et al. A revised European-American classification of lymphoid neoplasms: a proposal from the International Lymphoma Study Group. *Blood* 1994;84:1361–1392.
5. Gatter KC, Warnke RA. Diffuse large B-cell lymphoma. In: Jaffe ES, Harris NL, Stein H, et al., eds. *Pathology and genetics: tumours of haematopoietic and lymphoid tissues*. World Health Organization Classification of Tumours. Lyon: IARC Press, 2001:171–174.
6. The Non-Hodgkin's Lymphoma Classification Project. A clinical evaluation of the International Lymphoma Study Group classification of non-Hodgkin's lymphoma. *Blood* 1997;89:3909–3918.
7. Diebold J, Anderson JR, Armitage JO, et al. Diffuse large B-cell lymphoma: a clinicopathologic analysis of 444 cases classified according to the updated Kiel classification. *Leuk Lymphoma* 2002;43:97–104.
8. Nakamura S, Jaffe ES, Swerdlow SH. EBV positive diffuse large B-cell lymphoma of the elderly. In: Swerdlow SH, Campo E, Harris NL, et al., eds. *WHO classification of tumours of haematopoietic and lymphoid tissues*, 4th ed. Lyon: IARC, 2008:243–244.
9. Hummel M, Anagnostopoulos I, Korbjuhn P, et al. Epstein-Barr virus in B-cell non-Hodgkin's lymphomas: unexpected infection patterns and different infection incidence in low- and high-grade types. *J Pathol* 1995;175:263–271.
10. Armitage JO, Weisenburger DD. New approach to classifying non-Hodgkin's lymphomas: clinical features of the major histologic subtypes. Non-Hodgkin's Lymphoma Classification Project. *J Clin Oncol* 1998;16:2780–2795.
11. Conlan MG, Bast M, Armitage JO, et al. Bone marrow involvement by non-Hodgkin's lymphoma: the clinical significance of morphologic discordance between the lymph node and bone marrow. Nebraska Lymphoma Study Group. *J Clin Oncol* 1990;8:1163–1172.
12. Alizadeh AA, Eisen MB, Davis RE, et al. Distinct types of diffuse large B-cell lymphoma identified by gene expression profiling. *Nature* 2000;403:503–511.
13. Shipp MA, Ross KN, Tomayo P, et al. Diffuse large B-cell lymphoma outcome prediction by gene-expression profiling and supervised machine learning. *Nat Med* 2002;8(1):68–74.
14. Wang J, Chen C, Lau S, et al. CD3-positive large B-cell lymphoma. *Am J Surg Pathol* 2009;33:505–512.
15. Kennedy GA, Tey SK, Cobcroft R, et al. Incidence and nature of CD20-negative relapses following rituximab therapy in aggressive B-cell non-Hodgkin's lymphoma: a retrospective review. *Br J Haematol* 2002;119:412–416.
16. Barrans SL, O'Connor SJ, Evans PA, et al. Rearrangement of the *BCL6* locus at 3q27 is an independent poor prognostic factor in nodal diffuse large B-cell lymphoma. *Br J Haematol* 2002;117:322–332.
17. Barrans SL, Carter I, Owen RG, et al. Germinal center phenotype and bcl-2 expression combined with the International Prognostic Index improves patient risk stratification in diffuse large B-cell lymphoma. *Blood* 2002;99:1136–1143.
18. Huang JZ, Sanger WG, Greiner TC, et al. The t(14;18) defines a unique subset of diffuse large B-cell lymphoma with a germinal center B-cell gene expression profile. *Blood* 2002;99:2285–2290.
19. Onizuka T, Moriyama M, Yamochi T, et al. BCL-6 gene product, a 92- to 98-kD nuclear phosphoprotein, is highly expressed in germinal center B cells and their neoplastic counterparts. *Blood* 1995;86:28–37.
20. Falini B, Fizzotti M, Pucciarini A, et al. A monoclonal antibody (MUM1p) detects expression of the MUM1/IRF4 protein in a subset of germinal center B cells, plasma cells, and activated T cells. *Blood* 2000;95:2084–2092.
21. Miller TP, Grogan TM, Dahlberg S, et al. Prognostic significance of the Ki-67-associated proliferative antigen in aggressive non-Hodgkin's lymphomas: a prospective Southwest Oncology Group trial. *Blood* 1994;83:1460–1466.
22. Kreipe H, Wacker HH, Heidebrecht HJ, et al. Determination of the growth fraction in non-Hodgkin's lymphomas by monoclonal antibody Ki-S5 directed against a formalin-resistant epitope of the Ki-67 antigen. *Am J Pathol* 1993;142: 1689–1694.
23. Hans CP, Weisenburger DD, Greiner TC, et al. Confirmation of the molecular classification of diffuse large B-cell lymphoma by immunohistochemistry using a tissue microarray. *Blood* 2004;103:275–282.
24. Visco C, Li Y, Xu-Monette ZY, et al. Comprehensive gene expression profiling and immunohistochemical studies support application of immunophenotypic algorithm for molecular subtype classification in diffuse large B-cell lymphoma: a report from the International DLBCL Rituximab-CHOP Consortium Program Study. *Leukemia* 2012;26(9):2103–2113.
25. Choi WW, Weisenburger DD, Greiner TC, et al. A new immunostain algorithm classifies diffuse large B-cell lymphoma into molecular subtypes with high accuracy. *Clin Cancer Res* 2009;15:5494–5502.
26. Meyer PN, Fu K, Greiner TC, et al. Immunohistochemical methods for predicting cell of origin and survival in patients with diffuse large B-cell lymphoma treated with rituximab. *J Clin Oncol* 2011;29(2):200–207.
27. Perry AM, Cardesa-Salzmann TM, Meyer PN, et al. A new biologic prognostic model based on immunohistochemistry predicts survival in patients with diffuse large B-cell lymphoma. *Blood* 2012;120(11):2290–2296.
28. Monni O, Joensuu H, Franssila K, et al. DNA copy number changes in diffuse large B-cell lymphoma—comparative genomic hybridization study. *Blood* 1996;87:5269–5278.
29. Rao PH, Houldsworth J, Dyomina K, et al. Chromosomal and gene amplification in diffuse large B-cell lymphoma. *Blood* 1998;92:234–240.
30. Nanjangud G, Rao PH, Hegde A, et al. Spectral karyotyping identifies new rearrangements, translocations, and clinical associations in diffuse large B-cell lymphoma. *Blood* 2002;99:2554–2561.
31. Bea S, Zettl A, Wright G, et al. Diffuse large B-cell lymphoma subgroups have distinct genetic profiles that influence tumor biology and improve gene-expression-based survival prediction. *Blood* 2005;106:3183–3190.
32. Tagawa H, Suguro M, Tsuzuki S, et al. Comparison of genome profiles for identification of distinct subgroups of diffuse large B-cell lymphoma. *Blood* 2005;106:1770–1777.
33. Scandurra M, Mian M, Greiner TC, et al. Genomic lesions associated with a different clinical outcome in diffuse large B-cell lymphoma treated with R-CHOP-21. *Br J Haematol* 2010;151(3):221–231.
34. Lenz G, Wright GW, Emre NC, et al. Molecular subtypes of diffuse large B-cell lymphoma arise by distinct genetic pathways. *Proc Natl Acad Sci U S A* 2008;105(36):13520–13525.
35. Mian M, Scandurra M, Chigrinova E, et al. Clinical and molecular characterization of diffuse large B-cell lymphomas with 13q14.3 deletion. *Ann Oncol* 2012;23(3): 729–735.
36. Lossos S, kada CY, Tibshirani R, et al. Molecular analysis of immunoglobulin genes in diffuse large B-cell lymphomas. *Blood* 2000;95:1797–1803.
37. Kawasaki C, Ohshim K, Suzumiya J, et al. Rearrangements of bcl-1, bcl-2, bcl-6, and c-myc in diffuse large B-cell lymphomas. *Leuk Lymphoma* 2001;42: 1099–1106.
38. Visco C, Tzankov A, Xu-Monette ZY, et al. Patients with diffuse large B-cell lymphoma of germinal center origin with *BCL2* translocations have poor outcome, irrespective of *MYC* status: a report from an International DLBCL Rituximab-CHOP Consortium Program Study. *Haematologica* 2013;98:255–263.
39. Rosenwald A, Wright G, Chan WC, et al. The use of molecular profiling to predict survival after chemotherapy for diffuse large-B-cell lymphoma. *N Engl J Med* 2002;346:1937–1947.
40. Lossos IS, Alizadeh AA, Eisen MB, et al. Ongoing immunoglobulin somatic mutation in germinal center B cell-like but not in activated B cell-like diffuse large cell lymphomas. *Proc Natl Acad Sci U S A* 2000;97:10209–10213.
41. Lo Coco F, Ye BH, Lista F, et al. Rearrangements of the *BCL6* gene in diffuse large cell non-Hodgkin's lymphoma. *Blood* 1994;83:1757–1759.
42. Otsuki T, Yano T, Clark HM, et al. Analysis of LAZ3 (BCL-6) status in B-cell non-Hodgkin's lymphomas: results of rearrangement and gene expression studies and a mutational analysis of coding region sequences. *Blood* 1995;85:2877–2884.
43. Migliazza A, Martinotti S, Chen W, et al. Frequent somatic hypermutation of the 5′ noncoding region of the *BCL6* gene in B-cell lymphoma. *Proc Natl Acad Sci U S A* 1995;92:12520–12524.
44. Capello D, Vitolo U, Pasqualucci L, et al. Distribution and pattern of BCL-6 mutations throughout the spectrum of B-cell neoplasia. *Blood* 2000;95:651–659.
45. Pasqualucci L, Migliazza A, Fracchiolla N, et al. *BCL-6* mutations in normal germinal center B cells: evidence of somatic hypermutation acting outside Ig loci. *Proc Natl Acad Sci U S A* 1998;95:11816–11821.
46. Hummel M, Bentink S, Berger H, et al. A biologic definition of Burkitt's lymphoma from transcriptional and genomic profiling. *N Engl J Med* 2006;354:2419–2430.
47. Akasaka T, Akasaka H, Ueda C, et al. Molecular and clinical features of non-Burkitt's, diffuse large-cell lymphoma of B-cell type associated with the c-MYC/immunoglobulin heavy-chain fusion gene. *J Clin Oncol* 2000;18:510–518.
48. Aukema SM, Siebert R, Schuuring E, et al. Double-hit B-cell lymphomas. *Blood* 2011;117:2319–2331.
49. Xu-Monette ZY, Mederios LJ, Li Y, et al. Dysfunction of the *TP53* tumor suppressor gene in lymphoid malignancies. *Blood* 2012;119(16):3668–3683.
50. Young KH, Leroy K, Moller MB, et al. Structural profiles of *TP53* gene mutations predict clinical outcome in diffuse large B-cell lymphoma: an international collaborative study. *Blood* 2008;112:3088–3098.
51. Young KH, Weisenburger DD, Dave B, et al. Mutations in the DNA-binding codons of *TP53*, which are associated with decreased expression of *TRAIL* receptor-2, predict for poor survival in diffuse large B-cell lymphoma. *Blood* 2007;110:4396–4405.
52. Xu-Monette ZY, Wu L, Visco C, et al. Mutational profiles and prognostic significance of *TP53* gene predict clinical outcome in diffuse large B-cell lymphoma: a report from international R-CHOP consortium program study. *Blood* 2012;120(19):3986–3996.
53. Sander CA, Yano T, Clark HM, et al. p53 Mutation is associated with progression in follicular lymphomas. *Blood* 1993;82:1994–2004.
54. Pasqualucci L, Neumeister P, Goossens T, et al. Hypermutation of multiple proto-oncogenes in B-cell diffuse large-cell lymphomas. *Nature* 2001;412:341–346.
55. Pasqualucci L, Trifonov V, Fabbri G, et al. Analysis of the coding genome of diffuse large B-cell lymphoma. *Nat Genet* 2011;43(9):830–837.
56. Morin RD, Mendez-Lago M, Mungall AJ, et al. Frequent mutation of histone-modifying genes in non-Hodgkin lymphoma. *Nature* 2011;476:298–303.
57. Chen E, Staudt LM, Green AR. Janus kinase deregulation in leukemia and lymphoma. *Immunity* 2012;36(4):529–541.
58. Lee JW, Soung YH, Kim SY, et al. JAK2 V617F mutation is uncommon in non-Hodgkin lymphomas. *Leuk Lymphoma* 2006;47:313–314.
59. Hu G, Witzig TE, Gupta M. A novel STAT3 mutation associated with diffuse large B-cell lymphoma reregulates STAT3 signaling. *Blood* 2012;120–121: Abstract #2690.
60. Gupta M, Han JJ, Stenson M, et al. Elevated serum IL-10 levels in diffuse large B-cell lymphoma: a mechanism of aberrant JAK2 activation. *Blood* 2012;119:2844–2853.
61. Ochman M, Lemonnier F, Damotte D, et al. Mutation of STAT6 DNA binding domain are characteristic of PMBCL and belong to the genetic signature of this entity. *Blood* 2012;120–121: Abstract #2645.
62. Rimsza LM, Roberts RA, Miller TP, et al. Loss of *MHC* class II gene and protein expression in diffuse large B-cell lymphoma is related to decreased tumor immunosurveillance and poor patient survival regardless of other prognostic factors: a follow-up study from the Leukemia and Lymphoma Molecular Profiling Project. *Blood* 2004;103:4251–4258.
63. Steidl C, Shah SP, Woolcock BW, et al. MHC class II transactivator *CIITA* is a recurrent gene fusion partner in lymphoid cancers. *Nature* 2011;471(7338):377–381.
64. Lenz G, Wright G, Dave SS, et al. Stromal gene signatures in large-B-cell lymphomas. *N Engl J Med* 2008;359(22):2313–2323.
65. Slymen DJ, Miller TP, Lippman SM, et al. Immunobiologic factors predictive of clinical outcome in diffuse large-cell lymphoma. *J Clin Oncol* 1990;8:986–993.
66. Goto N, Tsurumi H, Shibata Y, et al. Prognostic impact of tumor-infiltrating FOXP3+ regulatory T-cells in DLBCL with R-CHOP. *Blood* 2012;120(21): Abstract #1555.
67. Bohn OL, Maragulia JC, Gonzalez C, et al. Tumor associated macrophage expression, CD163, is associated with poorer outcome in diffuse large B-cell lymphoma. *Blood* 2012;120(21): Abstract #1583.

68. Kiali S, Clear AJ, Gribben JG. Impact of tumor infiltrating T cells in patients with diffuse large B-cell lymphoma. *Blood* 2012;120(21): Abstract #1572.
69. Sonoki T, Harder L, Horsman DE, et al. Cyclin D3 is a target gene of t(6;14)(p21.1;q32.3) of mature B-cell malignancies. *Blood* 2001;98:2837–2844.
70. Di Lisio L, Martinez N, Montes-Moreno S, et al. The role of miRNAs in the pathogenesis and diagnosis of B-cell lymphomas. *Blood* 2012;120(9):1782–1790.
71. The International Non-Hodgkin's Lymphoma Prognostic Factors Project. A predictive model for aggressive non-Hodgkin's lymphoma. *N Engl J Med* 1993;329: 987–994.
72. Sehn LH, Berry B, Chhanabhai M, et al. The revised International Prognostic Index (R-IPI) is a better predictor of outcome than the standard IPI for patients with diffuse large B-cell lymphoma treated with R-CHOP. *Blood* 2007;109: 1857–1861.
73. Ott G, Ziepert M, Klapper W, et al. Immunoblastic morphology but not the immunohistochemical GCB/nonGCB classifier predicts outcome in diffuse large B-cell lymphoma in the RICOVER-60 trial of the DSHNHL. *Blood* 2010;116(23): 4916–4925.
74. Chung R, Lai R, Wei P, et al. Concordant but not discordant bone marrow involvement in diffuse large B-cell lymphoma predicts a poor clinical outcome independent of the International Prognostic Index. *Blood* 2007;110:1278–1282.
75. Colomo L, Lopez-Guillermo A, Perales M, et al. Clinical impact of the differentiation profile assessed by immunophenotyping in patients with diffuse large B-cell lymphoma. *Blood* 2003;101:78–84.
76. Chang CC, McClintock S, Cleveland RP, et al. Immunohistochemical expression patterns of germinal center and activation B-cell markers correlate with prognosis in diffuse large B-cell lymphoma. *Am J Surg Pathol* 2004;28:464–470.
77. Wilson WH, Grossbard ML, Pittaluga S, et al. Dose-adjusted EPOCH chemotherapy for untreated large B-cell lymphomas: a pharmacodynamic approach with high efficacy. *Blood* 2002;99:2685–2693.
78. Grogan TM, Lippman SM, Spier CM, et al. Independent prognostic significance of a nuclear proliferation antigen in diffuse large cell lymphomas as determined by the monoclonal antibody Ki-67. *Blood* 1988;71:1157–1160.
79. Bauer KD, Merkel DE, Winter JN, et al. Prognostic implications of ploidy and proliferative activity in diffuse large cell lymphomas. *Cancer Res* 1986;46:3173–3178.
80. Ruminy P, Etancelin P, Couronne L, et al. The isotype of the BCR as a surrogate for the GCB and ABC molecular subtypes in diffuse large B-cell lymphoma. *Leukemia* 2011;25:681–688.
81. Molina TJ, Briere J, Copie-Bergman C, et al. Expression of Myc, IgM, as well as non-germinal center center B-cell like immunophenotype and positive immunofish index predict a worse progression free survival and overall survival in a series of 670 de novo diffuse large B-cell lymphomas included in clinical trials: a GELA study of the 2003 program. *Blood* 2012;120(21): Abstract #1539.
82. Cox MC, Napoli AD, Scarpino S, et al. Diffuse large B-cell lymphoma patients with secretory IgM monoclonal component are a very poor prognostic subset. *Blood* 2012;120(21): Abstract #2659.
83. Adida C, Haioun C, Gaulard P, et al. Prognostic significance of survivin expression in diffuse large B-cell lymphomas. *Blood* 2000;96:1921–1925.
84. Filipits M, Jaeger U, Pohl G, et al. Cyclin D3 is a predictive and prognostic factor in diffuse large B-cell lymphoma. *Clin Cancer Res* 2002;8:729–733.
85. Hans CP, Weisenburger DD, Greiner TC, et al. Expression of PKC-beta or cyclin D2 predicts for inferior survival in diffuse large B-cell lymphoma. *Mod Pathol* 2005;18:1377–1384.
86. Muris JJ, Cillessen SA, Vos W, et al. Immunohistochemical profiling of caspase signaling pathways predicts clinical response to chemotherapy in primary nodal diffuse large B-cell lymphomas. *Blood* 2005;105:2916–2923.
87. Ferrajoli A, Faderl S, Ravandi F, et al. The JAK-STAT pathway: a therapeutic target in hematological malignancies. *Curr Cancer Drug Targets* 2006;6:671–679.
88. Ding BB, Yu JJ, Yu RY, et al. Constitutively activated STAT3 promotes cell proliferation and survival in the activated B-cell subtype of diffuse large B-cell lymphomas. *Blood* 2008;111:1515–1523.
89. Meier C, Hoeller S, Bourgau C, et al. Recurrent numerical aberrations of JAK2 and deregulation of the JAK2-STAT cascade in lymphomas. *Mod Pathol* 2009;22(3):476–487.
90. Sanchez-Aguilera A, Sanchez-Beato M, Garcia JF, et al. P14(ARF) nuclear overexpression in aggressive B-cell lymphomas is a sensor of malfunction of the common tumor suppressor pathways. *Blood* 2002;99:1411–1418.
91. Lossos IS, Czerwinski DK, Alizadeh AA, et al. Prediction of survival in diffuse large-B-cell lymphoma based on the expression of six genes. *N Engl J Med* 2004;350:1828–1837.
92. Rimsza LM, Leblanc ML, Unger JM, et al. Gene expression predicts overall survival in paraffin-embedded tissues of diffuse large B-cell lymphoma treated with R-CHOP. *Blood* 2008;112:3425–3433.
93. Tome ME, Johnson DB, Rimsza LM, et al. A redox signature score identifies diffuse large B-cell lymphoma patients with a poor prognosis. *Blood* 2005;106: 3594–3601.
94. Iqbal J, Sanger WG, Horsman DE, et al. *BCL2* translocation defines a unique tumor subset within the germinal center B-cell-like diffuse large B-cell lymphoma. *Am J Pathol* 2004;165:159–166.
95. Yunis JJ, Mayer MG, Arnesen MA, et al. Bcl-2 and other genomic alterations in the prognosis of large-cell lymphoma. *N Engl J Med* 1989;320:1047–1054.
96. Akasaka T, Ueda C, Kurata M, et al. Nonimmunoglobulin (non-Ig)/*BCL6* gene fusion in diffuse large B-cell lymphoma results in worse prognosis than Ig/BCL6. *Blood* 2000;96:2907–2909.
97. Lossos IS, Jones CD, Warnke R, et al. Expression of a single gene, *BCL-6*, strongly predicts survival in patients with diffuse large B-cell lymphoma. *Blood* 2001;98:945–951.
98. Iqbal J, Greiner TC, Patel K, et al. Distinctive patterns of *BCL6* molecular alterations and their functional consequences in different subgroups of diffuse large B-cell lymphoma. *Leukemia* 2007;21(11):2332–2343.
99. Vitolo U, Botto B, Capello D, et al. Point mutations of the BCL-6 gene: clinical and prognostic correlation in B-diffuse large cell lymphoma. *Leukemia* 2002;16: 268–275.
100. Alencar AJ, Malumbres R, Kozloski GA, et al. MicroRNAs are independent predictors of outcome in diffuse large B-cell lymphoma patients treated with R-CHOP. *Clin Cancer Res* 2011;17(12):4125–4135.
101. Roehle A, Hoefig KP, Repsilber D, et al. MicroRNA signatures characterize diffuse large B-cell lymphomas and follicular lymphomas. *Br J Haematol* 2008;142(5):732–744.
102. Jung I, Aguiar RCT. MicroRNA-155 expression and outcome in diffuse large B-cell lymphoma. *Br J Haematol* 2009;144(1):138–140.
103. Shaknovich R, Geng H, Johnson NA, et al. DNA methylation signatures define molecular subtypes of diffuse large B-cell lymphoma. *Blood* 2010;116(20): e81–e89.
104. Esteller M, Gaidano G, Goodman SN, et al. Hypermethylation of the DNA repair gene O(6)-methylguanine DNA methyltransferase and survival of patients with diffuse large B-cell lymphoma. *J Natl Cancer Inst* 2002;94:26–32.
105. Zhang YW, Xie HQ, Chen Y, et al. Loss of promoter methylation contributes to the expression of functionally impaired PRDM1β isoform in diffuse large B-cell lymphoma. *Int J Hematol* 2010;92(3):439–444.
106. Zainuddin N, Kanduri M, Berglund M, et al. Quantitative evaluation of p16(INK4a) promoter methylation using pyrosequencing in de novo diffuse large B-cell lymphoma. *Leuk Res* 2011;35(4):438–443.
107. Houldsworth J, Olshen AB, Cattoretti G, et al. Relationship between REL amplification, REL function, and clinical and biologic features in diffuse large B-cell lymphomas. *Blood* 2004;103:1862–1868.
108. Iqbal J, Meyer PN, Smith LM, et al. BCL2 predicts survival in germinal center B-cell-like diffuse large B-cell lymphoma treated with CHOP-like therapy and rituximab. *Clin Cancer Res* 2011;17(24):7785–7795.
109. Yang Y, Shaffer AL III, Emre NC, et al. Exploiting synthetic lethality for the therapy of ABC diffuse large B cell lymphoma. *Cancer Cell* 2012;21(6):723–737.
110. Leoncini L, Raphael M, Stein H, et al. Burkitt lymphoma. In: Swerdlow SH, Campo E, Harris NL, et al., eds. *WHO classification of tumours of haematopoietic and lymphoid tissues*, 4th ed. Lyon: IARC, 2008:262–264.
111. Kluin PM, Harris NL, Stein H, et al. B-cell lymphoma, unclassifiable, with features intermediate between diffuse large B-cell lymphoma and Burkitt lymphoma. In: Swerdlow SH, Campo E, Harris NL, et al., eds. *WHO classification of tumours of haematopoietic and lymphoid tissues*, 4th ed. Lyon: IARC, 2008:265–266.
112. Zoldan MC, Inghirami G, Masuda Y, et al. Large-cell variants of mantle cell lymphoma: cytologic characteristics and p53 anomalies may predict poor outcome. *Br J Haematol* 1996;93:475–486.
113. Ehinger M, Linderoth J, Christensson B, et al. A subset of CD5- diffuse large B-cell lymphomas expresses nuclear cyclin D1 with aberrations at the CCND1 locus. *Am J Clin Pathol* 2008;129:630–638.
114. Bernard M, Gressin R, Lefrere F, et al. Blastic variant of mantle cell lymphoma: a rare but highly aggressive subtype. *Leukemia* 2001;15:1785–1791.
115. Rodriguez-Justo M, Huang Y, Ye H, et al. Cyclin D1-positive diffuse large B-cell lymphoma. *Histopathology* 2008;52:900–903.
116. Stein H, Delsol G, Pileri S, et al. Classical Hodgkin lymphoma. In: Jaffe ES, Harris NL, Stein H, et al., eds. *Pathology and genetics: tumours of haematopoietic and lymphoid tissues*. World Health Organization classification of tumours. Lyon: IARC Press, 2001:244–253.
117. Stein H, Delsol G, Pileri S, et al. Nodular lymphocyte predominant Hodgkin lymphoma. In: Jaffe ES, Harris NL, Stein H, et al., eds. *Pathology and genetics: tumours of haematopoietic and lymphoid tissues*. Lyon: IARC Press, 2001: 240–243.
118. Lasota J, Hyjek E, Koo CH, et al. Cytokeratin-positive large-cell lymphomas of B-cell lineage. A study of five phenotypically unusual cases verified by polymerase chain reaction. *Am J Surg Pathol* 1996;20:346–354.
119. Childs CC, Parham DM, Berard CW. Infectious mononucleosis. The spectrum of morphologic changes simulating lymphoma in lymph nodes and tonsils. *Am J Surg Pathol* 1987;11:122–132.
120. Strickler JG, Fedeli F, Horwitz CA, et al. Infectious mononucleosis in lymphoid tissue. Histopathology, in situ hybridization, and differential diagnosis. *Arch Pathol Lab Med* 1993;117:269–278.
121. Anagnostopoulos I, Hummel M, Kreschel C, et al. Morphology, immunophenotype, and distribution of latently and/or productively Epstein-Barr virus-infected cells in acute infectious mononucleosis: implications for the interindividual infection route of Epstein-Barr virus. *Blood* 1995;85:744–750.
122. Kuo TT. Kikuchi's disease (histiocytic necrotizing lymphadenitis). A clinicopathologic study of 79 cases with an analysis of histologic subtypes, immunohistology, and DNA ploidy. *Am J Surg Pathol* 1995;19:798–809.
123. Sumiyoshi Y, Kikuchi M, Takeshita M, et al. Immunohistologic studies of Kikuchi's disease. *Hum Pathol* 1993;24:1114–1119.
124. Bouabdallah R, Mounier N, Guettier C, et al. T-cell/histiocyte-rich large B-cell lymphomas and classical diffuse large B-cell lymphomas have similar outcome after chemotherapy: a matched-control analysis. *J Clin Oncol* 2003;21: 1271–1277.
125. Rodriguez J, Pugh WC, Cabanillas F. T-cell-rich B-cell lymphoma. *Blood* 1993;82:1586–1589.
126. Greer JP, Macon WR, Lamar RE, et al. T-cell-rich B-cell lymphomas: diagnosis and response to therapy of 44 patients. *J Clin Oncol* 1995;13:1742–1750.
127. Loke SL, Ho F, Srivastava G, et al. Clonal Epstein-Barr virus genome in T-cell-rich lymphomas of B or probable B lineage. *Am J Pathol* 1992;140:981–989.
128. Fraga M, Sanchez-Verde L, Forteza J, et al. T-cell/histiocyte-rich large B-cell lymphoma is a disseminated aggressive neoplasm: differential diagnosis from Hodgkin's lymphoma. *Histopathology* 2002;41:216–229.
129. Mitterer M, Pescosta N, McQuain C, et al. Epstein-Barr virus related hemophagocytic syndrome in a T-cell rich B-cell lymphoma. *Ann Oncol* 1999;10:231–234.
130. Hodges E, Hamid Y, Quin CT, et al. Molecular analysis reveals somatically mutated and unmutated clonal and oligoclonal B cells in T-cell-rich B-cell lymphoma. *J Pathol* 2000;192:479–487.
131. Brauninger A, Kuppers R, Spieker T, et al. Molecular analysis of single B cells from T-cell-rich B-cell lymphoma shows the derivation of the tumor cells from mutating germinal center B cells and exemplifies means by which immunoglobulin genes are modified in germinal center B cells. *Blood* 1999;93:2679–2687.
132. Monti S, Savage KJ, Kutok JL, et al. Molecular profiling of diffuse large B-cell lymphoma identifies robust subtypes including one characterized by host inflammatory response. *Blood* 2005;105:1851–1861.
133. Larocca LM, Capello D, Rinelli A, et al. The molecular and phenotypic profile of primary central nervous system lymphoma identifies distinct categories of the disease and is consistent with histogenetic derivation from germinal center-related B cells. *Blood* 1998;92:1011–1019.
134. Thompsett AR, Ellison DW, Stevenson FK, et al. V(H) gene sequences from primary central nervous system lymphomas indicate derivation from highly mutated germinal center B cells with ongoing mutational activity. *Blood* 1999;94:1738–1746.

135. Weber T, Weber RG, Kaulich K, et al. Characteristic chromosomal imbalances in primary central nervous system lymphomas of the diffuse large B-cell type. *Brain Pathol* 2000;10(1):73–84.
136. Rijlaarsdam JU, Toonstra J, Meijer OW, et al. Treatment of primary cutaneous B-cell lymphomas of follicle center cell origin: a clinical follow-up study of 55 patients treated with radiotherapy or polychemotherapy. *J Clin Oncol* 1996;14:549–555.
137. Willemze R, Jaffe ES, Burg G, et al. WHO-EORTC classification for cutaneous lymphomas. *Blood* 2005;105(10):3768–3785.
138. Oyama T, Yamamoto K, Asano N, et al. Age-related EBV-associated B-cell lymphoproliferative disorders constitute a distinct clinicopathologic group: a study of 96 patients. *Clin Cancer Res* 2007;13:5124–5132.
139. Park S, Lee J, Ko YH, et al. The impact of Epstein-Barr virus status on clinical outcome in diffuse large B-cell lymphoma. *Blood* 2007;110:972–978.
140. Shimoyama Y, Yamamoto K, Asano N, et al. Age-related Epstein-Barr virus–associated B-cell lymphoproliferative disorders: special references to lymphomas surrounding this newly recognized clinicopathologic disease. *Cancer Sci* 2008;99:1085–1091.
141. Montes-Moreno S, Odqvist L, Diaz-Perez JA, et al. EBV+ DLBCL of the elderly is an aggressive post-germinal center B cell neoplasm characterized by prominent NF-kB activation. *Mod Pathol* 2012;25(7):968–982.
142. Yamaguchi M, Nakamura N, Suzuki R, et al. De novo CD5+ diffuse large B-cell lymphoma: results of a detailed clinicopathological review in 120 patients. *Haematologica* 2008;93:1195–1202.
143. Kume M, Suzuki R, Yatabe Y, et al. Somatic hypermutations in the VH segment of immunoglobulin genes of CD5-positive diffuse large B-cell lymphomas. *Jpn J Cancer Res* 1997;88:1087–1093.
144. Taniguchi M, Oka K, Hiasa A, et al. De novo CD5+ diffuse large B-cell lymphomas express VH genes with somatic mutation. *Blood* 1998;91:1145–1151.
145. Kobayashi T, Yamaguchi M, Kim S, et al. Microarray reveals differences in both tumors and vascular specific gene expression in de novo CD5+ and CD5– diffuse large B-cell lymphomas. *Cancer Res* 2003;63:60–66.
146. Suguro M, Tagawa H, Kagami Y, et al. Expression profiling analysis of the CD5+ diffuse large B-cell lymphoma subgroup: development of a CD5 signature. *Cancer Sci* 2006;97:868–874.
147. Ennishi D, Takeuchi K, Yokoyama M, et al. CD5 expression is potentially predictive of poor outcome among biomarkers in patients with diffuse large B-cell lymphoma receiving rituximab plus CHOP therapy. *Ann Oncol* 2008;19:1921–1926.
148. Tagawa H, Tsuzuki S, Suzuki R, et al. Genome-wide array-based comparative genomic hybridization of diffuse large B-cell lymphoma: comparison between CD5-positive and CD5-negative cases. *Cancer Res* 2004;64:5948–5955.
149. Matolcsy A, Chadburn A, Knowles DM. De novo CD5-positive and Richter's syndrome-associated diffuse large B cell lymphomas are genotypically distinct. *Am J Pathol* 1995;147:207–216.
150. Gaulard P, Harris NL, Pileri SA, et al. Primary mediastinal (thymic) large B-cell lymphoma. In: Swerdlow SH, Campo E, Harris NL, et al., eds. *WHO classification of tumours of haematopoietic and lymphoid tissues*, 4th ed. Lyon: IARC, 2008:250–251.
151. Levitt LJ, Aisenberg AC, Harris NL, et al. Primary non-Hodgkin's lymphoma of the mediastinum. *Cancer* 1982;50:2486–2492.
152. Addis BJ, Isaacson PG. Large cell lymphoma of the mediastinum: a B-cell tumour of probable thymic origin. *Histopathology* 1986;10:379–390.
153. Lazzarino M, Orlandi E, Paulli M, et al. Treatment outcome and prognostic factors for primary mediastinal (thymic) B-cell lymphoma: a multicenter study of 106 patients. *J Clin Oncol* 1997;15:1646–1653.
154. Isaacson PG, Norton AJ, Addis BJ. The human thymus contains a novel population of B lymphocytes. *Lancet* 1987;2:1488–1491.
155. Hofmann WJ, Momburg F, Moller P, et al. Intra- and extrathymic B cells in physiologic and pathologic conditions. Immunohistochemical study on normal thymus and lymphofollicular hyperplasia of the thymus. *Virchows Arch A Pathol Anat Histopathol* 1988;412:431–442.
156. Kimm LR, deLeeuw RJ, Savage KJ, et al. Frequent occurrence of deletions in primary mediastinal B-cell lymphoma. *Genes Chromosomes Cancer* 2007;46(12):1090–1097.
157. Cazals-Hatem D, Lepage E, Brice P, et al. Primary mediastinal large B-cell lymphoma. A clinicopathologic study of 141 cases compared with 916 nonmediastinal large B-cell lymphomas, a GELA (Groupe d'Etude des Lymphomes de l'Adulte) study. *Am J Surg Pathol* 1996;20:877–888.
158. Chan JK. Mediastinal large B-cell lymphoma, new evidence in support of its distinctive identity. *Adv Anat Pathol* 2000;7:201–209.
159. Pileri SA, Gaidano G, Zinzani PL, et al. Primary mediastinal B-cell lymphoma: high frequency of BCL-6 mutations and consistent expression of the transcription factors OCT-2, BOB.1, and PU.1 in the absence of immunoglobulins. *Am J Pathol* 2003;162:243–253.
160. Leithauser F, Bauerle M, Huynh MQ, et al. Isotype-switched immunoglobulin genes with a high load of somatic hypermutation and lack of ongoing mutational activity are prevalent in mediastinal B-cell lymphoma. *Blood* 2001;98:2762–2770.
161. Hsi ED, Sup SJ, Alemany C, et al. MAL is expressed in a subset of Hodgkin lymphoma and identifies a population of patients with poor prognosis. *Am J Clin Pathol* 2006;125:776–782.
162. Roberts RA, Wright G, Rosenwald AR, et al. Loss of major histocompatibility class II gene and protein expression in primary mediastinal large B cell lymphoma is highly coordinated and related to poor patient survival. *Blood* 2006;108:311–318.
163. de Leval L, Ferry JA, Falini B, et al. Expression of bcl-6 and CD10 in primary mediastinal large B-cell lymphoma: evidence for derivation from germinal center B cells. *Am J Surg Pathol* 2001;25:1277–1282.
164. Fraternali-Orcioni G, Falini B, Quaini F, et al. Beta-HCG aberrant expression in primary mediastinal large B-cell lymphoma. *Am J Surg Pathol* 1999;23:717–721.
165. Tsang P, Cesarman E, Chadburn A, et al. Molecular characterization of primary mediastinal B cell lymphoma. *Am J Pathol* 1996;148:2017–2025.
166. Scarpa A, Borgato L, Chilosi M, et al. Evidence of c-myc gene abnormalities in mediastinal large B-cell lymphoma of young adult age. *Blood* 1991;78:780–788.
167. Rosenwald A, Wright G, Leroy K, et al. Molecular diagnosis of primary mediastinal B cell lymphoma identifies a clinically favorable subgroup of diffuse large B cell lymphoma related to Hodgkin lymphoma. *J Exp Med* 2003;198:851–862.
168. Palanisamy N, Abou-Elella AA, Chaganti SR, et al. Similar patterns of genomic alterations characterize primary mediastinal large-B-cell lymphoma and diffuse large-B-cell lymphoma. *Genes Chromosomes Cancer* 2002;33:114–122.
169. Weniger MA, Gesk S, Ehrlich S, et al. Gains of REL in primary mediastinal B-cell lymphoma coincide with nuclear accumulation of REL protein. *Genes Chromosomes Cancer* 2007;46:406–415.
170. Savage KJ, Monti S, Kutok JL, et al. The molecular signature of mediastinal large B-cell lymphoma differs from that of other diffuse large B-cell lymphomas and shares features with classical Hodgkin lymphoma. *Blood* 2003;102:3871–3879.
171. van Besien K, Kelta M, Bahaguna P. Primary mediastinal B-cell lymphoma: a review of pathology and management. *J Clin Oncol* 2001;19:1855–1864.
172. Zinzani PL, Martelli M, Bertini M, et al. Induction chemotherapy strategies for primary mediastinal large B-cell lymphoma with sclerosis: a retrospective multinational study on 426 previously untreated patients. *Haematologica* 2002;87:1258–1264.
173. Chadburn A, Frizzera G. Mediastinal large B-cell lymphoma vs. classic Hodgkin lymphoma. *Am J Clin Pathol* 1999;112:155–158.
174. Traverse-Glehen A, Pittaluga S, Gaulard P, et al. Mediastinal gray zone lymphoma: the missing link between classical Hodgkin's lymphoma and mediastinal large B-cell lymphoma. *Am J Surg Pathol* 2005;29:1411–1421.
175. Gualco G, Natkunam Y, Bacchi. The spectrum of B-cell lymphoma, unclassifiable, with features intermediate between diffuse large B-cell lymphoma and classical Hodgkin lymphoma: a description of 10 cases. *Mod Pathol* 2012;25:661–674.
176. Jaffe ES, Stein H, Swerdlow SH, et al. B-cell lymphoma, unclassifiable, with features intermediate between diffuse large B-cell lymphoma and classical Hodgkin lymphoma. In: Swerdlow SH, Campo E, Harris NL, et al., eds. *WHO classification of tumours of haematopoietic and lymphoid tissues*, 4th ed. Lyon: IARC, 2008:87–88.
177. Eberle FC, Salaverria I, Steidl C, et al. Gray zone lymphoma: chromosomal aberrations with immunophenotypic and clinical correlations. *Mod Pathol* 2011;24:1586–1597.
178. Eberle FC, Rodriguez-Canales J, Wei L, et al. Methylation profiling of mediastinal gray zone lymphoma reveals a distinctive signature with elements shared by classical Hodgkin's lymphoma and primary mediastinal large B-cell lymphoma. *Haematologica* 2011;96:558–566.
179. Ponzoni M, Ferreri AJ, Campo E, et al. Definition, diagnosis, and management of intravascular large B-cell lymphoma: proposals and perspectives from an international consensus meeting. *J Clin Oncol* 2007;25:3168–3173.
180. Nakamura S, Ponzoni M, Campo E. Intravascular large B-cell lymphoma. In: Swerdlow SH, Campo E, Harris NL, et al., eds. *WHO classification of tumours of haematopoietic and lymphoid tissues*, 4th ed. Lyon: IARC, 2008:252–253.
181. Ponzoni M, Arrigoni G, Gould VE, et al. Lack of CD29 (beta1 integrin) and CD54 (ICAM-1) adhesion molecules in intravascular lymphomatosis. *Hum Pathol* 2000;31:220–226.
182. Ferreri AJ, Campo E, Seymour JF, et al. Intravascular lymphoma: clinical presentation, natural history, management and prognostic factors in a series of 38 cases, with special emphasis on the "cutaneous variant." *Br J Haematol* 2004;127:173–183.
183. Shimizu I, Ichikawa N, Yotsumoto M, et al. Asian variant of intravascular lymphoma: aspects of diagnosis and the role of rituximab. *Intern Med* 2007;46(17):1381–1386.
184. Estalilla OC, Koo CH, Brynes RK, et al. Intravascular large B-cell lymphoma: a report of five cases initially diagnosed by bone marrow biopsy. *Am J Clin Pathol* 1999;112(2):248–255.
185. Khalidi HS, Brynes RK, Browne P, et al. Intravascular large B-cell lymphoma: the CD5 antigen is expressed by a subset of cases. *Mod Pathol* 1998;11:983–988.
186. Murase T, Yamaguchi M, Suzuki R, et al. Intravascular large B-cell lymphoma (IVLBCL): a clinicopathologic study of 96 cases with special reference to the immunophenotypic heterogeneity of CD5. *Blood* 2007;109:478–485.
187. Au WY, Shek TW, Kwong YL. Epstein-Barr virus–related intravascular lymphomatosis. *Am J Surg Pathol* 2000;24:309–310.
188. Shimada K, Matsue K, Yamamoto K, et al. Retrospective analysis of intravascular large B-cell lymphoma treated with rituximab-containing chemotherapy as reported by the IVL study group in Japan. *J Clin Oncol* 2008;26:3189–3195.
189. Murase T, Nakamura S, Kawauchi K, et al. An Asian variant of intravascular large B-cell lymphoma: clinical, pathological and cytogenetic approaches to diffuse large B-cell lymphoma associated with haemophagocytic syndrome. *Br J Haematol* 2000;111:826–834.
190. Dufau JP, Le Tourneau A, Molina T, et al. Intravascular large B-cell lymphoma with bone marrow involvement at presentation and haemophagocytic syndrome: two Western cases in favour of a specific variant. *Histopathology* 2000;37:509–512.
191. Nakatsuka S, Yao M, Hoshida Y, et al. Pyothorax-associated lymphoma: a review of 106 cases. *J Clin Oncol* 2002;20:4255–4260.
192. Takakuwa T, Tresnasari K, Rahadiani N, et al. Cell origin of pyothorax-associated lymphoma: a lymphoma strongly associated with Epstein-Barr virus infection. *Leukemia* 2008;22:620–627.
193. Narimatsu H, Ota Y, Kami M, et al. Clinicopathological features of pyothorax-associated lymphoma; a retrospective survey involving 98 patients. *Ann Oncol* 2007;18:122–128.
194. Nishiu M, Tomita Y, Nakatsuka S, et al. Distinct pattern of gene expression in pyothorax-associated lymphoma (PAL), a lymphoma developing in long-standing inflammation. *Cancer Sci* 2004;95:828–834.
195. Loong F, Chan AC, Ho BC, et al. Diffuse large B-cell lymphoma associated with chronic inflammation as an incidental finding. *Mod Pathol* 2010;23:493–501.
196. Boroumand N, Ly TL, Sonstein J, et al. Microscopic diffuse large B-cell lymphoma (DLBCL) occurring in pseudocyst: do these tumors belong to the category of DLBCL associated with chronic inflammation? *Am J Surg Pathol* 2012;36:1074–1080.
197. Pittaluga S, Wilson WH, Jaffe ES. Lymphomatoid granulomatosis. In: Swerdlow SH, Campo E, Harris NL, et al., eds. *WHO classification of tumours of haematopoietic and lymphoid tissues*, 4th ed. Lyon: IARC, 2008:247–249.
198. Liebow AA, Carrington CR, Friedman PJ. Lymphomatoid granulomatosis. *Hum Pathol* 1972;3:457–558.
199. Katzenstein AL, Peiper SC. Detection of Epstein-Barr virus genomes in lymphomatoid granulomatosis: analysis of 29 cases by the polymerase chain reaction technique. *Mod Pathol* 1990;3:435–441.
200. Guinee DG Jr, Jaffe ES, Kingma D, et al. Pulmonary lymphomatoid granulomatosis. Evidence for a proliferation of Epstein-Barr virus infected B-lymphocytes with a prominent T-cell component and vasculitis. *Am J Surg Pathol* 1994;18:753–764.

201. Wilson WH, Kingma DW, Raffeld M, et al. Association of lymphomatoid granulomatosis with Epstein-Barr viral infection of B lymphocytes and response to interferon-alpha 2b. *Blood* 1996;87:4531–4537.
202. Delsol G, Campo E, Gascoyne RD. ALK-positive large B-cell lymphoma. In: Swerdlow SH, Campo E, Harris NL, et al., eds. *WHO classification of tumours of haematopoietic and lymphoid tissues*, 4th ed. Lyon: IARC, 2008:254–255.
203. Delsol G, Lamant L, Mariame B, et al. A new subtype of large B-cell lymphoma expressing the ALK kinase and lacking the 2;5 translocation. *Blood* 1997; 89:1483–1490.
204. Reichard KK, McKenna RW, Kroft SH. ALK-positive diffuse large B-cell lymphoma: report of four cases and review of the literature. *Mod Pathol* 2007;20:310–319.
205. Gascoyne RD, Lamant L, Martin-Subero JI, et al. ALK-positive diffuse large B-cell lymphoma is associated with Clathrin-ALK rearrangements: report of 6 cases. *Blood* 2003;102:2568–2573.
206. Valera A, Colomo L, Martinez, et al. ALK-positive large B-cell lymphomas express a terminal B-cell differentiation program and activated STAT3 but lack MYC rearrangement. Mod Pathol 2013 April 19 [Epub ahead of print].
207. Adam P, Katzenberger T, Seeberger H, et al. A case of a diffuse large B-cell lymphoma of plasmablastic type associated with the t(2;5)(p23;q35) chromosome translocation. *Am J Surg Pathol* 2003;27:1473–1476.
208. Onciu M, Behm FG, Downing JR, et al. ALK-positive plasmablastic B-cell lymphoma with expression of the NPM-ALK fusion transcript: report of 2 cases. *Blood* 2003;102:2642–2644.
209. Stein H, Harris NL, Campo E. Plasmablastic lymphoma. In: Swerdlow SH, Campo E, Harris NL, et al., eds. *WHO classification of tumours of haematopoietic and lymphoid tissues*, 4th ed. Lyon: IARC, 2008:256–257.
210. Delecluse HJ, Anagnostopoulos I, Dallenbach F, et al. Plasmablastic lymphomas of the oral cavity: a new entity associated with the human immunodeficiency virus infection. *Blood* 1997;89:1413–1420.
211. Colomo L, Loong F, Rives S, et al. Diffuse large B-cell lymphomas with plasmablastic differentiation represent a heterogeneous group of disease entities. *Am J Surg Pathol* 2004;28:736–747.
212. Dong HY, Scadden DT, de Leval L, et al. Plasmablastic lymphoma in HIV-positive patients: an aggressive Epstein-Barr virus–associated extramedullary plasmacytic neoplasm. *Am J Surg Pathol* 2005;29:1633–1641.
213. Vega F, Chang CC, Medeiros LJ, et al. Plasmablastic lymphomas and plasmablastic plasma cell myelomas have nearly identical immunophenotypic profiles. *Mod Pathol* 2005;18:806–815.
214. Oksenhendler E, Boulanger E, Galicier L, et al. High incidence of Kaposi sarcoma-associated herpesvirus-related non-Hodgkin lymphoma in patients with HIV infection and multicentric Castleman disease. *Blood* 2002;99:2331–2336.
215. D'Antonio A, Boscaino A, Addesso M, et al. KSHV- and EBV-associated germinotropic lymphoproliferative disorder: a rare lymphoproliferative disease of HIV patient with plasmablastic morphology, indolent course and favourable response to therapy. *Leuk Lymphoma* 2007;48:1444–1447.
216. Montes-Moreno S, Montalban C, Piris MA. Large B-cell lymphomas with plasmablastic differentiation: a biological and therapeutic challenge. *Leuk Lymphoma* 2012;53:185–194.
217. Nador RG, Cesarman E, Chadburn A, et al. Primary effusion lymphoma: a distinct clinicopathologic entity associated with the Kaposi's sarcoma-associated herpesvirus. *Blood* 1996;88:645–656.
218. Pan ZG, Zhang QY, Lu ZB, et al. Extracavitary KSHV-associated large B-cell lymphoma: a distinct entity or a subtype of primary effusion lymphoma? Study of 9 cases and review of an additional 43 cases. *Am J Surg Pathol* 2012;36:1129–1140.
219. Horenstein MG, Nador RG, Chadburn A, et al. Epstein-Barr virus latent gene expression in primary effusion lymphomas containing Kaposi's sarcoma–associated herpesvirus/human herpesvirus-8. *Blood* 1997;90:1186–1191.
220. Russo JJ, Bohenzky RA, Chien MC, et al. Nucleotide sequence of the Kaposi sarcoma-associated herpesvirus (HHV8). *Proc Natl Acad Sci U S A* 1996;93:14862–14867.
221. Moore PS, Boshoff C, Weiss RA, et al. Molecular mimicry of human cytokine and cytokine response pathway genes by KSHV. *Science* 1996;274:1739–1744.
222. Renne R, Zhong W, Herndier B, et al. Lytic growth of Kaposi's sarcoma-associated herpesvirus (human herpesvirus 8) in culture. *Nat Med* 1996;2:342–346.
223. Arvanitakis L, Geras-Raaka E, Varma A, et al. Human herpesvirus KSHV encodes a constitutively active G-protein-coupled receptor linked to cell proliferation. *Nature* 1997;385:347–350.
224. Matolcsy A, Nador RG, Cesarman E, et al. Immunoglobulin V$_H$ gene mutational analysis suggests that primary effusion lymphomas derive from different stages of B cell maturation [see comments]. *Am J Pathol* 1998;153:1609–1614.
225. Noorduyn LA, de Bruin PC, van Heerde P, et al. Relation of CD30 expression to survival and morphology in large cell B cell lymphomas. *J Clin Pathol* 1994;47:33–37.
226. Maes B, Anastasopoulou A, Kluin-Nelemans JC, et al. Among diffuse large B-cell lymphomas, T-cell-rich/histiocyte-rich BCL and CD30+ anaplastic B-cell subtypes exhibit distinct clinical features. *Ann Oncol* 2001;12:853–858.
227. de Leval L, Gaulard P. CD30+ lymphoproliferative disorders. *Haematologica* 2010;95:1627–1630.
228. Segal GH, Kjeldsberg CR, Smith GP, et al. CD30 antigen expression in florid immunoblastic proliferations. A clinicopathologic study of 14 cases. *Am J Clin Pathol* 1994;102:292–298.
229. Hu S, Xu-Monette ZY, Manyam GC, et al. CD30 expression defines a novel subset of diffuse large B-cell lymphoma with superior clinical outcome: a report from the International DLBCL Rituximab-CHOP Consortium Program Study. *Blood* 2013;121:2715–2724.
230. Jacobsen ED, Advani RH, Oki Y, et al. A phase 2 study of Brentuximab vedotin in patients with relapsed or refractory CD30 positive non-Hodgkin lymphomas: interim results. *Blood* 2012;120(21): Abstract #2746.
231. Steidl C, Lee T, Shah SP, et al. Tumor-associated macrophages and survival in classic Hodgkin's lymphoma. *N Engl J Med* 2010;362(10):875–885.
232. Younes A, Bartlett NL, Leonard JP, et al. Brentuximab vedotin (SGN-35) for relapsed CD30-positive lymphomas. *N Engl J Med* 2010;363:1812–1821.
233. Fanale MA, Forero-Torres A, Rosenblatt JD, et al. A phase I weekly dosing study of brentuximab vedotin in patients with relapsed/refractory CD30-positive hematologic malignancies. *Clin Cancer Res* 2012;18:248–255.
234. Perry AM, Mitrovic Z, Chan WC. Biological prognostic markers in diffuse large B-cell lymphoma. *Cancer Control* 2012;19(3):214–226.
235. Schneider C, Pasqualucci L, Dalla-Favera R. Molecular pathogenesis of diffuse large B cell lymphoma. *Semin Diagn Pathol* 2011;28:167–177.
236. Chin L, Gray JW. Translating insight from the cancer genome into clinical practice. *Nature* 2008;452:533–563.
237. Schmitz R, Young RM, Ceribelli M, et al. Burkitt lymphoma pathogenesis and therapeutic targets from structural and functional genomics. *Nature* 2012; 490(7418):116–120.
238. Green TN, Youn KH, Visco C, et al. Immunohistochemical double-hit score is a strong predictor of outcome in patients with diffuse large B-cell lymphoma treated with rituximab plus cyclophosphamide, doxorubicin, vincristine, and prednisone. *J Clin Oncol* 2012;30(28):3460–3467.
239. Johnson NA, Slack GW, Savage KJ, et al. Concurrent expression of MYC and BCL2 in diffuse large B-cell lymphoma treated with rituximab plus cyclophosphamide, doxorubicin, vincristine, and prednisone. *J Clin Oncol* 2012;30(28):3452–3459.
240. Hu S, Xu-Monette ZY, Tzankov A, et al. MYC/BCL2 protein co-expression is associated with high-risk gene signatures and contributes to the inferior prognosis of ABC subtype of diffuse large B-cell lymphoma: a report from the International DLBCL Rituximab-CHOP Consortium Program Study. *Blood* 2012; In Press.
241. Lawrie CH. MicroRNAs and lymphomagenesis: a functional review. *Br J Haematol* 2013;160(5):571–581. doi: 10.1111/bjh.12157.
242. Cesarman E, Chang Y, Moore PS, et al. Kaposi's sarcoma-associated herpesvirus-like DNA sequences in AIDS-related body-cavity-based lymphomas. *N Engl J Med* 1995;332:1186–1191.

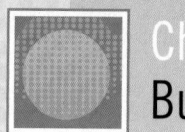

Chapter 24
Burkitt Lymphoma and Related Disorders

Philip M. Kluin • Stefano Rosati

Burkitt lymphoma (BL) was first described in 1958 by the British surgeon Denis P. Burkitt as a sarcoma presenting either in the jaw or in the abdomen of African children (1). In the same year, Jan Saave (2) described a similar case in the coastal regions of Papua New Guinea. In 1960, O'Conor and Davies (3) recognized this lesion as a lymphoma instead of a sarcoma. The first ideas on the pathogenesis of the disease came from an epidemiologic study. During a long safari expedition in 1961, Burkitt observed a relationship between the incidence of BL and certain geographic and climatic factors such as a limited altitude, high rainfall, and high humidity (4), which later appeared to match the distribution of malaria falciparum infection (5). Three years later, Epstein et al. (6) discovered the Epstein-Barr virus (EBV) in a large number of endemic BL cases and suggested a causative role of the virus in the pathogenesis of this lymphoma. However, the common presence of EBV infection in individuals without this lymphoma spoke against its role as a single cause for the lymphoma. Neither could the co-occurrence with malaria fully explain its pathogenesis (7).

Similar lymphomas arising in other tropical regions such as in Papua New Guinea were described shortly after the discovery in Africa, mostly by the same team of investigators (8,9). Occasional tumors with a similar morphology outside these endemic regions were later identified (often referred to as "sporadic" or "nonendemic" types of BL) (9–11). After the discovery of the human immunodeficiency virus (HIV) in 1983, a third category of similar lymphomas arising in immunodeficient patients was described, mostly in association with HIV infection but also as posttransplant lymphoproliferative disorders (12–15). In consequence, due to the partially overlapping geography of HIV infection and malaria infection, some countries in equatorial Africa are targeted by both a high incidence of typical endemic BL and immunodeficiency-related BL.

Additional information on the pathogenesis of the disease came from a genetic perspective in the early 1970s. In 1972, Manolov and Manolova (16) described a recurring genetic abnormality in BL cell lines involving an extra band on the telomeric end of the long arm of chromosome 14. Subsequently, several groups found that the telomeric region of the long arm of chromosome 8 translocated toward specific bands on chromosome 2, 14, or 22 in both endemic and sporadic BL cases (17–22). However, it was not before 1981 that the oncogene MYC was discovered to be the target of the recurrent translocations (23,24). In the following years it became clear that MYC overexpression plays a pivotal role in BL, but that additional oncogenic events are needed for the development of BL, as MYC overexpression alone is insufficient for tumorigenesis (25–31).

DEFINITION

BL represents a unique, extremely rapidly growing mature B-cell lymphoma derived from germinal center (GC) B-cell blasts. It has a highly characteristic, if not obligatory, reciprocal chromosomal translocation involving MYC at 8q24 and one of the immunoglobulin gene loci, whereas it harbors relatively few other genetic abnormalities (32). Three epidemiologic variants with a variable involvement of EBV are recognized. Most patients are young and present with a rapidly expanding extranodal mass. Few cases may present with a leukemic component. The histology, cytomorphology, and immunophenotype are relatively alike between all three subtypes, but some other aggressive mature B-cell lymphomas may mimic BL.

EPIDEMIOLOGY

Three distinct clinical variants of BL are recognized: the endemic, the sporadic, and the immunodeficiency-related variant. The endemic variant, almost exclusively occurring in equatorial Africa and Papua New Guinea, represents the most common form of pediatric lymphoma in these regions (33). Because of this association, and the fact that by far most epidemiologic and other studies have been done in African cases, endemic BL is often also called "African Burkitt lymphoma." However, in this chapter we refer to it as endemic Burkitt lymphoma (eBL). Sporadic Burkitt lymphoma (sBL) was previously also called "non-African Burkitt lymphoma," but after the discovery of immunodeficiency-associated BL, this name is no longer used. Finally, immunodeficiency-related BL is often called AIDS-related BL, which is due to the very close association between HIV infection and AIDS.

The peak incidence of eBL is at the age of 5 years with an estimated rate in children of around 1:10,000. The male:female ratio is about 2.5:1 (34–37). A complicating factor in recent decades is the high increase of AIDS-related lymphomas, including BL in almost the same regions of Africa. These lymphomas should not be considered as eBL, but on the other hand are very difficult to distinguish as they have many overlapping features, including involvement of the jaw in pediatric patients (38,39). This diagnostic difficulty is even more prominent since often a very limited diagnostic procedure is performed and many other lymphomas or other infectious conditions in these immunodeficient patients may mimic BL.

In children around the age of 5 years, eBL usually presents with a large extranodal mass either in the jaw or in the abdomen. At higher ages, the presentation may be more diverse. By definition, there is an almost complete association with EBV with over 95% of the cases being positive for EBV (40). Many epidemiologic studies have also shown a very strong relationship with malaria infection (5,36,39,41–43) and to a lesser extent with exposure to a domestic bush, *Euphorbia tirucalli* (44–48).

In Western countries, sBL is a rare tumor that occurs predominantly in the first two decades of life but it is observed at all ages. In the United States, the incidence is one to three per million inhabitants. In a Dutch study of 203 patients registered in the National Cancer Registry between 1994 and 1998 (34), the incidence was 3.5 per million Dutch inhabitants for males and 1.7 for females. It is generally stated that the male:female ratio is 2:1 or 3:1. However, in the Dutch study a very strong male

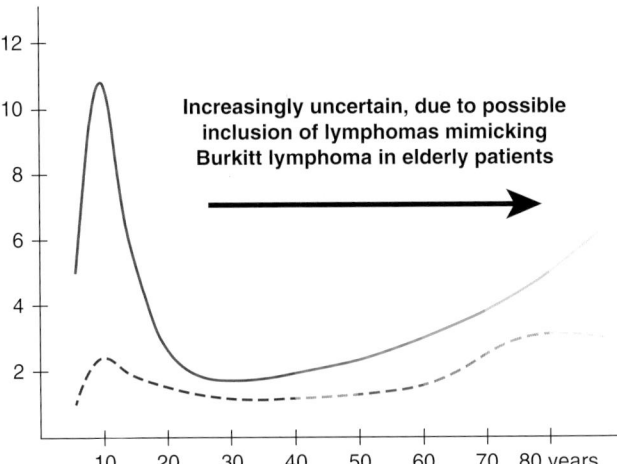

FIGURE 24.1. Age and gender distribution of sBL. Data are derived from (34) and (37). In pediatric patients, there is a very pronounced male predominance that is much less pronounced over the age of 15 years. The incidence of true BL may be much less certain in elderly patients, since mimics like double-hit lymphomas (see Differential Diagnosis of Burkitt Lymphoma in text) may have been included in epidemiologic studies.

preponderance was in particular found for patients younger than 15 years (80% boys), whereas the gender distribution was more balanced at higher ages (Fig. 24.1). Except for the very high peak incidence in young boys in the Netherlands, almost similar results were found in a SEER-based study on more than 3,000 BL patients from the United States for the period between 1972 and 2005 (37,49). A trimodal age distribution was suggested exclusively in male patients. Interestingly, BL was more frequently seen in whites than among blacks in the United States. However, all historical data should be interpreted cautiously because especially in the higher-age groups, lymphomas mimicking BL, in particular some diffuse large B-cell lymphomas (DLBCL) and double-hit lymphomas, may have been included (see Differential Diagnosis of Burkitt Lymphoma section). In contrast with endemic BL, EBV is only found in a minority of sporadic eBL (15% to 20%) (50).

The immunodeficiency-related variant is most commonly associated with HIV and often represents one of the first AIDS-defining symptoms (51). In Western countries, incidence rates vary between 2 in 1,000 in pediatric (52) and 1 in 1,000 in adult AIDS patients (53), with a male:female ratio of 2:1. Different from other AIDS related lymphomas, only a minority of these BL are EBV positive (~40%), which is related to relatively low copy numbers of HIV and concomitant high CD4 counts. In contrast with the other two variants, nodal presentation as well as bone marrow involvement is relatively common in this variant of BL. In regions in Africa where both endemic BL and HIV infection rates are high, the distinction between endemic and HIV-related BL is, however, much more difficult to make, the association with EBV being higher; also, more children may be affected. Furthermore, the clinical presentation is similar to endemic BL with frequent extranodal disease (38).

Interestingly, BL is only rarely seen in the context of other immunodeficiency states (e.g., as posttransplant lymphoproliferative disease [PTLD]). The presence of EBV in these tumors seems to be relatively more frequent than in AIDS-related BL, at least in pediatric patients (54).

CLINICAL FEATURES

Sites of Involvement

In general, the clinical presentation is highly dependent on the variant of BL (endemic, sporadic, or immunodeficiency-related),

as well as age. In endemic BL, involvement of the jaw (frequently of both the maxilla and the mandible) and orbital tumors are often seen, occurring in some 60% at presentation. Other sites are the abdomen, breasts, or, in adolescents, the ovaries. Lymph node involvement is uncommon. A primary bone marrow localization/leukemia is highly uncommon. Involvement of the jaw may present by early loss of teeth or a large intra-oral mass with necrosis, extension to the skin, or penetration through the floor of the orbit giving rise to exophthalmia and chemosis of the conjunctiva. Involvement of the cranial nerves or the paraspinal epidural space is also common. Interestingly, a study in different provinces of Kenya showed that these clinical features vary by geographical region (55). These differences have been suggested to be related to environmental factors.

In sBL, the disease is also primarily extranodal, and up to 90% of the patients within the United States and Europe present with abdominal pain or swelling that may be caused by a solid tumor mass, by ascites with tumor cells, or by secondary complications like invagination of the terminal ileum in the colon. Organs less commonly involved at presentation include the oropharynx, breasts (often bilateral), ovaries, lymph nodes, bone marrow, central nervous system (CNS), and pleural cavity. In patients with exclusive involvement of the bone marrow and blood, a diagnosis of Burkitt leukemia can be made. However, this term should not be used for cases with a typical extranodal or other mass in which the bone marrow is secondarily infiltrated. Of note, the extent of bone marrow involvement should not be used to distinguish between lymphoma and leukemia; however, it is an important prognostic factor used for therapy stratification (56,57). In some patients, the primary site is difficult to ascertain because of the massive involvement or multiple sites of involvement. Whereas jaw involvement is frequent in endemic regions and extremely rare in Europe and the United States, it occurs with intermediate frequency in some other parts of the world, such as in Turkey and Brazil (58–60).

Patients with AIDS-related BL more commonly present with nodal disease, involvement of the bone marrow, and a leukemic picture than patients with the other two variants (57). Of note, in a series of 11 pediatric patients with posttransplant BL (54), most patients presented with bulky extranodal masses, often intra-abdominal, and in contrast to other posttransplant lymphoproliferative disorders, only two times in the allograft itself.

Serious primary complications of the disease are mostly related to the expansion or infiltration of the rapidly growing tumor or tumor lysis and the complications thereof (61). These complications include gastrointestinal bleeding or perforation, invagination at the ileocecal valve, ureteric obstruction, intra-abdominal venous obstruction and obstructive jaundice, and paraplegia from epidural localizations. Mediastinal masses, as in precursor T-cell lymphoblastic lymphoma, with complications thereof are rarely seen in BL. A tumor lysis syndrome with rapid development of hyperuricemia, hyperkalemia, hyperphosphatemia, hypocalcemia, and acute renal failure may arise from the high cell turnover in patients who have a large tumor burden. If no or insufficient preventive measures are taken, such patients are at extremely high risk of death after start of chemotherapy.

Clinical Evaluation and Staging

The clinical evaluation and staging procedure is highly dependent on the socioeconomic conditions. In some endemic regions with poor health care, in particular when a child is presenting with a jaw tumor, the diagnosis is made on the basis of the clinical presentation and therapy is sometimes instituted without any further diagnostic or staging procedure. In countries with better health care conditions, including the Western countries, children are evaluated according to the Murphy/

St. Jude's system (62), whereas adult patients are mostly staged according to the Ann Arbor system. Using the St. Jude's system, patients can be assigned to distinct risk groups that form the basis of the various treatment protocols. According to this pediatric staging system, stage and prognosis are also predicted by the assessment of complete removal of the tumor. For instance, complete removal of an ileocecal mass as assessed by the pathologist together with the lack of any clinical evidence of residual lymphoma elsewhere indicates stage II disease, which is associated with a favorable prognosis. However, this association is likely related to a limited tumor mass, by itself a favorable prognostic indicator.

 ## MORPHOLOGY

Histology and Cytology

Histologically, BL is characterized by a diffuse growth pattern without any nodularity. No follicular dendritic cells are present in the tumor. Extremely exceptional cases may show a follicular growth pattern, which might reflect a possible GC origin or follicular colonization (Fig. 24.2). The interpretation of this pattern remains highly speculative since the extremely high growth rate of the tumor makes it very difficult to identify the origin of the tumor at the moment of surgery. In fact, in many cases preexistent lymph nodes are surrounded and entrapped by the tumor cells without any hint as to where the tumor has arisen. Also, in ileocaecal resection specimens the origin of the lymphoma remains obscure; the tumor shows just a heavy infiltration of all layers of the intestinal wall, often with a relatively modest infiltration and apparently secondary ulceration of the mucosa. Some authors believe that the frequent extranodal localization favors an origin from mucosa-associated lymphoid tissue tissue, but no cases have been described in which an inflammatory background or low-grade component supports such an origin.

In almost all cases the tumor cells are densely packed without any intervening reactive lymphoid cells and without any induction of stroma. The presence of reactive macrophages with phagocytosis of remnants of apoptotic tumor cells gives rise to a starry sky pattern at low power. However, this pattern is nonspecific as it may be seen in many lymphomas and myeloid leukemia/myeloid sarcoma with a high proliferation or apoptotic rate. Moreover, the presence of this pattern is

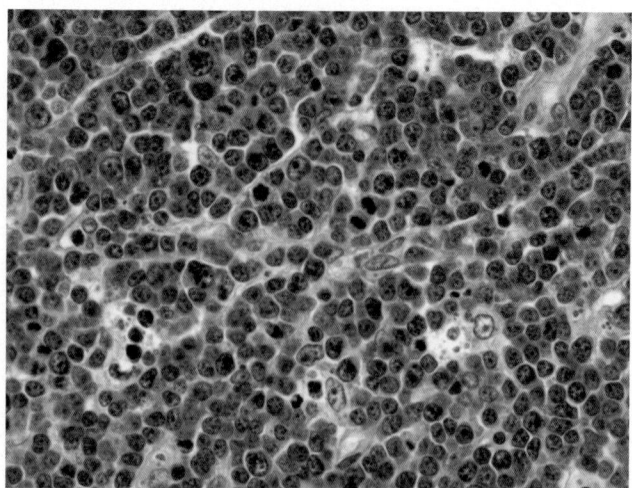

FIGURE 24.3. Burkitt lymphoma. Ileocecal lymphoma, boy, 15 years. Hematoxylin-and-eosin–stained section showing typical BL. Note the starry sky macrophages with nuclei that are larger than those of the lymphoma cells. Nucleoli are relatively small, but even in this field, some larger nuclei with more prominent nucleoli can be found. This variation should never rule out a diagnosis of BL. The "squaring-off" phenomenon can be appreciated in several areas.

not a prerequisite to diagnose BL. The combination of this high density of tumor cells without intercellular stroma and the absence of other intercellular structures or cells in combination with fixation (shrinkage) artifacts often gives rise to a "squared-off" phenomenon in tissue sections (Fig. 24.3).

Rare cases of exclusively EBV-positive sporadic BL have been described in which there is an overt granulomatous reaction in the tumor, sometimes even overshadowing the tumor cells (63–65). In these cases the BL cells have a classical morphology, phenotype, and MYC breakpoint. This granulomatous reaction may be related to a specific and HLA-dependent T-cell response to EBNA1-positive lymphoma cells, and has been associated with a very favorable outcome (65).

At closer look BL cells have medium-sized nuclei, the nuclei often being two times the size of normal lymphocytes but smaller than or of the same size as the nuclei of starry sky macrophages. In fact, in many cases these macrophages are the only cells available to calibrate for nuclear size. In principle the nucleus should be round; however, in many cases artifacts may be present, giving rise to wrinkled nuclear contours or some lobulation, both in histologic slides and in imprints. This phenomenon may be caused by *in vivo* mechanisms such as massive apoptosis or necrosis, but also by improper tissue handling after biopsy/surgical removal. The latter includes delayed fixation (many abdominal tumors being removed during acute interventions when a pathologist is not available for immediate tissue processing), fixation without appropriate slicing of the often bulky tumor and hence improper fixative penetration, a too short fixation, but also subsequent improper histotechnical handling including the use of too high temperatures to stretch and dry the tissue sections on the glass slides after cutting. Insufficient fixation may sometimes lead to an "explosion" artifact with nuclear blebbing, with the tumor cells looking bigger, mimicking centroblasts or immunoblasts. This may give rise to an erroneous diagnosis of DLBCL. An opposite artifact is shrinkage of nuclei, most often caused by massive ischemia or incipient cell death, for instance after initiation of steroid therapy before biopsy. Many of these problems can be avoided by examination of Giemsa-stained preparations of cytologic fine needle aspirations or imprints of fresh tumor tissue. The impact of these artifacts is illustrated by a study showing that interobserver agreement on the diagnosis amongst experienced hematopathologists is highly dependent on the quality of the tissue sections (66).

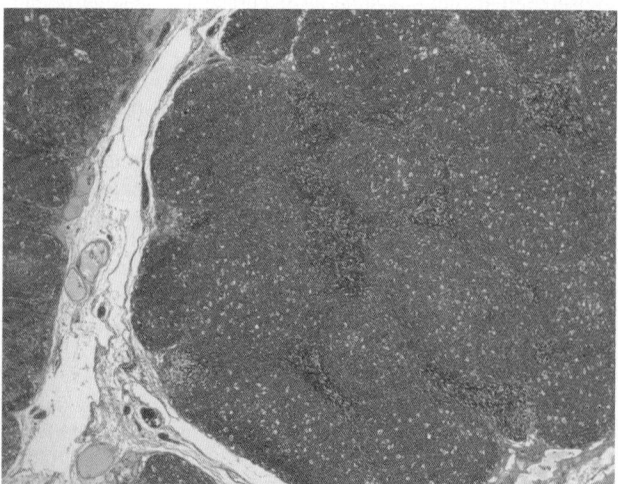

FIGURE 24.2. BL with a follicular growth pattern. This patient presented with an ileocecal mass and local lymph node involvement. The growth pattern was diffuse, except for one lymph node with a distinct follicular pattern, possibly reflecting a GC cell origin, or more likely reflecting follicular colonization by tumor cells.

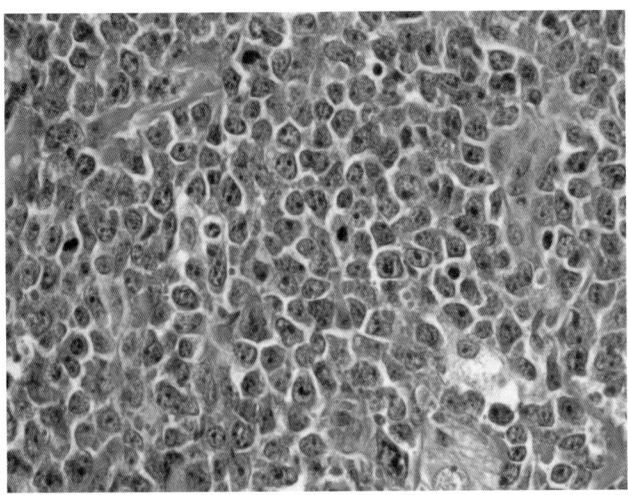

FIGURE 24.4. Atypical BL. Ileocecal tumor, 4-year-old boy, MYC-IGH breakpoint demonstrated by FISH. Hematoxylin-and-eosin–stained slide showing somewhat more variation in nuclear and nucleolar size than that shown in Figure 24.3. Many cells have one central nucleolus.

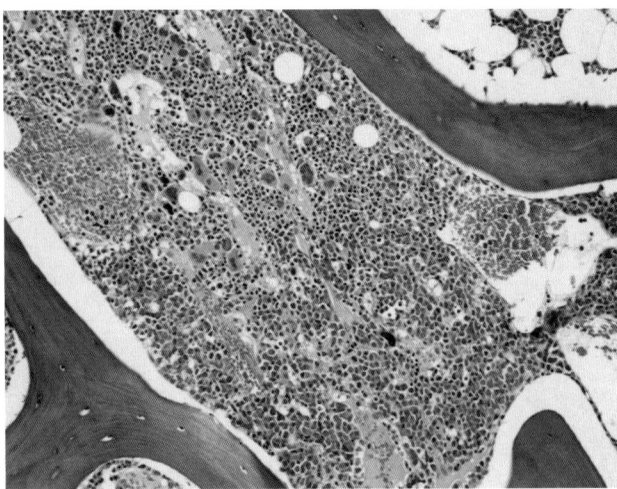

FIGURE 24.5. Bone marrow infiltration by BL. Bone marrow biopsy of BL patient with extensive disease. MYC-IGH breakpoint demonstrated by FISH. The pattern is typically interstitial/diffuse but not nodular. Preexistent hematopoietic cells may be hidden in between the neoplastic cells, just as in acute leukemia.

The chromatin of typical BL cells is granular, much different from that of lymphoblastic lymphoma (which is finer) and from that of most DLBCL (more open nucleus with condensation of heterochromatin along the nuclear membrane). Most BL contain small to medium-sized nucleoli; however, some contain a variable percentage of cells with one or two bigger nucleoli. In the past, the latter appearance was considered as atypical, and therefore such cases were called "atypical Burkitt lymphoma" or aBL (Fig. 24.4).

The cytoplasm of all variants of BL should be very basophilic in the Giemsa staining, again best appreciated in fine needle aspiration or imprint preparations. Most BL cells show a symmetrical configuration with a centrally positioned nucleus; however, some cases and in particular cases with plasmacytic differentiation, as may be observed in immunodeficiency-associated BL, may have a slightly eccentric nucleus. The cytoplasm often contains numerous punched-out vacuoles containing lipid. These vacuoles are typical but not entirely specific for this type of lymphoma, since some GC-derived DLBCL, in particular centroblastic lymphomas, may contain similar vacuoles.

Morphologic Variants of Burkitt Lymphoma

Originally, the morphologic definition of BL was mainly based on typical endemic BLs. However, with the recognition of similar sporadic cases in Western countries and the finding that similar lymphomas could also be found in elderly patients and/or immunodeficient patients, the entity was broadened (67). Since solid immunohistochemical and molecular tools such as fluorescent *in situ* hybridization (FISH) were not readily available or not reliable, the definition became increasingly indistinct. Thus, cases with a wider variation in nuclear size, the presence of one big nucleolus instead of multiple nucleoli and less granular heterochromatin than usually present, the presence of a more "secretory" appearance of the cytoplasm with an eccentric widening of the cytoplasm, or the absence of cytoplasmic vacuoles were all debated to be acceptable for or to be at odds with BL. In the latter case, they were attributed a variety of names, including small noncleaved non-BL (68), Burkitt-like lymphoma (69) and aBL (WHO classification 2001). This led to much confusion among pathologists and hematooncologists, also since it appeared that several of these patients had a clinically extremely aggressive disease and could not be

cured with the otherwise highly effective polychemotherapy regimens used in regular BL patients.

Two relatively recent developments contributed to a renovation of the definition of BL. First, two publications on gene expression profiling (GEP) of classical BL and related lymphomas showed that BL have a highly restricted and predictive molecular profile, quite different from that of DLBCL, including the DLBCL with a GC pattern of gene expression (43,70). Both studies indicated that some morphologic variants, in particular atypical BL with an otherwise classical immunophenotype and the presence of a MYC/8q24 breakpoint, invariably have a GEP similar to that of prototypic BL (the profile being called molecular Burkitt lymphoma or mBL). Moreover, both studies showed that a number of BL mimics had a "non-mBL" GEP or at least an intermediate profile, still much different from that of true BL. From one GEP study in which FISH analysis and array comparative genomic hybridization (CGH) were also applied (70), it appeared that mBL cases always have colocalization of the MYC gene and one of the immunoglobulin genes ("MYC-IG") whereas BL mimics more often had a breakpoint of MYC without such colocalization ("MYC-non IG") (Fig. 24.5). In addition, mBL cases have many fewer genetic abnormalities (gains or losses) than intermediate or non-mBL cases. Both observations are in agreement with older classical cytogenetic studies, showing that almost 40% of BL do not have any other chromosomal abnormality in addition to the t(8;14) or variant t(8;22) or t(2;8) translocations.

A second contribution to the redefinition of BL in the WHO classification system of 2008 was the routine introduction of FISH assays for MYC/8q24 as well for BCL2/18q21 and BCL6/3q27 breakpoints. In fact, a large number of publications (71–77) showed that many of these BL mimics either lack an 8q24 breakpoint or have a combination of the 8q24 breakpoint with an additional BCL2/18q21 or BCL6/3q27 breakpoint, representing a so-called double-hit lymphoma. In particular, these double-hit lymphomas, which are increasingly frequent at higher ages, have a very poor outcome (see Differential Diagnosis of Burkitt Lymphoma section). These observations led to the redefinition of BL in the 2008 WHO classification in which some variation in cytomorphology is accepted as long as a MYC/8q24 breakpoint and preferably also colocalization with one of the immunoglobulin loci can be demonstrated, whereas a double hit involving BCL2/18q21 or BCL6/3q27 is actively excluded.

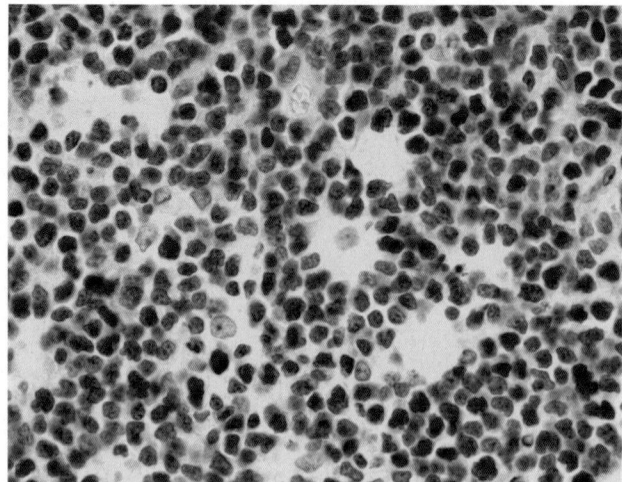

FIGURE 24.6. BCL6 expression in BL. Woman, 79 years, with tumor of the small intestine. BL with classical phenotype; however, FISH analysis was unsuccessful (no signals). All BLs are homogeneously bcl6 protein and CD10 positive, which likely reflects their origin from GCs.

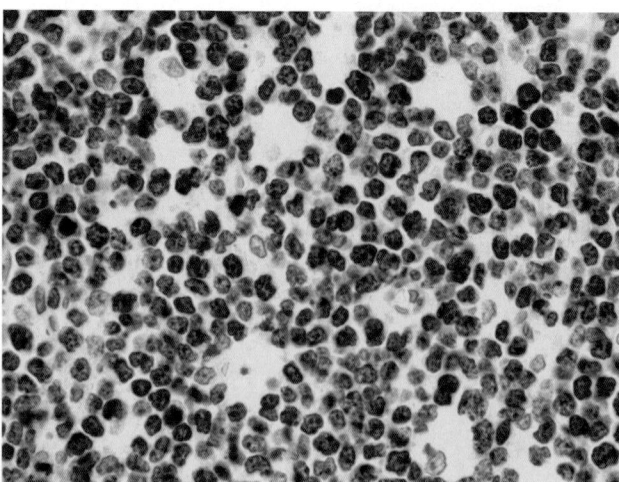

FIGURE 24.8. Ki67/MIB1 proliferation index in BL. Same patient as in Figures 24.6 and 24.7. The Ki67 staining is homogeneously positive in (almost) all tumor cells. A variable staining pattern should raise the possibility of a mimic of BL, even if an MYC breakpoint is demonstrable.

IMMUNOPHENOTYPE

The immunophenotype of BL is very consistent in the literature: The cells reflect mature GC B cells with expression of pan–B-cell markers such as CD19, CD20, CD79a, PAX5, homogeneous expression of the transcriptional repressor bcl6 (100% of the cases, Fig. 24.6), the functionally still enigmatic antigen CD10 (also 100% of the cases), and a rather strong expression of surface IgM with either kappa or lambda. A few cases with plasmacytic differentiation may show cytoplasmic immunoglobulin expression as well. In none of the cases has Ig class switching to IgG or IgA been described. As in normal GC B cells, there is no coexpression of IgD. Cases that lack expression of immunoglobulin heavy chains as assessed by flow cytometry or by immunofluorescence on frozen tissue sections should be strongly suspected for a double-hit lymphoma with concomitant translocations of both IGH alleles with involvement of a BCL2 or BCL6 (or even CCND1) gene on one allele and MYC on the other allele. Other markers, also expressed in normal GCs, that are positive in BL are TCL1, CD38, CD77, and GCET2.

CD44 expression should be low. Importantly, and also similar to normal GC B cells, bcl2 expression should be completely absent or very weak (Fig. 24.7). All cases with some expression of BCL2 protein should be tested for MYC, BCL2, and BCL6 breakpoints to exclude a double-hit lymphoma. MUM1/IRF4 expression was initially thought to be entirely negative in BL, but it now appears that approximately half of all BL show a weak and often homogeneous expression of the protein (78). Of note, this expression is not related to plasmacytoid differentiation in immunodeficiency-associated BL, nor with translocations involving the IRF4 gene as described in some cases of pediatric lymphomas (79). Finally, the proliferation index as determined by Ki67/MIB1 should be homogeneously approaching a 100% score, only some preexistent endothelial cells and other stromal cells being negative (Fig. 24.8). In fact, all cases with a lower or slightly heterogeneous proliferation index likely reflect mimics of BL such as double-hit lymphoma.

ETIOLOGY AND MOLECULAR PATHOGENESIS OF BURKITT LYMPHOMA

The Role of Epstein-Barr Virus in Burkitt Lymphoma

Since the discovery of EBV in endemic BL samples (6), much research has been done on the virus itself and its role in BL. EBV is present in more than 95% of all cases of endemic type BL, 30% to 40% of AIDS-associated BL, probably more than 50% of posttransplant BL, but only in 20% to 30% of sporadic cases arising in Western countries. Intermediate frequencies may be found in other countries (80–82). EBV is a complex virus with many genes involved in lytic cycles and various latency types. The virus was originally detected in an indirect way (6). In fact, the working hypothesis at that time was that a possible vector-mediated virus played a causative role in BL. However, using electron microscopy, Epstein et al. could not detect any virus particles in fresh tumor samples of BL. Instead, complete virus particles were observed in cultures derived from continuously growing cell lines derived from a case of BL. This was reproduced in other cultures; however, in all instances only a few cells showed virus particles (6).

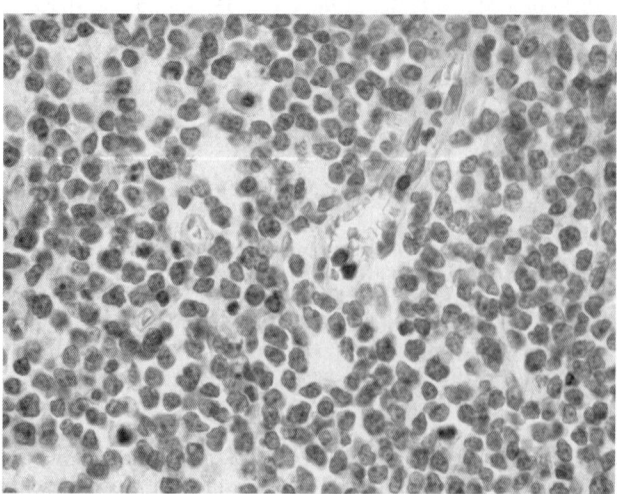

FIGURE 24.7. Absence of bcl2 expression in BL. Same patient as in Figure 24.6. Immunohistochemistry shows complete absence of protein expression in the tumor cells. Three residual cells show a perinuclear staining and serve as internal control cells, obligatory to exclude any possibility of false-negative staining.

In the same period, Henle et al. (83) made use of fluorescent-labeled antisera of EBV-infected patients, and could detect viral proteins (that later appeared to be the EBNAs) in the nuclei of EBV-infected BL cells. Essentially, this test—and in particular later developed tests specific for EBNA1—showed the presence of viral proteins in all tumor cells, including cells in which no virus particles were detectable. Anti-EBNA1 immunofluorescence assays have been used as the most sensitive test for many years until *in situ* hybridization tests for EBER1/2 RNA became available (84).

EBV is a gamma herpesvirus of the *Lymphocryptovirus* genus and is closely related to other viruses in nonhuman primates. The EBV genome is composed of linear double-stranded DNA, approximately 172 kb in length. EBV has a series of internal and terminal repeats (TRs; Fig. 24.9) that divide the genome into different domains. The complete sequences of the two strains of EBV suggest a coding for about 80 proteins. These proteins are involved in active replication and lysis of host cells as well as the maintenance of the virus inside host cells. Three major latency types exist, type III showing expression of most genes and type I cells showing the fewest being expressed. The latter situation is seen *in vivo* in BL cells (85,86). In fact, in most BL tumor cells, only the virus genome–maintenance protein EBNA1 is expressed via a unique transcript from the *Bam*HI Q promoter QpI (27,87). This contrasts with the latency III program in EBV-transformed B lymphoblastoid cell lines, and in early-onset PTLD lesions, in which multiple EBNAs and LMP1 are also expressed. It also differs from the latency pattern II with expression of EBNA1, LMP1, and LMP2 as seen in the Reed-Sternberg cells of Hodgkin lymphoma (28). Importantly, expression of cell surface adhesion molecules was shown to be associated with the latency type in BL cell lines, low levels of ICAM-1 and LFA-3 in latency group I/II BL cell lines being associated with an impaired ability to interact with EBV-specific cytotoxic T cells (88). In 2002, Kelly et al. (89) described a novel latency program in approximately 15% of endemic BLs. In these cases a deletion in EBNA-2 and expression of EBNA-3A, -3B, and -3C and of the viral BCL2 homologue BHRF1 is mediated by the use of the Wp promoter instead of the Qpl promoter. In these cases, EBNA-3 expression may lead to transcriptional repression of the antiapoptotic BH3-only protein (BCL2 family member) BIM and, therefore, may result in BL cells that are more resistant to drug-induced apoptosis. An alternative mechanism leading to BIM repression might be via BHRF-1.

EBNA-1 protein binds to a replication origin (oriP) within the viral genome and mediates replication and partitioning of the episome during division of the host cell. The EBNA1 protein contains a glycine-glycine-alanine (gly-gly-ala) repeat sequence, which varies in size in different EBV isolates. Interestingly, this repeat domain is an inhibitor of MHC class I-restricted presentation by inhibiting antigen processing via the ubiquitin-proteosome pathway (90). This failure to present EBNA1-derived peptides results in ineffective CD8+ T-cell responses. Other work (91) suggests that EBNA-1 activates the transcription of the catalytic subunit of the NADPH oxidase, NOX2/gp91Phox, and consequently increases the production of reactive oxygen species (ROS), thereby inducing genetic instability. This may be a cofactor in the induction of chromosomal translocation. Finally, at least theoretically, EBNA-1 may also act as a transcription factor, and is able to modulate the expression of RAG1 and RAG2, two important proteins involved in immunoglobulin heavy and light chain gene recombination in B cells, both in precursor B cells and later on in B cells that undergo reediting of the B-cell receptor (92).

EBER-1/EBER-2 are small nuclear RNAs, which bind to certain nucleoprotein particles, enabling binding to dsRNA-dependent serin/threonin protein kinase (PKR), thus inhibiting its function. EBER particles also induce the production of IL-10, which enhances growth and inhibits cytotoxic T cells (93,94).

Recently, EBV-coded viral microRNAs (miRs) also have been identified. They are arranged in two clusters: the BHRF1 cluster

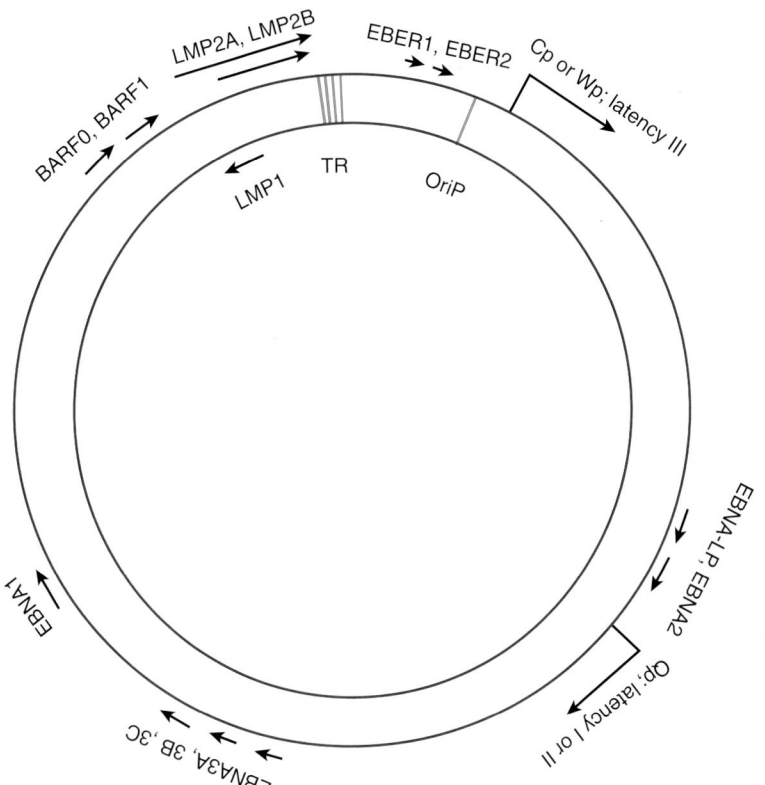

FIGURE 24.9. Structure of EBV. Only latency genes are shown in combination of the EBER genes and various promoters (Cp, WP for latency III vs. Qp for latency I or II). TR indicates the TRs necessary for circularization and the episomal state.

and the BART cluster, the latter comprising 20 miRs located in the introns of the BART transcripts (95,96). Interestingly, the BART cluster is expressed predominantly in both latency I and II, suggesting a functional role in BL as well.

In view of the very restricted pattern of viral gene expression in most BLs, and the fact that only a subset of all BL is EBV-related, there is an ongoing discussion on the role of the virus in the pathogenesis of BL. One idea is that the virus plays a major role in the very early initiation of the tumor but not thereafter ("hit and run" theory) (97). In particular, in young African children who may live in a relative state of immunodeficiency and who are frequently infected with malaria, the resulting massive expansion of B cells may lead to the circulation of a large number of EBV-infected B cells with a diverse latency state of the virus. These B cells may be susceptible to various attacks including DNA damage via somatic hypermutations (SHMs) of IG genes and other genes such as MYC. These mutations may be generated by virally (LMP1) induced activation-induced deaminase (AID) (27), but also via an EBNA1-mediated production of ROS (91).

The Role of Malaria and Other Cofactors in Burkitt Lymphoma

Endemic BL is particularly frequent in regions where infection with malaria falciparum is holoendemic; these areas are characterized by very early and chronic malaria infection at the age of 1 to 5 years. These children, however, also suffer from other infections such as early and often massive EBV infection. The importance of this association is illustrated by the fact that eradication of malaria from these regions or emigration of families to other regions without holoendemic malaria is associated with a shift to later EBV infection and to the less frequent occurrence of BL, with a later onset of disease between 5 and 15 years of age as is the case in sporadic BL in Western countries (98).

There are at least two mechanisms that may explain this association: The first explanation is that malaria itself is a powerful B-cell mitogen-inducing proliferation of B cells by the cysteine-rich interdomain region 1a (CIDR1a) domain of the *Plasmodium falciparum* erythrocyte membrane protein 1, preferentially targeting the activation of memory B cells, and providing protection against apoptosis. This may lead to a massively expanded pool of B-cells, which can harbor EBV. Some evidence exists that malaria infection may also directly lead to reactivation of EBV infection in B cells (99,100). The second and more widely accepted explanation is that malaria leads to a severe impairment of T-cell responses against EBV-infected cells (87,101–104). In fact, there is considerable experimental evidence that *P. falciparum* malaria coinfection may negatively impact EBV latent antigen-specific T-cell responses and that recurrent *P. falciparum* malaria infections as seen in holoendemic malaria infection may also impair EBV-lytic antigen-specific T cells.

Other Cofactors: *Euphorbium tirucalli*

Some epidemiologic evidence exists that BL is especially frequent in regions with holoendemic malaria infection and the use of a domestic bush, *E. tirucalli*. Extracts from this plant have been shown to induce a lytic cycle of EBV, to reduce cellular immunity and be able to induce chromosomal breaks in human B cells as well (44–48).

The Molecular Localization of Chromosomal Breakpoints in Burkitt Lymphoma

The first publication on the involvement of MYC in the characteristic translocation t(8;14) was by Dalla Favera in 1982 (23).

In classical BL, either endemic type or sporadic type, 90% to 95% of all cases show a breakpoint where both MYC and one of the IG loci are involved. The frequency of involvement of the IGH, IGL, and IGK loci is very consistently reported as 85% for t(8;14), 10% for t(8;22), and 5% or less for t(2;8), respectively (105,106). In 5% to 10% of otherwise typical BLs, no translocation can be detected, both by classical cytogenetics (karyotyping) and by molecular methods like FISH analysis. It is possible that this is due to technical failure of the assays, but some observations suggest the existence of alternative ways of activation of MYC, or even activation of other genes resulting in a similar phenotype and tumor. One possibility is that a very small excision of MYC and insertion of the gene into one of the IG loci takes place and is missed, because MYC is a very small gene of only 6 kb and excision of the gene from 8q24 and subsequent insertion elsewhere would be undetectable by these methods (71). Another explanation is that the breakpoint is missed because of a localization far outside the region covered by the currently available FISH probes that mostly span a region of 300 kb 5′ of MYC and more than 1,000 kb 3′ of MYC (Fig. 24.10) (107). However, such breakpoints should still be detectable by conventional karyotyping and in cases of juxtaposition to the IGH locus also by FISH in colocalization assays where a probe covering the MYC gene is used in combination with a probe covering IGH. Alternative mechanisms like deregulation of MYC caused by deregulation of micro RNAs (miRNAs) have been described (108) (see Gene expression and Micro RNA Expression Analysis of Burkitt Lymphoma section).

In all cases with a translocation of MYC to one of the IG loci, there is a wide variability in the exact localization of the breakpoints. Extensive molecular analyses, however, showed distinct patterns of these breakpoints, where distinct localizations of the MYC breakpoints are associated with the involvement of the different partner chromosomes (IGH, IGK, and IGL) and with the subtype of BL (endemic vs. sporadic and/or EBV-positive vs. -negative). A summary of these breakpoint associations is given in Figure 24.10. Most importantly, in sBL with a t(8;14), 90% of the breakpoints fall in two distinct clusters, one "immediately 5′ of MYC" and one in exon 1 or intron 1 (Fig. 24.10). In contrast, most (~75%) t(8;14) breakpoints in eBL are far more 5′ (centromeric) from MYC (81,114–116). Cases from Brazil, Argentina, and Chile showed less distinct clustering than African cases. In contrast, both in eBL and in sBL with a variant t(2;8) or t(8;22), the breakpoints with involvement of immunoglobulin light chain genes are at the 3′ side of the MYC gene. Apart from the various molecular mechanisms that may be involved in the generation of the actual breakpoints, the different patterns between cases with a classical t(8;14) and a variant t(2;8) or t(8;22) likely are also caused by selection, only a certain configuration resulting in appropriate IGH or IGL enhancer juxtaposition in relation to MYC, and consequently constitutional activation of MYC.

Interestingly, there are also major differences in the localization of the IGH breaks between BLs from Africa and Western countries. By far, most breakpoints in eBL are present in the telomeric VDJ region, whereas most sBL have breakpoints at the IGH switch sites. Based on these observations it was thought that the breakpoints in African cases have an origin from RAG1/2-mediated errors in precursor B cells and that the breakpoints in sporadic BL are generated during IGH class switch recombination. However, sequencing of the breakpoints showed that the telomeric junctions in the VDJ region do not carry any sign of RAG1/2-mediated breaks, that is, that they are not at or near nonamer-heptamer signal sequences (117). By far most breakpoints in sBL are at switch sites of the heavy chain genes, involved in physiologic class switch events. Sμ, Sγ, and Sα sites seem to be affected equally frequently (118).

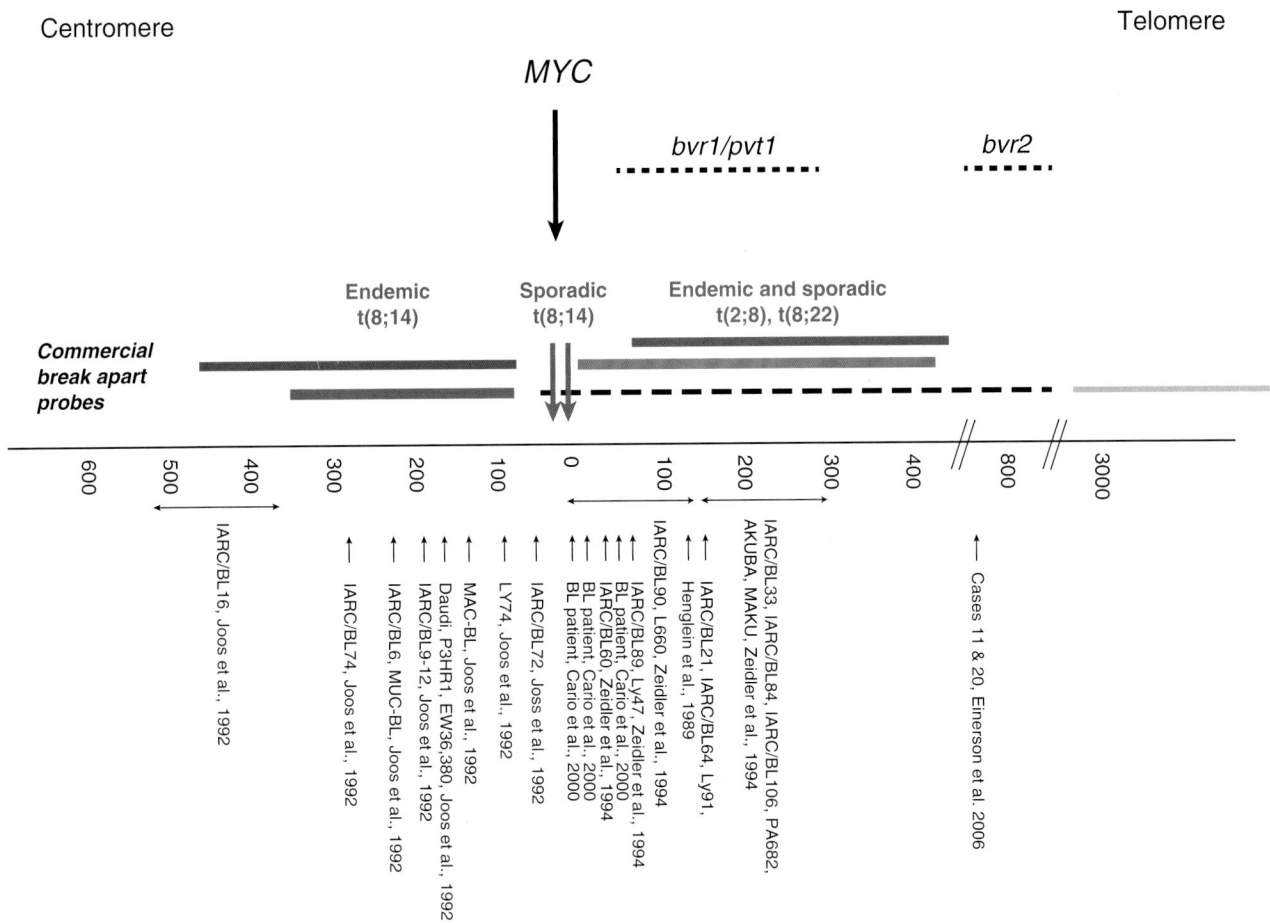

FIGURE 24.10. Distribution of breakpoints at 8q24 in BL. Chromosomal breakpoints are differently positioned, dependent on the partner involved (IGH or IGL and IGK locus), and the epidemiologic type of lymphoma. The individual breakpoints are indicated by *arrows* and references (107,109–113). The position by two commonly used probes in a break apart assay is indicated as well. Note that some breakpoints may be missed with the current FISH probes, as they may be positioned centromeric from the area covered by these probes.

Mechanisms of MYC Translocation

Based on the localization of breakpoints in eBL in VDJ regions of the IGH locus, it was previously assumed that these translocations were recombinase activating gene 1/2 (RAG1/2)-mediated, and thus had an origin from precursor B cells. More recent work on the exact localization of these breakpoints (117) and in particular much experimental work in murine B-cell models in particular the MYC breakpoints (119–125), however, clearly indicate that these breakpoints are AID-mediated, and therefore, likely originate from GC B cells. AID acts by deaminating cytosine residues in single-strand DNA during transcription. The resulting uracil:guanine mismatches are recognized by the uracil DNA glycosylase (UNG) or mismatch repair proteins and processed in an error-prone manner by DNA repair pathways leading either to mutations or to double-strand DNA breaks, which are intermediates in class switching (126–128). AID deaminates cytosines in nearly any DNA sequence context but has a preference for so-called RGYW motifs (127,129). Experiments with human and mouse B cells show that, in addition to *IG*, AID can mutate a large number of oncogenes, including *MYC, PIM1, PAX5*, and *RHOH*, as well as *BCL6*, IGα, IGβ, and *FAS* (130–133). More recent studies show that even many other genes can be mutated at low rates by AID as well (134,135). Mutations and translocations at *MYC* are detected at very low levels under physiologic conditions (133,135), but they accumulate in the absence of efficient base excision and mismatch repair pathways, for instance, in the absence

of NBS1, ATM, p53, and p19/ARF. In the same experimental models, down-regulation of PUMA, BIM, and PKCdelta also facilitates these translocations (136).

In spite of these novel findings, many questions still have to be answered, for instance, the high positional diversity of MYC/8q24 breakpoints in BL and the exact cell of origin of the different variants of BL. For instance, Bellan et al. (137) suggested that African BL and AIDS-related BL are derived from relatively late GC B cells since they carry more SHMs in the *IGH* genes than do sporadic cases. However, the load of SHM is more related to the functional state of the actual tumor cells (including levels of AID in these cells) than to the exact B-cell subset from which the tumor originally developed when the translocation did arise.

The Function of MYC

All translocations involving MYC/8q24 result in a constitutive overexpression of MYC. This is in strong contrast to normal GC B cells that, contrary to what might be thought for these rapidly proliferating cells, have very low levels of MYC expression (138). MYC is a transcription factor that regulates more than 15% of all cellular genes, controlling cell growth, progression through the cell cycle, survival, and metabolism. The N-terminus of MYC (Fig. 24.11) contains three conserved sequences, which are essential for protein stability, protein interaction, and transcriptional activation or repression of MYC target genes (139). A C-terminal basic helix-loop-helix leucine zipper domain allows dimerization of MYC with the partner protein MAX. Interaction with MAX is essential for the binding of MYC to specific DNA sequences (E-boxes) in the promoter regions of target genes. Here it can recruit chromatin remodeling proteins, such as histone acetyltransferases. Gene repression is mainly mediated through MYC/MAX heterodimers preventing the interaction with MIZ-1 and P300, allowing recruitment of the DNA methyltransferases DNMT3A and DNMT3B.

Using potential MYC binding sites and MYC-induced changes in gene expression in a human B-cell line as a model, Zeller et al. (140) identified more than 3,000 genes with potential MYC binding sites. Less than one quarter of these genes were differentially modulated in response to Myc in microarray analyses, two-thirds being up-regulated and one-third being down-regulated. Functional classification of these direct target genes based on gene ontology categorization revealed many categories, metabolism, cell cycle control, transcription regulation, intracellular signal cascade and biosynthesis being statistically overrepresented (see also http://www.myccancergene.org/site/mycTargetDB.asp). Well-known examples of genes that are up-regulated are p19/ARF, Cdc2, Cdc25A, cyclin A, cyclin D1, cyclin E, LDH-A, p53, telomerase (hTERT) (Table 24.1). In reverse, some genes are down-regulated, including the immunorecognition-associated genes LFA1 and MHC class I, as well as terminal deoxynucleotidyl transferase (TdT) (141). In a combined chromatin immunoprecipitation and deep sequencing study of all DNA fragments by Seitz et al. on five BL cell lines, even more (~7,000) MYC binding sites were found. Additional MYC siRNA experiments suggested that in addition to already known MYC targets, many B-cell–specific proteins such as CD20, PAX5, and CD79a are down-regulated by MYC (142). Alternatively, MYC may function as a more global transcriptional amplifier than activating specific genes (143).

One other aspect of MYC is its ability to induce DNA damage at the initiation of DNA replication. MYC interacts with the pre-replicative complex and localizes to early sites of DNA synthesis. Overexpression causes increased replication origin activity with DNA damage and checkpoint activation (144).

In conclusion, MYC both stimulates the cell cycle by enhancing metabolism and increases replication origin activity, but also causes DNA damage and in consequence activation of DNA damage repair or apoptosis. Indeed, acute induction of MYC has been shown to activate p14/ARF and p53 and consequently apoptosis, the latter being a hallmark of BL. The main question, therefore, is how this activated apoptotic pathway is counteracted in BL. This is described under Other Molecular Events in Burkitt Lymphoma.

Finally, recent studies also indicate that MYC drives the expression of a large number of miRNA, many of which are deregulated in BL (145–148). Most miRNAs are down-regulated, but in particular the members of the miRNA 17-92 family, also called "OncomiR-1," are up-regulated by MYC (Table 24.1). One interesting issue is that these miRNAs seem to affect many genes and pathways that are also directly affected by MYC. In conclusion, MYC plays a major role in many aspects of B cells and B-cell lymphomas, either directly as a transcriptional activator or repressor or indirectly via miRNAs.

Other Molecular Events in Burkitt Lymphoma

Classical karyotyping of regular BL in general reveals few genetic abnormalities in addition to the translocation involving MYC/8q24. In consequence, in up to 40% of all BL the t(8;14) or its variant t(2;8) or t(8;22) remains the single chromosomal abnormality (149–151). According to a systematic review of all cases reported in the literature (106), the most common aberrations in the remaining 60% of BL (occurring in >4% of the cases) are copy number gains involving 1q, 7, and 12, and losses involving 6q, 13q32-q34, and 17p. So far the only target gene in these regions that has been exactly defined is p53 on 17p. p53 Mutation on one allele and deletion of the other allele have been found in approximately half of all BL cell lines and in 30% of primary cases of BL (152–156). As described above, these deletions and mutations may efficiently counteract the proapoptotic effect of MYC. The clinical impact of the additional chromosomal alterations has been studied in a large cohort of 182 pediatric BL patients treated with the FAB/LMB6 protocol (157): whereas +1q or dup1q together present in 39% of the cases was not associated with outcome, +7q (present in 14%) as well as del13q (present in 14%) were both associated with poor outcome. Of note, del6q, a very common abnormality in DLBCL, was found in only 10% of the BL cases.

FIGURE 24.11. Structure of MYC. The figure shows an 8 kb area covering MYC with main protein domains, exons, promoter sites, and areas that are affected by AID and therefore susceptible for mutations and translocations.

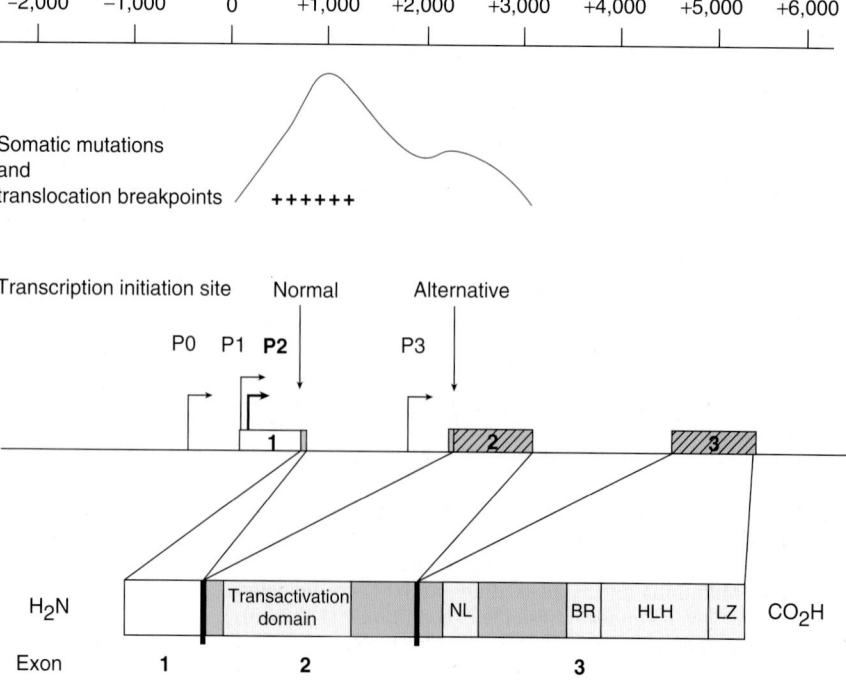

Table 24.1	EFFECTS OF MYC ON GENE EXPRESSION AND MICRO RNAs IN B CELLS
Category	**Specific Pathways/Genes**
Enhancement of metabolism	Activation of nucleotide and amino acid metabolism and telomere integrity (hTERT)
	Activation of mitochondrial biogenesis
	Activation of glycolysis (LDH-A, GLUT1)
	Iron metabolism (iron regulatory protein 2, H-ferritin)
Cell cycle progression	Activation of many proteins (cyclin D1 and 2, cyclin E1, CDK2, CDK4, E2F2); repression of p21, p27/KIP
	Simulation of origin of replication
Induction of apoptosis	Activation of p16/INK4a, p14/ARF and p53, Bim1, Bax, Fas/FasL
Induction of cellular senescence	Activation of p14, p53, p16/INK4a
Decrease of adhesion, migration, and matrix production (also relevant in stem cell pathophysiology)	Repression of N-Cadherin, LFA1, CD44, collagen production, fibronectin production
Decrease of T- and B-cell interaction	Repression of HLA-A,B,C etc.; CD40, CD80, CD86, LFA1
Induction of growth and differentiation	Activation of IRF4 (with autocrine loop) and downstream BLIMP1 in B cells
Induction of stem cell features	Chromatin modification: activation of HDAC2
miRNAs	Repression of relatively many miRNAs (miR-150, miR-155, miR-34a, etc.)
	Early B-cell formation, GC formation and B-cell maturation (miR-34A: FoxP1; miR-150: cMyb; miR-155: PU-1)
	Cell cycle: Let-7a: RAS, CCND2; miR-34A: CDK4&6, E2F
	Apoptosis: miR-15A/16-1: BCL2; miR34A: BCL2, BIRC3
	Activation of relatively few miRNAs (Mir17-92 cluster)
	Cell cycle: miR-17; 20a: E2F1-3, CDKN1A
	Survival: miR19a: PTEN, BIM

Shown are some of the targets and possible functional effects of MYC overexpression in human B cells.

Recent studies in which the genome of BL was explored by more refined methods such as high-resolution array/matrix CGH and single nucleotide polymorphism analysis did not reveal many novel alterations in BL. Moreover, in a group of BLs that were also studied by gene expression array analysis, the alterations were completely similar between pediatric and adult cases of molecularly defined cases of BL (158–160). This observation represents a biologic rationale for attempts to harmonize treatment protocols between pediatric and adult BL patients.

Apart from the gross genomic alterations found by karyotyping and (matrix) array CGH, no other structural translocations and only a few mutations in potential target genes have been identified so far at the molecular level. Apart from p53, another gene that is occasionally inactivated in BL is P16/INK4a, also called CDKN2A, a cell cycle inhibitor that interacts with CDK4/6 and thus interferes with cyclin D-mediated cell cycle progression (161–163). The alternative reading frame (ARF) transcript of the gene interferes with MDM2 and this complex stabilizes p53 (164). Microdeletions affecting P16/INK4a at 9p21 have been described in a low percentage of BL (161,165). However, the gene may be affected much more frequently by methylation than by deletion or mutation (166). In one study, another gene involved in the cell cycle, *RBL2/p130*, previously called pRb2 and mapped to chromosome 16q12, was often mutated in endemic BL (10/13 cases tested) but less frequently in sporadic and AIDS-related cases (167). In G0 cells, RBL2 complexes with E2F4/5 to repress many genes including E2F1/2 and RBL1/ p107. *RBL2* mutation leads to release of E2F4/5 from this complex and degradation of RBL2 with derepression of RBL1/ p107 and other genes. This facilitates the formation of E2F4/5, RBL1/p107, CDK2, and cyclin A complexes that induce cell cycle progression. Thus, mutations in RBL2/p130 may result in a constitutive cell cycle progression without the presence of any G0 phase, a hallmark of BL.

Applying integrative structural and functional genomics, three independent research groups very recently identified frequent inactivating mutations in *ID3*, an inhibitor of TCF3/ E2A in 34% to 68% of BL (168–170). In one of these studies

activating mutations of *TCF3* itself were also identified (170), albeit at a lower frequency than *ID3* mutations. The highest frequency of *ID3* mutations was found in sporadic BL. Interestingly, TCF3 enhances BCR signaling and in consequence B-cell survival via PI3K but also proliferation via CCND3, the latter gene itself being a target of activating mutations in some BL (169,170). These data strongly indicate that ID3 functions as a major tumor suppressor gene in BL. One group found evidence for AID-mediated mutagenesis of *ID3* (169). Apart from the possible clinical and therapeutical implications for new drugs that could target these pathways, the various groups also gave evidence that these mutations in *ID3* (and *TCF3*) are tumor specific and do occur much less frequently in DLBCL, including cases that carry MYC-IGH breakpoints. However, while the mutations may be promising markers for classification, it should be noted that ID3 protein expression is not, since the level is high in many BL, except for the cases with homozygous deletion/mutation (169,171).

Mutations in *MYC* in Burkitt Lymphoma

Between 1988 and 1995 several investigators identified frequent mutations within the *MYC* gene involved in the chromosomal translocation (115,172–176). These mutations cluster in the first two exons and the first intron, both in the translocated and actively transcribed as well as in the nontranslocated allele (see also Fig. 24.11). As explained above, MYC is one of the genes that is most susceptible to AID-mediated SHM in B-cell lymphomas. Mutations preferentially occur in a 2-kb region from the promoter sites and the so-called RGYW nucleotide sequence motifs, and almost completely overlap with the position of the t(8;14) MYC breakpoints as seen in sporadic BLs (133). These mutations may increase MYC stability and transforming activity or affect regulatory proteins that bind to MYC.

Interestingly, the already mentioned protein RBL1/p107 interacts with specific phosphorylation sites of MYC and is involved in a negative feedback of MYC itself. Mutations of a specific phosphorylation site to which RBL1/p107 binds therefore inhibit negative feedback and augment MYC activity (177,178). More recently, another consequence of these mutations was identified (179), because specific MYC mutations also inhibit the BH3 protein BIM, an antagonist of BCL2, thereby protecting the tumor cells against apoptosis. The exact mechanism is still unknown, one hypothesis being that this effect on BIM is mediated by p21. Thus, an intriguing model emerges (Fig. 24.12) where mutations in either the p53 pathway or the BIM pathway counteract MYC-induced apoptosis in BL, stabilizing the rapidly expanding tumor. This is supported by the analysis of a series of 31 human BL, in which Hemann et al. (179) found almost mutual mutations in p53 or MYC in the majority of BL cases. Notably, p53 mutations or MYC mutations with associated deregulation of BIM apparently do not lead to strong overexpression of bcl2 protein, since almost all BLs are bcl2 protein negative or only very weakly positive as assessed by immunohistochemistry (Figs. 24.7 and 24.12).

Somatic Hypermutations and Class Switching of the Immunoglobulin Genes

All studies so far show that BL carry a moderate number of SHMs within the immunoglobulin genes. In spite of the relatively high expression of AID in BL, most studies show no evidence for ongoing mutations (180,181). Interestingly, Bellan et al. (137) found significant differences in the load of SHM between eBL and AIDS-related BL (high) and sporadic BL (low) with an even stronger correlation with the EBV status of the lymphomas. Moreover, half of the cases of eBL and AIDS-related BL had evidence of antigen selection whereas sBL did not. One explanation for the apparent lack of detectable ongoing SHM in BL may be that—in contrast with, for example, follicular lymphoma with a very slow evolution over many years and readily detectable ongoing SHM—BL cells have a very short generation time, not allowing the tumor to diversify in a period comparable to that in follicular lymphoma. Interestingly, whereas the MYC and IG breaks in BL are now generally considered to be mediated by AID, all BL cases express IgM instead of IgG or IgA. Detailed analysis of the Ig genes has shown that the functional IGH allele does not undergo any class switch event and that the IGH allele involved in the translocation often shows aberrant,

incomplete recombinations not involving both Sμ and more downstream switch regions, suggesting that these translocations are induced in relatively early GC B cells, unlike the IGH translocations seen in plasmacytomas (182,183). An explanation for this absence of normal class switch recombination may be that BL lymphoma cells proliferate entirely independently of T cells or other immune cells and are therefore not exposed to significant level of the cytokines that are necessary to stimulate B cells to class switch.

Gene Expression and Micro RNA Expression Analysis of Burkitt Lymphoma

Three studies focused on gene expression analysis of BL (43,70,184). Interestingly, although all three studies completely differed in the way the profiles were built and the cases were analyzed, all studies showed a very distinct profile for BLs, called the "molecular BL" or "mBL profile." In general, this profile reflects the origin from GC B cells and the very high expression of MYC with its many target genes such as TERT, HDAC2, and DLEU1. Major differences were also found between BL and DLBCL, also when analyzing the separate categories of GC-type DLBCL and activated B-cell type DLBCL. Apart from MYC-associated genes, NFκB and associated genes such as CD40, CD44, IRF4, BCLA1, and PIM1 are strongly down-regulated in BL, as well as are most HLA class I genes (HLA-A, -B, -C, etc.). Subtle but significant differences between endemic, HIV-associated and sporadic BL were found in the study by Piccaluga et al. Interestingly, these differences seemed to be independent of the presence of EBV, again underlying that while EBV might have a major role in the early initiation of BL, the latency type I infection has only minor effects on the behavior of the mature tumor cells ("hit and run" theory).

More recent work also focused on miRNA expression patterns of BL. Comparing BL cells with normal B-cell subsets and various types of lymphomas, it appeared that the pattern in BL was dominated by MYC overexpression. Under experimental conditions MYC represses many miRNAs, including miR-34a, miR-150, miR-155, and let-7a, and indeed a large number of the miRNAs were also down-regulated in BL (148). Relatively few miRNAs are induced by MYC, including almost all members of the miRNA 17-92 family. These miRNAs were also

FIGURE 24.12. Possible mechanisms of inhibition of apoptosis in BL. A: Overexpression of MYC leads to enhanced proliferation and cell metabolism, but also to enhanced apoptosis. **B:** Apoptosis may be counteracted by several mechanisms, one being that mutations within MYC may affect p21/BIM and thereby increase BCL2 function. **C:** The other mechanism is via p53 mutation, as observed in more than half of the BL cell lines and one-third of the native samples.

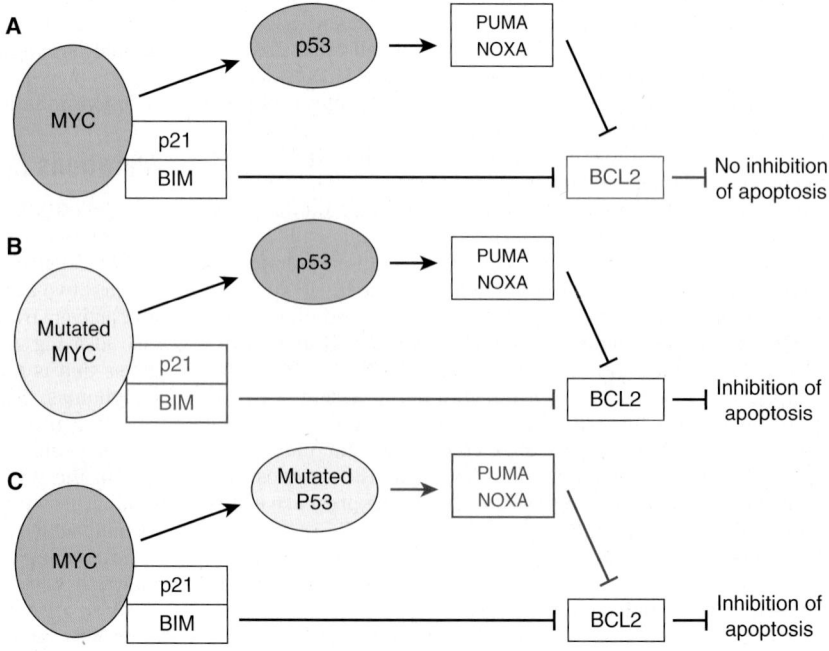

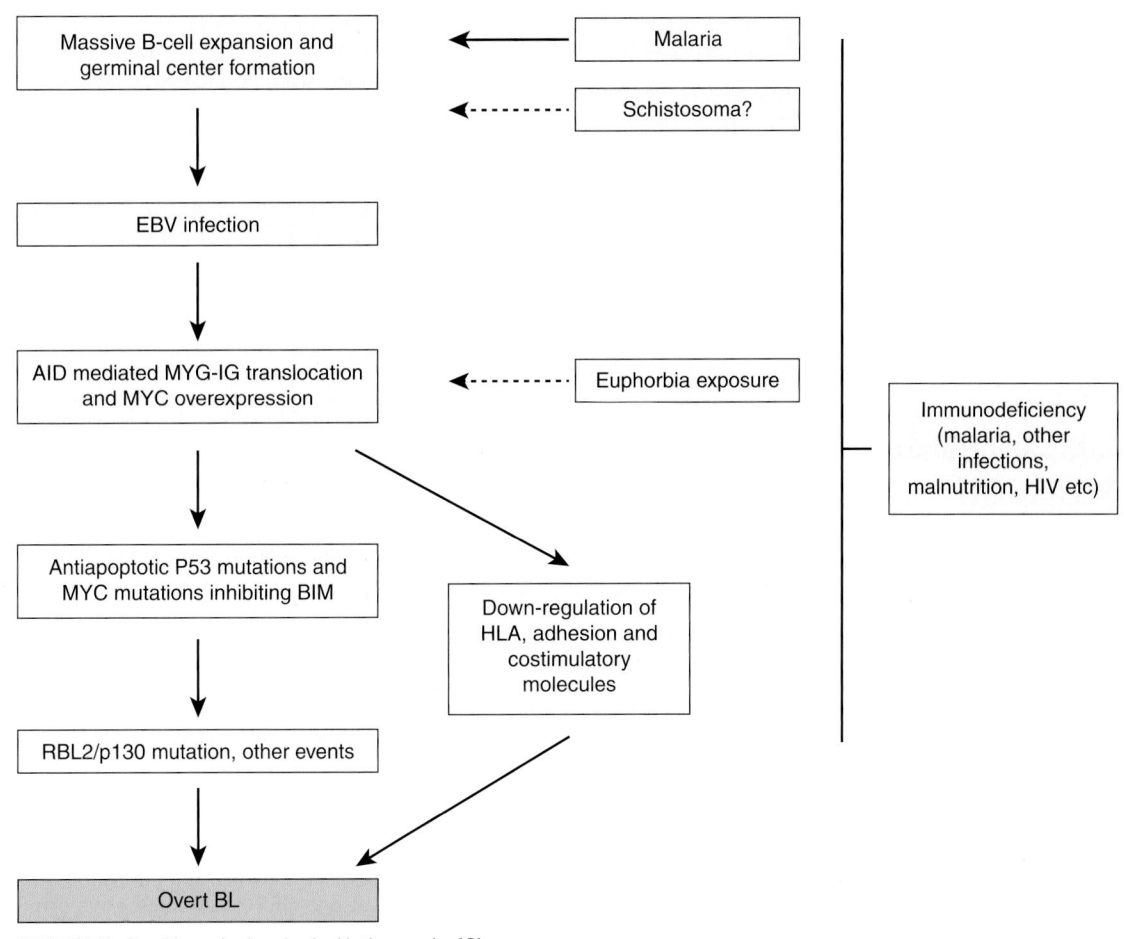

FIGURE 24.13. Possible mechanisms involved in the genesis of BL.

overexpressed in BL; however, this pattern was less consistent if comparing BL with other aggressive B-cell lymphomas, probably because of gain or amplification of the 13q31.3 chromosomal region in other lymphomas as well. Again, neither HIV nor EBV infection had a significant impact on the miRNA profile (185,186). In particular, the restriction to a latency 1 infection pattern might prevent a significant modification of the miRNA profile.

In summary, BL seems to arise from a limited but still not entirely clarified number of intrinsic and environmental factors, which likely differ between endemic and sporadic cases. A very simplified scheme is shown in Figure 24.12.

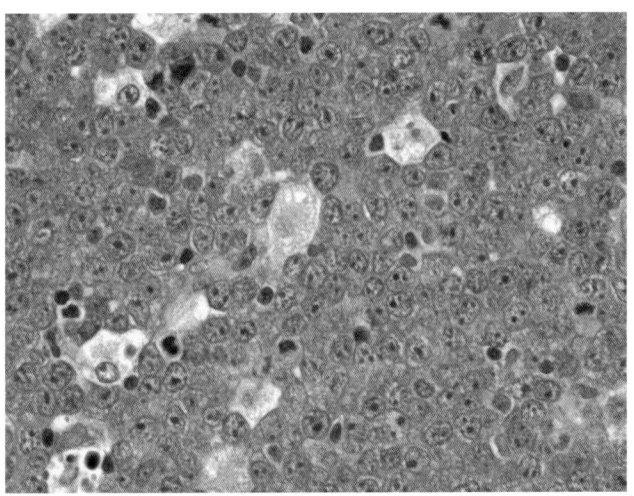

FIGURE 24.14. Morphology of double-hit lymphoma. Male patient, 78 years, cervical lymph node. Double-hit lymphoma with MYC and BCL6 breakpoint. This figure shows hematoxylin-and-eosin staining. Tumor cells are almost indistinguishable from atypical BL, however, with prominent nucleoli.

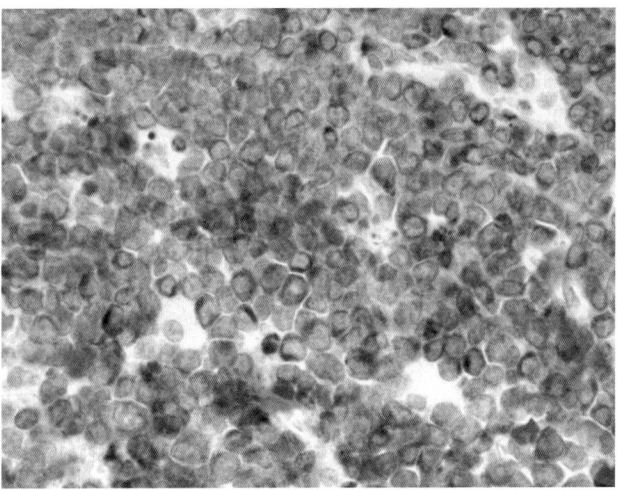

FIGURE 24.15. BCL2 immunohistochemistry of a double-hit lymphoma. This is the same case as shown in Figure 24.14. Note the very strong bcl2 staining, which is incompatible with true BL.

THE POSTULATED NORMAL COUNTERPART OF BURKITT LYMPHOMA

Based on the morphology of cells mimicking small centroblasts in the dark zone of normal GCs, the homogeneous phenotype of IgM+, CD10+, BCL6+, TCL1+, CD44−, and BCL2−, the SHM pattern with lack of normal class switching, AID expression, as well as the gene expression pattern (except for the MYC expression and the many downstream targets in BL, not seen in normal cells), it is generally accepted that the normal counterpart of BL cells are (early) GC B cells.

CLINICAL COURSE AND PROGNOSTIC ASSESSMENT

The natural clinical course of BL patients has been described at the moment of discovery of the disease for endemic cases. The descriptions showed a rapidly fatal course, which can be explained by the extremely rapid growth, with a tumor doubling time that can approach 1 day. Apart from local tumor growth leading to complications such as obstruction or invagination, spread in the body with the formation of ascitic and pleural effusions as well as CNS involvement is common. Ultimately, with large tumors, hyperuricemia and lactic acidemia may follow, and these are one of the major causes of death after therapy as well. Another complication is renal failure caused by ureteric compression or diffuse renal involvement. The prognosis depends primarily on the extent of tumor at the start of chemotherapy (and the complications thereof) rather than on the efficacy of the therapy itself, because almost all tumors respond very well to the initial therapy. Based on clinical parameters a risk score can be assessed, with involvement of the bone marrow and the CNS (stage IV disease in the St. Jude's system) carrying a worse prognosis. However, with modern high-intensity and short-duration polychemotherapy CNS localization is a relative risk factor, even in adult patients. This situation is therefore different from patients with DLBCL and CNS localization.

TREATMENT AND SURVIVAL

Prompt diagnosis, staging, and appropriate treatment are essential in BL because of the very short doubling time of the tumor. Surgery may be needed initially for diagnosis and to treat urgent complications such as gastrointestinal bleeding, invagination, or (less frequently) perforation of the bowel. Patients in whom all abdominal tumor has been resected (stage II in the St. Jude's staging system) have an excellent prognosis even if low-intensity chemotherapy regimens are used. It is likely that the good prognosis in these cases is related to the low tumor burden, rather than to the completeness of the surgical resection.

Effective combination chemotherapy regimens in pediatric patients of Western countries consist of a risk-dependent number of components that follow each other in a relatively short time. For instance, in the LMB89 study (57,187,188) patients with an intermediate risk (no resected tumor but also no CNS involvement and <70% blasts in the bone marrow) are first treated with low doses of vincristine, cyclophosphamide, and prednisone (COP) to induce tumor reduction without the generation of tumor lysis. After 1 week this is followed by induction therapy consisting of two courses of a combination of high-dose cyclophosphamide, methotrexate (MTX), vincristine,

doxorubicin, and prednisone (COPADM). This is followed by a short consolidation of cytarabine (Ara-C) and one cycle of maintenance therapy. CNS prophylaxis comprises high-dose MTX and intrathecal MTX plus Ara-C. In patients with CNS localization or >70% bone marrow blasts more chemotherapy cycles are given. In patients with resected tumor masses, the first week of preinduction therapy can be omitted. In consequence, patients with stage I or II disease had a 6-year EFS of 100%, with stage III disease of 92%, and with stage IV disease or leukemic BL of almost 88%. Comparable risk-dependent schemes with excellent outcome results are used in other countries (189,190).

In the past, adult patients with sporadic BL were treated with chemotherapy regimens directed against other mature B-cell lymphomas, like CHOP, or against precursor B-cell lymphoblastic leukemia, but the outcome of these cases was poor as compared with the results in pediatric BL patients. It is now well understood that BL patients need a different treatment, even if they present with a leukemic disease (26,191). Indeed, in 1996 Magrath et al. reported a dramatic improvement in survival of adult patients treated with short-duration and high-intensity protocols (26,192). Subsequently, several studies were initiated in adult patients; however, many studies failed because the inclusion criteria were not strict enough and many lymphomas other than BL were likely included. A cytogenetic reanalysis of all published karyotypes of 538 "Burkitt lymphomas" published before September 2007 showed that at least 25% of the lymphomas published as BL in patients over 60 years actually were MYC/BCL2 double-hit lymphomas (106), a bias that may have significantly influenced outcome results. Indeed, in a recent reanalysis of the effect of age on outcome, a significant difference was shown between studies published before and after 2000. In fact, after 2000 no significant age effect was noted anymore (193,194). This is likely due to both better classification and improved therapeutical options for these patients. Of note, this is likely not caused by addition of rituximab to the current chemotherapy regimens.

Studies in Africa on children with endemic BL are more difficult to evaluate, partially due to the limited facilities and drugs available, in particular leading to more toxic deaths if high-intensity protocols are used (195). Therefore, highly modified protocols have been introduced, up to the use of only cyclophosphamide. Using such a monotherapy in patients with stage I to III disease, a modest survival rate of approximately 50% still can be achieved (196). However, it should be realized that many survival data are uncertain, also because of the fact that many patients are lost to follow-up after some time.

In AIDS-related BL, the initial treatment results were extremely poor, mainly due to the dose reductions that were used. However, with the introduction of HAART therapy and the use of some high-intensity polychemotherapy protocols, major improvements in survival have been achieved (197).

DIFFERENTIAL DIAGNOSIS OF BURKITT LYMPHOMA

In hematoxylin and eosin-stained sections, BL should be distinguished from a variety of tumors including some nonhematologic malignancies, acute myeloid leukemia/myeloblastic sarcoma, and lymphoblastic lymphoma/acute lymphoblastic leukemia. Also, some blastic cases of mantle cell lymphoma and even transformed myelomas may mimic BL. This can all be resolved relatively simply with a small battery of antibodies applied on paraffin tissue sections. When a cell suspension is available, the distinction can be very easily made as well. As discussed before, each BL should be CD20+, CD10+, BCL6+, sIgM⁺, and MIB1/KI67 approximating 100%, whereas BCL2 should be negative or only weakly positive. All myeloid markers as well as markers for precursor B cells such as TdT and CD34 should be negative.

More challenging is the differential diagnosis from a small subset of mature B-cell lymphomas in adult patients. Approximately 10% of all DLBCL have a growth pattern that mimics BL, that is, the presence of sheets of relatively monomorphic and cohesive cells with few intermingling T cells and the presence of starry sky macrophages (although often less impressive than in some BL). The lymphoma cells have larger nuclei than classical BL cells and starry sky macrophages. The chromatin is often more condensed along the nuclear membrane than in BL. The cytoplasm may be basophilic, but this is often not as dark as in BL. This can be best appreciated in high-quality Giemsa stainings or Giemsa-stained fine needle aspirations or cytologic imprints. In most cases the distinction between DLBCL and BL is readily made, since the phenotype may be deviant: for instance, absence of CD10 expression, strong BCL2 expression, or a MIB1/Ki67 proliferation index below 90% all indicate that the lymphoma should not be classified as BL. These mimickers of BL were previously often diagnosed as "Burkitt-like lymphoma," "aggressive B-cell lymphoma NOS," or "gray-zone lymphoma" (198), and according to the 2008 version of the WHO classification often fall into the provisional category of "B-cell lymphoma unclassifiable, with features intermediate between DLBCL and BL." Thirty to fifty percent of such cases harbor a MYC breakpoint, and in approximately half of the cases with a MYC breakpoint no t(18;14), t(2;8), or t(8;22) but other translocations such as t(3;8)(q27;q24) are found. In many of these cases the karyotype is much more complex than in regular BL. Finally GEP shows considerable differences with BL (70).

An alternative, genetic, approach to identify lymphomas that mimic BL is by looking at the so-called double-hit lymphomas (32,198). These lymphomas share an 8q24 breakpoint involving MYC (this breakpoint is obligatory) with an 18q21 breakpoint involving BCL2, a 3q27 breakpoint involving BCL6 or any other recurrent breakpoint/translocation that could be considered as a primary lymphomagenic event. In some cases more than two breakpoints (for instance MYC, BCL2, and BCL6) can be detected in a single lymphoma case. Again, in roughly two-thirds of the cases MYC is involved in regular t(18;14), t(2;8), or t(8;22), as observed in BL, but in the remaining cases MYC is not juxtaposed to any of the immunoglobulin genes. The 18q21 breakpoint is almost always part of t(14;18)(q21;q32) as seen in follicular lymphoma. Like typical DLBCL, BCL6 at the 3q27 breakpoint may have different partners. In MYC/BCL2 double-hit lymphomas, the t(14;18)(q21;q32) is likely a primary event followed by the MYC breakpoint at 8q24, the latter therefore representing a secondary transformation event. Indeed, a considerable part of the double-hit lymphoma cases may have a history of follicular lymphoma. In these cases, the 8q24 break may affect the second IGH allele, a IG light chain allele, or the IGH allele that is already involved in the t(14;18) translocation, generating a t(8;14;18) that can be readily detected by FISH analysis but less easily by conventional cytogenetics (199).

The exact frequency of double-hit lymphomas is not known, because classical karyotyping or FISH analysis is not regularly performed in all patients, and single-center studies, in particular from tertiary centers, may show a considerable referral bias. This is likely also true for cases that have been submitted for karyotype analysis (more cases with blood and/or bone marrow involvement) and thus have been published and/or included in the Mitelman database (198).

In the 2008 WHO classification, these lymphomas were separated from regular BL and DLBCL and also included in the provisional category of "B-cell lymphoma unclassifiable, with features intermediate between DLBCL and Burkitt lymphoma."

Table 24.2	IMMUNOHISTOCHEMICAL MARKERS FOR FORMALIN-FIXED MATERIALS TO DIFFERENTIATE BL FROM ITS MIMICKERS			
	BL	DLBCL	DLBCL[a] with MYC/8q24 Break	Double-Hit Lymphoma[b]
CD20	++	++	++	Variable
CD10	+	40% + (GCB type)	+	Most +
Bcl6	+	50%–80% +	+	Most +
Bcl2	−/weak +	50%–60% +	Most +	Most +
MUM1/IRF4	50% weak +	50%–70% + (non GCB type)	−	Most −
CD38	+	Almost all −	+ (2 cases)	Unknown
CD44	−	65% +	− (2 cases)	Unknown
TCL1	+	<50% +	+ (2 cases)	Unknown
Cyclin H	−	Most +	Unknown	Unknown
Ki67/MIB1	95%–100%	Highly variable	Most 50%–100%	Most 50%–100%

[a]Plasmablastic lymphoma excluded.
[b]Cases (with features) of TdT⁺ precursor B-cell lymphoblastic lymphoma excluded.
BL, Burkitt's lymphoma; DLBCL, diffuse large B-cell lymphoma.

In fact, these double-hit lymphomas seem to constitute the major component of this category.

After the 2008 WHO classification many publications addressed these double-hit lymphomas, in particular lymphomas with a MYC and BCL2 breakpoint, and concluded that most patients have a very aggressive disease course (29,198,200–216). The problem is that the microscopic spectrum of these double-hit lymphomas is wide, ranging from follicular lymphoma up to cases that mimic BL. The histologic differences with regular BL may be subtle and the distinction may be hampered by (histologic) artifacts. Immunophenotypically, many of these cases have expression of CD10 and BCL6, which is similar to BL cases. In one single-institute study of 52 patients with a MYC/BCL2 double-hit lymphoma (216) 98% expressed CD10 and 96% BCL6, whereas the MIB1/Ki67 index ranged from 40% to 99%. In this study, an IG partner of MYC was found in 86% of all cases; however, the karyotype was complex in 100% of the cases. Histologically, 36% of the cases were diagnosed as DLBCL and 56% as a "gray-zone" lymphoma. Clinically, 81% of the patients had *de novo* disease and 74% had stage II to IV disease, with CNS involvement in 23%. This patient group had a poor course of the disease with a 1-year survival of 58%, despite aggressive polychemotherapy in 49/52 patients. Outcome was independent of the morphology of the tumor, although other studies suggest a superior outcome for double-hit lymphomas with DLBCL morphology (203).

Of note, newer antibodies such as against CD44 and TCL1 that have been used to distinguish BL from DLBCL have not systematically been tested on double-hit lymphomas (Table 24.2). Nonetheless, all the available data show that these lymphomas should be distinguished from typical BL.

SUMMARY AND CONCLUSIONS

BL is a distinct clinicobiologic entity that arises in three different epidemiologic (endemic/African, sporadic/non-African, and immunodeficiency/AIDS-related) settings. In spite of these different settings the disorder is remarkably homogeneous with respect to clinical presentation, behavior and response to chemotherapy, histology and immunophenotype, and gene expression as well as molecular genetics. At the genetic level it is characterized by the presence of MYC/IG breakpoints in almost all cases, a simple karyotype, and the absence of additional chromosomal breakpoints. BL mainly presents in children but can occur in adolescents and elderly patients as well; thus, age itself should never be used as an argument to reject the diagnosis. Recent clinical data suggest that like pediatric lymphomas, high-intensity, short-duration polychemotherapy schemes have a very favorable outcome, even in adult patients. Strict criteria should be used to distinguish BL from its mimickers, including the so-called double-hit lymphomas.

References

1. Burkitt D. A sarcoma involving the jaws in African children. *Br J Surg* 1958;46(197):218–223.
2. Saave JJ. Thesis. University of Edinburgh, 1958.
3. O'Conor GT, Davies JN. Malignant tumors in African children. With special reference to malignant lymphoma. *J Pediatr* 1960;56:526–535.
4. Burkitt D. Determining the climatic limitations of a children's cancer common in Africa. *Br Med J* 1962;2(5311):1019–1023.
5. Kafuko GW, Burkitt DP. Burkitt's lymphoma and malaria. *Int J Cancer* 1970; 6(1):1–9.
6. Epstein MA, Achong BG, Barr YM. Virus particles in cultured lymphoblasts from Burkitt's lymphoma. *Lancet* 1964;1(7335):702–703.
7. Burkitt DP. The discovery of Burkitt's lymphoma. *Cancer* 1983;51(10):1777–1786.
8. Booth K, Burkitt DP, Bassett DJ, et al. Burkitt lymphoma in Papua, New Guinea. *Br J Cancer* 1967;21(4):657–664.
9. Burkitt DP. Epidemiology of Burkitt's lymphoma. *Proc R Soc Med* 1971;64(9):909–910.
10. Arseneau JC, Canellos GP, Banks PM, et al. American Burkitt's lymphoma: a clinicopathologic study of 30 cases. I. Clinical factors relating to prolonged survival. *Am J Med* 1975;58(3):314–321.
11. Levine PH, Connelly RR, Berard CW, et al. The American Burkitt Lymphoma Registry: a progress report. *Ann Intern Med* 1975;83(1):31–36.
12. Radin DR, Rosenstein H, Boswell WD, et al. Burkitt lymphoma in acquired immune deficiency syndrome. *J Comput Assist Tomogr* 1984;8(1):173–174.
13. Chaganti RS, Jhanwar SC, Koziner B, et al. Specific translocations characterize Burkitt's-like lymphoma of homosexual men with the acquired immunodeficiency syndrome. *Blood* 1983;61(6):1265–1268.
14. Magrath I, Erikson J, Whang-Peng J, et al. Synthesis of kappa light chains by cell lines containing an 8;22 chromosomal translocation derived from a male homosexual with Burkitt's lymphoma. *Science* 1983;222(4628):1094–1098.
15. Whang-Peng J, Lee EC, Sieverts H, et al. Burkitt's lymphoma in AIDS: cytogenetic study. *Blood* 1984;63(4):818–822.
16. Manolov G, Manolova Y. Marker band in one chromosome 14 from Burkitt lymphoma. *Nature* 1972;237:33–34.
17. Miyoshi I, Hiraki S, Kimura I, et al. 2/8 translocation in a Japanese Burkitt's lymphoma. *Experientia* 1979;35(6):742–743.
18. Malcolm S, Barton P, Murphy C, et al. Localization of human immunoglobulin kappa light chain variable region genes to the short arm of chromosome 2 by in situ hybridization. *Proc Natl Acad Sci U S A* 1982;79(16):4957–4961.
19. Zech L, Haglund U, Nilsson K, et al. Characteristic chromosomal abnormalities in biopsies and lymphoid cell lines from patients with Burkitt and non-Burkitt lymphomas. *Int J Cancer* 1976;17:47.
20. Erikson J, Finan J, Nowell PC, et al. Translocation of immunoglobulin VH genes in Burkitt lymphoma. *Proc Natl Acad Sci U S A* 1982;79(18):5611–5615.
21. Berger R, Bernheim A, Weh HJ, et al. A new translocation in Burkitt's tumor cells. *Hum Genet* 1979;53(1):111–112.
22. De la Chapelle A, Lenoir G, Boue J, et al. Lambda Ig constant region genes are translocated to chromosome 8 in Burkitt's lymphoma with t(8;22). *Nucleic Acids Res* 1983;11(4):1133–1142.
23. Dalla-Favera R, Bregni M, Erikson J, et al. Human c-myc onc gene is located on the region of chromosome 8 that is translocated in Burkitt lymphoma cells. *Proc Natl Acad Sci U S A* 1982;79(24):7824–7827.
24. Taub R, Kirsch I, Morton C, et al. Translocation of the c-myc gene into the immunoglobulin heavy chain locus in human Burkitt lymphoma and murine plasmacytoma cells. *Proc Natl Acad Sci U S A* 1982;79(24):7837–7841.
25. Hecht JL, Aster JC. Molecular biology of Burkitt's lymphoma. *J Clin Oncol* 2000;18(21):3707–3721.
26. Blum KA, Lozanski G, Byrd JC. Adult Burkitt leukemia and lymphoma. *Blood* 2004;104(10):3009–3020.
27. Bornkamm GW. Epstein-Barr virus and the pathogenesis of Burkitt's lymphoma: more questions than answers. *Int J Cancer* 2009;124(8):1745–1755.
28. Allday MJ. How does Epstein-Barr virus (EBV) complement the activation of Myc in the pathogenesis of Burkitt's lymphoma? *Semin Cancer Biol* 2009;19(6):366–376.
29. Slack GW, Gascoyne RD. MYC and aggressive B-cell lymphomas. *Adv Anat Pathol* 2011;18(3):219–228.
30. Wolf J, Pawlita M, Bullerdiek J, et al. Suppression of the malignant phenotype in somatic cell hybrids between Burkitt's lymphoma cells and Epstein-Barr virus-immortalized lymphoblastoid cells despite deregulated c-*myc* expression. *Cancer Res* 1990;50:3095–3100.
31. Hotchin NA, Allday MJ, Crawford DH. Deregulated c-myc expression in Epstein-Barr-virus-immortalized B-cells induces altered growth properties and surface phenotype but not tumorigenicity. *Int J Cancer* 1990;45(3):566–571.
32. Swerdlow SH, Campo E, Harris NL, et al. *WHO classification of tumours of haematopoietic and lymphoid tissues,* 4th ed. Lyon: International Agency for Research on Cancer, 2008.
33. Magrath IT. Non-Hodgkin's lymphomas: epidemiology and treatment. *Ann N Y Acad Sci* 1997;824:91–106.
34. Boerma EG, van Imhoff GW, Appel IM, et al. Gender and age-related differences in Burkitt lymphoma—epidemiological and clinical data from The Netherlands. *Eur J Cancer* 2004;40(18):2781–2787.
35. Levine AM, Pavlova Z, Pockros AW, et al. Small noncleaved follicular center cell (Fcc) lymphoma—Burkitt and non-Burkitt variants in the United-States.1. Clinical-features. *Cancer* 1983;52(6):1073–1079.
36. Emmanuel B, Kawira E, Ogwang MD, et al. African Burkitt lymphoma: age-specific risk and correlations with malaria biomarkers. *Am J Trop Med Hyg* 2011;84(3):397–401.
37. Mbulaiteye SM, Anderson WF, Bhatia K, et al. Trimodal age-specific incidence patterns for Burkitt lymphoma in the United States, 1973–2005. *Int J Cancer* 2010;126(7):1732–1739.
38. Orem J, Maganda A, Mbidde EK, et al. Clinical characteristics and outcome of children with Burkitt lymphoma in Uganda according to HIV infection. *Pediatr Blood Cancer* 2009;52(4):455–458.
39. Orem J, Mbidde EK, Lambert B, et al. Burkitt's lymphoma in Africa, a review of the epidemiology and etiology. *Afr Health Sci* 2007;7(3):166–175.
40. Olweny CL, Atine I, Kaddu-Mukasa A, et al. Epstein-Barr virus genome studies in Burkitt's and non-Burkitt's lymphomas in Uganda. *J Natl Canc Inst* 1977;58(5):1191–1196.
41. Rochford R, Cannon MJ, Moormann AM. Endemic Burkitt's lymphoma: a polymicrobial disease? *Nat Rev Microbiol* 2005;3(2):182–187.
42. Rainey JJ, Mwanda WO, Wairiumu P, et al. Spatial distribution of Burkitt's lymphoma in Kenya and association with malaria risk. *Trop Med Int Health* 2007;12(8):936–943.
43. Dave SS, Fu K, Wright GW, et al. Molecular diagnosis of Burkitt's lymphoma. *N Engl J Med* 2006;354(23):2431–2442.
44. Osato T, Mizuno F, Imai S, et al. African Burkitt's lymphoma and an Epstein-Barr virus-enhancing plant *Euphorbia tirucalli. Lancet* 1987;1(8544):1257–1258.
45. Mizuno F, Osato T, Imai S, et al. Epstein-Barr virus-enhancing plant promoters in east Africa. *AIDS Res* 1986;2(Suppl 1):S151–S155.
46. MacNeil A, Sumba OP, Lutzke ML, et al. Activation of the Epstein-Barr virus lytic cycle by the latex of the plant *Euphorbia tirucalli. Br J Cancer* 2003;88(10):1566–1569.
47. Imai S, Sugiura M, Mizuno F, et al. African Burkitt's lymphoma: a plant, *Euphorbia tirucalli*, reduces Epstein-Barr virus-specific cellular immunity. *Anticancer Res* 1994;14(3A):933–936.
48. Aya T, Kinoshita T, Imai S, et al. Chromosome translocation and c-MYC activation by Epstein-Barr virus and *Euphorbia tirucalli* in B lymphocytes. *Lancet* 1991;337:1190.
49. Mbulaiteye SM, Biggar RJ, Bhatia K, et al. Sporadic childhood Burkitt lymphoma incidence in the United States during 1992–2005. *Pediatr Blood Cancer* 2009;53(3):366–370.
50. Magrath I. The pathogenesis of Burkitt's lymphoma. *Adv Cancer Res* 1990;55:134–270.
51. Ziegler JL, Drew WL, Miner RC, et al. Outbreak of Burkitt's-like lymphoma in homosexual men. *Lancet* 1982;2(8299):631–633.
52. Biggar RJ, Frisch M, Goedert JJ. Risk of cancer in children with AIDS. AIDS-Cancer Match Registry Study Group. *JAMA* 2000;284(2):205–209.
53. Patel P, Hanson DL, Sullivan PS, et al. Incidence of types of cancer among HIV-infected persons compared with the general population in the United States, 1992–2003. *Ann Intern Med* 2008;148(10):728–736.
54. Picarsic J, Jaffe R, Mazariegos G, et al. Post-transplant Burkitt lymphoma is a more aggressive and distinct form of post-transplant lymphoproliferative disorder. *Cancer* 2011;117(19):4540–4550.
55. Mwanda WO, Orem J, Remick SC, et al. Clinical characteristics of Burkitt's lymphoma from three regions in Kenya. *East Afr Med J* 2005;82(9 Suppl):S135–S143.
56. Patte C, Auperin A, Michon J, et al. The Societe Francaise d'Oncologie Pediatrique LMB89 protocol: highly effective multiagent chemotherapy tailored to the tumor burden and initial response in 561 unselected children with B-cell lymphomas and L3 leukemia. *Blood* 2001;97(11):3370–3379.
57. Patte C, Auperin A, Gerrard M, et al. Results of the randomized international FAB/LMB96 trial for intermediate risk B-cell non-Hodgkin lymphoma in children and adolescents: it is possible to reduce treatment for the early responding patients. *Blood* 2007;109(7):2773–2780.
58. Ertem U, Duru F, Pamir A, et al. Burkitt's lymphoma in 63 Turkish children diagnosed over a 10 year period. *Pediatr Hematol Oncol* 1996;13(2):123–134.
59. Cavdar AO, Yavuz G, Babacan E, et al. Burkitt's lymphoma in Turkish children: clinical, viral [EBV] and molecular studies. *Leuk Lymphoma* 1994;14(3-4):323–330.
60. Sandlund JT, Fonseca T, Leimig T, et al. Predominance and characteristics of Burkitt lymphoma among children with non-Hodgkin lymphoma in northeastern Brazil. *Leukemia* 1997;11(5):743–746.
61. Cohen LF, Balow JE, Magrath IT, et al. Acute tumor lysis syndrome. A review of 37 patients with Burkitt's lymphoma. *Am J Med* 1980;68(4):486–491.
62. Murphy SB. Classification, staging and end results of treatment of childhood non-Hodgkin's lymphomas: dissimilarities from lymphomas in adults. *Semin Oncol* 1980;7(3):332–339.
63. Hollingsworth HC, Longo DL, Jaffe ES. Small noncleaved cell lymphoma associated with florid epithelioid granulomatous response. A clinicopathologic study of seven patients. *Am J Surg Pathol* 1993;17(1):51–59.
64. Haralambieva E, Rosati S, van Noesel C, et al. Florid granulomatous reaction in Epstein-Barr virus-positive nonendemic Burkitt lymphomas—report of four cases. *Am J Surg Pathol* 2004;28(3):379–383.
65. Schrager JA, Pittaluga S, Raffeld M, et al. Granulomatous reaction in Burkitt lymphoma: correlation with EBV positivity and clinical outcome. *Am J Surg Pathol* 2005;29(8):1115–1116.
66. Lones MA, Raphael M, Perkins SL, et al. Mature B-cell lymphoma in children and adolescents: International group pathologist consensus correlates with histology technical quality. *J Pediatr Hematol Oncol* 2006;28(9):568–574.
67. Wright DH. What is Burkitt's lymphoma? *J Pathol* 1997;182(2):125–127.
68. Grogan TM, Warnke RA, Kaplan HS. A comparative study of Burkitt's and non-Burkitt's "undifferentiated" malignant lymphoma: immunologic, cytochemical, ultrastructural, cytologic, histopathologic, clinical and cell culture features. *Cancer* 1982;49:1817–1828.
69. Harris NL, Jaffe ES, Stein H, et al. A revised European-American classification of lymphoid neoplasms: a proposal from the International Lymphoma Study Group. *Blood* 1994;84:1361–1392.
70. Hummel M, Bentink S, Berger H, et al. A biologic definition of Burkitt's lymphoma from transcriptional and genomic profiling. *N Engl J Med* 2006;354(23):2419–2430.
71. Haralambieva E, Schuuring E, Rosati S, et al. Interphase fluorescence in situ hybridization for detection of 8q24/MYC breakpoints on routine histologic sections: Validation in Burkitt lymphomas from three geographic regions. *Genes Chromosome Cancer* 2004;40(1):10–18.

72. Barth TF, Muller S, Pawlita M, et al. Homogeneous immunophenotype and paucity of secondary genomic aberrations are distinctive features of endemic but not of sporadic Burkitt's lymphoma and diffuse large B-cell lymphoma with MYC rearrangement. *J Pathol* 2004;203(4):940–945.
73. McClure RF, Remstein ED, Macon WR, et al. Adult B-cell lymphomas with burkitt-like morphology are phenotypically and genotypically heterogeneous with aggressive clinical behavior. *Am J Surg Pathol* 2005;29(12):1652–1660.
74. Rodig SJ, Vergilio JA, Shahsafaei A, et al. Characteristic expression patterns of TCL1, CD38, and CD44 identify aggressive lymphomas harboring a MYC translocation. *Am J Surg Pathol* 2008;32(1):113–122.
75. May PC, Foot N, Dunn R, et al. Detection of cryptic and variant IGH-MYC rearrangements in high-grade non-Hodgkin's lymphoma by fluorescence in situ hybridization: implications for cytogenetic testing. *Cancer Genet Cytogenet* 2010;198(1):71–75.
76. Foot NJ, Dunn RG, Geoghegan H, et al. Fluorescence in situ hybridisation analysis of formalin-fixed paraffin-embedded tissue sections in the diagnostic work-up of non-Burkitt high grade B-cell non-Hodgkin's lymphoma: a single centre's experience. *J Clin Pathol* 2011;64(9):802–808.
77. Naresh KN, Ibrahim HA, Lazzi S, et al. Diagnosis of Burkitt lymphoma using an algorithmic approach—applicable in both resource-poor and resource-rich countries. *Br J Haematol* 2011;154(6):770–776.
78. Gualco G, Queiroga EM, Weiss LM, et al. Frequent expression of multiple myeloma 1/interferon regulatory factor 4 in Burkitt lymphoma. *Hum Pathol* 2009;40(4):565–571.
79. Salaverria I, Philipp C, Oschlies I, et al. Translocations activating IRF4 identify a subtype of germinal center-derived B-cell lymphoma affecting predominantly children and young adults. *Blood* 2011;118(1):139–147.
80. Chan JK, Tsang WY, Ng CS, et al. A study of the association of Epstein-Barr virus with Burkitt's lymphoma occurring in a Chinese population. *Histopathol* 1995;26(3):239–245.
81. Gutierrez MI, Bhatia K, Barriga F, et al. Molecular epidemiology of Burkitt's lymphoma from South America: differences in breakpoint location and Epstein-Barr virus association from tumors in other world regions. *Blood* 1992;79(12):3261–3266.
82. Klumb CE, Hassan R, De Oliveira DE, et al. Geographic variation in Epstein-Barr virus-associated Burkitt's lymphoma in children from Brazil. *Int J Cancer* 2004;108(1):66–70.
83. Henle G, Henle W. Immunofluorescence in cells derived from Burkitt's lymphoma. *J Bacteriol* 1966;91(3):1248–1256.
84. Howe JG, Steitz JA. Localization of Epstein-Barr virus-encoded small RNAs by in situ hybridization. *Proc Natl Acad Sci U S A* 1986;83(23):9006–9010.
85. Rowe M, Rowe DT, Gregory CD, et al. Differences in B cell growth phenotype reflect novel patterns of Epstein-Barr virus latent gene expression in Burkitt's lymphoma cells. *EMBO J* 1987;6(9):2743–2751.
86. Sample C, Kieff E. Molecular basis for Epstein-Barr virus induced pathogenesis and disease. *Springer Semin Immunopathol* 1991;13(2):133–146.
87. Young LS, Rickinson AB. Epstein-Barr virus: 40 years on. *Nat Rev Cancer* 2004;4(10):757–768.
88. Gregory CD, Murray RJ, Edwards CF, et al. Downregulation of cell adhesion molecules LFA-3 and ICAM-1 in Epstein-Barr virus-positive Burkitt's lymphoma underlies tumor cell escape from virus-specific T cell surveillance. *J Exp Med* 1988;167(6):1811–1824.
89. Kelly G, Bell A, Rickinson A. Epstein-Barr virus-associated Burkitt lymphomagenesis selects for downregulation of the nuclear antigen EBNA2. *Nat Med* 2002;8(10):1098–1104.
90. Levitskaya J, Coram M, Levitsky V, et al. Inhibition of antigen processing by the internal repeat region of the Epstein-Barr virus nuclear antigen-1. *Nature* 1995;375:685–688.
91. Gruhne B, Sompallae R, Marescotti D, et al. The Epstein-Barr virus nuclear antigen-1 promotes genomic instability via induction of reactive oxygen species. *Proc Natl Acad Sci U S A* 2009;106(7):2313–2318.
92. Kuhn-Hallek I, Sage DR, Stein L, et al. Expression of recombination activating genes (RAG-1 and RAG-2) in Epstein-Barr virus-bearing B cells. *Blood* 1995;85(5):1289–1299.
93. Kitagawa N, Goto M, Kurozumi K, et al. Epstein-Barr virus-encoded poly(A)(-) RNA supports Burkitt's lymphoma growth through interleukin-10 induction. *EMBO J* 2000;19(24):6742–6750.
94. Iwakiri D, Takada K. Role of EBERs in the pathogenesis of EBV infection. *Adv Cancer Res* 2010;107:119–136.
95. Walz N, Christalla T, Tessmer U, et al. A global analysis of evolutionary conservation among known and predicted gammaherpesvirus microRNAs. *J Virol* 2010;84(2):716–728.
96. Klapproth K, Wirth T. Advances in the understanding of MYC-induced lymphomagenesis. *Br J Haematol* 2010;149(4):484–497.
97. Jox A, Rohen C, Belge G, et al. Integration of Epstein-Barr virus in Burkitt's lymphoma cells leads to a region of enhanced chromosome instability. *Ann Oncol* 1997;8 Suppl 2:131–135.
98. Morrow RH, Jr. Epidemiological evidence for the role of falciparum malaria in the pathogenesis of Burkitt's lymphoma. *IARC Sci Publ* 1985;(60):177–186.
99. Donati D, Zhang LP, Chene A, et al. Identification of a polyclonal B-cell activator in *Plasmodium falciparum*. *Infect Immun* 2004;72(9):5412–5418.
100. Donati D, Mok B, Chene A, et al. Increased B cell survival and preferential activation of the memory compartment by a malaria polyclonal B cell activator. *J Immunol* 2006;177(5):3035–3044.
101. Moormann AM, Snider CJ, Chelimo K. The company malaria keeps: how co-infection with Epstein-Barr virus leads to endemic Burkitt lymphoma. *Curr Opin Infect Dis* 2011;24(5):435–441.
102. Njie R, Bell AI, Jia H, et al. The effects of acute malaria on Epstein-Barr virus (EBV) load and EBV-specific T cell immunity in Gambian children. *J Infect Dis* 2009;199(1):31–38.
103. Moormann AM, Chelimo K, Sumba PO, et al. Exposure to holoendemic malaria results in suppression of Epstein-Barr virus-specific T cell immunosurveillance in Kenyan children. *J Infect Dis* 2007;195(6):799–808.
104. Whittle HC, Brown J, Marsh K, et al. T-cell control of Epstein-Barr virus-infected B cells is lost during *P. falciparum* malaria. *Nature* 1984;312(5993):449–450.
105. Kornblau SM, Goodacre A, Cabanillas F. Chromosomal abnormalities in adult non-endemic Burkitt's lymphoma and leukemia: 22 new reports and a review of 148 cases from the literature. *Hematol Oncol* 1991;9:63–78.
106. Boerma EG, Siebert R, Kluin PM, et al. Translocations involving 8q24 in Burkitt lymphoma and other malignant lymphomas: a historical review of cytogenetics in the light of todays knowledge. *Leukemia* 2009;23(2):225–234.
107. Einerson RR, Law ME, Blair HE, et al. Novel FISH probes designed to detect IGK-MYC and IGL-MYC rearrangements in B-cell lineage malignancy identify a new breakpoint cluster region designated BVR2. *Leukemia* 2006;20(10):1790–1799.
108. Leucci E, Cocco M, Onnis A, et al. MYC translocation-negative classical Burkitt lymphoma cases: an alternative pathogenetic mechanism involving miRNA deregulation. *J Pathol* 2008;216(4):440–450.
109. Joos S, Haluska FG, Falk MH, et al. Mapping chromosomal breakpoints of Burkitt's t(8;14) translocations far upstream of c-*myc*. *Cancer Res* 1992;52:6547–6552.
110. Joos S, Falk MH, Lichter P, et al. Variable breakpoints in Burkitt lymphoma cells with chromosomal t(8;14) translocation separate c-myc and the IgH locus up to several hundred kb. *Hum Mol Genet* 1992;1(8):625–632.
111. Cario G, Stadt UZ, Reiter A, et al. Variant translocations in sporadic Burkitt's lymphoma detected in fresh tumour material: analysis of three cases. *Br J Haematol* 2000;110(3):537–546.
112. Zeidler R, Joos S, Delecluse H-J, et al. Breakpoints of Burkitt's lymphoma t(8;22) translocations map within a distance of 300 kb downstream of MYC. *Gen Chrom Canc* 1994;9:282–287.
113. Henglein B, Synovzik H, Groitl P, et al. Three breakpoints of variant t(2;8) translocations in Burkitt's lymphoma cells fall within a region 140 kilobases distal from c-*myc*. *Mol Cell Biol* 1989;9:2105–2113.
114. Shiramizu B, Barriga F, Neequaye J, et al. Patterns of chromosomal breakpoint locations in Burkitt's lymphoma: relevance to geography and Epstein-Barr virus association. *Blood* 1991;77:1516–1526.
115. Pelicci PG, Knowles DM2, Magrath I, et al. Chromosomal breakpoints and structural alterations of the c-myc locus differ in endemic and sporadic forms of Burkitt lymphoma. *Proc Natl Acad Sci U S A* 1986;83(9):2984–2988.
116. Neri A, Barriga F, Knowles DM, et al. Different regions of the immunoglobulin heavy-chain locus are involved in chromosomal translocations in distinct pathogenetic forms of Burkitt lymphomas. *Proc Natl Acad Sci U S A* 1988;85:2748–2752.
117. Goossens T, Klein U, Kuppers R. Frequent occurrence of deletions and duplications during somatic hypermutation: implications for oncogene translocations and heavy chain disease. *Proc Natl Acad Sci U S A* 1998;95(5):2463–2468.
118. Busch K, Keller T, Fuchs U, et al. Identification of two distinct MYC breakpoint clusters and their association with various IGH breakpoint regions in the t(8;14) translocations in sporadic Burkitt-lymphoma. *Leukemia* 2007;21(8):1739–1751.
119. Ramiro AR, Jankovic M, Callen E, et al. Role of genomic instability and p53 in AID-induced c-myc-Igh translocations. *Nature* 2006;440(7080):105–109.
120. Dorsett Y, Robbiani DF, Jankovic M, et al. A role for AID in chromosome translocations between c-myc and the IgH variable region. *J Exp Med* 2007;204(9):2225–2232.
121. Takizawa M, Tolarova H, Li Z, et al. AID expression levels determine the extent of cMyc oncogenic translocations and the incidence of B cell tumor development. *J Exp Med* 2008;205(9):1949–1957.
122. Robbiani DF, Bothmer A, Callen E, et al. AID is required for the chromosomal breaks in c-myc that lead to c-myc/IgH translocations. *Cell* 2008;135(6):1028–1038.
123. Pasqualucci L, Bhagat G, Jankovic M, et al. AID is required for germinal center-derived lymphomagenesis. *Nat Genet* 2008;40(1):108–112.
124. Robbiani DF, Bunting S, Feldhahn N, et al. AID produces DNA double-strand breaks in non-Ig genes and mature B cell lymphomas with reciprocal chromosome translocations. *Mol Cell* 2009;36(4):631–641.
125. Wang JH, Gostissa M, Yan CT, et al. Mechanisms promoting translocations in editing and switching peripheral B cells. *Nature* 2009;460(7252):231–236.
126. Di Noia JM, Rada C, Neuberger MS. SMUG1 is able to excise uracil from immunoglobulin genes: insight into mutation versus repair. *EMBO J* 2006;25(3):585–595.
127. Di Noia JM, Neuberger MS. Molecular mechanisms of antibody somatic hypermutation. *Annu Rev Biochem* 2007;76:1–22.
128. Stavnezer J, Guikema JE, Schrader CE. Mechanism and regulation of class switch recombination. *Annu Rev Immunol* 2008;26:261–292.
129. Peled JU, Kuang FL, Iglesias-Ussel MD, et al. The biochemistry of somatic hypermutation. *Annu Rev Immunol* 2008;26:481–511.
130. Gordon MS, Kanegai CM, Doerr JR, et al. Somatic hypermutation of the B cell receptor genes B29 (Igbeta, CD79b) and mb1 (Igalpha, CD79a). *Proc Natl Acad Sci U S A* 2003;100(7):4126–4131.
131. Muschen M, Re D, Jungnickel B, et al. Somatic mutation of the CD95 gene in human B cells as a side-effect of the germinal center reaction. *J Exp Med* 2000;192(12):1833–1840.
132. Pasqualucci L, Migliazza A, Fracchiolla N, et al. BCL-6 mutations in normal germinal center B cells: evidence of somatic hypermutation acting outside Ig loci. *Proc Natl Acad Sci U S A* 1998;95(20):11816–11821.
133. Pasqualucci L, Neumeister P, Goossens T, et al. Hypermutation of multiple proto-oncogenes in B-cell diffuse large-cell lymphomas. *Nature* 2001;412(6844):341–346.
134. Staszewski O, Baker RE, Ucher AJ, et al. Activation-induced cytidine deaminase induces reproducible DNA breaks at many non-Ig Loci in activated B cells. *Mol Cell* 2011;41(2):232–242.
135. Liu M, Duke JL, Richter DJ, et al. Two levels of protection for the B cell genome during somatic hypermutation. *Nature* 2008;451(7180):841–845.
136. Nussenzweig A, Nussenzweig MC. Origin of chromosomal translocations in lymphoid cancer. *Cell* 2010;141(1):27–38.
137. Bellan C, Lazzi S, Hummel M, et al. Immunoglobulin gene analysis reveals 2 distinct cells of origin for EBV-positive and EBV-negative Burkitt lymphomas. *Blood* 2005;106(3):1031–1036.
138. Klein U, Tu YH, Stolovitzky GA, et al. Transcriptional analysis of the B cell germinal center reaction. *Proc Natl Acad Sci U S A* 2003;100(5):2639–2644.
139. Adhikary S, Eilers M. Transcriptional regulation and transformation by Myc proteins. *Nat Rev Mol Cell Biol* 2005;6(8):635–645.
140. Zeller KI, Zhao X, Lee CW, et al. Global mapping of c-Myc binding sites and target gene networks in human B cells. *Proc Natl Acad Sci U S A* 2006;103(47):17834–17839.
141. Dang CV, O'donnell KA, Zeller KI, et al. The c-Myc target gene network. *Semin Cancer Biol* 2006;16(4):253–264.

142. Seitz V, Butzhammer P, Hirsch B, et al. Deep sequencing of MYC DNA-binding sites in Burkitt lymphoma. *PLoS One* 2011;6(11):e26837.
143. Nie Z, Hu G, Wei G, et al. c-Myc is a universal amplifier of expressed genes in lymphocytes and embryonic stem cells. *Cell* 2012;151(1):68–79.
144. Dominguez-Sola D, Ying CY, Grandori C, et al. Non-transcriptional control of DNA replication by c-Myc. *Nature* 2007;448(7152):445–451.
145. Green TM, de Stricker K, Moller MB. Validation of putative reference genes for normalization of Q-RT-PCR data from paraffin-embedded lymphoid tissue. *Diagn Mol Pathol* 2009;18(4):243–249.
146. Chang TC, Yu D, Lee YS, et al. Widespread microRNA repression by Myc contributes to tumorigenesis. *Nat Genet* 2008;40(1):43–50.
147. O'donnell KA, Wentzel EA, Zeller KI, et al. c-Myc-regulated microRNAs modulate E2F1 expression. *Nature* 2005;435(7043):839–843.
148. Robertus JL, Kluiver J, Weggemans C, et al. MiRNA profiling in B non-Hodgkin lymphoma: a MYC-related miRNA profile characterizes Burkitt lymphoma. *Br J Haematol* 2010;149(6):896–899.
149. Bernheim A, Berger R, Lenoir G. Cytogenetic studies on Burkitt's lymphoma cell lines. *Cancer Genet Cytogenet* 1983;8(3):223–229.
150. Berger R, Bernheim A. Cytogenetic studies on Burkitt's lymphoma-leukemia. *Cancer Genet Cytogenet* 1982;7(3):231–244.
151. Berger R, Bernheim A. Cytogenetics of Burkitt's lymphoma-leukaemia: a review. *IARC Sci Publ* 1985;(60):65–80.
152. Bhatia KG, Gutiérrez MI, Huppi K, et al. The pattern of *p53* mutations in Burkitt's lymphoma differs from that of solid tumors. *Cancer Res* 1992;52:4273–4276.
153. Farrell PJ, Allan GJ, Shanahan F, et al. p53 Is frequently mutated in Burkitt's lymphoma cell lines. *EMBO J* 1991;10:2879–2887.
154. Gaidano G, Ballerini P, Gong JZ, et al. p53 Mutations in human lymphoid malignancies: association with Burkitt lymphoma and chronic lymphocytic leukemia. *Proc Natl Acad Sci U S A* 1991;88:5413–5417.
155. Ramqvist T, Magnusson KP, Wang Y, et al. Wild-type p53 induces apoptosis in a Burkitt lymphoma (BL) line that carries mutant p53. *Oncogene* 1993;8: 1495–1500.
156. Wiman KG, Magnusson KP, Ramqvist T, et al. Mutant p53 detected in a majority of Burkitt lymphoma cell lines by monoclonal antibody PAb240. *Oncogene* 1991;6:1633–1639.
157. Poirel HA, Cairo MS, Heerema NA, et al. Specific cytogenetic abnormalities are associated with a significantly inferior outcome in children and adolescents with mature B-cell non-Hodgkin's lymphoma: results of the FAB/LMB 96 international study. *Leukemia* 2009;23(2):323–331.
158. Salaverria I, Zettl A, Bea S, et al. Chromosomal alterations detected by comparative genomic hybridization in subgroups of gene expression-defined Burkitt's lymphoma. *Haematologica* 2008;93(9):1327–1334.
159. Scholtysik R, Kreuz M, Klapper W, et al. Detection of genomic aberrations in molecularly defined Burkitt's lymphoma by array-based, high resolution, single nucleotide polymorphism analysis. *Haematologica* 2010;95(12):2047–2055.
160. Klapper W, Szczepanowski M, Burkhardt B, et al. Molecular profiling of pediatric mature B-cell lymphoma treated in population-based prospective clinical trials. *Blood* 2008;112(4):1374–1381.
161. Stranks G, Height SE, Mitchell P, et al. Deletions and rearrangement of CDKN2 in lymphoid malignancy. *Blood* 1995;85:893–901.
162. Wilda M, Bruch J, Harder L, et al. Inactivation of the ARF-MDM-2-p53 pathway in sporadic Burkitt's lymphoma in children. *Leukemia* 2004;18(3):584–588.
163. Lindstrom MS, Klangby U, Wiman KG. p14ARF homozygous deletion or MDM2 overexpression in Burkitt lymphoma lines carrying wild type p53. *Oncogene* 2001;20(17):2171–2177.
164. Zhang Y, Xiong Y, Yarbrough WG. ARF promotes MDM2 degradation and stabilizes p53: ARF-INK4a locus deletion impairs both the Rb and p53 tumor suppression pathways. *Cell* 1998;92(6):725–734.
165. Fernandez-Piqueras J, Santos J, Perez dC, I, et al. Frequent allelic losses of 9p21 markers and low incidence of mutations at p16(CDKN2) gene in non-Hodgkin lymphomas of B-cell lineage. *Cancer Genet Cytogenet* 1997;98(1):63–68.
166. Roberti A, Rizzolio F, Lucchetti C, et al. Ubiquitin-mediated protein degradation and methylation-induced gene silencing cooperate in the inactivation of the INK4/ARF locus in Burkitt lymphoma cell lines. *Cell Cycle* 2011;10(1):127–134.
167. Cinti C, Leoncini L, Nyongo A, et al. Genetic alterations of the retinoblastoma-related gene RB2/p130 identify different pathogenetic mechanisms in and among Burkitt's lymphoma subtypes. *Am J Pathol* 2000;156(3):751–760.
168. Love C, Sun Z, Jima D, et al. The genetic landscape of mutations in Burkitt lymphoma. *Nat Genet* 2012;44(12):1321–1325.
169. Richter J, Schlesner M, Hoffmann S, et al. Recurrent mutation of the ID3 gene in Burkitt lymphoma identified by integrated genome, exome and transcriptome sequencing. *Nat Genet* 2012;44(12):1316–1320.
170. Schmitz R, Young RM, Ceribelli M, et al. Burkitt lymphoma pathogenesis and therapeutic targets from structural and functional genomics. *Nature* 2012;490(7418):116–120.
171. Soldini D, Montagna C, Schuffler P, et al. A new diagnostic algorithm for Burkitt and diffuse large B-cell lymphomas based on the expression of CSE1L and STAT3 and on MYC rearrangement predicts outcome. *Ann Oncol* 2012.
172. Rabbitts TH, Hamlyn PH, Baer R. Altered nucleotide sequences of a translocated c-myc gene in Burkitt lymphoma. *Nature* 1983;306(5945):760–765.
173. Bhatia K, Huppi K, Spangler G, et al. Point mutations in the c-Myc transactivation domain are common in Burkitt's lymphoma and mouse plasmacytomas. *Nature Genet* 1993;5:56–61.
174. Smith-Sorensen B, Hijmans EM, Beijersbergen RL, et al. Functional analysis of Burkitt's lymphoma mutant c-Myc proteins. *J Biol Chem* 1996;271(10):5513–5518.
175. Cesarman E, Dalla-Favera R, Bentley D, et al. Mutations in the first exon are associated with altered transcription of c-myc in Burkitt lymphoma. *Science* 1987;238(4831):1272–1275.
176. Zajac-Kaye M, Gelmann EP, Levens D. A point mutation in the c-myc locus of a Burkitt lymphoma abolishes binding of a nuclear protein. *Science* 1988;240(4860):1776–1780.
177. Hoang AT, Lutterbach B, Lewis BC, et al. A link between increased transforming activity of lymphoma-derived MYC mutant alleles, their defective regulation by p107, and altered phosphorylation of the c-Myc transactivation domain. *Mol Cell Biol* 1995;15(8):4031–4042.
178. Raffeld M, Yano T, Hoang AT, et al. Clustered mutations in the transcriptional activation domain of Myc in 8q24 translocated lymphomas and their functional consequences. *Curr Top Microbiol Immunol* 1995;194:265–272.
179. Hemann MT, Bric A, Teruya-Feldstein J, et al. Evasion of the p53 tumour surveillance network by tumour-derived MYC mutants. *Nature* 2005;436(7052):807–811.
180. Tamaru J, Hummel M, Marafioti T, et al. Burkitt's lymphomas express VH genes with a moderate number of antigen-selected somatic mutations. *Am J Pathol* 1995;147:1398–1407.
181. Chapman CJ, Mockridge CI, Rowe M, et al. Analysis of VH genes used by neoplastic B cells in endemic Burkitt's lymphoma shows somatic hypermutation and intraclonal heterogeneity. *Blood* 1995;85:2176–2181.
182. Guikema JE, Schuuring E, Kluin PM. Structure and consequences of IGH switch breakpoints in Burkitt lymphoma. *J Natl Cancer Inst Monogr* 2008;(39):32–36.
183. Guikema JE, de Boer C, Haralambieva E, et al. IGH switch breakpoints in Burkitt lymphoma: exclusive involvement of noncanonical class switch recombination. *Genes Chromosomes Cancer* 2006;45(9):808–819.
184. Piccaluga PP, De FG, Kustagi M, et al. Gene expression analysis uncovers similarity and differences among Burkitt lymphoma subtypes. *Blood* 2011;117(13):3596–3608.
185. Lenze D, Leoncini L, Hummel M, et al. The different epidemiologic subtypes of Burkitt lymphoma share a homogenous micro RNA profile distinct from diffuse large B-cell lymphoma. *Leukemia* 2011;25(12):1869–1876.
186. Onnis A, De FG, Antonicelli G, et al. Alteration of microRNAs regulated by c-Myc in Burkitt lymphoma. *PLoS One* 2010;5(9):e12960.
187. Cairo MS, Gerrard M, Sposto R, et al. Results of a randomized international study of high-risk central nervous system B non-Hodgkin lymphoma and B acute lymphoblastic leukemia in children and adolescents. *Blood* 2007;109(7):2736–2743.
188. Patte C. Treatment of mature B-ALL and high grade B-NHL in children. *Best Pract Res Clin Haematol* 2002;15(4):695–711.
189. Pees HW, Radtke H, Schwamborn J, et al. The BFM-protocol for HIV-negative Burkitt's lymphomas and L3 ALL in adult patients: a high chance for cure. *Ann Hematol* 1992;65(5):201–205.
190. Reiter A, Schrappe M, Parwaresch R, et al. Non-Hodgkin's lymphomas of childhood and adolescence: results of a treatment stratified for biologic subtypes and stage—a report of the Berlin-Frankfurt-Munster Group. *J Clin Oncol* 1995;13(2):359–372.
191. Perkins AS, Friedberg JW. Burkitt lymphoma in adults. *Hematol Am Soc Hematol Educ Prog* 2008;341–348.
192. Magrath I, Adde M, Shad A, et al. Adults and children with small non-cleaved-cell lymphoma have a similar excellent outcome when treated with the same chemotherapy regimen. *J Clin Oncol* 1996;14(3):925–934.
193. Kelly JL, Toothaker SR, Ciminello L, et al. Outcomes of patients with Burkitt lymphoma older than age 40 treated with intensive chemotherapeutic regimens. *Clin Lymphoma Myeloma* 2009;9(4):307–310.
194. Todeschini G, Bonifacio M, Tecchio C, et al. Intensive short-term chemotherapy regimen induces high remission rate (over 90%) and event-free survival both in children and adult patients with advanced sporadic Burkitt lymphoma/leukemia. *Am J Hematol* 2012;87(1):22–25.
195. Magrath I. Lessons from clinical trials in African Burkitt lymphoma. *Curr Opin Oncol* 2009;21(5):462–468.
196. Traore F, Coze C, Atteby JJ, et al. Cyclophosphamide monotherapy in children with Burkitt lymphoma: a study from the French-African Pediatric Oncology Group (GFAOP). *Pediatr Blood Cancer* 2011;56(1):70–76.
197. Blinder VS, Chadburn A, Furman RR, et al. Improving outcomes for patients with Burkitt lymphoma and HIV. *AIDS Patient Care STDS* 2008;22(3):175–187.
198. Aukema SM, Siebert R, Schuuring E, et al. Double-hit B-cell lymphomas. *Blood* 2011;117(8):2319–2331.
199. Knezevich S, Ludkovski O, Salski C, et al. Concurrent translocation of BCL2 and MYC with a single immunoglobulin locus in high-grade B-cell lymphomas. *Leukemia* 2005;19(4):659–663.
200. Quintanilla-Martinez L, de JD, de MA, et al. Gray zones around diffuse large B cell lymphoma. Conclusions based on the workshop of the XIV meeting of the European Association for Hematopathology and the Society of Hematopathology in Bordeaux, France. *J Hematop* 2009;2(4):211–236.
201. Tomita N, Tokunaka M, Nakamura N, et al. Clinicopathological features of lymphoma/leukemia patients carrying both BCL2 and MYC translocations. *Haematologica* 2009;94(7):935–943.
202. de LL, Hasserjian RP. Diffuse large B-cell lymphomas and burkitt lymphoma. *Hematol Oncol Clin North Am* 2009;23(4):791–827.
203. Johnson NA, Savage KJ, Ludkovski O, et al. Lymphomas with concurrent BCL2 and MYC translocations: the critical factors associated with survival. *Blood* 2009;114(11):2273–2279.
204. Hasserjian RP, Ott G, Elenitoba-Johnson KS, et al. Commentary on the WHO classification of tumors of lymphoid tissues (2008): "Gray zone" lymphomas overlapping with Burkitt lymphoma or classical Hodgkin lymphoma. *J Hematop* 2009;2(2):89–95.
205. Snuderl M, Kolman OK, Chen YB, et al. B-cell lymphomas with concurrent IGH-BCL2 and MYC rearrangements are aggressive neoplasms with clinical and pathologic features distinct from Burkitt lymphoma and diffuse large B-cell lymphoma. *Am J Surg Pathol* 2010;34(3):327–340.
206. Tauro S, Cochrane L, Lauritzsen GF, et al. Dose-intensified treatment of Burkitt lymphoma and B-cell lymphoma unclassifiable, (with features intermediate between diffuse large B-cell lymphoma and Burkitt lymphoma) in young adults (<50 years): a comparison of two adapted BFM protocols. *Am J Hematol* 2010;85(4):261–263.
207. Carbone A, Gloghini A, Aiello A, et al. B-cell lymphomas with features intermediate between distinct pathologic entities. From pathogenesis to pathology. *Hum Pathol* 2010;41(5):621–631.
208. Wu D, Wood BL, Dorer R, et al. "Double-Hit" mature B-cell lymphomas show a common immunophenotype by flow cytometry that includes decreased CD20 expression. *Am J Clin Pathol* 2010;134(2):258–265.
209. Maruyama D, Watanabe T, Maeshima AM, et al. Modified cyclophosphamide, vincristine, doxorubicin, and methotrexate (CODOX-M)/ifosfamide, etoposide, and cytarabine (IVAC) therapy with or without rituximab in Japanese adult patients with Burkitt lymphoma (BL) and B cell lymphoma, unclassifiable, with features intermediate between diffuse large B cell lymphoma and BL. *Int J Hematol* 2010;92(5):732–743.
210. Thomas DA, O'Brien S, Faderl S, et al. Burkitt lymphoma and atypical Burkitt or Burkitt-like lymphoma: should these be treated as different diseases? *Curr Hematol Malig Rep* 2011;6(1):58–66.
211. Harrington AM, Olteanu H, Kroft SH, et al. The unique immunophenotype of double-hit lymphomas. *Am J Clin Pathol* 2011;135(4):649–650.

212. Salaverria I, Siebert R. The gray zone between Burkitt's lymphoma and diffuse large B-cell lymphoma from a genetics perspective. *J Clin Oncol* 2011;29(14): 1835–1843.
213. da Cunha SG, Ko HM, Saieg MA, et al. Cytomorphologic findings of B-cell lymphomas with concurrent IGH/BCL2 and MYC rearrangements (dual-translocation lymphomas). *Cancer Cytopathol* 2011;119(4):254–262.
214. Tomita N. BCL2 and MYC dual-hit lymphoma/leukemia. *J Clin Exp Hematop* 2011;51(1):7–12.

215. Lin P, Dickason TJ, Fayad LE, et al. Prognostic value of MYC rearrangement in cases of B-cell lymphoma, unclassifiable, with features intermediate between diffuse large B-cell lymphoma and Burkitt lymphoma. *Cancer* 2012;118(6):1566–1573.
216. Li S, Lin P, Fayad LE, et al. B-cell lymphomas with MYC/8q24 rearrangements and IGH@BCL2/t(14;18)(q32;q21): an aggressive disease with heterogeneous histology, germinal center B-cell immunophenotype and poor outcome. *Mod Pathol* 2012;25(1):145–156.

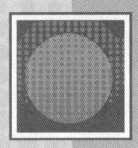

Chapter 25
Lymphadenopathy and the Lymphoid Neoplasms Associated with HIV Infection and Other Causes of Immunosuppression

Jonathan Said • Ethel Cesarman • Daniel M. Knowles

HIV-RELATED LYMPHOID PROLIFERATIONS

Introduction: HIV/AIDS 30 Years Later

The medical community was alerted to the existence of the acquired immunodeficiency syndrome (AIDS) in 1981 by a Morbidity and Mortality Weekly Report description of five cases of *Pneumocystis carinii* pneumonia in homosexual men in Los Angeles (1,2). Almost simultaneously, nine cases of Kaposi sarcoma (KS) were reported in young homosexual men as a preliminary communication (3), followed 4 months later by an article describing eight additional cases of KS in homosexual men (4). Within several months AIDS cases were reported in infants, female sex partners of men with AIDS, and an infant and adults who had received blood transfusions (5). Since these early reports HIV has spread throughout the world, resulting in the death of half of the 60 million people infected to date (6). About 2 million new HIV infections occur each year. The Centers for Disease Control (CDC) estimates 1.2 million people in the United States (US) are living with HIV infection, and one in five (20%) of those people are unaware of their infection. While men who have sex with men are responsible for the largest numbers of new HIV infections, it is estimated that heterosexual men and women account for 27% and 23%, respectively, of new infections in the United States (7). Regardless of the mode of transmission, blacks and Hispanics have been disproportionately affected by the epidemic in the United States.

Survival of HIV-infected individuals has been greatly impacted by modern combined antiretroviral therapy (cART), but a cure or effective immunization remains elusive. In recent years, increasing diversity due to circulating recombinant viral forms has become a major challenge to diagnosis, treatment, and vaccine production. At least 48 circulating recombinant forms of HIV have been identified (8), and HIV diversification has been aided by the increasing ease of worldwide travel. Moreover, the HIV/AIDS epidemic in Africa is growing increasingly dire; it is projected that the number of people living with HIV/AIDS could reach 70 million by 2050 in Africa alone (9).

The HIV Virus

The origin of HIV has now been traced to chimpanzees, and its most recent common ancestor to 1908 (8). HIV resembles other lentiviruses in that the RNA genome is reverse-transcribed into DNA, which is integrated into the cellular genome and encodes for the major common retroviral genes gag, pol, and env, and the HIV-specific genes like Tat and Nef (10). The HIV virus can be classified into two major types, HIV-1 and HIV-2. HIV-2 has been shown to be associated with the development of AIDS in a small number of patients and has a very low prevalence (11). Recombinant forms of HIV may have different serologic properties, which may complicate diagnosis. Infection by these retroviruses is spread most frequently by intimate sexual contact, by inoculation or infusion of infected blood and blood products, or perinatally from mother to child, and injection drug use (12). The epidemiologic patterns of the AIDS epidemic are diverse and vary according to geographic location. In the United States, the major groups at risk for AIDS are men who have sex with men (MSM) and injecting drug users (IDUs). Heterosexual transmission has been responsible for the largest proportionate increase in AIDS prevalence recently.

Pathogenesis

Although most viral infection occurs through sexual contact, the route of transmission does not appear to affect the subsequent course. Cell-free HIV has been found in semen, vaginal secretions, and blood, and infection also results from exposure to HIV-infected cells. Although the CD4+ T cell is the primary target for HIV infection, a large range of hematopoietic and other cells have been shown to be susceptible (6). These include dendritic cells, natural killer (NK) cells, B lymphocytes, macrophages, megakaryocytes, endothelial cells, Langerhans cells, and epithelial cells, including those in the bowel, liver, cervix, prostate, and testis. HIV has been shown to infect glial cells and capillary endothelial cells in the central nervous system (CNS). Immunosuppression with severely decreased circulating CD4+ T cells and neuropsychologic deficits are among the most devastating consequences for the host.

The main receptor for HIV on human cells is the CD4 molecule (13), which is expressed primarily by helper or inducer T lymphocytes and monocytes or dendritic cells, to which HIV binds through envelope gp120 (14). Langerhans cells are early targets of the virus, and other dendritic cells may play a role, although it is now believed that monocyte-derived macrophages are generally poor targets for infection (15). Alterations of myeloid and plasmacytoid dendritic cells play leading roles in inducing and sustaining the chronic immune activation associated with HIV infection (16–18).

Two viral co-receptors are required for viral growth. CXCR4 is the receptor for the CXCL12 chemokine (SDF-1), and CCR5 is a receptor for the CC chemokines CCL3 (MIP-1α), CCL4 (MIP-1β), and CCL5 (RANTES) (6). Individuals lacking CCR5 expression are long-term nonprogressors, and there is evidence that HIV infection can be controlled or even cured by transplantation with stem cells from a donor who is homozygous for CCR5 delta32 (19,20). HIV-1 can be assigned to one of three classes based on its ability to use the two co-receptors: class R5 comprises the viruses that only use CCR5 (previously called non–syncytia-inducing or M-tropic); the viruses that use only CXCR4 are in class X4 (previously called syncytia-inducing or T-tropic viruses); and viruses that can use either co-receptor are referred to as R5X4 or dual viruses (21). Primary lymphocytes and macrophages express both co-receptors, so co-receptor use does not strictly define cell tropism (22). Thus, while X4 virus infects T-cell lines, and R5 virus infects macrophage cell lines, in primary cells, these definitions are not as clear. CD4-positive T cells in lymphoid tissues can express both CCR5 and CXCR4 and are the main target for replication *in vivo*. CCR5 is expressed predominantly on the CD45R0$^+$ memory subset of CD4-positive T lymphocytes, while CXCR4 is expressed on CD4-positive CD45R0 and on CD4-positive CD45RAlow naive cells. The primary determinants of co-receptor tropism are located in the V3 region of the gp120 envelope protein and phenotypic assays and genotyping can be used to determine tropism. Most individuals have the R5 virus at the time of diagnosis, whereas the presence of the X4 and dual virus is associated with progression to AIDS (22).

Eighty percent of adults are infected with HIV-1 through exposure of mucosal surfaces to the virus; the remaining 20% are infected though percutaneous or intravenous inoculations (15). The virus then replicates in the mucosa, submucosa, or lymphoreticular tissues, and in this "eclipse phase," which lasts 7 to 21 days, the virus cannot be detected in the plasma (15). The stage that defines acute viral infection is characterized by sequential appearance of viral markers and antibodies in the blood. Regardless of the route of infection, within days the viral replication converges on the gut-associated lymphoid tissues (15). The severe immunodeficiency that develops in untreated individuals has a number of causations including chronic immune activation leading to telomere shortening and immune senescence, apoptotic cell death of infected and uninfected CD4$^+$ T cells, and CD8$^+$ T-cell activation. Impairment of the mucosal barrier also permits bacteria and toxins to enter the circulation. In addition to abnormalities affecting T cells and histiocytes, multiple B-cell defects have been documented in patients with HIV. These include polyclonal hypergammaglobulin with chronic B-cell activation and progressive loss of memory B cells. Defects in the innate immune response include a decrease in plasmacytoid dendritic cells and a reduction in cytokine production that restricts lymphoid and NK-cell activation.

Antiretroviral Therapy

While elimination of HIV from infected individuals remains elusive, control of the virus with cART, also referred to as highly active antiretroviral therapy (HAART), has been the major achievement in the past decades. These drugs inhibit viral enzymes (reverse transcriptase, integrase, and protease) and the cell binding steps required for the virus to enter the host cell and begin replication. The drugs have also been used as chemoprophylaxis to prevent infection in high-risk situations, or reduce virus transmission after exposure. Infected individuals are required to take the drugs for life, and potential long-standing side effects may involve the heart, liver, pancreas, kidney, muscle, and bone marrow, among other organs. The emergence of drug-resistant virus is also a concern. As the HIV-infected population continues to age on cART therapy, the long-term effects, including cognitive decline and cellular senescence, remain to be determined. While 6.6 million people with HIV are receiving ART, 9 million are waiting to receive it. It is estimated that treatment costs could reach $35 billion a year (23).

Pediatric HIV

Since the demonstration that antiretroviral therapy is remarkably efficient in reducing mother-to-child transmission of HIV, perinatal HIV has become virtually eliminated in high-income countries. However, in countries such as sub-Saharan Africa and Asia, prevention programs are inadequate, and it is estimated that more than 1,000 children are infected and 700 die of AIDS-related diseases each day (24). The

Table 25.1	DIAGNOSIS OF HIV INFECTION IN CHILDREN

HIV infected
A child <18 mo of age who is known to be HIV seropositive or born to an HIV-infected mother and
Has positive results on two separate determinations (excluding cord blood) from one or more of the following HIV detection tests:
HIV culture
HIV polymerase chain reaction
HIV antigen (p24) or
Meets criteria for AIDS diagnosis based on the 1987 AIDS surveillance case definition (61)
A child ≥18 mo of age born to an HIV-infected mother or any child infected by blood, blood products, or other known modes of transmission (e.g., sexual contact) who
Is HIV-antibody positive by repeatedly reactive EIA and confirmatory test (e.g., Western blot or IFA) or
Meets any of the criteria for children <18 mo
Perinatally exposed (prefix E)
A child who does not meet the criteria above who
Is HIV seropositive by EIA and confirmatory test (e.g., Western blot or IFA) and is <18 mo of age at the time of test or
Has unknown antibody status, but was born to a mother known to be infected with HIV
Seroreverter
A child who is born to an HIV-infected mother and who
Has been documented as HIV antibody negative (i.e., two or more negative EIA tests performed at 6–18 mo of age or one negative EIA test after 18 mo of age) and
Has had no other laboratory evidence of infection (has not had two positive viral detection tests, if performed) and
Has not had an AIDS-defining condition

clinical characteristics of AIDS in children differ from those in adults (25). In the 1994 Revised Classification System for HIV Infection in Children less than 13 years of Age, children are classified into mutually exclusive categories according to three parameters: infection status, clinical status, and immunologic status. Virtually all children born to HIV-infected women are HIV antibody–positive at birth, because maternal anti-HIV IgG antibodies cross the placenta. Only 15% to 30% children of untreated mothers actually acquire HIV infection. The HIV-uninfected children can remain HIV antibody positive up to 18 months of age (26). Standard anti-HIV IgG antibody tests cannot be relied upon to determine a child's HIV status until after this age. Consequently, it is difficult to diagnose HIV infection in children born to HIV-infected women (26). Criteria have been established for the diagnosis of pediatric HIV infection (Table 25.1). Children who are HIV infected or exposed to HIV perinatally may be classified into one of four mutually exclusive clinical categories based on signs, symptoms, or diagnoses related to HIV infection (Table 25.2). Lymphocytic interstitial pneumonitis (LIP) is a common complication of AIDS in children. LIP is characterized by diffuse infiltration of alveolar septa by mature lymphocytes with occasional plasma cells and immunoblasts. Nodular aggregates and granulomatous infiltrates are also encountered. The clinical course of LIP in children is variable. Progressive disease can lead to respiratory failure, but spontaneous resolution may also occur.

HIV-Related Disease
Acute HIV Infection

The first signal of an immune response to HIV-1 is the appearance of acute-phase reactants in plasma 3 to 5 days following transmission. There follows a rise in HIV-1 viral load (ramp-up viremia) accompanied by a shower of

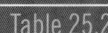

Table 25.2	CLINICAL CATEGORIES FOR CHILDREN WITH HIV INFECTION

Category N: Not symptomatic
Children who have no signs or symptoms considered to be the result of HIV infection or who have only one of the conditions listed in category A
Category A: Mildly symptomatic
Children with two or more of the conditions listed below but none of the conditions listed in categories B and C
Lymphadenopathy (≥0.5 cm at more than two sites; bilateral = one site)
Hepatomegaly
Splenomegaly
Dermatitis
Parotitis
Recurrent or persistent upper respiratory infection, sinusitis, or otitis media
Category B: Moderately symptomatic
Children who have symptomatic conditions other than those listed for category A or C that are attributed to HIV infection. Examples of conditions in clinical category B include but are not limited to
Anemia (<8 g/dL), neutropenia (<1,000/mm³), or thrombocytopenia (<100,000/mm³) persisting ≥30 days
Bacterial meningitis, pneumonia, or sepsis (single episode)
Candidiasis, oropharyngeal (thrush), persisting (>2 mo) in children >6 mo of age
Cardiomyopathy
Cytomegalovirus infection, with onset before 1 mo of age
Diarrhea, recurrent or chronic
Hepatitis
HSV stomatitis, recurrent (more than two episodes within 1 y)
HSV bronchitis, pneumonitis, or esophagitis with onset before 1 mo of age
Herpes zoster (shingles) involving at least two distinct episodes or more than one dermatome
Leiomyosarcoma
LIP or pulmonary lymphoid hyperplasia complex
Nephropathy
Nocardiosis
Persistent fever (lasting >1 mo)
Toxoplasmosis, onset before 1 mo of age
Varicella, disseminated (complicated chickenpox)
Category C: Severely symptomatic
Children who have any condition listed in the 1987 surveillance case definition for AIDS (254), with the exception of LIP. These conditions include a number of infections, wasting, KS, and lymphoma.

HSV, herpes simplex virus; LIP, lymphoid interstitial pneumonia.

microparticles derived from infected and activated CD4⁺ T cells undergoing apoptosis. Antibodies that neutralize the virus are not detected until 3 months or more after infection. Entry and replication of the virus is followed by a massive and rapid loss of CD4⁺ cells in lymphoid organs, which is poorly reflected in peripheral CD4⁺ T-cell counts. In the absence of seroconversion, confirmation of acute infection is detected by the presence of HIV-1 RNA or p24 antigen (15). Acute infection usually manifests within 6 weeks of infection. Constitutional symptoms include fever, lymphadenopathy, skin rash, headache, diarrhea, myalgia, and arthralgia, which may be associated with leucopenia and thrombocytopenia. Viral loads usually peak between 6 weeks to 6 months after infection, as the host is able to mount an effective immune response with symptoms subsiding. The typical asymptomatic period without therapy is about 9 years before the onset of opportunistic infections, neurologic disorders, and neoplastic conditions that characterize AIDS develop. The previously held view of HIV disease as a chronic and slowly progressive loss of function has been revised with newer evidence that the early events may cause irremediable damage to the immune system, which will gradually fail (16). Massive depletion of CD4⁺ T cells occurs during the course of HIV-1 infection, and maintenance of adequate T cells depends on the capacity to renew depleted lymphocytes (27).

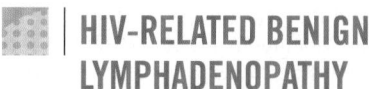

HIV-RELATED BENIGN LYMPHADENOPATHY

General Comments and Historical Context

In 1982, unexplained, persistent diffuse lymphadenopathy not attributable to previously known causes was reported in homosexual men in major metropolitan areas of the United States, especially New York and San Francisco, where cases of KS and opportunistic infections had been previously described (28). This was designated *persistent generalized lymphadenopathy syndrome* and was defined as lymphadenopathy of at least 3 months' duration involving two or more noncontiguous, extrainguinal sites in the absence of any illness or drug use known to cause lymphadenopathy and displaying hyperplastic histopathology on lymph node biopsy (28). Most patients were aware of the lymphadenopathy for 10 to 18 months before presentation (28–32). In some individuals, persistent generalized lymphadenopathy was accompanied by fever, night sweats, malaise, weight loss, diarrhea, cutaneous anergy, hypergammaglobulinemia, diminished CD4⁺ T-cell counts, and other phenomena associated with HIV infection; this was referred to as the *AIDS-related complex* (33,34). Although any lymph node or lymph node group might be enlarged, the lymphadenopathy often involved unusual sites, such as epitrochlear and submandibular lymph nodes (35). The enlarged lymph nodes usually were tender, and they sometimes fluctuated in size with illness or stress (35).

Biopsy examination of such lymph nodes frequently was performed in the early years of the AIDS epidemic to exclude AIDS-defining conditions such as KS, opportunistic infections, or non-Hodgkin lymphoma (NHL), as the cause of the enlargement. Consequently, many benign, reactive lymph nodes obtained from HIV-seropositive individuals who had varying levels of immunosuppression were biopsied. Some investigators noticed that certain histopathologic patterns appeared to correlate with peripheral blood CD4:CD8 T-cell ratios and the clinical stage of HIV infection (36–42). Patients who had florid follicular hyperplasia had a relatively stable clinical course, sometimes lasting for several years; those who had other histologies, such as follicular involution and lymphocyte depletion, rapidly developed some of the stigmata of AIDS (36,38,39,43,44). By examining sequential lymph node biopsies from HIV-infected persons, it has become known that lymph node histology transforms in a consistent pattern throughout the course of untreated HIV infection (38). The temporal progression of lymph node histopathology observed in routine histologic sections correlates with other features of HIV disease progression, such as peripheral blood CD4⁺ T-cell counts, viremia, and the development of opportunistic infections, and has prognostic implications for the HIV-infected patient (38).

Histopathology: Florid Follicular Hyperplasia

Grossly, most lymph nodes are soft and moderately enlarged (2 to 4 cm) and do not show evidence of necrosis (30,36). Histologically, they are composed of large, hyperplastic follicles, sometimes with serrated borders. The follicles may coalesce and become very large, forming "dumbbell" and other irregular shapes—hence the term *geographic follicles* (30,34,43,45) (Fig. 25.1). These hyperplastic follicles may be present in the medulla (45,46) as well as the cortex and may extend outside the lymph node capsule (35). In some instances, the follicles occupy more than two-thirds of the cross-sectional area of the lymph node (37). The reactive follicles contain various lymphoid cells; however, large centrocytes and small and large centroblasts predominate (36,38,45). In addition, numerous tingible body macrophages and abundant mitotic figures are usually present within the reactive follicles, giving them a starry-sky

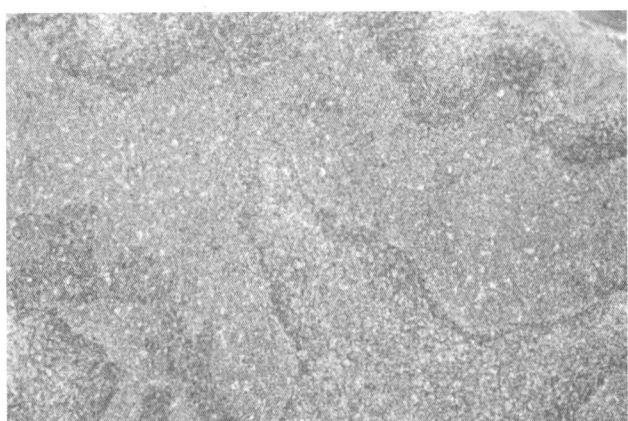

FIGURE 25.1. HIV-related florid follicular hyperplasia. The hyperplastic follicles coalesce to form extremely large and irregularly shaped follicles referred to as *geographic follicles* (hematoxylin and eosin stain, original magnification: 40× magnification).

FIGURE 25.3. HIV-related florid follicular hyperplasia. The large hyperplastic and coalescent follicles lack a mantle zone and appear to merge with the surrounding interfollicular lymphoid cells. The follicle appears disrupted, and there is focal hemorrhage (hematoxylin and eosin stain, original magnification: 100× magnification).

appearance (30,36,38,45,47) (Fig. 25.2). The surrounding mantle zones often exhibit disruption, extensive attenuation, or even total effacement (30,45,48), so that the germinal centers are poorly defined and appear to merge with the surrounding interfollicular area. In some instances the mantle zones are entirely absent, and only "naked" germinal centers are present (49) (Fig. 25.3).

Follicle lysis, also known as *follicular fragmentation*, is characterized by germinal centers transected by invaginating small lymphocytes, with or without erythrocytes (30,35,37,38,50–52). Follicle lysis is identified in a minority of follicles in approximately 50% of lymph nodes that exhibit florid follicular hyperplasia (50,52). The infiltrating small lymphocytes, which sometimes appear to track along small blood vessels (34,47), eventually break up the follicle into separate clusters of follicle center B cells (50) (Fig. 25.4). The combination of follicle lysis and mantle zone effacement obscures normal lymph node architecture and can cause confusion with lymphoma (35) (Fig. 25.5).

Collections of monocyte-like or marginal zone cells often are seen surrounding trabecular vessels in the sinusoids between the floridly hyperplastic germinal centers (30,43,45,50). These monocytoid cells possess bland, oval, slightly indented nuclei containing inconspicuous nucleoli and relatively abundant pale

to clear cytoplasm. Immunophenotypic studies have shown that these cells are polyclonal B lymphocytes (53). In HIV-related florid follicular hyperplasia, monocytoid B cells usually are seen in sinusoids associated with neutrophils (30,35,45,53,54); occasionally, monocytoid B cells also are seen partially encircling a reactive follicle (30,53). The interfollicular areas of lymph nodes exhibiting florid follicular hyperplasia contain numerous small blood vessels with prominent endothelium and a mixed population of small lymphocytes, immunoblasts, plasma cells, histiocytes, and sometimes eosinophils (35,36,43,46). Increased numbers of neutrophils also may be seen (37). The subcapsular sinuses are usually patent and contain histiocytes admixed with scattered neutrophils, lymphocytes, and erythrocytes. Multinucleated giant cells of the Warthin-Finkeldy type, which are identified in 9% to 25% of lymph nodes exhibiting florid follicular hyperplasia, are seen in the follicular or interfollicular areas (34,43,50). Hemophagocytosis also has been identified in lymph nodes displaying florid follicular hyperplasia (43). Rarely, foci of necrosis or noncaseating granulomas, with no organisms identified by special stains, have been identified (31). Some lymph nodes display the classic triad of toxoplasmic lymphadenitis comprising follicular hyperplasia, sinusoidal monocytoid B cells, and epithelioid histiocytes that encroach

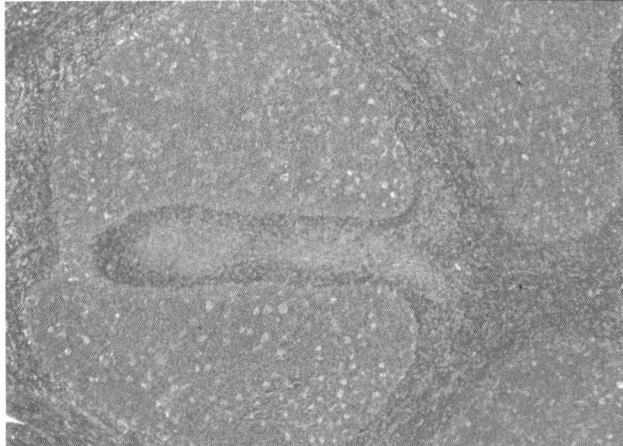

FIGURE 25.2. HIV-related florid follicular hyperplasia. The large hyperplastic follicles have a prominent starry-sky appearance caused by the presence of numerous tingible body macrophages and abundant mitotic figures, indicative of a high rate of proliferation. Adjacent to this hyperplastic follicle is a zone of monocytoid B cells (hematoxylin and eosin stain, original magnification: 40× magnification).

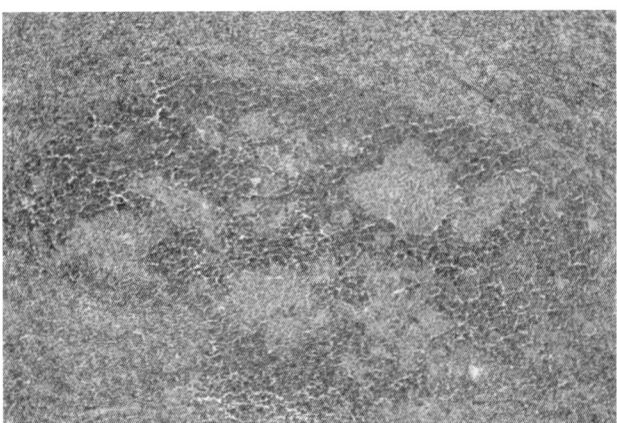

FIGURE 25.4. Follicular lysis. This hyperplastic follicle has undergone follicle lysis characterized by the infiltration of small lymphocytes into the germinal center, accompanied by hemorrhage, resulting in formation of irregularly shaped clusters of follicle center cells (hematoxylin and eosin stain, original magnification: 63× magnification).

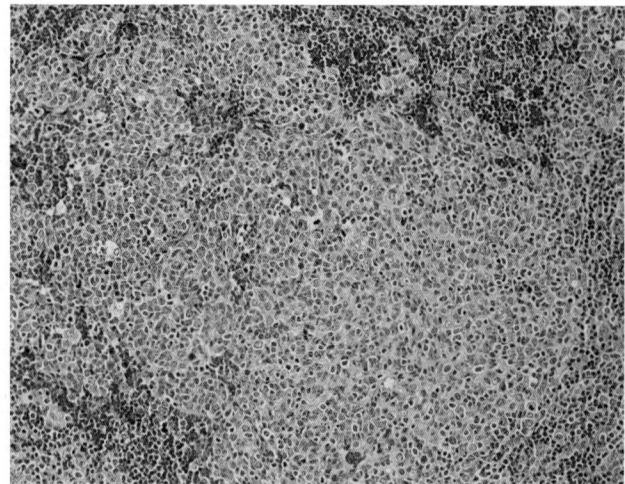

FIGURE 25.5. HIV-related florid follicular hyperplasia. The irregularly shaped clusters of large transformed follicle center B cells may be confused with malignant lymphoma (hematoxylin and eosin stain, original magnification: 250× magnification).

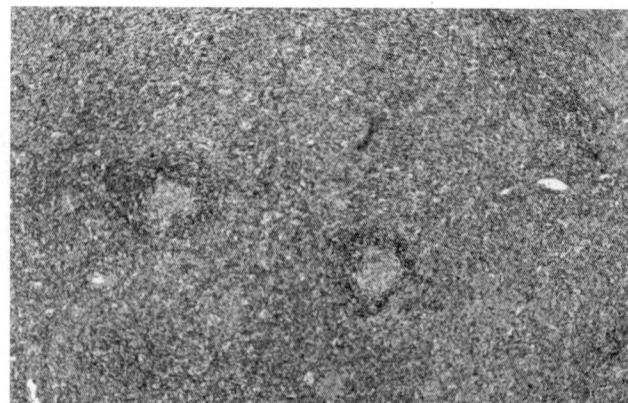

FIGURE 25.6. HIV-related follicular involution. The germinal centers are small, atrophic, and hypocellular (hematoxylin and eosin stain, original magnification: 100× magnification).

on the follicles (50). Focal dermatopathic change, with or without melanin pigment, has been seen in lymph nodes exhibiting florid follicular hyperplasia, even in patients without skin lesions (50). Lymph nodes displaying florid follicular hyperplasia also may have foci of KS. These can be focal, present only in the subcapsular sinuses or along the perivascular septa, or partially replace the lymph node parenchyma (30,34,38).

Several of the histologic features of lymph nodes exhibiting florid follicular hyperplasia have been thought to be highly characteristic of HIV-related lymphadenopathy (54–56). However, comparison of lymph nodes from patients at risk for AIDS with those from patients without AIDS risk factors has shown that few, if any, of these morphologic findings are specific for HIV-related lymphadenopathy (54–56). Polykaryocytes, large and irregularly shaped hyperplastic follicles, sinusoidal monocytoid B cells, and effaced mantle zones all have been reported to occur statistically significantly more often in patients who have AIDS risk factors (55,56). Studies also have found, however, that multinucleated cells in lymph nodes from HIV-infected persons are present too infrequently to be of much diagnostic significance. Although mantle zone effacement, sinusoidal monocytoid B cells, and large, irregularly shaped hyperplastic follicles occur more frequently in patients who have persistent generalized lymphadenopathy, these features are also seen in a significant number of lymph nodes from patients who have no AIDS risk factors. Monocytoid B cells, for example, represent one of the three diagnostic features of toxoplasmic lymphadenitis (57). Furthermore, follicle lysis, which was first described in patients at risk for AIDS (50), may occur in follicular hyperplasia not associated with HIV infection. Nonetheless, this constellation of histopathologic features, if present in the correct clinical and epidemiologic setting, can be considered highly suggestive of HIV-related lymphadenopathy (54,55).

Mixed Follicular Hyperplasia and Follicular Involution

Mixed follicular hyperplasia and follicular involution is histologically transitional between florid follicular hyperplasia and follicular involution (34,38,44). Grossly, the lymph nodes usually are enlarged (36). A combination of histopathologic features that encompasses those characteristic of florid follicular hyperplasia and follicular involution are observed (46,51,58). The lymph nodes contain distinct areas of florid follicular hyperplasia, with large, irregularly shaped germinal centers that account for less than two-thirds of the cross-sectional area

of the lymph node (37) and areas of follicular involution, with small, hyalinized follicles (46,51,58) (Fig. 25.6). The mantle zones surrounding the large follicles are effaced, as in florid follicular hyperplasia; those surrounding the involuted follicles may be thick, thin, or absent (58). In most patients, the percentage of involuted follicles does not exceed 50% of the total number of germinal centers (58). The interfollicular area appears expanded, compared with florid follicular hyperplasia, and widely separates the follicles (37,51,58). Vascular proliferation (which is most prominent around the germinal centers), lymphocytes, plasma cells, immunoblasts, and histiocytes are evident in the interfollicular area (37,44,51). In some patients, however, lymphocytes are relatively depleted throughout the lymph node, especially compared with patients with florid follicular hyperplasia (44,46). Foci of sinusoidal monocytoid B cells are seen in over 80% of cases (37). Warthin-Finkeldy–type giant cells also are seen occasionally (51).

Follicular Involution

In contrast to florid follicular hyperplasia, the germinal centers in lymph nodes exhibiting follicular involution are small, atrophic, and hypocellular (34,36,38,41,43,44,58) (Fig. 25.7). The involuted germinal centers are hyalinized or epithelialized and consist primarily of concentric layers of follicular dendritic cells and occasional follicle center cells (35,38,44,46,50,58). Sometimes, only a fibrous scar remains of what once was a follicle

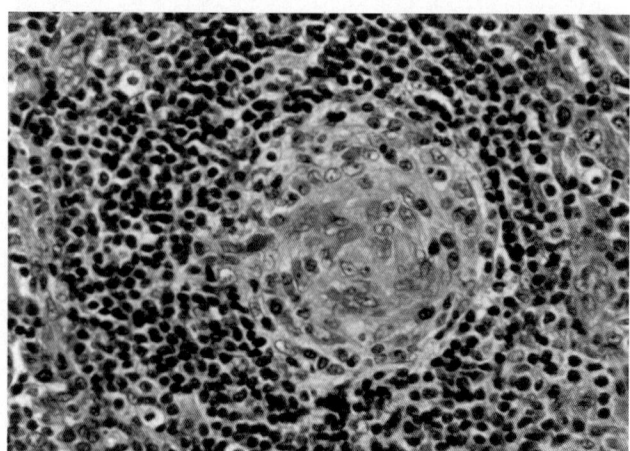

FIGURE 25.7. HIV-related follicular involution. This small atrophic germinal center contains a penetrating hyalinized blood vessel and is surrounded by a thin mantle zone (hematoxylin and eosin stain, original magnification: 250× magnification).

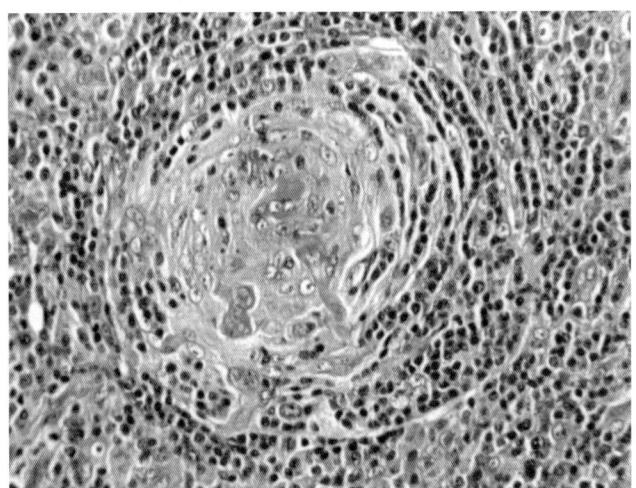

FIGURE 25.8. HIV-related follicular involution. The involuted germinal centers consist primarily of concentric layers of follicular dendritic cells, often contain penetrating hyalinized blood vessels, and are surrounded by concentric layers of small lymphocytes that mimic the appearance of the germinal centers frequently seen in Castleman disease (hematoxylin and eosin stain, original magnification: 250× magnification).

(43,51). Small hyalinized blood vessels penetrate the atrophic germinal centers, often at right angles, resembling those seen in Castleman disease (36,44,58) (Fig. 25.8). Some of the follicles have a rim of small mantle zone lymphocytes; others do not; the latter consist only of "naked" germinal centers (36). Extracellular hyalinized eosinophilic material that stains with the periodic acid-Schiff stain sometimes is associated with the atrophic follicles (34,36,41,44).

The interfollicular area is expanded widely and yet is lymphoid depleted (38,41,44,50,52). Although small lymphocytes remain the major cell type in the paracortical area, they are decreased in number and are associated with an increased number of histiocytes and plasma cells (34,38,41,44,45). Occasionally, Russell bodies are seen (43). Normal numbers of immunoblasts as well as mast cells, eosinophils, and scattered mitotic figures also are identified in the interfollicular areas (41,43,51). Warthin-Finkeldy–like polykaryocytes are identified in 50% to 70% of lymph nodes exhibiting HIV-related follicular involution (30,43,51). Vascular proliferation with endothelial cell hyperplasia and fibrous thickening of the vessel walls is prominent (41,43–45,51). Many of these vessels are the size of postcapillary venules, and the number of lymphocytes that traverses them is increased (43,45). Sinus histiocytosis may or may not be prominent (41,43,45,51); however, neutrophils as well as histiocytes can be identified within the sinuses (41). In some lymph nodes, increased amounts of background eosinophilic material, which may represent necrotic debris (35), are present, and there may be fibrosis of the medullary region (43). Fibrosis of the lymph node capsule is often present (43,45,51), and this occasionally extends down into and obliterates the subcapsular sinuses (30,45). Erythrophagocytosis has been identified in 13% of patients with follicular involution (43).

The histologic picture of HIV-related follicular involution may be confused with the hyaline vascular form of Castleman disease and angioimmunoblastic lymphadenopathy, because many of the morphologic features, such as hyalinized atrophic follicles, expanded interfollicular areas, and prominent vascular proliferation, are shared by all these entities. Furthermore, HIV-infected individuals who have the follicular involution phase of HIV-related lymphadenopathy and HIV-uninfected individuals who have Castleman disease or angioimmunoblastic lymphadenopathy share many clinical features (38,58–62).

For these reasons, it is not surprising that there have been several reports describing the occurrence of Castleman disease and angioimmunoblastic lymphadenopathy in young HIV-seropositive homosexual men, many of whom also have KS (63–68). Most of these cases were reported early in the AIDS epidemic, prior to widespread awareness of the follicular involution pattern of HIV-related lymphadenopathy. In all probability, most of these cases represent HIV-related follicular involution and not Castleman disease or angioimmunoblastic lymphadenopathy.

There is a strong association between the Kaposi sarcoma–associated herpesvirus (KSHV) and multicentric Castleman disease (MCD) in both HIV-infected and HIV-uninfected individuals, including those with and those without KS (69,70). Although the histologic features of HIV-related follicular involution and KSHV-associated MCD in HIV-seropositive individuals are very similar, morphologic differences between the two entities exist (71). Lack of concentric layers of mantle cells surrounding atrophic germinal centers and marked lymphoid depletion are more suggestive of HIV-related follicular involution, and increases in hyalinized blood vessels and plasma cells are more suggestive of KSHV-associated MCD in an HIV-infected individual (71). Many HIV-seropositive individuals who have benign lymphadenopathy exhibiting the follicular involution pattern are not infected with KSHV. These findings suggest that MCD is a separate entity, even if it occurs in HIV-seropositive individuals, and is distinct from the follicular involution and other histologic patterns of HIV-related lymphadenopathy. HIV-seropositive individuals in all stages of HIV disease may be KSHV-infected, and it is possible to identify KSHV-infected individuals who have HIV-related lymphadenopathy exhibiting any of the four histopathologic patterns, that is, florid follicular hyperplasia, mixed follicular hyperplasia and involution, follicular involution, or lymphocyte depletion. Both Castleman disease and angioimmunoblastic lymphadenopathy exhibit relatively constant histopathologic patterns in separate lymph node biopsies obtained several months apart from the same patient (59–61). In contrast, HIV-related lymphadenopathy is in dynamic evolution: Progressive changes in lymph node histopathology correlate with a constantly changing clinical picture that parallels the patient's deteriorating immune status. HIV-related follicular involution is only one of several histopathologic patterns seen in the dynamic continuum of HIV-related lymphadenopathy (38,44).

Lymphocyte Depletion

The lymph nodes in HIV-seropositive persons who exhibit lymphocyte depletion usually are obtained at autopsy (72). Grossly, the lymph nodes are small, usually measuring <1.0 cm in diameter (46). Histologically, the lymph nodes are characterized by severe lymphoid depletion and a complete loss of germinal centers (34,38,43,46,72). They are composed primarily of medullary cords and sinusoids (38,43,72). Subcapsular and sinusoidal fibrosis is present, with focal hyaline deposits in sites of degenerated follicles (34,38,72) (Fig. 25.9). The lymph nodes are populated primarily by histiocytes, plasma cells, and scattered immunoblasts (34,38,43). Some of the plasma cells are large and atypical; they may contain multiple nuclei and display bizarre shapes (43). Russell bodies sometimes are also seen (43,72). Sinus histiocytosis can be extensive (41). Phagocytosis of blood cells, including erythrocytes, neutrophils, and lymphocytes, by sinus histiocytes can be seen in up to 90% of lymphocyte-depleted lymph nodes (43). The venules are usually thin-walled and contain few, if any, transversing lymphocytes (43). Small lymphocytes, lying either singly or in small clusters, can be identified scattered diffusely throughout lymphocyte-depleted lymph nodes (41,43).

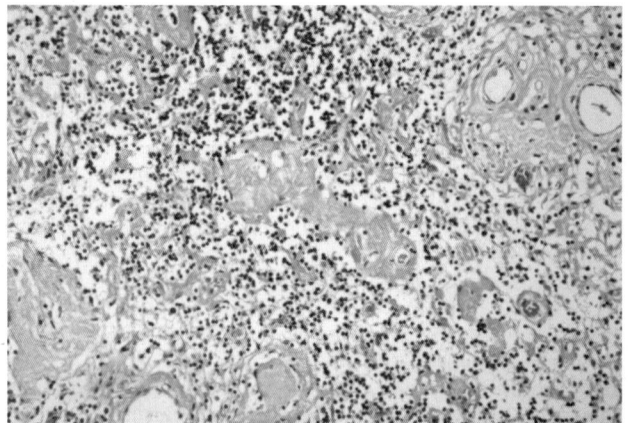

FIGURE 25.9. HIV-related lymphocyte depletion. The lymph node displays severe lymphoid depletion, a total loss of germinal centers, and focal hyaline deposits in sites of degenerated follicles. The cell population is composed largely of histiocytes and plasma cells, with scattered immunoblasts (hematoxylin and eosin stain, original magnification: 250× magnification).

Mycobacterial Lymphadenitis

Some investigators believe that lymph nodes that are totally replaced by infectious organisms, such as *Mycobacterium avium intracellulare*, should be classified as lymphocyte-depleted lymph nodes (41,46). In patients with HIV–associated atypical mycobacterial infection, particularly with *M. avium-intracellulare*, the infection may become disseminated and frequently involves lymph nodes. Numerous histiocytes are present, which do not form well-defined granulomas, and these contain large numbers of acid-fast bacteria easily identified with Ziehl-Neelsen and related stains. The histiocytes may become spindled and can be confused with soft tissue neoplasms, hence the descriptive term "spindle-cell pseudotumor" for this appearance (Fig. 25.10A and B).

Ultrastructure

The human immunodeficiency virions have been characterized ultrastructurally as 80- to 120-nm particles containing a central core composed of the viral p24 gag capsid protein. The majority of virions contain one cone-shaped core measuring 60 nm

at the broad end (which contains the viral RNA) and 20 nm at the narrow end (73,74). A small percentage of virions contain a single tubular-shaped core approximately 40 nm in diameter. Two to several cores, however, cone-shaped, tubular-shaped, or both, may be present in one virion (74). Irregularly shaped electron-dense masses, known as *lateral bodies*, are situated parallel to the long axis of the core and appear to be continuous with the membrane-associated matrix protein (MA) shell. This p17 MA, which is about 7 nm thick, is tightly bound to the inner layer of the viral envelope. This intimate attachment is necessary for viral budding (74). The HIV viral envelope is studded with 72 9- to 10-nm-long envelope glycoprotein projections, known as *knobs*, which are arranged symmetrically on the viral surface. The knobs consist of oligomers (probably trimers composed of the surface envelope glycoprotein, gp120, and the transmembrane protein, gp41) (74–76). Progressive loss of these knobs, which are shed from the viral surface at a rate dependent on strain, virion age, and temperature, is associated with a gradual decrease in infectivity. It is thought that a minimal number of knobs are necessary for a virion to be infectious (74,77). The mechanism by which HIV actually enters the cell is still unclear. Thin-section electron microscopic studies have demonstrated both direct fusion and receptor-mediated uptake of the virus into the cell (74,76). In addition, HIV can be transmitted either by syncytium formation or by cell-to-cell contact without cell membrane fusion.

Systemic dissemination occurs during the acute phase of HIV infection, which covers a period of approximately 3 to 6 weeks after initial infection (78). Virus has been found in lymphoid organs within 1 week of infection and prior to seroconversion in animal models of simian immunodeficiency virus (SIV) infection (78). Human immunodeficiency virus has been identified in a variety of lymphoid organs, including lymph nodes, tonsils, spleen, and thymus, as early as 2 weeks after seroconversion (79,80). During the early and clinically latent stages of the disease, viral particles have been found primarily in the germinal centers of lymph nodes, in which they have been identified most commonly along the cellular processes of the follicular dendritic cells (78,80–86). During the latent stage the viral load associated with follicular dendritic cells is thought to be 100- to 10,000-fold greater than in the peripheral blood. Most studies examining lymph nodes obtained from HIV-infected individuals have identified virions in the extracellular spaces between the dendritic cells, usually complexed with antibody and complement. Some studies have reported viral budding from follicular

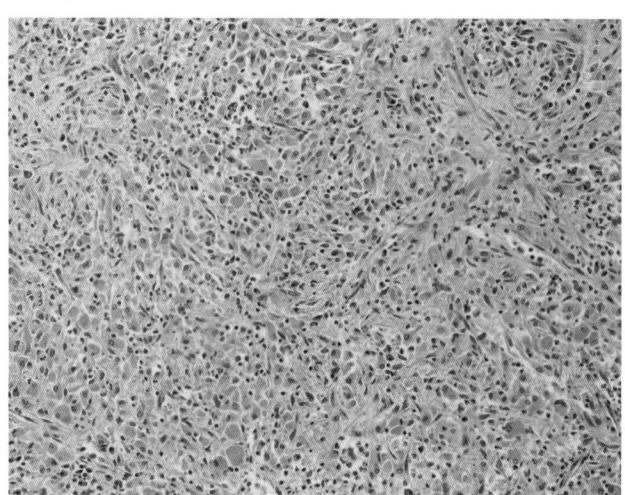
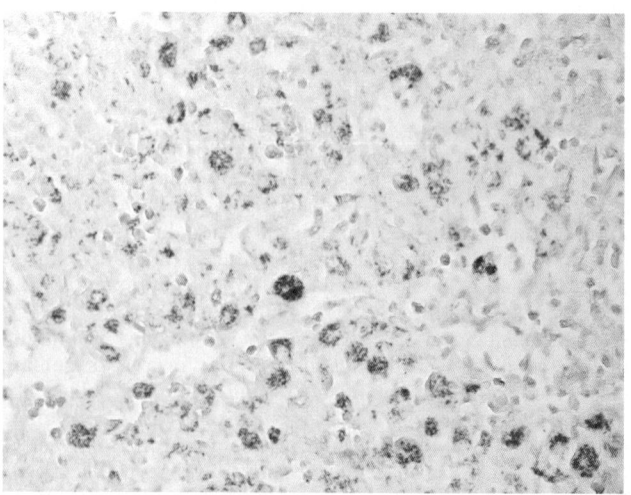

FIGURE 25.10 A,B: Lymph node is replaced by histiocytes and spindle cells imparting a lymphocyte depleted and pseudosarcomatous appearance **(A)**. The acid-fast stain reveals that the histiocytes are filled with bacilli **(B)**. **(A**, hematoxylin and eosin, 200× magnification; **B**, acid-fast stain, 400×).

dendritic cells; others have found immune-complexed viral proteins or complete virus within these cells (80–89). Whether the follicular dendritic cells are infected by HIV directly or only trap the virus, it is clear that the destruction of these cells, as demonstrated by ultrastructural studies, is an important factor in the pathobiology and clinical behavior of HIV disease. Early in HIV infection the follicular dendritic cells may resemble those seen in the hyperplastic follicles of lymph nodes obtained from HIV-uninfected individuals. In most lymph nodes morphologically classified as representing florid follicular hyperplasia, however, the labyrinthine structure is expanded and may be composed of hyperplastic follicular dendritic cells. The follicular dendritic cell cytoplasmic extensions are more voluminous and extensive than those found in most reactive lymph nodes in HIV-uninfected individuals. In addition, the dendritic meshwork often contains relatively large groups of blast cells between the cellular extensions. Within the cells the rough endoplasmic reticulum cisterns are often swollen, and increased numbers of lysosomes are present (90). Numerous viral particles are seen in association with the dendritic processes (82,86,91). At this stage there is little or no evidence of cytolysis of the follicular dendritic cells (90,92–94). As HIV disease progresses, fragmentation, degeneration, and lysis of the follicular dendritic cells occur (85,88). The cause of follicular dendritic cell destruction is unclear. Several hypotheses have been suggested, including HIV-mediated mitochondrial damage, abnormal cytokine production, viral or viral product toxicity, and cytotoxic T-cell destruction (80,86,89,95–97). The ultrastructural destruction of the follicular dendritic cells, however, is associated with disease progression, follicle involution, and loss of virus-trapping capability (78,85,88). The stage of lymphocyte depletion is associated with virtual loss of follicular dendritic cells (85).

Although the majority of HIV has been identified ultrastructurally within germinal centers associated with follicular dendritic cells, HIV has been identified in other cell types within lymph nodes, primarily by *in situ* hybridization (ISH) or immunohistochemistry (78,79,88,98). Prior to destruction of the follicular dendritic cells, HIV is only rarely, if ever, identified ultrastructurally outside of the germinal center (84,85). Once the dendritic meshwork has been destroyed, however, HIV particles often are observed scattered throughout the lymph node, where they are found most frequently in macrophages (99). Viral particles also have been seen rarely within endothelial cells and mononuclear cells, often associated with the endoplasmic reticulum (10,97). Tubuloreticular structures and test tube– and ring-shaped forms, also known as *cylindric conformational cisternae*, have been identified frequently in cells populating the lymph nodes of HIV-infected individuals (47,82,84,100). The percentage of cells containing these structures and forms appears to increase with HIV disease progression (100). The tuboreticular structures seen in HIV-infected patients are intracellular structures composed of anastomosing tubules measuring 24 nm in diameter, and are located within the cisternae of the endoplasmic reticulum (100). These structures also have been associated with other viral infections and autoimmune diseases (100–102). The test tube– and ring-shaped forms are observed less commonly than tuboreticular structures (100). They are tubal in appearance on longitudinal section and ring-shaped on cross section. They are composed of two or more cisternae of endoplasmic reticulum, one inside the other, separated by a 24-nm layer of electron-dense material (100). The tuboreticular structures and test tube– and ring-shaped forms are found most frequently in lymphocytes, monocytes, and endothelial cells, but they also have been identified in macrophages, plasma cells, interdigitating dendritic cells, and follicular dendritic cells (84,100). Initially, they were thought to represent viral constituents and to possess diagnostic significance (100); it is now believed that they arise from

the rough endoplasmic reticulum membrane in the setting of elevated interferon-α levels (103,104). They are mentioned here primarily for historical interest.

Immunoarchitecture

The immunoarchitecture of lymph nodes exhibiting florid follicular hyperplasia in HIV-infected persons in some ways is similar to, and in other ways is distinctly different from, that of lymph nodes exhibiting follicular hyperplasia attributable to other causes. In both HIV-seropositive and HIV-uninfected individuals the transformed germinal center B (GCB) cells present in such lymph nodes are polyclonal (34,52,105). In HIV-seropositive individuals, however, the germinal centers of such lymph nodes contain increased numbers of T cells, in contrast to those in HIV-negative persons (40,47,106–108). These T cells, nearly all of which are CD8 positive, are present in small clusters around small penetrating blood vessels or are scattered diffusely throughout the follicles (51,107–112). The CD8 T cells present within the germinal centers almost exclusively represent CD45RO$^+$ memory T cells (113). Early reports suggested that these cells are suppressor T cells, based on their lack of CD28 expression (106). More recent studies, however, have demonstrated increased levels of cytotoxic T-cell–associated enzymes and proteins such as TIA-1, serine esterase B, granzyme B, and perforin in the follicles of HIV-positive individuals compared with HIV-uninfected persons, indicating that they most likely are cytotoxic CD8 T cells (96,107,108,110). The lack of CD28 expression by intrafollicular cytotoxic CD8 T cells may be explained in part by the progressive down-regulation and eventual loss of surface CD28 antigen expression by both CD4 and CD8 T cells during the course of HIV infection (114,115). The increase in CD8 T cells results in a marked decrease in the intrafollicular CD4:CD8 T-cell ratio from the normal range of >10:1 to not more than 2.5:1 (48,106,109,112,116). The number of CD4$^+$ T cells present within the germinal centers has been reported to be approximately the same, slightly increased, or decreased compared with non–HIV-related follicular hyperplasia (34,47,48,106,112,116–118). Approximately 30% to 50% of these CD4$^+$ T cells express CD57 (116,118). These CD4$^+$CD57$^+$ T cells appear to be the most abundant productively HIV-infected cells within the germinal centers of lymph nodes exhibiting florid follicular hyperplasia (118).

The destruction of the follicular dendritic cell meshwork is a consistent immunoarchitectural feature of HIV-related lymphadenopathy. Immunostaining with a variety of monoclonal antibodies such as anti-DRC-1, anti-CD21, and anti-CD35 shows that the usual interwoven concentric pattern of the follicular dendritic cell meshwork is lost (34,36,51,52,87,88,94,108,111, 117,119). In HIV-related florid follicular hyperplasia this meshwork is disrupted extensively with focal areas of negative staining that correspond to areas infiltrated by small lymphocytes as seen in routine histologic sections (34,36,41,52,86,94,98,111, 117,120). In other germinal centers, the follicular dendritic cell meshwork is destroyed completely, leaving behind only residual small clusters of cells exhibiting loss of their cytoplasmic dendritic extensions (51,118). It is not completely clear why or how the follicular dendritic cell meshwork is destroyed during the course of HIV infection (107,108). Both a direct cytolytic effect of the virus, either by lytic infection of the follicular dendritic cells or by the lytic action of entrapped viral antigens, and lysis by cytotoxic T cells have been suggested as mechanisms of follicular dendritic cell destruction (36,87,96,107,108,110,113,121). Some investigators have suggested that HIV, through a complex and incompletely understood mechanism, is directly responsible for the death of the follicular dendritic cells and dissolution of the meshwork (36,51,80,105,117,118). Within weeks of seroconversion, scattered viral particles are seen within germinal centers (80), and immunostaining for HIV p17 and p24 proteins and follicular dendritic cell–associated antigens has shown identical staining patterns within the germinal centers (98,110, 111,116,118,120,122,123), indicating an intimate relationship between the virus and the follicular dendritic cells. Although follicular dendritic cells generally are CD4 negative (124), they occasionally express CD4 (52,105,125) and can be infected by HIV *in vitro* (126,127). Along with the identification of budding viral particles by electron microscopy and the localization of viral DNA and mRNA by ISH within the cells, this suggests that follicular dendritic cells can be productively infected by HIV (80,82,86,87,107,128). In time, this may lead to direct cell lysis. Furthermore, the association of free cytoplasmic virus and the presence of cellular degenerative changes, particularly involving the mitochondria, suggests that HIV directly damages follicular dendritic cells (86,97). However, arguing against the notion that a direct cytopathic effect of HIV significantly contributes to the destruction of follicular dendritic cells in most instances, HIV is more frequently found in the intrafollicular dendritic cell spaces and not within the follicular dendritic cells themselves (34,84,88,92,117,122). In addition, recent studies have identified a second, much smaller population of dendritic cells within lymph node germinal centers that expresses CD4 and is thought to be derived from peripheral blood dendritic cells (129).

In HIV infection, there is a significant increase in the number of intrafollicular CD8 T cells, which frequently are found in clusters in the areas of negative immunostaining within the follicular dendritic cell meshwork, suggesting that the follicular dendritic cells are destroyed by these cells (34,80,116). The follicular dendritic cells most likely are destroyed as innocent bystanders. The intrafollicular CD8 T cells, the majority of which are cytotoxic T cells based on the expression of TIA-1, perforin, serine esterase B, and granzyme (95,96,108,110,113), are thought to be recruited to the germinal center by a chemotactic effect of HIV or specific HIV components (130). These clusters of cytotoxic T cells often contain HIV p24 antigen–positive cells (116). The cytotoxic CD8 T cells may exert lysis through class I restricted lysis after antigen recognition (130). Alternatively, because there is a high degree of similarity between HIV gp41 and gp120 and human class II major histocompatibility complex (MHC) β1 domain and β chain, resulting in a large number of pseudo–class II determinants, the CD8 T-cells may destroy HIV-containing immune complexes attached to the follicular dendritic cells by antibody-dependent cell-mediated cytotoxicity or lysis (130–132). In this instance, follicular dendritic cells theoretically are damaged and eventually destroyed in a retrograde manner, resulting in dissolution of the meshwork (130). Circulating plasmacytoid dendritic cells are major interferon-producing cells in response to viral infections, and these cells have been shown to decrease in patients infected with HIV (133). Clusters of plasmacytoid dendritic cells may be seen in lymph nodes in interfollicular and perivascular locations, and these are increased with decreasing CD4 cell counts and later stages of HIV-related lymphadenopathy (133).

The presence of HIV in the follicular dendritic cell meshwork and its subsequent destruction is a critical component in the pathogenesis of HIV disease. The follicular dendritic cells trap HIV in the form of immune complexes on the surface of the cell membrane (81,88,94,116,123,128,134). This trapped virus is highly infectious and can readily infect CD4$^+$ T cells forming a syncytium, further propagating the infection. Once the follicular dendritic cell meshwork is destroyed, the germinal center no longer has the capability to trap HIV, resulting in a marked increase in the number of circulating virions and the onset of more severe symptoms (78,88). Furthermore, electron microscopic studies have shown that in the majority of lymph nodes displaying florid follicular hyperplasia, the follicular dendritic cells exhibit undifferentiated and regressive morphology that is associated with an inversion in the ratio of GCB-cell blasts (centroblasts to centrocytes) (90). The destruction of the

follicular dendritic cell meshwork and associated imbalance of the microenvironment in the germinal center may contribute to the B-cell dysregulation and functional abnormalities seen in HIV-infected individuals (80,118,135).

HIV has been documented to have direct effects on the B-cell milieu through production of viral proteins, including Nef, and the envelope protein gp120. Nef can suppress activation-induced cytidine deaminase (AID) and antigen-dependent class switching in germinal centers, thereby inhibiting a productive humoral response. In contrast, gp120 can induce B-cell hyperactivation with polyclonal IgG and IgA responses contributing to hypergammaglobulinemia, and possibly causing immune exhaustion. B cells represent the most common cell within the germinal centers of lymph nodes exhibiting florid follicular hyperplasia. These B cells express CD19, CD20, CD22, and IgM or IgG but not IgD (32,36,111,120) and are polyclonal with respect to immunoglobulin light chain determinants (34,52,109,136). These cells also express class II MHC antigens, CD10, CD21, CD38 (weakly), and CD71 (weakly) (52,105,111,120,136). The GCB cells are highly proliferative, with more than 90% in the G_1 or G_2 phases of the cell cycle, as measured by Ki-67 expression (116,117). As the follicular dendritic cell meshwork is destroyed, the number of total B cells and proliferating B cells within the germinal center is reduced (118–120,136). In addition, a significant number of cytoplasmic immunoglobulin-containing follicular center cells (centroblasts and plasma cells) are found within the germinal centers (86,120).

In HIV-related florid follicular hyperplasia, as in other types of follicular hyperplasia, the mantle zone lymphocytes surrounding the germinal centers are polyclonal B cells that express both IgM and IgD (34,35,52,105,136). These mantle zone B cells also express HLA-DR and CD62L and lack CD38 and CD71 (52,105). Mirroring the architectural features of the mantle zones observed on routine histologic sections, immunohistochemical staining shows that these IgM$^+$ and IgD$^+$ B-cell mantle zones are usually disrupted, attenuated, or even focally absent in cases of HIV-related florid follicular hyperplasia (35,36,48,51,105). Small lymphocytes invaginate into the germinal centers, often along small penetrating blood vessels, into areas of negative staining with anti-DRC-1, anti-CD21, or anti-CD35 antibodies (36,52,86,94,111,116). These invaginating lymphocytes are thought by some investigators to be mantle zone B cells associated with a variable number of CD4 or CD8 T cells (41,51,52,111). Other investigators have suggested that most, if not all, of the cells that infiltrate into areas devoid of follicular dendritic cells are T cells (34,36,80,86,111,120). There are decreased numbers of CD4 helper T cells and increased numbers of CD8 suppressor T cells in the mantle cell zone (35,106,137).

Immunophenotypic analysis of the paracortical regions of lymph nodes exhibiting HIV-related florid follicular hyperplasia may show a decrease in the overall number of T cells (106) as a result of the decrease in the number of CD4 helper T cells (106). Although there may be a decrease in the number of CD8$^+$CD28$^+$ cytotoxic T cells, there is usually a significant increase in CD8$^+$CD28$^-$ suppressor T cells, resulting in an overall increase in the number of CD8 T cells in the paracortex (35,40,48,106,108,112,119,138). Increased numbers of serine esterase B–positive and TIA-1$^+$ cells also are found in the paracortex in comparison with HIV-negative control subjects (110), again suggesting that at least some of the CD8 T cells are cytotoxic in nature. It may be that these CD8$^+$CD28$^-$ T cells, similar to those in the follicle, are actually cytotoxic cells that have down-regulated and lost surface CD28 antigen expression secondary to HIV infection (114,115). Only a relatively small increase in the number of granzyme B–positive cells, however, is seen in the paracortical area of lymph nodes exhibiting florid follicular hyperplasia (108).

Early in HIV disease the CD4:CD8 T-cell ratio in lymph nodes may be relatively normal (43). In most cases, the

CD4:CD8 T-cell ratio in the paracortex is decreased or inverted compared with that in HIV-negative control subjects (34,106,109,111,112,117,119). The CD4:CD8 T-cell ratio in the lymph nodes is usually not as low as that in the peripheral blood (36,40,41,94,116). In addition, the number of paracortical CD62L-positive cells is reduced (106). The CD62L antigen is expressed by a wide variety of cell types, including some CD4 and CD8 T cells, NK cells, monocytes, and granulocytes (106). It is the expression of CD62L by the CD4$^+$ T cells, however, that separates the helper T-cell population into two main functional groups: CD4$^+$CD62L$^-$ T cells that help B cells to differentiate and CD4$^+$CD62L$^+$ T cells that are involved in other types of inducer functions (106,138). This relative loss of one of the CD4 T-cell subsets (inducer) and the relative excess of the other subset (helper) may account at least partially for the florid follicular hyperplasia and hypergammaglobulinemia that occurs in HIV-infected individuals (31,106,139).

The sinusoidal monocytoid B cells are polyclonal B cells (53). Interdigitating dendritic cells, as identified by immunostaining with antibodies to CD1 and S-100 protein, are increased in the paracortical regions of lymph nodes from HIV-infected patients (34,40,51,94,111,116,119). These cells may be seen in clusters (36,51) or associated with cytoplasmic IgG-containing CD38$^+$ lymphocytes, immunoblasts, and plasma cells (111,119). This increase may be caused by an influx of interdigitating dendritic cells that present antigen to CD4$^+$ T cells (41,94,123). This is thought by some to indicate the continuous exposure of antigen to T cells that have lost the capacity of adequate responsiveness (94). This increase may not be caused by HIV infection itself but may be secondary to dermatopathic lymphadenopathy attributable to other HIV-related diseases such as dermatopathic KS or HIV-related dermatitis (50,105,138). In addition, the number of NK cells and histiocytes usually are increased in the interfollicular areas of lymph nodes that exhibit HIV-related florid follicular hyperplasia (105,106,119). There is also an increase in the numbers of polyclonal plasma cells in the paracortex (119) and arborizing HLA-DR$^-$, factor VIII$^-$, and ulex-positive blood vessels (111,119).

Immunohistochemistry, ISH, and ISH polymerase chain reaction (PCR) studies have helped localize HIV to specific areas and cells within lymph nodes exhibiting florid follicular hyperplasia. Immunohistochemical staining for the HIV p24 core protein shows a pattern of positive staining in the germinal center that parallels that of immunostaining for follicular dendritic cells using the anti-DRC-1 antibody (86,87,98,110, 111,116,120,123,128,140). A similar pattern and intensity of reactivity in the germinal center can be seen using antibodies to HIV-related core and envelope antigens p15, p17, p18, and gp120 (87,94,116,120,123,128). Immunostaining for gp41 in the germinal center, however, is somewhat less extensive and less intense (87,94,123). Immunostaining for HIV-related antigens outside of the germinal center shows scattered positive cells in the paracortical area, which occasionally are seen in a perivascular location (98). Furthermore, a few p24$^+$ and gp41$^+$ endothelial cells have been observed (94,98,111,123). ISH studies for viral RNA, identifying cells that are infected productively, have demonstrated two patterns of reactivity in lymph nodes displaying HIV-related florid follicular hyperplasia: a diffuse or reticular pattern in the germinal centers (38,81,88,92,110,121,128), which is thought to correlate with the HIV particles present in the extracellular space between the follicular dendritic cells (38,81,92), and an intense, dot-like labeling of scattered individual cells in both the follicular and paracortical areas (38,88,91,94,110,121,123,128). In the majority of studies, the individual positive germinal center cells, which represent the actively replicating HIV-infected cells, have been found to be CD4$^+$CD45RO$^+$CD57$^+$ T cells (81,118,121). The scattered individual viral RNA–positive cells in the paracortical area appear to be CD4$^+$, S-100 protein–positive interdigitating

dendritic cells, or rarely macrophages (81,121). In tonsils and benign lymphoepithelial cysts of the parotid salivary gland, the number of productively infected dendritic cells and macrophages, located primarily in and beneath the epithelium, is increased (121,141), and rare positive marginal sinus cells also have been identified using ISH (116). Although the number of productively infected cells appears to be relatively small as determined using ISH PCR, which identifies viral DNA, and limiting dilution assays, the number of latently infected cells is much higher (81,142). The latently infected CD4$^+$ T cells appear to be present most frequently in and around germinal centers and paracortical regions and around blood vessels (81). In addition, scattered latently infected monocytes and macrophages are also present (81).

Immunohistochemical staining of lymph nodes exhibiting mixed follicular hyperplasia and involution demonstrates a decrease in the number of, and area covered by, follicles, as seen by staining for follicular dendritic cells and B cells (51,119,136). In addition, there is often a decrease in the number and percentage of CD4$^+$ T cells and an increase in the number and percentage of CD8 T cells in the germinal centers, mantle zones, and interfollicular areas, compared with these same areas in lymph nodes exhibiting florid follicular hyperplasia attributable to HIV or other causes (51,119,136). Overall, the percentage of CD3 T cells is increased in the mixed follicular hyperplasia and involution pattern of HIV-related lymphadenopathy, compared with florid follicular hyperplasia (136).

In HIV-related lymph nodes exhibiting follicular involution, immunohistochemical studies show that the follicular remnants consist of only a small number of follicular dendritic cells present in small shrunken nests, associated with few, if any, IgM$^+$ B cells (34,36,51,119,120,143). The number of proliferating cells in the germinal center is low (51,116,120). The number of such lymph nodes containing plasma cells in the germinal centers is increased compared with HIV-related lymph nodes exhibiting florid follicular hyperplasia (120,140). In comparison with lymph nodes from both HIV-negative and HIV-positive individuals who exhibit follicular hyperplasia, the number of CD4$^+$ T cells is decreased and the number of CD8 T cells is increased within the germinal centers (116,119,120). CD68$^+$ macrophages also have been identified within the atrophic germinal centers (119). Furthermore, the expanded interfollicular region contains decreased numbers of T cells based on CD3 expression compared with HIV-negative individuals who have follicular hyperplasia (143). In addition, there is a relative depletion of CD4$^+$ T cells with increased or normal numbers of CD8 T cells (36,41,119) in the interfollicular area, leading to an inverted CD4:CD8 T-cell ratio that varies between 0.6 and 1.1 (112,143). Numerous CD1$^+$ or S-100 protein–positive interdigitating dendritic cells usually are identified, often in the subcapsular area of the paracortex (34,41,51). Histiocytes are present in increased numbers in the interfollicular area (143). Cytoplasmic immunoglobulin-positive plasma cells are seen in aggregates and diffusely scattered throughout the lymph nodes but are most prominent in the medullary area; these cells usually contain polyclonal IgG and only rarely IgM. The number of CD57$^+$ NK cells is not increased over that in control subjects (143), but the number of TIA-1$^+$ CD8$^+$ cells in the interfollicular area is greater than that seen in lymph nodes from HIV-negative individuals (113).

Overall, the percentage of B cells, based on immunostaining for pan–B-cell antigens or surface immunoglobulin, present in cases of follicular involution is approximately the same as in both the florid follicular hyperplasia and mixed follicular hyperplasia and involution patterns of HIV-related lymphadenopathy (120,144). Furthermore, based on morphometric studies, the total B-cell area does not decrease in follicular involution, because the B cells are often present in small clusters or scattered diffusely throughout the lymph nodes (120).

In comparison with florid follicular hyperplasia, however, in which the B cells (follicle center cells) usually express CD10, the B cells present in follicular involution express only pan–B-cell antigens or surface immunoglobulin (120). The overall percentage of T cells, based on CD3 expression, is somewhat increased; the overall percentage of CD4+ cells is decreased or approximately the same (140,142,144) compared with that seen in florid follicular hyperplasia and mixed follicular hyperplasia and involution (120,144).

Viral proteins, as determined by immunohistochemical staining for the p17 and p24 gag proteins, have been identified in at least 80% of lymph nodes exhibiting follicular involution (123); however, the density of these viral proteins is less than in florid follicular hyperplasia (123). ISH for viral RNA shows that the majority of the cells with a positive signal are present in the interfollicular areas of the lymph node (88,123). The number of positive cells in the interfollicular areas is increased compared with that in patients showing florid follicular hyperplasia (88). Furthermore, in contrast with the predominantly diffuse extracellular pattern of reactivity seen in the germinal centers of florid follicular hyperplasia and mixed follicular hyperplasia and involution, only scattered individual positive cells are identified by ISH in the atrophic follicles of follicular involution (145). There is an overall decrease in the number of productively infected cells per area compared with lymph nodes exhibiting florid follicular hyperplasia (99).

Immunohistochemical studies of lymph nodes exhibiting lymphocyte depletion reveal their lymphocyte-depleted state. Variable numbers of T cells are present, either scattered singly or in small groups (41). Most of them are CD8+ T cells; CD4+ T cells are virtually absent (36,41,142). Collections of B cells expressing pan–B-cell markers or immunoglobulin are also present (36,41,123) and may be the predominant cell population (142). In some cases there are numerous polyclonal IgG+ plasma cells, including those cells with Russell bodies (146). In others, the lymph nodes are characterized by fibrosis (146). Immunostaining with anti-DRC-1 demonstrates that virtually no follicular dendritic cells are present (41,87,145). Immunostaining for p17, p24, and gp41 HIV proteins identifies scattered positive cells in the interfollicular area (123); however, they are present in smaller numbers than in lymph nodes displaying florid follicular hyperplasia (123). ISH and ISH PCR studies show that lymphocyte depletion lymph nodes generally contain fewer HIV-positive cells than do lymph nodes that exhibit the other three patterns of HIV-related lymphadenopathy (99,147). The positive cells are dispersed throughout the lymph node but tend to be more concentrated near the subcapsular sinuses (147). Serial section immunostaining, ISH, and ISH PCR indicate that virtually all of the CD4+ cells in lymphocyte depletion lymph nodes are infected productively with HIV (147), reflecting the CD4 T cell and follicular dendritic cell loss characteristic of this stage.

Clinical Correlations

Relatively early in the AIDS epidemic it was realized that the incubation period between initial HIV infection and seroconversion and the development of AIDS can be quite long (148). The institution of antiretroviral therapy and the use of prophylactic medications for a variety of opportunistic infections has been changing the natural history of HIV-related disease (149). Because of these therapeutic advances, the time from seroconversion to the development of opportunistic infections and other HIV-related illnesses has and likely will continue to become even longer (149).

Between 40% and 90% of individuals who are acutely infected with HIV become clinically ill within days to weeks of their initial exposure (78,150). The most common symptoms are fever, fatigue, a maculopapular rash, myalgias, and, in up to 70% of patients, lymphadenopathy (150,151). Following infection,

there is a rapid increase in plasma viremia, which results in dissemination of the virus to the lymphoid tissues (78,150). Dendritic cells are thought to be the initial cellular target of HIV, and lymphoid tissues such as tonsils and adenoids, which are rich in these cells, are thought to facilitate the transmission of the virus to the CD4+ T cells (141,150). The virus is cleared from the blood relatively rapidly by cytotoxic T cells and by follicular dendritic cells that trap viral particles (78,150,151). After the acute infection stage, lymphoid tissue serves as the primary reservoir for HIV and as one of the principal sites for the progressive infection and death of CD4+ T cells (81,88,89,142).

Lymph node histology in HIV-related lymphadenopathy is progressive over the course of HIV-related disease (38,44,61,88,136,144). As the lymph node histology progresses from florid follicular hyperplasia to mixed follicular hyperplasia and follicular involution, to follicular involution, and finally to lymphocyte depletion, there is a progressive loss of follicles and lymphocytes, which can be observed histologically and immunohistochemically. In addition, accompanying the progressive destruction of the follicles, there is a loss of viral trapping by the follicular dendritic cells, resulting in higher levels of circulating virus (78,88) and the redistribution of HIV outside of the lymphoid system (152). It appears that the baseline for this temporal progression is determined early in HIV infection by the level of viremia and CD4 T-cell count after the acute HIV infection stage (153). Specifically, patients who have higher plasma levels of virus and lower CD4 T-cell counts progress more rapidly to AIDS (150,153–156). It is believed that the natural course of the disease can be altered by lowering the viral load and raising the peripheral blood CD4 T-cell count with antiretroviral therapy (150,157,158).

That the histopathologic patterns in the lymph nodes of HIV-seropositive individuals are progressive and predictive of their clinical status was suggested by several studies (34–36,39,42,43,119,159). Only by examining multiple, sequential lymph node biopsy specimens obtained from patients at risk for HIV infection, however, has it been shown definitively that, with only rare exceptions, lymph node histology changes over time in a consistent pattern, from florid follicular hyperplasia to mixed follicular hyperplasia and follicular involution, to follicular involution, to lymphocyte depletion (38,61,136,144). The clinical course of the patients parallels this dynamic morphologic transformation, indicative of the prognostic significance of lymph node histopathology (38,44,119,136). Persons whose lymph nodes display florid follicular hyperplasia or mixed follicular hyperplasia and follicular involution appear to have the best prognosis (38,44,119); they do not appear to develop opportunistic infections or die as long as their lymph nodes display these early histologies. It appears that HIV-infected patients only develop the complications of AIDS after their lymph node histology has progressed to either follicular involution or lymphocyte depletion (38,119,159). No matter how long the lymph node pattern of florid follicular hyperplasia persists in an HIV-infected person, however, at some point the lymph node pattern changes, signaling progression of the disease (38,42). In the era before cART for all patients who had persistent generalized lymphadenopathy, the incidence of AIDS increased after 3 years of lymphadenopathy, leading to a cumulative incidence progression to AIDS of approximately 30% within 5 years (160,161). For those patients who had no other symptoms except persistent generalized lymphadenopathy and who had CD4 T cell counts >400/mm³, the 5-year incidence of developing AIDS was 19%, with none developing AIDS until the 4th year after the onset of lymphadenopathy (161). The lymph nodes of HIV-infected individuals diagnosed with AIDS usually show follicular involution or lymphocyte depletion, especially in those who have opportunistic infections. The impact of cART on this time course of disease progression with respect to type of lymphadenopathy has yet to be determined.

It is often years before HIV-infected individuals whose lymph nodes display florid follicular hyperplasia progress histologically and clinically to AIDS. None of 57 HIV-infected persons who had florid follicular hyperplasia or mixed follicular hyperplasia and follicular involution histologies followed for 1 to 53 months developed AIDS (38,44,144). With longer clinical follow-up (up to 7.2 years after lymph node biopsy), however, 40% to 50% of those whose lymph nodes displayed florid follicular hyperplasia and 65% to 80% of those whose lymph nodes displayed mixed follicular hyperplasia and follicular involution progressed to AIDS (38,44). In addition, the patients whose lymph node histology showed florid follicular hyperplasia had a median duration of survival that varied from 30 to 54 months after lymph node biopsy, whereas the median survival was 30 to 35 months for those who had mixed follicular hyperplasia and follicular involution histology (38,44). The mixed follicular hyperplasia and follicular involution pattern most likely represents a transition from the immunosuppressed florid follicular hyperplasia stage to the immunodeficient follicular involution stage (34,38,46,162). Although most patients are not ill with full-blown AIDS, HIV-infected patients whose lymph nodes display florid follicular hyperplasia and mixed follicular hyperplasia and follicular involution histologies have decreased CD4:CD8 T-cell ratios in both the peripheral blood (0.2 to 1.0) and lymph nodes (0.4 to 3.7) (40–42,44,72,112,142,144). In patients with florid follicular hyperplasia, plasma viremia is at levels that are low or undetectable using coculture techniques (155). A significant amount of virus, however, is detected in the plasma by reverse transcriptase-PCR, although in general the viral load is less than in patients with follicular involution (142).

Histologic progression to follicular involution signals a marked change not only in histology, as evidenced by the loss of hyperplastic germinal centers that have become hyalinized atrophic follicles, but also in the immunologic and clinical status of the HIV-infected person (38,42,44,142,144). A significantly higher percentage of patients who are symptomatic (AIDS-related complex) have follicular involution rather than florid follicular hyperplasia or mixed follicular hyperplasia and follicular involution (36,38,42); the majority of the remaining patients with follicular involution, including 20% to 40% with opportunistic infections, have AIDS at the time of lymph node biopsy (36,38,42,43,142,159,162). Immunologic studies indicate marked immunodeficiency with peripheral blood CD4:CD8 T-cell ratios lower than 0.5 (36,41,42,44,49,142,144) and absolute CD4 T-cell counts that average <400/mm^3 and are frequently <200/mm^3 (44,49,142,144). There is an increase in viral load in the peripheral blood during this stage (88). This plasma viremia is thought to be secondary to the loss of follicular dendritic cells, which trap HIV particles within germinal centers and thereby effectively remove virus from the circulation (78,88). It is also during this stage of histologic progression of HIV-related lymphadenopathy that HIV-infected individuals develop opportunistic infections, with 65% to 95% of patients developing an opportunistic infection a median of <1 year after a lymph node biopsy exhibiting follicular involution. The median duration of survival for patients with follicular involution is also <1 year (38,44). The lymphocyte depletion pattern is seen most commonly in lymph nodes obtained at autopsy but occasionally is seen in *antemortem* lymph node biopsies as well (34,38,41,43,44,146). This pattern appears to reflect the near-complete destruction of the immune system.

Although the development of opportunistic infections and length of survival are predicted by the histopathologic pattern of the lymph nodes, the development of KS and malignant lymphoma are not (38). HIV-infected patients who develop KS can exhibit any one of the four histologic patterns of HIV-related lymphadenopathy (34,38,49). Malignant lymphoma also has been identified in association with all four histologic patterns of HIV-related lymphadenopathy (38,61). Although

HIV-seropositive patients who have KS and florid follicular hyperplasia do not usually live as long as HIV-seropositive patients who have only florid follicular hyperplasia, they live nearly twice as long as those patients diagnosed with AIDS on the basis of an opportunistic infection (38). The immunologic status of AIDS patients who have florid follicular hyperplasia and KS is more like that of HIV-infected individuals who have only florid follicular hyperplasia, as reflected by peripheral blood CD4:CD8 T-cell ratios of 0.7 and 0.5, respectively (48,49,109,142,144). AIDS patients who have opportunistic infections and, therefore, usually follicular involution often have a CD4:CD8 T-cell ratio of <0.2 (142,163). Lymph node histology may be a more important prognostic indicator than the diagnosis of AIDS. The institution of cART in the later stages of HIV disease, however, also can increase CD4 T-cell counts significantly and lower the viral load in both the peripheral blood and lymphoid tissues, resulting in at least partial reconstitution of the immune system (78,164–168) and potentially influencing the temporal progression of the disease and the histologic features of the lymph nodes.

OTHER HIV-ASSOCIATED LESIONS THAT MAY INVOLVE LYMPH NODES

Benign Lymphoepithelial Lesion

The benign lymphoepithelial lesion (BLEL) is a nodular or diffuse salivary gland enlargement characterized histologically by atrophy of salivary gland parenchyma, replacement of ducts by collections of epithelial and myoepithelial cells, and lymphocytic infiltration (169). It occurs most frequently in patients who have autoimmune diseases such as Sjögren syndrome or as an isolated salivary gland lesion caused by periductal sialadenitis, localized autoimmune sialadenitis, or reactive lymphoid proliferation of intraglandular or periglandular lymph nodes (169).

Salivary gland enlargement as a result of apparent BLEL was first recognized in HIV-infected individuals by Ryan et al. (170) in 1985. We now know that this lesion, designated *BLEL* by Smith et al. (169) in 1988, occurs in a small percentage of HIV-infected patients; its significance is unknown. Initially, it was hypothesized that HIV-associated BLELs are related to Sjögren syndrome (171); however, HIV-infected patients who have this lesion lack the signs, symptoms, and laboratory abnormalities of Sjögren syndrome, including antinuclear SS-A and SS-B antibodies as well as rheumatoid factor (172–174). The BLELs occurring in association with HIV infection are bilateral, multiple, and cystic far more frequently than those occurring in Sjögren syndrome (175); HIV-associated BLEL appears to represent a distinctive clinicopathologic subtype of BLEL related to HIV infection. Most investigators believe that HIV-associated BLELs actually arise in incompletely encapsulated intraglandular lymph nodes that contain salivary ducts or acinar inclusions. It is believed that the progressive lymphoid hyperplasia causes obstruction, squamous metaplasia, and cystification of the intranodal ductal structures, eventually resulting in the BLEL (169,173,176–178). According to this hypothesis, HIV-associated BLELs are a localized manifestation of persistent generalized lymphadenopathy. The presence of *EBER1* expression, indicative of latent Epstein-Barr virus (EBV) infection, in the lymphocyte nuclei of HIV-associated BLELs, but not of Sjögren syndrome–related or other BLELs, has been cited in support of this hypothesis (179). Some authors have referred to HIV-associated BLELs as *cystic BLELs* (180) or prefer the term *benign lymphoepithelial cyst* (172,178,181) because of the prominent cyst formation in these cases and their distinction from the BLELs occurring in Sjögren syndrome.

The gross specimens of HIV-associated BLELs are usually 2 to 5 cm in diameter and consist of one or multiple tan, fleshy,

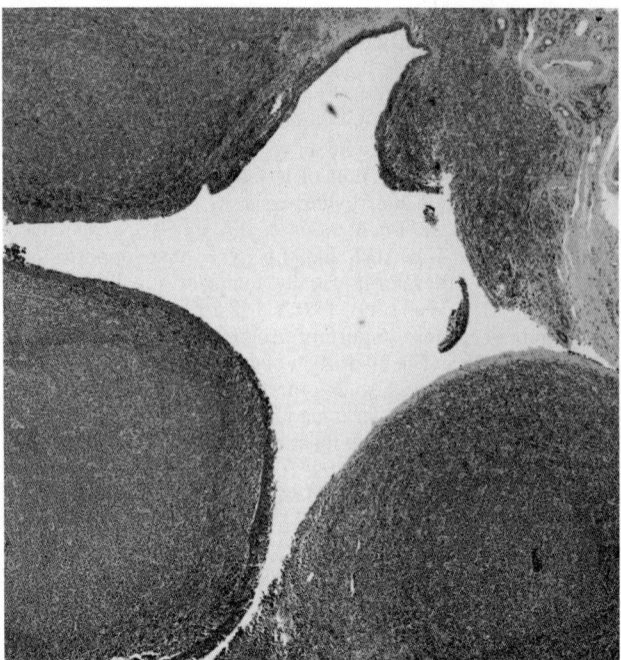

FIGURE 25.11. Salivary gland cyst with epithelial lining and marked lymphoid hyperplasia in the wall. Abnormal germinal centers are noted with attenuated follicular mantles (magnification: 63×).

or rubbery nodules surrounded by varying amounts of salivary gland tissue. Multiple cysts ranging from a few millimeters to 3 cm and containing clear yellow to turbid, watery to gelatinous material are present within the nodules in many of the specimens (169,171,172,177). Stensen duct is normal, without evidence of sialolithiasis or periductal fibrosis in most, if not all, patients (170,177).

Histologically, the nodules are partially to completely delimited by fibrous capsules, beneath which a peripheral sinus may be present focally (169,172). The nodules consist of masses of lymphoid tissue containing epithelial structures of ductal origin embedded within them (169–171,177) (Fig. 25.11). The ducts often are dilated cystically and lined by cuboidal, columnar, or variably keratinized stratified squamous epithelium (169,170,172). The cysts contain pale, eosinophilic homogeneous material (172). Epimyoepithelial islands are present in the majority of patients (169,171–173,177). The lymphoid tissue usually exhibits the histologic features of HIV-related florid follicular hyperplasia: large, irregularly shaped hyperplastic follicles, mantle zone effacement, follicle lysis, interfollicular monocytoid B cells, and Warthin-Finkeldey cells (169,171,173,176). In occasional patients, the lymphoid tissue displays the small shrunken follicles and other histologic features of HIV-related follicular involution (169,170,172). Immunohistochemical studies demonstrate an increase in CD8 T cells, including their presence within germinal centers, and a decrease in CD4 T cells (173,182), similar to HIV-related benign lymphadenopathy (34,40,106,109,119). In addition, CD8 T cells predominate within the epimyoepithelial islands (173). This is in contrast with Sjögren syndrome, in which CD4 T cells predominate (183). The adjacent salivary gland tissue is usually unremarkable, except for interstitial and periductal lymphoid infiltration that appears to represent expansion of the lymphoid cell population and extension through capsular defects (169,173). The intraglandular and periglandular lymph nodes in BLELs exhibit histologic features identical to those of the lymphoid tissue comprising the BLEL nodules (169).

Virtually all the patients who develop HIV-related BLELs are adults, predominantly men and mostly IDUs, with an average age in the late thirties (169,172,174,175,177,184). Members of all AIDS risk groups (169,175,177,184,185), however, apparently even children born to HIV-infected women (185), may develop BLELs. The patients are usually in the early stages of HIV infection, possess CD4 T-cell counts >200/µL, and only rarely have received a prior diagnosis of AIDS (169,175,177,184). BLELs often are the initial manifestation of HIV infection in these individuals (169,177). The patients are usually asymptomatic except for dull aching pain and mild tenderness in the affected area (172,174,175,184). The HIV-infected individuals described as having persistent generalized lymphadenopathy, salivary gland lymphocytic infiltration, and the sicca complex (186,187) likely have the CD8 lymphocytosis syndrome described by Itescu et al. (137,188), and not HIV-associated BLELs. Patients usually complain of unilateral or sometimes bilateral parotid salivary gland enlargement (169,172,177,189,190). Computed tomographic (CT) and magnetic resonance imaging (MRI) demonstrates multiple intraparotid cystic lesions bilaterally, accompanied by bilateral cervical lymphadenopathy in the majority of patients (189,190). The submandibular and submaxillary glands also may be involved (169–171,177). Salivary gland enlargement usually evolves slowly, often over 1 to 4 years (169,177). The majority of the patients have the persistent generalized lymphadenopathy syndrome as well (169,171,173,177), and BLELs develop and persist concurrently with persistent generalized lymphadenopathy in most of them.

A uniform set of recommendations concerning the management of HIV-associated BLELs has not been accepted universally. Superficial parotidectomy (174) or local excision of the lesions (184), which predominantly are located in the tail of the parotid gland (172,184), has been recommended to exclude malignant lymphoma unequivocally and to provide cosmetic improvement and pain relief to the patient. These patients appear to have an indolent clinical course, however. In the largest series with long-term follow-up, almost 50% of patients developed AIDS, at a median interval of 4 years following the diagnosis of HIV-associated BLELs (175). Very few patients develop AIDS-defining conditions within the first 2 years following diagnosis of BLELs (169,170,172,174,175,177). For this reason, observation and periodic fine needle aspiration biopsy has been advocated in the diagnosis and management of asymptomatic lesions that are cosmetically acceptable (175,177). Zidovudine therapy may be helpful in some instances (175). Even if surgically excised, these lesions may recur on the same or on the opposite side (175,176). Malignant lymphoma, and rarely even KS, may originate or present within a HIV-associated BLEL (172,176), and Knowles (unpublished observations, 2001).

Opportunistic Infections

Various opportunistic infectious agents have been identified within the lymph nodes of HIV-infected patients (34,72,191–193). Among the most common infectious agents are *M. avium complex*, *Cryptococcus neoformans*, *Histoplasmosis capsulatum*, and cytomegalovirus. Many other organisms may be seen (34,50,72,191–193). Opportunistic infections are identified in approximately 5% of lymph nodes from HIV-infected persons who have persistent generalized lymphadenopathy and who undergo lymph node biopsy (194). If tissue biopsy and cytology specimens from all sites are evaluated, approximately 42% of HIV-seropositive patients are diagnosed with opportunistic infections prior to death (192). Autopsy studies indicate that up to 95% of the AIDS population has at least one opportunistic infection at death (194,195). The development of opportunistic infections occurs relatively late in the course of HIV infection, when the patients usually have CD4 T-cell counts lower than 400/µL and CD4:CD8 T-cell ratios lower than 0.5 (36,41,42,49,163). In addition, there frequently is clinical regression of the lymphadenopathy 6 to 11 months before the diagnosis of an opportunistic infection (29). Histologically, the lymph nodes in the areas not replaced by organisms usually exhibit either the follicular involution or lymphocyte depletion pattern (30,38,42,43). Prior to the cART era, patients who developed an opportunistic infection, whether in a lymph node or elsewhere in the body, had a median duration of survival of approximately 1 year (46,48).

Grossly, the lymph nodes may be enlarged (34,43) and may be necrotic (34). Histologically, lymph nodes involved by acid-fast bacilli or fungus usually contain poorly formed granulomas consisting of ill-defined collections of histiocytes possessing relatively abundant eosinophilic cytoplasm that, in heavy infections, may replace the entire lymph node (50,194). Granulomas with multinucleated giant cells, palisading histiocytes, caseous necrosis, and other characteristic tissue responses to mycobacteria or fungi occasionally are seen but usually are absent (36,194). Fungal organisms often can be identified on routine tissue sections, with or without a granulomatous response. Special stains, such as methanamine silver, periodic acid-Schiff, and mucicarmine, highlight their presence. Cytomegalovirus inclusions also can be identified within lymph nodes, often within endothelial cells (36,72,194).

It appears that the natural history of at least some opportunistic infections, including their clinical presentation and possibly the histopathologic appearance of the involved lymph nodes, is impacted substantially by cART (149). It was found recently that within a few weeks of initiation of cART some patients who have extremely low CD4 T-cell counts develop fever and lymphadenopathy in the setting of a substantial increase in the CD4 T-cell count and a decrease in the viral load (168,196,197). Lymph node biopsies in these patients, many of whom have no prior history of *M. avium complex*, show the presence of granulomatous inflammation consisting primarily of histiocytes accompanied by a variable number of acute and chronic inflammatory cells (168,196,197). Some of these lymph nodes contain many acid-fast bacilli; others do not. This onset of symptomatic *M. avium complex* infection in patients with improved CD4 T-cell counts is thought to be a result of cART-induced immunorestoration, which results in an inflammatory response to a previously clinically silent infectious organism (149,168,197). A similar phenomenon has been described in cytomegalovirus-related retinitis (149,166). How cART impacts other opportunistic infections, particularly with respect to the presentation and histopathology of opportunistic infection-related lymphadenopathy, has not yet been delineated.

Bacillary Angiomatosis

Bacillary angiomatosis is an uncommon pseudoneoplastic vasoproliferative disorder with an infectious cause. It was first recognized in 1983 by Stoler et al. (198), who observed bacteria within subcutaneous lesions that mimicked KS in an HIV-seropositive man. Four years later, unaware of Stoler's report, Cockerell et al. (199) described the same lesions but failed to recognize their infectious nature, designating them "epithelioid angiomatosis," emphasizing their distinction from KS. LeBoit et al. (200) identified the relationship between these lesions and a cat-scratch disease bacillus–like organism in 1988. One year later they defined the entity histopathologically and coined the term *bacillary angiomatosis* to reflect the infectious and proliferative nature of the lesions (201). This term has been generally accepted as the preferred designation.

Bacillary angiomatosis occurs primarily in HIV-infected individuals (198–203) but has been described in other immunocompromised individuals, including organ transplant recipients (204–206) and individuals who have an underlying malignancy (207–209), and rarely in some apparently healthy immunocompetent hosts (210–213). Bacillary angiomatosis results

from infection by *Bartonella henselae* and *Bartonella quintana* (204,214,215), small Gram-negative bacilli previously classified among the genus *Rochalimaea* (216). These and other organisms belonging to this genus have been associated with an array of diseases besides bacillary angiomatosis, including bacillary peliosis of the liver and spleen, a bacteremic syndrome, cat-scratch disease, and trench fever (217). Bacillary peliosis hepatitis and splenitis are now believed to represent visceral manifestations of bacillary angiomatosis (218). The domestic cat is a reservoir for *B. henselae* (219,220); as many as 40% of cats have been documented to be bacteremic with this organism (220). Exposure to cats and a history of a cat scratch or bite is associated with a significant proportion, although not all, of the cases of bacillary angiomatosis (217,220).

Cutaneous disease is the most frequent clinical manifestation of bacillary angiomatosis (198–201,209,210,213,217,220). Patients usually have multiple and sometimes large numbers, >1,000, of variably sized, superficial, cutaneous red to purple or flesh-colored papules that may mimic pyogenic granulomas and dermal and subcutaneous nodules that may be misinterpreted as KS (198–201,217). Indurated hyperpigmented plaquelike lesions also have been described (221). An occasional patient, especially one who is immunocompetent, may have a solitary or only a few skin lesions (210,213,222,223). The lesions may occur anywhere on the skin surface including on the scalp (223), the palmar and plantar surfaces (220), and the penis (224). They range from 1 mm to several centimeters in diameter. The lesions may be tender or even painful and tend to bleed (217,221). Usually, they increase rapidly in size and number (199,217,221); rarely, they may undergo spontaneous regression (199). Patients often have associated constitutional signs and symptoms, such as fever, chills, malaise, headache, and anorexia, sometimes accompanied by weight loss (203,217,221).

Cutaneous bacillary angiomatosis may be accompanied by mucosal and visceral involvement. Conversely, extracutaneous bacillary angiomatosis often is accompanied by multiple cutaneous lesions, although it may occur in the absence of skin involvement (217). For example, approximately 20% of patients present with lymphadenopathy alone (225). The gastrointestinal and respiratory mucosal surfaces (201,204,214,226–230) and most organ systems have been reported to be involved by bacillary angiomatosis. These include the heart (231), liver and spleen (203–205,211,226,227), bone marrow and lymph nodes (203–206,228–230,232), bones (202), muscles and soft tissues (203,230), female genital tract (233), and even the CNS (203,234). Patients with extracutaneous disease usually have constitutional symptoms, including fever, anorexia, nausea, vomiting, and weight loss (202,217,225,235). They usually suffer from marked immunodeficiency, manifested by severely depressed CD4 T-cell counts (225); some patients have concomitant AIDS-associated opportunistic infections (202,217,225,227,233,236). These findings suggest that bacillary angiomatosis occurs late in the course of HIV infection, and consequently it has been suggested that bacillary angiomatosis should be considered an AIDS-defining opportunistic infection (225). There does not appear to be a predominant AIDS risk factor among individuals who have bacillary angiomatosis (199,225).

The peripheral, mediastinal, and abdominal lymph nodes are the ones most commonly involved by bacillary angiomatosis (203,235). The involved lymph nodes usually are enlarged, firm in consistency, and pale brown to red brown in color (206). Bacillary angiomatosis involves lymph nodes as discrete, variably sized nodules, some of which may coalesce to form large masses. The underlying lymph node architecture may survive intact (206). Cutaneous and extracutaneous bacillary angiomatosis are essentially identical histopathologically. Bacillary angiomatosis characteristically consists of variably sized, circumscribed lobules of small blood vessels, some well-formed, some barely canalized, and some ectatic, that are situated in an alternately mucinous

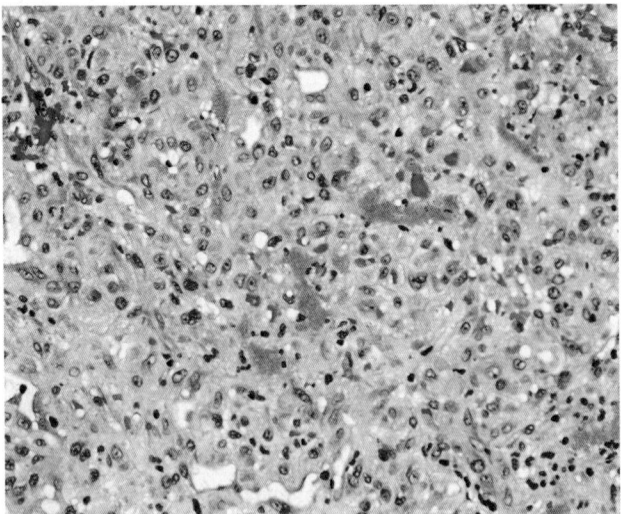

FIGURE 25.12. Bacillary angiomatosis characterized by circumscribed lobules of small blood vessels, some well formed, some barely canalized, and some ectatic. The vessels are lined by protuberant, plump, polygonal endothelial cells with pale cytoplasm, and there are clumps of the causative bacteria (hematoxylin and eosin stain, original magnification: 250× magnification).

and fibrotic stroma. The vessels are lined by protuberant, plump, polygonal endothelial cells that contain abundant pale cytoplasm, and ovoid nuclei containing one to several small nucleoli. They sometimes exhibit mild nuclear pleomorphism and mitotic figures. Occasional polygonal cells exhibiting similar cytologic features, and probably also of endothelial origin, lie between the vessels. Aggregates of granular acidophilic to amphophilic material, which represent clumps and tangled masses of the causative bacteria, lie in the interstitium separating the vessels. Numerous neutrophils, accompanied by leukocytoclastic debris (nuclear dust), usually are scattered throughout the lesions and frequently aggregate around the bacterial clumps (198,199,201,206,209, 217,230,233,237) (Fig. 25.12).

The bacteria can be visualized with the Warthin-Starry stain but not with Gram, methenamine silver, periodic acid-Schiff, or Ziehl-Neelsen stains (198,200,201,206). Electron microscopy can be used to identify the bacteria, which are located extracellularly and exhibit an electron-dense core surrounded by a trilaminar cell wall (198,200,206,230), characteristic of Gram-negative bacilli. *B. henselae* and *B. quintana* are fastidious organisms. They can be cultured from tissue lesions or from the peripheral blood, but this is often technically difficult and time-consuming (210,215,231); this approach is utilized infrequently for clinical diagnosis. Definitive identification of these organisms also can be made by PCR amplification of characteristic genetic sequences (204,215).

The principal differential diagnosis of bacillary angiomatosis involving a lymph node includes KS (206,217), with which it can occur simultaneously in the same patient (202,227,234,237), epithelioid hemangioma, and angiosarcoma (206). Careful assessment of the clinical features of the patient and of the gross appearance and histopathology of the lesions, however, should lead to suspicion of bacillary angiomatosis (217), which can be confirmed readily by Warthin-Starry stain or electron microscopic demonstration of the bacteria (198,200,201,206,217,230). The accurate recognition of bacillary angiomatosis is important because appropriate antibiotic therapy, erythromycin or deoxycycline, leads to regression of both the cutaneous and extracutaneous lesions and resolution of the disease in virtually all patients (217). If bacillary angiomatosis remains undiagnosed or untreated, death may result from local complications, such as laryngeal obstruction (199), or overwhelming disseminated infection (199,203,236).

HIV-RELATED LYMPHOMAS

A long-standing recognition of the relationship between immune deficiency and neoplasia predated infection with HIV (238–240). The incidence of cancer is 100 times greater than expected in individuals who have congenital immune deficiency states such as ataxia-telangiectasia and the Wiscott-Aldrich syndrome; malignant lymphomas comprise the majority of these malignancies (240–242). A spectrum of lymphoproliferative disorders (LPDs), including high-grade malignant lymphomas, also occurs with greatly increased incidence in solid organ transplant recipients, in the setting of iatrogenic immunosuppression and chronic antigenic stimulation (243–245). Malignant lymphomas occur with increased frequency among individuals with acquired autoimmune disorders such as collagen vascular diseases, Sjögren syndrome, and Hashimoto thyroiditis (238,246,247). Recurrent themes among these immunodeficiency-associated malignant lymphomas include origination in or involvement of extranodal and unusual anatomic sites, high-grade histopathology with a tendency toward plasmacytoid differentiation, aggressive clinical behavior, B-cell lineage derivation, and a frequent association with EBV infection (241,243,245).

A broad spectrum of lymphomas may be associated with HIV, usually high-grade B-cell lymphomas of diffuse large B-cell, immunoblastic, or plasmablastic type, Burkitt lymphoma (BL), or Hodgkin lymphoma. These lymphomas naturally occur in the immunocompetent population, but have characteristic features in the setting of HIV. The occurrence of lymphomas in patients with HIV infection relates to the underlying immune suppression and the patient's CD4 T-cell counts. Since the advent of cART the incidence of lymphoma, particularly CNS lymphoma, has declined with improvements in CD4 T-cell counts. Prognosis has also improved with the use of combination chemotherapy in conjunction with antiretroviral treatment. The WHO has classified HIV-associated lymphomas into those also occurring in immunocompetent patients, those occurring more specifically in HIV-positive patients, and those occurring in other immunodeficient states (248) (Table 25.3).

Epidemiology

In May 1982, approximately 1 year after the initial cases of AIDS were described, Doll and List (249) reported an immunocompromised young homosexual man who had BL. A few months later, Ziegler et al. (250–252) reported four additional cases of what was termed Burkitt-like lymphoma occurring in immunocompromised homosexual men. At that time, the relationship between malignant lymphoma and AIDS was

Table 25.3	CLASSIFICATION OF LYMPHOMAS ASSOCIATED WITH HIV INFECTION

Lymphomas also occurring in immunocompetent patients
BL
Diffuse large B-cell lymphoma
Hodgkin lymphoma

Lymphomas occurring more specifically in HIV-positive patients
Primary effusion lymphoma
Plasmablastic lymphoma
Lymphoma arising in HHV8-associated multicentric Castleman disease

Lymphomas occurring in other immunodeficiency states
Polymorphic lymphoid proliferations resembling PTLD

From Raphael M, Said J, Borisch B, et al. Lymphomas associated with HIV infection. In: Swerdlow SH, Campo E, Harris NL, et al., eds. *WHO Classification of tumours of haematopoietic and lymphoid tissues*. Geneva: WHO Press, 2008:340–342.

uncertain. The CDC, however, included the occurrence of primary CNS NHL in persons younger than 60 years of age without a known cause of immunosuppression as an additional criterion for the diagnosis of AIDS in 1982 (253). The CDC excluded NHLs occurring in other sites from the criteria at that time, because malignant lymphoma is known to cause immunosuppression (253). The incidence of clinically aggressive, high-grade NHL in persons at risk for AIDS, however, increased in parallel with the AIDS epidemic. This led the CDC to revise their criteria for the diagnosis of AIDS in 1985 to include HIV-seropositive persons who had diffuse, undifferentiated (Burkitt and Burkitt-like) lymphoma occurring in all anatomic sites (254). A multiinstitutional study of 90 MSM who had malignant lymphoma (252), several large clinical series of AIDS-related malignant lymphoma reported from the endemic areas of Los Angeles (255), Houston (256), and New York City (257–259), and numerous additional reports of smaller numbers of cases of AIDS-related NHL (260–270) led to widespread recognition of this new AIDS-defining malignancy. These reports prompted the CDC to expand its criteria for the diagnosis of AIDS again in 1987 to include all HIV-seropositive persons who had intermediate- or high-grade NHLs of B cell or indeterminate phenotype (254). AIDS-related NHLs displaying comparable clinical, pathologic, and immunologic characteristics were observed with similarly increasing frequency worldwide (271–275). NHL now is recognized widely as the second most common neoplasm occurring among HIV-infected individuals and the most common neoplasm occurring among HIV-infected IDUs and hemophiliacs (270,276). The CDC has calculated the risk of NHL among individuals in the United States to be 60 times greater among those who have AIDS than among those in the general population, and the incidence of NHL in AIDS to be 2.9% (276). This is based on reports of 2,824 NHLs occurring among 97,258 patients with AIDS in the United States reported to the CDC between 1981 and mid-1989 (276). A similar percentage has been reported from Europe (277). Although primary CNS lymphoma and BL have been reportable conditions since 1981, immunoblastic lymphoma has been a reportable condition only since 1985 (254). Immunoblastic lymphoma frequently occurs as a secondary manifestation of AIDS late in the course of HIV infection (278). Once an individual has been diagnosed with the initial AIDS-defining illness, notification regarding subsequent AIDS-defining illnesses is not required by the CDC (276). For this reason, the subsequent development of malignant lymphoma following the initial notification of an AIDS case frequently is not reported to the CDC (276). The magnitude of this underreporting is unclear. Within a cohort of 60 patients reported by Levine et al. (279), for example, 75% of the patients with primary CNS lymphoma and 37% of the patients with systemic lymphoma had been diagnosed with AIDS prior to the development of lymphoma. None of these cases would have been reported to the CDC. In one large teaching hospital in the United Kingdom, malignant lymphoma has accounted for 12% to 16% of all AIDS-related deaths (280), suggesting that the true incidence is higher than 3%. The overall incidence may be further underestimated because the spectrum of AIDS-related illnesses may reduce the likelihood that the diagnosis of malignant lymphoma will be pursued. In several autopsy series of AIDS patients, relatively high rates of previously undiagnosed NHLs, especially primary CNS lymphoma, were identified (281–283). Presumably, many other AIDS-related NHLs go unrecognized because of the failure to perform *postmortem* examinations. Data collected from cohort studies and cancer registries may be more informative regarding the true incidence and risk factors for AIDS-related NHL (284). For these and other reasons, it is clear that the true incidence of AIDS-related NHL has been substantially underestimated. The incidence is more likely to be about 200-fold in excess of expected rates (285), and estimates placing the overall incidence of NHL in AIDS between 4% and 10% probably are more accurate (275,286–288).

Malignant lymphoma appears to be a relatively late manifestation of HIV infection. Epidemiologic studies have demonstrated that the increased incidence of NHL actually lagged behind the emergence of epidemic KS among the young homosexual male population in San Francisco at high risk for AIDS by 1 to 2 years (289). The incidences of KS and opportunistic infections were increased statistically as early as 1981; a true lymphoma epidemic was not defined until 1985 (290). Comparable studies have demonstrated that NHL frequently occurs after KS in immunosuppressed renal allograft recipients. KS and NHL develop in these patients at 16 and 30 months after transplantation, respectively (290). The delay in recognizing NHL as an AIDS-related phenomenon was probably secondary to its delay in presentation relative to other AIDS-defining illnesses. Among a cohort of 1,065 HIV-infected patients with hemophilia, the incidence of NHL increased exponentially as the duration of HIV infection increased, with the risk doubling every 2.4 years (291). These observations support the contention that the incidence of NHL in AIDS has risen steadily as other AIDS-related illnesses have become better controlled and the length of survival following HIV seroconversion has increased (292). Currently, about 10% of all NHLs occurring in the United States are thought to be AIDS-related (287).

In the United States, approximately 3% of patients with AIDS present with malignant lymphoma (287,290,293). In addition to MSM and IDUs, AIDS-related NHLs may develop in individuals of all ages who have been transfused with HIV-infected blood and blood products (251,259,263,276), children born to HIV-infected mothers (276), and the heterosexual partners of HIV-infected persons (276,294,295). The risk of developing NHLs is relatively consistent among all population groups at risk for AIDS (294,295), without regard for geography (276,287), although it is highest in hemophiliacs (276). In the United States, approximately 80% of persons who develop AIDS-related NHLs are MSM, and the majority of the remainder are IDUs, once again predominantly men (259,296). In Western Europe, approximately two-thirds of persons who develop AIDS-related NHLs are IDUs (274,297). This is because MSM and IDUs represent the principal populations at risk for AIDS. The differences between their representation in the United States and Europe reflect the epidemiologic variations in the spread of the AIDS epidemic in these different regions. Similar to the distribution of conventional NHLs occurring in the HIV-uninfected general population, the incidence of AIDS-related NHL appears to be higher in men than in women (276,287), and in whites than in blacks (276). The incidence of AIDS-related NHL appears to increase with age among MSM and hemophiliacs, although not in IDUs (287). The clinicopathologic features of AIDS-related NHLs occurring in the various AIDS risk groups appear to be similar, based on data collected on MSM, IDUs, hemophiliacs, and transfusion recipients from the United States and Europe (252,255,259,276,298–302). One possible exception is that primary oral and anorectal NHLs appear to occur preferentially in MSM (251,255,276,297–300,302).

The AIDS status of patients at the time of diagnosis of AIDS-related NHL has changed over the course of the AIDS epidemic. In the multiinstitutional study published by Ziegler et al. (252) in 1984, 47% of the patients with NHL carried a prior diagnosis of AIDS, based on the presence of severe opportunistic infections, KS, or both. In contrast, in results from a series in San Francisco published in 1989 (299) and a Washington-area study published in 1990 (303), only 27% and 25% of patients, respectively, had received a prior diagnosis of AIDS. These changes may be because of earlier recognition of HIV infection status, changes in risk factors, or the impact of antiretroviral therapy on the natural history of the disease (293,303).

Lymphomas More Specifically Associated with HIV

These include plasmablastic lymphoma of the oral cavity type, primary effusion lymphoma (PEL), the extra cavitary (solid) variant of PEL, and lymphoma arising in KSHV/HHV-8-associated MCD.

Plasmablastic Lymphoma of the Oral Cavity Type

In 1997, Delecluse et al. (304) described a subset of NHLs that displays blastoid morphology and plasma cell–like immunophenotypic features and preferentially occurs in the oral cavity of HIV-infected individuals. They designated these cases *plasmablastic lymphomas* (304) (Fig. 25.13). Among 16 cases, 15 occurred in HIV-infected individuals, consisting of 12 MSM, 1 male IDU, 1 female IDU, and 1 male whose risk factors were unknown. The sole HIV-uninfected individual was an elderly woman. The median age of the patients was 39 years. About one-third of the patients had B symptoms. None had a monoclonal gammopathy. The tumors were localized in the mucosa of the oral cavity, usually in the gingiva but sometimes in the floor of the mouth or the palate. Jaw bone infiltration occurred in one patient. At the time of diagnosis 11 patients had stage IE disease, and the remaining 5 patients had stage IV disease. The lymphoma sometimes extended to involve the abdomen, retroperitoneum, soft tissues of the extremities, and bone marrow. Because this type of plasmablastic lymphoma also occurs outside of the oral cavity in the 2008 WHO classification of HIV-related lymphomas they were classified as plasmablastic lymphoma of the oral cavity type (248,305). Occasional patients who had lymphoma limited to the oral cavity responded well to radiation therapy, but despite multidrug chemotherapy most patients died in 7 months on average, often of unrelated or multiple causes (304).

Most plasmablastic lymphoma associated with HIV infection are extramedullary, clinically aggressive EBV-positive tumors (306). The median age at presentation is 38 years (307). The plasmablastic lymphomas grow diffusely with frequent apoptotic cells or single cell necrosis, but a starry-sky pattern is unusual (306). The lymphoma cells are large and possess abundant, deeply basophilic cytoplasm, eccentrically placed nuclei, and a paranuclear clearing or "hof." The nuclei are round to ovoid and possess little chromatin and either a single prominent, centrally placed nucleolus or several peripherally located nucleoli. The proliferation index is very high, as evidenced by numerous apoptotic figures, single cell necrosis, and mitotic figures with >90% positivity with MAb MIB-1 detecting the Ki-67 protein (304). Some plasmablastic lymphomas have a centroblastic appearance, but exhibit a distinctive immunophenotype characterized by diminished or absent CD45 or CD20 expression and strong immunoreactivity with the monoclonal antiplasma cell antibody VS38c. Approximately one-half of patients display complete absence of CD45 and B-cell lineage–associated antigen CD20. In the remaining one-half of patients, variable proportions of the lymphoma cells weakly express cytoplasmic CD45 or CD20, sometimes accompanied by weak surface membrane expression in a small number of cells. A variable proportion, 5% to 90%, of the lymphoma cells express CD79a. Intracytoplasmic IgG, but not other heavy chain isotypes, is detectable in about one-half of patients. Sometimes this is accompanied by monotypic light chain expression. In all patients, the lymphoma cells exhibit strong immunoreactivity with VS38c. Occasional patients express BCL-6 protein (304). In keeping with the late stages of B-cell differentiation they are usually negative for PAX5 and positive for BLIMP1 (Fig. 25.14). In summary, the plasmablastic lymphomas express immunophenotypic features closer to plasma cells.

About 60% of plasmablastic lymphomas exhibit EBV-encoded nuclear RNA transcripts (EBER), in the absence of EBNA-2 expression, and only extremely small numbers of cells express LMP-1 or BZLF-1 (304). The plasmablastic lymphomas appear to be unrelated to follicular center cell lymphomas and those large cell lymphomas of follicular center cell origin. Approximately 50% are positive for MYC by immunohistochemical stains (Fig. 25.15) and more recently 49% of 42 cases evaluated by fluorescence *in situ* hybridization (FISH) were shown to have MYC translocations, largely involving the Ig genes (308). No translocations of BCL2, BCL6, MALT1, or PAX5 were found.

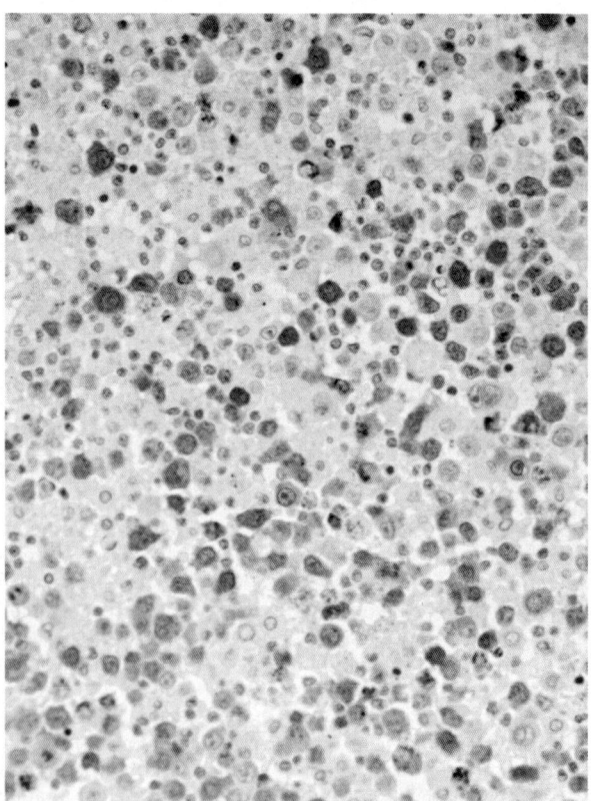

FIGURE 25.14. Plasmablastic lymphoma of the oral cavity type staining for BLIMP1, which is associated with plasma cell differentiation (magnification: 250×.)

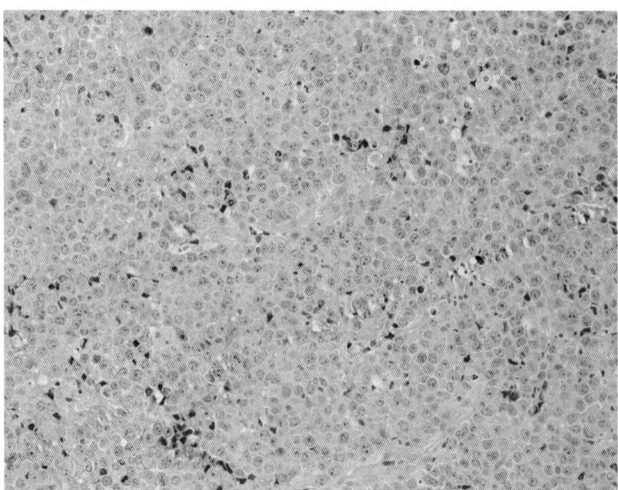

FIGURE 25.13. Plasmablastic lymphoma of the oral cavity type. There are sheets of large lymphoid cells that resemble plasmablasts. The phenotype is that of plasmablasts, negative for CD20 and 45 and positive for CD138 and IRF4/MUM1 (magnification: 250×.)

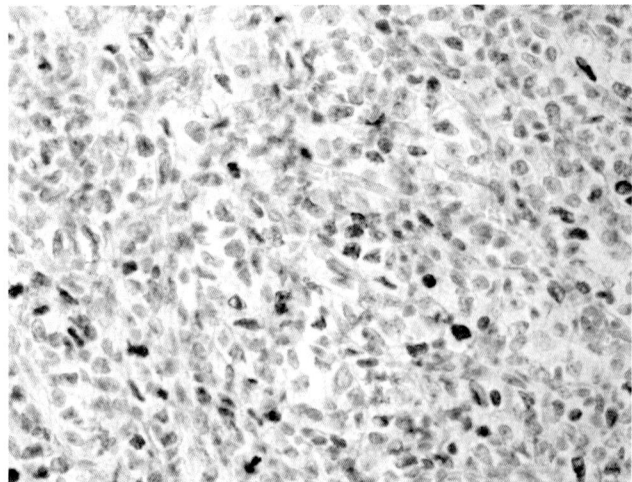

FIGURE 25.15 Plasmablastic lymphoma of the oral cavity type staining for MYC (magnification: 250×.)

The plasmablastic lymphomas appear to exhibit a unique constellation of clinical, morphologic, and immunophenotypic characteristics and represent a distinct clinicopathologic and biologic category of NHLs that is preferentially, but not entirely, associated with AIDS. The blastoid morphology and immunophenotype of these lymphomas suggest that they most closely resemble plasmablasts, cells that still retain the blastoid feature of immunoblasts but already have acquired the antigen profile of plasma cells—hence the designation *plasmablastic lymphoma* (304). These lymphomas may be mistaken for diffuse large B-cell lymphomas with plasmacytoid differentiation or plasmacytomas, but careful attention to their distinctive clinical, morphologic, and immunophenotypic features should result in an accurate diagnosis. Factors that contribute especially to the pathogenesis of these lymphomas are unclear. Not all cases involve EBV, and those that do exhibit an EBV latent gene pattern of expression that is inconsistent with EBV-driven LPDs seen in the posttransplantation setting. The plasmablastic lymphomas also lack KSHV (304). Other than FISH, molecular studies are limited to array comparative genomic hybridization (aCGH) on 16 cases of plasmablastic lymphoma, where multiple segmental gains and some losses were reported (309). Additional molecular genetic analyses of these lymphomas should contribute to our understanding of their pathogenesis and relationship to other categories of NHL.

Primary Effusion Lymphoma

After the discovery of KSHV (310), Cesarman et al. (311) examined DNA extracted from a clinically and pathologically diverse panel of 42 patients with AIDS-related NHLs and 151 with conventional lymphoid neoplasms occurring in HIV-uninfected individuals for the presence of KSHV by Southern blotting, PCR, or both. They discovered KSHV sequences in only eight patients with AIDS-related NHLs. All eight, and only these eight, cases had been classified as body cavity–based lymphomas, subsequently designated PELs. These eight cases included ones that had been reported previously by Knowles et al. (312), Walts et al. (313), and Chadburn et al. (314). None of the remaining 185 DNA samples from patients with AIDS-related and non–AIDS-related NHL, Hodgkin disease (HD), or lymphoid leukemia contained KSHV. Between 40 and 80 copies of KSHV were present per lymphoma cell, in comparison with an average of one copy of KSHV per cell in KS tissue (311). Other investigators from the United States and Europe later confirmed the unique association between KSHV and those AIDS-related NHLs arising as

lymphomatous effusions (315–318). In addition, KSHV-positive PELs were reported in HIV-negative individuals, including women (319,320). Rarely, it has been claimed that KSHV is present in other malignant lymphomas including primary CNS lymphomas (321–323). However, there was a lack of epidemiologic and serologic support for these associations, and dozens of subsequent studies were unable to confirm them. The association of KSHV with hematologic malignancies other than PEL has been attributed to technical artifacts, such as PCR contamination, or the presence of very low copy number resulting from a few KSHV-positive cells infiltrating the tumors (324–326). Some lymphoma associations with KSHV that go beyond classical PEL have stood the power of time: those with features that are very similar to those of PEL, but occurring as solid tumor masses (extracavitary PEL or solid PEL) (327), plasmablastic lymphomas arising in MCD, and the very rare KSHV-associated germinotropic LPD (328). Taken together, these findings underscore the unique nature of PELs and strongly suggest that KSHV plays a role in their pathogenesis. These KSHV-positive lymphomas appear to account for about 3% of all AIDS-related NHLs (316). They also rarely occur in the HIV-uninfected general population, in which they comprise far <1% of all conventional NHLs.

Another infrequently occurring subset of NHLs also arises in the pleural cavity and can be considered body cavity–based lymphomas. These are the pyothorax-associated lymphomas, which have been reported largely from Japan (329,330). The pyothorax-associated lymphomas arise in the pleural cavity following a multiyear history of pyothorax resulting from artificially induced pneumothorax for the treatment of pulmonary tuberculosis or tuberculous pleuritis (329,330). Although they exhibit immunoblastic morphology, are of B-cell origin, and contain EBV, they grow as solid tumor masses instead of as lymphomatous effusions (329–331). However, the pyothorax-associated lymphomas do not contain KSHV (332); thus, the KSHV-containing body cavity–based lymphomas and the pyothorax-associated lymphomas are distinct clinicopathologic entities. This study led to replacing the term *body cavity–based lymphoma* used initially with the term *primary effusion lymphoma*, because the latter term described these KSHV-containing lymphomas more accurately given the known associations at the time and avoided their confusion with other lymphomas that arise in the body cavities, including the pyothorax-associated lymphomas (332,333).

The accepted nomenclature for KSHV-associated lymphomas in body cavities is now PEL, which is clearly a distinct clinicopathologic entity (333) and recognized by the WHO Classification of Tumors of Haematopoietic and Lymphoid Tissues (334,335). However, not all lymphomatous effusions occurring in the absence of a tumor mass necessarily contain KSHV and represent PELs (336). In our experience, those cases presenting as lymphomatous effusions that exhibit Burkitt morphology and contain *MYC* gene rearrangements lack KSHV and probably represent an unusual presentation of BL (333). Currently, the presence of KSHV in the lymphoma cells is a diagnostic criterion for PEL. So, by definition, lymphomatous effusions lacking this virus should be classified according to their morphologic, phenotypic, and molecular features as large cell lymphoma, BL, and so on.

Since our initial studies, several groups had the opportunity to investigate many AIDS-related and non–AIDS-related lymphoid malignancies for the presence of KSHV and to evaluate the clinical, morphologic, immunologic, and molecular features of those lymphoid neoplasms that contain KSHV (319,320,333,337–339). These studies have confirmed that the PELs exhibit a unique and unusual constellation of characteristics that distinguish them from all other categories of malignant lymphoma, establishing them as a distinct clinicopathologic and biologic entity (Table 25.4). These characteristics include an

Table 25.4	CLINICOPATHOLOGIC, IMMUNOLOGIC, AND MOLECULAR CHARACTERISTICS OF KSHV-POSITIVE LYMPHOMAS		
Parameter	n	Total No.	Percentage
Epidemiology similar to KS			
HIV positive 42 years of age, HIV negative 73 Years			
Male predominance	29	32	91
HIV seropositive	28	32	88
Homosexuality as a risk factor	28	28	100
Initial presentation as an effusion	24	32	75
Disease remains restricted to the body cavity	21	24	88
Initially solid, subsequently develop effusion	4	8	50
Presence of KS	9	27	33
Median survival 5 mo			
CD45 expression	29	31	94
Absence of B-cell–associated antigens	27	30	90
Lack of immunoglobulin expression	19	22	86
Clonal immunoglobulin gene rearrangements	27	27	100
EBV genome	27	32	84
Absence of MYC gene rearrangements	23	24	96
Absence of other genetic alterations	18	20	90

epidemiology similar to KS, that is, a younger median age at presentation in HIV-infected than in HIV-uninfected individuals (42 years vs. 73 years) and a vast predominance in men. The majority of the men are HIV-seropositive and homosexuality is the most common risk factor, except in southern Europe, where injecting drug use is often also a risk factor. HIV-seropositive MSM are the AIDS group at highest risk for the development of KS, in which KSHV is also consistently present. KSHV-containing PELS have also been diagnosed in HIV-seronegative men or women without AIDS risk factors (319,320,324,340). Among HIV-seropositive individuals, the median CD4 T-cell count has been reported to be 84 and 203 cells/µL in two series (333,341). Approximately one-third of individuals who have PELs also have

KS. Most patients present initially with a malignant lymphomatous effusion in the peritoneal, pleural, or abdominal cavity, usually in the absence of a contiguous tumor mass and without associated lymphadenopathy or organomegaly. These lymphomas can also present in unusual cavities, such as in an artificial cavity related to the capsule of a breast implant (319). In most patients, the lymphoma presents in the body cavity of origin and remains restricted to this site, but in approximately 15% there is subsequent dissemination, and in another 15%, there is a history of a previous lymphoma in another site (339,342). The median survival is only about 5 months (311,319,320,333,338,339). However, more recently, a few case reports have documented clinical responses with the use of antivirals (343–345).

In Wright-Giemsa–stained air-dried cytocentrifuge preparations, the malignant cells display cytomorphologic features that appear to bridge those of immunoblastic and anaplastic large cell lymphoma (Figs. 25.16 and 25.17). The majority of the malignant cells are large, sometimes extremely large, and are round or ovoid to polygonal. They contain moderate to abundant amphophilic to deeply basophilic cytoplasm and nuclei ranging from large, round, and regular to highly irregular and pleomorphic. The nuclei possess coarsely reticular chromatin and one to four large prominent nucleoli. Most cells display plasmacytoid or immunoblastic features. Some of the cells are binucleated or multinucleated and resemble Reed-Sternberg cells. Mitotic figures, sometimes atypical, are numerous. The lymphoma cells appear somewhat more uniform in size and shape in cell block sections and in hematoxylin and eosin–stained tissue sections. They possess moderate to abundant lightly eosinophilic cytoplasm and round to slightly irregular nuclei that contain one or more prominent nucleoli. Occasional large pleomorphic cells are present. Some of these resemble Reed-Sternberg cells, and others have wreathlike nuclei, reminiscent of anaplastic large cell lymphoma (333,338) (Fig. 25.18).

In nearly all patients, the lymphoma cells express CD45 and a variety of activation-associated antigens, most commonly HLA-DR, CD30, CD38, CD71, and epithelial membrane antigen. In most but not all patients, the lymphoma cells lack surface immunoglobulin and B-cell lineage–associated antigens, as well as T-cell, myeloid, and monocyte- or macrophage-associated antigens (311,315,319,320,333,338,339). Some investigators

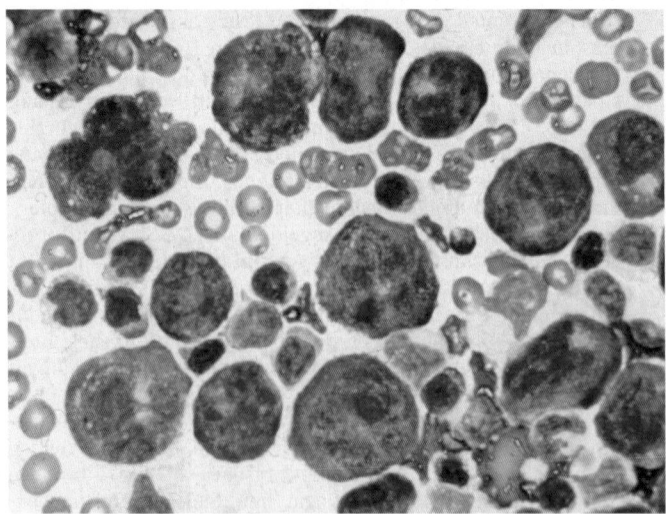
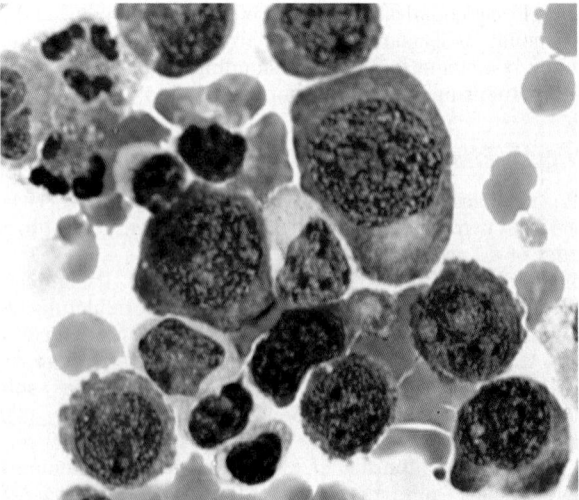

FIGURE 25.16 and 25.17. Air-dried cytocentrifuge preparation of a PEL containing Kaposi sarcoma–associated herpesvirus. The cells are considerably larger than normal benign lymphocytes and red blood cells and exhibit cytomorphologic features that bridge immunoblastic large cell lymphoma and anaplastic large cell lymphoma. The cells display variable polymorphism and generally possess moderately abundant amphophilic to deeply basophilic cytoplasm. A prominent clear perinuclear Golgi zone is frequently present. Small cytoplasmic vacuoles are occasionally present. The nuclei vary from large and round to highly irregular, multilobated, and pleomorphic and often contain one or more large prominent nucleoli (Wright stain, original magnification: 630×).

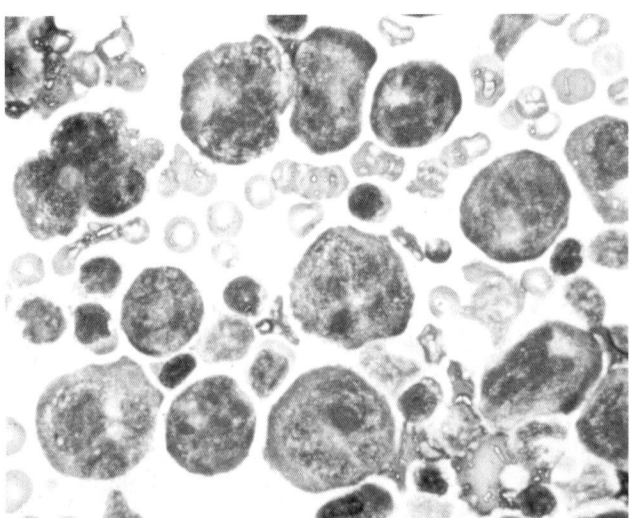

FIGURE 25.18. Kaposi sarcoma–associated herpesvirus (KSHV) in primary effusion lymphomas. Air-dried cytocentrifuge preparation of a KSHV-positive PEL. The cells are considerably larger than normal benign lymphocytes and exhibit cytomorphologic features that appear to bridge immunoblastic lymphoma and anaplastic large cell lymphoma. The cells display significant polymorphism and possess moderately abundant amphophilic to deeply basophilic cytoplasm. A prominent clear perinuclear Golgi zone is frequently present. The nuclei vary from large and round to highly irregular, multilobated, and pleomorphic and often contain one or more prominent nucleoli (Wright-Giemsa stain, original magnification: 1,000×).

have detected monotypic cytoplasmic immunoglobulin in some patients, but levels of immunoglobulin expression are low, if at all detectable (315,316,346). All patients exhibit clonal immunoglobulin heavy chain gene rearrangements, and most also exhibit κ light chain gene rearrangements, indicating a B-cell derivation (333). Rare patients also display clonal T-cell receptor gene rearrangements and are biphenotypic or bigenotypic (316,347). The PELs uniformly contain KSHV and nearly always contain clonal EBV. They consistently lack *MYC* gene rearrangements and mutations and usually also lack *RAS* and *P53* gene mutations and *BCL1*, *BCL2*, and *BCL6* gene rearrangements (333,348) (Table 25.4). In contrast, approximately 60% of all PELs, irrespective of EBV content and occurring in both HIV-infected and HIV-uninfected individuals, exhibit mutations involving the 5′ noncoding region of the *BCL6* gene (348). They display a hyperdiploid karyotype with numerous chromosomal abnormalities (338,348). Partial or complete trisomy 12, complete trisomy 7, and abnormalities of 1q21-q25 are observed frequently (348).

The consistent presence of clonal immunoglobulin gene rearrangements in conjunction with the expression of cell surface antigens associated with the late stages of B-cell differentiation or activation, in the absence of antigens associated with the early and middle stages of B-cell differentiation, strongly suggest that PELs represent the malignant counterpart of a mature stage of B-cell ontogeny. Because the lymphoma cells usually also lack surface immunoglobulin but sometimes express cytoplasmic immunoglobulin, this would appear to be a stage following antigenic stimulation and lying somewhere between a mature B cell and a plasma cell. Because a germinal center reaction in B cells involves somatic hypermutation of the nucleotide sequences of immunoglobulin heavy chain variable region (IgHV) genes, as well as class switch recombination, genetic analysis of the Ig genes can provide insight into the stage of B-cell development at which clonal expansion occurred. Pre–GCB cells contain IgHV genes with a germ line sequence; post–GCB cells contain mutated IgHV genes. Antigen-selected post–GCB cells display somatic mutations clustered in the complementary determining region sequences. GCB cells are characterized by ongoing mutation, which is absent in post–GCB cells (232,349). Nucleotide sequences of the IgHV region genes

expressed by several PELs showed that all the EBV-positive PELs obtained from HIV-infected individuals contained somatic hypermutation of IgHV genes (350,351). Only two of four of the EBV-negative cases had somatic hypermutation. This indicates that the tumor cells of most cases of PEL have been selected by antigen, or, in other words, have undergone affinity maturation, and this implies a post–germinal center cell origin. The lack of somatic hypermutation in some EBV-negative cases implies that these may be more like the lymphomas arising in MCD, which lack EBV infection and where there is no somatic hypermutation, indicating that they arose from cells that underwent some sort of extrafollicular differentiation (351). The molecular observation that PEL is derived from post–GCB cells is also consistent with a differentiation status defined by gene expression profiling as plasmablastic or plasma cell–like (352,353). The PEL transcriptome is very specific and clearly distinguishable from other AIDS and non–AIDS-related lymphomas, and has features of both immunoblasts identified by EBV-positive lymphoblastoid cell lines and AIDS immunoblastic lymphoma, and multiple myeloma cell lines.

It is rather remarkable in this regard that most PELs contain clonal EBV genome in addition to KSHV (311,333,338). This remains the only example of a consistent dual herpesviral infection in a human neoplasm. A critical question is the relative contribution of each virus to the pathogenesis of these lymphomas. It is well known, for example, that EBV is capable of immortalizing B cells *in vitro* but alone may be insufficient for tumorigenesis, as exemplified by the complementation of EBV and an activated *MYC* gene in BL (354). Genetic complementation can occur *in vitro* with dual viral infections, an example of which is activation of the EBV replicative cycle by human herpesvirus-6 (355). In fact, while KSHV and HIV do not infect the same cell, complementation *in vitro* has also been documented, where these viruses can enhance each other's replication (356–359). In order to better appreciate the respective contributions of KSHV and EBV to the pathogenesis of the PELs, EBV latent gene expression was analyzed (360). In PELs EBV was found to have a restricted latency pattern (i.e., type I latency), with low if any expression levels of EBV genes other than EBNA1 and EBERs, suggesting that EBV is not solely responsible for their malignant transformation and that KSHV plays the major role in the pathogenesis of the PELs. This conclusion is supported by a considerable body of evidence, including the existence of PELs that contain KSHV but lack EBV (319,320,333).

The presence of KSHV in the PELs and its conspicuous absence from all other categories of lymphoid neoplasia strongly suggest that this virus plays an important role in the pathogenesis of PEL. The accumulated evidence suggests that KSHV is an oncogenic herpesvirus that is important in malignant lymphoid transformation in these lymphomas: First, KSHV belongs to the *Gammaherpesvirinae* subfamily of herpesvirus, which is characterized by the ability to replicate in lymphoblastoid cells (361). Herpesvirus saimiri (a squirrel monkey virus) and EBV are the two herpesviruses first recognized to have the most structural homology to KSHV, and both possess the ability to induce latent infection of peripheral lymphocytes of their natural host, immortalize lymphocytes *in vitro*, and lead to the development of malignant lymphomas (361–363). Additional simian viruses have since been identified that have more extensive homology with KSHV, including the rhesus rhadinovirus (364,365), which can cause multicentric Castleman-like disease and lymphomas in rhesus macaques coinfected with SIV (366).

Additional evidence implicating KSHV as an oncogenic virus is the presence in its genome of a number of homologues to known viral and cellular genes, some of which are homologous to know cellular oncogenes, for example, a cyclin D homolog and a BCL-2 homolog, and others that have been documented to be oncogenic *in vitro* and *in vivo* in different experimental systems (367,368). It is important to distinguish the large number of genes expressed during lytic replication from those expressed during latency. While there are genes with clear oncogenic potential that are more highly expressed during lytic replication, these are thought to play a role in the pathogenesis of KS and MCD. In this section we focus on viral gene products for which there is evidence indicating a pathogenic role in PELs. These are the following:

i.   *LANA-1*. This protein has been shown to be important to segregate the KSHV genome, that is episomal, during cell division (369). In addition, it has the ability to affect several pathways with a likely role in tumorigenesis, such as binding and activation of the retinoblastoma (Rb) protein (370) and p53 (371). LANA-1 has also been shown to bind and inactivate GSK3β, which results in activation of the β-catenin pathway, which is involved in solid tumors (372), and via this pathway stabilize the CMYC protein (373). Other activities of LANA-1 are transcriptional effects on a variety of viral and cellular genes, including IL-6, hTERT, Pim1, and the TGFbeta type II receptor (374–378). The utility of LANA for diagnosis of KSHV-associated disease using immunohistochemistry thanks to a commercially available monoclonal antibody is clear (379).

ii. *vFLIP (K13)*. The KSHV-encoded vFLIP protein is homologous to cellular FLICE/caspase 8 inhibitory proteins (cFLIPs) (380), which inhibit death receptor–mediated apoptosis. In addition to a direct antiapoptotic function, vFLIP has the ability to activate NF-κB through both the classical and alternative pathways by binding to IKKγ and TRAF2 (381–384). Thus, vFLIP has developed an additional mechanism to promote cell growth and protect the cells from apoptosis by inducing the expression of a panel of pro-survival genes (384,385). vFLIP protects PEL cells from spontaneous apoptosis and is essential for tumor cell survival *in vitro* (386,387). vFLIP can also bind Atg3 and inhibit autophagy in B cells (388). Transgenic mice engineered to express vFLIP in B cells develop B-cell malignancies, which are accelerated in the context of a cMYC transgene (389–391). vFLIP is also involved in maintaining viral latency, since NF-κB activity prevents lytic reactivation (392,393).

iii. *vCYC (v-cyclin)*. This protein is homologous to the cellular cyclin D family of proteins. It has been shown to be functional, since it associates with CDK6 and induces phosphorylation of Rb protein and overcomes Rb-mediated cell-cycle arrest (394,395). However, in contrast to the cellular cyclin Ds, vCYC is able to induce degradation of the CDK inhibitor p27Kip when complexed with CDK6 (396,397). This results in the ability of vCYC to avoid the normal regulatory cell-cycle checkpoints in PEL cells. On its own, while altering the cell cycle, vCYC triggers a DNA damage response associated with genomic instability, resulting in autophagy and senescence, which in turn is inhibited by vFLIP in the context of virus infection (398–400). Consistent with an oncogenic role for vCYC only in the context of other oncogenic events that protect the cell from DNA damage response–associated cell death is the observation that transgenic mice with vCYC develop lymphomas, but only in the absence of p53 (401,402).

iv. *LANA-2 (vIRF-3)*. This protein is expressed in PELs, although not in KS, and has been shown to inhibit the tumor suppressor protein p53 (403). This protein is recruited to the interferon promoters via its interaction with cellular IRF-3 and IRF-7, stimulating their transcriptional activity (404).

v.   *vIL-6*. Interleukin 6 (IL-6) is an important cytokine centrally involved in immunologic responses, including B-cell differentiation to plasma cells. KSHV encodes a viral homolog of IL-6, simply called viral IL-6 (vIL-6). It differs from the cellular IL-6 in receptor binding and activation; while IL-6 requires two receptor chains for its activity, the gp130 glycoprotein plus the high-affinity IL-6 receptor, only the former is involved in vIL-6 signaling, and thus vIL-6 can activate IL-6-responsive genes and promote B-cell survival in cells that lack expression of the IL-6 receptor, providing it with the ability to affect a broader range of cell types (405–407). vIL-6 is expressed by a variable but significant proportion of latently infected PEL cells and in MCD, although it is considered a lytic gene. Taking into account the fact that this protein can be secreted, it may affect other tumor and reactive cells that don't express it in a paracrine fashion, and play a role in their proliferation and clinical manifestations.

vi. *K1*. Like the B-cell antigen receptor alpha and beta chains (CD79a and CD79b), the K1 protein encoded by KSHV has an ITAM motif that can activate cytoplasmic tyrosine kinases and the Akt pathway and affect cellular proliferation (408–410). While this protein is considered a lytic viral protein because its expression is much higher when the virus is replicating, it has been also reported to be expressed at low levels during latency (411). K1 has been shown to be tumorigenic in a simian model where it was found to induce lymphomas in common marmosets when replaced for the saimiri transforming protein (408), and is also tumorigenic in transgenic mice (412).

vii. *Kaposins*. KSHV contains a genomic region with great complexity that includes two families of direct repeats (DR1 and DR2) followed by a small coding region designated open reading frame (ORF) K12. Transcription from this region results in mRNAs that potentially encode three proteins, called kaposin A, B, and C (413). Kaposin B encompasses DR1 and DR2, and appears to be expressed in KS and some PEL cells (413), but not others (414). This protein is potentially transforming; it can activate the p38 pathway and stabilize cytokine mRNAs containing AU-rich elements in their 3′ untranslated regions, resulting in an increase in the production of pro-inflammatory cytokines (415).

viii. *K15*. At the end of the KSHV genome lies an ORF that encodes a protein with complex splicing and multiple transmembrane motifs, structurally resembling EBV LMP-2A (416). Also, like EBV LMP-2A, K15 can inhibit B-cell receptor signaling (416). It has SH2 and SH3 motifs, and also a TRAF binding motif, and thus can activate signaling cascades that include MAP kinases and NF-κB resulting potentially have significant effects on KSHV-infected B-cells, including inhibition of apoptosis (417,418). However, it is unclear whether this protein is expressed in latently infected PEL cells. One group reported expression of the K15 protein in most latently infected cells (418), but the RNA expression data is controversial, with most studies arguing for lytic expression.

ix. *KSHV microRNAs*. Like other herspesviruses including EBV, KSHV encodes at least 12 miRNAs, which cluster in the K12/kaposin genomic locus and are expressed in latently infected cells (419–422). Like cellular microRNAs, these viral products appear to fine-tune many different cellular regulatory pathways, and our specific understanding of the functions of each of these is rapidly growing. Some interesting observations have emerged so far. miR-K1 targets IκBα, an inhibitor of NF-κB, so it may strengthen the NF-κB activity induced by vFLIP, and thus promote cellular survival (423). miR-K1 has also been shown to prevent cell-cycle arrest by targeting cellular mRNAs encoding the cellular cyclin-dependent kinase inhibitor p21 (424). Another KSHV-encoded microRNA is miR-K12-11, which is an ortholog of cellular miR-155, which plays an important role in B-cell transformation and differentiation (425,426).

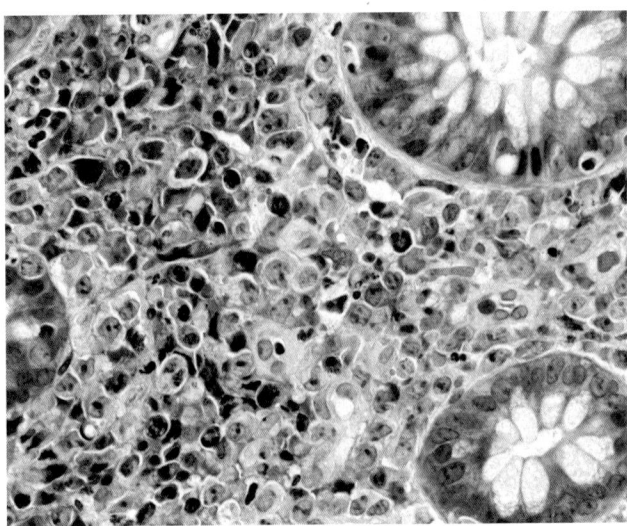

FIGURE 25.19. Solid PEL presenting as a large mass in the colon. The malignant cells are large and pleomorphic and infiltrate between residual glands (hematoxylin and eosin, magnification: 400×).

In summary, PELs represent a distinct clinicopathologic entity with a very specific gene expression signature and are defined by the presence of KSHV. The molecular details of how this virus induces lymphomagenesis are beginning to be understood, but all the evidence is consistent with this virus being the causal agent of PEL. Our understanding of the molecular pathogenesis of KSHV has revealed cellular signaling pathways that are activated by the virus that may be targeted for treatment, and in the future, specific agents that inhibit viral genes involved in lymphomagenesis may contribute to improved treatment (368).

Extracavitary (Solid) Primary Effusion Lymphoma

It has become evident that not all KSHV-associated lymphomas involve body cavities. The first report of a series of cases where KSHV was found in solid lymphomas was a study of NHL cases occurring in patients with AIDS and KS. In this study, three of seven evaluable cases of AIDS-related diffuse large B-cell lymphoma (DLBCL) with immunoblastic morphology were found to be positive for KSHV by immunohistochemistry for LANA (Figs. 25.19 and 25.20) (327,334). Approximately 4%

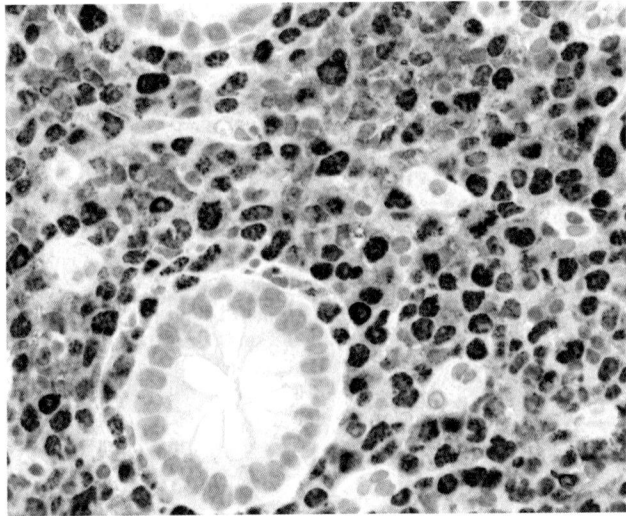

FIGURE 25.20. Solid PEL with malignant cells showing nuclear staining for KSHV LANA (hematoxylin and eosin, magnification: 400×).

of all AIDS-related lymphomas contain KSHV, and since most of these lymphomas have molecular and immunophenotypic features that resemble PEL, with the exception of presentation as a lymphomatous effusion, they have been called extracavitary or solid variants of PEL (327,334). Other investigators have since confirmed the existence of this entity, which is now accepted by the WHO (248,305). Features of extracavitary PEL that are similar to those of PEL include an immunoblastic to anaplastic morphology, CD45, CD30, EMA, and CD138 expression but lack of expression of T-cell antigens, CD10, CD15, or BCL6. Genotypically, extracavitary PEL has been shown to contain clonal immunoglobulin gene rearrangements, with no identifiable abnormalities in C-MYC, BCL6, BCL1, BCL2, and to be uniformly EBV positive (327,334). The only identifiable phenotypic difference reported is that the KSHV-positive solid lymphomas express B-cell–associated antigens and immunoglobulin in 25% of the cases, which is more frequent than in PEL (<5% and 15%, respectively) (327,334). The clinical presentation and course of patients with extracavitary PEL is similar, although those lacking an effusion were reported to have a somewhat better survival (median 11 months vs. 3 months).

Large B-cell Lymphoma Arising in KSHV-Associated Multicentric Castleman Disease

This entity has been described mainly as occurring in HIV-positive patients (427), and has also been called plasmablastic lymphoma. However, it differs from the conventional plasmablastic lymphoma category in that it is associated with KSHV, rather than with EBV. Lymphomas arising in KSHV-associated MCD are different from extracavitary (solid) PEL in a number of ways. They are EBV negative, they do not contain mutations in the immunoglobulin genes, and they are thought to arise from naive IgM lambda-expressing B cells rather than terminally differentiated B cells.

Histologically, clusters or sheets of KSHV-positive plasmablasts are seen in lymph nodes with classic histologic features of MCD, with variable hyalinization of follicle centers, mantle zone expansion, and abundant polytypic plasma cells in the interfollicular regions (428). Like KSHV-positive MCD, these cases contain KSHV-positive plasmablasts that are positive for cytoplasmic IgMλ. These plasmablasts can form microscopic lymphomas that are adjacent to or partially replace the follicles. These microlymphomas are frequently polyclonal, as seen by immunoglobulin gene rearrangement analysis, and probably do not represent a true malignancy. However, confluent sheets of plasmablasts that are monoclonal can be found (428). The terminology of "large B-cell lymphoma arising in KSHV-associated MCD" should probably be restricted to cases with these sheets of plasmablasts, which in some instances may completely efface the lymph node. Sheets of plasmablasts can also be seen in the spleen, and lead to massive splenomegaly, as well as to infiltrates in the lung and GI tract (71,427,429). Leukemic involvement has also been described (427).

Germinotropic Lymphoproliferative Disorder

Another entity that has been reported is germinotropic LPD, in which GCB cells are coinfected with EBV and KSHV (328). Reported cases occur in HIV-negative individuals, who lack a history of KS or immunodeficiency (328,430). Histologically, the lymph node has preservation of the architecture, but germinal centers are partially or completely replaced by large cells containing moderately abundant amphophilic cytoplasm and large eccentric vesicular nuclei containing one or two prominent nucleoli. Morphologic features range from those of plasmablasts associated with KSHV-positive MCD to cells with more anaplastic features. Infected cells are monotypic but can express kappa or lambda light chains, but lack expression of CD20 and other B-cell–associated antigens. Genotypically, they appear to be polyclonal and to be of germinal center cell origin (328).

Lymphomas Occurring in Other Immunodeficiency States

Polymorphic Lymphoid Proliferations Resembling Post–Transplant–Associated Lymphoproliferative Disorder

The clinically and histopathologically heterogeneous group of EBV-driven lymphoid proliferations that arise following solid organ transplantation are referred to collectively as *post-transplant lymphoproliferative disorders* (PTLD) (431). Many PTLDs comprise polymorphous cell populations of varying clonal composition (243,431–434). These features often make it difficult to determine their benign or malignant nature, classify those thought to be malignant by the standard lymphoma classifications, or reliably predict their clinical behavior (431,432,435,436). This is in marked contrast with the vast majority of AIDS-related NHLs, which are monomorphic, high-grade, monoclonal B-cell tumors; are easily recognized as malignant; and are usually readily classifiable, and whose aggressive clinical behavior is predictable. Furthermore, unlike AIDS-related NHLs, the polymorphic PTLDs consistently lack *MYC* gene rearrangements, *P53* gene mutations, *BCL6* gene rearrangements, and *RAS* gene mutations (245). These clinical, morphologic, and molecular differences between the PTLDs and the AIDS-related NHLs suggest that distinct mechanisms are operational in their pathogenesis.

Reviewing a large collection of cases previously classified as AIDS-related NHL, however, Chadburn, Knowles, and colleagues identified a subset displaying morphologic features resembling the polymorphic PTLDs in 10 HIV-infected individuals (437). They designated these cases *polymorphic lymphoproliferative disorders*. These lesions appear to arise in both men and women who have acquired HIV infection through various routes, including homosexual and heterosexual contact and blood transfusion. The 10 patients ranged in age from 28 to 55 years, with a mean of 38 years, similar to patients who have AIDS-related NHLs. None of the 10 individuals had a history of KS or opportunistic infections. The lesions developed in lymph nodes as well as in extranodal sites. Seven of the ten individuals had only clinical stage I or IE disease at presentation; two patients presented with generalized lymph node involvement (clinical stage III). Information regarding therapy and outcome was limited. Four patients received chemotherapy, one of whom died disease-free 28 months later and one of whom was alive with recurrent disease 7 months later. Histologically, the lesions exhibit a diffuse growth pattern. They consist of a polymorphic cell population consisting of lymphocytes, plasmacytoid lymphocytes, plasma cells, immunoblasts, and histiocytes. The lesions display variable degrees of plasmacytoid differentiation and cytologic atypia and variable numbers of atypical immunoblasts (Fig. 25.21).

Immunophenotypic analysis demonstrated a monotypic B-cell population in six of the eight patients in whom immunoglobulin expression was evaluated. A clonal B-cell population was detected in 7 of 10 patients by immunoglobulin heavy and light chain gene rearrangement analysis, and in 1 additional patient by EBV terminal repeat analysis. This included all six patients having significant monotypic B-cell populations, and the two in whom immunoglobulin expression was not assessed but who had large numbers of B cells. The non-germ line hybridizing bands were usually faint, indicating that the clonal B-cell population represented only a subset of the total cells in each lesion. This finding is consistent with the

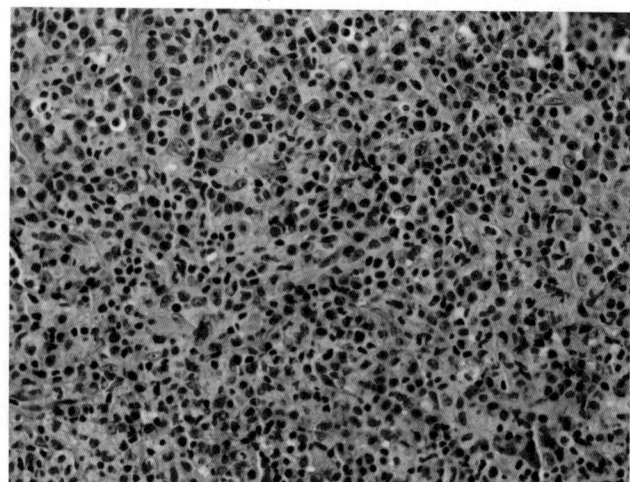

FIGURE 25.21. Polymorphous lymphoid proliferation resembling PTLD, with numerous small and large lymphoid cells as well as plasma cells and immunoblasts (magnification: 250×.)

histopathologic appearance of the lesions, which suggests the presence of variable numbers of cytologically atypical cells within a polymorphic cellular background, which includes many benign-appearing lymphoid cells. Strong immunoglobulin gene rearrangement bands were present in one patient in whom there was clear morphologic evidence of transformation to diffuse large B-cell lymphoma. They were unable to detect a clonal B-cell population in the two patients who expressed a polyclonal immunophenotypic profile.

Clonal EBV infection was demonstrable in 4 of the 10 patients, and type A EBV was identified in all 4 of those. EBV was identified in two additional lesions by ISH. The exclusive presence of type A EBV in these patients is analogous to the PTLDs (438) and contrasts with AIDS-related systemic NHLs, in which type B EBV is often present (439). KSHV, which is highly associated with PELs and not with solid lymphomas (311,333) or HIV-associated lymphadenopathy (142), was detectable in two cases by PCR but not by Southern blotting. ISH demonstrated KSHV in some of the benign, reactive cells and in some of the cytologically malignant-appearing cells in both lesions. The two cases containing KSHV occurred in MSM. Conceivably, herpesviruses may play a role in the development of these polymorphic LPDs. The one patient with polymorphic LPD who had focal areas of morphologic transformation to diffuse large B-cell lymphoma exhibited mutations involving the *MYC*, *BCL6*, and *P53* genes. One additional patient also displayed *P53* gene mutation. The remaining eight patients lacked structural alterations of the *MYC*, *BCL6*, *RAS*, or *P53* genes (437). Once again, these molecular features resemble those of the polymorphic PTLDs more closely than those of most AIDS-related systemic NHLs.

The malignant nature of the polymorphic PTLDs is unclear. Their morphologic appearance is atypical for a conventional malignant lymphoma, and a significant proportion of the lesions regress following a reduction in immunosuppressive therapy (431,440). One possible explanation for the development of these lesions is strong antigenic stimulation attributable to EBV infection, resulting in sequential polyclonal and oligoclonal lymphoid proliferations, which sometimes eventuate into monoclonal B-cell lymphomas (431). The lack of oncogene and tumor suppressor gene alterations in these lesions, however, suggests that the clonal, cytologically atypical B cells in these lesions are not fully transformed (245,431).

Somatic mutations involving the 5′ noncoding region of the *BCL6* gene occur independent of translocation of the *BCL6* gene (441). They are present in about 70% of diffuse large B-cell lymphomas (441) and 60% of AIDS-related NHLs (348). They have been identified in that subset of polymorphic PTLDs exhibiting unresponsiveness to immune reconstitution. In our experience, none of the PTLDs that regress following reduction of immune suppression exhibit *BCL6* gene mutation, whereas all of the PTLDs that fail to regress exhibit *BCL6* gene mutation (442). Mutational analysis of the *BCL6* gene appears to be a reliable predictor of the biologic behavior of polymorphic PTLDs. The fact that monoclonal *BCL6* gene mutation was identified only in the one patient with AIDS-related polymorphic LPD in transformation to diffuse large B-cell lymphoma, and not in other patients, supports the hypothesis that structural alteration of this gene may represent one of the earliest indicators of full malignant transformation and progression identified thus far. Like the polymorphic PTLDs, AIDS-related polymorphic LPDs display a histologic spectrum ranging from polymorphic hyperplasia to malignant lymphoma, and the distinction between the two may be difficult at the morphologic level. The presence or absence of *BCL6* gene mutations in these lesions may serve to subdivide them into distinct biologic categories, analogous to the polymorphic PTLDs. This hypothesis is supported by the fact that the one patient whose lesion contained a *BCL6* gene mutation developed recurrent and disseminated disease, but many of the other patients exhibited only localized disease. The lack of *BCL6* gene mutation may represent a favorable prognostic indicator for these AIDS-related polymorphic LPDs. More detailed clinical information concerning additional cases of AIDS-related polymorphic LPDs clearly is needed, however, to substantiate this hypothesis.

These polymorphic LPDs appear to represent a small but distinct subset of HIV-related lymphoid proliferations that are distinguishable from the traditional pathologic categories of AIDS-related NHL based on their morphologic and molecular characteristics and probably their clinical features as well. The polymorphic histopathology, the low "clonal strength," the general lack of oncogene and tumor suppressor gene alterations, the ability to transform to a high-grade malignant lymphoma, and the apparently lower disease load and better outcome suggest that these lymphoid proliferations resemble the polymorphic PTLDs more closely than they resemble the common categories of AIDS-related NHL. As in the case of the polymorphic PTLDs, the malignant nature and biologic significance of these lesions and their relationship to monomorphic B-cell lymphomas remains to be determined.

The remaining AIDS-associated lymphomas also occur in the immunocompetent population, but have characteristic clinical and histologic features in the setting of HIV.

Lymphomas Also Occurring in Immunocompetent Patients

Burkitt Lymphoma

BL accounts for up to 20% of AIDS-related NHL, and is more commonly seen with HIV infection than with other forms of immunodeficiency (443). BL typically occurs in less immunosuppressed patients with HIV, peaking at CD4 lymphocyte counts well above the laboratory cutoff for AIDS onset (200 cells/μL) (444). This suggests that the onset of BL may require functional CD4 T cells. BL cells are derived from GCB cells, and the Ig/c-myc translocation is considered to be an error in activation-induced cytidine deaminase (AID)-mediated immunoglobulin class switch recombination requiring activation by exposure to antigen and CD4 lymphocyte help (444). In support of this hypothesis, expression of AID has been shown to increase in peripheral blood mononuclear cells prior to the development of BL (444,445). There appears to be a bi- or trimodal peak for BL in persons with AIDS, and the risk of BL is independent of the HIV transmission category and antiretroviral therapy (446). The relative risk of NHL other than BL increases with declining CD4 T-cell counts (444).

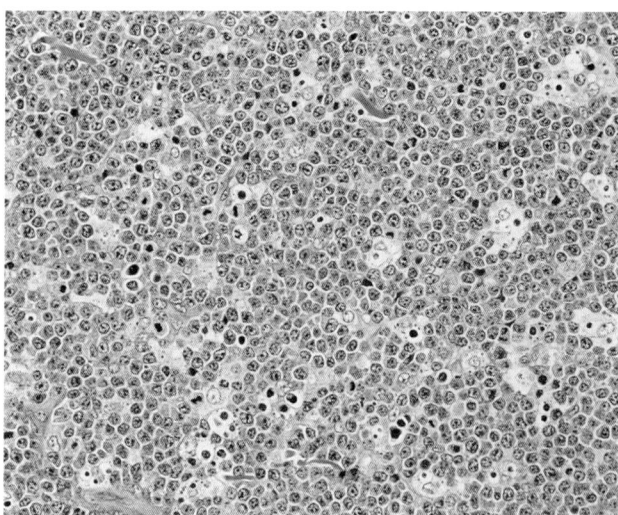

FIGURE 25.22. AIDS-related Burkitt lymphoma. Note the prominent starry-sky pattern, which is distributed evenly throughout the entire tumor (hematoxylin and eosin stain, original magnification: 100× magnification).

BL frequently involves the gastrointestinal tract but may present in unusual sites including the bone marrow. BL characteristically contains numerous, evenly distributed tingible body macrophages possessing abundant clear cytoplasm that impart a prominent starry-sky pattern (Fig. 25.22). It is characterized by a diffuse, monotonous proliferation of small- to intermediate-sized neoplastic lymphoid cells containing moderately abundant basophilic cytoplasm and round, regular nuclei possessing two to five distinct nucleoli (Fig. 25.23). These cohesive sheets of malignant cells are uniform and intermediate in size with small nucleoli. There is a rim of cytoplasm that appears blue with the Giemsa stain. The cells frequently have cytoplasmic vacuoles on touch preparations or bone marrow smears, which can be seen with oil red O stain in air-dried Romanowsky-stained imprints (Fig. 25.24). Characteristically, in BL associated with AIDS the cells have a more plasmacytoid cytoplasmic appearance with somewhat eccentric amphophilic cytoplasm. Tumor cells resemble noncleaved germinal center cells in that they are positive for CD20, CD10, and BCL6,

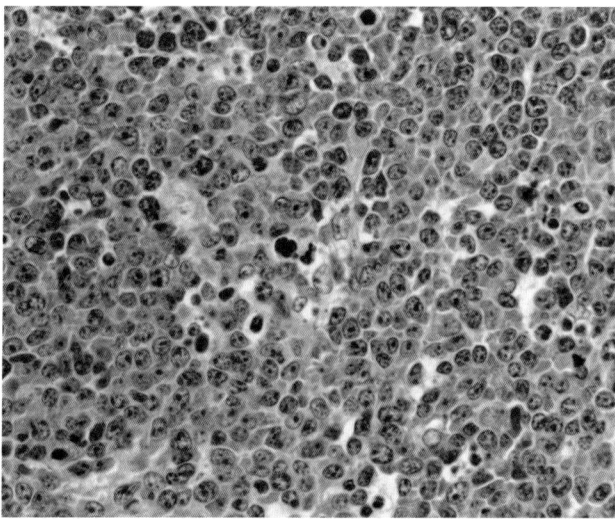

FIGURE 25.23. AIDS-related Burkitt lymphoma. There is a monotonous proliferation of uniformly sized neoplastic cells containing round regular nuclei and generally two to four nucleoli. The nuclei are surrounded by a small rim of cytoplasm. Numerous tingible body macrophages impart a starry-sky pattern (magnification: 400×.)

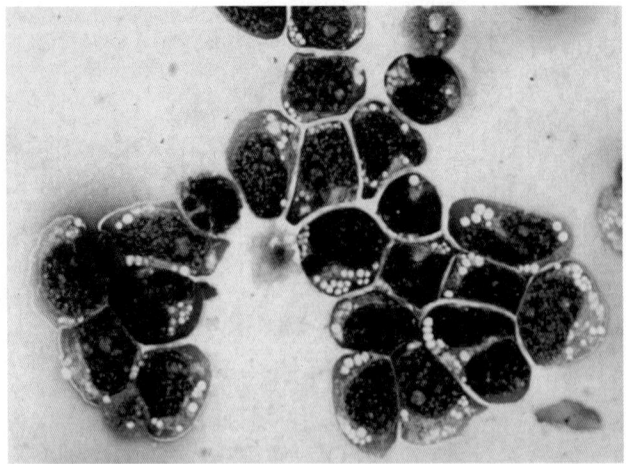

FIGURE 25.24. Cytospin preparation of an AIDS-related BL that presented as a massive abdominal effusion. The neoplastic cells possess abundant cytoplasm containing numerous small, round vacuoles. The nuclei contain one or more nucleoli (Wright stain, original magnification: 630×).

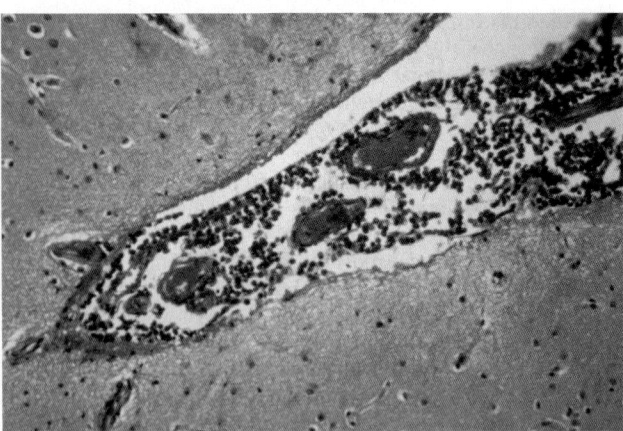

FIGURE 25.25. An HIV-positive heterosexual woman presented with massive bone marrow replacement and peripheral blood involvement by BL/leukemia, accompanied by meningeal signs. Malignant lymphoid cells were identified in a cerebrospinal fluid sample. Examination at autopsy revealed extensive infiltration of the leptomeninges by neoplastic lymphoid cells but no solid parenchymal masses, consistent with secondary involvement of the CNS (hematoxylin and eosin stain, original magnification: 100×).

but negative for BCL2. The Ki67 proliferation rate approaches 100%. Molecular studies reveal a translocation for C-MYC, and nuclear staining for MYC can also be demonstrated with immunohistochemical stains. Because a significant proportion have atypical cytologic features, they have been termed Burkitt-like lymphomas in the past. More appropriately, they have been referred to as *Burkitt's lymphoma with plasmablastic differentiation* by Hui et al. (447). The macrophages contain phagocytosed remnants of neoplastic cell debris, indicative of the high proliferation index of the lymphoma. Mitotic figures are extremely numerous, scattered nuclear debris is abundant, and there is a tendency for these lymphomas to undergo necrosis.

Prior to antiretroviral therapy infectious deaths made intensive chemotherapy regimens difficult to deliver. In the era of cART, intensive regimens for BL have been used with success similar to that of the nonimmunocompromised population. Newer combination chemotherapy approaches include the McGrath regimen (CODOX-M/IVAC) with or without added rituximab (448).

Diffuse Large B-Cell Lymphoma, Not Otherwise Specified

The AIDS patients with DLBCL present with extranodal or disseminated disease; presentation with localized lymph node–based disease is less common (252,255,259,274,296,297,301). Approximately 65% of these individuals have clinical stage III or IV disease, and another 20% have clinical stage IE disease initially (259,274,297,301). Even the patients with clinical stage IE disease often have large bulky tumors, however (259). All together, about 85% of the patients have extranodal involvement at presentation (251,255,258,259,274,288,297,299,449). The CNS, the gastrointestinal tract, the bone marrow, and the liver are the most common sites of extranodal disease at presentation (252,255,259,274,296,299,301,450). Furthermore, certain extranodal locations that uncommonly serve as primary sites of conventional lymphoma in the HIV-uninfected general population, such as the CNS, the anorectal region, and the heart, among others, have become recognized as frequent sites of origin for AIDS-related NHL (252,259,286,451–455). An extranodal biopsy is used to make the initial diagnosis of malignant lymphoma in approximately two-thirds of patients (259). Not infrequently, the diagnosis is based on the biopsy of a particularly unusual extranodal site, such as the gingiva, anorectal region, mandible, or orbit, or the cytologic examination of an abdominal or pleural effusion (259). Cases of AIDS-related diffuse large B-cell lymphoma, not otherwise specified (DLBCL-NOS) may be of GCB or non-GCB types. In one clinical trial of 33 patients from the National Cancer Institute there were 72% and 28% GCB and non-GCB cases. The outcome was less favorable in the non-GCB group with 44% 5 year survival compared with 95% for the GCB group (456). However, another study from the AIDS Malignancy Consortium that included 81 patients from two different trials failed to find any significant difference in outcome between GCB and non-GCB subtypes, while confirming that the GC subtype is more common than the non-GC subtype (59% vs. 41%) (457).

The CNS is the most common extranodal site of involvement by AIDS-related NHL (288). Approximately 20% to 40% of patients who have AIDS-related systemic lymphoma, especially those who have bone marrow infiltration, have CNS infiltration at presentation (252,255,259,296,449). The majority of patients who have systemic NHL accompanied by secondary CNS involvement have leptomeningeal infiltration (Fig. 25.25) and not solid parenchymal masses (281). These patients usually present with lymphomatous meningitis and commonly have nuccal rigidity, headaches, cranial neuropathies, or numbness of the chin (275), although they may be asymptomatic (451). Cerebrospinal fluid samples obtained from these patients may contain neoplastic cells. Therefore, cytologic examination of the cerebrospinal fluid should be performed as part of the initial staging evaluation of all patients with AIDS-related systemic lymphoma, in order to rule out CNS involvement (286).

The second most common extranodal site of involvement by AIDS NHL is the gastrointestinal tract (288) (Fig. 25.26). Of the patients who had AIDS-related NHL reported from the Los Angeles County–University of Southern California (LAC-USC) (286) and New York University (259) Medical Centers, 27% and 28%, respectively, had gastrointestinal tract involvement initially. In addition, 10% and 16% of the patients, respectively, had liver involvement initially (259,286). The majority of patients who have AIDS-related systemic NHL are discovered to have gastrointestinal tract and liver involvement at the time of *postmortem* examination (281).

The gastrointestinal tract is also a common primary extranodal site of AIDS-related NHL (259,286). The most frequent sites of origin within the gastrointestinal tract are the stomach and the small intestine (286); however, any region from the oropharynx to the rectum and anus, including the liver

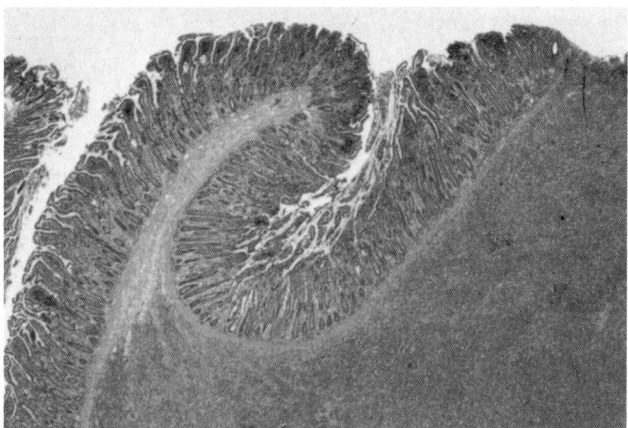

FIGURE 25.26. AIDS-related NHL occurring in the small bowel, in which it forms a large, bulky tumor mass. The gastrointestinal tract is the second most common extranodal site of origin for AIDS-related NHL. (From Knowles DM, Chamulak GA, Subar M, et al. Clinicopathologic, immunophenotypic, and molecular genetic analysis of AIDS-associated lymphoid neoplasia. In: Rosen PP, Fechner RE, eds. *Pathology annual 1988, part 2.* East Norwalk, CT: Appleton and Lange, 1988:33–67, with permission.)

(458,459), may serve as the primary site of NHL. Alternatively, patients may have extensive lymphomatous involvement of the entire gastrointestinal tract (286).

The signs and symptoms may be related to primary gastrointestinal tract involvement or result from extension into abdominal lymph nodes. Patients initially may complain of gingival swelling and bleeding, dysphagia, abdominal pain, symptoms related to ulceration, obstipation, bowel obstruction, abdominal swelling because of ascites or a palpable mass, jaundice or perirectal abscess, and ulceration (259). Organomegaly with or without ascites, abdominal masses, retroperitoneal lymphadenopathy, and nonhealing perirectal ulcers or abscesses should prompt a tissue biopsy to rule out malignant lymphoma (426).

NHL arising or presenting in the anus or rectum of homosexual men is recognized as a frequent manifestation of AIDS (286,453–455). Primary anorectal lymphoma occurs infrequently in the general population. Malignant lymphomas of all histologic types comprise only 0.1% to 1.3% of all malignant tumors of the rectum (453,460), and rectal lymphomas represent only approximately 5% of all gastrointestinal tract lymphomas (460–462). Burkes et al. (453) and Ioachim et al. (455) reported series of four patients who had primary anorectal lymphoma diagnosed within brief time spans at the Los Angeles County–University of Southern California Medical Center and Lenox Hill Hospital in New York City, respectively. The patients usually are young MSM between 22 and 45 years of age (median 35) who have a history of practicing passive rectal intercourse with multiple anonymous sexual partners. They usually complain of rectal bleeding, pain on defecation, or a mucoid rectal discharge and B symptoms and have a palpable rectal mass on examination. The lymphomas tend to occur in the lower rectum and anal canal and display intermediate- and high-grade histologies. Although most patients present with clinical stage IE disease, nearly all of them develop disseminated lymphoma shortly thereafter. The median duration of survival has been approximately 7 months, with only rare patients sustaining a complete remission (CR) (453–455). In contrast, primary anorectal lymphomas occurring in the HIV-uninfected general population affect men and women equally, usually occur in the sixth and seventh decades of life, generally develop higher up in the rectum, and often exhibit low-grade histology (455,460). The significance of the development of anorectal lymphoma in MSM in association with AIDS at a specific site of sexual activity is unknown. Anal intercourse has been shown to be a risk factor, however, for the development of

anal carcinoma (463,464) and, by analogy, may play a contributory role in the development of anorectal lymphoma as well.

AIDS-related systemic NHLs may originate or present in virtually any extranodal site, regardless of how isolated or obscure. They have been reported, for example, in the orbit (258,259,465), oropharynx (252,259,466), mandible (258,259,265), heart (467,468), lungs (258,259,466), skin (258,259,469), salivary glands (176,259), common bile duct (470), muscles (466), bones (364,435), kidneys (252,274), gonads (259,301,466), and adrenal glands (259) and even in the placenta and products of conception (471). Neoplastic cells may even circulate in the peripheral blood (259). In many instances, involvement of these extranodal sites is the result of extensive, widely disseminated disease; however, the malignant lymphoma often appears to have originated in the extranodal site. For example, Constantino et al. (467) described a malignant lymphoma arising in, and remaining limited to, the heart of a 34-year-old IDU; we have observed similar cases (Fig. 25.27). Levecq et al. (472) described a histologic high-grade B-cell lymphoma arising in an ileostomy stoma in a 73-year-old heterosexual man who apparently acquired HIV infection following transfusion. Kaplan et al. (470) described a BL originating in the common bile duct that subsequently spread to the bone marrow and CNS. Malignant lymphoma should be considered if an individual at risk for AIDS presents with a tumor, regardless of the mode of presentation. The atypical presentation of a diffuse aggressive NHL involving an unusual extranodal site should raise suspicion of HIV infection. The factors that influence the development of malignant lymphoma in a particular location are unclear but may include site-specific chronic antigenic stimulation (473) and trauma (474).

Cases of AIDS-related diffuse large B-cell lymphoma usually lack a prominent starry-sky pattern because of the presence of fewer tingible body macrophages. Mitotic figures are less numerous, scattered nuclear debris is less abundant, and necrosis occurs less frequently than in Burkitt and immunoblastic lymphomas. The neoplastic cells are intermediate in size between those of Burkitt and immunoblastic lymphoma and usually are round to slightly ovoid. They generally possess scant to moderately abundant acidophilic cytoplasm, without a paranuclear hof or other evidence of plasmacytoid differentiation. The nuclei tend to be round and regular and contain one to several small, but distinct, nucleoli adjacent to the nuclear membrane (208,209) (Fig. 25.28). When the bone marrow is involved the cells are large with round or oval nuclei and

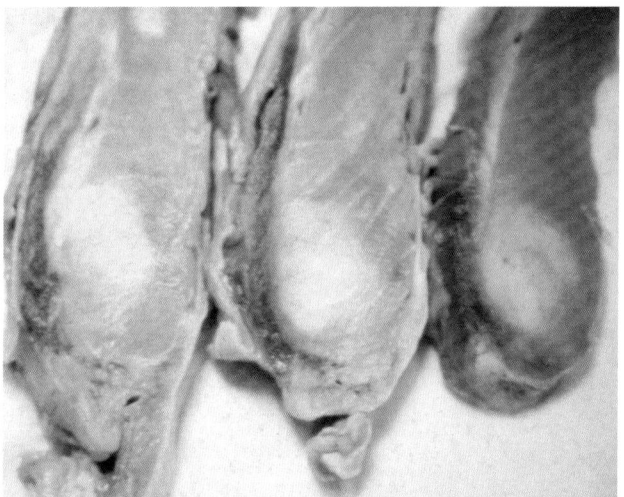

FIGURE 25.27. Primary cardiac NHL occurring in an HIV-positive 34-year-old IDU. Autopsy examination failed to demonstrate any evidence of lymphoma beyond the heart. (From Constantino A, West TE, Gupta M, et al. Primary cardiac lymphoma in a patient with acquired immune deficiency syndrome. *Cancer* 1987;60:2801–2805, with permission.)

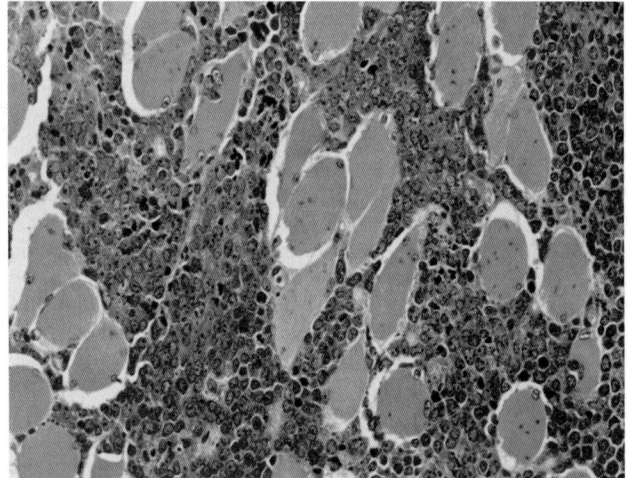

FIGURE 25.28. AIDS-related diffuse large B-cell lymphoma with sheets of large centroblasts infiltrating skeletal muscle (magnification: 400×).

frequent cytoplasmic vacuolation (Fig. 25.29). Some large cell lymphomas contain variable proportions or are even composed entirely of neoplastic cells containing cleaved or multilobated nuclei (466).

Diffuse Large B-Cell Lymphoma—Immunoblastic

Immunoblastic lymphomas also often exhibit a starry-sky pattern, although it is usually less prominent than in BL. Mitotic figures are extremely numerous, scattered nuclear debris is abundant, and these lymphomas also have a tendency to undergo necrosis. The neoplastic cells are larger than those comprising Burkitt or large cell lymphomas. They are round, ovoid, or polygonal and often contain abundant, deeply basophilic cytoplasm, sometimes with a paranuclear hof indicative of their plasmacytoid differentiation. The nuclei are round to ovoid and often contain a solitary prominent, centrally placed nucleolus (Fig. 25.30). Binucleate and even multinucleate cells are often present (417,418). Occasional immunoblastic lymphomas exhibit marked cellular pleomorphism (312). These cases are composed of large, pleomorphic tumor cells that contain abundant acidophilic to amphophilic cytoplasm and large, round, and regular to highly irregular and hyperconvoluted

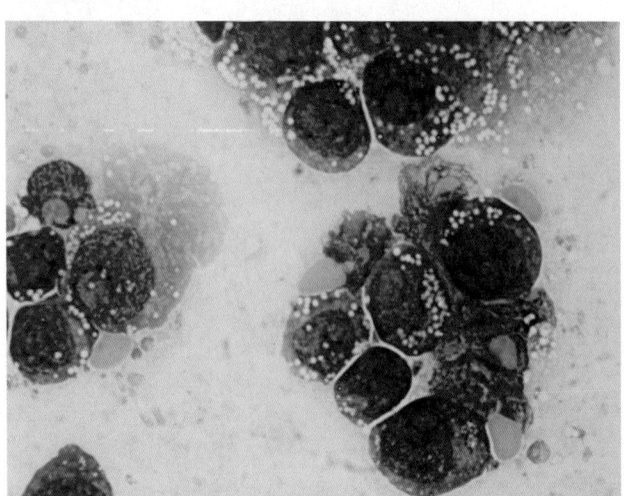

FIGURE 25.29. Diffuse large B-cell lymphoma infiltrating the marrow. Aspirate shows large malignant cells with vacuolated cytoplasm (Giemsa stain, magnification: 400×).

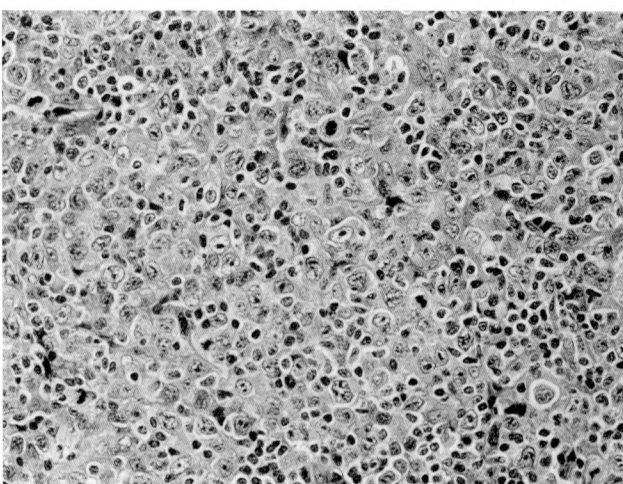

FIGURE 25.30. AIDS-related immunoblastic lymphoma. The neoplastic cells are larger and show more variability in size and shape than those of Burkitt and large cell lymphomas. The nuclei sometimes are placed eccentrically, have prominent central nucleoli, and are surrounded by more abundant cytoplasm (hematoxylin and eosin stain, original magnification: 400×).

nuclei containing one or more prominent nucleoli, sometimes reminiscent of Reed-Sternberg cells (259,312) (Fig. 25.31).

Primary Central Nervous System Lymphoma

In addition to the high frequency of secondary lymphomatous involvement of the CNS, approximately 20% of all AIDS-related NHLs are primary CNS lymphomas, that is, present as intracranial parenchymal mass lesions limited to the CNS (252,258,270,281,296,297,465). Before the emergence of AIDS, primary CNS lymphomas occurred rarely, constituting <1.5% of all primary brain tumors (475). In a study of 12,000 patients who had malignant lymphoma, involvement was limited to the brain in only 0.2% of the patients (476), and this usually occurred in the elderly (475) and among patients who had collagen vascular disorders (477) and various congenital and acquired immune deficiencies, including renal transplant recipients (436), Louie et al. (473). Data collected by the CDC

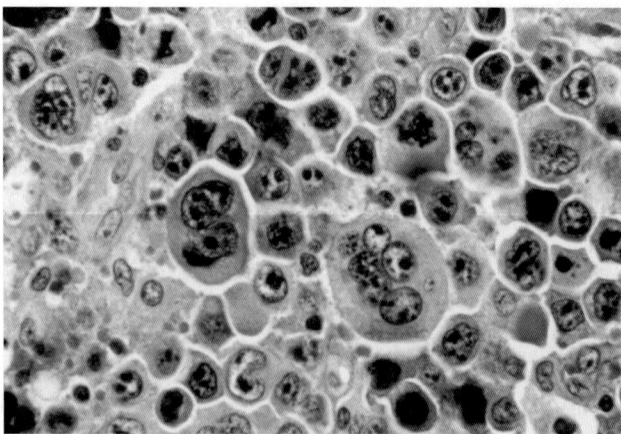

FIGURE 25.31. AIDS-related immunoblastic lymphoma. This neoplasm is composed of large, pleomorphic tumor cells, many of which are binucleated and even multinucleated. Some resemble the pleomorphic Reed-Sternberg cells of HD. The tumor cells expressed CD45 and a variety of activation-associated antigens but lacked B-cell lineage–restricted antigens. They displayed clonal immunoglobulin heavy and light chain gene rearrangements, consistent with a B-cell derivation, and contained EBV (hematoxylin and eosin stain, original magnification: 630× magnification). (From Knowles DM, Dalla-Favera R. AIDS-associated malignant lymphoma. In: Broder S, Merigan TC, Bolognesi D, editors. *Textbook of AIDS medicine.* Baltimore: Williams & Wilkins, 1994:431–464, with permission.)

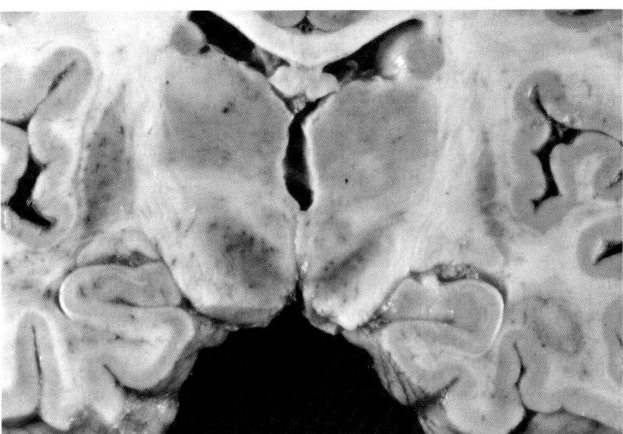

FIGURE 25.32. AIDS-related central nervous system lymphoma. The infiltrative nature of this lymphoma is manifested on the left by the uniform enlargement of the thalamus and subthalamic areas bilaterally. (Courtesy of Dr. James Powers, University of Rochester, Rochester, NY.)

suggest that primary CNS lymphomas occur about 1,000 times more frequently in AIDS patients than in the general population (276). AIDS now represents the most common risk factor, by far, for the development of primary CNS lymphoma.

AIDS-related primary CNS lymphomas are intracranial parenchymal tumors. They are often large, sometimes larger than 3 cm, and frequently are multifocal (452,478,479). Grossly, they are characterized by indistinct borders and a granular surface (452) (Fig. 25.32). At autopsy, they nearly always are discovered to be multicentric, especially on microscopic examination (281,452). They occur most commonly in the cerebrum but also occur frequently in the cerebellum, basal ganglia, and brainstem (452,478–480). The lymphoma cells tend to be distributed along vascular channels as perivascular cuffs (452,479,480) (Fig. 25.33). Because the lesions are primarily intracranial, cerebrospinal fluid samples often do not contain diagnostic malignant cells (452); however, concurrent leptomeningeal involvement accompanied by malignant cells within the cerebrospinal fluid sometimes is observed (451,452). The lymphomas are of B-cell origin and display large cell and immunoblastic histologies (259,281,451,452,465,466,479,480).

The majority of patients who have AIDS-related primary CNS NHL are profoundly immunocompromised young homosexual

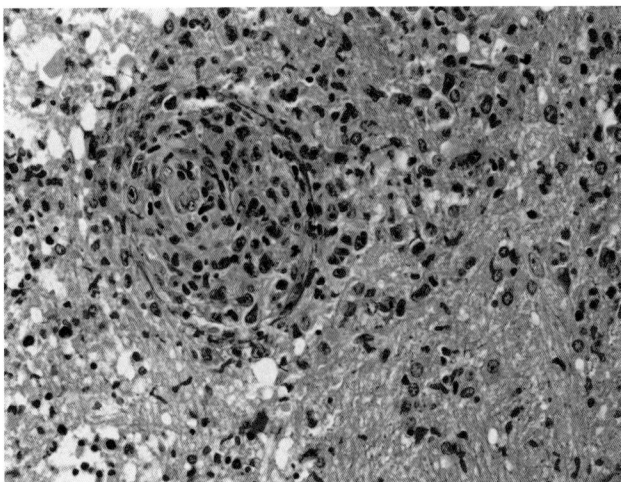

FIGURE 25.33. Diffuse large B-cell lymphoma of the brain showing cuffing of large lymphoid cells around a blood vessel, and admixed small lymphocytes and glial cells (magnification: 240×).

men with very advanced HIV disease who have CD4 T-cell counts below 50 per microliter (281,296,451,452,465). Approximately two-thirds or more of them have AIDS-defining conditions, often severe opportunistic infections, or KS, before the development of primary CNS lymphoma (252,279,296,452,465,479,481). Approximately one-half of patients experience focal seizures and a subacute progression of focal neurologic symptoms over days or weeks (452). Occasionally, clinical progression may be strikingly rapid, causing difficulty in distinguishing neoplastic, vascular, and infectious causes (452). Headaches, confusion, lethargy, and memory loss are other common symptoms, and subtle changes in behavior and personality may be seen (286,451,452,465,479,481). Many patients eventually show signs suggesting an intracranial mass lesion; however, because many of them are seriously ill from their underlying systemic illness, these relatively nonspecific symptoms may not raise suspicion of such a lesion, and primary CNS lymphoma may not be diagnosed until after death (259,281,296,301,452). Only 11 of 20 patients who had AIDS-related primary CNS lymphoma at the University of California at San Francisco were diagnosed correctly prior to death; the remaining nine patients were correctly diagnosed only at autopsy (452).

The majority of persons who have AIDS-related primary CNS lymphoma exhibit abnormalities on CT scans consistent with an intracranial mass lesion (452,482). Solitary discrete and multiple discrete lesions are seen in equal proportions (452). CT scans have been widely used to distinguish between intracranial lymphoma and toxoplasmosis, based on the belief that malignant lymphoma exhibits a homogeneous, isodense, or hyperdense pattern, and toxoplasmosis displays a ring-enhancing pattern (451,483). This is generally true of conventional primary CNS lymphomas occurring in the general population, because these lymphomas usually consist of tightly packed tumor cells without necrosis (482). AIDS-related primary CNS lymphomas, however, frequently contain extensive necrosis and show some degree of enhancement, although the pattern is variable. This often makes it difficult or impossible to distinguish between AIDS-related primary CNS lymphoma and toxoplasmosis by CT scan (452,482). Brain biopsy is essential for accurate diagnosis in these patients (261,452,479,482,484–487).

Lineage and Clonality

Many investigators have demonstrated that the more than 90% of AIDS-related systemic and primary CNS lymphomas that display Burkitt, immunoblastic, and large cell morphology are of B-cell derivation. This conclusion is based on their expression of monotypic surface immunoglobulin or B-cell lineage–associated antigens CD19, CD20, and CD22, in the absence of T-cell lineage–associated antigens (252,255,259, 286,300,337,450,466,488,489). Most of the remaining small proportion, approximately 3%, of AIDS-related NHLs, represent PELs. These tumors often express indeterminate phenotypes, that is, lack surface immunoglobulin and B-cell– and T-cell–associated antigens, and express non–lineage-specific antigens associated with activation (311–313,490). Occasional T-cell lineage–derived NHLs and lymphoid leukemias have been reported in HIV-infected individuals, but their relationship to HIV infection and the AIDS epidemic remains unclear (288). AIDS lymphomagenesis can be regarded as a B-cell phenomenon. Nearly all AIDS-related BL express surface immunoglobulin, most commonly IgMκ, and approximately 75% express CD10. They express CD21 (the C3d-EBV receptor) uncommonly. Only about 50% of large cell and immunoblastic lymphomas express monotypic surface immunoglobulin, and the isotype is variable. The large cell and immunoblastic lymphomas express CD10 and CD21 heterogeneously (259). AIDS-related B-cell NHLs appear to express immunophenotypes that are similar to those expressed by conventional B-cell NHLs of comparable morphology occurring in the immunocompetent, HIV-uninfected general population (259,337).

Numerous investigators have demonstrated that most AIDS-related NHLs, including those with indeterminate immunophenotypes, display clonal immunoglobulin heavy and light gene chain rearrangements in the absence of clonal T-cell receptor gene rearrangements, thus confirming their B-cell derivation (259,311,337,488,491–493). These malignant lymphomas appear to contain one dominant clonal B-cell population, based on the presence of one or two non–germ line hybridizing bands of high intensity on Southern blotting. This dominant clonal B-cell population, representing the malignant lymphoma, sometimes is accompanied by additional minor B-cell clones that are detectable as additional faint bands following prolonged exposure on Southern blotting (488). Minor B-cell clones lacking evidence of malignant transformation have been identified in about 20% of hyperplastic lymph nodes obtained from HIV-infected patients (488). Possibly, these clones persist in some lymph nodes that become replaced by malignant lymphoma, thus accounting for the additional faint rearranged bands observed in these cases.

A conspicuous exception to these findings are the studies published by McGrath, Herndier, and colleagues (494–497). These investigators reported that approximately one-third of all AIDS-related lymphomas from the San Francisco Bay area that they studied are polyclonal. This conclusion was based on their inability to detect clonal immunoglobulin heavy chain gene rearrangements in biopsy specimens by Southern blotting or in some instances by reverse transcriptase-PCR (494–496). These lymphoid proliferations were described as exhibiting large cell morphology and expressing a spectrum of mixed immunophenotypes based on the presence of variable numbers of B cells, T cells, and macrophages (494–496). These "polyclonal lymphomas" were reported to lack EBV and MYC gene rearrangements and to have a more favorable clinical outcome than other AIDS-related NHLs (497). It was suggested by these investigators that these polyclonal lymphomas represent a new category of AIDS-related lymphoma. These findings are unusual in that they are at odds with the vast literature concerning AIDS-related NHL, as well as with the widely held concept of monoclonality in lymphomagenesis. The explanation for these discordant findings is unclear. McGrath et al. may have identified a novel subset of AIDS-related NHLs. Alternatively, tissue sampling or other technical factors may explain their findings. For example, these investigators often failed to analyze their cases for immunoglobulin light chain gene rearrangements (494–496). Furthermore, the absence of clonal immunoglobulin gene rearrangements by Southern blotting does not necessarily indicate polyclonality. Other scientific explanations can be offered to account for such findings (498).

In order to resolve the controversy surrounding the clonal nature of AIDS-related NHLs, we performed a comprehensive correlative molecular genetic and morphologic analysis of 74 AIDS-related systemic NHLs originating from the east and west coasts (37 cases each) of the United States (259,499,500). We were able to detect a solitary, dominant monoclonal B-cell population in 66 (89%) of the 74 patients by Southern blot immunoglobulin heavy chain gene rearrangement analysis, using two probes specific to different segments of the immunoglobulin heavy chain gene joining region. We were able to determine the monoclonal B-cell nature of 71 (96%) of the 74 cases if immunoglobulin heavy chain gene, immunoglobulin κ and λ light chain genes, and EBV terminal repeat analyses were used in conjunction. The occasional AIDS-related NHLs that apparently lack clonal immunoglobulin heavy chain gene rearrangements usually exhibit clonal immunoglobulin light chain gene rearrangements. Furthermore, many of the AIDS-related NHLs that apparently lack clonal immunoglobulin heavy and light chain gene rearrangements contain evidence of clonal

EBV infection. We failed to determine a clonal nature in only 1 (3%) of 37 east coast cases and 2 (6%) of 37 west coast cases, employing multiple approaches (259,499,500). None of these three cases resembled morphologically the so-called polyclonal lymphomas reported by McGrath et al. (494–497).

Our findings confirm that AIDS-related systemic NHLs exhibiting a germ line immunoglobulin gene configuration exist but clearly demonstrate that such cases are quite uncommon. The results of Raphael et al. (337), who reported only rare cases of AIDS-related NHLs exhibiting a germ line immunoglobulin gene configuration on Southern blot hybridization, are consistent with our findings. Whether these germ line cases are truly polyclonal or clonality is not detectable with the methods employed remains to be determined.

Finally, studies concerning structural alterations of protooncogenes and tumor suppressor genes have provided considerable additional evidence in support of the widely held belief that most AIDS-related NHLs are monoclonal neoplasms. For example, the fact that only one rearranged MYC allele is detectable in each AIDS-related NHL (488,492,493) also supports the concept that each malignant lymphoma contains one vastly predominant clone, that is, is monoclonal. This conclusion is further supported by the presence of a solitary P53 gene mutation, a solitary BCL6 gene rearrangement, and so on in AIDS-related NHLs (493,501). Additional studies are necessary to confirm the authenticity of so-called polyclonal AIDS-related NHLs, as well as the significance of the observation that some AIDS-related NHLs apparently lack evidence of clonal immunoglobulin gene rearrangements. We have failed to find evidence to support the contention that true polyclonal lymphomas, those in which the neoplastic cell population is derived from multiple clones, exist.

Molecular Genetics

Several dominantly acting protooncogenes, MYC, BCL1, BCL2, and BCL6, are believed to play roles in lymphomagenesis in the immunocompetent host through chromosomal translocation or point mutation. The structural alterations involving these oncogenes occur nonrandomly in association with specific histopathologic categories of conventional NHL. Also, it is believed that inactivation of the P53 and the Rb tumor suppressor genes are involved in lymphomagenesis (see Chapter 8). Structural alterations in some of these genes, and also in the RAS gene family, variably occur among AIDS-related NHLs as well.

Reciprocal chromosomal translocations occurring between the MYC oncogene on chromosome 8 and the immunoglobulin heavy chain, κ light chain, or λ light chain gene on chromosomes 14, 2, and 22, respectively, are associated highly with endemic (African) and sporadic (Western) BL (502–504). These translocations are observed infrequently in other categories of conventional NHL occurring in the HIV-uninfected general population (504). The initial cytogenetic studies performed in the early years of the AIDS epidemic revealed the frequent occurrence of chromosomal translocations involving band 8q24, the site of the MYC gene, in AIDS-related NHLs, suggesting their molecular similarity to BL occurring in immunocompetent hosts (262,265,266). These findings were confirmed and expanded by molecular analysis of the MYC locus in AIDS-related NHLs. Pelicci et al. (488) and Subar et al. (492) identified MYC gene rearrangements in approximately 75% of AIDS-related NHLs. These included most patients exhibiting Burkitt morphology and, surprisingly, some exhibiting large cell and immunoblastic morphology. In addition, conventional BLs carrying the t(2;8) translocation usually express kappa light chains, and those carrying the t(8;22) translocation usually express λ light chains (505). A lack of correlation between the type of translocation and light chain expression has been described in AIDS-related BL (506,507).

With respect to those AIDS-related DLBCLs carrying *MYC* gene rearrangements, Delecluse et al. (508) proposed that they actually represent a subset of AIDS-related BLs that have adopted large cell or immunoblastic morphology in the context of impaired immune surveillance. These investigators have suggested that severe perturbation of the immune system acts as a permissive factor for the morphologic switch of Burkitt to large cell or immunoblastic histology and maintains the genetic distinction of BL, namely, *MYC* gene activation (508). Supporting this hypothesis, AIDS-related NHLs displaying cytomorphologic features intermediate between those of BL and large cell or immunoblastic lymphoma have been observed (337,509). Conventional BL cells, especially if infected by EBV, often undergo immunoblastic transformation during serial passages in culture *in vitro*. This may be accompanied by immunophenotypic variations and by a change in the pattern of EBV latent gene expression (510–512). It has been suggested that AIDS-related large cell lymphomas exhibiting *MYC* gene activation display hybrid clinical features, namely, the host immunosuppression typical of AIDS-related large cell lymphoma and the preferential association with preexistent persistent generalized lymphadenopathy often seen in AIDS-related BL (497). Another hypothesis that has been suggested is that the *MYC* gene activation observed in these cases may simply reflect the pathogenetic heterogeneity of AIDS lymphomagenesis (513).

Several differences exist between endemic and sporadic BL. In nearly all patients with endemic BL, the tumor cells contain the EBV genome, express Fc receptors and CD21 (the EBV receptor), lack CD10, and do not secrete IgM. Only a small proportion of sporadic BLs contain the EBV genome, and the tumor cells usually lack Fc receptors and CD21, express CD10, and secrete IgM. Dalla-Favera and others have demonstrated that the translocations involving chromosome 8 lead to *MYC* gene deregulation by molecular mechanisms that vary according to the geographic origin of the BL (514,515). The *MYC* gene is activated by point mutations or small rearrangements occurring within regulatory regions spanning its first exon-first intron border in the translocation t(8;14) associated with endemic BL and the variant translocations t(2;8) and t(8;22) associated with both endemic and sporadic BL. In contrast, the *MYC* gene is activated by truncations occurring within its first exon, first intron, or 5′ flanking sequences in the translocation t(8;14) associated with sporadic BL (514–517). The pattern of chromosome 14 involvement in t(8;14) is also heterogeneous. *MYC* recombines preferentially with the joining region of the immunoglobulin heavy chain gene in all BLs, but more often with the switch region of the immunoglobulin heavy chain gene in sporadic BL than in endemic BL (514–517). The pathogeneses of endemic and sporadic BL appear to differ, probably as a consequence of differences in the differentiation state of the target cells in which the translocational events occur (515) (see Chapter 27).

Most AIDS-related systemic BLs exhibit *MYC* gene rearrangement, but many of them do not contain EBV, and the tumor cells lack Fc and EBV receptors (CD21) but express CD10 (259,488,492), analogous to sporadic BL (501). In addition, the molecular mechanisms leading to *MYC* gene activation in these lymphomas are similar to those operational in sporadic BL (492,493,516). The bulk of the accumulated immunologic and molecular genetic data suggests that most AIDS-related systemic BLs resemble sporadic rather than endemic BL.

The *BCL6* gene is located on 3q27 (518), the site of frequent chromosomal breaks in conventional and some AIDS-related NHLs (519,520). The *BCL6* gene encodes a zinc finger protein that shares homologies with several transcription factors (521–523). The BCL-6 protein normally is expressed at high levels by mature GCB cells (524) and is believed to control germinal center formation (525). Chromosomal translocations between 3q27 and a heterogeneous chromosomal partner cause the truncation of the *BCL6* gene within its 5′ noncoding

regulatory sequences (521) in about 40% of diffuse large B-cell lymphomas occurring in immunocompetent hosts (526). *BCL6* gene rearrangements generally are not found in other categories of NHL, except for a small proportion of follicular center cell lymphomas (526). *BCL6* gene rearrangements are detectable in approximately 20% of AIDS-related systemic NHLs, including both EBV-positive and EBV-negative cases (501). As in the case of conventional NHLs, however, they are associated overwhelmingly with those AIDS-related NHLs exhibiting large cell and immunoblastic morphology and are absent from those exhibiting classic Burkitt morphology (501). *BCL6* and *MYC* gene rearrangements do not occur in the same tumor, suggesting that these genetic lesions represent mutually exclusive molecular pathways in lymphomagenesis. It has been suggested that *BCL6* gene rearrangement occurs preferentially among extranodal large cell lymphomas and is a favorable prognostic indicator for these lymphomas (527). Whether this holds true for *BCL6* gene rearrangement in AIDS-related NHLs has not been determined.

Activation of the *RAS* family of genes by single nucleotide substitutions at codons 12, 13, and 61 has been associated with a variety of human malignancies (528). Mutations involving *NRAS* gene codons 12 or 13 are detectable in almost 20% of precursor B-cell acute lymphoblastic leukemias (ALLs), and mutations involving *NRAS* gene codon 61 are detectable in approximately one-third of cases of multiple myeloma and plasmacytoma (529). *RAS* gene mutations are not detectable in conventional NHLs occurring in the HIV-uninfected general population, however, including those exhibiting Burkitt, large cell, or immunoblastic morphology (529). In contrast, activating point mutations involving *NRAS* or, less commonly, *KRAS*, are detectable in about 15% of AIDS-related systemic lymphomas (493). *RAS* gene mutations are more likely to be distinctive features in AIDS-related NHLs than in conventional NHLs of comparable morphology arising in immunocompetent persons. The biologic significance of this association is unknown. It is likely, however, that the mutated *RAS* genes contribute to the pathogenesis of those AIDS-related lymphomas in which they are present, because their role in the tumorigenic conversion of EBV-infected B-cells *in vitro* is established (530).

Rearrangements of the *BCL1* gene, associated with translocation t(11;14), are associated preferentially with mantle cell lymphoma and occur in about 50% of these lymphomas (531). Rearrangements of the *BCL2* gene, associated with t(14;18), are associated highly with malignant lymphomas of follicular center cell origin. They occur in more than 80% of such cases displaying a follicular growth pattern and in the 20% of diffuse large B-cell lymphomas preceded by a follicular phase (532,533). AIDS-related NHLs consistently lack *BCL1* and *BCL2* gene rearrangements (312,492,534). These findings strongly suggest that AIDS-related NHLs are not derived from mantle or follicular center B cells and that they originate *de novo* and are not preceded by a follicular phase, as is a subset of conventional diffuse large B-cell lymphomas (533).

Certain tumor suppressor genes, including the *P53* gene, the Rb gene, and putative genes on chromosome 6q, are believed to play an important role in the development and progression of human neoplasia if deletions or mutations in these loci relieve cells from normal negative regulatory signals (535–538). The *P53* gene, mapping to 17p13, encodes a nuclear phosphoprotein that is believed to play an essential role in cell-cycle control (536,537). Inactivation of the *P53* gene is usually the result of point mutations in the coding sequence of exons 5 through 8 in one allele, with or without loss of the corresponding allele (536,537). Mutations of the *P53* gene occur relatively frequently in many categories of human malignancy (539,540). Among lymphoid neoplasms, *P53* gene mutations are highly associated with BL, large cell transformation of B-cell chronic lymphocytic leukemia (Richter syndrome), and adult T-cell lymphoma/leukemia (541,542). Overexpression of MDM2, and negative regulators of P53, also occurs in BL. *P53* gene mutations occur uncommonly among other categories of conventional NHL (541). Mutations involving the *P53* gene occur in about 37% of AIDS-related systemic NHLs (493) but are associated preferentially with Burkitt morphology (493). This includes both EBV-positive and EBV-negative tumors (493). The frequent association between *P53* gene mutation and *MYC* gene deregulation in both AIDS-related and non–AIDS-related BLs suggest a pathogenetic relationship between these two genetic lesions that may have a synergistic effect on the development of these tumors. This hypothesis is supported by the finding that the MYC protein may be involved in the regulation of *P53* gene expression (543). The mutations similarly occur in exons 5 through 8 in AIDS-related NHLs. The most frequently encountered mutations are transitions at CpG dinucleotides (493), as is the case for conventional NHLs and some other tumors (536,537). This type of mutation is believed to occur as a DNA replication error, with no direct causal relationship with any known carcinogen (536). In some instances, *P53* gene mutations are accompanied by loss of the corresponding allele (493). The molecular mechanisms of *P53* gene inactivation in AIDS-related systemic NHLs are similar to those occurring in other human tumors (537), and the mutational spectrum is comparable to that of conventional NHLs occurring in immunocompetent hosts (541).

Deletions of the long arm of chromosome 6 have been long recognized as one of the predominant genetic lesions, as well as an indicator of poor prognosis, among B-cell lymphomas (538). Deletions of 6q are present in approximately 25% of AIDS-related NHLs and may play a role in their pathogenesis (535). The 6q deletions cluster in two discrete regions along the long arm of chromosome 6 mapping to 6q27 (region of minimal deletion-1 [*RMD1*]) and 6q21-23 (*RMD2*). These two regions represent the sites of two putative tumor suppressor genes, which appear to be relevant to lymphomagenesis, leukemiagenesis, and tumorigenesis (544–546). *RMD1* and *RMD2* exhibit preferential association with low- and high-grade B-cell lymphomas, respectively (547). It is thought that *RMD2* lesions participate in AIDS lymphomagenesis, although the precise mechanism is unclear.

The Rb gene, located on chromosome 13q14 (548), encodes 110- to 114-kd phosphorylated proteins that are normally present in all human tissues and are believed to inhibit cell growth (549). Mutational inactivation of the Rb gene has been documented in a large variety of malignant tumors, suggesting that functional loss of this gene is involved in the initiation or progression of many human malignancies (535). Point mutations, encountered in 80% of lesions, represent the most frequent mechanism of Rb gene inactivation; gross rearrangements or large intragenic deletions occur much less commonly (550). A small proportion of diffuse aggressive conventional NHLs occurring in the HIV-uninfected general population exhibit Rb gene mutations or deletions (546). Investigators have failed to find evidence of Rb gene inactivation in AIDS-related NHLs (493,551), suggesting that this gene does not play a role in AIDS lymphomagenesis.

These molecular genetic alterations do not appear to occur entirely randomly among the AIDS-related NHLs, however. Previous molecular genetic analyses have suggested that distinct molecular differences exist among AIDS-related NHLs according to their histopathologic categories and anatomic sites of origin, that is, systemic versus primary CNS (300,301,480,492,493,501). These studies have suggested that virtually 100% of patients with BL exhibit *MYC* gene rearrangements, two-thirds display *P53* gene mutations, one-third have EBV, and essentially none exhibit *BCL6* gene rearrangements. In the case of immunoblastic lymphoma, these studies have suggested that nearly 100% of patients have EBV, 25% display *MYC* gene rearrangements, 20%

display *BCL6* gene rearrangements, and very few exhibit *P53* gene mutations. *RAS* gene mutations occur in a comparable proportion, about 20%, of patients with Burkitt and immunoblastic lymphomas. These studies also have suggested, in the case of large cell lymphoma, that about 25% contain EBV, 50% exhibit *MYC* gene rearrangements, 25% exhibit *BCL6* gene rearrangements, and none contain *P53* or *RAS* gene mutations (493,501). Most of these studies, however, have involved only a small number of patients, often seen at a single institution where some but not all of the parameters were investigated.

A comprehensive analysis of the viral content and the oncogene and tumor suppressor gene status of a cohort of 64 AIDS-related systemic NHLs originating on the east and west coasts of the United States was performed by our group, and findings were correlated with the histopathology of the lesions (259,499,500). The incidence, type, and clonal pattern of EBV infection and the type and frequency of molecular genetic lesions were similar among the east and west coast cases, suggesting no evidence of geographic distinctions. Clonal EBV infection was seen in 41% of the AIDS-related systemic NHLs by Southern blot hybridization analysis of the EBV terminal repeat region, consistent with previous studies (492,493). Type A EBV was found in two-thirds of the patients, and type B in the remaining one-third. *MYC* gene rearrangements, *P53* gene mutations or deletions, *BCL6* gene rearrangements, and *RAS* gene mutations were seen in 44%, 30%, 17%, and 6% of patients with these AIDS-related systemic NHLs, respectively. No *BCL1* or *BCL2* gene rearrangements or Rb gene mutations or deletions were found among these patients. More than 80% of the patients with BL were found to have EBV and *MYC* gene rearrangements, and approximately one-half have *P53* gene mutations in the absence of *BCL6* gene rearrangements and *RAS* gene mutations. The Burkitt-like lymphomas exhibited a comparable constellation of genetic alterations, except that a smaller proportion of patients have EBV infection, *MYC* gene rearrangements, and *P53* gene mutations, and that *BCL6* gene rearrangements occur in a small percentage of patients. Among the large cell lymphomas, only very few patients were found to have EBV, approximately one-half had *MYC* gene rearrangements, a small percentage had *P53* gene mutations, and approximately 25% exhibited *BCL6* gene rearrangements. Comprehensive molecular genetic analysis of AIDS-related primary CNS lymphomas has not been performed. We know that they uniformly contain the EBV genome and lack *MYC* gene rearrangements (480).

More recent genomic studies have been performed on AIDS-related lymphomas, albeit on smaller cohorts. Comparative genomic hybridization single nucleotide polymorphism–based microarrays were reported by Capello et al. on 57 cases, and compared to 105 DLBCL cases occurring in immunocompetent individuals. BLs were reported to have less alterations and HIV-related DLBCLs, and, among the latter, the EBV+ cases had fewer alterations. Specific deletions were reported to occur in AIDS-related NHLs, including those in the following genes: FHIT (FRA3B), WWOX (FRA16D), DCC (FRA18B), and PARK2 (FRA6E), which were also frequently found to be suppressed through aberrant methylation of regulative regions (552). Deffenbacher et al. (553) compared DNA copy number and gene expression in 20 cases. Again, differences between BL and DLBCL were noted, as well as recurrent losses and gains. Specifically, this study documented gain of 19p13.2 and loss of 16q23; the latter region includes the WW domain–containing oxidoreductase (WWOX) tumor suppressor gene also reported by Capello et al. The WWOX gene is present in a chromosomal fragile site and has been shown to interact with a variety of proteins involved in growth, differentiation, apoptosis, and tumor suppression, and is deleted in a variety of different malignancies. Deffenbacher et al. (553) reported that WWOX is silenced or encodes truncated transcript in 9 of 16 cases of AIDS-related lymphoma.

These findings indicate that AIDS-related lymphomas are characterized by the accumulation of multiple distinct genetic lesions, involving viruses, protooncogenes, and tumor suppressor genes. These genetic lesions apparently accrue rather quickly, during the brief 4- to 6-year period between HIV infection and the development of malignant lymphoma (276,288). This contrasts sharply with the widely held belief that multistep tumorigenesis occurs over a long period of time, perhaps as long as 30 years (554,555). These findings also support the contention that multiple alternative molecular pathways operate in AIDS lymphomagenesis, and that some of these pathways may be associated preferentially with specific histopathologic categories or anatomic sites of origin. Although EBV infection and certain molecular genetic alterations are associated with distinct histopathologic categories, the correlations do not appear to be as specific as previously suggested. AIDS-related NHLs appear to represent a morphologic and molecular genetic spectrum of high-grade lymphoid neoplasia. Future clinical studies, including therapeutic trials, should include a comprehensive correlative morphologic and molecular genetic analysis of the lymphomas in order to verify and extend these findings. Such studies eventually may yield a classification, based at least partially on genetic features, that is clinically and prognostically more relevant than the current classification of AIDS-related lymphomas, which is based largely on histopathologic evaluation alone.

Clinical Characteristics Including Correlations with Anatomic Site of Origin and Histopathology

Approximately 95% of AIDS-related NHLs occur in adult men (252,255,257–259,270,276,278,288,449). This is largely because adult men predominate among the principal AIDS risk groups, that is, MSM and IDUs. The median age of patients is between 37 and 38 years in the largest clinical series reported from the United States (255,259,296) and 27 and 29 years in the largest Western European series (274,297); however, AIDS-related NHLs occasionally occur in the very young or in the elderly who have other AIDS risk factors. The age distribution for patients with AIDS-related NHL conforms closely to that of AIDS in general (252). Approximately 50% of patients develop one or more severe opportunistic infections, and as many as 25% of patients (primarily MSM) have been reported to develop KS before, concurrent with, or after the onset of NHL (252,259,296,449). The majority of patients exhibit the alterations in cellular immunity commonly associated with HIV infection, including cytopenias, cutaneous anergy, polyclonal hypergammaglobulinemia, and greatly decreased numbers of peripheral blood CD4 T cells, resulting in markedly reduced CD4:CD8 T-cell ratios (252,255,259,449). The majority of patients also have serologic evidence of preceding or active cytomegalovirus or EBV infection (255,296,301,449).

Approximately 75% or more of patients who have AIDS-related NHLs complain of B symptoms as defined by the Ann Arbor staging system (556): unexplained fever, night sweats, or weight loss in excess of 10% of usual body weight (255,279,286,288,301). The B symptoms are secondary to malignant lymphoma in the majority of patients (286). Aside from B symptoms, patient complaints at initial presentation are variable because of the diverse and multiple organ systems involved by malignant lymphoma. The complaints may be local or systemic and usually depend on the principal location of lymphomatous disease (426).

AIDS-related NHLs belonging to all histopathologic categories were lumped together initially in most clinical studies for purposes of management, therapy, and clinicopathologic analysis. Knowles et al. (259) demonstrated that each histopathologic category of AIDS-related NHL actually exhibits distinctive clinical characteristics, including specific associations with clinical stage, preferential involvement of certain extranodal sites,

and perhaps even statistically significant differences in median survival. For example, approximately two-thirds of patients who have BL, but only approximately 40% of patients who have immunoblastic or large cell lymphoma, present with clinical stage IV disease. This is partially because AIDS-related NHLs differ in their propensity to involve the bone marrow according to their histopathology. In a series of 89 patients with AIDS-related NHLs, 39% of those who had BL, only 16% of those who had immunoblastic lymphoma, and none of the 25 patients who had large cell lymphoma had bone marrow involvement at initial presentation (259). AIDS-related NHLs differ in their propensity to involve the gastrointestinal tract according to their histopathology. In that same series, 48% of immunoblastic, 36% of large cell, but only 8% of BLs involved the gastrointestinal tract initially (259). The French Study Group, based on an analysis of 113 AIDS-related NHLs, confirmed and extended these findings (466). They demonstrated that BL more frequently involves lymph nodes, the bone marrow, and skeletal muscles; that immunoblastic lymphoma and large cell lymphoma more frequently involve the oral cavity, the gastrointestinal tract, and the CNS; and that these associations are statistically significant (466). The vast majority of primary CNS lymphomas express immunoblastic or large cell morphology (278,279,301,466,480). It appears that AIDS-related BLs usually originate in lymph nodes and then rapidly disseminate to involve distant lymph node groups, the bone marrow, and obscure extranodal sites; AIDS-related immunoblastic and large cell lymphomas more often originate in extranodal sites such as the gastrointestinal tract, grow to a large size at the primary site of origin, spread to regional lymph nodes, and subsequently disseminate to other lymph node groups and extranodal sites (259).

Other significant clinical distinctions exist among AIDS-related NHLs according to their histopathologic category and anatomic site of origin. For example, those individuals who develop AIDS-related BL tend to be younger, usually do not have a prior diagnosis of AIDS, and tend to have higher mean CD4 T-cell counts at the time of diagnosis. In contrast, those individuals who develop AIDS-related immunoblastic lymphoma tend to be older, frequently have a prior diagnosis of AIDS, and tend to have lower mean CD4 T-cell counts at diagnosis (276,278,301). BL tends to be an earlier manifestation of HIV infection than does immunoblastic lymphoma, which represented a secondary AIDS diagnosis in 87% of patients in one study (278). Immunodeficiency appears to be more severe and the HIV-associated illnesses appear to be more extensive in HIV-infected individuals who develop primary CNS lymphoma than in those who develop systemic lymphoma. In one study, the median CD4 T-cell count in patients with primary CNS lymphoma was only 30 cells/μL; it was 189 cells/μL in those patients who developed systemic lymphoma (279). In that same study, more than 70% of the patients who developed primary CNS lymphoma had a prior diagnosis of AIDS; only 37% of those who developed systemic lymphoma had documented AIDS (279).

The PELs more closely resemble immunoblastic lymphoma than BL and primary CNS lymphomas than systemic lymphomas, with respect to these various clinical characteristics. The PELs tend to occur in slightly older HIV-infected individuals (median age 42 years), who are usually severely immunodeficient (median CD4 T-cell count 84 cells/μL) and two-thirds of whom have prior diagnoses of AIDS (333).

The therapeutic response and eventual outcome appear to differ according to the histopathologic category of NHL (259). In a clinicopathologic study of 89 patients who had AIDS-related NHL, Knowles et al. (259) found that 52% of patients who had large cell, 26% of patients who had Burkitt, and 21% of patients who had immunoblastic lymphoma achieved complete responses. The patients who had large cell, Burkitt, and immunoblastic lymphoma had median durations of survival of 7.5, 5.5, and 2.0 months, respectively (259). These survival rates are significantly shorter than those of HIV-uninfected patients in the general population who have histologically identical conventional NHLs (557). These findings strongly suggest that patients who have AIDS-related immunoblastic lymphoma fare the worst. These conclusions were based on a retrospective series of patients who had been treated with a variety of chemotherapeutic regimens and who were not stratified in terms of prognostic factors, however. More recent clinical trials have shown better clinical outcomes, where accrual was based on specific histologic subtype, and rituximab was included (558,559). It is now thought that therapy should largely be similar to that of HIV-uninfected individuals based on subclassification, including autologous stem cell transplantation when indicated, with adequate supportive care for other complications of AIDS, appropriate antiretroviral therapy, and consideration of all the possible pharmacologic interactions.

It is likely that the significance of these clinical observations will be solidified, and other distinctions having etiologic, therapeutic, and prognostic significance will become evident as more data are accumulated.

Prognostic Factors

Several factors are associated with shorter durations of survival among HIV-uninfected individuals who have conventional intermediate and high-grade NHL. These include older age, the presence of systemic B symptoms, increased tumor burden, and lower patient performance status (560,561). These factors, however, have not been uniformly applicable to patients who have AIDS-related NHL, among whom prognostic factors related to HIV infection and associated illnesses appear to be more important than those related to malignant lymphoma *per se*. For example, no correlation was found between clinical stage or histologic grade and complete response in the first large multiinstitutional series (252). In a multivariate analysis of 49 patients with AIDS-related systemic NHL from a single institution, Levine et al. (279) found that a prior history of AIDS, a Karnofsky performance status <70%, and bone marrow involvement each predicted shorter survival. Lower CD4 T-cell counts also appeared to imply shorter duration of survival (279). Systemic B symptoms, tumor size, histopathologic category, elevated lactic dehydrogenase levels, and leptomeningeal disease did not predict shorter survival (279).

A series of 84 patients with AIDS-related NHL reported from San Francisco (299) confirmed the dominance of prognostic factors related to HIV infection and AIDS. In that series, the total number of CD4 T cells was the most important predictor of survival. Patients who had a total CD4 T-cell count >100 cells/μL had a median duration of survival of 24 months; for those whose CD4 T-cell count was <100 cells/μL, the duration of survival was only 4.1 months. If CD4 T-cell counts were available, no other factors contributed prognostic information. More recent studies using current therapies have confirmed that patients have an improved CR rate and improved event-free survival and overall survival when they have a low aaIPI score and a baseline CD4 count $\geq$100/μL (562,563). In the absence of CD4 T-cell counts, however, the best predictor of survival was a prior diagnosis of AIDS. The median survival of those patients without a prior AIDS diagnosis was 8.3 months, versus 2.2 months for those patients with a prior AIDS diagnosis. Less important prognostic factors were the Karnofsky performance status and the presence of extranodal disease. A Karnofsky performance status >70% was associated with a median duration of survival of 6.8 months; one <70% was associated with a median duration of survival of 3.8 months. The median survival of those patients with extranodal disease was only 3.4 months, versus 12.2 months for those patients who had lymphadenopathy alone. Survival was not influenced by the specific extranodal site or the total number of extranodal

sites. In this series, the use of more intensive chemotherapy regimens also correlated with decreased duration of survival (299). The survival of patients who have AIDS-related NHL appears to be most dependent on their level of immunodeficiency. The prognostic significance of the histopathologic category of AIDS-related NHL within the context of this immunodeficiency was evaluated in a more recent clinical trial of R-CHOP: the response rate for DLBCL was 81% (95% CI, 79% to 82%) and the response rate for BL was 73%, but these survival data were not statistically different (562).

Clinical Evaluation, Treatment, and Survival

The staging procedures routinely employed in the evaluation of patients who have AIDS-related NHLs are the same as those for HIV-uninfected patients who have conventional NHLs. They include a complete blood count; serum biochemistry studies, including liver function tests and creatinine and lactic acid dehydrogenase measurements; chest radiograph; bone marrow aspiration and biopsy; and CT of the chest, abdomen, and pelvis, with oral and intravenous contrast administration. In addition, a diagnostic lumbar puncture should be performed and the cerebrospinal fluid checked for cytology, cell count, and protein and glucose levels. Other workup depends on whether or not there are other unusual extranodal sites of involvement. It is desirable to check on the status of the HIV infection with CD4 T-cell counts and measurements of HIV load with plasma RNA levels (564).

The diagnosis of primary CNS lymphoma usually is established firmly by brain biopsy performed at craniostomy or with a CT–guided stereotactic procedure. Some clinicians are reluctant to perform these diagnostic procedures, however, because of the associated risks and the poor therapeutic outcome (565). For this reason, noninvasive diagnostic procedures that may obviate the need for brain biopsy in some patients are being investigated. For example, one universal and potentially diagnostic feature of AIDS-related primary CNS lymphoma is the presence of the EBV genome (480). Cinque et al. (566) investigated as a possible diagnostic test a PCR assay of EBV in the cerebrospinal fluid of patients with AIDS-related primary CNS lymphoma. They reported that EBV DNA is consistently present in the cerebrospinal fluid of patients who have AIDS-related primary CNS lymphoma before the lesions can be visualized by CT scan or by MRI, and that it is consistently absent from the cerebrospinal fluid of HIV-infected patients who die with other neurologic disorders, including toxoplasmosis and other infections. De Luca et al. (567) reported similar findings.

Sometimes, the diagnosis of AIDS-related NHL is made first at autopsy, especially in the case of primary CNS lymphoma (252,258,259,301,452). In other instances, malignant lymphoma is so widespread at initial presentation and the patient is so ill that death occurs almost immediately following diagnosis, before therapy can be initiated (252,259,296,301). In approximately 85% of patients, however, a tissue diagnosis of AIDS-related NHL is established *antemortem*, and the patient is treated. The treatment of AIDS-related systemic NHL is complicated by the fact that most patients have high- or intermediate-grade NHL and present with clinical stage III or IV disease, and many patients have secondary lymphomatous involvement of the bone marrow or the CNS. With these factors in mind, early treatment strategies employed dosage-intensive chemotherapeutic regimens comparable to those used to treat HIV-uninfected patients in the general population who have high- or intermediate-grade NHL (259,296). These approaches generally achieved dismal results, however. In one study, those patients who were treated more intensively actually experienced a significantly shorter duration of survival than those who were treated less intensively (299). HIV-infected patients often tolerate systemic chemotherapy poorly because of the severe underlying immune deficiency, recurring opportunistic infections, and leukopenia (426,568).

Complete response rates to the various, often dosage-intensive, chemotherapy regimens utilized in these early treatment strategies ranged between 20% and 67% (259,274,296,301,568–570). CR occurred primarily in those patients who presented with clinical stage I or II disease, without bone marrow or CNS involvement, and who had not experienced AIDS-related symptomatology (296). Even those responses were usually of short duration, and second-line chemotherapeutic regimens were rarely effective in inducing a second remission (259). CNS relapses were particularly problematic, and the use of prophylactic intrathecal chemotherapy did not prevent this phenomenon consistently (259,286,296,569). The median duration of survival usually was brief, ranging from 5 to 11 months (255,259,270,296,568–570).

Based on this information, the AIDS Clinical Trials Group initiated a prospective multiinstitutional trial using a low-dosage modification of the M-BACOD regimen (571), accompanied by early CNS prophylaxis with intrathecal cytosine arabinoside, and zidovudine at the completion of chemotherapy (563). A CR rate of approximately 50%, including long-term lymphoma-free survival in 75% of complete responders, was achieved among all patients, including those with poor prognostic indicators. Intrathecal CNS prophylaxis was effective; no patient experienced isolated CNS relapse. The median duration of survival was 6.5 months for all patients and 15 months for complete responders (572). Shortly thereafter, the availability of hematopoietic growth factors permitted the AIDS Clinical Trials Group (573) and Kaplan et al. (574), among others, to abrogate leukopenia and administer full doses of chemotherapy.

These and other therapeutic trials have led to some progress in achieving longer survival among patients who have AIDS-related systemic NHL (288). For example, it is now known that very low-dosage multiagent chemotherapy may be effective in achieving long-term, lymphoma-free survival; CNS prophylaxis is necessary and intrathecal chemotherapy is effective in this regard (563,575); and hematopoietic growth factors may ameliorate the hematologic toxicity of chemotherapy in these patients (573,574). Individuals who have AIDS-related systemic NHL should receive antilymphoma therapy, because relatively long-lasting remissions can be obtained even in those who have poor prognostic indicators. Successful salvage therapy, however, has not been achieved in patients who fail initial therapy or who experience relapse after initial remission, even among those who have undergone bone marrow transplantation (BMT) (288). Only occasional patients during the earlier trials were long-term survivors (259,296,449), with patients usually dying from progressive lymphoma, opportunistic infections, or a combination of the two (252,258,259,274,296,301). More recent clinical trials have resulted in much better outcomes. The addition of rituximab to the CHOP regimen (cyclophosphamide, doxorubicin, vincristine, and prednisone) has resulted in improved outcome albeit with inclusion of prophylactic antibiotics because of the potential for increased risk from infection (563,576). Infusional chemotherapy with EPOCH (etoposide, vincristine, doxorubicin, cyclophosphamide, and prednisone) given concurrently with rituximab has resulted in the most promising progression-free and overall survivals, with 73% of patients achieving a complete response (576). Autologous stem cell transplantation has also been successful in patients on antiretroviral therapy (577).

Patients who have AIDS-related primary CNS lymphoma usually are treated with intracranial irradiation, sometimes in combination with intrathecal chemotherapy (452,465). This approach often leads to regression of the lesions (451,465). These patients generally have very severe immune deficiency, however, as manifested by CD4 T-cell counts below 50 cells/μL and multiple prior or concurrent opportunistic infections (279,302). They often die as a result of severe opportunistic infections (465,481).

Some patients have a fulminant course and die within weeks following diagnosis (452). The mean duration of survival of patients following the onset of CNS symptoms was shorter than 2 months for those diagnosed and cared for at both the LAC-USC and University of California at San Francisco Medical Centers (451,452). In the largest clinical series of such patients reported to date, the median duration of survival was about 1 month for those patients who received no treatment and 4 months for those patients who received radiation therapy (481). Only rare patients survive for longer than 1 year (465,578,579), and these are usually the ones who have CD4 T-cell counts >200 cells/μL (578). This is substantially worse than the prognosis for conventional primary CNS lymphoma occurring in the HIV-uninfected general population (580). It has been suggested that the use of systemic chemotherapy in addition to intracranial radiation may be helpful in patients who have AIDS-related primary CNS lymphoma (579). Historically, the severe immune deficiency in these individuals, however, usually rendered them unable to tolerate the additional immune suppression caused by systemic chemotherapy. The optimal therapeutic approach for these patients remains undefined, and recent prospective clinical trials have not been done because of the dramatic decrease in the incidence of AIDS-related primary CNS lymphoma since the onset of cART, making this a rather rare disease.

Pathogenesis of HIV-related Non-Hodgkin Lymphomas

The increased risk of lymphoma in patients with HIV is multifactorial and may be related to the transforming properties of the retrovirus, the resulting immunosuppression and cytokine dysregulation caused by the virus, and opportunistic infections with lymphotropic viruses such as EBV and KSHV (581). Initially, it was thought that HIV might be directly responsible for the B-cell NHLs that develop in HIV-infected patients, because HIV can infect EBV-transformed cells (582) and is endemic in regions of Africa in which BL is common (583). Laurence and Astrin (584) provided some experimental support for this hypothesis when they were able to infect peripheral blood B cells obtained from HIV-seronegative, EBV-seropositive donors with HIV and derive continuously proliferating cell lines. If inoculated into severe combined immune deficiency (SCID) or nude mice, the HIV-transformed B cells gave rise to lymphoid proliferations resembling malignant lymphomas (584). These findings led these investigators to conclude that HIV may play a direct role in AIDS lymphomagenesis. Numerous other investigators, however, consistently have failed to find evidence of HIV DNA by Southern blot hybridization analysis in the genomes of freshly isolated AIDS-related lymphomas and lymphoma cell lines established *in vitro* (252,312,488,492,506,521,585). PCR analysis of AIDS-related lymphoma tissues has demonstrated HIV levels consistent with the presence of infiltrating benign T cells within the tissues and inconsistent with HIV infection of the malignant lymphoma B cells (586). It is now thought that HIV is not involved directly in the *in vivo* malignant transformation of B cells or, consequently, in the direct induction of AIDS-related B-cell lymphomas. High-grade B-cell lymphomas develop in a similar setting in a primate model 5 to 15 months after infection by SIV and coincidentally with the onset of severe immune deficiency (587). These SIV–associated lymphomas are devoid of SIV genomes (587), consistent with the absence of HIV genome from AIDS-related lymphomas. It is more likely that the NHLs arising in HIV-infected individuals are the consequence of the immunosuppression and lack of immunosurveillance that develops in these individuals. HIV may play an indirect role in AIDS lymphomagenesis by inducing cytokine deregulation of the microenvironment (588) or by chronic antigen stimulation by HIV antigens (589–591).

Impaired Immune Surveillance

Diffuse aggressive B-cell NHLs, many of which share clinical and morphologic characteristics with AIDS-related NHLs, occur with an increased incidence in individuals who have congenital or acquired immune defects (244,473). HIV infection is associated with a variety of immunologic observations, including quantitative changes and functional defects in the CD4 T-cell population (592,593). Several investigators have demonstrated that the greatest risk for the development of AIDS-related NHLs occurs when CD4 T-cell counts are $<50/\mu L$ (279,594,595), as is often the case in patients who have AIDS-related systemic immunoblastic lymphomas and primary CNS lymphomas (277–279). Prolonged exposure to immunosuppression appears to be another critical factor. Pluda et al. (595) estimated that the risk of individuals who have <50 CD4 T cells per microliter for 24 months developing an AIDS-related NHL is more than double that of individuals with AIDS who are not selected for their CD4 T-cell counts. HIV-infected individuals suffer from selective impairment of immune surveillance against EBV-infected B cells, which are present in increased numbers in the peripheral blood and lymphoid tissues and may be responsible for minor clonal B-cell expansions that precede malignant transformation (596). Some investigators have suggested that these clonal expansions represent the precursors of AIDS-related NHLs (535).

AIDS lymphomagenesis likely also is affected by a failed local T-cell response *in situ*. The magnitude of the local response by tumor-infiltrating T cells has been suggested as an independent predictor of clinical outcome (597). Fewer tumor-infiltrating T cells are present in biopsy specimens from large cell lymphomas occurring in patients who have AIDS than in those from immunocompetent hosts (598). This is consistent with the description of profound functional defects of CD8 T cells in HIV-infected persons (588).

Cytokines and Growth Factors

Although it is unlikely that HIV participates in AIDS lymphomagenesis directly, it may participate indirectly by inducing the release of cytokines. Numerous cytokines and growth factors, including IL-1, IL-2, IL-4, IL-6, IL-7, IL-10, interferon-γ, tumor necrosis factor, lymphotoxin, and B-cell growth factors of 25 and 50 kDa, are responsible for B-cell differentiation and proliferation (599–605). The ongoing activation of various cytokine networks and the release of these stimuli contributes to the state of chronic B-cell proliferation that characterizes HIV-induced immunosuppression (288). Experimental evidence suggests that at least some of these factors may play roles in the development and growth of malignant lymphoma. Additionally, cytokines known to be able to stimulate B cells, as well as markers of immune activation, can be found to be elevated in HIV-infected patients several years before the diagnosis of AIDS-related NHL (606).

Deregulation of the normal cytokine networks is a key feature of HIV infection (588). This may contribute to AIDS lymphomagenesis in two ways: First, cytokine deregulation may assist in maintaining HIV infection, or even making it more severe, in turn worsening immune function and facilitating the development of AIDS-related NHL (535). For example, in persons who have AIDS, the intense antigenic exposure of B cells *in vivo* directly activates IL-6 and tumor necrosis factor-α production. In turn, IL-6 and tumor necrosis factor-α induce HIV expression, maintaining viral infection (588). Second, deregulation by HIV of the numerous cytokines that normally control B-cell differentiation and proliferation may induce or sustain the growth of B-cell malignancies (535). For example, B cells from HIV-infected individuals who have hypergammaglobulinemia constitutively secrete high levels of tumor necrosis factor-α and IL-6 *in vitro* in the absence of exogenous stimuli (588).

There is considerable experimental evidence to support a role for IL-6 and IL-10 in AIDS lymphomagenesis. It is known that IL-6 potentiates the tumorigenicity of EBV-infected B cells (607,608) and plays a role in the development of B-cell lymphomas in immunocompetent hosts (609–612). IL-6 functions as an autocrine growth factor in tumor cell lines derived from non–AIDS-related, EBV-negative NHLs (613) and in multiple myeloma (609). Constitutive expression of the *IL6* gene has been demonstrated in chronic lymphocytic leukemia (614). With respect to AIDS lymphomagenesis, HIV directly stimulates IL-6 production by monocytes and macrophages (615), which in turn promotes the chronic proliferation of activated B cells, thereby driving immunoglobulin synthesis and causing the nonspecific hypergammaglobulinemia commonly seen in early HIV infection (616–618). IL-6 also is produced by activated B cells, which further contributes to the relatively high IL-6 serum levels observed in HIV-infected persons (619). Once a malignant lymphoma is established firmly, its continuous growth and expansion may be driven by IL-6 through paracrine loops (620). Macrophages and endothelial cells intermingled with the tumor cells release IL-6, which acts on IL-6 receptors expressed at high levels on the tumor cells (620). Consistent with this hypothesis, high levels of IL-6 have been demonstrated in both AIDS-related and non–AIDS-related immunoblastic and large cell lymphomas, independent of their EBV status (620). The number of IL-6 expressing cells has been found to be substantially higher in large cell lymphomas containing a high proportion of immunoblasts than in BLs, in which immunoblasts are absent (620), consistent with the purported role of IL-6 in the terminal stages of B-cell differentiation. Finally, clinical support for the role of IL-6 in the development of AIDS-related NHL comes from Pluda et al. (403,595) who discovered that elevated IL-6 serum levels may predict the future development of malignant lymphoma among individuals with symptomatic HIV infection.

Interleukin-10 is a pleiotropic cytokine with striking homology to BCRF-1, an EBV protein, and is a potent EBV stimulator (621). IL-10 production is absent from endemic and sporadic BL occurring in non–HIV-infected individuals (622). Benjamin et al. (622), however, demonstrated that B-cell lines derived from AIDS-related BL constitutively express IL-10 in large amounts, suggesting that IL-10 production is especially associated with AIDS lymphomagenesis. These findings were confirmed by Masood et al. (623) who also showed that IL-10 acts as an autocrine growth factor in these cell lines. It has been suggested that IL-10 contributes to AIDS lymphomagenesis by impairing immune surveillance against EBV-infected B cells through inhibition of T-cell production of IL-2 and interferon-α (624,625), by inhibiting B-cell apoptosis (626), or through its B-cell–differentiating activity (627).

Other B-cell stimulatory cytokines and molecules associated with immune activation that have been found to be elevated in patients with AIDS-related NHL, when compared with HIV+ controls or with AIDS controls, and after adjusting for CD4 T-cell number, are C-reactive protein, soluble CD23, soluble CD27, soluble CD30, and CXCL13 (606,628,629).

Epstein-Barr Virus

EBV initially was implicated as a cause of endemic BL. It was theorized that a compromised immune system permits EBV infection, resulting in polyclonal B-cell activation in the context of aberrant B-cell regulation, and that the inherent genetic instability of the EBV-immortalized B cells eventually leads to *MYC* gene rearrangement and the development of malignant lymphoma (630,631). Support for this hypothesis includes the facts that EBV infection occurs prior to the development of endemic BL (632) and that the EBV genome is found consistently in endemic BL cells (633). Subsequently, EBV has been implicated in the pathogenesis of an array of LPDs occurring in individuals who have congenital, acquired, and iatrogenic immunodeficiency. For example, boys who have the X-linked lymphoproliferative (XLP) disorder develop malignant lymphoma after primary EBV infection (634,635). The majority of LPDs occurring in solid organ and bone marrow transplant recipients, in the setting of iatrogenic immunosuppression, contain the EBV genome (245,438) (see Chapter 16).

More than 90% of HIV-infected individuals are EBV-infected, and reactivation of EBV infection is a common occurrence in AIDS (636). HIV-infected individuals often suffer from a profound defect in T-cell immunity to EBV and possess abnormally high numbers of circulating EBV-infected B cells (596). EBV-infected B cells are long-lived and are capable of replicating *in vivo* and *in vitro*, where they can be established readily as long-term cell lines (637). It has been suggested frequently that EBV plays a role in AIDS lymphomagenesis; however, the precise nature of that role remains unclear.

Many investigators, including us, have identified EBV DNA or nuclear antigen in AIDS-related lymphomas (268,275,300,301,312,337,491–493,506). Within an individual EBV-positive AIDS-related NHL, essentially all the tumor cells carry the EBV genome and express viral genes (638). Neri et al. (639) demonstrated that each EBV-containing AIDS-related NHL is infected by a single form of EBV, suggesting that EBV infection occurs prior to clonal expansion, and that the malignant lymphoma represents the clonally expanded progeny of a single EBV-infected cell. This concept has been corroborated by Shibata et al. (640), who detected a single identical form of EBV in multiple sites of involvement by a disseminated AIDS-related NHL. This is strong evidence in support of an important role for EBV in AIDS lymphomagenesis.

Based on these observations and findings, Pelicci et al. (488) and others (262,268) have suggested that AIDS lymphomagenesis is a multistep process that shares pathogenetic mechanisms with endemic BL and other immunodeficiency-associated lymphomas. The hypothesis that has been advanced is that the immunosuppression induced by HIV infection permits frequent, continuous, and massive EBV infections, leading to polyclonal B-cell activation and the development of EBV-infected and immortalized B-cell clones. Such clones would be unstable and susceptible to genetic alterations, that is, the reciprocal chromosomal translocations associated with *MYC* gene rearrangement, resulting in the emergence of a fully transformed monoclonal B-cell population that contains EBV sequences in its genome and the development of a clinically overt B-cell NHL. This hypothesis is supported by studies showing that the introduction of an activated *MYC* gene into EBV-infected lymphoblasts obtained from AIDS patients leads to their malignant conversion (354).

The existence of two distinct EBV strains has been established on the basis of differences in the *EBNA* coding regions (438,641). Type A EBV can be identified in the oropharynx and peripheral blood B cells of immunocompetent individuals worldwide and is associated with efficient B-cell immortalization. Type B EBV initially was identified in individuals from central Africa, is present only rarely in peripheral blood B cells, and is associated with poor B-cell immortalization (431). An increased incidence of peripheral blood B cells infected with EBV type B has been identified in immunosuppressed individuals, especially in those who are HIV-infected or who have undergone solid organ transplantation (642). Many AIDS-related NHLs contain type B EBV (439). These findings suggest that type B EBV may play a role in the pathogenesis of LPDs associated with immune suppression.

Nonetheless, a significant proportion of AIDS-related NHLs lack EBV. EBV DNA sequences are detected in only about 40% of AIDS-related systemic NHLs by Southern blot hybridization analysis (492,493). Utilizing the more sensitive technique of ISH for EBERs, Hamilton-Dutoit et al. (275) demonstrated EBV in

about 50% of patients, and more recent studies have found EBV in close to 30% of AIDS-related DLBCL (457). Many of the AIDS-related lymphoma cell lines established *in vitro* also lack EBV (551,585). Even if the model that has been proposed to explain the role of EBV in EBV-containing AIDS-related systemic NHLs is valid, alternative models must be formulated to explain those lymphomas lacking EBV. Ganser et al. (585) have speculated that these lymphomas occur through a different although comparable mechanism from that proposed by Pelicci et al. (488). They suggested that nonspecific B-cell activation caused by chronic antigenic stimulation by bacterial, fungal, or viral agents, which occurs in persons who have AIDS-induced immune alterations (22,474), results in monoclonal B-cell expansions (488), increasing the risk of a chromosomal translocation and rearrangement of *MYC* and immunoglobulin loci at the time of immunoglobulin gene rearrangement. It has also been shown that AIDS-related lymphomas that lack EBV may have more genetic alterations as determined by genomic gains and losses (552).

In contrast with the presence of EBV in only about 30% of AIDS-related systemic lymphomas, virtually all AIDS-related primary CNS lymphomas contain EBV. MacMahon et al. (480) detected EBV early region (EBER-1) transcripts, indicative of latent EBV infection, by ISH in 100% of the 21 AIDS-related primary CNS lymphomas that they studied. They found EBER-1 in only 43% of AIDS-related systemic lymphomas (as expected) and in only 7% of non–AIDS-related primary CNS lymphomas. In addition, they found that 45% of the AIDS-related, but none of the non–AIDS-related, primary CNS lymphomas expressed EBV LMP-1 (480), which is known to have transforming and oncogenic properties (643). It is possible that the pathogenesis of AIDS-related systemic and primary CNS lymphomas differ. Evidence has accumulated to suggest that AIDS-related NHLs exhibit distinct clinical and biologic differences according to their anatomic sites of origin and histopathologic categories. Most AIDS-related primary CNS lymphomas, including those analyzed by MacMahon et al. (480), exhibit large cell or immunoblastic morphology (278,279,301,466), and EBV is preferentially associated with these histopathologic categories. Whether the difference in EBV content between AIDS-related systemic and primary CNS lymphomas is a function of the anatomic site or the histopathologic category has been debated.

The role of EBV in AIDS lymphomagenesis and its preferential association with certain anatomic sites or histopathologic categories actually may be determined by the level of host immune surveillance (535). The highest frequency of EBV infection among AIDS-related NHLs occurs in the primary CNS lymphomas (480), which are associated with the lowest CD4 T-cell counts (279) and the lowest level of host immune function. Among AIDS-related systemic lymphomas, EBV occurs more frequently in immunoblastic lymphomas than in BLs (493,638). The former are associated with significantly lower CD4 T-cell counts than the latter (276). In addition, Pedersen et al. (301) have shown that among all AIDS-related systemic NHLs, the EBV-infected instances are associated with significantly lower CD4 T-cell counts and lower CD8 T-cell counts as well. Expression of the highly immunogenic EBV transforming antigens EBNA-2 and LMP-1 is restricted to AIDS-related lymphomas arising in the context of severely impaired immunity (509,638). The accumulated data strongly suggests that the involvement of EBV in AIDS lymphomagenesis is dependent on the level of immunity against EBV and requires highly permissive immunologic conditions (535).

Other Viruses

In addition to EBV, a number of viruses, including human T-cell lymphotrophic virus type 1 (HTLV-1), HTLV-2, human herpesvirus-6, and cytomegalovirus, have been claimed to be associated with AIDS-related NHLs (644–647). Aside from

KSHV, however, which is highly associated with the PELs (333), there is no definitive evidence for the presence of these viruses within the actual lymphoma cells and, hence, their involvement in AIDS lymphomagenesis.

Chronic B-Cell Stimulation and Proliferation

HIV infection also is characterized by a state of chronic stimulation of B cells by various environmental antigens and self-antigens (588), mitogens, and viruses, including EBV (596,635) and HIV itself (589). This leads to polyclonal hypergammaglobulinemia (588,589) and florid follicular (B-cell) hyperplasia (593) within enlarged, reactive lymph nodes, which is referred to as the *persistent generalized lymphadenopathy syndrome* (29,31). That HIV is one direct cause of polyclonal B-cell activation is evidenced by the frequent oligoclonal bands displaying anti-HIV reactivity that accompany the hypergammaglobulinemia (648,649). Furthermore, HIV can produce proteins that, while suppressing specific antigen responses in the follicles, can induce polyclonal B-cell activation.

The crucial role of antigens in normal B-cell development is well documented (650). A role for antigen stimulation in B-cell expansion and selection associated with the development of malignant lymphoma in immunocompetent hosts has been established (651,652). The studies performed by Riboldi et al. (653) provide evidence that chronic antigenic stimulation is involved in AIDS lymphomagenesis as well. These investigators discovered that some AIDS-related BLs produce autoantibodies. Furthermore, they demonstrated somatic hypermutation of the immunoglobulin gene hypervariable regions utilized by these lymphoma cells. An antigen-driven process of clonal selection may play a role in the emergence or expansion of a neoplastic B-cell clone in AIDS lymphomagenesis.

The persistent generalized lymphadenopathy syndrome precedes the development of AIDS-related NHL in as many as one-third of individuals (252,259,466). This is of particular interest in view of the previously mentioned model of AIDS lymphomagenesis and the long-held belief that chronic antigenic stimulation is associated with the development of B-cell lymphoma (473). One report suggested that malignant lymphoma develops 850 times more frequently than expected in individuals who have persistent generalized lymphadenopathy (654). These observations suggest that a pathogenetic relationship may exist between B-cell hyperplasia and the development of B-cell lymphoma in HIV-infected individuals.

Pelicci et al. (488) investigated that relationship by performing a correlative immunophenotypic and molecular genetic analysis of hyperplastic lymph nodes obtained from HIV-infected individuals. They discovered that about 20% of the lymph nodes exhibiting polyclonal florid follicular hyperplasia contained one or more discrete immunoglobulin heavy chain gene rearrangements as determined by Southern blot hybridization, indicating the presence of one or more clonal B-cell expansions. The new rearranged bands often were of low intensity and sometimes were accompanied by a hybridization smear, suggesting the presence of additional oligoclonal B-cell populations. These results suggest that the hyperplastic lymph nodes of HIV-infected patients often contain occult clonal B-cell populations that are not identifiable by morphologic examination or by immunophenotypic analysis. Comparable analysis of hyperplastic lymph nodes obtained from HIV-uninfected individuals generally fails to demonstrate the presence of clonal B-cell expansions, suggesting that the presence of oligoclonal B-cell expansions is preferentially associated with the immunosuppressed state of AIDS. Pelicci et al. (488) demonstrated that these B-cell clones do not carry *MYC* gene rearrangements, suggesting that they are immortalized but not yet fully transformed. They hypothesized that these oligoclonal B-cell populations represent the EBV-infected and immortalized B-cell clones in their proposed multistep process of AIDS

lymphomagenesis. The investigators theorized that the oligoclonal B-cell expansions occurring in these hyperplastic lymph nodes may represent a premalignant condition for the future development of AIDS-related B-cell lymphoma, but the clonal relationship between clones present in reactive lymph nodes and subsequent lymphoma has not been evaluated.

Some experimental evidence is available to support the hypothesis that oligoclonal expansions precede lymphoma development. Shibata et al. (655) identified EBV DNA in 37% of reactive lymph nodes obtained from HIV-infected individuals. They demonstrated a statistically significant positive correlation between the presence of detectable amounts of EBV DNA in these reactive lymph nodes and the concurrent occurrence or subsequent development of EBV-containing malignant lymphoma (655). In addition, chromosomal abnormalities have been identified in hyperplastic lymph nodes obtained from HIV-infected individuals who later developed malignant lymphoma (656). However, hyperplastic lymphadenopathy precedes the development of AIDS-related lymphoma in only approximately one-third of individuals (252,259). Only about 5% to 10% of patients who have persistent generalized lymphadenopathy actually develop malignant lymphoma (29,657). It has been reported that HIV-infected individuals who previously have had persistent generalized lymphadenopathy have NHL restricted to lymph nodes significantly more frequently (466). Nevertheless, a high proportion of those lymphomas originate outside of lymph nodes, often in obscure extranodal sites (259). Once again, only about 30% of AIDS-related systemic NHLs contain EBV (275,300,492,493). AIDS-related NHL clearly occurs in a large number of individuals at risk for AIDS who do not have a prior history of persistent generalized lymphadenopathy and who develop AIDS-related systemic lymphomas that do not contain EBV. For all these reasons, the precise relationship among EBV infection, the persistent generalized lymphadenopathy syndrome, and the eventual development of AIDS-related lymphoma remains unclear.

Hodgkin Lymphoma

Background
The initial cases of HL occurring in individuals at risk for AIDS were reported from the United States in 1984 and 1985 (257,658–661), as early as 3 years after the AIDS epidemic was recognized by the CDC (1,2). Since then, numerous cases of HIV-associated HL have been reported, including isolated incidents (662–664), those collected as small series from a single institution (259,270,296,297,450,665–672), and most gathered through national AIDS registries worldwide (274,302,673–680). These reports have served to characterize HIV-associated HL, including its often atypical clinical features and frequently aggressive biologic behavior, which distinguish it from conventional HL occurring in the HIV-uninfected general population. These reports, however, have not determined unequivocally whether HIV infection truly promotes the development of HL or merely modifies its course; they have not fully clarified the relationship among HIV infection, AIDS, and HL. Paradoxically, the incidence of HL appears to have increased with the introduction of cART suggesting that immune reconstitution may have played a role in some cases and that a threshold of CD4 T cells may be required for the pathogenesis (681,682). In one series the highest incidence of HL was found to occur with CD4 T-cell counts in the range of 50 to 99 cells/mm^3 (682). Regional differences may occur but other studies, such as the Swiss HIV consort study, did not demonstrate increased HL risk in the setting of cART therapy and improved immunity (683).

Epidemiology
Many investigators have suggested that the atypical manifestations peculiar to HL occurring in HIV-infected individuals justifies its recognition as an AIDS-related neoplasm

(667,668,684,685). HL occurring in individuals who have primary immunodeficiency (PID) and in solid organ transplant recipients, however, similarly display a preponderance of unfavorable histopathologic subtypes and aggressive clinical behavior (241,686), although its incidence is not increased in these patient populations (687,688). Therefore, alternatively, the atypical clinical features and aggressive biologic behavior of HIV-associated HL may simply represent an epiphenomenon of the underlying immunodeficiency state induced by HIV infection. AIDS-related neoplasms have been defined as those occurring in statistically increased numbers in HIV-infected persons compared with the general population (294). Currently, these include KS, diffuse aggressive B-cell NHL, and invasive cervical carcinoma, each of which has been accepted by the CDC as an AIDS-defining condition (62). Although innumerable cases of HL occurring in patients at risk for AIDS have been reported, the relationship between HL and HIV infection has been difficult to evaluate because of the relatively high incidence of HL in the age group at greatest risk for HIV infection. The initial population-based studies of AIDS-associated neoplasms conducted in the 1980s failed to detect a statistically significant increase in the incidence of HL among young, never married men in San Francisco, New York, and Los Angeles, the epicenters of the then-emerging AIDS epidemic (289,295,654,689). For this reason, it was concluded that the relationship between HL and HIV infection is merely coincidental (286,689). Consequently, the CDC has never accepted HL as an AIDS-defining malignancy. Two critical issues require consideration in this regard, however.

First, the decision to investigate young, never married men as a surrogate population for homosexual men at risk for AIDS rather than HIV-infected individuals in these studies may have limited the ability of these studies to detect subtle increases in the incidence of HL. Alternatively, the failure of these studies to detect an increased incidence of HL in the first 5 years of the AIDS epidemic may reflect the requirement for a longer latency period for the development of HIV-associated HL. In any case, Hessol et al. (690) reported an excess risk of HL of 19.3 cases per 100,000 person years attributable to HIV infection among 6,704 homosexual men residing in the San Francisco area from 1978 through 1989. By linking the California Tumor Registry and the San Francisco AIDS Surveillance Registry, Reynolds et al. (691) similarly discovered a significantly increased incidence of HL among HIV-positive men with AIDS in the San Francisco area between 1980 and 1987. More recently, Lyter et al. (692) detected a statistically significant, nearly 20-fold increased risk of developing HL (85 cases/100,000 person years) among the HIV-infected homosexual male cohort registered at the Pittsburgh site of the Multicenter AIDS Cohort Study between 1984 and 1993. Despite the fact that the actual number of cases of HL identified in these epidemiologic studies was small, these findings suggest that the incidence of HL has increased among HIV-infected persons in the United States.

Second, determination of the incidence of HL in HIV-infected individuals has been based largely on epidemiologic data gathered from the United States, which is based primarily on homosexual men and not on IDUs. Although Ahmed et al. (270) failed to detect a significant increase in the overall incidence of HL among HIV-infected New York City prisoners from 1981 through 1984, they found that the incidence was 3 to 10 times higher among prisoners who were IDUs than among those who were not. Since then, National Registry surveys from Italy (274,680), France (674,676,678), and Spain (679) and several other studies (668,690) have shown that the ratio of NHL to HL is significantly lower in HIV-infected IDUs than in HIV-infected homosexual men, suggesting that HIV-associated HL occurs significantly more frequently among HIV-infected IDUs than among HIV-infected homosexual men. Despite these findings, HIV-associated HL does not appear to have a restricted distribution among AIDS risk groups. HIV-associated HL has been described in HIV-infected hemophiliacs (298,670,679,693) and in women who have apparently acquired HIV infection through heterosexual contact with IDUs (667,675,678,679), in addition to MSM (450,666,669,675), although the incidence does not appear to be increased in these latter groups (291). Regardless of whether the CDC considers HL an AIDS-related neoplasm versus an AIDS-defining condition, this neoplasm is clearly increased in HIV-infected individuals and some unique features in this population merit special attention.

Pathology

The pathologic spectrum of conventional HL varies in different parts of the world and in different socioeconomic groups within the United States. Large referral centers in the United States and Western Europe have reported the following approximate histopathologic distribution of types of conventional HL: nodular sclerosis, 52% to 62%; mixed cellularity, 24% to 27%; lymphocytic depletion, 3% to 6%; and lymphocyte predominance, the remaining 7% to 11% (694,695). In contrast, mixed cellularity and lymphocytic depletion are the most common histologic subtypes in underdeveloped countries (696,697). Similar increases in mixed cellularity and lymphocytic depletion HL have been observed in minority populations of lower socioeconomic status within the United States (698).

The pathologic spectrum of HIV-associated HL is similar to that of underdeveloped countries and patients of lower socioeconomic status within the United States. The approximate histopathologic distribution is mixed cellularity, 50%; nodular sclerosis, 28%; lymphocytic depletion, 14%, and unclassified, 5% (257,259,274,296,302,658–660,662,665–668,670–680,684). Only rare cases of lymphocyte predominance HL have been reported (668,679,680). The mixed cellularity and lymphocytic depletion subtypes of HL occur significantly more frequently among HIV-infected than among HIV-uninfected individuals. Increases in the incidence of unfavorable histopathologic subtypes and a corresponding decrease in the prevalence of the more favorable nodular sclerosis subtype similarly is found in HL occurring in patients who have PID (241,686,699).

Cases of HIV-associated HL exhibit morphologic features comparable to those of conventional HL of corresponding histopathologic subtype (Fig. 25.34). Frequently, however, cases of HIV-associated HL display a distinct decrease in the number of benign lymphocytes making up the background host response cell population (670). This imparts a relative lymphocyte-depleted appearance compared with cases of conventional HL. The relative lymphocytic depletion probably reflects the decrease in CD4 T cells associated with HIV infection

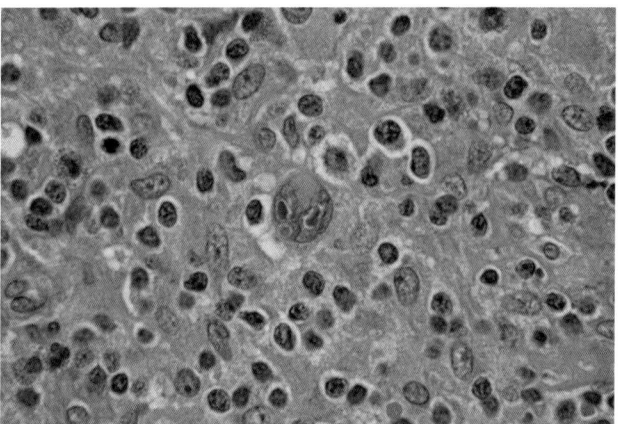

FIGURE 25.34. AIDS related classical Hodgkin lymphoma. The background is relatively depleted and contains relatively few CD4+ small lymphoid cells. Classical Reed-Sternberg cells are identified in a mixed background, which includes eosinophils. (magnification: 400×.)

(259,665,670). Reed-Sternberg cells and variants sometimes are particularly numerous and may appear even more so against a relatively lymphocyte-depleted background. Histiocytes are often abundant, as is multifocal necrosis (670). These slightly atypical features sometimes render the histopathologic diagnosis of HL problematic in the setting of HIV infection. For example, these features may cause some cases of HIV-associated HL to be misinterpreted as diffuse large B-cell lymphoma or peripheral T-cell lymphoma. This diagnostic problem may be compounded by the presence of the HL lesion in the bone marrow or in another, often unusual, extranodal site. Bone marrow involvement by HIV-associated HL often is confluent, but it may be focal and patchy (450,670,671). In the latter cases, diagnostic Reed-Sternberg cells may be sparse and difficult to identify. In these instances, the bone marrow lesions of HIV-associated HL may be overlooked as benign lymphohistiocytic aggregates or thought to have an infectious cause (671). This is especially true in the absence of documented lymph node involvement and clinical suspicion of HL. Recognition of these histopathologic features of HIV-associated HL and the appropriate use of immunohistochemical studies as adjuncts to morphologic interpretation should prevent misdiagnosis in these cases.

Immunophenotypic and Immunogenotypic Characteristics

HIV-associated and non–HIV-associated HL share similar immunophenotypic and immunogenotypic characteristics. In each instance, the lesions contain a variable mixture of CD4 and CD8 T cells, polyclonal B cells, histiocytes, Reed-Sternberg cells, and Reed-Sternberg cell variants (259,670). The Reed-Sternberg cells in HIV-associated HL similarly lack CD45 and usually express CD30 and CD15 when immunostained in paraffin tissue sections (259,670). The benign host response T-cell populations present within the HL lesions usually differ, however. The majority of T cells in most cases of non–HIV-associated HL belong to the CD4+CD8− subset (700). In contrast, fewer than usual numbers of T cells, reduced numbers of CD4 T cells, and increased numbers of CD8 T cells are often present in the lesions of HIV-associated HL (259,665,670). These differences are probably a consequence of the progressive depletion of the CD4 T-cell subset in HIV-infected patients caused by the cytopathic effect of HIV on CD4 T cells (592,701). It has been suggested that the presence of an inappropriate T-cell population and altered immunity in the HL lesions contributes to their biologic aggressiveness and the poor prognosis of patients who have HIV-associated HL (665,670).

Epstein-Barr Virus

It has been suggested that EBV may be involved in the pathogenesis of conventional HL, because early EBV RNAs, LMP-1, or both are detectable in the Reed-Sternberg cells of almost 50% of such patients using ISH and immunohistochemical techniques (664,702). EBV is preferentially associated with the mixed cellularity and lymphocytic depletion subtypes (664,702,703), and is found far less commonly in the nodular sclerosis subtype (664,702,703). EBV is frequently present in the Reed-Sternberg cells of HL occurring in developing countries where these histopathologic subtypes and peripheral HL are more prevalent (704). It is not altogether surprising that the Reed-Sternberg cells contain EBER or LMP-1 in a significantly higher percentage (approximately 80% to 100%) of patients with HIV-associated HL than of those with conventional HL (680,705). This finding partially reflects the significantly higher frequency of these unfavorable histopathologic subtypes in HIV-infected individuals (667,668,677–680,685). Even in cases of HIV-associated nodular sclerosis HL, however,

the Reed-Sternberg cells consistently contain the EBV genome (705,706). The presence of clonal EBV genomes in a very high proportion of cases of HIV-associated HL, in comparison with conventional HL (680), and the same EBV genome in multiple metachronous HL lesions in some HIV-seropositive individuals (680) further suggests an etiologic role for EBV in the pathogenesis of HIV-associated HL. These findings suggest that in at least a subset of cases of HL, the Reed-Sternberg cells represent a clonal expansion of a single EBV-infected cell, which continues to express EBV latent gene products. In contrast with EBV-containing, non–HIV-associated HL, in which type B EBV is present uncommonly (680,702), type A and type B EBV have approximately equal distributions in EBV-containing, HIV-associated HL (680,707). This finding suggests that type B EBV may be involved in the pathogenesis of HL in the setting of HIV infection, analogous to AIDS-related NHL. In support for role for EBV in the pathogenesis of HIV-related HL is expression of LMP-1, as well as LMP-2 in the Hodgkin/Reed Sternberg cells, as both of these proteins have important biologic and transforming functions, including activation of the NF-κB pathway, known to be important in lymphomagenesis.

Clinical Features

Individuals who develop HIV-associated HL display a distinct constellation of clinical features that is remarkably consistent among all AIDS risk groups, regardless of geographic location (259,274,296,450,666,667,669,670,675,677–680). These features contrast sharply with those of conventional HL occurring in the HIV-uninfected general population. In the United States, only approximately 30% of newly diagnosed patients with conventional HL, or 60% in the case of those of low socioeconomic status, complain of B symptoms (695,698), only 30% lack mediastinal disease, and only 40% have stage III or IV disease at presentation (694,695). Extranodal involvement is uncommon; bone marrow infiltration occurs in <5% of patients overall (694) and only approaches 30% even in those patients who have the mixed cellularity or lymphocytic depletion subtypes. Comparable findings have been reported in Western European patients who have conventional HL (668,680,708).

Approximately 90% or more of the patients who have HIV-associated HL are adult men (296,297,450,665–670, 675,677–680). In the United States, the majority are MSM (259,296,665,666,669,670,675), but in Western Europe most are male IDUs (274,302,667,668,677–680). Initially, this difference was believed to reflect the epidemiologic patterns of the AIDS epidemic, since the majority of patients with AIDS in the United States are MSM, but in Europe they are IDUs (302,668,678,679). Many investigators, however, now believe that this difference reflects a genuine predilection for HIV-associated HL to occur in IDUs. The median ages of patients who have HIV-associated HL are about 35 years in the United States (259,450,669,675) and about 28 years in Western Europe (274,302,668,677–680), comparable to the median ages of patients in these regions who have AIDS-related NHL (259,274).

HIV-associated HL usually occurs prior to an AIDS-defining illness and thus usually is the first manifestation of HIV infection in these individuals (274,296,679). Among 114 patients with HIV-associated HL studied by the Italian Cooperative Group on AIDS and Tumors, 33% were asymptomatic, 28% had persistent generalized lymphadenopathy, 22% had AIDS-related complex, and only 17% had a diagnosis of AIDS (680). Only 11% of patients with HIV-associated HL in the French Registry had been diagnosed previously with AIDS (678). As many as 60% to 70% of individuals, especially IDUs, who develop HIV-associated HL have histories of persistent generalized lymphadenopathy (274,302). The persistent generalized lymphadenopathy precedes the diagnosis of HL by between 1 month and more than 3 years, although the median is 8 months (302). The clinical presentations of HIV-associated HL and persistent generalized lymphadenopathy, that is, enlarged peripheral lymph nodes accompanied by malaise, fever, night sweats, weight loss, and splenomegaly, may overlap significantly. In a European series of IDUs with HIV-associated HL, the diagnosis of HL was made in lymph nodes already known to exhibit persistent generalized lymphadenopathy in almost 40% of cases (302). HL may even coexist with the florid follicular hyperplasia (659) or follicular involution (450,670) phase of HIV-associated lymphadenopathy in individual lymph nodes. Accurate diagnosis and distinction between persistent generalized lymphadenopathy and HL requires a tissue biopsy. An increase in the size of persistently enlarged lymph nodes or the development of B symptoms warrants biopsy evaluation, possibly of multiple sites.

Patients who have HIV-associated HL exhibit a variable spectrum of the laboratory findings associated with HIV infection, that is, cutaneous anergy, polyclonal hypergammaglobulinemia, cytopenias, and a reduction in the number of peripheral blood CD4 T cells (259,667,669,679). Approximately 30% have active opportunistic infections at the time of diagnosis of HL (677,680). KS occurs infrequently in patients who have HIV-associated HL (678,679) and only rarely prior to the diagnosis of HL (678). This may relate partially to the lesser degree of immune suppression and higher CD4 T-cell counts in these individuals than in those who have AIDS-related NHL. Median CD4 T-cell counts of between 201 and 306/μL have been reported in multiple series of patients with HIV-associated HL (302,675,677,678,680). Like BL, HIV-associated HL appears to occur relatively early in the clinical course of HIV infection, prior to the onset of severe immunodeficiency and the development of AIDS-related illnesses. This finding is consistent with the fact that, like BL, HL occurs infrequently in other immunodeficiency states (687,688). Factors other than HIV-induced immunosuppression may be involved in the development of HIV-associated HL.

Approximately 80% to 90% of patients who have HIV-associated HL complain of B symptoms (fever, drenching night sweats, or weight loss in excess of 10% of normal body weight) at presentation (667,668,677–680). Other symptomatic complaints are variable, because of the diverse and multiple organ systems involved by HIV-associated HL, and usually depend on the principal location of disease. These individuals normally already possess widely disseminated disease at the time of initial presentation. Approximately 75% to 90% have clinical stage III or IV disease (259,274,296,658–660,662,665–670,675,677–680,684) and about two-thirds have extranodal involvement (259,274,667,668,675,679,680) at diagnosis. The most common extranodal site is the bone marrow, which is involved in up to 40% to 50% of cases in some series (667,668,675,679). Not infrequently, this is the first indication of the presence of HL in these individuals (450,670,675). About one-third of patients have involvement of other extranodal sites initially, most commonly the liver, spleen, and lungs (259,274,668,677,679). Lung involvement in the absence of mediastinal lymphadenopathy, which is observed regularly in North American MSM, appears to occur less commonly among European IDUs, however (302). HIV-associated HL often involves unusual extranodal sites (675,677), including even the CNS (709). HIV-associated HL has been reported to originate or present in the oropharynx (296,675), the anorectal region (663,710) the skin (659,711), and even the bone marrow (712). As in AIDS-related NHL, the diagnosis of HIV-associated HL often is established on the basis of the biopsy of an extranodal site (259,675).

HIV-associated HL often has an atypical presentation and spreads in a random, noncontiguous fashion. There is a conspicuous absence of the classic presentation of supradiaphragmatic peripheral as well as mediastinal and hilar lymph node disease (259,296,659,678,680). Patients often have involvement of multiple, noncontiguous lymph node groups, extensive liver or bone marrow disease in the absence of splenic involvement,

widespread disease with sparing of the mediastinum and hilar lymph nodes, and involvement of unusual extranodal sites (259,296,659). Mediastinal lymph node involvement occurs infrequently in HIV-associated HL (668,678,680). Only 23% of the Italian cohort (680) and only 13% of the French cohort (678) with HIV-associated HL had mediastinal involvement, and these generally were individuals who had clinical stage IV disease. A very high frequency of the peripheral form of HL (absence of mediastinal involvement) is a specific feature of HIV-associated HL. Andrieu et al. (678) have pointed out that the mixed cellularity subtype occurs in 37% of patients with conventional HL lacking mediastinal involvement, and in 48% of such patients if only men aged 23 to 50 years are considered. The mixed cellularity subtype is highly associated with peripheral HL in both HIV-infected and HIV-uninfected individuals. An increase in the incidence of the peripheral but not the central form of HL may account for the higher incidence of HL among HIV-infected individuals. HIV seropositivity should be suspected in patients with HL who exhibit atypical clinical manifestations or a hyperaggressive disease course. The identification of patients who have HIV-associated HL rather than conventional HL has significant therapeutic, managerial, and prognostic implications.

Treatment and Survival

Most patients who have HIV-associated HL are treated with standard mechlorethamine, Oncovin (vincristine), procarbazine, prednisone/Adriamycin (doxorubicin), bleomycin, vinblastine, decarbizine protocols that are employed in treating patients with conventional HL (713). These protocols may be administered alone or followed by radiation therapy. These protocols achieve a CR in almost 90% of patients who have conventional HL (714) and render more than 70% of all patients who have conventional HL permanently disease-free (713,715). They are associated with CR in 70% to 80% of patients and with long-term disease-free survival in 60% to 70% of patients with stage III or IV conventional HL (713). Conventional HL is considered curable even in the presence of widely disseminated disease.

The prognosis of patients who have HIV-associated HL is significantly worse than that of those who have conventional HL, however. CR rates of only about 40% to 70% (296,302,668,677,679,680) and median durations of survival of only 8 to 18 months (274,302,668,669,675,677,679,680) have been reported in virtually all large series of HIV-associated HL when these chemotherapeutic protocols have been employed. One problem is that these regimens often cause significant hematologic toxicity, including further cytopenias, disproportionate to the dosages employed if they are administered to HIV-infected patients, who often have extensive bone marrow disease and are already cytopenic (259,659,667,668,678–680). The increased hematologic toxicity and the propensity of these patients to develop multiple severe opportunistic infections often delays or necessitates dosage reductions of scheduled chemotherapy, compromising therapy and management (302,668,675,677). Errante et al. (716) discovered that the addition of antiretroviral therapy to standard antineoplastic chemotherapy regimens significantly decreased the occurrence of opportunistic infections both during and after chemotherapy, although it did not significantly increase the CR rate or the median survival. Newcom et al. (672), however, achieved a CR rate of 100% and a median duration of survival of 38 months in a small group of patients with HIV-associated HL by employing truncated standard chemotherapy regimens individualized to induce a clinical remission in conjunction with *P. carinii* pneumonia prophylaxis. The optimal therapeutic approach for treating HIV-associated HL is evolving, and prospective clinical trials are ongoing in patients with cART to define better therapeutic strategies for these patients, and to determine whether they should be treated like HL in immunocompetent individuals.

Historically, patients who have HIV-associated HL experience a high incidence of severe, life-threatening opportunistic infections during and after chemotherapy, often in the terminal phase in which HL relapses (302,667,668,677,678,680,717). These infections include *P. carinii* pneumonia, Legionella pneumonia, cerebral toxoplasmosis, cryptococcal meningitis, cryptosporidiosis, and disseminated cytomegalovirus, candidiasis, and *M. avium complex* infections (666,667,675,678,679). These severe opportunistic infections occur only rarely in conventional HL, in which bacterial infections predominate (668,718,719). The predilection for individuals with HIV-associated HL to develop serious opportunistic infections is related to the underlying HIV-induced immunodeficiency. Patients who have HIV-associated HL occasionally develop KS, either during or after therapy (259,662,678,679,720,721). Rarely, an HIV-seropositive individual develops HL prior to (722), concurrent with (723), or after development of an AIDS-related NHL (724). Approximately one-third of patients who have HIV-associated HL die as a direct result of tumor progression. All the earlier studies showed that the majority of patients die as a result of opportunistic infections, either alone or in conjunction with tumor progression, and a minority die as a result of severe cytopenias (274,302,668,675,677,678,680). However, the outcome appears to have been better since the implementation of cART (725).

Little is known about prognostic factors for survival in HIV-associated HL. A prior diagnosis of AIDS, pretreatment cytopenias, failure to attain CR, and CD4 T-cell counts lower than 250/μL have been found to be associated with a significantly shorter duration of survival (668,677,680). AIDS risk group, stage of disease, histologic subtype, bone marrow involvement, therapeutic regimen, and presence of opportunistic infections have not proven to be significant prognostic factors (668,680), but multivariate analysis of large numbers of uniformly treated patients has not been performed (717).

OTHER HEMATOPOIETIC NEOPLASMS

A variety of other hematopoietic neoplasms occurring in HIV-infected persons, some of whom have AIDS, have been reported. These include B-cell ALL (721,726–735), plasma cell tumors (260,736–750), histologic low-grade B-cell leukemias and lymphomas (252,255,257,296,751–753), an array of T-cell neoplasms (259,314,754–770), angiocentric immunoproliferative lesions (771–773), and a spectrum of myeloproliferative disorders, including various subtypes of acute myeloid leukemia (AML) (732,774–787). The true incidence of these neoplasms in individuals at risk for AIDS is uncertain and may be underestimated because these cases are not reported to the CDC. Nonetheless, these neoplasms only appear to occur sporadically in these individuals, and there is no definitive epidemiologic evidence to suggest that their incidence has increased in parallel with the AIDS epidemic. Because the relationship of these hematologic neoplasms to HIV infection and AIDS is generally unclear, these neoplasms are not recognized as meeting the criteria for the diagnosis of AIDS in HIV-infected individuals by the CDC at the present time. Low-grade lymphomas, however, although not characteristically associated with HIV, are being observed more often in patients with prolonged survivals maintained on cART therapy. These include extranodal marginal zone (MALT) lymphomas that may be seen in the lungs and at other sites. Cases of primary mediastinal large B-cell lymphoma have rarely been reported in HIV-infected patients as well (788).

Cases of plasma cell neoplasia, including extramedullary plasmacytoma, occurring in AIDS risk persons have been described in the literature (789–793). Patients were men who ranged in age from 22 to 65 years, with a median of 34 years. Most of them were severely immunosuppressed and had CD4:CD8 T-cell ratios of 1.0 or lower. AIDS risk factors were

homosexuality (794), injecting drug use (795), transfused blood products (2), and unknown (795). All patients tested were HIV-seropositive. Only four patients fulfilled the CDC criteria for AIDS on the basis of severe opportunistic infections or KS; the remaining patients had the AIDS-related complex, the persistent generalized lymphadenopathy syndrome, or otherwise asymptomatic HIV infection. The neoplasms included solitary and disseminated extramedullary plasmacytomas and secretory and nonsecretory myelomas associated with osteolytic bone disease and marrow plasmacytosis. Some extramedullary plasmacytomas arose in unusual anatomic sites including the skin (747), the oropharynx (741), and the penis (742). In two instances, myeloma involved the serous cavities and presented as massive peritoneal effusions (748), which is very rare in conventional multiple myeloma (789). Many of the patients exhibited elevated serum lactate dehydrogenase levels and, despite chemotherapy, experienced disease progression and died within a few months of presentation. It is difficult to prove that the occurrence of plasmacytomas and multiple myeloma in persons at risk for AIDS is related specifically to HIV infection and is not merely coincidental. Plasma cell malignancies, however, generally occur in the sixth decade and beyond; <2% of all patients who have conventional myeloma are younger than 40 years of age (790,791). The frequent development of multiple extramedullary plasmacytomas in individuals at risk for AIDS represents an unusual clinical course for conventional plasma cell neoplasia. HIV is capable of infecting B cells directly (792), and retroviral infection has been shown to promote the growth of murine plasmacytomas (793). Konrad et al. (746) reported an HIV-seropositive man with multiple myeloma whose IgGγ paraprotein specifically recognized the HIV p24 *gag* antigen. This plasma cell neoplasm may have developed at least in part because of an antigen-driven response to circulating p24 antigen, suggesting a direct pathogenetic role for HIV. Also, the EBV genome has been detected in several AIDS-associated myelomas (685,748,749), and clonal EBV populations have been demonstrable in some of these tumors (748), analogous to AIDS-related B-cell NHLs (488,492). These plasma cell neoplasms may have similar pathogeneses and fall within the spectrum of HIV-associated aggressive B-cell neoplasia. The definition of AIDS eventually may be expanded to include plasma cell malignancies.

The sporadic occurrence of B-cell chronic lymphocytic leukemia and histologic low-grade B-cell NHLs, including small lymphocytic lymphoma (SLL), follicle center cell lymphoma, marginal zone (monocytoid B-cell) lymphoma, and mantle cell lymphoma, in MSM and IDUs has been reported (252,255,296,751–753,796). Some of these patients have been HIV seronegative, and many of those who were HIV infected lacked evidence of severe immune deficiency and AIDS-defining illnesses. Some of these patients have even enjoyed prolonged survival with no or minimal therapy, as would be expected in similar patients who are not HIV-infected (797). No evidence currently exists to suggest that these low-grade B-cell neoplasms are specifically associated with HIV infection or that their incidence has increased in parallel with the AIDS epidemic. It is likely that their occurrence in this patient population is merely coincidental, and that their pathogenesis is similar to that of comparable neoplasms occurring in the general population unassociated with HIV infection.

Several well-documented cases of precursor T-cell lymphoblastic lymphoma (754, 758) and adult T-cell lymphoma/leukemia (755,759) and a minimum of 34 cases of cutaneous T-cell lymphoma (760–763,767,769,770) and peripheral T-cell lymphoma (756,757,762,766) occurring in HIV-infected persons have been described in the literature. Of the latter 34 cases, 21 were reported from a single institution, the University of California at San Francisco (770). Several cases of HIV-associated T cell–derived anaplastic large cell lymphoma have been reported (314,764,765,768). Other cases of purported

HIV-associated T-cell lymphoma described in the literature (798–801) are poorly documented or unconvincing. Several cases of so-called lymphomatoid granulomatosis and lethal midline granuloma have been reported in persons at risk for AIDS (771–773). These cases appear to represent a heterogeneous group of neoplasms whose precise histopathologic classification and lineage derivation is unclear.

All 34 HIV-seropositive individuals who developed cutaneous or peripheral T-cell lymphoma were men. They ranged in age from 23 to 62 years. The mean age of the 20 University of California at San Francisco patients was 39 years and of the 13 literature cases was 42 years. AIDS risk factors were homosexuality (802), injecting drug use (2), and unknown or unstated (756,757,760–763). Kerschmann et al. (770) suggested that the individuals who have cutaneous presentations are divisible into two distinct clinical groups: those who have epidermatropic mycosis fungoides–like patches and plaques or Sezary syndrome–like exfoliative erythroderma, early HIV disease without AIDS, relative immunocompetence, and an indolent clinical course with a mean duration of survival longer than 3 years; and those who have nonepidermatropic large cell or immunoblastic lymphoma manifesting as papules or nodules, advanced HIV disease and often AIDS, significant immunosuppression, and a rapid clinical course, with a mean duration of survival of <7 months. The other literature reports generally support these findings. The epidermatropic mycosis fungoides, like cutaneous T-cell lymphomas, are CD30 negative, and lack EBV; a majority of the nonepidermatropic cutaneous T-cell lymphomas express CD30 and may contain EBV. Many of the CD30-positive tumors might be considered anaplastic large cell lymphomas. Unlike in conventional cutaneous anaplastic large cell lymphoma (803), however, CD30 expression did not correlate with survival among these patients. Those HIV-infected individuals who have peripheral T-cell lymphoma generally possess advanced HIV disease, have severe immunosuppression and sometimes AIDS, often exhibit disseminated lymphoma at presentation, and experience a rapidly fatal course (Fig. 25.35). The HIV-infected individuals who have anaplastic large cell lymphoma similarly have been severely immunosuppressed MSM or male IDUs in the third to fifth decades of life. They present with localized or extensive cutaneous disease, which sometimes is accompanied by disseminated lymph node and organ involvement. The clinical course has varied from sustained CR following chemotherapy to a rapidly fatal outcome because of disease progression or other AIDS-related illnesses (314,764,765,768). T-cell subset antigen expression was not studied in the University of California at San Francisco cohort. Among six cutaneous T-cell lymphomas, six peripheral

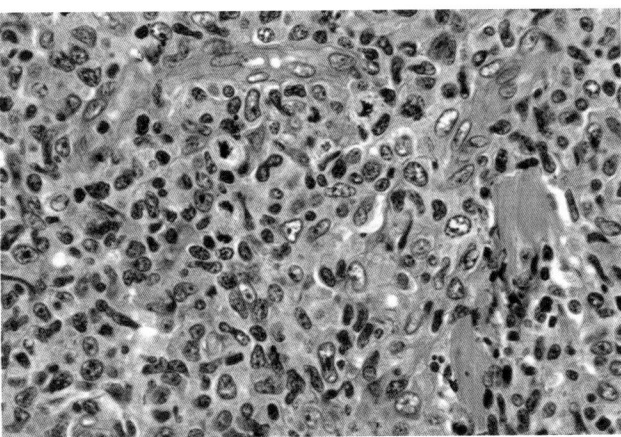

FIGURE 25.35. Peripheral T-cell lymphoma, NOS in a patient with AIDS. The infiltrate consists of pleomorphic intermediate and large lymphoid cells (hematoxylin and eosin, original magnification: 150×).

T-cell lymphomas, and two anaplastic large cell lymphomas analyzed, eight expressed the CD4+CD8- (helper-inducer) phenotype, four expressed the CD4-CD8+ (suppressor-cytotoxic) phenotype, and two expressed the CD4-CD8- phenotype (756,757,760–762,764,766–769). Some of these lesions exhibited clonal T-cell receptor β chain gene rearrangements.

Several cases of apparent T-cell prolymphocytic leukemia occurring in HIV-infected persons have been reported (259,260). In the three cases described by Knowles et al. (259), the lymphoid cells resembled small mature lymphocytes; expressed the mature peripheral suppressor-cytotoxic (CD4-CD8+) T-cell subset phenotype; lacked the azurophilic granule-rich basophilic cytoplasm characteristic of large granular lymphocytes and NK cells and their associated antigens CD16 and CD57, said to be characteristic of Tγ lymphoproliferative disease (804); and exhibited clonal T-cell receptor β chain gene rearrangements (259). These findings are indicative of a clonal expansion of the mature CD4-CD8+ (suppressor-cytotoxic) T-cell subset. They detected a single specific HTLV-1 hybridizing band in one of these clonal T-cell proliferations (259), strongly suggesting clonal integration of the HTLV-1 genome. The significance of a solitary report of CD3- Tγ lymphoproliferative disease occurring in an HIV-seropositive, HTLV-1-seronegative MSM following an acute viral illness (805) is not certain. Other peripheral T-cell lymphomas rarely encountered in the setting of HIV include anaplastic large cell lymphomas. More recent series report HIV+ T-cell lymphomas in men and women in nodal and extranodal sites, including bone marrow, skin, spleen, lung, eye, breast, gastrointestinal tract, nasal cavity, bone, and soft tissue (806). PTCL-NOS remains the most common type, and the majority have a cytotoxic T-cell phenotype and variable association with EBV. Because cases of PEL may have aberrant expression of CD3, HHV8-related PEL should be considered in the differential.

In addition to these T-cell malignancies, nonneoplastic CD8 lymphocytoses occurring in HIV-infected persons have been described (137,188,805,807). Itescu et al. have described "diffuse infiltrative CD8 lymphocytosis syndrome" associated with the HLA-DR5 haplotype (137,188). These patients are predominantly black men who characteristically have persistent peripheral blood CD8 lymphocytosis accompanied by clinically significant diffuse visceral CD8 infiltration, most commonly involving the salivary glands, lungs, and lymph nodes and sometimes the gastrointestinal tract, the nervous system, and other viscera. The most common clinical manifestations are bilateral salivary gland and lymph node enlargement, sicca symptoms, and LIP leading to dyspnea (307). The patients have polyclonal hypergammaglobulinemia but usually lack the rheumatoid factors and antinuclear antibodies associated with Sjögren syndrome. They generally have borderline normal or slightly subnormal CD4 T-cell counts, lack AIDS-defining illnesses, and do not appear to develop lymphoproliferative malignancies. A small number of African children displaying some or all of these clinical features has been reported as well (808).

Oksenhendler et al. (807) have described a clinical syndrome involving CD8 lymphocytosis associated with the HLA-DR3 haplotype. The patients are Caucasian and have peripheral blood and bone marrow CD8 lymphocytosis, marked hypergammaglobulinemia, and massive pseudotumoral splenomegaly. The CD8 lymphocytes are activated suppressor T cells that exhibit the germ line T-cell receptor gene configuration, consistent with the polyclonal expansion of a CD8 T-cell population aimed at suppressing viral replication. The association with specific haplotypes suggests that these clinical syndromes represent genetically determined distinct immune host responses to HIV. These systemic CD8 lymphocytoses should not be misinterpreted as T-cell malignancies.

Whether the occurrence of some or all of the various T-cell neoplasms reported in HIV-infected persons is directly related to HIV infection or is merely coincidental is unclear. Precursor T-cell lymphoblastic lymphomas and peripheral T-cell lymphomas, however, have been described in renal transplant recipients (809–813), another immunosuppressed patient population with an increased incidence of lymphoid neoplasia (402). It has been suggested that HIV itself may be a causal agent in the development of T-cell neoplasia, based on similarities between the transactivator genes in HIV, HTLV-1, and HTLV-2 (756). The transactivator gene product in HTLV-1 and HTLV-2 is believed to activate the expression of growth-promoting genes, which in turn may lead ultimately to the immortalization and malignant transformation of the infected cells (756). Southern blot hybridization studies have identified clonal integration of HIV provirus only in the neoplastic T cells of a single HIV-associated T-cell neoplasm (766), however; all the other T-cell neoplasms examined have been negative (259,754,756–758). HTLV-1, whose mode of transmission is similar to HIV, also has been suggested as a causal agent, and rare cases of adult T-cell lymphoma/leukemia occurring in individuals coinfected with HIV and HTLV-1 have been reported (755,759). Knowles et al. (259) described HIV-seropositive persons who had CD8 lymphocytosis with clonal integration of HTLV-1 in the CD8 T cells. HTLV-1 rarely may contribute to the development of clinically indolent, clonal CD4$^-$CD8$^+$ T-cell proliferations in HIV-infected patients depleted of CD4 T cells. These clonal CD8 proliferations could develop as the result of destruction of CD4 T cells by HIV and the subsequent loss of control over a group of CD8 T cells infected with HTLV-1 caused by the immunosuppression induced by HIV. Alternatively, prior infection with HTLV-1 and subsequent destruction of CD4 T cells may select for a CD8 T-cell population that is transformed more easily on subsequent exposure to HTLV-1. Dual infection by HIV and HTLV-1 has been documented frequently in populations at risk for AIDS worldwide, especially in IDUs (813–816). None of the HIV-seropositive patients who developed T-cell lymphomas, however, has been discovered to have serum antibodies to HTLV-1, and Southern blot hybridization analyses have failed to find HTLV-1 in the majority of HIV-associated T-cell neoplasms (754,756–758,760,761,763,766,767,769,770). EBV has been suggested as a possible causative factor in HIV-associated T-cell neoplasia (762). Human T cells may be immortalized following transfection with EBV DNA (817). Furthermore, Harabuchi et al. (818) described five angiocentric immunoproliferative lesions containing EBV, and Jones et al. (819) described two peripheral T-cell lymphomas exhibiting clonal integration of EBV DNA. Some AIDS-associated T-cell lymphomas contain EBV (768,770), and EBV may contribute to the pathogenesis of T-cell neoplasms in HIV-infected individuals who are known to experience severe, massive, and continuous EBV infections. Additional studies, however, are needed to clarify the relationship between HIV infection and the development of T-cell neoplasia.

The occurrence of various myeloproliferative disorders in HIV-seropositive individuals also has been reported. AIDS risk factors for these individuals primarily have been homosexuality, injecting drug use, and transfusion of HIV-contaminated blood products. Only a few of these individuals meet the CDC criteria for AIDS. Myelodysplasia similar to that observed in the myelodysplastic or preleukemic syndromes has been described frequently in HIV-infected persons (820). AML arising in myelodysplastic syndrome (289), de novo AML (732,775,777–787), chronic myeloid leukemia (781), and agnogenic myeloid metaplasia (776) have been described. One individual developed NHL 4 months after chemotherapy-induced remission of AML (787). Among the 12 cases of AML reported in HIV-infected persons for which information is available, 5 were classified as FAB M2 (732,774,779,780,787), 4 as FAB M4 (acute myelomonocytic leukemia) (781–783), and 3 as FAB M5 (acute monocytic leukemia) (784–786).

The significance of the association between these myeloproliferative disorders and HIV infection is uncertain. Two patients who had transfusion-associated AIDS and AML were 58 and 62 years old (774). Nearly all the MSM and IDUs with myeloproliferative disorders, however, have been in the third and fourth decades of life. The incidence of myelodysplasia and AML in men younger than 45 years of age is low, and it is possible that these disorders, rather than merely being coincidental, are a consequence of the severe T-cell immunodeficiency caused by HIV infection, either because of a failure of immune surveillance or because of defective T-cell control of hematopoiesis. The incidence of AML equals or exceeds that of ALL in at least two immunodeficiencies associated with chronic T-cell abnormalities, the Wiskott-Aldrich syndrome (WAS) and severe combined immunodeficiency (SCID) (821). HIV has been shown to infect the HL-60 promyelocytic cell line and other myelomonocytic cell lines expressing the CD4 antigen (822,823), bone marrow myeloid precursors in AIDS patients, and myeloid progenitor cells lacking CD4 (824). In one HIV-infected patient with AML, the circulating myelomonocytic leukemia cells were found to be infected productively by HIV (783). These observations suggest that HIV may play a direct, or at least an indirect, role in the malignant transformation of these cell populations. Additional studies, however, are necessary to explain the relationships among HIV infection, immunodeficiency, myelodysplasia, and leukemiagenesis.

NONHEMATOPOIETIC NEOPLASMS

Kaposi Sarcoma

Between the time of its discovery by Moritz Kaposi (825) in 1872, and the recognition of its epidemic spread among homosexual men in the early 1980s heralding the AIDS epidemic (2,826), KS largely was considered an enigmatic dermatologic curiosity whose incidence and natural history varied geographically (368). Four clinicoepidemiologic forms of KS are now recognized. These are classic Mediterranean KS, which occurs rarely in elderly individuals, predominantly men, of Mediterranean and Eastern Europe descent, in whom it usually exhibits benign, indolent clinical behavior; endemic African KS, which occurs frequently in HIV-uninfected patients in equatorial Africa, in whom it often exhibits aggressive clinical behavior; iatrogenic KS, which occurs relatively frequently in solid organ transplant recipients, in whom it often undergoes spontaneous regression following the withdrawal of immunosuppressive therapy (368); and AIDS epidemic KS, which is a defining condition for the diagnosis of AIDS in HIV-infected individuals (254,827). While the incidence of KS varies widely, it is now one of the most common cancers in several subequatorial African countries where it is associated with significant morbidity and mortality and that increases when individuals are coinfected with HIV (828). In the mid 1990s, the reported incidence of KS was approximately 1:100,000 in the general population, while in HIV-infected individuals it was around 1:20 (829,830), and up to 1:3 in HIV-infected homosexual men prior to the introduction of cART, or an increased risk of 73,000-fold compared with the general population (294,831). Since the widespread implementation of cART, the incidence of AIDS-KS in the Western world has declined, but it remains increased compared to the pre-AIDS era and now occurs in the presence of high CD4 T-cell counts and low HIV viral load (832).

In all the epidemiologic subtypes of KS, there is a range and overlap in clinical presentation, with the exception of pediatric KS that, with very rare exceptions, only occurs in Africa. KS exhibits a variable clinical course, ranging from minimal disease presenting as an incidental finding and exhibiting slow progression over many years, to the explosive onset of widespread, rapidly progressive disease resulting in significant injury and high mortality (833,834). Both corticosteroid therapy and opportunistic infections have been associated with the *de novo* appearance of KS and with the exacerbation of preexisting KS in HIV-infected persons (269,275,834).

The most frequent site of involvement is the skin (834,835), although lesions can occur anywhere. They are concentrated on the face, genitalia, and lower extremities in many patients (834). Cutaneous KS lesions are usually multifocal and may be seen as papules, patches, plaques, or nodules, but there can be fungating lesions and tumors as well. The patch lesions are considered the earlier stage lesions, and other forms are considered more advanced. However, while these definitions are useful as dermatologic descriptors, in practice these distinctions commonly do not accurately reflect disease progression and several forms can appear simultaneously (368). In addition, there can be patch-type lesions comprising large areas, or nodules with limited disease. Lymphedema may be extensive. KS can also involve noncutaneous sites. Extracutaneous spread of AIDS epidemic KS is very common (836,837). The oral cavity, especially the palate and gingiva, frequently is involved (834,838). Pulmonary and gastrointestinal tract involvement are also quite common; the latter is highly associated with oral KS and is detectable in 40% of patients who have KS at initial diagnosis and in as many as 80% at autopsy and both may occur in the absence of mucocutaneous disease (834). No organ has been spared from involvement by AIDS epidemic KS. Investigators have described invasion by KS into solid organs such as the heart, liver, pancreas, testis, and bone marrow (836), and metastasis to the brain (195). Extracutaneous involvement by AIDS epidemic KS ranges from a solitary small nodule to multiple, variably sized nodules, to a large confluent hemorrhagic tumor mass of 10 cm or even greater in size (836).

Lymph node involvement by AIDS epidemic KS is also common and may occur in the absence of mucocutaneous disease (834). AIDS epidemic KS may occur in benign lymph nodes exhibiting any of the histopathologic patterns: florid follicular hyperplasia, mixed follicular hyperplasia and involution, follicular involution, or lymphocyte depletion (30,34,38,49,50,63–68,192,193), as well as in lymph nodes containing malignant lymphoma (260). Early in the clinical course, lymph nodes involved by AIDS epidemic KS are usually between 1 and 2 cm in diameter and are discrete, mobile, firm or fleshy, and nontender (839). On cross section, foci of purple or red-brown discoloration as well as firm, white to tan areas sometimes are grossly discernible (63,67). Early lesions as well as small foci of involvement usually are seen in or adjacent to the capsule, in the hilum, or occasionally in the perinodal adipose tissue (Fig. 25.36) (30,50,63,193). Diagnosis of these early lesions and small foci of KS can be difficult in the absence of immunohistochemistry, especially if they involve only the pericapsular tissue. They can be easily overlooked or may be dismissed as areas of fibrosis (34). Late in the clinical course, lymph nodes involved by AIDS epidemic KS may appear grossly as hemorrhagic tumors measuring several centimeters in diameter (836).

AIDS epidemic KS generally is histopathologically indistinguishable from the other clinicoepidemiologic forms of the disease (840). KS comprises a variable mixture of ectatic, irregularly shaped, round capillary and slitlike endothelial-lined vascular spaces and spindle-shaped cells accompanied by a variable mixed mononuclear inflammatory cell infiltrate. The endothelial cells may be thin and spindle-shaped or oval to round (Fig. 25.37). They generally lack cytologic atypia and mitotic activity. Erythrocytes and hemosiderin pigment are frequently present, often extravasated between the spindle cells. Small refractile, eosinophilic, hyaline globules that stain with the periodic acid-Schiff stain, representing the breakdown products of phagocytosed erythrocytes, may be present extracellularly or within macrophages. The earliest patch and plaque

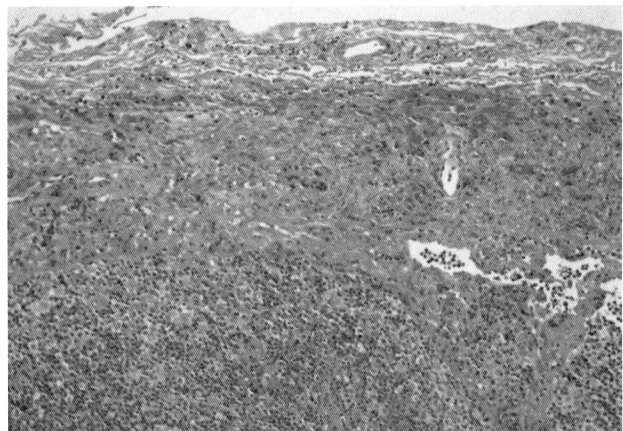

FIGURE 25.36. Lymphadenopathic KS showing involvement of the capsule and subcapsular sinus (hematoxylin and eosin b120).

stage lesions sometimes may be difficult to distinguish from granulation tissue. The spindle cells increasingly become the predominant cell population, forming fascicles that compress the vascular slits, and the lesions may progress to form nodules and tumors. The latter consist primarily of interwoven fascicles of spindle cells displaying prominent cytologic atypia, numerous mitotic figures, and often striking pleomorphism (34,50,63,840).

Extracutaneous KS may differ slightly histologically from, and may exhibit a different developmental chronology than, cutaneous KS (840). The earliest histopathologic changes in lymph nodes involved by KS are those that have been referred to as *hypervascular follicular hyperplasia* (841). Vascular channels within the lymph node are prominent, increased in number, and associated with increased numbers of plasma cells (842). Over time, these areas may develop the classical histopathologic features of KS, including interwoven fascicles of spindle cells, vascular slits, and extravasated erythrocytes (840,842). KS involving lymph nodes extends along the sinusoids, infiltrates the interfollicular areas (63,193), and eventually may replace the entire lymph node (30,34).

The histogenesis of the spindle cell component of KS, believed to be the "tumor cell," was initially difficult to determine. With

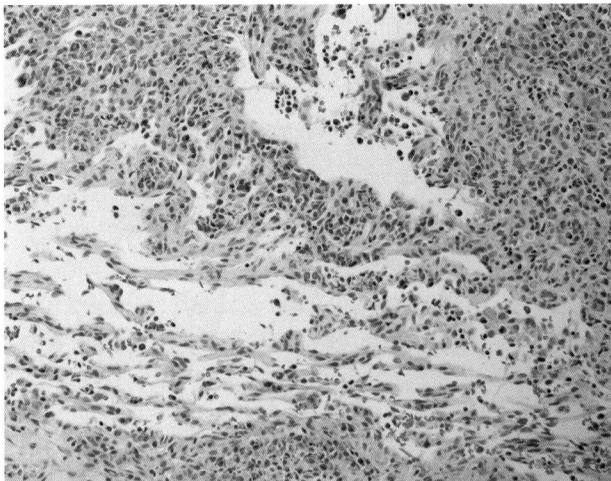

FIGURE 25.37. Lymphadenopathic Kaposi sarcoma. The lesion comprises a variable mixture of ectatic, irregularly shaped, round capillary and slitlike endothelial-lined vascular spaces and spindle-shaped cells accompanied by a variable mixed mononuclear inflammatory cell infiltrate. The endothelial cells range from thin and spindle-shaped to oval to round. They generally lack cytologic atypia and mitotic activity. Erythrocytes and hemosiderin pigment are frequently present, often extravasated between the spindle cells (hematoxylin and eosin stain, original magnification: 250×).

increasing antibody panels available for immunohistochemistry, investigators first documented a vascular endothelial cell origin for the spindle cells as well as the vascular lining cells of KS (285–287,843,844). Several investigators reported that these spindle cells were more closely related to lymphatic endothelium (845–848), but the specific cell of origin remained controversial until gene expression analysis revealed a transcriptional signature more like that of lymphatic endothelial cells (849). In actuality, most spindle cells express endothelial lineage markers including factor VIII, CD34, and PECAM/CD31, as well as lymphatic endothelial markers such as VEGFR3, Podoplanin, D2-40, and LYVE (850,851). In addition, KS spindle cells have long been known to express mesenchymal markers such as vimentin. In addition, KS spi and recently molecular reprograming was documented indicating that there is an endothelial to mesenchymal transition (EnMT) occurring in KS, which explains the expression of endothelial and mesenchymal antigens. This EnMT is analogous to an epithelial mesenchymal transition documented in carcinomas.

Our entire understanding of the pathogenesis of KS changed with the discovery of its etiologic agent, the KSHV, also called human herpesvirus 8 (HHV-8), in 1994 (310) (Fig. 25.38). Observations that led to this discovery include a considerable body of clinical observations and epidemiologic data suggesting that KS had an infectious cause and was spread most frequently by sexual transmission of this infectious agent to an immunocompromised host, independent of HIV transmission (831,852). Compelling epidemiologic evidence included the much higher frequency of KS in MSM than in IDUs and hemophiliacs with AIDS. Herpes-type virus particles were identified electron microscopically in cultured cells derived from KS lesions in African patients as early as 1972 (853). In search of the elusive cause of KS, Chang and collaborators utilized representational difference analysis to identify unique nonhuman, herpesvirus-like DNA sequences in a KS lesion obtained from a homosexual man who had died from AIDS (310). They showed that these sequences belong to a novel, previously unidentified herpesvirus exhibiting homology with herpesvirus saimiri and EBV. We now know that KSHV is a transmissible, B-cell lymphotropic herpesvirus belonging to the γ2 sublineage (genus *Rhadinovirus*) of the *Gammaherpesvirinae* subfamily (368,850). KSHV was shown to be detectable by PCR in virtually all KS lesions of individuals who have any of the four clinicoepidemiologic forms of the disease (310,854,855). This virus was first visualized in the nuclei of the spindle cells and the flat vascular lining cells of KS lesions by *in situ* techniques (856,857). Now, immunohistochemistry using commercially

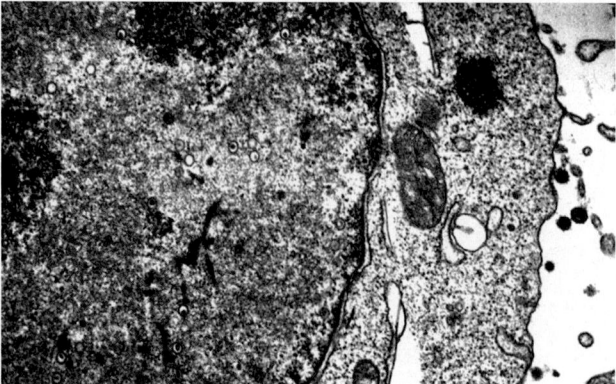

FIGURE 25.38. Kaposi sarcoma–associated herpesvirus (human herpesvirus-8). A PEL cell containing nuclear capsids and a cytoplasmic virion within the dilated endoplasmic reticulum (uranyl acetate, lead acetate stain, original magnification: 44,000×). (From Said JW, Chien K, Takeuchi S, et al. Kaposi sarcoma–associated herpesvirus (KSHV or HHV-8) in primary effusion lymphoma: ultrastructural demonstration of herpesvirus in lymphoma cells. *Blood* 1996;87:4937–4943.)

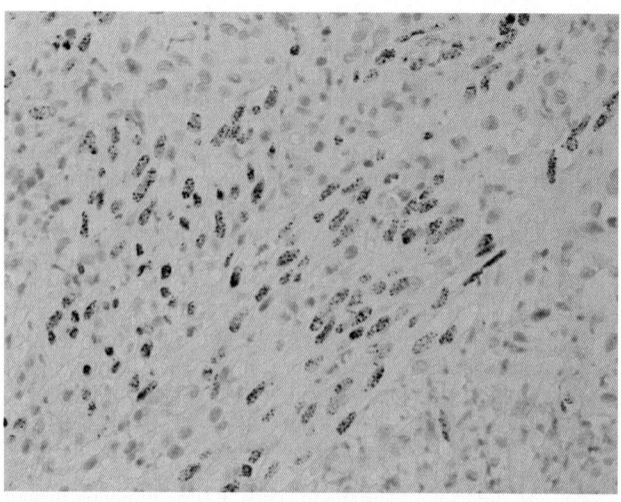

FIGURE 25.39. Kaposi sarcoma stained for HHV8 LANA. The neoplastic spindle cells reveal granular nuclear staining for LANA. (Immunoperoxidase, hematoxylin counterstain, magnification: 240×.)

available antibodies to the KSHV latency-associated antigen LANA-1 (also called LNA and encoded by ORF73) is most commonly used for identification of the virus and confirmation of a diagnosis of KS (379,858) (Fig. 25.39).

All evidence points to a causal role for KSHV in the pathogenesis of KS (368,850). Detection of an infectious agent in a particular tumor is not sufficient to establish causality and Koch postulates established in 1884 cannot be applied to oncogenic agents in humans (these postulates included isolation of a parasite, growth in culture, and induction of disease anew) (859). Helpful updated guidelines were provided in 1965 by Austin Bradford Hill. These include strength of the association, consistency of disease association, analogy, specificity of the association, temporality, biologic plausibility, coherence, and experimental evidence (860). According to all of these criteria, KSHV qualifies as the etiologic agent of KS (861). KSHV is absent, according to most studies, from the wide array of vascular tumors and inflammatory conditions that resemble KS in their cellular composition (310,368,850). Further support for a causal relationship between KSHV and KS comes from studies showing that the presence of KSHV DNA sequences in the peripheral blood often antedates, and may predict, the subsequent development of KS (405,830). Seroconversion to positivity for antibodies against KSHV-related nuclear antigens has been found to occur before the clinical appearance of KS in a significant proportion of patients who have AIDS-related KS (862). Biologic plausibility also has been clearly established. KSHV encodes a large array of genes that are homologous to cellular genes involved in cellular proliferation, immune evasion, and antiapoptotic functions, consistent with an oncogenic role. The function of some of these genes is described in more detail in the section on PELs. Briefly, among these are proteins expressed during latent infection encoding a viral cyclin homologous to cellular cyclin D, and vFLIP, which like cellular FLIP proteins, can inhibit caspase-mediated apoptosis and induce spindling of endothelial cells in culture, a feature of KS (863–865). In KS, it appears that lytic genes that are expressed in a very small subset of tumor cells may play a role by providing powerful paracrine signals inducing inflammation and angiogenesis (866). Among these lytic genes are vIL-6, the viral chemokines, and the viral G protein coupled receptor (vGPCR), all of which can induce inflammation and angiogenesis (867–869). The KSHV vGPCR has received particular attention because it has been shown to induce KS-like vascular tumors in transgenic mice, when only expressed by a few cells in the lesions (870,871). However, in spite of the evidence supporting KSHV as the causal agent of KS, infection by this virus is necessary, but not sufficient for KS development. This is probably a multistep process that involves the interplay of KSHV with impaired immune surveillance, immune stimulation, and multiple genetic, environmental, behavioral, and other factors. Nevertheless, the discovery of KSHV and the elucidation of its precise role in the complex development of KS has facilitated the diagnosis of this disease, and work is under way to develop prevention and targeted treatment strategies.

Summary and Conclusions

Since AIDS was described initially in 1981, it has spread as a fatal epidemic among high-risk groups—MSM, IDUs, and recipients of HIV-infected blood products—and its incidence has increased steadily among the heterosexual contacts of HIV-infected persons and among children born to woman who have AIDS. The causal agent of AIDS is HIV-1. The main receptor for HIV on human cells is the CD4 molecule, which is expressed primarily by helper-inducer T cells and monocytes or macrophages. The HIV infection and subsequent cytopathic destruction of CD4 helper T cells results in their progressive depletion, progressively worsening immune deficiency, and eventually the collapse of the immune system. Most AIDS-defining conditions, especially opportunistic infections, occur if the level of CD4 T cells in a HIV-infected patient falls below 200/μL. For this reason, measurements of CD4 T cells have been used to guide the clinical and therapeutic management of HIV-infected persons in the United States. The progressive depletion of the CD4 T-cell population is reflected in the shifting cell populations and consequent changing histopathologic appearance of the lymph nodes of HIV-infected individuals in different clinical stages of the disease. Since the beginning of the AIDS epidemic the clinical indications to biopsy HIV-infected patients have changed to only include patients with suspected malignancy. Therefore, there are no large studies evaluating lymph node histology in the era of cART. Four distinct histopathologic patterns of HIV-related lymphadenopathy have been described; these are now commonly designated *florid follicular hyperplasia*, *mixed follicular hyperplasia and involution*, *follicular involution*, and *lymphocyte depletion*. The HIV-associated BLEL occurring in the salivary glands may be a localized manifestation of persistent generalized lymphadenopathy and usually exhibit florid follicular hyperplasia. HIV-related lymphadenopathy is in a state of dynamic evolution. Over time, the lymph nodes consistently and progressively transform histologically from florid follicular hyperplasia to mixed follicular hyperplasia and involution to follicular involution and, finally, to lymphocyte depletion. The temporal progression of HIV-related lymphadenopathy parallels the patient's deteriorating immune status and has clinical prognostic implications. In general, patients who have the histologic patterns of florid follicular hyperplasia or mixed follicular hyperplasia and involution appear to have the best prognosis because they do not seem to develop severe opportunistic infections or die from HIV-associated illnesses as long as they display these "early" histologies. HIV-infected patients develop the complications of AIDS only after the lymph node histology has progressed to either follicular involution or lymphocyte depletion. Although the development of severe opportunistic infections and length of survival are predicted by the histopathologic pattern of the lymph nodes, the development of KS and malignant lymphoma are not. HIV-infected persons who have KS or malignant lymphoma may exhibit any one of these four histopathologic patterns in their lymph nodes, including those lymph nodes actually involved by KS or malignant lymphoma.

Various severe opportunistic infections, which represent AIDS-defining conditions, frequently are identified within the lymph nodes of HIV-infected patients who are severely immune deficient. The most common infectious agents identified within

the lymph nodes of these individuals are *M. avium complex*, *C. neoformans*, *H. capsulatum*, and cytomegalovirus. Opportunistic infections are identified in approximately 5% of lymph nodes from HIV-infected persons who have persistent generalized lymphadenopathy exhibiting florid follicular hyperplasia, but in up to 95% of AIDS patients at the time of autopsy. Bacillary angiomatosis is a rare pseudoneoplastic vasoproliferative disorder of infectious origin that occurs primarily in HIV-infected individuals. It is caused by *B. henselae* and *B. quintana*, cat-scratch disease bacillus-like organisms. Cutaneous disease is the most frequent clinical manifestation of bacillary angiomatosis, but this may be accompanied by mucosal, visceral, and lymph node involvement. Clumps and tangled masses of the causative organisms can be identified within the lesions with a Warthin-Starry stain. Bacillary angiomatosis must not be mistaken for KS clinically or histopathologically. Appropriate antibiotic therapy leads to regression of the lesions and resolution of the disease.

KS is the most common neoplasm occurring in association with HIV infection and is an AIDS-defining condition. KS occurs most frequently in MSM and uncommonly in persons in other AIDS risk groups. AIDS-related KS exhibits a variable clinical course ranging from an asymptomatic incidental finding to the explosive onset of widespread, rapidly progressive disease resulting in significant illness and even death. The lesions occur most commonly on the skin but can occur anywhere, particularly in the lungs and gastrointestinal tract. Lymph node involvement by AIDS-related KS is also common and may occur in the absence of mucocutaneous disease. KS often involves lymph nodes as small foci in or adjacent to the capsule, in the hilum, or occasionally in the perinodal adipose tissue. These lesions may be overlooked by an inexperienced observer. AIDS-related KS is histopathologically indistinguishable from the other clinicoepidemiologic forms of the disease. The many special clinical, epidemiologic, and pathologic peculiarities of KS, including the presence of a mixed cell population in the lesions, have led to controversy concerning the cell of origin, nature, and cause of the disease. There is now strong evidence indicating that the spindle cells of KS are of lymphatic endothelial cell origin and that the disease is caused by KSHV, also known as human herpesvirus-8, which is detectable in virtually all KS lesions occurring in individuals who have any of the four clinicoepidemiologic forms of the disease. The use of antibodies to this virus, specifically to the LANA protein, can greatly help confirm the diagnosis. The development of KS is probably a multistep process involving the interplay of KSHV with impaired immune surveillance, immune stimulation, and multiple genetic environmental, behavioral, and other factors.

Malignant lymphoma is the second most common neoplasm occurring in association with HIV infection and AIDS. The CDC has adopted the occurrence of intermediate - or high-grade NHL of B-cell or indeterminate phenotype in a HIV-seropositive person as a criterion for the diagnosis of AIDS. NHLs occur in persons who belong to all AIDS risk groups worldwide, although the majority of the patients are MSM and male IDUs. The clinical and pathologic characteristics of the NHLs occurring in these various AIDS risk groups are similar, although primary oral and anorectal NHLs appear to preferentially occur in MSM. AIDS-related NHLs are divisible into three broad categories according to their anatomic site of origin: those arising systemically (nodal or extranodal), those arising in the CNS, and those arising in the body cavities. Approximately 80% of all NHLs arise systemically. At initial presentation, approximately two-thirds of patients who have systemic NHL already have widely disseminated disease, including a high frequency of extranodal involvement; the majority of the remaining patients have clinical stage IE disease but have large bulky tumor masses in these sites. The CNS and the gastrointestinal tract are the most common extranodal sites of primary and secondary involvement by NHL, respectively. AIDS-related NHLs, however, may arise or present at virtually any anatomic site, including, for example, the anorectal region and the heart. AIDS-related NHL should always be given diagnostic consideration in an individual at risk for AIDS who presents with a tumor mass, regardless of the site or mode of presentation, and the atypical presentation of diffuse, aggressive NHLs involving unusual extranodal sites should raise suspicion of HIV infection. Approximately 20% of all AIDS-related NHLs arise in the CNS; AIDS now represents the most common risk factor, by far, for the development of primary CNS lymphoma, although these have declined since the introduction of cART. The majority of these patients are profoundly immunocompromised young MSM with far advanced HIV disease. Primary CNS lymphoma is often a secondary manifestation of AIDS in these patients. Less than five percent of all AIDS-related NHLs arise in the body cavities as lymphomatous effusions in the absence of a tumor mass. These are now designated PELs; they exhibit a unique constellation of clinical, morphologic, immunophenotypic, and molecular characteristics, including the presence of KSHV, and represent a distinct clinopathologic entity. A proportion of KSHV-positive lymphomas occur as solid masses with no evidence of body cavity involvement, and have been called extracavitary or solid variants of PEL. Investigators also have described a distinct subset of AIDS-related NHLs designated *plasmablastic lymphoma* that preferentially occur in the oral cavity, and a group of HIV-associated lymphoid proliferations of uncertain malignant potential referred to as *polymorphic lymphoproliferative disorders*.

The histopathologic distribution of NHLs occurring in HIV-infected persons differs from that of conventional NHLs occurring in the HIV-uninfected general population, and also from that of NHLs occurring in other immune-deficient states. Approximately 40% of AIDS-related NHLs are BLs, and the remainder is evenly divided between immunoblastic lymphomas and large cell lymphomas. Some patients exhibit transitional morphologic features. Each of these histopathologic categories of AIDS-related NHL exhibits distinctive clinical characteristics. The prognostic significance of the histopathologic category of AIDS-related NHL within the context of this immune deficiency remains unclear. The survival of patients who have AIDS-related NHLs appears to be most dependent on their levels of immune deficiency.

Generally speaking, the treatment of AIDS-related NHL is complicated by the fact that most patients have widely disseminated disease, including CNS and bone marrow involvement; have intermediate - and high-grade histologies; and have an underlying immune deficiency. The original notion that less intensive chemotherapy was beneficial has evolved, with improved antiretroviral therapy, leading to better immunologic performance. More aggressive regimens are now recommended in patients with cART therapy and immune reconstitution. The addition of rituximab to the CHOP regimen has resulted in improved outcome (872), and infusional chemotherapy with R-EPOCH as well as autologous stem cell transplantation have led to good clinical results, in particular in patients with CD4 T-cell counts of more than $100/\mu L$ (563,576,577). The prognosis and clinical outcomes in patients with HIV-related diffuse large B-cell lymphoma is approaching the outcomes of patients with *de novo* lymphoma (873).

More than 95% of AIDS-related NHLs express B-cell immunophenotypes comparable to those expressed by B-cell NHLs of similar morphology occurring in the general population. Most of the remaining cases are PELs, which characteristically often express indeterminate immunophenotypes. More than 95% of AIDS-related NHLs, including those displaying indeterminate immunophenotypes, exhibit clonal immunoglobulin gene rearrangements. Structural alterations involving several protooncogenes and tumor suppressor genes occur nonrandomly in

association with specific histopathologic categories of conventional NHL and are believed to play a role in their pathogenesis. Structural alterations of some of these genes—*MYC*, *BCL6*, *RAS*, and *P53*—occur in AIDS-related NHLs as well. Infection by EBV can be seen in approximately one-third of AIDS-related lymphomas, including both BL and DLBCL. In addition to the molecular analysis relying on Southern blotting, cytogenetics, ISH and PCR, more detailed genomic and epigenomic studies are beginning to emerge with the development of microarray and high-throughput sequencing technologies. While the depth of our understanding of the molecular mechanisms of AIDS-related lymphoma pathogenesis is rapidly expanding, we now know that they are characterized by the accumulation of multiple distinct genetic lesions, which apparently accrue quickly. Diverse molecular genetic pathways are likely to operate in AIDS lymphomagenesis.

More than 400 cases of HL occurring in HIV-infected persons, many collected through national AIDS registries, have been reported. These reports have not determined unequivocally whether HIV infection truly promotes the development of HL or merely modifies its course, and thus they have not fully clarified the relationship among HIV infection, AIDS, and HL. Although the incidence of HL apparently is not increased among MSM or individuals who have acquired HIV infection through heterosexual contact, it may be significantly increased among IDUs. Nonetheless, the occurrence of HL in a HIV-seropositive person has not been accepted by the CDC as an AIDS-defining condition. HL occurring in association with HIV infection displays distinctive clinical pathologic characteristics. The pathologic spectrum of HIV-associated HL, that is, a significant increase in the proportion of the unfavorable histologic subtypes (mixed cellularity and lymphocytic depletion), is similar to that of underdeveloped countries and patients of lower socioeconomic status in the United States. The lesions of HIV-associated and non–HIV-associated HL share similar immunophenotypic and genotypic characteristics, although the lesions of HIV-associated HL contain diminished numbers of CD4 T cells, and the Reed-Sternberg cells of HIV-associated HL of all histologic subtypes more frequently contain EBV. HIV-infected individuals belonging to any AIDS risk group who develop HL display a distinct constellation of clinical features that contrast sharply with those of conventional HL. These features include a significantly higher frequency of B symptoms, a higher propensity for advanced stage (III or IV) disease, and bone marrow and other extranodal involvement at initial presentation; random, noncontiguous spread of the disease; a high incidence of the peripheral form of the disease (absent mediastinal disease); an atypical and particularly aggressive clinical course; poor response to and enhanced hematologic toxicity from chemotherapy; and shortened duration of survival, often because of the development of severe opportunistic infections associated with the underlying HIV-induced immune deficiency.

A variety of other neoplasms occurring in HIV-infected persons, some of whom have AIDS, have been reported. These include B-cell ALL, plasmacytomas, and multiple myeloma, histologic low-grade NHLs and lymphoid leukemias, an array of T-cell neoplasms, and a spectrum of subtypes of AML. The cases of B-cell ALL essentially represent BL in the leukemic phase; their development is most likely HIV related and not merely coincidental. The other neoplasms apparently only occur sporadically in HIV-seropositive individuals, and there is no epidemiologic evidence to suggest that their incidence has increased in parallel with the AIDS epidemic. It is likely, for example, that the occurrence of low-grade NHLs and lymphoid leukemias in this patient population is merely coincidental. The CDC does not recognize the occurrence of any of these neoplasms in HIV-seropositive individuals as an AIDS-defining condition. Their relationship to HIV infection and the development of AIDS remains to be determined.

The spread of HIV infection and the consequent increase in the number of patients with AIDS worldwide ensures an increase in the overall occurrence of AIDS-related pathology and the likelihood that pathologists, hematologists, oncologists, and other physicians will come into frequent contact with patients who have HIV-related illnesses.

Taking the next step: In three decades the AIDS epidemic has provided unprecedented insights into the role of the immune system and viral agents in the pathogenesis of malignancy, particularly malignant lymphoma. There have been remarkable scientific achievements with regard to HIV diagnostics, antiretroviral agents, and prevention including the use of male circumcision and preexposure prophylaxis. Global resources are limited, however, and a substantial percentage of infected individuals are unaware of their status. Control of HIV infection and the diagnosis and treatment of AIDS-related malignancies worldwide continues to pose an enormous challenge.

POSTTRANSPLANTATION LYMPHOPROLIFERATIVE DISORDERS

Introduction

PTLDs are a heterogeneous group of lymphoid proliferations that occur in patients who are immunosuppressed following transplantation (solid organ, bone marrow, or stem cell). Although morphologically diverse, they have a number of features in common, including frequent association with EBV. The degree of immunosuppression and EBV status prior to transplantation appears to be the most important factors that determine susceptibility to PTLD. Patients more heavily immunosuppressed following multiorgan transplants may have greater incidence. PTLD following BMT is rare, but is associated with characteristic clinical and pathologic features described below.

Historical Background

Since the original reports of McKhann (874) and Penn et al. (239) in 1969, it has been well established that there is an increased incidence of neoplasms, especially skin and lip carcinomas and lymphoid lesions, in transplant recipients (875,876). The other key relationship between PTLDs and EBV infection became evident shortly thereafter (877,878). The PTLDs were initially thought of as malignancies associated with high mortality (879). It became evident that these lesions represented a more complex group of B-cell proliferations, covering a spectrum from reactive lymphoid hyperplasias to lymphoma, had a unique morphology in some cases referred to as *polymorphic*, and were different from sporadic NHL (432,880).

The existence of a pathologic spectrum fitted well the pathogenetic scenario proposed by Purtilo in 1980 and since then generally accepted: "Defective immune responses to EBV permit persistence of polyclonal proliferation of B cells. Conversion from polyclonal to monoclonal proliferation is probably the result of a cytogenetic error in a B cell" (881). The Pittsburgh group later showed that some of these lesions are reversible with reduction of immunosuppression and therefore arguably nonneoplastic (882). This concept opened the way to modern therapeutic strategies, which aim at restoring the patient's immune response to the EBV-driven proliferation. It also presents pathologists with a double challenge. The first is to provide as precise as possible a set of criteria that guide early recognition of these disorders in terms of allograft rejection or other unrelated inflammatory responses; underdiagnosis or delay in diagnosis allows the proliferation to progress, and overdiagnosis can lead to unnecessary or excessive therapy. The second is to establish criteria to discern which lesions

are likely to regress with immunologic intervention and which are likely to progress as *bona fide* lymphomas.

Clinical Findings

PTLD is variable in its clinical presentation. It is the second most common malignancy after skin cancer in adult transplant recipients. It may be nodal but is frequently extranodal or in the transplanted organ, and can affect any organ system including the gastrointestinal tract, lung, kidney, and liver. The PTLD risk is greatest in the first 12 to 18 months after the transplant, but can occur at any time. The incidence varies according to the type of organ transplanted and the degree of immunosuppression. Patients who are EBV negative at the time of transplantation are at greatest risk for developing EBV-driven PTLD. The frequency of PTLD is low in renal transplants, but in lung transplants that may require increased immunosuppression due to the higher risk of graft rejection the incidence is reported as 2.5% to 8% (883). Primary CNS PTLD is rare, but the incidence is increased in small bowel transplants and in children. The time from transplantation to diagnosis of primary CNS PTLD ranges from 12 months to 4 years in most cases. The CNS may also be involved as a site of multiorgan PTLD. Early PTLD lesions such as plasmacytic hyperplasia and infectious mononucleosis-like lymphoid proliferations are more common in children, particularly in tonsillar biopsies. This form of PTLD is usually associated with primary EBV infection in children without prior exposure to EBV, and is becoming less common with modern preventive strategies. These early lesions are polyclonal and generally regress with conservative treatment. Monomorphic PTLD more often involves extranodal sites and are more frequent in older individuals. EBV-negative and T-/NK-cell PTLD usually present longer after transplantation (4 to 6 years).

Bone Marrow and Stem Cell Transplants

This risk of PTLD is low with stem cell and bone marrow transplants, and is generally of donor origin (884–891), because the immune system of these patients is disproportionately of foreign origin (892), including B cells that are not removed by many T-cell depletion methods. In bone marrow allograft recipients PTLD usually presents early in the first 6 months, and is often disseminated involving nodal and extranodal sites including the gastrointestinal tract, liver, and lungs.

In BMT, several risk factors are consistently detected by multivariate analysis, although not in the same order of statistical relevance: T-cell depletion of the grafted marrow, human leukocyte antigen (HLA) disparity between donor and host, use of anti-CD3 (or ATG), and primary immune deficiency in the host and acute graft-versus-host disease grades 3 or 4 (893–895). The methods used for T-cell depletion of the donor marrow have been found to be relevant. Although the incidence of PTLD using unmanipulated bone marrow is 0.45% when HLA-identical and 1.4% when HLA-mismatched (885), the incidence remains similar (1.3%) with marrows treated with the CAMPATH (CD52) antibodies or elutriation, which also remove B cells (896), but it rises up to 8%, 11%, 14%, and 26% with other protocols for T-cell depletion (896,897). A detailed evaluation of these risk factors can be found in several excellent reviews (897,898).

PTLD Incidence

The incidence of lymphoid lesions, as reported in the literature, varies depending on the type of organ transplanted, the age of the recipient, and the immunosuppressive regimen used. In cases of solid organ transplantation, the overall incidence of PTLDs is 1.4% to 1.7% of all patients transplanted (899,900). The variable figures given for the various organs (as number of cases per number of patients transplanted) are 0.6% for pancreas (901); 1% to 2% for liver (435,901,902); 0.3% to 3% for kidney (900–908); 1.8% to 9.8% for heart (435,900,902–905,909,910); 3.7% to 7.9% for lung (900,903,910,911); 4.6% to 12.5% for heart and lung (435,903,912); and 32% for transplantation of pancreas alone and with other viscera (913).

Comparison within the same institution (University of Pittsburgh) of the experience with pediatric and adult transplantation reveals consistently a higher frequency of PTLD among children: 4% (vs. 0.8%, $p < 0.005$) among all organ transplants (914) and 9.7% (vs. 3.5%) among all thoracic organ transplants (910,915). This is probably because children are more often EBV seronegative before transplantation and seroconvert after transplantation (914,915). For BMT, the overall frequency of PTLD in recipients of allogeneic grafts varies from 0.4% up to 7.4% (884,885,893,894,916–919). The striking differences in incidence depend on the type of bone marrow grafted: 0% to 0.4% for recipients of unmanipulated marrow (884,885,919) but 6% to 9% for those with T-cell–depleted marrow (885,918,919) and 16% to 24% for those with mismatched and T-cell–depleted marrow (884,918–920). Among recipients of autologous bone marrow, there are no cases of LPDs reported in several studies (893,918,921), but two cases have been described in a small series of T-cell–depleted autologous grafts (14%) (922) in addition to other sporadic reports (897,923).

The variations in the incidence of PTLDs in relation to the diverse immunosuppressive regimens used have received much attention; the risk is related to the aggressiveness of the regimen (905,924,925). The incidence of LPDs in patients treated with conventional immunosuppression (such as antilymphocyte globulin, steroids, and azathioprine [AZT]) was from about 1% (902,926) to 4.9% (927). Initial reports on patients treated with cyclosporine A (CSA) suggested a much higher incidence of LPDs (9% to 13%) (928), but later figures are between 0% and 1.5% (905,929–931) as a result of dose reduction and careful monitoring of serum levels of the drug. There has been also an increase in PTLDs reported in patients treated with FK506 (tacrolimus), an immunosuppressant that is about 100 times more potent than CSA (907,913,932). There is mounting evidence about the risk of using multiple agents. A significantly increased incidence of PTLDs has been associated with the use of triple therapy (CSA in combination with AZT and prednisone) in several studies (905,906,933,934), and an even higher incidence with the further addition of OKT3 (i.e., "quadruple therapy") (935).

The statistics given for the overall incidence of PTLD are only a general indication of the risk of this complication in transplantation. In addition to the influence of the different immunosuppressive regimens, other very important risk factors have been reported. A first encounter with EBV after transplantation has emerged as the major risk factor for the development of PTLD. The incidence of this complication is many times higher among seronegative than seropositive patients, such as 33% versus <2% among recipients of lung transplants (911); 50% versus 0.8% among adult recipients of nonrenal organs (936); or 25% versus 0% among children receiving transplantation of solid organs (937). Unrelated to EBV, and contributing additional significant immune dysregulation (924), a CMV infection adds to the risk of PTLD. A history of symptomatic CMV disease in a recipient (924) and a CMV seromismatch (host⁻/donor⁺) (938) are important risk factors for this complication in two studies.

Pathologic Features

Grossly, PTLDs form tumoral masses or infiltrate the organ diffusely (435). Multiple lesions are common in the same patient and in the same organ, especially in lymph nodes, lungs (912), the CNS, and the gastrointestinal tract, where several small ulcers leading to perforation are often observed (939). Histologically,

the lymphoid proliferations observed in transplant recipients are quite heterogeneous, and the distinctions between these forms are not always sharp. Overlapping patterns may be observed, and more than one of these patterns may be observed simultaneously at different sites (435,442,884,940) or consecutively in the same patient (440,941,942). Polymorphic PTLDs account for 46% to 69% of the PTLDs, and the monomorphic cases for 16% to 48% in different series of organ transplant patients (440,900,901,943–945). In BMT recipients, 68% to 70% of the lesions have been classified as polymorphic and 14% to 30% as monomorphic (884,919).

Classification of PTLD

PTLD can be classified into early lesions that are polyclonal and generally reversible, although they may progress to more aggressive forms of PTLD (946). These include plasmacytic hyperplasia and infectious mononucleosis-like PTLD (Table 25.5).

Polymorphic PTLD has variable morphology but is monoclonal and has a variable clinical course. Monomorphic PTLD resemble lymphomas in the immunocompetent population, and are classified according to the lymphomas they resemble. They are usually of B-cell type, but T-cell lymphomas including peripheral T-cell lymphoma NOS and hepatosplenic T-cell lymphoma may also occur. Although rare, there are cases in which T-cell PTLD occur in association with or subsequent to B-cell PTLD.

Early Lesions in PTLD

Clinically early lesions are more common in younger individuals and children involving the head and neck lymph nodes, tonsils, or Waldeyer ring (440). They occur relatively soon after transplantation. Although they usually regress either spontaneously or following reduction of immunosuppressive regimens, they can progress to more advanced forms of PTLD. The pattern of EBV infection varies from polyclonal to oligoclonal and rarely monoclonal, but they are not associated with structural alterations in oncogenes or tumor suppressor genes.

In plasmacytic hyperplasia the architecture is preserved, but there is a proliferation of polyclonal plasma cells as well as admixed small T and B lymphocytes (Fig. 25.40) (947). The infectious mononucleosis–like PTLD resembles an accelerated form of mononucleosis with expanded paracortical regions

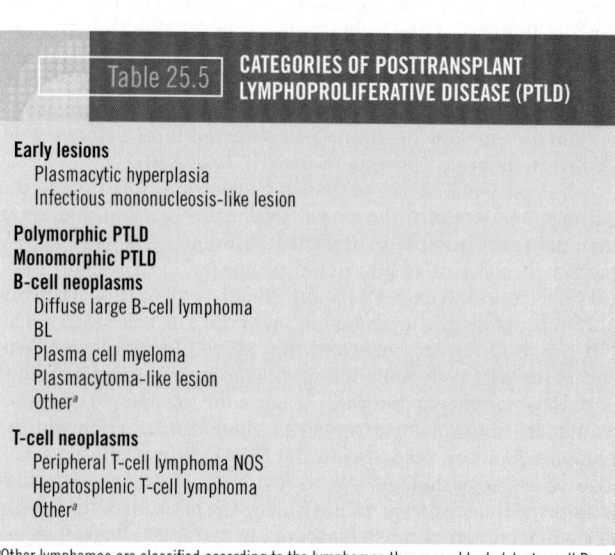

Table 25.5	CATEGORIES OF POSTTRANSPLANT LYMPHOPROLIFERATIVE DISEASE (PTLD)

Early lesions
  Plasmacytic hyperplasia
  Infectious mononucleosis-like lesion

Polymorphic PTLD
Monomorphic PTLD
B-cell neoplasms
  Diffuse large B-cell lymphoma
  BL
  Plasma cell myeloma
  Plasmacytoma-like lesion
  Other[a]

T-cell neoplasms
  Peripheral T-cell lymphoma NOS
  Hepatosplenic T-cell lymphoma
  Other[a]

[a]Other lymphomas are classified according to the lymphomas they resemble. Indolent small B-cell lymphomas are not included as PTLD.
Swerdlow SH, Webber SA, Chadburn A, et al. WHO classification of tumours of haematopoietic and lymphoid tissues. In: Swerdlow, SH, Campo E, Harris NL, eds., eds. *WHO Classification of Tumours of Haematopoietic and Lymphoid Tissues*. Geneva: WHO Press, 2008.

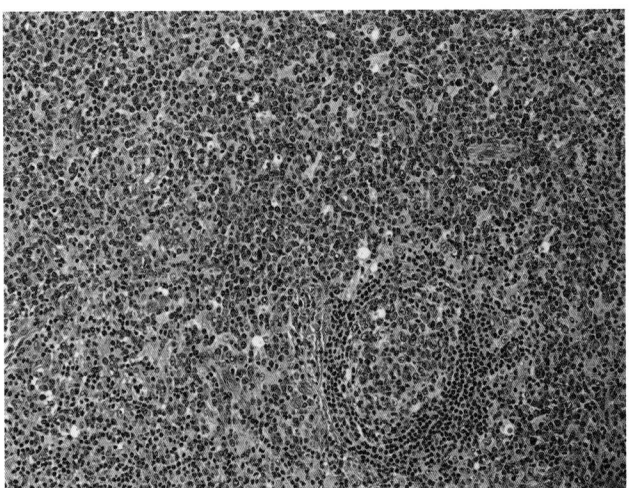

FIGURE 25.40. Early lesion PTLD with plasma cell hyperplasia. Architecture is retained with normal germinal center surrounded by sheets of polyclonal plasma cells. (Magnification: 120×.)

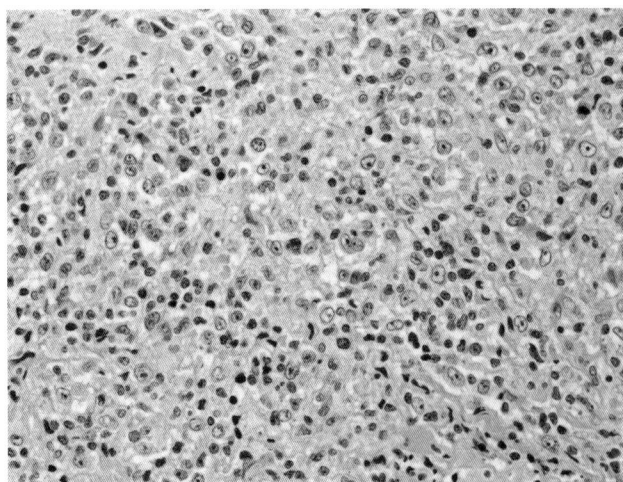

FIGURE 25.41. Polymorphous PTLD showing effacement of architecture by a mixed infiltrate of small lymphocytes, plasma cells, and large immunoblasts. (Magnification: 120×.)

and a marked immunoblastic proliferation (942). There may be foci of necrosis, but the overall architecture is preserved. Cases of infectious mononucleosis like PTLD are EBV⁺ including the presence of EBV⁺ immunoblasts, which are also positive for EBV-LMP1. Early PTLD should be differentiated from other causes of lymphoid hyperplasia of infectious or inflammatory nature. Florid follicular hyperplasia may also be seen in lymph node or tonsillar biopsies in the posttransplantation setting, and is considered by some authors to be a precursor lesion (948). However, cases of follicular hyperplasia are usually EBV negative. Rare EBV EBER-positive cells can commonly be identified in the posttransplantation setting and are not necessarily indicative of PTLD. Molecular genetics characteristically confirm a polyclonal B-cell proliferation, although oligoclonal populations may be present (947). Occasionally, and more often in the IM-like lesions, there may be small clonal populations, usually in an oligoclonal background.

Polymorphic PTLD

Polymorphic PTLD is associated with effacement of nodal architecture, and a proliferation that is mixed, including small and intermediate-sized lymphocytes, plasma cells, and immunoblasts including atypical forms (949) (Fig. 25.41). Necrosis as well as numerous mitoses may be present. Multinucleated cells and large mononuclear cells that resemble Hodgkin or Reed-Sternberg cells may be seen and some cases can resemble classical Hodgkin lymphoma (CHL). However, the spectrum of abnormal cells including immunoblasts seen in PTLD is not present in CHL. They may involve lymph nodes or form masslike lesions at extranodal sites. In the pediatric age group polymorphic lesions comprise the most common form of PTLD. Clinically these may respond to reduced immunosuppression or require addition treatment such as rituximab or chemotherapy. Immunophenotypic studies reveal a spectrum of B cells including immunoblasts positive for CD20 as well as cells with plasmacytic differentiation. Light chain restriction may be present. They are invariably monoclonal despite the polymorphous histologic appearance, although the peaks may be less prominent than those associated with monomorphic PTLD. Clonality can also be demonstrated in most cases using Southern blots, PCR, and/or EBV long terminal repeats (see Discussion below) (243,434). Most but not all cases of polymorphic PTLD are EBV⁺, and EBV EBER staining cells are usually numerous. The Hodgkin and Reed-Sternberg–like cells are usually positive for

EBV LMP1 (Fig. 25-42). They may be positive for CD20 as well as CD30, but negative for CD15.

Monomorphic PTLD

Monomorphic PTLD resemble B- and T-cell lymphomas seen in the immunocompetent population (950). Monomorphic PTLD are more often associated with abnormalities in oncogenes and tumor suppressor genes. Small B-cell lymphomas such as follicular lymphomas and small lymphocytic lymphoma (CLL/SLL) are not considered within the spectrum of PTLD. Cases of EBV extranodal marginal zone (MALT) lymphoma that are EBV positive and respond to immune reconstitution have been described, and these may also form part of the spectrum of PTLD although not recognized as such by the WHO.

Most case of monomorphic PTLD resemble diffuse large B-cell lymphoma NOS (Fig. 25.43), although plasmablastic lymphomas and BLs may also occur as well as high-grade unclassifiable lymphomas(950). As in cases of polymorphic PTLD, cases of DLBCL can include large pleomorphic or Hodgkin-like cells, but the range of plasmacytic differentiation seen in polymorphic PTLD is not present. Some cases resemble myeloma or extramedullary plasmacytoma, with sheets of mature or blastic plasma cells. The lymphoma cells generally

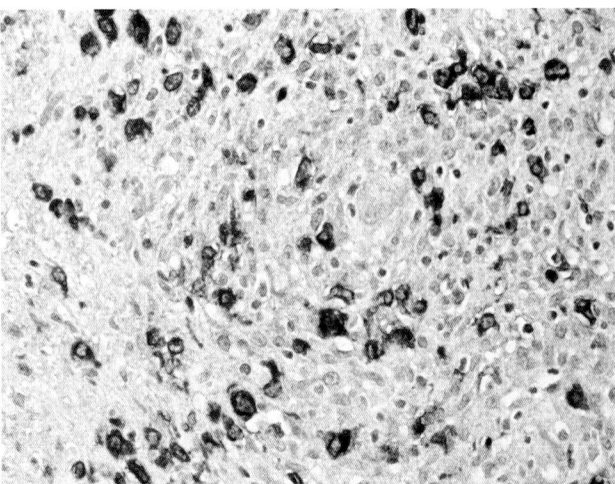

FIGURE 25.42. Polymorphous PTLD showing large immunoblasts positive for EBV LMP1. (Immunoperoxidase, hematoxylin counterstain, magnification: 240×.)

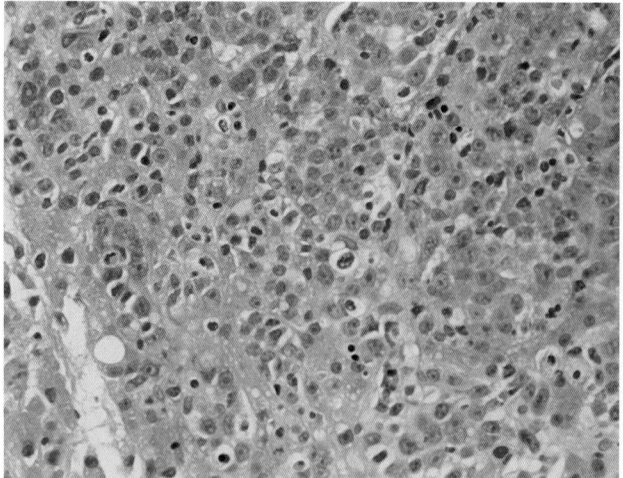

FIGURE 25.43. Monomorphous PTLD with features of diffuse large B-cell lymphoma. (Magnification: 240×.)

express B-cell markers including CD20 and CD79a, although cases with plasmacytic differentiation may show loss of B-cell markers and may express CD38, CD138, and BLIMP1. They are invariably monoclonal, and immunoglobulin light chain restriction can often be demonstrated. Most of these cases are postfollicular or non-GCB type DLBCL, positive for IRF4/MUM1 and negative for CD10, although GCB-type DLBCL may be encountered particularly in the EBV-negative cases. In an international multicenter trial sequential treatment with rituximab followed by CHOP chemotherapy in adult PTLD cases achieved a 68% complete response supporting this therapeutic approach (951).

The plasmacytoma/myeloma cases are similar to those in the immunocompetent cases and can be EBV positive or negative (Fig. 25.44) (952). The plasmacytomas may be nodal or extranodal, and characteristically arise late after transplantation (mean 7.0 years). Patients with plasmacytoma usually do not develop lytic bone lesions or have bone marrow involvement (953), and they may respond to reduction of immunosuppression (954). Molecular studies reveal clonal immunoglobulin gene rearrangements and EBV in clonal episomal form when present. Abnormalities in oncogenes including TP53 mutations, RAS, MYC, and BCL6 may also be found.

BL is a form of PTLD more common in the pediatric age group. Most patients are EBV negative pretransplant, and there is a high incidence of EBV infection in the lymphoma compared with sporadic and other immunodeficiency-associated cases. The median time from transplantation to diagnosis is 52 months. The disease tends to be aggressive and it has been suggested that immediate lymphoma-specific chemotherapy may be required for treatment (955). They are EBV EBER+ and negative for EBV LMP (viral latency pattern I).

T-/NK-cell lymphomas comprise 15% or less of PTLD cases in the West. Rarely can they occur subsequent to or in association with B-cell PTLD. T-/NK-cell PTLD is always clonal, and tends to occur later, with the median time from transplantation to development of PTLD at 66 months. They are often extranodal and less likely to involve the allograft. Less than thirty percent are EBV associated (956), and EBV+ cases are reported to have a longer survival following treatment (957). Sites of involvement include the peripheral blood and bone marrow, spleen, skin, liver, gastrointestinal tract, lung, and kidney although involvement of other sites including the heart, brain, and bladder have been described (956).

Monomorphic T-/NK-cell PTLD resembles T-cell lymphoma in the immunocompetent population and are usually extranodal (957). Most resemble peripheral T-cell lymphoma not otherwise specified (PTCL-NOS) (Fig. 25.45), but less common types are also encountered. Hepatosplenic gamma-delta T-cell lymphoma develops late after transplantation (up to 10 years) and pathologic features are similar to those in the nontransplant population. EBV is usually negative and patients do not respond to reduction of immunosuppression (958). Angioimmunoblastic T-cell lymphoma (AITL) is rarely associated with immunosuppression, and care must be taken to exclude EBV lymphadenitis, which can have a similar histologic appearance (959). Characteristic features of AITL including the presence of clear cells and staining for CD10 may be helpful in making the diagnosis (960). NK-/T-cell large granular lymphocytic leukemia, extranodal NK-/T-cell lymphoma nasal type, and anaplastic large cell lymphomas have also been reported. Lymphocytosis with T-large granular lymphocytes (TLGL) may persist for a long duration following hematopoietic stem cell transplantation, but most cases are polyclonal and have an indolent clinical course without symptoms of TLGL leukemia. Cutaneous T-cell lymphomas that may occur in the posttransplantation setting include mycosis fungoides and primary cutaneous anaplastic large cell lymphoma.

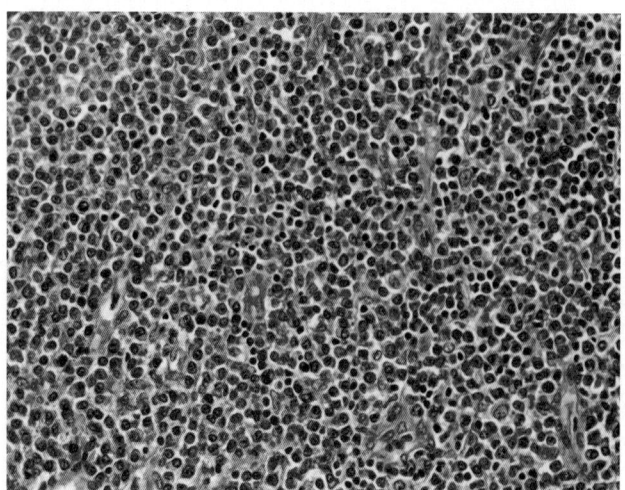

FIGURE 25.44. Monomorphous PTLD plasmacytoma type with sheets of plasma cells. (Magnification: 240×.)

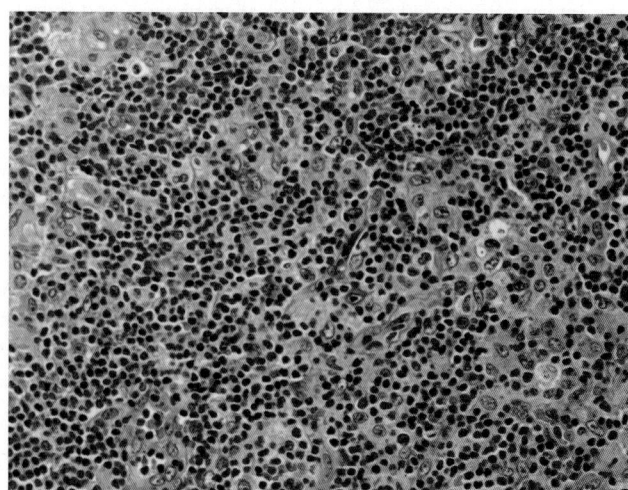

FIGURE 25.45. Monomorphous PTLD with features of peripheral T-cell lymphoma NOS. The proliferation consists of small irregular lymphoid cells of T-cell phenotype admixed with histiocytes and scattered large lymphoid cells with prominent nucleoli. Molecular studies revealed clonal T-cell gene rearrangement. (Magnification: 120×.)

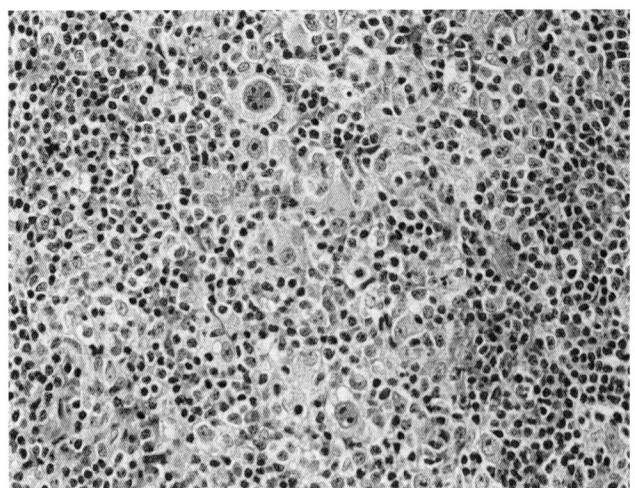

FIGURE 25.46. PTLD with features of CHL. (Magnification: 120×.)

Classical Hodgkin's Lymphoma Type PTLD

CHL is a rare form of PTLD that tends to occur late after transplantation, >2.5 years (961). Diagnosis requires the characteristic histologic and immunophenotypic features of Hodgkin lymphoma, including the presence of diagnostic Hodgkin and Reed-Sternberg (H-RS) cells in the appropriate background of small lymphocytes, histiocytes, plasma cells, and eosinophils (Fig. 25.46) (962). In some forms of monomorphic or polymorphic B-cell PTLD there may be Reed-Sternberg–like cells resembling Hodgkin lymphoma, but these cases should be separated from CHL for classification and treatment (963). Cases of true CHL posttransplant should be negative or only weakly expressive of CD20, lack a full complement of B-cell transcription factors including coexpression of OCT2 and BOB.1, and preferably be positive for CD30 and CD15. The H-RS are EBV positive, including expression of EBV EBER and EBV LMP1.

Immunophenotypic Features

The EBV-induced LPDs that occur in transplant recipients are mostly B-cell proliferations and express variable clonality patterns (243,435,884,885,902,912,916,919,964–967). Polyclonal and monoclonal lesions may be found at different sites in the same patient (435,884,926,940) and clones might be identical or different at different sites. In a compilation of studies, 63% of PTLDs were immunophenotypically monoclonal, 28% were polyclonal, and 9% were immunoglobulin negative (900,919,940,965,966).

The expression of the classic B-cell–associated antigens such as CD19, CD20, CD21, CD22 by neoplastic cells is heterogeneous (965,966); CD21, in particular, is expressed uncommonly (965) or in a small proportion of cells (919,964). The cells variably express antigens suggestive of germinal center cells, such as CD38 and CD10, and activation antigens, such as CD23, CD30, CD39, and CDw70 (919,964–968), and cell adhesion molecules, such as CD11a, CD54, and CD58 (964–966,968). They express MHC class I and II antigens and strongly immunoregulatory markers (CD80, CD86) (964). Most cases of PTLD strongly express BCL-2 (969,970). P53 expression was detected in a variable proportion of cells in 50% of cases of PTLD in one study (919) and 86% of cases in another (971).

The proliferating B lymphocytes are associated with a variable proportion of mature T cells, usually limited (902,965), but at times prominent (972). These cells may be more numerous in polymorphic than in monomorphic lesions (925). The T cells are a mixture of CD4+ and CD8+ cells (902,964,965). The ratio of the two subsets in the tissue of PTLD is 2:1, in contrast to the predominant CD8+ response to EBV in the peripheral blood and lymph nodes of immunocompetent patients with IM (964). Although CD4+ cells may have cytolytic functions, they "may also encourage tumor proliferation by providing inappropriate signals for B-cell activation and growth by the production of cytokines" (964). The T-cell microenvironment in PTLDs is poor in cells efficient in killing EBV-infected cells and rich in cells that facilitate B-cell growth. However, in that study, there is no definite correlation between the degree of T-cell infiltration and clinical outcome (964). No CD56+ cells were detected within PTLDs, in contrast to the tissues of IM (973).

Etiology and Pathogenesis

It has been said that PTLDs "straddle the borderland between infection and neoplasia" (925) and evidence has been presented throughout this section indicating that EBV infection of B cells is usually the starting point, that the proliferation of the infected cells is not controlled by an inefficient immune response, and that genomic changes may occur within such proliferations that give rise to *bona fide* neoplasms. Some PTLDs, independent of their clonal status, should be regarded as an exaggerated response to EBV infection and treated as such, while others are true neoplasms capable of autonomous growth (974). With the exception of the bone marrow transplant population, most PTLD are of recipient origin (892).

Role of EBV in the Pathogenesis of LPDs

Many different methods, molecular and immunohistochemical, have documented the presence of EBV in the tissue of PTLDs, the former including the detection of viral DNA by slot-blot (975) Southern blot (434,436,886,900,976–979), PCR (438,886,919,980–982), or ISH techniques (976,983–986); EBER by ISH (886,900,966,975,987,988); viral mRNA by reverse transcriptase (RT)–PCR (987,988); or proteins by Western blot (979). With one or more of these techniques, EBV has been detected in most cases of PTLD, from a low of 68% to 75% (900,982) to 87% to 90% (438,886,902,919,975,986), or 94% to 97% (886).

Two main types (1 and 2) of EBV are distinguished on the basis of sequence variations in the EBNA-2 proteins and, in the West, more than 90% of people carry type 1 (989). In up to 33% of transplant recipients and other immunosuppressed individuals (vs. 3% of the general population), the peripheral blood lymphocytes are infected with EBV of type 2 (438). Despite this, it is type 1 EBV that is most often detected in the tissues of PTLD by molecular techniques, with an incidence of 83% (945), 98% (990), and 100% (438,991), or by immunohistochemistry (100%, with monoclonal antibodies R3 and 3E9) (987). This is thought to reflect the greater efficiency of type 1 in transforming B cells (989). Special variants of EBV that carry a specific 30-base pair deletion of the *LMP1* gene (del-LMP1 variants) and have been previously reported in Hodgkin lymphoma, undifferentiated nasopharyngeal carcinoma, peripheral T-cell lymphomas, and other lymphomas, as well as in benign EBV-driven lesions (945), were also found initially in the aggressive, but not in the "reactive," histologic forms of PTLD and were thought to contribute to the lymphomatous process (991). However, such variants were later detected in 41% to 44% (945,990) of PTLDs and in a similar proportion of reactive EBV lesions (945). No correlation was found between the presence of the 30-bp deletion (or point mutations (945)) of *LMP1* and the histologic type of the lesions or patients' survival in these two studies (945,990). The wild or deleted type of LMP-1 was the same in the same patient, in multiple lesions, and in tissues not involved by PTLD (990). These data lead to the conclusion that the EBV strain in a PTLD depends on the one that the patient is carrying (990).

Most EBV-encoded proteins expressed in infected tissues can be detected by immunohistochemistry in frozen and paraffin-embedded material (313,919,965,966,968,970,971,979,982,987,988). There are 10 main products of the latent cycle genes (2 RNA species, EBER-1 and EBER-2; 6 EBV nuclear antigens [EBNA-1 through EBNA-6]; and 3 latent membrane proteins [LMP-1, LMP-2A, LMP-2B]), as well as several products of the lytic cycle genes. It is the former that are relevant to the transformation of B cells, and they are differently expressed in cell lines and human EBV-related proliferations (989). EBER1and EBER2 are small noncoding RNAs and present in abundance in EBV-infected cells, and are therefore an excellent screening test to identify EBV in tissue sections using ISH techniques. The function of these EBV-encoded RNAS has not been completely established. EBV-related microRNAs (miRs) have also been identified and appear to be involved in both oncogenesis and modulation of the immune response (992).

Patterns of EBV latency

EBV in LPDs is usually in its latent form. Although there may be a spectrum of viral latency there are three main patterns of viral latency. EBNA1 is required for maintaining episomal EBV and is the major viral protein expressed in latency pattern 1. This latency pattern may be found in few B cells in healthy individuals, which may also be positive for EBV EBER. In latency pattern III by contrast there is expression of EBV-encoded nuclear antigens (EBNA1-6) and EBV latent membrane proteins LMP1, LMP2A, and LMP2B. In latency pattern II there is expression of EBNA1 and variable expression of other latent proteins but, there is no expression of one of the two EBV transforming proteins (EBNA2 in type IIa latency pattern and LMP1 in type IIb latency). Latency pattern I is associated with BL, pattern II is seen in Hodgkin lymphoma, and most PTLDs are characterized by type III viral latency (993).

In addition to proteins of the latent cycle, lytic cycle products can be detected immunohistochemically in PTLDs (as well as by RT-PCR) (988), by ISH (986), and by Southern blot (989). The immediately early BZLF1 gene was found to be expressed in 55% to 95% (966,970,986) of cases; EA-D in 54%, and EA-R in 52% of cases (986); MA and VCA were found in 33% of cases (966). In one of these studies, 92% of all cases expressed at least one of three proteins (BZLF1, EA-D, EA-R) and 29% all three (986). However, the proportion of cells entering the lytic cycle is very small (<5%) (988). Although this has raised questions about the relevance of EBV replication in the pathogenesis of PTLDs (989), the presence of active EBV infection may explain why some patients benefit from treatment with acyclovir (908,941,986), which inhibits EBV DNA replication. It has been commented that, although the number of cells in replicative cycle at any given time might be small, "the additional viral burden produced during the lifetime of LPD" might be considerable and pathogenetically important (908).

Molecular Genetic Features of PTLD

B-cell PTLDs are heterogenous at the genomic level (243,435, 436,885,900,909,919,945,966,967,990,994–996). In some of these lesions, no rearrangement of the Ig genes is detected (polyclonal lesions). In others, clonal Ig gene rearrangement bands are found, which may be weakly or strongly hybridizing (monoclonal lesions) (435,436). Rarely, multiple rearrangement bands have been observed, which are interpreted as representing multiple minor emerging clones (oligoclonal lesions) (945,967,988,997). In a compilation of cases (885,900,909,919, 945,966,967,988,990,994,996), 76% (132 of 174) of cases were monoclonal, 21% (22 of 105) were polyclonal, and 12% (4 of 34) were oligoclonal. Although there has been poor correlation between histologic type and Ig genomic pattern in some studies, particularly with regard to the polymorphic lesions (435,

900,945,966,988,990), this may be as a result of differences in classification as understanding of these lesions has evolved over time. Cases of PH are polyclonal (245,990), and 80% to 100% of monomorphic lesions (435,900,945,966) or immunoblastic lymphoma/multiple myeloma (990) are monoclonal.

In studies in which multiple lesions in the same patient were evaluated, different clonal bands can be found (up to 24 clones in 24 separate tumor masses (939)), indicating the presence of multiclonal proliferations (243,245,995,996), or the same band is observed, suggesting the metastatic dissemination of one clone from one to another site (245,322,996,998). Similarly, different genomic patterns can be detected in consecutive lesions of the same patient (245,925,942): a germ line pattern followed by a clonal lesion, same clone, or different clones in consecutive lesions. Clinical "recurrence" of PTLD "cannot be assumed to represent pathologic recurrence of the original tumor" (925). There are occasional reports of PTLDs in which T-cell clones were found, in addition to B-cell clones (945,999–1001), with one case showing a predominance of the T-cell clone in an early lesion and of the B-cell clone in a later one (1001).

Clonality patterns of PTLD have also been studied by using the molecular configuration of the fused termini of the EBV genome in its circular (or episomal) form within latently infected cells (434,436,945,977,990,996). This configuration is unique for each episome and is transmitted by the infected cell to its progeny. Southern blot analyses of PTLDs using probes for the fused termini demonstrated, as for the Ig genes, polyclonal (smear), monoclonal, or oligoclonal patterns; the latter were observed in isolation or coexistent with a smear, indicative of the emergence of clones from a polyclonal B-cell proliferation (434,945,990,996). In the same patients, different or identical bands can be found at different sites (434,996). Consecutive lesions in two patients demonstrated the same EBV clonal band but different rearrangement bands of the Ig gene, suggesting that the pattern of EBV termini is a more stable marker of clonality, because "additional rearrangement or somatic hypermutation of Ig genes following primary rearrangement" is possible (996). As is the case for Ig genes, the correlation between histologic type and EBV genomic pattern is variable, with PH mainly polyclonal, and polymorphic lesions showing a smear with one clonal band or definite clonal bands; however, all monomorphic lesions have a monoclonal pattern (990).

Genomic abnormalities have been looked for in PTLDs in an attempt to better understand the pathogenesis of these disorders. In a pivotal study, alterations of one or more oncogenes or tumor suppressor genes (i.e., NRAS gene codon 61 point mutation, TP53 gene mutation, or MYC gene rearrangement) were found only in the immunoblastic lymphoma/multiple myeloma histologic category and therefore were taken as indicating the emergence of a fully neoplastic clone (245). These data are in agreement with the finding of MYC gene rearrangement in monomorphic lymphomas (436) and one of three PT plasmacytomas (994), but in contrast to the lack of TP53 gene mutations in the PTLD of another study (1002). Other important genomic abnormalities of PTLD are those of the BCL6 gene, located on 3q27. Clonal rearrangements of BCL6, which are found in about 40% of diffuse large B-cell lymphoma and 20% of AIDS-related large B-cell lymphomas, are rare (7%) (1003) or lacking (442) in PTLDs. However, BCL6 point mutations are detected in these disorders, by single-strand conformation polymorphism and sequence analysis, in 44% of cases, as frequently as in large cell lymphomas of AIDS patients or the general population (442). In patients with multiple lesions, the same or different mutations of the gene are present (442). Importantly, there is a statistically significant difference in the incidence of BCL6 gene mutations in different histologic types: 0% of PH, 37% of polymorphic B-cell hyperplasia [PBCH], 48% of polymorphic B-cell lymphoma [PBCL], and 87% of monomorphic lymphomas/multiple myeloma (442). The presence of mutations correlates with shorter survival and resistance of the lesions to discontinuation of immunosuppression or surgical excision (442). Whether *BCL6* mutations are a cause in the pathogenesis of PTLD or reflect a genetic instability secondary to malignant transformation is unclear: however, they may be the first genetic abnormality in these processes, because they precede mutations or rearrangements of other genes (442).

Cytogenetic Features

There are only sparse cytogenetic data on the PTLDs and they show no specific karyotypic pattern. From a compilation of the reported findings (884,914,919,926,935,999,1004–1009), the most common changes are two of the classic translocations of BL [t(8;14) and t(8;22)], observed mostly in neoplasms with Burkitt morphology; and abnormalities of chromosome 11 (trisomy 11 or dup11q). These latter changes, as well as monosomy 21 and a break at 1q21, which have been observed in two cases of PTLD (1004,1005), are rare in primary NHLs and have been thought to be characteristic chromosomal alterations of secondary (posttherapy) lymphomas (1005,1006). Less common recurrent abnormalities in PTLDs are trisomy 9; translocations involving chromosome 1, 3, or 14; and monosomy 6. Most often, these changes occur as part of very complex karyotypes. The occurrence of unrelated clones (884,1006) and nonclonal abnormalities (354,1005,1007,1008) has also been reported, supporting the multiclonal origin of these processes, as well as the presence of many normal metaphases associated with abnormal clones (919). Some cases of PTLD have shown a normal karyotype (919,1008,1010).

The correlation of histologic or immunologic types and cytogenetic pattern is poor. In the original studies, all PBCH were cytogenetically normal, but so were 6 of 10 PBCLs (977,995) and, in another study, there were two additional cases of PBCL (919). In two other series, however, clonal abnormalities were detected in 83% of the monomorphic, but in none of the 10 polymorphic (oligoclonal or polyclonal) cases (1008), and in all four immunohistochemically monoclonal cases, but in none of the five polyclonal lesions (1004).

Cytokines

Several studies have addressed the role of cytokines and chemokines in the development of PTLDs (1011,1012). Most of the evidence, both at the level of involved tissues and in the patients' serum, seems to indicate the predominance of a T_H2 over a T_H1 environment (904,925,1013,1014). The former, characterized by high levels of IL-4, IL-6, and IL-10, is geared to provide help to B cells and favors B-cell growth (1015). In particular, IL-6 is a B-cell growth factor; suppresses NK cell cytotoxicity; promotes the EBV lytic cycle, increasing the number of infected cells; and promotes neovascularization, helping local tumor growth (1011,1016). IL-10, produced by EBV-infected cells, promotes proliferation and differentiation of B cells and inhibits T_H1 cytokines (908,1011). The T_H1 environment, characterized by high levels of IFN-γ and IL-2, provides help for cytotoxic T cells and NK cells (1015). In particular, IL-2 is the main autocrine factor for T cells and stimulates growth and cytotoxic activity of NK cells. IFN-α is the first cytokine released by B and NK cells, in response to EBV infection and favors the production of T_H1 cytokines (1012). As Faro states about EBV infection, "EBV induces B cells to secrete cytokines that produce an environment that the virus can thrive in, a T_H2 environment. The immune system's response is for T cells to release IL-2 and IFN-γ and NK cells to release IFN-α and establish a T_H1 environment that will allow CTLs and NK cells to thrive and successfully combat the virus" (1012).

An alteration of this equilibrium, expressed in an imbalance of circulating cytokines that favors B-cell proliferation,

has been demonstrated in many studies of patients with PTLD. These show an increase in serum levels of IL-4 (1013,1017), IL-6 (1018,1019), and IL-10 (908,1018), as well as a decrease of serum levels of IL-2 (1017) and IFN-α (1013). Similar findings have been reported in the tissues involved by PTLDs. In an evaluation by semiquantitave RT-PCR, a pattern of increased mRNA expression of IL-4 and IL-10 and decreased expression of IFN-γ and IL-2 was found in these tissues that was not detected in tissues of transplant recipients without LPDs or normal lymph nodes (1014). That pattern was also present in the normal spleen of one patient with PTLD, indicating a systemic phenomenon, and it disappeared, in two patients, with resolution of their PTLD (1014). In a later study (973) using the same technique, IFN-γ and another lymphokine, IL-18 (known to promote the expression of IFN-γ), were found significantly reduced in the tissues of PTLD compared with lymphoid tissues of patients with IM, suggesting again that T_H1 factors important in an effective response to EBV are missing in PTLDs. In this study, however, the level of expression of IL-10 was actually decreased as compared with tissues of IM.

Clinicopathologic Correlations

The striking heterogeneity of PTLDs at all levels (histologic, immunophenotypic, genomic, EBV expression patterns) presents pathologists with the difficult challenge of determining which pathologic features are relevant in helping oncologists with the treatment of these patients. In reviewing the literature, as well as in dealing with a specific patient's disease, it is important to consider the variations in any pathologic parameters that are common at different sites of involvement; in either situation, the evaluation of the disease based on a single lesion "may lead to failure to assess accurately the pathobiologic nature and clinical aggressiveness of the patient's disease" and helps explain, in part, the lack of correlation between pathologic parameters and outcome in some cases (974). In the original Pittsburgh series, there was no correlation between the histologic subdivision of the lesions into minimally polymorphic, polymorphic, and monomorphic and response to therapy (435). However, later studies have shown a striking correlation between histologic and clinical aggressiveness, with a mortality rate of 0% for PH, 13% for polymorphic lesions, and 67% for monomorphic tumors (440). Molecular clonality of the PTLD may not predict outcome (435,886), but other genomic changes have been shown to have prognostic value. Abnormalities of oncogenes and tumor suppressor genes are poor prognostic factors (436,440,442). The presence of *NRAS* or *TP53* gene mutations or *MYC* gene rearrangement was associated with 67% mortality (440), and *BCL6* gene mutations were correlated with shorter survival and refractoriness to therapy (442).

Among clinical parameters, the extent of disease at presentation (localized vs. disseminated) has long been recognized as an important prognostic factor in PTLD; localization to a single organ is associated with a good prognosis (1020,1021), and mortality is higher for patients with disseminated disease (943,1022). The correlation of time of onset of the PTLD with outcome is a disputed issue. Although in most studies late-onset PTLDs have a worse prognosis than those of early onset (900,910,943,1010,1021,1023), the difference, when evaluated statistically, may not be significant (900,943).

Correlating this wealth and variety of pathologic and clinical features with outcome to provide meaningful categorization to guide oncologists in the management of PTLDs has proven difficult, but a picture is emerging that may begin clarifying some of this complexity (245). Three groups of lesions are recognized (Table 25.6): PHs are polyclonal and contain multiple EBV infection events or only a minor cell population infected by a single form of EBV and lack alterations of oncogenes or tumor suppressor genes (*MYC*, *BCL6*, *NRAS*, *TP53*); polymorphic lesions

Table 25.6	POSTTRANSPLANTATION LPDS: RELATION OF PATHOLOGIC PARAMETERS WITH RESPONSE TO REDUCED IMMUNOSUPPRESSION		
Pathologic Parameter	**Early Lesions (Plasmacytic Hyperplasia or Infectious Mononucleosis-Like Lesion)**	**Polymorphic PTLD**	**Monomorphic PTLD**
Involved Sites	Oropharynx or cervical nodes	Lymph nodes or extranodal	Often extranodal or disseminated
Oncogene or tumor suppressor gene alterations	No	No	Yes
Immunoglobulin genes	Polyclonal	Monoclonal	Monoclonal
Response to reduced immunosuppression	Regress	Variable	Progress

Modified from Knowles DM, Cesarman E, Chadburn A, et al. Correlative morphologic and molecular genetic analysis demonstrates three distinct categories of posttransplantation lymphoproliferative disorders. *Blood* 1995;85:552–565, with permission.

are nearly always monoclonal, usually contain a single form of EBV, and lack alterations of oncogenes or tumor suppressor genes (except for *BCL6* mutations, detected in one-half of them); and monomorphic lymphomas or multiple myeloma, which are monoclonal, contain a single form of EBV, and usually show alterations of oncogenes or tumor suppressor genes (245,990). Clinically, PH corresponds to a localized (stage I) lesion, usually in the tonsils and lymph nodes of younger patients; it is controlled by reduced immunosuppression or surgical excision, without any fatality in this series (440). At the opposite extreme, monomorphic lymphoma/multiple myeloma are disseminated lesions (stages III and IV) that develop in older people, do not respond to RIS and respond poorly to medical treatment, and are associated with a high mortality. The polymorphic lesions remain a somewhat heterogeneous category presenting at different sites and in different stages and have a relatively unpredictable clinical course. In this last group, the detection of the wild or mutant type of *BCL6* gene may be able to separate those patients who respond to RIS or surgical excision from those who require aggressive medical treatment (442,974).

EBV-Negative PTLDs

EBV-negative PTLD are more common in adults and include most cases of T-cell PTLD and a variable percentage (3% to 28%) of B-cell PTLDs (688,1024). EBV-negative PTLD are less likely to respond to decreased immunosuppression, and the etiologic factors are largely unknown. They usually occur at long intervals from transplantation. With the increasing experience in the management of PTLDs and the longer survivals obtained the incidence of EBV-negative lesions appears to be increasing with time (688,1024). Histologically most EBV-negative PTLDs are monomorphic and unlikely to respond to RIS. Different and multiple causes may be at play in different cases; chronic antigenic stimulation and deficient immune surveillance may produce mutations in critical genes (1024), or alternative viral causes can be considered (1025), such as HHV-8 documented in patients with PT-PEL (1026,1027).

KSHV-Related Disease in Posttransplant Patients

Both neoplastic and nonneoplastic KSHV-related disease have been reported in the posttransplantation setting (1028) These include KS, multicentric Castleman disease (MCD), and PEL. MCD presents with lymphadenopathy and inflammatory symptoms, with histologic features typical of MCD previously described, as well as KSHV LANA-positive plasmablasts surrounding germinal centers. Treatment has included antivirals and rituximab, and prognosis is relatively favorable compared with PEL (1028). Other benign complications of KSHV infection in this setting include plasmacytic B-cell hyperplasia, bone marrow failure, and hepatitis.

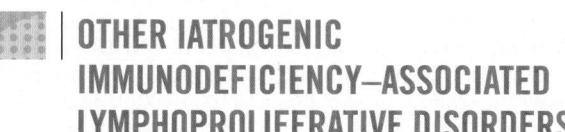

OTHER IATROGENIC IMMUNODEFICIENCY–ASSOCIATED LYMPHOPROLIFERATIVE DISORDERS

Introduction

"Other iatrogenic lymphoproliferative disorders" is a term adopted by the WHO to define lymphoid proliferations or lymphomas that arise in patients treated with immunosuppressive drugs for autoimmune disease or conditions other than in the allograft/autograft transplant setting (946) Similar to PTLDs they include a spectrum ranging form polymorphic proliferations to DLBCL, CHL, and T-/NK-cell lymphomas. Iatrogenic immunodeficiency lymphoid proliferations are becoming more prominent with the increasing use of immunosuppressive drugs for the treatment of patients with autoimmune diseases. The association with EBV is not as strong as with other immunodeficiency LPDs. However, there is a higher incidence of EBV (up to 80%) in patients who develop CHL. The EBV status is important to determine since there is greater likelihood of regression in the EBV-positive cases. The prototype for this type of proliferation is lymphoid proliferation in patients treated with methotrexate for rheumatoid arthritis (RA).

Lymphoproliferative Disorders Arising in Patients Treated with Methotrexate for Rheumatoid Arthritis

RA has a 2- to 20-fold increased risk of lymphoma in the absence of methotrexate, and the interval between diagnosis of RA and development of lymphoma is a mean of 15 years (1029–1035). The mean duration of methotrexate therapy is 3 years (0.5 to 5.5 years). The most prevalent lymphoma in patients not treated with immunosuppressive agents is extranodal marginal zone lymphoma (MALT) of the salivary glands. Marginal zone lymphoma is often associated with Sjögren syndrome and is negative for EBV. Since patients with rheumatoid arthritis and other autoimmune conditions are at increased risk for developing malignant lymphoma it may be difficult to assess the contribution of immunomodulatory therapeutic agents. Regression of the LPD occurs in up to 60% of patients on withdrawal of the immunosuppressive therapy, and this is more likely to occur in cases that are EBV positive.

Risk of Lymphoma in Patients Receiving Anti–Tumor Necrosis Factor α Antagonists

TNFα is a proinflammatory cytokine that is critical in inflammatory synovitis, articular matrix degeneration, and bony erosions in RA. TNFα antagonists include etanercept, adalimumab, and infliximab. Etanercept is a dimeric fusion protein of the extracellular ligand binding portion of the human TNF receptor linked to the Fc portion of the IgG molecule (1036). Infliximab is a chimeric monoclonal antibody that specifically binds to human TNFa and neutralizes its biologic activity (1037), and has been used for treatment of Crohn disease and RA. Adalimumab is the first human anti-TNFa monoclonal antibody that blocks p55 and p75 TNF surface receptors. Since anti-TNF agents are used to treat patients with more aggressive autoimmune disease and those who have failed first-line therapies, these patients are at an increased risk of developing lymphomas. In a study of over 18,000 patients the standardized incidence ratios (SIR) for lymphomas in patients with RA were 2.6 and 3.8 for the use of infliximab and etanercept, respectively, compared with methotrexate alone where the SIR was 1.7 (1038). We performed an analysis of 14 studies with over 5,000 patients who received anti-TNFα and 2000 controls to determine the incidence of LPDs (1036). Although it did not reach statistical significance the results suggest an excess in the number of lymphomas in the treated group with a rate of 1.65 versus 0.36 in the untreated group. In addition to B-cell lymphomas there was one case of T-cell lymphoma and one case of Hodgkin lymphoma. Also, an association between hepatosplenic T-cell lymphoma in young patients (usually males) with Crohn disease treated with infliximab has been reported (1039). Hepatosplenic T-cell lymphoma has also been reported in association with azathioprine therapy suggesting the association of a particular immunosuppressive agent and a tumor type (1040).

Pathogenesis

EBV is frequently found in the synovium of RA patients who may have impaired immunologic control of EBV. RA patients also have abnormally high numbers of circulating EBV⁺ B cells (1041). Latent infection genes of EBV, especially LMP1 and EBNA-2, have transforming activity in infected cells. EBV latency patterns II or III have been described (1042). Infected lymphoid cells can escape from the host cytotoxic T-cell response and studies have shown a reduced ability of T cells to control EBV infection in patients with RA and related rheumatic diseases including Sjögren and Felty syndrome (1043). The frequency of EBV infection is variable, however, with only about 40% of LPD associated with RA treated with methotrexate being positive. The association with EBV is stronger in cases of CHL and polymorphic LPD.

Pathologic Features:

The lymphoid proliferations may be nodal or extranodal in up to 50% of cases, involving multiple extranodal sites including the gastrointestinal tract, skin, lung, liver, spleen, kidney, CNS, and bone marrow among others (1044). The most common type of LPD seen in this setting is DLBCL in about 50% of the cases (Fig. 25.47) (1042), but polymorphic lymphoid proliferations resembling those seen in PTLD are also encountered (Fig. 25.48). Cases of DLBCL may be of GCB or non-GCB type (1042). Other types of lymphoma reported include follicular lymphoma, BT, lymphoplasmacytic lymphoma, and small lymphocytic lymphoma (CLL/SLL). A case of a composite T- and B-cell lymphoma was described in the skin in a patient treated with methotrexate for RA (1045). Although salivary extranodal marginal zone lymphoma (MALT) is not typically associated with methotrexate therapy or EBV, there is a report of EBV⁺ polymorphic LPD and MALT lymphoma coexistent in the thymus of a patient treated with methotrexate for RA (1046).

T-cell lymphomas may occur but are rare and include cases of PTCL NOS and anaplastic large cell lymphoma (1047). They are usually EBV negative. There is an association between

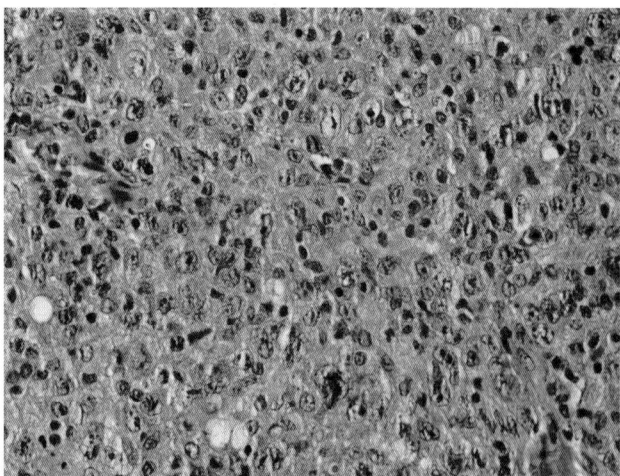

FIGURE 25.47. Diffuse large B-cell lymphoma in a patient treated with methotrexate for rheumatoid disease. (Magnification: 120×.)

hepatosplenic T-cell lymphoma and young patients with Crohn disease receiving infliximab in combination with azathioprine and/or 6-mercaptopurine (1039).

CHL may also be seen in this setting and comprises up to 25% of cases. Even without immunosuppressive therapy, a personal or family history of autoimmune disease is associated with increased risk of CHL (1048). CHL is usually of mixed cellularity type and EBV⁺. Cases that resemble Hodgkin lymphoma because of the presence of Hodgkin or RS-like cells should be considered variants of B-cell LPD. Classical HL cases should have typical histologic and phenotypic features of CHL with absent or weak staining for CD20.

Clinical Course

Abnormal lymphoid proliferations in this setting may respond to withdrawal of the immunosuppressive agent, particularly in those cases that are EBV⁺ (1043). Cases that do not respond may require chemotherapy, particularly cases of DLBCL and CHL. The overall 5-year survival in treated patients with DLBCL was 74% in one recent series (1042). LMO2 protein expression may predict survival in patients with DLBCL treated with anthracycline-based chemotherapy with and without rituximab (1049,1050). Cases of hepatosplenic T-cell lymphoma in patients treated with infliximab have been refractory to therapy.

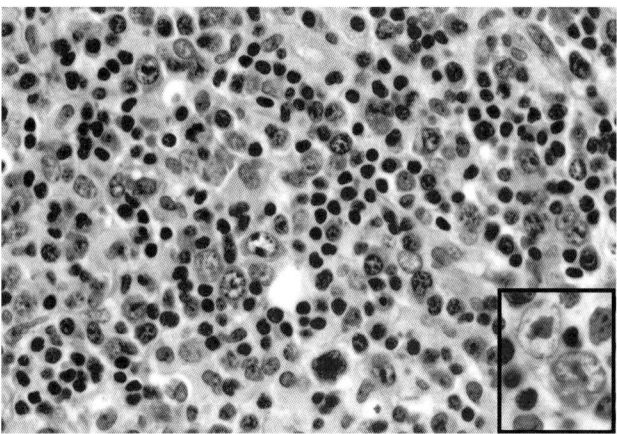

FIGURE 25.48. Polymorphic LPD resembling polymorphous PTLD in a patient treated with methotrexate for rheumatoid arthritis. Note the presence of Reed-Sternberg–like cells (**inset**). (Magnification: 120×.)

LYMPHOPROLIFERATIVE DISEASES AND PRIMARY IMMUNODEFICIENCY

Introduction

Children and adults with a PID carry an increased risk of developing LPDs, which may be associated with EBV. Like AIDS-related lymphomas and PTLDs, these may arise as a result of a lack of immunologic control of EBV-driven B-cell expansions, or in some instances, a consequence of immunologic dysregulation and lymphoid hyperactivation. Over 175 different PIDs are now recognized, making each of these quite rare (1051). Specifically, as the genetic causes have been discovered, several previously described syndromes have been subdivided into individual disease entities. The clinical presentation and immunologic defects are very heterogeneous among PIDs, and with the exception of some very well-defined syndromes, precise diagnosis can be challenging, and relies on the assessment of numbers of circulating lymphoid subpopulations, antibody classes produced, and sometimes molecular studies of affected families. Over the past few decades, identification of the specific genetic alterations in these patients has led to greater understanding of the molecular pathogenesis of PID and LPD.

All PIDs predispose affected individuals to recurrent infections and/or autoimmunity. In addition, children and adults with PID have an overall risk for developing malignancies of 4% to 25% (1052–1054); cancer is the second most common cause of death in children and adults with PID. NHL is the most common malignancy in patients with PID, with an overall eight-fold increased risk over the general population (1055). Lymphomas represent close to 60% of all cancers in patients with PID according to the Immunodeficiency Cancer Registry (1053), with approximately 50% being NHL and close to 8% reported as Hodgkin lymphoma. Leukemias are also increased in the setting of PID. Some subtypes of PID are known to be commonly associated with LPD and lymphoma, but for all there is very little information in the literature regarding the features of the specific lymphoma subtypes and frequency of viral association. The largest studies were done without a complete pathologic analysis using current classification methods, immunohistochemistry, and molecular tools. Thus, much of our understanding comes from large registries (with limited pathologic analysis), and small series or case reports.

According to the Immunodeficiency Cancer Registry data, over 80% of cancers in individuals with PID occur in patients with one of the following syndromes: ataxia talengiectasia (AT, 30%), common variable immunodeficiency (CVID, 24%), Wiskott-Aldrich syndrome (WAS, 16%), severe combined immunodeficiency (SCID, 8%), and selective IgA deficiency (8%) (1054), while the more rare XLP disorder and autoimmune lymphoproliferative syndrome (ALPS) are notable for their strong association with LPDs (1053,1055,1056). These PIDs with well-documented increased risk for hematologic malignancy are reviewed in the following paragraphs and Table 25.7.

Common Variable Immunodeficiency

This is a heterogenous disorder characterized by low IgG and IgA and/or IgM. It is considered the most common clinically significant form of PID, with an incidence of 1 in 25,000 to 50,000. The disease usually manifests itself between 20 and 40 years of age, although it can also present in children, with recurrent bacterial infections, autoimmunity, granulomatous diseases, LPD, or lymphoma (1057).

Several different genetic alterations have been identified in CVID, and genetic alterations previously ascribed to this syndrome have now been classified as separate individual disease entities. CVID currently remains a diagnosis of exclusion within the category of syndromes with deficient humoral immunity. According to the newest classification from the International Union of Immunological Societies Expert Committee for Primary Immunodeficiency (1051), the class of PIDs characterized by predominantly antibody deficiencies include those with (a) severe reduction in all serum Ig isotypes with profound decreases or absent B cells (including deficiencies of BTK, BLNK, ∞ heavy chain, $\lambda5$, Igα and Igβ); (b) severe reduction in at least two serum Ig isotypes with normal or low number of B cells (this class includes CVID, as well as specific genetic alterations causing deficiency of CD19, CD81, CD20, ICOS, TNFRSF13B/TACI, and TNFRSF13B/BAFF receptor); (c) severe reduction in serum IgG and IgA with normal/elevated IgM and normal numbers of B cells (including CD40L, CD40, AID, and UNG deficiencies); (d) isotype or light chain deficiencies with normal numbers of B cells (caused by Ig heavy chain mutations and deletions, and deficiencies of κ light chain, deficiency of isolated IgG subclasses, IgA with IgG subclass deficiency, and selective IgA deficiency); (e) specific antibody deficiency with normal Ig concentrations and normal numbers of B cells; and (f) transient hypogammaglobulinemia of infancy with normal numbers of B cells.

All the studies evaluating the incidence of cancer in CVID were done prior to the most recent classification and subdivision of syndromes with low IgG and IgA and/or IgM into different genetic categories, so the risk for lymphoma and LPD in each distinct entity is unclear. Nevertheless, under the umbrella of what has been classically called CVID, reactive lymphoid hyperplasias are common and far exceed cases of malignant lymphoma. Lymphadenopathy is most common in the cervical, mediastinal, or abdominal regions, and lymphoid infiltrates may extend to involve extranodal sites including the liver, lung, gastrointestinal tract, skin, and spleen. Hypersplenism may also be due to immune thrombocytopenia or autoimmune hemolytic anemia (1058). Lymphoid proliferations may cause architectural distortion due to florid expansions of the B or T zones (Fig. 25.49), and care must be taken to avoid the overdiagnosis of lymphoma in these patients. There is usually polytypic kappa and lambda expression, consistent with polyclonality by Ig gene rearrangement analysis (1059). One study of 30 lesions from 17 patients with CVID found reactive lymphoid hyperplasia in 47%, atypical lymphoid hyperplasia in 27%, and chronic granulomatous inflammation in 20% (1059). EBV was found in 25% of cases with atypical lymphoid hyperplasia. While lymphoma was suspected in three cases, in this study a lymphoma diagnosis was not confirmed with immunohistochemical and molecular analysis, and the authors concluded that the majority of lymphoproliferative lesions in patients with CDIV are benign. However, lymphomas have been reported by others in 1% to 9% of CVID patients, more frequently in women (1060). These occurred most frequently in the fourth to seventh decade of life and were more frequently EBV-negative (1058). Extranodal marginal zone lymphoma, small lymphocytic lymphoma, lymphoplasmacytic lymphoma, and peripheral T-cell lymphoma can occur, but these are rare (1056). Patients with CVID have also been identified with other malignancies, including gastric cancer, as well as a variety of tumors including breast cancer and melanoma (1060,1061).

Together with CVID, selective IgA deficiency falls within the category of PIDs with defective antibody production. This is a common entity, thought to affect approximately 1 in 600 individuals, with very variable clinical impact, many being asymptomatic and unrecognized. While it is not clear if there is a true increase in malignancies in these patients, because of the its high prevalence, cancer occurring in these individuals has been documented (1054). Lymphoid hyperplasia has also been observed in individuals with IgA deficiency, and changes reported relate mostly to infections (1062).

Table 25.7	PRIMARY IMMUNODEFICIENCIES ASSOCIATED WITH LPDs		
Primary Immunodeficiency	**Genes Implicated (Inheritance)**	**Most Common Lymphoproliferative Disorders**	**Approximate Percentage of Lymphoid Tumors**
PIDs Resulting in Antibody Defects			
Antibody deficiencies including common variable immunodeficiency disorders	TNFRSF13B (AR) ICOS (AR) CD19 (AR) CD20 (AR) C81 (AR) TNFRSF13B/TACI (AD or AR or complex) TNFRSF13B/BAFF receptor (AR)	Reactive lymphoid hyperplasia atypical lymphoid hyperplasia chronic granulomatous inflammation NHL	LPD 47% NHL 1%–8%
Combined Immunodeficiencies			
Severe combined immunodeficiency (SCID)	T⁻B⁺ γc (XL) JAK3 (AR) IL7Rα (AR) CD45 (AR) CD3δ/CD3ε/CD3ζ (AR) Coronin-1a (AR) T⁻B⁻ RAG 1/2 (AR) DCLRE1C (Artemis) (AR) DNA-PKcs (AR) AK2 (AR) ADA (AR)	NHL HL Leukemia	NHL 1%–5%
Well-Defined Syndromes with Immunodeficiency			
Wiskott-Aldrich syndrome	WAS (XL)	DLBCL HL Leukemia	NHL 9%
Defects in DNA Repair			
Ataxia Telangiectasia	ATM (AR)	B cell NHL HL T-ALL T-cell lymphomas	Lymphoid malignancy 16%
Disorders with Immune Dysregulation			
X-linked lymphoproliferative disorder	SH2D1A (XLP1) (XL) XIAP (XLP2) (XL)	BL DLBCL	NHL 30%
Autoimmune lymphoproliferative syndrome	FAS (AD; AR cases are rare and severe) FASLG (AD, AR) CASP10 (AD) CASP8 (AD) N-RAS or K-RAS (activating mutations) (Sporadic) FADD (AR)	HL NHL	HL 8% NHL 7%

AR, autosomal recessive; AD, autosomal dominant; XL, X-linked; DLBCL, diffuse large B-cell lymphoma; HL, Hodgkin lymphoma; BL, Burkitt lymphoma; NHL, non-Hodgkin lymphoma; LPD, lymphoproliferative disease.

Severe Combined Immunodeficiency

This is the most severe type of congenital immunodeficiency. It encompasses several genetically distinct syndromes that lead to profound impairment of cellular and humoral immune responses. Patients present early in life with recurrent, persistent, and severe infections that may be bacterial, viral, or fungal. Affected children have failure to thrive, diarrhea, and rashes (1063). These disorders were uniformly fatal until the advent of BMT and for some, such as those with ADA deficiency, gene therapy has been possible and successful.

SCID has been divided into T⁻B⁺ and T⁻B⁻ subtypes (1051). The first class of patients have markedly decreased numbers of T cells but normal or increased B cells, and include those with genetic alterations of γc, *JAK3, IL7Rα, CD45 CD3δ/CD3ε/CD3ζ,* and *CORO1A* (Coronin-1a). In the second group, patients have absent or markedly decreased numbers of circulating B and T cells, and include those with genetic deficiencies of *RAG 1/2,*

DCLRE1C (Artemis), *DNA-PKcs, AK2* (reticular dysgenesis), and *ADA* (adenosine deaminase). Twenty additional syndromes also fall into the category of combined immunodeficiencies; these include Omenn syndrome, CD3γ deficiency, CD8 deficiency, ZAP-70 deficiency and Ca²⁺ channel deficiencies, among other genetic alterations (1051).

The histologic appearance of nonneoplastic lymphoid tissues may depend on the type and severity of SCID, but in general lymph nodes are reduced in number and size. Often only a marginal sinus and reticular framework devoid of lymphocytes is seen. Mucosa-associated lymphoid tissues are atrophic. Lymphoid depletion can also be seen in the spleen, and in T⁺B⁻ SCID, B cells may localize around the central arteriole instead of T cells. Thymic involution with paucity of lymphoid cells has also been described (1062,1064).

Malignancies occur in 1% to 5% of patients with SCID, which are primarily NHL, but Hodgkin lymphoma and leukemia have also been reported (1061). The Immunodeficiency

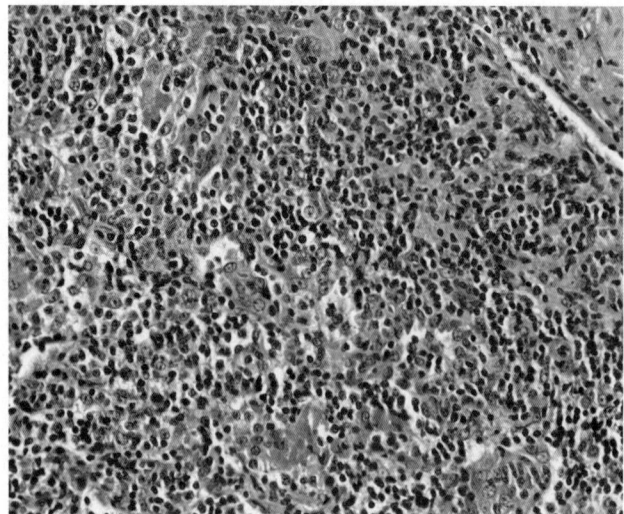

FIGURE 25.49. Atypical lymphoid hyperplasia in a patient with generalized lymphade-nopathy and CVID. The architecture is effaced and there is a polymorphic infiltrate that includes large immunoblasts. This type of lymphoid hyperplasia is far more common than lymphoma that should be diagnosed with caution in patients with CVID. (Hematoxylin and eosin, original magnification: 150×.)

Cancer Registry listed 31 patients with SCID and NHL, 4 with Hodgkin disease, and 5 with leukemia (1053). These occur in very young children (under 2 years of age) and are usually extranodal. Complete pathologic descriptions of lymphomas occurring in patients with SCID are very few in the literature. One report indicated the presence of EBV in two cases of B-cell NHL that presented in a series of four patients with SCID due to an Artemis deficiency (1065). A case series of eight autopsies from patients with ADA deficiency reported one patient with an immunoblastic B-cell lymphoma, but the presence of EBV was not assessed (1064). One case of BT has also been reported in a patient with ADA deficiency (1066). Fatal infectious mono-nucleosis can also occur (1056).

Ataxia Telangiectasia

This is an autosomal recessive disorder of DNA repair. It is caused by mutations in the *ATM* gene, presenting with progres-sive ataxia (because of progressive cerebellar degeneration), oculocutanous telangiectasia, and dysarthria, usually between the age of 1 and 4 years. Children present with recurrent bacte-rial infections, and frequently thymic hypoplasia, growth retar-dation, hypogonadism, and elevated levels of alpha fetoprotein. There is a progressive decrease in the numbers of circulating T cells, and often decreased IgA, IgE, and IgG, with increased IgM monomers (1051).

The ATM protein is a member of the phosphatidyl inositol kinase (PI3K) family, which normally acts as a sensor of dou-ble-stranded DNA breaks. It functions as a regulator of many downstream proteins, including the tumor suppressor proteins p53 and BRCA1, checkpoint kinase CHK2, checkpoint proteins RAD17 and RAD9, and DNA repair protein NBS1. The ATM proteins, as well as the closely related kinase ATR, are thought to be master controllers of cell-cycle checkpoint signaling pathways that are required for cell response to DNA damage and for genome stability. Therefore, cells in these patients are defective in their ability to activate cell-cycle arrest following radiation exposure or other types of DNA damage, explaining their high incidence of cancer.

Approximately 22% of individuals with ataxia telangiectasia (AT) have been reported to develop malignancies (1067,1068). Interestingly, lymphoid leukemias and lymphomas occur, with

a notable paucity of myeloid neoplasms (1069). Patients with null mutations in *ATM* that cause total loss of expression or function of the gene have a lower life expectancy than those with hypomorphic mutations because of earlier onset of can-cer, which are mainly lymphoid malignancies (1068). In fact, cancer is the major risk for mortality in AT patients with null *ATM* mutations.

The ATM protein has been found to play a role in antigen receptor gene rearrangement, and specifically in v(D)J recom-bination. This is consistent with the tumors that occur in individuals with AT. While in the general population the most common early childhood leukemia is B-cell ALL involving a differentiation stage before V(D)J recombination, this type of leukemia is not increased in children with AT. Furthermore, myeloid tumors do not occur. Patients with AT develop mostly lymphoid malignancies at differentiation stages that follow antigen receptor rearrangements, with translocations of the TCR or Ig genes to various oncogenes (1069). Lymphoid malig-nancies in patients with AT include T-ALL, T-cell lymphomas including AITL, ALCL, B-cell DLBCL, HL, and BT (1067,1070). One recent study divided cases into those with no ATM activity and those with residual (partial) ATM function, and determined the tumor types in these two subgroups (1067). Children with absent ATM were more likely to develop cancer before 16 years of age. In this study, the incidence rate for lymphoid tumors was significantly lower in those with some residual ATM kinase activity than in those without. Nonlymphoid tumors can be seen in about 6% of individuals with AT; in those with null *ATM* mutations these are more frequently brain tumors occurring in childhood, and in individuals with some ATM kinase activity, they occur in affected adults, where breast cancer is the most common in affected women.

Wiskott-Aldrich Syndrome

WAS is an X-linked PID caused as a result of mutations in the *WAS* gene (also called WASP, IMD2, and THC). This disease is characterized clinically by immunodeficiency, bleeding ten-dency with microthrombocytopenia, and severe eczema (1071). The immunodeficiency is characterized by progressive decrease of circulating T cells and abnormal responses to anti-CD3, with normal numbers of circulating B cells. There is a decrease in IgM with antibodies to polysaccharides being particularly decreased, often accompanied by increased IgA and IgE. Patients may also have autoimmunity, IgA nephropathy, bacte-rial and viral infections, and lymphoid malignancies. X-linked thrombocytopenia is a mild form of WAS and X-linked neutro-penia is another related disease caused by missense mutations in the GTPases binding domain of the WAS protein (1051).

The function of the WAS family of proteins is transduction of signals from receptors, including the T-cell receptor, and integrins on the cell surface to the actin cytoskeleton. These proteins associate directly or indirectly with the small GTPase Cdc42, known to regulate the formation of actin filaments, and the cytoskeletal organizing complex Arp2/3. The WAS gene product is a cytoplasmic protein, expressed exclusively in hematopoietic cells, explaining the signaling and cytoskel-etal abnormalities responsible for altered immune responses in WAS patients. This protein is also important for the function of regulatory T-cells and in TCR-induced apoptosis, two negative mechanisms of immune regulation that maintain peripheral immune tolerance, thus explaining the simultaneous immuno-deficiency and autoimmunity seen in these patients (1072).

Children with WAS have an increased incidence of malig-nancy, ranging between 12% and 33%, with an approximately 9% incidence of lymphoma (1073,1074). The median age of presentation is 6 years. The most common lymphoma sub-type is DLBCL (75%), followed by Hodgkin lymphoma (4%) and leukemia (10%) (1062). Cases of fatal EBV+ LPDs as well as

EBV⁺ Hodgkin's and NHLs as well as lymphomatoid granulomatosis have been reported (1075–1079). One of the contributing factors for this increased incidence is the observation that
cytotoxic T cells (CTLs) from patients with WAS are deficient
in their ability to kill lymphoma cells, at least *in vitro* using
cytotoxicity assays against the EBV⁺ B-cell lines (Daudi and Raji
(1080)).

X-linked Lymphoproliferative Disorders

Two genetic alterations are known as causes of this syndrome:
Mutations in *SH2D1A* causes XLP type 1, and alterations on
the *XIAP/BIRC4* gene is the cause of XLP type 2. XLP1 disease
is characterized by extreme susceptibility to EBV infection,
including life-threatening fulminant infectious mononucleosis,
which is accompanied by hemophagocytosis and liver failure
(1054). The *SH2D1A* gene encodes a protein containing an SH2
domain, also called SAP for " signaling lymphocyte-activation
molecule (SLAM) associated protein." The binding of SH2D1A/
SAP with SLAM initiates signaling mostly in T and NK cells, so
a deletion in the *SH2D1A* gene leads to defective activation of T
and NK cells impairing their ability to control the proliferation
of EBV-infected B cells. Lately, one of the members of the SLAM
protein family, called 2B4 or CD244, has received particular
attention for its role in signaling that is essential for the effective immune control of chronic viral infections (1081).

XLP2 is caused by mutations in the *XIAP* gene, which encodes
a protein that acts as an inhibitor of apoptosis. While XIAP deficiency has been described in patients with XLP, this syndrome is
associated with a high incidence of hemophagocytic lymphohistiocytosis, but no lymphomas. Therefore, it has been proposed
that this disease be reclassified as X-linked familial hemophagocytic lymphohistiocytosis, rather than XLP (1082).

Histologically, lymphoid proliferations in XLP1 patients that
occur as a response to EBV infection can vary from a reactive
lymphocytic vasculitis to extensive involvement of multiple tissues by lymphocytes, plasma cells, and histiocytes. There may
be extensive tissue destruction of the liver and bone marrow,
which may result from an abnormal CTL response. Hemophagocytic lymphohistiocytosis can be seen in some patients
(1062). Approximately one-third of children with XLP1 develop
lymphomas or other LPDs. The mean age of onset for these
is 6 years. Lymphomas are most frequently extranodal high-
grade B-cell NHL. A common extranodal site of involvement
is the intestine and approximately 75% of lymphomas were
reported to occur in the ileocecal region in one study (1083).
The lymphomas have been histologically classified as BTs
(approximately 40%) or DLBCL (35%), of which close to half
have immunoblastic features (1084). Interestingly, EBV can be
found in some, but not all, of the B-cell lymphomas in patients
with XLP1 (1083).

Autoimmune Lymphoproliferative Syndromes

Several different genetic alterations (Table 25.7) can lead
to defects in apoptosis that fall into the clinical definition of
ALPS, characterized by early-onset lymphoproliferation, autoimmune cytopenias, expansion of double-negative T cells, and
increased incidence of lymphoma (1052). The most common
form of inheritance is autosomal dominant germ line mutations of the *FAS* gene. The FAS protein is a member of the
tumor necrosis factor (TNF) superfamily, specifically involved
in induction of apoptotic (programmed) cell death, and other
genetic alterations causing ALPS also affect apoptosis in lymphoid cells. Apoptosis is an important mechanism for limiting
lymphoid expansions after an infection, so it is thought that
defective apoptosis leads to lymphoproliferative disease.

Chronic lymphoproliferation and lymphadenopathy is seen
in the majority of individuals with ALPS. Lymph nodes are

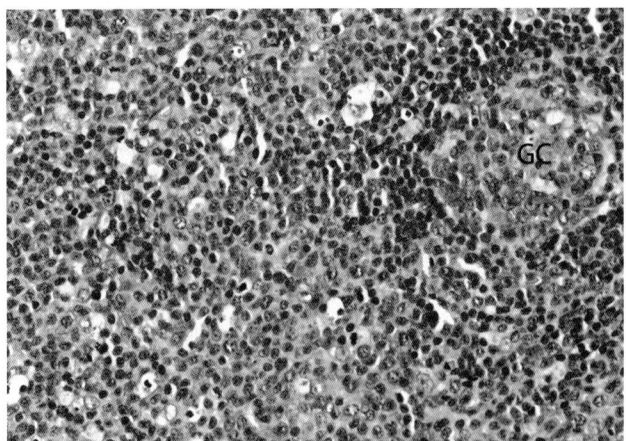

FIGURE 25.50. Lymph node biopsy from a patient with ALPS. There is paracortical expansion by small to intermediate-sized lymphoid cells that consist of T cells double negative for
CD4 and CD8. (GC, Germinal center; hematoxylin and eosin: 120×.)

enlarged and may display follicular hyperplasia, with follicles
ranging from those with hyperplastic germinal center to others
with atrophic features. There may be expansion of the paracortex with small- to medium-sized T cells that are CD3⁺ and
CD45RA⁺ but double negative for CD4 and CD8 (Fig. 25.50).
These cells may have cytologic atypia and should not be confused with lymphoma (1062). Approximately 15% of patients
develop classical Hodgkin or non-Hodgkin B-cell lymphomas (about 55% and 45%, respectively) before the age of 30
(1085–1087). The NHLs appear to be include cases of DLBCL,
as well as individual cases of histiocyte-rich, T-cell–rich large
B-cell lymphoma, BT, follicular lymphoma, EBV-positive T-cell
lymphoma, marginal zone lymphoma, and nodular lymphocyte-predominant Hodgkin lymphoma (1086–1088). In a few
of these cases the presence of EBV was determined, and both
positive and negative cases were found.

Other Primary Immunodeficiencies

Additional primary immunodeficiencies have also been documented to be associated with an increased risk of hematologic malignancies, although these are very rare. These PIDs
include Chediak-Higashi syndrome, cartilage hair hypoplasia,
DiGeorge syndrome, MonoMAC syndrome, hyper IgM syndrome, X-linked agammaglobulinemia and Nijmegen breakage
syndrome (1052).

 ## ACKNOWLEDGMENTS

The authors thank Drs. Amy Chadburn, Yuan Chang, Riccardo
Dalla-Favera, Giorgio Inghirami, Patrick Moore, Roland Nador,
Pier-Giuseppe Pelicci, Bruce Raphael, and Milayna Subar for
their collaborative participation in portions of the studies summarized here.

References

1. Pneumocystis pneumonia—Los Angeles. *MMWR Morb Mortal Wkly Rep* 1981;
   30:250–252.
2. Kaposi's sarcoma and *Pneumocystis* pneumonia among homosexual men—New
   York City and California. *MMWR Morb Mortal Wkly Rep* 1981;30:305–308.
3. Gottlieb MS, Schroff R, Schanker HM, et al. *Pneumocystis carinii* pneumonia and
   mucosal candidiasis in previously healthy homosexual men: evidence of a new
   acquired cellular immunodeficiency. *N Engl J Med* 1981;305:1425–1431.
4. Hymes KB, Cheung T, Greene JB, et al. Kaposi's sarcoma in homosexual men-a
   report of eight cases. *Lancet* 1981;2:598–600.
5. Curran JW, Jaffe HW. AIDS: the early years and CDC's response. *MMWR Surveill
   Summ* 2011;60(Suppl 4):64–69.

6. Killian MS, Levy JA. HIV/AIDS: 30 years of progress and future challenges. *Eur J Immunol* 2011;41:3401–3411.

7. HIV surveillance—United States, 1981–2008. *MMWR Morb Mortal Wkly Rep* 2011;60:689–693.

8. Tebit DM, Arts EJ. Tracking a century of global expansion and evolution of HIV to drive understanding and to combat disease. *Lancet Infect Dis* 11:45–56.

9. Quinn TC, Serwadda D. The future of HIV/AIDS in Africa: a shared responsibility. *Lancet* 377:1133–1134.

10. Barre-Sinoussi F, Chermann JC, Rey F, et al. Isolation of a T-lymphotropic retrovirus from a patient at risk for acquired immune deficiency syndrome (AIDS). *Science* 1983;220:868–871.

11. De Cock KM, Adjorlolo G, Ekpini E, et al. Epidemiology and transmission of HIV-2. Why there is no HIV-2 pandemic. *JAMA* 1993;270:2083–2086.

12. Curran JW, Jaffe HW, Hardy AM, et al. Epidemiology of HIV infection and AIDS in the United States. *Science* 1988;239:610–616.

13. Dalgleish AG, Beverley PC, Clapham PR, et al. The CD4 (T4) antigen is an essential component of the receptor for the AIDS retrovirus. *Nature* 1984;312:763–767.

14. Robey WG, Safai B, Oroszlan S, et al. Characterization of envelope and core structural gene products of HTLV-III with sera from AIDS patients. *Science* 1985;228:593–595.

15. Cohen MS, Shaw GM, McMichael AJ, et al. Acute HIV-1 Infection. *N Engl J Med* 2011;364:1943–1954.

16. Boasso A. HIV and DC: hate at first sight. *Blood* 2010;116:3687–3689.

17. Sabado RL, O'Brien M, Subedi A, et al. Evidence of dysregulation of dendritic cells in primary HIV infection. *Blood* 2010;116:3839–3852.

18. Boasso A, Royle CM, Doumazos S, et al. Overactivation of plasmacytoid dendritic cells inhibits antiviral T-cell responses: a model for HIV immunopathogenesis. *Blood* 2011;118:5152–5162.

19. Hutter G, Nowak D, Mossner M, et al. Long-term control of HIV by CCR5 Delta32/Delta32 stem-cell transplantation. *N Engl J Med* 2009;360:692–698.

20. Allers K, Hutter G, Hofmann J, et al. Evidence for the cure of HIV infection by CCR5Delta32/Delta32 stem cell transplantation. *Blood* 2011;117:2791–2799.

21. Coakley E, Petropoulos CJ, Whitcomb JM. Assessing chemokine co-receptor usage in HIV. *Curr Opin Infect Dis* 2005;18:9–15.

22. Goodenow MM, Collman RG. HIV-1 coreceptor preference is distinct from target cell tropism: a dual-parameter nomenclature to define viral phenotypes. *J Leukoc Biol* 2006;80:965–972.

23. Shattock RJ, Warren M, McCormack S, et al. AIDS. Turning the tide against HIV. *Science* 333:42–43.

24. Lallemant M, Chang S, Cohen R, et al. Pediatric HIV—a neglected disease? *N Engl J Med* 2011;365:581–583.

25. Unexplained immunodeficiency and opportunistic infections in infants—New York, New Jersey, California. *MMWR Morb Mortal Wkly Rep* 1982;31:665–667.

26. Simpson BJ, Andiman WA. Difficulties in assigning human immunodeficiency virus-1 infection and seroreversion status in a cohort of HIV-exposed in children using serologic criteria established by the Centers for Disease Control and Prevention. *Pediatrics* 1994;93:840–842.

27. Sauce D, Larsen M, Fastenackels S, et al. HIV disease progression despite suppression of viral replication is associated with exhaustion of lymphopoiesis. *Blood* 2011;117:5142–5151.

28. Centers for Disease Control (CDC). Persistent, generalized lymphadenopathy among homosexual males. *MMWR Morb Mortal Wkly Rep* 1982;31:249–251.

29. Metroka CE, Cunningham-Rundles S, Pollack MS, et al. Generalized lymphadenopathy in homosexual men. *Ann Intern Med* 1983;99:585–591.

30. Ioachim HL, Lerner CW, Tapper ML. Lymphadenopathies in homosexual men. Relationships with the acquired immune deficiency syndrome. *JAMA* 1983;250:1306–1309.

31. Mathur-Wagh U, Enlow RW, Spigland I, et al. Longitudinal study of persistent generalised lymphadenopathy in homosexual men: relation to acquired immunodeficiency syndrome. *Lancet* 1984;1:1033–1038.

32. Fishbein DB, Kaplan JE, Spira TJ, et al. Unexplained lymphadenopathy in homosexual men. A longitudinal study. *JAMA* 1985;254:930–935.

33. Recommendations: diagnosis of AIDS used by the Centers for Disease Control. *Eur J Cancer Clin Oncol* 1984;20:169–173.

34. Diebold J, Marche C, Audouin J, et al. Lymph node modification in patients with the acquired immunodeficiency syndrome (AIDS) or with AIDS related complex (ARC). A histological, immuno-histopathological and ultrastructural study of 45 cases. *Pathol Res Pract* 1985;180:590–611.

35. Said JW. AIDS-related lymphadenopathies. *Semin Diagn Pathol* 1988;5:365–375.

36. Biberfeld P, Ost A, Porwit A, et al. Histopathology and immunohistology of HTLV-III/LAV related lymphadenopathy and AIDS. *Acta Pathol Microbiol Immunol Scand A* 1987;95:47–65.

37. Pileri S, Rivano MT, Raise E, et al. The value of lymph node biopsy in patients with the acquired immunodeficiency syndrome (AIDS) and the AIDS-related complex (ARC): a morphological and immunohistochemical study of 90 cases. *Histopathology* 1986;10:1107–1129.

38. Chadburn A, Metroka C, Mouradian J. Progressive lymph node histology and its prognostic value in patients with acquired immunodeficiency syndrome and AIDS-related complex. *Hum Pathol* 1989;20:579–587.

39. Fernandez R, Mouradian J, Metroka C, et al. The prognostic value of histopathology in persistent generalized lymphadenopathy in homosexual men. *N Engl J Med* 1983;309:185–186.

40. Chan WC, Brynes RK, Spira TJ, et al. Lymphocyte subsets in lymph nodes of homosexual men with generalized unexplained lymphadenopathy. Correlation with morphology and blood changes. *Arch Pathol Lab Med* 1985;109:133–137.

41. Schuurman HJ, Kluin PM, Gmelig Meijling FH, et al. Lymphocyte status of lymph node and blood in acquired immunodeficiency syndrome (AIDS) and AIDS-related complex disease. *J Pathol* 1985;147:269–280.

42. Gerstoft J, Pallesen G, Mathiesen L, et al. Stages in LAV/HTLV-III lymphadenitis. II. Correlation with clinical and immunological findings. *Scand J Immunol* 1987;25:93–99.

43. Ewing EP Jr, Chandler FW, Spira TJ, et al. Primary lymph node pathology in AIDS and AIDS-related lymphadenopathy. *Arch Pathol Lab Med* 1985;109:977–981.

44. Ioachim HL, Cronin W, Roy M, et al. Persistent lymphadenopathies in people at high risk for HIV infection. Clinicopathologic correlations and long-term follow-up in 79 cases. *Am J Clin Pathol* 1990;93:208–218.

45. Brynes RK, Chan WC, Spira TJ, et al. Value of lymph node biopsy in unexplained lymphadenopathy in homosexual men. *JAMA* 1983;250:1313–1317.

46. Marche C, Kernbaum S, Saimot AG, et al. Histopathological study of lymph nodes in patients with lymphadenopathy or acquired immune deficiency syndrome. *Eur J Clin Microbiol* 1984;3:75–76.

47. Baroni CD, Pezzella F, Stoppacciaro A, et al. Systemic lymphadenopathy (LAS) in intravenous drug abusers. Histology, immunohistochemistry and electron microscopy: pathogenic correlations. *Histopathology* 1985;9:1275–1293.

48. Raphael M, Pouletty P, Cavaille-Coll M, et al. Lymphadenopathy in patients at risk for acquired immunodeficiency syndrome. Histopathology and histochemistry. *Arch Pathol Lab Med* 1985;109:128–132.

49. Meyer PR, Yanagihara ET, Parker JW, et al. A distinctive follicular hyperplasia in the acquired immune deficiency syndrome (AIDS) and the AIDS related complex. A pre-lymphomatous state for B cell lymphomas? *Hematol Oncol* 1984;2:319–347.

50. Burns BF, Wood GS, Dorfman RF. The varied histopathology of lymphadenopathy in the homosexual male. *Am J Surg Pathol* 1985;9:287–297.

51. Pallesen G, Gerstoft J, Mathiesen L. Stages in LAV/HTLV-III lymphadenitis. I. Histological and immunohistological classification. *Scand J Immunol* 1987;25:83–91.

52. Wood GS, Garcia CF, Dorfman RF, et al. The immunohistology of follicle lysis in lymph node biopsies from homosexual men. *Blood* 1985;66:1092–1097.

53. Sohn CC, Sheibani K, Winberg CD, et al. Monocytoid B lymphocytes: their relation to the patterns of the acquired immunodeficiency syndrome (AIDS) and AIDS-related lymphadenopathy. *Hum Pathol* 1985;16:979–985.

54. Butler JJ, Osborne BM. Lymph node enlargement in patients with unsuspected human immunodeficiency virus infections. *Hum Pathol* 1988;19:849–854.

55. Stanley MW, Frizzera G. Diagnostic specificity of histologic features in lymph node biopsy specimens from patients at risk for the acquired immunodeficiency syndrome. *Hum Pathol* 1986;17:1231–1239.

56. O'Murchadha MT, Wolf BC, Neiman RS. The histologic features of hyperplastic lymphadenopathy in AIDS-related complex are nonspecific. *Am J Surg Pathol* 1987;11:94–99.

57. Miettinen M. Histological differential diagnosis between lymph node toxoplasmosis and other benign lymph node hyperplasias. *Histopathology* 1981;5:205–216.

58. Turner RR, Levine AM, Gill PS, et al. Progressive histopathologic abnormalities in the persistent generalized lymphadenopathy syndrome. *Am J Surg Pathol* 1987;11:625–632.

59. Frizzera G, Moran EM, Rappaport H. Angio-immunoblastic lymphadenopathy. Diagnosis and clinical course. *Am J Med* 1975;59:803–818.

60. Frizzera G, Banks PM, Massarelli G, et al. A systemic lymphoproliferative disorder with morphologic features of Castleman's disease. Pathological findings in 15 patients. *Am J Surg Pathol* 1983;7:211–231.

61. Weisenburger DD, Nathwani BN, Winberg CD, et al. Multicentric angiofollicular lymph node hyperplasia: a clinicopathologic study of 16 cases. *Hum Pathol* 1985;16:162–172.

62. Tirelli U, Vaccher E, Carbone A, et al. Persistent generalized lymphadenopathy: clinical characteristics of a lymphadenopathy syndrome in intravenous drug abusers. *AIDS Res* 1986;2:227–230.

63. Finkbeiner WE, Egbert BM, Groundwater JR, et al. Kaposi's sarcoma in young homosexual men: a histopathologic study with particular reference to lymph node involvement. *Arch Pathol Lab Med* 1982;106:261–264.

64. Perlow LS, Taff ML, Orsini JM, et al. Kaposi's sarcoma in a young homosexual man. Association with angiofollicular lymphoid hyperplasia and a malignant lymphoproliferative disorder. *Arch Pathol Lab Med* 1983;107:510–513.

65. Blumenfeld W, Beckstead JH. Angioimmunoblastic lymphadenopathy with dysproteinemia in homosexual men with acquired immune deficiency syndrome. *Arch Pathol Lab Med* 1983;107:567–569.

66. Harris NL. Hypervascular follicular hyperplasia and Kaposi's sarcoma in patients at risk for AIDS. *N Engl J Med* 1984;310:462–463.

67. Lachant NA, Sun NC, Leong LA, et al. Multicentric angiofollicular lymph node hyperplasia (Castleman's disease) followed by Kaposi's sarcoma in two homosexual males with the acquired immunodeficiency syndrome (AIDS). *Am J Clin Pathol* 1985;83:27–33.

68. Lowenthal DA, Filippa DA, Richardson ME, et al. Generalized lymphadenopathy with morphologic features of Castleman's disease in an HIV-positive man. *Cancer* 1987;60:2454–2458.

69. Soulier J, Grollet L, Oksenhendler E, et al. Kaposi's sarcoma-associated herpesvirus-like DNA sequences in multicentric Castleman's disease. *Blood* 1995;86:1276–1280.

70. Chadburn A, Cesarman E, Nador RG, et al. Kaposi's sarcoma-associated herpesvirus sequences in benign lymphoid proliferations not associated with human immunodeficiency virus. *Cancer* 1997;80:788–797.

71. Oksenhendler E, Duarte M, Soulier J, et al. Multicentric Castleman's disease in HIV infection: a clinical and pathological study of 20 patients. *AIDS* 1996;10:61–67.

72. Ambros RA, Lee EY, Sharer LR, et al. The acquired immunodeficiency syndrome in intravenous drug abusers and patients with a sexual risk: clinical and post-mortem comparisons. *Hum Pathol* 1987;18:1109–1114.

73. Gallo RC, Salahuddin SZ, Popovic M, et al. Frequent detection and isolation of cytopathic retroviruses (HTLV-III) from patients with AIDS and at risk for AIDS. *Science* 1984;224:500–503.

74. Gelderblom HR. Assembly and morphology of HIV: potential effect of structure on viral function. *AIDS* 1991;5:617–637.

75. Gelderblom HR, Hausmann EH, Ozel M, et al. Fine structure of human immunodeficiency virus (HIV) and immunolocalization of structural proteins. *Virology* 1987;156:171–176.

76. Ozel M, Pauli G, Gelderblom HR. The organization of the envelope projections on the surface of HIV. *Arch Virol* 1988;100:255–266.

77. McKeating JA, McKnight A, Moore JP. Differential loss of envelope glycoprotein gp120 from virions of human immunodeficiency virus type 1 isolates: effects on infectivity and neutralization. *J Virol* 1991;65:852–860.

78. Cohen OJ, Pantaleo G, Schwartzentruber DJ, et al. Pathogenic insights from studies of lymphoid tissue from HIV-infected individuals. *J Acquir Immune Defic Syndr Hum Retrovirol* 1995;10(Suppl 1):S6–S14.

79. Pekovic DD, Gornitsky M, Ajdukovic D, et al. Pathogenicity of HIV in lymphatic organs of patients with AIDS. *J Pathol* 1987;152:31–35.

80. Tenner-Racz K. Human immunodeficiency virus associated changes in germinal centers of lymph nodes and relevance to impaired B-cell function. *Lymphology* 1988;21:36–43.

81. Embretson J, Zupancic M, Ribas JL, et al. Massive covert infection of helper T lymphocytes and macrophages by HIV during the incubation period of AIDS. *Nature* 1993;362:359–362.

82. Armstrong JA, Horne R. Follicular dendritic cells and virus-like particles in AIDS-related lymphadenopathy. *Lancet* 1984;2:370–372.
83. Tenner-Racz K, Racz P, Dietrich M, et al. Altered follicular dendritic cells and virus-like particles in AIDS and AIDS-related lymphadenopathy. *Lancet* 1985;1:105–106.
84. Le Tourneau A, Audouin J, Diebold J, et al. LAV-like viral particles in lymph node germinal centers in patients with the persistent lymphadenopathy syndrome and the acquired immunodeficiency syndrome-related complex: an ultrastructural study of 30 cases. *Hum Pathol* 1986;17:1047–1053.
85. Cameron PU, Dawkins RL, Armstrong JA, et al. Western blot profiles, lymph node ultrastructure and viral expression in HIV-infected patients: a correlative study. *Clin Exp Immunol* 1987;68:465–478.
86. Tacchetti C, Favre A, Moresco L, et al. HIV is trapped and masked in the cytoplasm of lymph node follicular dendritic cells. *Am J Pathol* 1997;150:533–542.
87. Parmentier HK, van Wichen D, Sie-Go DM, et al. HIV-1 infection and virus production in follicular dendritic cells in lymph nodes. A case report, with analysis of isolated follicular dendritic cells. *Am J Pathol* 1990;137:247–251.
88. Pantaleo G, Graziosi C, Demarest JF, et al. HIV infection is active and progressive in lymphoid tissue during the clinically latent stage of disease. *Nature* 1993;362:355–358.
89. Heath SL, Tew JG, Szakal AK, et al. Follicular dendritic cells and human immunodeficiency virus infectivity. *Nature* 1995;377:740–744.
90. Rademakers LH, Schuurman HJ, de Frankrijker JF, et al. Cellular composition of germinal centers in lymph nodes after HIV-1 infection: evidence for an inadequate support of germinal center B lymphocytes by follicular dendritic cells. *Clin Immunol Immunopathol* 1992;62:148–159.
91. Schmitz J, van Lunzen J, Tenner-Racz K, et al. Follicular dendritic cells (FDC) are not productively infected with HIV-1 in vivo. *Adv Exp Med Biol* 1994;355:165–168.
92. Schmitz J, van Lunzen J, Tenner-Racz K, et al. Follicular dendritic cells retain HIV-1 particles on their plasma membrane, but are not productively infected in asymptomatic patients with follicular hyperplasia. *J Immunol* 1994;153:1352–1359.
93. Rademakers LH, Schuurman HJ, de Frankrijker JF. Ultrastructural analysis of human lymph node follicles after HIV-1 infection. *Adv Exp Med Biol* 1993;329:359–363.
94. Schuurman HJ, Joling P, van Wichen DF, et al. Follicular dendritic cells and infection by human immunodeficiency virus type 1—a crucial target cell and virus reservoir. *Curr Top Microbiol Immunol* 1995;201:161–188.
95. Laman JD, van den Eertwegh AJ. Cytotoxic potential of CD8+ T-cells in lymphoid follicles during HIV-1 infection. *AIDS* 1992;6:333–335.
96. Sunila I, Vaccarezza M, Pantaleo G, et al. Activated cytotoxic lymphocytes in lymph nodes from human immunodeficiency virus (HIV) 1-infected patients: a light and electronmicroscopic study. *Histopathology* 1997;30:31–40.
97. Carbonari M, Pesce AM, Cibati M, et al. Death of bystander cells by a novel pathway involving early mitochondrial damage in human immunodeficiency virus-related lymphadenopathy. *Blood* 1997;90:209–216.
98. Baroni CD, Pezzella F, Pezzella M, et al. Expression of HIV in lymph node cells of LAS patients. Immunohistology, in situ hybridization, and identification of target cells. *Am J Pathol* 1988;133:498–506.
99. Orenstein JM, Fox C, Wahl SM. Macrophages as a source of HIV during opportunistic infections. *Science* 1997;276:1857–1861.
100. Sidhu GS, Stahl RE, el-Sadr W, et al. The acquired immunodeficiency syndrome: an ultrastructural study. *Hum Pathol* 1985;16:377–386.
101. Helder AW, Feltkamp-Vroom TM. Tubuloreticular structures and antinuclear antibodies in autoimmune and non-autoimmune diseases. *J Pathol* 1976;119:49–56.
102. Jackson D, Tabor E, Gerety RJ. Acute non-A, non-B hepatitis: specific ultrastructural alterations in endoplasmic reticulum of infected hepatocytes. *Lancet* 1979;1:1249–1250.
103. Grimley PM, Davis GL, Kang YH, et al. Tubuloreticular inclusions in peripheral blood mononuclear cells related to systemic therapy with alpha-interferon. *Lab Invest* 1985;52:638–649.
104. Luu JY, Bockus D, Remington F, et al. Tubuloreticular structures and cylindrical confronting cisternae: a review. *Hum Pathol* 1989;20:617–627.
105. Wood GS, Burns BF, Dorfman RF, et al. The immunohistology of non-T cells in the acquired immunodeficiency syndrome. *Am J Pathol* 1985;120:371–379.
106. Wood GS, Burns BF, Dorfman RF, et al. In situ quantitation of lymph node helper, suppressor, and cytotoxic T cell subsets in AIDS. *Blood* 1986;67:596–603.
107. Parmentier HK, Van Wichen DF, Peters PJ, et al. No histological evidence for cytotoxic T cells in destruction of lymph-node follicle centres after HIV infection? *AIDS* 1991;5:778–780.
108. Koopman G, Wever PC, Ramkema MD, et al. Expression of granzyme B by cytotoxic T lymphocytes in the lymph nodes of HIV-infected patients. *AIDS Res Hum Retroviruses* 1997;13:227–233.
109. Carbone A, Manconi R, Poletti A, et al. Lymph node immunohistology in intravenous drug abusers with persistent generalized lymphadenopathy. *Arch Pathol Lab Med* 1985;109:1007–1012.
110. Devergne O, Peuchmaur M, Crevon MC, et al. Activation of cytotoxic cells in hyperplastic lymph nodes from HIV-infected patients. *AIDS* 1991;5:1071–1079.
111. Baroni CD, Vitolo D, Uccini S. Immunohistopathogenesis of persistent generalized lymphadenopathy in HIV-positive patients. *Ric Clin Lab* 1990;20:1–10.
112. Said JW, Shintaku IP, Teitelbaum A, et al. Distribution of T-cell phenotypic subsets and surface immunoglobulin-bearing lymphocytes in lymph nodes from male homosexuals with persistent generalized adenopathy: an immunohistochemical and ultrastructural study. *Hum Pathol* 1984;15:785–790.
113. Tenner-Racz K, Racz P, Thome C, et al. Cytotoxic effector cell granules recognized by the monoclonal antibody TIA-1 are present in CD8+ lymphocytes in lymph nodes of human immunodeficiency virus-1-infected patients. *Am J Pathol* 1993;142:1750–1758.
114. Choremi-Papadopoulou H, Viglis V, Gargalianos P, et al. Downregulation of CD28 surface antigen on CD4+ and CD8+ T lymphocytes during HIV-1 infection. *J Acquir Immune Defic Syndr* 1994;7:245–253.
115. Borthwick NJ, Bofill M, Gombert WM, et al. Lymphocyte activation in HIV-1 infection. II. Functional defects of CD28 - T cells. *AIDS* 1994;8:431–441.
116. Tenner-Racz K, Racz P. Follicular dendritic cells initiate and maintain infection of the germinal centers by human immunodeficiency virus. *Curr Top Microbiol Immunol* 1995;201:141–159.
117. Piris MA, Rivas C, Morente M, et al. Persistent and generalized lymphadenopathy: a lesion of follicular dendritic cells? An immunohistologic and ultrastructural study. *Am J Clin Pathol* 1987;87:716–724.
118. Mori S, Ezaki Y, Mori M, et al. Deterioration of B cell proliferation correlates with dendritic reticulum cell destruction in germinal centers of an AIDS patient. Case study. *Acta Pathol Jpn* 1988;38:1205–1214.
119. Muller H, Falk S, Schmidts HL, et al. In situ immunophenotyping of lymphocytes/macrophages: grading of lymphadenopathy, staging and pathophysiology of HIV infection. *Res Virol* 1990;141:171–184.
120. Porwit A, Bottiger B, Pallesen G, et al. Follicular involution in HIV lymphadenopathy. A morphometric study. *APMIS* 1989;97:153–165.
121. Tenner-Racz K, von Stemm AM, Guhlk B, et al. Are follicular dendritic cells, macrophages and interdigitating cells of the lymphoid tissue productively infected by HIV? *Res Virol* 1994;145:177–182.
122. Tenner-Racz K, Racz P, Bofill M, et al. HTLV-III/LAV viral antigens in lymph nodes of homosexual men with persistent generalized lymphadenopathy and AIDS. *Am J Pathol* 1986;123:9–15.
123. Schuurman HJ, Krone WJ, Broekhuizen R, et al. Expression of RNA and antigens of human immunodeficiency virus type-1 (HIV-1) in lymph nodes from HIV-1 infected individuals. *Am J Pathol* 1988;133:516–524.
124. Schriever F, Freedman AS, Freeman G, et al. Isolated human follicular dendritic cells display a unique antigenic phenotype. *J Exp Med* 1989;169:2043–2058.
125. Wood GS, Turner RR, Shiurba RA, et al. Human dendritic cells and macrophages. In situ immunophenotypic definition of subsets that exhibit specific morphologic and microenvironmental characteristics. *Am J Pathol* 1985;119:73–82.
126. Parravicini CL, Vago L, Costanzi GC, et al. Follicle lysis in lymph nodes from homosexual men. *Blood* 1986;68:595–597.
127. Stahmer I, Zimmer JP, Ernst M, et al. Isolation of normal human follicular dendritic cells and CD4-independent in vitro infection by human immunodeficiency virus (HIV-1). *Eur J Immunol* 1991;21:1873–1878.
128. Spiegel H, Herbst H, Niedobitek G, et al. Follicular dendritic cells are a major reservoir for human immunodeficiency virus type 1 in lymphoid tissues facilitating infection of CD4+ T-helper cells. *Am J Pathol* 1992;140:15–22.
129. Grouard G, Durand I, Filgueira L, et al. Dendritic cells capable of stimulating T cells in germinal centres. *Nature* 1996;384:364–367.
130. Laman JD, Claassen E, Van Rooijen N, et al. Immune complexes on follicular dendritic cells as a target for cytolytic cells in AIDS. *AIDS* 1989;3:543–544.
131. Golding H, Robey FA, Gates FT III, et al. Identification of homologous regions in human immunodeficiency virus I gp41 and human MHC class II beta 1 domain. I. Monoclonal antibodies against the gp41-derived peptide and patients' sera react with native HLA class II antigens, suggesting a role for autoimmunity in the pathogenesis of acquired immune deficiency syndrome. *J Exp Med* 1988;167:914–923.
132. Young JA. HIV and HLA similarity. *Nature* 1988;333:215.
133. Dave B, Kaplan J, Gautam S, et al. Plasmacytoid dendritic cells in lymph nodes of patients with human immunodeficiency virus. *Appl Immunohistochem Mol Morphol* 2012;20:566–572.
134. Grouard G, Clark EA. Role of dendritic and follicular dendritic cells in HIV infection and pathogenesis. *Curr Opin Immunol* 1997;9:563–567.
135. Gerdes J, Flad HD. Follicular dendritic cells and their role in HIV infection. *Immunol Today* 1992;13:81–83.
136. Turner RR, Meyer PR, Taylor CR, et al. Immunohistology of persistent generalized lymphadenopathy. Evidence for progressive lymph node abnormalities in some patients. *Am J Clin Pathol* 1987;88:10–19.
137. Itescu S, Brancato LJ, Winchester R. A sicca syndrome in HIV infection: association with HLA-DR5 and CD8 lymphocytosis. *Lancet* 1989;2:466–468.
138. Lash RH, Tubbs RR, Calabrese LH. Paracortical immunoregulatory subpopulations in lymph nodes from homosexual men with persistent generalized lymphadenopathy. *Hum Pathol* 1988;19:419–422.
139. Nicholson JK, McDougal JS, Spira TJ, et al. Immunoregulatory subsets of the T helper and T suppressor cell populations in homosexual men with chronic unexplained lymphadenopathy. *J Clin Invest* 1984;73:191–201.
140. Burke AP, Anderson D, Mannan P, et al. Systemic lymphadenopathic histology in human immunodeficiency virus-1-seropositive drug addicts without apparent acquired immunodeficiency syndrome. *Hum Pathol* 1994;25:248–256.
141. Frankel SS, Wenig BM, Burke AP, et al. Replication of HIV-1 in dendritic cell-derived syncytia at the mucosal surface of the adenoid. *Science* 1996;272:115–117.
142. Rosok B, Brinchmann JE, Voltersvik P, et al. Correlates of latent and productive HIV type-1 infection in tonsillar CD4(+) T cells. *Proc Natl Acad Sci U S A* 1997;94:9332–9336.
143. Wood GS, Burns BF, Dorfman RF, et al. Fatal post-transfusion acquired immunodeficiency in a heterosexual man: quantitative lymph node immunopathology. *Hum Pathol* 1988;19:236–238.
144. Turner RR, Boone DC, Levine AM, et al. Flow cytometric lymphocyte immunophenotyping in homosexual men with the persistent generalized lymphadenopathy syndrome: a longitudinal study of lymph nodes and blood. *Diagn Clin Immunol* 1987;5:194–200.
145. Fox CH, Tenner-Racz K, Racz P, et al. Lymphoid germinal centers are reservoirs of human immunodeficiency virus type 1 RNA. *J Infect Dis* 1991;164:1051–1057.
146. Walewska-Zielecka B, Nowoslawski A. HIV lymphadenopathy—a histopathological and immunomorphological study of 65 cases. *Pol J Pathol* 1995;46:211–217.
147. Nuovo GJ, Becker J, Burk MW, et al. In situ detection of PCR-amplified HIV-1 nucleic acids in lymph nodes and peripheral blood in patients with asymptomatic HIV-1 infection and advanced-stage AIDS. *J Acquir Immune Defic Syndr* 1994;7:916–923.
148. Anderson RM, May RM. Epidemiological parameters of HIV transmission. *Nature* 1988;333:514–519.
149. Sepkowitz KA. Effect of HAART on natural history of AIDS-related opportunistic disorders. *Lancet* 1998;351:228–230.
150. Kahn JO, Walker BD. Acute human immunodeficiency virus type 1 infection. *N Engl J Med* 1998;339:33–39.
151. Saag MS. Evolving understanding of the immunopathogenesis of HIV. *AIDS Res Hum Retroviruses* 1994;10:887–892.
152. Donaldson YK, Bell JE, Ironside JW, et al. Redistribution of HIV outside the lymphoid system with onset of AIDS. *Lancet* 1994;343:383–385.
153. Mellors JW, Kingsley LA, Rinaldo CR, Jr, et al. Quantitation of HIV-1 RNA in plasma predicts outcome after seroconversion. *Ann Intern Med* 1995;122:573–579.
154. Schechter MT, Craib KJ, Le TN, et al. Susceptibility to AIDS progression appears early in HIV infection. *AIDS* 1990;4:185–190.

155. Lafeuillade A, Tamalet C, Pellegrino P, et al. High viral burden in lymph nodes during early stages of HIV-1 infection. *AIDS* 1993;7:1527–1528.
156. Mellors JW, Rinaldo CR Jr, Gupta P, et al. Prognosis in HIV-1 infection predicted by the quantity of virus in plasma. *Science* 1996;272:1167–1170.
157. Fischl MA, Richman DD, Grieco MH, et al. The efficacy of azidothymidine (AZT) in the treatment of patients with AIDS and AIDS-related complex. A double-blind, placebo-controlled trial. *N Engl J Med* 1987;317:185–191.
158. Jacobson MA, Bacchetti P, Kolokathis A, et al. Surrogate markers for survival in patients with AIDS and AIDS related complex treated with zidovudine. *BMJ* 1991;302:73–78.
159. Paiva DD, Morais JC, Pilotto J, et al. Spectrum of morphologic changes of lymph nodes in HIV infection. *Mem Inst Oswaldo Cruz* 1996;91:371–379.
160. Kaplan JE, Spira TJ, Fishbein DB, et al. Lymphadenopathy syndrome in homosexual men. Evidence for continuing risk of developing the acquired immunodeficiency syndrome. *JAMA* 1987;257:335–337.
161. Kaplan JE, Spira TJ, Fishbein DB, et al. A six-year follow-up of HIV-infected homosexual men with lymphadenopathy. Evidence for an increased risk for developing AIDS after the third year of lymphadenopathy. *JAMA* 1988;260:2694–2697.
162. Diebold J, Audouin J, Le Tourneau A. Lymphoid tissue changes in HIV-infected patients. *Lymphology* 1988;21:22–27.
163. Formenti SC, Turner RR, de Martini RM, et al. Immunophenotypic analysis of peripheral blood leukocytes at different stages of HIV infection. An analysis of asymptomatic, ARC, and AIDS populations. *Am J Clin Pathol* 1989;92:300–307.
164. Cavert W, Notermans DW, Staskus K, et al. Kinetics of response in lymphoid tissues to antiretroviral therapy of HIV-1 infection. *Science* 1997;276:960–964.
165. Lafeuillade A, Chouraqui M, Hittinger G, et al. Lymph node expansion of CD4+ lymphocytes during antiretroviral therapy. *J Infect Dis* 1997;176:1378–1382.
166. Jacobson MA, Zegans M, Pavan PR, et al. Cytomegalovirus retinitis after initiation of highly active antiretroviral therapy. *Lancet* 1997;349:1443–1445.
167. Tenner-Racz K, Stellbrink HJ, van Lunzen J, et al. The unenlarged lymph nodes of HIV-1-infected, asymptomatic patients with high CD4 T cell counts are sites for virus replication and CD4 T cell proliferation. The impact of highly active antiretroviral therapy. *J Exp Med* 1998;187:949–959.
168. Race EM, Adelson-Mitty J, Kriegel GR, et al. Focal mycobacterial lymphadenitis following initiation of protease-inhibitor therapy in patients with advanced HIV-1 disease. *Lancet* 1998;351:252–255.
169. Smith FB, Rajdeo H, Panesar N, et al. Benign lymphoepithelial lesion of the parotid gland in intravenous drug users. *Arch Pathol Lab Med* 1988;112:742–745.
170. Ryan JR, Ioachim HL, Marmer J, et al. Acquired immune deficiency syndrome—related lymphadenopathies presenting in the salivary gland lymph nodes. *Arch Otolaryngol* 1985;111:554–546.
171. Ulirsch RC, Jaffe ES. Sjogren's syndrome-like illness associated with the acquired immunodeficiency syndrome-related complex. *Hum Pathol* 1987;18:1063–1068.
172. Finfer MD, Schinella RA, Rothstein SG, et al. Cystic parotid lesions in patients at risk for the acquired immunodeficiency syndrome. *Arch Otolaryngol Head Neck Surg* 1988;114:1290–1294.
173. Kornstein MJ, Parker GA, Mills AS. Immunohistology of the benign lymphoepithelial lesion in AIDS-related lymphadenopathy: a case report. *Hum Pathol* 1988;19:1359–1361.
174. Tunkel DE, Loury MC, Fox CH, et al. Bilateral parotid enlargement in HIV-seropositive patients. *Laryngoscope* 1989;99:590–595.
175. Terry JH, Loree TR, Thomas MD, et al. Major salivary gland lymphoepithelial lesions and the acquired immunodeficiency syndrome. *Am J Surg* 1991;162:324–329.
176. Ioachim HL, Ryan JR, Blaugrund SM. Salivary gland lymph nodes. The site of lymphadenopathies and lymphomas associated with human immunodeficiency virus infection. *Arch Pathol Lab Med* 1988;112:1224–1228.
177. Sperling NM, Lin PT, Lucente FE. Cystic parotid masses in HIV infection. *Head Neck* 1990;12:337–341.
178. Som PM, Brandwein MS, Silvers A. Nodal inclusion cysts of the parotid gland and parapharyngeal space: a discussion of lymphoepithelial, AIDS-related parotid, and branchial cysts, cystic Warthin's tumors, and cysts in Sjogren's syndrome. *Laryngoscope* 1995;105:1122–1128.
179. DiGiuseppe JA, Wu TC, Corio RL. Analysis of Epstein-Barr virus-encoded small RNA 1 expression in benign lymphoepithelial salivary gland lesions. *Mod Pathol* 1994;7:555–559.
180. Labouyrie E, Merlio JP, Beylot-Barry M, et al. Human immunodeficiency virus type 1 replication within cystic lymphoepithelial lesion of the salivary gland. *Am J Clin Pathol* 1993;100:41–46.
181. Cleary KR, Batsakis JG. Lymphoepithelial cysts of the parotid region: a "new face" on an old lesion. *Ann Otol Rhinol Laryngol* 1990;99:162–164.
182. Poletti A, Manconi R, Volpe R, et al. Study of AIDS-related lymphadenopathy in the intraparotid and perisubmaxillary gland lymph nodes. *J Oral Pathol* 1988;17:164–167.
183. Fox RI, Howell FV, Bone RC, et al. Primary Sjogren syndrome: clinical and immunopathologic features. *Semin Arthritis Rheum* 1984;14:77–105.
184. Shaha AR, DiMaio T, Webber C, et al. Benign lymphoepithelial lesions of the parotid. *Am J Surg* 1993;166:403–406.
185. de Vries EJ, Kapadia SB, Johnson JT, et al. Salivary gland lymphoproliferative disease in acquired immune disease. *Otolaryngol Head Neck Surg* 1988;99:59–62.
186. Gordon JJ, Golbus J, Kurtides ES. Chronic lymphadenopathy and Sjogren's syndrome in a homosexual man. *N Engl J Med* 1984;311:1441–1442.
187. Couderc LJ, D'Agay MF, Danon F, et al. Sicca complex and infection with human immunodeficiency virus. *Arch Intern Med* 1987;147:898–901.
188. Itescu S, Brancato LJ, Buxbaum J, et al. A diffuse infiltrative CD8 lymphocytosis syndrome in human immunodeficiency virus (HIV) infection: a host immune response associated with HLA-DR5. *Ann Intern Med* 1990;112:3–10.
189. Holliday RA, Cohen WA, Schinella RA, et al. Benign lymphoepithelial parotid cysts and hyperplastic cervical adenopathy in AIDS-risk patients: a new CT appearance. *Radiology*, 1988;168:439–441.
190. Shugar JM, Som PM, Jacobson AL, et al. Multicentric parotid cysts and cervical adenopathy in AIDS patients. A newly recognized entity: CT and MR manifestations. *Laryngoscope* 1988;98:772–775.
191. Niedt GW, Schinella RA. Acquired immunodeficiency syndrome. Clinicopathologic study of 56 autopsies. *Arch Pathol Lab Med* 1985;109:727–734.
192. Welch K, Finkbeiner W, Alpers CE, et al. Autopsy findings in the acquired immune deficiency syndrome. *JAMA* 1984;252:1152–1159.
193. Amberson JB, DiCarlo EF, Metroka CE, et al. Diagnostic pathology in the acquired immunodeficiency syndrome. Surgical pathology and cytology experience with 67 patients. *Arch Pathol Lab Med* 1985;109:345–351.
194. Levine AM, Meyer PR, Gill PS, et al. Results of initial lymph node biopsy in homosexual men with generalized lymphadenopathy. *J Clin Oncol* 1986;4:165–169.
195. Gorin FA, Bale JF Jr, Halks-Miller M, et al. Kaposi's sarcoma metastatic to the CNS. *Arch Neurol* 1985;42:162–165.
196. Dworkin MS, Fratkin MD. *Mycobacterium avium* complex lymph node abscess after use of highly active antiretroviral therapy in a patient with AIDS. *Arch Intern Med* 1998;158:1828.
197. Ball SC, Chadburn A. HAART-associated lymphadenopathy. *AIDS Read* 1999;9:11–12, 17.
198. Stoler MH, Bonfiglio TA, Steigbigel RT, et al. An atypical subcutaneous infection associated with acquired immune deficiency syndrome. *Am J Clin Pathol* 1983;80:714–718.
199. Cockerell CJ, Whitlow MA, Webster GF, et al. Epithelioid angiomatosis: a distinct vascular disorder in patients with the acquired immunodeficiency syndrome or AIDS-related complex. *Lancet* 1987;2:654–656.
200. LeBoit PE, Berger TG, Egbert BM, et al. Epithelioid haemangioma-like vascular proliferation in AIDS: manifestation of cat scratch disease bacillus infection? *Lancet* 1988;1:960–963.
201. LeBoit PE, Berger TG, Egbert BM, et al. Bacillary angiomatosis. The histopathology and differential diagnosis of a pseudoneoplastic infection in patients with human immunodeficiency virus disease. *Am J Surg Pathol* 1989;13:909–920.
202. Baron AL, Steinbach LS, LeBoit PE, et al. Osteolytic lesions and bacillary angiomatosis in HIV infection: radiologic differentiation from AIDS-related Kaposi sarcoma. *Radiology* 1990;177:77–81.
203. Moore EH, Russell LA, Klein JS, et al. Bacillary angiomatosis in patients with AIDS: multiorgan imaging findings. *Radiology* 1995;197:67–72.
204. Relman DA, Loutit JS, Schmidt TM, et al. The agent of bacillary angiomatosis. An approach to the identification of uncultured pathogens. *N Engl J Med* 1990;323:1573–1580.
205. Kemper CA, Lombard CM, Deresinski SC, et al. Visceral bacillary epithelioid angiomatosis: possible manifestations of disseminated cat scratch disease in the immunocompromised host: a report of two cases. *Am J Med* 1990;89:216–222.
206. Chan JK, Lewin KJ, Lombard CM, et al. Histopathology of bacillary angiomatosis of lymph node. *Am J Surg Pathol* 1991;15:430–437.
207. Myers SA, Prose NS, Garcia JA, et al. Bacillary angiomatosis in a child undergoing chemotherapy. *J Pediatr* 1992;121:574–578.
208. Torok L, Viragh SZ, Borka I, et al. Bacillary angiomatosis in a patient with lymphocytic leukaemia. *Br J Dermatol* 1994;130:665–658.
209. Milde P, Brunner M, Borchard F, et al. Cutaneous bacillary angiomatosis in a patient with chronic lymphocytic leukemia. *Arch Dermatol* 1995;131:933–936.
210. Cockerell CJ, Bergstresser PR, Myrie-Williams C, et al. Bacillary epithelioid angiomatosis occurring in an immunocompetent individual. *Arch Dermatol* 1990;126:787–790.
211. Tappero JW, Koehler JE, Berger TG, et al. Bacillary angiomatosis and bacillary splenitis in immunocompetent adults. *Ann Intern Med* 1993;118:363–365.
212. Paul MA, Fleischer AB Jr, Wieselthier JS, et al. Bacillary angiomatosis in an immunocompetent child: the first reported case. *Pediatr Dermatol* 1994;11:338–341.
213. Smith KJ, Skelton HG, Tuur S, et al. Bacillary angiomatosis in an immunocompetent child. *Am J Dermatopathol* 1996;18:597–600.
214. Welch DF, Pickett DA, Slater LN, et al. *Rochalimaea henselae* sp. nov., a cause of septicemia, bacillary angiomatosis, and parenchymal bacillary peliosis. *J Clin Microbiol* 1992;30:275–280.
215. Koehler JE, Quinn FD, Berger TG, et al. Isolation of Rochalimaea species from cutaneous and osseous lesions of bacillary angiomatosis. *N Engl J Med*, 1992;327:1625–1631.
216. Brenner DJ, O'Connor SP, Winkler HH, et al. Proposals to unify the genera *Bartonella* and *Rochalimaea*, with descriptions of *Bartonella quintana* comb. nov., *Bartonella vinsonii* comb. nov., *Bartonella henselae* comb. nov., and *Bartonella elizabethae* comb. nov., and to remove the family Bartonellaceae from the order Rickettsiales. *Int J Syst Bacteriol*, 1993;43:777–786.
217. Adal KA, Cockerell CJ, Petri WA Jr. Cat scratch disease, bacillary angiomatosis, and other infections due to *Rochalimaea*. *N Engl J Med* 1994;330:1509–1515.
218. Perkocha LA, Geaghan SM, Yen TS, et al. Clinical and pathological features of bacillary peliosis hepatis in association with human immunodeficiency virus infection. *N Engl J Med* 1990;323:1581–1586.
219. Regnery R, Martin M, Olson J. Naturally occurring "*Rochalimaea henselae*" infection in domestic cat. *Lancet* 1992;340:557–558.
220. Koehler JE, Glaser CA, Tappero JW. *Rochalimaea henselae* infection. A new zoonosis with the domestic cat as reservoir. *JAMA* 1994;271:531–535.
221. Webster GF, Cockerell CJ, Friedman-Kien AE. The clinical spectrum of bacillary angiomatosis. *Br J Dermatol* 1992;126:535–541.
222. Bastug DF, Ness DT, DeSantis JG. Bacillary angiomatosis mimicking pyogenic granuloma in the hand: a case report. *J Hand Surg Am* 1996;21:307–308.
223. Malane MS, Laude TA, Chen CK, et al. An HIV-1-positive child with fever and a scalp nodule. *Lancet* 1995;346:1466.
224. Eden CG, Marker A, Pryor JP. Human immunodeficiency virus-related bacillary angiomatosis of the penis. *Br J Urol* 1996;77:323–324.
225. Mohle-Boetani JC, Koehler JE, Berger TG, et al. Bacillary angiomatosis and bacillary peliosis in patients infected with human immunodeficiency virus: clinical characteristics in a case-control study. *Clin Infect Dis* 1996;22:794–800.
226. Slater LN, Welch DF, Min KW. *Rochalimaea henselae* causes bacillary angiomatosis and peliosis hepatis. *Arch Intern Med* 1992;152:602–606.
227. Steeper TA, Rosenstein H, Weiser J, et al. Bacillary epithelioid angiomatosis involving the liver, spleen, and skin in an AIDS patient with concurrent Kaposi's sarcoma. *Am J Clin Pathol* 1992;97:713–718.
228. Milam MW, Balerdi MJ, Toney JF, et al. Epithelioid angiomatosis secondary to disseminated cat scratch disease involving the bone marrow and skin in a patient with acquired immune deficiency syndrome: a case report. *Am J Med* 1990;88:180–183.
229. Krekorian TD, Radner AB, Alcorn JM, et al. Biliary obstruction caused by epithelioid angiomatosis in a patient with AIDS. *Am J Med* 1990;89:820–822.
230. Schinella RA, Greco MA. Bacillary angiomatosis presenting as a soft-tissue tumor without skin involvement. *Hum Pathol* 1990;21:567–569.

231. Spach DH, Callis KP, Paauw DS, et al. Endocarditis caused by *Rochalimaea quintana* in a patient infected with human immunodeficiency virus. *J Clin Microbiol* 1993;31:692–694.
232. Kuppers R, Zhao M, Hansmann ML, et al. Tracing B cell development in human germinal centres by molecular analysis of single cells picked from histological sections. *EMBO J* 1993;12:4955–4967.
233. Long SR, Whitfeld MJ, Eades C, et al. Bacillary angiomatosis of the cervix and vulva in a patient with AIDS. *Obstet Gynecol* 1996;88:709–711.
234. Spach DH, Panther LA, Thorning DR, et al. Intracerebral bacillary angiomatosis in a patient infected with human immunodeficiency virus. *Ann Intern Med* 1992;116:740–742.
235. Haught WH, Steinbach J, Zander DS, et al. Case report: bacillary angiomatosis with massive visceral lymphadenopathy. *Am J Med Sci* 1993;306:236–240.
236. Slater LN, Min KW. Polypoid endobronchial lesions. A manifestation of bacillary angiomatosis. *Chest* 1992;102:972–974.
237. Walford N, Van der Wouw PA, Das PK, et al. Epithelioid angiomatosis in the acquired immunodeficiency syndrome: morphology and differential diagnosis. *Histopathology* 1990;16:83–88.
238. Miller DG. The association of immune disease and malignant lymphoma. *Ann Intern Med* 1967;66:507–521.
239. Penn I, Hammond W, Brettschneider L, et al. Malignant lymphomas in transplantation patients. *Transplant Proc* 1969;1:106–112.
240. Penn I. Occurrence of cancer in immune deficiencies. *Cancer* 1974;34:(Suppl):858–866.
241. Frizzera G, Rosai J, Dehner LP, et al. Lymphoreticular disorders in primary immunodeficiencies: new findings based on an up-to-date histologic classification of 35 cases. *Cancer* 1980;46:692–699.
242. Morrell D, Cromartie E, Swift M. Mortality and cancer incidence in 263 patients with ataxia-telangiectasia. *J Natl Cancer Inst* 1986;77:89–92.
243. Cleary ML, Warnke R, Sklar J. Monoclonality of lymphoproliferative lesions in cardiac-transplant recipients. Clonal analysis based on immunoglobulin-gene rearrangements. *N Engl J Med* 1984;310:477–482.
244. Penn I. Cancers complicating organ transplantation. *N Engl J Med* 1990;323:1767–1769.
245. Knowles DM, Cesarman E, Chadburn A, et al. Correlative morphologic and molecular genetic analysis demonstrates three distinct categories of posttransplantation lymphoproliferative disorders. *Blood* 1995;85:552–565.
246. Burke JS, Butler JJ, Fuller LM. Malignant lymphomas of the thyroid: a clinical pathologic study of 35 patients including ultrastructural observations. *Cancer* 1977;39:1587–1602.
247. Zulman J, Jaffe R, Talal N. Evidence that the malignant lymphoma of Sjogren's syndrome is a monoclonal B-cell neoplasm. *N Engl J Med* 1978;299:1215–1220.
248. Raphael M, Said J, Borisch B, et al. Lymphomas associated with HIV infection. In: Swerdlow SH, Campo E, Harris NL, et al., eds. *WHO Classification of tumours of haematopoietic and lymphoid tissues.* Geneva: WHO Press, 2008:340–342.
249. Doll DC, List AF. Burkitt's lymphoma in a homosexual. *Lancet* 1982;1:1026–1027.
250. Centers for Disease Control. Diffuse, undifferentiated non-Hodgkins lymphoma among homosexual males—United States. *MMWR Morb Mortal Wkly Rep* 1982;31:277–279.
251. Ziegler JL, Drew WL, Miner RC, et al. Outbreak of Burkitt's-like lymphoma in homosexual men. *Lancet* 1982;2:631–633.
252. Ziegler JL, Beckstead JA, Volberding PA, et al. Non-Hodgkin's lymphoma in 90 homosexual men. Relation to generalized lymphadenopathy and the acquired immunodeficiency syndrome. *N Engl J Med* 1984;311:565–570.
253. Update on acquired immune deficiency syndrome (AIDS)—United States. *MMWR Morb Mortal Wkly Rep* 1982;31:507–508, 513–514.
254. Revision of the CDC surveillance case definition for acquired immunodeficiency syndrome. Council of State and Territorial Epidemiologists; AIDS Program, Center for Infectious Diseases. *MMWR Morb Mortal Wkly Rep* 1987;36(Suppl 1):1S–15S.
255. Levine AM, Meyer PR, Begandy MK, et al. Development of B-cell lymphoma in homosexual men. Clinical and immunologic findings. *Ann Intern Med* 1984;100:7–13.
256. Levine AM, Gill PS, Meyer PR, et al. Retrovirus and malignant lymphoma in homosexual men. *JAMA* 1985;254:1921–1925.
257. Ioachim HL, Cooper MC, Hellman GC. Lymphomas in men at high risk for acquired immune deficiency syndrome (AIDS). A study of 21 cases. *Cancer* 1985;56:2831–2842.
258. Di Carlo EF, Amberson JB, Metroka CE, et al. Malignant lymphomas and the acquired immunodeficiency syndrome. Evaluation of 30 cases using a working formulation. *Arch Pathol Lab Med* 1986;110:1012–1016.
259. Knowles DM, Chamulak GA, Subar M, et al. Lymphoid neoplasia associated with the acquired immunodeficiency syndrome (AIDS). The New York University Medical Center experience with 105 patients (1981–1986). *Ann Intern Med* 1988;108:744–753.
260. Kaplan MH, Susin M, Pahwa SG, et al. Neoplastic complications of HTLV-III infection. Lymphomas and solid tumors. *Am J Med* 1987;82:389–396.
261. Snider WD, Simpson DM, Aronyk KE, et al. Primary lymphoma of the nervous system associated with acquired immune-deficiency syndrome. *N Engl J Med* 1983;308:45.
262. Chaganti RS, Jhanwar SC, Koziner B, et al. Specific translocations characterize Burkitt's-like lymphoma of homosexual men with the acquired immunodeficiency syndrome. *Blood* 1983;61:1265–1268.
263. Gordon EM, Berkowitz RJ, Strandjord SE, et al. Burkitt lymphoma in a patient with classic hemophilia receiving factor VIII concentrates. *J Pediatr* 1983;103:75–77.
264. Shibuya A, Saitoh K, Tsuneyoshi H, et al. Burkitt's lymphoma in a haemophiliac. *Lancet* 1983;2:1432.
265. Whang-Peng J, Lee EC, Sieverts H, et al. Burkitt's lymphoma in AIDS: cytogenetic study. *Blood* 1984;63:818–822.
266. Petersen JM, Tubbs RR, Savage RA, et al. Small noncleaved B cell Burkitt-like lymphoma with chromosome t(8;14) translocation and Epstein-Barr virus nuclear-associated antigen in a homosexual man with acquired immune deficiency syndrome. *Am J Med* 1985;78:141–148.
267. Ragni MV, Lewis JH, Bontempo FA, et al. Lymphoma presenting as a traumatic hematoma in an HTLV-III antibody-positive hemophiliac. *N Engl J Med* 1985;313:640.
268. Groopman JE, Sullivan JL, Mulder C, et al. Pathogenesis of B cell lymphoma in a patient with AIDS. *Blood* 1986;67:612–615.
269. Mernick MH, Malamud SC, Haubenstock A, et al. Non-Hodgkin's lymphoma in AIDS: report of 11 cases and literature review. *Mt Sinai J Med* 1986;53:664–667.
270. Ahmed T, Wormser GP, Stahl RE, et al. Malignant lymphomas in a population at risk for acquired immune deficiency syndrome. *Cancer* 1987;60:719–723.
271. Payan MJ, Gambarelli D, Routy JP, et al. Primary lymphoma of the brain associated with AIDS. A study of one case. *Acta Neuropathol* 1984;64:78–80.
272. Casadei GP, Arrigoni GL, Versari P, et al. Central neurocytoma. A clinico-pathologic study of five cases. *Tumori* 1991;77:323–327.
273. Raphael M, Tulliez M, Bellefqih S, et al. [Lymphomas and AIDS]. *Ann Pathol* 1986;6:278–281.
274. Monfardini S. Malignant lymphomas in patients with or at risk for AIDS in Italy. *Recent Results Cancer Res* 1988;112:37–45.
275. Hamilton-Dutoit SJ, Pallesen G, Karkov J, et al. Identification of EBV-DNA in tumour cells of AIDS-related lymphomas by in-situ hybridisation. *Lancet* 1989;1:554–552.
276. Beral V, Peterman T, Berkelman R, et al. AIDS-associated non-Hodgkin lymphoma. *Lancet* 1991;337:805–809.
277. Casabona J, Melbye M, Biggar RJ. Kaposi's sarcoma and non-Hodgkin's lymphoma in European AIDS cases. No excess risk of Kaposi's sarcoma in Mediterranean countries. *Int J Cancer* 1991;47:49–53.
278. Roithmann S, Tourani JM, Andrieu JM. AIDS-associated non-Hodgkin lymphoma. *Lancet* 1991;338:884–885.
279. Levine AM, Sullivan-Halley J, Pike MC, et al. Human immunodeficiency virus-related lymphoma. Prognostic factors predictive of survival. *Cancer* 1991;68:2466–2472.
280. Peters BS, Beck EJ, Coleman DG, et al. Changing disease patterns in patients with AIDS in a referral centre in the United Kingdom: the changing face of AIDS. *BMJ* 1991;302:203–207.
281. Loureiro C, Gill PS, Meyer PR, et al. Autopsy findings in AIDS-related lymphoma. *Cancer* 1988;62:735–739.
282. Klatt EC. Diagnostic findings in patients with acquired immune deficiency syndrome (AIDS). *J Acquir Immune Defic Syndr* 1988;1:459–465.
283. Wilkes MS, Fortin AH, Felix JC, et al. Value of necropsy in acquired immunodeficiency syndrome. *Lancet* 1988;2:85–88.
284. Rabkin CS. Epidemiology of AIDS-related malignancies. *Curr Opin Oncol* 1994;6:492–496.
285. Biggar RJ, Curtis RE, Cote TR, et al. Risk of other cancers following Kaposi's sarcoma: relation to acquired immunodeficiency syndrome. *Am J Epidemiol* 1994;139:362–368.
286. Levine AM, Gill PS. AIDS-related malignant lymphoma: clinical presentation and treatment approaches. *Oncology (Williston Park)* 1987;1:41–46.
287. Biggar RJ, Rabkin CS. The epidemiology of acquired immunodeficiency syndrome-related lymphomas. *Curr Opin Oncol* 1992;4:883–893.
288. Levine AM. Acquired immunodeficiency syndrome-related lymphoma. *Blood* 1992;80:8–20.
289. Harnly ME, Swan SH, Holly EA, et al. Temporal trends in the incidence of non-Hodgkin's lymphoma and selected malignancies in a population with a high incidence of acquired immunodeficiency syndrome (AIDS). *Am J Epidemiol* 1988;128:261–267.
290. Ross R, Dworsky R, Paganini-Hill A, et al. Non-Hodgkin's lymphomas in never married men in Los Angeles. *Br J Cancer* 1985;52:785–787.
291. Pluda JM, Yarchoan R, Jaffe ES, et al. Development of non-Hodgkin lymphoma in a cohort of patients with severe human immunodeficiency virus (HIV) infection on long-term antiretroviral therapy. *Ann Intern Med* 1990;113:276–282.
292. Bernstein L, Hamilton AS. The epidemiology of AIDS-related malignancies. *Curr Opin Oncol* 1993;5:822–830.
293. Obrams GI, Grufferman S. Epidemiology of HIV associated non-Hodgkin lymphoma. *Cancer Surv* 1991;10:91–102.
294. Biggar RJ, Rabkin CS. The epidemiology of AIDS-related neoplasms. *Hematol Oncol Clin North Am* 1996;10:997–1010.
295. Rabkin CS, Biggar RJ, Horm JW. Increasing incidence of cancers associated with the human immunodeficiency virus epidemic. *Int J Cancer* 1991;47:692–696.
296. Lowenthal DA, Straus DJ, Campbell SW, et al. AIDS-related lymphoid neoplasia. The Memorial Hospital experience. *Cancer* 1988;61:2325–2337.
297. Carbone A, Tirelli U, Vaccher E, et al. A clinicopathologic study of lymphoid neoplasias associated with human immunodeficiency virus infection in Italy. *Cancer* 1991;68:842–852.
298. Rabkin CS, Hilgartner MW, Hedberg KW, et al. Incidence of lymphomas and other cancers in HIV-infected and HIV-uninfected patients with hemophilia. *JAMA* 1992;267:1090–1094.
299. Kaplan LD, Abrams DI, Feigal E, et al. AIDS-associated non-Hodgkin's lymphoma in San Francisco. *JAMA* 1989;261:719–724.
300. Hamilton-Dutoit SJ, Pallesen G, Franzmann MB, et al. AIDS-related lymphoma. Histopathology, immunophenotype, and association with Epstein-Barr virus as demonstrated by in situ nucleic acid hybridization. *Am J Pathol* 1991;138:149–163.
301. Pedersen C, Gerstoft J, Lundgren JD, et al. HIV-associated lymphoma: histopathology and association with Epstein-Barr virus genome related to clinical, immunological and prognostic features. *Eur J Cancer* 1991;27:1416–1423.
302. Monfardini S, Tirelli U, Vaccher E, et al. Hodgkin's disease in 63 intravenous drug users infected with human immunodeficiency virus. Gruppo Italiano Cooperativo AIDS & Tumori (GICAT). *Ann Oncol* 1991;2(Suppl 2):201–205.
303. Freter CE. Acquired immunodeficiency syndrome-associated lymphomas. *J Natl Cancer Inst Monogr* 1990;45–54.
304. Delecluse HJ, Anagnostopoulos I, Dallenbach F, et al. Plasmablastic lymphomas of the oral cavity: a new entity associated with the human immunodeficiency virus infection. *Blood* 1997;89:1413–1420.
305. Schichman SA, McClure R, Schaefer RF, et al. HIV and plasmablastic lymphoma manifesting in sinus, testicles, and bones: a further expansion of the disease spectrum. *Am J Hematol* 2004;77:291–295.
306. Dong HY, Scadden DT, de Leval L, et al. Plasmablastic lymphoma in HIV-positive patients: an aggressive Epstein-Barr virus-associated extramedullary plasmacytic neoplasm. *Am J Surg Pathol* 2005;29:1633–1641.
307. Castillo J, Pantanowitz L, Dezube BJ. HIV-associated plasmablastic lymphoma: lessons learned from 112 published cases. *Am J Hematol* 2008;83:804–809.
308. Valera A, Balague O, Colomo L, et al. IG/MYC rearrangements are the main cytogenetic alteration in plasmablastic lymphomas. *Am J Surg Pathol* 2010;34:1686–1694.

309. Chang CC, Zhou X, Taylor JJ, et al. Genomic profiling of plasmablastic lymphoma using array comparative genomic hybridization (aCGH): revealing significant overlapping genomic lesions with diffuse large B-cell lymphoma. *J Hematol Oncol* 2009;2:47.

310. Chang Y, Cesarman E, Pessin MS, et al. Identification of herpesvirus-like DNA sequences in AIDS-associated Kaposi's sarcoma. *Science* 1994;266:1865–1869.

311. Cesarman E, Chang Y, Moore PS, et al. Kaposi's sarcoma-associated herpesvirus-like DNA sequences in AIDS-related body-cavity-based lymphomas. *N Engl J Med* 1995;332:1186–1191.

312. Knowles DM, Inghirami G, Ubriaco A, et al. Molecular genetic analysis of three AIDS-associated neoplasms of uncertain lineage demonstrates their B-cell derivation and the possible pathogenetic role of the Epstein-Barr virus. *Blood* 1989;73:792–799.

313. Walts AE, Shintaku IP, Said JW. Diagnosis of malignant lymphoma in effusions from patients with AIDS by gene rearrangement. *Am J Clin Pathol* 1990;94:170–175.

314. Chadburn A, Cesarman E, Jagirdar J, et al. CD30 (Ki-1) positive anaplastic large cell lymphomas in individuals infected with the human immunodeficiency virus. *Cancer* 1993;72:3078–3090.

315. Carbone A, Tirelli U, Gloghini A, et al. Herpesvirus-like DNA sequences selectively cluster with body cavity-based lymphomas throughout the spectrum of AIDS-related lymphomatous effusions. *Eur J Cancer* 1996;32A:555–556.

316. Otsuki T, Kumar S, Ensoli B, et al. Detection of HHV-8/KSHV DNA sequences in AIDS-associated extranodal lymphoid malignancies. *Leukemia* 1996;10:1358–1362.

317. Karcher DS, Alkan S. Herpes-like DNA sequences, AIDS-related tumors, and Castleman's disease. *N Engl J Med* 1995;333:797–798; author reply 798–799.

318. Pastore C, Gloghini A, Volpe G, et al. Distribution of Kaposi's sarcoma herpesvirus sequences among lymphoid malignancies in Italy and Spain. *Br J Haematol* 1995;91:918–920.

319. Said JW, Tasaka T, Takeuchi S, et al. Primary effusion lymphoma in women: report of two cases of Kaposi's sarcoma herpes virus-associated effusion-based lymphoma in human immunodeficiency virus-negative women. *Blood* 1996;88:3124–3128.

320. Nador RG, Cesarman E, Knowles DM, et al. Herpes-like DNA sequences in a body-cavity-based lymphoma in an HIV-negative patient. *N Engl J Med* 1995;333:943.

321. Robert C, Agbalika F, Blanc F, et al. HIV-negative patient with HHV-8 DNA follicular B-cell lymphoma associated with Kaposi's sarcoma. *Lancet* 1996;347:1042–1043.

322. Luppi M, Barozzi P, Marasca R, et al. HHV-8-associated primary cerebral B-cell lymphoma in HIV-negative patient after long-term steroids. *Lancet* 1996;347:980.

323. Corboy JR, Garl PJ, Kleinschmidt-DeMasters BK. Human herpesvirus 8 DNA in CNS lymphomas from patients with and without AIDS. *Neurology* 1998;50:335–340.

324. Tarte K, Chang Y, Klein B. Kaposi's sarcoma-associated herpesvirus and multiple myeloma: lack of criteria for causality. *Blood* 1999;93:3159–3163; discussion 3163–3164.

325. Gaidano G, Capello D, Pastore C, et al. Analysis of human herpesvirus type 8 infection in AIDS-related and AIDS-unrelated primary central nervous system lymphoma. *J Infect Dis* 1997;175:1193–1197.

326. Feuillard J, Aubin JT, Poirel L, et al. Detection rate and intratumoral virus load of human herpesvirus-8 in immunodeficiency-related B-cell lymphoid malignancies. *J Med Virol* 1997;53:277–281.

327. Chadburn A, Hyjek E, Mathew S, et al. KSHV-positive solid lymphomas represent an extra-cavitary variant of primary effusion lymphoma. *Am J Surg Pathol* 2004;28:1401–1416.

328. Du MQ, Diss TC, Liu H, et al. KSHV- and EBV-associated germinotropic lymphoproliferative disorder. *Blood* 2002;100:3415–3418.

329. Iuchi K, Ichimiya A, Akashi A, et al. Non-Hodgkin's lymphoma of the pleural cavity developing from long-standing pyothorax. *Cancer* 1987;60:1771–1775.

330. Iuchi K, Aozasa K, Yamamoto S, et al. Non-Hodgkin's lymphoma of the pleural cavity developing from long-standing pyothorax. Summary of clinical and pathological findings in thirty-seven cases. *Jpn J Clin Oncol* 1989;19:249–257.

331. Fukayama M, Ibuka T, Hayashi Y, et al. Epstein-Barr virus in pyothorax-associated pleural lymphoma. *Am J Pathol* 1993;143:1044–1049.

332. Cesarman E, Nador RG, Aozasa K, et al. Kaposi's sarcoma-associated herpesvirus in non-AIDS related lymphomas occurring in body cavities. *Am J Pathol* 1996;149:53–57.

333. Nador RG, Cesarman E, Chadburn A, et al. Primary effusion lymphoma: a distinct clinicopathologic entity associated with the Kaposi's sarcoma-associated herpes virus. *Blood* 1996;88:645–656.

334. Engels EA, Pittaluga S, Whitby D, et al. Immunoblastic lymphoma in persons with AIDS-associated Kaposi's sarcoma: a role for Kaposi's sarcoma-associated herpesvirus. *Mod Pathol* 2003;16:424–429.

335. Said J, Cesarman E. Primary effusion lymphoma. In: Swerdlow SH, Campo E, Harris NL, et al., eds. *WHO classification of tumours of haematopoietic and lymphoid tissues*. Lyon: IARC Press, 2008:260–261.

336. Hermine O, Michel M, Buzyn-Veil A, et al. Body-cavity-based lymphoma in an HIV-seronegative patient without Kaposi's sarcoma-associated herpesvirus-like DNA sequences. *N Engl J Med* 1996;334:272–273.

337. Raphael MM, Audouin J, Lamine M, et al. Immunophenotypic and genotypic analysis of acquired immunodeficiency syndrome-related non-Hodgkin's lymphomas. Correlation with histologic features in 36 cases. French Study Group of Pathology for HIV-associated tumors. *Am J Clin Pathol* 1994;101:773–782.

338. Ansari MQ, Dawson DB, Nador R, et al. Primary body cavity-based AIDS-related lymphomas. *Am J Clin Pathol* 1996;105:221–229.

339. DePond W, Said JW, Tasaka T, et al. Kaposi's sarcoma-associated herpesvirus and human herpesvirus 8 (KSHV/HHV8)-associated lymphoma of the bowel. Report of two cases in HIV-positive men with secondary effusion lymphomas. *Am J Surg Pathol* 1997;21:719–724.

340. Said W, Chien K, Takeuchi S, et al. Kaposi's sarcoma-associated herpesvirus (KSHV or HHV8) in primary effusion lymphoma: ultrastructural demonstration of herpesvirus in lymphoma cells. *Blood* 1996;87:4937–4943.

341. Mbulaiteye SM, Biggar RJ, Goedert JJ, et al. Pleural and peritoneal lymphoma among people with AIDS in the United States. *J Acquir Immune Defic Syndr* 2002;29:418–421.

342. Cesarman E, Knowles DM. The role of Kaposi's sarcoma-associated herpesvirus (KSHV/HHV-8) in lymphoproliferative diseases. *Semin Cancer Biol* 1999;9:165–174.

343. Tanaka PY, Atala MM, Pereira J, et al. Primary effusion lymphoma with cardiac involvement in HIV positive patient-complete response and long survival with chemotherapy and HAART. *J Clin Virol* 2009;44:84–85.

344. Simonelli C, Tedeschi R, Gloghini A, et al. Characterization of immunologic and virological parameters in HIV-infected patients with primary effusion lymphoma during antiblastic therapy and highly active antiretroviral therapy. *Clin Infect Dis* 2005;40:1022–1027.

345. Ghosh SK, Wood C, Boise LH, et al. Potentiation of TRAIL-induced apoptosis in primary effusion lymphoma through azidothymidine-mediated inhibition of NF-kappa B. *Blood* 2003;101:2321–2327.

346. Di Bartolo DL, Hyjek E, Keller S, et al. Role of defective Oct-2 and OCA-B expression in immunoglobulin production and Kaposi's sarcoma-associated herpesvirus lytic reactivation in primary effusion lymphoma. *J Virol* 2009;83:4308–4315.

347. Said JW, Shintaku IP, Asou H, et al. Herpesvirus 8 inclusions in primary effusion lymphoma: report of a unique case with T-cell phenotype. *Arch Pathol Lab Med* 1999;123:257–260.

348. Gaidano G, Capello D, Cilia AM, et al. Genetic characterization of HHV-8/KSHV-positive primary effusion lymphoma reveals frequent mutations of BCL6: implications for disease pathogenesis and histogenesis. *Genes Chromosomes Cancer* 1999;24:16–23.

349. Pascual V, Liu YJ, Magalski A, et al. Analysis of somatic mutation in five B cell subsets of human tonsil. *J Exp Med* 1994;180:329–339.

350. Matolcsy A, Nador RG, Cesarman E, et al. Immunoglobulin VH gene mutational analysis suggests that primary effusion lymphomas derive from different stages of B cell maturation. *Am J Pathol* 1998;153:1609–1614.

351. Hamoudi R, Diss TC, Oksenhendler E, et al. Distinct cellular origins of primary effusion lymphoma with and without EBV infection. *Leuk Res* 2004;28:333–338.

352. Klein U, Gloghini A, Gaidano G, et al. Gene expression profile analysis of AIDS-related primary effusion lymphoma (PEL) suggests a plasmablastic derivation and identifies PEL-specific transcripts. *Blood* 2003;101:4115–4121.

353. Jenner RG, Maillard K, Cattini N, et al. Kaposi's sarcoma-associated herpesvirus-infected primary effusion lymphoma has a plasma cell gene expression profile. *Proc Natl Acad Sci U S A* 2003;100:10399–10404.

354. Lombardi L, Newcomb EW, Dalla-Favera R. Pathogenesis of Burkitt lymphoma: expression of an activated c-myc oncogene causes the tumorigenic conversion of EBV-infected human B lymphoblasts. *Cell* 1987;49:161–170.

355. Flamand L, Stefanescu I, Ablashi DV, et al. Activation of the Epstein-Barr virus replicative cycle by human herpesvirus 6. *J Virol* 1993;67:6768–6777.

356. Varthakavi V, Smith RM, Deng H, et al. Human immunodeficiency virus type-1 activates lytic cycle replication of Kaposi's sarcoma-associated herpesvirus through induction of KSHV Rta. *Virology* 2002;297:270–280.

357. Aoki Y, Tosato G. HIV-1 Tat enhances Kaposi sarcoma-associated herpesvirus (KSHV) infectivity. *Blood* 2004;104:810–814.

358. Caselli E, Galvan M, Cassai E, et al. Human herpesvirus 8 enhances human immunodeficiency virus replication in acutely infected cells and induces reactivation in latently infected cells. *Blood* 2005;106:2790–2797.

359. Mercader M, Nickoloff BJ, Foreman KE. Induction of human immunodeficiency virus 1 replication by human herpesvirus 8. *Arch Pathol Lab Med* 2001;125:785–789.

360. Horenstein MG, Nador RG, Chadburn A, et al. Epstein-Barr virus latent gene expression in primary effusion lymphomas containing Kaposi's sarcoma-associated herpesvirus/human herpesvirus-8. *Blood* 1997;90:1186–1191.

361. Pellett PE, Roizman B. The family *Herpesviridae*: a brief introduction. In: Knipe DM, Griffin DE, Lamb RA, et al., eds. *Fields' virology*, New York: Lippincott-Williams and Wilkins, 2007:2479–2499.

362. Klein G, Dombos L, Gothoskar B. Sensitivity of Epstein-Barr virus (EBV) producer and non-producer human lymphoblastoid cell lines to superinfection with EB-virus. *Int J Cancer* 1972;10:44–57.

363. Biesinger B, Muller-Fleckenstein I, Simmer B, et al. Stable growth transformation of human T lymphocytes by herpesvirus saimiri. *Proc Natl Acad Sci U S A* 1992;89:3116–3119.

364. Rose TM, Strand KB, Schultz ER, et al. Identification of two homologs of the Kaposi's sarcoma-associated herpesvirus (human herpesvirus 8) in retroperitoneal fibromatosis of different macaque species. *J Virol* 1997;71:4138–4144.

365. Damania B, Desrosiers RC. Simian homologues of human herpesvirus 8. *Philos Trans R Soc Lond B Biol Sci* 2001;356:535–543.

366. Orzechowska BU, Powers MF, Sprague J, et al. Rhesus macaque rhadinovirus-associated non-Hodgkin lymphoma: animal model for KSHV-associated malignancies. *Blood* 2008;112:4227–4234.

367. Cesarman E. Gammaherpesvirus and lymphoproliferative disorders in immunocompromised patients. *Cancer Lett* 2011;305:163–174.

368. Damania B, Cesarman E. Kaposi's sarcoma-associated herpesvirus. In: David M, Knipe PMH, Diane E, et al., eds. *Field's virology*, 6th ed. Philadelphia: Lippincott Williams & Wilkins, 2013.

369. Ballestas ME, Chatis PA, Kaye KM. Efficient persistence of extrachromosomal KSHV DNA mediated by latency-associated nuclear antigen. *Science* 1999;284:641–644.

370. Radkov SA, Kellam P, Boshoff C. The latent nuclear antigen of Kaposi sarcoma-associated herpesvirus targets the retinoblastoma-E2F pathway and with the oncogene Hras transforms primary rat cells. *Nat Med* 2000;6:1121–1127.

371. Friborg J Jr, Kong W, Hottiger MO, et al. p53 inhibition by the LANA protein of KSHV protects against cell death. *Nature* 1999;402:889–894.

372. Fujimuro M, Hayward SD. Manipulation of glycogen-synthase kinase-3 activity in KSHV-associated cancers. *J Mol Med (Berl)* 2004;82:223–231.

373. Bubman D, Guasparri I, Cesarman E. Deregulation of c-Myc in primary effusion lymphoma by Kaposi's sarcoma herpesvirus latency-associated nuclear antigen. *Oncogene* 2007;26:4979–4986.

374. Renne R, Barry C, Dittmer D, et al. Modulation of cellular and viral gene expression by the latency-associated nuclear antigen of Kaposi's sarcoma-associated herpesvirus. *J Virol* 2001;75:458–468.

375. Bajaj BG, Verma SC, Lan K, et al. KSHV encoded LANA upregulates Pim-1 and is a substrate for its kinase activity. *Virology* 2006;351:18–28.

376. Verma SC, Borah S, Robertson ES. Latency-associated nuclear antigen of Kaposi's sarcoma-associated herpesvirus up-regulates transcription of human telomerase reverse transcriptase promoter through interaction with transcription factor Sp1. *J Virol* 2004;78:10348–10359.

377. An J, Lichtenstein AK, Brent G, et al. The Kaposi sarcoma-associated herpesvirus (KSHV) induces cellular interleukin 6 expression: role of the KSHV latency-associated nuclear antigen and the AP1 response element. *Blood* 2002;99:649–654.

378. Di Bartolo DL, Cannon M, Liu YF, et al. KSHV LANA inhibits TGF-beta signaling through epigenetic silencing of the TGF-beta type II receptor. *Blood* 2008;111: 4731–4740.
379. Rainbow L, Platt GM, Simpson GR, et al. The 222 - to 234-kilodalton latent nuclear protein (LNA) of Kaposi's sarcoma-associated herpesvirus (human herpesvirus 8) is encoded by orf73 and is a component of the latency-associated nuclear antigen. *J Virol* 1997;71:5915–5921.
380. Thome M, Schneider P, Hofmann K, et al. Viral FLICE-inhibitory proteins (FLIPs) prevent apoptosis induced by death receptors. *Nature* 1997;386:517–521.
381. Chaudhary PM, Jasmin A, Eby MT, et al. Modulation of the NF-kappa B pathway by virally encoded death effector domains-containing proteins. *Oncogene* 1999;18: 5738–5746.
382. Matta H, Chaudhary PM. Activation of alternative NF-kappa B pathway by human herpes virus 8-encoded Fas-associated death domain-like IL-1 beta-converting enzyme inhibitory protein (vFLIP). *Proc Natl Acad Sci U S A* 2004;101:9399–9404.
383. Guasparri I, Wu H, Cesarman E. The KSHV oncoprotein vFLIP contains a TRAF-interacting motif and requires TRAF2 and TRAF3 for signalling. *EMBO Rep* 2006;7:114–119.
384. Field N, Low W, Daniels M, et al. KSHV vFLIP binds to IKK-gamma to activate IKK. *J Cell Sci* 2003;116:3721–3728.
385. Djerbi M, Screpanti V, Catrina AI, et al. The inhibitor of death receptor signaling, FLICE-inhibitory protein defines a new class of tumor progression factors. *J Exp Med* 1999;190:1025–1032.
386. Guasparri I, Keller SA, Cesarman E. KSHV vFLIP is essential for the survival of infected lymphoma cells. *J Exp Med* 2004;199:993–1003.
387. Godfrey A, Anderson J, Papanastasiou A, et al. Inhibiting primary effusion lymphoma by lentiviral vectors encoding short hairpin RNA. *Blood* 2005;105: 2510–2518.
388. Lee JS, Li Q, Lee JY, et al. FLIP-mediated autophagy regulation in cell death control. *Nat Cell Biol* 2009;11:1355–1362.
389. Ballon G, Chen K, Perez R, et al. Kaposi sarcoma herpesvirus (KSHV) vFLIP oncoprotein induces B cell transdifferentiation and tumorigenesis in mice. *J Clin Invest* 2011;121:1141–1153.
390. Chugh P, Matta H, Schamus S, et al. Constitutive NF-kappaB activation, normal Fas-induced apoptosis, and increased incidence of lymphoma in human herpes virus 8 K13 transgenic mice. *Proc Natl Acad Sci U S A* 2005;102:12885–12890.
391. Ahmad A, Groshong JS. Kaposi's sarcoma associated herpesvirus-encoded viral FLICE inhibitory protein (vFLIP) K13 cooperates with Myc to promote lymphoma in mice. *Cancer Biol Ther* 2010;10:1033–1040.
392. Brown HJ, Song MJ, Deng H, et al. NF-kappaB inhibits gammaherpesvirus lytic replication. *J Virol* 2003;77:8532–8540.
393. de Oliveira DE, Ballon G, Cesarman E. NF-kappaB signaling modulation by EBV and KSHV. *Trends Microbiol* 2010;18:248–257.
394. Godden-Kent D, Talbot SJ, Boshoff C, et al. The cyclin encoded by Kaposi's sarcoma-associated herpesvirus stimulates cdk6 to phosphorylate the retinoblastoma protein and histone H1. *J Virol* 1997;71:4193–4198.
395. Li M, Lee H, Yoon DW, et al. Kaposi's sarcoma-associated herpesvirus encodes a functional cyclin. *J Virol* 1997;71:1984–1991.
396. Ellis M, Chew YP, Fallis L, et al. Degradation of p27(Kip) cdk inhibitor triggered by Kaposi's sarcoma virus cyclin-cdk6 complex. *EMBO J* 1999;18:644–653.
397. Mann DJ, Child ES, Swanton C, et al. Modulation of p27(Kip1) levels by the cyclin encoded by Kaposi's sarcoma-associated herpesvirus. *EMBO J* 1999;18:654–663.
398. Cuomo ME, Knebel A, Morrice N, et al. p53-Driven apoptosis limits centrosome amplification and genomic instability downstream of NPM1 phosphorylation. *Nat Cell Biol* 2008;10:723–730.
399. Sarek G, Jarviluoma A, Moore HM, et al. Nucleophosmin phosphorylation by v-cyclin-CDK6 controls KSHV latency. *PLoS Pathog* 2010;6:e1000818.
400. Leidal AM, Cyr DP, Hill RJ, et al. Subversion of autophagy by Kaposi's sarcoma-associated herpesvirus impairs oncogene-induced senescence. *Cell Host Microbe* 2012;11:167–180.
401. Verschuren EW, Hodgson JG, Gray JW, et al. The role of p53 in suppression of KSHV cyclin-induced lymphomagenesis. *Cancer Res* 2004;64:581–589.
402. Verschuren EW, Klefstrom J, Evan GI, et al. The oncogenic potential of Kaposi's sarcoma-associated herpesvirus cyclin is exposed by p53 loss in vitro and in vivo. *Cancer Cell* 2002;2:229–241.
403. Rivas C, Thlick AE, Parravicini C, et al. Kaposi's sarcoma-associated herpesvirus LANA2 is a B-cell-specific latent viral protein that inhibits p53. *J Virol* 2001;75:429–438.
404. Lubyova B, Kellum MJ, Frisancho AJ, et al. Kaposi's sarcoma-associated herpesvirus-encoded vIRF-3 stimulates the transcriptional activity of cellular IRF-3 and IRF-7. *J Biol Chem* 2004;279:7643–7654.
405. Moore PS, Boshoff C, Weiss RA, et al. Molecular mimicry of human cytokine and cytokine response pathway genes by KSHV. *Science* 1996;274:1739–1744.
406. Molden J, Chang Y, You Y, et al. A Kaposi's sarcoma-associated herpesvirus-encoded cytokine homolog (vIL-6) activates signaling through the shared gp130 receptor subunit. *J Biol Chem* 1997;272:19625–19631.
407. Nicholas J, Ruvolo VR, Burns WH, et al. Kaposi's sarcoma-associated human herpesvirus-8 encodes homologues of macrophage inflammatory protein-1 and interleukin-6. *Nature Med* 1997;3:287–292.
408. Lee H, Veazey R, Williams K, et al. Deregulation of cell growth by the K1 gene of Kaposi's sarcoma-associated herpesvirus. *Nat Med* 1998;4:435–440.
409. Tomlinson CC, Damania B. The K1 protein of Kaposi's sarcoma-associated herpesvirus activates the Akt signaling pathway. *J Virol* 2004;78:1918–1927.
410. Prakash O, Swamy OR, Peng X, et al. Activation of Src kinase Lyn by the Kaposi sarcoma-associated herpesvirus K1 protein: implications for lymphomagenesis. *Blood* 2005;105:3987–3994.
411. Chandriani S, Ganem D. Array-based transcript profiling and limiting-dilution reverse transcription-PCR analysis identify additional latent genes in Kaposi's sarcoma-associated herpesvirus. *J Virol* 84:5565–5573.
412. Prakash O, Tang ZY, Peng X, et al. Tumorigenesis and aberrant signaling in transgenic mice expressing the human herpesvirus-8 K1 gene. *J Natl Cancer Inst* 2002;94:926–935.
413. Sadler R, Wu L, Forghani B, et al. A complex translational program generates multiple novel proteins from the latently expressed kaposin (K12) locus of Kaposi's sarcoma-associated herpesvirus. *J Virol* 1999;73:5722–5730.
414. Li H, Komatsu T, Dezube BJ, et al. The Kaposi's sarcoma-associated herpesvirus K12 transcript from a primary effusion lymphoma contains complex repeat elements, is spliced, and initiates from a novel promoter. *J Virol* 2002;76:11880–11888.
415. McCormick C, Ganem D. The kaposin B protein of KSHV activates the p38/MK2 pathway and stabilizes cytokine mRNAs. *Science* 2005;307:739–741.
416. Choi JK, Lee BS, Shim SN, et al. Identification of the novel K15 gene at the rightmost end of the Kaposi's sarcoma-associated herpesvirus genome. *J Virol* 2000;74: 436–446.
417. Brinkmann MM, Glenn M, Rainbow L, et al. Activation of mitogen-activated protein kinase and NF-kappaB pathways by a Kaposi's sarcoma-associated herpesvirus K15 membrane protein. *J Virol* 2003;77:9346–9358.
418. Sharp TV, Wang HW, Koumi A, et al. K15 protein of Kaposi's sarcoma-associated herpesvirus is latently expressed and binds to HAX-1, a protein with antiapoptotic function. *J Virol* 2002;76:802–816.
419. Cai X, Lu S, Zhang Z, et al. Kaposi's sarcoma-associated herpesvirus expresses an array of viral microRNAs in latently infected cells. *Proc Natl Acad Sci U S A* 2005;102:5570–5575.
420. Samols MA, Hu J, Skalsky RL, et al. Cloning and identification of a microRNA cluster within the latency-associated region of Kaposi's sarcoma-associated herpesvirus. *J Virol* 2005;79:9301–9305.
421. Pfeffer S, Sewer A, Lagos-Quintana M, et al. Identification of microRNAs of the herpesvirus family. *Nat Methods* 2005;2:269–276.
422. Grundhoff A, Sullivan CS, Ganem D. A combined computational and microarray-based approach identifies novel microRNAs encoded by human gamma-herpesviruses. *RNA* 2006;12:733–750.
423. Lei X, Bai Z, Ye F, et al. Regulation of NF-kappaB inhibitor IkappaBalpha and viral replication by a KSHV microRNA. *Nat Cell Biol* 12:193–199.
424. Gottwein E, Cullen BR. A human herpesvirus microRNA inhibits p21 expression and attenuates p21-mediated cell cycle arrest. *J Virol* 84:5229–5237.
425. Gottwein E, Mukherjee N, Sachse C, et al. A viral microRNA functions as an orthologue of cellular miR-155. *Nature* 2007;450:1096–1099.
426. Skalsky RL, Samols MA, Plaisance KB, et al. Kaposi's sarcoma-associated herpesvirus encodes an ortholog of miR-155. *J Virol* 2007;81:12836–12845.
427. Dupin N, Diss TL, Kellam P, et al. HHV-8 is associated with a plasmablastic variant of Castleman disease that is linked to HHV-8-positive plasmablastic lymphoma. *Blood* 2000;95:1406–1412.
428. Du MQ, Liu H, Diss TC, et al. Kaposi sarcoma-associated herpesvirus infects monotypic (IgM lambda) but polyclonal naive B cells in Castleman disease and associated lymphoproliferative disorders. *Blood* 2001;97:2130–2136.
429. Isaacson PG, Campo E. Large B-cell lymphoma arising in HHV8-associated multicnetric Castleman disease. In: Swerdlow SH, Campo E, Harris NL, et al., eds. *WHO classification of tumours of haematopoietic and lymphoid tissues*. Lyon: IARC Press, 2008:258–259.
430. D'Antonio A, Boscaino A, Addesso M, et al. KSHV- and EBV-associated germinotropic lymphoproliferative disorder: a rare lymphoproliferative disease of HIV patient with plasmablastic morphology, indolent course and favourable response to therapy. *Leuk Lymphoma* 2007;48:1444–1447.
431. Chadburn A, Cesarman E, Knowles DM. Molecular pathology of posttransplantation lymphoproliferative disorders. *Semin Diagn Pathol* 1997;14:15–26.
432. Frizzera G, Hanto DW, Gajl-Peczalska KJ, et al. Polymorphic diffuse B-cell hyperplasias and lymphomas in renal transplant recipients. *Cancer Res* 1981;41: 4262–4279.
433. Cleary ML, Sklar J. Lymphoproliferative disorders in cardiac transplant recipients are multiclonal lymphomas. *Lancet* 1984;2:489–493.
434. Cleary ML, Nalesnik MA, Shearer WT, et al. Clonal analysis of transplant-associated lymphoproliferations based on the structure of the genomic termini of the Epstein-Barr virus. *Blood* 1988;72:349–352.
435. Nalesnik MA, Jaffe R, Starzl TE, et al. The pathology of posttransplant lymphoproliferative disorders occurring in the setting of cyclosporine A-prednisone immunosuppression. *Am J Pathol* 1988;133:173–192.
436. Locker J, Nalesnik M. Molecular genetic analysis of lymphoid tumors arising after organ transplantation. *Am J Pathol* 1989;135:977–987.
437. Nador RG, Chadburn A, Gundappa G, et al. Human immunodeficiency virus (HIV)-associated polymorphic lymphoproliferative disorders. *Am J Surg Pathol* 2003;27:293–302.
438. Frank D, Cesarman E, Liu YF, et al. Posttransplantation lymphoproliferative disorders frequently contain type A and not type B Epstein-Barr virus. *Blood* 1995;85:1396–1403.
439. Boyle MJ, Sewell WA, Sculley TB, et al. Subtypes of Epstein-Barr virus in human immunodeficiency virus-associated non-Hodgkin lymphoma. *Blood* 1991; 78:3004–3011.
440. Chadburn A, Chen JM, Hsu DT, et al. The morphologic and molecular genetic categories of posttransplantation lymphoproliferative disorders are clinically relevant. *Cancer* 1998;82:1978–1987.
441. Migliazza A, Martinotti S, Chen W, et al. Frequent somatic hypermutation of the 5′ noncoding region of the BCL6 gene in B-cell lymphoma. *Proc Natl Acad Sci U S A* 1995;92:12520–12524.
442. Cesarman E, Chadburn A, Liu YF, et al. BCL-6 gene mutations in posttransplantation lymphoproliferative disorders predict response to therapy and clinical outcome. *Blood* 1998;92:2294–2302.
443. Rodrigo JA, Hicks LK, Cheung MC, et al. HIV-associated Burkitt lymphoma: good efficacy and tolerance of intensive chemotherapy including CODOX-M/IVAC with or without Rituximab in the HAART era. *Adv Hematol* 2012;2012:735392.
444. Guech-Ongey M, Simard EP, Anderson WF, et al. AIDS-related Burkitt lymphoma in the United States: what do age and CD4 lymphocyte patterns tell us about etiology and/or biology? *Blood* 2010;116:5600–5604.
445. Epeldegui M, Breen EC, Hung YP, et al. Elevated expression of activation induced cytidine deaminase in peripheral blood mononuclear cells precedes AIDS-NHL diagnosis. *AIDS* 2007;21:2265–2270.
446. Smith SM. AIDS-related BL and CD4 count: a clue? *Blood* 2010;116:5435–5436.
447. Hui PK, Feller AC, Lennert K. High-grade non-Hodgkin's lymphoma of B-cell type. I. Histopathology. *Histopathology* 1988;12:127–143.
448. Mohamedbhai SG, Sibson K, Marafioti T, et al. Rituximab in combination with CODOX-M/IVAC: a retrospective analysis of 23 cases of non-HIV related B-cell non-Hodgkin lymphoma with proliferation index >95%. *Br J Haematol* 2011;152:175–181.
449. Kalter SP, Riggs SA, Cabanillas F, et al. Aggressive non-Hodgkin's lymphomas in immunocompromised homosexual males. *Blood* 1985;66:655–659.
450. Ioachim HL, Dorsett B, Cronin W, et al. Acquired immunodeficiency syndrome-associated lymphomas: clinical, pathologic, immunologic, and viral characteristics of 111 cases. *Hum Pathol* 1991;22:659–673.

451. Gill PS, Levine AM, Meyer PR, et al. Primary central nervous system lymphoma in homosexual men. Clinical, immunologic, and pathologic features. *Am J Med* 1985;78:742–748.
452. So YT, Beckstead JH, Davis RL. Primary central nervous system lymphoma in acquired immune deficiency syndrome: a clinical and pathological study. *Ann Neurol* 1986;20:566–572.
453. Burkes RL, Meyer PR, Gill PS, et al. Rectal lymphoma in homosexual men. *Arch Intern Med* 1986;146:913–915.
454. Lee MH, Waxman M, Gillooley JF. Primary malignant lymphoma of the anorectum in homosexual men. *Dis Colon Rectum* 1986;29:413–416.
455. Ioachim HL, Weinstein MA, Robbins RD, et al. Primary anorectal lymphoma. A new manifestation of the acquired immune deficiency syndrome (AIDS). *Cancer* 1987;60:1449–1453.
456. Dunleavy K, Little RF, Pittaluga S, et al. The role of tumor histogenesis, FDG-PET, and short-course EPOCH with dose-dense rituximab (SC-EPOCH-RR) in HIV-associated diffuse large B-cell lymphoma. *Blood* 2010;115:3017–3024.
457. Chadburn A, Chiu A, Lee JY, et al. Immunophenotypic analysis of AIDS-related diffuse large B-cell lymphoma and clinical implications in patients from AIDS Malignancies Consortium clinical trials 010 and 034. *J Clin Oncol* 2009;27:5039–5048.
458. Reichert CM, O'Leary TJ, Levens DL, et al. Autopsy pathology in the acquired immune deficiency syndrome. *Am J Pathol* 1983;112:357–382.
459. Caccamo D, Pervez NK, Marchevsky A. Primary lymphoma of the liver in the acquired immunodeficiency syndrome. *Arch Pathol Lab Med* 1986;110:553–555.
460. Vanden Heule B, Taylor CR, Terry R, et al. Presentation of malignant lymphoma in the rectum. *Cancer* 1982;49:2602–2607.
461. Loehr WJ, Mujahed Z, Zahn FD, et al. Primary lymphoma of the gastrointestinal tract: a review of 100 cases. *Ann Surg* 1969;170:232–238.
462. Dragosics B, Bauer P, Radaszkiewicz T. Primary gastrointestinal non-Hodgkin's lymphomas. A retrospective clinicopathologic study of 150 cases. *Cancer* 1985;55:1060–1073.
463. Daling JR, Weiss NS, Klopfenstein LL, et al. Correlates of homosexual behavior and the incidence of anal cancer. *JAMA* 1982;247:1988–1990.
464. Peters RK, Mack TM. Patterns of anal carcinoma by gender and marital status in Los Angeles County. *Br J Cancer* 1983;48:629–636.
465. Formenti SC, Gill PS, Lean E, et al. Primary central nervous system lymphoma in AIDS. Results of radiation therapy. *Cancer* 1989;63:1101–1107.
466. Raphael M, Gentilhomme O, Tulliez M, et al. Histopathologic features of high-grade non-Hodgkin's lymphomas in acquired immunodeficiency syndrome. The French Study Group of Pathology for Human Immunodeficiency Virus-Associated Tumors. *Arch Pathol Lab Med* 1991;115:15–20.
467. Constantino A, West TE, Gupta M, et al. Primary cardiac lymphoma in a patient with acquired immune deficiency syndrome. *Cancer* 1987;60:2801–2805.
468. Gill PS, Chandraratna PA, Meyer PR, et al. Malignant lymphoma: cardiac involvement at initial presentation. *J Clin Oncol* 1987;5:216–224.
469. Brooks HL Jr, Downing J, McClure JA, et al. Orbital Burkitt's lymphoma in a homosexual man with acquired immune deficiency. *Arch Ophthalmol* 1984;102:1533–1537.
470. Kaplan LD, Kahn J, Jacobson M, et al. Primary bile duct lymphoma in the acquired immunodeficiency syndrome (AIDS). *Ann Intern Med* 1989;110:161–162.
471. Pollack RN, Sklarin NT, Rao S, et al. Metastatic placental lymphoma associated with maternal human immunodeficiency virus infection. *Obstet Gynecol* 1993;81:856–857.
472. Levecq H, Hautefeuille M, Hoang C, et al. Primary stomal lymphoma. An unusual complication of ileostomy in a patient with transfusion-related acquired immune deficiency syndrome. *Cancer* 1990;65:1028–1032.
473. Louie S, Daoust PR, Schwartz RS. Immunodeficiency and the pathogenesis of non-Hodgkin's lymphoma. *Semin Oncol* 1980;7:267–284.
474. Krivitzky A, Bentata-Pessayre M, Lejeune F, et al. [Malignant lymphoma initially of the buttocks: possible role of repeated intramuscular injections]. *Ann Med Interne (Paris)* 1984;135:205–207.
475. Henry JM, Heffner RR Jr, Dillard SH, et al. Primary malignant lymphomas of the central nervous system. *Cancer* 1974;34:1293–1302.
476. Freeman C, Berg JW, Cutler SJ. Occurrence and prognosis of extranodal lymphomas. *Cancer* 1972;29:252–260.
477. Good AE, Russo RH, Schnitzer B, et al. Intracranial histiocytic lymphoma with rheumatoid arthritis. *J Rheumatol* 1978;5:75–78.
478. Gill PS, Graham RA, Boswell W, et al. A comparison of imaging, clinical, and pathologic aspects of space-occupying lesions within the brain in patients with acquired immune deficiency syndrome. *Am J Physiol Imaging* 1986;1:134–141.
479. Goldstein JD, Dickson DW, Moser FG, et al. Primary central nervous system lymphoma in acquired immune deficiency syndrome. A clinical and pathologic study with results of treatment with radiation. *Cancer* 1991;67:2756–2765.
480. MacMahon EM, Glass JD, Hayward SD, et al. Epstein-Barr virus in AIDS-related primary central nervous system lymphoma. *Lancet* 1991;338:969–973.
481. Baumgartner JE, Rachlin JR, Beckstead JH, et al. Primary central nervous system lymphomas: natural history and response to radiation therapy in 55 patients with acquired immunodeficiency syndrome. *J Neurosurg* 1990;73:206–211.
482. Lee YY, Bruner JM, Van Tassel P, et al. Primary central nervous system lymphoma: CT and pathologic correlation. *AJR Am J Roentgenol* 1986;147:747–752.
483. Kelly WM, Brant-Zawadzki M. Acquired immunodeficiency syndrome: neuroradiologic findings. *Radiology* 1983;149:485–491.
484. Edwards KR, Pendlebury WW. Central nervous system lymphomas versus toxoplasmosis in a patient with AIDS. *N Engl J Med* 1987;317:1540.
485. Levine AM. AIDS-related malignancies: the emerging epidemic. *J Natl Cancer Inst* 1993;85:1382–1397.
486. Bishburg E, Eng RH, Slim J, et al. Brain lesions in patients with acquired immunodeficiency syndrome. *Arch Intern Med* 1989;149:941–943.
487. Ciricillo SF, Rosenblum ML. Use of CT and MR imaging to distinguish intracranial lesions and to define the need for biopsy in AIDS patients. *J Neurosurg* 1990;73:720–724.
488. Pelicci PG, Knowles DM II, Arlin ZA, et al. Multiple monoclonal B cell expansions and c-myc oncogene rearrangements in acquired immune deficiency syndrome-related lymphoproliferative disorders. Implications for lymphomagenesis. *J Exp Med* 1986;164:2049–2060.
489. Egerter DA, Beckstead JH. Malignant lymphomas in the acquired immunodeficiency syndrome. Additional evidence for a B-cell origin. *Arch Pathol Lab Med* 1988;112:602–606.
490. Green I, Espiritu E, Ladanyi M, et al. Primary lymphomatous effusions in AIDS: a morphological, immunophenotypic, and molecular study. *Mod Pathol* 1995;8:39–45.
491. Barriga F, Whang-Peng J, Lee E, et al. Development of a second clonally discrete Burkitt's lymphoma in a human immunodeficiency virus-positive homosexual patient. *Blood* 1988;72:792–795.
492. Subar M, Neri A, Inghirami G, et al. Frequent c-myc oncogene activation and infrequent presence of Epstein-Barr virus genome in AIDS-associated lymphoma. *Blood* 1988;72:667–671.
493. Ballerini P, Gaidano G, Gong JZ, et al. Multiple genetic lesions in acquired immunodeficiency syndrome-related non-Hodgkin's lymphoma. *Blood* 1993;81:166–176.
494. McGrath MS, Shiramizu B, Meeker TC, et al. AIDS-associated polyclonal lymphoma: identification of a new HIV-associated disease process. *J Acquir Immune Defic Syndr* 1991;4:408–415.
495. Meeker TC, Shiramizu B, Kaplan L, et al. Evidence for molecular subtypes of HIV-associated lymphoma: division into peripheral monoclonal, polyclonal and central nervous system lymphoma. *AIDS* 1991;5:669–674.
496. Shiramizu B, Herndier B, Meeker T, et al. Molecular and immunophenotypic characterization of AIDS-associated, Epstein-Barr virus-negative, polyclonal lymphoma. *J Clin Oncol* 1992;10:383–389.
497. Kaplan LD, Shiramizu B, Herndier B, et al. Influence of molecular characteristics on clinical outcome in human immunodeficiency virus-associated non-Hodgkin's lymphoma: identification of a subgroup with favorable clinical outcome. *Blood* 1995;85:1727–1735.
498. Seiden M, Sklar J. AIDS and non-Hodgkin's lymphoma: a pre-pre-B-cell monoclonal lymphoma versus a novel mechanism of polyclonality? *J Clin Oncol* 1992;10:1650–1651.
499. Knowles DM. Biologic aspects of AIDS-associated non-Hodgkin's lymphoma. *Curr Opin Oncol* 1993;5:845–851.
500. Knowles DM, Chamulak G, Subar M, et al. Clinicopathologic, immunophenotypic, and molecular genetic analysis of AIDS-associated lymphoid neoplasia. Clinical and biologic implications. *Pathol Annu* 1988;23(Pt 2):33–67.
501. Gaidano G, Lo Coco F, Ye BH, et al. Rearrangements of the BCL-6 gene in acquired immunodeficiency syndrome-associated non-Hodgkin's lymphoma: association with diffuse large-cell subtype. *Blood* 1994;84:397–402.
502. Dalla-Favera R, Bregni M, Erikson J, et al. Human c-myc onc gene is located on the region of chromosome 8 that is translocated in Burkitt lymphoma cells. *Proc Natl Acad Sci U S A* 1982;79:7824–7827.
503. Dalla-Favera R, Martinotti S, Gallo RC, et al. Translocation and rearrangements of the c-myc oncogene locus in human undifferentiated B-cell lymphomas. *Science* 1983;219:963–967.
504. Croce CM. Molecular genetics of human B cell neoplasia. *Horiz Biochem Biophys* 1986;8:545–570.
505. Lenoir GM, Preud'homme JL, Bernheim A, et al. Correlation between immunoglobulin light chain expression and variant translocation in Burkitt's lymphoma. *Nature* 1982;298:474–476.
506. Rechavi G, Ben-Bassat I, Berkowicz M, et al. Molecular analysis of Burkitt's leukemia in two hemophilic brothers with AIDS. *Blood* 1987;70:1713–1717.
507. Magrath I, Erikson J, Whang-Peng J, et al. Synthesis of kappa light chains by cell lines containing an 8;22 chromosomal translocation derived from a male homosexual with Burkitt's lymphoma. *Science* 1983;222:1094–1098.
508. Delecluse HJ, Raphael M, Magaud JP, et al. Variable morphology of human immunodeficiency virus-associated lymphomas with c-myc rearrangements. The French Study Group of Pathology for Human Immunodeficiency Virus-Associated Tumors, I. *Blood* 1993;82:552–563.
509. Carbone A, Tirelli U, Gloghini A, et al. Human immunodeficiency virus-associated systemic lymphomas may be subdivided into two main groups according to Epstein-Barr viral latent gene expression. *J Clin Oncol* 1993;11:1674–1681.
510. Rooney CM, Gregory CD, Rowe M, et al. Endemic Burkitt's lymphoma: phenotypic analysis of tumor biopsy cells and of derived tumor cell lines. *J Natl Cancer Inst* 1986;77:681–687.
511. Rowe DT, Rowe M, Evan GI, et al. Restricted expression of EBV latent genes and T-lymphocyte-detected membrane antigen in Burkitt's lymphoma cells. *EMBO J* 1986;5:2599–2607.
512. Rowe M, Rowe DT, Gregory CD, et al. Differences in B cell growth phenotype reflect novel patterns of Epstein-Barr virus latent gene expression in Burkitt's lymphoma cells. *EMBO J* 1987;6:2743–2751.
513. Gaidano G, Dalla-Favera R. Molecular pathogenesis of AIDS-related lymphomas. *Antibiot Chemother* 1994;46:117–124.
514. Pelicci PG, Knowles DM II, Magrath I, et al. Chromosomal breakpoints and structural alterations of the c-myc locus differ in endemic and sporadic forms of Burkitt lymphoma. *Proc Natl Acad Sci U S A* 1986;83:2984–2988.
515. Shiramizu B, Barriga F, Neequaye J, et al. Patterns of chromosomal breakpoint locations in Burkitt's lymphoma: relevance to geography and Epstein-Barr virus association. *Blood* 1991;77:1516–1526.
516. Lanfrancone L, Pelicci PG, Dalla-Favera R. Structure and expression of translocated c-myc oncogenes: specific differences in endemic, sporadic and AIDS-associated forms of Burkitt lymphomas. *Curr Top Microbiol Immunol* 1986;132:257–265.
517. Neri A, Barriga F, Knowles DM, et al. Different regions of the immunoglobulin heavy-chain locus are involved in chromosomal translocations in distinct pathogenetic forms of Burkitt lymphoma. *Proc Natl Acad Sci U S A* 1988;85:2748–2752.
518. Ye BH, Rao PH, Chaganti RS, et al. Cloning of bcl-6, the locus involved in chromosome translocations affecting band 3q27 in B-cell lymphoma. *Cancer Res* 1993;53:2732–2735.
519. Offit K, Jhanwar S, Ebrahim SA, et al. t(3;22)(q27;q11): a novel translocation associated with diffuse non-Hodgkin's lymphoma. *Blood* 1989;74:1876–1879.
520. Bastard C, Tilly H, Lenormand B, et al. Translocations involving band 3q27 and Ig gene regions in non-Hodgkin's lymphoma. *Blood* 1992;79:2527–2531.
521. Ye BH, Lista F, Lo Coco F, et al. Alterations of a zinc finger-encoding gene, BCL-6, in diffuse large-cell lymphoma. *Science* 1993;262:747–750.
522. Kerckaert JP, Deweindt C, Tilly H, et al. LAZ3, a novel zinc-finger encoding gene, is disrupted by recurring chromosome 3q27 translocations in human lymphomas. *Nat Genet* 1993;5:66–70.
523. Baron BW, Nucifora G, McCabe N, et al. Identification of the gene associated with the recurring chromosomal translocations t(3;14)(q27;q32) and t(3;22)(q27;q11) in B-cell lymphomas. *Proc Natl Acad Sci U S A* 1993;90:5262–5266.

524. Cattoretti G, Chang CC, Cechova K, et al. BCL-6 protein is expressed in germinal-center B cells. *Blood* 1995;86:45–53.
525. Ye BH, Cattoretti G, Shen Q, et al. The BCL-6 proto-oncogene controls germinal-centre formation and Th2-type inflammation. *Nat Genet* 1997;16:161–170.
526. Lo Coco F, Ye BH, Lista F, et al. Rearrangements of the BCL6 gene in diffuse large cell non-Hodgkin's lymphoma. *Blood* 1994;83:1757–1759.
527. Offit K, Lo Coco F, Louie DC, et al. Rearrangement of the bcl-6 gene as a prognostic marker in diffuse large-cell lymphoma. *N Engl J Med* 1994;331:74–80.
528. Bos JL. ras oncogenes in human cancer: a review. *Cancer Res* 1989;49:4682–4689.
529. Neri A, Knowles DM, Greco A, et al. Analysis of RAS oncogene mutations in human lymphoid malignancies. *Proc Natl Acad Sci U S A* 1988;85:9268–9272.
530. Seremetis S, Inghirami G, Ferrero D, et al. Transformation and plasmacytoid differentiation of EBV-infected human B lymphoblasts by ras oncogenes. *Science* 1989;243:660–663.
531. Raffeld M, Jaffe ES. bcl-1, t(11;14), and mantle cell-derived lymphomas. *Blood* 1991;78:259–263.
532. Tsujimoto Y, Cossman J, Jaffe E, et al. Involvement of the bcl-2 gene in human follicular lymphoma. *Science* 1985;228:1440–1443.
533. Weiss LM, Warnke RA, Sklar J, et al. Molecular analysis of the t(14;18) chromosomal translocation in malignant lymphomas. *N Engl J Med* 1987;317: 1185–1189.
534. Athan E, Foitl DR, Knowles DM. bcl-1 rearrangement. Frequency and clinical significance among B-cell chronic lymphocytic leukemias and non-Hodgkin's lymphomas. *Am J Pathol* 1991;138:591–599.
535. Goodrich DW, Lee WH. The molecular genetics of retinoblastoma. *Cancer Surv* 1990;9:529–554.
536. Hollstein M, Sidransky D, Vogelstein B, et al. p53 mutations in human cancers. *Science* 1991;253:49–53.
537. Levine AJ, Momand J, Finlay CA. The p53 tumour suppressor gene. *Nature* 1991;351:453–456.
538. Offit K, Wong G, Filippa DA, et al. Cytogenetic analysis of 434 consecutively ascertained specimens of non-Hodgkin's lymphoma: clinical correlations. *Blood* 1991;77:1508–1515.
539. Baker SJ, Fearon ER, Nigro JM, et al. Chromosome 17 deletions and p53 gene mutations in colorectal carcinomas. *Science* 1989;244:217–221.
540. Nigro JM, Baker SJ, Preisinger AC, et al. Mutations in the p53 gene occur in diverse human tumour types. *Nature* 1989;342:705–708.
541. Gaidano G, Ballerini P, Gong JZ, et al. p53 mutations in human lymphoid malignancies: association with Burkitt lymphoma and chronic lymphocytic leukemia. *Proc Natl Acad Sci U S A* 1991;88:5413–5417.
542. Cesarman E, Chadburn A, Inghirami G, et al. Structural and functional analysis of oncogenes and tumor suppressor genes in adult T-cell leukemia/lymphoma shows frequent p53 mutations. *Blood* 1992;80:3205–3216.
543. Ronen D, Rotter V, Reisman D. Expression from the murine p53 promoter is mediated by factor binding to a downstream helix-loop-helix recognition motif. *Proc Natl Acad Sci U S A* 1991;88:4128–4132.
544. Hayashi Y, Raimondi SC, Look AT, et al. Abnormalities of the long arm of chromosome 6 in childhood acute lymphoblastic leukemia. *Blood* 1990;76:1626–1630.
545. Millikin D, Meese E, Vogelstein B, et al. Loss of heterozygosity for loci on the long arm of chromosome 6 in human malignant melanoma. *Cancer Res* 1991;51: 5449–5453.
546. Morita R, Saito S, Ishikawa J, et al. Common regions of deletion on chromosomes 5q, 6q, and 10q in renal cell carcinoma. *Cancer Res* 1991;51:5817–5820.
547. Offit K, Parsa NZ, Gaidano G, et al. 6q deletions define distinct clinico-pathologic subsets of non-Hodgkin's lymphoma. *Blood* 1993;82:2157–2162.
548. Dryja TP, Rapaport JM, Joyce JM, et al. Molecular detection of deletions involving band q14 of chromosome 13 in retinoblastomas. *Proc Natl Acad Sci U S A* 1986;83: 7391–7394.
549. Ludlow JW, Shon J, Pipas JM, et al. The retinoblastoma susceptibility gene product undergoes cell cycle-dependent dephosphorylation and binding to and release from SV40 large T. *Cell* 1990;60:387–396.
550. Yandell DW, Campbell TA, Dayton SH, et al. Oncogenic point mutations in the human retinoblastoma gene: their application to genetic counseling. *N Engl J Med* 1989;321:1689–1695.
551. Gaidano G, Parsa NZ, Tassi V, et al. In vitro establishment of AIDS-related lymphoma cell lines: phenotypic characterization, oncogene and tumor suppressor gene lesions, and heterogeneity in Epstein-Barr virus infection. *Leukemia* 1993;7:1621–1629.
552. Capello D, Scandurra M, Poretti G, et al. Genome wide DNA-profiling of HIV-related B-cell lymphomas. *Br J Haematol* 2010;148:245–255.
553. Deffenbacher KE, Iqbal J, Liu Z, et al. Recurrent chromosomal alterations in molecularly classified AIDS-related lymphomas: an integrated analysis of DNA copy number and gene expression. *J Acquir Immune Defic Syndr* 2010;54:18–26.
554. Weinberg RA. Oncogenes, antioncogenes, and the molecular bases of multistep carcinogenesis. *Cancer Res* 1989;49:3713–3721.
555. Fearon ER, Vogelstein B. A genetic model for colorectal tumorigenesis. *Cell* 1990;61:759–767.
556. Carbone PP, Kaplan HS, Musshoff K, et al. Report of the committee on Hodgkin's disease staging classification. *Cancer Res* 1971;31:1860–1861.
557. National Cancer Institute sponsored study of classifications of non-Hodgkin's lymphomas: summary and description of a working formulation for clinical usage. The Non-Hodgkin's Lymphoma Pathologic Classification Project. *Cancer* 1982;49: 2112–2135.
558. Oriol A, Ribera JM, Bergua J, et al. High-dose chemotherapy and immunotherapy in adult Burkitt lymphoma: comparison of results in human immunodeficiency virus-infected and noninfected patients. *Cancer* 2008;113:117–125.
559. Re A, Michieli M, Casari S, et al. High-dose therapy and autologous peripheral blood stem cell transplantation as salvage treatment for AIDS-related lymphoma: long-term results of the Italian Cooperative Group on AIDS and Tumors (GICAT) study with analysis of prognostic factors. *Blood* 2009;114:1306–1313.
560. Shipp MA, Harrington DP, Klatt MM, et al. Identification of major prognostic subgroups of patients with large-cell lymphoma treated with m-BACOD or M-BACOD. *Ann Intern Med* 1986;104:757–765.
561. Hoskins PJ, Ng V, Spinelli JJ, et al. Prognostic variables in patients with diffuse large-cell lymphoma treated with MACOP-B. *J Clin Oncol* 1991;9:220–226.
562. Boue F, Gabarre J, Gisselbrecht C, et al. Phase II trial of CHOP plus rituximab in patients with HIV-associated non-Hodgkin's lymphoma. *J Clin Oncol* 2006;24: 4123–4128.
563. Barta SK, Lee JY, Kaplan LD, et al. Pooled analysis of AIDS malignancy consortium trials evaluating rituximab plus CHOP or infusional EPOCH chemotherapy in HIV-associated non-Hodgkin lymphoma. *Cancer* 2012;118:3977–3983.
564. Straus DJ. Human immunodeficiency virus-associated lymphomas. *Med Clin North Am* 1997;81:495–510.
565. Galetto G, Levine A. AIDS-associated primary central nervous system lymphoma. Oncology Core Committee, AIDS Clinical Trials Group. *JAMA* 1993;269:92–93.
566. Cinque P, Brytting M, Vago L, et al. Epstein-Barr virus DNA in cerebrospinal fluid from patients with AIDS-related primary lymphoma of the central nervous system. *Lancet* 1993;342:398–401.
567. De Luca A, Antinori A, Cingolani A, et al. Evaluation of cerebrospinal fluid EBV-DNA and IL-10 as markers for in vivo diagnosis of AIDS-related primary central nervous system lymphoma. *Br J Haematol* 1995;90:844–849.
568. Raphael BG, Knowles DM. Acquired immunodeficiency syndrome-associated non-Hodgkin's lymphoma. *Semin Oncol* 1990;17:361–366.
569. Gill PS, Levine AM, Krailo M, et al. AIDS-related malignant lymphoma: results of prospective treatment trials. *J Clin Oncol* 1987;5:1322–1328.
570. Bermudez MA, Grant KM, Rodvien R, et al. Non-Hodgkin's lymphoma in a population with or at risk for acquired immunodeficiency syndrome: indications for intensive chemotherapy. *Am J Med* 1989;86:71–76.
571. Skarin AT, Canellos GP, Rosenthal DS, et al. Improved prognosis of diffuse histiocytic and undifferentiated lymphoma by use of high dose methotrexate alternating with standard agents (M-BACOD). *J Clin Oncol* 1983;1:91–98.
572. Levine AM, Wernz JC, Kaplan L, et al. Low-dose chemotherapy with central nervous system prophylaxis and zidovudine maintenance in AIDS-related lymphoma. A prospective multi-institutional trial. *JAMA* 1991;266:84–88.
573. Walsh C, Wernz JC, Levine A, et al. Phase I trial of m-BACOD and granulocyte macrophage colony stimulating factor in HIV-associated non-Hodgkin's lymphoma. *J Acquir Immune Defic Syndr* 1993;6:265–271.
574. Kaplan LD, Kahn JO, Crowe S, et al. Clinical and virologic effects of recombinant human granulocyte-macrophage colony-stimulating factor in patients receiving chemotherapy for human immunodeficiency virus-associated non-Hodgkin's lymphoma: results of a randomized trial. *J Clin Oncol* 1991;9:929–940.
575. Haddy TB, Adde MA, Magrath IT. CNS involvement in small noncleaved-cell lymphoma: is CNS disease per se a poor prognostic sign? *J Clin Oncol* 1991;9: 1973–1982.
576. Sparano JA, Lee JY, Kaplan LD, et al. Rituximab plus concurrent infusional EPOCH chemotherapy is highly effective in HIV-associated B-cell non-Hodgkin lymphoma. *Blood* 2010;115:3008–3016.
577. Diez-Martin JL, Balsalobre P, Re A, et al. Comparable survival between HIV+ and HIV- non-Hodgkin and Hodgkin lymphoma patients undergoing autologous peripheral blood stem cell transplantation. *Blood* 2009;113:6011–6014.
578. Chamberlain MC. Long survival in patients with acquired immune deficiency syndrome-related primary central nervous system lymphoma. *Cancer* 1994;73: 1728–1730.
579. Forsyth PA, Yahalom J, DeAngelis LM. Combined-modality therapy in the treatment of primary central nervous system lymphoma in AIDS. *Neurology* 1994;44:1473–1479.
580. Woodman R, Shin K, Pineo G. Primary non-Hodgkin's lymphoma of the brain. A review. *Medicine (Baltimore)* 1985;64:425–430.
581. Grogg KL, Miller RF, Dogan A. HIV infection and lymphoma. *J Clin Pathol* 2007;60:1365–1372.
582. Montagnier L, Gruest J, Chamaret S, et al. Adaptation of lymphadenopathy associated virus (LAV) to replication in EBV-transformed B lymphoblastoid cell lines. *Science* 1984;225:63–66.
583. Saxinger WC, Levine PH, Dean AG, et al. Evidence for exposure to HTLV-III in Uganda before 1973. *Science* 1985;227:1036–1038.
584. Laurence J, Astrin SM. Human immunodeficiency virus induction of malignant transformation in human B lymphocytes. *Proc Natl Acad Sci U S A* 1991;88:7635–7639.
585. Ganser A, Carlo-Stella C, Bartram CR, et al. Establishment of two Epstein-Barr virus negative Burkitt cell lines from a patient with AIDS and B-cell lymphoma. *Blood* 1988;72:1255–1260.
586. Shibata D, Brynes RK, Nathwani B, et al. Human immunodeficiency viral DNA is readily found in lymph node biopsies from seropositive individuals. Analysis of fixed tissue using the polymerase chain reaction. *Am J Pathol* 1989;135:697–702.
587. Feichtinger H, Putkonen P, Parravicini C, et al. Malignant lymphomas in cynomolgus monkeys infected with simian immunodeficiency virus. *Am J Pathol* 1990;137:1311–1315.
588. Fauci AS, Schnittman SM, Poli G, et al. NIH conference. Immunopathogenic mechanisms in human immunodeficiency virus (HIV) infection. *Ann Intern Med* 1991;114:678–693.
589. Schnittman SM, Lane HC, Higgins SE, et al. Direct polyclonal activation of human B lymphocytes by the acquired immune deficiency syndrome virus. *Science* 1986;233:1084–1086.
590. Amariglio N, Vonsover A, Hakim I, et al. Immunoglobulin VH3-positive AIDS-related Burkitt's lymphoma: a possible role for the HIV gp120 superantigen. *Acta Haematol* 1994;91:103–105.
591. Ng VL, Hurt MH, Fein CL, et al. IgMs produced by two acquired immune deficiency syndrome lymphoma cell lines: Ig binding specificity and VH-gene putative somatic mutation analysis. *Blood* 1994;83:1067–1078.
592. Fauci AS. The human immunodeficiency virus: infectivity and mechanisms of pathogenesis. *Science* 1988;239:617–622.
593. Pantaleo G, Graziosi C, Fauci AS. New concepts in the immunopathogenesis of human immunodeficiency virus infection. *N Engl J Med* 1993;328:327–335.
594. Moore RD, Kessler H, Richman DD, et al. Non-Hodgkin's lymphoma in patients with advanced HIV infection treated with zidovudine. *JAMA* 1991;265:2208–2211.
595. Pluda JM, Venzon DJ, Tosato G, et al. Parameters affecting the development of non-Hodgkin's lymphoma in patients with severe human immunodeficiency virus infection receiving antiretroviral therapy. *J Clin Oncol* 1993;11:1099–1107.
596. Birx DL, Redfield RR, Tosato G. Defective regulation of Epstein-Barr virus infection in patients with acquired immunodeficiency syndrome (AIDS) or AIDS-related disorders. *N Engl J Med* 1986;314:874–879.
597. Ramsay AD, Smith WJ, Isaacson PG. T-cell-rich B-cell lymphoma. *Am J Surg Pathol* 1988;12:433–443.
598. List AF, Spier CM, Miller TP, et al. Deficient tumor-infiltrating T-lymphocyte response in malignant lymphoma: relationship to HLA expression and host immunocompetence. *Leukemia* 1993;7:398–403.

599. Hirano T, Yasukawa K, Harada H, et al. Complementary DNA for a novel human interleukin (BSF-2) that induces B lymphocytes to produce immunoglobulin. *Nature* 1986;324:73–76.
600. Jelinek DF, Splawski JB, Lipsky PE. The roles of interleukin 2 and interferon-gamma in human B cell activation, growth and differentiation. *Eur J Immunol* 1986;16:925–932.
601. Jelinek DF, Lipsky PE. Enhancement of human B cell proliferation and differentiation by tumor necrosis factor-alpha and interleukin 1. *J Immunol* 1987;139: 2970–2976.
602. Paul WE. Interleukin 4/B cell stimulatory factor 1: one lymphokine, many functions. *FASEB J* 1987;1:456–461.
603. Sharma S, Mehta S, Morgan J, et al. Molecular cloning and expression of a human B-cell growth factor gene in *Escherichia coli*. *Science* 1987;235:1489–1492.
604. Saeland S, Duvert V, Pandrau D, et al. Interleukin-7 induces the proliferation of normal human B-cell precursors. *Blood* 1991;78:2229–2238.
605. Zlotnik A, Moore KW. Interleukin 10. *Cytokine* 1991;3:366–371.
606. Breen EC, Hussain SK, Magpantay L, et al. B-cell stimulatory cytokines and markers of immune activation are elevated several years prior to the diagnosis of systemic AIDS-associated non-Hodgkin B-cell lymphoma. *Cancer Epidemiol Biomarkers Prev* 2011;20:1303–1314.
607. Scala G, Quinto I, Ruocco MR, et al. Expression of an exogenous interleukin 6 gene in human Epstein Barr virus B cells confers growth advantage and in vivo tumorigenicity. *J Exp Med* 1990;172:61–68.
608. Tanner J, Tosato G. Impairment of natural killer functions by interleukin 6 increases lymphoblastoid cell tumorigenicity in athymic mice. *J Clin Invest* 1991;88: 239–247.
609. Kawano M, Hirano T, Matsuda T, et al. Autocrine generation and requirement of BSF-2/IL-6 for human multiple myelomas. *Nature* 1988;332:83–85.
610. Kishimoto T. The biology of interleukin-6. *Blood* 1989;74:1–10.
611. Levy Y, Tsapis A, Brouet JC. Interleukin-6 antisense oligonucleotides inhibit the growth of human myeloma cell lines. *J Clin Invest* 1991;88:696–699.
612. Schwab G, Siegall CB, Aarden LA, et al. Characterization of an interleukin-6-mediated autocrine growth loop in the human multiple myeloma cell line, U266. *Blood* 1991;77:587–593.
613. Yee C, Biondi A, Wang XH, et al. A possible autocrine role for interleukin-6 in two lymphoma cell lines. *Blood* 1989;74:798–804.
614. Biondi A, Rossi V, Bassan R, et al. Constitutive expression of the interleukin-6 gene in chronic lymphocytic leukemia. *Blood* 1989;73:1279–1284.
615. Nakajima K, Martinez-Maza O, Hirano T, et al. Induction of IL-6 (B cell stimulatory factor-2/IFN-beta 2) production by HIV. *J Immunol* 1989;142:531–536.
616. Emilie D, Peuchmaur M, Maillot MC, et al. Production of interleukins in human immunodeficiency virus-1-replicating lymph nodes. *J Clin Invest* 1990;86: 148–159.
617. Birx DL, Redfield RR, Tencer K, et al. Induction of interleukin-6 during human immunodeficiency virus infection. *Blood* 1990;76:2303–2310.
618. Amadori A, Zamarchi R, Veronese ML, et al. B cell activation during HIV-1 infection. II. Cell-to-cell interactions and cytokine requirement. *J Immunol* 1991;146:57–62.
619. Keyserlingk H, Ludwig WD, Seibt H, et al. Atypical presentation of Hodgkin's disease in a patient at risk for the acquired immunodeficiency syndrome. *Cancer Detect Prev* 1988;12:243–248.
620. Emilie D, Coumbaras J, Raphael M, et al. Interleukin-6 production in high-grade B lymphomas: correlation with the presence of malignant immunoblasts in acquired immunodeficiency syndrome and in human immunodeficiency virus-seronegative patients. *Blood* 1992;80:498–504.
621. Vieira P, de Waal-Malefyt R, Dang MN, et al. Isolation and expression of human cytokine synthesis inhibitory factor cDNA clones: homology to Epstein-Barr virus open reading frame BCRFI. *Proc Natl Acad Sci U S A* 1991;88:1172–1176.
622. Benjamin D, Knobloch TJ, Dayton MA. Human B-cell interleukin-10: B-cell lines derived from patients with acquired immunodeficiency syndrome and Burkitt's lymphoma constitutively secrete large quantities of interleukin-10. *Blood* 1992;80:1289–1298.
623. Masood R, Zhang Y, Bond MW, et al. Interleukin-10 is an autocrine growth factor for acquired immunodeficiency syndrome-related B-cell lymphoma. *Blood* 1995;85:3423–3430.
624. Fiorentino DF, Zlotnik A, Vieira P, et al. IL-10 acts on the antigen-presenting cell to inhibit cytokine production by Th1 cells. *J Immunol* 1991;146:3444–3451.
625. de Waal Malefyt R, Haanen J, Spits H, et al. Interleukin 10 (IL-10) and viral IL-10 strongly reduce antigen-specific human T cell proliferation by diminishing the antigen-presenting capacity of monocytes via downregulation of class II major histocompatibility complex expression. *J Exp Med* 1991;174:915–924.
626. Go NF, Castle BE, Barrett R, et al. Interleukin 10, a novel B cell stimulatory factor: unresponsiveness of X chromosome-linked immunodeficiency B cells. *J Exp Med* 1990;172:1625–1631.
627. Rousset F, Garcia E, Defrance T, et al. Interleukin 10 is a potent growth and differentiation factor for activated human B lymphocytes. *Proc Natl Acad Sci U S A* 1992;89:1890–1893.
628. Breen EC, Fatahi S, Epeldegui M, et al. Elevated serum soluble CD30 precedes the development of AIDS-associated non-Hodgkin's B cell lymphoma. *Tumour Biol* 2006;27:187–194.
629. Widney DP, Gui D, Popoviciu LM, et al. Expression and function of the chemokine, CXCL13, and its receptor, CXCR5, in aids-associated non-Hodgkin's lymphoma. *AIDS Res Treat* 2010;2010:164586.
630. de-The G, Geser A, Day NE, et al. Epidemiological evidence for causal relationship between Epstein-Barr virus and Burkitt's lymphoma from Ugandan prospective study. *Nature* 1978;274:756–761.
631. Klein G, Klein E. Evolution of tumours and the impact of molecular oncology. *Nature* 1985;315:190–195.
632. Geser A, de The G, Lenoir G, et al. Final case reporting from the Ugandan prospective study of the relationship between EBV and Burkitt's lymphoma. *Int J Cancer* 1982;29:397–400.
633. Lindahl T, Klein G, Reedman BM, et al. Relationship between Epstein-Barr virus (EBV) DNA and the EBV-determined nuclear antigen (EBNA) in Burkitt lymphoma biopsies and other lymphoproliferative malignancies. *Int J Cancer* 1974;13:764–772.
634. Purtilo DT. Opportunistic non-Hodgkin's lymphoma in X-linked recessive immunodeficiency and lymphoproliferative syndromes. *Semin Oncol* 1977;4:335–343.
635. Purtilo DT, Klein G. Introduction to Epstein-Barr virus and lymphoproliferative diseases in immunodeficient individuals. *Cancer Res* 1981;41:4209.
636. Peiper SC, Myers JL, Broussard EE, et al. Detection of Epstein-Barr virus genomes in archival tissues by polymerase chain reaction. *Arch Pathol Lab Med* 1990;114:711–714.
637. Tosato G, Blaese RM. Epstein-Barr virus infection and immunoregulation in man. *Adv Immunol* 1985;37:99–149.
638. Hamilton-Dutoit SJ, Raphael M, Audouin J, et al. In situ demonstration of Epstein-Barr virus small RNAs (EBER 1) in acquired immunodeficiency syndrome-related lymphomas: correlation with tumor morphology and primary site. *Blood* 1993;82:619–624.
639. Neri A, Barriga F, Inghirami G, et al. Epstein-Barr virus infection precedes clonal expansion in Burkitt's and acquired immunodeficiency syndrome-associated lymphoma. *Blood* 1991;77:1092–1095.
640. Shibata D, Weiss LM, Hernandez AM, et al. Epstein-Barr virus-associated non-Hodgkin's lymphoma in patients infected with the human immunodeficiency virus. *Blood* 1993;81:2102–2109.
641. Sample J, Young L, Martin B, et al. Epstein-Barr virus types 1 and 2 differ in their EBNA-3A, EBNA-3B, and EBNA-3C genes. *J Virol* 1990;64:4084–4092.
642. Kyaw MT, Hurren L, Evans L, et al. Expression of B-type Epstein-Barr virus in HIV-infected patients and cardiac transplant recipients. *AIDS Res Hum Retroviruses* 1992;8:1869–1874.
643. Wang D, Liebowitz D, Kieff E. An EBV membrane protein expressed in immortalized lymphocytes transforms established rodent cells. *Cell* 1985;43:831–840.
644. Borisch B, Ellinger K, Neipel F, et al. Lymphadenitis and lymphoproliferative lesions associated with the human herpes virus-6 (HHV-6). *Virchows Arch B Cell Pathol Incl Mol Pathol* 1991;61:179–187.
645. Karp JE, Broder S. Acquired immunodeficiency syndrome and non-Hodgkin's lymphomas. *Cancer Res* 1991;51:4743–4756.
646. Torelli G, Marasca R, Luppi M, et al. Human herpesvirus-6 in human lymphomas: identification of specific sequences in Hodgkin's lymphomas by polymerase chain reaction. *Blood* 1991;77:2251–2258.
647. Paulus W, Jellinger K, Hallas C, et al. Human herpesvirus-6 and Epstein-Barr virus genome in primary cerebral lymphomas. *Neurology* 1993;43:1591–1593.
648. Ng VL, Hwang KM, Reyes GR, et al. High titer anti-HIV antibody reactivity associated with a paraprotein spike in a homosexual male with AIDS related complex. *Blood* 1988;71:1397–1401.
649. Ng VL, Chen KH, Hwang KM, et al. The clinical significance of human immunodeficiency virus type 1-associated paraproteins. *Blood* 1989;74:2471–2475.
650. Berek C, Milstein C. Mutation drift and repertoire shift in the maturation of the immune response. *Immunol Rev* 1987;96:23–41.
651. Bahler DW, Levy R. Clonal evolution of a follicular lymphoma: evidence for antigen selection. *Proc Natl Acad Sci U S A* 1992;89:6770–6774.
652. Zelenetz AD, Chen TT, Levy R. Clonal expansion in follicular lymphoma occurs subsequent to antigenic selection. *J Exp Med* 1992;176:1137–1148.
653. Riboldi P, Gaidano G, Schettino EW, et al. Two acquired immunodeficiency syndrome-associated Burkitt's lymphomas produce specific anti-i IgM cold agglutinins using somatically mutated VH4-21 segments. *Blood* 1994;83: 2952–2961.
654. Bernstein L, Levin D, Menck H, et al. AIDS-related secular trends in cancer in Los Angeles County men: a comparison by marital status. *Cancer Res* 1989;49: 466–470.
655. Shibata D, Weiss LM, Nathwani BN, et al. Epstein-Barr virus in benign lymph node biopsies from individuals infected with the human immunodeficiency virus is associated with concurrent or subsequent development of non-Hodgkin's lymphoma. *Blood* 1991;77:1527–1533.
656. Alonso ML, Richardson ME, Metroka CE, et al. Chromosome abnormalities in AIDS-associated lymphadenopathy. *Blood* 1987;69:855–858.
657. Mathur-Wagh U, Mildvan D, Senie RT. Follow-up at 41/2 years on homosexual men with generalized lymphadenopathy. *N Engl J Med* 1985;313:1542–1543.
658. Robert NJ, Schneiderman H. Hodgkin's disease and the acquired immunodeficiency syndrome. *Ann Intern Med* 1984;101:142–143.
659. Schoeppel SL, Hoppe RT, Dorfman RF, et al. Hodgkin's disease in homosexual men with generalized lymphadenopathy. *Ann Intern Med* 1985;102:68–70.
660. Scheib RG, Siegel RS. Atypical Hodgkin's disease and the acquired immunodeficiency syndrome. *Ann Intern Med* 1985;102:554.
661. Moore GE, Cook DD. AIDS in association with malignant melanoma and Hodgkin's disease. *J Clin Oncol* 1985;3:1437.
662. Baer DM, Anderson ET, Wilkinson LS. Acquired immune deficiency syndrome in homosexual men with Hodgkin's disease. Three case reports. *Am J Med* 1986;80:738–740.
663. Ranganathan V. Primary rectal Hodgkin's lymphoma: initial manifestation of HIV. *Am J Gastroenterol* 1996;91:180–181.
664. Pallesen G, Hamilton-Dutoit SJ, Rowe M, et al. Expression of Epstein-Barr virus latent gene products in tumour cells of Hodgkin's disease. *Lancet* 1991;337: 320–322.
665. Unger PD, Strauchen JA. Hodgkin's disease in AIDS complex patients. Report of four cases and tissue immunologic marker studies. *Cancer* 1986;58:821–825.
666. Prior E, Goldberg AF, Conjalka MS, et al. Hodgkin's disease in homosexual men. An AIDS-related phenomenon? *Am J Med* 1986;81:1085–1088.
667. Alfonso PG, Sanudo EF, Carretero JM, et al. Hodgkin's disease in HIV-infected patients. *Biomed Pharmacother* 1988;42:321–325.
668. Serrano M, Bellas C, Campo E, et al. Hodgkin's disease in patients with antibodies to human immunodeficiency virus. A study of 22 patients. *Cancer* 1990;65:2248–2254.
669. Gold JE, Altarac D, Ree HJ, et al. HIV-associated Hodgkin disease: a clinical study of 18 cases and review of the literature. *Am J Hematol* 1991;36:93–99.
670. Pelstring RJ, Zellmer RB, Sulak LE, et al. Hodgkin's disease in association with human immunodeficiency virus infection. Pathologic and immunologic features. *Cancer* 1991;67:1865–1873.
671. Karcher DS. Clinically unsuspected Hodgkin disease presenting initially in the bone marrow of patients infected with the human immunodeficiency virus. *Cancer* 1993;71:1235–1238.
672. Newcom SR, Ward M, Napoli VM, et al. Treatment of human immunodeficiency virus-associated Hodgkin disease. Is there a clue regarding the cause of Hodgkin disease? *Cancer* 1993;71:3138–3145.
673. Tirelli U, Vaccher E, Rezza G, et al. Hodgkin disease and infection with the human immunodeficiency virus (HIV) in Italy. *Ann Intern Med* 1988;108:309–310.
674. Roithmann S, Tourani JM, Andrieu JM. Hodgkin's disease in HIV-infected intravenous drug abusers. *N Engl J Med* 1990;323:275–276.

675. Ames ED, Conjalka MS, Goldberg AF, et al. Hodgkin's disease and AIDS. Twenty-three new cases and a review of the literature. *Hematol Oncol Clin North Am* 1991;5:343–356.

676. Garnier G, Taillan B, Michiels JF. HIV-associated Hodgkin disease. *Ann Intern Med* 1991;115:233.

677. Tirelli U, Errante D, Vaccher E, et al. Hodgkin's disease in 92 patients with HIV infection: the Italian experience. GICAT (Italian Cooperative Group on AIDS & Tumors). *Ann Oncol* 1992;3(Suppl 4):69–72.

678. Andrieu JM, Roithmann S, Tourani JM, et al. Hodgkin's disease during HIV1 infection: the French registry experience. French registry of HIV-associated tumors. *Ann Oncol* 1993;4:635–641.

679. Rubio R. Hodgkin's disease associated with human immunodeficiency virus infection. A clinical study of 46 cases. Cooperative Study Group of Malignancies Associated with HIV Infection of Madrid. *Cancer* 1994;73:2400–2407.

680. Tirelli U, Errante D, Dolcetti R, et al. Hodgkin's disease and human immunodeficiency virus infection: clinicopathologic and virologic features of 114 patients from the Italian Cooperative Group on AIDS and Tumors. *J Clin Oncol* 1995;13:1758–1767.

681. Biggar RJ, Jaffe ES, Goedert JJ, et al. Hodgkin lymphoma and immunodeficiency in persons with HIV/AIDS. *Blood* 2006;108:3786–3791.

682. Lanoy E, Rosenberg PS, Fily F, et al. HIV-associated Hodgkin lymphoma during the first months on combination antiretroviral therapy. *Blood* 2011;118:44–49.

683. Clifford GM, Rickenbach M, Lise M, et al. Hodgkin lymphoma in the Swiss HIV Cohort Study. *Blood* 2009;113:5737–5742.

684. Temple JJ, Andes WA. AIDS and Hodgkin's disease. *Lancet* 1986;2:454–455.

685. Serraino D, Carbone A, Franceschi S, et al. Increased frequency of lymphocyte depletion and mixed cellularity subtypes of Hodgkin's disease in HIV-infected patients. Italian Cooperative Group on AIDS and Tumours. *Eur J Cancer* 1993;29A:1948–1950.

686. Doyle TJ, Venkatachalam KK, Maeda K, et al. Hodgkin's disease in renal transplant recipients. *Cancer* 1983;51:245–247.

687. Elenitoba-Johnson KS, Jaffe ES. Lymphoproliferative disorders associated with congenital immunodeficiencies. *Semin Diagn Pathol* 1997;14:35–47.

688. Swerdlow SH. Classification of the posttransplant lymphoproliferative disorders: from the past to the present. *Semin Diagn Pathol* 1997;14:2–7.

689. Biggar RJ, Burnett W, Mikl J, et al. Cancer among New York men at risk of acquired immunodeficiency syndrome. *Int J Cancer* 1989;43:979–985.

690. Hessol NA, Katz MH, Liu JY, et al. Increased incidence of Hodgkin disease in homosexual men with HIV infection. *Ann Intern Med* 1992;117:309–311.

691. Reynolds P, Saunders LD, Layefsky ME, et al. The spectrum of acquired immunodeficiency syndrome (AIDS)-associated malignancies in San Francisco, 1980–1987. *Am J Epidemiol* 1993;137:19–30.

692. Lyter DW, Bryant J, Thackeray R, et al. Incidence of human immunodeficiency virus-related and nonrelated malignancies in a large cohort of homosexual men. *J Clin Oncol* 1995;13:2540–2546.

693. Bello JL, Magallon M, Villar JM. Hodgkin disease in hemophilia. *Ann Intern Med* 1987;107:257.

694. Colby TV, Hoppe RT, Warnke RA. Hodgkin's disease: a clinicopathologic study of 659 cases. *Cancer* 1982;49:1848–1858.

695. Davis S, Dahlberg S, Myers MH, et al. Hodgkin's disease in the United States: a comparison of patient characteristics and survival in the Centralized Cancer Patient Data System and the Surveillance, Epidemiology, and End Results Program. *J Natl Cancer Inst* 1987;78:471–478.

696. Correa P, O'Conor GT. Epidemiologic patterns of Hodgkin's disease. *Int J Cancer* 1971;8:192–201.

697. Riyat MS. Hodgkin's disease in Kenya. *Cancer* 1992;69:1047–1051.

698. Hu E, Hufford S, Lukes R, et al. Third-World Hodgkin's disease at Los Angeles County-University of Southern California Medical Center. *J Clin Oncol* 1988;6:1285–1292.

699. Robison LL, Stoker V, Frizzera G, et al. Hodgkin's disease in pediatric patients with naturally occurring immunodeficiency. *Am J Pediatr Hematol Oncol* 1987;9:189–192.

700. Knowles DM II, Halper JP, Jakobiec FA. T-lymphocyte subpopulations in B-cell-derived non-Hodgkin's lymphomas and Hodgkin's disease. *Cancer* 1984;54:644–651.

701. Greene WC. The molecular biology of human immunodeficiency virus type 1 infection. *N Engl J Med* 1991;324:308–317.

702. Armstrong AA, Weiss LM, Gallagher A, et al. Criteria for the definition of Epstein-Barr virus association in Hodgkin's disease. *Leukemia* 1992;6:869–874.

703. Carbone A, Gloghini A, Zanette I, et al. Co-expression of Epstein-Barr virus latent membrane protein and vimentin in "aggressive" histological subtypes of Hodgkin's disease. *Virchows Arch A Pathol Anat Histopathol* 1993;422:39–45.

704. Glaser SL. Hodgkin's disease in black populations: a review of the epidemiologic literature. *Semin Oncol* 1990;17:643–659.

705. Uccini S, Monardo F, Stoppacciaro A, et al. High frequency of Epstein-Barr virus genome detection in Hodgkin's disease of HIV-positive patients. *Int J Cancer* 1990;46:581–585.

706. Audouin J, Diebold J, Pallesen G. Frequent expression of Epstein-Barr virus latent membrane protein-1 in tumour cells of Hodgkin's disease in HIV-positive patients. *J Pathol* 1992;167:381–384.

707. De Re V, De Vita S, Dolcetti R, et al. Association between B-type Epstein-Barr virus and Hodgkin's disease in immunocompromised patients. *Blood* 1993;82:328–330.

708. Errante D, Zagonel V, Vaccher E, et al. Hodgkin's disease in patients with HIV infection and in the general population: comparison of clinicopathological features and survival. *Ann Oncol* 1994;5(Suppl 2):37–40.

709. Hair LS, Rogers JD, Chadburn A, et al. Intracerebral Hodgkin's disease in a human immunodeficiency virus-seropositive patient. *Cancer* 1991;67:2931–2934.

710. Picard O, de Gramont A, Krulik M, et al. Rectal Hodgkin disease and the acquired immunodeficiency syndrome. *Ann Intern Med* 1987;106:775.

711. Shaw MT, Jacobs SR. Cutaneous Hodgkin's disease in a patient with human immunodeficiency virus infection. *Cancer* 1989;64:2585–2587.

712. Shah BK, Subramaniam S, Peace D, et al. HIV-associated primary bone marrow Hodgkin's lymphoma: a distinct entity? *J Clin Oncol* 2010;28:e459–e460.

713. Canellos GP, Anderson JR, Propert KJ, et al. Chemotherapy of advanced Hodgkin's disease with MOPP, ABVD, or MOPP alternating with ABVD. *N Engl J Med* 1992;327:1478–1484.

714. Bonadonna G, Valagussa P, Santoro A. Alternating non-cross-resistant combination chemotherapy or MOPP in stage IV Hodgkin's disease. A report of 8-year results. *Ann Intern Med* 1986;104:739–746.

715. Urba WJ, Longo DL. Hodgkin's disease. *N Engl J Med* 1992;326:678–687.

716. Errante D, Tirelli U, Gastaldi R, et al. Combined antineoplastic and antiretroviral therapy for patients with Hodgkin's disease and human immunodeficiency virus infection. A prospective study of 17 patients. The Italian Cooperative Group on AIDS and Tumors (GICAT). *Cancer* 1994;73:437–444.

717. Levine AM. HIV-associated Hodgkin's disease. Biologic and clinical aspects. *Hematol Oncol Clin North Am* 1996;10:1135–1148.

718. Notte, DT, Grossman PL, Rosenberg SA, et al. Infections in patients with Hodgkin's disease: a clinical study of 300 consecutive adult patients. *Rev Infect Dis* 1980;2:761–800.

719. Coker DD, Morris DM, Coleman JJ, et al. Infection among 210 patients with surgically staged Hodgkin's disease. *Am J Med* 1983;75:97–109.

720. Mitsuyasu RT, Colman MF, Sun NC. Simultaneous occurrence of Hodgkin's disease and Kaposi's sarcoma in a patient with the acquired immune deficiency syndrome. *Am J Med* 1986;80:954–958.

721. Ernberg I, Bjorkholm M, Zech L, et al. An EBV genome carrying pre-B cell leukemia in a homosexual man with characteristic karyotype and impaired EBV-specific immunity. *J Clin Oncol* 1986;4:1481–1488.

722. Lichtman SM, Brody J, Kaplan MH, et al. Hodgkin's disease and non-Hodgkin's lymphoma in an HIV positive patient. *Leuk Lymphoma* 1993;9:393–398.

723. de Mascarel A, Merlio JP, Laborie V, et al. Hodgkin's disease and malignant lymphoma in acquired immunodeficiency syndrome. *Arch Pathol Lab Med* 1989;113:328.

724. Senaldi E, Lee MH, Toth I, et al. Hodgkin's disease after non-Hodgkin's malignant lymphoma in acquired immune deficiency syndrome. *Cancer* 1990;66:960–964.

725. Carbone A, Gloghini A, Serraino D, et al. HIV-associated Hodgkin lymphoma. *Curr Opin HIV AIDS* 2009;4:3–10.

726. Berman M, Minowada J, Loew JM, et al. Burkitt cell acute lymphoblastic leukemia with partial expression of T-cell markers and subclonal chromosome abnormalities in a man with acquired immunodeficiency syndrome. *Cancer Genet Cytogenet* 1985;16:341–347.

727. Gill PS, Meyer PR, Pavlova Z, et al. B cell acute lymphocytic leukemia in adults. Clinical, morphologic, and immunologic findings. *J Clin Oncol* 1986;4:737–743.

728. Rossi G, Gorla R, Cadeo GP, et al. Acute lymphoblastic leukaemia of B cell origin in an anti-HIV positive intravenous drug abuser. *Br J Haematol* 1988;68:140–141.

729. Flanagan P, Chowdhury V, Costello C. HIV-associated B cell ALL. *Br J Haematol* 1988;69:287.

730. Milpied N, Bourhis JH, Garand R, et al. B cell ALL in an anti-HIV positive patient: achievement of a complete response with aggressive chemotherapy. *Br J Haematol* 1988;70:501–502.

731. Bernheim A, Berger R. Cytogenetic studies of Burkitt lymphoma-leukemia in patients with acquired immunodeficiency syndrome. *Cancer Genet Cytogenet* 1988;32:67–74.

732. Garavelli PL, Azzini M. [Leukosis in HIV infections]. *Minerva Med* 1988;79:105–107.

733. Gold JE, Castella A, Zalusky R. B-cell acute lymphocytic leukemia in HIV-antibody-positive patients. *Am J Hematol* 1989;32:200–204.

734. Gold JE, Babu A, Penchaszadeh V, et al. Hybrid acute leukemia in an HIV-antibody-positive patient. *Am J Hematol* 1989;30:240–247.

735. Arico M, Caselli D, D'Argenio P, et al. Malignancies in children with human immunodeficiency virus type 1 infection. The Italian Multicenter Study on Human Immunodeficiency Virus Infection in Children. *Cancer* 1991;68:2473–2477.

736. Israel AM, Koziner B, Straus DJ. Plasmacytoma and the acquired immunodeficiency syndrome. *Ann Intern Med* 1983;99:635–636.

737. Vandermolen LA, Fehir KM, Rice L. Multiple myeloma in a homosexual man with chronic lymphadenopathy. *Arch Intern Med* 1985;145:745–746.

738. Gold JW, Weikel CS, Godbold J, et al. Unexplained persistent lymphadenopathy in homosexual men and the acquired immune deficiency syndrome. *Medicine (Baltimore)* 1985;64:203–213.

739. Thomas MA, Ibels LS, Wells JV, et al. IgA kappa multiple myeloma and lymphadenopathy syndrome associated with AIDS virus infection. *Aust N Z J Med* 1986;16:402–404.

740. Karnad AB, Martin AW, Koh HK, et al. Nonsecretory multiple myeloma in a 26-year-old man with acquired immunodeficiency syndrome, presenting with multiple extramedullary plasmacytomas and osteolytic bone disease. *Am J Hematol* 1989;32:305–310.

741. Voelkerding KV, Sandhaus LM, Kim HC, et al. Plasma cell malignancy in the acquired immune deficiency syndrome. Association with Epstein-Barr virus. *Am J Clin Pathol* 1989;92:222–228.

742. Gold JE, Schwam L, Castella A, et al. Malignant plasma cell tumors in human immunodeficiency virus-infected patients. *Cancer* 1990;66:363–368.

743. von Keyserlingk H, Baur R, Stein H, et al. Multiple myeloma in a patient at risk for AIDS. *Cancer Detect Prev* 1990;14:403–404.

744. Nogues X, Supervia A, Knobel H, et al. Multiple myeloma and AIDS. *Am J Hematol* 1996;53:210–211.

745. Shokunbi WA, Okpala IE, Shokunbi MT, et al. Multiple myeloma co-existing with HIV-1 infection in a 65-year-old Nigerian man. *AIDS* 1991;5:115–116.

746. Konrad RJ, Kricka LJ, Goodman DB, et al. Brief report: myeloma-associated paraprotein directed against the HIV-1 p24 antigen in an HIV-1-seropositive patient. *N Engl J Med* 1993;328:1817–1819.

747. Pizarro A, Gamallo C, Sanchez-Munoz JF, et al. Extramedullary plasmacytoma and AIDS-related Kaposi's sarcoma. *J Am Acad Dermatol* 1994;30:797–800.

748. Kumar S, Kumar D, Schnadig VJ, et al. Plasma cell myeloma in patients who are HIV-positive. *Am J Clin Pathol* 1994;102:633–639.

749. Ventura G, Lucia MB, Damiano F, et al. Multiple myeloma associated with Epstein-Barr virus in an AIDS patient: a case report. *Eur J Haematol* 1995;55:332–334.

750. Nosari AM, Landonio G, Cantoni S, et al. Multiple myeloma associated to HIV infection: report of two patients. *Eur J Haematol* 1996;56:98–99.

751. Sewell HF, Walker F, Bennett B, et al. Chronic lymphocytic leukaemia contemporaneous with HIV infection. *Br Med J (Clin Res Ed)* 1987;294:938–939.

752. Sheibani K, Ben-Ezra J, Swartz WG, et al. Monocytoid B-cell lymphoma in a patient with human immunodeficiency virus infection. Demonstration of human immunodeficiency virus sequences in paraffin-embedded lymph node sections by polymerase chain reaction amplification. *Arch Pathol Lab Med* 1990;114:1264–1267.

753. Bilgrami S, Shafi N, Pesanti EL, et al. Mantle-cell lymphoma in a patient with human immunodeficiency viral infection. *Acta Haematol* 1995;93:101–104.
754. Presant CA, Gala K, Wiseman C, et al. Human immunodeficiency virus-associated T-cell lymphoblastic lymphoma in AIDS. *Cancer* 1987;60:1459–1461.
755. Baurmann H, Miclea JM, Ferchal F, et al. Adult T-cell leukemia associated with HTLV-I and simultaneous infection by human immunodeficiency virus type 2 and human herpesvirus 6 in an African woman: a clinical, virologic, and familial serologic study. *Am J Med* 1988;85:853–857.
756. Nasr SA, Brynes RK, Garrison CP, et al. Peripheral T-cell lymphoma in a patient with acquired immune deficiency syndrome. *Cancer* 1988;61:947–951.
757. Lust JA, Banks PM, Hooper WC, et al. T-cell non-Hodgkin lymphoma in human immunodeficiency virus-1-infected individuals. *Am J Hematol* 1989;31:181–187.
758. Ruff P, Bagg A, Papadopoulos K. Precursor T-cell lymphoma associated with human immunodeficiency virus type 1 (HIV-1) infection. First reported case. *Cancer* 1989;64:39–42.
759. Shibata D, Brynes RK, Rabinowitz A, et al. Human T-cell lymphotropic virus type I (HTLV-I)-associated adult T-cell leukemia-lymphoma in a patient infected with human immunodeficiency virus type 1 (HIV-1). *Ann Intern Med* 1989;111: 871–875.
760. Parker SC, Fenton DA, McGibbon DH. Homme rouge and the acquired immunodeficiency syndrome. *N Engl J Med* 1989;321:906–907.
761. Goldstein J, Becker N, DelRowe J, et al. Cutaneous T-cell lymphoma in a patient infected with human immunodeficiency virus type 1. Use of radiation therapy. *Cancer* 1990;66:1130–1132.
762. Crane GA, Variakojis D, Rosen ST, et al. Cutaneous T-cell lymphoma in patients with human immunodeficiency virus infection. *Arch Dermatol* 1991;127: 989–994.
763. Nahass GT, Kraffert CA, Penneys NS. Cutaneous T-cell lymphoma associated with the acquired immunodeficiency syndrome. *Arch Dermatol* 1991;127:1020–1022.
764. Gonzalez-Clemente JM, Ribera JM, Campo E, et al. Ki-1+ anaplastic large-cell lymphoma of T-cell origin in an HIV-infected patient. *AIDS* 1991;5:751–755.
765. Diekman MJ, Bresser P, Noorduyn LA, et al. Spontaneous regression of Ki-1 positive T-cell non-Hodgkin's lymphoma in a patient with HIV infection. *Br J Haematol* 1992;82:477–478.
766. Herndier BG, Shiramizu BT, Jewett NE, et al. Acquired immunodeficiency syndrome-associated T-cell lymphoma: evidence for human immunodeficiency virus type 1-associated T-cell transformation. *Blood* 1992;79:1768–1774.
767. Burns MK, Cooper KD. Cutaneous T-cell lymphoma associated with HIV infection. *J Am Acad Dermatol* 1993;29:394–399.
768. Dreno B, Milpied-Homsi B, Moreau P, et al. Cutaneous anaplastic T-cell lymphoma in a patient with human immunodeficiency virus infection: detection of Epstein-Barr virus DNA. *Br J Dermatol* 1993;129:77–81.
769. Berger TG, Kerschmann RL, Roth R, et al. Sezary's syndrome and human immunodeficiency virus infection. *Arch Dermatol* 1995;131:739–741.
770. Kerschmann RL, Berger TG, Weiss LM, et al. Cutaneous presentations of lymphoma in human immunodeficiency virus disease. Predominance of T cell lineage. *Arch Dermatol* 1995;131:1281–1288.
771. Montilla P, Dronda F, Moreno S, et al. Lymphomatoid granulomatosis and the acquired immunodeficiency syndrome. *Ann Intern Med* 1987;106:166–167.
772. Anders KH, Latta H, Chang BS, et al. Lymphomatoid granulomatosis and malignant lymphoma of the central nervous system in the acquired immunodeficiency syndrome. *Hum Pathol* 1989;20:326–334.
773. Gold JE, Ghali V, Gold S, et al. Angiocentric immunoproliferative lesion/T-cell non-Hodgkin's lymphoma and the acquired immune deficiency syndrome: a case report and review of the literature. *Cancer* 1990;66:2407–2413.
774. Napoli VM, Stein SF, Spira TJ, et al. Myelodysplasia progressing to acute myeloblastic leukemia in an HTLV-III virus-positive homosexual man with AIDS-related complex. *Am J Clin Pathol* 1986;86:788–791.
775. Darne C, Solal-Celigny P, Herrera A, et al. Acute myelofibrosis and infection with the lymphadenopathy-associated virus/human T-lymphotropic virus type III. *Ann Intern Med* 1986;104:130–131.
776. Solal-Celigny P, Leporrier, M, Brousse N, et al. [Myeloid splenomegaly and LAV/HTLVIII virus infection]. *Nouv Rev Fr Hematol* 1986;28:163–169.
777. Willumsen L, Ellegaard J, Pedersen B. HIV infection in acute myeloblastic leukemia: a similar case. *Am J Clin Pathol* 1987;88:536–537.
778. Diebold J, Audouin J. [Malignant lymphomas and other malignant proliferations in hematopoietic organs in HIV-positive patients]. *Arch Anat Cytol Pathol* 1988;36:5–11.
779. Monfardini S, Vaccher E, Pizzocaro G, et al. Unusual malignant tumours in 49 patients with HIV infection. *AIDS* 1989;3:449–452.
780. Wijermans PW, ten Kate RW. Successful chemotherapy for acute myeloid leucaemia in HIV-infected patients. *Eur J Haematol* 1990;44:136–138.
781. Peters BS, Matthews J, Gompels M, et al. Acute myeloblastic leukaemia in AIDS. *AIDS* 1990;4:367–368.
782. Puppo F, Scudeletti M, Murgia L, et al. Acute myelomonocytic leukaemia in an HIV-infected patient. *AIDS* 1992;6:136–137.
783. Murthy AR, Ho D, Goetz MB. Relationship between acute myelomonoblastic leukemia and infection due to human immunodeficiency virus. *Rev Infect Dis* 1991;13:254–256.
784. Mansberg R, Rowlings PA, Yip MY, et al. First and second complete remissions in a HIV positive patient following remission induction therapy for acute non-lymphoblastic leukaemia. *Aust N Z J Med* 1991;21:55–57.
785. Rivers JK, Laubenstein LJ, Postel AH. Acute monocytic leukaemia in a HIV-seropositive man. *Clin Exp Dermatol* 1992;17:203–205.
786. De la Salmoniere P, Janier M, Gilquin J, et al. Chicken pox and acute monocytic leukaemia skin lesions in an HIV-seropositive man. *Clin Exp Dermatol* 1994;19:505–506.
787. Rabaud C, Dorvaux V, May T, et al. Acute myelogenous leukaemia followed by non-Hodgkin's lymphoma in a patient with AIDs. *J Infect* 1995;31:69–70.
788. Milling DL, Lazarchick J, Chaudhary UB. Primary mediastinal large B-cell lymphoma in an HIV-infected patient. *Am J Med Sci* 2005;329:136–138.
789. Sasser RL, Yam LT, Li CY. Myeloma with involvement of the serous cavities. Cytologic and immunochemical diagnosis and literature review. *Acta Cytol* 1990;34:479–485.
790. Kyle RA. Multiple myeloma: review of 869 cases. *Mayo Clin Proc* 1975;50:29–40.
791. Meis JM, Butler JJ, Osborne BM, et al. Solitary plasmacytomas of bone and extramedullary plasmacytomas. A clinicopathologic and immunohistochemical study. *Cancer* 1987;59:1475–1485.
792. Salahuddin SZ, Ablashi DV, Hunter EA, et al. HTLV-III infection of EBV-genome-positive B-lymphoid cells with or without detectable T4 antigens. *Int J Cancer* 1987;39:198–202.
793. Potter M, Mushinski JF, Mushinski EB, et al. Avian v-myc replaces chromosomal translocation in murine plasmacytomagenesis. *Science* 1987;235:787–789.
794. Blum S, Singh TP, Gibbons J, et al. Trends in survival among persons with acquired immunodeficiency syndrome in New York City. The experience of the first decade of the epidemic. *Am J Epidemiol* 1994;139:351–361.
795. Update: trends in AIDS incidence, deaths, and prevalence—United States, 1996. *MMWR Morb Mortal Wkly Rep* 1997;46:165–173.
796. Arcaini L, Sacchi P, Jemos V, et al. Splenic marginal zone B-cell lymphoma in a HIV-positive patient: a case report. *Ann Hematol* 2009;88:379–381.
797. Horning SJ, Rosenberg SA. The natural history of initially untreated low-grade non-Hodgkin's lymphomas. *N Engl J Med* 1984;311:1471–1475.
798. Ciobanu N, Andreeff M, Safai B, et al. Lymphoblastic neoplasia in a homosexual patient with Kaposi's sarcoma. *Ann Intern Med* 1983;98:151–155.
799. Kobayashi M, Yoshimoto S, Fujishita M, et al. HTLV-positive T-cell lymphoma/leukaemia in an AIDS patient. *Lancet* 1984;1:1361–1362.
800. Howard MR, McVerry BA. T-cell lymphoma in a haemophiliac positive for antibody to HIV. *Br J Haematol* 1987;67:115.
801. Sternlieb J, Mintzer D, Kwa D, et al. Peripheral T-cell lymphoma in a patient with the acquired immunodeficiency syndrome. *Am J Med* 1988;85:445.
802. Taylor JM, Fahey JL, Detels R, et al. CD4 percentage, CD4 number, and CD4:CD8 ratio in HIV infection: which to choose and how to use. *J Acquir Immune Defic Syndr* 1989;2:114–124.
803. Beljaards RC, Kaudewitz P, Berti E, et al. Primary cutaneous CD30-positive large cell lymphoma: definition of a new type of cutaneous lymphoma with a favorable prognosis. A European Multicenter Study of 47 patients. *Cancer* 1993;71: 2097–2104.
804. Reynolds CW, Foon KA. T gamma-lymphoproliferative disease and related disorders in humans and experimental animals: a review of the clinical, cellular, and functional characteristics. *Blood* 1984;64:1146–1158.
805. Ghali V, Castella A, Louis-Charles A, et al. Expansion of large granular lymphocytes (natural killer cells) with limited antigen expression (CD2+, CD3-, CD4-, CD8-, CD16+, NKH-1-) in a human immunodeficiency virus-positive homosexual man. *Cancer* 1990;65:2243–2247.
806. Copie-Bergman C, Megnin V, Gilardin L, et al. The distribution of peripheral T-cell lymphoma in the context of HIV infection differs from that seen in non-immunocompromised patients: a retrospective study of 32 cases. *J Hematopathol* 2012;5:235.
807. Oksenhendler E, Autran B, Gorochov G, et al. CD8 lymphocytosis and pseudotumoral splenomegaly in HIV infection. *Lancet* 1992;340:207–208.
808. Goddart D, Francois A, Ninane J, et al. Parotid gland abnormality found in children seropositive for the human immunodeficiency virus (HIV). *Pediatr Radiol* 1990;20:355–357.
809. Lippman SM, Grogan TM, Carry P, et al. Post-transplantation T cell lymphoblastic lymphoma. *Am J Med* 1987;82:814–816.
810. Garvin AJ, Self S, Sahovic EA, et al. The occurrence of a peripheral T-cell lymphoma in a chronically immunosuppressed renal transplant patient. *Am J Surg Pathol* 1988;12:64–70.
811. Ulrich W, Chott A, Watschinger B, et al. Primary peripheral T cell lymphoma in a kidney transplant under immunosuppression with cyclosporine A. *Hum Pathol* 1989;20:1027–1030.
812. Griffith RC, Saha BK, Janney CM, et al. Immunoblastic lymphoma of T-cell type in a chronically immunosuppressed renal transplant recipient. *Am J Clin Pathol* 1990;93:280–285.
813. Kemnitz J, Cremer J, Gebel M, et al. T-cell lymphoma after heart transplantation. *Am J Clin Pathol* 1990;94:95–101.
814. De Rossi A, Gassa OD, del Mistro A, et al. HTLV-III and HTLV-I infection in populations at risk in the Veneto region of Italy. *Eur J Cancer Clin Oncol* 1986;22: 411–418.
815. Bartholomew C, Saxinger WC, Clark JW, et al. Transmission of HTLV-I and HIV among homosexual men in Trinidad. *JAMA* 1987;257:2604–2608.
816. Cortes E, Detels R, Aboulafia D, et al. HIV-1, HIV-2, and HTLV-I infection in high-risk groups in Brazil. *N Engl J Med* 1989;320:953–958.
817. Stevenson M, Volsky B, Hedenskog M, et al. Immortalization of human T lymphocytes after transfection of Epstein-Barr virus DNA. *Science* 1986;233:980–984.
818. Harabuchi Y, Yamanaka N, Kataura A, et al. Epstein-Barr virus in nasal T-cell lymphomas in patients with lethal midline granuloma. *Lancet* 1990;335: 128–130.
819. Jones JF, Shurin S, Abramowsky C, et al. T-cell lymphomas containing Epstein-Barr viral DNA in patients with chronic Epstein-Barr virus infections. *N Engl J Med* 1988;318:733–741.
820. Schneider DR, Picker LJ. Myelodysplasia in the acquired immune deficiency syndrome. *Am J Clin Pathol* 1985;84:144–152.
821. Spector BD, Perry GS III, Kersey JH. Genetically determined immunodeficiency diseases (GDID) and malignancy: report from the immunodeficiency—cancer registry. *Clin Immunol Immunopathol* 1978;11:12–29.
822. Levy JA, Shimabukuro J, McHugh T, et al. AIDS-associated retroviruses (ARV) can productively infect other cells besides human T helper cells. *Virology* 1985;147: 441–448.
823. Clapham PR, Weiss RA, Dalgleish AG, et al. Human immunodeficiency virus infection of monocytic and T-lymphocytic cells: receptor modulation and differentiation induced by phorbol ester. *Virology* 1987;158:44–51.
824. Folks TM, Kessler SW, Orenstein JM, et al. Infection and replication of HIV-1 in purified progenitor cells of normal human bone marrow. *Science* 1988;242: 919–922.
825. Kaposi M. Idiopatisches multiples Pigmentsarkom der Haut. *Arch Dermatol Syphillis* 1872;4:265–273.
826. Friedman-Kien AE, Laubenstein LJ, Rubinstein P, et al. Disseminated Kaposi's sarcoma in homosexual men. *Ann Intern Med* 1982;96:693–700.
827. 1993 revised classification system for HIV infection and expanded surveillance case definition for AIDS among adolescents and adults. *MMWR Recomm Rep* 1992;41:1–19.
828. Sinfield RL, Molyneux EM, Banda K, et al. Spectrum and presentation of pediatric malignancies in the HIV era: experience from Blantyre, Malawi, 1998–2003. *Pediatr Blood Cancer* 2007;48:515–520.
829. Gallo RC. The enigmas of Kaposi's sarcoma. *Science* 1998;282:1837–1839.

830. Whitby D, Howard MR, Tenant-Flowers M, et al. Detection of Kaposi's sarcoma associated herpesvirus in peripheral blood of HIV-infected individuals and progression to Kaposi's sarcoma. *Lancet* 1995;346:799–802.

831. Beral V, Peterman TA, Berkelman RL, et al. Kaposi's sarcoma among persons with AIDS: a sexually transmitted infection? *Lancet* 1990;335:123–128.

832. Eltom MA, Jemal A, Mbulaiteye SM, et al. Trends in Kaposi's sarcoma and non-Hodgkin's lymphoma incidence in the United States from 1973 through 1998. *J Natl Cancer Inst* 2002;94:1204–1210.

833. Krown SE. AIDS-associated Kaposi's sarcoma: pathogenesis, clinical course and treatment. *AIDS* 1988;2:71–80.

834. Dezube BJ. Clinical presentation and natural history of AIDS—related Kaposi's sarcoma. *Hematol Oncol Clin North Am* 1996;10:1023–1029.

835. Gill PS, Loureiro C, Bernstein-Singer M, et al. Clinical effect of glucocorticoids on Kaposi sarcoma related to the acquired immunodeficiency syndrome (AIDS). *Ann Intern Med* 1989;110:937–940.

836. Ioachim HL, Adsay V, Giancotti FR, et al. Kaposi's sarcoma of internal organs. A multiparameter study of 86 cases. *Cancer* 1995;75:1376–1385.

837. Rabkin CS, Bedi G, Musaba E, et al. AIDS-related Kaposi's sarcoma is a clonal neoplasm. *Clin Cancer Res* 1995;1:257–260.

838. Nichols CM, Flaitz CM, Hicks MJ. Treating Kaposi's lesions in the HIV-infected patient. *J Am Dent Assoc* 1993;124:78–84.

839. Steis RG, Longo DL. Clinical, biologic, and therapeutic aspects of malignancies associated with the acquired immunodeficiency syndrome: Part I and Part II. *Ann Allergy* 1988;60:310–323.

840. Cockerell CJ. Histopathological features of Kaposi's sarcoma in HIV infected individuals. *Cancer Surv* 1991;10:73–89.

841. Lubin J, Rywlin AM. Lymphoma-like lymph node changes in Kaposi's sarcoma. Two additional cases. *Arch Pathol* 1971;92:338–341.

842. Amazon K, Rywlin AM. Subtle clues to diagnosis by conventional microscopy. Lymph node involvement in Kaposi's sarcoma. *Am J Dermatopathol* 1979;1:173–176.

843. Rutgers JL, Wieczorek R, Bonetti F, et al. The expression of endothelial cell surface antigens by AIDS-associated Kaposi's sarcoma. Evidence for a vascular endothelial cell origin. *Am J Pathol* 1986;122:493–499.

844. Scully PA, Steinman HK, Kennedy C, et al. AIDS-related Kaposi's sarcoma displays differential expression of endothelial surface antigens. *Am J Pathol* 1988;130:244–251.

845. Beckstead JH, Wood GS, Fletcher V. Evidence for the origin of Kaposi's sarcoma from lymphatic endothelium. *Am J Pathol* 1985;119:294–300.

846. Dorfman RF. Kaposi's sarcoma: evidence supporting its origin from the lymphatic system. *Lymphology* 1988;21:45–52.

847. Jussila L, Valtola R, Partanen TA, et al. Lymphatic endothelium and Kaposi's sarcoma spindle cells detected by antibodies against the vascular endothelial growth factor receptor-3. *Cancer Res* 1998;58:1599–1604.

848. Weninger W, Partanen TA, Breiteneder-Geleff S, et al. Expression of vascular endothelial growth factor receptor-3 and podoplanin suggests a lymphatic endothelial cell origin of Kaposi's sarcoma tumor cells. *Lab Invest* 1999;79:243–251.

849. Wang HW, Trotter MW, Lagos D, et al. Kaposi sarcoma herpesvirus-induced cellular reprogramming contributes to the lymphatic endothelial gene expression in Kaposi sarcoma. *Nat Genet* 2004;36:687–693.

850. Mesri EA, Cesarman E, Boshoff C. Kaposi's sarcoma and its associated herpesvirus. *Nat Rev Cancer* 2010;10:707–719.

851. Mesri EA, Cesarman E. Kaposi's sarcoma herpesvirus oncogenesis is a notch better in 3D. *Cell Host Microbe* 2011;10:529–531.

852. Beral V, Bull D, Darby S, et al. Risk of Kaposi's sarcoma and sexual practices associated with faecal contact in homosexual or bisexual men with AIDS. *Lancet* 1992;339:632–635.

853. Giraldo G, Beth E, Haguenau F. Herpes-type virus particles in tissue culture of Kaposi's sarcoma from different geographic regions. *J Natl Cancer Inst* 1972;49:1509–1526.

854. Huang YQ, Li JJ, Kaplan MH, et al. Human herpesvirus-like nucleic acid in various forms of Kaposi's sarcoma. *Lancet* 1995;345:759–761.

855. Schalling M, Ekman M, Kaaya EE, et al. A role for a new herpes virus (KSHV) in different forms of Kaposi's sarcoma. *Nat Med* 1995;1:707–708.

856. Boshoff C, Schulz TF, Kennedy MM, et al. Kaposi's sarcoma-associated herpesvirus infects endothelial and spindle cells. *Nat Med* 1995;1:1274–1278.

857. Reed JA, Nador RG, Spaulding D, et al. Demonstration of Kaposi's sarcoma-associated herpes virus cyclin D homolog in cutaneous Kaposi's sarcoma by colorimetric in situ hybridization using a catalyzed signal amplification system. *Blood* 1998;91:3825–3832.

858. Kellam P, Bourboulia D, Dupin N, et al. Characterization of monoclonal antibodies raised against the latent nuclear antigen of human herpesvirus 8. *J Virol* 1999;73:5149–5155.

859. Fredericks DN, Relman DA. Sequence-based identification of microbial pathogens: a reconsideration of Koch's postulates. *Clin Microbiol Rev* 1996;9:18–33.

860. Hill AB. The Environment and Disease: Association or Causation? *Proc R Soc Med* 1965;58:295–300.

861. Sarid R, Gao SJ. Viruses and human cancer: from detection to causality. *Cancer Lett* 305:218–227.

862. Gao SJ, Kingsley L, Hoover DR, et al. Seroconversion to antibodies against Kaposi's sarcoma-associated herpesvirus-related latent nuclear antigens before the development of Kaposi's sarcoma. *N Engl J Med* 1996;335:233–241.

863. Grossmann C, Podgrabinska S, Skobe M, et al. Activation of NF-kappaB by the latent vFLIP gene of Kaposi's sarcoma-associated herpesvirus is required for the spindle shape of virus-infected endothelial cells and contributes to their proinflammatory phenotype. *J Virol* 2006;80:7179–7185.

864. Glykofrydes D, Niphuis H, Kuhn EM, et al. Herpesvirus saimiri vFLIP provides an antiapoptotic function but is not essential for viral replication, transformation, or pathogenicity. *J Virol* 2000;74:11919–11927.

865. Efklidou S, Bailey R, Field N, et al. vFLIP from KSHV inhibits anoikis of primary endothelial cells. *J Cell Sci* 2008;121:450–457.

866. Cesarman E, Mesri EA, Gershengorn MC. Viral G protein-coupled receptor and Kaposi's sarcoma: a model of paracrine neoplasia? *J Exp Med* 2000;191:417–422.

867. Boshoff C, Endo Y, Collins PD, et al. Angiogenic and HIV-inhibitory functions of KSHV-encoded chemokines. *Science* 1997;278:290–294.

868. Aoki Y, Jaffe ES, Chang Y, et al. Angiogenesis and hematopoiesis induced by Kaposi's sarcoma-associated herpesvirus-encoded interleukin-6. *Blood* 1999;93:4034–4043.

869. Bais C, Santomasso B, Coso O, et al. G-protein-coupled receptor of Kaposi's sarcoma-associated herpesvirus is a viral oncogene and angiogenesis activator. *Nature* 1998;391:86–89.

870. Yang TY, Chen SC, Leach MW, et al. Transgenic expression of the chemokine receptor encoded by human herpesvirus 8 induces an angioproliferative disease resembling Kaposi's sarcoma. *J Exp Med* 2000;191:445–454.

871. Montaner S, Sodhi A, Molinolo A, et al. Endothelial infection with KSHV genes in vivo reveals that vGPCR initiates Kaposi's sarcomagenesis and can promote the tumorigenic potential of viral latent genes. *Cancer Cell* 2003;3:23–36.

872. Levine AM. HIV-associated lymphoma. *Blood* 2010;115:2986–2987.

873. Lim ST, Karim R, Tulpule A, et al. Prognostic factors in HIV-related diffuse large-cell lymphoma: before versus after highly active antiretroviral therapy. *J Clin Oncol* 2005;23:8477–8482.

874. McKhann CF. Primary malignancy in patients undergoing immunosuppression for renal transplantation. *Transplantation* 1969;8:209–212.

875. Hoover R, Fraumeni JF Jr. Risk of cancer in renal-transplant recipients. *Lancet* 1973;2:55–57.

876. Penn I. Cancer is a complication of severe immunosuppression. *Surg Gynecol Obstet* 1986;162:603–610.

877. Crawford DH, Thomas JA, Janossy G, et al. Epstein Barr virus nuclear antigen positive lymphoma after cyclosporin A treatment in patient with renal allograft. *Lancet* 1980;1:1355–1356.

878. Nagington J, Gray J. Cyclosporin A immunosuppression, Epstein-Barr antibody, and lymphoma. *Lancet* 1980;1:536–537.

879. Penn I. Malignancies associated with immunosuppressive or cytotoxic therapy. *Surgery* 1978;83:492–502.

880. Hanto DW, Frizzera G, Purtilo DT, et al. Clinical spectrum of lymphoproliferative disorders in renal transplant recipients and evidence for the role of Epstein-Barr virus. *Cancer Res* 1981;41:4253–4261.

881. Purtilo DT. Epstein-Barr-virus-induced oncogenesis in immune-deficient individuals. *Lancet* 1980;1:300–303.

882. Starzl TE, Nalesnik MA, Porter KA, et al. Reversibility of lymphomas and lymphoproliferative lesions developing under cyclosporin-steroid therapy. *Lancet* 1984;1:583–587.

883. Kremer BE, Reshef R, Misleh JG, et al. Post-transplant lymphoproliferative disorder after lung transplantation: a review of 35 cases. *J Heart Lung Transplant* 2012;31:296–304.

884. Shapiro RS, McClain K, Frizzera G, et al. Epstein-Barr virus associated B cell lymphoproliferative disorders following bone marrow transplantation. *Blood* 1988;71:1234–1243.

885. Zutter MM, Martin PJ, Sale GE, et al. Epstein-Barr virus lymphoproliferation after bone marrow transplantation. *Blood* 1988;72:520–529.

886. Benkerrou M, Jais JP, Leblond V, et al. Anti-B-cell monoclonal antibody treatment of severe posttransplant B-lymphoproliferative disorder: prognostic factors and long-term outcome. *Blood* 1998;92:3137–3147.

887. Le Frere-Belda MA, Martin N, Gaulard P, et al. Donor or recipient origin of post-transplantation lymphoproliferative disorders: evaluation by in situ hybridization. *Mod Pathol* 1997;10:701–707.

888. Lones MA, Kirov I, Said JW, et al. Post-transplant lymphoproliferative disorder after autologous peripheral stem cell transplantation in a pediatric patient. *Bone Marrow Transplant* 2000;26:1021–1024.

889. Schouten HC, Hopman AH, Haesevoets AM, et al. Large-cell anaplastic non-Hodgkin's lymphoma originating in donor cells after allogenic bone marrow transplantation. *Br J Haematol* 1995;91:162–166.

890. Trimble MS, Waye JS, Walker IR, et al. B-cell lymphoma of recipient origin 9 years after allogeneic bone marrow transplantation for T-cell acute lymphoblastic leukaemia. *Br J Haematol* 1993;85:99–102.

891. O'Riordan JM, Molloy K, O'Briain DS, et al. Localized, late-onset, high-grade lymphoma following bone marrow transplantation: response to combination chemotherapy. *Br J Haematol* 1994;86:183–186.

892. Chadburn A, Suciu-Foca N, Cesarman E, et al. Post-transplantation lymphoproliferative disorders arising in solid organ transplant recipients are usually of recipient origin. *Am J Pathol* 1995;147:1862–1870.

893. Bhatia S, Ramsay NK, Steinbuch M, et al. Malignant neoplasms following bone marrow transplantation. *Blood* 1996;87:3633–3639.

894. Micallef IN, Chhanabhai M, Gascoyne RD, et al. Lymphoproliferative disorders following allogeneic bone marrow transplantation: the Vancouver experience. *Bone Marrow Transplant* 1998;22:981–987.

895. Witherspoon RP, Fisher LD, Schoch G, et al. Secondary cancers after bone marrow transplantation for leukemia or aplastic anemia. *N Engl J Med* 1989;321:784–789.

896. Hale G, Waldmann H. Risks of developing Epstein-Barr virus-related lymphoproliferative disorders after T-cell-depleted marrow transplants. CAMPATH Users. *Blood* 1998;91:3079–3083.

897. Aguilar LK, Rooney CM, Heslop HE. Lymphoproliferative disorders involving Epstein-Barr virus after hemopoietic stem cell transplantation. *Curr Opin Oncol* 1999;11:96–101.

898. Deeg HJ, Socie G. Malignancies after hematopoietic stem cell transplantation: many questions, some answers. *Blood* 1998;91:1833–1844.

899. Penn I. The problem of cancer in organ transplant recipients: an overview. *Transplant Sci* 1994;4:23–32.

900. Leblond V, Sutton L, Dorent R, et al. Lymphoproliferative disorders after organ transplantation: a report of 24 cases observed in a single center. *J Clin Oncol* 1995;13:961–968.

901. Morrison VA, Dunn DL, Manivel JC, et al. Clinical characteristics of post-transplant lymphoproliferative disorders. *Am J Med* 1994;97:14–24.

902. Ferry JA, Jacobson JO, Conti D, et al. Lymphoproliferative disorders and hematologic malignancies following organ transplantation. *Mod Pathol* 1989;2:583–592.

903. Mihalov ML, Gattuso P, Abraham K, et al. Incidence of post-transplant malignancy among 674 solid-organ-transplant recipients at a single center. *Clin Transplant* 1996;10:248–255.

904. Nalesnik MA. Clinical and pathological features of post-transplant lymphoproliferative disorders (PTLD). *Springer Semin Immunopathol* 1998;20:325–342.

905. Opelz G, Henderson R. Incidence of non-Hodgkin lymphoma in kidney and heart transplant recipients. *Lancet* 1993;342:1514–1516.

906. Melosky B, Karim M, Chui A, et al. Lymphoproliferative disorders after renal transplantation in patients receiving triple or quadruple immunosuppression. *J Am Soc Nephrol* 1992;2:S290–S294.

907. Ciancio G, Siquijor AP, Burke GW, et al. Post-transplant lymphoproliferative disease in kidney transplant patients in the new immunosuppressive era. *Clin Transplant* 1997;11:243–249.

908. Birkeland SA, Bendtzen K, Moller B, et al. Interleukin-10 and posttransplant lymphoproliferative disorder after kidney transplantation. *Transplantation* 1999;67:876–881.

909. Swinnen LJ, Mullen GM, Carr TJ, et al. Aggressive treatment for postcardiac transplant lymphoproliferation. *Blood* 1995;86:3333–3340.

910. Armitage JM, Kormos RL, Stuart RS, et al. Posttransplant lymphoproliferative disease in thoracic organ transplant patients: ten years of cyclosporine-based immunosuppression. *J Heart Lung Transplant* 1991;10:877–886; discussion 886–887.

911. Aris RM, Maia DM, Neuringer IP, et al. Post-transplantation lymphoproliferative disorder in the Epstein-Barr virus-naive lung transplant recipient. *Am J Respir Crit Care Med* 1996;154:1712–1717.

912. Randhawa PS, Yousem SA, Paradis IL, et al. The clinical spectrum, pathology, and clonal analysis of Epstein-Barr virus-associated lymphoproliferative disorders in heart-lung transplant recipients. *Am J Clin Pathol* 1989;92:177–185.

913. Finn L, Reyes J, Bueno J, et al. Epstein-Barr virus infections in children after transplantation of the small intestine. *Am J Surg Pathol* 1998;22:299–309.

914. Ho M, Jaffe R, Miller G, et al. The frequency of Epstein-Barr virus infection and associated lymphoproliferative syndrome after transplantation and its manifestations in children. *Transplantation* 1988;45:719–727.

915. Boyle GJ, Michaels MG, Webber SA, et al. Posttransplantation lymphoproliferative disorders in pediatric thoracic organ recipients. *J Pediatr* 1997;131:309–313.

916. Davey DD, Kamat D, Laszewski M, et al. Epstein-Barr virus-related lymphoproliferative disorders following bone marrow transplantation: an immunologic and genotypic analysis. *Mod Pathol* 1989;2:27–34.

917. Deeg HJ, Socie G, Schoch G, et al. Malignancies after marrow transplantation for aplastic anemia and fanconi anemia: a joint Seattle and Paris analysis of results in 700 patients. *Blood* 1996;87:386–392.

918. Gross TG, Steinbuch M, DeFor T, et al. B cell lymphoproliferative disorders following hematopoietic stem cell transplantation: risk factors, treatment and outcome. *Bone Marrow Transplant* 1999;23:251–258.

919. Orazi A, Hromas RA, Neiman RS, et al. Posttransplantation lymphoproliferative disorders in bone marrow transplant recipients are aggressive diseases with a high incidence of adverse histologic and immunobiologic features. *Am J Clin Pathol* 1997;107:419–429.

920. Lucas KG, Small TN, Heller G, et al. The development of cellular immunity to Epstein-Barr virus after allogeneic bone marrow transplantation. *Blood* 1996;87:2594–2603.

921. Peniket AJ, Perry AR, Williams CD, et al. A case of EBV-associated lymphoproliferative disease following high-dose therapy and CD34-purified autologous peripheral blood progenitor cell transplantation. *Bone Marrow Transplant* 1998;22:307–309.

922. Anderson KC, Soiffer R, DeLage R, et al. T-cell-depleted autologous bone marrow transplantation therapy: analysis of immune deficiency and late complications. *Blood* 1990;76:235–244.

923. Shepherd JD, Gascoyne RD, Barnett MJ, et al. Polyclonal Epstein-Barr virus-associated lymphoproliferative disorder following autografting for chronic myeloid leukemia. *Bone Marrow Transplant* 1995;15:639–641.

924. Basgoz N, Preiksaitis JK. Post-transplant lymphoproliferative disorder. *Infect Dis Clin North Am* 1995;9:901–923.

925. Nalesnik MA, Starzl TE. Epstein-Barr virus, infectious mononucleosis, and post-transplant lymphoproliferative disorders. *Transplant Sci* 1994;4:61–79.

926. Hanto DW, Gajl-Peczalska KJ, Frizzera G, et al. Epstein-Barr virus (EBV) induced polyclonal and monoclonal B-cell lymphoproliferative diseases occurring after renal transplantation. Clinical, pathologic, and virologic findings and implications for therapy. *Ann Surg* 1983;198:356–369.

927. Weintraub J, Warnke RA. Lymphoma in cardiac allotransplant recipients. Clinical and histological features and immunological phenotype. *Transplantation* 1982;33:347–351.

928. Calne RY, Rolles K, White DJ, et al. Cyclosporin A initially as the only immunosuppressant in 34 recipients of cadaveric organs: 32 kidneys, 2 pancreases, and 2 livers. *Lancet* 1979;2:1033–1036.

929. Cockburn I. Assessment of the risks of malignancy and lymphomas developing in patients using Sandimmune. *Transplant Proc* 1987;19:1804–1807.

930. Boubenider S, Hiesse C, Goupy C, et al. Incidence and consequences of post-transplantation lymphoproliferative disorders. *J Nephrol* 1997;10:136–145.

931. Kahan BD, Flechner SM, Lorber MI, et al. Complications of cyclosporin therapy. *World J Surg* 1986;10:348–360.

932. Praghakaran K, Wise B, Chen A, et al. Rational management of posttransplant lymphoproliferative disorder in pediatric recipients. *J Pediatr Surg* 1999;34:112–115; discussion 115–116.

933. Wilkinson AH, Smith JL, Hunsicker LG, et al. Increased frequency of posttransplant lymphomas in patients treated with cyclosporine, azathioprine, and prednisone. *Transplantation* 1989;47:293–296.

934. Smith JL, Wilkinson AH, Hunsicker LG, et al. Increased frequency of posttransplant lymphomas in patients treated with cyclosporin, azathioprine, and prednisone. *Transplant Proc* 1989;21:3199–200.

935. Swinnen LJ, Costanzo-Nordin MR, Fisher SG, et al. Increased incidence of lymphoproliferative disorder after immunosuppression with the monoclonal antibody OKT3 in cardiac-transplant recipients. *N Engl J Med* 1990;323:1723–1728.

936. Walker RC, Paya CV, Marshall WF, et al. Pretransplantation seronegative Epstein-Barr virus status is the primary risk factor for posttransplantation lymphoproliferative disorder in adult heart, lung, and other solid organ transplantations. *J Heart Lung Transplant* 1995;14:214–221.

937. Savoie A, Perpete C, Carpentier L, et al. Direct correlation between the load of Epstein-Barr virus-infected lymphocytes in the peripheral blood of pediatric transplant patients and risk of lymphoproliferative disease. *Blood* 1994;83:2715–2722.

938. Walker RC, Marshall WF, Strickler JG, et al. Pretransplantation assessment of the risk of lymphoproliferative disorder. *Clin Infect Dis* 1995;20:1346–1353.

939. Chadburn A, Cesarman E, Liu YF, et al. Molecular genetic analysis demonstrates that multiple posttransplantation lymphoproliferative disorders occurring in one anatomic site in a single patient represent distinct primary lymphoid neoplasms. *Cancer* 1995;75:2747–2756.

940. d'Amore ES, Manivel JC, Gajl-Peczalska KJ, et al. B-cell lymphoproliferative disorders after bone marrow transplant. An analysis of ten cases with emphasis on Epstein-Barr virus detection by in situ hybridization. *Cancer* 1991;68:1285–1295.

941. Hanto DW, Frizzera G, Gajl-Peczalska KJ, et al. Epstein-Barr virus-induced B-cell lymphoma after renal transplantation: acyclovir therapy and transition from polyclonal to monoclonal B-cell proliferation. *N Engl J Med* 1982;306:913–918.

942. Wu TT, Swerdlow SH, Locker J, et al. Recurrent Epstein-Barr virus-associated lesions in organ transplant recipients. *Hum Pathol* 1996;27:157–164.

943. Chen JM, Barr ML, Chadburn A, et al. Management of lymphoproliferative disorders after cardiac transplantation. *Ann Thorac Surg* 1993;56:527–538.

944. Koeppen H, Newell K, Baunoch DA, et al. Morphologic bone marrow changes in patients with posttransplantation lymphoproliferative disorders. *Am J Surg Pathol* 1998;22:208–214.

945. Smir BN, Hauke RJ, Bierman PJ, et al. Molecular epidemiology of deletions and mutations of the latent membrane protein 1 oncogene of the Epstein-Barr virus in posttransplant lymphoproliferative disorders. *Lab Invest* 1996;75:575–588.

946. Swerdlow SH, Webber SA, Chadburn A, et al. WHO classification of tumours of haematopoietic and lymphoid tissues. In: Swerdlow, SH, Campo E, Harris NL, eds. *WHO classification of tumours of haematopoietic and lymphoid tissues.* Geneva: WHO Press, 2008.

947. Lones MA, Mishalani S, Shintaku IP, et al. Changes in tonsils and adenoids in children with posttransplant lymphoproliferative disorder: report of three cases with early involvement of Waldeyer's ring. *Hum Pathol* 1995;26:525–530.

948. Vakiani E, Nandula SV, Subramaniyam S, et al. Cytogenetic analysis of B-cell posttransplant lymphoproliferations validates the World Health Organization classification and suggests inclusion of florid follicular hyperplasia as a precursor lesion. *Hum Pathol* 2007;38:315–325.

949. Webber SA, Naftel DC, Fricker FJ, et al. Lymphoproliferative disorders after paediatric heart transplantation: a multi-institutional study. *Lancet* 2006;367:233–239.

950. Harris NL, Ferry JA, Swerdlow SH. Posttransplant lymphoproliferative disorders: summary of Society for Hematopathology Workshop. *Semin Diagn Pathol* 1997;14:8–14.

951. Trappe R, Oertel S, Leblond V, et al. Sequential treatment with rituximab followed by CHOP chemotherapy in adult B-cell post-transplant lymphoproliferative disorder (PTLD): the prospective international multicentre phase 2 PTLD-1 trial. *Lancet Oncol* 2012;13:196–206.

952. Tcheng WY, Said J, Hall T, et al. Post-transplant multiple myeloma in a pediatric renal transplant patient. *Pediatr Blood Cancer* 2006;47:218–223.

953. Trappe R, Zimmermann H, Fink S, et al. Plasmacytoma-like post-transplant lymphoproliferative disorder, a rare subtype of monomorphic B-cell post-transplant lymphoproliferation, is associated with a favorable outcome in localized as well as in advanced disease: a prospective analysis of 8 cases. *Haematologica* 2011;96:1067–1071.

954. Richendollar BG, Hsi ED, Cook JR. Extramedullary plasmacytoma-like posttransplantation lymphoproliferative disorders: clinical and pathologic features. *Am J Clin Pathol* 2009;132:581–588.

955. Picarsic J, Jaffe R, Mazariegos G, et al. Post-transplant Burkitt lymphoma is a more aggressive and distinct form of post-transplant lymphoproliferative disorder. *Cancer* 2011;117:4540–4550.

956. Arora N, Nair S, Srivastava A. T/NK-cell post-transplant lymphoproliferative disorder of the urinary bladder: a case report. *J Clin Pathol* 2010;63:1042.

957. Swerdlow SH. T-cell and NK-cell posttransplantation lymphoproliferative disorders. *Am J Clin Pathol* 2007;127:887–895.

958. Wu H, Wasik MA, Przybylski G, et al. Hepatosplenic gamma-delta T-cell lymphoma as a late-onset posttransplant lymphoproliferative disorder in renal transplant recipients. *Am J Clin Pathol* 2000;113:487–496.

959. Steciuk MR, Massengill S, Banks PM. In immunocompromised patients, Epstein-Barr virus lymphadenitis can mimic angioimmunoblastic T-cell lymphoma morphologically, immunophenotypically, and genetically: a case report and review of the literature. *Hum Pathol* 2012;43:127–133.

960. Attygalle AD, Kyriakou C, Dupuis J, et al. Histologic evolution of angioimmunoblastic T-cell lymphoma in consecutive biopsies: clinical correlation and insights into natural history and disease progression. *Am J Surg Pathol*, 2007;31:1077–1088.

961. Rowlings PA, Curtis RE, Passweg JR, et al. Increased incidence of Hodgkin's disease after allogeneic bone marrow transplantation. *J Clin Oncol* 1999;17:3122–3127.

962. Said JW. Immunodeficiency-related Hodgkin lymphoma and its mimics. *Adv Anat Pathol* 2007;14:189–194.

963. Pitman SD, Huang Q, Zuppan CW, et al. Hodgkin lymphoma-like posttransplant lymphoproliferative disorder (HL-like PTLD) simulates monomorphic B-cell PTLD both clinically and pathologically. *Am J Surg Pathol* 2006;30:470–476.

964. Perera SM, Thomas JA, Burke M, et al. Analysis of the T-cell micro-environment in Epstein-Barr virus-related post-transplantation B lymphoproliferative disease. *J Pathol* 1998;184:177–184.

965. Thomas JA, Hotchin NA, Allday MJ, et al. Immunohistology of Epstein-Barr virus-associated antigens in B cell disorders from immunocompromised individuals. *Transplantation* 1990;49:944–953.

966. Rea D, Fourcade C, Leblond V, et al. Patterns of Epstein-Barr virus latent and replicative gene expression in Epstein-Barr virus B cell lymphoproliferative disorders after organ transplantation. *Transplantation* 1994;58:317–324.

967. Quintanilla-Martinez L, Lome-Maldonado C, Schwarzmann F, et al. Post-transplantation lymphoproliferative disorders in Mexico: an aggressive clonal disease associated with Epstein-Barr virus type A. *Mod Pathol* 1998;11:200–208.

968. Young L, Alfieri C, Hennessy K, et al. Expression of Epstein-Barr virus transformation-associated genes in tissues of patients with EBV lymphoproliferative disease. *N Engl J Med* 1989;321:1080–1085.

969. Chetty R, Biddolph S, Gatter K. An immunohistochemical analysis of Reed-Sternberg-like cells in posttransplantation lymphoproliferative disorders: the possible pathogenetic relationship to Reed-Sternberg cells in Hodgkin's disease and Reed-Sternberg-like cells in non-Hodgkin's lymphomas and reactive conditions. *Hum Pathol* 1997;28:493–498.

970. Murray PG, Swinnen LJ, Constandinou CM, et al. BCL-2 but not its Epstein-Barr virus-encoded homologue, BHRF1, is commonly expressed in posttransplantation lymphoproliferative disorders. *Blood* 1996;87:706–711.

971. Chetty R, Biddolph S, Kaklamanis L, et al. bcl-2 protein is strongly expressed in post-transplant lymphoproliferative disorders. *J Pathol* 1996;180:254–258.

972. Kowal-Vern A, Swinnen L, Pyle J, et al. Characterization of postcardiac transplant lymphomas. Histology, immunophenotyping, immunohistochemistry, and gene rearrangement. *Arch Pathol Lab Med* 1996;120:41–48.
973. Setsuda J, Teruya-Feldstein J, Harris NL, et al. Interleukin-18, interferon-gamma, IP-10, and Mig expression in Epstein-Barr virus-induced infectious mononucleosis and posttransplant lymphoproliferative disease. *Am J Pathol* 1999;155: 257–265.
974. Knowles DM. The molecular genetics of post-transplantation lymphoproliferative disorders. *Springer Semin Immunopathol* 1998;20:357–373.
975. Davis CL, Wood BL, Sabath DE, et al. Interferon-alpha treatment of posttransplant lymphoproliferative disorder in recipients of solid organ transplants. *Transplantation* 1998;66:1770–1779.
976. Berg LC, Copenhaver CM, Morrison VA, et al. B-cell lymphoproliferative disorders in solid-organ transplant patients: detection of Epstein-Barr virus by in situ hybridization. *Hum Pathol* 1992;23:159–163.
977. Patton DF, Wilkowski CW, Hanson CA, et al. Epstein-Barr virus—determined clonality in posttransplant lymphoproliferative disease. *Transplantation* 1990;49: 1080–1084.
978. Ho M, Miller G, Atchison RW, et al. Epstein-Barr virus infections and DNA hybridization studies in posttransplantation lymphoma and lymphoproliferative lesions: the role of primary infection. *J Infect Dis* 1985;152:876–886.
979. Cen H, Williams PA, McWilliams HP, et al. Evidence for restricted Epstein-Barr virus latent gene expression and anti-EBNA antibody response in solid organ transplant recipients with posttransplant lymphoproliferative disorders. *Blood* 1993;81:1393–1403.
980. Lager DJ, Burgart LJ, Slagel DD. Epstein-Barr virus detection in sequential biopsies from patients with a posttransplant lymphoproliferative disorder. *Mod Pathol* 1993;6:42–47.
981. Hoffmann DG, Gedebou M, Jimenez A, et al. Detection of Epstein-Barr virus by polymerase chain reaction in transbronchial biopsies of lung transplant recipients: evidence of infection? *Mod Pathol* 1993;6:555–559.
982. Liebowitz D. Epstein-Barr virus and a cellular signaling pathway in lymphomas from immunosuppressed patients. *N Engl J Med* 1998;338:1413–1421.
983. Randhawa PS, Jaffe R, Demetris AJ, et al. The systemic distribution of Epstein-Barr virus genomes in fatal post-transplantation lymphoproliferative disorders. An in situ hybridization study. *Am J Pathol* 1991;138:1027–1033.
984. Weiss LM, Movahed LA. In situ demonstration of Epstein-Barr viral genomes in viral-associated B cell lymphoproliferations. *Am J Pathol* 1989;134:651–659.
985. Borisch-Chappuis B, Nezelof C, Muller H, et al. Different Epstein-Barr virus expression in lymphomas from immunocompromised and immunocompetent patients. *Am J Pathol* 1990;136:751–758.
986. Montone KT, Hodinka RL, Salhany KE, et al. Identification of Epstein-Barr virus lytic activity in post-transplantation lymphoproliferative disease. *Mod Pathol* 1996;9:621–630.
987. Brink AA, Dukers DF, van den Brule AJ, et al. Presence of Epstein-Barr virus latency type III at the single cell level in post-transplantation lymphoproliferative disorders and AIDS related lymphomas. *J Clin Pathol* 1997;50:911–918.
988. Oudejans JJ, Jiwa M, van den Brule AJ, et al. Detection of heterogeneous Epstein-Barr virus gene expression patterns within individual post-transplantation lymphoproliferative disorders. *Am J Pathol* 1995;147:923–933.
989. Rowe M, Niedobitek G, Young LS. Epstein-Barr virus gene expression in post-transplant lymphoproliferative disorders. *Springer Semin Immunopathol*, 1998;20:389–403.
990. Scheinfeld AG, Nador RG, Cesarman E, et al. Epstein-Barr virus latent membrane protein-1 oncogene deletion in post-transplantation lymphoproliferative disorders. *Am J Pathol* 1997;151:805–812.
991. Kingma DW, Weiss WB, Jaffe ES, et al. Epstein-Barr virus latent membrane protein-1 oncogene deletions: correlations with malignancy in Epstein-Barr virus—associated lymphoproliferative disorders and malignant lymphomas. *Blood* 1996;88:242–251.
992. Swaminathan S. Noncoding RNAs produced by oncogenic human herpesviruses. *J Cell Physiol* 2008;216:321–326.
993. Klein E, Kis LL, Klein G. Epstein-Barr virus infection in humans: from harmless to life endangering virus-lymphocyte interactions. *Oncogene* 2007;26:1297–1305.
994. Delecluse HJ, Kremmer E, Rouault JP, et al. The expression of Epstein-Barr virus latent proteins is related to the pathological features of post-transplant lymphoproliferative disorders. *Am J Pathol* 1995;146:1113–1120.
995. Hanto DW, Birkenbach M, Frizzera G, et al. Confirmation of the heterogeneity of posttransplant Epstein-Barr virus-associated B cell proliferations by immunoglobulin gene rearrangement analyses. *Transplantation* 1989;47:458–464.
996. Kaplan MA, Ferry JA, Harris NL, et al. Clonal analysis of posttransplant lymphoproliferative disorders, using both episomal Epstein-Barr virus and immunoglobulin genes as markers. *Am J Clin Pathol* 1994;101:590–596.
997. Shearer WT, Ritz J, Finegold MJ, et al. Epstein-Barr virus-associated B-cell proliferations of diverse clonal origins after bone marrow transplantation in a 12-year-old patient with severe combined immunodeficiency. *N Engl J Med* 1985;312:1151–1159.
998. Brown NA, Liu C, Garcia CR, et al. Clonal origins of lymphoproliferative disease induced by Epstein-Barr virus. *J Virol* 1986;58:975–978.
999. Dror Y, Greenberg M, Taylor G, et al. Lymphoproliferative disorders after organ transplantation in children. *Transplantation* 1999;67:990–998.
1000. Hollingsworth HC, Stetler-Stevenson M, Gagneten D, et al. Immunodeficiency-associated malignant lymphoma. Three cases showing genotypic evidence of both T - and B-cell lineages. *Am J Surg Pathol* 1994;18:1092–1101.
1001. Nelson BP, Locker J, Nalesnik MA, et al. Clonal and morphological variation in a posttransplant lymphoproliferative disorder: evolution from clonal T-cell to clonal B-cell predominance. *Hum Pathol* 1998;29:416–421.
1002. Edwards RH, Raab-Traub N. Alterations of the p53 gene in Epstein-Barr virus-associated immunodeficiency-related lymphomas. *J Virol* 1994;68:1309–1315.
1003. Delecluse HJ, Rouault JP, Jeammot B, et al. Bcl6/Laz3 rearrangements in post-transplant lymphoproliferative disorders. *Br J Haematol* 1995;91:101–103.
1004. Fischer A, Blanche S, Le Bidois J, et al. Anti-B-cell monoclonal antibodies in the treatment of severe B-cell lymphoproliferative syndrome following bone marrow and organ transplantation. *N Engl J Med* 1991;324:1451–1456.
1005. Cabanillas F, Pathak S, Zander A, et al. Monosomy 21, partial duplication of chromosome 11, and structural abnormality of chromosome 1q21 in a case of lymphoma developing in a transplant recipient: characteristic abnormalities of secondary lymphoma? *Cancer Genet Cytogenet* 1987;24:7–10.
1006. Olopade OL, Anastasi J, Thangavelu M, et al. Cytogenetic abnormalities in a secondary lymphoma complicating cardiac transplantation. *Leukemia* 1989;3: 303–304.
1007. Forman SJ, Sullivan JL, Wright C, et al. Epstein-Barr-virus-related malignant B cell lymphoplasmacytic lymphoma following allogeneic bone marrow transplantation for aplastic anemia. *Transplantation* 1987;44:244–249.
1008. Lyons SF, Liebowitz DN. The roles of human viruses in the pathogenesis of lymphoma. *Semin Oncol* 1998;25:461–475.
1009. Delecluse HJ, Rouault JP, Ffrench M, et al. Post-transplant lymphoproliferative disorders with genetic abnormalities commonly found in malignant tumours. *Br J Haematol* 1995;89:90–97.
1010. Hanto DW, Frizzera G, Gajl-Peczalska KJ, et al. Epstein-Barr virus, immunodeficiency, and B cell lymphoproliferation. *Transplantation* 1985;39:461–472.
1011. Tosato G, Teruya-Feldstein J, Setsuda J, et al. Post-transplant lymphoproliferative disease (PTLD): lymphokine production and PTLD. *Springer Semin Immunopathol* 1998;20:405–423.
1012. Faro A. Interferon-alpha and its effects on post-transplant lymphoproliferative disorders. *Springer Semin Immunopathol* 1998;20:425–436.
1013. Mathur A, Kamat DM, Filipovich AH, et al. Immunoregulatory abnormalities in patients with Epstein-Barr virus-associated B cell lymphoproliferative disorders. *Transplantation* 1994;57:1042–1045.
1014. Nalesnik MA, Zeevi A, Randhawa PS, et al. Cytokine mRNA profiles in Epstein-Barr virus-associated post-transplant lymphoproliferative disorders. *Clin Transplant* 1999;13:39–44.
1015. Morel PA, Oriss TB. Crossregulation between Th1 and Th2 cells. *Crit Rev Immunol* 1998;18:275–303.
1016. Tanner JE, Alfieri C. Interactions involving cyclosporine A, interleukin-6, and Epstein-Barr virus lead to the promotion of B-cell lymphoproliferative disease. *Leuk Lymphoma* 1996;21:379–390.
1017. Burke GW, Cirocco R, Hensley G, et al. The rapid development of a fatal, disseminated B cell lymphoma following liver transplantation—serial changes in levels of soluble serum interleukin 2 and interleukin 4 (B cell growth factor). *Transplantation* 1992;53:1148–1150.
1018. Birkeland SA, Hamilton-Dutoit S, Sandvej K, et al. EBV-induced post-transplant lymphoproliferative disorder (PTLD). *Transplant Proc* 1995;27:3467–3472.
1019. Tosato G, Jones K, Breinig MK, et al. Interleukin-6 production in posttransplant lymphoproliferative disease. *J Clin Invest* 1993;91:2806–2814.
1020. Penn I. Cancers following cyclosporine therapy. *Transplant Proc* 1987;19:2211–2213.
1021. Cohen JI. Epstein-Barr virus lymphoproliferative disease associated with acquired immunodeficiency. *Medicine (Baltimore)* 1991;70:137–160.
1022. Benkerrou M, Durandy A, Fischer A. Therapy for transplant-related lymphoproliferative diseases. *Hematol Oncol Clin North Am* 1993;7:467–475.
1023. Alfrey EJ, Friedman AL, Grossman RA, et al. A recent decrease in the time to development of monomorphous and polymorphous posttransplant lymphoproliferative disorder. *Transplantation* 1992;54:250–253.
1024. Leblond V, Davi F, Charlotte F, et al. Posttransplant lymphoproliferative disorders not associated with Epstein-Barr virus: a distinct entity? *J Clin Oncol* 1998;16:2052–2059.
1025. Haque T, Crawford DH. Role of donor versus recipient type Epstein-Barr virus in post-transplant lymphoproliferative disorders. *Springer Semin Immunopathol* 1998;20:375–387.
1026. Jones D, Ballestas ME, Kaye KM, et al. Primary-effusion lymphoma and Kaposi's sarcoma in a cardiac-transplant recipient. *N Engl J Med* 1998;339:444–449.
1027. Dotti G, Fiocchi R, Motta T, et al. Primary effusion lymphoma after heart transplantation: a new entity associated with human herpesvirus-8. *Leukemia* 1999;13:664–670.
1028. Riva G, Luppi M, Barozzi P, et al. How I treat HHV8/KSHV-related diseases in posttransplant patients. *Blood* 2012;120:4150–4159.
1029. Rheumatoid arthritis and the lymphoma link. It's the disease's chronic, severe inflammation, not the treatment, that causes the risk. *Health News* 2006;12: 8–9.
1030. Bachman TR, Sawitzke AD, Perkins SL, et al. Methotrexate-associated lymphoma in patients with rheumatoid arthritis: report of two cases. *Arthritis Rheum* 1996;39:325–329.
1031. Baecklund E, Ekbom A, Sparen P, et al. Disease activity and risk of lymphoma in patients with rheumatoid arthritis: nested case-control study. *BMJ* 1998;317:180–181.
1032. Baecklund E, Sundstrom C, Ekbom A, et al. Lymphoma subtypes in patients with rheumatoid arthritis: increased proportion of diffuse large B cell lymphoma. *Arthritis Rheum* 2003;48:1543–1550.
1033. Cobeta-Garcia JC, Ruiz-Jimeno MT, Fontova-Garrofe R. Non-Hodgkin's lymphoma, rheumatoid arthritis and methotrexate. *J Rheumatol* 1993;20:200–202.
1034. Georgescu L, Quinn GC, Schwartzman S, et al. Lymphoma in patients with rheumatoid arthritis: association with the disease state or methotrexate treatment. *Semin Arthritis Rheum* 1997;26:794–804.
1035. Taillan B, Garnier G, Castanet J, et al. Lymphoma developing in a patient with rheumatoid arthritis taking methotrexate. *Clin Rheumatol* 1993;12:93–94.
1036. Wong AK, Kerkoutian S, Said J, et al. Risk of lymphoma in patients receiving antitumor necrosis factor therapy: a meta-analysis of published randomized controlled studies. *Clin Rheumatol* 2012;31:631–636.
1037. Elliott MJ, Maini RN, Feldmann M, et al. Repeated therapy with monoclonal antibody to tumour necrosis factor alpha (cA2) in patients with rheumatoid arthritis. *Lancet* 1994;344:1125–1127.
1038. Wolfe F, Michaud K. Lymphoma in rheumatoid arthritis: the effect of methotrexate and anti-tumor necrosis factor therapy in 18,572 patients. *Arthritis Rheum* 2004;50:1740–1751.
1039. Rosh JR, Gross T, Mamula P, et al. Hepatosplenic T-cell lymphoma in adolescents and young adults with Crohn's disease: a cautionary tale? *Inflamm Bowel Dis* 2007;13:1024–1030.
1040. Rashidi A, Lee ME, Fisher SI. Hepatosplenic alpha beta T-cell lymphoma associated with azathioprine therapy. *Int J Hematol* 2012;95:592–594.
1041. Balandraud N, Roudier J, Roudier C. What are the links between Epstein-Barr virus, lymphoma, and tumor necrosis factor antagonism in rheumatoid arthritis? *Semin Arthritis Rheum* 2005;34:31–33.
1042. Niitsu N, Okamoto M, Nakamine H, et al. Clinicopathologic correlations of diffuse large B-cell lymphoma in rheumatoid arthritis patients treated with methotrexate. *Cancer Sci* 2010;101:1309–1313.

1043. Salloum E, Cooper DL, Howe G, et al. Spontaneous regression of lymphoproliferative disorders in patients treated with methotrexate for rheumatoid arthritis and other rheumatic diseases. *J Clin Oncol* 1996;14:1943–1949.

1044. Migita K, Miyashita T, Mijin T, et al. Epstein-Barr virus and methotrexate-related CNS lymphoma in a patient with rheumatoid arthritis. *Mod Rheumatol* 2012.

1045. Huwait H, Wang B, Shustik C, et al. Composite cutaneous lymphoma in a patient with rheumatoid arthritis treated with methotrexate. *Am J Dermatopathol* 2010;32:65–70.

1046. Fujimoto M, Yuba Y, Huang CL, et al. Coexistence of Epstein-Barr virus-associated lymphoproliferative disorder and marginal zone B-cell lymphoma of the thymus in a patient with rheumatoid arthritis treated with methotrexate. *Histopathology* 2012;61:1230–1232.

1047. De Angelis F, Di Rocco A, Minotti C, et al. Atypical presentation of anaplastic large T-cell lymphoma mimicking an articular relapse of rheumatoid arthritis in a patient treated with etanercept. A case report and literature review. *Leuk Res* 2012;36:e199–e201.

1048. Landgren O, Engels EA, Pfeiffer RM, et al. Autoimmunity and susceptibility to Hodgkin lymphoma: a population-based case-control study in Scandinavia. *J Natl Cancer Inst* 2006;98:1321–1330.

1049. Baecklund E, Backlin C, Mansouri M, et al. LMO2 protein expression predicts survival in patients with rheumatoid arthritis and diffuse large B-cell lymphoma. *Leuk Lymphoma* 2011;52:1146–1149.

1050. Natkunam Y, Farinha P, Hsi ED, et al. LMO2 protein expression predicts survival in patients with diffuse large B-cell lymphoma treated with anthracycline-based chemotherapy with and without rituximab. *J Clin Oncol* 2008;26:447–454.

1051. Al-Herz W, Bousfiha A, Casanova JL, et al. Primary immunodeficiency diseases: an update on the classification from the international union of immunological societies expert committee for primary immunodeficiency. *Front Immunol* 2011;2:54.

1052. Leechawengwongs E, Shearer WT. Lymphoma complicating primary immunodeficiency syndromes. *Curr Opin Hematol* 2012;19:305–312.

1053. Filipovich AH, Mathur A, Kamat D, et al. Primary immunodeficiencies: genetic risk factors for lymphoma. *Cancer Res* 1992;52:5465s–5467s.

1054. Shapiro RS. Malignancies in the setting of primary immunodeficiency: implications for hematologists/oncologists. *Am J Hematol* 2011;86:48–55.

1055. Vajdic CM, Mao L, van Leeuwen MT, et al. Are antibody deficiency disorders associated with a narrower range of cancers than other forms of immunodeficiency? *Blood* 2010;116:1228–1234.

1056. Van Krieken JH, Onciu M, Elenitoba-Johnson KS, et al. Lymphoproliferative diseases associated with primary immune disorders. In: Swerdlow SH, Campo E, Harris NL, et al., eds. *WHO classification of tumours of haematopoietic and lymphoid tissues.* Lyon: IARC Press, 2008:336–339.

1057. Cunningham-Rundles C. How I treat common variable immune deficiency. *Blood* 2010;116:7–15.

1058. Cunningham-Rundles C. The many faces of common variable immunodeficiency. *Hematology Am Soc Hematol Educ Program* 2012;2012:301–305.

1059. Sander CA, Medeiros LJ, Weiss LM, et al. Lymphoproliferative lesions in patients with common variable immunodeficiency syndrome. *Am J Surg Pathol* 1992;16:1170–1182.

1060. Resnick ES, Moshier EL, Godbold JH, et al. Morbidity and mortality in common variable immune deficiency over 4 decades. *Blood* 2012;119:1650–1657.

1061. Mueller BU, Pizzo PA. Cancer in children with primary or secondary immunodeficiencies. *J Pediatr* 1995;126:1–10.

1062. Lim MS, Elenitoba-Johnson KS. The pathology of primary immunodeficiencies. In: Jaffe ES, Harris NL, Vardiman JW, et al., eds. *Hematopathology.* Philadelphia: Elsevier, 2011:839–853.

1063. Aloj G, Giardino G, Valentino L, et al. Severe combined immunodeficiences: new and old scenarios. *Int Rev Immunol* 2012;31:43–65.

1064. Ratech H, Hirschhorn R, Greco MA. Pathologic findings in adenosine deaminase deficient-severe combined immunodeficiency. II. Thymus, spleen, lymph node, and gastrointestinal tract lymphoid tissue alterations. *Am J Pathol* 1989;135:1145–1156.

1065. Moshous D, Pannetier C, Chasseval Rd R, et al. Partial T and B lymphocyte immunodeficiency and predisposition to lymphoma in patients with hypomorphic mutations in Artemis. *J Clin Invest* 2003;111:381–387.

1066. Husain M, Grunebaum E, Naqvi A, et al. Burkitt's lymphoma in a patient with adenosine deaminase deficiency-severe combined immunodeficiency treated with polyethylene glycol-adenosine deaminase. *J Pediatr* 2007;151:93–95.

1067. Reiman A, Srinivasan V, Barone G, et al. Lymphoid tumours and breast cancer in ataxia telangiectasia; substantial protective effect of residual ATM kinase activity against childhood tumours. *Br J Cancer* 2011;105:586–591.

1068. Micol R, Ben Slama L, Suarez F, et al. Morbidity and mortality from ataxia-telangiectasia are associated with ATM genotype. *J Allergy Clin Immunol* 2011;128:382.e1–389.e1.

1069. Taylor AM, Metcalfe JA, Thick J, et al. Leukemia and lymphoma in ataxia telangiectasia. *Blood* 1996;87:423–438.

1070. Seidemann K, Henze G, Beck JD, et al. Non-Hodgkin's lymphoma in pediatric patients with chromosomal breakage syndromes (AT and NBS): experience from the BFM trials. *Ann Oncol* 2000;11(Suppl 1):141–145.

1071. Ariga T. Wiskott-Aldrich syndrome; an x-linked primary immunodeficiency disease with unique and characteristic features. *Allergol Int* 2012;61:183–189.

1072. Cleland SY, Siegel RM. Wiskott-Aldrich Syndrome at the nexus of autoimmune and primary immunodeficiency diseases. *FEBS Lett* 2011;585:3710–3714.

1073. Sullivan KE, Mullen CA, Blaese RM, et al. A multiinstitutional survey of the Wiskott-Aldrich syndrome. *J Pediatr* 1994;125:876–885.

1074. Imai K, Morio T, Zhu Y, et al. Clinical course of patients with WASP gene mutations. *Blood* 2004;103:456–464.

1075. Sasahara Y, Fujie H, Kumaki S, et al. Epstein-Barr virus-associated hodgkin's disease in a patient with Wiskott-Aldrich syndrome. *Acta Paediatr* 2001;90:1348–1351.

1076. Sebire NJ, Haselden S, Malone M, et al. Isolated EBV lymphoproliferative disease in a child with Wiskott-Aldrich syndrome manifesting as cutaneous lymphomatoid granulomatosis and responsive to anti-CD20 immunotherapy. *J Clin Pathol* 2003;56:555–557.

1077. Gulley ML, Chen CL, Raab-Traub N. Epstein-Barr virus-related lymphomagenesis in a child with Wiskott-Aldrich syndrome. *Hematol Oncol* 1993;11:139–145.

1078. Okano M, Osato T, Koizumi S, et al. Epstein-Barr virus infection and oncogenesis in primary immunodeficiency. *AIDS Res* 1986;2(Suppl 1):S115–S119.

1079. Nakanishi M, Kikuta H, Tomizawa K, et al. Distinct clonotypic Epstein-Barr virus-induced fatal lymphoproliferative disorder in a patient with Wiskott-Aldrich syndrome. *Cancer* 1993;72:1376–1381.

1080. De Meester J, Calvez R, Valitutti S, et al. The Wiskott-Aldrich syndrome protein regulates CTL cytotoxicity and is required for efficient killing of B cell lymphoma targets. *J Leukoc Biol* 2010;88:1031–1040.

1081. Waggoner SN, Kumar V. Evolving role of 2B4/CD244 in T and NK cell responses during virus infection. *Front Immunol* 2012;3:377.

1082. Marsh RA, Madden L, Kitchen BJ, et al. XIAP deficiency: a unique primary immunodeficiency best classified as X-linked familial hemophagocytic lymphohistiocytosis and not as X-linked lymphoproliferative disease. *Blood* 2010;116:1079–1082.

1083. Filipovich A, Johnson J, Zhang K, et al. Lymphoproliferative Disease, X-Linked. 1993;

1084. Harrington DS, Weisenburger DD, Purtilo DT. Malignant lymphoma in the X-linked lymphoproliferative syndrome. *Cancer* 1987;59:1419–1429.

1085. Rao VK, Oliveira JB. How I treat autoimmune lymphoproliferative syndrome. *Blood* 2011;118:5741–5751.

1086. Neven B, Magerus-Chatinet A, Florkin B, et al. A survey of 90 patients with autoimmune lymphoproliferative syndrome related to TNFRSF6 mutation. *Blood* 2011;118:4798–4807.

1087. Straus SE, Jaffe ES, Puck JM, et al. The development of lymphomas in families with autoimmune lymphoproliferative syndrome with germline Fas mutations and defective lymphocyte apoptosis. *Blood* 2001;98:194–200.

1088. Boulanger E, Rieux-Laucat F, Picard C, et al. Diffuse large B-cell non-Hodgkin's lymphoma in a patient with autoimmune lymphoproliferative syndrome. *Br J Haematol* 2001;113:432–434.

Chapter 26

Peripheral T-Cell Lymphomas

Andrew L. Feldman • Ahmet Dogan

Peripheral T-cell lymphomas (PTCLs) are neoplasms derived from mature (peripheral) T cells; the term typically also includes neoplasms of mature natural killer (NK) cell origin. PTCLs present considerable challenges to both the pathologist and the treating oncologist. Though incidence appears to be increasing in the United States (1), PTCLs are relatively uncommon. PTCLs account for only 10% to 15% of non-Hodgkin lymphomas worldwide and are less common in the United States than in some other countries. Despite the relative rarity of PTCLs as a group, the WHO classification of PTCLs includes more than 20 established or provisional entities, making each individual entity still less common (Table 26.1) (2). The relative distributions of T-cell neoplasms seen in a referral practice are shown in Figure 26.1. As a further challenge to diagnosis, PTCLs have a morphologic spectrum that overlaps considerably with reactive lymphoid hyperplasias, B-cell lymphomas, and Hodgkin lymphomas. Challenges to the clinician include the relatively poor prognosis of PTCLs overall, though some specific subtypes behave indolently. In addition, in part due to the relative rarity of these tumors, less is known about the genetics and molecular pathogenesis of most PTCL subtypes than B-cell non-Hodgkin lymphomas. Thus, fewer data exist to suggest promising molecular targets for newer therapies than for more common malignancies, and accrual to clinical trials of new agents is more challenging. This chapter addresses the most common PTCL subtypes with typical presentation in lymph nodes and noncutaneous extranodal sites (Table 26.1). Primary cutaneous PTCLs and T-/NK-cell neoplasms typically presenting with leukemic or disseminated involvement are addressed in other chapters.

Early immature T-cell precursors are generated in the bone marrow from pluripotential hematopoietic stem cells. These early precursors travel to the thymus, where most of the T-cell development occurs. In the thymus, naïve T cells are formed after a series of complex biologic processes. These include rearrangement of T-cell receptor (TCR) genes, positive selection for ability to generate a TCR-mediated immune response, and negative selection to avoid autoimmunity. During TCR gene rearrangement in the thymus, each T cell is genetically programmed to recognize a specific peptide via its TCR. Thus, the peripheral T-cell pool constitutes a repertoire capable of recognizing a very large number of peptides. This extensive TCR diversity is a product of somatic rearrangement of multiple segments of the TCR genes (known as V, D, and J regions) and addition of random nucleotides during the joining of different segments. This unique property is the basis of clonality determination in the diagnosis of T-cell neoplasms. Once differentiation in the thymus is completed, mature/naïve T cells join the peripheral blood circulation, where they account for 60% to 70% of all lymphocytes. Naïve T cells express a set of molecules that enable to them to traffic through organized lymphoid structures, including the lymph nodes, the spleen, and the Peyer patches. In the lymph nodes, the naïve T-cell trafficking occurs through the high endothelial venules (HEVs), and, histologically, these cells are found in the paracortex of the lymph node surrounding the HEV.

A brief discussion of normal T-cell subsets is important for understanding the phenotype and classification of the T-cell neoplasms derived from them (Table 26.2). T cells carry two different types of TCR, each formed by two different polypeptide chains. Approximately 95% of all T cells carry the $\alpha\beta$ TCR and the rest carry the $\gamma\delta$ TCR. Both $\alpha\beta$ and $\gamma\delta$ TCRs are attached to a downstream signal transduction complex, which includes CD3 polypeptide chains. Unlike B cells, which can recognize whole antigens, T cells require processing of antigens to smaller 8 to 12-amino acid peptides. This processing occurs in antigen-presenting cells such as B cells, dendritic cells, and, under certain circumstances, epithelial cells. The peptides generated by antigen processing are presented to T cells via major histocompatibility complex (MHC) molecules. MHC class I molecules (e.g., HLA-A, -B, -C) present peptides derived from the intracellular compartment (e.g., viral antigens), whereas the MHC class II molecules (e.g., HLA-DR, DQ) present peptides derived from the extracellular compartment (e.g., bacterial antigens). In addition to TCR, CD4 molecules expressed on the surface of T cells are required for MHC class II–mediated antigen presentation; CD8 plays a similar role for MHC class I–mediated antigen presentation. This subspecialization of CD4+ and CD8+ T cells in antigen recognition also is reflected in their functional differentiation. CD4+ T cells typically play a significant role in regulation of the immune response, in particular by interacting with B cells and providing help for B-cell responses. Immunologists have identified different functional subsets of CD4+ T-helper (Th) cells. For example, Th1 cells secrete the cytokines IL-2 and interferon-γ and help with IgG-mediated responses and cell-mediated immunity. Th2 cells produce IL-4, IL-5, and IL-13 but not IL-2 or IFN-γ and are critical in IgE-mediated immunity such as responses against helminths, as well as in a number of hypersensitivity reactions. Another functional subset of CD4+ T cells is the regulatory T (T_{reg}) cells, which typically express the transcription factor FoxP3 and the IL2 receptor, CD25. These cells are important in down-regulating immune responses. Follicular helper T (T_{FH}) cells are a specific subtype of CD4+ Th cells that provide help for follicular B-cell function. In contrast to CD4+ Th cells, most CD8+ T cells have cytotoxic function and play roles in killing virally infected cells and in transplant rejection. Human peripheral blood and organized lymphoid tissues, in particular the spleen, contain another population of lymphoid cells, the NK cells. Like T cells, NK cells are derived from lymphoid precursors in the bone marrow but do not go through TCR gene rearrangement process or thymic selection. Whereas the vast majority of T cells are part of the adoptive immune system, NK cells, some $\gamma\delta$ T cells, and a minor subset of CD8+ $\alpha\beta$ T cells confer innate immunity. These cells recognize antigens through cell surface receptors that recognize common structures shared by bacteria and viruses as well as other cell stress signals. These receptors include the toll-like receptor family and NK-cell receptors.

Careful histologic examination remains the mainstay of pathologic diagnosis of reactive and neoplastic T-cell proliferations. The histologic features of PTCLs demonstrate marked

Table 26.1	WHO CLASSIFICATION OF MATURE T- AND NK-CELL NEOPLASMS, STRATIFIED BY TYPICAL CLINICAL PRESENTATION

Lymph Node Presentation
PTCL, not otherwise specified (NOS)[a]
AITL[a]
ALCL, ALK[+a]
ALCL, ALK[−a]

Extranodal Presentation
Extranodal NKTL[a]
EATL[a]
Hepatosplenic T-cell lymphoma[a]
Subcutaneous panniculitis-like T-cell lymphoma
MF
Primary cutaneous PTCLs
    Primary cutaneous γδ T-cell lymphoma
    Primary cutaneous CD8[+] aggressive epidermotropic cytotoxic T-cell lymphoma
    Primary cutaneous CD4[+] small/medium T-cell lymphoma
Primary cutaneous CD30[+] lymphoproliferative disorders
    Primary cutaneous ALCL
    Lymphomatoid papulosis
Hydroa vacciniforme–like lymphoma

Blood/Bone Marrow and/or Disseminated Presentation
T-PLL
T-cell large granular lymphocytic leukemia
Chronic lymphoproliferative disorder of NK cells
Aggressive NK-cell leukemia
Systemic EBV[+] T-cell lymphoproliferative disease of childhood
ATLL
SS

[a]Entity discussed primarily in this chapter.

than in B-cell lymphomas. Thus, cytologic grading generally plays a minimal role in diagnosis and subclassification, though in some entities the occurrence of histologic transformation in sequential biopsies is well documented and clinically relevant (e.g., the cutaneous T-cell lymphoma, mycosis fungoides, discussed in Chapter 29). The neoplastic T cells in PTCLs range from small cells with minimal cytologic atypia to large, anaplastic cells with multilobated nuclei, including cells resembling Reed-Sternberg cells. Cells with moderate-to-abundant clear cytoplasm may be seen and are particularly common in angioimmunoblastic T-cell lymphoma (AITL). A background of nonneoplastic inflammatory cells is common in PTCLs, typically consisting of varying numbers of histiocytes, plasma cells, and eosinophils. Increased vascularity also is common and is particularly pronounced in AITL. Necrosis is not a common feature in most PTCL types but often is seen in extranodal NK/T-cell lymphoma, nasal type (NKTL). The architectural features in PTCLs with lymph node involvement may give clues to their T-cell origin, with predominant paracortical (T zone) or interfollicular involvement and preservation of residual lymphoid follicles. However, many cases demonstrate complete architectural effacement. Occasionally, involvement limited to the follicles may be seen, mimicking follicular B-cell lymphoma. Subcapsular and sinusoidal involvement is common in anaplastic large cell lymphoma (ALCL).

Ancillary studies including immunophenotyping and molecular genetic analysis to complement the morphologic opinion have become necessary in most cases. For many years, flow cytometric immunophenotyping was the main ancillary technique for diagnosing T-cell proliferations. This method permits rapid analysis of large numbers of cells for virtually any cytoplasmic or surface antigens on either peripheral blood white cells or cell suspensions prepared from solid tissues. Typically an aberrant T-cell phenotype infers T-cell clonality (e.g., loss of T-cell antigens normally expressed or expression of antigens not usually present). An abnormal phenotype by flow cytometry is seen in nearly one-half of PTCLs, with loss of CD3 and/or CD7 being the most common abnormalities; CD2 expression is the most stable. NK-cell–associated antigen (such as CD16, CD56, and CD57) expression is important in the diagnosis of T-cell large granular lymphocytic leukemias and various NK-like lymphoid proliferations and is easily accomplished by flow cytometry. Immunohistochemistry (IHC) allows the use of a wide variety of antibodies, similar to those used in flow

heterogeneity, making diagnosis and classification challenging, particularly given the overall infrequency with which these tumors are encountered in general pathology practice. Specific histologic features of each subtype are given in the remaining sections of this chapter. In general, PTCLs tend to exhibit more cytologic heterogeneity within a given tumor than B-cell lymphomas, and the presence of a cytologic spectrum of neoplastic lymphoid cells is common. However, monotonous neoplastic lymphoid populations can be seen in some subtypes. Cytologic features are less predictive of clinical aggressiveness in PTCLs

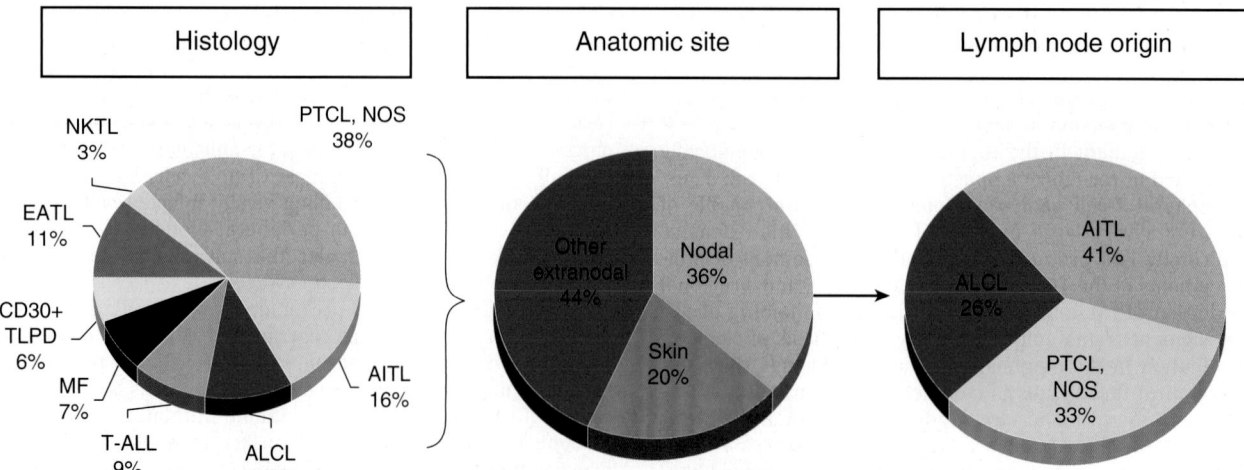

FIGURE 26.1. Distribution of T-cell neoplasms by histologic subtype and anatomic site, based on 468 cases seen in a referral practice (University College London Hospital) between 1998 and 2002. PTCL, peripheral T-cell lymphoma; NOS, not otherwise specified; AITL, angioimmunoblastic T-cell lymphoma; ALCL, anaplastic large cell lymphoma; T-ALL, T-cell acute leukemia/lymphoma; MF, mycosis fungoides; CD30[+] TLPD, primary cutaneous CD30[+] T-cell lymphoproliferative disorder (primary cutaneous ALCL, lymphomatoid papulosis); EATL, enteropathy-associated T-cell lymphoma; NKTL, extranodal NK/T-cell lymphoma, nasal type.

Table 26.2	HYPOTHETICAL PHYSIOLOGIC NORMAL COUNTERPARTS OF PTCLs				
Lymphoma	**Adoptive Immunity**				**Innate Immunity**
	Activated	T_{FH}	T_{REG}	**Cytotoxic**	**NK/T**
Peripheral T-cell lymphoma, NOS	X	X	X	X	X
Anaplastic large cell lymphoma, ALK+	X				
Anaplastic large cell lymphoma, ALK−	X				
Cutaneous anaplastic large cell lymphoma	X				
Angioimmunoblastic T-cell lymphoma		X			
Adult T-cell leukemia/lymphoma			X		
Mycosis fungoides/Sézary syndrome			?		
T-cell large granular lymphocytic leukemia				X	
Subcutaneous panniculitis-like T-cell lymphoma				X	
Enteropathy-associated T-cell lymphoma				X	X
Hepatosplenic T-cell lymphoma				X	X
Extranodal NK/T-cell lymphoma, nasal type					X
Cutaneous $\gamma\delta$ T-cell lymphoma					X

T_{FH}, follicular T-helper cell; T_{reg}, regulatory T cell.

cytometry, and is currently the most commonly used ancillary method for diagnosis. IHC initially required frozen tissue, but morphologic and cytologic detail suffered. Additionally, most biopsy specimens are fixed before any fresh tissue is apportioned for flow cytometry or frozen IHC. In recent years, a new generation of antibodies reactive with the vast majority of many of the surface and cytoplasmic targets used by flow cytometry or frozen IHC for diagnosis of T-cell proliferations has become available for paraffin sections, and paraffin IHC has replaced flow cytometry and frozen section IHC as the main method of immunophenotyping in solid tissues. The IHC

markers most frequently used in the diagnosis of PTCL are summarized in Table 26.3.

The role of molecular studies in evaluation of T-cell proliferations is evolving. In B-cell neoplasms, light chain restriction has been used extensively as a surrogate for clonality. In T-cell neoplasms, however, phenotypic assessment of possible clonality is considerably more challenging. TCR-β chain family typing and expression of killer cell immunoglobulin–like receptors (KIRs) have found some use in flow cytometric evaluation of T-cell proliferations, particularly those involving the peripheral blood. However, proof of clonality in T-cell proliferation

Table 26.3	IMMUNOPHENOTYPIC MARKERS USED IN DIAGNOSIS OF PTCL	
Target	**Cellular Reactivity**	**Reactivity in PTCLs**
ALK	ALCL	ALCL
CD2	T cells, NK cells	Most PTCLs
CD3	T cells, NK cells (cytoplasmic only)	Most PTCLs
CD4	T-helper cells, macrophages	AITL; PTCL, NOS; ALCL; ATLL
CD5	T cells, subset of B cells	Most PTCLs; negative in $\gamma\delta$ PTCLs, NK-cell lymphomas
CD7	T cells	Subset of PTCLs
CD8	T-suppressor/cytotoxic cells, some NK cells	PTCL-NOS
CD10	T_{FH} cells, follicle center B cells	AITL
CD21	FDCs, subset of B cells	AITL (FDCs)
CD23	FDCs, subset of B cells	AITL (FDCs)
CD25	Activated B and T cells, T_{reg} cells	ATLL, ALCL
CD30	Activated B and T cells, Reed-Sternberg cells	ALCL; some PTCLs, NOS
CD43	T cells, subset of B cells	Most PTCLs
CD45	Pan-leukocyte	Most PTCLs, may be negative in ALCL
CD45RO	T cells, macrophages	Most PTCLs
CD56	Cytotoxic T cells, NK cells	Cytotoxic PTCLs, NK lymphomas
CXCL13	T_{FH} cells	AITL
EMA	Epithelial cells, plasma cells	ALCL
FOXP3	T_{reg} cells	ATLL
Granzyme B	Activated cytotoxic T cells, NK cells	Cytotoxic PTCLs, NK lymphomas
PD1 (CD279)	T_{FH} cells	AITL
TCL1	B cells	T-PLL
TCR-β chain	$\alpha\beta$ T cells	Most PTCLs (ALCL usually negative)
TCR-γ chain	$\gamma\delta$ T cells	HSTCL, other $\gamma\delta$ PTCLs
TIA-1	Cytotoxic T cells, NK cells	Cytotoxic PTCLs, NK lymphomas

PTCL, peripheral T-cell lymphoma; ALCL, anaplastic large cell lymphoma; NOS, not otherwise specified; AITL, angioimmunoblastic T-cell lymphoma; ATLL, adult T-cell leukemia/lymphoma; T_{FH} cell, T-follicular helper cell; FDC, follicular dendritic cell; T_{reg} cell, regulatory T cell; T-PLL, T-cell prolymphocytic leukemia; HSTCL, hepatosplenic T-cell lymphoma.

Table 26.4	GENE-SPECIFIC RECURRENT GENETIC ABNORMALITIES IN PTCL
Genetic Abnormality	PTCL Subtype(s)
ALK translocation	ALK⁺ ALCL (100%)
CDK6 amplification	PTCL, NOS (23%)
DUSP22 or *IRF4* rearrangements	Cutaneous ALCL (28%); ALK⁻ ALCL (18%); PTCL, NOS (rare)
IDH2 mutation	AITL (20%–45%)
ITK/SYK translocation	PTCL, NOS (rare)
TET2 mutation	AITL (33%), PTCL, NOS (20%)
MYC amplification	EATL (73% in type II)
TRA@/BCL3 translocation	PTCL, NOS (rare)
TRA@/TCL1A/B translocation	T-PLL (80%)

PTCL, peripheral T-cell lymphoma; ALCL, anaplastic large cell lymphoma; NOS, not otherwise specified; AITL, angioimmunoblastic T-cell lymphoma; T-PLL, T-cell prolymphocytic leukemia.

relies heavily on molecular genetic analysis. Current techniques rely on detecting the unique TCR gene rearrangement present in each T cell to establish a monoclonal expansion. The gold standard for determination of T-cell clonality remains the Southern blotting technique. However, this method requires large amounts of high molecular weight DNA (and thus fresh material) and is cumbersome for routine diagnostic testing. Currently, most laboratories use polymerase chain reaction (PCR)–based methodologies. PCR methods work on most formalin-fixed, paraffin-embedded tissues, require smaller amounts of tissues than Southern blotting, and are easily applicable in a routine diagnostic setting. Until recently, reproducibility between laboratories has been poor due to differences of primers used for PCR amplification. To overcome this, a European consortium (BIOMED-2 Concerted Action) developed standardized primers and protocols and validated these in multiple laboratories. Using BIOMED-2 primers, clonality of T-cell populations can be demonstrated in 99% of all T-cell lymphomas, suggesting that PCR methodology will replace Southern blotting as the most sensitive and specific test in the diagnosis of T-cell neoplasms. With a few important exceptions, little is known about the gene-specific recurrent genetic abnormalities among the PTCL subtypes (Table 26.4). Molecular testing for genetic abnormalities currently plays a limited role in diagnosis and subclassification of PTCLs because the abnormalities are rare, because they have unknown clinical significance, or because they have acceptable immunohistochemical surrogates (e.g., anaplastic lymphoma kinase [ALK]). With new genetic discoveries from next-generation sequencing data and increasing use of individualized, targeted therapeutic approaches, the importance of molecular testing is likely to increase dramatically in the near future.

PERIPHERAL T-CELL LYMPHOMAS PRESENTING WITH PREDOMINANTLY LYMPH NODE INVOLVEMENT

Peripheral T-cell Lymphoma, Not Otherwise Specified (PTCL, NOS)

Definition

PTCL, NOS is a heterogeneous group of lymphomas derived from mature T lymphocytes that do not meet criteria for any of the other, specific PTCL entities defined in the WHO classification system (2). This category includes both nodal and extranodal lymphomas and encompasses a variety of morphologic and phenotypic findings. PTCL, NOS has considerable morphologic and phenotypic overlap with more specific entities such as AITL and ALCL; cases resembling these entities but without sufficient features for definitive classification as such may be diagnosed as PTCL, NOS to keep the more specific categories "pure." The borders between PTCL, NOS and these other entities are in evolution and are likely to change significantly with increasing genetic data using new sequencing technologies. While PTCL, NOS has been considered a "wastebasket" category, it can also be considered the prototype of PTCLs in general, based on its commonness (see below) and the present lack of clinically meaningful approaches to subclassify these tumors further (3).

Epidemiology

PTCL, NOS is the most common PTCL subtype in Western countries, representing from 30% to 60% of PTCLs (1,4–6). It is relatively less common in Asia due to the prevalence in those countries of the virus-associated PTCLs, adult T-cell leukemia/lymphoma (ATLL), and extranodal NKTL (4). PTCL, NOS affects mostly adults, with a median age of about 60 years and a male:female ratio of about 2:1 (1,4–6). Data from Surveillance, Epidemiology and End Results (SEER) registries show an apparent recent increase in the incidence of PTCL, NOS in the United States (1), though the influence of advancing diagnostic modalities and changes in lymphoma classification on these data is unclear. The etiology of PTCL, NOS is unknown.

Clinical Features

Sites of Involvement

Because PTCL, NOS is an intentionally heterogeneous category, there is not a characteristic presentation. However, most patients have lymphadenopathy, with or without involvement of extranodal sites (6). Bone marrow and skin are the most commonly involved extranodal sites (5). Neoplastic infiltrates in the liver and spleen also are relatively common. Peripheral blood may be involved, but is rarely the presenting site.

Clinical Evaluation and Staging

Most cases are disseminated, with 40% to 60% of patients presenting with stage IV disease (1,5,6). B symptoms are seen in about 40% of patients, elevated lactate dehydrogenase (LDH) levels in about 60%, and a nonambulatory performance status in about 30% (5,6). Some patients have eosinophilia, sometimes accompanied by pruritis, and occasional patients present with hemophagocytic syndrome (7). Unfavorable international prognostic index (IPI) scores (3–5) are seen in 60% of patients (6). In addition to the importance of staging for prognosis and treatment stratification, staging data and a thorough clinical history are necessary to distinguish PTCL, NOS from more specific extranodal PTCL subtypes, such as some of the primary cutaneous PTCLs.

Morphology

Cytologic Composition

By definition, PTCL, NOS is a heterogeneous category of PTCLs that do not meet criteria for another of the specifically defined entities within the WHO classification (Fig. 26.2) (2). Therefore, pathologic findings vary widely. In most cases, the tumor cells are medium sized to large, though a minority of cases consist predominantly of small cells (8). Cells with clear cytoplasm as seen in AITL may be seen in the follicular variant or in cases with other AITL-like features but insufficient overall findings for a diagnosis of AITL (see below). Marked nuclear pleomorphism and cases with Reed-Sternberg–like cells may be seen

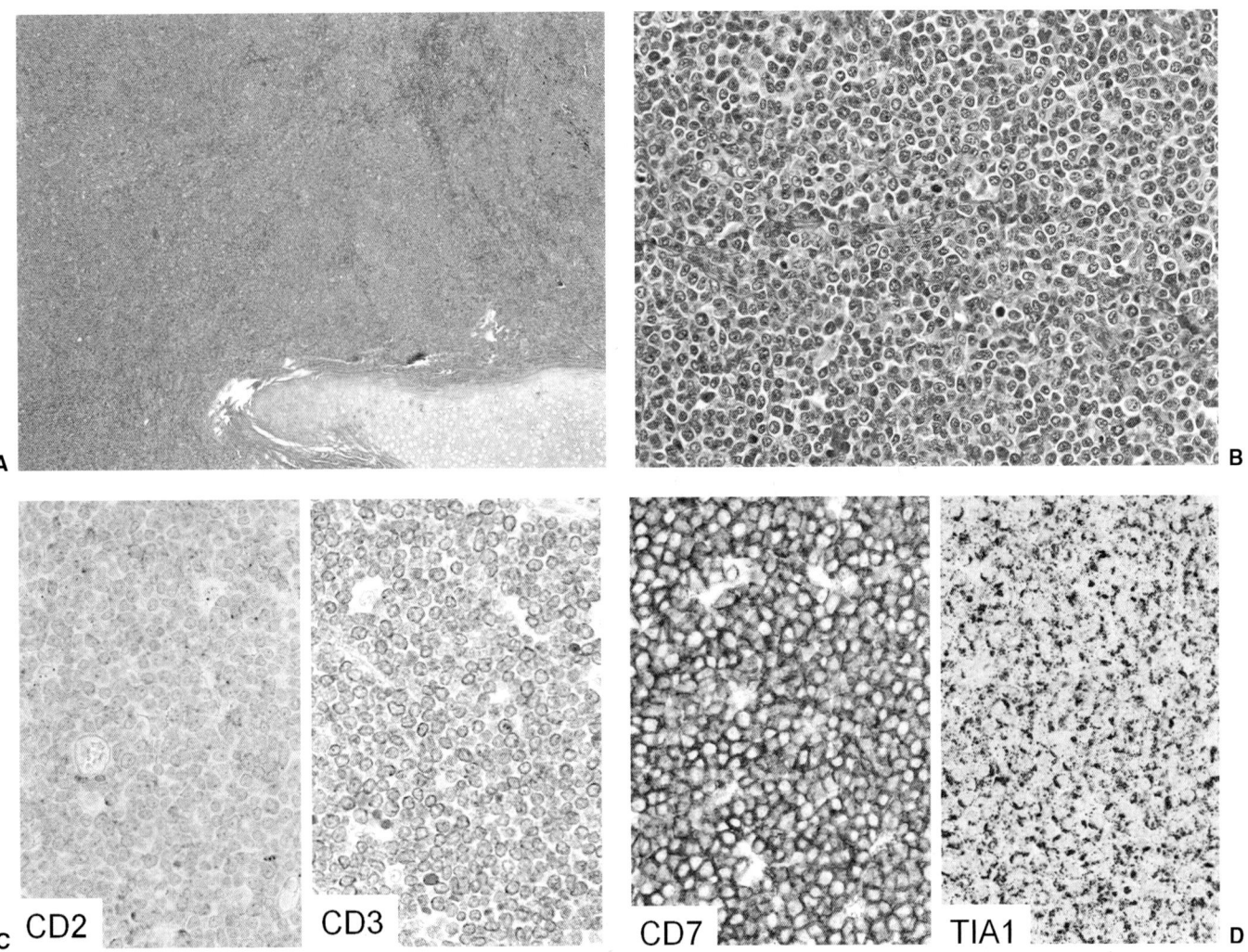

FIGURE 26.2. PTCL, NOS involving the lymph node with a diffuse pattern. The neoplastic lymphocytes are mostly medium in size. They express CD3 (weak), CD7, and the cytotoxic granule marker TIA1, but show aberrant loss of CD2 expression.

(9). The cellular background is variable but may contain small lymphocytes, plasma cells, eosinophils, histiocytes, large B cells, and/or vascular proliferation.

Grading
PTCL, NOS is not graded.

Proliferative Pattern
Typically, the lymph node shows effacement of the normal architecture, with either a diffuse or paracortical pattern. Predominant follicular and/or perifollicular patterns are seen in the follicular and T-zone variants (see below). Prominent sinusoidal involvement should raise the possibility of ALCL.

Histologic Progression/Transformation
No criteria exist for the diagnosis of histologic progression or transformation.

Histologic Variants
The WHO classification recognizes lymphoepithelioid, follicular, and T-zone variants of PTCL, NOS (2). The lymphoepithelioid variant (Lennert lymphoma) is characterized by mostly small neoplastic cells with extensive clusters of epithelioid histiocytes (Fig. 26.3) (8,10). The neoplastic lymphoid cells typically are oval in shape and show mild nuclear irregularities. Often, there are scattered, admixed larger cells, which may have

RS-like features (11). The epithelioid histiocytes usually are mononucleate and most commonly are seen in small clusters, but also may appear as single cells or large sheets. Scattered eosinophils and plasma cells may be seen in the background. The follicular variant typically shows expanded, occasionally confluent follicles containing an intrafollicular population of atypical, medium-sized lymphoid cells with only slight nuclear irregularities and clear cytoplasm (12). Normal follicle center lymphocytes typically are lost, but follicular dendritic cells (FDCs) may be seen in the background. Other cases may show features resembling progressive transformation of germinal centers (PTGC) or a perifollicular growth pattern (Fig. 26.4) (13). The T-zone variant of PTCL, NOS shows an extensive perifollicular infiltrate surrounding residual intact follicles, often containing germinal centers demonstrating regressive changes (13). The infiltrate is composed of small to medium-sized cells that often lack significant cytologic atypia, but may demonstrate clear cytoplasm. Eosinophils and histiocytes may be seen in the background, but typically are not prominent; a marked plasmacytosis may be present.

Morphology in Sites Other Than Lymph Node
Morphologic features in extranodal sites are nonspecific, given the heterogeneous nature of this category. In the skin, cases diagnosed as PTCL, NOS typically show a predominantly dermal infiltrate lacking the epidermotropism seen in

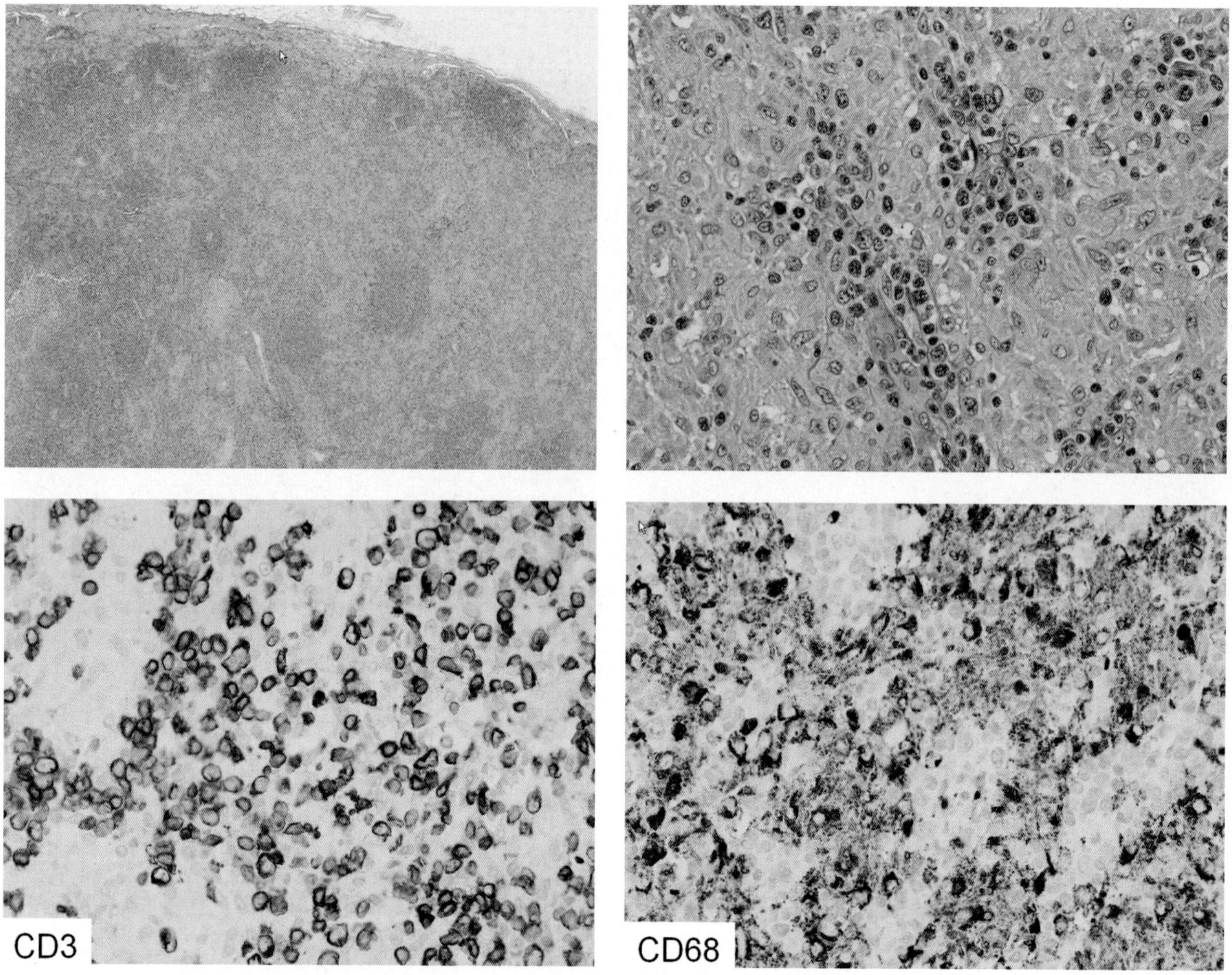

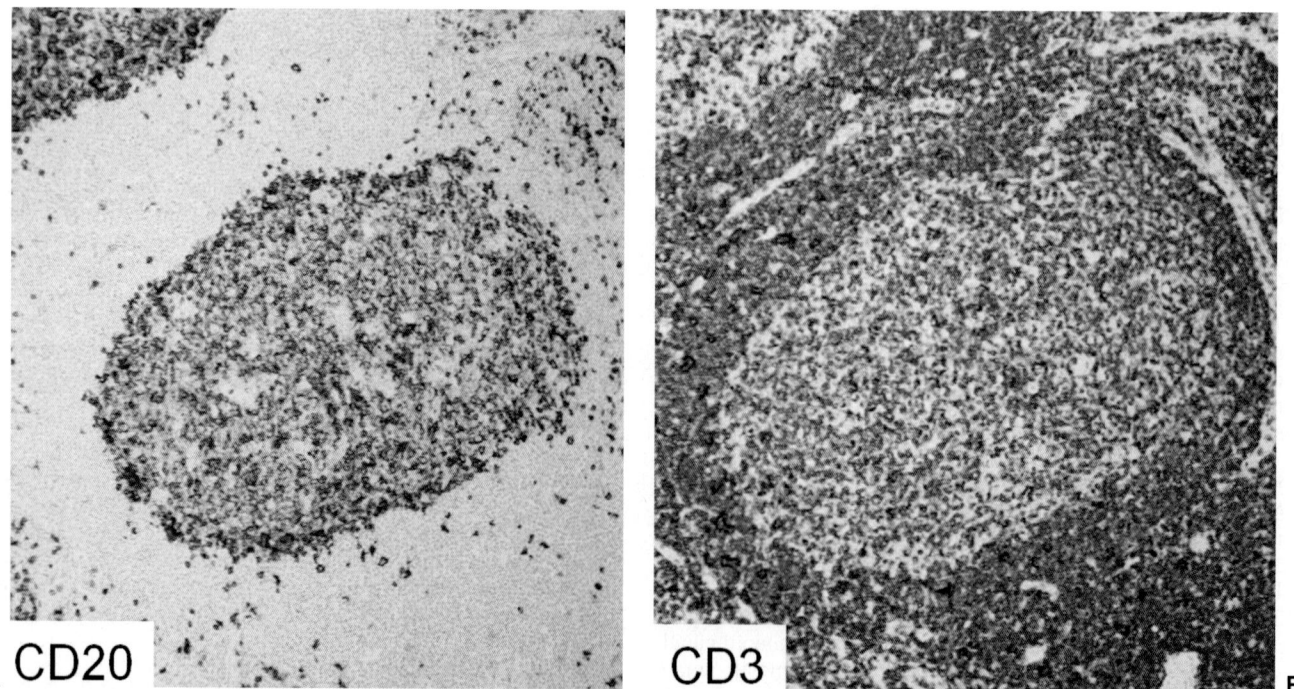

FIGURE 26.3. PTCL, NOS, lymphoepithelioid variant (Lennert lymphoma). The lymph node architecture is effaced and shows a vaguely granulomatous appearance. The atypical lymphocytes are mostly small to medium in size, with occasional larger cells. There are abundant epithelioid histiocytes in the background. CD3 highlights the tumor cells. CD68 stains the background histiocytes.

FIGURE 26.4. PTCL, NOS, with a perifollicular growth pattern. A residual germinal center is highlighted by CD20. The neoplastic cells surround the germinal center, as seen on the stain for CD3. They are positive for CD4 and negative for CD7 and CD8. The neoplastic cells also express the T$_{FH}$ marker, BCL6; this case was negative for CD10 (not shown).

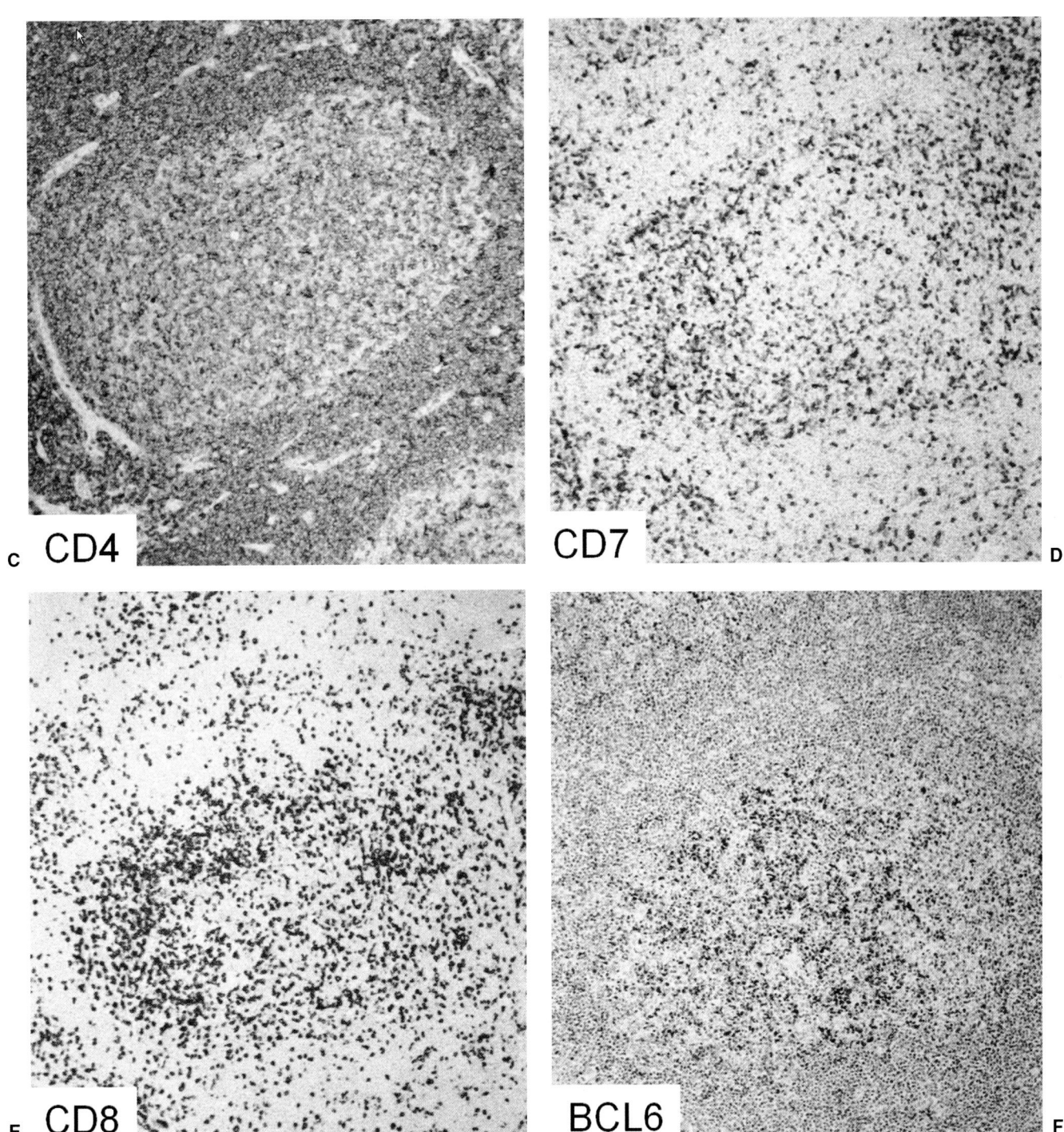

FIGURE 26.4. *(continued)*

mycosis fungoides (MF) and the chiefly panniculitic pattern of subcutaneous panniculitic-like T-cell lymphoma (SCPTCL). The presence of peripheral blood involvement and a sinusoidal pattern of bone marrow involvement can be seen, but should raise the question of T-cell LGL or another more specific extranodal PTCL subtype (see below).

Immunophenotype

IHC is essential for proper diagnosis and subclassification of PTCLs. The typical immunophenotypic features of PTCL, NOS involving the lymph nodes and the more specific entities in its differential diagnosis are summarized in Table 26.5. PTCL, NOS

often shows an aberrant immunophenotype with loss of one or more T-cell antigens, most commonly CD3, CD5, or CD7. Most cases are CD4+, though some may express CD8, particularly the lymphoepithelioid variant (11,14). Cases double-positive or double-negative for CD4 and CD8 may be seen. Most cases are positive for the TCR-β chain. Recent development of a $\gamma\delta$ TCR antibody for use in paraffin sections is generating new data on the expression of this marker; early findings suggest (a) lack of beta-F1 positivity does not imply $\gamma\delta$ T-cell origin; (b) occasional PTCLs are positive for both beta-F1 and $\gamma\delta$ TCR; and (c) a small but significant subset of PTCL, NOS may be of $\gamma\delta$ T-cell origin. Cytotoxic markers and/or CD56 may occasionally be expressed in PTCL, NOS. A subset of PTCLs, NOS expresses CD30 and

Table 26.5	COMPARISON OF TYPICAL IMMUNOPHENOTYPIC FINDINGS IN PTCLs INVOLVING THE LYMPH NODES							
	PTCL, NOS	AITL	ALCL, ALK±	ALCL, ALK⁻	ATLL	MF	T-PLL	EATL
ALK	−	−	+	−	−	−	−	−
CD2	+	+	−/+	−/+	+	+	+	+
CD3	+	+	−/+	−/+	+	+	+	+
CD4	+/−	+	−/+	−/+	+	+	+/−	−
CD5	+/−	+	−	−	+	+	+	−
CD7	+/−	−/+			−	−	+	−
CD8	−/+	−	−	−	−	−	−/+	−/+
CD10	−	+/−	−	−	−	−		
CD25	−/+	−	+	+	+	−/+	−	−/+
CD30	−/+	−	+	+	−/+	−/+	−	−/+
CD45RO	+	+	+	+	+	+	+	+
CD56	−/+	−	−/+	−	−	−		−/+
CXCL13	−	+/−	−	−	−	−	−	−
EMA	−	−	+/−	+/−	−	−	−	−
FOXP3	−/+	−	−	−	+/−	+	−/+	−
Granzyme B	−/+	−	+/−	+/−	−	−	−	+
PD1 (CD279)	−/+	+	−	−	−	−	−	−
TCL1	−	−	−	−	−	−	+	−
TCR-β chain	+/−	+	−	−	+	+	+	+/−
TCR-γ chain	−/+	−	−	−	−	−	−	−
TIA-1	−/+	−	+/−	+/−	−	−	−	+

+, expressed.
+/−, frequently expressed.
−/+, occasionally expressed.
−, not expressed.
PTCL, peripheral T-cell lymphomas; NOS, not otherwise specified; AITL, angioimmunoblastic T-cell lymphoma; ALCL, anaplastic large cell lymphoma; ATLL, adult T-cell leukemia/lymphoma; MF, mycosis fungoides; T-PLL, T-cell prolymphocytic leukemia; EATL, enteropathy-associated T-cell lymphoma.

occasionally may coexpress both CD30 and CD15 (9). A follicle center T-cell (T_FH) phenotype, including expression of CD10, Bcl6, CXCL13, and/or CD279 (PD1), may be seen in the follicular variant of PTCL, NOS.

Flow cytometry may be helpful in the evaluation of lymph nodes for PTCLs by recognizing aberrant antigenic loss, particularly in cases with subtle involvement. Marked alterations in the CD4:CD8 ratio can be seen in reactive conditions and are nonspecific. Because of the importance of morphology and newer immunohistochemical markers, flow cytometry is rarely sufficient for definitive diagnosis and subclassification of PTCLs.

Cytogenetics

Though PTCLs, NOS typically have complex karyotypes, specific recurrent abnormalities are uncommon. A subset of cases with a follicular growth pattern has a t(5;9)(q33;q22) translocation that fuses the tyrosine kinase genes, *ITK* and *SYK* (15). The resultant fusion protein has transforming properties *in vitro*, suggesting the translocation may be important in the pathogenesis of these cases (16). The incidence of *ITK/SYK* translocations is low in PTCLs, NOS overall, but a larger proportion of PTCLs aberrantly express the SYK tyrosine kinase, which promotes growth and inhibits apoptosis in PTCL cells and may represent a therapeutic target (17,18). Rare cases of PTCL, NOS carry a t(6;14)(p25.3;q11.2) translocation involving the *IRF4* gene encoding interferon regulatory factor-4 and the *T-cell receptor alpha* (*TRA@*) locus (Fig. 26.5) (19). Reported cases have had a CD5⁻ cytotoxic phenotype, coexpressed the IRF4/MUM1 protein, and showed marked bone marrow involvement with peripheral cytopenias. Amplifications at 7q22 targeting *CDK6* have been demonstrated in 23% of PTCLs, NOS (20). Rare cases have rearrangements of *BCL3* (21). Recently, mutations in the *TET2* gene were demonstrated in 20% of PTCLs,

NOS (22). Comparative genomic hybridization (CGH) and gene expression profiling (GEP) studies have identified other potential therapeutic targets and differences among PTCL, NOS, AITL, and ALCL (23–27), but the clinical utility of these findings remains unclear.

Molecular Characteristics

Evaluation for Epstein-Barr virus (EBV) by IHC or *in situ* hybridization (ISH) may be helpful. Most cases of PTCL, NOS are negative for EBV. Diffuse positivity may raise the possibility of rare nodal involvement by extranodal NKTL. Scattered EBV⁺ B cells may be seen in both PTCL, NOS and AITL. Clonal rearrangements of TCR genes are seen in the majority of PTCLs, NOS, and PCR for TCR and/or immunoglobulin (IG) gene rearrangement is important in the distinction from atypical reactive hyperplasias and B-cell lymphomas.

Postulated Normal Counterpart

The majority of PTCLs, NOS are thought to derive from CD4⁺ Th2 cells. The follicular variant is believed to derive from T_FH cells, sharing features with AITL. Cases with a cytotoxic phenotype likely derive from αβ or γδ cytotoxic T cells.

Clinical Course and Prognostic Assessment

Most cases of PTCL, NOS present with advanced clinical stage (stage III or IV) and pursue an aggressive course. Progressive lymphadenopathy and extensive solid organ involvement is common. Stage and the IPI score are the best validated prognostic factors (1,4–6). A more favorable prognosis has been reported in the follicular and T-zone variants, as well as in cases with deletions of 5q, 10q, and 12q (24). Features reported to have an adverse influence on prognosis include high proliferative rate or

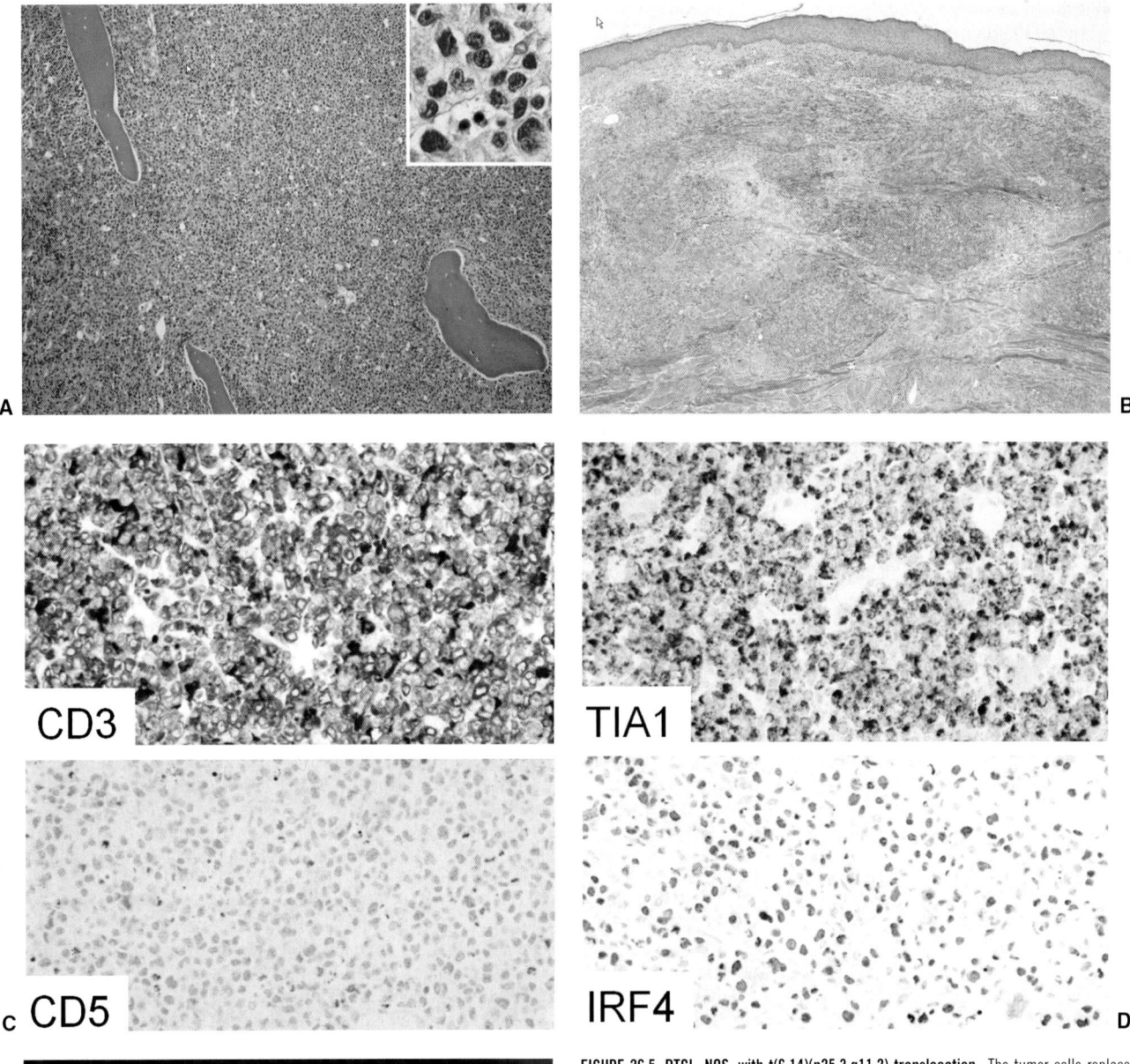

FIGURE 26.5. PTCL, NOS, with t(6;14)(p25.3;q11.2) translocation. The tumor cells replace the bone marrow and involve the skin. Most are medium sized with irregular or slightly folded nuclei. They have a cytotoxic T-cell phenotype, with positivity for CD3 and TIA1, but lack CD5 expression. BetaF1 was positive (not shown), indicating an $\alpha\beta$ T-cell phenotype. Tumor cell nuclei are positive for IRF4 (MUM1). FISH with a breakapart probe demonstrated separation of the *red* and *green* signals flanking the *IRF4* gene region. Further studies in this case confirmed an *IRF4/TRA@* fusion involving the *TCR@* locus.

proliferation signature by GEP, expression of cytotoxic markers, EBV, or CD30, and reduced expression of NFκB genes (28,29).

Treatment and Survival

Patients with PTCL, NOS typically receive combination chemotherapy regimens such as cyclophosphamide, doxorubicin, vincristine, and prednisone (CHOP), with response rates of 50% to 60% (28,30). However, the long-term prognosis of PTCL, NOS is poor, with 5-year overall survival (OS) rates of 20% to 30%. High-intensity chemotherapy regimens have not yielded results superior to CHOP. Durable responses have been reported after high-dose chemotherapy with stem cell transplantation, but experience is limited (31). Experimental therapies using single-agent therapies (e.g., gemcitabine), recombinant proteins (e.g., denileukin diftitox), monoclonal antibodies (e.g., alemtuzumab), and histone deacetylase inhibitors (e.g., depsipeptide) have been utilized, but none has achieved widespread acceptance (31). Recently, pralatrexate has been approved as second-line therapy for PTCL, NOS, and clinical trials of its use in other clinical settings are under way (32).

Differential Diagnosis

Angioimmunoblastic T-Cell Lymphoma
The follicular variant of PTCL, NOS and the follicular phase of AITL show overlapping features (33,34). These entities have similar phenotypes based on their common T_{FH} cell origin, though CD10 expression is more common in AITL. Distinction is primarily based on the degree of the follicular pattern morphologically. Other PTCLs have a more widespread, paracortical pattern of distribution but lack sufficient features for a definitive diagnosis of AITL (see section on AITL below). These cases should be classified as PTCL, NOS at present; this distinction does not necessarily impact the clinical management or prognosis.

ALK⁻ ALCL
Recent data have provided evidence that distinction of CD30⁺ PTCL, NOS from ALK⁻ ALCL is important based on the significantly poor OS rates seen in the former entity (19% at 5 years) compared with 49% 5-year OS in the latter (29). Nevertheless, this distinction can be challenging; current recommendations suggest limiting ALK⁻ ALCL to cases that morphologically resemble ALK⁺ ALCL but lack ALK protein expression or *ALK* translocations, with the goal of keeping the ALK⁻ ALCL designation "pure" (see section below). Thus, even the subset of PTCLs, NOS that express CD30 may be somewhat heterogeneous. Cases without clear evidence of characteristic hallmark cells seen in ALCL and those with weak or nonuniform staining for CD30 should be classified as PTCL, NOS. While the presence of markers such as EMA, clusterin, CD56, and cytotoxic markers help support a diagnosis of ALK⁻ ALCL, it is not clear that their absence should be grounds for a diagnosis of PTCL, NOS. Recurrent translocations involving the *DUSP22-IRF4* locus on 6p25.3 have been reported in 18% of systemic ALK⁻ ALCLs but only in approximately 1% of PTCLs, NOS (19,35); fluorescence *in situ* hybridization (FISH) testing for this abnormality therefore might be helpful in this differential diagnosis, pending the results of larger studies.

Other Specific PTCL Subtypes and T-Cell Leukemias
PTCL, NOS involving the lymph nodes needs to be differentiated from extranodal PTCLs and T-cell leukemias that secondarily involve the lymph node. This clinical information may not always be available. When the neoplastic cells are predominantly small to medium sized, consideration should be given to lymph node involvement by ATLL, MF, or T-cell prolymphocytic leukemia (T-PLL). These entities are covered briefly here and described in more detail in other chapters.

ATLL is a peripheral T-cell neoplasm caused by human T-cell leukemia virus-1 (HTLV-1) infection. Four clinical variants with different risks for disease progression and death are recognized, including smoldering, chronic, acute and lymphomatous variants (36). The acute variant is the most common form and is characterized by systemic disease with involvement of blood, bone marrow, lymph node, spleen, and frequently extranodal sites. Lymph node involvement has either a diffuse or a paracortical pattern. The neoplastic cells are medium to large in size and have characteristic pleomorphic, hyperlobated nuclei (37). Rarely, ATLL may have morphologic features reminiscent of AITL (38), and EBV⁺ B cells resembling Reed-Sternberg cells can be seen. By flow cytometry and IHC, the tumor cells express CD2, CD3, TCR-β, CD4, CD5, and CD25, but not CD7 or CD8. Cells with large cell anaplastic morphology may be positive for CD30. Around half of the cases express FOXP3, a transcription factor expressed by T_{reg} cells (39,40), which have proposed as the cell of origin of ATLL (41). The differential diagnosis of ATLL includes PTCL, NOS; TPLL; AITL; and ALK⁻ ALCL. In addition to morphologic and phenotypic evaluation, serologic testing for HTLV-1 is important in distinguishing ATLL from other PTCLs.

MF is a primary cutaneous lymphoproliferative disorder characterized by an epidermotropic infiltrate of small to medium-sized T cells with cerebriform nuclei (2). MF may involve lymph nodes and/or peripheral blood. Sézary syndrome (SS) is a leukemic disease composed of a similar neoplastic cell population involving the skin, lymph nodes, and peripheral blood. Lymph nodes involved by MF/SS typically show paracortical expansion and dermatopathic lymphadenopathy, with abundant interdigitating cells and histiocytes containing melanin (42). Cytologically, the tumor cells in lymph nodes involved by MF/SS have features similar to those in skin and are small to medium in size and have cerebriform nuclei. Cases of transformed MF may have large, pleomorphic tumor cells. Clinical history and staging is critical in distinguishing nodal involvement by MF/SS from PTCL, NOS and other PTCLs. Phenotyping often is not helpful in this distinction. MF/SS often show retained expression of CD2, CD3, and CD5, usually with loss of CD7 expression (43). Most cases are CD4⁺, but occasional cases express CD8. The T cells are of $\alpha\beta$ type (positive for βF1). Whether MF and SS are derived from T_{reg} cells is controversial. Transformed MF may express CD30 and occasionally cytotoxic markers (44).

T-PLL is a clinically aggressive peripheral T-cell neoplasm involving peripheral blood, bone marrow, spleen, the lymph nodes, and the skin. The neoplastic cells are relatively uniform, small-to-medium in size with basophilic cytoplasm, an oval nucleus, and a prominent nucleolus. The diagnosis often is made on peripheral blood smears, but occasionally a lymph node biopsy may be the first diagnostic specimen. In the lymph nodes, involvement is diffuse, but occasional trapped reactive follicles can be seen. Immunophenotypically, the neoplastic T cells express CD2, CD3, CD5, CD7, and TCR-β. Most cases are CD4⁺, and the finding of coexpression of CD4 and CD8 in about 25% of cases is helpful in suggesting the diagnosis (45,46). A translocation involving the *TCL1* locus at 14q31 and *TRA@* locus at 14q11 is seen in 80% of the cases and leads to overexpression of TCL1A in the neoplastic T cells (45). Since TCL1A expression is restricted to B cells under physiologic conditions, the immunohistochemical detection of TCL1A is a useful diagnostic marker for T-PLL (46).

Several other T-cell neoplasms enter the differential diagnosis of PTCLs with specific features. Cases of PTCL, NOS with a true $\gamma\delta$ TCR phenotype need to be distinguished from other more specific entities, including primary cutaneous $\gamma\delta$ T-cell lymphoma and hepatosplenic T-cell lymphoma of the $\gamma\delta$ type. In abdominal lymph nodes, involvement by enteropathy-associated T-cell lymphoma (EATL) should be considered. Occasionally, the neoplastic cells of PTCL, NOS will have a blastlike appearance, raising

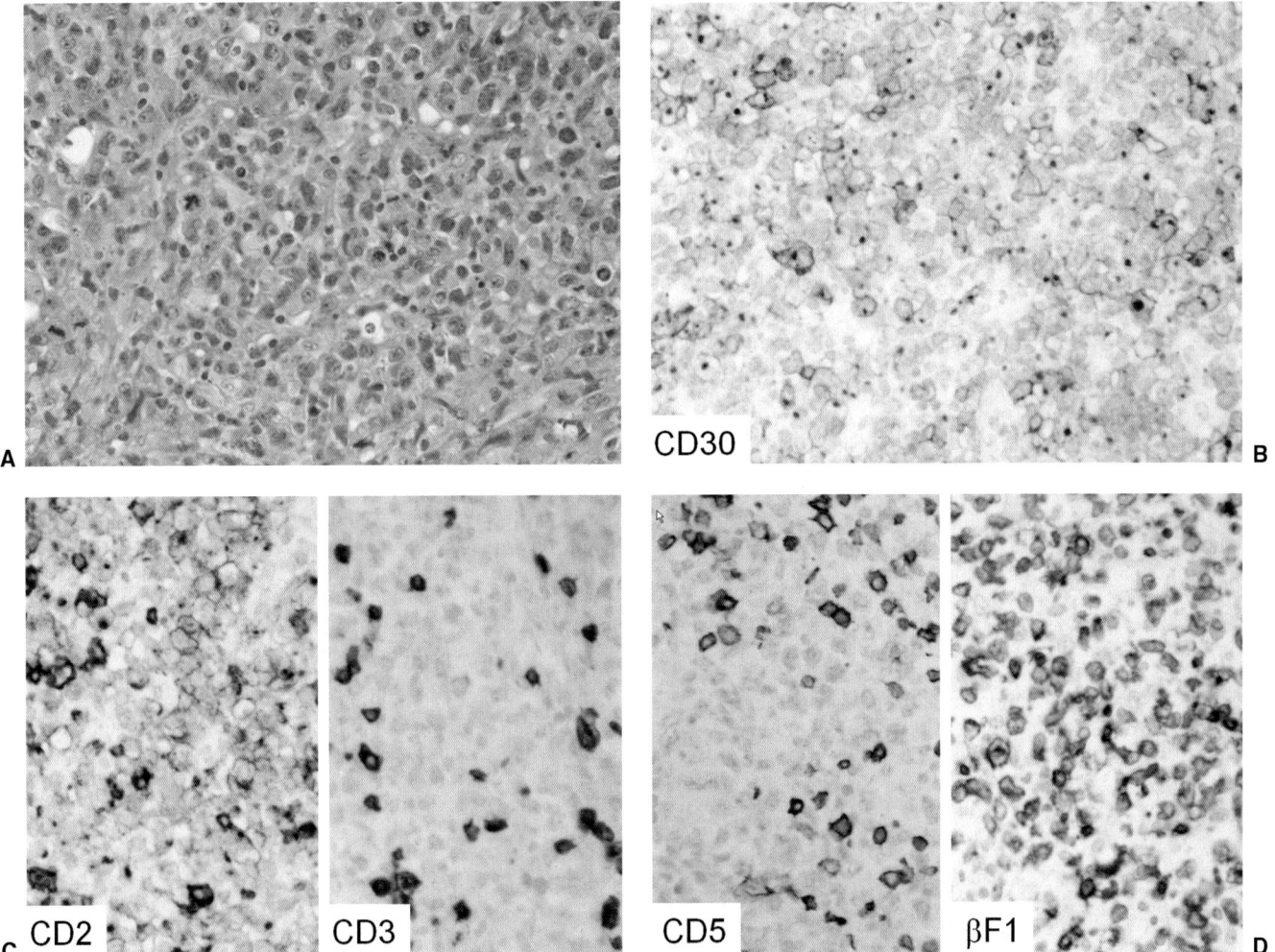

FIGURE 26.6. PTCL, NOS expressing CD30. The differential diagnosis in this case was with ALK⁻ ALCL. The lymph node is diffusely infiltrated by large atypical lymphoid cells. The expression of CD30 is somewhat weak and variable. The tumor cells weakly express CD2, show loss of CD3 and CD5, and strongly express TCR-β chain (βF1). The variable CD30 expression and strong βF1 expression are features favoring a diagnosis of PTCL, NOS over ALK⁻ ALCL in this case.

the possibility of T-lymphoblastic lymphoma. IHC for TdT, CD99, CD34, and CD1a is helpful in this differential. Extranodal NKTLs may involve lymph nodes and resemble PTCL, NOS.

PTCL, NOS should be diagnosed at extranodal sites when the overall features support a mature T-cell neoplasm but are insufficient for a more specific PTCL subtype associated with those sites. In the skin, this designation should be used both for systemic PTCLs, NOS with secondary cutaneous involvement and for primary cutaneous PTCLs where MF/SS, SCPTCL, primary cutaneous γδ T-cell lymphoma, and other specific entities have been excluded both pathologically and clinically. Nasal PTCLs resembling NKTL but lacking both a definite NK-cell phenotype and EBV are best classified as PTCL, NOS (Figs. 26.5 and 26.6).

Hodgkin and B-Cell Non-Hodgkin Lymphomas

B-cell lymphomas may be mistaken for PTCL, NOS. The follicular variant of PTCL, NOS may mimic follicular lymphoma or, sometimes, marginal zone lymphoma (12,13). T-cell/histiocyte-rich large B-cell lymphomas show a predominance of small reactive T cells; the key to this distinction is recognition of the scattered large, CD20⁺, neoplastic B cells, and the lack of cytologic atypia or phenotypic aberrancy in the reactive T-cell infiltrate. Recently, cases of nodular lymphocyte predominant Hodgkin lymphomas with atypical T cells mimicking PTCL have

been reported (47). Upon further evaluation, these T cells show neither aberrant T-cell antigen loss nor clonal TCR gene rearrangements, and scattered lymphocyte predominant cells can be found. Conversely, occasional cases of PTCL, NOS with a nodular pattern with PTGCs may resemble nodular lymphocyte predominant Hodgkin lymphoma.

PTCLs, NOS occasionally may mimic classical Hodgkin lymphoma (CHL). Some of these cases have EBV⁺, B-lineage Reed-Sternberg–like cells accompanying the neoplastic T-cell infiltrate, though these more commonly are classified as AITL than as PTCL, NOS (48). In other cases, the neoplastic T cells themselves resemble Reed-Sternberg cells cytologically and/ or phenotypically (with coexpression of CD30 and CD15) (9). An extended panel of immunohistochemical stains and gene rearrangement studies are needed to arrive at the correct diagnosis in these cases. PTCL, NOS occasionally may express B-cell antigens, raising the possibility of a B-lineage lymphoma. Most of these cases also express T-cell antigens, while the number of B-cell antigens expressed typically is limited; PAX5 is one of the most specific B-cell antigens in such cases, but gene rearrangement studies typically are recommended. Various B-cell lymphomas also can coexpress T-cell antigens. Though CD5 expression in mantle cell lymphoma and chronic lymphocytic leukemia/small lymphocytic leukemia rarely causes confusion, most B-cell non-Hodgkin lymphomas have been reported to express CD5 at least occasionally. Down-regulation of CD20 associated with monoclonal antibody therapy can present a diagnostic challenge in these cases. Other T-cell antigens and cytotoxic proteins occasionally may be expressed in diffuse large B-cell lymphomas (DLBCL) and other B-lineage neoplasms. Plasmablastic lymphomas, primary effusion lymphomas, and CHL express T-cell antigens somewhat more commonly and often lack many B-cell antigens. Negativity for CD43 and weak positivity for PAX5 are fairly consistent features of CHL that aid in the differential diagnosis from PTCLs.

Nonlymphoid Neoplasms

Nonlymphoid hematopoietic neoplasms may resemble PTCL, NOS. Systemic mast cell disease typically shows a paracortical pattern of distribution when it involves lymph nodes; the clear tumor cell cytoplasm and accompanying eosinophils are additional features of mast cell disease that also may be seen in PTCLs (34). The neoplastic mast cells typically express CD43, often express CD2 and CD25, and may coexpress CD30. Stains for mast cell tryptase and CD117 are helpful when mast cell disease is in the differential diagnosis. Extramedullary myeloid tumors and cases of acute myeloid leukemia (AML) typically have blastic cytologic features and a "leukemic" pattern of lymph node involvement; however, they may be morphologically indistinguishable from PTCL, NOS in cases with complete architectural effacement. AMLs typically express CD43 and may express CD2, CD4, CD7, and/or CD56. Stains for myeloperoxidase, CD33, and CD34 are helpful in establishing this diagnosis, as well as stains for lysozyme and CD68 in cases with monocytic differentiation. Blastic plasmacytoid dendritic cell neoplasms also have a blastic appearance; typically express CD4, CD43, and CD56; and may express CD2 and CD7. Though this tumor characteristically involves skin and bone marrow, lymph node involvement is seen in about 25% of cases (49). Staining for the plasmacytoid dendritic cell marker, CD123, is helpful in such cases; most cases also express TCL1 and about one-third express TdT.

Immunodeficiency Disorders and Other Reactive Conditions

In children, consideration must be given to autoimmune lymphoproliferative syndrome (ALPS); this primary immune disorder is characterized by an apoptotic defect, usually due to mutations in the *FAS* or *FASL* gene, which causes a marked paracortical expansion by double-negative (CD4−/CD8−) T cells (Fig. 26.7) (50). Occasionally, other types of immune dysregulation may mimic PTCL, NOS, including common variable immunodeficiency, chronic active EBV infection, and systemic EBV+ T-cell lymphoproliferative disease of childhood (34). The last is a fulminant, clonal cytotoxic T-cell lymphoproliferative disorder often accompanied by hemophagocytic syndrome, sepsis, and death (51). Monomorphic T/NK-cell post-transplant lymphoproliferative disease can present as any of the PTCL subtypes seen in immunocompetent hosts, including PTCL, NOS; about one-third of these cases are EBV+. Lymph node involvement is relatively rare (52).

PTCL, NOS may appear similar to a variety of benign processes. The T-zone variant may resemble T-zone hyperplasia. A marked paracortical immunoblastic proliferation may be seen in response to phenytoin and other anticonvulsants, mimicking PTCL (53). In some cases of PTCL, NOS, the reactive inflammatory background may be so pronounced so as to obscure the neoplastic cell population; this may occur particularly in the

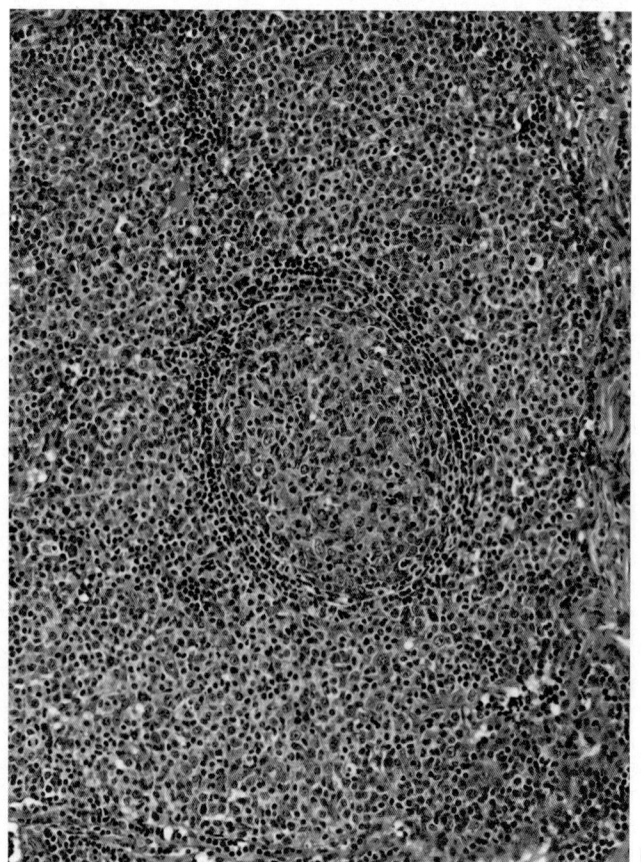

A   B

FIGURE 26.7. Lymph node appearances of ALPS. Although the overall architecture is preserved, there is a marked expansion of the paracortex. Perifollicular areas contain numerous large atypical T cells mimicking PTCL.

Table 26.6	EXAMPLES OF BENIGN MALIGNANT CONDITIONS THAT COULD HISTOLOGICALLY MIMIC PTCLs
Entity	**Mimic**
Benign	
Paracortical lymph node hyperplasia	PTCL, NOS, T-zone variant; AITL; ALCL; MF
Infectious mononucleosis, lymph nodes	PTCL, NOS; ALCL
Infectious mononucleosis, spleen and liver	PTCL, NOS; HSTCL
Autoimmune lymphoproliferative syndrome	PTCL, NOS
Castleman disease	AITL
Traumatic ulcerative granuloma with stromal eosinophilia	ALCL
Celiac disease	EATL
NK-cell enteropathy	EATL
Malignant	
Carcinoma	ALCL, NKTL
THRLBCL	PTCL, NOS
Granulocytic sarcoma	PTCL, NOS; NKTL
Systemic mastocytosis	PTCL, NOS; AITL
Follicular dendritic cell sarcoma	AITL
Plasmablastic lymphoma	ALCL; PTCL, NOS; NKTL
Blastic plasmacytoid dendritic cell neoplasm	PTCL, NOS; NKTL
Classical Hodgkin lymphoma	ALCL; PTCL, NOS

PTCL, peripheral T-cell lymphomas; NOS, not otherwise specified; AITL, angioimmunoblastic T-cell lymphoma; ALCL, anaplastic large cell lymphoma; HSTCL, hepatosplenic T-cell lymphoma; MF, mycosis fungoides; EATL, enteropathy-associated T-cell lymphoma; THRLBCL, T-cell/histiocyte-rich large B-cell lymphoma; NKTL, NK/T-cell lymphoma.

lymphoepithelioid variant of PTCL, NOS, in which the numerous epithelioid histiocytes may resemble reactive granulomatous inflammation. Kikuchi lymphadenitis may show marked paracortical expansion characterized by a prominent atypical lymphohistiocytic infiltrate with areas of geographical necrosis. Examples of benign and neoplastic conditions that could mimic PTCLs is listed in Table 26.6.

ALK⁺ Anaplastic Large Cell Lymphoma

Definition

ALK⁺ ALCL is a neoplasm of mature T cells that usually are large, with abundant cytoplasm and characteristic nuclear pleomorphism. By definition, the tumor cells express CD30 and ALK

and have translocations involving the *ALK* gene. These tumors were originally known as Ki-1 antibody based on their positivity for CD30 using the Ki-1 antibody, developed in 1982 as a result of a search for Hodgkin lymphoma–related antigens (54). In addition to staining Reed-Sternberg cells, Ki-1 subsequently was found to stain a group of large cell lymphomas with "histiocytic" features and sinusoidal involvement (55). The updated Kiel classification included these tumors, which could be of either B- or T-cell origin, under the designation of "large cell anaplastic lymphoma" (56). The Revised European-American Lymphoma (REAL) classification introduced the current nomenclature of ALCL and restricted the entity to tumors with a T- or null-cell phenotype (57). The association of a t(2;5) translocation with cases designated "malignant histiocytosis" was identified in 1989, leading to subsequent cloning of the *ALK* gene in 1994 (58–60). The third edition of the WHO classification considered ALK⁺ and ALK⁻ ALCLs part of the same disease spectrum, but the fourth edition lists ALK⁺ ALCL as a distinct entity, with ALK⁻ ALCL listed as a provisional entity (see the next section).

Epidemiology

ALCL is the second most common subtype of PTCL in the Western world, representing about 25% of PTCLs and about 5% of all non-Hodgkin lymphomas. The distribution between ALK⁺ and ALK⁻ cases varies somewhat by study and geographic region, but on average 50% to 60% of cases are ALK⁺ (4,5,29,61). ALK⁺ ALCL occurs mostly in children and young adults and has a male predominance (male:female ratio of about 2:1) (4,5,62). ALK⁺ ALCL is the most common type of PTCL in children and represents 10% to 30% of all lymphomas in children. The etiology of ALK⁺ ALCL is unknown. An association with insect bites has been reported.

Clinical Features

Sites of Involvement

Most patients present with peripheral lymphadenopathy. Involvement of the mediastinum is uncommon. The most common extranodal site of involvement is the skin (Fig. 26.8); other common sites include bone, lung, liver, and soft tissues (62). Gastrointestinal and central nervous system involvement may occur but are rare (Fig. 26.9). Occasionally, cases present with a leukemic picture, often associated with the small cell histologic variant (see below) (63). The bone marrow is

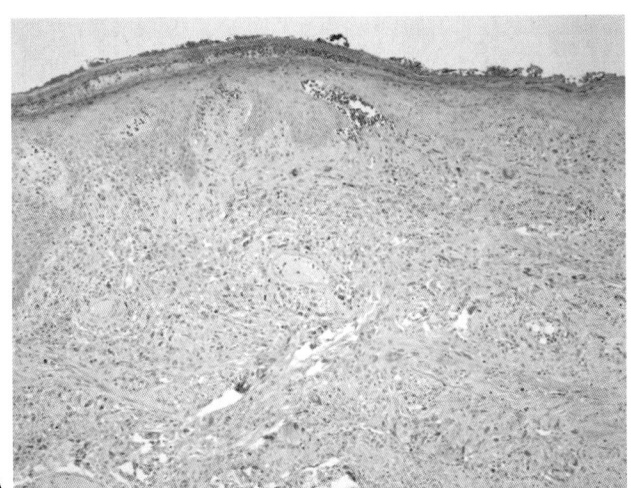

A

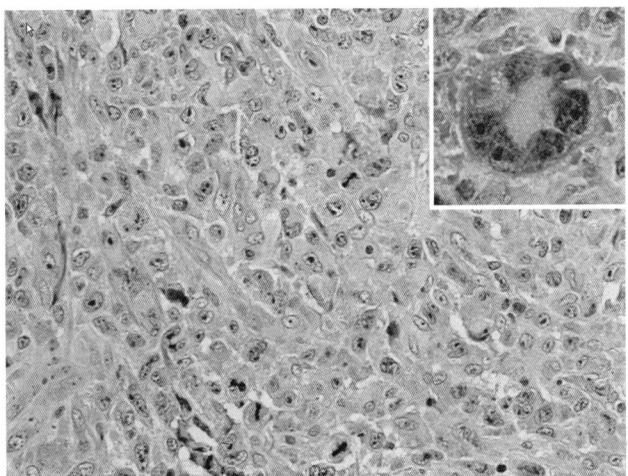

B

FIGURE 26.8. ALK⁺ ALCL secondarily involving skin. This patient also had nodal disease. There is an extensive dermal infiltrate of large tumor cells, including occasional pleomorphic giant cells. The cells are positive for CD30 and ALK. The staining for ALK is cytoplasmic only, without nuclear staining, suggestive of a variant *ALK* translocation (i.e., not involving *NPM*). This case also expressed multiple T-cell antigens, including CD3, CD5, CD43, and CD45RO (not shown).

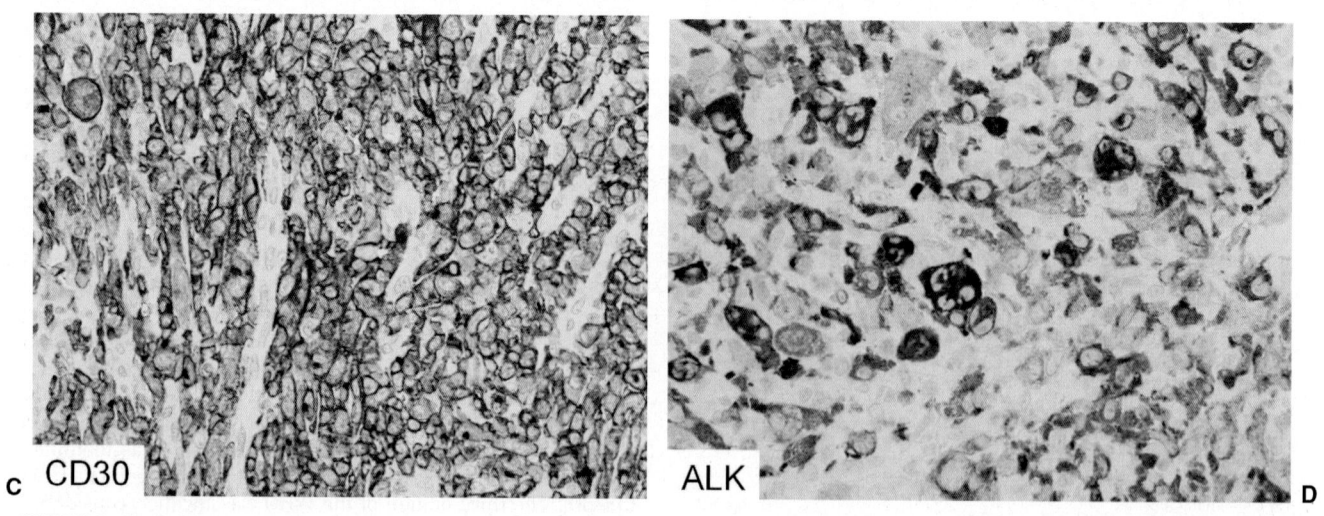

c CD30

ALK D

FIGURE 26.8. *(Continued)*

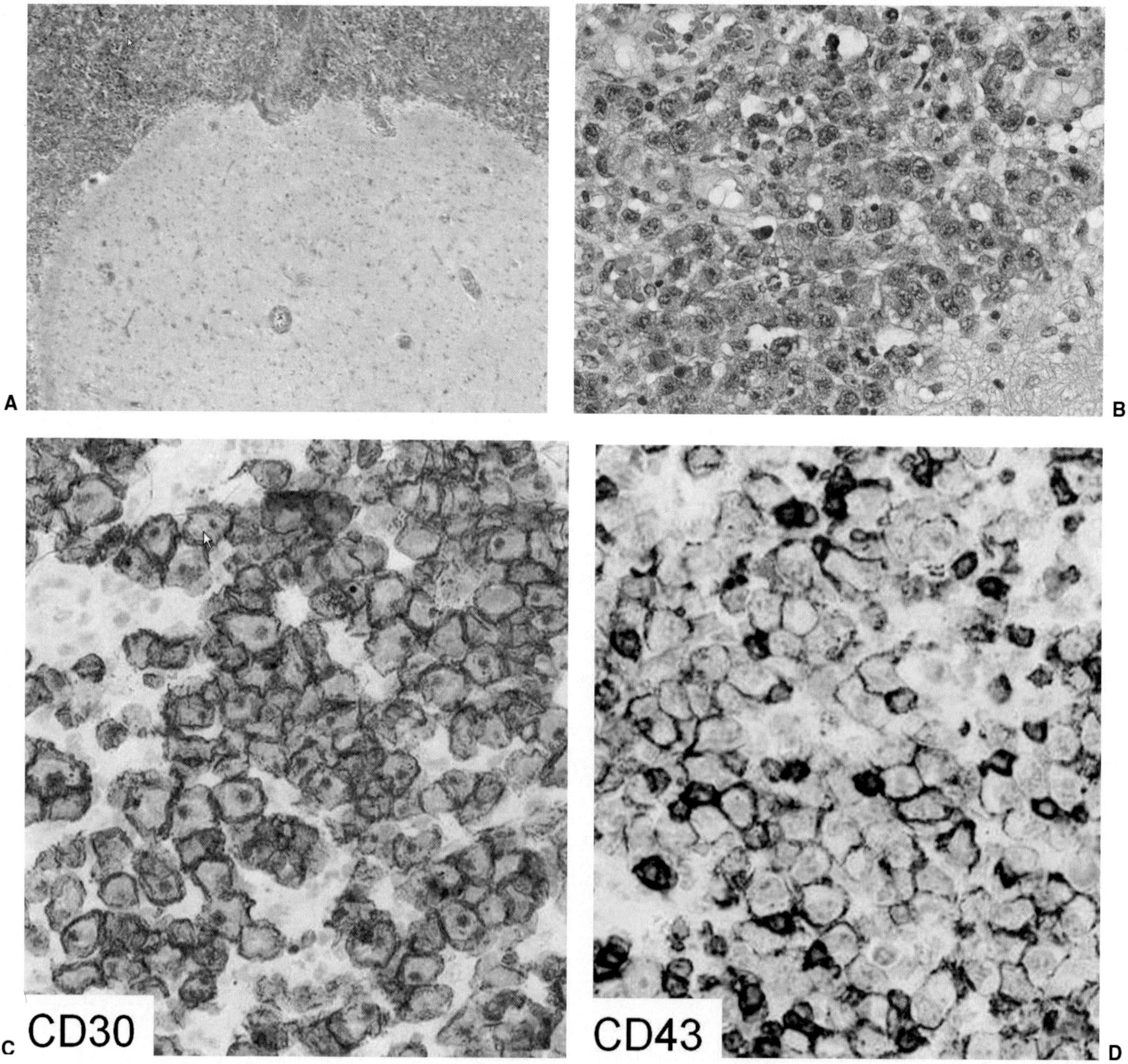

A

B

c CD30

CD43 D

FIGURE 26.9. ALK+ ALCL with unusual presentation in the brain. The biopsy shows sheets of hallmark cells. The tumor cells are positive for CD30, CD43, and ALK. The staining for ALK is both nuclear and cytoplasmic, suggestive of an *NPM/ALK* translocation. CD45RO was the only other T-cell antigen expressed (not shown).

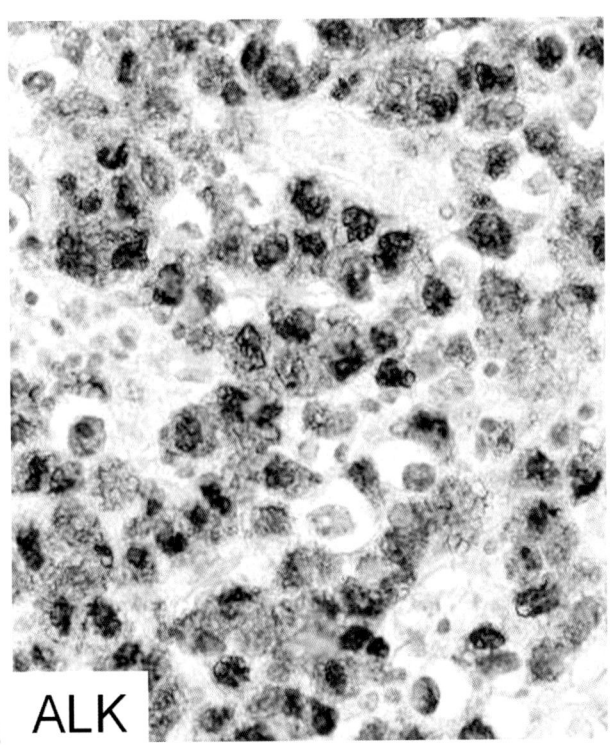

E   ALK

FIGURE 26.9. *(Continued)*

involved in between 10% and 30% of cases, depending on whether or not special studies are used to determine tumor involvement (64).

Clinical Evaluation and Staging
Most patients with ALK⁺ ALCL have B symptoms, particularly fever (5,29,62). Routine lymphoma staging procedures typically are performed. Involvement of bone marrow and sometimes lymph node may not be apparent without the use of special stains. Antibodies to the NPM-ALK fusion protein have been demonstrated in serum from patients with ALK⁺ ALCL but their detection is not used in routine clinical practice.

Morphology

Cytologic Composition
All histologic variants have in common the so-called "hallmark" cell, a large cell with a pleomorphic, often horseshoe-shaped nucleus, a prominent central Golgi zone, and abundant cytoplasm (65). In some cases, the nuclei may show only mild indentation and in others it may be extensively lobated. In some cuts, the nuclei may appear to entirely encircle the Golgi zone ("wreath-like"). In the small cell variant (see below), typical hallmark cells usually represent the minority of the tumor cell population, with small to medium-sized cells without distinct horseshoe-shaped nuclei predominating. The cellular background of the tumor cells varies by histologic subtype and is discussed further below.

Grading
ALCLs are not graded.

Proliferative Pattern
ALK⁺ ALCL typically effaces the lymph node architecture, with sheets of tumor cells that may surround residual lymphoid follicles and characteristically show infiltration of the sinusoids. In some cases, only the sinusoidal distribution may be present, and some nodes may show minimal involvement, occasionally only detectable with the use of special stains.

Histologic Progression/Transformation
Changes in the morphologic patterns seen over time in sequential biopsies may be seen (65). However, histologic features may remain constant over the course of the disease, and criteria for histologic progression have not been formulated. Occasional cases may develop leukemic involvement later in the course of the disease, and this event has a poor prognosis.

Histologic Variants
The current WHO classification considers several morphologic patterns in addition to the most common one described above (Fig. 26.10) (2). The lymphohistiocytic pattern is seen in about 10% of cases and shows numerous reactive histiocytes in the background; the histiocytic infiltrate may be so prominent as to obscure the tumor cells (66). Erythrophagocytosis by the histiocytes may be seen. The tumor cells may be somewhat smaller than those seen in the common pattern, but not as small as those seen in the "small cell" pattern (see below). Clustering of the neoplastic cells around vessels may aid recognition. The "small cell" pattern or variant is seen in 5% to 10% of cases and is characterized by mostly small- to medium-sized tumor cells with nuclear pleomorphism (Fig. 26.11) (67). Typical hallmark cells are nonetheless present on careful examination, particularly surrounding vessels. The "Hodgkin-like" pattern is seen in about 3% of cases and shows features resembling those seen in the nodular sclerosis type of CHL, including tumor cells resembling Reed-Sternberg cells and a polymorphous inflammatory background containing eosinophils (68). Even in Hodgkin-like cases of ALCL, however, the tumor cells typically lack the large, inclusion-like eosinophilic nucleoli of true Reed-Sternberg cells (69). About 15% of cases of ALK⁺ ALCL have a mixture of the above morphologic features ("composite pattern"), particularly cases with a mixture of the lymphohistiocytic and small cell patterns. Rarer features include tumor cells that are predominantly multinucleated giant cells, smaller cells with round nuclei, or spindled ("sarcomatoid") cells (70). Some cases are relatively hypocellular, with an edematous or myxoid background.

Morphology in Sites Other Than Lymph Node
The cytologic features and background inflammatory cell populations seen in extranodal sites often are similar to those seen in the lymph nodes. In the skin, secondary involvement by ALK⁺ ALCL typically takes the form of dermal nodules that morphologically resemble primary cutaneous ALCL (see below). Bone marrow involvement may be subtle and require special stains for detection.

Immunophenotype

IHC is essential for the diagnosis of ALK⁺ ALCL, including demonstration of expression of CD30 and ALK (or demonstration of an *ALK* gene translocation). Expression of both these antigens is almost always uniform, with the exception of some cases of the small cell variant (see below), in which strong staining may be seen only in the true hallmark cells, often surrounding blood vessels. The cellular localization of ALK staining correlates with the partner gene involved in the *ALK* translocation (see the next section), but is of unknown clinical significance (61). Most cases show loss of some or all (so-called "null" type) T-cell antigens (65,71). However, at least the vast majority of these are considered to be of T-cell origin. CD2 and CD4 are the T-cell antigens that are most commonly preserved. Rare

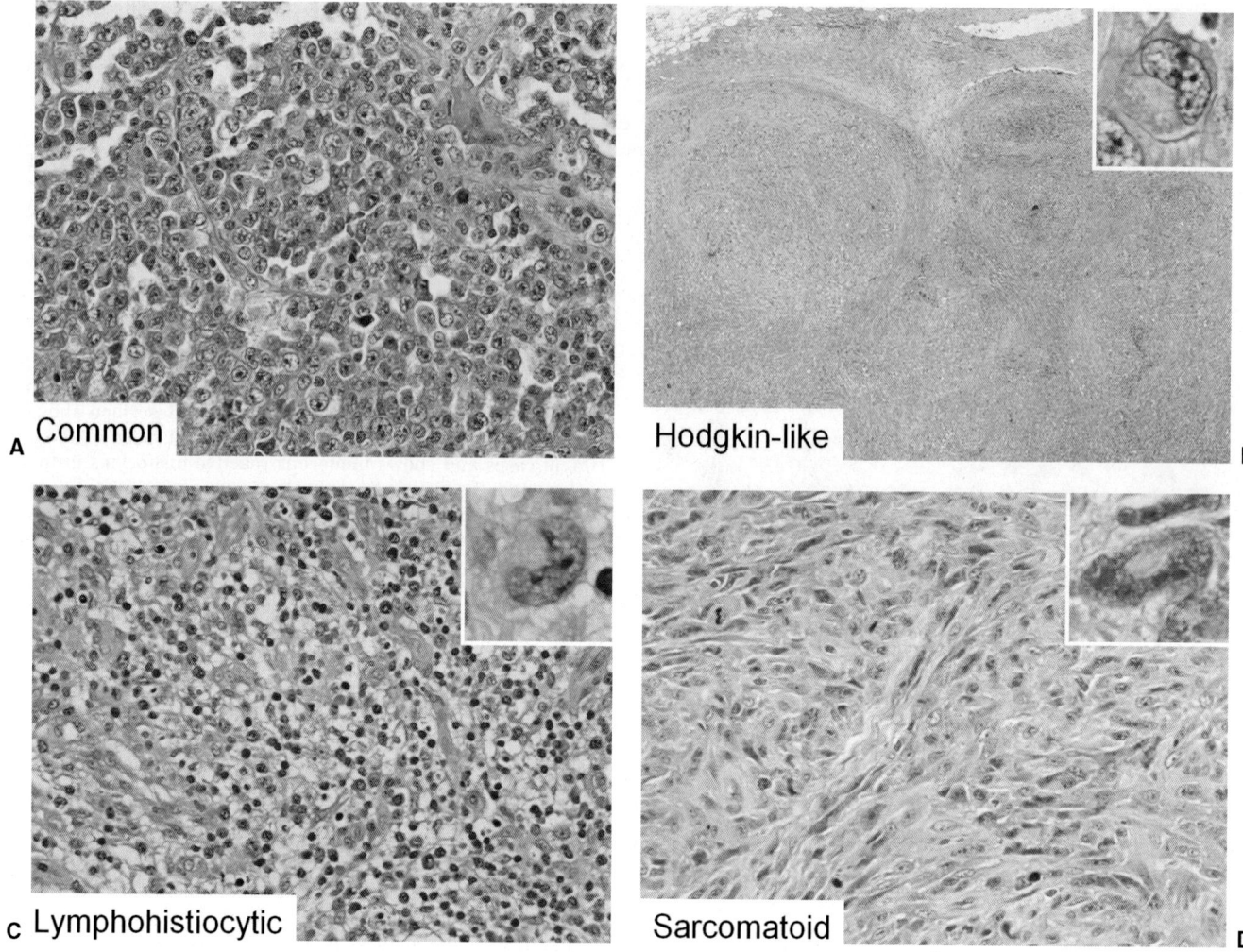

FIGURE 26.10. Morphologic patterns in ALK⁺ ALCL. The common pattern consists of sheets of easily recognizable hallmark cells, often with sinusoidal involvement. The Hodgkin-like case shown here had low-power features resembling the nodular sclerosis type of CHL; there was a mixed inflammatory background, including the presence of eosinophils, but the scattered tumor cells resembled hallmark cells rather than classic Reed-Sternberg cells. In the lymphohistiocytic pattern, tumor cells may be difficult to identify due to the numerous background reactive cells; hallmark cells are present on close examination, but these cases may be mistaken for reactive lymphohistiocytic infiltrates. The sarcomatoid pattern is rare as a sole histologic pattern; this case had other areas with more recognizable hallmark cells.

cases are CD8⁺. Antibodies against TCR proteins such as beta-F1 often are negative, corresponding to lack of TCR expression in most cases. Using a recently developed antibody to the γδ TCR in paraffin material, occasional cases have been shown to be positive, sometimes with coexpression of TCR-βF1. Cytotoxic proteins such as perforin, TIA-1, and granzyme B typically are present (71). Most cases express EMA (65); clusterin and CD56 also may be expressed (72,73). Though typically negative, occasional cases may express CD15 (74). In addition, rare cases may express the B-lineage transcription factor, PAX5, a finding associated with additional copies of the *PAX5* gene locus (75). Rare cases may express keratins. Myeloid markers such as CD13 and CD33 occasionally may be expressed by ALK⁺ ALCLs and should not be interpreted as evidence of an extramedullary myeloid tumor (76). Flow cytometry has been evaluated for immunophenotyping of ALCL, but is not used routinely.

Cytogenetics

All cases of ALK⁺ ALCL have translocations involving *ALK* on 2p23 and one of various partner genes, most commonly the nucleophosmin gene *NPM* on 5q35 (77). Most of these are seen in karyotypic studies, though some may be cryptic

(e.g., *ALK-ATIC*). The fusion partner determines the localization of the fusion protein in the cell, and differences can be seen by IHC. Presence of the *NPM/ALK* translocation leads to both nuclear and cytoplasmic staining for ALK by IHC (Fig. 26.9). Less common partners lead to diffuse cytoplasmic staining only (Fig. 26.8; *TPM3, ATIC, TFG, TPM4, MYH9, ALO17*), granular cytoplasmic staining (*CLTC*), or membranous staining (*MSN*). Identification of the *ALK* partner gene in a given case currently is not necessary for diagnosis or management. FISH can be used to confirm the presence of *ALK* translocations, most commonly used as a breakapart probe spanning the *ALK* locus. Typically, neither FISH nor karyotyping is necessary for diagnosis if ALK protein expression is demonstrated by IHC (see also discussion under *Differential Diagnosis*, below). Secondary chromosomal imbalances have been identified in ALK⁺ ALCLs using CGH. Gains on 17p and losses on 4q and 11q were seen specifically in ALK⁺ ALCLs compared with ALK⁻ ALCLs (78).

Molecular Characteristics

ALCLs lack EBV as detected by either IHC or ISH (79). TCR genes are clonally rearranged in the majority of cases,

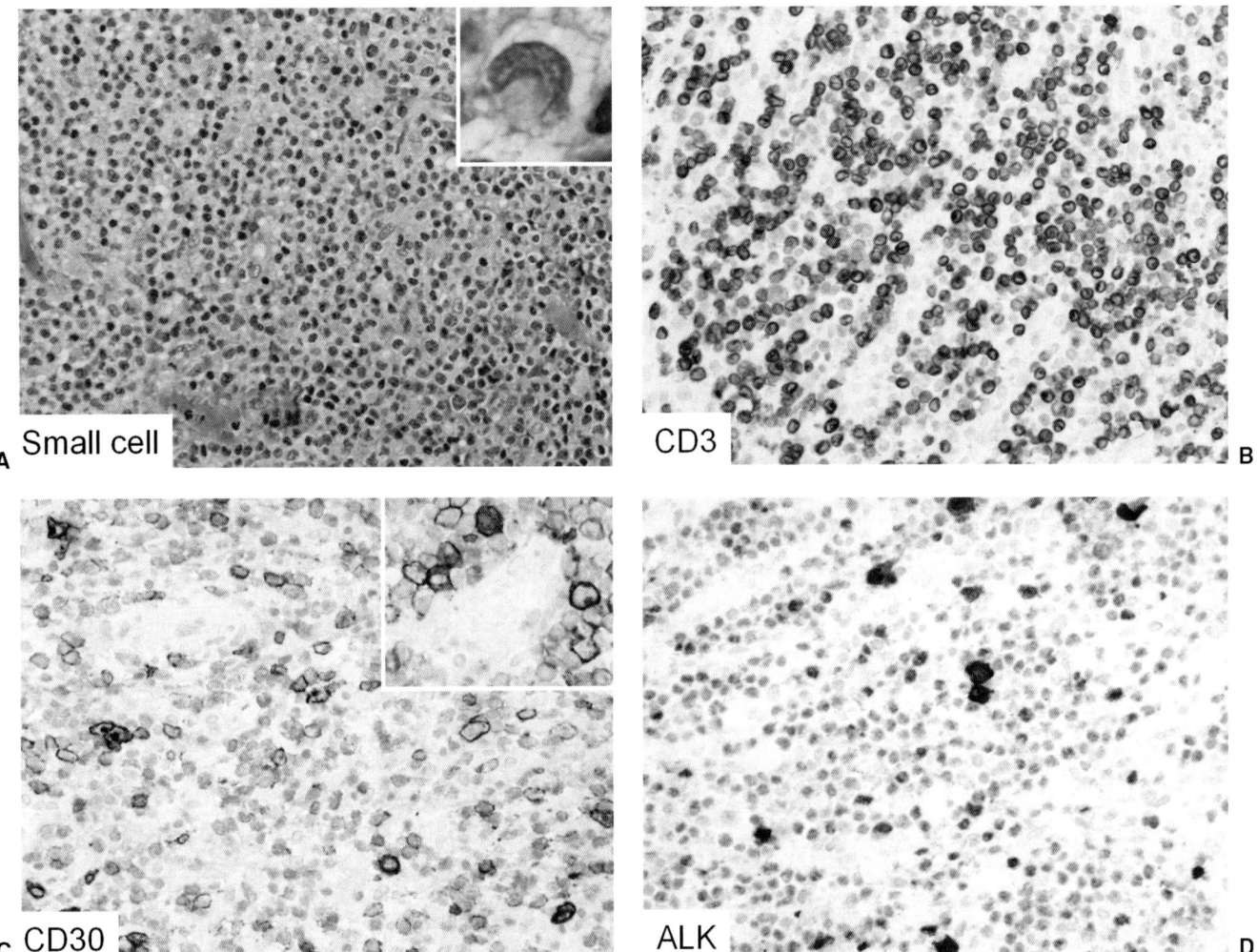

FIGURE 26.11. ALK⁺ ALCL, small cell pattern. There is a diffuse infiltrate of mostly small to medium-sized atypical cells with a moderate amount of cytoplasm. Occasional larger cells with cytologic features of hallmark cells can be seen. The atypical cells are positive for CD3. They are variably positive for CD30, with the strongest staining seen in the larger cells, particularly surrounding vessels. ALK shows cytoplasmic and nuclear staining in both the small cell component and the occasional larger cells.

including those that lack expression of T-cell antigens ("null-cell" cases) (71). IG genes are germline. GEP also has identified differences between ALK⁺ and ALK⁻ ALCLs, including overexpression of the genes encoding BCL6 and C/EBPβ (80). The function of ALK fusion proteins, particularly NPM-ALK, has been studied extensively and includes cellular activation via the AKT and MAP kinase signaling pathways (81).

Postulated Normal Counterpart

The normal counterpart is believed to be an activated CD4⁺ T lymphocyte. Recent data have suggested similarities with Th17 cells, but it is not known whether these represent the cell of origin (82).

Clinical Course and Prognostic Assessment

ALK⁺ ALCL generally has a favorable outcome. The most important prognostic feature is the expression of ALK itself, which distinguishes this entity from ALK⁻ ALCL (see the next section) and other CD30⁺ PTCLs. Among ALK⁺ cases, low IPI scores and limited stage disease are associated with better prognosis (29,62), and these data should be obtained. Patients with leukemic presentation tend to follow

a particularly aggressive clinical course. Additional prognostic factors have not been introduced into routine clinical practice. Antibodies to the NPM-ALK fusion protein have been detected in the sera of patients with ALK⁺ ALCL, even following complete clinical responses to therapy. However, the prognostic significance of the presence or levels of these antibodies is unknown.

Treatment and Survival

Most adult patients with ALK⁺ ALCL are treated with CHOP-like chemotherapy regimens; pediatric patients have responded to short-pulse chemotherapy regimens modeled after high-grade B-cell lymphoma protocols (61). Retreatment often is effective for relapses; refractory cases also may respond to allogeneic bone marrow transplantation (83). Several targeted therapies have been explored in clinical trials, including therapies utilizing monoclonal antibodies against the CD30 molecule and small-molecule inhibitors of the ALK tyrosine kinase (31,84). Recently, a toxin linked to an anti-CD30 monoclonal antibody (SGN-35) has shown promising results (85). The prognosis of ALK⁺ ALCL is one of the most favorable among PTCLs, with a 5-year OS rate of 70% to 80%, with the lower end of the spectrum reflecting studies that exclude children (29,62). These outcomes are significantly better than those for either ALK⁻ ALCL (see below) or PTCL, NOS.

Differential Diagnosis

ALK⁻ and Primary Cutaneous ALCL
The common pattern of ALK⁺ ALCL usually has characteristic morphologic features, in which the major differential diagnosis is ALK⁻ ALCL. This differential is resolved by IHC for ALK protein or genetic studies confirming a translocation involving the *ALK* gene. In the skin, the morphologic and phenotypic features of secondary involvement by ALK⁺ ALCL often resemble those of primary cutaneous ALCL (Fig. 26.8). Thus, IHC for ALK always should be performed in the evaluation of cutaneous CD30⁺ T-cell lymphoproliferative disorders. Cutaneous presentation of ALK⁺ ALCL has been associated with insect bites, possibly due to the effects of local cytokine release on T cells already bearing *ALK* translocations (86). These patients typically develop systemic disease. Primary cutaneous ALCLs traditionally have been considered ALK⁻, allowing ALK IHC to differentiate between these entities. Recently, however, it has been appreciated that occasional ALK⁺ lesions present in, and are anatomically limited to, the skin, suggesting that ALK⁺ variants of primary cutaneous ALCL exist (87). Therefore, the clinical history and staging

data are important before assigning a diagnosis of systemic ALK⁺ ALCL based on a skin biopsy.

Classical Hodgkin Lymphoma
Hodgkin-like ALCL must be differentiated from CHL, which is treated differently. The diagnosis is not difficult once an ALK immunostain has been performed; for this reason, awareness of the considerable morphologic and phenotypic overlap between these two entities is critical (68). Occasional expression of CD15 and rarely PAX5 by ALCL may lead to a mistaken diagnosis of CHL; conversely, CHL may occasionally express T-cell antigens and/or cytotoxic proteins.

Reactive Conditions
The lymphohistiocytic pattern occasionally may have sufficient inflammatory cells so as to obscure the tumor cells and mimic a reactive process. A careful search for hallmark cells is necessary to prompt IHC, which will secure the correct diagnosis.

Other CD30⁺ PTCLs
The small cell pattern may be mistaken for PTCL, NOS if testing for ALK is not performed, since the majority of tumor cells in this pattern do not have the cytologic features of hallmark cells (Fig. 26.11). A careful search for the latter, particularly around blood vessels, is the key to identifying this pattern. In some

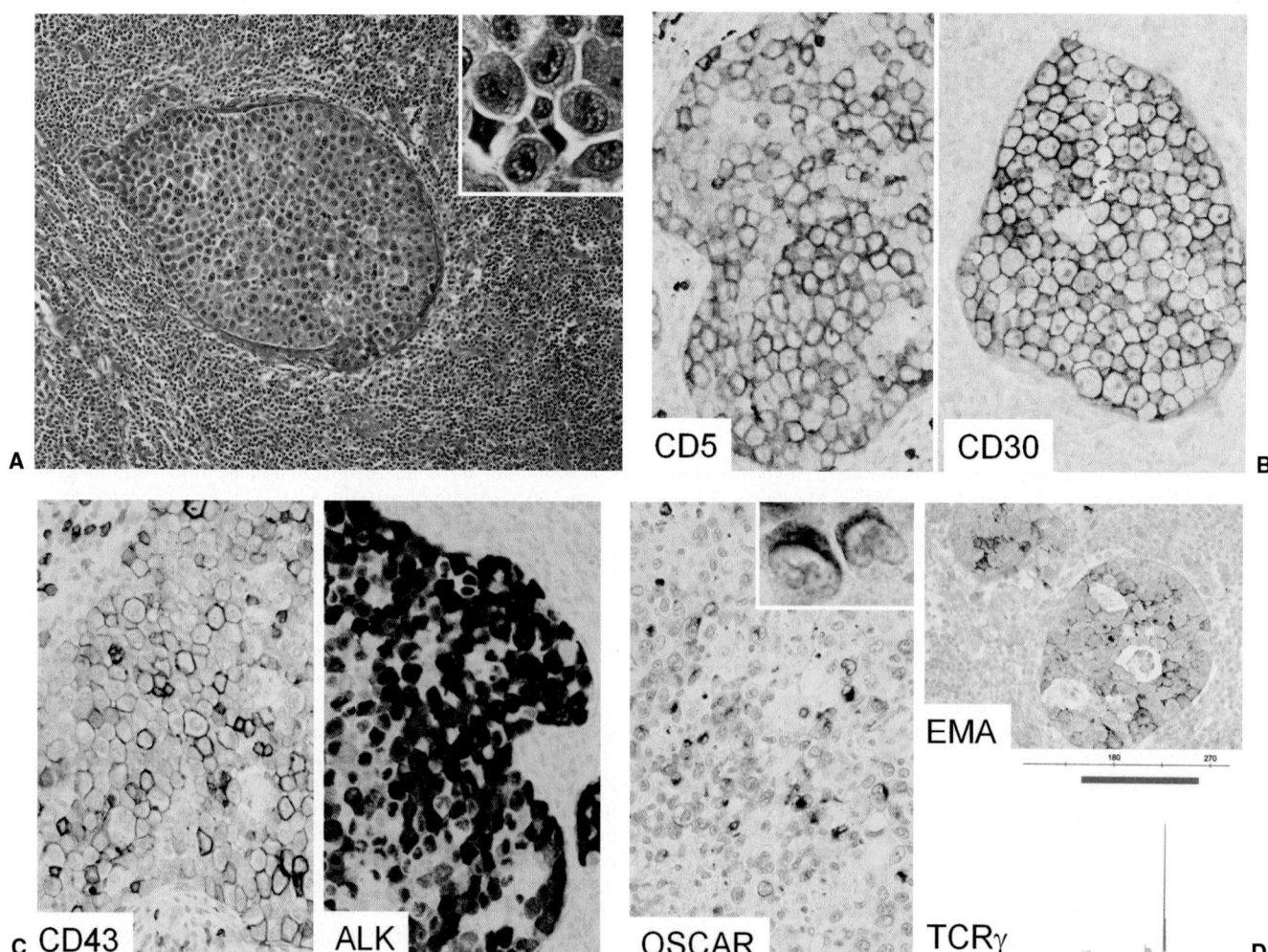

FIGURE 26.12. ALK⁺ ALCL mimicking metastatic carcinoma. Tumor cells are nearly exclusively within sinusoids. This case was originally interpreted as metastatic carcinoma based on the expression of EMA and the broad-spectrum keratin stain, OSCAR. Other keratins were negative (not shown). Additional stains were performed. The tumor expresses the T-cell antigens CD5, CD43, and CD45RO (not shown), as well as nuclear and cytoplasmic ALK. A clonal *TCR* (gamma and beta, not shown) gene rearrangement pattern is seen by PCR.

cases, these larger perivascular hallmark cells may be the only tumor cells to show reactivity for CD30.

ALK⁺ Diffuse Large B-Cell Lymphoma

A subset of DLBCLs express ALK (as well as EMA, see below) and have *ALK* translocations. These may show a sinusoidal pattern of distribution; in addition, ALK⁺ DLBCLs often lack CD20 expression and may coexpress CD4 (88). In contrast to ALCL, however, hallmark cells are absent and the tumor cells are negative for CD30 (88). Most ALK⁺ DLBCLs demonstrate plasmablastic cytologic features and typically are positive for CD138, IgA, and either kappa or lambda IG light chain. Further studies such as TCR and IG gene rearrangement studies rarely are necessary.

Carcinomas and Other Solid Tumors

Cases of ALK⁺ ALCL with infiltration of the sinusoids and minimal nodal effacement can resemble metastatic tumors, but cytologic and phenotypic features usually are distinct. In the differential diagnosis between ALK⁺ ALCL and carcinoma, keratins should be used instead of EMA. It should be noted, however, that rarely ALCL may express keratins (Fig. 26.12). In addition, a subset of lung carcinomas (89) and rare other carcinomas carry *ALK* translocations and express ALK protein. Neuroblastomas also may express ALK (90). These tumors generally are distinguishable morphologically, and a complete immunohistochemical panel will lead to the correct diagnosis. Some nonhematologic tumors, including germ cell tumors and occasional soft tissue sarcomas, express CD30. The sarcomatoid pattern of ALK⁺ ALCL also may mimic soft tissue sarcomas morphologically (Fig. 26.10). Awareness of this pattern and performance of ALK IHC resolves this issue. Inflammatory myofibroblastic tumors also carry *ALK* translocations and express ALK protein (91). These typically have a distinctly benign morphologic appearance compared to the rare cases of sarcomatoid ALCL.

ALK⁻ Anaplastic Large Cell Lymphoma

Definition

ALK⁻ ALCL is listed provisionally as a distinct entity in the fourth edition of the WHO classification for the first time (2). This distinction was made based on differences in demographics, biology, and outcome between ALK⁻ ALCL and either ALK⁺ ALCL or CD30⁺ PTCL, NOS. ALK⁻ ALCL is a neoplasm of mature T cells that express CD30 and is morphologically indistinguishable from ALK⁺ ALCL but lacks expression of ALK protein and translocations of the *ALK* gene. These tumors previously were included in the general designation, Ki-1 lymphoma, based on their immunoreactivity for CD30 using the Ki-1 antibody. In general, the designation ALK⁻ ALCL is used to define cases with a narrower morphologic spectrum than the range of histologic variants seen in ALK⁺ ALCL; the border between ALK⁻ ALCL and CD30⁺ PTCL, NOS continues to be refined.

Epidemiology

ALK⁻ ALCL represents about 40% to 50% of ALCLs, depending on the study. ALK⁻ ALCL is a disease of adults, with a peak incidence in the sixth decade (29). In this regard, it differs from ALK⁺ ALCL, which is primarily a disease of the young. The male:female ratio of ALK⁻ ALCL is about 1.5:1.

Clinical Features

Sites of Involvement

ALK⁻ ALCL typically presents with lymphadenopathy. Extranodal involvement occurs, but is less common than in ALK⁺ ALCL; the most common extranodal sites are skin, lung, and liver (29).

Clinical Evaluation and Staging

Most patients present with advanced (stage III or IV) disease, and most have B symptoms (29). Because secondary cutaneous involvement shows considerable morphologic and phenotypic overlap with primary cutaneous ALCL, which is a distinct entity, staging and clinical history are critical to distinguish these entities. Primary cutaneous ALCL may involve local lymph nodes, so the distribution of lymph node involvement relative to the skin lesions and the order of appearance of the cutaneous and nodal sites of disease in the evolution of the process are important for correct classification.

Morphology

Cytologic Composition

The cytologic features of the neoplastic cells in ALK⁻ ALCL are similar to those of most ALK⁺ ALCLs, including the presence of hallmark cells. In general, the cells in ALK⁻ ALCL tend to be larger and more pleomorphic than in ALK⁺ ALCL (Fig. 26.13) (92). Multinucleated cells with wreath-like nuclei are common. A small-cell variant is not recognized. Varying numbers of inflammatory cells may be seen in the background, including small lymphocytes, histiocytes, plasma cells, and eosinophils; however, histologic patterns such as the lymphohistiocytic and Hodgkin-like patterns are not strictly defined.

Grading

ALK⁻ ALCL is not graded.

Proliferative Pattern

ALK⁻ ALCL has similar morphologic features to its ALK⁺ counterpart. Typically, it effaces the lymph node architecture, often with sheet-like growth sparing residual lymphoid follicles. Cases with less architectural effacement may predominantly involve the sinuses and may mimic metastatic tumors.

Histologic Progression/Transformation

Cases of ALK⁻ ALCL tend to have similar histologic features over the entire disease course. Histologic features of transformation have not been described.

Histologic Variants

The WHO classification does not include distinct variants or patterns of ALK⁻ ALCL as it does for ALK⁺ ALCL (2). This may be partly due to differing biology, but also based on the provisional nature of ALK⁻ ALCL as a distinct entity in the WHO classification and the lack of ALK positivity to assist in differentiating it from CD30⁺ cases of PTCL, NOS. However, cases with relatively numerous small lymphocytes and histiocytes exist, analogous to the lymphohistiocytic variant of ALK⁺ ALCL. Other cases have a mixed inflammatory background, including eosinophils and Reed-Sternberg–like cells, analogous to the Hodgkin-like variant of ALK⁺ ALCL (Fig. 26.14). Based on strict definition of the morphology of this entity to keep this provisional category pure, cases with features analogous to the small-cell variant of ALK⁺ ALCL probably should be classified as PTCL, NOS. Better understanding of genetic differences between ALK⁻ ALCL and PTCL, NOS may allow expansion of the morphologic criteria for ALK⁻ ALCL and the ability to characterize histologic variants more accurately.

Morphology in Sites Other Than Lymph Node

The morphology of ALK⁻ ALCL involving extranodal sites is similar to that seen in lymph nodes and that seen in ALK⁺ ALCL. In the skin, ALK⁻ ALCL typically forms dermal nodules or diffuse infiltrates that often are morphologically and phenotypically indistinguishable from primary cutaneous

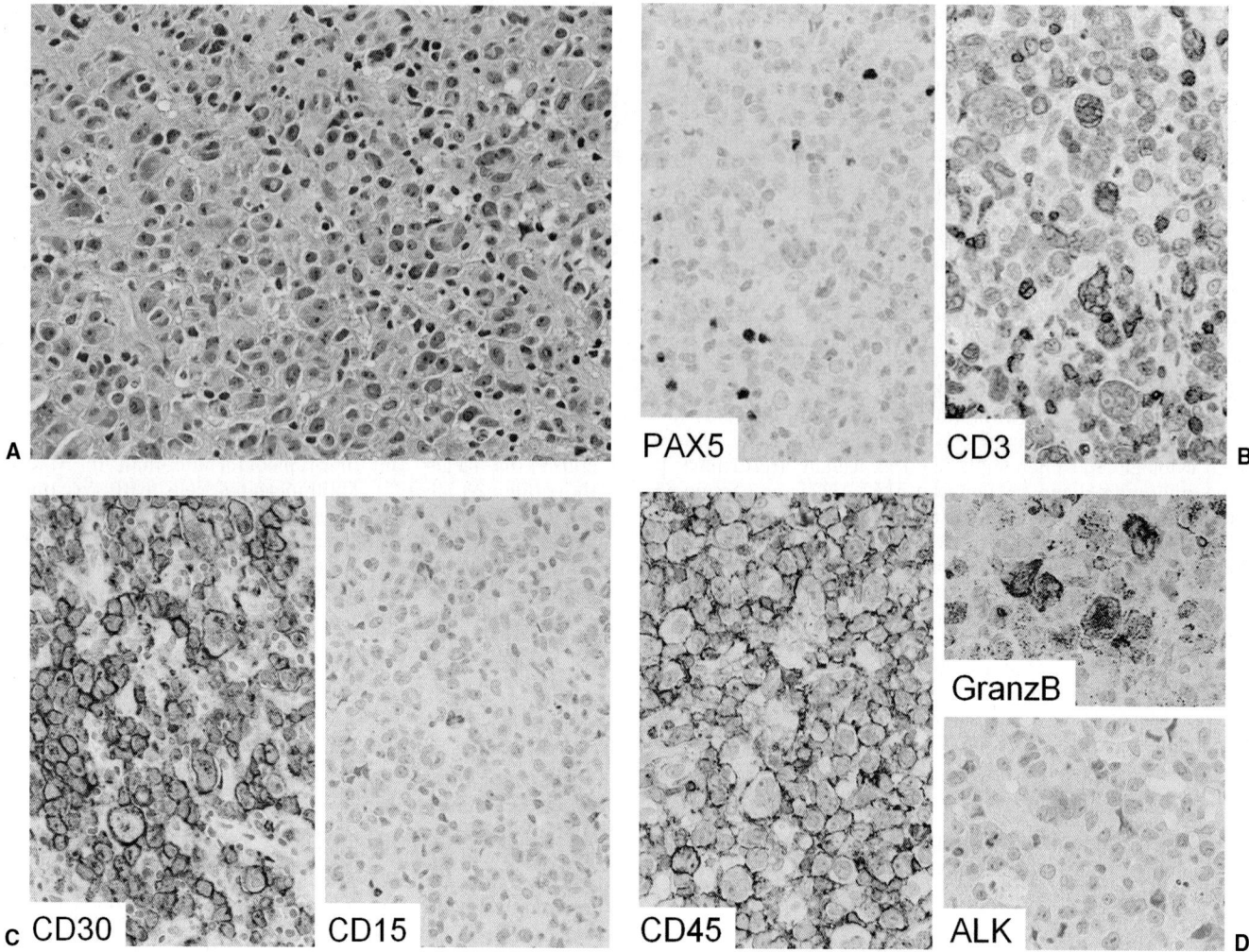

FIGURE 26.13. ALK⁻ anaplastic large cell lymphoma. The tumor cells are large and pleomorphic, including some cells with cytologic features of hallmark cells and some with wreath-like nuclei. The tumor cells form sheets with minimal inflammatory background. They lack expression of PAX5 and other B-cell markers (not shown) and are positive for CD3. They express CD30 but not CD15. This case uniformly expressed CD45 and was positive for the cytotoxic marker, granzyme B. ALK was negative.

ALCL. Occasional cases with similar morphologic and phenotypic features may be seen involving mucosal surfaces of the head and neck, including oral cavity, respiratory mucosa, and conjunctiva/orbit (Fig. 26.15). Though these cases do not meet the criteria for primary cutaneous ALCL based on site, they share similarities with that entity, and it is not clear they should be classified as systemic ALK⁻ ALCL when limited to mucosal sites, based on overall indolent clinical behavior (93). Recently, neoplasms with the cytologic and immunophenotypic features of ALK⁻ ALCL have been reported in the seroma fluid and fibrous capsule surrounding breast implants (Fig. 26.15). Most such cases have an indolent clinical course and may represent a distinct entity; however, occasional seroma-associated ALCLs have been associated with systemic disease and aggressive clinical behavior (94,95).

Immunophenotype

IHC is essential for the diagnosis of ALK⁻ ALCL, including demonstration of expression of CD30 and confirming negativity for ALK. CD30 staining should be strong and uniform, with membranous, Golgi, and sometimes cytoplasmic staining. Weak or partial CD30 expression may suggest PTCL, NOS. Like its ALK⁺ counterpart, ALK⁻ ALCL may lack expression of

multiple T-cell antigens, so its T-cell lineage may not be initially apparent. Cytotoxic markers often are expressed even when surface T-cell antigens are absent. EMA and/or clusterin may be expressed, but this is less common than in ALK⁺ ALCL (29). ALK⁻ ALCLs may demonstrate aberrant expression of myeloid markers, but this is less common than in ALK⁺ ALCL (96).

Cytogenetics

Genetic studies to exclude *ALK* translocations generally are not necessary if reliable IHC for ALK protein is available. Recently, recurrent rearrangements of the *DUSP22-IRF4* locus on 6p25.3 with non-*TCR* gene partners have been described in ALCL (19,35,97). The most common partner is a nongenic region on 7q32.3 near the DNA fragile site, *FRA7H* (Fig. 26.16). These rearrangements should not be confused with the *IRF4/TRA@* translocations seen in rare PTCLs, NOS, which are CD30⁻ (19). To date, 6p25.3 rearrangements in ALCL are mutually exclusive of *ALK* translocations; they are most common in primary cutaneous ALCL, where they occur in about 28% of cases, but also may be seen in up to 18% of systemic ALK⁻ ALCLs and occasional ALK⁻ ALCLs with disease limited to mucosal sites (93). As discussed in the section on genetics of ALK⁺ ALCL, various studies using CGH and GEP have identified differences between ALK⁻ and ALK⁺ ALCLs; however, the clinical utility of these differences remains unclear.

Molecular Characteristics

EBV typically is absent in ALK⁻ ALCLs; its presence may suggest the possibility of CHL. TCR genes are clonally rearranged in the majority of cases; IG genes are germline. PCR may help distinguish ALK⁻ ALCL from CHL. It should be noted, however, that (a) ALCL, ALK⁻ may rarely lack clonal TCR gene rearrangements; (b) IG gene rearrangements are not always detected by PCR in CHL; and (c) rare cases of CHL may be of T-cell origin, though this is controversial. Cases with rearrangements of 6p25.3 demonstrate down-regulated expression of the *DUSP22* gene encoding a dual-specificity phosphatase; those with the 7p32.3 partner show overexpression of micro-RNAs in the *MIR29* cluster (35).

Postulated Normal Counterpart

Like ALK⁺ ALCL, ALK⁻ ALCL is believed to derive from an activated CD4⁺ T cell.

Clinical Course and Prognostic Assessment

Patients with ALK⁻ ALCL typically present with advanced stage (III or IV) disease and have a more aggressive clinical course than patients with ALK⁺ ALCL (29). Aside from confirming negativity for ALK, prognostic assessment currently is limited to clinical features, principally stage and IPI. The presence of 6p25.3 rearrangements may be associated with favorable prognosis (98), but this has not been confirmed in larger studies.

Treatment and Survival

Like patients with other PTCLs, patients with ALK⁻ ALCL typically receive cytotoxic chemotherapy such as CHOP. Refractory cases may be transplanted. No therapeutic modalities specific for this entity have been identified; however, patients with ALK⁻ ALCL have been included in various experimental approaches for treatment of PTCL in general, including those targeting CD30. The prognosis of ALK⁻ ALCL is poorer than that of its ALK⁺ counterpart in most studies, with a 5-year OS rate of 49% (vs. 80%) (29). This difference appears independent

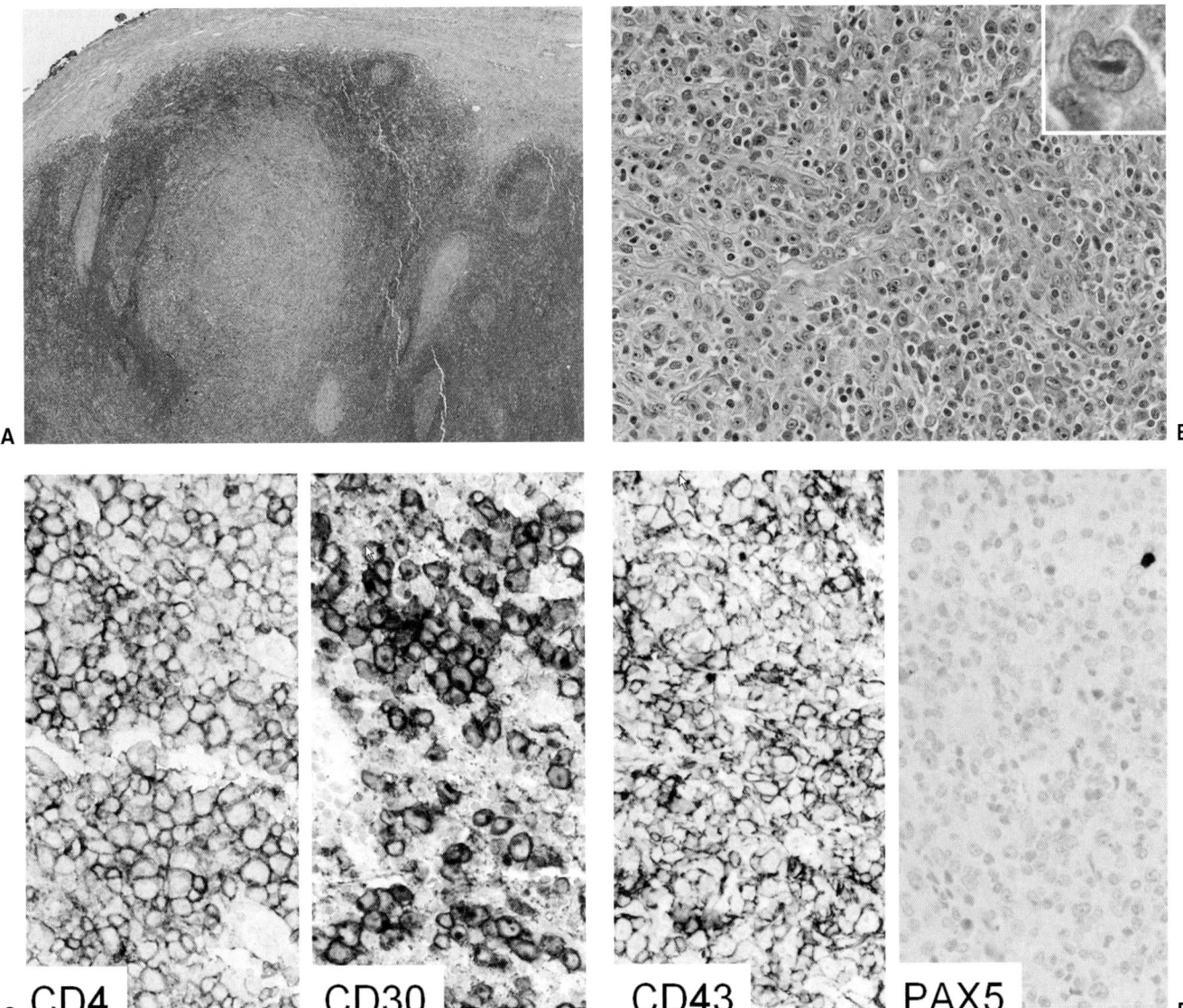

FIGURE 26.14. ALK⁻ ALCL mimicking the nodular sclerosis type of CHL. The lymph node shows a nodular lymphohistiocytic infiltrate with a thickened, sclerotic capsule. There are large tumor cells in a background of small lymphocytes, histiocytes, and eosinophils. While some of the tumor cells have Reed-Sternberg–like cytologic features, hallmark cells are present. The tumor cells expressed CD4, CD30, and CD43. They were negative for other T-cell antigens and cytotoxic markers, as well as CD15 (not shown). PAX5 and ALK were negative. PCR showed a clonal T-cell gene rearrangement; no clonal IG gene rearrangement was detected (not shown).

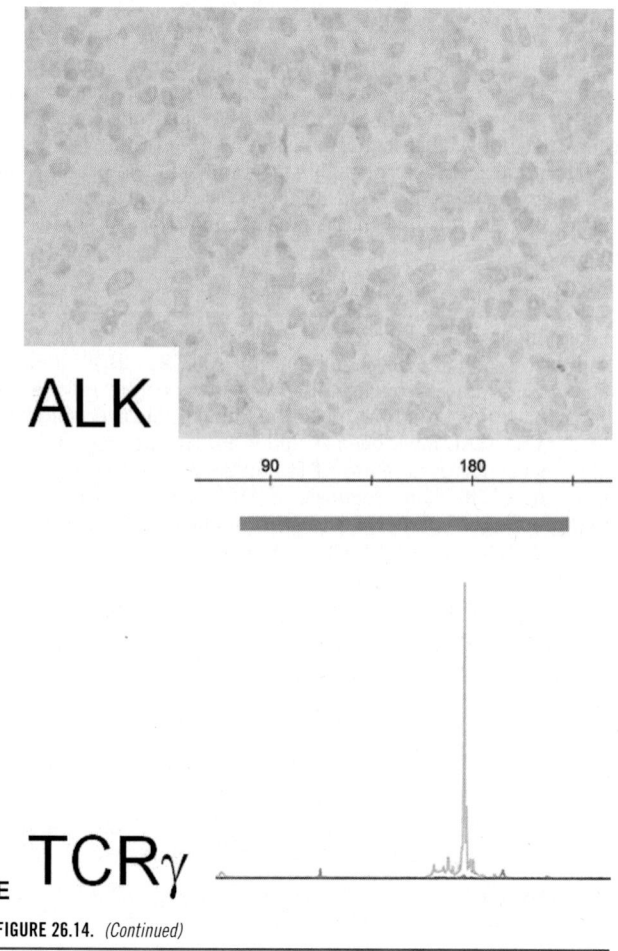

ALK

TCRγ

E

FIGURE 26.14. *(Continued)*

difference that is even more pronounced when ALK⁻ ALCL is compared to the subset of PTCL, NOS that is CD30⁺ (49% vs. 19%) (29). Together, these data provide a rationale for considering ALK⁻ ALCL a separate disease entity, distinct from both ALK⁺ ALCL and PTCL, NOS.

Differential Diagnosis

ALK⁺ ALCL

The morphologic features of ALK⁻ ALCL resemble those of ALK⁺ ALCL by definition. Therefore, ALK⁻ ALCL must be distinguished from ALK⁺ ALCL by IHC for an ALK fusion protein or FISH or other genetic analysis for *ALK* translocations.

Primary Cutaneous ALCL

Secondary cutaneous involvement by systemic ALK⁻ ALCL has virtually identical morphologic and phenotypic features as primary cutaneous ALCL. Clinical history and staging data are paramount in this distinction when only a skin biopsy is available for examination. Reliable immunohistochemical markers to distinguish cutaneous from systemic ALK⁻ ALCL in lymph nodes have not been established, though it has been suggested that in skin the cells of primary cutaneous ALCL express cutaneous lymphocyte antigen and lack expression of EMA (31,100). While rearrangements of the *DUSP22-IRF4* locus on 6p25.3 are more common in primary cutaneous ALCL, they also may occur in systemic ALK⁻ ALCL (35). Extracutaneous spread occurs in about 10% of cases of primary cutaneous ALCL, usually to regional lymph nodes. The histologic manifestations of lymph node involvement have not been studied comprehensively, but in most cases they resemble the findings in systemic ALCLs. Sheets of large, neoplastic cells efface the lymph node architecture. Cases with a lesser degree of nodal effacement may show a predominant sinusoidal pattern. Cytologically, tumor cells are pleomorphic and may have features of hallmark cells; distinct variants or patterns (small-cell, lymphohistiocytic, etc.) have not been described in the lymph node. When lymph node involvement is present, the anatomic relationship of the involved nodes to the skin lesion(s) and the sequence of presentation are important considerations in distinguishing involvement by primary cutaneous ALCL from systemic ALK⁻ ALCL. Primary cutaneous ALCL with locoregional lymph node involvement has a favorable prognosis nearly identical to that observed in primary cutaneous ALCL limited to the skin, and significantly better than that seen in systemic ALK⁻ ALCL (101). When only a

of the older median age of patients with ALK⁻ ALCL. Initially, it was thought that ALK⁻ ALCL had a prognosis similar to that of PTCL, NOS (99), raising the question of whether distinction between these two entities was clinically important. Recent data, however, show that ALK⁻ ALCL has a 5-year OS rate better than that of PTCL, NOS (49% vs. 32%, respectively), a

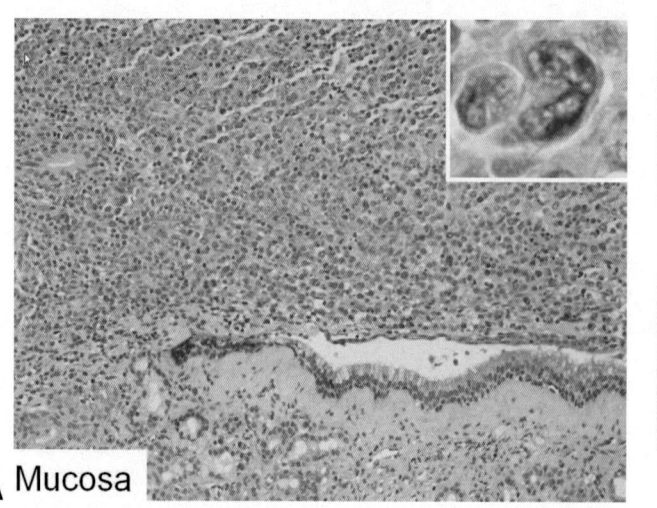

Mucosa

A

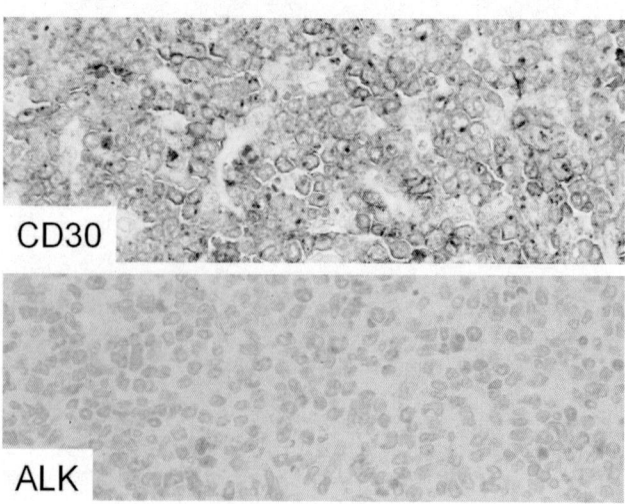

CD30

ALK

B

FIGURE 26.15. ALK⁻ ALCLs in the nasal mucosa and in a breast implant-associated seroma. The cytologic and immunophenotypic features of these tumors are similar to other ALK⁻ ALCLs. However, most cases occurring in these sites without systemic disease have indolent clinical behavior more akin to primary cutaneous ALCL than to most cases of systemic ALK⁻ ALCL.

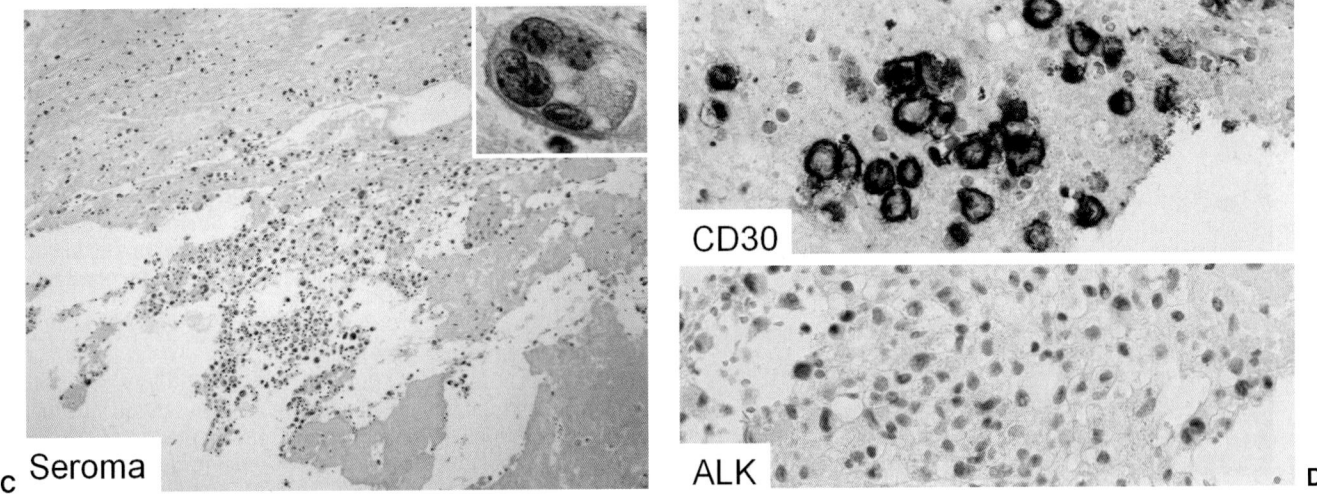

C Seroma

CD30

ALK   D

FIGURE 26.15. *(Continued)*

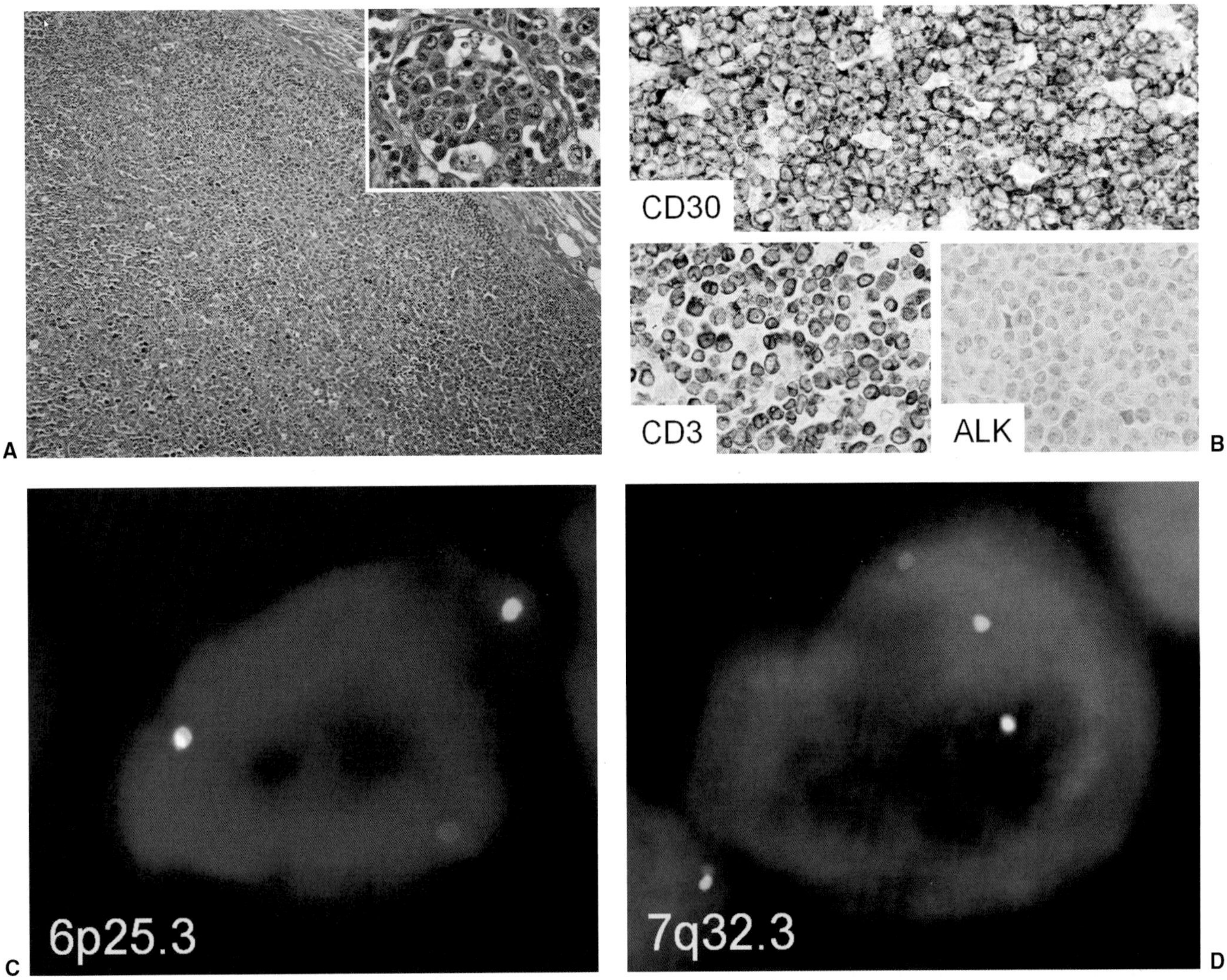

A   B

CD30

CD3   ALK

C 6p25.3   7q32.3   D

FIGURE 26.16. ALK⁻ ALCL with t(6;7)(p25.3;q32.3). The lymph node architecture is effaced by the tumor cells, many of which have cytologic features of hallmark cells. Sinusoidal involvement was present. The tumor cells expressed CD3 and CD30 and were negative for ALK. Breakapart FISH probes for the *DUSP22-IRF4* locus on 6p25.3 and the *FRA7H* locus on 7q32.3 each showed abnormal separation of red and green signals. Dual-fusion FISH confirmed t(6;7)(p25.3;q32.3).

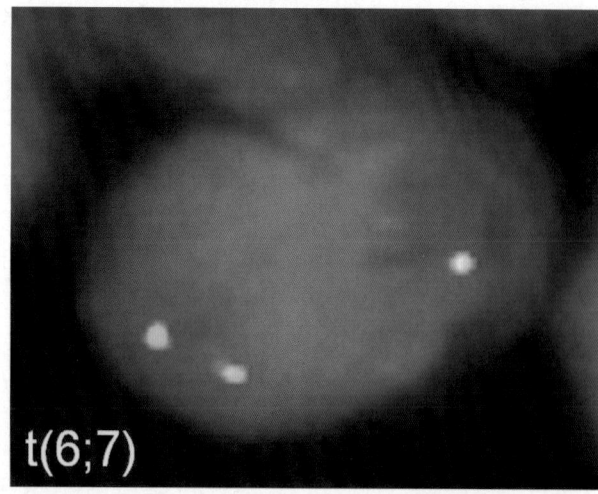

t(6;7)

E

FIGURE 26.16. *(Continued)*

lymph node is available for examination, secondary lymph node involvement by primary cutaneous ALCL should be considered, even when a clinical history of skin involvement is not available.

Classical Hodgkin Lymphoma and Other B-Cell Lineage Lymphomas

Although a Hodgkin-like variant of ALK⁻ ALCL is not formally recognized in the WHO classification, cases with morphologic and phenotypic overlap with CHL exist, and accurate diagnosis is critical due to differing treatments. The approach to this distinction was discussed in the section on ALK⁺ ALCL; however, the distinction is more difficult for ALK⁻ ALCL without the ability to rely on ALK staining to aid in diagnosis. Positivity for EMA, clusterin, or CD56 help support a diagnosis of ALK⁻ ALCL, as they are consistently absent in CHL; however, these markers are expressed less frequently in ALK⁻ ALCL than in ALK⁺ ALCL. Strong, uniform expression of CD45 (Fig. 26.13) or CD43 (Fig. 26.14) favors ALK⁻ ALCL over CHL. The presence of EBV favors CHL. It should be noted that CHL may occasionally express cytotoxic markers and/or T-cell antigens (102). Conversely, ALK⁻ ALCL may express CD15 and lack expression of CD45. PAX5 is weakly positive in most CHLs and negative in most ALK⁻ ALCLs (103); however, weak PAX5 staining may be seen in rare ALK⁻ ALCLs (75). Gene rearrangement studies are helpful, but not entirely sensitive as discussed above. Occasionally, other B-lineage lymphomas may enter the differential diagnosis. Both plasmablastic lymphomas and primary effusion lymphomas (and rare cases of DLBCL, NOS) may express CD30 and EMA, lack multiple B-cell antigens, and may aberrantly express T-cell antigens. Clinical presentation, IG expression, demonstration of EBV and/or human herpesvirus-8 (HHV8), and gene rearrangement studies are important in distinguishing these lymphomas from ALK⁻ ALCL.

Other CD30⁺ PTCLs

ALK⁻ ALCL must be differentiated from CD30⁺ PTCL, NOS, particularly in light of recent data suggesting inferior outcomes in the latter (29). This distinction is primarily morphologic, based on the cytologic features consistent with hallmark cells in a majority of tumor cells, but IHC also is helpful. The WHO recommends a conservative approach to classification, reserving the term ALK⁻ ALCL for cases with morphology and phenotype similar to ALK⁺ ALCL except for the absence of ALK expression (2). Cases diagnosed as ALK⁻ ALCL should have uniform, strong CD30 expression and preferably expression of cytotoxic markers. In addition to the cytologic features of the tumor cells, architectural features, particularly the presence

of sinusoidal involvement, are helpful. In the gastrointestinal tract, it is not clear whether tumors resembling ALK⁻ ALCL should be diagnosed as such or considered EATLs (type 2), which may express CD30. When only abdominal lymph nodes are available for examination, nodal involvement by CD30⁺ EATL should be considered. In lymph nodes at any site, transformed MF may enter the differential diagnosis. Transformed MF may express CD30 and cytotoxic proteins. However, (a) CD30 expression in transformed MF often is less uniform than in ALCL; (b) cell size often is more variable in MF, including the presence of smaller cerebriform cells; and (c) hallmark cells typically are absent.

Carcinomas and Other Solid Tumors

Like ALK⁺ ALCL, ALK⁻ ALCLs may show a primarily sinusoidal pattern with minimal architectural effacement, mimicking metastatic tumors including carcinoma, melanoma, and germ cell tumors. The last may express CD30. A comprehensive immunophenotyping panel generally resolves these issues.

Angioimmunoblastic T-Cell Lymphoma

Definition

AITL is a PTCL characterized by systemic disease invariably involving lymph nodes but also frequently extranodal sites. The disease currently recognized as AITL was first described in the 1970s as a clinical syndrome characterized by generalized lymphadenopathy, hepatosplenomegaly, anemia, and hypergammaglobulinemia (104–106). The lymph node histology showed a number of distinctive features including partial effacement of normal architecture by a polymorphic inflammatory infiltrate containing large immunoblasts and marked vascular proliferation (107). Based on these histologic features, the disease was initially known by a variety of terms, including immunoblastic lymphadenopathy, lymphogranulomatosis X, and angioimmunoblastic lymphadenopathy with dysproteinemia (AILD). Of these, AILD was the term most consistently associated with the clinical syndrome, and originally was thought to represent a reactive, albeit atypical, lymphoid hyperplasia with increased risk of progressing to frank malignancy. Subsequently, most cases were shown to have clonal TCR gene rearrangements and cytogenetic abnormalities, and the condition was included as a type of T-cell lymphoma in the updated Kiel classification of non-Hodgkin lymphomas (56).

Epidemiology

AITL is one of the most common types of PTCL, accounting for 15% to 20% of all T-cell lymphomas and 1% to 2% of all non-Hodgkin lymphomas. AITL affects males more than females (male/female:1.5/1) (108). Patients typically present in the seventh decade (median age of presentation, 52 years), but cases in patients as young as 20 have been described. No geographical or race bias has been identified.

Clinical Features

Sites of Involvement

Virtually all cases of AITL present with generalized lymphadenopathy and advanced stage. Extranodal sites such as the lungs, skin, or bone marrow frequently are involved at presentation.

Clinical Evaluation and Staging

Laboratory investigations show anemia with a positive Coombs test and hypergammaglobulinemia in over half of the patients. LDH levels are typically elevated.

Morphology

Cytologic Composition

The neoplastic T cells of AITL are typically intermediate in size with round, centroblast-like nuclei and abundant pale/clear cytoplasm. In about half of cases, they readily can be seen as perivascular or perifollicular collections of atypical medium-large lymphoid cells with clear or pale cytoplasm (109). In other cases, cytologic features of malignancy may not be apparent. In approximately one third of cases, the neoplastic T cells are accompanied by a B-cell component. The B-cell component may have morphologic features of reactive immunoblastic hyperplasia and/or plasmacytosis, or may have Reed-Sternberg–like cytologic features mimicking CHL.

Grading

AITL is not graded.

Proliferative Pattern

AITL is characterized by partial effacement of the lymph node architecture by a polymorphic infiltrate, predominantly within paracortical areas. In the original descriptions of AITL, absence of reactive hyperplastic B-cell follicles was considered to be a characteristic feature. It is now recognized that the architectural changes in AITL fall into a spectrum that has been categorized into three patterns (107). In pattern I (15% of the cases), there is partial preservation of the lymph node architecture (Fig. 26.17). Hyperplastic B-cell follicles with poorly developed mantle zones and ill-defined borders are easily identifiable in the cortex of the lymph node. These merge into the expanded paracortex containing a polymorphic infiltrate of lymphocytes, immunoblasts, plasma cells, macrophages, and eosinophils within a prominent vascular network. Pattern II (25% of the cases) is characterized by loss of normal architecture except for the presence of occasional depleted follicles with concentrically arranged FDCs. FDC proliferation extending beyond the follicles can be identified in some cases. The remaining node shows a polymorphic infiltrate with increased numbers of immunoblasts and vascular proliferation similar to pattern I. In pattern III (60% of the cases), the normal architecture is completely effaced and B-cell follicles are not identified (Fig. 26.18). Prominent, irregular proliferation of FDCs can be seen in H&E-stained sections in some cases; this is accompanied by extensive vascular proliferation and a polymorphic infiltrate similar to that seen in patterns I and II.

Histologic Progression/Transformation

A transition from architectural pattern I to pattern III occasionally has been observed in consecutive biopsies from the same

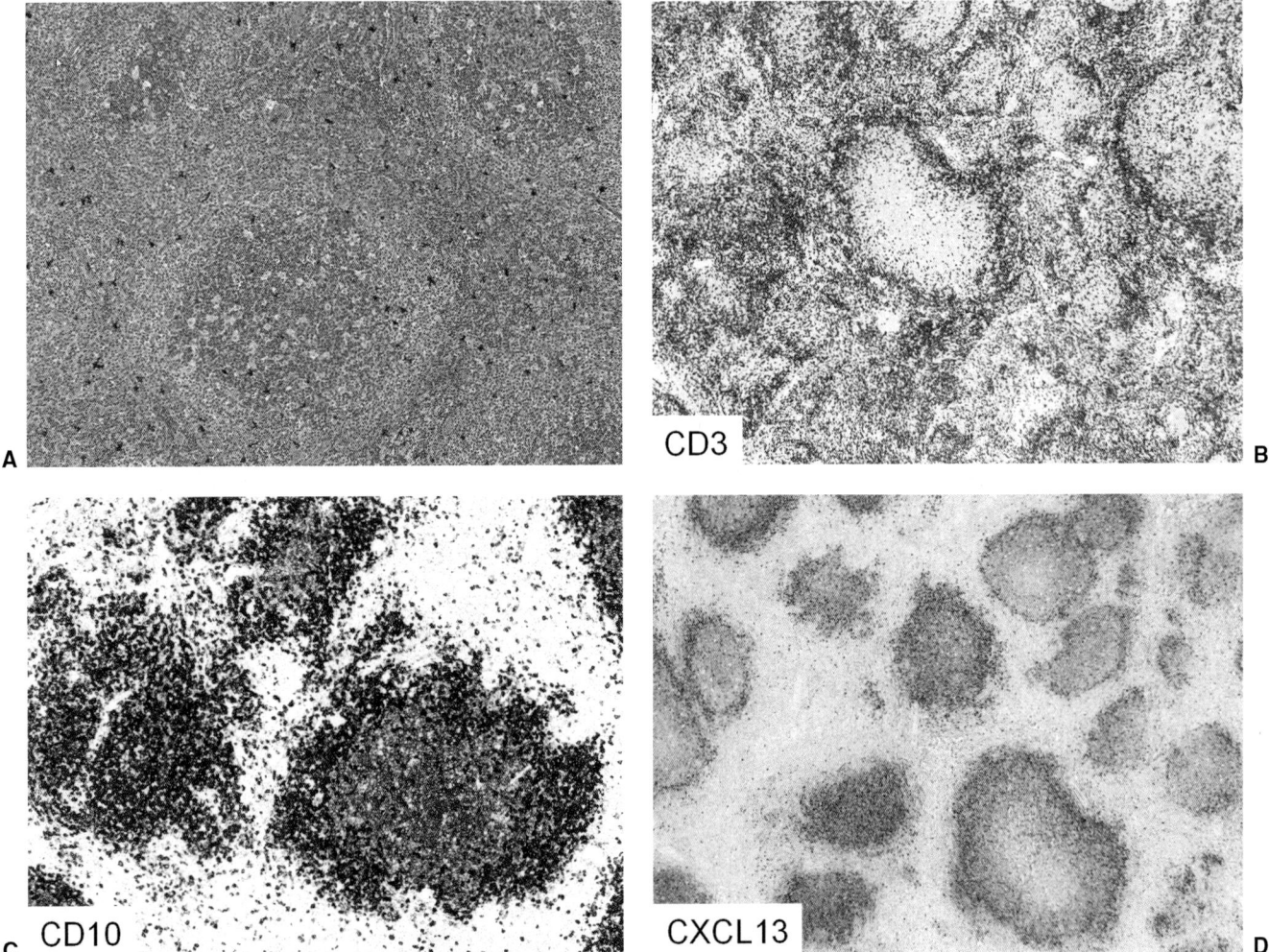

FIGURE 26.17. Angioimmunoblastic T-cell lymphoma, pattern I. The overall lymph node architecture is preserved. However, there is a monotonous perifollicular infiltrate of small lymphoid cells with clear cytoplasm. The paracortex shows proliferation of HEVs, a characteristic feature of AITL. The neoplastic cells are positive for CD3, and the T_FH markers for CD10 and CXCL13. The germinal center B cells are negative for CD3 and show weaker expression of CD10 than the surrounding neoplastic T cells.

patient, suggesting that pattern III may represent advanced disease. However, designation of the pattern type is not part of routine diagnostic practice.

Histologic Variants
Aside from the three histologic patterns described above, distinct variants are not recognized. It has been suggested that the follicular variant of PTCL, NOS might be considered a variant of AITL based on similar immunophenotypic features and proposed cell of origin (T_{FH}), but at present this entity remains classified within the spectrum of PTCL, NOS.

Morphology in Sites Other Than Lymph Node
Although generalized lymphadenopathy is the main presenting sign and the diagnosis of AITL rests on histologic examination of the lymph node, many patients have evidence of extranodal involvement at the time of diagnosis. The histologic appearance of AITL in extranodal sites often is nonspecific, but may mimic some of the features described in the lymph node including increased vascularity and a polymorphic inflammatory infiltrate. Cytologic features of malignancy are identified only rarely and tumor involvement often is shown only by IHC and/or molecular assessment of clonality (110,111).

Immunophenotype

IHC shows the expansion of the interfollicular areas by a diffuse infiltrate of CD3+ T cells. CD4+ T cells dominate in most cases, but there usually is an intermixed population of CD8+ cells. B-cell markers such as CD20 and CD79a highlight the residual germinal center and mantle zone B cells as well as many of the immunoblasts in the interfollicular areas. In some instances,

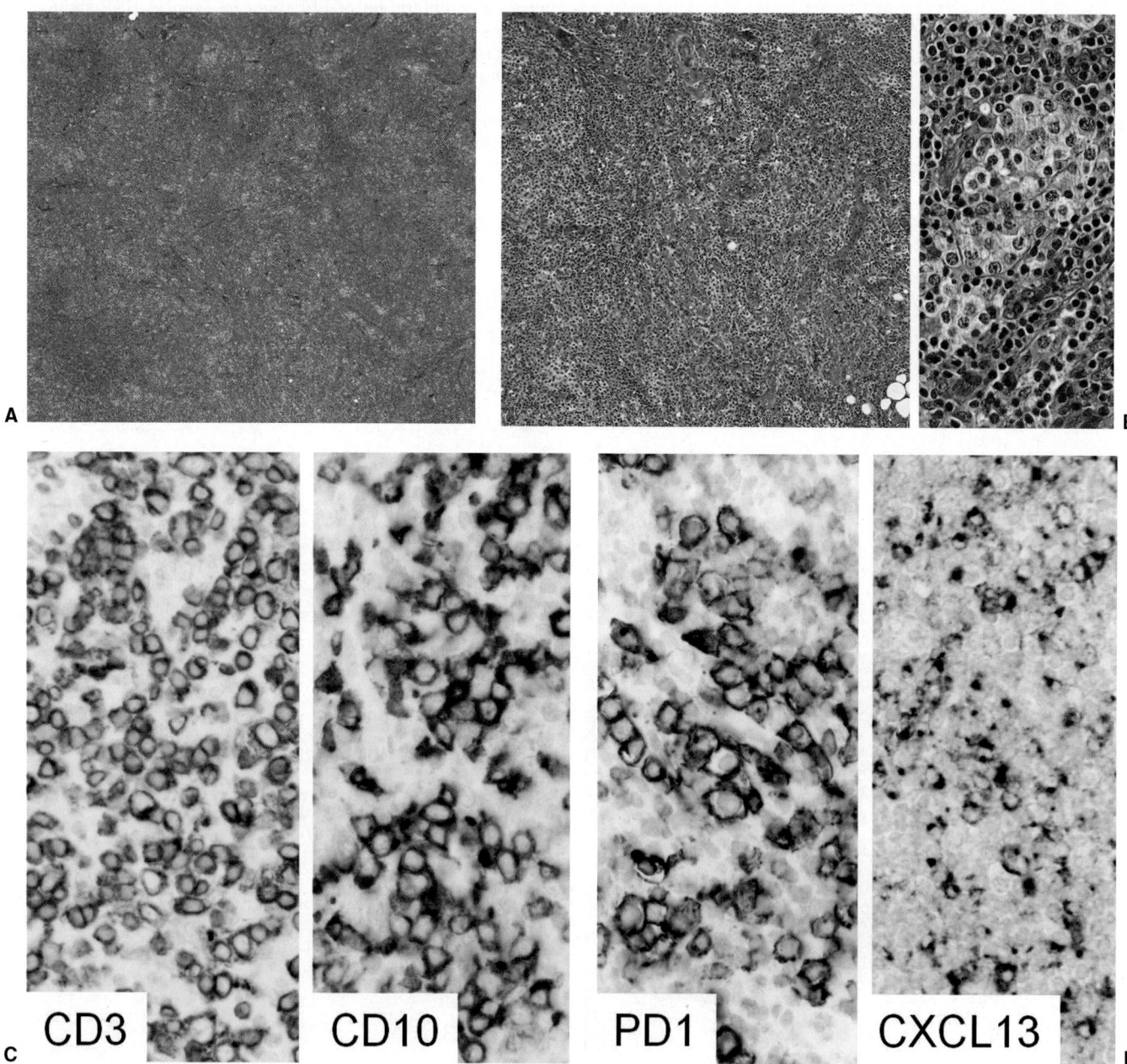

FIGURE 26.18. Angioimmunoblastic T-cell lymphoma, pattern III. The lymph node architecture is completely effaced by a polymorphic lymphoid infiltrate associated with marked proliferation of small vessels. The small vessels have an arborizing pattern and prominent basement membranes. They are surrounded by numerous atypical T cells with clear cytoplasm. The neoplastic T cells express CD3 and the T_{FH} markers CD10, PD1 (CD279), and CXCL13. CD21 highlights marked expansion of FDC meshworks.

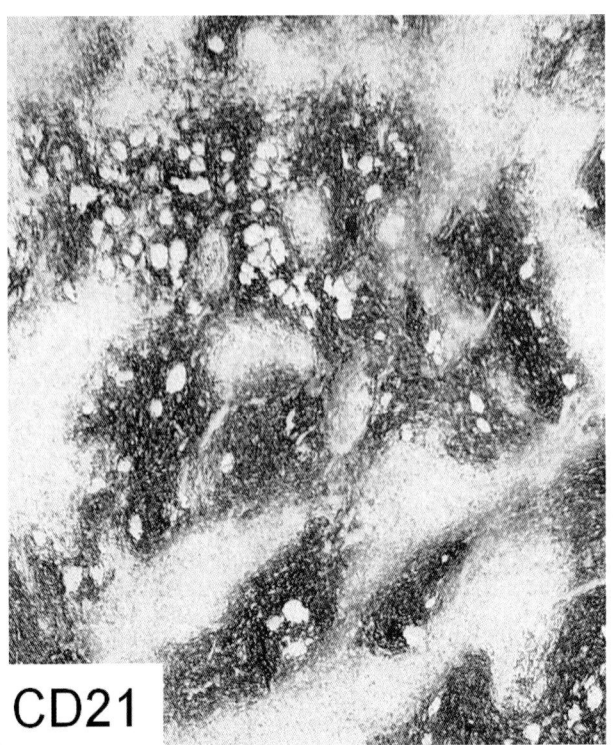

CD21

E

FIGURE 26.18. *(Continued)*

these can be numerous, mimicking a large B-cell lymphoma or CHL, though they typically demonstrate polytypic light chain expression. One of the most important immunophenotypic features in AITL is the expansion of FDC meshworks, which typically surround the paracortical small vessels. Although this is sometimes visible on H&E sections, it is best demonstrated by staining for FDC markers such as CD21 (Fig. 26.18).

GEP studies recently have shown that the neoplastic cells of AITL express a number of markers characteristic of T$_{FH}$ cells, including CD10, CXCL13, and PD1 (CD279; Figs. 26.17 and 26.18) (27,112,113). CD10 is not expressed by normal peripheral T cells except for a minority of T$_{FH}$ cells; thus, extensive CD10 expression is highly specific for AITL, with other nodal PTCLs only rarely expressing this antigen (109,114). CXCL13 and PD1 have broader expression patterns. CXCL13 is expressed not only by T$_{FH}$ cells but also by FDCs (112). PD1 is strongly expressed by most T$_{FH}$ cells but also is weakly expressed by paracortical T cells (115). In practice, CD10 provides the highest specificity but lower sensitivity, whereas PD1 provides the highest sensitivity but lower specificity for identifying the neoplastic cells of AITL. Therefore, using at least two of these T$_{FH}$ markers in combination is recommended. Using T$_{FH}$ markers, the tumor cells account for only a small fraction of the whole infiltrate in pattern I cases (Fig. 26.18). The cells are intimately related to the residual reactive B-cell follicles and the expanded FDC meshworks, some being located within the follicle centers and others surrounding the follicles. In patterns II and III, the tumor cells spill into the interfollicular area but retain the intimate association with FDC meshworks. This suggests that the FDC microenvironment may be important for tumor growth.

Cytogenetics

Recurrent mutations of the *TET2* and *IDH2* genes recently have been reported in AITL. However, mutations in these genes are not specific for AITL and are seen in other PTCLs as well as nonlymphoid malignancies. CGH studies have shown that a

subset of AITLs show gains of chromosomes X, 3, 5, 11q13, 13q, 19, and 22q. The genes in these areas that are potentially relevant in the biology of AITL remain undetermined.

Molecular Characteristics

Virtually all cases of AITL contain increased numbers of EBV-infected cells with immunoblastic or Reed-Sternberg–like morphology. Thus, assessment of EBV by IHC or ISH is an important part of the diagnosis of AITL. Double immunolabeling studies suggest that the EBV$^+$ cells in AITL are B cells; there is no convincing evidence that the neoplastic T cells are infected.

The vast majority of AITLs contain a monoclonal T-cell population that can be demonstrated by southern blotting or PCR-based molecular methods. Interestingly, the presence of a B-cell clone can also be demonstrated in about one quarter of the cases. These are thought to be expanded EBV-infected B-cell clones, possibly secondary to underlying immunodeficiency/immune activation (116). In some cases, this clonal B-cell expansion is extensive enough to warrant a diagnosis of DLBCL in addition to AITL.

Postulated Normal Counterpart

AITL is believed to derive from T$_{FH}$ cells.

Clinical Course and Prognostic Assessment

Most cases of AITL present with advanced stage disease and follow an aggressive clinical course. Prognostic markers specific to AITL have not been characterized.

Treatment and Survival

No specific therapy is available. Most patients initially are treated with CHOP-based regimens with variable responses. Some sustained responses have been achieved using high-dose therapy with peripheral blood stem cell transplantation. A role for immunoregulatory drugs such as cyclosporine is under investigation. Most patients still have poor outcomes, with a median survival of around 3 years.

Differential Diagnosis

Other PTCLs

As discussed previously, other PTCLs involving the lymph node—particularly PTCL, NOS—may have overlapping features with AITL. The presence of morphologic and immunophenotypic characteristics of AITL, including vascular proliferation, clear cell cytology, FDC proliferation, EBV$^+$ B cells, and expression of T$_{FH}$ differentiation markers favor AITL. Nevertheless, approximately 10% of all nodal PTCLs show features overlapping with both PTCL, NOS, and AITL, and definitive subclassification may not be possible (33,117).

B-Cell Neoplasms

One of the most important pitfalls in the diagnosis of AITL remains CHL. As discussed, most AITLs contain EBV$^+$ B-cell proliferations. These B cells sometimes acquire the morphologic appearance of Reed-Sternberg cells and variants. Furthermore, the cellular background of AITL may resemble that of CHL, including the presence of eosinophils, histiocytes, and plasma cells. Clues for the presence of an underlying PTCL include the presence of not only EBV$^+$ Reed-Sternberg cells but also a wider range of EBV$^+$ cells including typical immunoblasts, cytologic atypia and an aberrant phenotype in the T-cell compartment, and expansion of FDC meshworks. Occasionally, the EBV$^+$ B-cell proliferation may be so extensive as to mimic or truly represent a DLBCL (118,119). Diagnosis of a true DLBCL accompanying AITL is supported by the presence of sheets of EBV+ large B cells with a dominant B-cell clone by IG gene rearrangement studies (120). Rarely, EBV- DLBCL may accompany AITL (120). In addition to DLBCL, a spectrum of clonal B-cell and plasma cell proliferations, both EBV+ and EBV-, has been reported in association with AITL. Identification of the underlying AITL, which may represent a relatively small proportion of the total cellularity, can be very difficult in such cases and requires a high index of suspicion (121).

Nonlymphoid Neoplasms

In occasional cases of AITL, the FDC proliferation may be so prominent as to raise the possibility of a spindle cell neoplasm, particularly an FDC sarcoma. Careful attention to the cellular background, immunophenotyping, and molecular testing is important in establishing the diagnosis in such cases.

Reactive Conditions

Early AITL cases showing pattern I histology appear very similar to reactive lymphoid hyperplasia with a marked paracortical component, and may be very difficult to diagnose. The clues indicating AITL include markedly increased vascularity in paracortical areas, the presence of aggregates of atypical lymphoid cells with clear cytoplasm in perifollicular areas, the presence of a mixture of hyperplastic and depleted follicles, and the presence of CD10+, PD1+, and/or CXCL13+ T cells in perifollicular areas. However, in most instances, the final diagnosis may be only reached after molecular analysis of clonality and additional biopsies. Occasionally, AITL may resemble Castleman disease, particularly the plasma cell variant. Both these conditions may demonstrate depleted follicles with prominent FDC whorls. However, the interfollicular areas in the plasma cell variant of Castleman disease contain a monotonous infiltrate of plasma cells and small lymphoid cells without cytologic atypia, and the vascularity is typically not as prominent as in AITL.

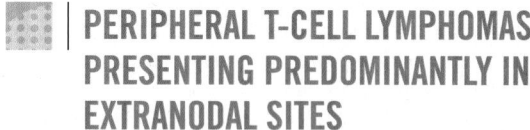

PERIPHERAL T-CELL LYMPHOMAS PRESENTING PREDOMINANTLY IN EXTRANODAL SITES

Extranodal NK/T-Cell Lymphoma, Nasal Type

Definition

Extranodal NKTL, nasal type, is a lymphoma characterized by predominantly extranodal location, a tendency for angiocentricity and necrosis, and EBV infection. Most cases appear to be of NK-cell origin, but phenotypic and genetic evidence of T-cell origin is present occasionally. The nasal location of most cases, the aggressive clinical behavior, and resemblance to necrotizing granulomatous processes led to the previous designations of lethal midline granuloma or malignant midline reticulosis. It is clear, however, that not all cases occur in the nasal region or in midline structures. The previous terms angiocentric T-cell lymphoma and angiocentric immunoproliferative lesion also are not preferred, since not all cases of NKTL exhibit an angiocentric growth pattern and because angiocentricity may seen in other lymphoma types. The previous term polymorphic reticulosis is similarly nonspecific.

Epidemiology

NKTL is most common in areas with endemic EBV infection, particularly among Asians and native populations of Central and South America (122,123). It is predominantly an adult disease, with a slight male predominance. The etiology is

unknown, but the association with EBV is strong, suggesting a possible viral pathogenetic mechanism (124). The EBV in NKTLs is clonal, often contains a deletion in the latent membrane protein-1 gene, and most commonly is of EBV subtype type A (125).

Clinical Features

Sites of Involvement

The nasal cavity and upper respiratory tract are the most common sites of involvement. Nasal obstruction and/or epistaxis may be the presenting signs. Additional cases are seen in the gastrointestinal tract, lung, skin, and testis. Lymph nodes rarely are involved (see below). Bone marrow involvement may be seen, but marked peripheral blood involvement should raise the differential diagnosis of aggressive NK-cell leukemia (described in Chapter 38).

Clinical Evaluation and Staging

Endoscopic evaluation and biopsy of the respiratory or gastrointestinal tract usually provides sufficient material for diagnosis. Routine lymphoma staging studies and clinical assessment for IPI risk factors should be obtained. Quantification of circulating EBV DNA at presentation may have prognostic significance and serves as a baseline for further studies later in the clinical course (126). The possibility of hemophagocytic syndrome, which may accompany NKTL, should be considered (127).

Morphology

Cytologic Composition

In most cases, the neoplastic cells of NKTL are medium sized to large, with mildly irregular nuclei and a modest amount of cytoplasm (Fig. 26.19). Histiocytes and acute inflammatory cells often are seen accompanying areas of necrosis.

Grading

NKTL is not graded.

Proliferative Pattern

NKTL typically shows an angiocentric pattern of distribution, often with extensive areas of geographic necrosis. Occasionally, a monotonous infiltrate without these features can be seen. At mucosal sites in the respiratory or gastrointestinal tract, the tumor often extensively ulcerates the overlying epithelial surface.

Histologic Progression/Transformation

No criteria for histologic progression or transformation have been established.

Histologic Variants

No histologic variants are recognized.

Morphology in Lymph Node

NKTL primarily is an extranodal disease. Lymph node involvement occasionally may be seen in addition to extranodal sites, and very rarely may occur in the absence of documented extranodal disease (128). When nodal involvement occurs, the tumor typically shows sheet-like growth with necrosis, often partially effacing the lymph node architecture.

Immunophenotype

NKTLs typically have the immunophenotype of NK cells, including expression of CD2; cytoplasmic CD3, CD7, CD56; and cytotoxic markers including TIA-1, granzyme B, and perforin.

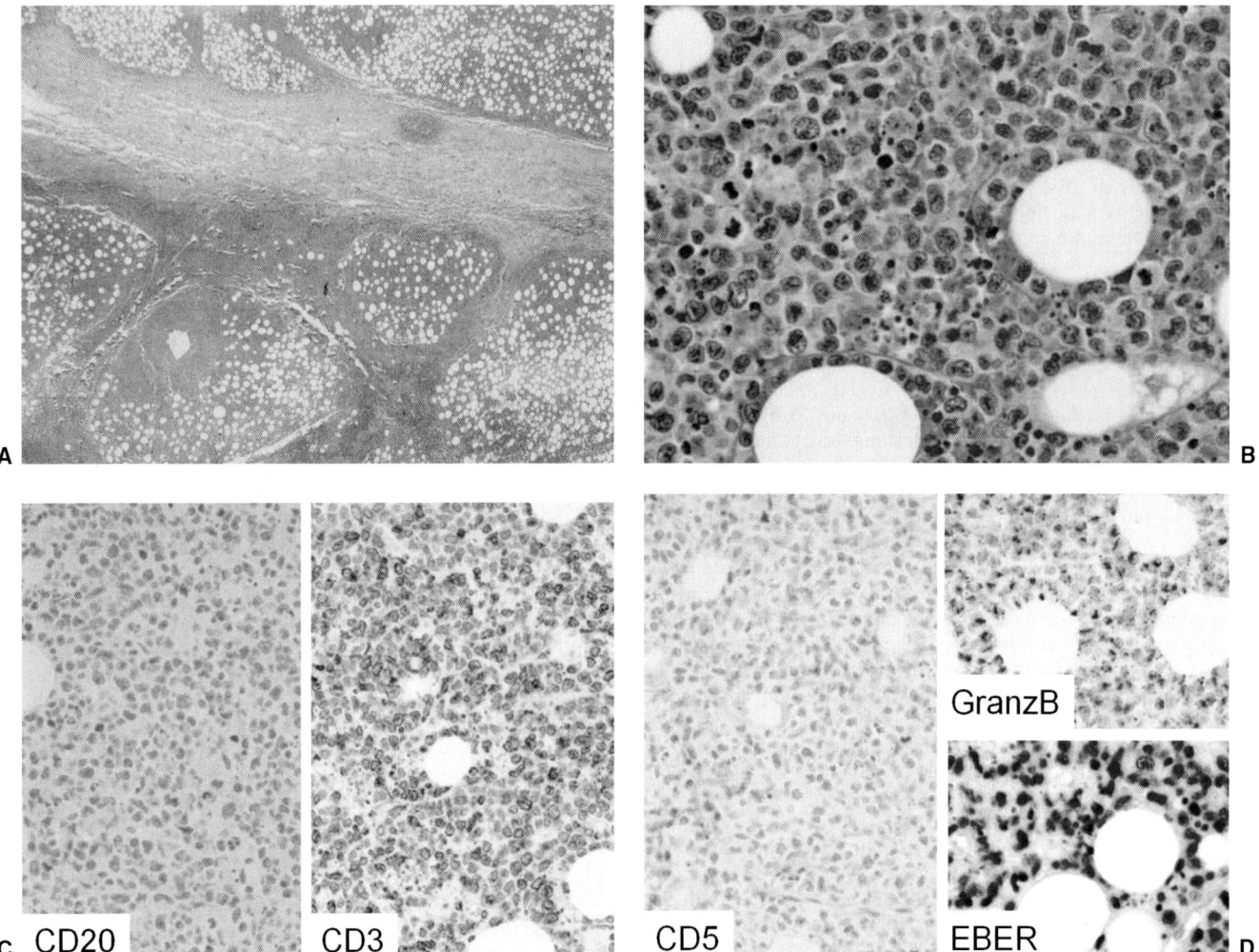

FIGURE 26.19. Extranodal NKTL, involving the subcutaneous tissue of the arm. The biopsy shows a panniculitic pattern of involvement. The tumor cells are medium to large in size and show abundant apoptotic debris in the background. The neoplastic cells are negative for CD20 and positive for CD3, with a cytoplasmic staining pattern. CD2 also is expressed (not shown), but the tumor cells lack expression of CD5, as well as CD4 and CD8 (not shown). They are positive for granzyme B and TIA1 (not shown), as well as for EBV by EBER ISH.

Other T-cell antigens may be expressed, sometimes in association with clonally rearranged TCR genes (see below). A subset of cases expresses CD30.

Cytogenetics

Characteristic recurrent karyotypic abnormalities have not been identified.

Molecular Characteristics

EBV is present in nearly all cases (see *Epidemiology*, above). Otherwise typical cases without EBV may be diagnosed as NKTL, but unusual clinical or pathologic features accompanied by the absence of EBV should suggest another entity, often PTCL, NOS. Most commonly, TCR and IG genes are germline, but occasional cases have clonally rearranged TCR genes (129).

Postulated Normal Counterpart

NKTLs are believe to derive from NK cells in the majority of cases, but occasional cases with a more complete T-cell antigen profile and clonally rearranged TCR genes may derive from cytotoxic T cells. Recent data suggest that up to 10% of cases

may be of T-cell origin, including cases expressing $\alpha\beta$, $\gamma\delta$, and mixed-phenotype TCR receptors (129).

Clinical Course and Prognostic Assessment

NKTL is a clinically aggressive disease. Overall, extranasal disease has a poorer prognosis than nasal disease; however, extranasal cases also present at more advanced stage (130). Prognostic markers appear to be most helpful in nasal disease and include stage, IPI, and the Korean NK/T-cell prognostic index. Prognostic features in extranasal disease are less well established. The copy number of circulating EBV DNA parallels the clinical course in many patients and may serve as a prognostic biomarker (126).

Treatment and Survival

Patients treated with CHOP and similar regimens have poor OS, prompting development and testing of other regimens. The SMILE regimen (steroid [dexamethasone], methotrexate, ifosfamide, L-asparaginase, and etoposide) has shown promising results in Asia and has been recently introduced in the West (131). Radiotherapy plays an important role in the locoregional control of patients with early-stage nasal disease (130,132).

Differential Diagnosis

PTCL, NOS, and Other T/NK-Cell Neoplasms

As discussed above and in the section on PTCL, NOS, cases with morphology similar to NKTL but with phenotypic and genetic features suggesting a T-cell origin and lacking EBV usually should be diagnosed as PTCL, NOS. Though NKTLs are associated with EBV, patients typically do not have an underlying clinical cause for immunosuppression. Post-transplant and other immunosuppression-related T-cell lymphoproliferative disorders should be considered in EBV+ tumors in immunosuppressed patients. Patients from EBV-endemic areas also may develop EBV-associated T-cell lymphoproliferative disorder of childhood and the spectrum of hydroa-like EBV-associated T-cell lymphomas. While these typically do not have clinical features overlapping NKTL, hydroa vacciniforme-like lymphomas may be confused with cutaneous NKTL pathologically. Clinical appearance of the lesions and patient age are helpful in this differential.

Aggressive NK-cell leukemia is an EBV+ leukemic disorder that may occasionally involve solid tissues. The characteristic angiocentric pattern with necrosis is often absent in these cases. Occasionally, a biopsy may contain such extensive necrosis that the tumor cells are difficult to find; thus, rebiopsy should be recommended when the clinical features are suspicious but tumor cells are not identified (e.g., an erosive mass lesion). Cases with smaller tumor cells and without much necrosis may be difficult to distinguish from other PTCL subtypes if NKTL is not suspected based on site and EBV studies are not carried out. Thus, EBV studies should be applied more liberally in patients from EBV-endemic areas.

Nasopharyngeal and Other Carcinomas

Because of the nasal site, positivity for EBV, and extensive necrosis, NKTL may mimic nasopharyngeal carcinoma. Usually the cytologic features are sufficient to distinguish these entities, but in difficult cases a broader immunohistochemical panel is useful. In addition, NKTLs in the upper respiratory tract may be accompanied by marked pseudoepitheliomatous hyperplasia of the overlying epithelium, occasionally leading to the impression of squamous cell carcinoma if the neoplastic lymphoid cells are not recognized.

Reactive Conditions

Occasionally, NKTL may mimic reactive conditions. Cases with a relative paucity of tumor cells may suggest necrotizing granulomatous inflammation, while cases with a monomorphic population of smaller tumor cells may overlap with reactive lymphoid hyperplasia. Generally, the clinical presentation is helpful in prompting immunohistochemical workup or another biopsy if necessary.

Enteropathy-Associated T-Cell Lymphoma

Definition

EATL is a subtype of PTCL occurring in the intestines believed to derive from intraepithelial T cells. Two types are recognized. The classical type is strongly associated with celiac disease and typically contains numerous large transformed cells. The so-called monomorphic variant (type II EATL) contains a monomorphic population of medium-sized cells and often occurs in the absence of celiac disease.

Epidemiology

The incidence of EATL is low overall, but in classical EATL, it parallels the relative prevalence of celiac disease and is relatively more common in Northern Europe. EATL is additionally associated with the HLA class II subtypes commonly associated with celiac disease, DQA1*0501 and DQB*0201 (133). Other HLA genotypes (e.g., DRB1*03,04) may be specific risk factors for development of EATL. Geographic distribution of type II EATL appears to be independent of celiac disease prevalence.

Clinical Features

Sites of Involvement

The most commonly involved sites are the jejunum and ileum. Involvement of more proximal or distal gastrointestinal sites is unusual but may be seen. The disease is multifocal at presentation in 10% to 25% of patients.

Clinical Evaluation and Staging

Most patients with classical EATL have a known history of celiac disease at the time of presentation with lymphoma. Occasionally, celiac disease is diagnosed only at the time of lymphoma presentation. In other patients, episodes of refractory celiac disease may precede the time of lymphoma diagnosis. Patients with type II EATL typically lack celiac disease. The most common presenting symptom is abdominal pain, and there may be a history of weight loss, diarrhea, and/or symptoms associated with bowel obstruction. Intestinal perforation, most often in the jejunum, is common. As such, the disease often is diagnosed at laparotomy, and abdominal staging is performed at that time. In the remaining patients, combined radiographic and endoscopic study of the entire small and large intestine is recommended to determine the extent of disease and the presence of multifocality. Ann Arbor staging is not well suited to the staging of EATL, and alternative systems have been proposed (134).

Morphology

Cytologic Composition

In classical EATL, most of the tumor cells are medium to large in size, have moderately atypical cytologic features, and demonstrate high mitotic activity (Fig. 26.20). Occasionally, markedly pleomorphic nuclear features may be seen (so-called anaplastic variant). There typically is a rich inflammatory background, often including histiocytes and eosinophils (Fig. 26.21); at times, these may outnumber the tumor cells. Type II EATL is characterized by a more monomorphic infiltrate of medium-sized cells with hyperchromatic nuclei and pale cytoplasm (Fig. 26.22). Type II EATL often lacks the prominent inflammatory background seen in classical EATL.

Grading

EATL is not graded.

Proliferative Pattern

EATL typically shows a mass-forming lesion invading the intestinal wall with overlying mucosal ulceration. Often an intraepithelial component may be seen within intestinal crypts. Mucosa adjacent to the tumor typically shows enteropathic changes, including villous blunting and an increase in intraepithelial lymphocytes (Fig. 26.23). Necrosis is more common in classical EATL than in type II EATL. Early cases may not present with a mass and may be predominantly intraepithelial (so-called intraepithelial or "in situ" EATL).

Histologic Progression/Transformation

EATL typically is an aggressive disease at presentation, and criteria for progression or transformation have not been formulated. Conversely, EATL itself has been proposed in some cases to represent progression from a precursor lesion, namely refractory celiac disease. Some of these cases are complicated

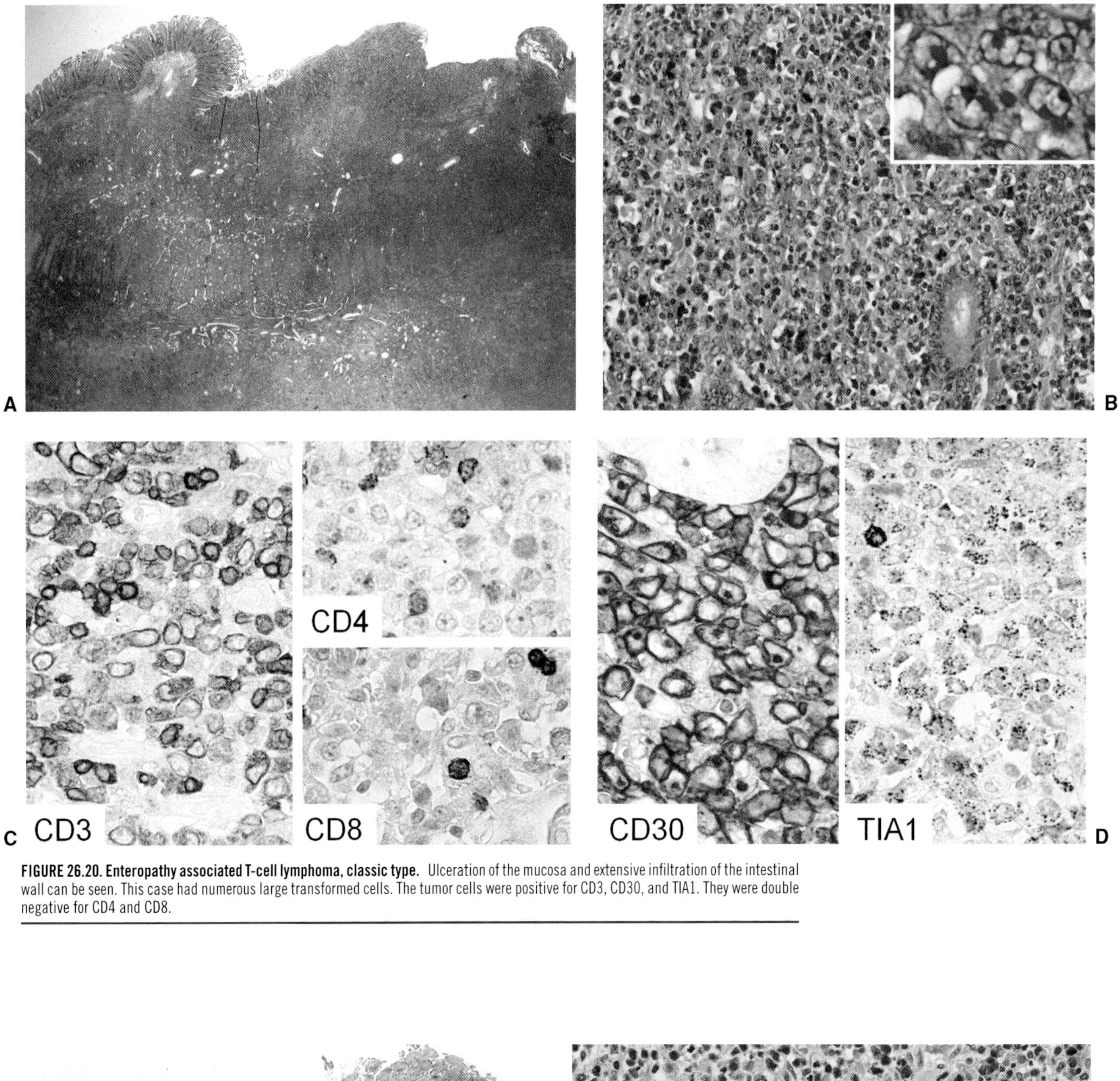

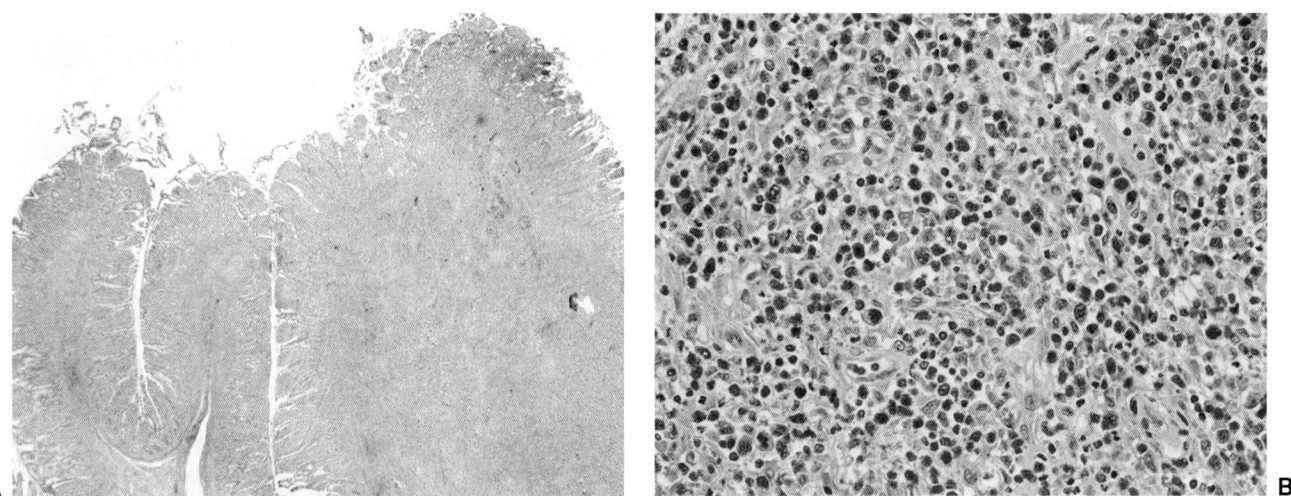

FIGURE 26.20. Enteropathy associated T-cell lymphoma, classic type. Ulceration of the mucosa and extensive infiltration of the intestinal wall can be seen. This case had numerous large transformed cells. The tumor cells were positive for CD3, CD30, and TIA1. They were double negative for CD4 and CD8.

FIGURE 26.21. EATL with marked inflammatory infiltrate. The resection specimen shows numerous eosinophils with scattered histiocytes and plasma cells in addition to the atypical lymphoid cells. Immunohistochemical stains showed an aberrant T-cell phenotype with loss of CD2. This case also focally expressed CD30.

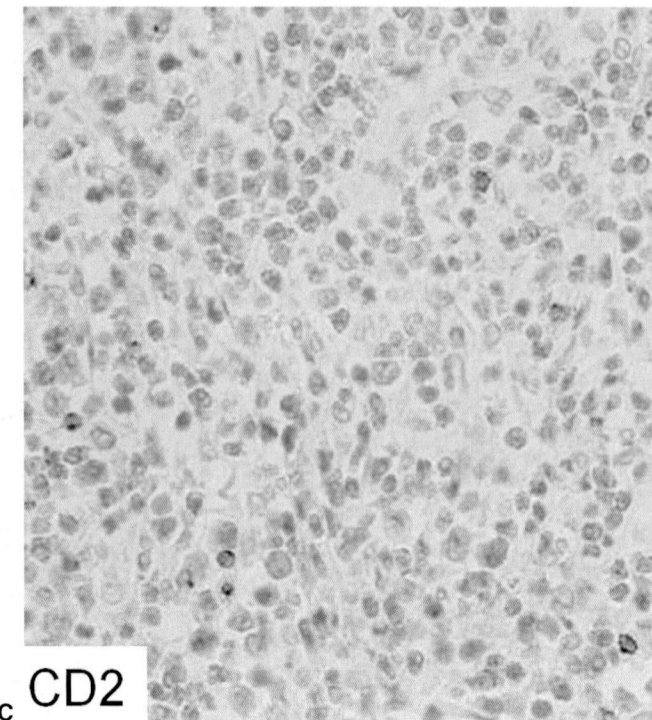

CD2

C

CD3

D

FIGURE 26.21. *(Continued)*

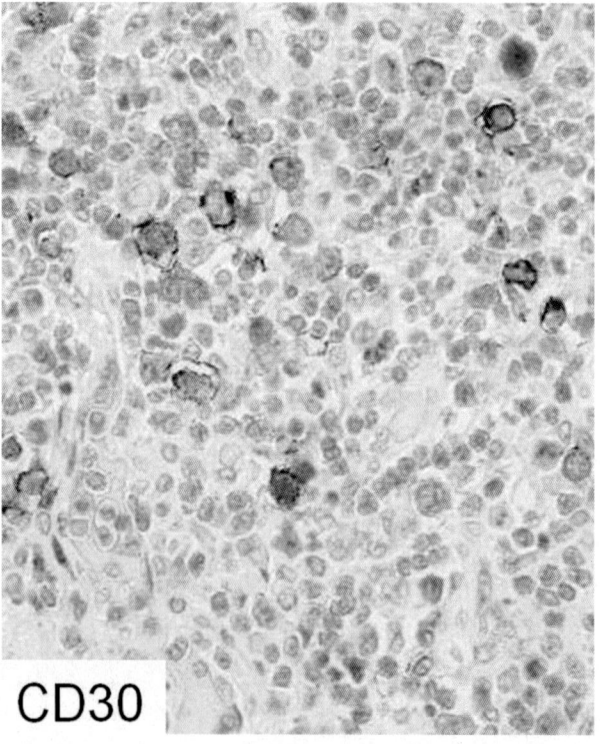

CD30

E

by multiple ulcers in the small intestinal mucosa (ulcerative jejunitis) (135). In some cases of refractory celiac disease associated with subsequent EATL, the intestinal intraepithelial cells of the refractory celiac disease have the same aberrant T-cell phenotype and the same clonal TCR gene rearrangement as the subsequent EATL (136). Such cases can be considered intraepithelial or "*in situ*" EATL.

Histologic Variants

While classic-type EATL and type II EATL could be considered histologic variants, these may represent two distinct entities with different clinical, pathologic, and genetic features. The so-called "anaplastic" variant may be considered a histologic variant.

Morphology in Sites Other Than the Gastrointestinal Tract

The mesenteric lymph nodes are the most common extraintestinal sites involved by EATL. Nodal involvement by EATL may mimic other PTCLs, from which it must be distinguished. Other extranodal sites, in particular skin and the central nervous system, can be involved. Occasionally, extranodal site involvement may be the first sign of disease.

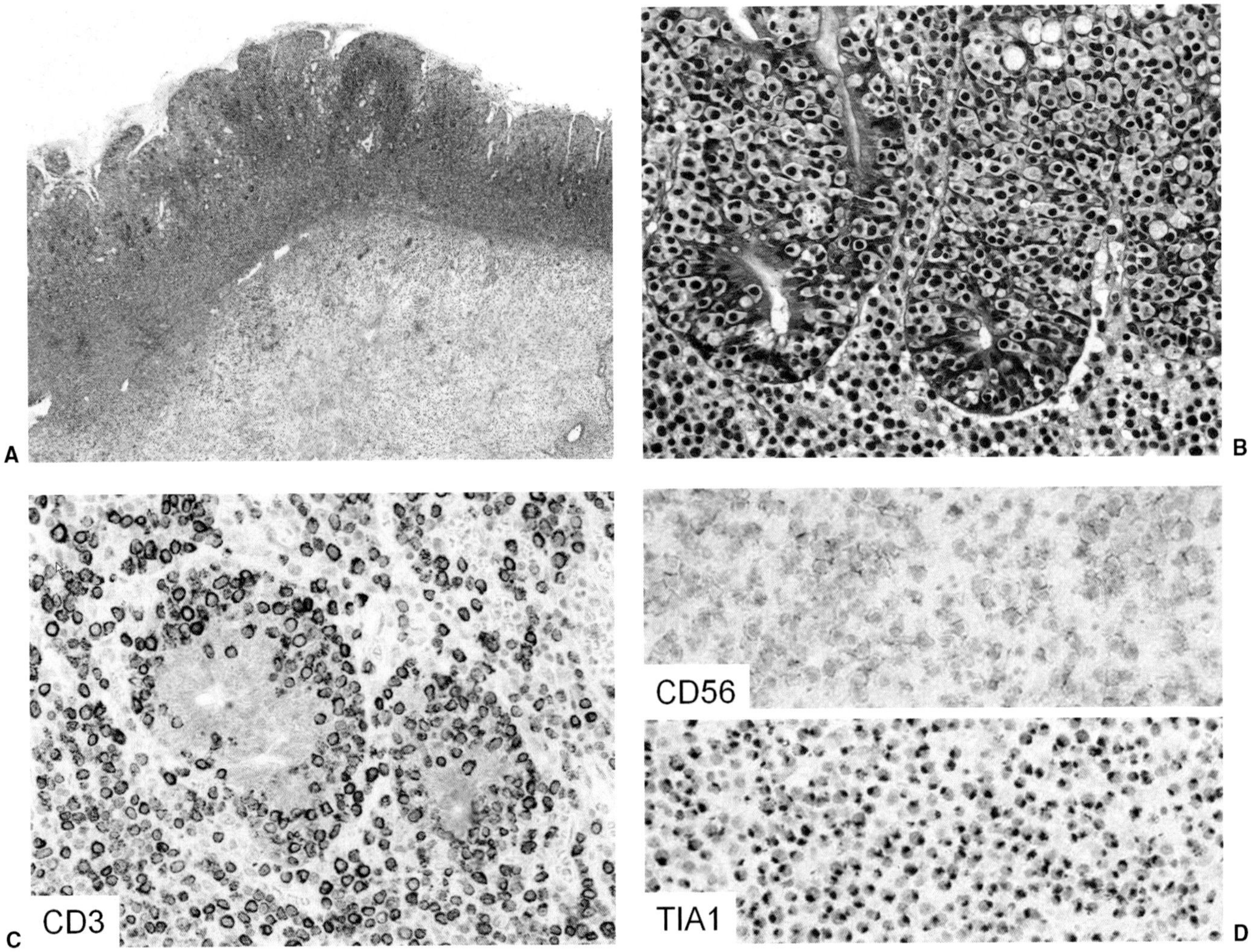

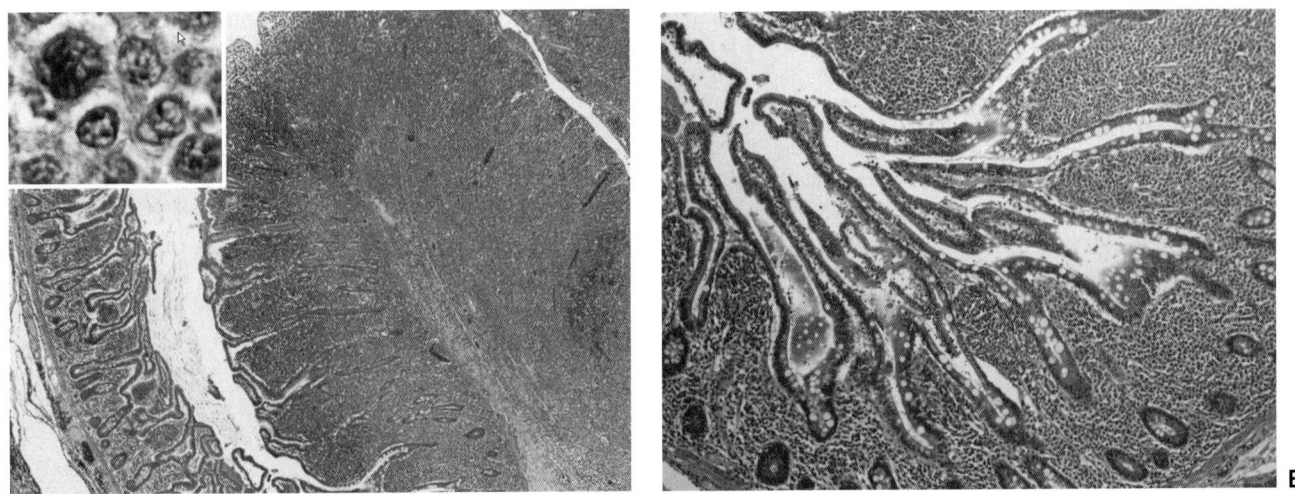

FIGURE 26.22. Enteropathy associated T-cell lymphoma, type II. Colon resection demonstrated a monotonous population of medium-sized lymphoid cells with marked epitheliotropism. The tumor cells in this case have particularly abundant pale cytoplasm. They expressed CD3, CD8 (not shown), CD56 (weak), and TIA1. CD5 was negative (not shown).

FIGURE 26.23. EATL with adjacent area of intraepithelial lymphocytosis. This jejunal resection showed extensive involvement by tumor (**right side** of panels), while adjacent bowel showed a marked increase in intraepithelial T cells (**left side** of panels). This case was positive for CD8, as well as for CD3 and TIA1 (not shown). The intraepithelial T cells in the adjacent bowel had a similar phenotype but retained expression of CD2, which was lost in the tumor cells.

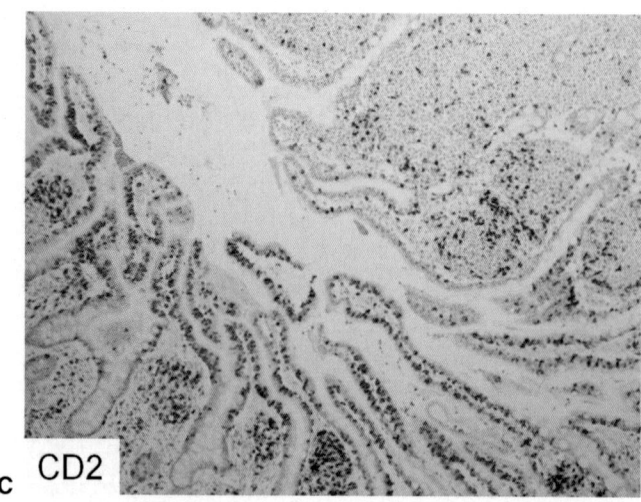

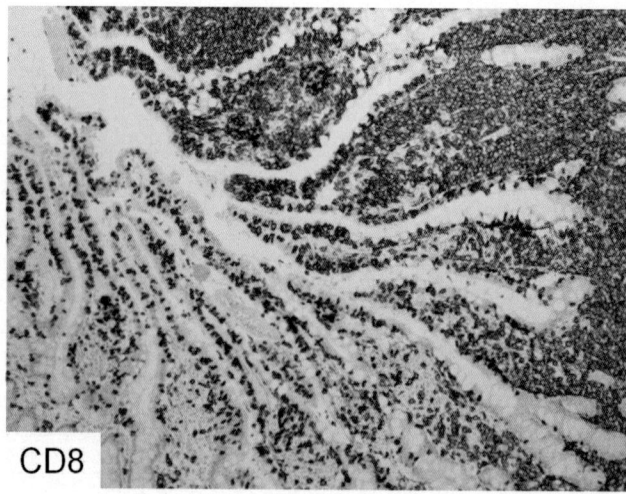

FIGURE 26.23. *(Continued)*

Immunophenotype

By IHC, the tumor cells of classic-type EATL typically are positive for CD3, CD7, CD103, and cytotoxic granule-associated proteins, but negative for CD4, CD5, and CD8. Most cases lack expression of CD56. They show variable expression of TCR-β chain and CD30. Intraepithelial lymphocytes in the neighboring mucosa may show a similar phenotype. The tumor cells in type II EATL typically express CD3, CD56, CD8, and TCR-β chain in both the tumoral mass and the neighboring mucosa (137). When mesenteric lymph nodes are involved by EATL, the phenotype seen in the main mucosal tumor typically is retained.

Cytogenetics

Both classic-type EATL and type II EATL frequently have 9q31.3-qter amplifications or 16q12.1 deletions. In addition, gains in 1q32.2-q41 and 5q34-q35.2 often are seen in classic-type EATL, whereas type II EATL often shows amplifications of 8q24, including the *MYC* locus (138).

Molecular Characteristics

EATL demonstrates clonal TCR gene rearrangements. EBV is absent. Similar to the findings in patients with celiac disease in general, the HLA haplotypes HLADQA1*0501 and HLADQB1*0201 are common.

Postulated Normal Counterpart

EATL is believed to derive from intestinal intraepithelial $\alpha\beta$ T cells.

Clinical Course and Prognostic Assessment

Most cases of EATL (both classic type and type II) follow an aggressive clinical course, and specific prognostic tools beside stage are of limited value. Patients often present after a prodromal period of refractory celiac disease and may be significantly malnourished, limiting their ability to tolerate complications (e.g., intestinal perforation) or aggressive therapies.

Treatment and Survival

No standard treatment approach for EATL patients has been determined, and prognosis is poor, with 5-year OS of <20% (139). Most patients require resection of severely affected or perforated bowel. In addition, CHOP or similar chemotherapy regimens often are used. Many patients are unable to complete planned courses of chemotherapy, often due to severe nutritional compromise. Radiation therapy may be indicated for bulky disease or rectal involvement. Patients able to withstand more aggressive therapy may derive benefit from high-dose chemotherapy with autologous stem cell transplantation.

Differential Diagnosis

Other PTCLs

NKTLs may involve the gastrointestinal tract and share some morphologic features with EATL. Such patients typically lack a history of celiac disease, and biopsies do not show the epitheliotropism of EATL or intraepithelial lymphocytosis in the adjacent bowel. While there is phenotypic overlap between these two entities, demonstration of EBV in NKTL but not in EATL is a critical distinguishing feature. The differential diagnosis with other PTCLs is most challenging in cases where local mesenteric lymph nodes are involved. At times, these may be biopsied in isolation and/or adequate clinical history may not be available. Such cases may prompt a diagnosis of PTCL, NOS or, occasionally, ALK⁻ ALCL when anaplastic cytologic features and CD30 expression are present.

Reactive Conditions and Benign Lymphoproliferations

EATL must be distinguished from the reactive lymphocytic infiltrate seen in the intestinal mucosa of conventional (i.e., not refractory) celiac disease, which is composed predominantly of CD8⁺, polyclonal T cells. Occasionally, cases of true EATL may be difficult to identify when infiltrating eosinophils and macrophages are so abundant that they obscure the tumor cell population. The diagnosis may be particularly challenging when a superficial biopsy is taken near a site of ulceration. Recently, cases of so-called NK-cell enteropathy have been described that have a benign clinical course (140). Such cases may have significant cytologic atypia and may be mistaken for EATL. Features that assist in the diagnosis of NK-cell enteropathy include the mature NK-cell phenotype, the general lack of epithelial infiltration or deep invasion of the intestinal wall, and the absence of clonally rearranged TCR genes.

Hepatosplenic T-Cell Lymphoma

Definition

Hepatosplenic T-cell lymphoma (HSTCL) is a cytotoxic T-cell lymphoma that typically involves the sinusoids of the liver, spleen, and often bone marrow. Most cases are of γδ T-cell origin, but occasional αβ cases exist with otherwise similar clinicopathologic features.

Epidemiology

HSTCL is rare. It is most common in adolescents and young adults (median age, ~35 years) and shows a male predominance. HSTCL is associated with underlying immunodeficiency, most commonly due to solid organ transplantation or immunosuppressive therapies for inflammatory bowel disease (141). HSTCL also has been reported to occur in pediatric patients, particularly in children with Crohn disease treated with infliximab (142,143).

Clinical Features

Sites of Involvement
Involvement of the liver, spleen, and bone marrow are seen in nearly all cases. Peripheral blood involvement may be seen occasionally, usually as a late finding. Lymphadenopathy is very rare, though the sinuses of splenic hilar lymph nodes may be involved without marked lymph node enlargement.

Clinical Evaluation and Staging
Patients typically present with hepatosplenomegaly. Lymphadenopathy is absent. Most patients have B symptoms. The majority have thrombocytopenia, which may be accompanied by anemia and/or leukopenia. Because bone marrow involvement is usually present, most patients have stage IV disease.

Morphology

Cytologic Composition
The tumor cells of HSTCL typically are medium in size and have a moderate amount of pale cytoplasm (Figs. 26.24 and 26.25). Cytologic atypia often is minimal, but occasional cases may contain large transformed or blastlike cells.

Grading
HSTCL is not graded.

Proliferative Pattern
In the spleen, the tumor cells diffusely involve the red pulp and are contained within intact sinuses and cords. The white pulp is generally atrophied or completely absent. If perihilar lymph nodes are involved, the tumor cells are usually limited to the sinuses without effacement of the nodal architecture. The liver is diffusely enlarged without mass lesions. The tumor cells are predominantly confined to the sinusoids.

Histologic Progression/Transformation
Though occasional advanced cases may have large transformed cells, criteria for histologic progression or transformation have not been established.

Histologic Variants
Histologic variants have not been defined.

Morphology in Sites Other Than Liver and Spleen
Involvement of the bone marrow is common and also shows a sinusoidal pattern (Fig. 26.26). However, the degree of marrow involvement may be minimal, requiring special stains for detection.

Immunophenotype

The tumor cells of HSTCL are most frequently of γδ origin (Fig. 26.24), but cases of αβ origin positive for βF1 may be seen (Fig. 26.25) (144). Most cases express CD3, are variably positive for CD8 and CD56, and are negative for CD4 and CD5. The tumor cells express TIA1 and granzyme M, but lack expression of granzyme B and perforin, indicative of a nonactivated cytotoxic phenotype (145). KIRs often are expressed. Flow cytometry may be helpful in identifying the aberrant phenotype of HSTCL, particularly in bone marrow specimens with minimal involvement.

Cytogenetics

Most cases demonstrate i(7)(q10), though this finding is not specific to HSTCL (146). Trisomy 8 also may be present.

Molecular Characteristics

HSTCLs have clonal rearrangements of the TCR-γ genes. TCR-β genes are rearranged in cases of αβ origin. EBV is usually negative.

Postulated Normal Counterpart

Cytotoxic T cells of the innate immune system, usually of γδ origin.

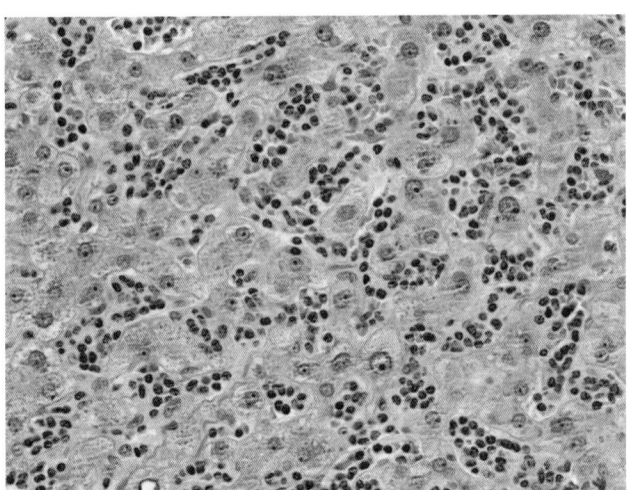 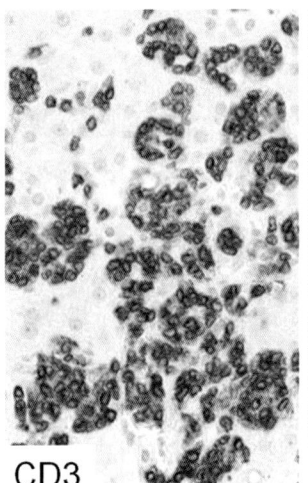 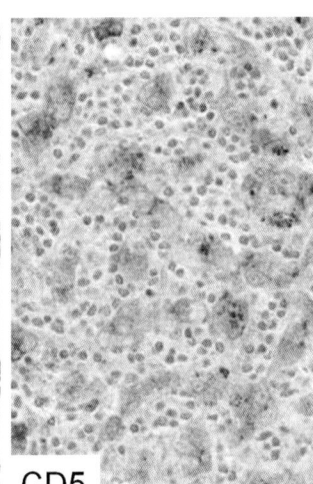

FIGURE 26.24. Hepatosplenic T-cell lymphoma, γδ type. There is a marked sinusoidal infiltrate of small lymphocytes. These express CD3 as well as CD2 and CD7 (not shown). They are negative for CD4, CD5, and CD8, as well as the TCR-β chain (βF1). They express TIA1 but not granzyme B, indicating a nonactivated cytotoxic phenotype.

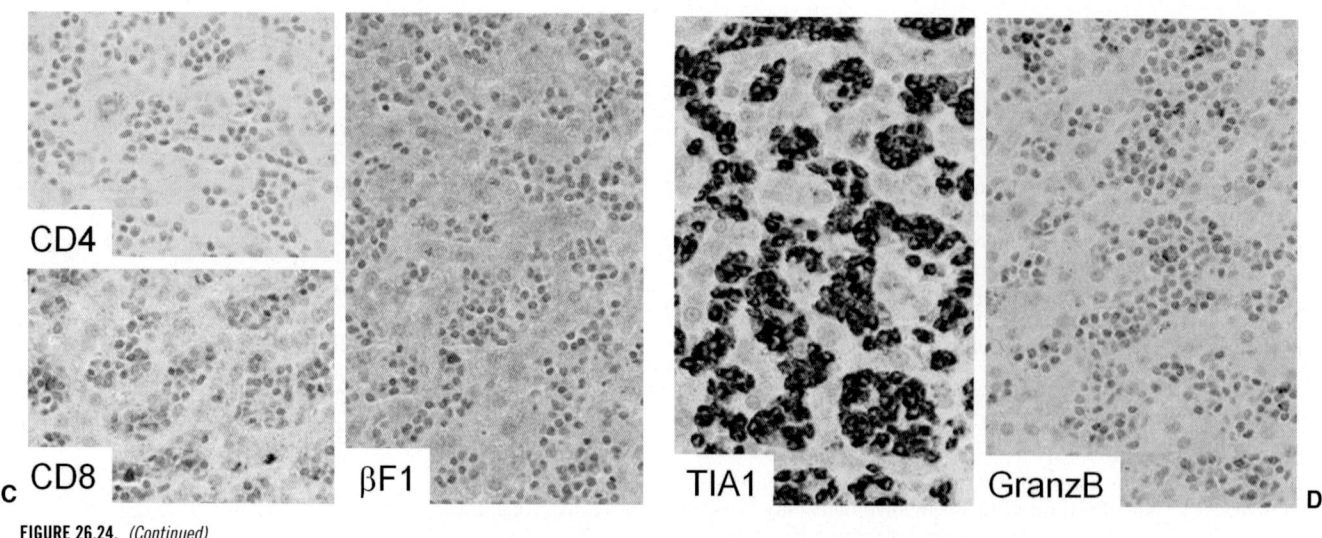

CD4

CD8

βF1

TIA1

GranzB

FIGURE 26.24. *(Continued)*

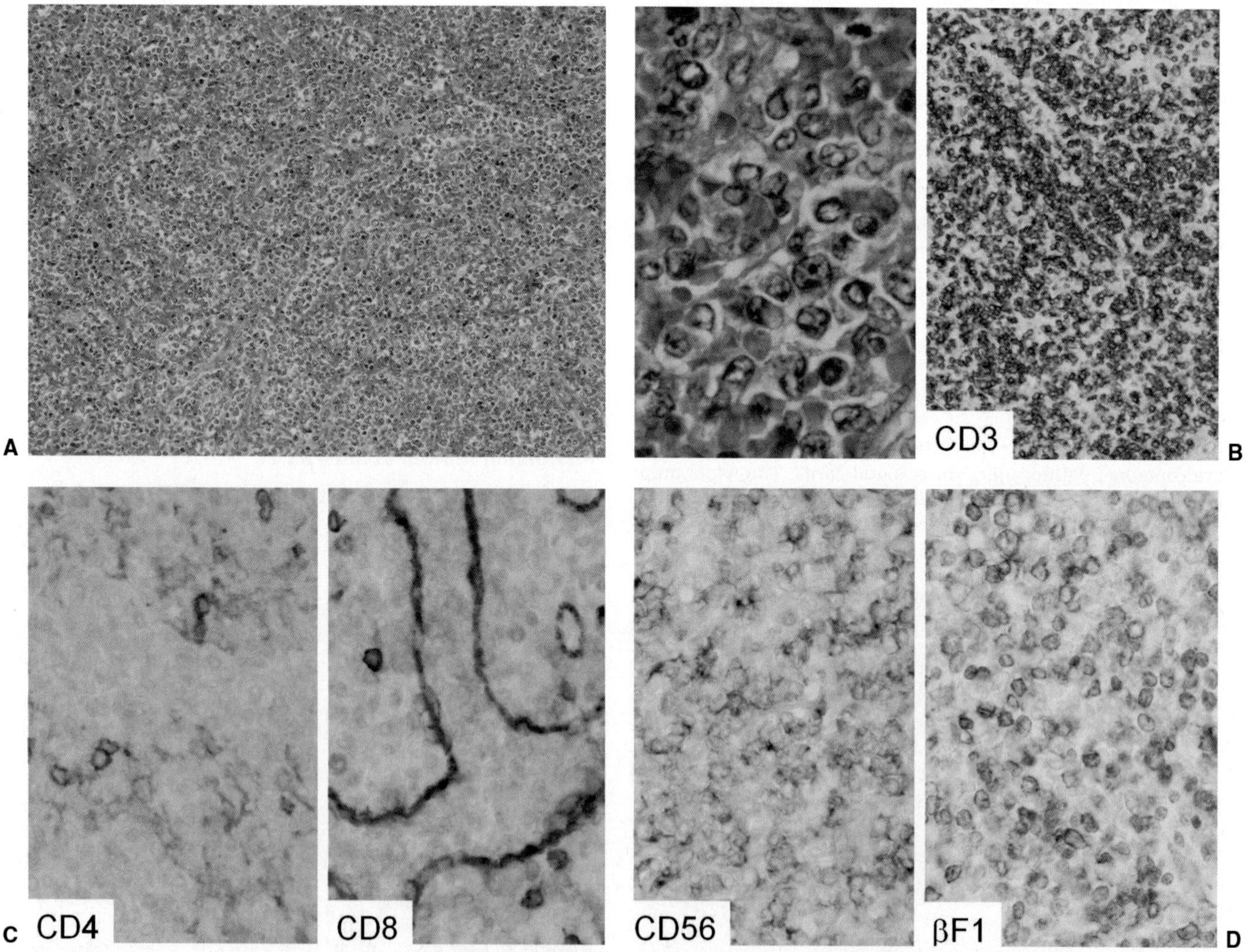

A

CD3

B

CD4

CD8

CD56

βF1

D

FIGURE 26.25. Hepatosplenic T-cell lymphoma, αβ type. The red pulp of the spleen shows an extensive atypical lymphoid infiltrate within the cords and sinuses. The tumor cells express CD3, CD56, and TCR-β (βF1), but are negative for CD4 and CD8.

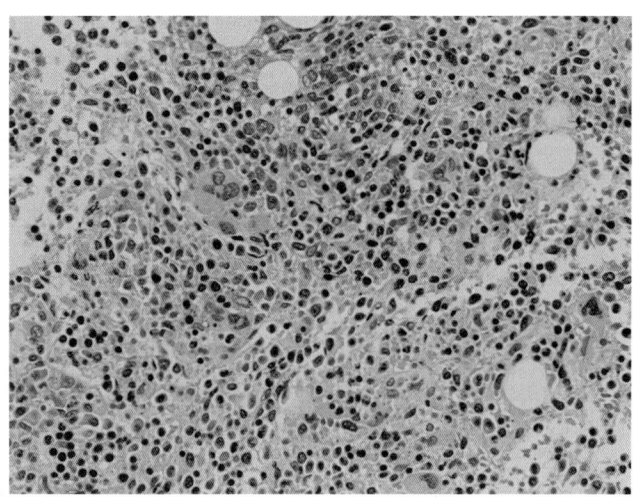
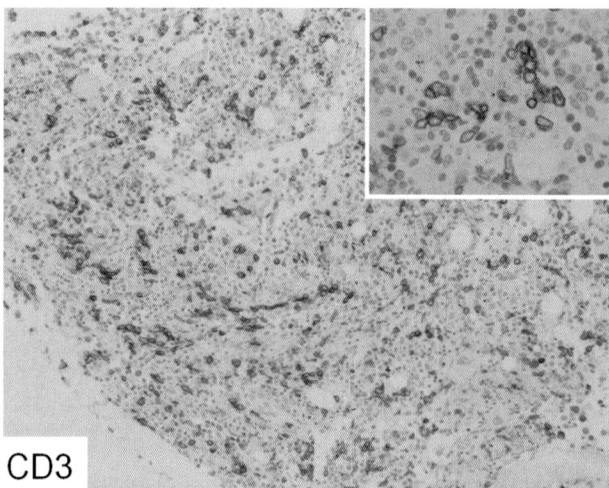

FIGURE 26.26. Hepatosplenic T-cell lymphoma involving the bone marrow. The infiltrating tumor cells can be difficult to appreciate on H&E sections. The sinusoidal pattern can be appreciated on CD3 stains.

Clinical Course and Prognostic Assessment

HSTCL is a clinically aggressive disease. Most patients experience relapse even if early responses to therapy are seen. Prognostic tools specific to HSTCL have not been adopted.

Treatment and Survival

HSTCL most commonly has been treated with CHOP-like chemotherapy, though long-term responses are rare and numerous combinations have been tried. Single-agent 2′-deoxycoformycin may have specific activity in this disease (147). OS rates are poor (median, <2 years).

Differential Diagnosis

Other PTCLs

The differential diagnosis typically is with other cytotoxic PTCLs. In cases of γδ origin, the anatomic sites of involvement usually are helpful in excluding diseases such as primary cutaneous (or mucosal) γδ T-cell lymphoma or PTCL, NOS of γδ origin. Specimens from the bone marrow or occasionally peripheral blood or unusual sites may be encountered without good clinical history. Aggressive NK-cell leukemia and T-LGL may have clinical presentation and immunophenotypic features similar to HSTCL. The former is associated with EBV. T-LGL typically is an indolent disease and has characteristic cytologic features. Both diseases show an activated cytotoxic T-cell phenotype, in contrast to HSTCL; occasionally studies for i(7)(q10) and/or trisomy 8 may be helpful.

For further discussion of the differential diagnosis of HSTCL, see Chapter 50.

▦ | SUMMARY AND CONCLUSIONS

PTCL is not a single disease, but rather a heterogeneous group of non-Hodgkin lymphomas of T- and NK-cell derivation that differ markedly in their clinical, pathologic, and molecular features. PTCL, NOS is the most common subtype, representing cases that cannot be classified as one of the more specific entities. This fact underscores the need for improved understanding of the molecular pathogenesis of PTCLs in general to facilitate clinically meaningful classification. Most subtypes of PTCL are clinically aggressive and have been associated with poor outcomes. Recently, however, targeted agents have been shown to have efficacy in some PTCLs.

Furthermore, new sequencing technologies are just beginning to identify previously unknown recurrent genetic abnormalities in these diseases. These advances suggest that the near future holds promise for improved molecular classification of PTCLs by pathologists, an expanding armamentarium of new drugs available to clinicians, and—hopefully—improved outcomes for patients.

References

1. Abouyabis AN, Shenoy PJ, Lechowicz MJ, et al. Incidence and outcomes of the peripheral T-cell lymphoma subtypes in the United States. *Leuk Lymphoma* 2008;49:2099–2107.
2. Swerdlow S, Campo E, Harris N, et al., eds. WHO Classification of tumours of haematopoietic and lymphoid tissues. In: Bosman F, Jaffe E, Lakhani S, et al., eds. *World health organization classification of tumours*, 4th ed. Lyon: International Agency for Research on Cancer, 2008.
3. Macon WR. Peripheral T-cell lymphomas. *Hematol Oncol Clin North Am* 2009;23: 829–842.
4. Vose J, Armitage J, Weisenburger D. International peripheral T-cell and natural killer/T-cell lymphoma study: pathology findings and clinical outcomes. *J Clin Oncol* 2008;26:4124–4130.
5. Savage KJ, Chhanabhai M, Gascoyne RD, et al. Characterization of peripheral T-cell lymphomas in a single North American institution by the WHO classification. *Ann Oncol* 2004;15:1467–1475.
6. Rudiger T, Weisenburger DD, Anderson JR, et al. Peripheral T-cell lymphoma (excluding anaplastic large-cell lymphoma): results from the non-Hodgkin's Lymphoma Classification Project. *Ann Oncol* 2002;13:140–149.
7. Falini B, Pileri S, De Solas I, et al. Peripheral T-cell lymphoma associated with hemophagocytic syndrome. *Blood* 1990;75:434–444.
8. Suchi T, Lennert K, Tu L-Y. Histopathology and immunohistochemistry of peripheral T-cell lymphomas: a proposal for their classification. *J Clin Pathol* 1987;40: 995–1015.
9. Barry TS, Jaffe ES, Sorbara L, et al. Peripheral T-cell lymphomas expressing CD30 and CD15. *Am J Surg Pathol* 2003;27:1513–1522.
10. Patsouris E, Noel H, Lennert K. Histological and immunohistological findings in lymphoepithelioid cell lymphoma (Lennert's lymphoma). *Am J Surg Pathol* 1988;12:341–350.
11. Yamashita Y, Nakamura S, Kagami Y, et al. Lennert's lymphoma: a variant of cytotoxic T-cell lymphoma? *Am J Surg Pathol* 2000;24:1627–1633.
12. de Leval L, Savilo E, Longtine J, et al. Peripheral T-cell lymphoma with follicular involvement and a CD4+/bcl-6+ phenotype. *Am J Surg Pathol* 2001;25:395–400.
13. Rudiger T, Ichinohasama R, Ott MM, et al. Peripheral T-cell lymphoma with distinct perifollicular growth pattern: a distinct subtype of T-cell lymphoma? *Am J Surg Pathol* 2000;24:117–122.
14. Geissinger E, Odenwald T, Lee SS, et al. Nodal peripheral T-cell lymphomas and, in particular, their lymphoepithelioid (Lennert's) variant are often derived from CD8(+) cytotoxic T-cells. *Virchows Arch* 2004;445:334–343.
15. Streubel B, Vinatzer U, Willheim M, et al. Novel t(5;9)(q33;q22) fuses ITK to SYK in unspecified peripheral T-cell lymphoma. *Leukemia* 2006;20:313–318.
16. Rigby S, Huang Y, Streubel B, et al. The lymphoma-associated fusion tyrosine kinase ITK-SYK requires pleckstrin homology domain-mediated membrane localisation for activation and cellular transformation. *J Biol Chem* 2009;284(39): 26871–26881.
17. Feldman AL, Sun DX, Law ME, et al. Overexpression of Syk tyrosine kinase in peripheral T-cell lymphomas. *Leukemia* 2008;22:1139–1143.
18. Wilcox RA, Sun DX, Novak A, et al. Inhibition of Syk protein tyrosine kinase induces apoptosis and blocks proliferation in T-cell non-Hodgkin's lymphoma cell lines. *Leukemia* 2010;24:229–232.
19. Feldman AL, Law M, Remstein ED, et al. Recurrent translocations involving the IRF4 oncogene locus in peripheral T-cell lymphomas. *Leukemia* 2009;23:574–580.

20. Nagel S, Leich E, Quentmeier H, et al. Amplification at 7q22 targets cyclin-dependent kinase 6 in T-cell lymphoma. *Leukemia* 2008;22:387–392.
21. Martin-Subero JI, Wlodarska I, Bastard C, et al. Chromosomal rearrangements involving the BCL3 locus are recurrent in classical Hodgkin and peripheral T-cell lymphoma. *Blood* 2006;108:401–402; author reply 402–403.
22. Quivoron C, Couronne L, Della Valle V, et al. TET2 inactivation results in pleiotropic hematopoietic abnormalities in mouse and is a recurrent event during human lymphomagenesis. *Cancer Cell* 2011;20:25–38.
23. Piccaluga PP, Agostinelli C, Califano A, et al. Gene expression analysis of angioimmunoblastic lymphoma indicates derivation from T follicular helper cells and vascular endothelial growth factor deregulation. *Cancer Res* 2007;67:10703–10710.
24. Zettl A, Rudiger T, Konrad MA, et al. Genomic profiling of peripheral T-cell lymphoma, unspecified, and anaplastic large T-cell lymphoma delineates novel recurrent chromosomal alterations. *Am J Pathol* 2004;164:1837–1848.
25. Thorns C, Bastian B, Pinkel D, et al. Chromosomal aberrations in angioimmunoblastic T-cell lymphoma and peripheral T-cell lymphoma unspecified: a matrix-based CGH approach. *Genes Chromosomes Cancer* 2007;46:37–44.
26. Martinez-Delgado B, Cuadros M, Honrado E, et al. Differential expression of NF-kappaB pathway genes among peripheral T-cell lymphomas. *Leukemia* 2005;19:2254–2263.
27. de Leval L, Rickman DS, Thielen C, et al. The gene expression profile of nodal peripheral T-cell lymphoma demonstrates a molecular link between angioimmunoblastic T-cell lymphoma (AITL) and follicular helper T (TFH) cells. *Blood* 2007;109:4952–4963.
28. Savage KJ. Prognosis and primary therapy in peripheral T-cell lymphomas. *Hematol Am Soc Hematol Educ Prog* 2008:280–288.
29. Savage KJ, Harris NL, Vose JM, et al. ALK$^-$ anaplastic large-cell lymphoma is clinically and immunophenotypically different from both ALK$^+$ ALCL and peripheral T-cell lymphoma, not otherwise specified: report from the International Peripheral T-Cell Lymphoma Project. *Blood* 2008;111:5496–5504.
30. Vose JM. Peripheral T-cell non-Hodgkin's lymphoma. *Hematol Oncol Clin North Am* 2008;22:997–1005, x.
31. Savage KJ. Peripheral T-cell lymphomas. *Blood Rev* 2007;21:201–216.
32. O'Connor OA, Pro B, Pinter-Brown L, et al. Pralatrexate in patients with relapsed or refractory peripheral T-cell lymphoma: results from the pivotal PROPEL study. *J Clin Oncol* 2011;29:1182–1189.
33. Huang Y, Moreau A, Dupuis J, et al. Peripheral T-cell lymphomas with a follicular growth pattern are derived from follicular helper T cells (TFH) and may show overlapping features with angioimmunoblastic T-cell lymphomas. *Am J Surg Pathol* 2009;33:682–690.
34. Warnke RA, Jones D, Hsi ED. Morphologic and immunophenotypic variants of nodal T-cell lymphomas and T-cell lymphoma mimics. *Am J Clin Pathol* 2007;127:511–527.
35. Feldman AL, Dogan A, Smith DI, et al. Discovery of recurrent t(6;7)(p25.3;q32.3) translocations in ALK-negative anaplastic large cell lymphomas by massively-parallel genomic sequencing. *Blood* 2011;117:915–919.
36. Shimoyama M. Diagnostic criteria and classification of clinical subtypes of adult T-cell leukaemia-lymphoma. A report from the Lymphoma Study Group (1984–87). *Br J Haematol* 1991;79:428–437.
37. Matutes E. Adult T-cell leukaemia/lymphoma. *J Clin Pathol* 2007;60: 1373–1377.
38. Karube K, Suzumiya J, Okamoto M, et al. Adult T-cell lymphoma/leukemia with angioimmunoblastic T-cell lymphomalike features: report of 11 cases. *Am J Surg Pathol* 2007;31:216–223.
39. Karube K, Aoki R, Sugita Y, et al. The relationship of FOXP3 expression and clinicopathological characteristics in adult T-cell leukemia/lymphoma. *Mod Pathol* 2008;21:617–625.
40. Roncador G, Garcia JF, Garcia JF, et al. FOXP3, a selective marker for a subset of adult T-cell leukaemia/lymphoma. *Leukemia* 2005;19:2247–2253.
41. Kohno T, Yamada Y, Akamatsu N, et al. Possible origin of adult T-cell leukemia/lymphoma cells from human T lymphotropic virus type-1-infected regulatory T cells. *Cancer Sci* 2005;96:527–533.
42. Burke J, Khalil S, Rappaport H. Dermatopathic lymphadenopathy. An immunophenotypic comparison of cases asssociated and unassociated with mycosis fungoides. *Am J Pathol* 1986;123:256–263.
43. Ralfkiaer E. Immunohistological markers for the diagnosis of cutaneous lymphomas. *Semin Diagn Pathol* 1991;8:62–72.
44. Vermeer MH, Geelen FA, Kummer JA, et al. Expression of cytotoxic proteins by neoplastic T cells in mycosis fungoides increases with progression from plaque stage to tumor stage disease. *Am J Pathol* 1999;154:1203–1210.
45. Dungarwalla M, Matutes E, Dearden CE. Prolymphocytic leukaemia of B- and T-cell subtype: a state-of-the-art paper. *Eur J Haematol* 2008;80:469–476.
46. Herling M, Khoury JD, Washington LT, et al. A systematic approach to diagnosis of mature T-cell leukemias reveals heterogeneity among WHO categories. *Blood* 2004;104:328–335.
47. Sohani AR, Jaffe ES, Harris NL, et al. Nodular lymphocyte-predominant hodgkin lymphoma with atypical T cells: a morphologic variant mimicking peripheral T-cell lymphoma. *Am J Surg Pathol* 2011;35:1666–1678.
48. Quintanilla-Martinez L, Fend F, Moguel LR, et al. Peripheral T-cell lymphoma with Reed-Sternberg-like cells of B-cell phenotype and genotype associated with Epstein-Barr virus infection. *Am J Surg Pathol* 1999;23:1233–1240.
49. Petrella T, Bagot M, Willemze R, et al. Blastic NK-cell lymphomas (agranular CD4$^+$CD56$^+$ hematodermic neoplasms): a review. *Am J Clin Pathol* 2005;123: 662–675.
50. Lim M, Straus SE, Dale J, et al. Pathologic findings in human autoimmune lymphoproliferative syndrome. *Am J Pathol* 1998;153:1541–1550.
51. Quintanilla-Martinez L, Kumar S, Fend F, et al. Fulminant EBV(+) T-cell lymphoproliferative disorder following acute/chronic EBV infection: a distinct clinicopathologic syndrome. *Blood* 2000;96:443–451.
52. Lundell R, Elenitoba-Johnson KS, Lim MS. T-cell posttransplant lymphoproliferative disorder occurring in a pediatric solid-organ transplant patient. *Am J Surg Pathol* 2004;28:967–973.
53. Abbondazo SL, Irey NS, Frizzera G. Dilantin-associated lymphadenopathy. Spectrum of histopathologic patterns. *Am J Surg Pathol* 1995;19:675–686.
54. Schwab U, Stein H, Gerdes J, et al. Production of a monoclonal antibody specific for Hodgkin and Reed-Sternberg cells of Hodgkin's disease and a subset of normal lymphoid cells. *Nature* 1982;299:65–67.
55. Stein H, Mason D, Gerdes J, et al. The expression of the Hodgkin's disease associated antigen Ki-1 in reactive and neoplastic lymphoid tissue: evidence that Reed-Sternberg cells and histiocytic malignancies are derived from activated lymphoid cells. *Blood* 1985;66:848–858.
56. Stansfeld A, Diebold J, Kapanci Y, et al. Updated Kiel classification for lymphomas. *Lancet* 1988;1:292–293.
57. Harris NL, Jaffe ES, Stein H, et al. A revised European-American classification of lymphoid neoplasms: a proposal from the International Lymphoma Study Group. *Blood* 1994;84:1361–1392.
58. Rimokh R, Magaud JP, Berger F, et al. A translocation involving a specific breakpoint (q35) on chromosome 5 is characteristic of anaplastic large cell lymphoma ('Ki-1 lymphoma'). *Br J Haematol* 1989;71:31–36.
59. Kaneko Y, Frizzera G, Edamura S, et al. A novel translocation, t(2;5)(p23;q35), in childhood phagocytic large T-cell lymphoma mimicking malignant histiocytosis. *Blood* 1989;73:806–813.
60. Morris SW, Kirstein MN, Valentine MB, et al. Fusion of a kinase gene, ALK, to a nucleolar protein gene, NPM, in non-Hodgkin's lymphoma. *Science* 1994;263:1281–1284.
61. Rizvi MA, Evens AM, Tallman MS, et al. T-cell non-Hodgkin lymphoma. *Blood* 2006;107:1255–1264.
62. Falini B, Pileri S, Zinzani PL, et al. ALK+ lymphoma: clinico-pathological findings and outcome. *Blood* 1999;93:2697–2706.
63. Bayle C, Charpentier A, Duchayne E, et al. Leukaemic presentation of small cell variant anaplastic large cell lymphoma:report of four cases. *Br J Haematol* 1999;104:680–688.
64. Fraga M, Brousset P, Schlaifer D, et al. Bone marrow involvement in anaplastic large cell lymphoma. Immunohistochemical detection of minimal disease and its prognostic significance. *Am J Clin Pathol* 1995;103:82–89.
65. Benharroch D, Meguerian-Bedoyan Z, Lamant L, et al. ALK-positive lymphoma: a single disease with a broad spectrum of morphology. *Blood* 1998;91:2076–2084.
66. Pileri S, Falini B, Delsol G, et al. Lymphohistiocytic T-cell lymphoma (anaplastic large cell lymphoma CD30+/Ki-1+ with a high content of reactive histiocytes). *Histopathology* 1990;16:383–391.
67. Kinney M, Collins R, Greer J, et al. A small-cell-predominant variant of primary Ki-1 (CD30)+ T-cell lymphoma. *Am J Surg Pathol* 1993;17:859–868.
68. Vassallo J, Lamant L, Brugieres L, et al. ALK-positive anaplastic large cell lymphoma mimicking nodular sclerosis Hodgkin's lymphoma: report of 10 cases. *Am J Surg Pathol* 2006;30:223–229.
69. Nakamura S, Shiota M, Nakagawa A, et al. Anaplastic large cell lymphoma: a distinct molecular pathologic entity: a reappraisal with special reference to p80(NPM/ALK) expression. *Am J Surg Pathol* 1997;21:1420–1432.
70. Chan JK, Buchanan R, Fletcher CD. Sarcomatoid variant of anaplastic large-cell Ki-1 lymphoma. *Am J Surg Pathol* 1990;14:983–988.
71. Foss HD, Anagnostopoulos I, Araujo I, et al. Anaplastic large-cell lymphomas of T-cell and null-cell phenotype express cytotoxic molecules. *Blood* 1996;88:4005–4011.
72. Wellmann A, Thieblemont C, Pittaluga S, et al. Detection of differentially expressed genes in lymphomas using cDNA arrays: identification of clusterin as a new diagnostic marker for Anaplastic Large Cell Lymphomas (ALCL). *Blood* 2000;96:398–404.
73. Dunphy CH, DeMello DE, Gale GB. Pediatric CD56+ anaplastic large cell lymphoma: a review of the literature. *Arch Pathol Lab Med* 2006;130:1859–1864.
74. Rosso R, Paulli M, Magrini U, et al. Anaplastic large cell lymphoma, CD30/Ki-1 positive, expressing the CD15/Leu-M1 antigen. Immunohistochemical and morphological relationships to Hodgkin's disease. *Virchows Arch A Pathol Anat Histopathol* 1990;416:229–235.
75. Feldman AL, Law ME, Inwards DJ, et al. PAX5-positive T-cell anaplastic large cell lymphomas associated with extra copies of the PAX5 gene locus. *Mod Pathol* 2010;23:593–602. PMCID: PMC2848697.
76. Juco J, Holden JT, Mann KP, et al. Immunophenotypic analysis of anaplastic large cell lymphoma by flow cytometry. *Am J Clin Pathol* 2003;119:205–212.
77. de Leval L, Bisig B, Thielen C, et al. Molecular classification of T-cell lymphomas. *Crit Rev Oncol Hematol* 2009;72(2):125–143.
78. Salaverria I, Bea S, Lopez-Guillermo A, et al. Genomic profiling reveals different genetic aberrations in systemic ALK-positive and ALK-negative anaplastic large cell lymphomas. *Br J Haematol* 2008;140:516–526.
79. Brousset P, Rochaix P, Chittal S, et al. High incidence of Epstein-Barr virus detection in Hodgkin's disease and absence of detection in anaplastic large-cell lymphoma in children. *Histopathology* 1993;23:189–191.
80. Lamant L, de Reynies A, Duplantier MM, et al. Gene-expression profiling of systemic anaplastic large-cell lymphoma reveals differences based on ALK status and two distinct morphologic ALK+ subtypes. *Blood* 2007;109:2156–2164.
81. Amin HM, Lai R. Pathobiology of ALK+ anaplastic large-cell lymphoma. *Blood* 2007;110:2259–2267.
82. Matsuyama H, Suzuki HI, Nishimori H, et al. miR-135b mediates NPM-ALK-driven oncogenicity and renders IL-17-producing immunophenotype to anaplastic large cell lymphoma. *Blood* 2011;118:6881–6892.
83. Liso A, Tiacci E, Binazzi R, et al. Haploidentical peripheral-blood stem-cell transplantation for ALK-positive anaplastic large-cell lymphoma. *Lancet Oncol* 2004;5:127–128.
84. Li R, Morris SW. Development of anaplastic lymphoma kinase (ALK) small-molecule inhibitors for cancer therapy. *Med Res Rev* 2008;28:372–412.
85. Minich SS. Brentuximab vedotin: a new age in the treatment of hodgkin lymphoma and anaplastic large cell lymphoma. *Ann Pharmacother* 2012;46:377–383.
86. Lamant L, Pileri S, Sabattini E, et al. Cutaneous presentation of ALK-positive anaplastic large cell lymphoma following insect bites: evidence for an association in five cases. *Haematologica* 2010;95:449–455.
87. Kadin ME, Pinkus JL, Pinkus GS, et al. Primary cutaneous ALCL with phosphorylated/activated cytoplasmic ALK and novel phenotype: EMA/MUC1+, cutaneous lymphocyte antigen negative. *Am J Surg Pathol* 2008;32:1421–1426.
88. Delsol G, Lamant L, Mariame B, et al. A new subtype of large B-cell lymphoma expressing the ALK kinase and lacking the 2;5 translocation. *Blood* 1997;89:1483–1490.
89. Soda M, Choi YL, Enomoto M, et al. Identification of the transforming EML4-ALK fusion gene in non-small-cell lung cancer. *Nature* 2007;448:561–566.
90. Chen Y, Takita J, Choi YL, et al. Oncogenic mutations of ALK kinase in neuroblastoma. *Nature* 2008;455:971–974.
91. Griffin CA, Hawkins AL, Dvorak C, et al. Recurrent involvement of 2p23 in inflammatory myofibroblastic tumors. *Cancer Res* 1999;59:2776–2780.

92. Pittaluga S, Wlodarska I, Pulford K, et al. The monoclonal antibody ALK1 identifies a distinct morphological subtype of anaplastic large cell lymphoma associated with 2p23/ALK rearrangements. *Am J Pathol* 1997;151:343–351.

93. Sciallis AP, Law ME, Inwards DJ, et al. Mucosal CD30-positive T-cell lymphoproliferations of the head and neck show a clinicopathologic spectrum similar to cutaneous CD30-positive T-cell lymphoproliferative disorders. *Mod Pathol* 2012;25(7):983–992.

94. Roden AC, Macon WR, Keeney GL, et al. Seroma-associated primary anaplastic large-cell lymphoma adjacent to breast implants: an indolent T-cell lymphoproliferative disorder. *Mod Pathol* 2008;21:455–463.

95. Popplewell L, Thomas SH, Huang Q, et al. Primary anaplastic large-cell lymphoma associated with breast implants. *Leuk Lymphoma* 2011;52:1481–1487.

96. Bovio IM, Allan RW. The expression of myeloid antigens CD13 and/or CD33 is a marker of ALK+ anaplastic large cell lymphomas. *Am J Clin Pathol* 2008; 130:628–634.

97. Wada DA, Law ME, His ED, et al. Specificity of IRF4 translocations for primary cutaneous anaplastic large cell lymphoma: a multicenter study of 204 skin biopsies. *Mod Pathol* 2011;24:596–605.

98. Parrilla Castellar ER, Grogg KL, Law ME, et al. Rearrangements of the 6p25.3 locus identify a subset of systemic ALK-negative anaplastic large cell lymphomas with favorable prognosis. *Mod Pathol* 2012;25:359A (abst 1508).

99. ten Berge RL, de Bruin PC, Oudejans JJ, et al. ALK-negative anaplastic large-cell lymphoma demonstrates similar poor prognosis to peripheral T-cell lymphoma, unspecified. *Histopathology* 2003;43:462–469.

100. de Bruin PC, Beljaards RC, van Heerde P, et al. Differences in clinical behaviour and immunophenotype between primary cutaneous and primary nodal anaplastic large cell lymphoma of T-cell or null cell phenotype. *Histopathology* 1993;23:127–135.

101. Bekkenk MW, Geelen FA, van Voorst Vader PC, et al. Primary and secondary cutaneous CD30(+) lymphoproliferative disorders: a report from the Dutch Cutaneous Lymphoma Group on the long-term follow-up data of 219 patients and guidelines for diagnosis and treatment. *Blood* 2000;95:3653–3661.

102. Asano N, Oshiro A, Matsuo K, et al. Prognostic significance of T-cell or cytotoxic molecules phenotype in classical Hodgkin's lymphoma: a clinicopathologic study. *J Clin Oncol* 2006;24:4626–4633.

103. Feldman AL, Dogan A. Diagnostic uses of Pax5 immunohistochemistry. *Adv Anat Pathol* 2007;14:323–334.

104. Lennert K. Nature, prognosis and nomenclature of angioimmunoblastic lymphadenopathy (lymphogranulomatosis X or T-zone lymphoma). *Dtsch Med Wochenschr* 1979;104:1246–1247.

105. Frizzera G, Moran EM, Rappaport H. Angio-immunoblastic lymphadenopathy with dysproteinaemia. *Lancet* 1974;1:1070–1073.

106. Lukes RJ, Tindle BH. Immunoblastic lymphadenopathy. A hyperimmune entity resembling Hodgkin's disease. *N Engl J Med* 1975;292:1–8.

107. Dogan A, Gaulard P, Jaffe ES, et al. Angioimmunoblastic T-cell lymphoma. In: Swerdlow SH, ed. *WHO classification of tumours of haematopoietic and lymphoid tissues*. Lyon: International Agency for Research on Cancer (IARC), 2008:309–311.

108. Mourad N, Mounier N, Briere J, et al. Clinical, biologic, and pathologic features in 157 patients with angioimmunoblastic T-cell lymphoma treated within the Groupe d'Etude des Lymphomes de l'Adulte (GELA) trials. *Blood* 2008;111:4463–4470.

109. Attygalle AD, Chuang SS, Diss TC, et al. Distinguishing angioimmunoblastic T-cell lymphoma from peripheral T-cell lymphoma, unspecified, using morphology, immunophenotype and molecular genetics. *Histopathology* 2007;50:498–508.

110. Attygalle AD, Diss TC, Munson P, et al. CD10 expression in extranodal dissemination of angioimmunoblastic T-cell lymphoma. *Am J Surg Pathol* 2004;28:54–61.

111. Ortonne N, Dupuis J, Plonquet A, et al. Characterization of CXCL13+ neoplastic t cells in cutaneous lesions of angioimmunoblastic T-cell lymphoma (AITL). *Am J Surg Pathol* 2007;31:1068–1076.

112. Grogg KL, Attygalle AD, Macon WR, et al. Angioimmunoblastic T-cell lymphoma: a neoplasm of germinal-center T-helper cells? *Blood* 2005;106:1501–1502.

113. Attygalle A, Al-Jehani R, Diss TC, et al. Neoplastic T cells in angioimmunoblastic T-cell lymphoma express CD10. *Blood* 2002;99:627–633.

114. Grogg KL, Attygalle AD, Macon WR, et al. Expression of CXCL13, a chemokine highly upregulated in germinal center T-helper cells, distinguishes angioimmunoblastic T-cell lymphoma from peripheral T-cell lymphoma, unspecified. *Mod Pathol* 2006;19:1101–1107.

115. Dorfman DM, Brown JA, Shahsafaei A, et al. Programmed death-1 (PD-1) is a marker of germinal center-associated T cells and angioimmunoblastic T-cell lymphoma. *Am J Surg Pathol* 2006;30:802–810.

116. Dogan A, Attygalle AD, Kyriakou C. Angioimmunoblastic T-cell lymphoma. *Br J Haematol* 2003;121:681–691.

117. Attygalle AD, Kyriakou C, Dupuis J, et al. Histologic evolution of angioimmunoblastic T-cell lymphoma in consecutive biopsies: clinical correlation and insights into natural history and disease progression. *Am J Surg Pathol* 2007;31:1077–1088.

118. Zettl A, Lee SS, Rudiger T, et al. Epstein-Barr virus-associated B-cell lymphoproliferative disorders in angioimmunoblastic T-cell lymphoma and peripheral T-cell lymphoma, unspecified. *Am J Clin Pathol* 2002;117:368–379.

119. Willenbrock K, Brauninger A, Hansmann ML. Frequent occurrence of B-cell lymphomas in angioimmunoblastic T-cell lymphoma and proliferation of Epstein-Barr virus-infected cells in early cases. *Br J Haematol* 2007;138:733–739.

120. Attygalle AD, Kyriakou C, Dupuis J, et al. Histologic evolution of angioimmunoblastic T-cell lymphoma in consecutive biopsies: clinical correlation and insights into natural history and disease progression. *Am J Surg Pathol* 2007;31:1077–1088.

121. Huppmann AR, Roullet MR, Raffeld M, et al. Angioimmunoblastic T-cell lymphoma partially obscured by an epstein-barr virus-negative clonal plasma cell proliferation. *J Clin Oncol* 2013;31:e28–e30.

122. Au WY, Ma SY, Chim CS, et al. Clinicopathologic features and treatment outcome of mature T-cell and natural killer-cell lymphomas diagnosed according to the World Health Organization classification scheme: a single center experience of 10 years. *Ann Oncol* 2005;16:206–214.

123. Gualco G, Domeny-Duarte P, Chioato L, et al. Clinicopathologic and molecular features of 122 Brazilian cases of nodal and extranodal NK/T-cell lymphoma, nasal type, with EBV subtyping analysis. *Am J Surg Pathol* 2011;35:1195–1203.

124. Chan JK, Yip TT, Tsang WY, et al. Detection of Epstein-Barr viral RNA in malignant lymphomas of the upper aerodigestive tract. *Am J Surg Pathol* 1994;18:938–946.

125. Elenitoba-Johnson KSJ, Zarate-Osorno A, Meneses A, et al. Cytotoxic granular protein expression, Epstein-Barr virus strain type, and latent membrane protein-1 oncogene deletions in nasal T-lymphocyte/natural killer cell lymphomas from Mexico. *Mod Pathol* 1998;11:754–761.

126. Au WY, Pang A, Choy C, et al. Quantification of circulating Epstein-Barr virus (EBV) DNA in the diagnosis and monitoring of natural killer cell and EBV-positive lymphomas in immunocompetent patients. *Blood* 2004;104:243–249.

127. Takahashi N, Miura I, Chubachi A, et al. A clinicopathological study of 20 patients with T/natural killer (NK)-cell lymphoma-associated hemophagocytic syndrome with special reference to nasal and nasal-type NK/T-cell lymphoma. *Int J Hematol* 2001;74:303–308.

128. Chim CS, Ma ES, Loong F, et al. Diagnostic cues for natural killer cell lymphoma: primary nodal presentation and the role of in situ hybridisation for Epstein-Barr virus encoded early small RNA in detecting occult bone marrow involvement. *J Clin Pathol* 2005;58:443–445.

129. Pongpruttipan T, Sukpanichnant S, Assanasen T, et al. Extranodal NK/T-cell lymphoma, nasal type, includes cases of natural killer cell and alphabeta, gammadelta, and alphabeta/gammadelta T-cell origin: a comprehensive clinicopathologic and phenotypic study. *Am J Surg Pathol* 2012;36:481–499.

130. Au WY, Weisenburger DD, Intragumtornchai T, et al. Clinical differences between nasal and extranasal natural killer/T-cell lymphoma: a study of 136 cases from the International Peripheral T-Cell Lymphoma Project. *Blood* 2009;113:3931–3937.

131. Yamaguchi M, Kwong YL, Kim WS, et al. Phase II study of SMILE chemotherapy for newly diagnosed stage IV, relapsed, or refractory extranodal natural killer (NK)/T-cell lymphoma, nasal type: the NK-Cell Tumor Study Group study. *J Clin Oncol* 2011;29:4410–4416.

132. Li YX, Liu QF, Wang WH, et al. Failure patterns and clinical implications in early stage nasal natural killer/T-cell lymphoma treated with primary radiotherapy. *Cancer* 2011;117:5203–5211.

133. Howell WM, Leung ST, Jones DB, et al. HLA-DRB, -DQA, and -DQB polymorphism in celiac disease and enteropathy-associated T-cell lymphoma. Common features and additional risk factors for malignancy. *Hum Immunol* 1995;43:29–37.

134. Rohatiner A, d'Amore F, Coiffier B, et al. Report on a workshop convened to discuss the pathological and staging classifications of gastrointestinal tract lymphoma. *Ann Oncol* 1994;5:397–400.

135. Ashton-Key M, Diss TC, Pan L, et al. Molecular analysis of T-cell clonality in ulcerative jejunitis and enteropathy-associated T-cell lymphoma. *Am J Pathol* 1997;151:493–498.

136. Cellier C, Delabesse E, Helmer C, et al. Refractory sprue, coeliac disease, and enteropathy-associated T-cell lymphoma. French Coeliac Disease Study Group. *Lancet* 2000;356:203–208.

137. Chott A, Haedicke W, Mosberger I, et al. Most CD56+ intestinal lymphomas are CD8+CD5-T-cell lymphomas of monomorphic small to medium size histology. *Am J Pathol* 1998;153:1483–1490.

138. Deleeuw RJ, Zettl A, Klinker E, et al. Whole-genome analysis and HLA genotyping of enteropathy-type T-cell lymphoma reveals 2 distinct lymphoma subtypes. *Gastroenterology* 2007;132:1902–1911.

139. Gale J, Simmonds PD, Mead GM, et al. Enteropathy-type intestinal T-cell lymphoma: clinical features and treatment of 31 patients in a single center. *J Clin Oncol* 2000;18:795–803.

140. Mansoor A, Pittaluga S, Beck PL, et al. NK-cell enteropathy: a benign NK-cell lymphoproliferative disease mimicking intestinal lymphoma: clinicopathologic features and follow-up in a unique case series. *Blood* 2011;117:1447–1452.

141. Kotlyar DS, Osterman MT, Diamond RH, et al. A systematic review of factors that contribute to hepatosplenic T-cell lymphoma in patients with inflammatory bowel disease. *Clin Gastroenterol Hepatol* 2011;9:36–41 e1.

142. Rosh JR, Gross T, Mamula P, et al. Hepatosplenic T-cell lymphoma in adolescents and young adults with Crohn's disease: a cautionary tale? *Inflamm Bowel Dis* 2007;13:1024–1030.

143. Mackey AC, Green L, Liang LC, et al. Hepatosplenic T cell lymphoma associated with infliximab use in young patients treated for inflammatory bowel disease. *J Pediatr Gastroenterol Nutr* 2007;44:265–267.

144. Macon WR, Levy NB, Kurtin PJ, et al. Hepatosplenic alphabeta T-cell lymphomas: a report of 14 cases and comparison with hepatosplenic gammadelta T-cell lymphomas. *Am J Surg Pathol* 2001;25:285–296.

145. Cooke CB, Krenacs M, Stetler-Stevenson M, et al. Hepatosplenic gamma/delta T-cell lymphoma: a distinct clinicopathologic entity of cytotoxic gamma/delta T-cell origin. *Blood* 1996;88:4265–4274.

146. Feldman AL, Law M, Grogg KL, et al. Incidence of TCR and TCL1 gene translocations and isochromosome 7q in peripheral T-cell lymphomas using fluorescence in situ hybridization. *Am J Clin Pathol* 2008;130:178–185.

147. Corazzelli G, Capobianco G, Russo F, et al. Pentostatin (2′-deoxycoformycin) for the treatment of hepatosplenic gammadelta T-cell lymphomas. *Haematologica* 2005;90:ECR14.

Chapter 27
Nonhematopoietic Elements in Lymph Nodes

Julia Turbiner Geyer • Daniel M. Knowles

The pathologist is frequently asked to evaluate a lymph node biopsy specimen to determine the presence of any one of a wide spectrum of benign and malignant lymphoid proliferations that commonly involve lymph nodes. Various nonhematopoietic elements and nonlymphoid hematopoietic proliferations may be encountered in lymph nodes, and some of them may mimic benign or malignant lymphoid proliferations to an extraordinary degree.

Nonhematopoietic elements that occur in lymph nodes may be benign or malignant. The benign elements include a variety of congenital malformations and inclusions that may be misinterpreted as malignant neoplasms metastatic to lymph nodes. Rarely, a nonhematopoietic neoplasm may even originate from these ectopic elements, giving rise to a nonhematopoietic neoplasm primary in a lymph node. Malignant nonhematopoietic proliferations that involve lymph nodes include a large number of epithelial and mesenchymal proliferations that may mimic malignant lymphoma. Several nonlymphoid hematopoietic processes (e.g., myeloid sarcoma, mast cell disease) may occur in lymph nodes and be mistaken for malignant lymphoma.

The recognition and correct interpretation of these nonhematopoietic elements and nonlymphoid hematopoietic proliferations often carry considerable clinical significance. The proper management, treatment, and prognosis of the patient may depend entirely on the pathologist's diagnosis. Fortunately, in recent years, the sometimes difficult pathologic differential diagnosis caused by these lesions has been aided by the application of immunohistochemistry that uses panels of antibodies whose reactivity patterns characterize specific clinicopathologic entities.

In this chapter, we describe the morphologic features of the nonhematopoietic developmental ectopias and the benign and malignant nonhematopoietic and nonlymphoid hematopoietic proliferations that involve lymph nodes, and we discuss their differential diagnosis with lymphoid proliferations, including the contribution of immunohistochemistry (Table 27.1).

APPROACH TO DIAGNOSIS

A variety of clinical and morphologic clues may enable the pathologist to distinguish benign and malignant nonhematolymphoid elements from hematolymphoid proliferations and to categorize further the nonhematolymphoid neoplasms. However, the histopathologic features of malignant lymphomas and nonlymphoid neoplasms occasionally overlap. When confronted with the difficult histopathologic differential diagnosis of a poorly differentiated malignant neoplasm of unknown origin compared with malignant lymphoma, multiple sections should be obtained to ensure that areas of specific cellular differentiation (i.e., squamous, glandular, and melanocytic) can be demonstrated. Histochemical stains can be performed for reticulin fibers, mucin, glycoprotein, glycogen, melanin, and endocrine granules (1). Even these approaches still leave many diagnostic dilemmas unresolved, however.

Electron Microscopy

In the past, ultrastructural studies were used frequently and widely to classify neoplasms that could not be identified by light microscopy. For example, the presence of desmosomal junctions and tonofilaments was taken to indicate a squamous epithelial origin, well-developed cell junctions and microvilli to indicate glandular derivation, melanosomes or premelanosomes to indicate a melanocytic proliferation, neurosecretory granules to indicate a neuroendocrine tumor such as neuroblastoma, and actin-myosin complexes to indicate rhabdomyosarcoma (1). Malignant lymphomas do not possess distinctive ultrastructural features (1). Moreover, many undifferentiated neoplasms cannot be classified on the basis of electron microscopic examination (1). These factors, in addition to the requirement for costly facilities, specially trained personnel, and the large amount of time necessary to actually perform ultrastructural studies, render them neither practical nor cost-effective in routine diagnosis. Such studies are now almost exclusively reserved for research.

Immunohistochemistry

Immunohistochemistry has become the principal method employed by pathologists to resolve difficult histopathologic dilemmas in the diagnosis and classification of neoplasms. Immunohistochemistry obviates all the disadvantages of electron microscopy. Extensive panels of well-characterized polyclonal and monoclonal antibodies that recognize a wide range of surface membrane and cytoplasmic structural proteins and cellular products are now available commercially. Nearly every major category of malignant neoplasia, including the most undifferentiated tumors, exhibits a constellation of immunohistochemical markers that permits diagnosis and classification (2,3) (Table 27.2). The malignant lymphomas express specific markers that readily permit their separation from the large variety of epithelial and other neoplasms that may simulate them (see Chapter 3). Moreover, this technology does not require costly or extensive facilities or specially trained and skilled laboratory personnel. The technical protocols must be followed carefully and the actual procedures performed meticulously. In general, however, the techniques are easy to teach to even inexperienced personnel. Most assays can be performed on routinely prepared paraffin tissue sections, are relatively inexpensive to perform, and can be completed within a few hours (4).

Whenever possible, the pathologic material subjected to immunostaining should be collected, stored, and processed under optimal conditions. Standard formalin fixation and paraffin embedding are the optimum methods of handling tissue to demonstrate most antigens in routine diagnostic pathology. However, certain antigens expressed by hematolymphoid neoplasms are still best detected in unfixed tissue (see Chapter 3). Fresh tissue can be used for ancillary cytogenetic and molecular diagnostic procedures. Ideally, in the case of all pathologic specimens of neoplasms but especially those that may require immunohistochemical examination, the specimens should be

698

Table 27.1	NONHEMATOPOIETIC ELEMENTS IN LYMPH NODES

Congenital malformations and inclusions
   Ectopic nevus cells
   Ectopic mesothelial cells
   Ectopic müllerian and celomic epithelium
   Ectopic salivary gland
   Ectopic thyroid gland
   Ectopic breast and sweat gland tissue
Epithelial lesions primary in lymph nodes
   Malignant melanoma
   Warthin tumor
   Acinic cell and mucoepidermoid carcinoma
   Thyroid carcinoma
   Breast carcinoma
Mesenchymal lesions primary in lymph nodes
   Lipomatosis of lymph nodes
   Fibrosis of lymph nodes
   Vascular transformation
   Nodal angiomatosis
   Angiomyomatous hamartoma
   Angiolipomatous hamartoma
   Hemangioma
   Vascular neoplasm of Castleman disease
   Lymphangioma
   Lymphangiomyomatosis
   Lymphangioleiomyomatosis
   Epithelioid hemangioendothelioma
   Kaposi sarcoma
   Angiomyolipoma
   Bacillary angiomatosis

Inflammatory pseudotumor of lymph node
Palisaded myofibroblastoma
Mycobacterial spindle cell pseudotumor
Leiomyomatosis
Deciduosis
Other sarcomas
Metastatic neoplasms in lymph nodes
   Poorly differentiated carcinomas
      Undifferentiated nasopharyngeal carcinoma
      Poorly differentiated neuroendocrine carcinoma
      Mammary lobular carcinoma
      Signet ring cell lesions
      Other poorly differentiated carcinomas
   Differentiated adenocarcinomas
   Malignant melanoma
   Germ cell tumors
   Small round cell sarcomas
      Ewing sarcoma
      Primitive neuroectodermal tumor
      Rhabdomyosarcoma
      Desmoplastic small round cell tumor
   Synovial sarcoma and epithelioid sarcoma
   Clear cell sarcoma
   Metastatic sarcoma with glandular differentiation
   Myeloid sarcoma

collected fresh and unfixed and some representative portions should be snap-frozen and cryopreserved while other representative portions should be fixed and processed in the usual manner. This approach permits reliable immunohistochemical demonstration of the greatest range of antigenic markers.

The demonstration of a single antigenic marker should never be relied on to determine the histogenesis of a particular neoplasm or to make a definitive diagnosis. A carefully selected panel of antibody reagents that reflects positive and negative staining results of entities in the differential diagnosis should be used. This maximizes the specificity of the immunodiagnosis and minimizes the possibility of diagnostic error. Interpretation of immunophenotypic data should also include attention to the intensity and distribution of immune reactivity and the morphology of the immunoreactive cells. For example, mCEA positivity is commonly found in neutrophils (5), which does not

have a bearing on the immunophenotype of the neoplasm in question. Paranuclear cytoplasmic "dot" positivity is characteristic of anticytokeratin antibodies in neuroendocrine tumors (6). Rare cytokeratin-positive cells may indicate epithelial differentiation in the appropriate setting, but only strong and diffuse nuclear and cytoplasmic S-100 protein expression permits the identification of melanocytic differentiation (7). The results of immunohistochemical studies should be used as an adjunct to histopathologic diagnosis; all diagnostic conclusions should be based on correlation of the immunohistochemical findings with careful examination of the histopathologic sections.

For the initial evaluation of neoplasms that appear undifferentiated on routine hematoxylin and eosin sections, we recommend an antibody panel capable of identifying the following antigens: leukocyte common antigen (LCA; CD45), cytokeratins (i.e., CAM 5.2, AE1/AE3, or both), and S-100 protein. In most

Table 27.2	IMMUNOHISTOCHEMICAL STAINING PROFILES OF NEOPLASMS

Stain	Non-Hodgkin Lymphoma	Carcinoma	Neuroendocrine Carcinoma	Malignant Melanoma	Germ Cell Tumor	ES/PNET	Rhabdo-myosarcoma	Sarcomas with Epithelial Differentiation
CD45	+	−	−	−	−	−	−	−
Cytokeratin	−	+	+	−	+/−	−	−	+
EMA	−/+	+	+	−	+/−	−	−	+
S-100	−	−/+	−	+	−	−/+	−	−/+
Chromogranin/synaptophysin	−	−/+	+	−	−	+/−	−	−
CD99	−/+	−	−/+	−	−	+	−/+	−/+
HMB-45	−	−	−	+/−	−	−	−	−
AFP/PLAP	−	−	−	−	+/−	−	−	−
Desmin/SMA	−	−	−	−	−	−	+	−
CD34	−/+[a]	−	−	−	−	−	−	−/+

ES, Ewing sarcoma; PNET, primitive neuroectodermal tumor.
[a]CD34 expression is limited to lymphoblastic lymphoma.

cases, this antibody panel permits distinction among malignant lymphoma, carcinoma, and malignant melanoma (8). However, uniformly negative or unanticipated results should prompt the use of relevant "backup" antibodies, which is discussed in the context of the lesions discussed later in this chapter.

A brief discussion of the antigens recognized by the most commonly employed antibodies follows. These antigens represent an abbreviated list; Table 27.2 and the discussion of individual lesions provide a more comprehensive treatment of other important antigens and antibodies.

Leukocyte Common Antigen

The LCA (CD45) represents a family of surface membrane glycoproteins, ranging in size from 180 to 240 kd, that are found on all hematopoietic cells except erythrocytes and their precursors (9). Six to eight isoforms of LCA are expressed differentially on leukocyte subpopulations (9); B and T lymphocytes express LCA strongly, whereas macrophages and histiocytes express LCA variably and neutrophils express LCA very weakly (9). LCA is a remarkably specific and sensitive marker for hematopoietic neoplasms and should be used in evaluating all morphologically undifferentiated neoplasms to rule out the possibility of malignant lymphoma (10–14). The neoplastic cells that comprise most B- and T-cell non-Hodgkin lymphomas and lymphoid leukemias express LCA (CD45) (10–14) (Fig. 27.1). Notable exceptions are plasmablastic lymphomas, anaplastic lymphoma kinase (ALK)-positive diffuse large B-cell lymphoma, ALK-positive and ALK-negative anaplastic large cell lymphomas (ALCLs), and plasmacytoma/plasma cell myeloma, which may be CD45-negative (15–17). Reed-Sternberg cells diagnostic of classical Hodgkin lymphoma and the neoplastic cells of myeloid and erythroid origin are also typically negative for CD45 (9) (see Chapter 3). Nonhematopoietic neoplasms, including those most commonly mistaken for hematopoietic neoplasms histopathologically, that is, poorly differentiated carcinomas, malignant melanoma, neuroblastoma, and Ewing sarcoma, are CD45 negative (10–14). However, exceptionally rare cases of primitive sarcoma, undifferentiated carcinoma, and neuroendocrine carcinoma with aberrant expression of CD45 expression have been reported (18–21). All patients had evidence of metastatic disease with lymphadenopathy at presentation. Three of five reported cases of carcinoma were diagnosed on a lymph node excision (19,21). These rare cases highlight the importance of a wide panel of immunohistochemical stains to include various lineage-specific leukocyte, mesenchymal and epithelial antibodies so as to avoid misdiagnosis.

Cytokeratins

Cytokeratins are the cytoskeletal intermediate filament proteins characteristic of almost all epithelial cells (22,23). There are at least 54 distinct functional keratin subsets that are divisible into 2 families—I (acidic) or II (basic)—according to their molecular weights and isoelectric points (22,24). Low molecular weight keratins are typical of simple, nonstratified epithelia. High molecular weight keratins are found in stratified epithelia whose keratin composition is more complex (22–24). Cytokeratin staining is routinely used to exclude malignant lymphoma. It should be noted that rare cases of B-cell and T-cell lymphomas have been found to contain keratins (25–28). Thus, Gustmann and colleagues reported cytokeratin expression in 27% of cases of ALCL (28). Several cases of cytokeratin-positive plasmacytoma have also been reported (29). In contrast, virtually all carcinomas, except adrenal cortical carcinoma, regularly contain keratins (22). Biphasic tumors, such as synovial sarcomas and epithelioid sarcomas, also show immunoreactivity for keratins, but this is usually limited to the glandular elements, although the spindle cell component occasionally may express keratin (22,30). Thirty to forty percent of leiomyosarcomas at all locations are immunopositive for cytokeratin with a focal, dotlike, or diffuse staining pattern (31–34). The exact nature of this finding is not well understood, but normal myometrium has been shown to contain keratin (35). Several other sarcomas (i.e., Ewing sarcoma, rhabdomyosarcoma, and malignant fibrous histiocytoma) and malignant melanomas rarely have been reported to express cytokeratins (22,31,36,37). Although most adenocarcinomas do not demonstrate specific immunophenotypes, the use of antibodies against cytokeratins 7 and 20 permits separation into groups used to narrow the differential diagnosis.

Epithelial Membrane Antigen

Epithelial membrane antigen (EMA) is the name given to the incompletely characterized glycoprotein of apocrine cells. EMA is located in the milk fat globules, where it originally was identified with an antiserum (38,39); hence, it has been also called milk fat globule protein (38). For the most part, monoclonal

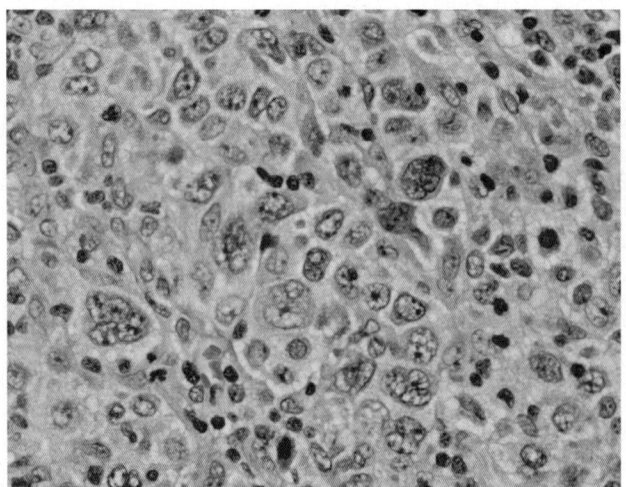
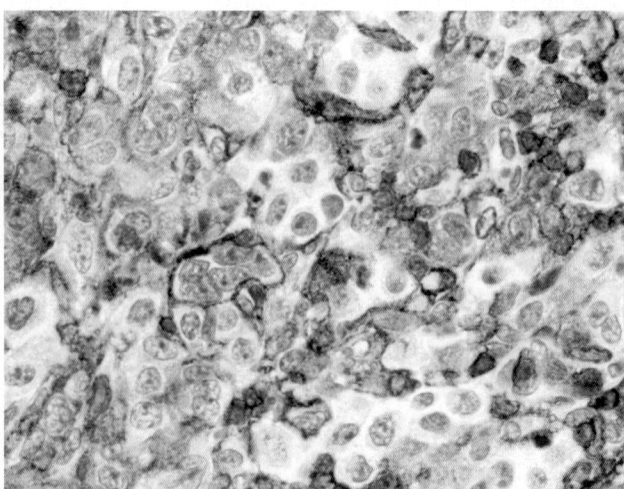

A   B

FIGURE 27.1. Anaplastic variant of diffuse large B-cell lymphoma. A: The tumor cells are large and are markedly atypical. **B:** Immunostaining performed in paraffin tissue sections demonstrates that the pleomorphic tumor cells express CD45 (i.e., LCA), consistent with a hematopoietic neoplasm. Additional immunophenotypic and genotypic studies demonstrated that this tumor represents a diffuse large B-cell lymphoma (immunoperoxidase stain, original magnification: 400×).

antibodies are now used to demonstrate EMA, which is found on almost all benign and malignant epithelial cells (38,40,41); however, EMA is not specific for epithelial neoplasms, and it can be found in mesotheliomas (42), synovial sarcomas (43), leiomyosarcomas (34), perineural epithelium and their neoplasms (44), plasma cells and plasmacytoid neoplasms (45), meningiomas (43), and ALCLs (46). The frequent expression of EMA and lack of CD45 by ALCLs probably accounts for their occasional misdiagnosis as poorly differentiated carcinomas or other nonhematopoietic neoplasms.

Vimentin

Vimentin is a cytoskeletal intermediate filament protein with a molecular mass of 57,000 Da (47). Vimentin is present in mesenchymal cells, fibroblasts, endothelial cells, chondrocytes, histiocytes, lymphocytes, melanocytes, many glial cells, and some smooth muscle cells, especially vascular smooth muscle (22). It has been used as a general marker for sarcomas (22). Many poorly differentiated carcinomas, especially those of renal, thyroid, and endometrial origin, and malignant melanomas and lymphomas also express vimentin (22,48). Its utility in the differential diagnosis of human neoplasms is very limited.

Desmin- and Muscle-Associated Antigens

Desmin is an intermediate filament protein with a molecular mass of 53,000 Da, which is believed to link myofilaments together (49). Desmin is almost always expressed by smooth muscle cells and skeletal and cardiac muscle cells and their neoplastic counterparts (50). Numerous other tumors also have been reported to be desmin positive, including liposarcomas, Schwann cell tumors, desmoplastic melanoma, fibromatosis, and malignant fibrous histiocytomas (50,51). Desmin positivity also has been described in squamous cell carcinomas and small cell carcinomas of the lung in frozen section material (50). Malignant lymphomas are desmin negative.

Actins that measure 6 nm in diameter are found in all cell types (52). α-Actins are present in muscle cells, β-actins are present in nonmuscle cells, and γ-actins are found in muscle and in some nonmuscle cells (52,53). The HHF-35 antibody to muscle actin selectively reacts with the α- and γ-actins of muscle cells and immunoreacts with all striated muscle cells as does desmin. It also reacts with all smooth muscle cells, including the desmin-negative subsets of vascular smooth muscle cells (54,55). Pericytes and myoepithelial cells of salivary gland, skin, and breast are also HHF-35-positive, although they do not contain desmin (55). In general, myofibroblasts are desmin negative but positive for HHF-35 (55). Muscle actins are typically found in leiomyosarcomas, rhabdomyosarcomas, and benign mixed tumors of salivary gland and skin adnexal origin (53,55).

Myogenin and MYO-D1 are myogenic transcriptional regulatory proteins expressed early in skeletal muscle differentiation and are two of the other widely used muscle-specific immunohistochemical markers. They appear to have a higher sensitivity and specificity for rhabdomyosarcoma, compared to desmin and actin (56,57). Their expression has not been reported in hematopoietic tumors.

Factor VIII– and Endothelial-Associated Antigens

Factor VIII–related antigen (factor VIIIRAg), also called von Willebrand factor, is part of the factor VIII complex of the clotting system and is produced by vascular endothelial cells (58). Factor VIIIRAg is a very specific marker for endothelial cells and vascular neoplasms of endothelial cell origin (59). It is helpful for distinguishing angiosarcoma and occasionally Kaposi sarcoma (KS) from other pleomorphic and spindle cell tumors

of nonendothelial cell origin, for example, fibrosarcomas, leiomyosarcomas, and malignant fibrous histiocytomas (60,61). Factor VIIIRAg is consistently expressed by well-differentiated angiosarcomas that possess vasoformative papillary patterns. Less well-differentiated solid tumors are weakly or not at all immunoreactive for factor VIIIRAg (61); therefore, factor VIIIRAg is not a very sensitive marker for endothelial cells (59).

In contrast, CD31, also known as platelet/endothelial cell adhesion molecule-1, is a very useful marker because it is extremely sensitive for endothelial differentiation. It is expressed in the lateral borders between endothelial cells, on platelets, neutrophils, monocytes and subpopulations of T cells (62). Although it is not entirely specific for endothelial differentiation, it is only rarely expressed in neoplasms that resemble those with endothelial properties.

Antibodies against CD34, a transmembrane cell surface glycoprotein, are also useful in the identification of endothelial differentiation (63). However, the utility of this antibody is limited by its very broad range of reactivity. In addition to endothelial cells, anti-CD34 antibodies recognize hematopoietic stem cells, immature thymocytes, a subpopulation of blasts in acute lymphoblastic and myeloid leukemias, interstitial dendritic cells, and numerous spindle cell proliferations and neoplasms (31,63,64) (see Chapter 3).

S-100 Protein

S-100 protein is a calcium-binding protein of unknown function that originally was described in bovine brain extract and is 100% soluble in neutral ammonium sulfate (65), hence, its name. The S-100 protein is present in glial cells, Schwann cells, melanocytes, epidermal Langerhans cells, interdigitating dendritic cells, chondrocytes, adipocytes, and myoepithelial cells (66). Schwann cell tumors, granular cell tumors, benign and malignant melanocytic proliferations, salivary gland myoepitheliomas, cartilaginous tumors, lipomatous tumors, interdigitating dendritic cell sarcoma, indeterminate cell tumor, and Langerhans cell histiocytosis (histiocytosis X) all are S-100 protein positive (15,66–71). Weak or focal S-100 expression can be seen in cases of follicular dendritic cell sarcoma and histiocytic sarcoma (15). Many carcinomas are also S-100 positive (72,73). The sustentacular or supportive cells in pheochromocytomas, ganglioneuroblastomas, and paragangliomas are S-100 positive, but the predominant neuroendocrine component of these tumors is S-100 negative (74). The monoclonal antibodies HMB-45, Melan-A, and microphthalmia transcription factor (MITF) are more specific but less sensitive for melanocytic differentiation.

Neuron-Specific Enolase and Neuroendocrine/Neural-Associated Antigens

Neuron-specific enolase (NSE) designates the γ subunit of the dimeric enzyme enolase typical of neural cells (75). Initial studies suggested a high cell-type specificity for NSE (75), hence the name. Later studies on a wide spectrum of tumors, however, revealed NSE positivity in numerous nonneural and nonneuroendocrine tumors (76), limiting its use in diagnostic pathology. In general, NSE should be used in conjunction with more specific neural/neuroendocrine markers such as chromogranin, synaptophysin, nerve growth factor receptor protein, and neurofilament proteins. Synaptophysin is a protein found in the membranes of neuronal cell vesicles (77). It is present in peripheral nerves, in central and peripheral nervous system neurons, and in neuroendocrine cells (77). Synaptophysin is consistently positive in neuroendocrine tumors, paragangliomas, and neuroblastomas (77). Nerve growth factor receptor is consistently positive in Schwann cell neoplasms, although some nonneural tumors have been reported to be positive; these include synovial sarcomas and hemangiopericytomas (78).

CONGENITAL MALFORMATIONS AND INCLUSIONS

Ectopic Nevus Cells

Not uncommonly, nevus cell aggregates occur in peripheral lymph nodes, most often those in the axillary region, and less frequently in the cervical and inguinal regions (79–82). The overall incidence of benign nevus cell aggregates ranged from 0.33% to 6.2% in patients who had undergone axillary lymph node dissections for breast carcinoma and malignant melanoma, respectively (79,80). The presence of ectopic nevus cells is significantly correlated with patients' history of melanoma or cutaneous nevi, especially nevi with congenital features (83–85). A large recent study conducted by Carson and associates demonstrated that only 1 of 1,071 lymph nodes from 50 patients with breast cancer (0.1%) and none of 521 nodes from 50 patients with pelvic cancer contained nevus cells, as opposed to 49 of 226 (22%) lymph nodes in patients with melanoma (84).

In 1977, Azzopardi et al. (81) described the occurrence of blue nevi in lymph nodes. About 10 cases have been reported; they occur in both sexes and most commonly involve axillary lymph nodes (81,82). Intranodal blue nevi, in contrast to ectopic nevus cell aggregates, have not been identified in patients who have cutaneous malignant melanoma. Intranodal nevus cell aggregates and blue nevi morphologically resemble their dermal counterparts, intradermal nevi and common blue nevi, respectively. Both lesions are discovered incidentally in peripheral lymph nodes, where they occur predominantly in the capsular and pericapsular tissues (81,82,84) (Fig. 27.2). These cells can also be seen around small vessels, and even can occasionally be encountered within the substance of a lymph node (84,86). The presence of cells thought to be benign nevus cells within a lymph node should lead to careful study of the cell population. Some malignant melanoma cells show only slight atypia and few mitotic figures. For a diagnosis of benign ectopia of nevus cells, the cells should not show any cytologic atypia, nuclear pleomorphism, or mitotic activity. Rarely, these cells may contain small amounts of melanin. Carson and associates could identify nevus cells in hematoxylin and eosin-stained sections in 78% of the cases, while the remaining cases were diagnosed exclusively by immunohistochemical staining with S-100 protein (84). S-100-positive ectopic nevus cells may be distinguished from the presence of melanoma metastasis in

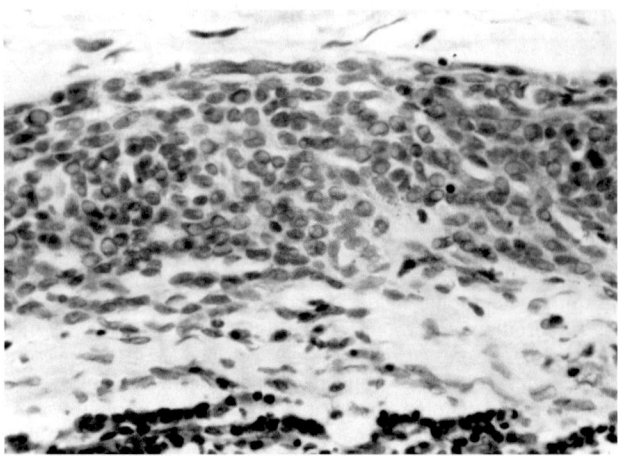

FIGURE 27.2. Intranodal nevus cells. An aggregate of bland nevus cells without significant cytologic atypia or mitotic activity is situated in the lymph node capsule (hematoxylin and eosin, original magnification: 400×).

intracapsular lymphatic vessels with the help of CD31, CD34, and D2-40 antibodies, which would detect the rim of lining endothelial cells around the melanoma cell clusters (87). Ki-67 immunostaining may be performed in problematic cases, since capsular nevi have a very low Ki-67 expression as opposed to melanoma cells (86,88).

Benign metastasis of cutaneous nevi and arrested migration of neural crest cells are the most appealing hypotheses advanced to explain the presence of nevus cell aggregates and blue nevi in lymph nodes. The occurrence of these benign nevus cells in lymph node capsules suggests that these cells migrate into the capsules of lymph nodes during embryonic migration of neural crest cells (85,89). The presence of benign nevus cells in the lymph node itself and their association with cutaneous nevi and melanoma would suggest mechanical transport or *benign metastasis* (83–85,89).

Ectopic Mesothelial Cells

The occurrence of mesothelial cell inclusions in lymph nodes is rare (90–92). Brooks et al. (91) described benign mesothelial cell aggregates in mediastinal lymph nodes that mimic metastatic carcinoma. Both patients had histories of pleuritis and pleural effusion with mediastinal widening. Subsequently, several case series and case reports have described benign mesothelial cell aggregates in cervical, hilar, mediastinal, intra-abdominal, and pelvic lymph nodes (92–98). It has been postulated that benign mesothelial cells embolize to regional lymph nodes in association with effusion or inflammation of serosal surfaces. In most cases, these cells are few and undetectable on routine sections. Rarely, hyperplastic mesothelial cells may be present and must be distinguished from metastatic carcinoma, mesothelioma, and melanoma. Recognition of this rare entity in the appropriate clinical setting may avoid the misdiagnosis of carcinoma of unknown origin and false upstaging of known tumors.

The mesothelial cells, which were cytologically benign and mitotically inactive, occurred as individual cells and in small clusters and appeared only in the lymph node sinuses. On immunohistochemical examination, these cells were found to contain cytokeratin or calretinin and lack EMA, CD15, and carcinoembryonic antigen and, for the most part, were negative for B72.3 (91). The cells appeared to be mesothelial cells morphologically and immunohistochemically.

Ectopic Müllerian and Celomic Epithelium

Benign glandular inclusions that occur in pelvic and periaortic lymph nodes have been described almost exclusively in women (99–101). These inclusions have been referred to as *endometriosis, endometriosis-like inclusions, müllerian epithelial inclusions, endosalpingiosis,* and *mesothelial cell inclusions.* Endosalpingiosis refers to ectopic epithelium that resembles benign tubal epithelium (Fig. 27.3). In contrast to endometriosis, endosalpingiosis is usually found incidentally, especially in the setting of pelvic inflammatory disease and ovarian neoplasms. The most important differential diagnostic concern is to distinguish endosalpingiosis from a serous neoplasm, especially implants of serous borderline tumors (serous tumors of low malignant potential and atypically proliferating serous tumors). Endosalpingiosis lacks the tufting, stratification, and arborizing architecture that characterizes serous borderline tumors. Rare cases of benign müllerian-type inclusions have been also described in supradiafragmatic lymph nodes (102–104). Immunohistochemical staining for WT-1 and PAX-8 can be performed in difficult cases in order to confirm the müllerian origin of the ectopic epithelium (102).

Ectopic endometrium has been attributed to several mechanisms, including müllerian and wolffian duct rests (101). Such rests, however, are a less likely explanation than the theory

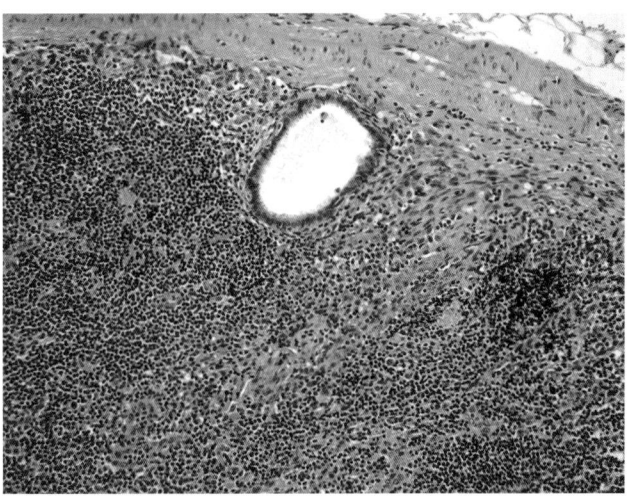

FIGURE 27.3. Endosalpingiosis. Tubular and cystically dilated glands with cytologic features of endosalpingiosis: a monolayer of bland ciliated columnar cells without apparent endometrial stroma, intracytoplasmic mucin, or squamous metaplasia (hematoxylin and eosin, original magnification: 200×). (Photomicrograph courtesy of Dr. Esther Oliva, Massachusetts General Hospital, Boston, MA.)

of celomic metaplasia of mesothelial cell inclusions (100) or the regurgitation theory (105). In the metaplastic theory, these inclusions are believed to occur as the result of a metaplastic proliferation of peritoneal mesothelial implants within lymph nodes. Because peritoneal and müllerian epithelium derive from the embryonic celomic epithelium, it is not surprising that metaplastic mesothelium can resemble müllerian epithelium. According to the regurgitation hypothesis, endometrial tissue is believed to be released through the fallopian tubes during menstruation and then implants on pelvic organs or travels through lymphatic or venous channels to distant organs and lymph nodes (106).

Intranodal endometrial gland inclusions have been found in 14% of women in surgical and autopsy series alike (107). Infrequent case reports have identified similar benign glandular inclusions in mediastinal and perinephric lymph nodes in men (108,109). These benign inclusions potentially could be misinterpreted as metastases to regional lymph nodes. On histologic examination, however, these inclusions are composed of small tubular structures lined by a single layer of cuboidal to columnar cells that contain round uniform nuclei. Occasionally, cilia may be found on their luminal surfaces, and endometrial-type stroma may accompany these glandular or tubular structures. The endometrial stroma may undergo a decidual reaction; this may be misinterpreted as a metastatic tumor, especially on a frozen section. The stromal cells become large but have abundant cytoplasm and uniform nuclei.

Ectopic Salivary Gland

Salivary gland elements frequently are found in intraparotid lymph nodes and, to a lesser degree, in nearby upper cervical lymph nodes (110,111). This tissue most often consists of striated ducts, intercalated ducts, and less commonly, acini (110). Parotid glandular tissue normally becomes incorporated into these lymph nodes during embryologic development. The parotid salivary gland develops from an outpouching of the primitive oral cavity while lymphoid tissue is condensing into parotid lymph nodes. Most of the intranodal glandular tissue fails to develop as the lymphoid tissue enlarges, but many of these lymph nodes retain small islands of the glandular tissue. All this is functioning salivary gland tissue connected to the adjacent parotid gland; occasionally, a fortuitous section or

serial section shows the connection between the parotid gland and the intranodal glandular tissue. This ectopic tissue is subject to the same disease processes as the normal salivary gland. Salivary gland ductal inclusions can give rise to proliferative sialometaplasia (112) and lymphoepithelial cysts, a condition that has been frequently identified in human immunodeficiency virus (HIV)–infected patients (113,114) (see Chapter 25). Many lymphoepithelial cysts positioned in the high neck and in the parotid salivary gland are thought to arise from these intranodal glandular inclusions rather than from the branchial cleft apparatus, as previously believed. These inclusions occasionally also produce salivary gland tumors, both benign and malignant.

Ectopic Thyroid Gland

Small clusters of microscopically normal-appearing thyroid follicles may be encountered rarely within cervical lymph nodes (115–117). These thyroid follicles probably become incorporated inside lymph nodes during the migration of thyroid tissue from the foramen cecum of the tongue to its final midline location and, perhaps, from the primitive intestinal tract in the area of the pharyngobranchial pouches. The occurrence of thyroid tissue in the lateral neck should not be automatically assumed to represent heterotopic or "lateral aberrant thyroid" tissue (118,119). Whereas midline thyroid rests seldom represent metastatic thyroid carcinoma, intranodal thyroid tissue in the lateral cervical chains should be considered to be metastatic carcinoma until proven otherwise (118). Unfortunately, the location of thyroid follicles within a lymph node, such as in the capsule, subcapsular sinus, or the medullary portion, does not help in distinguishing benign ectopic thyroid follicles from metastatic thyroid carcinoma. Even when intranodal thyroid follicles appear well formed, with cytologically benign cuboidal cells containing colloid, and having the appearance of normal thyroid follicles (117), the possibility of a malignancy cannot be entirely excluded. The thyroid carcinomas that spread to regional lymph nodes include papillary carcinomas and their variants and mixed papillary and follicular carcinoma. These neoplastic follicles contain papillary structures, psammoma bodies, or cells with optically clear nuclei and nuclear grooves, and often do not contain colloid (Fig. 27.4). Pure follicular carcinomas only rarely metastasize to cervical lymph nodes; in these cases, the cells have cytologically malignant nuclei.

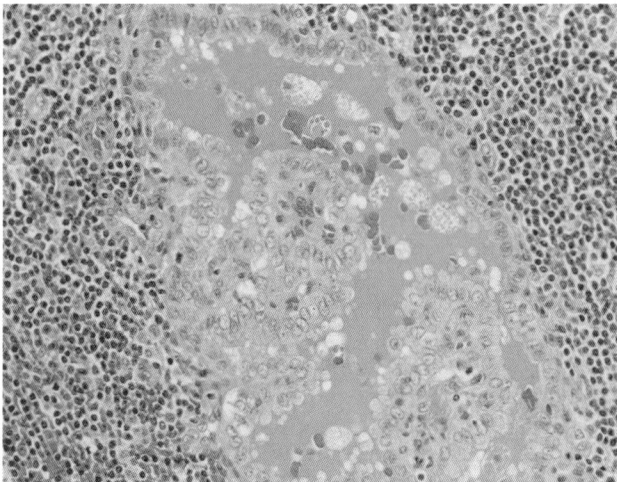

FIGURE 27.4. Metastatic papillary thyroid carcinoma. This papillary thyroid carcinoma metastatic to a lymph node shows neoplastic follicles that contain colloid and have a papillary architecture. The nuclei overlap and appear optically clear and grooved (hematoxylin and eosin, original magnification: 200×).

There are rare reports of primary intranodal papillary thyroid carcinoma (119–121). In the presence of a presumed intranodal thyroid inclusion, the patient should undergo a thorough thyroid evaluation, including a technetium thyroid scan and ultrasound examination, to search for a primary thyroid carcinoma. If no thyroid lesion is found and the intranodal lesion fulfills the morphologic criteria for ectopic thyroid tissue, then no further treatment is likely to be required.

Ectopic Breast and Sweat Gland Tissue

Ectopic ducts and acini that have the appearance of normal breast or sweat gland tissue rarely may be found in axillary lymph nodes (122,123) (Fig. 27.5). Because breast tissue represents a modified sweat gland, it may be difficult to distinguish between the two when they are present in axillary lymph nodes. The possible presence of these benign glandular inclusions should be kept in mind when evaluating axillary node dissections for the presence of metastatic carcinoma (124–126). Ectopic glandular tissue usually has a double-cell layer, which is cytologically benign and does not resemble breast carcinoma. Immunohistochemical stains can help in identifying the myoepithelial cell component, consistently present in the benign ectopic breast tissue and absent in the metastatic lesions (126).

EPITHELIAL LESIONS PRIMARY IN LYMPH NODES

Malignant Melanoma

When malignant melanoma occurs in a lymph node, it is presumed to be a metastasis, and the primary cutaneous or mucosal process is discovered to be active, previously excised, spontaneously regressed, or occult (127,128). Intranodal nevus cell aggregates and blue nevi, as already described, are well-documented lesions that occur in lymph nodes. It has been hypothesized that these intranodal nevoid inclusions may serve as progenitors of primary intranodal malignant melanoma (129). A malignant melanoma that occurs in an axillary lymph node in conjunction with an intranodal blue nevus has been described; no other evidence of melanoma was found in this patient (129). As many as 4% of patients who show nodal involvement by malignant melanoma have no known primary

lesion (130). The lymph nodes most often involved are axillary or cervical in men and inguinal in women. Spontaneous regression of a cutaneous primary malignant melanoma—always a possibility—can be demonstrated in some patients (127,130). When a primary melanoma cannot be found elsewhere, however, the possibility exists that a malignant melanoma has developed primarily in ectopic intranodal nevus cells.

Warthin Tumor

Warthin tumor occurs most often in intraparotid lymph nodes but occasionally also may be seen in extraparotid cervical lymph nodes (131). These tumors are composed of cystic and papillary structures lined by oncocytic epithelial cells, histologically similar to striated duct cells. The lymphoid component represents the residual or hyperplastic lymphoid tissue of the lymph node in which the tumor arose, presumably from ectopic salivary gland tissue normally found in these lymph nodes (132). In resection specimens of the parotid salivary gland, other intraparotid lymph nodes may contain incidental microscopic Warthin tumors. These are commonly found in patients who have clinically evident Warthin tumors and, occasionally, in specimens resected for other lesions.

Warthin tumor is seen most frequently in men older than 50 years of age and may be bilateral, occurring synchronously or metachronously (132). Primary Hodgkin and non-Hodgkin lymphomas have developed in Warthin tumors (133–136); the presence of one lesion does not preclude the occurrence of a second lesion. Rarely, poorly differentiated carcinomas have developed in lymph nodes that contain Warthin tumor (137,138). Whether these carcinomas arose in the Warthin tumor cell population or in other ectopic salivary gland tissue cannot be determined conclusively.

Acinic Cell and Mucoepidermoid Carcinoma

Occasionally, other types of salivary gland tumors, including acinic cell carcinomas and mucoepidermoid carcinomas, may occur in ectopic salivary gland tissue in cervical nodes (139–142). These well-documented cases can only be accepted as primary tumors if thorough histologic evaluation of the salivary gland shows the tumor to be limited to lymph nodes. If neoplastic tissue is identified outside of lymph nodes, then the lesion may have developed in extranodal tissue and extended secondarily into lymph nodes.

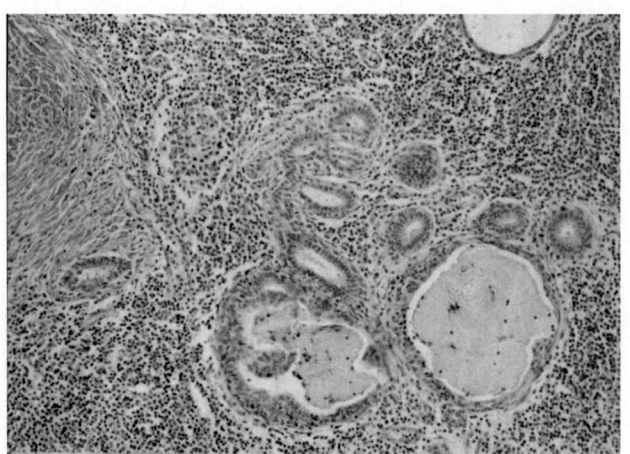
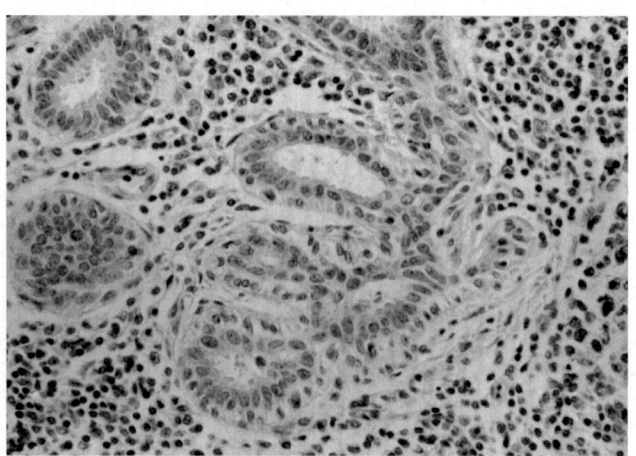

A   B

FIGURE 27.5. Intranodal ectopic breast tissue. A: This microscopic focus of intranodal ectopic breast tissue was discovered as an incidental finding in a lymph node removed as part of an axillary dissection in the treatment of breast cancer. The patient had no evidence of carcinoma metastatic to lymph nodes and had no clinical evidence of metastatic disease (hematoxylin and eosin, original magnification: 100×). **B:** Higher magnification demonstrates that the ducts are lined by a double-cell layer and that the cells show bland cytologic features and possess apocrine snouts (hematoxylin and eosin, original magnification: 250×).

Thyroid Carcinoma

Rare case reports have described intranodal papillary thyroid carcinoma with no apparent evidence of a primary carcinoma in a total thyroidectomy specimen (120,121). Of course, the possibility always remains that the thyroid tissue was examined or sampled incompletely, or that the primary carcinoma developed in ectopic thyroid tissue that occurred elsewhere, such as in the mediastinum (143) or as a component of a thyroglossal duct cyst (119) or a branchial cleft cyst (144,145).

Breast Carcinoma

A single case of primary intranodal breast carcinoma in an axillary lymph node has been reported (122). The tumor was a cystic, micropapillary carcinoma that also contained cytologically benign glandular inclusions. Although this must be an extraordinarily rare event, epithelial inclusions in lymph nodes should be examined carefully with the possibility of malignant transformation in mind. When a carcinoma with the histologic features of a breast carcinoma is discovered in an axillary lymph node, however, in almost all cases the tumor has arisen in the breast and secondarily involved the axillary lymph node. In some of these cases, the tumor can be shown to have developed in nearby breast tissue, such as in the axillary tail. In other cases, careful examination of a mastectomy specimen demonstrates the primary lesion in the breast.

 MESENCHYMAL LESIONS PRIMARY IN LYMPH NODES

Lipomatosis of Lymph Nodes

Much of the normal architecture of a lymph node may be obscured by mature adipose tissue. Fatty replacement of nodal tissue has been called *lipomatosis, adipose metaplasia,* and *"lipo lymph node."* This is most frequently observed in the axillary lymph nodes that accompany breast resections for carcinoma. These lymph nodes can be recognized clinically and on gross examination as lymph nodes, but on histologic examination, only a rim of lymphoid tissue surrounds mature adipose tissue, which compresses the bulk of the lymph node. The fat probably extends into and compresses the lymph node from the hilar region. This fatty infiltration can be considered a normal finding associated with advancing age, obesity, and lymphoid depletion. This common finding should not mislead the pathologist into thinking that there may not be a lymphoma or metastatic neoplasm involving the lymph node as well, because fat does not appear to be a protective phenomenon.

Fibrosis of Lymph Nodes

Diffuse fibrosis of a lymph node usually involves the hilar region but may advance into the medullary and subcapsular sinuses, eventually separating the lymph node into regions or nodules. The observer should take special care not to misdiagnose such lesions as nodular sclerosis Hodgkin lymphoma. Fibrosis is found frequently in the inguinal and obturator lymph nodes and, most likely, represents the end-stage process of a nodal inflammatory lesion. Other processes that can commonly lead to areas of lymph node fibrosis include resolved granulomatous diseases, inflammatory pseudotumor of lymph nodes, and chronic lymphadenitis of any cause. Previous treatment of lymph nodes for malignant lymphoma or nonlymphoid

malignancies may lead to fibrosis, especially if radiation has been used in the therapy.

Benign Vascular Lesions

Vascular Transformation

Vascular transformation of lymph nodes superficially resembles a hemangioma. This lesion is characterized, however, by congestion and striking reorganization of all subcapsular and medullary sinuses, the normal sinusoidal structure being replaced by an anastomosing network of small vascular channels lined by reactive endothelial cells (Fig. 27.6). The hilar and perinodal veins tend to be obliterated (146,147). This nonneoplastic lesion can easily be mistaken for Kaposi sarcoma (KS). The absence of capsular involvement and the periodic acid–Schiff (PAS)–positive hyaline globules frequently observed in KS help in the differential diagnosis (148,149).

Nodal Angiomatosis

In nodal angiomatosis, the cortical and medullary sinuses are replaced by irregular cords of proliferating endothelial cells, but the underlying lymph node architecture remains intact. In pannodal hemangiomatoid lesions, vessels radially fan out around a central fibrovascular core and involve perinodal tissues; this architecture is the most prominent feature of this lesion (150). Like vascular transformation, nodal angiomatosis probably represents a reactive process rather than a true neoplasm (147).

Angiomyomatous Hamartoma

This innocuous lesion is characterized by a proliferation of thick-walled blood vessels and bland smooth muscle cells centered on the lymph node hilum (151). It is believed to occur almost exclusively in inguinal lymph nodes (151).

Angiolipomatous Hamartoma

Angiolipomatous hamartoma is a rare lesion that may accompany lymph nodes involved by the hyaline-vascular form of Castleman disease. Well-developed blood vessels are interspersed between mature adipocytes in extranodal soft tissue (152,153).

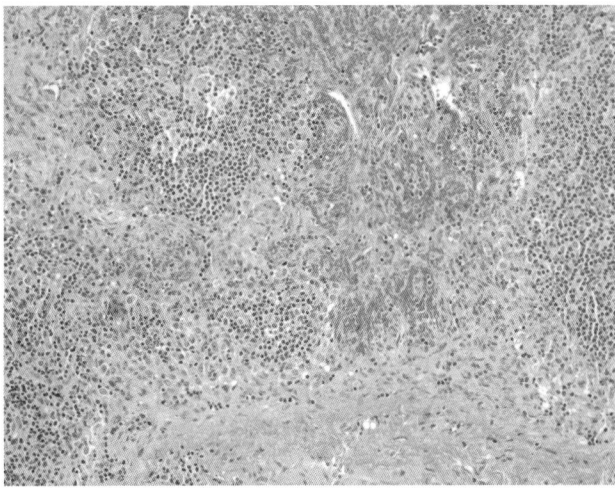

FIGURE 27.6. Vascular transformation of a lymph node. It consists of cytologically bland endothelial cells present in the subcapsular and intermediate sinuses without involvement of the capsule. The latter finding is helpful in excluding KS (hematoxylin and eosin, original magnification: 100×).

Hemangiomas

Hemangiomas occur in lymph nodes uncommonly, but several well-characterized intranodal hemangiomas have been reported (154–156). These lesions frequently demonstrate distinct feeder vessels, as seen in hemangiomas in other sites. The space-occupying effect, shown by the displacement of normal lymph nodal tissue to the periphery, supports the neoplastic nature of these lesions. Epithelioid hemangioma, also known as angiolymphoid hyperplasia with eosinophilia, is now considered a hemangioma variant instead of analogous to Kimura disease (157). This proliferation shows well-formed vascular channels lined by epithelioid endothelium. The interstitium is frequently rich in chronic inflammatory cells, including lymphocytes and eosinophils.

Vascular Neoplasm of Castleman Disease

The vascular neoplasm that arises in the setting of Castleman disease is a proliferation of blood vessels, some of which resemble high endothelial venules and others that appear to be branching capillaries (158,159) (Fig. 27.7). Staghorn-shaped blood vessels may also be encountered. This vascular proliferation distorts and obscures the underlying lymph node architecture, and frequently, it may be difficult to identify the hyalinized follicles that are characteristic of hyaline-vascular Castleman disease. The cytologic features range from bland to overtly malignant. This may have some bearing on the biologic behavior of the lesion because recurrence and metastasis have been reported (158,159).

Lymphangiomas

Intranodal lymphangiomas occur not infrequently and most commonly affect cervical and axillary lymph nodes. They are histologically identical to their soft tissue counterparts and are composed of vascular channels lined by flattened endothelium, resembling normal lymphatics (160). Lymphangiomas are benign, well-delimited, space-occupying lesions. The lymphatic channels occasionally are cystically dilated; the cysts may be recognized grossly. Little or no smooth muscle is found in the walls of these lymphatic-like channels, which usually are filled with eosinophilic proteinaceous fluid, lymphocytes, and scattered red blood cells. Intranodal lymphangiomas displace the normal lymph node architecture as would a neoplasm, distinguishing them from the vascular transformation and reactive lesions of lymph nodes (160).

Lymphangioleiomyomatosis

Lymphangiomyomatosis is a rare disorder characterized by a proliferation of lymphatic channels and smooth muscle cells, which affects women primarily of reproductive age and is frequently associated with tuberous sclerosis. Although it classically involves the lungs, it has also been found in mediastinal, supraclavicular, intra-abdominal, retroperitoneal, and pelvic lymph nodes (161–163). These lesions tend to dissect lymph nodes into compartments because they initially develop in the subcapsular and medullary sinuses (Fig. 27.8). They do not usually represent a solitary lesion but, rather, a multifocal process that eventually can obliterate the lymph node. Compared with lymphangiomas, the smooth muscle component of their vascular walls is prominent (164,165). Intranodal lymphangiomyomatosis that occurs in patients who have tuberous sclerosis is thought by some investigators to be a precursor of intranodal angiomyolipoma (166,167). In contrast to angiomyomatous hamartoma, lymphangioleiomyomatosis occurs exclusively in females, is not limited to inguinal lymph nodes, does not show significant sclerosis, and expresses HMB-45 (168,169).

Epithelioid Hemangioendothelioma

Epithelioid hemangioendothelioma is a malignant endothelial-derived tumor that may originate in lymph nodes or present as a metastasis from another site, including the skin, soft tissue, and visceral organs (170,171). The spindled and epithelioid cells are arranged singly, in cords and trabeculae, and occasionally, in poorly formed nests. The stroma ranges from hyalinized to myxomatous. The identification of intracellular lumens that entrap blood cells and cellular aggregates around vascular channels are morphologic clues to the diagnosis. The nuclear features are usually bland to moderately atypical. Although the boundary between epithelioid hemangioendothelioma and epithelioid angiosarcoma is not strictly defined, severe atypia with brisk mitotic activity, in combination with a paucity of intracellular lumens, is more in keeping with a diagnosis of epithelioid angiosarcoma. Like epithelioid angiosarcoma, epithelioid hemangioendothelioma expresses the endothelial cell–associated markers CD31, CD34, and factor VIIIRAg (170). Because there are numerous reports of epithelioid vascular tumors that express cytokeratins, it is important

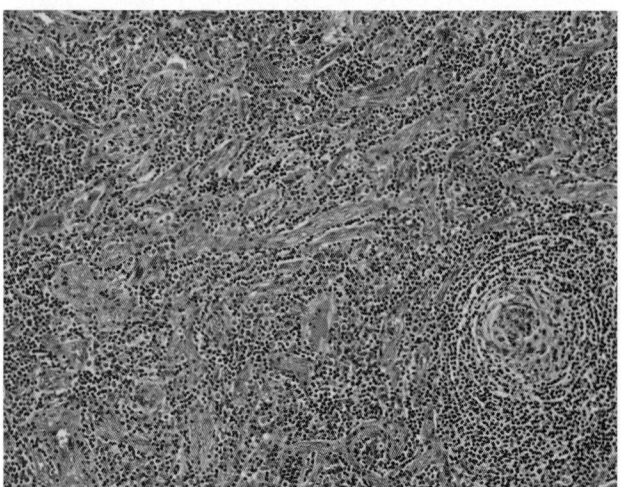

FIGURE 27.7. Vascular neoplasm of Castleman disease. The affected lymph node shows a hyaline-vascular follicle, lymphoid depletion, and a prominent endothelial cell proliferation (hematoxylin and eosin, original magnification: 100×).

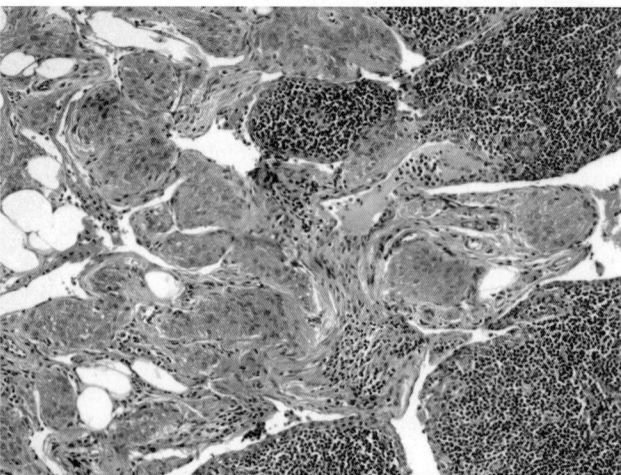

FIGURE 27.8. Intranodal lymphangioleiomyomatosis. This entity is best known as a pulmonary and thoracic lesion but occasionally affects pelvic and abdominal retroperitoneal lymph nodes, causing clinical confusion with a primary gynecologic neoplasm and/or a retroperitoneal sarcoma. This lesion is composed of fascicles and small bundles of cytologically innocuous smooth muscle cells derived from lymphatic vessels (hematoxylin and eosin, original magnification: 100×).

to use an immunohistochemical panel that includes endothelial markers to make the correct diagnosis. Recently, a characteristic chromosomal translocation involving chromosomes 1 and 3, t(1;3)(p36.3;q25) with a subsequent WWTR1-CAMTA1 fusion product was detected in most cases of epithelioid hemangioendothelioma (172–174).

The polymorphous hemangioendothelioma is characterized by a low-power variegated appearance: solid nests and primitive vascular structures lined by endothelial cells (151). There may be evidence of incomplete or primitive angiomatous differentiation in the form of cytoplasmic vacuoles, slitlike clefts, anastomosing vascular channels, and papillary structures. The tumor cells are positive for *Ulex europaeus* but not factor VIIIRAg. This is an uncommon tumor about which little is known. The lesion is considered a low-grade malignancy and has the capability of metastasis (151).

Kaposi Sarcoma

Between the time of its discovery in 1872 and the recognition of its epidemic spread among homosexual men in the early 1980s heralding the AIDS epidemic (175,176), KS was largely considered an enigmatic dermatologic curiosity whose incidence and natural history varied geographically (177,178). Four clinical-epidemiologic forms of KS are now recognized; these are classic Mediterranean, endemic African, iatrogenic, and AIDS-epidemic KS (177,178). The classic Mediterranean form of KS occurs in the United States uncommonly, having an incidence of only approximately 0.02% in the general population. This form of KS usually occurs as an indolent, nonprogressive neoplasm that primarily affects the skin of the lower extremities of the elderly, particularly those of Mediterranean descent (179). This form usually only involves lymph nodes secondarily and generally late in the course of the disease (179,180).

AIDS-epidemic KS is by far the most common clinical-epidemiologic form of the disease occurring in the United States at the present time (177,181). The presence of KS in an HIV-infected individual is an AIDS-defining condition; it remains the most common neoplasm overall in this patient population (181). However, while all AIDS-risk groups possess an extraordinary risk of developing KS, the risk among homosexual men is astronomical; therefore, these individuals represent the vast majority of patients who have AIDS-epidemic KS (181) (see Chapter 25). The introduction of effective antiretroviral therapies in the mid-1990s led to a sharp decrease in the incidence of KS in HIV-infected subjects in developed countries; however, the risk of KS remains substantially increased and further decreases have not been observed (182,183). KS has recently been reported in subjects with well-controlled HIV infection and CD4 counts >200 (184).

The many special clinical, epidemiologic, and pathologic features of KS have led to significant debate concerning its cell of origin, its hyperplastic versus neoplastic nature, and its cause, infectious or otherwise (177,178,185,186). It is now accepted that Kaposi sarcoma–associated herpesvirus (KSHV), also called human herpesvirus-8 (HHV-8), infects both lymphatic and blood vascular endothelial cells, causing the production of lymphangiogenic growth factors that are involved in the pathogenesis of the KS lesion and resulting in a lymphatic reprogramming of the vascular endothelial cells (187). Gene expression profiles of infected cells have shown that both lymphatic and blood vascular endothelial cells undergo a shift in their gene expression profile to a cell type that closely resembles lymphatic endothelial cells (187). The frequent clinical presentation of KS with multiple lesions has raised questions about the clonality of this disease (188). Studies based upon X chromosome inactivation have yielded conflicting results although at least some cutaneous nodular tumor masses of KS have been

shown to be clonal (186,189,190). It has been hypothesized that the significantly higher incidence of KS among homosexual men is because of the preferential or enhanced transmissibility of an infectious agent related to the sexual practices of this group, especially those involving oral-fecal and orogenital contact (191,192).

In 1994, Chang, Moore, Cesarman, Knowles, and collaborators identified a novel, previously unidentified herpesvirus exhibiting homology with herpesvirus saimiri and Epstein-Barr virus (EBV) (193–196), in a KS lesion obtained from a homosexual man who had died from AIDS (193). They named the virus descriptively Kaposi sarcoma–associated herpesvirus (193). We now know that KSHV is a transmissible, B-cell lymphotropic herpesvirus belonging to the γ2 sublineage (genus Rhadinovirus) of the Gammaherpesvirinae subfamily (194,196,197), which are characterized by their ability to replicate in lymphoblastoid cells. This virus is detectable in virtually all KS lesions occurring in more than 90% of individuals who have any of the four clinical-epidemiologic forms of the disease (194). It can be visualized in the nuclei of the spindle cells and the flat vascular lining cells of KS lesions by *in situ* techniques and immunohistochemistry (198,199). According to most studies, KSHV is absent from the wide array of vascular tumors and inflammatory conditions that resemble KS (193,194,200). The development of KS is probably a multistep process that involves the interplay of KSHV with impaired immune surveillance, immune stimulation and multiple genetic, environmental, behavioral, and other factors.

In all forms of the disease, the skin is the most frequent site of involvement (176,177,201). Among individuals who have AIDS-epidemic KS, the lesions are often concentrated on the face, genitalia, and lower extremities (201). However, extracutaneous spread is very common among individuals who have AIDS-epidemic KS (185,202); frequent sites of involvement include the oral cavity, the lungs, and the gastrointestinal tract (201,203), all of which may be involved in the absence of mucocutaneous disease (201).

Lymph node involvement by AIDS-epidemic KS is also common and, similarly, may occur in the absence of mucocutaneous disease (201). AIDS-epidemic KS may occur in benign lymph nodes exhibiting florid follicular hyperplasia, follicular involution, and lymphocyte depletion (204–208), as well as in lymph nodes containing malignant lymphoma (209). Early lesions as well as small foci of involvement are usually observed in or adjacent to the capsule, in the hilum, or, occasionally, in the perinodal adipose tissue (204,206,210,211) (Fig. 27.9). Diagnosis of these early lesions and small foci of KS can be difficult, particularly when they only involve the pericapsular tissue. They can be easily overlooked or may be dismissed as an area of fibrosis (204). Late in the clinical course, lymph nodes involved by AIDS-epidemic KS may appear grossly as hemorrhagic tumors measuring several centimeters in diameter (185).

AIDS-epidemic KS generally is histopathologically indistinguishable from the other clinical-epidemiologic forms of the disease (212) (see Chapter 25). KS consists of a variable mixture of ectatic, irregularly shaped, round capillary, and slitlike endothelial-lined vascular spaces and spindle-shaped cells accompanied by a variable, mixed mononuclear cell infiltrate. The endothelial cells may be thin and spindle-shaped or oval to round; they generally lack cytologic atypia and mitotic activity. Erythrocytes and hemosiderin pigment are frequently present, often extravasated between the spindle cells. Small refractile, eosinophilic, PAS-positive hyaline globules, representing the breakdown products of phagocytosed erythrocytes, may be present extracellularly or within macrophages. The latter are highly associated with KS and assist in its differential diagnosis with angiosarcoma and other vascular proliferations (148). The spindle cells increasingly become the predominant

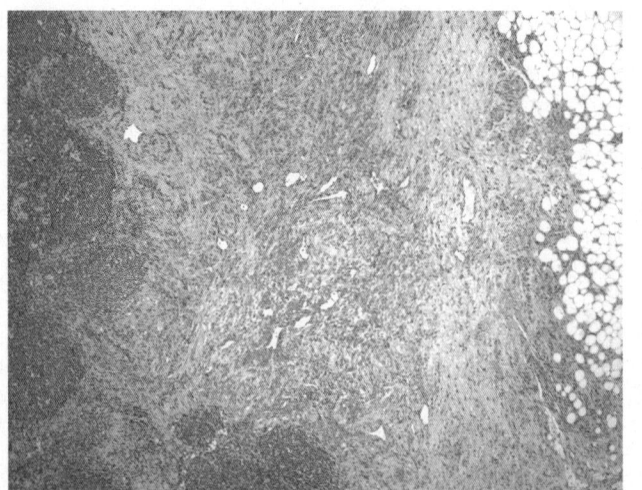
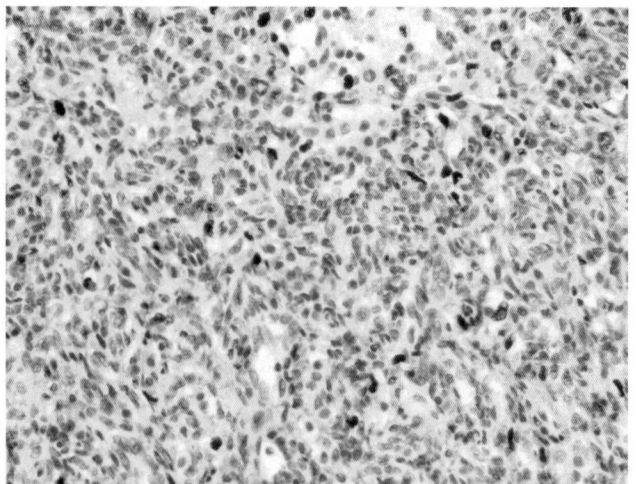

FIGURE 27.9. Intranodal Kaposi sarcoma. A: The lesion involves the lymph node capsule and extends into the perinodal adipose tissue. It consists of interwoven bundles of spindle cells that extend in various directions and produce cleftlike vascular channels. Red blood cells sometimes percolate through these vascular channels, and extravasated erythrocytes and hemosiderin are frequently present in the surrounding tissue (hematoxylin and eosin, original magnification: 40×). **B:** Immunohistochemical stain for HHV-8 (LANA) (original magnification: 200×).

cell population, forming fascicles that compress the vascular slits, and the lesions may progress to form nodules and tumors. The latter consist primarily of interwoven fascicles of spindle cells displaying prominent cytologic atypia, numerous mitotic figures, and often striking pleomorphism (180,204,206,212).

Extracutaneous KS may differ slightly histologically and may exhibit a different developmental chronology than cutaneous KS (212). The earliest histopathologic changes in lymph nodes involved by KS have been referred to as "hypervascular follicular hyperplasia" (213). Vascular channels within the lymph node are prominent, increased in number, and are associated with increased numbers of plasma cells (214). Over time, these areas may develop the classic histopathologic features of KS, including interwoven fascicles of spindle cells, vascular slits, and extravasated erythrocytes (212,214). KS involving lymph nodes extends along the sinusoids, infiltrates the interfollicular areas (206,211), and eventually may replace the entire lymph node (204,210).

Immunohistochemical studies demonstrate that the spindle cells and the vascular lining cells of KS express a variety of endothelial cell–associated antigens. These include factor VIIIRAg, CD34, and CD31 (215–217). The most useful means of diagnosis is immunohistochemistry for HHV-8 latency-associated nuclear antigen (LANA), which is expressed in nearly all cases of KS and is absent in all its mimickers (218–222) (Fig. 27.9). Ultrastructural studies demonstrate Weibel-Palade bodies in the cytoplasm of some KS cells (223,224).

Angiomyolipoma

Renal angiomyolipomas that also involve lymph nodes are rare (225). The regional periaortic lymph nodes are the nodes typically involved (165). Histologically, this lesion is composed of a mixture of adipose tissue, smooth muscle arranged in fascicles, and thick-walled blood vessels. Focally, the smooth muscle cells may have mildly to moderately atypical nuclei; however, mitoses are found only infrequently (165). Nonetheless, because nodal involvement by a tumor implies malignancy, some investigators have raised the possibility of malignant transformation of this tumor (225). It is generally accepted, however, that nodal involvement by a renal angiomyolipoma most likely represents a multicentric growth pattern and not a true nodal metastasis (165). Follow-up studies in 12 cases show that the patients

were well from 1 to 15 years (median, 3 years) after excision (225). This finding supports the interpretation that these lesions are benign. DNA analysis of nodal angiomyolipoma in three cases demonstrated a diploid DNA content (225), further supporting the benign nature of these lesions. The perivascular myoid cells in angiomyolipoma express HMB-45, a phenotype shared by lymphangioleiomyomatosis (169).

Bacillary Angiomatosis

Bacillary angiomatosis is an uncommon pseudoneoplastic vasoproliferative disorder resulting from infection by *Bartonella henselae* and *Bartonella quintana* (226–228). The lesion was first described by Stoler et al. in 1983 (229). LeBoit et al. (230,231) defined the entity histopathologically, identified the relationship between the lesions and the cat scratch bacillus-like organisms found within them, and coined the term bacillary angiomatosis to reflect their infectious as well as their proliferative nature. The disease generally occurs in immunocompromised individuals, predominantly those who are HIV-infected and have AIDS (226,230–235) (see Chapter 25).

Cutaneous disease is the most frequent clinical manifestation of bacillary angiomatosis (229–232,236–238). The patients usually have multiple variably sized, superficial cutaneous papules that may mimic pyogenic granuloma to dermal and subcutaneous nodules that may be misinterpreted as KS (229–232,236). Cutaneous disease may be accompanied by mucosal, visceral, or lymph node involvement (232,234–235,238–241). The peripheral, mediastinal, and abdominal lymph nodes are the ones most commonly involved by bacillary angiomatosis (234).

Bacillary angiomatosis involves lymph nodes as discrete, variably sized nodules, some of which may coalesce to form large masses. The underlying lymph node architecture may survive intact. Bacillary angiomatosis is composed of variably sized, circumscribed lobules of small blood vessels (some well formed, some barely canalized, and some ectatic) that are situated in an alternately mucinous and fibrotic stroma. The vessels are lined by protuberant plump, polygonal endothelial cells containing abundant pale cytoplasm and ovoid nuclei that contain one to several small nucleoli. They sometimes exhibit mild nuclear pleomorphism and mitotic figures. Aggregates of granular acidophilic to amphophilic material, representing clumps of the causative bacteria, lie in the interstitium separating the vessels (239). The bacteria can be visualized with the Warthin-Starry stain (229–231,239). Numerous neutrophils accompanied by "nuclear dust" usually are scattered throughout the lesions and frequently aggregate around the bacterial clumps (229,231–232,239–240) (see Chapter 25).

The principal differential diagnosis of bacillary angiomatosis involving a lymph node includes KS (236,239), with which it can occur simultaneously in the same patient (233,240,241); epithelioid hemangioma; and angiosarcoma (239). Careful assessment of the clinical features of the patient and of the gross appearance and histopathology of the lesions should lead to suspicion of bacillary angiomatosis (236), which can be readily confirmed by a Warthin-Starry stain (230,231,239,240). The accurate recognition of bacillary angiomatosis is important because appropriate antibiotic therapy leads to regression of the lesions and resolution of the disease in virtually all patients (236).

Inflammatory Pseudotumor of Lymph Node

The main histologic feature of this lesion is a spindle cell proliferation arranged in a storiform pattern, accompanied by proliferating small blood vessels and inflammatory cells (242,243). This proliferation predominantly involves the connective tissue framework of the lymph node that results in expansion of the hilum, trabeculae, and capsule. Frequently, this proliferation extends into the paracortical region and the perinodal soft tissues (Fig. 27.10). As in nodular fasciitis that involves soft tissues, myxoid as well as fibrotic areas may be identified. The spindle cells appear to be a mixture of fibroblasts and myofibroblasts, as shown by their positivity for muscle actin. However, some investigators have reported inflammatory pseudotumors that exhibit the immunophenotypic features of follicular dendritic cells (244). The proliferating vessels are usually straight, rarely ramifying. The vessels are lined by plump, reactive-appearing endothelial cells and are surrounded by one or two layers of spindle cells. In the paracortical region, these vessels are mixed with postcapillary venules. Small benign lymphocytes, immunoblasts, histiocytes, and many plasma cells are present (Fig. 27.10). Neutrophils may be seen infrequently, and some cases may have a prominent eosinophilic infiltrate. Multinucleated giant cells also can be found. Necrosis and a high mitotic rate are not usual features of inflammatory pseudotumors (243).

Moran and colleagues emphasized the heterogeneity of these lesions and histologically classified them into three different stages: stage I, small nodules with partial involvement of the lymph node; stage II, more diffuse fibroblastic proliferation causing marked distortion of the lymph node often with secondary spread into the extranodal adipose tissue; and stage III, almost complete sclerosis of the lymph node with scant residual inflammatory elements (245).

There is controversy surrounding the nomenclature of histologically similar lesions that have been reported to recur, metastasize, and involve extranodal tissues. When these lesions extend into the perinodal soft tissue and irregularly entrap normal structures, they may be considered "inflammatory myofibroblastic tumors" that have recurring potential (246). As opposed to inflammatory myofibroblastic tumors of soft tissue, inflammatory pseudotumors of lymph node are not associated with ALK translocations and therefore are not considered to be neoplastic (247). Some investigators have reported histologically similar lesions in visceral organs and have used the term "inflammatory fibrosarcoma" to describe those with cytologic atypia and an aggressive clinical course (246,248).

A recent study by Facchetti and associates reported that four of nine examined cases of nodal inflammatory pseudotumor had large numbers of spirochetes that reacted positively with an anti–*Treponema pallidum* serum (249). These cases were accompanied by pronounced follicular hyperplasia in the residual lymphoid parenchyma, and plasma cell infiltrate in the fibrotic capsule. The authors recommend investigating a spirochetal etiology in all cases of nodal inflammatory pseudotumors (249). Other microorganisms have also been found to be associated with this distinctive pattern of nodal reaction, such as atypical mycobacteria (250–252) and more rarely *Pseudomonas veronii* (253), *Pseudomonas psittaci* (243), *Actinomyces* (254,255), and EBV (247,256).

Finally, the newly described spectrum of IgG4-related sclerosing disease has to be considered in the differential diagnosis. The morphologic features of IgG4-related lymphadenopathy differs from IgG4-related involvement of other sites in that in general there is no sclerosis or phlebitis (257–260). Thus, the fibroinflammatory lesions typical of this entity are unusual in the lymph nodes; however, a nodal inflammatory pseudotumor-like pattern has been described (257–261). The diagnosis is based on the presence of increased numbers of

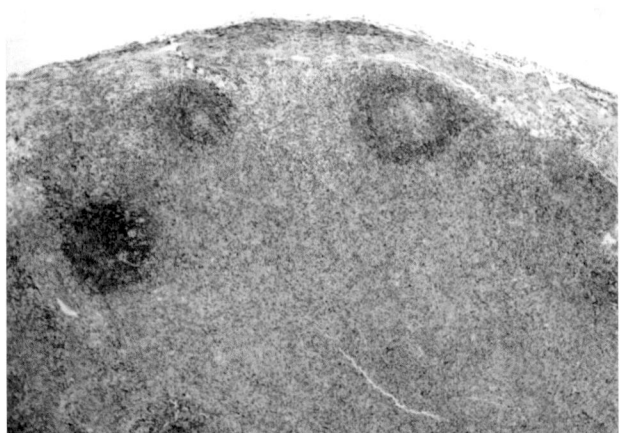
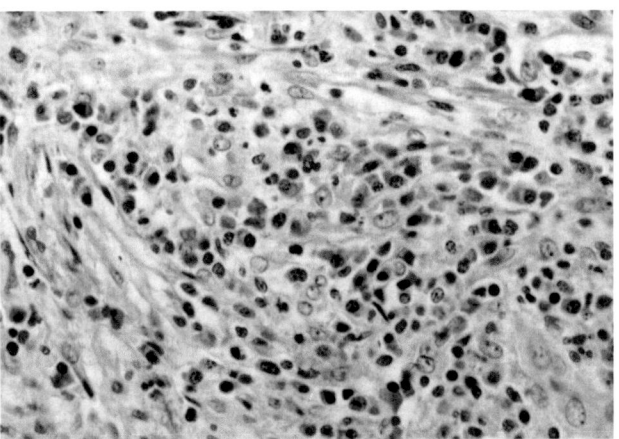

FIGURE 27.10. Inflammatory pseudotumor of lymph node. A: Low-power examination of this lymph node demonstrates the presence of residual benign germinal centers, which are largely surrounded by an interfollicular spindle cell and inflammatory cell proliferation. This process extends focally into the paracortical region and into the perinodal tissue (hematoxylin and eosin, original magnification: 40×). **B:** Higher magnification demonstrates that the proliferation consists of spindle cells, blood vessels, and a mixed inflammatory cell population. Cellular pleomorphism, necrosis, and frequent mitotic figures are absent (hematoxylin and eosin, original magnification: 400×).

IgG4-positive plasma cells and an increased IgG4/IgG ratio (257,260,261). Therefore, immunohistochemical staining for IgG and IgG4 should be performed on all cases morphologically consistent with an inflammatory pseudotumor.

Mycobacterial Spindle Cell Pseudotumor

This proliferation shows a significant degree of histologic overlap with inflammatory pseudotumor; one can observe short fascicles and storiform arrangements of spindle cells admixed with capillaries and chronic inflammatory cells, including plasma cells (250,262) (Fig. 27.11). Evaluation with a histochemical stain for acid-fast bacilli permits the correct diagnosis (250,262) (Fig. 27.11). The mycobacterial spindle cell tumor characteristically arises in the setting of *Mycobacterium avium-intracellulare* infection in immunocompromised patients. The spindle cell population is thought to be histiocytic; however, immunoreactivity with antidesmin antibodies has been reported (262).

Palisaded Myofibroblastoma

Palisaded myofibroblastoma is also known as *hemorrhagic spindle cell tumor with amainthoid fibers*. As the names imply, this rare tumor is composed of myofibroblasts with interstitial hemorrhage and amainthoid fibers (263,264). This benign lesion occurs predominantly in the inguinal lymph nodes, although presentation in other sites has also been reported. The constituent spindle cells appear bland and mitotically inactive. The so-called amainthoid fibers are ovoid and stellate regions of collagen deposition that may be calcified. The myofibroblast nuclei appear to palisade around the amainthoid fibers. The tumor cells express antigens shared with myofibroblasts in other lesions: vimentin, muscle-specific actin, but not desmin or S-100 protein. The morphologic and immunophenotypic features permit distinction from other lesions in the differential diagnosis, including KS, true dendritic cell sarcoma, and smooth muscle lesions such as metastatic leiomyosarcoma and leiomyomatosis.

Leiomyomatosis

Tumor-forming nodules of smooth muscle without the cytologic features of malignancy are occasionally encountered in lymph nodes (265–268). These proliferations should not be considered metastatic leiomyosarcoma unless there is significant nuclear pleomorphism and necrosis. The distinction between an intranodal tumor and a primary soft tissue tumor is important because even small and cytologically bland smooth muscle tumors of the soft tissue can recur and metastasize. Nodal leiomyomatosis can result from deposits of benign metastasizing leiomyoma and leiomyomatosis peritonealis disseminata, or may represent a primary nodal lesion (265–268). The differential diagnosis is lengthy, and includes most of the spindle cell lesions discussed in this chapter. In contrast to the other spindle cell lesions, nodal leiomyomatosis is a homogeneous-appearing lesion that is indistinguishable from uterine leiomyoma (265–268).

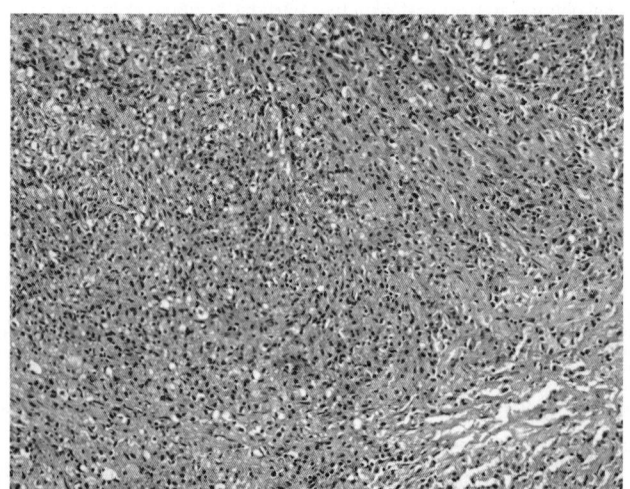

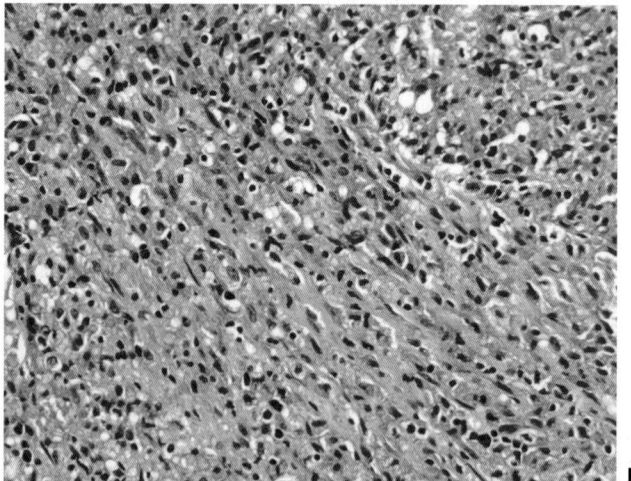

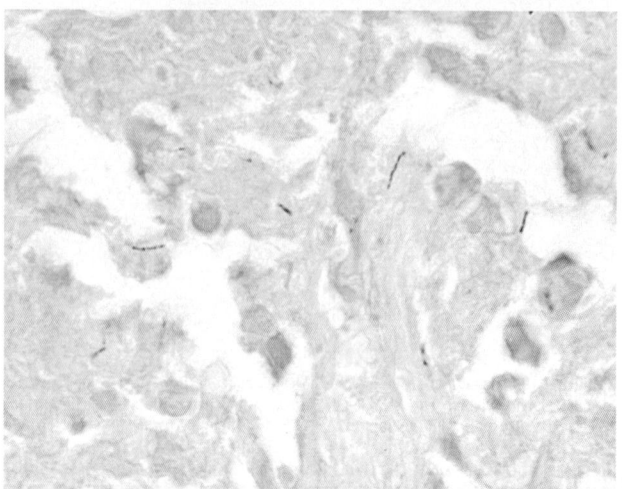

FIGURE 27.11. Mycobacterial spindle cell pseudotumor. A: This patient with newly diagnosed HIV infection presented with mesenteric lymph node enlargement. The lymph node was replaced by fascicles of spindle cells. The patient was subsequently found to have disseminated *Mycobacterium avium-intracellulare* infection (hematoxylin and eosin, original magnification: 100×). **B:** The spindle cells are admixed with small lymphocytes and plasma cells (hematoxylin and eosin, original magnification: 200×). **C:** Acid-fast stain shows numerous mycobacteria (Ziehl-Neelsen stain, original magnification: 1,000×).

Deciduosis

Intranodal, tumor-forming decidual cells can occur during pregnancy. They may be associated with endometriosis, although decidual deposits outside of the setting of endometriosis have been well described (100,269). The constituent cells are morphologically similar to decidual cells found within the endometrium. However, because of their intra-abdominal or retroperitoneal distribution, there is often concern about the possibility of metastatic carcinoma, especially squamous cell carcinoma. The relatively bland cytologic appearance of the decidual cells and the absence of immunoreactivity for cytokeratins permit distinction from metastatic carcinoma.

Other Sarcomas

Rare cases have been reported in which an intranodal sarcoma, that is, leiomyosarcoma, rhabdomyosarcoma, or malignant fibrous histiocytoma, has been found with no other evidence of disease elsewhere (270). The extreme rarity of such lesions, however, should always prompt a thorough clinical investigation for a primary lesion. Diagnostically, the possibility should always be left open of a primary lesion that has occurred in some other site.

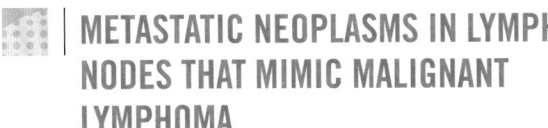

METASTATIC NEOPLASMS IN LYMPH NODES THAT MIMIC MALIGNANT LYMPHOMA

Poorly Differentiated Carcinomas

Metastatic carcinomas that involve lymph nodes secondarily often recapitulate features of their primary lesion, displaying squamous, glandular, or transitional cell differentiation and therefore are readily recognizable. In cases in which it is unknown, the primary site sometimes can be inferred from the histologic features of the metastasis. In other instances, the clinical history, including the age and sex of the patient, can be used as well as the anatomic location of the involved lymph node to develop a likely differential diagnosis. Not infrequently, however, metastatic carcinomas may present a diagnostic problem in that they occasionally lack any obvious

morphologic features of differentiation and thus mimic other malignant neoplasms. For example, they may simulate a malignant lymphoma if they are poorly differentiated and the cells lack cohesion; a sarcoma, if the cells undergo spindle cell metaplasia; and a melanoma, if the cells are characterized by solitary, prominent, centrally placed nucleoli.

The most common situation is one in which a poorly differentiated carcinoma replaces a lymph node in a diffuse sheetlike matter, mimicking a diffuse large cell lymphoma. The clinical history and a thorough clinical evaluation may distinguish between these two diagnostic possibilities and ascertain the primary site of metastatic carcinoma. Several histopathologic criteria may be helpful in distinguishing carcinoma from malignant lymphoma. In malignant lymphomas, the interface between the neoplastic cells and the uninvolved lymph node tissue is often indiscrete, with lymphoma cells infiltrating freely into the adjacent benign lymph node parenchyma. In contrast, in carcinomas, prominent sinusoidal involvement results in large islands of neoplastic cells that often form a broad, clearly distinct border that appears to push against the benign residual lymphoid tissue (1).

Epithelial cells tend to be cohesive; epithelial neoplasms are frequently characterized by the formation of nests of cells. These cell nests may be well defined and readily apparent in routine histologic sections. In contrast to malignant lymphomas, poorly differentiated carcinomas are more likely to exhibit a greater degree of cellular anaplasia and pleomorphism, a higher frequency of multiple nuclei, and larger, more prominent nucleoli (1) (Fig. 27.12).

If necrosis is present, the pattern may serve as an additional feature to help establish a differential diagnosis. Carcinomas display areas of necrosis that are zonal and well demarcated from surrounding viable tumor. In contrast, individual cell necrosis is more common in malignant lymphomas. The single cell necrosis of lymphomas is associated with the presence of numerous phagocytic tingible body macrophages, resulting in a starry-sky pattern. Even in very aggressive carcinomas with extensive necrosis, broad areas of well-delimited necrosis are usually found and a starry-sky pattern is not seen.

Carcinomas metastatic to lymph nodes may mimic malignant lymphoma if the tumor cells lack cohesiveness (Fig. 27.12). In cervical lymph nodes, metastatic carcinomas from the nasopharynx and occasionally from other areas of Waldeyer ring are prime suspects in this differential diagnosis. Occasionally,

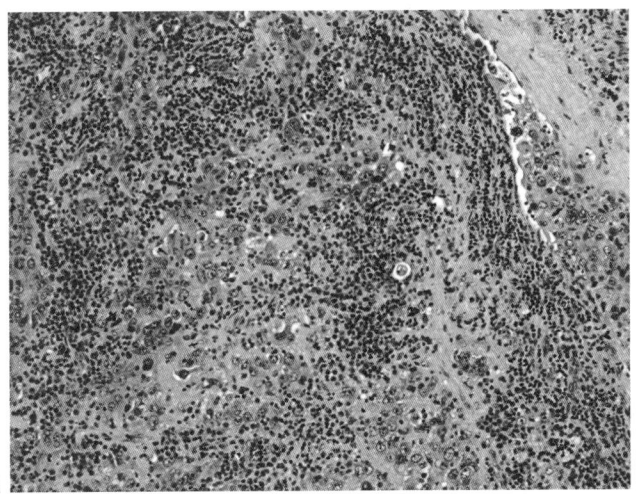
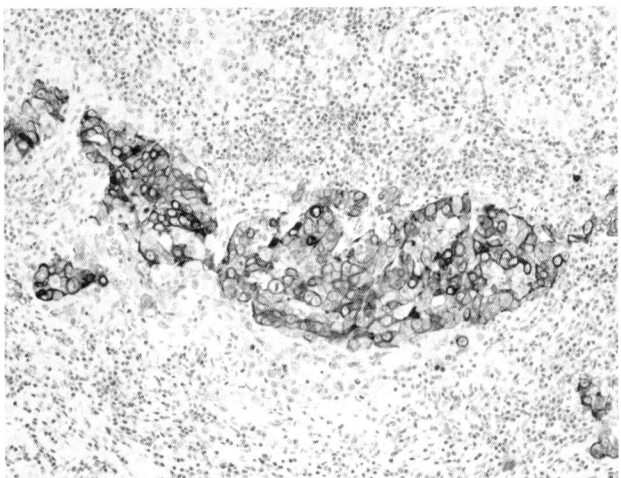

FIGURE 27.12. Poorly differentiated metastatic carcinoma. A: The tumor cells display prominent sinusoidal involvement and no definite formation of cohesive cell nests. The cells are large and pleomorphic with vesicular chromatin and prominent central nucleoli, mimicking a large cell lymphoma (hematoxylin and eosin, original magnification: 100×). **B:** Immunohistochemical stain for pan-cytokeratin is positive in the tumor cells and highlights a cohesive cell growth pattern (original magnification: 200×).

only a few carcinoma cells may be present, and these may be obscured even more by a marked histiocytic and lymphocytic proliferation. An obvious nesting pattern is frequently absent (Fig. 27.12). Such lesions may be diagnosed incorrectly as large cell lymphoma or mixed small and large cell lymphoma. Medullary and apocrine breast carcinomas may also resemble large cell lymphomas. Small cell carcinomas of the breast and lung may mimic small lymphocytic lymphoma, Burkitt lymphoma, and lymphoblastic lymphoma, depending on their particular cytologic features.

ALCL represents one category of malignant lymphoma that frequently has been misdiagnosed in the past because these lymphoid neoplasms often exhibit the growth pattern and cellular characteristics of epithelial neoplasms (15,271). ALCL exhibits a marked predilection for sinusoidal infiltration and, hence, often grows in an epithelial pattern (15,271) (Fig. 27.13). Moreover, the neoplastic cells of ALCL often exhibit marked pleomorphism and have one to many large, prominent nucleoli (15) (Fig. 27.13) (see Chapter 26).

In all these situations, immunohistochemical staining of routinely prepared paraffin tissue sections for CD45, cytokeratins, EMA, CD15, CD30, ALK-1 and B- and T-cell–associated antigens usually leads to the correct diagnosis (Figs. 27.12 and 27.13).

The most common poorly differentiated carcinomas that may be confused with malignant lymphoma are undifferentiated nasopharyngeal carcinoma (UNC), pulmonary small cell undifferentiated carcinoma, and mammary lobular carcinoma. Signet ring cell carcinomas also enter into the differential diagnosis, but less commonly.

Undifferentiated Nasopharyngeal Carcinoma

Because of its peculiar epidemiology and usual site of presentation, the diagnosis of UNC may be suspected before morphologic examination. Occurrence in young to middle-aged Southern Chinese is typical, as is dissemination to cervical and mediastinal lymph nodes. However, other presentations are not uncommon (272).

Morphologically, UNC is a tumor composed of single or aggregated large cells possessing scanty cytoplasm, and vesicular nuclei containing a single prominent eosinophilic nucleolus. Because these lesional cells may be rare, one's low power impression is often that of a "blue" tumor, with a dense background of small, round lymphocytes. Despite a superficial resemblance to small lymphocytic lymphoma, T-cell–rich diffuse large B-cell lymphoma, and lymphocyte-predominant

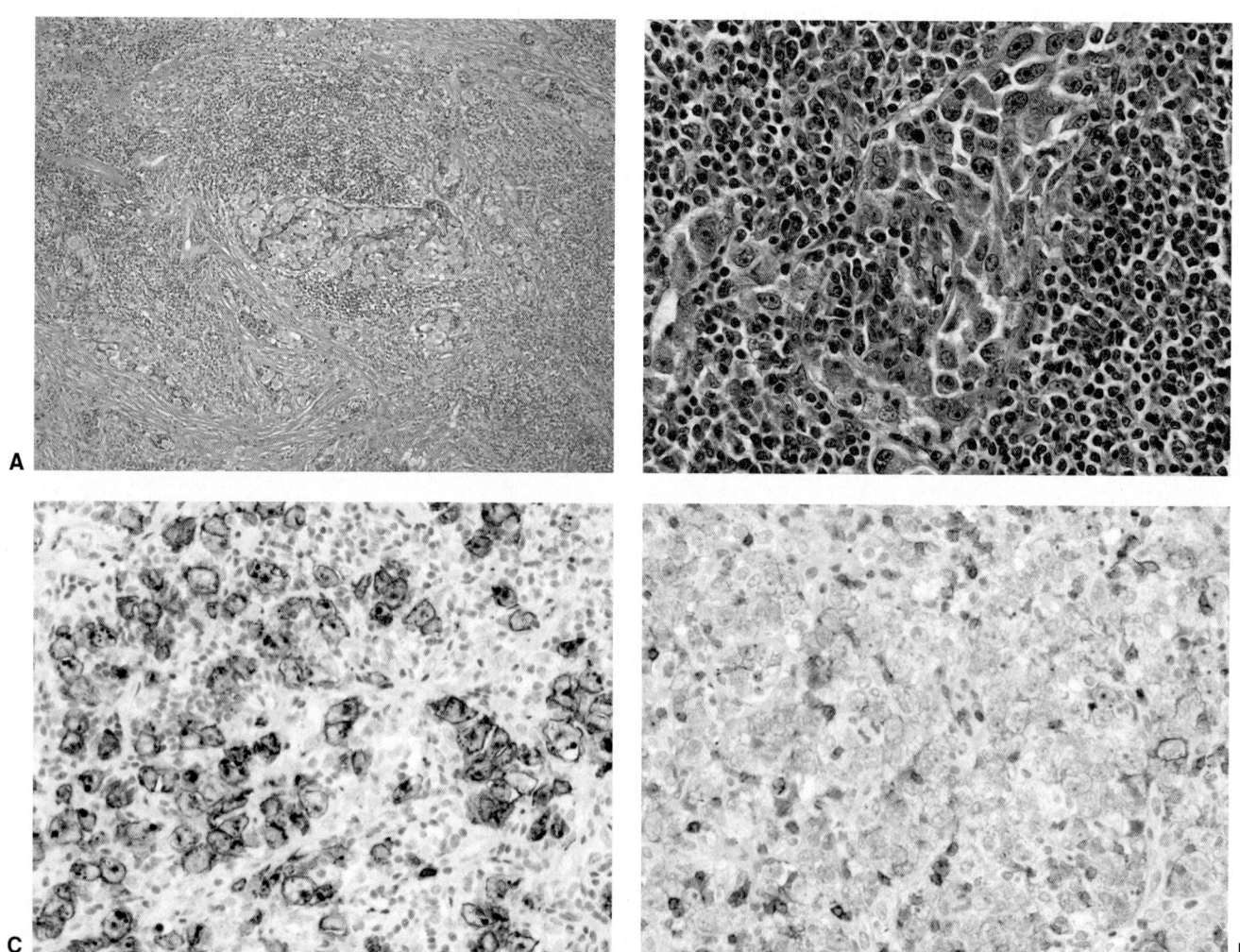

FIGURE 27.13. Anaplastic large cell lymphoma, ALK-negative. This category of non-Hodgkin lymphoma frequently exhibits the growth pattern and cellular characteristics of epithelial neoplasms. **A:** The neoplastic cells show a marked predilection for sinusoidal infiltration, hence mimicking metastatic carcinoma (hematoxylin and eosin, original magnification: 100×). **B:** The neoplastic cells exhibit considerable pleomorphism and have prominent nucleoli (hematoxylin and eosin, original magnification: 400×). **C:** Immunoperoxidase staining demonstrates that these large neoplastic cells strongly express CD30 (original magnification: 200×). **D:** Additional immunostaining demonstrates that these neoplastic cells express T-cell-associated antigen CD2 (original magnification: 200×).

classical Hodgkin lymphoma, UNC is an epithelial tumor that expresses cytokeratins and lacks CD45. One should be cautious about the interpretation of CD45 positivity in UNC, however. One may encounter the CD45-negative UNC cells ringed by background CD45-positive lymphocytes, which may confer on them the false appearance of CD45 expression. Determination of CD45 status in UNC should probably only be performed in clusters of cohesive UNC cells, thereby lessening the chance for misinterpretation.

UNC is associated with EBV infection (273,274). Although detection of EBV genome and virus-associated proteins is straightforward in UNC, it is probably not contributory to its distinction from malignant lymphoma, as a variety of malignant lymphomas are also associated with EBV infection (15).

Poorly Differentiated Neuroendocrine Carcinoma

Poorly differentiated neuroendocrine carcinoma (PDNC) represents a spectrum of related tumors that encompasses small cell carcinoma, neuroendocrine carcinoma not otherwise specified, and large cell neuroendocrine carcinoma. The most common PDNC is the pulmonary small cell carcinoma, which in many cases may be correctly recognized in lymph nodes on the basis of the history of a pulmonary mass. When the history is not forthcoming or when a PDNC originates in an extrapulmonary organ, diagnosis can be difficult, however.

Small cell carcinoma may be easily mistaken for malignant lymphoma because the constituent cells possess inapparent cytoplasm and small, hyperchromatic nuclei. Other carcinomas in this spectrum contain nuclei with finely stippled chromatin and small nucleoli. Cohesive, nestlike growth favors the diagnosis of carcinoma over lymphoma, but this finding is not specific (Fig. 27.14). Smudged nuclear chromatin, including the well-recognized *Azzopardi* effect, may be present, but this feature is shared in part by some lymphoid proliferations, including in the setting of systemic lupus erythematosus (275).

When PDNC is a possibility, immunohistochemical evaluation may aid in its distinction from malignant lymphoma and, perhaps, in tumor subtyping. Most PDNCs express cytokeratin and many demonstrate a characteristic paranuclear "dot" staining pattern for cytokeratin (276). EMA expression may be seen in the absence of cytokeratin expression and may be considered supportive of epithelial differentiation, especially when CD45 is absent and ALCL is not a consideration (277). Many small cell carcinomas also express neuroendocrine-associated and neural markers, such as chromogranin, synaptophysin, CD56, and CD99 (MIC-2 antigen) (276–279) (Fig. 27.14). It should be noted that evidence of neuroendocrine differentiation is less prominent than in well or moderately differentiated neuroendocrine carcinoma and may be difficult to document.

The use of antibodies to cytokeratins 7 and 20 (CK7 and CK20) may aid in the separation of cutaneous neuroendocrine carcinoma (i.e., Merkel cell carcinoma) from other PDNCs. In addition to the expression of pancytokeratins and neuroendocrine antigens, Merkel cell carcinoma is apparently unique among the PDNCs in the expression of CK20; many other PCNCs express only CK7 (280).

Mammary Lobular Carcinoma

Isolated axillary lymphadenopathy in a postpubertal woman should be considered likely to represent metastatic breast carcinoma until proven otherwise (281). Although the distinction from malignant lymphoma is not always straightforward, infiltrating ductal carcinomas often form glands or large, cohesive tumor cell clusters in lymph nodes, which is typical of epithelial neoplasms. In contrast, however, metastatic lobular carcinoma of the breast is generally a small cell neoplasm that can infiltrate the lymph node parenchyma in single cells and form vague, confluent masses that mimic malignant lymphoma and sinus histiocytosis at low power (Fig. 27.15).

The first challenge confronted by the morphologist is determining that a lesion actually exists at all. Any low-power abnormality that suggests a mass lesion or prominent sinuses should be examined at high magnification. Sinus histiocytosis should not form a mass lesion. Its high-power morphology includes a moderate amount of vacuolated cytoplasm and small nuclei with reniform or oval shapes with nuclear grooves. This appearance is also shared, in part, by sinus histiocytosis with massive lymphadenopathy (Rosai-Dorfman disease) and Langerhans cell histiocytosis (see Chapter 49). In contrast, lobular carcinoma of the breast usually demonstrates monotonous, round nuclei of small to intermediate size, with small or inapparent nucleoli. The cytoplasm is generally scant; however, at low power, a mass of lobular carcinoma cells may impart the impression of a pink mass, generally because of the contrast between its epithelioid features and those of lymphocytes and histiocytes. Both these epithelioid characteristics and the fact that metastases are frequently focal may permit distinction from malignant lymphoma.

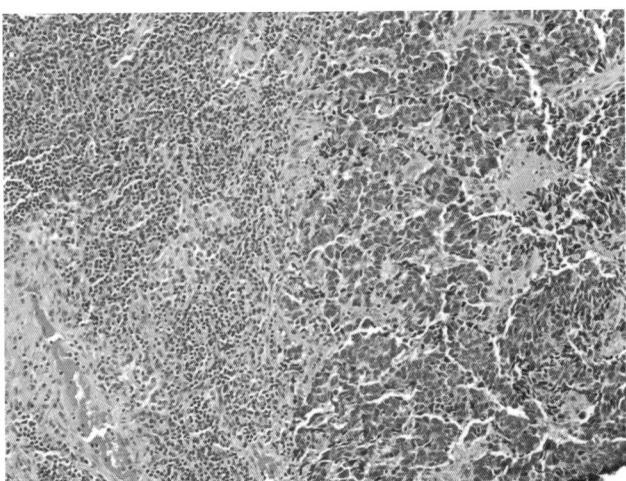 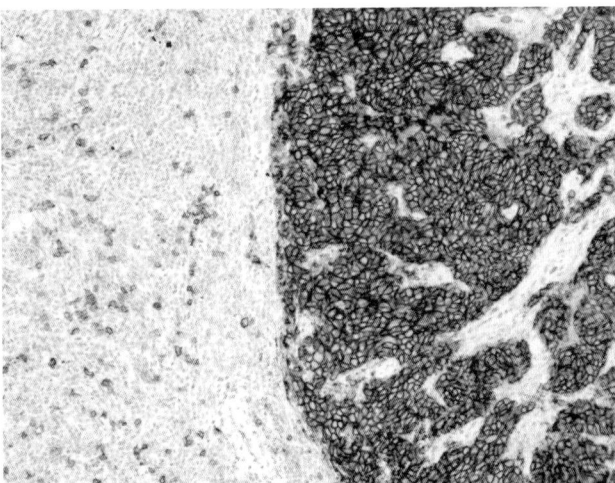

A **B**

FIGURE 27.14. Metastatic pulmonary small cell carcinoma. A: Cohesive tumor cell nests with focal necrosis (hematoxylin and eosin, original magnification: 100×). **B:** Immunohistochemical stain for CD56 is positive in the tumor cells, suggestive of neuroendocrine differentiation (original magnification: 100×).

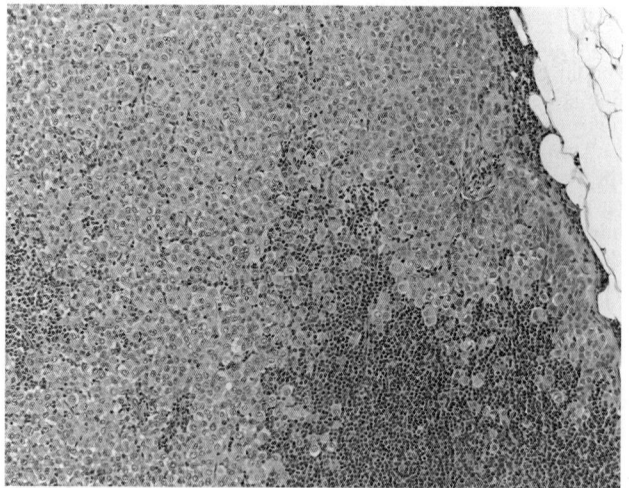

FIGURE 27.15. Metastatic lobular carcinoma of breast. Metastatic lobular breast carcinoma can be overlooked because of its histologic similarity to sinus histiocytosis. The keys to diagnosis in this case are the nested pattern of growth, the relatively large nuclear size, and the absence of twisted, bean-shaped, and reniform nuclei (hematoxylin and eosin, original magnification: 100×). (Photomicrograph courtesy of Dr. Syed Hoda, Weill Cornell Medical College, New York, NY.)

However, these features are neither specific nor exclusive; immunohistochemical evaluation may be helpful. The screening panel (i.e., CD45, cytokeratin, and S-100) enables distinction from malignant lymphoma and a histiocytic proliferation. Lobular carcinoma expresses pancytokeratins, and as many as 50% of cases express the S-100 protein (282). Malignant lymphoma demonstrates the expected CD45-positive, S-100, and cytokeratin-negative phenotype, and the histiocytes of sinus histiocytosis may express CD45 but are more likely to express CD68.

The morphologic appearance of lobular carcinoma may be heterogeneous. Lobular carcinoma variants include the alveolar, solid, pleomorphic, and signet ring cell subtypes (283). Awareness of these lobular carcinoma variants may help in the distinction from malignant lymphoma and other metastatic neoplasms.

Once the correct diagnosis of metastatic carcinoma has been made, it may become necessary to determine the primary site of origin, especially when a complete physical examination and mammogram have not been performed. Using antibodies to estrogen and progesterone receptors, human cystic disease fluid protein (HCDFP/brst-2), mCEA, CK7, and CK20, it may be possible to distinguish a breast primary from an extramammary primary. Expression of estrogen, progesterone, or both receptors and brst-2 expression with negative or focally reactive mCEA are characteristic of breast carcinoma (284). The CK7+CK20− phenotype is also supportive, although not entirely specific, of a mammary primary. Because the immunohistochemical results should not be considered diagnostic, but merely confirmatory of a type of differentiation, one should interpret the results in light of the clinical and light microscopic findings. For example, estrogen and progesterone receptors have been reported in numerous neoplasms (285) and the phenotype, as well as the morphology, of breast carcinoma may be indistinguishable from skin adnexal and salivary gland neoplasms (286).

Signet Ring Cell Lesions

The presence of vacuolated signet ring cells should not automatically lead to a diagnosis of adenocarcinoma. In some instances, the vacuoles may not represent intracellular mucin but instead may contain immunoglobulin. The tumor may be an uncommon variety of follicular lymphoma, so-called signet ring cell lymphoma, in which lymphoma cells produce and retain immunoglobulin in large intracytoplasmic vacuoles (287,288) (see Chapter 22). Demonstration of intracellular mucin with an appropriate histochemical stain suggests epithelial differentiation, but is not specific for it. Evaluation with antibodies to cytokeratin, CD45, and immunoglobulin light chains may also be useful, especially when intracytoplasmic mucin is not readily identified. Rarely, liposarcomas, epithelioid hemangioendotheliomas, malignant melanomas, and rhabdoid carcinomas may contain cytoplasmic inclusions with eccentric, deformed nuclei (289). Nodal muciphages (290) and macrophages that contain mucicarmine-positive polyvinyl-pyrrolidone (291) may also mimic metastatic poorly differentiated carcinoma. Attention to the clinical history and immunophenotype prevents misdiagnosis.

Other Poorly Differentiated Carcinomas

Adrenal cortical carcinoma can be difficult to diagnose because of its histologic overlap with renal clear cell carcinomas, hepatocellular carcinomas (HCCs), pheochromocytomas, and melanomas. Its very frequent lack of expression of cytokeratin and EMA (292) may even cause confusion with a mesenchymal neoplasm. Useful diagnostic markers include Melan-A (MART-1), inhibin, and calretinin (293,294). Immunostaining for synaptophysin is positive in a subset of the cases (295).

Metastatic carcinosarcomas, also known as malignant mixed müllerian tumors when they occur in the female genital tract, are relatively uncommon tumors. They can sometimes be distinguished from metastatic carcinoma because they usually demonstrate malignant mesenchymal and malignant epithelial differentiation, at least focally. However, it is not uncommon for the metastases of carcinosarcoma to fail to show biphasic (mixed epithelial and mesenchymal) characteristics. That is, carcinosarcoma may be associated with metastatic deposits that appear carcinomatous or sarcomatous only (296).

It is well known that carcinomas can exhibit spindle cell morphology. In these instances, in addition to a thorough clinical history, immunohistochemical evaluation can be very informative. Cytokeratin expression is usually supportive of epithelial differentiation. Although this usually indicates carcinoma, carcinosarcoma, or sarcomatous carcinoma, one should not exclude primary soft tissue tumors that show epithelial differentiation, such as monophasic synovial sarcoma, based on the immunohistochemistry results alone. Most primary soft tissue spindle cell sarcomas also express cytokeratin (297). In these tumors, cytokeratin expression is generally not strong or diffuse or detectable with numerous cytokeratin antibodies. If a primary soft tissue spindle cell sarcoma is considered, one should be in the possession of a complete and supportive clinical history and should be aware of the fact that nodal metastasis of primary soft tissue spindle cell sarcomas is rare. S-100 protein expression supports the diagnosis of metastatic melanoma, although it does not exclude soft tissue spindle cell sarcoma, especially metastatic malignant peripheral nerve sheath tumor. Knowledge of the patient's clinical history is particularly important in such distinctions.

Differentiated Adenocarcinoma

The most common and most important obviously glandular lesion to recognize in lymph nodes is metastatic adenocarcinoma. Because of the presence of glands, this entity should not be confused with malignant lymphoma unless the lymphoma demonstrates numerous pseudorosettes, which may simulate glands (298,299). We include a discussion of these well- and moderately differentiated adenocarcinomas in this chapter to outline effective ways of determining the primary site of origin. A complete clinical history is often contributory, of course. When the clinical history and the morphologic features of the lesion in question do not aid in determination of the primary site of origin, immunohistochemical analysis may be beneficial.

Some metastatic adenocarcinomas, such as prostatic and well-differentiated thyroid carcinoma, exhibit very characteristic immunophenotypes that aid in their correct identification. More than 90% of prostatic adenocarcinomas express prostate-specific antigen, prostatic acid phosphatase (PSAP), or both (300,301). However, because very poorly differentiated prostatic carcinomas may not express these antigens, other antibodies should be included in the panel; strong expression of CK7 and CK20, mCEA, and CA 19-9 are unusual in prostate carcinoma (302). Hindgut carcinoids may express PSAP as well (303). If carcinoid tumor is in the differential diagnosis, the appropriate neuroendocrine markers should be included in the panel, but caution is advised because some aggressive prostate cancers express neuroendocrine markers (304).

Papillary and follicular carcinomas of the thyroid gland express thyroglobulin and thyroid transcription factor 1 (TTF-1). Many papillary carcinomas express S-100 protein (305). Caution should be used with TTF-1 interpretation, as it is frequently positive in nonsquamous lung carcinomas and extrapulmonary small cell carcinomas. Medullary carcinomas express calcitonin in addition to neuroendocrine markers. Anaplastic carcinomas frequently lack thyroglobulin, TTF-1, and cytokeratin expression (306).

Although most of the other adenocarcinomas do not demonstrate specific immunophenotypes, the use of cytokeratins 7 and 20 permits separation into groups used to narrow the differential diagnosis. The CK7+CK20+ phenotype is characteristic of transitional cell carcinoma, pancreatic/biliary adenocarcinoma, and ovarian mucinous adenocarcinoma; these tumors often express mCEA and CA 19-9 as well (307,308). Antibodies against estrogen and progesterone receptors and CA 125 may permit separation of ovarian mucinous tumors from the others, although none of these markers is specific. Pulmonary, breast, nonmucinous ovarian, and endometrial carcinomas, as well as mesotheliomas, demonstrate a CK7+CK20- phenotype. Some subtypes of renal cell carcinomas also exhibit the CK7+CD20- phenotype. The expression of TTF-1 supports the diagnosis of a pulmonary carcinoma in the CK7+CK20- category (309). Cytokeratin 5/6, calretinin, WT-1, D2-40, and podoplanin expression, in addition to lack of TTF-1, mCEA, Ber-EP4, and B72.3 expression, helps separate pulmonary adenocarcinomas from mesothelioma (310,311). Breast, ovarian, and endometrial carcinomas frequently express estrogen, progesterone, or both receptors. At least 40% to 50% of breast carcinomas express GCDFP-15 (BRST-2) (312,313). Colorectal adenocarcinoma is predominantly CK7-CK20+. Other tumors that are less commonly CK7-CK20+ include gastric and, rarely, prostatic adenocarcinomas.

HCC and prostatic adenocarcinomas, as well as some renal cell carcinomas, are characteristically predominantly CK7-CK20-. Because a significant minority of HCC and pancreaticobiliary carcinomas may express the CK7+CK20- phenotype, use of additional antibodies is necessary for a precise diagnosis. Hep Par 1 is currently considered the most sensitive and specific marker for HCC (314,315).

Malignant Melanoma

Malignant melanomas often exhibit an intrasinusoidal distribution within lymph nodes (Fig. 27.16). The cells tend to be less cohesive then those that comprise epithelial neoplasms. Moreover, melanoma cells often possess abundant eosinophilic

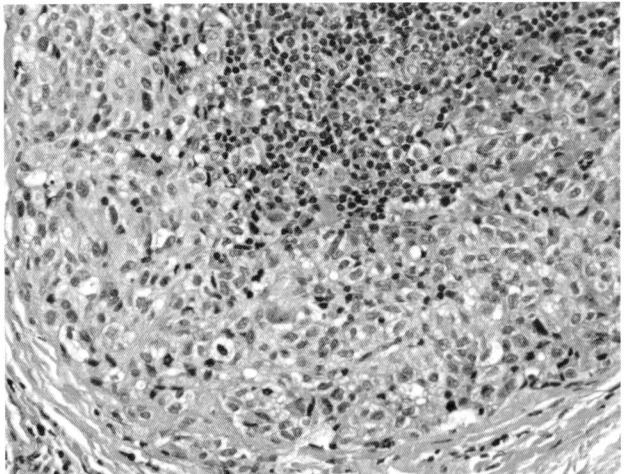

FIGURE 27.16. Malignant melanoma metastatic to lymph node. The malignant melanoma cells are filling the subcapsular sinus. They possess abundant eosinophilic cytoplasm and large irregular nuclei. The nucleoli are inconspicuous in this particular example. However, focally melanin pigment is present, providing evidence of the melanocytic nature of the neoplasm (hematoxylin and eosin, original magnification: 200×).

cytoplasm and large vesicular nuclei that contain large prominent, centrally placed nucleoli (316). For these reasons, malignant melanomas may closely resemble malignant lymphomas in their growth pattern and cytomorphologically. They may be confused easily with immunoblastic diffuse large B-cell lymphoma and ALCLs. Malignant melanoma is also well known for its propensity to recur and metastasize after a prolonged asymptomatic period. For all these reasons a complete clinical history may aid in the diagnosis of malignant melanoma that is metastatic to lymph nodes.

Identification of melanin pigment in a malignant neoplasm is generally considered confirmatory of malignant melanoma, although many melanomas are not pigmented, and other neoplasms, such as psammomatous melanotic schwannoma (317) and pheochromocytoma (318), may contain melanin. Benign melanocytic nevi of lymph nodes also may be pigmented (79–82). Attention to morphologic detail and clinical history is useful. The classic morphologic appearance of metastatic malignant melanoma is an epithelioid neoplasm comprising round to polygonal cells with large nucleoli that contain prominent nucleoli. However, melanoma may assume other appearances, including spindle cell and rhabdoid morphology (319). Rarely, melanomas may contain vacuolated cytoplasm similar to that seen in signet ring cells (289). Because of these features, the differential diagnosis of malignant melanoma is lengthy and includes poorly differentiated carcinoma, malignant lymphoma, and certain sarcomas.

Malignant melanoma is almost always negative for cytokeratins and CD45 (13,320). More than 90% of malignant melanomas express the S-100 protein (321). However, because S-100 protein expression is not specific for melanocytic differentiation, one must interpret S-100 expression in combination with the results of other immunohistochemical studies and the morphologic impression. Carcinomas (66,72,322), various sarcomas (e.g., clear cell sarcoma, malignant peripheral nerve sheath sarcoma), and some hematolymphoid neoplasms, including histiocytic (323,324) and dendritic cell tumors (325), may express the S-100 protein. HMB-45 is also expressed in more than 50% of melanomas and is more specific for melanocytic differentiation than S-100 (326,327). However, melanomas with spindle-shaped cells rarely express HMB-45 (328). HMB-45 may be expressed in angiomyolipoma and lymphangioleiomyomatosis, benign lesions that rarely involve lymph nodes (329,330). Expression of Melan-A, recognized by monoclonal antibody A103, may be more sensitive for melanocytic differentiation than HMB-45 (331). MITF with nuclear positivity is another marker for metastatic melanoma with high specificity and moderate sensitivity (332–334). Since it is positive in nonmelanocytic cells, such as lymphocytes and histiocytes, it should only be used in combination with other markers (335). Rare melanomas with rhabdoid cytoplasm have been reported to express desmin (319). Malignant melanomas also have been reported to express CD10, CD30 and CD57 (336).

Germ Cell Tumors

Seminomas and other germ cell tumors may be mistaken for malignant lymphoma morphologically because the tumor cells possess abundant, often clear, cytoplasm and large vesicular nuclei containing prominent nucleoli; exhibit frequent mitotic figures; and grow diffusely (337) (Fig. 27.17). They are most commonly mistaken for immunoblastic lymphoma, ALCL, or even Hodgkin lymphoma. The distinction between seminoma and malignant lymphoma is often straightforward, however, given a complete clinical history and careful morphologic examination. It may be more difficult to distinguish between germ cell tumors, especially seminoma, and malignant lymphoma when disease is limited to the mediastinum. Evaluation for α-fetoprotein (AFP) and β-human chorionic gonadotrophin (β-HCG) may aid in the differential diagnosis between germ cell tumors and malignant lymphomas in some instances.

The malignant cells comprising seminoma in the male and dysgerminoma in the female may occur in variably sized nests that may be separated by aggregates of small lymphocytes and even by fibrous strands. These benign small lymphocyte aggregates are absent from immunoblastic lymphomas. The sinusoidal architecture of ALCL is absent as are large malignant cells with wreathlike nuclei. Conceivably, some seminoma cells may be mistaken for mononuclear Reed-Sternberg cell variants, but classic Reed-Sternberg cells should be absent. Lacunae are distinctly uncommon as are well-developed fibrous septa. Occasionally, granulomatous inflammation can obscure the classic histopathologic features of seminoma, resulting in misdiagnosis (338).

Immunohistochemical studies may be of additional help in distinguishing between these entities. In general, seminoma cells do not express CD45 (339) or other lymphoid cell antigens but do express placental alkaline phosphatase (PLAP) (340,341). Although PLAP was once thought to be specific for seminoma, trophoblasts, and the cells of intratubular germ cell neoplasms, it has become clear that PLAP expression alone is insufficient to support an unequivocal diagnosis of seminoma because it is expressed in carcinomas and other germ cell tumors (342,343). If metastatic carcinoma is a possibility, immunohistochemical staining for cytokeratin may be helpful. However, although seminoma was once considered to be a cytokeratin-negative neoplasm, there are numerous reports of cytokeratin expression in seminoma (344,345). Cytokeratin expression in seminoma is probably not common, however, and when it occurs, it is usually weak and patchy in distribution. Strong, diffuse cytokeratin expression in a lesion thought to be seminoma is unusual, and it should prompt the pathologist to consider metastatic carcinoma or another germ cell tumor. The syncytiotrophoblastic giant cells in seminoma express β-HCG; choriocarcinoma should not be diagnosed unless a biphasic proliferation of both cytotrophoblasts and syncytiotrophoblasts is identified. β-HCG is also expressed by a variety of poorly differentiated carcinomas (346). Identification of AFP in the serum or in sections from a lesion thought to be a pure seminoma should probably prompt a search for a yolk sac tumor. Other markers that have recently gained popularity in the diagnosis of seminoma are CD117 (positive in most cases) (347) and OCT4, a transcription factor expressed in embryonic stem cells and germ cells and positive in seminoma nuclei (Fig. 27.17) (348,349).

Yolk sac tumors, choriocarcinoma, and embryonal carcinoma may share many features with other carcinomas, including cellular cohesion and growth in nests, tubules, trabeculae, and sheets. These features, in addition to expression of cytokeratins, aid in the distinction from malignant lymphoma. However, embryonal carcinoma, like some lymphomas, including Hodgkin lymphoma, express CD30 (350). Expression of CD30 in nonhematopoietic tumors is unusual and, for the most part, limited to embryonal carcinoma. There are rare reports of CD30 expression in other carcinomas (350). At the same time, metastatic embryonal carcinomas after chemotherapy have frequent loss of CD30 expression (351).

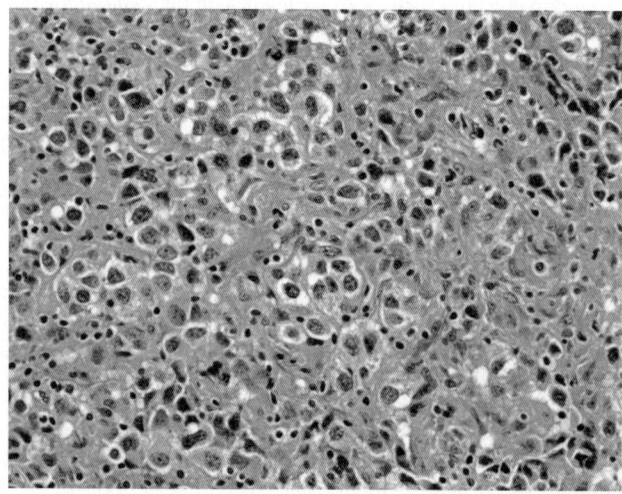
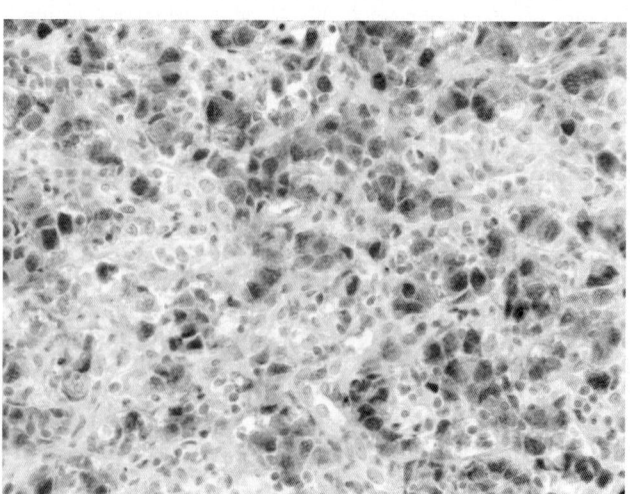

A

B

FIGURE 27.17. Metastatic seminoma. A: The neoplastic cells characteristically possess clear cytoplasm and round vesicular nuclei containing a prominent, centrally placed nucleolus. On occasion, the neoplastic cells do not have prominent central nucleoli and may be partially obscured by a prominent granulomatous response with scattered eosinophils, as illustrated here. This 24-year-old man presented with a large anterior mediastinal mass, clinically suspicious for lymphoma (hematoxylin and eosin, original magnification: 200×). **B:** Immunohistochemical staining demonstrates that the tumor cells express Oct-4 (magnification: 200×).

Sarcomas

Sarcomas arising in the soft tissues metastasize infrequently to lymph nodes (270). Recognition of metastatic sarcoma is usually relatively straightforward. As in the case of poorly differentiated carcinomas, malignant melanomas, and other neoplasms, sarcomas occasionally may be incorrectly diagnosed as malignant lymphoma and vice versa. Those sarcomas that resemble malignant lymphoma and therefore most commonly lead to difficulties in differential diagnosis are the small round cell sarcomas, such as Ewing sarcoma, synovial sarcoma, and epithelioid sarcoma. In a background of diffuse fibrosis, some sarcomatous spindle cell proliferations may mimic lymphocyte-depleted Hodgkin lymphoma. Cases of Hodgkin lymphoma that contain numerous neutrophils may mimic inflammatory fibrous histiocytoma. Focal cellular areas of malignant fibrous histiocytoma may simulate a large cell lymphoma, just like those sarcomas in which the malignant cells lack cohesion.

Small Round Cell Sarcomas

Ewing sarcoma/primitive neuroectodermal tumor, embryonal and alveolar rhabdomyosarcoma, and desmoplastic small round cell tumor (DSRCT) occur most commonly in children and young adults (31). They may mimic a small cell carcinoma, neuroblastoma, lymphoblastic lymphoma, or a large cell lymphoma. Clinical features may help in the differential diagnosis. Morphologic features, such as the presence of rosette formation, rhabdomyoblasts, or desmoplastic stroma, for example, may be helpful; however, these tumors often have cells with scant cytoplasm and small- to moderate-sized nuclei with finely dispersed chromatin, features that may result in the mistaken diagnosis of lymphoblastic lymphoma. In these instances, the presence of glycogen in the cytoplasm may lead to a diagnosis of Ewing sarcoma, although this is not, by any means, specific for Ewing sarcoma. The identification of cytoplasmic cross-striations justifies the diagnosis of rhabdomyosarcoma; unfortunately, this finding is uncommon (31). Overall, the diagnosis of small round cell sarcoma has been radically transformed, with immunohistochemistry and especially molecular genetics superseding morphology.

In most instances, immunohistochemical studies should be performed to provide a definitive answer. Ewing sarcoma may be distinguished from all malignant lymphomas by its lack of CD45 and B- and T-cell–associated antigens. A potential pitfall is Ewing sarcoma cells expression of CD99 (352,353), a product of the *MIC2* pseudoautosomal gene (354), which is also expressed by lymphoblastic lymphomas (355,356). Immunostains for terminal deoxynucleotidyl transferase (TdT) (positive in lymphoblastic lymphoma) (357) and desmin (positive in rhabdomyosarcoma) (50) should be performed in addition to CD99 when confronted with this differential diagnosis. Ewing sarcoma is currently considered to be a form of primitive neuroectodermal tumor; thus expression of neural markers may be present (31,358). Both tumors demonstrate the reciprocal translocations t(11;22)(q24;q12) and t(21;22)(q22q12) involving the *EWS*, the *FLI-1*, and the *ERG* genes, and are treated with the same protocol (31,359,360).

Rhabdomyosarcomas are characteristically positive for desmin, myogenin, and MyoD1 (31,50,361). NSE and CD57 can be detected in myogenic tumors. There are only rare reports of CD99 expression in rhabdomyosarcoma (352,353,356). Rhabdomyosarcomas consistently lack S-100 and HMB-45 and similarly lack CD45 and B- and T-cell–associated antigens. Because the prognosis and therapy for embryonal rhabdomyosarcomas and alveolar rhabdomyosarcomas differ significantly (362), attention to morphologic detail is important. No consistent immunohistochemical differences have been described. The characteristic presence of a reproducible, specific chromosome translocation t(2;13)(q35;q14) resulting in *PAX3-FOXO1*

fusion and, rarely, a variant translocation t(1;13)(p36;q14) that results in *PAX7-FOXO1* fusion in alveolar rhabdomyosarcomas permits their distinction from embryonal rhabdomyosarcomas, which typically have deletions of the short arm of chromosome 11 (31,363).

DSRCT shares the translocation t(11;22) with Ewing sarcoma/primitive neuroectodermal tumor, although the fusion protein differs (364). DSRCT is also immunohistochemically distinct from these neoplasms; DSRCT expresses cytokeratins, desmin, and S-100 protein and lacks CD99 (365).

Neuroblastoma can mimic lymphoblastic lymphoma histologically. Both of these lesions are characterized by a sheetlike growth pattern of small- to medium-sized cells that possess scanty cytoplasm, nuclei containing finely stippled nuclear chromatin, and abundant mitotic figures. Rosettes are not always a conspicuous feature of neuroblastoma (366). Clinical correlation sometimes may be useful in distinguishing between these two entities; however, clinical correlation often does not provide a definitive answer, and immunohistochemical studies should then be used. Neuroblastoma cells frequently express NSE, synaptophysin, chromogranin, beta catenin, CD56, CD57, S-100, and neural filaments. They consistently lack CD45, TdT, and B- and T-cell–associated antigens (366,367), associated with lymphoblastic lymphoma. CD99 is not expressed, making the distinction from Ewing sarcoma/primitive neuroectodermal tumor and lymphoblastic lymphoma relatively straightforward (352,353,356). Neuroblastoma also has characteristic chromosomal abnormalities, such as *N-myc* oncogene amplification, loss of chromosome 1, deletion of the short arm of chromosome 1, and extra copies of chromosome 17 (368–370).

Synovial Sarcoma and Epithelioid Sarcoma

These sarcomatous lesions infrequently involve lymph nodes and therefore only occasionally present a diagnostic problem to the pathologist. If the epithelial component predominates or is the exclusive component in the lymph node metastasis, the possibility of confusing either of these with a carcinoma or malignant lymphoma becomes evident. The features previously attributed to undifferentiated carcinomas hold true for the epithelial components of both of these biphasic sarcomas. Immunohistochemically, they usually express cytokeratin and EMA, but they consistently lack CD45 and B- and T-cell–associated antigens (371). To help in the distinction from carcinoma, many epithelioid sarcomas express CD34 (372), and many synovial sarcomas express CD99; both of these markers are only rarely expressed in carcinoma (64,373). Synovial sarcoma possesses a distinctive genotype with a reciprocal translocation t(X;18) (p11.2;q11.2) (374).

Clear Cell Sarcoma

Clear cell sarcoma is similarly a neoplasm of young adults and frequently involves lymph nodes (375,376). It is characterized by aggregates of tumor cells that possess clear cytoplasm and prominent, centrally placed nucleoli (376). Clear cell sarcoma was previously known as malignant melanoma of soft parts (376). Reports confirm a unique genotype with translocation t(12;22)(q13;12) that has not been identified in malignant melanomas (377). Like malignant melanoma, clear cell sarcomas almost uniformly express S-100 protein, HMB-45, Melan-A, and MITF (375,378).

Metastatic Sarcoma with Glandular Differentiation

Rarely, sarcomas demonstrating glandular differentiation can metastasize to lymph nodes. These sarcomas include synovial sarcoma, malignant peripheral nerve sheath tumor, and endometrial stromal sarcoma.

NONLYMPHOID HEMATOPOIETIC DISORDERS THAT MIMIC MALIGNANT LYMPHOMA

Myeloid Sarcoma

Myeloid sarcoma is a localized, tumor-like proliferation of immature cells that belongs to the myeloid lineage (379). Myeloid sarcoma may occur as a localized tissue manifestation in patients who have acute myeloid leukemia, as a sign of impending blast crisis in chronic myelogenous leukemia or leukemic transformation in patients who have myelodysplastic disorders, or as a forerunner of acute myeloid leukemia in nonleukemic patients (379). Myeloid sarcomas most frequently involve soft tissues, lymph nodes, and skin or occur as isolated lytic bone lesions (379).

Myeloid sarcomas exhibit a spectrum of histopathologic features. Most cases are composed of myeloblasts with or without features of promyelocytic or neutrophilic maturation (15). The blasts are characterized by the presence of round, ovoid, or reniform nuclei that possess finely stippled chromatin and one or two small nucleoli (379,380) (Fig. 27.18). These cells may be mistaken for those comprising diffuse large B- and T-cell lymphomas, Burkitt lymphoma, or lymphoblastic lymphoma (379,380). Consequently, granulocytic sarcomas are frequently misinterpreted as non-Hodgkin lymphomas. Alternatively, especially in children, these lesions sometimes may be misinterpreted histopathologically as rhabdomyosarcoma, neuroblastoma, or various other nonhematopoietic neoplasms (381). Other cases of myeloid sarcoma are characterized by a diffuse monotonous proliferation of myelomonocytic or monoblastic cells. Rarely, tumors with trilineage hematopoiesis or tumors composed of erythroblasts or megakaryoblasts are seen (15,382).

The histopathologic differential diagnosis of myeloid sarcoma from malignant lymphoma and nonhematopoietic neoplasms is greatly aided by immunohistochemical studies. Approximately 90% or more of granulocytic sarcomas express CD45 (LCA) (383). CD68/KP1 is the most commonly expressed marker (100%) in myeloid sarcomas, followed by myeloperoxidase (83.6%), CD117 (80.4%), and CD99 (54.3%) (384). It is also important to remember that CD43, commonly thought of as a T-cell–associated antigen, is expressed by myeloid cells (see Chapter 3). Approximately 50% of myeloid sarcomas express CD43 (383); these cases should not be misdiagnosed as T-cell lymphoma.

Mast Cell Disease

An uncontrolled proliferation of mast cells that occurs locally or systemically is usually referred to as mastocytosis or mast cell disease. Mast cell proliferations most commonly involve the dermis, where they form small, localized tumors (mastocytomas) or disseminate throughout the dermis, resulting in urticaria pigmentosa (15). Mast cell proliferations may involve multiple organs, however, including lymph nodes, whether accompanied by cutaneous manifestations or not. These are referred to as systemic mastocytosis (SM) (15,385).

Lymph nodes appear to be involved in about 25% or more of cases of SM (386). The mast cells preferentially infiltrate the paracortical areas where they surround and partially infiltrate the follicles and vessels. Most mast cells are round, have abundant clear cytoplasm, and contain only a few metachromatic granules; fusiform mast cells are usually infrequent. Even when present, however, spindle mast cells cannot be distinguished from connective tissue fibroblasts without special stains. These morphologic features, combined with the failure to consider SM in the differential diagnosis, may lead to the mistaken diagnosis of malignant lymphoma or sometimes hairy cell leukemia (386). Rare patients present with marked lymphadenopathy accompanied by significant blood eosinophilia. Such cases are called "lymphadenopathic SM with eosinophilia" and belong to the category of aggressive SM (387,388). Cytogenetic analysis of the *FIP1L1-PDGFRA* fusion gene should be performed in order to rule out a myeloid neoplasm with eosinophilia and *PDGFRA* rearrangement (15).

The clinical findings may be helpful in pointing the pathologist toward the correct diagnosis. Histologically, the dimorphic nature of the infiltrate, when present, is helpful, as is the frequent accompaniment of the mast cells by clusters of eosinophils. Wright-Giemsa–stained touch preparations of the lymph node biopsy provide an excellent means of identifying the mast cells. Toluidine blue stains of paraffin tissue sections are useful in highlighting the metachromatic granules (1). Immunophenotypic analysis highlights the proliferation of CD117-positive, mast cell tryptase-positive mast cells with aberrant expression of CD2 and CD25 (15).

Dendritic Cell Neoplasms

It is extremely uncommon to encounter a neoplasm derived from follicular dendritic cells, interdigitating dendritic cells, and fibroblastic reticular cells. These neoplasms all share storiform and interlacing fascicular growth. The constituent ovoid and spindle cells contain nuclei with smooth nuclear membranes and small central eosinophilic nucleoli (Fig. 27.19). Cytologically, atypical multinucleate cells with prominent nuclear pseudoinclusions have also been reported. Admixed lymphocytes and plasma cells are common. These tumors may also show hemorrhage and necrosis as well as significant mitotic indices (389–392).

The distinction among follicular dendritic cell, interdigitating dendritic cell, and fibroblastic reticular cell neoplasms depends primarily on the immunohistochemical profile and the ultrastructural features. Follicular dendritic cells express vimentin, CD21, CD23, and CD35 and, occasionally, CD68 and S-100 (15,393). The EBV genome has been found in a subset of follicular dendritic cell tumors (244). Interdigitating dendritic cell tumors express vimentin and S-100, but they lack CD21, CD23, and CD35 (15,393). The fibroblastic reticular cell tumor

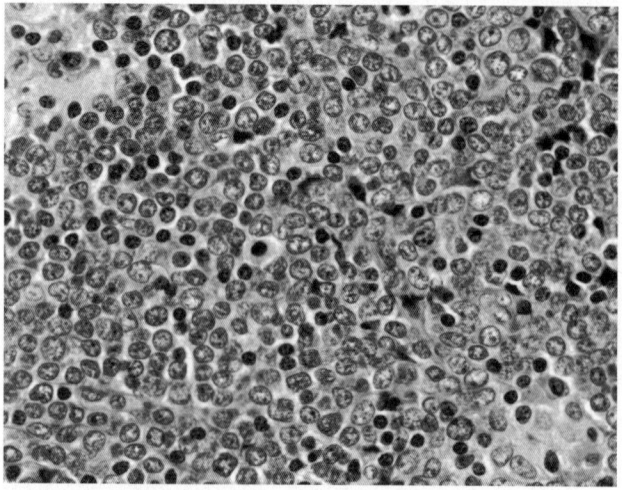

FIGURE 27.18. Myeloid sarcoma in lymph node. This 55-year-old man with history of myeloproliferative neoplasm presented with cervical lymphadenopathy, suspicious for lymphoma. The lymph node biopsy showed a monotonous population of neoplastic cells that contained moderately abundant cytoplasm and round to irregularly shaped nuclei with fine chromatin and small nucleoli. These neoplastic cells expressed myeloperoxidase, CD117, CD68, and CD43. (hematoxylin and eosin, original magnification: 400×).

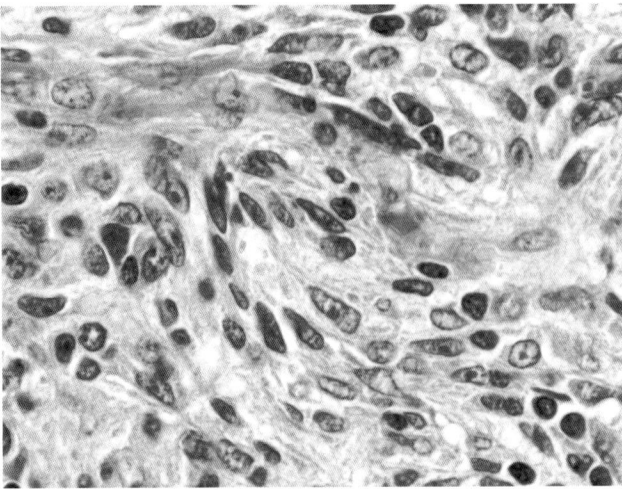

FIGURE 27.19. Follicular dendritic cell sarcoma. The histologic appearance of the follicular dendritic cell sarcoma is reminiscent of other spindle cell proliferations such as neoplasms exhibiting fibroblastic, smooth muscle, or metaplastic epithelial differentiation. Follicular dendritic cell sarcoma is composed of fascicles of spindle cells possessing pointed and elongated hyperchromatic nuclei (hematoxylin and eosin, original magnification: 400×). (Photomicrographs courtesy of Dr. Lawrence Weiss, Clarient, Aliso Viejo, CA.)

expresses vimentin, CD68, smooth muscle actin or desmin, and factor XIII (15,393).

The prognosis of these tumors can be difficult to predict because of the variation in morphologic appearance from case to case and the paucity of large clinicopathologic studies with adequate follow-up data. The follicular dendritic cell tumor, often referred to as *follicular dendritic sarcoma,* is capable of recurrence and metastasis, resulting in death (389–391,394). Significant cytologic atypia, necrosis, and an elevated mitotic index are features that have been suggested to indicate the possibility of an aggressive clinical course. Follicular dendritic cell tumors may coexist with Castleman disease of the hyaline-vascular, plasma cell, and mixed types (395). Interdigitating dendritic cell tumors are said to be more aggressive than follicular dendritic cell tumors (391–392,396). The patients with fibroblastic reticular cell tumors of lymph node appear to have pursued a benign clinical course (393) (see Chapter 48).

One must consider numerous entities in the differential diagnosis of dendritic cell neoplasms. If metastatic carcinoma, malignant melanoma, and other primary and metastatic sarcomas are excluded with attention to clinical history, morphologic detail, and immunophenotype, palisaded myofibroblastoma, true histiocytic lymphoma, and thymoma should also be considered. The distinction between reticulum cell tumors and carcinomas can be difficult, especially given the report of cytokeratin-positive tumors with reticulum cell morphology (397).

 SUMMARY AND CONCLUSIONS

A large and diverse variety of benign and malignant nonhematopoietic elements and proliferations may be encountered in lymph nodes. The benign elements include epithelial and mesenchymal congenital malformations, inclusions, and proliferations that must be distinguished from malignant neoplasms that secondarily involve lymph nodes. The malignant elements include a spectrum of primary and secondary epithelial and mesenchymal neoplasms that must be distinguished from a lymphoproliferative disorder, usually malignant lymphoma. Several nonlymphoid hematopoietic proliferations also may occur in lymph nodes and can be confused with malignant lymphoma. These pathologic processes usually can be recognized and interpreted correctly, based on careful evaluation of their

histopathologic features in conjunction with the clinical findings. The judicious use of immunohistochemistry serves as a useful adjunct to diagnosis and may contribute significantly to the accurate diagnosis of poorly differentiated neoplasms difficult to classify by histopathologic criteria alone.

References

1. Kant J, Jaffe ES. The interpretation of non-lymphoid elements in lymph node biopsy specimens. In: Jaffe ES, ed. *Surgical pathology of the lymph nodes and related organs.* Philadelphia: W.B. Saunders, 1985:412–437.
2. Ramaekers FC, Puts JJ, Moesker O, et al. Antibodies to intermediate filament proteins in the immunohistochemical identification of human tumours: an overview. *Histochem J* 1983;15:691–713.
3. Miettinen M. Immunohistochemistry of soft-tissue tumors. Possibilities and limitations in surgical pathology. *Pathol Annu* 1990;25(Pt 1):1–36.
4. Sheibani K, Tubbs RR. Enzyme immunohistochemistry: technical aspects. *Semin Diagn Pathol* 1984;1:235–250.
5. Kuroki M, Yamanaka T, Matsuo Y, et al. Immunochemical analysis of carcinoembryonic antigen (CEA)-related antigens differentially localized in intracellular granules of human neutrophils. *Immunol Invest* 1995;24:829–843.
6. Alvarez-Gago T, Bullon MM, Rivera F, et al. Intermediate filament aggregates in mitoses of primary cutaneous neuroendocrine (Merkel cell) carcinoma. *Histopathology* 1996;28:349–355.
7. Blessing K, Sanders DS, Grant JJ. Comparison of immunohistochemical staining of the novel antibody melan-A with S100 protein and HMB-45 in malignant melanoma and melanoma variants. *Histopathology* 1998;32:139–146.
8. Michie SA, Spagnolo DV, Dunn KA, et al. A panel approach to the evaluation of the sensitivity and specificity of antibodies for the diagnosis of routinely processed histologically undifferentiated human neoplasms. *Am J Clin Pathol* 1987;88:457–462.
9. Thomas ML, Lefrancois L. Differential expression of the leucocyte-common antigen family. *Immunol Today* 1988;9:320–326.
10. Pizzolo G, Sloane J, Beverley P, et al. Differential diagnosis of malignant lymphoma and nonlymphoid tumors using monoclonal anti-leucocyte antibody. *Cancer* 1980;46:2640–2647.
11. Battifora H, Trowbridge IS. A monoclonal antibody useful for the differential diagnosis between malignant lymphoma and nonhematopoietic neoplasms. *Cancer* 1983;51:816–821.
12. Warnke RA, Gatter KC, Falini B, et al. Diagnosis of human lymphoma with monoclonal antileukocyte antibodies. *N Engl J Med* 1983;309:1275–1281.
13. Kurtin PJ, Pinkus GS. Leukocyte common antigen—a diagnostic discriminant between hematopoietic and nonhematopoietic neoplasms in paraffin sections using monoclonal antibodies: correlation with immunologic studies and ultrastructural localization. *Hum Pathol* 1985;16:353–365.
14. Mason DY, Gatter KC. The role of immunocytochemistry in diagnostic pathology. *J Clin Pathol* 1987;40:1042–1054.
15. Swerdlow S, Campo E, Harris NL, et al., eds. *WHO classification of tumours of haematopoietic and lymphoid tissues,* 4th ed. IARC: Lyon, 2008.
16. Leoncini L, Del Vecchio MT, Kraft R, et al. Hodgkin's disease and CD30-positive anaplastic large cell lymphomas—a continuous spectrum of malignant disorders. A quantitative morphometric and immunohistologic study. *Am J Pathol* 1990;137:1047–1057.
17. Strickler JG, Audeh MW, Copenhaver CM, et al. Immunophenotypic differences between plasmacytoma/multiple myeloma and immunoblastic lymphoma. *Cancer* 1988;61:1782–1786.
18. McDonnell JM, Beschorner WE, Kuhajda FP, et al. Common leukocyte antigen staining of a primitive sarcoma. *Cancer* 1987;59:1438–1441.
19. Nandedkar MA, Palazzo J, Abbondanzo SL, et al. CD45 (leukocyte common antigen) immunoreactivity in metastatic undifferentiated and neuroendocrine carcinoma: a potential diagnostic pitfall. *Mod Pathol* 1998;11:1204–1210.
20. Ngo N, Patel K, Isaacson PG, et al. Leucocyte common antigen (CD45) and CD5 positivity in an "undifferentiated" carcinoma: a potential diagnostic pitfall. *J Clin Pathol* 2007;60:936–938.
21. Houreih MA, Eyden BP, Reeve N, et al. Aberrant leukocyte common antigen expression in metastatic small cell lung carcinoma: a rare finding and a potential diagnostic pitfall. *Appl Immunohistochem Mol Morphol* 2007;15:236–238.
22. Azumi N, Battifora H. The distribution of vimentin and keratin in epithelial and nonepithelial neoplasms. A comprehensive immunohistochemical study on formalin- and alcohol-fixed tumors. *Am J Clin Pathol* 1987;88:286–296.
23. Thomas P, Battifora H. Keratins versus epithelial membrane antigen in tumor diagnosis: an immunohistochemical comparison of five monoclonal antibodies. *Hum Pathol* 1987;18:728–734.
24. Moll R, Divo M, Langbein L. The human keratins: biology and pathology. *Histochem Cell Biol* 2008;129:705–733.
25. de Mascarel A, Merlio JP, Coindre JM, et al. Gastric large cell lymphoma expressing cytokeratin but no leukocyte common antigen. A diagnostic dilemma. *Am J Clin Pathol* 1989;91:478–481.
26. McCluggage WG, el-Agnaff M, O"Hara MD. Cytokeratin positive T cell malignant lymphoma. *J Clin Pathol* 1998;51:404–406.
27. Lasota J, Hyjek E, Koo CH, et al. Cytokeratin-positive large-cell lymphomas of B-cell lineage. A study of five phenotypically unusual cases verified by polymerase chain reaction. *Am J Surg Pathol* 1996;20:346–354.
28. Gustmann C, Altmannsberger M, Osborn M, et al. Cytokeratin expression and vimentin content in large cell anaplastic lymphomas and other non-Hodgkin's lymphomas. *Am J Pathol* 1991;138:1413–1422.
29. Wotherspoon AC, Norton AJ, Isaacson PG. Immunoreactive cytokeratins in plasmacytomas. *Histopathology* 1989;14:141–150.
30. Miettinen M, Virtanen I, Damjanov H. Coexpression of keratin and vimentin in epithelioid sarcoma. *Am J Surg Pathol* 1985;9:460–463.
31. Fletcher CDM. Soft tissue tumors. In: Fletcher CDM, ed. *Diagnostic histopathology of tumors,* 3rd ed. Philadelphia: Churchill Livingstone Elsevier, 2007:1527–1593.

32. Brown DC, Theaker JM, Banks PM, et al. Cytokeratin expression in smooth muscle and smooth muscle tumours. *Histopathology* 1987;11:477–486.
33. Norton AJ, Thomas JA, Isaacson PG. Cytokeratin-specific monoclonal antibodies are reactive with tumours of smooth muscle derivation. An immunocytochemical and biochemical study using antibodies to intermediate filament cytoskeletal proteins. *Histopathology* 1987;11:487–499.
34. Miettinen M. Immunoreactivity for cytokeratin and epithelial membrane antigen in leiomyosarcoma. *Arch Pathol Lab Med* 1988;112:637–640.
35. Huitfeldt HS, Brandtzaeg P. Various keratin antibodies produce immunohistochemical staining of human myocardium and myometrium. *Histochemistry* 1985;83:381–389.
36. Miettinen M, Franssila K. Immunohistochemical spectrum of malignant melanoma. The common presence of keratins. *Lab Invest* 1989;61:623–628.
37. Zarbo RJ, Gown AM, Nagle RB, et al. Anomalous cytokeratin expression in malignant melanoma: one- and two-dimensional western blot analysis and immunohistochemical survey of 100 melanomas. *Mod Pathol* 1990;3:494–501.
38. Ceriani RL, Thompson K, Peterson JA, et al. Surface differentiation antigens of human mammary epithelial cells carried on the human milk fat globule. *Proc Natl Acad Sci U S A* 1977;74:582–586.
39. Heyderman E, Steele K, Ormerod MG. A new antigen on the epithelial membrane: its immunoperoxidase localisation in normal and neoplastic tissue. *J Clin Pathol* 1979;32:35–39.
40. Heyderman E, Strudley I, Powell G, et al. (EMA)-E29. A comparison of its immunocytochemical reactivity with polyclonal anti-EMA antibodies and with another monoclonal antibody, HMFG-2. *Br J Cancer* 1985;52:355–361.
41. Mattes MJ, Major PP, Goldenberg DM, et al. Patterns of antigen distribution in human carcinomas. *Cancer Res* 1990;50:880s–884s.
42. Strickler JG, Herndier BG, Rouse RV. Immunohistochemical staining in malignant mesotheliomas. *Am J Clin Pathol* 1987;88:610–614.
43. Pinkus GS, Kurtin PJ. Epithelial membrane antigen—a diagnostic discriminant in surgical pathology: immunohistochemical profile in epithelial, mesenchymal, and hematopoietic neoplasms using paraffin sections and monoclonal antibodies. *Hum Pathol* 1985;16:929–940.
44. Ariza A, Bilbao JM, Rosai J. Immunohistochemical detection of epithelial membrane antigen in normal perineurial cells and perineurioma. *Am J Surg Pathol* 1988;12:678–683.
45. Delsol G, Gatter KC, Stein H, et al. Human lymphoid cells express epithelial membrane antigen. Implications for diagnosis of human neoplasms. *Lancet* 1984;2:1124–1129.
46. Delsol G, Al Saati T, Gatter KC, et al. Coexpression of epithelial membrane antigen (EMA), Ki-1, and interleukin-2 receptor by anaplastic large cell lymphomas. Diagnostic value in so-called malignant histiocytosis. *Am J Pathol* 1988;130:59–70.
47. Franke WW, Schmid E, Osborn M, et al. Different intermediate-sized filaments distinguished by immunofluorescence microscopy. *Proc Natl Acad Sci U S A* 1978;75:5034–5038.
48. Dabbs DJ, Geisinger KR, Norris HT. Intermediate filaments in endometrial and endocervical carcinomas. The diagnostic utility of vimentin patterns. *Am J Surg Pathol* 1986;10:568–576.
49. Miettinen M, Lehto VP, Badley RA, et al. Alveolar rhabdomyosarcoma. Demonstration of the muscle type of intermediate filament protein, desmin, as a diagnostic aid. *Am J Pathol* 1982;108:246–251.
50. Truong LD, Rangdaeng S, Cagle P, et al. The diagnostic utility of desmin. A study of 584 cases and review of the literature. *Am J Clin Pathol* 1990;93:305–314.
51. Seidal T, Kindblom LG, Angervall L. Myoglobin, desmin and vimentin in ultrastructurally proven rhabdomyomas and rhabdomyosarcomas. An immunohistochemical study utilizing a series of monoclonal and polyclonal antibodies. *Appl Pathol* 1987;5:201–219.
52. Miller F, Lazarides E, Elias J. Application of immunologic probes for contractile proteins to tissue sections. *Clin Immunol Immunopathol* 1976;5:416–428.
53. Miettinen M. Antibody specific to muscle actins in the diagnosis and classification of soft tissue tumors. *Am J Pathol* 1988;130:205–215.
54. Tsukada T, Tippens D, Gordon D, et al. HHF35, a muscle-actin-specific monoclonal antibody. I. Immunocytochemical and biochemical characterization. *Am J Pathol* 1987;126:51–60.
55. Tsukada T, McNutt MA, Ross R, et al. HHF35, a muscle actin-specific monoclonal antibody. II. Reactivity in normal, reactive, and neoplastic human tissues. *Am J Pathol* 1987;127:389–402.
56. Morotti RA, Nicol KK, Parham DM, et al. An immunohistochemical algorithm to facilitate diagnosis and subtyping of rhabdomyosarcoma: the Children's Oncology Group experience. *Am J Surg Pathol* 2006;30:962–968.
57. Cessna MH, Zhou H, Perkins SL, et al. Are myogenin and myoD1 expression specific for rhabdomyosarcoma? A study of 150 cases, with emphasis on spindle cell mimics. *Am J Surg Pathol* 2001;25:1150–1157.
58. Ozge-Anwar AH, Connell GE, Mustard JF. The activation of factor 8 by thrombin. *Blood* 1965;26:500–509.
59. McComb RD, Jones TR, Pizzo SV, et al. Specificity and sensitivity of immunohistochemical detection of factor VIII/von Willebrand factor antigen in formalin-fixed paraffin-embedded tissue. *J Histochem Cytochem* 1982;30:371–377.
60. Mukai K, Rosai J, Burgdorf WH. Localization of factor VIII-related antigen in vascular endothelial cells using an immunoperoxidase method. *Am J Surg Pathol* 1980;4:273–276.
61. Ordonez NG, Batsakis JG. Comparison of Ulex europaeus I lectin and factor VIII-related antigen in vascular lesions. *Arch Pathol Lab Med* 1984;108:129–132.
62. Miettinen M, Lindenmayer AE, Chaubal A. Endothelial cell markers CD31, CD34, and BNH9 antibody to H- and Y-antigens—evaluation of their specificity and sensitivity in the diagnosis of vascular tumors and comparison with von Willebrand factor. *Mod Pathol* 1994;7:82–90.
63. Traweek ST, Kandalaft PL, Mehta P, et al. The human hematopoietic progenitor cell antigen (CD34) in vascular neoplasia. *Am J Clin Pathol* 1991;96:25–31.
64. Ramani P, Bradley NJ, Fletcher CD. QBEND/10, a new monoclonal antibody to endothelium: assessment of its diagnostic utility in paraffin sections. *Histopathology* 1990;17:237–242.
65. Moore BW. A soluble protein characteristic of the nervous system. *Biochem Biophys Res Commun* 1965;19:739–744.
66. Nakajima T, Watanabe S, Sato Y, et al. An immunoperoxidase study of S-100 protein distribution in normal and neoplastic tissues. *Am J Surg Pathol* 1982;6:715–727.
67. Cocchia D, Lauriola L, Stolfi VM, et al. S-100 antigen labels neoplastic cells in liposarcoma and cartilaginous tumours. *Virchows Arch A Pathol Anat Histopathol* 1983;402:139–145.
68. Watanabe S, Nakajima T, Shimosato Y, et al. Neoplasms of T-zone histiocyte with S100 protein. *Cancer* 1983;51:1412–1424.
69. Cochran AJ, Wen DR. S-100 protein as a marker for melanocytic and other tumours. *Pathology* 1985;17:340–345.
70. Kawahara E, Oda Y, Ooi A, et al. Expression of glial fibrillary acidic protein (GFAP) in peripheral nerve sheath tumors. A comparative study of immunoreactivity of GFAP, vimentin, S-100 protein, and neurofilament in 38 schwannomas and 18 neurofibromas. *Am J Surg Pathol* 1988;12:115–120.
71. Mazur MT, Shultz JJ, Myers JL. Granular cell tumor. Immunohistochemical analysis of 21 benign tumors and one malignant tumor. *Arch Pathol Lab Med* 1990;114:692–696.
72. Drier JK, Swanson PE, Cherwitz DL, et al. S100 protein immunoreactivity in poorly differentiated carcinomas. Immunohistochemical comparison with malignant melanoma. *Arch Pathol Lab Med* 1987;111:447–452.
73. Herrera GA, Turbat-Herrera EA, Lott RL. S-100 protein expression by primary and metastatic adenocarcinomas. *Am J Clin Pathol* 1988;89:168–176.
74. Lloyd RV, Blaivas M, Wilson BS. Distribution of chromogranin and S100 protein in normal and abnormal adrenal medullary tissues. *Arch Pathol Lab Med* 1985;109:633–635.
75. Tapia FJ, Polak JM, Barbosa AJ, et al. Neuron-specific enolase is produced by neuroendocrine tumours. *Lancet* 1981;1:808–811.
76. Leader M, Collins M, Patel J, et al. Antineuron specific enolase staining reactions in sarcomas and carcinomas: its lack of neuroendocrine specificity. *J Clin Pathol* 1986;39:1186–1192.
77. Wiedenmann B, Franke WW. Identification and localization of synaptophysin, an integral membrane glycoprotein of Mr 38,000 characteristic of presynaptic vesicles. *Cell* 1985;41:1017–1028.
78. Trojanowski J. Immunohistochemistry of neural filament proteins and their diagnostic applications. In: DeLellis RA, ed. *Advances in immunohistochemistry*. New York: Raven Press, 1988:237–260.
79. Ridolfi RL, Rosen PP, Thaler H. Nevus cell aggregates associated with lymph nodes: estimated frequency and clinical significance. *Cancer* 1977;39:164–171.
80. Gadaleanu V, Muresan R. Inclusions of benign nevus cells in the capsule of axillary lymph nodes in three cases of breast cancer. *Morphol Embryol (Bucur)* 1984;30:137–139.
81. Azzopardi JG, Ross CM, Frizzera G. Blue naevi of lymph node capsule. *Histopathology* 1977;1:451–461.
82. Bansal RK, Bhaduri AS, Pancholi YJ, et al. Cellular blue nevus with nevus cells in regional lymph nodes: a lesion that mimics melanoma. *Indian J Cancer* 1989;26:145–150.
83. Holt JB, Sangueza OP, Levine EA, et al. Nodal melanocytic nevi in sentinel lymph nodes. Correlation with melanoma-associated cutaneous nevi. *Am J Clin Pathol* 2004;121:58–63.
84. Carson KF, Wen DR, Li PX, et al. Nodal nevi and cutaneous melanomas. *Am J Surg Pathol* 1996;20:834–840.
85. Fontaine D, Parkhill W, Greer W, et al. Nevus cells in lymph nodes: an association with congenital cutaneous nevi. *Am J Dermatopathol* 2002;24:1–5.
86. Biddle DA, Evans HL, Kemp BL, et al. Intraparenchymal nevus cell aggregates in lymph nodes: a possible diagnostic pitfall with malignant melanoma and carcinoma. *Am J Surg Pathol* 2003;27:673–681.
87. Prieto VG. Sentinel lymph nodes in cutaneous melanoma. *Clin Lab Med* 2011;31:301–310.
88. Lohmann CM, Iversen K, Jungbluth AA, et al. Expression of melanocyte differentiation antigens and ki-67 in nodal nevi and comparison of ki-67 expression with metastatic melanoma. *Am J Surg Pathol* 2002;26:1351–1317.
89. Johnson WT, Helwig EB. Benign nevus cells in the capsule of lymph nodes. *Cancer* 1969;23:747–753.
90. Hsu YK, Parmley TH, Rosenshein NB, et al. Neoplastic and non-neoplastic mesothelial proliferations in pelvic lymph nodes. *Obstet Gynecol* 1980;55:83–88.
91. Brooks JS, LiVolsi VA, Pietra GG. Mesothelial cell inclusions in mediastinal lymph nodes mimicking metastatic carcinoma. *Am J Clin Pathol* 1990;93:741–748.
92. Argani P, Rosai J. Hyperplastic mesothelial cells in lymph nodes: report of six cases of a benign process that can stimulate metastatic involvement by mesothelioma or carcinoma. *Hum Pathol* 1998;29:339–346.
93. Clement PB, Young RH, Oliva E, et al. Hyperplastic mesothelial cells within abdominal lymph nodes: mimic of metastatic ovarian carcinoma and serous borderline tumor—a report of two cases associated with ovarian neoplasms. *Mod Pathol* 1996;9:879–886.
94. Suarez Vilela D, Izquierdo Garcia FM. Embolization of mesothelial cells in lymphatics: the route to mesothelial inclusions in lymph nodes? *Histopathology* 1998;33:570–575.
95. Parkash V, Vidwans M, Carter D. Benign mesothelial cells in mediastinal lymph nodes. *Am J Surg Pathol* 1999;23:1264–1269.
96. Rutty GN, Lauder I. Mesothelial cell inclusions within mediastinal lymph nodes. *Histopathology* 1994;25:483–487.
97. Colby TV. Benign mesothelial cells in lymph node. *Adv Anat Pathol* 1999;6:41–48.
98. Kir G, Eren S, Kir M. Hyperplastic mesothelial cells in pelvic and abdominal lymph node sinuses mimicking metastatic ovarian microinvasive serous borderline tumor. *Eur J Gynaecol Oncol* 2004;25:236–238.
99. Schnurr RC, Delgado G, Chun B. Benign glandular inclusions in para-aortic lymph nodes in women undergoing lymphadenectomies. *Am J Obstet Gynecol* 1978;130:813–816.
100. Mills SE. Decidua and squamous metaplasia in abdominopelvic lymph nodes. *Int J Gynecol Pathol* 1983;2:209–215.
101. Clement PB. Diseases of the peritoneum (including endometriosis). In: Kurman RJ, ed. *Blaustein's pathology of the female genital tract*. New York: Springer-Verlag, 1995:647–782.
102. Corben AD, Nehhozina T, Garg K, et al. Endosalpingiosis in axillary lymph nodes: a possible pitfall in the staging of patients with breast carcinoma. *Am J Surg Pathol* 2010;34:1211–1216.
103. Henley JD, Michael HB, English GW, et al. Benign mullerian lymph node inclusions. An unusual case with implications for pathogenesis and review of the literature. *Arch Pathol Lab Med* 1995;119:841–844.
104. Piana S, Asioli S, Cavazza A. Benign Mullerian inclusions coexisting with breast metastatic carcinoma in an axillary lymph node. *Virchows Arch* 2005;446:467–469.

105. Sampson JA. Metastatic or embolic endometriosis, due to the menstrual dissemination of endometrial tissue into the venous circulation. *Am J Pathol* 1927;3:93–110.
106. Javert CT. Pathogenesis of endometriosis based on endometrial homeoplasia, direct extension, exfoliation and implantation, lymphatic and hematogenous metastasis, including five case reports of endometrial tissue in pelvic lymph nodes. *Cancer* 1949;2:399–410.
107. Karp LA. Czernobilsky B. Glandular inclusions in pelvic and abdominal para-aortic lymph nodes. A study of autopsy and surgical material in males and females. *Am J Clin Pathol* 1969;52:212–218.
108. Huntrakoon M. Benign glandular inclusions in the abdominal lymph nodes of a man. *Hum Pathol* 1985;16:644–646.
109. Zanetti G. Epithelial inclusions and Tamm-Horsfall protein in paranephric lymph nodes. A light microscopy and immunocytochemical study. *Virchows Arch A Pathol Anat Histopathol* 1986;408:593–601.
110. Micheau C. [Salivary ectopia. General review]. *Arch Anat Pathol (Paris)* 1969;17:179–186.
111. Gricouroff G. Epithelial inclusions in the lymph nodes. Diagnostic, histogenetic, and prognostic problems. *Diagn Gynecol Obstet* 1982;4:285–293.
112. Goldman RL, Klein HZ. Proliferative sialometaplasia arising in an intraparotid lymph node. *Am J Clin Pathol* 1986;86:116–119.
113. Ryan JR, Ioachim HL, Marmer J, et al. Acquired immune deficiency syndrome—related lymphadenopathies presenting in the salivary gland lymph nodes. *Arch Otolaryngol* 1985;111:554–556.
114. Smith FB, Rajdeo H, Panesar N, et al. Benign lymphoepithelial lesion of the parotid gland in intravenous drug users. *Arch Pathol Lab Med* 1988;112:742–745.
115. Ansari-Lari MA, Westra WH. The prevalence and significance of clinically unsuspected neoplasms in cervical lymph nodes. *Head Neck* 2003;25:841–847.
116. Niwayama G. Inclusions of non-neoplastic thyroid tissue within cervical lymph nodes. *Tohoku J Exp Med* 1968;96:45–62.
117. Ibrahim NB, Milewski PJ, Gillett R, et al. Benign thyroid inclusions within cervical lymph nodes: an alarming incidental finding. *Aust N Z J Surg* 1981;51:188–189.
118. Batsakis JG, El-Naggar AK, Luna MA. Thyroid gland ectopias. *Ann Otol Rhinol Laryngol* 1996;105:996–1000.
119. LiVolsi VA, Perzin KH, Savetsky L. Carcinoma arising in median ectopic thyroid (including thyroglossal duct tissue). *Cancer* 1974;34:1303–1315.
120. Wang Z, Qiu S, Eltorky MA, et al. Histopathologic and immunohistochemical characterization of a primary papillary thyroid carcinoma in the lateral cervical lymph node. *Exp Mol Pathol* 2007;82:91–94.
121. Sampson RJ, Oka H, Key CR, et al. Metastases from occult thyroid carcinoma. An autopsy study from Hiroshima and Nagasaki, Japan. *Cancer* 1970;25:803–811.
122. Walker AN, Fechner RE. Papillary carcinoma arising from ectopic breast tissue in an axillary lymph node. *Diagn Gynecol Obstet* 1982;4:141–145.
123. Mesa-Tejada R, Palakodety RB, Leon JA, et al. Immunocytochemical distribution of a breast carcinoma associated glycoprotein identified by monoclonal antibodies. *Am J Pathol* 1988;130:305–314.
124. Zynger DL, McCallum JC, Everton MJ, et al. Paracortical axillary sentinel lymph node ectopic breast tissue. *Pathol Res Pract* 2009;205:427–432.
125. Kadowaki M, Nagashima T, Sakata H, et al. Ectopic breast tissue in axillary lymph node. *Breast Cancer* 2007;14:425–428.
126. Maiorano E, Mazzarol GM, Pruneri G, et al. Ectopic breast tissue as a possible cause of false-positive axillary sentinel lymph node biopsies. *Am J Surg Pathol* 2003;27:513–518.
127. Baab GH, McBride CM. Malignant melanoma: the patient with an unknown site of primary origin. *Arch Surg* 1975;110:896–900.
128. Cochran AJ, Wen DR, Morton DL. Occult tumor cells in the lymph nodes of patients with pathological stage I malignant melanoma. An immunohistological study. *Am J Surg Pathol* 1988;12:612–618.
129. Shenoy BV, Fort L III, Benjamin SP. Malignant melanoma primary in lymph node. The case of the missing link. *Am J Surg Pathol* 1987;11:140–146.
130. Jonk A, Kroon BB, Rumke P, et al. Lymph node metastasis from melanoma with an unknown primary site. *Br J Surg* 1990;77:665–668.
131. Nishikawa H, Kirkham N, Hogbin BM. Synchronous extra-parotid Warthin's tumour. *J Laryngol Otol* 1989;103:792–793.
132. Luna MA. Salivary glands. In: Pilch BZ, ed. *Head and neck surgical pathology*. Philadelphia: Lippincott Williams & Wilkins, 2001:284–350.
133. Miller R, Yanagihara ET, Dubrow AA, et al. Malignant lymphoma in the Warthin's tumor. Report of a case. *Cancer* 1982;50:2948–2950.
134. Bunker ML, Locker J. Warthin"s tumor with malignant lymphoma. DNA analysis of paraffin-embedded tissue. *Am J Clin Pathol* 1989;91:341–344.
135. Medeiros LJ, Rizzi R, Lardelli P, et al. Malignant lymphoma involving a Warthin's tumor: a case with immunophenotypic and gene rearrangement analysis. *Hum Pathol* 1990;21:974–977.
136. Melato M, Falconieri G, Fanin R, et al. Hodgkin's disease occurring in a Warthin's tumor: first case report. *Pathol Res Pract* 1986;181:615–620.
137. Morrison GA, Shaw HJ. Squamous carcinoma arising within a Warthin's tumour of the parotid gland. *J Laryngol Otol* 1988;102:1189–1191.
138. Onder T, Tiwari RM, van der Waal I, et al. Malignant adenolymphoma of the parotid gland: report of carcinomatous transformation. *J Laryngol Otol* 1990;104:656–661.
139. Healey WV, Perzin KH, Smith L. Mucoepidermoid carcinoma of salivary gland origin. Classification, clinical-pathologic correlation, and results of treatment. *Cancer* 1970;26:368–388.
140. Perzin KH, Livolsi VA. Acinic cell carcinoma arising in ectopic salivary gland tissue. *Cancer* 1980;45:967–972.
141. Smith A, Winkler B, Perzin KH, et al. Mucoepidermoid carcinoma arising in an intraparotid lymph node. *Cancer* 1985;55:400–403.
142. Adkins GF, Hinckley DM. Primary muco-epidermoid carcinoma arising in a parotid lymph node. *Aust N Z J Surg* 1989;59:433–435.
143. Zapatero J, Baamonde C, Gonzalez Aragoneses F, et al. Ectopic goiters of the mediastinum: presentation of two cases and review of the literature. *Jpn J Surg* 1988;18:105–109.
144. Matsumoto K, Watanabe Y, Asano G. Thyroid papillary carcinoma arising in ectopic thyroid tissue within a branchial cleft cyst. *Pathol Int* 1999;49:444–446.
145. Mehmood RK, Basha SI, Ghareeb E. A case of papillary carcinoma arising in ectopic thyroid tissue within a branchial cyst with neck node metastasis. *Ear Nose Throat J* 2006;85:675–676.
146. Haferkamp O, Rosenau W, Lennert K. Vascular transformation of lymph node sinuses due to venous obstruction. *Arch Pathol* 1971;92:81–813.
147. Bedrosian SA, Goldman RL. Nodal angiomatosis: relationship to vascular transformation of lymph nodes. *Arch Pathol Lab Med* 1984;108:864–845.
148. Dorfman RF. Kaposi's sarcoma revisited. *Hum Pathol* 1984;15:1013–1017.
149. Chan JK, Warnke RA, Dorfman R. Vascular transformation of sinuses in lymph nodes. A study of its morphological spectrum and distinction from Kaposi's sarcoma. *Am J Surg Pathol* 1991;15:732–743.
150. Fayemi AO, Toker C. Nodal angiomatosis. *Arch Pathol* 1975;99:170–172.
151. Chan JK, Frizzera G, Fletcher CD, et al. Primary vascular tumors of lymph nodes other than Kaposi's sarcoma. Analysis of 39 cases and delineation of two new entities. *Am J Surg Pathol* 1992;16:335–350.
152. Al-Jabi M, Tolnai G, McCaughey WT. Angiofollicular lymphoid hyperplasia in an angiolipomatous mass. *Arch Pathol Lab Med* 1980;104:313–315.
153. Madero S, Onate JM, Garzon A. Giant lymph node hyperplasia in an angiolipomatous mediastinal mass. *Arch Pathol Lab Med* 1986;110:853–855.
154. Gupta IM. Haemangioma in a lymph node. *Indian J Pathol Bacteriol* 1964;55:110–111.
155. Almagro UA, Choi H, Rouse TM. Hemangioma in a lymph node. *Arch Pathol Lab Med* 1985;109:576–578.
156. Kasznica J, Sideli RV, Collins MH. Lymph node hemangioma. *Arch Pathol Lab Med* 1989;113:804–807.
157. Urabe A, Tsuneyoshi M, Enjoji M. Epithelioid hemangioma versus Kimura's disease. A comparative clinicopathologic study. *Am J Surg Pathol* 1987;11:758–766.
158. Gerald W, Kostianovsky M, Rosai J. Development of vascular neoplasia in Castleman's disease. Report of seven cases. *Am J Surg Pathol* 1990;14:603–614.
159. Tsang WY, Chan JK, Dorfman RF, et al. Vasoproliferative lesions of the lymph node. *Pathol Annu* 1994;29(Pt 1):63–133.
160. Williams HB. Hemangiomas and lymphangiomas. *Adv Surg* 1981;15:317–349.
161. Iwasa Y, Tachibana M, Ito H, et al. Extrapulmonary lymphangioleiomyomatosis in pelvic and paraaortic lymph nodes associated with uterine cancer: a report of 3 cases. *Int J Gynecol Pathol* 2011;30:470–475.
162. Kebria M, Black D, Borelli C, et al. Primary retroperitoneal lymphangioleiomyomatosis in a postmenopausal woman: a case report and review of the literature. *Int J Gynecol Cancer* 2007;17:528–532.
163. Kamitani T, Yabuuchi H, Soeda H, et al. A case of lymphangioleiomyomatosis affecting the supraclavicular lymph nodes. *J Comput Assist Tomogr* 2006;30:279–282.
164. Wolff M. Lymphangiomyoma: clinicopathologic study and ultrastructural confirmation of its histogenesis. *Cancer* 1973;31:988–1007.
165. McIntosh GS, Dutoit SH, Chronos NV, et al. Multiple unilateral renal angiomyolipomas with regional lymphangioleiomyomatosis. *J Urol* 1989;142:1305–1307.
166. Monteforte WJ Jr, Kohnen PW. Angiomyolipomas in a case of lymphangiomyomatosis syndrome: relationships to tuberous sclerosis. *Cancer* 1974;34:317–321.
167. Kaku T, Toyoshima S, Enjoji M, et al. Tuberous sclerosis with pulmonary and lymph node involvement. Relationship to lymphangiomyomatosis. *Acta Pathol Jpn* 1983;33:395–401.
168. Corrin B, Liebow AA, Friedman PJ. Pulmonary lymphangiomyomatosis. A review. *Am J Pathol* 1975;79:348–382.
169. Chan JK, Tsang WY, Pau MY, et al. Lymphangiomyomatosis and angiomyolipoma: closely related entities characterized by hamartomatous proliferation of HMB-45-positive smooth muscle. *Histopathology* 1993;22:445–455.
170. van Haelst UJ, Pruszczynski M, ten Cate LN, et al. Ultrastructural and immunohistochemical study of epithelioid hemangioendothelioma of bone: coexpression of epithelial and endothelial markers. *Ultrastruct Pathol* 1990;14:141–149.
171. Weiss SW, Enzinger FM. Epithelioid hemangioendothelioma: a vascular tumor often mistaken for a carcinoma. *Cancer* 1982;50:970–981.
172. Mendlick MR, Nelson M, Pickering D, et al. Translocation t(1;3)(p36.3;q25) is a nonrandom aberration in epithelioid hemangioendothelioma. *Am J Surg Pathol* 2001;25:684–687.
173. Woelfel C, Liehr T, Weise A, et al. Molecular cytogenetic characterization of epithelioid hemangioendothelioma. *Cancer Genet* 2011;204:671–676.
174. Errani C, Zhang L, Sung YS, et al. A novel WWTR1-CAMTA1 gene fusion is a consistent abnormality in epithelioid hemangioendothelioma of different anatomic sites. *Genes Chromosomes Cancer* 2011;50:644–653.
175. Epidemiologic aspects of the current outbreak of Kaposi's sarcoma and opportunistic infections. *N Engl J Med* 1982;306:248–252.
176. Friedman-Kien AE, Laubenstein LJ, Rubinstein P, et al. Disseminated Kaposi's sarcoma in homosexual men. *Ann Intern Med* 1982;96:693–700.
177. Beral V. Epidemiology of Kaposi's sarcoma. *Cancer Surv* 1991;10:5–22.
178. Peterman TA, Jaffe HW, Friedman-Kien AE, et al. The aetiology of Kaposi's sarcoma. *Cancer Surv* 1991;10:23–37.
179. Safai B, Good RA. Kaposi's sarcoma: a review and recent developments. *Clin Bull* 1980;10:62–69.
180. Santucci M, Pimpinelli N, Moretti S, et al. Classic and immunodeficiency-associated Kaposi's sarcoma. Clinical, histologic, and immunologic correlations. *Arch Pathol Lab Med* 1988;112:1214–1220.
181. Biggar RJ, Rabkin CS. The epidemiology of AIDS—related neoplasms. *Hematol Oncol Clin North Am* 1996;10:997–1010.
182. Franceschi S, Maso LD, Rickenbach M, et al. Kaposi sarcoma incidence in the Swiss HIV Cohort Study before and after highly active antiretroviral therapy. *Br J Cancer* 2008;99:800–804.
183. Uldrick TS. Whitby D. Update on KSHV epidemiology, Kaposi sarcoma pathogenesis, and treatment of Kaposi sarcoma. *Cancer Lett* 2011;305:150–162.
184. Maurer T, Ponte M, Leslie K. HIV-associated Kaposi's sarcoma with a high CD4 count and a low viral load. *N Engl J Med* 2007;357:1352–1353.
185. Ioachim HL, Adsay V, Giancotti FR, et al. Kaposi's sarcoma of internal organs. A multiparameter study of 86 cases. *Cancer* 1995;75:1376–1385.
186. Rabkin CS, Bedi G, Musaba E, et al. AIDS-related Kaposi's sarcoma is a clonal neoplasm. *Clin Cancer Res* 1995;1:257–260.
187. Hong YK, Foreman K, Shin JW, et al. Lymphatic reprogramming of blood vascular endothelium by Kaposi sarcoma-associated herpesvirus. *Nat Genet* 2004;36:683–685.
188. Gill PS. The origin of Kaposi sarcoma. *J Natl Cancer Inst* 2007;99:1063.
189. Gill PS, Tsai YC, Rao AP, et al. Evidence for multiclonality in multicentric Kaposi's sarcoma. *Proc Natl Acad Sci U S A* 1998;95:8257–8261.
190. Rabkin CS, Janz S, Lash A, et al. Monoclonal origin of multicentric Kaposi's sarcoma lesions. *N Engl J Med* 1997;336:988–993.
191. Dukers NH, Renwick N, Prins M, et al. Risk factors for human herpesvirus 8 seropositivity and seroconversion in a cohort of homosexual men. *Am J Epidemiol* 2000;151:213–224.

192. Beral V, Bull D, Darby S, et al. Risk of Kaposi's sarcoma and sexual practices associated with faecal contact in homosexual or bisexual men with AIDS. *Lancet* 1992;339:632–635.
193. Chang Y, Cesarman E, Pessin MS, et al. Identification of herpesvirus-like DNA sequences in AIDS-associated Kaposi's sarcoma. *Science* 1994;266:1865–1869.
194. Cesarman E, Knowles DM. Kaposi's sarcoma-associated herpesvirus: a lymphotropic human herpesvirus associated with Kaposi's sarcoma, primary effusion lymphoma, and multicentric Castleman's disease. *Semin Diagn Pathol* 1997;14:54–66.
195. Moore PS, Gao SJ, Dominguez G, et al. Primary characterization of a herpesvirus agent associated with Kaposi's sarcomae. *J Virol* 1996;70:549–558.
196. Cesarman E, Nador RG, Bai F, et al. Kaposi's sarcoma-associated herpesvirus contains G protein-coupled receptor and cyclin D homologs which are expressed in Kaposi's sarcoma and malignant lymphoma. *J Virol* 1996;70:8218–8223.
197. Mesri EA, Cesarman E, Arvanitakis L, et al. Human herpesvirus-8/Kaposi's sarcoma-associated herpesvirus is a new transmissible virus that infects B cells. *J Exp Med* 1996;183:2385–2390.
198. Boshoff C, Schulz TF, Kennedy MM, et al. Kaposi's sarcoma-associated herpesvirus infects endothelial and spindle cells. *Nat Med* 1995;1:1274–1278.
199. Reed JA, Nador RG, Spaulding D, et al. Demonstration of Kaposi's sarcoma-associated herpes virus cyclin D homolog in cutaneous Kaposi's sarcoma by colorimetric *in situ* hybridization using a catalyzed signal amplification system. *Blood* 1998;91:3825–3832.
200. Knowles DM, Cesarman E. The Kaposi's sarcoma-associated herpesvirus (human herpesvirus-8) in Kaposi's sarcoma, malignant lymphoma, and other diseases. *Ann Oncol* 1997;8(Suppl 2):123–129.
201. Dezube BJ. Clinical presentation and natural history of AIDS—related Kaposi's sarcoma. *Hematol Oncol Clin North Am* 1996;10:1023–1029.
202. Niedt GW, Schinella RA. Acquired immunodeficiency syndrome. Clinicopathologic study of 56 autopsies. *Arch Pathol Lab Med* 1985;109:727–734.
203. Nichols CM, Flaitz CM, Hicks MJ. Treating Kaposi's lesions in the HIV-infected patient. *J Am Dent Assoc* 1993;124:78–84.
204. Diebold J, Marche C, Audouin J, et al. Lymph node modification in patients with the acquired immunodeficiency syndrome (AIDS) or with AIDS related complex (ARC). A histological, immuno-histopathological and ultrastructural study of 45 cases. *Pathol Res Pract* 1985;180:590–611.
205. Chadburn A, Metroka C, Mouradian J. Progressive lymph node histology and its prognostic value in patients with acquired immunodeficiency syndrome and AIDS-related complex. *Hum Pathol* 1989;20:579–587.
206. Finkbeiner WE, Egbert BM, Groundwater JR, et al. Kaposi's sarcoma in young homosexual men: a histopathologic study with particular reference to lymph node involvement. *Arch Pathol Lab Med* 1982;106:261–264.
207. Perlow LS, Taff ML, Orsini JM, et al. Kaposi's sarcoma in a young homosexual man. Association with angiofollicular lymphoid hyperplasia and a malignant lymphoproliferative disorder. *Arch Pathol Lab Med* 1983;107:510–513.
208. Harris NL. Hypervascular follicular hyperplasia and Kaposi's sarcoma in patients at risk for AIDS. *N Engl J Med* 1984;310:462–463.
209. Kaplan MH, Susin M, Pahwa SG, et al. Neoplastic complications of HTLV-III infection. Lymphomas and solid tumors. *Am J Med* 1987;82:389–396.
210. Ioachim HL, Lerner CW, Tapper ML. Lymphadenopathies in homosexual men. Relationships with the acquired immune deficiency syndrome. *JAMA* 1983;250:1306–1309.
211. Amberson JB, DiCarlo EF, Metroka CE, et al. Diagnostic pathology in the acquired immunodeficiency syndrome. Surgical pathology and cytology experience with 67 patients. *Arch Pathol Lab Med* 1985;109:345–351.
212. Cockerell CJ. Histopathological features of Kaposi's sarcoma in HIV infected individuals. *Cancer Surv* 1991;10:73–89.
213. Lubin J, Rywlin AM. Lymphoma-like lymph node changes in Kaposi's sarcoma. Two additional cases. *Arch Pathol* 1971;92:338–341.
214. Amazon K, Rywlin AM. Subtle clues to diagnosis by conventional microscopy. Lymph node involvement in Kaposi's sarcoma. *Am J Dermatopathol* 1979;1:173–176.
215. Beckstead JH, Wood GS, Fletcher V. Evidence for the origin of Kaposi's sarcoma from lymphatic endothelium. *Am J Pathol* 1985;119:294–300.
216. Schulze HJ, Rutten A, Mahrle G, et al. Initial lesions of HIV-related Kaposi's sarcoma—a histological, immunohistochemical, and ultrastructural study. *Arch Dermatol Res* 1987;279:499–503.
217. Russell Jones R, Orchard G, Zelger B, et al. Immunostaining for CD31 and CD34 in Kaposi sarcoma. *J Clin Pathol* 1995;48:1011–1016.
218. Cheuk W, Wong KO, Wong CS, et al. Immunostaining for human herpesvirus 8 latent nuclear antigen-1 helps distinguish Kaposi sarcoma from its mimickers. *Am J Clin Pathol* 2004;121:335–342.
219. Robin YM, Guillou L, Michels JJ, et al. Human herpesvirus 8 immunostaining: a sensitive and specific method for diagnosing Kaposi sarcoma in paraffin-embedded sections. *Am J Clin Pathol* 2004;121:330–334.
220. Schwartz EJ, Dorfman RF, Kohler S. Human herpesvirus-8 latent nuclear antigen-1 expression in endemic Kaposi sarcoma: an immunohistochemical study of 16 cases. *Am J Surg Pathol* 2003;27:1546–1550.
221. Patel RM, Goldblum JR, Hsi ED. Immunohistochemical detection of human herpes virus-8 latent nuclear antigen-1 is useful in the diagnosis of Kaposi sarcoma. *Mod Pathol* 2004;17:456–460.
222. Hammock L, Reisenauer A, Wang W, et al. Latency-associated nuclear antigen expression and human herpesvirus-8 polymerase chain reaction in the evaluation of Kaposi sarcoma and other vascular tumors in HIV-positive patients. *Mod Pathol* 2005;18:463–468.
223. Dictor M, Carlen B, Bendsoe N, et al. Ultrastructural development of Kaposi's sarcoma in relation to the dermal microvasculature. *Virchows Arch A Pathol Anat Histopathol* 1991;419:35–43.
224. Marquart KH. Weibel-Palade bodies in Kaposi's sarcoma cells. *J Clin Pathol* 1987;40:933.
225. Ro JY, Ayala AG, el-Naggar A, et al. Angiomyolipoma of kidney with lymph node involvement. DNA flow cytometric analysis. *Arch Pathol Lab Med* 1990;114:65–67.
226. Relman DA, Loutit JS, Schmidt TM, et al. The agent of bacillary angiomatosis. An approach to the identification of uncultured pathogens. *N Engl J Med* 1990;323:1573–1580.
227. Welch DF, Pickett DA, Slater LN, et al. Rochalimaea henselae sp. nov., a cause of septicemia, bacillary angiomatosis, and parenchymal bacillary peliosis. *J Clin Microbiol* 1992;30:275–280.
228. Koehler JE, Quinn FD, Berger TG, et al. Isolation of Rochalimaea species from cutaneous and osseous lesions of bacillary angiomatosis. *N Engl J Med* 1992;327:1625–1631.
229. Stoler MH, Bonfiglio TA, Steigbigel RT, et al. An atypical subcutaneous infection associated with acquired immune deficiency syndrome. *Am J Clin Pathol* 1983;80:714–718.
230. LeBoit PE, Berger TG, Egbert BM, et al. Epithelioid haemangioma-like vascular proliferation in AIDS: manifestation of cat scratch disease bacillus infection? *Lancet* 1988;1:960–963.
231. LeBoit PE, Berger TG, Egbert BM, et al. Bacillary angiomatosis. The histopathology and differential diagnosis of a pseudoneoplastic infection in patients with human immunodeficiency virus disease. *Am J Surg Pathol* 1989;13:909–920.
232. Cockerell CJ, Whitlow MA, Webster GF, et al. Epithelioid angiomatosis: a distinct vascular disorder in patients with the acquired immunodeficiency syndrome or AIDS-related complex. *Lancet* 1987;2:654–656.
233. Baron AL, Steinbach LS, LeBoit PE, et al. Osteolytic lesions and bacillary angiomatosis in HIV infection: radiologic differentiation from AIDS-related Kaposi sarcoma. *Radiology* 1990;177:77–81.
234. Moore EH, Russell LA, Klein JS, et al. Bacillary angiomatosis in patients with AIDS: multiorgan imaging findings. *Radiology* 1995;197:67–72.
235. Kemper CA, Lombard CM, Deresinski SC, et al. Visceral bacillary epithelioid angiomatosis: possible manifestations of disseminated cat scratch disease in the immunocompromised host: a report of two cases. *Am J Med* 1990;89:216–222.
236. Adal KA, Cockerell CJ, Petri WA Jr. Cat scratch disease, bacillary angiomatosis, and other infections due to Rochalimaea. *N Engl J Med* 1994;330:1509–1515.
237. Tappero JW, Mohle-Boetani J, Koehler JE, et al. The epidemiology of bacillary angiomatosis and bacillary peliosis. *JAMA* 1993;269:770–775.
238. Szaniawski WK, Don PC, Bitterman SR, et al. Epithelioid angiomatosis in patients with AIDS. Report of seven cases and review of the literature. *J Am Acad Dermatol* 1990;23:41–48.
239. Chan JK, Lewin KJ, Lombard CM, et al. Histopathology of bacillary angiomatosis of lymph node. *Am J Surg Pathol* 1991;15:430–437.
240. Walford N, Van der Wouw PA, Das PK, et al. Epithelioid angiomatosis in the acquired immunodeficiency syndrome: morphology and differential diagnosis. *Histopathology* 1990;16:83–88.
241. Steeper TA, Rosenstein H, Weiser J, et al. Bacillary epithelioid angiomatosis involving the liver, spleen, and skin in an AIDS patient with concurrent Kaposi's sarcoma. *Am J Clin Pathol* 1992;97:713–718.
242. Perrone T, De Wolf-Peeters C, Frizzera G. Inflammatory pseudotumor of lymph nodes. A distinctive pattern of nodal reaction. *Am J Surg Pathol* 1988;12:351–361.
243. Davis RE, Warnke RA, Dorfman RF. Inflammatory pseudotumor of lymph nodes. Additional observations and evidence for an inflammatory etiology. *Am J Surg Pathol* 1991;15:744–756.
244. Selves J, Meggetto F, Brousset P, et al. Inflammatory pseudotumor of the liver. Evidence for follicular dendritic reticulum cell proliferation associated with clonal Epstein-Barr virus. *Am J Surg Pathol* 1996;20:747–753.
245. Moran CA, Suster S, Abbondanzo SL. Inflammatory pseudotumor of lymph nodes: a study of 25 cases with emphasis on morphological heterogeneity. *Hum Pathol* 1997;28:332–338.
246. Coffin CM, Watterson J, Priest JR, et al. Extrapulmonary inflammatory myofibroblastic tumor (inflammatory pseudotumor). A clinicopathologic and immunohistochemical study of 84 cases. *Am J Surg Pathol* 1995;19:859–872.
247. Kutok JL, Pinkus GS, Dorfman DM, et al. Inflammatory pseudotumor of lymph node and spleen: an entity biologically distinct from inflammatory myofibroblastic tumor. *Hum Pathol* 2001;32:1382–1387.
248. Meis JM, Enzinger FM. Inflammatory fibrosarcoma of the mesentery and retroperitoneum. A tumor closely simulating inflammatory pseudotumor. *Am J Surg Pathol* 1991;15:1146–1156.
249. Facchetti F, Incardona P, Lonardi S, et al. Nodal inflammatory pseudotumor caused by luetic infection. *Am J Surg Pathol* 2009;33:447–453.
250. Chen KT. Mycobacterial spindle cell pseudotumor of lymph nodes. *Am J Surg Pathol* 1992;16:276–281.
251. Logani S, Lucas DR, Cheng JD, et al. Adsay NV. Spindle cell tumors associated with mycobacteria in lymph nodes of HIV-positive patients: 'Kaposi sarcoma with mycobacteria' and 'mycobacterial pseudotumor'. *Am J Surg Pathol* 1999;23:656–661.
252. Wolf DA, Wu CD, Medeiros LJ. Mycobacterial pseudotumors of lymph node. A report of two cases diagnosed at the time of intraoperative consultation using touch imprint preparations. *Arch Pathol Lab Med* 1995;119:811–814.
253. Cheuk W, Woo PC, Yuen KY, et al. Intestinal inflammatory pseudotumour with regional lymph node involvement: identification of a new bacterium as the aetiological agent. *J Pathol* 2000;192:289–292.
254. Das N, Lee J, Madden M, et al. A rare case of abdominal actinomycosis presenting as an inflammatory pseudotumour. *Int J Colorectal Dis* 2006;21:483–484.
255. Sweis RF, Propes MJ, Hyjek E. Actinomyces-induced inflammatory pseudotumor of the lymph node mimicking scrofula. *Ann Intern Med* 2011;155:66–67.
256. Arber DA, Kamel OW, van de Rijn M, et al. Frequent presence of the Epstein-Barr virus in inflammatory pseudotumor. *Hum Pathol* 1995;26:1093–1098.
257. Cheuk W, Chan JK. IgG4-related sclerosing disease: a critical appraisal of an evolving clinicopathologic entity. *Adv Anat Pathol* 2010;17:303–332.
258. Cheuk W, Yuen HK, Chu SY, et al. Lymphadenopathy of IgG4-related sclerosing disease. *Am J Surg Pathol* 2008;32:671–681.
259. Sato Y, Kojima M, Takata K, et al. Systemic IgG4-related lymphadenopathy: a clinical and pathologic comparison to multicentric Castleman's disease. *Mod Pathol* 2009;22:589–599.
260. Sato Y, Notohara K, Kojima M, et al. IgG4-related disease: historical overview and pathology of hematological disorders. *Pathol Int* 2010;60:247–258.
261. Sato Y, Kojima M, Takata K, et al. Immunoglobulin G4-related lymphadenopathy with inflammatory pseudotumor-like features. *Med Mol Morphol* 2011;44:179–182.
262. Umlas J, Federman M, Crawford C, et al. Spindle cell pseudotumor due to Mycobacterium avium-intracellulare in patients with acquired immunodeficiency syndrome (AIDS). Positive staining of mycobacteria for cytoskeleton filaments. *Am J Surg Pathol* 1991;15:1181–1187.
263. Weiss SW, Gnepp DR, Bratthauer GL. Palisaded myofibroblastoma. A benign mesenchymal tumor of lymph node. *Am J Surg Pathol* 1989;13:341–346.
264. Suster S, Rosai J. Intranodal hemorrhagic spindle-cell tumor with "amianthoid" fibers. Report of six cases of a distinctive mesenchymal neoplasm of the inguinal region that simulates Kaposi's sarcoma. *Am J Surg Pathol* 1989;13:347–357.

265. Abell MR, Littler ER. Benign metastasizing uterine leiomyoma. Multiple lymph nodal metastases. *Cancer* 1975;36:2206–2213.
266. Hsu YK, Rosenshein NB, Parmley TH, et al. Leiomyomatosis in pelvic lymph nodes. *Obstet Gynecol* 1981;57:91S–93S.
267. Mazzoleni G, Salerno A, Santini D, et al. Leiomyomatosis in pelvic lymph nodes. *Histopathology* 1992;21:588–589.
268. Fujii S, Okamura H, Nakashima N, et al. Leiomyomatosis peritonealis disseminata. *Obstet Gynecol* 1980;55:79S–83S.
269. Zaytsev P, Taxy JB. Pregnancy-associated ectopic decidua. *Am J Surg Pathol* 1987;11:526–530.
270. Mazeron JJ, Suit HD. Lymph nodes as sites of metastases from sarcomas of soft tissue. *Cancer* 1987;60:1800–1808.
271. Kinney MC, Greer JP, Glick AD, et al. Anaplastic large-cell Ki-1 malignant lymphomas. Recognition, biological and clinical implications. *Pathol Annu* 1991;26(Pt 1):1–24.
272. Coffin CM, Rich SS. Dehner LP. Familial aggregation of nasopharyngeal carcinoma and other malignancies. A clinicopathologic description. *Cancer* 1991;68:1323–1328.
273. Ambinder RF, Mann RB. Detection and characterization of Epstein-Barr virus in clinical specimens. *Am J Pathol* 1994;145:239–252.
274. Raab-Traub N. Epstein-Barr virus and nasopharyngeal carcinoma. *Semin Cancer Biol* 1992;3:297–307.
275. Medeiros LJ, Kaynor B, Harris NL. Lupus lymphadenitis: report of a case with immunohistologic studies on frozen sections. *Hum Pathol* 1989;20:295–299.
276. van Muijen GN, Ruiter DJ, van Leeuwen C, et al. Cytokeratin and neurofilament in lung carcinomas. *Am J Pathol* 1984;116:363–369.
277. Guinee DG Jr, Fishback NF, Koss MN, et al. The spectrum of immunohistochemical staining of small-cell lung carcinoma in specimens from transbronchial and open-lung biopsies. *Am J Clin Pathol* 1994;102:406–414.
278. Loy TS, Darkow GV, Quesenberry JT. Immunostaining in the diagnosis of pulmonary neuroendocrine carcinomas. An immunohistochemical study with ultrastructural correlations. *Am J Surg Pathol* 1995;19:173–182.
279. Lumadue JA, Askin FB, Perlman EJ. MIC2 analysis of small cell carcinoma. *Am J Clin Pathol* 1994;102:692–694.
280. Moll I, Kuhn C, Moll R. Cytokeratin 20 is a general marker of cutaneous Merkel cells while certain neuronal proteins are absent. *J Invest Dermatol* 1995;104:910–915.
281. Rosen PP, Kimmel M. Occult breast carcinoma presenting with axillary lymph node metastases: a follow-up study of 48 patients. *Hum Pathol* 1990;21:518–523.
282. Matsushima S, Mori M, Adachi Y, et al. S100 protein positive human breast carcinomas: an immunohistochemical study. *J Surg Oncol* 1994;55:108–113.
283. Fechner RE. Histologic variants of infiltrating lobular carcinoma of the breast. *Hum Pathol* 1975;6:373–378.
284. Brown RW, Campagna LB, Dunn JK, et al. Immunohistochemical identification of tumor markers in metastatic adenocarcinoma. A diagnostic adjunct in the determination of primary site. *Am J Clin Pathol* 1997;107:12–19.
285. Su JM, Hsu HK, Chang H, et al. Expression of estrogen and progesterone receptors in non-small-cell lung cancer: immunohistochemical study. *Anticancer Res* 1996;16:3803–3806.
286. Wallace ML, Longacre TA, Smoller BR. Estrogen and progesterone receptors and anti-gross cystic disease fluid protein 15 (BRST-2) fail to distinguish metastatic breast carcinoma from eccrine neoplasms. *Mod Pathol* 1995;8:897–901.
287. Coffing BN, Lim MS. Signet ring cell lymphoma in a patient with elevated CA-125. *J Clin Oncol* 2011;29:e416–e418.
288. Kim H, Dorfman RF, Rappaport H. Signet ring cell lymphoma. A rare morphologic and functional expression of nodular (follicular) lymphoma. *Am J Surg Pathol* 1978;2:119–132.
289. LiVolsi VA, Brooks JJ, Soslow R, et al. Signet cell melanocytic lesions. *Mod Pathol* 1992;5:515–520.
290. De Petris G, Lev R, Siew S. Peritumoral and nodal muciphages. *Am J Surg Pathol* 1998;22:545–549.
291. Kuo TT, Hsueh S. Mucicarminophilic histiocytosis. A polyvinylpyrrolidone (PVP) storage disease simulating signet-ring cell carcinoma. *Am J Surg Pathol* 1984;8:419–428.
292. Sheahan K, O'Brien MJ, Burke B, et al. Differential reactivities of carcinoembryonic antigen (CEA) and CEA-related monoclonal and polyclonal antibodies in common epithelial malignancies. *Am J Clin Pathol* 1990;94:157–164.
293. Loy TS, Phillips RW, Linder CL. A103 immunostaining in the diagnosis of adrenal cortical tumors: an immunohistochemical study of 316 cases. *Arch Pathol Lab Med* 2002;126:170–172.
294. Zhang PJ, Genega EM, Tomaszewski JE, et al. The role of calretinin, inhibin, melan-A, BCL-2, and C-kit in differentiating adrenal cortical and medullary tumors: an immunohistochemical study. *Mod Pathol* 2003;16:591–597.
295. Miettinen M. Neuroendocrine differentiation in adrenocortical carcinoma. New immunohistochemical findings supported by electron microscopy. *Lab Invest* 1992;66:169–174.
296. Clement PB, Scully RE. Uterine tumors with mixed epithelial and mesenchymal elements. *Semin Diagn Pathol* 1988;5:199–222.
297. Swanson PE. Heffalumps, jagulars, and cheshire cats. A commentary on cytokeratins and soft tissue sarcomas. *Am J Clin Pathol* 1991;95:S2–S7.
298. Tsang WY, Chan JK, Tang SK, et al. Large cell lymphoma with fibrillary matrix. *Histopathology* 1992;20:80–82.
299. Frizzera G, Gajl-Peczalska K, Sibley RK, et al. Rosette formation in malignant lymphoma. *Am J Pathol* 1985;119:351–356.
300. Bates RJ, Chapman CM, Prout GR Jr, et al. Immunohistochemical identification of prostatic acid phosphatase: correlation of tumor grade with acid phosphatase distribution. *J Urol* 1982;127:574–580.
301. Nadji M, Tabei SZ, Castro A, et al. Prostatic-specific antigen: an immunohistologic marker for prostatic neoplasms. *Cancer* 1981;48:1229–1232.
302. Loy TS, Sharp SC, Andershock CJ. Craig SB. Distribution of CA 19-9 in adenocarcinomas and transitional cell carcinomas. An immunohistochemical study of 527 cases. *Am J Clin Pathol* 1993;99:726–728.
303. Azumi N, Traweek ST, Battifora H. Prostatic acid phosphatase in carcinoid tumors. Immunohistochemical and immunoblot studies. *Am J Surg Pathol* 1991;15:785–790.
304. di Sant''Agnese PA, Cockett AT. Neuroendocrine differentiation in prostatic malignancy. *Cancer* 1996;78:357–361.
305. McLaren KM, Cossar DW. The immunohistochemical localization of S100 in the diagnosis of papillary carcinoma of the thyroid. *Hum Pathol* 1996;27:633–636.
306. Carcangiu ML, Steeper T, Zampi G, et al. Anaplastic thyroid carcinoma. A study of 70 cases. *Am J Clin Pathol* 1985;83:135–158.
307. Jautzke G, Altenaehr E. Immunohistochemical demonstration of carcinoembryonic antigen (CEA) and its correlation with grading and staging on tissue sections of urinary bladder carcinomas. *Cancer* 1982;50:2052–2056.
308. Soslow RA, Rouse RV, Hendrickson MR, et al. Transitional cell neoplasms of the ovary and urinary bladder: a comparative immunohistochemical analysis. *Int J Gynecol Pathol* 1996;15:257–265.
309. Tan J, Sidhu G, Greco MA, et al. Villin, cytokeratin 7, and cytokeratin 20 expression in pulmonary adenocarcinoma with ultrastructural evidence of microvilli with rootlets. *Hum Pathol* 1998;29:390–396.
310. Ordonez NG. The immunohistochemical diagnosis of mesothelioma: a comparative study of epithelioid mesothelioma and lung adenocarcinoma. *Am J Surg Pathol* 2003;27:1031–1051.
311. Betta PG, Magnani C, Bensi T, et al. Immunohistochemistry and molecular diagnostics of pleural malignant mesothelioma. *Arch Pathol Lab Med* 2012;136:253–261.
312. Monteagudo C, Merino MJ, LaPorte N, et al. Value of gross cystic disease fluid protein-15 in distinguishing metastatic breast carcinomas among poorly differentiated neoplasms involving the ovary. *Hum Pathol* 1991;22:368–372.
313. Wick MR, Lillemoe TJ, Copland GT, et al. Gross cystic disease fluid protein-15 as a marker for breast cancer: immunohistochemical analysis of 690 human neoplasms and comparison with alpha-lactalbumin. *Hum Pathol* 1989;20:281–287.
314. Minervini MI, Demetris AJ, Lee RG, et al. Utilization of hepatocyte-specific antibody in the immunocytochemical evaluation of liver tumors. *Mod Pathol* 1997;10:686–692.
315. Fan Z, van de Rijn M, Montgomery K, et al. Hep par 1 antibody stain for the differential diagnosis of hepatocellular carcinoma: 676 tumors tested using tissue microarrays and conventional tissue sections. *Mod Pathol* 2003;16:137–144.
316. Murphy GF, Mihm MC Jr. Histologic reporting of malignant melanoma. *Monogr Pathol* 1988;30:79–93.
317. Carney JA. Psammomatous melanotic schwannoma. A distinctive, heritable tumor with special associations, including cardiac myxoma and the Cushing syndrome. *Am J Surg Pathol* 1990;14:206–222.
318. Unger PD, Hoffman K, Thung SN, et al. HMB-45 reactivity in adrenal pheochromocytomas. *Arch Pathol Lab Med* 1992;116:151–153.
319. Chang ES, Wick MR, Swanson PE, et al. Metastatic malignant melanoma with "rhabdoid" features. *Am J Clin Pathol* 1994;102:426–431.
320. Spagnolo DV, Michie SA, Crabtree GS, et al. Monoclonal anti-keratin (AE1) reactivity in routinely processed tissue from 166 human neoplasms. *Am J Clin Pathol* 1985;84:697–704.
321. Argenyi ZB, Cain C, Bromley C, et al. S-100 protein-negative malignant melanoma: fact or fiction? A light-microscopic and immunohistochemical study. *Am J Dermatopathol* 1994;16:233–240.
322. Schmitt FC, Bacchi CE. S-100 protein: is it useful as a tumour marker in diagnostic immunocytochemistry? *Histopathology* 1989;15:281–288.
323. Soslow RA, Davis RE, Warnke RA, et al. True histiocytic lymphoma following therapy for lymphoblastic neoplasms. *Blood* 1996;87:5207–5212.
324. Writing Group of the Histiocyte Society. Histiocytosis syndromes in children. *Lancet* 1987;1:208–209.
325. Pallesen G, Myhre-Jensen O. Immunophenotypic analysis of neoplastic cells in follicular dendritic cell sarcoma. *Leukemia* 1987;1:549–557.
326. Gown AM, Vogel AM, Hoak D, et al. Monoclonal antibodies specific for melanocytic tumors distinguish subpopulations of melanocytes. *Am J Pathol* 1986;123:195–203.
327. Fernando SS, Johnson S, Bate J. Immunohistochemical analysis of cutaneous malignant melanoma: comparison of S-100 protein, HMB-45 monoclonal antibody and NKI/C3 monoclonal antibody. *Pathology* 1994;26:16–19.
328. Anstey A, Cerio R, Ramnarain N, et al. Desmoplastic malignant melanoma. An immunocytochemical study of 25 cases. *Am J Dermatopathol* 1994;16:14–22.
329. Pea M, Bonetti F, Zamboni G, et al. Melanocyte-marker-HMB-45 is regularly expressed in angiomyolipoma of the kidney. *Pathology* 1991;23:185–188.
330. Bonetti F, Chiodera PL, Pea M, et al. Transbronchial biopsy in lymphangiomyomatosis of the lung. HMB45 for diagnosis. *Am J Surg Pathol* 1993;17:1092–1102.
331. Jungbluth AA, Busam KJ, Gerald WL, et al. A103: An anti-melan-a monoclonal antibody for the detection of malignant melanoma in paraffin-embedded tissues. *Am J Surg Pathol* 1998;22:595–602.
332. Miettinen M, Fernandez M, Franssila K, et al. Microphthalmia transcription factor in the immunohistochemical diagnosis of metastatic melanoma: comparison with four other melanoma markers. *Am J Surg Pathol* 2001;25:205–211.
333. Busam KJ, Iversen K, Coplan KC, et al. Analysis of microphthalmia transcription factor expression in normal tissues and tumors, and comparison of its expression with S-100 protein, gp100, and tyrosinase in desmoplastic malignant melanoma. *Am J Surg Pathol* 2001;25:197–204.
334. Granter SR, Weilbaecher KN, Quigley C, et al. Role for microphthalmia transcription factor in the diagnosis of metastatic malignant melanoma. *Appl Immunohistochem Mol Morphol* 2002;10:47–51.
335. Carlson JA, Ross JS, Slominski AJ. New techniques in dermatopathology that help to diagnose and prognosticate melanoma. *Clin Dermatol* 2009;27:75–102.
336. Duray PH, Ernstoff MS, Titus-Ernstoff L. Immunohistochemical phenotyping of malignant melanoma. A procedure whose time has come in pathology practice. *Pathol Annu* 1990;25(Pt 2):351–377.
337. Mostofi FK, Sesterhenn IA. Pathology of germ cell tumors of testes. *Prog Clin Biol Res* 1985;203:1–34.
338. Richter HJ, Leder LD. Lymph node metastases with PAS-positive tumor cells and massive epithelioid granulomatous reaction as diagnostic clue to occult seminoma. *Cancer* 1979;44:245–249.
339. Mostofi FK, Sesterhenn IA, Davis CJ Jr. Immunopathology of germ cell tumors of the testis. *Semin Diagn Pathol* 1987;4:320–341.
340. Manivel JC, Jessurun J, Wick MR, et al. Placental alkaline phosphatase immunoreactivity in testicular germ-cell neoplasms. *Am J Surg Pathol* 1987;11:21–29.
341. Ramaekers F, Feitz W, Moesker O, et al. Antibodies to cytokeratin and vimentin in testicular tumour diagnosis. *Virchows Arch A Pathol Anat Histopathol* 1985;408:127–142.
342. Bailey D, Marks A, Stratis M, et al. Immunohistochemical staining of germ cell tumors and intratubular malignant germ cells of the testis using antibody to placental alkaline phosphatase and a monoclonal anti-seminoma antibody. *Mod Pathol* 1991;4:167–171.

343. Wick MR, Swanson PE, Manivel JC. Placental-like alkaline phosphatase reactivity in human tumors: an immunohistochemical study of 520 cases. *Hum Pathol* 1987;18:946–954.

344. Miettinen M, Virtanen I, Talerman A. Intermediate filament proteins in human testis and testicular germ-cell tumors. *Am J Pathol* 1985;120:402–410.

345. Suster S, Moran CA, Dominguez-Malagon H, et al. Germ cell tumors of the mediastinum and testis: a comparative immunohistochemical study of 120 cases. *Hum Pathol* 1998;29:737–742.

346. Kuida CA, Braunstein GD, Shintaku P, et al. Human chorionic gonadotropin expression in lung, breast, and renal carcinomas. *Arch Pathol Lab Med* 1988;112:282–285.

347. McIntyre A, Summersgill B, Grygalewicz B, et al. Amplification and overexpression of the KIT gene is associated with progression in the seminoma subtype of testicular germ cell tumors of adolescents and adults. *Cancer Res* 2005;65: 8085–8089.

348. Jones TD, Ulbright TM, Eble JN, et al. OCT4 staining in testicular tumors: a sensitive and specific marker for seminoma and embryonal carcinoma. *Am J Surg Pathol* 2004;28:935–940.

349. Looijenga LH, Stoop H, de Leeuw HP, et al. POU5F1 (OCT3/4) identifies cells with pluripotent potential in human germ cell tumors. *Cancer Res* 2003;63: 2244–2250.

350. Pallesen G, Hamilton-Dutoit SJ. Ki-1 (CD30) antigen is regularly expressed by tumor cells of embryonal carcinoma. *Am J Pathol* 1988;133:446–450.

351. Berney DM, Shamash J, Hendry WF, et al. Prediction of relapse after lymph node dissection for germ cell tumours: can salvage chemotherapy be avoided? *Br J Cancer* 2001;84:340–343.

352. Ambros IM, Ambros PF, Strehl S, et al. MIC2 is a specific marker for Ewing's sarcoma and peripheral primitive neuroectodermal tumors. Evidence for a common histogenesis of Ewing's sarcoma and peripheral primitive neuroectodermal tumors from MIC2 expression and specific chromosome aberration. *Cancer* 1991;67:1886–1893.

353. Fellinger EJ, Garin-Chesa P, Triche TJ, et al. Immunohistochemical analysis of Ewing's sarcoma cell surface antigen p30/32MIC2. *Am J Pathol* 1991;139: 317–325.

354. Smith MJ, Goodfellow PJ, Goodfellow PN. The genomic organisation of the human pseudoautosomal gene MIC2 and the detection of a related locus. *Hum Mol Genet* 1993;2:417–422.

355. Levy R, Dilley J, Fox RI, et al. A human thymus-leukemia antigen defined by hybridoma monoclonal antibodies. *Proc Natl Acad Sci U S A* 1979;76:6552– 6556.

356. Ramani P, Rampling D, Link M. Immunocytochemical study of 12E7 in small round-cell tumours of childhood: an assessment of its sensitivity and specificity. *Histopathology* 1993;23:557–561.

357. Soslow RA, Bhargava V, Warnke RA. MIC2, TdT, bcl-2, and CD34 expression in paraffin-embedded high-grade lymphoma/acute lymphoblastic leukemia distinguishes between distinct clinicopathologic entities. *Hum Pathol* 1997;28: 1158–1165.

358. Parham DM, Hijazi Y, Steinberg SM, et al. Neuroectodermal differentiation in Ewing's sarcoma family of tumors does not predict tumor behavior. *Hum Pathol* 1999;30:911–918.

359. Delattre O, Zucman J, Melot T, et al. The Ewing family of tumors—a subgroup of small-round-cell tumors defined by specific chimeric transcripts. *N Engl J Med* 1994;331:294–299.

360. Ladanyi M, Lewis R, Garin-Chesa P, et al. EWS rearrangement in Ewing's sarcoma and peripheral neuroectodermal tumor. Molecular detection and correlation with cytogenetic analysis and MIC2 expression. *Diagn Mol Pathol* 1993;2:141–146.

361. Dias P, Parham DM, Shapiro DN, et al. Myogenic regulatory protein (MyoD1) expression in childhood solid tumors: diagnostic utility in rhabdomyosarcoma. *Am J Pathol* 1990;137:1283–1291.

362. Wijnaendts LC, van der Linden JC, van Unnik AJ, et al. Histopathological classification of childhood rhabdomyosarcomas: relationship with clinical parameters and prognosis. *Hum Pathol* 1994;25:900–907.

363. Downing JR, Khandekar A, Shurtleff SA, et al. Multiplex RT-PCR assay for the differential diagnosis of alveolar rhabdomyosarcoma and Ewing's sarcoma. *Am J Pathol* 1995;146:626–634.

364. Gerald WL, Rosai J, Ladanyi M. Characterization of the genomic breakpoint and chimeric transcripts in the EWS-WT1 gene fusion of desmoplastic small round cell tumor. *Proc Natl Acad Sci U S A* 1995;92:1028–1032.

365. Gerald WL, Miller HK, Battifora H, et al. Intra-abdominal desmoplastic small round-cell tumor. Report of 19 cases of a distinctive type of high-grade polyphenotypic malignancy affecting young individuals. *Am J Surg Pathol* 1991;15:499–513.

366. Triche TJ, Askin FB. Neuroblastoma and the differential diagnosis of small-, round-, blue-cell tumors. *Hum Pathol* 1983;14:569–595.

367. Oppedal BR, Brandtzaeg P, Kemshead JT. Immunohistochemical differentiation of neuroblastomas from other small round cell neoplasms of childhood using a panel of mono- and polyclonal antibodies. *Histopathology* 1987;11:363–374.

368. Taylor CP, McGuckin AG, Bown NP, et al. Rapid detection of prognostic genetic factors in neuroblastoma using fluorescence *in situ* hybridisation on tumour imprints and bone marrow smears. United Kingdom Children's Cancer Study Group. *Br J Cancer* 1994;69:445–451.

369. Caron H, van Sluis P, de Kraker J, et al. Allelic loss of chromosome 1p as a predictor of unfavorable outcome in patients with neuroblastoma. *N Engl J Med* 1996;334:225–230.

370. Attiyeh EF, London WB, Mosse YP, et al. Chromosome 1p and 11q deletions and outcome in neuroblastoma. *N Engl J Med* 2005;353:2243–2253.

371. du Boulay CE. Immunohistochemistry of soft tissue tumours: a review. *J Pathol* 1985;146:77–94.

372. Arber DA, Kandalaft PL, Mehta P, et al. Vimentin-negative epithelioid sarcoma. The value of an immunohistochemical panel that includes CD34. *Am J Surg Pathol* 1993;17:302–307.

373. Weidner N, Tjoe J. Immunohistochemical profile of monoclonal antibody O13: antibody that recognizes glycoprotein p30/32MIC2 and is useful in diagnosing Ewing's sarcoma and peripheral neuroepithelioma. *Am J Surg Pathol* 1994;18: 486–494.

374. Dal Cin P, Rao U, Jani-Sait S, et al. Chromosomes in the diagnosis of soft tissue tumors. I. Synovial sarcoma. *Mod Pathol* 1992;5:357–362.

375. Hocar O, Le Cesne A, Berissi S, et al. Clear cell sarcoma (malignant melanoma) of soft parts: a clinicopathologic study of 52 cases. *Dermatol Res Pract* 2012: 2012;984096.

376. Chung EB. Enzinger FM. Malignant melanoma of soft parts. A reassessment of clear cell sarcoma. *Am J Surg Pathol* 1983;7:405–413.

377. Bridge JA, Borek DA, Neff JR, et al. Chromosomal abnormalities in clear cell sarcoma. Implications for histogenesis. *Am J Clin Pathol* 1990;93:26–31.

378. Swanson PE, Wick MR. Clear cell sarcoma. An immunohistochemical analysis of six cases and comparison with other epithelioid neoplasms of soft tissue. *Arch Pathol Lab Med* 1989;113:55–60.

379. Meis JM, Butler JJ, Osborne BM, et al. Granulocytic sarcoma in nonleukemic patients. *Cancer* 1986;58:2697–2709.

380. Neiman RS, Barcos M, Berard C, et al. Granulocytic sarcoma: a clinicopathologic study of 61 biopsied cases. *Cancer* 1981;48:1426–1437.

381. Zimmerman LE. Font RL. Ophthalmologic manifestations of granulocytic sarcoma (myeloid sarcoma or chloroma). The third Pan American Association of Ophthalmology and American Journal of Ophthalmology Lecture. *Am J Ophthalmol* 1975;80:975–990.

382. Campidelli C, Agostinelli C, Stitson R, et al. Myeloid sarcoma: extramedullary manifestation of myeloid disorders. *Am J Clin Pathol* 2009;132:426–437.

383. Davey FR, Olson S, Kurec AS, et al. The immunophenotyping of extramedullary myeloid cell tumors in paraffin-embedded tissue sections. *Am J Surg Pathol* 1988;12:699–707.

384. Pileri SA, Ascani S, Cox MC, et al. Myeloid sarcoma: clinico-pathologic, phenotypic and cytogenetic analysis of 92 adult patients. *Leukemia* 2007;21:340–350.

385. Travis WD, Li CY, Bergstralh EJ, et al. Systemic mast cell disease. Analysis of 58 cases and literature review. *Medicine (Baltimore)* 1988;67:345–368.

386. Travis WD, Li CY. Pathology of the lymph node and spleen in systemic mast cell disease. *Mod Pathol* 1988;1:4–14.

387. Miranda RN, Esparza AR, Sambandam S, et al. Systemic mast cell disease presenting with peripheral blood eosinophilia. *Hum Pathol* 1994;25:727–730.

388. Valent P, Horny HP, Escribano L, et al. Diagnostic criteria and classification of mastocytosis: a consensus proposal. *Leuk Res* 2001;25:603–625.

389. Chan JK, Fletcher CD, Nayler SJ, et al. Follicular dendritic cell sarcoma. Clinicopathologic analysis of 17 cases suggesting a malignant potential higher than currently recognized. *Cancer* 1997;79:294–313.

390. Perez-Ordonez B, Erlandson RA, Rosai J. Follicular dendritic cell tumor: report of 13 additional cases of a distinctive entity. *Am J Surg Pathol* 1996;20:944–955.

391. Weiss LM, Berry GJ, Dorfman RF, et al. Spindle cell neoplasms of lymph nodes of probable reticulum cell lineage. True reticulum cell sarcoma? *Am J Surg Pathol* 1990;14:405–414.

392. Chan WC, Zaatari G. Lymph node interdigitating reticulum cell sarcoma. *Am J Clin Pathol* 1986;85:739–744.

393. Andriko JW, Kaldjian EP, Tsokos M, et al. Reticulum cell neoplasms of lymph nodes: a clinicopathologic study of 11 cases with recognition of a new subtype derived from fibroblastic reticular cells. *Am J Surg Pathol* 1998;22:1048–1058.

394. Hollowood K, Pease C, Mackay AM, et al. Sarcomatoid tumours of lymph nodes showing follicular dendritic cell differentiation. *J Pathol* 1991;163:205–216.

395. Chan JK, Tsang WY, Ng CS. Follicular dendritic cell tumor and vascular neoplasm complicating hyaline-vascular Castleman's disease. *Am J Surg Pathol* 1994;18:517–525.

396. Nakamura S, Hara K, Suchi T, et al. Interdigitating cell sarcoma. A morphologic, immunologic, and enzyme-histochemical study. *Cancer* 1988;61:562–568.

397. Chan AC, Serrano-Olmo J, Erlandson RA, et al. Cytokeratin-positive malignant tumors with reticulum cell morphology: a subtype of fibroblastic reticulum cell neoplasm? *Am J Surg Pathol* 2000;24:107–116.

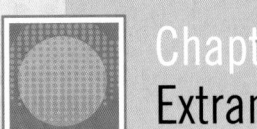

Chapter 28
Extranodal Lymphoid Proliferations: General Principles

Jerome S. Burke

Many pathologists and clinicians have the misconception that extranodal lymphomas are an uncommon and exotic category of malignant lymphomas. Only extranodal presentation of Hodgkin lymphoma is rare; among non-Hodgkin lymphomas, extranodal presentations are relatively common, as reflected by the multiple and different extranodal lymphomas categorized in the current World Health Organization (WHO) lymphoma classification (1). The WHO classification includes not only extranodal marginal zone lymphoma of mucosa-associated lymphoid tissue (MALT) type (2) but other specific extranodal B-cell lymphomas encompassing primary diffuse large B-cell lymphoma (DLBCL) of the mediastinum/thymus, central nervous system (CNS), and skin of leg, as well as lymphomatoid granulomatosis, primary effusion lymphoma, and primary cutaneous follicle center lymphoma. Extranodal lymphomas of T-cell lineage equally are detailed entities in the WHO system, particularly extranodal natural killer (NK)/T-cell lymphoma of nasal type (see Chapter 26), enteropathy-associated T-cell lymphoma, hepatosplenic T-cell lymphoma, and a host of skin lymphomas such as mycosis fungoides, primary cutaneous CD30+ lymphoproliferative disorder, and subcutaneous panniculitis-like T-cell lymphoma (1) (see Chapter 29).

The definition of extranodal lymphoma generally includes cases that present in certain extranodal lymphoid tissue–bearing sites, such as Waldeyer ring, but not those cases of lymphoma that present in mediastinum (see Chapter 23), bone marrow (see Chapter 35), and spleen (see Chapter 50). Up to 42% of non-Hodgkin lymphomas present in extranodal locations (3–8), and the incidence is mounting. Based on Surveillance, Epidemiology, and End Results (SEER) data from the National Cancer Institute of the United States, the incidence rate for extranodal lymphomas increased 4.1% per year from 1975 to 2003 as opposed to an increase of 1.4% per year for node-based non-Hodgkin lymphomas (7). Some histologic categories of malignant lymphoma, specifically Burkitt lymphoma and DLBCL, consistently arise in extranodal locations, and other histologic forms are inclined to arise in a specific geographic region or ethnic group, as for example Epstein-Barr virus (EBV)–associated NK/T-cell lymphoma of nasal type in the Far East and in aboriginal people in both Central and South America (1). Extranodal lymphomas may present or originate in any site, but according to SEER data, the gastrointestinal tract, mainly the stomach, is the most common location followed by skin, oral cavity, and pharynx (4,7) (Table 28.1). The incidence of primary lymphomas of stomach, expressly extranodal marginal zone lymphomas of MALT type, has fluctuated, with a peak reached in the 1990s as a consequence of the increasing recognition of MALT lymphoma as a precise diagnostic entity followed by a persistent decline in the past decade; this decline is likely related to the improved clinical management and reduction of *Helicobacter pylori* infection (9). Primary lymphomas of the CNS are escalating with an age-adjusted threefold increase that surpassed that of systemic lymphoma, with the enhancement evident in all age groups and both genders and apparently independent from lymphomas presenting in the

CNS secondary to the acquired immunodeficiency syndrome (AIDS) (10). AIDS is the best known of the immunodeficiency states associated with the onset of extranodal lymphomas. Up to 80% of patients who have AIDS and who develop malignant lymphoma have extranodal presentations, and the extranodal site is frequently unusual, such as the brain, or the type of extranodal lymphoma is unusual, such as plasmablastic lymphoma of the oral cavity (11,12) (see Chapter 25).

To be categorized as having an extranodal lymphoma, the patient must present with localized, clinical stage IE or IIE disease (13). Patients who have clinical stage IIIE or IV disease and who are diagnosed in an extranodal site are not included as cases of extranodal lymphoma, because the extranodal site is assumed to be a manifestation of disseminated and frequently occult lymphoma. Patients with known lymphoma who relapse in an extranodal site also are excluded.

The past three decades have witnessed an increasing interest in extranodal lymphomas, particularly since the advent of immunologic cell marker and molecular genetic techniques to analyze lymphomas. The most obvious source of an increasing awareness of extranodal lymphomas is the numerous publications about extranodal lymphomas and their relationship to MALT (14–17). The varying proposals, nomenclature, and merits of MALT and its association with extranodal lymphomas are not addressed in this chapter. This chapter develops the general diagnostic principles employed in separating extranodal malignant lymphomas from extranodal lymphoid hyperplasias, or so-called *pseudolymphomas*, as well as from other lymphoid and nonlymphoid entities that simulate extranodal malignant lymphoma, such as undifferentiated carcinoma. The histologic criteria that allow this distinction are emphasized here, and the role of immunophenotypic and genotypic studies in the refinement and alteration of these histologic criteria is analyzed.

TRADITIONAL DIAGNOSTIC CRITERIA

In establishing a histologic diagnosis of an extranodal lymphoma, pathologists are aware that various reactive lymphoid hyperplasias exist that mimic extranodal lymphomas clinically and pathologically. Examples of extranodal florid lymphoid hyperplasias that simulate extranodal lymphomas include lymphoid hyperplasia of the ileocecal region, lymphoepithelial sialadenitis (LESA) of salivary glands, chronic lymphocytic thyroiditis, and the many types of cutaneous lymphoid hyperplasia. To complicate matters, malignant lymphomas may develop in association with some of these reactive and autoimmune conditions (18). Patients who have Sjögren syndrome or chronic lymphocytic thyroiditis (Hashimoto thyroiditis) have increased risk of developing malignant lymphoma (19,20). One explanation for the predisposition of patients with Sjögren syndrome or Hashimoto thyroiditis to develop malignant lymphoma is the observation that many histologically benign lymphoid infiltrates in the salivary and thyroid glands represent occult monoclonal and oligoclonal B-cell proliferations

Table 28.1	EXTRANODAL LYMPHOMAS: INCIDENCE RATE IN MEN PER 100,000, 1999–2003	
	Number of Cases	**%**
Skin	5,560	18.3
Stomach	4,714	15.5
Oral cavity/pharynx	2,314	7.6
Small intestine	2,103	6.9
Colon/rectum	1,804	5.9
Brain	1,706	5.6
Soft tissue	1,224	4.0
Lung/bronchus	1,209	4.0
Testis	1,061	3.5
Orbit/eye	1,055	3.5
Bone/joints	986	3.2
Nose/nasal cavity	623	2.0
Liver	521	1.7
Thyroid	424	1.4
Other sites	5,081	16.7

Adapted from Wu XC, Andrews P, Chen VW, et al. Incidence of extranodal non-Hodgkin's lymphomas among whites, blacks, and Asian/Pacific Islanders in the United States; anatomic site and histology differences. *Cancer Epidemiol* 2009;33:337–346, with permission.

(21–23). As well as autoimmune disorders, extranodal lymphomas, mainly those of MALT type, frequently develop in a setting of chronic inflammation often due to infection (2,24). The best example is gastric MALT lymphoma in association with *H. pylori* infection (25), but other connections have been reported such as immunoproliferative small intestinal disease with *Campylobacter jejuni* (26), and, depending on the geographic region, certain MALT lymphomas especially of the ocular region and lung with *Chlamydia psittaci* (27,28) and a small subset of cutaneous MALT lymphomas with *Borrelia burgdorferi* infection (29,30). Chronic and sustained stimulation of the immune system by the infectious agent is thought to result in protracted lymphoid proliferation with the eventual development of extranodal lymphoma (24).

The morphologic criteria for distinguishing extranodal lymphoma from extranodal lymphoid hyperplasia historically were extrapolated from those used to distinguish malignant lymphoma from lymphoid hyperplasia in lymph nodes (31). The major criteria that allowed this distinction included monomorphic lymphocytic infiltrates, cellular atypia, and disruption of the normal architecture. Identical criteria have been used as the histologic standards for the diagnosis of extranodal lymphomas (Table 28.2). Because the majority of all extranodal lymphomas are DLBCL (7,8), as for example almost 60% of cases originating in stomach (32), with associated monomorphism, cellular atypia, and architectural destruction of the extranodal site (e.g., obliteration of glands or follicles), these traditional criteria generally have proven to be reliable and applicable. Reactive lymphoid conditions that are at the opposite end of

the spectrum also do not pose diagnostic problems. Lymphocytic infiltrates that are polymorphous, that display a range of mature lymphocytes (including plasma cells and immunoblasts), that are associated with well-defined germinal centers, and that do not destroy completely the architectural landmarks of an extranodal site can be diagnosed confidently as benign and reactive.

The main difficulty in the separation of extranodal lymphomas from lymphoid hyperplasia concerns MALT lymphomas, such as those in the stomach, ocular adnexa, and lung, that are composed of small lymphocytes and frequently associated with germinal center formation (17,33–37). In such cases, the traditional histologic criteria are not fully applicable (38). Modern studies have revealed that many histologically ambiguous extranodal small lymphocytic proliferations are monoclonal and consequently are presumed to be malignant lymphomas (23,39). The application of immunologic and molecular genetic analyses to extranodal small lymphocytic proliferations has altered the traditional histologic criteria and has revealed myriad inconsistencies in these criteria (Table 28.3). For example, in a review of 97 cases originally diagnosed as gastric pseudolymphoma between 1970 and 1985, 79% were reclassified as malignant lymphoma, with fully two-thirds of the newly classified lymphomatous cases interpreted as lymphomas of MALT type (40). The remaining cases were regarded as examples of lymphoid hyperplasia or atypical lymphocytic infiltrates. Similarly, many cases previously interpreted as LESA or as Hashimoto thyroiditis also are low-grade lymphomas and commonly arise secondary to "acquired" MALT (16,22,41,42). Consequently, the term *pseudolymphoma* is regarded as imprecise and anachronistic and no longer is acceptable as a diagnostic category (38,43).

Cases in which extranodal lymphoma coexists with reactive lymphoid hyperplasia and technical artifacts, found mainly in small biopsy specimens, are other common factors that lead to diagnostic problems in the evaluation of extranodal lymphocytic infiltrates.

MODIFICATIONS OF THE TRADITIONAL HISTOLOGIC CRITERIA FOR THE DIAGNOSIS OF EXTRANODAL LYMPHOMAS

Polymorphous Extranodal Lymphomas

A polymorphous or mixed lymphoid proliferation in an extranodal site usually infers a benign reactive state. In extranodal lymphoid hyperplasia, the polymorphous cell population exhibits a spectrum of lymphocytic transformation, including small lymphocytes, intermediate-sized lymphocytes, plasma cells,

Table 28.2	TRADITIONAL HISTOLOGIC CRITERIA FOR DISTINGUISHING EXTRANODAL LYMPHOMAS FROM LYMPHOID HYPERPLASIAS	
Extranodal Lymphomas		**Lymphoid Hyperplasias**
Infiltrate monomorphous		Infiltrate polymorphous (lymphocytes in stages of transformation)
Cytologic atypia		Cytologic maturity (lymphocytes, plasma cells, and immunoblasts)
Germinal centers uncommon		Germinal centers common (usually in center of infiltrate)
Massive infiltration with architectural destruction		Random infiltration with architectural retention

Table 28.3	MODIFICATIONS OF THE TRADITIONAL HISTOLOGIC CRITERIA FOR DISTINGUISHING EXTRANODAL LYMPHOMAS FROM LYMPHOID HYPERPLASIA

- Extranodal lymphomas may be polymorphous (including PTCL)
- Extranodal lymphomas may be composed of cytologically mature-appearing lymphocytes (extranodal marginal zone lymphoma of MALT and other low-grade lymphomas with or without plasma cell differentiation)
- Germinal centers may be observed at the periphery of extranodal lymphomas and in the centers of many low-grade extranodal lymphomas, especially those extranodal marginal zone lymphoma of MALT type
- Degree of infiltration and architectural and epithelial destruction highly variable in benign and malignant extranodal lymphocytic infiltrates

and large cells or immunoblasts. This proliferation frequently is accompanied by germinal centers. If there are no germinal centers, it is the *range* of lymphocytic transformation and its orderliness that indicate that the lymphocytic population is hyperplasia and not lymphoma.

The morphologic interpretation of extranodal florid immunoblastic hyperplasia may be demanding, because florid hyperplasia often leads to obliteration of the normal histologic landmarks of that extranodal site (Fig. 28.1). In this setting, the immunoblasts may appear atypical, with increased mitotic activity that results from an antigenic stimulus. Distinction from malignant lymphoma relies on recognizing that the lymphocytes have some symmetry in their proliferative activity, even if dominated by immunoblasts (Fig. 28.2). Unlike malignant lymphoma, the small lymphocytes in extranodal reactive lymphoid hyperplasia are round and appear mature. Chronic lymphocytic leukemia/small lymphocytic lymphoma (CLL/SLL) that contains admixed large cells or paraimmunoblasts and marginal zone lymphoma of MALT type dominated by small lymphocytes with some associated large cells are exceptions; the small lymphocytes have no significant cytologic atypia (37,38). Such cases can be distinguished from reactive states because the cellular proliferation in the lymphomas usually is dense and destructive, and there often is an abrupt transition from the small lymphocytes to the large cells. In cases in which frank DLBCL has developed, the large cells are monomorphous and form microscopic sheets or masses. In some extranodal sites, such as the stomach, however, the malignant large B cells are arcane and may form only small clusters or diffusely intermingle with the small lymphocytes of a MALT lymphoma. In this setting, there is no existing consensus as to the number or pattern of large cells required to establish the evolution from gastric MALT lymphoma to one of DLBCL. In one study, the observation of a diffuse large cell component in the range of 1% to 10% with and without nonconfluent clusters of large cells predicted a significantly worse prognosis in an otherwise MALT lymphoma (44). Another report, however, documented that the presence of scattered large cells that constituted 5% to 10% of the gastric MALT lymphoma cell population was prognostically irrelevant, whereas compact clustered large cells that represented more than 10% of the MALT lymphoma proved significant, as they were associated with a worse survival (45).

Hodgkin lymphoma is another malignant lymphoma with a polymorphous cell population and without atypia among the small lymphocytes; however, primary extranodal Hodgkin

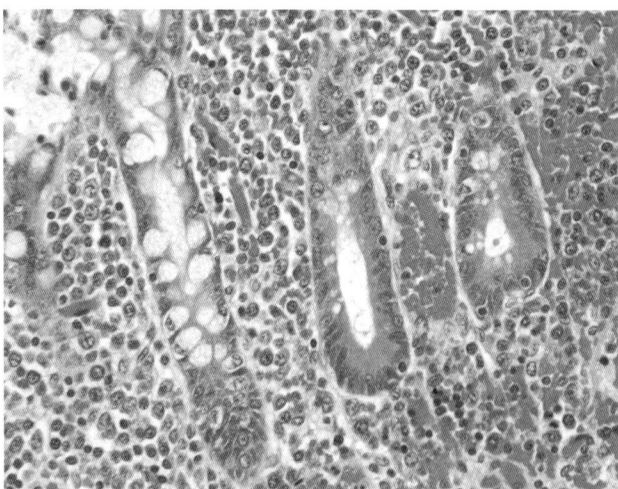

FIGURE 28.2. Although numerous large immunoblasts appear in the lamina propria of the ileum, there is an orderly range of lymphocytic transformation indicative of florid reactive hyperplasia (hematoxylin and eosin stain, original magnification: 300× magnification).

lymphoma is uncommon. Hodgkin lymphoma that presents in an extranodal site usually is a consequence of direct invasion from adjacent lymph nodes or by retrograde lymphatic spread (see Chapter 15). For example, genuine cases of primary Hodgkin lymphoma of skin are exceedingly rare and must be viewed with skepticism. Most instances likely are cases of primary cutaneous CD30+ T-cell lymphoproliferative disorders with Reed-Sternberg–like cells (46) or possibly EBV+ mucocutaneous ulcer (47). In EBV+ mucocutaneous ulcer, Reed-Sternberg–like cells that coexpress both CD15 and CD30 are common so that the distinction from Hodgkin lymphoma is difficult; however, awareness that primary cutaneous stage IE Hodgkin lymphoma is so extraordinary should allow for the strong possibility of another condition. Of most significance and like patients with lymphomatoid papulosis, patients with EBV+ mucocutaneous ulcer frequently exhibit spontaneous regression without therapy (47).

Most extranodal polymorphous or mixed small to medium-sized and large cell lymphomas are characterized by nuclear membrane irregularities and atypia in the small lymphocytes (Fig. 28.3). This includes the peripheral T-cell lymphomas (PTCL) and NK/T-cell lymphomas of extranodal sites. Fortunately,

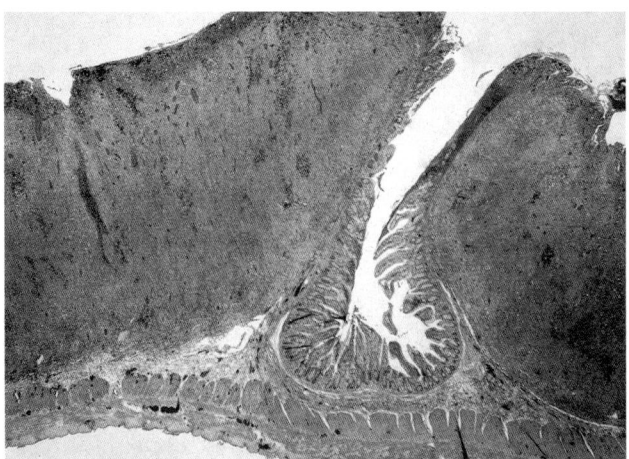

FIGURE 28.1. Florid lymphoid hyperplasia of the terminal ileum results in a tumor mass that obliterates the mucosa and submucosa. Despite the massive size of the hyperplastic process, the proliferating lymphocytes do not invade the muscularis propria (hematoxylin and eosin stain, original magnification: 15× magnification).

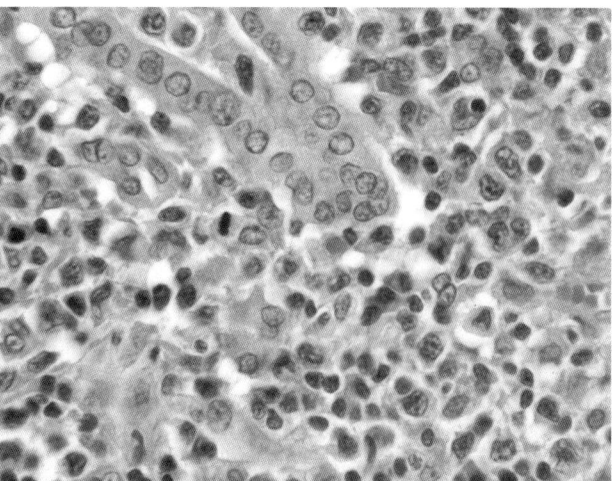

FIGURE 28.3. Large B-cell lymphoma with a polymorphous cell population displays nuclear membrane irregularities in small and large lymphocytes alike. Note the residual thyroid follicle with lymphomatous cells in the lumen (hematoxylin and eosin stain, original magnification: 600× magnification).

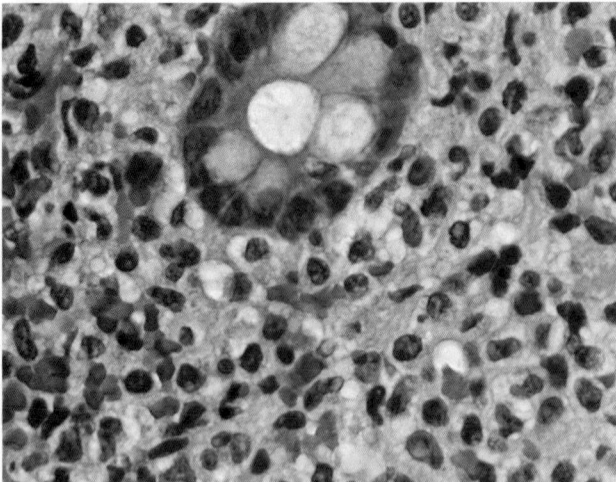

FIGURE 28.4. In NK-cell enteropathy of the intestinal tract, atypical lymphocytes invade the lamina propria and surround residual glands to mimic lymphoma. Unlike NK/T-cell lymphoma, EBV is not present, and the patients pursue a benign clinical course (hematoxylin and eosin stain, original magnification: 300× magnification). (Reproduced from Mansoor A, Pittaluga S, Beck PL, et al. NK-cell enteropathy: a benign NK-cell lymphoproliferative disease mimicking intestinal lymphoma: clinicopathological features and follow-up in a unique case series. *Blood* 2011;117:1447–1452, with permission and courtesy of Elaine S. Jaffe, MD.)

noncutaneous extranodal PTCL and NK/T-cell lymphomas are uncommon, except in the Far East where NK/T-cell lymphomas of nasal type are frequent and involve not only the upper nasal air passages but also extranasal sites such as the gastrointestinal tract (48–50). Occasionally, the distinction of a polymorphous lymphoma from extranodal florid lymphoid hyperplasia may not be possible using only histologic criteria; immunologic and, at times, gene rearrangement studies are required for a definite diagnosis (18,39). In some instances, however, such studies may not allow for this distinction. For example, extranodal NK/T-cell lymphoma of the gastrointestinal tract must be distinguished from two seemingly identical, recently reported entities, *lymphomatoid gastropathy* or *NK-cell enteropathy* (51,52). In the latter condition, patients present with multiple superficial, discrete, flat lesions or small, <1 cm, patchy superficial hemorrhagic ulcers that involve either single or multiple sites, including stomach, duodenum, small intestine, and colon. The lesions form diffuse, well-circumscribed, mucosal infiltrates composed of a polymorphous population of atypical medium to large lymphocytes with invasion or obliteration of mucosal glands (Fig. 28.4). The atypical lymphocytes are cytoplasmic CD3$^+$ as well as CD56$^+$ and TIA-1$^+$. Similar to true NK-cell lymphomas of extranodal nasal type, the T-cell receptor in the gastropathy/enteropathy cases is germline, but, in contrast to NK nasal-type lymphomas, studies for EBV are negative (51,52). Of most significance and clinically parallel to patients with EBV$^+$ mucocutaneous ulcer, patients with lymphomatoid gastropathy or NK-cell enteropathy exhibit a benign clinical course.

Cytologically Mature Extranodal Lymphomas

The conventional view is that extranodal lymphomas are characterized by nuclear membrane irregularities or atypia. Extranodal marginal zone lymphomas of MALT type, however, are cytologically mutable (37). Although MALT lymphomas typically are composed of marginal zone cells with centrocyte-like features, they also may have a monocytoid appearance, or they may be composed of plasma cells or have no or only subtle nuclear membrane irregularities, similar to the cells of CLL/SLL (2,15,37,38); the latter variant often is confused with extranodal lymphoid hyperplasia. With the widespread use of immunologic markers, it now is established that many extranodal small lymphocytic proliferations, such as those in the

ocular adnexa, lung, and gastrointestinal tract, are malignant lymphomas, mainly extranodal marginal zone lymphomas of MALT type (2,33–38,53,54).

Small biopsy specimens, such as endoscopic or needle core, that contain a predominance of small lymphocytes represent the most difficult problem in the diagnosis of extranodal lymphocytic lesions (17,36,38,55). A small lymphocytic proliferation that appears mature is the histologic norm in cases of extranodal lymphoid hyperplasia, but cytologic maturity or minimal atypia also is the histologic hallmark of most low-grade malignant lymphomas. How can these two groups be distinguished in a small biopsy specimen? In many cases, this is impossible if only histologic criteria are applied. At one point, this histologic dilemma prompted the use of the noncommittal term *extranodal small lymphocytic proliferation* to describe histologically ambiguous or indeterminate extranodal lymphocytic infiltrates (56). Morphologic criteria currently used to separate benign from extranodal malignant small lymphocytic infiltrates include whether the infiltrate is monomorphous, is dense, or exhibits cytologic atypia or Dutcher bodies, and whether this results in destruction of glands, follicles, or other structures indigenous to that extranodal site (2,33,38,39,48,57) (Fig. 28.5). If these morphologic features are unequivocally present, then the lymphocytic infiltrate likely is malignant lymphoma. In the stomach, a histologic scoring system for MALT has been proffered, in which invasion of epithelial structures ("lymphoepithelial lesions" of MALT) is considered essential to the diagnosis (25). Employing the scoring system, a definite diagnosis of low-grade B-cell lymphoma of MALT is based on the presence of a dense diffuse infiltrate of marginal zone-type cells in the lamina propria, with prominent lymphoepithelial lesions. Cases regarded as suspicious lymphocytic infiltrates are those in which reactive follicles are surrounded by marginal zone cells that diffusely infiltrate into the lamina propria and into epithelium in small groups (25). Nonetheless, dense infiltrates, slight cytologic atypia, and lymphoepithelial-like lesions may be observed in cases of lymphoid hyperplasia in many extranodal sites, including stomach (38,42,58,59). As a mark of the diagnostic difficulty that can occur even with the apparent prudent application of the scoring system for gastric MALT lymphoma, an international study by 17 pathologists, including hematopathologists, gastrointestinal pathologists, and general pathologists, histologically reviewed 41 stomach specimens encompassing cases from simple gastritis to lymphoma (60). Interobserver reproducibility was poor and the scale of disagreement was dependent on the familiarity of

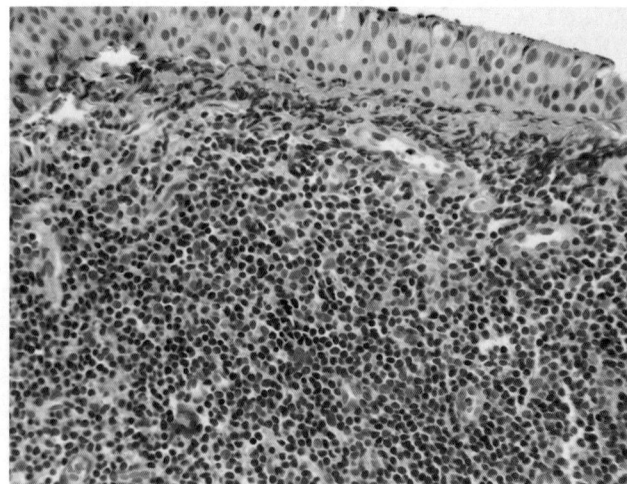

FIGURE 28.5. An extranodal marginal zone lymphoma composed of small lymphocytes in the conjunctiva is characterized by a dense uniform infiltrate of the subepithelial connective tissue with destruction of accessory lacrimal glands (hematoxylin and eosin stain, original magnification: 300× magnification).

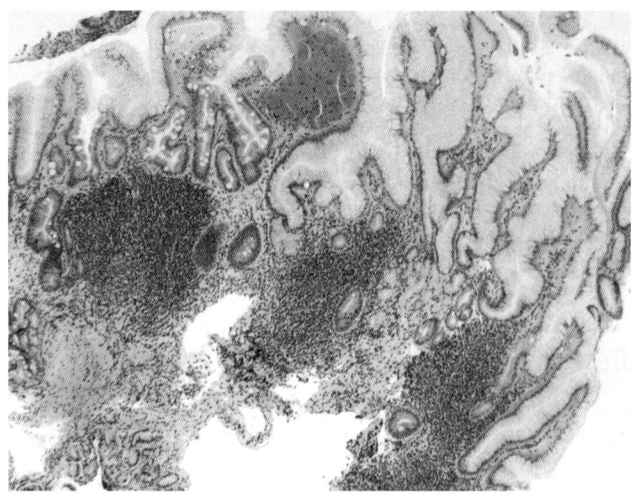

FIGURE 28.6. This gastric biopsy specimen contains patchy, variably dense lymphocytic infiltrates composed of small lymphocytes without cytologic atypia. The morphologic and immunophenotypic features were not regarded as completely diagnostic of malignant lymphoma, but a subsequent biopsy demonstrated monoclonal B lymphocytes (hematoxylin and eosin stain, original magnification: 60× magnification).

the pathologist in evaluating gastric biopsies for MALT lesions. In order to enhance diagnostic accuracy, clinical information, extensive sampling, recognition of lymphoepithelial lesions, immunophenotypic data, and cytogenetic results were recommended (60).

The application of immunologic markers to analyze the clonality of extranodal small lymphocytic proliferations that appear mature has revised dramatically our perspective of these lesions (2,38,39). Immunologic studies have indicated that many extranodal small lymphocytic proliferations that fulfill the current histologic criteria are monoclonal B-cell proliferations; such cases usually are equated with marginal zone lymphomas of MALT type (2,15–17,53,55). Correlative immunopathologic studies of monoclonal B-cell lymphoproliferative lesions, such as those in the ocular adnexa, have reduced the number of cases regarded as atypical or indeterminate (33,34). Naturally, cases persist, especially small biopsy specimens, in which the histologic features or immunologic findings remain equivocal (Fig. 28.6); these cases should receive not only a

descriptive diagnosis but also a request for a repeat biopsy with reservation of fresh tissue to determine clonality, by immunohistochemistry, flow cytometry, molecular techniques, or a combination thereof (23,37,38,61,62). If the only available tissue is fixed and paraffin embedded, a consistent determination of clonality in a biopsy specimen dominated by small lymphocytes usually is not possible in most laboratories. In some cases, immunologic studies of paraffin-embedded tissue can reveal an aberrant phenotype in the suspicious small lymphocytic population, such as the coexpression of B-cell antigen CD20 and T-cell antigen CD43 (63,64) (Fig. 28.7). For example, up to 50% of gastric MALT lymphoma cases demonstrate coexpression of CD43 and rare examples of nongastric MALT lymphoma coexpress CD5 (64,65). Obviously, in a suspected case of extranodal marginal zone lymphoma, coexpression of CD5 requires staining for cyclin D1 to exclude extranodal mantle cell lymphoma. Prudence is necessary in the evaluation of immunoglobulin gene rearrangement studies employing polymerase chain reaction (PCR) techniques in fixed paraffin-embedded tissues (39); small monoclonal bands may occur in extranodal reactive lymphoid hyperplasias, as for example in chronic active gastritis associated with *H. pylori* (66,67). Monoclonal B-cell and/or T-cell receptor gene rearrangements equally are encountered in a variety of benign reactive cutaneous lesions (68,69). Therefore, if PCR for gene rearrangement is to be performed, the procedure should be limited to those cases with strong morphologic suspicion for actual lymphoma (17,62,69).

In addition to mature-appearing small lymphocytes, some cases of extranodal marginal zone lymphoma of MALT type are dominated by plasma cells, such as in the salivary gland, ocular region, lung, thyroid, and skin (2,22,33,35,42,69). Plasma cells also may predominate occasionally in gastric marginal zone lymphomas, but are especially prevalent in cases following treatment with rituximab (Fig. 28.8) (70). Many plasma cell–rich extranodal MALT cases may be confused with a benign inflammatory process, as for example IgG4-related disease or another lymphoma apart from one of MALT type, such as lymphoplasmacytic lymphoma or even extraosseous plasmacytoma. IgG4-related disease can affect a variety of extranodal sites and the diagnostic microscopic features encompass a dense lymphoplasmacytic infiltrate (Fig. 28.9), storiform-type fibrosis, and obliterative phlebitis coupled with increased IgG4+ plasma cells with an elevated IgG4:IgG ratio of more than 40% (71). The diagnosis of IgG4-related disease is especially

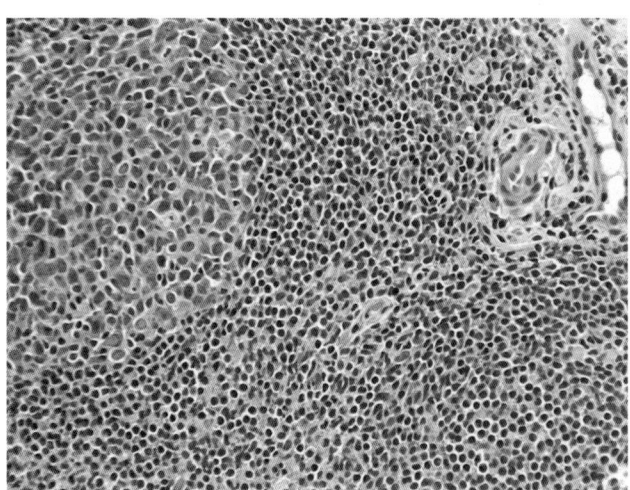

A

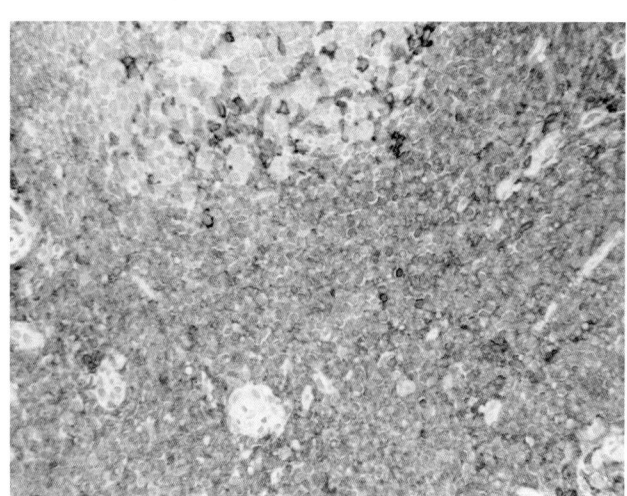

B

FIGURE 28.7. A: A histologically suspicious small lymphocytic infiltrate in a stomach biopsy is adjacent to a germinal center on the left (hematoxylin and eosin stain, original magnification: 300× magnification). **B:** Both the germinal center and the surrounding lymphocytes expressed B-cell antigen CD20, but in contrast to the germinal center on the **top left**, the infiltrating small lymphocytes coexpressed T-cell–associated antigen CD43, supporting a diagnosis of MALT lymphoma (immunoperoxidase stain, original magnification: 300× magnification).

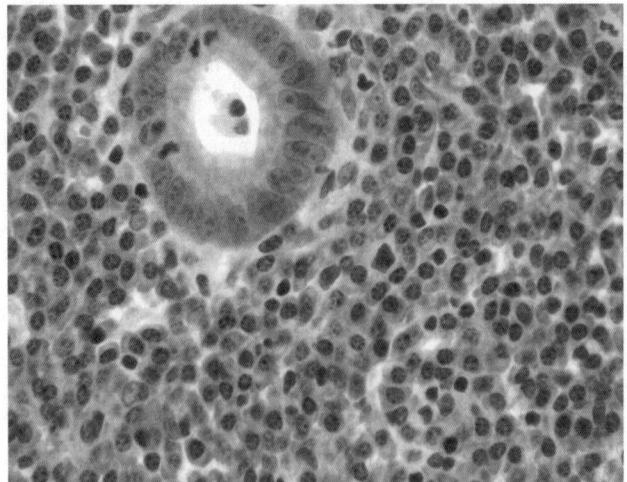

FIGURE 28.8. Follow-up gastric biopsy from patient with established extranodal marginal zone lymphoma of MALT type exhibits a loss of B lymphocytes and replacement by a monomorphous infiltrate of plasma cells that were shown to be of monoclonal κ type. Plasma cell–rich extranodal MALT cases in stomach are reported in patients after treatment with rituximab (hematoxylin and eosin stain, original magnification: 600× magnification).

challenging in small biopsy specimens, such as the ocular region, where it may mimic lymphoma (72). Equally vexing is the distinction of extramedullary, extranodal lymphoplasmacytic lymphoma from extranodal marginal zone lymphoma with plasmacytic differentiation. Whereas lymphoplasmacytic lymphoma usually is associated with a monoclonal gammopathy, mainly IgM, extranodal marginal zone lymphoma similarly may be associated with an IgM paraprotein, particularly in cases with conspicuous plasmacytic features (73,74). Both lymphomas also exhibit morphologic and immunophenotypic overlap with common lack of CD5 and CD10 expression. The distinction of lymphoplasmacytic lymphoma from extranodal marginal zone lymphoma rich in plasma cells may require ancillary studies, such as fluorescence *in situ* hybridization to determine whether a translocation, such as *AP12-MLT1,* is present to indicate extranodal marginal zone lymphoma (74). Translocations, however, are discovered in only a minority of MALT lymphomas, and in some cases the difference between these two lymphomas is ambiguous, leading to a descriptive diagnosis, such as "small B-cell lymphoma with plasmacytic differentiation" (73,75). The differential diagnosis of extraosseous

plasmacytoma from extranodal marginal zone lymphoma with sheets of plasma cells likewise may be difficult. Extraosseous plasmacytoma is rare, and although it may occur in a variety of extranodal sites, approximately 80% affect the upper respiratory tract with a classic plasma cell immunophenotype including expression of CD138 and monoclonal light chain restriction (54). The documentation of a B-cell component coupled with the presence of invasion of germinal centers and epithelium by the neoplastic marginal zone cells generally allows for the distinction of plasmacytic extranodal marginal zone lymphoma from extraosseous plasmacytoma (74).

Germinal Centers in Extranodal Lymphomas

The presence of germinal centers is a commonly accepted histologic attribute of extranodal lymphoid hyperplasias. Germinal centers, however, are regular constituents of many extranodal lymphomas. Germinal centers often are observed at the periphery of large cell lymphomas, such as those in the thyroid (42,76). In the thyroid, a histologic continuum frequently occurs between areas of chronic lymphocytic thyroiditis with germinal centers and areas of adjacent large cell lymphoma, usually devoid of germinal centers (42) (Fig. 28.10); this finding has suggested that thyroid lymphomas evolve from chronic lymphocytic (Hashimoto) thyroiditis (76).

There now is unequivocal acceptance that germinal centers also may be identified in the middle of an aggressive lymphoma, for example, lymphoblastic lymphomas of the scalp and mantle cell lymphomas of intestinal multiple lymphomatous polyposis (38,77,78). Frequently, in cases of multiple lymphomatous polyposis due to mantle cell lymphoma, the germinal centers appear atrophic and are encircled by dense, monomorphous neoplastic lymphocytes (38,77) (Fig. 28.11). Germinal centers also are an integral component of the center of many extranodal marginal zone lymphomas of MALT type. The essential morphologic characteristic of MALT lymphomas is their emulation of normal MALT, as typified by Peyer patches found in the terminal ileum (15). The neoplastic B cells of MALT lymphomas are found in marginal-type zones surrounding reactive follicles, and frequently in attenuated rims of mantle zone lymphocytes. In MALT lymphomas of the lung, for example, germinal centers frequently are observed in the expanded alveolar walls surrounded by the proliferating neoplastic small lymphocytes (35–37) (Fig. 28.12). The germinal centers vary in appearance but commonly appear atrophic as a result of impingement by

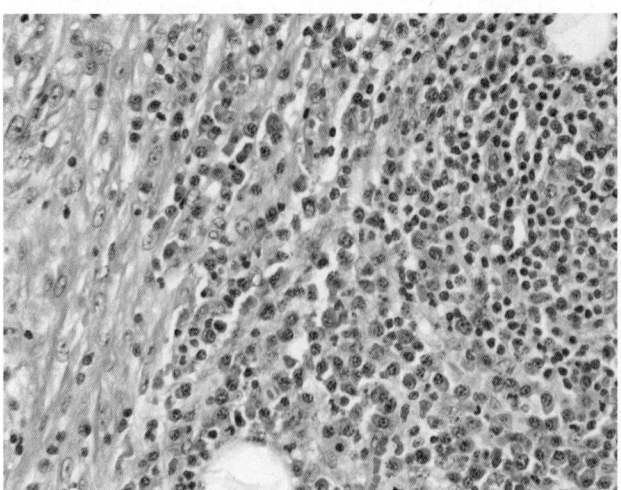

FIGURE 28.9. A compact lymphoplasmacytic infiltrate in breast due to IgG4-related disease can simulate an extranodal marginal zone lymphoma, especially in core biopsy specimens (hematoxylin and eosin stain, original magnification: 300× magnification).

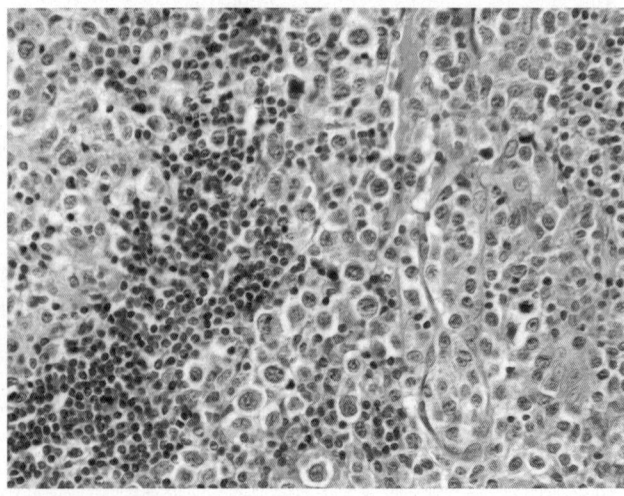

FIGURE 28.10. A reactive germinal center on the left that reflects chronic lymphocytic thyroiditis merges with large B-cell lymphoma in the thyroid gland (hematoxylin and eosin stain, original magnification: 300× magnification).

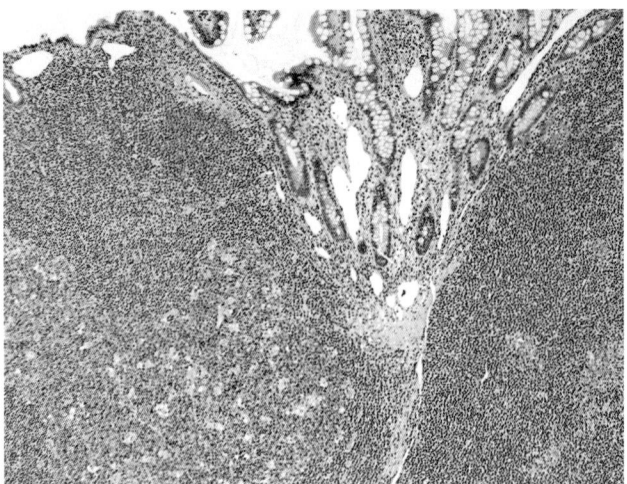

FIGURE 28.11. Mantle cell lymphoma of the small intestine surrounds germinal centers in a case of multiple lymphomatous polyposis (hematoxylin and eosin stain, original magnification: 60× magnification).

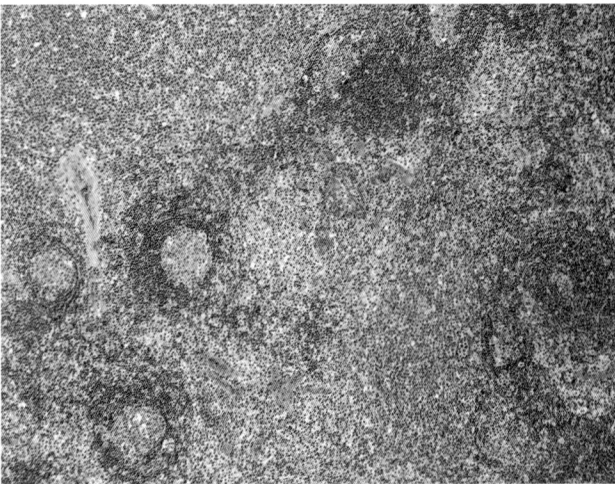

FIGURE 28.13. Extranodal marginal zone lymphoma in the parotid gland composed mainly of monocytoid B cells that developed in a setting of LESA. The monocytoid cells form interconnecting strands. The residual germinal centers contain variably intact mantle zones, distinct from the light staining cytoplasm of the monocytoid cells (hematoxylin and eosin stain, original magnification: 60× magnification).

the surrounding small lymphocytes. In marginal zone MALT lymphomas of the stomach associated with peptic ulceration, germinal centers tend to occur at the base of the ulcer and in the adjacent mucosa, in which they seem encroached on and entrapped by the monotonous marginal zone lymphomatous population (53,59). In some cases, the neoplastic B cells in the marginal zone invade the germinal centers in a process referred to as *follicular colonization* (59,79). Follicular colonization may simulate follicular lymphoma in patients in whom there are numerous follicles. At times, the lymphomatous proliferation may be so extensive as to result in architectural obliteration with masking of any residual germinal centers; however, the presence of former germinal centers can be highlighted by the immunohistochemical demonstration of follicular dendritic cells employing an antibody against CD21 or CD23 (37,38,59).

The finding of germinal centers in a small lymphocytic infiltrate in either the lung or stomach could be construed as examples of extranodal lymphoid hyperplasia; however, in both extranodal sites, replacement of the mantle zones is a histologic indication that the small lymphocytes likely are neoplastic. The mantle zones often are intact in MALT lymphomas dominated by monocytoid-like cells that affect salivary glands,

but in such patients the mantle zones and the germinal centers appear attenuated by the surrounding monocytoid cells (22,41) (Fig. 28.13). The characteristic, well-developed lucent cytoplasm in the monocytoid cells contrasts with the lack of visible cytoplasm in residual small lymphocytes (Fig. 28.14).

Incomplete Architectural Effacement in Extranodal Lymphomas

Architectural effacement as a consequence of malignant lymphoma is a standard diagnostic tenet. Extranodal lymphomas usually obliterate and destroy normal epithelial structures and extend beyond the margins of that organ. For example, in the gastrointestinal tract, most aggressive lymphomas invade beyond the muscularis propria to the serosa and often into adjacent mesenteric fat. Gastrointestinal lymphoid hyperplasia generally is restricted to the mucosa or submucosa, with conservation of mucosal glands and crypts. Gastrointestinal lymphoid hyperplasia and malignant lymphomas, however, can deviate from these norms (59,80). Gastrointestinal

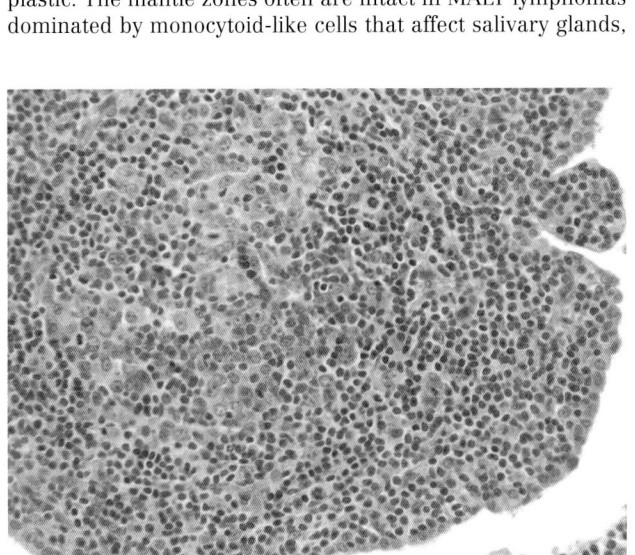

FIGURE 28.12. In extranodal marginal zone lymphoma of the lung, a germinal center is entrapped and the follicles infiltrated or "colonized" by the neoplastic small lymphocytes with obliteration of the mantle zone. The small lymphocytes proved to be monoclonal B cells of IgMλ type (hematoxylin and eosin stain, original magnification: 300× magnification).

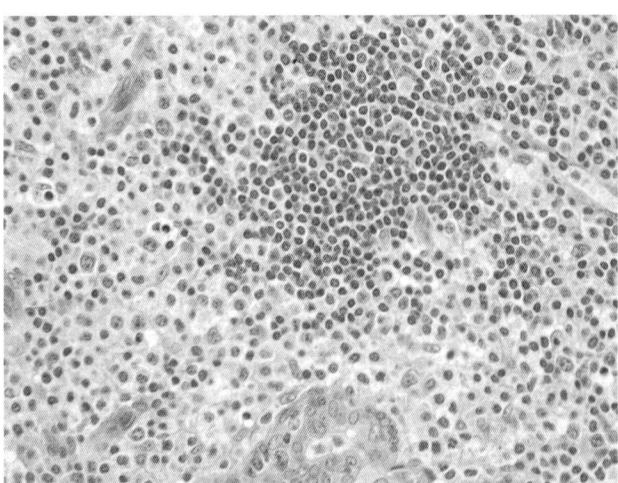

FIGURE 28.14. The pale, almost lucent cytoplasm of the monocytoid cells contrasts with the small lymphocytes in a residual lymphoid island in the parotid gland (hematoxylin and eosin stain, original magnification: 300× magnification).

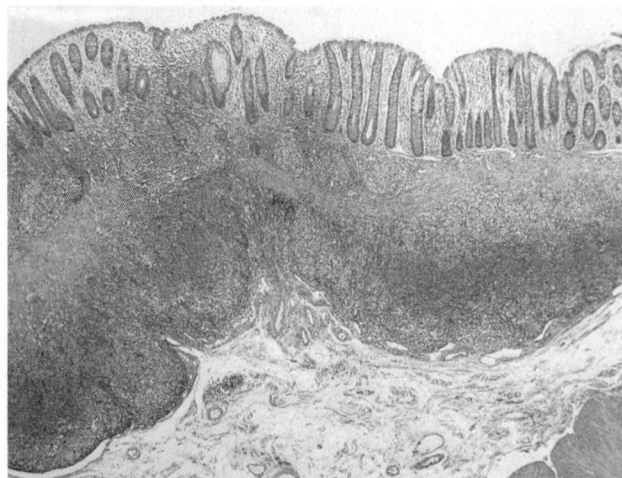

FIGURE 28.15. An extranodal marginal zone monoclonal B-cell lymphoma forms a localized polyp in the colon without destruction of the mucosa. The pattern mimics gastrointestinal lymphoid hyperplasia (hematoxylin and eosin stain, original magnification: 30× magnification).

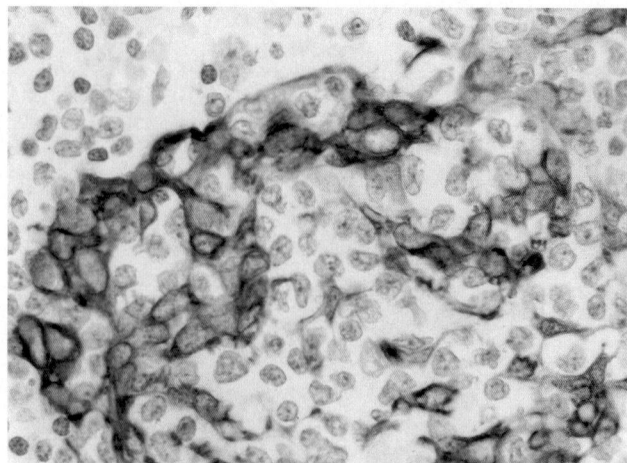

FIGURE 28.16. In LESA, invasion of epimyoepithelial islands may be observed; in this case it is highlighted with a stain for cytokeratin. Epithelial invasion or a lymphoepithelial-like lesion is not an absolute diagnostic criterion for extranodal lymphoma (immunoperoxidase stain, original magnification: 900× magnification).

lymphomas, particularly of MALT type, may be exceedingly subtle and confined to the mucosa and submucosa, without violation of the muscularis propria and with preservation of most mucosal glands (53,59) (Fig. 28.15). Alternatively, rare cases of lymphoid hyperplasia may be florid and involve the entire depth of the gastrointestinal wall (80). In skin, malignant lymphomas may have a patchy, perivascular distribution in early lesions, may surround cutaneous adnexa, and even may be "top heavy," similar to cutaneous lymphoid hyperplasia (81,82). Conversely, cases of cutaneous lymphoid hyperplasia may invade cutaneous adnexa and be "bottom heavy," with infiltration into subcutaneous fat (68,83).

Invasion of epithelial structures, or "lymphoepithelial lesions" in the context of lymphomas of MALT, is an architectural feature purported to be significant in the diagnosis of extranodal lymphomas (14–17). However, epithelial invasion by neoplastic lymphocytes actually may be difficult to identify, especially in the assessment of a small biopsy specimen when the differential diagnosis rests between a marginal zone lymphoma of MALT type and lymphoid hyperplasia. In both conditions, epithelial structures are reduced by the lymphoid proliferation, but frank epithelial infiltration may not be prominent even with the use of a cytokeratin stain, which accentuates a lymphoepithelial lesion (42). Epithelial invasion virtually indistinguishable from a lymphoepithelial lesion may be found in various extranodal lymphoid hyperplasias, such as in the lung, salivary gland, thyroid, ileocecal region, and skin (36,41,42,58,83) (Fig. 28.16). Lymphoepithelial lesions are thought to be most significant as a diagnostic criterion of MALT lymphomas in the stomach where a lymphoepithelial lesion is defined as invasion of gastric epithelium by three or more neoplastic B lymphocytes (64); however, even in the stomach, lymphoid hyperplasia associated with *H. pylori* infection can exhibit infiltration of gastric epithelium and resemble a lymphomatous lymphoepithelial lesion (43,59). Vascular invasion is a more consistent morphologic feature of lymphomas than of extranodal lymphoid hyperplasias. In the rare cases of intravascular lymphomatosis, such as those in the skin and CNS, vascular involvement may be the only sign of extranodal lymphoma (84).

Although massive infiltration with architectural destruction is the general rule for most extranodal lymphomas, each case and each specific site must be assessed independently. Interpretation of architectural features in extranodal lymphocytic infiltrates depends on knowledge of the topography and histologic uniqueness of a specific site, in addition to a thorough evaluation of the cytologic composition of the lymphocytic infiltrate.

JUXTAPOSITION OF EXTRANODAL LYMPHOMA AND LYMPHOID HYPERPLASIA

One idiosyncrasy that results in diagnostic problems in the pathologic evaluation of extranodal lymphoid proliferations is that lymphomas commonly are juxtaposed with areas of lymphoid hyperplasia (41,42,59,76). This problem is accentuated in small biopsy specimens, in which it may prove impossible to sort out the reactive from the neoplastic areas. Frequently, the sample is delusive and contains only the hyperplastic area. In the skin, for example, reactive T cells often proliferate in the superficial dermis, with lymphoma confined to the deeper portion of the dermis (81) (Fig. 28.17). In this setting, a thin shave biopsy specimen is inadequate.

In large surgical resections of extranodal lymphoid lesions, a continuous spectrum between areas of lymphoid hyperplasia and malignant lymphoma frequently is discovered. This is especially true in the salivary and thyroid glands and correlates with the observation that patients who have Sjögren syndrome and Hashimoto disease have an increased risk of developing malignant lymphoma (19–22,41,42,76). The propensity for malignant lymphoma in the salivary and thyroid glands, as well as in other extranodal sites, likely parallels those associated with infectious agents, as for example *H. pylori*, and is a probable multistage process tacitly related to abnormal immune surveillance, possible decreased normal suppressor T-cell modulation, and development of a neoplastic clone that follows persistent antigenic B-cell stimulation by exoantigens or autoantigens that generate lymphoid hyperplasia with immunoglobulin gene hypermutation, encompassing aberrant somatic hypermutation (16,24,64,85–89). In the salivary glands of patients with Sjögren syndrome, for example, LESA–associated clonal infiltrates derived from different patients bind the identical or similar antigens to suggest that LESA clones begin as nonmalignant antigen-selected B-cell expansions (90). These investigations and hypotheses support molecular genetic studies that have detected clonal immunoglobulin gene rearrangements in patients who have clinical Sjögren syndrome and Hashimoto disease and who do not have histologic evidence of malignant lymphoma (21–23,91,92). For those patients with Hashimoto disease who evolve to thyroid lymphoma, clonality and sequence similarity ensues between the Hashimoto and lymphomatous components (93), whereas the lymphomas

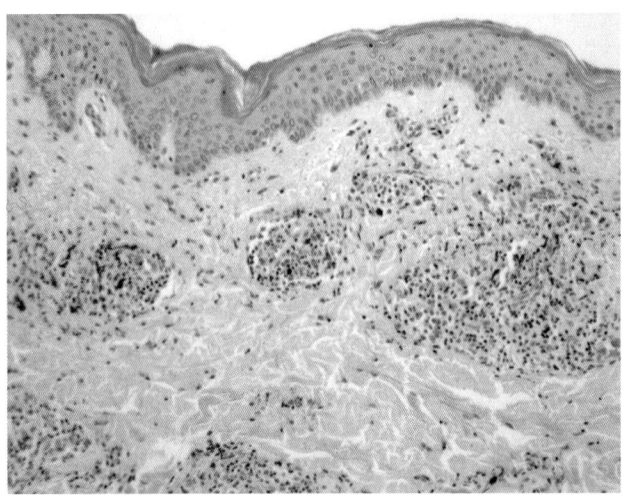
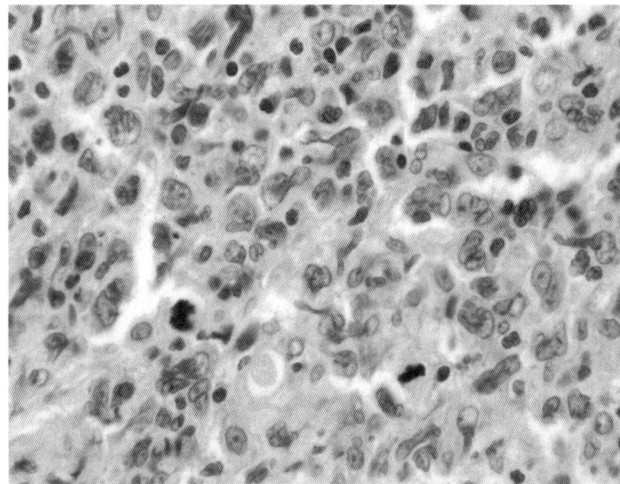

A   B

FIGURE 28.17. A: The superficial dermis in this skin biopsy specimen contains merely a reactive T-cell population (hematoxylin and eosin stain, original magnification: 150× magnification). **B:** The areas diagnostic of large B-cell lymphoma were present only in the deeper dermis (hematoxylin and eosin stain, original magnification: 600× magnification).

that develop secondary to the reactive salivary gland infiltrates of Sjögren syndrome express a restricted immunoglobulin V_H gene repertoire that differs from MALT lymphomas of other sites (87,94).

Although an extranodal lymphoma may be relatively straightforward to diagnose, even if found contiguous to lymphoid hyperplasia, lymphoma may be masked when it is focal and the hyperplasia prolific. An unequivocal diagnosis of malignant lymphoma in this setting rests on the conviction that a discrete homogeneous zone of lymphoid cells appears malignant. This zone must be more than the small cluster or aggregate of atypical lymphocytes that can be present in cases of lymphoid hyperplasia.

The most demanding diagnostic problem occurs when the malignant lymphoma that develops in the setting of lymphoid hyperplasia is not an aggressive but an indolent lymphoma. This situation is best exemplified in patients who have Sjögren syndrome and histologic LESA in a salivary gland. In LESA, multiple confluent lymphocytic aggregates that include germinal centers and surrounding mantle zones are present (41). Epimyoepithelial islands are observed with partial destruction and obliteration of salivary gland ducts and acini. The malignant lymphomas that arise in this background frequently are subtle and histologically are lymphomas of MALT that usually are dominated by monocytoid-type cells and often display some plasma cell differentiation (22,37,41). The recognition of concentrated monomorphous areas of monocytoid cells sufficient to be morphologically diagnostic of malignant lymphoma is frequently problematic, and immunologic confirmation is important. If the histologic features are equivocal, such as the formation of nonconfluent monocytoid or clear cell "halos" (Fig. 28.18), a diagnosis of focal malignant lymphoma is controversial and may not be justifiable even if a monoclonal cell population can be demonstrated with the use of molecular methods (22,91,92). Moreover, clonality does not necessarily predict progression to the eventual development of clinically overt lymphoma (92).

TECHNICAL CONSIDERATIONS

In the assessment of extranodal lymphomas, technical considerations are a common and vexing problem (95). An accurate histologic diagnosis depends on the nature and quality of the tissue sample. Many initial biopsy specimens of extranodal lesions are small, such as shave and punch biopsies of skin;

incisional biopsies of ocular lesions; and bronchoscopic, gastroscopic, and endoscopic biopsies; in addition to needle core biopsy specimens from any site. These specimens often are subject to various alterations, including crush artifact and smudging (Fig. 28.19), as well as the fact that a small sample may not be representative of the extranodal infiltrate.

If the extranodal lesion is composed mainly of large cells, these may be insufficient in quantity, and the pattern may be developed inadequately to exclude absolutely the possibility of another large cell malignant neoplasm, for example carcinoma. In small biopsy specimens that contain a malignant large cell neoplasm, an immunoperoxidase panel for cytokeratin, pan–B cell and pan–T cell antigens such as CD20 and CD3, and possibly S-100 protein should be performed routinely (18,95) (Fig. 28.20). Should reactivity for these markers be negative, the differential diagnostic possibilities broaden and for cases in which a malignant hematopoietic neoplasm is suspected, appropriate stains with antimyeloid antibodies, such as myeloperoxidase, ought to follow (Fig. 28.21).

Some extranodal large cell proliferations are not neoplastic and are mere clusters of reactive immunoblasts or stimulated

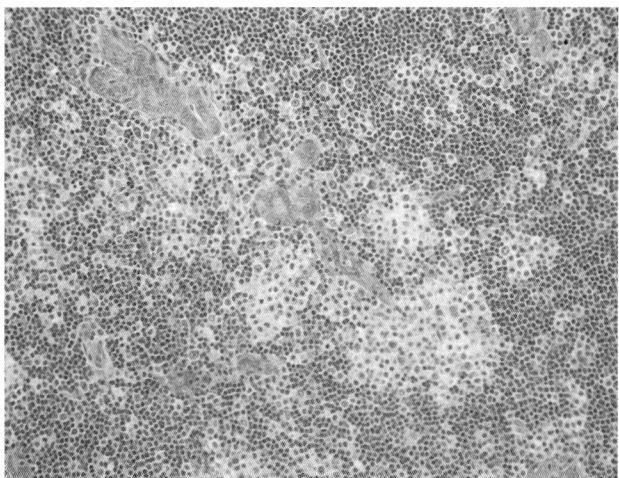

FIGURE 28.18. A halo-like lesion composed of pale-staining monocytoid cells forms against a background of LESA in a salivary gland. Many such halos prove to be monoclonal, but there is no consensus as to whether these cases should be interpreted as early extranodal marginal zone lymphomas (hematoxylin and eosin stain, original magnification: 150× magnification).

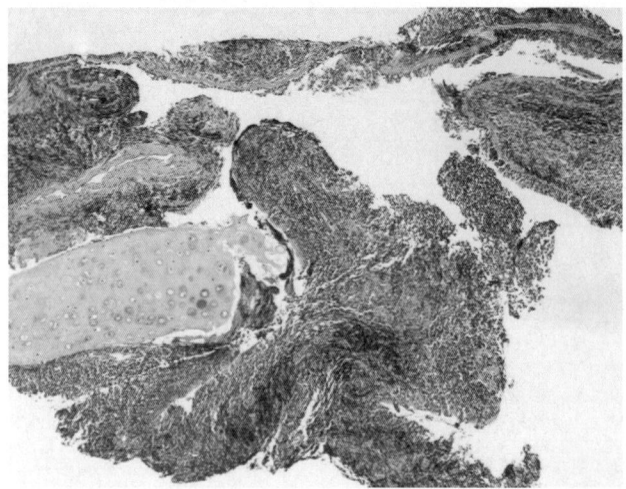

FIGURE 28.19. A bronchial biopsy specimen of the right middle lobe is not diagnostic because of severe crush artifact. An immunoperoxidase panel revealed that the crushed cells were CD20⁺ B cells, but due to the distortion only a descriptive diagnosis of "lymphocytic infiltrate, predominately B cell" was rendered. A subsequent excisional specimen disclosed unequivocal extranodal marginal zone lymphoma of MALT type (hematoxylin and eosin stain, original magnification: 60× magnification).

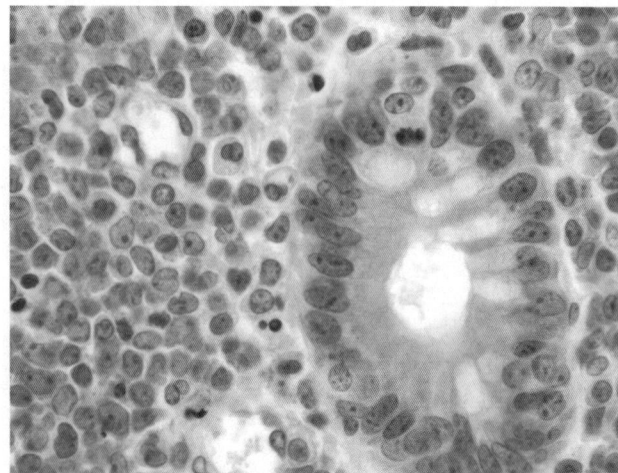

FIGURE 28.21. A large cell malignant neoplasm in the small intestine did not express B- or T-cell lineage–specific antigens or cytokeratin; however, the neoplastic cells subsequently were shown to express myeloperoxidase to justify a diagnosis of myeloid sarcoma (hematoxylin and eosin stain, original magnification: 600× magnification).

centroblasts in germinal centers of patients with florid lymphoid hyperplasia (Fig. 28.22). Reactive immunoblasts or centroblasts in hyperplastic germinal centers may appear monomorphous and do not always exhibit a range of lymphocytic transformation in a small biopsy specimen. Should a diagnosis of large cell lymphoma in this setting be at odds with the clinical setting, or if there is any suggestion of a reactive condition, it is sensible to offer a diagnosis, such as "atypical," and to request a second biopsy including fresh tissue for clonality studies. Similar discretion should be used for small biopsy specimens that contain only small lymphocytes, particularly if the infiltrate is focal or insufficiently dense or monomorphous, to be absolutely certain about whether the small lymphocytes are reactive or neoplastic. Both reactive and neoplastic small lymphocytes may mask an underlying, deeper aggressive lymphoma, such as in stomach or skin (59,81); only the small lymphocytic, often reactive component may be submitted for pathologic examination in a gastroscopic or superficial shave biopsy specimen. If the morphologic features tally best with a marginal zone lymphoma of

MALT type, yet are not completely absolute, an immunoperoxidase panel is required, primarily CD20 and CD3, as well as CD43 and/or CD5, CD21, possibly cytokeratin, and, if plasma cells are numerous, stains for κ and λ light chains (38). These stains will determine if an aberrant immunophenotype exists, such as a predominance of CD20⁺ B cells, if the B lymphocytes exhibit aberrant coexpression with CD43 or CD5, if the cytokeratin stain accentuates lymphoepithelial lesions, if cryptic germinal centers are present by reactivity for CD21 to indicate follicular colonization, and if a plasma cell population is monoclonal with κ or λ light chain restriction (37,59,64,79). Providing that the morphologic and immunophenotypic studies in this setting are strongly suspicious, but not absolutely indicative, of MALT lymphoma, molecular studies employing PCR also can be employed (22,35,36,55,62,91,93). Under these circumstances, interpretation of the histologic, immunophenotypic, and molecular studies must be placed in the context of the clinical setting, especially with the awareness that benign entities, such as chronic active gastritis and LESA, may exhibit immunoglobulin gene rearrangements without necessarily developing clinical

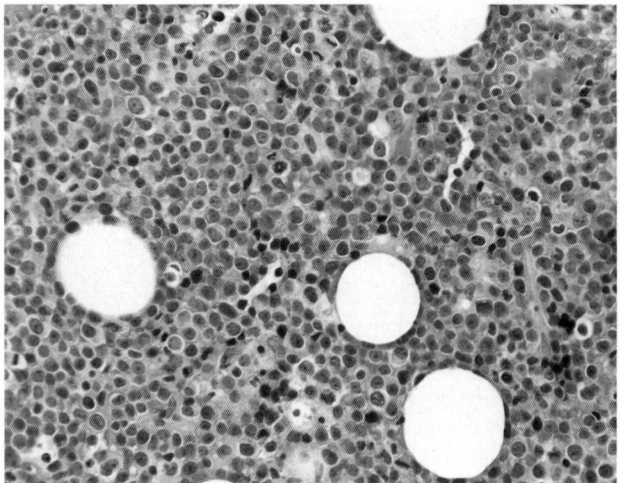

FIGURE 28.20. A large cell malignant neoplasm suspicious for lymphoma was found in a small core biopsy from breast. The diagnosis of lymphoma was verified by positive reactivity for the CD20 antigen coupled with a negative stain for cytokeratin (hematoxylin and eosin stain, original magnification: 300× magnification).

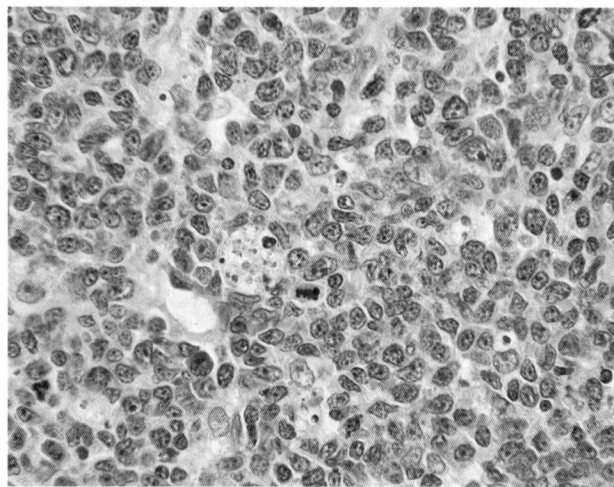

FIGURE 28.22. Stimulated centroblasts in a hyperplastic germinal center easily may be confused with malignant lymphoma in a small colonoscopic biopsy specimen, despite the presence of a tingible body macrophage (hematoxylin and eosin stain, original magnification: 600× magnification).

malignant lymphoma in follow-up studies (66,67,92). Should the PCR study prove negative, the possibility of lymphoma in the ambiguous lymphocytic infiltrate remains, resulting in a descriptive diagnosis and, depending on the clinical features, another biopsy with reservation of fresh tissue to determine clonality, such as by flow cytometry (38,61). Molecular studies also can be requested at this stage if the new biopsy remains suspicious and flow cytometry and other investigations prove unproductive.

IMPLICATIONS OF IMMUNOLOGIC CELL MARKER AND MOLECULAR GENETIC STUDIES ON EXTRANODAL LYMPHOID PROLIFERATIONS

The use of immunologic cell marker and molecular genetic studies has offered an entirely new perspective for the interpretation of lymphoid lesions, including those in extranodal sites (16,17,23,39,64). With simple, readily accessible immunoperoxidase techniques, an extranodal large cell neoplasm can be classified definitively as malignant lymphoma, as opposed to undifferentiated carcinoma, malignant melanoma, or myeloid sarcoma (18,96). In addition, the B- or T-cell lineage of a malignant lymphoma can be ascertained in both fixed and fresh tissues (22,33–36,41,42,53,76–78,81–83). Extranodal B-cell small lymphocytic lesions that formerly were regarded as histologically indeterminate can be phenotyped precisely as polyclonal, and therefore reactive or monoclonal. The demonstration of monoclonality in an extranodal small lymphocytic proliferation generally has been equated with malignant lymphoma and has reduced the number of cases that are interpreted as extranodal lymphoid hyperplasia or pseudolymphoma (16,17,40). As discussed earlier, judicious use of PCR also can be employed to determine clonality with the proviso that patients with a variety of histologically benign and immunologically polyclonal extranodal lymphoid hyperplasias, including chronic active gastritis, LESA, and various cutaneous disorders, may reveal immunoglobulin gene rearrangements yet not histologically display, or progress to, overt malignant lymphoma (17,21–23,55,62,66–69,92). Nonetheless, B-cell monoclonality may have clinical ramifications in some patients with extranodal lymphoid hyperplasia, and such lesions could be viewed as prelymphomatous or borderline; for example, clonality in *H. pylori*–associated chronic gastritis may precede the onset of gastric MALT lymphoma by 3 to 4 years (97,98).

The biologic significance of finding a clonal B- or T-cell population in the setting of a histologically reactive and clinically benign extranodal lymphocytic proliferation is uncertain. Because many extranodal clonal B-cell populations are antigen driven, early clonal lesions are reversible and susceptible to antibiotic therapy, such as *H. pylori*–related clonal gastric lymphocytic infiltrates, *C. jejuni*–associated MALT lymphomas of the intestine, and *C. psittaci*–positive ocular adnexal MALT lymphomas (25,26,28,85); successful antibiotic treatment additionally has been reported for early-stage *H. pylori*–positive DLBCL of stomach (99). Antibiotics, as well as use of rituximab, an anti-CD20 antibody, also may prove effective in the early lymphoid infiltrates associated with autoimmune-related marginal zone lymphomas, as seen in Sjögren syndrome (28,89).

The events that trigger the transformation of extranodal lymphoid hyperplasia to extranodal lymphoma, specifically MALT type, in a block of cases commence with the onset of cytogenetic alterations. The genetic abnormalities encompass trisomies 3, 12, and 18, as well as balanced translocations, expressly t(11;18)(q21;q21), t(14;18)(q32;q21), t(1;14)

(p22;q32), and t(3;14)(p14;q32) (16,17,55,64,100–105). The most frequent translocation in gastric MALT lymphoma arising in approximately 20% to 30% of cases (though lower in North America) is t(11;18)(q21;q21), in which the t(11;18) fuses with amino terminal of the inhibitor of apoptosis *API2* at 11q21 to the carboxyl terminal of *MALT1* at 18q21, leading to a chimeric fusion product (55,101,105). MALT1 is involved in antigen receptor-mediated nuclear factor (NF)-κB activation, and MALT lymphomas that express the translocation exhibit enhanced expression of NF-κB target genes, although MALT lymphomas without t(11;18)(q21;q21) support active inflammatory and immune responses (106). The t(11;18)(q21;q21) is limited to extranodal MALT lymphomas, mainly gastrointestinal tract and lung (64,107), and has not been reported in other forms of marginal zone lymphoma, specifically splenic or nodal, or in chronic gastritis associated with *H. pylori* (108,109). Gastric MALT lymphomas devoid of t(11;18)(q21;q21) frequently demonstrate aneuploidy, as for example trisomy 3, 12, or 18 (103,104,110). Pulmonary MALT lymphomas may exhibit *API-MALT1* fusion, trisomy, or no detectable gene abnormality (111). Although the *API-MALT1* fusion and trisomy 3 cases may be mutated, others are unmutated to suggest that T-cell–independent extrafollicular B-cell maturation could be significant in the pathogenesis of pulmonary MALT lymphoma.

For gastric MALT lymphoma, the discovery of t(11;18)(q21;q21) in some patients has prompted stimulating clinicopathologic correlations. Patients with gastric MALT lymphoma who express t(11;18)(q21;q21) commonly do not respond to *H. pylori* therapy, and this translocation frequently develops in patients who are *H. pylori* negative (17,55,112,113). Endosonographic staging reveals that t(11;18)(q21;q21)-positive patients who are refractory to antibiotic *H. pylori* eradication often have lymphoma that has extended beyond the gastric submucosa into muscularis and/or serosa as opposed to patients with lymphoma restricted to the mucosa and submucosa who usually are t(11;18)(q21;q21) negative (17,37,102). Additionally, t(11;18)(q21;q21) is rare in extranodal DLBCL, and patients with this translocation usually do not transform to DLBCL (55,103,104). In contrast, patients with aneuploidy, who are t(11;18)(q21;q21) negative and unresponsive to *H. pylori* eradication, are in jeopardy to progress to DLBCL.

The remaining three translocations are far less common than t(11;18)(q21;q21), with a dearth of statistics regarding their prevalence and specificity (105,114). Translocation t(14;18)(q32;q21) deregulates *MALT1* expression by juxtaposing the immunoglobulin heavy chain (*IGH*) gene enhancer region to *MALT1* at 18q21 and has been reported in MALT lymphoma in various sites including skin, ocular adnexa, salivary gland, and liver, but rarely in the gastrointestinal tract and lung and not in thyroid (64,105,114,115). The t(1;14)(p22;q32) deregulates *BCL10* expression with the combination of the *IGH* enhancer region at 14q32 to *BCL10* on 1p22 leading to overexpression of BCL10 (64,105,116); in one study, this translocation was discovered in only 1.6% of 252 primary lymphomas of MALT (114). The translocation t(3;14)(p14;q32) deregulates the expression of the *FOXP1* gene and is found in lymphomas of the thyroid, ocular adnexa, and skin (117). Most MALT lymphomas with t(3;14)(p14;q32) harbor further genetic abnormalities, as for example trisomy 3. Trisomies also are common in association with t(14;18)(q32;q21) and t(1;14)(p22;q32) (115,118).

Translocations t(11;18)(q21;q21), t(14;18)(q32;q21), and t(1;14)(p22;q32) are connected by the functions of MALT1 and BCL10 in stimulating the canonical NF-κB pathway and aberrant deregulated NF-κB activation signifies their crucial role in lymphomagenesis (105,106,118,119). MALT lymphoma cases with t(3;14)(p14;q32) also may impact the NF-κB pathway through various FOXP1 isoforms (119). In addition to aberrant

NF-κB signaling, and as noted earlier, translocation-positive extranodal marginal zone lymphomas of MALT are characterized by enhanced expression of NF-κB target genes, including toll like receptor 6, CD69, and BCL2 (106). Translocation-negative cases exhibit enhanced expression of genes associated with active inflammatory and immune responses, as for example interleukin-8, CD28, CD86, and inducible T-cell costimulator. Translocation-negative MALT lymphomas also may impact the NF-κB pathway through A20, an essential global NF-κB inhibitor; A20 is inactivated by somatic deletions and/or mutations in some translocation-negative cases, mainly in the ocular adnexa (119). In MALT lymphomas of the ocular adnexa, A20 inactivation is associated with poor disease-free survival and a correlative need for higher radiation dosages to achieve complete remission in contrast to those patients without A20 abnormalities (119,120). In patients with autoimmune-associated MALT lymphomas of salivary gland and thyroid, the incidence of A20 abnormalities is low (121).

Notwithstanding the clinicopathologic correlations associated with cytogenetic and other molecular abnormalities in patients with extranodal marginal lymphomas of MALT type, the overall prognosis of this lymphoma is excellent, despite a propensity for dissemination in one-third of cases (122). For example, in one study of gastric MALT lymphomas treated by various modalities, the 5-year projected overall survival was 82% (123). Extranodal marginal zone lymphomas originating extrinsic to the stomach likewise are indolent with a reported 5-year overall survival of 90% (124). In a report of 211 extranodal marginal zone lymphomas from any site, the 5-year overall survival was documented at 87% (125). In that series, for extranodal sites with more than five cases, the 5-year overall survival rates were salivary gland 96%, intestine 91%, orbit 90%, skin 84%, lung 84%, stomach 83%, and Waldeyer ring 80%; the 5-year overall survival for the remaining sites encompassing connective tissue, breast kidney, thyroid, larynx, and dura was 100% (125). According to two well-documented studies, histologic progression to DLBCL develops in 3% to 8% of cases without statistical differences between patients with localized or disseminated disease at presentation (122,124). Clearly, patients who transform to DLBCL, or who present with extranodal DLBCL or who are diagnosed with noncutaneous extranodal T-cell lymphomas, such as nasal type NK/T-cell lymphoma, have a more guarded prognosis and usually require aggressive therapy.

SUMMARY AND CONCLUSIONS

The pathologic interpretation of a lymphoid proliferation in an extranodal site is demanding, particularly with the many exceptions and pitfalls in the histologic norms traditionally used to separate extranodal malignant lymphoma from lymphoid hyperplasia. Despite these exceptions, most extranodal lymphoid proliferations are readily diagnosable. The diagnosis of extranodal marginal zone lymphomas of MALT, or other lymphoma subtypes, depends not on the discovery of an occult clonal cell population but on strict histopathologic criteria augmented by immunophenotypic and prudent molecular genetic studies. Moreover, traditional morphologic perceptions must be tempered by and integrated into the evolving concepts discovered as a result of immunopathologic and molecular genetic correlations and viewed in the context of the clinical setting. The initiation of long-term clinical studies and the continually rapid discovery of new genetic and biologic markers to precisely determine malignant transformation of extranodal lymphoid proliferations will define further their natural history and increase the accuracy of distinguishing between extranodal lymphoid hyperplasia and malignant lymphoma.

References

1. Swerdlow SH, Campo E, Harris NL, et al., eds. *WHO classification of tumours of haematopoietic and lymphoid tissues*, 4th ed. Lyon: IARC, 2008.
2. Isaacson PG, Chott A, Nakamura S, et al. Extranodal marginal zone lymphoma of mucosa-associated lymphoid tissue (MALT lymphoma). In: Swerdlow SH, Campo E, Harris NL, et al., eds. *WHO classification of tumours of haematopoietic and lymphoid tissues*, 4th ed. Lyon: IARC, 2008:214–217.
3. D'Amore F, Christensen BE, Brincker H, et al. Clinicopathological features and prognostic factors in extranodal non-Hodgkin lymphomas. *Eur J Cancer* 1991;27:1201–1208.
4. Greiner TC, Medeiros JL, Jaffe ES. Non-Hodgkin's lymphoma. *Cancer* 1995;75:370–380.
5. Groves FD, Linet MS, Travis LB, et al. Cancer surveillance series: non-Hodgkin's lymphoma incidence by histologic subtype in the United States from 1978 through 1995. *J Natl Cancer Inst* 2000;92:1240–1251.
6. Krol AD, le Cessie S, Snijder S, et al. Primary extranodal non-Hodgkin's lymphomas (NHL): the impact of alternative definitions tested in the Comprehensive Cancer Centre West population-based NHL registry. *Ann Oncol* 2003;14:131–139.
7. Wu XC, Andrews P, Chen VW, et al. Incidence of extranodal non-Hodgkin lymphomas among whites, blacks, and Asian/Pacific Islanders in the United States; anatomic site and histology differences. *Cancer Epidemiol* 2009;33:337–346.
8. Yang QP, Zhang WY, Yu JB, et al. Subtype distribution of lymphomas in southwest China: analysis of 6,382 cases using WHO classification in a single institution. *Diagn Pathol* 2011;6:77–83.
9. Luminari S, Cesaretti M, Marcheselli L, et al. Decreasing incidence of gastric MALT lymphomas in the era of anti-*Helicobacter pylori* interventions: results from a population-based study on extranodal marginal zone lymphomas. *Ann Oncol* 2010;21:855–859.
10. Olson JE, Janney CA, Rao RD, et al. The continuing increase in the incidence of primary central nervous system non-Hodgkin lymphoma: a surveillance, epidemiology, and end results analysis. *Cancer* 2002;95:1504–1510.
11. Knowles DM. Etiology and pathogenesis of AIDS-related non-Hodgkin's lymphomas. *Hematol Oncol Clin North Am* 2003;17:785–820.
12. Delecluse HJ, Anagnostopoulos I, Dallenbach F, et al. Plasmablastic lymphomas of the oral cavity: a new entity associated with the human immunodeficiency virus infection. *Blood* 1997;89:1413–1420.
13. Gospodarowicz MK, Sutcliffe SB. The extranodal lymphomas. *Semin Radiat Oncol* 1995;4:281–300.
14. Isaacson P, Wright DH. Extranodal malignant lymphoma arising from mucosa-associated lymphoid tissue. *Cancer* 1984;53:2515–2524.
15. Isaacson PG, Spencer J. Malignant lymphoma of mucosa-associated lymphoid tissue. *Histopathology* 1987;11:445–462.
16. Isaacson PG, Du MQ. MALT lymphoma: from morphology to molecules. *Nat Rev Cancer* 2004;4:644–653.
17. Bacon CM, Du MQ, Dogan A. Mucosa-associated lymphoid tissue (MALT) lymphoma: a practical guide for pathologists. *J Clin Pathol* 2007;60:361–372.
18. Burke JS. Extranodal hematopoietic/lymphoid disorders: an introduction. *Am J Clin Pathol* 1999;111(Suppl 1):S40–S45.
19. Ekström Smedby K, Vajdic CM, Falster M, et al. Autoimmune disorders and risk of non-Hodgkin lymphoma subtypes: a pooled analysis within the Inter Lymph Consortium. *Blood* 2008;111:4029–4038.
20. Holm LE, Blomgren H, Lowhagen T. Cancer risks in patients with chronic lymphocytic thyroiditis. *N Engl J Med* 1985;312:601–604.
21. Fishleder A, Tubbs R, Hesse B, et al. Uniform detection of immunoglobulin-gene rearrangement in benign lymphoepithelial lesions. *N Engl J Med* 1987;316:1118–1121.
22. Quintana PG, Kapadia SB, Bahler DW, et al. Salivary gland lymphoid infiltrates associated with lymphoepithelial lesions: a clinicopathologic, immunophenotypic, and genotypic study. *Hum Pathol* 1997;28:850–861.
23. Knowles DM, Athan E, Ubriaco A, et al. Extranodal noncutaneous lymphoid hyperplasias represent a continuous spectrum of B-cell neoplasia: demonstration by molecular genetic analysis. *Blood* 1989;73:1635–1645.
24. Suarez F, Lortholary O, Hermine O, et al. Infection-associated lymphomas derived from marginal zone B cells: a model of antigen-driven lymphoproliferation. *Blood* 2006;107:3034–3044.
25. Wotherspoon AC, Doglioni C, Diss TC, et al. Regression of primary low-grade B-cell gastric lymphoma of mucosa-associated lymphoid tissue type after eradication of *Helicobacter pylori*. *Lancet* 1993;342:575–577.
26. Lecuit M, Abachin E, Matin A, et al. Immunoproliferative small intestinal disease associated with *Campylobacter jejuni*. *N Engl J Med* 2004;350:239–248.
27. Ferreri AJ, Guidoboni M, Ponzoni M, et al. Evidence for an association between *Chlamydia psittaci* and ocular adnexal lymphomas. *J Natl Cancer Inst* 2004;96:586–594.
28. Aigelsreiter A, Gerlza T, Deutsch AJ, et al. *Chlamydia psittaci* infection in non-gastrointestinal extranodal MALT lymphomas and their precursor lesions. *Am J Clin Pathol* 2011;135:70–75.
29. Goodlad JR, Davidson MM, Hollowood K, et al. *Borrelia burgdorferi*–associated cutaneous marginal zone lymphoma: a clinicopathological study of two cases illustrating the temporal progression of *B. burgdorferi*–associated B-cell proliferation in the skin. *Histopathology* 2000;37:501–508.
30. Ponzoni M, Ferreri AJ, Mappa S, et al. Prevalence of *Borrelia burgdorferi* infection in a series of 98 primary cutaneous lymphomas. *Oncologist* 2011;16:1582–1588.
31. Saltzstein SL. Extranodal malignant lymphomas and pseudolymphomas. *Pathol Annu* 1969;4:159–184.
32. Koch P, Probst A, Berdel W, et al. Treatment results in localized primary gastric lymphoma: data of patients registered within the German multicenter study (GIT NHL 02/96). *J Clin Oncol* 2005;23:7050–7059.
33. Ferry JA, Fung CY, Zukerberg L, et al. Lymphoma of the ocular adnexa: a study of 353 cases. *Am J Surg Pathol* 2007;31:170–174.
34. Ruiz A, Reischl U, Swerdlow SH, et al. Extranodal marginal zone B-cell lymphoma of the ocular adnexa: multiparameter analysis of 34 cases including interphase molecular cytogenetics and PCR for *Chlamydia psittaci*. *Am J Surg Pathol* 2007;31:792–802.
35. Kurtin PJ, Myers JL, Adlakha H, et al. Pathologic and clinical features of primary pulmonary extranodal marginal zone lymphoma of MALT type. *Am J Surg Pathol* 2001;25:997–1008.

36. Bégueret H, Vergier B, Parrens M, et al. Primary lung small B-cell lymphoma versus lymphoid hyperplasia. *Am J Surg Pathol* 2002;26:76–81.
37. Burke JS. Are there site-specific differences among the MALT lymphomas: morphologic, clinical? *Am J Clin Pathol* 1999;111(Suppl 1):S133–S143.
38. Burke JS. Lymphoproliferative disorders of the gastrointestinal tract: a review and pragmatic guide to diagnosis. *Arch Pathol Lab Med* 2011;135:1283–1297.
39. Kurtin PJ. How do you distinguish benign from malignant extranodal small B-cell proliferations? *Am J Clin Pathol* 1999;111(Suppl 1):S119–S126.
40. Abbondanzo SL, Sobin LH. Gastric "pseudolymphoma:" a retrospective morphologic and immunophenotypic study of 97 cases. *Cancer* 1997;79:1656–1663.
41. Hyjek E, Smith WJ, Isaacson PG. Primary B-cell lymphoma of salivary glands and its relationship to myoepithelial sialadenitis. *Hum Pathol* 1988;19:766–776.
42. Hyjek E, Isaacson PG. Primary B cell lymphoma of the thyroid and its relationship to Hashimoto's thyroiditis. *Hum Pathol* 1988;19:1315–1326.
43. Isaacson PG. Lymphomas of mucosa-associated lymphoid tissue (MALT). *Histopathology* 1990;16:617–619.
44. de Jong D, Boot H, Taal B. Histological grading with clinical relevance in gastric mucosa-associated lymphoid tissue (MALT) lymphoma. *Cancer Res* 2000;156: 27–32.
45. Ferreri AJ, Freschi M, Dell'Oro S, et al. Prognostic significance of the histopathologic recognition of low- and high-grade components in stage I-II B-cell gastric lymphomas. *Am J Surg Pathol* 2001;25:95–102.
46. Eberle FC, Song JY, Xi L, et al. Nodal involvement by cutaneous CD30-positive T-cell lymphoma mimicking classical Hodgkin lymphoma. *Am J Surg Pathol* 2012;36: 716–725.
47. Dojcinov SD, Venkataraman G, Raffeld M, et al. EBV positive mucocutaneous ulcer–a study of 26 cases associated with various sources of immunosuppression. *Am J Surg Pathol* 2010;34;405–417.
48. Jaffe ES, Krenacs L, Kumar S, et al. Extranodal peripheral T-cell and NK-cell neoplasms. *Am J Clin Pathol* 1999;111(Suppl 1):S46–S55.
49. Au WY, Weisenburger DD, Intragumtornchai T, et al. Clinical differences between nasal and extranasal natural killer/T-cell lymphoma: a study of 136 cases from the International Peripheral T-Cell Lymphoma Project. *Blood* 2009;113:3931–3937.
50. Chuang SS, Chang ST, Chuang WY, et al. NK-cell lineage predicts poor survival in primary intestinal NK-cell and T-cell lymphomas. *Am J Surg Pathol* 2009;33: 1230–1240.
51. Takeuchi K, Yokoyama M, Ishizawa S, et al. Lymphomatoid gastropathy: a distinct clinicopathologic entity of self-limited pseudomalignant NK-cell proliferation. *Blood* 2010;116:5631–5637.
52. Mansoor A, Pittaluga S, Beck PL, et al. NK-cell enteropathy: a benign NK-cell lymphoproliferative disease mimicking intestinal lymphoma: clinicopathological features and follow-up in a unique case series. *Blood* 2011;117:1447–1452.
53. Burke JS, Sheibani K, Nathwani BN, et al. Monoclonal small (well-differentiated) lymphocytic proliferations of the gastrointestinal tract resembling lymphoid hyperplasia: a neoplasm of uncertain malignant potential. *Hum Pathol* 1987;18:1238–1245.
54. Rao DS, Said JW. Small lymphoid proliferations in extranodal locations. *Arch Pathol Lab Med* 2007;131:383–396.
55. Ruskone-Fourmestraux A, Fischbach W, Aleman BMP, et al. EGILS consensus report. Gastric extranodal marginal zone B-cell lymphoma of MALT. *Gut* 2011;60: 747–758.
56. Evans HL. Extranodal small lymphocytic proliferation: a clinicopathologic and immunocytochemical study. *Cancer* 1982;49:84–96.
57. Zukerberg LR, Ferry JA, Southern JF, et al. Lymphoid infiltrates of the stomach: evaluation of histologic criteria for the diagnosis of low-grade gastric lymphoma on endoscopic biopsy specimens. *Am J Surg Pathol* 1990;14:1087–1099.
58. Rubin A, Isaacson PG. Florid reactive lymphoid hyperplasia of the terminal ileum in adults: a condition bearing a close resemblance to low-grade malignant lymphoma. *Histopathology* 1990;17:19–26.
59. Isaacson PG. Gastrointestinal lymphomas of T- and B-cell types. *Mod Pathol* 1999; 12:151–158.
60. El-Zimaity HM, Wotherspoon A, de Jong D. Interobserver variation in the histopathological assessment of malt/malt lymphoma: towards a consensus. *Blood Cells Mol Dis* 2005;34:6–16.
61. Almasri NM, Zaer FS, Iturraspe JA, et al. Contribution of flow cytometry to the diagnosis of gastric lymphomas in endoscopic biopsy specimens. *Mod Pathol* 1997;10: 650–656.
62. Hummel M, Oeschger S, Barth TF, et al. Wotherspoon criteria combined with B cell clonality analysis by advanced polymerase chain reaction technology discriminates covert gastric marginal zone lymphoma from chronic gastritis. *Gut* 2006;55:782–787.
63. de Leon ED, Alkan S, Huang JC, et al. Usefulness of an immunohistochemical panel in paraffin-embedded tissues for the differentiation of B-cell non-Hodgkin's lymphomas of small lymphocytes. *Mod Pathol* 1998;11:1046–1051.
64. Isaacson PG, Du MQ. Gastrointestinal lymphoma; where morphology meets molecular biology. *J Pathol* 2005;205;255–274.
65. Jaso J, Chen L, Li S, et al. CD5-positive mucosa-associated lymphoid tissue (MALT) lymphoma: a clinicopathologic study of 14 cases. *Hum Pathol* 2012;43: 1436–1443.
66. Hsi ED, Greenson JK, Singleton TP, et al. Detection of immunoglobulin heavy chain gene rearrangement by polymerase chain reaction in chronic active gastritis associated with *Helicobacter pylori. Hum Pathol* 1996;27:290–296.
67. Wündisch T, Neubauer A, Stolte M, et al. B-cell monoclonality is associated with lymphoid follicles in gastritis. *Am J Surg Pathol* 2003;27:882–887.
68. Nihal M, Mikkola D, Horvath N, et al. Cutaneous lymphoid hyperplasia: a lymphoproliferative continuum with lymphomatous potential. *Hum Pathol* 2003;34:617–622.
69. Sproul AM, Goodlad JR. Clonality testing of cutaneous lymphoid infiltrates: practicalities, pitfalls and potential uses. *J Hematopathol* 2012;5:69–82.
70. Troch M, Kiesewetter B, Dolak W, et al. Plasmacytic differentiation in MALT lymphomas following treatment with rituximab. *Ann Hematol* 2012;91:723–728.
71. Deshpande V, Zen Y, Chan JKC, et al. Consensus statement on the pathology of IgG4-realted disease. *Mod Pathol* 2012;25:1181–1192.
72. Karamchandani JR, Younes SF, Warnke RA, et al. IgG4-realted systemic sclerosing disease of the ocular adnexa: a potential mimic of ocular lymphoma. *Am J Clin Pathol* 2012;137:699–711.
73. Lin P, Molina TJ, Cook JR, et al. Lymphoplasmacytic lymphoma and other nonmarginal zone lymphomas with plasmacytic differentiation. *Am J Clin Pathol* 2011;136:195–210.
74. Molina TJ, Lin P, Swerdlow SH, et al. Marginal zone lymphomas with plasmacytic differentiation and related disorders. *Am J Clin Pathol* 2011;136:211–225.
75. Swerdlow SH, Berger F, Pileri SA, et al. Lymphoplasmacytic lymphoma. In: Swerdlow SH, Campo E, Harris NL, et al., eds. *WHO classification of tumours of haematopoietic and lymphoid tissues,* 4th ed. Lyon: IARC, 2008:194–195.
76. Derringer GA, Thompson LDR, Frommelt RA, et al. Malignant lymphoma of the thyroid gland: a clinicopathologic study of 108 cases. *Am J Surg Pathol* 2000;24:623–639.
77. Moynihan MJ, Bast MA, Chan WC, et al. Lymphoid polyposis: a neoplasm of either follicular mantle or germinal center cell origin. *Am J Surg Pathol* 1996;20: 442–452.
78. Ruskoné-Fourmestraux A, Audouin J. Primary gastrointestinal tract mantle cell lymphoma as multiple lymphomatous polyposis. *Best Pract Res Clin Gastroenterol* 2010;24:35–42.
79. Isaacson PG, Wotherspoon AC, Pan L. Follicular colonization in B-cell lymphoma of mucosa-associated lymphoid tissue. *Am J Surg Pathol* 1991;15:819–828.
80. Ranchod M, Lewin KJ, Dorfman RF. Lymphoid hyperplasia of the gastrointestinal tract: a study of 26 cases and review of the literature. *Am J Surg Pathol* 1978;2:383–400.
81. Gilliam AC, Wood GS. Primary cutaneous lymphomas other than mycosis fungoides. *Semin Oncol* 1999;26:290–306.
82. Edinger JT, Kant JA, Swerdlow SH. Cutaneous marginal zone lymphomas have distinctive features and include 2 subsets. *Am J Surg Pathol* 2010;34: 1830–1841.
83. Baldassano MF, Bailey EM, Ferry JA, et al. Cutaneous lymphoid hyperplasia and cutaneous marginal zone lymphoma: comparison of morphologic and immunophenotypic features. *Am J Surg Pathol* 1999;23:88–96.
84. Orwat DE, Batalis NI. Intravascular large B-cell lymphoma. *Arch Pathol Lab Med* 2012;136:333–338.
85. Hussell T, Isaacson PG, Crabtree JE, et al. The response of cells from low-grade B-cell gastric lymphomas of mucosa-associated lymphoid tissue to *Helicobacter pylori. Lancet* 1993;342:571–574.
86. Du M, Diss TC, Xu C, et al. Ongoing mutation in MALT lymphoma immunoglobulin gene suggests that antigen stimulation plays a role in the clonal expansion. *Leukemia* 1996;10:1190–1197.
87. Bahler DW, Miklos JA, Swerdlow SH. Ongoing Ig gene hypermutation in salivary gland mucosa-associated lymphoid tissue-type lymphomas. *Blood* 1997;89: 3335–3344.
88. Deutsch AJA, Aigelsreiter A, Staber PB, et al. MALT lymphoma and extranodal diffuse large B-cell lymphoma are targeted by aberrant hypermutation. *Blood* 2007;109:3500–3504.
89. Voulgarelis M, Skopouli FN. Clinical, immunologic and molecular factors predicting lymphoma development in Sjögren's syndrome patients. *Clin Rev Allergy Immunol* 2007;32:265–274.
90. Bahler DW, Swerdlow SH. Clonal salivary gland infiltrates associated with myoepithelial sialadenitis (Sjögren's syndrome) begin as nonmalignant antigen-selected expansions. *Blood* 1998;91:1864–1872.
91. Diss TC, Wotherspoon AC, Speight P, et al. B-cell monoclonality, Epstein Barr virus, and t(14;18) in myoepithelial sialadenitis and low-grade B-cell MALT lymphoma of the parotid gland. *Am J Surg Pathol* 1995;19:531–536.
92. Hsi ED, Siddiqui J, Schnitzer B, et al. Analysis of immunoglobulin heavy chain gene rearrangement in myoepithelial sialadenitis by polymerase chain reaction. *Am J Clin Pathol* 1996;106:498–503.
93. Moshynska OV, Saxena A. Clonal relationship between Hashimoto thyroiditis and thyroid lymphoma. *J Clin Pathol* 2008;61:438–444.
94. Miklos JA, Swerdlow SH, Bahler DW. Salivary gland mucosa-associated lymphoid tissue lymphoma immunoglobulin V_H genes show frequent use of *V1-69* with distinctive CDR3 features. *Blood* 2000;95:3878–3884.
95. Burke JS. Histologic criteria for distinguishing between benign and malignant extranodal lymphoid infiltrates. *Semin Diagn Pathol* 1985;2:152–162.
96. Campidelli C, Agostinelli C, Stitson R, et al. Myeloid sarcoma: extramedullary manifestation of myeloid disorders. *Am J Clin Pathol* 2009;132:426–437.
97. Zucca E, Bertoni F, Roggero E, et al. Molecular analysis of the progression from *Helicobacter pylori*-associated chronic gastritis to mucosa-associated lymphoid-tissue lymphoma of the stomach. *N Engl J Med* 1998;338:804–810.
98. Nakamura S, Aoyagi K, Furuse M, et al. B-cell monoclonality precedes the development of gastric MALT lymphoma in *Helicobacter pylori*-associated chronic gastritis. *Am J Pathol* 1998;152:1271–1279.
99. Kuo SH, Yeh KH, Wu MS, et al. *Helicobacter pylori* eradication therapy is effective in the treatment of early-stage *H. pylori*–positive gastric diffuse large B-cell lymphomas. *Blood* 2012;119:4838–4844.
100. Wotherspoon AC, Finn TM, Isaacson PG. Trisomy 3 in low-grade B-cell lymphomas of mucosa-associated lymphoid tissue. *Blood* 1995;85:2000–2004.
101. Auer IA, Gascoyne RD, Connors JM, et al. t(11;18)(q21;q21) is the most common translocation in MALT lymphomas. *Ann Oncol* 1997;8:979–985.
102. Liu H, Ye H, Dogan A, et al. t(11;18)(q21;q21) is associated with advanced mucosa-associated lymphoid tissue lymphoma that expresses nuclear BCL10. *Blood* 2001;98:1182–1187.
103. Remstein ED, Kurtin PJ, James CD, et al. Mucosa-associated lymphoid tissue lymphomas with t(11;18)(q21;q21) and mucosa-associated lymphoid tissue lymphomas with aneuploidy develop along different pathogenetic pathways. *Am J Pathol* 2002;161:63–71.
104. Starostik P, Patzner J, Greiner A, et al. Gastric marginal zone B-cell lymphomas of MALT type develop along 2 distinct pathogenetic pathways. *Blood* 2002; 99:3–9.
105. Remstein ED, Dogan A, Einerson RR, et al. The incidence and anatomic site specificity of chromosomal translocations in primary extranodal marginal zone B-cell lymphoma of mucosa-associated lymphoid tissue (MALT lymphoma) in North America. *Am J Surg Pathol* 2006;30:1546–1553.
106. Hamoudi RA, Appert A, Ye H, et al. Differential expression of NF-κB target genes in MALT lymphoma with and without chromosome translocation: insights into molecular mechanism. *Leukemia* 2010;24:1487–1497.
107. Ye H, Liu H, Attygalle A, et al. Variable frequencies of t(11;18)(q21;q21) in MALT lymphomas of different sites: significant association with CagA strains of *H. pylori* in gastric MALT lymphoma. *Blood* 2003;102:1012–1018.
108. Rosenwald A, Ott G, Stilgebauer S, et al. Exclusive detection of the t(11;18)(q21;21) in extranodal marginal zone B cell lymphomas (MZBL) of MALT type in contrast to other MZBL and extranodal large B cell lymphomas. *Am J Pathol* 1999;155:1817–1821.

109. Remstein ED, James CD, Kurtin PJ. Incidence and subtype specificity of *API2-MALT1* fusion transcripts in extranodal, nodal, and splenic marginal zone lymphomas. *Am J Pathol* 2000;156:1183–1188.
110. Rinaldi A, Mian M, Chigrinova E, et al. Genome-wide DNA profiling of marginal zone lymphomas identifies subtype-specific lesions with an impact on the clinical outcome. *Blood* 2011;117:1595–1604.
111. Xia H, Nakayama T, Sakuma H, et al. Analysis of *API-MALT1* fusion, trisomies, and immunoglobulin *VH* genes in pulmonary mucosa-associated lymphoid tissue lymphoma. *Hum Pathol* 2011;42:1297–1304.
112. Wündisch T, Thiede C, Morgner A, et al. Long-term follow-up of gastric MALT lymphoma after *Helicobacter pylori* eradication. *J Clin Oncol* 2005;23:8018–8024.
113. Ye H, Liu H, Raderer M, et al. High incidence of t(11;18)(q21;q21) in *Helicobacter pylori*–negative gastric MALT lymphoma. *Blood* 2003;101(7):2547–2550.
114. Streubel B, Simonitsch-Klupp I, Müllauer L, et al. Variable frequencies of MALT lymphoma-associated genetic aberrations in MALT lymphomas of different sites. *Leukemia* 2004;18:1722–1726.
115. Streubel B, Lambrecht A, Dierlamm J, et al. T(14;18)(q32;q21) involving *IGH* and *MALT1* is a frequent chromosomal aberration in MALT lymphoma. *Blood* 2003;101:2335–2339.
116. Sagaert X, Laurent M, Baens M, et al. *MALT1* and *BCL10* aberrations in MALT lymphomas and their effect on the expression of BCL10 in the tumor cells. *Mod Pathol* 2006;19:225–232.
117. Streubel B, Vinatzner U, Lamprecht A, et al. T(3;14)(p14.1;q32) involving *IGH* and *FOXP1* is a novel recurrent chromosomal aberration in MALT lymphoma. *Leukemia* 2005;19:652–658.
118. Kuper-Hommel MJJ, van Krieken HJM. Molecular pathogenesis and histologic and clinical features of extranodal marginal zone lymphomas of mucosa-associated lymphoid tissue type. *Leuk Lymphoma* 2012;53:1032–1045.
119. Du MQ. MALT lymphoma: many roads lead to nuclear factor-κb activation. *Histopathology* 2011;58:26–38.
120. Bi Y, Zeng N, Chanudet E, et al. A20 inactivation in ocular adnexal lymphoma. *Haematologica* 2012;97:926–930.
121. Chanudet E, Huang Y, Zeng N, et al. TNFAIP3 abnormalities in MALT lymphoma with autoimmunity. *Br J Haematol* 2011;154:535–539.
122. Thieblemont C, Berger F, Dumontet C, et al. Mucosa-associated lymphoid tissue lymphoma is a disseminated disease in one third of 158 patients. *Blood* 2000;95:802–806.
123. Zucca E, Bertoni F, Roggero E, et al. The gastric marginal zone B-cell lymphoma of MALT type. *Blood* 2000;96:410–419.
124. Zucca E, Conconi A, Pedrinis E, et al. Nongastric marginal zone B-cell of mucosa-associated lymphoid tissue. *Blood* 2003;101:2489–2495.
125. Mazloom A, Medeiros J, McLaughlin PW, et al. Marginal zone lymphoma: factors that affect the final outcome. *Cancer* 2010;116:4291–4298.

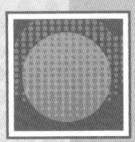

Chapter 29
Benign and Malignant Cutaneous Lymphoproliferative Disorders Including Mycosis Fungoides

Cynthia Magro

THE NEOPLASTIC DIFFUSE AND NODULAR LYMPHOCYTIC INFILTRATES: B-CELL LYMPHOPROLIFERATIVE DISORDERS

Introduction

The spectrum of lymphocytic infiltrates that can involve the skin is a broad one of varied etiologies ranging from purely reactive infiltrates to overt T- and/or B-cell neoplasia. As well, an indeterminate category may presage B- and T-cell lymphoma, respectively. The focus of this chapter is to consider the more common lymphoid malignancies that present primarily in the skin. The lymphomas that secondarily involve the skin such as lymphomatoid granulomatosis, adult T-cell leukemia/lymphoma, T-cell prolymphocytic leukemia, and angioimmunoblastic lymphadenopathy are considered in the respective chapters devoted to the topic. The vast majority of lymphocytic infiltrates of the skin are reactive, albeit they may exhibit features that could create a diagnostic conundrum with respect to their distinction from the malignant counterpart. Cutaneous lymphocytic infiltrates can be broadly categorized as follows:

1. T-cell–dominant reactive lymphoid infiltrates including immunologic responses to exogenous triggers including drug, light, an infectious stimulus and/or contactant, collagen vascular disease, and idiopathic: B-cell–dominant infiltrates in the skin do not typically occur except in rare examples of reactive cutaneous polytypic plasmacytosis.
2. Preneoplastic lymphoproliferative disorders such as lymphocytoma cutis and Castleman disease as a precursor lesion to low-grade B-cell lymphoma and the various T-cell dyscrasias that may presage mycosis fungoides (MF) including large plaque parapsoriasis, pityriasis lichenoides chronica (PLC), pigmentary purpura, alopecia mucinosis, and folliculotropic T-cell lymphocytosis.
3. B-cell lymphoma/leukemia including primary cutaneous B-cell lymphoma (marginal zone lymphoma [MZL], primary cutaneous follicle center cell lymphoma, diffuse large cell B-cell lymphoma of leg type, intravascular B-cell lymphoma, T-cell–rich CD30+ B-cell lymphoma, and lymphoblastic lymphoma), and extracutaneous B-cell lymphoma secondarily involving the skin most frequently represented by nodal follicular lymphoma, mantle cell lymphoma, Hodgkin lymphoma, double-hit lymphoma, Burkitt lymphoma, and chronic lymphocytic leukemia (CLL).
4. T-cell lymphoma comprising those that are primary in the skin; the commonest of these being MF while less common forms include primary cutaneous pleomorphic CD4+ small-/medium-sized T-cell lymphoma, primary cutaneous epidermotropic aggressive cytotoxic CD8+ T-cell lymphoma, natural killer (NK)/T-cell lymphoma and gamma delta T-cell lymphoma versus secondary T-cell malignancies exhibiting a propensity to involve the skin such as T-cell prolymphocytic leukemia, adult T-cell leukemia/lymphoma, and angioimmunoblastic lymphadenopathy
5. CD30-positive lymphoproliferative disease encompassing a spectrum of lesions comprising lymphomatoid papulosis (LYP), borderline C30+ lymphoproliferative disease, and anaplastic large cell lymphoma (ALCL)
6. CD4+CD56+ hematodermic neoplasm, a tumor of plasmacytoid dendritic cell origin

To understand the significance of cutaneous T- and B-cell neoplasia, it is important to consider the baseline features clinically and histologically, which define the reactive lymphocytic infiltrates. However, a review of inflammatory dermatoses is not possible due to space constraints and hence a standard dermatopathology textbook should be consulted. Instead, the focus in this chapter is on infiltrates that mimic lymphoma such as lymphocytoma cutis and other forms of pseudolymphomas including drug-associated reversible T-cell dyscrasias along with a comprehensive review of primary cutaneous T- and B-cell lymphoma.

LYMPHOCYTOMA CUTIS

Introduction/Clinical Features

Lymphocytoma cutis represents one of the classic forms of well-differentiated diffuse and nodular lymphocytic infiltrates of the skin, a common diagnostic dilemma for the dermatopathologist due to their inherent morphologic similarity to certain low-grade cutaneous lymphomas (1–4). The lesions present as solitary plaques with a head and neck and truncal predisposition. The absolute distinction morphologically from low-grade B-cell lymphoma is problematic especially in those cases that are recurrent. As well, low-grade B-cell lymphoma may arise in a background of lymphocytoma cutis (1,2). One should consider lymphocytoma cutis as an initial step in cutaneous B-cell lymphomagenesis. There are variants of benign reactive lymphoid hyperplasia that exhibit distinctive features such as angiolymphoid hyperplasia with eosinophilia/Kimura disease and Castleman disease (3); they are considered elsewhere in the textbook.

Light Microscopic Findings

There is a diffuse and/or nodular pan dermal lymphocytic infiltrate. The infiltrate may be accentuated superficially with a gradual diminution as the base of the biopsy is approached or, less often, is dominant in the deep dermis or subcutis (Figs. 29.1A and 29.2B). Small mature lymphocytes, scattered granulomata, and germinal centers of variable size with many tingible body macrophages are frequent; mitoses are seen within the germinal centers (Figs. 29.1B and 29.2B). The infiltrate shows accentuation around adnexal structures and blood vessels. As an immune-based trigger can be implicated in certain cases, epidermal changes of hypersensitivity such as concomitant eczematous changes and/or interface dermatitis may be observed. Tissue eosinophilia can be seen especially in those cases triggered by an arthropod. There may be some permeation of the germinal center by peripherally disposed small lymphocytes, but it is not prominent (1–4).

An additional variant of lymphocytoma cutis is one characterized by a T-cell–rich nodular and diffuse lymphocytic infiltrate. There is concomitant B-cell hyperplasia; however, well-formed germinal centers are not seen. A few scattered CD30-positive activated T cells may be seen. Such cases become very difficult to distinguish from primary cutaneous CD4+ small-/medium-sized pleomorphic T-cell lymphoma. Possible discriminating features include the well-differentiated appearance of the dominant small lymphocyte population (i.e., the lymphocytes do not show the inherent atypicality seen in

primary cutaneous CD4+ small-/medium-sized pleomorphic T-cell lymphoma), the absence of a severely atypical large cell infiltrate, a relatively normal phenotypic profile, and polyclonality. In the vast majority of cases of primary cutaneous CD4+ pleomorphic small-/medium-sized T-cell lymphoma, hallmark larger atypical cells that really defy categorization as a reactive lymphocyte are noted, defining 30% or less of the infiltrate.

Progressive transformation of the germinal center characterized by infiltration of the germinal center by small B lymphocytes is a feature that has been reported in the context of reactive cutaneous lymphoid hyperplasia (Fig. 29.2C) (5). However, at extracutaneous sites, this finding can signify MZL. For example, progressive transformation of germinal centers is a feature of pediatric MZL of lymph nodes (6). When this phenomenon occurs in extranodal tissue, there is no definitive association with MZL. In my own experience, I have seen progressive transformation of the germinal center as part of the morphologic spectrum of cutaneous MZL especially in those cases without a significant dysplastic plasmacytic component. I have adopted the appellation of a small

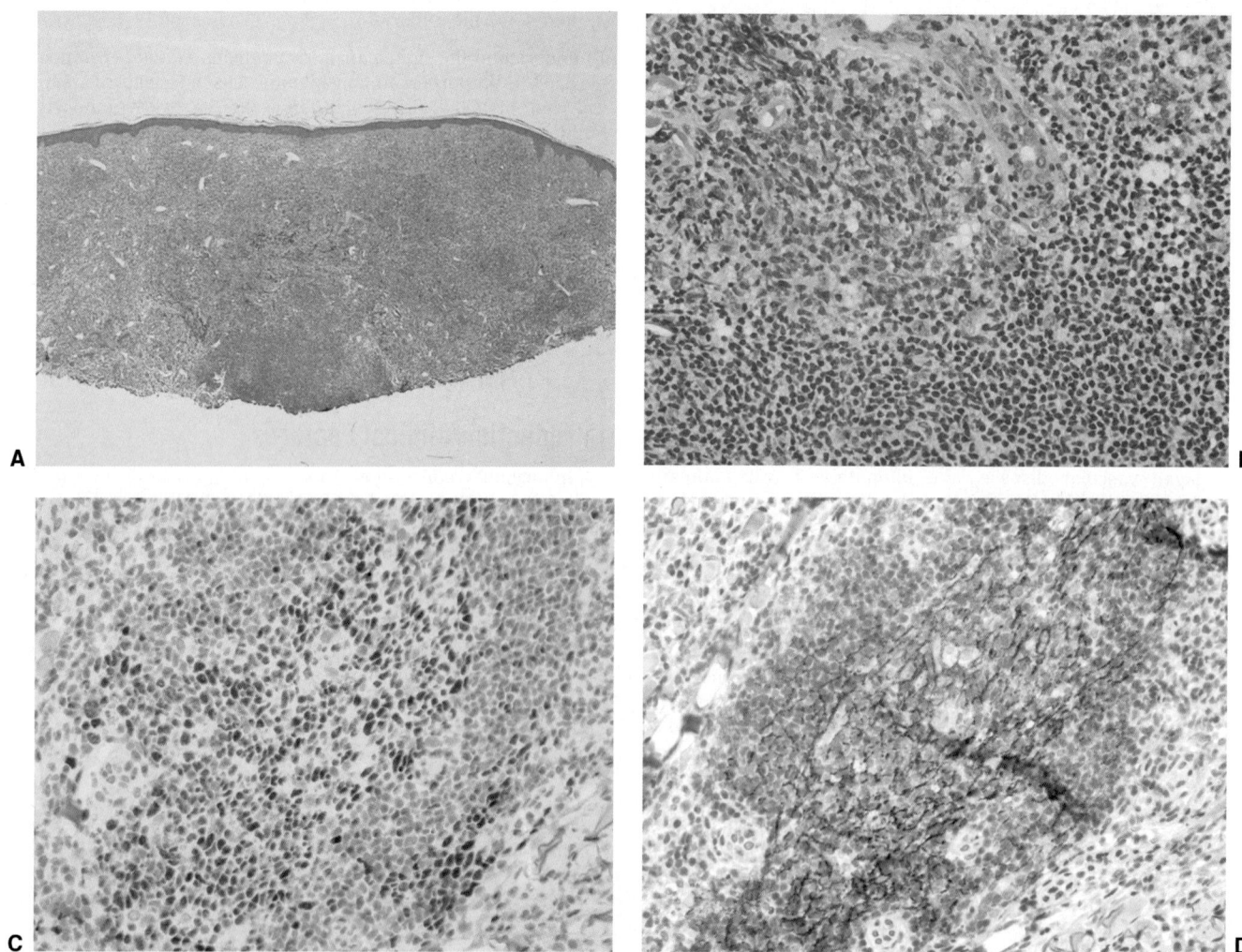

FIGURE 29.1. A: The biopsy shows a dense diffuse and nodular lymphocytic infiltrate that demonstrates enhanced cellularity at the base. This finding of a bottom-heavy infiltrate is more commonly seen in low-grade B-cell lymphoma but can also be seen in cases of reactive lymphoid hyperplasia (hematoxylin and eosin, magnification: 100×). **B:** Reactive germinal centers are a frequent finding in lesions of lymphocytoma cutis. However, benign germinal centers can also be observed in MZL, although usually the germinal center is disrupted and infiltrated by neoplastic small B cells, defining the concept of progressive transformation of the germinal center (hematoxylin and eosin, magnification: 400×). **C:** The reactive germinal centers are highlighted by Bcl-6 and CD10. Illustrated is the nuclear marker Bcl-6 (400× diaminobenzidine). **D:** A CD21 preparation shows the relatively well-preserved follicular dendritic cell network that is in contradistinction to the dendritic cell lysis that can be observed in the setting of either MZL or follicle center cell lymphoma (diaminobenzidine, magnification: 400×).

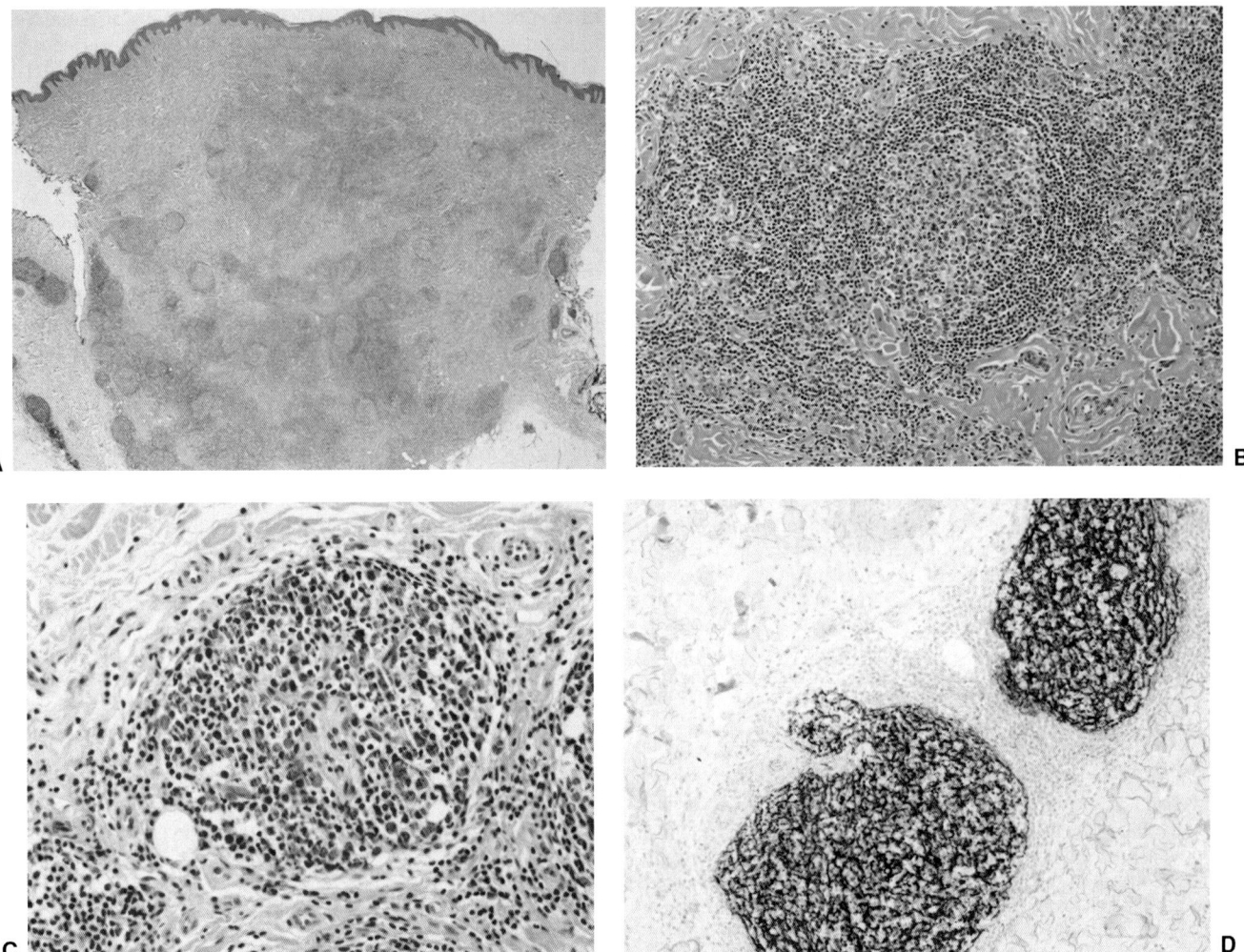

FIGURE 29.2. A: In this additional case of lymphocytoma cutis, one observes very striking nodular lymphocytic infiltration. The infiltrate spans the entire thickness of the dermis. At low power, the differential diagnosis encompasses low-grade B-cell lymphoma (hematoxylin and eosin, magnification: 40×). **B:** The germinal center–like foci have a somewhat castlemanoid appearance. In particular, they appear atrophic, hypervascular, and surrounded by a laminated onionskin-like arrangement of small lymphocytes without obvious atypia (hematoxylin and eosin, magnification: 200×). **C:** Higher magnification of the germinal center shows its atrophic quality and hypervascularity reminiscent therefore of the changes seen in hyaline vascular Castleman disease, a distinct form of reactive lymphoid hyperplasia (hematoxylin and eosin, magnification: 400×). **D:** The follicular dendritic cell network highlighted by CD21 is very extensive. Dendritic cell lysis typical of low-grade B-cell lymphoma is not observed (hematoxylin and eosin, magnification: 200×).

lymphocytic variant of MZL. Those cases may not have an obvious light chain restriction when examining kappa and lambda although a reduction in CD79A amidst the B cells may be observed; in addition, the small B cells are frequently CD23 positive (7).

Phenotypic Profile

In classic lesions of lymphocytoma cutis, there is a dominance of T cells over B cells. There is a zonation to the distribution of T and B cells. The B-cell component is characteristically disposed centrally in a nodular fashion surrounded by zones of diffuse T-cell infiltration. A dominance of B cells over T cells would be indicative of an evolving low-grade B-cell lymphoproliferative disorder as either a precursor state to low-grade B-cell lymphoma or representing low-grade B-cell lymphoma. Cases in which the B- to T-cell ratio is very high (i.e., in excess of 3:1) likely represent B-cell lymphoma. The T cells most often show a normal phenotype without loss of CD2, CD3, CD7, and CD62L expression. In the setting of drug therapy, I have seen cases showing diminution in expression of CD7 and CD62L although only rarely to the degree observed

in primary cutaneous CD4+ pleomorphic small/medium-sized cell lymphoma (1–5,8). The B cells demonstrate a normal phenotype including expression of both CD20 and CD79 without any reduction of CD79 compared to CD20; the germinal centers exhibit positivity of centrocytes and centroblasts for both CD10 and Bcl6 (Fig. 29.1C), and there is no expression of Bcl2 in centrocytes and centroblasts. Of course Bcl2 expression can be seen in follicular helper T cells and possibly reactive small postgerminal B cells within the germinal center. An extensive well-formed dendritic cell network, highlighted by CD23 and CD21 (Figs. 29.1D and 29.2D), is observed. Significant zones of dendritic cell lysis should not be seen (9). Extensive staining of the B-cell component for CD23 would be very unusual and is a finding more commonly seen with low-grade B-cell lymphoma.

In situ hybridization studies for kappa and lambda are an important part of the evaluation. If kappa and lambda show an equal number of positive-staining cells and/or if there is a dominance of lambda over kappa such findings could signify an emerging lambda light chain–restricted infiltrate. A normal kappa to lambda ratio is 3:1 up to 5:1 (10). Conversely, a high kappa to lambda ratio in excess of 5:1 suggests an emerging kappa light chain–restricted infiltrate. The presence of kappa and/or lambda light chain restriction is a feature of MZL. At times, a select phenotypic aberration amidst a lesion otherwise typical for lymphocytoma cutis can be seen. This concept is perhaps best exemplified by a mild reduction of CD79A. Such findings and/or clonality in a lesion otherwise typical for lymphocytoma cutis would be indicative of an evolving low-grade B-cell lymphoproliferative disorder albeit not diagnostic of B-cell lymphoma.

Molecular Profile

It is reasonable to obtain both immunoglobulin heavy chain and T cell receptor (TCR) studies. T-cell clonality can occur in lesions of lymphocytoma cutis especially if there is a substantial polyclonal background, but such cases must be carefully evaluated and followed. A heavy chain immunoglobulin rearrangement would be worrisome for a B-cell lymphoproliferative disorder; either the lesions are better reclassified as B-cell lymphomas or it is stated that a diagnosis of low-grade B-cell lymphoproliferative disease cannot be excluded if there are no unequivocal light microscopic and/or phenotypic abnormalities. Drs. Guitart and Gerami (11) recently introduced the concept of marginal zone hyperplasia as a precursor lesion to MZL. The authors described cutaneous lymphocytic and plasmacytic infiltrates with evidence of lambda light chain restriction in the absence of heavy chain immunoglobulin gene rearrangements.

Pathogenetic Basis of Lymphocytoma Cutis

The pathogenetic basis of classic lymphocytoma cutis can be viewed as an exuberant immunologic response to a variety of antigenic triggers (4). The excessive nature of the immune response may reflect a state of underlying iatrogenic and/or endogenous immune dysregulation. There are certain drugs that have been implicated etiologically in the pathogenesis of lymphocytoma cutis of which the most common are antidepressants, anticonvulsants, antihistamines, statins, and calcium channel blockers (6,12–16). Certain infectious triggers have been proposed including Borrelia, hepatitis C, and attenuated virus used at sites of vaccination. Arthropod bites can evoke prominent lymphoid hyperplasia. Most of these infiltrates are dominated by predominantly dermal-based T cells most commonly of the CD4 subset. The B-cell component is typically minor and is frequently in the context of reactive germinal centers.

Differential Diagnosis of Lymphocytoma Cutis

Most lesions of lymphocytoma can be distinguished from marginal zone or follicle center cell lymphoma since the infiltrate is without significant cytologic and architectural atypia. The phenotypic profile of the B cells is usually normal, and polyclonality is characteristic. However, there are cases with light microscopic features typical of lymphocytoma cutis but in which there may be a dominance of B cells, B-cell clonality, and/or isolated phenotypic aberrations such as light chain restriction or a diminution in CD79a. Since low-grade B-cell lymphoma can arise in a background of lymphocytoma cutis, cases with these aforesaid atypical features are more likely to represent an evolving B-cell lymphoproliferative disorder although not diagnostic of overt lymphoma (1,2). Specific abnormalities pointing toward a diagnosis of MZL include dysplastic-appearing plasma cells exhibiting light chain restriction, a reduction in the expression of CD79a in a significant component of the infiltrate, and an effacing architectural growth pattern exhibiting enhanced cellularity at the base of the biopsy. Another important clue signifying low-grade B-cell lymphoproliferative disease and possibly early MZL is one of progressive transformation of the germinal center (17). The latter is characterized by infiltration

of the germinal center by small B cells. Certain abnormalities in the germinal center such as BCL2 staining in larger centroblastic appearing cells, a reduction in the expression of CD10, and marked dendritic cell lysis could signify incipient primary cutaneous follicle center cell lymphoma. We have seen cases of T-cell–rich B-cell lymphoma that may be very difficult to distinguish from lymphocytoma cutis since most of the infiltrate is reactive.

In those cases of T-cell–rich lymphocytoma cutis exhibiting T-cell clonality, distinction from primary cutaneous CD4+ small-/medium-sized pleomorphic T-cell lymphoma is problematic especially if there is a reduction in CD62L and CD7. One may have to rebiopsy the patient and send the tissue for cytogenetic studies to discriminate between these two diagnostic possibilities. In classic primary cutaneous CD4+ pleomorphic small/medium-sized T-cell lymphoma, a significant reduction can be seen in the expression of other pan T-cell markers including CD2, CD5, and CD3 in addition to the more commonly reduced ones (i.e., CD7 and CD62L). It has also been suggested that these lymphomas are derived from follicular helper T cells (8); the subset of cells exhibiting a follicular helper T-cell phenotype as revealed by staining for CXCL13, PD1, BCL6, and CD10 is the larger atypical one. While a reduction of CD7 and CD62L can be seen in the setting of lymphocytoma cutis, a diminution in the expression of other pan T-cell markers such as CD5 would be extremely uncommon and would point toward a diagnosis of neoplasia. In addition, the extent of reduction of CD7 is important. A marked reduction in CD7 in excess of 75% would be very unusual in the setting of benign reactive lymphoid hyperplasia and could support a diagnosis of T-cell neoplasia.

MIMICS OF T-CELL LYMPHOMA

The Lymphomatoid Drug Reaction/Drug-Associated Reversible T-Cell Dyscrasia

Drug therapy can be associated with T-cell–rich cutaneous infiltrates that resemble certain endogenous lymphoproliferative disorders including patch and plaque-stage MF, granulomatous MF, LYP, pityriasis lichenoides, and pigmented purpuric dermatosis (PPD). The main implicated drugs are those with immune dysregulating properties such as antihistamines, antidepressants, statins, benzodiazepines, calcium channel blockers, and angiotensin-converting enzyme inhibitors (6,12–18). As these infiltrates have an atypical clinical presentation and as well demonstrate a number of abnormal features from a morphologic, phenotypic, and molecular perspective, this type of drug reaction falls under the designation of drug-associated reversible T-cell dyscrasia.

In the setting of drug-associated reversible T-cell dyscrasia, it is important to remember that there is typically no temporal association between lesional onset and duration of drug therapy. Characteristically, the patients have been on the drug for months to years likely reflecting a cumulative effect of iatrogenic immune dysregulation. Any atypical epitheliotropic lymphocytic infiltrate resembling MF could potentially be related to immune dysregulatory drug therapy.

Features supportive of a drug-associated reversible T-cell dyscrasia include (i) an eruption of recent onset, (ii) a positive drug history, and (iii) an atypical clinical presentation for MF such as involvement of photodistributed areas. In the classic endogenous T-cell dyscrasia, the eruption follows a waxing and waning course over years as opposed to the recent and abrupt onset seen in drug-associated reversible T-cell dyscrasia. From a morphologic perspective, the additional features that could point toward a drug-based etiology include a true cytotoxic interface dermatitis with keratinocyte injury,

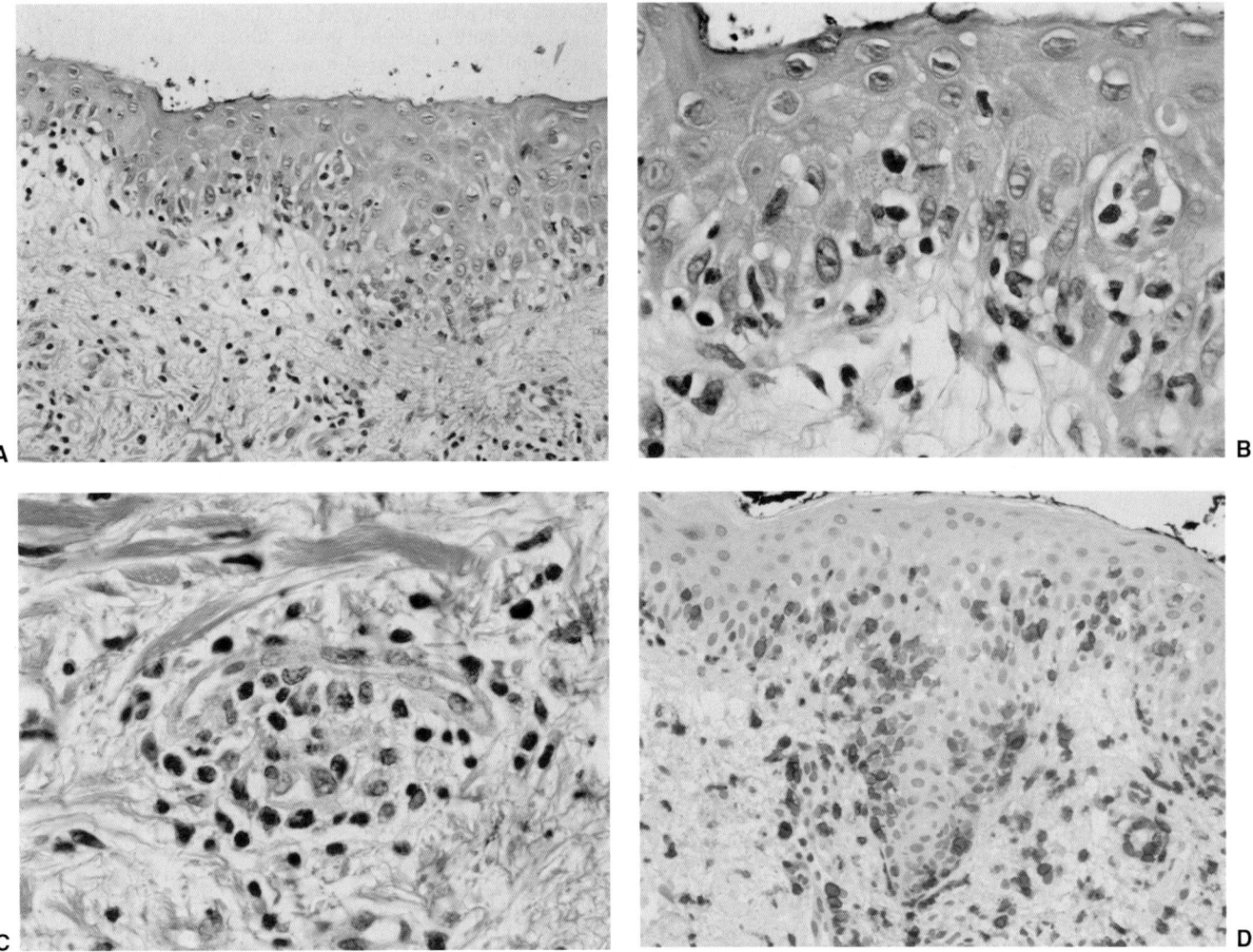

FIGURE 29.3. A: In this case, of Dilantin pseudolymphoma, the patient presented with erythroderma, lymphadenopathy, and peripheral blood eosinophilia. There is an interface dermatitis accompanied by basilar vacuolar change and dyskeratosis along with papillary dermal edema (hematoxylin and eosin, magnification: 200×). **B:** Higher power magnification shows low-grade lymphoid atypia. However, a differentiating point from MF is one of lymphocyte satellitosis around necrotic keratinocytes, indicative of a true immunologically mediated interface dermatitis (hematoxylin and eosin, magnification: 400×). **C:** There is a lymphomatoid vascular reaction characterized by many transformed lymphocytes surrounding and permeating the cutaneous vasculature. A few of the cells have an immunoblastic appearance. This type of vascular reaction is common within the morphologic realm of drug-associated pseudolymphoma and defines an important differentiating point from MF (hematoxylin and eosin, magnification: 400×). **D:** Unlike MF, there is relative preservation of CD7. In classic MF, there is an obvious reduction in the expression of CD7 oftentimes in excess of 70% when comparing intraepidermal CD7 expression to other pan T-cell markers such as CD2 and CD3 (diaminobenzidine, magnification: 400×). The acrosyringeal accentuation of the infiltrate is a characteristic finding in drug reactions and reflects the role of the acrosyringium in antigenic processing.

supervening eczematoid changes, eosinophilic spongiosis, a dominant angiocentric disposition within the dermis, and a directed pattern of migration into the epidermis (Fig. 29.3A–C). In regard to the latter, it is characterized by foci of lymphocytic infiltration into the epidermis at sites of critical antigenic processing including the suprapapillary plates, hair follicle, and acrosyringium (Fig. 29.3D).

From a phenotypic perspective, significant reductions can occur in the expression of both CD7 and CD62L; there may be a greater extent of reduction of CD62L compared to CD7. A diminution in the expression of CD5 and CD3 would be very unusual and more in keeping with MF. We have observed clonality in drug-associated reversible T-cell dyscrasia. It is possible that cases accompanied by clonality and significant phenotypic abnormalities could progress to an endogenous T-cell dyscrasia. In such cases a reasonable therapeutic approach would comprise topical therapy such as narrow-band UVB along with drug modulation similar to that given for an endogenous T-cell dyscrasia.

Drug Reaction with Peripheral Blood Eosinophilia and Systemic Symptoms (DRESS Syndrome)

A distinct subset of the drug-associated reversible T-cell dyscrasia/lymphomatoid drug reaction is DRESS syndrome. Patients with DRESS syndrome present with erythroderma, peripheral blood eosinophilia, and lymphadenopathy. Constitutional symptoms are present.

While the biopsies can exhibit features reminiscent of those potentially encountered in Sezary syndrome (SS) including epitheliotropism of somewhat cerebriform lymphocytes, the flow cytometry studies are not diagnostic of SS. In fact, there may be a reversal of the CD4 to CD8 ratio with a predominance of circulating CD8 lymphocytes. There may be a marked reduction in the expression of CD7 adding to the diagnostic conundrum in such cases. As well, clonality can be seen in skin biopsies and in the peripheral blood. In addition, there may be a similar predominance of CD8 lymphocytes within the epidermis. Angiocentricity of the dermal infiltrate including an admixture of transformed lymphocytes lying in apposition to vessels of the superficial dermis is a common feature.

The drug history may not be revealing as the inciting agent may have only been ingested briefly such as a short course of minocycline (19). In certain cases an antecedent viral illness may play a contributing a role as demonstrated by elevations of antibody titers of IgM isotype to human herpes type VI (20). In this regard, virally triggered immune dysregulation may be pathogenetically relevant. The pathogenetic basis of DRESS syndrome is an excessive and at times clonally restricted T-lymphocyte response to a drug-based antigen. The process differs from toxic epidermal necrolysis by virtue of the lack of epithelial necrosis in concert with extensive lymphocytic infiltration. In TEN, also a severe drug reaction, the drug functions as a hapten binding to epithelial cells rendering the cell antigenic. A systemic dysregulated cytotoxic immune response associated with high levels of circulating CD8 lymphocyte–derived FAS binds to FAS ligand on keratinocytes. The result is systemic cytokine-driven epithelial necrosis where the striking extent of epithelial necrosis far exceeds the degree of *in vivo* lymphocytic infiltration.

CD8+ PSEUDOLYMPHOMA OF HUMAN IMMUNODEFICIENCY DISEASE

Patients with advanced human immunodeficiency virus disease exhibit a marked reduction in the CD4 to CD8 ratio as a direct consequence of viral-induced injury of CD4-positive lymphocytes. This alteration in the cytokine milieu triggers an accumulation of CD8 lymphocytes in various organ sites including the lung and skin. A reduction in the CD4+ regulatory cell populations such as FoxP3 CD4+CD25+ T cells may play a role in this distinct reactive CD8+ lymphocyte influx (21,22).

CD30+ LYMPHOMATOID HYPERSENSITIVITY REACTIONS

Certain viruses preferentially processed through the follicle such as molluscum contagiosum and herpes can be accompanied by a striking interstitial and perivascular activated appearing lymphocytic infiltrate including many transformed immunoblastic forms that express CD30. Differentiating points include viral cytopathic changes but as well the activated CD30-positive cells while exhibiting CD4 positivity do not show cytotoxic protein expression as revealed by a lack of staining for granzyme, TIA-1, and perforin.

A similar CD30+ reaction is observed in the setting of drug therapy. In our experience, the main implicated drugs are those with immune dysregulating properties such as antidepressants, statins, and chemotherapy drugs (manuscript in preparation). The infiltrates are superficially confined and a dominant angiocentric disposition is observed as opposed to the deeper-seated eccrinotropic and neurotropic extension observed in the setting of LYP (23).

MARGINAL ZONE LYMPHOMA OF THE SKIN

Clinical Features

Primary cutaneous MZL is an indolent low-grade B-cell lymphoma of the skin representing 2% to 16% of all cutaneous lymphomas. It is associated with an excellent prognosis (98% 5-year survival rate) (24–26). This low-grade B-cell lymphoma

was recognized by the WHO-EORTC as a distinct entity in 2005 and is currently included in the 2008 WHO classification as extranodal MZL of mucosa-associated lymphoid tissue (MALT) lymphoma. While MZL is rarely curable, dissemination to extracutaneous sites is uncommon (2% to 8%). Lymph nodes, bone marrow, and orbit are among potential organs that can be involved secondarily. MZL of the skin may present as a *de novo* lymphoma unassociated with extracutaneous disease at the time of presentation, with concurrent disease involving the breast, orbit, and lung or as a secondary lymphoma if it is previously established that the patient has MALT-like lymphoma elsewhere (typically of the orbit, breast, lung, or parotid). While there is a tendency for relapse, progression to a higher-grade lymphoma is uncommon although it has been described and may portend a worse prognosis (27). MZL is most common in middle-aged women. The entity of primary cutaneous immunocytoma shares many clinical and morphologic features with MZL such that primary cutaneous immunocytoma is considered a plasmacytic variant/counterpart of low-grade MZL (see Fig. 29.5A–D). However, at variance with classic MZL is the multiplicity of the lesions clinically while histologically one observes a predominance of plasma cells and a noneffacing angiocentric pattern of infiltration potentially mimicking an inflammatory dermatosis such as secondary syphilis (28–30).

For localized disease, treatment includes excision and/or radiotherapy. For disseminated disease and/or disease, which includes both extracutaneous and cutaneous lymphoma, systemic chemotherapy is indicated. For solitary lesions, many oncologists do not treat the lymphoma.

Pathology

Morphology

Biopsies demonstrate a sheetlike and nodular superficial and deep growth of small lymphocytes comprising a mixture of reactive T cells and atypical B cells showing a centrocytic slightly grooved, small rounded, and/or monocytoid morphology. A few larger immunoblastic cells can be seen. The morphologic distinction between T and B cells is very difficult and must be made via immunohistochemical assessment as discussed below. The infiltrates assume a disposition around adnexal structures but also manifest an interstitial and angiocentric pattern. The infiltrates are dense and exhibit areas of both diffuse and nodular growth, frequently demonstrating a greater intensity of infiltration at the base (Fig. 29.4A). Also characteristic are dysplastic plasma cells manifested by a larger size and less condensed heterochromatin with or without Dutcher bodies, oftentimes most apparent around vessels of the superficial dermis and within the adventitial dermis of the eccrine coil (Fig. 29.5A and B). The cells are light chain restricted (Fig. 29.5C and D). Reactive germinal centers are infiltrated by small neoplastic lymphocytes, defining the concept of progressive transformation of the germinal center (Fig. 29.4B). Subcutaneous involvement is more typical of patients who have secondary MALT or present with concurrent disease involving extracutaneous sites (28–32).

Phenotypic Profile

The two most critical markers that must be obtained in evaluating any well-differentiated small cell–dominant lymphocytic infiltrate are CD20 and CD3, staining B and T cells, respectively. In most cases of MZL, there is a dominance of B cells over T cells; however, it should be emphasized that MZL can on occasion exhibit striking reactive T-cell lymphoid hyperplasia whereby the T- to B-cell ratio is more in keeping with a reactive process (i.e., lymphocytoma cutis). Such disorders are very difficult to differentiate from lymphocytoma cutis, and

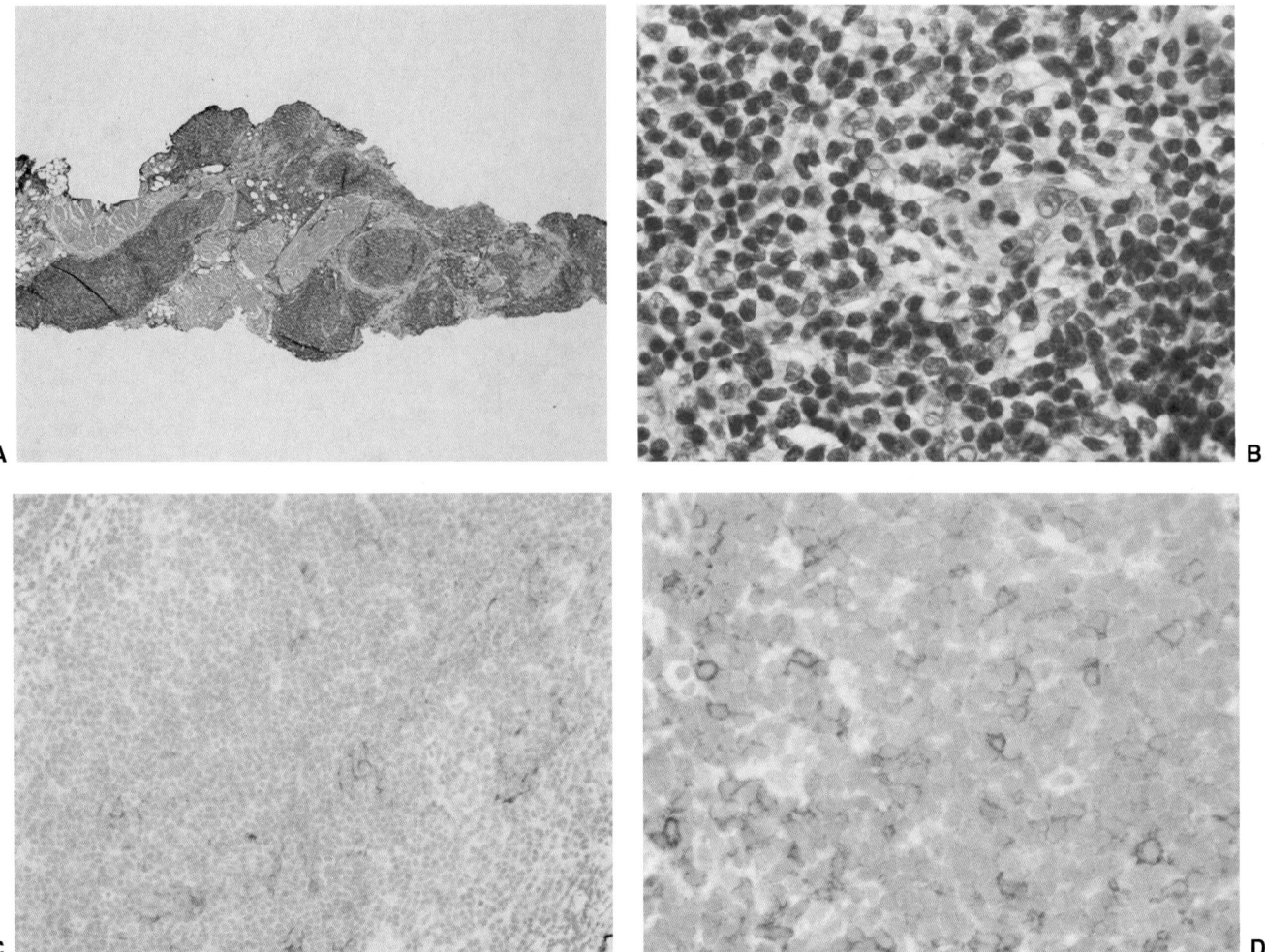

FIGURE 29.4. A: In this case of MZL, one observes a well-differentiated nodular lymphocytic infiltrate predominated by small lymphocytes infiltrating skeletal muscle of the periorbital area. This infiltrative growth pattern into muscle would be very unusual in the realm of reactive lymphoid hyperplasia (hematoxylin and eosin, magnification: 40×). **B:** Higher magnification shows the small monotonous lymphocytic infiltrate with slight lymphoid atypia. Dysplastic plasmacytic elements, a frequent feature of MZL, are not observed in this photograph. If present, they are a useful morphologic clue and are oftentimes times accentuated around blood vessels and the eccrine coil (hematoxylin and eosin, magnification: 1,000×). **C:** Reactive germinal centers can be identified with CD21, CD23, Bcl6, and CD10. In this photomicrograph, there is disruption of the CD21 follicular dendritic cell network attributable to infiltration of the germinal center by neoplastic post–germinal center B cells consistent with progressive transformation of the germinal center (diaminobenzidine, magnification: 200×). **D:** The neoplastic cells express CD5, a potential risk factor for blastic transformation (diaminobenzidine, magnification: 1,000×).

only select subtle phenotypic abnormalities such as a reduction in CD79A may suggest a diagnosis of evolving low-grade B-cell lymphoproliferative disorder. In most cases of MZL, there are reactive germinal centers. It is important to perform stains to highlight the germinal centers including Bcl6, CD10, CD21, CD23, and Bcl2. In the benign germinal center of MZL, the centrocytes and centroblasts stain positively for CD10 and Bcl6 and negativity for Bcl2 (26). The follicular dendritic cell network is highlighted by CD21 and CD23. However, there may be focal irregular areas of dendritic cell lysis reflective of infiltration of the germinal center by small neoplastic B cells (Fig. 29.4C). This particular finding is an important clue in regard to a diagnosis of MZL (11). The lymphocytes can be CD23 negative typical of a post–germinal center B cell; however, CD23 positivity can be seen especially in recurrent MZL and would be considered an aberrant phenotype supportive of a diagnosis of lymphoma (12).

Dysplastic plasma cells are a critical clue to the diagnosis of MZL; they are invariably light chain restricted be it in the context of kappa and/or lambda light chain restriction. The normal kappa to lambda ratio is 3:1 up to 5:1. Any equalization of the kappa and lambda ratio and/or a dominance of lambda over kappa however slight would signify light chain restriction, an important phenotypic feature supportive of MZL (Fig. 29.5C and D). In the same vein, a very high kappa to lambda ratio typically higher than 10:1 would suggest a kappa light chain–restricted infiltrate. Neoplastic plasma cells may express cyclin D1 and CD56 (28–30).

A reduction in the expression of CD79 amidst the small post–germinal center nonplasmacytic B cells would also be a phenotypic clue favoring MZL. In a minority of cases the neoplastic cells will express CD5 and CD43 (Fig. 29.4D).

Molecular Profile Studies

PCR analysis will demonstrate a heavy chain immunoglobulin rearrangement. The automated Ventanna RT mRNA analysis will invariably show kappa or lambda light chain restriction in diagnostic cases. However, there are small cell nonplasmacytic variants of MZL with very few plasma cells, and hence a meaningful assessment regarding light chain restriction is not possible.

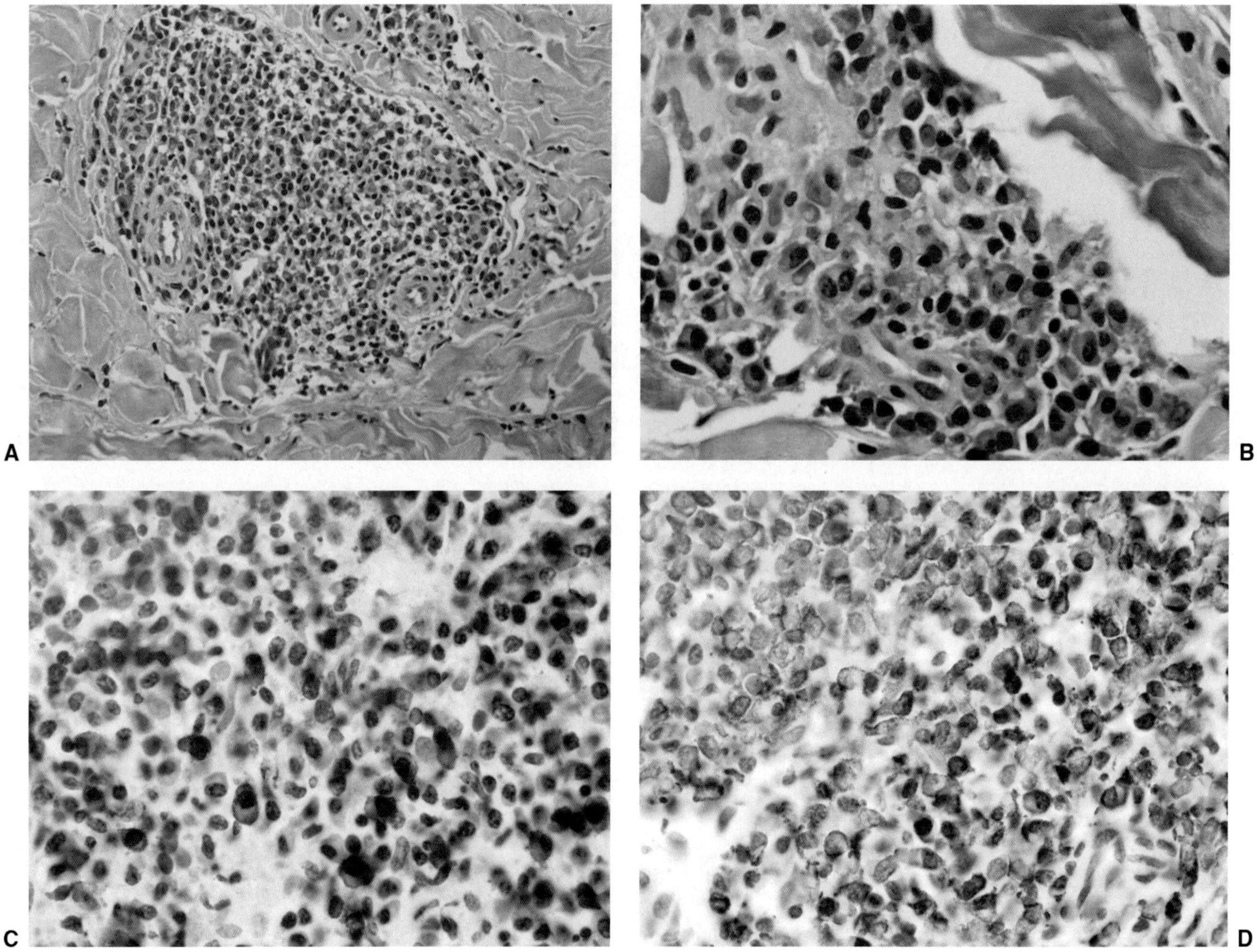

FIGURE 29.5. **A:** In this case of plasmacytic MZL one sees a number of atypical plasma cells arranged around blood vessels (hematoxylin and eosin, magnification: 200×). **B:** The dysplastic quality of the plasma cells is revealed by significant size heterogeneity and as well, the nuclei show a finely dispersed chromatin with somewhat angulated nuclear contours. In contrast, the reactive plasma cell demonstrates a round nucleus with a clock face distribution of chromatin (hematoxylin and eosin, magnification: 1,000×). **C:** There are a few positive-staining kappa light chain–restricted plasma cells (diaminobenzidine, magnification: 1,000×). **D:** The dominant infiltrate, however, is lambda positive indicative of a lambda light chain–restricted dysplastic plasmacytic infiltrate consistent with immunocytoma/marginal zone lymphoma (diaminobenzidine, magnification: 1,000×).

Pathogenesis

A preexisting state of benign lymphoid hyperplasia presumably exists. Various antigen triggers could stimulate B-cell hyperplasia including *Borrelia burgdorferi* and certain lymphotropic viral infections including hepatitis C and Epstein-Barr virus (EBV). We have also encountered cases of MZL developing in the setting of immune dysregulatory therapy specifically in the context of antidepressant and antihistamine administration (31–34).

The exact cell of origin is a post–germinal center B cell. Overall, the phenotype most closely resembles the post–germinal center memory B cells. Analysis of Ig gene rearrangements shows the presence of ongoing hypermutations associated with a (post) follicle center cell genotype (31–34).

Differential Diagnosis

The main differential diagnosis is with reactive cutaneous lymphoid hyperplasia. The characteristic features of lymphocytoma cutis have already been considered. In brief a dominance of T cells over B cells, reactive germinal centers without progressive transformation (for definition see above), the lack of cytologic atypia amidst the plasma cells, and a polytypic plasma cell infiltrate are important features. Molecular studies typically show a polyclonal result.

PLASMACYTOMA

Plasmacytomas are now considered under the same rubric as MZL. The lesions present in a fashion similar to a MZL, manifesting as a solitary or few lesions involving the arms and trunk. The biopsies typically show a diffuse infiltrate of differentiated plasma cells without other admixed inflammatory cell elements including small lymphocytes (Fig. 29.6A–C). There may be concomitant paraproteinemia. A bone marrow biopsy may be warranted to rule out an underlying systemic plasma cell dyscrasia. From a histomorphologic perspective, the main differentiating point from MZL is the absence of small lymphocytes (35). Amyloid production can be observed. Kappa or light chain restriction is invariably present (Fig. 29.6D). The main differential diagnosis comprises reactive cutaneous plasmacytic infiltrates as those seen in the setting of cutaneous Rosai-Dorfman disease and reactive systemic plasmacytosis. Plasmacytomas can show significant atypia, and hence the distinction from plasmablastic lymphoma can be difficult. In plasmablastic lymphoma, a trabeculated architecture is observed with nests of large plasmablastic cells demarcated by a hyalinized stromal network. Atypia is striking and includes many transformed cells. Plasmablastic lymphoma exhibits HHV8 and Epstein Barr virus- encoded small RNAs (EBER) positivity (36).

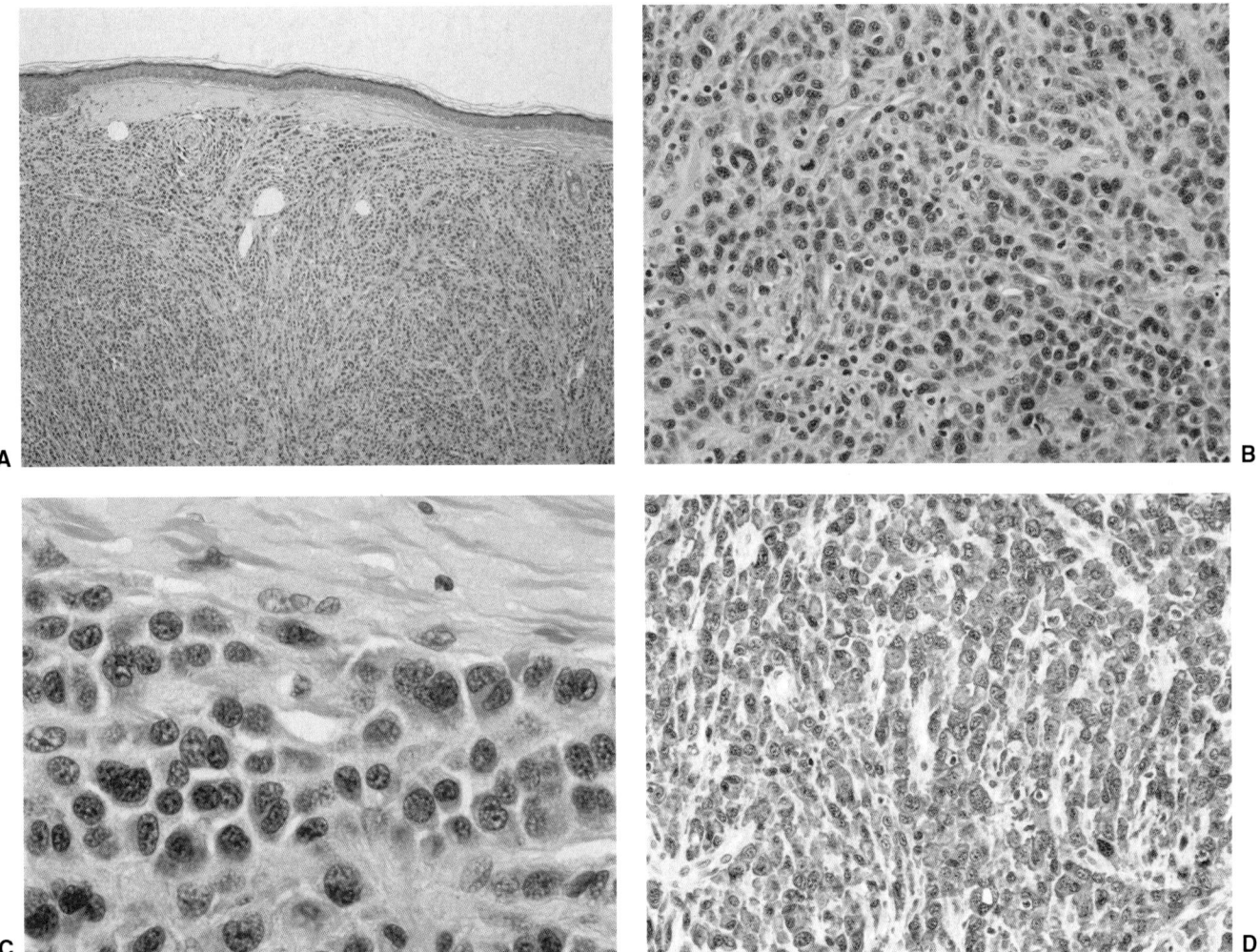

FIGURE 29.6. A: In this case of plasmacytoma one observes a sheetlike infiltrate of atypical plasma cells (hematoxylin and eosin, magnification: 200×). **B:** Higher magnification shows that the dominant infiltrate is of plasmacytic origin with marked atypia. The background population of small nonplasmacytic neoplastic B cells warranting categorization as an immunocytoma/plasmacytic MZL is not identified (hematoxylin and eosin, magnification: 400×). **C:** The extent of plasma cell atypia is quite prominent. Most plasmacytomas do not show this degree of plasma cell atypia although the cells still have a differentiated plasmacytic quality and do not exhibit an immunoblastic morphology, hence precluding categorization as a true plasmablastic lymphoma (hematoxylin and eosin, magnification: 1,000×). **D:** In this plasmacytoma the cells exhibit lambda light chain restriction (diaminobenzidine, magnification: 400×).

PRIMARY CUTANEOUS FOLLICLE CENTER CELL LYMPHOMA

Clinical Features and Pathology

Primary cutaneous follicle center cell lymphoma is another low-grade B-cell lymphoma, representing the most common form of B-cell lymphoma. The most characteristic presentation is in the context of solitary nodules and/or plaques with a predilection to involve the head and neck area (see Fig. 29.12). Like MZL, extracutaneous dissemination is rare. Patients affected with this form of lymphoma have an excellent prognosis (>95% survival at 5 years). A younger patient population is affected compared to those patients who develop large cell lymphoma of the legs. After appropriate treatment, relapses are very uncommon (37–39).

Light Microscopic Findings

The most common morphologic expression closely recapitulates lymphocytoma cutis. In this scenario, there is a superficial and deep nodular lymphocytic infiltrate exhibiting a zonation pattern characterized by small lymphocytes located peripheral to germinal center–like foci (Fig. 29.7A and B). The germinal centers exhibit considerable variation in size. The germinal centers show enhanced atypia among the centroblasts and centrocytes. Other admixed cellular elements most notably tingible body macrophages are absent. As these lesions typically arise in a background of lymphocytoma cutis, it is common to see reactive germinal centers as well as those that are neoplastic. Another important feature signifying malignant transformation is the infiltrative quality of the germinal center. Specifically the borders of the germinal centers are irregular and merge with the surrounding small reactive lymphocytes. As well, autonomous small neoplastic collections of centroblasts can be observed throughout the infiltrate. The far end of the spectrum would be a follicle center cell lymphoma dominated by a diffuse infiltrate of neoplastic large lymphocytes, hence falling under the rubric of diffuse large cell B-cell lymphoma (see Figs. 29.8 and 29.9A, B).

As with nodal follicular lymphoma, there are two main cell types. The first cell type is a small to medium-sized cell in the 7- to 9-µm size range with angulated twisted cleaved nuclei and inconspicuous nucleoli, referred to as centrocytes or cleaved follicle center cells. The second cell type is large transformed

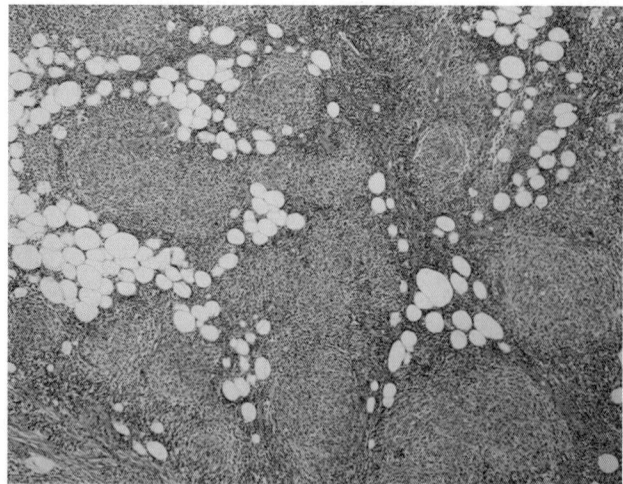 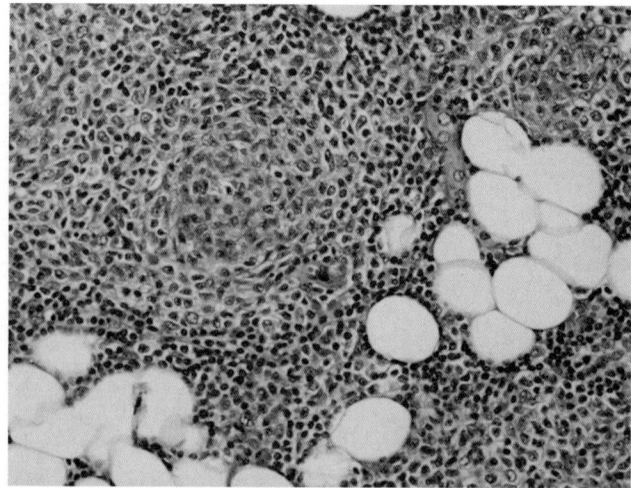

FIGURE 29.7. A: In this case of follicle center cell lymphoma, one sees neoplastic germinal centers extending into fat (hematoxylin and eosin, magnification: 100×). **B:** This higher magnification reveals the composition of the germinal center, being that of small to intermediate-sized centrocytes with a minor larger cell centroblastic component without an admixture of tingible body macrophages and therefore compatible with a grade 1 follicle center cell lymphoma (hematoxylin and eosin, magnification: 400×). Follicle center lymphomas of the skin are not typically graded since they all represent indolent forms of lymphoma independent of the grade.

cells manifesting round to oval nuclei with one to three peripherally disposed nucleoli. These cells are referred to as centroblasts. A designation as small cell dominant, mixed, and/ or large cell dominant is made based on the number of centroblasts identified. Hence, a small cell–dominant lymphoma has 1 to 5 centroblasts per high power field (grade I), a mixed lymphoma exhibits 6 to 15 centroblasts per high power field (grade II), and a large cell lymphoma manifests >15 centroblasts per high power field (grade III) (see Fig. 29.9A and B). Neither the architectural growth pattern nor the percent of large atypical cells alters the prognosis in this low-grade B-cell lymphoma.

Phenotypic Profile

The classic phenotypic profile is one in which the neoplasm exhibits lineage fidelity with respect to being of germinal center cell origin demonstrating Bcl-6 and CD10 positivity (Figs. 29.10A, C, 29.11A–D, and 29.12A, see Fig. 29.9D). Other markers to highlight germinal centers include CD21 and CD23

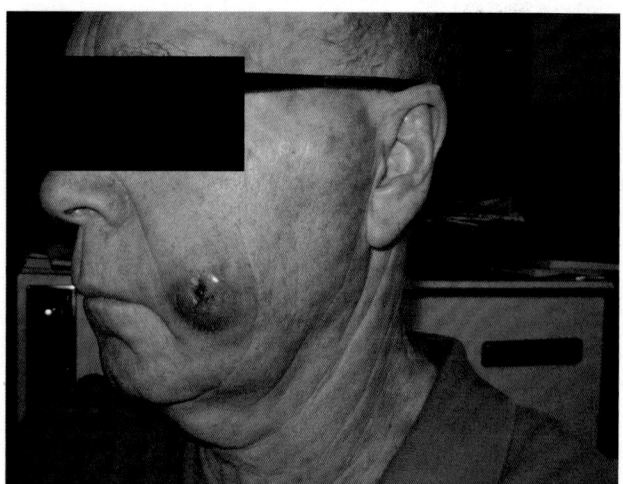

FIGURE 29.8. In this patient with grade 3 follicle center cell lymphoma, despite the sheet-like growth of large immunoblastic cells and the enormous size of the tumor the clinical course was relatively indolent with the patient demonstrating an excellent response to radiation therapy. The localization to the head and neck area is typical for this form of B-cell lymphoma.

(Figs. 29.10B and 29.12B). These markers highlight the follicular dendritic cell network. In classic follicle center cell lymphoma, the follicular dendritic cell network is irregular with significant zones of dendritic cell lysis. In the extreme case, there may be dendritic cell lysis/loss whereby the germinal center is completely negative for either of these markers (Fig. 29.12B). Although CD23 typically highlights follicular dendritic cells, it can show positivity amidst the centroblasts and centrocytes, a phenotypic aberration that could be helpful in establishing a diagnosis of follicle center cell lymphoma since reactive centrocytes and centroblasts are typically negative.

In approximately 30% of cases, the neoplastic germinal centers stain positively for Bcl2, mirroring the phenotypic profile encountered in nodular follicular lymphoma (Fig. 29.10D). CD10 positivity can be variable ranging from normal expression to enhanced expression to one of deletion. In primary cutaneous follicle center cell lymphoma, a neoplastic germinal center may exhibit variable expression of CD10 ranging from positivity in a subset of neoplastic cells to cells devoid of staining. Heterogeneity in CD10 expression (Fig. 29.12C) and Bcl2 negativity distinguish primary cutaneous follicle center cell lymphoma from nodal follicular lymphoma secondarily involving the skin. MUM1 staining is typically absent in lower-grade follicle center cell lymphomas (i.e., grade I and grade II follicle center cell lymphomas) but can be observed in higher-grade follicle center cell lymphomas (i.e., grade III) (40) (Figs.29.9C and 29.12D).

Molecular studies

In those cases, PCR analysis to assess for heavy chain immunoglobulin rearrangement will show a clonal result.

 ## PRIMARY CUTANEOUS DIFFUSE LARGE CELL LYMPHOMA OF LEG TYPE

Primary cutaneous diffuse large cell B-cell lymphoma has a variable prognosis that relates to specific variables including site localization, extent of disease, and phenotypic profile. In earlier published studies, it was established that patients who presented with diffuse large cell B-cell lymphomas primarily involving the lower extremities appeared to have a worse prognosis than those patients with localization of similar neoplasms at other sites (41).

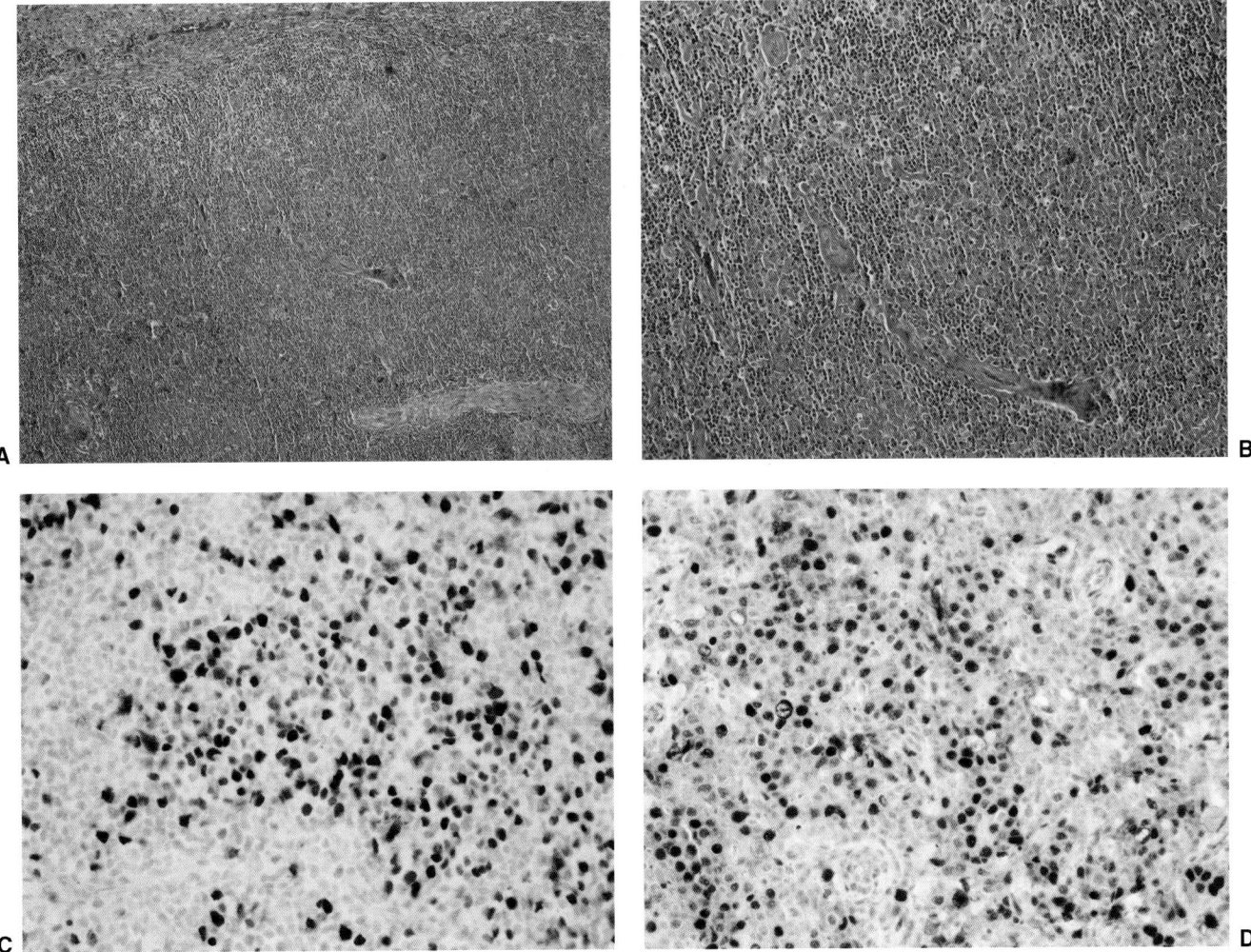

FIGURE 29.9. A: In this patient with follicle center cell lymphoma there are areas of both diffuse and nodular lymphocytic infiltration (hematoxylin and eosin, magnification: 100×). **B:** Higher power magnification demonstrates a vague nodularity to the infiltrate. The nodular foci are predominated by large atypical cells compatible with a grade 3 follicle center cell lymphoma while there is a background of small mature lymphocytes (hematoxylin and eosin, magnification: 200×). Despite the higher grade, this lymphoma would be considered as indolent as a lower grade follicle center cell lymphoma. **C:** Extensive MUM1 staining was seen, a finding observed in the higher-grade follicle center cell lymphomas (diaminobenzidine, magnification: 400×). **D:** The follicle center cell nature of the neoplasm was revealed by the positivity for Bcl6 (diaminobenzidine, magnification: 400×).

The combination of a large cell diffuse morphology, the location on the leg, and the more aggressive clinical course was sufficiently distinctive to warrant the designation of diffuse large cell B-cell lymphoma of the legs. It later became apparent that a subset of patients with lesions located outside of the leg may have an aggressive clinical course, hence supplanting the former designation with diffuse large cell lymphoma of leg type (42,43).

The designation of leg type lymphoma is now largely based on the phenotypic profile, as will be discussed presently. Furthermore, recent literature suggests the cytogenetic profile may be a further prognostic determinant. Even when considering those lymphomas that have a more "aggressive" phenotype, limited disease cases always fair better than cases with a similar morphology and phenotypic profile when disseminated disease is present (43–45). This type of lymphoma is relatively uncommon, representing 5% to 10% of all cutaneous B-cell lymphomas (38,44,45).

Pathology

A dominant diffuse pan dermal infiltrate effacing the dermal architecture is characteristic. Zones of nodular infiltration with some angiocentric accentuation may also be seen. Mitotic activity is brisk and there are numerous apoptotic cells. If the infiltrate contains a higher proportion of small cells, consideration should be given to alternative categories of primary cutaneous B-cell lymphoma such as follicle center cell lymphoma or MZL with blastic foci (Fig. 29.13A and B). The large cells are in the 15- to 20-μm size range exhibiting an immunoblastic and/or pleomorphic large cell morphology. There may be a background of small T lymphocytes representing part of an immune response to the neoplastic B-cell populace. Some cases of diffuse large cell B-cell lymphoma of leg type show a paucicellular necrobiotic process demarcated by sheets and nodules of neoplastic cells. Angioinvasion and recurrent disease manifesting as an angiotropic B-cell lymphoma can be seen (46).

Phenotype

In evaluating any lymphocytic infiltrate, the relative CD3 to CD20 ratio is a critical determinant in diagnostic assessment. In leg type lymphoma, as with other types of B-cell lymphoma, there is characteristically a dominance of B cells over T cells. A reduction in the expression of CD79 defines a phenotypic aberration indicative of B-cell lymphoma (45). Cytoplasmic expression of IgM is characteristic and provides a differentiating point that separates this lymphoma from the more indolent diffuse large cell follicle center cell counterpart (47).

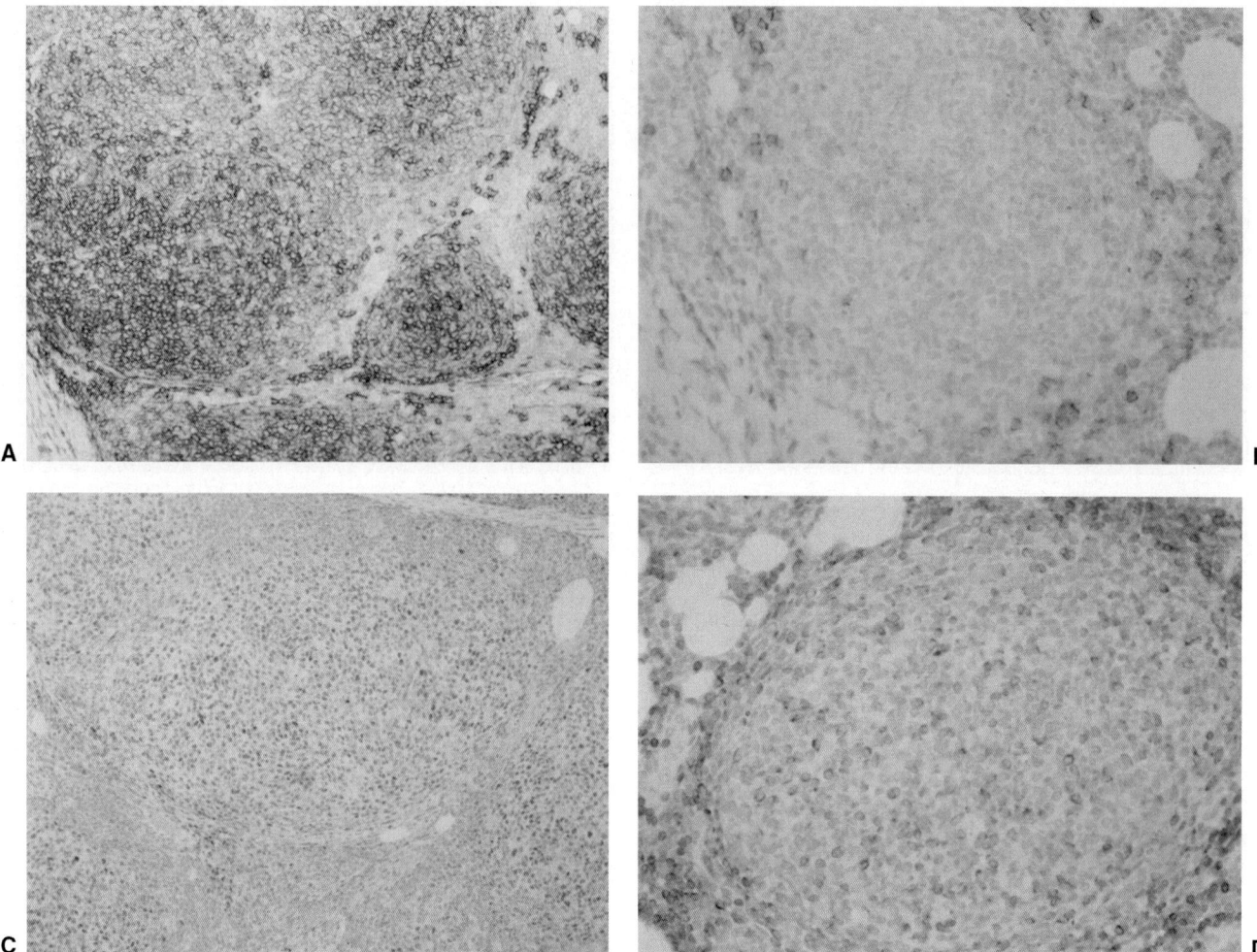

FIGURE 29.10. A: The germinal center–like foci are strongly positive for CD10 (diaminobenzidine, magnification: 200×). **B:** Neoplastic germinal centers may show minimal reactivity for the follicular dendritic cell marker CD23 indicative of extensive dendritic cell lysis, a characteristic finding in primary cutaneous follicle center cell lymphoma (diaminobenzidine, magnification: 200×). **C:** The germinal center–like foci are highlighted by Bcl6 (diaminobenzidine, magnification: 400×). **D:** Thirty percent of primary cutaneous follicle center cell lymphomas show Bcl2 staining in the neoplastic germinal center. In this case there is focal staining for bcl2 although the majority of the neoplastic cells are Bcl2 negative. It is quite characteristic in primary cutaneous follicle center cell lymphoma to see variation in staining with respect to CD10 and Bcl2, ranging from cells that may overexpress Bcl2 and CD10 to cells that do not exhibit any immunoreactivity for either CD10 or bcl2 (diaminobenzidine, magnification: 400×).

In those patients with recurrent tumors treated with rituximab, diminution in CD20 expression compared to pretreatment biopsies may be observed (48,49). Lineage infidelity may be seen with CD43, a marker that characteristically stains T cells and monocytes. The neoplastic cells demonstrate positivity for BCL2, Oct2, and MUM1 and are usually BCL6 positive. They do not show any significant immunoreactivity with CD10 and CD138. (Fig. 29.13C and D) (48,49). The tumors are characteristically CD23, CD30, and CD5 negative. It has been our experience that CD30-positive large cell B-cell lymphomas that can be Bcl2 positive may be associated with underlying iatrogenic and/or endogenous immune dysregulation and define a form of indolent B-cell lymphoma distinct from the leg type lymphoma. CD30+ B-cell lymphomas are a defined entity discussed in further detail elsewhere in the chapter (50).

Cytogenetics

In one study an interphase fluorescence *in situ* hybridization (FISH) technique was employed to assess for structural aberrations of the genes BCL2, BCL6, and MYC, and numerical aberrations of the chromosomes 3, 7, 8, 11, 12, 13, 17, 18q, RB1, and P53. Genetic aberrations are observed in 76% of cases

(51,52). The most frequent numerical abnormalities are gains of chromosome 12, 7, 3, 18q, 11, and X while losses of genes encoding p53 are observed very infrequently. BCL2, MYC, and BCL6 are rearranged with the IGH gene either in a very small number of cases or not at all. The most significant genetic difference separating diffuse large cell B-cell lymphoma of the skin from the nodal counterpart and extracutaneous diffuse large cell B-cell lymphoma is the absence of Bcl6 rearrangement (51). Overall, the cytogenetic abnormalities were uniform among all cases of diffuse large cell B-cell lymphoma of the skin independent of site and of Bcl2 expression (51).

In another study significant differences using array-based comparative genomic hybridization was established between primary cutaneous follicle center cell lymphomas and diffuse large cell B-cell lymphomas of leg type. The recurrent alterations in primary cutaneous follicle center cell lymphoma were high-level DNA amplifications at 2p16.1 and deletion of chromosome 14q32.33. FISH analysis demonstrated c-REL amplification in patients with gains at 2p16.1. In primary cutaneous large cell B-cell lymphoma of the leg type, the most striking abnormalities were characterized by a high-level DNA amplification of 18q21.31-q21.33 to include the BCL2 and MALT1 genes. As well, deletions of a small region within 9p21.3

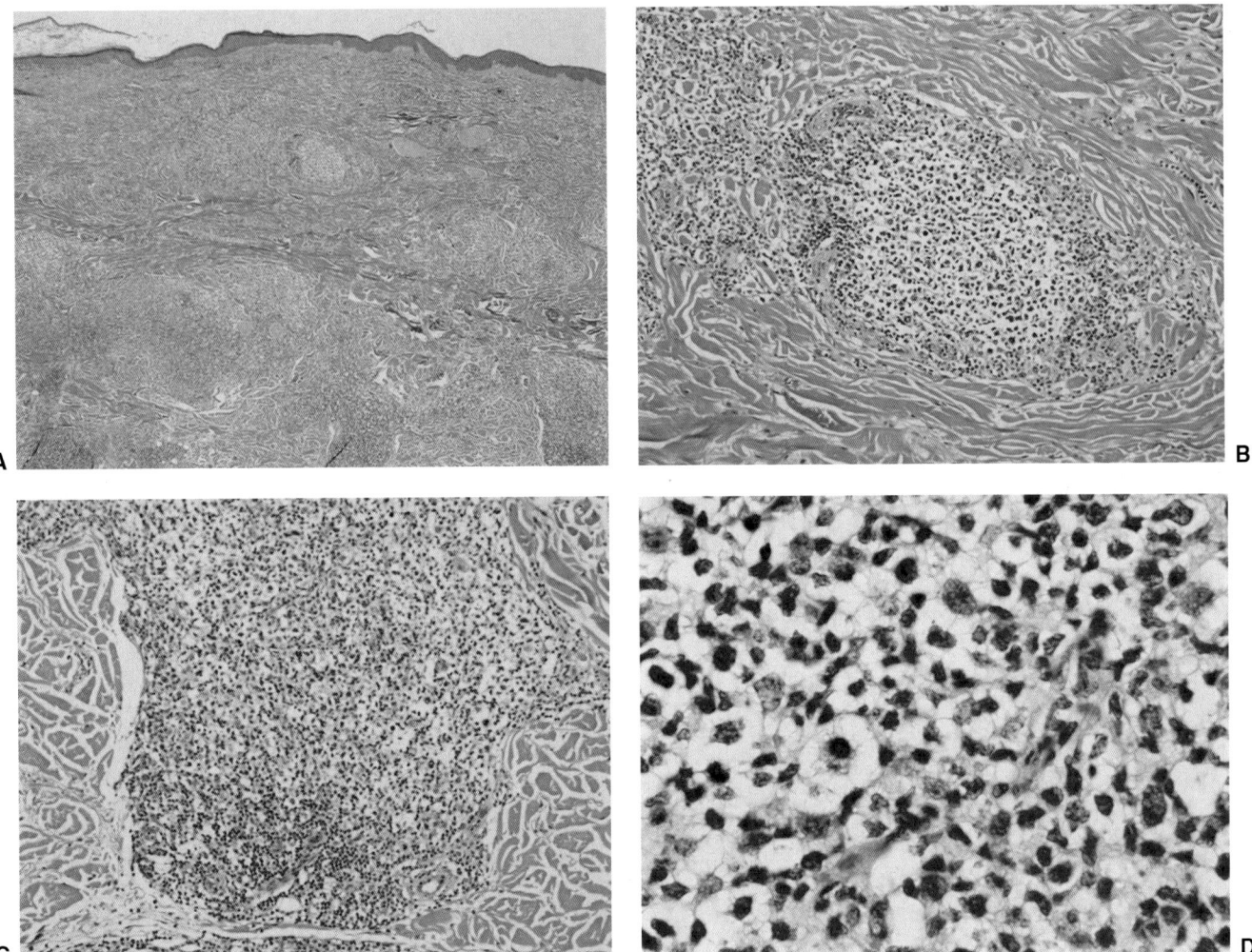

FIGURE 29.11. A: There are a number of nodular lymphocytic foci present throughout the dermis with enhanced cellularity toward the base (hematoxylin and eosin, magnification: 200×). **B:** Higher magnification of the germinal center shows that it is surrounded by small lymphocytes. Without higher power magnification and more importantly immunohistochemical assessment, it may be difficult to discriminate between a neoplastic germinal center and a reactive one. Reactive germinal centers are seen in MZL. Unlike MZL, there is no infiltration of the germinal center by neoplastic post–germinal center B cells (hematoxylin and eosin, magnification: 200×). **C:** One of the characteristic features of the neoplastic germinal center is a relative lack of tingible body macrophages. As well, there is enhanced atypia amidst the centrocytes and/or centroblasts. In this case the dominant composition, being that of a small centrocytic cell, is abnormal and signifies a neoplastic process. In reactive germinal centers, a more heterogeneous mixture of cell types is seen (hematoxylin and eosin, magnification: 200×). **D:** From a cytomorphologic perspective, the majority of the atypical cells in the germinal center are small centrocytes. Less than ten centroblastic forms are noted per high power field, hence defining a grade 1 follicle center cell lymphoma (hematoxylin and eosin, magnification: 1,000×). From a practical diagnostic perspective the case would be signed out as a primary cutaneous follicle center cell lymphoma without the grade.

containing the CDKN2A, CDKN2B, and NSG-x genes were observed. Homozygous deletion of 9p21.3 was detected in almost 50% of patients with diffuse large cell B-cell lymphomas of leg type but in none of the patients with primary cutaneous follicle center cell lymphoma (51,52). Complete methylation of the promoter region of the CDKN2A gene was demonstrated only in the leg type B-cell lymphomas (53–55). Only those patients harboring a 9p21 deletion had a worse prognosis. Cases of leg type lymphoma without a 9p21 deletion had a prognosis similar to other more indolent forms of cutaneous B-cell lymphoma (53).

Pathogenesis

The leg type lymphomas are held to be of later-stage germinal center cell origin, reflected phenotypically by the Bcl6 positivity along with CD10 negativity in most neoplasms. The expression of Mum1/IRF4 protein is a feature of leg type lymphoma in contrast with the observed negativity in primary cutaneous follicle center cell lymphoma (56). DNA tissue microarray studies

have shown increased expression of genes associated with cell proliferation, namely, the protooncogenes PIM-1, PIM-2, and c-MYC and the transcription factors Mum1/IRF4 and Oct-2 in lymphomas of leg type with their absence in primary cutaneous follicle center cell lymphoma. Primary cutaneous follicle center cell lymphoma shows high expression of SPINK2 (57). Deletion or promoter region hypermethylation of the p16INK4a gene and a higher level of retinoblastoma protein expression are greater in diffuse large B-cell lymphoma of the skin (>50%) compared to MZL or follicle center cell lymphoma (<10%) (42). Nevertheless, only those tumors of leg type are associated with an intermediate prognosis while the other forms of diffuse large cell B-cell lymphoma, despite adverse molecular and genetic markers, have a relatively indolent clinical course.

The location-dependent difference in prognosis has been a source of investigation by many authors although now there is more of a trend to consider these neoplasms from a phenotypic as opposed to site perspective. Endothelial expression of ICAM-3 is associated with a more aggressive clinical course (58). ICAM-1 and leukocyte function–associated antigen-1 (LFA-1)

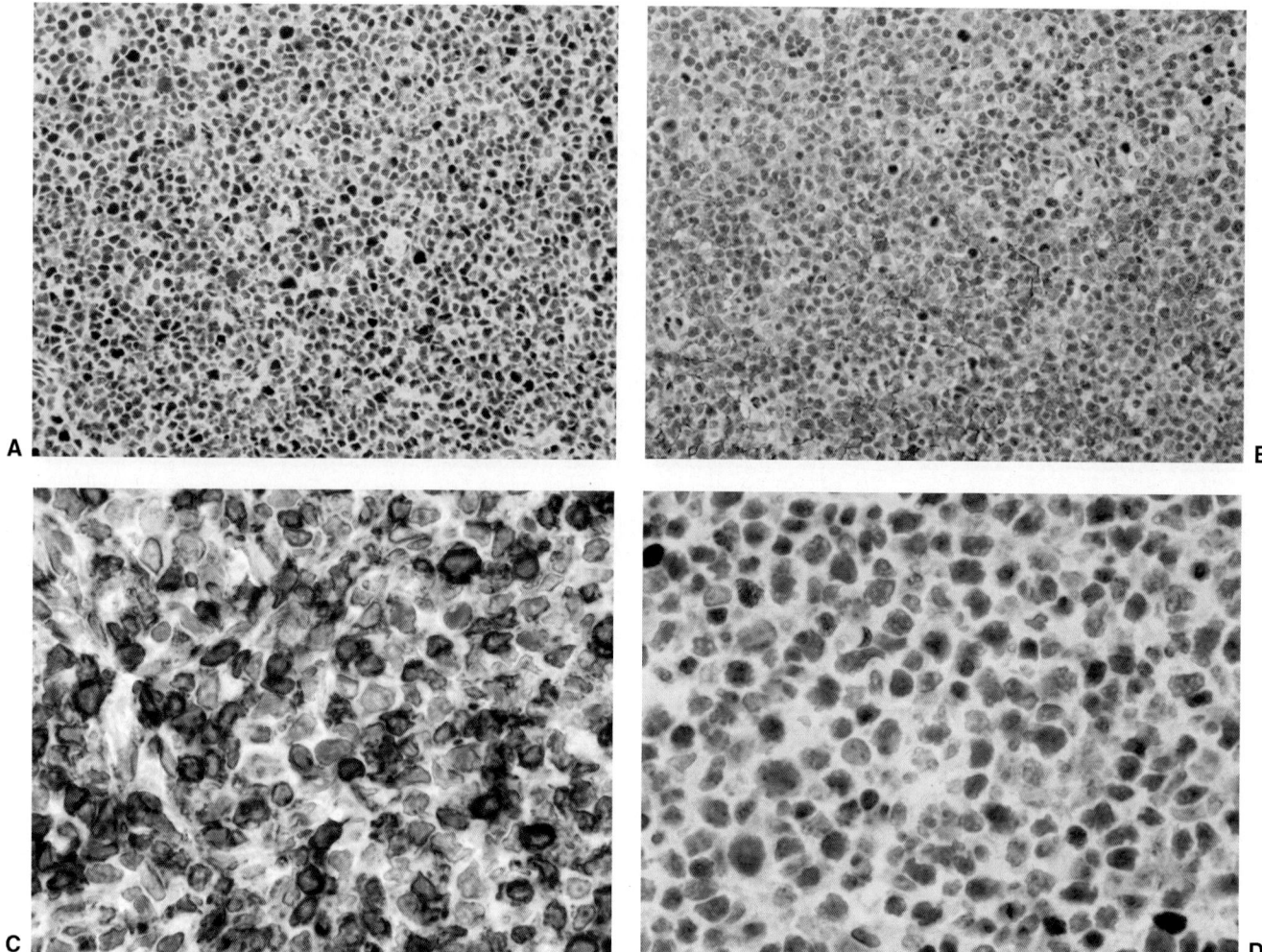

FIGURE 29.12. A: The follicle center cell marker Bcl6 is positive (diaminobenzidine, magnification: 400×). **B:** A CD21 preparation highlights some residuum of the follicular dendritic cell network; most of the dendritic cell network however is absent (diaminobenzidine, magnification: 400×). **C:** Like nodal follicular lymphoma, strong expression of CD10 can be observed. However, a lack of staining of CD10 in a germinal center would be considered an aberrant phenotype (diaminobenzidine, magnification: 1,000×). **D:** Illustrated is MUM1. Lower-grade follicle center cell lymphomas as noted here are characteristically MUM1 negative (diaminobenzidine, magnification: 1,000×).

were expressed in a high percentage of primary cutaneous large cell lymphomas of the head and neck as opposed to those tumors of the leg that had significantly lower levels of expression of these adhesion molecules (59). Dissemination of disease and death directly attributable to the lymphoma only occurred in those patients whose tumors lacked expression of the adhesion markers ICAM-1 and LFA-1 (59). In cases where the tumor expressed ICAM-1 and LFA-1, death from lymphoma was not documented (59). Tissue-specific migration is mediated by the interaction of adhesion molecules on the lymphocyte surface (i.e., lymphocyte homing receptors) and endothelial cell ligands. Hence, the difference in expression of adhesion molecules may be of importance in determining clinical behavior (59–61). In the same vein, differential integrin expression may be of pathogenetic importance (62,63).

INTRAVASCULAR B-CELL LYMPHOMA

Intravascular lymphoma is a rare lymphoma that exhibits a peculiar intravascular localization and hence signs and symptoms associated with this tumor are primarily in the context of ischemic sequel. Elderly individuals are more commonly affected. Constitutional symptoms are frequent (63–65). When the entity was first recognized, the actual cell of origin was

unclear and it was assumed to be of endothelial cell origin, hence the former designation of malignant angioendotheliomatosis. The essence of intravascular B-cell lymphoma is one of a microvascular occlusive lesion attributable to proliferating neoplastic B cells largely confined to the endoluminal aspect of vessels; there is an unusual predilection to involve the skin and central nervous system (65). The spleen and marrow can be involved in one-third of cases. Lymph node involvement is very uncommon. In a minority of cases, the process is confined to the skin; such patients do have a much better prognosis compared to patients with multiorgan involvement.

A variant of intravascular B-cell lymphoma that primarily affects patients of Asian descent falls under the designation of the so-called Asian variant of intravascular B-cell lymphoma. The patients may have a clinical course complicated by hemophagocytic syndrome (HPS); the extent of cutaneous and skin involvement is less. Intravascular B-cell lymphoma has been described in patients with underlying immune dysregulation potentially linked with a relative CD4 T-cell lymphopenia typified by rheumatoid arthritis, human immunodeficiency virus infection, and Sjögren syndrome (66). Intravascular colonization of benign vascular tumors by intravascular B-cell lymphoma has been described (66–70). A single report with a patient presenting with fever of unknown origin has been described. The rare T-cell variant shows dominant involvement of the lung without

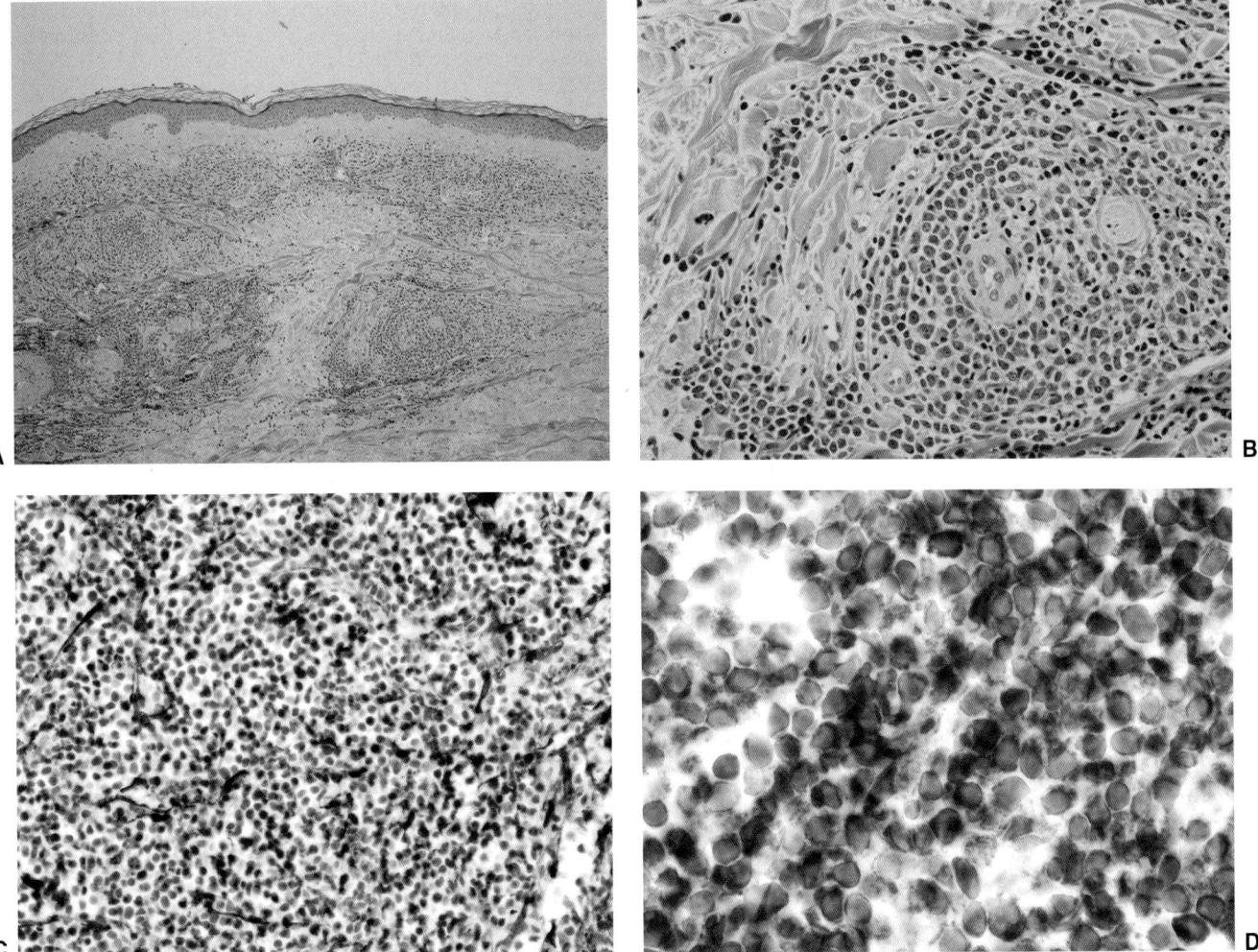

FIGURE 29.13. A: In this case of diffuse large cell B-cell lymphoma of leg type, one observes both a diffuse and angiocentric nodular pattern. At times the interstitial scaffolding resembles a palisading granulomatous dermatitis (hematoxylin and eosin, magnification: 100×). **B:** Although one assumes that the lymphoma is diffuse, it can show a nodular pattern, exhibiting angiocentricity as noted here. The dominant cytology is that of a large centroblast and/or immunoblast. The smaller lymphocytes are reactive (hematoxylin and eosin, magnification: 400×). **C:** In leg type lymphomas, the CD10 preparation is negative (diaminobenzidine, magnification: 400×). **D:** Bcl2 is characteristically positive and in fact is an immunophenotypic requirement to render a diagnosis of diffuse large cell lymphoma of leg type (diaminobenzidine, magnification: 1,000×).

skin and central nervous system disease (68). There are recent reports regarding other lymphomas presenting as recurrent "secondary" intravascular lymphoma. I have encountered cases of primary cutaneous ALCL and follicular lymphoma that have recurred as an intravascular lymphoma (71).

Light Microscopic Findings

The hallmark is one of large atypical cells found within the vascular lumens of capillaries and venules throughout the dermis. The process does not elicit a secondary inflammatory response nor are the cells present in the surrounding tissue. The occlusive vascular foci are most apparent in the deeper aspects of the biopsy.

Phenotypic Studies

The cells will exhibit pan B-cell marker positivity including CD20 and CD79A staining. The cells can show positive staining for CD5 (72). CD29 and CD54 are markedly diminished and/or absent. In secondary intravascular lymphoma (i.e., recurrent lymphoma presenting in an intravascular fashion) we have not encountered a similar reduction in CD29 and CD54 (71), hence indicative of other mechanisms of intravascular localization.

Molecular Studies

Heavy chain immunoglobulin rearrangement will be identified as long as there are sufficient neoplastic cells to allow adequate DNA amplification.

CHRONIC LYMPHOCYTIC LEUKEMIA

Clinical Features

Chronic lymphocytic leukemia (CLL)/small lymphocytic lymphoma (SLL) represents a form of low-grade B-cell lymphoproliferative disease that can involve the skin but always in the context of systemic disease. I have seen several cases over the years where the initial diagnosis of CLL was based on passive colonization of a skin excision specimen with neoplastic B cells in an otherwise asymptomatic patient (73).

CLL is the most common leukemia in adults. The designation of CLL is used when the peripheral blood lymphocyte count is in excess of 5,000/mm³. There is a predilection toward CLL in elderly males. Among the potential symptoms are fatigue, generalized lymphadenopathy, and hepatosplenomegaly. The implicated neoplastic cell is a naive B cell showing CD23 and

CD5 positivity; the benign counterpart is an autoreactive B cell. It is unusual for CLL to infiltrate the skin as the sole process. In the majority of cases, however the neoplastic infiltrates represent passenger lymphocytes colonizing surgical sites and lesions of cutaneous herpes. The identification of chronic lymphocytic leukemic infiltrates in the skin does not adversely affect prognosis.

Light Microscopic Findings

The most frequently encountered pattern in skin specimens is in the context of an incidental finding in skin specimens procured for other reasons, most commonly represented by re-excision specimens. The classic morphology is a nodular lymphocytic infiltrate involving the deeper dermis and subcutaneous tissue. Unlike the typical inflammatory cell infiltrate that is found in the immediate vicinity of the tumor or surgical site, the nodular infiltrates are discontinuous from the main surgical site and neoplasm, appearing as autonomous small lymphocytic clusters in the deeper aspects of the specimen, oftentimes with subcutaneous localization. The cells have a small monomorphic appearance; they are in the 7-μm size range, exhibiting a condensed chromatin with rounded nuclear contours. Rarely CLL presents as a *de novo* process similar to other forms of extracutaneous lymphoma secondarily involving the skin. In this latter scenario, the infiltrates are dense and pan dermal exhibiting both an interstitial and a nodular growth pattern. Foci of proliferation centers can be observed characterized by structures that are vaguely reminiscent of a germinal center; however, rather than exhibiting a mixed centrocytic and centroblastic composition with admixed tingible body macrophages, nodular collections of monotypic round to oval intermediate-sized neoplastic cells are noted, with the cells exhibiting a less condensed chromatin than the smaller neoplastic counterpart.

Phenotype

Neoplastic B lymphocytes are CD5[+], CD23[+], and CD43[+] although there are rare cases where there is no expression of CD23 or CD5 (74). When one encounters clonal B-cell lymphocytosis associated with a lack of staining for CD5 and CD23, an important diagnostic consideration is one of monoclonal lymphocytosis of undetermined significance (75). While CD38 expression in peripheral blood samples of patients with CLL has been correlated with a more aggressive clinical course, there has been no application to date of this marker in the evaluation of cutaneous CLL infiltrates (76).

Molecular Studies

Polymerase chain reaction performed on paraffin-embedded tissues using consensus primers for immunoglobulin heavy chain genes demonstrates rearrangement of the immunoglobulin heavy chain immunoglobulin (76).

DIFFUSE LARGE CELL B-CELL LYMPHOMA OTHER

A distinct subset of diffuse large cell B-cell lymphoma is one that from a phenotypic perspective does not exhibit features supportive of its categorization as either the leg type lymphoma by virtue of the lack of staining for Bcl2 and Mum1 or as a follicle center cell lymphoma as the neoplastic cells are typically negative for Bcl6 and CD10. There is a further lymphoma subset in which only a minor malignant large cell component is observed. There is a dominant reactive

infiltrate comprising T cells and granulomatous foci. The large cell component commonly expresses CD30 despite the lack of expression for Bcl2, CD10, and Bcl6 (50,77,78). T-cell–rich CD30[+] B-cell lymphoma of the skin is an indolent form of cutaneous lymphoma that occurs most commonly in elderly women presenting as solitary nodules with trunk, arm, and head localization. Underlying autoimmune disease, therapy with immunosuppressive, and/or immunomodulatory drugs (i.e., methotrexate) indicate that altered immunity may play a role in lesional propagation. Positivity for EBV is observed in the neoplastic cells in some cases. (78).

Light Microscopic Findings

In T-cell–rich large cell B-cell lymphoma, the neoplastic large cell populace is typically obscured by a reactive T-cell and granulomatous infiltrate. The differential diagnosis is primarily with lymphocytoma cutis. In reactive lymphoid hyperplasia, scattered activated CD30-positive immunoblasts can also be seen; the large cells exhibit round to oval nuclei demonstrating a typical nondysplastic centroblastic and immunoblastic morphology. In contrast the CD30[+] lymphoma cells manifest significant nuclear contour irregularity with thickened nuclear membranes and large basophilic to eosinophilic nucleoli defying categorization as a reactive transformed lymphocyte.

Phenotypic Profile

The cells exhibit CD43, CD30, and Bcl2 positivity without positivity for the follicle center cell markers Bcl6 and CD10. There may be positivity for EBER in those cases associated with chronic methotrexate therapy. In lesions of lymphocytoma cutis, phenotypic studies do not show lineage infidelity with CD43 nor is there Bcl-2 expression.

CUTANEOUS T-CELL LYMPHOMA

Mycosis Fungoides

Clinical Features

Jean-Louis Alibert first described MF, the first recognized cutaneous lymphoma, in 1806. It was established to be a lymphoma of T-cell phenotype in the 1970s based on a distinctive pattern of rosetting of the neoplastic T cells with sheep red blood cells (79–81). MF represents the most common form of cutaneous lymphoma in the skin, whereby it presents to the dermatologist as a chronic recalcitrant dermatitis slowly progressive over several years. A few years typically have transpired between lesional onset and confirmatory tissue diagnosis. According to the World Health Organization, MF is a neoplastic skin growth of mature lymphocytes, representing the most common type of cutaneous T-cell lymphoma (CTCL). MF is categorized into three phases: patch-stage MF, plaque-stage MF, and tumor-stage MF (Fig. 29.14). The male-to-female ratio is approximately 2:1. It is a T-cell lymphoma of mature/postthymic T cells, usually of CD4 phenotype, although less common phenotypes include double-negative CD45 RA, CD8, and/or CD56 variants (82,83). Untreated, patients may undergo a slow evolutionary progression of their disease from patch- to plaque- to tumor-stage MF. In some cases, however, despite the absence of any therapeutic intervention, the clinical course may be stable. When progression to tumor stage occurs, there may be dissemination to other organ sites such as the lymph nodes, bone marrow, central nervous system, and peripheral blood (84). The time course that passes from the inception of the

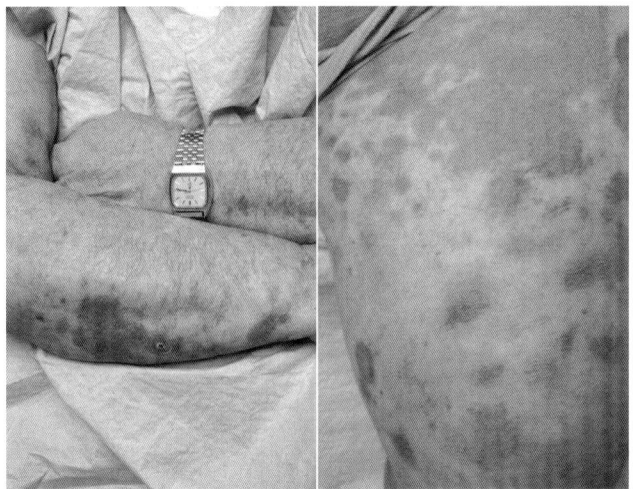

FIGURE 29.14. This patient with MF shows raised somewhat purpuric irregular plaques with areas of coalescence. The purpuric quality with a supervening bronze discoloration is compatible with a purpuric variant of MF, which likely arose in a background of pigmented purpuric dermatosis. (Photo courtesy of Dr. Lindsay Ackerman, Medical Dermatology Specialists, Phoenix, AZ.)

disease process to extracutaneous dissemination is usually one of several years. At times after a several-year history of an apparently stable plaque- and patch-stage form of the disease, the patient may become erythrodermic with generalized lymphadenopathy and atypical circulating Sézary cells, hence defining Sézary syndrome (85). SS may also develop in the absence of known MF as a *de novo* malignancy or in the setting of idiopathic erythroderma. We will consider SS in further detail.

MF is very uncommon in childhood but can occur (86–90). In childhood the disease presents in a very early stage, namely, as patches and plaques without any evidence of peripheral blood or lymph node involvement. Hypopigmented MF is a form of CTCL that appears more commonly among younger patients compared to the older adult counterpart (87,88). This variant of patch-stage CTCL is more common among young black children or those with darker skin types.

In general, one of the most critical clues to the diagnosis of MF is the protracted history. If the eruption is of recent onset a more plausible basis is one induced by drug therapy, defining what is in essence a *drug-associated reversible T-cell dyscrasia*. This topic has been previously discussed (5,7,8,13).

A prelymphomatous T-cell dyscrasia may presage overt MF by many years and includes large plaque parapsoriasis, PPD, folliculotropic T-cell lymphocytosis, alopecia mucinosis, and pityriasis lichenoides. It would be unusual for MF to develop in the absence of a prelymphomatous T-cell dyscrasia (89).

Morphology

Histologically most cases of biopsied MF represent patch-stage/early plaque-stage MF; a superficial bandlike epitheliotropic lymphocytic infiltrate with variable epitheliotropism is characteristic (91). If the infiltrate within the dermis assumes a predominantly angiocentric pattern rather than the aforesaid bandlike pattern, a hypersensitivity-based etiology should be considered even in the presence of lymphoid atypia. An additional clue that the lymphocytic infiltrate is of reactive-based etiology is the directed pattern of lymphocyte migration into the epidermis, characteristically involving the suprapapillary plates, rete ridges, and adnexal epithelium. In early patch-stage MF, the density of lymphocytic infiltration into the epidermis can be low. The epidermotropism of lymphocytes is very

distinctive with cells lining up in a passive fashion along the dermal epidermal junction but also migrating in a haphazard fashion into the spinous layer of the epidermis (Fig. 29.15A and B). Another cardinal hallmark is the Pautrier microabscess, which is a cohesive collection of cerebriform lymphocytes within the parabasilar epidermis. The presence of Pautrier microabscesses typically signifies transition into plaque-stage MF. In the appropriate clinical setting, the designation of patch stage is characterized by significantly atypical epitheliotropic lymphocytic infiltrates with noticeable severe cerebriform lymphoid atypia; the density of infiltration is low to intermediate. The lesion is clinically detectable but not indurated. In plaque-stage MF, Pautrier microabscesses are common. The density of infiltration in the superficial dermis is dense and accompanied by laminated pattern of sclerosis. The constellation of these findings would translate clinically into an infiltrative plaque. In tumor-stage MF, a tumefactive infiltrate of neoplastic lymphocytes develops and may no longer be epidermotropic. There are certain variants of MF such as granulomatous and follicular MF in which there is a greater propensity for this pattern of progressive dermal and subcutaneous infiltration to occur. In most instances of tumor-stage MF, the cells are large blastic-appearing tumor cells; however, small cell variants of tumor-stage MF exist. The diagnosis of tumor-stage MF rests on clinical exam showing palpable tumor nodules while histologically one observes a dense nodular and/or diffuse lymphocytic infiltrate. The cytomorphologic composition *per se* is not a specific determinant in rendering a diagnosis of tumor-stage MF.

As already alluded to, the cells of MF have a characteristic cerebriform cytomorphology. The extent of cytologic atypia intrinsic to MF requires examination under oil. The cells within the epidermis are more atypical than those cells within the dermis. Collections of cerebriform cells within the epidermis would be the characteristic hallmarks of a Pautrier microabscess (92). Langerhans cells are present and are intimately apposed to cerebriform lymphocytes although the cerebriform atypical lymphocytes exceed the extent of Langerhans cell hyperplasia. Unlike a spongiotic microvesicle of eczema, the neoplastic cellular collection defined by the Pautrier microabscess is typically found adjacent to areas of basilar colonization, assuming a parabasilar distribution. Basilar colonization without true destructive interface dermatitis is also a common finding; the lymphocytes assume an almost perfect alignment along the dermal epidermal junction. The foci of basilar colonization can be small and discontinuous (92). In areas of dermal infiltration, there may be laminated dermal fibroplasia. Papillary dermal edema, basilar vacuolar alterations, and eosinophilic spongiosis are exceptional findings and would be more commonly seen in the realm of a hypersensitivity reaction (93,94).

Phenotypic Profile

The lymphoid cells are CD3+/CD4+/CD45 RO+; a few of the larger atypical cells can be CD30+. Only rarely is a naive CD5 RA phenotype observed. There is a reduction in the expression of certain pan T-cell markers, most commonly CD7 and CD62L (95,96) (Fig. 29.15C and D). In many cases, the extent of reduction for CD7 and CD62L is in the realm of 90% amidst lymphocytes within the epidermal compartment compared to lymphocytes in the dermis where the reduction is significantly less, typically more in the range of 50% (96). This likely reflects the greater admixture of reactive lymphocytes in the dermal infiltrate compared to the intraepidermal lymphoid populace. Specifically in any given lesion of MF, there are many reactive cells representing regulatory T cells and benign cytotoxic CD8 T cells. At times the cytologic and phenotypic aberration may only be apparent in the intraepidermal lymphocytes.

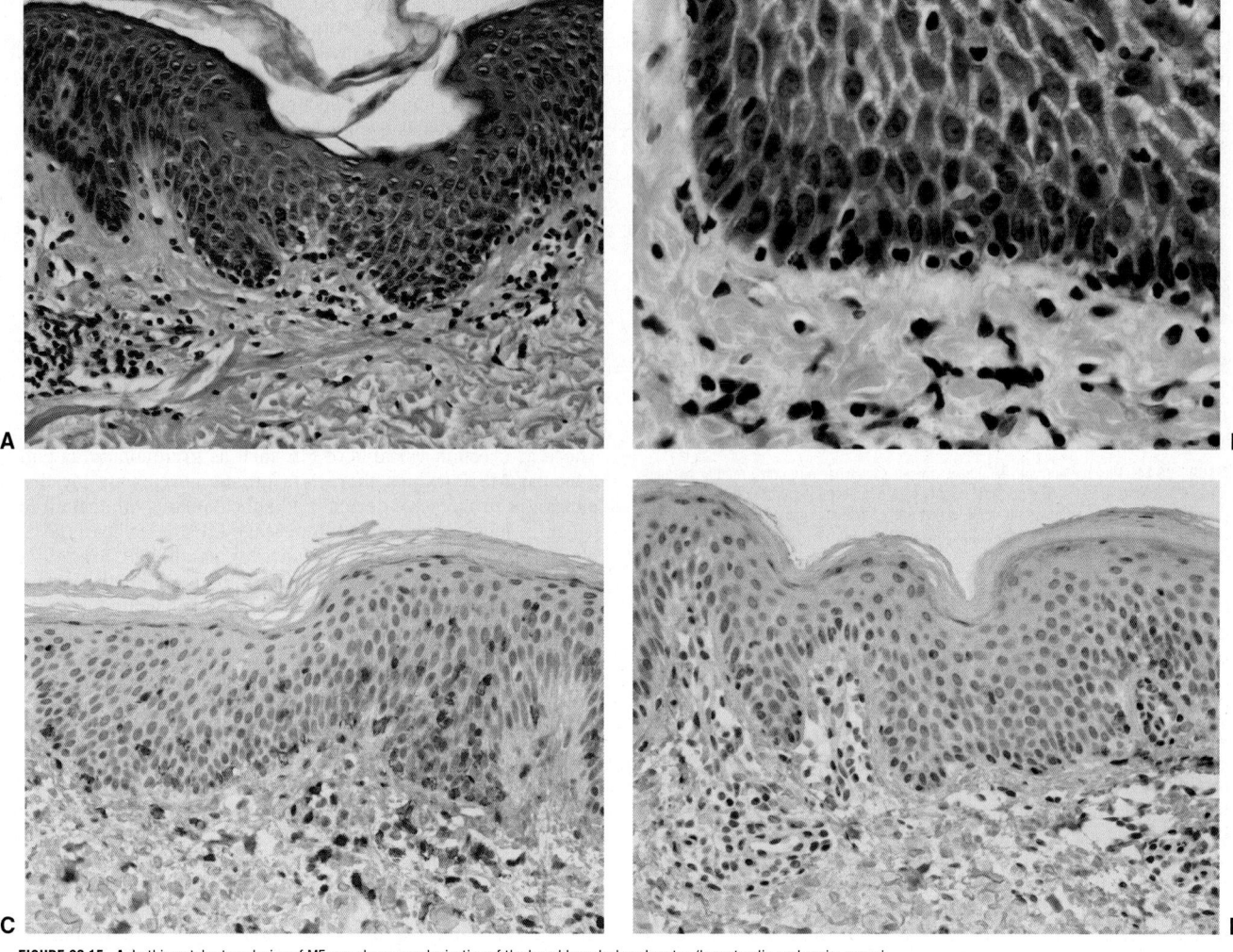

FIGURE 29.15. A: In this patch-stage lesion of MF, one observes colonization of the basal layer by lymphocytes (hematoxylin and eosin, magnification: 400×). **B:** The pattern of lymphocyte migration into the epidermis is a passive one. While there is lymphocyte apposition to basal layer keratinocytes, significant destructive epithelial changes are not seen (hematoxylin and eosin, magnification: 1,000×). **C:** In this CD2 stain, one can see a number of intraepidermal and dermal lymphocytes that are highlighted by CD2. Note the number of lymphocytes colonizing the basal layer of the epidermis (diaminobenzidine, magnification: 400×). **D:** In contrast, the CD7 preparation shows a marked reduction positivity. There is minimal staining of lymphocytes within the epidermis and dermis. The reduction is in the realm of 90% and is a highly characteristic finding in MF (diaminobenzidine, magnification: 400×).

Any persistent inflammatory condition can be accompanied by a mild to moderate reduction in CD7. Furthermore, significant reductions of CD7 can be observed in the drug-associated reversible T-cell dyscrasias and in the prelymphomatous T-cell dyscrasias. Hence, the significance of a CD7 reduction should be correlated with other aspects of the biopsy and clinical presentation. The same pattern of reduction can be observed with CD62L in the nonneoplastic setting. In contrast, a diminution in the expression of CD5 and CD3 would point toward a diagnosis of T-cell lymphoma (95,97).

CD103 (i.e., alpha E beta 7 integrin), the epithelium lymphocyte homing receptor, is expressed on epidermotropic lymphocytes and to a lesser extent on dermal infiltrating cells. CD103 is noted in early stages of the disease (i.e., patch- and plaque-stage MF) while the loss of this marker is associated with disease progression. In tumor-stage MF, the neoplastic lymphocytes may acquire a cytotoxic phenotype characterized by positivity for granzyme, TIA, and perforin (98,99). There may also be a marked reduction in the number of regulatory T cells in the infiltrate. CD26 is characteristically diminished in neoplastic T cells found within the skin but also circulating in the peripheral blood in patients with SS. CD26 is a dipeptidyl peptidase IV that is expressed on normal T cells (100).

Molecular Studies

Molecular studies in early lesions of MF may be negative, reflecting the low density of the neoplastic infiltrate. One study examined T-cell rearrangement by polymerase chain reaction and denaturing gradient gel electrophoresis in archival specimens of patients with CTCL and found an overall positivity rate of 75% (101). PCR is preferred over Southern blot because of greater sensitivity. Specifically, clonality is detected in 59% of cases CTCL examined by Southern blot analysis while it is present in over 75% of cases by PCR (102).

Tax and/or Pol have been detected in 30% to 90% of patients in the United states with MF; however, none of these patients has PCR positivity with respect to HTLV-1-associated proteins (103).

Pathogenesis

MF typically develops in the background of a precursor T-cell dyscrasia such as PPD, pityriasis lichen ides, and parapsoriasis. The evolution to fully evolved CTCL is revealed by commonality of T-cell clones between the precursor lesions and overt MF (89). As well, MF may arise in a setting of chronic antigen stimulation with features of eczematous dermatitis. I have seen cases of long-standing atopic dermatitis evolve into MF. It is also likely that drug-associated reversible T-cell dyscrasia could eventuate in a state of endogenous irreversible T-cell dyscrasia especially in those cases of drug-associated reversible T-cell dyscrasia where clonality is identified.

As mentioned above, the implicated neoplastic cell is most commonly of the CD4 subset. In the earlier phases of the illness a TH1-dominant cytokine profile is observed; however, with disease progression, the cells may elaborate interleukin 10, interleukin 5, and interleukin 6, all of which define a Th2 cytokine milieu (104–106). The result of this altered skewed cytokine milieu is one associated with depletion of critical immune cells including CD8 cells, NK/T cells, and dendritic cells. This leads to a relative state of immunosuppression resulting in tumor progression and the development of secondary malignancies, rendering the host susceptible to infection especially from viruses. In the initial phases of the disease, the neoplastic lymphocytes are heavily dependent on the epidermal milieu for sustained growth and proliferation. This reflects the interplay between CCL17 and CCL27 on the neoplastic cells with their natural ligands being that of CXCR4 and CXCR10 expressed on keratinocytes. In addition, Langerhans cells are an important source of interleukin 15 that encourages and sustains neoplastic T-cell growth. Finally, intraepidermal Langerhans cells present apoptotic antigen fragments derived from dead neoplastic T cells to viable intraepidermal resident neoplastic T cells, providing a stimulus for further clonal expansion (107,108).

The counterregulatory T cells are important for controlling tumor progression. The main reactive T cells that have antitumor effects are regulatory CD4+CD25+ T cells and cytotoxic CD8 T cells. With transformation into tumor-stage MF, diminished regulatory T-cell and CD8 infiltration is seen. The acquisition of cytotoxic properties by the transformed tumor cells as revealed by variable staining for perforin and granzyme may contribute to the diminished local reservoir of regulatory CD4 and CD8 T cells. MF remains an indolent disease as long as the intraepidermal growth dependency and preservation of counterregulatory T cells are maintained.

Prognostic Variables

A recent study analyzed 1,502 patients with MF. The study demonstrated specific clinical and pathologic features, which significantly influence patient survival. Disease progression was observed in 34% of cases while patients died of MF in 26% of cases. In patients with early limited patch-stage MF, there was no overall difference in survival compared to the general population.

Factors adversely affecting outcome included increasing age, male sex, increased lactate dehydrogenase levels, and large cell transformation (109). Folliculotropic variants were also associated with an increased risk for disease progression. An important predictor of poor survival and increased risk for disease progression included the presence of a peripheral blood T-cell clone identical to that identified in the skin. The extent of peripheral blood involvement is also an important factor with Sezary counts of more than 10,000/µL correlating with a worse outcome (109). Improved survival was observed in the setting of poikilodermatous MF and hypopigmented MF (109).

MORPHOLOGIC VARIANTS OF MYCOSIS FUNGOIDES

The main morphologic variants of MF considered in the EORTC-WHO classification scheme include MF exhibiting a predilection to involve the hair follicles and eccrine apparatus. There is also a diffuse interstitial granulomatous form of MF and finally Woringer-Kolopp disease (25). Less common additional variants, although not considered separately in the EORTC-WHO classification scheme, are vesicular, lichenoid, pustular, and hypopigmented MF.

Adnexaltropic Mycosis Fungoides

Recently, a variant of MF has been described that manifests dominant tropism of lymphocytes to adnexal structures. One falls under the designation of follicular MF/pilotropic MF while the other has been described under the term of syringotropic CTCL.

In pilotropic/follicular MF, the patient presents with clinical lesions suggestive of a pilotropic process including the presence of dissecting cellulitis (110), follicular papules, comedones, and cysts (Figs. 29.16 and 29.17). The follicular-based lesions precede, develop concurrently, or occur subsequent to lesions more typical of MF (111). Two closely related pilotropic T-cell dyscrasias fall under the designation of folliculotropic T-cell lymphocytosis and alopecia mucinosis and can presage follicular MF; they have been discussed in a different section of this chapter. The follicular variant of MF is an independent predictor of disease progression and overall reduced patient survival (111). In one recent study, the overall survival rates were 96% and 62%, respectively, with a 3.2:1.0 predominance of males over females (112). Another study suggests a clinical

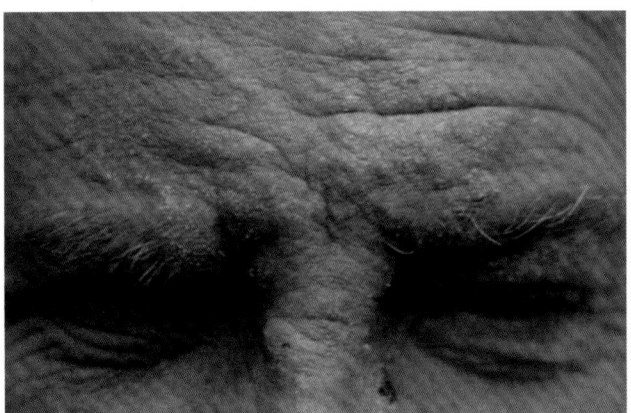
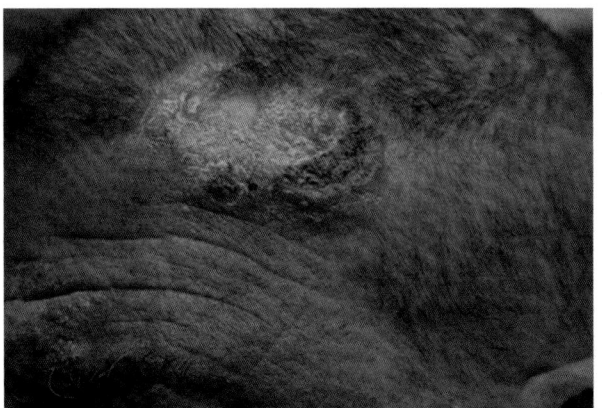

FIGURE 29.16. A,B: Follicular MF represents a distinct clinical variant of MF characterized by infiltrative indurated plaques with a predilection to involve the head and neck area due to the sequel of the follicle infiltration by neoplastic lymphocytes. Follicular dilatation with comedones as well as hair loss are among the more common features that one observes clinically. As well there is a higher incidence of tumor-stage transformation. Tumor-stage lesions will exhibit an infiltrative nodular and ulcerating quality. (Photos courtesy of Dr. Michael K. Jacobs, Skin Pathology Associates Inc., Birmingham, AL.) Follicular MF has a worse prognosis than conventional MF reflective of a greater tendency toward large cell transformation and the development of tumor stage MF.

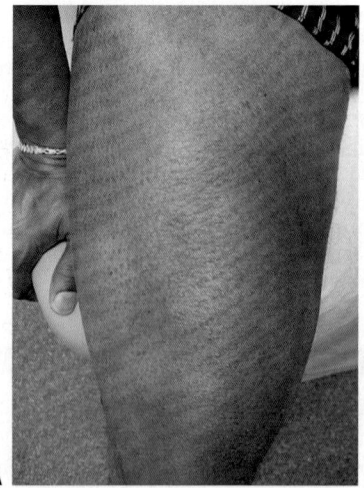

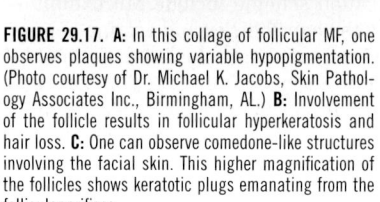

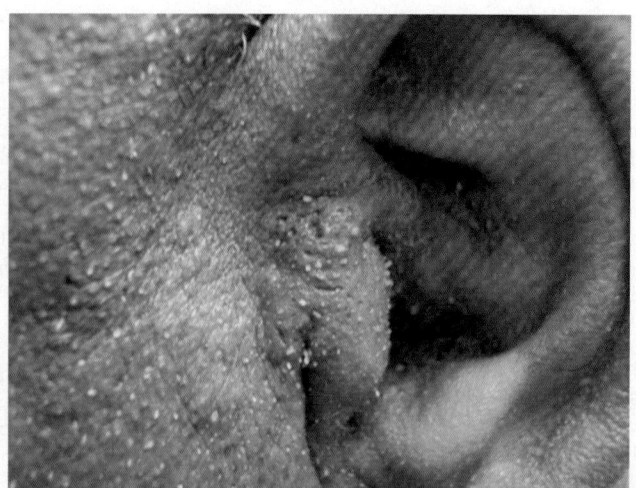

FIGURE 29.17. A: In this collage of follicular MF, one observes plaques showing variable hypopigmentation. (Photo courtesy of Dr. Michael K. Jacobs, Skin Pathology Associates Inc., Birmingham, AL.) **B:** Involvement of the follicle results in follicular hyperkeratosis and hair loss. **C:** One can observe comedone-like structures involving the facial skin. This higher magnification of the follicles shows keratotic plugs emanating from the follicular orifices.

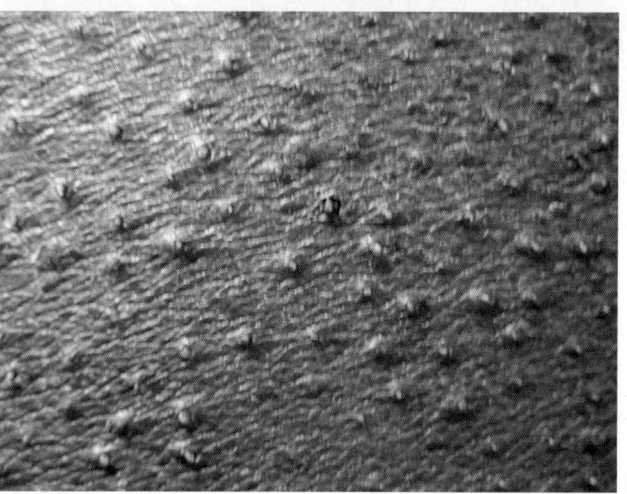

course that is more indolent. However, some cases categorized as follicular MF may represent a prelymphomatous T-cell dyscrasia, namely, alopecia mucinosis and/or folliculotropic T-cell lymphocytosis, which does exhibit a very benign course. Intense pruritus is a characteristic feature, and as well hair loss was among the most common symptoms; in some patients mucinous material can be expressed from the ostium of the follicle consistent with mucorrhea (112). Syringotropic MF is oftentimes accompanied by follicular involvement. The classic presentation is less dramatic than follicular MF. A large anhidrotic alopecic plaque is typical; in other cases, concomitant lesions of conventional MF may be observed (113).

Pathology

Histologic features include the presence of mononuclear cell infiltrates in close apposition to the outer root sheath epithelium with permeation of the wall by lymphocytes. There may be concomitant attenuation of the outer root sheath epithelium and follicular plugging (Fig. 29.18). The follicular hyperkeratosis can be striking. In regressed lesions, the morphology may resemble a comedone. Another cardinal hallmark is an unusual complex hyperplasia of the follicular epithelium reminiscent of that seen in a basaloid follicular hamartoma. As well, conspicuous follicular mucinosis can be observed. It is very characteristic for the infiltrate to extend deep to involve the lower third of the follicle. Tissue eosinophilia can be striking (112). The cytomorphology of the lymphocytes includes small and intermediate-sized cerebriform lymphocytes but it is also common

to see larger atypical transformed elements. The larger cells are frequently found in an extrafollicular disposition with significant extension into the interstitium. Some degree of interfollicular epidermotropism may be observed. Careful assessment of the interfollicular compartment reveals low-density haphazard infiltration of the epidermis by atypical lymphocytes in a fashion reminiscent of an early T-cell dyscrasia (111) (Fig. 29.19). An aberrant phenotype similar to that of classic MF is observed in follicular MF. Not every case of follicular MF exhibits follicular mucinosis (Fig. 29.20A–D). In many cases there will be concomitant interfollicular epidermotropism resembling conventional MF. In syringotropic MF, a striking epithelial response occurs and defines the entity of syringometaplasia resulting in a morphologic appearance resembling the lymphoepithelial lesion of Sjögren syndrome.

Differential Diagnosis

The differential diagnosis encompasses folliculotropic T-cell lymphocytosis and alopecia mucinosis. In brief, from a clinical perspective in neither of these prelymphomatous T-cell dyscrasias is the clinical extent of the lesions that typify follicular MF observed. The nodularity and extensive plaque-like infiltrates involving the head and neck are not seen. From a light microscopic perspective, the degree of lymphoid atypia is less. In folliculotropic T-cell lymphocytosis, the infiltrate is more superficial, largely confined to the superficial and midisthmic part of the follicle. The oftentimes striking polymorphous inflammatory cell infiltrate seen in follicular MF is not seen.

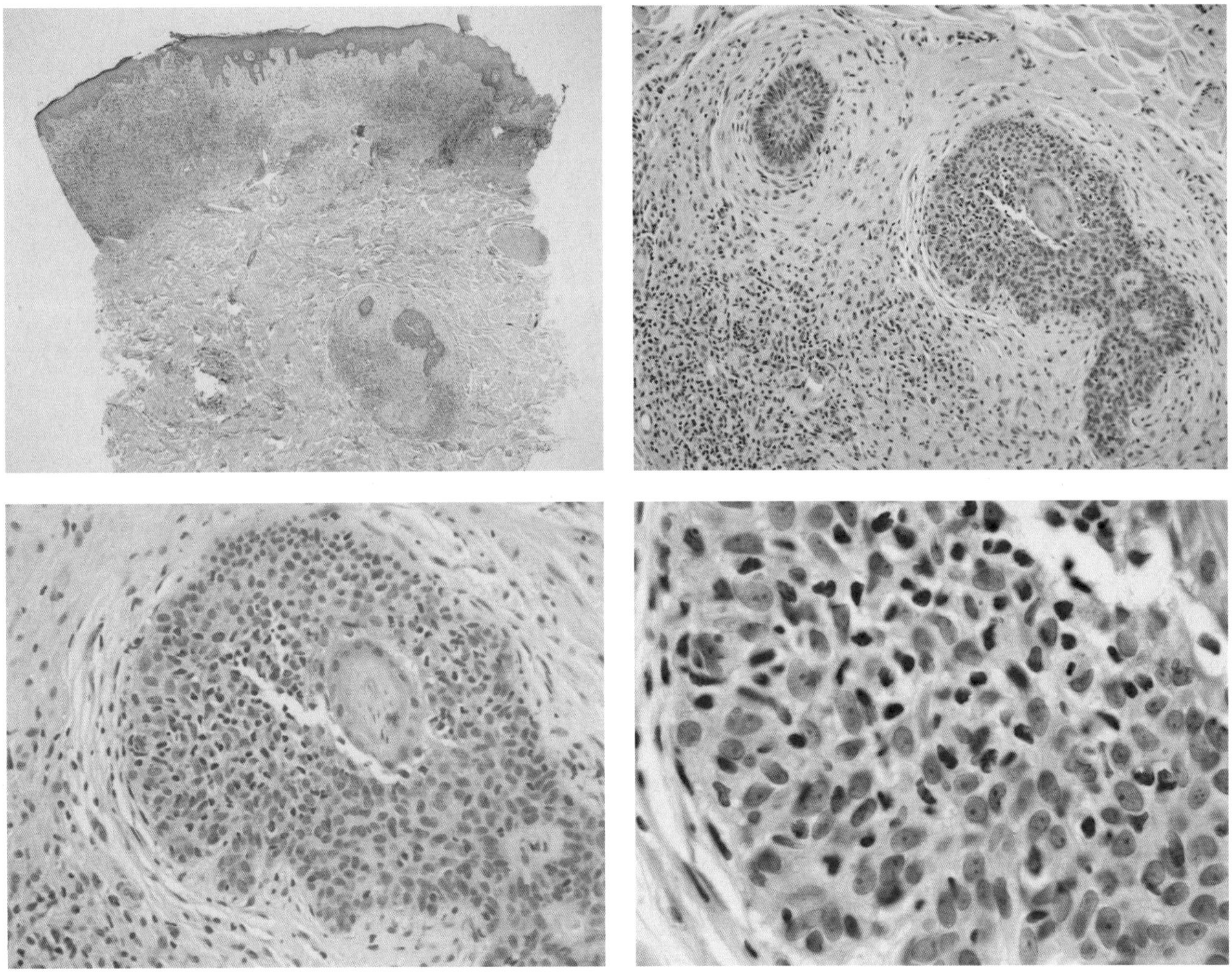

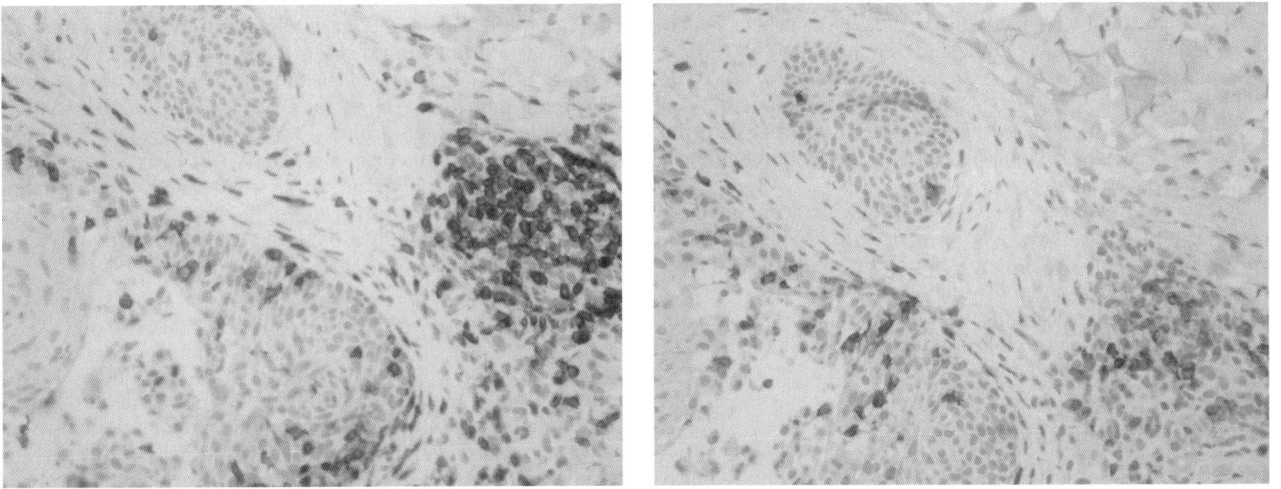

FIGURE 29.18. **A:** More superficially the process resembles plaque-stage MF with a dense bandlike lymphocytic infiltrate lying in apposition to the epidermis (hematoxylin and eosin, magnification: 40×). **B:** One observes significant follicular involvement with infiltration of the adventitial dermis and outer root sheath epithelium by atypical cerebriform lymphocytes (hematoxylin and eosin, magnification: 200×). **C:** The pattern of lymphocyte migration into the outer root sheath epithelium is a passive one unaccompanied by significant destructive epithelial changes (hematoxylin and eosin, magnification: 400×). **D:** Higher power magnification shows the atypical morphology of the lymphocytes. The lymphocytes appear angulated and hyperchromatic (hematoxylin and eosin, magnification: 1,000×).

FIGURE 29.19. **A:** The lymphocytes infiltrating the follicle are highlighted by CD3 (diaminobenzidine, magnification: 400×). **B:** One can see a significant reduction in the expression of CD7 compared to CD3, an important clue regarding categorization as a form of pilotropic T cell dyscrasia (diaminobenzidine, magnification: 400×).

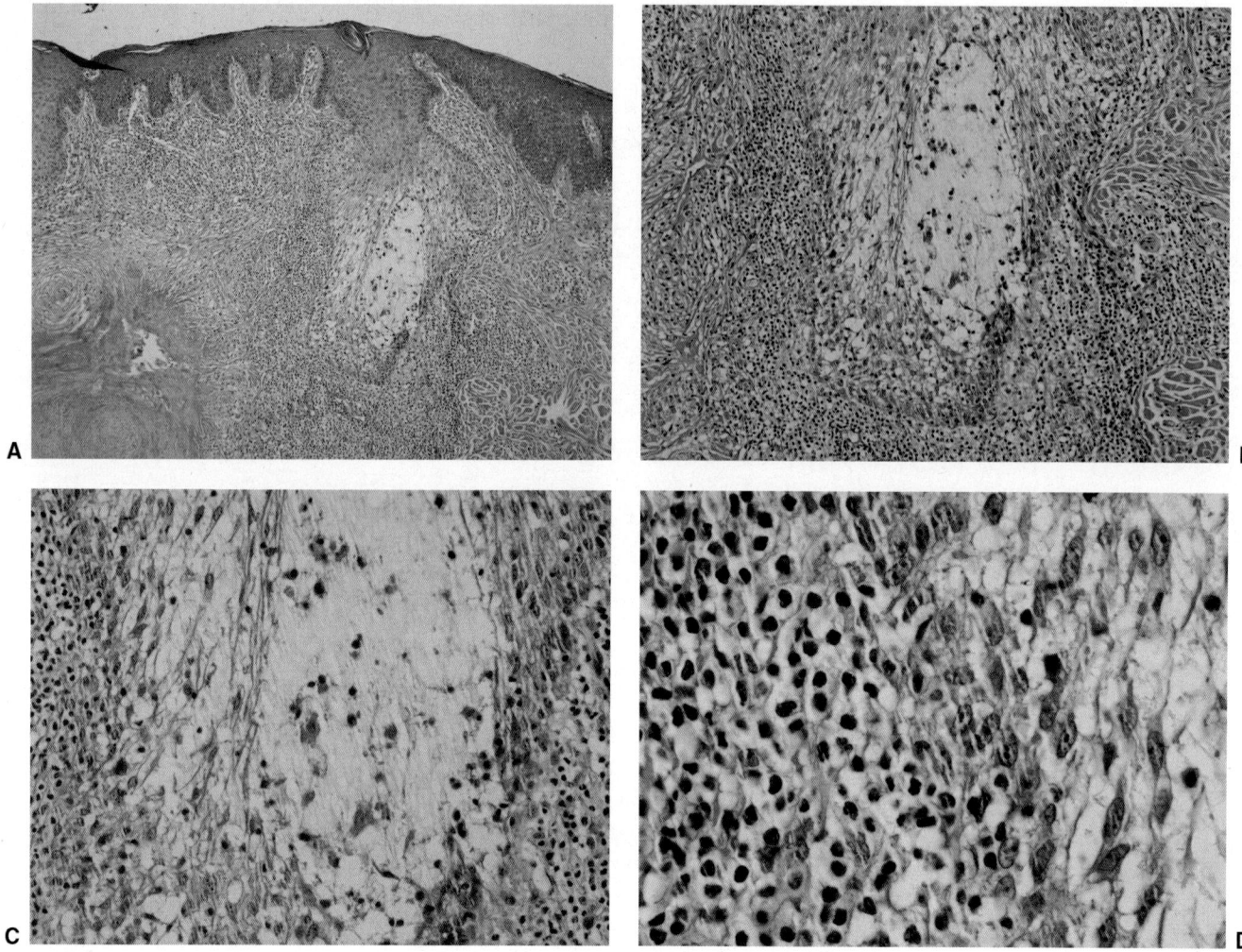

FIGURE 29.20. A: Follicular mucinosis can be seen in follicular MF but is not a *sine qua non* of follicular MF and can be seen in the precursor prelymphomatous pilotropic T-cell dyscrasia designated alopecia mucinosis but also in other reactive settings such as discoid lupus erythematosus and eczema although uncommonly. In this figure, one observes very striking follicular mucinosis with a dense lymphocytic infiltrate within and around the follicle. In addition, there is a necrotizing palisading granulomatous response noted adjacent to the involved follicle (hematoxylin and eosin, magnification: 100×). **B:** Higher power magnification shows the prominent mucin deposition within the follicle. The intrafollicular mononuclear cells comprise atypical lymphocytes as well as Langerhans cells (hematoxylin and eosin, magnification: 200×). **C:** Higher power magnification shows the many atypical cerebriform lymphocytes and Langerhans cells with concomitant mucin deposition (hematoxylin and eosin, magnification: 400×). **D:** This higher power magnification shows splaying of the follicular keratinocytes by mucin and as well highlights the atypical hyperconvoluted nature of the lymphocytes within and around the follicle (hematoxylin and eosin, magnification: 1,000×).

In syringotropic MF, one of the cardinal hallmarks is hyperplasia of the eccrine ducts and glands somewhat similar to the hyperplasia that accompanies follicular variants of MF. The term syringometaplasia has been applied to this epithelial response. The pattern of epitheliotropism in concert with the marked hyperplastic response resembles the lymphoepithelial lesions of Sjögren syndrome.

We have previously reported on folliculotropic atypical lymphocytic infiltrates as a form of drug-associated pseudolymphoma. As well, prominent lymphocytic infiltrates can infiltrate the follicular outer root sheath epithelium in the setting of Jessner lymphocytic infiltrate of skin, nonscarring discoid lupus erythematosus, and follicular eczema, and hence any of these disorders may be confused with MF (5).

Woringer-Kolopp Disease

Woringer-Kolopp disease also falls under the alternative designations of unilesional MF and pagetoid reticulosis (93,114–116). It is a unique form of CTCL with an unusual predilection to involve acral sites, most commonly the finger, wrist, and knee. However, other reported sites include the thigh and

buttocks. It is considered an indolent form of CTCL. A disseminated variant falls under the designation of Ketron-Goodman variant of pagetoid reticulosis (117). However, many of these cases are thought to represent an aggressive form of CTCL in the context of either primary cutaneous aggressive cytotoxic CD8 T-cell lymphoma or gamma delta T-cell lymphoma. Unilesional Woringer-Kolopp disease is treated with local radiation (118). It has been reported in young children (119). A spider bite has been isolated as a potential trigger in certain cases of Woringer-Kolopp disease (115,120).

Light Microscopic Findings

There is striking epitheliotropism whereby the dominant localization of the neoplastic infiltrate is within the epidermis with a minimal dermal infiltrate. The infiltrate tends to involve the lower two-thirds of the epidermis. The epitheliotropism is relatively confluent without any evidence of directed migration typical for a reactive lymphomatoid process. The main epidermal response is hyperplasia (121). There is a disparity between the marked extent of epithelotropism and a lesser degree of dermal inflammation.

Phenotypic Profile

The profile does not differ from that seen in more common forms of MF. The neoplastic cell is typically of the CD4 subset. The uncommon subsets that express CD8 or are double negative do not differ prognostically from the more common CD4 variant and should not be equated with primary cutaneous aggressive cytotoxic CD8⁺ T-cell lymphoma.

Differential Diagnosis

As mentioned, primary cutaneous aggressive cytotoxic CD8-positive T-cell lymphoma is an important diagnostic consideration in cases showing a CD8⁺ phenotype. However, in the setting of this aggressive form of cutaneous lymphoma, the onset is abrupt, presenting as multiple nodules. Light microscopically angioinvasion with secondary ischemic sequelae is characteristic. Phenotypically, the cells in primary cutaneous aggressive cytotoxic CD8-positive T-cell lymphoma exhibit a CD45 RA phenotype. Another important consideration diagnostically is a lymphomatoid drug reaction/drug-associated reversible T-cell dyscrasia. Such lesions can present as a solitary lesion comprising superficially disposed cerebriform lymphocytes with epitheliotropism (115). However, localization to acral surfaces would be uncommon. As well, a significant component of the infiltrate is found within the dermis in the context of a lichenoid reaction.

In the same vein, benign lichenoid keratoses can exhibit lymphoid atypia; however, the nonacral localization along with the dominant localization of the infiltrate to involve the dermis with attendant destructive epithelial changes defines a constellation of findings that allows easy distinction.

Granulomatous Mycosis Fungoides

Granulomatous MF represents a distinct subtype of MF exhibiting a diffuse pattern of dermal infiltration comprising neoplastic lymphocytes and histiocytes whereby histiocytes represent at least 30% of the infiltrate. In the majority of cases, the presentation does not differ from classic plaque-stage MF. The lesions are large violaceous plaques with a predilection to involve photoprotected areas. In this variant of MF, there is accentuation in the intertriginous areas and as well involving the posterior aspect of the arm and thigh (Fig. 29.21A and B). In one study, the majority of patients were male and the average time of onset was in the sixth decade (122). The lesions had been present for several years before the correct diagnosis was made. There is a unique variant of interstitial granulomatous MF associated with extensive elastolysis involvement of the intertriginous areas manifesting as pendulous skin folds; it is indolent without the biologic progression seen in conventional granulomatous MF. This variant is designated granulomatous slack skin. An important differential diagnosis of granulomatous

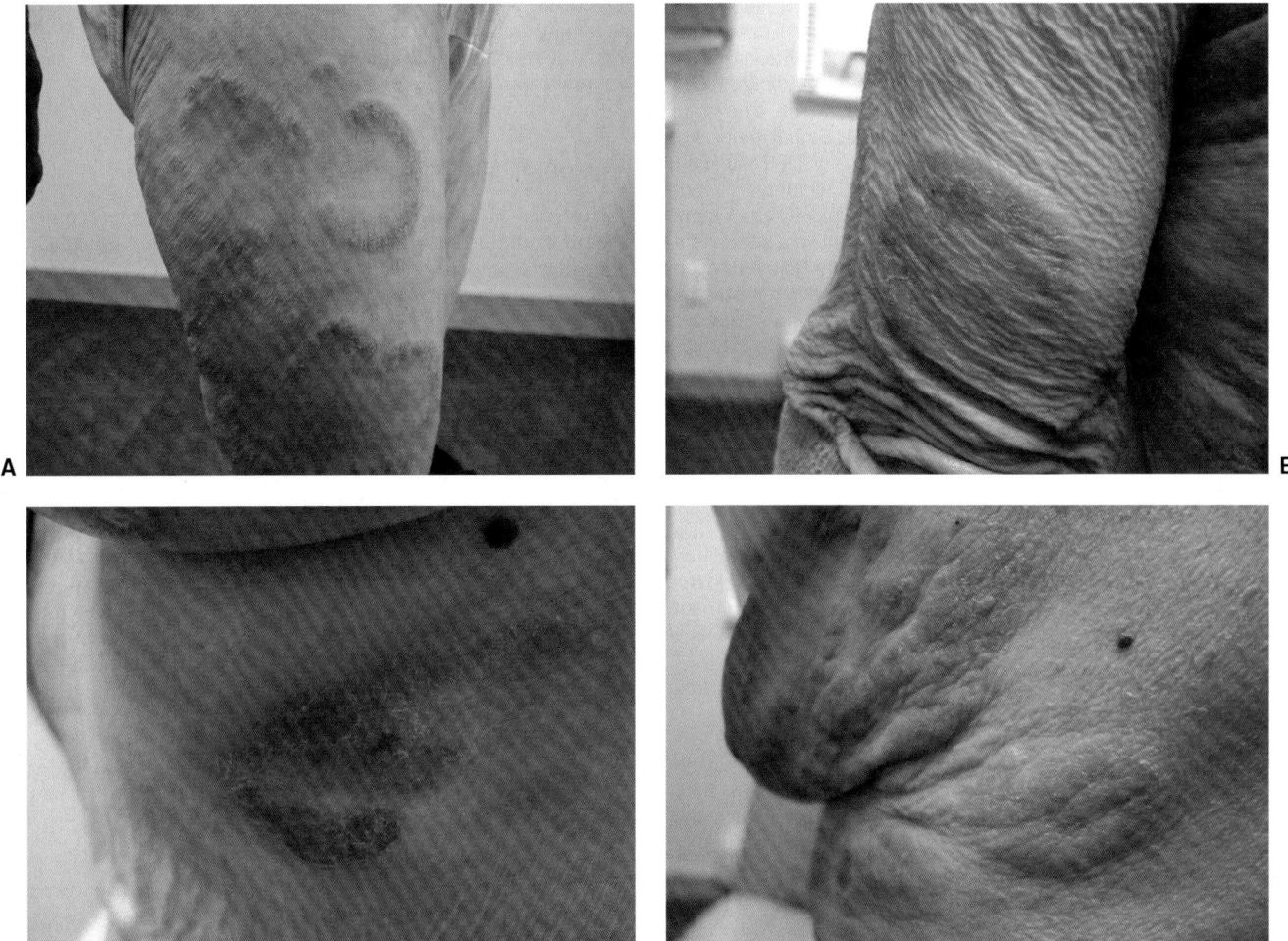

FIGURE 29.21. A: In this case of granulomatous MF, one sees very striking annular plaques reminiscent of granuloma annulare. Granulomatous MF show an unusual predilection to involve intertriginous areas as well as the thigh. **B:** The raised infiltrative quality of the annular plaques differentiates the lesions from granuloma annulare. **C:** The patient has progressive disease with ensuing areas of raised plaques and nodules. **D:** There is the residuum of annular lesions typical of granulomatous MF; a supervening tumorous nodular component is observed. (Photos courtesy of Dr. Ty Hanson, Aberdeen Dermatology Associates, Aberdeen, SD.)

MF is the interstitial granulomatous drug reaction (123,124). In cases of drug-based etiology the clinical presentation, phenotypic profile, and molecular studies may closely resemble those of classic interstitial granulomatous MF, and hence they have been referred to as drug-associated reversible granulomatous T-cell dyscrasia (Fig. 29.21A–C) (124). One potential variation phenotypically is in the dominance of CD8 lymphocytes in the epidermis in the setting of drug-associated reversible granulomatous T-cell dyscrasia (Fig. 29.21D). In addition, peripheral blood assessment may disclose a reduction in the CD4 to CD8 ratio potentially reflective of a relative peripheral blood CD8+ lymphocytosis. It has been suggested that the clinical course in granulomatous MF is more indolent albeit due to the depth of the infiltrate the process may be more refractory to topical therapies and hence the natural course is one of slow biologic progression (Fig. 29.21C and D) (125). Cases of MF resembling granulomatous MF but where the histiocytes are less than 30% of the infiltrate fall under the designation of interstitial MF. Interstitial MF follows an indolent course without the insidious biologic progression of classic granulomatous MF.

Light Microscopic Findings

Granulomatous MF does share in common with other forms of MF epitheliotropism of atypical lymphocytes; however, the degree of epitheliotropism is typically less. The dominant infiltrate is found within the superficial and deep dermis. Lymphocytes may dominate within the dermis, however, at least 30% of the infiltrate is histiocytic in nature; the pattern of infiltration is one characterized by scaffolding of mononuclear cells of lymphocytic and histiocytic derivation along collagen and elastic fibers (125). Variable adnexal tropism is seen. The giant cells are frequently bizarre with many nuclei. Emperipolesis of lymphocytes by multinucleated histiocytes is a characteristic finding. There can be other inflammatory cell elements including eosinophils and plasma cells although typically the extent of tissue eosinophilia is not prominent. One does not see vasculitis nor are there zones of complete collagen necrobiosis typical of granuloma annulare; neutrophils would be exceptional. Sarcoidal granulomas and foci of lichenoid and granulomatous inflammation can be seen. In rare cases there may be a supervening sclerosing reaction reminiscent of morphea. Under oil examination, the cerebriform nature of the abnormal lymphocyte is apparent.

Phenotypic Profile

There is a dominance of CD4 T cells over those of the CD8 subset. The apparent CD4 to CD8 ratio is very high reflecting not only the dominant CD4+ lymphocyte population but also the concomitant positivity amid histiocytes, an integral component of the background infiltrates in granulomatous MF. There is a reduction in the expression of CD7 that can be significant (i.e., potentially in excess of 70%), and as well there is a marked diminution in the expression of CD62L typically in excess of 90%. A similar decrement in staining is noted within the epidermis. Comparing the intraepidermal and dermal compartments for CD7 and CD62L must be done in conjunction with the other pan T-cell markers CD3 and CD2. There may be some diminution in CD5 as well although not typically of the quantity seen with CD7 and CD62L. A Th1 cytokine profile dominates. Neoplastic T cells express CCR4 and CXCR3 (126).

As mentioned, the phenotypic profile in the setting of the interstitial granulomatous drug reaction can resemble that seen in interstitial granulomatous MF. The cells may show significant phenotypic abnormalities by virtue of the extent of diminution in the expression of the pan-T-cell markers CD7 and CD62L amidst atypical lymphocytes in the epidermis and dermis. Finally, we have identified T-cell clonality in this unique form of drug reaction (124).

Papular Mycosis Fungoides

There is a very rare variant of MF characterized by a generalized disseminated papular eruption. The individual lesions appear very monomorphic and raise diagnostic consideration in regard to disseminated lichen nitidus.

Light Microscopic Findings

There is an area of epitheliotropism of cerebriform lymphocytes. It is a circumscribed discrete focus whereby there is an unusual predilection for the epitheliotropic lymphocytic infiltrate to involve the hair follicle and/or acrosyringium. There may be a paucity of other inflammatory cell elements. The phenotypic profile is not different from that of conventional MF. In particular most commonly there is a dominant infiltrate of CD4+ T cells that exhibit a characteristic reduction in the expression of CD7, CD5, and CD62L; some reduction can be seen in CD5 (127).

Lichenoid Mycosis Fungoides

Lichenoid MF exhibits clinical features typical for MF and not lichen planus. Histologically, there are areas of destructive interface dermatitis resembling lichen planus; however, the granular cell layer is diminished and there is parakeratosis. More importantly are foci of passive epitheliotropism of atypical cerebriform lymphocytes juxtaposed to the zones of destructive lichenoid inflammation. It may occur more frequently in African American patients and can be associated with leukoderma. In addition, it has been suggested that this variant of MF may follow a more aggressive clinical course (128).

Vesicular Mycosis Fungoides

In vesicular MF, the apparent spongiotic vesicles contain mucin defining an intraepidermal equivalent reaction to follicular mucinosis, and as well there is basilar colonization, which would be unusual for a reactive eczematous process (129).

Purpuric Mycosis Fungoides

MF can arise in a background of PPD. When this occurs, there is typically prominent accompanying red cell extravasation along with hemosiderin deposition (Fig. 29.14). It is unusual for purpuric MF to occur in the absence of prior PPD, one of the prototypic prelymphomatous T-cell dyscrasias. The question arises regarding the distinction of purpuric MF from its precursor state, namely, PPD. Perhaps the most critical distinguishing feature is the extent of the eruption clinically. In classic purpuric MF, the lesions are large plaques that involve the upper legs, buttocks, and trunks. Upper extremity involvement is also seen. Since epitheliotropism, cerebriform atypia, loss of pan T-cell markers and clonality can be seen in PPD, it is important to correlate the morphologic findings with the clinical presentation (130,131).

UNUSUAL PHENOTYPIC VARIANTS OF MYCOSIS FUNGOIDES

A number of unusual phenotypic profiles can be observed in the setting of MF, none of which has any prognostic impact. These less common profiles include CD8+ MF, double-negative MF, a variant of MF that shows a naive phenotype by virtue of CD45 RA positivity, and a form of MF derived from gamma delta T cells. These variants can resemble more traditional MF although CD8 forms of MF can be hypopigmented due to the destruction of melanocytes by cytotoxic CD8 lymphocytes.

There are many faces of double-negative MF including ichthyotic MF and hypopigmented MF. Pigmented purpuric MF can also be double-negative (132–134). In the study by Fierro et al. (135), 8.7% of cases of MF showed intraepidermal CD45RA+ lymphocytes. It has been hypothesized that CD45 RO+ memory T cells can revert to a CD45 RA phenotype, a so-called memory revertant that does not require constant antigen stimulation.

Sezary Syndrome

Historically, SS) is an aggressive form of CTCL characterized by the triad of erythroderma, generalized lymphadenopathy, and the presence of neoplastic cerebriform T cells in the skin, lymph nodes, and peripheral blood. The hematologic criteria for diagnosis of SS described by the International Society for Cutaneous Lymphoma include T-cell clonality and two or more of an absolute Sézary cell count of 2292/μL (with minimal diagnostic cutoff being >1,000/μL), a high CD4 to CD8 ratio in excess of 10:1, a loss of the pan T-cell marker CD7, and/or CD26 in a subset of circulating T cells (136). It is a rare form of malignancy accounting for only 2.5% of all CTCLs (137). There are two main variants of SS: *de novo* SS and SS arising in a background of either MF or idiopathic erythroderma. The latter (i.e., idiopathic erythroderma) may be difficult to distinguish from primary *de novo* SS. The main differentiating point is the lack of sufficient diagnostic peripheral blood criteria to warrant categorization as SS.

The extent of peripheral blood involvement has been stratified into B0, B1, and B2 by the presence or absence of circulating Sezary cells. B0 and B1 are then subcategorized as *a* or *b* according to the molecular detection of a T-cell clone. In order to be designated as the B2 stage, detection of a T-cell clone either by PCR or by Southern blot analysis is required in addition to high tumor burden (≥1,000/μL of Sezary cells) (138).

Light Microscopic Findings

The diagnosis can be very difficult to make. In many cases only a psoriasiform epidermal hyperplasia unaccompanied by significant lymphocytic epitheliotropism is observed. Due to the pruritic nature of the eruption the morphology will be further obscured by impetiginization resulting in neutrophil-imbued parakeratosis. A common pattern is one characterized by eczematous changes and a prominent angiocentric lymphomatoid vascular reaction. The adjectival modifier of lymphomatoid denotes the atypical nature of the lymphocytes surrounding the blood vessels. There may be a disparity between the extent of blood vessel infiltration and lack of epitheliotropism. Such cases serve to emphasize the critical role of peripheral blood assessment.

Phenotypic Profile

The malignant cells in SS are characterized as atypical skin-homing CD4+CD45RO+ T cells that lack certain pan T-cell markers including CD7, CD62L, CD5, and CD26. While the vast majority of MF and SS cases are of the CD4 subset, occasionally the neoplastic cells are CD8 positive (139). A T helper 1 (Th1) cytokine profile characterizes earlier phases of MF. In contrast, progressive disease in the setting of MF and SS is associated with a T helper 2 (Th2) cytokine profile with increased levels of IL-4, -5, -7, -10, and -18. A dysregulated Th2-dominant profile contributes to the poor prognosis associated with SS and advanced MF via multiple mechanisms (140). The chronic local overproduction of IL-4, -5, and -10 decreases recruitment of reactive CD8+ T cells, allowing tumor cells to evade the host antitumor immune response.

Pathogenesis/Pathophysiologic Considerations

The diminished Th1 cytokine production in the peripheral blood in patients with SS is associated with a decrease in IL-12 and IFN-γ, which causes a decline in myeloid and plasmacytoid dendritic cells, as well as CD56+ NK cells (133), contributing further to deterioration in both immune function against microbial organisms and host antitumor immunity. Therefore, SS patients have a high incidence of bacterial, herpetic, and secondary malignant processes leading to significant mortality and morbidity (141–143). Peripheral eosinophilia and high levels of IgE are independent markers for poor prognosis and disease progression reflective of another Th2 cytokine, namely, interleukin 5 (144). An additional hypothesis explaining the immunosuppression seen in advanced disease comes from *in vitro* findings that have shown that immature dendritic cells can induce Sézary cells to develop T-regulatory activity. The result of this conversion to a regulatory T-cell phenotype is one of diminution of CD8+ T-cell effector function against microbial pathogens and tumor cells (137,145,146).

CD30-POSITIVE LYMPHOPROLIFERATIVE DISORDERS

The classic CD30-positive lymphoproliferative disorders of the skin encompass LYP and ALCL. There are other lymphomas associated with CD30 expression best exemplified by CD30-positive large cell B-cell lymphoma and Hodgkin lymphoma; however, for purposes of this discussion, the primary focus is one of LYP and ALCL, the prototypic CD30-positive lymphoproliferative disorders of T-cell derivation. In one study that addressed the spectrum of all CD30-positive cutaneous lymphoproliferative lesions, ALCL, LYP including type C LYP/borderline CD30+ lymphoproliferative disease, non-Hodgkin B-cell lymphoma, and Hodgkin disease were represented by 45%, 33%, 19.8%, and 1% of all cases, respectively (147). In addition, lymphomatoid drug reactions frequently exhibit angiocentric CD30+ activated T cells, and as well specific lymphomatoid hypersensitivity reactions including persistent arthropod bite reactions and aberrant immunologic responses to viruses such as cutaneous herpes and molluscum contagiosum can mimic endogenous CD30+ lymphoproliferative disease (148).

The somewhat diverse spectrum of cutaneous lesions associated with CD30 expression reflects the nature of the CD30 molecule and the inherent diversity of cells that can express the molecule including the apparent expression of the molecule on mitotically active cells of monocytic, B-cell or T-cell lineage (149). It does not necessarily equate with a neoplastic event. A minority of reactive T or B lymphocytes and lymphocytes exposed to transforming viruses such as EBV and HTLV1 can exhibit CD30 positivity. It was first detected on Reed-Sternberg cells of Hodgkin disease but has since been observed in stimulated or transformed peripheral blood T or B cells, T-cell and B-cell lymphoma lines, and myeloid cell lines (150,151).

On paraffin-embedded tissue, an epitope of the CD30 molecule, which is preserved following formalin fixation, is detected with the BerH2 antibody. The Ki antibody detects a much greater proportion of the CD30 molecule on frozen tissue and hence is a more sensitive assay for assessing CD30 expression. Anti-Ki-1 was raised against a Hodgkin disease cell line in 1982 and subsequently shown to be expressed by the malignant cells in Hodgkin disease as well as by a small percentage of smaller lymphoid cells found in the parafollicular regions of normal lymph nodes. The Ki-1 antigen subsequently designated the CD30 cluster was identified as an activation antigen that could be expressed on T cells, B cells, and activated histiocytes (151). It is part of the growth factor tumor necrosis factor (TNF) family and the gene encoding the CD30 molecule is found on chromosome 1p36 (152,153).

I first consider LYP, the benign end of the primary CD30 positive of lymphoproliferative disorders followed by a discussion of ALCL, its malignant counterpart.

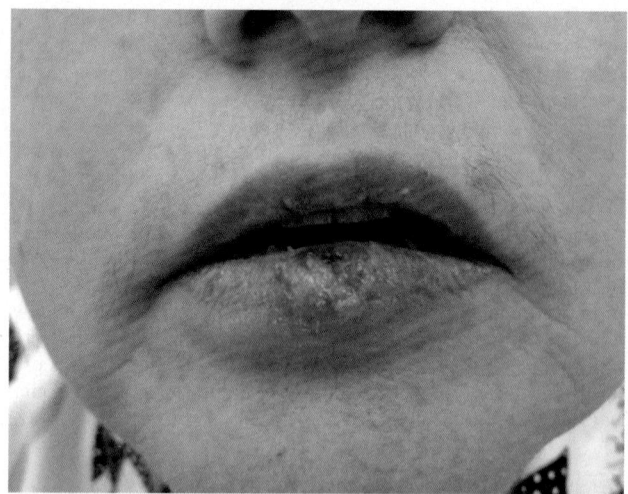

FIGURE 29.22. In this case, borderline CD30 positive lymphoproliferative disease/type C LYP, the cells were primarily of the CD8 subset. The patient presents with recurrent swelling and ulceration of her lip. Despite the diffuse effacing quality of the infiltrate a diagnosis of type C LYP was rendered given the clinical circumstances, being that of a lesion that has followed a waxing and waning course over years in a patient who is otherwise well. (Photo courtesy of Dr. Noah S. Heftler, New York, NY.)

LYMPHOMATOID PAPULOSIS

First described by McCauley in 1968, LYP is a distinctive syndrome characterized by recrudescent eruption of nodules or papules that clinically follow a benign course despite a worrisome histology (154,155). Since its original description the morphologic and phenotypic spectrum of LYP has expanded to include type A, type B, type C, and type D variants (156–158). Clinical criteria currently used to diagnose LYP are (i) multiple papules or nodules, (ii) spontaneous regression or waxing and waning of lesions that often heal with a scar (Fig. 29.22), (iii) no evidence that skin lesions progressively grow to a diameter larger than 3 cm during 3 months of observation without treatment, and (iv) absence of lymphadenopathy (157). Significant advances in the understanding of this disorder have been made over the last decade. Willemze first recognized that there were two distinct variants: type A and type B. Five variants are now recognized: A, B, C, D and E. The morphologic, immunophenotypic, and genotypic differences

are alluded to presently. Many articles suggest that in 10% to 20% of cases, concurrent or subsequent development of lymphoma occurs; the lymphomas include MF, ALCL, and Hodgkin lymphoma (159–161). Lesions manifest no sex predilection and can occur at any age from infancy to the eighth decade with the median age being in the fourth or fifth decades (162,163). The incidence ranges from 1.2 to 1.9 per million in New England (162). The most common lymphomas that develop in the setting of LYP are MF and primary cutaneous ALCL. Less common are Hodgkin lymphoma and CLL (164). It appears that progression of LYP to malignant lymphoma is a more frequent occurrence in males (165). Those patients who have or subsequently develop MF may exhibit lesions of type B LYP (Fig. 29.23) while those patients with ALCL or Hodgkin disease characteristically demonstrate type A LYP (165).

Pathology

The histology of LYP depends on the subtype of LYP (i.e., A, B, C, D and E) and upon the age of the lesion biopsied (163). Early lesions show only a sparse, nondescript perivascular lymphoid infiltrate, while the characteristic atypical morphology is seen in the fully developed, mature lesion (156,164).

In type A LYP, one observes a wedge-shaped superficial and deep perivascular infiltrates that include both small lymphoid forms and atypical large lymphocytes mimicking Reed-Sternberg cells and their variants. The angiocentric infiltrate is expansile and is associated with luminal attenuation. Ischemic alterations of the overlying epidermis may be seen. Mural or luminal fibrin deposition is seen (160). There is concomitant erythrocyte extravasation within the dermis and epidermis. In the type A lesion the dominant cell around and within the vessel walls is a large lymphoreticular cell in the 20- to 30-μm range with abundant lightly eosinophilic cytoplasm; the cells have round, oval, and/or reniform nuclei with an open chromatin pattern and a prominent basophilic to eosinophilic nucleolus. Most of the cells are mononuclear although occasional binucleated cells can be seen. Mitoses are numerous. An almost ubiquitous finding is a concomitant polymorphous inflammatory defined by neutrophils, eosinophils, and a few plasma cells. The infiltrate extends deep and characteristically expands the adventitial dermis of the eccrine coil. While epidermotropism of atypical lymphocytes is minimal to absent, a psoriasiform pattern of epidermal hyperplasia with prominent spongiform pustulation mimicking psoriasis is very characteristic (159).

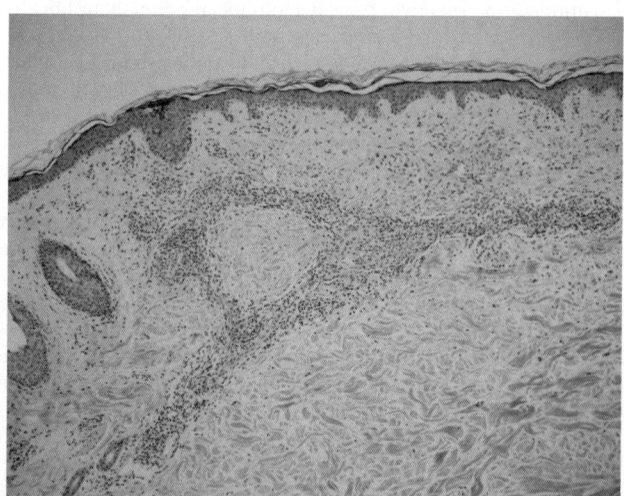

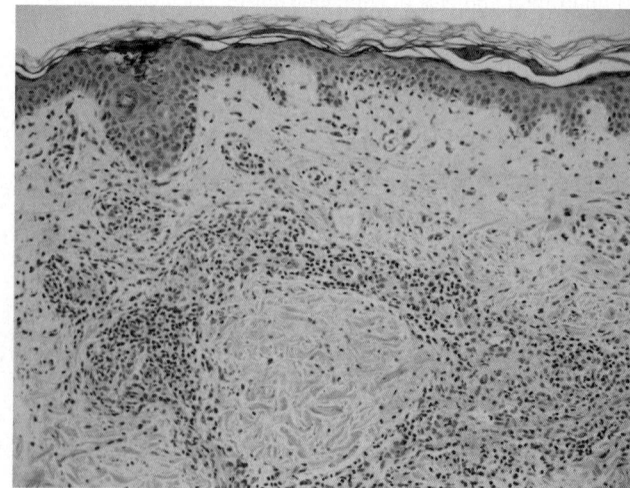

A   **B**

FIGURE 29.23. A: In this case, of type B LYP, one observes an epitheliotropic lymphocytic infiltrate accompanied by a perivascular lymphocytic infiltrate (hematoxylin and eosin, magnification: 100×). **B:** Higher power magnification shows focal colonization of the epidermis by lymphocytes in a fashion reminiscent of early mycosis fungoides and as well there is accentuation of lymphocytes around blood vessels (hematoxylin and eosin, magnification: 200×).

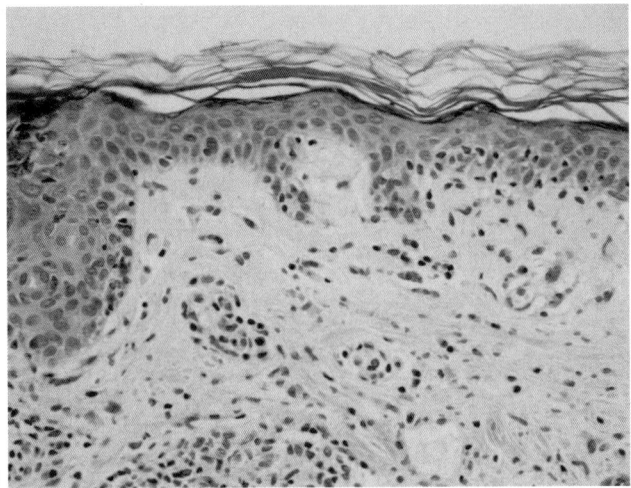
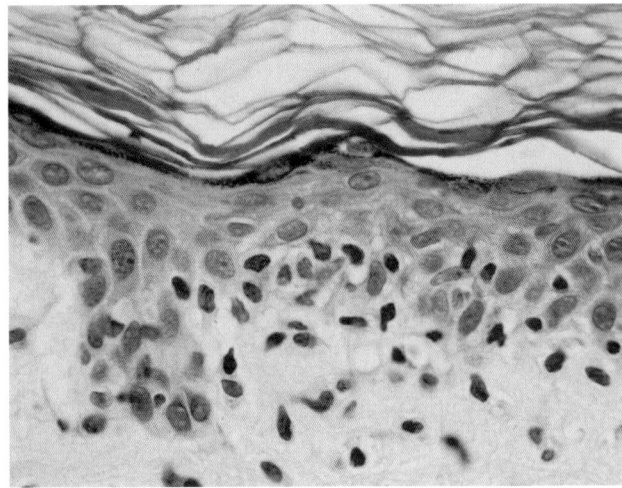

C   D

FIGURE 29.23. *(Continued)* **C:** However, the infiltrate in this case of type B LYP is predominated by small lymphocytes within the epidermis and dermis (hematoxylin and eosin, magnification: 400×). **D:** The epidermotropic lymphocytes bear a striking morphologic resemblance to the cytomorphology as well as architectural disposition within the epidermis that is encountered in MF (hematoxylin and eosin, magnification: 1,000×).

The so-called type B lesions of LYP more closely mimic MF histologically, with bandlike infiltrates of small, irregularly contoured lymphoid forms in close apposition to the undersurface of the epidermis (Fig. 29.23). The CD30 stain may be negative especially if there is no significant admixture of larger atypical cells. It is very difficult to distinguish type B LYP from PLC. Pautrier microabscesses are unusual in type B LYP; their presence is highly suggestive of MF (166). Most important, however, in the distinction of type LYP from MF is the clinical presentation. While the histology may resemble MF, the clinical features are those of small papular nodular lesions that undergo spontaneous regression. Likely a subset of type LYP lesions represent PLC given the similarities histologically and clinically between type B LYP and PLC. The deeper extent of the infiltrate and the presence of a few atypical larger cells that stain for CD30 would define potential features useful in the separation of type B LYP from PLC.

In type C LYP, it is common to see areas of cellular effacing sheetlike growth of large transformed cells resulting in a morphology that is indistinguishable from ALCL (Figs. 29.22 and 29.24) (164). Type C LYP also falls under the alternative designation borderline CD30+ lymphoproliferative disease and will be considered separately along with the recently described types D and E LYP.

Phenotypic and Molecular Studies in Type A and Type B LYP

Immunophenotypically, the large atypical lymphocytes of type A LYP exhibit pan T-cell antigen expression demonstrating positivity for CD2, CD3, and CD5. Both the large atypical cells of type A LYP and the large cerebriform cells of type B LYP show positivity for activation markers including HLADR, TAC (the antigen for the interleukin-2 receptor), transferring receptor (T9), and Ki-67. An aberrant phenotypic profile is revealed in both subtypes of LYP by virtue of diminished expression in the pan T-cell markers CD62L, CD7, and at times CD5. The large atypical cells are CD30 positive and typically express cytotoxic proteins including perforin, T-cell intracellular antigen (TIA) and granzyme (Fig. 29.25). They are most frequently of the CD4 subset although in a minority of cases the atypical cells are positive for CD8 and CD56, as will be discussed below (167). The chemokine receptor CCR3 is held to be negative in the neoplastic lymphocytes in lesions of MF while CCR3 is expressed in about 40% of cases of LYP. This phenotypic finding could be of value in the potential distinction of type B LYP from MF (168). MUM1 translocations have been observed in a spectrum of T-cell lymphoproliferative

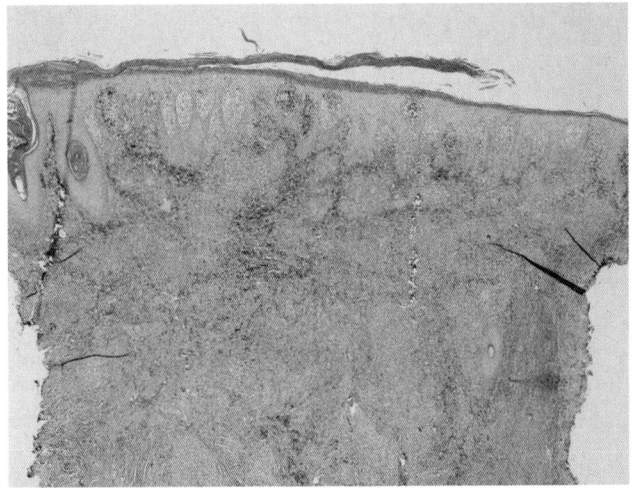
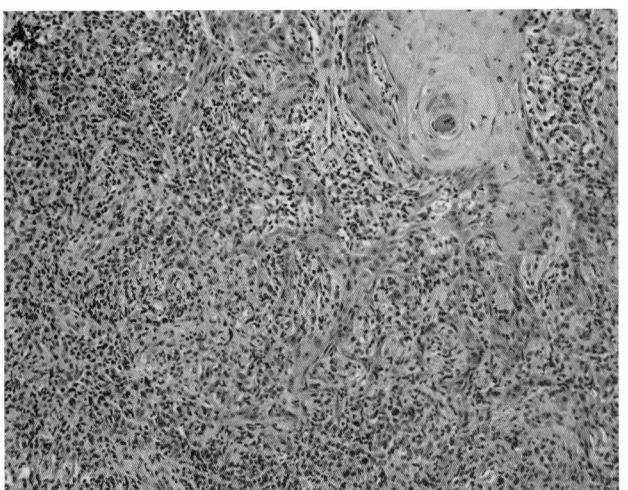

A   B

FIGURE 29.24. *(Continued)* **A:** In this case of borderline CD30-positive lymphoproliferative disease one observes an effacing diffuse and nodular lymphocytic infiltrate spanning the entire sampled thickness of the dermis (diaminobenzidine, magnification: 100×). **B:** A characteristic finding observed in type C LYP as well as ALCL is pseudoepitheliomatous hyperplasia mimicking squamous cell carcinoma (hematoxylin and eosin, magnification: 200×).

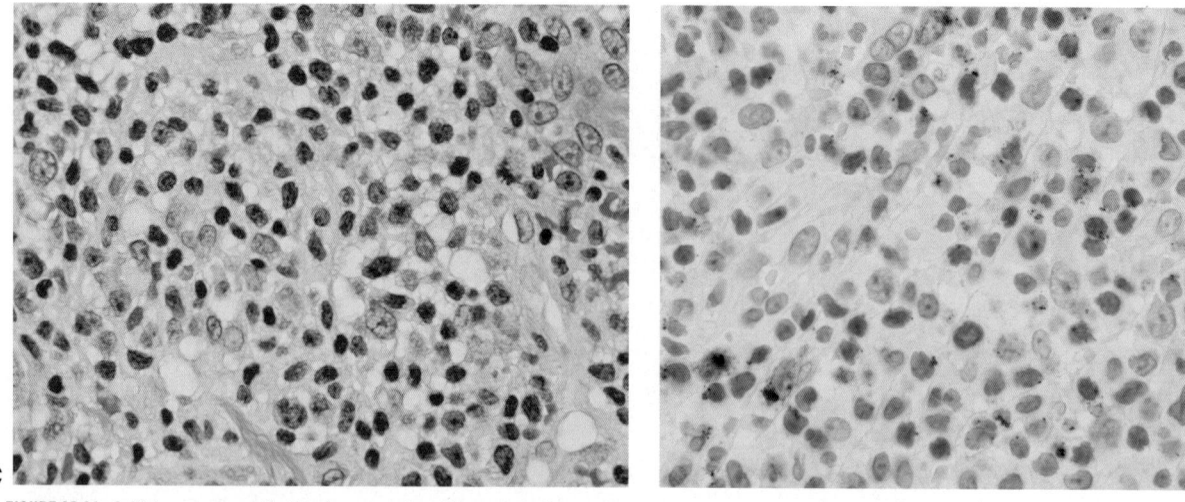

FIGURE 29.24. C: Higher power magnification shows a number of larger atypical immunoblastic-appearing cells in a background of small lymphocytes (hematoxylin and eosin, magnification: 1,000×). **D:** The neoplastic cells implicated in CD30-positive lymphoproliferative disease expresses the cytotoxic protein granzyme (diaminobenzidine, magnification: 1,000×).

disorders including LYP (169). Small atypical cerebriform lymphocytes of type B LYP will have a phenotypic profile similar to MF; the cells do not express CD30. Twenty percent of ALCL cases and three percent of LYP cases exhibited IR4/Mum1 translocation (169). One study by Kempf et al. suggested that MUM1 was expressed in the atypical cells of LYP as well as secondary ALCL. In contrast, Mum1 expression was not observed in the setting of primary cutaneous ALCL (157). However, we have found expression of MUM1 in the large atypical cells in LYP as well as primary and secondary ALCL. Others have found similar results suggesting that Mum1 is not useful in the morphologic distinction of LYP from ALCL (170,171).

The chemokine profile of LYP and ALCL has been extensively studied by Yamaguchi et al. They discovered that there was strong expression of CCR3 and CCR4 in atypical cells of primary cutaneous ALCL while <50% of cases of LYP showed

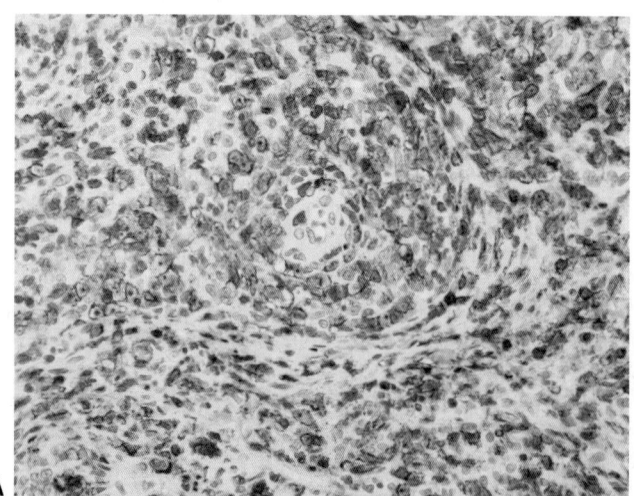

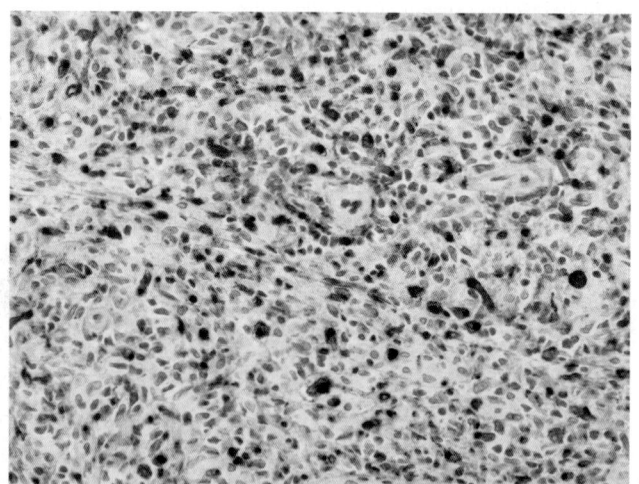

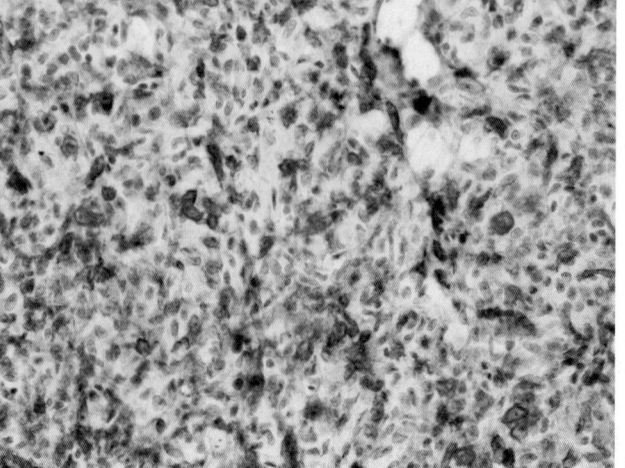

FIGURE 29.25. A: Uncommonly CD30-positive lymphoproliferative disease can be of the CD8 subset. There is extensive staining of the lymphocytes for CD8 (diaminobenzidine, magnification: 400×). **B:** The cells show prominent staining with granzyme (diaminobenzidine, magnification: 400×). **C:** The atypical lymphocytes are positive for CD30. Given the extensive nature of the infiltrate, the process resembles ALCL. However, the small size of the lesions along with the tendency toward spontaneous regression was more in keeping with a diagnosis of type C LYP (diaminobenzidine, magnification: 400×).

CCR3 and CCR4 staining. In addition, the ligand RANTES/CCL5 was strongly expressed by atypical cells of ALCL with weak or no expression in lesions of LYP (168). An additional anecdotal case report describes CCR3 expression in a lesion of LYP while a concurrent lesion of MF was CCR3 negative (172).

Differential Diagnosis

I have encountered cases of LYP in which the biopsy has been previously interpreted as psoriasis and/or a psoriasiform drug reaction due to the extent of epidermal infiltration by neutrophils. One of the most useful clues in establishing a diagnosis of LYP is the deep extent of the angiocentric lymphomatoid infiltrate within the dermis. Most superficial lymphomatoid vascular reactions including those containing CD30-positive T cells are forms of hypersensitivity in contrast to classic type A LYP that assumes a deeper-seated pattern of lymphocytic infiltration most notably around the eccrine coil and nerves.

Type B LYP has many morphologic similarities with PLC. Both are characterized by a small lymphocytic epitheliotropic lymphocytic infiltrate accompanied by a low-grade lymphocytic vasculitis. In both, the lymphocytes have a mildly atypical cerebriform morphology. Phenotypic abnormalities including a diminution of CD7 and CD62L and clonality can be observed in both type B LYP and PLC. There may be some differentiating points including the lack of eosinophils and plasma cells in PLC and the deeper-seated extent of the infiltrate in lesions of type B LYP. As well, the patient may have other biopsies showing a more common morphology, namely, type A LYP (148).

Treatment

Methotrexate appears to the treatment of choice for moderately severe cases of LYP. The effectiveness of methotrexate relates to its inhibitory effect on DNA synthesis, its anti-inflammatory effects, or both. The atypical lymphocytes seen in LYP and ALCL manifest high mitotic activity and hence it would seem likely that methotrexate significantly inhibits the proliferation of these cells especially during the initial phase of lesional development. The recommended dosage is 10 to 25 mg given every 1 to 4 weeks. The major side effect of importance is hepatic fibrosis. Liver biopsies with guidelines similar to that implemented for patients with psoriasis should be used (173).

TYPE C LYPHOMATOID PAPULOSIS/ BORDERLINE CD30-POSITIVE LYMPHOPROLIFERATIVE DISORDERS

There are cases that manifest a morphology more in keeping with ALCL although the clinical presentation is consistent with LYP based on a lesional size <3 cm and a tendency toward spontaneous remission. The characteristic hallmarks light microscopically include a sheetlike growth of large atypical cells exhibiting the typical phenotypic profile that one encounters in ALCL. The epidermis oftentimes appears hyperplastic with infiltration of the epidermis by neutrophils. The changes within the epidermis can resemble psoriasis albeit the infiltrate in the dermis defies categorization as a reactive one. The absolute distinction between borderline type C LYP and spontaneously regressing lesions of ALCL can be impossible. Both lesions can show a striking pattern of pseudoepitheliomatous hyperplasia (Fig. 29.24B). One could use size as a determinant and any history of concurrent and/or prior biopsies compatible with ALCL. Overall, if the lesion is <3 cm and spontaneously regresses, regardless of the extent and degree of large cell infiltration, the process is still best treated and categorized as LYP. It has not been established that type C LYP is at greater risk for disease progression to ALCL.

Phenotypic Profile

The dominant infiltrate is one comprising a CD30+ T cell exhibiting granzyme, TIA and perforin positivity in two thirds of cases. In general, the absolute distinction between ALCL and borderline LYP is difficult. Such lesions therefore fall under the general rubric of borderline C30-positive lymphoproliferative disease. A loss of CD62L and CD7 amidst the larger atypical cells is characteristic. The cells may not express CD3. The cells are most frequently of the CD4 subset or may exhibit a null phenotype (i.e., CD4 and CD8 negative); however, CD8 positivity with or without expression of CD56 can be seen in a minority of cases. Such cases pose a diagnostic problem in regard to the aggressive counterparts, as is discussed below (160).

CD8-POSITIVE LYMPHOMATOID PAPULOSIS/TYPE D/E LYMPHOMATOID PAPULOSIS

In a minority of cases of LYP, the neoplastic/clonally restricted T cell can be of the CD8 subset. There are certain distinguishing features that would favor a diagnosis of CD8-positive LyP over one of the more characteristic CD4 subtypes. Firstly, eosinophils and neutrophils characteristic of classic CD4+ LyP are frequently absent in this variant. Secondly, striking vasculitic changes are common, possibly reflective of the concomitant cytokine milieu. Finally, a granulomatous eccrine hidradenitis is common. The excessive atypia and significant pleomorphism, which characterizes type A LYP, may not be apparent (174).

In CD8-positive LyP, the cytokine milieu will dictate the pattern of inflammation and vascular injury. There are two functional CD8 subsets based on a distinctive cytokine profile. One referred to as Tc1 produces high levels of interferon (IFN)-gamma while the other is designated as Tc2, producing interleukin (IL)-4, -5, -10, and -13 and reciprocally low levels of IFN-gamma. The CD8 T cells of the Tc1 subset are held to be mediators of transplant vasculopathy (174). In our series, the paucity of eosinophils along with the presence of vascular injury suggested that the Tc1 subset might be implicated.

The differential diagnosis of this variant of LYP is one of primary cutaneous aggressive epidermotropic CD8-positive cytotoxic T-cell lymphoma (174–176). Those cases that resemble this lymphoma on a light microscopic and phenotypic perspective have been designated as so-called type D LYP (175) (Fig. 29.26). When there is an usual degree of angiotropism with angiodestruction the designation of type E LYP is used (176). Despite significant histologic dissimilarities, clinical pathologic correlation remains the cornerstone for distinguishing between primary cutaneous aggressive cytotoxic CD8-positive T-cell lymphoma and CD8-positive LYP. The waxing and waning clinical behavior of LYP allows this distinction to be made. The latter is crucial in sparing the patient the cost and toxicity of inappropriately administered chemotherapy (174,176).

CUTANEOUS ANAPLASTIC LARGE CELL LYMPHOMA

Clinical Features

At the opposite end of the CD30-positive lymphoproliferative disorders is ALCL. This lymphoma was first recognized by Stein et al. in 1985. They described a distinctive large cell hematopoietic neoplasm associated with extensive lymph node effacement manifesting sinusoidal accentuation; the neoplastic cell population was held to be of the T-cell or null-cell phenotype expressing CD30 (aka Ki-1 antigen) (177). There

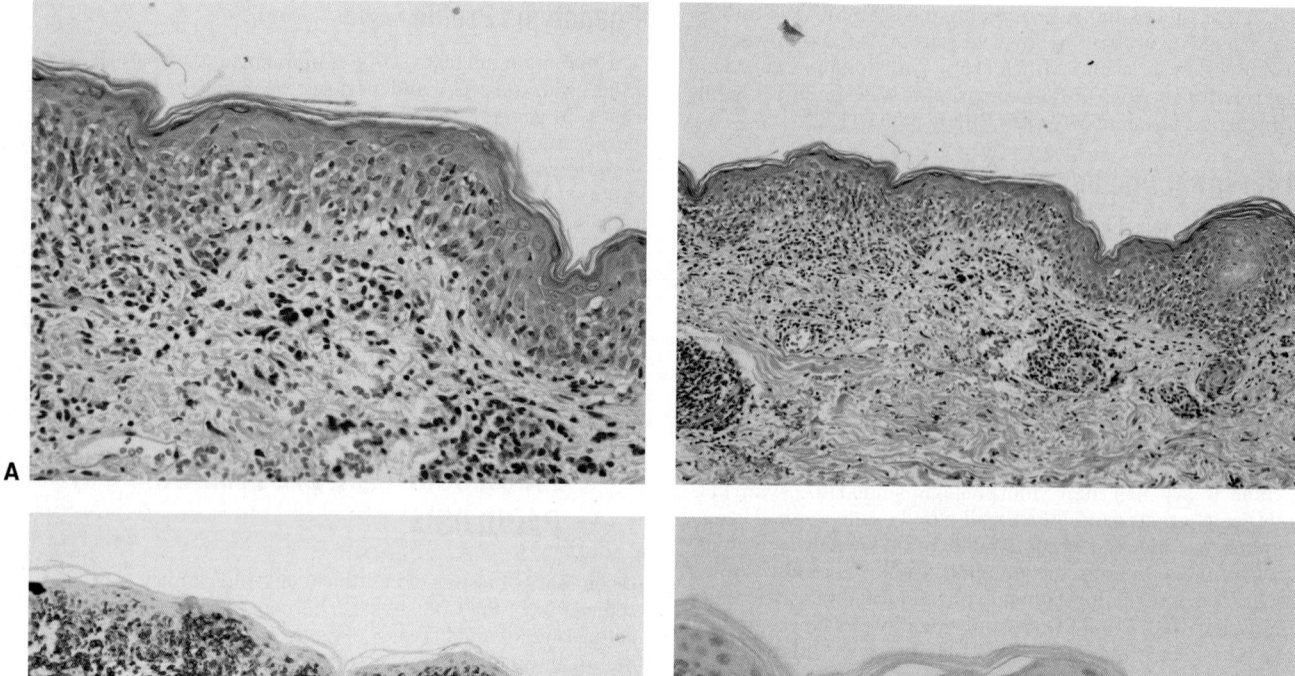

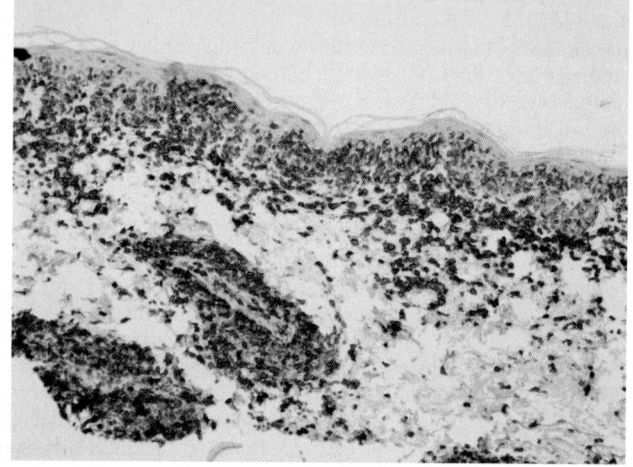

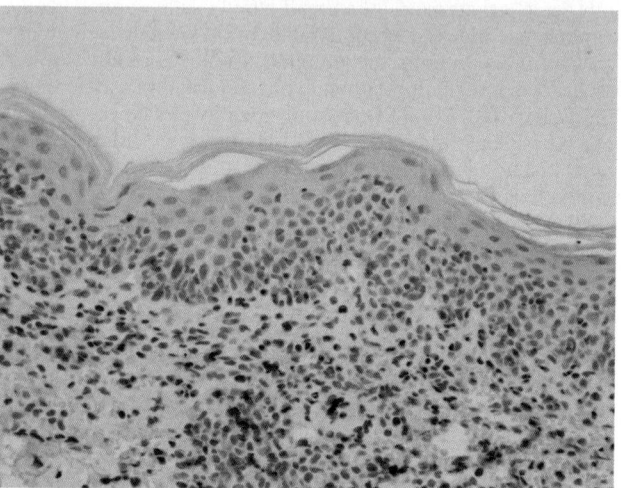

FIGURE 29.26. **A:** In this case of type D LYP, one observes an epidermotropic lymphocytic infiltrate resembling what can be encountered in primary cutaneous aggressive cytotoxic CD8-positive T-cell lymphoma (diaminobenzidine, magnification: 200×). **B:** The infiltrate shows prominent epitheliotropism along with a perivascular lymphocytic infiltrate accompanied by red cell extravasation. An epitheliotropic lymphocytic infiltrate accompanied by red cell extravasation would also raise diagnostic consideration in regard to pigmented purpuric dermatosis and pityriasis lichenoides chronica. (hematoxylin and eosin, magnification: 100×). **C:** The cells are extensively CD8 positive with very prominent marked infiltration of the epidermis. Given the angiocentricity with hemorrhage along with the extensive degree of epidermotropism, it is very easy to misinterpret this case as a primary cutaneous aggressive cytotoxic CD8-positive T-cell lymphoma (diaminobenzidine, magnification: 200×). **D:** The aberrant nature of the lymphocytic infiltrate is revealed by the marked degree of reduction in CD7, a common finding in the realm of cutaneous T-cell dyscrasias (diaminobenzidine, magnification: 200×).

is heterogeneity in terms of the morphologic spectrum of the lesion with cells ranging from small forms to large highly atypical sarcomatoid variants. There are four main variants: the common type (classic), giant cell rich, small cell, lymphohistiocytic, and finally Hodgkin disease–like. There are other unusual variants including neutrophil rich, eosinophil rich, sarcomatoid, and signet ring (177,178). Although one recognizes these morphologic subtypes, there is no clear-cut clinical difference between the various morphologic subtypes except the small cell variant. Specifically, this subtype of ALCL may be associated with a leukemic picture and hence a more aggressive clinical course (179). An alternative classification scheme is according to the anaplastic lymphoma kinase (ALK) result. Specifically the lymphomas are now categorized according to the presence or absence of ALK expression. The vast majority of primary cutaneous ALCL are ALK negative. However, in the context of extracutaneous ALCL, ALCL without ALK expression tends to occur in older individuals and has a much worse prognosis compared to ALK-positive forms of ALCL (178).

ALCL of the skin was described first by Kaudewitz et al. (180) and then by Berti et al. in 1988 and 1989, respectively. There are three primary forms of ALCL: primary cutaneous

ALCL, secondary ALCL developing in the setting of known lymphoma, and finally nodal ALCL secondarily involving the skin in the context of stage IV disease (179). Primary cutaneous ALCL develops *de novo* in the skin and/or in the setting of LYP with a median age of presentation of 60 years. It is considered an indolent form of T-cell lymphoproliferative disease. Certain cases designated as ALCL likely represent type C LYP/borderline CD30+ lymphoproliferative disease. In 30% of cases, the lesions spontaneously regress. The most common presentation is in the context of solitary tumors manifesting variable ulceration; however, at times the lesions may exhibit multicentricity. Patients with more disseminated disease would likely benefit from systemic polychemotherapy.

Clinically the distinction of ALCL from LYP is important. Some authors note that the presence of a solitary lesion >3 cm, persistence without spontaneous regression, and the presence of significant lymphadenopathy are probably indicative of malignant lymphoma and/or a progression of lesions of LYP into ALCL. Such criteria might be construed as rather stringent in that there are published series addressing the clinical features of ALCL whereby lesions smaller than 2 cm occur in over 63% of patients; 63% had a solitary lesion. Regression is a helpful feature but it is not an absolute finding diagnostic of LYP since 25% of cases of ALCL undergo spontaneous regression (181).

Secondary ALCL develops in the setting of a known prior history of lymphoma and may signify tumor progression in the setting of MF. It is the general consensus that the subsequent acquisition of CD30 expression in the setting of MF may have the same prognostic significance as tumor-stage MF (178).

ALCL of the skin has also been described in the posttransplant setting. While the vast majority of posttransplant lymphoproliferative disorders are of B-cell derivation, there is an increasing body of literature that describes monomorphic T-cell variants of posttransplant lymphoproliferative disease (PTLD). Among these are primary CTCLs including MF, Sézary syndrome, primary cutaneous pleomorphic T-cell lymphoma, subcutaneous panniculitis-like T-cell lymphoma, LYP, and ALCL. The most common T-cell variant is ALCL. A direct role for EBV in lesional propagation usually cannot be demonstrated. Cutaneous PTLD typically develop several years after the solid organ transplant. In contradistinction, extracutaneous PTLD usually develop within 1 to 2 years after transplantation (182,183).

One of the distinctive features of ALCL is the tendency toward regression in only a minority of cases. The pathogenetic basis of the regression is of interest. The question arises as to molecular events that are responsible for the spontaneous regression of some cases of CD30-positive lymphoma and what events lead to lesional persistence. Transforming growth factor receptor B, designated TBRII, is a multifunctional polypeptide that regulates cell proliferation and differentiation; its main affect is one of growth inhibition. In one study, cell culture lines derived from a lesion of ALCL did not show any inhibitory growth response to TGB. The basis was a point mutation in TBRII, leading to inhibition of the wild-type receptor, hence rendering the cell resistant to the inhibitory effects of TBRII (184).

Lymph node–based CD30-positive large cell lymphomas of either T-cell or null-cell lineage manifest a very characteristic translocation, namely, t(2;5)(p23;q35), and express the NPM-ALK hybrid protein detected by the antibody ALK1 (185) In 1994, the translocation was cloned by Steve Morris and others at St. Jude Children's Research Hospital in Memphis, Tennessee. The translocation was found to involve a receptor tyrosine kinase designated *ALK*. ALK is found on 2p23 and nucleophosmin (*NPM*) on 5q35. Because ALK is not normally expressed in lymphoid tissue, anti-ALK antibodies can be used as a surrogate method for detecting t(2;5) cloning of the translocation breakpoints. The incidence of positivity for translocation ranges from 15% to 80% (186). Furthermore, the translocation has been detected in some peripheral T-cell lymphomas other than classical ALCL and some diffuse large cell B-cell lymphoma. In addition, a cryptic abnormality has been detected that is easily recognized using FISH inv(2) (p23q35). The result is a distinctive ALK protein expression restricted to the cytoplasm of the neoplastic cells. ALK protein expression is held to be an independent prognostic variable predicting good patient outcome. The principal methods of detection of ALK are RT *in situ* PCR, cytogenetics, and finally immunohistochemistry. There are two genes involved in this translocation: the nucleophosmin gene on chromosome 5 and the ALK gene on chromosome 2. They are present in a small minority of cases of LYP and primary cutaneous CD30-positive large cell lymphoma (i.e., 10% to 20% of cases) with some studies not detecting any translocation. In contrast, the rate of t(2;5) is higher in nodal CD30-positive lymphomas with a prevalence rate of about 40% of primary nodal cases. The t(2;5) is more common in cases affecting younger patients. The findings suggest that lymph node–based CD30-positive lymphoproliferative disease may be cytogenetically distinct from cutaneous CD30-positive lymphoproliferative disorders (186).

Light Microscopic Findings

Pathologically ALCL differs from LYP by virtue of a predominance of CD30-positive staining cells with >75% of cells exhibiting a large anaplastic morphology. In contrast, in LYP the CD30-positive cells are noted amidst a dominant polymorphous inflammatory cell background. Features suggestive of evolution from LYP into CD30-positive lymphoma include a further loss of pan T-cell marker expression, extension into the subcutis, and a greater proportion of atypical cells relative to the inflammatory cell background with focal effacement of the dermal architecture by sheets of atypical cells. In addition to the sheetlike pattern of growth, there is a striking tendency for angiocentricity. Typically, a polymorphous inflammatory cell infiltrate comprising neutrophils and eosinophils is identified. A striking pattern of psoriasiform epidermal hyperplasia with extensive spongiform pustulation is common, defining a pattern reminiscent of that also encountered in type A LYP (187).

In the small cell variant of ALCL, there are scattered large atypical hallmark cells as described above; however, the dominant cell population is an abnormal small to intermediate-sized lymphocyte. The cells demonstrate nuclear contour irregularities including the presence of cells with polylobated cells with a florette-like morphology. The cells have clear cytoplasm with distinct cytoplasmic membranes. The cells can be mistaken for representing histiocytes especially when the neoplastic cells are negative for CD3 and CD45 Ro (179).

Additional morphologic variants of ALCL have been described including a form that mimics a low-grade myxoid sarcoma. In the myxoid variant of ALCL, an exuberant pattern of pseudoepitheliomatous hyperplasia mimicking squamous cell carcinoma is seen (188). The two cases we have encountered of myxoid ALCL had concomitant lymph node involvement. In both cases, the lymph node architecture was not discernible, which added to the diagnostic confusion. A diagnosis of myxoid ALCL can be difficult to make due to the degree of myxomatous stromal change, the supervening inflammatory cell infiltrate, and neovascularization, hence producing a morphology reminiscent of granulation tissue. An important caveat is to at least consider the diagnosis of myxoid ALCL when confronted with a highly inflammatory myxomatous process. In cases associated with MF (a variant of secondary ALCL), a small cerebriform epidermotropic T-cell lymphocytic infiltrate can be observed.

Phenotypic Profile

Immunophenotypically most cases of ALCL are CD45 RO positive and exhibit CD4 positivity. However, less common variants exist including CD8+ ALCL and those in which the neoplastic cells are negative for CD3, CD4, and CD8, although other pan T-cell markers such as CD2 may be observed. It has been suggested that a small percentage of cases of ALCL may be of B-cell phenotype. The basis of their classification as ALCL is due to CD30, EMA, and ALK positivity. These lymphomas exhibit a male predominance and typically occur in middle age (189). This particular phenotypic variant of ALCL has not been described in the skin however. The expression of activation antigens is very common in ALCL including T9 (transferrin receptor), HLA-DR, and Tac. ALCL may show an aberrant T-cell phenotype by virtue of CD3, CD4, and CD8 negativity defining a null phenotype. As well, loss of CD7, CD62L, and CD5 may be seen especially amidst the larger cells. Unlike Hodgkin disease, the cells are leukocyte antigen positive and CD15 negative (178,190).

One of the unique phenotypic features of ALCL is the presence of perforin and TIA-1 expression in the tumor cells. TIA-1 is a 15-kDa cytotoxic granule associated membrane protein expressed in NK cells and cytotoxic T lymphocytes. TIA-1 was first produced and characterized by Anderson et al. in 1990.

TIA-1 reacted with 20% to 36% of peripheral blood T lymphocytes. It reacted strongly with NK cells and CD8+ cytolytic T cells and less strongly with CD4-activated cells. This suggested a preferential expression in cells possessing cytotoxic potential. Since then several studies have shown that the expression of these cytotoxic proteins are seen in a spectrum of lymphoma including NK-cell lymphomas, rare cases of Hodgkin lymphoma, ALCL, and certain distinctive forms of peripheral T-cell lymphoma including subcutaneous T-cell, hepatosplenic, and intestinal lymphoma (191). In primary cutaneous ALCL, granzyme B- and T-cell–restricted intracellular antigens have been observed while in CD30-negative primary cutaneous large T-cell lymphomas the neoplastic cells usually do not express these proteins. CD56 positivity can be seen on rare occasions in primary cutaneous ALCL. While it may portend a worse prognosis in nodal sites, this finding in the context of primary cutaneous ALCL is usually not associated with a more aggressive clinical course. This CD56+ variant occurs both in the transplant setting and in previously healthy adults (192,193). In the small cell variant, the smaller lymphoid cells are typically CD30 negative. In those cases of null phenotype, expression of CD11b and CD13 has been observed (179,187).

The profile of primary cutaneous ALCL is unique in light of the lack of ALK, epithelial membrane antigen, and clusterin staining. MUM1 positivity is held to be more frequent in LYP compared to ALCL although there are conflicting reports in this regard (122). This point has already been discussed.

PRIMARY CUTANEOUS CD4+ SMALL/MEDIUM-SIZED PLEOMORPHIC T-CELL LYMPHOMA

Clinical Features

Primary cutaneous CD4+ small/medium-sized pleomorphic T-cell lymphoma is a rare subtype of peripheral T-cell lymphoma that unlike MF is not preceded by a waxing and waning prelymphomatous phase (25,194–198). The lesions consist of a sudden onset of plaques, papules, or tumors, some of which show central ulceration without scaling. The most common presentation is in the context of solitary lesions involving the upper trunk and face (Fig. 29.27) (25). The lesions are more commonly seen in patients in the fifth through sixth decades of life with a male predominance. However, pediatric cases

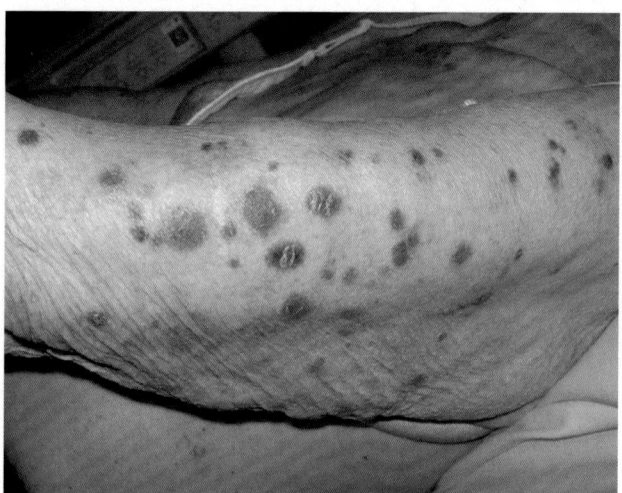

FIGURE 29.27. This patient with primary cutaneous pleomorphic T-cell lymphoma developed an abrupt onset of multiple infiltrative violaceous plaques and nodules.

have been described (195). In the EORTC WHO classification of lymphoma, this lymphoma is considered an indolent lymphoproliferative disorder along with MF, CD30+ lymphoproliferative disease, and subcutaneous panniculitis-like T-cell lymphoma (25). When the disease is localized to a small area, the treatment of choice is one of radiation while more disseminated disease might require systemic therapy. Not surprisingly the prognosis is much better with limited disease (essentially 100% 5-year survival) compared to a more disseminated presentation (199). Although the infiltrates are characteristically CD4 positive, an analogous indolent form of lymphoproliferative disease resembling the localized variants of this lymphoma can be composed of neoplastic CD8-positive lymphocytes (200). This form of T-cell lymphoproliferative disease has an unusual predilection to involve the face, most notably the ears, eyelid, and nose, and falls under the designation of indolent CD8+ lymphoid proliferation of the face and will be discussed separately.

Light Microscopic Findings

In earlier-stage lesions, a distinct pattern of dermal infiltration may be seen whereby the tumor cells surround and permeate nerves, pilosebaceous units, and blood vessels. The infiltrate frequently lies in intimate apposition to the dermoepidermal junction whereby the superficial aspect of the infiltrate coalesces to produce a bandlike pattern of infiltration (Fig. 29.28A–D). At disparity with the striking infiltrate within the dermis is only minimal epidermotropism, although folliculotropism can be seen. The distinctive pattern of epidermotropism observed in MF including Pautrier microabscesses is not seen. Unlike MF, there is invariably deep dermal involvement in the initial phase of the disease. There may even be extension into the subcutaneous fat. In contrast, in MF the lesions are confined to the epidermis and superficial dermis for years. Only after a protracted history of untreated disease does a deep dermal infiltrate develop, potentially signifying tumor stage progression. One of the cardinal hallmarks is the absence of germinal centers even though there can be striking B-cell hyperplasia; the B-cell component is primarily in the context of post–germinal center B cells disposed singly and in small aggregates amidst the T-cell infiltrate. There may be prominent involvement of adnexal structures including epitheliotropism; adnexal destruction has been described (194–198,201,202).

Histologically the characteristic cerebriform cells of MF are absent. However, the nuclei of the lymphocytes are irregular and variable in appearance with multilobation, nuclear angulation, transverse nuclear grooves, and irregular nuclear blebs. The heterochromatin is less condensed than in the Sézary cell of MF. Nucleoli are not prominent except in large atypical cells. There may be a variable admixture of eosinophils, plasma cells, and epithelioid histiocytes. The extent of granulomatous inflammation can be significant (203,204).

Even though the lymphoma is designated as one composed of small and medium-sized cells, large atypical cells are an integral component of the infiltrate. The large cell component defies categorization as a reactive lymphocyte, showing an excessive degree of nuclear enlargement and hyperchromasia with nuclear contour irregularity amidst the more monotypic effacing small and intermediate-sized cell populace. This large cell populace can exhibit CD30 positivity that can be of sufficient magnitude to suggest CD30-positive lymphoproliferative disease. This large cell component does not exceed 30% of the infiltrate.

Phenotypic Profile

Immunophenotypic studies have shown that most CTCLs exhibit a mature T-cell phenotype, expressing CD45 RO. There may be a diminution in the expression of certain pan

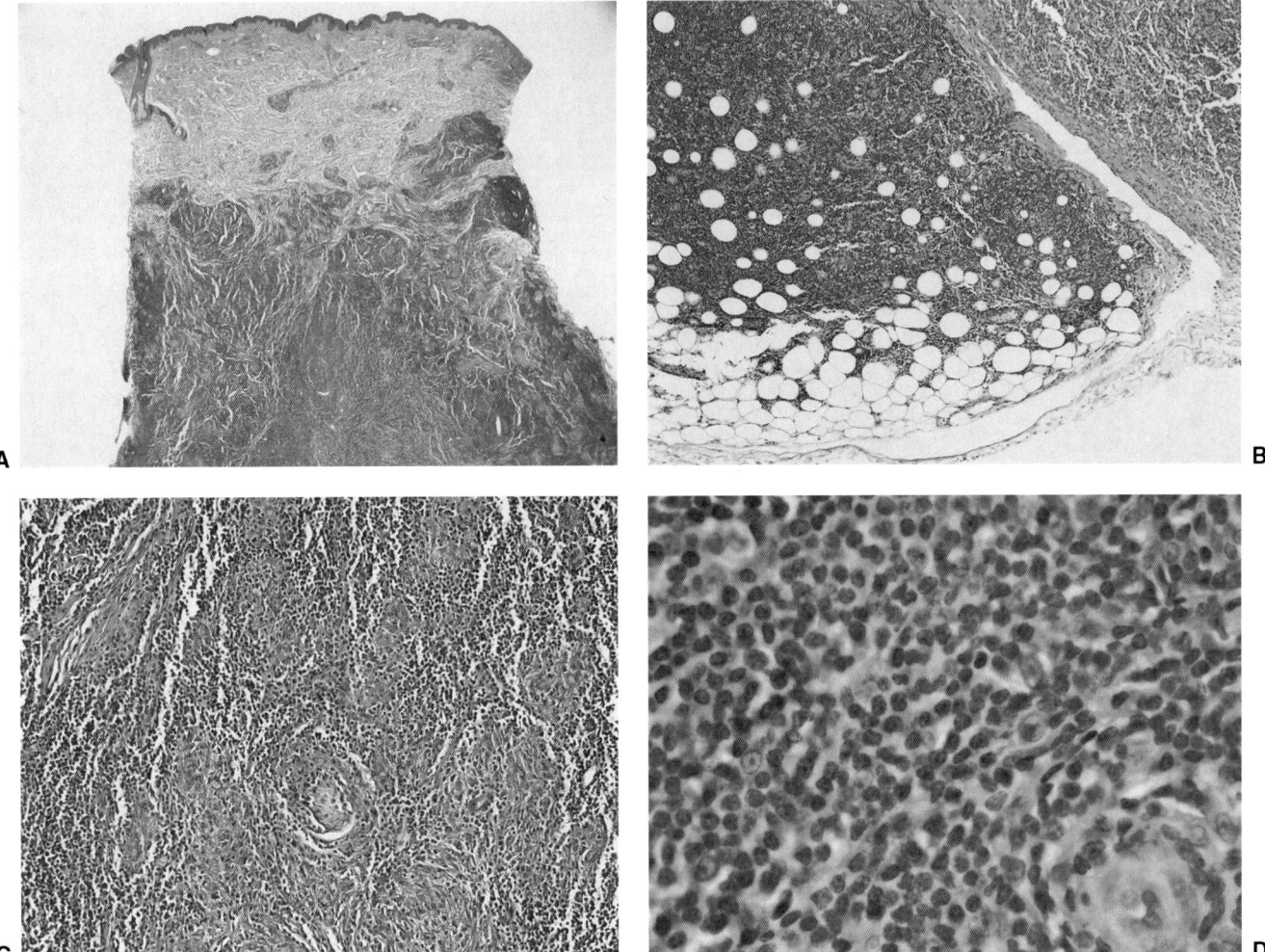

FIGURE 29.28. A: In this biopsy of primary cutaneous pleomorphic CD4-positive small-/medium-sized T-cell lymphoma, one observes a dense diffuse and nodular lymphocytic infiltrate that essentially effaces the dermal architecture. The lower power differential diagnosis would encompass lymphocytoma cutis and low-grade forms of B-cell lymphoma (hematoxylin and eosin, magnification: 40×). **B:** The infiltrate extends into the subcutaneous fat, defining a form of lymphomatoid panniculitis. The extent of necrosis within the fat lobule that one observes in subcutaneous panniculitis-like T-cell lymphoma is not seen. In addition in subcutaneous panniculitis-like T-cell lymphoma, the extent of superficial and middermal infiltration is not observed (hematoxylin and eosin, magnification: 100×). **C:** Supervening granulomas within the infiltrate can be seen, likely representing a paraneoplastic reactive process to the neoplastic lymphocytes. When extensive one can use the designation of Lennert's lymphoma (hematoxylin and eosin, magnification: 200×). **D:** This oil emersion image shows the standard morphology of the lymphocytes that define this tumor. They are relatively small. They do not exhibit a cerebriform outline but demonstrate other nuclear contour aberrations. The chromatin is finely dispersed and as well there are discernible nucleoli (hematoxylin and eosin, magnification: 1,000×).

T-cell markers including CD5, CD7, and CD62L (194–199) (Fig. 29.29A–C). The most common markers to show a reduction are CD7 and CD62L. In addition, the larger atypical cells can show a reduction in several pan T-cell markers including CD2, CD3, and CD5. Recent studies suggest that these neoplasms may be of follicular helper cell origin based on the expression of PD1, CXCL13, and BCL6 in the large neoplastic component of these lymphomas (8). It has been hypothesized that the invariable B-cell hyperplasia observed in this lymphoma is due to the presence of neoplastic follicular helper T cells. The B-cell infiltrate is in the context of postgerminal B cells and may occupy a significant component of the infiltrate (Fig. 29.29D). The identification of germinal centers favors a diagnosis of lymphocytoma cutis and is not a feature of this lymphoma. As already mentioned, a number of CD30-positive cells can be observed in this lymphoma although not of the magnitude to warrant categorization as ALCL. The cells that show positivity for CD30 are frequently the severely atypical large cells that defy categorization as a reactive infiltrate, also showing the aforesaid

follicular helper T-cell phenotype. The extent of positivity is typically not in excess of 30%.

Differential Diagnosis

Primary cutaneous CD4⁺ small/medium-sized pleomorphic T-cell lymphoma is very difficult to distinguish from a T-cell–rich lymphocytoma cutis, and it is likely that cases reported in the literature as representing primary cutaneous CD4⁺ small/medium-sized pleomorphic T-cell lymphoma represent lymphocytoma cutis. Both share a similar architectural growth pattern being that of a dermal-based diffuse and nodular lymphocytic infiltrate, a cytomorphology dominated by small lymphocytes, and a mixture of T and B cells. Even reactive T cells can be cytomorphologically atypical; hence separating the two based on cytology adds to the diagnostic conundrum. In many cases, this diagnosis is made with some hesitation. That said, integrating certain aspects of light microscopy and phenotypic profile can lead to the correct diagnosis. Among the clues that favor a diagnosis of primary cutaneous pleomorphic T-cell lymphoma over

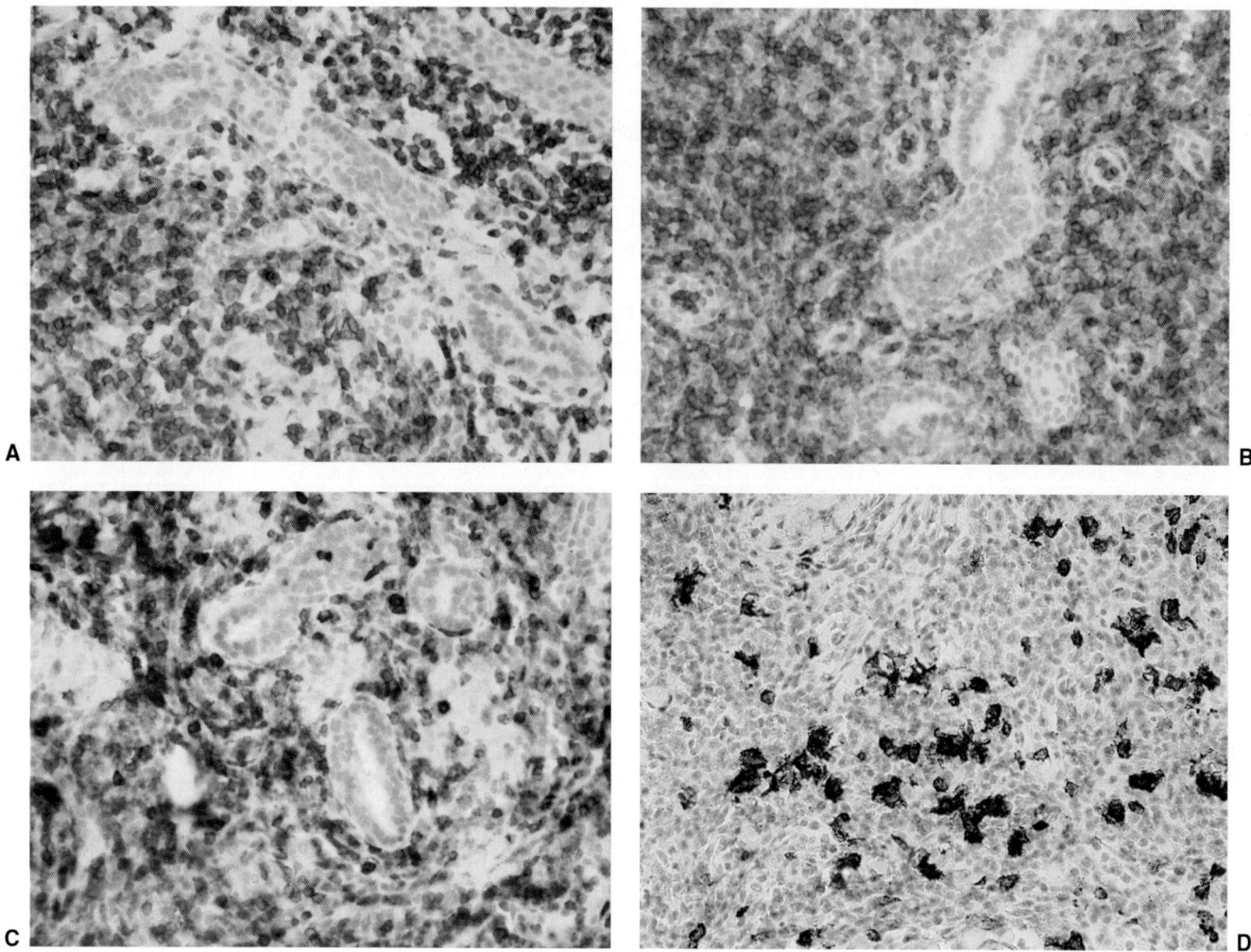

FIGURE 29.29. A: The phenotypic profile shows extensive positivity for CD3 (diaminobenzidine, magnification: 400×). **B:** The neoplastic cell in this lymphoma is a CD4-positive T cell (diaminobenzidine, magnification: 400×). **C:** Compared to the pan T-cell marker CD3, there is a reduction in the expression of CD7. In some instances, the CD7 can be relatively preserved as noted here. It becomes very difficult to render a definitive diagnosis in the absence of an aberrant phenotypic profile (diaminobenzidine, magnification: 400×). **D:** One of the cardinal hallmarks of this lymphoma is a post–germinal center B-cell hyperplasia. B lymphocytes are disposed singly and in small clusters. Germinal centers are not observed (hematoxylin and eosin, magnification: 400×).

T-cell–rich pseudolymphoma/lymphocytoma cutis is the quality of the B-cell hyperplasia. The B-cell hyperplasia that invariably accompanies this lymphoma is in the context of small clusters and singly disposed postgerminal B cells distributed throughout the lesion without distinct germinal centers. Identifying a minor cell populace of severely atypical large hyperchromatic angulated lymphocytes that exhibit an aberrant phenotype including a loss of CD2, CD7, and CD5 and positivity for PD1 would point toward a diagnosis of primary cutaneous CD4+ small/medium-sized pleomorphic T-cell lymphoma. A truly effacing growth pattern with extension into the subcutaneous fat may be an important clue favoring a diagnosis of lymphoma assuming the biopsy is deep enough. Finally, an aberrant phenotype in the smaller cells especially in regard to reductions of CD7, CD5, CD3, and/or CD2 would favor a diagnosis of lymphoma over lymphocytoma cutis. That said, there are diffuse variants of T-cell–rich lymphocytoma cutis that may be difficult to distinguish from this rare form of lymphoma because some reduction in CD7 and the identification of T-cell clonality can be observed.

Primary cutaneous CD4+ small/medium-sized pleomorphic T-cell lymphoma must be distinguished from peripheral T-cell lymphoma secondarily involving the skin. In regard to the latter, the patient is usually known to have a preexisting lymphoma. Peripheral T-cell lymphomas are those postthymic T-cell lymphomas that generally present in a lymph node or other lymphoid organs such as the spleen and Waldeyer ring. Most patients with nodal PTL present with generalized lymphadenopathy and have stage IV disease by virtue of involvement of the skin (50%), liver (50%), peripheral blood (30%), and lungs and/or pleura (20%).

In regard to low-grade B-cell lymphoma, germinal centers are a critical diagnostic feature since they are seen in both MZLs where they are reactive and in follicular lymphoma. In the latter scenario, they define the neoplastic component of the infiltrate exhibiting certain phenotypic abnormalities including dendritic cell lysis highlighted by CD21, coexpression of CD23, a reduction in the expression of CD79, positivity of centrocytes and centroblasts for Bcl-2, and a potential diminution in the expression of CD79 and CD10. As a point of reiteration, germinal centers are not a feature of primary cutaneous CD4+ small/medium-sized pleomorphic T-cell lymphoma. Identifying a dysplastic light chain–restricted plasmacytic infiltrate favors a diagnosis of MZL.

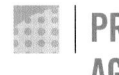 PRIMARY CUTANEOUS EPIDERMOTROPIC AGGRESSIVE CD8-POSITIVE CYTOTOXIC T-CELL LYMPHOMA

Clinical Features

The majority of CTCLs are of the CD4 subset. However, a small minority of cutaneous T-cell lymphoproliferative disorders are CD8 positive. Most of these are in the context of representing the CD8 variant of MF including unilesional variants CD8[+] ALCL and CD8[+] LYP (25,174). There are additional CTCLs in which the neoplastic cell population is exclusively of the CD8 subset represented by primary cutaneous aggressive CD8[+] cytotoxic CD8[+] T-cell lymphoma (205–207) and indolent CD8[+] lymphoid proliferation of the face (200,208). Primary cutaneous aggressive CD8[+] epidermotropic T-cell lymphoma was first recognized as a distinct entity in 1999 by Berti et al. although there were prior reports describing cytotoxic CD8[+] cutaneous lymphomas exhibiting epidermotropism in which the clinical course was aggressive (209,210). In this unique form of cutaneous lymphoma, the extent of intraepidermal infiltration resembles MF. However, prominent angiotropism with associated angiodestruction and the noncerebriform quality of the neoplastic cell are distinguishing features. The clinical course is one of abrupt onset without any antecedent history of a waxing and waning dermatosis. This lymphoma typically occurs in patients in the fifth through seventh decades of life. Metastatic disease to uncommon sites such as the liver, testes, and lung is characteristic. Some studies have shown a male predominance. While responding initially to therapy most patients have succumbed to the disease within 3 years following the initial presentation (205–207). There is no known viral trigger although a recently described fatal case in an HTLV1-positive patient has been described (123).

Light Microscopic Findings

The epidermis may exhibit acanthosis and pseudoepitheliomatous hyperplasia of the epidermis. It is common to see diffuse spongiosis. A striking angiocentric infiltrate is observed. There is concomitant angiodestruction with mural and luminal fibrin deposition.

Due to the extent of vascular injury, it is characteristic to see ischemic alterations of the overlying epidermis. Ulceration can occur and it usually attributable to ischemia reflective of angioinvasion. From a cytomorphologic perspective, the lymphocytes are intermediate in size and exhibit a noncerebriform atypical nuclear outline accompanied by marked nuclear hyperchromasia. Basophilic nucleoli and discernible eosinophilic cytoplasm are characteristic.

Phenotypic Profile

The abnormal cells are highlighted by CD8. They are typically of the alpha beta subset despite their aggressive course and hence are beta F1 positive. In some cases, there will be a relative preservation of CD7 although with a loss of CD2. The cytoxic molecules TIA, granzyme, and perforin are characteristically positive. Unlike MF, the neoplastic cells are CD45RA positive indicative of a naive phenotype (205). The CLA preparation shows diminished staining whereby the positive-staining cells exhibit a punctuate cytoplasmic pattern of staining typical of aggressive hematologic dyscrasias (211).

Differential Diagnosis

The two main diagnostic considerations are CD8[+] MF and type D CD8[+] LYP. Most cases of CD8[+] LYP resemble other forms of LYP especially the more common type A and type C variants. However, there is a distinctive variant where the epidermotropism is very extensive. The extent of infiltration in the epidermis exactly recapitulates the findings in primary cutaneous aggressive cytotoxic CD8-positive T-cell lymphoma. The key distinguishing features lies in the clinical presentation. In type D LYP, the lesions are relatively small and undergo spontaneous regression. As well, the patient is typically asymptomatic. In contrast in this lymphoma, the lesions undergo progressive enlargement and ulceration; constitutional symptoms reflective of extracutaneous dissemination occur (174,175). In CD8[+] variants of MF, a young patient presents with indolent waxing and waning disease over years characterized by hypopigmented patches and plaques with a truncal predilection. The lesions may clinically resemble vitiligo (212,213).

INDOLENT CD8-POSITIVE LYMPHOID PROLIFERATION OF THE FACE

There is a spectrum of neoplastic CD8 lymphocytic infiltrates of the skin with a variant prognosis including primary cutaneous aggressive cytotoxic CD8-positive T-cell lymphoma, subcutaneous panniculitis-like lymphoma (214), pagetoid reticulosis (121). Also, uncommonly MF (212,213), Sézary syndrome, CD30-positive lymphomas (215), and nasal-type NK/T-cell lymphomas (25,207,216) can exhibit a CD8-positive phenotype. While the classic gamma delta T cell is negative for CD4 and CD8, there is a subset of cutaneous gamma delta T-cell lymphomas in which there is expression of beta F1 (217,218).

An emerging concept in the field of CD8[+] lymphoproliferative disease is one of indolent CD8-positive lymphoproliferative disorders involving the ear and other anatomic sites of the face. I have also encountered its localization to involve the eyelid over and above the classic anatomic locations on the ear and nose (201). PCR studies revealed T-cell receptor-γ gene rearrangements in the majority of the reported cases of indolent CD8-positive lymphoproliferative disease (200,208,219,220). The two cases that have been encountered in this medical practice exhibited T-cell monoclonality.

Some authors have argued that these indolent CD8-positive lymphoid proliferation of the face represent an immunophenotypic variant of primary cutaneous CD4[+] small/medium-sized pleomorphic T-cell lymphoma (204,220). Several reports of CD8-positive small/medium-sized pleomorphic T-cell lymphoma exist in the literature with a variety of clinical presentations, including one involving the eyelid showing epidermotropism and recurrence in the lip following radiotherapy (197,221). Because of these observations, it has been argued that these rare cases of indolent CD8-positive disease represent part of the phenotypic spectrum of primary cutaneous pleomorphic small/medium-sized T-cell lymphoma. Given the localization to specific sites on the face and lack of multiplicity of lesions and/or dissemination to other areas of the skin, it is perhaps best to consider this entity as a distinct one. By using the designation of CD8[+] indolent lymphoproliferative disease of the face, the stigma associated with the designation of lymphoma is not present.

In early reports, an association was suggested between a history of *B. burgdorferi* or *Epstein-Barr* virus infections and patients who went on to develop an indolent CD8-positive lymphoid proliferation; however, no evidence was found for such a connection in the majority of patients tested.

Light Microscopic Findings

The biopsy shows a dense typically effacing lymphocytic infiltrate. The infiltrate assumes a nodular disposition within the dermis without epidermotropism. The lymphocytes are small to medium in size with an open chromatin and small basophilic nucleoli; nuclear contours exhibit irregular lobations. There is discrete pericellular clearing seemingly separating adjacent lymphocytes from one another. A significant large cell populace is not seen. A polymorphous inflammatory cell infiltrate is not seen.

Phenotypic Studies

The cells are CD8 positive and show positive staining for cytotoxic proteins including granzyme, TIA, and perforin. The neoplastic cells express beta F1 and CD45RO. CD45RA and CD11 c are negative. Significant reductions in CD7 are noted. CD5 may also be diminished.

Clonality Studies

T-cell clonality is a characteristic finding (219,220).

Treatment

Concerning treatment, local radiotherapy or surgery has been shown to be effective in preventing recurrence in the majority of indolent CD8-positive lymphoid proliferation cases (219,220).

Differential Diagnosis

Over and above the aggressive lymphomas already considered, the differential diagnosis is primarily with a pseudolymphoma. The classic CD8-positive pseudolymphoma is one associated with underlying human immunodeficiency virus infection. In pseudolymphoma, the B-cell component is characteristically in the context of well-formed germinal centers as opposed to singly disposed or small clusters of post–germinal center B cells as noted in other reported cases of the entity. However, it is worth emphasizing that clonality is not the *sine que non* of malignancy. Nevertheless, polyclonality is more common in the pseudolymphoma setting. In the same vein, while reactive infiltrates are most characteristically without significant phenotypic aberrations, some loss of CD7 has been described in reactive infiltrates; in certain cases especially those associated with immune dysregulatory drug therapy, the CD7 reduction can be substantial. Pseudolymphoma tends to reflect an overzealous response to various antigenic triggers in the setting of iatrogenic and endogenous immune dysregulation. Hence, a very critical aspect in the evaluation of such infiltrates is the clinical history in regard to immune status of the patient, drug history, and any possible inciting trigger such as an arthropod insult.

SUBCUTANEOUS PANNICULITIS-LIKE T-CELL LYMPHOMA

Clinical Features

Subcutaneous panniculitis-like T-cell lymphoma is a primary form of CTCL that shows dominant localization within the fat. It has a predilection for females in the third to fourth decades of life although pediatric cases have been described (222). This condition exhibits many overlapping features with lupus profundus (223–225). We postulated that the basis of the similarities might reflect a pathogenic commonality with both conditions representing forms of panniculitic T-cell dyscrasia (223). There are indeed recent reports of combined features of dermatomyositis or lupus erythematosus with subcutaneous panniculitis-like T-cell lymphoma, suggesting an underlying systemic connective tissue disease diathesis as a potential

precursor event (225,226). According to the WHO-EORTC classification of lymphoma the neoplastic cells of subcutaneous panniculitis-like T-cell lymphoma are of the alpha beta subset (227). Those subcutaneous lymphomas comprising cells of the gamma delta subset are categorized as primary cutaneous gamma delta T-cell lymphoma despite many overlapping features clinically and pathologically with the classic alpha beta variant (224,228). The basis for this separation was suggested by virtue of the more aggressive clinical course associated with gamma delta forms of subcutaneous panniculitis-like T-cell lymphoma (214,229). However, a more indolent course can be observed in the setting of gamma delta T-cell lymphoma, which therefore questions the validity of this separation (230).

In both lupus profundus and subcutaneous panniculitis-like T-cell lymphoma, there is an unusual predilection to involve the thigh and proximal arms, and as well, there is a female preponderance. As is often the case in the setting of lupus erythematosus, exacerbation of the disease by pregnancy has been documented. Connective tissue disease-like symptoms such as fever, anorexia, and leucopenia are frequent. Pathologically subcutaneous panniculitis-like T-cell lymphoma shares with lupus profundus infiltration of the fat lobule by a pleomorphic and polymorphous lymphoid populace, karyorrhexis, phagocytosis of debris by histiocytes, fat necrosis, vascular thrombosis, and a lymphomatoid vascular reaction (223). In this regard, it is not surprising then that many patients with subcutaneous panniculitis-like T-cell lymphoma are initially diagnosed with lupus profundus. Patients with subcutaneous panniculitis-like T-cell lymphoma untreated will die while those treated can achieve remission. Those who die succumb to HPS, either initially or after several years rather than one related to extracutaneous dissemination. Due to the inherent cytopenia associated with HPS, the terminal event is typically one of bacterial or fungal sepsis (231,232).

Extracutaneous dissemination is very uncommon and usually occurs late in the disease course. While the natural history is indeed aggressive, most patients respond to combination chemotherapy (233,234). The lymphoma remains largely confined to the subcutaneous fat; however, systemic stigmata can occur including cytopenias and fever due to neoplastic cytokine-driven macrophage activation (235).

Pathogenesis

Both local and systemic macrophage activation are a cardinal manifestation of subcutaneous panniculitis-like T-cell lymphoma. The basis of the hemophagocytosis is the production of a phagocytosis-inducing factor by neoplastic T lymphocytes. The main microbial pathogens implicated in nonneoplastic HPS are EBV, adenovirus, and herpes virus (236). While some patients with subcutaneous panniculitis-like T-cell lymphoma present very acutely, other patients report a waxing and waning course of several years before being diagnosed with subcutaneous panniculitis-like T-cell lymphoma. It is likely that such patients have a preneoplastic indeterminate lymphocytic panniculitis during this initial phase of their disease falling under the designation of atypical lymphocytic lobular panniculitis (223,237).

Histology

Histomorphologically biopsies of subcutaneous panniculitis-like T-cell lymphoma exhibit a variable admixture of pleomorphic small, medium, and/or large lymphocytes and histiocytes infiltrating the subcutis in a lobular pattern. Erythrophagocytosis is a frequent finding although the degree with which this phenomenon is observed is variable. In some instances it can be striking while in other cases erythrocyte phagocytosis is quite scarce although discernible after careful analysis.

Karyorrhexis and necrosis within the fat lobule is present in most cases. The necrosis is in the context of adipocyte necrosis as well necrosis of the neoplastic lymphocytes (228). Accelerated apoptosis driven by the cytokine milieu along with ischemic changes induced by the vasculopathy are likely integral factors in the pathogenesis of the necrosis.

The cells exhibit pleomorphic nuclear contours with many cells showing irregular nuclear blebs and polylobated nuclear contours. Striking vasculopathic changes are observed and range from a pauci-inflammatory thrombogenic vasculopathy to one characterized by prominent lymphocytic angioinvasion with variable mural and luminal fibrin deposition within vessels. One of the characteristic hallmarks is apparent colonization of the adipocyte by lymphocytes. The lymphocytes are internalized within the adipocyte that imparts an effect that is referred to as adipocyte rimming (personal observations). Our own studies have show disruption of the adipocyte membrane with true internalization of lymphocytes to assume an internal disposition. There is typically extension into the overlying dermis whereby the dominant infiltrate is localized primarily to the eccrine coil. The degree of adventitial dermal infiltration can be striking. Throughout the dermis there is a subtle single-cell infiltrate of histiocytes accompanied by an increase in hyaluronic acid. The cells have abundant cytoplasm and may contain erythrocytes (214,224,228).

There is usually a low-density epitheliotropic infiltrate of atypical lymphocytes within the epidermis. However, a grenz of relatively uninvolved papillary and superficial reticular dermis is seen. Phenotypic studies have shown that intraepidermal lymphoid populace is likely neoplastic based on the dominant CD8 lymphoid populace within the epidermis.

An additional distinctive feature of subcutaneous panniculitis-like T-cell lymphoma is the presence of large polyhedral macrophages with abundant eosinophilic cytoplasm unaccompanied by other inflammatory cells exhibiting a single-cell pattern of infiltration amidst a mucinous dermis and within the septa of the fat.

The most important morphologic clues, which serve to distinguish subcutaneous panniculitis-like T-cell lymphoma from lupus profundus, include erythrocyte phagocytosis and the absence of a destructive atrophying interface dermatitis with hyperkeratosis; dermal mucin deposition is not a discriminating feature as this phenomenon can be observed in both disorders.

Phenotype

Immunophenotypically primary subcutaneous panniculitis-like T-cell lymphoma frequently are found to express a CD3⁺CD8⁺ phenotype along with cytotoxic proteins such as granzyme B, T-cell intracellular antigen 1 (TIA-1), and perforin (224,228). The cells frequently manifest a deletion of CD5 and CD7 with variable diminution in CD3 expression. The mature counterpart is a cytotoxic CD8 T cell. The prominent tissue necrosis probably results from the cytotoxic properties of the tumor cells. Tumor cell apoptosis is also characteristic and likely reflects the enhanced and constitutive expression of the Fas ligand (FasL), a member of the TNF family. The ki67 proliferation index is intermediate to high. The neoplastic cells typically exhibit positivity for CCL5; the natural ligand for CCL5 is CCR5. CCR5 is naturally expressed by adipocytes and may account for the inherent tropism of the lymphocytes for the fat (24). Cutaneous lymphocyte antigen is either negative or only weakly expressed (238).

Molecular Studies

The cases will show a T-cell receptor gene rearrangement. There is no compelling evidence, which points toward a role of EBV genome in the propagation of lesions of subcutaneous T-cell lymphoma (228).

Differential Diagnosis

Two other conditions morphologically resembling subcutaneous panniculitis-like T-cell lymphoma are atypical lymphocytic lobular panniculitis and lupus profundus (223). With respect to atypical lymphocytic lobular panniculitis, I consider this entity a form of panniculitic T-cell dyscrasia that may correspond to the waxing and waning phase that frequently is observed in subcutaneous panniculitis-like T-cell lymphoma. Atypical lymphocytic lobular panniculitis shares with subcutaneous panniculitic-like T-cell lymphoma lymphocytic infiltration of the fat lobule, lymphoid atypia, erythrocyte phagocytosis, variable CD5 and CD7 deletion, increased numbers of CD8 lymphocytes, and clonality. However, distinguishing clinical features from panniculitic T-cell lymphoma include the lack of any constitutional symptoms, the tendency for spontaneous resolution, and the absence of cytopenia while light microscopically the density of infiltration, cytologic atypia, and erythrocyte phagocytosis is less and necrosis is typically absent (223,237).

With respect to lupus profundus, this condition also presents with waxing and waning plaques and nodules involving the proximal extremities; however, either there are overlying skin changes diagnostic of lupus erythematosus or the patient has a known history of lupus erythematosus. Useful discriminating light microscopic features include an atrophying interface dermatitis, plasmacellular infiltration, germinal centers within the fat, a positive lupus band test, the absence of red cell phagocytosis, and a dominance of CD4 lymphocytes over those of the CD8 subset (223). A deletion of CD5 or CD7 and clonality can be seen in lupus profundus although not to the magnitude of that observed in subcutaneous panniculitis-like T-cell lymphoma (223). We find two additional immunohistochemical stains helpful, namely, MXA and CCL5 (24). MXA is strongly upregulated in biopsies of lupus profundus and is not expressed significantly in the setting of subcutaneous panniculitis-like T-cell lymphoma (238). CCL5 is extensively positive in the neoplastic cells of subcutaneous panniculitis-like T-cell lymphoma while CCL5 expression is expressed at significantly lower levels in the setting of subcutaneous panniculitis-like T-cell lymphoma (239).

Not all lymphomas showing subcutaneous localization represent subcutaneous panniculitis like T-cell lymphoma. Other forms of peripheral T- cell lymphoma can exhibit a panniculitic presentation. For example, a small cell variant of ALCL localized to the fat has been described and as well I have encountered rare tumor-stage presentations of MF predominantly involving the subcutaneous fat (240).

In any case of subcutaneous panniculitis-like T-cell lymphoma appropriate phenotypic studies are necessary to exclude gamma delta T-cell lymphoma involving the subcutaneous fat. The clinical presentation and light microscopic findings are essentially identical although constitutional symptoms, more pronounced cytopenias, and features of HPS would be more commonly observed n the setting of gamma delta T-cell lymphoma. Phenotypically the cells do not express beta F1, there is no significant staining for CD4 and CD8, and CD56 positivity is frequent (224).

NK/T-Cell Lymphoma

The NK and NK-like T-cell (i.e., collectively now designated as NK/T-cell) lymphomas are aggressive lymphomas with a propensity to involve extra nodal sites including the gastrointestinal tract, skin, and nasal cavities. The 5-year survival rate is 30%. Bone marrow involvement at initial presentation is uncommon. The nasal variant results in lethal midline destruction and is associated with EBV infection. It is more common in men and range of ages affected is in the fifth through seventh decades of life. Subsequent dissemination to the skin is common with other sites of involvement including gastrointestinal tract, testis, and cervical lymph nodes. The angiocentricity of the neoplasm results in tissue destruction manifesting as facial destruction, cutaneous ulceration, and intestinal perforation. The clinical course may be complicated by HPS (191,241–254).

In the nonnasal category, the main categories of lymphoma are nasal type, aggressive, and blastoid. *Nasal type* is a confusing term as it suggests an initial presentation in the sinonasal region when in fact this tumor does not present initially in the sinonasal area, but instead in extranasal sites. However, from a morphologic perspective the lesions resemble nasal NK/T-cell lymphoma (207,242–248). Aggressive NK/T-cell lymphoma does not involve the skin; bone marrow, peripheral blood, and lymph node involvement are common. Blastoid NK lymphoma is a tumor of plasmacytoid dendritic cells and will be considered separately under the topic of CD4⁺ CD56⁺ hematodermic neoplasm (193,247,248).

EBV is implicated in true NK lymphomas particularly among patients of Asiatic extraction as opposed to the infrequency with which EBV is detected in the setting of the closely related NK-like T-cell lymphomas. The prognosis is very guarded with many patients succumbing to disease within 12 months of initial presentation. There may be preceding chronic peripheral blood NK cell lymphocytosis associated with neutropenia (250).

Light Microscopic Findings

The infiltrates are dense and assume a variably angiocentric and effacing pattern within the dermis. The angiocentric nature of the infiltrate results in vascular compromise including frank vasculitic changes as revealed by mural and/or luminal fibrin deposition. Ischemic alterations primarily in the context of ulceration are usually seen. From a cytomorphologic perspective, the cells are intermediate in size and show nuclear contour irregularity but characteristically do not exhibit the cerebriform morphology typical of MF. The cells appear hyperchromatic largely attributable to nuclear membrane thickening. Nucleoli are deeply basophilic in quality. There may be discernible rims of eosinophilic cytoplasm (246).

Phenotypic Profile

NK- like T cells perform a similar function to the NK cells and share with true NK cells CD56 and cytoplasmic CD3 positivity; however, they demonstrate a rearrangement of the TCR and express CD3 on the surface.

Both NK cells and NK-like cytotoxic T lymphocytes are phenotypically mature lymphocytes whose cytoplasmic granules contain cytotoxic proteins that are capable of mediating cellular lysis *in vitro*. Among the cytolytic proteins are perforin (cytolysin), granzyme, and Fas ligand (CD95L) and TIA-1 (191,242,255). Lymphomas that manifest surface CD3 expression and TCRβ or gamma gene rearrangement are considered to represent NK-like T-cell lymphomas. The NK and NK-like T-cell lymphomas typically do not express either CD4 or CD8 (191,242–248).

CD30-NEGATIVE LARGE CELL T-CELL LYMPHOMA

An important subset of peripheral T-cell lymphoma is CD30-negative large cell T-cell lymphoma. Unlike the CD30⁺ counterpart, this tumor is associated with a poor prognosis. The 5-year survival is <10%. The aggressive nature of this tumor

with its natural tendency toward extracutaneous dissemination is unclear. A further category of this lymphoma is one associated with positivity for CD20. B-cell lineage infidelity is a curious finding that is not limited to CD30-negative large cell T-cell lymphoma but has also been described in MF (256).

The prognosis in CD30-negative large cell T-cell lymphoma is grim regardless of its presentation as a solitary lesion or one exhibiting multifocal cutaneous disease. There is a male to female ratio of 2.5 to 1 with a median age of 68 years. The overall 5-year survival is 24% with patients dying of complications related to disseminated disease (197, 257–261).

Light Microscopic Findings

In the study by Bekkenk et al. the infiltrates could be diffuse, nodular, and/or bandlike with pronounced epidermotropism being observed in 27% of cases. In a minority of cases folliculotropism can be observed; angiocentricity with angiodestruction is very uncommon, being a more frequent observation in the setting of the smaller cell counterpart (i.e., primary cutaneous pleomorphic small/medium-sized T-cell lymphoma). Pronounced epidermotropism was noted in 27% of cases (197). Although there may be reactive and/or smaller neoplastic cellular elements at least 30% of the infiltrate is one comprising large neoplastic lymphocytes. The large atypical cells are in the 15- to 20-μm size range and exhibit variable hyperchromasia albeit they do not exhibit a cerebriform morphology. In one study, cytomorphology was most characteristically pleomorphic with less common morphologic expressions being in the context of a monomorphic immunoblastic cytology and rarely one resembling ALCL. There is typically a paucity of other inflammatory cells with a relative dearth of plasma cells and eosinophils.

Phenotypic Studies

There is a mixture of T and B cells although with a clear-cut dominance of T cells. There are no germinal centers highlighted by markers such as Bcl6 and CD10. An important finding is an aberrant phenotype characterized by variable losses of CD5, CD7, and CD2. A reduction of CD2 with a relative preservation of CD7 can be observed. This expanded phenotypic expression includes a profile that may potentially mimic that encountered in T lymphocytes at an earlier stage of differentiation. This concept is best exemplified by those postthymic T-cell lymphomas that express CD10 and/or in which there may be dual expression of CD4 and CD8 or an absence of CD4 and CD8 expression, hence mimicking the profile of a cortical thymocyte (257–261). The CD30 stain is negative although rare cells might express CD30.

PRIMARY CUTANEOUS GAMMA DELTA T-CELL LYMPHOMA

Gamma delta T-cell lymphoma represents an uncommon form of primary CTCL, representing <1% of all forms of CTCL. There are no known predisposing factors. Unlike MF, there is no long waxing and waning phase (217,218,262). This lymphoma is considered an aggressive lymphoma; the survival at 5 years is <5% although ablative chemotherapy and allogenic stem cell transplantation may induce remission and possibly enhance disease-free survival. The presentation may be in the context of solitary or multiple plaques and nodules associated with variable ulceration. There are two primary morphologic variants. One is characterized by striking epidermotropism resembling the pattern of epitheliotropic growth that one can observe in MF although typically accompanied by significant dermal involvement with marked angiotropism. In this variant of gamma delta T-cell lymphoma, rapid dissemination to extracutaneous sites is seen, although lymph node, spleen and bone marrow involvement is uncommon (218). Such cases have also fallen under the alternative designation of disseminated pagetoid reticulosis (263). The other demonstrates dominant localization to the subcutaneous fat whereby the morphology is indistinguishable from that seen with the alpha beta CD8 variant of subcutaneous panniculitis-like T-cell lymphoma.

The differential diagnosis of gamma delta T-cell lymphoma includes other atypical lymphocytic infiltrates that can be composed of gamma delta T cells. For example, there are rare cases of double-negative MF whereby the defining neoplastic cell is a gamma delta T cell. The clinical course, however, would be typical for MF, comprising waxing and waning patches and plaques primarily involving photoprotected areas of the skin. The rash has typically been present for years before the patient is biopsied. The subcutaneous presentation of gamma delta T-cell lymphoma cannot be distinguished from subcutaneous panniculitis-like T-cell lymphoma and the distinction really rests on the phenotypic profile. As well, there is considerable clinical and pathologic overlap with lupus profundus, a reactive lymphocytic lobular panniculitis in the setting of lupus erythematosus. Distinguishing features light microscopically separating gamma delta T-cell lymphoma from lupus profundus are discussed below; we have found MXA and CCL5 immunostains to be of value diagnostically in cases of lymphomatoid panniculitis (264).

While many primary cutaneous gamma delta T-cell lymphomas follow an aggressive clinical course, there is literature precedent indicative of a clinical course that is less fulminant (221,264,265). This concept is perhaps best exemplified by gamma delta variants of MF, which do not appear to follow a more aggressive clinical course compared to the more common form of MF comprising cells of the alpha beta subset (128). One must make the distinction from other forms of epidermotropic gamma delta T-cell lymphoma that can be aggressive. In one study by Salhany et al. (224) of 11 cases reported, two were of the gamma delta subtype and both died of their disease within 3 to 25 months. In a comprehensive study addressing SPTCL, Willemze et al. (214) examined clinicopathologic features, immunophenotype, treatment, and survival in 63 alpha beta and 20 gamma delta forms of SPTCL at a workshop of the EORTC Cutaneous Lymphoma Group. The alpha beta form was generally confined to the subcutis, had a CD4⁻, CD8⁺, CD56⁻, βF1⁺ phenotype, was uncommonly associated with a HPS (17%), and had a favorable prognosis (5-year OS: 82%). Patients with this variant of SPTCL without HPS had a significantly better survival than patients with HPS (5-year OS: 91% vs. 46%; $P < 0.001$). The gamma delta form often showed epidermal involvement and/or ulceration, a CD4⁻, CD8⁻, CD56⁺/⁻, βF1⁻ T-cell phenotype, and poor prognosis (5-year OS: 11%), irrespective of the presence of HPS or type of treatment. These results indicate that the alpha beta versus gamma delta forms of SPTCL are distinct entities, and justify that the term SPTCL should further be used only for the alpha beta variant. However, in that same series, 3 out of 14 patients with gamma delta form of SPTCL treated with multiagent chemotherapy achieved complete remission. One patient unresponsive to chemotherapy reached complete remission following an allo stem cell transplant. Among the responsive patients, two were still in complete remission at 38 and 108 months after initial diagnosis at the end of follow-up. In addition, there is one prior report of a patient with a 15-year history of panniculitis (230). Following several years of indolent behavior, the disease underwent an aggressive turn and she was diagnosed with

gamma delta T-cell lymphoma. We have recently reported a series of patients with gamma delta T-cell lymphoma exhibiting dominant subcutaneous localization in which the clinical course was more indolent with all patients alive after 5 years from the initial presentation (266). We have seen three cases of subcutaneous gamma delta T-cell lymphoma in which an earlier waxing and waning phase compatible with atypical lymphocytic lobular panniculitis was observed. All three cases had striking dermal mucin deposition leading to an initial erroneous diagnosis of lupus profundus. In all three cases, the cytologic atypia was minimal although the phenotypic profile was identical to subsequent biopsies that demonstrated changes of fully evolved gamma delta T-cell lymphoma (266).

Light Microscopic Findings

As already mentioned, there are two main morphologic forms of gamma delta T-cell lymphoma of the skin, namely, one characterized by prominent epidermotropism and another one showing dominant subcutaneous localization. With respect to the epidermotropic variant, the cells infiltrating the epidermis are atypical but without a classic cerebriform morphology that typifies MF. A more acute epidermal reaction characterized by spongiosis and serum-imbued parakeratosis can be observed. In fact, such features could be misleading and suggest a reactive eczematous process. A reproducible finding is one of an atypical angiocentric lymphocytic infiltrate. Atypical lymphocytes surround and permeate vessels of the superficial and deep dermis. There may be frank vasculitis with mural and luminal fibrin deposition and associated ischemic alterations of the epidermis. The neoplastic cells are quite large with an activated morphology oftentimes in the 15-μm size range. The cells appear hyperchromatic with thick nuclear membranes and prominent basophilic nucleoli. A cerebriform morphology is not identified. The laminated pattern of fibrosis typical for plaque and patch-stage MF is not seen.

The other main morphologic expression of gamma delta T-cell lymphoma is in the context of a lymphomatoid panniculitis. Discriminating light microscopic features separating panniculitis-like T-cell lymphoma from lupus profundus include erythrocyte phagocytosis and the absence of a destructive atrophying interface dermatitis and true cell necrosis accompanied by striking apoptotic debris as opposed to the mucinous hyaline-like acellular degeneration observed in the subcutaneous as in cases of LP. Dermal mucin deposition *per se* is not a useful morphologic criterion. Cases of SPTCL can exhibit dermal and subcuticular mucin deposition (267). Gamma delta T-cell lymphoma showing subcutaneous localization can exhibit very striking pan dermal mucin deposition. The "bean bag histiocyte" is seen with great regularity in both panniculitis-like T-cell lymphoma and lupus profundus, and reflects the phagocytosis of cellular debris (268) (Fig. 29.30A–D).

Phenotypic Studies

From a phenotypic perspective, the cells are double-negative for CD4 and CD8. The cells express CD56 and also cytotoxic proteins granzyme and Tia-1 (Figs. 29.31 and 29.32). We have also found that strong expression of MXA, an interferon alpha marker, is characteristically upregulated within biopsies of lupus profundus while significant MXA staining is not seen and/or is significantly less in the setting of gamma delta T-cell lymphoma (238). CCL5 is strongly expressed within the cytoplasm of the neoplastic lymphocytes and may account for the adipotropism given its known ligand being CCR5 expressed on adipocytes (24).

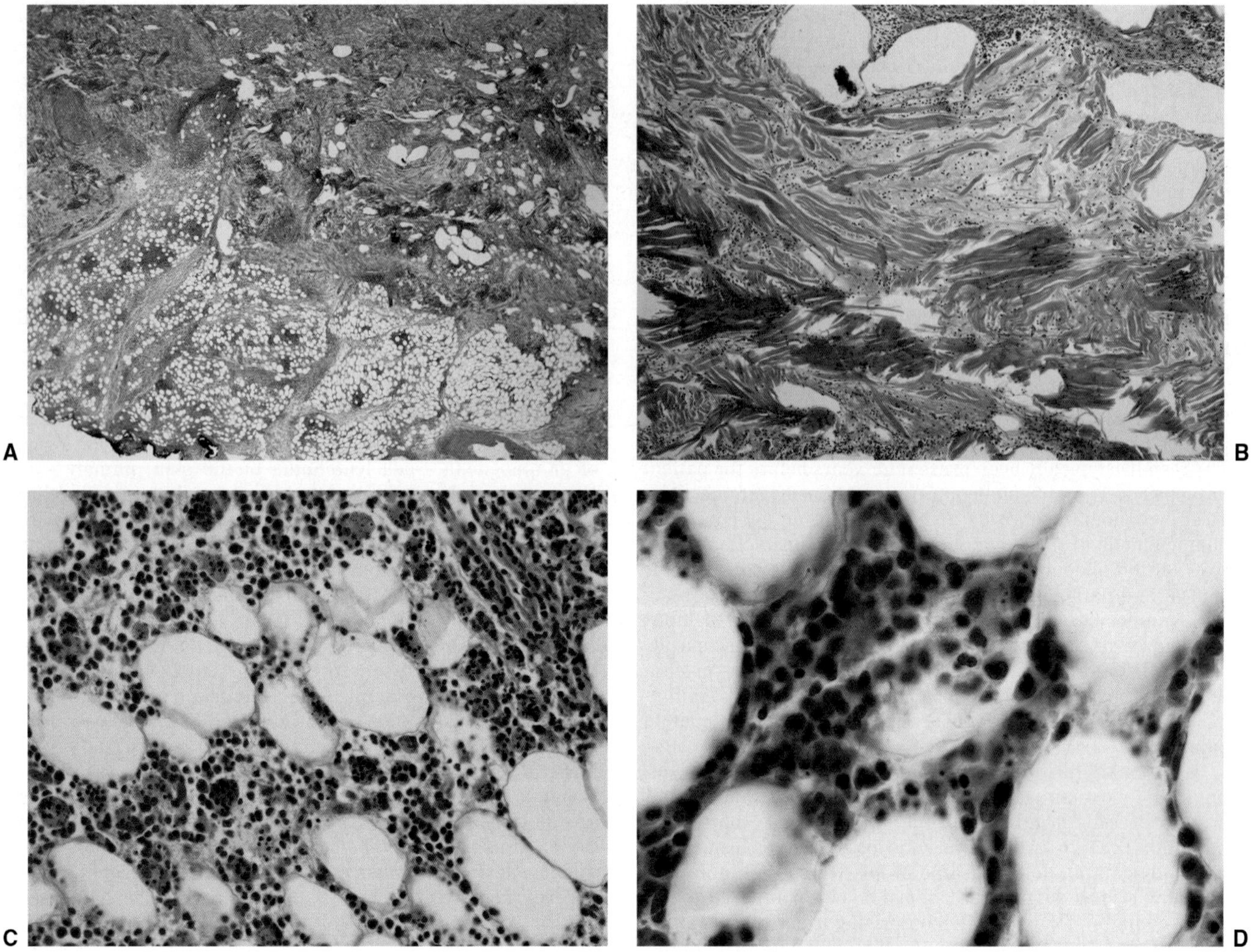

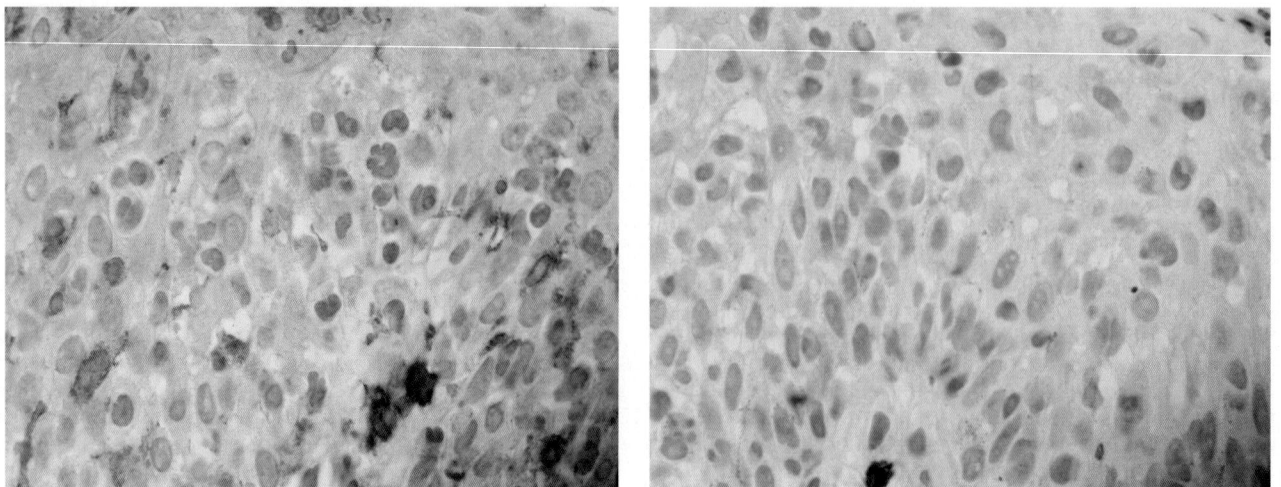

FIGURE 29.30. A: The biopsy shows a deep dermal and subcutaneous nodular and diffuse lymphocytic infiltrate. The nodular disposition in the dermis is attributable to accentuation of infiltration of neoplastic lymphocytes around the eccrine coil. This low-power architecture is a characteristic one for subcutaneous panniculitis-like T-cell lymphoma (hematoxylin and eosin, magnification: 40×). **B:** A characteristic feature in subcutaneous panniculitis-like T-cell lymphoma is dermal mucin with infiltration of the interstitium by activated-appearing macrophages. Extensive dermal mucin deposition can lead to a misdiagnosis of lupus profundus (hematoxylin and eosin, magnification: 100×). **C:** The macrophages show very striking engulfment of nuclear debris. In panniculitis-like T-cell lymphoma there is both enhanced apoptosis of neoplastic cells and prominent macrophage activation (hematoxylin and eosin, magnification: 200×). **D:** The tropism of the lymphocytes for the adipocyte leads to disruption of the adipocyte membrane with colonization of the adipocyte by neoplastic T cells (hematoxylin and eosin, magnification: 1,000×).

FIGURE 29.31. A: In this case of primary cutaneous epidermotropic gamma delta T-cell lymphoma, the neoplastic cells do not express CD4 (diaminobenzidine, magnification: 1,000×). **B:** The neoplastic cells are CD8 negative (diaminobenzidine, magnification: 1,000×).

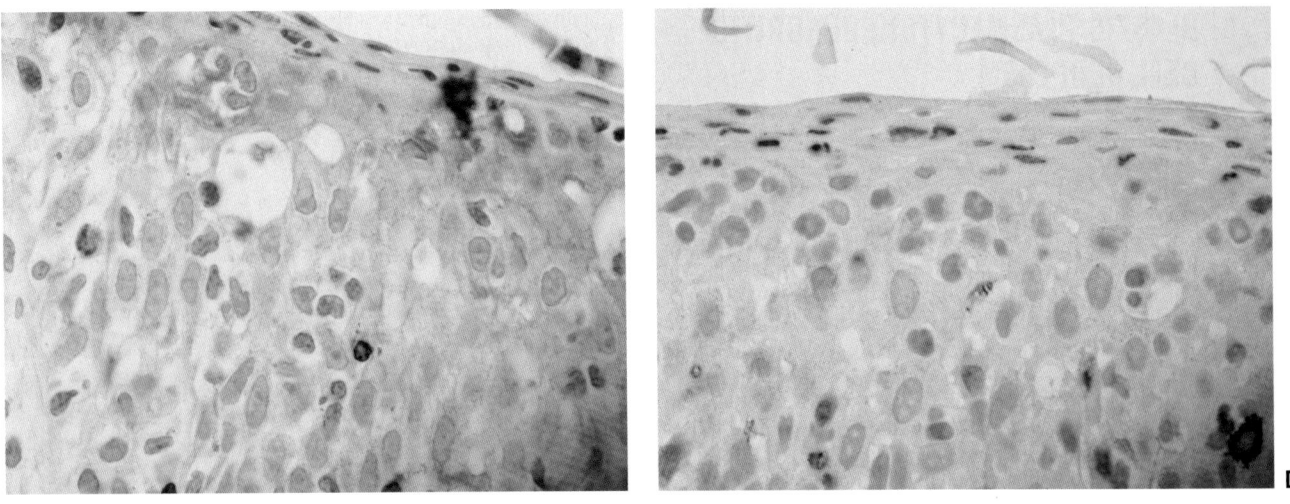

FIGURE 29.31. *(Continued)* **C:** The neoplastic cell populace does not show immunoreactivity for beta F1 (diaminobenzidine, magnification: 1,000×). **D:** In more aggressive CTCLs, a loss of CD5 is common (diaminobenzidine, magnification: 1,000×).

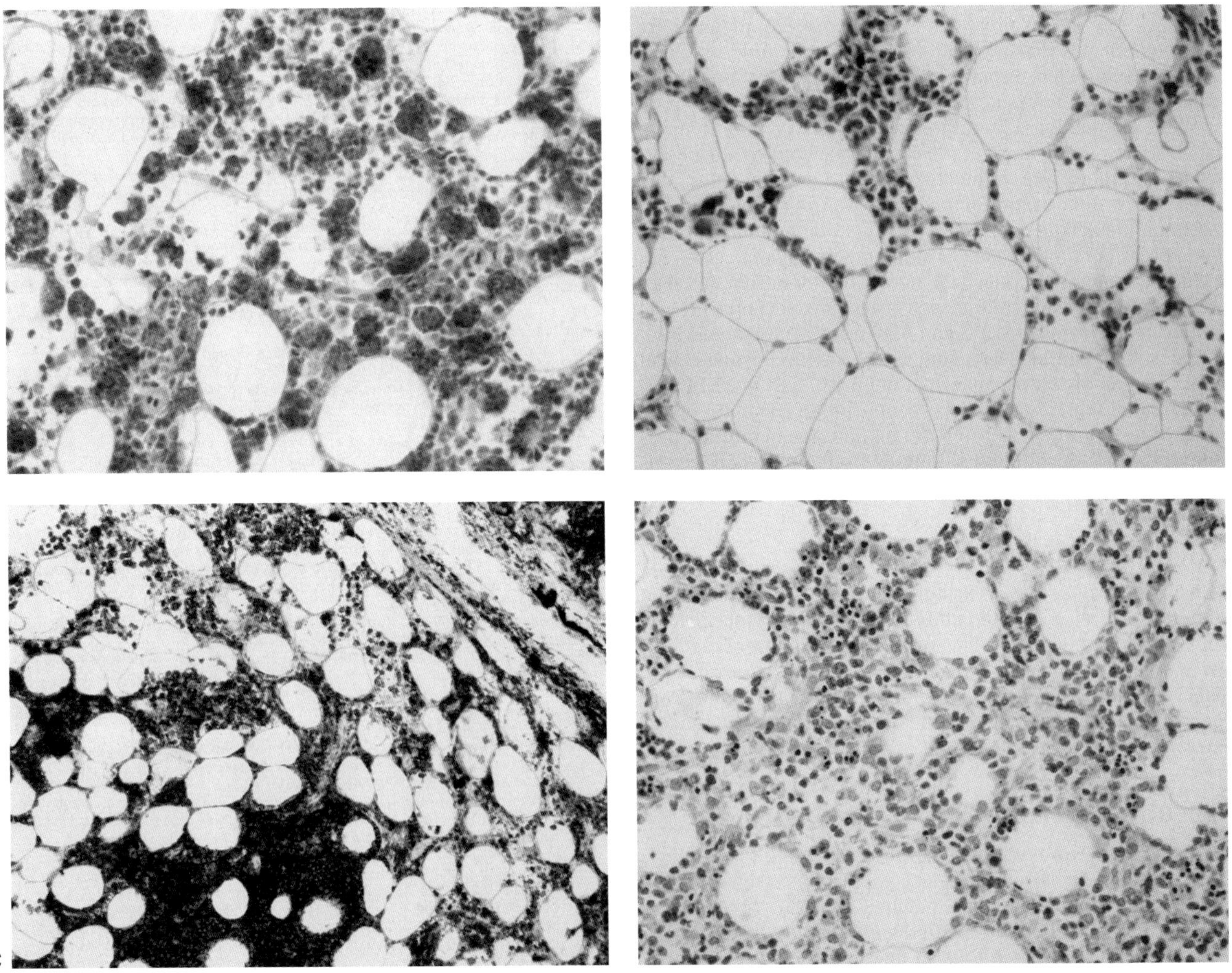

FIGURE 29.32. **A:** The lymphocytes are negative for CD4 (diaminobenzidine, magnification: 200×). **B:** The lymphocytes are negative for CD8 (diaminobenzidine, magnification: 200×). **C:** The lymphocytes are extensively positive for CD56 (diaminobenzidine, magnification: 200×). **D:** The lymphocytes are beta F1 negative (diaminobenzidine, magnification: 200×).

BLASTIC PLASMACYTOID DENDRITIC CELL NEOPLASM

In the original classification scheme, there was a distinctive CD56+ NK neoplasm phenotypically different from the other reported NK and NK-like T-cell lymphomas based on its CD4 positivity. This tumor fell under the designation of blastic NK-like T- cell lymphoma. In the revised World Health Organiza-tion-European Organization for Research and Treatment of Cancer (WHO-EORTC) classification, blastic NK-cell lymphoma was considered a clinically aggressive T-cell neoplasm; skin involvement typically occurred concurrently with leukemic dis-semination (255). A blastic cytomorphology and expression of CD56 were held to be evidence of an NK-precursor cell origin. The designation of this neoplasm as CD4+CD56+ hematoder-mic neoplasm was by Kato and coworkers in 2001 although it was not until 2002 when a plasmacytoid dendritic cell origin for this neoplasm was proposed (247). Consequently the term blastic NK-like T-cell lymphoma was supplanted by the term CD4+CD56+ hematodermic neoplasm and now more recently blastic plasmacytoid dendritic cell neoplasm (247,269), and has more recently been renamed as blastic plasmcytoid den-dritic cell neoplasm (270). In those neoplasms categorized as true NK lymphomas, there is a frequent association with EBV, especially in Asian patients with nasopharyngeal involvement (241,271); EBV has not been pathogenetically implicated in blastic plasmacytoid dendritic cell neoplasm. Most patients die within 12 months of initial presentation. Elderly patients are characteristically affected, and there is a male predominance (193). Disseminated disease is common involving peripheral blood and lymph nodes and bone marrow.

While the dominant literature addressing CD4+CD56+ malig-nancies is in the context of blastic plasmcytoid dendritic cell neoplasm, there are other hematologic malignancies that may express this particular phenotypic profile including MF, ALCL, and leukemia cutis (193). It should be emphasized that the expression of other pan T-cell markers, however, does not exclude a diagnosis of blastic plasmacytoid dendritic cell neo-plasm. In particular while blastic plasmacytoid dendritic cell neoplasms are typically CD2 and CD7 negative, CD7 and focal CD2 positivity can be seen. The classic immunohistochemical stains for identifying plasmacytoid dendritic cells are BDCA-2, CD123, and TCL1. CD123 represents the alpha chain of the interleukin-3 receptor. This 60- to 70-kDa transmembrane pro-tein binds to IL-3 with low affinity by itself, and when associ-ated with CD131 (common β chain) binds IL-3 with high affinity.

Light Microscopic Findings

Biopsies typically show a striking effacing nonepitheliotropic mononuclear cell infiltrate exhibiting variable angiocentricity. The cells have a lymphoid-like appearance and are of medium size (i.e., in the 9-μm size range). The chromatin is more finely dispersed than in a mature lymphocyte. The cells demonstrate conspicuous nucleoli. In foci of angiocentric infiltration, red cell extravasation is observed (193).

Phenotypic Profile

The infiltrate expresses CD4 CD56+ and CD123+. As well, there is positivity for cutaneous lymphocyte antigen. Other markers that may be positive include CD2, CD7, MxA, CD83, and TCL1. The cells do not express granzyme and TIA. TCR clonality studies revealed a germ line configuration and/or a polyclonal T-cell population (193). Markers of myeloid differ-entiation including CD11c, lysozyme, myeloperoxidase, CD14, and CD68 are negative (193). A few cases of purported blastic

plasmacytoid dendritic cell neoplasm do not express CD4. The vast majority of cases reported in the literature, however, describe CD4 staining (272).

References

1. Rijlaarsdam JU, Willemze R. Cutaneous pseudolymphomas: classification and differential diagnosis.*Semin Dermatol* 1994;13:187–196.
2. Burg G, Braun Falco O, Hoffmann-Fezer Schmoeckel C. Differentiation between pseudolymphomas and malignant B-cell lymphomas of the skin. In: Goos M, Christophers E, eds. *Lymphoproliferative diseases of the skin*. Berlin: Springer Verlag, 1982:101–134.
3. Askew FC, Greer KE, Legum LL. Lymphomatoid papulosis and other pseudoma-lignancies of the skin. *South Med J* 1977;70(1):57–61.
4. van Vloten WA, Willemze R. The many faces of lymphocytoma cutis. *J Eur Acad Dermatol Venereol* 2003;17(1):3–6.
5. Kojima M, Sakurai S, Shimizu K, et al. B-cell cutaneous lymphoid hyperplasia representing progressive transformation of germinal center: a report of 2 cases. *Int J Surg Pathol* 2010;18(5):429–432.
6. Magro CM, Crowson AN. Drug-induced immune dysregulation as a cause of atypical cutaneous lymphoid infiltrates: a hypothesis. *Hum Pathol* 1996;27(2):125–132.
7. Magro C. The expression of CD23 and CD40 in primary cutaneous B-cell lympho-mas. *J Cutan Pathol* 2007;34(6):461–466.
8. Rodríguez Pinilla SM, Roncador G, Rodríguez-Peralto JL, et al. Primary cutane-ous CD4+ small/medium-sized pleomorphic T- cell lymphoma expresses follicular T-cell markers. *Am J Surg Pathol* 2009;33(1):81–90.
9. Arai E, Shimizu M, Hirose T. A review of 55 cases of cutaneous lymphoid hyper-plasia: reassessment of the histopathologic findings leading to reclassification of 4 lesions as cutaneous marginal zone lymphoma and 19 as pseudolymphomatous folliculitis. *Hum Pathol* 2005;36(5):505–511
10. Magro C, Crowson AN, Porcu P, et al. Automated kappa and lambda light chain mRNA expression for the assessment of B-cell clonality in cutaneous B-cell infil-trates: its utility and diagnostic application. *J Cutan Pathol* 2003;30(8):504–511.
11. Guitart J, Gerami P. Is there a cutaneous variant of marginal zone hyperplasia? *Am J Dermatopathol* 2008;30(5):494–496.
12. Crowson AN, Magro CM. Antidepressant therapy. A possible cause of atypical cutaneous lymphoid hyperplasia. *Arch Dermatol* 1995;131(8):925–929.
13. Magro CM, Crowson AN. Drugs with antihistaminic properties as a cause of atyp-ical cutaneous lymphoid hyperplasia. *J Am Acad Dermatol* 1995;32(3):419–428.
14. Magro CM, Schaefer JT. T and B cell clonally restricted pseudolymphoma in the setting of phytoestrogen therapy. *J Eur Acad Dermatol Venerol* 2008;22:642–643.
15. Magro CM, Crowson AN, Kovatich AJ, et al. Drug-induced reversible lymphoid dyscrasia: a clonal lymphomatoid dermatitis of memory and activated T cells. *Hum Pathol* 2003;34(2):119–129.
16. Brady SP, Magro CM, Diaz-Cano SJ, et al. Analysis of clonality of atypical cutane-ous lymphoid infiltrates associated with drug therapy by PCR/DGGE. *Hum Pathol* 1999;30:130–136.
17. Gitelson E, Al-Saleem T, Robu V, et al. Pediatric nodal marginal zone lymphoma may develop in the adult population. *Leuk Lymphoma* 2010;51(1):89–94.
18. Magro CM, Nuovo GJ, Crowson AN. The utility of the in situ detection of T-cell receptor Beta rearrangements in cutaneous T-cell-dominant infiltrates. *Diagn Mol Pathol* 2003;12:133–141.
19. Cacoub P, Musette P, Descamps V, et al. The DRESS syndrome: a literature review. *Am J Med* 2011;124(7):588–597.
20. Mardivirin L, Valeyrie-Allanore L, Branlant-Redon E, et al. Amoxicillin-induced flare in patients with DRESS (Drug Reaction with Eosinophilia and Systemic Symptoms): report of seven cases and demonstration of a direct effect of amoxi-cillin on Human Herpesvirus 6 replication in vitro. *Eur J Dermatol* 2010;20(1):68–73.
21. Muche JM, Toppe E, Sterry W, et al. Palpable arciform migratory erythema in an HIV patient, a CD8+ pseudolymphoma. *J Cutan Pathol* 2004;31(5):379–382.
22. Bachelez H, Hadida F, Parizot C, et al. Oligoclonal expansion of HIV-specific cyto-toxic CD8 T lymphocytes in the skin of HIV-1-infected patients with cutaneous pseudolymphoma. *J Clin Invest* 1998;101(11):2506–2516.
23. Werner B, Massone C, Kerl H, et al. Large CD30-positive cells in benign, atypical lymphoid infiltrates of the skin. *J Cutan Pathol* 2008;35(12):1100–1107.
24. Hoefnagel JJ, Vermeer MH, Jansen PM, et al. Primary cutaneous marginal zone B-cell lymphoma: clinical and therapeutic features in 50 cases. *Arch Dermatol* 2005;141(9):1139–1145.
25. Willemze R, Jaffe ES, Burg G, et al. WHO-EORTC classification for cutaneous lymphomas. *Blood* 2005;105(10):3768–3785.
26. Cho-Vega JH, Vega F, Rassidakis G, et al. Primary cutaneous marginal zone B-cell lymphoma. *Am J Clin Pathol* 2006;125(Suppl):S38–S49.
27. Magro CM, Yang A, Fraga G. Blastic marginal zone lymphoma: a clinical and pathological study of 8 cases and review of the literature. *Am J Dermatopathol* 2013;35(3):319–326.
28. Bailey E, Ferry J, Harris N, et al. Marginal zone lymphoma (Low-grade B cell lymphoma of mucosa-associated lymphoid tissue type) of skin and subcutaneous tissue. *Am J Surg Pathol* 1996;20(8):1011–1023.
29. Cerroni L, Signoretti S, Höfler G, et al. Primary cutaneous marginal zone B-cell lymphoma: a recently described entity of low-grade malignant cutaneous B-cell lymphoma. *Am J Surg Pathol* 1997;21(11):1307–1315.
30. Magro CM, Porcu P, Ahmad N, et al. Cutaneous immunocytoma: a clinical, his-tologic, and phenotypic study of 11 cases. *Appl Immunohistochem Mol Morphol* 2004;12(3):216–224.
31. Breza TS Jr, Zheng P, Porcu P, et al. Cutaneous marginal zone B-cell lym-phoma in the setting of fluoxetine therapy: a hypothesis regarding pathogenesis based on in vitro suppression of T-cell-proliferative response. *J Cutan Pathol* 2006;33(7):522–528.
32. Sroa N, Magro CM. Pediatric primary cutaneous marginal zone lymphoma: in association with chronic antihistamine use. *J Cutan Pathol* 2006;33(Suppl 2):1–5.
33. Cerroni L, Zihling N, Ptz B, et al. Infection by *Borrelia burgdorferi* and cutaneous B-cell lymphoma. *J Cutan Pathol* 1997;24:457–461.

34. Silvestri F, Barillari G, Fanin R, et al. Hepatitis C virus infection among cryoglobulinemic and non-cryoglobulinemic B-cell non-Hodgkin's lymphomas. *Haematologica* 1997;82(3):314–317.
35. Fitzhugh VA, Siegel D, Bhattacharyya PK. Multiple primary cutaneous plasmacytomas [Review]. *J Clin Pathol* 2008;61(6):782–783.
36. Verma S, Nuovo GJ, Porcu P, et al. Epstein-Barr virus- and human herpesvirus 8-associated primary cutaneous plasmablastic lymphoma in the setting of renal transplantation. *J Cutan Pathol* 2005;32(1):35–39.
37. Cerroni L, Kerl H. Primary cutaneous follicle center cell lymphoma. *Leuk Lymphoma* 2001;42(5):891–900.
38. Cerroni L, Kerl H. Cutaneous follicle center cell lymphoma, follicular type. *Am J Dermatopathol* 2001;23(4):370–373.
39. Franco R, Fernandez-Vazquez A, Rodriguez-Peralto JL, et al. Cutaneous follicular B-cell lymphoma: description of a series of 18 cases. *Am J Surg Pathol* 2001;25(7):875–883.
40. Naresh KN. MUM1 expression dichotomises follicular lymphoma into predominantly, MUM1-negative low-grade and MUM1-positive high-grade subtypes. *Haematologica* 2007;92(2):267–26.
41. Vermeer MH, Geelen FA, van Haselen CW, et al. Primary cutaneous large B-cell lymphomas of the legs. A distinct type of cutaneous B-cell lymphoma with an intermediate prognosis. Dutch Cutaneous Lymphoma Working Group. *Arch Dermatol* 1996;132(11):1304–1308.
42. Grange F, Bekkenk MW, Wechsler J, et al. Prognostic factors in primary cutaneous large B-cell lymphomas: a European multicenter study. *J Clin Oncol* 2001;19(16):3602–3610.
43. Grange F, Petrella T, Beylot-Barry M, et al. Bcl-2 protein expression is the strongest independent prognostic factor of survival in primary cutaneous large B-cell lymphomas. *Blood* 2004;103:3662–3668.
44. Fernandez-Vazquez A, Rodriguez-Peralto JL, Martinez MA, et al. Primary cutaneous large B-cell lymphoma: the relation between morphology, clinical presentation, immunohistochemical markers, and survival. *Am J Surg Pathol* 2001;25:307–315.
45. Brogan BL, Zic JA, Kinney MC, et al. Large B-cell lymphoma of the leg: clinical and pathologic characteristics in a North American series. *J Am Acad Dermatol* 2003;49(2):223–238.
46. Kamath NV, Gilliam AC, Nihal M, et al. Primary cutaneous large B-cell lymphoma of the leg relapsing as cutaneous intravascular large B-cell lymphoma. *Arch Dermatol* 2001;137(12):1657–1658.
47. Koens L, Vermeer MH, Willemze R, et al. IgM expression on paraffin sections distinguishes primary cutaneous large B-cell lymphoma, leg type from primary cutaneous follicle center lymphoma. *Am J Surg Pathol* 2010;34(7):1043–108.
48. Hembury TA, Lee B, Gascoyne RD, et al. Primary cutaneous diffuse large B-cell lymphoma: a clinicopathologic study of 15 cases. *Am J Clin Pathol* 2002;117(4):574–580.
49. Hoefnagel JJ, Vermeer MH, Jansen PM, et al. Bcl-2, Bcl-6 and CD10 expression in cutaneous B-cell lymphoma: further support for a follicle centre cell origin and differential diagnostic significance. *Br J Dermatol* 2003;149(6):1183–1191.
50. Magro CM, Nash JW, Werling RW, Porcu P, Crowson N. Primary cutaneous CD30+ large cell B-cell lymphoma: a series of 10 cases. *Appl Immunohistochem Mol Morphol* 2006;14(1):7–11.
51. Wiesner T, Streubel B, Huber D, et al. Genetic aberrations in primary cutaneous large B-cell lymphoma: a fluorescence in situ hybridization study of 25 cases. *Am J Surg Pathol* 2005;29(5):666–673.
52. Sánchez-Beato M, Sáez AI, Navas IC, et al. Overall survival in aggressive B-cell lymphomas is dependent on the accumulation of alterations in p53, p16, and p27. *Am J Pathol* 2001;159(1):205–213.
53. Senff NJ, Zoutman WH, Vermeer MH, et al. Fine-mapping chromosomal loss at 9p21: correlation with prognosis in primary cutaneous diffuse large B-cell lymphoma, leg type. *J Invest Dermatol* 2009;129(5):1149–1155.
54. Wiesner T, Obenauf AC, Geigl JB, et al. 9p21 deletion in primary cutaneous large B-cell lymphoma, leg type, may escape detection by standard FISH assays. *J Invest Dermatol* 2009;129(1):238–240.
55. Kaune KM, Neumann C, Hallermann C, et al. Simultaneous aberrations of single CDKN2A network components and a high Rb phosphorylation status can differentiate subgroups of primary cutaneous B-cell lymphomas. *Exp Dermatol* 2011;20(4):331–335.
56. Belaud-Rotureau MA, Marietta V, Vergier B, et al. Inactivation of p16INK4a/CDKN2A gene may be a diagnostic feature of large B cell lymphoma leg type among cutaneous B cell lymphomas. *Virchows Arch* 2008;452(6):607–620.
57. Paulli M, Viglio A, Vivenza D, et al. Primary cutaneous large B-cell lymphoma of the leg: histogenetic analysis of a controversial clinicopathologic entity. *Hum Pathol* 2002;33(9):937–943.
58. Hoefnagel JJ, Dijkman R, Basso K, et al. Distinct types of primary cutaneous large B-cell lymphoma identified by gene expression profiling. *Blood* 2005;105(9):3671–3678.
59. Beljaards RC, Van Beek P, Willemze R. Relation between expression of adhesion molecules and clinical behavior in cutaneous follicle center cell lymphomas. *J Am Acad Dermatol* 1997;37(1):34–40.
60. Pham-Ledard A, Prochazkova-Carlotti M, Vergier B, et al. IRF4 expression without IRF4 rearrangement is a general feature of primary cutaneous diffuse large B-cell lymphoma, leg type. *J Invest Dermatol* 2010;130(5):1470–1472.
61. Dommann SN, Dommann-Scherrer CC, Ziegler T, et al. Expression of intercellular adhesion molecule 3 (CDw50) on endothelial cells in cutaneous lymphomas. A comparative study between nodal and cutaneous lymphomas. *Am J Dermatopathol* 1997;19(4):391–395.
62. Lair G, Parant E, Tessier MH, et al. Primary cutaneous B-cell lymphomas of the lower limbs: a study of integrin expression in 11 cases. *Acta Derm Venereol* 2000;80(5):367–369.
63. Willemze R, Meijer CJ, Scheffer E, et al. Diffuse large cell lymphomas of follicular center cell origin presenting in the skin. A clinicopathologic and immunologic study of 16 patients. *Am J Pathol* 1987;126(2):325–333.
64. Wick MR, Rocamora A. Reactive and malignant "angioendotheliomatosis": a discriminant clinicopathological study. *J Cutan Pathol* 1988;15(5):260–271.
65. Erös N, Károlyi Z, Kovács A, et al. Intravascular B-cell lymphoma. *J Am Acad Dermatol* 2002;47(5 Suppl):S260–S262.
66. Chakravarty K, Goyal M, Scott DG, et al. Malignant 'angioendotheliomatosis'—(intravascular lymphomatosis) an unusual cutaneous lymphoma in rheumatoid arthritis. *Br J Rheumatol* 1993;32(10):932–934.
67. Ozguroglu E, Buyulbabani N, Ozguroglu M, et al. Generalized telangiectasia as the major manifestation of angiotropic (intravascular) lymphoma. *Br J Dermatol* 1997;137(3):422–425.
68. Suh CH, Kim SK, Shin DH, et al. Intravascular lymphomatosis of the T cell type presenting as interstitial lung disease—a case report. *J Korean Med Sci* 1997;12(5):457–460.
69. Rubin MA, Cossman J, Freter CE, et al. Intravascular large cell lymphoma coexisting within hemangiomas of the skin. *Am J Surg Pathol* 1997;21(7):860–864.
70. Smith ME, Stamatakos MD, Neuhauser TS. Intravascular lymphomatosis presenting within angiolipomas. *Ann Diagn Pathol* 2001;5(2):103–106.
71. Panzoni M, Arrigoni G, Gould VE, et al. Lack of CD 29 (beta1 integrin) and CD 54 (ICAM-1) adhesion molecules in intravascular lymphomatosis. *Hum Pathol* 2000;31(2):220–226.
72. Khalidi HS, Brynes RK, Browne P, et al. Intravascular large B-cell lymphoma: the CD5 antigen is expressed by a subset of cases. *Mod Pathol* 1998;11(10):983–988.
73. Khandelwal A, Seilstad KH, Magro CM. Subclinical chronic lymphocytic leukaemia associated with a 13q deletion presenting initially in the skin: apropos of a case. *J Cutan Pathol* 2006;33(3):256–259.
74. Kaddu S, Smolle J, Cerroni L, et al. Prognostic evaluation of specific cutaneous infiltrates in B-chronic lymphocytic leukemia. *J Cutan Pathol* 1996;23(6):487–494.
75. Wang C, Amato D, Fernandes B. CD5-negative phenotype of monoclonal B-lymphocytosis of undetermined significance (MLUS). *Am J Hematol* 2002;69(2):147–149.
76. Mulligan CS, Thomas ME, Mulligan SP. Monoclonal B-lymphocytosis: demographics, nature and subclassification in 414 community patients. *Leuk Lymphoma* 2011;52(12):2293–2298.
77. Starostik P, O'Brien S, Ching-Yang C, et al. The prognostic significance of 13q14 deletions in chronic lymphocytic leukemia. *Leuk Res* 1993;23:795.
78. Oguz O, Engin B, Demirkesen C. Primary cutaneous CD30-positive large B-cell lymphoma associated with Epstein-Barr virus. *Int J Dermatol* 2003;42(9):718–720.
79. Alibert JL. Description des maladies de la peau. Observees a l'hopital St. Louis et exposition des meilleures methodes suivries pour leur traitement. Paris: Barrois L'Aine & Fils, 1806:167.
80. Clendenning WE, Brecher G, Vanscott EJ. Mycosis fungoides. Relationship to malignant cutaneous reticulosis and the S'ezary syndrome. *Arch Dermatol* 1964;89:785–792.
81. Zucker-Franklin D. Properties of the Sezary lymphoid cell. An ultrastructural analysis. *Mayo Clin Proc* 1974;49(8):567–574.
82. Sawada Y, Sugita K, Kabashima R, et al. CD8+ CD56+ mycosis fungoides with an indolent clinical behaviour: case report and literature review. *Acta Derm Venereol* 2010;90(5):525–526.
83. Horst BA, Kasper R, LeBoit PE. CD4+, CD56+ mycosis fungoides: case report and review of the literature. *Am J Dermatopathol* 2009;31(1):74–76.
84. Zinzani PL, Ferreri AJ, Cerroni L. Mycosis fungoides. *Crit Rev Oncol Hematol* 2008;65(2):172–182.
85. Arulogun SO, Prince HM, Ng J, et al. Long-term outcomes of patients with advanced-stage cutaneous T-cell lymphoma and large cell transformation. *Blood* 2008 15;112(8):3082–3087.
86. Garzon M. Cutaneous T cell lymphoma in children. *Semin Cutan Med Surg* 1999;18:226–232.
87. Pope E, Weitzman S, Ngan B, et al. Mycosis fungoides in the pediatric population: report from an international Childhood Registry of Cutaneous Lymphoma. *J Cutan Med Surg* 2010;14(1):1–6.
88. Ngo JT, Trotter MJ, Haber RM. Juvenile-onset hypopigmented mycosis fungoides mimicking vitiligo. *J Cutan Med Surg* 2009;13(4):230–233.
89. Guitart J, Magro C. Cutaneous T-cell lymphoid dyscrasia: a unifying term foridiopathic chronic dermatoses with persistent T-cell clones. *Arch Dermatol* 2007;143(7):921–932. Review.
90. Quaglino P, Zaccagna A, Verrone A et al. Mycosis fungoides in patients under 20 years of age: Report of 7 cases, Review of the literature and study of the clinical course. *Dermatology* 1999;199:8–14.
91. Glusac EJ, Shapiro PE, McNiff JM. Cutaneous T-cell lymphoma. Refinement in the application of controversial histologic criteria [Review]. *Dermatol Clin* 1999;17(3):601–614, ix.
92. Shapiro PE, Pinto FJ. The histologic spectrum of mycosis fungoides/Sézary syndrome (cutaneous T-cell lymphoma). A review of 222 biopsies, including newly described patterns and the earliest pathologic changes. *Am J Surg Pathol* 1994;18(7):645–667.
93. Magro CM, Crowson AN, Mihm MC. *The Cutaneous Lymphoid Proliferation: a comprehensive text book of lymphocytic infiltrates*. New York: John Wiley & Sons, 2007.
94. Smoller BR, Bishop K, Glusac E, et al. Reassessment of histologic parameters in the diagnosis of mycosis fungoides. *Am J Surg Pathol* 1995;19(12):1423–1430.
95. Lindae ML, Abel EA, Hoppe RT, et al. Poikilodermatous mycosis fungoides and atrophic large-plaque parapsoriasis exhibit similar abnormalities of T-cell antigen expression. *Arch Dermatol* 1988;124:366–372.
96. Ormsby A, Bergfeld WF, Tubbs RR, et al. Evaluation of a new paraffin-reactive CD7 T-cell deletion marker and a polymerase chain reaction–based T-cell receptor gene rearrangement assay: implications for diagnosis of mycosis fungoides in community clinical practice. *J Am Acad Dermatol* 2001;45:405–413.
97. Bakels V, van Oostveen JW, van der Putte SC, et al. Immunophenotyping and gene rearrangement analysis provide additional criteria to differentiate between cutaneous T-cell lymphomas and pseudo-T-cell lymphomas. *Am J Pathol* 1997;150:1941–1949.
98. Vermeer M, Geelen F, Kummer J, et al. Expression of cytotoxic proteins by neoplastic T cells in mycosis fungoides increases with progression from plaque stage to tumor stage disease. *Am J Pathol* 1999;154;1203–1209.
99. Simonitsch I, Volc-Platzer B, Mosberger I, et al. Expression of monoclonal antibody HML-1-defined alpha E beta 7 integrin in cutaneous T cell lymphoma. *Am J Pathol* 1994;145(5):1148–1158.
100. Jones D, Dang NH, Duvic M, et al. Absence of CD26 expression is a useful marker for diagnosis of T-cell lymphoma in peripheral blood. *Am J Clin Pathol* 2001;115(6):885–892.
101. Xu C, Tang Y, Wang L, et al. [Significance of TCR gene clonal rearrangement analysis in diagnosis of mycosis fungoides]. *Zhonghua Zhong Liu Za Zhi* 2010;32(9):685–689.

102. Guitart J, Camisa C, Ehrlich M, et al. Long-term implications of T-cell receptor gene rearrangement analysis by Southern blot in patients with cutaneous T-cell lymphoma. *J Am Acad Dermatol* 2003;48(5):775–779.
103. Lessin SR, Vowels BR, Rook AH. Retroviruses and cutaneous T-cell lymphomas. *Dermatol Clin* 1994;112:243–253.
104. Yamaguchi T, Ohshima K, Tsuchiya T, et al. The comparison of expression of cutaneous lymphocyte-associated antigen (CLA), and Th1- and Th2-associated antigens in mycosis fungoides and cutaneous lesions of adult T-cell leukemia/lymphoma. *Eur J Dermatol* 2003;13(6):553–559.
105. Papadavid E, Economidou J, Psarra A, et al. The relevance of peripheral blood T-helper 1 and 2 cytokine pattern in the evaluation of patients with mycosis fungoides and Sézary syndrome. *Br J Dermatol* 2003;148(4):709–718.
106. Savvateeva MV, Savina MI, Markusheva LI, et al. Relative content of cytokines in different tissues in mycosis fungoides. *Bull Exp Biol Med* 2002;134(2):175–176.
107. Wu XS, Lonsdorf AS, Hwang ST. Cutaneous T-cell lymphoma: roles for chemokines and chemokine receptors. *J Invest Dermatol* 2009;129(5):1115–1119.
108. Kallinich T, Muche JM, Qin S, et al. Chemokine receptor expression on neoplastic and reactive T cells in the skin at different stages of mycosis fungoides. *J Invest Dermatol* 2003;121(5):1045–102.
109. Agar NS, Wedgeworth E, Crichton S, et al. Survival outcomes and prognostic factors in mycosis fungoides/Sézary syndrome: validation of the revised International Society for Cutaneous Lymphomas/European Organisation for Research and Treatment of Cancer staging proposal. *J Clin Oncol* 2010;28(31):4730–4739.
110. Gilliam AC, Lessin SR, Wilson DM, et al. Folliculotropic mycosis fungoides with large-cell transformation presenting as dissecting cellulitis of the scalp. *J Cutan Pathol* 1997;24(3):169–175.
111. Pereyo NG, Requena L, Galloway J, et al. Follicular mycosis fungoides: a clinicohistopathologic study. *J Am Acad Dermatol* 1997;36(4):563–568.
112. Lehman JS, Cook-Norris RH, Weed BR, et al. Folliculotropic mycosis fungoides: single-center study and systematic review. *Arch Dermatol* 2010;146(6):607–613.
113. Pileri A, Facchetti F, Rütten A, et al. Syringotropic mycosis fungoides: a rare variant of the disease with peculiar clinicopathologic features. *Am J Surg Pathol* 2011;35(1):100–109.
114. Lichte V, Ghoreschi K, Metzler G, et al. Pagetoid reticulosis (Woringer-Kolopp disease). *J Dtsch Dermatol Ges* 2009;7(4):353–354.
115. Crowson AN, Magro CM. Woringer-Kolopp disease. A lymphomatoid hypersensitivity reaction. *Am J Dermatopathol* 1994;16(5):542–548.
116. Sedghizadeh PP, Allen CM, Kalmar JR, et al. Pagetoid reticulosis: a case report and review of the literature. *Oral Surg Oral Med Oral Pathol Oral Radiol Endod* 2003;95:318–323.
117. Skiljevic D, Bogdanovic Z, Vesic S, et al. Pagetoid reticulosis of Woringer-Kolopp. *Dermatol Online J* 2008;14(1):18.
118. Zengin AY, Topkan E, Cimsit G, et al. Woringer-Kolopp disease coexpressing CD4 and CD8 treated with radiation therapy: a case report. *Tumori* 2008;94(5):754–757.
119. Matsuzaki Y, Kimura K, Nakano H, et al. Localized pagetoid reticulosis (Woringer-Kolopp disease) in early childhood. *J Am Acad Dermatol* 2009;61(1):120–123.
120. Gorpelioglu C, Sarifakioglu E, Haltas H. Spider bite-induced pagetoid reticulosis? *J Eur Acad Dermatol Venereol* 2009;23(4):446–447.
121. Haghighi B, Smoller BR, LeBoit PE, et al. Pagetoid reticulosis (Woringer-Kolopp disease): an immunophenotypic, molecular, and clinicopathologic study. *Mod Pathol* 2000;13(5):502–510.
122. Kempf W, Ostheeren-Michaelis S, Paulli M, et al.; Cutaneous Lymphoma Histopathology Task Force Group of the European Organization for Research and Treatment of Cancer. Granulomatous mycosis fungoides and granulomatous slack skin: a multicenter study of the Cutaneous Lymphoma Histopathology Task Force Group of the European Organization For Research and Treatment of Cancer (EORTC). *Arch Dermatol* 2008;144(12):1609–1617.
123. Magro CM, Crowson AN, Schapiro BL. The interstitial granulomatous drug reaction: a distinctive clinical and pathological entity. *J Cutan Pathol* 1998;25:72–78.
124. Magro CM, Cruz-Inigo AE, Votava H, et al. Drug-associated reversible granulomatous T cell dyscrasia: a distinct subset of the interstitial granulomatous drug reaction. *J Cutan Pathol* 2010;37 (Suppl 1):96–111.
125. Ferrara G, Crisman G, Zalaudek I, et al. Free-floating collagen fibers in interstitial mycosis fungoides. *Am J Dermatopathol* 2010;32(4):352–356.
126. Shimauchi T, Kabashima K, Tokura Y. CXCR3 and CCR4 double positive tumor cells in granulomatous mycosis fungoides. *J Am Acad Dermatol* 2006;54(6):1109–1111.
127. Martorell-Calatayud A, Botella-Estrada R, Sanmartín-Jimenez O, et al. Papular mycosis fungoides: two new cases of a recently described clinicopathological variant of early mycosis fungoides. *J Cutan Pathol* 2010;37(3):330–335.
128. Guitart J, Peduto M, Caro WA, et al. Lichenoid changes in mycosis fungoides. *J Am Acad Dermatol* 1997;36(3 Pt 1):417–422.
129. Bittencourt AL, Mota K, Oliveira RF, et al. A dyshidrosis-like variant of adult T-cell leukemia/lymphoma with clinicopathological aspects of mycosis fungoides. A case report. *Am J Dermatopathol* 2009;31(8):834–837.
130. Barnhill RL, Braverman IM. Progression of pigmented purpura-like eruptions to mycosis fungoides: report of three cases. *J Am Acad Dermatol* 1988;19(1 Pt 1):25–31.
131. Lipsker D. The pigmented and purpuric dermatitis and the many faces of mycosis fungoides. *Dermatology* 2003;207(3):246–247.
132. El-Shabrawi-Caelen L, Cerroni L, Medeiros LJ, et al. Hypopigmented mycosis fungoides: frequent expression of a CD8+ T-cell phenotype. *Am J Surg Pathol* 2002;26(4):450–457.
133. Magro CM, Schaefer JT, Crowson AN, et al. Pigmented purpuric dermatosis: classification by phenotypic and molecular profiles. *Am J Clin Pathol* 2007;128(2):218–229.
134. Toro JR, Sander CA, LeBoit PE. Persistent pigmented purpuric dermatitis and mycosis fungoides: simulant, precursor, or both? A study by light microscopy and molecular methods. *Am J Dermatopathol* 1997;19(2):108–118.
135. Fierro MT, Novelli M, Savoia P, et al. CD45RA+ immunophenotype in mycosis fungoides: clinical, histological and immunophenotypical features in 22 patients. *J Cutan Pathol* 2001;28(7):356–362.
136. Vonderheid EC, Bernengo MG, Burg G, et al.; ISCL. Update on erythrodermic cutaneous T-cell lymphoma: report of the International Society for Cutaneous Lymphomas. *J Am Acad Dermatol* 2002;46(1):95–106.
137. Hwang ST, Janik JE, Jaffe ES, et al. Mycosis fungoides and Sézary syndrome. *Lancet* 2008;371:945–957.
138. Hutchinson CB, Stoecker M, Wang FF, et al. Molecular detection of circulating Sezary cells in patients with mycosis fungoides: Could it predict future development of secondary Sezary syndrome? A single institution experience. *Leuk Lymphoma* 2012;53:868–877.
139. Hoppe RT, Wood GS, Abel EA. Mycosis fungoides and the Sézary syndrome: pathology, staging, and treatment. *Curr Probl Cancer* 1990;14:293.
140. Clark RA. Regulation gone wrong; a subset of Sezary patients have malignant regulatory T cells. *J Invest Dermatol* 2009;129:2747–2750.
141. Vonderheid EC, Diamond LW, van Vloten WA, et al. Lymph node classification systems in cutaneous T-cell lymphoma. Evidence for the utility of the Working Formulation of Non-Hodgkin's Lymphomas for Clinical Usage. *Cancer* 1994;73:207.
142. Gardner JM, Evans KG, Musiek A, et al. Update on treatment of cutaneous T-cell lymphoma. *Curr Opin Oncol* 2009;21:131–137.
143. Kim EJ, Hess S, Richardson SK, et al. Immunopathogenesis and therapy of cutaneous T-cell lymphoma. *J Clin Invest* 2005;115:798–812.
144. Saed G, Fivenson DP, Naidu Y, et al. Mycosis fungoides exhibits a Th1-type cell-mediated cytokine profile whereas Sézary syndrome expresses a Th2-type profile. *J Invest Dermatol* 1994;103:29–33.
145. Wysocka M, Zaki MH, French LE, et al. Sézary syndrome patients demonstrate a defect in dendritic cell populations: effects of CD40 ligand and treatment with GM-CSF on dendritic cell numbers and the production of cytokines. *Blood* 2002;100:3287–3294.
146. Axelrod PI, Lorber B, Vonderheid EC. Infections complicating mycosis fungoides and Sézary syndrome. *JAMA* 1992;267:1354–1358.
147. Paulli M, Berti E, Rosso R, et al. CD30/Ki-1-positive lymphoproliferative disorders of the skin—clinicopathologic correlation and statistical analysis of 86 cases: a multicentric study from the European Organization for Research and Treatment of Cancer Cutaneous Lymphoma Project Group. *J Clin Oncol* 1995;13(6):1343–1354.
148. Kempf W. CD30+ lymphoproliferative disorders: histopathology, differential diagnosis, new variants, and simulators. *J Cutan Pathol* 2006;33(Suppl 1):58–70.
149. Granados S, Hwang ST. Roles for CD30 in the biology and treatment of CD30 lymphoproliferative diseases. *J Invest Dermatol* 2004;122(6):1345–1347.
150. Weiss LM, Movahed LA, Warnke RA, et al. Detection of Epstein-Barr viral genomes in Reed-Sternberg cells of Hodgkin's disease. *N Engl J Med* 1989;320(8):502–506.
151. Froese P, Lemke H, Gerdes J, et al. Biochemical characterization and biosynthesis of the Ki-1 antigen in Hodgkin-derived and virus-transformed human B and T lymphoid cell lines. *J Immunol* 1987;139(6):2081–2087
152. Gruss HJ, Ulrich D, Braddy S, et al. Recombinant CD30 ligand and CD40 ligand share common biological activities on Hodgkin and Reed-Sternberg cells. *Eur J Immunol* 1995;25(7):2083–2089.
153. Ralfkiaer E, Bosq J, Gatter KC, et al. Expression of a Hodgkin and Reed-Sternberg cell associated antigen (Ki-1) in cutaneous lymphoid infiltrates. *Arch Dermatol Res* 1987;279(5):285–292.
154. Macauley WL. In defense of lymphomatoid papulosis. *Arch Dermatol* 1971; 104(4):434.
155. Macauley WL. Lymphomatoid papulosis. *Am J Dermatopathol* 1980;2(1):93–94.
156. Borchmann P. CD30+ diseases: anaplastic large-cell lymphoma and lymphomatoid papulosis. *Cancer Treat Res* 2008;142:349–365. Review.
157. Kempf W, Pfaltz K, Vermeer MH, et al. EORTC, ISCL, and USCLC consensus recommendations for the treatment of primary cutaneous CD30-positive lymphoproliferative disorders: lymphomatoid papulosis and primary cutaneous anaplastic large-cell lymphoma. *Blood* 2011;118(15):4024–4035.
158. Crowson AN, Baschinsky DY, Kovatich A, et al. Granulomatous eccrinotropic lymphomatoid papulosis. *Am J Clin Pathol* 2003;119:731–739.
159. Willemze R, Scheffer E, Van Vloten W, et al. Lymphomatoid papulosis and Hodgkin's disease: are they related? *Arch Dermatol Res* 1982;275:159–167.
160. El Shabrawi-Caelen L, Kerl H, Cerroni L. Lymphomatoid papulosis: reappraisal of clinicopathologic presentation and classification into subtypes A, B, and C. *Arch Dermatol* 2004;140(4):441–447.
161. Cabanillas F, Armitage J, Pugh WC, et al. Lymphomatoid papulosis: a T-cell dyscrasia with a propensity to transform into malignant lymphoma. *Ann Intern Med* 1995;122(3):210–217.
162. Wang HH, Lach L, Kadin ME. Epidemiology of lymphomatoid papulosis. *Cancer* 1992;70(12):2951–2957.
163. Kadin M, Nasu K, Sako D, et al. Lymphomatoid papulosis. A cutaneous proliferation of activated helper T cells expressing Hodgkin's disease-associated antigens. *Am J Pathol* 1985;119(2):315–325.
164. Willemze R, Meijer CJ. Primary cutaneous CD30-positive lymphoproliferative disorders. *Hematol Oncol Clin North Am* 2003;17(6):1319–1332, vii–viii.
165. Beljaards RC, Willemze R. The prognosis of patients with lymphomatoid papulosis associated with malignant lymphomas. *Br J Dermatol* 1992;126(6):596–602.
166. Paulli M, Berti E, Rosso R, et al. CD30/Ki-1-positive lymphoproliferative disorders of the skin—clinicopathologic correlation and statistical analysis of 86 cases: a multicentric study from the European Organization for Research and Treatment of Cancer Cutaneous Lymphoma Project Group. *J Clin Oncol* 1995;13(6):1343–1354.
167. Wood GS, Stricker JG, Denea D, et al. Lymphomatoid papulosis expresses immunophenotypes associated with T cell lymphoma but not inflammation. *J Am Acad Dermatol* 1986;15:444–458.
168. Yamaguchi T, Ohshimia K, Karube K, et al. Expression of chemokines and chemokine receptors in cutaneous CD30+ lymphoproliferative disorders. *Br J Dermatol* 2006;904–909
169. Wada DA, Law ME, Hsi ED, et al. Specificity of IRF4 translocations for primary cutaneous anaplastic large cell lymphoma: a multicenter study of 204 skin biopsies. *Mod Pathol* 2011;24(4):596–605.
170. Wasco MJ, Fullen D, Su L, et al. The expression of MUM1 in cutaneous T-cell lymphoproliferative disorders. *Hum Pathol* 2008;39(4):557–563.
171. Hernandez-Machin B, de Misa RF, Montenegro T, et al. MUM1 expression does not differentiate primary cutaneous anaplastic large-cell lymphoma and lymphomatoid papulosis. *Br J Dermatol* 2009;160(3):713.
172. Suga H, Sugaya M, Sato S. C-C chemokine receptor type 3 expression in lymphomatoid papulosis, but not in mycosis fungoides lesions from the same patient. *Clin Exp Dermatol* 2012;37(1):75–77.
173. Vonderheid EC, Sajjadian A, Kadin ME. Methotrexate is effective therapy for lymphomatoid papulosis and other primary cutaneous CD30-positive lymphoproliferative disorders. *J Am Acad Dermatol* 1996;34(3):470–481.
174. Magro CM, Crowson AN, Morrison C, et al. CD8+ lymphomatoid papulosis and its differential diagnosis. *Am J Clin Pathol* 2006;125(4):490–501.
175. Saggini A, Gulia A, Argenyi Z, et al. A variant of lymphomatoid papulosis simulating primary cutaneous aggressive epidermotropic CD8+ cytotoxic T-cell lymphoma. Description of 9 cases. *Am J Surg Pathol* 2010;34(8):1168–1175.
176. Kempf W, Kazakov DV, Schärer L, et al. Angioinvasive lymphomatoid papulosis: a new variant simulating aggressive lymphomas. *Am J Surg Pathol* 2013;37(1): 1–13. doi: 10.1097/PAS.0b013e3182648596.

177. Stein H, Mason DY, Gerdes J, et al. The expression of the Hodgkin's disease associated antigen Ki-1 in reactive and neoplastic lymphoid tissue: evidence that Reed-Sternberg cells and histiocytic malignancies are derived from activated lymphoid cells. *Blood* 1985;66(4):848–858.
178. Diamantidis MD, Myrou AD. Perils and pitfalls regarding differential diagnosis and treatment of primary cutaneous anaplastic large-cell lymphoma. *Scientific World J* 2011;11:1048–1055.
179. Kinney MC, Collins RD, Greer JP, et al. A small-cell-predominant variant of primary Ki-1 (CD30)+ T-cell lymphoma. *Am J Surg Pathol* 1993;17(9):859–868.
180. Kaudewitz P, Stein H, Dallenbach F, et al. Primary and secondary cutaneous Ki-1+ (CD30+) anaplastic large cell lymphomas. Morphologic, immunohistologic, and clinical-characteristics. *Am J Pathol* 1989;135(2):359–367.
181. Demierre MF, Goldberg LJ, Kadin ME, et al. Is it lymphoma or lymphomatoid papulosis? *J Am Acad Dermatol* 1997;36(5 Pt 1):765–772.
182. Reams BD, McAdams HP, Howell DN, et al. Posttransplant lymphoproliferative disorder: incidence, presentation, and response to treatment in lung transplant recipients. *Chest* 2003;124(4):1242–1249.
183. Magro CM, Weinerman DJ, Porcu PL, et al. Post-transplant EBV negative anaplastic large cell lymphoma with dual rearrangement: a propos of two cases and review of the literature. *J Cutan Pathol* 2007;34(Suppl 1):1–8.
184. Knaus PI, Lindemann D, DeCoteau JF, et al. A dominant inhibitory mutant of the type II transforming growth factor beta receptor in the malignant progression of a cutaneous T-cell lymphoma. *Mol Cell Biol* 1996;16(7): 3480–3489.
185. Falini B. Anaplastic large cell lymphoma: pathological, molecular and clinical features. *Br J Haematol* 2001;114(4):741–760.
186. Pittaluga S, Wlodarska I, Pulford K, et al. The monoclonal antibody ALK1 identifies a distinct morphological subtype of anaplastic large cell lymphoma associated with 2p23/ALK rearrangements. *Am J Pathol* 1997;151(2): 343–351.
187. Stein H, Foss HD, Dürkop H, et al. CD30(+) anaplastic large cell lymphoma: a review of its histopathologic, genetic, and clinical features. *Blood* 2000;96(12): 3681–3695.
188. Chan JK, Buchanan R, Fletcher CD. Sarcomatoid variant of anaplastic large-cell Ki-1 lymphoma. *Am J Surg Pathol* 1990;14(10):983–938.
189. Laurent C, Do C, Gascoyne RD, et al. Anaplastic lymphoma kinase-positive diffuse large B-cell lymphoma: a rare clinicopathologic entity with poor prognosis. *J Clin Oncol* 2009;27(25):4211–4216.
190. Medeiros LJ, Elenitoba-Johnson KS. Anaplastic Large Cell Lymphoma. Am *J Clin Pathol* 2007;127(5):707–722.
191. Jaffe ES, Krenacs L, Raffeld M. Classification of T-cell and NK-cell neoplasms based on the REAL classification. *Ann Oncol* 1997;8(Suppl 2):17–24.
192. Suzuki R, Kagami Y, Takeuchi K, et al. Prognostic significance of CD56 expression for ALK-positive and ALK-negative anaplastic large-cell lymphoma of T/null cell phenotype. *Blood* 2000;96(9):2993–3000.
193. Magro CM, Porcu P, Schaefer J, et al. Cutaneous CD4+ CD56+ hematologic malignancies. *J Am Acad Dermatol* 2010;63(2):292–308.
194. Cetinözman F, Jansen PM, Willemze R. Expression of programmed death-1 in primary cutaneous CD4-positive small/medium-sized pleomorphic T-cell lymphoma, cutaneous pseudo-T-cell lymphoma, and other types of cutaneous T-cell lymphoma. *Am J Surg Pathol* 2012;36(1):109–116.
195. Baum CL, Link BK, Neppalli VT, et al. Reappraisal of the provisional entity primary cutaneous CD4+ small/medium pleomorphic T-cell lymphoma: a series of 10 adult and pediatric patients and review of the literature. *J Am Acad Dermatol* 2011;65(4):739–748.
196. Bekkenk MW, Vermeer MH, Jansen PM, et al. Peripheral T-cell lymphomas unspecified presenting in the skin: analysis of prognostic factors in a group of 82 patients. *Blood* 2003;102(6):2213–2219.
197. Montalbán C, Obeso G, Gallego A, et al. Peripheral T-cell lymphoma: a clinicopathological study of 41 cases and evaluation of the prognostic significance of the updated Kiel classification. *Histopathology* 1993;22(4):303–310.
198. Grogg KL, Jung S, Erickson LA, et al. Primary cutaneous CD4-positive small/medium-sized pleomorphic T-cell lymphoma: a clonal T-cell lymphoproliferative disorder with indolent behavior. *Mod Pathol* 2008;21(6):708–715.
199. Friedmann D, Wechsler J, Delfau MH, et al. Primary cutaneous pleomorphic small T-cell lymphoma. A review of 11 cases. The French Study Group of Cutaneous Lymphomas. *Arch Dermatol* 1995;131:1009–1015.
200. Petrella T, Maubec E, Cornillet-Lefebvre P, et al. Indolent CD8-positive lymphoid proliferation of the ear: a distinct primary cutaneous T-cell lymphoma? *Am J Surg Pathol* 2007;31(12):1887–1892.
201. Williams VL, Torres-Cabala CA, Duvic M. Primary cutaneous small- to medium-sized CD4+ pleomorphic T-cell lymphoma: a retrospective case series and review of the provisional cutaneous lymphoma category. *Am J Clin Dermatol* 2011;12:389–401.
202. Beltraminelli H, Leinweber B, Kerl H, et al. Primary cutaneous CD4+ small-/medium-sized pleomorphic T-cell lymphoma: a cutaneous nodular proliferation of pleomorphic T lymphocytes of undetermined significance? A study of 136 cases. *Am J Dermatopathol* 2009;31(4):317–322.
203. Scarabello A, Leinweber B, Ardigó M, et al. Cutaneous lymphomas with prominent granulomatous reaction. A potential pitfall in the histopathologic diagnosis of cutaneous T- and B-celllymphomas. *Am J Surg Pathol* 2002;26:1259–1268.
204. Gallardo F, García-Muret MP, Servitje O, et al. Cutaneous lymphomas showing prominent granulomatous component: clinicopathological features in a series of 16 cases. *J Eur Acad Dermatol Venereol* 2009;23(6):639–647.
205. Berti E, Tomasini D, Vermeer MH, et al. Primary cutaneous CD8-positive epidermotropic cytotoxic T cell lymphomas. A distinct clinicopathological entity with an aggressive clinical behavior. *Am J Pathol* 1999;155(2):483–492.
206. Gormley RH, Hess SD, Anand D, et al. Primary cutaneous aggressive epidermotropic CD8+ T-cell lymphoma. *J Am Acad Dermatol* 2010;62(2):300–307.
207. Santucci M, Pimpinelli N, Massi D, et al.; EORTC Cutaneous Lymphoma Task Force. Cytotoxic/natural killer cell cutaneous lymphomas. Report of EORTC Cutaneous Lymphoma Task Force Workshop. *Cancer* 2003;97(3):610–627.
208. Suchak R, O'Connor S, McNamara C, et al. Indolent CD8-positive lymphoid proliferation on the face: part of the spectrum of primary cutaneous small-/medium-sized pleomorphic T-cell lymphoma or a distinct entity? *J Cutan Pathol* 2010;37(9):977–981.
209. Fujiwara T, Abe Y, Kuyama M, et al. CD8 positive cutaneous T-cell lymphoma with pagetoid epidermotropism and angiocentric and angiodestructive infiltration. *Arch Dermatol* 1990;126:801–804.
210. Agnarsson B, Vonderheid E, Kadin M. Cutaneous T cell lymphoma suppressor/cytotoxic phenotype: identification of rapidly progressive and chronic subtypes. *J Am Acad Dermatol* 1990;22:569–577.
211. Magro CM, Dyrsen ME. Cutaneous lymphocyte antigen expression in benign and neoplastic cutaneous B- and T-cell lymphoid infiltrates. *J Cutan Pathol* 2008;35(11):1040–1049.
212. Diwan H, Ivan D. CD8-positive mycosis fungoides and primary cutaneous aggressive epidermotropic CD8-positive cytotoxic T-cell lymphoma. *J Cutan Pathol* 2009;36(3):390–392.
213. Nikolaou VA, Papadavid E, Katsambas A, et al. Clinical characteristics and course of CD8+ cytotoxic variant of mycosis fungoides: a case series of seven patients. *Br J Dermatol* 2009;161(4):826–830.
214. Willemze R, Jansen PM, Cerroni L, et al.; EORTC Cutaneous Lymphoma Group. Subcutaneous panniculitis-like T-cell lymphoma: definition, classification, and prognostic factors: an EORTC Cutaneous Lymphoma Group Study of 83 cases. *Blood* 2008;111(2):838–845.
215. Boulland ML, et al. Primary CD30-positive cutaneous T-cell lymphomas and lymphomatoid papulosis frequently express cytotoxic proteins. *Histopathology* 2000;36(2):136–144.
216. Jaffe ES, et al. Classification of lymphoid neoplasms: the microscope as a tool for disease discovery. *Blood* 2008;112(12):4384–4399.
217. Toro JR, Beaty M, Sorbara L, et al. Gamma delta T-cell lymphoma of the skin: a clinical, microscopic, and molecular study. *Arch Dermatol* 2000;136(8): 1024–1032.
218. Toro JR, Liewehr DJ, Pabby N, et al. Gamma-delta T-cell phenotype is associated with significantly decreased survival in cutaneous T-cell lymphoma. *Blood* 2003;101(9):3407–3412.
219. Petrella T, et al. Indolent CD8-positive lymphoid proliferation of the ear: a distinct primary cutaneous T-cell lymphoma? *Am J Surg Pathol* 2007;31(12):1887–1892.
220. Beltraminelli H, Mullegger R, Cerroni L. Indolent CD8+ lymphoid proliferation of the ear: a phenotypic variant of the small-medium pleomorphic cutaneous T-cell lymphoma? *J Cutan Pathol* 2010;37(1):81–84.
221. Hagiwara M, et al. Primary cutaneous T-cell lymphoma of unspecified type with cytotoxic phenotype: clinicopathological analysis of 27 patients. *Cancer Sci* 2009; 100(1):33–41.
222. Kawachi Y, Furuta JI, Fujisawa Y, et al. Indolent subcutaneous panniculitis-like T cell lymphoma in a 1-year-old child. *Pediatr Dermatol* 2012;29:374–377.
223. Magro CM, Crowson AN, Kovatich AJ, et al. Lupus profundus, indeterminate lymphocytic lobular panniculitis and subcutaneous T-cell lymphoma: a spectrum of subcuticular T-cell lymphoid dyscrasia. *J Cutan Pathol* 2001;28(5):235–247.
224. Salhany KE, Macon WR, Choi JK, et al. Subcutaneous panniculitis-like T-cell lymphoma: clinicopathologic, immunophenotypic, and genotypic analysis of alpha/beta and gamma/delta subtypes. *Am J Surg Pathol* 1998;22(7):881–893.
225. Pincus LB, LeBoit PE, McCalmont TH, et al. Subcutaneous panniculitis-like T-cell lymphoma with overlapping clinicopathologic features of lupus erythematosus: coexistence of 2 entities? *Am J Dermatopathol* 2009;31(6):520–526.
226. Chiu HY, He GY, Chen JS, et al. Subcutaneous panniculitis-like T-cell lymphoma presenting with clinicopathologic features of dermatomyositis. *J Am Acad Dermatol* 2011;64(6):e121–e123.
227. Parveen Z, Thompson K. Subcutaneous panniculitis-like T-cell lymphoma: redefinition of diagnostic criteria in the recent World Health Organization-European Organization for Research and Treatment of Cancer classification for cutaneous lymphomas. *Arch Pathol Lab Med* 2009;133(2):303–308.
228. Go RS, Wester SM. Immunophenotypic and molecular features, clinical outcomes, treatments, and prognostic factors associated with subcutaneous panniculitis-like T-cell lymphoma: a systematic analysis of 156 patients reported in the literature. *Cancer* 2004;101(6):1404–1413.
229. Kao GF, Resh B, McMahon C, et al. Fatal subcutaneous panniculitis-like T-cell lymphoma gamma/delta subtype (cutaneous gamma/delta T-cell lymphoma): report of a case and review of the literature. *Am J Dermatopathol* 2008;30(6): 593–599.
230. Hosler GA, Liegeois N, Anhalt GJ, et al. Transformation of cutaneous gamma/delta T-cell lymphoma following 15 years of indolent behavior. *J Cutan Pathol* 2008;35(11):1063.
231. Mizutani S, Kuroda J, Shimura Y, et al. Cyclosporine A for chemotherapy-resistant subcutaneous panniculitis-like T cell lymphoma with hemophagocytic syndrome. *Acta Haematol* 2011;126(1):8–12.
232. Tzeng HE, Teng CL, Yang Y, et al. Occult subcutaneous panniculitis-like T-cell lymphoma with initial presentations of cellulitis-like skin lesion and fulminant hemophagocytosis. *J Formos Med Assoc* 2007;106(2 Suppl):S55–S59.
233. Au WY, Ng WM, Choy C, et al. Aggressive subcutaneous panniculitis-like T-cell lymphoma: complete remission with fludarabine, mitoxantrone and dexamethasone. *Br J Dermatol* 2000;143(2):408–410.
234. Mehta N, Wayne AS, Kim YH, et al. Bexarotene is active against subcutaneous panniculitis-like T-cell lymphoma in adult and pediatric populations. *Clin Lymphoma Myeloma Leuk* 2012;12(1):20–25.
235. Teruya-Feldstein J, Setsuda J, Yao X, et al. MIP-1alpha expression in tissues from patients with hemophagocytic syndrome. *Lab Invest* 1999;79(12):1583–1590.
236. Craig AJ, Cualing H, Thomas G, et al. Cytophagic histiocytic panniculitis–a syndrome associated with benign and malignant panniculitis: case comparison and review of the literature. *J Am Acad Dermatol* 1998;39(5 Pt 1):721–736.
237. Magro CM, Schaefer JT, Morrison C, et al. Atypical lymphocytic lobular panniculitis: a clonal subcutaneous T-cell dyscrasia. *J Cutan Pathol* 2008;35(10): 947–954.
238. Wang X, Magro CM. Human myxovirus resistance protein 1 (MxA) as a useful marker in the differential diagnosis of subcutaneous lymphoma vs. lupus erythematosus profundus. *Eur J Dermatol* 2012;22(5):629–633.
239. Magro CM, Wang X. CCL5 expression in panniculitic T-cell dyscrasias and its potential role in adipocyte tropism. *Am J Dermatopathol* 2013;35(3):332–337.
240. Wang E, Papalas J, Siddiqi I, et al. A small cell variant of ALK-positive, CD8-positive anaplastic large cell lymphoma with primary subcutaneous presentation mimicking subcutaneous panniculitis-like T-cell lymphoma. *Pathol Res Pract* 2011;207(8):522–526.
241. Greer JP, Kinney MC, Loughran TP Jr. T cell and NK cell lymphoproliferative disorders. *Hematology Am Soc Hematol Educ Program* 2001;259–281.
242. Hirakawa S, Kuyama M, Takahashi S, et al. Nasal and nasal-type natural killer/T-cell lymphoma. *J Am Acad Dermatol* 1999;40(2 Pt 1):268–272.
243. Kato N, Yasukawa K, Onozuka T, et al. Nasal and nasal-type T/NK-cell lymphoma with cutaneous involvement. *J Am Acad Dermatol* 1999;40(5 Pt 2):850–856
244. Miyamoto T, Yoshino T, Takehisa T, et al. Cutaneous presentation of nasal/nasal type T/NK cell lymphoma: clinicopathological findings of four cases. *Br J Dermatol* 1998;139(3):481–487.

245. Ansai S, Maeda K, Yamakawa M, et al. CD56-positive (nasal-type T/NK cell) lymphoma arising on the skin. Report of two cases and review of the literature. *J Cutan Pathol* 1997;24(8):468–476.

246. Cheung MM, Chan JK, Wong KF. Natural killer cell neoplasms: a distinctive group of highly aggressive lymphomas/leukemias. *Semin Hematol* 2003;40(3):221–232.

247. Petrella T, Comeau MR, Maynadie M, et al. Agranular CD41 CD561 hematodermic neoplasm (blastic NK-cell lymphoma) originates from a population of CD561 precursor cells related to plasmacytoid monocytes. *Am J Surg Pathol* 2002;26:852–862.

248. Petrella T, Bagot M, Willemze R, et al. Blastic NK-cell lymphomas (agranular CD4+CD56+ hematodermic neoplasms): a review. *Am J Clin Pathol* 2005;123(5):662–675.

249. Aviles A, Diaz NR, Neri N, et al. Angiocentric nasal T/natural killer cell lymphoma: a single centre study of prognostic factors in 108 patients. *Clin Lab Haematol* 2000;22(4):215–220.

250. De Lord C, Mercieca J, Ashton-Key M, et al. Aggressive NK cell lymphoma preceded by a ten year history of neutropenia associated with large granular lymphocyte lymphocytosis. *Leuk Lymphoma* 1998;31(3–4):417–421.

251. Hallett WH, Murphy WJ. Natural killer cells: biology and clinical use in cancer therapy. *Cell Mol Immunol* 2004;1(1):12–21.

252. Farag SS, Caligiuri MA. Human natural killer cell development and biology. *Blood Rev* 2006;20:123–137.

253. Yok-Lam K. The diagnosis and management of extranodal NK/T-cell lymphoma, nasal-type and aggressive NK-cell leukemia [Review]. *J Clin Exp Hematop* 2011;51(1):21–28.

254. Harabuchi Y, Takahara M, Kishibe K, et al. Nasal natural killer (NK)/T-cell lymphoma: clinical, histological, virological, and genetic features. *Int J Clin Oncol* 2009;14(3):181–190.

255. Jaffe ES, Chan JK, Su IJ, et al. Report of the workshop on nasal and related extranodal angiocentric T/natural killer cell lymphomas; definitions, differential diagnosis, and epidemiology. *Am J Surg Pathol* 1996;20:103–111.

256. Rahemtullah A, Longtine JA, Harris NL, et al. CD20+ T-cell lymphoma: clinicopathologic analysis of 9 cases and a review of the literature. *Am J Surg Pathol* 2008;32(11):1593–1607.

257. Magro CM, Seilstad KH, Procu P, et al. Primary CD20+CD10+CD8+ T-cell lymphoma of the skin with IgH and TCR beta gene rearrangement. *Am J Clin Pathol* 2006;126:14–22.

258. Vermeer MH, Tensen CP, van der Stoop PM, et al. Absence of T(H)2 cytokine messenger RNA expression in CD30-negative primary cutaneous large T-cell lymphomas. *Arch Dermatol* 2001;137(7):901–905.

259. Murakami T, Fukasawa T, Fukayama M, et al. Gene expression profile in a case of primary cutaneous CD30-negative large T-cell lymphoma with a blastic phenotype. Clin *Exp Dermatol* 2001;26(2):201–214.

260. Nishio M, Koizumi K, Endo T, et al. Effective high-dose chemotherapy combined with CD34+-selected autologous peripheral blood stem cell transplantation in a patient with cutaneous CD30-negative large T cell lymphoma. *Bone Marrow Transplant* 2000;25(12):1315–1317.

261. Nishio M, Sawada K, Koizumi K, et al. Recurrence with histological transformation 40 days after autologous peripheral blood stem cell transplantation (APBSCT) for cutaneous CD30-negative large T cell lymphoma. *Bone Marrow Transplant* 1998;22(12):1211–1214.

262. Tripodo C, Iannitto E, Florena AM, et al. Gamma-delta T-cell lymphomas. *Nat Rev Clin Oncol* 2009;6(12):707–717.

263. Berti E, Cerri A, Cavicchini S, et al. Primary cutaneous gamma/delta T-cell lymphoma presenting as disseminated pagetoid reticulosis. *J Invest Dermatol* 1991;96:718–723.

264. Guitart J. Subcutaneous lymphoma and related conditions. *Dermatol Ther* 2010;23(4):350.

265. Thomson AB, McKenzie KJ, Jackson R, et al. Subcutaneous panniculitic T-cell lymphoma in childhood: successful response to chemotherapy. *Med Pediatr Oncol* 2001;37(6):549.

266. Magro CM, Wang X. Indolent Primary Cutaneous γ/δ T-Cell Lymphoma Localized to the Subcutaneous Panniculus and Its Association With Atypical Lymphocytic Lobular Panniculitis. Am *J Clin Pathol* 2012;138(1):50–56.

267. Ma L, Bandarchi B, Glusac EJ. Fatal subcutaneous panniculitis-like T-cell lymphoma with interface change and dermal mucin, a dead ringer for lupus erythematosus. *J Cutan Pathol* 2005;32(5):360.

268. Ikeda E, Endo M, Uchigasaki S, et al. Phagocytized apoptotic cells in subcutaneous panniculitis-like T-cell lymphoma. *J Eur Acad Dermatol Venereol* 2001;15(2):159–162.

269. Khoury JD, Medeiros LJ, Manning JT, et al. CD561 TdT1 blastic natural killer cell tumor of the skin. *Cancer* 2002;94:2401–2408.

270. Facchetti F, Jones DM, Petrella T. Blastic plasmacytoid dendritic cells neoplasm. In: Swerdlow SH, Campo E, Harris NL, et al., eds. WHO classification of tumours of haematopoietic and lymphoid tissues, 4th ed. Lyon: International Agency for Research on Cancer, 2008:145–147.

271. Hamadani M, Magro CM, Porcu P. CD4 CD56 hematodermic tumor (plasmacytoid dendritic cell neoplasm). *Br J Haematol* 2008;140:122.

272. Ascani S, Massone C, Ferrara G, et al. CD4-negative variant of CD4+/CD56+ hematodermic neoplasm: description of three cases. *J Cutan Pathol* 2008;35(10):911–915.

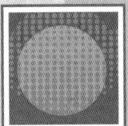

Chapter 30
Gastrointestinal Lymphomas and Lymphoid Hyperplasias

Ming-Qing Du • Andrew C. Wotherspoon

The gastrointestinal tract (GIT) is frequently involved as a secondary event by node-based non-Hodgkin lymphoma. In these situations, it is not possible to distinguish primary from secondary lymphoma on the basis of tissue morphology, immunophenotype, or molecular studies at the present time. Clinical information supported by radiology is the only way to distinguish between these two situations. Early definitions of primary gastrointestinal lymphoma required the extranodal site to be the sole site of involvement by lymphoma (1). This definition was restrictive and implied that all primary gastrointestinal lymphomas were low stage and would imply a better prognosis dictated by disease definition rather than by biology. More recently, it has become accepted that a lymphoma can be considered to be primary if the GIT is the dominant site of disease.

Almost all lymphomas arising in the GIT are non-Hodgkin lymphoma. Primary gastrointestinal Hodgkin lymphoma is almost never encountered. Primary gastrointestinal lymphomas account for approximately 30% of all extranodal lymphomas, but there is a geographical variation in the proportion of non-Hodgkin lymphomas that arise at this site with these lymphomas accounting for about 4% to 18% of all lymphoma cases in the Western world compared to 25% in the Middle East (2).

The site of involvement of gastrointestinal lymphoma also shows geographic variation with the stomach being the commonest location for lymphoma to arise in the Western countries while, in the Middle East, lymphomas are more frequently encountered in the small intestine (2). In all areas, lymphomas arising in other regions (the esophagus, colon, and rectum) are rarer than those arising in the stomach and small intestine.

LYMPHOMA OF THE GASTROINTESTINAL TRACT

The majority of lymphomas arising in the GIT are B-cell lymphomas. Most of the B-cell lymphomas are extranodal marginal zone (mucosa-associated lymphoid tissue [MALT]) type, with gastric MALT lymphoma the most frequent and the most intensely studied. This forms the paradigm of MALT lymphoma at any site. Immunoproliferative small intestinal disease (IPSID) is a specific subtype of MALT lymphoma that has many unique features and a characteristic geographic distribution. Other indolent, histologically low-grade B-cell lymphomas that occur in the GIT include mantle cell lymphoma and follicular lymphoma, both of which recapitulate the morphologic and immunophenotypic characteristics of their nodal counterparts but differ slightly in their clinical behavior. Aggressive B-cell lymphomas arising in the GIT are either diffuse large B-cell lymphoma (DLBCL) or Burkitt lymphoma. As with other extranodal sites, the GIT is a frequent site of origin for lymphomas that develop in a background of immunodeficiency.

The majority of T-cell lymphomas in the GIT are in the category of enteropathy-associated T-cell lymphoma (EATL). Other types of T-cell lymphoma can arise in the GIT, including extranodal NK/T-cell lymphoma, which is indistinguishable morphologically and immunophenotypically from similar lymphomas arising in the upper aerodigestive tract/nose. Other peripheral T-cell lymphomas (PTCL) are very rare and recapitulate the morphologic and immunophenotypic features of their nodal counterparts.

EXTRANODAL MARGINAL ZONE LYMPHOMA OF MUCOSA-ASSOCIATED LYMPHOID TISSUE (MALT LYMPHOMA)

Normal Mucosa-Associated Lymphoid Tissue

The majority of sites in which MALT lymphomas develop are normally devoid of lymphoid tissue. While some areas of the intestine have scattered foci of normal lymphoid tissue in the form of lymphoid follicles, the highest concentration of constitutive normal organized extranodal lymphoid tissue is found in the terminal ileum in the form of Peyer patches. These are therefore considered to be the best example of MALT. This gut-associated lymphoid tissue (GALT) is a specially adapted component of the immune system that governs the appropriate response to luminal antigen, tolerance of food and commensal flora, and maintenance of the integrity of the epithelial barrier. Peyer patches are unencapsulated areas of lymphoid tissue that, in some ways, resemble the components and normal architecture of lymph nodes (Fig. 30.1). There are secondary lymphoid follicles that rest on the muscularis mucosae. The germinal center shows a normal zoned pattern with the dark zone in the deeper part of the follicle. The germinal center is surrounded by a mantle zone similar to that seen in the lymph node, showing variable thickness. It is greatest in the subluminal area and thinnest at the point of contact with the muscularis. In contrast to the normal follicle in peripheral lymph nodes, there is a further B-cell zone outside the mantle. This is the marginal zone and is composed of slightly larger cells with small nuclei and moderately abundant pale eosinophilic cytoplasm, resembling the marginal zone that is seen in splenic white pulp and occasionally in mesenteric lymph nodes. Like the mantle, the marginal zone is also thicker in the subluminal area where, at the periphery, marginal zone cells can be seen to enter the overlying (dome) epithelium to form a lymphoepithelium. Mucosal crypts are absent from this area. Plasma cells are present in the subepithelial lamina propria, the majority of which secrete IgA. Around the lateral margin of the follicle is a T-cell area that resembles the T zone of the paracortex with prominent high endothelial venules. Accessory cells and

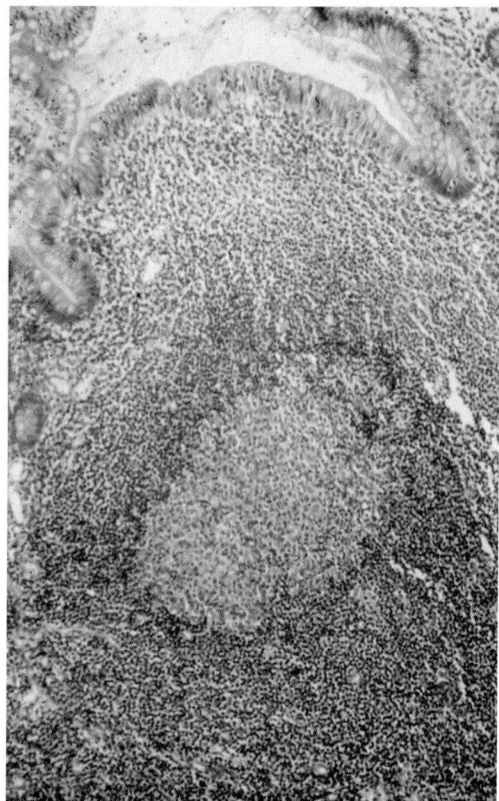

FIGURE 30.1. Ileal Peyer patch. The central germinal center is surrounded by a rim of small lymphocytes with scanty cytoplasm forming the mantle zone. This in turn is surrounded by a zone of cells with more abundant cytoplasm forming the marginal zone. Marginal zone cells enter the dome epithelium above the follicle to form a lymphoepithelium.

macrophages are also present. Within the dome epithelium, there is a population of epithelial cells, M cells. These cells have adapted to facilitate the transport of macromolecules from the lumen, so they can be presented to the lymphoid tissue beneath. As in the lymph node and spleen, MALT provides the niche for T-dependent B-cell maturation at the mucosal sites. The resulting memory B and T cells may migrate from GALT to the mesenteric lymph nodes, join blood circulation, and subsequently home back to mucosal effector sites as directed by their surface adhesion molecules.

Immunohistochemistry has shown that the B cells in the germinal center and mantle have an identical phenotype to their nodal counterparts. The cells within the marginal zone express CD21 and CD35 in addition to the pan B-cell antigens, but lack CD23, giving an identical immunoprofile to the cells in the marginal zone of the spleen. Most of plasma cells produce IgA and to a less extent IgM, and the secretory immunoglobulin is taken up by secretory epithelial cells via the polymeric Ig receptor and exported to the lumen (3). The T cells in the paracortex are predominantly CD4+. The epithelium away from the dome contains T cells that are present in the entire surface epithelium of the intestine with a ratio to enterocytes in the range of 1:5 to 10 in the small intestine, and 1:40 in the colon. These intraepithelial lymphocytes (IEL) are a phenotypically heterogeneous unconventional T-cell population, which are distinctive from T cells in other peripheral tissues. The vast majority of IEL express T-cell receptor (TCR) $\alpha\beta$, with approximately 10% positive for TCR $\gamma\delta$ (4,5). The majority of IEL are CD8+ cytotoxic T cells, predominately expressing the CD8$\alpha\alpha$ homodimer, with a small proportion of TCR $\alpha\beta$+ and TCR $\gamma\delta$+ T cells lacking expression of both CD4 and CD8 (4,5). IEL also express CD103, an integrin protein important for T-cell homing to the intestinal sites.

Mesenteric lymph nodes are considered to be a part of the mucosal lymphoid complex. These nodes vary slightly from peripheral lymph nodes. The sinuses are more widely patent, and the paracortex is less developed. In the B-cell areas, secondary follicles have typical germinal centers and mantles, but there is frequently a marginal zone similar to that seen in the mucosa.

Epidemiology

The GIT is the commonest site for the origin of MALT lymphoma with about 85% of these arising in the stomach (6). Most occur in adults over the age of 50, with a median age of 61 and is slightly more common in females (male:female, 0.9:1). There is geographical variation with a 13-fold higher incidence reported in Northeastern Italy compared to the United Kingdom (7).

Etiology and Pathogenesis

MALT lymphomas arise from native MALT only very rarely, so the terminal ileum is a rare site for development of these lymphomas. In most circumstances, the lymphoma develops in areas devoid of constitutive MALT. This may be due to disorganized antigen presentation in acquired lymphoid tissue, as no M cells have been demonstrated in the epithelium around the acquired lymphoid tissue. The initial step on the path to the development of MALT lymphoma is therefore the acquisition of organized lymphoid tissue within which the neoplastic transformation can develop. Stimuli for the acquisition of lymphoid tissue in the GIT, and particularly in the stomach, appear quite limited. In the stomach, this is most frequently seen in the context of *Helicobacter pylori*–associated gastritis but can be seen in autoimmune conditions such as Sjögren syndrome. For the intestine, the stimuli remain largely unknown.

Helicobacter pylori and Gastric MALT Lymphoma

The normal gastric mucosa is devoid of organized lymphoid tissue. Many series have demonstrated that lymphoid tissue in the stomach is acquired as part of the inflammatory response to infection by *H. pylori* (8–10), and similar inflammatory responses are seen in the rarer infection by *Helicobacter heilmannii* (11). The acquired lymphoid tissue recapitulated the organization of constitutive MALT with lymphoid follicles that are composed of reactive germinal centers, mantles, and a marginal zone (Fig. 30.2). Individual small B cells from the marginal zone can be seen in the adjacent epithelial structures forming a lymphoepithelium, although specialist M cells have not been described.

Evidence has accumulated to suggest that the majority of gastric MALT lymphomas derive from the lymphoid tissue acquired in association with *H. pylori* infections. Firstly, it has been shown that gastric MALT lymphoma is particularly common in one area of Northeastern Italy compared to other geographical areas, and this is in the background of a similarly high prevalence of *H. pylori* (7). Secondly, many studies have demonstrated the presence of *H. pylori* organisms on the mucosa of cases of gastric MALT lymphoma (12). Initial studies suggested that the organism was present in up to 90% of cases, but subsequent studies found a lower association. This may be due to geographic variation, decreased organism density in mucosa around the lymphoma, unintentional partial eradication in patients on proton pump inhibitor therapy, or due to the detection technique. Serologic studies for anti-*Helicobacter* antibodies appear the most reliable detection method in these

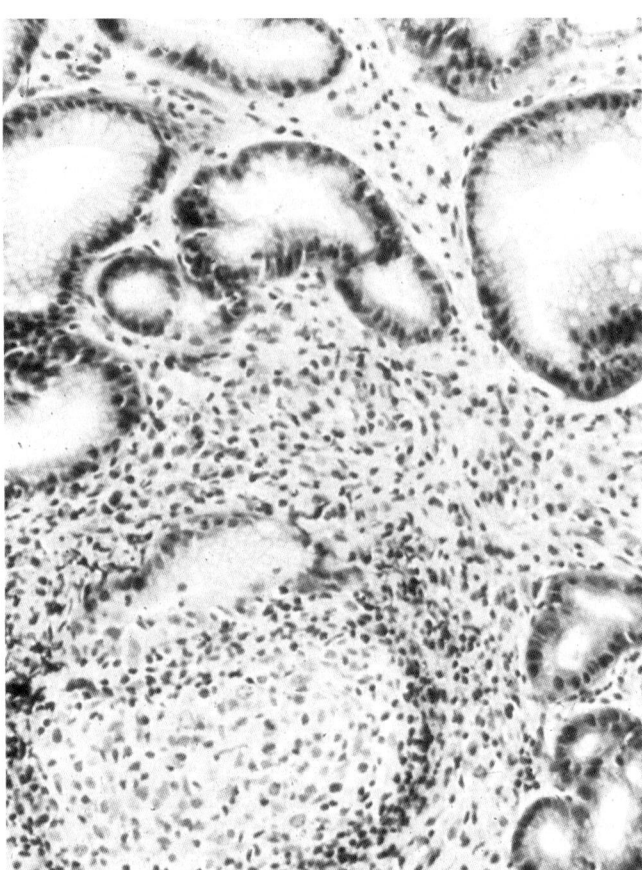
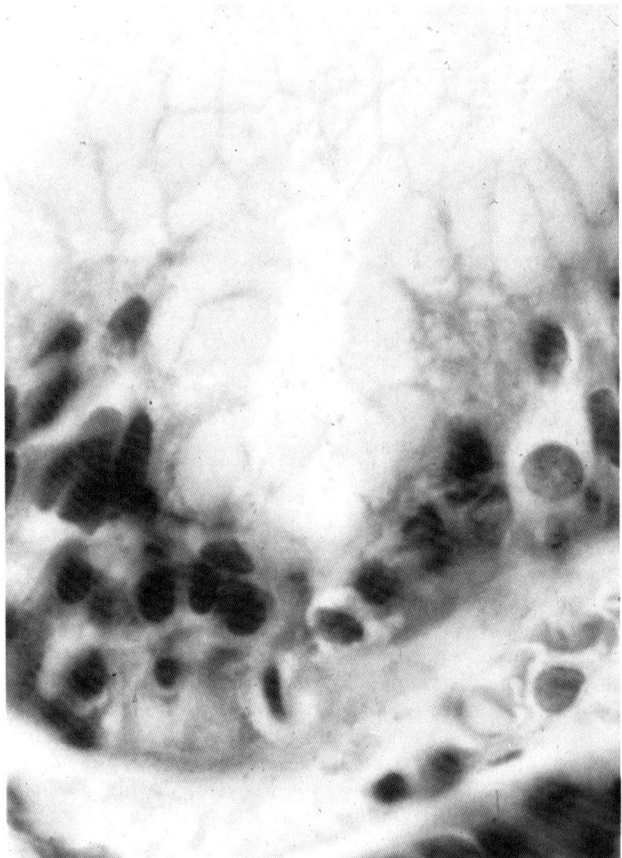

FIGURE 30.2. *Helicobacter pylori*–associated gastritis. A lymphoid follicle is present with benign lymphocytes entering the gland epithelium to form lymphoepithelial lesions. Organisms are present in the lumen of the glands.

circumstances and have shown a higher detection of infection in cases otherwise thought to be *Helicobacter negative* by histology or other locally directed detection methods (13). Thirdly, studies have shown a close association between prior infection by *H. pylori* and a risk of development of MALT lymphoma (14–16).

In vitro studies have provided further evidence to support the association between *H. pylori* infection and development of gastric MALT lymphoma. Culture-based studies have shown that MALT lymphoma cells can be stimulated *in vitro* by coculturing with *H. pylori* organisms (17). This proliferative drive was only achieved in culture systems that included tumor-infiltrating T cells from the original lymphoma, suggesting that the growth stimulation was conditional on the contact-dependent signaling between the T cells and the neoplastic B cells (18). Removal of one of the components of this culture system resulted in lack of growth, a feature recapitulated *in vivo* by the finding that many gastric MALT lymphomas regress following *H. pylori* eradication therapy (19–27).

Clinical Presentation

Presenting symptoms of gastrointestinal MALT lymphoma are frequently nonspecific and, in the stomach, may be more related to the associated *Helicobacter* gastritis with dyspepsia, nausea and, occasionally, vomiting. The presence of more severe epigastric pain or a mass lesion is rare. MALT lymphomas in the colorectum present with nonspecific features, including rectal bleeding and obstruction, and may simulate adenocarcinoma.

Macroscopic/Endoscopic Appearances

The findings at endoscopy are variable and nonspecific and may be minimal but include gastritis, which may be erosive, and thickened gastric folds (28). Polypoid masses and malignant-appearing ulcers may be seen. In the stomach, the lymphoma is most frequently encountered in the antrum, but any area may be involved, and macroscopic lesions may be multiple. Depth of invasion of the wall in the stomach and regional nodal involvement are best assessed by endoscopic ultrasound.

For the most part, gastrointestinal MALT lymphomas are diagnosed on endoscopic biopsy material, and resection specimens are usually confined to cases of surgical emergency, which are rare in this disease.

Histology

The morphologic features of MALT lymphoma (29,30) closely recapitulate the organization of native MALT as exemplified by the histology of Peyer patches. In the earliest lesions, the neoplastic cell infiltrate is present in the marginal zone around reactive follicles, separated from the germinal center by an intact mantle. The infiltrate extends out around crypts/glands with extension of the infiltrate away from the normal confines of the marginal zone into the upper part of the mucosa (Fig. 30.3). With advancing disease, the infiltrate extends through the muscularis mucosae, expanding the submucosa and eventually through to the serosa.

In the mucosa, the neoplastic cells infiltrate epithelial structures to recapitulate the lymphoepithelium of native MALT. In its earliest form, these lymphoepithelial lesions consist of

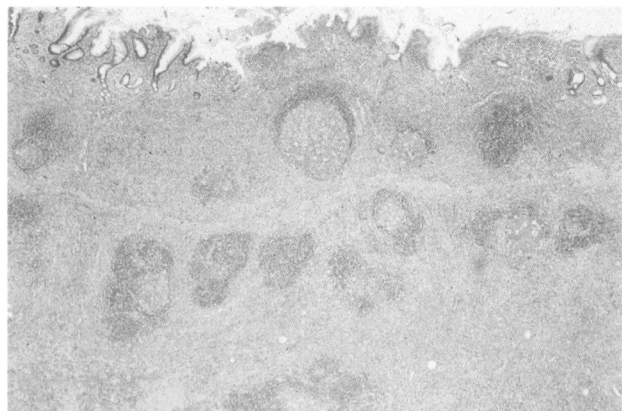

FIGURE 30.3. Gastric MALT lymphoma. The cells extend around residual reactive follicles to expand the mucosa and extend into the submucosa.

aggregates of three or more neoplastic cells within the epithelial structure, associated with distortion of the gland/crypt architecture. As the lesion develops, there is progressive destruction of the gland/crypt architecture with the cells expanding and developing more eosinophilic cytoplasm (Fig. 30.4). This is due to sublethal/lethal effects of the neoplastic cells on the normal glandular epithelial cells resulting in swelling of mitochondria and loss of intracellular organelles (31) (Fig. 30.5). The neuroendocrine cells appear to be more resistant and can be seen as single cells within the diffuse neoplastic cell infiltrate in some cases (32).

The cytology of MALT lymphoma cells can be variable. The cells are typically intermediate to small with moderate amounts of pale eosinophilic cytoplasm and slightly irregular nuclei that overall give a vague resemblance to the centrocyte in the germinal center, leading to these being termed "centrocyte-like" (CCL) cells (33) (Fig. 30.6). The cells may have more abundant cytoplasm with sharply defined cell borders resembling monocytoid cells (Fig 30.6) or, in some cases, they may be more reminiscent of typical small lymphocytes. A mixture of all these cytologic variants can be seen in an individual case. Plasma cell differentiation is frequently seen and is prominent in about a third of cases (Fig. 30.7). The plasma cells are most dense beneath the luminal epithelium. In some of these cases, plasma cell differentiation is extreme, and there may be associated

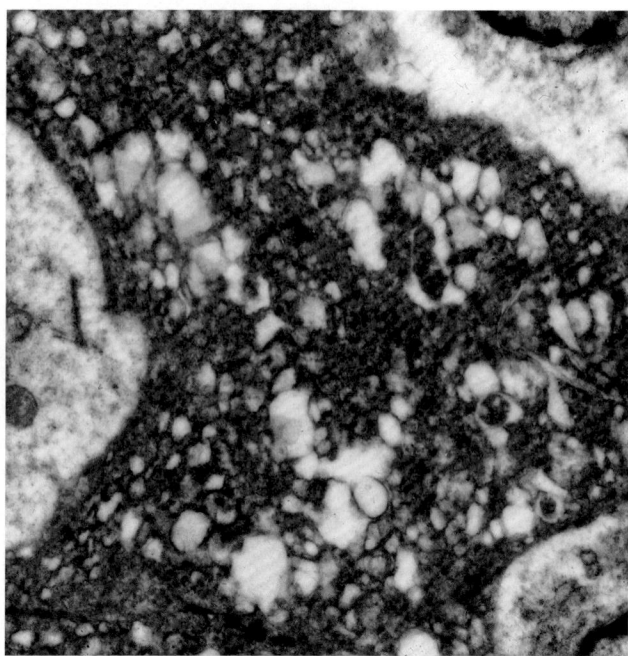

FIGURE 30.5. Lymphoepithelial lesion. Electron micrograph showing swollen mitochondria in the epithelial cell cytoplasm.

extracellular deposition of immunoglobulin (Fig. 30.7). Scattered large transformed cells with abundant cytoplasm and vesicular nuclei that contain nucleoli are a ubiquitous finding. If these are seen in sheets, then the lesion is best considered to be an associated component of large B-cell lymphoma.

Lymphoid follicles are ubiquitous to MALT lymphoma. There may be easily identifiable residual reactive lymphoid follicles within the lymphomatous infiltrate (34) (Fig. 30.3). They are present deep in the wall in more advanced cases and are not confined to the mucosa. In some cases, the follicles may have been overrun by the neoplastic infiltrate, resulting in only a vague nodular appearance to the infiltrate (Fig. 30.8) with the preexistence of follicles only demonstrated by the presence of disrupted follicular dendritic cells highlighted by immunohistochemical staining with antibodies to CD21 or CD23. Occasionally, the neoplastic cells appear to specifically colonize the germinal centers. In some of these cases, the colonizing cells become enlarged with a more activated appearance compared to the extrafollicular component from which it is separated by an intact mantle. In extreme cases, the degree of follicular colonization may result in an appearance that closely resembles follicular lymphoma (Fig. 30.9). In other cases, the intrafollicular cells may show plasma cell differentiation (Fig. 30.10).

Examination of entire resection specimens from gastric MALT lymphoma cases has shown that the infiltrate is multifocal (35) (Figs. 30.11 and 30.12). Away from the main area of infiltration, neoplastic cells can be demonstrated around lymphoid follicles in the adjacent mucosa. In the smallest microlymphoma, this can be in the form of a small rim of neoplastic cells in the marginal zone of a single follicle, occasionally associated with a lymphoepithelial lesion (Fig. 30.13). The cells are monotypic and have been shown to be clonal and derived from the main lymphomatous infiltrate (36). It is assumed that similar intraorgan multifocality is present in all MALT lymphomas.

When MALT lymphoma disseminates to lymph nodes, the infiltrate of CCL cells extends in a marginal zone or interfollicular pattern. There may be follicular colonization. With increasing degree of infiltration, there is effacement of the nodal architecture, and the infiltrate becomes diffuse.

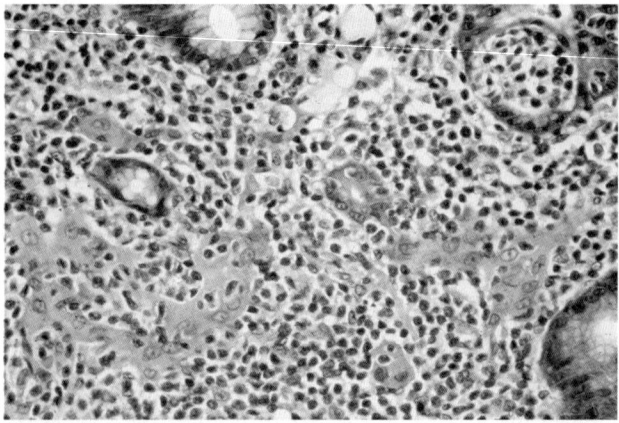

FIGURE 30.4. Lymphoepithelial lesion. Variable nature of the lymphoepithelial lesion. In one area, the neoplastic CCL cells enter the epithelium in clusters (**top right**) while in more advanced lesions (**bottom left**), the epithelial cells are swollen and have abundant eosinophilic cytoplasm.

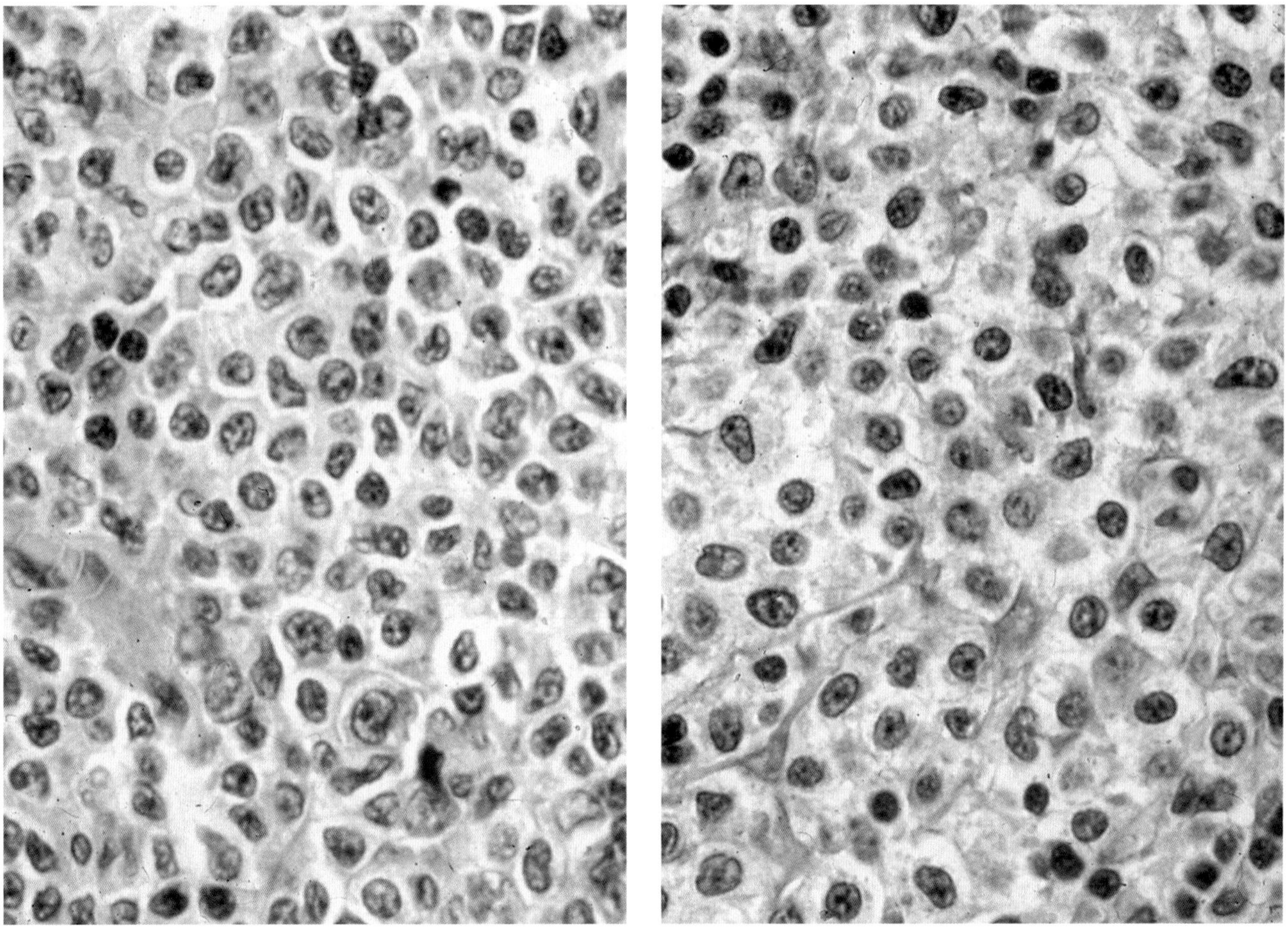

FIGURE 30.6. CCL cell morphology. The neoplastic cells may resemble centrocytes with irregular nuclear contours and scanty cytoplasm (**left**) or have more abundant cytoplasm with sharp cytoplasmic borders (**right**).

Immunophenotype

MALT lymphomas express pan B-cell markers CD19, CD20, CD22, CD79a, and PAX5. They express surface immunoglobulin, which is most commonly IgM or IgA with IgG expression being rare. There is light chain restriction, kappa > lambda. The cells are typically negative for CD5, CD23, CD10, BCL6, and cyclinD1. There is expression of BCL2 protein. There is expression of CD43 in up to 50% of cases, which may be helpful in distinguishing the infiltrate from CD43-negative reactive B-cell infiltrates. A small proportion of cases are positive for CD5, and these appear to have a propensity for the leukemic phase and earlier dissemination. Staining for cytokeratin is helpful in identifying lymphoepithelial lesions (Fig. 30.14). Antibodies against CD21 and/or CD23 can be used to highlight follicular dendritic cells. Staining for CD10 and BCL6 can help identify residual germinal center cells and distinguish clusters of normal residual follicle center cells from aggregates of transformed neoplastic cells when a diagnosis of associated large B-cell lymphoma is being considered.

Molecular Genetics

Immunoglobulin heavy chain and light chain genes are clonally rearranged, and show a high load of somatic hypermutation with features of antigen selection. These, together with the immunophenotype, suggest that MALT lymphomas are derived from post–germinal center marginal zone B cells. But unlike other memory B-cell–derived lymphomas, a high proportion of MALT lymphomas show ongoing mutations (intraclonal variations) in their rearranged immunoglobulin genes (37,38), which are most likely the result of their colonization of reactive B-cell follicles.

For diagnostic biopsies, clonality analysis of the rearranged immunoglobulin genes may help to establish or refute a diagnosis of lymphoma. Nonetheless, this should be performed

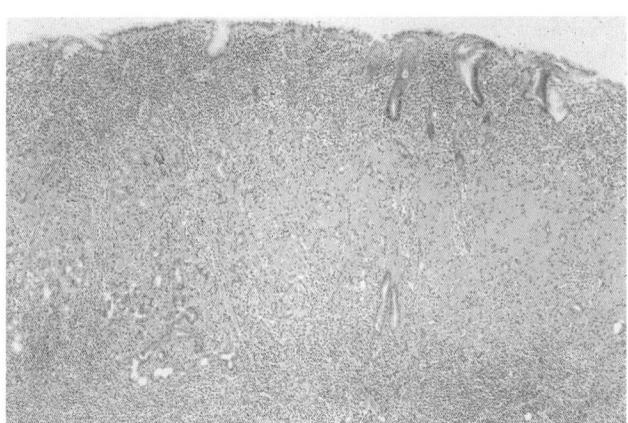

FIGURE 30.7. Plasma cell differentiation. This may be extreme with deposition of extracellular immunoglobulin.

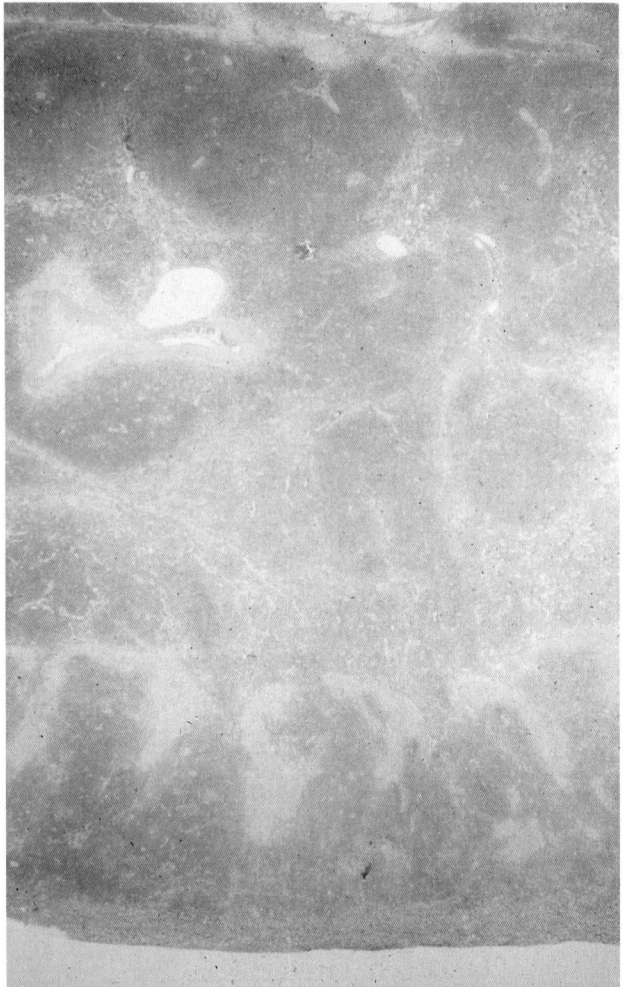

FIGURE 30.8. Follicles have been overrun or colonized by neoplastic CCL cells, giving a nodular appearance to the infiltrate within the wall.

only when histologic and immunophenotypic features are suspicious but not diagnostic of lymphoma. Clonality analyses by polymerase chain reaction (PCR) can be readily performed on formalin-fixed and paraffin-embedded tissue biopsies using the well-established European BIOMED-2 protocols, which are

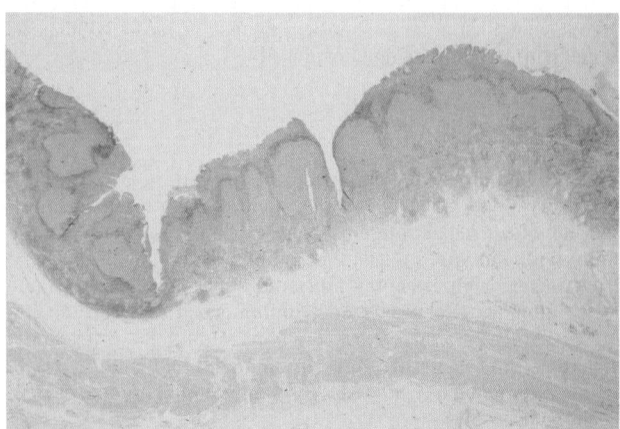

FIGURE 30.9. Follicular colonization. In some cases, the colonization of the follicles can be so extreme as to resemble follicular lymphoma.

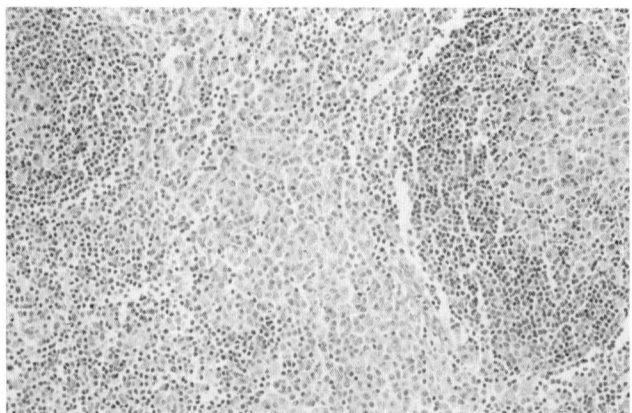

FIGURE 30.10. Follicular colonization. In cases with plasma cell differentiation, the intrafollicular component may be rich in plasma cells.

capable of demonstrating clonally rearranged immunoglobulin genes in 95% of B-cell lymphomas (39,40).

In general, MALT lymphoma is characterized by several recurrent chromosome translocations, copy number alterations, and somatic mutations, which involve the NF-κB pathway regulators. Intriguingly, these genetic abnormalities occur

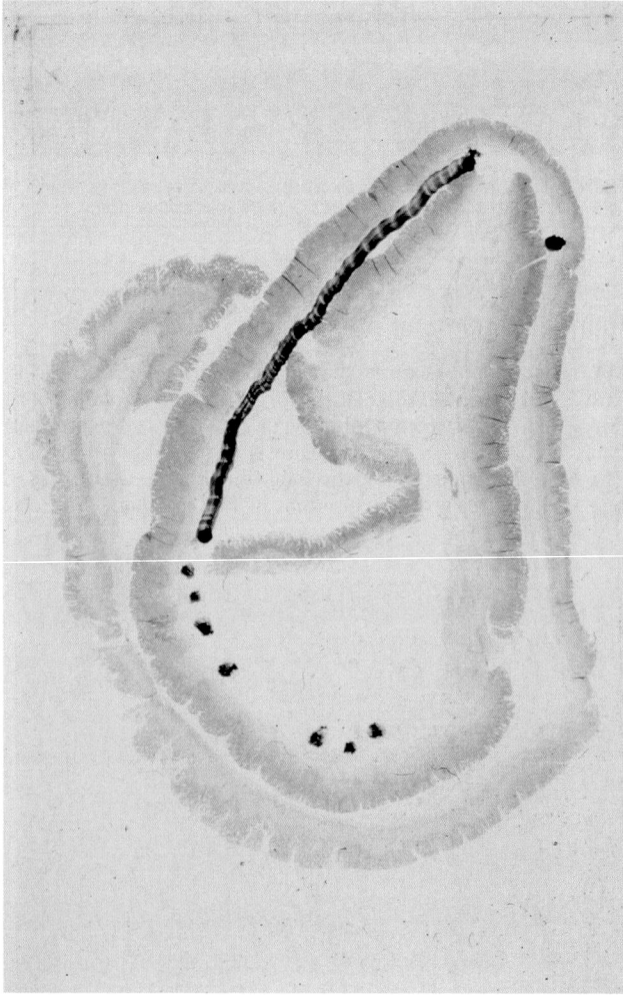

FIGURE 30.11. Examination of entire gastrectomy specimens show small tumor deposits away from the main area of lymphoma.

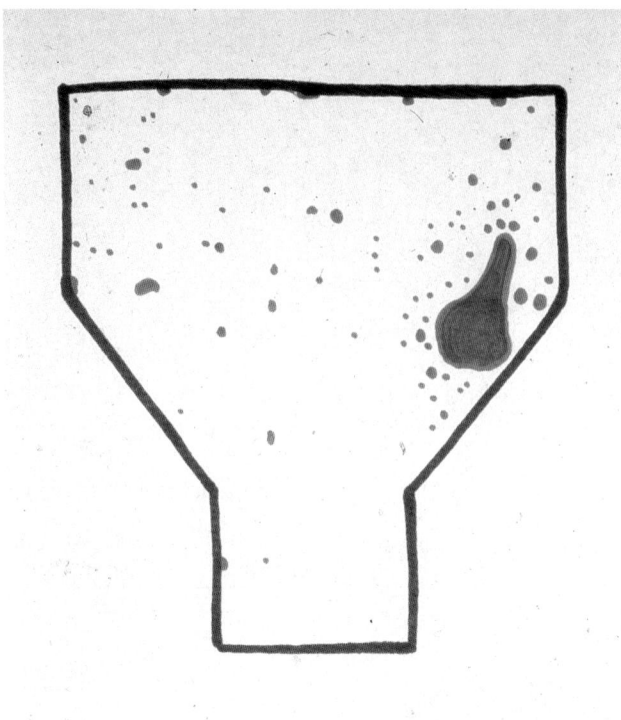

FIGURE 30.12. Virtual map of the distribution of lymphoma within a distal partial gastrectomy specimen performed for gastric MALT lymphoma.

at variable frequencies in MALT lymphoma of different anatomic sites with the gastric form featured by t(11;18)(q21;q21) and t(1;14)(p22;q32).

t(11;18)(q21;q21)

The translocation fuses the amino terminus of the *API2* gene to the carboxyl terminus of the *MALT1* gene and generates a functional *API2-MALT1* fusion product (41–43). It has been shown that the fusion product gains ability to activate both the canonical and noncanonical NF-κB activation pathways (Fig. 30.15). Through heterotypic interaction between the BIR1 of the API2 moiety and the C-terminal region of MALT1, the fusion product forms an oligomer in absence of any upstream stimulation, and this oligomerization is critical for API2-MALT1–mediated NF-κB activation (44). The API2-MALT1 fusion product binds

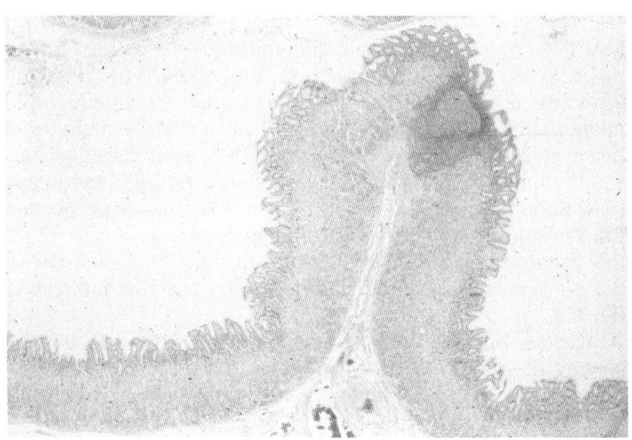

FIGURE 30.13. Microlymphoma. The smallest lesion in the mucosa distant from the main lesion is composed of a perifollicular infiltration by CCL cells.

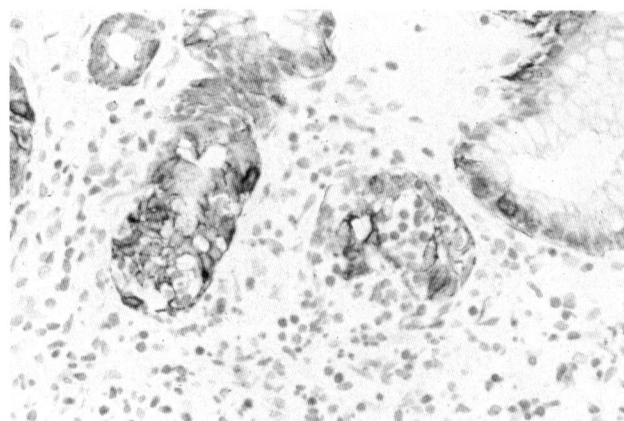

FIGURE 30.14. Staining for cytokeratin highlights the lymphoepithelial lesions (CAM5.2).

directly to TRAF2 and TRAF6, and their interaction likely mediates TRAF6 oligomerization, consequently triggering the activation of the IKK complex, hence the canonical NF-κB pathway (45). In addition, API2-MALT1 binds to NIK (NF-κB–inducing kinase) via the API2 moiety, and causes its cleavage through the MALT1 moiety that possesses protease activities (46). This NIK cleavage generates a C-terminal NIK fragment that retains kinase activity but resists to proteasome degradation, thus can cause constitutive activation of the noncanonical NF-κB pathway (46). Finally, the API2-MALT1 fusion product is also capable of proteolytic inactivation of A20 (also known as TNF-α–inducible protein 3), which is a transcriptional target of NF-κB and serves as an autonegative regulator of the NF-κB activation pathways (47). Through the above molecular mechanisms, API2-MALT1 can cause constitutive NF-κB activation.

T(11;18) (q21;q21) is specifically associated with the MALT lymphoma entity, not found in other low-grade B-cell lymphomas and chronic inflammatory conditions associated with MALT lymphoma development. The translocation is seen in 25% of gastric MALT lymphoma, more frequent in cases at stage II$_E$ or above than those at stage I$_E$ (48–53). At the genetic level, MALT lymphoma with t(11;18)(q21;q21) infrequently shows genomic copy number changes as shown by conventional cytogenetic and array comparative genomic hybridization studies (54,55). At the cellular level, MALT lymphoma with t(11;18)(q21;q21) appears to be more monotonous, lacking prominent transformed blasts, and shows moderately intense aberrant nuclear immunostaining for BCL10 (56). However, these histologic and immunophenotypic features are not reliable surrogate markers for the translocation.

t(1;14)(p22;q32)/t(1;2)(p22;p12)

These translocations juxtapose the entire *BCL10* gene under the regulatory control of the *IG* gene enhancer and hence cause its overexpression (57,58). BCL10 is a critical component of the CBM (CARMA1/BCL10/MALT1) complex that links the antigen receptor signaling to the canonical NF-κB activation pathway (59). Overexpression of BCL10 results in its oligomerization through interaction of its CARD domain, and this leads to constitutive activation of the canonical NF-κB pathway (60–64).

T(1;14)(p22;q32) or its variant is only found in MALT lymphoma, approximately in 4% of gastric cases, and often in association with advanced stages of the disease (65). MALT lymphoma with t(1;14)(p22;q32) often shows trisomies 3, 12, and 18 (57,58). The lymphoma cells are characterized by strong aberrant nuclear BCL-10 immunostaining, much more intense than that seen in cases with t(11;18)(q21;q21) (56,66).

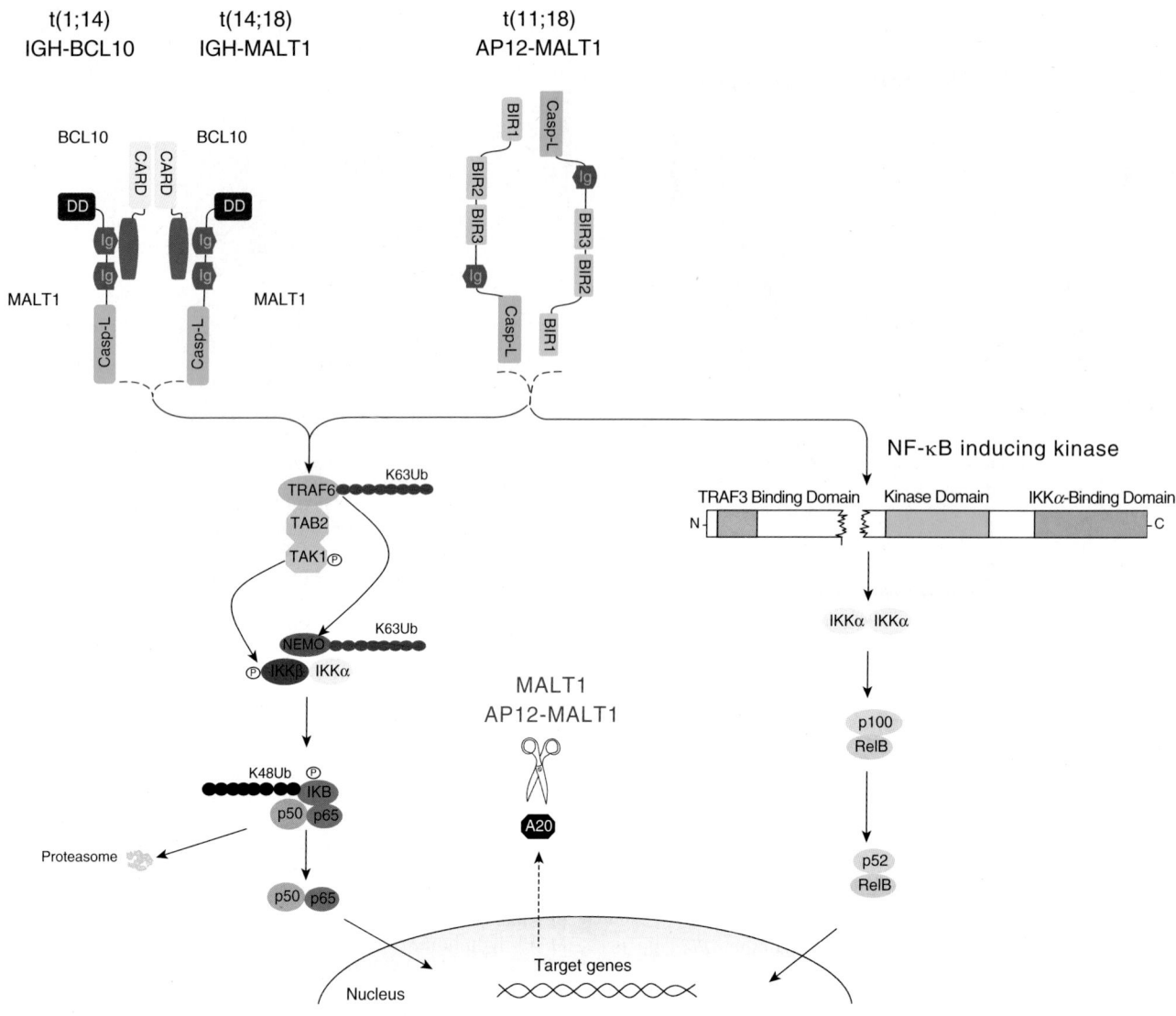

FIGURE 30.15. Constitutive NF-κB activation by chromosome translocation in MALT lymphoma. Overexpression of BCL10 and MALT1 by respective t(1;14)(p22;q32) and t(14;18)(q32;q21) results in its oligomerization through CARD-CARD interaction, and this leads to constitutive activation of the canonical NF-κB pathway. The chimeric API2-MALT1 fusion product by t(11;18)(q21;q21) gains novel functional properties and is capable of activating both the canonical and noncanonical NF-κB pathways. In addition, these oncogenic products may also obliterate the negative regulator A20 through MALT1 proteolytic activity.

Nonetheless, a diagnosis of the translocation should be established by interphase fluorescence *in situ* hybridization (FISH) with *BCL10* dual-color break-apart probe, followed by *BCL10/IGH* dual-color dual-fusion probes where indicated.

t(14;18)(q32;q21)/*IGH-MALT1* and t(3;14)(p14;q32)/*FOXP1-IGH* are only rarely found in gastric MALT lymphoma (49,67–69), and the clinical significance of these translocations remains to be investigated. Recent studies show frequent inactivation of *A20* by deletion and somatic mutation in ocular adnexal MALT lymphoma (70–73). However, these *A20* genetic changes are only infrequently seen in gastric cases.

Cell of Origin of MALT Lymphoma

The architectural organization of MALT lymphoma, the cellular morphology, and the immunophenotype all point to the marginal zone B cell as the cell of origin of MALT lymphoma. The phenomenon of follicular colonization adds support to this theory, as migration into the germinal center is a feature of marginal zone B cells after exposure to antigen (74).

Staging

MALT lymphomas are rarely disseminated at the time of diagnosis. When dissemination occurs, this is more frequently to other mucosal sites rather than showing disseminated lymphadenopathy. Staging procedures should include evaluation of these sites, including evaluation of the upper aerodigestive tract, mouth, thyroid, and salivary glands and panendoscopy (75). Bone marrow infiltration is seen in a smaller proportion than in other indolent B-cell lymphomas (~10% of cases), but the presence of a subtle CD20-positive B-cell population in the marrow should not be interpreted as marrow infiltration (76,77).

Various staging procedures have been proposed for the staging of gastrointestinal lymphoma. Initial systems recommended use of a conventional system based on stages I to IV (78). More recently, the importance of local factors such as depth of wall involvement in predicting for response of gastric MALT lymphoma to eradication therapy has led to one group suggesting that a system indicating degree of local spread,

| Table 30.1 | LUGANO (78) AND PARIS (79) STAGING SYSTEMS FOR GASTROINTESTINAL LYMPHOMAS | |

Lugano Staging	Paris Staging	Extent of Tumor Spread
Stage I	T1-3 N0 M0	Tumor confined to the GIT (single primary site or multiple noncontiguous lesions)
I$_1$	T1 N0 M0	Infiltration limited to mucosa and/or submucosa
I$_2$	T2-T3 N0 M0	Tumor extends into muscularis propria and/or subserosa and/or serosa
Stage II	T1-3 N0-N2 M0	Tumor extending into abdomen from primary GI site (nodal involvement)

II$_1$	T1-3 N1 M0	Local
		    Perigastric nodes in gastric lymphoma
		    Mesenteric in small and large bowel lymphoma

II$_2$	T1-3 N2 M0	Distant
		    Mesenteric in gastric lymphoma
		    Para-aortic, paracaval, pelvic, inguinal

Stage IIE	T4N0-2M0	Penetration of serosa with involvement of adjacent organs/tissues (Enumerate the actual site of involvement, e.g., IIE$_{(pancreas)}$, IIE$_{(large intestine)}$) Where there is both nodal involvement and penetration into adjacent organs, stage should be denoted using both subscript and E, e.g., II$_1$E$_{(pancreas)}$
Stage IV	T1-4 N3M0	GIT lesion with supradiaphragmatic or extra-abdominal nodal involvement
	T1-4 N0-3 M1-2	Disseminated extranodal involvement (M1, noncontiguous separate site in GIT; M2, noncontiguous other organs)
	B1	Bone marrow involved

nodal status, distant spread, and marrow involvement (TNMB) would be more appropriate (Table 30.1) (79).

Treatment

In the majority of cases of gastric MALT lymphoma, eradication of *H. pylori* alone results in regression of the lymphomatous infiltrate (19–27). Time to regression of the lymphoma following eradication therapy can be variable with total regression seen after 1 month in some cases, while other cases may show no change for months or years before eventual response. The interval before more conventional antilymphoma therapy is instituted remains controversial, but careful evaluation of posteradication biopsies may help to determine when further therapy is required.

There is anecdotal evidence of intestinal MALT lymphomas responding to anti-*Helicobacter*–type therapy or other antibiotics (80–85). Even if *H. pylori* is demonstrated in the stomach, this may not indicate a direct link between the organism and the lymphoma, as other bacteria will respond to combinations of antimicrobials.

Prediction of Response to Eradication Therapy

Absence of *Helicobacter* infection at diagnosis is associated with lack of response to eradication therapy. Deep submucosal invasion, or beyond by endoscopic ultrasonography (EUS), and advanced stage (involvement of regional lymph node or beyond) are significantly and independently associated with increased resistance to *H. pylori* eradication (20,22,26,86–88).

Among the genetic abnormalities seen in gastric MALT lymphoma, only t(11;18)(q21;q21) and, potentially, t(1;14) (p22;q32) are valuable in guiding treatment choice.

As shown by a number of retrospective studies, t(11;18) (q21;q21) is present in a high proportion (~50% in cases at stage I$_E$; ~70% in those at stage II$_E$ or above) of gastric MALT lymphomas that do not respond to *H. pylori* eradication. In contrast, the translocation is only seen in approximately 3% of those that respond to the antibiotic therapy, and these translocation-positive cases often show a late response and/or lymphoma relapse in absence of *H. pylori* reinfection (22,89–93). Thus, t(11;18)(q21;q21) is highly valuable in prediction of the treatment response of gastric MALT lymphoma to *H. pylori* eradication; particularly, this is independent of the clinical stage.

In addition, t(11;18)(q21;q21) was significantly associated with treatment failure of gastric MALT lymphoma by single oral alkylating agents (chlorambucil or cyclophosphamide) (94) or thalidomide (95). Despite the strong association of t(11;18) (q21;q21) with adverse clinical features, the translocation-positive cases rarely undergo high-grade transformation (96–98). For the reasons above, detection of t(11;18)(q21;q21) is valuable in patient management.

T(11;18)(q21;q21) is commonly detected by interphase FISH with *MALT1* dual-color break-apart and *API2-MALT1* dual-color dual-fusion probes or reverse transcription-PCR of the *API2-MALT1* fusion transcript. Both methods can be readily applied to routine formalin-fixed paraffin-embedded tissue biopsies with high sensitivity and specificity when appropriately performed. Nonetheless, interphase FISH offers several distinct advantages, including requirement of only small amounts of tissue, permission of histologic correlation, and minimal risk of false-positive results.

The prognostic value of t(1;14)(p22;q32) in gastric MALT lymphoma is less established. Nonetheless, a retrospective study showed that t(1;14)–positive gastric MALT lymphomas are typical of advanced stages, and cases with strong BCL10 nuclear expression or t(1;14)(p22;q32) did not respond to *H. pylori* eradication (65). T(1;14)(p22;q32) and its variant may be screened first by BCL10 immunohistochemistry to identify those with strong nuclear BCL10 expression, followed by confirmation with interphase FISH.

When a more conventional therapy is required, there are several options (75). Surgery is no longer considered appropriate, as the multifocal nature of the disease would necessitate resection of the entire organ to avoid subsequent relapse. Targeted radiotherapy is a reasonable option for localized disease. MALT lymphomas respond well to chemotherapy and immunotherapy either alone or in combination, and many regimens have equal efficacy. Of note, however, is the fact that patients with the t(11;18) are significantly less responsive to alkylating agents alone (94). No single chemotherapeutic approach has been shown to be superior.

Assessment of Posteradication Biopsies

Assessment of posteradication biopsies for the presence of lymphoma is crucial to the management of gastric MALT lymphoma. While a scheme that was designed to illustrate

	Table 30.2	WOTHERSPOON HISTOLOGIC SCORE FOR THE ASSESSMENT OF CONFIDENCE FOR A DIAGNOSIS OF MALT LYMPHOMA

Grade	Description	Histologic features
0	Normal	Scattered plasma cells in LP. No lymphoid follicles
1	Chronic active gastritis	Small clusters of lymphocytes in lamina propria. No lymphoid follicles. No LELs
2	Chronic active gastritis with florid lymphoid follicle formation	Prominent lymphoid follicles with surrounding mantle zone and plasma cells. No LELs
3	Suspicious lymphoid infiltrate in LP, probably reactive	Lymphoid follicles surrounded by small lymphocytes that infiltrate diffusely in LP and occasionally into epithelium
4	Suspicious lymphoid infiltrate in LP, probably lymphoma	Lymphoid follicles surrounded by CCL cells that infiltrate diffusely in LP and into epithelium in small groups
5	Low-grade B-cell lymphoma of MALT	Presence of dense diffuse infiltrate of CCL cells in LP with prominent LELs

LP, lamina propria; LEL, lymphoepithelial lesions; CCL, centrocyte-like.
Data from Wotherspoon AC, Doglioni C, Diss TC, et al. Regression of primary low grade B cell gastric lymphoma of mucosa associated lymphoid tissue after eradication of *Helicobacter pylori*. *Lancet* 1993;342:575–577.

confidence of a primary diagnosis of MALT lymphoma was used in initial studies (Wotherspoon score) (Table 30.2) (19,99), this alone was not seen as ideal as there was considerable interobserver variability. The GELA group recommends an assessment that included changes in density of lymphoid infiltrate, stromal changes, and presence of lymphoepithelial lesions (Table 30.3) (100). This scheme identified four categories of response and has been shown to have low interobserver variability (101). At one extreme, there is no change with persistence of the lymphoma with a dense infiltrate indistinguishable from the diagnostic material. At the other extreme is complete histologic remission with no significant lymphoid infiltrate. Between these two extremes, there are two categories that indicate responsive disease. Responding disease implies a partial regression of the lymphoid infiltrate, but persistence of overt lymphomatous infiltrate, and indicates response to therapy that may be ongoing with the implication that further intervention is not an immediate requirement, and follow-up remains the option of preference. The final category reflects the finding of lymphoid aggregates in the base of the mucosa (Fig. 30.16). While clinically these are probably of no significance and in the absence of endoscopically demonstrable disease should be considered as remission, it has been demonstrated that, in many cases,

these aggregates harbor residual clonal lymphoma cells. This has been designated probable minimal residual disease but, while these areas may harbor neoplastic B cells, clinically this should not indicate a need for further intervention.

Although clonality analysis may be valuable in assessment of the diagnostic biopsies, particularly those of suspicious lymphoma on a histologic and immunophenotypic ground, studies to date do not support a significant role of this molecular analysis in routine assessment of follow-up biopsies after treatments. First, the follow-up biopsies show presence of the tumor clone by PCR in approximately 50% of cases despite of absence of any macroscopic and histologic evidence of lymphoma (21,89,91,102–105). Second, the monoclonality is persistently present in a high proportion (~40%) of cases, with the basal lymphoid aggregates being the source of the clonal B cells (89,91,102,104,105). Finally, there was only a slightly higher risk of lymphoma relapse in the cases with persistent monoclonality than those without persistent monoclonality (89,91,102,104,105).

Similarly, there is no evidence suggesting a role of monitoring t(11;18)(q21;q21) during follow-up in guiding clinical management.

Clinical Behavior

Local recurrences may occur. In the stomach, these may be associated with recrudescence or reinfection with *H. pylori*. Follow-up biopsies may reveal isolated foci of lymphoma in the absence of endoscopically obvious relapse (105). Such foci may show spontaneous regression, and an abnormal infiltrate can be undetectable in subsequent biopsies (105). Relatively few patients die of gastric MALT lymphoma with a 90% 5-year survival and 75% 10-year survival. High-grade transformation can occur.

Differential Diagnosis

MALT Lymphoma Versus Reactive Lymphoid Infiltrates in the Stomach

In the early stages of lymphoma evolution, distinction between lymphoma and reactive infiltrates can be difficult. The presence of a significant B-cell infiltrate outside the mantle zone should be viewed as suspicious, particularly if there is extension of the B cells around glands and into the superficial lamina propria. The identification of true lymphoepithelial lesions is highly suspicious for lymphoma, but these have to be distinguished from the lymphoepithelium that can be seen with reactive

	Table 30.3	GELA SCHEME FOR ASSESSMENT OF GASTRIC BIOPSIES IN PATIENTS WITH GASTRIC MALT LYMPHOMA FOLLOWING ERADICATION THERAPY

GELA Category	Histology
CR (complete histologic response)	Absent or scattered plasma cells and small lymphoid cells in the LP. No LELs. Normal or empty LP and/or fibrosis
pMRD (probable minimal residual disease)	Aggregates of lymphoid cells or lymphoid nodules in the LP/muscularis mucosa and/or submucosa. No LELs. Empty LP and/or fibrosis
rRD (responding residual disease)	Dense, diffuse, or nodular extending around glands in the LP Focal or no LELs. Focal empty LP and/or fibrosis
NC (no change)	Dense, diffuse, or nodular LELs present (may be absent). No changes

LP, lamina propria; LEL, lymphoepithelial lesions; CCL, centrocyte-like.
Data from Copie-Bergman C, Wotherspoon AC, Capella C, et al. GELA histological scoring system for post-treatment biopsies of patients with gastric MALT lymphoma is feasible and reliable in routine practice. *Br J Hematol* 2013;160:47–52.

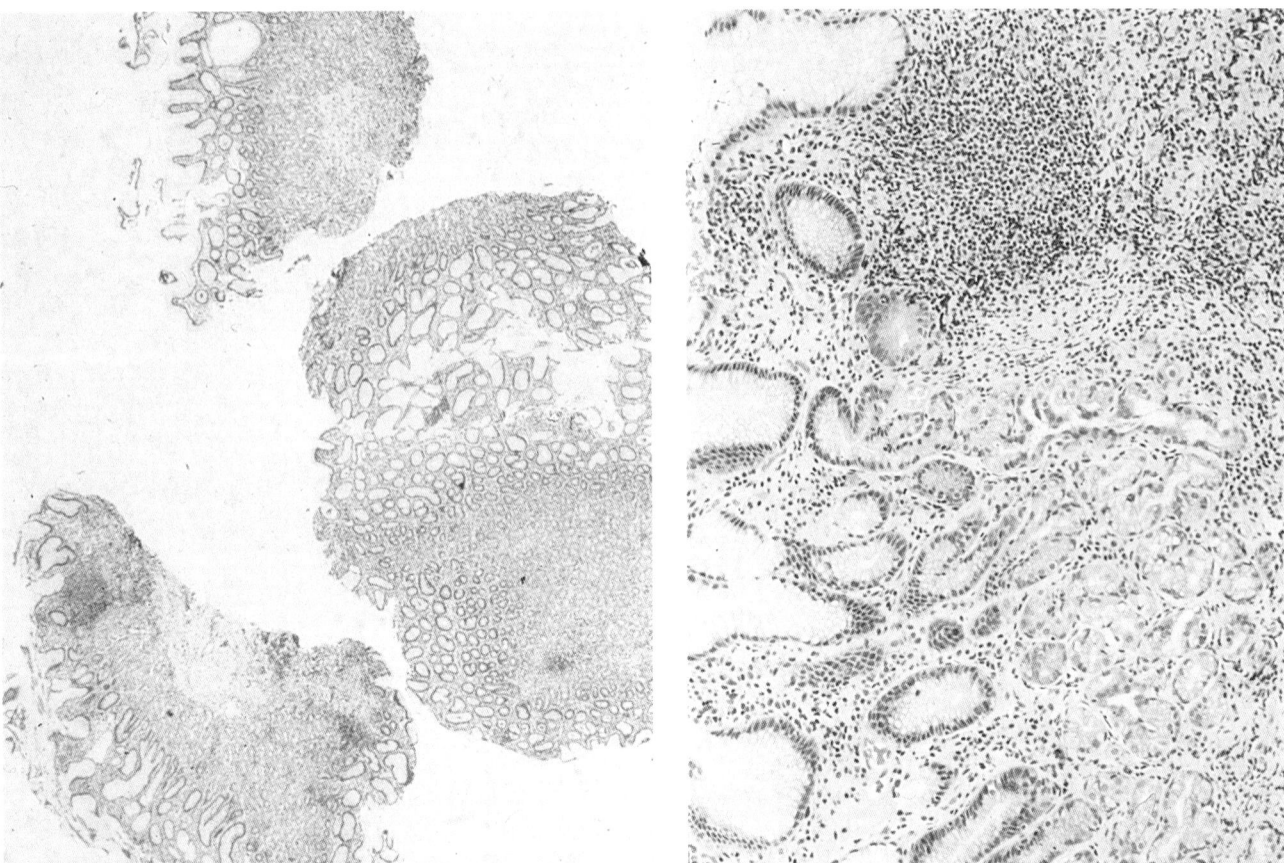

FIGURE 30.16. Posteradication biopsy. Probable minimal residual disease—presence of lymphoid nodules that in many cases harbor a small number of neoplastic cells that can be detected at the molecular level. This appearance has no clinical significance and should not, on its own, instigate further therapy.

proliferations and infiltration of the epithelium by clusters of small T cells that can also be encountered as a reactive process. Zukerberg et al. (106) suggest that the presence of prominent lymphoepithelial lesions, Dutcher bodies, and moderate cytologic atypia were features present in neoplastic infiltrates but absent in reactive proliferations.

Demonstration of light chain restriction is good evidence for lymphoma, but this may be difficult in small or distorted endoscopic biopsies. The presence of CD43 coexpression on the B cells is an indication of a neoplastic phenotype. The role of molecular studies using PCR is controversial. Several studies have suggested that clonal populations can be detected in reactive proliferations. These studies were conducted before the development of the European BIOMED-2 primer/protocol. With the optimized protocol/heteroduplex analysis, false-positive results from gastric biopsies are very rare if the assay is conducted correctly. The detection of clear clonal population should therefore be considered highly suspicious for the diagnosis of lymphoma in cases with equivocal histology. The detection of clonal populations in endoscopic biopsies has been shown to correlate well with higher Wotherspoon scores (107).

Lymphoid Hyperplasia of the Intestine

Focal Nodular Hyperplasia
This is a condition occurring at the ileocecal junction that is most common in children and young adults with a male preponderance (108). In the childhood variant, the presentation may be with intussusception. There is preservation of the normal architecture with hyperplastic follicles and edema of the submucosa.

The adult variant (109) often presents with a prolonged history of abdominal pain, sometimes with an associated mass in the right iliac fossa. There may be surface ulceration. There is marked follicular hyperplasia with expansion of the marginal zone. Cells from the marginal zone may enter the adjacent/overlying epithelium. There is a marked expansion of lymphoplasmacytoid cells in the bowel wall with deep extension that may extend to the serosa. This needs to be distinguished from MALT lymphoma, which can be achieved by demonstration of the polyclonal nature of this disorder with lack of monotypic light chain expression and absence of clonal gene rearrangement.

Diffuse Nodular Lymphoid Hyperplasia
This is a rare condition that affects long segments of the small bowel, colon, or both. In some cases, it is associated with acquired hypogammaglobulinemia (110). There are hyperplastic follicles in the mucosa with an intact mantle and indistinct marginal zone and an inconspicuous interfollicular infiltrate. In cases associated with hypogammaglobulinemia, there is no associated risk for development of lymphoma, but in other cases, there is a risk of progression to MALT lymphoma (111).

MALT Lymphoma Versus Other Indolent B-cell Lymphomas

Distinction between MALT lymphomas and other lymphomas composed mainly of small cells, principally mantle cell lymphoma, small lymphocytic lymphoma/chronic lymphocytic leukemia (SLL/CLL), and follicular lymphoma, is important as the management of these lymphomas will vary significantly.

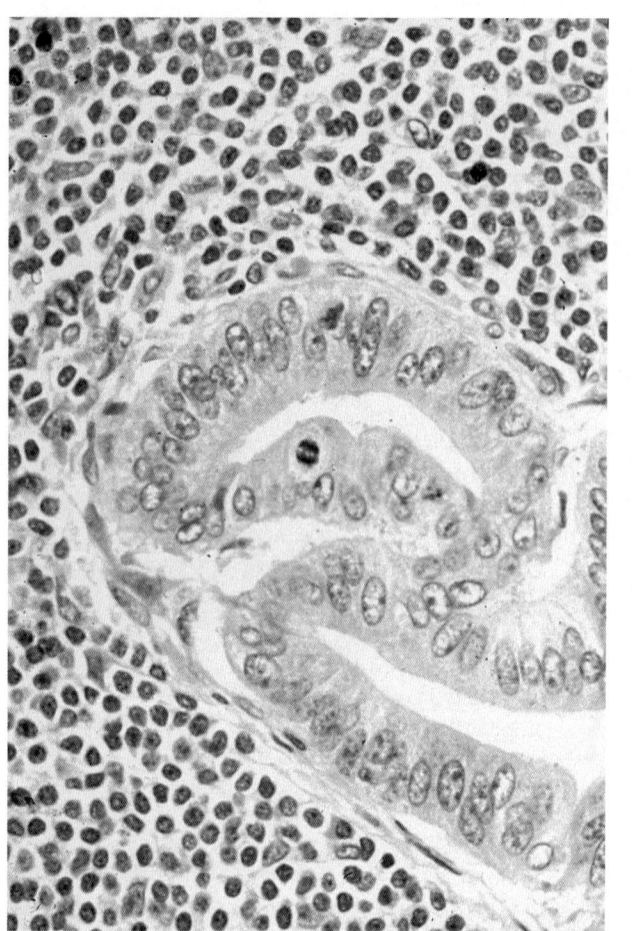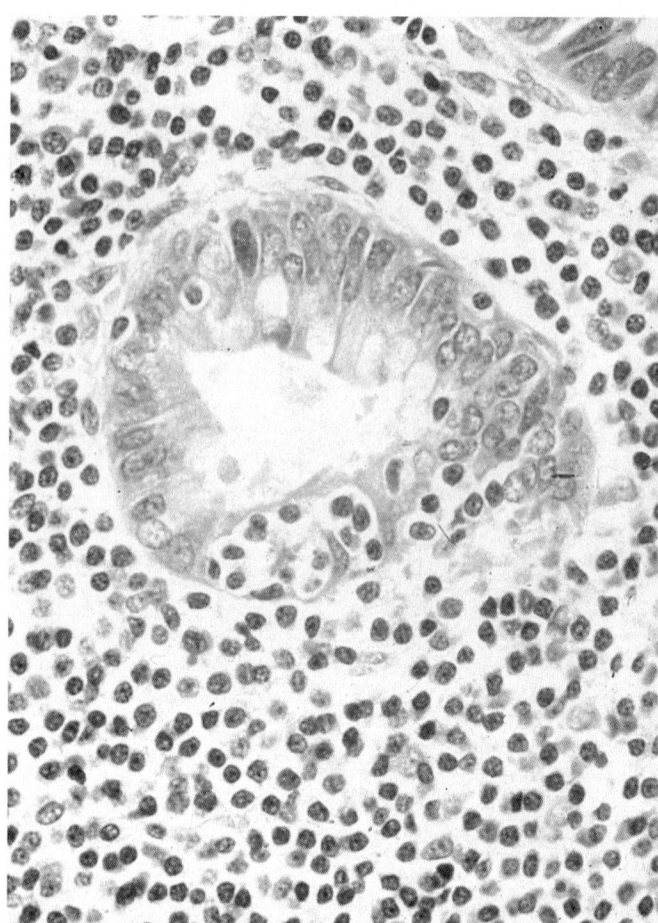

FIGURE 30.17. Gastric MALT lymphoma and adenocarcinoma. The neoplastic lymphoma cells do not infiltrate the neoplastic gland (**left**), while lymphoepithelial lesions are seen with normal glands (**right**).

MALT lymphoma cells can resemble the neoplastic cells of mantle cell lymphoma. Scattered transformed cells are seen in MALT lymphoma but are typically absent in mantle cell lymphoma. Immunophenotypically, mantle lymphoma characteristically expresses IgD, CD5, and, crucially, nuclear cyclinD1, which distinguishes it from MALT lymphoma.

The architectural organization also helps distinguish MALT lymphoma from SLL/CLL. There are no proliferation centers in MALT lymphoma, which is also characteristically strongly positive for CD20 and lacks staining for CD5 and CD23.

Distinction between MALT lymphoma with follicular colonization and follicular lymphoma can be problematic. In most cases, MALT lymphomas lack expression of CD10 and BCL6 in the follicles, while follicular lymphomas express these antigens in the neoplastic population within and between the follicles. Detection of t(14;18)(q32;q21) is characteristic of follicular lymphoma.

Gastric MALT Lymphoma and Adenocarcinoma

There are numerous reports of synchronous or metachronous gastric lymphoma and carcinoma (112,113) (Fig. 30.17). An epidemiologic study showed that patients with gastric MALT lymphoma had six times increased risk of developing gastric carcinoma as compared with the general control population (114) although there is no difference in the presence of premalignant lesions at the time of diagnosis between those who subsequently developed adenocarcinoma compared to those who did not (115). Thus, surveillance for gastric carcinoma should

be considered as a part of the routine in assessment of gastric biopsies in diagnosis and follow-up of gastric lymphoma.

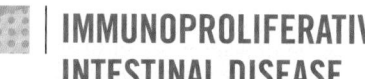 **IMMUNOPROLIFERATIVE SMALL INTESTINAL DISEASE**

IPSID is a specific subtype of MALT lymphoma characterized by pronounced lymphoplasmacytic and plasmacytic differentiation and is encountered in the upper intestine.

Epidemiology

IPSID is most frequently encountered in the Middle East and countries bordering the Mediterranean Sea, parts of the Indian subcontinent, and in the Cape region of South Africa and is very rare outside these regions. It most frequently occurs in young adults.

Clinical Presentation

IPSID presents at any age but mainly in young adults of low socioeconomic status. It presents with symptoms associated with malabsorption, diarrhea, obstruction and, in more advanced cases, a mass lesion and/or ascites. The disease runs a prolonged clinical course remaining confined to the abdomen until the terminal stages. In about two-thirds of cases, alpha-heavy chain can be detected in the serum or duodenal juice.

Macroscopic Appearance

As with other types of MALT lymphoma, the endoscopic/macroscopic appearance of IPSID depends on the degree of infiltration and stage. There is thickening of the small bowel wall in most cases, although more circumscribed areas can be encountered. Multiple polyps may be seen. Spread outside the small intestine is uncommon although the stomach may rarely be involved. Mesenteric lymph nodes are often enlarged.

IPSID and *Campylobacter jejuni* Infection

A number of studies attempted to identify the causative agent underlying the development of IPSID. An early case report showed the presence of *H. pylori* infection in the gastric metaplasia of the duodenum in a patient with chemotherapy refractory IPSID and complete regression of the lymphoma following antibiotic treatment (116). However, a subsequent study did not show any evidence of association between *H. pylori* infection and IPSID (117). In 2004, Lecuit and colleagues identified *C. jejuni* infection in the jejunal biopsy of a patient with IPSID by a PCR-based bacterial screening and reported a dramatic response of the lymphoma to eradication of *C. jejuni* (118). In addition, these authors further demonstrated the presence of the bacterium in 4/6 archival cases investigated (118). A later unpublished investigation showed *C. jejuni* in 12/27 (47%) cases of IPSID and 14/87 (16%) cases of other intestinal lymphomas, but not in nonintestinal lymphoma and normal/reactive intestinal biopsies (Diss TC, Personal communication, 2007). These results therefore support an association between IPSID and *C. jejuni* infection. However, unlike *H. pylori*, *C. jejuni* infection is not persistent in human, with the median duration of shedding in stools being only 1 month (119). It remains to be investigated whether *C. jejuni* has a causative role in the development of IPSID.

Histology

IPSID has a very characteristic appearance with the presence of sheets of plasma cells and very scanty lymphocytes (Fig. 30.18). The infiltrate causes widening of the villi. Plasma cells may colonize follicles in a similar fashion to classical MALT lymphoma.

Three stages are recognized (120,121). In stage A, the disease is confined to the mucosa with infiltration of the mesenteric nodes. Stage B is characterized by extension of the infiltrate through the muscularis mucosae, and the mucosal infiltrate is nodular. In stage C, there are lymphomatous masses and transformation to large cell lymphoma. The small lymphocytes have features of CCL cells and are typically seen around epithelial structures with lymphoepithelial lesions. These may be hard to detect and may only be seen with the assistance of immunostaining for CD20 but are more numerous in stage B than stage A.

Immunophenotype

The CCL cells of IPSID show a similar phenotype to classical MALT lymphoma occurring at other sites. The neoplastic cells show synthesis of IgA (usually IgA1), best demonstrated in the plasma cells (121,122). Light chain synthesis is not normally seen, although light chain restriction can be demonstrated in a few cases.

Molecular Genetics

The vast majority of IPSID are characterized by the synthesis of Ig-α1 heavy chain without the light chain by the neoplastic cells, with occasional cases showing the production of Ig-γ

heavy chain in absence of the light chain (123,124). Sequence analyses of the *IG* heavy chain gene derived from the neoplastic cells of IPSID show noncontiguous deletion that involves most of the VH/JH (heavy chain variable/joining) segments and the switch/CH1 (heavy chain constant region domain 1) sequence (125,126). The deletion often spares JH6, thus permitting demonstration of clonal *IGH* gene rearrangement by Southern blot with the *JH* probe (127). In addition, the deletion is commonly accompanied by inframe insertion of a sequence of unknown origin between the leader and *JH6*, *JH6*, and *CH2*, or between the leader and CH2 in cases with complete deletion of the *VH/JH* regions (125,126). The newly synthesized, truncated Ig heavy chains lacking the VH/JH and CH1 region most likely lose the ability to interact with BiP (the H-chain–binding protein), a chaperon protein that facilitates the nascent polypeptide folding and assembly, thus are secreted or expressed on the cell surface in the absence of the light chains. In some cases, additional deletion involves the 3′ region of CH3, which contains the polyadenylation site for secretory-form Ig-α mRNA, and this produces the nonsecretory phenotype of IPSID (126,128,129).

The genetic and molecular mechanisms underlying the absence of Ig light chain expression in IPSID are poorly understood. Truncated *IGκ* mRNA and *IGκ* rearrangement involving the κ deletion element have been described in cases of IPSID (128,129), and these genetic findings indicate functional inactivation of the *IGκ* allele. In addition, the lack of the Ig light chain expression may be due to transcriptional repression (130).

With the exception of a case report (128), there is hardly any PCR-based clonality study of IPSID. In view of the deletion seen in the *IGH* locus, the *IGH* PCR assays that use primers targeting the various frameworks (*Fr1*, *Fr2*, and *Fr3*) and *JH* regions offer no value in demonstration of monoclonality in IPSID. The value of *IG* light chain PCR in demonstration of monoclonality in IPSID remains to be investigated.

Despite being the prototype of MALT lymphoma, IPSID lacks the chromosome translocations associated with the MALT lymphoma entity (48). However, several chromosome translocations have been described in IPSID, and they include t(9;14)(p11;q32), t(2;14)(p12;q32), t(5;9)(q13;q31), t(1;20)(p36;q13), t(15;x)(p11;q11), and t(21;22)(q22;q11) (131–133). Later breakpoint analysis reveals that t(9;14)(p11;q32) juxtaposes the *PAX5* gene to the *IGH* locus and deregulates its expression (134). It remains to be investigated whether any of the above chromosome translocation is recurrent in IPSID. The genetic bases and molecular mechanisms underlying the development of IPSID also remain unknown.

Clinical Behavior

The disease usually has a prolonged course with rare dissemination outside the abdomen. In stage A disease, there may be regression following administration of broad-spectrum antibiotics (135). High-grade transformation can occur.

PRIMARY FOLLICULAR LYMPHOMA OF THE GIT

While follicular lymphoma is most commonly associated with nodal disease with frequent presentation in stage III to IV, often with bone marrow disease, the recent WHO classification of hemopoietic and lymphoid tumors has recognized the possibility of follicular lymphoma presenting with a primary extranodal location. It is recognized that primary intestinal follicular lymphoma differs in some respects from the nodal counterpart, principally in respect to clinical course and frequency of dissemination.

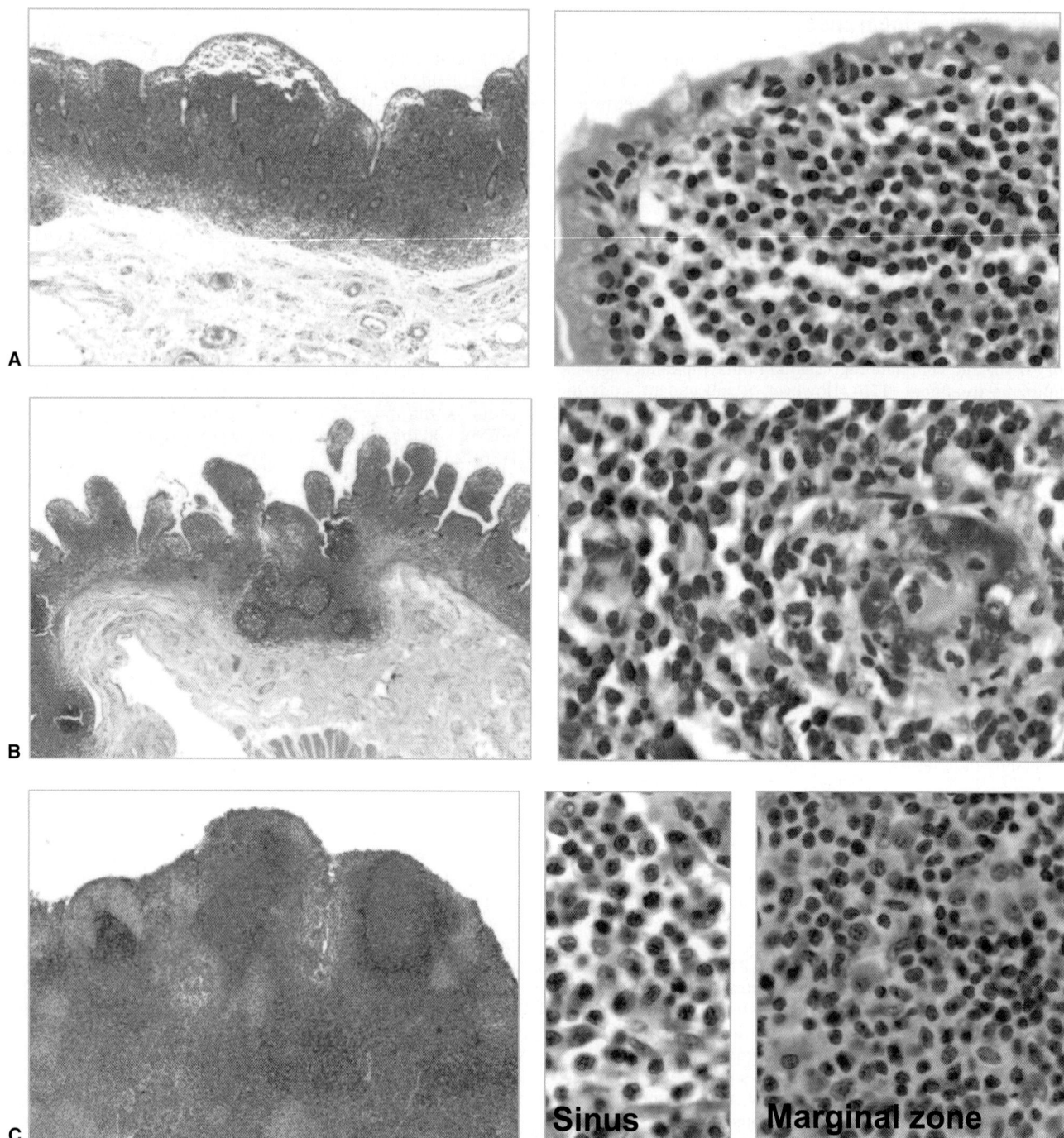

FIGURE 30.18. Histologic presentation of IPSID. Panel A shows diffuse infiltration of mature-looking neoplastic plasma cells in the mucosa; **Panel B** displays nodular lymphoid infiltrates extending through the muscularis mucosae and lymphoepithelial lesion; **Panel C** demonstrates the effacement of a mesenteric lymph node by the neoplastic cells, with diffuse infiltrate of plasma cells in the sinus and mixed infiltrate of plasma cells and CCL cells in the marginal zone.

Clinical Presentation

The demographics of patients developing primary intestinal follicular lymphoma are similar to those developing nodal disease (M:F 1:1; median age 56 years). Patients often have nonspecific symptoms, but may have abdominal pain or discomfort. The duodenum is the most frequent region involved although any part of the intestine can be involved.

Macroscopic Appearance

Endoscopically, there may be small nodules or polyps. In some cases, the lymphoma may be more advanced with deep infiltration of the wall. Although early studies suggested that a high proportion of cases were unifocal in the GIT, the introduction of wireless capsule endoscopy and double-balloon endoscopy has suggested that up to 73% may be multifocal (136).

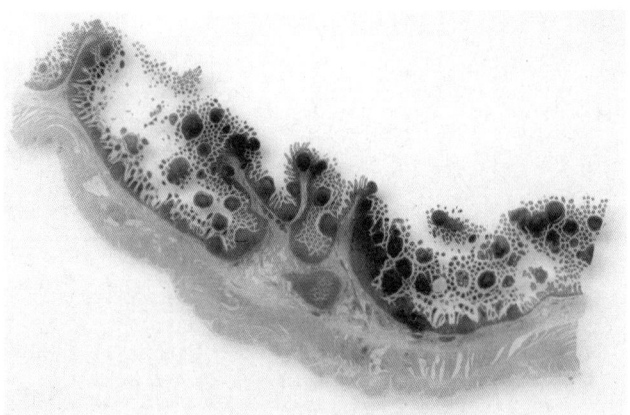

FIGURE 30.19. Primary follicular lymphoma of the intestine. Small intestine showing multiple neoplastic follicles in the mucosa.

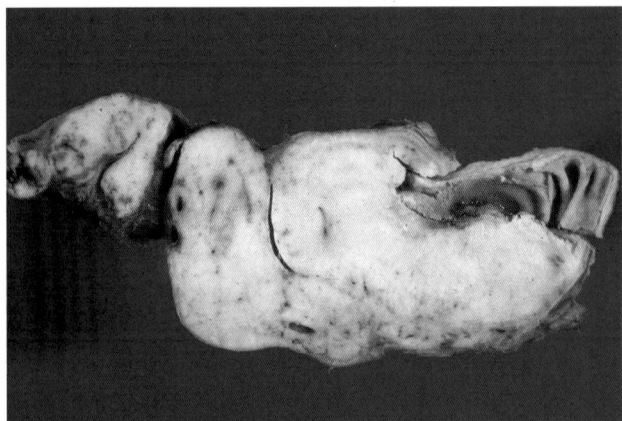

FIGURE 30.20. Resection of colonic lesion. Mantle cell lymphoma extending through the entire bowel wall.

Histology and Genetics

The morphology of GI follicular lymphoma is identical to the nodal counterpart with a mixture of centroblasts and centrocytes within the neoplastic follicles, but the majority of cases are grade 1 or 2 with only 4.3% being grade 3 (compared to around 20% for nodal follicular lymphoma) (137,138) (Fig. 30.19).

The immunophenotype of GI follicular lymphoma is identical to that of the nodal counterpart with the cells expressing CD19, CD20, CD22, PAX5, CD10, and BCL6. The vast majority are positive for BCL2. They are negative for CD5 and cyclinD1. Many cases express IgA. Studies have shown expression of $\alpha 4\beta 7$ integrin, which mediates migration to intestinal mucosa by binding to Mad-CAM-1 on mucosal vascular endothelium (139,140). This may explain the tendency for these tumors to remain localized to the GIT.

Genetic studies have shown the presence of the typical t(14;18)(q32;q21) in a similar proportion of cases to nodal lymphoma (137).

Clinical Behavior

In contrast to nodal follicular lymphoma where about a third of cases are low stage at presentation, the majority of GI follicular lymphomas present in clinical stage I/II (93.2%). It has been suggested that extraduodenal intestinal follicular lymphoma may show wider dissemination, but this may not always be the case (141).

The prognosis is good with few patients dying of disease and a median relapse-free survival of 63 months following therapy (142,143).

MANTLE CELL LYMPHOMA

Clinical Presentation

The majority of cases are encountered in patients over the age of 50 with an equal male-to-female ratio. Presenting symptoms are usually nonspecific, including abdominal pain and occasionally rectal bleeding.

Macroscopic Appearance

In the intestine, the lymphoma may present as discrete mass lesions (Figs. 30.20 and 30.21) or in the form of multiple small polyps. The most frequent site of involvement is the terminal ileum, although any part of the GIT can be involved.

Histology and Immunophenotype

Primary intestinal mantle cell lymphoma shows essentially identical features to its nodal counterpart. The cytology is usually that of typical mantle cell lymphoma with irregular/clefted nuclei and scanty cytoplasm (Fig. 30.22). The nuclei have absent or indistinct nucleoli. Immunophenotypically, the cells express CD19, CD20, CD22, CD5, CD43, and cyclinD1. SOX11 is also expressed. The cells are more frequently lambda-light chain restricted. Staining for CD21 or CD23 can highlight expanded follicular dendritic cell meshworks as seen in nodal cases. At the genetic level, the extranodal lymphomas show the same t(11;14)(q13;q32) as the nodal counterpart.

Clinical Behavior

There is usually involvement of mesenteric lymph nodes, and wider dissemination is frequent. The intestinal tract is frequently a secondary site of involvement from nodal mantle cell lymphoma. Almost all cases of stage IV disease (mainly by virtue of blood or bone marrow involvement) show infiltration of the stomach and intestine, even in areas with normal endoscopic appearance (144,145).

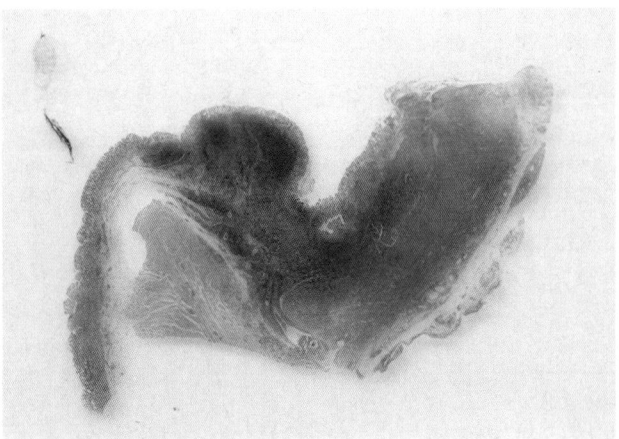

FIGURE 30.21. Mantle cell lymphoma. Low power showing extension of the lymphoid infiltrate through the gastric wall.

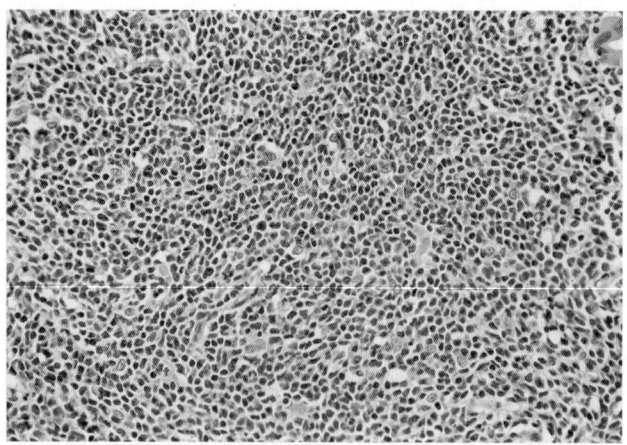

FIGURE 30.22. Mantle cell lymphoma. High power showing morphology of mantle cell lymphoma with features similar to nodal counterpart. Infiltrate is monotonous with cells having scanty cytoplasm and indented/clefted nuclei with indistinct nucleoli.

 ## MULTIPLE LYMPHOMATOUS POLYPOSIS

First described in 1961 (146), this condition was initially considered almost synonymous with mantle cell lymphoma (Fig. 30.23). However, it is now evident that follicular hyperplasia, follicular lymphoma, and MALT lymphoma may have indistinguishable endoscopic appearances with multiple small polyp/mucosal nodules over long segments of intestine (147,148).

 ## TRANSFORMED MALT LYMPHOMA AND DIFFUSE LARGE B-CELL LYMPHOMA OF THE STOMACH

Scattered transformed centroblast- or immunoblast-like cells are commonly found in gastric MALT lymphoma, but when they appear as solid or sheetlike proliferation, a diagnosis of DLBCL with accompanying MALT lymphoma should be made. The term "high-grade MALT lymphoma" should not be used. When solid or sheetlike large B cells are present in absence of

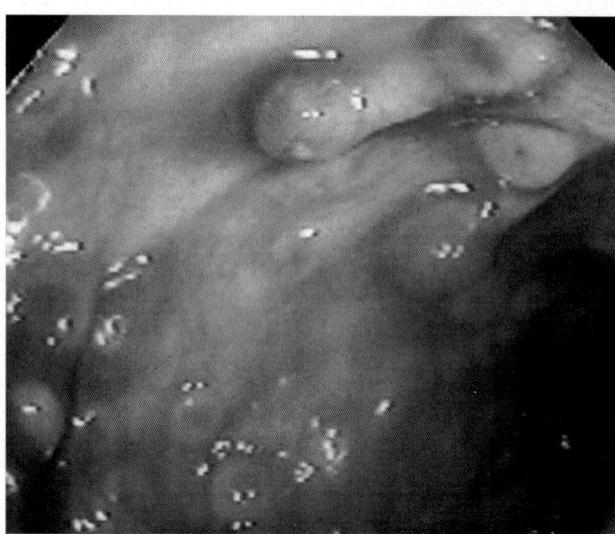

FIGURE 30.23. Endoscopic appearance of multiple lymphomatous polyposis. Multiple polyps are seen. The appearance is not specific to mantle cell lymphoma.

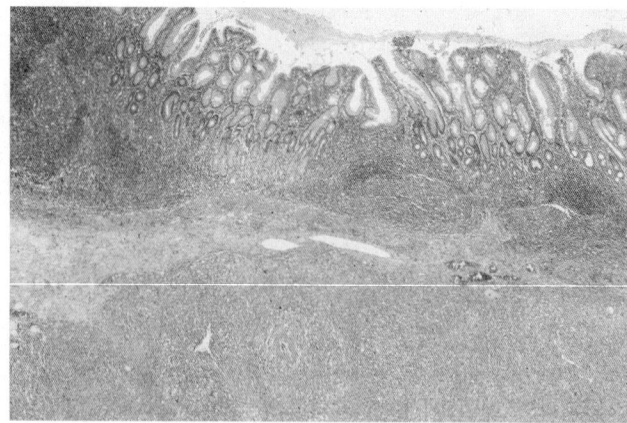

FIGURE 30.24. Gastric MALT lymphoma left with associated diffuse large B-cell lymphoma (**right**) composed of sheets of large cells.

MALT lymphoma component, the term DLBCL should be used (Figs. 30.24 and 30.25).

Clinical Presentation

The age and sex distribution of patients with DLBCL are similar to those of gastric MALT lymphoma, although a slightly increased age and male-to-female ratio are noted in some studies. The clinical symptoms are nonspecific, similar to those of gastric MALT lymphoma or carcinoma, and include dyspepsia, weight loss, and bleeding. Endoscopic features are variable but, unlike gastric MALT lymphoma, are often characterized by the presence of a tumor mass, particularly in patients with *de novo* DLBCL. Similar to gastric MALT lymphoma, the depth of lymphoma invasion and perigastric lymph node involvement are best to be assessed by EUS.

Histology and Immunophenotype

The cells resemble centroblasts or immunoblasts with moderately abundant cytoplasm and prominent nucleoli (Fig. 30.26). Multinucleated cells may be seen, and there may be infiltration of the epithelium (Fig. 30.27). Proliferation is high.

Molecular Genetics

The presence of coexisting MALT lymphoma and DLBCL does not necessarily indicate a clonal relationship between the two tumors. PCR and sequencing analyses of the rearranged

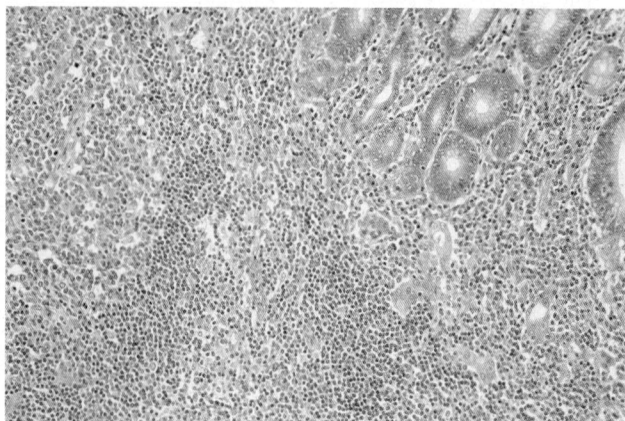

FIGURE 30.25. High power of combined gastric MALT lymphoma (**right**) with diffuse large B-cell lymphoma (**left**) showing a sheet of cells with centroblast-type morphology.

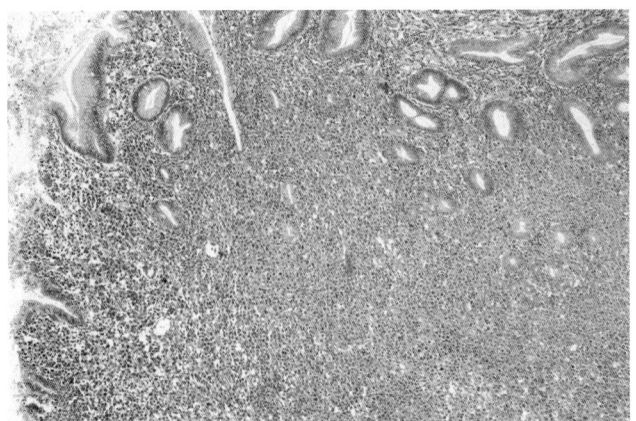

FIGURE 30.26. Diffuse large B-cell lymphoma. Diffuse infiltration of the lamina propria by a proliferation of large cells with abundant cytoplasm and vesicular nuclei with nucleoli.

IG gene of both lymphoma components indicate that DLBCL may derive from a MALT lymphoma or develop independently (149–151). Despite that a proportion of gastric DLBCL is the result of transformation of MALT lymphoma, the chromosome translocations that characterize MALT lymphoma are rarely seen in gastric DLBCL. Similar to nodal DLBCL, gastric DLBCL are heterogeneous in their genetic makeup and are featured by a range of common genetic abnormalities. The *BCL6*- and *MYC*-involved translocations are seen in approximately 20% and approximately 10% of gastric DLBCL (152–154), comparable to those observed in nodal DLBCL. However, unlike nodal DLBCL, gastric DLBCL rarely show the *BCL2*-involved translocation or presence of double chromosome translocations (152,154). The *FOXP1*- and *CD44*-involved translocations are infrequently seen in gastric DLBCL (67,152,155). Gains of 18q21 (*MALT1* and *BCL2*), 3q (*FOXP1* and *BCL6*), and 8q24 (*MYC*) are frequently observed in gastric DLBCL (67,152). In general, there is no significant difference in the frequencies of the above genetic abnormalities between gastric DLBCL with and without accompanying MALT lymphoma component (152).

A wide spectrum of somatic mutations has been reported in nodal DLBCL, particularly propelled by the recent studies using the massive parallel sequencing technology. These somatic changes affect several distinct cellular pathways, including the p53 pathway (156), the NF-κB activation pathway (157–163), the plasma cell differentiation program (164), the epigenetic program (157,165), and the antigen presentation machinery (166). Up to now, most of the above genetic changes have not

been investigated in gastric DLBCL (167). An early study demonstrated *TP53* mutation in 33% of cases of gastric DLBCL (168), and a recent study showed *TNFAIP3* (also known as *A20*, an NF-κB inhibitor) inactivation and *CARD11* (a positive NF-κB regulator) activation by somatic mutation in 17% and 10% of gastric DLBCL, respectively (167), which are similar to those seen in nodal DLBCL. It remains to be investigated to what extent the genetics of gastric DLBCL is similar or different from those of its nodal counterpart.

Clinical Behavior

Many cases present in stage I/II. Several independent studies have demonstrated that a high proportion (~65%) of early-stage gastric DLBCL with or without accompanying MALT lymphoma showed complete lymphoma remission after *H. pylori* eradication (169–174). The prognostic value of immunophenotypic features and genetic abnormalities in this clinical setting has not been investigated.

The conventional therapeutic options are similar to those for nodal DLBCL. Local resection can be undertaken to remove areas of bulk disease if clinically indicated, and this is often the case where patients have presented with an acute surgical emergency. In the setting of chemo- and radiation therapy, the prognostic value of immunophenotype and chromosome translocations has been evaluated only in retrospective studies, and the results are largely controversial. For example, the *MYC*-involved translocation was associated with low stage and better outcome in one study (154), but with aggressive disease in another (175). Among somatic mutations investigated so far, *TP53* and *A20* inactivation appears to be associated with poor overall survival (167,176).

Addition of rituximab to CHOP therapy clearly improves the survival of patients with gastric DLBCL (177,178), with the prognostic factors other than the clinical stage and IPI to be investigated.

DIFFUSE LARGE B-CELL LYMPHOMA OF THE INTESTINE

Clinical Presentation

The majority of cases are seen in older individuals, usually seventh decade or older with a slight male preponderance. Some cases are seen in children, and these are mostly located in the

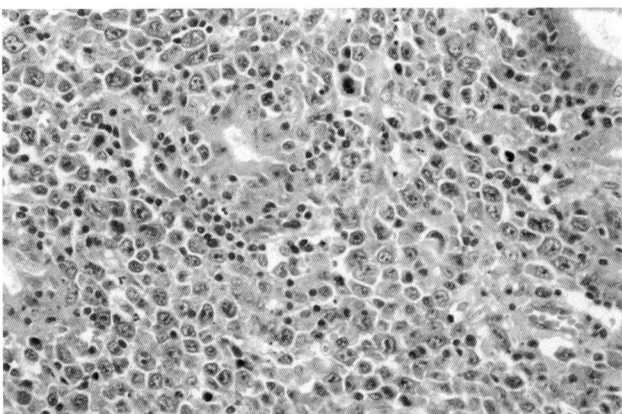

FIGURE 30.27. Diffuse large B-cell lymphoma of the stomach. In some cases, the neoplastic cells infiltrate and destroy the epithelial structures.

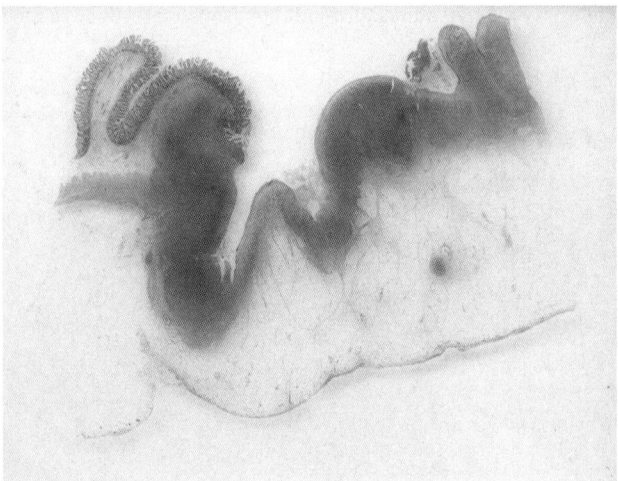

FIGURE 30.28. Low-power image of diffuse large B-cell lymphoma of the intestine. Tumor extends just beyond the muscularis propria.

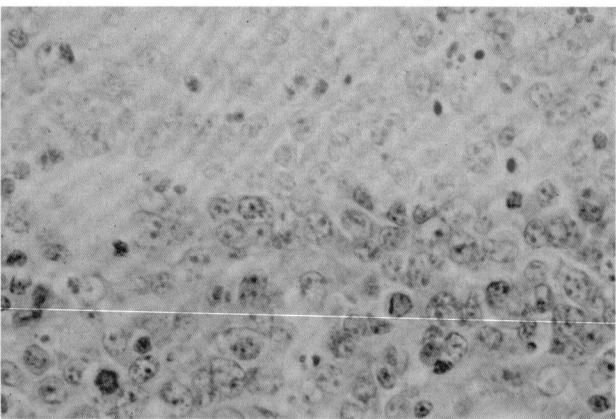

FIGURE 30.29. Diffuse large B-cell lymphoma. High power cytology is similar to nodal large B-cell lymphoma with large cells having nuclei with open chromatin and multiple nucleoli.

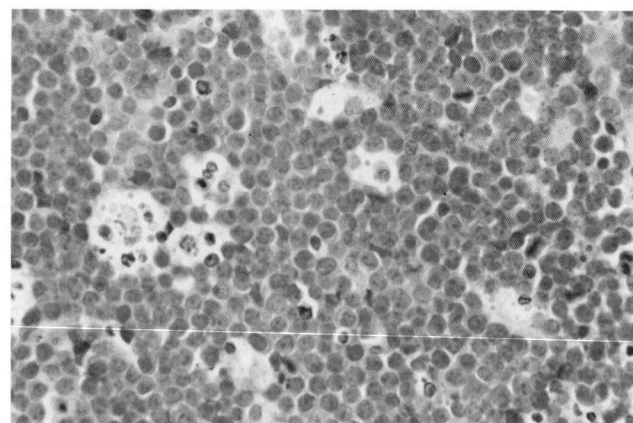

FIGURE 30.31. Burkitt lymphoma. High-power image showing the typical starry sky appearance. The cells are of intermediate size with regular round nuclei and small nucleoli.

terminal ileum. The lesions are usually single and mass forming, although multiple sites of involvement can be seen in some cases. There is a slightly higher incidence of intestinal large B-cell lymphoma in patients with ulcerative colitis with lesions more frequent in the distal colon/rectum (179–182).

Histology, Immunophenotype, and Genetics

The morphology is essentially identical to similar lymphomas encountered in lymph nodes with sheets of large cells expanding the wall (Figs. 30.28 and 30.29). The cells express pan B-cell markers and may show either germinal center or activated B-cell immunophenotype. Rearrangements of *BCL6* are more frequent and *BCL2* less frequent than seen in the nodal counterpart.

Clinical Behavior

Many cases present in stage I/II. Therapeutic options are similar to nodal large B-cell lymphoma. Local resection can be undertaken to remove areas of bulk disease if clinically indicated, but combination chemotherapy remains the main therapeutic option.

 BURKITT LYMPHOMA

Clinical Presentation

The majority of patients are male, and they usually present as children or young adults. Presentation is with intestinal-related

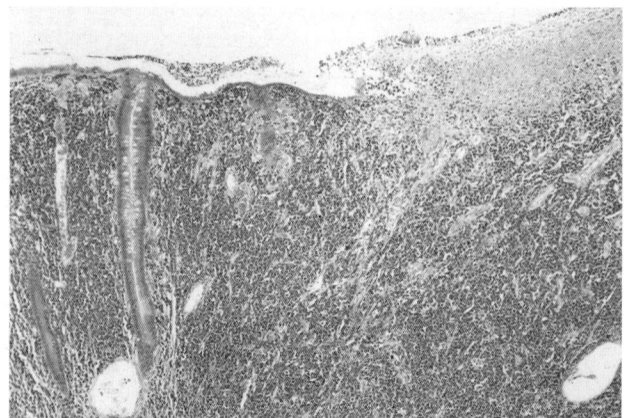

FIGURE 30.30. Burkitt lymphoma. Low-power image of intestinal Burkitt lymphoma showing diffuse infiltration of the lamina propria.

symptoms usually due to the effect of a mass lesion. Symptoms of intussusception may occur in patients with bulky lesions at the ileocecal valve.

Involvement of the intestinal tract is common in endemic and sporadic Burkitt lymphoma but less frequent in immunodeficiency-associated cases. The ileocecal valve is the most frequently involved region with the stomach and other parts of the intestine, rarely the site of origin for these tumors.

Tumors are frequently in the form of obstructing tumors or large masses with extension through the bowel wall. In spite of the extensive local spread, mesenteric nodal disease is not common.

Histology, Immunophenotype, and Genetics

The histology, immunophenotype, and cytogenetics of intestinal Burkitt lymphoma are identical to those seen elsewhere (Figs. 30.30 and 30.31). The cells are of intermediate size with a nucleus that is the same size or small than that of a histiocyte and shows minimal pleomorphism. The nuclear chromatin is finely clumped, and there are multiple small nucleoli. Mitoses are frequent. There is a sheetlike growth pattern with interspersed macrophages that contain apoptotic nuclear debris.

The cells express pan B-cell markers (CD19, CD20, CD22, and PAX5) with coexpression of CD10 and BCL6. Staining for BCL2 is characteristically negative. Proliferation is high (essentially 100% in most cases). The presence of EBV is seen in endemic cases, but the association is less common in sporadic and immunodeficiency cases.

Intestinal Burkitt lymphoma shows a similar genetic profile to lymphomas encountered elsewhere with translocations that involve *MYC* with t(8:14)(q24:q32) involving the heavy chain gene most frequently, while the kappa– or lambda–light chain genes are much less frequent translocation partners.

Clinical Behavior

The clinical behavior and treatment options are similar to those for Burkitt lymphoma encountered at other sites.

 T- AND NK-CELL LYMPHOMAS

Any T-cell lymphoma can develop or involve the GIT. In particular, extranodal NK/T-cell lymphoma of nasal type can be encountered. Few T- and NK-cell proliferations appear to be specific to this area.

ENTEROPATHY-ASSOCIATED T-CELL LYMPHOMA

EATL is a group of rare lymphomas that arise primarily in the small intestine with two variants that appear to have distinct epidemiologic, morphologic, and immunophenotypic features that suggest that they may represent two distinct pathologic entities (183). EATL accounts for about 5.4% of all PTCL being more common in Europe (9.1% of PTCL) than North America (5.8% of PTCL) and rare in Asia (1.9% of PTCL) (184). There is a slight male preponderance (184).

CLASSICAL EATL

Clinical Presentation

Classical EATL has a strong association with celiac disease (CD), although this is not absolute. Presentation is commonest in the sixth or seventh decade with an equal gender distribution. While the lymphoma may develop in the context of long-standing CD, often with poor dietary control, it is more frequent in cases with adult onset. This suggests that chronic antigen stimulation in subclinical CD may predispose to the development of lymphoma. The presence of the human leukocyte antigen (HLA) DQ2 or DQ8 in EATL and CD supports the association between the two conditions (185).

The most common presentation is malabsorption. In patients with established CD, EATL may manifest itself by reemergence of symptoms with failure to respond to a gluten-free diet. There may be accompanying abdominal pain and, in some cases, presentation is as a surgical emergence with perforation.

The disease is most often centered on the jejunum although any part of the small intestine can be affected and, occasionally, the stomach or colon. Rarely, patients present with extraintestinal manifestations as the first indication of disease. There is usually multifocal disease with ulcerating lesions, but there may be plaques or fissures. Mesenteric lymph nodes are frequently enlarged.

Histology, Immunophenotype, and Genetics

The characteristic appearance is of an infiltrate of pleomorphic cells often with numerous bizarre giant cells that are multinucleated (Fig. 30.32). In other cases, the cells may be more monotonous with abundant cytoplasm and large nuclei with nucleoli. Associated inflammatory cells and eosinophils are present in a variable density but, on occasion, may be so pronounced as to obscure the neoplastic population. These cases are frequently associated with extensive necrosis. The mucosa away from the lymphoma usually shows features characteristic of CD with villous atrophy, crypt hyperplasia and increased intraepithelial lymphocytes, and increased plasma cells in the lamina propria.

The neoplastic cells express T-cell antigen CD3 and CD7, but often lack CD5 (Fig. 30.32). Expression of CD3 may be cytoplasmic or may be absent in some cases. The cells are typically negative for both CD4 and CD8 (Fig. 30.32). Cytotoxic granule–associated proteins can be detected. In cases with large cells, these are frequently positive for CD30. There may be expression of TCR-alpha/beta, but expression of TCR-gamma/delta is not seen. Detection of CD103, a specific marker of intestinal intraepithelial lymphocytes, can be detected, but this requires unfixed material.

The mucosa away from EATL often shows marked villous atrophy and increased IEL, which are CD8 negative and have been shown to be clonally related to the main tumor (Fig. 30.32).

There is rearrangement of the TCR-beta and gamma genes (186). The vast majority (>90%) have the HLA DQA1'0501, DBQ1'0201 haplotype (187). There may be chromosomal gains at 9q33-q34, 7q, 5q34-q35, and 1q21-q23 and losses at 8p, 13q21, and 9p21, deletions in 16q12.1 or gains in 1q or 5q (183,188).

Clinical Behavior

Classical EATL generally has a dismal prognosis. The overall survival is around 10 months with a median failure-free survival of 6 months (184). The involvement of multiple segments of the bowel makes resection impossible in most cases. Patients are frequently severely debilitated by malabsorption, making administration of chemotherapy impossible.

TYPE II EATL

Clinical Presentation

Patients present with similar symptoms to the classical variant with abdominal pain and diarrhea, intestinal obstruction, or perforation. There is no specific association with CD, and the lymphoma develops in geographic areas where CD is not seen. It has recently been shown that all cases of EATL in the Chinese population fall into this group (189). The disease usually arises in the small intestine, although isolated involvement of other areas can be seen.

Histology, Immunophenotype, and Genetics

The infiltrate is usually transmural. There is frequently very marked intraepithelial lymphocytosis. The cells are intermediate sized and monotonous with central round hyperchromatic nuclei and pale cytoplasm (Fig. 30.33).

The cells express CD3, CD8, and CD56 with cytotoxic granule–associated proteins (Fig. 30.33). They are negative for CD5, CD4, and CD30. A study of EATL in a Chinese population has shown that the majority (78%) express the gamma/delta-TCR (189). A minority may express both gamma/delta- and alpha/beta-receptors and, occasionally, both receptors are absent (189). The majority of cases are not associated with EBV, although the virus may be detected in a small minority of cases.

There is no association with the HLA characteristics of CD but, in common with the classical variant gain of 9q31.1 or loss of 16q12.1, is frequently seen (188). Gain in 1q and 5q is less commonly seen in this variant.

Clinical Behavior

The outlook for type II EATL is similar to the classical variant (184).

REFRACTORY COELIAC DISEASE

Refractory celiac disease (RCD) may be considered as a smoldering premalignant state before the development of overt EATL (190,191). Clinically, RCD is defined either by the presence of persistent diarrhea, abdominal pain, and involuntary loss of weight, with demonstration of villous atrophy or deterioration on biopsies despite a strict gluten-free diet for more than 12 months, or where symptoms recur after a former period of response to a gluten-free diet (190,191). Based on the immunophenotypic and genotypic investigations, RCD is subdivided into two subtypes: RCD-I and RCD-II.

RCD-I is featured by IEL that are polyclonal and show no evidence of aberrant immunophenotype, while RCD-II is

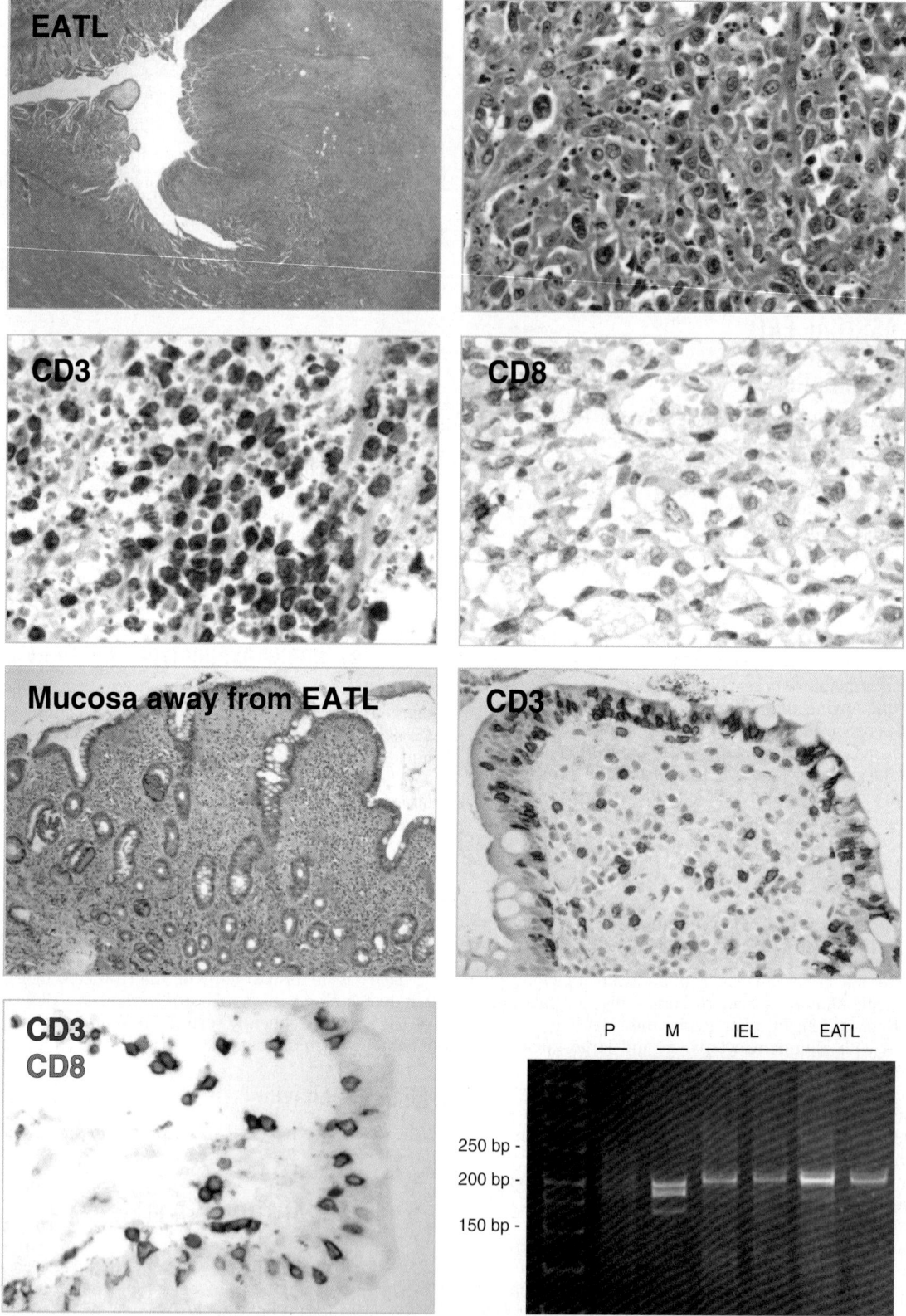

FIGURE 30.32. **An example of classical EATL and the jejunal mucosa away from the tumor.** Low-power image (**top left**) shows extensive ulceration and lymphoid infiltration of the intestinal wall. High-power image (**top right**) displays the pleomorphic neoplastic T cells, which are CD3 positive and CD8 negative by immunohistochemistry. The mucosa away from EATL shows severe villous trophy and increased IELs, which are negative for CD8. Clonality analysis of the rearranged TCR genes demonstrates the clonal link between EATL and IELs in the mucosa away from the lymphoma. P, polyclonal control; M, monoclonal control; IEL, intraepithelial lymphocyte.

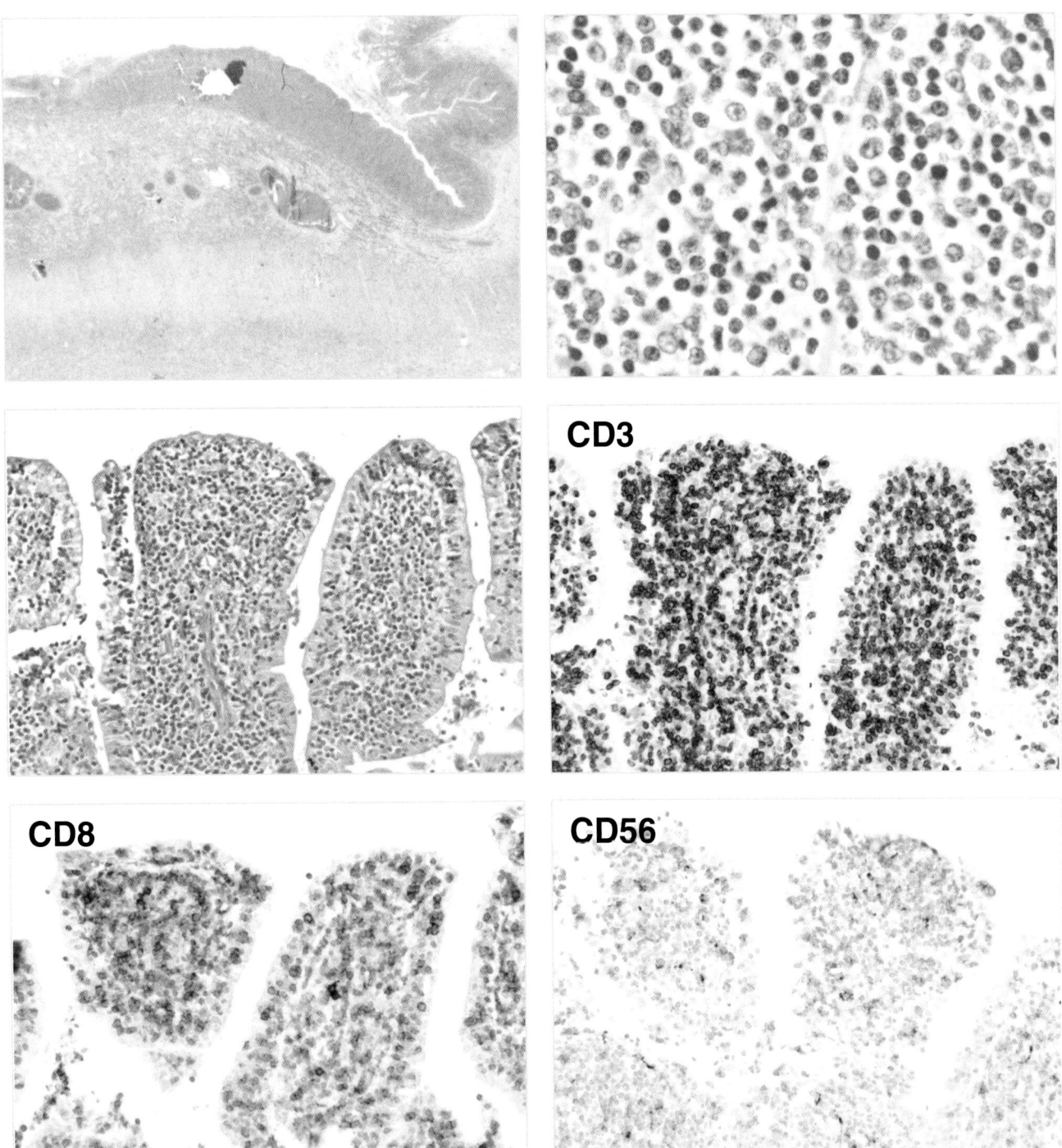

FIGURE 30.33.   An example of Type II EATL. Top panel shows extensive mucosal infiltration by small round monomorphic cells. The adjacent mucosa displays very marked intraepithelial lymphocytosis. The IELs are positive for CD3, CD8, and CD56 by immunohistochemistry.

characterized by IEL that are clonal and exhibit an aberrant immunophenotype (Fig. 30.34). The majority of RCD-II show IEL expressing CD103 and cytoplasmic CD3, but not surface CD3, CD4, CD8, TCR $\alpha\beta$, and TCR $\gamma\delta$ (190–194). A proportion of IEL in RCD-II may express CD30 (195). The phenotypically aberrant and monoclonal IEL population is frequently present throughout the GIT (196), and occasionally involves skin (197). In patients with RCD-II, ulcerative jejunitis is common (195,198). Approximately 50% of patients with RCD-II develop EATL, which shows an identical aberrant immunophenotype

and TCR rearrangement to those of the preceding RCD (186,191,193,199,200,201). It is generally accepted that RCD-II is in fact a cryptic T-cell lymphoma, an early manifestation of EATL (202). Not surprisingly, patients with RCD-II have a poor prognosis, with a 5-year survival being 40% to 50%, in comparison with over 90% survival rate for patients with RCD-I (194,201).

The diagnosis of RCD can be a challenge. Although several clinical, histologic/immunophenotypic, and molecular features point to the diagnosis of RCD, none of these features alone is

Duodenal biopsy

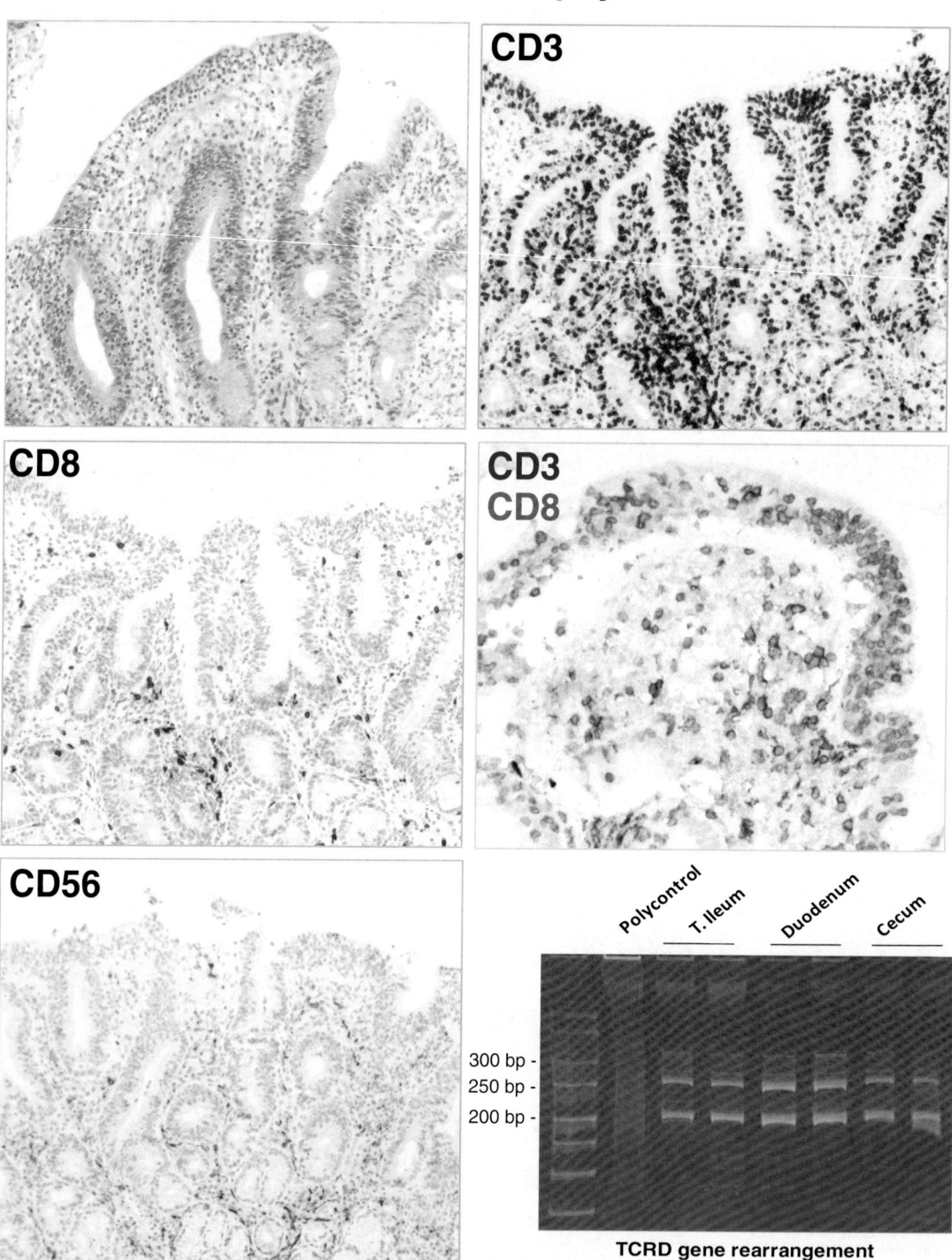

FIGURE 30.34. An example of RCD-II. The duodenal biopsy shows villous atrophy and marked intraepithelial lymphocytosis, which is highlighted by CD3 immunohistochemistry. The IELs are negative for CD8 and CD56. Clonality analysis of the rearranged TCR-delta genes using the BIOMED-2 protocol demonstrates the presence of an identical clonal T-cell population among the duodenal, terminal ileal, and cecal biopsies in this case.

sufficiently sensitive or specific to support a definite diagnosis. The interpretation of clinical and histologic features is often complicated by lack of strict compliance with a gluten-free diet. Thus, an integrate assessment of clinical presentation, dietary compliance, serologic, histologic, immunophenotypic, and genetic findings is critical for final diagnosis.

For RCD-II, demonstration of monoclonality and aberrant immunophenotype is essential for diagnosis (Fig. 30.34). T-cell clonality analysis is now commonly carried out using the standardized BIOMED2 protocols (39). The IEL immunophenotype is conventionally analyzed by single immunohistochemistry, but increasingly double immunohistochemistry or flow cytometry is employed (203). Flow cytometry analysis is more objective, but requires fresh tissue biopsies and does not offer a direct correlation with histologic features. In general, an aberrant immunophenotype is considered when flow cytometry shows >20% of CD103$^+$, CD7$^+$, surface CD3$^-$, and CD8$^-$ T cells (203). Double immunohistochemistry is amenable to routine formalin-fixed paraffin-embedded tissue biopsies and allows direct correlation with histologic features but suffers from imprecision, as interpretation can be subjective. Nonetheless, when it is appropriately performed, it is highly valuable in RCD-II diagnosis (193,198,199). In general, an aberrant immunophenotype is considered when CD3/CD8 double immunohistochemistry shows CD3$^+$CD8$^-$ IEL above 40%.

The aberrant immunophenotype and monoclonality of IEL may be seen during the celiac disease stage, but they are often transient and associated with gluten-free diet noncompliance, and rarely occur concurrently (199). In contrast, the aberrant immunophenotype and monoclonality are nearly always persistent and often concurrent in RCD-II, and the extent of CD3$^+$CD8$^-$ IEL also increases during the disease progression (199). The presence of persistent concurrent aberrant IEL (especially >80% CD3$^+$CD8$^-$) and monoclonality is a strong predictor of EATL development (199).

A small proportion of RCD-II shows either a loss of CD8 or monoclonality (191,192,196,199,203,204). Such inconsistency may be due to limitation of sensitivity of the methodologies used. Nonetheless, rare cases of clonal RCD-II showing an aberrant IEL immunophenotype other than loss of CD8$^+$ have been reported (203,204).

The genetic basis of RCD is unknown. Several clonal genetic abnormalities, including partial trisomy 1q22-q44 and chromosome translocation, have been reported in the immunophenotypically abnormal T-cell clones isolated from patients with RCD by conventional cytogenetic analysis (205).

 ## CD4-POSITIVE SMALL T-CELL LYMPHOMA OF THE INTESTINE

There have been several recent reports of a distinctive T-cell lymphoma that arises in the intestine of patients who present with malabsorptive features (206–209). The infiltrate is composed of small lymphoid cells that fill the lamina propria with a minor infiltration of the epithelium (Fig. 30.35). There is mild villous shortening without crypt hyperplasia. The T cells express CD4 without CD8 and express TCR-beta (Fig. 30.35). They do not stain with antibodies to CD56 (Fig. 30.35) and show clonal TCR gene rearrangement. In one case, a novel translocation, t(4:16)(q26;p13), which involves the interleukin-2 gene, has been demonstrated (209). The clinical course is slowly progressive with prolonged survival but a poor response to therapy (206).

 ## INTESTINAL NK/T-CELL LYMPHOMA

Clinical Features

Primary intestinal NK/T-cell lymphoma is mainly reported in the Southeast Asia where extranodal NK/T-cell lymphoma, nasal type, is more prevalent. The lymphoma occurs in a wide range of age, but often in 30s to 40s with a significant male predominance (210–213). The most common symptoms are abdominal pain, followed by fever, weight loss, diarrhea, and hematochezia, but no history of celiac disease (210–213). Patients with primary intestinal NK/T-cell lymphoma are often complicated by intestinal perforation and obstruction (210–213).

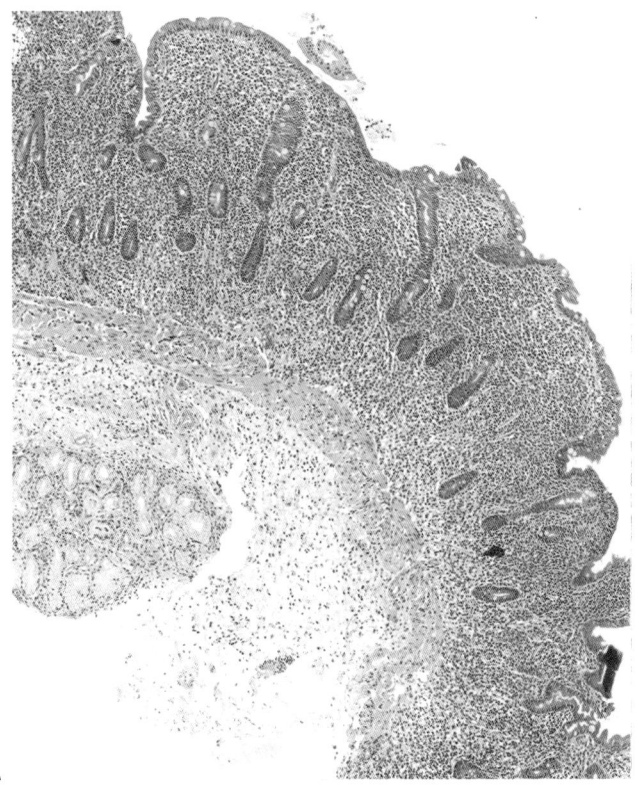
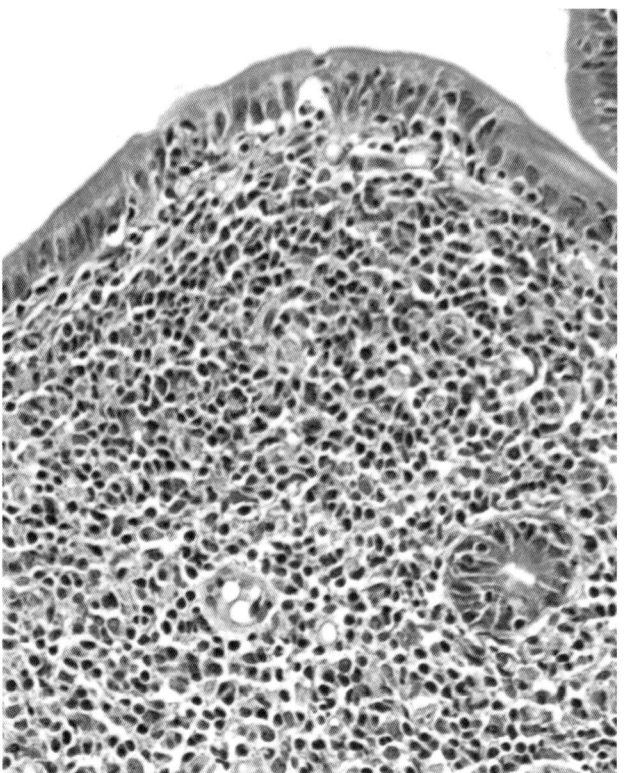

A   **B**

FIGURE 30.35. CD4$^+$ small T-cell lymphoma of the intestine. There is expansion of the lamina propria by a population of small mature lymphocytes that express CD4 and TCR-beta but are negative for CD8 and CD56. (**A, B**) H&E,

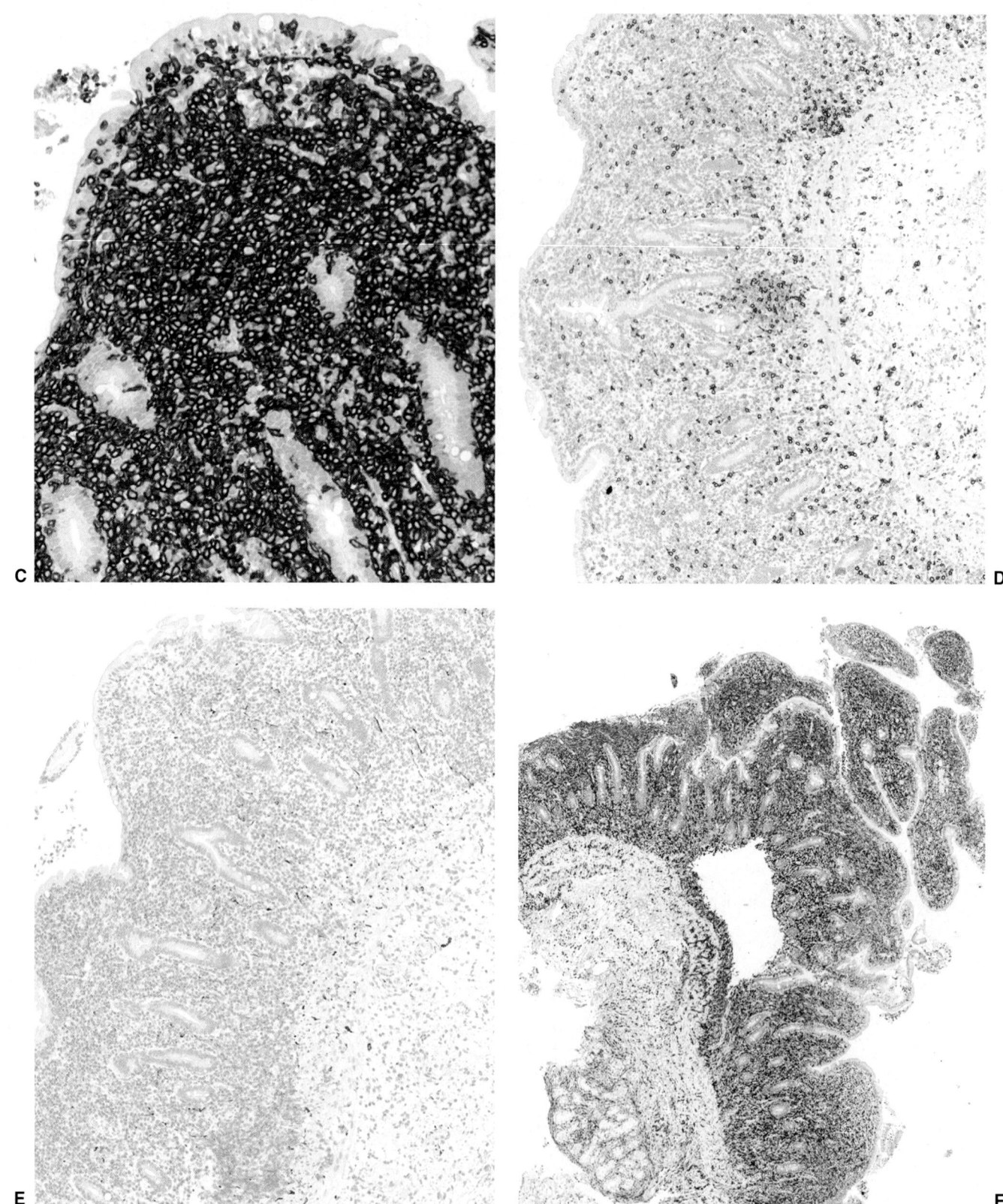

FIGURE 30.35. *(Continued)* **(C)** CD4, **(D)** CD8, **(E)** CD56, **(F)** TCR-beta.

Macroscopic Appearance

Primary intestinal NK/T-cell lymphoma may occur in any part of the intestine, but commonly involves the jejunum, followed by the ileum and cecum, and is frequently multicentric (210–213). The tumor is commonly featured by diffuse irregular ulcers, followed by tumor masses, which are frequently accompanied by stricture.

Histology, Immunophenotype, and Genetics

The tumor is characterized by mucosal ulceration and diffuse lymphomatous infiltration, often involving the deep layers of the intestinal wall. The tumor cells are medium-to-large pleomorphic lymphoid cells with angulated nuclei and moderate cytoplasm (Fig. 30.36). In the vast majority of cases, there are prominent necrosis and infiltration by inflammatory cells, including small lymphocytes, neutrophils, and plasma cells.

There is no evidence of increased IEL and villous atrophy in the mucosa adjacent and distant to the main tumor mass (210–213).

The tumor cells are typically positive for CD56 and cytotoxic markers (TIA1 and granzyme B), and also variably express CD3, but are CD5⁻, CD4⁻, CD8⁻, and βF1⁻ (210–213) (Fig. 30.36). The tumor cells are diffusely positive for EBV by EBER *in situ* hybridization (210–213) (Fig. 30.36).

The TCR and immunoglobulin genes are in germline configuration. The genetic bases of primary intestinal NK/T-cell lymphoma are unknown. Nonetheless, studies of extranodal NK/T-cell lymphoma, nasal type, show recurrent gain of 7q and recurrent loss of 6q16-q27 (214,215).

Clinical Behavior

This is a very aggressive lymphoma with short survival and poor response to therapy.

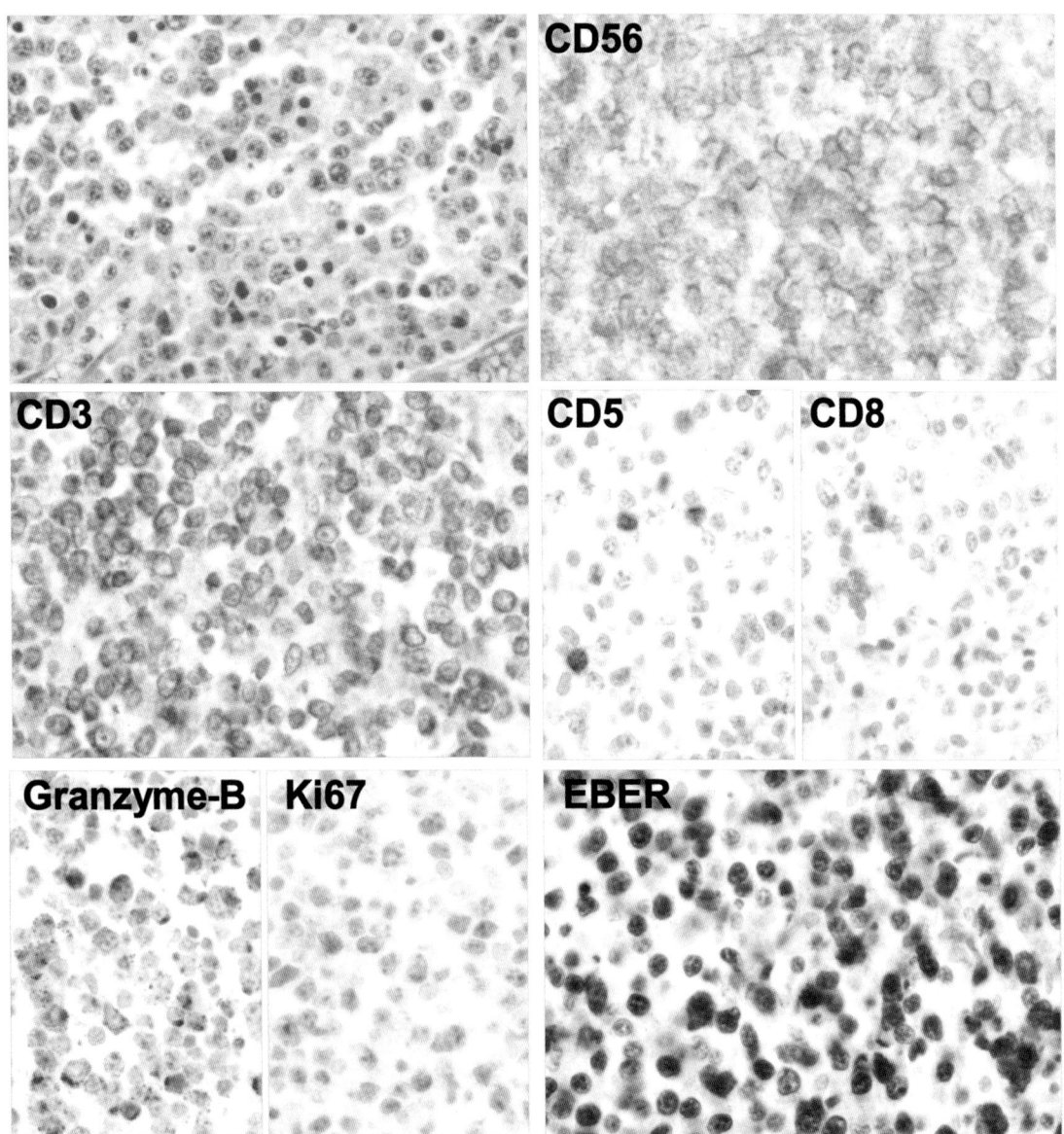

FIGURE 30.36. An example of intestinal NK/T-cell lymphoma. The neoplastic cells are medium-to-large–sized lymphoid cells with one or two nucleoli and moderate cytoplasm, expressing CD56 and CD3, but not CD5 and CD8. The neoplastic cells are positive for granzyme B and highly proliferative as shown by Ki67 immunohistochemistry. All tumor cells are EBV positive by EBER *in situ* hybridization.

PERIPHERAL T-CELL LYMPHOMA NOT OTHERWISE SPECIFIED

There are also cases of primary intestinal T-cell lymphomas that are clearly different from the above entities and commonly reported under the term of peripheral T-cell lymphoma not otherwise specified (PTCL NOS). These lymphomas are heterogeneous in their cytologic appearances and immunophenotype. They show variable expression of T-cell markers (CD3, CD4, CD8, and βF1) and CD56, and are often positive for cytotoxic markers. A small proportion of these cases are EBV positive, but all cases show clonally rearranged TCR genes.

NK-CELL ENTEROPATHY

It has recently been recognized that reactive proliferations of NK cells can occur in the stomach and intestines (216,217). These are rare but need to be distinguished from neoplastic infiltrates to avoid overtreatment.

Clinical Presentation and Macroscopic Appearance

This is a rare entity that is more common in patients over 45 years with a possible slight female preponderance (216,217). Patients present with vague intestinal symptoms. Endoscopy shows variable appearance with mainly small lesions that may be hemorrhagic or small (<10 mm) ulcers that may be single or multiple (216,217).

Histology and Immunophenotype

The infiltrate is generally circumscribed and confined to the mucosa with no loss of villous height in small intestinal cases. The cells have a diffuse growth pattern and are intermediate to large with moderate amounts of cytoplasm that may contain eosinophilic granules. The nuclei are round or mildly irregular with clumped chromatin and indistinct nucleoli. There is no angiocentricity or angiodestruction. The periphery of the lesion contains an infiltrate of small lymphocytes, plasma cells, and histiocytes.

The cells express CD56 and CD7 with cytoplasmic CD3 and presence of cytotoxic granules identified by staining for perforin, TIA1, or granzyme B. There is variable staining for CD2 and CD45. The cells are negative for cytoplasmic CD3 and do not express CD16. Proliferation is low, and EBV is not detected.

Clinical Behavior

This is a benign proliferation characterized by persistence of the lesions with occasional spontaneous remissions (216,217). The lesions need to be distinguished from aggressive lymphomas.

HISTIOCYTIC AND MYELOPROLIFERATIVE LESIONS IN THE INTESTINAL TRACT

Neoplastic histiocytic and myeloid proliferations are rare in the GIT, although histiocytic tumors, when they occur, are frequently encountered as primary intestinal tumors. Histiocytic sarcoma in the GIT has similar morphology, immunophenotype, and behavior to those tumors occurring at other sites (Fig. 30.37).

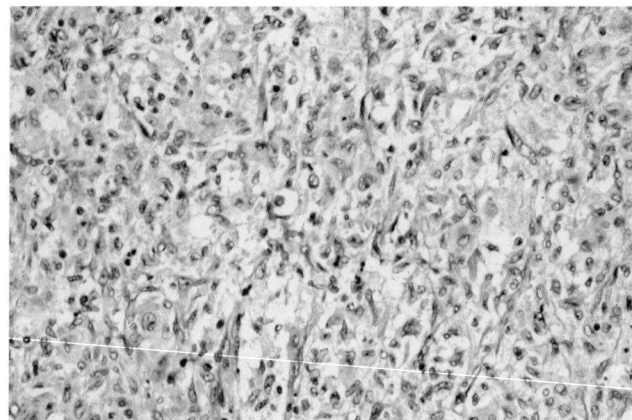
FIGURE 30.37. Histiocytic lymphoma (sarcoma). The tumor consists of a sheet of pleomorphic large cells with abundant pale eosinophilic cytoplasm.

SUMMARY AND CONCLUSIONS

There is a group of lymphomas of both B- and T-cell type that occur specifically at extranodal sites, and these account for the majority of the lymphomas in the GIT. When lymphomas are mainly encountered in GIT, particularly follicular lymphoma, the clinical features and natural history may vary from their nodal counterparts. Recognition of the different behavior of these primary gastrointestinal lymphomas and correct diagnosis of these entities are important for the selection of appropriate and often less intensive therapies.

References

1. Dawson IMP, Cornes JS, Morson BC. Primary malignant tumour of the intestinal tract. *Br J Surg* 1962;49:80–89.
2. Salem P, El-Hashimi L, Anaissie E, et al. Primary small intestinal lymphoma in adults: a comparative study of IPSID in the Middle East. *Cancer* 1987;59:1670–1676.
3. Brandtzaeg P. Mucosal immunity: induction, dissemination and effector functions. *Scand J Immunol* 2009;70:505–515.
4. Sheridan BS, Lefrancois L. Intraepithelial lymphocytes: to serve and protect. *Curr Gastroenterol Rep* 2010;12:513–521.
5. Gibbons DL, Sencer J. Mouse and human intestinal immunity: same ballpark, different players; different rules, same score. *Mucosal Immunol* 2011;4:148–157.
6. Radaszkiewicz T, Dragosics B, Bauer P. Gastrointestinal malignant lymphomas of the mucosa-associated lymphoid tissue: factors relevant to prognosis. *Gastroenterology* 1992;102:1628–1638.
7. Doglioni C, Wotherspoon AC, Moschini A, et al. High incidence of primary gastric lymphoma in Northeastern Italy. *Lancet* 1992;33:834–835.
8. Genta RM, Hamner HW, Graham DY. Gastric lymphoid follicles in *Helicobacter pylori* infection: frequency, distribution and response to triple therapy. *Hum Pathol* 1993;24:577–583.
9. Wyatt JL, Rathbone BJ. Immune response of the gastric mucosa to *Campylobacter pylori*. *Scand J Gastroenterol Suppl* 1988;142:44–49.
10. Stolte M, Eidt S. Lymphoid follicles in antral mucosa: immune response to *Campylobacter pylori*? *J Clin Pathol* 1989;42:1269–1271.
11. Joo M, Kwak JE, Chang SH, et al. *Helicobacter heilmannii*-associated gastritis: clinicopathologic findings and comparison with *Helicobacter pylori*-associated gastritis. *J Korean Med Sci* 2007;22:63–69.
12. Wotherspoon AC, Ortiz Hidalgo C, Falzon MR, et al. *Helicobacter pylori*–associated gastritis and primary B cell gastric lymphoma. *Lancet* 1991;338:1175–1176.
13. Eck M, Greiner A, Schmausser B, et al. Evaluation of *Helicobacter pylori* in gastric MALT-type lymphoma: differences between histologic and serologic diagnosis. *Mod Pathol* 1999;12:1148–1151.
14. Zucca E, Bertoni F, Roggero E, et al. Molecular analysis of the progression from *Helicobacter pylori*-associated chronic gastritis to mucosa-associated lymphoid-tissue lymphoma of the stomach. *N Engl J Med* 1998;338:804–810.
15. Nakamura S, Aoyagi K, Furuse M, et al. B-cell monoclonality precedes the development of gastric MALT lymphoma in *Helicobacter pylori*-associated chronic gastritis. *Am J Pathol* 1998;152:1271–1279.
16. Parsonnet J, Freidman GD, Vandersteen DP, et al. *Helicobacter pylori* infection and the risk of gastric carcinoma. *N Engl J Med* 1991;325:1127–1131.
17. Hussell T, Isaacson PG, Crabtree JE, et al. The response of cells from low grade B cell gastric lymphomas of mucosa associated lymphoid tissue to *Helicobacter pylori*. *Lancet* 1993;342:571–574.
18. Hussell T, Isaacson PG, Crabtree JE, et al. *Helicobacter pylori*–specific tumour infiltrating T cells provide contact dependent help for the growth of malignant B cells in low grade gastric lymphoma of mucosa associated lymphoid tissue. *J Pathol* 1996;178:122–127.

19. Wotherspoon AC, Doglioni C, Diss TC, et al. Regression of primary low grade B cell gastric lymphoma of mucosa associated lymphoid tissue after eradication of *Helicobacter pylori*. *Lancet* 1993;342:575–577.
20. Bayerdorffer E, Neubauer A, Rudolph B, et al. Regression of primary gastric lymphoma of mucosa associated lymphoid tissue type after cure of *Helicobacter pylori* infection. *Lancet* 1995;345:1591–1594.
21. Savio A, Franzin G, Wotherspoon AC, et al. Diagnosis and post treatment follow up of *Helicobacter pylori*-positive gastric lymphoma of mucosa associated lymphoid tissue: histology, polymerase chain reaction, or both? *Blood* 1996;87:1255–1260.
22. Nakamura S, Sugiyama T, Matsumoto T, et al. Long-term clinical outcome of gastric MALT lymphoma after eradication of *Helicobacter pylori*: a multicentre cohort follow-up study of 420 patients in Japan. *Gut* 2012;61:507–513.
23. Wotherspoon AC, Doglioni C, de Boni M, et al. Antibiotic treatment for low grade gastric MALT lymphoma. *Lancet* 1994;343:1503.
24. Weber DM, Dimopoulos MA, Anandu MA, et al. Regression of gastric lymphoma of mucosa associated lymphoid tissue with antibiotic therapy for *Helicobacter pylori*. *Gastroenterology* 1994;107:1835–1838.
25. Roggero E, Zucca E, Pinotti G, et al. Eradication of *Helicobacter pylori* infection in primary low grade gastric lymphoma of mucosa associated lymphoid tissue. *Ann Intern Med* 1995;122:767–769.
26. Montalban C, Castrillo JM, Abraira V, et al. Gastric B cell mucosa associated lymphoid tissue (MALT) lymphoma: clinicopathological study and evaluation of the prognostic factors in 143 patients. *Ann Oncol* 1995;6:355–362.
27. Blecker U, McKeithan TW, Hart J, et al. Resolution of *Helicobacter pylori*–associated gastric lymphoproliferative disease in a child. *Gastroenterology* 1995;109:973–977.
28. Taal BG, Boot H, van Heerde P, et al. Primary non Hodgkin's lymphoma of the stomach: endoscopic pattern and prognosis in low versus high grade malignancy in relation to the MALT concept. *Gut* 1996;39:556–561.
29. Isaacson PG, Spencer J. Malignant lymphoma of mucosa associated lymphoid tissue. *Histopathology* 1987;11:445–462.
30. Myhre MJ, Isaacson PG. Primary B cell gastric lymphoma—a reassessment of its histogenesis. *J Pathol* 1987;152:1–11.
31. Papadaki L, Wotherspoon AC, Isaacson PG. The lymphoepithelial lesion of gastric low-grade B-cell lymphoma of mucosa-associated lymphoid tissue (MALT): an ultrastructural study. *Histopathology* 1992;21:415–421.
32. Sutak J, Stoddard C, Smith ME. Solitary epithelial cells in B cell gastric MALT lymphoma. *J Clin Pathol* 2005;58:1226–1228.
33. Isaacson P, Wright DH. Malignant lymphoma of mucosa-associated lymphoid tissue. A distinctive type of B-cell lymphoma. *Cancer* 1983;52:1410–1416.
34. Isaacson PG, Wotherspoon AC, Diss TC, et al. Follicular colonization in B cell lymphoma of mucosa associated lymphoid tissue. *Am J Surg Pathol* 1991;15:819–828.
35. Wotherspoon AC, Doglioni C, Isaacson PG. Low grade gastric B cell lymphoma of mucosa associated lymphoid tissue (MALT) a multifocal disease. *Histopathology* 1992;20:29–34.
36. Du MQ, Diss TC, Dogan A, et al. Clone-specific PCR reveals wide dissemination of gastric MALT lymphoma to the gastric mucosa. *J Pathol* 2000;192:488–493.
37. Du MQ, Diss TC, Xu CF, et al. Ongoing mutation in MALT lymphoma immunoglobulin VH gene suggests that antigen stimulation plays a role in the clonal expansion. *Leukemia* 1996;10:1190–1197.
38. Thiede C, Alpen B, Morgner A, et al. Ongoing somatic mutations and clonal expansions after cure of *Helicobacter pylori* infection in gastric mucosa-associated lymphoid tissue B-cell lymphoma. *J Clin Oncol* 1998;19:1600–1609.
39. Van Dongen JJ, Langerak AW, Bruggemann M, et al. Design and standardization of PCR primers and protocols for detection of clonal immunoglobulin and T-cell receptor gene recombinations in suspect lymphoproliferations: report of the BIOMED-2 Concerted Action BMH4-CT98-3936. *Leukemia* 2003;17:2257–2317.
40. Liu H, Bench AJ, Bacon CM, et al. A practical strategy for the routine use of BIOMED-2 PCR assays for detection of B- and T-cell clonality in diagnostic haematopathology. *Br J Haematol* 2007;138:31–43.
41. Dierlamm J, Baens M, Wlodarska I, et al. The apoptosis inhibitor gene *API2* and a novel 18q gene, *MLT*, are recurrently rearranged in the t(11;18)(q21;q21) associated with mucosa-associated lymphoid tissue lymphomas. *Blood* 1999;93:3601–3609.
42. Akagi T, Motegi M, Tamura A, et al. A novel gene, *MALT1* at 18q21 is involved in t(11;18)(q21;q21) found in low-grade B-cell lymphoma of mucosa-associated lymphoid tissue. *Oncogene* 1999;18:5785–5794.
43. Morgan JA, Yin Y, Borowsky AD, et al. Breakpoints of the t(11;18)(q21;q21) in mucosa-associated lymphoid tissue (MALT) lymphoma lie within or near the previously undescribed gene *MALT1* in chromosome 18. *Cancer Res* 1999;59:6205–6213.
44. Lucas PC, Kuffa P, Gu S, et al. A dual role for the API2 moiety in API2-MALT1-dependant NK-kappaB activation: heterotypic oligomerization and TRAF2 recruitment. *Oncogene* 2007;26:5643–5654.
45. Noels H, Van Loo G, Hagens S, et al. A novel TRAF6 binding site in MALT1 defines distinct mechanisms of NF-kappaB activation by API2middle dotMALT1 fusion. *J Biol Chem* 2007;282:10180–10189.
46. Rosebeck S, Madden L, Jin X, et al. Cleavage of NIK by the API2-MALT1 fusion oncoprotein leads to noncanonical NF-kappaB activation. *Science* 2011;331:468–472.
47. Coornaert B, Baens M, Heyninck K, et al. T cell antigen receptor stimulation induces MALT1 paracaspase-mediated cleavage of the NF-kappaB inhibitor A20. *Nat Immunol* 2008;9:263–271.
48. Ye H, Liu H, Attygalle A, et al. Variable frequencies of t(11;18)(q21;q21) in MALT lymphomas of different sites: significant association with CagA strains of H. pylori in gastric MALT lymphoma. *Blood* 2003;102:1012–1018.
49. Streubel B, Simonitsch-Klupp I, Mullauer L, et al. Variable frequencies of MALT lymphoma-associated genetic aberrations in MALT lymphomas of different sites. *Leukaemia* 2004;18:1722–1726.
50. Ye H, Liu H, Raderer M, et al. High incidence of t(11;18)(q21;q21) in *Helicobacter pylori*-negative gastric MALT lymphoma. *Blood* 2003;101:2547–2550.
51. Murga Penas EM, Hinz K, Roser K, et al. Translocations t(11;18)(q21;q21) and t(14;18)(q32;q21) are the main chromosomal abnormalities involving *MLT/MALT1* in MALT lymphomas. *Leukaemia* 2003;17:2225–2229.
52. Remstein ED, Dogan A, Einerson RR, et al. The incidence and anatomic site specificity of chromosomal translocations in primary extranodal marginal zone B-cell lymphoma of mucosa-associated lymphoid tissue (MALT lymphoma) in North America. *Am J Surg Pathol* 2006;30:1546–1553.
53. Nakamura S, Ye H, Bacon CM, et al. Clinical impact of genetic aberrations in gastric MALT lymphoma: a comprehensive analysis using interphase fluorescence in situ hybridisation. *Gut* 2007;56:1358–1363.
54. Ott G, Katzenberger T, Greiner, et al. The t(11;18)(q21;q21) chromosome translocation is a frequent and specific aberration in low-grade but not high-grade malignant non-Hodgkin's lymphoma of mucosa-associated lymphoid tissue (MALT-) type. *Cancer Res* 1997;57:3944–3948.
55. Zhou Y, Ye H, Martin-Subero JI, et al. Distinct comparative genomic hybridisation profiles in gastric mucosa-associated lymphoid tissue lymphomas with and without t(11;18)(q21;q21). *Br J Haematol* 2006;133:35–42.
56. Liu H, Ye H, Dogan A, et al. T(11;18)(q21;q21) is associated with advanced mucosa-associated lymphoid tissue lymphoma that express nuclear BCL10. *Blood* 2001;98:1182–1187.
57. Willis TG, Jadayel DM, Du MQ, et al. *BCL-10* is involved in t(1;14)(p22;q32) of MALT B-cell lymphoma and mutated in multiple tumour types. *Cell* 1999;96:35–45.
58. Zhang Q, Siebert R, Yan M, et al. Inactivating mutations and overexpression of BCL10, a caspase recruitment domain-containing gene in MALT lymphoma with t(1;14)(p22;q32). *Nat Genet* 1999;22:63–68.
59. Thome M, Weil R. Post-translational modifications regulate distinct functions of CARMA1 and BCL10. *Trend Immunol* 2007;28:281–288.
60. Koseki T, Inohara N, Chen S, et al. CIPER, a novel NF kappaB-activating protein containing a caspase recruitment domain with homology to Herpesvirus-2 protein E10. *J Biol Chem* 1999;274:9955–9961.
61. Thome M, Martinon F, Hofmann K, et al. Equine herpesvirus-2 E10 gene product, but not its cellular homologue, activates NF-kappaB transcription factor and c-jun N-terminal kinase. *J Biol Chem* 1999;274:9962–9968.
62. Yan M, Lee J, Schilbach S, et al. mE10, a novel caspase recruitment domain-containing proapoptotic molecule. *J Biol Chem* 1999;274:10287–10292.
63. Srinivasula SM, Ahmad M, Lin JH, et al. CLAP, a novel caspase recruitment domain-containing protein in the tumour necrosis factor receptor pathway, regulates NF-kappaB activation and apoptosis. *J Biol Chem* 1999;274:17946–17954.
64. Tian MT, Gonzalez G, Scheer B, et al. BCL-10 can promote survival of antigen-stimulated B lymphocytes. *Blood* 2005;106:2105–2112.
65. Ye H, Gong L, Liu H, et al. Strong BCL10 nuclear expression identifies gastric MALT lymphomas that do not respond to *H. pylori* eradication. *Gut* 2006;55:137–138.
66. Ye H, Dogan A, Karran L, et al. BCL10 expression in normal and neoplastic lymphoid tissue: nuclear localization in MALT lymphoma. *Am J Pathol* 2000;157:1147–1154.
67. Goatly A, Bacon CM, Nakamura S, et al. *FOXP1* abnormalities in lymphoma: translocation breakpoint mapping reveals insights into deregulated transcriptional control. *Mod Pathol* 2008;21;902–911.
68. Ye H, Gong L, Liu H, et al. MALT lymphoma with t(14;18)(q32;q21)/IGH-MALT1 is characterised by strong cytoplasmic MALT1 and BCL10 expression. *J Pathol* 2005;205:293–301.
69. Haralambieva E, Adam P, Ventura R, et al. Genetic rearrangement of FOXP1 is predominantly detected in a subset of diffuse large B cell lymphomas with extranodal presentation. *Leukemia* 2006;20:1300–1303.
70. Bi Y, Zeng N, Chanudet E, et al. A20 inactivation in ocular adnexal MALT lymphoma. *Haematologica* 2012;97:926–930.
71. Chanudet E, Huang Y, Ichimura K, et al. *A20* is targeted by promotor methylation, deletion and inactivating mutation in MALT lymphoma. *Leukemia* 2010;24:483–487.
72. Chanudet E, Ye H, Ferry J, et al. *A20* deletion is associated with copy number gain at the *TNFA/B/C* locus and occurs preferentially in translocation-negative MALT lymphoma of the ocular adnexa and salivary glands. *J Pathol* 2009;217:420–430.
73. Honma K, Tsuzuki S, Nakagawa M, et al. *TNFAIP3* is the target gene of chromosomal band 6q23.3-q24.1 loss in ocular adnexal marginal zone B cell lymphoma. *Genes Chromosomes Cancer* 2008;47:1–7.
74. MacLennan IC, Liu YJ. Marginal zone B cells respond both to polysaccharide antigens and protein antigens. *Res Immunol* 1991;142:346–351.
75. Dreyling M, Thieblemont C, Gallamini A, et al. ESMO consensus conferences: guidelines on malignant lymphoma. Part 2: marginal zone lymphoma, mantle cell lymphoma, peripheral T cell lymphoma. *Ann Oncol* 2013;24:857–877.
76. Thieblemont C, Coiffier B. MALT lymphomas: sites of presentation, clinical features and staging procedures. In: Zucca E, Bertoni F, eds. *MALT lymphoma*. New York: Kluwer Academic/Plenem Publishers, 2004:60–80.
77. Won D, Park C-J, Shim H, et al. Subtle CD20 positivity in the bone marrow of a patient who has a mucosa-associated lymphoid tissue lymphoma should not be regarded as evidence of involvement in the bone marrow. *Histopathology* 2013;62:397–405.
78. Rohatiner A, d'Amore F, Coiffier B, et al. Report on a workshop convened to discuss the pathological and staging classifications of gastrointestinal tract lymphoma. *Ann Oncol* 1994;5:397–400.
79. Ruskoné-Fourmestraux A, Dragosics B, Morgner A, et al. Paris staging system for primary gastrointestinal lymphomas. *Gut* 2003;52:912–913.
80. De Sanctis V, Marignani M, Angeletti S, et al. Anti-*Helicobacter pylori* therapy in primary MALT lymphoma of rectum. *Tumori* 2012;98:e105–e110.
81. Nakamura S, Matsumoto T, Nakamura S, et al. Duodenal mucosa-associated lymphoid tissue lymphoma treated by eradication of *Helicobacter pylori*: report of 2 cases including EUS findings. *Gastrointest Endosc* 2001;54:772–775.
82. Niino D, Yamamoto K, Tsuruta O, et al. Regression of rectal mucosa-associated lymphoid tissue (MALT) lymphoma after antibiotic treatments. *Pathol Int* 2010;60:438–442.
83. Ahlawat S, Kanber Y, Charabaty-Pishvaian A, et al. Primary mucosa-associated lymphoid tissue (MALT) lymphoma occurring in the rectum: a case report and review of the literature. *South Med J* 2006;99:1378–1384.
84. Dohden K, Kaizaki Y, Hosokawa O, et al. Regression of rectal mucosa-associated lymphoid tissue lymphoma but persistence of *Helicobacter pylori* infection of gastric mucosa after administration of levofloxacin: report of a case. *Dis Colon Rectum* 2004;47:1544–1546.
85. Matsumoto T, Iida M, Shimizu M. Regression of mucosa-associated lymphoid-tissue lymphoma of rectum after eradication of *Helicobacter pylori*. *Lancet* 1997;350:115–116.
86. Fischbach W, Goebeler-Kolve ME, Greiner A. Diagnostic accuracy of EUS in the local staging of primary gastric lymphoma: results of a prospective, multicenter study comparing EUS with histopathologic stage. *Gastrointest Endosc* 2002;56:696–700.

87. Ruskoné-Fourmestraux A, Lavergne A, Aegerter PH, et al. Predictive factors for regression of gastric MALT lymphoma after anti-*Helicobacter pylori* treatment. *Gut* 2001;48:297–303.
88. Sackmann M, Morgner A, Rudolph B, et al. Regression of gastric MALT lymphoma after eradication of *Helicobacter pylori* is predicted by endosonographic staging. MALT Lymphoma Study Group. *Gastroenterology* 1997;113:1087–1090.
89. Wündisch T, Thiede C, Morgner A, et al. Long-term follow-up of gastric MALT lymphoma after *Helicobacter pylori* eradication. *J Clin Oncol* 2005;23:8018–8024.
90. Liu H, Ye H, Ruskone-Fourmestraux A, et al. T(11;18) is a marker for all stage gastric MALT lymphomas that will not respond to *H. pylori* eradication. *Gastroenterology* 2002;122:1286–1294.
91. Montalban C, Santón A, Redondo C, et al. Long-term persistence of molecular disease after histological remission in low-grade gastric MALT lymphoma treated with *H. pylori* eradication. Lack of association with translocation t(11;18): a 10-year updated follow-up of a prospective study. *Ann Oncol* 2005;16:1539–1544.
92. Inagaki H, Nakamura T, Li C, et al. Gastric MALT lymphomas are divided into three groups based on responsiveness to *Helicobacter pylori* eradication and detection *of API2*-MALT1 fusion. *Am J Surg Pathol* 2004;28:1560–1567.
93. Alpen B, Neubauer A, Dierlamm J, et al. Translocation t(11;18) absent in early gastric marginal zone B-cell lymphoma of MALT type responding to eradication of *Helicobacter pylori* infection. *Blood* 2000;95:4014–4015.
94. Lévy M, Copie-Bergman C, Gameiro C, et al. Prognostic value of translocation t(11;18) in tumoral response of low-grade gastric lymphoma of mucosa-associated lymphoid tissue type to oral chemotherapy. *J Clin Oncol* 2005;23:5061–5066.
95. Kuo SH, Cheng AL, Lin CW, et al. t(11;18)(q21;q21) translocation as predictive marker for non-responsiveness to salvage thalidomide therapy in patients with marginal zone B-cell lymphoma with gastric involvement. *Cancer Chemother Pharmacol* 2011;68:1387–1395.
96. Tan SY, Ye H, Liu H, et al. t(11;18)(q21;q21)-positive transformed MALT lymphoma. *Histopathology* 2008;52:777–780.
97. Remstein ED, Kurtin PJ, James CD, et al. Mucosa-associated lymphoid tissue lymphomas with t(11;18)(q21;q21) and mucosa-associated lymphoid tissue lymphomas with aneuploidy develop along different pathogenetic pathways. *Am J Pathol* 2002;161:63–71.
98. Starostik P, Patzner J, Greiner A, et al. Gastric marginal zone B-cell lymphomas of MALT type develop along 2 distinct pathogenetic pathways. *Blood* 2002;99:3–9.
99. Shiozawa E, Norose T, Kaneko K, et al. Clinicopathological comparison of the World Health Organization/Wotherspoon score to the Groupe d'Etude des Lymphomes de l'Adult grade for the post-treatment evaluation of gastric mucosa-associated lymphoid tissue lymphoma. *J Gastroenterol Hepatol* 2009;24:307–315.
100. Copie-Bergman C, Gaulard P, Lavergne-Slove A, et al. Proposal for a new histological grading system for post-treatment evaluation of gastric MALT lymphoma. *Gut* 2003;52:1656.
101. Copie-Bergman C, Wotherspoon AC, Capella C, et al. GELA histological scoring system for post-treatment biopsies of patients with gastric MALT lymphoma is feasible and reliable in routine practice. *Br J Hematol* 2013;160:47–52.
102. Thiede C, Wündisch T, Alpen B, et al. Long-term persistence of monoclonal B cells after cure of *Helicobacter pylori* infection and complete histologic remission in gastric mucosa-associated lymphoid tissue B-cell lymphoma. *J Clin Oncol* 2001;19:1600–1609.
103. Santón A, García-Cosio M, Bellosillo B, et al. Persistent monoclonality after histological remission in gastric mucosa-associated lymphoid tissue lymphoma treated with chemotherapy and/or surgery: influence of t(11;18)(q21;q21). *Leuk Lymph* 2008;49:1516–1522.
104. Noy A, Yahalom J, Zaretsky L, et al. Gastric mucosa-associated lymphoid tissue lymphoma detected by clonotypic polymerase chain reaction despite continuous pathologic remission induced by involved-field radiotherapy. *J Clin Oncol* 2005;23:3768–3772.
105. Bertoni F, Conconi A, Capella C, et al. Molecular follow-up in gastric mucosa-associated lymphoid tissue lymphomas: early analysis of the LY03 cooperative trial. *Blood* 2002;99:2541–2544.
106. Zukerberg LR, Ferry JA, Southern JF, et al. Lymphoid infiltrates of the stomach. Evaluation of histologic criteria for the diagnosis of low-grade gastric lymphoma on endoscopic biopsy specimens. *Am J Surg Pathol* 1990;14:1087–1099.
107. Hummel M, Oeschger S, Barth TF, et al. Wotherspoon criteria combined with B cell clonality analysis by advanced polymerase chain reaction technology discriminates covert gastric marginal zone lymphoma from chronic gastritis. *Gut* 2006;55:782–787.
108. Fieber SS, Schaefer HJ. Lymphoid hyperplasia of the terminal ileum—a clinical entity? *Gastroenterology* 1961;50:83–98.
109. Rubin A, Isaacson PG. Florid reactive lymphoid hyperplasia of the terminal ileum in adults: a condition bearing a close resemblance to low grade malignant lymphoma. *Histopathology* 1990;17:19–26.
110. Matuchansky C, Touchard G, Lemoire M, et al. Malignant lymphoma of the small bowel associated with diffuse nodular lymphoid hyperplasia. *N Engl J Med* 1985;313:166–171.
111. Rambaud JC, Saint Louvent P, Mati R, et al. Diffuse follicular lymphoid hyperplasia of the small intestine without primary immunoglobulin deficiency. *Am J Med* 1982;73:125–132.
112. Hamaloglu E, Topaloglu S, Ozdemir A, et al. Synchronous and metachronous occurrence of gastric adenocarcinoma and gastric lymphoma: a review of the literature. *World J Gastroenterol* 2006;12:3564–3574.
113. Wotherspoon AC, Isaacson PG. Synchronous adenocarcinoma and low grade B-cell lymphoma of mucosa associated lymphoid tissue (MALT) of the stomach. *Histopathology* 1995;27:325–331.
114. Capelle LG, de Vries AC, Looman CW, et al. Gastric MALT lymphoma: epidemiology and high adenocarcinoma risk in a nation-wide study. *Eur J Cancer* 2008;44:2470–2476.
115. Capelle LG, den Hoed CM, de Vries AC, et al. Premalignant gastric lesions in patients with gastric mucosa-associated lymphoid tissue lymphoma and metachronous gastric adenocarcinoma: a case-control study. *Eur J Gastroenterol Hepatol* 2012;24:42–47.
116. Fischbach W, Tacke W, Greiner A, et al. Regression of immunoproliferative small intestinal disease after eradication of *Helicobacter pylori. Lancet* 1997;349:31–32.
117. Malekzadeh R, Kaviani MJ, Tabei SZ, et al. Lack of association between *Helicobacter pylori* infection and immunoproliferative small intestinal disease. *Arch Iran Med* 1999;2:1–4.
118. Lecuit M, Abachin E, Martin A, et al. Immunoproliferative small intestinal disease associated with *Campylobacter jejuni. N Engl J Med* 2004;350:239–248.
119. Parsonnet J, Isaacson PG. Bacterial infection and MALT lymphoma. *N Engl J Med* 2004;350:213–215.
120. Galian A, Lecester MJ, Scott J, et al. Pathological study of alpha chain disease, with special emphasis on evolution. *Cancer* 1977;39:2081–2101.
121. Isaacson PG, Dogan A, Price SK, et al. Immunoproliferative small intestinal disease: an immunohistochemical study. *Am J Surg Pathol* 1989;13:1023–1033.
122. Price SK. Immunoproliferative small intestinal disease: a study of 13 cases with alpha heavy chain disease. *Histopathology* 1990;17:7–17.
123. Bender SW, Danon F, Preud'homme JL, et al. Gamma heavy chain disease simulating alpha chain disease. *Gut* 1978;19:1148–1152.
124. Kopeć M, Swierczyñska Z, Pazdur J, et al. Diffuse lymphoma of the intestines with a monoclonal gammopathy of IgG3 kappa type. *Am J Med* 1974;56:381–385.
125. Al-Saleem T, Al-Mondhiry H. Immunoproliferative small intestinal disease (IPSID): a model for mature B-cell neoplasms. *Blood* 2005;105:2274–2280.
126. Cogné M, Silvain C, Khamlichi AA, et al. Structurally abnormal immunoglobulins in human immunoproliferative disorders. *Blood* 1992;79:2181–2195.
127. Smith WJ, Price SK, Isaacson PG. Immunoglobulin gene rearrangement in immunoproliferative small intestinal disease (IPSID). *J Clin Pathol* 1987;40:1291–1297.
128. Pai RK, Snider WK, Starkey CR, et al. Nonsecretory variant of immunoproliferative small intestinal disease: a case report with pathologic, immunophenotypic, and molecular findings. *Arch Pathol Lab Med* 2005;129:1487–1490.
129. Matuchansky C, Cogné M, Lemaire M, et al. Nonsecretory alpha-chain disease with immunoproliferative small-intestinal disease. *N Engl J Med* 1989;320:1534–1539.
130. Teng MH, Rosen S, Gorny MK, et al. Gamma heavy chain disease in man: independent structural abnormalities and reduced transcription of a functionally rearranged lambda L-chain gene result in the absence of L-chains. *Blood Cells Mol Dis* 2000;26:1771–1785.
131. Berger R, Bernheim A, Tsapis A, et al. Cytogenetic studies in four cases of alpha chain disease. *Cancer Genet Cytogenet* 1986;22;219–223.
132. Pellet P, Tsapis A, Brouet JC. Alpha heavy chain disease of patient MAL: structure of the non-functional rearranged alpha gene translocated on chromosome 9. *Eur J Immunol* 1990;20:2731–2735.
133. Chang CS, Lin SF, Chen TP, et al. Leukemic manifestation in a case of alpha-chain disease with multiple polypoid intestinal lymphocytic lymphoma. *Am J Hematol* 1992;41:209–214.
134. Iida S, Rao PH, Nallasivam P, et al. The t(9;14)(p13;q32) chromosomal translocation associated with lymphoplasmacytoid lymphoma involves the PAX-5 gene. *Blood* 1996;88:4110–4117.
135. Ben Ayed F, Halphen M, Najjar T, et al. Treatment of alpha chain disease—results of a prospective study in 21 Tunisian patients by the Tunisian French intestinal lymphoma study group. *Cancer* 1989;63:1251–1256.
136. Nakamura M, Ohmiya N, Hirooka Y, et al. Endoscopic diagnosis of follicular lymphoma with small-bowel involvement using video capsule endoscopy and double-balloon endoscopy: a case series. *Endoscopy* 2013;45:67–70.
137. Yamamoto S, Nakase H, Yamashita K, et al. Gastrointestinal follicular lymphoma: review of the literature. *J Gastroenterol* 2010;45:370–388.
138. Schmatz AI, Streubel B, Kretschmer-Chott E, et al. Primary follicular lymphoma of the duodenum is a distinct mucosal/submucosal variant of follicular lymphoma: a retrospective study of 63 cases. *J Clin Oncol* 2011;29:1445–1451.
139. Drillenburg P, van der Voort R, Koopman G, et al. Preferential expression of the mucosal homing receptor integrin alpha 4 beta 7 in gastrointestinal non-Hodgkin's lymphomas. *Am J Pathol* 1997;150:919–927.
140. Bende RJ, Smit LA, Bossenbroek JG, et al. Primary follicular lymphoma of the small intestine: alpha4beta7 expression and immunoglobulin configuration suggest an origin from local antigen-experienced B cells. *Am J Pathol* 2003;162:105–113.
141. Jain VK, Bystricky B, Wotherspoon AC, et al. Primary follicular lymphoma of the GI tract: an increasingly recognized entity. *J Clin Oncol* 2012;30:e370–e372.
142. Damaj G, Verkarre V, Delmer A, et al. Primary follicular lymphoma of the gastrointestinal tract: a study of 25 cases and a literature review. *Ann Oncol* 2003;14:623–629.
143. Shia J, Teruya-Feldstein J, Pan D, et al. Primary follicular lymphoma of the gastrointestinal tract: a clinical and pathologic study of 26 cases. *Am J Surg Pathol* 2002;26:216–224.
144. Salar A, Juanpere N, Bellosillo B, et al. Gastrointestinal involvement in mantle cell lymphoma: a prospective clinic, endoscopic, and pathologic study. *Am J Surg Pathol* 2006;30:1274–1280.
145. Romaguera JE, Medeiros LJ, Hagemeister FB, et al. Frequency of gastrointestinal involvement and its clinical significance in mantle cell lymphoma. *Cancer* 2003;97:586–591.
146. Cornes JS. Multiple lymphomatous polyposis of the gastrointestinal tract. *Cancer* 1961;14:249–257.
147. Ruskoné-Fourmestraux A, Delmer A, Lavergne A, et al. Multiple lymphomatous polyposis of the gastrointestinal tract: prospective clinicopathologic study of 31 cases. *Gastroenterology* 1997;112:7–16.
148. Kodama T, Ohshima K, Nomura K, et al. Lymphomatous polyposis of the gastrointestinal tract, including mantle cell lymphoma, follicular lymphoma and mucosa-associated lymphoid tissue lymphoma. *Histopathology* 2005;47:467–478.
149. Kuo SH, Chen LT, Wu MS, et al. Differential response to *H. pylori* eradication therapy of co-existing diffuse large B-cell lymphoma and MALT lymphoma of stomach-significance of tumour cell clonality and BCL10 expression. *J Pathol* 2007;211:296–304.
150. Peng H, Du M, Diss TC, et al. Genetic evidence for a clonal link between low and high-grade components in gastric MALT B-cell lymphoma. *Histopathology* 1997;30(5):425–429.
151. De Wolf-Peeters C, Tierens A. Controversies in MALT lymphoma classification, low and high grade. *Histopathology* 1998;32:277–278.
152. Nakamura S, Ye H, Bacon CM, et al. Translocations involving the immunoglobulin heavy chain gene locus predict better survival in gastric diffuse large B-cell lymphoma. *Clin Cancer Res* 2008;14:3002–3010.
153. Chen YW, Hu XT, Liang AC, et al. High BCL6 expression predicts better prognosis, independent of BCL6 translocation status, translocation partner, or BCL6-deregulating mutations, in gastric lymphoma. *Blood* 2006;108:2373–2383.

154. Kramer MH, Hermans J, Parker J, et al. Clinical significance of bcl2 and p53 protein expression in diffuse large B-cell lymphoma: a population-based study. *J Clin Oncol* 1996;14:2131–2138.
155. Hu XT, Chen YW, Liang AC, et al. CD44 activation in mature B-cell malignancies by a novel recurrent IGH translocation. *Blood* 2010;115:2458–2461.
156. Young KH, Leroy K, Møller MB, et al. Structural profiles of TP53 gene mutations predict clinical outcome in diffuse large B-cell lymphoma: an international collaborative study. *Blood* 2008;112:3088–3098.
157. Pasqualucci L, Trifonov V, Fabbri G, et al. Analysis of the coding genome of diffuse large B-cell lymphoma. *Nat Genet* 2011;43:830–837.
158. Pasqualucci L, Dominguez-Sola D, Chiarenza A, et al. Inactivating mutations of acetyltransferase genes in B-cell lymphoma. *Nature* 2011;471:189–195.
159. Ngo VN, Young RM, Schmitz R, et al. Oncogenically active MYD88 mutations in human lymphoma. *Nature* 2011;470:115–119.
160. Davis RE, Ngo VN, Lenz G, et al. Chronic active B-cell-receptor signalling in diffuse large B-cell lymphoma. *Nature* 2010;463:88–92.
161. Compagno M, Lim WK, Grunn A, et al. Mutations of multiple genes cause deregulation of NF-kappaB in diffuse large B-cell lymphoma. *Nature* 2009;459:717–721.
162. Honma K, Tsuzuki S, Nakagawa M, et al. TNFAIP3/A20 functions as a novel tumor suppressor gene in several subtypes of non-Hodgkin lymphomas. *Blood* 2009;114:2467–2475.
163. Lenz G, Davis RE, Ngo VN, et al. Oncogenic CARD11 mutations in human diffuse large B cell lymphoma. *Science* 2008;319:1676–1679.
164. Pasqualucci L, Compagno M, Houldsworth J, et al. Inactivation of the PRDM1/BLIMP1 gene in diffuse large B cell lymphoma. *J Exp Med* 2006;203:311–317.
165. Morin RD, Johnson NA, Severson TM, et al. Somatic mutations altering EZH2 (Tyr641) in follicular and diffuse large B-cell lymphomas of germinal-center origin. *Nat Genet* 2010;42:181–185.
166. Challa-Malladi M, Lieu YK, Califano O, et al. Combined genetic inactivation of β2-Microglobulin and CD58 reveals frequent escape from immune recognition in diffuse large B cell lymphoma. *Cancer Cell* 2011;20:728–740.
167. Dong G, Chanudet E, Zeng N, et al. A20, ABIN-1/2, and CARD11 mutations and their prognostic value in gastrointestinal diffuse large B-cell lymphoma. *Clin Cancer Res* 2011;17:1440–1451.
168. Du M, Peng H, Singh N, et al. The accumulation of p53 abnormalities is associated with progression of mucosa-associated lymphoid tissue lymphoma. *Blood* 1995;86:4587–4593.
169. Kuo SH, Yeh KH, Wu MS, et al. *Helicobacter pylori* eradication therapy is effective in the treatment of early-stage *H. pylori*-positive gastric diffuse large B-cell lymphomas. *Blood* 2012;119:4838–4844.
170. Chen LT, Lin JT, Tai JJ, et al. Long-term results of anti-*Helicobacter pylori* therapy in early-stage gastric high-grade transformed MALT lymphoma. *J Natl Cancer Inst* 2005;97:1345–1353.
171. Tari A, Asaoku H, Kashiwado K, et al. Predictive value of endoscopy and endoscopic ultrasonography for regression of gastric diffuse large B-cell lymphomas after *Helicobacter pylori* eradication. *Dig Endosc* 2009;21:219–227.
172. Cavanna L, Pagani R, Seghini P, et al. High grade B-cell gastric lymphoma with complete pathologic remission after eradication of *Helicobacter pylori* infection: report of a case and review of the literature. *World J Surg Oncol* 2008;6:35.
173. Morgner A, Miehlke S, Fischbach W, et al. Complete remission of primary high-grade B-cell gastric lymphoma after cure of *Helicobacter pylori* infection. *J Clin Oncol* 2001;19:2041–2048.
174. Montalban C, Santon A, Boixeda D, et al. Regression of gastric high grade mucosa associated lymphoid tissue (MALT) lymphoma after *Helicobacter pylori* eradication. *Gut* 2001;49:584–587.
175. Akasaka T, Akasaka H, Ueda C, et al. Molecular and clinical features of non-Burkitt's, diffuse large-cell lymphoma of B-cell type associated with the c-MYC/immunoglobulin heavy-chain fusion gene. *J Clin Oncol* 2000;18:510–518.
176. Krugmann J, Dirnhofer S, Gschwendtner A, et al. Primary gastrointestinal B-cell lymphoma. A clinicopathological and immunohistochemical study of 61 cases with an evaluation of prognostic parameters. *Pathol Res Pract* 2001;197:385–393.
177. Tanaka T, Shimada K, Yamamoto K, et al. Retrospective analysis of primary gastric diffuse large B cell lymphoma in the rituximab era: a multicenter study of 95 patients in Japan. *Ann Hematol* 2012;91:383–390.
178. Avilés A, Castañeda C, Cleto S, et al. Rituximab and chemotherapy in primary gastric lymphoma. *Cancer Biother Radiopharm* 2009;24:25–28.
179. Lenzen R, Borchard F, Lubke H, et al. Colitis ulserosa complicated by malignant lymphoma: case report and analysis of published works. *Gut* 1995;36:306–310.
180. Abulafi AM, Fiddian RV. Malignant lymphoma in ulcerative colitis. *Dis Colon Rectum* 1990;33:615–618.
181. Shepherd NA, Hall PA, Williams GT, et al. Primary malignant lymphoma of the large intestine complicating chronic inflammatory bowel disease. *Histopathology* 1989;15:325–337.
182. Baker D, Chiprut RO, Rimer D, et al. Colonic lymphoma in ulcerative colitis. *J Clin Gastroenterol* 1985;7:379–386.
183. Deleeuw RJ, Zettl A, Klinker E, et al. Whole-genome analysis and HLA genotyping of enteropathy-type T-cell lymphoma reveals 2 distinct lymphoma subtypes. *Gastroenterology* 2007;132:1902–1911.
184. Delabie J, Holte H, Vose JM, et al. Enteropathy-associated T-cell lymphoma: clinical and histological findings from the International Peripheral T-Cell Lymphoma Project. *Blood* 2011;118:148–155.
185. O'Driscoll BRC, Stevens FM, O'Gorman TA, et al. HLA type of patients with coeliac disease and malignancy in the west of Ireland. *Gut* 1982;23:662–665.
186. Murray A, Cuevas D, Jones B, et al. Study of the immunohistochemistry and T-cell clonality of enteropathy-associated T-cell lymphoma. *Am J Pathol* 1995;146:509–519.
187. Howell WM, Leung ST, Jones DB, et al. HLA-DRB, DQA and DQB polymorphism in celiac disease and enteropathy-associated T-cell lymphoma. Common features and additional risk factors for malignancy. *Hum Immunol* 1995;43:29–37.
188. Zettl A, Ott G, Makulik A, et al. Chromosomal gains at 9q characterize enteropathy-type T-cell lymphoma. *Am J Pathol* 2002;161:1635–1645.
189. Chan JKC, Chan ACL, Cheuk W, et al. Type II enteropathy-associated T-cell lymphoma: A distinct aggressive lymphoma with frequent γδ T-cell receptor expression. *Am J Surg Pathol* 2011;35:1557–1569.
190. Daum S, Cellier C, Mulder CJ. Refractory coeliac disease. *Best Pract Res Clin Gastroenterol* 2005;19:413–424.
191. Cellier C, Delabesse E, Helmer C, et al. Refractory sprue, coeliac disease and enteropathy-associated T-cell lymphoma. *Lancet* 2000;356:203–208.
192. Daum S, Weiss D, Hummel M, et al. Frequency of clonal intraepithelial T lymphocyte proliferations in enteropathy-type intestinal T cell lymphoma, coeliac disease and refractory sprue. *Gut* 2001;49:804–812.
193. Bagdi E, Diss TC, Munson P, et al. Mucosal intra-epithelial lymphocytes in enteropathy-associated T-cell lymphoma, ulcerative jejunitis, and refractory celiac disease constitute a neoplastic population. *Blood* 1999;94:260–264.
194. Cellier C, Patey N, Mauvieux L, et al. Abnormal intestinal intraepithelial lymphocytes in refractory sprue. *Gastroenterology* 1998;114:471–481.
195. Malamut G, Afchain P, Verkarre V, et al. Presentation and long-term follow-up of refractory celiac disease: comparison or type I with type II. *Gastroenterology* 2009;136:81–90.
196. Verkarre V, Asnafi V, Lecomte T, et al. Refractory coeliac disease is a diffuse gastrointestinal disease. *Gut* 2003;52:205–211.
197. Verbeek WH, von Blomberg BM, Coupe VM, et al. Aberrant T-lymphocytes in refractory coeliac disease are not strictly confined to a small intestinal intraepithelial location. *Cytom Part B: Clin Cytom* 2009;76:367–374.
198. Rubio-Tapia A, Kelly DG, Lahr BD, et al. Clinical staging and survival in refractory celiac disease: a single center experience. *Gastroenterology* 2009;136:99–107.
199. Liu H, Brais R, Lavergne-Slove A, et al. Continual monitoring of intraepithelial lymphocyte immunophenotype and clonality is more important than snapshot analysis in the surveillance of refractory coeliac disease. *Gut* 2010;59:452–460.
200. Ashton Key M, Diss TC, Pan L, et al. Molecular analysis of T-cell clonality in ulcerative jejunitis and enteropathy-associated T-cell lymphoma. *Am J Pathol* 1997;151:493–498.
201. Al Toma A, Verbeek WH, Hadithi M, et al. Survival in refractory coeliac disease and enteropathy-associated T-cell lymphoma: retrospective evaluation of a single-centre experience. *Gut* 2007;56:1373–1378.
202. Isaacson PG, Du MQ. Gastrointestinal lymphoma: where morphology meets molecular biology. *J Pathol* 2005;205:255–274.
203. Verbeek WH, Goerres MS, von Blomberg BM, et al. Flow cytometric determination of aberrant intra-epithelial lymphocytes predicts T-cell lymphoma development more accurately than T-cell clonality analysis in refractory celiac disease. *Clin Immunol* 2008;126:48–56.
204. de Masceral A, Belleannee G, Stanislas S, et al. Mucosal intraepithelial T-lymphocytes in refractory celiac disease: a neoplastic population with a variable CD8 phenotype. *Am J Surg Pathol* 2008;32:744–751.
205. Verkarre V, Romana SP, Cellier C, et al. Recurrent partial trisomy 1q22-q44 in clonal intraepithelial lymphocytes in refractory celiac sprue. *Gastroenterology* 2003;125:40–46.
206. Svrcek M, Garderet L, Sebbagh V, et al. Small intestinal CD4+ T-cell lymphoma: a rare distinctive clinicopathological entity associated with prolonged survival. *Virch Arch* 2007;451:1091–1093.
207. Zivny J, Banner BF, Agrawal S, et al. CD4+ T-cell lymphoproliferative disorder of the gut clinically mimicking celiac sprue. *Dig Dis Sci* 2004;49:551–555.
208. Carbonnel F, d'Almagne H, Lavergne A, et al. The clinicopathological features of extensive small intestinal CD4 T cell infiltration. *Gut* 1999;45:662–667.
209. Carbonnel F, Lavergne A, Messing B, et al. Extensive small intestinal T-cell lymphoma of low-grade malignancy associated with a new chromosomal translocation. *Cancer* 1994;73:1286–1291.
210. Sun J, Lu Z, Yang D, et al. Primary intestinal T-cell and NK-cell lymphomas: a clinicopathological and molecular study from China focused on type II enteropathy-associated T-cell lymphoma and primary intestinal NK-cell lymphoma. *Mod Pathol* 2011;24:983–992.
211. Tung CL, Hsieh PP, Chang JH, et al. Intestinal T-cell and natural killer-cell lymphomas in Taiwan with special emphasis on 2 distinct types: natural killer-like cytotoxic T cell and true natural killer cell. *Hum Pathol* 2008;39:1081–1025.
212. Zheng S, Ouyang Q, Li G, et al. Primary intestinal NK/T cell lymphoma: a clinicopathologic study of 25 Chinese cases. *Arch Iran Med* 2012;15:L36–L42.
213. Chuang SS, Chang ST, Chuang WY, et al. NK-cell lineage predicts poor survival in primary intestinalNK-cell and T-cell lymphomas. *Am J Surg Pathol* 2009;33:1230–1240.
214. Nakashima Y, Tagawa H, Suzuki R, et al. Genome-wide array-bases comparative genomic hybridization of natural killer cell lymphoma/leukemia: different genomic alteration patterns of aggressive NK-cell leukemia and extranodal NK/T-cell lymphoma, nasal type. *Genes Chromosomes Cancer* 2005;44:247–255.
215. Ko YH, Cho EY, Kim JE, et al. NK and NK-like T-cell lymphoma in extranodal sites: a comparative clinicopathological study according to site and EBV status. *Histopathology* 2004;44:739–746.
216. Takeuchi K, Yokoyama M, Ishizawa S, et al. Lymphomatoid gastropathy: a distinct clinicopathologic entity of self-limited pseudomalignant NK-cell proliferation. *Blood* 2010;116:5631–5637.
217. Mansoor A, Pittaluga S, Beck PL, et al. NK-cell enteropathy: a benign NK-cell lymphoproliferative disease mimicking intestinal lymphoma: clinicopathologic features and follow-up in a unique case series. *Blood* 2011;117:1447–1452.

Chapter 31
Hematolymphoid Lesions of the Lung and Pleura

Gerald J. Berry

Surgical pathologists not infrequently encounter lung biopsies containing lymphocytes or other hematolymphoid elements as conspicuous histopathologic findings. For example, interstitial processes such as hypersensitivity pneumonitis (HP), viral pneumonia, nonspecific interstitial pneumonia/fibrosis (NSIP), usual interstitial pneumonia, and pulmonary involvement by connective tissue disorders all display lymphoid or lymphoplasmacytic infiltrates as part of their morphologic constituency. On the other hand, primary hematolymphoid disorders of the lung are infrequent and uniformly challenging even for experienced pulmonary pathologists. Moreover, they require an ever-expanding and complicated array of ancillary testing for accurate diagnosis and classification. In addition to flow cytometry and/or immunohistochemistry (IHC), cytogenetics and molecular testing for specific translocations are routinely employed in the diagnostic evaluation and classification of malignant lymphomas. In many cases, these provide both diagnostic and prognostic information that is essential for treatment planning (1–4). A multidisciplinary approach including Tumor Boards is now common in both academic and community practices. Open communication between clinicians and pathologists is a mainstay of excellent patient management. Further, thoracic radiologists provide an invaluable resource in the preoperative assessment of pulmonary disorders and often guide surgeons and pulmonologists to the optimal regions for tissue sampling and provide a focused differential diagnosis on the basis of radiologic findings (5–6).

The concept of lymphoproliferative disorders of the lung encompasses a broad assortment of benign and malignant processes, ranging from reactive to neoplastic lesions. A variety of classifications are available, but central to all of them is the recognition that the lung normally contains a rich environment of both lymphoid elements and lymphatics. Therefore, a general understanding of the normal anatomy of the lymphatic system and normal immunoarchitecture of the lung is a prerequisite to assessing morphologic abnormalities. The classifications have undergone substantial changes over the last two decades and continue to evolve as newer immunologic concepts, and molecular tests replace older doctrines. For example, the most recent *WHO Classification of Tumors of Hematopoietic and Lymphoid Tissues* enumerated new types of mature B-cell neoplasms and refined others (7). It continues to serve as the most widely accepted and utilized paradigm for the clinicopathologic classification of malignant neoplasms. The purpose of this discussion is to update benign and malignant hematolymphoid lesions of the lung and to provide a practical diagnostic approach for pathologists.

SPECIMEN HANDLING AND PROCESSING

The accurate diagnosis and classification of this confounding group of lesions mandates that optimal specimen handling and processing are established at the outset. Currently, a variety of diagnostic modalities are available, and it is the responsibility of the multidisciplinary team to select the technique that will ensure that sufficient material is procured for all interpretative and ancillary studies. Careful elucidation of both systemic and pulmonary symptoms and clarification of the radiologic patterns and extent of the disease process within the lung and mediastinum are vital. The list of potential approaches includes fine needle aspiration (FNA) with core biopsy, endoscopic bronchial ultrasound (EBUS) sampling, fiberoptic bronchoscopy with transbronchial biopsy (TBBx), and open lung biopsy/video-assisted thoracoscopic biopsy (OLB/VATS).

Fine Needle Aspiration Biopsy with Core Needle Biopsy

For more than 25 years now, bronchoalveolar lavage and FNA cytology have been recognized as an excellent, minimally invasive methodology in the evaluation of thoracic lesions (8–13). Transthoracic intervention under ultrasound, fluoroscopic, or computerized tomography (CT) guidance is commonly performed. Diagnostic material for cytomorphologic assessment, microbiologic studies, flow cytometry, and cell block preparations can be obtained. Immediate assessment in the interventional radiology suite or operating room permits the integrated allotment of material into appropriate solutions such as RPMI for flow cytometry or cytogenetics, alcohol-based media for cytopathology, 10% neutral-buffered formalin or other fixatives for cell blocks, and core needle samples for immunohistochemical and molecular testing. Historically, these procedures have been limited by the absence of architectural integrity on account of tissue fragmentation, rendering subclassification of lymphoma challenging. The implementation of flow cytometry, tissue immunophenotyping, fluorescence *in situ* hybridization (FISH), and molecular analysis has improved the diagnostic accuracy (14–17). More recently, the addition of 18 gauge biopsy-cut needle to the diagnostic armamentarium provides intact cores of tissue measuring up to 2 cm in length that preserves both cytologic and architectural components (18). In our experience, ancillary techniques such as IHC, FISH, and molecular genetics can be performed on both cell block samples and core needle specimens.

Endobronchial Ultrasound Techniques

Over the last decade, the role of cervical mediastinoscopy and biopsy and transbronchial needle aspiration (TBNA) in the evaluation of lung cancer has changed. It has been due, in part, to the introduction of the EBUS technique of visualization and sampling of hilar (N1) and mediastinal (N2) lymph nodes and masses. The nodal stations that are accessible to EBUS sampling include the N1 nodes—hilar (station 10), interlobar (station 11), and lobar (station 12)—and N2 nodes—highest mediastinal (station 1), upper (station 2) and lower (station 4) paratracheal, and subcarinal (station 7) (19). The technique of

EBUS-directed TBNA (EBUS-TBNA) has resulted in improved diagnostic yields in the staging of lung cancer (20–23).

The role of EBUS-TBNA in the evaluation of lymphoproliferative lesions in mediastinal and pulmonary hilar lymph nodes is less well defined. A number of recent studies have reported a sensitivity range of 57% to 91%; some have recommended the technique as an initial diagnostic modality over mediastinoscopy (24–27). A more detailed analysis by Iqbal et al. (28) of their experience at the Mayo Clinic offered a less enthusiastic recommendation. The overall sensitivity in their study for the diagnosis of lymphoproliferative disorder defined as a variety of neoplastic hematolymphoid lesions (B-cell chronic lymphocytic leukemia [CLL], T-cell prolymphocytic leukemia, Hodgkin lymphoma [HL], and B-cell or T-cell non-Hodgkin lymphoma [NHL]) was 38%. The technique was more useful for the diagnosis of recurrence (sensitivity 55%) compared to the initial diagnosis (sensitivity 22%). Further experience with EBUS-TBNA will be required to determine its primary role in the evaluation of lymphoproliferative disorders.

Fiberoptic Bronchoscopy with Transbronchial Biopsy

Fiberoptic bronchoscopy with TBBx is an established technique to visualize the divisions of the bronchial tree of the lung and provide tissue for histopathologic assessment. The role of TBBx in the primary evaluation of lymphoproliferative disorders has traditionally been limited. In our experience, this is generally limited to lymphomas with characteristic cytomorphology such as large cell lymphoma or lesions that can be established and confirmed by IHC or other ancillary methods such as large cell lymphoma or HL (29). Here again the importance of clinical and radiologic correlation must be reiterated. More importantly, TBBx and BAL are essential tools in the work-up of patients with known lymphoproliferative disorders who develop infiltrates or nodular lesions following therapeutic interventions. The distinction of recurrent or persistent disease from infection or drug toxicity is critical for proper treatment and for prognostic implications.

From a practical perspective, the TBBx provides both interpretative challenges and technical problems related to procurement of the tissue. Tissue atelectasis and artifactual distortion are found to varying degrees with every sample. Gentle swirling agitation of the biopsy pieces in formalin fixative can reduce the degree of atelectasis. The liberal use of leveled sections and connective tissue stains can resolve crush artifact and render a biopsy fragment interpretable in some cases. Although there are no guidelines established for the number of tissue samples, we encourage at least five pieces of alveolated pieces that are not completely collapsed. They should be immediately fixed in a standard fixative such as 10% neutral buffered formalin. Other fixatives such as B5 or Bouin may interfere with IHC or other ancillary studies, and each laboratory should carefully establish their optimal thresholds. Additional tissue pieces can be set aside for microbiologic cultures, genetic studies, etc. as needed. The histologic assessment requires optimum handling and processing. Overnight processing in an automated processor is desirable, but a variety of rapid processing programs are available for handling emergent biopsies or clinically indicated biopsies that yield slides in 3 to 4 hours. Following embedding in paraffin wax, a minimum of three "leveled" sections each with multiple ribbons are prepared at 4 to 5 μm thickness and routinely stained with hematoxylin and eosin (H&E). A connective tissue stain such as Masson trichrome and/or an elastic stain is helpful for assessing airway and vascular integrity. We routinely perform a silver stain such as Gomori-methenamine-silver (GMS) for fungal organisms especially in the setting of posttreatment infiltrates. Additional histochemical stains, IHC,

and molecular techniques are advocated on a case-by-case basis, for example, for viral infections such as cytomegalovirus (CMV) or for the diagnosis and classification of lymphoproliferative disorders.

Open Lung Biopsy/Video-Assisted Thoracoscopic Biopsy

OLB and VATS biopsy are both invasive procedures requiring general anesthesia and the entire attendant risks associated with the procedure. Nonetheless, they remain the most common diagnostic interventions for the evaluation of lymphoproliferative disorders in most centers. Preoperative selection of site(s) for sampling should involve discussions with clinicians and radiologists. We recommend intraoperative involvement of the pathologist to determine appropriate tissue handing. The wedge-shaped piece or pieces of lung tissue should be sent on saline-soaked gauze to the laboratory. The need for microbiologic cultures should be assessed in each case and, when indicated, should be harvested in the operating room to preserve sterile conditions. We encourage intraoperative consultation as there is a limited role for frozen section examination. Both touch imprints stained with Diff-Quik (Dade Behring, Newark, NJ) and frozen sections H&E slides can confirm that diagnostic material has been obtained and suggest alternative diagnoses such as infection, nonspecific organizing pneumonia, or non-hematolymphoid malignancy. It can also be used to direct the handling of tissue for special studies such as cytogenetics and molecular analysis. Further, the sample used for frozen section analysis can be kept frozen and set aside for future genetic analysis as the quality of the morphology in formalin-fixed paraffin-embedded slides after snap-freezing is often suboptimal for detailed assessment. We do not render a definitive diagnosis or subclassification on the basis of frozen section interpretation but indicate to the surgeons that "diagnostic material has been obtained." We routinely prepare additional unstained touch imprints for rapid histochemical staining if there is a suggestion of an infectious etiology. Complications from the procedure range from minor issues such as wound infection, postoperative pain, and prolonged air-leaks to more serious but uncommon problems such as respiratory failure and intrathoracic bleeding requiring surgical re-exploration.

Once tissue has been procured for the necessary ancillary studies, we gently inflate the wedge biopsy specimen with formalin using a 25- or 27-guage needle (Fig. 31.1). This promotes tissue expansion of the airspaces and airways and prevents

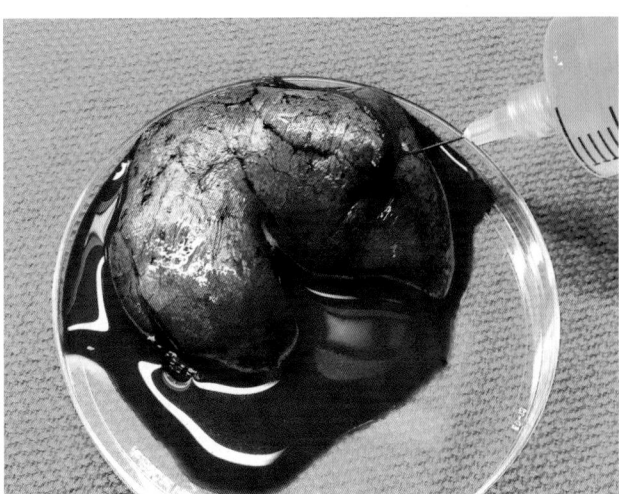

FIGURE 31.1.   Inflation of VATS lung biopsy with formalin through a 25-guage needle.

tissue atelectasis and architectural distortion. Following adequate fixation time of at least 3 hours, the wedge is thinly sectioned and submitted for overnight processing. Five-micron sections are cut and H&E-stained slides and unstained slides are prepared for morphologic and immunohistochemical study, respectively. The number of monoclonal antibodies available for diagnostic application on formalin-fixed paraffin-embedded slides continues to expand. Our approach based on an initial histopathologic assessment is to apply a panel of B-cell and T-cell lineage markers that is further refined in follow-up staining profiles dependent on cellular distribution and composition. These are discussed in detail in the sections that follow.

NORMAL DISTRIBUTION OF LYMPHOID ELEMENTS AND A PATTERN APPROACH TO MORPHOLOGIC EVALUATION

The lung, rich in both lymphoid elements and lymphatics, serves as an interesting model for understanding the concept of mucosa-associated lymphoid tissue (MALT). The recognition of the important role of the lymphoid component goes back over 40 years to the work of Bienenstock and colleagues among others (30–32). Pulmonary MALT or the more specific designation of bronchus-associated lymphoid tissue (BALT) in the lung is inconspicuous in lung tissue of adults and tends to be more frequent in the upper lung zones. It is more common in smokers than nonsmokers (33). BALT is arranged as nodular aggregates at distal bronchial and bronchiolar division points and is composed of poorly formed primary follicles, mantle and marginal zones, and interfollicular regions (34) (Fig. 31.2). Plasma cells are infrequently sprinkled in the interfollicular regions. In response to airway antigenic or infectious stimuli, all the attributes of reactive lymphoid changes are found including polarization within the secondary follicles, conspicuous mantle zones, and an expanded interfollicular region. Scattered lymphocytes and other inflammatory cells are also found as scattered cells in the walls of airways particularly of the lower lung zones and appear to lack any specific organization. These likely serve in the capacity of "lymphoid first defense" following antigenic inhalation. Another component of BALT is the specialized airway epithelium overlying the lymphoid elements or "lymphoepithelium." These follicle-associated epithelial cells or M cells are arranged as a uniquely adapted pseudostratified

mucosal layer of attenuated epithelial cells lacking cilia and diminished numbers of goblet cells. They have the ability to selectively phagocytose and pinocytose and are critical to the formulation of an immune response (32). This compilation of specialized epithelium, underlying BALT, and nearby efferent lymphatic vessels that drain to hilar nodes constitute what was formerly known as the "pulmonary sump," an environment tailored to inhaled antigen-host immune interactions (35).

Another constituent of the "normal" lymphoid elements of the lung is intraparenchymal lymph nodes (IPLNs). These are infrequent but are not uncommonly surgically removed in patients suspected of metastatic disease. This is due largely to the ever-enhancing resolution of imaging studies such as CT scan. They are discussed in detail below. Importantly, the scattered lymphoid aggregates that are found in the pleura or the septa are not currently recognized as part of BALT.

There is an abundant but delicate network of lymphatic channels within the lung that serve to drain fluid away from the airspaces toward hilar and mediastinal lymph nodes and ultimately into the thoracic duct or right bronchomediastinal lymphatic trunk. Within the lung, the lymphatics are classically distributed within and around bronchovascular bundles, within the interlobular septa, and in the pleural tissues. The lymphoproliferative disorders, both reactive and neoplastic that will be discussed commonly demonstrate a classic lymphangitic pattern of distribution. Centered on the lymphatics, these can assume a variety of morphologic patterns ranging from focal, nodular collections to diffuse interstitial or airway patterns. The distribution, density, and cellular composition of the infiltrates determine in large part the classification of the process and serve as the paradigm for the histopathologic approach to the classification of these lesions (Table 31.1).

REACTIVE LYMPHOPROLIFERATIVE LESIONS

There are a variety of published classifications of reactive processes within the lung. The classification used in previous editions of this book serves as a comprehensive consideration (36) (Table 31.2). Primary reactive processes can be further separated into focal/nodular patterns and diffuse patterns recognizing that there can be an overlap of patterns. In this situation, we classify the process on the basis of the dominant architectural pattern.

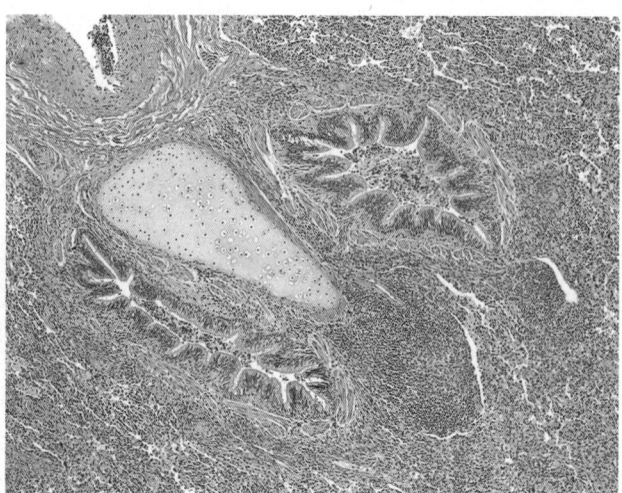

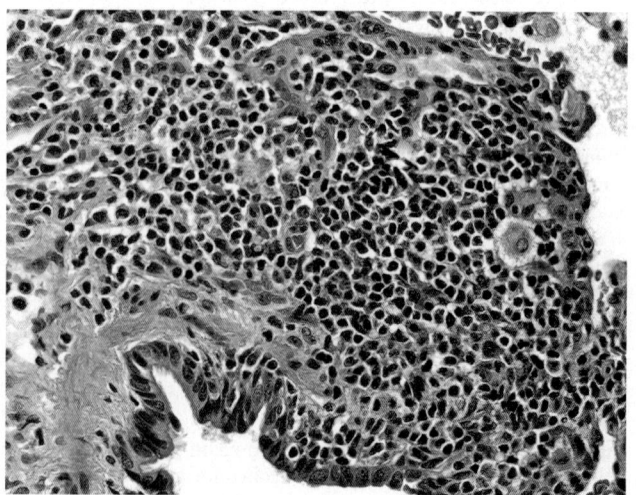

FIGURE 31.2. A: Low-power magnification of BALT in the wall of a small cartilaginous bronchus (H&E, magnification: 40×). **B:** High-power magnification showing discrete nodule composed of small lymphocytes, with focal extension into specialized airway epithelium (H&E, magnification: 400×).

Table 31.1	HEMATOLYMPHOID LESIONS OF THE LUNG AND PLEURA

Benign Lymphoid Proliferations
1. **Nodular Disorders**
   Intraparenchymal lymph node
   Nodular lymphoid hyperplasia
   Intraparenchymal/hilar Castleman disease
   Pulmonary hyalinizing granuloma
   Inflammatory pseudotumor including IgG4-related sclerosing disease
2. **Multifocal/diffuse disorders**
   Follicular bronchitis/bronchiolitis
   Lymphoid interstitial pneumonia

Malignant Lymphoid Proliferations
1. **Primary Pulmonary Neoplasms**
   Extranodal MZL
   Diffuse large B-cell lymphoma
   Lymphomatoid granulomatosis
   Other EBV-associated lymphomas and lymphoproliferative disorders
      EBV+ diffuse large cell lymphoma of the elderly
      DLBCL associated with chronic inflammation
      Posttransplant lymphoproliferative disorder
   Intravascular large B-cell lymphoma
   Primary HL
   Primary effusion lymphoma
   Plasmacytoma
   Other neoplasms with infrequent primary presentation in the lung
      Peripheral T-cell lymphoma
      T-cell ALCL
2. **Secondary Pulmonary Involvement**
   Small mature B-cell lymphomas/leukemias
      Chronic lymphocytic leukemia/small lymphocytic lymphoma
      Mantle cell lymphoma
      Follicular lymphoma
   Mature T-cell and NK-cell neoplasms
      Mycosis fungoides
   Myeloid proliferations
      Acute myeloid leukemias
      Idiopathic myelofibrosis

Histiocytic Proliferations
Primary Histiocytic Lesions
Pulmonary Langerhans cell histiocytosis
Erdheim-Chester disease
Rosai-Dorfman disease
True histiocytic sarcoma
Langerhans cell sarcoma
Follicular and interdigitating dendritic cell tumor

Table 31.2	REACTIVE LYMPHOPROLIFERATIVE LESIONS

Focal/Nodule Reactive Processes
Intraparenchymal lymph node
Nodular lymphoid hyperplasia
Intraparenchymal/hilar CD
Pulmonary hyalinizing granuloma
IPT including ISD

Multifocal/Diffuse Disorders
Follicular bronchitis/bronchiolitis
Lymphoid interstitial pneumonia

are enveloped within the visceral pleura or fissure or in close proximity to either structure (within 1 cm) (37–45) (Fig. 31.3).

Macroscopically, they are solitary, round-to-ovoid nodules within the pleura or fissures. In adults, the majority are blackened by anthracotic pigment. Under the microscope, the subpleural or septa localization is confirmed, and most display a fibrous capsule with subcapsular sinuses. Primary and reactive follicles along with variable amounts of fibrosis, calcifications, anthracotic pigment, silica and silicate particles, and sinus histiocytes are observed. In some cases, fibrosis obliterates the cortical and medullary compartments (Fig. 31.3).

The primary differential diagnostic considerations are intraparenchymal metastasis with a host lymphoid response and nodular lymphoid hyperplasia (NLH). The presence of normal nodal cytoarchitecture and absence of atypical cells are helpful clues.

Nodular Lymphoid Hyperplasia

Few entities in pulmonary lymphoproliferative disorders have stirred as vigorous an existential debate as pulmonary NLH or "pseudolymphoma" as it was originally named by Saltzstein in 1963. He described this collection of "lymphocytic tumors" as "an infiltrate of mature lymphocytes and other inflammatory cells, true germinal centers, and lymph nodes free of lymphoma" (46). Over the ensuing years, the introduction of IHC, molecular techniques to establish clonality, and careful long-term follow-up of patient populations revealed that cases that were initially thought to be "pseudolymphoma" on morphologic grounds were low-grade lymphomas. Kradin and Mark (47) introduced the term "nodular lymphoid hyperplasia" and emphasized the importance of detailed immunohistochemical studies to distinguish NLH from malignant lymphoma. Thereafter, the diagnosis of NLH was rarely made as most cases were shown to be low-grade lymphomas, usually of the extranodal marginal zone type (48,49). Abbondanzo et al. (50) reported a small series of bono vide cases of NLH utilizing strict histopathologic, immunophenotypic, and genotypic criteria. Specifically, all of their 14 cases demonstrated preservation of the normal immunoarchitecture and absence of a molecular rearrangement of the immunoglobulin heavy chain gene or the minor or major break-point region of the t(14;18), supporting the concept of NLH as a definitive, albeit rare lesion. There was a broad age range (19 to 80 years) with an average age at presentation of 60 years and a slight female predominance (4:3). Most were asymptomatic, and two-thirds of patients had a solitary pulmonary lesion without hilar or mediastinal adenopathy. CT imaging reveals a discrete solitary or less commonly coalescence of one or more nodules or multiple nodules (two to three) with focal, limited lymphangitic extension adjacent to the mass (6) (Fig. 31.4). Surgical excision is curative, and recurrences have not been reported to date.

Focal/Nodular Reactive Lymphoid Processes
Intrapulmonary Lymph Node

The recognition of IPLNs dates back well over a century. An argument can still be made as to whether this category truly represents a "disorder" or not. In our experience, they are typically found in VATS biopsy specimens obtained in the metastatic workup or metastasectomy for osteosarcoma in children and teens and colorectal carcinoma in adults. Others are captured as part of a screening practice for patients at risk for lung cancer, during the evaluation of nonneoplastic lung disease, or as an incidental postmortem finding. On CT imaging, they are usually solitary (2+ in up to a third of cases), measuring <1.0 cm in greatest dimension, and display sharply delineated borders, but on occasion they are speculated, irregular, or poorly defined prompting concern for neoplasia. Most are angular in shape, but round-to-oval shapes are also reported. The majority are solid and homogeneous, but cases with a ground-glass internal composition are reported. They are located below the level of the carina in either lower lobe or right middle lobe and

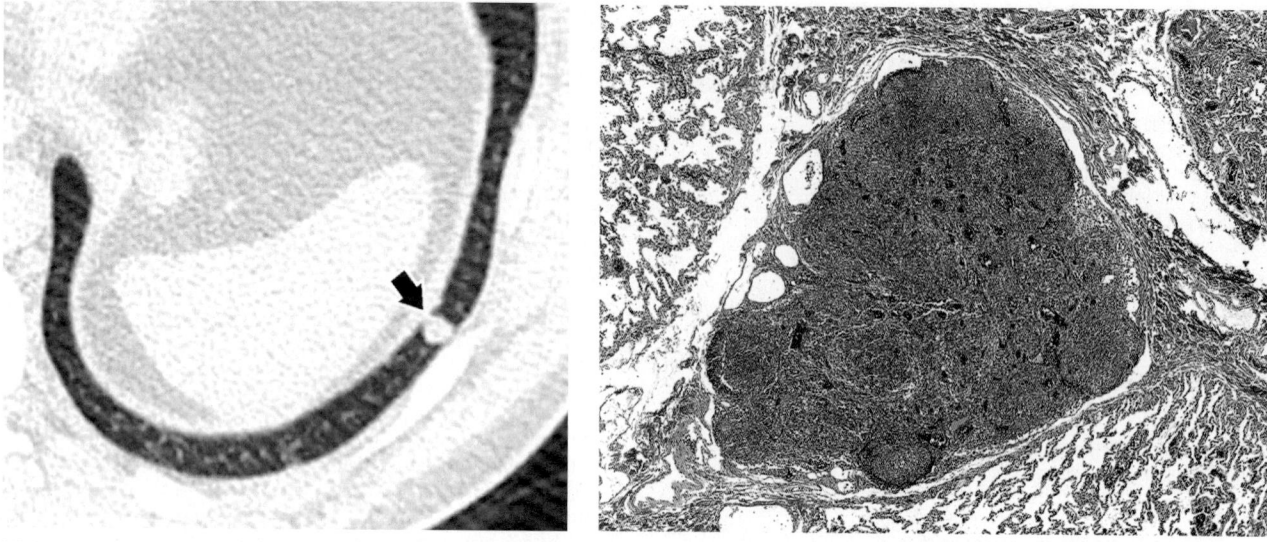

FIGURE 31.3. Intraparenchymal lymph node. A: CT image of IPLN in subpleural region of lung (*arrow*). **B:** Low-power magnification showing constituents of normal lymph node embedded within subpleural fibrous tissue (H&E, magnification: 40×).

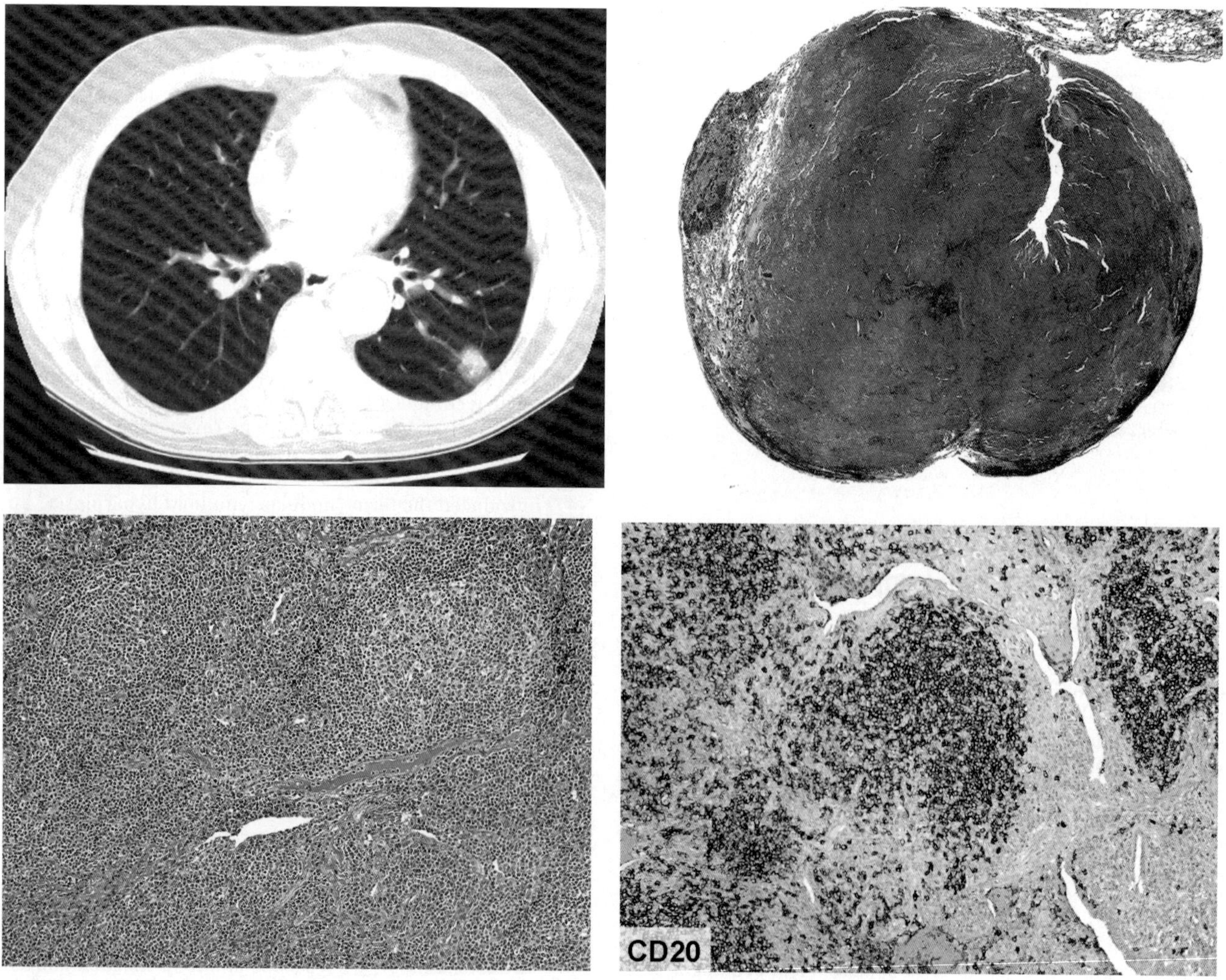

FIGURE 31.4. Nodular lymphoid hyperplasia. A: HRCT showing subpleural, discrete nodule. **B:** Low-power magnification showing nonencapsulated, circumscribed lesion composed of lymphocytes (H&E, magnification: 15×). **C:** Numerous reactive germinal centers with delineated mantle zone and interfollicular regions (H&E, magnification: 100×). **D:** CD20 highlights germinal centers (magnification: 60×).

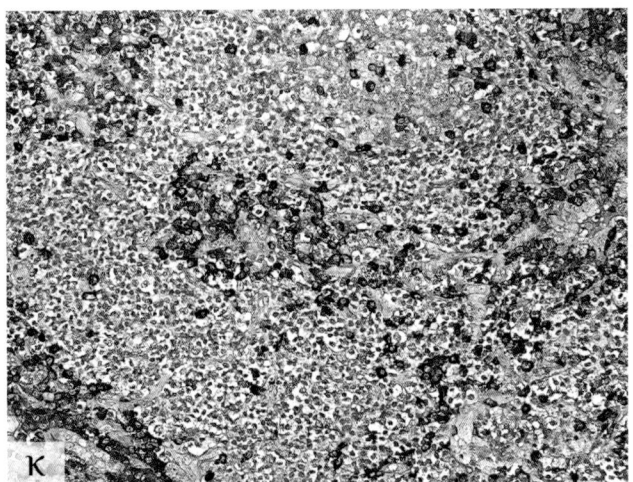
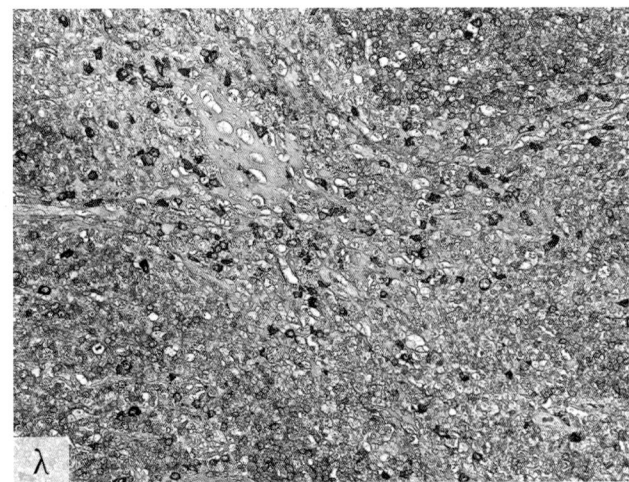

E   K   λ   F

FIGURE 31.4. *(Continued)* **E:** Polytypic kappa light chain staining of plasma cells (magnification: 200×). **F:** Polytypic lambda light chain staining of plasma cells (magnification: 200×).

Grossly, the lesions are gray, tan, or white and rubbery, fleshy, or firm in consistency and measure 0.06 to 6.0 cm in diameter with the majority in 2 to 4 cm range (average 2.1 cm) (50). The classic histopathologic features include a sharply delineated, unencapsulated lesion. Reflecting the radiologic findings, the edge of the lesion can exhibit minimal extension along alveolar septa, creating an irregular border at low-power magnification. The mass is composed of reactive germinal centers containing immunoblasts, tingible-body macrophages, and mitotic figures (Fig. 31.4). The secondary follicles are surrounded by discrete mantle zones and sheets of plasma cells and lymphocytes within the interfollicular regions. Central foci of sclerosis within the lesion and collections of Russell bodies can be found. Dutcher bodies, lymphoepithelial lesions (LEL), conspicuous deposits of amyloid, and infiltration of adjacent structures such as the visceral pleura or large airways are absent in NLH and are useful morphologic clues in distinguishing it from malignant lymphoma. By definition, immunohistochemical and polymerase chain reaction (PCR) yield a polyclonal lesion characterized by CD20+ germinal centers, CD3+ and CD5+ T cells within the interfollicular regions, absence of anomalous CD43 or CD5 coexpression of B cells, polytypic plasma cells, and restriction of Bcl-2 staining to mantle zone cells and interfollicular lymphocytes (50). By definition, cyclin D1 is negative.

The differential diagnosis includes intrapulmonary lymph node, lymphocytic interstitial pneumonia (LIP), follicular bronchitis/bronchiolitis (FB), inflammatory myofibroblastic tumor (IMT), plasmacytoma, and MALT lymphoma (Table 31.3). Both LIP and FB are diffuse rather than nodular proliferations, and IMT displays a spindle cell component, at least focally. As mentioned, the presence of Dutcher bodies, parenchymal invasion, prominent alveolar extension, LEL, amyloid deposits, or colonization of the follicles by marginal zone cells are useful histopathologic clues for identifying MALT lymphoma. Further, immunohistochemical staining and molecular studies support a polyclonal process in NLH versus a monoclonal lesion in MALT lymphoma. Ultimately, both careful attention to the histologic composition and ancillary studies are required to confidently distinguish these entities (51,52).

Intrapulmonary Castleman Disease (Angiofollicular/ Giant Lymph Node Hyperplasia)

Castleman disease (CD) is a rare benign lymphoid proliferation that primarily involves cervical, hilar, and mediastinal lymph

chains and occasionally the lung itself. It has a number of synonyms that are solely of historical curiosity including angiomatous lymphoid hyperplasia, Castleman tumor, giant benign lymphoma, and hamartoma of the lymphatics (53). As originally described, the group consisted of two main histopathologic patterns: the hyaline vascular type and the plasma cell type. In the original report by Castleman et al. (54), all 13 cases were localized to mediastinal or hilar lymph nodes and most presented as asymptomatic masses (54). In an expanded series of cases, Keller described 74 cases of the hyaline vascular variant, 2 of which were intrapulmonary lesions and 8 cases were of the nodal plasma cell type (55). In light of molecular and clinicopathologic discoveries, the concept of CD has evolved over the last 25 years, and there are now four recognized subtypes of CD: *hyaline vascular type of CD (HVCD), plasma cell variant of CD (PVCD)*, human herpesvirus 8 (*HHV8)–associated CD*, and *multicentric CD, not otherwise specified (NOS)* (56). The HVCD classically presents in young adults as an asymptomatic mass ranging from 1 to 16 cm in diameter. In a minority of cases, signs and symptoms attributable to compressive effects on adjacent airways or vascular structures occur. The CT manifestations are a solid, sharply delineated mass with soft tissue attenuation (57–59). Calcifications are absent or infrequent and are punctate or arborizing in distribution. The limited experience with ^{18}F-FDG PET imaging suggests that radiotracer uptake is less intense in most cases of CD than malignant lymphomas and other neoplastic processes but exceptions occur (60). Surgical excision is curative. The key histopathologic findings are described in detail in another section of this book. Briefly, the germinal centers appear diminutive and are laced with fibrous bands that envelop capillary vessels. The follicles are "transfixed by radially penetrating capillaries" (55), and the mantle zone is expanded by small lymphocytes (both CD20+ B cells and CD4+ CD68+ plasmacytoid monocytes) arranged in laminar circular arrays (Fig. 31.5). The dendritic cell network within the follicles is not normal, and there are reported associations of HVCD and follicular dendritic cell proliferations or tumors.

The PCVCD represents only 10% of cases of CD. The localized form has demographics similar to the hyaline vascular type. The *multicentric variant, NOS* typically presents in an older patient population. It may be localized (thorax or abdomen lymph nodes) or multicentric in distribution; the multicentric type is often associated with systemic signs and symptoms such as fever, cough, shortness of breath, splenomegaly, hepatomegaly, lymphadenopathy, polyclonal hypergammaglobulinemia, anemia, and elevated erythrocyte sedimentation

Table 31.3   CLINICAL, PATHOLOGIC, AND IMMUNOPHENOTYPIC FEATURES OF REACTIVE AND NEOPLASTIC PULMONARY LYMPHOPROLIFERATIVE LESIONS

	Nodule Lymphoid Hyperplasia	Pulmonary Castleman Disease	Pulmonary Hyalinizing Granuloma	Inflammatory Myofibroblastic Tumor	Follicular Bronchiolitis	Lymphoid Interstitial Pneumonia	Extranodal Marginal Zone Lymphoma	Diffuse Large B-cell Lymphoma	Lymphomatoid Granulomatosis
Age	19–80 y; median 65 y	HVCD: young adults; PCVD: young adults; Multicentric CD: variable; median sixth decade	Adults; median fifth decade	Infants-Elderly (most <40 y)	Children-Adults (median 44 y)	Children with HIV infection; Adults with median age sixth decade	Adults in sixth and seventh decades	Adults sixth and seventh decades up to 50% arise from MZL	Adults (rare in children); often in immunocompromised patients; Median age 60
Clinical Presentation	Majority Asymptomatic Minority: cough, dyspnea, chest pain	HVCD: asymptomatic; Other types: frequently have constitutional symptoms, hematologic and/or immunologic abnormalities	Majority asymptomatic or mild pulmonary symptoms	Majority: asymptomatic	Dyspnea, cough, fever ± weight loss	Dry cough, dyspnea, fatigue, dysproteinemias	Majority are asymptomatic	Cough, dyspnea, fever, weight loss, hemoptysis	Cough, dyspnea, chest pain and B symptoms
Chest Radiograph	Solitary lesion without adenopathy	HVCD: solitary lesion without adenopathy; Other Types: multifocal lesions ± generalized adenopathy	Poorly delineated homogeneous nodules or infiltrates	Solitary lesion (bilateral or multifocal in 15%) with lower lobe predilection	Bilateral reticular or reticulonodular infiltrates	Bilateral predominantly lower zone reticular or reticulonodular infiltrates	Solitary or multiple nodules	Single or multiple opacities	Diffuse reticulonodular opacities to rounded opacities
CT Features	Solitary, nodular mass; 2–4 cm	HVCD: solid, delineated mass ± rare calcifications; Other types: interstitial thickening, centrilobular nodules, septal thickening, subpleural cysts, GGO	1+ centrally located solid nodules with discrete edges; <1–15 cm (mean 2 cm)	Varies from sharply delineated to irregular and spiculated	Bilateral centrilobular and peribronchial nodules; 1–3 mm	Bilateral GGO, centrilobular nodules, thin-walled cysts, thickened peribronchovascular interstitium	Nodular or consolidative opacities ± air bronchograms	Single or multiple nodules or masses ±cavitation	Nodular lesions 0.5–8.0 cm along bronchovascular bundles and interlobular septa; basilar predominance; cavitation common
Macroscopic Findings	Gray, tan, white fleshy mass; 0.06–6.0 cm in diameter	Solid, circumscribed, tan firm masses; Other types: multinodular lesions		White or yellow-tan, nonencapsulated; 1–25 cm (most < 8 cm)	Nodular thickening of distal bronchi & bronchioles	Nondescript	Single or multiple white, fleshy nodules 2–20 cm; less commonly parenchymal consolidation with poorly defined borders	Parenchymal or endobronchial fleshy masses	Yellow-white nodules with central necrosis

Microscopic Findings Localization/Distribution	Circumscribed nonencapsulated cellular mass with minimal extension along adjacent alveolar septa	Circumscribed nodule(s)	Delineated lesions	Peripheral lung or endobronchial	Broncho and bronchiolocentric	Interstitial; especially alveolar septa	Lymphatic routes; disruption of architecture with invasion of pleura and bronchi	Nodular consolidations with parenchyma destruction & pleural invasion, ±necrosis	Lymphatic distribution
Cellular Composition	Reactive germinal centers with discrete mantle zones; No tissue destruction or pleural invasion	HVCD: diminutive GC with radially penetrating vessels; mantle zone expansion by lymphocytes and plasmacytoid monocytes; Other types: hyperplastic GC with expanded mantle zones and paracortical plasmacytosis	Densely collagenized bands admixed with plasma cells and small lymphocytes; GC and lymphoid follicles at periphery	Plasma Cell Type: plasma cells and lymphocytes with scattered spindle cells and collagen bundles; Spindle Cell Type: bundles of uniform spindle cells with foamy macrophages; Touton giant cells and mononuclear inflammatory cells	Prominent peribronchiolar reactive germinal centers with scattered lymphoid aggregates along other lymphatic routes	Mixed infiltrates of small lymphocytes, immunoblasts, plasma cells and histiocytes; Occasional epithelioid granulomas and giant cells	Monotonous monocytoid, atypical small lymphocytes or plasmacytoid cells along lymphatic routes; colonization of germinal centers, lymphoepithelial cells; Occasionally multinucleated giant cells, amyloid deposits, giant cells	Monotonous atypical large cells with vesicular nuclei, 1+ nucleoli	Angiocentric polymorphous infiltrates of small lymphocytes, plasma cells, histiocytes & large atypical lymphocytes and immunoblasts; Usually conspicuous infarctive necrosis (LYG 3)
Immunophenotype	CD20+ germinal centers surrounded by CD3+ T cells in interfollicular zones	CD20+ in GC and CD20+ B cells & CD4+CD68+ plasmacytoid monocytes in mantle zones	Polytypic plasma cells and T cells	Polytypic plasma cells, CD20+ B cells and CD3+ T cells	CD20+ B cells lacking Bcl-2 in follicles	Polytypic plasma cells and CD3+ T cells; CD20+ B cells restricted to follicles	CD20+, CD79a+, CD5-, Cd10-, CD23-, Bcl-1-, CD43±	CD20+, CD79a+, CD19+; with either GC-(72%) or ABC-(29%) subtype; High proliferation rate	Large cells are CD20+, EBV+ B cells
Clonality	Polyclonal	Polyclonal	Polyclonal	Polyclonal	Polyclonal	Polyclonal	monoclonal	monoclonal	monoclonal large B cells

Abbreviations: HVCD, hyaline vascular castleman disease; PCVCD, plasma cell variant Castleman disease; GC, germinal center; GGO, ground-glass opacities; MZL, marginal zone lymphoma.

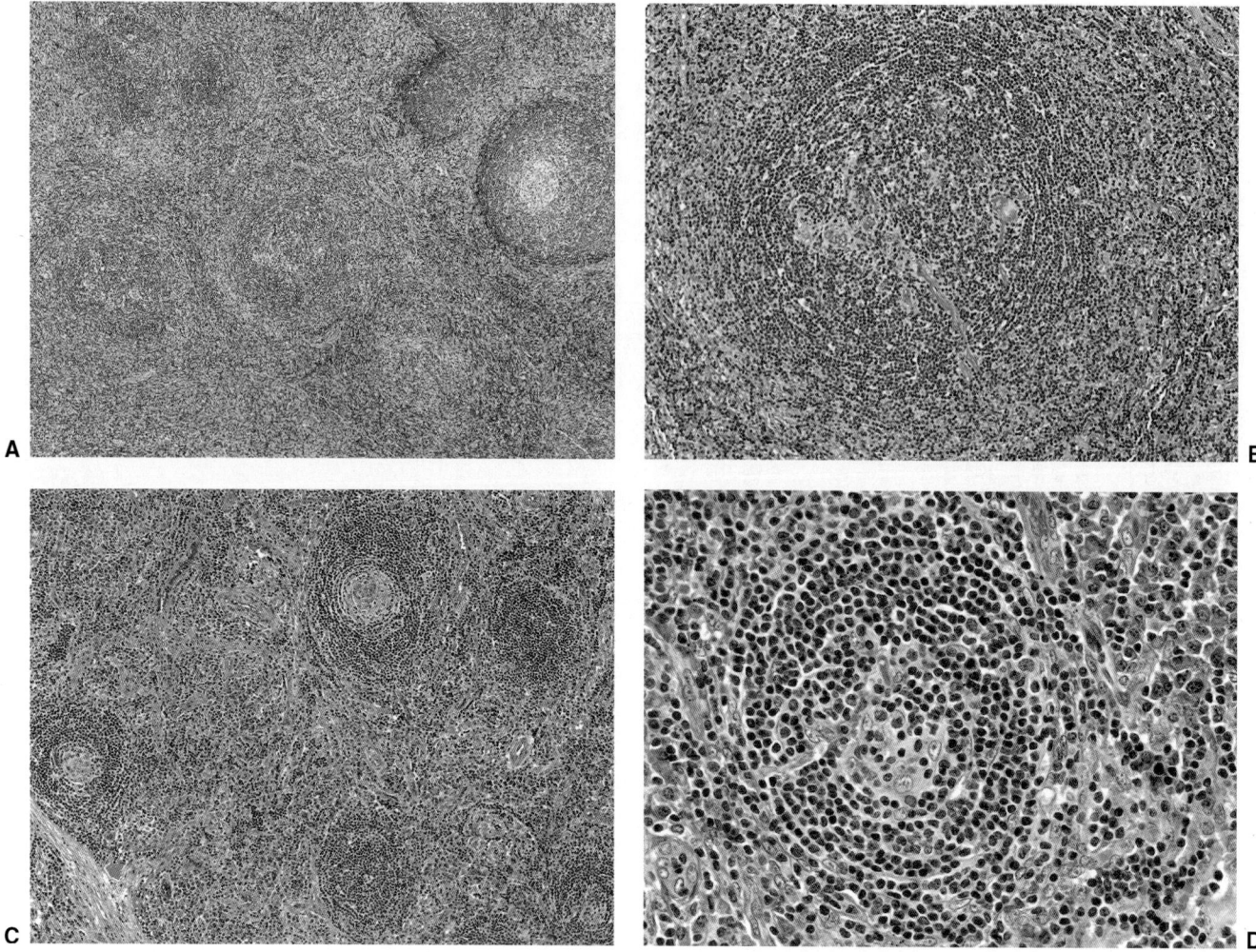

FIGURE 31.5. Thoracic Castleman disease. A: Hyaline vascular type showing diminutive follicles and expanded mantle zones and interfollicular regions (H&E, magnification: 40×). **B:** HVCD characterized by radially penetrating capillaries and laminar array of lymphocytes in the mantle zone (H&E, magnification: 125×). **C:** Plasma cell variant of CD can be either localized or multicentric. Hyperplasia of germinal centers, expanded mantle zones, and plasmacytosis in the interfollicular zones are noted (H&E, magnification: 100×). **D:** High-power magnification showing laminar arrangement of lymphocytes around the follicles and numerous plasma cells in the interfollicular zones (H&E, magnification: 400×).

rate and elevated interleukin-6 (IL-6) (61,62). Recently, an association of the multicentric variant with HHV8 has been reported (63,64). This group includes cases of multicentric CD occurring in HIV-infected patients. Other associations have included POEMS syndrome, pulmonary hyalinizing granulomas (PHGs), and LIP (65–67). The radiologic patterns of pulmonary involvement include peribronchovascular interstitial thickening, centrilobular nodules, interlobular septal thickening, thin-walled cysts, subpleural nodules, ground-glass attenuation, airspace consolidation, and bronchiectasis (58,68,69). Treatment typically includes systemic therapy with corticosteroids, single-agent or combination chemotherapy, rituximab or immunotherapy (interferon-alpha, anti-IL-6 receptor antibodies), thalidomide. Multicentric CD has a poorer prognosis compared to HVCD (61,70). There is an increased risk of relapses and the development of malignancies such as Kaposi sarcoma, primary effusion lymphoma (PEL), medullary plasmablastic lymphoma, and cardiac diffuse large cell lymphoma (66). The cardinal histopathologic findings include hyperplasia of the germinal centers with expansion of the mantle zones and a brisk paracortical plasmacytosis (56) (Fig. 31.5). The primary differential diagnostic considerations are extranodal marginal zone lymphoma (MZL), plasmacytoma, and other reactive lymphoid processes.

Pulmonary Hyalinizing Granuloma

PHG is an uncommon fibrosclerotic and inflammatory lesion of the lung of unknown etiology that presents as multiple parenchymal lesions mimicking pulmonary metastases. Originally described by Engleman et al. in 1977, it shares a number of features with other parenchymal disease such as plasma cell–rich variant of inflammatory pseudotumor (IPT)/IMT and IgG4-related (systemic) sclerosing disease (ISD) (52,71,72). Recently, Chapman et al. (73) reported a case of PHG associated with elevated serum and tissue IgG4 and suggested that PHG falls within the spectrum of ISD. Less than 100 cases are reported in the literature and the 2 largest series account for almost half the cases (71,74). At presentation, most patients are adults (mean age early 40s) relaying minimal or no respiratory symptoms (mild cough, dyspnea on exertion, or pleuritic chest pain), with radiographic studies revealing either solitary or more commonly multiple bilateral lung infiltrates or nodules. The constellation of radiologic findings include slowly growing centrally located solid nodules (one or more) ranging from few mm to 15 cm (average 2 cm) with discrete contours (75–77). Less common findings are lesions with cystic or cavitary components, irregular outlines, or calcifications (78,79). At resection, the nodules are solid, circumscribed, tan and firm, and lack hemorrhagic or caseating necrosis. Microscopically, the lesion is composed of dense, collagenous bands of fibrous tissue resembling cutaneous keloid arranged randomly and whorled and interspersed and rimmed by collections of polytypic plasma cells and small lymphocytes that are predominantly T cells (Fig. 31.6). The densely eosinophilic bands are concentrically arranged around small arteries and arterioles. In distinction to amyloid, the lamellar bands of collagen stain strongly with Masson trichrome and lack apple-green birefringence under polarized microscopy on the Congo red stain. Further, punctate foci of ischemic necrosis, calcification, or even ossification may be present, but necrotizing granulomatous inflammation and fibrinoid necrosis of vessels are, by definition, absent. The lesion is surrounded by lymphoplasmacytic collections, and the small vessels often show transmural inflammation and endothelialitis without medial disruption (74). The adjacent pulmonary parenchyma can show a variety of inflammatory changes such as hyperplasia of BALT/peribronchiolitis, interstitial inflammation, organizing pneumonia with loose fibromyxoid plugs (73). Surgical excision and in some cases corticosteroids lead to a good clinical outcome.

The major diagnostic considerations in the differential diagnosis include nodular infectious and noninfectious granulomatous diseases, pulmonary granulomatosis and angiitis (formerly Wegener granulomatosis), rheumatoid nodules,

nodular amyloidosis, HL, and low-grade lymphoplasmacytic lymphoma. Appropriate microbiologic, serologic, histochemical, and immunohistochemical studies are required to distinguish these lesions.

Inflammatory Pseudotumor Including IgG4-Related Sclerosing Disease

Pulmonary IPT and the vast number of names that have been ascribed to it is another uncommon but confusing fibroinflammatory lesion that can have an exclusive pulmonary presentation or be part of a multisystem disorder. The terms that have been ascribed include plasma cell granuloma, IMT, fibroxanthoma, xanthogranuloma, fibrous histiocytoma, plasma cell granuloma-histiocytoma complex, and inflammatory myofibrohistiocytic proliferation, which reflect in part the spectrum of morphologic patterns and the conceptual heterogeneity of etiologies and pathogenesis. At one end of the spectrum is the concept of IPT as a reactive lesion in response to infectious or unknown injurious antigens. Recently, a number of studies linking ISD to a subset of IMT have been published (80–85). At the other end of the spectrum is the group of lesions that morphologically and clinically resemble neoplastic proliferations. The most recent WHO classification of pulmonary neoplasms

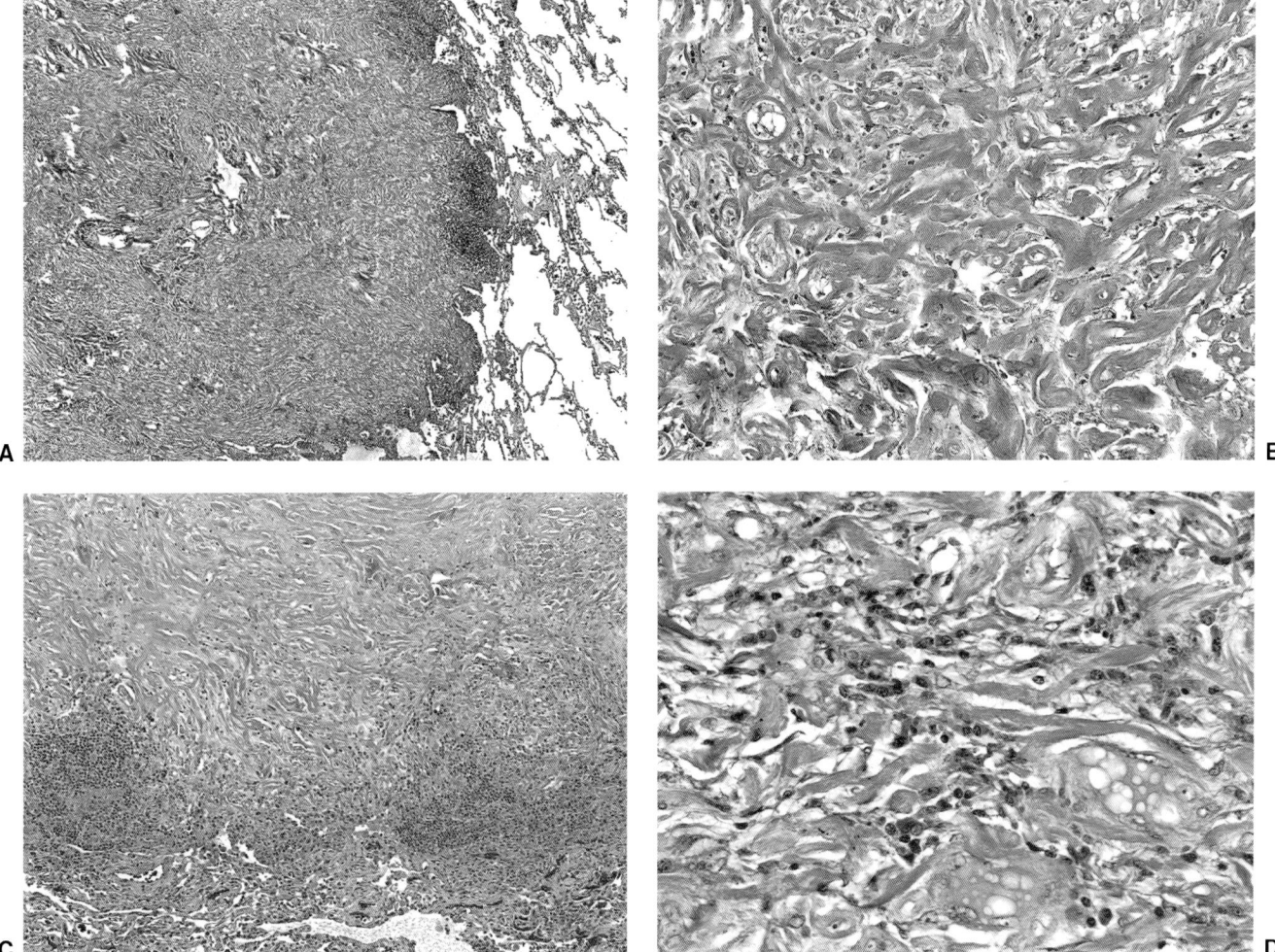

FIGURE 31.6. Pulmonary hyalinizing granuloma. A: Low-power magnification showing nonencapsulated mass composed of dense collagenous connective tissue and rimmed by lymphoid aggregates (H&E, magnification: 15×). **B:** Dense bands of collagen resembling keloid separated by fibroblasts (H&E, magnification: 200×). **C:** The edge of the lesion containing small aggregates of chronic inflammatory cells (H&E, magnification: 100×). **D:** Sparse collections of small lymphocytes and plasma cells are interspersed throughout the hyalinized matrix (H&E, magnification: 400×).

classifies this group as IMT and defines them as a subgroup of IPTs characterized by a variable mixture of collagen, inflammatory cells (plasma cells and lymphocytes) and cytologically bland spindle cells exhibiting myofibroblastic differentiation (86). As these represent differing clinicopathologic entities, they will be discussed separately.

Patients with IPT present across a broad age range from infants to the elderly, but the majority are under the age of 40 years. Many are asymptomatic and the lesion is found incidentally on thoracic imaging, while others have cough, chest pain, hemoptysis, recurrent infections, fever, and other systemic symptoms. Radiographically, the majority are solitary lesions, but bilateral or multifocal lesions are found in up to 15% of cases and there is a predilection for the lower lung zones. In some cases, the lesions are sharply delineated from the adjacent lung, and in others the margins are irregular or speculated and the lesions poorly circumscribed (87,88). Kim et al. (89) reported that the majority of their cases have a proximal endobronchial component, with only a few cases of peripheral nodules. Central cavitation and calcifications within the masses and postobstructive parenchymal changes are uncommon (90). [18]FDG-PET imaging shows increased update and mimics malignant neoplasms such as carcinomas and malignant lymphomas.

At resection, the lesions range in size from 1 to >25 cm but the majority <8 cm. Endobronchial lesions present as polypoid masses while the parenchymal lesions are nonencapsulated, discrete masses. The cut surface is white to yellow-tan in color, firm, and whorled in consistency. There are a number of classifications used for IPT (91–93). The two-pattern scheme (spindle cell and plasma cell types) of Moran and Suster based on morphologic growth patterns provides a practical paradigm for IPT (94). It is important to emphasis that overlap of patterns can be found in any lesion. The *plasma cell type* is characterized by a predominance of polytypic plasma cells and lymphocytes, often obscuring the myofibroblastic cells (Fig. 31.7). The borders of these lesions may be less defined than in the spindle cell type. The inflammatory cells are admixed with entrapped alveolar and bronchiolar structures and variable amounts of collagenous bundles. In some cases, the fibroinflammatory process extends into and beyond the boundaries of the visceral pleura. In the IgG4-related lesions (also called "inflammatory pseudotumor with IgG4+ plasma cells") presenting as the solid nodular pattern, the mass is composed of a connective tissue matrix, lymphoplasmacytic infiltrates and nodules, and obliterative phlebitis (Fig. 31.8). In addition to increased numbers of IgG4+ plasma cells and elevated IgG4+/IgG+ ratios, many cases also display interstitial infiltrates at the edges of the lesions, lymphoplasmacytic bronchiolitis with airway narrowing, postobstructive pneumonia, scattered multinucleated giant cells and neutrophils, and arterial endothelialitis +/− obliteration

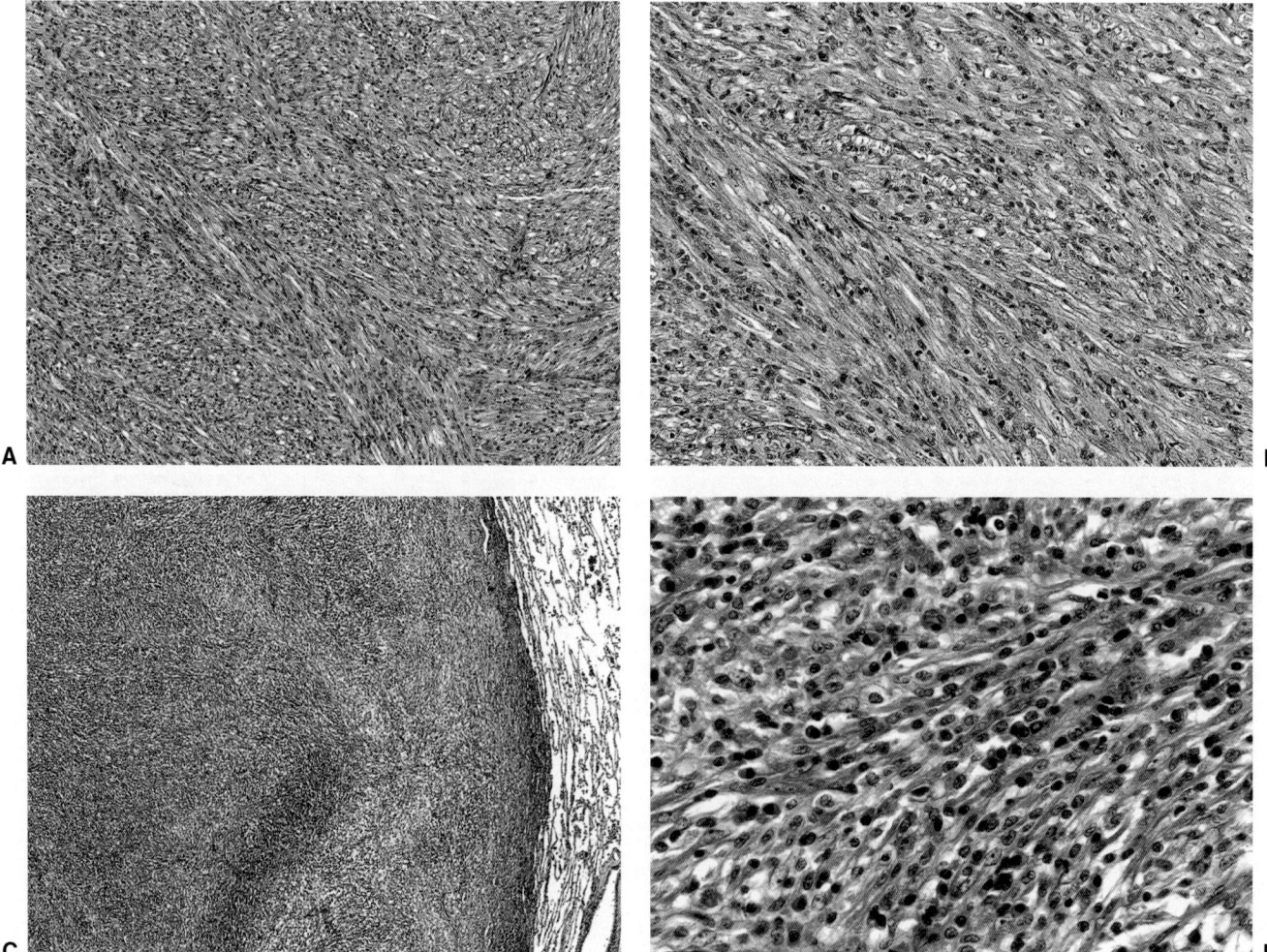

FIGURE 31.7. Inflammatory myofibroblastic tumor. A: Spindle cell type is characterized by bundles of bland spindle (H&E, magnification: 100×). **B:** High-power magnification showing uniform cells with elongated oval nuclei and fine chromatin (H&E, magnification: 200×). **C:** Plasma cell type showing nonencapsulated, sharply circumscribed cellular lesion (H&E, magnification: 40×). **D:** This type is composed of numerous plasma cells and lymphocytes often obscuring the scattered spindle cells (H&E, magnification: 400×).

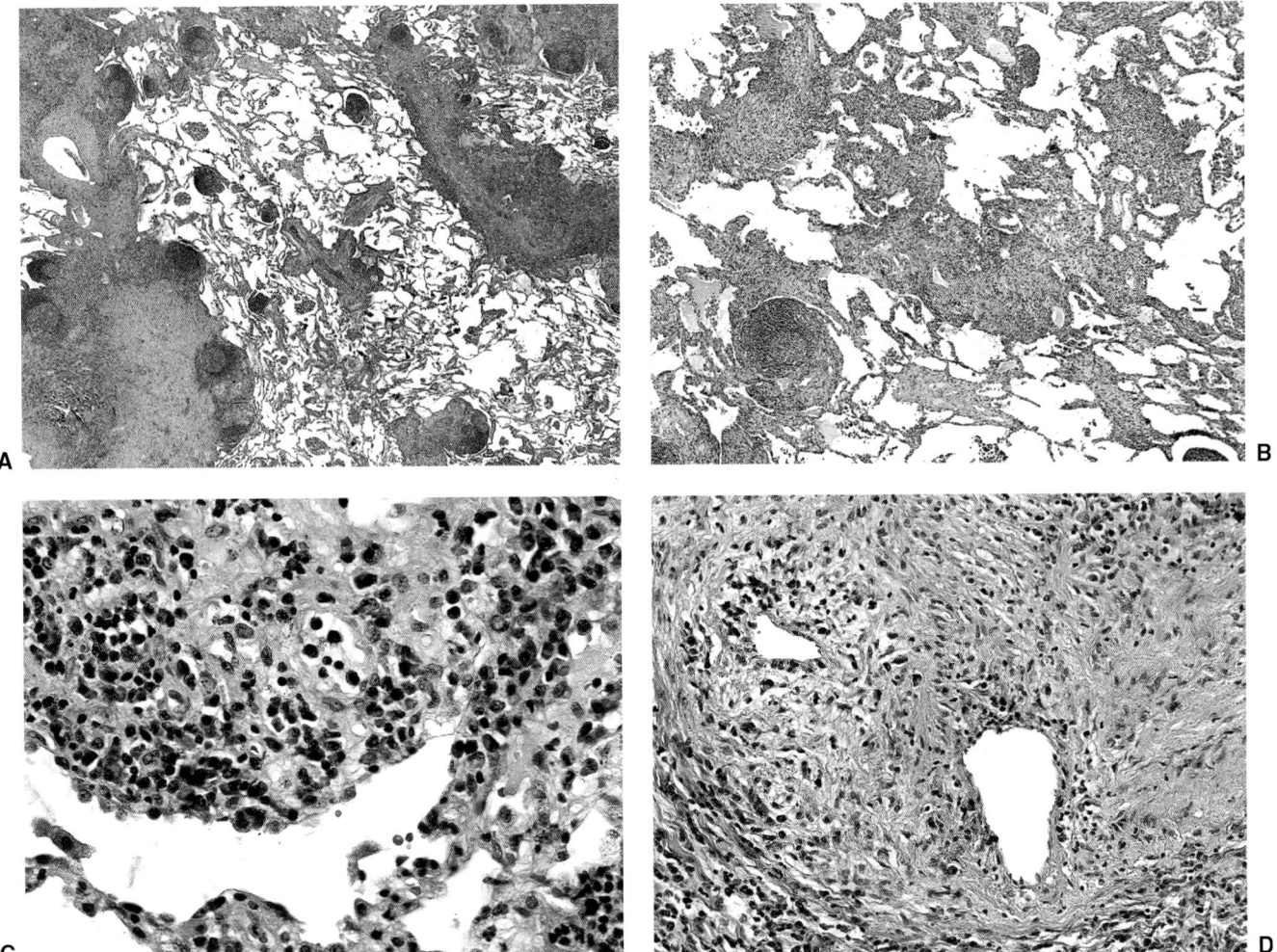

FIGURE 31.8. IgG4-related sclerosing lesion. A: Low-power magnification showing lymphatic distribution of fibroinflammatory process along interlobular septa and bronchovascular bundles (H&E, magnification: 15×). **B:** Lymphoid aggregates and interstitial infiltrates expanding the perivascular spaces (H&E, magnification: 40×). **C:** High-power magnification showing admixture of plasma cells, lymphocytes, and scattered eosinophils and a variable background of fibrosis (H&E, magnification: 400×). **D:** Fibroinflammatory process involving parenchymal vessels (H&E, magnification: 200×).

(52,84). The differential diagnostic considerations are reviewed in detail in a number of recent publications (82–84).

The *spindle cell or fibrohistiocytic type* is thought to more closely mirror a neoplastic proliferation. It occurs more frequently in young patients, grossly resembles a solid mass, and demonstrates clonal cytogenetic abnormalities. In particular, a number of studies have shown clonal alterations at the encoding site for the ALK gene on chromosome 2p23 (95–98). These translocations are found in 20% to 50% of cases. Microscopically, they display cellular storiform arrangements at scanning magnification and are composed of uniform spindle cells with elongated nuclei, inconspicuous nucleoli, and limited eosinophilic to clear cytoplasm (Fig. 31.7). They are typically reactive against vimentin and smooth muscle actin but are negative for desmin, myogenin, myoglobin, S100, CD117, and high molecular weight cytokeratin. Loose aggregates of foamy macrophages are sprinkled throughout the lesion, especially around the periphery. In addition, Touton-type multinucleated giant cells and mononuclear inflammatory cells are seen.

The diagnosis and treatment involves surgical resection. The plasma cell variant, and the IgG4-related type in particular, is responsive to corticosteroid therapy. There have been reports of recurrences, and close follow-up is recommended for patients.

Multifocal/Diffuse Reactive Lymphoid Processes

The list of entities within the multifocal and diffuse patterns of reactive lymphoid hyperplasia is limited to FB and LIP. These represent architectural variations of hyperplasia of BALT, with FB centered on the airways and LIP centered on the interstitium. Each has unique clinical, morphologic, and prognostic features that warrant separate discussions. Parenthetically, there is often an overlap of patterns in patients (99,100).

Follicular Bronchitis/Bronchiolitis

FB is defined as reactive lymphoid nodules, often with germinal centers, within the walls of small airways. It is a relatively common histopathologic finding in lung biopsy specimens and resection specimens removed for tumor, abscess, chronic obstructive lung disease, infection, asthma, and bronchiectasis (101,102). After excluding these associated conditions, Yousem and colleagues classified FB into three distinct clinicopathologic categories: (i) collagen vascular diseases, especially rheumatoid arthritis or Sjögren syndrome, (ii) congenital or acquired immunodeficiency syndromes and conditions such as HIV and lung transplantation, and (iii) hypersensitivity reactions including drug reactions with peripheral eosinophilia (103). Presenting symptoms include dyspnea, cough, and fever, and some patients also have weight loss and recurrent infections. Pulmonary function studies range from normal to restrictive, obstructive, or mixed patterns (103–109). The main high-resolution CT (HRCT) findings are bilateral small centrilobular and peribronchial nodules measuring 1 to 3 mm, and foci of ground-glass opacification. Less frequently, thickening of bronchial walls and interlobular septa, "tree-in-bud" nodularity, peribronchovascular airspace consolidation, and bronchial dilation can be seen (5,6,110,111).

The key histopathologic finding in FB is the peribronchiolar distribution of lymphoid nodules containing reactive germinal centers. The nodules are located between the bronchiole and the muscular pulmonary artery and cause impingement or narrowing of airway lumens (Fig. 31.9). In addition to the peribronchiolar localization, there are usually similar lymphoid aggregates distributed in a lymphatic distribution along the interlobular septa and subpleural tissues (103). The follicles are composed of CD20+ B cells lacking Bcl-2 and other immunohistochemical evidence of malignant lymphoma. The differential diagnosis includes LIP, MALT lymphoma, and other low-grade lymphomas/leukemias such as CLL and NLH. LIP displays an alveolar interstitial distribution rather than peribronchiolar pattern of FB, and NLH is typically presents as a mass lesion. The immunophenotypic profile allows the discrimination of FB from low-grade lymphoid malignancies (Table 31.3).

The treatment and prognosis depend in large part on the presence or absence of an underlying disorder such as rheumatoid arthritis. Corticosteroids are given with variable results.

Lymphocytic Interstitial Pneumonia

Liebow and Carrington (112) first described LIP over 40 years ago as a form of idiopathic interstitial pneumonia (IIP). Since then, it has been removed and then added back into the different revisions of the IIP and is currently recognized as a rare type (113,114). With the application of IHC, some of the cases originally classified as LIP have been reclassified as extranodal forms of low-grade B-cell lymphoma such as MZL/MALT lymphoma or recognized as cellular variants of nonspecific interstitial pneumonia (NSIP). Further, the majority of cases are associated with an underlying systemic disorder such as a collagen vascular disease (e.g., Sjögren syndrome, rheumatoid arthritis, systemic lupus erythematosus) or congenital or acquired immunodeficiency states including HIV infection, common variable immunodeficiency, post allogeneic bone marrow transplantation. Less common associations include viral infections such as Epstein-Barr virus (EBV) and HTLV-1, *Legionella, Mycoplasma, Chlamydia pneumoniae*, tuberculosis, drug reaction (e.g., diphenylhydantoin), and pulmonary alveolar proteinosis (35,115). As a result, the number of idiopathic

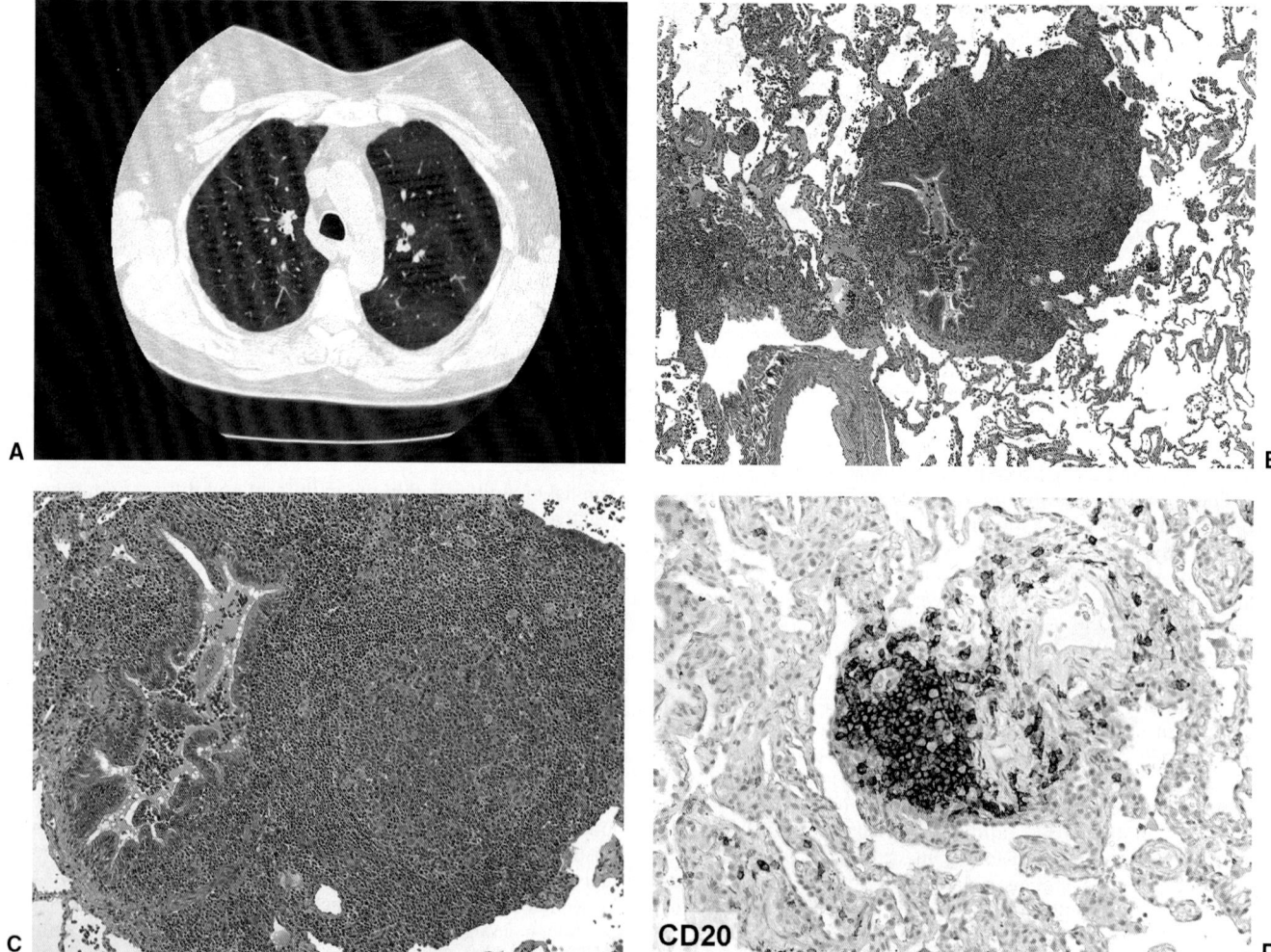

FIGURE 31.9. Follicular bronchiolitis. A: HRCT showing bilateral small peribronchial and centrilobular nodules. **B:** Prominent reactive germinal centers centered on membranous bronchiole. There is a slight interstitial expansion of chronic inflammatory cells in the adjacent peribronchiolar interstitium (H&E, magnification: 40×). **C:** High-power magnification showing reactive follicle and mantle zone, creating narrowing of the bronchiolar lumen (H&E, magnification: 100×). **D:** CD20 stain highlighting the germinal center component of FB (magnification: 400×).

LIP cases is now thought to be very few. There is a wide age range from infants to the elderly with the mean age at diagnosis in the sixth decade. At presentation, signs and symptoms include dry cough, dyspnea, and fatigue with bibasilar "Velcro" crackles on auscultation. Most patients have serum dysproteinemias, most commonly polyclonal hypergammaglobulinemia. Pulmonary function studies show a restrictive defect with diminished forced vital capacity, forced expiratory volume in 1 second, total lung capacity, and diffusing capacity of the lung for carbon monoxide. The chest radiograph shows bilateral, predominantly lower lung zone fine reticular, or reticulonodular opacities. HRCT features include uniform or patchy areas of bilateral ground-glass opacity (GGO), poorly defined centrilobular nodules, thin-walled cystic airspaces measuring 1 to 30 mm, thickened peribronchovascular interstitium, and mild interlobular septal thickening (5,6,35).

Microscopically, LIP displays diffuse interstitial cellular infiltrates that expand interlobular and alveolar septa (Fig. 31.10). The infiltrates are composed of small lymphocytes, immunoblasts, plasma cells, and histiocytes, including occasional epithelioid and giant cell types. Generally, lymphocytes predominate over plasma cells, but in some cases the pattern is reversed, giving rise to older terms such as lymphoplasmacytic pneumonia, plasmacytic interstitial pneumonia, and plasma cell interstitial pneumonitis. In most cases, there is uniform involvement of the parenchyma, but foci of interstitial sparing

may be found. Less common findings are small non-necrotizing granulomas, intraepithelial lymphocytes, "spillage" of inflammatory cells into the adjacent airspaces along with proteinaceous collections, foci of amyloid deposition, and interstitial fibrosis (35,51,52,99,116). In most cases, a component of FB is notable. The plasma cells demonstrate polytypic expression of kappa and lambda light chains, and the interstitial lymphocytes are predominantly CD3+ T cells (Fig. 31.10). The B cells are isolated to the foci of FB.

The differential diagnosis includes a variety of infectious, inflammatory, and neoplastic disorders. *Pneumocystis jiroveci* pneumonia (PJP) and a variety of viral infections such as EBV or CMV can closely mimic LIP, and we routinely perform a silver stain such as GMS to exclude PJP. Other patterns of interstitial lung disease (ILD) should be considered. The cellular type of NSIP exhibits mild-to-moderate interstitial expansion by lymphocytic or lymphoplasmacytic cells and not the dense infiltrates of LIP (Fig. 31.11). Further, FB is a common finding in LIP and is unusual or minimal in NSIP. HP shows mononuclear bronchiolitis, cellular interstitial pneumonitis, and poorly formed nonnecrotizing granulomas (Fig. 31.11). Unlike LIP, it is patchy in distribution, less intense than in LIP, and often has an organizing pneumonia component with loose fibromyxoid plugs. Cases of interstitial pneumonia with IgG4+ plasma cells have been reported. In those cases the overall morphologic pattern more closely resembles NSIP than LIP (80,81,116). As alluded

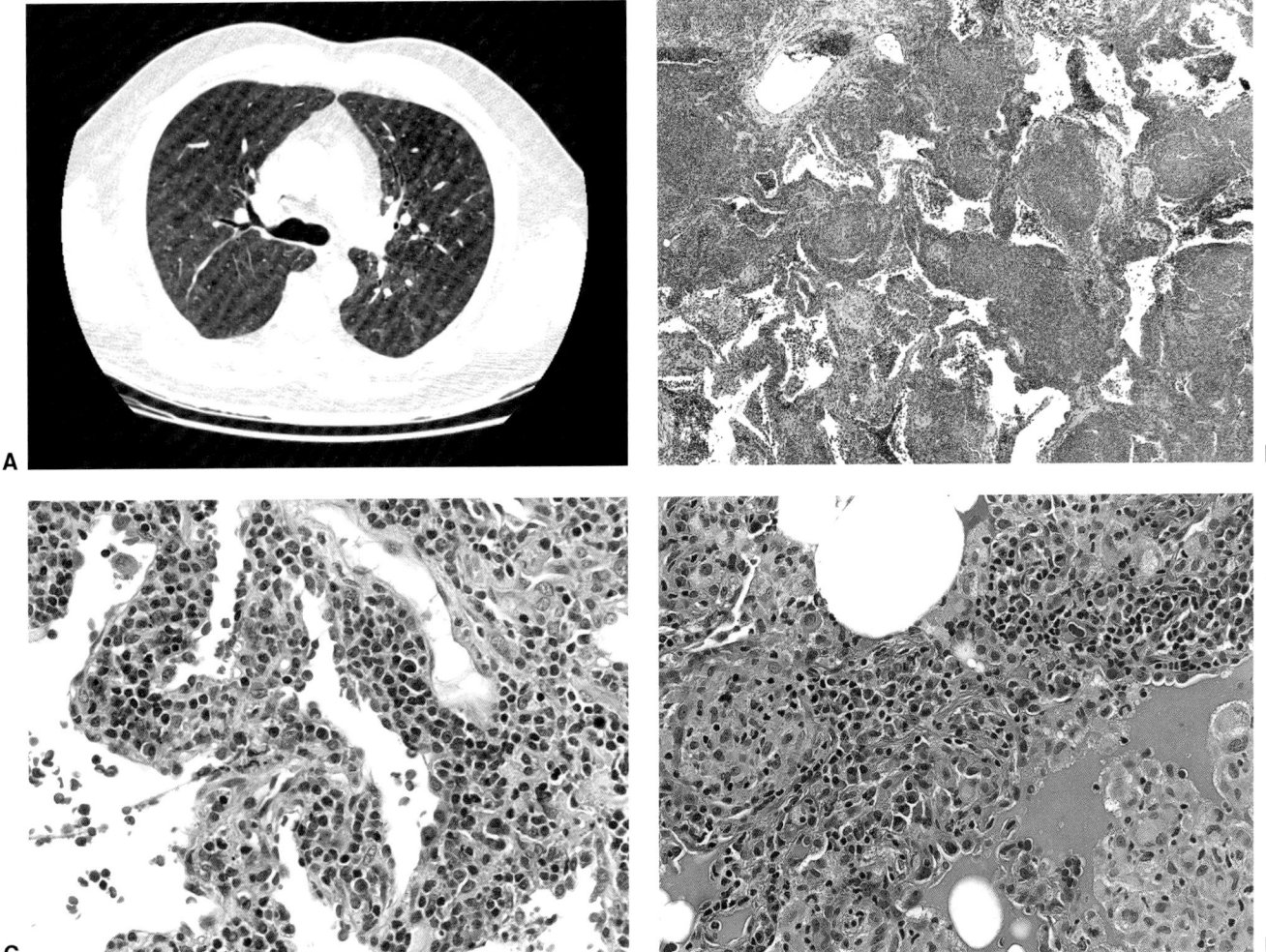

FIGURE 31.10. Lymphocytic interstitial pneumonia. A: HRCT patchy, bilateral ground-glass opacities and centrilobular and peribronchovascular nodules. **B:** Prominent diffuse expansion of alveolar interstitium by cellular process in association with hyperplasia of BALT (H&E, magnification: 40×). **C:** Widening of alveolar septa by lymphoplasmacytic infiltrates (H&E, magnification: 400×). **D:** Scattered loosely formed granulomas admixed with interstitial inflammation are also seen in LIP (H&E, magnification: 400×).

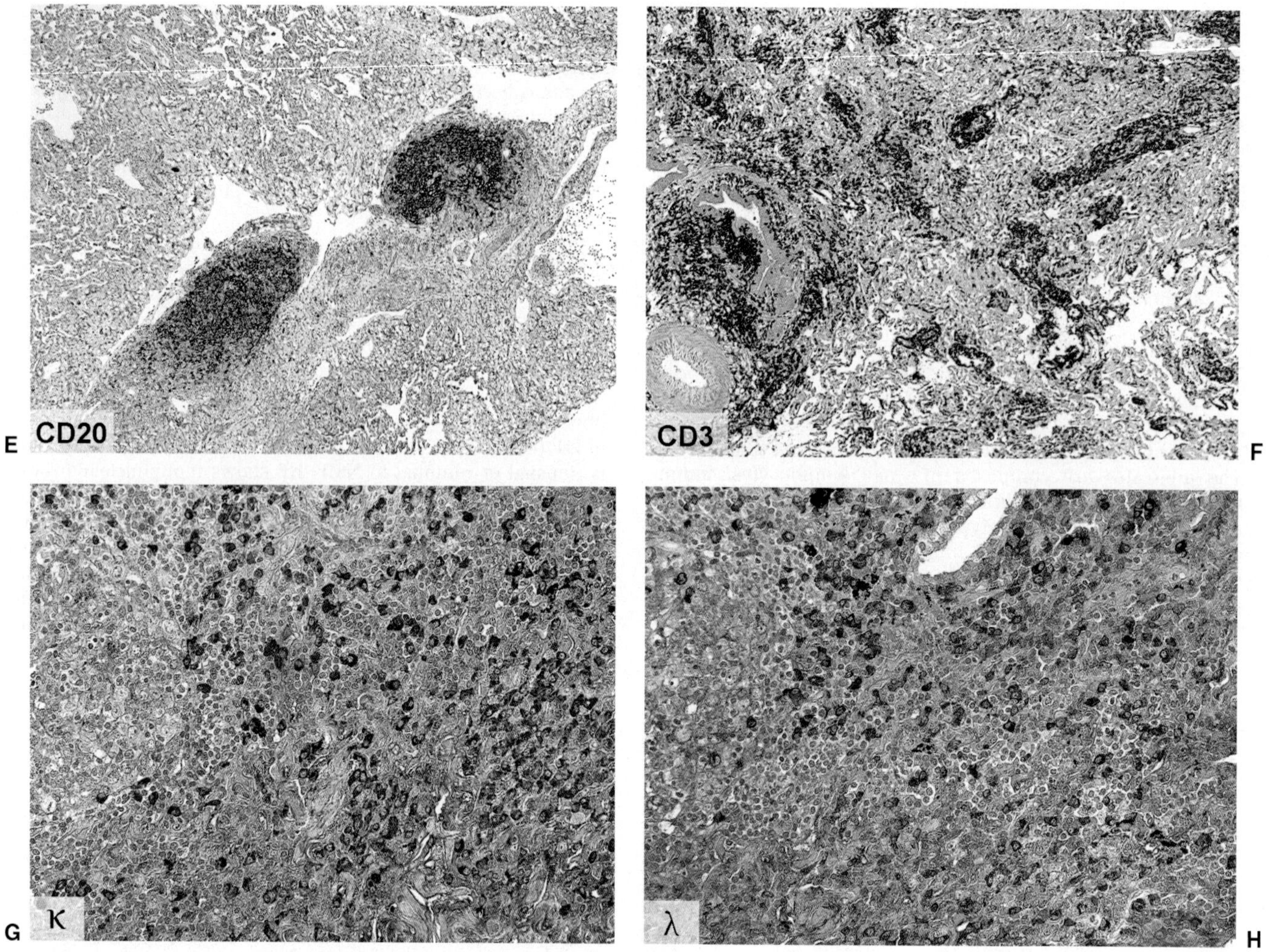

FIGURE 31.10. *(Continued)* **E:** CD20 staining highlights the reactive germinal centers (magnification: 40×). **F:** The interstitial infiltrates are composed of CD3+ T cells (magnification: 100×). **G,H:** The plasma cells are polytypic in LIP (magnification: 200×).

to earlier in the discussion of LIP, it must be distinguished from pulmonary involvement by low-grade malignant lymphoid neoplasms such as small lymphocytic lymphoma (SLL)/CLL, extranodal MZL/MALT lymphoma, and mantle cell lymphoma. Histopathologic clues that suggest malignant lymphoma include a monotonous population of lymphoid cells centered on a lymphatic distribution (bronchovascular structures, subpleural tissue, and interlobular septa), infiltration of pleural and bronchial structures, the formation of parenchymal nodules, and the presence of Dutcher bodies (Table 31.3). Immunohistochemical staining or flow cytometry in LIP shows a predominance of interstitial T cells, whereas the low-grade malignant neoplasms show a predominance of B cells with or without light chain restriction. A clonal rearrangement of immunoglobulin heavy chain can be detected by PCR in malignant lymphoma.

The diagnosis of LIP should prompt a careful clinical assessment for associated conditions, as these will impact treatment and prognosis. Controlled treatment trials have not been performed, and most protocols are based on anecdotal reports. From these reports, corticosteroid therapy has been the primary treatment modality, with cyclophosphamide and chlorambucil reserved as secondary options. Treatment response is variable, and generally a third of patients respond and improve, a third develop stable disease, and the remainder progress and die of infectious complications or progressive restrictive lung disease. Transformation to malignant lymphoma is uncommon (35).

NEOPLASTIC HEMATOLYMPHOID LESIONS

The number of entities within the group of neoplastic pulmonary lesions continues to undergo refinement and clarification. In the most recent *WHO Classification of Tumors of Hematopoietic and Lymphoid Tissues*, the clinicopathologic entities with primary or frequent thoracic involvement has expanded beyond the traditional lesions of primary extranodal MZL (MALT lymphoma), diffuse aggressive large B-cell lymphoma, and lymphomatoid granulomatosis (LYG) to include diffuse large B-cell lymphoma (DLBCL) of the elderly, DLBCL associated with chronic inflammation, intravascular large B-cell lymphoma, and posttransplant lymphoproliferative disorders (PTLDs) (1,7,118) (Table 31.4). These are described in detail in other chapters in this book, and the thoracic aspects are highlighted herein.

Saltzstein originally defined primary pulmonary lymphoma as a malignant lymphoma of the histicytic type that "involves only the lung or the lung and its regional lymph nodes, and in which there is no evidence of dissemination of the tumor for at least 3 months after the diagnosis is established" (46). This definition has been modified over the last five decades, but the general concepts of unilateral or bilateral parenchymal

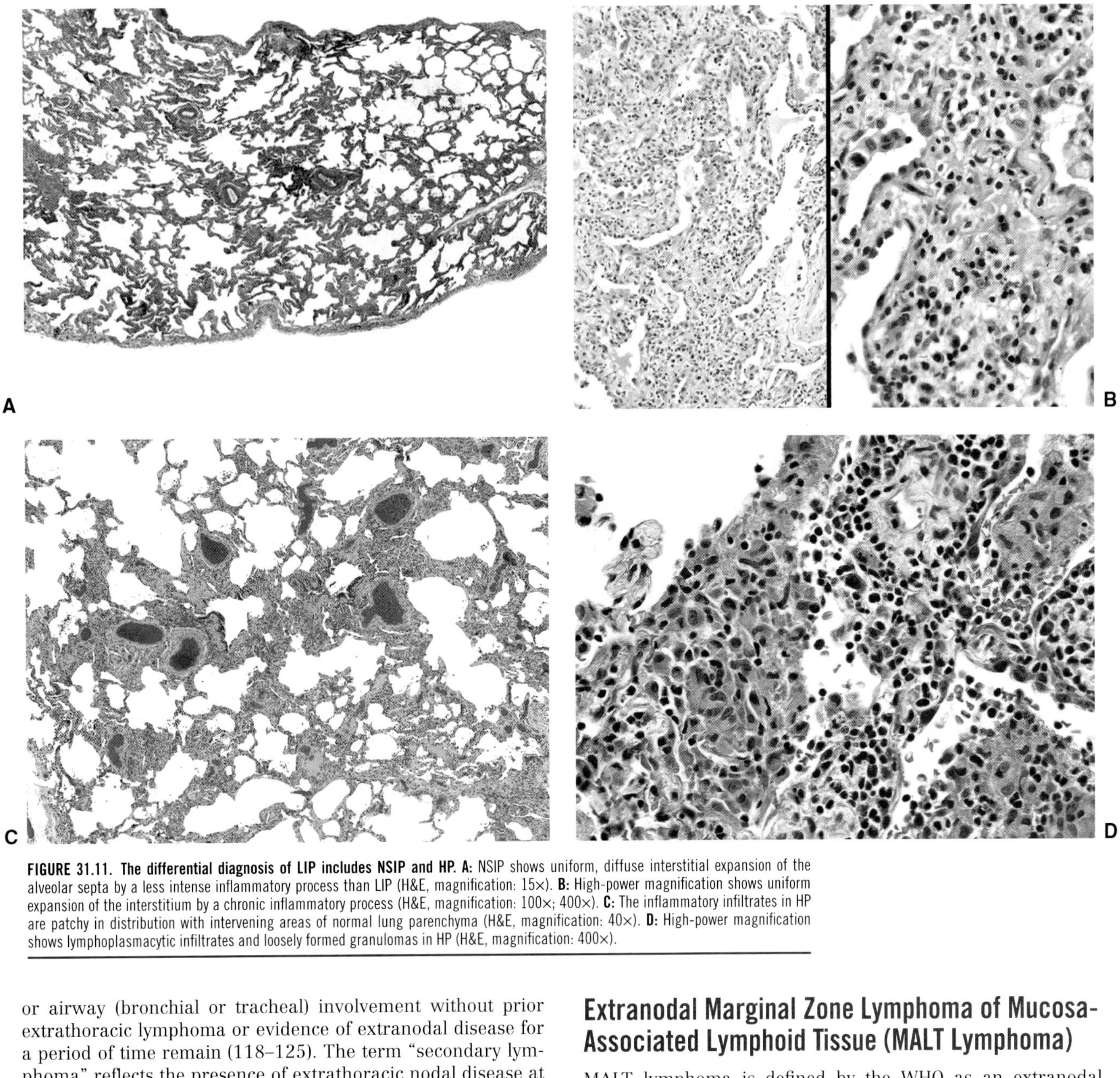

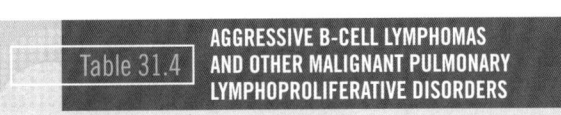

FIGURE 31.11. The differential diagnosis of LIP includes NSIP and HP. A: NSIP shows uniform, diffuse interstitial expansion of the alveolar septa by a less intense inflammatory process than LIP (H&E, magnification: 15×). **B:** High-power magnification shows uniform expansion of the interstitium by a chronic inflammatory process (H&E, magnification: 100×; 400×). **C:** The inflammatory infiltrates in HP are patchy in distribution with intervening areas of normal lung parenchyma (H&E, magnification: 40×). **D:** High-power magnification shows lymphoplasmacytic infiltrates and loosely formed granulomas in HP (H&E, magnification: 400×).

or airway (bronchial or tracheal) involvement without prior extrathoracic lymphoma or evidence of extranodal disease for a period of time remain (118–125). The term "secondary lymphoma" reflects the presence of extrathoracic nodal disease at the time of diagnosis, pulmonary involvement during relapse of lymphoma, or systemic involvement shortly following the initial pulmonary involvement or at autopsy (2,116).

Table 31.4	AGGRESSIVE B-CELL LYMPHOMAS AND OTHER MALIGNANT PULMONARY LYMPHOPROLIFERATIVE DISORDERS

DLBCL, not otherwise specified
EBV⁺ diffuse large cell lymphoma of the elderly
DLBCL associated with chronic inflammation
Intravascular large B-cell lymphoma
Primary effusion lymphoma
Extranodal MZL
Lymphomatoid granulomatosis
Posttransplant lymphoproliferative disorder
Primary HL
Plasmacytoma
Peripheral T-cell lymphoma
T-cell ALCL

Extranodal Marginal Zone Lymphoma of Mucosa-Associated Lymphoid Tissue (MALT Lymphoma)

MALT lymphoma is defined by the WHO as an extranodal lymphoma composed of a heterogeneous population of small B cells including centrocyte-like marginal cells, small lymphocytes, plasma cells and plasmacytoid cells, occasional immunoblasts, and centroblast-like cells (126). They occur in a variety of sites including the gastrointestinal tract, thyroid, salivary gland and other head and neck structures, ocular structures, and the lung. The gastrointestinal tract is the most common site and the lungs constitute about 15% of MALT lymphomas (127). Moreover, MALT lymphoma is the most common form of primary pulmonary lymphoma accounting for up to 90% of cases. Unlike its counterparts in other organs that are associated with chronic infectious etiologies such as *Helicobacter pylori* in the stomach, *Chlamydia psittaci* in ocular MALT lymphoma, *Campylobacter jejuni* in immunoproliferative small intestinal disease, and hepatitis C in the liver or spleen, pulmonary MALT lymphoma does not have an identified infectious agent (128–131). It does share similarity with thyroid MALT lymphoma as associations with chronic inflammatory and autoimmune disorders such as Sjögren syndrome, primary biliary cirrhosis, rheumatoid arthritis, and others have been reported (125,132).

The pathogenesis of MALT lymphoma including its molecular biology and complex evolution is slowly evolving. Classical cytogenetics and locus-specific FISH studies have identified three chromosomal translocations in this group: t(11;18)(q21;q21), t(1;14)(p22;q32), and t(14;18)(q32;q21), all of which result in the activation of NF-κB, a transcription factor with an essential function in immunity, inflammation, and apoptosis in normal cells (133,134). Abnormal signaling is thought to play a role in promoting tumor cell growth, survival, and resistance to chemotherapy (135). These translocations are found in up to 50% of cases and result in overexpression of Bcl-10 or MALT1 or production of a fusion product, cIAP2-MALT1. A recent gene-expression study of pulmonary MALT lymphomas revealed the important role that the T-cell–dependent immune response plays in the development of this neoplasm (136). Two genes were highly expressed: matrix metalloproteinase 7 *MMP7/matrilysin* gene (which is known to decrease tumor cell apoptosis) and *sialic acid–binding Ig-like lectin 6/SIGLEC6* genes (which are involved in regulating cell activation), and both may play a role in homing of lymphocytes to normal BALT. Gene-profiling studies also demonstrated that morphologic subtypes of MALT lymphoma were characterized by distinct groups of deregulated genes. Three groups were classified: the subtype with plasmacytic differentiation exhibited high FKBP11 expression, the group with high RGS13 expression usually had trisomy 3, and the group with MALT1 translocations had high expression of MALT1 and RARA.

Patients with MALT lymphoma typically present in the sixth and seventh decades of life (range second to ninth). Up to two-thirds of patients are asymptomatic at the time of diagnosis, with the remainder presenting with cough, dyspnea, or rarely chest pain and hemoptysis. Constitutional symptoms are also uncommon (125,137–139). The laboratory studies are usually either negative or nonspecific. Up to a third of patients will have a serum monoclonal IgM spike. Interestingly, some patients present with concurrent involvement of other sites of MALT lymphoma or develop recurrence at those sites. These are usually separate and unrelated clonal proliferations, suggesting multifocal rather than disseminated disease (140). Common patterns on CT imaging are either a single nodular or consolidative opacity containing air bronchograms or multiple nodules; bronchiectasis, bronchiolitis, and diffuse ILD are less frequent (5,6,141). Currently, the diagnosis is established by FNA cytology with flow cytometry or TBBx with paraffin section IHC in some cases. VATS biopsy is reserved for complicated cases, although in some older published series the

diagnosis was established by lobectomy and open lung biopsies in the majority of cases (125).

The macroscopic findings are either discrete white, fleshy nodules measuring 2.0 to 20 cm in diameter or diffuse consolidations with ill-defined borders but preservation of bronchovascular structures. Microscopic examination at low and scanning magnification yields important diagnostic clues such as disruption of the lung architecture, invasion of the visceral pleural and cartilaginous bronchi, and a beaded alignment along a lymphatic distribution of monotonous-appearing atypical lymphoid cells (Fig. 31.12). Obliteration of alveolar structures and expansion and filling of airspaces produce consolidative masses containing entrapped vessels and larger airways without hemorrhage or necrosis (142,143). Parenthetically, this morphologic sequence produces the air bronchograms observed on imaging studies. At low-power magnification, numerous germinal centers are observed either distributed throughout the lesions or at the periphery in some cases (Fig. 31.12). Venous structures are often permeated or obliterated by lymphoid cells, but arteries are rarely involved. Less common growth patterns are lymphomatous extension along the perivascular, peribronchiolar, or interstitial structures and randomly scattered foci of lymphoma surrounded by normal lung tissue. The neoplastic infiltrates are composed of lymphoid cells with small- to medium-sized nuclei, inconspicuous nucleoli, and dispersed chromatin (Fig. 31.13). In some cases, the cells resemble small lymphocytes, while those with small rims of clear cytoplasm resemble centrocytes and the neoplastic cells with more abundant pale eosinophilic cytoplasm resemble monocytoid cells. Plasmacytoid cells with Russell and/or Dutcher bodies can also be found. In many cases, there is a heterogeneous admixture of these different neoplastic cell types with variation from region to region. Plasma cells and small lymphocytes are present in variable numbers, but immunoblasts and centroblasts are infrequent. If solid or sheetlike regions of large transformed cells are present, the diagnosis of MALT lymphoma with DLBCL should be considered (125). LEL are present in the vast majority of cases and are characterized by infiltration and sometimes destruction of the bronchiolar epithelium by clusters of lymphoid cells (Fig. 31.12). LEL should be distinguished from the normal configuration of mucosa-associated lymphoid elements composed of isolated B cells within the epithelium and from intraepithelial T cells that are constituents of reactive airway processes (144).

The reactive germinal centers in MALT lymphoma often lack well-developed mantle zones; in some cases, they are absent.

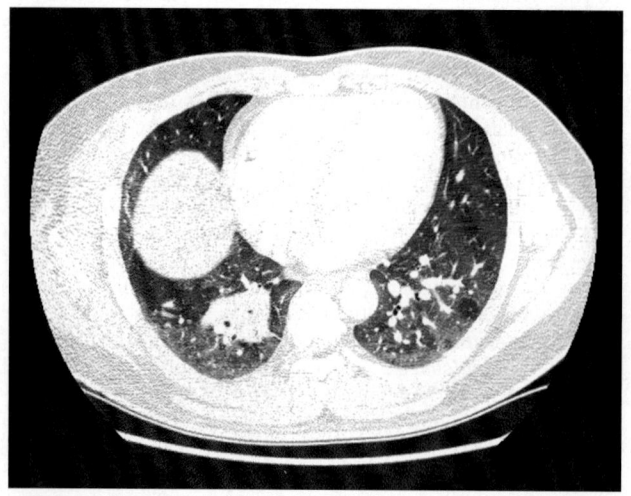

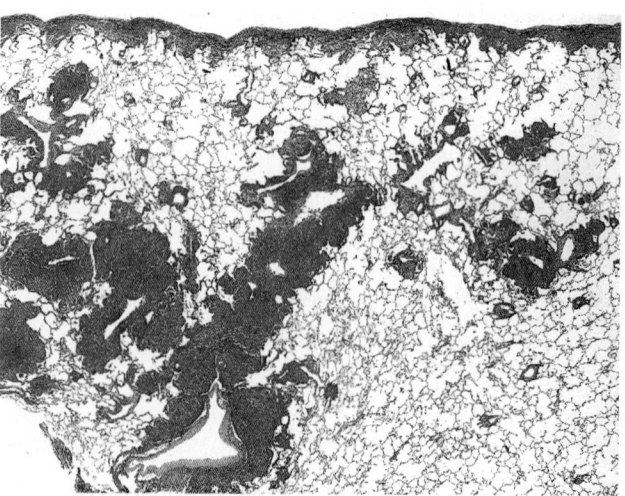

A   B

FIGURE 31.12. Extranodal marginal zone lymphoma. A: HRCT showing bilateral nodules and masses centered on the airways. **B:** Low-power magnification showing lymphatic distribution of pleural, interlobular septal, and bronchovascular infiltrates (H&E, magnification: 10×).

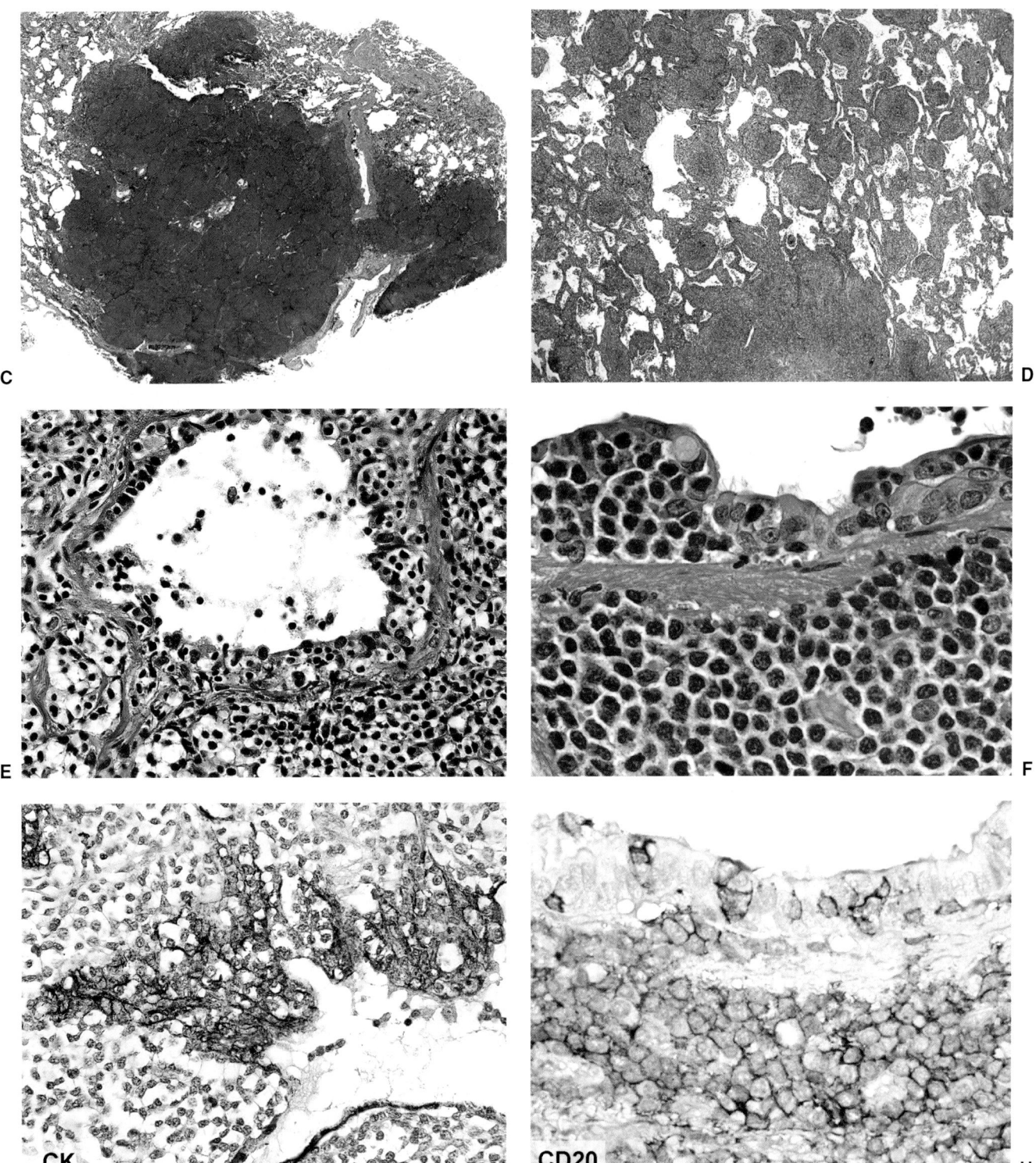

FIGURE 31.12. *(Continued)* **C:** Another pattern in pulmonary MZL is discrete nodular lesions (H&E, magnification: 15×). **D:** Interstitial and bronchovascular collections of neoplastic lymphocytes is another pattern of involvement (H&E, magnification: 100×). **E:** LEL characterized by lymphomatous infiltration of bronchioles (H&E, magnification: 200×). **F:** High-power magnification showing monotonous lymphoid cells within the mucosal and submucosal layers of the airway (H&E, magnification: 400×). **G:** Cytokeratin stain highlighting the LEL (magnification: 200×). **H:** CD20 stain showing transmural infiltration of the airway by neoplastic B cells (magnification: 400×).

Infiltration of the germinal centers or so-called "follicular colonization" creates the appearance of attenuated follicles that are overrun by the neoplastic cells; a finding highlighted by CD21 or other dendritic markers (126) (Fig. 31.12). Other features found in MALT lymphomas include areas of central parenchymal sclerosis, sarcoid-like non-necrotizing granulomas, giant

lamellar bodies, massive crystal storing histiocytosis, nodular or interstitial amyloid deposition, and multinucleated giant cells (145–149).

The neoplastic cells of MALT lymphoma express IgM or IgA heavy chain, and the majority show light chain restriction. In distinction to other small lymphoid neoplasms, the cells are

CD20+, CD79a+, CD5− (vast majority), CD10−, CD23−, Bcl-1/cyclin D1−, CD43+/−, and CD11c+/(weak). PCR studies demonstrate immunoglobulin heavy- and light chain rearrangements (Fig. 31.13).

The differential diagnosis includes a number of benign and malignant lymphoproliferative disorders such as NLH, LIP, and pulmonary involvement by other small lymphoid lymphomas

(Table 31.3). The presence of parenchymal destruction, pleural infiltration, pleural effusions, lymphangitic growth pattern, conspicuous LEL, colonization of follicles, Dutcher bodies, anomalous coexpression CD43 or CD5 B cells, and light chain–restricted plasma cells and plasmacytoid cells support MALT lymphoma and not NLH. As previously noted, there can be

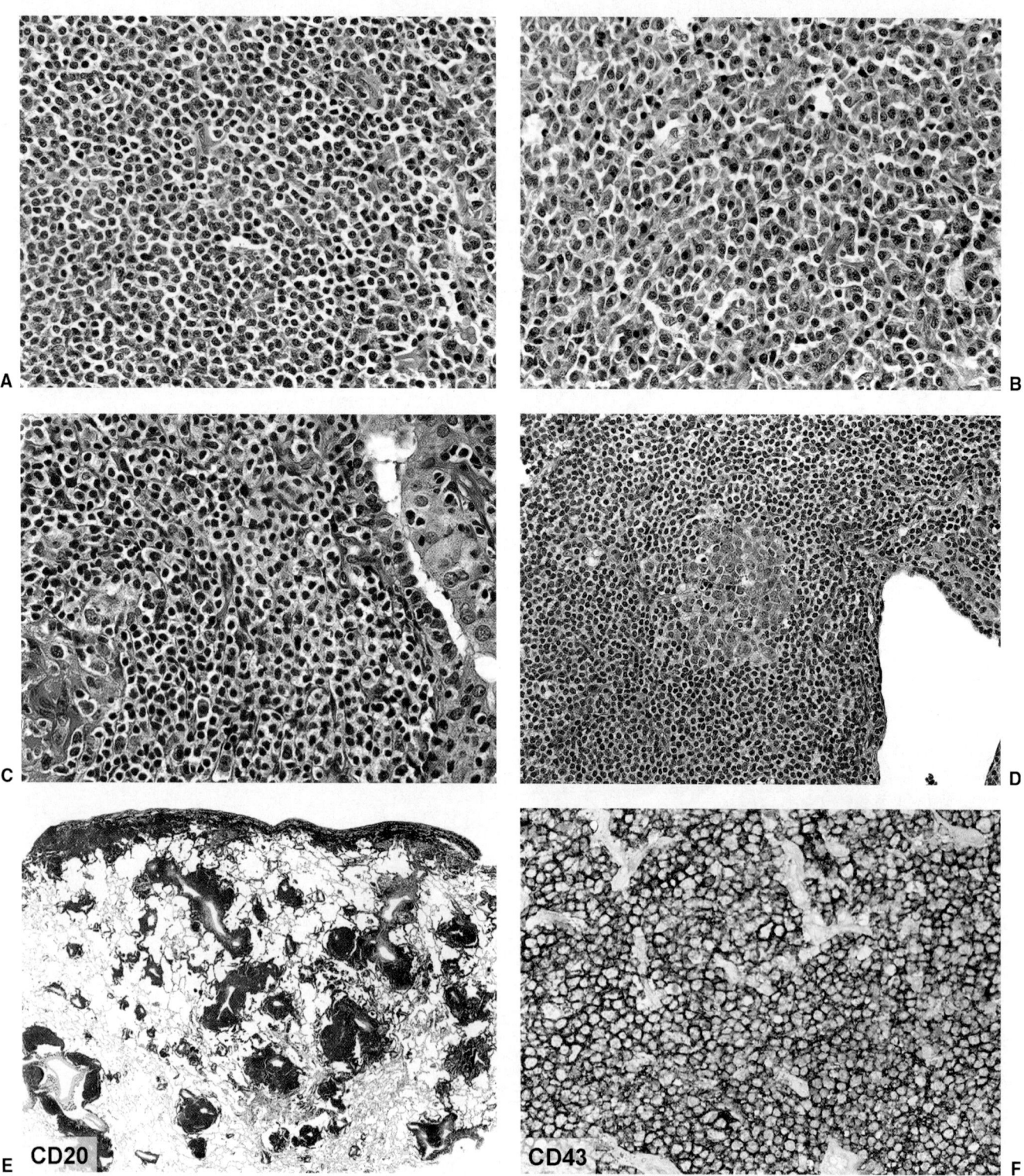

FIGURE 31.13. Extranodal MZL. A: Histopathologic patterns in MZL including a predominance of atypical small lymphocytes (H&E, magnification: 400×). **B:** Another pattern showing plasmacytoid differentiation (H&E, magnification: 400×). **C:** Another pattern composed of cells with abundant cell cytoplasm resembling monocytoid cells (H&E, magnification: 400×). **D:** "Follicular colonization" is characterized by germinal centers overrun by neoplastic cells (H&E, magnification: 200×). **E:** Low-power magnification staining with CD20 showing lymphatic distribution of neoplastic infiltrates (H&E, magnification: 10×). **F:** Anomalous coexpression of CD43 is seen in MZL (magnification: 400×).

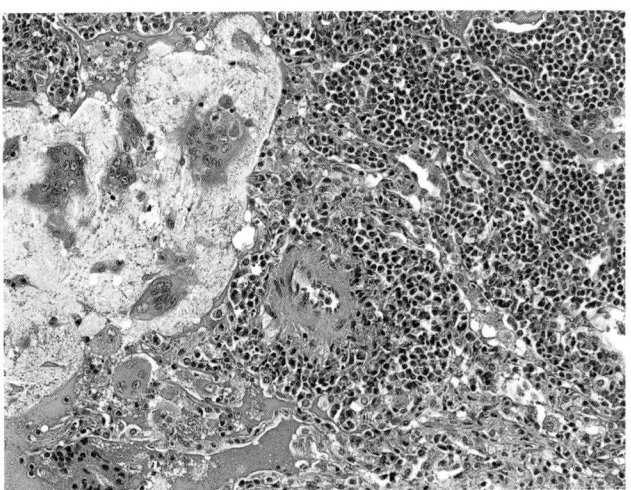

G

FIGURE 31.13. *(Continued)* **G:** Other findings in MZL include the presence of multinucleated giant cells, amyloid deposits, sclerotic bands, and giant lamellar bodies (H&E, magnification: 200×).

overlap of morphologic findings in MALT lymphoma with LIP. The presence of broad invasion of the visceral pleura or bronchial cartilage, infiltration of the parietal pleura, monotonous lymphoid cells with centrocyte or monocytoid features, and monotypic plasma cells and other evidence of clonality are seen in lymphoma and not LIP. Finally, pulmonary involvement by small lymphoid lymphomas such as CLL/SLL, mantle cell lymphoma, follicular lymphoma, and lymphoplasmacytic lymphoma is variable. Flow cytometry/IHC and careful attention to the morphologic appearance of the lymphomatous infiltrate are necessary (150) (Table 31.4). The tumor cells of CLL/SLL are composed of small round lymphocytes and are CD20+, CD79a+, CD5+, CD10−, CD23+, and Bcl-2+ and show monoclonal surface Ig. In follicular lymphoma, the atypical lymphoid cells resemble centrocytes and centroblasts and are CD20+, CD5− CD10+, CD23−, Bcl-2+, and Bcl-6+ and show monoclonal surface Ig. Mantle cell lymphoma shows small- to medium-sized round and angulated cells with inconspicuous nucleoli and the immunophenotypic profile of CD20+, CD5+, CD10−, CD23−, Bcl-1+/cyclin D1+, Bcl-2+, Bcl-6−, and monoclonal surface Ig. Cytogenetic analysis may show a t(11:14)(q13;q32) translocation. Lymphoplasmacytic lymphoma is composed of small lymphocytes, plasmacytoid lymphocytes, and plasma cells and usually involves lymph nodes, spleen, and bone marrow and can be associated with macroglobulinemia, hyperviscosity, and cryoglobulinemia. The lung is an uncommon extranodal site of involvement. The tumor cells are CD20+, IgM+, CD5−, CD10−, CD23−, and CD138+ (plasma cells). Extraosseous plasmacytoma is composed of mature plasma cells and shows CD38+, VS38c, CD138+, CD19−, CD20−, CD79a+, and monoclonal cytoplasmic

Ig (Table 31.5). Finally, the recently described entity of atypical marginal zone hyperplasia of MALT of the tonsil and appendix has not been described in the lung (151).

The current treatment options for MALT lymphoma include a number of choices from careful clinical observation to surgical resection, to antibiotic therapy with clarithromycin, radiation therapy, single-agent therapy such as rituximab, combination chemotherapy, or chemoimmunotherapy. While the prognosis depends in large part on the stage of disease, overall this form of extranodal lymphoma has an excellent prognosis. Five- and ten-year survival rates of over 80% are reported, and most recurrences occur in the lung or other sites of MALT (125,152,153).

Diffuse Large B-Cell Lymphoma

Primary DLBCL of the lung is less common than MALT lymphoma and accounts for 10% to 15% of primary pulmonary lymphomas. While some cases arise *de novo*, up to half develop in the setting of MALT lymphoma or other low-grade lymphomas (49). It is defined as a diffuse neoplastic proliferation composed of atypical lymphoid cells with nuclei comparable in size or larger than normal macrophage nuclei or approximately twice the size of normal lymphocytes (154). In addition to numerous morphologic subtypes, recent immunophenotypic and molecular investigations have delineated different pathways of transformation and molecular translocations that produce distinct subtypes of DLBCL (153–160). Molecular alterations may involve *BCL6, MYC,* or *BCL2* genes. Two subtypes have been delineated by gene-expression profiling analysis with corresponding immunophenotypic profiles: those resembling germinal center B cells (CD10+, Bcl-6+, and IRF4/MUM1−) and the activated (nongerminal center) B-cell subtype (CD10−, Bcl-6−, and IRF4/MUM1+).

The age at presentation of primary pulmonary DLBCL is similar to patients with MALT lymphoma and typically affects older individuals in their sixth or seventh decade of life. However, unlike the MALT lymphoma group, most patients with DLBCL are symptomatic with cough, dyspnea, fever, weight loss, and on occasion, hemoptysis (49,119–122,142,145,161). Chest CT imaging reveals peripheral solitary or multiple nodules or masses; cavitation is not infrequent (6). Endobronchial masses causing lobar collapse have also been reported (162). In resection specimens, one or more circumscribed white, fleshy masses are seen. Foci of hemorrhage and necrosis can be present. Microscopically, the characteristic large vesicular nuclei with multiple nucleoli, often aligned near or along the nuclear membrane, are observed in sheets and groups infiltrating and disrupting the lung parenchyma and visceral pleura (Fig. 31.14). Punctate foci of necrosis are found in many lesions, but LELs are rare. Li et al. (49) also reported the presence of airspace accumulations of large cells or "neoplastic pneumonia" and mural infiltration of vessel walls. Strong B-cell

Table 31.5	IMMUNOPHENOTYPIC PROFILE OF EXTRANODAL LOW-GRADE SMALL LYMPHOID PROLIFERATIONS			
	Extranodal MZL	**CLL/SLL**	**Mantle Cell Lymphoma**	**Grade 1 Follicular Lymphoma**
CD20	Positive	Positive	Positive	Positive
PAX5	Positive	Positive	Positive	Positive
CD43	Positive/negative	Positive	Positive	Negative
CD5	Negative	Positive	Positive	Negative
CD10	Negative	Negative	Negative	Positive
CD23	Negative	Positive	Negative	Negative
Bcl-1/cyclin D1	Negative	Negative	Positive	Negative

MZL, marginal zone lymphoma; CLL/SLL, chronic lymphocytic leukemia/small lymphocytic lymphoma.

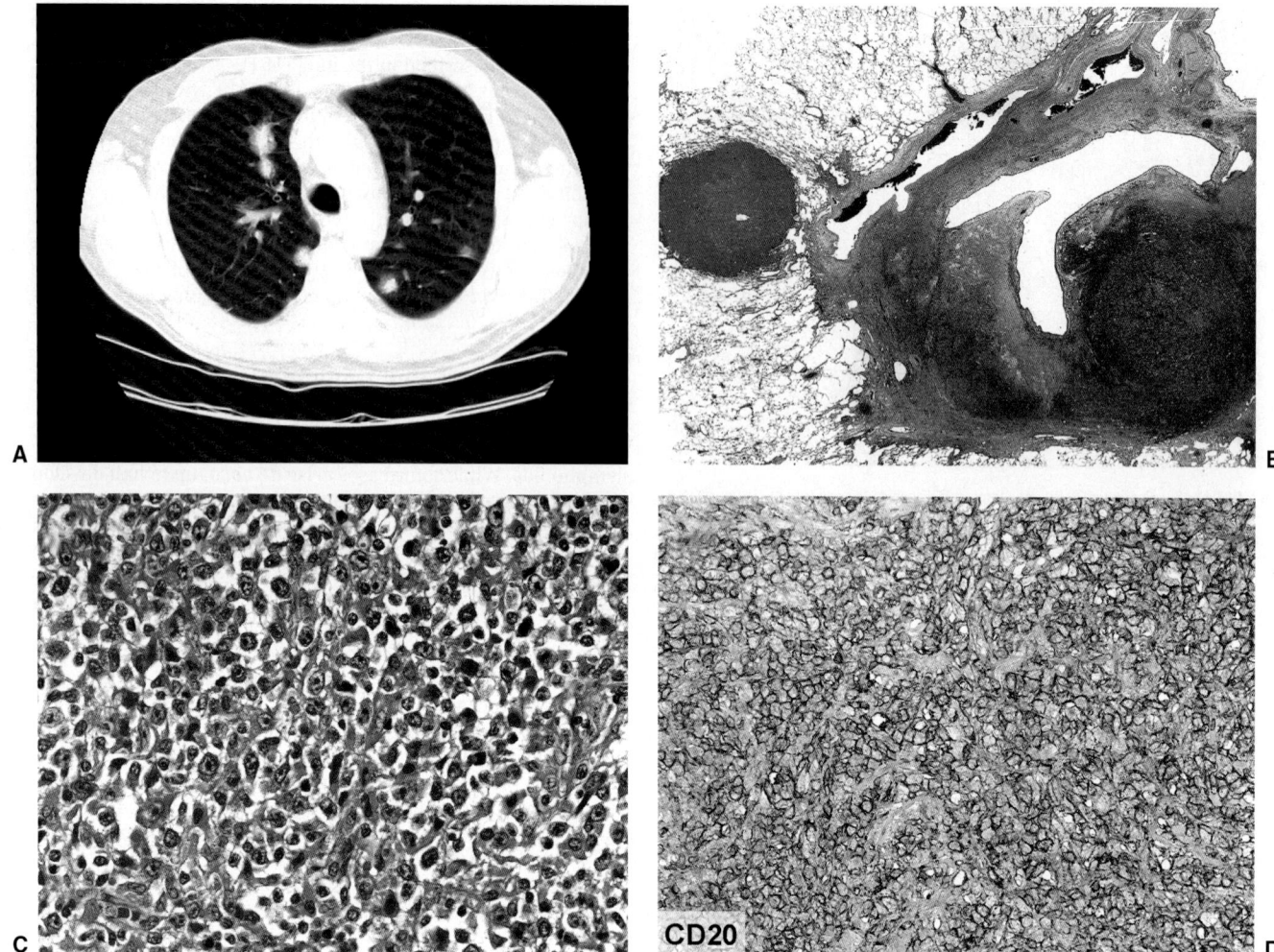

FIGURE 31.14. Diffuse large B-cell lymphoma. A: CT imaging showing well-defined nodules adjacent to airway structures. **B:** Low-power magnification showing multilobated mass centered on a cartilaginous bronchus (H&E, magnification: 15×). **C:** DLBCL is composed of monotonous lymphoid cells with large vesicular nuclei and one or more nucleoli (H&E, magnification: 400×). **D:** Diffuse staining of neoplastic cells with CD20 (magnification: 400×).

immunophenotypic staining with pan-B markers such as CD19, CD20, and CD79a is typical (Fig. 31.14). In a study of 82 cases of pulmonary DLBCL by Neri et al. (163), 59 (72%) cases were classified as germinal center subtype and 23 as activated B-cell phenotype. Variable numbers of host CD3+ T cells are admixed with the neoplastic cells. The proliferation rate as detected by Ki67 staining is high and ranges from 40% to 90%. Light chain restriction can be shown by IHC. Heavy chain genes are clonally rearranged by PCR analysis. While earlier studies showed a poor prognosis following surgery and chemotherapy, more recent studies demonstrate improved survival rates. Neri et al. reported complete responses, and overall survival rates of >90% are 10 years utilizing conventional chemotherapy. No difference in response rates, event free, or overall survival between patients with germinal center phenotype and activated B-cell phenotype was demonstrated (163).

The differential diagnosis of DLBCL includes a variety of epithelioid neoplasms, either primary or metastatic to lung. Malignant melanoma, germ cell neoplasms, large cell neuroendocrine carcinoma, and other primary bronchogenic carcinomas and metastatic lymphoepithelioma of the nasopharynx are readily distinguished by paraffin IHC. Anaplastic large cell lymphoma (ALCL) is characterized by pleomorphic cells and CD30 and ALK1 expression while LYG displays conspicuous angiocentricity and the presence of EBV+ large B cells.

Lymphomatoid Granulomatosis

LYG is a rare but distinct clinicopathologic disorder. Originally described by Liebow et al. in 1972 as "an angiocentric and angiodestructive lymphoreticular proliferative and granulomatous disease involving predominantly the lungs," it has undergone numerous revisions and pathogenetic evolutions over the last four decades (164,165). It is defined by the WHO as an extranodal lymphoproliferative disease characterized by the histopathologic features described by Liebow et al. and composed of variable numbers of EBV+ B cells admixed with numerous reactive T cells (166). Far more common in men than women (2:1), it commonly presents as multiple, bilateral mid-, and lower lung zone pulmonary nodules (>90%), with concurrent and/or subsequent extranodal sites of involvement such as skin (25% to 50%), central nervous system (CNS) (25% to 50%), peripheral nervous system (15% to 20%), kidney (40% to 50%), but infrequently the liver, lymph nodes, or spleen (165–168). Most are adults, although rare cases of LYG in children are reported. Further, most patients are suspected to harbor an underlying immunologic defect resulting in insufficient regulation of EBV-infected B cells. There are reported associations with recurrent infections, collagen vascular disorders, congenital and acquired immunodeficiency disorders such as Wiskott-Aldrich syndrome, common variable immunodeficiency, human immunodeficiency syndrome (HIV), following solid organ transplantation, and treatment for acute leukemia. Like pulmonary DLBCL patients are usually symptomatic at presentation with cough, dyspnea, chest pain and constitutional systems of fever, weight loss, and malaise. Often

confused with pulmonary infection, ILD, abscess, or bronchogenic malignancy, the diagnosis may be delayed until a tissue biopsy is procured (169–173). The radiologic manifestations range from diffuse reticulonodular opacities to rounded, irregular but well-defined nodular opacifications measuring

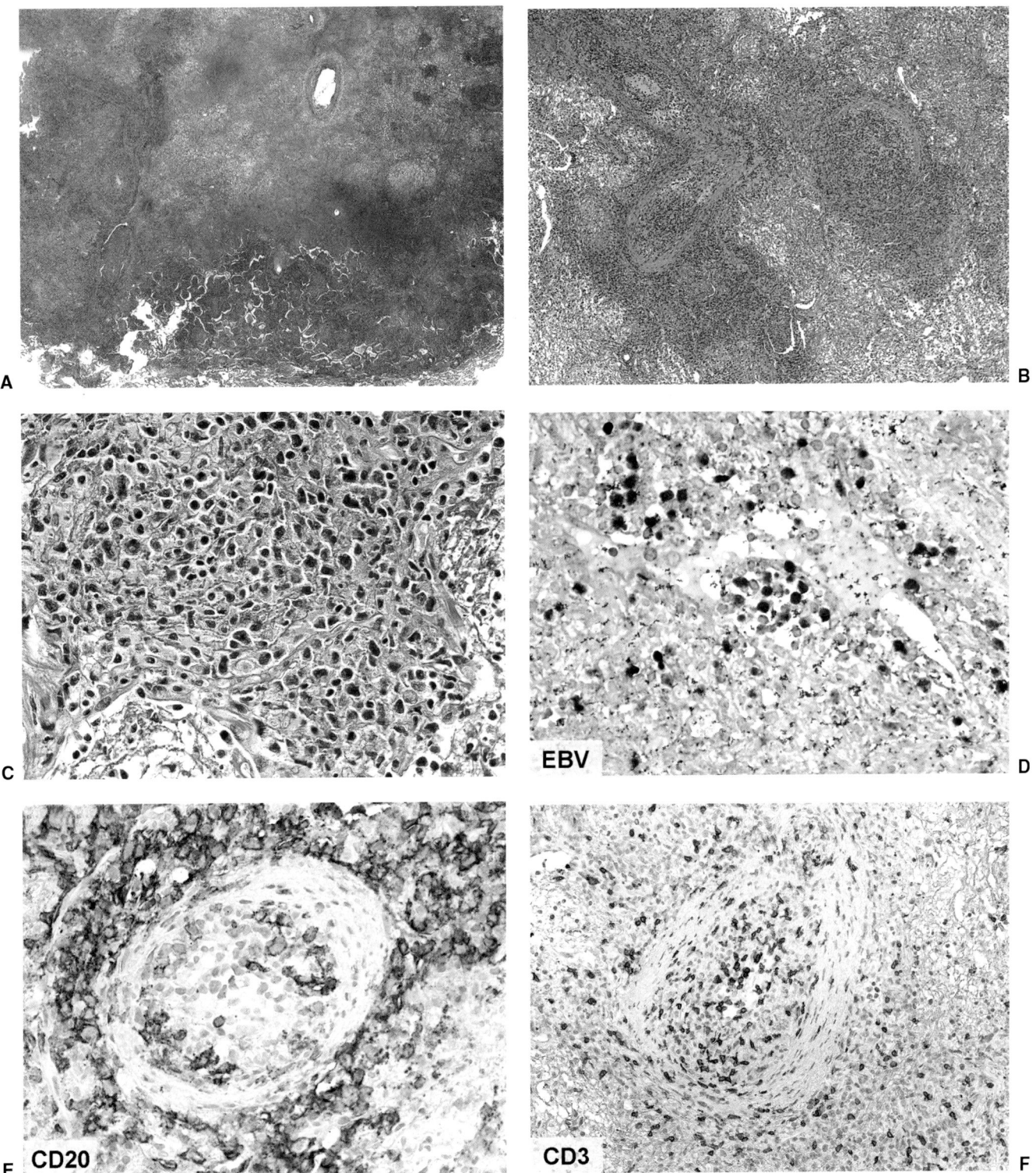

FIGURE 31.15. Grade 3 lymphomatoid granulomatosis. A: Low-power magnification showing extensive hemorrhagic central necrosis (H&E, magnification: 10×). **B:** The muscular pulmonary arteries are filled and expanded by mononuclear cells in LYG (H&E, magnification: 40×). **C:** High-power magnification showing an admixture of small and large lymphocytes including atypical large cells (H&E, magnification: 400×). **D:** Numerous EBV+ cells within and around a vessel demonstrated by ISH for EBER (magnification: 400×). **E:** CD20+ atypical large cells in classic angiocentric distribution (magnification: 400×). **F:** Numerous CD3+ host T cells admixed with the neoplastic cells (magnification: 400×).

0.5 to 8.0 cm. They are distributed along the bronchovascular bundles and interlobular septa with a basilar predominance. Coalescence of tumor nodules and cavitation are frequently observed. Less common patterns include thin-walled cysts and central GGO surrounded by a denser consolidation (the non-specific "reversed halo sign") (6,174,175). There is avid FDG uptake on FDG-PET imaging, a finding similar to DLBCL but generally not MALT lymphoma (176). Mediastinal adenopathy is usually not present.

The macroscopic appearance reflects the radiologic findings. In surgical specimens, the nodules are yellow-white, often with central softening reflecting necrosis. Cavitation may be present. Smaller nodules are uniformly white and firm. At low-power magnification, the lymphatic distribution along bronchovascular structures, subpleural structures, and interlobular septa is recognized (Fig. 31.15). As the nodular infiltrates coalesce and enlarge, areas of central necrosis and parenchymal destruction become apparent. The muscular pulmonary arteries and veins are enveloped by a polymorphous infiltrate and mural infiltration, and damage is noted. The infiltrates are composed of small lymphocytes, plasma cells, histiocytes, and large transformed lymphocytes and immunoblasts including atypical large cells (164,177–179) (Fig. 31.15). The atypical large cells have round or indented nuclei; coarsely clumped chromatin; one or more nucleoli; and amphophilic, clear, or basophilic cytoplasm. Multinucleated giant cells, clusters of epithelioid histiocytes, eosinophils, and neutrophils are rarely present; the term "granulomatosis" reflects the increased numbers of macrophages or spindled histiocytes in the infiltrates. In some cases, the large immunoblastic cells can resemble Reed-Sternberg (RS-like) cells, but by definition classic RS cells are absent. The majority of the small lymphocytes are CD3+ T cells, the majority of which are CD8+ cytotoxic cells (180). The atypical large cells are CD20+ B cells. Katzenstein and Peiper and other investigators have shown that the B cells and not T cells are infected by EBV, supporting the concept of LYG as a "T-cell–rich EBV-driven B-cell proliferation" and not a T-cell lymphoma (167,181–184).

The number of atypical large cells in LYG varies considerably and is associated with clinical behavior and prognosis (177). Lipford et al. (185) first proposed a three-tiered system on the basis of degree of atypia of the small cells and the overall number of large cells. This has undergone a number of modifications, and the current WHO scheme is based on the number of atypical large EBV-infected cells (166). Grade 1 LYG

lesions are defined as few or no EBV-infected cells or as <5 per high-power field (HPF) (Fig. 31.14). Grade 2 LYG lesions have scattered EBV+ cells in the range of 5 to 20 per HPF. Unlike grade 1 lesions, these usually have foci of necrosis (Fig. 31.16). Grade 3 LYG are characterized by sheets of monomorphous atypical large EBV-infected cells (>50 cells per HPF) and conspicuous necrosis. This pattern is recognized as a subtype of DLBCL. It should be cautioned that in any LYG lesion, there can be variation in cellular patterns, and multiple sections should be examined, stained for EBV by *in situ* hybridization (ISH), and assessed for the highest grade. In general, this requires surgical biopsies and classification cannot be confidently established on TBBx specimens. There remains some degree of controversy about the diagnostic criteria for LYG. The WHO defines LYG as EBV-associated B-cell proliferation producing angiocentric/angiodestructive lesions. Katzenstein et al. (168) recently proposed a two-tiered series of morphologic and immunophenotypic criteria:

Findings Necessary for Diagnosis; Always Present:

1. Nodular lesions composed of polymorphous infiltrates of large and small lymphoid cells, plasma cells, and histiocytes with associated mural infiltration of blood vessels
2. Variable numbers of CD20+ large cells, often with cytologic atypia associated with reactive small CD3+ cells.

Findings Supporting the Diagnosis; Usually, but not Always Present:

3. Necrosis within the cellular infiltrate
4. EBV+ cells by ISH
5. The presence of multiple pulmonary nodules or skin or CNS involvement

The relationship between the different grades of LYG and their association with malignant lymphoma has been addressed by a number of studies. As noted previously, grade 3 LYG is considered to be a subtype of DLBCL on the basis of morphologic, immunophenotypic, and genotypic data. It is distinct, however, from DLBCL, not otherwise specified on account of the EBV positivity and the polymorphous mononuclear cell background in LYG. At the other end of the spectrum are grade 1 LYG lesions that appear to be polyclonal, contain few atypical cells, often lack necrosis, and may be EBV-. In some cases, a transition to a higher grade is found in subsequent biopsies,

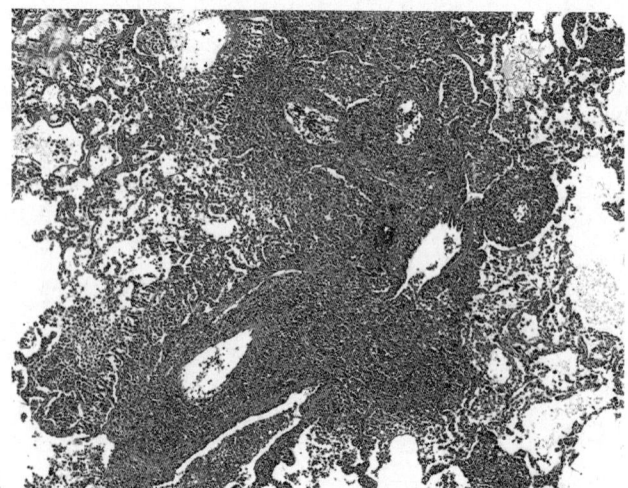

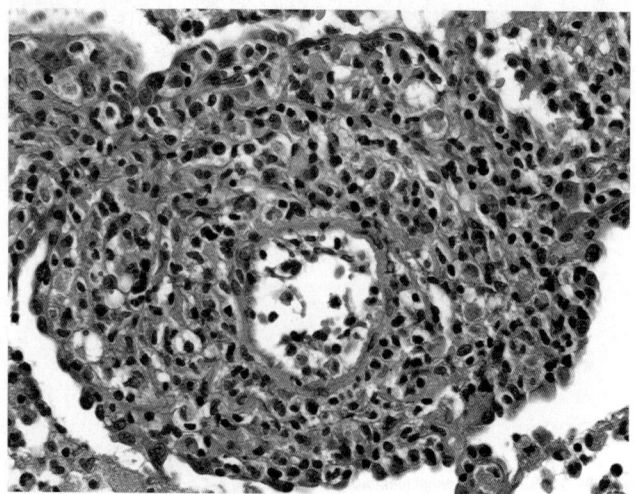

FIGURE 31.16. Low-grade lymphomatoid granulomatosis (grade 1). A: Angiocentric distribution is observed at scanning magnification (H&E, magnification: 60×). **B:** The small vessel is enveloped by small lymphocytes and histiocytes. Atypical large cells are not seen. Only rare EBV+ cells were found by ISH (H&E, magnification: 400×).

suggesting either transformation to a higher grade or sampling limitations (186). Interestingly, there have also been recent reports of IgG4-related disease resembling low-grade LYG (81,187).

Katzenstein et al. (168) recently proposed new terminology for LYG lesions to emphasize the neoplastic nature of grade 2 and 3 lesions. Grade 1 lesions in the WHO classification are retained as LYG, grade 1. WHO grade 2 lesions are defined as polymorphous mononuclear cell infiltrates with easily identified large, often atypical B cells arranged in monomorphous clusters and small sheets, usually with EBV RNA demonstrable by ISH. They are classified as EBV+, T-cell–rich large B-cell lymphoma (LYG, grade 2). WHO grade 3 LYG is characterized by numerous large B cells forming sheets and only focal polymorphous infiltrates with EBV RNA usually present in numerous cells. The corresponding nomenclature is EBV+ DLBCL (LYG, grade 3). The utility of this proposed scheme will require multicenter studies.

The treatment and prognosis in LYG depends on the grading. Grade 1 and grade 2 lesions are rare and there are limited anecdotal reports of response to interferon alpha-2b (167). Corticosteroids have transient utility in low-grade pulmonary LYG as relapses are common. Likewise rituximab monoclonal therapy is considered to be of limited utility or, at best, a temporizing intervention. Patients with grade 3 LYG currently receive combination chemotherapy consisting of rituximab, prednisone, etoposide, vincristine, cyclophosphamide, and adriamycin and may achieve a complete response, but unfortunately there is limited progression-free survival of 40% at a median follow-up of <2.5 years (165). Importantly, there is a strong recommendation to biopsy all recurrences of LYG as some may show progression from low-grade to a higher-grade LYG while the converse is also found.

The differential diagnosis includes peripheral T-cell lymphoma, extranodal T/natural killer (NK)-cell lymphoma, pulmonary granulomatosis, and angiitis and infection. As noted, LYG represents a T-cell–rich B-cell proliferation that is associated with EBV, while the atypical large cells in peripheral T-cell lymphoma are T lineage and generally EBV− (Fig. 31.17). Both display a polymorphous background of inflammatory cells. These aggressive neoplasms arise in the upper aerodigestive tract, and pulmonary involvement by NK/T-cell lymphoma is uncommon. It shares a number of findings with LYG including angiocentricity and angiodestructive morphology, the polymorphous cellular infiltrates, and EBV+ neoplastic cells, but the classic profile of NK/T-cell lymphoma is CD2+, CD56+, and granzyme+ (Fig. 31.18). Pulmonary granulomatosis and angiitis show abundant geographic necrosis and vascular damage but lack the atypical large cells of LYG.

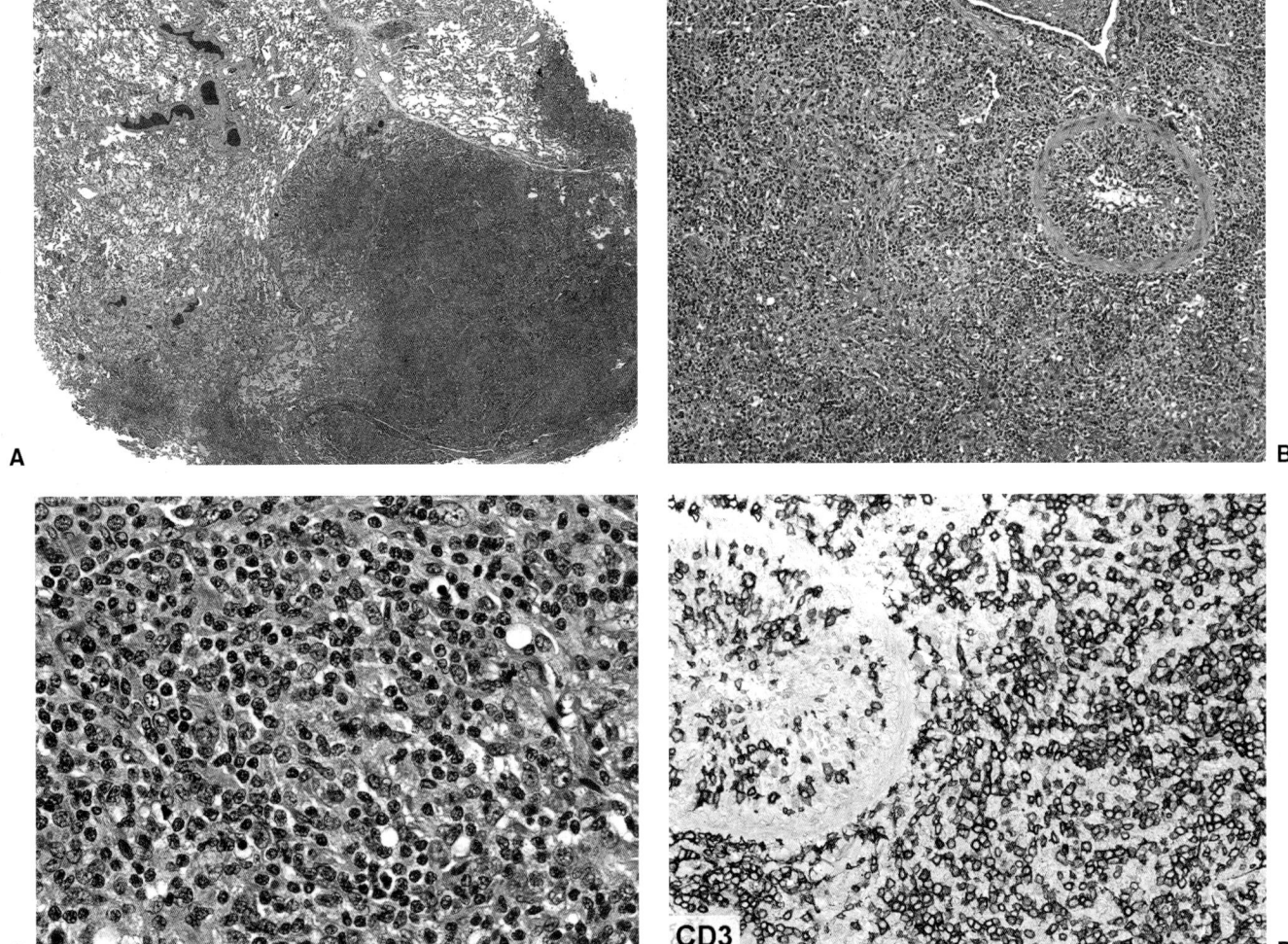

FIGURE 31.17. Pulmonary involvement by peripheral T-cell lymphoma. A: Cellular lesion delineated by interlobular septa (H&E, magnification: 10×). **B:** Parenchymal and vascular invasion by atypical lymphoid infiltrate creating parenchymal consolidation (H&E, magnification: 100×). **C:** High-power magnification showing admixture of atypical small and large lymphocytes (H&E, magnification: 400×). **D:** CD3 staining the majority of cells including the atypical lymphocytes indicative of T lineage (magnification: 300×).

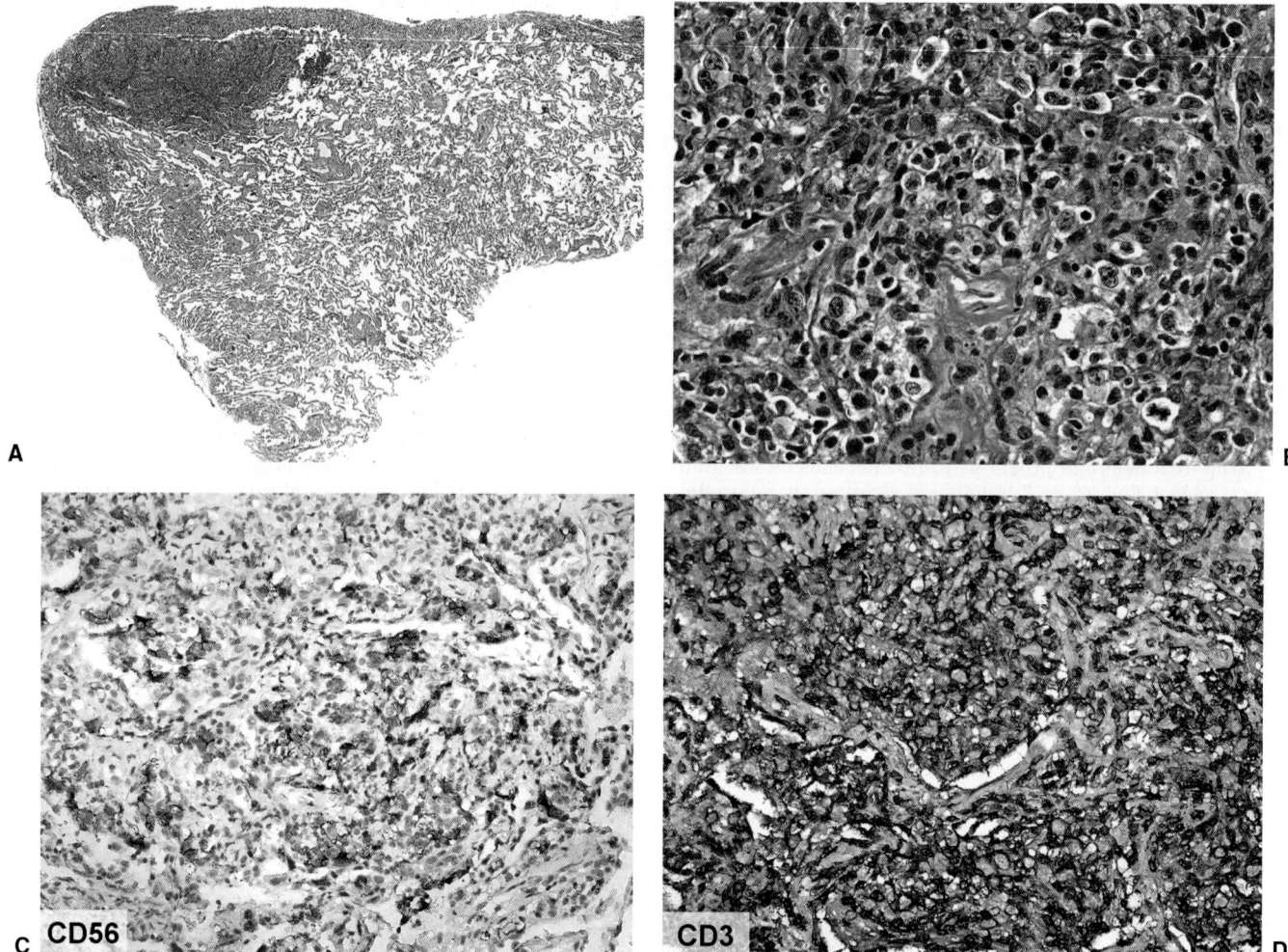

FIGURE 31.18. NK/T-cell lymphoma in a patient with multiorgan involvement. A: Sharply delineated mass centered on lymphatic distribution (H&E, magnification: 7.5×). **B:** The neoplastic cells are medium- to large-sized irregular, folded nuclei admixed with small lymphocytes (H&E, magnification: 400×). **C:** CD56 stains numerous large atypical cells (magnification: 400×). **D:** CD3 stains numerous small cells (magnification: 400×).

Other EBV-Associated Lymphomas and Lymphoproliferative Disorders

EBV⁺ Diffuse Large B-Cell Lymphoma of the Elderly

EBV⁺ DLBCL of the elderly is defined by the WHO as an EBV clonal proliferation occurring in patients >50 years of age and without any known immunodeficiency or prior lymphoma (188). It commonly presents in extranodal sites such as the lung (10%), pleural effusion (10%), skin (13%), tonsil (8%), and stomach (9%) and may have concurrent nodal involvement (189–192). The majority of patients are elderly Japanese, but recently Dojcinov et al. (193) reported a series of 122 patients in Western populations and showed similar demographics and poor clinical outcomes. Microscopically, the pulmonary parenchyma is effaced by either a polymorphous or a monomorphous infiltrate of atypical large cells composed predominantly of large transformed cells/immunoblasts along with scattered Hodgkin-Reed-Sternberg (HRS)–like cells (Fig. 31.19). Areas of geographic necrosis are common, and vascular intrusion may be seen. The large cells are positive for CD20 or CD79a, and MUM1, and EBV by ISH or LMP staining but are CD10⁻ and BCL-6⁻. In some cases, CD30 positivity is seen but the HRS-like cells are CD15⁻. PCR analysis shows clonality of the immunoglobulin genes and EBV. Despite combination chemotherapy, the prognosis is poor with median survival of 2 years or less. The mechanism is not well established but is associated with immunologic senescence.

Diffuse Large B-cell Lymphoma Associated with Chronic Inflammation

DLBCL associated with chronic inflammation is an EBV-associated lymphoproliferative disorder arising in the setting of prolonged localized inflammation. Pyothorax-associated lymphoma (PAL) was described by Iuchi et al. (194) in patients with longstanding pyothorax secondary to artificial pneumothorax for the treatment of pulmonary or pleural tuberculosis. The majority of cases are reported in patients from Japan, but small series of patients in Western populations have also been reported (195–199). There is a prolonged latent period of pyothorax prior to presentation of PAL, ranging from 20 to 60+ years (mean 35+ years). Most patients present with chest or back pain, fever, respiratory symptoms of cough, dyspnea, and hemoptysis. CT imaging shows a pleural-based mass usually >10 cm in size with invasion of adjacent structures. In biopsy specimens, marked fibrous pleural thickening containing small lymphocytes and plasma cells is observed adjacent to the collections of large atypical lymphoid cells (Fig. 31.20). In some cases, immunoblastic morphology predominates. On occasion,

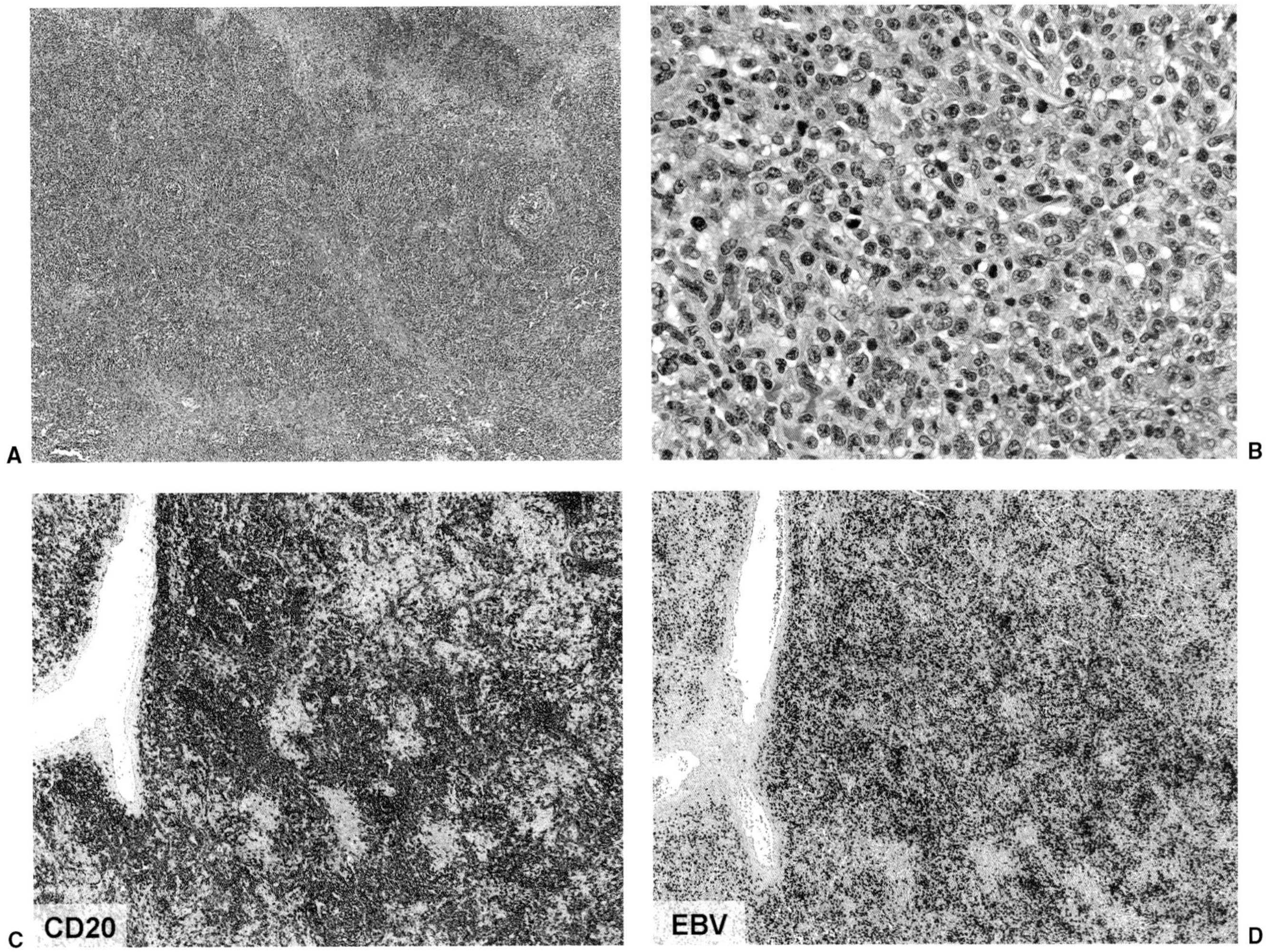

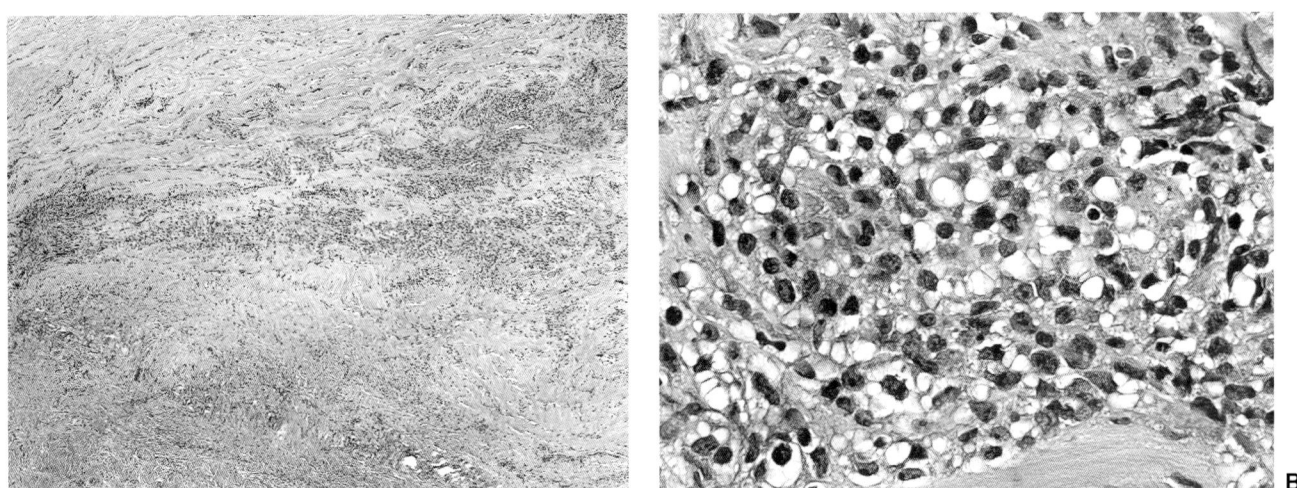

FIGURE 31.19. **EBV⁺ diffuse large B-cell lymphoma of the elderly. A:** Extensive parenchymal involvement with areas of geographic necrosis (H&E, magnification: 40×). **B:** The lesion is composed of medium-sized lymphoid cells and small lymphocytes (H&E, magnification: 400×). **C:** CD20 shows sheets of B cells at low magnification (magnification: 40×). **D:** ISH for EBV RNA (EBER) shows numerous positive cells (magnification: 40×).

FIGURE 31.20. **Diffuse large B-cell lymphoma associated with chronic inflammation. A:** Densely fibrotic pleural and chest wall tissue containing scattered islands of lymphoid cells (H&E, magnification: 10×). **B:** Nodular collections of typical large lymphoid cells including immunoblastic forms (H&E, magnification: 600×).

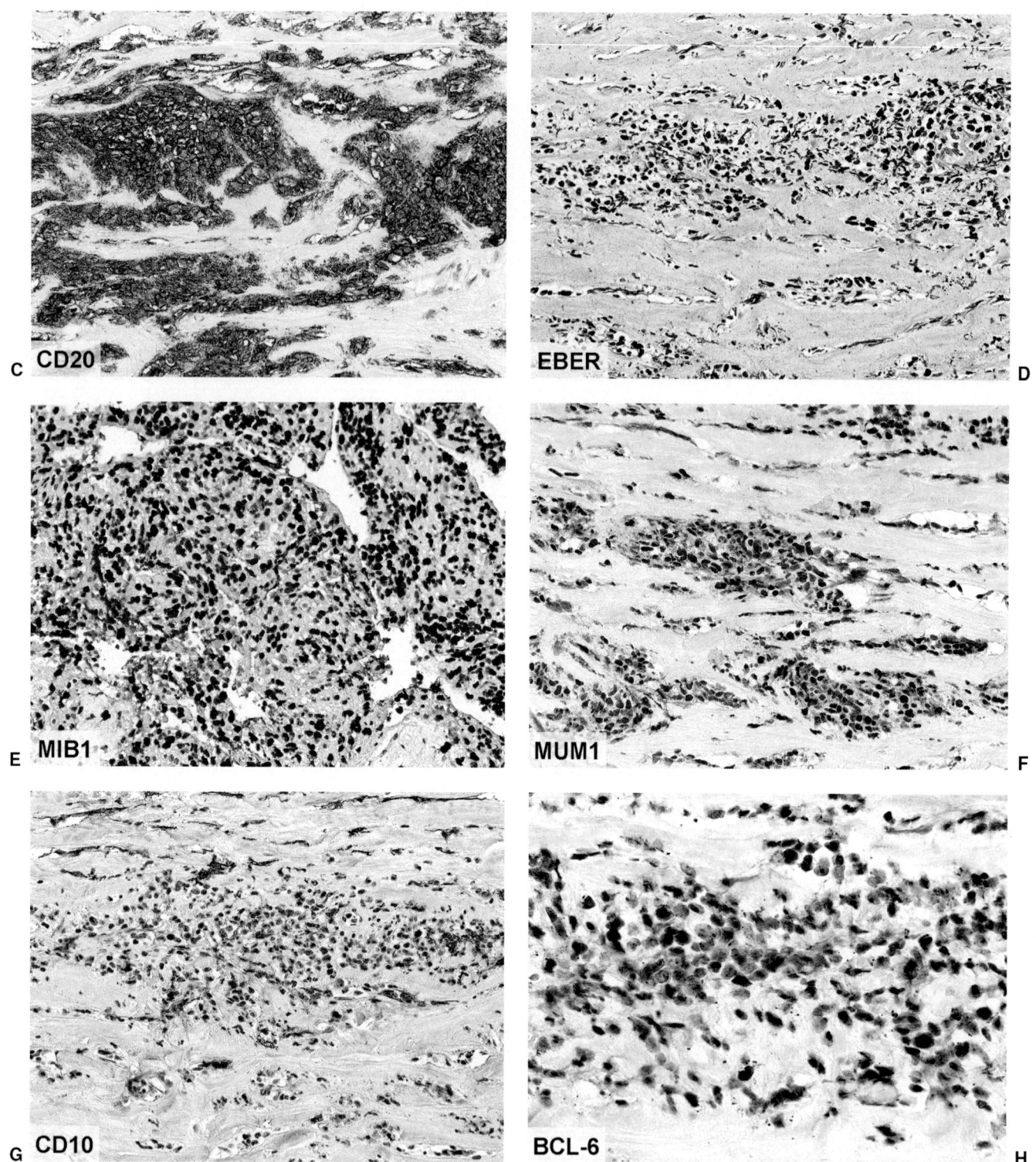

FIGURE 31.20. *(Continued)* **C:** CD20 staining of the large cells (magnification: 200×). **D:** The majority of the tumor cells show EBV by ISH with EBER probe (magnification: 200×). **E:** There is a high proliferation rate of 90% by MIB1 (magnification: 200×). **F–H:** The tumor cells exhibit activated B-cell subtype with MUM1+, CD10−, and Bcl-6− profile.

a conspicuous angiocentric and angiodestructive pattern can be seen, but this is uncommon. The large cells are positive for CD20 and CD79a, and a subset of cases showing plasmacytoid differentiation can also express CD138. In the majority of cases, EBV-encoded RNA (EBER) expression is demonstrated by ISH. Mechanistically, the role of viruses such as EBV and in some cases HHV8 along with chronic inflammation produce a

distinct form of DLBCL. Recently gene-expression profiling has shown higher expression level of interferon-inducible genes (200–201). PAL is an aggressive form of DLBCL with poor outcomes. The 5-year overall survival rates are well below 50% even with chemotherapy; some report the median survival of <6 months. In some cases, pleuropneumonectomy has been attempted.

Posttransplant Lymphoproliferative Disorder

PTLD is defined in the *WHO Classification of Tumours of Hematopoietic and Lymphoid Tissues* as "lymphoid or plasmacytic proliferations that develop as a consequence of immunosuppression in a recipient of a solid organ, bone marrow (BM) or stem cell allograft" (202). Lung transplant recipients continue to have a high incidence of PTLD among the different solid organ groups. Wudhikarn and colleagues report an incidence of 5% in heart-lung and lung recipients over a 20-year period, but older series have reported rates closer to 10% (203,204). Over the last decade, the median interval to PTLD has increased from 6 months (80% within the first year) to approximately 3 years (205). This increase is due in part to the increase in EBV⁻ PTLD cases. Previously 80% to 90% of PTLD were EBV associated, but currently up to 40% of cases are EBV⁻. The risk factors for developing PTLD include seronegative allograft recipients (which includes a significant proportion of children), intensity and duration of immunosuppression, CMV disease, and the degree of donor/recipient HLA mismatch (206,207). Treatment protocols have changed, although reduction in immunosuppression remains the central component. More recently, the introduction of the rituximab has expanded the therapeutic options, and systemic chemotherapy is generally reserved for cases that fail to respond to these two approaches or for patients with CNS involvement. Conventional antiviral therapy alone with acyclovir and ganciclovir has not been shown to be of therapeutic benefit, but clinical trials are currently evaluating the efficacy of antiviral drugs in combination with arginine butyrate, a drug that induces EBV thymidine kinase transcription (208,209). Other novel modalities include infusion of EBV-specific cytotoxic T cells to help reestablish immunologic control of EBV-infected B-cell activation and proliferation (210).

There is tremendous heterogeneity in both the clinical presentation and histopathologic appearance of PTLD. Diagnostic modalities include image-guided needle core biopsy, TBBx, and open biopsy. Flow cytometry, immunohistochemical, and molecular studies are required to determine clonality and other diagnostic, potential therapeutic, and prognostic information. Currently, the WHO grading scheme is used by most centers and is divided into four patterns (Table 31.6).

Early Lesions Including Plasmacytic Hyperplasia and Infectious Mononucleosis–Like PTLD

These patterns are characterized by the formation of mass lesions with lymphoid or lymphoplasmacytic proliferation but preservation of architecture of lymph nodes or extranodal sites such as tonsils and adenoids. These typically occur in EBV-seronegative recipients (children and occasionally adults) and represent primary EBV infections. In tissue sections, plasmacytic hyperplasia (PH) exhibits numerous plasma cells and small lymphocytes with occasional immunoblasts in a background of follicular hyperplasia while infectious mononucleosis (IM)-like lesions display paracortical expansion and immunoblasts admixed with plasma cells and T cells (Fig. 31.21).

Immunostaining reveals polytypic B cells and plasma cells with variable detection of EBV by EBER ISH.

Polymorphous PTLD

This pattern is characterized by architectural effacement of nodal or extranodal structures by a mixture of cell types including small and transformed lymphocytes, immunoblasts, and plasma cells (Fig. 31.21). In some cases, cells resembling HRS-like cells are present, and necrosis and division figures can be variable. It is the most common pattern reported in pediatric PTLD and usually represents primary EBV infection rather than reactivation. A range of clonality results have been found including polyclonal, oligoclonal, and monoclonal cases. The HRS-like cells are usually CD30⁺ and CD20⁺ but CD15⁻ and generally EBV⁺ by ISH.

Monomorphic PTLD

Monomorphic PTLD resembles the classic forms of B-cell and NK/T-cell lymphomas encountered in immunocompetent patients. The B-cell lesions are usually DLBCL, but Burkitt-like lymphomas and plasma cell neoplasms are also included in this group (Fig. 31.21). Both nodal and extranodal lesions are reported, and the lung is a common site of involvement presenting as endobronchial or parenchymal nodular masses. The B-cell lesions are monoclonal, and cytogenetic abnormalities are common but the presence of EBV is less consistent than in polymorphous PTLD.

Monomorphic NK/T-cell PTLD is less common than the B-cell type and are frequently extranodal. Numerous patterns have been described including peripheral T-cell lymphoma, hepatosplenic T-cell lymphoma, T-cell large granular lymphocytic leukemia, adult T-cell leukemia/lymphoma, extranodal NK/T-cell lymphoma, nasal type, and the spectrum of T-cell cutaneous lymphoid neoplasms (202). Up to a third are EBV⁺.

Classical Hodgkin Lymphoma-Type PTLD

This is the least common pattern of PTLD and the most diagnostically challenging for pathologists. It must be distinguished from the polymorphous PTLD group and requires both the morphology and immunophenotype of classical HD such as CD30⁺ and CD15⁺ immunostaining.

In the setting of diffuse alveolar consolidative rather than nodular distribution of PTLD or with small biopsy specimens, the distinction of PTLD from acute cellular rejection, infection, and drug toxicity can be challenging. The liberal use of leveled tissue sections, IHC, and ISH and careful attention to the morphologic findings can usually resolve the problems. Findings that favor PTLD include monomorphic and atypical lymphoid cells, necrosis, and numerous mitotic figures (211).

Intravascular Large B-Cell Lymphoma

Intravascular large B-cell lymphoma (IVLBCL) or angiotropic large cell lymphoma is a rare extranodal type of aggressive B-cell lymphoma in the current WHO classification. It is characterized by the presence of luminal plugs of neoplastic cells with a predilection for capillaries, arterioles, and postcapillary venules. Presentation as primary cutaneous or CNS disorders is more common in Western populations than pulmonary conditions. Patients from Asian countries often present with hemophagocytic syndrome. The nonspecific nature of the pulmonary symptoms often leads to a delay in diagnosis. IVLBCL usually occurs in adults (median age 67 years), but isolated cases in adolescents and young adults have been reported (212–214). Pulmonary symptoms of dyspnea and cough reflect vascular obstruction, but a wide range of presentations including pulmonary arterial hypertension, ILD, adult respiratory distress syndrome, and congestive heart failure are reported (215–218). Most patients have constitutional symptoms such as fever, weight loss, malaise, and fatigue. Laboratory abnormalities include elevated lactate dehydrogenase B2-microglobulin

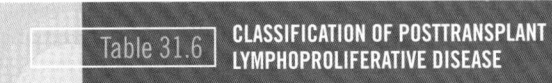

Table 31.6	CLASSIFICATION OF POSTTRANSPLANT LYMPHOPROLIFERATIVE DISEASE

1. Early lesions (PH and IM-like PTLD)
2. Polymorphous PTLD
3. Monomorphic PTLD (including diffuse large B-cell, Burkitt-like, plasma cell lesions and NK/T-cell lymphoma)
4. Classical HL-like PTLD
5. Other (including cutaneous and PELs)

Modified from Swerdlow SH, Webber SA, Chadburn A, et al. Post-transplant lymphoproliferative disorders. In: Swerdlow SH, Campo E, Harris NL, et al., eds. *WHO classification of tumours of haematopoietic and lymphoid tissues*, 4th ed. Lyon: IARC Press, 2008:343–349.

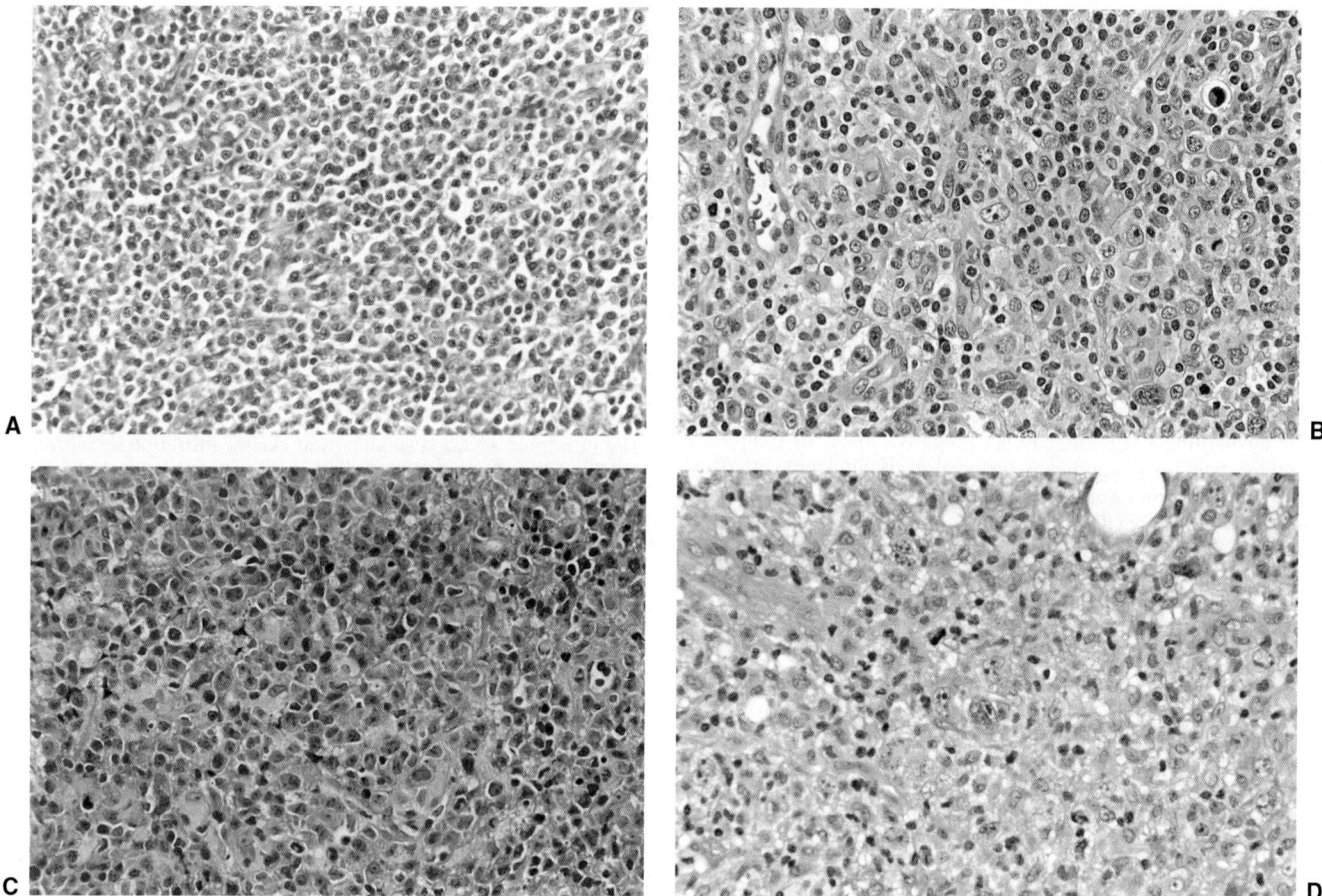

FIGURE 31.21. Posttransplant lymphoproliferative disorder. A: Reactive lymphoid hyperplasia showing small and transformed lymphocytes without necrosis or atypia. **B:** Polymorphous PTLD showing an admixture of small and large lymphocytes and plasma cells. This pattern can be found in either polytypic or monotypic PTLD. **C:** Monomorphic PTLD showing a uniform population of atypical large lymphocytes resembling diffuse aggressive large B-cell lymphoma. **D:** Hodgkin-like PTLD showing an admixture of cell types including a central RS cell. (All H&E, magnification: 400×).

levels (>80%), anemia (65%), and high levels of soluble interleukin-2 receptor (sIL2-R) (212,213). Profound hypoxemia and increased alveolar-arterial oxygen difference (A-aDO$_2$) are common. Chest CT abnormalities include interstitial infiltrates, patchy parenchymal consolidations, or ground-glass opacities, but in some cases no abnormalities are seen (217). FDG-PET imaging and 67Ga scintigraphy are useful techniques and show diffuse accumulation of tracers in the lungs (219,220).

In older published series, the diagnosis was established at postmortem (221). Random transbronchial and VATS biopsy now are routinely used to confirm the clinical diagnosis (217). At scanning magnification, patchy thickening of the alveolar septa is noted by a cellular rather than fibrotic process (Fig. 31.22). The interstitium is expanded, creating a "serpentine of string of beads" appearance (222). The lumens of small vessels are uniformly filled by monomorphic cells with the typical appearance of DLBCL. Large atypical lymphocytes display vesicular nuclei, one or more conspicuous nucleoli, and scant-to-moderate amounts of pale cytoplasm. Mitotic figures, necrosis, and hyaline membranes are absent, but alveolar congestion and hemorrhage, atelectasis, patchy organizing pneumonia, and focal interstitial scarring are reported. The perivascular spaces are also cellular, but the predominant cell types are small lymphocytes, plasma cells, and histiocytes. The pulmonary arterioles may show concentric fibroelastotic intimal thickening reflecting hypertensive alterations. The cells in IVLBCL are CD20$^+$, CD79a$^+$, and CD19$^+$. Murase et al. (213) reported the following phenotype in IVLBCL: CD10$^+$ 13%, MUM1$^+$ 95%, cyclin D1 0%,

Bcl-2$^+$ 91%, EBER$^-$ by ISH 0% and coexpression of CD5 38%. The activated B-cell phenotype is the most common type, but neither phenotype nor expression of CD5 affects outcome.

The underlying mechanism of IVLBCL is complex and involves defective interactions between the lymphocytes and vascular structures. Diminished levels of the proteins responsible for lymphocytes tracking and migration across blood vessels such as CD29 (Beta1-integrin), CD54 (ICAM) adhesion B-molecules, and CD18 of the CD18/CD11a complex (lymphocyte function-associated antigen-1) promote intravascular localization of the tumor cells (223,224). Recently, Kato et al. (225) reported the presence of the chemokine receptor CXCR3 on the lymphocytes in IVLBCL and its ligand, CXCL9 on blood vessels, suggesting that the combination may promote intravascular localization.

Patients with IVLBCL are treated with combination chemotherapy, but the prognosis remains poor (214). The differential diagnosis includes other intravascular malignancies such as malignant melanoma, angiosarcoma and carcinoma, and other hematolymphoid malignancies like leukemia and secondary involvement by lymphoma (Fig. 31.23). Careful attention to the cytologic appearance of the neoplastic cells and immunohistochemical profiles resolves the diagnostic difficulties.

Primary Pulmonary Hodgkin Lymphoma

HL presenting exclusively in the lung (or with minimal hilar nodal involvement) is rare; secondary pulmonary involvement

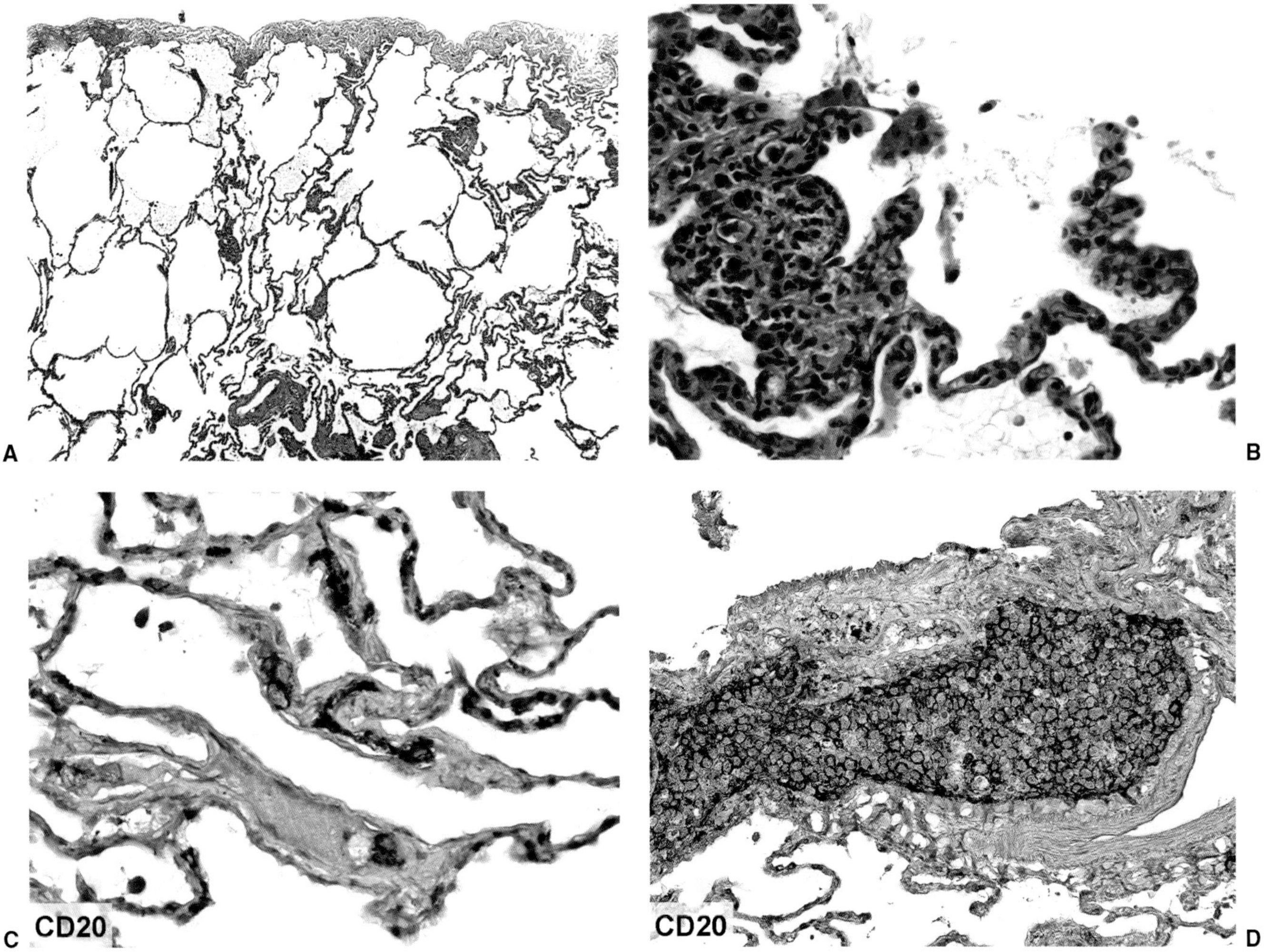

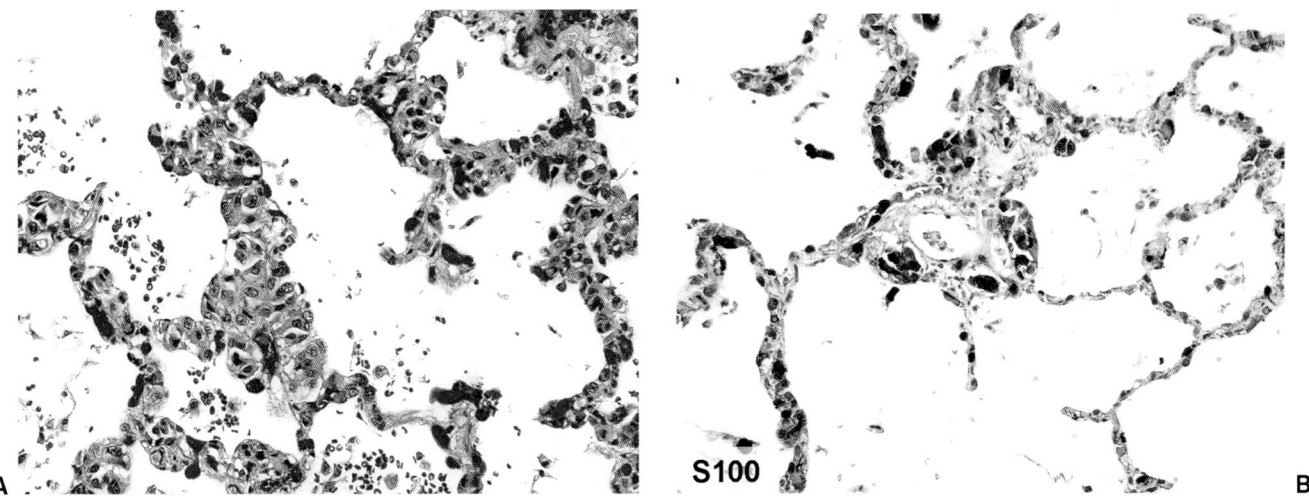

FIGURE 31.22. Intravascular large B-cell lymphoma. A: Low-power magnification shows preservation of the lung parenchyma (H&E, magnification: 10×). **B:** High-power magnification showing filling and expansion of small vasculature by atypical large lymphocytes (H&E, magnification: 400×). **C:** The intravascular tumor cells are highlighted by staining for CD20 (magnification: 400×). **D:** Lymphatics in bronchovascular bundle are filled with CD20⁺ tumor cells (magnification: 400×).

FIGURE 31.23. Mimics of intravascular lymphoma. A: Diffuse intravascular plugs of malignant melanoma within the alveolar septa (H&E, magnification: 400×). **B:** The neoplastic cells strongly express S100 protein (magnification: 400×).

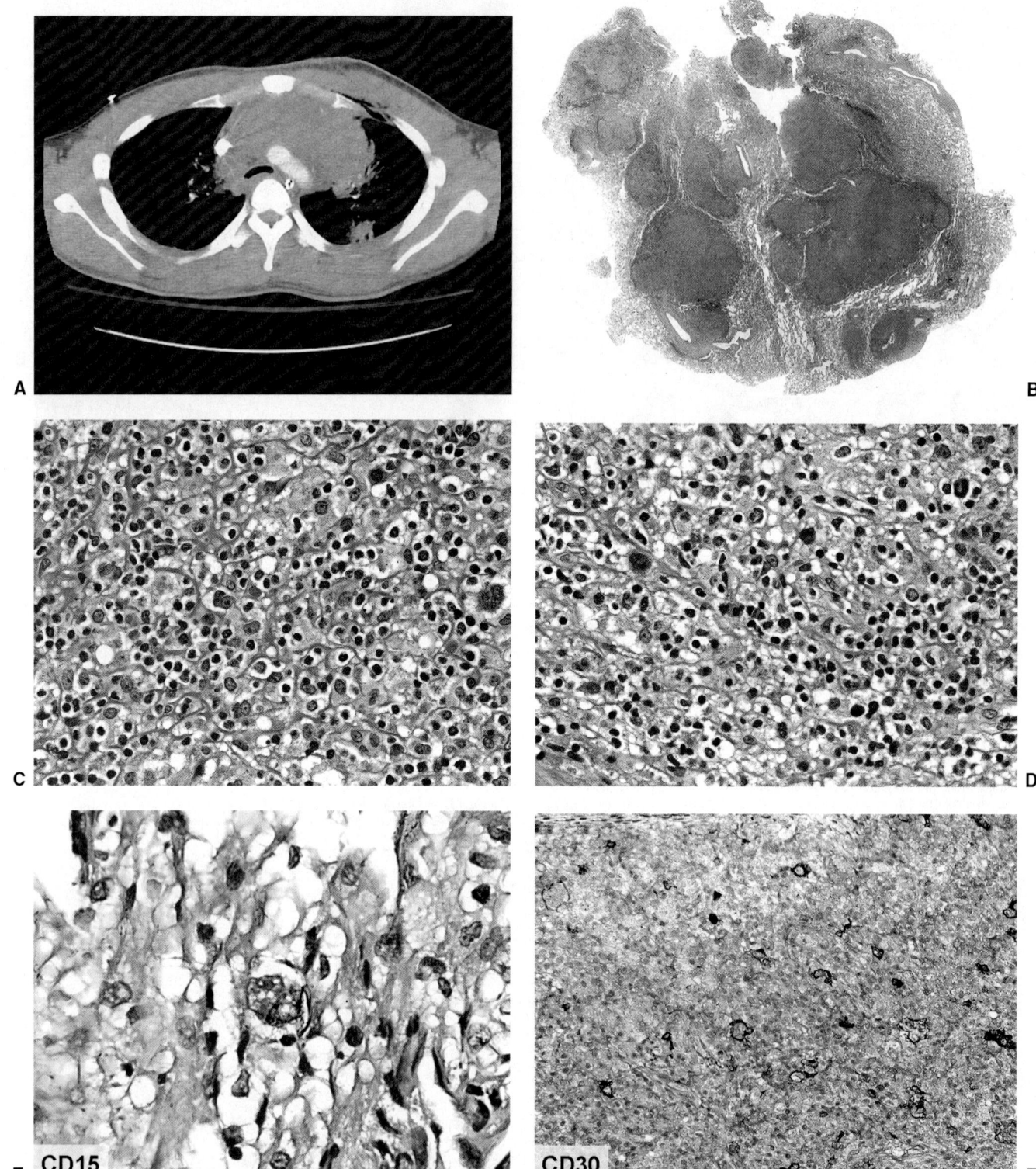

FIGURE 31.24. Primary pulmonary Hodgkin lymphoma. A: CT image exhibiting peripherally located mass with irregular borders. **B:** VATS specimen showing coalescence of nodules sharply separated from the adjacent lung parenchyma (H&E, magnification: 5×). **C,D:** The nodules are composed of polymorphous infiltrates with scattered diagnostic RS cells (magnification: 400×). **E:** Membrane and paranuclear staining of RS cell for CD15 (magnification: 600×). **F:** CD30 membrane expression is noted in scattered HRS cells (magnification: 200×).

at the time of diagnosis with mediastinal nodal involvement or at postmortem examination is much more common (226–231). With fewer than 100 cases of primary pulmonary HL reported in the literature, there are no recent large series of patients to assess patient outcomes with current treatment regimens. The diagnosis is often delayed or complicated by the clinical or radiologic findings at presentation. There is a broad age range from adolescents to the elderly, with a mean age in the fifth decade in most series; others suggest a bimodal distribution similar to nodal HL. A minority of patients present with asymptomatic lesions while the majority have respiratory and accompanying B symptoms. Solitary or multiple upper lobe-predominant nodules or masses are seen on chest radiographs, with a third showing central cavitation; pleural effusions are uncommon. Less common findings are reticulonodular infiltrates or pneumonic consolidations (227,228). Cartier et al. (232) describe the CT findings in primary pulmonary HL and note that the pattern (central cavitation more common in HL) and distribution (upper lung zone predominance in HL) differ from primary pulmonary NHL. The pathologic diagnosis can be established by a variety of diagnostic techniques with immunohistochemical support, but in many cases VATS biopsy is required. In a limited number of cases, the lesions are endobronchial in location, and fiberoptic bronchoscopy with biopsy yields sufficient material for diagnosis (10,233,234). The nodular lesions are distributed along lymphatic routes. The majority of cases are classified as classical HL, with most cases representing either nodular sclerosing or mixed cellularity subtypes; a handful of lymphocyte-predominant HL cases are documented. The cellular composition is similar to nodal HL with HRS cells, lymphocytes, plasma cells, eosinophils, and histiocytes (Fig. 31.24). The HRS cells are distributed within or at the periphery of the nodules, around the edges of necrotic lesions or admixed within the cellular infiltrates in the interstitium (227). The patterns of necrosis include geographic and infarct-like patterns. Granulomas, including nonnecrotizing sarcoid-like types, are reported in half of the cases. Infiltration and destruction of cartilaginous bronchi by the inflammatory cells (including HRS cells) is also observed, but the mural infiltration of arteries and veins does not harbor HRS cells. Secondary patterns such as acute, obstructive, or organizing pneumonia are also present in some cases. HRS cells typically are positive for CD30 (>95%), CD15 (75% to 85%), CD20 (30% to 40%, weak), and PAX5 (95%, weak) and negative for CD79a, CD45, and CD138 (235). The EBV-staining profile supports latency type II EBV infection and is seen in the mixed cellularity and nodular sclerosis subtypes (236).

Treatment is centered on chemotherapy and/or radiation therapy. In two published series, a 50% 2-year disease-free survival was reported; the presence of B symptoms, the extent of parenchymal involvement, and cavitary disease were associated with a poor outcome (227,228). The differential diagnosis includes NHL including T-cell ALCL and peripheral T-cell lymphoma, LYG, granulomatosis with polyangiitis (formerly Wegener granulomatosis), metastatic nasopharyngeal carcinoma, and infectious granulomatous disease. As noted previously, RS-like cells can be seen in a variety of NHL including LYG and EBV+ DLBCL of the elderly. Classic HL lacks the characteristic angiocentric and angiodestructive patterns of LYG and stains strongly for CD30 and CD15; CD20 shows weak staining of scattered HRS cells. Most cases of T-cell ALCL of the lung represent secondary involvement, although a few cases of primary pulmonary and tracheal ALCL have been reported (237,238). ALCL occurs in both children and adults and has been reported in both immunocompetent patients and in immunosuppressed patients with acquired immunodeficiency syndrome or PTLD (238–245). Extranodal involvement is more common in ALK+ ALCL than ALK− ALCL (7). Pulmonary symptoms include cough, fever, weight loss, and night sweats. In four of the five cases reported by Rush

et al. (237), solitary lesions were found, two of which had an endobronchial localization. Microscopically, the normal alveolar parenchyma was disrupted by a nodular lesion measuring 1.1 to 5.0 cm in size. In one case, the neoplastic proliferation extended into the alveolar spaces producing "tumoral pneumonia." The tumor cells varied from monomorphic large cells with vesicular nuclei, inconspicuous nucleoli, and pale cytoplasm to large cells with pleomorphic nuclei, one or more prominent nucleoli, and abundant eosinophilic cytoplasm resembling HRS cells (246). In some cases, vascular intrusion is observed. The tumor cells are admixed with variable numbers of lymphocytes, eosinophils, and neutrophils. A number of patterns have been delineated in most recent *WHO Classification of Tumours of Haematopoietic and Lymphoid Tissues*, reflecting the heterogeneous morphologic patterns (247). The tumor cells are CD30+, CD15−, EMA+, and CD45+, and most are positive for one or more pan T-cell markers such as CD2, CD3, or CD5; the null-cell phenotype is characterized by negative T-cell staining. ALK immunostaining is correlated with the t(2;5)/*NPM-ALK* translocation and therefore may not be found in all cases of ALK+ ALCL. They are also negative for EBV by IHC or ISH.

The distinction of HL from pulmonary granulomatosis with angiitis (formerly Wegener granulomatosis) is usually not difficult. Although zones of necrosis, polymorphous cell types, and "granulomatous" features can be seen in both lesions, HRS cells are not seen in the granulomatosis and angiitis. Serologic studies such as c-ANCA are helpful in the diagnosis of granulomatosis with angiitis. Infectious granulomatous should always be considered, and appropriate histochemical stains and cultures are important. The diagnosis of metastatic neoplasms with abundant inflammatory cells such as metastatic nasopharyngeal carcinoma can be distinguished by clinical history and IHC.

Primary Effusion Lymphoma

PEL is another uncommon aggressive B-cell lymphoma that is defined by the WHO as a large B-cell lymphoma presenting as a serous effusion in the pleural, pericardial, or peritoneal cavities in the absence of a solid tumor mass (248). By definition, it is associated with HHV8 (also called Kaposi sarcoma-associated herpesvirus/KSHV), and in two thirds of cases there is also an associated EBV infection. In most cases, an underlying immunodeficiency condition such as HIV infection, solid organ or bone marrow transplantation, cirrhosis, or elderly men of Mediterranean origin has been documented. The majority of EBV+ cases occur in HIV+ patients (249–253). Other HHV8-related conditions such as Kaposi sarcoma and less commonly multicentric CD have been reported in the setting of PEL (254). The pleural cavity is the most common site of involvement, but more than one site can present concurrently or during disease progression. Moreover, solid tumors with similar morphology and phenotype can develop in extra-cavity sites such as the gastrointestinal tract or lungs either with evolution of the disease or may precede PEL. The cytologic appearance of the tumor cells can vary, but most cytologic preparations display large cells with immunoblastic or plasmablastic morphology or cells resembling ALCL (253,254). The large cells usually have a single eccentrically placed nucleus with round or irregular contours, one or multiple nucleoli, coarse chromatin, and moderate-to-abundant basophilic cytoplasm (Fig. 31.25). Numerous division figures, apoptotic bodies, and nuclear debris are found. Tumor cells with a plasmacytoid appearance may display a perinuclear hof, but this finding and cytoplasmic vacuoles are only seen in a minority of cases. In the majority of published series, the tumor cells express CD45 (93%) but typically lack B-lineage markers CD20, CD79a, and CD19 and surface and cytoplasmic

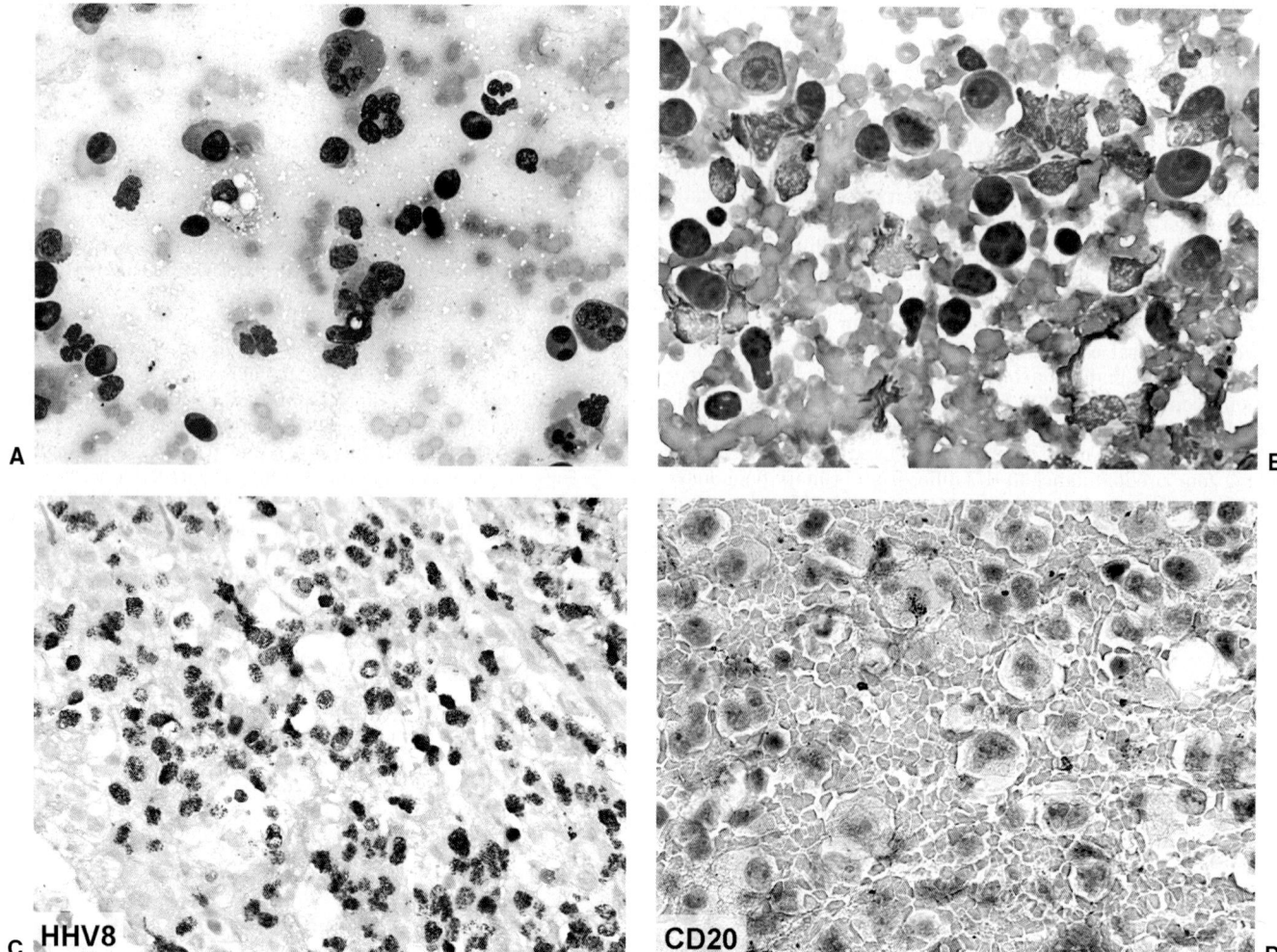

FIGURE 31.25. Primary effusion lymphoma. A,B: Cytologic preparations from pleural effusions showing markedly pleomorphic cells with prominent macronucleoli (Diff-Quik, magnification: 600×). **C:** Cell block sections showing strong nuclei staining for HHV8 (magnification: 400×). **D:** The tumor cells lack CD20 expression (magnification: 600×).

immunoglobulin. Activation and plasma cell markers (CD30, EMA, HLA-DR, CD38, and CD138) are reported in more than 70% of cases, and aberrant T-cell expression (CD3, CD43) is seen occasionally. HHV8-associated latent protein LANA shows strong nuclear staining of tumor cells in cell block and tissue sections. B lineage is confirmed by clonal rearrangement of immunoglobulin genes. The major differential diagnosis rests on HHV8-negative effusion-based B-cell lymphoma which has different clinical, immunophenotypic, and clinical outcomes and is often associated with fluid overload conditions (255,256). The prognosis in PEL is dismal, with median survival rates of <6 months.

Plasmacytoma

Primary pulmonary plasmacytoma is a rare example of an extraosseous plasma cell neoplasm; the majority of these pulmonary disorders arise in the setting of multiple myeloma as secondary involvement or as primary neoplasms in upper airways. Only a handful of published series are reported, with most reports representing case reports (257–263). The tumor masses are located either in the hilum, as endobronchial lesions, as parenchymal infiltrates or consolidation, or as solitary or multiple nodules or masses. Symptoms at presentation range from absent to cough and dyspnea. The chest

CT findings are homogeneous, well-delineated lesions that can be sampled by percutaneous FNA and core needle biopsy (264–266). Sheets and clusters of plasma cells with few or no small lymphocytes are observed. In resection specimens, the masses range up to 10 cm in diameter, but most are <5 cm and are peribronchial or involve large proximal bronchi. The cut surface is white to tan-brown. Microscopically, sheets of plasma cells with or without zones of amyloid deposition are observed (Fig. 31.26). Germinal centers are absent. The differentiation of the plasma cells can range from mature cells to binucleated forms to poorly differentiated or anaplastic variants. Kazzaz et al. (267) reported an unusual case that showed intracytoplasmic paraprotein crystalloid deposition in plasma cells, macrophages, and epithelial cells. The classic immunophenotype of plasmacytomas is CD45-, CD20-, CD19-, PAX5-, and CD138+. Kappa or lambda light chain restriction is readily demonstrable by IHC. Amyloid deposits or collections of neoplastic cells can also be found in hilar or mediastinal lymph nodes.

The major diagnostic considerations include extranodal MZL, SLL/CLL, and lymphoplasmacytic lymphoma. As previously discussed, MZL can have a conspicuous plasmacytic component, and the presence of small lymphocytes within the tumor should raise the possibility of a diagnosis other than plasmacytoma. Further, the immunophenotype of all three disorders

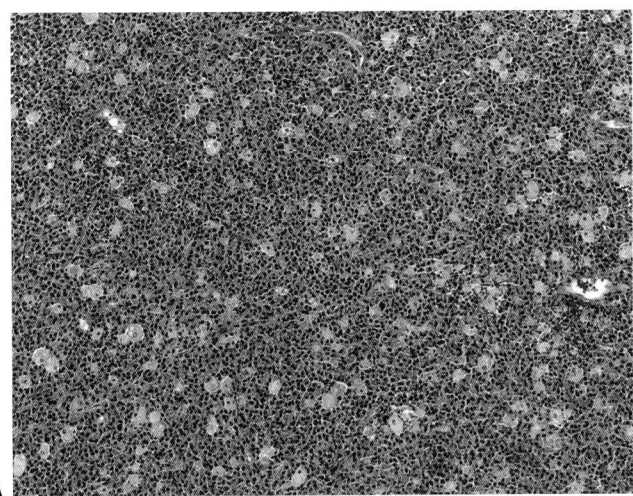
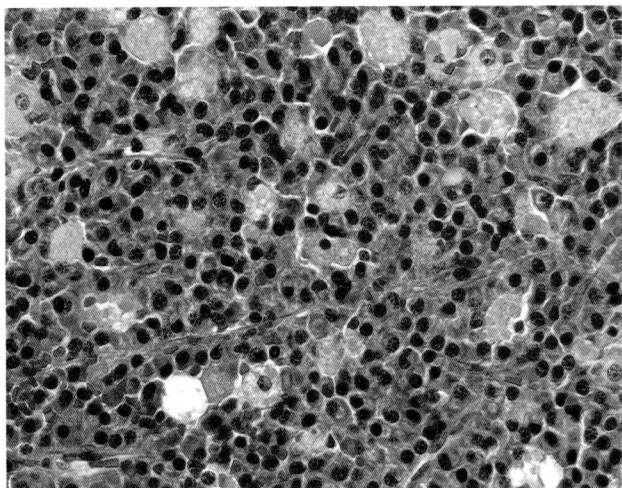

FIGURE 31.26. Pulmonary plasmacytoma. A: Low-power magnification showing sheets of mononuclear cells with sprinkling of foamy macrophages (H&E, magnification: 100×). **B:** Mature plasma cells with eccentrically placed nuclei (H&E, magnification: 400×).

differs from plasmacytoma as the tumor cells are CD45[+] and CD20[+] and express surface immunoglobulin (268). The diagnosis of primary pulmonary plasmacytoma is one of exclusion, and thorough radiologic, serologic, and marrow assessment is required to exclude the diagnosis of multiple myeloma. The treatment is primarily surgical with 2-year and 5-year survival rates of 66% and 40%, respectively reported by Koss et al. (257).

Secondary Pulmonary Involvement in Lymphoma and Leukemia

As previously mentioned in an earlier segment, the lung is a common site of involvement by lymphoma or leukemia at postmortem examination but less commonly at presentation or during relapses (226,230,269,270). The differential diagnosis of infiltrates, nodules, and masses in this population is broad and also includes infection, heart failure, radiation injury, disorders of hemostasis, PTLD, and drug toxicity. BAL and TBBx or VATS biopsy are commonly utilized to differentiate these processes. The radiologic appearance of recurrent lymphoma is variable but usually includes multilobar multiple nodules (>10), lymphadenopathy, and parenchymal consolidation (271,272). Awareness of the clinical history and treatment regimens, laboratory data, radiologic findings and review of prior diagnostic histopathologic material together with communication with clinicians and radiologists are important measures and provide helpful clinical clues. Any type of lymphoma or acute or chronic leukemia can have a pulmonary component, and we will restrict the discussion to two lesions that illustrate key diagnostic points (Table 31.1). Common to all the hematolymphoid neoplasms, they display a lymphatic distribution.

Chronic Lymphocytic Leukemia

Patients with CLL are at risk for a variety of pulmonary complications including infection (75%), malignant pleural effusion or parenchymal infiltrates (9%), pulmonary leukostasis (4%), Richter transformation or nonsmall cell carcinoma (3%), and upper airway obstruction (2%) (273). Alveolar hemorrhage and edema secondary to leukostasis occur but are less common than in other forms of leukemic infiltration of the lung. Following treatment, drug toxicity secondary to chlorambucil is another documented complication (274). Direct involvement of the lung by CLL is more common than other leukemic infiltration, and

patients commonly complain of dry cough, progressive dyspnea, and low-grade fever. Chest radiographs show unilateral or bilateral diffuse interstitial or reticulonodular infiltrates, hilar adenopathy, and/or effusions. Centrilobular nodularity in a "tree-in-bud" pattern can be seen on CT imaging. Mosaic perfusion, expiratory airtrapping, and centrilobular nodules reflect the bronchiolocentric distribution of CLL (275,276). Abnormal pulmonary function studies can also demonstrate small airway dysfunction (277). Rollins and Colby described the histopathologic changes in nine patients and noted the presence of dense lymphocytic infiltrates that traversed along the bronchovascular bundles (Fig. 31.27). Coalescence of the infiltrates can lead to the development of discrete nodules, and "spillage" of tumor cells into expanded airspaces produces "tumoral pneumonia" (278,279). Viral and fungal infections are uncommon in CLL patients unless they have received corticosteroids; the most common infections are gram-positive organisms, *Nocardia* spp., and *Haemophilus influenzae*. Flow cytometry or IHC rapidly confirms the diagnosis of CLL as the small lymphocytes are CD20[+], CD5[+], CD23[+], CD10[-], and Bcl-1/cyclin D1[-]. Rare cases of T-cell CLL have been reported (280).

Mycosis Fungoides

Mycosis fungoides (MF) is the most common form of cutaneous T-cell lymphoma and is generally considered to be an indolent disease. Extracutaneous involvement occurs in advanced "tumor" stages of the disease. Pulmonary involvement by MF is a common site of involvement at the time of postmortem examination (281). In some patients, the onset of pulmonary involvement is abrupt, and its rapid progression mimics infection and other conditions. In slowly progressive involvement, the clinical symptoms are nonspecific cough and dyspnea, but rapid dissemination produces ARDS-like symptoms. The reported chest radiographic findings include multiple bilateral parenchymal nodular densities, patchy foci of airspaces consolidation, diffuse reticulonodular or interstitial infiltrates, and isolated pleural effusions (282). HRCT findings reflect the lymphatic distribution with thickened bronchovascular bundles and interlobular septa surrounded by ground-glass opacities and central traction bronchiectasis (283,284). Diagnostic interventions include FNA of nodular densities, fiberoptic bronchoscopy with TBBx, and VATS biopsy (285). Microscopically, the interlobular septa and/or bronchovascular bundles are expanded by small- to medium-sized lymphocyte with indented and convoluted or cerebriform nuclei (Fig. 31.28). Kitching and

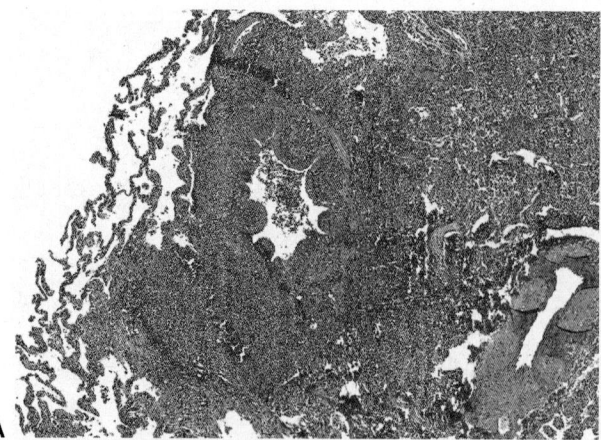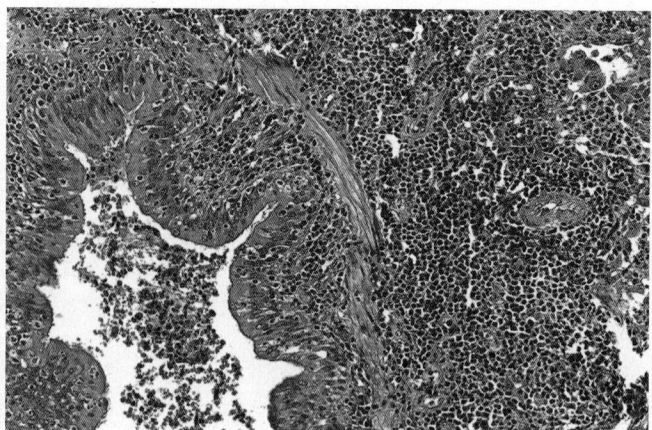

A

B

FIGURE 31.27. Bronchiolocentric chronic lymphocytic leukemia. A: The membranous bronchiole shows extensive transmural infiltration by a monotonous lymphoid process (magnification: 150×). **B:** The small lymphocytic cells extend from the peribronchiolar and interstitial regions and permeate the mucosal and submucosal layers with luminal narrowing (H&E, magnification: 400×).

Gibbs (286) reported an unusual case of disseminated MF with an angiocentric distribution that was associated with numerous epithelioid granulomas in the lung.

Histiocytic Proliferations

Histiocytic neoplasms such as true histiocytic sarcoma, interdigitating and follicular dendritic cell sarcoma, Langerhans cell histiocytosis (LCH), and Langerhans cell sarcoma rarely involve the lung except in the setting of widespread metastasis or multiorgan involvement. The subject has been recently discussed in detail in a number of excellent review articles (287,288). The current discussion focuses on three different types of primary pulmonary nonneoplastic histiocytic proliferation (Table 31.1).

Pulmonary Langerhans Cell Histiocytosis

Pulmonary Langerhans cell histiocytosis (PLCH) is a smoking-related ILD characterized by a proliferation of Langerhans cells (289). It has been called pulmonary histiocytosis X, eosinophilic granuloma, and Langerhans cell granulomatosis in older published literature. In contrast to the childhood LCH that represents a clonal proliferation of neoplastic histiocytes, PLCH is thought to be a complex reactive proliferation characterized by a "nonlethal, nonmalignant clonal evolution of LCH" evolving from monoclonal LCH hyperplasia. Yousem et al. (290) utilized the X-linked polymorphic human androgen receptor assay technique on 24 microdissected nodules from 13 patients and found that seven (29%) were clonal and 17 (71%) were nonclonal. Additional molecular studies support the concept of a reactive process (291). Clinically, PLCH presents with cough and progressive dyspnea in most patients; systemic symptoms of malaise, fever, and weight loss may accompany the respiratory conditions. Most patients have restrictive or mixed restrictive-obstructive defects and reduced diffusing capacity on PFTs. Small (2 to 5 mm) nodules with or without cystic changes in the mid- and upper lung zones are seen on chest HRCT imaging. Microscopically, a host of smoking-related changes are usually observed including centrilobular emphysema and respiratory bronchiolitis along with bronchiolocentric collections of Langerhans cells admixed with eosinophils, lymphocytes, and mast cells (Fig. 31.29). They progress from cellular nodules rich in Langerhans cells to stellate scars to cystic spaces. Reflecting the smoking-related etiology, it is common to see lesions in various stages of development in a VATS biopsy specimen. The classic

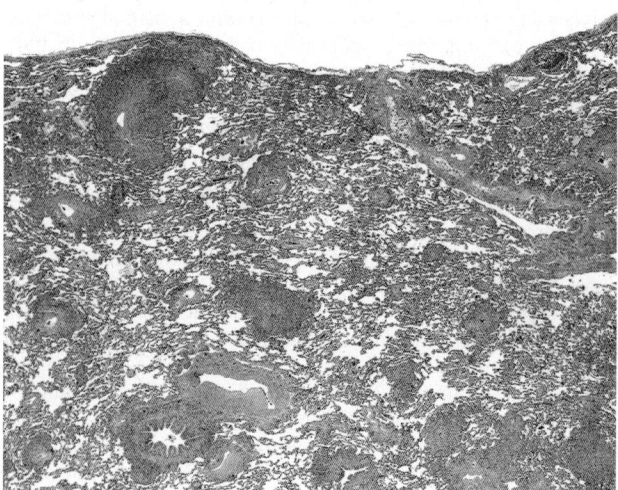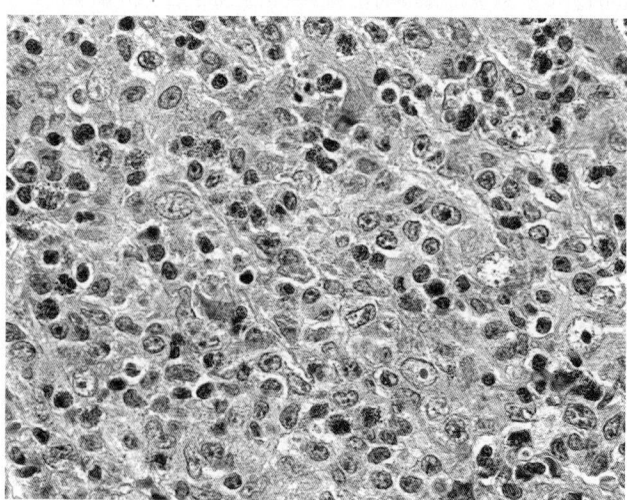

A

B

FIGURE 31.28. Pulmonary involvement by mycosis fungoides. A: Lymphatic distribution along the pleural, interlobular septal lymphatics and around the bronchovascular bundles (H&E, magnification: 80×). **B:** The infiltrates are composed of eosinophils and medium-sized lymphocytes with twisted, cerebriform nuclei typical of MF (H&E, magnification: 600×).

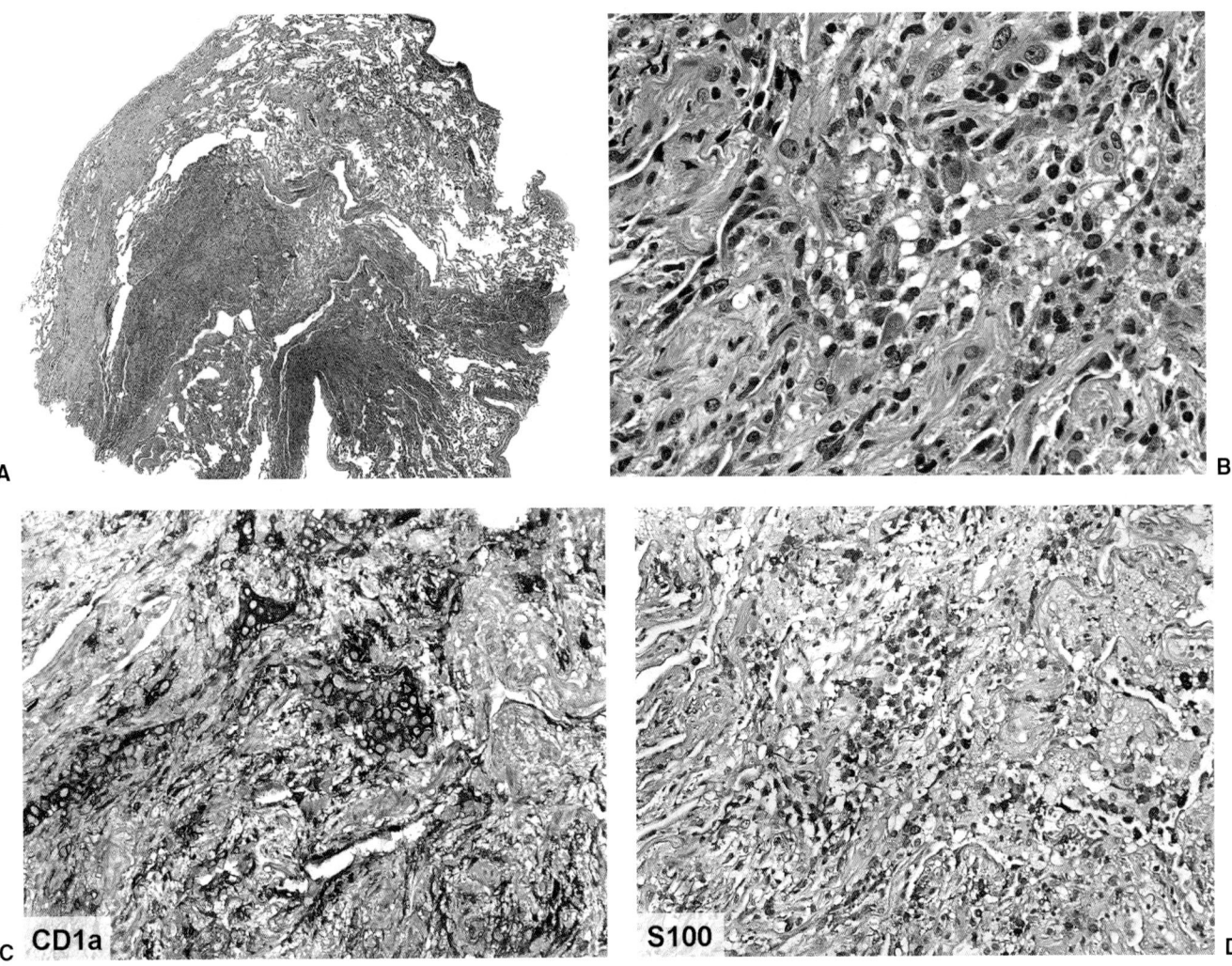

FIGURE 31.29. Pulmonary Langerhans cell histiocytosis. A: VATS biopsy showing bronchiolocentric nodular lesions (H&E, magnification: 15×). **B:** Langerhans cells characterized by oval nuclei with central clefting and abundant eosinophilic to clear cytoplasm are admixed with eosinophils and chronic inflammatory cells (H&E, magnification: 400×). **C,D:** The Langerhans cells stain positively for CD1a (magnification: 300×) and express S100 protein (magnification: 200×).

Langerhans cell displays abundant eosinophilic cytoplasm with central, ovoid nuclei with indentation and grooves, fine chromatin, and inconspicuous nucleoli. They express S100 protein, CD1a, and Langerin (292–294). The primary treatment modality is smoking cessation together with corticosteroids. A subset of patients progress to advanced pulmonary fibrosis requiring lung transplantation; recurrence of PLCH has been reported in this group.

Erdheim-Chester Disease

Erdheim-Chester disease (ECD) is another uncommon pulmonary histiocytic proliferation characterized by the proliferation of non-Langerhans-type histiocytes in the setting of classic osteosclerotic long bone disease. The molecular mechanisms of the disease are unclear, but the clinical behavior ranges from slowly progressive disease to aggressive clinical disease in a limited number of patients. It is thought that the histiocytic cell of origin belongs to the dendritic family. The diagnosis is usually made by the characteristic radiologic findings of symmetrical, bilateral cortical sclerosis of the metaphyseal and diaphyseal regions of the long bones of the extremities. Up to 40% of patients may have pulmonary manifestations

and other extranodal sites of involvement have been reported (295–297). Patients present with signs and symptoms of ILD. Radiographic and CT findings include smooth interlobular septal thickening, centrilobular nodules, ground-glass opacities, thickening of interlobular fissures, pleural thickening or effusions, and parenchymal consolidation (298,299). The histopathologic findings have been described in detail in a number of published reports (295–297). Collections of histiocytes with abundant pale, finely granular eosinophilic or foamy cytoplasm are distributed along lymphatic routes (Fig. 31.30). The histiocytes are admixed with lymphocytes, histiocytes, and Touton-type giant cells and are embedded within variable amounts of fine fibrillary fibrosis. IHC shows strong positivity for CD68 and factor XIIIa and S100 is positive in a subset of cases, but the cells are uniformly negative for the Langerhans cell markers, CD1a, and Langerin.

Rosai-Dorfman Disease

Originally described as sinus histiocytosis with massive lymphadenopathy by Rosai and Dorfman in 1969, Rosai-Dorfman disease (RDD) is a reactive histiocytic proliferation that is encountered in extranodal sites as well (300–302). The lung and

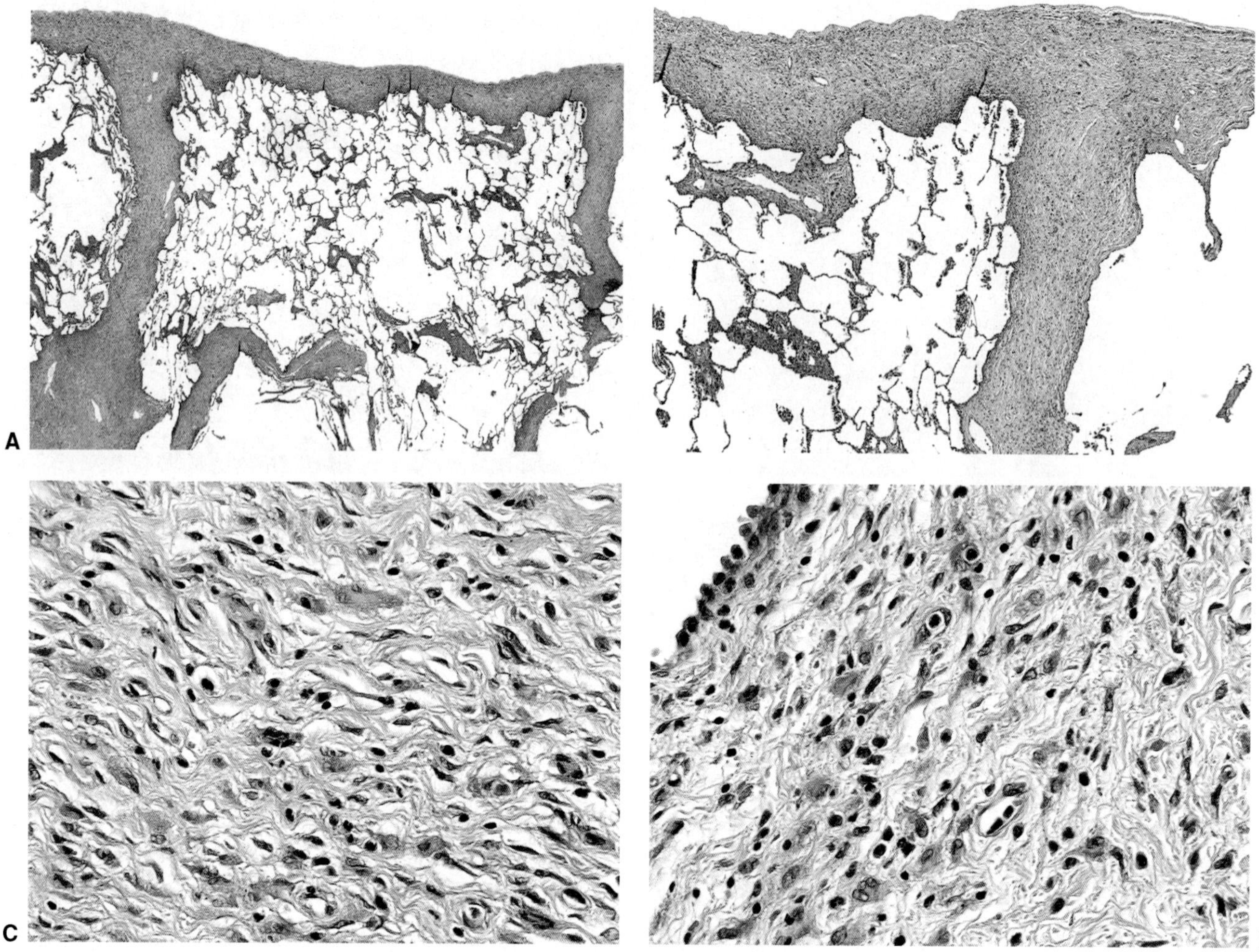

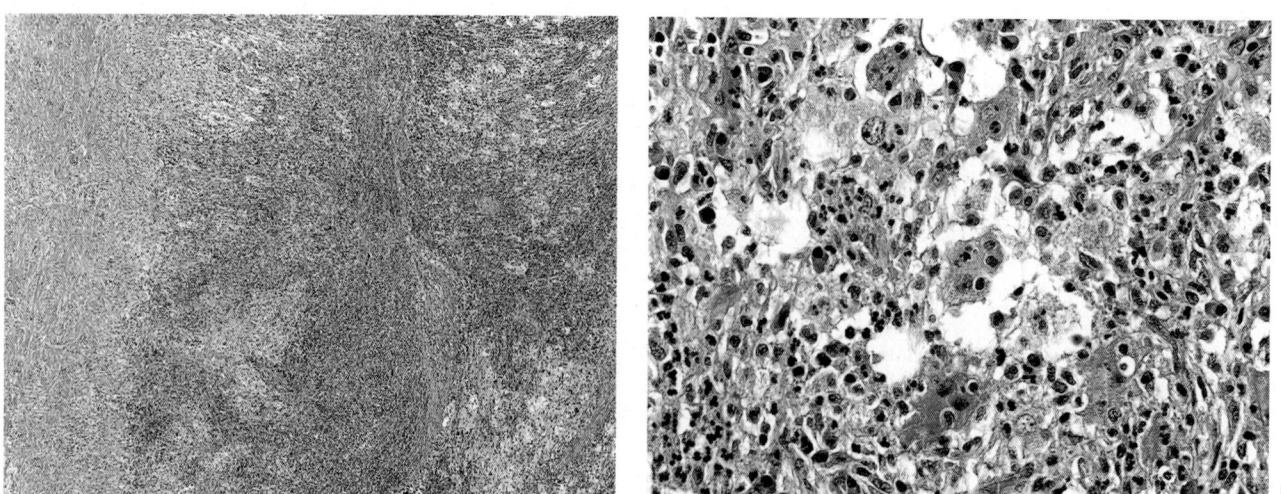

FIGURE 31.30. Pulmonary involvement by Erdheim-Chester disease. A: The lymphatics expanded by a fibroinflammatory process creating thickening of the pleura and interlobular septa (H&E, magnification: 15×). **B:** The alveolar parenchyma is preserved, but there is marked distortion of the pulmonary lymphatic routes (H&E, magnification: 40×). **C,D:** Admixed with fibroblasts, plasma cells and lymphocytes are histiocytes with abundant pale, finely granular cytoplasm (H&E, magnification: 400×).

FIGURE 31.31. Pulmonary involvement by Rosai-Dorfman disease. A: A fibroinflammatory lesion showing numerous histiocytes with abundant clear cytoplasm and chronic inflammatory cells (H&E, magnification: 40×). **B:** Emperipolesis of small lymphocytes within the histiocytes is observed (H&E, magnification: 400×).

pleural (2% to 9% of cases) are not common sites of extranodal involvement, but the clinical presentation in adults and radiologic manifestations mimicking high-stage pulmonary neoplasia warrants discussion. Cartin-Ceba et al. (303) reported mediastinal adenopathy as the predominant thoracic finding in nine patients. Others have described endotracheal or endobronchial mass involving large airways, cystic lung, ILD, air trapping and bronchiectasis, pleural effusion, or parenchymal disease (303–307). A lymphatic distribution is encountered in lung biopsy specimens. The lesion is composed of histiocytic cells with abundant pale cytoplasm and conspicuous emperipolesis of small lymphocytes (Fig. 31.31). These diagnostic cells are admixed with plasma cells and lymphocytes in a background of fibrous connective tissue. The histiocytes are S100[+] and CD68[+], suggesting a mixed macrophage/dendritic lineage. They are CD1a[−], Langerin[−], Factor XIIIa[−], and usually EBV[−] and can be distinguished from PLCH and ECD on the basis of the histopathologic and immunophenotypic findings. Although earlier reports suggested that RDD with extranodal involvement had a more aggressive behavior, recent reports suggest a benign course with benefit from corticosteroid therapy.

SUMMARY AND FUTURE DIRECTIONS

The last decade has witnessed tremendous strides in our understanding of hematolymphoid lesions of the lung and pleura. Molecular analysis has provided clarification and refinement of established inflammatory, reactive, and neoplastic lesions and enumerated the clinicopathologic distinction of others. An understanding of the normal immunologic mechanisms and immunoarchitecture of the lung provides the basis for the macroscopic and microscopic assessment and classification of these processes. Further advances are fully expected in the near future, and the surgical pathologist will continue to play an essential role in this endeavor.

References

1. Cadranel J, Wislez M, Antoine M. Primary pulmonary lymphoma. *Eur Respir J* 2002;20:750–762.
2. Chilosi M, Zinzani PL, Poletti V. Lymphoproliferative lung disorders. *Semin Respir Crit Care Med* 2005;26:490–501.
3. Dillman RO. Cancer immunotherapy. *Cancer Biother Radiopharm* 2011;26:1–64.
4. Merkel O, Hamacker F, Sifft E, et al. Novel therapeutic options in anaplastic large cell lymphoma: molecular targets and immunological tools. *Mol Cancer Ther* 2011;10:1127–1136.
5. Do K-H, Lee JS, Seo JB, et al. Pulmonary parenchymal involvement of low-grade lymphoproliferative disorders. *J Comput Assist Tomogr* 2005;29:825–830.
6. Hare SS, Souza CA, Bain G, et al. The radiological spectrum of pulmonary lymphoproliferative disease. 2012;85:848–864.
7. Swerdlow SH, Campo E, Harris NL, et al. *WHO classification of tumours of haematopoietic and lymphoid tissues*, 4th ed. Lyon: IARC Press, 2008.
8. Bonfiglio TA, Dvoretsky PM, Piscioli F, et al. Fine needle aspiration biopsy in the evaluation of lymphoreticular tumors of the thorax. *Acta Cytol* 1985;29:548–553.
9. Davis WB, Gadek JE. Detection of pulmonary lymphoma by bronchoalveolar lavage. *Chest* 1987;91:787–790.
10. Flint A, Kumar NB, Naylor B. Pulmonary Hodgkin's disease. Diagnosis by fine needle aspiration. *Acta Cytol* 1988;32:221–225.
11. Poletti V, Romagna M, Gasponi A, et al. Bronchoalveolar lavage in the diagnosis of low-grade, MALT type, B-cell lymphoma in the lung. *Monaldi Arch Chest Dis* 1995;50:191–194.
12. Gattuso P, Castelli MJ, Peng Y, et al. Post-transplant lymphoproliferative disorders: a fine needle aspiration study. *Diagn Cytopathol* 1997;16:392–395.
13. Zaer FS, Braylan RC, Zander DS, et al. Multiparametric flow cytometry in the diagnosis and characterization of low-grade pulmonary mucosa-associated lymphoid tissue lymphomas. *Mod Pathol* 1998;11:525–532.
14. Meda BA, Buss DH, Woodruff RD, et al. Diagnosis and subclassification of primary and recurrent lymphoma. The usefulness and limitations of combined fine-needle aspiration cytomorphology and flow cytometry. *Am J Clin Pathol* 2000;113:688–699.
15. Nicol TL, Silberman M, Rosenthal DL, et al. The accuracy of combined cytopathologic and flow cytometric analysis of fine-needle aspirates of lymph nodes. *Am J Clin Pathol* 2000;114:18–28.
16. Ali AE, Morgen EK, Geddie WR, et al. Classifying B-cell non-Hodgkin lymphoma by using MIB-1 proliferative index in fine-needle aspirates. *Cancer Cytopathol* 2010;118:166–172.
17. da Cunha Santos G, Ko HM, Geddie WR, et al. Targeted use of fluorescent in situ hybridization (FISH) in cytospin preparations: results of 298 fine needle aspirates of B-cell non-Hodgkin lymphoma. *Cancer Cytopathol* 2010;118:250–258.
18. Wang Z, Li X, Chen J, et al. Value of computed tomography-guided core needle biopsy in diagnosis of primary pulmonary lymphomas. *J Vasc Interv Radiol* 2013;24:97–102.
19. Herth FJF. Endobronchial and endoesophageal ultrasound techniques. In: Spiro SG, Silvestri GA, Agusti A, eds. *Clinical respiratory medicine*, 4th ed. Philadelphia: Elsevier Saunders, 2012:174–179.
20. Talebian M, von Bartheld MB, Braun J, et al. EUS-FNA in the preoperative staging of non-small cell lung cancer. *Lung Cancer* 2010;69:60–65.
21. Chrissian A, Misselhorn D, Chen A. Endobronchial-ultrasound guided mini-forceps biopsy of mediastinal and hilar lesions. *Ann Thorac Surg* 2011;92:284–289.
22. Khoo K-L, Ho K-Y. Endoscopic mediastinal staging of lung cancer. *Respir Med* 2011;105:515–518.
23. Lee BE, Kletsman E, Rutledge JR, et al. Utility of endobronchial ultrasound–guided mediastinal lymph node biopsy in patients with non–small cell lung cancer. *J Thorac Cardiovasc Surg* 2012;143:585–590.
24. Kennedy M, Jimenez C, Bruzzi J, et al. Endobronchial ultrasound-guided transbronchial needle aspiration in the diagnosis of lymphoma. *Thorax* 2008;63:360–365.
25. Steinfort D, Conron M, Tsui A, et al. Endobronchial ultrasound-guided transbronchial needle aspiration for the evaluation of suspected lymphoma. *J Thorac Oncol* 2010;5:804–809.
26. Ko HM, da Cunha Santos G, Darling G, et al. Diagnosis and subclassification of lymphomas and non-neoplastic lesions involving mediastinal lymph nodes using endobronchial-ultrasound-guided transbronchial needle aspiration. *Diagn Cytopathol* 2011 DOI: 10.1002/dc.21741.
27. Marshall C, Jacob B, Patel S, et al. The utility of endobronchial ultrasound-guided transbronchial needle aspiration biopsy in the diagnosis of mediastinal lymphoproliferative disorders. *Cancer Cytopathol* 2011;119:118–126.
28. Iqbal S, DePew ZS, Kurtin PJ, et al. Endobronchial ultrasound and lymphoproliferative disorders: a retrospective study. *Ann Thorac Surg* 2012;94:1830–1834.
29. Colby TV, Koss MN, Travis WD. Tumors of the lower respiratory tract. *Atlas of Tumor Pathology*, 3rd Series, Fascicle 13. Washington: Armed Forces Institute of Pathology, 1994:419–464.
30. Bienenstock J, Johnston N, Perey DY. Bronchial lymphoid tissue. I. Morphologic characteristics. *Lab Invest* 1973;28:686–692.
31. Bienenstock J. Bronchus-associated lymphoid tissue. *Int Arch Allergy Appl Immunol* 1985;76(Suppl 1):62–69.
32. Bienenstock J, McDermott MR. Bronchus- and nasal-associated lymphoid tissues. *Immunol Rev* 2005;206:22–31.
33. Richmond I, Pritchard GE, Ashcroft T, et al. Bronchus associated lymphoid tissue (BALT) in human lung: its distribution in smokers and non-smokers. *Thorax* 1993;48:1130–1134.
34. Leslie KO, Yousem SA, Colby TV. Lungs. In: Mills SE, ed. *Histology for pathologists*, 4th ed. Philadelphia: Lippincott Williams and Wilkins, 2012:505–529.
35. Swigris JJ, Berry GJ, Raffin TA, et al. Lymphoid interstitial pneumonia: a narrative review. *Chest* 2002;122:2150–2164.
36. Flieder DB, Yousem SA. Pulmonary lymphomas and lymphoid hyperplasias. In: Knowles DM, ed. *Neoplastic hematopathology*. Philadelphia: Lippincott Williams and Wilkins, 2001:1263–1301.
37. Kradin RL, Spirn PW, Mark EJ. Intrapulmonary lymph nodes. Clinical, radiologic, and pathologic features. *Chest* 1985;87(5):662–667.
38. Miyake H, Yamada Y, Kawagoe T, et al. Intrapulmonary lymph nodes: CT and pathological features. *Clin Radiol* 1999;54:640–643.
39. Tsunezuka Y, Sato H, Hiranuma C, et al. Intrapulmonary lymph nodes detected by exploratory video-assisted thoracoscopic surgery: appearance of helical computed tomography. *Ann Thorac Cardiovasc Surg* 2000;6:369–372.
40. Matsuki M, Noma S, Kuroda Y, et al. Thin-section CT features of intrapulmonary lymph nodes. *J Comput Assist Tomogr* 2001;25:753–756.
41. Oshiro Y, Kusumoto M, Moriyama N, et al. Intrapulmonary lymph nodes: thin-section features of 19 nodules. *J Comput Assist Tomogr* 2002;26:553–557.
42. Sykes AMG, Swensen SJ, Tazelaar HD, et al. Computed tomography of intrapulmonary lymph nodes: retrospective comparison with sarcoma metastases. *Mayo Clin Proc* 2002;77:329–333.
43. Hyodo T, Kanazawa S, Dendo S, et al. Intrapulmonary lymph nodes: thin-section CT findings, pathological findings, and CT differential diagnosis from pulmonary metastatic nodules. *Acta Med Okayama* 2004;58:235–240.
44. Shaham D, Vazquez M, Bogot NR, et al. CT features of intrapulmonary lymph nodes confirmed by cytology. *Clin Imaging* 2010;34:185–190.
45. Wang C-W, Teng Y-H, Huang C-C, et al. Intrapulmonary lymph nodes: computed tomography findings with histopathologic correlations. *Clin Imaging* 2013;37:487–492.
46. Saltzstein SL. Pulmonary malignant lymphomas and pseudolymphomas: classification, therapy, and prognosis. *Cancer* 1963;16:928–955.
47. Kradin RL, Mark EJ. Benign lymphoid disorders of the lung, with a theory regarding their development. *Hum Pathol* 1983;14:857–867.
48. Addis BJ, Hyjek E, Isaacson PG. Primary pulmonary lymphoma: a re-appraisal of its histogenesis and its relationship to pseudolymphoma and lymphoid interstitial pneumonia. *Histopathology* 1988;13:1–17.
49. Li G, Hansmann ML, Zwingers T, et al. Primary lymphomas of the lung: morphological, immunohistochemical and clinical features. *Histopathology* 1990;16:519–531.
50. Abbondanzo SL, Rush W, Bijwaard KE, et al. Nodular lymphoid hyperplasia of the lung: a clinicopathologic study of 14 cases. *Am J Surg Pathol* 2000;24:587–597.
51. Travis WD, Galvin JR. Non-neoplastic lymphoid lesions. *Thorax* 2001;56:964–971.
52. Guinee DG. Update on nonneoplastic pulmonary lymphoproliferative disorders and related entities. *Arch Pathol Lab Med* 2010;134:691–701.
53. Yeh CM, Chou C-M, Wong LC. Castleman's disease mimicking intrapulmonary malignancy. *Ann Thorac Surg* 2007;84:e6–e7.
54. Castleman B, Iverson L, Menendex V. Localized mediastinal lymph node hyperplasia resembling thymoma. *Cancer* 1956;9:822–830.
55. Keller AR, Hochholzer L, Castleman B. Hyaline-vascular and plasma-cell types of giant lymph node hyperplasia of the mediastinum and other locations. *Cancer* 1972;29:670–682.
56. Cronin DMP, Warnke RA. Castleman disease: an update on classification and the spectrum of associated lesions. *Adv Anat Pathol* 2009;16:236–246.

57. Gupta NK, Torigian DA, Gefter WB, et al. Mediastinal Castleman disease mimicking mediastinal pulmonary sequestration. *J Thorac Imaging* 2005;20:229–232.
58. Gunluoglu G, Olcmen A, Sokucu SN, et al. Intrapulmonary-located Castleman's disease which was surgically resected without pulmonary resection. *Ann Thorac Cardiovasc Surg* 2011;17:580–583.
59. Madan R, Chen J-H, Trotman-Dickenson B, et al. The spectrum of Castleman's disease: mimics, radiologic pathologic correlation and role of imaging in patient management. *Eur J Radiol* 2012;81:123–131.
60. Reddy MP, Graham MM. FDG positron emission tomographic imaging of thoracic Castleman disease. *Clin Nucl Med* 2003;28:325–326.
61. Frizzera G, Banks PM, Massarelli G, et al. A systemic lymphoproliferative disorder with morphologic features of Castleman's disease: pathologic findings in 15 patients. *Am J Surg Pathol* 1983;7:211–231.
62. Iyonaga K, Ichikado K, Muranaka H, et al. Multicentric Castleman's disease manifesting in the lung: clinical, radiographic and pathologic findings and successful treatment with corticosteroid and cyclophosphamide. *Int Med* 2003;42:182–186.
63. Soulier J, Grollet L, Oksenhendler E, et al. Kaposi's sarcoma-associated herpesvirus-like DNA sequences in multicentric Castleman's disease. *Blood* 1995;86:1276–1280.
64. Uldrick TS, Polizzotto MN, Yarchoan R. Recent advances in Kaposi sarcoma herpesvirus-associated multicentric Castleman disease. *Curr Opin Oncol* 2012;24:495–505.
65. Kirsch CF, Webb EM, Webb WR. Multicentric Castleman's disease and POEMS syndrome: CT findings. *J Thorac Imaging* 1997;12:75–77.
66. Atagi S, Sakatani M, Akira M, et al. Pulmonary hyalinizing granuloma with Castleman's disease. *Int Med* 1994;33:689–691.
67. Guihot A, Couderc LJ, Agbalika F, et al. Pulmonary manifestations of multicentric Castleman's disease in HIV infection: a clinical, biological and radiological study. *Eur Respir J* 2005;26:118–125.
68. Barrie JR, English JC, Muller N. Castleman's disease of the lung: radiographic, high-resolution CT, and pathologic findings. *Am J Roentgenol* 1996;166:1055–1056.
69. Johkoh T, Muller NL, Ichikado K, et al. Intrathoracic multicentric Castleman disease: CT findings in 12 patients. *Radiology* 1998;209:477–481.
70. Dispenzieri A, Gertz MA. Treatment of Castleman's disease. *Curr Treat Options Oncol* 2005;6(3):255–266.
71. Engleman P, Liebow AA, Gmelich J, et al. Pulmonary hyalinizing granuloma. *Am Rev Respir Dis* 1977;115:997–1008.
72. Schlosnagle DC, Check IJ, Sewell CW, et al. Immunologic abnormalities in two patients with pulmonary hyalinizing granuloma. *Am J Clin Pathol* 1982;78:231–235.
73. Chapman EM, Gown A, Mazziotta R, et al. Pulmonary hyalinizing granuloma with associated elevation in serum and tissue IgG4 occurring in a patient with a history of sarcoidosis. *Am J Surg Pathol* 2012;36:774–778.
74. Yousem SA, Hochholzer L. Pulmonary hyalinizing granuloma. *Am J Clin Pathol* 1987;37:91–95.
75. Chalaoui J, Gregoire P, Sylvestre J, et al. Pulmonary hyalinizing Granuloma: a cause of pulmonary nodules. *Radiology* 1984;152:23–26.
76. Patel Y, Ishikawa S, MacDonnell KF. Pulmonary hyalinizing granuloma presenting as multiple cavitary calcified nodules. *Chest* 1991;100:1720–1721.
77. Shibata Y, Kobayashi T, Hattori Y, et al. High resolution CT findings in pulmonary hyalinizing granuloma. *J Thorac Imaging* 2007;22:374–377.
78. Fujishima N, Takada T, Moriyama H, et al. Pulmonary hyalinizing granuloma with massive infiltration of lymphocytes. *Nihon Kokyuki Gakkai Zasshi* 2001;39:924–929.
79. Kihara Y, Koizumi N, Sakai K, et al. Pulmonary hyalinizing granuloma. *Gazoushindan* 2000;20:1322–1323.
80. Zen Y, Kitagawa S, Minato H, et al. IgG4-positive plasma cells in inflammatory pseudotumor (plasma cell granuloma) of the lung. *Hum Pathol* 2005;36:710–717.
81. Yamashita K, Haga H, Kobashi Y, et al. Lung involvement in IgG4-related lymphoplasmacytic vasculitis and interstitial fibrosis: report of 3 cases and review of the literature. *Am J Surg Pathol* 2008;32:1620–1626.
82. Shrestha B, Sekiguchu H, Colby TV, et al. Distinctive pulmonary histopathology with increased IgG4-positive plasma cells in patients with autoimmune pancreatitis: report of 6 and 12 cases with similar histopathology. *Am J Surg Pathol* 2009;33:1450–1462.
83. Zen Y, Inoue D, Kitao A, et al. IgG4-related lung and pleural disease: a clinicopathologic study of 21 cases. *Am J Surg Pathol* 2009;33:1886–1893.
84. Cheuk W, Chan JKC. IgG4-related sclerosing disease: a critical appraisal of an evolving clinicopathologic entity. *Adv Anat Pathol* 2010;17:303–332.
85. Stone JH, Zen Y, Deshpande V. IgG4-related disease. *N Engl J Med* 2012;366:539–551.
86. Travis WD, Brambilla E, Muller-Hermelink HK, et al. WHO Classification of Tumours. *Pathology and genetics of tumours of the lung, pleura, thymus and heart*. Lyon: IARC Press, 2004:105–106.
87. Kotoulas C, Konstantinou M, Fotinou M, et al. Inflammatory pseudotumor of the lung: our experience. *Pneumonology* 2006;19:54–58.
88. Kakitsubata Y, Theodorou SJ, Theodorou DJ, et al. Myofibroblastic inflammatory tumor of the lung: CT findings with pathologic correlation. *Comput Med Imaging Graph* 2007;31:607–613.
89. Kim TS, Han J, Kim GY, et al. Pulmonary inflammatory pseudotumor (inflammatory myofibroblastic tumor): CT features with pathologic correlation. *J Comput Assist Tomogr* 2005;29:633–639.
90. Fornell-Perez R, Santana-Montesdeoca JM, Garcia-Villar C, et al. Two types of presentation of pulmonary inflammatory pseudotumors. *Arch Bronconeumol* 2012;48:296–299.
91. Matsubara O, Tan-Liu NS, Kenney RM, et al. Inflammatory pseudotumors of the lung: progression from organizing pneumonia to fibrous histiocytoma or to plasma cell granuloma in 32 cases. *Hum Pathol* 1988;19:807–814.
92. Gal AA, Koss MN, McCarthy WF, et al. Prognostic factors in pulmonary fibrohistiocytic lesions. *Cancer* 1994;73:1817–1824.
93. Coffin CM, Dehner LP, Meis-Kindblom JM. Inflammatory myofibroblastic tumor, inflammatory fibrosarcoma, and related lesions: an historical review with differential diagnostic considerations. *Semin Diagn Pathol* 1998;15:102–110.
94. Moran CA, Suster S. Unusual non-neoplastic lesions of the lung. *Sem Diag Pathol* 2007;24:199–208.
95. Snyder CS, Dell'Aquila M, Haghighi P, et al. Clonal changes in inflammatory pseudotumor of the lung: a case report. *Cancer* 1995;76:1545–1549.
96. Yousem SA, Shaw H, Cieply K. Involvement of 2p23 in pulmonary inflammatory pseudotumors. *Hum Pathol* 2001;32:428–433.
97. Gomez-Roman JJ, Sanchez-Velazco P, Ocejo-Vinyals G, et al. Human herpesvirus-8 genes expressed in pulmonary inflammatory myofibroblastic tumor (inflammatory pseudotumor). *Am J Surg Pathol* 2001;25:624–629.
98. Alaggio R, Cecchetto G, Bisogno G, et al. Inflammatory myofibroblastic tumors in childhood: a report from the Italian Cooperative Group studies. *Cancer* 2010;116:216–226.
99. Nicholson AG, Wotherspoon AC, Diss TC, et al. Reactive pulmonary lymphoid disorders. *Histopathology* 1995;26:405–412.
100. Terada T. Follicular bronchiolitis and lymphocytic interstitial pneumonia in a Japanese man. *Diag Pathol* 2011;6:85–89.
101. Masuda T, Ishikawa Y, Akasaka Y, et al. Follicular bronchiolitis (FBB) associated with *Legionella pneumophilia* infection. *Ped Pathol Mol Med* 2002;21:517–524.
102. Shimizu K, Konno S, Nashuhara Y, et al. A case of follicular bronchiolitis associated with asthma, eosinophilia, and increased immunoglobulin E. *J Asthma* 2010;47:1161–1164.
103. Yousem SA, Colby TV, Carrington CB. Follicular bronchitis/bronchiolitis. *Hum Pathol* 1985;16:700–706.
104. Sato A, Hayakawa H, Uchiyama H, et al. Cellular distribution of bronchus-associated lymphoid tissue in rheumatoid arthritis. *Am J Respir Crit Care Med* 1996;154:1903–1907.
105. Hayakawa H, Sato A, Imokawa S, et al. Bronchiolar disease in rheumatoid arthritis. *Am J Respir Crit Care Med* 1996;154:1531–1536.
106. Romero S, Barroso E, Gil J, et al. Follicular bronchiolitis: clinical and pathologic findings in six patients. *Lung* 2003;181:309–319.
107. Theron S, Goussard P. Follicular bronchiolitis in an HIV-positive child. *Pediatr Radiol* 2008;38:1031.
108. Vos R, Vanaudenaerde BM, De Vleeschauwer SI, et al. Follicular bronchiolitis: a rare cause of bronchiolitis obliterans syndrome after lung transplantation: a case report. *Am J Transplant* 2009;9:644–650.
109. Larsen BT, Vaszar L, Colby TV, et al. Lymphoid hyperplasia and eosinophilic pneumonia as histologic manifestations of amiodarone lung toxicity. *Am J Surg Pathol* 2012;36:509–516.
110. Howling SJ, Hansell DM, Wells AU, et al. Follicular bronchiolitis: thin-section CT and histology findings. *Radiology* 1999;212:637–642.
111. Kang E-Y, Woo OH, Shin BK, et al. Bronchiolitis: classification, computed tomographic and histopathologic features, and radiologic approach. *J Comput Assist Tomogr* 2009;33:32–41.
112. Liebow AA, Carrington CB. The interstitial pneumonia. In: Simon M, Potchen EJ, LeMay M, eds. *Frontiers of pulmonary radiology: pathophysiologic, roentgenographic and radioisotpic considerations: proceedings of the symposium sponsored by Harvard Medical School, April 21–22, 1967*, 1st ed. New York: Grune & Stratton, 1969:102–141.
113. American Thoracic Society; European Respiratory Society. American Thoracic Society/European Respiratory Society international multidisciplinary consensus classification of the idiopathic interstitial pneumonias. *Am J Respir Crit Care Med* 2002;165:277–304.
114. Larsen BT, Colby TV. Update for pathologists on idiopathic interstitial pneumonias. *Arch Pathol Lab Med* 2012;136:1234–1241.
115. Cha S-I, Fessler MB, Cool CD, et al. Lymphoid interstitial pneumonia: clinical features, associations and prognosis. *Eur Respir J* 2006;28:364–369.
116. Nicholson AG, Lymphocytic interstitial pneumonia and other lymphoproliferative disorders in the lung. *Semin Respir Crit Care Med* 2001;22:409–422.
117. Takato H, Yasui M, Ichikawa Y, et al. Nonspecific interstitial pneumonia with abundant IgG4-positive cells infiltration, which was thought as pulmonary involvement of IgG4-related autoimmune disease. *Intern Med* 2008;47:291–294.
118. Thieblemont C, Berger F, Dumontet C, et al. Mucosa-associated lymphoid tissue lymphoma is a disseminated disease in one third of 158 patients analyzed. *Blood* 2000;95:802–806.
119. L'Hoste RJ, Filippa DA, Lieberman PH, et al. Primary pulmonary lymphomas: a clinicopathologic analysis of 36 cases. *Cancer* 1984;54:1397–1406.
120. Cordier JF, Chailleux E, Lauque D, et al. Primary pulmonary lymphoma: a clinical study of 70 cases in nonimmunocompromised patients. *Chest* 1993;103:201–208.
121. Ferraro P, Trastek VF, Adlakha H, et al. Primary non-Hodgkin's lymphoma of the lung. *Ann Thorac Surg* 2000;69:993–997.
122. Graham BB, Mathisen DJ, Mark EJ, et al. Primary pulmonary lymphoma. *Ann Thorac Surg* 2005;80:1248–1253.
123. Hu YH, Hsiao LT, Yang CF, et al. Prognostic factors of Chinese patients with primary pulmonary non-Hodgkin's lymphoma: the single-institute experience in Taiwan. *Ann Hematol* 2009;88:839–846.
124. Parissis H. Forty years literature review of primary lung lymphoma. *J Cardiothorac Surg* 2011;6:23–32.
125. Kurtin PJ, Myers JL, Adlakha H, et al. Pathologic and clinical features of primary pulmonary extranodal marginal zone B-cell lymphoma of MALT type. *Am J Surg Pathol* 2001;25:997–1008.
126. Isaacson PG, Chott, Nakamura S, et al. Extranodal marginal zone lymphoma of mucosa-associated lymphoid tissue (MALT lymphoma). In: Swerdlow SH, Campo E, Harris NL, et al., eds. *WHO classification of tumours of haematopoietic and lymphoid tissues*, 4th ed. Lyon: IARC Press, 2008:214–219.
127. Freeman C, Berg JW, Cutler SJ. Occurrence and prognosis of extranodal lymphomas. *Cancer* 1972;29:252–260.
128. Wotherspoon AC, Ortiz-Hidalgo C, Falzon MR, et al. *Helicobacter pylori*-associated gastritis and primary B-cell gastric lymphoma. *Lancet* 1991;338:1175–1176.
129. Hermine O, Lefrere F, Bronowicki JP, et al. Regression of splenic lymphoma with villous lymphocytes after treatment of hepatitis C virus infection. *N Engl J Med* 2002;347:89–94.
130. Ferreri AJ, Guidoboni M, Ponzoni M, et al. Evidence for an association between *Chlamydia psittaci* and ocular adnexal lymphomas. *J Natl Cancer Inst* 2004;96:586–594.
131. Lecuit M, Abachin E, Martin A, et al. Immunoproliferative small intestinal disease associated with *Campylobacter jejuni*. *N Engl J Med* 2004;350:239–248.
132. Ahmed S, Kussick SJ, Siddiqui AK, et al. Bronchial-associated lymphoid tissue lymphoma: a study of a rare disease. *Eur J Cancer* 2004;40:1320–1326.
133. Farinha P, Gascoyne RD. Molecular pathogenesis of mucosa-associated lymphoid tissue lymphoma. *J Clin Oncol* 2005;23:6370–6378.

134. Bertoni F, Zucca E. Delving deeper into MALT lymphoma biology. *J Clin Invest* 2006;116:22–26.
135. Karin M. Nuclear factor-kB in cancer development and progression. *Nature* 2006;441:431–436.
136. Chng WJ, Remstein ED, Fonseca R, et al. Gene expression profiling of pulmonary mucosa-associated lymphoid tissue lymphoma identifies new biologic insights with potential diagnostic and therapeutic applications. *Blood* 2009;113:635–645.
137. Borie R, Wislez M, Thabut G, et al. Clinical characteristics and prognostic factors of pulmonary MALT lymphoma. *Eur Respir J* 2009;34:1408–1416.
138. Imai H, Sunaga N, Kaira K, et al. Clinicopathological features of patients with bronchial-associated lymphoid tissue lymphoma. *Intern Med* 2009;48:301–306.
139. Ogusa E, Tomita N, Takasaki H, et al. Clinical manifestations of primary pulmonary extranodal marginal zone lymphoma of mucosa-associated lymphoid tissue in Japanese population. *Hematol Oncol* 2013;31:18–21.
140. Konoplev S, Lin P, Qiu X, et al. Clonal relationship of extranodal marginal zone lymphomas of mucosa-associated lymphoid tissue involving different sites. *Am J Clin Pathol* 2010;134:112–118.
141. King LJ, Padley SP, Wotherspoon AC, et al. Pulmonary MALT lymphoma: imaging findings in 24 cases. *Eur Radiol* 2000;10:1932–1938.
142. Nicholson AG, Wotherspoon AC, Diss TC, et al. Pulmonary B-cell non-Hodgkin's lymphoma. The value of immunohistochemistry and gene analysis in diagnosis. *Histopathology* 1995;26:395–403.
143. Koss M, Zeren EH. Low grade B-cell lymphomas of lung and lymphomatoid granulomatosis. *Pathology (Phila)* 1996;4:125–139.
144. Bacon CM, Du MQ, Dogan A. Mucosa-associated lymphoid tissue (MALT) lymphoma: a practical guide for pathologists. *J Clin Pathol* 2007;60:361–372.
145. Koss MN, Hochholzer L, Nichols PW, et al. Primary non-Hodgkin's lymphoma and pseudolymphoma of lung: a study of 161 patients. *Hum Pathol* 1983;14: 1024–1028.
146. Perry L, Florio R, Dewar A, et al. Giant lamellar bodies as a feature of pulmonary low-grade MALT lymphomas. *Histopathology* 2000;36:240–244.
147. Nakamura N, Yamada G, Itoh T, et al. Pulmonary MALT lymphoma with amyloid production in a patient with primary Sjögren's syndrome. *Intern Med* 2002;41:309–311.
148. Fairweather PM, Williamson R, Tsikleas G. Pulmonary extranodal marginal zone lymphoma with massive crystal storing histiocytosis. *Am J Surg Pathol* 2006;30:262–267.
149. Grogg KL, Aubry MC, Vrana JA, et al. Nodular pulmonary amyloidosis is characterized by localized immunoglobulin deposition and is frequently associated with an indolent B-cell lymphoproliferative disorder. *Am J Surg Pathol* 2013;37: 406–412.
150. Rao DS, Said JW. Small lymphoid proliferations in extranodal locations. *Arch Pathol Lab Med* 2007;131:383–396.
151. Attygalle AD, Liu H, Shirali S, et al. Atypical marginal zone hyperplasia of mucosa-associated lymphoid tissue: a reactive condition of childhood showing immunoglobulin lambda light-chain restriction. *Blood* 2004;104:3343–3348.
152. Troch M, Kiesewetter B, Raderer. Recent developments in nongastric mucosa-associated lymphoid tissue lymphoma. *Curr Hematol Malig Rep* 2011;6:216–221.
153. Zinzani PL, Pellegrini C, Gandolfi L, et al. Extranodal marginal zone B-cell lymphoma of the lung: experience with fludarabine and mitoxantrone-containing regimens. *Hematol Oncol* 2012. Epub ahead of print.
154. Stein H, Warnke RA, Jaffe ES, et al. Diffuse large B-cell lymphoma, not otherwise specified. In: Swerdlow SH, Campo E, Harris NL, et al., eds. *WHO classification of tumours of haematopoietic and lymphoid tissues*, 4th ed. Lyon: IARC Press, 2008:233–237.
155. Hans CP, Weisenburger DD, Greiner TC, et al. Confirmation of the molecular classification of diffuse large B-cell lymphoma by immunohistochemistry using a tissue microarray. *Blood* 2004;103:275–282.
156. Gleissner B, Kuppers R, Siebert R, et al. Report of a workshop on malignant lymphoma: a review of molecular and clinical risk profiling. *Br J Haematol* 2008;142:166–178.
157. Choi WW, Weisenburger DD, Greiner TC, et al. A new immunostain algorithm classifies diffuse large B-cell lymphoma into molecular subtypes with high accuracy. *Clin Cancer Res* 2009;15:5494–5502.
158. Meyer PN, Fu K, Greiner TC, et al. Immunohistochemical methods for predicting cell of origin and survival in patients with diffuse large B-cell lymphoma treated with rituximab. *J Clin Oncol* 2011;29:200–207.
159. Salles G, de Jong D, Xie W, et al. Prognostic significance of immunohistochemical biomarkers in diffuse large B-cell lymphoma: a study from the Lunenburg Lymphoma Biomarker Consortium. *Blood* 2011;117:7070–7078.
160. Jaffe ES, Pittaluga S. Aggressive B-cell lymphomas: a review of new and old entities in the WHO classification. *Hematology Am Soc Hematol Educ Program* 2011;2011:506–514.
161. Weiss LM, Yousem SA, Warnke RA. Non-Hodgkin's lymphomas of the lung. A study of 19 cases emphasizing the utility of frozen section immunologic studies in differential diagnosis. *Am J Surg Pathol* 1985;9:480–490.
162. Solomonov A, Zuckerman T, Goralnik L, et al. Non-Hodgkin's lymphoma presenting as an endobronchial tumor: report of eight cases and literature review. *Am J Hematol* 2008;83:416–419.
163. Neri N, Nambo MJ, Aviles A. Diffuse large B-cell lymphoma primary of lung. *Hematology* 2011;16:110–112.
164. Liebow AA, Carrington CB, Friedman PJ. Lymphomatoid granulomatosis. *Cancer* 1972;3:457–558.
165. Roschewski M. Wilson WH. Lymphomatoid granulomatosis. *Cancer J* 2012;18: 469–474.
166. Pittaluga S, Wilson WH, Jaffe ES. Lymphomatoid granulomatosis. In: Swerdlow SH, Campo E, Harris NL, et al., eds. *WHO classification of tumours of haematopoietic and lymphoid tissues*, 4th ed. Lyon: IARC Press, 2008:247–249.
167. Wilson WH, Kingma DW, Raffeld M, et al. Association of lymphomatoid granulomatosis with Epstein-Barr viral infection of B lymphocytes and response to interferon-alpha 2b. *Blood* 1996;87:4531–4537.
168. Katzenstein A-LA, Doxtader E, Narendra S. Lymphomatoid granulomatosis: insights gained over 4 decades. *Am J Surg Pathol* 2010;34:e35–e48.
169. McCloskey M, Catherwood M, McManus D, et al. A case of lymphomatoid granulomatosis masquerading as a lung abscess. *Thorax* 2004;59:818–819.
170. Makol A, Kosuri K, Tamkus D, et al. Lymphomatoid granulomatosis masquerading as an interstitial pneumonia in a 66-year-old man: a case report and review of the literature. *J Hematol Oncol* 2009;2:39–44.
171. Wu SM, Min Y, Ostrzega N, et al. Lymphomatoid granulomatosis: a rare mimicker of vasculitis. *J Rheumatol* 2005;32:2242–2245.
172. Braham E, Ayadi-Kaddour A, Smati B, et al. Lymphomatoid granulomatosis mimicking interstitial lung disease. *Respirology* 2008;13:1085–1087.
173. Bartosik W, Raza A, Kalimuthu S, et al. Pulmonary lymphomatoid granulomatosis mimicking lung cancer. *Interact Cardiovasc Thorac Surg* 2012;14:662–624.
174. Dee PM, Arora NS, Innes DJ Jr. The pulmonary manifestations of lymphomatoid granulomatosis. *Radiology* 1982;143:613–618.
175. Lee JS, Tuder R, Lynch DA. Lymphomatoid granulomatosis: radiologic features and pathologic correlation. *AJR Am J Roentgenol* 2000;175:1335–1339.
176. Chung JH, Wu CC, Gilman WD, et al. Lymphomatoid granulomatosis: CT and FDG-PET findings. *Korean J Radiol* 2011;12:671–678.
177. Katzenstein A-LA, Carrington CB, Liebow AA. Lymphomatoid granulomatosis: a clinicopathologic study of 152 cases. *Cancer* 1979;43:360–373.
178. Koss MN, Hochholzer L, Langloss JM, et al. Lymphomatoid granulomatosis: a clinicopathologic study of 42 patients. *Pathology* 1986;18:283–288.
179. Nicholson AG, Wotherspoon AC, Diss TC, et al. Lymphomatoid granulomatosis: evidence that some cases represent Epstein-Barr virus-associated B-cell lymphoma. *Histopathology* 1996;29:317–324.
180. Morice WG, Kurtin PJ, Myers JL. Expression of cytolytic lymphocyte-associated antigens in pulmonary lymphomatoid granulomatosis. *Am J Clin Pathol* 2002;118:391–398.
181. Katzenstein A-LA, Peiper SC. Detection of Epstein-Barr virus genomes in lymphomatoid granulomatosis: analysis of 29 cases by the polymerase chain reaction technique. *Mod Pathol* 1990;3:435–441.
182. Myers JL, Kurtin PJ, Katzenstein A-LA, et al. Lymphomatoid granulomatosis. Evidence of immunophenotypic diversity and relationship to Epstein-Barr virus infection. *Am J Surg Pathol* 1995;19:1300–1312.
183. Guinee D Jr, Jaffe E, Kingma D, et al. Pulmonary lymphomatoid granulomatosis. Evidence for a proliferation of Epstein-Barr virus infected B-lymphocytes with a prominent T-cell component and vasculitis. *Am J Surg Pathol* 1994;18:753–764.
184. Taniere PH, Thivolet-Bejui F, Vitrey D, et al. Lymphomatoid granulomatosis: a report on four cases: evidence for B phenotype of the tumoral cells. *Eur Respir J* 1998;12:102–106.
185. Lipford EH, Margolick JB, Longo DL, et al. Angiocentric immunoproliferative lesions: a clinicopathologic spectrum of postthymic T-cell proliferations. *Blood* 1988;72:1674–1681.
186. Colby TV. Current histological diagnosis of lymphomatoid granulomatosis. *Mod Pathol* 2012;25:S39–S42.
187. Miyashita T, Yoshioka K, Nakamura T, et al. A case of lymphomatoid granulomatosis-like lung lesions with abundant infiltrating IgG4-positive plasma cells whose serum IgG4 levels became higher following the start of corticosteroid therapy. *Intern Med* 2010;49:2007–2011.
188. Nakamura S, Jaffe ES, Swerdlow SH. EBV positive diffuse large B-cell lymphoma of the elderly. In: Swerdlow SH, Campo E, Harris NL, et al., eds. *WHO classification of tumours of haematopoietic and lymphoid tissues*, 4th ed. Lyon: IARC Press, 2008:243–244.
189. Shimoyama Y, Oyama T, Asano N, et al. Senile EBV+ B-cell lymphoproliferative disorders: a clinicopathologic study of 22 patients. *J Clin Exp Hematop* 2006; 46:1–4.
190. Oyama T, Ichimura K, Suzuki R, et al. Senile EBV+ B-cell lymphoproliferative disorders: a clinicopathologic study of 22 patients. *Am J Surg Pathol* 2003;27:16–26.
191. Oyama T, Yamamoto K, Asano N, et al. Age-related EBV-associated B-cell lymphoproliferative disorders constitute a distinct clinicopathologic group: a study of 96 patients. *Clin Cancer Res* 2007;13:5124–5132.
192. Asano N, Yamamoto K, Tamaru J, et al. Age-related Epstein-Barr virus (EBV)-associated B-cell lymphoproliferative disorders: comparison with EBV-positive classic Hodgkin lymphoma in elderly patients. *Blood* 2009;113:2629–2636.
193. Dojcinov SD, Venkataraman G, Pittaluga S, et al. Age-related EBV-associated lymphoproliferative disorders in the Western population: a spectrum of reactive lymphoid hyperplasia and lymphoma. *Blood* 2011;117:4726–4735.
194. Iuchi K, Ichimiya A, Akashi A, et al. Non-Hodgkin's lymphoma of the pleural cavity developing from long-standing pyothorax. *Cancer* 1987;60:1771–1775.
195. Martin A, Capron F, Lignory-Brunaud MD, et al. Epstein-Barr virus-associated primary lymphomas of the pleural cavity occurring in longstanding pleural chronic inflammation. *Hum Pathol* 1994;25:1314–1318.
196. Molinie V, Pouchot J, Navratil E, et al. Primary Epstein-Barr virus-related non-Hodgkin's lymphoma of the pleural cavity following long-standing tuberculous emphysema. *Arch Pathol Lab Med* 1996;120:288–291.
197. Petitjean B, Jardin F, Joly B, et al. Pyothorax-associated lymphoma. A peculiar clinicopathologic entity derived from B cells at late stage of differentiation and with occasional aberrant dual B- and T-cell phenotype. *Am J Surg Pathol* 2002;26:724–732.
198. Androulaki A, Drakos E, Hatzianastassiou D, et al. Pyothorax-associated lymphoma (PAL): a western case with marked angiocentricity and review of the literature. *Histopathology* 2004;44:69–76.
199. Saint-Blancard P, Harket A, Defuentes G, et al. Primary pleural lymphoma: a late complication of pleural decortication for tuberculosis: two cases in western countries. *Rev Pneumol Clin* 2007;63:277–281.
200. Nakatsuka S, Yao M, Hoshida Y, et al. Pyothorax-associated lymphoma: a review of 106 cases. *J Clin Oncol* 2002;20:4255–4260.
201. Aozasa K. Pyothorax-associated lymphoma. *J Clin Exp Hematop* 2006;46:5–10.
202. Swerdlow SH, Webber SA, Chadburn A, et al. Post-transplant lymphoproliferative disorders. In: Swerdlow SH, Campo E, Harris NL, et al., eds. *WHO classification of tumours of haematopoietic and lymphoid tissues*, 4th ed. Lyon: IARC Press, 2008:343–349.
203. Wudhikarn K, Holman CJ, Linan M, et al. Post-transplant lymphoproliferative disorders in lung transplant recipients: 20-yr experience at the University of Minnesota. *Clin Transplant* 2011;25:705–713. DOI: 10.1111/j.1399–0012.2010.01332.x
204. Yousem SA, Randhawa P, Locker J, et al. Posttransplant lymphoproliferative disorders in heart-lung transplant recipients: Primary presentation in the allograft. *Hum Pathol* 1989;20:361–369.
205. Walker RC, Paya CV, Marshall WF, et al. Pretransplantation seronegative Epstein–Barr virus status is the primary risk factor for posttransplantation lymphoproliferative disorder in adult heart, lung, and other solid organ transplantations. *J Heart Lung Transplant* 1995;14:214–221.
206. Walker RC, Marshall WF, Strickler JG, et al. Pretransplantation assessment of the risk of lymphoproliferative disorder. *Clin Infect Dis* 1995;20:1346–1353.

207. Knight JS, Tsodikov A, Cibrik DM, et al. Lymphoma after solid organ transplantation: risk, response to therapy, and survival at a transplantation center. *J Clin Oncol* 2009;27:3354–3362.
208. Perrine SP, Hermine O, Small T, et al. A phase I/II trial of arginine butyrate and ganciclovir in patients with Epstein-Barr-virus-associated lymphoid malignancies. *Blood* 2007;109:2571–2578.
209. DiNardo CD, Tsai DE. Treatment advances in posttransplant lymphoproliferative disease. *Curr Opin Hematol* 2010;17:368–374.
210. Haque T, Wilkie GM, Jones MM, et al. Allogeneic cytotoxic T-cell therapy for EBV-positive posttransplantation lymphoproliferative disease: results of a phase 2 multicenter clinical trial. *Blood* 2007;110:1123–1131.
211. Rosendale B, Yousem SA. Discrimination of Epstein-Barr virus-related posttransplant lymphoproliferations from acute rejection in lung allograft recipients. *Arch Pathol Lab Med* 1995;119:418–423.
212. Ferreri AJM, Campo E, Seymour JF. Intravascular lymphoma: clinical presentation, natural history, management and prognostic factors in a series of 38 cases with special emphasis on the 'cutaneous variant'. *Br J Haematol* 2004;127: 173–183.
213. Murase T, Yamaguchi M, Suzuki R, et al. Intravascular large B-cell lymphoma (IVLBCL): a clinicopathologic study of 96 cases with special reference to the immunophenotypic heterogeneity of CD5. *Blood* 2007;109:478–485.
214. Ponzoni M, Ferreri AJM, Campo E, et al. Definition, diagnosis, and management of intravascular large B-cell lymphoma: proposals and perspectives from an international consensus meeting. *J Clin Oncol* 2007;25:3168–3178.
215. Fujiwara A, Azuma T, Yamanouchi J, et al. Intravascular large B-cell lymphoma presenting as interstitial lung disease. *Nihon Naika Gakkai Zasshi* 2007;96: 2783–2785.
216. Kotake T, Kosugi S, Takimoto T, et al. Intravascular large B-cell lymphoma presenting as pulmonary arterial hypertension as an initial manifestation. *Intern Med* 2010;49:51–54.
217. Kaku N, Seki M, Doi S, et al. A case of intravascular large B-cell lymphoma (IVLBCL) with no abnormal findings on chest computed tomography diagnosed by random transbronchial lung biopsy. *Intern Med* 2010;49:2697–2701.
218. Yu H, Chen G, Zhang R, et al. Primary intravascular large B-cell lymphoma of lung: a report of one case and review. *Pathology* 2012;7:70–74.
219. Shinoda H, Maejima A, Shimizu K. A case of intravascular lymphoma with diffuse centrilobular opacities. *Nihon Kokyuki Gakkai Zasshi* 2010;48(1):76–80.
220. Yamashita H, Suzuki A, Takahashi Y, et al. Intravascular large B-cell lymphoma with diffuse FDG uptake in the lung by ^{18}FDG-PET/CT without chest CT findings. *Ann Nucl Med* 2012;26:515–521.
221. Wick MR, Mills SE, Scheithauer BW, et al. Malignant "angioendotheliomatosis": Evidence in favor of its reclassification as "intravascular lymphomatosis." *Am J Surg Pathol* 1986;10:112–123.
222. Yousem SA, Colby TV. Intravascular lymphomatosis presenting in the lung. *Cancer* 1990;65:349–353.
223. Jalkanen S, Aho R, Kallajoki M, et al. Lymphocyte homing receptors and adhesion molecules in intravascular malignant lymphomatosis. *Int J Cancer* 1989;44: 777–782.
224. Ponzoni M, Arrigoni G, Gould VE, et al. Lack of CD29 (beta 1 integrin) and CD54 (ICAM-1) adhesion molecules in intravascular lymphomatosis. *Hum Pathol* 2000;31:220–226.
225. Kato M, Ohshima K, Mizuno M, et al. Analysis of CXCL9 and CXCR3 expression in a case of intravascular large B-cell lymphoma. *J Am Acad Dermatol* 2009;61:888–891.
226. Colby TV, Hoppe RT, Warnke R. Hodgkin's disease at autopsy: 1972–1977. *Cancer* 1981;47:1852–1862.
227. Yousem SA, Weiss LM, Colby TV. Primary pulmonary Hodgkin's disease: a clinicopathologic study of 15 patients. *Cancer* 1986;57:1217–1224.
228. Radin AI. Primary pulmonary Hodgkin's disease. *Cancer* 1990;65:550–563.
229. Berkman N, Breuer R, Kramer MR, et al. Pulmonary involvement in lymphoma. *Leuk Lymphoma* 1996;20:229–237.
230. Costa MBG, Siqueira SAC, Saldiva PHN, et al. Histologic patterns of lung infiltration of B-cell. T-cell and Hodgkin lymphomas. *Am J Clin Pathol* 2004;121: 718–726.
231. Rodriguez J, Tirabosco R, Pizzolitto S, et al. Hodgkin lymphoma presenting with exclusive or preponderant pulmonary involvement: a clinicopathologic study of 5 new cases. *Ann Diagn Pathol* 2006;10:83–88.
232. Cartier Y, Johkoh T, Honda O, et al. Primary pulmonary Hodgkin's disease: Ct findings in three patients. *Clin Radiol* 1999;54:182–184.
233. Trédaniel J, Peillon I, Fermé C, et al. Endobronchial presentation of Hodgkin's disease: a report of nine cases and review of the literature. *Eur Respir J* 1994;7:1852–1855.
234. Kiani B, Magro CM, Ross P. Endobronchial presentation of Hodgkin lymphoma: a review of the literature. *Ann Thorac Surg* 2003;76:967–972.
235. Chetty R, Slavin JL, O'Leary JJ, et al. Primary Hodgkin's disease of the lung. *Pathology* 1995;27:111–114.
236. Delsol G, Broussett P, Chittal S, et al. Correlation of the expression of Epstein-Barr virus latent membrane protein and in situ hybridization with biotinylated BamH1-W probes in Hodgkin's disease. *Am J Pathol* 1992;140:247–253.
237. Rush WL, Andriko JAW, Taubenberger JK, et al. Primary anaplastic large cell lymphoma of the lung: a clinicopathologic study of five patients. *Mod Pathol* 2000;13:1285–1292.
238. Close PM, Macrae MB, Hammond JM, et al. Anaplastic large-cell Ki-1 lymphoma. Pulmonary presentation mimicking miliary tuberculosis. *Am J Clin Pathol* 1993;99:631–636.
239. Rubie H, Gladieff L, Robert A, et al. Childhood anaplastic large cell lymphoma: Ki-1/CD30: clinicopathologic features of 19 cases. *Med Pediatr Oncol* 1994;22:155–161.
240. Tilly H, Gaulard P, Lepage E, et al. Primary anaplastic large-cell lymphoma in adults: clinical presentation, phenotype, and outcome. *Blood* 1997;90:3727–3734.
241. Guerra J, Echevarria-Escudero M, Barrios N, et al. Primary endobronchial anaplastic large cell lymphoma in a pediatric patient. *P R Health Sci J* 2006;25:159–161.
242. Campo E, Chott A, Kinney MC, et al. Update on extranodal lymphomas. Conclusions of the Workshop held by the EAHP and the SH in Thessaloniki, Greece. *Histopathology* 2006;48:481–504.
243. Sevilla DW, Choi JK, Gong JZ. Mediastinal adenopathy, lung infiltrates and hemophagocytosis: unusual manifestations of pediatric anaplastic large cell lymphoma: report of two cases. *Am J Clin Pathol* 2007;127:458–464.
244. Medeiros LJ, Elenitoba-Johnson KSJ. Anaplastic large cell lymphoma. *Am J Clin Pathol* 2007;127:707–722.
245. D'amore ESG, Menin A, Bonoldi E, et al. Anaplastic large cell lymphomas: a study of 75 pediatric patients. *Pediatr Dev Pathol* 2007;10:181–191.
246. Falini B, Bigema B, Fizzotti M, et al. ALK expression defines a distinct group of T/null lymphomas ("ALK" lymphomas) with a wide morphological spectrum. *Am J Pathol* 1998;153:875–886.
247. Delsol G, Falini B, Muller-Hermelink HK, et al. Anaplastic large cell lymphoma (ALCL), ALK-positive. In: Swerdlow SH, Campo E, Harris NL, et al., eds. *WHO classification of tumours of haematopoietic and lymphoid tissues*, 4th ed. Lyon: IARC Press, 2008:312–316.
248. Said J, Cesarman E. Primary effusion lymphoma. In: Swerdlow SH, Campo E, Harris NL, et al., eds. *WHO classification of tumours of haematopoietic and lymphoid tissues*, 4th ed. Lyon: IARC Press, 2008:260–261.
249. Cesarman E, Chang Y, Moore PS, et al. Kaposi's sarcoma-associated herpesvirus-like DNA sequences are present in AIDS-related body cavity-based lymphomas. *N Engl J Med* 1995;332:1186–1191.
250. Nador RG, Cesarman E, Chadburn A, et al. Primary effusion lymphoma: a distinct clinicopathologic entity associated with the Kaposi's sarcoma-associated herpesvirus. *Blood* 1996;88:645–656.
251. Carbone A, Blochii A, Vacher E, et al. Kaposi's sarcoma-associated herpesvirus DNA sequences in AIDS-related and AIDS-unrelated lymphomatous effusion. *Br J Haematol* 1996;94:533–543.
252. Karcher DS, Alkan S. Human herpesvirus-8-associated body cavity-based lymphoma in human immunodeficiency virus-infected patients: a unique B-cell neoplasm. *Hum Pathol* 1997;28:801–808.
253. Brimo F, Michel RP, Khetani K, et al. Primary effusion lymphoma: a series of 4 cases and review of the literature with emphasis on cytomorphologic and immunocytochemical differential diagnosis. *Cancer* 2007;111:224–233.
254. Lobo C, Amin S, Ramsay A, et al. Serous fluid cytology of multicentric Castleman's disease and other lymphoproliferative disorders associated with Kaposi sarcoma-associated herpesvirus: a review with case reports. *Cytopathology* 2012;23:76–85.
255. Kobayashi Y, Kamitsuji Y, Kuroda J, et al. Comparison of human herpes virus 8 related primary effusion lymphoma with human herpes virus 8 unrelated primary effusion lymphoma-like lymphoma on the basis of HIV: report of 2 cases and review of 212 cases in the literature. *Acta Haematol* 2007;117:132–144.
256. Alexanian S, Said J, Lones M, et al. KSHV/HHV8-negative effusion-based lymphoma, a distinct entity associated with fluid overload states. *Am J Surg Pathol* 2013;37:241–249.
257. Koss MN, Hochholzer L, Moran CA, et al. Pulmonary plasmacytomas: a clinicopathologic and immunohistochemical study of five cases. *Ann Diagn Pathol* 1998;2:1–11.
258. Horiuchi T, Hirokawa M, Omyama Y, et al. Diffuse pulmonary infiltrates as a Roentgenographic manifestation of primary pulmonary plasmacytoma. *Am J Med* 1998; 105:72–74.
259. Chang C-C, Chang Y-L, Lee L-N, et al. Primary pulmonary plasmacytoma with immunoglobulin G/lambda light chain monoclonal gammopathy. *J Thorac Cardiovasc Surg* 2006;132:984–985.
260. Montero C, Souto A, Vidal I, et al. Three cases of primary pulmonary plasmacytoma. *Arch Bronconeumol* 2009;45(11):564–566.
261. Wei S, Li X, Song Z, et al. Primary endobronchial plasmacytoma involving local lymph nodes and presenting with rare immunoglobulin G lambda monoclonal gammopathy. *Can Respir J* 2012;19:e28–e30.
262. Tiaheri M. Mohammadi F, Karbasi M, et al. Primary pulmonary plasmacytoma with diffuse alveolar consolidation: a case report. *Pathol Res Int* 2010;2010: 463–465.
263. Kim S-H, Kim TH, Sohn JW, et al. Primary pulmonary plasmacytoma presenting as multiple lung nodules. *Korean J Intern Med* 2012;27:111–113.
264. Kaneko Y, Satoh H, Haraguchi N, et al. Radiologic findings in primary pulmonary plasmacytoma. *J Thorac Imaging* 2005;20:53–54.
265. Egashira K, Hirakata K, Nakata H, et al. CT and MRI manifestations of primary pulmonary plasmacytoma. *Clin Imaging* 1995;19:17–19.
266. Husain M, Nguyen GK. Primary pulmonary plasmacytoma diagnosed by transthoracic needle aspiration cytology and immunocytochemistry. *Acta Cytol* 1996;40:622–624.
267. Kazzaz B, Dewar A, Corrin B. An unusual pulmonary plasmacytoma. *Histopathology* 1992;21:285–287.
268. Niitsu N, Kohri M, Hayama M, et al. Primary pulmonary plasmacytoma involving bilateral lungs and marked hypergammaglobulinemia: differentiation from extranodal marginal zone B-cell lymphoma of mucosa-associated lymphoid tissue. *Leuk Res* 2005;29:1361–1364.
269. Risdall R, Hoppe RT, Warnke R. Non-Hodgkin's lymphoma: a study of the evolution of the disease based upon 92 autopsied cases. *Cancer* 1979;44:529–542.
270. Doran HM, Sheppard MN, Collins PW, et al. Pathology of the lung in leukaemia and lymphoma: a study of 87 autopsies. *Histopathology* 1991;18:211–219.
271. Hwang GL, Leung AN, Zinck SE, et al. Recurrent lymphoma of the lung: computed tomography appearance. *J Comput Assist Tomogr* 2005;29:228–230.
272. Vargas HA, Hampson FA, Baba JL, et al. Imaging the lungs in patients treated for lymphoma. *Clin Radiol* 2009;64:1048–1055.
273. Ahmed S, Siddiqui AK, Rossoff L, et al. Pulmonary complications in chronic lymphocytic leukemia. *Cancer* 2003;98:1912–1917.
274. Khong HT, McCarthy J. Chlorambucil-induced pulmonary disease: a case report and review of the literature. *Ann Hematol* 1998;7:85–87.
275. Trisolini R, Agli LL, Poletti V. Bronchiolocentric pulmonary involvement due to chronic lymphocytic leukemia. *Haematologica* 2000;85:1097.
276. Moore W, Baram D, Hu Y. Pulmonary infiltration from chronic lymphocytic leukemia. *J Thorac Imaging* 2006;21:172–175.
277. Rollo G, Bucca C, Chiampo F, et al. Respiratory symptoms, lung function tests, airway responsiveness, and bronchoalveolar lymphocyte subsets in B-Chronic lymphocytic leukemia. *Lung* 1993;171:265–275.
278. Rollins SD, Colby TV. Lung biopsy in chronic lymphocytic leukemia. *Arch Pathol Lab Med* 1988;112:607–611.
279. Hill BT, Weil AC, Kalaycio M, et al. Pulmonary involvement by chronic lymphocytic leukemia/small lymphocytic lymphoma is a specific pathologic finding independent of inflammatory infiltration. *Leuk Lymphoma* 2012;53:589–595.
280. Vaiman E, Odeh M, Attias D, et al. T-cell chronic lymphocytic leukaemia with pulmonary involvement and relapsing BOOP. *Eur Respir J* 1999;14:471–474.

281. Rappaport H, Thomas LB. Mycosis fungoides: the pathology of extracutaneous involvement. *Cancer* 1974;34:1198–1229.
282. Stokar LM, Vonderheid EC, Abell E, et al. Clinical manifestations of Intrathoracic cutaneous T-cell lymphoma. *Cancer* 1985;56:2694–2702.
283. Ueda T, Hosoki N, Isobe K, et al. Diffuse pulmonary involvement by mycosis fungoides: high-resolution computed tomography and pathologic findings. *J Thorac Imaging* 2002;17:157–159.
284. Tamai K, Koyama T, Kondo T, et al. High-resolution computed tomography findings of diffuse pulmonary involvement by mycosis fungoides. *J Thorac Imaging* 2007;22:366–368.
285. Rosen SE, Vonderheid EC, Koprowska I. Mycosis fungoides with pulmonary involvement. Cytopathologic findings. *Acta Cytol* 1984;28:51–57.
286. Kitching PA, Gibbs AR. Pulmonary involvement by mycosis fungoides. A case showing angiocentric lesions and granulomas. *Pathol Res Pract* 1993;189:594–596.
287. Wang C-W, Colby TV. Histiocytic lesions and proliferations in the lung. *Semin Diagn Pathol* 2007;24:162–182.
288. Rao RN, Moran CA, Suster S. Histiocytic disorders of the lung. *Adv Anat Pathol* 2010;17:12–22.
289. Colby TV, Travis WD. Pulmonary Langerhans cell histiocytosis. In: Travis WD, Brambilla E, Muller-Hermelink HK, et al., eds. *World Health Organization classification of tumours of the lung, pleura, thymus and heart*. Lyon: IARC Press, 2004:95–96.
290. Yousem SA, Colby TV, Chen YY, et al. Pulmonary Langerhans' cell histiocytosis: molecular analysis of clonality. *Am J Surg Pathol* 2001;25:630–636.
291. Dacic S, Trusky C, Bakker A, et al. Genotypic analysis of pulmonary Langerhans cell histiocytosis. *Hum Pathol* 2003;34:1345–1349.
292. Travis WD, Borok Z, Roum JH, et al. Pulmonary Langerhans cell granulomatosis (histiocytosis X) a clinicopathologic study of 48 cases. *Am J Surg Pathol* 1993;17:971–986.
293. Lieberman PH, Jones CR, Steinman RM, et al. Langerhans cell (eosinophilic) granulomatosis: a clinicopathologic study encompassing 50 years. *Am J Surg Pathol* 1996;20:519–522.
294. Allen TC. Pulmonary Langerhans cell histiocytosis and other pulmonary histiocytic diseases: a review. *Arch Pathol Lab Med* 2008;132:1171–1181.
295. Egan AJM, Boardman LA, Tazelaar HD, et al. Erdheim-Chester disease: clinical, radiologic, and histopathologic findings in five patients with interstitial lung disease. *Am J Surg Pathol* 1999;23:17–26.
296. Rush WL, Andriko JAW, Galateau-Salle F, et al. Pulmonary pathology of Erdheim-Chester disease. *Mod Pathol* 2000;13:747–754.
297. Arnaud L, Pierre I, Beigelman-Aubry C, et al. Pulmonary involvement in Erdheim-Chester disease: a single-center study of thirty-four patients and a review of the literature. *Arthritis Rheum* 2010;62:3504–3512.
298. Wittenberg KH, Swensen SJ, Myers JL. Pulmonary involvement with Erdheim-Chester disease: radiographic and CT findings. *AJR Am J Roentgenol* 2000;174:1327–1331.
299. Brun A-L, Touitou-Gottenberg D, Haroche J, et al. Erdheim-Chester disease: CT findings of thoracic involvement. *Eur Radiol* 2010;20:2579–2587.
300. Rosai J, Dorfman RF. Sinus histiocytosis with massive lymphadenopathy: a newly recognized benign clinicopathological entity. *Arch Pathol* 1969;87:63–70.
301. Rosai J, Dorfman RF. Sinus histiocytosis with massive lymphadenopathy: a pseudolymphomatous benign disorder. Analysis of 34 cases. *Cancer* 1972;30:1174–1188.
302. Foucar E, Rosai J, Dorfman R. Sinus histiocytosis with massive lymphadenopathy (Rosai-Dorfman disease): review of the entity. *Semin Diagn Pathol* 1990;7:19–73.
303. Cartin-Ceba R, Golbin JM, Yi ES, et al. Intrathoracic manifestations of Rosai-Dorfman disease. *Respir Med* 2010;104:1344–1349.
304. Zander MP, Foster RA, Ohori P, et al. Pulmonary parenchymal sinus histiocytosis with massive lymphadenopathy (Rosai Dorfman disease). *Mod Pathol* 1997;10:174A.
305. Ohori NP, Yu J, Landreneau RJ, et al. Rosai-Dorfman disease of the pleura: a rare extranodal presentation. *Hum Pathol* 2003;c34:1210e1.
306. Ali A, Mackay D. Rosai-Dorfman disease of the lung. *Thorax* 2009;64:908–909.
307. Ji H, Zhang B, Tian D, et al. Rosai-Dorfman disease of the lung. *Respir Care* 2012;57:1679–1681.

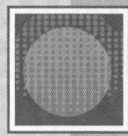

Chapter 32

Malignant Lymphomas and Lymphoid Hyperplasias that Occur in the Ocular Adnexa (Orbit, Conjunctiva, and Eyelids)

Julia Turbiner Geyer • Daniel M. Knowles

Lymphoid infiltrates occurring in the ocular adnexa (i.e., orbit, conjunctiva, and eyelid) have traditionally posed a formidable clinical and histopathologic dilemma. In the past, the rate of error in the accuracy of histopathologic diagnosis and ability to predict clinical outcome were estimated to lie between 20% and 50%. Some patients diagnosed with malignant lymphoma of the ocular adnexa enjoyed disease-free survival despite minimal therapy, whereas some patients diagnosed with lymphoid hyperplasia of the ocular adnexa developed systemic lymphoma (1–3). Several factors contributed to diagnostic error and inaccurate prognostication:

1. Difficulties inherent in the histopathologic evaluation of extranodal lymphoid proliferations, particularly those predominantly composed of small lymphocytes (1–6)
2. Lack of histopathologic criteria to recognize the existence of extranodal small lymphocytic lymphomas, mantle cell lymphomas, and extranodal marginal zone lymphomas (5)
3. Indiscriminate consideration of all lymphoid proliferations that occur in or about the eye together, disregarding the fact that the conjunctiva contains indigenous lymphoid tissue, whereas the orbit normally does not (7,8)
4. Lack of a large clinical series of patients whose lesions were diagnosed and categorized according to an acceptable standard histopathologic classification and who were systematically evaluated using modern staging practices
5. Lack of access to immunologic and molecular biologic techniques capable of delineating lymphoid cell subpopulations and determining their monoclonal or polyclonal nature

Thirty years ago, Knowles and Jakobiec demonstrated that the diagnostic dilemma posed by ocular adnexal and other extranodal lymphoid infiltrates often may be resolved by immunophenotypic analysis of their constituent lymphoid subpopulations (3,9,10). Immunophenotypic analysis is capable of determining the immunologic polyclonality or B-cell monoclonality and presumably the benign or malignant nature of lymphoid proliferations that cannot be deciphered morphologically (11) (see Chapter 3). The inclusion of these immunologic criteria in the evaluation of ocular adnexal and other extranodal lymphoid infiltrates substantially altered many of the traditional beliefs concerning these lymphoid proliferations. In particular, multiple investigators demonstrated by immunophenotypic analysis that most extranodal diffuse, monomorphic small lymphoid cell infiltrates are monoclonal B-cell proliferations (3,9,10,12–17). Application of immunologic criteria resulted in the reclassification as small B-cell lymphomas of many ocular adnexal lymphoid proliferations formerly classified as benign lymphoid hyperplasia by traditional morphologic criteria (6). Lymphoid hyperplasias of the ocular adnexa occur far less commonly than previously believed (6,14,16–18). This reclassification also resulted in a dramatic shift in the distribution of ocular adnexal malignant lymphomas according to histopathologic category.

Nonetheless, results of some studies suggested that immunophenotypic analysis also might be limited in its ability to prognosticate reliably for patients who have ocular adnexal lymphoid proliferations (6,17). In the early 1980s, several scientists discovered that the antigen recognition molecules of B and T cells, immunoglobulin and T-cell receptors, were encoded by genetic loci that undergo somatic recombination (i.e., rearrangement) to become functionally active in mature lymphocytes (19–21). Clonal rearrangements of the immunoglobulin and T-cell receptor genes have proved to be accurate and objective molecular genetic markers of the lineage and clonality of B and T cells, respectively (11). The demonstration of clonal immunoglobulin and T-cell receptor gene rearrangements by Southern blot hybridization analysis and by polymerase chain reaction analysis has been used successfully to determine the lineage and clonality of lymphoproliferative disorders and has become an important adjunct in the diagnosis, classification, and investigation of lymphoid neoplasia (see Chapter 6). This approach is capable of determining the presence of clonal B- and T-cell populations that are not detectable by morphologic examination or by immunophenotypic analysis (22–24). Southern blot hybridization and polymerase chain reaction analysis are also capable of detecting viral sequences, chromosomal translocations, and structural alterations of protooncogenes and tumor suppressor genes, and thereby investigating pathogenetic mechanisms of neoplasia as well (see Chapters 7 and 8).

Correlative multiparametric clinical, morphologic, immunophenotypic, cytogenetic, and molecular genetic analysis has provided considerable insight into the origin, nature, and natural history of the ocular adnexal lymphoid proliferations, transcending what was historically attainable by light microscopic examination alone. This chapter is largely devoted to a review of our current knowledge and understanding of the clinical, morphologic, and biologic characteristics of the ocular adnexal lymphoid proliferations. Other hematopoietic disorders involve the eye and the ocular adnexa less commonly; these are summarized briefly here as well.

TERMINOLOGY

The often indiscriminate use of a wide variety of terms to refer to the lymphoid proliferations that involve the orbit, conjunctiva, and eyelid over the years contributed significantly to the long-standing failure to delineate the clinical, pathologic, and biologic features of these lesions. It also engendered confusion about these entities among ophthalmologists and pathologists alike, much of which remains to this day.

The term *pseudotumor* was originally introduced to designate the wide spectrum of local and systemic inflammatory conditions affecting the orbital contents that produce proptosis and the false clinical impression of a neoplasm

(25). Orbital reactive lymphoid hyperplasia was initially thought to be a specific hypercellular type of orbital pseudotumor (26,27) and was referred to as *orbital lymphoid pseudotumor* by Hogan and Zimmerman (28). In 1963, the term *pseudolymphoma* was introduced by Saltzstein (29) to designate the extranodal benign lymphoid infiltrates that mimic malignant lymphoma clinically and histopathologically. Consequently, orbital reactive lymphoid hyperplasias and orbital pseudotumors came to be categorized as benign lymphoid tumors (30) and called orbital *pseudolymphomas* (2,9). The terms orbital pseudotumor, orbital lymphoid pseudotumor, orbital reactive lymphoid hyperplasia, and orbital pseudolymphoma often were used interchangeably (31,32). In recent years, the widespread use of a multiparameter diagnostic approach that combines morphology with immunohistochemistry, flow cytometry and molecular analysis has helped clarify the etiology of many of these lesions, thus dramatically decreasing the use of the term *orbital pseudotumor*. Importantly, recent studies have suggested that a substantial proportion of the cases previously classified as *orbital pseudotumor* are part of the spectrum of IgG4-related disease (33–35).

The term *pseudolymphoma*, generally considered to be confusing and misleading, has been largely abandoned. The equally ambiguous term *lymphoid pseudotumor* similarly should be discarded (36). It is further recommended that the term *lymphoid hyperplasia* replace the term *reactive lymphoid hyperplasia*, because the word reactive implies a response to an exogenous stimulus, which may not be the case. It is widely recognized that the generally hypocellular, lymphoid cell–poor orbital pseudotumors and the usually hypercellular, lymphoid cell–rich lymphoid hyperplasias represent distinct entities. They differ with respect to clinical presentation, natural history, histopathology, treatment, management, and prognosis, as well as pathogenesis (17,36–38) and should therefore be clearly distinguished from one another. It is recommended that the term *orbital pseudotumor* be used to denote those benign, hypocellular, lymphoid cell–poor orbital inflammatory conditions that are without evidence of a specific local or systemic cause and that the term *lymphoid hyperplasia* be used to denote those hypercellular, lymphoid cell–rich lesions that mimic malignant lymphomas clinically and histopathologically.

The term *histologically indeterminate* has been used by some investigators (14,16,39,40) to refer to those lesions that cannot be assigned with certainty to the category of lymphoid hyperplasia or malignant lymphoma. This term is acceptable only when the morphology of such lesions has been studied and they are truly indeterminate histologically. However, use of this term is inappropriate if such a lesion still defies classification after immunophenotypic or molecular genetic analysis. In these instances, the term *atypical lymphoid hyperplasia*, recommended by Knowles and Jakobiec (2,17), is clearly more appropriate.

The term *ocular adnexal lymphoid proliferation* is used to encompass all the hypercellular, lymphoid cell–rich lymphoid hyperplasias, atypical lymphoid hyperplasias, and malignant lymphomas that occur in the ocular adnexa (i.e., the orbit, conjunctiva, and eyelids). The intraocular lymphoid proliferations include the same categories but involve the choroid, retina, and vitreous body. In addition to the orbital pseudotumors, the other hematopoietic disorders, such as plasmacytomas, myeloid sarcomas, and Langerhans cell histiocytosis, that involve the ocular adnexa represent distinct clinicopathologic entities. They exhibit fundamental clinical, pathologic, and biologic differences from the ocular adnexal lymphoid proliferations (36) and therefore should be distinguished from them.

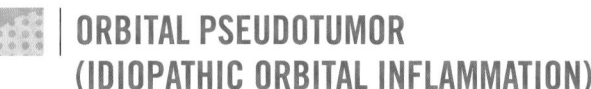

ORBITAL PSEUDOTUMOR (IDIOPATHIC ORBITAL INFLAMMATION)

Birch-Hirschfeld is credited with coining the term *inflammatory orbital pseudotumor* in 1905 to describe a mysterious orbital mass that was discovered to be inflammatory in nature (25). Inflammatory orbital pseudotumor soon became a diagnostic term used to encompass a wide array of poorly understood inflammatory disorders that are now recognized as specific disease entities (41). Unfortunately, the term *inflammatory orbital pseudotumor* also was sometimes used for poorly understood lymphoid proliferations, probably even including some malignant lymphomas (41). Older studies and literature reports of inflammatory orbital pseudotumors include examples of syphilis, tuberculosis, sarcoidosis, infectious cellulitis, Graves' ophthalmopathy, polyarteritis nodosa, and Wegener granulomatosis (41). Over time, conditions with a known infectious or immune cause were recognized and separated, and misuse of the term *inflammatory orbital pseudotumor* gradually diminished (41). As a result, the definition of inflammatory orbital pseudotumor has evolved to denote the benign, nonspecific, orbital inflammatory processes that have no evidence of a specific local or systemic origin (38,42). Thus, the diagnosis of orbital pseudotumor is one of exclusion.

The term *pseudotumor* has been attacked over the years, because it defines what this entity is not, rather than what it is (43). Many investigators have proposed alternative names. Unfortunately, this practice often merely engendered further confusion surrounding the definition of orbital pseudotumor. Some of the recommended names in the older literature include orbital granuloma, nonspecific orbital granuloma, orbital lipogranuloma (41), inflammatory nonneoplastic orbital pseudotumor (28), *idiopathic inflammatory orbital pseudotumor* (26), *idiopathic orbital inflammation* (42), and, more recently, *fibroinflammatory disease* (44–46). *Orbital pseudotumor* and *idiopathic orbital inflammation* appear to be the most favored terms in the recent literature and are used interchangeably by many ophthalmologists, internists, and radiologists. Unfortunately, the interpretation of older studies of orbital pseudotumor is complicated by these terminologic difficulties. Moreover, the multiple early descriptions and subclassifications of orbital pseudotumor are largely unhelpful in delineating a histopathologic spectrum of orbital pseudotumor in the modern sense of the term. With these caveats, in order to avoid further confusion, we continue the use of the term *orbital pseudotumor* in this chapter.

Orbital pseudotumor accounts for approximately 5% of all orbital disorders (47). Orbital pseudotumor usually occurs in adults but may also affect children. Pediatric orbital pseudotumor encompasses about 6% to 16% of orbital pseudotumors (48,49). Men and women are affected equally (38). Orbital pseudotumor is protean in its clinical and radiologic presentation (26). Except for myositic pseudotumor, only one orbit is almost always affected (38). The clinical presentation ranges from that of orbital inflammation with an abrupt onset of periocular discomfort or pain accompanied by epibulbar injection, erythema of the lid skin, chemosis, ptosis, and diplopia to that of a space-occupying or infiltrating orbital lesion with proptosis, motility disturbances, and optic nerve compression, varying according to the location and extent of the mass in the orbit (47) and to the extent of the fibrotic component of the lesion (50,51). Symptoms usually develop over the course of days (acute pseudotumor) to weeks (subacute pseudotumor) but sometimes occur insidiously over a period of months (chronic pseudotumor). The patient may complain of generalized malaise but is usually afebrile (36,47,48,51).

Orbital pseudotumor may manifest as a focal or diffuse mass, which is poorly demarcated and enhances with contrast on computed tomography (CT) (52,53). Lesions located anteriorly may have sharply defined borders (38). Sinus involvement (54,55) or intracranial extension (56,57), with or without bone erosion, is seen rarely. This clinicoradiologic picture is shared with a number of other orbital disorders, however (58).

Orbital pseudotumor is a benign lesion and is believed to be a self-limited disorder (27,59). However, the natural history and evolution of orbital pseudotumor is unknown. It has been generally accepted that orbital pseudotumors are sensitive to systemic corticosteroids (42,59). We now know that a large subset of cases previously called orbital pseudotumor correspond to examples of ocular adnexal IgG4-related disease, thus validating this observation because cases of IgG4-related disease are known to be exquisitely sensitive to steroids. Historically, a prompt favorable clinical response within days of corticosteroid administration has been advocated as evidence for orbital pseudotumor, even in the absence of histopathologic confirmation (42,60). Consequently, the working diagnosis of orbital pseudotumor based on clinical and radiologic findings and a favorable response to corticosteroids, without histopathologic support (53,60), has been widely adopted. However, steroid-nonresponsive orbital pseudotumors have been described in many series (31,53,61–63). Many orbital lesions, including malignant lymphomas, may be steroid responsive transiently (58,62,63). Consequently, steroid responsiveness does not in itself represent a valid criterion for the reliable diagnosis of orbital pseudotumor (58,62,63). A biopsy is necessary for a definitive diagnosis of orbital pseudotumor and to exclude many other entities from consideration (41). A biopsy should be obtained in all cases of suspected orbital pseudotumor (30,57,58,63,64), except in pure myositic locations in which the clinicoradiologic picture is distinctive and a surgical biopsy may damage the muscle (30,65,66) and except in posterior locations in which the optic nerve may be at risk during surgery (30,47,63). Fine needle aspiration biopsy is not helpful in the differential diagnosis of orbital pseudotumor, because a nonspecific cytologic smear of inflammatory cells does not exclude an underlying malignancy or an IgG4-related disease (67–69).

Although orbital pseudotumors are benign, they may pursue a malignant clinical course in which the eye, extraocular muscles, and optic nerve are endangered (38). Therapy is advised to relieve discomfort during the active phase to preserve visual and motility functions and to prevent sequelae in a later stage (41). Since corticosteroids are not always effective, low-dose irradiation has been administered with various degrees of success in steroid-dependent and steroid-nonresponsive cases (32,60,61,70). Combined therapy with other immunosuppressive drugs, including cyclosporine, cyclophosphamide, azathioprine, or methotrexate, may be successful in the case of some aggressive orbital pseudotumors (50,71,72).

Grossly, orbital pseudotumors appear as firm, rubbery, yellowish gray to pink lesions (38). Pseudotumors can affect any orbital structure. The lesion may be confined to one structure, such as the lacrimal gland, the orbital fat, or extraocular muscle (i.e., myositic pseudotumor), but often more than one of these structures are involved in a localized or diffuse pattern (59), thereby simulating a tumor mass. They are generally hypocellular, lymphoid cell–poor lesions that consist of a variably dense connective tissue stroma (38). The stromal changes range from edema to proliferative fibrosis and sclerosis to marked hyalinization (42) (Fig. 32.1). Eosinophil degranulation has been found in the areas of fibrosis and contributes to fibrosis formation in orbital pseudotumors (73). It had been long assumed that the fibrosis and sclerosis that develops in orbital pseudotumors is the result of long-standing inflammation (38,42,49,51). However, it has been suggested that fibrosis

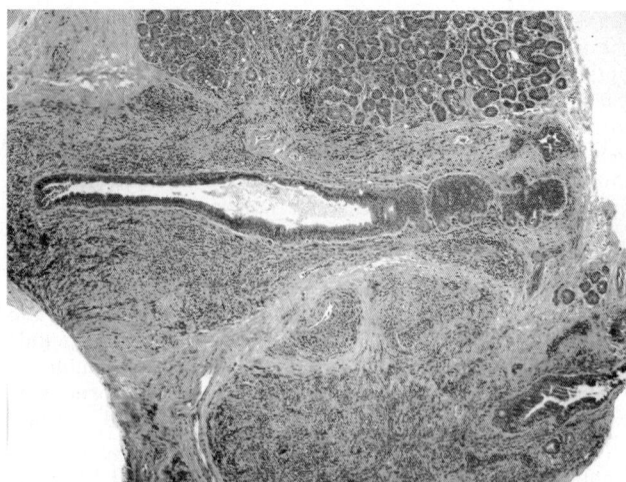

FIGURE 32.1.   Orbital pseudotumor involving lacrimal gland. There is a dense inflammatory infiltrate accompanied by fibrous connective tissue stroma, with periductal and periacinar fibrosis, ductal dilatation, and focal acinar atrophy (hematoxylin and eosin stain, original magnification: 40× magnification).

formation in orbital pseudotumors is an immune-mediated process and that the fibrosis forms early in the development of the lesion (50). Orbital pseudotumors contain a variable but generally sparse polymorphous cellular infiltrate that may be diffuse or multifocal. It is primarily composed of chronic inflammatory cells (i.e., small lymphocytes and plasma cells) accompanied by variable numbers of immunoblasts, histiocytes, and eosinophils and sometimes by neutrophils (38,42,51,59) (Fig. 32.2). Most of the lymphocytes are T cells, with helper T cells predominating over suppressor or cytotoxic T cells (74). The B cells are polyclonal (9,38). Mitotic figures are infrequent. Variable numbers of lymphoid follicles, some containing germinal centers, may be present (38,74). They are usually surrounded by abundant, dense, fibrous connective tissue (Fig. 32.1). In some pediatric orbital pseudotumors, eosinophils represent the majority cell population (49). Orbital pseudotumors may be highly vascularized because of capillary proliferation (38). The endothelial cells are increased in number and swollen and hypertrophic (38). The most common vascular change is perivasculitis presenting as angiocentric lymphocytic cuffing (38). The hypocellular and inflammatory histopathologic

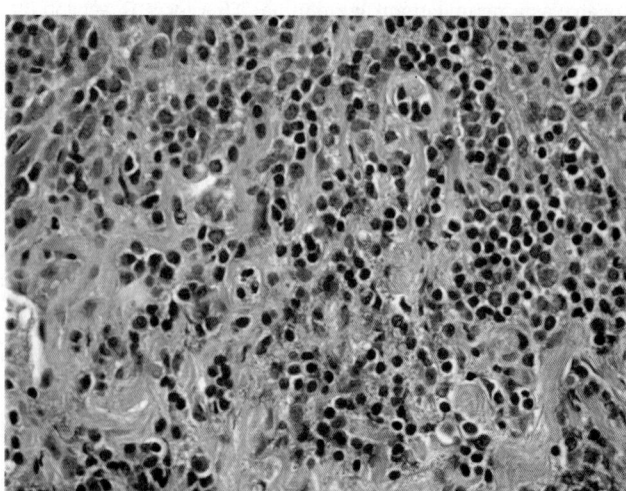

FIGURE 32.2. Orbital pseudotumors are generally composed of a polymorphous cellular infiltrate containing predominantly small lymphocytes, plasma cells, immunoblasts, and histiocytes. Eosinophils and neutrophils also may be present. Mitotic figures are uncommon (hematoxylin and eosin stain, original magnification: 400× magnification).

appearance of these lesions nearly always allows them to be readily distinguished from ocular adnexal lymphoid hyperplasias and malignant lymphomas.

The involvement of specific orbital structures (i.e., orbital fat, lacrimal gland, and extraocular muscle) by orbital pseudotumor is associated with additional histopathologic changes (41). For example, orbital pseudotumor involving the orbital fat appears as a mixed inflammatory cell infiltrate with increased supportive fibrous tissue. The delicate interlobular septa of the adipose tissue become thickened and accentuated and become confluent (49). Lipogranuloma formation may occur (38,42,75). Involvement of the lacrimal gland by pseudotumor results in periductal and periacinar fibrosis, ductal dilatation, and acinar atrophy (42). When extraocular muscle is involved by orbital pseudotumor, the muscle fibers become swollen, the normal striations are lost, and the fibers degenerate; they become separated by edema and fibrosis (41).

Occasionally, the stromal, cellular, or vascular component of orbital pseudotumor deviates significantly from the classic histopathologic pattern (41). This has led to the recognition of four histopathologic subtypes of orbital pseudotumor: sclerosing, granulomatous, vasculitic, and eosinophilic (41). The principal features of these lesions have been reviewed in detail elsewhere (41).

The etiology and pathogenesis of orbital pseudotumor are unknown. Many theories have been suggested (41). Originally, it was thought that orbital pseudotumor is infectious in origin. However, an infectious cause appears inconsistent with the fact that orbital pseudotumor may improve with immunosuppressive therapies. Many years ago, Easton and Smith (76) suggested an autoimmune pathogenesis for orbital pseudotumor. This theory fits with the occasional observation of a coexistent autoimmune disorder, such as diabetes mellitus, rheumatoid arthritis, or systemic lupus erythematosus, in patients who have orbital pseudotumor (42,50). That an immunologic process is central to the pathogenesis of orbital pseudotumor is also strongly supported by the fact that these lesions are often treated successfully with corticosteroids and other immunosuppressive agents (41). The fact that orbital pseudotumor is commonly unilateral seems incongruous with an autoimmune basis, however. Orbital pseudotumor shares histopathologic similarities with idiopathic mediastinal fibrosclerosis (77) and idiopathic retroperitoneal fibrosis (74). For this reason, Barrett (77) proposed many years ago that orbital pseudotumors result from a fibroproliferative disorder. Studies by McCarthy and Rootman and colleagues (50,74) support this theory by providing evidence that fibrosis formation in at least some orbital pseudotumors is an immunologically mediated process. Orbital pseudotumor has been rarely reported to occur in association with retroperitoneal fibrosis (78,79), mediastinal fibrosclerosis (80), and other fibroproliferative disorders (81–83). It has been suggested that all of these entities may be a manifestation of a single generalized disorder called multifocal fibrosclerosis (75). It has also been suggested that development of orbital pseudotumor should be considered a form of aberrant wound healing with cytokine-driven fibroblastic proliferation and collagen synthesis as a final common pathway provoked by damage (e.g., infectious, autoimmune) (41). However, all of the above-mentioned studies were conducted before the description of IgG4-related disease, thus complicating their interpretation since IgG4-related sclerosing disease is known to coexist with autoimmune conditions, is successfully treated with steroids, and is part of the spectrum of sclerosing conditions involving other organs, such as mediastinal fibrosclerosis and retroperitoneal fibrosis. It is possible that as our awareness and knowledge of the rapidly emerging IgG4-related disease spectrum increases, most if not all cases of orbital pseudotumor will become absorbed into this category and the use of the term will be abandoned.

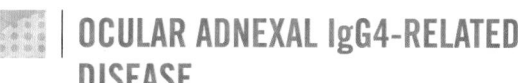

OCULAR ADNEXAL IgG4-RELATED DISEASE

IgG4 isoform is the rarest of immunoglobulin G subtypes and represents 3% to 6% of total IgG in the serum of normal subjects. IgG4 differs from other IgG isoforms in the composition of the hinge region, with a 25% to 75% loss of covalent interaction between the heavy chains. This intrinsic weakness leads to a dynamic exchange between FAB arms with the resultant formation of bispecific, functionally monovalent antibodies (84,85). The exchange of half-molecules decreases the effectiveness of the antibodies with poor ability to induce complement, activate cells, and cross-link identical antigens (85). In 2001, high serum and tissue levels of IgG4 were reported in patients with autoimmune pancreatitis in the landmark study by Hamano et al. (86,87). Autoimmune pancreatitis is an idiopathic, mass-forming inflammatory lesion of the pancreas that was initially recognized in the early 1960s (88). In 1995, a case report by Yoshida et al. (89) rekindled interest in the entity. In recent years these patients have been extensively studied, and it has been recognized that patients who present with autoimmune pancreatitis may in addition have involvement of numerous extrapancreatic sites, such as the ocular adnexa, salivary glands, kidney, lung, liver, gallbladder, and lymph nodes (90–96). On the other hand, some patients may present with primary extrapancreatic disease and have no evidence of a concurrent pancreatic lesion (97,98). Thus, it was postulated that autoimmune pancreatitis is part of a disease spectrum variably named *IgG4-related sclerosing disease, IgG4-related systemic disease, multifocal fibrosclerosis,* or *IgG4-multiorgan lymphoproliferative disorder* (91,99–101). In 2010, Japanese investigators reached a consensus to refer to this new disease entity as *IgG4-related disease.* This term has also been provisionally accepted by North American researchers (102).

The etiology of IgG4-related disease is unknown, but is currently under intense investigation. One hypothesis states that an increase in IgG4 is an autoimmune response, induced by activated type 2 helper T cells and associated with elevated IL-2 receptors (103,104). A recent case report described a 64-year-old female patient who developed dacryoadenitis and chronic sclerosing sialadenitis with histologically proven abundant IgG4-positive plasma cells at presentation and during treatment for cervical lymph node tuberculosis (105). Thus, an abnormal immunologic reaction to an infectious agent has been postulated as one of the etiologic candidates for IgG4-related disease.

Histologic features of IgG4-related disease are very similar independent of the location of the lesion. In exocrine glands, such as lacrimal glands, salivary glands, and the pancreas, the sections show preservation of the lobular architecture, marked lymphoplasmacytic inflammation, large irregular lymphoid follicles with expanded germinal centers, acinar atrophy, obliterative phlebitis, absence of prominent lymphoepithelial lesions, and, characteristically, the presence of prominent cellular interlobular fibrosis, composed of activated fibroblasts, lymphocytes, and plasma cells (87,90,99,106–112) (Fig. 32.3). An elastic stain helps unmask obliterative phlebitis (107,113,114). The inflammatory infiltrate is dominated by lymphocytes and plasma cells. The plasma cells are polyclonal. The inflammatory infiltrate is composed of an admixture of T cells and B cells; the latter are organized predominantly in aggregates and germinal centers. Large numbers of IgG4-positive plasma cells are invariably noted (Fig. 32.3).

Diagnostic criteria for IgG4-related disease are still evolving. In 2011, Okazaki et al. (115,116) suggested to base the diagnosis on the following features: diffuse or focal enlargement or mass lesions in one or more organs; elevated levels of serum IgG4 (>135 mg/dL) and the histologic presence of a prominent lymphoplasmacytic infiltrate; abundant IgG4-positive plasma

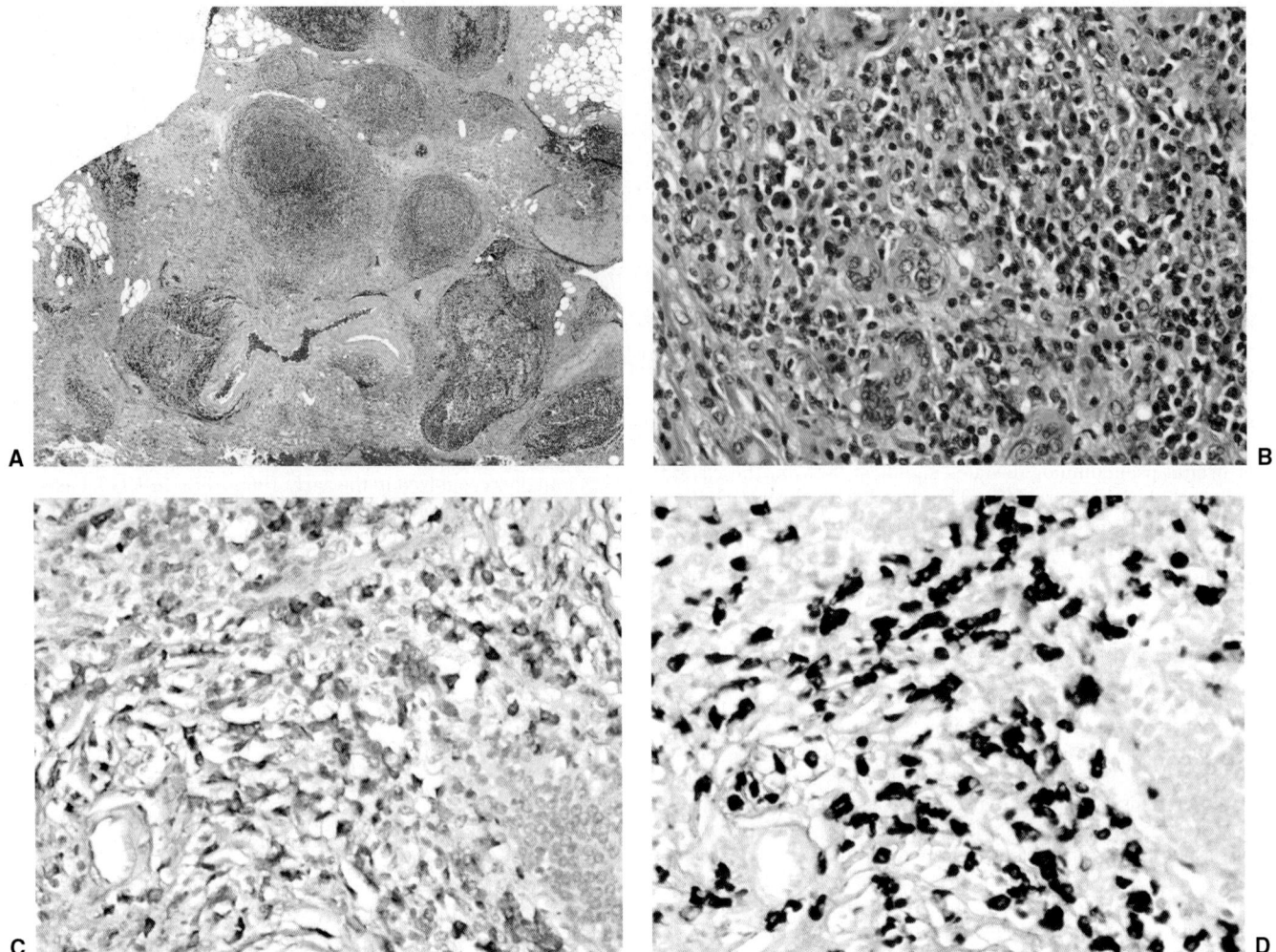

FIGURE 32.3.   IgG4-related ocular adnexal sclerosing disease. A: There are large irregular lymphoid follicles, some with expanded germinal centers and prominent cellular interlobular fibrosis, composed of activated fibroblasts, lymphocytes, and plasma cells (hematoxylin and eosin stain, original magnification: 40× magnification). **B:** Numerous plasma cells admixed with small lymphocytes and scattered eosinophils are noted (hematoxylin and eosin stain, original magnification: 200× magnification). **C:** The plasma cells express IgG (IgG immunostain, original magnification: 400x magnification). **D:** Numerous IgG4-positive plasma cells are present. There are >10 IgG4-positive cells per high power field. The IgG4/IgG ratio is approximately 60% (IgG4 immunostain, original magnification: 400x magnification).

cells (>10 cells per high power field and/or IgG4 to IgG ratio of >40%); storiform swirling fibrosis and obliterative phlebitis. In 2012, Carruthers et al. (102) suggested the following potential criteria: dysfunction in one or more of the characteristic organs for IgG4-related disease; typical radiographic evidence of IgG4-related disease; IgG4 serum level of more than 1.5 times the normal upper limit and characteristic histopathologic features such as a lymphoplasmacytic infiltrate, storiform fibrosis, tissue eosinophilia, obliterative or nonobliterative phlebitis, and abundant IgG4-positive plasma cells (>10 cells per high power field and/or IgG4 to IgG ratio of >50%).

Several retrospective case series have been performed in order to study the manifestations of IgG4-related disease in the orbit. An increased number of IgG4-positive plasma cells was noted in 19% of all orbital lymphoproliferative lesions (35) and in 44% to 60% of patients with benign orbital inflammation (117–119). Lacrimal gland involvement was the most commonly reported site of ocular adnexal IgG4-related disease, followed by lesions centered in the orbital and periocular soft tissue. Wallace et al. (34) described one patient with orbital myositis and IgG4-related disease. No cases of conjunctival involvement have yet been reported (35,118–120).

Histologically, IgG4-related disease of the orbit may be broadly divided into lacrimal gland–based lesions characterized

by prominent lymphoid hyperplasia and sclerosing lesions similar to the sclerosing variant of orbital pseudotumor. While there are no unified criteria specific to orbital adnexal IgG4-related disease, the general approach has been to consider positive cases as those with >10 IgG4-positive plasma cells per high power field (35,117–119), an IgG4/IgG ratio of >30% to 40% (117,118), and/or a serum level of IgG4 of >135 mg/dL (117).

In the orbit, IgG4-related disease most frequently involves the lacrimal glands causing chronic sclerosing dacryoadenitis, usually in bilateral fashion (35,92,121,122). In 2007, Cheuk et al. (92) and, independently, Takahira et al. (122) reported on six and four patients, respectively, with chronic sclerosing dacryoadenitis and an increased number of IgG4-positive cells, suggesting that lacrimal gland involvement was part of the spectrum of IgG4-related disease. Subsequently, several groups have confirmed this observation (35,118–120). The number of male and female patients was approximately equal, with ages ranging from 24 to 86 years. A subset of the patients showed evidence of salivary gland involvement (part of a syndrome historically called "Mikulicz disease"). Serum IgG4 was elevated in 77% of patients (35). The histologic features were similar to those seen in cases of IgG4-related disease in other anatomical sites, although obliterative phlebitis was generally absent. A small subset of patients had an increased number of eosinophils. Immunohistochemical stains for IgG4 revealed an elevated number of IgG4-positive plasma cells (>10 per high power field), with an elevated IgG4 to IgG ratio (29% to 78%).

Mehta et al. (45) reported a case of a man with massive facial swelling and a fibroinflammatory process centering on periorbital fibrous membrane (periosteum) and the soft tissue of the eyelids. Histologically, most of the lesion had fibrosclerosis with sparse inflammatory cells and rare lymphoplasmacytic aggregates. IgG4-positive plasma cells were numerous and were greater than 35/high power field in the more cellular areas. The authors concluded that the lesion was an example of sclerosing orbital pseudotumor-like IgG4-related disease, different from the more common cases of chronic sclerosing dacryoadenitis described above.

A study by Kubota et al. (117) compared cases of orbital adnexal IgG4-related disease with extensive sclerosis to cases of orbital adnexal IgG4-related disease with significant lymphoplasmacytic infiltrate and prominent lymphoid follicles and found that they had similar levels of serum IgG4 and a similar IgG4-to-IgG ratio.

Sato et al. and Kubota et al. have also performed polymerase chain reaction for B-cell clonality and found that 3 of 27 patients (11%) had a clonal immunoglobulin heavy chain gene rearrangement. These patients were diagnosed as having extranodal marginal B-cell lymphoma of mucosa-associated lymphoid tissue (MALT lymphoma), suggesting that MALT lymphoma may arise from a background of IgG4-related disease (35,117). In a separate study, Kubota et al. (123) examined 114 cases of ocular adnexal MALT lymphoma and found that 10 cases (9%) had an increased number of infiltrating IgG4-positive plasma cells.

The patients with IgG4-related ocular adnexal disease had more frequent bilateral involvement, higher prevalence of allergic diseases, polyclonal hypergammaglobulinemia, and evidence of systemic organ involvement compared to patients with ocular adnexal lesions unrelated to IgG4 (117–119). Extraocular involvement included the parotid glands, pancreas, liver, biliary tree, lung, thyroid, and lymph nodes (118–120). Morphologically, while some studies have not found significant differences between the two groups (117,118), others have described that marked follicular hyperplasia, background fibrosis, and presence of increased plasma cells and eosinophils may help in identifying cases of orbital IgG4-related disease (119).

Treatment for IgG4-related orbital adnexal disease is similar to that of orbital pseudotumor and systemic IgG4-related disease. The patients frequently require repeated courses of high-dose corticosteroids that sometimes become less effective over time (35,117,124,125). Local radiotherapy is occasionally used. More recently, patients have been treated with rituximab, with promising results (34,119,126–128).

In conclusion, while it is clear that a significant proportion of nonclonal sclerosing and inflammatory diseases involving the lacrimal gland are IgG4-related, the relationship of IgG4-related disease to the other fibroinflammatory diseases of the orbit, such as orbital pseudotumor (idiopathic orbital inflammation), idiopathic orbital sclerosing disease, orbital myositis, and Tolosa-Hunt syndrome is still uncertain (35). However, many of these fibroinflammatory processes are steroid responsive, and thus are likely to belong to the spectrum of IgG4-related disease.

OCULAR ADNEXAL LYMPHOID PROLIFERATIONS

Introduction

Much of the current knowledge of ocular adnexal lymphoid proliferations is based on the seminal studies performed by Knowles and Jakobiec between 1977 and 1987. Knowles and Jakobiec (17) prospectively evaluated 108 patients who had lymphoid proliferations (i.e., lymphoid hyperplasia, atypical lymphoid hyperplasia, and malignant lymphoma) that originated or presented in the ocular adnexa. They examined the histopathology and analyzed the immunophenotypic characteristics of 117 ocular adnexal and 9 nonocular lymphoid proliferations obtained from these 108 patients during that time. After these studies were completed, the patients were referred to a hematologist-oncologist for systemic evaluation, including radiologic survey and bone marrow examination, before therapy. The patients were followed carefully and periodically underwent reexamination. Complete clinical information concerning each patient was collected; this included age, sex, past medical history, presenting complaints, duration of symptoms, principal clinical findings, precise anatomic location of the lesion, results of laboratory and radiologic studies, extent of disease, type and extent of therapy, therapeutic response, duration of survival, and outcome. In 1988, Knowles and Jakobiec correlated the clinical, histopathologic, and immunophenotypic findings and critically reviewed them. The results of this prospective multiparametric analysis (17) and the numerous other studies performed by Knowles and Jakobiec during the 1980s (2,3,9,10,12,15,23,129–134) have served as the basis for much of our modern understanding of the ocular adnexal lymphoid proliferations.

Since the time of those studies, two important developments have taken place that have contributed significantly to our further understanding of lymphoid neoplasia, especially that involving the ocular adnexa. The first is the recognition of MALT and the special characteristics of MALT and the malignant lymphomas that arise within MALT (135); the second is the development of the Revised European-American Lymphoma (REAL) classification, followed by the creation of the World Health Organization (WHO) classification of tumors of hematopoietic and lymphoid tissues, currently in its fourth edition—the only standard lymphoma classification that is relevant for nodal and extranodal lymphomas (136,137). These highly significant contributions provided the scientific underpinnings to support and extend many of the notions of Knowles and Jakobiec, but they also challenged many others, especially the classification of ocular adnexal malignant lymphomas. Other large clinicopathologic studies of the ocular adnexal lymphoid proliferations that have incorporated these developments (40,138) have built on the classic studies of Knowles and Jakobiec to provide us with a better understanding of these lesions.

Definition

Nearly every malignant lymphoid neoplasm originating in the ocular adnexa and most that involve the ocular adnexa secondarily are B-cell lymphomas (18), predominately small B-cell lymphomas (16,17,40,138). High-grade (immunoblastic and Burkitt) lymphomas may arise or manifest in the ocular adnexa of adults in the setting of the acquired immunodeficiency syndrome (AIDS) (139,140) (see Chapter 25). Rarely, sporadic (Western) Burkitt lymphoma may involve the ocular adnexa in children (141,142) (see Chapter 24). Peripheral T-cell lymphomas frequently involve the ocular adnexa and nearly always represent systemic disease (40,143); very few cases of primary ocular adnexal T-cell lymphoma have been described (144,145). Mycosis fungoides occasionally involves the skin of the eyelid (146), and, much less commonly, other adnexal locations (147), usually in the late plaque or tumor stage of the disease. Rarely, the ocular adnexa may serve as the initial site of presentation of disseminated mycosis fungoides (148). Lastly, Hodgkin lymphoma of the ocular adnexa is extraordinarily rare (149). All of these lymphoid neoplasms differ clinically and biologically from conventional ocular adnexal B-cell lymphomas. Consequently, the discussion that follows concerning the clinical, radiologic, histopathologic, immunophenotypic, immunogenotypic, and molecular genetic features of ocular adnexal lymphoid proliferations excludes the B-cell neoplasms arising in association with AIDS and other immunodeficiency states, T-cell neoplasms, and Hodgkin lymphoma.

Epidemiology and Etiology

A series of 1,264 consecutive patients who presented to an ocular oncology service because of a space-occupying orbital lesion demonstrated that the most common diagnosis was that of a "lymphoid tumor" (11% of the cases) with the vast majority of these patients receiving a diagnosis of non-Hodgkin lymphoma (73%), followed by atypical lymphoid hyperplasia (9%) and benign lymphoid hyperplasia (7%) (18). Overall, lymphomas of the ocular adnexa represent approximately 1% to 2% of all non-Hodgkin lymphomas and approximately 8% of all extranodal lymphomas (150,151). An autopsy series of 1,269 patients with systemic lymphoma described that 0.24% of the patients presented with ocular adnexal lymphoma, while 1.3% of all patients had evidence of ocular adnexal lymphoma involvement at the time of death (152). In the United States, the incidence of ocular adnexal lymphoma has increased more rapidly than that of any other non-Hodgkin lymphoma at extranodal sites, by 6.3% per year between 1971 and 2001 with no evidence of peaking, as opposed to lymphomas of other sites (153).

In the experience of Knowles and Jakobiec (17), the patients with ocular adnexal lymphoid proliferations range in age from 17 to 93 years. About 85% of patients are 50 years of age or older, and the median age is 61 years, regardless of the anatomic site of disease. Other investigators agree. For example, Coupland et al. (40) reported that 112 patients collected from Germany and Scotland ranged in age from 14 to 91 years (median, 61 years). Ocular adnexal lymphoid proliferations occur very uncommonly in children. Many of the childhood orbital "histiocytic lymphomas" reported many years ago probably represent myeloid sarcomas, embryonal rhabdomyosarcomas, or other neoplasms and not malignant lymphomas (36). Knowles and Jakobiec (17) and Coupland et al. (40) reported a male-to-female ratio of 1:1.4 and 1:2.5, respectively, for all lymphoid proliferations occurring in all adnexal locations.

In the experience of Knowles and Jakobiec (17), lymphoid proliferations occurring within the ocular adnexa are distributed as follows: orbit, 64%; conjunctiva, 28%; and eyelids, 8%. Coupland et al. (40) reported a slightly lower proportion of orbital, a slightly higher proportion of eyelid, and an identical proportion of conjunctival lesions. Among persons who have orbital lesions, about 46% have lacrimal gland involvement and 54% have involvement of the non–lacrimal gland orbital soft tissues. All orbital lesions may be considered together, however, because their clinical and other characteristics are virtually identical (17).

Lymphoid proliferations involve the right and left adnexa about equally and are bilateral in about 15% of cases. Approximately 80% of patients with bilateral ocular adnexal lymphoid proliferations have simultaneous bilateral disease; the remaining patients initially present with a unilateral lesion and subsequently develop a lesion in the contralateral eye. Equal proportions of patients with orbital, conjunctival, and eyelid lesions develop bilateral disease (17,134). In most cases, bilateral orbital, bilateral conjunctival, or bilateral eyelid lesions occur (17,134). Rarely, for example, does a bilateral lesion develop that involves the conjunctiva in one eye and the orbit in the other eye (154).

A subset of patients with MALT lymphoma of the ocular adnexa have an associated autoimmune disorder, such as Sjögren disease, Hashimoto thyroiditis, myasthenia gravis, Grave disease or rheumatoid arthritis (120,155–160). A prospective, case-controlled study from Italy showed a significant association between exposure to household animals, rural residence, and history of chronic conjunctivitis in patients with ocular adnexal MALT lymphoma (161). The same authors found that 80% of patients with ocular MALT lymphoma had *Chlamydia psittaci* (currently classified as *Chlamydophila psittaci*) DNA; some of these patients responded to antibiotic therapy (161,162). These findings were confirmed in a study from Korea, where *C. psittaci* DNA was found in 78% of cases (163). A follow-up large multi-institutional study demonstrated the presence of *C. psittaci* DNA in MALT lymphoma samples from Germany (47%), the United States (35%), and the Netherlands (29%), with a lower frequency found in Italy (13%), the United Kingdom (12%), and Southern China (11%) (164). However, these results have not been replicated in several other studies (164–168). A meta-analysis of 11 studies, which included 458 patients from 10 countries, showed that *C. psittaci* was identified in 25% of MALT lymphoma specimens (169). However, 90% of the positive cases came from 3 of the 11 studies (169). Incidentally, a similarly discrepant geographic distribution has been reported regarding the association between cutaneous MALT lymphoma and infection with *Borrelia burgdorferi* (170). Thus, while the reported geographic variation may represent a true phenomenon, it may also, at least in part, be due to differences in diagnostic criteria and PCR technique. In contrast with MALT lymphoma, *C. psittaci* DNA has been detected in only a low number of other lymphoid and nonlymphoid conditions involving the orbit (163,164). Other infectious agents that have been anecdotally implicated in the pathogenesis of ocular adnexal MALT lymphoma include HIV (40), HCV (171,172), *Chlamydia pneumonia* (173,174), and *Helicobacter pylori* (173,175,176). No such associations have been found for other ocular adnexal lymphomas.

Ocular adnexal IgG4-related disease has been associated with several cases of lymphoma, including marginal zone lymphoma and follicular lymphoma (35,121,123,160). Additional studies are required in order to confirm this association.

Clinical Features

Sites of Involvement

Knowles and Jakobiec (17) suggested that the proportion of ocular adnexal lymphoid proliferations classified as lymphoid hyperplasia and malignant lymphoma and their natural history, including the development of systemic lymphoma, varies according to their location within the ocular adnexa (i.e., orbit, conjunctiva, or eyelid). Although not all investigators agree (39,40), it is important that the patient who has an ocular adnexal lymphoid proliferation receive a careful clinical ocular examination, usually in conjunction with imaging studies, so that the precise anatomic location of the lesion can be determined. The following guidelines can be used in this determination.

Lesions should be designated as orbital if the lacrimal gland is involved or if any aspect of the retroorbital soft tissue, including the muscles, is involved (Fig. 32.4). Lesions that manifest subconjunctivally or in the lids whose epicenters obviously are within the orbit also should be categorized among the orbital lesions (Fig. 32.5). Most orbital lesions occur superiorly or in the retrobulbar tissues (Fig. 32.6); fewer than 5% are located predominantly in the inferior orbit. Lesions should be designated as conjunctival if they occur as freely movable salmon patches on the epibulbar, forniceal, caruncular, or palpebral surfaces without infiltrating the eyelid skin or encroaching on the orbit (Figs. 32.7 and 32.8). Lesions should be designated as occurring primarily in the eyelids if the dermis or orbicularis muscle of the anterior eyelid skin is infiltrated and if they are located anterior to the orbital septum (found by physical examination or imaging studies) (Figs. 32.9 and 32.10).

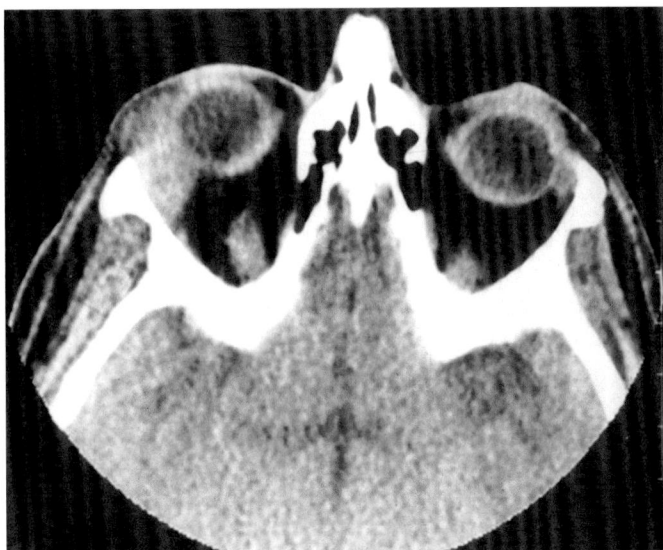
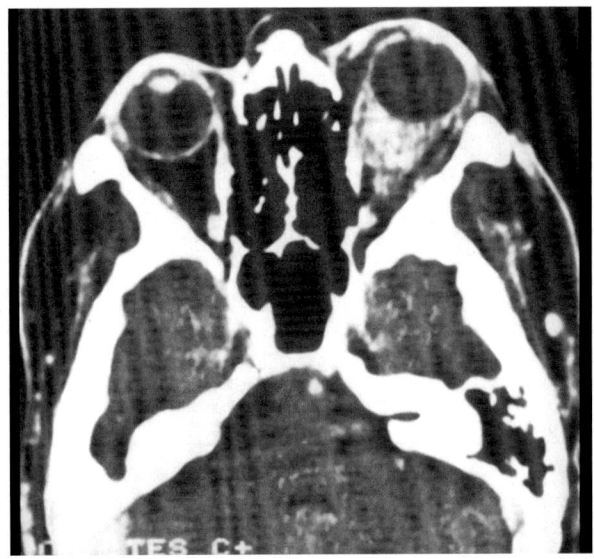

A   B

FIGURE 32.4.   CT scan of orbital lymphoid proliferation. A: A lymphoid proliferation occupies the lacrimal gland on the left. Approximately 45% of orbital lymphoid proliferations involve the lacrimal gland. **B:** A lymphoid proliferation molded to the posterior sclera occurs in the retrobulbar orbital soft tissues on the right. (From Knowles DM, Jakobiec FA, McNally L, et al. Lymphoid hyperplasia and malignant lymphoma occurring in the ocular adnexa [orbit, conjunctiva, and eyelids]: a prospective multiparametric analysis of 108 cases during 1977–1987. *Hum Pathol* 1990;21:959–973, with permission.)

Clinical Evaluation

Patients who have ocular adnexal lymphoid proliferations, regardless of histopathology (i.e., lymphoid hyperplasia, atypical lymphoid hyperplasia, or malignant lymphoma) or bilaterality, do not appear to differ significantly with respect to age, sex, presenting complaints, duration of symptoms, or ophthalmic findings (1–3,17,36,134). The one exception is pain associated with bone erosion on radiologic examination, which apparently is only observed in malignant lymphoma (2,40,177), primarily large B-cell lymphomas (40,178). Otherwise, clinical evaluation alone usually is of little value in distinguishing benign and malignant ocular adnexal lymphoid proliferations. For this reason, these proliferations are grouped together for the purpose of discussing their clinical characteristics (Table 32.1).

Approximately 90% of patients who present with an orbital lymphoid proliferation complain of a mass or swelling, proptosis or ocular displacement, diplopia, or ptosis. Less common

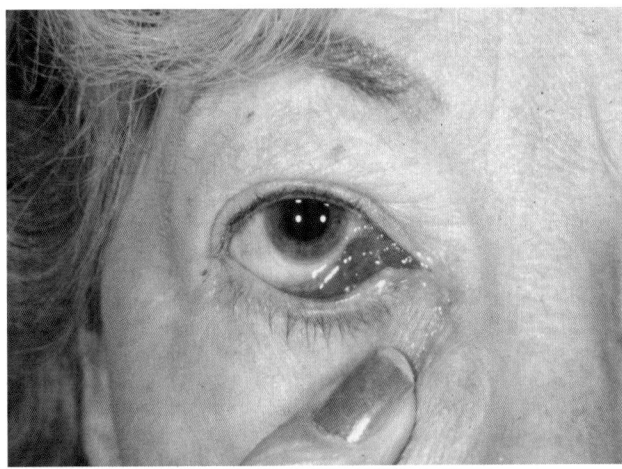

A

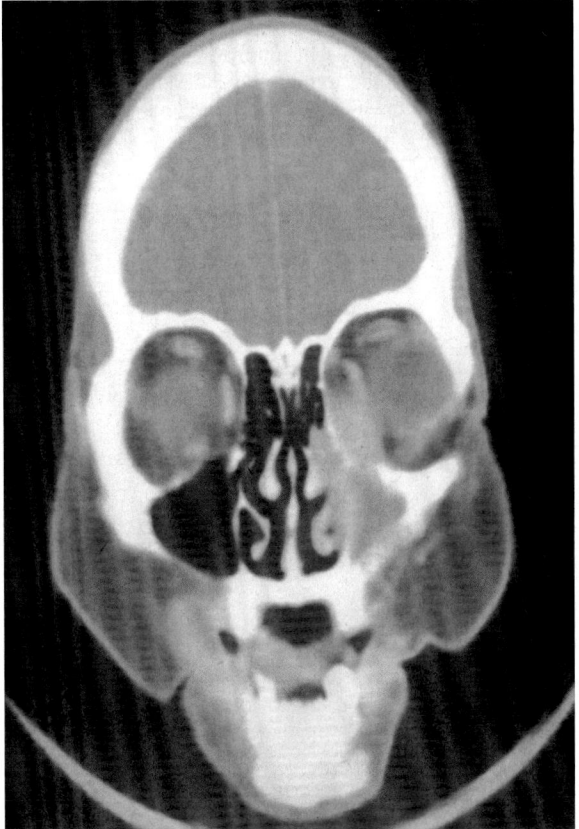

B

FIGURE 32.5.   An orbital large B-cell lymphoma is beneath the nasal conjunctiva. A: There is some displacement of the globe, suggesting that the lesion extends beyond the conjunctiva. **B:** CT scan of the patient shown in (**A**). The lesion involved the inferonasal orbit and caused bone destruction inferonasally by extending into the contiguous maxillary sinus. The patient had no evidence of systemic lymphoma. Local radiation therapy was administered, with resolution of the process.

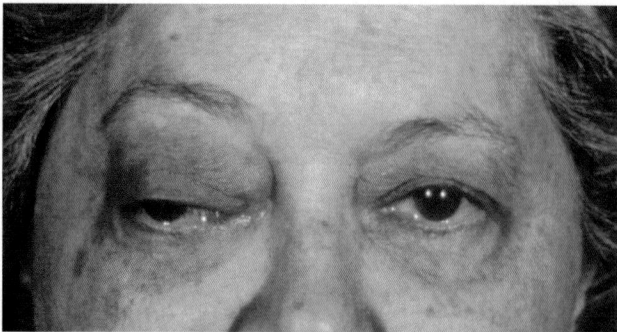

FIGURE 32.6.   Orbital malignant lymphoma. This woman presented with a superior and superonasal orbital B-cell lymphoma that caused proptosis and lateral displacement of the globe. On evaluation, the patient was found to have no evidence of systemic lymphoma. The lesion was treated with local radiation therapy and regressed.

secondary complaints include redness, irritation, and pain. Nearly all of these patients have a palpable mass, proptosis, ocular displacement, diplopia, or decreased ocular motility on physical examination. The mass usually is firm to rubbery (Fig. 32.6). About 20% of patients are discovered to have a history or concurrent evidence of extraocular lymphoma (17,178).

Approximately 80% of patients who present with a conjunctival lymphoid proliferation complain of a mass or swelling. These lesions are situated in the substantia propria of the conjunctiva and do not infiltrate the anterior orbital tissues or the anterior eyelid skin. They do not cause proptosis, ocular displacement, or diplopia. Essentially every patient is discovered to have a palpable mass on physical examination, by palpating a fullness through the lid or by everting the eyelid and finding the typical thickening on the forniceal, epibulbar, or palpebral conjunctiva. The mass typically is salmon or pink to flesh colored, sausage shaped, and freely movable (Figs. 32.7 and 32.8). Only about 10% of patients are discovered to have a history or concurrent evidence of extraocular lymphoma (17).

Essentially all patients who present with an eyelid lymphoid proliferation complain of ptosis and a mass or swelling of the eyelid. These lesions represent infiltrations of the dermis and orbicularis muscle of the anterior eyelid skin in front of the orbital septum. This results in a palpable mass with a firm to rubbery consistency that causes ptosis (Figs. 32.9 and 32.10).

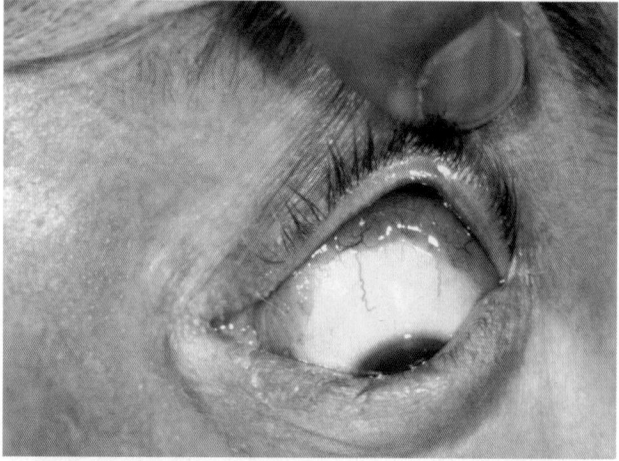

FIGURE 32.7.   Conjunctival lymphoid proliferation. A typical sausage-shaped swelling of the superofornix occurred in a patient with a lymphoid lesion confined to the substantia propria of the conjunctiva. These lesions are sometimes referred to as salmon patches by clinical ophthalmologists. (From Knowles DM, Jakobiec FA, McNally L, et al. Lymphoid hyperplasia and malignant lymphoma occurring in the ocular adnexa [orbit, conjunctiva, and eyelids]: a prospective multiparametric analysis of 108 cases during 1977–1987. *Hum Pathol* 1990;21:959–973, with permission.)

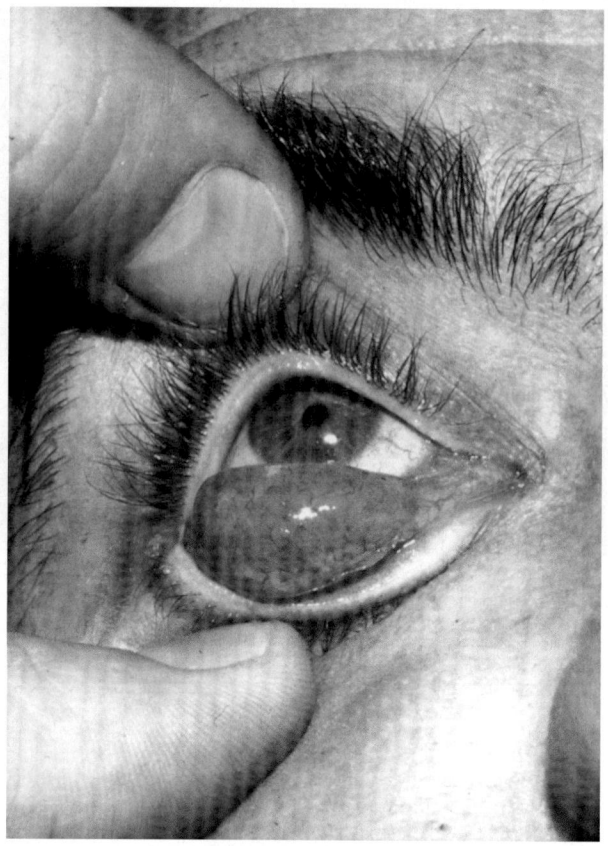

FIGURE 32.8.   Conjunctival lymphoid proliferation. This 39-year-old man presented with a 2-month history of increasing fullness of the right lower lid unaccompanied by diplopia, proptosis, or displacement of the globe. The lymphoid lesion is exposed by eversion of the right lower eyelid. The lesion is restricted to the tarsal and inferior forniceal conjunctiva, making this a conjunctival rather than an eyelid lymphoid proliferation. Excisional biopsy demonstrated a polyclonal follicular lymphoid hyperplasia. No additional therapy was administered. The patient was alive and well without evidence of ocular adnexal or systemic lymphoma 115 months later. (From Knowles DM, Jakobiec FA, Halper JP. Immunologic characterization of ocular adnexal lymphoid neoplasms. *Am J Ophthalmol* 1979;87:603–619, with permission.)

They frequently are discovered to have a history or concurrent evidence of extraocular lymphoma (17).

The duration of symptoms varies markedly, from as short as 1 week to as long as 10 years. The median duration of symptoms is approximately 4 months, however, regardless of the anatomic location of the lesion within the ocular adnexa (17).

The nonophthalmic findings discovered on general physical examination depend on the presence or absence of systemic malignant lymphoma and vary according to the anatomic location of the lesion within the ocular adnexa. Knowles and Jakobiec found that 90% of patients with conjunctival, 81% with orbital, and 78% with eyelid lymphoid proliferations have a negative nonophthalmic physical examination. Most of the remaining patients have lymphadenopathy, hepatomegaly, or splenomegaly (17). However, biopsy examination often reveals that the lymphadenopathy is merely reactive and not the result of involvement by malignant lymphoma (17,179). Fewer than 10% of patients are found to have peripheral blood or bone marrow involvement by malignant lymphoma (17,167,178). A small subset of lymphoplasmacytic lymphomas may be associated with a monoclonal gammopathy and systemic disease (40). These lymphomas also may be associated with the local or systemic deposition of amyloid (180–182).

Staging

Staging of patients with ocular adnexal lymphoma includes ophthalmologic and clinical examination, routine laboratory

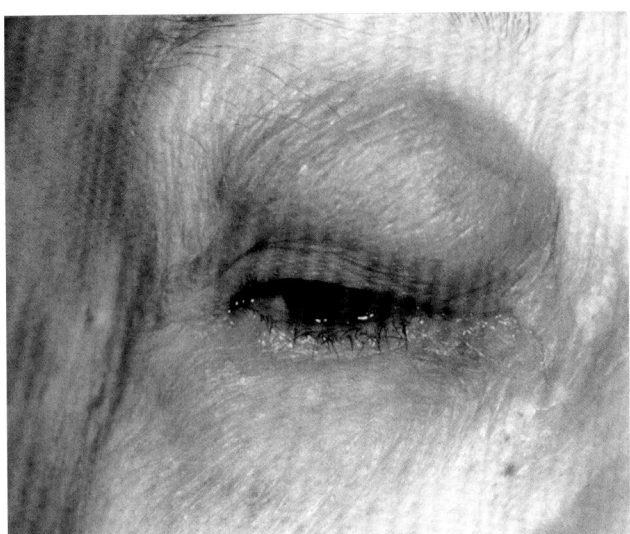 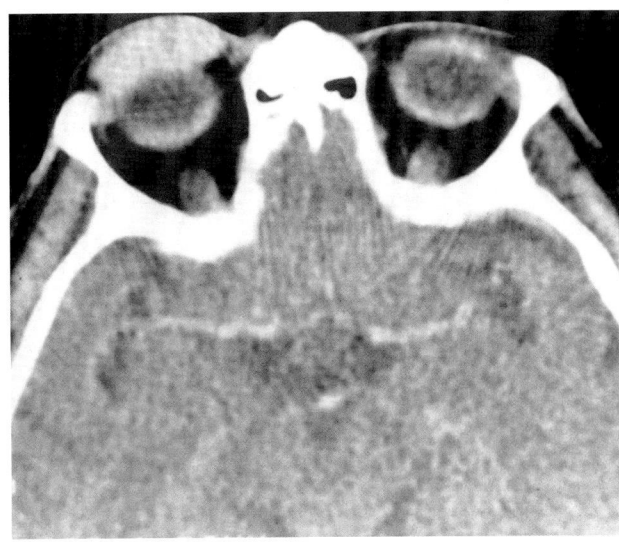

A   B

FIGURE 32.9.   Eyelid lymphoid proliferation.   A: The clinical appearance of an elderly patient presenting with a lymphoid proliferation of the upper eyelid that infiltrated the dermis of the eyelid skin and the orbicularis striated muscle. **B:** The CT scan indicates that the mass is confined to the lid tissues and occupies the lid space anterior to the orbital septum. The retroseptal orbital tissues are not infiltrated, and there were no orbital findings on physical examination (e.g., absence of proptosis, ocular displacement, or diplopia). The patient was discovered to have systemic lymphoma on further evaluation. (From Knowles DM, Jakobiec FA, McNally L, et al. Lymphoid hyperplasia and malignant lymphoma occurring in the ocular adnexa [orbit, conjunctiva, and eyelids]: a prospective multiparametric analysis of 108 cases during 1977–1987. *Hum Pathol* 1990;21:959–973, with permission.)

studies, serum lactate dehydrogenase (LDH), serum protein electrophoresis, β2-microglobulin, CT scan of head and paranasal sinuses, chest, abdomen and pelvis, magnetic resonance imaging (MRI) with contrast enhancement, as well as a bone marrow biopsy. Positron emission tomography (PET) imaging may be a valuable adjunct to conventional imaging in the initial staging as well as in the evaluation of response to therapy (183). However, FDG uptake is only present in approximately 45% of cases of ocular adnexal MALT lymphoma, similar to MALT lymphomas in other sites (184).

The traditional Ann Arbor staging system was first used for Hodgkin lymphoma and has serious shortcomings when used for extranodal lymphomas, since their pattern of dissemination is typically different from that of a nodal lymphoma (185). Thus, ocular adnexal lymphoma has a disproportionate staging distribution with two-thirds of cases classified as stage IE (extranodal) by the Ann Arbor system. In addition, it does not address the issues of specific anatomic location in the orbital region,

multicentric or bilateral disease, as well as involvement of other extranodal sites. Therefore, a new TNM-based staging system has been developed specifically for ocular adnexal lymphomas (186). It classifies the cases according to their location in the orbit as follows: T1 represents conjunctival lymphoma, T2 is lymphoma with orbital involvement, T3 is lymphoma with preseptal eyelid involvement, and T4 is reserved for lymphoma extending beyond the orbit to adjacent structures (186). This TNM staging system has been based on both published studies and its authors' experience. Validation studies are currently in progress.

Radiologic Characteristics

CT greatly assists in the preoperative evaluation of patients who have orbital lesions, including determination of the location, size, and extent of a lesion, which are essential factors in planning the surgical approach and treatment (187,188) (Figs. 32.4, 32.5, and 32.9). CT also can provide a strong presumptive diagnosis of a lymphoid proliferation within the orbit. However, CT reveals no known characteristic features that permit this technique to discriminate reliably, much less definitively, between benign and malignant orbital lymphoid proliferations (36,177,187,189).

Orbital lymphoid hyperplasias and malignant lymphomas are nearly always unifocal mass lesions, in contrast to orbital pseudotumors, which frequently are multifocal. Most are located in the orbital fat and soft tissues. Most of the remaining lesions are represented by diffuse, oblong, molded expansions of the lacrimal gland (36,187). Rarely, a lymphoid proliferation may be situated predominantly within an extraocular muscle (187,190).

CT demonstrates the distinctive tendency of orbital lymphoid proliferations to mold or plaster themselves along preexisting orbital structures (187). They may contour to the globe, lacrimal gland, optic nerve, extraocular muscles, and orbital bones, but they do not enlarge the orbit and only rarely cause bone destruction (36,187) (Figs. 32.11 to 32.13).

Typical MRI features of ocular adnexal lymphoma consist of an ill-defined lesion with intermediate signal intensity on T1- and T2-weighted images with moderate enhancement with gadolinium (191). PET imaging has a low sensitivity in the detection of orbital tumors, but is recommended for

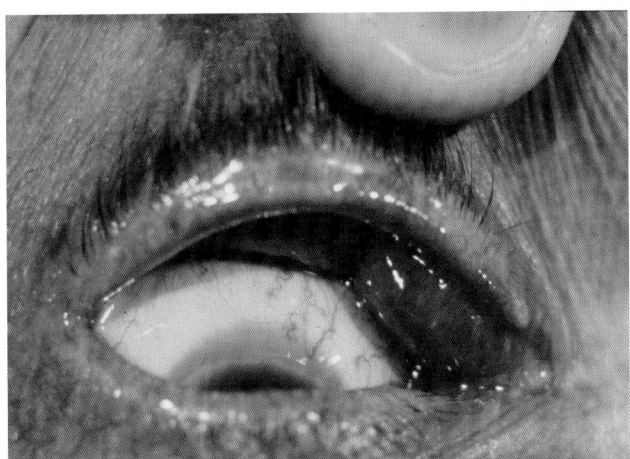

FIGURE 32.10.   Eyelid lymphoid proliferation. This lymphoid tumor with a rounded appearance affected the upper eyelid and penetrated through the tarsus to beneath the palpebral conjunctiva. The lesion was a diffuse large B-cell lymphoma. Systemic evaluation revealed evidence of systemic malignant lymphoma.

Table 32.1	CLINICAL CHARACTERISTICS OF 108 PATIENTS PRESENTING WITH OCULAR ADNEXAL LYMPHOID PROLIFERATIONS			
Parameter	Orbit	Conjunctiva	Eyelid	Total
Patients (no.)	69	30	9	108
Age range (y)	17–93	29–89	48–85	17–93
Median (y)	63	60	63	61
Male-to-female ratio	35:34	7:23	3:6	45:63
Location				
Right	29	12	7	48
Left	31	12	1	44
Bilateral	9	6	1	16
Chief complaint				
Mass/swelling	59	24	9	92
Ptosis	6	1	9	16
None—incidental finding	0	3	0	3
Other	4	2	0	6
Secondary complaints				
Diplopia	9	0	0	9
Ptosis	5	0	0	5
Pain	1	0	0	1
Other	3	4	0	7
Duration of symptoms				
Range (mo)	1–72	0.25–120	2–36	0.25–120
Median (mo)	4	4	4	4
Physical findings				
Ocular				
Palpable mass	56	30	9	95
Proptosis	34	0	0	34
Ptosis	13	1	9	23
Diplopia	9	0	0	9
Decreased motility	8	0	0	8
Other	1	0	0	1
Extraocular				
Negative	56	27	7	90
Lymphadenopathy	11	2	2	15
Hepatomegaly	3	0	0	3
Splenomegaly	4	1	0	5
Other	1	0	0	1
Number of patients with concurrent extraocular lymphoma	13	3	4	20
Locations				
Lymph nodes	12	2	4	18
Bone marrow	8	1	0	9
Peripheral Blood	2	1	0	3
Other	6	2	1	9

From Knowles DM, Jakobiec FA, McNally FA, et al. Lymphoid hyperplasia and malignant lymphoma occurring in the ocular adnexa (orbit, conjunctiva, and eyelids): a prospective multiparametric analysis of 108 cases during 1977–1987. *Hum Pathol* 1990;21:959–973, with permission.

staging as it appears superior in the detection of systemic disease compared to the traditional CT and MRI (192,193).

Morphology

Classification

Previously, Knowles and Jakobiec (194) proposed a histopathologic classification system for the ocular adnexal lymphoid proliferations that divided them into three broad categories: lymphoid hyperplasia (follicular or diffuse), atypical lymphoid hyperplasia, and malignant lymphoma (Table 32.2). The term *lymphoid hyperplasia* was used to designate the hypercellular, lymphoid cell–rich lesions that mimic malignant lymphoma clinically and histopathologically. The term *atypical lymphoid hyperplasia* was used to designate those lymphoid proliferations that cannot be categorized unequivocally as lymphoid hyperplasia or malignant lymphoma. Knowles and Jakobiec subclassified the malignant lymphomas according to the then widely accepted Working Formulation (195).

It is recommended that the terms *lymphoid hyperplasia* and *atypical lymphoid hyperplasia* be retained but that the malignant lymphomas be classified according to the WHO classification (137) (Table 32.2). This is especially important because such a large proportion of the ocular adnexal malignant lymphomas have been shown to represent MALT (extranodal marginal zone) lymphomas (40,138,196) and because of the greater prognostic value of the WHO classification when applied to ocular adnexal malignant lymphomas.

Lymphoid Hyperplasia

Knowles and Jakobiec (17) were the first to demonstrate by immunophenotypic analysis that most of the conjunctival small lymphocytic proliferations represent monoclonal small B-cell lymphomas. They showed that 30% of orbital, 26% of conjunctival, and 10% of eyelid lymphoid proliferations represent lymphoid hyperplasias (17). Regardless of location, most lymphoid hyperplasias are follicular (17).

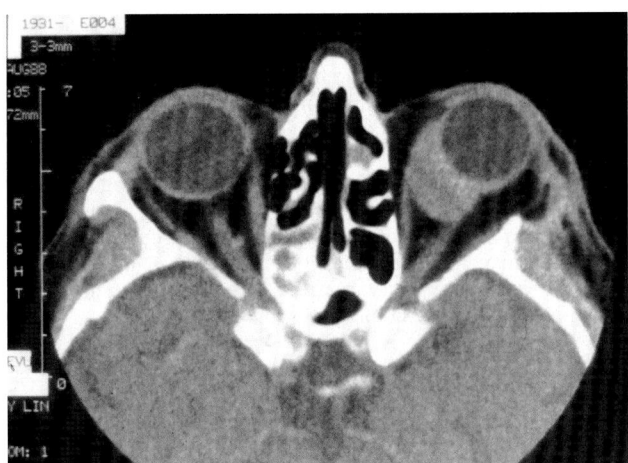

FIGURE 32.11.   CT scan of an orbital lymphoid proliferation. A retrobulbar nasal lymphoid proliferation molded to the posterior sclera of the globe. Despite its size, this lesion produced only minimal proptosis.

In some studies, lymphoid hyperplasias constitute an even lower proportion of ocular adnexal lymphoid proliferations, however. For example, Coupland et al. (40) classified only 12 of 102 (12%) and White et al. (197) classified even fewer ocular adnexal lymphoid proliferations as lymphoid hyperplasia. It is likely that patient referral patterns or case selection bias account in part for this discrepancy. However, the lower percentage of lymphoid hyperplasias in recent series also reflects increased histopathologic sophistication, an awareness

of MALT lymphomas, and an enhanced ability to detect clonality because of technologic advances in immunohistochemical, flow cytometric, and molecular genetic methods. Knowles and Jakobiec (23,133) and, later, other investigators (198,199) detected small clonal B-cell populations by molecular genetic techniques in some ocular adnexal lymphoid proliferations that were otherwise considered to be lymphoid hyperplasias (primarily diffuse) morphologically and immunophenotypically. Today, many investigators would interpret at least some of those lesions as malignant lymphomas, primarily belonging to the MALT category.

Lymphoid hyperplasias are hypercellular, lymphoid cell–rich lesions that can mimic malignant lymphomas clinically and histopathologically, sometimes to an extraordinary degree. In contrast to pseudotumors, but like malignant lymphomas, they lack a significant connective tissue stroma. The term *follicular* is used for lymphoid hyperplasias that contain prominent reactive germinal centers, and the term *diffuse* is used for lymphoid hyperplasias devoid of reactive germinal centers. Some follicular lymphoid hyperplasias are composed predominantly of reactive germinal centers that lie almost back to back. Reactive germinal centers usually are easily distinguished from neoplastic follicles by their polymorphous cell population, high mitotic rate, and numerous tingible body macrophages. The diffuse lymphoid hyperplasias are composed largely of a densely cellular, sometimes seemingly monomorphous, infiltrate of small lymphocytes. Dutcher bodies are absent. Occasional immunoblasts, plasma cells, and histiocytes are almost invariably present, however, imparting a subtle yet detectable polymorphous appearance. This cellular polymorphism greatly assists in distinguishing diffuse lymphoid hyperplasias from

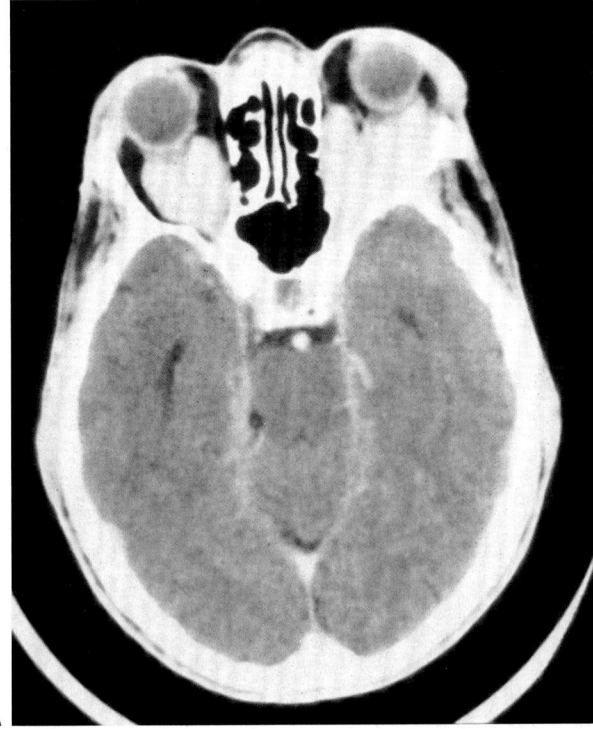

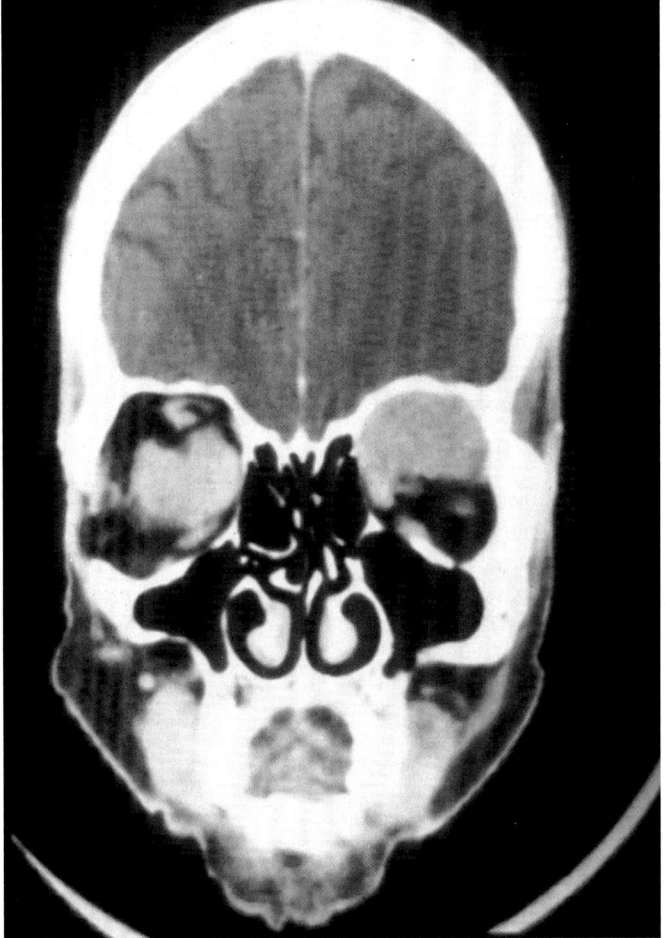

FIGURE 32.12.   CT scan of a bilateral orbital malignant lymphoma. A: Bilateral orbital malignant lymphoma occurring in an elderly patient surrounds the optic nerve bilaterally, conferring a bilobed appearance. Particularly on the left, the negative optic nerve shadow can be seen running down the middle of the lesion. Despite the presence of tumor tissue surrounding the optic nerve, vision was well preserved because of absence of compression as a result of the stroma-free nature of the lymphoid proliferation. **B:** A coronal projection of the axial depiction of the lesion shown in (**A**). There is no bone destruction, which is typical of most orbital lymphoid proliferations. There is also molding of the lesional tissue to the bone of the roof of the orbit.

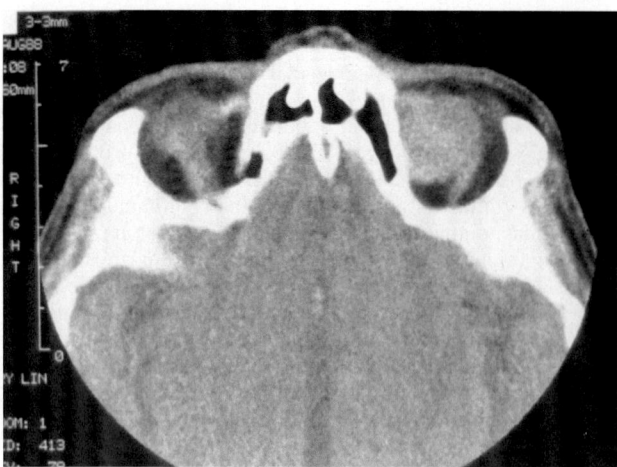

FIGURE 32.13.   CT scan of an orbital lymphoid proliferation. A superior orbital lymphoid proliferation molding as a *straight line* to the bone of the medial orbital wall without bone destruction.

small B-cell lymphomas that usually are monomorphic. Neutrophils and eosinophils are absent. Mitotic figures are infrequent. Numerous vessels lined by prominent hypertrophic endothelial cells are often present. Hemosiderin may be present (17,194). The lymphoepithelial lesions characteristically seen in MALT lymphomas (135) are absent (17,40).

Atypical Lymphoid Hyperplasia

Atypical lymphoid hyperplasias are those lymphoid proliferations that cannot be categorized unequivocally as lymphoid hyperplasia or malignant lymphoma. Most are predominantly diffuse, densely cellular lymphoid proliferations that fail to display a sufficiently obvious degree of cellular polymorphism or monomorphism to permit definitive classification as lymphoid hyperplasia or malignant lymphoma. At one time, Knowles and Jakobiec (2) classified as many as 10% of all ocular adnexal lymphoid proliferations as atypical lymphoid hyperplasia. Since then, extensive correlative histopathologic and immunophenotypic studies, many supported by antigen receptor

gene rearrangement analyses, have taught us that the diffuse, densely cellular, monomorphic ocular adnexal small lymphocytic proliferations, including those cases that contain reactive germinal centers or in which most of the cells display plasmacytoid differentiation, represent small B-cell lymphomas (3,9,10,13,15–17,24,39,40,131,178,197,200). Most ocular adnexal lymphoid proliferations not readily categorized as lymphoid hyperplasia or malignant lymphoma by morphologic criteria alone usually can be classified after immunophenotypic or molecular genetic analysis. Only about 5% or less of ocular adnexal lymphoid proliferations are classified as atypical lymphoid hyperplasia at the present time (40,138,197).

Malignant Lymphoma

Most malignant lymphomas occurring in the ocular adnexa are diffuse, densely cellular proliferations composed predominantly of small lymphoid cells superimposed on a sparse connective tissue stroma (Fig. 32.14). MALT lymphomas were initially recognized by Isaacson and Wright (201,202) in the gastrointestinal tract in 1983 and in the lung, salivary gland, and thyroid gland shortly thereafter. Over time, the breadth of distribution and the frequency of occurrence of MALT lymphomas became increasingly appreciated. In the early to mid-1990s investigators began to recognize that the clinicopathologic features of some malignant lymphomas arising in the ocular adnexa resemble those of MALT lymphomas arising at other extranodal sites (15,16,178,200,203,204). It is now known that MALT lymphomas are ubiquitous and comprise a significant proportion of the malignant lymphomas arising in the gastrointestinal tract and in all other extranodal locations where MALT is acquired. This includes the skin, breast, urinary bladder, kidney, and many other sites in addition to the ones already mentioned (205). In the Non-Hodgkin Lymphoma Classification Project, MALT lymphomas ranked third, constituting almost 8% of all non-Hodgkin lymphomas, behind diffuse large B-cell and follicle center lymphomas (206). The MALT lymphomas of the orbit and conjunctiva are classified among the extranodal marginal zone lymphoma of MALT in the WHO classification (137). The wide cytologic spectrum of MALT lymphomas and their consequent misclassification among numerous histologic categories before their recognition accounts for the multiple additional diagnostic categories used by Knowles and Jakobiec (17) and others (16,39) to classify the ocular adnexal malignant lymphomas in the past. It is now recognized that a large

Table 32.2	HISTOPATHOLOGIC CLASSIFICATION OF OCULAR ADNEXAL LYMPHOID PROLIFERATIONS
Former Classification (194)	**Current Classification**

Lymphoid hyperplasia
  Diffuse
  Follicular
	Lymphoid Hyperplasia
	  Diffuse
	  Follicular

Atypical lymphoid hyperplasia	Atypical lymphoid hyperplasia
Malignant lymphoma subclassified according to the Working Formulation	Malignant lymphoma subclassified according to the 2008 WHO classification (137)
Small lymphocytic, diffuse Small lymphocytic, plasmacytoid, diffuse	Chronic lymphocytic leukemia/small lymphocytic lymphoma
Intermediate lymphocytic, diffuse	Lymphoplasmacytic lymphoma
Small cleaved cell, diffuse, or follicular	Mantle cell lymphoma
Mixed small and large cell, diffuse, or follicular	Follicular lymphoma
Large cell, diffuse, or follicular	
Lymphoblastic lymphoma	Extranodal marginal zone lymphoma (MALT lymphoma)
Small, noncleaved cell, diffuse	Diffuse large B-cell lymphoma
Plasmacytoma, including myeloma	

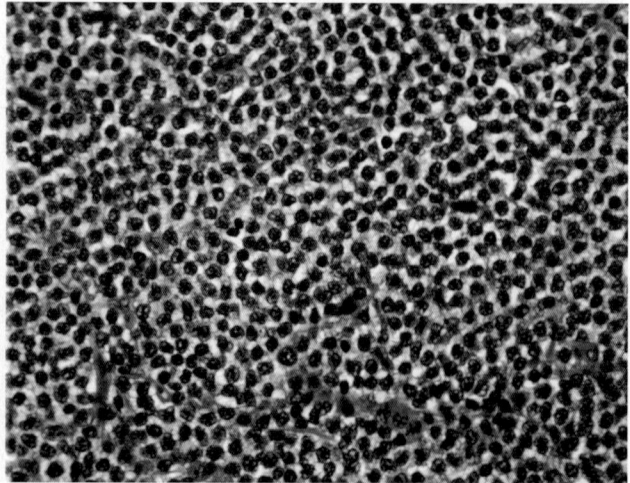

FIGURE 32.14. Most malignant lymphomas occurring in the ocular adnexa are diffuse, densely cellular proliferations composed predominately of small lymphoid cells superimposed on a sparse connective tissue stroma (hematoxylin and eosin stain, original magnifications: 400× magnification).

proportion of ocular adnexal malignant lymphomas previously classified otherwise instead represent MALT lymphomas.

The most important recent study is that by Ferry et al. (157), who analyzed 353 cases of ocular adnexal lymphoma based on the WHO classification. The authors classified the lymphomas as follows: marginal zone lymphoma, 52% (11% bilateral and 8% with a prior lymphoma diagnosis); follicular lymphoma, 23% (12.5% bilateral and 31% with a prior lymphoma diagnosis); diffuse large B-cell lymphoma, 8% (11% bilateral and 19% with a prior lymphoma); mantle cell lymphoma, 5% (32% bilateral and 63% with a prior lymphoma); chronic lymphocytic leukemia/small lymphocytic lymphoma, 4% (15% bilateral and 69% with prior lymphoma) and lymphoplasmacytic lymphoma, 1% (25% bilateral and 100% with prior lymphoma), in addition to other, more rare neoplasms, described in the study. Lagoo et al. (207) categorized 115 lymphomas of the ocular adnexa based on the WHO classification and have similarly found that marginal zone lymphoma represented 54% of the cases. A smaller study by Rosado et al. (167) diagnosed 89% MALT lymphomas among 62 ocular adnexal lymphomas. Of all ocular adnexal lymphomas, MALT lymphoma was the best candidate for the category of primary lymphoma (15,157,167,208,209), while mantle cell lymphoma, CLL/SLL, and lymphoplasmacytic lymphoma were rarely if ever primary (157). Approximately 50% of diffuse large B-cell lymphomas appeared to originate in the ocular adnexa (157,167,210).

The essential morphologic characteristics of MALT lymphomas is their emulation of normal MALT as exemplified by Peyer patches found in the terminal ileum (135). MALT lymphomas are characterized by the presence of neoplastic centrocyte-like cells distributed in a marginal zone pattern around reactive follicles and frequently attenuated rims of mantle zone lymphocytes (211) (Figs. 32.15 and 32.16). The neoplastic cells are believed to originate from benign equivalents that normally reside in the marginal zone around the mantle zone and the germinal centers (212). The neoplastic centrocyte-like cells may infiltrate into the follicles, at times entirely overtaking them, a process called *follicle colonization* (213). Sometimes, the neoplastic proliferation may be sufficiently extensive to result in architectural obliteration and masking of the residual benign germinal centers. In these instances, the preexisting benign follicles can be highlighted by the immunohistochemical demonstration of CD21-positive follicular dendritic cells (135). The neoplastic cells also infiltrate the surrounding tissue where they characteristically invade the overlying epithelium to form lymphoepithelial lesions (211), which are associated with epithelial destruction (214).

FIGURE 32.15.   MALT lymphoma arising in the conjunctiva. A benign germinal center is surrounded by a dense, monomorphic small lymphocytic proliferation (hematoxylin and eosin stain, original magnification: 40× magnification).

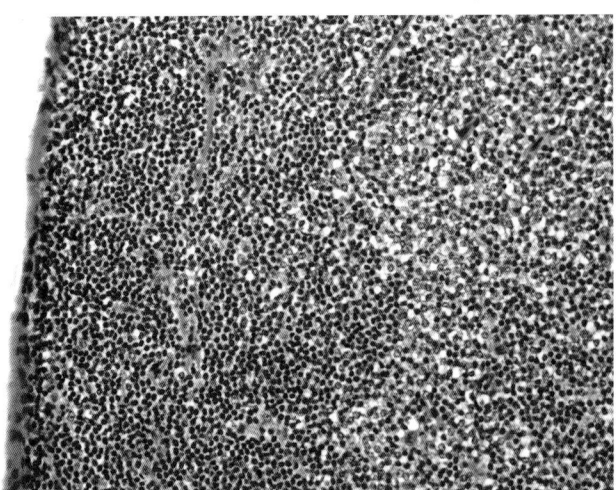

FIGURE 32.16.   Conjunctival MALT lymphoma. MALT lymphomas are characterized by the presence of a dense, monomorphic proliferation of neoplastic centrocyte-like cells distributed in a marginal zone pattern around benign germinal centers (hematoxylin and eosin stain, original magnification: 200× magnification).

Their presence can be highlighted by the immunohistochemical demonstration of cytokeratin-positive epithelium in which the neoplastic lymphoid cells lie (135). Coupland et al. (40) found lymphoepithelial lesions in the conjunctival or lacrimal gland epithelium in 70% of the ocular adnexal MALT lymphomas in their series. However, a significantly lower proportion was identified by Ferry et al. (157) (13% of all cases). Lymphoepithelial lesions were also rare to absent in a study by Rawal et al. (215) and White et al. (178). The neoplastic cells may also migrate into the same organ at different locations or into other mucosal sites (205). These properties probably account for the high frequency of multiple localizations of MALT lymphoma in the same organ (i.e., the stomach, at diagnosis [216,217]) as well as recurrences in other organs that harbor MALT (202,218). The latter explains the synchronous and dysynchronous occurrence of MALT lymphoma in the ocular adnexa and other mucosal sites (178,196,219,220).

The neoplastic cells of MALT lymphoma have been called centrocyte-like because of their resemblance to follicle center centrocytes. These cells characteristically are small to medium-sized and contain moderately abundant cytoplasm and irregularly shaped nuclei that bear a close resemblance to those of centrocytes (small cleaved cells) (135) (Fig. 32.17). They exhibit greater cytologic variability than centrocytes, however. Scattered large cells, resembling centroblasts or immunoblasts, are usually present (Fig. 32.18). Sometimes, the marginal zone B cells have minimal nuclear membrane irregularities and closely resemble small lymphocytes (Fig. 32.19). Other times, they contain abundant pale-staining to clear cytoplasm and resemble monocytoid B cells (Fig. 32.17). They frequently exhibit plasmacytoid differentiation (135,205,211,215). As opposed to MALT lymphomas in other sites, ocular adnexal tumors rarely contain monocytoid cells with abundant clear cytoplasm (160,166). Similarly, numerous plasma cells are present in only 10% to 30% of the ocular adnexal MALT lymphoma cases (160,215). Coupland and Ferry identified Dutcher bodies in 20% and 27% of the ocular adnexal MALT lymphomas in their series, respectively (40,157). The latter finding suggests that many cases formerly classified as lymphoplasmacytic lymphomas and immunocytomas represent MALT lymphomas. Polykaryocytes (multinucleated cells, which probably represent modified follicular dendritic cells) are a frequent feature of ocular adnexal MALT lymphoma, where they are seen in nearly half of the cases (46,157) (Fig. 32.19). A small subset of ocular adnexal MALT lymphomas may be associated with amyloid

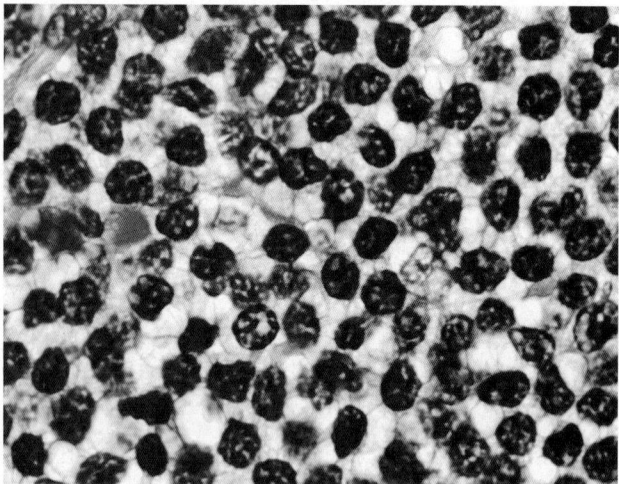

FIGURE 32.17.   Ocular adnexal MALT lymphoma. The malignant lymphoid cells that make up MALT lymphomas have been called centrocyte-like because of their close resemblance to follicle center centrocytes (small cleaved cells). These cells characteristically are small to medium sized and contain moderately abundant cytoplasm and irregularly shaped nuclei (hematoxylin and eosin stain, original magnification: 1,000× magnification).

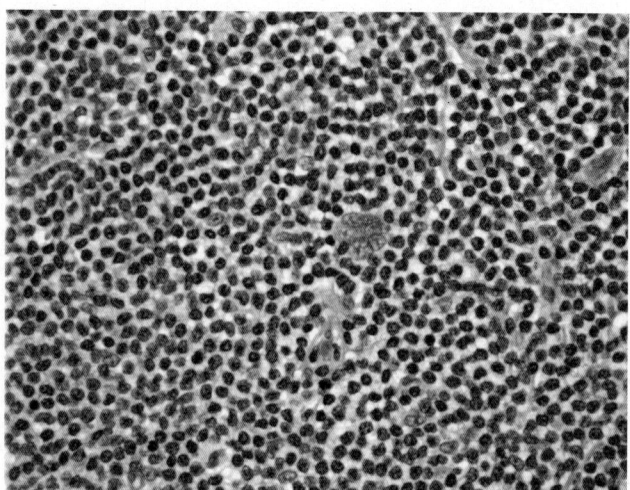

FIGURE 32.19.   Ocular adnexal MALT lymphoma. The centrocyte-like neoplastic cells that make up MALT lymphomas exhibit greater cytologic variability than centrocytes. Sometimes, as in this case, they possess minimal nuclear membrane irregularities and closely resemble the neoplastic cells of small lymphocytic lymphoma. For this reason, many MALT lymphomas were previously included within the small lymphocytic lymphoma category of the Working Formulation. A multinucleated polykaryocyte is seen in the center of the image (hematoxylin and eosin stain, original magnification: 400× magnification).

deposition (2% of all MALT lymphoma cases in the study by Ferry et al. [157]). A separate study by Ryan and Ferry showed that these patients may have amyloid in other sites involved by MALT lymphoma but do not have systemic amyloidosis (221). Lastly, ocular adnexal MALT lymphomas are capable of undergoing large cell transformation, which is associated with more aggressive clinical behavior (135,157,216,222).

Follicular lymphoma is the distant second most common lymphoma of the ocular adnexa (40,135,157,178,207,223,224) (Fig. 32.20). The study by Ferry et al. (157) included 80 patients with ocular adnexal follicular lymphoma. There were 30 males and 50 females with an age range of 11 to 92 years. Twenty-five patients (31%) had a prior diagnosis of lymphoma. The interval to the development of ocular manifestations was 2 to 228 months (median, 72 months). Bilateral involvement was seen in 10 patients. Most follicular lymphomas of the ocular adnexa were low-grade (grade 1–2 of 3) and were predominantly follicular (157) (Fig. 32.20). One patient had a "pediatric-type" follicular lymphoma. In addition, cases of ocular adnexal follicular lymphoma arising in association with IgG4-related sclerosing disease have been described (121,160).

Diffuse large B-cell lymphoma was the third most common ocular adnexal lymphoma in many of the larger recent case series (40,157,224). Ferry et al. (157) have described 27 cases of ocular adnexal DLBCL. Fourteen patients were men and thirteen were women with an age range of 21 to 88 years. Five patients (36%) had a prior lymphoma, initially arising in bone, liver, spleen, lymph node, and testis, respectively. Three patients had bilateral orbital involvement. Morphologically, the lymphomas were predominantly centroblastic, although some cases were composed of large multilobated cells or immunoblasts (157).

Ocular adnexal mantle cell lymphoma is less common than the previously described entities. The study by Ferry et al. included 19 patients with ocular adnexal mantle cell lymphoma. There were 13 men and 6 women, aged 51 to 91 years. Sixteen patients (84%) had either a history of lymphoma or widespread systemic disease at the time of the diagnosis. Bilateral ocular adnexal involvement was seen in six patients. The morphology and immunophenotype were typical of mantle cell lymphoma (157). Similar results were obtained by Rasmussen et al. (225) who studied 21 patients with ocular adnexal mantle cell lymphoma.

Differential Diagnosis

The histopathologic criteria that traditionally have been used to distinguish between benign and malignant extranodal lymphoid infiltrates emphasize that minimal architectural effacement, the presence of germinal centers, and cytologic maturity and polymorphism favor benignancy, whereas extensive architectural effacement, the absence of germinal centers, cytologic atypia, and monomorphism favor malignancy (29). These criteria often are not only not helpful in evaluating ocular adnexal small lymphocytic proliferations but may be misleading in some instances (4–6). Criteria that sometimes are useful in evaluating nodal lymphoid proliferations, such as effacement of the preexisting lymph node architecture and capsular invasion, are not useful in evaluating ocular adnexal lymphoid proliferations. Lymphoid hyperplasias and malignant lymphomas may infiltrate into the adipose and fibrous connective tissue of the ocular adnexa without regard for anatomic boundaries (2,5,207). Definitive diagnosis usually depends on careful

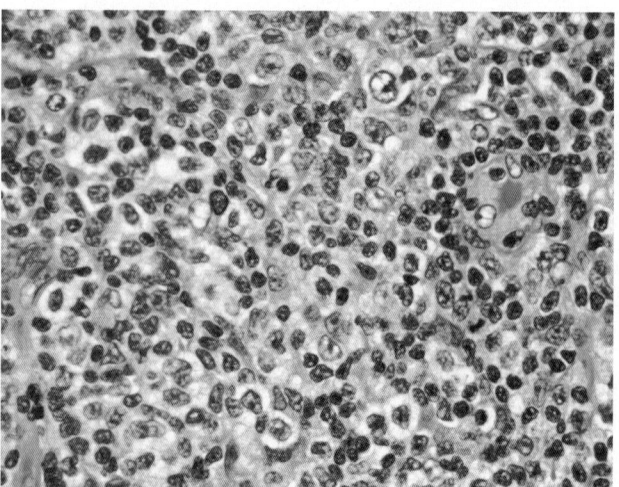

FIGURE 32.18.   Conjunctival MALT lymphoma. The tumor cells are composed of variable numbers of marginal zone cells, plasma cells, and scattered large transformed B cells (hematoxylin and eosin stain, original magnification: 400× magnification).

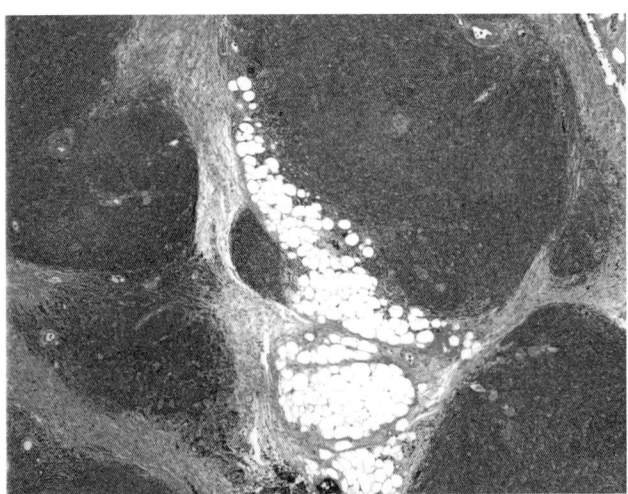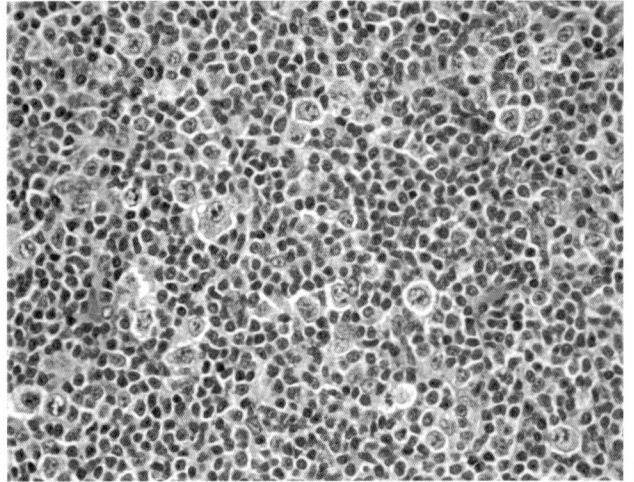

A   B

FIGURE 32.20.   **Follicular lymphoma of the periorbital soft tissue. A:** There is a nodular infiltrate with lymphoid follicles of variable size and shape (hematoxylin and eosin stain, original magnification: 40× magnification). **B:** The follicles consist of a mixture of small centrocytes with irregular, cleaved nuclei and larger centroblasts with cleaved or noncleaved nuclei (hematoxylin and eosin stain, original magnification: 400× magnification).

evaluation of the cytomorphology of the cell populations that comprise the lymphoid proliferation, despite the shortcomings inherent in the application of solely cytologic criteria to proliferations of small lymphocytic cells with a relatively bland cytologic appearance occurring in an extranodal location.

The several parameters that are important to evaluate in the differential diagnosis of ocular adnexal lymphoid proliferations include the presence or absence of reactive germinal centers and pseudofollicular proliferation centers, the relationship between the germinal centers and the interfollicular cells, the density, monomorphic versus polymorphic nature, the degree of cytologic atypia of the cellular proliferation, and the presence or absence of lymphoepithelial lesions and Dutcher bodies.

Lymphoid hyperplasias generally contain one to several reactive germinal centers. These usually are surrounded by well-defined mantle zones of small lymphocytes and are separated by an interfollicular polymorphous cell population (17,194). MALT lymphomas also may contain reactive germinal centers. These may be circumscribed by a thin zone of mantle cells but are characteristically surrounded by a diffuse, relatively monomorphic proliferation of centrocyte-like cells, which sometimes may infiltrate and even colonize the follicles (135) (Fig. 32.16). Mantle cell lymphomas, similarly, may contain reactive germinal centers, which may range from small and atrophic to large and hyperplastic. They usually are devoid of mantle zones and characteristically are surrounded and separated by a dense, monotonous, small- to medium-sized lymphoid cell proliferation exhibiting variable but obvious cytologic atypia. The reactive germinal centers in lymphoid hyperplasias, MALT lymphomas, and mantle cell lymphomas are distinguishable from the neoplastic follicles of follicular lymphoma by their polymorphous cell population, numerous tingible body macrophages, and high mitotic index. In addition, follicular lymphoma has been shown to have a propensity for the lacrimal gland, while cases of reactive lymphoid follicular hyperplasia preferentially involve the conjunctiva (226). Some lymphoid hyperplasias are diffuse. These usually are less densely cellular than small B-cell lymphomas and nearly always exhibit polymorphous cytomorphology because of the admixture of distinct cell populations, namely, cytologically benign small lymphocytes, mature plasma cells, immunoblasts, and histiocytes (17,194). In contrast, small lymphocytic lymphomas are strikingly monomorphic because of the presence of a dense, diffuse proliferation of monotonous-appearing small lymphoid

cells. Plasmacytoid small lymphocytic lymphomas, currently referred to as lymphoplasmacytic lymphomas (137,180,182), often retain this homogeneous appearance because of the presence of a diffuse proliferation of small lymphocytes, plasmacytoid lymphocytes, and plasma cells. A variable proportion of the neoplastic cells in these cases contain Dutcher bodies, eosinophilic periodic acid-Schiff–positive, diastase-resistant intranuclear inclusions of immunoglobulin or Russell bodies, cytoplasmic globules of immunoglobulin (180,182) (Figs. 32.21 and 32.22). Lymphoid hyperplasias lack the pseudofollicular proliferation centers comprising large, variably transformed lymphoid cells that are characteristically observed in small lymphocytic lymphomas (136,195). Lymphoepithelial lesions are present in many MALT lymphomas (135,211). However, they are less relevant as a diagnostic criterion outside of the stomach because they may be observed in nonlymphomatous extranodal lymphocytic infiltrates (227). Dutcher bodies are only rarely, if ever, identified in lymphoid hyperplasias, but they are found relatively frequently in MALT lymphomas and lymphoplasmacytic lymphomas (16,40). Recognition of these subtle morphologic differences usually permits most ocular

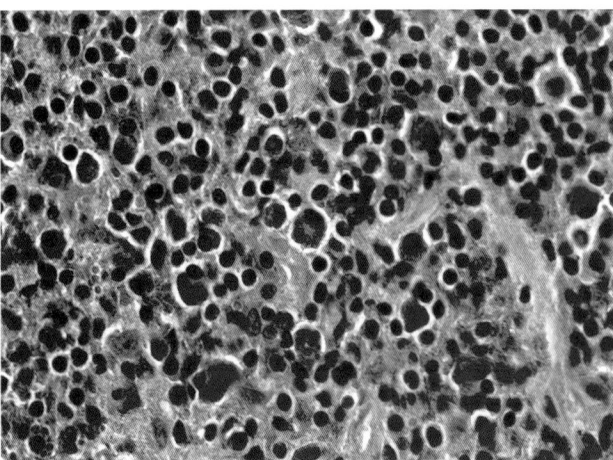

FIGURE 32.21.   **Lymphoplasmacytic lymphoma of the orbit.** In this instance, many of the neoplastic cells contain abundant cytoplasmic globules of immunoglobulin, so-called Russell bodies (hematoxylin and eosin stain, original magnification: 400× magnification).

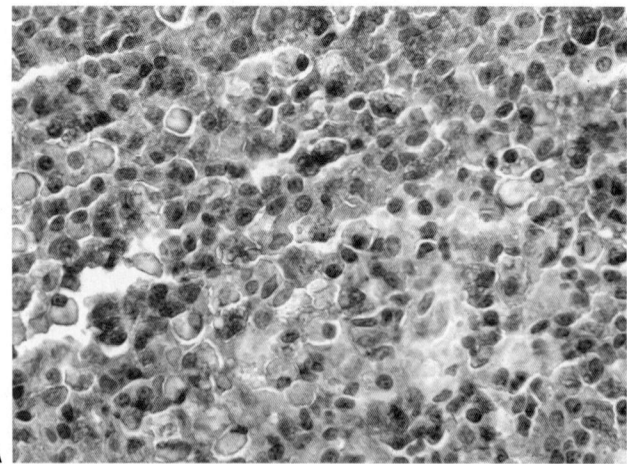

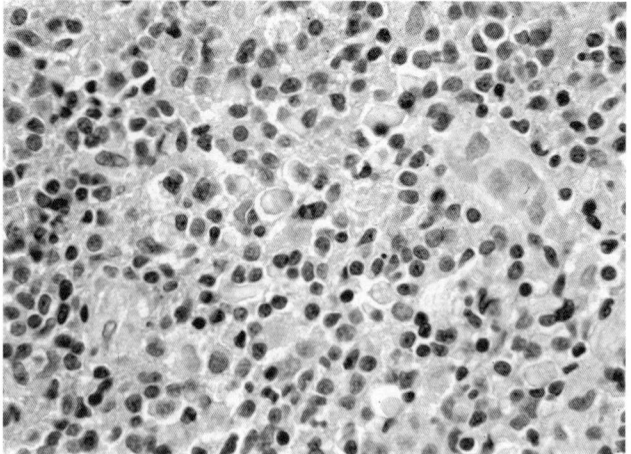

FIGURE 32.22. Paraffin sections of the orbital lymphoplasmacytic lymphoma illustrated in Figure 32.21 stained for cytoplasmic immuno-globulin by immunoperoxidase. This technique demonstrates that most of these immunoglobulin inclusions are κ light-chain positive **(A)** and λ light-chain negative **(B)**, consistent with a clonal B-cell derivation (original magnification: 630× magnification).

adnexal lymphoid hyperplasias and malignant lymphomas to be distinguished from one another. However, immunopheno-typic and, if necessary, molecular analysis serve as the final arbiters.

Immunophenotype

More than 90% of all ocular adnexal lymphoid proliferations can be categorized as polyclonal lymphoid hyperplasias or monoclonal B-cell lymphomas based on the results of immu-nophenotypic analysis; the remaining cases generally are con-sidered indeterminate because of various technical problems encountered during immunophenotypic analysis (17,135,178).

Immunophenotypic analysis of isolated cells in suspension by flow cytometry offers the advantage of precise quantitation of lymphoid cell subpopulations and the ability to perform pref-erential gated and rare event analysis, sometimes permitting the detection of a small clonal B-cell population in the middle of a large polyclonal cell population (see Chapter 4). Immuno-histochemical analysis of frozen and paraffin tissue sections allows precise localization of lymphoid cell subpopulations *in situ* and avoids the possible loss of selected cell populations during cell isolation (see Chapter 3). Maximum information is derived by performing flow cytometric and immunohisto-chemical analysis in each case and then correlating the results in conjunction with morphologic examination of the histologic sections. Knowles and Jakobiec collected immunophenotypic data on more than 150 ocular adnexal lymphoid proliferations analyzed in this manner during the 1980s (3,17,131,132,134). They based many of their conclusions concerning the ocular adnexal lymphoid proliferations on these data, which are sub-sequently described.

In the experience of Knowles and Jakobiec (3,17,131,132,134), diffuse and follicular lymphoid hyperplasias of the ocular adnexa contain between 38% and 73% (mean, 55%) T cells. The one case of lymphoid hyperplasia that contained only 38% T cells was the only one they encountered in which T cells accounted for <40% of the total cell population. In tissue sections, T cells usually appear to represent between 50% and 75% of the total cell population. This varies, however, with the number and size of the reactive germinal centers (B-cell zones) present in the lesion. The ratio of CD4 (helper) to CD8 (suppressor or cytotoxic) T cells ranges from 2.2 to 14.4 (mean, 5.6) based on flow cyto-metric analysis. Polyclonal lymphoid hyperplasias contain from 4% to 57% (mean, 35%) B cells based on the flow cytometric detection of cells that express pan-B-cell–associated antigens

CD20 or CD22. The ratio of κ to λ light-chain–positive B cells ranges from 0.3 to 6.3 (mean, 2.0). Most of the remaining cells express HLA-DR (Ia) antigens and represent small numbers of surface immunoglobulin–negative B cells and tissue monocytes (17). Ocular adnexal polyclonal lymphoid hyperplasias reca-pitulate the immunophenotypic profiles of benign and reactive lymph nodes, except for a generally higher CD4 to CD8 ratio.

Knowles and Jakobiec (3,17,131,132) found that the ocular adnexal B-cell lymphomas contain 48% to 96% (mean, 78%) B cells based on the flow cytometric detection of cells that express surface immunoglobulin or B-cell–associated antigen CD20. B cells constituted <60% of the total cell population in only 3 of 65 B-cell lymphomas that they examined. In tissue sections, B cells always appear to represent the majority cell population, constituting from about 60% to 90% of the total cell population. Approximately 95% of these B-cell lymphomas express monotypic surface immunoglobulin. The most common surface immunoglobulin isotypes are IgMκ, IgMDκ, IgMλ, and IgMDλ; these account for about 85% of the immunoglobulin isotypes expressed by ocular adnexal B-cell lymphomas. Ocu-lar adnexal lymphomas infrequently express IgA, even though IgA B cells, IgA plasma cells, and IgA secretory antibody are present in the MALT of the conjunctiva (8) and lacrimal gland (228). The ratio of κ to λ light-chain–positive B cells was ≤0.1 or ≥13.8 in 56 (92%) of 61 B-cell lymphomas and between 6.9 and 9.5 in the remaining 5 cases that they studied. The inten-sity of staining for surface immunoglobulin is sometimes faint, as in the case of chronic lymphocytic leukemia, but usually is moderate to bright, as in the case of most B-cell non-Hodgkin lymphomas (11). Monoclonal B-cell lymphomas contain 1% to 46% (mean, 18%) T cells. Only 3 of 65 monoclonal B-cell lym-phomas that Knowles and Jakobiec studied contained >40% T cells. In contrast with lymphoid hyperplasias, the CD4 to CD8 ratio among monoclonal B-cell lymphomas ranges from 0.8 to 5.7 (mean, 2.5) and is virtually identical to that of systemic B-cell lymphomas (229).

The neoplastic cells of ocular adnexal MALT lymphoma, which represent most primary ocular adnexal malignant lym-phomas, express B-cell–associated antigens CD19, CD20, CD22, and CD79a, and monotypic surface immunoglobulin, usually IgM, followed by IgG with only rare cases of IgA(+) or IgD(+) cells (160,205) (Fig. 32.23). They usually also express CD21 and CD35 and usually lack CD5, CD10, and CD23 (205). Bcl-2 is aberrantly expressed in up to 95% of the cases (157) (Fig. 32.23). CD43 reactivity is seen less often than in other MALT lympho-mas, in 12% to 25% of the cases (160,166). Nearly all cases

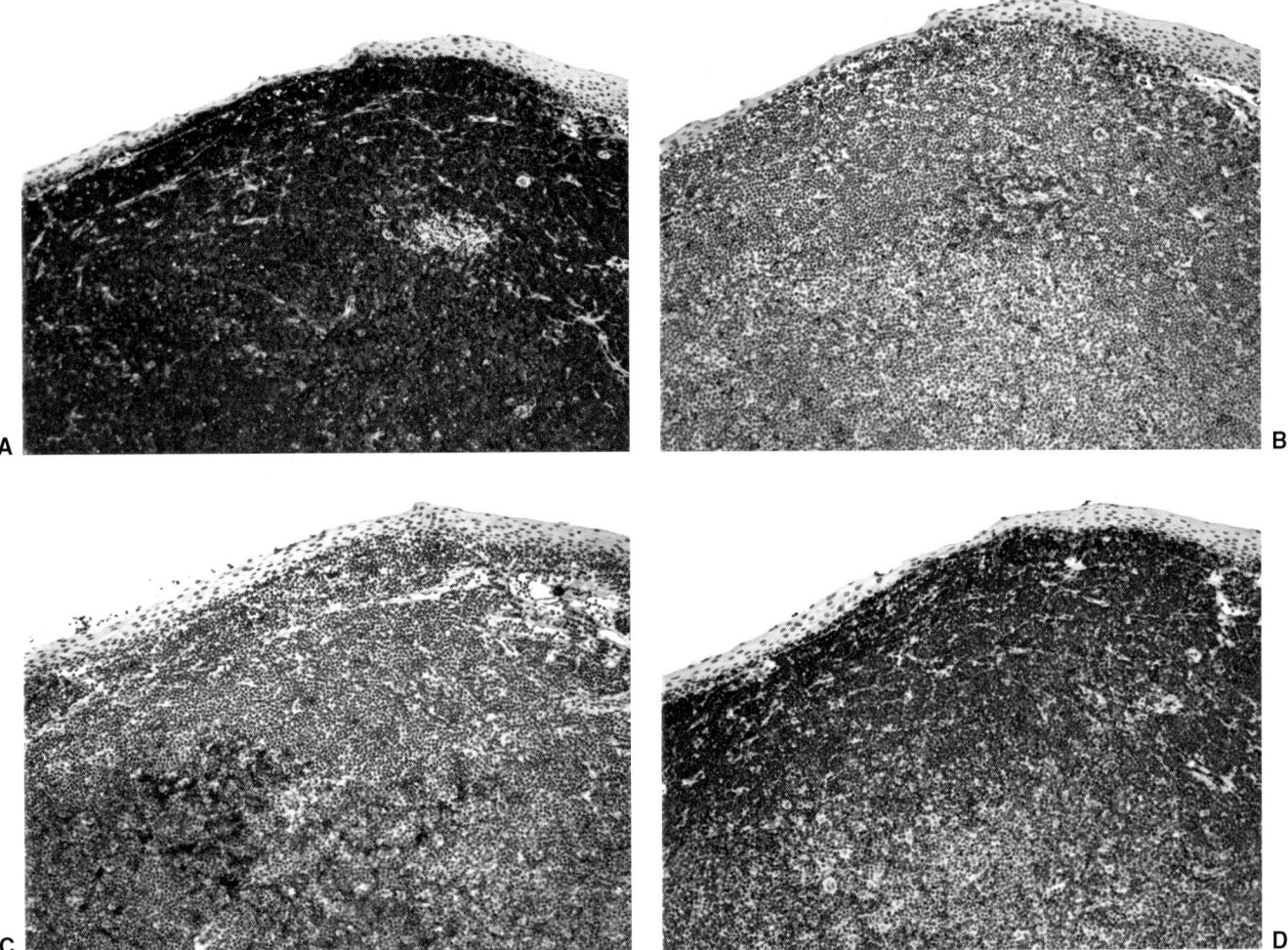

FIGURE 32.23.   Immunostaining of an orbital marginal zone lymphoma of MALT. A: Approximately 90% of the cells are B cells, based on the expression of CD20. **B:** fewer than 10% of the cells are T cells, based on the expression of CD3. **C:** CD21 highlights disrupted follicular dendritic cell meshworks, consistent with a colonized reactive lymphoid follicle. **D:** The neoplastic B lymphocytes aberrantly express Bcl-2.

have residual follicular dendritic cell meshworks, which may be highlighted by CD21 and CD23 (160) (Fig. 32.23). They also usually exhibit a low proliferation index based on monoclonal antibody Ki-67 reactivity (205).

In this regard, it may be considered somewhat surprising that Knowles and Jakobiec found variable populations of CD5+ neoplastic B cells in 22% of their cases, primarily those that they classified as small lymphocytic or mantle cell lymphoma (17). However, although there is no doubt about the appropriateness of the histopathologic classification of most of these lesions, at least in some instances, they represented systemic lymphomas secondarily involving the ocular adnexa. Ferry et al. (230) have since described cases of apparent CD5+ MALT lymphoma. They further suggested that CD5 expression in MALT lymphomas occurring in all sites, including the ocular adnexa, is a prognostic marker for persistent or recurrent disease, for dissemination to the bone marrow and other extranodal sites, and for leukemic involvement of the peripheral blood (230). Some of the cases reported by Knowles and Jakobiec may fall into this category. Several studies have also identified a CD5-positive subtype of splenic marginal zone lymphoma. These cases appeared clinically different from chronic lymphocytic leukemia and were similar to CD5-positive cases of marginal zone lymphoma found elsewhere (231,232). Rarely, cases of apparent CD5+ ocular adnexal MALT lymphoma have been described (40,135,157,166,178,233–236). Some of the

latter patients, uncharacteristically for MALT lymphoma, also had advanced-stage disease and died from their disease within 5 years after diagnosis (40,230,236). Further and larger studies are necessary to determine the prognostic value of CD5 expression among ocular adnexal and other MALT lymphomas.

These results provide some useful guidelines for employing immunophenotypic analysis as an adjunct in the differential diagnosis of lymphoid hyperplasia versus malignant lymphoma in the ocular adnexa. First, Knowles and Jakobiec found that 24 (96%) of 25 polyclonal lymphoid hyperplasias contained more than 40% T cells and fewer than 60% B cells, whereas 62 (95%) of 65 monoclonal B-cell lymphomas contained more than 60% B cells and fewer than 40% T cells. Merely determining the proportion of T and B cells resulted in accurately predicting the histopathologic diagnosis and the polyclonal or monoclonal B-cell nature of 86 of 90 (96%) ocular adnexal lymphoid proliferations. Second, they found that the κ to λ light-chain ratio ranged between 0.3 and 6.3 (mean, 2.0) among 25 polyclonal lymphoid hyperplasias but was $\leq$0.1 and $\geq$13.8 among 56 (92%) of 61 B-cell lymphomas and between 6.9 and 9.5 in the remaining five cases. Precise quantitation of the ratio of κ to λ light chains by flow cytometric analysis of isolated cells in suspension is extremely useful for distinguishing reliably between lymphoid hyperplasia and malignant lymphoma. Third, they found that approximately 25% of B-cell lymphomas express anomalous immunophenotypic profiles (i.e., CD5 expression or absence of surface immunoglobulin) (17). In conclusion, the judicious application of these immunophenotypic criteria usually permits an ocular adnexal lymphoid proliferation to be classified as polyclonal lymphoid hyperplasia or monoclonal B-cell lymphoma.

Cytogenetics

The principal genes involved among the major clinicopathologic categories of B-cell non-Hodgkin lymphomas, and therefore believed to play a role in their pathogenesis, are *BCL1*, *BCL2*, *BCL6*, *MYC*, and *TP53* (see Chapter 7). The MALT lymphomas characteristically lack rearrangements of the *BCL1*, *BCL2*, *BCL6*, and *MYC* genes (237,238); a *MYC* gene rearrangement has only been described in some high-grade MALT lymphomas (239).

Cytogenetic studies have revealed several recurrent translocations in a significant proportion of ocular adnexal MALT lymphomas. The most common abnormalities are trisomy of chromosome 3 observed in up to 68% of the patients and trisomy of chromosome 18 seen in up to 57% of the patients (166,240–242). In a study by Ruiz et al. (166), gain of chromosome 3 was significantly more frequent in cases of MALT lymphoma of the orbit (81%), compared with lacrimal gland (40%) and conjunctiva (12%). Tanimoto et al. (241) studied 34 Japanese patients and showed that trisomy 18 was present predominantly in the conjunctival lesions of young females. The authors also demonstrated that all cases of recurrent lymphoma harbored trisomy 18 (241).

Four major translocations have been identified in MALT lymphomas from various sites. They include the t(11;18)(q21;q21), which results in chimeric fusion protein (API2-MALT1) by juxtaposing the API2 (apoptosis inhibitor 2) gene on chromosome 11 to the MALT1 gene on chromosome 18. The three remaining translocations involve the immunoglobulin heavy chain gene on chromosome 14 and include t(1;14)(p22;q32), which results in the transcriptional deregulation of BCL10 protein, t(14;18) (q32;q21), which deregulates the MALT1 protein, and t(3;14) (p14.1;q32), which increases the expression of FOXP1 protein. These translocations appear to be mutually exclusive (243). All the translocations affect the common signaling pathway, which results in activation of the NF-κB complex, leading to lymphomatous cell transformation, proliferation, and an antiapoptotic phenotype (166). The presence of these abnormalities correlates with the site of lymphoma (243). Thus, ocular adnexal marginal zone lymphoma harbors t(14;18) in approximately 25% of the cases, while this translocation is very rare in the stomach (243,244). It is largely specific to MALT lymphoma and so far has only been reported in rare cases of extranodal diffuse large B-cell lymphoma (245). This translocation may be associated with trisomy 3 (244). Alternatively, t(11;18) is more frequent in the stomach and lung MALT lymphoma compared to lymphoma of the ocular adnexa (34%, 24%, and 16% of the patients, respectively) based on a large multicentric study of 417 patients (246,247). It was present in only 3% of cases in the study of 252 patients by Streubel et al. (243). A Japanese study of 51 cases of ocular adnexal MALT lymphoma did not identify t(11;18) in any of the cases (248). The t(3;14) has been identified in approximately 20% of the patients (249). This translocation has also been identified in diffuse large B-cell lymphomas and transformed MALT lymphomas (249,250). The t(1;14) is rare or absent in ocular adnexal lymphoma (243,251).

Immunohistochemistry with BCL10 has been investigated as a surrogate marker for several translocations. BCL10 is normally expressed in the cytoplasm of germinal center and marginal zone B cells (252). Several studies have found that the presence of t(11;18) and t(1;14) correlated with nuclear BCL10 expression, while cases with t(14;18) had perinuclear staining (251,253), However, nuclear staining has also been found in

cases of MALT lymphoma and lymphoplasmacytic lymphoma that lack these translocations, limiting its usefulness (246,248).

Only a few investigators have studied the molecular genetic characteristics of the ocular adnexal lymphoid proliferations. Knowles et al. failed to detect evidence of *BCL1*, *BCL2*, or *MYC* gene rearrangements among more than 20 primary ocular adnexal malignant lymphomas that they studied (unpublished observations). Wotherspoon et al. similarly failed to detect rearrangements of these genes among several primary conjunctival malignant lymphomas (200,203), as did Baldini et al. (254). The latter investigators also failed to detect *BCL6* gene rearrangements among these cases (254). These negative findings reflect the fact that most of the cases studied by all these investigators are MALT lymphomas. Unfortunately, only very few additional studies have been performed. Coupland et al. (40), for example, identified p53 protein overexpression in occasional malignant cells in 11% of their ocular adnexal MALT lymphomas. Although p53 protein overexpression does not consistently correlate with *TP53* gene mutation (255), this finding may have prognostic significance.

Recently, array-comparative genomic hybridization (array-CGH) of ocular adnexal and pulmonary MALT lymphomas revealed recurrent 6q23 losses and 6p21.2-6p22.1 gains exclusive to ocular cases (256). High-resolution chromosome 6 tile-path array-CGH identified NF-κB inhibitor A20 as the target of 6q23.3 deletion and the TNFA/B/C locus as a putative target of 6p21.2-22.1 gain. Interphase fluorescence *in situ* hybridization showed that A20 deletion occurred in MALT lymphoma of the ocular adnexa (8/42 = 19%), salivary gland (2/24 = 8%), thyroid (1/9 = 11%), and liver (1/2), but not that of the lung (26), stomach (45), and skin (13) (256). Inactivation of A20 has been shown to occur by deletion, mutation, and promoter methylation (257). In the largest study to date of 105 cases of ocular adnexal MALT lymphoma somatic mutation of A20 was seen in almost one-third of cases (28.6%) (258). A20 mutations were significantly associated with A20 heterozygous deletion. These abnormalities appear to occur exclusively in translocation-negative cases. A20 mutation/deletion was also significantly associated with increased expression of the NF-κB target genes CCR2, TLR6, and BCL2. Clinically, A20 deletion was associated with concurrent involvement of different adnexal tissues or extraocular sites at diagnosis, a higher proportion of relapse (67% vs. 37%), and a shorter relapse-free survival (256). These cases have also required significantly higher radiation dosages to achieve complete remission (258).

Further insight into the pathogenesis of the ocular adnexal malignant lymphomas awaits more extensive investigation of their molecular genetic basis.

Molecular Characteristics

Ocular adnexal MALT lymphomas have been shown to have a clonal immunoglobulin heavy chain variable region PCR product in 60% to 70% of cases, which is similar to the rate of B-cell clonality in other extranodal MALT lymphomas (259–261). The inability to detect monoclonal IGH gene sequences in some of the cases may be due to technical artifact, somatic mutations of the PCR primer-binding region, or absence of immunoglobulin gene rearrangement, which has rarely been observed in lymphoma (262). Biased use of IGHV families and genes (in particular the IGHV4 family in US patients and the IGHV3 family in non-US patients) has been demonstrated in a significant proportion of patients with MALT lymphoma, highlighting B-cell receptor-mediated antigen stimulation in the pathogenesis of these lymphomas (260,263–267).

The ocular adnexal B-cell lymphomas consistently exhibit monoallelic or biallelic clonal immunoglobulin heavy- and light-chain gene rearrangements by Southern blot hybridization analysis (23). This finding is consistent with the clonal

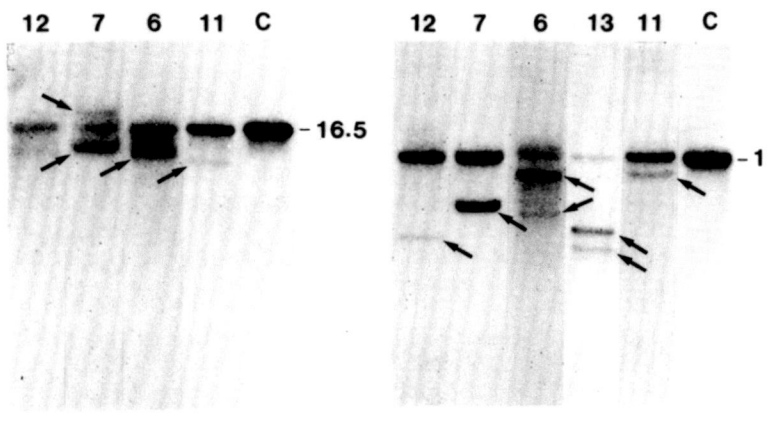

FIGURE 32.24. Southern blot hybridization analysis of ocular adnexal lymphoid proliferations for immunoglobulin gene rearrangements. The DNA extracted from ocular adnexal lymphoid proliferations classified as B-cell lymphomas according to histopathologic and immunophenotypic criteria and from human fibroblasts (control [C]) were digested with *Eco*RI or *Hind*III and hybridized to an immunoglobulin heavy-chain joining region (J_H) probe. Rearrangement bands are indicated by *arrows*. Lane C displays the immunoglobulin gene germ line configuration. Each ocular adnexal lymphoid proliferation exhibits clonal immunoglobulin heavy chain gene rearrangements consistent with a clonal B-cell derivation. (Modified from Neri A, Jakobiec FA, Pelicci PG, et al. Immunoglobulin and T cell receptor beta chain gene rearrangement analysis of ocular adnexal lymphoid neoplasms: clinical and biologic implications. *Blood* 1987;70:1519–1529, with permission.)

expansion of a mature B-cell population (11). The hybridization signals usually are clear and intense because the clonal B-cell population nearly always represents at least 60% of the total cell population in the lesion. The presence of more than two new hybridizing bands—suggesting biclonality, somatic mutation, or clonal evolution—is uncommon (Fig. 32.24). They almost never are bigenotypic (i.e., exhibit clonal T-cell receptor gene and clonal immunoglobulin gene rearrangements) (23).

Simultaneous bilateral ocular adnexal B-cell lymphomas usually exhibit identical clonal immunoglobulin gene rearrangements (23,134,200,203) (Fig. 32.25). This finding strongly suggests that, in these instances, both lesions are derived from the identical B-cell clone and represent the same B-cell neoplasm. In these cases, it would appear that the lymphoma arose on one side and subsequently spread to the other side. That this can occur without systemic dissemination is a property of mucosal B lymphocytes and reflects their known behavior to home back to their parent tissue after passage through the

general circulation (268). Such a pattern of spread is observed in MALT lymphomas in other sites, resulting, for example, in multifocal deposits in primary gastric lymphoma (216) and the high incidence of bilateral involvement in cases of parotid gland MALT lymphoma (135). Ocular adnexal and extraocular lymphomas that occur concurrently in the same patient may exhibit identical clonal immunoglobulin gene rearrangements, suggesting that they are derived from the identical B-cell clone, or distinct clonal immunoglobulin gene rearrangements, suggesting that they are derived from the identical B-cell clone but have undergone clonal evolution or somatic mutation or, alternatively, are derived from unique B-cell clones and represent the synchronous occurrence of separate B-cell neoplasms (23,134,269,270).

Immunogenotypic analysis has demonstrated that some unilateral and bilateral ocular adnexal polyclonal lymphoid hyperplasias are polyclonal at the molecular genetic level (23,133,134,197). These lesions appear to represent truly reactive proliferations of lymphoid cells, perhaps occurring in response to an as yet unidentified antigenic stimulus. An unanticipated finding, however, was the demonstration many years ago by Knowles and Jakobiec that many ocular adnexal lymphoid proliferations classified as polyclonal lymphoid hyperplasias histopathologically exhibit clonal immunoglobulin gene rearrangements (23,24,133). Among these cases, the patterns of immunoglobulin gene rearrangement included solitary and multiple, barely perceptible to faint bands, solitary clear and easily recognizable bands, and solitary high-intensity bands superimposed on a background of multiple less intense bands (23,24) (Fig. 32.26). These lesions contain oligoclonal or monoclonal B-cell populations that have escaped recognition by morphologic examination and immunophenotypic analysis. These lesions consistently lack clonal T-cell receptor gene rearrangements, indicating that the constituent T cells are truly polyclonal (23,24,133,134). Similar results have been obtained when immunogenotypic analysis has been applied to lymphoid hyperplasias occurring in other extranodal sites in which B-cell lymphomas frequently arise, such as the salivary gland, gastrointestinal tract, and skin (24,271–273). These findings suggest that extranodal lymphoid hyperplasias and B-cell lymphomas are pathogenetically related. They suggest that the ocular adnexal and other extranodal lymphoid hyperplasias represent a continuous and progressive spectrum of B-cell neoplasia, up to and including the earliest identifiable stages of malignant lymphoma (24).

The frequent detection of clonal immunoglobulin gene rearrangements in ocular adnexal lymphoid proliferations otherwise classified as polyclonal lymphoid hyperplasias has also

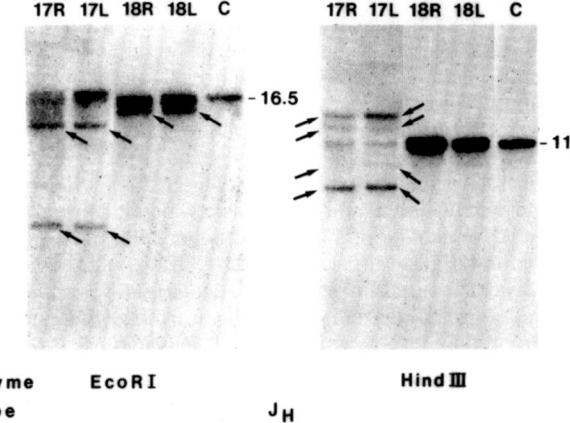

FIGURE 32.25. Southern blot hybridization analysis of two pairs of bilateral ocular adnexal monoclonal B-cell lymphomas for immunoglobulin gene rearrangements. The DNA extracted from the right (R)- and left (L)-sided neoplasms occurring in two patients (lanes 17 and 18) and from human fibroblasts (control [C]) were digested with *Eco*RI or *Hind*III and were hybridized to an immunoglobulin heavy chain joining region (J_H) probe. Rearrangement bands are indicated by *arrows*. Lane C shows the immunoglobulin heavy chain gene germ line configuration. The bilateral ocular adnexal monoclonal B-cell lymphomas that occur simultaneously in each patient exhibited identical clonal immunoglobulin heavy chain gene rearrangement patterns. This finding suggests that the two neoplasms were derived from the same B-cell clone and do not represent separate primary neoplasms. (Modified from Neri A, Jakobiec FA, Pelicci PG, et al. Immunoglobulin and T cell receptor beta chain gene rearrangement analysis of ocular adnexal lymphoid neoplasms: clinical and biologic implications. *Blood* 1987;70:1519–1529, with permission.)

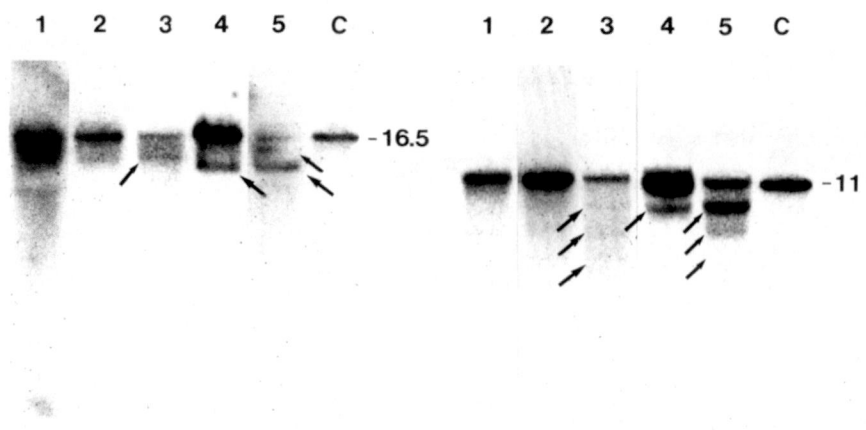

FIGURE 32.26. Southern blot hybridization analysis of ocular adnexal lymphoid proliferations exhibiting seemingly benign histopathology and a polyclonal cell marker profile for immunoglobulin gene rearrangements. The DNA extracted from the indicated cases (lanes 1–5) and human fibroblasts (control [C]) were digested with *Eco*RI or *Hind*III and hybridized to an immunoglobulin heavy chain joining region (J_H) probe. *Arrows* indicate rearrangement bands. Lane C displays the immunoglobulin heavy chain gene germ line configuration. Four of the five apparently benign polyclonal ocular adnexal lymphoid proliferations exhibit one or more rearrangement bands. The hybridization patterns include solitary to multiple faint and barely perceptible bands, solitary clearly visible bands, and a solitary clearly visible band associated with multiple faint bands. These findings suggest the presence of monoclonal and oligoclonal B-cell populations that have escaped recognition by morphologic examination and immunophenotypic analysis. At least some of these lesions probably represent MALT lymphomas whose histopathologic features were not appreciated in the past and whose monoclonal nature cannot be determined immunophenotypically because of numerous benign polyclonal lymphoid cells or for various technical reasons. (Modified from Neri A, Jakobiec FA, Pelicci PG, et al. Immunoglobulin and T cell receptor beta chain gene rearrangement analysis of ocular adnexal lymphoid neoplasms: clinical and biologic implications. *Blood* 1987;70:1519–1529, with permission.)

raised important practical questions concerning the role of immunogenotypic analysis in the diagnosis and classification of these and other extranodal lymphoid proliferations. In this regard, it is important to remember that the molecular determination of clonality does not necessarily imply malignancy or aggressive clinical behavior. Clonal immunoglobulin and T-cell receptor gene rearrangements have been detected in many lymphoproliferative disorders that are not overt malignant lymphomas and are not inevitably associated with the development of malignant lymphoma (11,22,24,271–277). Most patients who possess apparently morphologically benign and immunophenotypically polyclonal ocular adnexal and other extranodal lymphoid proliferations but contain immunogenotypically detectable clonal B-cell populations do not develop disseminated lymphoma despite conservative therapy (23,24,135,271). For these reasons, Knowles and Jakobiec recommended against classifying ocular adnexal lymphoid proliferations as malignant lymphomas merely based on the detection of occult clonal B-cell populations by immunogenotypic analysis. However, many of these lesions represent MALT lymphomas whose histopathologic features were not appreciated in the past and whose monoclonal nature sometimes cannot be determined immunophenotypically because of the presence of large numbers of benign polyclonal lymphoid cells or for various technical reasons (40,197,200,203).

Postulated Normal Counterpart (Mucosa-Associated Lymphoid Tissue)

In the mid-1980s, Isaacson et al. brought attention to the characteristic arrangement of lymphoid tissue underlying certain mucosal surfaces, for which the term *mucosa-associated lymphoid tissue* (MALT) was employed (278). The arrangement of MALT consists of the following characteristic histologic and immunologic features: submucosal B-cell follicles composed of reactive germinal centers containing a network of CD21-positive (CD21⁺) follicular dendritic cells and a surrounding mantle zone of small CD20⁺ B cells expressing immunoglobulin M (IgM) and IgD, and a region of larger, centrocyte-like CD20⁺ B cells expressing IgM, which extend from the mantle zone into the overlying epithelium to form a characteristic lymphoepithelium. Scattered plasma cells may be observed around and above the lymphoid follicles. CD3⁺ T cells are seen within and around the germinal centers, condensing at the base of the follicle farthest from the surface epithelium (203,279).

In humans, most of the organized MALT is located in the terminal ileum, whereas other mucosal sites are apparently normally devoid of organized MALT (279). However, MALT may be acquired in these other mucosal sites, particularly the bronchus, stomach, salivary gland, and thyroid gland, as a result of antigenic stimulation (222,279). Bronchus-associated lymphoid tissue is absent in the newborn but is acquired in early childhood in response to antigenic stimulation (280–282). In the stomach, MALT is acquired specifically in response to local infection by *H. pylori* (283). In the case of the salivary and thyroid glands, the antigenic stimulation may be a component of autoimmune disease, Sjögren syndrome (284), and Hashimoto thyroiditis (285), respectively. Once acquired, subsequent oncogenic events, occurring in a small number of cases, may eventually result in the development of a distinctive type of B-cell non-Hodgkin lymphoma that morphologically and immunologically resembles the MALT from which it arises (135).

Morphologic and functional studies in animals suggest that MALT is variably present in the conjunctiva of normal turkey, rabbit, mouse, rat, and guinea pig (286–290). In the guinea pig, MALT displays structural organization similar to that of the human Peyer patch (290). Examination of conjunctival MALT in animals raised in a bacteria-free environment shows that for-nix follicle size and the number of lymphocytes in the conjunctival lamina propria, although present, remain lower than in animals reared conventionally (286). Other experimental studies performed in animals suggest that conjunctival MALT can be induced and stimulated by external antigenic stimuli (288,289).

Knowles et al. showed that the lamina propria of the normal human conjunctiva contains a mixed lymphoid cell infiltrate in which T cells outnumber B cells and occasional intraepithelial T cells are present (8). This was later confirmed by Wotherspoon et al. (279). Jakobiec and associates also described the presence of organized MALT, including the formation of lymphoid follicles, in the forniceal region of the apparently normal conjunctiva of some individuals (291). In a carefully conducted investigation of representative strips of superior and inferior forniceal conjunctiva obtained during the autopsy examination of 90 individuals with no known history of ocular or conjunctival disease, Wotherspoon et al. (279) found organized MALT in about 30% of the cases, the youngest one being 28 years old. This finding suggests that conjunctival MALT, like that of other mucosal surfaces, is not found in the normal human conjunctiva but is acquired during life in response to external antigenic stimulation (279). In support of these findings and this conclusion, it is known that conjunctival folliculosis, a common childhood condition of limited clinical significance (292), has an appearance consistent with that of exuberant MALT (279). In adults, follicular conjunctivitis may be observed in response to infection by *Chlamydia*, adenovirus, and Epstein-Barr virus or a chemically induced allergic reaction (279). Regardless of the natural history of conjunctival MALT, once acquired, it provides the cellular milieu from which primary conjunctival B-cell MALT lymphomas may arise, analogous to MALT in other locations.

Clinical Course and Prognostic Assessment

The latest available literature review shows that the 5-year survival for all types of ocular adnexal lymphoma varies from 50% to 94% (293). The survival of patients with low-grade lymphoma, particularly MALT lymphoma, is significantly better than those with high-grade lymphoma (167,178,209,223,224, 294–297). The outcome for patients with MALT lymphoma is very good, with 84% to 100% of the patients presenting with stage I disease, indolent clinical course, and disease-free survival. Lymphoma-related mortality for patients with ocular adnexal MALT ranges from 0% to 16% (167,178,209,223,224, 295,297,298).

Approximately 80% to 90% of patients with ocular adnexal marginal zone lymphoma have disease confined to the ocular adnexa, either unilaterally or bilaterally (168,299). Other types of lymphoma are more frequently disseminated (300). Raderer et al. (301) reported that 6 out of 12 patients with ocular adnexal MALT lymphoma who had achieved complete remission after initial therapy subsequently relapsed (301). Preliminary data from a large study conducted by Ferry et al. (299) showed that 42 of 106 (40%) patients with primary MALT lymphoma and 15 of 40 (38%) patients with primary follicular lymphoma relapsed. The most common sites of relapse are the ocular adnexa (same side or opposite side), skin, and soft tissue (299,301). Occasionally, patients develop extraocular lymphoma as long as 4 years and sometimes even later after presentation (17). Thus, lifelong observation of all patients with lymphoma is recommended.

Effect of Anatomic Location

Knowles and Jakobiec suggested that the precise anatomic location of a lymphoid proliferation within the ocular adnexa has a significant bearing on its natural history, including the development of extraocular lymphoma. They found that approximately 35%, 20%, and 67% of patients who present with lymphoid proliferations of the orbit, conjunctiva, and eyelids, respectively,

have prior, concurrent, or subsequent extraocular lymphoma (statistical significance, $p < 0.03$) (17). Based on these findings, Knowles and Jakobiec (17) concluded that the conjunctiva is the most favorable prognostic location within the ocular adnexa. White et al. (197) confirmed that extraocular lymphoma is significantly more likely to develop in patients who have orbital rather than conjunctival lymphoma. Knowles and Jakobiec postulated that this is because the conjunctiva, unlike the orbit, contains its own indigenous lymphoid tissue that is capable of undergoing hyperplasia or developing primary localized malignant lymphoma (36). We now know that the conjunctiva contains MALT (279), that most malignant lymphomas originating in the conjunctiva arise in this MALT (36,135,178,196), and that MALT lymphomas characteristically tend to remain localized to the mucosal surface where they develop and do not disseminate systemically (134,206,302). Wotherspoon et al. also found that malignant lymphomas arising in the conjunctiva are MALT lymphomas and tend not to disseminate, even when they are bilateral (200,203).

In contrast, some other investigators have failed to identify prognostic differences among adnexal locations (39,40). However, these series included cases of both primary and secondary ocular adnexal malignant lymphoma. These differences may also be explained by differing patient referral patterns and case selection bias. It is important to point out that the precise anatomic site of origination of an ocular adnexal lymphoid proliferation often may not be appreciated clinically by the examining ophthalmologist. In one series, no effort was even made to distinguish between eyelid and conjunctival lesions, for example, and so they were lumped together for purposes of analysis (138). It is important that the precise anatomic location of a lymphoid proliferation occurring within the ocular adnexa be determined. For this reason, the patient should receive a careful clinical ocular examination in conjunction with orbital imaging studies. This was done in all of the patients included in the series reported by Knowles and Jakobiec (17).

Relation of Histopathology and Immunophenotype

Knowles and Jakobiec found that the histopathologic subclassification of ocular adnexal monoclonal B-cell lymphomas is helpful in predicting eventual outcome. They reported that although identical proportions (27%) of patients who had ocular adnexal lymphoid proliferations that they classified as lymphoid hyperplasia and small lymphocytic or intermediate lymphocytic lymphoma developed extraocular lymphoma, a significantly higher proportion (46%) of patients who had lesions that they classified as follicle center and large cell lymphomas developed extraocular lymphoma ($p < 0.09$) (17). Based on these findings, they suggested that the prior, concurrent, or future development of extraocular lymphoma varies according to the histopathologic category of the ocular adnexal lymphoid proliferation (17). These findings have been subsequently corroborated by other investigators (157,160,299).

In retrospect, we now know that most of the small B-cell lymphomas classified in this manner represented MALT lymphomas. The behavior of MALT lymphomas is distinctly nonaggressive and differs from that of all other extranodal B-cell lymphomas (206,302). MALT lymphomas generally remain localized to the mucosal surface where they originate and do not disseminate systemically (135,206,302). Patients who have MALT lymphomas usually do not have adverse prognostic factors such as high tumor burden, disseminated disease, bone marrow involvement, poor performance status, or high LDH levels (303). Patients who have MALT lymphoma have a high response rate with local treatment (i.e., surgery or radiotherapy) or with single-agent chemotherapy, and enjoy a long survival. These patients have a better prognosis than patients who have a non-MALT lymphoma arising at the same site (304).

Recurrences may appear several years after therapy (303,305) in the same organ or in other extranodal sites (299,306). Histologic transformation to a more aggressive lymphoma may occur in association with recurrence (205,222,299).

Role of Systemic Evaluation and Relationship with Clinical Stage

Knowles and Jakobiec uncovered that about 24% of patients who presented with an ocular adnexal lymphoid proliferation (20% orbital, 10% conjunctiva, and 44% eyelid) were discovered to have had prior or concurrent extraocular lymphoma. The remaining 76% of patients did not have a past history of lymphoma and did not develop evidence of extraocular lymphoma within 6 months after ocular presentation (17). Coupland et al. (40) similarly found that 76% of their patients who had ocular adnexal B-cell lymphoma had disease limited to the ocular adnexa (e.g., had stage IE disease). In a similar fashion, the study of 353 patients with ocular adnexal lymphoma conducted by Ferry et al. (157) revealed that 78% of the patients had no prior history of lymphoma. In a follow-up study, these authors found that 40% of patients with MALT lymphoma and 38% of patients with follicular lymphoma had a subsequent relapse (299).

The results of these studies (17,40,299) suggest that patients who present with ocular adnexal lymphoid proliferations should be subdivided into two broad categories: those with and those without a past history or evidence of extraocular lymphoma within 6 months after ocular presentation. Many, if not the majority, of the approximately 25% of patients who belong to the former category probably already had disseminated extraocular lymphoma with secondary involvement of the ocular adnexa at the time of presentation. Most of the approximately 75% of patients who belong to the latter category probably have stage IE primary ocular adnexal lymphoid proliferations.

According to Knowles and Jakobiec, these two patient groups exhibit several important clinical differences. First, the anatomic sites of involvement appear to differ. They found that approximately 90% of patients who have conjunctival, but only 74% who have orbital, and 44% who have eyelid, lymphoid proliferations have stage IE disease. Second, the histopathology apparently differs. Among the patients who had stage IE disease, they classified 72% of the lesions as small B-cell lymphomas and the remaining 28% as follicle center or diffuse large B-cell lymphomas. In contrast, among patients who had past or concurrent extraocular lymphoma, they classified 52% of the lesions as small B-cell lymphomas and the remaining 48% as follicle center cell or large B-cell lymphomas (17). The studies by Coupland and Ferry et al. reported similar findings (40,299). This is consistent with studies showing that most malignant lymphomas involving the ocular adnexa secondarily are follicle center and large cell lymphomas (150,157,178). Third, and most important, prognosis and outcome apparently differ according to stage at the time of ocular presentation ($p < 0.001$). In the experience of Knowles and Jakobiec, approximately 86% of patients who presented with a stage IE ocular adnexal lymphoid proliferation, unilateral or bilateral (78% with polyclonal lymphoid hyperplasia and 90% with monoclonal B-cell lymphoma), remained alive and well and were disease free, despite conservative therapy, at a median follow-up of 51 months. In contrast, only 20% of patients who presented with an ocular adnexal lymphoid proliferation and who had past or current extraocular lymphoma remained alive and well and were disease free at a mean follow-up of 57 months after ocular presentation. The remaining 80% of these patients were alive with disease or had died from progressive lymphoma with a median survival of only 19 months (17). Knowles and

Table 32.3	EVENTUAL OUTCOME OF 108 PATIENTS PRESENTING WITH OCULAR ADNEXAL LYMPHOID PROLIFERATIONS			
Characteristic	Orbit	Conjunctiva	Lid	Total
No evidence of disease				
Patients (no.)	50[a]	24	3[b]	77
Follow-up, range (mo)	4–113	8–115	11–46	4–115
Follow-up, median (mo)	54	56	21	53
Alive with disease				
Patients (no.)	14[c]	3	2	19
Follow-up, range (mo)	6–108	18–62	22–42	6–108
Follow-up, median (mo)	58	43	32	51
Dead because of lymphoma				
Patients (no.)	4	2	2	8
Follow-up, range (mo)	12–28	8–67	23–79	8–79
Follow-up, median (mo)	15	38	51	19
Lost to follow-up	1	1	2	4
Patients (total)	69	30	9	108

From Knowles DM, Jakobiec FA, McNally FA, et al. Lymphoid hyperplasia and malignant lymphoma occurring in the ocular adnexa (orbit, conjunctiva and eyelids): a prospective multiparametric analysis of 108 cases during 1977–1987. *Hum Pathol* 1990;21:959–973, with permission.
[a]Two patients died of other causes and had no evidence of lymphoma at the time of death.
[b]One patient died of carcinoma and had no evidence of lymphoma at the time of death.
[c]One patient died of carcinoma but had systemic lymphoma at the time of death.

Jakobiec found that the single most important and statistically significant prognostic factor among patients who present with ocular adnexal lymphoid proliferations is the extent of disease determined after a thorough clinical staging. In their experience, most patients who present with a lymphoid proliferation limited to the ocular adnexa (stage IE), regardless of histopathology, immunophenotype, or bilaterality, have a benign indolent clinical course (17) (Table 32.3). Other investigators have reported a similar experience (40,138). On the other hand, a recent study of 326 patients by Jenkins et al. has challenged the widely recognized concept that bilaterality does not affect prognosis. In this study, patients with bilateral disease were at a significantly greater risk for developing systemic lymphoma and lymphoma-related death (307).

Extensive staging using radiographic imaging and endoscopy of the gastrointestinal tract is often performed in patients with the diagnosis of MALT lymphoma. These methods have shown that up to 46% of patients with extragastric lymphoma have at least two sites of disease at diagnosis (308,309). Presence of trisomy 18 has been associated with multifocality (309). The bone marrow is involved in <10% of patients (17,167,178,309). Bone marrow involvement or multifocal lymphoma involvement of MALT regions does not appear to impact patient survival (308–311).

Other Prognostic Factors

Studies have identified a number of additional parameters that may have prognostic value among the ocular adnexal malignant lymphomas. For example, Coupland et al. (40) suggested that the immunohistochemical demonstration of MIB-1 (Ki-67) and p53 have prognostic significance. They found the average MIB-1 proliferation rate for the MALT lymphomas to be 15%, which correlated with stage IE disease. They also found that 14 of the 15 cases that had a MIB-1 proliferation rate >20% had at least stage II disease. They further found that high proliferation rates corresponded positively with stage of disease at presentation, stage of disease at final follow-up, and the occurrence of lymphoma-related death ($p < 0.001$). They observed similar statistically significant correlations with respect to tumor subdivision, stage of disease at presentation and at final follow-up, and occurrence of lymphoma-related death with tumor cell p53 positivity (40). In a follow-up study of 230 patients, the authors confirmed that a Ki-67 proliferation index of >10% had a significantly increased risk of developing systemic disease and lymphoma-related death both in stage IE MALT lymphoma and in stage IE non-MALT lymphoma (312). They also demonstrated that an increased tumor cell positivity for BCL-6 (defined as >10% of the cells) was statistically associated with an increased risk of relapse (312).

Nakata et al. (138) analyzed the survival data of 57 patients who had ocular adnexal malignant lymphoma with a median follow-up period of 5 years. Statistical analysis of the prognostic factors influencing the cause-specific survival of these patients revealed that histopathology, LDH levels, and clinical stage were statistically significant (138). These findings largely reflect the fact that most ocular adnexal lymphomas are MALT lymphomas, which are usually localized lesions unassociated with adverse prognostic factors.

CD5-positive MALT lymphoma was associated with a poorer outcome in one series (230). Similarly, the presence of trisomy 18 has been found to be associated with a risk of dissemination of MALT lymphoma in a small number of patients (309). Larger studies are needed to confirm these findings.

Therapy and Management

If the patient is found to have a lymphoid proliferation limited to the ocular adnexa (unilateral or bilateral) after a careful and thorough systemic evaluation, local radiation therapy is recommended (40,70,138,178,188,196,254,313). A surgical approach is not recommended because of the infiltrative nature of lymphoid proliferations. Complete surgical excision of these lesions usually is not possible without causing severe functional deficiencies (36). Some physicians have adopted a "watch and wait" policy and have treated patients who have asymptomatic MALT lymphoma restricted to the ocular adnexa with "observation only" after excisional biopsy (138,314). However, disease recurs locally or develops systemically in a significant proportion of these individuals (178,196,254,300,314). For these reasons, surgery alone is suboptimal. Even polyclonal lymphoid hyperplasias are capable of recurrence (40,197) and therefore should be ablated by radiation therapy (36,315). Systemic corticosteroids usually are only useful in treating orbital pseudotumors. They generally produce only a temporary clinical suppression of ocular adnexal lymphoid proliferations that rebound on cessation of the drug (36). There is no consensus on the optimal radiation dose for treating ocular adnexal lymphomas (188,313). The current National Cancer Center network guidelines recommend radiotherapy of 20 to 30 Gy for initial treatment of early-stage nongastric extranodal marginal zone lymphoma of all sites and reirradiation for locally recurrent disease (316). Stefanovic and Lossos (168) consider 30 Gy to be the optimal dose for patients with ocular adnexal lymphoma but state that reirradiation should be avoided. Bayraktar et al. (317) have conducted one of the largest studies to date and have concluded that a dose >30.6 Gy is crucial for optimal local treatment outcome. The specifics of ocular radiation therapy are discussed in detail elsewhere (188,313,318). Virtually 100% of patients who have stage IE disease treated with local radiation therapy alone undergo complete remission (40,178,188,196,254,313,319–321).

The presence of bilateral adnexal lesions or of follicular or diffuse large B-cell lymphoma in the ocular adnexa does not necessarily imply the existence or the eventual development of systemic disease. A few of these lesions appear to represent truly localized disease. Perhaps some of the large B-cell lymphomas arise from low-grade MALT lymphomas. Some data suggest that high-grade MALT lymphomas arising in other sites are associated with a better prognosis than for non-MALT types

(304). For these reasons, it is recommended that patients who have lymphoid proliferations—even follicular and large B-cell lymphomas limited to the ocular adnexa (unilateral or bilateral)—be subjected to local ocular radiation therapy, which may be curative, rather than to systemic chemotherapy. Since radiation treatment is considered a gold standard, data on chemotherapy for patients with ocular adnexal lymphoma is very limited. When chemotherapy has been used, regimens included single-agent chemotherapy with chlorambucil or fludarabine for low-grade lymphoma and combined protocols such as cyclophosphamide, doxorubicin, vincristine, and prednisone (CHOP) for high-grade lymphomas (196,322–325). Chlorambucil was the most widely used single agent for MALT lymphoma. There are no accepted practical recommendations based on the available data (168).

Several pilot studies have examined the usefulness of intralesional or intravenous administration of rituximab, a chimeric monoclonal antibody that targets the CD20 antigen (326–336). Single-agent rituximab achieved complete remission in 50% to 87% of patients with ocular adnexal lymphoma. However, many patients had evidence of an early relapse (336). One study of orbital pseudolymphoma demonstrated successful treatment with rituximab in 10 of 11 patients (337). Treatment was well tolerated with no side effects reported except for pain at the injection site, mild neutropenia, and mild thrombocytopenia. Additional larger studies are necessary in order to validate this approach.

If extraocular lymphoma is discovered, systemic chemotherapy can be administered and the effect on the ocular adnexal lymphoid proliferation awaited. Generally, ocular adnexal malignant lymphoma is sensitive to radiation therapy and systemic chemotherapy and so only one and not both modalities are necessary (150,196). The patient should be carefully followed (e.g., by repeat CT scanning) by an ophthalmologist to determine the adequacy of local ocular regression. If the ocular response to chemotherapy is suboptimal, adjunctive local ocular radiation therapy can be administered. If the ocular adnexal lesion is bulky or causing a threat to vision, radiation therapy can be administered when systemic chemotherapy is given (17).

Ferreri et al. (161) found evidence of *Chlamydophila* (formerly known as *Chlamydia*) *psittaci* infection in 80% of the DNA samples in a group of European patients affected by ocular adnexal lymphoma. Subsequently, the same authors investigated the efficacy of bacteria-eradicating therapy with doxycycline (338). A group of 27 patients affected by ocular adnexal lymphoma—11 *C. psittaci* DNA-positive and 16 *C. psittaci* DNA-negative—were treated with a 3-week course of doxycycline. The authors observed a complete response in 6 patients and a partial response in 7, with a total of 13 patients (45%) that responded to the treatment. In particular, 64% of *C. psittaci* DNA-positive patients responded positively (338). These results have not yet been replicated by others, probably due to the wide geographic and laboratory detection variability of *C. psittaci* infection. A meta-analysis of the response of ocular adnexal lymphoma to antibiotic treatment included four studies from Italy, Austria, Taiwan, and the United States and included 42 patients (169). Twenty patients (48%) achieved some response (complete response in eight patients, partial response in eight patients, and minimal response in four patients). Twenty patients had stable disease, and two patients progressed during antibiotic therapy. Objective documentation of response was available for only 3 of the 42 patients. Seven additional patients developed disease recurrence after their initial response or stable disease after antibiotic therapy; six of these cases occurred during the first 12 months of follow-up. The study concluded that antibiotics have variable efficacy against ocular adnexal lymphoma (169). Coleman et al. reported a case series of three patients from the New York area with low-grade B-cell lymphoma who were treated with clarithromycin (one patient) and doxycycline (two patients). All patients achieved complete remission and had no evidence of relapse after follow-up ranging from 16 to 46 months (339). More recently, Govi et al. (340) reported their results concerning long-term use (6 months) of clarithromycin in relapsed or refractory MALT lymphoma. Clarithromycin was chosen due to its broad antimicrobial activity but also its immunomodulatory effects with suggested activity in other lymphoid malignancies. Of 11 patients with ocular adnexal MALT lymphoma, 5 had an objective response, 3 had stable disease, and 3 had progressed. The patients who responded to treatment did so in spite of being refractory to doxycycline. Large prospective trials are needed to further evaluate the role of antibiotics in the treatment of ocular adnexal lymphoma from different geographic regions.

OTHER HEMATOPOIETIC DISORDERS

Sinus Histiocytosis with Massive Lymphadenopathy (Rosai-Dorfman Disease)

Sinus histiocytosis with massive lymphadenopathy (SHML), also called Rosai-Dorfman disease, is a rare histiocytic proliferative disorder that exhibits distinctive clinical and pathologic features and usually resolves spontaneously (341–343). SHML is discussed in detail in Chapter 48. This discussion is limited primarily to ocular adnexal and ocular globe involvement by SHML.

SHML occurs in individuals belonging to all racial groups, regardless of socioeconomic status, worldwide. It occurs in all age groups; the youngest reported patient had congenital SHML and the oldest reported patient was 74 years old. The mean age at onset of symptoms is 21 years. The male-to-female ratio is about 1.5:1. Rarely, SHML occurs among family members (341).

Lymph node involvement occurs in nearly all cases. Approximately 87% of patients have cervical lymphadenopathy, which is usually bilateral. Axillary, inguinal, and mediastinal lymph nodes are commonly affected as well. Although SHML is considered a lymph node–based disease, at least one extranodal site is involved in 25% to 43% of cases (344). Extranodal SHML may occur as part of a generalized disease process involving lymph nodes or may involve extranodal sites independent of lymph node involvement. The most common sites of extranodal involvement are, in order of frequency: skin, upper respiratory tract, soft tissue, orbit, bone, salivary gland, central nervous system, breast, and pancreas (344). Within the head and neck region, SHML has a predilection for the nasal cavity and paranasal sinuses (341). Among 423 well-documented cases of SHML collected by Rosai and Dorfman over a 20-year period, orbital or eyelid involvement was described in 36 cases (8.5%), and ocular globe involvement was described in six cases (1.4%) (341). Of the 36 cases, 22 had only orbital, 5 had only eyelid, and 9 had both orbital and eyelid involvement. In two of the cases, involvement of all four eyelids was described (341). Since this review, 34 additional cases involving the ocular adnexa have been reported in the English literature (345). Twenty-four patients had an orbital mass, with six cases confined to the lacrimal gland, and seven involving the eyelids alone. Two patients had corneal involvement, and one had involvement of the lacrimal sac and duct. One patient had intraocular involvement with choroidal mass secondary to aggressive infiltration of the sclera and choroid (345). Two patients had involvement of all four eyelids but not the orbits (346,347).

Among persons who have SHML involving the orbit or eyelids, approximately 67% are men and 75% are black. The mean age at onset of symptoms is 17 years. Most patients present with an orbital or eyelid mass or swelling associated with proptosis, ocular displacement, decreased ocular motility, or ptosis. In addition, uveitis and, rarely, serous retinal detachment have been described (345). The masses usually are firm and rubbery to palpation. Bilateral disease exists in 22% of patients. Approximately 57% of patients have additional sites of extranodal involvement, most commonly the nasal cavity and paranasal sinuses. Lymphadenopathy is absent in 17% of patients, suggesting that the disease is entirely extranodal in some individuals (341).

The ocular globe is very rarely involved by SHML. The mean age of onset of symptoms is 6 years. Males outnumber females by 2 to 1. Blacks are affected more often than whites. The patients present with conjunctivitis, photophobia, and loss of visual acuity. Nearly all of them have additional sites of extranodal disease, and most of them have lymph node involvement as well (341).

The pathology of SHML occurring in extranodal sites, including the ocular adnexa, is highly distinctive (341,348,349) and is overall similar to that of SHML occurring in lymph nodes. Grossly, the lesions may be polypoid, nodular, or exophytic, depending on the site of origin, and are tan-white to yellow. Microscopically, nests, clusters, and sheets of loosely aggregated histiocytes alternate with trabecular collections of mature plasma cells and small, benign, and mature-appearing lymphocytes, mimicking the dilated sinuses and medullary cords of lymph nodes involved by SHML. In some instances, the lymphocytes and especially the plasma cells predominate, obscuring the histiocytes. Germinal centers are generally absent. The histiocytes are usually large and contain abundant pale eosinophilic cytoplasm with indistinct borders. Most nuclei are round to oval, vesicular, and contain a single small nucleolus, but some contain a prominent nucleolus or multiple nucleoli. Nuclear atypia and mitotic figures within the histiocytes are infrequent. Foamy histiocytes may be present. A variable number of the histiocytes contain well-preserved lymphocytes and, occasionally, plasma cells, neutrophils, and erythrocytes in their cytoplasm, a phenomenon called emperipolesis (341,348,349). The histiocytes characteristically strongly express S-100 protein, CD11c, CD14, CD33, CD68, and CD163, variably express lysozyme, CD11b, and CD36, and generally lack CD1a and HLA-DR (344,348,350–353). They may express CD30 in up to one-half of the cases (350). Recent reports have documented an increased number of IgG4-positive plasma cells in some cases (354–356). However, other investigators have not confirmed this relationship (357). In general, extranodal SHML exhibits more fibrosis, fewer typical histiocytes, and smaller numbers of histiocytes displaying emperipolesis than lymph nodal SHML (341,349). Consequently, the diagnosis of SHML is often more difficult when it occurs in an extranodal site.

Most patients have stable, persistent disease or eventually enter remission; progression to death is uncommon. Consequently, therapy is not necessary for most patients. When the manifestations of the disease are severe or progressive, therapeutic intervention in the form of corticosteroids in conjunction with cytotoxic drugs is often offered, although the response is not always dramatic. Thus, nearly half of patients treated with chemotherapy do not respond or relapse (345). Although some patients who have massive ocular adnexal disease may require enucleation, involvement of the orbit or eyelid *per se* does not have an adverse effect on prognosis. In contrast, all known patients who have ocular globe involvement have died from their disease or are alive with persistent disease (341).

Langerhans Cell Histiocytosis

Langerhans cell histiocytosis (i.e., histiocytosis X) is an uncommonly occurring multisystem disease that has a broad spectrum of clinical and pathologic presentations (358). Lichtenstein introduced the generic term histiocytosis X in 1953 to encompass three clinicopathologic syndromes: eosinophilic granuloma of bone, Hand-Schüller-Christian syndrome (i.e., triad of exophthalmos, diabetes insipidus, and osteolytic bone lesions), and Letterer-Siwe disease (359). The disease is further described clinically as unifocal or multifocal, localized or disseminated, and with or without systemic involvement (360,361). These disorders are discussed in detail in Chapter 48. They are summarized briefly here, primarily as they relate to the ocular adnexa.

In general, the younger the patient who has Langerhans cell histiocytosis, the greater is the likelihood of multifocal disease (359,362). Letterer-Siwe disease is the acute disseminated form of Langerhans cell histiocytosis; it accounts for approximately 10% of all cases. Letterer-Siwe disease occurs in infants and very young children (<2 years). It is characterized by fever, anemia, thrombocytopenia, failure to thrive, and multisystem (i.e., cutaneous, lymph node, and visceral) involvement. Death usually occurs within 2 years after diagnosis (363). Hand-Schüller-Christian disease is the chronic disseminated form of Langerhans cell histiocytosis. It occurs in children and is characterized by chronic, progressive, remitting, and relapsing lesions of the skull bones, especially the orbit, jaw, and mastoid, and frequently is accompanied by skin and pulmonary involvement (362). Eosinophilic granuloma is the localized form of Langerhans cell histiocytosis. It usually occurs in older children and adolescents and rarely in adults. It occurs primarily as solitary osseous lesions or in the lungs. This is the most common form of the disease and carries the best prognosis (362). No satisfactory explanation exists to account for the various clinical courses observed among patients who have Langerhans cell histiocytosis, but young age, multifocal disease, and organ dysfunction appear to indicate a poor prognosis (364,365).

Intraocular involvement by Langerhans cell histiocytosis is rare; it usually occurs as part of the acute disseminated form of the disease (i.e., Letterer-Siwe disease) (365). In these cases, the uveal tract, particularly the choroid, is affected (366–368), although involvement of the retina and sclera also has been described (369,370). Orbital involvement occurs in about 25% of cases of Langerhans cell histiocytosis, overall (365). The most common form of Langerhans cell histiocytosis involving the orbit is the localized form (i.e., eosinophilic granuloma), which usually is associated with an osteolytic lesion of the orbit (365). Orbital soft tissue involvement without a bony defect is uncommon and should raise the suspicion of an alternative disease process, such as a pseudotumor or myeloid sarcoma (36).

Orbital involvement by Langerhans cell histiocytosis accounts for <1% of all orbital tumors (365). The most common sign and symptom is proptosis; other signs and symptoms include erythema of the eyelids, edema, ptosis, and periorbital pain (365,371). Typical findings include a unifocal osteolytic lesion of the frontal bone or the lateral wall of the orbit with erosion of the greater wing of the sphenoid bone accompanied by a large soft tissue mass that extends into the extraconal space of the orbit, the infratemporal fossa, middle cranial fossa, and the ocular adnexa. Intraocular and brain parenchymal involvement are rare (365,372). Occasionally, additional osteolytic lesions may be present in the region, but the radiographic skeletal survey is usually otherwise normal (372,373). Radiologic evidence of disease may be present without clinical signs (365). Nonophthalmic findings and laboratory studies are generally unremarkable (372).

Grossly, the lesions are described as soft, friable, hemorrhagic tan-yellow tissue. The unifying histopathologic feature of Langerhans cell histiocytosis is the presence of organ infiltration by dendritic cells related to the normally occurring Langerhans cell population. Langerhans cells are weakly phagocytic, antigen-presenting dendritic cells (see Chapters 2 and 3). These cells are large and contain abundant, ill-defined acidophilic cytoplasm. Peculiar cytoplasmic organelles called Birbeck (Langerhans) granules may be identified in the cytoplasm of many, although not all, of these cells by electron microscopy. The nuclei are pale, vesicular, and oval to irregular in shape,

often having an indented, folded, or creased appearance. Many nuclei exhibit a longitudinal groove resulting in a "coffee-bean" appearance (Fig. 32.27). They contain stippled chromatin and nucleoli are inconspicuous. Phagocytosis is not seen and mitoses are uncommon. Some of the cells may become foamy. Multinucleated giant cells containing "coffee-bean" nuclei may be present. The cells characteristically express S-100 protein, langerin (CD207), CD45, CD1a, perinuclear CD68, HLA-DR, ATPase, and α-D-mannosidase and lack nonspecific esterase, lysozyme, and α_1-antichymotrypsin, analogous to normal Langerhans cells (374) (Fig. 32.27). Variable numbers of inflammatory cells, especially eosinophils, usually are present in the lesions (36,358,361,362,375) (Fig. 32.27). There are no obvious histopathologic differences among lesions occurring in patients who have localized disease compared with multisystem involvement (375). The histopathologic features cannot be used to predict clinical behavior or determine prognosis (375).

The treatment for orbital Langerhans cell histiocytosis is controversial because of the unpredictable outcome following therapy and occurrence of spontaneous healing in some cases (365,376,377). The unifocal lesions often respond well to curettage with or without low-dose irradiation or local injection of corticosteroids (359,365,373). Other treatment options include close observation, high-dose systemic corticosteroids, chemotherapy, and, for more recalcitrant cases, bone marrow transplantation and antibody therapy (378). The choice of therapeutic regimen is based ultimately on disease severity, and the number of systems involved.

Plasma Cell Myeloma and Plasmacytoma

Plasma cell myeloma is a systemic malignant plasma cell proliferation. It is characterized by the presence of multiple "punched-out" osteolytic lesions, particularly in the skull and vertebrae, caused by tumor-like collections of neoplastic plasma cells within the bone and bone marrow. Cases of plasma cell myeloma comprise most plasma cell neoplasms (379,380) (see Chapter 37).

A plasmacytoma is a solitary, localized tumor-like collection of clonal neoplastic plasma cells that are capable of synthesizing and secreting a specific monoclonal immunoglobulin. Plasmacytomas constitute <5% of all plasma cell tumors (137,379,380). Plasmacytomas may occur within bone (i.e., solitary plasmacytoma of bone [osseous plasmacytoma]) or outside of bone (i.e., extramedullary plasmacytoma) (379). Solitary osseous plasmacytomas manifest as lytic bone lesions, most commonly in the femur, pelvis, and spine. They commonly represent an early manifestation of plasma cell myeloma with eventual evolution to additional solitary or multiple plasmacytomas or to generalized plasma cell myeloma in two-thirds of patients (137,379,381). The median time to dissemination occurs within 2 to 3 years in most cases (379,381). Solitary extramedullary plasmacytomas occur most frequently in the head and neck, especially in the sinonasal or nasopharyngeal regions (379,380,382). Radiologic surveys of the skeleton are normal (379,381). Dissemination is far less common than with solitary osseous plasmacytomas (~15% of the patients) (137). Solitary extramedullary plasmacytomas are considered to be a separate disease process, whereas solitary osseous plasmacytomas are probably in a continuum toward plasma cell myeloma (137,379,381).

The ocular adnexa rarely are the site of involvement by systemic plasma cell myeloma, a solitary osseous plasmacytoma, or an extramedullary plasmacytoma. In a compilation of four series of orbital tumors, only four of almost 2,000 such tumors were plasmacytomas (383). The orbital roof and frontal bones are most often affected; occasionally, tumors erode upward from the floor of the orbit. As of 2011, fewer than 50 cases of solitary extramedullary plasmacytoma of the ocular adnexa had been reported (384–386). Some of these cases represent involvement by known plasma cell myeloma, while others

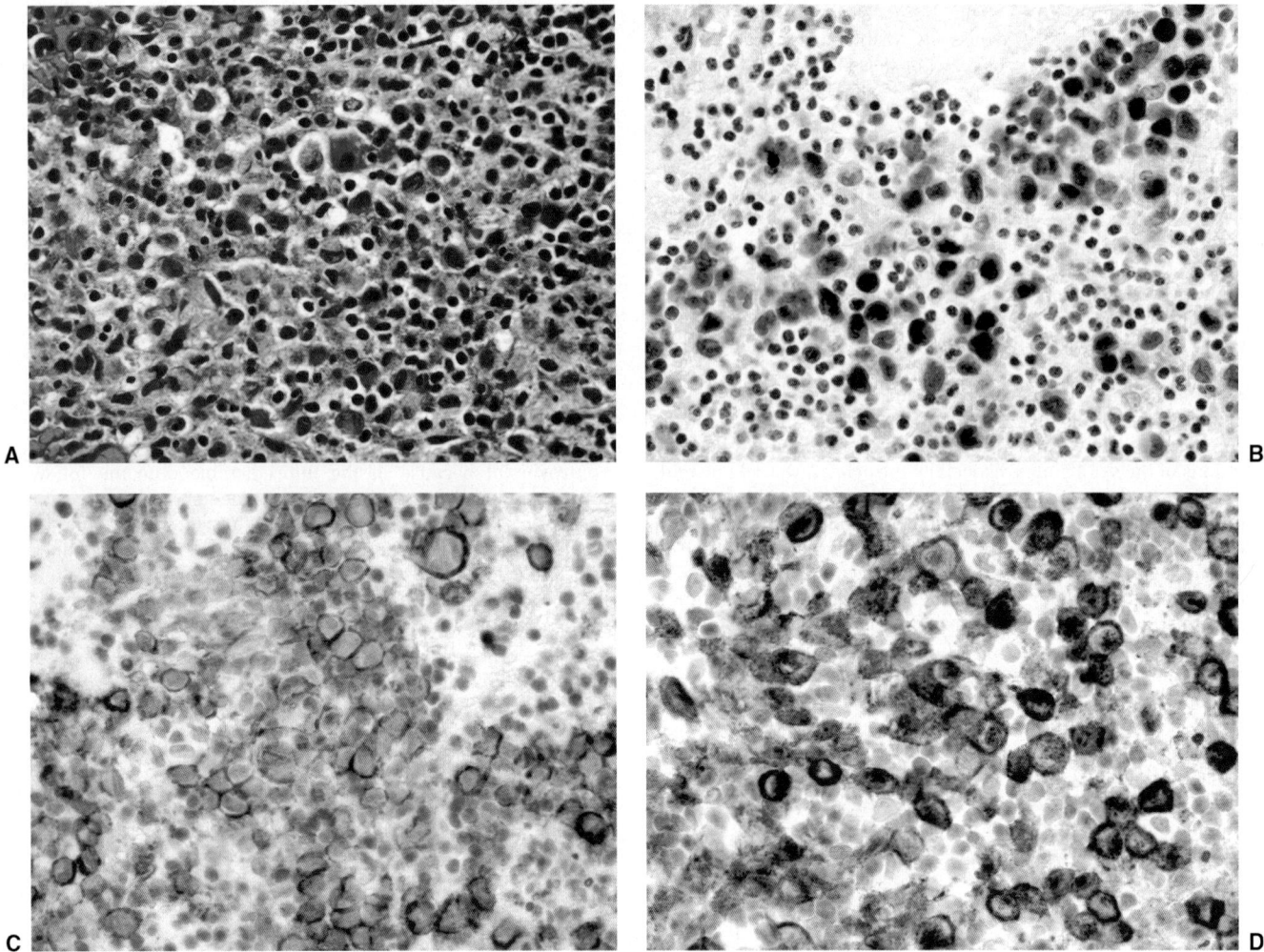

FIGURE 32.27. Langerhans cell histiocytosis. A: The lesion is composed of large histiocytoid cells containing abundant, ill-defined acidophilic cytoplasm and pale nuclei that often have an indented, folded, or creased appearance. Numerous eosinophils are scattered throughout. Immunoperoxidase staining demonstrates that many of these large histiocytoid cells contain **B:** S-100 protein, **C:** CD1a and **D:** Langerin (hematoxylin and eosin stain, original magnification: 400× magnification; immunostains, original magnification: 400× magnification).

appeared *de novo* (384,385). Rarely, orbital myeloma plasma cell infiltrates and plasmacytomas are associated with the local deposition of amyloid (387–389).

Most patients who have orbital involvement present with slowly progressive proptosis over weeks to months, often accompanied by vision loss, diplopia, disturbances in ocular motility, and sometimes by ptosis, similar to patients who present with orbital lymphoid proliferations. Patients also may complain of pain, particularly if there is bone destruction (390,391). The presence of one or more osteolytic lesions is helpful in the differential diagnosis because inflammatory pseudotumors are not associated, and lymphoid proliferations rarely are associated with bone destruction (17,36,48,49).

Microscopically, the lesions consist of a diffuse, sheetlike proliferation of neoplastic plasma cells supported by a sparse fibrous connective tissue stroma. The immunohistochemical demonstration of monotypic cytoplasmic immunoglobulin within the cells confirms their plasma cell lineage, clonal origin, and neoplastic nature (11,392).

It is important to distinguish a solitary extramedullary plasmacytoma from plasma cell myeloma because of the difference in therapy, management, and prognosis. Most patients found to have a malignant plasma cell tumor involving the orbit or orbital bones are discovered to have plasma cell myeloma on systemic evaluation or develop disseminated disease shortly

thereafter (36,391–393). Solitary osseous and extramedullary plasmacytomas are highly radiosensitive and usually can be managed successfully with localized radiation therapy; surgery and chemotherapy are generally reserved for recurrent or persistent disease (379,390,391). Systemic disease generally is treated with chemotherapy (379,380).

Myeloid Sarcoma

Myeloid sarcoma is a localized extramedullary tumor consisting of malignant cells of myeloid-lineage derivation (137). It occurs in the following clinical situations:

1. As a localized tissue manifestation in patients who have acute myeloid leukemia
2. As an initial manifestation of relapse in a previously treated acute myeloid leukemia in remission (394,395)
3. As a sign of acute blast crisis in chronic myelogenous leukemia and other myeloproliferative neoplasms or leukemic transformation in patients who have myelodysplastic syndromes or myelodysplastic syndrome/myeloproliferative neoplasms (137)
4. As a forerunner of acute myeloid leukemia in nonleukemic patients (396)
5. Less commonly, as an isolated neoplasm without progression to systemic acute myeloid leukemia (397)

Myeloid sarcoma is observed in only about 3% to 7% of cases of myeloid leukemia overall (398). In the largest study to date, Pileri et al. (395) studied 92 patients with myeloid sarcoma classified based on the WHO classification. Chromosomal aberrations were detected in about 54% of cases; monosomy 7 (10.8%), trisomy 8 (10.4%), and mixed lineage leukemia gene rearrangements (8.5%) were the most common abnormalities (395). The t(8;21) was rare (2.2%). However, only one of the 92 studied myeloid sarcoma cases was localized to the orbit. Several case series and case reports have demonstrated a close association between t(8;21) and periorbital involvement by myeloid sarcoma in the pediatric population (399–402).

Myeloid sarcomas have been described in almost every site of the body, but occur most frequently in the skin, soft tissues, lymph nodes, gastrointestinal tract, testis and as isolated lytic bone lesions (137,396). They also may arise in the orbital bones or the soft tissues of the orbit and eyelids (403). The most common presentation is that of a tumor confined to a single location (396). A disproportionate number of ophthalmic myeloid sarcomas appear to occur in children from Asia, the South Pacific, Latin America, and Africa (400,401,404). The incidence of ophthalmic myeloid sarcoma also appears to be remarkably high among Turkish children (405).

Myeloid sarcomas may involve the ocular adnexa of persons of all ages, but predominantly occur in the pediatric population. Presentation in adults is extremely uncommon (400). Males predominate over females by a ratio of about 1.5:1. Unlike nonophthalmic cases, when myeloid sarcoma occurs in the orbit or eyelids, it usually represents the initial clinical manifestation of an as yet undiagnosed underlying leukemia (404). Most patients have simultaneous evidence of bone marrow and peripheral blood involvement by acute myeloid leukemia or their leukemia manifests itself within 6 months after the ocular presentation (403,404). Occasionally, however, myeloid sarcoma occurs late in the course of disease. Most patients present with an orbital or eyelid mass or swelling associated with proptosis, ocular displacement, diplopia, or ptosis. Often, patients have bilateral disease (403,404,406). Other patients have diffuse disease, including involvement of the paranasal sinuses and other skull bones (403). Consequently, myeloid sarcoma should be strongly considered when an intraorbital mass, especially if bilateral, is encountered in a child.

The differential diagnosis of a retrobulbar orbital soft tissue mass in a child includes, in addition to myeloid sarcoma, inflammatory pseudotumor, African Burkitt lymphoma, rhabdomyosarcoma, and metastatic neuroblastoma (404). Inflammatory pseudotumors more commonly present as extraocular polymyositis or optic nerve inflammation rather than as a focal orbital tumor mass (404). African Burkitt lymphoma characteristically involves the maxillary bone, and orbital involvement is secondary. Other non-Hodgkin lymphomas of the orbit and eyelids generally occur in older persons (404). Moreover, unlike orbital lymphomas, orbital myeloid sarcomas frequently are associated with destruction of the bony walls of the orbit (404). Myeloid sarcomas have a predilection for the lateral orbit (406), which differs from the more common location of rhabdomyosarcoma in the superior orbit (404). Bilateral disease or multiple intraorbital and extraorbital soft tissue masses mitigate strongly against rhabdomyosarcoma (404). Metastatic neuroblastoma more commonly causes concomitant osteolytic defects (404). Radiographically, myeloid sarcoma lesions tend to mold to contiguous structures, including the sclera and the orbital bones, in patterns that mimic orbital lymphomas in adults (17,187,189), and only the medial wall is likely to show dissolution with sinus involvement (404).

Myeloid sarcomas exhibit a spectrum of histopathologic features. Most cases are composed of myeloblasts with or without features of promyelocytic or neutrophilic maturation (137). The blasts are characterized by the presence of round, ovoid, or reniform nuclei that possess finely stippled chromatin and one or two small nucleoli (396,397). These cells may be mistaken for those comprising diffuse large B- and T-cell lymphomas, Burkitt lymphoma, or lymphoblastic lymphoma (396,397). Consequently, granulocytic sarcomas are frequently misinterpreted as non-Hodgkin lymphomas. Alternatively, especially in children, these lesions sometimes may be misinterpreted histopathologically as rhabdomyosarcoma, neuroblastoma, or various other nonhematopoietic neoplasms (403). Other cases of myeloid sarcoma are characterized by a diffuse monotonous proliferation of myelomonocytic or monoblastic cells. Rarely, tumors with trilineage hematopoiesis or tumors composed of erythroblasts or megakaryoblasts are seen (137,407).

The histopathologic differential diagnosis of myeloid sarcoma from malignant lymphoma and nonhematopoietic neoplasms is greatly aided by immunohistochemical studies. Approximately 90% or more of granulocytic sarcomas express CD45 (leukocyte common antigen) (408), indicative of their hematopoietic origin, which greatly assists in distinguishing them from various nonhematopoietic neoplasms. Pileri and associates have demonstrated that CD68/KP1 is the most commonly expressed marker (100%) in myeloid sarcomas, followed by myeloperoxidase (83.6%), CD117 (80.4%), CD99 (54.3%), CD68/PG-M1 (51%), CD34 (43.4%), TdT (31.5%), CD56 (13%), CD61/linker for activation of T cells (2.2%), CD30 (2.2%) and CD4 (1.1%) (395). Foci of CD123-positive plasmacytoid dendritic cells are occasionally observed in cases carrying inv(16) (137). It is also important to remember that CD43, commonly thought of as a T-cell–associated antigen, is expressed by myeloid cells (see Chapter 3). Approximately 50% of myeloid sarcomas express CD43 (408); these cases should not be misdiagnosed as T-cell lymphoma.

The prognosis of patients who have myeloid sarcoma is poor (409). The clinical behavior and response to therapy does not seem to be influenced by age, sex, anatomical site involved, *de novo* presentation, morphology, immunophenotype, or cytogenetics (137,395). Most cases of myeloid sarcoma occurring in nonleukemic patients progress to acute myeloid leukemia within months (409). The median interval from diagnosis to acute myeloid leukemia has been reported to be about 10 months and the median survival 22 months (396,409). Among patients who have orbital myeloid sarcoma, the interval to death secondary to overt leukemia has been reported to vary from 1 to 30 months after the onset of tumor symptoms (403). The prevailing opinion is that myeloid sarcoma should be treated as acute myeloid leukemia, even in the absence of clinically detectable leukemia (410). Among those patients who have overt acute myeloid leukemia, the presence of myeloid sarcoma does not alter the rate of remission after chemotherapy (411). Although the results of some studies suggest that the presence of myeloid sarcoma adversely affects the prognosis of patients with t(8;21)-positive acute myeloid leukemia (402,412), other reports indicate that myeloid sarcoma does not influence their outcome (401,413,414). Allogeneic or autologous bone marrow transplant is associated with a higher probability of prolonged survival (395).

SUMMARY AND CONCLUSIONS

Lymphoid infiltrates occurring in the ocular adnexa have traditionally posed a formidable clinical and histopathologic dilemma. In the past, the rate of error in accuracy of histopathologic diagnosis and ability to predict clinical outcome were estimated to lie between 20% and 50%. Significant advances in our understanding of these lesions has occurred because of improvements in histopathologic criteria; the development of immunodiagnostic criteria; the correlative clinical, histopathologic, and immunophenotypic analysis of large patient cohorts; and the application of molecular genetic techniques. The recognition of MALT lymphomas and the development of the WHO classification have contributed to our further understanding of the ocular adnexal lymphoid proliferations.

Patients who have ocular adnexal lymphoid proliferations, regardless of histopathology (i.e., lymphoid hyperplasia, atypical lymphoid hyperplasia, or malignant lymphoma), or bilaterality, do not appear to differ significantly with respect to age, sex, presenting complaints, duration of symptoms, or ophthalmic findings, with the possible exception of orbital bone erosion, which is highly associated with malignant lymphoma. Clinical evaluation alone usually is of little value in distinguishing benign and malignant ocular adnexal lymphoid proliferations. CT similarly reveals no known characteristic features that permit this technique to discriminate reliably between benign and malignant orbital lymphoid proliferations. Consequently, the accurate diagnosis of ocular adnexal lymphoid proliferations requires histopathologic examination assisted by ancillary techniques such as immunophenotypic and molecular genetic analysis.

Most lymphoid proliferations occurring in the ocular adnexa are malignant lymphomas. It is now widely recognized that most ocular adnexal malignant lymphomas arise in MALT, represent MALT lymphomas, and display the morphologic spectrum observed in MALT lymphomas originating in other extranodal sites. The MALT lymphomas share common histopathologic characteristics that include a marginal zone-type distribution and a variable cytologic composition, dominated by centrocyte-like cells, monocytoid cells, small lymphocytes, or plasmacytoid cells. The neoplastic cells often surround, and sometimes infiltrate into, benign reactive follicles and infiltrate the overlying epithelium, resulting in so-called lymphoepithelial lesions. MALT lymphomas and nearly all other categories of malignant lymphoma occurring in the ocular adnexa are B-cell neoplasms. Consequently, they express a variety of pan-B-cell–associated antigens and monotypic surface immunoglobulin and exhibit clonal immunoglobulin heavy- and light-chain gene rearrangements. Ocular adnexal MALT lymphomas have site-specific cytogenetic changes. Up to two-thirds of the patients have trisomy 3 and more than half of the patients have trisomy 18. In addition, about 25% of the patients have t(14;18)(q32;q21) and up to 20% of the patients have t(3;14) (p14.1;q32). Most patients who present with a lymphoid proliferation limited to the ocular adnexa (stage IE), regardless of the histopathology, immunophenotype, or bilaterality, appear to have a benign, relatively indolent clinical course.

ACKNOWLEDGMENTS

Dr. Knowles thanks his longtime friend and colleague, Dr. Frederick Jakobiec, for his collaborative participation in many of the studies cited here. The authors also thank Ida Nathan and Al Lamme for preparing the excellent photomicrographs.

References

1. Jakobiec FA, McLean I, Font RL. Clinicopathologic characteristics of orbital lymphoid hyperplasia. *Ophthalmology* 1979;86:948–966.
2. Knowles DM II, Jakobiec FA. Orbital lymphoid neoplasms: a clinicopathologic study of 60 patients. *Cancer* 1980;46:576–589.
3. Knowles DM II, Jakobiec FA. Ocular adnexal lymphoid neoplasms: clinical, histopathologic, electron microscopic, and immunologic characteristics. *Hum Pathol* 1982;13:148–162.
4. Knowles DM II. The extranodal lymphoid infiltrate: a diagnostic dilemma. *Semin Diagn Pathol* 1985;2:147–151.
5. Burke JS. Histologic criteria for distinguishing between benign and malignant extranodal lymphoid infiltrates. *Semin Diagn Pathol* 1985;2:152–162.
6. Knowles DM II, Jakobiec FA. Cell marker analysis of extranodal lymphoid infiltrates: to what extent does the determination of mono- or polyclonality resolve the diagnostic dilemma of malignant lymphoma v pseudolymphoma in an extranodal site? *Semin Diagn Pathol* 1985;2:163–168.
7. Jakobiec FA, Iwamoto T. The ocular adnexa: introduction to lids, conjunctiva, and orbit. In: Jakobiec FA, ed. *Ocular anatomy, embryology and teratology.* Philadelphia: Harper and Row, 1982:677–732.
8. Sacks EH, Wieczorek R, Jakobiec FA, et al. Lymphocytic subpopulations in the normal human conjunctiva. A monoclonal antibody study. *Ophthalmology* 1986;93:1276–1283.
9. Knowles DM II, Jakobiec FA, Halper JP. Immunologic characterization of ocular adnexal lymphoid neoplasms. *Am J Ophthalmol* 1979;87:603–619.
10. Knowles DM II, Halper JP, Jakobiec FA. The immunologic characterization of 40 extranodal lymphoid infiltrates: usefulness in distinguishing between benign pseudolymphoma and malignant lymphoma. *Cancer* 1982;49:2321–2335.
11. Knowles DM. Immunophenotypic and immunogenotypic approaches useful in distinguishing benign and malignant lymphoid proliferations. *Semin Oncol* 1993;20:583–610.
12. Jakobiec FA, Iwamoto T, Knowles DM II. Ocular adnexal lymphoid tumors. Correlative ultrastructural and immunologic marker studies. *Arch Ophthalmol* 1982;100:84–98.
13. Harmon DC, Aisenberg AC, Harris NL, et al. Lymphocyte surface markers in orbital lymphoid neoplasms. *J Clin Oncol* 1984;2:856–860.
14. Harris NL, Pilch BZ, Bhan AK, et al. Immunohistologic diagnosis of orbital lymphoid infiltrates. *Am J Surg Pathol* 1984;8:83–91.
15. Jakobiec FA, Iwamoto T, Patell M, et al. Ocular adnexal monoclonal lymphoid tumors with a favorable prognosis. *Ophthalmology* 1986;93:1547–1557.
16. Medeiros LJ, Harris NL. Lymphoid infiltrates of the orbit and conjunctiva. A morphologic and immunophenotypic study of 99 cases. *Am J Surg Pathol* 1989;13:459–471.
17. Knowles DM, Jakobiec FA, McNally L, et al. Lymphoid hyperplasia and malignant lymphoma occurring in the ocular adnexa (orbit, conjunctiva, and eyelids): a prospective multiparametric analysis of 108 cases during 1977 to 1987. *Hum Pathol* 1990;21:959–973.
18. Shields JA, Shields CL, Scartozzi R. Survey of 1264 patients with orbital tumors and simulating lesions: the 2002 Montgomery Lecture, part 1. *Ophthalmology* 2004;111:997–1008.
19. Seidman JG, Leder P. The arrangement and rearrangement of antibody genes. *Nature* 1978;276:790–795.
20. Tonegawa S. Somatic generation of antibody diversity. *Nature* 1983;302:575–581.
21. Yanagi Y, Yoshikai Y, Leggett K, et al. A human T cell-specific cDNA clone encodes a protein having extensive homology to immunoglobulin chains. *Nature* 1984;308:145–149.
22. Pelicci PG, Knowles DM II, Arlin ZA, et al. Multiple monoclonal B cell expansions and c-myc oncogene rearrangements in acquired immune deficiency syndrome-related lymphoproliferative disorders. Implications for lymphomagenesis. *J Exp Med* 1986;164:2049–2060.
23. Neri A, Jakobiec FA, Pelicci PG, et al. Immunoglobulin and T cell receptor beta chain gene rearrangement analysis of ocular adnexal lymphoid neoplasms: clinical and biologic implications. *Blood* 1987;70:1519–1529.
24. Knowles DM, Athan E, Ubriaco A, et al. Extranodal noncutaneous lymphoid hyperplasias represent a continuous spectrum of B-cell neoplasia: demonstration by molecular genetic analysis. *Blood* 1989;73:1635–1645.
25. Birch-Hirschfeld A. Zur Diagnostik und Pathologie der Orbital tumoren. *Ber Dtsch Ophthalmol Ges* 1905;32:127–135.
26. Jakobiec FA, Jones IS. Orbital inflammations. In: Jones I, Jakobiec FA, eds. *Diseases of the orbit.* Hagertown: Harper & Row, 1979:187–205.
27. Henderson J. *Orbital tumors.* New York: Decker, Thieme-Statton, 1980.
28. Hogan M, Zimmerman LE. *Ophtalmic pathology: an atlas and textbook.* Philadelphia: WB Saunders, 1962.
29. Saltzstein SL. Pulmonary malignant lymphomas and pseudolymphomas: classification, therapy, and prognosis. *Cancer* 1963;16:928–955.
30. Char D. *Clinical ocular pathology.* New York: Churchill Livingstone, 1989.
31. Fujii H, Fujisada H, Kondo T, et al. Orbital pseudotumor: histopathological classification and treatment. *Ophthalmologica* 1985;190:230–242.
32. Lanciano R, Fowble B, Sergott RC, et al. The results of radiotherapy for orbital pseudotumor. *Int J Radiat Oncol Biol Phys* 1990;18:407–411.
33. Geyer JT, Deshpande V. IgG4-associated sialadenitis. *Curr Opin Rheumatol* 2011;23:95–101.
34. Wallace ZS, Khosroshahi A, Jakobiec FA, et al. IgG4-related systemic disease as a cause of "idiopathic" orbital inflammation, including orbital myositis, and trigeminal nerve involvement. *Surv Ophthalmol* 2012;57:26–33.
35. Sato Y, Ohshima K, Ichimura K, et al. Ocular adnexal IgG4-related disease has uniform clinicopathology. *Pathol Int* 2008;58:465–470.
36. Jakobiec FA, Font RL. Orbit: lymphoid tumors. In: Spencer W, Font RL, Green WR, et al., eds. *Ophtalmic pathology: an atlas and textbook.* 3rd ed. Philadelphia: WB Saunders, 1986:2663–2737.
37. Garner A. Orbital lymphoproliferative disorders. *Br J Ophthalmol* 1992;76:47–48.
38. Henderson J. *Orbital tumors.* New York: Raven Press, 1994.
39. Medeiros LJ, Harmon DC, Linggood RM, et al. Immunohistologic features predict clinical behavior of orbital and conjunctival lymphoid infiltrates. *Blood* 1989;74:2121–2129.
40. Coupland SE, Krause L, Delecluse HJ, et al. Lymphoproliferative lesions of the ocular adnexa. Analysis of 112 cases. *Ophthalmology* 1998;105:14301441.
41. Mombaerts I, Goldschmeding R, Schlingemann RO, et al. What is orbital pseudotumor? *Surv Ophthalmol* 1996;41:66–78.
42. Jakobiec F, Font RL. Noninfectious orbital inflammations. In: Spencer W, ed. *Ophtalmic pathology: an atlas and textbook.* 3rd ed. Philadelphia: WB Saunders, 1986: 2777–2795.
43. Garner A. Pathology of 'pseudotumours' of the orbit: a review. *J Clin Pathol* 1973;26:639–648.
44. Jakobiec F. Orbit. In: Spencer W, ed. *Ophtalmic pathology: an atlas and textbook.* 4th ed. Philadelphia: WB Saunders, 1996:2822–2844.
45. Mehta M, Jakobiec F, Fay A. Idiopathic fibroinflammatory disease of the face, eyelids, and periorbital membrane with immunoglobulin G4-positive plasma cells. *Arch Pathol Lab Med* 2009;133:1251–1251.
46. Jakobiec FA. Ocular adnexal lymphoid tumors: progress in need of clarification. *Am J Ophthalmol* 2008;145:941–950.
47. Rootman J, Nugent R. The classification and management of acute orbital pseudotumors. *Ophthalmology* 1982;89:1040–1048.
48. Mottow LS, Jakobiec FA. Idiopathic inflammatory orbital pseudotumor in childhood. I. Clinical characteristics. *Arch Ophthalmol* 1978;96:1410–1417.

49. Mottow-Lippa L, Jakobiec FA, Smith M. Idiopathic inflammatory orbital pseudotumor in childhood. II. Results of diagnostic tests and biopsies. *Ophthalmology* 1981;88:565–574.
50. Rootman J, McCarthy M, White V, et al. Idiopathic sclerosing inflammation of the orbit. A distinct clinicopathologic entity. *Ophthalmology* 1994;101:570–584.
51. Snebold N. Noninfectious orbital inflammations and vasculitis. In: Albert DM, Jakobiec FA, eds. *Principles and practice of ophthalmology: clinical practice*. Philadelphia: WB Saunders, 1994:1923–1942.
52. Nugent RA, Rootman J, Robertson WD, et al. Acute orbital pseudotumors: classification and CT features. *AJR Am J Roentgenol* 1981;137:957–962.
53. McNicholas MM, Power WJ, Griffin JF. Idiopathic inflammatory pseudotumour of the orbit: CT features correlated with clinical outcome. *Clin Radiol* 1991;44:3–7.
54. Edwards MK, Zauel DW, Gilmor RL, et al. Invasive orbital pseudotumor–CT demonstration of extension beyond orbit. *Neuroradiology* 1982;23:215–217.
55. Weissler MC, Miller E, Fortune MA. Sclerosing orbital pseudotumor: a unique clinicopathologic entity. *Ann Otol Rhinol Laryngol* 1989;98:496–501.
56. Frohman LP, Kupersmith MJ, Lang J, et al. Intracranial extension and bone destruction in orbital pseudotumor. *Arch Ophthalmol* 1986;104:380–384.
57. Clifton AG, Borgstein RL, Moseley IF, et al. Intracranial extension of orbital pseudotumour. *Clin Radiol* 1992;45:23–26.
58. Moseley IF, Wright JE. Orbital pseudotumour. *Clin Radiol* 1992;45:67.
59. Rootman J, Robertson W, Lapointe JS. Inflammatory diseases. In: Rootman J, ed. *Diseases of the orbit: a multidisciplinaty approach*. Philadelphia: JB Lippincott, 1988: 159–179.
60. Leone CR Jr, Lloyd WC III. Treatment protocol for orbital inflammatory disease. *Ophthalmology* 1985;92:1325–1331.
61. Hsuan JD, Selva D, McNab AA, et al. Idiopathic sclerosing orbital inflammation. *Arch Ophthalmol* 2006;124:1244–1250.
62. Char DH, Miller T. Orbital pseudotumor. Fine-needle aspiration biopsy and response to therapy. *Ophthalmology* 1993;100:1702–1710.
63. Mombaerts I, Schlingemann RO, Goldschmeding R, et al. Are systemic corticosteroids useful in the management of orbital pseudotumors? *Ophthalmology* 1996;103:521–528.
64. Wright JE, Stewart WB, Krohel GB. Clinical presentation and management of lacrimal gland tumours. *Br J Ophthalmol* 1979;63:600–606.
65. Bullen CL, Younge BR. Chronic orbital myositis. *Arch Ophthalmol* 1982;100: 1749–1751.
66. Mauriello JA Jr, Flanagan JC. Management of orbital inflammatory disease. A protocol. *Surv Ophthalmol* 1984;29:104–116.
67. van der Gaag R, Koornneef L, van Heerde P, et al. Lymphoid proliferations in the orbit: malignant or benign? *Br J Ophthalmol* 1984;68:892–900.
68. Kennerdell JS, Slamovits TL, Dekker A, et al. Orbital fine-needle aspiration biopsy. *Am J Ophthalmol* 1985;99:547–551.
69. Tijl JW, Koornneef L. Fine needle aspiration biopsy in orbital tumours. *Br J Ophthalmol* 1991;75:491–492.
70. Austin-Seymour MM, Donaldson SS, Egbert PR, et al. Radiotherapy of lymphoid diseases of the orbit. *Int J Radiat Oncol Biol Phys* 1985;11:371–379.
71. Paris GL, Waltuch GF, Egbert PR. Treatment of refractory orbital pseudotumors with pulsed chemotherapy. *Ophthal Plast Reconstr Surg* 1990;6:96–101.
72. Shah SS, Lowder CY, Schmitt MA, et al. Low-dose methotrexate therapy for ocular inflammatory disease. *Ophthalmology* 1992;99:1419–1423.
73. Noguchi H, Kephart GM, Campbell RJ, et al. Tissue eosinophilia and eosinophil degranulation in orbital pseudotumor. *Ophthalmology* 1991;98:928–932.
74. McCarthy JM, White VA, Harris G, et al. Idiopathic sclerosing inflammation of the orbit: immunohistologic analysis and comparison with retroperitoneal fibrosis. *Mod Pathol* 1993;6:581–587.
75. Comings DE, Skubi KB, Van Eyes J, et al. Familial multifocal fibrosclerosis. Findings suggesting that retroperitoneal fibrosis, mediastinal fibrosis, sclerosing cholangitis, Riedel's thyroiditis, and pseudotumor of the orbit may be different manifestations of a single disease. *Ann Intern Med* 1967;66:884–892.
76. Easton JA, Smith WT. Non-specific granuloma of orbit ("orbital pseudotumour"). *J Pathol Bacteriol* 1961;82:345–354.
77. Barrett NR. Idiopathic mediastinal fibrosis. *Br J Surg* 1958;46:207–218.
78. Richards AB, Shalka HW, Roberts FJ, et al. Pseudotumor of the orbit and retroperitoneal fibrosis. A form of multifocal fibrosclerosis. *Arch Ophthalmol* 1980;98:1617–1620.
79. Schonder AA, Clift RC, Brophy JW, et al. Bilateral recurrent orbital inflammation associated with retroperitoneal fibrosclerosis. *Br J Ophthalmol* 1985;69: 783–787.
80. DuPont HL, Varco RL, Winchell CP. Chronic fibrous mediastinitis simulating pulmonic stenosis, associated with inflammatory pseudotumor of the orbit. *Am J Med* 1968;44:447–452.
81. Andersen SR, Seedorff HH, Halberg P. Thyroiditis with myxoedema and orbital pseudotumour. *Acta Ophthalmol (Copenh)* 1963;41:120–125.
82. Arnott EJ, Greaves DP. Orbital involvement in Riedel's thyroiditis. *Br J Ophthalmol* 1965;49:1–5.
83. Wenger J, Gingrich GW, Mendeloff J. Sclerosing cholangitis—a manifestation of systemic disease. Increased serum gamma-globulin, follicular lymph node hyperplasia, and orbital pseudotumor. *Arch Intern Med* 1965;116:509–514.
84. Aalberse RC, Schuurman J. IgG4 breaking the rules. *Immunology* 2002;105:9–19.
85. van der Neut Kolfschoten M, Schuurman J, Losen M, et al. Anti-inflammatory activity of human IgG4 antibodies by dynamic Fab arm exchange. *Science* 2007;317:1554–1557.
86. Hamano H, Kawa S, Horiuchi A, et al. High serum IgG4 concentrations in patients with sclerosing pancreatitis. *N Engl J Med* 2001;344:732–738.
87. Deshpande V, Chicano S, Finkelberg D, et al. Autoimmune pancreatitis: a systemic immune complex mediated disease. *Am J Surg Pathol* 2006;30:1537–1545.
88. Sarles H, Sarles JC, Muratore R, et al. Chronic inflammatory sclerosis of the pancreas—an autoimmune pancreatic disease? *Am J Dig Dis* 1961;6:688–698.
89. Yoshida K, Toki F, Takeuchi T, et al. Chronic pancreatitis caused by an autoimmune abnormality. Proposal of the concept of autoimmune pancreatitis. *Dig Dis Sci* 1995;40:1561–1568.
90. Hamano H, Arakura N, Muraki T, et al. Prevalence and distribution of extrapancreatic lesions complicating autoimmune pancreatitis. *J Gastroenterol* 2006;41:1197–1205.
91. Deshpande V, Mino-Kenudson M, Brugge W, et al. Autoimmune pancreatitis: more than just a pancreatic disease? A contemporary review of its pathology. *Arch Pathol Lab Med* 2005;129:1148–1154.
92. Cheuk W, Yuen HK, Chan JK. Chronic sclerosing dacryoadenitis: part of the spectrum of IgG4-related Sclerosing disease? *Am J Surg Pathol* 2007;31:643–645.
93. Cornell LD, Chicano SL, Deshpande V, et al. Pseudotumors due to IgG4 immune-complex tubulointerstitial nephritis associated with autoimmune pancreatocentric disease. *Am J Surg Pathol* 2007;31:1586–1597.
94. Zen Y, Fujii T, Harada K, et al. Th2 and regulatory immune reactions are increased in immunoglobin G4-related sclerosing pancreatitis and cholangitis. *Hepatology* 2007;45:1538–1546.
95. Masaki Y, Dong L, Kurose N, et al. Proposal for a new clinical entity, IgG4-positive multiorgan lymphoproliferative syndrome: analysis of 64 cases of IgG4-related disorders. *Ann Rheum Dis* 2009;68:1310–1315.
96. Yamamoto M, Takahashi H, Ohara M, et al. A new conceptualization for Mikulicz's disease as an IgG4-related plasmacytic disease. *Mod Rheumatol* 2006;16: 335–340.
97. Ghazale A, Chari ST, Zhang L, et al. Immunoglobulin G4-associated cholangitis: clinical profile and response to therapy. *Gastroenterology* 2008;134:706–715.
98. Cheuk W, Yuen HK, Chu SY, et al. Lymphadenopathy of IgG4-related sclerosing disease. *Am J Surg Pathol* 2008;32:671–681.
99. Kamisawa T, Nakajima H, Egawa N, et al. IgG4-related sclerosing disease incorporating sclerosing pancreatitis, cholangitis, sialadenitis and retroperitoneal fibrosis with lymphadenopathy. *Pancreatology* 2006;6:132–137.
100. Kamisawa T, Okamoto A. Autoimmune pancreatitis: proposal of IgG4-related sclerosing disease. *J Gastroenterol* 2006;41:613–625.
101. Kamisawa T, Funata N, Hayashi Y, et al. A new clinicopathological entity of IgG4-related autoimmune disease. *J Gastroenterol* 2003;38:982–984.
102. Carruthers MN, Stone JH, Khosroshahi A. The latest on IgG4-RD: a rapidly emerging disease. *Curr Opin Rheumatol* 2012;24:60–69.
103. Genton C, Wang Y, Izui S, et al. The Th2 lymphoproliferation developing in LatY136F mutant mice triggers polyclonal B cell activation and systemic autoimmunity. *J Immunol* 2006;177:2285–2293.
104. Rubin LA, Nelson DL. The soluble interleukin-2 receptor: biology, function, and clinical application. *Ann Intern Med* 1990;113:619–627.
105. Kawano M, Yamada K, Kakuchi Y, et al. A case of immunoglobulin G4-related chronic sclerosing sialadenitis and dacryoadenitis associated with tuberculosis. *Mod Rheumatol* 2009;19:87–90.
106. Chan JK. Kuttner tumor (chronic sclerosing sialadenitis) of the submandibular gland: an underrecognized entity. *Adv Anat Pathol* 1998;5:239–251.
107. Kitagawa S, Zen Y, Harada K, et al. Abundant IgG4-positive plasma cell infiltration characterizes chronic sclerosing sialadenitis (Kuttner's tumor). *Am J Surg Pathol* 2005;29:783–791.
108. Geyer JT, Ferry JA, Harris NL, et al. Chronic sclerosing sialadenitis (Kuttner tumor) is an IgG4-associated disease. *Am J Surg Pathol* 2010;34:202–210.
109. Finkelberg DL, Sahani D, Deshpande V, et al. Autoimmune pancreatitis. *N Engl J Med* 2006;355:2670–2676.
110. Masaki Y, Sugai S, Umehara H. IgG4-related diseases including Mikulicz's disease and sclerosing pancreatitis: diagnostic insights. *J Rheumatol* 2010;37: 1380–1385.
111. Takano KI, Yamamoto M, Takahashi H, et al. Clinicopathologic similarities between Mikulicz disease and Kuttner tumor. *Am J Otolaryngol* 2010;31:429–434.
112. Yamamoto M, Harada S, Ohara M, et al. Clinical and pathological differences between Mikulicz's disease and Sjogren's syndrome. *Rheumatology (Oxford)* 2005;44:227–234.
113. Kawaguchi K, Koike M, Tsuruta K, et al. Lymphoplasmacytic sclerosing pancreatitis with cholangitis: a variant of primary sclerosing cholangitis extensively involving pancreas. *Hum Pathol* 1991;22:387–395.
114. Zen Y, Harada K, Sasaki M, et al. IgG4-related sclerosing cholangitis with and without hepatic inflammatory pseudotumor, and sclerosing pancreatitis-associated sclerosing cholangitis: do they belong to a spectrum of sclerosing pancreatitis? *Am J Surg Pathol* 2004;28:1193–1203.
115. Okazaki K, Uchida K, Koyabu M, et al. Recent advances in the concept and diagnosis of autoimmune pancreatitis and IgG4-related disease. *J Gastroenterol* 2011;46:277–288.
116. Okazaki K, Uchida K, Miyoshi H, et al. Recent concepts of autoimmune pancreatitis and IgG4-related disease. *Clin Rev Allergy Immunol* 2011;41:126–138.
117. Kubota T, Moritani S, Katayama M, et al. Ocular adnexal IgG4-related lymphoplasmacytic infiltrative disorder. *Arch Ophthalmol* 2010;128:577–584.
118. Matsuo T, Ichimura K, Sato Y, et al. Immunoglobulin G4 (IgG4)-positive or -negative ocular adnexal benign lymphoid lesions in relation to systemic involvement. *J Clin Exp Hematop* 2010;50:129–142.
119. Plaza JA, Garrity JA, Dogan A, et al. Orbital inflammation with IgG4-positive plasma cells: manifestation of IgG4 systemic disease. *Arch Ophthalmol* 2011;129:421–428.
120. Kubota T, Moritani S, Yoshino T, et al. Ocular adnexal mucosa-associated lymphoid tissue lymphoma with polyclonal hypergammaglobulinemia. *Am J Ophthalmol* 2008;145:1002–1006.
121. Cheuk W, Yuen HK, Chan AC, et al. Ocular adnexal lymphoma associated with IgG4+ chronic sclerosing dacryoadenitis: a previously undescribed complication of IgG4-related sclerosing disease. *Am J Surg Pathol* 2008;32:1159–1167.
122. Takahira M, Kawano M, Zen Y, et al. IgG4-related chronic sclerosing dacryoadenitis. *Arch Ophthalmol* 2007;125:1575–1578.
123. Kubota T, Moritani S, Yoshino T, et al. Ocular adnexal marginal zone B cell lymphoma infiltrated by IgG4-positive plasma cells. *J Clin Pathol* 2010;63: 1059–1065.
124. Cheuk W, Chan JK. IgG4-related sclerosing disease: a critical appraisal of an evolving clinicopathologic entity. *Adv Anat Pathol* 2010;17:303–332.
125. Espinoza GM. Orbital inflammatory pseudotumors: etiology, differential diagnosis, and management. *Curr Rheumatol Rep* 2010;12:443–437.
126. Khosroshahi A, Bloch DB, Deshpande V, et al. Rituximab therapy leads to rapid decline of serum IgG4 levels and prompt clinical improvement in IgG4-related systemic disease. *Arthritis Rheum* 2010;62:1755–1762.
127. Topazian M, Witzig TE, Smyrk TC, et al. Rituximab therapy for refractory biliary strictures in immunoglobulin G4-associated cholangitis. *Clin Gastroenterol Hepatol* 2008;6:364–346.
128. Khosroshahi A, Carruthers MN, Deshpande V, et al. Rituximab for the treatment of IgG4-related disease: lessons from 10 consecutive patients. *Medicine (Baltimore)* 2012;91:57–66.
129. Jakobiec FA, Gibralter RA, Knowles DM II, et al. Ocular pathology for clinicians. 6. Lymphoid tumor of the lid. *Ophthalmology* 1980;87:1058–1064.

130. Knowles DM II, Jakobiec FA. Quantitative determination of T cells in ocular lymphoid infiltrates. An indirect method for distinguishing between pseudolymphomas and malignant lymphomas. *Arch Ophthalmol* 1981;99:309–316.
131. Knowles DM II, Jakobiec FA, Wang CY. The expression of surface antigen Leu 1 by ocular adnexal lymphoid neoplasms. *Am J Ophthalmol* 1982;94:246–254.
132. Knowles DM II, Jakobiec FA. Identification of T lymphocytes in ocular adnexal neoplasms by hybridoma monoclonal antibodies. *Am J Ophthalmol* 1983;95: 233–242.
133. Jakobiec FA, Neri A, Knowles DM II. Genotypic monoclonality in immunophenotypically polyclonal orbital lymphoid tumors. A model of tumor progression in the lymphoid system. The 1986 Wendell Hughes lecture. *Ophthalmology* 1987;94:980–994.
134. McNally L, Jakobiec FA, Knowles DM II. Clinical, morphologic, immunophenotypic, and molecular genetic analysis of bilateral ocular adnexal lymphoid neoplasms in 17 patients. *Am J Ophthalmol* 1987;103:555–568.
135. Isaacson PG, Nortan AJ. *Extranodal lymphomas*. Edinbirgh: Churchill Livingstone, 1994.
136. Harris NL, Jaffe ES, Stein H, et al. A revised European-American classification of lymphoid neoplasms: a proposal from the International Lymphoma Study Group. *Blood* 1994;84:1361–1392.
137. Swerdlow S, Campo E, Harris NL, et al., eds. *WHO classification of tumours of haematopoietic and lymphoid tissues*. 4th ed. Lyon: IARC, 2008.
138. Nakata M, Matsuno Y, Katsumata N, et al. Histology according to the Revised European-American Lymphoma Classification significantly predicts the prognosis of ocular adnexal lymphoma. *Leuk Lymphoma* 1999;32:533–543.
139. Knowles DM, Chamulak GA, Subar M, et al. Lymphoid neoplasia associated with the acquired immunodeficiency syndrome (AIDS). The New York University Medical Center experience with 105 patients (1981–1986). *Ann Intern Med* 1988;108:744–753.
140. Reifler DM, Warzynski MJ, Blount WR, et al. Orbital lymphoma associated with acquired immune deficiency syndrome (AIDS). *Surv Ophthalmol* 1994;38: 371–380.
141. Weisenthal RW, Streeten BW, Dubansky AS, et al. Burkitt lymphoma presenting as a conjunctival mass. *Ophthalmology* 1995;102:129–134.
142. Edelstein C, Shields JA, Shields CL, et al. Non-African Burkitt lymphoma presenting with oral thrush and an orbital mass in a child. *Am J Ophthalmol* 1997;124:859–861.
143. Sherman MD, Van Dalen JT, Conrad K. Bilateral orbital infiltration as the initial sign of a peripheral T-cell lymphoma presenting in a leukemic phase. *Ann Ophthalmol* 1990;22:93–95.
144. Henderson JW, Banks PM, Yeatts RP. T-cell lymphoma of the orbit. *Mayo Clin Proc* 1989;64:940–944.
145. Leidenix MJ, Mamalis N, Olson RJ, et al. Primary T-cell immunoblastic lymphoma of the orbit in a pediatric patient. *Ophthalmology* 1993;100:998–1002.
146. Stenson S, Ramsay DL. Ocular findings in mycosis fungoides. *Arch Ophthalmol* 1981;99:272–277.
147. Zucker JL, Doyle MF. Mycosis fungoides metastatic to the orbit. *Arch Ophthalmol* 1991;109:688–691.
148. Meekins B, Proia AD, Klintworth GK. Cutaneous T-cell lymphoma presenting as a rapidly enlarging ocular adnexal tumor. *Ophthalmology* 1985;92:1288–1293.
149. Jakobiec F. Orbital Hodgkin's disease: clinicopathological conference. *N Engl J Med* 1989;320:447–457.
150. Bairey O, Kremer I, Rakowsky E, et al. Orbital and adnexal involvement in systemic non-Hodgkin's lymphoma. *Cancer* 1994;73:2395–2399.
151. Freeman C, Berg JW, Cutler SJ. Occurrence and prognosis of extranodal lymphomas. *Cancer* 1972;29:252–260.
152. Rosenberg SA, Diamond HD, Jaslowitz B, et al. Lymphosarcoma: a review of 1269 cases. *Medicine (Baltimore)* 1961;40:31–84.
153. Moslehi R, Devesa SS, Schairer C, et al. Rapidly increasing incidence of ocular non-hodgkin lymphoma. *J Natl Cancer Inst* 2006;98:936–939.
154. Mamalis N, Mackman G, Holds JB, et al. Simultaneous bilateral conjunctival and orbital lymphoma presenting as a conjunctival lesion. *Ophthalmic Surg* 1988;19:662–663.
155. Nutting CM, Shah-Desai S, Rose GE, et al. Thyroid orbitopathy possibly predisposes to late-onset of periocular lymphoma. *Eye (Lond)* 2006;20:645–648.
156. Gruenberger B, Woehrer S, Troch M, et al. Assessment of the role of hepatitis C, *Helicobacter pylori* and autoimmunity in MALT lymphoma of the ocular adnexa in 45 Austrian patients. *Acta Oncol* 2008;47:355–359.
157. Ferry JA, Fung CY, Zukerberg L, et al. Lymphoma of the ocular adnexa: a study of 353 cases. *Am J Surg Pathol* 2007;31:170–184.
158. Lauer SA. Ocular adnexal lymphoid tumors. *Curr Opin Ophthalmol* 2000;11: 361–366.
159. Streubel B, Chott A, Huber D, et al. Lymphoma-specific genetic aberrations in microvascular endothelial cells in B-cell lymphomas. *N Engl J Med* 2004;351: 250–259.
160. Ferry J. *Extranodal lymphomas*. Philadelphia: Elsevier Saunders, 2011.
161. Ferreri AJ, Guidoboni M, Ponzoni M, et al. Evidence for an association between *Chlamydia psittaci* and ocular adnexal lymphomas. *J Natl Cancer Inst* 2004;96:586–594.
162. Ferreri AJ, Ponzoni M, Guidoboni M, et al. Regression of ocular adnexal lymphoma after *Chlamydia psittaci*-eradicating antibiotic therapy. *J Clin Oncol* 2005;23:5067–5073.
163. Yoo C, Ryu MH, Huh J, et al. *Chlamydia psittaci* infection and clinicopathologic analysis of ocular adnexal lymphomas in Korea. *Am J Hematol* 2007;82: 821–823.
164. Chanudet E, Zhou Y, Bacon CM, et al. *Chlamydia psittaci* is variably associated with ocular adnexal MALT lymphoma in different geographical regions. *J Pathol* 2006;209:344–351.
165. Zhang GS, Winter JN, Variakojis D, et al. Lack of an association between *Chlamydia psittaci* and ocular adnexal lymphoma. *Leuk Lymphoma* 2007;48: 577–583.
166. Ruiz A, Reischl U, Swerdlow SH, et al. Extranodal marginal zone B-cell lymphomas of the ocular adnexa: multiparameter analysis of 34 cases including interphase molecular cytogenetics and PCR for *Chlamydia psittaci*. *Am J Surg Pathol* 2007;31:792–802.
167. Rosado MF, Byrne GE Jr, Ding F, et al. Ocular adnexal lymphoma: a clinicopathologic study of a large cohort of patients with no evidence for an association with *Chlamydia psittaci*. Blood 2006;107:467–472.
168. Stefanovic A, Lossos IS. Extranodal marginal zone lymphoma of the ocular adnexa. *Blood* 2009;114:501–510.
169. Husain A, Roberts D, Pro B, et al. Meta-analyses of the association between *Chlamydia psittaci* and ocular adnexal lymphoma and the response of ocular adnexal lymphoma to antibiotics. *Cancer* 2007;110:809–815.
170. Wood GS, Kamath NV, Guitart J, et al. Absence of *Borrelia burgdorferi* DNA in cutaneous B-cell lymphomas from the United States. *J Cutan Pathol* 2001;28:502–507.
171. Arcaini L, Burcheri S, Rossi A, et al. Prevalence of HCV infection in nongastric marginal zone B-cell lymphoma of MALT. *Ann Oncol* 2007;18:346–350.
172. Ferreri AJ, Viale E, Guidoboni M, et al. Clinical implications of hepatitis C virus infection in MALT-type lymphoma of the ocular adnexa. *Ann Oncol* 2006;17: 769–772.
173. Chan CC, Shen D, Mochizuki M, et al. Detection of *Helicobacter pylori* and *Chlamydia pneumoniae* genes in primary orbital lymphoma. *Trans Am Ophthalmol Soc* 2006;104:62–70.
174. Shen D, Yuen HK, Galita DA, et al. Detection of *Chlamydia pneumoniae* in a bilateral orbital mucosa-associated lymphoid tissue lymphoma. *Am J Ophthalmol* 2006;141:1162–1163.
175. Lee SB, Yang JW, Kim CS. The association between conjunctival MALT lymphoma and *Helicobacter pylori*. *Br J Ophthalmol* 2008;92:534–536.
176. Decaudin D, Ferroni A, Vincent-Salomon A, et al. Ocular adnexal lymphoma and *Helicobacter pylori* gastric infection. *Am J Hematol* 2010;85:645–649.
177. Westacott S, Garner A, Moseley IF, et al. Orbital lymphoma versus reactive lymphoid hyperplasia: an analysis of the use of computed tomography in differential diagnosis. *Br J Ophthalmol* 1991;75:722–725.
178. White WL, Ferry JA, Harris NL, et al. Ocular adnexal lymphoma. A clinicopathologic study with identification of lymphomas of mucosa-associated lymphoid tissue type. *Ophthalmology* 1995;102:1994–2006.
179. Sigelman J, Jakobiec FA. Lymphoid lesions of the conjunctiva: relation of histopathology to clinical outcome. *Ophthalmology* 1978;85:818–843.
180. Jampol LM, Marsh JC, Albert DM, et al. IgA associated lymphoplasmacytic tumor involving the conjunctiva, eyelid, and orbit. *Am J Ophthalmol* 1975;79:279–284.
181. Knowles DM II, Jakobiec FA, Rosen M, et al. Amyloidosis of the orbit and adnexae. *Surv Ophthalmol* 1975;19:367–384.
182. Brisbane JU, Lessell S, Finkel HE, et al. Malignant lymphoma presenting in the orbit: a clinicopathologic study of a rare immunoglobulin-producing variant. *Cancer* 1981;47:548–553.
183. Gayed I, Eskandari MF, McLaughlin P, et al. Value of positron emission tomography in staging ocular adnexal lymphomas and evaluating their response to therapy. *Ophthalmic Surg Lasers Imaging* 2007;38:319–325.
184. Hoffmann M, Kletter K, Diemling M, et al. Positron emission tomography with fluorine-18-2-fluoro-2-deoxy-D-glucose (F18-FDG) does not visualize extranodal B-cell lymphoma of the mucosa-associated lymphoid tissue (MALT)-type. *Ann Oncol* 1999;10:1185–1189.
185. Carbone PP, Kaplan HS, Musshoff K, et al. Report of the committee on Hodgkin's disease staging classification. *Cancer Res* 1971;31:1860–1861.
186. Coupland SE, White VA, Rootman J, et al. A TNM-based clinical staging system of ocular adnexal lymphomas. *Arch Pathol Lab Med* 2009;133:1262–1267.
187. Yeo JH, Jakobiec FA, Abbott GF, et al. Combined clinical and computed tomographic diagnosis of orbital lymphoid tumors. *Am J Ophthalmol* 1982;94: 235–245.
188. Chao CK, Lin HS, Devineni VR, et al. Radiation therapy for primary orbital lymphoma. *Int J Radiat Oncol Biol Phys* 1995;31:929–934.
189. Jakobiec FA, Yeo JH, Trokel SL, et al. Combined clinical and computed tomographic diagnosis of primary lacrimal fossa lesions. *Am J Ophthalmol* 1982;94:785–807.
190. Hornblass A, Jakobiec FA, Reifler DM, et al. Orbital lymphoid tumors located predominantly within extraocular muscles. *Ophthalmology* 1987;94:688–697.
191. Bernardini FP, Bazzan M. Lymphoproliferative disease of the orbit. *Curr Opin Ophthalmol* 2007;18:398–401.
192. Roe RH, Finger PT, Kurli M, et al. Whole-body positron emission tomography/computed tomography imaging and staging of orbital lymphoma. *Ophthalmology* 2006;113:1854–1858.
193. Valenzuela AA, Allen C, Grimes D, et al. Positron emission tomography in the detection and staging of ocular adnexal lymphoproliferative disease. *Ophthalmology* 2006;113:2331–2337.
194. Knowles DM Jakobiec FA. Malignant lymphoma and lymphoid hyperplasias that occur in the ocular adnexa (orbit, conjunctiva and eyelids). In: Knowles DM, ed. *Neoplastic hematopathology*. Baltimore: Williams & Wilkins, 1992:1009–1046.
195. National Cancer Institute sponsored study of classifications of non-Hodgkin's lymphomas: summary and description of a working formulation for clinical usage. The Non-Hodgkin's Lymphoma Pathologic Classification Project. *Cancer* 1982;49:2112–2135.
196. Galieni P, Polito E, Leccisotti A, et al. Localized orbital lymphoma. *Haematologica* 1997;82:436–439.
197. White VA, Gascoyne RD, McNeil BK, et al. Histopathologic findings and frequency of clonality detected by the polymerase chain reaction in ocular adnexal lymphoproliferative lesions. *Mod Pathol* 1996;9:1052–1061.
198. Chen PM, Liu JH, Lin SH, et al. Rearrangements of immunoglobulin gene and oncogenes in ocular adnexal pseudolymphoma. *Curr Eye Res* 1991;10:547–555.
199. Ohshima K, Kikuchi M, Sumiyoshi Y, et al. Clonality of benign lymphoid hyperplasia in orbit and conjunctiva. *Pathol Res Pract* 1994;190:436–443.
200. Wotherspoon AC, Diss TC, Pan LX, et al. Primary low-grade B-cell lymphoma of the conjunctiva: a mucosa-associated lymphoid tissue type lymphoma. *Histopathology* 1993;23:417–424.
201. Isaacson P, Wright DH. Extranodal malignant lymphoma arising from mucosa-associated lymphoid tissue. *Cancer* 1984;53:2515–2524.
202. Isaacson P, Wright DH. Malignant lymphoma of mucosa-associated lymphoid tissue. A distinctive type of B-cell lymphoma. *Cancer* 1983;52:1410–1416.
203. Hardman-Lea S, Kerr-Muir M, Wotherspoon AC, et al. Mucosal-associated lymphoid tissue lymphoma of the conjunctiva. *Arch Ophthalmol* 1994;112:1207–1212.
204. Petrella T, Bron A, Foulet A, et al. Report of a primary lymphoma of the conjunctiva. A lymphoma of MALT origin? *Pathol Res Pract* 1991;187:78–84.
205. Thieblemont C, Berger F, Coiffier B. Mucosa-associated lymphoid tissue lymphomas. *Curr Opin Oncol* 1995;7:415–420.
206. A clinical evaluation of the International Lymphoma Study Group classification of non-Hodgkin's lymphoma. The Non-Hodgkin's Lymphoma Classification Project. *Blood* 1997;89:3909–3918.

207. Lagoo AS, Haggerty C, Kim Y, et al. Morphologic features of 115 lymphomas of the orbit and ocular adnexa categorized according to the World Health Organization classification: are marginal zone lymphomas in the orbit mucosa-associated lymphoid tissue-type lymphomas? *Arch Pathol Lab Med* 2008;132:1405–1416.
208. Sharara N, Holden JT, Wojno TH, et al. Ocular adnexal lymphoid proliferations: clinical, histologic, flow cytometric, and molecular analysis of forty-three cases. *Ophthalmology* 2003;110:1245–1254.
209. Auw-Haedrich C, Coupland SE, Kapp A, et al. Long term outcome of ocular adnexal lymphoma subtyped according to the REAL classification. Revised European and American Lymphoma. *Br J Ophthalmol* 2001;85:63–69.
210. Jakobiec FA, Knowles DM. An overview of ocular adnexal lymphoid tumors. *Trans Am Ophthalmol Soc* 1989;87:420–442; discussion 442–444.
211. Isaacson PG. Gastrointestinal lymphoma. *Hum Pathol* 1994;25:1020–1029.
212. Spencer J, Finn T, Pulford KA, et al. The human gut contains a novel population of B lymphocytes which resemble marginal zone cells. *Clin Exp Immunol* 1985; 62:607–612.
213. Isaacson PG, Wotherspoon AC, Diss T, et al. Follicular colonization in B-cell lymphoma of mucosa-associated lymphoid tissue. *Am J Surg Pathol* 1991;15: 819–828.
214. Papadaki L, Wotherspoon AC, Isaacson PG. The lymphoepithelial lesion of gastric low-grade B-cell lymphoma of mucosa-associated lymphoid tissue (MALT): an ultrastructural study. *Histopathology* 1992;21:415–421.
215. Rawal A, Finn WG, Schnitzer B, et al. Site-specific morphologic differences in extranodal marginal zone B-cell lymphomas. *Arch Pathol Lab Med* 2007;131: 1673–1678.
216. Wotherspoon AC, Doglioni C, Isaacson PG. Low-grade gastric B-cell lymphoma of mucosa-associated lymphoid tissue (MALT): a multifocal disease. *Histopathology* 1992;20:29–34.
217. Morel P, Quiquandon I, Janin A. Involvement of minor salivary glands in gastric lymphomas. *Lancet* 1994;344:139–140.
218. Hernandez JA, Sheehan WW. Lymphomas of the mucosa-associated lymphoid tissue. Signet ring cell lymphomas presenting in mucosal lymphoid organs. *Cancer* 1985;55:592–597.
219. Kurz-Levin MM, Flury R, Bernauer W. Diagnosis of MALT lymphoma by conjunctival biopsy: a case report. *Graefes Arch Clin Exp Ophthalmol* 1997;235: 606–609.
220. Cahill MT, Moriarty PA, Kennedy SM. Conjunctival 'MALToma' with systemic recurrence. *Arch Ophthalmol* 1998;116:97–99.
221. Ryan RJ, Sloan JM, Collins AB, et al. Extranodal marginal zone lymphoma of mucosa-associated lymphoid tissue with amyloid deposition: a clinicopathologic case series. *Am J Clin Pathol* 2012;137:51–64.
222. Isaacson PG. The MALT lymphoma concept updated. *Ann Oncol* 1995;6:319–320.
223. Jenkins C, Rose GE, Bunce C, et al. Histological features of ocular adnexal lymphoma (REAL classification) and their association with patient morbidity and survival. *Br J Ophthalmol* 2000;84:907–913.
224. McKelvie PA, McNab A, Francis IC, et al. Ocular adnexal lymphoproliferative disease: a series of 73 cases. *Clin Exp Ophthalmol* 2001;29:387–393.
225. Rasmussen P, Sjo LD, Prause JU, et al. Mantle cell lymphoma in the orbital and adnexal region. *Br J Ophthalmol* 2009;93:1047–1051.
226. Stacy RC, Jakobiec FA, Schoenfield L, et al. Unifocal and multifocal reactive lymphoid hyperplasia vs follicular lymphoma of the ocular adnexa. *Am J Ophthalmol* 2010;150:412.e1–426 e1.
227. Isaacson PG. Lymphomas of mucosa-associated lymphoid tissue (MALT). *Histopathology* 1990;16:617–619.
228. Wieczorek R, Jakobiec FA, Sacks EH, et al. The immunoarchitecture of the normal human lacrimal gland. Relevancy for understanding pathologic conditions. *Ophthalmology* 1988;95:100–109.
229. Knowles DM II, Halper JP, Jakobiec FA. T-lymphocyte subpopulations in B-cell-derived non-Hodgkin's lymphomas and Hodgkin's disease. *Cancer* 1984;54: 644–651.
230. Ferry JA, Yang WI, Zukerberg LR, et al. CD5+ extranodal marginal zone B-cell (MALT) lymphoma. A low grade neoplasm with a propensity for bone marrow involvement and relapse. *Am J Clin Pathol* 1996;105:31–37.
231. Baseggio L, Traverse-Glehen A, Petinataud F, et al. CD5 expression identifies a subset of splenic marginal zone lymphomas with higher lymphocytosis: a clinico-pathological, cytogenetic and molecular study of 24 cases. *Haematologica* 2010;95:604–612.
232. Kojima M, Sato E, Oshimi K, et al. Characteristics of CD5-positive splenic marginal zone lymphoma with leukemic manifestation; clinical, flow cytometry, and histopathological findings of 11 cases. *J Clin Exp Hematop* 2010;50:107–112.
233. Tasaki K, Shichishima A, Furuta M, et al. CD5-positive mucosa-associated lymphoid tissue (MALT) lymphoma of ocular adnexal origin: usefulness of fluorescence in situ hybridization for distinction between mantle cell lymphoma and MALT lymphoma. *Pathol Int* 2007;57:101–107.
234. Ballesteros E, Osborne BM, Matsushima AY. CD5+ low-grade marginal zone B-cell lymphomas with localized presentation. *Am J Surg Pathol* 1998;22:201–207.
235. Heuring AH, Franke FE, Hutz WW. Conjunctival CD5+ MALT lymphoma. *Br J Ophthalmol* 2001;85:498–499.
236. Wenzel C, Dieckmann K, Fiebiger W, et al. CD5 expression in a lymphoma of the mucosa-associated lymphoid tissue (MALT)-type as a marker for early dissemination and aggressive clinical behaviour. *Leuk Lymphoma* 2001;42:823–829.
237. Pan L, Diss TC, Cunningham D, et al. The bcl-2 gene in primary B cell lymphoma of mucosa-associated lymphoid tissue (MALT). *Am J Pathol* 1989;135:7–11.
238. Wotherspoon AC, Pan LX, Diss TC, et al. A genotypic study of low grade B-cell lymphomas, including lymphomas of mucosa associated lymphoid tissue (MALT). *J Pathol* 1990;162:135–140.
239. Raghoebier S, Kramer MH, van Krieken JH, et al. Essential differences in oncogene involvement between primary nodal and extranodal large cell lymphoma. *Blood* 1991;78:2680–2685.
240. Schiby G, Polak-Charcon S, Mardoukh C, et al. Orbital marginal zone lymphomas: an immunohistochemical, polymerase chain reaction, and fluorescence in situ hybridization study. *Hum Pathol* 2007;38:435–442.
241. Tanimoto K, Sekiguchi N, Yokota Y, et al. Fluorescence in situ hybridization (FISH) analysis of primary ocular adnexal MALT lymphoma. *BMC Cancer* 2006;6:249.
242. Wotherspoon AC, Finn TM, Isaacson PG. Trisomy 3 in low-grade B-cell lymphomas of mucosa-associated lymphoid tissue. *Blood* 1995;85:2000–2004.
243. Streubel B, Simonitsch-Klupp I, Mullauer L, et al. Variable frequencies of MALT lymphoma-associated genetic aberrations in MALT lymphomas of different sites. *Leukemia* 2004;18:1722–1726.
244. Streubel B, Lamprecht A, Dierlamm J, et al. T(14;18)(q32;q21) involving IGH and MALT1 is a frequent chromosomal aberration in MALT lymphoma. *Blood* 2003;101:2335–2339.
245. Cook JR, Sherer M, Craig FE, et al. T(14;18)(q32;q21) involving MALT1 and IGH genes in an extranodal diffuse large B-cell lymphoma. *Hum Pathol* 2003;34: 1212–1215.
246. Ye H, Liu H, Attygalle A, et al. Variable frequencies of t(11;18)(q21;q21) in MALT lymphomas of different sites: significant association with CagA strains of *H. pylori* in gastric MALT lymphoma. *Blood* 2003;102:1012–1018.
247. Streubel B, Ye H, Du MQ, et al. Translocation t(11;18)(q21;q21) is not predictive of response to chemotherapy with 2CdA in patients with gastric MALT lymphoma. *Oncology* 2004;66:476–480.
248. Adachi A, Tamaru J, Kaneko K, et al. No evidence of a correlation between BCL10 expression and API2-MALT1 gene rearrangement in ocular adnexal MALT lymphoma. *Pathol Int* 2004;54:16–25.
249. Streubel B, Vinatzer U, Lamprecht A, et al. T(3;14)(p14.1;q32) involving IGH and FOXP1 is a novel recurrent chromosomal aberration in MALT lymphoma. *Leukemia* 2005;19:652–658.
250. Goatly A, Bacon CM, Nakamura S, et al. FOXP1 abnormalities in lymphoma: translocation breakpoint mapping reveals insights into deregulated transcriptional control. *Mod Pathol* 2008;21:902–911.
251. Ye H, Gong L, Liu H, et al. MALT lymphoma with t(14;18)(q32;q21)/IGH-MALT1 is characterized by strong cytoplasmic MALT1 and BCL10 expression. *J Pathol* 2005;205:293–301.
252. Ye H, Dogan A, Karran L, et al. BCL10 expression in normal and neoplastic lymphoid tissue. Nuclear localization in MALT lymphoma. *Am J Pathol* 2000;157:1147–1154.
253. Sagaert X, Laurent M, Baens M, et al. MALT1 and BCL10 aberrations in MALT lymphomas and their effect on the expression of BCL10 in the tumour cells. *Mod Pathol* 2006;19:225–232.
254. Baldini L, Blini M, Guffanti A, et al. Treatment and prognosis in a series of primary extranodal lymphomas of the ocular adnexa. *Ann Oncol* 1998;9:779–781.
255. Cesarman E, Inghirami G, Chadburn A, et al. High levels of p53 protein expression do not correlate with p53 gene mutations in anaplastic large cell lymphoma. *Am J Pathol* 1993;143:845–856.
256. Chanudet E, Ye H, Ferry J, et al. A20 deletion is associated with copy number gain at the TNFA/B/C locus and occurs preferentially in translocation-negative MALT lymphoma of the ocular adnexa and salivary glands. *J Pathol* 2009;217:420–430.
257. Chanudet E, Huang Y, Ichimura K, et al. A20 is targeted by promoter methylation, deletion and inactivating mutation in MALT lymphoma. *Leukemia* 2010;24: 483–487.
258. Bi Y, Zeng N, Chanudet E, et al. A20 inactivation in ocular adnexal MALT lymphoma. *Haematologica* 2012;97:926–930.
259. Bertoni F, Cotter FE, Zucca E. Molecular genetics of extranodal marginal zone (MALT-type) B-cell lymphoma. *Leuk Lymphoma* 1999;35:57–68.
260. Zhu D, Lossos C, Chapman-Fredricks JR, et al. Biased use of the IGHV4 family and evidence for antigen selection in *Chlamydophila psittaci*-negative ocular adnexal extranodal marginal zone lymphomas. *PLoS One* 2011;6:e29114.
261. Servitje O, Gallardo F, Estrach T, et al. Primary cutaneous marginal zone B-cell lymphoma: a clinical, histopathological, immunophenotypic and molecular genetic study of 22 cases. *Br J Dermatol* 2002;147:1147–1158.
262. Lossos IS, Okada CY, Tibshirani R, et al. Molecular analysis of immunoglobulin genes in diffuse large B-cell lymphomas. *Blood* 2000;95:1797–1803.
263. Bahler DW, Szankasi P, Kulkarni S, et al. Use of similar immunoglobulin VH gene segments by MALT lymphomas of the ocular adnexa. *Mod Pathol* 2009;22: 833–838.
264. Coupland SE, Foss HD, Anagnostopoulos I, et al. Immunoglobulin VH gene expression among extranodal marginal zone B-cell lymphomas of the ocular adnexa. *Invest Ophthalmol Vis Sci* 1999;40:555–562.
265. Hara Y, Nakamura N, Kuze T, et al. Immunoglobulin heavy chain gene analysis of ocular adnexal extranodal marginal zone B-cell lymphoma. *Invest Ophthalmol Vis Sci* 2001;42:2450–2457.
266. Mannami T, Yoshino T, Oshima K, et al. Clinical, histopathological, and immunogenetic analysis of ocular adnexal lymphoproliferative disorders: characterization of malt lymphoma and reactive lymphoid hyperplasia. *Mod Pathol* 2001;14:641–649.
267. Adam P, Haralambieva E, Hartmann M, et al. Rare occurrence of IgVH gene translocations and restricted IgVH gene repertoire in ocular MALT-type lymphoma. *Haematologica* 2008;93:319–320.
268. Goudie RB, Macfarlane PS, Lindsay MK. Homing of lymphocytes to non-lymphoid tissues. *Lancet* 1974;1:292–293.
269. Lasota J, Miettinen MM. Coexistence of different B-cell clones in consecutive lesions of low-grade MALT lymphoma of the salivary gland in Sjogren's disease. *Mod Pathol* 1997;10:872–878.
270. Konoplev S, Lin P, Qiu X, et al. Clonal relationship of extranodal marginal zone lymphomas of mucosa-associated lymphoid tissue involving different sites. *Am J Clin Pathol* 2010;134:112–118.
271. Fishleder A, Tubbs R, Hesse B, et al. Uniform detection of immunoglobulin-gene rearrangement in benign lymphoepithelial lesions. *N Engl J Med* 1987;316: 1118–1121.
272. Wood GS, Ngan BY, Tung R, et al. Clonal rearrangements of immunoglobulin genes and progression to B cell lymphoma in cutaneous lymphoid hyperplasia. *Am J Pathol* 1989;135:13–19.
273. Spencer J, Diss TC, Isaacson PG. Primary B cell gastric lymphoma. A genotypic analysis. *Am J Pathol* 1989;135:557–564.
274. Geyer JT, Ferry JA, Harris NL, et al. Florid reactive lymphoid hyperplasia of the lower female genital tract (lymphoma-like lesion): a benign condition that frequently harbors clonal immunoglobulin heavy chain gene rearrangements. *Am J Surg Pathol* 2010;34:161–168.
275. Weiss LM, Wood GS, Trela M, et al. Clonal T-cell populations in lymphomatoid papulosis. Evidence of a lymphoproliferative origin for a clinically benign disease. *N Engl J Med* 1986;315:475–479.
276. Kadin ME, Vonderheid EC, Sako D, et al. Clonal composition of T cells in lymphomatoid papulosis. *Am J Pathol* 1987;126:13–17.
277. Hanson CA, Frizzera G, Patton DF, et al. Clonal rearrangement for immunoglobulin and T-cell receptor genes in systemic Castleman's disease. Association with Epstein-Barr virus. *Am J Pathol* 1988;131:84–91.
278. Spencer J, Finn T, Isaacson PG. Gut associated lymphoid tissue: a morphological and immunocytochemical study of the human appendix. *Gut* 1985;26:672–679.

279. Wotherspoon AC, Hardman-Lea S, Isaacson PG. Mucosa-associated lymphoid tissue (MALT) in the human conjunctiva. *J Pathol* 1994;174:33–37.
280. Emery JL, Dinsdale F. The postnatal development of lymphoreticular aggregates and lymph nodes in infants' lungs. *J Clin Pathol* 1973;26:539–545.
281. Pabst R, Gehrke I. Is the bronchus-associated lymphoid tissue (BALT) an integral structure of the lung in normal mammals, including humans? *Am J Respir Cell Mol Biol* 1990;3:131–135.
282. Gould SJ, Isaacson PG. Bronchus-associated lymphoid tissue (BALT) in human fetal and infant lung. *J Pathol* 1993;169:229–234.
283. Wotherspoon AC, Ortiz-Hidalgo C, Falzon MR, et al. *Helicobacter pylori*-associated gastritis and primary B-cell gastric lymphoma. *Lancet* 1991;338:1175–1176.
284. Hyjek E, Smith WJ, Isaacson PG. Primary B-cell lymphoma of salivary glands and its relationship to myoepithelial sialadenitis. *Hum Pathol* 1988;19:766–776.
285. Hyjek E, Isaacson PG. Primary B cell lymphoma of the thyroid and its relationship to Hashimoto's thyroiditis. *Hum Pathol* 1988;19:1315–1326.
286. McMaster PR, Aronson SB, Bedford MJ. Mechanisms of the host response in the eye. IV. The anterior eye in germ-free animals. *Arch Ophthalmol* 1967;77:392–399.
287. Franklin RM, Remus LE. Conjunctival-associated lymphoid tissue: evidence for a role in the secretory immune system. *Invest Ophthalmol Vis Sci* 1984;25:181–187.
288. Fix AS, Arp LH. Conjunctiva-associated lymphoid tissue (CALT) in normal and *Bordetella avium*-infected turkeys. *Vet Pathol* 1989;26:222–230.
289. Khatami M, Donnelly JJ, Haldar JP, et al. Massive follicular lymphoid hyperplasia in experimental allergic conjunctivitis. Local antibody production. *Arch Ophthalmol* 1989;107:433–438.
290. Latkovic S. Ultrastructure of M cells in the conjunctival epithelium of the guinea pig. *Curr Eye Res* 1989;8:751–755.
291. Jakobiec FA, Lefkowitch J, Knowles DM II. B- and T-lymphocytes in ocular disease. *Ophthalmology* 1984;91:635–654.
292. Duke-Elder S. Disease of the outer eye, part I. In: Duke-Elder S, ed. *System of ophtalmology*. London: Henry Kempton, 1965:102–103.
293. Decaudin D, de Cremoux P, Vincent-Salomon A, et al. Ocular adnexal lymphoma: a review of clinicopathologic features and treatment options. *Blood* 2006;108:1451–1460.
294. Meunier J, Lumbroso-Le Rouic L, Vincent-Salomon A, et al. Ophthalmologic and intraocular non-Hodgkin's lymphoma: a large single centre study of initial characteristics, natural history, and prognostic factors. *Hematol Oncol* 2004;22:143–158.
295. Coupland SE, Hellmich M, Auw-Haedrich C, et al. Plasmacellular differentiation in extranodal marginal zone B cell lymphomas of the ocular adnexa: an analysis of the neoplastic plasma cell phenotype and its prognostic significance in 136 cases. *Br J Ophthalmol* 2005;89:352–359.
296. Cho EY, Han JJ, Ree HJ, et al. Clinicopathologic analysis of ocular adnexal lymphomas: extranodal marginal zone B-cell lymphoma constitutes the vast majority of ocular lymphomas among Koreans and affects younger patients. *Am J Hematol* 2003;73:87–96.
297. Tanimoto K, Kaneko A, Suzuki S, et al. Primary ocular adnexal MALT lymphoma: a long-term follow-up study of 114 patients. *Jpn J Clin Oncol* 2007;37:337–344.
298. Zucca E, Conconi A, Pedrinis E, et al. Nongastric marginal zone B-cell lymphoma of mucosa-associated lymphoid tissue. *Blood* 2003;101:2489–2495.
299. Ferry JA, Hasserjian R, Lucarelli MJ, et al. Ocular adnexal lymphoma: outcome in 254 patients with evaluation of patterns of failure and prognostic factors. 2013, manuscript in preparation.
300. Bennett CL, Putterman A, Bitran JD, et al. Staging and therapy of orbital lymphomas. *Cancer* 1986;57:1204–1208.
301. Raderer M, Streubel B, Woehrer S, et al. High relapse rate in patients with MALT lymphoma warrants lifelong follow-up. *Clin Cancer Res* 2005;11:3349–3352.
302. Thieblemont C, Bastion Y, Berger F, et al. Mucosa-associated lymphoid tissue gastrointestinal and nongastrointestinal lymphoma behavior: analysis of 108 patients. *J Clin Oncol* 1997;15:1624–1630.
303. Berger F, Felman P, Sonet A, et al. Nonfollicular small B-cell lymphomas: a heterogeneous group of patients with distinct clinical features and outcome. *Blood* 1994;83:2829–2835.
304. Cogliatti SB, Schmid U, Schumacher U, et al. Primary B-cell gastric lymphoma: a clinicopathological study of 145 patients. *Gastroenterology* 1991;101:1159–1170.
305. Montalban C, Castrillo JM, Abraira V, et al. Gastric B-cell mucosa-associated lymphoid tissue (MALT) lymphoma. Clinicopathological study and evaluation of the prognostic factors in 143 patients. *Ann Oncol* 1995;6:355–362.
306. Radaszkiewicz T, Dragosics B, Bauer P. Gastrointestinal malignant lymphomas of the mucosa-associated lymphoid tissue: factors relevant to prognosis. *Gastroenterology* 1992;102:1628–1638.
307. Jenkins C, Rose GE, Bunce C, et al. Clinical features associated with survival of patients with lymphoma of the ocular adnexa. *Eye (Lond)* 2003;17:809–820.
308. Raderer M, Vorbeck F, Formanek M, et al. Importance of extensive staging in patients with mucosa-associated lymphoid tissue (MALT)-type lymphoma. *Br J Cancer* 2000;83:454–457.
309. Raderer M, Wohrer S, Streubel B, et al. Assessment of disease dissemination in gastric compared with extragastric mucosa-associated lymphoid tissue lymphoma using extensive staging: a single-center experience. *J Clin Oncol* 2006;24:3136–3141.
310. Zinzani PL, Magagnoli M, Galieni P, et al. Nongastrointestinal low-grade mucosa-associated lymphoid tissue lymphoma: analysis of 75 patients. *J Clin Oncol* 1999;17:1254.
311. Thieblemont C, Berger F, Dumontet C, et al. Mucosa-associated lymphoid tissue lymphoma is a disseminated disease in one third of 158 patients analyzed. *Blood* 2000;95:802–806.
312. Coupland SE, Hellmich M, Auw-Haedrich C, et al. Prognostic value of cell-cycle markers in ocular adnexal lymphoma: an assessment of 230 cases. *Graefes Arch Clin Exp Ophthalmol* 2004;242:130–145.
313. Smitt MC, Donaldson SS. Radiotherapy is successful treatment for orbital lymphoma. *Int J Radiat Oncol Biol Phys* 1993;26:59–66.
314. Tanimoto K, Kaneko A, Suzuki S, et al. Long-term follow-up results of no initial therapy for ocular adnexal MALT lymphoma. *Ann Oncol* 2006;17:135–140.
315. Jereb B, Lee H, Jakobiec FA, et al. Radiation therapy of conjunctival and orbital lymphoid tumors. *Int J Radiat Oncol Biol Phys* 1984;10:1013–1019.
316. McKelvie PA. Ocular adnexal lymphomas: a review. *Adv Anat Pathol* 2010;17:251–261.
317. Bayraktar S, Bayraktar UD, Stefanovic A, et al. Primary ocular adnexal mucosa-associated lymphoid tissue lymphoma (MALT): single institution experience in a large cohort of patients. *Br J Haematol* 2011;152:72–80.
318. Durkin SR, Roos D, Higgs B, et al. Ophthalmic and adnexal complications of radiotherapy. *Acta Ophthalmol Scand* 2007;85:240–250.
319. Bischof M, Karagiozidis M, Krempien R, et al. Radiotherapy for orbital lymphoma: outcome and late effects. *Strahlenther Onkol* 2007;183:17–22.
320. De Cicco L, Cella L, Liuzzi R, et al. Radiation therapy in primary orbital lymphoma: a single institution retrospective analysis. *Radiat Oncol* 2009;4:60.
321. Platanias LC, Putterman AM, Vijayakumar S, et al. Treatment and prognosis of orbital non-Hodgkin's lymphomas. *Am J Clin Oncol* 1992;15:79–83.
322. Ben Simon GJ, Cheung N, McKelvie P, et al. Oral chlorambucil for extranodal, marginal zone, B-cell lymphoma of mucosa-associated lymphoid tissue of the orbit. *Ophthalmology* 2006;113:1209–1213.
323. Charlotte F, Doghmi K, Cassoux N, et al. Ocular adnexal marginal zone B cell lymphoma: a clinical and pathologic study of 23 cases. *Virchows Arch* 2006;448:506–516.
324. Song EK, Kim SY, Kim TM, et al. Efficacy of chemotherapy as a first-line treatment in ocular adnexal extranodal marginal zone B-cell lymphoma. *Ann Oncol* 2008;19:242–246.
325. Rigacci L, Nassi L, Puccioni M, et al. Rituximab and chlorambucil as first-line treatment for low-grade ocular adnexal lymphomas. *Ann Hematol* 2007;86:565–568.
326. Lossos IS, Morgensztern D, Blaya M, et al. Rituximab for treatment of chemoimmunotherapy naive marginal zone lymphoma. *Leuk Lymphoma* 2007;48:1630–1632.
327. Benetatos L, Alymara V, Asproudis I, et al. Rituximab as first line treatment for MALT lymphoma of extraocular muscles. *Ann Hematol* 2006;85:625–626.
328. Conconi A, Martinelli G, Thieblemont C, et al. Clinical activity of rituximab in extranodal marginal zone B-cell lymphoma of MALT type. *Blood* 2003;102:2741–2745.
329. Heinz C, Merz H, Nieschalk M, et al. Rituximab for the treatment of extranodal marginal zone B-cell lymphoma of the lacrimal gland. *Br J Ophthalmol* 2007;91:1563–1564.
330. Nuckel H, Meller D, Steuhl KP, et al. Anti-CD20 monoclonal antibody therapy in relapsed MALT lymphoma of the conjunctiva. *Eur J Haematol* 2004;73:258–262.
331. Esmaeli B, Murray JL, Ahmadi MA, et al. Immunotherapy for low-grade non-hodgkin secondary lymphoma of the orbit. *Arch Ophthalmol* 2002;120:1225–1227.
332. Savino G, Battendieri R, Balia L, et al. Evaluation of intraorbital injection of rituximab for treatment of primary ocular adnexal lymphoma: a pilot study. *Cancer Sci* 2011;102:1565–1567.
333. Laurenti L, De Padua L, Battendieri R, et al. Intralesional administration of rituximab for treatment of CD20 positive orbital lymphoma: safety and efficacy evaluation. *Leuk Res* 2011;35:682–684.
334. Bilgir O, Bilgir F, Calan M, et al. Treatment of a patient with adnexal lymphoma with Rituximab. *Transfus Apher Sci* 2011;44:135–137.
335. Sullivan TJ, Grimes D, Bunce I. Monoclonal antibody treatment of orbital lymphoma. *Ophthal Plast Reconstr Surg* 2004;20:103–106.
336. Ferreri AJ, Ponzoni M, Martinelli G, et al. Rituximab in patients with mucosal-associated lymphoid tissue-type lymphoma of the ocular adnexa. *Haematologica* 2005;90:1578–1579.
337. Witzig TE, Inwards DJ, Habermann TM, et al. Treatment of benign orbital pseudolymphomas with the monoclonal anti-CD20 antibody rituximab. *Mayo Clin Proc* 2007;82:692–699.
338. Ferreri AJ, Ponzoni M, Guidoboni M, et al. Bacteria-eradicating therapy with doxycycline in ocular adnexal MALT lymphoma: a multicenter prospective trial. *J Natl Cancer Inst* 2006;98:1375–1382.
339. Abramson DH, Rollins I, Coleman M. Periocular mucosa-associated lymphoid/low grade lymphomas: treatment with antibiotics. *Am J Ophthalmol* 2005;140:729–730.
340. Govi S, Dognini GP, Licata G, et al. Six-month oral clarithromycin regimen is safe and active in extranodal marginal zone B-cell lymphomas: final results of a single-centre phase II trial. *Br J Haematol* 2010;150:226–229.
341. Foucar E, Rosai J, Dorfman R. Sinus histiocytosis with massive lymphadenopathy (Rosai-Dorfman disease): review of the entity. *Semin Diagn Pathol* 1990;7:19–73.
342. Rosai J, Dorfman RF. Sinus histiocytosis with massive lymphadenopathy. A newly recognized benign clinicopathological entity. *Arch Pathol* 1969;87:63–70.
343. Rosai J, Dorfman RF. Sinus histiocytosis with massive lymphadenopathy: a pseudolymphomatous benign disorder. Analysis of 34 cases. *Cancer* 1972;30:1174–1188.
344. Rezk AR, Sullivan JL, Woda BA. Nonneoplstic histiocytic proliferations of lymph node and bone marrow. In: Jaffe ES, Harris NL, Vardiman JW, et al., eds. *Hematopathology*. St. Louis: Elsevier Saunders, 2011:801–836.
345. Mohadjer Y, Holds JB, Rootman J, et al. The spectrum of orbital Rosai-Dorfman disease. *Ophthal Plast Reconstr Surg* 2006;22:163–168.
346. Zimmerman LE, Hidayat AA, Grantham RL, et al. Atypical cases of sinus histiocytosis (Rosai-Dorfman disease) with ophthalmological manifestations. *Trans Am Ophthalmol Soc* 1988;86:113–135.
347. Levinger S, Pe'er J, Aker M, et al. Rosai-Dorfman disease involving four eyelids. *Am J Ophthalmol* 1993;116:382–384.
348. Sacchi S, Artusi T, Torelli U, et al. Sinus histiocytosis with massive lymphadenopathy. *Leuk Lymphoma* 1992;7:189–194.
349. Wenig BM, Abbondanzo SL, Childers EL, et al. Extranodal sinus histiocytosis with massive lymphadenopathy (Rosai-Dorfman disease) of the head and neck. *Hum Pathol* 1993;24:483–492.
350. Weiss L. *Lymph nodes*. New York: Cambridge University Press, 2008.
351. Bonetti F, Chilosi M, Menestrina F, et al. Immunohistological analysis of Rosai-Dorfman histiocytosis. A disease of S-100 + CD1-histiocytes. *Virchows Arch A Pathol Anat Histopathol* 1987;411:129–135.
352. Eisen RN, Buckley PJ, Rosai J. Immunophenotypic characterization of sinus histiocytosis with massive lymphadenopathy (Rosai-Dorfman disease). *Semin Diagn Pathol* 1990;7:74–82.
353. Paulli M, Rosso R, Kindl S, et al. Immunophenotypic characterization of the cell infiltrate in five cases of sinus histiocytosis with massive lymphadenopathy (Rosai-Dorfman disease). *Hum Pathol* 1992;23:647–654.
354. Kuo TT, Chen TC, Lee LY, et al. IgG4-positive plasma cells in cutaneous Rosai-Dorfman disease: an additional immunohistochemical feature and possible relationship to IgG4-related sclerosing disease. *J Cutan Pathol* 2009;36:1069–1073.

355. Roberts SS, Attanoos RL. IgG4+ Rosai-Dorfman disease of the lung. *Histopathology* 2010;56:662–664.
356. Chen TD, Lee LY. Rosai-Dorfman disease presenting in the parotid gland with features of IgG4-related sclerosing disease. *Arch Otolaryngol Head Neck Surg* 2011;137:705–708.
357. Richter JT, Strange RG Jr, Fisher SI, et al. Extranodal Rosai-Dorfman disease presenting as a cardiac mass in an adult: report of a unique case and lack of relationship to IgG4-related sclerosing lesions. *Hum Pathol* 2010;41:297–301.
358. Cline MJ. Histiocytes and histiocytosis. *Blood* 1994;84:2840–2853.
359. Lichtenstein L. Histiocytosis X; integration of eosinophilic granuloma of bone, Letterer-Siwe disease, and Schuller-Christian disease as related manifestations of a single nosologic entity. *AMA Arch Pathol* 1953;56:84–102.
360. McLelland J, Pritchard J, Chu AC. Current controversies. Histiocytosis-X. *Hematol Oncol Clin North Am* 1987;1:147–162.
361. Favara BE, Jaffe R. Pathology of Langerhans cell histiocytosis. *Hematol Oncol Clin North Am* 1987;1:75–97.
362. Favara BE, McCarthy RC, Mierau GW. Histiocytosis X. *Hum Pathol* 1983;14:663–676.
363. Raney RB Jr, D'Angio GJ. Langerhans' cell histiocytosis (histiocytosis X): experience at the Children's Hospital of Philadelphia, 1970–1984. *Med Pediatr Oncol* 1989;17:20–28.
364. Nezelof C, Frileux-Herbet F, Cronier-Sachot J. Disseminated histiocytosis X: analysis of prognostic factors based on a retrospective study of 50 cases. *Cancer* 1979;44:1824–1838.
365. Moore AT, Pritchard J, Taylor DS. Histiocytosis X: an ophthalmological review. *Br J Ophthalmol* 1985;69:7–14.
366. Mittelman D, Apple DJ, Goldberg MF. Ocular involvement in Letterer-Siwe disease. *Am J Ophthalmol* 1973;75:261–265.
367. Lahav M, Albert DM. Unusual ocular involvement in acute disseminated histiocytosis X. *Arch Ophthalmol* 1974;91:455–458.
368. MacCumber MW, Hoffman PN, Wand GS, et al. Ophthalmic involvement in aggressive histiocytosis X. *Ophthalmology* 1990;97:22–27.
369. Heath P. The ocular features of a case of acute reticuloendotheliosis (Letterer-Siwe type). *Trans Am Ophthalmol Soc* 1959;57:290–302.
370. Mozziconacci P, Offret G, Forest A, et al. [Histiocytosis-X with ocular lesions. Anatomical study]. *Ann Pediatr (Paris)* 1966;13:348–355.
371. Hidayat AA, Mafee MF, Laver NV, et al. Langerhans' cell histiocytosis and juvenile xanthogranuloma of the orbit. Clinicopathologic, CT, and MR imaging features. *Radiol Clin North Am* 1998;36:1229–1240, xii.
372. Erly WK, Carmody RF, Dryden RM. Orbital histiocytosis X. *AJNR Am J Neuroradiol* 1995;16:1258–1261.
373. LaBorwit SE, Karesh JW, Hirschbein MJ, et al. Multifocal Langerhans' cell histiocytosis involving the orbit. *J Pediatr Ophthalmol Strabismus* 1998;35:234–236.
374. Jaffe R. Langerhans cell histiocytosis and Langerhans cell sarcoma. In: Jaffe ES, ed. *Hematopathology*. St. Louis: Elsevier, 2011:811–826.
375. Malone M. The histiocytoses of childhood. *Histopathology* 1991;19:105–119.
376. Kramer TR, Noecker RJ, Miller JM, et al. Langerhans cell histiocytosis with orbital involvement. *Am J Ophthalmol* 1997;124:814–824.
377. Glover AT, Grove AS Jr. Eosinophilic granuloma of the orbit with spontaneous healing. *Ophthalmology* 1987;94:1008–1012.
378. Levy J, Monos T, Kapelushnik J, et al. Ophthalmic manifestations in Langerhans cell histiocytosis. *Isr Med Assoc J* 2004;6:553–555.
379. Kyle RA. Diagnosis and management of multiple myeloma and related disorders. *Prog Hematol* 1986;14:257–282.
380. Osserman EF, Merlini G, Butler VP Jr. Multiple myeloma and related plasma cell dyscrasias. *JAMA* 1987;258:2930–2937.
381. Knowling MA, Harwood AR, Bergsagel DE. Comparison of extramedullary plasmacytomas with solitary and multiple plasma cell tumors of bone. *J Clin Oncol* 1983;1:255–262.
382. Miller FR, Lavertu P, Wanamaker JR, et al. Plasmacytomas of the head and neck. *Otolaryngol Head Neck Surg* 1998;119:614–618.
383. Mewis-Levin L, Garcia CA, Olson JD. Plasma cell myeloma of the orbit. *Ann Ophthalmol* 1981;13:477–481.
384. Pan SW, Wan Hitam WH, Mohd Noor RA, et al. Recurrence of multiple myeloma with soft tissue plasmacytoma presenting as unilateral proptosis. *Orbit* 2011;30:105–107.
385. Chin KJ, Kempin S, Milman T, et al. Ocular manifestations of multiple myeloma: three cases and a review of the literature. *Optometry* 2011;82:224–230.
386. Adkins JW, Shields JA, Shields CL, et al. Plasmacytoma of the eye and orbit. *Int Ophthalmol* 1996;20:339–343.
387. Goshe JM, Schoenfield L, Emch T, et al. Myeloma-associated orbital amyloidosis. *Orbit* 2010;29:274–277.
388. Levine MR, Buckman G. Primary localized orbital amyloidosis. *Ann Ophthalmol* 1986;18:165–167.
389. Yakulis R, Dawson RR, Wang SE, et al. Fine needle aspiration diagnosis of orbital plasmacytoma with amyloidosis. A case report. *Acta Cytol* 1995;39:104–110.
390. de Smet MD, Rootman J. Orbital manifestations of plasmacytic lymphoproliferations. *Ophthalmology* 1987;94:995–1003.
391. Knapp AJ, Gartner S, Henkind P. Multiple myeloma and its ocular manifestations. *Surv Ophthalmol* 1987;31:343–351.
392. Knowles DM II, Halper JA, Trokel S, et al. Immunofluorescent and immunoperoxidase characteristics of IgDlambda myeloma involving the orbit. *Am J Ophthalmol* 1978;85:485–494.
393. Ryder C, Naclerio RM. Multiple myeloma presenting as proptosis. *Ann Otol Rhinol Laryngol* 1999;108:211–213.
394. Maeng H, Cheong JW, Lee ST, et al. Isolated extramedullary relapse of acute myelogenous leukemia as a uterine granulocytic sarcoma in an allogeneic hematopoietic stem cell transplantation recipient. *Yonsei Med J* 2004;45:330–333.
395. Pileri SA, Ascani S, Cox MC, et al. Myeloid sarcoma: clinico-pathologic, phenotypic and cytogenetic analysis of 92 adult patients. *Leukemia* 2007;21:340–350.
396. Neiman RS, Barcos M, Berard C, et al. Granulocytic sarcoma: a clinicopathologic study of 61 biopsied cases. *Cancer* 1981;48:1426–1437.
397. Meis JM, Butler JJ, Osborne BM, et al. Granulocytic sarcoma in nonleukemic patients. *Cancer* 1986;58:2697–2709.
398. Liu PI, Ishimaru T, McGregor DH, et al. Autopsy study of granulocytic sarcoma (chloroma) in patients with myelogenous leukemia, Hiroshima-Nagasaki 1949–1969. *Cancer* 1973;31:948–955.
399. Bonig H, Gobel U, Nurnberger W. Bilateral exophthalmus due to retro-orbital chloromas in a boy with t(8;21)- positive acute myeloblastic acute leukemia. *Pediatr Hematol Oncol* 2002;19:597–600.
400. Lee SG, Park TS, Cheong JW, et al. Preceding orbital granulocytic sarcoma in an adult patient with acute myelogenous leukemia with t(8;21): a case study and review of the literature. *Cancer Genet Cytogenet* 2008;185:51–54.
401. Rubnitz JE, Raimondi SC, Halbert AR, et al. Characteristics and outcome of t(8;21)-positive childhood acute myeloid leukemia: a single institution's experience. *Leukemia* 2002;16:2072–2077.
402. Tallman MS, Hakimian D, Shaw JM, et al. Granulocytic sarcoma is associated with the 8;21 translocation in acute myeloid leukemia. *J Clin Oncol* 1993;11:690–697.
403. Zimmerman LE, Font RL. Ophthalmologic manifestations of granulocytic sarcoma (myeloid sarcoma or chloroma). The Third Pan American Association of Ophthalmology and American Journal of Ophthalmology Lecture. *Am J Ophthalmol* 1975;80:975–990.
404. Jakobiec FA. Granulocytic sarcoma. *AJNR Am J Neuroradiol* 1991;12:263–264.
405. Cavdar AO, Ozger Topuz U, Erten J, et al. Effect of human serum thymic factor on immature T lymphocytes in acute leukemia and other hematologic malignancies. *Isr J Med Sci* 1978;14:1216–1220.
406. Banna M, Aur R, Akkad S. Orbital granulocytic sarcoma. *AJNR Am J Neuroradiol* 1991;12:255–258.
407. Campidelli C, Agostinelli C, Stitson R, et al. Myeloid sarcoma: extramedullary manifestation of myeloid disorders. *Am J Clin Pathol* 2009;132:426–437.
408. Davey FR, Olson S, Kurec AS, et al. The immunophenotyping of extramedullary myeloid cell tumors in paraffin-embedded tissue sections. *Am J Surg Pathol* 1988;12:699–707.
409. Imrie KR, Kovacs MJ, Selby D, et al. Isolated chloroma: the effect of early antileukemic therapy. *Ann Intern Med* 1995;123:351–353.
410. Hutchison RE, Kurec AS, Davey FR. Granulocytic sarcoma. *Clin Lab Med* 1990;10:889–901.
411. Cavdar AO, Arcasoy A, Babacan E, et al. Ocular granulocytic sarcoma (chloroma) with acute myelomonocytic leukemia in Turkish children. *Cancer* 1978;41:1606–1609.
412. Byrd JC, Weiss RB, Arthur DC, et al. Extramedullary leukemia adversely affects hematologic complete remission rate and overall survival in patients with t(8;21)(q22;q22): results from Cancer and Leukemia Group B 8461. *J Clin Oncol* 1997;15:466–475.
413. Felice MS, Zubizarreta PA, Alfaro EM, et al. Good outcome of children with acute myeloid leukemia and t(8;21)(q22;q22), even when associated with granulocytic sarcoma: a report from a single institution in Argentina. *Cancer* 2000;88:1939–1944.
414. Bisschop MM, Revesz T, Bierings M, et al. Extramedullary infiltrates at diagnosis have no prognostic significance in children with acute myeloid leukaemia. *Leukemia* 2001;15:46–49.

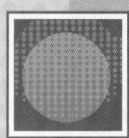

Chapter 33

Extranodal Lymphomas and Lymphoid Hyperplasias of Waldeyer Ring, Sinonasal Region, Salivary Gland, Thyroid Gland, Central Nervous System, and Other Less Common Sites

Jerome S. Burke

The incidence of extranodal lymphomas in specific anatomic sites is relatively consistent. In the United States, most extranodal lymphomas occur in the gastrointestinal tract, predominantly stomach and small intestine, and are followed in frequency by lymphomas of the skin and head and neck region, including Waldeyer ring (1) (see Chapter 28). Involvement of other locations is variable and frequently dependent on the environment. For example, among sites of extranodal lymphomas in Southwest China, Waldeyer ring ranks first followed closely by the gastrointestinal tract, sinonasal region, and skin (2). Despite the relative rarity of primary extranodal lymphomas in some anatomic areas, they form a fascinating group of neoplasms and are interesting to epidemiologists, pathologists, immunologists, and oncologists. This interest stems in some cases from the prevalence of extranodal lymphomas at one specific site in a specific geographic region; in other cases, the interest stems from the association of extranodal lymphomas with autoimmune disorders and immunodeficiency states; in still other cases, the interest revolves around the relationship to infectious agents, as, for example, *Chlamydia psittaci* (3). In all sites, extranodal lymphomas represent a challenge in the establishment of an accurate diagnosis, specifically in the distinction of extranodal lymphoma from undifferentiated carcinoma, malignant melanoma, myeloid sarcoma, or various forms of extranodal lymphoid hyperplasia and unusual reactive states, such as IgG4-related disease, Epstein-Barr virus (EBV)[+] mucocutaneous ulcer, and natural killer (NK)–cell enteropathy (4–6). The general principles of extranodal lymphomas and the differential diagnosis are discussed in Chapter 28. The characteristics of lymphomas of skin, gastrointestinal tract, lung, and ocular adnexa are described in Chapters 29 through 32. In this chapter, lymphomas of other extranodal sites are reviewed. Table 33.1 provides a summary of the predominant lymphomas and their immunophenotype that arise in these different extranodal sites.

WALDEYER RING

Waldeyer ring refers to the lymphoid tissues of the faucial tonsils, nasopharynx, and base of tongue. As described in the introduction to this chapter, Waldeyer ring comes third in the United States and first in Southwest China in the incidence of extranodal non-Hodgkin lymphomas (1,2). From 5% to 15% of all non-Hodgkin lymphomas originate in Waldeyer ring, and Waldeyer ring constitutes more than 50% of lymphomas of the head and neck region (7–9). The faucial tonsils are the most common sites of involvement in Waldeyer ring, followed by the nasopharynx with base of tongue barely involved in up to 7% of cases (7,10).

A tentative link between Waldeyer ring lymphomas and those of the gastrointestinal tract exists either at diagnosis or at relapse, despite the lack of direct lymphatic communication between these two sites (7,11). There is greater than expected incidence of gastrointestinal involvement in patients who have lymphomas of Waldeyer ring, and, conversely, there is increased risk of involvement of Waldeyer ring in patients who have gastrointestinal lymphomas (7–9). The association between lymphomas of Waldeyer ring and the gastrointestinal tract is considered a result of the homing tendency of common mucosa-associated lymphoid tissue (MALT) (12). This homing pattern is offered as an explanation for the tendency of some lymphomas that originate in extranodal sites to relapse in other extranodal sites, such as Waldeyer ring and the gastrointestinal tract (12); however, the clonal relationship between concomitant lymphomas in both sites is inconsistent with cases either clonally linked or unrelated and independent (13,14). Paradoxically, the incidence of extranodal marginal zone lymphomas of MALT type in Waldeyer ring is low (1.3% to 3.6%) (15–17), but many of the more prevalent large B-cell lymphomas of Waldeyer ring may originate as MALT type (11).

Patients who have lymphomas that arise in Waldeyer ring generally are in their sixth and seventh decades of life, and they frequently present with symptoms of local swelling, pain and/or dysphagia; constitutional symptoms are uncommon (7–9). A fleshy, tan tumor mass usually is discovered on clinical examination (Fig. 33.1).

All varieties of non-Hodgkin lymphomas are seen in Waldeyer ring, but from 66% to 85% of the lymphomas are diffuse and of large B-cell type (8–10,15). Most examples of diffuse large B-cell lymphoma (DLBCL) in this region are composed of centroblasts with <10% of cases dominated by immunoblasts (18) (Fig. 33.2). Employing immunohistochemistry and the Hans algorithm (19), more than 60% of DLBCL cases in Waldeyer ring exhibit a germinal center immunophenotype (18,20). By *in situ* hybridization for EBV-encoded RNA (EBER), up to 6% of Waldeyer DLBCL cases are positive (18,21).

The main differential diagnosis of DLBCL of Waldeyer ring concerns poorly differentiated squamous carcinoma of the nonkeratinizing or lymphoepithelial type. Histologically, the distinction of carcinoma from large cell lymphoma relies on the observation of cellular cohesion or a syncytial growth pattern in carcinoma; however, the nonkeratinizing type of squamous carcinoma occasionally occurs in diffuse sheets and is accompanied by inflammation and fibrosis. This results in difficulty in the distinction of carcinoma from lymphoma. Immunohistochemical studies that use antibodies directed against cytokeratin and pan-B-cell and pan-T-cell antigens almost always resolve this diagnostic problem (see Chapter 27). Florid immunoblastic hyperplasia in the tonsils, such as found in infectious mononucleosis, also may simulate DLBCL. Although infectious mononucleosis often leads to architectural distortion, germinal centers usually persist and the proliferating lymphocytes are histologically heterogeneous (Fig. 33.3). In this setting, however, immunoblastic proliferation can be profound with the presence of Reed-Sternberg–like cells and areas of necrosis (22). Despite areas of relatively monomorphous-appearing

Table 33.1	PREDOMINANT HISTOLOGIC TYPE AND IMMUNOPHENOTYPE OF VARIOUS EXTRANODAL LYMPHOMAS	
Site	Predominant Lymphoma	Immunophenotype
Waldeyer ring	Large cell	B
Sinonasal region	Large cell/polymorphous	NK/T
Salivary gland	Marginal zone (MALT) (LESA-associated)	B
	Follicular (non-LESA)	B
Thyroid gland	Large cell	B
Central nervous system	Large cell	B
Testis	Large cell	B
Ovary	Large cell /Burkitt	B
Uterus and Cervix	Large cell	B
Bone	Large cell (multilobated)	B
Breast	Large cell/Burkitt	B
Miscellaneous	Large cell/marginal zone (MALT)	B

B, B cell; NK, natural killer cell; T, T cell; MALT, mucosa-associated lymphoid tissue LESA, lymphoepithelial sialadnitis.

immunoblasts, the recognition of an overall orderly range of lymphocytic transformation should aid in the distinction of florid hyperplasia from lymphoma. Immunophenotypic studies also assist in diagnosis as the B immunoblasts in mononucleosis are polyclonal and, whereas those simulating Reed-Sternberg cells frequently express CD30, the reactive immunoblasts are negative for CD15 and positive for B-cell transcription factors, Oct2 and BOB.1 (22).

In some examples of DLBCL involving Waldeyer ring, follicular areas may be identified that often are due to residual germinal centers with CD21⁺ follicular dendritic cell meshworks consistent with follicular invasion or colonization (18,23). This observation suggests that such cases of DLBCL may have transformed from extranodal marginal zone lymphoma of MALT type (23,24). As noted earlier, classic extranodal marginal zone lymphoma of MALT type is very uncommon in Waldeyer ring (15–17). Other examples of DLBCL with a partial follicular architectural pattern suggest genuine focal follicular lymphoma due to sharp demarcation of the follicles (18) (Fig. 33.4). Waldeyer ring is a common site for pediatric follicular lymphoma, which mainly is grade 3 type, dominated by centroblasts or intermediate-sized blastoid cells (25,26). In contrast with most pediatric follicular lymphomas involving lymph nodes, those in tonsil frequently express BCL-2 protein and are positive for MUM1 (26).

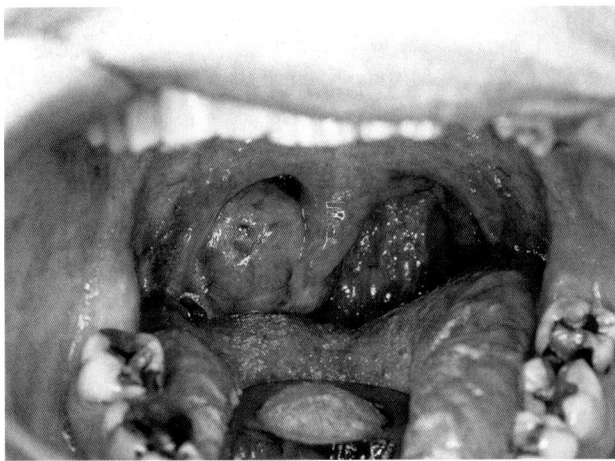

FIGURE 33.1. Malignant lymphoma of the tonsil results in a fleshlike, tan tumor mass that often is associated with pain and the sensation of a foreign body in the throat.

Mantle cell lymphoma is another lymphoma that may be encountered in Waldeyer ring, as a primary malignant lymphoma or as a manifestation of disseminated disease (15,25) (Fig 33.5). Waldeyer ring is involved in 20% of patients who have mantle cell lymphoma at presentation, although, like the gastrointestinal tract, the incidence may be greater by obtaining multiple blind biopsies of the seemingly clinically benign foci in the nasopharynx (25,27). In any primary lymphoma of Waldeyer ring that is composed of small lymphocytes, mantle cell lymphoma requires to be excluded by appropriate immunophenotypic studies mainly by determining whether there is aberrant coexpression of CD5 and nuclear reactivity for cyclin D1.

Hodgkin lymphoma that manifests in Waldeyer ring is uncommon and, parallel to lymph nodes, many such cases likely represent examples of T-cell/histiocyte-rich large B-cell lymphoma or various forms of peripheral T-cell lymphoma (PTCL) including cases with a high content of epithelioid histiocytes (Lennert lymphoma) (28). When rare cases of Hodgkin lymphoma primarily affect Waldeyer ring, they mainly are either nodular sclerosis or lymphocyte-rich classical type (Fig. 33.6) and frequently express EBV (29,30) (see Chapter 15).

In the Far East, where T-cell lymphomas are more common, from 70% to 100% of lymphomas of Waldeyer ring are found to be of B-cell origin, mainly DLBCL (21,31,32). In one study from Japan, all 25 cases of non-Hodgkin lymphoma of Waldeyer ring from an adult T-cell leukemia/lymphoma (ATLL) nonendemic area were B-cell malignancies and, with one exception, were DLBCL (31). Of 37 cases from an ATLL endemic area, 20 (54%) were also B-cell lymphomas (75% large cell) with the remaining 17 cases exhibiting a T-cell phenotype. From 6% to 19% of lymphomas of Waldeyer ring are of T-cell lineage, including those of nasal NK-/T-cell type (9). In a report from China, 91 of 785 patients (11.6%) with lymphomas of Waldeyer ring were regarded as nasal NK-/T-cell lymphoma (NKTCL) (32). In Waldeyer ring, most cases of this form of lymphoma engage the nasopharynx or upper part of the ring and occur predominantly in young males. Such patients have a low-risk International Prognostic Index (IPI) and, with combined radiation and chemotherapy, the 5-year overall survival is 65% (32).

In general, for patients who have malignant lymphomas that manifest in Waldeyer ring, the most important prognostic factors are the IPI score, clinical stage, and tumor bulk (10,17,18,33). Patients with stage I or IIE DLBCL of Waldeyer ring, who generally are treated by combined modality therapy, with or without rituximab, exhibit a good prognosis with a reported 5-year survival rate ranging from 77% to 96% (7,18,20,33,34). A germinal center immunophenotype is associated with a superior overall survival (18). Compared to patients with lymph node–based DLBCL, those with Waldeyer ring DLBCL more often present with early-stage disease; absence of "B" symptoms, bulky disease, and bone marrow involvement; lower IPI scores; and a superior survival rate (18,20,33,34).

SINONASAL REGION

Non-Hodgkin lymphomas of the sinonasal region form an extraordinary group of extranodal lymphomas because they are more prevalent in specific geographic regions, mainly the Far East and Latin America, where they predominately are of NK-/T-cell immunophenotype associated with EBV (35). As corroboration of their uniqueness, sinonasal malignant lymphomas constitute a separate category, referred to as *extranodal NKTCLs, nasal type*, in the World Health Organization (WHO) classification of malignant lymphomas (36).

Malignant lymphomas of the sinonasal region, including those in the hard palate and specifically NKTCL, are uncommon neoplasms in the United States and Europe and account for <1.5% of non-Hodgkin lymphomas, whereas they are much

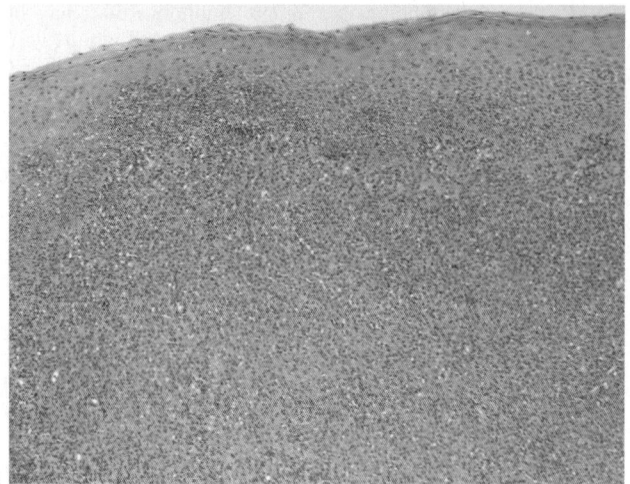

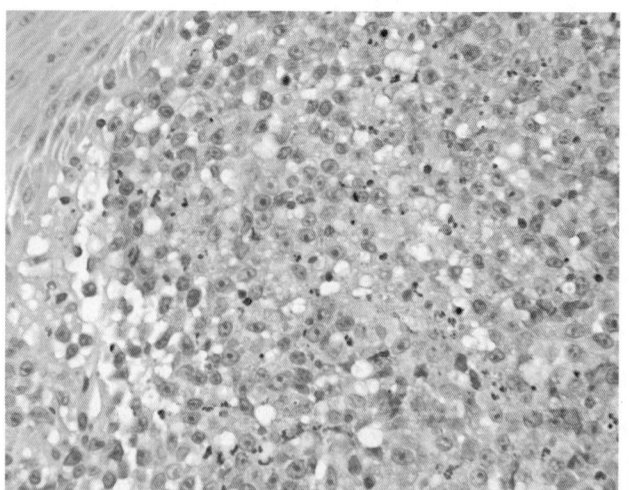

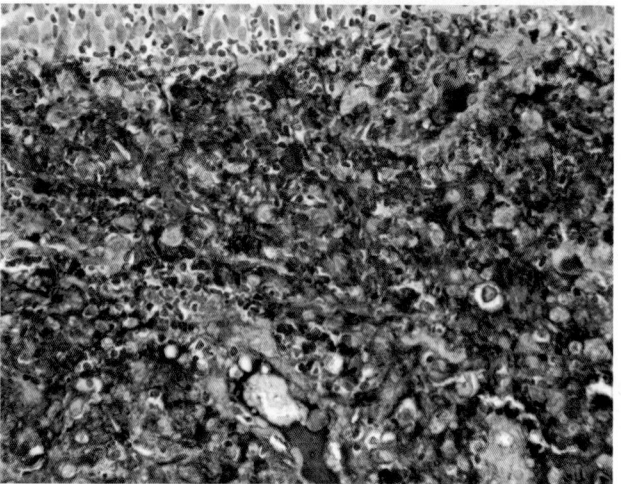

FIGURE 33.2. **A:** DLBCL is found adjacent to tonsillar squamous epithelium. At this magnification, lymphoma may be difficult to distinguish from nonkeratinizing squamous carcinoma (hematoxylin and eosin stain, original magnification: 60× magnification). **B:** In this case, the large cells conform to immunoblasts with conspicuous central nucleoli (hematoxylin and eosin stain, original magnification: 300× magnification). **C:** As well as expressing B-cell antigens with a non–germinal center immunophenotype (*not shown*), the immunoblasts are monoclonal with lambda light chain restriction (immunoperoxidase stain, original magnification: 300× magnification).

more widespread in the Far East, particularly China, where such neoplasms comprise up to 10.9% of all non-Hodgkin lymphomas (2,37,38). They also are more frequent in Latin America, for example, in Chile, Peru, Guatemala, and Mexico, where they primarily affect individuals of Native American descent (39–43). Of interest, in the United States extranodal

NKTCL mainly affects those of Asian ethnicity with an Asian-to-Caucasian incidence rate ratio of 2.91 (44). The predisposition for sinonasal lymphomas among Asians and Latin Americans of Native American origin indicates that shared host susceptibility is a probable factor in the pathogenesis of these lymphomas (39). Environmental influences, such as exposure to

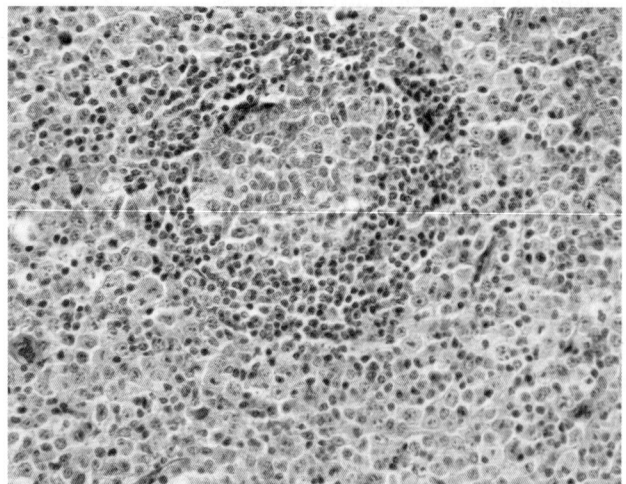

FIGURE 33.3. Florid lymphoid hyperplasia of the tonsil in infectious mononucleosis. Surrounding a germinal center, a polymorphous proliferation of lymphocytes dominated by immunoblasts is present. Unlike malignant lymphoma, the lymphocytes exhibit a relatively orderly range of transformation (hematoxylin and eosin stain, original magnification: 300× magnification).

FIGURE 33.4. In some cases of DLBCL originating in Waldeyer ring, a partial follicular pattern may be present. Unlike possible marginal zone lymphoma with follicular colonization, in this example the follicles are well demarcated to tally with focal follicular lymphoma; the follicles constituted no more than 5% of the lymphoma and were of grade 3 type (hematoxylin and eosin stain, original magnification: 60× magnification).

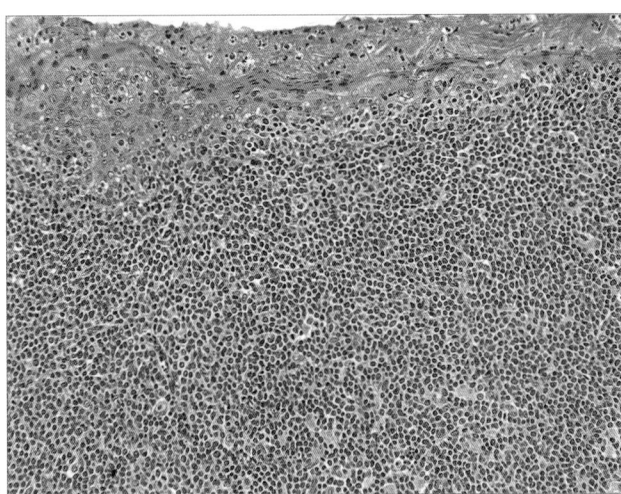
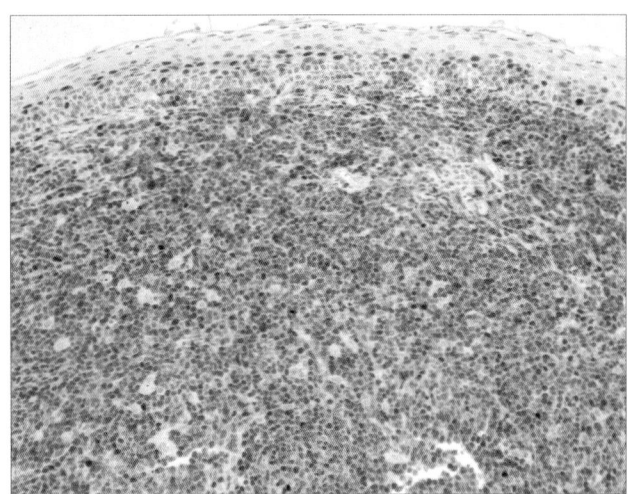

A

B

FIGURE 33.5. A: Mantle cell lymphoma frequently involves Waldeyer ring at presentation and is required to be excluded in any small lymphocytic infiltrate in this site (hematoxylin and eosin stain, original magnification: 150× magnification). **B:** The demonstration of cyclin D1 reactivity validates the diagnosis of mantle cell lymphoma (immunoperoxidase stain, original magnification: 150× magnification).

pesticides and chemical solvents, also could contribute to the causation of NKTCL (45).

Sinonasal malignant lymphomas often are confusing because historically many cases were included in the clinical spectrum of the midline granuloma syndrome (46). This unusual clinical syndrome is characterized by slowly progressive ulceration and destruction of the nose and paranasal sinuses, with frequent erosion of the soft tissues, bone, and cartilage. In fact, virtually all cases with this form of presentation currently are regarded as NKTCL so that the term *midline granuloma syndrome* as well as the terms *idiopathic midline destructive disease, polymorphic reticulosis,* and *midline malignant reticulosis* are passé. The major clinical symptom associated with malignant lymphoma of the sinonasal region is nasal obstruction; however, depending on the extent of the disease, epistaxis, nasal discharge, repeated infections, ozena, facial swelling, and cranial nerve palsy may ensue (7,36,47). However, clinically advanced midline facial destruction is far less common today, likely a result of early disposition (47).

Pathologic assessment of a biopsy specimen from the sinonasal region frequently is problematic, particularly in the setting of severe inflammation. With extensive inflammatory changes, it always is speculative whether the biopsy specimen is truly representative or whether neoplastic cells have been obscured by the inflammation and the commonly accompanying necrosis. A diagnosis of lymphoma depends on the recognition of atypical lymphoid cells against the background of severe inflammation, necrosis, and cellular degeneration (Fig. 33.7). To identify the frequently obscure neoplastic lymphoid cells in this environment, the biopsy must be not only of sufficient size but also of adequate technical quality, and multiple biopsy specimens may be required to establish the diagnosis (47). In some cases, reactive T-cell infiltrates, such as observed in association with Herpes simplex virus, may mimic NKTCL (48), whereas in other cases, the NKTCL may be composed of small, subtle lymphocytes to mimic an inflammatory process (49).

Nasal NKTCL frequently exhibits a wide morphologic spectrum with a predominant mixed or polymorphous cellular composition including atypical large lymphocytes (Fig. 33.8) and occasional epithelioid histiocytes, as well as monomorphous cell infiltrates usually dominated by large cells, but also cases with a small or medium-sized cellularity (35,41,50–52).

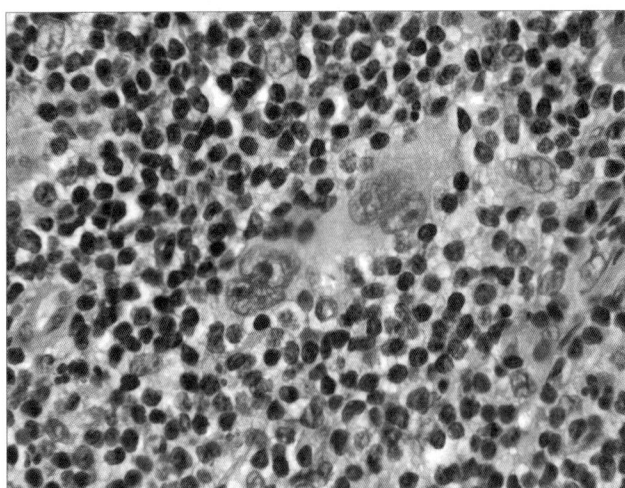

FIGURE 33.6. Hodgkin lymphoma rarely presents in Waldeyer ring and must be distinguished from T-cell-/histiocyte-rich large B-cell lymphoma and a PTCL. In this case, Reed-Sternberg cells are readily apparent and they displayed the characteristic immunophenotype of classical Hodgkin lymphoma (CD15+, CD30+, PAX5+, fascin+) to conform to the lymphocyte-rich classical type (hematoxylin and eosin stain, original magnification: 600× magnification).

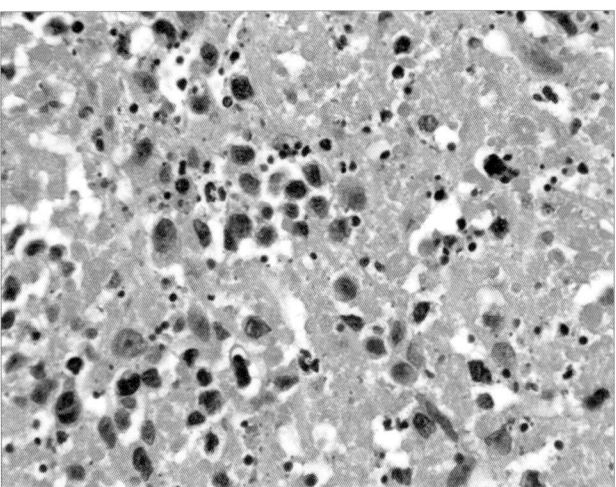

FIGURE 33.7. Extensive necrosis and degeneration is common in malignant lymphoma of the nasal cavity and may mask a large cell polymorphous lymphoma of NK-/T-cell type (hematoxylin and eosin stain, original magnification: 600× magnification).

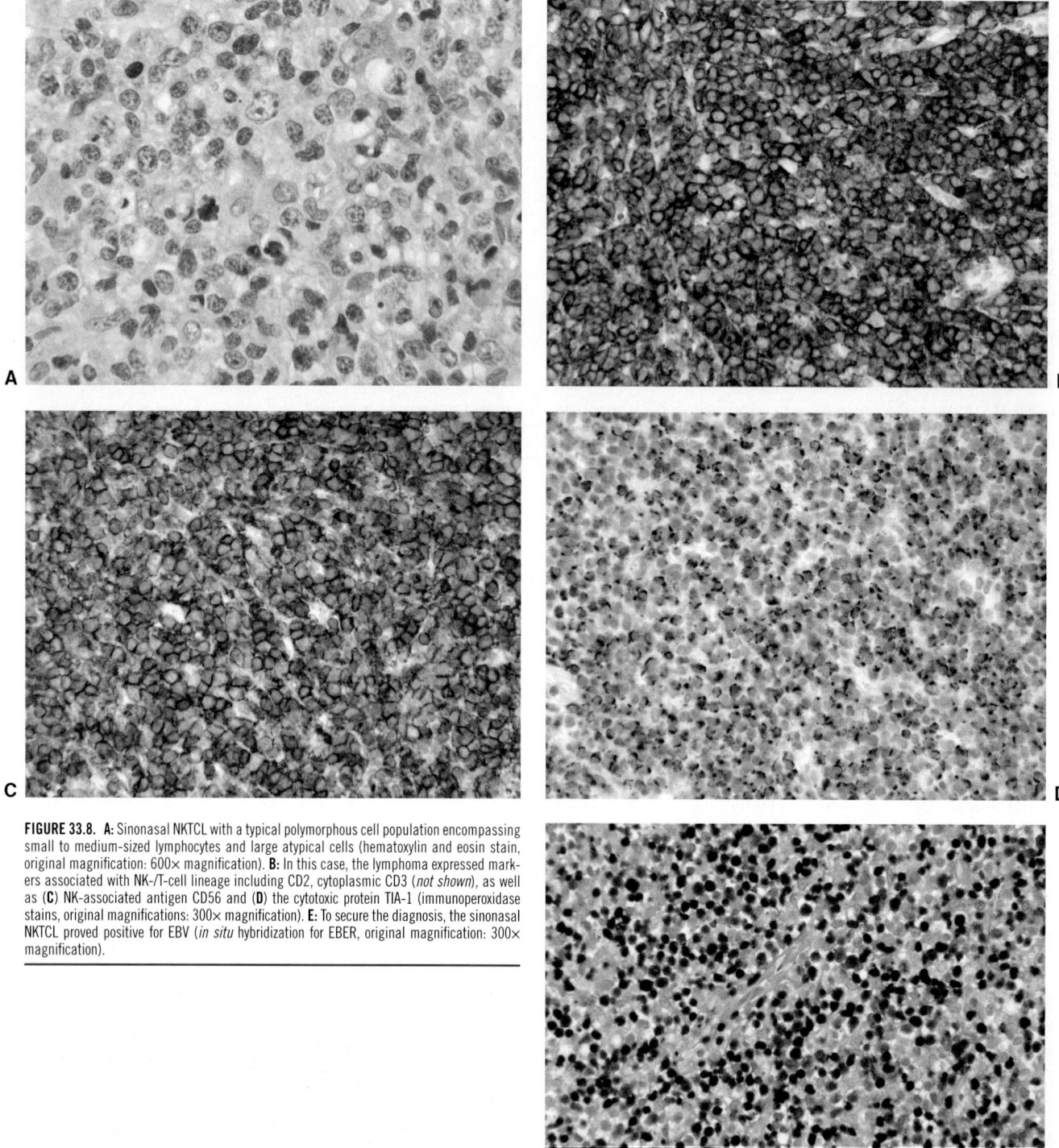

FIGURE 33.8. A: Sinonasal NKTCL with a typical polymorphous cell population encompassing small to medium-sized lymphocytes and large atypical cells (hematoxylin and eosin stain, original magnification: 600× magnification). **B:** In this case, the lymphoma expressed markers associated with NK-/T-cell lineage including CD2, cytoplasmic CD3 (*not shown*), as well as (**C**) NK-associated antigen CD56 and (**D**) the cytotoxic protein TIA-1 (immunoperoxidase stains, original magnifications: 300× magnification). **E:** To secure the diagnosis, the sinonasal NKTCL proved positive for EBV (*in situ* hybridization for EBER, original magnification: 300× magnification).

As noted above, the lymphoma often is accompanied by extensive inflammation and coagulative necrosis. The necrosis often has a zonal distribution to suggest a vascular cause, but chemokines and cytokines may play a role (35,36,53,54). Many polymorphous NKTCL in the sinonasal region encircle vessels and frequently are angioinvasive, raising the spectrum of Wegener granulomatosis (35,36,55) (Fig. 33.9). An absolute diagnosis of Wegener granulomatosis requires the presence of granulomatous inflammation, necrosis, and vasculitis (56). In contrast, NKTCL does not exhibit granulomatous angiitis or fibrinoid necrosis, but rather concentrates around

and within blood vessels with lymphomatous infiltration and destruction of the vessel walls (35,55,57–59). In addition to frequent necrosis and an angiocentric growth pattern, NKTCL may exhibit epitheliotropism similar to that seen in the skin in mycosis fungoides (60) (Fig. 33.10) and an intramucosal variant has been described (61). In Wright-Giemsa–stained touch imprint preparations, azurophilic granules often are observed in tumor cells (36,47).

The prevalent polymorphous NKTCL of the sinonasal region share many pathologic features with lymphomatoid granulomatosis of the lung, including the tendency to be angiocentric

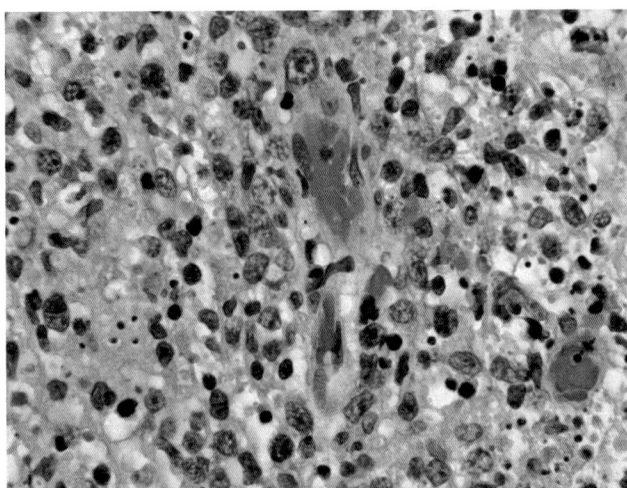

FIGURE 33.9. Angioinvasion with angiodestruction by NKTCL in the sinonasal region is a frequent occurrence (hematoxylin and eosin stain, original magnification: 600× magnification).

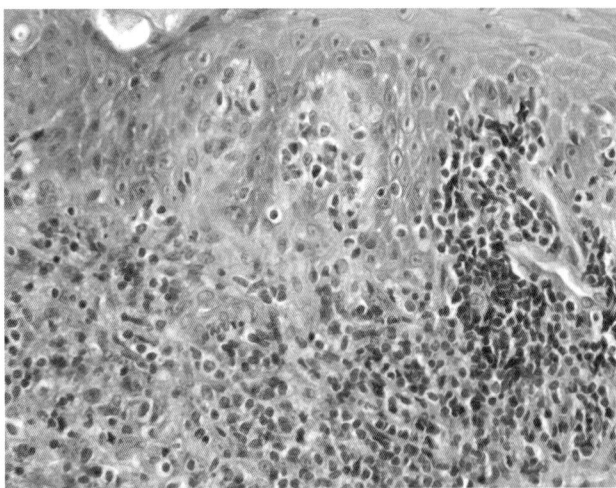

FIGURE 33.10. An NK-/T-cell lymphoma of the palate invades the overlying squamous mucosa (epitheliotropism) and parallels the epidermotropism common in mycosis fungoides (hematoxylin and eosin stain, original magnification: 300× magnification).

and angiodestructive with associated necrosis, as well as to be related to EBV infection (62,63). The current consensus is that lymphomatoid granulomatosis is an EBV-linked B-cell lymphoma with a vigorous T-cell reaction or, in other words, a distinct type of T-cell–rich large B-cell lymphoma (63). Notwithstanding, cases of *bona fide* nasal-type NKTCL can arise external to the sinonasal region, especially in extranodal sites such as skin, upper respiratory tract, testis, gastrointestinal tract, soft tissue, adrenal gland, and brain (32,64–66); curiously, sinonasal NKTCL tends to disseminate to these same sites. The extranasal NKTCL cases are demographically, morphologically, and phenotypically identical to the cases in the sinonasal region, but the extranasal cases exhibit more adverse clinical features (see Chapter 26).

Immunophenotypic studies have confirmed the NK-/T-cell nature of most malignant lymphomas of the sinonasal region. In one study of 80 patients with sinonasal malignant lymphoma from Korea, 42.5% had an NK-/T-cell (CD56$^+$) immunophenotype, 33.8% were PTCL, not otherwise specified (NOS) (CD56$^-$), and 23.7% were B-cell lymphomas (CD20$^+$) (67). Although there is heterogeneity, the commonest immunophenotype of sinonasal NKTCL is CD2$^+$, membranous CD3$^-$, cytoplasmic CD3ε^+, and CD56$^+$ (35,36,40,47,51,55,58,68,69). This immunophenotypic profile is found not only in the Far East and Latin America but also in sinonasal malignant lymphoma cases originating in patients from the United States and Europe (52,57,70–72). The malignant lymphomas with the CD2$^+$, membranous CD3$^-$, cytoplasmic CD3ε^+, and CD56$^+$ immunophenotype may express other T-cell–associated antigens, such as CD43 and CD45RO and occasionally CD4, CD5, CD7, and CD8 (35,36,40,43,52,68,70,71). CD30 expression is found in up to 43% of cases and p53 in as many as 86% (40,52,55,70,73); the transcription factor T-bet and its cofactor ETS-1 also are positive in the majority of cases (52,61). NKTCL consistently expresses cytotoxic proteins TIA-1 and granzyme B, as well as perforin (36,43,53,59,69,72,74). NKTCL, including those in the sinonasal region, also express CD95 (Fas) and CD95 ligand (74,75). The release of cytotoxic proteins probably leads to zonal tumor cell death and likely contributes to the necrosis seen in cases of sinonasal NKTCL that are without an angiocentric growth pattern (53).

Notwithstanding that these sinonasal malignant lymphomas are usually negative for NK-cell markers CD16 and CD57, the reactivity for CD56 in frozen and paraffin-embedded tissues with lack of expression of surface membranous CD3, but presence of cytoplasmic CD3ε and sporadic expression of T-lineage

antigens other than CD2, connotes that the CD56$^+$ sinonasal malignant lymphomas are derived from NK cells rather than T cells (40,59,68,72). In concert with the putative NK lineage, such sinonasal malignant lymphomas do not exhibit clonal T-cell receptor (TCR) gene rearrangements or express βF1 and TCRδ (55,59,68,69,71). Alternatively, a minority of the sinonasal malignant lymphoma cases are of T-cell derivation exhibiting clonal TCR gene rearrangements and originating from $\gamma\delta$, $\alpha\beta$, or $\alpha\beta/\gamma\delta$ T cells (52,55,59,71,76). Although the presumptive NK cases more often express CD56, Oct2, CDXCL13, and MUM1, and less often PD-1, than those of T-cell lineage, the sinonasal T-cell cases are similar to the NK-cell cases in that they are pleomorphic tumors with frequent angiocentricity and epitheliotropism with expression of cytotoxic molecules and EBV (36,55,59). The T-cell cases, therefore, are coupled with the NK-cell cases as extranodal NKTCL, nasal type; however, sinonasal cases with the identical immunophenotype, but lacking EBV and cytoxic molecules, are best classified as PTCL, NOS (36).

Clearly, EBV positivity is essential for the diagnosis of sinonasal NKTCL and is best demonstrated by employing *in situ* hybridization to detect EBER. Moreover, the finding of EBER$^+$ cells may be beneficial in diagnosis, particularly in cases with small numbers of lymphomatous cells and in the distinction of NKTCL from Wegener granulomatosis (35,77); EBER positivity is not found in Wegener granulomatosis. The intimate association of EBER to NKTCL of nasal type has suggested the etiologic role of EBV in the pathogenesis of this lymphoma (40,43,64,71,76). In sinonasal NKTCL, EBV generally exhibits a 30–base pair deletion of the *LMP1* gene and EBV exists in a clonal episomal form with a type II latency pattern that is LMP1$^+$, EBNA1$^+$, and EBNA2$^-$ (36,43,58,69,71,73,78,79). In this lymphoma, EBV is most commonly subtype A, especially in Asia and in other regions such as Mexico, but subtype B has been reported in Europe, Peru, and southern Brazil (41,43,58,79,80). EBV infection is significant, not only for the diagnosis of NKTCL but also as a clinical biomarker. Measurement of circulating EBV-DNA in plasma tallies with disease activity as a high viral load conforms to a higher clinical stage and an inferior prognosis (81,82). In tissue samples of NKTCL, EBV tumor viral load also is important; employing real-time quantitative polymerase chain reaction (PCR) for EBV, patients with a low EBV viral load (<1 copy per cell) exhibit a better overall survival than patients with high viral loads (83). EBV in bone marrow is equally significant in NKTCL. Histologic involvement of the bone marrow by nasal NKTCL is uncommon at diagnosis, but the detection of EBER transcripts in the marrow in the absence of morphologic evidence correlates with a poor prognosis (84,85).

Because of necrosis and adulteration by inflammatory cells, cytogenetic studies of NKTCL are problematic and no specific genetic abnormality has been recognized (86). The most frequent recurrent cytogenetic abnormalities among sinonasal NKTCL involve deletions of chromosome 6 at around the q21-q23 region, and fluorescence *in situ* hybridization (FISH) studies have confirmed the existence of deletions at 6q22-q23 in the CD56+CD3− lymphoma cells (87). By genome-wide array-based comparative genomic hybridization (CGH) technology, NKTCL, nasal type, most frequently exhibits loss of 6q21-q22, 6q22.33-q23.2, 6q25.3, and 6q26-q27 (88). Gene expression profiling (GEP) of nasal NKTCL reveals enrichment for cell cycle–related genes and pathways including PLK1, CDK1, and Aurora-A, and a proproliferative and antiapoptotic phenotype with activation of Myc and nuclear factor kappa B (NF-κB) with deregulation of p53 (89). In tandem with the GEP results, by immunohistochemistry many NKTCL cases overexpress c-Myc, NF-κB p50, and also survivin. These results suggest that the lymphomagenesis of NKTCL may involve deregulation of p53 in association with Myc and NF-κB activation, possibly driven by EBV, leading to the cumulative up-regulation of survivin and an antiapoptotic effect on the neoplastic NK-/T-cells (89).

As indicated earlier, studies from the United States and Europe have documented cases of sinonasal malignant lymphomas that are of NK-/T-cell lineage (52,57,71,72,90). Reports from these areas, however, have shown a preponderance of sinonasal malignant lymphomas that are of B-cell lineage (50,90); moreover, B-cell lymphomas constitute almost a quarter of the sinonasal malignant lymphomas in Korea (67). The B-cell sinonasal malignant lymphomas, regardless of geographic origin, tend to be DLBCL and usually are composed of relatively monomorphous centroblasts or immunoblasts (50,67,90) (Fig. 33.11). The DLBCL cases predominately involve the paranasal sinuses, whereas those limited to the nasal cavity are mainly NKTCL (67,90). Patients with paranasal sinus DLBCL exhibit a 5-year overall survival of 54% and disease-specific survival of 67% that is superior to patients with an NK-/T-cell immunophenotype (91). Because of the risk of central nervous system (CNS) relapse in patients with DLBCL of this region, CNS prophylaxis is advised (91,92).

Historically, the clinical prognosis of patients with sinonasal NKTCL was inconstant and difficult to evaluate, possibly because the polymorphous forms of NKTCL went unrecognized

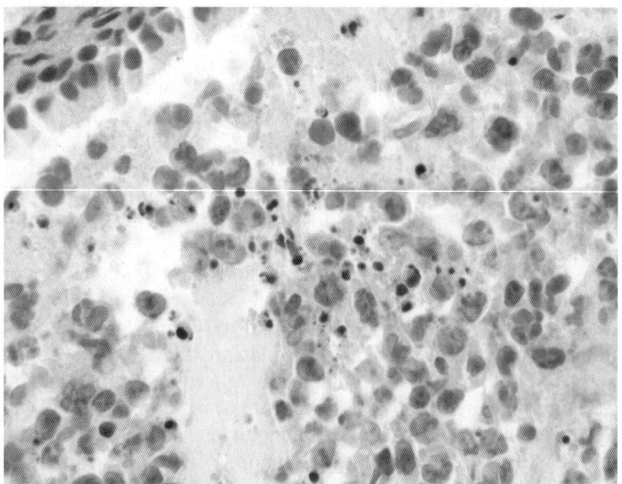

FIGURE 33.11. A "conventional" lymphoma of large cell type is discovered in a paranasal sinus. Despite degeneration, the large cells expressed B-cell antigens. While most lymphomas of the nasal cavity are NKTCLs, those in paranasal sinuses are mainly large B-cell lymphomas (hematoxylin and eosin stain, original magnification: 600× magnification).

for prolonged periods, and many patients were not treated by conventional lymphoma protocols. According to a study from the International Peripheral T-Cell Lymphoma Project based on cases accrued between 1990 and 2002, the median overall survival of nasal NKTCL was 2.96 years for patients with early-stage disease, whereas for those with late-stage disease the median survival was only 0.8 years (66). Unfavorable prognostic factors include an elevated IPI score, Ki-67 proliferation rate >50%, tumor cell transformation of more than 40%, elevated C-reactive protein level, anemia, and thrombocytopenia (66). In a study from Hong Kong of 67 patients with well-characterized sinonasal NKTCL, 84% had stage I/II disease with an IPI score of 1 or less (93). Patients with an IPI score of <1 fared superiorly to those with an IPI score of 2 or more with a 20-year overall survival of 57.4% versus 27.6%. For patients with nasal NKTCL and stage IE disease or contiguous stage IIE with cervical lymph node involvement, the current therapeutic recommendation is concurrent chemoradiotherapy with non–multidrug-resistant agents plus etoposide; in clinical trials, the 5-year overall survival with this regimen is 70% (94). For the other patients with NKTCL, chemotherapy incorporating L-asparaginase, such as SMILE (steroid, methotrexate, ifosfamide, L-asparaginase, etoposide), is advised as induction therapy (95); in a phase II study of this protocol, the overall response rate was 79%, which was far superior to the historical control using conventional chemotherapy (94,95). Sinonasal NKTCL tends to relapse in other extranodal sites such as the skin, lung, liver, gastrointestinal tract, testis, and brain (7). Some patients develop a terminal hemophagocytic syndrome (35).

SALIVARY GLAND

Malignant lymphomas that manifest initially in salivary glands are uncommon and are estimated to constitute only 1.7% of all reported salivary gland tumors (96). The parotid gland is the salivary gland most frequently involved by malignant lymphoma; malignant lymphoma is discovered in 4% of patients who undergo parotid gland surgery (97,98). Among patients with extragastric marginal zone lymphoma of MALT type, salivary gland comprised 26% of cases and was the most common initial site of primary extranodal marginal zone lymphoma (99).

It is convenient to separate lymphomas of the salivary gland that develop in patients who have no prior history of antecedent disease from those that develop in patients who have a history of Sjögren syndrome, another autoimmune disease, or what has been historically known as *myoepithelial sialadenitis* or *benign lymphoepithelial lesion* (100,101) (Table 33.2). The term *lymphoepithelial sialadenitis* (LESA) has supplanted these older terms to reflect the fact that the cells in so-called *epimyoepithelial islands* may not be myoepithelial but of basal epithelial origin, and even include vascular endothelium, and that many cases that formerly were coded as benign lymphoepithelial lesion may represent low-grade malignant lymphomas (102,103).

Sjögren syndrome, or sicca syndrome, is a multisystem autoimmune disorder in which the salivary and lacrimal glands are damaged, resulting in keratoconjunctivitis sicca, xerostomia, lymphoid infiltrates in the minor salivary glands of the lip, and bilateral parotid enlargement (7). Classic Sjögren syndrome is indistinguishable from LESA; patients with Sjögren syndrome all have LESA, but not all patients with LESA have Sjögren syndrome. In LESA, there is a histologic spectrum that ranges from focal lymphocytic infiltrates associated with mild acinar atrophy to a fully developed reactive process in which the lymphocytic infiltrates are dense and confluent and are associated with germinal center formation, extensive acinar atrophy, disruption of ducts,

	COMPARISON OF MALIGNANT LYMPHOMAS OF SALIVARY GLANDS THAT DEVELOP IN PATIENTS WITH OR WITHOUT LESA	
Table 33.2		
Characteristic	**LESA**	**Non-LESA**
Age/sex	Elderly/female	Elderly/female
Antecedent disease	With or without Sjögren syndrome or other autoimmune disorder	None
Symptoms	Pain, swelling, not fixed to adjacent tissues	Pain, mass, often fixed to adjacent tissues
Lymphoma type	MZL/MALT (monocytoid and plasmacytic variants)	All types—follicular (most common)
Lymphoma extent	Often focal	Usually diffuse replacement of gland
Immunophenotype	B cell	B cell
BCL2 rearrangements	No	Yes
Clinical course	Indolent, potential for extrasalivary presentation (lymph nodes, lungs) and histologic transformation	Similar to nodal counterpart

LESA, lymphoepithelial sialadenitis; MZL, marginal zone lymphoma; MALT, mucosa-associated lymphoid tissue.

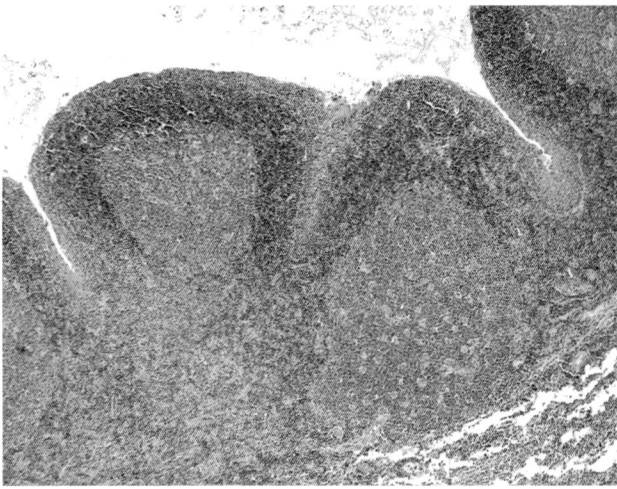

FIGURE 33.13. Lymphoid hyperplasia with cyst formation may mimic LESA in the salivary gland including in patients infected with the human immunodeficiency virus (HIV) (hematoxylin and eosin stain, original magnification: 60× magnification).

and the presence of numerous epimyoepithelial islands (Fig. 33.12); monocytoid B cells often are in the epimyoepithelial islands (102). The lymphocytes between the germinal centers mainly are small lymphocytes with scattered plasma cells, immunoblasts, and occasional monocytoid B cells. Morphologic changes similar to LESA have been described in salivary glands and intrasalivary gland lymph nodes in patients who have acquired immunodeficiency syndrome (AIDS) and in intravenous drug users (104,105); cystically dilated salivary gland ducts with squamous metaplasia are observed in these cases, as well as in patients without AIDS (106,107) (see Chapter 25) (Fig. 33.13). The lymphoepithelial cysts mainly are in the parotid gland and probably form secondary to the obstruction of parotid ducts by the florid reactive lymphocytic infiltrate (106); they are not regarded as originating from intraparotid lymph nodes (107). Occasionally, in the salivary gland from a patient with AIDS, the degree of lymphoid and immunoblastic hyperplasia may be so prolific as to mimic malignant lymphoma (Fig. 33.14).

Like patients who have AIDS, patients who have actual Sjögren syndrome have a predisposition to develop malignant lymphoma, which most recently has been reported as 6.5 times more than expected with a dramatic 1,000-fold increased risk of marginal zone lymphoma in the parotid gland, as well as increased risk for DLBCL and follicular lymphoma (108). Cases of LESA are characterized by a predominance of CD4+ T-helper cells, and the general consensus is that the increased risk of malignant lymphoma in Sjögren syndrome is a consequence of T helper cell–dependent chronic antigenic stimulation of B cells with eventual immunoglobulin gene hypermutation, including aberrant somatic hypermutation, and escape of a malignant B-cell clone (109–112). The growth of early clones in LESA is thought to initiate as nonmalignant antigen-selected expansions (113). Genotypic studies have documented rearrangement of immunoglobulin genes in salivary gland tissues from patients who have LESA, including patients who show none of the usual morphologic characteristics of malignant lymphoma (114–116). The marginal zone lymphomas of MALT that can develop in a background of the reactive lymphocytic infiltrates of Sjögren syndrome represent a highly selected B-cell population that expresses a restricted immunoglobulin V_H gene repertoire that differs from MALT lymphomas of other sites (110,117).

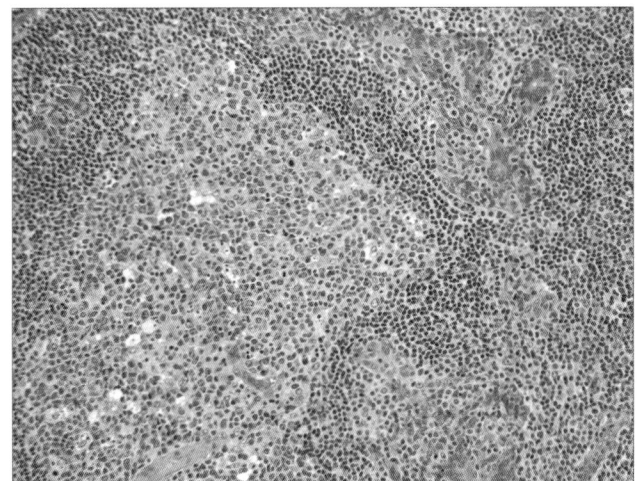

FIGURE 33.12. In LESA, there frequently is florid lymphoid hyperplasia associated with germinal centers, dense lymphocytic infiltrates, atrophy of salivary gland acini, and the formation of epimyoepithelial islands (hematoxylin and eosin stain, original magnification: 150× magnification).

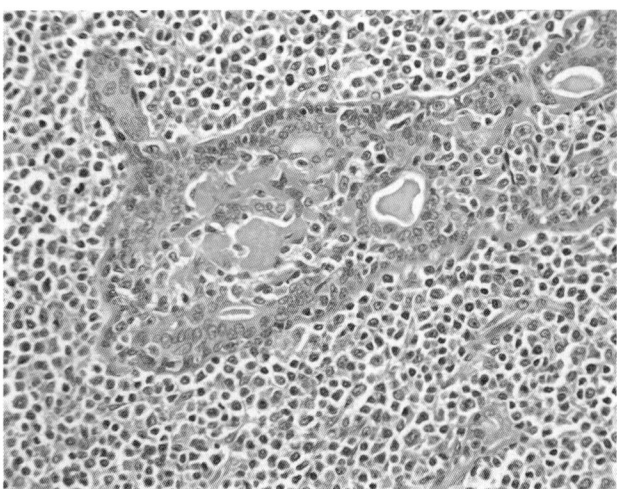

FIGURE 33.14. Florid immunoblastic hyperplasia in the salivary gland of a patient infected with the HIV is indistinguishable from LESA. Notice the invasion of the epimyoepithelial islands by the proliferating small lymphocytes and immunoblasts despite the reactive nature of this process (hematoxylin and eosin stain, original magnification: 300× magnification).

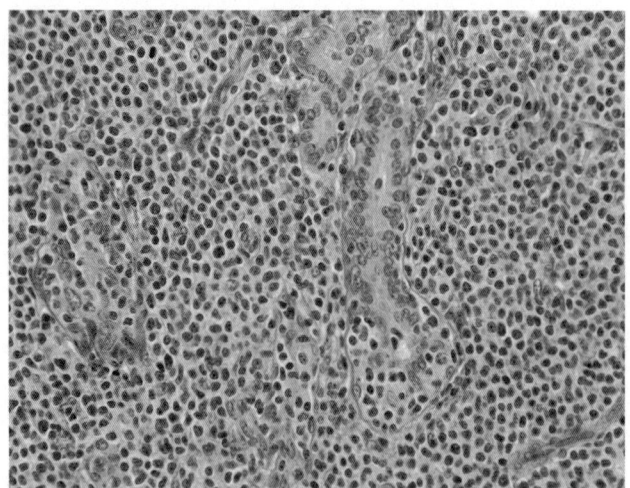

FIGURE 33.15. Marginal zone lymphoma of MALT type in a salivary gland is characterized by a dense, monotonous pattern of infiltration with invasion of residual salivary gland ducts. The neoplastic lymphocytes are monocytoid with slight nuclear membrane irregularities and abundant lucent cytoplasm. Immunophenotypic studies demonstrated κ light chain restriction (hematoxylin and eosin stain, original magnification: 300× magnification).

EBV rarely plays a role in the pathogenesis of malignant lymphoma occurring in the setting of Sjögren syndrome (117a), and in some cases, hepatitis C virus may be involved and is particularly relevant in patients with positive rheumatoid factor and mixed cryoglobulinemia (114,118–120). Curiously, although patients who have Sjögren syndrome may develop clinically overt lymphoma in the salivary gland, most patients who do have this syndrome evince their lymphoma clinically in extrasalivary gland sites, particularly marginal zone lymphomas in lymph nodes and lung (96,118,121,122). A prediction model for lymphoma development in primary Sjögren syndrome has been proposed based on clinical and serologic disease variables; enlargement of salivary glands, low serum C3 and/or C4 levels, and disease duration are independent risk factors for B-cell lymphoma in patients with Sjögren syndrome (123). Foxp3⁺ T-regulatory cells also may play a role in foretelling lymphoma in Sjögren syndrome with lower levels of Foxp3⁺ cell incidence correlating with C4 hypocomplementemia and salivary gland enlargement (124).

Despite the fact that clinically obvious malignant lymphoma is relatively uncommon in the salivary glands of patients who have Sjögren syndrome, immunophenotypic and genotypic studies have served to refine the histologic criteria of LESA and have led to the discovery of subtle malignant lymphoma in this setting (101,114–116,122,125). Frequently, a histologic and immunologic continuum develops from areas of benign polyclonal lymphocytic infiltrates to monoclonal B-cell lymphoma (101,114–116,125); this continuum has implied that malignant lymphomas of salivary gland form part of the spectrum of lymphomas of MALT (125). The MALT lymphomas of salivary gland conform to the general morphologic features of extranodal marginal zone lymphomas with the exception that their marginal zone cells have a distinct monocytoid or clear cell appearance or have plasmacytic characteristics (116,122,125). The neoplastic monocytoid-type B cells in the salivary gland have a marginal zonelike distribution, encircling reactive follicles and the adjacent rims of attenuated mantle zone lymphocytes. The unequivocal salivary gland marginal zone lymphomas exhibit coalescence of monocytoid cells to form broad, interconnecting strands that surround and invade epimyoepithelial islands, displace germinal centers, and eventually produce sheetlike masses resulting in destruction of the acinar architecture of the gland (116,122,125,126). In contrast to a reactive process, these extranodal marginal zone lymphomas of MALT type usually are dense and have monotonous cytologic features (Fig. 33.15). The presence of wide strands of coalescing monocytoid B cells correlates with monoclonality and the development of extrasalivary gland malignant lymphomas, all of which exhibit the same light chain restriction as the corresponding neoplastic B cells in the salivary gland (101,122). The demonstration of monoclonality also is important in the plasmacytic variant of extranodal marginal zone lymphoma, which aids in the differentiation from chronic sclerosing sialadenitis (Küttner tumor), an IgG4-related disease (127–129). The marked lymphoplasmacytic infiltrate with architectural destruction of the salivary gland found in chronic sclerosing sialadenitis could be misconstrued as marginal zone lymphoma, but in chronic sclerosing sialadenitis the plasma cells are polyclonal, in addition to expressing high levels of IgG4 (127–129) (Fig. 33.16). Nevertheless, marginal zone lymphoma of the salivary gland rarely may arise in association with chronic sclerosing sialadenitis (130).

The immunophenotypic profile of salivary gland MALT lymphomas replicates the established B-cell immunophenotype

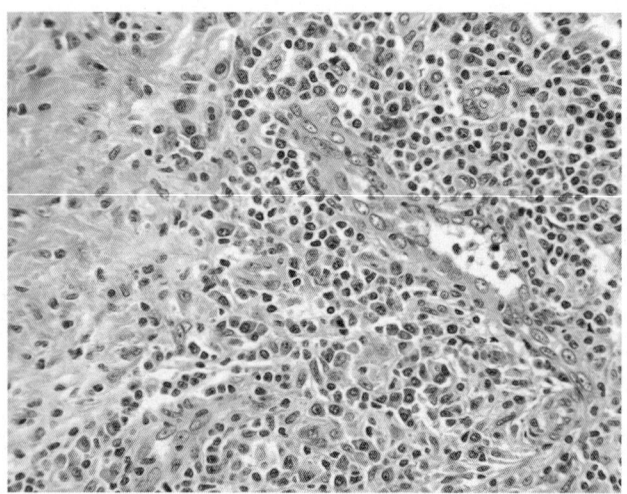
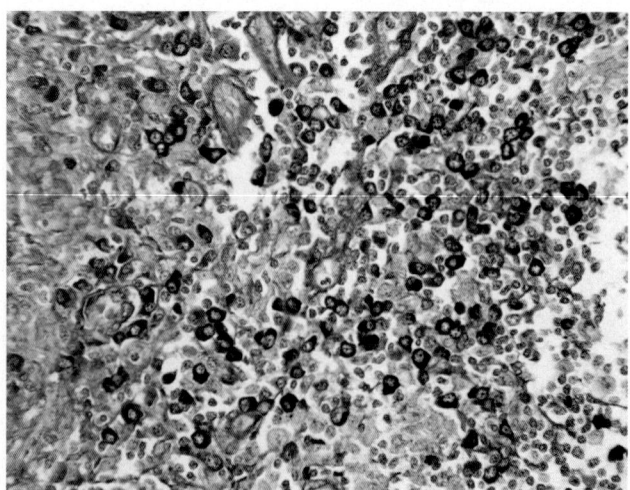

FIGURE 33.16. A: In chronic sclerosing sialadenitis, the dense plasma cell and lymphocytic infiltrate with associated architectural destruction of the salivary gland could be mistaken for lymphoma (hematoxylin and eosin stain, original magnification: 300× magnification). **B:** Chronic sclerosing sialadenitis is an IgG4-related disease with increased IgG4⁺ plasma cells (immunoperoxidase stain, original magnification: 300× magnification).

of marginal zone lymphomas in other extranodal sites and in many cases the neoplastic monocytoid/marginal zone B cells coexpress CD43 (12,116,122,131). In the salivary gland, the neoplastic B cells of extranodal marginal zone lymphoma often exhibit trisomy 3 and to a lesser extent trisomy 18, but only rarely the t(11;18) chromosomal translocation (132,133); however, 12% of cases exhibit the t(14;18) chromosomal translocation due to fusion of the *IGH* gene to the *MALT1* gene at 18q21 (132). For the translocation-negative marginal zone lymphomas in salivary gland, the global NF-κB inhibitor A20 shows deletion in a minority of cases (134).

The main contention in salivary gland MALT lymphomas concerns the morphologic threshold for interpreting cases as malignant lymphoma (126). With PCR techniques, for example, clonality has been demonstrated across the full spectrum of lymphoid infiltrates in the salivary gland including cases regarded as reactive LESA, cases with halos of monocytoid cells surrounding epimyoepithelial islands, and cases with unequivocal confluent-type MALT lymphomas (114–116). The difficulty concerns the cases containing monocytoid or clear cell halos (Fig. 33.17). In some instances, cases with focal or halo-type monocytoid B-cell proliferations in the salivary gland are ignored or simply misconstrued as hyperplastic and as variants of LESA because of their juxtaposition to benign reactive areas, including germinal centers and mantle zone cells. Nonetheless, the abundant, pale, often clear cytoplasm with well-defined cytoplasmic borders of the monocytoid cells in the halos is morphologically distinct and should assist in distinguishing them from the adjacent reactive small lymphocytes and associated germinal centers (Fig. 33.18). The monocytoid halos that are recognized in salivary glands with LESA are analogous to the circumscribed pale-staining "proliferation areas" that previously were reported and some investigators consider clonal halo-type cases as examples of early MALT lymphoma, whereas others regard the halo-type cases as indeterminate, borderline, or perhaps as examples of disorders of "uncertain malignant potential" (101,114,116,125,135).

This issue is not resolved readily because clonality does not appear to predict progression of lymphoid lesions in the salivary gland to clinically overt lymphoma (115). For example, Quintana et al. (116) examined 61 salivary gland

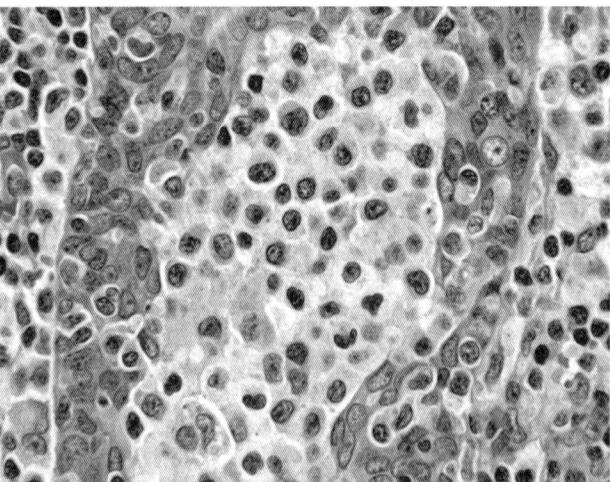

FIGURE 33.18. Detail of neoplastic monocytoid cells with disruption of an epimyoepithelial island in the parotid salivary gland. The cytoplasm is characteristically pale staining, and the nuclei frequently are reniform (hematoxylin and eosin stain, original magnification: 600× magnification).

specimens with lymphoid infiltrates and histologically classified them as equivalent to LESA, LESA with monocytoid B-cell halos, unequivocal malignant lymphomas of MALT type with confluent monocytoid B-cell zones, MALT lymphomas with monoclonal plasma cells, and DLBCL in association with lymphomas of MALT type. As demonstrated by others, CD43 coexpression on monocytoid B cells did not correlate with the histologic category, clonality, or with extrasalivary gland malignant lymphoma (122). Employing PCR, clonal B cells were identified across the entire morphologic spectrum of salivary gland lymphoid infiltrates, including 42% of the cases that were regarded as histologically classic benign LESA and 65% of the cases with halos of monocytoid B cells (116); yet, most patients pursued an indolent clinical course. The investigators concluded that two types of borderline lesions exist within the context of salivary gland lymphoid infiltrates (116) (Table 33.3). One has the morphologic appearance of benign LESA but with demonstrable B-cell clonality, and the other is LESA that has halos of monocytoid B cells that extend beyond the confines of the epimyoepithelial islands or lymphoepithelial lesions. With either of these lesions, the term *borderline* portends that there is morphologic or clonal documentation that is suggestive of malignant lymphoma, but that there is limited chance of dissemination unless histologic progression develops (116). However, this viewpoint is contentious and others signify that the emergence of a monoclonal B-cell population in a setting of LESA with monocytoid B-cell halo-type lesions heralds the onset of frank malignant lymphoma, although genetic alterations may be required for progression and dissemination (114). Regardless of whether clonality is interpreted as tantamount to malignant lymphoma in cases of LESA with halos, patients with such lesions require careful clinical monitoring. Patients who have salivary gland marginal zone lymphoma are at risk to develop a synchronous or a subsequent aggressive lymphoma (116,131) (Fig. 33.19).

Malignant lymphomas of salivary gland associated with Sjögren syndrome or LESA, specifically marginal zone lymphomas of MALT, usually are relatively indolent (125). Although some patients may develop extrasalivary gland lymphoma in months instead of years, most patients behave similarly to patients who have equivalent extranodal marginal zone lymphomas of MALT and have a predilection for localized disease (12,101,114,122). The onset of progressive malignant lymphoma can vary and if extrasalivary gland lymphoma does develop, it usually exhibits the identical histologic and

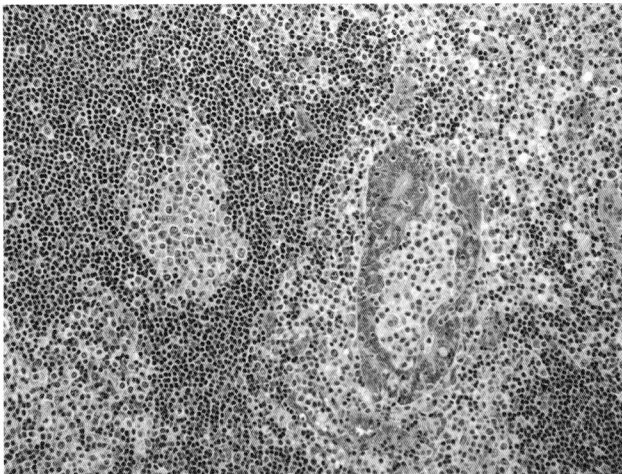

FIGURE 33.17. Monocytoid B cells concentrate around and invade epimyoepithelial islands to form a halo pattern. The pale-staining cytoplasm of the monocytoid cells contrasts with the darker-staining small lymphocytes of the adjacent mantle zone surrounding a germinal center. Despite the presence of frequent monoclonality, there is no agreement on whether cases with monocytoid halos are an early form of extranodal marginal zone lymphoma or a borderline lesion (hematoxylin and eosin stain, original magnification: 150× magnification).

Table 33.3	SYNOPSIS OF LYMPHOID INFILTRATES OF THE SALIVARY GLAND ASSOCIATED WITH LESA

Benign
  LESA, polyclonal
Borderline (clonal or morphologic features suggesting malignant lymphoma but with little risk of dissemination)
  LESA, monoclonal
  LESA with halos of monocytoid-like B cells
Lymphoma, low-grade (risk for spread to extrasalivary lymph nodes)
  MZL/MALT type (LESA with wide interconnecting strands of monocytoid-like B cells, with or without plasmacytic differentiation)
Lymphoma, high-grade (primary or secondary to MZL/MALT)
  Large B-cell type

LESA, lymphoepithelial sialadenitis; MZL, marginal zone lymphoma; MALT, mucosa-associated lymphoid tissue.
Adapted with permission from Quintana PG, Kapadia SB, Bahler DW, et al. Salivary gland lymphoid infiltrates associated with lymphoepithelial lesions: a clinicopathologic, immunophenotypic, and genotypic study. *Hum Pathol* 1997;28:850–861. Copyright © 1997, Elsevier.

immunohistochemical features of the initial marginal zone lymphoma in the salivary gland (114,136).

The management of patients who have marginal zone lymphoma of MALT type in the salivary gland associated with LESA still is evolving, but the patients require appropriate staging followed in most instances by moderate-dose radiation therapy as the recommended therapy (7,137). With this modality, a minority of patients develop recurrent marginal zone lymphoma, often to the contralateral salivary gland; however, these patients usually achieve remission following resection and/or radiation therapy of the recurrent lymphoma (137). In one study of 23 patients with lymphoma of the salivary gland, including patients with DLBCL as well as marginal zone lymphoma of MALT, the overall survival at 5 years was 94.7% (138). Because many cases of MALT lymphoma of the salivary gland are discovered after retrospective review of cases originally regarded as benign LESA, and because these patients have not received therapy except for surgical biopsy, they may not require any therapy and need only careful follow-up (116,125).

Malignant lymphomas that arise in the salivary glands of patients who have no history of antecedent disease are,

paradoxically, more common than the better-known lymphomas of salivary glands that develop in patients who have Sjögren syndrome or LESA (96,139). Patients who have overt lymphoma that arise in the salivary gland generally present with a firm, bulging mass that may be fixed to superficial or deep structures and occasionally is associated with nerve palsy (96). Grossly, malignant lymphomas of the salivary gland appear gray-tan to pink, bulge on cut section, and often are circumscribed (139).

In contrast to the diffuse, indolent MALT lymphomas characteristic of the salivary gland in patients who have Sjögren syndrome or LESA, patients who have no autoimmune disorder develop all histologic types of salivary gland non-Hodgkin lymphomas, but follicular lymphomas are the most common (96,98,100,131,140) (Fig. 33.20). Many such lymphomas, including those with a follicular architectural pattern, probably originate in lymph nodes attached to the capsule or entrapped within the involved gland, for example, intraparotid lymph nodes (98,102). Diagnosis in these cases is usually not a problem, although occasional follicular large cell lymphomas may be difficult to differentiate from florid reactive follicular hyperplasia with so-called giant follicles (141). The distinction of follicular lymphoma from reactive follicular hyperplasia with giant follicles in the salivary gland depends on the application of criteria identical to those used to separate these two lesions in lymph nodes. The same criteria are equally applicable to the diagnosis of rare follicular lymphomas that arise in salivary glands involved by Warthin tumor (142). Histologically and immunologically, no differences are apparent between a follicular lymphoma that arises in a salivary gland and one in a lymph node. For example, studies have demonstrated that follicular lymphomas that present in the salivary gland have molecular evidence of the *IGH/BCL2* translocation (140). This contrasts with the MALT lymphomas of salivary gland that lack *BCL2* gene rearrangements (114,118). One exception involved a patient who had salivary gland marginal zone lymphoma in association with Sjögren syndrome and who later developed follicular lymphoma (143). PCR analysis of the t(14;18) translocation demonstrated an identical-sized band from both the marginal zone and follicular lymphoma components, and sequencing indicated a common clonal lineage. The prognosis of patients with follicular lymphoma of salivary glands may be superior to those arising in the lymph node. In one report the 5-year overall survival was comparable to the survival of the indolent marginal zone cases that presented in the salivary gland (131).

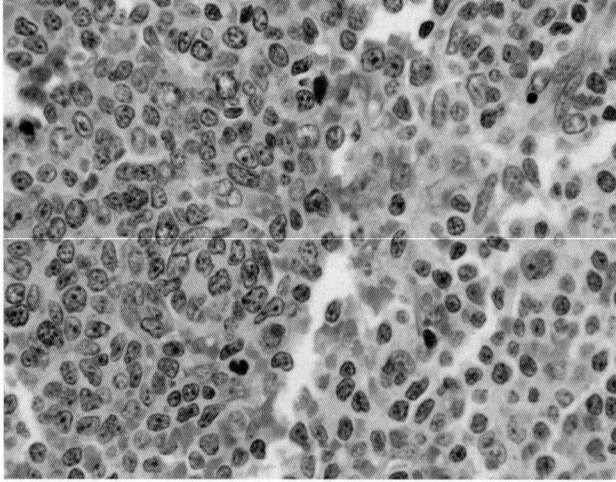

FIGURE 33.19. Interface of large B-cell lymphoma on the left and marginal zone lymphoma of MALT type composed of smaller monocytoid-type B cells on the right. The large B-cell lymphoma was focal and developed in a background of a lymphoma of MALT in the parotid gland. The monocytoid B cells and the large cells expressed identical immunoglobulin heavy and light chains (IgMλ) (hematoxylin and eosin stain, original magnification: 600× magnification).

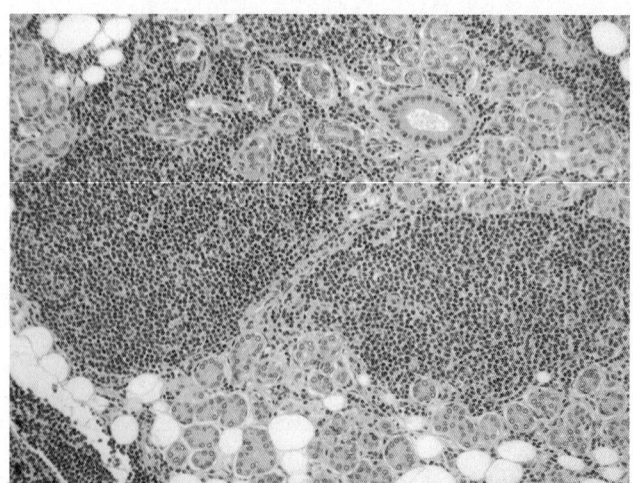

FIGURE 33.20. Follicular lymphoma, grade 1, is the most common malignant lymphoma that occurs in the salivary gland of patients who do not have Sjögren syndrome or LESA (hematoxylin and eosin stain, original magnification: 150× magnification).

Although most primary malignant lymphomas of the salivary gland are B-cell malignancies, rare cases of PTCL, including anaplastic large cell lymphoma (ALCL) and NKTCL, also may primarily involve the salivary glands (144). The PTCL and NKTCL cases are characterized by polymorphous infiltrates of small, medium-sized, or large lymphocytes and by invasion of salivary gland ducts and acini to form lymphoepithelial lesions; angioinvasion also may develop. Similar to NKTCL of the sinonasal region, the cases in the salivary gland exhibit reactivity for EBER (144). Patients who have PTCL or NKTCL of the salivary gland have an aggressive clinical behavior, similar to comparable cases presenting in lymph nodes or other extranodal sites.

THYROID GLAND

Malignant lymphomas of the thyroid gland share many features with those that manifest in the salivary glands in that they almost always are associated with an immunologically mediated, extranodal lymphoid infiltrate, specifically chronic lymphocytic thyroiditis or Hashimoto thyroiditis (145–148). Between 80% and 100% of patients who have malignant lymphoma of the thyroid exhibit chronic lymphocytic thyroiditis in the adjacent tissue and 67% to 80% have thyroid antibodies (148,149). The chance of developing malignant lymphoma of the thyroid gland in patients who have chronic lymphocytic thyroiditis is greatly increased, with an estimated relative risk of 67 in a seminal study from Sweden, and in Japan, the frequency of thyroid lymphomas in patients with Hashimoto thyroiditis is 80 times greater than expected (150,151). A more recent analysis from a Japanese hospital that specializes in thyroid disease reports that the incidence rate of primary lymphomas of thyroid in patients with Hashimoto thyroiditis is 16 persons/year per 10,000 persons, which is about 10 times higher than in the previous Swedish study (152). The dramatic increase in cases of lymphomas of thyroid may be a consequence of selection bias, but advances in imaging studies as well as in pathologic concepts and diagnostic criteria for extranodal lymphomas likely play a significant role (152).

The predisposition among patients who have chronic lymphocytic thyroiditis to develop malignant lymphoma is analogous to the proposed pathways in patients with Sjögren syndrome. As in Sjögren syndrome, the lymphocytes infiltrating the thyroid in chronic lymphocytic thyroiditis mainly are activated T helper cells that are specific for thyroid antigens (149). The T helper cells stimulate autoreactive B cells. The onset of malignant lymphoma likely is a consequence of the chronic antigenic stimulation of B lymphocytes that take place in this autoimmune disorder; this chronic stimulation probably leads to a population of lymphocytes that are more susceptible to neoplastic transformation, possibly as a result of a disorder of immune surveillance related to B cells with aberrant somatic hypermutation and associated cytogenetic changes that triggers histologic progression (149,150,153,154). Sequence similarity has been reported in the clonal bands in Hashimoto thyroiditis and the ensuing malignant lymphoma in the thyroid (155). Moreover, a significant proportion of patients with primary thyroid lymphomas of marginal zone and DLBCL types exhibit common homologous germline V_H genes used by antithyroid antibody to further implicate derivation of thyroid lymphomas from Hashimoto thyroiditis (156,157). Activation of EBV is uncommon in chronic lymphocytic thyroiditis and malignant lymphomas of the thyroid and EBV probably is not a significant factor in the pathogenesis of malignant lymphomas (158).

Unlike in patients who have morphologically benign LESA, clonal immunoglobulin gene rearrangements usually are not detected or are present only in a minority of patients

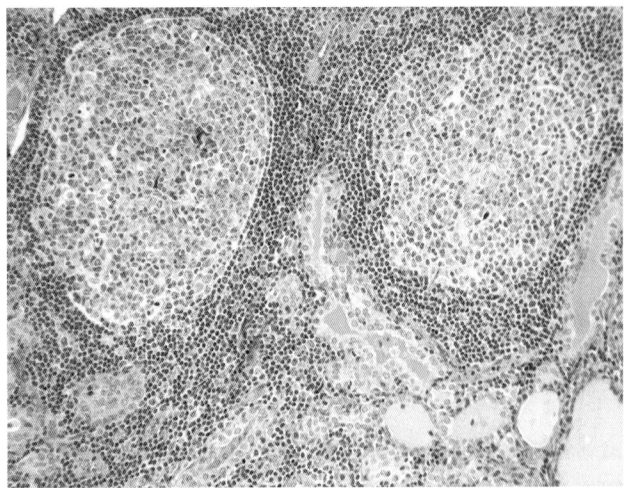

FIGURE 33.21. Reactive lymphoid follicles with germinal center formation and Hürthle cell change in the thyroid follicles characterize chronic lymphocytic thyroiditis. These lesions often are encountered adjacent to malignant lymphomas in the thyroid gland (hematoxylin and eosin stain, original magnification: 150× magnification).

who have chronic lymphocytic thyroiditis despite a skewed κ:λ light chain ratio in comparison to reactive lymph nodes (159–162). Most cases of chronic lymphocytic thyroiditis that have immunoglobulin gene rearrangements probably are malignant lymphomas at the outset and the low frequency of monoclonality in chronic lymphocytic thyroiditis compared with LESA reflects the relative rarity of malignant lymphomas of the thyroid as opposed to those in the salivary gland (160). Notwithstanding, histologic studies have demonstrated that there is a histologic gradation between chronic lymphocytic thyroiditis (Fig. 33.21), marginal zone lymphomas of MALT that resemble chronic lymphocytic thyroiditis, and the more common DLBCL of the thyroid (145–147). This morphologic spectrum between reactive and neoplastic lymphoid infiltrates has boosted the evidence that most thyroid lymphomas are derived from MALT (145,146,163), as has the observation that a significant proportion of cases of DLBCL of thyroid exhibit features of preexisting or associated marginal zone lymphoma of MALT (147,164).

Like patients who have Hashimoto thyroiditis, patients who have malignant lymphoma of the thyroid gland are predominantly female and in the sixth and seventh decades of life (147,152,164,165). Patients generally present with complaints of a painless neck mass. They also may have a history of rapid growth of the mass and compression symptoms, including dysphagia, dyspnea, pain, and hoarseness (146,147,154,165). The clinical diagnosis generally is a possible primary thyroid malignancy, but malignant lymphoma usually is not suspected except in patients with a history of Hashimoto thyroiditis who have rapid thyroid enlargement (165). In cases of malignant lymphoma, the use of fine needle aspiration (FNA) of the thyroid has yielded mixed results particularly in the distinction of marginal zone lymphoma of MALT from chronic lymphocytic thyroiditis so that ancillary methods, such as immunohistochemistry and/or flow cytometry, are required in order to detect monoclonality in the thyroid FNA cytology specimen (165,166). Most cases generally are diagnosed by an open biopsy or surgical resection. On gross examination, the resected thyroid gland often is replaced by a fleshy, pink-tan tumor mass similar to lymphoma in a lymph node (Fig. 33.22).

Malignant lymphoma usually is morphologically distinguishable from chronic lymphocytic thyroiditis, and morphologic features that specifically aid in the diagnosis of malignant lymphoma include those that are obvious, as for example, invasion of blood vessel walls and extension of the lymphocytic infiltrate

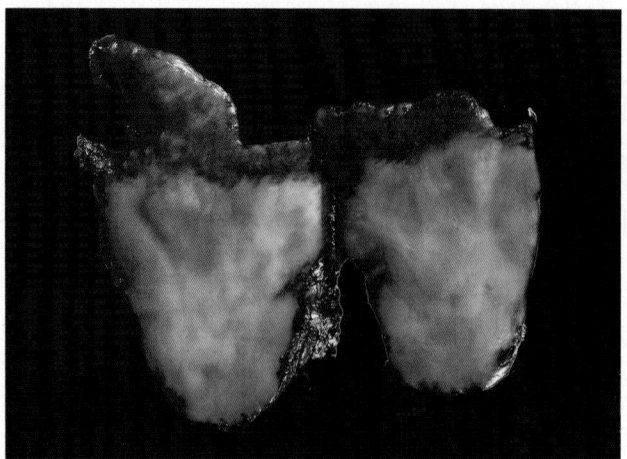

FIGURE 33.22. DLBCL of the thyroid gland forms a large, fleshy mass and virtually replaces the thyroid parenchyma.

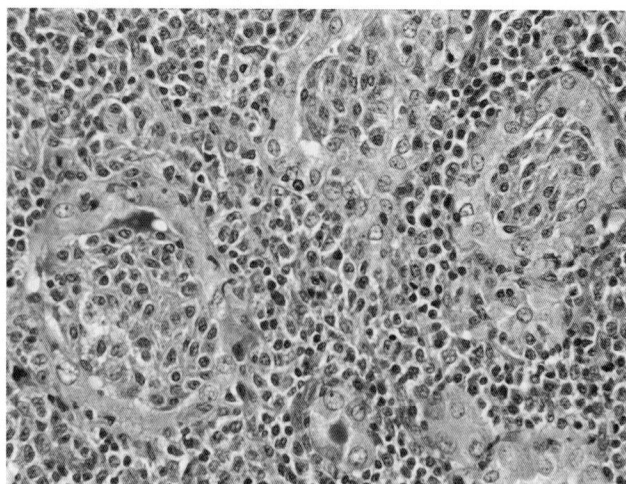

FIGURE 33.24. Marginal zone lymphoma of MALT type stuffs and expands thyroid follicles to form another type of lymphoepithelial lesion, referred to as a "MALT ball" (hematoxylin and eosin stain, original magnification: 300× magnification).

beyond the thyroid capsule into the surrounding perithyroidal soft tissues that are common to DLBCL (147). Invasion by lymphocytes into residual thyroid follicles that result in lymphoepithelial lesions is another morphologic feature important in the distinction of malignant lymphoma from thyroiditis (145,167). In lymphomas of the thyroid, lymphoepithelial lesions chiefly are characterized by invasion within and between thyroid follicles (Fig. 33.23) or less commonly, and especially in marginal zone lymphomas of MALT, the lymphoepithelial lesions are categorized by rounded masses of lymphocytes that expand and fill the thyroid follicles, in a manner termed a "MALT ball" (147,164) (Fig. 33.24); a cytokeratin stain can accentuate lymphoid invasion of thyroid follicles including the "MALT ball" (145,147,160,167) (Fig. 33.25). The finding of thyroid follicular infiltration by lymphocytes, however, is not an absolute diagnostic criterion for malignancy because similar infiltration by benign, reactive B lymphocytes has been described in cases of chronic lymphocytic thyroiditis (145,168). Nonetheless, there are quantitative and qualitative differences in so far as the lymphoepithelial lesions in MALT lymphomas of the thyroid are more common, larger, and more destructive (160).

The issue of whether a lymphocytic infiltrate is benign or malignant generally only pertains to marginal zone lymphomas of MALT. The incidence of marginal zone lymphoma of the thyroid is variable. For example, in three series of primary

malignant lymphomas of the thyroid comprising 23, 47, and 53 patients, marginal zone lymphomas of MALT represented 4 (17.3%), 8 (17%), and 3 (5.6%) of the cases, respectively (146,158,164). Data from the Surveillance, Epidemiology, and End Results (SEER) program of the National Cancer Institute from 1973 to 2005 indicate that 10% of 1,408 patients with primary lymphoma of the thyroid were coded as marginal zone lymphoma (169); however, this demographic study lacked pathologic confirmation. Other studies have documented increased percentages of marginal zone lymphoma cases among primary lymphomas of the thyroid ranging from 23% to as high as 72% (147,148,152,170); in the series of 171 patients from the hospital in Japan specializing in diseases of thyroid, 80 (47%) were diagnosed as marginal zone lymphoma (152). When present, marginal zone lymphomas of MALT in the thyroid reiterate the morphologic features of MALT lymphomas in other sites with confluent dense lymphocytic infiltrates surrounding residual germinal centers resulting in effacement of the thyroid architecture, except for scattered remaining thyroid follicles with Hürthle cell changes (126,145,147) (Fig. 33.26). Follicular colonization of the germinal centers may be florid and may impart a follicular-like pattern (147,171). The cytologic features of MALT lymphomas of the thyroid can be variable,

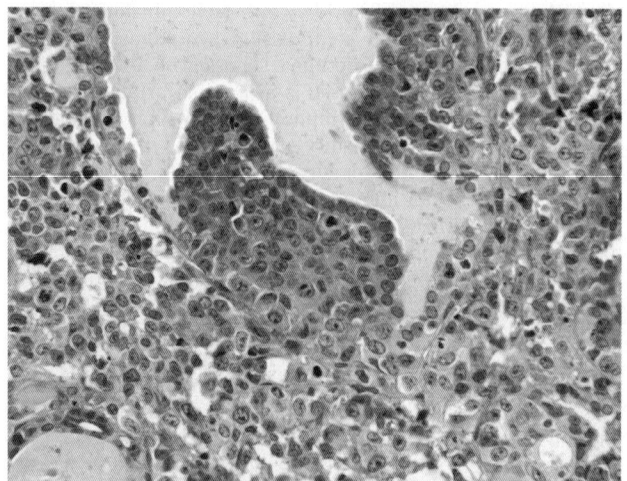

FIGURE 33.23. DLBCL invades residual thyroid follicles to form a typical lymphoepithelial lesion, a frequent observation in malignant lymphomas of the thyroid gland (hematoxylin and eosin stain, original magnification: 300× magnification).

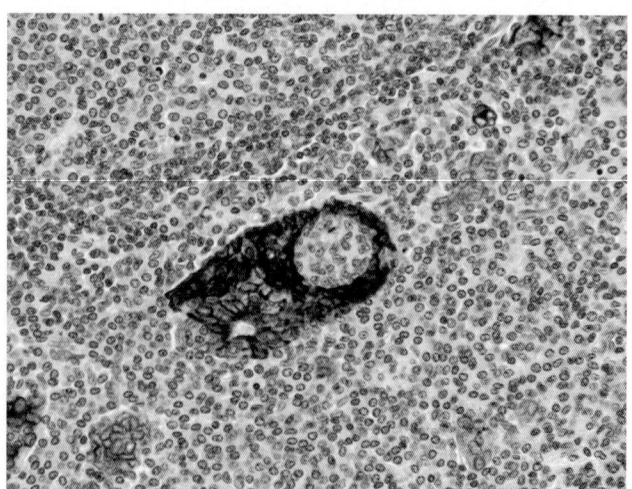

FIGURE 33.25. An immunoperoxidase stain for cytokeratin highlights the invasion of residual thyroid follicles by marginal zone lymphoma and the so-called MALT ball (immunoperoxidase stain, original magnification: 300× magnification).

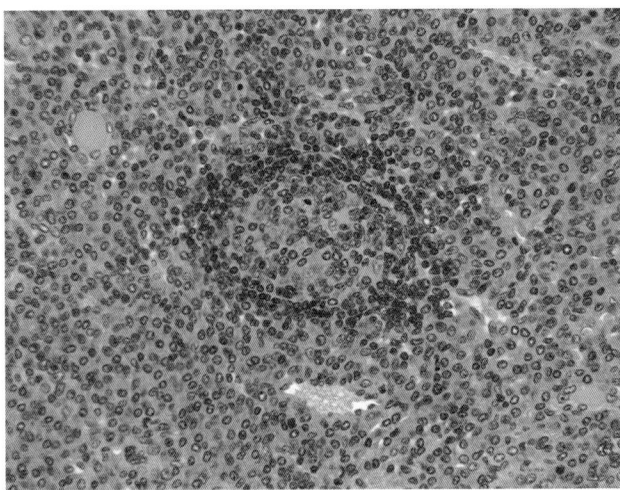
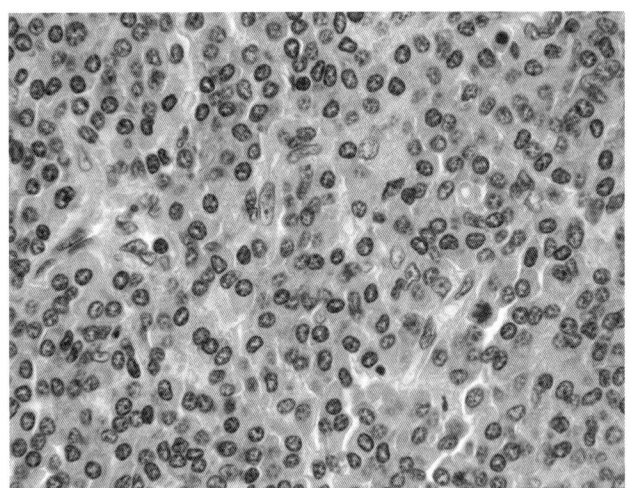

FIGURE 33.26. A: The thyroid parenchyma is practically obliterated by a marginal zone lymphoma of MALT type, which surrounds a germinal center and attenuated corona of mantle cells (hematoxylin and eosin stain, original magnification: 300× magnification). **B:** The neoplastic cells of MALT lymphomas in the thyroid often display plasmacytic features (hematoxylin and eosin stain, original magnification: 600× magnification).

but many cases have a plasmacytic appearance and in such cases monoclonality is readily demonstrable (145,147). In a small biopsy specimen, the plasma cell–rich cases of marginal zone lymphoma could be confused histologically with the sclerosing and IgG4 variants of Hashimoto thyroiditis (172,173).

The majority of lymphomas of the thyroid gland are DLBCL cases (Fig. 33.27) including immunoblastic types (147,152,158,164,169). In the SEER study, 68% of registered cases were DLBCL and in two pathology-oriented series of 108 and 53 cases of primary thyroid lymphoma, 71% and 85% of cases, respectively, were classified as DLBCL (152,164,169). As noted previously, many DLBCL cases are thought to have transformed from lymphomas of MALT based largely on a residual marginal zone component or a pattern that conforms to a marginal zone distribution (147,152,158,164,167,174). The DLBCL cases are not difficult to separate from lymphocytic thyroiditis, but they may be difficult to distinguish from carcinomas, specifically cases that in the past were interpreted as "small cell" carcinoma of thyroid. The existence of small cell undifferentiated carcinoma of the thyroid is mute, because currently almost all cases diagnosed as small cell carcinoma in the thyroid

have been reclassified retrospectively as lymphoma (175). The question of whether a thyroid neoplasm is carcinoma or lymphoma can be resolved readily with a combination of appropriate immunohistochemical studies that use antibodies directed against cytokeratin, B-cell (CD20), and T-cell (CD3) lineage antigens (Fig. 33.28).

In addition to the dominant DLBCL and marginal zone lymphomas of MALT, other categories of lymphoma may present in the thyroid including rare examples of PTCL (152,176) and occasional instances of follicular lymphoma, which, according to the SEER data, comprise 10% of thyroid lymphoma cases (147,164,169,170). In a collaborative study of 22 cases of follicular lymphoma in the thyroid, many cases exhibited concomitant chronic lymphocytic thyroiditis, contained lymphoepithelial lesions, and displayed conspicuous interfollicular lymphomatous infiltrates (177). Two groups of follicular lymphoma were identified, one of which was similar to conventional node-based follicular lymphoma of grade 1 or 2 type (Fig. 33.29); these cases mainly were CD10+ with BCL-2 expression and carried t(14;18)/*IGH/BCL2*. The second group primarily was grade 3 follicular lymphoma, often CD10-, and

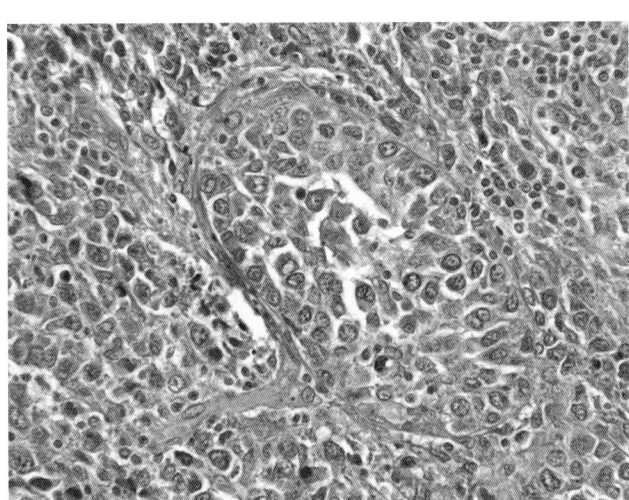

FIGURE 33.27. DLBCLs form the major histologic category of lymphoma in the thyroid gland. The infiltration and replacement of thyroid follicles by the large cells may be misinterpreted as carcinoma (hematoxylin and eosin stain, original magnification: 300× magnification).

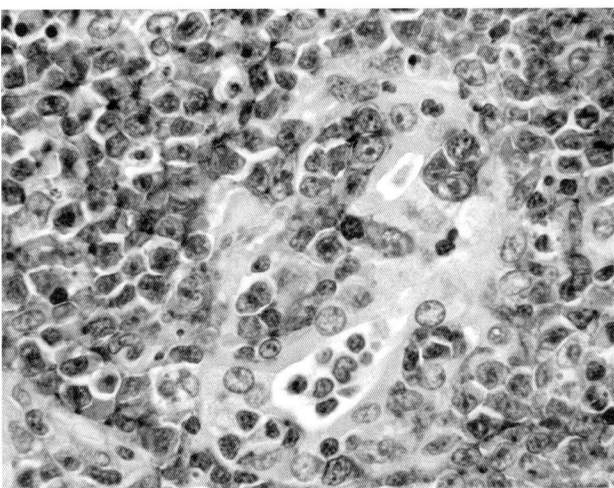

FIGURE 33.28. The neoplastic lymphoid cells express B-cell antigen CD20 to distinguish large B-cell lymphoma of the thyroid from undifferentiated carcinoma. Note that the residual thyroid follicular cells are nonreactive (immunoperoxidase stain, original magnification: 600× magnification).

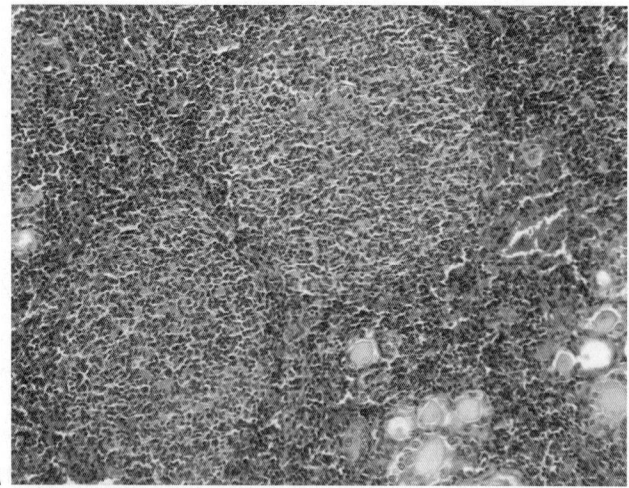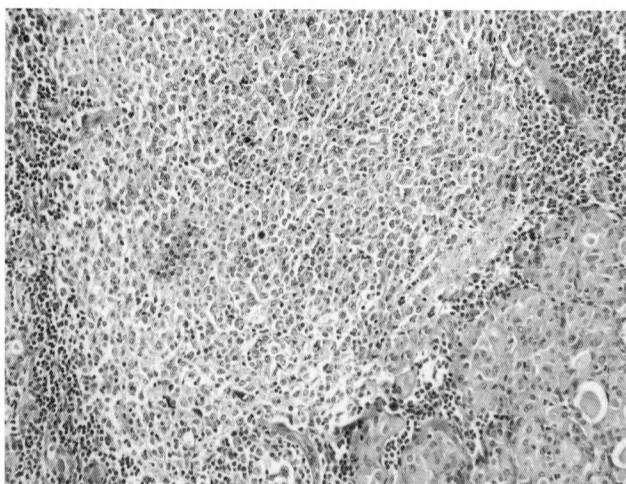

A   B

FIGURE 33.29. A: Follicular lymphoma, grade 1, in the thyroid is histologically and phenotypically similar to its nodal counterpart and generally is associated with extrathyroid disease, so as not to qualify as primary thyroid lymphoma (hematoxylin and eosin stain, original magnification: 150× magnification). **B:** In contrast, cases of follicular lymphoma, grade 3, usually lack the characteristic phenotype of follicular lymphoma (CD10⁻ and BCL2⁻), but are localized to the thyroid to correlate with primary thyroid lymphoma (hematoxylin and eosin stain, original magnification: 150× magnification).

lacked BCL-2 expression or *IGH/BCL2* (177). The latter group tally with primary lymphoma of thyroid as they tend to have localized, stage I disease, whereas the former group is associated with higher-stage disseminated lymphoma.

Immunophenotypic analysis of malignant lymphomas of the thyroid gland clearly demonstrates a preponderance of B-cell lymphomas that react with monoclonal antibodies directed against B-cell-associated antigens, such as CD20 and CD79a (145–147,158,164,175,178). Most marginal zone lymphomas of MALT in the thyroid can be differentiated from other B-cell lymphomas of small lymphocytes by using an immunohisto-chemical panel incorporating antibodies to CD5, CD10, CD20, CD23, CD43, and cyclin D1 (179). With this panel, the lymphomas of MALT in the thyroid consistently only express CD20, but, in comparison to gastric marginal zone lymphoma, exhibit limited aberrant coexpression of CD43 (147). In the thyroid, the neoplastic B cells of extranodal marginal zone lymphoma rarely display trisomy 3 and/or trisomy 18 and, like MALT lymphomas of salivary glands, the t(11;18) chromosomal translocation is uncommon (132,156,180); however, about 50% of cases harbor the t(3;14)(p14;q32) chromosomal translocation due to merging of the *IGH* gene to the *FOXP1* gene (181). These findings imply that the molecular pathogenesis of MALT lymphomas of the thyroid may be organ specific (157,181). With respect to the more prevalent DLBCL of thyroid, the genetic lesions parallel those discovered in nodal DLBCL and DLBCL in other extranodal sites and comprise trisomy 18, t(14;18) (q24;q32), 3q27 translocations with BCL-6 expression, 17p11 abnormalities, and *c-MYC/IGH* (178,180). Using the Hans algorithm, most thyroid DLBCL cases are of germinal center type and have a more favorable clinical outcome than those cases of DLBCL in the thyroid with a non–germinal center immunophenotype (19,152,178).

Patients who have malignant lymphomas of the thyroid gland have a relatively good prognosis. In the SEER report of 1,408 patients, the median overall survival was 9.3 years and the 5-year disease-specific survival was 79% (169). For patients with thyroid DLBCL, the 5-year disease-specific survival rate was 75%, whereas for those with marginal zone lymphoma, the rate was 96% (169). Similarly, other studies have described the excellent prognosis of patients who develop marginal zone lymphoma in the thyroid with disease-specific survivals at 5 years ranging from 89% to 100% (147,152,170).

Radiation therapy usually is recommended for patients who have stage IE small bulk marginal zone lymphomas of MALT in the thyroid, but these patients require close clinical follow-up due to the potential risk of recurrence and/or dissemination (154). Localized therapy usually is not an option for patients who have DLBCL of thyroid; combined modality therapy is the treatment of choice (158,165). According to an international study of patients with primary thyroid DLBCL, combined modality treatment was superior with a 90% complete remission rate compared to 76% for patients who received other forms of therapy (182); in the same study, the 5-year estimated disease-free survival was 89%. Poor performance status and advanced age correlated with decreased survival (182). Other prognostic factors include tumor stage and bulk, presence of retrosternal extension, extracapsular spread, and vascular invasion (147,165). Cases of DLBCL of the thyroid that disseminate often involve the gastrointestinal tract and this pattern of spread likely is another example of the homing tendency of lymphomas of MALT (12,165).

CENTRAL NERVOUS SYSTEM

Malignant lymphomas that originate in the CNS are relatively uncommon and represent approximately 4% of all primary brain tumors (183). Data from the SEER program from 1980 to 2008 indicate that the overall incidence rate of primary CNS lymphoma (PCNSL) was 0.47 per 100,000 person-years (183). The average annual age-adjusted incidence rate significantly increased through the mid 1990s, presumably largely due to the onset of the AIDS epidemic, but has since decreased with the advent of highly active antiretroviral therapy (184). Since then and for unknown reasons, the incidence of PCNSL is increasing among men and women alike in the immunocompetent population of the United States. SEER statistics documented a more than threefold increase in PCNSL that exceeded that of systemic lymphoma with elevation in all age groups and both genders (185); the increase has been especially dramatic in patients aged over 75 (183). Immunocompromise, however, is a predisposing factor for the development of PCNSL including those who have AIDS, congenital immunodeficiency syndromes, and organ transplantation (186–188) (see Chapter 25). EBV is implicated in the pathogenesis of PCNSL in immunocompromised patients (187–189). Employing *in situ* hybridization techniques, EBV sequences are detected in almost all PCNSL from immunocompromised patients, but are uncommon in immunocompetent patients who have PCNSL (189,190).

By definition, PCNSL arises in the brain parenchyma, spinal cord, eyes, cranial nerves, and/or meninges (191). Spinal cord lymphoma is a rare expression of PCNSL and *neurolymphomatosis*, referring to lymphoma arising in spinal nerve roots, cranial nerves, and plexus, is exceedingly rare (191,192). The typical immunocompetent patient with PCNSL is from 42 to 60 years of age. The patients often present with nonfocal and nonspecific symptoms related to elevated intracranial pressure and there frequently are general complaints of headache, lethargy, nausea, confusion, personality changes, and seizures (186,191,193). Antemortem diagnosis of lymphoma in the brain has been facilitated greatly by contrast-enhanced magnetic resonance imaging (MRI) that demonstrates an often isointense to hypointense intracranial space-occupying lesion with inconstant surrounding edema and a homogeneous diffuse pattern of enhancement (191,193). The diagnosis also is enabled by stereotactic-guided core biopsies coupled with the use of immunohistochemistry to demonstrate cell lineage and clonality (186,194); immunocytochemical studies and molecular genetic analysis of cerebrospinal fluid (CSF) lymphocytes using PCR and/or microRNAs also complement conventional cytology and allow for the accurate detection of occult PCNSL (195,196). Most PCNSL are supratentorial with a periventricular distribution, usually involving the corpus callosum, basal ganglia, or fornix (191,197). PCNSL tend to be solitary bulky tumors, immediately adjacent to the meningeal or the ventricular surfaces, and with indistinct margins that merge with the surrounding normal or edematous brain (198). Many lymphomas that are associated with AIDS have a multifocal distribution in the brain, and the lesions are dark to pale gray with indistinct borders and a granular texture (187).

The histopathologic diagnosis of PCNSL by stereotactic-guided core biopsy may be hampered by prior steroid therapy that can result in tumor lysis so that steroids need to be avoided in patients with a presumptive diagnosis of PCNSL (191,193). On microscopic examination, the typical finding is dense, concentric cuffing of lymphocytes in the perivascular spaces with diffuse centrifugal invasion into the adjacent parenchyma (190,191,198) (Fig. 33.30). Associated necrosis is frequent, and there may be extensive areas of confluent

malignant lymphoma with no perivascular relationship (198). PCNSL also may invade the dura and blood vessels, and at the periphery, a glial reaction may ensue. DLBCL and variants, including immunoblastic lymphomas, constitute the most common PCNSL and comprise up to 95% of cases so that CNS DLBCL forms a distinct subcategory in the WHO lymphoma classification scheme (191,198–200). CNS DLBCL commonly has a polymorphous appearance and exhibits variability in nuclear size and shape (199–201). Slightly more than a third of CNS DLBCL cases are associated with a reactive perivascular T-cell infiltrate that either occurs independently or is located between the vascular wall and the large lymphoma cells; such cases are reported to exhibit a significantly better overall survival than cases without a perivascular T-cell infiltrate (202). Occasionally, CNS DLBCL presents as a diffuse, infiltrating lymphoma of white matter and without formation of a cohesive mass or significant leptomeningeal involvement, a pattern referred to as *lymphomatosis cerebri* (203). Rare cases in the CNS are purely intravascular large B-cell lymphoma and these constitute a separate category in the WHO classification, distinct from CNS DLBCL (198,204,205); patients with intravascular lymphomatosis have neurologic manifestations that reflect vascular occlusive disease.

The CNS DLBCL cases express pan B-cell antigens including CD19, CD20, CD22, and CD79a with the majority also positive for BCL-2, BCL-6, and MUM1, but CD10 is expressed only in approximately 10% to 20% of cases (200). A staining panel for CD20, CD10, BCL-2, Ki-67, TdT, and EBER has been proposed to differentiate CNS DLBCL cases from other aggressive lymphomas affecting the CNS, such as lymphoblastic lymphoma, Burkitt lymphoma, and immunodeficiency-related DLBCL (193) (Table 33.4). The immunophenotypic profile of CNS DLBCL, coupled with analysis of the immunoglobulin variable region genes that demonstrate high levels of somatic mutations with intraclonal heterogeneity, indicates that the majority of cases are derived from late activated germinal center B lymphocytes (206–209). Despite this activated profile of CNS DLBCL, BCL-6 expression is regarded as a favorable prognostic factor (210,211).

The past decade has witnessed an avalanche of studies concerning the molecular pathogenesis of PCNSL, specifically CNS DLBCL, engendering excellent reviews (184,193,212). For example, chromosomal analysis of PCNSL by CGH reports frequent deletion of the long arm of chromosome 6, primarily involving 6q21-q23 (213,214) and loss of heterozygosity mapping discloses loss of one or more loci at 6q21-q23 in

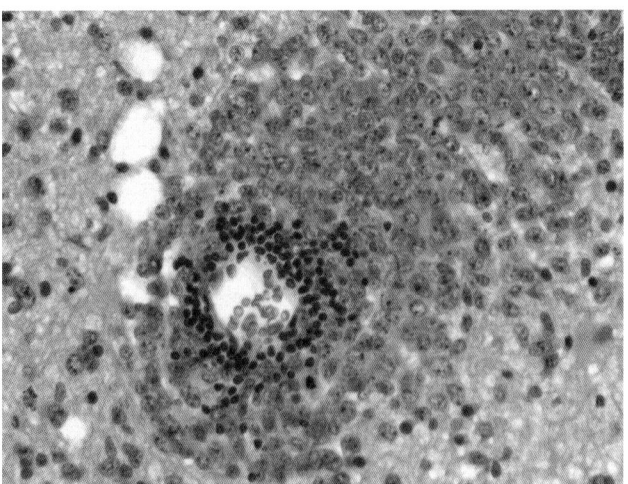

FIGURE 33.30. Primary DLBCL of the CNS characteristically concentrates around blood vessels. The perivascular small lymphocytes interposed between the vessel wall and the large lymphoma cells are reactive T cells, which are reported to be associated with a better survival in this lymphoma (hematoxylin and eosin stain, original magnification: 300× magnification).

Table 33.4	PRIMARY DLBCL OF THE CNS: PROPOSED PRIMARY STAINING PANEL FOR DIFFERENTIAL DIAGNOSIS			
Staining Panel	CNS DLBCL	Lymphoblastic Lymphoma	Burkitt Lymphoma[a]	DLBCL, Immunodeficiency Related
CD20	+	−/+	+	+
CD10	−/+	+/−	+	−/+
BCL-2	+/−	+	−[b]	+/−
Ki-67	>80%	>50%	>90%	>80%
TdT	−	+	−	−
EBER	−	−	−	+/−

[a] Staining for MYC should distinguish Burkitt lymphoma from the other entities, but the incidence of MYC positivity by immunoperoxidase in CNS DLBCL is not yet established.
[b] Partial and weak staining can be present in a minority of Burkitt lymphoma.
CNS, central nervous system; DLBCL, diffuse large B-cell lymphoma; EBER, Epstein-Barr virus encoded RNA.
Adapted with permission from Deckert M, Engert A, Brück W, et al. Modern concepts in the biology, diagnosis, differential diagnosis and treatment of primary central nervous system lymphoma. *Leukemia* 2011;25:1797–1807. Copyright © 2011. Reprinted by permission from Macmillan Publishers Ltd.

two-thirds of cases (215); the deletion incriminates the putative tumor suppressor gene *PTPRK*. Another relatively common chromosomal abnormality in PCNSL involves translocations of the *BCL6* gene, but as opposed to nodal DLBCL, the *BCL6* translocations in PCNSL engage nonimmunoglobulin partners (216,217). In PCNSL, deletions of 6q22 and *BCL6* translocations are adverse prognostic factors (218). Molecular analyses of PCNSL describe aberrant activation of the NF-κB pathway with increased expression of NF-κB regulating genes, genes of the NF-κB complex, and NF-κB target genes (219,220). *MALT1* gene amplification and activating mutations of the oncogene *CARD11* in a minority of PCNSL cases likely contribute to the NF-κB activation (216,220). In comparison to nodal DLBCL, PCNSL exhibits a distinct pattern of microRNA expression with up-regulation of the Myc pathway, blocking of terminal B-cell differentiation, or up-regulation by inflammatory cytokines, whereas putative tumor suppressor microRNAs are down-regulated (221). Using GEP, one report verified that PCNSL cases are derived from a late germinal center B cell (222). In another GEP study, high expression of activated STAT6 was associated with a short survival in patients who were treated with high-dose intravenous methotrexate (223). Two other analyses described that, among others, extracellular matrix and cell adhesion–related pathways are important in the pathogenesis of PCNSL (224,225); up-regulation of the extracelluar matrix gene osteopontin (*SPP1*) can be demonstrated by immunohistochemistry in the malignant cells of PCNSL (224,226). In addition, JAK-1 displays increased expression by GEP to also significantly implicate the JAK-STAT pathway in the pathogenesis of PCNSL (223,225). Notwithstanding this impressive body of investigation, the exact pathogenesis of PCNSL remains unresolved (193).

In addition to DLBCL, Burkitt lymphoma occurs in the CNS, but Hodgkin lymphoma rarely is encountered as a PCNSL (198,199,201,227) (see Chapter 15). T-cell lymphomas also are uncommon in the CNS, and most examples are reported in series of PCNSL from the Far East where CNS DLBCL still predominates (197,198,228). Paradoxically, the largest series of T-cell PCNSL comprising 45 patients is a multi-institutional study from North America and Europe (229). Like CNS DLBCL, the T-cell cases tend to be angiocentric, but most examples consist of small or small to medium-sized lymphocytes (228) (Fig. 33.31). The remaining T-cell

cases are constituted by pleomorphic or medium to large cells encompassing cases of ALCL (229). Rare examples of primary NKTCL of the CNS also are described (230). Even less common are reports of primary histiocytic sarcoma of the CNS (231); the latter entity evokes a broad differential diagnosis necessitating a thorough immunohistochemical panel for diagnosis (193).

Primary low-grade lymphomas of the CNS likewise are exceptional and the B-cell cases mainly include those classified as lymphoplasmacytic lymphoma and small lymphocytic lymphoma, not otherwise classified (232). Extranodal marginal zone lymphoma of MALT type also arises in the CNS, but these mainly are dura-based (233–235). Morphologically, the cases in the dura are similar to MALT lymphomas in other regions as they are composed of small lymphocytes with admixed centrocyte-like or monocytoid cells and variable numbers of germinal centers; moreover, the cases in dura chiefly are rich in plasma cells (Fig. 33.32). The plasma cells are clonal and associated amyloid deposition may be observed (233,235). With the exception of one report of *IgH/MALT1* translocation (236), cases presenting in dura do not exhibit the translocations associated with extranodal marginal zone lymphoma; by FISH, however, trisomies arise, mainly trisomy 3 (233,235). In marginal zone lymphoma of dura, the predominant plasma cell population raises the differential diagnosis with IgG4-related disease (4). IgG4-related disease rarely can manifest in the CNS, as, for example, in the thoracic dura as IgG4-related sclerosing pachymeningitis (237). Immunoperoxidase staining of plasma cells in extranodal marginal zone lymphoma of dura reveals numerous IgG4+ cells, but unlike IgG4-related disease, the IgG4+ plasma cells in the marginal zone lymphoma cases are monoclonal (235). Although the IgG4+ marginal zone lymphoma cases could indicate antecedent IgG4-related disease, they more likely represent pristine IgG4+ extranodal marginal zone lymphoma. Clinically, primary extranodal marginal zone MALT-type lymphomas of dura usually affect females who present with localized intracranial masses that often mimic a meningioma (233–235). Similar to other MALT lymphomas, the prognosis is favorable with few recurrences; surgery plus radiation and/or chemotherapy allows for complete remission (233–235).

Although primary lymphomas of the CNS are increasing in frequency, secondary lymphomatous involvement in patients who have systemic lymphoma is more common. Secondary lymphomas of the CNS tend to infiltrate the leptomeninges and

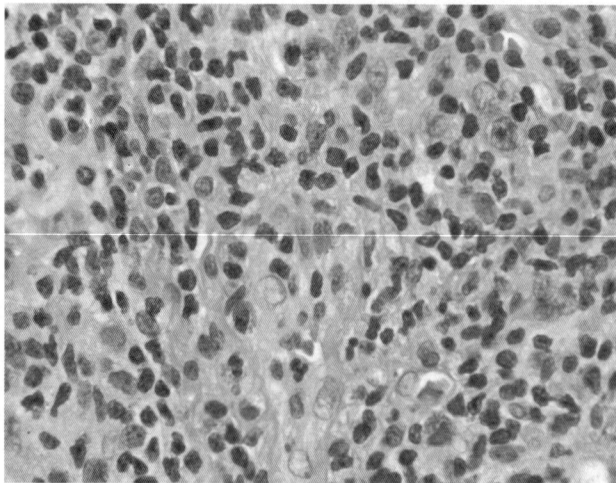

FIGURE 33.31. Primary PTCL in the frontal lobe exhibits an angiocentric distribution identical to the more common large B-cell lymphomas of the CNS. In contrast to large B-cell lymphoma, the neoplastic T cells are small to medium sized with distinct nuclear membrane irregularities. In this case, the diagnosis was supported by the demonstration of a T-cell gene rearrangement (hematoxylin and eosin stain, original magnification: 600× magnification).

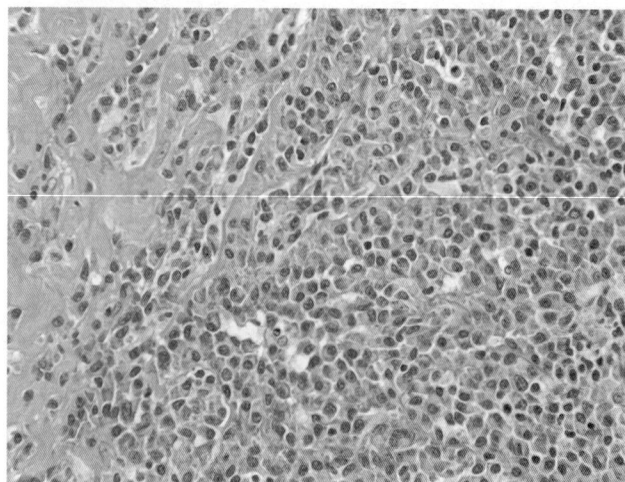

FIGURE 33.32. In the dura, a marginal zone lymphoma of MALT forms a dense infiltrate and is dominated by plasma cells. The plasma cells in MALT lymphomas of the dura may be chiefly IgG4+, but unlike IgG4-related disease, the plasma cells are monoclonal (hematoxylin and eosin stain, original magnification: 300× magnification).

involve the CSF, but otherwise their distribution is similar to that of PCNSL. Although conventional cytologic examination of the CSF is used to diagnose secondary CNS lymphoma, flow cytometry analysis improves sensitivity and needs to be performed in conjunction with cytology to augment the diagnosis (238). Almost all secondary lymphomas are aggressive forms of malignant lymphoma and the risk is greatest for patients who have lymphoblastic and Burkitt lymphoma with a 24% incidence of CNS recurrence (239). DLBCL is the most frequent lymphoma to secondarily affect the CNS and in a collaborative study of 113 patients, the median time from systemic lymphoma to CNS relapse was 1.8 years (240). An elevated serum lactate dehydrogenase, involvement of more than one extranodal site, advanced stage, high IPI score, and involvement of specific extranodal sites, mainly testes, orbit, and paranasal sinuses, prove to be risk factors for CNS recurrence among patients who have DLBCL (239). Because CNS prophylaxis carries the hazard of neurotoxicity, prophylactic chemotherapy is required only for those patients at greatest risk. As expected, the prognosis of secondary CNS dissemination of lymphoma is dismal with a median survival of 4 to 5 months (239). Historically, the prognosis of PCNSL is similarly poor. Using SEER statistics from 1975 to 1999, the median survival for an immunocompetent cohort of 1,565 patients with PCNSL was 9 months (241). Rather than exclusive treatment with intracranial radiation therapy, the current use of antimetabolites, such as methotrexate and cytarabine, has evolved as the mainstay of therapy of PCNSL. In contemporary trials employing this form of chemotherapy, with or without radiation therapy, the overall survival of PCNSL at 5 years ranges from 25% to 56% (191).

TESTIS

Malignant lymphomas of the testis represent approximately 0.6% of all non-Hodgkin lymphoma cases in the United States and comprise up to 9% of testicular neoplasms, but they are the most common testicular malignancy after the age of 60 years with a raising incidence (242,243). Although some patients who have testicular lymphoma are discovered to have widespread disease at the time of presentation, almost 80% of patients have localized stage IE and IIE primary testicular lymphoma (244,245). Approximately 20% of patients have initial involvement of both testes (243). The most common presenting symptom is painless testicular enlargement of generally short duration (243,246). Some patients present with constitutional symptoms at the time of diagnosis and this is associated with more aggressive disease (246). There are no known predisposing causes for primary lymphomas of the testis, including no known association with an undescended testis.

Testicular lymphomas range from <1 to 16 cm in diameter with an average of 4 to 6 cm (246–248). The tumors are almost always covered by an attenuated, but intact, tunica vaginalis. Involvement of the epididymis is common, as is invasion of the tunica albuginea, and in some patients, the lymphomas extend to the spermatic cord (246,248). In rare instances, the lymphoma is confined to the epididymis or to the spermatic cord (249). On cut section of the cases arising in the testis, the parenchyma is diffusely replaced by a circumscribed tumor mass that varies from gray to light tan (Fig. 33.33); in some cases, there may be foci of hemorrhage and necrosis.

Usually, no difficulty arises in distinguishing a lymphoma in the testis from reactive lymphoid hyperplasia because testicular low-grade lymphomas are uncommon, and most reactive lymphocytic infiltrates conform to the appearance of granulomatous or nongranulomatous lymphocytic orchitis. Granulomatous orchitis is an uncommon inflammatory condition of unknown etiology typified by extensive destruction of seminiferous tubules due to tubular and interstitial granulomatous

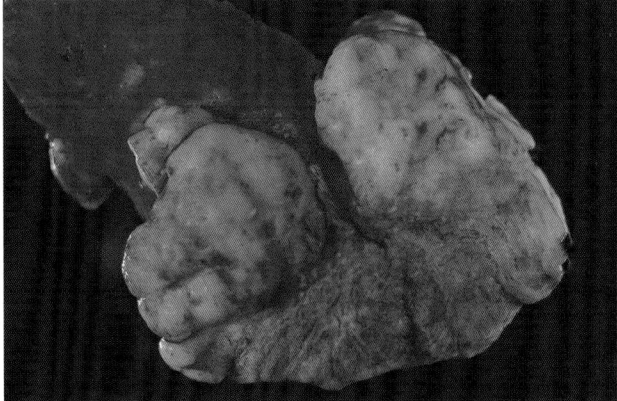

FIGURE 33.33. The bisected testis contains a large, bulky, nodular lymphomatous tumor mass that replaces most of the testicular stroma.

inflammation with multinucleated giant cells and fibrosis (250). Lymphocytic orchitis is an inflammatory lymphocytic infiltrate composed of small lymphocytes with scattered germinal centers (251). Like most reactive lymphoid proliferations and inflammatory pseudotumors, nongranulomatous lymphocytic orchitis is associated with a polymorphous cell population, including plasma cells and macrophages, and with fibrosis. The fibrosis tends to be in the interstitium and the infiltrate encases the seminiferous tubules (251) (Fig. 33.34). Viral-type orchitis is another process that can mimic lymphoma because of a lymphohistiocytic infiltrate that involves seminiferous tubules and the interstitium (252). Testicular lymphoma also may be simulated by rare examples of Rosai-Dorfman disease that present as a testicular mass (253).

Up to 90% of malignant lymphomas of the testis display large cell (including immunoblastic) histologies and are of B-cell origin (246–248,254,255). Although myeloid sarcoma and perhaps plasmacytoma should be considered in the diagnosis, the main differential diagnosis is seminoma (243,248,256–258). In contrast with seminoma, the margins of an aggressive lymphoma are infiltrative and without a pushing border. DLBCL exhibits a diffuse intertubular growth pattern and tends to surround and invade seminiferous tubules with frequent disruption of the basement membranes (247,248) (Fig. 33.35). Sclerosis and tubular atrophy are common and vascular invasion by lymphoma can be highlighted with the use of an elastic

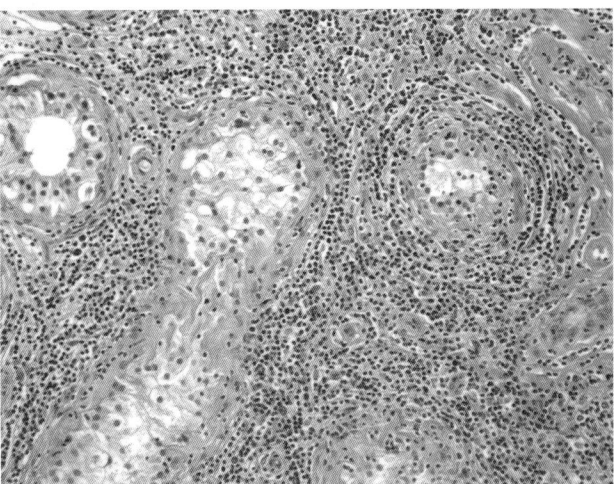

FIGURE 33.34. Lymphocytic orchitis of the nongranulomatous type forms a dense infiltrate and surrounds seminiferous tubules (hematoxylin and eosin stain, original magnification: 150× magnification).

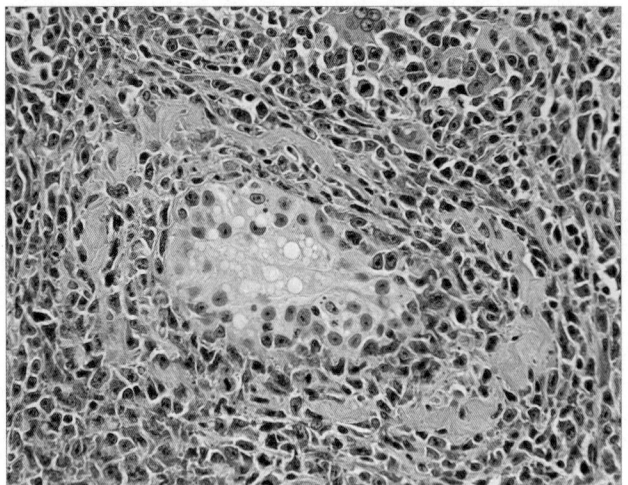

FIGURE 33.35. Primary DLBCL of the testis encircles and invades seminiferous tubules, leading to disruption of the basement membranes (hematoxylin and eosin stain, original magnification: 300× magnification).

stain or an appropriate marker for endothelial cells, such as CD31. Often, the periphery of the lymphoma contains a benign-appearing lymphocytic infiltrate composed of small lymphocytes and plasma cells.

Testicular DLBCL cases express the usual complement of B-cell antigens, such as CD20 (248,254,255). Using CD10, BCL-6, and MUM1, immunohistochemical studies reveal that DLBCL of the testis conforms to the non–germinal center group and displays a high proliferative rate with Ki-67 (19,255,259,260). GEP studies corroborate the immunohistochemical results by demonstrating an activated B-cell gene expression pattern (261). As well, most examples of testicular DLBCL demonstrate molecular evidence of ongoing mutations, as indicated by intraclonal variation in immunoglobulin heavy chain gene sequences (254); this observation supports the contention that large B-cell lymphomas of the testis are related to other antigen exposure, or postgerminal center cell lymphocytes.

Like DLBCL of the CNS, DLBCL cases in the testis are regarded as inhabiting an immunoprivileged site and cases in both CNS and testis exhibit decrease or loss of HLA class I and II expression, which may aid the lymphoma to escape immune attack (262,263). Using array CGH, loss of 6p21.3-p25.3,

including the *HLA* genes, was shown to be linked with DLBCL of both CNS and testis, in contrast to node-based DLBCL (264). Unlike CNS DLBCL, testicular cases were associated with gain of 19q13.12-q13.43 and analysis of candidate genes in site-specific regions uncovered two major gene groups—one involved in the immune response, including regulation of HLA expression, and the second involved in apoptosis, including the p53 pathway (264). Although DLBCL of both the CNS and testis share aberrations, these results indicate that site-specific aberrations also develop and that they do not form a single entity. For DLBCL of the testis, moreover, numerical aberrations, specifically trisomy 1, 3, and/or 18, are frequent and one case has been described with both trisomy 3 and t(14;18)(q32;q21) with breakpoints in *IGH* and *MALT1* to suggest that some cases of testicular DLBL are linked to extranodal marginal zone lymphoma (180).

In addition to the more prevalent DLBCL, a variety of other non-Hodgkin lymphomas manifest in the testis. Like Waldeyer ring, primary follicular lymphoma, grade 3, can arise localized to the testis of children (26,265). The neoplastic centroblasts in the follicles invade between seminiferous tubules and lack complete mantle cell cuffs. Despite the follicular architecture and B-cell immunophenotype, the pediatric cases do not express BCL-2 protein or have demonstrable *IgH/BCL2* gene rearrangements; in contrast, the childhood testicular lymphoma cases are positive for CD10 and BCL-6 and may show a *BCL6* gene rearrangement, implying that pediatric follicular lymphomas in the testis are distinct (26,265). Rare cases of adult testicular follicular lymphoma that are virtually identical to the examples of pediatric follicular lymphoma also have been described (266); the adult patients tend to be age 35 or younger and, like the pediatric cases, have localized and clinically indolent lymphoma. Occasionally, T-cell lymphomas primarily occur in the testis, comprising ALCL (Fig. 33.36) and NKTCL types (64,65,267,268). NKTCL of the testis is histologically and immunophenotypically similar to those in the sinonasal region, including the tendency for angiocentric growth and necrosis (268). They also have an aggressive clinical course.

Historically, primary lymphomas of the testis, specifically DLBCL, have been considered to have a particularly ominous prognosis. Despite localized disease at presentation, in one study 80% of patients experienced recurrence, including late recurrence, that was unaffected by treatment (244). Recurrences tend to involve extranodal sites including CNS, Waldeyer ring, skin, lung, and the contralateral testis (243,244); the CNS often

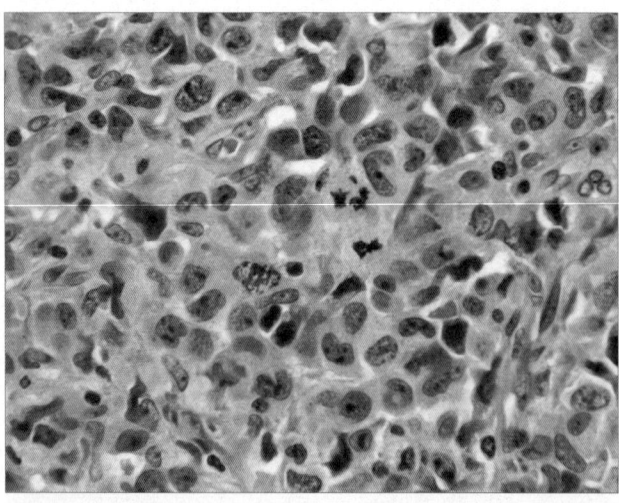

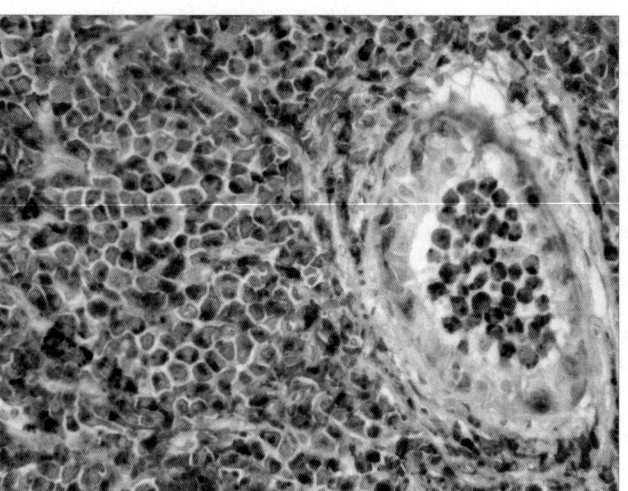

A   **B**

FIGURE 33.36. A: Markedly pleomorphic large cells are evident in ALCL of the testis. Some large cells conform to "hallmark" cells (hematoxylin and eosin stain, original magnification: 600× magnification). **B:** In addition to expressing T-cell antigens (*not shown*), the ALCL exhibits characteristic reactivity for CD30; however, ALK was not expressed (immunoperoxidase stain, original magnification: 300× magnification).

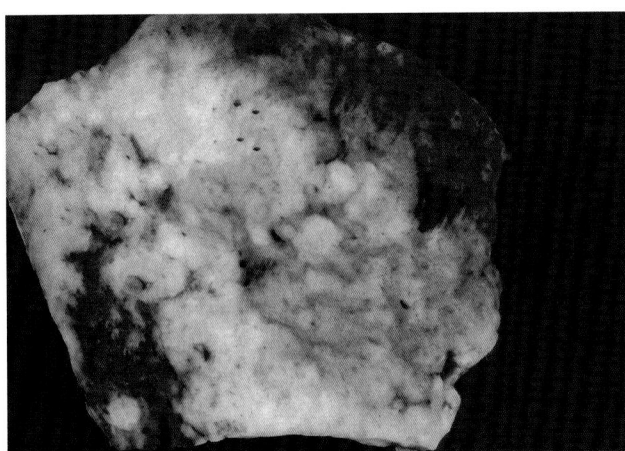

FIGURE 33.37. Malignant lymphoma in the ovary forms a large fleshy mass with areas of hemorrhage and degeneration.

is an isolated site of recurrence. However, recent advances in therapy have resulted in dramatic improvement in prognosis. For example, in an analysis of 75 patients with primary testicular DLBCL who were diagnosed between 1964 and 2008, and who underwent pathologic confirmation of diagnosis, the 5-year overall survival for patients treated prior to 1977 was 15.4%, whereas patients who were treated between 1997 and 1999 and mainly received combination chemotherapy with cyclophosphamide, doxorubicin, vincristine, and prednisone (CHOP) had a 5-year overall survival of 56.3% (269). In comparison, for those patients treated after 2000 and who received rituximab in addition to CHOP (R-CHOP) plus intrathecal chemotherapy and scrotal radiotherapy, the 5-year overall survival was 86.6%. An international trial of 53 patients with untreated stage I and II testicular DLBCL that employed a similar modern therapeutic regimen reported an essentially identical 5-year overall survival rate of 85% (270); the 5-year cumulative incidence of CNS relapse was 6%, but no contralateral testicular relapses developed.

FEMALE GENITAL TRACT

Malignant lymphomas that manifest in the female genital tract are exceedingly unusual, with the ovary being the most frequently involved site. In a study from the Armed Forces

Institute of Pathology, only 19 of 9,500 women (0.2%) who had lymphoma initially manifested the disease in the ovary (271). An exception to the rarity of lymphomas in the ovary is found in African countries in which Burkitt lymphoma is endemic (272); in these areas, the ovaries are second only to the jaw in frequency of presentation. Involvement of the ovary by lymphoma can be a result of primary ovarian lymphoma, the initial manifestation of clinically occult disease in lymph nodes, or as a late complication of widespread lymphoma (246). The definition of primary includes not only stage IE cases but also cases limited to the female genital tract irrespective of involvement of more than one genital tract site (273). A report from the combined files of two major American lymphoma treatment centers found only eight cases that were regarded as primary ovarian stage IE ovarian lymphoma (274). However, a recent study from a major lymphoma repository center discovered 186 cases of lymphoma in the female genital tract over a 30-year period of which 117 (63%) were considered primary (273). In that series, the ovary/adnexa was the most common site of lymphoma, with 45 cases limited to that organ. This figure far surpasses other studies, many of which include cases of lymphoma that present in the ovary, but actually have disseminated disease (246,271,275).

An ovary involved by lymphoma may be massive and measure more than 20 cm in diameter and frequently there is bilateral ovarian lymphoma (246,273,275,276). The capsule usually is intact, but, on the cut surface, the ovarian stroma is replaced by a lobulated, often bosselated gray-tan fleshy mass with frequent areas of necrosis and cystic degeneration (246,271,276) (Fig. 33.37). Although follicular lymphomas and lymphoblastic lymphomas can manifest in the ovary, most are DLBCL and Burkitt lymphoma (246,273–276) (Fig. 33.38); the latter tend to predominate in patients younger than 20 years of age. The corpora lutea and albicantes often are spared and the lymphomas surround rather than replace these structures (246,271). Primary follicular lymphomas in the ovary parallel those in the thyroid and testis (177,266,277). These follicular lymphomas mainly are grade 3, are negative or weakly positive for BCL-2 protein expression, lack *IGH/BCL2* translocations, and are confined to the ovary (277). Alternatively, and like the thyroid, follicular lymphomas of grade 1 type in the ovary express BCL-2, exhibit *IGH/BCL* translocations, and have advanced-stage disease, so that they are unlikely to originate in the ovary (177,277).

Diffuse lymphomas in the ovary have a curious tendency to grow in cords with almost a linear pattern of infiltration (271,275,276) (Fig. 33.39). This linear pattern raises the

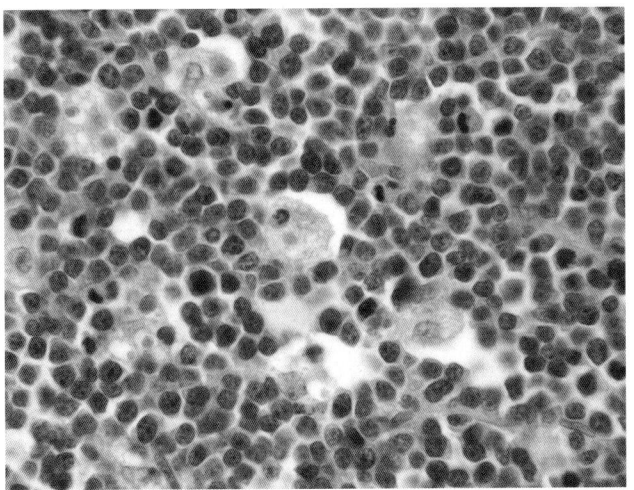

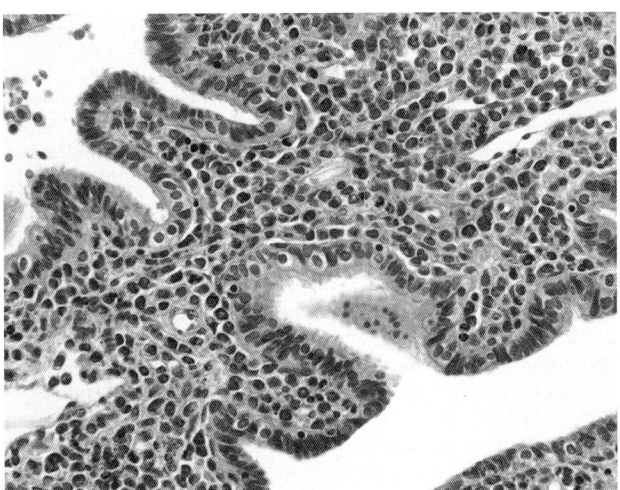

FIGURE 33.38. A: Burkitt-type lymphoma is the most common malignant lymphoma to involve the ovary in young women (hematoxylin and eosin stain, original magnification: 600× magnification). **B:** In this case, the adjacent fallopian tube also was involved by Burkitt lymphoma (hematoxylin and eosin stain, original magnification: 300× magnification).

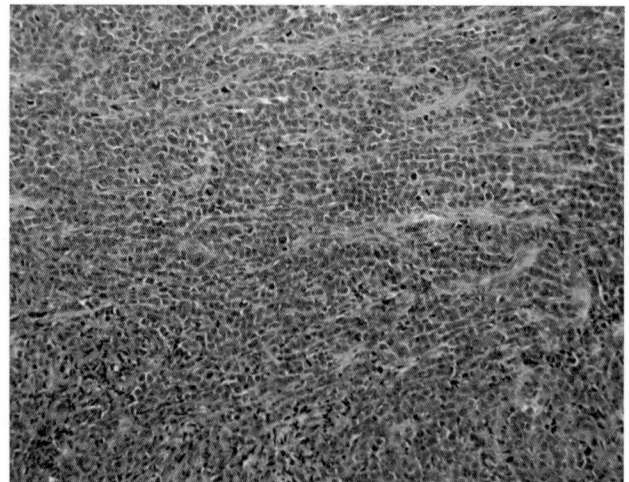

FIGURE 33.39. Ovarian lymphomas occasionally have a cordlike pattern of infiltration and resemble an epithelial malignancy or myeloid sarcoma (hematoxylin and eosin stain, original magnification: 150× magnification).

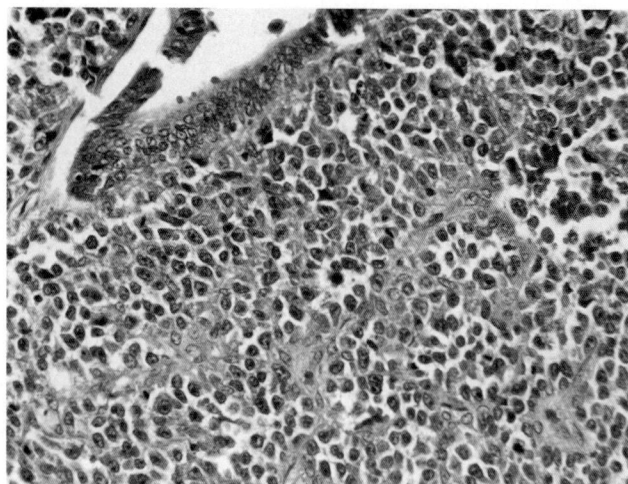

FIGURE 33.40. DLBCL is the most common primary lymphoma of the cervix (hematoxylin and eosin stain, original magnification: 300× magnification).

differential diagnosis of myeloid sarcoma, which also may manifest initially in the ovary as well as in other sites of the female genital tract (271,276,278); the recognition of eosinophilic myelocytes is helpful in the diagnosis, but most cases do not exhibit myeloid differentiation histologically and are characterized by primitive, blastlike nuclear features. The use of the naphthol–ASD–chloracetate esterase stain and immunoperoxidase stains for myeloperoxidase, lysozyme, and CD117, as well as reactivity for B- and T-cell antigens, are valuable in separating myeloid sarcoma from malignant lymphoma (278). Immunologic studies on lymphomas of the ovary have demonstrated that almost all the lymphomas have a B-cell immunophenotype (273,275). In addition to myeloid sarcoma, the major differential diagnosis of ovarian lymphomas includes dysgerminoma, undifferentiated carcinoma, metastatic carcinoma, especially those from the breast, primary small cell carcinoma, and adult granulosa cell tumor (276). Careful examination of the morphologic characteristics of the neoplasm and employment of immunohistochemical studies, such as antibodies against B- and T-cell antigens, as well as cytokeratin, should resolve this differential diagnosis. Unlike patients with disseminated disease at the time of diagnosis of ovarian lymphoma, those with actual primary lymphoma of the ovary appear to have an excellent prognosis irrespective of the histologic classification of the lymphoma (274,275,277).

Malignant lymphomas that arise in other sites of the female genital tract, including the cervix, uterine corpus, vagina, and vulva, are less common than those in the ovary, although these sites frequently are involved in cases of disseminated lymphoma (279–281). Patients regularly present with vaginal bleeding and the cervix is engaged more often than the other genital sites. In the cervix, the tumors may appear sessile or polypoid or may manifest as diffuse circumferential enlargement to assume a barrel shape, without evident mucosal abnormalities (276,282,283). DLBCL predominates (Fig. 33.40), and includes the sarcomatoid variant, but, unlike primary lymphomas of the ovary, lymphomas in the cervix, uterine corpus, and vagina encompass marginal zone lymphomas of MALT type (273,279,280,282–287). The marginal zone cases are more prevalent in the endometrium where they generally are discovered as incidental microscopic findings without grossly evident tumors (285,286). They largely are confined to the endometrium, but may obliterate endometrial glands and extend to the fallopian tube and/or invade myometrium (273,286). The lymphomas, composed of marginal zone-type B cells, form nodular aggregates without visible germinal centers. Staining with CD21 identifies remnants

of follicular dendritic networks in the nodular aggregates to suggest colonization of preexisting follicles by the neoplastic marginal zone cells (286). The marginal zone lymphomas of endometrium exhibit CD43 coexpression and proliferative activity with Ki-67 is low (273,285). In the one case that was examined for chromosomal abnormalities, translocations associated with lymphomas of MALT were absent (286). Nonetheless, the lymphoma presumably arises from endometrial lymphatic tissue or MALT and, parallel to marginal zone lymphoma of MALT in other sites, the clinical course appears indolent. Rarely, other low-grade lymphomas arise in the female genital tract, such as primary lymphoplasmacytic lymphoma that have been reported in the vagina and vulva in patients over 60 years of age (273).

The marginal zone and lymphoplasmacytic lymphomas of the lower female genital tract, especially cervix, must be separated from chronic inflammatory reactions including chronic endometritis, severe chronic cervicitis, and florid reactive lymphoid hyperplasia (lymphoma-like lesion) (288,289). The reactive lesions are characterized by a mixed lymphocytic infiltrate, including varying numbers of immunoblasts, with frequent accompanying erosion and ulceration of cervical squamous mucosa (288,289) (Fig. 33.41). Unlike malignant lymphomas,

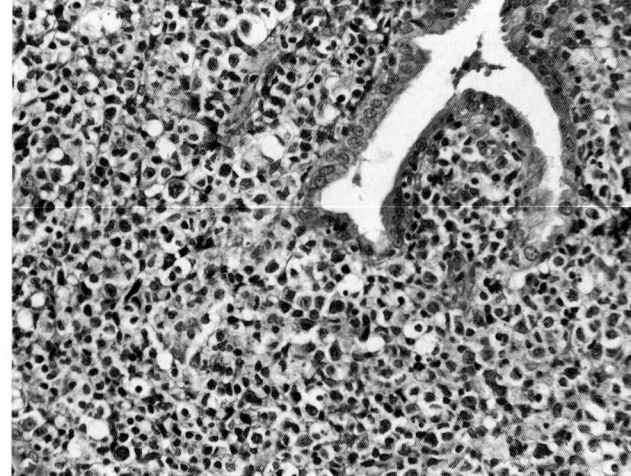

FIGURE 33.41. Biopsy of a weeping lesion of the uterine cervix in a 19-year-old patient with known infectious mononucleosis results in florid reactive lymphoid hyperplasia. The reactive immunoblasts could be confused with malignant lymphoma, but the infiltrate is polymorphous and exhibits an orderly range of lymphocytic transformation (hematoxylin and eosin stain, original magnification: 300× magnification).

florid reactive lymphoid hyperplasias in the lower female genital tract are superficial and do not form tumor masses. As opposed to the monomorphous infiltrates of marginal zone lymphomas, the lymphocytic infiltrates in the florid reactive hyperplasia cases are polymorphous and similar to other extranodal reactive lymphoid proliferations. The reactive cases are composed of a mixture of B and T cells, although the B cells may form aggregates and in some cases EBER is positive (289). By immunohistochemistry, there is no immunoglobulin light chain restriction, but, by PCR, monoclonal immunoglobulin heavy chain gene rearrangements are detectable in a subset of cases (288,289). Nonetheless, follow-up studies have not shown the development of lymphoma. The etiology is uncertain, but might be related to infection or reaction to prior surgery (289).

Many patients who have lymphomas of the cervix have stage IE disease; in one review, there was only one treatment failure among 28 patients whose treatment included radiation therapy and whose cases were followed for at least 2 years (283). This experience suggests that most patients who have stage IE lymphomas of the cervix are amenable to cure and, because the site of lymphoma is so unusual, an individualized approach to therapy is required (290).

 | # BONE

Malignant lymphomas that arise in bone are uncommon neoplasms, and any one institution requires long periods to accumulate sufficient cases for morphologic and clinical analysis. In the biggest published series, 422 cases were collected over a 76-year span (291). On review, the largest group (42%) had apparent primary lymphoma of bone, but other patients had multifocal osseous lymphoma, and others had evidence of extraosseous lymphoma. Patients with multiple sites of bone involvement are included as primary lymphomas of bone, stage IV, but those with extraosseous disease at presentation are not included (292). The definition of primary lymphomas of bone also does not encompass those uncommon cases that are limited to the bone marrow and are without features of a localized bone tumor and destruction of bone trabeculae (293). The peak incidence of bone lymphoma is in the fifth decade, but the age range is wide and bone lymphomas can occur in pediatric patients (291,294,295). Various sites are involved, with the most prevalent being the femur and other tubular long bones, maxilla and mandible, pelvic bones, and spine (291,294,296).

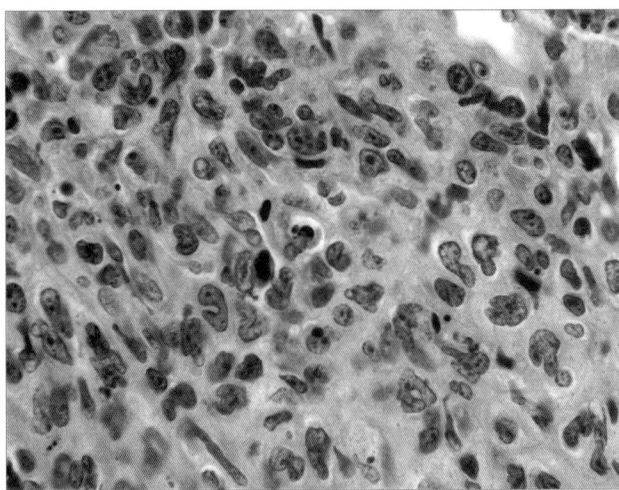

FIGURE 33.43. DLBCL is the most common type of primary lymphoma of bone and, as in this case, the large cells often have irregular nuclear contours, including multilobated shapes (hematoxylin and eosin stain, original magnification: 600× magnification).

The most common symptoms are local pain with occasional associated soft tissue swelling, a mass, or both (291,295,297). Radiologic studies show variable changes, but predominately destructive osteolytic lesions and, in some instances, cortical breakthrough, pathologic fracture, and soft tissue masses may develop (294,297,298) (Fig. 33.42). In the assessment of primary lymphoma of bone, MRI is the more accurate modality, typically registering marrow replacement, and is especially valuable in the evaluation of an accompanying soft tissue mass, spine involvement, and spinal cord compression (294,297).

Most bone lymphomas are classified as DLBCL, including those from the Far East (292,295–303). The large cells chiefly are centroblasts, but some cases may be composed of large clear cells (299,300). The lymphoma may be monomorphous or polymorphous. A curious feature of DLBCL of bone, which has not been widely described in DLBCL that occur in other extranodal sites, is the presence of complex nuclear contours; the large cells frequently are portrayed as multilobated (298–301) (Fig. 33.43). Fibrosis that ranges from delicate reticulin fibrosis to dense sclerosis with osteoid formation commonly occurs in association with DLBCL of bone (291). The lymphoma cells often are entrapped within the fibrous connective tissue and

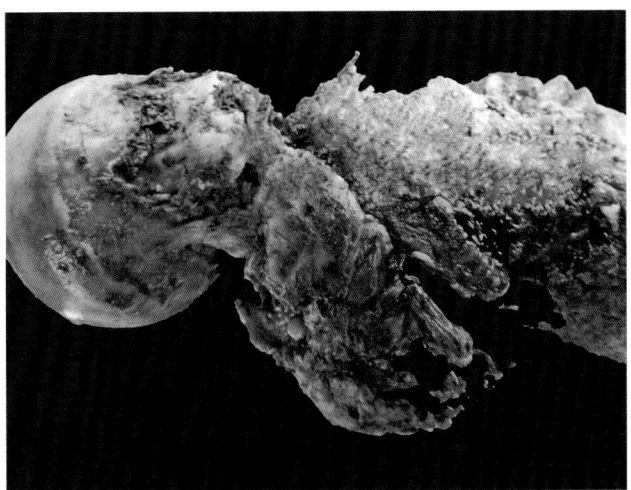

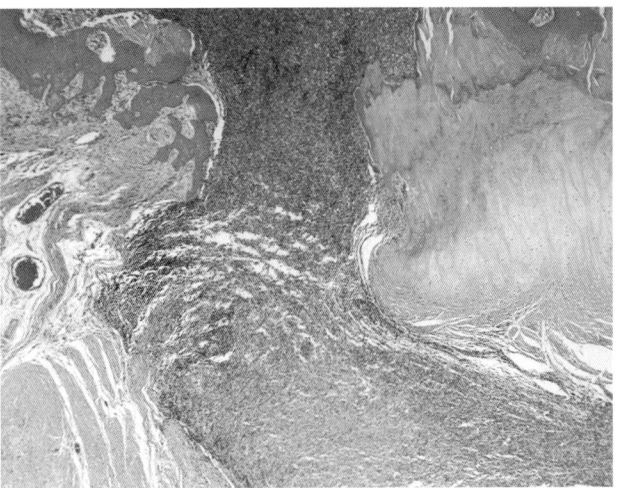

FIGURE 33.42. A: Resection of proximal femur with a pathologic fracture due to DLBCL of bone. **B:** Microscopic equivalent of **(A)** with invasion by the large B-cell lymphoma through the bone cortex into soft tissue (hematoxylin and eosin stain, original magnification: 30× magnification).

may appear spindled or may form small clusters that resemble carcinoma. An accurate diagnosis can be hampered not only because of the fibrosis but also because of decalcification and crush artifact (304); therefore, to establish the diagnosis more than one biopsy procedure may be required (294).

Immunologic studies indicate that cases of DLBCL of bone exhibit the immunophenotype of either germinal center or non–germinal center types and that, in general, the germinal center–like cases have the more favorable prognosis, whereas the non–germinal cases are characterized by an adverse prognosis to correlate with the proposition of the Hans algorithm (19,299,300); however, one study of 36 cases reported that survival of DLBCL of bone was independent of the germinal center or non–germinal center phenotype (305). By FISH, slightly more than a quarter of bone DLBCL cases show a BCL2 rearrangement to parallel that found in DLBCL of lymph nodes, but higher than found in other extranodal sites (306). Rearrangement of c-MYC is detected in fewer than 10% of cases, but to date, there are no correlative studies between c-MYC rearrangement and clinical outcome. Genetic studies using array-based CGH and FISH identify recurrent genomic aberrations including loss of 14q32, trisomy 7, gain of 1q, and amplification of 2p16.1 (307). These chromosomal aberrations differ from those found in other extranodal lymphomas and support the perception that DLBCL of bone is a distinct entity (307).

In addition to large B-cell lymphomas, ALCL may manifest in bone, as can cases of Hodgkin lymphoma (see Chapter 15), and precursor B-cell lymphoblastic lymphomas (298,302,303,308–312). The cases of osseous precursor B-cell lymphoblastic lymphoma often present as a lytic lesion and must be differentiated from other small round cell tumors of bone including Ewing sarcoma. Osteolytic lesions also are common in ALCL of bone, which develop in children as well as adults (302,303,308,309). Ewing sarcoma forms part of the clinical differential diagnosis, as does osteomyelitis and a metastatic lesion (308,309). The anaplastic cases almost always are composed of pleomorphic large cells that express CD30 and epithelial membrane antigen, and the majority have a demonstrable T-cell phenotype; however, anaplastic lymphoma kinase (ALK) expression is inconsistent (302,308,309). Most patients with ALCL of bone pursue an aggressive clinical course (302,308).

According to SEER figures, 1,500 adult patients were identified with primary lymphoma of bone from 1973 through 2005; the 5- and 10-year survival rates were 58% and 45%, respectively (313). DLBCL comprised 70.6% of the cases and multivariate analysis revealed that younger age and localized disease were independent predictors of survival (313). Younger age, combined with the IPI score, also were significant prognostic factors in a more controlled study from a single institution that analyzed 103 patients with DLBCL of bone (292). The 5-year overall survival of the 103 patients was 62%, but for patients under age 60 with an IPI of 1 to 3, the 5-year overall survival was 90%. Patients 60 years and older with an IPI of 0 to 3 or the same age range with an IPI of 4 to 5 had 5-year overall survivals of 61% and 25%, respectively (292). The more recent use of R-CHOP has furthered the response and survival of patients with primary DLBCL of bone (292,314).

BREAST

Although well recognized, primary malignant lymphomas of breast are rare and constitute <0.5% of primary malignant mammary tumors and fewer than 2% of all primary extranodal lymphomas (304,315). One major issue concerns the definition of primary malignant lymphomas of the breast. Most investigators include all cases in which the breast is the first site of presentation and with no evidence of extramammary lymphoma with the exception of ipsilateral axillary lymph node involvement (316). Patients with more advanced or disseminated disease, despite initial presentation in the breast, are designated as secondary lymphomas of breast (317).

Patients who have primary lymphomas in the breast range from teenagers to those in their ninth decade; the median age is between 53 and 65 years (318–320). Most patients present with a breast mass and clinically are diagnosed as possible carcinoma of breast. Inexplicably, the right breast often is reported to be more commonly involved than the left (319,321). Some patients have bilateral tumor masses and some are pregnant (318–321).

Lymphomas of the breast usually are well circumscribed on gross examination and are composed of white or gray-white firm tissue (315,322). Most lymphomas of the breast are DLBCL (Fig. 33.44) and, to a lesser extent, marginal zone lymphomas of MALT (315,317–327). Cases of Burkitt and lymphoblastic lymphoma also have been described as originating in the breast, as have examples of T-cell lymphoma, mainly ALCL (315,321,325–328). There are reports of follicular lymphomas in the breast, but they are uncommon as a primary breast neoplasm. For example, three pathology-emphasized series of primary lymphomas of the breast embraced a total of 93 cases, but only two cases were classified as follicular lymphoma (325–327). A clinically based multi-institutional study, however, collected data on 36 alleged primary follicular lymphomas of breast, but the study lacked central pathology review (320).

Historically, low-grade malignant lymphomas are uncommon, and some series do not contain any cases of low-grade malignant lymphomas, including marginal zone lymphomas of MALT type (317,323). Nonetheless, cases of primary lymphoma of breast classified as marginal zone lymphomas of MALT type are well documented, although the incidence is inconsistent (321,325–327,329). Two large series, comprising 29 and 50 cases of primary breast lymphomas, classified 21% and 28% of the lymphomas, respectively, as marginal zone lymphoma (326,327); in two smaller series, the marginal zone lymphomas represented up to 50% of the cases (325,329). Mammary MALT lymphomas contain randomly scattered germinal centers and are composed mainly of monocytoid-appearing cells with admixed plasma cells (326,329); Dutcher bodies often are present and follicular colonization can occur (325). Lymphoepithelial lesions are observed in ductal epithelium, but these may not be conspicuous because the tumor often is extensive, leading to architectural obliteration of the normal breast lobules (329) (Fig. 33.45); some intraepithelial lymphocytes are reactive T cells (329). Biologically, marginal zone lymphomas

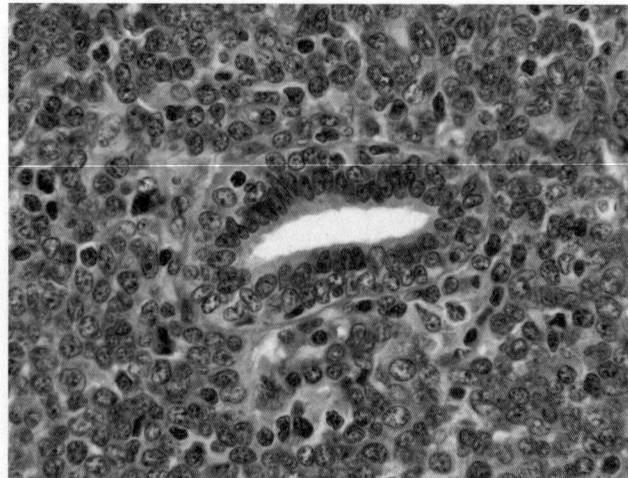

FIGURE 33.44. In the breast, most lymphomas are aggressive types, such as this DLBCL. Lymphomas of the breast frequently encase and invade residual ducts to form lymphoepithelial lesions (hematoxylin and eosin stain, original magnification: 600× magnification).

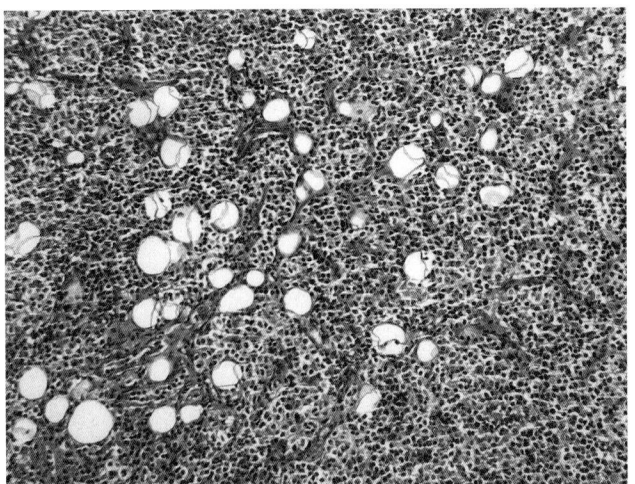

FIGURE 33.45. Marginal zone lymphoma dominated by monocytoid B cells may occur in the breast and in this example eradicates breast lobular units. The monocytoid cells are recognizable on low-power magnification by the wide separation of the nuclei caused by the relatively abundant, pale-staining cytoplasm (hematoxylin and eosin stain, original magnification: 150× magnification).

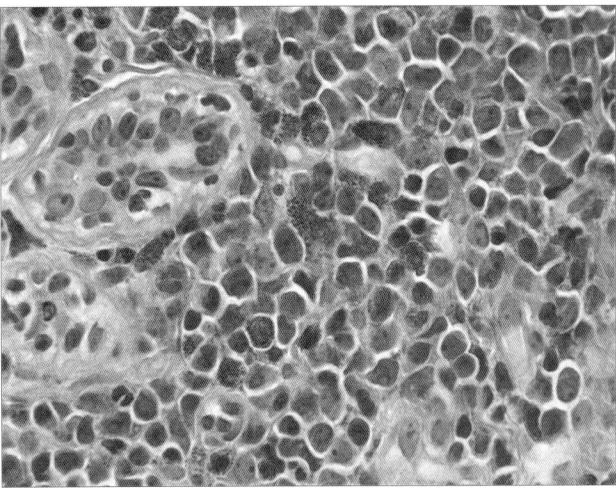

FIGURE 33.46. The diagnosis of myeloid sarcoma in the breast is facilitated in this example by the many eosinophilic myelocytes. Otherwise, the mononuclear cell infiltrate adjacent to breast ductules resembles large cell lymphoma. Immunohistochemical stains confirmed that the mononuclear cells were myeloid in origin (hematoxylin and eosin stain, original magnification: 600× magnification).

of breast do not show *MALT1* gene rearrangements by FISH and using nuclear staining for p65 and p50, NF-κB activation cannot be demonstrated (330).

Like marginal zone lymphomas of MALT, some DLBCL breast cases invade and disrupt breast ducts to create lymphoepithelial lesions (315,317,321,324). Frequently, DLBCL of the breast infiltrates the lobules or surrounds and separates individual ducts and lobules that may not be infiltrated but are compressed; this pattern of infiltration may impart a targetoid arrangement (317). The presence of a targetoid configuration and a frequent single-file pattern of infiltration with accompanying sclerosis or lymphomatous signet ring cells mimic infiltrating lobular carcinoma. Unlike lobular carcinoma, lymphomas of breast do not exhibit carcinoma *in situ*, cellular cohesion, or syncytial aggregation but may display lymphoepithelial lesions and associated karyorrhexis (317). Similar to other extranodal sites, DLBCL in the breast also may be confused with myeloid sarcoma because these cases may manifest as a solitary mass in the breast (317,331). As in the female genital tract, the use of histochemical stains and a succession of immunoperoxidase stains, as, for example, myeloperoxidase, coupled with the possible detection of eosinophilic myelocytes, should distinguish myeloid sarcoma from malignant lymphoma (278,331) (Fig. 33.46).

Immunohistochemical studies reveal that primary DLBCL of the breast predominately exhibits a non–germinal center immunophenotype and a high proliferative index of almost 80% to suggest an unfavorable clinical course in the context of DLBCL (326,332,333). As opposed to the marginal zone cases in breast, the DLBCL cases react for p65 and exhibit inconsistent expression of p50, indicative of NF-κB activation (330). In the same study, and identical to the marginal zone cases, 14 DLBCL cases did not have evident *MALT1* gene rearrangements (330). Nonetheless, in a different analysis of 15 cases of DLBCL of breast using FISH, two cases harbored t(14;18)(q32;q21) involving *IGH* and *MALT1* genes (180). Moreover, 60% of the breast lymphomas had numerical aberrations, primarily trisomy 18. These results suggest that a subset of DLBCL of breast cases form part of the spectrum of extranodal marginal zone lymphoma (180).

As noted above, T-cell lymphomas also can present primarily in the breast, most often ALCL (327,328). More recently, ALCL has been identified in association with breast implants, and this phenomenon is evolving as a new clinicopathologic entity, despite the lack of corroborative epidemiologic data (334,335).

Breast implant–associated ALCL is not strictly a lymphoma of breast, but rather a lymphoma of the fibrous capsule and the seroma, or effusion, that surround the silicone or saline implant (334). Patients commonly present because of an effusion around the implant or because of contracture of the fibrous capsule (335). Although thick, the fibrous capsule does not contain a discrete gross tumor mass, but cytologic examination of the effusion fluid and/or microscopic sections of the fibrous capsule disclose ALCL (336,337). The lymphomatous cells are present in fibrinoid material and in the fibrous capsule, but without invasion through the capsule (337) (Fig. 33.47). Characteristic of ALCL, the neoplastic cells are large, pleomorphic, and encompass some "hallmark" cells. The lymphomas are of T-cell lineage, express CD30 and commonly epithelial membrane antigen and cytotoxic granule-associated proteins, but are negative for ALK (334–337). The clinical course is indolent and analogous to primary cutaneous CD30⁺ lymphoproliferative disorders (334,336,337); the term *CD30-positive lymphoproliferative disorder associated with breast implant* has been proposed for these cases (337). Alternatively, a minority of patients present with a distinct capsular mass and often more advanced lymphoma with a less favorable prognosis and for these patients the diagnosis of ALCL appears justified (337). In addition to ALCL, a case of nasal-type NKTCL presenting in the capsule of breast implant was described (338); although the clinical follow-up was short, the case increases the scope of implant-associated T-cell lymphomas.

The differential diagnosis of primary lymphoma in breast from lymphoid hyperplasia usually is not an issue. Lymphoid hyperplasia in the breast is uncommon and is differentiated from lymphoma by the innocuous cytologic features (Fig. 33.48), the polymorphous cell population, and the finding of germinal centers. If the histologic features are ambiguous and difficult to differentiate from marginal zone lymphoma, demonstration of polyclonality by immunoperoxidase techniques, flow cytometry, or molecular analysis may be required (316). One form of lymphoid hyperplasia referred to as *lymphocytic mastopathy* is morphologically similar to a process known as *diabetic mastopathy* that has been described in patients with diabetes mellitus (316,339,340). In these conditions, the breast develops intralobular, perilobular, and perivascular lymphocytic infiltrates associated with germinal center formation, lymphoepithelial-type lesions, lobular atrophy, and stromal keloid-like fibrosis (229,340). Diabetic or lymphocytic mastopathy may represent an

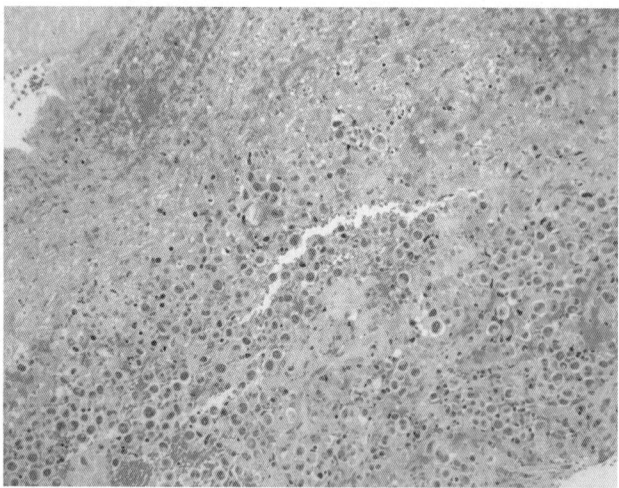

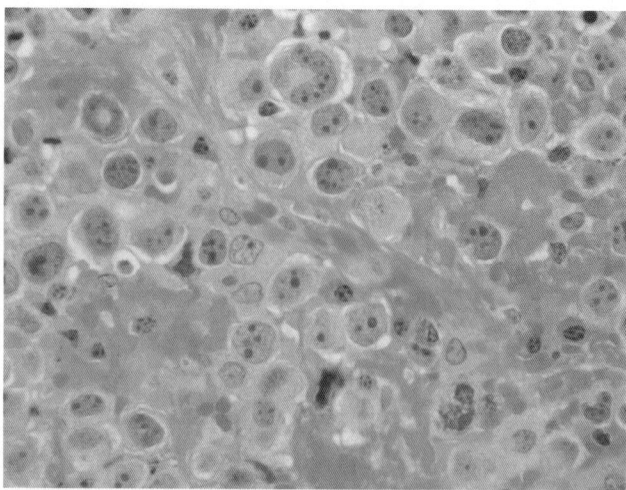

A

B

FIGURE 33.47. **A:** Breast implant–associated ALCL is present in the capsule of the implant with shedding of neoplastic cells into the hemorrhagic effusion adjacent to the implant (hematoxylin and eosin stain, original magnification: 150× magnification). **B:** Detail of the ALCL, including a "hallmark" cell. The ALCL cases associated with breast implants are ALK-negative and pursue an indolent clinical course (hematoxylin and eosin stain, original magnification: 600× magnification).

autoimmune disease because of morphologic and immunologic similarities to LESA of salivary glands or Hashimoto thyroiditis. B cells dominate the infiltrates and, although lymphoepithelial lesions may be observed, CD43 is not coexpressed and no B-cell clonal gene rearrangements are present (340). Diabetic mastopathy differs from IgG4-related disease affecting the breast in that the fibrosis usually predominates over the lymphocytic infiltrates and plasma cells are scarce (341). Rosai-Dorfman disease rarely may present in the breast, and one report describes overlapping features with IgG4-related disease (342).

Analysis of breast lymphomas in the literature suggests that there are two clinicopathologic types of primary lymphoma of the breast (304,316,321,322). One type affects younger patients under 40 years who frequently are pregnant and often have bilateral diffuse disease. These patients have a higher proportion of Burkitt lymphoma and a rapidly fatal clinical course. The second and more common group, which represents up to 80% of cases, involves a broad age range of patients but is mainly limited to older women who have unilateral breast lymphoma. These patients have a variable clinical course that is affected by the histologic grade of lymphoma. Treatment of breast lymphomas

has been inconstant, but treatment generally parallels that given for nodal lymphomas of similar morphologic type. For example, patients who have DLBCL of the breast receive CHOP-type chemotherapy and often involved field radiation therapy (318,319). In one retrospective study, the 5-year overall survival and progression-free survival for 18 patients with primary DLBCL of the breast was 82% and 61%, respectively (318). The IPI score is a statistically significant factor in overall survival (319). In contrast to patients with nodal DLBCL, those in breast tend to recur in the same breast, opposite breast, and in other extranodal sites (319); relapse in the CNS is uncommon (318). Survival statistics for primary DLBCL of breast obviously should improve with current R-CHOP therapy. Patients who have marginal zone lymphoma of the breast are treated by surgical excision, radiation therapy, and/or chemotherapy (316,320). Comparable with marginal zone lymphoma of other extranodal locations, mammary MALT lymphomas are clinically indolent with a 92% survival rate at 5 years (320).

MISCELLANEOUS SITES

Primary malignant lymphomas may involve virtually any anatomic site, but, with the exception of the extranodal lymphomas discussed in this and previous chapters, primary extranodal lymphomas that involve other organs are rare and generally account for <1% of extranodal lymphomas (1,2). Lymphomas that apparently arise in the adrenals, pancreas, urethra, peripheral nerve, and spinal cord are considered pathologically novel and generally are the subject of single case reports or derived from review of cases gleaned from the literature, multi-institutional collaborative studies, and cases accumulated over considerable time in lymphoma referral centers serving a broad catchment area (192,343–347). In many instances, the lymphomas in these extranodal sites are encountered in patients who develop rapid progression of disease within 3 to 6 months after diagnosis. In this vein, a retrospective study of primary lymphomas of the adrenal was based on 10 cases gathered from nine medical centers in Taiwan, Spain, and Great Britain (343). Eight of the ten lymphomas were DLBCL with a non–germinal center phenotype and, despite stage IE disease at presentation, the majority of patients died of lymphoma at a median follow-up of 4.5 months.

The incidence of primary lymphomas that affects these unusual and miscellaneous sites increased at the height of the AIDS epidemic (see Chapter 25). For example, malignant

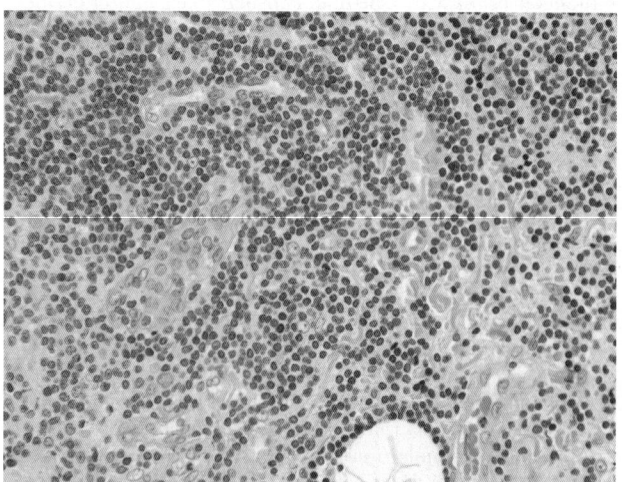

FIGURE 33.48. Lymphoid hyperplasia of the breast is a relatively infrequent pathologic finding but is distinguished from malignant lymphoma by the bland cytologic features of the lymphocytes and the variation in cellular density. Despite the benign infiltrate, there is focal invasion of ductal epithelium (hematoxylin and eosin stain, original magnification: 300× magnification).

lymphomas of the heart are very rare, but one study described nine cardiac lymphoma cases found in a single institution over an 8-year period (348); four of the patients fulfilled the criteria for AIDS. Since then, descriptions of primary cardiac lymphomas largely have been restricted to immunocompetent patients as case reports or in small series (349). Almost all cardiac lymphomas are DLBCL with a proclivity for the right atrium. Classically, the cardiac lymphomas invade the myometrium, but a significant number of cases are noninvasive and limited to fibrinous material either overlying cardiac prostheses or in fibrin thrombi involving cardiac chambers (350,351). The noninvasive cases are of non–germinal center B-cell type and are predominately EBV⁺ and, where tested, of latency III type; patients appear amenable to cure by cardiac repair with removal of the offending fibrin. Despite the favorable outcomes, it has been proposed that such cases should be included in the WHO category of DLBCL with chronic inflammation (350–352). The prototype of the latter category is EBV-associated extranodal lymphomas of the pleural cavity known as pyothorax-associated lymphoma, an aggressive lymphoma (352–354). Pyothorax-associated lymphomas arise in the pleural cavity after a prolonged (20 years and longer) history of pyothorax resulting from therapeutic artificial pneumothorax for pleural or pulmonary tuberculosis. Unlike primary effusion lymphomas, pyothorax-associated lymphomas are accompanied by contiguous tumor masses and are not related to AIDS or Kaposi sarcoma–associated herpes virus (355) (see Chapter 25). Other extranodal cases purported to be in the chronic inflammatory DLBCL class are those associated with chronic suppurative osteomyelitis, with metallic implants and with pseudocysts, including hydrocele sacs (356–359); because of a lack of prominent inflammation; however, the pseudocyst group may not strictly belong to the chronic inflammatory DLBCL category (359).

Several series have been published of lymphomas that clinically arise in other uncommon extranodal sites including the liver, gallbladder and extrahepatic bile ducts, urinary tract, prostate, oral cavity, and soft tissue. Although PTCL and marginal zone lymphoma may arise in the liver, the vast majority of cases are DLBCL in which a subset is associated with the hepatitis C virus (360–362). DLBCL in liver mainly exhibits a dense, nodular growth pattern leading to obliteration of hepatic acini (Fig. 33.49); the majority of DLBCL cases are of the non–germinal center type, based on the Hans algorithm (19,362). DLBCL also can present in the gallbladder (Fig. 33.50), but a variety of other lymphoma types affect this organ, most commonly

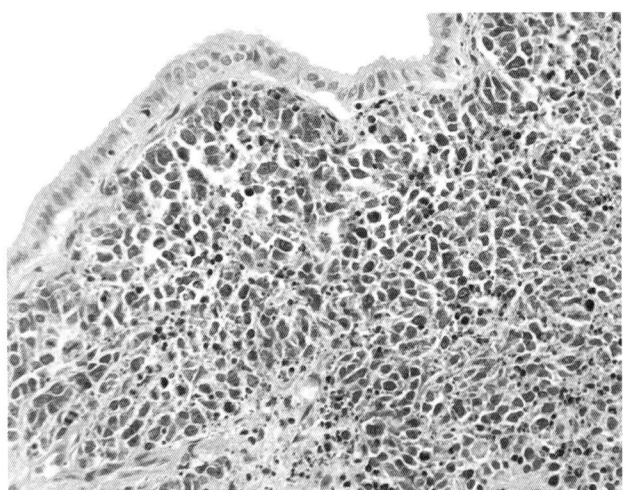

FIGURE 33.50. In the gallbladder, a large B-cell lymphoma infiltrates and expands the lamina propria beneath the intact surface epithelium. Primary lymphoma of the gallbladder is rare and includes cases classified as marginal zone lymphoma and follicular lymphoma, in addition to DLBCL (hematoxylin and eosin stain, original magnification: 300× magnification).

extranodal marginal zone lymphoma and follicular lymphoma (363). DLBCL, Burkitt lymphoma, and marginal zone lymphoma predominate in the kidney, whereas those that are primary in the urinary bladder are most commonly marginal zone lymphoma followed by DLBCL (364–366). Occasionally, lymphomas of the urinary bladder may contain signet ring cells to simulate carcinoma, and, conversely, carcinomas of the urinary bladder, specifically plasmacytoid urothelial carcinoma, simulate plasmablastic lymphoma and plasmacytoma (367,368). Lymphomas in the prostate tend to be DLBCL that distort the architecture with compression of acini and ducts (365,369). Primary lymphomas of the oral cavity are uncommon, but in a review of cases from an oral pathology referral service over a 26-year period, 73 cases were collected with the majority classified as DLBCL (68%), followed by marginal zone lymphoma of MALT (15%) and PTCL (8%) (370); 14% of the B-cell cases were EBV⁺. The association with EBV is more prevalent in plasmablastic lymphomas of the oral cavity discovered in patients with immunodeficiency virus infection (371) (see Chapter 25). With immunohistochemistry, a slight majority of oral DLBCL cases exhibit a non–germinal center phenotype (372). Lymphomas presenting in soft tissue are another example of a rare extranodal lymphoma site. The largest retrospective series of 75 cases were selected from the files of the Department of Soft Tissue Pathology of the Armed Forces Institute of Pathology (373). The lesions were most common in the thigh and chest wall, but no area was spared and, with the exception of lymphoblastic lymphoma, all types of non-Hodgkin lymphoma were identified; diffuse large cell lymphomas, including immunoblastic lymphomas, predominated and many stage IE patients successfully responded to therapy (373). That study antedated the widespread use of immunophenotypic markers, but subsequent reports with more limited numbers of cases verified the prevalence of DLBCL (374,375). Most cases of DLBCL in soft tissue have a non–germinal center phenotype (375). Unusual examples of soft tissue B-cell lymphomas include two cases that arose in the context of chronic postmastectomy lymphedema and three cases that originated in the soft tissue of the extremities near joints affected by rheumatoid arthritis (376,377). Conceivably, the latter cases could be included in the chronic inflammatory group of DLBCL, but are excluded as they lack EBV expression (352,377). Because of the dominance of DLBCL in soft tissue, distinguishing them from the rare examples of florid lymphoid hyperplasia of soft tissue ought not to be an issue (378).

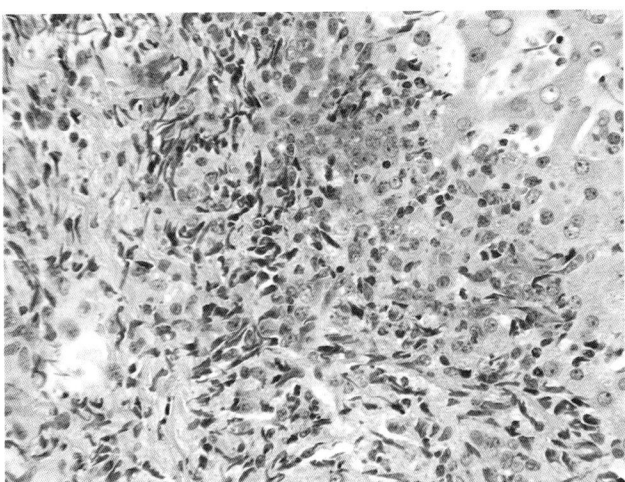

FIGURE 33.49. Although this core biopsy of liver is altered by crush artifact, neoplastic large lymphocytes are recognizable that invade and distort hepatic acini. The lymphoma proved to be B-cell type (CD20⁺), and additional immunoperoxidase stains demonstrated that the large B-cell lymphoma fit the non–germinal center category (CD10⁻, BCL-6⁻, MUM1⁺) (*not shown*) (hematoxylin and eosin stain, original magnification: 300× magnification).

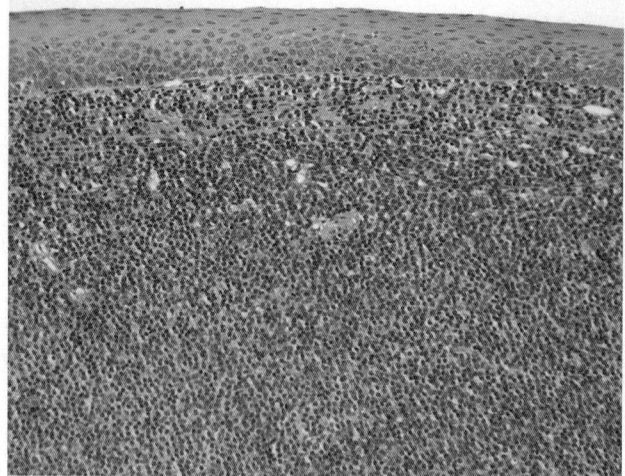
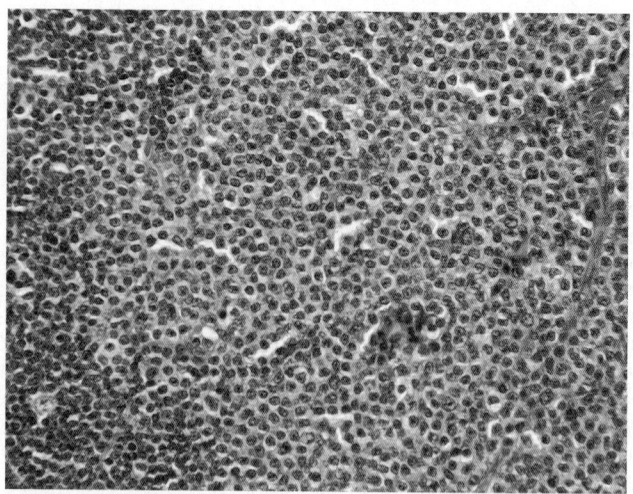

FIGURE 33.51. A: Primary lymphoma of the larynx is very rare, and this example is marginal zone lymphoma of MALT type. At this magnification, the lymphocytic nuclei are discrete to impart the impression of monocytoid-like cells (hematoxylin and eosin stain, original magnification: 150× magnification). **B:** At higher magnification, the monocytoid character of the neoplastic lymphocytes is apparent, and they contrast with the small darker lymphocytes on the left, which are part of the mantle of a residual germinal center (hematoxylin and eosin stain, original magnification: 300× magnification).

The mediastinum, specifically thymus, is another site of extranodal lymphoma and best known for primary mediastinal large B-cell lymphoma (see Chapter 23); however, some cases in the thymus have features of marginal zone lymphomas of MALT (379–381). In thymus, the marginal zone lymphomas often are associated with cysts and reactive lymphoid follicles together with a lymphocytic infiltrate composed of a varying population of small lymphocytes, monocytoid cells, and plasma cells that invade and expand Hassall corpuscles and the epithelial lining of cysts to form lymphoepithelial lesions. Differentiation of thymic marginal zone lymphoma from thymic reactive lymphoid hyperplasia can be challenging, especially as reactive follicles are found in both conditions and some hyperplastic cases form cysts and may bear an uncanny resemblance to LESA of salivary glands (382,383). In hyperplasia, a network of thymic cytokeratin⁺ epithelium surrounds the reactive follicles which is lacking in lymphoma. Alternatively, marginal zone lymphoma is characterized by an abnormal B-cell infiltrate that disrupts the cytokeratin⁺ epithelial network and that is absent in hyperplasia (382,383). Marginal zone lymphomas in the thymus do not exhibit *MALT1* gene abnormalities, including an absence of t(11;18), but, parallel to marginal zone lymphoma of salivary gland, the thymic cases have a high frequency of trisomy 3 (132,379,380,384); deletion of A20, the global NF-κB inhibitor, was reported in one thymic marginal zone lymphoma, a feature also described in a minority of salivary gland marginal zone lymphomas (134,380). The comparison to the salivary gland also is clinically apt since patients with thymic marginal zone lymphomas of MALT have a raised association with autoimmune disease, mainly Sjögren syndrome, and derivation from preexisting thymic lymphoid hyperplasia or MALT is conceivable (379,380,382,383). In addition to a link with autoimmune disease, thymic marginal zone lymphomas exhibit a predilection for middle-aged Asian females and, similar to extranodal marginal zone lymphomas at other sites, the clinical course is excellent with a very low incidence of recurrence (379–381). Extranodal marginal zone lymphomas of MALT are ubiquitous and originate not only in the thymus but, as noted earlier, in other uncommon locations, including endometrium, liver, gall bladder, kidney and urinary bladder, as well as exotic sites, such as urethra, larynx (Fig. 33.51), trachea, and even joint synovia (285,286,361–363,365,366,385–388). For completeness, another pervasive extranodal lymphoma is

intravascular large B-cell lymphoma that can present in any organ, but as opposed to marginal zone lymphomas of MALT, the intravascular cases are clinically aggressive with a poor prognosis (204) (see Chapter 23).

SUMMARY AND CONCLUSIONS

The extranodal lymphomas discussed in this chapter are relatively uncommon malignant tumors compared with other neoplasms or even other lymphomas, but they provide provocative insights into the pathogenesis of extranodal lymphomas and perhaps lymphomas in general. For example, many malignant lymphomas that arise in the salivary gland, and almost all of those in the thyroid gland, are closely linked to autoimmune disorders, namely, Sjögren syndrome or LESA and Hashimoto or chronic lymphocytic thyroiditis. In these conditions, the lymphomas are of B-cell origin and are thought to evolve secondary to chronic antigenic stimulation of B lymphocytes, because of unrestricted T-helper activity leading to immunoglobulin gene hypermutation or because of a disorder of immune surveillance with subsequent onset of cytogenetic aberrations. Curiously, the malignant lymphomas that develop from these altered immune states are morphologically and clinically distinctive. In patients who have Sjögren syndrome or LESA, the lymphomas commonly develop in extrasalivary gland lymph nodes rather than within the salivary gland. When lymphomas do occur within the salivary gland, they usually are clinically and pathologically occult lymphomas of marginal zone type and they often require verification by immunologic and molecular genetic techniques. In contrast, lymphomas of the thyroid gland associated with Hashimoto or chronic lymphocytic thyroiditis may be marginal zone lymphomas, but generally are clinically obvious malignancies and usually are morphologically aggressive DLBCL that occur within the thyroid gland. The clinical and histologic discrepancies between those lymphomas of the salivary and the thyroid glands associated with a predisposing autoimmune disorder may be consequence of differing genetic scenarios. Common to marginal zone lymphomas of other extranodal sites, those in salivary gland and thyroid are often translocation negative, such as for t(11;18). Both locations may exhibit trisomy 3 and/or 18, but a minority of marginal zone cases in salivary gland has chromosomal translocation t(14;18)(q32;q21) due to fusion of the *IGH* and *MALT1* genes. As well, a small number of translocation-negative salivary gland cases contain deletions of A20, an inhibitor of NF-κB. The less common marginal zone lymphomas of thyroid do not encompass t(14;18)(q32;q21), but 50% of cases exhibit chromosomal translocation t(3;14)(p14;q32) as result of an *IGH* and *FOXP1* gene combination to imply that the molecular pathogenesis of marginal zone lymphomas of thyroid is organ particular. Curiously, despite the well-established association of chronic lymphocytic thyroiditis and the more prevalent DLBCL cases in the thyroid, the genetic abnormalities discovered in thyroid cases of DLBCL match those of node-based DLBCL and not those associated with extranodal marginal zone lymphomas. Alternatively, and notwithstanding the virtual absence of testicular marginal zone lymphoma and the relative paucity of such cases in breast, DLBCL in both testis and breast may harbor t(14;18)(q32;q21) with breakpoints in *IGH* and *MALT1* to signify that some DLBCL cases are part of the continuum of extranodal marginal zone lymphoma. Other extranodal DLBCL cases that have no known association with extranodal marginal zone lymphoma, such as those in bone and particularly CNS, display chromosomal abnormalities that differ from those in other sites to indicate that DLBCL of bone and CNS are distinctive.

EBV plays a role in the pathogenesis of some extranodal lymphomas and has been implicated particularly in lymphomas of the sinonasal region, in extranodal lymphomas associated with immunodeficiency, such as the CNS and in the rare cases of lymphoma associated with chronic inflammation, as, for example, pyothorax-associated lymphoma. Unlike the B-cell lymphomas affiliated with immunodeficiency and chronic inflammation, lymphomas of the sinonasal region associated with EBV are polymorphous NKTCL. These cases are found in the United States and Europe but are far more prevalent in the Far East and Latin America, and almost half or more of the cases exhibit an NK-cell immunophenotype (CD2$^+$, membranous CD3$^-$, cytoplasmic CD3ε$^+$, CD56$^+$). In comparison, almost all malignant lymphomas of other extranodal sites discussed in this chapter express B-cell markers. Moreover, the B-cell lymphomas virtually are all aggressive malignancies of DLBCL type. The extranodal low-grade lymphomas covered in this chapter, especially the marginal zone lymphomas of MALT, are prevalent only in salivary glands associated with LESA or are found occasionally in the thyroid gland and breast and in a variety of miscellaneous organs, such as endometrium, urinary bladder, and thymus. The extranodal marginal zone lymphomas of MALT reflect a continuum of neoplastic evolution from polyclonal reactive hyperplasia to monoclonal malignant lymphoma (see Chapter 28).

The clinical course of extranodal lymphomas varies, but, in general, the extranodal marginal zone lymphomas of MALT lymphomas have an excellent prognosis and often are clinically occult. The more common extranodal DLBCL cases are clinically aggressive, but are responsive to modern therapy, including the addition of rituximab to the therapeutic regimen, and particularly if the lesion is confined to the extranodal site (stage IE). The division of extranodal DLBCL cases into germinal center (CD10$^+$, BCL-6$^+$, MUM1$^-$) and non–germinal center (CD10$^-$, BCL-6$^{+/-}$, MUM1$^+$) types appears to be prognostically relevant for most extranodal sites. Whether immunoperoxidase testing for BCL-2 and MYC expression in DLBCL cases of specific extranodal sites will be prognostically significant is currently unknown.

ACKNOWLEDGMENT

The author thanks Linda Cork for assistance with references.

References

1. Wu XC, Andrews P, Chen VW, et al. Incidence of extranodal non-Hodgkin lymphomas among whites, blacks, and Asian/Pacific Islanders in the United States; anatomic site and histology differences. *Cancer Epidemiol* 2009;33:337–346.
2. Yang QP, Zhang WY, Yu JB, et al. Subtype distribution of lymphomas in Southwest China: analysis of 6,382 cases using WHO classification in a single institution. *Diagn Pathol* 2011;6:77–83.
3. Aigelsreiter A, Gerlza T, Deutsch AJA, et al. *Chlamydia psittaci* infection in non-gastrointestinal extranodal MALT lymphomas and their precursor lesions. *Am J Clin Pathol* 2011;135:70–75.
4. Deshpande V, Zen Y, Chan JKC, et al. Consensus statement on the pathology of IgG4-related disease. *Mod Pathol* 2012;25:1181–1192.
5. Dojcinov SD, Venkataraman G, Raffeld M, et al. EBV positive mucocutaneous ulcer –a study of 26 cases associated with various sources of immunosuppression. *Am J Surg Pathol* 2010;34:405–417.
6. Mansoor A, Pittaluga S, Beck PL, et al. NK-cell enteropathy: a benign NK-cell lymphoproliferative disease mimicking intestinal lymphoma: clinicopathological features and follow-up in a unique case series. *Blood* 2011;117:1447–1452.
7. Yuen A, Jacobs C. Lymphomas of the head and neck. *Semin Oncol* 1999;26:338–345.
8. Krol ADG, Le Cessie S, Snuder S, et al. Waldeyer's ring lymphomas: a clinical study from the Comprehensive Cancer Center West population based NHL registry. *Leuk Lymphoma* 2001;42:1005–1013.
9. Laskar S, Mohindra P, Gupta S, et al. Non-Hodgkin lymphoma of the Waldeyer's ring: clinicopathologic and therapeutic issues. *Leuk Lymphoma* 2008;49:2263–2271.
10. Ezzat AA, Ibrahim EM, El Weshi AN, et al. Localized non-Hodgkin's lymphoma of Waldeyer's ring: clinical features, management, and prognosis of 130 adult patients. *Head Neck* 2001;23:547–558.
11. Wright DH. Lymphomas of Waldeyer's ring. *Histopathology* 1994;24:97–99.
12. Isaacson PG, Du MQ. Gastrointestinal lymphoma; where morphology meets molecular biology. *J Pathol* 2005;205:255–274.
13. Bertoni F, Sanna P, Tinguely M, et al. Association of gastric and Waldeyer's ring lymphoma: a molecular study. *Hematol Oncol* 2000;18:15–19.
14. Konoplev S, Lin P, Qiu X, et al. Clonal relationship of extranodal marginal zone lymphomas of mucosa-associated lymphoid tissue involving different sites. *Am J Clin Pathol* 2010;134:112–118.
15. Menárguez J, Mollejo M, Carrión R, et al. Waldeyer ring lymphomas: a clinicopathological study of 79 cases. *Histopathology* 1994;24:13–22.
16. Paulsen J, Lennert K. Low-grade B-cell lymphoma of mucosa-associated lymphoid tissue type in Waldeyer's ring. *Histopathology* 1994;24:1–11.
17. Oh SY, Kim WS, Kim JS, et al. Waldeyer's ring marginal zone lymphoma: are the clinical and prognostic features nodal or extranodal? A study by the Consortium for Improving Survival of Lymphoma (CISL). *Int J Hematol* 2012;96:631–637.
18. de Leval L, Bonnet C, Copie-Bergman C, et al. Diffuse large B-cell lymphoma of Waldeyer's ring has distinct clinicopathologic features: a GELA study. *Ann Oncol* 2012;23:3143–3151.
19. Hans CP, Weisenburger DD, Greiner TC, et al. Confirmation of the molecular classification of diffuse large B-cell lymphoma by immunohistochemistry using a tissue microarray. *Blood* 2004;103:275–282.
20. López-Guillermo A, Colomo L, Jiménez M, et al. Diffuse large B-cell lymphoma: clinical and biological characterization and outcome according to the nodal or extranodal primary origin. *J Clin Oncol* 2005;23:2797–2804.
21. Wada N, Ham MF, Fujita S, et al. Malignant lymphomas in Waldeyer's ring in Asian countries: association with histologic types and Epstein-Barr virus. *Mol Med Report* 2008;1:651–655.
22. Louissaint A, Ferry JA, Soupir CP, et al. Infectious mononucleosis mimicking lymphoma: distinguishing morphological and immunophenotypic features. *Mod Pathol* 2012;25:1149–1159.
23. Ree HJ, Kikuchi M, Lee SS, et al. Focal follicular features in tonsillar diffuse large B-cell lymphomas: follicular lymphoma with diffuse areas or follicular colonization. *Hum Pathol* 2002;33:732–740.
24. Kojima M, Nakamura N, Shimizu K, et al. Marginal zone B-cell lymphoma among primary B-cell lymphoma of Waldeyer's ring: histopathologic and immunohistochemical study of 16 tonsillectomy specimens. *Int J Surg Pathol* 2008;16:164–178.
25. Jaffe ES. Lymphoid lesions of the head and neck: a model of lymphocytes homing and lymphomagenesis. *Mod Pathol* 2002;15:255–263.
26. Liu Q, Salaverria I, Pittaluga S, et al. Follicular lymphomas in children and young adults: a comparison of the pediatric variant with usual follicular lymphoma. *Am J Surg Pathol* 2013;37:333–343.
27. Romaguera JE, Medeiros LJ, Hagemeister FB, et al. Frequency of gastrointestinal involvement and its clinical significance in mantle cell lymphoma. *Cancer* 2003;97:586–691.
28. Hartmann S, Agostinelli C, Klapper W, et al. Revising the historical collection of epithelioid cell-rich lymphomas of the Kiel Lymph Node Registry: what is Lennert's lymphoma nowadays? *Histopathology* 2011;59:1173–1182.
29. Kapadia SB, Roman LN, Kingma DW, et al. Hodgkin's disease of Waldeyer's ring: clinical and histoimmunophenotypic findings and association with Epstein-Barr virus in 16 cases. *Am J Surg Pathol* 1995;19:1431–1439.
30. Quiñones-Avila Mdel P, Gonzalez-Longoria AA, Admirand JH, et al. Hodgkin lymphoma involving Waldeyer ring: a clinicopathologic study of 22 cases. *Am J Clin Pathol* 2005;123:651–656.
31. Tomita Y, Ohsawa M, Mishiro Y, et al. Non-Hodgkin's lymphoma of Waldeyer's ring as a manifestation of lymphoproliferative diseases associated with human T-cell leukemia virus type 1 in southwestern Japan. *Mod Pathol* 1997;10:933–938.
32. Li, YX, Fang H, Liu QF, et al. Clinical features and treatment outcome of nasal-type NK/T-cell lymphoma of Waldeyer ring. *Blood* 2008;112:3057–3064.
33. Laskar S, Bahl G, Muckaden MA, et al. Primary diffuse large B-cell lymphoma of the tonsil: is a higher radiotherapy dose required? *Cancer* 2007;110:816–823.
34. Takahashi H, Tomita N, Yokoyama M, et al. Prognostic impact of extranodal involvement in diffuse large B-cell lymphoma in the rituximab era. *Cancer* 2012;118:4166–4172.

35. Jaffe ES, Chan JKC, Su IH, et al. Report of the workshop on nasal and related extranodal angiocentric T/natural killer cell lymphomas: definitions, differential diagnosis, and epidemiology. *Am J Surg Pathol* 1996;20:103–111.
36. Chan JKC, Quintanilla-Martinez L, Ferry JA, et al. Extranodal NK/T-cell lymphoma, nasal type. In: Swerdlow SH, Campo E, Harris NL, et al., eds. *WHO classification of tumours of haematopoietic and lymphoid tissues*, 4th ed. Lyon: IARC, 2008:285–288.
37. Vose J, Armitage J, Weisenburger D. International peripheral T-cell and natural killer/T-cell lymphoma study: pathology findings and clinical outcome. International T-cell lymphoma project. *J Clin Oncol* 2008;26:4124–4130.
38. Sun J, Yang Q, Lu Z, et al. Distribution of lymphoid neoplasms in China: analysis of 4,638 cases according to the World Health Organization classification. *Am J Clin Pathol* 2012;138:429–434.
39. Laurini JA, Perry AM, Boilesen E, et al. Classification of non-Hodgkin lymphoma in Central and South America: a review of 1028 cases. *Blood* 2012;120:4795–4801.
40. Quintanilla-Martinez L, Franklin JL, Guerrero I, et al. Histological and immunophenotypic profile of nasal NK/T cell lymphomas from Peru: high prevalence of p53 overexpression. *Hum Pathol* 1999;30:849–855.
41. Barrionuevo C, Zaharia M, Martinez MT, et al. Extranodal NK-T-cell lymphoma, nasal type: study of clinicopathologic and prognosis factors in a series of 78 cases from Peru. *Appl Immunohistochem Mol Morphol* 2007;15;38–44.
42. van de Rijn M, Bhargava V, Molina-Kirsch H, et al. Extranodal head and neck lymphomas in Guatemala: high frequency of Epstein-Barr virus-associated sinonasal lymphomas. *Hum Pathol* 1997;28:834–839.
43. Elenitoba-Johnson KSJ, Zarate-Osorno A, Meneses A, et al. Cytotoxic granular cell protein expression, Epstein-Barr virus strain type, and latent membrane protein-1 oncogene deletions in nasal T-lymphocyte/natural killer cell lymphomas from Mexico. *Mod Pathol* 1998;11:754–761.
44. Abouyabis AN, Shenoy PJ, Lechowicz MJ, et al. Incidence and outcomes of peripheral T-cell lymphoma subtypes in the United States. *Leuk Lymphoma* 2008;49:2099–2107.
45. Xu JX, Hoshida Y, Yang WI, et al. Life-style and environmental factors in the development of nasal NK/T-cell lymphoma: a case-control study in East Asia. *Int J Cancer* 2006;120:406–410.
46. Costa J, Delacretaz F. The midline granuloma syndrome. *Pathol Annu* 1986; 21:159–171.
47. Cheung MMC, Chan JKC, Wong KF. Natural killer cell neoplasms: a distinctive group of highly aggressive lymphomas/leukemias. *Semin Hematol* 2003;40:221–232.
48. Taddesse-Heath L, Feldman JI, Fahle GA, et al. Florid CD4+, CD56+ T-cell infiltrate associated with *herpes simplex* infection simulating nasal NK-/T-cell lymphoma. *Mod Pathol* 2003;16:166–172.
49. Hasserjian R, Harris N. NK-cell lymphomas and leukemias: a spectrum of tumors with variable manifestations and immunophenotype. *Am J Clin Pathol* 2007;127:860–868.
50. Abbondanzo SL, Wenig BM. Non-Hodgkin's lymphoma of the sinonasal tract: a clinicopathologic and immunophenotypic study of 120 cases. *Cancer* 1995;75: 1281–1291.
51. Kitamura A, Yamashita Y, Hasegawa Y, et al. Primary lymphoma arising in the nasal cavity among Japanese. *Histopathology* 2005;47:523–532.
52. Li S, Feng X, Li T, et al. Extranodal NK/T-cell lymphoma, nasal type: a report of 73 cases at MD Anderson Cancer Center. *Am J Surg Pathol* 2013;37:14–23.
53. Ng CS, Lo STH, Chan JKC, et al. CD56+ putative natural killer cell lymphomas: production of cytolytic effectors and related proteins mediating tumor cell apoptosis? *Hum Pathol* 1997;28:1276–1282.
54. Teruya-Feldstein J, Jaffe ES, Burd PR, et al. The role of Mig, the monokine induced by interferon-γ, and IP-10, the interferon-γ-inducible protein-10, in tissue necrosis and vascular damage associated with Epstein-Barr virus-positive lymphoproliferative disease. *Blood* 1997;90:4099–4105.
55. Ng SB, Lai KW, Murugaya, S, et al. Nasal-type extranodal natural killer/T-cell lymphomas: a clinicopathologic and genotypic study of 42 cases in Singapore. *Mod Pathol* 2004;17:1097–1107.
56. Yi ES, Colby TV. Wegener's granulomatosis. *Semin Diagn Pathol* 2001;18:34–46.
57. Gaal K, Sun NCJ, Hernandez AM, et al. Sinonasal NK/T-cell lymphoma in the United States. *Am J Surg Pathol* 2000;25:1511–1517.
58. Gualco G, Domeny-Duarte P, Chioato L, et al. Clincopathologic and molecular features of 122 Brazilian cases of nodal and extranodal NK/T-cell lymphoma, nasal type, with EBV subtyping analysis. *Am J Surg Pathol* 2011;35:1195–1203.
59. Pongpruttipan T, Sukpanichnant S, Assanasen T, et al. Extranodal NK/T-cell lymphoma, nasal type, includes cases of natural killer cell and $\alpha\beta$, $\gamma\delta$ and $\alpha\beta/\gamma\delta$ T-cell origin: a comprehensive clinicopathologic and phenotypic study. *Am J Surg Pathol* 2012;36:481–499.
60. Ko YH, Ree HJ, Kim WS, et al. Clinicopathologic and genotypic study of extranodal nasal-type natural killer/T-cell lymphoma and natural killer precursor lymphoma among Koreans. *Cancer* 2000;89:2106–2116.
61. Lin TC, Chen SU, Chen YF, et al. Intramucosal variant of nasal natural killer (NK)/T cell lymphoma has a better survival than does invasive variant: implication on loss of E26 transformation-specific sequence 1 (ETS-1) and T-box expressed in T cells (T-bet) with invasion. *Histopathology* 2012;60:287–295.
62. Katzenstein ALA, Doxtader E, Narendra S. Lymphomatoid granulomatosis: insights gained over 4 decades. *Am J Surg Pathol* 2010;34:e35–e48.
63. Colby TV. Current histological diagnosis of lymphomatoid granulomatosis. *Mod Pathol* 2012;25:S39–S42.
64. Chan JKC, Sin VC, Wong KF, et al. Nonnasal lymphoma expressing the natural killer cell marker CD56: a clinicopathologic study of 49 cases of an uncommon aggressive neoplasm. *Blood* 1997;89:4501–4513.
65. Ko YH, Cho EY, Kim JE, et al. NK and NK-like T-cell lymphoma in extranasal sites: a comparative clinicopathological study according to site and EBV status. *Histopathology* 2004;44:480–489.
66. Au WY, Weisenburger DD, Intragumtornchai T, et al. Clinical differences between nasal and extranasal natural killer/T-cell lymphoma: a study of 136 cases from the International Peripheral T-Cell Lymphoma Project. *Blood* 2009;113: 3931–3937.
67. Kim GE, Koom WS, Yang WI, et al. Clinical relevance of three subtypes of primary sinonasal lymphoma characterized by immunophenotypic analysis. *Head Neck* 2004;26:584–593.
68. Chan JKC, Ng CS, Tsang WYW. Nasal/nasopharyngeal lymphomas: an immunohistochemical analysis of 57 cases on frozen tissues. *Mod Pathol* 1993;6:87A(abst).
69. Piccaluga PP, Gazzola A, Agostinelli C, et al. Pathobiology of Epstein-Barr virus-driven peripheral T-cell lymphomas. *Semin Diagn Pathol* 2011;28:234–244.
70. Schwartz EJ, Molina-Kirsch H, Zhao S, et al. Immunohistochemical characterization of nasal-type extranodal NK/T-cell lymphoma using a tissue microarray. *Am J Clin Pathol* 2008;130:343–351.
71. Kanavaros P, Lescs M-C, Brière J, et al. Nasal T-cell lymphoma: a clinicopathologic entity associated with peculiar phenotype and with Epstein-Barr virus. *Blood* 1993;81:2688–2695.
72. Van Gorp J, De Bruin PC, Sie-Go DMDS, et al. Nasal T-cell lymphoma: a clinicopathological and immunophenotypic analysis of 13 cases. *Histopathology* 1995;27:139–148.
73. Kuo TT, Shih LY, Tsang NM. Nasal NK/T cell lymphoma in Taiwan: a clinicopathologic study of 22 cases, with analysis of histologic subtypes, Epstein-Barr virus *LMP-1* gene association, and treatment modalities. *Int J Surg Pathol* 2004;12:375–387.
74. Ohshima K, Suzumiya J, Shimazaki K, et al. Nasal T/NK cell lymphomas commonly express perforin and Fas ligand: important mediators of tissue damage. *Histopathology* 1997:31:444–450.
75. Ng CS, Lo STH, Chan JKC. Peripheral T and putative natural killer cell lymphomas commonly coexpress CD95 and CD95 ligand. *Hum Pathol* 1999;30:48–53.
76. Harabuchi Y, Imai S, Wakashima J, et al. Nasal T-cell lymphoma causally associated with Epstein-Barr virus: clinicopathologic, phenotypic, and genotypic studies. *Cancer* 1996;77:2137–2149.
77. Dictor M, Cervin A, Kalm O, et al. Sinonasal T-cell lymphoma in the differential diagnosis of lethal midline granuloma using in situ hybridization for Epstein-Barr virus RNA. *Mod Pathol* 1996;9:7–14.
78. Chiang AKS, Wong KY, Liang ACT, et al. Comparative analysis of Epstein-Barr virus gene polymorphisms in nasal T/NK-cell lymphomas and normal nasal tissues: implications on virus strain selection in malignancy. *Int J Cancer* 1999;80:356–364.
79. Suzumiya J, Ohshima K, Takeshita M, et al. Nasal lymphomas in Japan: a high prevalence of Epstein-Barr virus type A and deletion within the latent membrane protein gene. *Leuk Lymphoma* 1999;35:567–578.
80. Borisch B, Hennig I, Laeng RH, et al. Association of the subtype 2 of the Epstein-Barr virus with T-cell non-Hodgkin's lymphoma of the midline granuloma type. *Blood* 1993;82:858–864.
81. Au WY, Pang A, Choy C, et al. Quantification of circulating Epstein-Barr virus (EBV) DNA in the diagnosis and monitoring of natural killer cell and EBV-positive lymphomas in immunocompetent patients. *Blood* 2004;104:243–249.
82. Suzuki R, Yamaguchi M, Izutsu K, et al. Prospective measurement of Epstein-Barr virus-DNA in plasma and peripheral blood mononuclear cells of extranodal NK/T-cell lymphoma, nasal type. *Blood* 2011;118:6018–6022.
83. Hsieh PP, Tung CL, Chan ABW, et al. EBV viral load in tumor tissue is an important prognostic indicator for nasal NK/T-cell lymphoma. *Am J Clin Pathol* 2007;128:579–584.
84. Wong KF, Chan JKC, Cheung MMC, et al. Bone marrow involvement by nasal NK cell lymphoma at diagnosis is uncommon. *Am J Clin Pathol* 2001;115:266–270.
85. Huang WT, Chang KC, Huang GC, et al. Bone marrow that is positive for Epstein-Barr virus encoded RNA-1 by *in situ* hybridization is related with a poor prognosis in patients with extranodal natural killer/T-cell lymphoma, nasal type. *Haematologica* 2005;90:1063–1069.
86. Schmitt C, Sako N, Bagot M, et al. Extranodal NK/T-cell lymphoma: toward the identification of clinical molecular targets. *J Biomed Biotechnol* 2011;2011:790871.
87. Wong KF, Zhang YM, Chan JK. Cytogenetic abnormalities in natural killer cell lymphoma/leukemia: is there a consistent pattern? *Leuk Lymphoma* 1999;34:241–250.
88. Nakashima Y, Tagawa H, Suzuki, R et al. Genome-wide array-based comparative genomic hybridization of natural killer cell lymphoma/leukemia: different genomic alteration patterns of aggressive NK-cell leukemia and extranodal NK-T-cell lymphoma, nasal type. *Genes Chromosomes Cancer* 2005;44:247–255.
89. Ng SB, Selvarajan V, Huang G, et al. Activated oncogenic pathways and therapeutic targets in extranodal nasal-type NK/T cell lymphoma revealed by gene expression profiling. *J Pathol* 2011;223:496–510.
90. Cuadra-Garcia I, Proulx GM, Wu CL, et al. Sinonasal lymphoma: a clinicopathologic analysis of 58 cases from the Massachusetts General Hospital. *Am J Surg Pathol* 1999;23:1356–1369.
91. Laskin JJ, Savage KJ, Voss N, et al. Primary paranasal sinus lymphoma: natural history and improved outcome with central nervous system chemoprophylaxis. *Leuk Lymphoma* 2005;46:1721–1727.
92. Oprea C, Cainap C, Azoulay R, et al. Primary diffuse large B-cell non-Hodgkin lymphoma of the paranasal sinuses: a report of 14 cases. *Br J Haematol* 2005;131:468–471.
93. Chim CS, Ma SY, Au WY, et al. Primary nasal natural killer cell lymphoma: long-term treatment outcome and relationship with the International Prognostic Index. *Blood* 2004;103:216–221.
94. Yamaguchi M. Current and future management of NK/T-cell lymphoma based on clinical trials. *Int J Hematol* 2012;96:562–571.
95. Yamaguchi M, Kwong YL, Kim WS, et al. Phase II study of SMILE chemotherapy for newly diagnosed stage IV, relapsed, or refractory extranodal natural killer (NK)/T-cell lymphoma, nasal type: the NK-Cell Tumor Study Group study. *J Clin Oncol* 2011;29:4410–4416.
96. Gleeson MJ, Bennett MH, Cawson RA. Lymphomas of salivary glands. *Cancer* 1986;58:699–704.
97. Mehle ME, Kraus DH, Wood BG, et al. Lymphoma of the parotid gland. *Laryngoscope* 1993;103:17–21.
98. Barnes L, Myers EN, Prokopakis EP. Primary malignant lymphoma of the parotid gland. *Arch Otolaryngol Head Neck Surg* 1998;124:573–577.
99. Zucca E, Conconi A, Pedrinis E, et al. Nongastric marginal zone B-cell of mucosa-associated lymphoid tissue. *Blood* 2003;101:2489–2495.
100. Schmid U, Helbron D, Lennert K. Primary malignant lymphomas localized in salivary glands. *Histopathology* 1982;6:673–687.
101. Schmid U, Helbron D, Lennert K. Development of malignant lymphoma in myoepithelial sialadenitis (Sjögren's syndrome). *Virchows Arch Path Anat* 1982;395:11–43.

102. Harris NL. Lymphoid proliferations of the salivary glands. *Am J Clin Pathol* 1999;111(Suppl 1):S94–S103.
103. Metwaly H, Cheng J, Ida-Yonemochi H, et al. Vascular endothelial cell participation in formation of lymphoepithelial lesions (epi-myoepithelial islands) in lymphoepithelial sialadenitis (benign lymphoepithelial lesion). *Virchows Arch* 2003;443:17–27.
104. Ulirsch RC, Jaffe ES. Sjögren's syndrome-like illness associated with the acquired immunodeficiency syndrome-related complex. *Hum Pathol* 1987;18:1063–1068.
105. Smith FB, Rajdeo H, Panesar N, et al. Benign lymphoepithelial lesion of the parotid gland in intravenous drug users. *Arch Pathol Lab Med* 1988;112:742–745.
106. Maiorano E, Favia G, Viale G. Lymphoepithelial cysts of salivary glands: an immunohistochemical study of HIV-related and HIV-unrelated lesions. *Hum Pathol* 1998;29:260–265.
107. Wu L, Cheng J, Maruyama S, et al. Lymphoepithelial cyst of the parotid gland: its possible histopathogenesis based on clinicopathologic analysis of 64 cases. *Hum Pathol* 2009;40:683–692.
108. Ekström Smedby K, Vajdic CM, Falster M, et al. Autoimmune disorders and risk of non-Hodgkin lymphoma subtypes: a pooled analysis within the InterLymph Consortium *Blood* 2008;111:4029–4038.
109. Yamamoto K. Pathogenesis of Sjogren's syndrome. *Autoimmun Rev* 2003:2:13–18.
110. Bahler DW, Miklos JA, Swerdlow SH. Ongoing Ig gene hypermutation in salivary gland mucosa-associated lymphoid tissue-type lymphomas. *Blood* 1997;89:3335–3344.
111. Deutsch A, Airelsreiter A, Staber P, et al. MALT lymphoma and extranodal diffuse large B-cell lymphoma are targeted by aberrant somatic hypermutation. *Blood* 2007;109:3500–3504.
112. Voulgarelis M, Skopouli FN. Clinical, immunologic and molecular factors predicting lymphoma development in Sjogren's syndrome patients. *Clinic Rev Allerg Immunol* 2007;32:265–274.
113. Bahler DW, Swerdlow SH. Clonal salivary gland infiltrates associated with myoepithelial sialadenitis (Sjögren's syndrome) begin as nonmalignant antigen-selected expansions. *Blood* 1998;91:1864–1872.
114. Diss TC, Wotherspoon AC, Speight P, et al. B-cell monoclonality, Epstein Barr virus, and t(14;18) in myoepithelial sialadenitis and low-grade B-cell MALT lymphoma of the parotid gland. *Am J Surg Pathol* 1995;19:531–536.
115. Hsi ED, Siddiqui J, Schnitzer B, et al. Analysis of immunoglobulin heavy chain gene rearrangement in myoepithelial sialadenitis by polymerase chain reaction. *Am J Clin Pathol* 1996;106:498–503.
116. Quintana PG, Kapadia SB, Bahler DW, et al. Salivary gland lymphoid infiltrates associated with lymphoepithelial lesions: a clinicopathologic, immunophenotypic, and genotypic study. *Hum Pathol* 1997;28:850–861.
117. Miklos JA, Swerdlow SH, Bahler DW. Salivary gland mucosa-associated lymphoid tissue lymphoma immunoglobulin V_H genes show frequent use of *V1-69* with distinctive CDR3 features. *Blood* 2000;95:3878–3884.
117a. Strunk JE, Schüttler C, Ziebuhr J, et al. Epstein-Barr virus-induced secondary high-grade transformation of Sjögren's syndrome–related mucosa-associated lymphoid tissue lymphoma. *J Clin Oncol* 2013;31:e265–e268.
118. Royer B, Cazals-Hatem D, Sibilia J, et al. Lymphomas in patients with Sjögren's syndrome are marginal zone B-cell neoplasms, arise in diverse extranodal and nodal sites, and are not associated with viruses. *Blood* 1997;90:766–775.
119. Ramos-Casals M, La Civita L, De Vita S, et al. Characterization of B cell lymphoma in patients with Sjögren's syndrome and hepatitis C virus infection. *Arthritis Rheum* 2007;57:161–170.
120. Carrozzo M. Oral diseases associated with hepatitis C virus infection. Part 1: sialadenitis and salivary glands lymphoma. *Oral Dis* 2008;14:123–130.
121. McCurley TL, Collins RD, Ball E, et al. Nodal and extranodal lymphoproliferative disorders in Sjögren's syndrome: a clinical and immunopathologic study. *Hum Pathol* 1990;21:482–492.
122. Hsi ED, Zukerberg LR, Schnitzer B, et al. Development of extrasalivary gland lymphoma in myoepithelial sialadenitis. *Mod Pathol* 1995;8:817–824.
123. Baldini C, Pepe P, Luciano N, et al. A clinical prediction rule for lymphoma development in primary Sjögren's syndrome. *J Rheumatol* 2012;39:804–808.
124. Christodoulou MI, Kapsogeorgou EK, Moutsopoulos NM, et al. Foxp3+ T-regulatory cells in Sjögren's syndrome: correlation with the grade of the autoimmune lesion and certain adverse prognostic factors. *Am J Pathol* 2008;173:1389–1396.
125. Hyjek E, Smith WJ, Isaacson PG. Primary B-cell lymphoma of salivary glands and its relationship to myoepithelial sialadenitis. *Hum Pathol* 1988;19:766–776.
126. Burke JS. Are there site-specific differences among the MALT lymphomas-morphologic, clinical? *Am J Clin Pathol* 1999;111(Suppl 1):S133–S143.
127. Kojima M, Nakamura S, Itoh H, et al. Küttner's tumor of salivary glands resembling marginal zone B-cell lymphoma of the MALT type: a histopathologic and immunohistochemical study of 7 cases. *Int J Surg Pathol* 2004;12:389–393.
128. Kitagawa S, Zen Y, Harada K, et al. Abundant IgG4-positive plasma cells infiltration characterizes chronic sclerosing sialadenitis (Küttner's tumor). *Am J Surg Pathol* 2005;29:783–791.
129. Geyer JT, Ferry JA, Harris NL, et al. Chronic sclerosing sialadenitis (Küttner tumor) is an IgG4-associated disease. *Am J Surg Pathol* 2010;34:202–210.
130. Ochoa ER, Harris NL, Pilch BZ. Marginal zone B-cell lymphoma of the salivary gland arising in chronic sclerosing sialadenitis (Küttner Tumor). *Am J Surg Pathol* 2001;25:1546–1550.
131. Kojima M, Shimizu K, Nishikawa M, et al. Primary salivary gland lymphoma among Japanese: a clinicopathological study of 30 cases. *Leuk Lymphoma* 2007;48:1793–1798.
132. Streubel B, Simonitsch-Klupp I, Müllauer L, et al. Variable frequencies of MALT lymphoma associated genetic aberrations in MALT lymphomas of different sites. *Leukemia* 2004;18:1722–1726.
133. Remstein ED, Dogan A, Einerson RR, et al. The incidence and anatomic site specificity of chromosomal translocations in primary extranodal marginal zone B-cell lymphoma of mucosa-associated lymphoid tissue (MALT lymphoma) in North America. *Am J Surg Pathol* 2006;30:1546–1553.
134. Chanudet E, Ye H, Ferry J, et al. A20 deletion is associated with copy number gain at the TNFA/B/C locus and occurs preferentially in translocation-negative MALT lymphoma of the ocular adnexa and salivary glands. *J Pathol* 2009;217:420–430.
135. Collins RD. Is clonality equivalent to malignancy: specifically, is immunoglobulin gene rearrangement diagnostic of malignant lymphoma? *Hum Pathol* 1997;28:757–759.
136. Falzon M, Isaacson PG. The natural history of benign lymphoepithelial lesion of the salivary gland in which there is a monoclonal population of B cells: a report of two cases. *Am J Surg Pathol* 1991;15:59–65.
137. Goda JS, Gospodarowicz M, Pintilie M, et al. Long-term outcome in localized extranodal mucosa-associated lymphoid tissue lymphomas treated with radiotherapy. *Cancer* 2010;116:3815–3824.
138. Dunn P, Kuo TT, Shih LY, et al. Primary salivary gland lymphoma: a clinicopathologic study of 23 cases in Taiwan. *Acta Haematol* 2004;112:203–208.
139. Hyman GA, Wolff M. Malignant lymphomas of the salivary glands: review of the literature and report of 33 new cases, including four cases associated with the lymphoepithelial lesion. *Am J Clin Pathol* 1976;65:421–438.
140. Nakamura S, Ichimura K, Sato Y, et al. Follicular lymphoma frequently originates in the salivary gland. *Pathol Int* 2006;56:576–583.
141. Osborne BM, Butler JJ, Variakojis D, et al. Reactive lymph node hyperplasia with giant follicles. *Am J Clin Pathol* 1982;78:493–499.
142. Park CK, Manning JT, Battifora H, et al. Follicle center lymphoma and Warthin tumor involving the same anatomic site: report of two cases and review of the literature. *Am J Clin Pathol* 2000;113:113–119.
143. Aiello A, Du MQ, Diss TC, et al. Simultaneous phenotypically distinct but clonally identical mucosa-associated lymphoid tissue and follicular lymphoma in a patient with Sjögren's syndrome. *Blood* 1999;94:2247–2251.
144. Chan JKC, Tsang WYW, Hui P-K, et al. T- and T/natural killer-cell lymphomas of the salivary gland: a clinicopathologic, immunohistochemical and molecular study of six cases. *Hum Pathol* 1997;28:238–245.
145. Hyjek E, Isaacson PG. Primary B cell lymphoma of the thyroid and its relationship to Hashimoto's thyroiditis. *Hum Pathol* 1988;19:1315–1326.
146. Pedersen RK, Pedersen NT. Primary non-Hodgkin's 's lymphoma of the thyroid gland: a population based study. *Histopathology* 1996;28:25–32.
147. Derringer GA, Thompson LDR, Frommelt RA, et al. Malignant lymphoma of the thyroid gland: a clinicopathologic study of 108 cases. *Am J Surg Pathol* 2000;24:623–639.
148. Cho JH, Park YH, Kim WS, et al. High incidence of mucosa-associated lymphoid tissue in primary thyroid lymphoma: a clinicopathologic study of 18 cases in the Korean population. *Leuk Lymphoma* 2006;47:2128–2131.
149. Dayan CM, Daniels GH. Chronic autoimmune thyroiditis. *N Engl J Med* 1996;335:99–107.
150. Holm L-E, Blomgren H, Löwhagen T. Cancer risks in patients with chronic lymphocytic thyroiditis. *N Engl J Med* 1985;312:601–604.
151. Kato I, Tajima K, Suchi T, et al. Chronic thyroiditis as a risk factor for B-cell lymphoma in the thyroid gland. *Jpn J Cancer Res* 1985;76:1085–1090.
152. Watanabe N, Noh JY, Narimatsu H, et al. Clinicopathological features of 171 cases of primary thyroid lymphoma: a long-term study involving 24553 patients with Hashimoto's disease. *Br J Haematol* 2011;153:236–243.
153. Takakuwa T, Miyauchi A, Aozasa K. Aberrant hypermutations in thyroid lymphomas. *Leuk Res* 2009;22:649–654.
154. Graff-Baker A, Sosa JA, Roman SA. Primary thyroid lymphoma: a review of recent developments in diagnosis and histology-driven treatment. *Curr Opin Oncol* 2010;22:17–22.
155. Moshynska OV, Saxena A. Clonal relationship between Hashimoto thyroiditis and thyroid lymphoma. *J Clin Pathol* 2008;61:438–444.
156. Sato Y, Nakamura N, Nakamura S, et al. Deviated VH4 immunoglobulin gene usage is found among thyroid mucosa-associated lymphoid tissue lymphomas, similar to the usage at other sites, but is not found in thyroid diffuse large B-cell lymphomas. *Mod Pathol* 2006;19:1578–1584.
157. Rossi D. Thyroid lymphomas: beyond antigen recognition. *Leuk Res* 2009;33:607–609.
158. Lam KY, Lo CY, Kwong DLW, et al. Malignant lymphoma of the thyroid: a 30-year clinicopathologic experience and an evaluation of the presence of Epstein-Barr virus. *Am J Clin Pathol* 1999;112:263–270.
159. Knowles DM, Athan E, Ubriaco A, et al. Extranodal noncutaneous lymphoid hyperplasias represent a continuous spectrum of B-cell neoplasia: demonstration by molecular genetic analysis. *Blood* 1989;73:1635–1645.
160. Hsi ED, Singleton TP, Svoboda SM, et al. Characterization of the lymphoid infiltrate in Hashimoto's thyroiditis by immunohistochemistry and polymerase chain reaction for immunoglobulin heavy chain gene rearrangement. *Am J Clin Pathol* 1998;110:327–333.
161. Saxena A, Alport EC, Moshynska O, et al. Clonal B cell populations in a minority of patients with Hashimoto's thyroiditis. *J Clin Pathol* 2004;57:1258–1263.
162. Chen HI, Akpolat I, Mody DR, et al. Restricted κ/λ light chain ratio by flow cytometry in germinal center B cells in Hashimoto thyroiditis. *Am J Clin Pathol* 2006;125:42–48.
163. Isaacson PG, Spencer J. Malignant lymphoma and autoimmune disease. *Histopathology* 1993;22:509–510.
164. Skacel M, Ross CW, His ED. A reassessment of primary thyroid lymphoma: high-grade MALT-type lymphoma as a distinct subtype of diffuse large B-cell lymphoma. *Histopathology* 2000;37:10–18.
165. Ansell SM, Grant CS, Habermann TM. Primary thyroid lymphoma. *Semin Oncol* 1999;26:316–323.
166. Morgen EK, Geddie W, Boerner S, et al. The role of fine-needle aspiration in the diagnosis of thyroid lymphoma: a retrospective study of nine cases and review of the literature. *J Clin Pathol* 2010;63:129–133.
167. Bateman AC, Wright DH. Epitheliotropism in high-grade lymphomas of mucosa-associated lymphoid tissue. *Histopathology* 1993;23:409–415.
168. Matias-Guiu X, Esquius J. Lymphoepithelial lesion in the thyroid: a non-specific histological finding. *Pathol Res Pract* 1991;187:296–300.
169. Graff-Baker A, Roman SA, Thomas DC, et al. Prognosis of primary thyroid lymphoma: demographic, clinical, and pathologic predictors of survival in 1,408 cases. *Surgery* 2009;146:1105–1115.
170. Thieblemont C, Mayer A, Dumontet C, et al. Primary thyroid lymphoma is a heterogeneous disease. *J Clin Endocrinol Metab* 2002;87:105–111.
171. Isaacson PG, Androulakis-Papachristou A, Diss TC, et al. Follicular colonization in thyroid lymphoma. *Am J Pathol* 1992;41:43–52.
172. Kojima M, Nakamura N, Shimizu K, et al. MALT type lymphoma demonstrating prominent plasma cell differentiation resembling fibrous variant of Hashimoto's thyroiditis: a three case report. *Pathol Oncol Res* 2009;15:285–289.
173. Li Y, Zhou G, Ozaki T, et al. Distinct histopathological features of Hashimoto's thyroiditis with respect to IgG4-related disease. *Mod Pathol* 2012;25:1086–1097.
174. Higgins JPT, Warnke R. Large B-cell lymphoma of thyroid: two cases with a marginal zone distribution of the neoplastic cells. *Am J Clin Pathol* 2000;114:264–270.

175. Wolf BC, Sheahan K, DeCoste D, et al. Immunohistochemical analysis of small cell tumors of the thyroid gland: an Eastern Cooperative Oncology Group study. *Hum Pathol* 1992;23:1252–1261.
176. Kim NR, Ko YH, Lee YD. Primary T-cell lymphoma of the thyroid associated with Hashimoto's thyroiditis, histologically mimicking MALT-lymphoma. *J Korean Med Sci* 2010;25:481–484.
177. Bacon CM, Diss TC, Ye H, et al. Follicular lymphoma of the thyroid gland. *Am J Surg Pathol* 2009;33:22–34.
178. Niitsu N, Okamoto M, Nakamura H, et al. Clinicopathologic correlations of stage IE/IIE primary thyroid diffuse large B-cell lymphoma. *Ann Oncol* 2007;18: 1203–1208.
179. Diaz de Leon E, Alkan S, Huang JC, et al. Usefulness of an immunohistochemical panel in paraffin-embedded tissues for the differentiation of B-cell non-Hodgkin's lymphomas of small lymphocytes. *Mod Pathol* 1998;11:1046–1051.
180. Kuper-Hommel MJJ, Schreuder MI, Gemmink AH, et al. T(14;18)(q32;q21) involving *MALT1* and *IGH* genes occurs in extranodal diffuse large B-cell lymphomas of the breast and testis. *Mod Pathol* 2013;26:421–427.
181. Streubel B, Vinatzner U, Lamprecht A, et al. T(3;14)(p14.1;q32) involving *IGH* and *FOXP1* is a novel recurrent chromosomal aberration in MALT lymphoma. *Leukemia* 2005;19:652–658.
182. Mian M, Gaidano G, Conconi A, et al. High response rate and improvement of long-term survival with combined treatment modalities in patients with poor-risk primary thyroid diffuse large B-cell lymphoma: an International Extranodal Lymphoma Study Group and Intergruppo Italiano Linfomi study. *Leuk Lymphoma* 2011;52:823–832.
183. Villano JL, Koshy M, Shaikh H, et al. Age, gender, and racial differences in incidence and survival in primary CNS lymphoma. *Br J Cancer* 2011;105: 1414–1418.
184. Rubenstein J, Ferreri AJM, Pittaluga S. Primary lymphoma of the central nervous system: epidemiology, pathology and current approaches to diagnosis, prognosis and treatment. *Leuk Lymphoma* 2008;49:43–51.
185. Olson JE, Janney CA, Rao RD, et al. The continuing increase in the incidence of primary central nervous system non-Hodgkin lymphoma: a surveillance, epidemiology, and end results analysis. *Cancer* 2002;95:1504–1510.
186. Maher EA, Fine HA. Primary CNS lymphoma. *Semin Oncol* 1999;26:346–356.
187. Camilleri-Broët S, Davi F, Feuillard J, et al. AIDS-related primary brain lymphomas: histopathologic and immunohistochemical study of 51 cases. *Hum Pathol* 1997;28:367–374.
188. Cavaliere R, Petroni G, Lopes MB, et al. Primary central nervous system post-transplantation lymphoproliferative disorder: an International Primary Central Nervous System Lymphoma Collaborative Group Report. *Cancer* 2010;116: 863–870.
189. Chang KL, Flaris N, Hickey WF, et al. Brain lymphoma of immunocompetent and immunocompromised patients: study of the association with Epstein-Barr virus. *Mod Pathol* 1993;6:427–432.
190. Nuckols JD, Liu K, Burchette JL, et al. Primary central nervous system lymphomas: a 30-year experience at a single institution. *Mod Pathol* 1999;12: 1167–1173.
191. Ferreri AJM. How I treat primary CNS lymphoma. *Blood* 2011;118:510–522.
192. Grisariu S, Avni B, Batchelor TT, et al. Neurolymphomatosis: an International Primary CNS Lymphoma Collaborative Group report. *Blood* 2010;115:5005–5011.
193. Deckert M, Engert A, Brück W, et al. Modern concepts in the biology, diagnosis, differential diagnosis and treatment of primary central nervous system lymphoma. *Leukemia* 2011;25:1797–1807.
194. Sherman ME, Erozan YS, Mann RB, et al. Stereotactic brain biopsy in the diagnosis of malignant lymphoma. *Am J Clin Pathol* 1991:95:878–883.
195. Rhodes CH, Glantz MJ, Glantz L, et al. A comparison of polymerase chain reaction examination of cerebrospinal fluid and conventional cytology in the diagnosis of lymphomatous meningitis. *Cancer* 1996;77:543–548.
196. Baraniskin A, Kuhnhenn J, Schlegel U, et al. Identification of microRNAs in the cerebrospinal fluid as marker for primary diffuse large B-cell lymphoma of the central nervous system. *Blood* 2011;117:3140–3146.
197. Bataille B, Delwail V, Menet E, et al. Primary intracerebral malignant lymphoma: report of 248 cases. *J Neurosurg* 2000;92:261–266.
198. Miller DC, Hochberg FH, Harris NL, et al. Pathology with clinical correlations of primary central nervous system non-Hodgkin's lymphoma: the Massachusetts General Hospital experience 1958–1989. *Cancer* 1994;74:1383–1397.
199. Camilleri-Broët S, Martin A, Moreau A, et al. Primary central nervous system lymphomas in 72 immunocompetent patients: pathologic findings and clinical correlations. *Am J Clin Pathol* 1998;110:607–612.
200. Kluin PM, Deckert M, Ferry JA. Primary diffuse large B-cell lymphoma of the CNS. In: Swerdlow SH, Campo E, Harris NL, et al., eds. *WHO classification of tumours of haematopoietic and lymphoid tissues*, 4th ed. Lyon: IARC, 2008: 240–241.
201. Schwechheimer K, Braus DF, Schwarzkopf G, et al. Polymorphous high-grade B cell lymphoma is the predominant type of spontaneous primary cerebral malignant lymphomas: histological and immunomorphological evaluation of computed tomography-guided stereotactic brain biopsies. *Am J Surg Pathol* 1994;18:931–937.
202. Ponzoni M, Berger F, Chassagne-Clement C, et al. Reactive perivascular T-cell infiltrate predicts survival in primary central nervous system B-cell lymphomas. *Br J Haematol* 2007;138:316–323.
203. Rollins KE, Kleinschmidt-DeMasters BK, Corboy JR, et al. Lymphomatosis cerebri as a cause of white matter dementia. *Hum Pathol* 2005;36:282–290.
204. Nakamura S, Ponzoni M, Campo E. Intravascular large B-cell lymphoma. In: Swerdlow SH, Campo E, Harris NL, et al., eds. *WHO classification of tumours of haematopoietic and lymphoid tissues*, 4th ed. Lyon: IARC, 2008:252–253.
205. Shimada K, Murase T, Matsue K, et al. Central nervous system involvement in intravascular large B-cell lymphoma: a retrospective analysis of 109 patients. *Cancer Sci* 2010;101:1480–1486.
206. Thompsett AR, Ellison DW, Stevenson FK, et al. V_H gene sequences from primary central nervous system lymphomas indicate derivation from highly mutated germinal center B cells with ongoing mutational activity. *Blood* 1999;94:1738–1746.
207. Montesinos-Rongen M, Küppers R, Schlüter D, et al. Primary central nervous system lymphomas are derived from germinal-center B cells and show a preferential usage of the *V4–34* gene segment. *Am J Pathol* 1999;155:2077–2086.
208. Camilleri-Broët S, Crinière E, Broët P, et al. A uniform activated B-cell–like immunophenotype might explain the poor prognosis of primary central nervous system lymphomas: analysis of 83 cases. *Blood* 2006;107:190–196.
209. Hattab EM, Martin SE, Al-Khatib S, et al. Most primary central nervous system diffuse large B-cell lymphomas occurring in immunocompetent individuals belong to the nongerminal center subtype: a retrospective analysis of 31 cases. *Mod Pathol* 2010;23:235–243.
210. Braaten KM, Betensky RA, de Leval L, et al. BCL-6 expression predicts improved survival in patients with primary central nervous system lymphoma. *Clin Cancer Res* 2003;9:1063–1069.
211. Lin CH, Kuan-Ting K, Chuang SS, et al. Comparison of the expression and prognostic significance of differentiation markers between diffuse large B-cell lymphoma of central nervous system origin and peripheral nodal origin. *Clin Cancer Res* 2006;12:1152–1156.
212. Ferreri AJM, Marturano E. Primary CNS lymphoma. *Best Pract Res Clin Haematol* 2012;25:119–130.
213. Rickert CH, Dockhorn-Dworniczak B, Simon R, et al. Chromosomal imbalances in primary lymphomas of the central nervous system. *Am J Pathol* 1999;155:1445–1451.
214. Weber T, Weber RG, Kaulich K, et al. Characteristic chromosomal imbalances in primary central nervous system lymphomas of the diffuse large B-cell type. *Brain Pathol* 2000;10:73–84.
215. Nakamura M, Kishi M, Sakaki T, et al. Novel tumor suppressor loci on 6q22-23 in primary central nervous system lymphomas. *Cancer Res* 2003;63:737–741.
216. Montesinos-Rongen M, Zühlke-Jenisch R, Gesk S, et al. Interphase cytogenetic analysis of lymphoma-associated chromosomal breakpoints in primary diffue large B-cell lymphomas of the central nervous system. *J Neuropathol Exp Neurol* 2002;61:926–933.
217. Schwindt H, Akasaka T, Zühlke-Jenisch R, et al. Chromosomal translocations fusing the *BCL6* gene to different partner loci are recurrent in primary central nervous system lymphoma and may be associated with aberrant somatic hypermutation or defective class switch recombination. *J Neuropathol Exp Neurol* 2006;65:776–782.
218. Cady FM, O'Neill BP, Law ME, et al. Del(6)(q22) and *BCL6* rearrangements in primary CNS lymphoma are indicators of an aggressive clinical course. *J Clin Oncol* 2008;26:4814–4819.
219. Courts C, Montesinos-Rongen M, Martin-Subero JI, et al. Transcriptional profiling of the nuclear factor-κB pathway identifies a subgroup of primary lymphoma of the central nervous system with low BCL10 expression. *J Neuropathol Exp Neurol* 2007;66:230–237.
220. Montesinos-Rongen M, Schmitz R, Brunn A, et al. Mutations of *CARD11* but not *TNFAIP3* may activate the NF-κB pathway in primary CNS lymphoma. *Acta Neuropathol* 2010;120:529–535.
221. Fischer, L, Hummel M, Korfel A, et al. Differential micro-RNA expression in primary CNS and nodal diffuse large B-cell lymphomas. *Neuro Oncol* 2011;13:1090–1098.
222. Montesinos-Rongen M, Brunn A, Bentink S, et al. Gene expression profiling suggests primary central nervous system lymphomas to be derived from a late germinal center B cell. *Leukemia* 2008;22:400–405.
223. Rubenstein JL, Fridlyand J, Shen A, et al. Gene expression and angiotropism in primary CNS lymphoma. *Blood* 2006;107:3716–3723.
224. Tun, HW, Personett D, Baskerville KA, et al. Pathway analysis of primary central nervous system lymphoma. *Blood* 2008;111:3200–3210.
225. Sung CO, Kim SC, Karnan S, et al. Genomic profiling combined with gene expression profiling in primary central nervous system lymphoma. *Blood* 2011;117:1291–1300.
226. Yuan J, Gu K, He J, et al. Preferential up-regulation of osteopontin in primary central nervous system lymphoma does not correlate with putative receptor CD44v6 or CD44H expression. *Hum Pathol* 2013;44:606–611.
227. Gerstner ER, Abrey LE, Schiff D, et al. CNS Hodgkin lymphoma. *Blood* 2008;112:1658–1661.
228. Choi JS, Nam DH, Ko YH, et al. Primary central nervous system lymphoma in Korea: comparison of B- and T-cell lymphomas. *Am J Surg Pathol* 2003;17: 919–928.
229. Shenkier TN, Blay JY, O'Neill BP, et al. Primary CNS lymphoma of T-cell origin: a descriptive analysis from the International Primary CNS Lymphoma Collaborative Group. *J Clin Oncol* 2005;23:2233–2239.
230. Guan H, Huang Y, Wen W, et al. Primary central nervous system extranodal NK/T-cell lymphoma, nasal type: case report and review of the literature. *J Neurooncol* 2011;103:387–391.
231. Wu W, Tanrivermis Sayit A, Vinters HV, et al. Primary central nervous system histiocytic sarcoma presenting as a postradiation sarcoma: case report and literature review. *Hum Pathol* 2013;44:1177–1183.
232. Jahnke K, Korfel A, O'Neill BP, et al. International study on low-grade primary central nervous system lymphoma. *Ann Neurol* 2006;59:755–762.
233. Tu PH, Giannini C, Judkins AR, et al. Clinicopathologic and genetic profile of intracranial marginal zone lymphoma: a primary low-grade CNS lymphoma that mimics meningioma. *J Clin Oncol* 2005;23:5718–5727.
234. Iwamoto FM, DeAngelis LM, Abrey LE. Primary dural lymphomas: a clinicopathologic study of treatment and outcome in eight patients. *Neurology* 2006;66:1763–1765.
235. Venkataraman G, Rizzo KA, Chavez JJ, et al. Marginal zone lymphomas involving meningeal dura: possible link to IgG4-related diseases. *Mod Pathol* 2011;24:355–366.
236. Bhagavathi S, Greiner TC, Kazmi SA, et al. Extranodal marginal zone lymphoma of the dura mater with IgH/MALT1 translocation and review of literature. *J Hematopathol* 2008;1:131–137.
237. Chan SK, Cheuk W, Chan KT, et al. IgG4-related sclerosing pachymeningitis: a previously unrecognized form of central nervous system involvement in IgG4-related related sclerosing disease. *Am J Surg Pathol* 2009;33:1249–1252.
238. Benevolo G, Stacchini A, Spina M, et al. Final results of a multicenter trial addressing role of CSF flow cytometric analysis in NHL patients at high risk for CNS dissemination. *Blood* 2012;120:3222–3228.
239. Ferreri AJM, Assanelli A, Crocchiolo R, et al. Central nervous system dissemination in immunocompetent patients with aggressive lymphomas: incidence, risk factors and therapeutic options. *Hematol Oncol* 2009;27:61–70.
240. Doolittle ND, Abrey LE, Shenkier TN, et al. Brain parenchyma involvement as isolated central nervous system relapse of systemic non-Hodgkin lymphoma: an International Primary CNS Lymphoma Collaborative Group Report. *Blood* 2008;111:1085–1093.
241. Panageas KS, Elkin EB, DeAngelis LM, et al. Trends in survival from primary central nervous system lymphoma, 1975–1999: a population-based analysis. *Cancer* 2005;104:2466–2472.

242. Gundrum JD, Mathiason MA, Moore DB, et al. Primary testicular diffuse large B-cell lymphoma: a population-based study on the incidence, natural history, and survival comparison with primary nodal counterpart before and after the introduction of rituximab. *J Clin Oncol* 2009;27:5227–5232.
243. Shahab N, Doll DC. Testicular lymphoma. *Semin Oncol* 1999;26:259–269.
244. Fonseca R, Habermann TM, Colgan JP, et al. Testicular lymphoma is associated with a high incidence of extranodal recurrence. *Cancer* 2000;88:154–161.
245. Zucca E, Conconi A, Mughal TI, et al. Patterns of outcome and prognostic factors in primary large-cell lymphoma of the testis in a survey by the International Extranodal Lymphoma Study Group. *J Clin Oncol* 2003;21:20–27.
246. Paladugu RR, Bearman RM, Rappaport H. Malignant lymphoma with primary manifestation in the gonad: a clinicopathologic study of 39 patients. *Cancer* 1980;45:561–571.
247. Turner RR, Colby TV, MacKintosh FR. Testicular lymphomas: a clinicopathologic study of 35 cases. *Cancer* 1981;48:2095–2102.
248. Ferry JA, Harris NL, Young RH, et al. Malignant lymphoma of the testis, epididymis, and spermatic cord: a clinicopathologic study of 69 cases with immunophenotypic analysis. *Am J Surg Pathol* 1994;18:376–390.
249. Vega F, Medeiros LJ, Abruzzo LV. Primary paratesticular lymphoma: a report of 2 cases and review of the literature. *Arch Pathol Lab Med* 2001;125:428–432.
250. Roy S, Hooda S, Parwani AV. Idiopathic granulomatous orchitis. *Pathol Res Pract* 2011;207:275–278.
251. Agarwal V, Li JKH, Bard R. Lymphocytic orchitis: a case report. *Hum Pathol* 1990;21:1080–1082.
252. Braaten KM, Young RH, Ferry JA. Viral-type orchitis: a potential mimic of testicular neoplasia. *Am J Surg Pathol* 2009;33:1477–1484.
253. Fernandopulle SM, Hwang JS, Kuick CH, et al. Rosai-Dorfman disease of the testis: an unusual entity that mimics testicular malignancy. *J Clin Pathol* 2006;59:325–327.
254. Hyland J, Lasota J, Jasinski M, et al. Molecular pathological analysis of testicular diffuse large cell lymphomas. *Hum Pathol* 1998;29:1231–1239.
255. Hasselblom S, Ridell B, Wedel H, et al. Testicular lymphoma: a retrospective, population-based, clinical and immunohistochemical study. *Acta Oncol* 2004;43:758–765.
256. Valbuena JR, Admirand JH, Lin P, et al. Myeloid sarcoma involving the testis. *Am J Clin Pathol* 2005;124:445–452.
257. Ferry JA, Young RH, Scully RE. Testicular and epididymal plasmacytoma: a report of 7 cases, including three that were the initial manifestation of plasma cell myeloma. *Am J Surg Pathol* 1997;21:590–598.
258. Ubright TM. The most common, clinically significant misdiagnoses in testicular tumor pathology, and how to avoid them. *Adv Anat Pathol* 2008;15:18–27.
259. Al-Abbadi MA, Hattab EM, Tarawneh MS, et al. Primary testicular diffuse large B-cell lymphoma belongs to the nongerminal center B-cell-like subgroup: a study of 18 cases. *Mod Pathol* 2006;19:1521–1527.
260. Li D, Xie P, Mi C. Primary testicular diffuse large B-cell lymphoma shows an activated B-cell-like phenotype. *Pathol Res Pract* 2010;206:611–615.
261. Booman M, Douwes J, Glas AM, et al. Primary testicular diffuse large B-cell lymphomas have activated B-cell-like subtype characteristics. *J Pathol* 2006;210:163–171.
262. Riemersma SA, Jordanova ES, Schop RFJ, et al. Extensive genetic alterations of the HLA region, including homozygous deletions of HLA class II genes in B-cell lymphomas arising in immune-privileged sites. *Blood* 2000;96:3569–3577.
263. Booman M, Douwes J, Glas AM, et al. Mechanisms and effects of loss of human leukocyte antigen class II expression in immune-privileged site-associated B-cell lymphoma. *Clin Cancer Res* 2006;12:2698–2705.
264. Booman M, Szuhai K, Rosenwald A, et al. Genomic alterations and gene expression in primary diffuse large B-cell lymphomas of immune-privileged sites: the importance of apoptosis and immunomodulatory pathways. *J Pathol* 2008;216:209–217.
265. Finn LS, Viswanatha DS, Belasco JB, et al. Primary follicular lymphoma of the testis in childhood. *Cancer* 1999;85:1626–1635.
266. Bacon CM, Ye H, Diss TC, et al. Primary follicular lymphoma of the testis and epididymis in adults. *Am J Surg Pathol* 2007;31:1050–1058.
267. Azúa-Romeo J, Alvarez-Alegret R, Serrano P, et al. Primary anaplastic large cell lymphoma of the testis. *Int Urol Nephrol* 2004;36:393–396.
268. Liang DN, Yang ZR, Wang WY, et al. Extranodal nasal type natural killer/T-cell lymphoma of testis: report of seven cases with review of literature. *Leuk Lymphoma* 2012;53:1117–1123.
269. Mazloom A, Fowler N, Medeiros LJ, et al. Outcome of patients with diffuse large B-cell lymphoma of the testis by era of treatment: the M. D. Anderson Cancer Center experience. *Leuk Lymphoma* 2010;51:1217–1224.
270. Vitolo U, Chiappella A, Ferreri AJM, et al. First-line treatment for primary testicular diffuse large B-cell lymphoma with rituximab-CHOP, CNS prophylaxis, and contralateral testis irradiation: final results of an international phase II trial. *J Clin Oncol* 2011;29:2766–2772.
271. Chorlton I, Norris HJ, King FM. Malignant reticuloendothelial disease involving the ovary as a primary manifestation: a series of 19 lymphomas and 1 granulocytic sarcoma. *Cancer* 1974;34:397–407.
272. Leoncini L, Raphaël M, Stein H, et al. Burkitt lymphoma In: Swerdlow SH, Campo E, Harris NL, et al., eds. *WHO classification of tumours of haematopoietic and lymphoid tissues*, 4th ed. Lyon: IARC, 2008:262–264.
273. Kosari F, Daneshbod Y, Parwaresch R, et al. Lymphomas of the female genital tract: a study of 186 cases and review of the literature. *Am J Surg Pathol* 2005;29:1512–1520.
274. Vang R, Medeiros LJ, Warnke RA, et al. Ovarian non-Hodgkin's lymphoma: a clinicopathologic study of eight primary cases. *Mod Pathol* 2001;14:1093–1099.
275. Monterroso V, Jaffe ES, Merino MJ, et al. Malignant lymphomas involving the ovary: a clinicopathologic analysis of 39 cases. *Am J Surg Pathol* 1993;17:154–170.
276. Lagoo AS, Robboy SJ. Lymphoma of the female genital tract: current status. *Int Gynecol Pathol* 2005;25:1–21.
277. Özsan N, Bedke BJ, Law ME, et al. Clinicopathologic and genetic characterization of follicular lymphomas presenting in the ovary reveals 2 distinct subgroups. *Am J Surg Pathol* 2011;35:1691–1699.
278. Garcia MG, Deavers MT, Knoblock RJ, et al. Myeloid sarcoma involving the gynecologic tract: a report of 11 cases and review of the literature. *Am J Clin Pathol* 2006;125:783–790.
279. Vang R, Medeiros LJ, Ha CS, et al. Non-Hodgkin's lymphomas involving the uterus: a clinicopathologic analysis of 26 cases. *Mod Pathol* 2000;13:19–28.
280. Vang R, Medeiros LJ, Silva EG, et al. Non-Hodgkin's lymphoma involving the vagina: a clinicopathologic analysis of 14 patients. *Am J Surg Pathol* 2000;24:719–725.
281. Vang R, Medeiros LJ, Malpica A, et al. Non-Hodgkin's lymphoma involving the vulva. *Int J Gynecol Pathol* 2000;19:236–242.
282. Harris NL, Scully RE. Malignant lymphoma and granulocytic sarcoma of the uterus and vagina: a clinicopathologic analysis of 27 cases. *Cancer* 1984;53:2530–2545.
283. Muntz HG, Ferry JA, Flynn D, et al. Stage IE primary malignant lymphomas of the uterine cervix. *Cancer* 1991;68:2023–2032.
284. Kahlifa M, Buckstein R, Perez-Ordoñez B. Sarcomatoid variant of B-cell lymphoma of the uterine cervix. *Int J Gynecol Pathol* 2003;22:289–293.
285. van de Rijn M, Kamel OW, Chang PP, et al. Primary low-grade endometrial B-cell lymphoma. *Am J Surg Pathol* 1997;21:187–194.
286. Wright TM, Rule S, Liu H, et al. Extranodal marginal zone lymphoma of the uterine corpus. *Leuk Lymphoma* 2012;53:1831–1834. [Letter].
287. Yoshinaga K, Akahira JI, Niikura H, et al. A case of primary mucosa-associated lymphoid tissue lymphoma of the vagina. *Hum Pathol* 2004;35:1164–1166.
288. Geyer JT, Ferry JA, Harris NL, et al. Florid reactive lymphoid hyperplasia of the lower female genital tract (lymphoma-like lesion): a benign condition that frequently harbors clonal immunoglobulin heavy chain gene rearrangements. *Am J Surg Pathol* 2010;34:161–168.
289. Ramalingam P, Zoroquiain P, Valbuena JR, et al. Florid reactive lymphoid hyperplasia (lymphoma-like lesion) of the uterine cervix. *Ann Diagn Pathol* 2012;16:21–28.
290. Frey NV, Svoboda J, Andreadis C, et al. Primary lymphomas of the cervix and uterus: the University of Pennsylvania's experience and a review of the literature. *Leuk Lymphoma* 2006;47:1894–1901.
291. Ostrowski ML, Unni KK, Banks PM, et al. Malignant lymphoma of bone. *Cancer* 1986;58:2646–2655.
292. Ramadan KM, Shenkier T, Sehn LH, et al. A clinicopathological retrospective study of 131 patients with primary bone lymphoma: a population-based study of successively treated cohorts from the British Columbia Cancer Agency. *Ann Oncol* 2007;18:129–135.
293. Martinez A, Ponzoni M, Agostinelli C, et al. Primary bone marrow lymphoma: an uncommon extranodal presentation of aggressive non-Hodgkin lymphomas. *Am J Surg Pathol* 2012;36:296–304.
294. Baar J, Burkes RL, Gospodarowicz M. Primary non-Hodgkin's lymphoma of bone. *Semin Oncol* 1999;26:270–275.
295. Zhao XF, Young KH, Frank D, et al. Pediatric primary bone lymphoma-diffuse large B-cell lymphoma: morphologic and immunohistochemical characteristics of 10 cases. *Am J Clin Pathol* 2007;127:47–54.
296. Beal K, Allen L, Yahalom J, et al. Primary bone lymphoma: treatment results and prognostic factors with long-term follow-up of 82 patients. *Cancer* 2006;106:2652–2656.
297. Mikhaeel NG. Primary bone lymphoma. *Clin Oncol (R Coll Radiol)* 2012;24:366–370.
298. Jones D, Kraus MD, Dorfman DM. Lymphoma presenting as a solitary bone tumor. *Am J Clin Pathol* 1999;111:171–178.
299. de Leval L, Braaten KM, Ancukiewicz M, et al. Diffuse large B-cell lymphoma of bone: an analysis of differentiation-associated antigens with clinical correlation. *Am J Surg Pathol* 2003;27:1269–1277.
300. Adams H, Tzankov A, d'Hondt S, et al. Primary diffuse large B-cell lymphomas of the bone: prognostic relevance of protein expression and clinical factors. *Hum Pathol* 2008;39:1323–1330.
301. Bhagavathi S, Micale MA, Les K, et al. Primary bone diffuse large B-cell lymphoma: clinicopathologic study of 21 cases and review of literature. *Am J Surg Pathol* 2009;33:1463–1469.
302. Hsieh PP, Tseng HH, Chang ST, et al. Primary non-Hodgkin's lymphoma of bone: a rare disorder with high frequency of T-cell phenotype in southern Taiwan. *Leuk Lymphoma* 2006;47:65–70.
303. Maruyama D, Watanabe T, Beppu Y, et al. Primary bone lymphoma: a new and detailed characterization of 28 patients in a single-institution study. *Jpn J Clin Oncol* 2007;37:216–223.
304. Mann RB. Are there site-specific differences among extranodal aggressive B-cell neoplasms? *Am J Clin Pathol* 1999;111(Suppl 1):S144–S150.
305. Heyning FH, Hogendoorn PCW, Kramer MHH, et al. Primary lymphoma of bone: extranodal lymphoma with favorable survival independent of germinal centre, post-germinal centre or indeterminate phenotype. *J Clin Pathol* 2009;62:820–824.
306. Lima FP, Bousquet M, Gomez-Brouchet A, et al. Primary diffuse large B-cell lymphoma of bone displays preferential rearrangements of the c-*MYC* or *BCL2* gene. *Am J Clin Pathol* 2008;129:723–726.
307. Heyning FH, Jansen PM, Hogendoorn PCW, et al. Array-based comparative genomic hybridization analysis reveals recurrent chromosomal alterations in primary diffuse large B cell lymphoma of bone. *J Clin Pathol* 2010;63:1095–1100.
308. Nagasaka T, Nakamura S, Medeiros LJ, et al. Anaplastic large cell lymphomas presented as bone lesions: a clinicopathologic study of six cases and review of the literature. *Mod Pathol* 2000;10:1143–1149.
309. Bakshi NA, Ross CW, Finn WG, et al. ALK-positive anaplastic large cell lymphoma with primary bone involvement in children. *Am J Clin Pathol* 2006;125:57–63.
310. Ostrowski ML, Inwards CY, Strickler JG, et al. Osseous Hodgkin's disease. *Cancer* 1999;85:1166–1178.
311. Ozdemirli M, Fanburg-Smith JC, Hartmann D-P, et al. Precursor B-lymphoblastic lymphoma presenting as a solitary bone tumor and mimicking Ewing's sarcoma: a report of four cases and review of the literature. *Am J Surg Pathol* 1998;22:795–804.
312. Iravani S, Singleton TP, Ross CW, et al. Precursor B-lymphoblastic lymphoma presenting as lytic bone lesions. *Am J Clin Pathol* 1999;112:836–843.
313. Jawad MU, Schneiderbauer MM, Min ES, et al. Primary lymphoma of bone in adult patients. *Cancer* 2010;116:871–879.
314. Pellegrini C, Gandolfi L, Quirini F, et al. Primary bone lymphoma: evaluation of chemoimmunotherapy as front-line treatment in 21 patients. *Clin Lymphoma Myeloma Leuk* 2011;11:321–325.
315. Giardini R, Piccolo C, Rilke F. Primary non-Hodgkin's lymphomas of the female breast. *Cancer* 1992;69:725–735.
316. Brogi E, Harris NL. Lymphomas of the breast: pathology and clinical behavior. *Semin Oncol* 1999;26:357–364.
317. Lin Y, Govindan R, Hess JL. Malignant hematopoietic breast tumors. *Am J Clin Pathol* 1997;107:177–186.

318. Ganjoo K, Advani R, Mariappan MR, et al. Non-Hodgkin lymphoma of breast. *Cancer* 2007;110:25–30.
319. Ryan G, Martinelli G, Kuper-Hommel M, et al. Primary diffuse large B-cell lymphoma of the breast: prognostic factors and outcomes of a study by the International Extranodal Lymphoma Study Group. *Ann Oncol* 2008;19:233–241.
320. Martinelli G, Ryan G, Seymour JF, et al. Primary follicular and marginal-zone lymphoma of the breast: clinical features, prognostic factors and outcome: a study by the International Extranodal Lymphoma Study Group. *Ann Oncol* 2009;20:1993–1999.
321. Arber DA, Simpson JF, Weiss LM, et al. Non-Hodgkin's lymphoma involving the breast. *Am J Surg Pathol* 1994;18:288–295.
322. Jeon HJ, Akagi T, Hoshida Y, et al. Primary non-Hodgkin's malignant lymphoma of the breast: an immunohistochemical study of seven patients and literature review of 152 patients with breast lymphoma in Japan. *Cancer* 1992;70: 2451–2459.
323. Borbrow LG, Richards MA, Happerfield LC, et al. Breast lymphomas: a clinicopathologic review. *Hum Pathol* 1993;24:274–278.
324. Abbondanzo SL, Seidman JD, Lefkowitz M, et al. Primary diffuse large B-cell lymphoma of the breast: a clinicopathologic study of 31 cases. *Pathol Res Pract* 1996;192:37–43.
325. Farinha P, André S, Cabeçadas J, et al. High frequency of MALT lymphoma in a series of 14 cases of primary breast lymphoma. *Appl Immunohistochem Morphol* 2002;10:115–120.
326. Talwalkar SS, Miranda RN, Valbuena JR, et al. Lymphomas involving the breast: a study of 106 cases comparing localized and disseminated neoplasms. *Am J Surg Pathol* 2008;32:1299–1309.
327. Gualco G, Bacchi CE. B-cell and T-cell lymphomas of the breast: clinical–pathological features of 53 cases. *Int J Surg Pathol* 2008;16:407–413.
328. Aguilera NSI, Tavassoli FA, Chu WS, et al. T-cell lymphoma presenting in the breast: a histologic, immunophenotypic and molecular genetic study of four cases. *Mod Pathol* 2000;13:599–605.
329. Mattia AR, Ferry JA, Harris NL. Breast lymphoma: a B-cell spectrum including the low grade B-cell lymphoma of mucosa associated lymphoid tissue. *Am J Surg Pathol* 1993;17:574–587.
330. Talwalkar SS, Valbuena JR, Abruzzo LV, et al. *MALT* gene rearrangements and NF-κB activation involving p65 and p50 are absent or rare in primary MALT lymphomas of the breast. *Mod Pathol* 2006;19:1402–1408.
331. Valbuena JR, Admirand JH, Gualco G, et al. Myeloid sarcoma involving the breast. *Arch Pathol Lab Med* 2005;129:32–38.
332. Yoshida S, Nakamura N, Sasaki Y, et al. Primary breast diffuse large B-cell lymphoma shows a non-germinal center B-cell phenotype. *Mod Pathol* 2005;18: 398–405.
333. Li D, Deng J, He H, et al. Primary breast diffuse large B-cell lymphoma shows an activated B-cell-like phenotype. *Ann Diagn Pathol* 2012;16:335–343.
334. Thompson PA, Lade S, Webster H, et al. Effusion-associated anaplastic large cell lymphoma of the breast: time for it to be defined as a distinct clinico-pathological entity [Letter]. *Haematologica* 2010;98:1977–1979.
335. Lazzeri D, Agostini T, Bocci G, et al. ALK-1-negative anaplastic large cell lymphoma associated with breast implants: a new clinical entity. *Clin Breast Cancer* 2011;11:283–296.
336. Roden, AC, Macon WR, Keeney GL, et al. Seroma-associated primary anaplastic large-cell lymphoma adjacent to breast implants: an indolent T-cell lymphoproliferative disorder. *Mod Pathol* 2008;21:455–463.
337. Aladily TN, Medeiros LJ, Amin MB, et al. Anaplastic large cell lymphoma associated with breast implants: a report of 13 cases. *Am J Surg Pathol* 2012;36:1000–1008.
338. Aladily TN, Nathwani BN, Miranda RN, et al. Extranodal NK/T-cell lymphoma, nasal type, arising in association with saline breast implant; expanding the spectrum of breast implant-associated lymphomas. *Am J Surg Pathol* 2012;36: 1729–1734.
339. Schwartz IS, Strauchen JA. Lymphocytic mastopathy: an autoimmune disease of the breast? *Am J Clin Pathol* 1990;93:725–730.
340. Valdez R, Thorson J, Finn WG et al. Lymphocytic mastitis and diabetic mastopathy: a molecular, immunophenotypic, and clinicopathologic evaluation of 11 cases. *Mod Pathol* 2003;16:223–228.
341. Cheuk W, Chan ACL, Lam WL, et al. IgG4-related sclerosing mastitis: description of a new member of the IgG4-related sclerosing diseases. *Am J Surg Pathol* 2009;33:1058–1064.
342. Cha YJ, Yang WI, Park SH, et al. Rosai-Dorfman disease in the breast with increased IgG4 expressing plasma cells: a case report. *Korean J Pathol* 2012;46:489–493.
343. Mozos A, Ye H, Chuang WY, et al. Most primary adrenal lymphomas are diffuse large B-cell lymphomas with non-germinal center B-cell phenotype, *BCL6* gene rearrangement and poor prognosis. *Mod Pathol* 2009;22:1210–1217.
344. Rock J, Bloomston M, Lozanski G, et al. The spectrum of hematologic malignancies involving the pancreas: potential clinical mimics of pancreatic adenocarcinoma. *Am J Clin Pathol* 2012;137:414–422.
345. Zahrani AA, Abdelsalam M, Fiaar AA, et al. Diffuse large B-cell lymphoma transformed from mucosa-associated lymphoid tissue lymphoma arising in a female urethra treated with rituximab for the first time. *Case Rep Oncol* 2012;5:238–245.
346. Misdraji J, Ino Y, Louis DN, et al. Primary lymphoma of peripheral nerve: report of four cases. *Am J Surg Pathol* 2000;24:1257–1265.
347. Flanagan EP, O'Neill BP, Porter AB, et al. Primary intramedullary spinal cord lymphoma. *Neurology* 2011;77:784–791.
348. Gill PS, Chandraratna AN, Meyer PR, et al. Malignant lymphoma: cardiac involvement at initial presentation. *J Clin Oncol* 1987;5:216–224.
349. Nascimento AF, Winters GL, Pinkus GS. Primary cardiac lymphoma: clinical, histologic, immunophenotypic, and genotypic features of 5 cases of a rare disorder. *Am J Surg Pathol* 2007;31:1344–1350.
350. Miller DV, Firchau DJ, McClure RF, et al. Epstein-Barr virus-associated diffuse large B-cell lymphoma arising on cardiac prostheses. *Am J Surg Pathol* 2010;34:377–384.
351. Gruver AM, Huba MA, Dogan A, et al. Fibrin-associated large B-cell lymphoma: part of the spectrum of cardiac lymphomas. *Am J Surg Pathol* 2012;36:1527–1537.
352. Chan JKC, Aozasa K, Gaulard P. DLBCL associated with chronic inflammation. In: Swerdlow SH, Campo E, Harris NL, et al., eds. *WHO classification of tumours of haematopoietic and lymphoid tissues*, 4th ed. Lyon: IARC, 2008:245–246.
353. Petitjean B, Jardin F, Joly B, et al. Pyothorax-associated lymphoma: a peculiar clinicopathologic entity derived from B cells at late stage of differentiation and with occasional aberrant dual B- and T-cell phenotype. *Am J Surg Pathol* 2002;26:724–732.
354. Narimatsu H, Ota Y, Kami M, et al. Clinicopathological features of pyothorax-associated lymphoma; a retrospective survey involving 98 patients. *Ann Oncol* 2007;18:122–128.
355. Cesarman E, Nador RG, Aozasa K, et al. Kaposi's sarcoma-associated herpesvirus in non-AIDS-related lymphomas occurring in body cavities. *Am J Pathol* 1996;149:53–57.
356. Copie-Bergman C, Niedobitek G, Mangham DC, et al. Epstein-Barr virus in B-cell lymphomas associated with chronic suppurative inflammation. *J Pathol* 1997;183:287–292.
357. Cheuk W, Chan ACL, Chan JKC, et al. Metallic implant-associated lymphoma: a distinct subgroup of large B-cell lymphoma related to pyothorax-associated lymphoma? *Am J Surg Pathol* 2005;29:832–836.
358. Loong F, Chan ACL, Ho BCS, et al. Diffuse large B-cell lymphoma associated with chronic inflammation as an incidental finding and new clinical scenarios. *Mod Pathol* 2010;23:493–501.
359. Boroumand N, Ly L, Sonstein J, et al. Microscopic diffuse large B-cell lymphomas (DLBCL) occurring in pseudocysts: do these tumors belong to the category of DLBCL associated with chronic inflammation? *Am J Surg Pathol* 2012;36: 1074–1080.
360. Stancu M, Jones D, Vega F, et al. Peripheral T-cell lymphoma arising in the liver. *Am J Clin Pathol* 2002;118:574–581.
361. Page RD, Romaguera JE, Osborne B, et al. Primary hepatic lymphoma: favorable outcome after combination chemotherapy *Cancer* 2001;92:2023–2029.
362. Loddenkemper C, Longerich T, Hummel M, et al. Frequency and diagnostic patterns of lymphomas in liver biopsies with respect to the WHO classification. *Virchows Arch* 2007;450:493–502.
363. Mani H, Climent F, Colomo L, et al. Gall bladder and extrahepatic bile duct lymphomas: clinicopathological observations and biological implications. *Am J Surg Pathol* 2010;34:1277–1286.
364. Ferry JA, Harris NL, Papanicolaou N, et al. Lymphoma of the kidney: a report of 11 cases. *Am J Surg Pathol* 1995;19:134–144.
365. Schniederjan SD, Osunkoya AO. Lymphoid neoplasms of the urinary tract and male genital organs: a clinicopathological study of 40 cases. *Mod Pathol* 2009;22:1057–1065.
366. Kempton CL, Kurtin PJ, Inwards DJ, et al. Malignant lymphoma of the bladder: evidence from 36 cases that low-grade lymphoma of the MALT-type is the most common primary bladder lymphoma. *Am J Surg Pathol* 1997;21:1324–1333.
367. Siegel RJ, Napoli VM. Malignant lymphoma of the urinary bladder: a case with signet-ring cells simulating urachal adenocarcinoma. *Arch Pathol Lab Med* 1991;115:635–637.
368. Nigwekar P, Tamboli P, Amin MB, et al. Plasmacytoid urothelial carcinoma: detailed analysis of morphology with clinicopathologic correlation in 17 cases. *Am J Surg Pathol* 2009;33:417–424.
369. Bostwick DG, Iczkowski KA, Amin MB, et al. Malignant lymphoma involving the prostate: report of 62 cases. *Cancer* 1998;83:732–738.
370. Solomides CC, Miller AS, Christman RA, et al. Lymphomas of the oral cavity:1histology, immunologic type, and incidence of Epstein-Barr virus infection. *Hum Pathol* 2002;33:153–157.
371. Delecluse HJ, Anagnostopoulos I, Dallenbach F, et al. Plasmablastic lymphomas of the oral cavity: a new entity associated with the human immunodeficiency virus infection. *Blood* 1997;89:1413–1420.
372. Bhattacharyya I, Chehal HK, Cohen DM, et al. Primary diffuse large B-cell lymphoma of the oral cavity: germinal center classification. *Head Neck Pathol* 2010;4:181–191.
373. Lanham GR, Weiss SW, Enzinger FM. Malignant lymphoma: a study of 75 cases presenting in soft tissue. *Am J Surg Pathol* 1989;13:1–10.
374. Salomao DR, Nascimento AG, Lloyd RV, et al. Lymphoma in soft tissue: a clinicopathologic study of 19 cases. *Hum Pathol* 1996:27:253–257.
375. Yang J, Zhang F, Fang H, et al. Clinicopathologic features of primary lymphoma in soft tissue. *Leuk Lymphoma* 2010;51:2039–2046.
376. d'Amore ESG, Wick MR, Geisinger KR, et al. Primary malignant lymphoma arising in postmastectomy lymphedema: another facet of the Stewart-Treves syndrome. *Am J Surg Pathol* 1990;14:456–463.
377. Goodlad JR, Hollowood K, Smith MA, et al. Primary juxtaarticular soft tissue lymphoma arising in the vicinity of inflamed joints in patients with rheumatoid arthritis. *Histopathology* 1999;34:199–204.
378. McElroy MK, Kulidjian AA, Sumit R, et al. Benign lymphoid hyperplasia (pseudolymphoma) of soft tissue. *Hum Pathol* 2011;42:1813–1818.
379. Inagaki H, Chan JKC, Ng JWM, et al. Primary thymic extranodal marginal-zone B-cell lymphoma of mucosa-associated lymphoid tissue type exhibits distinctive clinicopathological and molecular features. *Am J Pathol* 2002;160:1435–1443.
380. Go H, Cho HJ, Paik JH, et al. Thymic extranodal marginal zone B-cell lymphoma of mucosa-associated lymphoid tissue: a clinicopathological and genetic analysis of six cases. *Leuk Lymphoma* 2011;52:2276–2283.
381. Weissferdt A, Moran CA. Primary MALT-type lymphoma of the thymus: a clinicopathological and immunohistochemical study of six cases. *Lung* 2011;189:461–466.
382. Parrens M, Dubus P, Danjoux M, et al. Mucosa-associated lymphoid tissue of the thymus: hyperplasia vs lymphoma. *Am J Clin Pathol* 2002;117:51–56.
383. Weissferdt A, Moran CA. Thymic hyperplasia with lymphoepithelial sialadenitis (LESA)-like features: a clinicopathologic and immunohistochemical study of 4 cases. *Am J Clin Pathol* 2012;138:816–822.
384. Kominato S, Nakayama T, Sato F, et al. Characterization of chromosomal aberrations in thymic MALT lymphoma. *Pathol Int* 2012;62:93–98.
385. Masuda A, Tsujii T, Kojima M, et al. Primary mucosa-associated lymphoid tissue (MALT) lymphoma arising from the male urethra: a case report and review of the literature. *Pathol Res Pract* 2002;198:571–575.
386. Yilmaz M, Ibrahimov M, Mamanov M, et al. Primary marginal zone B-cell lymphoma of the larynx. *J Craniofac Surg* 2012;23:e1–e2.
387. Luick M, Hansen EK, Greenberg MS, et al. Primary tracheal non-Hodgkin's lymphoma. *J Clin Oncol* 2012;29:e193–e195.
388. Ikeda J, Morii E, Yamauchi A, et al. Extranodal marginal zone B-cell lymphoma of mucosa-associated lymphoid tissue type developing in gonarthritis deformans. *J Clin Oncol* 2007;25:4310–4312.

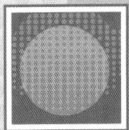

Chapter 34
Bone Marrow Specimen Procurement and Processing

Yi-Hua Chen • LoAnn Peterson

A comprehensive bone marrow examination includes review of peripheral blood, bone marrow aspirates, and core biopsies so that a maximum diagnostic information can be obtained (1–5). Although the evaluation usually begins with morphologic review, additional studies appropriate for the disease process, such as cytochemistry, immunohistochemistry, flow cytometric immunophenotyping, molecular analysis, and cytogenetic studies, are often included (6–10). This thorough assessment requires adequate sampling and appropriate specimen processing to ensure not only that the morphologic details can be appreciated but also that appropriate materials are available for ancillary studies. This chapter focuses on general approaches to the bone marrow sampling and processing; the step-by-step procedures are at the discretion of each institution and beyond the scope of the chapter.

INDICATIONS FOR BONE MARROW BIOPSY

Bone marrow examination is indicated in the evaluation of a large number of nonneoplastic and neoplastic diseases (4,11,12). The common indications for bone marrow biopsy are listed in Table 34.1. The decision to perform a bone marrow biopsy is made on a case-to-case basis after all available clinical and laboratory information has been considered. Bone marrow biopsies are frequently performed in workup of patients with unexplained cytopenias or elevated blood counts, abnormal peripheral blood findings (e.g., circulating blasts, teardrop-shaped red blood cells), abnormal laboratory results (e.g., monoclonal proteins), unexplained clinical findings (e.g., splenomegaly or systemic symptoms), and mass lesions inaccessible for biopsy. Bone marrow evaluation is an integral component in diagnosis, staging, and therapeutic monitoring of hematopoietic malignancies. It is also utilized in workup of patients with nonneoplastic hematopoietic disorders such as aplastic anemia and nonhematopoietic diseases such as storage diseases, metastatic carcinoma, and suspected systemic infections, particularly in immunocompromised patients. Knowledge of the indication for a bone marrow biopsy and the specific questions expected to be answered by the procedure is important in acquisition, triaging, and best utilization of bone marrow samples for various studies.

COMPONENTS OF BONE MARROW EXAMINATION

Peripheral Blood

Evaluation of peripheral blood is an important component of the bone marrow examination. Review of the peripheral blood smears in conjunction with a complete blood count (CBC)

provides important diagnostic information and may even avert the need for a bone marrow biopsy. For example, the finding of oval macrocytes and hypersegmented neutrophils in a patient with pancytopenia may lead to a diagnosis of megaloblastic anemia secondary to B12 or folate deficiency. Circulating blasts are common findings in hematologic malignancies, but even this observation does not always necessitate a bone marrow biopsy; for instance, circulating blasts in a small percentage are commonly seen in patients receiving growth factor therapy. Many neoplastic diseases are often first recognized from a CBC and peripheral blood smear examination; these include myeloproliferative neoplasms (MPNs), acute leukemia, myelodysplastic syndromes (MDSs), chronic lymphoproliferative disorders, and occasionally lymphomas. In addition, subtle morphologic features of hematopoietic cells such as dysplastic features of neutrophils are often best appreciated in a well-stained peripheral blood smear (Fig. 34.1). In some diseases such as hairy cell leukemia, peripheral blood may become the only source to identify the characteristic cytologic features of the neoplastic cells because of the frequent inability to aspirate cells from bone marrow.

Peripheral blood is also a convenient source for ancillary studies, including flow cytometric immunophenotyping, molecular analysis, fluorescence *in situ* hybridization (FISH), and cytogenetic studies, especially when there is disease involvement in the blood such as chronic lymphocytic leukemia or if no bone marrow aspirate is obtained. However, it should be recognized that if peripheral blood is used for cytogenetic studies, the yield of sufficient metaphases for chromosomal analysis is usually lower than that from bone marrow aspirate (13). Molecular analysis can also be performed on a peripheral blood sample and is commonly used for diagnosis and follow-up of patients with hematologic malignancies, for example, molecular analysis of *JAK-2* V617F mutation for diagnosis of MPNs, qualitative or quantitative analysis of *BCR-ABL 1* for diagnosis and follow-up of patients with chronic myelogenous leukemia and *PML-RARα* fusion for acute promyelocytic leukemia (APL) (14–18).

Bone Marrow Aspirate

Well-prepared and well-stained bone marrow aspirate smears are critical in evaluation of hematologic diseases as they provide excellent cytologic details of a variety of cell types in the marrow. Aspirate smears are routinely used for cytomorphologic evaluation and bone marrow differential count. Morphologic features of blasts and other precursor cells can usually be appreciated in more detail in the aspirate smears than a core biopsy section. For example, dysplasia of erythroid precursors is best assessed in optimally prepared aspirate smears (Fig. 34.2). In some circumstances, diagnostic clues are present only in the bone marrow aspirate. For example, the presence of cytoplasmic vacuoles in both granulocytes and erythroid precursors is a critical morphologic clue to copper deficiency,

Table 34.1	INDICATIONS FOR BONE MARROW EXAMINATION

Workup for abnormal clinical and laboratory findings
- Unexplained peripheral cytopenias or elevated counts
- Abnormal peripheral blood findings (e.g., circulating blasts or other abnormal leukocytes, teardrop-shaped red blood cells, leukoerythroblastic reaction)
- Abnormal laboratory results (e.g., serum or urine monoclonal proteins)
- Unexplained organomegaly or systemic symptoms
- Mass lesion inaccessible for biopsy
- Suspected systemic infections
- Unexplained radiographic findings

Diagnosis and monitoring of malignancies
- Marrow-based hematopoietic malignancies: acute leukemia, MDS, MPN, MDS/MPN, plasma cell myeloma, lymphoplasmacytic lymphoma, hairy cell leukemia, chronic lymphocytic leukemia/small lymphocytic lymphoma
- Systemic hematopoietic malignancies: lymphoma, systemic mastocytosis, primary amyloidosis

Staging of malignancies
- Lymphoma at initial diagnosis and follow-up
- Some carcinomas and sarcomas

Workup of nonneoplastic disorders
- Aplastic anemia
- Paroxysmal nocturnal hemoglobinuria
- Hemophagocytic syndrome
- Storage diseases
- Evaluation of congenital hematologic disorders (e.g., congenital dyserythropoietic anemia)
- Infection

Follow-up
- Low-grade hematopoietic malignancies suspicious for progression or transformation to high-grade disease
- Assessment of response to treatment
- Post–bone marrow transplant evaluation

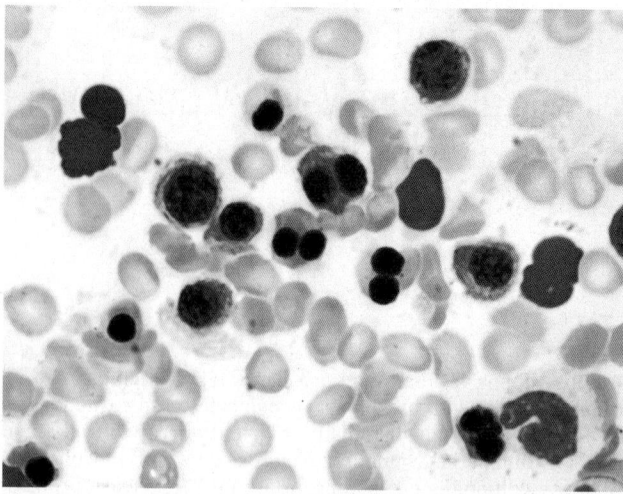

FIGURE 34.2. Dysplastic erythroid precursors in the bone marrow aspirate smear of a patient with congenital dyserythropoietic anemia, type II (CDA II). The aspirate smear shows numerous binucleated erythroid precursors with equal-sized nuclei, a characteristic feature for CDA II (Wright-Giemsa; 1,000×).

a condition that may be misdiagnosed as MDS because both diseases can present as unexplained cytopenias and exhibit ring sideroblasts (Fig. 34.3A and B) (19–21). The aspirate smears are also the most common preparations for iron stain and cytochemical studies. In addition, a fresh bone marrow aspirate serves as the optimal specimen for flow cytometric immunophenotyping, molecular analysis, FISH, and cytogenetic studies. It is superior to peripheral blood in yielding sufficient metaphases for chromosomal analysis (13). In our experience, the air-dried aspirate smears can also serve as an excellent alternative to a core biopsy for molecular analysis because DNA extracted from these preparations is free of fixative insult.

Bone Marrow Core Biopsy and Touch Imprint

Touch imprints made from the fresh, unfixed bone marrow core biopsies can be used for various purposes, including routine Wright-Giemsa staining for morphologic examination, cytochemical stains, and FISH analysis. In cases with unsuccessful aspiration, the touch imprint becomes an important substitute for cytomorphologic evaluation (Fig. 34.4).

A bone marrow core biopsy is crucial in evaluation of bone marrow. It may be the only source for evaluation if an aspirate cannot be obtained or if there is a focal bone marrow process that is not represented in the aspirate (e.g., lymphoma, carcinoma, granuloma). Core biopsies provide topographic information that cannot be observed in the aspirate smears, such as cellularity, cell distribution, presence or absence of an infiltrative process, patterns of infiltration, and extent of infiltration. For example, intravascular or paratrabecular infiltration of neoplastic lymphocytes can only be appreciated in the core biopsy sections (Figs. 34.5 and 34.6). Paraffin-embedded core biopsies are commonly used for special studies such as special stains (e.g., reticulin stain, Congo red stain, GMS and AFB stains), immunohistochemical stains, *in situ* hybridization, or molecular analysis (10). When a bone marrow aspirate is not available, single-cell suspensions can be prepared from a fresh core biopsy and used for flow cytometric immunophenotyping or cytogenetic studies (22–24).

Particle Clot

Particle clot sections are made from aggregated bone marrow aspirate particles processed and sectioned similar to the core biopsy but without decalcification. Particle clot sections that contain adequate bone marrow are complementary resource to the core biopsy or be the only specimen for histologic examination when the core biopsy is inadequate or unavailable. These sections may also provide additional morphologic findings that are not present in the core biopsy as they represent a different part of the bone marrow. However, one should be aware that particle clot sections may not be entirely representative of the overall bone marrow, for example, the abnormal infiltrates associated with fibrosis (e.g., Hodgkin lymphoma) or focal paratrabecular diseases (e.g., follicular lymphoma) may not be present in the particle clot section due to the difficulty in aspiration. Therefore, particle clot sections should not be

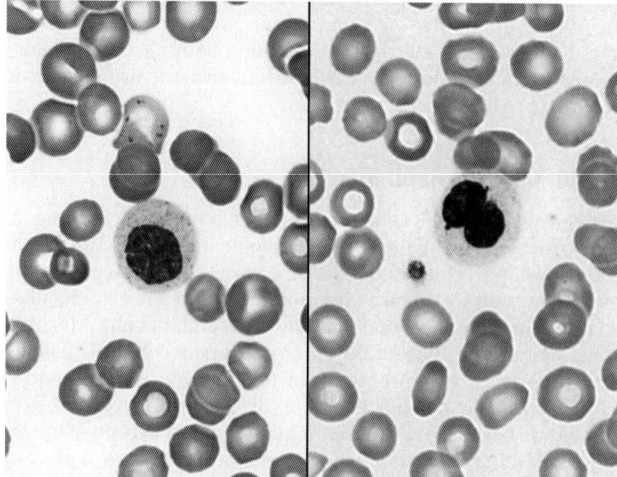

FIGURE 34.1. Dysplastic neutrophils in the peripheral blood smear. Left: A dysplastic neutrophil with monolobated nucleus. **Right:** A dysplastic neutrophil with hypogranulation and hyposegmented nucleus (Wright-Giemsa; 1,000×).

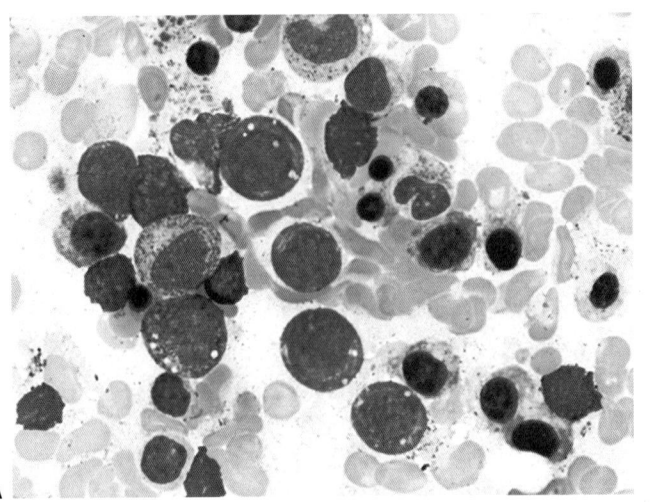
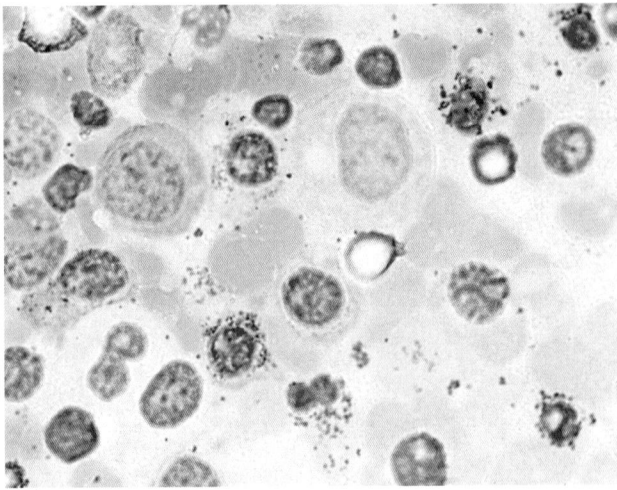

FIGURE 34.3. Bone marrow aspirate in a patient with copper deficiency. A: The aspirate smears show distinct cytoplasmic vacuoles in both granulocytes and erythroid precursors (Wright-Giemsa; 1,000×). **B:** Frequent ring sideroblasts are present (Prussian blue stain; 1,000×).

considered and used as substitute for core biopsies. However, since these specimens have not been decalcified, they can be used for molecular tests.

PROCUREMENT OF BONE MARROW SAMPLES

Advance Preparation

Before a bone marrow biopsy is performed, it is important to assess each case to ensure that adequate samples are obtained and properly prepared so that a comprehensive evaluation can be done. For example, if an acute leukemia is a diagnostic consideration, peripheral blood, bone marrow aspirate, and core biopsy should all be obtained for morphologic evaluation, and additional anticoagulated aspirate samples should be collected for flow cytometry immunophenotyping, cytogenetic studies, and molecular analysis, as indicated. For lymphoma staging or other lesions with frequent focal involvement of bone marrow, bilateral iliac crest biopsies rather than a unilateral biopsy are

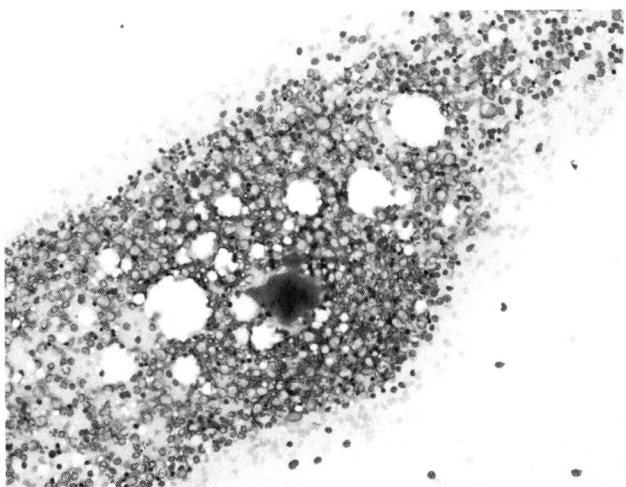

FIGURE 34.4. Touch imprint of bone marrow core biopsy. In cases with unsuccessful aspiration, the touch imprint becomes an important substitute for cytomorphologic evaluation of bone marrow cells (Wright-Giemsa; 100×).

optimal since this approach increases the yield of detection (25–28). The collection of additional samples for specialized testing should be based on the indications for the bone marrow biopsy, including details of the clinical history and laboratory findings. In our institution, specific guidelines for workup of patients with various categories of hematologic malignancies have been developed by consensus decisions of pathologists and clinicians. Each guideline specifies what types of samples are needed and what ancillary tests are required at various time points of the disease, for example, acute leukemia at diagnosis, nadir, remission, and relapse. This approach helps to streamline the bone marrow biopsy and evaluation process, making it more efficient and cost-effective.

Biopsy Site

The posterior superior iliac crest is the most common biopsy site for both adults and children. This site is easily assessable and relatively remote from vital areas, minimizing the potential for complications. It also provides the least discomfort to the patient compared with other potential sites. If the posterior iliac crest is not accessible because of morbid obesity or infection of the overlying skin or other local factors, the anterior iliac crest is a suitable alternative. However, this crest is narrow with a dense cortical layer; therefore, the biopsy may be more difficult to obtain. The sternum may be used in patients older than 12 years but only for bone marrow aspiration and should be performed by an experienced operator; core biopsy of sternum is contraindicated to prevent possible serious complications that may result from injury of the underlying vital organs (29,30). Sampling from the medial aspect of the proximal tibia is reserved for infants <18 months old and is restricted to aspiration only. Another consideration in the selection of biopsy site is to avoid areas with previous radiotherapy because radiation may induce bone marrow hypocellularity that can persist for years (31).

Complications of Bone Marrow Biopsy

Bone marrow aspirate and core biopsy can be safely performed on virtually all patients. Potential complications of the procedure are usually minor consisting mainly of hemorrhage and infection (32–34). Patient with coagulopathy should be assessed prior to the biopsy, and severe coagulopathy may need to be corrected prior to the procedure (11,12). Thrombocytopenia, even profound thrombocytopenia, is usually not a

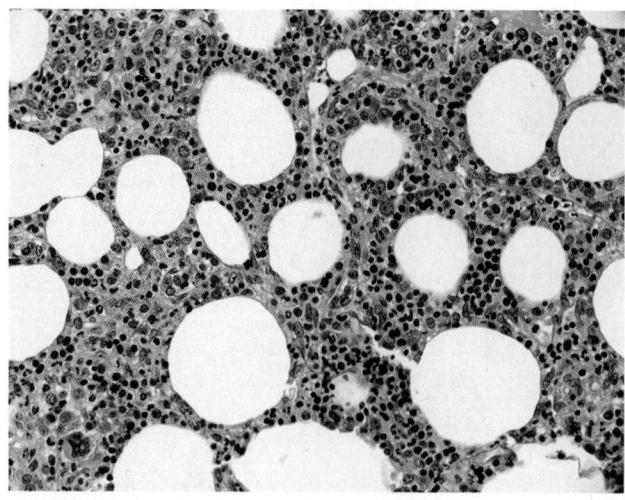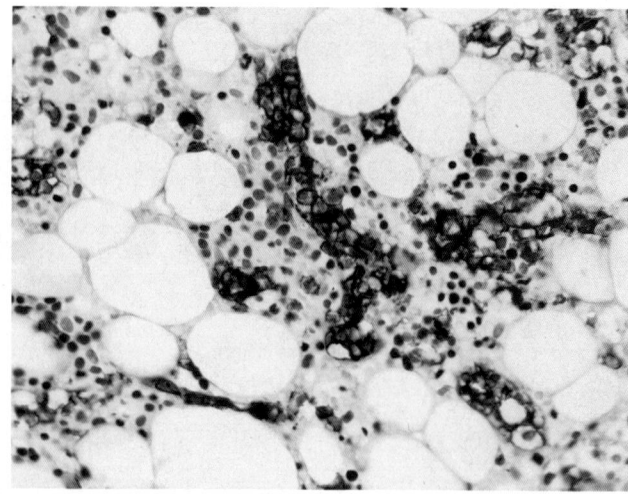

FIGURE 34.5. Intravascular large B-cell lymphoma. A: The intravascular pattern of infiltration can only be observed on the bone marrow core sections (H&E; 200×). **B:** The infiltration is better appreciated by immunohistochemical staining for CD20 (400×).

contraindication for bone marrow biopsy as long as adequate pressure is applied after the procedure to attain hemostasis (11). Wound infections following bone marrow biopsy are generally minor, usually requiring only topical medication. Sterile technique minimizes infectious complication.

Collection of Samples

Before bone marrow biopsy, the necessity of the biopsy for diagnosis and the steps of the procedure should be discussed and explained to the patient, and a consent form should be signed by the patient or the patient's legal guardians. Sterile techniques should be used, and the bone marrow tray should be prepared with the essential elements including various anticoagulated tubes appropriate for the anticipated studies. The items in the tray should be organized in a way that they can be easily located and reached.

The best sequence to obtain a bone marrow aspirate and core biopsy is controversial. Some authors recommend that the core biopsy be performed first as this minimizes the distortion of the marrow architecture resulting from aspiration.

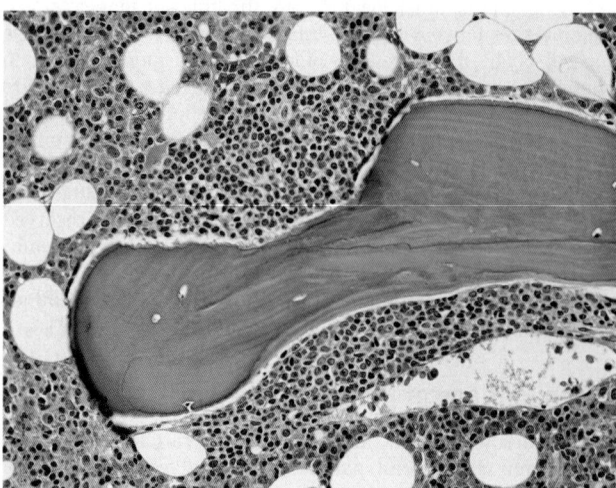

FIGURE 34.6. Mantle cell lymphoma with paratrabecular infiltration. Distinct paratrabecular lymphoid aggregates are almost always neoplastic, most commonly seen in follicular lymphoma but can also be observed in mantle cell lymphoma. This infiltration pattern can only be appreciated in the core biopsy sections (H&E; 200×).

Others argue that the aspirated sample may clot faster if it is obtained after the core biopsy; thus, the aspiration should be performed prior to the biopsy. Despite these issues, it is generally agreed that the order of aspiration and trephine biopsy is not critical as long as the samples are obtained with separate needles through separate (1 to 2 cm apart) punctures along the iliac crest (1,12,35).

Peripheral blood smears can be prepared as part of the bone marrow procedure by finger stick or by venipuncture into EDTA-anticoagulated tube. A finger puncture is performed by a quick single puncture to the finger pad using a sterile, disposable lancet. The first drop of blood should be wiped away, and gentle pressure should be applied to obtain free flow of blood. A small drop of blood is applied to the glass slide either directly from the finger puncture or from a capillary tube containing the collected blood. The slides are air-dried before staining.

Bone marrow aspiration is most commonly performed on the posterior iliac crest with local anesthesia. An Illinois needle or one of its modifications is most commonly used for the procedure. These needles are ideal for aspiration of the fluid portion of the specimen and cause less discomfort to the patient than the larger core biopsy needles. The needle is inserted through the same skin incision used for the core biopsy. After the needle has penetrated the cortex and advanced approximately 1 cm into the marrow cavity, a rapid aspiration of 0.5 to 1.0 mL bone marrow should be obtained for morphologic studies. A volume >1.0 mL is not recommended for morphology as it will cause dilution of the bone marrow particles by peripheral blood. It is important to proceed quickly and efficiently to minimize the patient's discomfort and clotting of the specimen. This initial aspirate should be collected in a syringe free of anticoagulant and immediately used for preparation of slides. If needed, a portion of the aspirate can be placed into a tube with EDTA anticoagulant to delay clotting, but the slides must be made immediately to avoid artifacts induced by EDTA. Additional samples should then be aspirated for special studies, including flow cytometric immunophenotyping, cytogenetic studies, molecular analysis, and cultures, as indicated. The aspirated samples for these studies should be collected in tubes containing anticoagulant that is appropriate for the anticipated study, for example, heparin or EDTA for flow cytometric immunophenotyping, preservative-free heparin for cytogenetic studies, and EDTA for molecular analysis. In rare cases when electron microscopic examination is needed, the aspirate immediately after the initial aliquot should be used

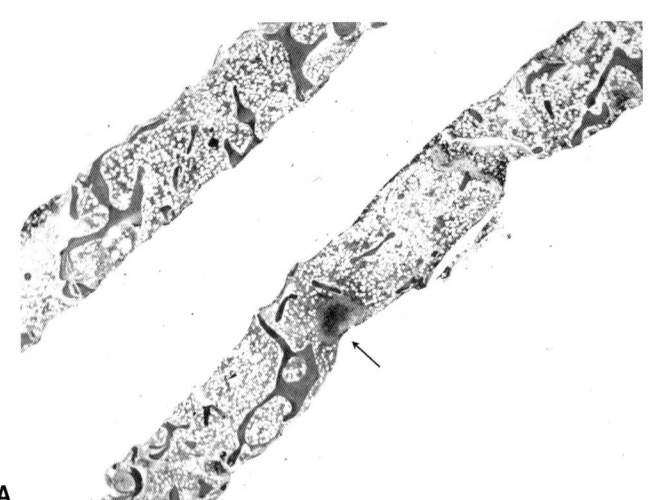
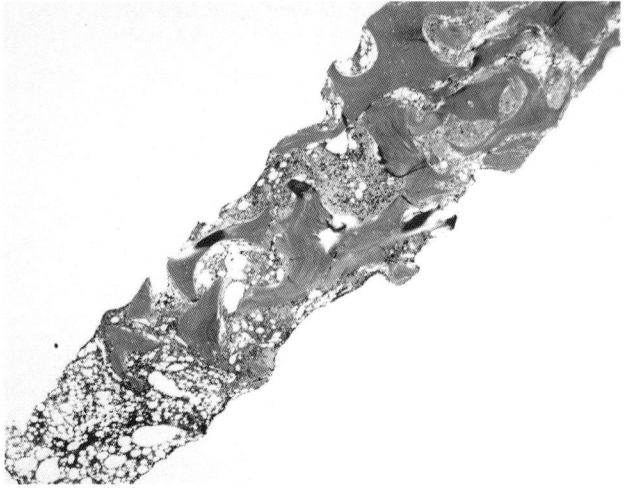

A   **B**

FIGURE 34.7. Adequacy of bone marrow core biopsy. A: An adequate core biopsy is critical for lymphoma staging or other processes that are often focal. This is a case of nodular lymphocyte–predominant Hodgkin lymphoma with very focal bone marrow involvement (H&E; 100×). **B:** The core biopsy consisting mainly of cortical bone and subcortical marrow should not be considered adequate for diagnosis (H&E; 200×).

and collected in a glutaraldehyde-containing tube. If samples are to be sent to reference laboratories or other off-site laboratories for testing, it is important to know sample requirements for each of the specific tests.

A "dry tap" may occur and no bone marrow is obtained by aspiration. It may be caused by technical problems, most commonly the tip of the aspiration needle is not within the marrow cavity. More often, it is due to an inherent bone marrow pathology associated with diffuse fibrosis or infiltration, such as MPNs, hairy cell leukemia, or extensive metastatic carcinoma. In such cases, touch preparations of the core biopsy can be used as an alternative for cytomorphologic evaluation.

The *bone marrow core biopsy* is obtained using the same site as aspiration but at a slightly different entry point in the cortical bone. Biopsy needles patterned after the needles introduced by Jamshidi and Swaim (36) are most commonly used for the procedure. Many different biopsy needles are available in various sizes designed for adult and pediatric patients. A specific type of biopsy needles should be evaluated before its institution to ensure that it yields adequate biopsies with no technical artifact and causes minimal discomfort to the patient. Proper technique with careful attention to appropriate landmark locations for the biopsy and adequate local anesthesia cannot be overemphasized. Once local anesthesia is assured, the biopsy needle is advanced through a small skin incision to the cortical bone. After being firmly lodged into the cortex, the needle is advanced into the medullary cavity. The central stylet is removed, and the needle is slowly advanced in a rotating movement for another 1.5 to 2 cm into the marrow cavity. When a bone marrow core is obtained, the needle is rotated in full circles to separate the biopsy specimen from the surrounding tissue and then advanced a small distance before removal. Once the core biopsy is expelled from the needle, the adequacy of the core biopsy should be inspected. Grossly, the marrow is usually dark red with a gritty texture unless there is a diffuse abnormal process. The cortex is white, while the cartilage is white and glistening. Before placing the core biopsy into fixative, several touch imprints should be prepared. Less damage to the core biopsy occurs when the imprint is prepared by gently touching a glass slide to the specimen rather than by holding the specimen with a forceps and touching it to a slide. If an aspirate cannot be obtained, cells can be disaggregated from fresh extra core biopsies and used for flow cytometric immunophenotyping or cytogenetic studies; cores

for these purposes should be placed in RPMI. If the core is collected for bacterial or fungal cultures, it should be placed in a dry, sterile container.

The optimal size of a core biopsy should be at least 1.5 to 2.0 cm in length for lymphoma staging or other processes that are often focal in the marrow (1,4,12,37). A smaller core may be adequate for evaluation of acute leukemia, MPN, or other diseases that generally have a diffuse bone marrow involvement. The core biopsy should contain sufficient bone marrow with intact architecture; specimens consisting mainly cortical bone and subcortical marrow that is normally hypocellular or disrupted bone marrow should not be considered adequate for diagnosis (Fig. 34.7A and B).

PREPARATION OF BONE MARROW ASPIRATE

Types of Preparations

Various techniques can be used to prepare satisfactory smears from the aspirated bone marrow samples. The two most common preparations are the direct smear and the particle crush smear. Buffy coat smears are not commonly performed because it is relatively time-consuming and does not add substantial information to that obtained from direct or particle crush smears. An adequate number of smears should be made for morphologic examination as well as for other studies, as indicated.

Direct smears of the bone marrow aspirate should be prepared immediately before clotting occurs. One drop of the aspirate is placed at one end of a slide and smeared with a pusher slide, as illustrated in Figure 34.8; the smear is then air-dried. The direct smear is an excellent preparation for examination of nuclear and cytoplasmic details as the cells are uniformly spaced, free of anticoagulant artifact, and have least cell damage caused by crush artifact. However, since the direct smear does not concentrate particles, certain cell types, such as megakaryocytes or mast cells, may not be well represented.

Particle crush smears are made by picking up the bone marrow particles and gently crushing between two slides (Fig. 34.9). A "flat-push-pull" motion should be used for smear

FIGURE 34.8. Preparation of direct aspirate smears. A: A single drop of the marrow aspirate from the syringe is placed on a clean slide. **B:** The drop is smeared by using a pusher slide. **C:** The pusher slide is prepared by placing a hemacytometer cover glass held in a Dieffenbach serrefine forceps. **D:** The result is a thin smear that is narrower than the width of the slide. The slide should be air-dried immediately after being made.

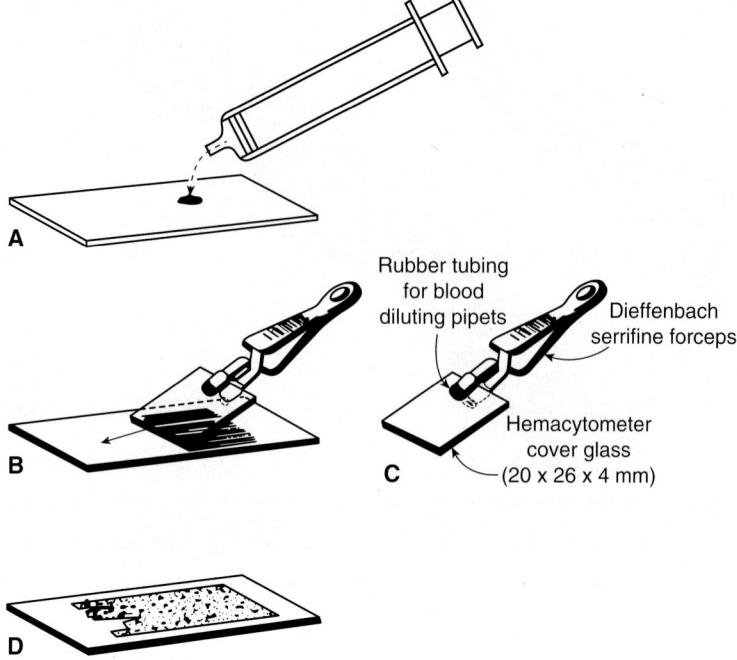

preparation to ensure that most cellular elements remain intact. It is important to include a small amount of blood from the aspirate to spread the particles. If an inadequate amount of blood is used, the cells will be ruptured during the preparation,

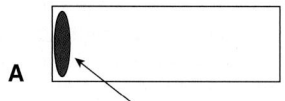

Bone marrow particles and a small amount of blood picked up by a slide

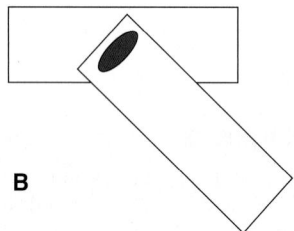

Bone marrow particles are placed onto the center of another slide

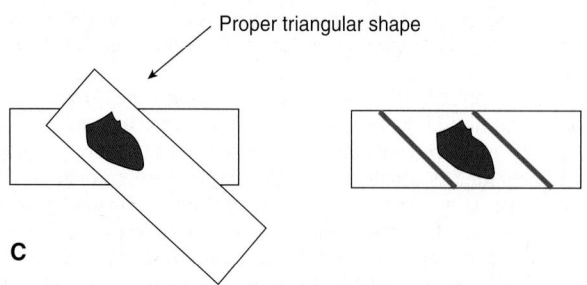

Particle crush smear is made by gently crushing the bone marrow particles between two slides in a "flat-push-pull" motion

FIGURE 34.9. Preparation of aspirate crush smears. A: Use the edge of one slide to pick up a small portion of blood and bone marrow particles in the aspirate sample. **B:** Place the blood with bone marrow particles near the center of another slide. **C:** Applying gentle pressure, use "flat-push-pull" technique to crush and spread the particles onto the bottom slide.

whereas if an excess amount of blood is used, the smear will be too thick, making it difficult to identify the individual cells. Particle crush smears are usually excellent for cytologic examination, but some features may be obscured due to uneven distribution, crowding, or disruption of cells.

Buffy coat smears have been used in the past but are rarely used at present for morphologic evaluation of bone marrow aspirate (1,38). Briefly, the EDTA-anticoagulated bone marrow aspirate is poured into a Petri dish. The fluid component is aspirated and transferred into a Wintrobe tube and then centrifuged. After centrifugation, the marrow specimen is layered into four major components, one of which has a buff color (buffy coat) that contains concentrated nucleated cells from the bone marrow aspirate. This layer is then aspirated and used to prepare smears for routine morphologic examination and special stains. Buffy coat smear is particularly useful in patients with hypoplastic or aplastic marrows where nucleated cells are markedly decreased in direct or particle crush smears.

Particle clots are made by aggregating the particles that remain after the preparation of aspirate smears. If the specimen is anticoagulated, addition of two to three drops of 0.015 M $CaCl_2$ can facilitate the clotting of the particles. The clotted particles are then fixed and processed in a manner similar to that of core biopsy except that the decalcification step is omitted.

Staining for Morphologic Review

The Wright-Giemsa stain, a Romanowsky-type stain, is most commonly used for staining of freshly made, air-dried peripheral blood smears, bone marrow aspirate smears, and touch imprints for morphologic evaluation. Romanowsky-type stains facilitate the distinction of different cell types in the blood and bone marrow. The main components of these stains include oxidized methylene blue, azure B, and eosin Y dyes (39,40). The eosin Y stains the cytoplasm of cells an orange to pink color, and the methylene blue and azure B stain the nucleus varying shades of blue to purple. The importance of well-prepared and well-stained samples cannot be overemphasized in bone marrow evaluation. The staining should be assessed for consistent high-quality staining that allows clear distinction of each cell type and cellular details such as nuclear chromatin patterns and cytoplasmic granules (Fig. 34.10).

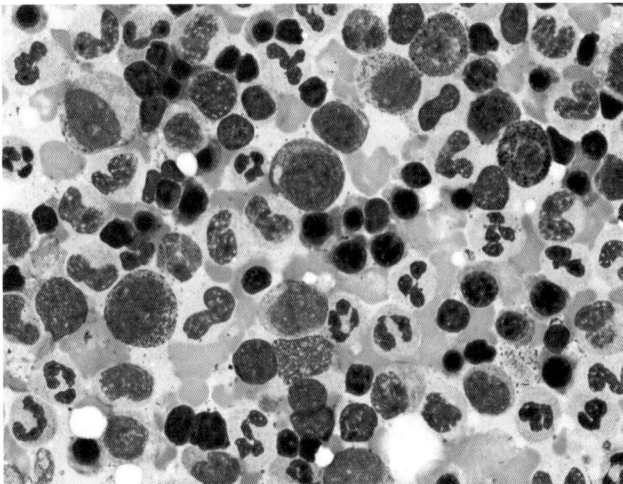

FIGURE 34.10. Bone marrow aspirate smears. Optimal staining of bone marrow aspirate smear allows clear distinction of each cell type and cellular details such as nuclear chromatin patterns and cytoplasmic granules (Wright-Giemsa; 600×).

PREPARATION AND PROCESSING OF BONE MARROW CORE BIOPSY

Fixation

Several choices of fixative are available for bone marrow core biopsies. Mercury-based fixatives, such as Zenker and B5 solutions, provide excellent morphologic details and have long been used for fixation of hematopoietic tissues. However, several drawbacks are associated with these fixatives including environmental concerns, strict control of fixation time, and compromising of the preservation of antigens and DNA quality that may affect immunohistochemical staining and molecular analysis. Because of these issues, neutral buffered formalin or other mercury-free fixatives have been increasingly used. Acetic acid-zinc formalin (AZF) and B-Plus have been reported to be viable alternatives to B5 (41,42). Tissues with AZF fixation have adequate staining quality and antigen preservation equivalent or superior for immunohistochemistry, and the DNA quality is adequate for successful amplification by polymerase chain reaction (PCR).

A core biopsy of 1 to 2 cm in length should be placed in approximately 20 mL of fixative. The optimal fixation period for bone marrow biopsy is as follows: B5, 1 to 2 hours; Zenker, at least 4 hours (no adverse effect if left in the fixative overnight or over the weekend); 10% neutral buffered formalin, at least 18 to 24 hours; and zinc formalin, 3 to 4 hours.

Decalcification

After removal from the fixative, the bone marrow core is subjected to decalcification. There are two primary methods used for decalcification: simple acids (e.g., hydrochloric acid, formic acid, acetic acid, picric acid, nitric acid) and chelating agents (e.g., EDTA). The most commercial decalcification agents are buffered simple acids. Decalcification time varies significantly depending on the type of decalcifying agent used and the size of the biopsy. Inappropriately prolonged decalcification not only affects the preservation of morphology but also the quality of histochemical or immunohistochemical staining as well as the potential for molecular analysis. It may be necessary to experiment with different agents and durations of decalcification process to obtain the best results with the material and staining methods used in each individual laboratory.

Sectioning and Staining for Morphologic Review

After processing and embedding in paraffin, the core biopsy should be sectioned at 3 to 4 μm with a knife blade that is free of defects. Adequate sampling of the core biopsy is critical for morphologic examination, particularly in diseases that often have focal involvement in the bone marrow, such as lymphoma, granuloma, and metastatic carcinoma. Several step sections should be prepared and examined. In our institution, 12 consecutive sections are cut from each core biopsy. Sections from step 1, 3, and 5 are routinely stained with H&E for morphologic examination, and the remaining unstained sections are stored for possible special stains and/or immunohistochemical staining.

The hematoxylin and eosin (H&E) stain provides excellent histology details and is the most widely used routine staining for bone marrow core biopsies and particle clot sections. Stains should be evaluated prior to institution to ensure properly differentiated staining of cells that allows assessment of cytologic details. Several other stains can also be applied to the core biopsy for morphologic examination, including periodic acid–Schiff (PAS) and Giemsa stains. PAS stain is useful in the identification of maturing granulocytes and megakaryocytes and can also be used as an initial screening procedure for detection of fungal organisms. The Giemsa stain may be used to accentuate granules in maturing neutrophils, eosinophils, and basophils; it also highlights the mast cells in the lesions of mastocytosis.

SPECIAL STAINS

Special stains constitute an important component in bone marrow evaluation. These stains are relatively simple and easily applied to the bone marrow specimens and can contribute significantly to an accurate diagnosis of a bone marrow process. Cytochemical stains of peripheral blood and aspirate smears include enzymatic stains (e.g., myeloperoxidase [MPO] and nonspecific esterase) and nonenzymatic stains (e.g., Prussian blue for iron). The general principles of the commonly used special stains in bone marrow evaluation is discussed in this chapter, and the bone marrow specimen types feasible for the stains and general considerations in the interpretation of the results are summarized in Tables 34.2 and 34.3.

An *iron stain* is commonly performed on the bone marrow particle crush smears to assess storage iron and sideroblasts. In the absence of a particle smear, an iron stain can be performed on a bone marrow core section to evaluate storage iron; however, caution should be taken in interpretation of the staining because the absence of iron may be secondary to chelation during decalcification of the core biopsy rather than true iron depletion (43,44). Prussian blue staining is the classic method used for demonstrating iron in tissues. The slide is treated with dilute hydrochloric acid to release ferric ions from binding proteins. These ions then react with potassium ferrocyanide to produce an insoluble blue compound that is visible under the light microscope. An adequate number of particles, ideally seven or more, should be examined to reliably evaluate the status of storage iron (45). It should be kept in mind that although storage iron cannot be assessed in a hemodiluted bone marrow aspirate smear due to lack of particles, evaluation of sideroblasts may still be possible as long as there are adequate numbers of erythroid precursors present, even scattered singly in the smears.

The *MPO* stain is helpful in identifying cytoplasmic granules characteristic of myeloid cells. The peroxidase activity in the azurophilic granules of myeloid cells transfers hydrogen from benzidine dihydrochloride to hydrogen peroxidase yielding a blue precipitate at the site of activity. Cytochemical stains for MPO can be performed on air-dried nonanticoagulated or anticoagulated (EDTA, heparin) aspirate smears, touch

Table 34.2	BONE MARROW SAMPLE TYPES AND APPLICABLE STUDIES

Samples	Preparations	Applicable Studies	Utility	Comment
Peripheral blood	Fresh peripheral blood	Flow cytometric immunophenotyping Cytogenetic analysis if blasts present FISH PCR	– Convenient source for ancillary studies when peripheral blood is involved – Useful in monitoring of diseases such as CML (BCR-ABL) and APL (PML-RARα) by PCR	– Lower yield of sufficient metaphases for chromosomal analysis than bone marrow aspirate
	Peripheral blood smear	Wright-Giemsa stain for morphology Differential count Cytochemical stains	– Provides complementary information to bone marrow aspirate and biopsy – Optimal for evaluation of some morphologic details such as dysplasia in neutrophils	– Peripheral blood may not be involved by the infiltrative process.
Bone marrow aspirate	Fresh aspirate	Flow cytometric immunophenotyping Cytogenetic analysis PCR	– Optimal for ancillary studies – Higher yield of metaphases for cytogenetic analysis than peripheral blood	– Appropriate anticoagulated tubes should be used for collection of samples for various ancillary studies.
	Direct smear	Wright-Giemsa stain for morphology Differential count Cytochemical stains FISH	– Excellent cytomorphology with least artifact	– Differential may not be representative because of lack of cellular particles.
	Particle crush smear	Wright-Giemsa stain for morphology Differential count Cytochemical stains FISH PCR using cells scraped from slide	– Closest representation of bone marrow cellular components and ideal for differential count – Best for assessing storage iron and other cytochemical studies – Valuable source for PCR when fresh aspirate is no longer available	– Cells may be damaged in smear preparation if handled inappropriately. – Cells may not be aspirated due to diffuse fibrosis or extensive abnormal infiltrate.
	Particle clot section	H&E stain for histology Immunohistochemistry Histochemical stains In situ hybridization PCR	– Provides similar information to core biopsy if adequate particles present – May be better than core biopsy for histochemical stains and immunohistochemistry because of absence of decalcification	– May not have adequate particles – Lesions with fibrosis or paratrabecular localization often not present due to difficulty in aspiration of cells from these areas
Bone marrow core biopsy	Touch imprint	Wright-Giemsa stain for morphology Differential count Cytochemical stains FISH PCR if cellular	– Serves as an substitute to aspirate smear for cytologic examination if aspirate is not available – Optimal for FISH	– Cells may be selectively touched from core; megakaryocytes are often sparse. – Cellular details are often less clear than aspirate smears.
	Core biopsy	H&E stain for histology Immunohistochemistry Histochemical stains In situ hybridization PCR	– Evaluation of bone marrow cellularity and topographic information – Best for focal processes (e.g., lymphoma, granuloma, and carcinoma) that may not be present in the aspirate; bilateral biopsies enhance the detection rate. – Optimal for immunohistochemistry – Best for evaluation of some diseases, for example, MF, amyloidosis, systemic mastocytosis	– Limitation in evaluation of subtle cytologic details. – Enzymatic cytochemical stains do not work. – Iron stain may not be accurate due to decalcification.

PCR, polymerase chain reaction; FISH, fluorescence *in situ* hybridization; CML, chronic myelogenous leukemia; APL, acute promyelocytic leukemia.

imprints, and peripheral blood smears. However, the slides should be <2 weeks old because prolonged storage will decrease peroxidase activity in the cells. A positive stain indicates cells of myeloid lineage. The staining process takes only about 3 to 5 minutes, and a STAT staining may be indicated in the peripheral blood smear under certain clinical scenarios, for example, a suspected microgranular (hypogranular) variant of APL. Morphologic distinction of this variant of APL from acute myelomonocytic leukemia may not always be possible in a peripheral blood smear; however, a strong MPO staining in virtually all blasts makes APL more likely. The STAT assessment of MPO in this clinical situation is helpful for patient management since the current recommendation for patients with suspected APL is to give urgent therapy with all-transretinoic acid to decrease the early mortality of the disease (46).

The *nonspecific esterase* (NSE) stain includes α-naphthyl acetate esterase (ANA) and α-naphthyl acetate butyrate esterase (ANB). ANA was initially used for identification of monocytes but now has been largely replaced by ANB since it is easier to perform and more specific for monocytes or cells with monocytic differentiation. NSE stain can be performed on air-dried aspirate smears, touch imprints, and peripheral blood smears. A positive staining is seen in monocytes, cells with monocytic differentiation, and platelets. Staining in the platelets serves as an internal positive control in the sample. This staining is commonly used to evaluate acute leukemia with monocytic differentiation, such as myelomonocytic or acute monocytic leukemia (Fig. 34.11A and B).

The *PAS stain* can be performed on the bone marrow aspirate smears, touch imprints, as well as core biopsies. This stain is based on the oxidation of glycol to aldehyde groups by periodic acid and the subsequent reaction of aldehyde groups with the chromophores in Schiff reagent that produces a bright pinkish-red color (Fig. 34.12). The PAS stain demonstrates glycogen, neutral mucosubstances, and basement membranes. This stain has been used in the past to help with diagnosis of acute erythroid leukemia and lymphoblastic leukemia in which the blasts may show "beaded" or "blocklike" cytoplastic staining,

Table 34.3   SPECIAL STAINS COMMONLY USED IN BONE MARROW EXAMINATION

Special Stain	Specimen	Utility	Comment
Prussian blue	Aspirate smear Core biopsy Particle clot section	– Used to evaluate for storage iron and sideroblasts	– An adequate number of bone marrow particles (ideally ≥7) should be examined to reliably evaluate the status of storage iron. – Evaluation of storage iron in bone marrow core biopsy may not be reliable due to chelating during decalcification.
Myeloperoxidase	Peripheral blood smear Aspirate smear Touch imprint	– Positivity in blasts indicates myeloid lineage.	– The preparation should be <2 weeks old. Prolonged storage may decrease peroxidase activity in the cells.
α-naphthyl acetate butyrate esterase	Peripheral blood smear Aspirate smear Touch imprint	– Positivity indicates monocytes or cells with monocytic differentiation including blasts.	– Staining in the platelets serves as an internal positive control.
Periodic acid-Schiff	Aspirate smear Touch imprint Core biopsy	– Highlights granulocytes and megakaryocytes in the core biopsy – Stains fungal organisms	– It has been used historically to help with the diagnosis of acute erythroid leukemia and lymphoblastic leukemia in which the neoplastic cells may show blocklike cytoplasmic staining.
Reticulin	Core biopsy	– Used to evaluate the presence and degree of reticulin fibrosis	– Especially useful in evaluation of MPN
Congo red	Core biopsy	– Stains amyloid deposition	– Blood vessel wall is the common site for amyloid deposition.
Grocott methenamine silver	Core biopsy	– Highlights fungal organisms	– PAS can also be used for this purpose.
Acid-fast bacillus stain	Core biopsy	– Highlights mycobacteria or other acid-fast bacteria	– Immunodeficient patients may not have granulomas.

while the normal erythroid precursors and lymphocytes are negative. However, it is rarely used at present for diagnosis of acute leukemia owing to the widespread application of flow cytometric immunophenotyping and cytogenetic studies in the evaluation of hematopoietic malignancies. PAS stain is useful in highlighting maturing granulocytes and megakaryocytes in the core biopsy and may also be used as an initial screening procedure for the detection of fungal organisms.

A *reticulin stain* is performed on the bone marrow core biopsy to evaluate reticulin fiber content that is best appreciated with silver stains. The two most common silver stains are the Gomori stain and Gordon and Sweet stain. One of the most common applications of reticulin stain in bone marrow biopsy is in the evaluation of patients with MPNs. Several scoring systems have been used in the past to semiquantitatively grade myelofibrosis (MF). The most recent European consensus guidelines define reticulin fiber content into four grades (MF-0, MF-1, MF-2, MF-3), with normal reticulin content as MF-0 and increasing degrees of fibrosis from MF-1 to MF-3 (47). These guidelines help with more precise and reproducible grading of MF during the disease process. Adequate staining is essential, and the staining in vessel walls can be used as an internal positive control.

IMMUNOHISTOCHEMISTRY

A large number of monoclonal or polyclonal antibodies can be used for immunohistochemical stains on fixed and decalcified bone marrow core biopsies (9). The majority of antibodies used for flow cytometric immunophenotyping can also be applied for immunohistochemistry. The immunoperoxidase technique

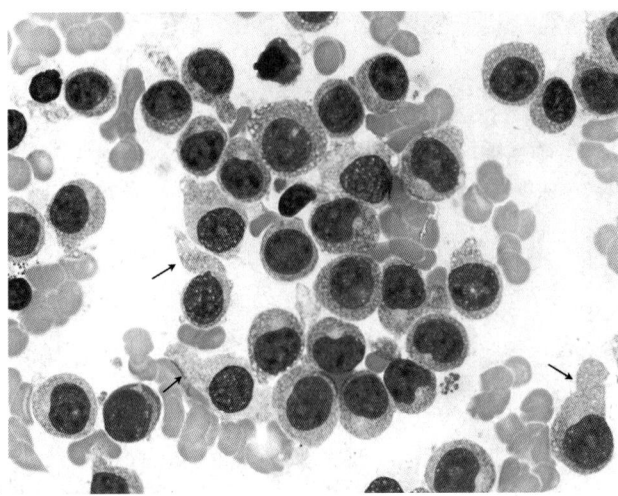
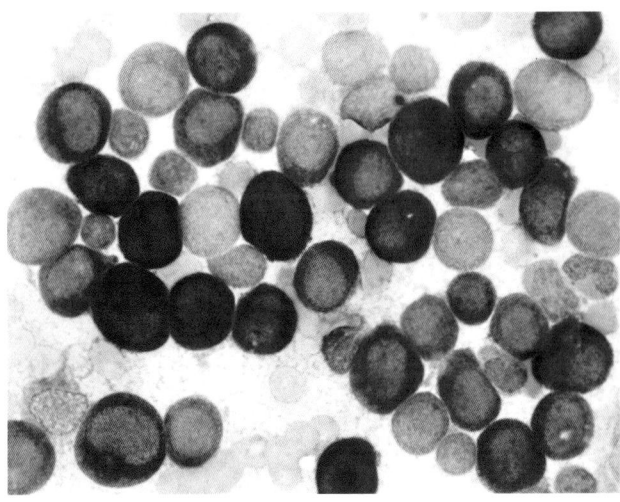

FIGURE 34.11. Bone marrow aspirate smears from a patient with acute monoblastic leukemia. A: The aspirate smears show sheets of blasts with round or slightly indented nuclei, delicate lacy chromatin, and prominent nucleoli. Cytoplasmic pseudopods are readily appreciated in this smear (*arrows*; Wright-Giemsa; 600×). **B:** The ANB stain is positive in the blasts, confirming monocytic lineage of the blasts (600×).

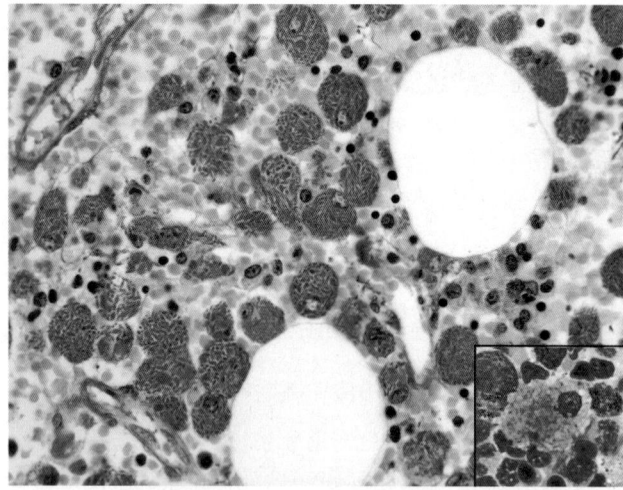

FIGURE 34.12. A periodic acid–Schiff (PAS) stain of the bone marrow core biopsy from a patient with chronic myelogenous leukemia (CML). This case has numerous sea-blue histiocytes that are positive for PAS stain (600×). **Inset:** Sea-blue histiocyte in aspirate smear (Wright-Giemsa).

is most commonly employed for immunohistochemical staining in clinical laboratories. Immunohistochemistry is generally performed by an automated instrument, and the process includes antigen retrieval, blocking endogenous peroxidase activity, a specific antigen-antibody (conjugated with peroxidase) reaction, and a color-producing enzymatic reaction. The sections are then counterstained with hematoxylin and mounted for microscopic examination.

Immunohistochemical staining is particularly valuable when flow cytometry analysis cannot be performed due to dry tap or hemodilution. It helps to determine the lineages of blasts, lymphoma cells, or other abnormal infiltrates; evaluate "clonality" of plasma cells; and assess the expression of various antigens that have diagnostic or therapeutic implications. Immunohistochemistry also helps to highlight subtle infiltrates that may be missed on routine H&E-stained bone marrow sections (Fig. 34.5) (48–50). Immunostaining for CD30 and ALK-1 is particularly valuable for detection of anaplastic large cell lymphoma with low-level bone marrow involvement (51). In addition, some diagnostically important antigens can only be examined by immunohistochemistry in the clinical laboratory, for example, ALK-1 and BCL-1 (Fig. 34.13A–C). It is important to realize that mercury-based fixatives or prolonged decalcification may compromise the preservation of certain antigens and lead to a false-negative result. The application of immunohistochemical staining in bone marrow evaluation is discussed in detail in Chapter 3.

 SUMMARY

Adequate bone marrow sampling and proper processing cannot be overemphasized in bone marrow examination. Knowledge of the patient's clinical history and indication for a bone marrow biopsy, optimal collection and preparation of the specimens, familiarity with various sample types and their applicable tests,

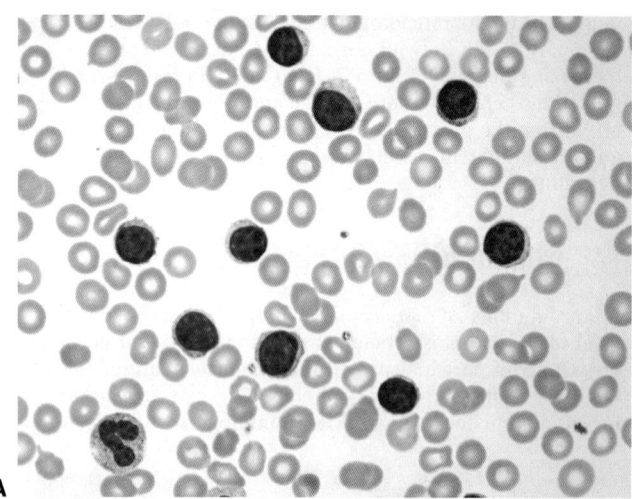

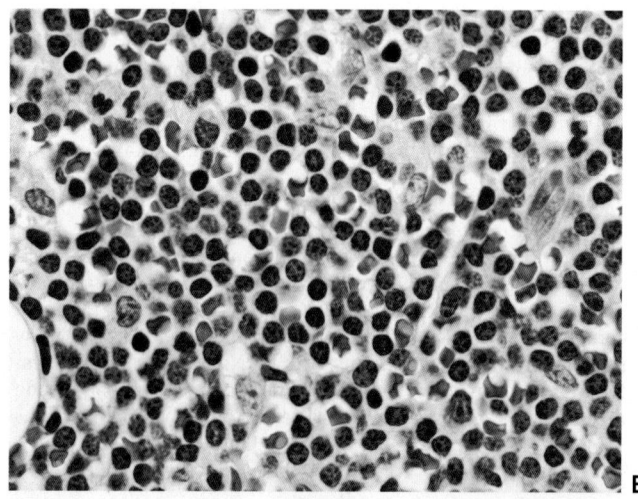

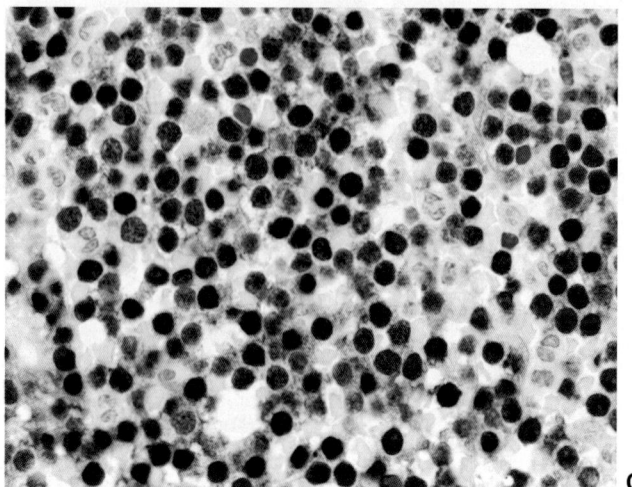

FIGURE 34.13. Mantle cell lymphoma. A: The peripheral blood smear shows marked lymphocytosis composed of small lymphocytes with round nuclei, condensed chromatin, and scant cytoplasm, morphologically indistinguishable from chronic lymphocytic leukemia (Wright-Giemsa; 600×). **B:** The core biopsy shows extensive infiltration by neoplastic lymphocytes (H&E, 600×). **C:** The neoplastic lymphocytes are positive for BCL-1 by immunohistochemical staining (600×). This case was also positive for t(11;14)-CCND1/IgH fusion by FISH analysis.

and appropriate triaging for ancillary tests all play important roles in bone marrow evaluation. Morphologic information derived from peripheral blood, bone marrow aspirates, and core biopsies is complementary and should all be correlated with each other. Specialized techniques, including flow cytometric immunophenotyping, molecular analysis, FISH, and cytogenetic studies, should be used when indicated, correlated with the morphologic findings, and interpreted in clinical context. The specific application of these specialized techniques in evaluation of hematopoietic disease is discussed in Chapters 3, 4, 8, and 9.

References

1. Brynes RK, McKenna RW, Sundberg RD. Bone marrow aspiration and trephine biopsy. An approach to a thorough study. *Am J Clin Pathol* 1978;70(5):753–759.
2. Hyun BH, Gulati GL, Ashton JK. Bone marrow examination: techniques and interpretation. *Hematol Oncol Clin North Am* 1988;2(4):513–523.
3. Hyun BH, Stevenson AJ, Hanau CA. Fundamentals of bone marrow examination. *Hematol Oncol Clin North Am* 1994;8(4):651–663.
4. Lee SH, Erber WN, Porwit A, et al. ICSH guidelines for the standardization of bone marrow specimens and reports. *Int J Lab Hematol* 2008;30(5):349–364.
5. Peterson LC, Agosti SJ, Hoyer JD. Protocol for the examination of specimens from patients with hematopoietic neoplasms of the bone marrow: a basis for checklists. *Arch Pathol Lab Med* 2002;126(9):1050–1056.
6. Vardiman JW, Thiele J, Arber DA, et al. The 2008 revision of the World Health Organization (WHO) classification of myeloid neoplasms and acute leukemia: rationale and important changes. *Blood* 2009;114(5):937–951.
7. Campo E, Swerdlow SH, Harris NL, et al. The 2008 WHO classification of lymphoid neoplasms and beyond: evolving concepts and practical applications. *Blood* 2011;117(19):5019–5032.
8. McGregor S, McNeer J, Gurbuxani S. Beyond the 2008 World Health Organization classification: the role of the hematopathology laboratory in the diagnosis and management of acute lymphoblastic leukemia. *Semin Diagn Pathol* 2012; 29(1):2–11.
9. Kremer M, Quintanilla-Martinez L, Nahrig J, et al. Immunohistochemistry in bone marrow pathology: a useful adjunct for morphologic diagnosis. *Virchows Arch* 2005;447(6):920–937.
10. Fend F, Bock O, Kremer M, et al. Ancillary techniques in bone marrow pathology: molecular diagnostics on bone marrow trephine biopsies. *Virchows Arch* 2005;447(6):909–919.
11. Bain BJ. Bone marrow aspiration. *J Clin Pathol* 2001;54(9):657–663.
12. Bain BJ. Bone marrow trephine biopsy. *J Clin Pathol* 2001;54(10):737–742.
13. Cherry AM, Slovak ML, Campbell LJ, et al. Will a peripheral blood (PB) sample yield the same diagnostic and prognostic cytogenetic data as the concomitant bone marrow (BM) in myelodysplasia? *Leuk Res* 2012;36(7):832–840.
14. Tefferi A. A refined diagnostic algorithm for polycythemia vera that incorporates mutation screening for JAK2(V617F). *Curr Hematol Malig Rep* 2006;1(2):81–86.
15. Tefferi A. JAK2 mutations and clinical practice in myeloproliferative neoplasms. *Cancer J* 2007;13(6):366–371.
16. Klco JM, Vij R, Kreisel FH, et al. Molecular pathology of myeloproliferative neoplasms. *Am J Clin Pathol* 2010;133(4):602–615.
17. Lima L, Bernal-Mizrachi L, Saxe D, et al. Peripheral blood monitoring of chronic myeloid leukemia during treatment with imatinib, second-line agents, and beyond. *Cancer* 2011;117(6):1245–1252.
18. Chendamarai E, Balasubramanian P, George B, et al. Role of minimal residual disease monitoring in acute promyelocytic leukemia treated with arsenic trioxide in frontline therapy. *Blood* 2012;119(15):3413–3419.
19. Summerfield AL, Steinberg FU, Gonzalez JG. Morphologic findings in bone marrow precursor cells in zinc-induced copper deficiency anemia. *Am J Clin Pathol* 1992;97(5):665–668.
20. Willis MS, Monaghan SA, Miller ML, et al. Zinc-induced copper deficiency: a report of three cases initially recognized on bone marrow examination. *Am J Clin Pathol* 2005;123(1):125–131.
21. Halfdanarson TR, Kumar N, Li CY, et al. Hematological manifestations of copper deficiency: a retrospective review. *Eur J Haematol* 2008;80(6):523–531.
22. Pihan GA, Woda BA. Immunophenotypic analysis of cells isolated from bone marrow biopsies in patients with failed bone marrow aspiration ('dry tap'). *Am J Clin Pathol* 1990;93(4):545–548.
23. Dunphy CH, Dunphy FR, Visconti JL. Flow cytometric immunophenotyping of bone marrow core biopsies: report of 8 patients with previously undiagnosed hematologic malignancy and failed bone marrow aspiration. *Arch Pathol Lab Med* 1999;123(3):206–212.
24. Novotny JR, Schmucker U, Staats B, et al. Failed or inadequate bone marrow aspiration: a fast, simple and cost-effective method to produce a cell suspension from a core biopsy specimen. *Clin Lab Haematol* 2005;27(1):33–40.
25. Brunning RD, Bloomfield CD, McKenna RW, et al. Bilateral trephine bone marrow biopsies in lymphoma and other neoplastic diseases. *Ann Intern Med* 1975;82(3): 365–366.
26. Menon NC, Buchanan JG. Bilateral trephine bone marrow biopsies in Hodgkin's and non-Hodgkin's lymphoma. *Pathology* 1979;11(1):53–57.
27. Juneja SK, Wolf MM, Cooper IA. Value of bilateral bone marrow biopsy specimens in non-Hodgkin's lymphoma. *J Clin Pathol* 1990;43(8):630–632.
28. Wang J, Weiss LM, Chang KL, et al. Diagnostic utility of bilateral bone marrow examination: significance of morphologic and ancillary technique study in malignancy. *Cancer* 2002;94(5):1522–1531.
29. van Marum RJ, te Velde L. Cardiac tamponade following sternal puncture in two patients. *Neth J Med* 2001;59(1):39–40.
30. Polverino M, Schiavo A, Fiorenzano G, et al. 1st reported case of pneumothorax caused by sternal puncture. *Minerva Med* 1989;80(6):611–613.
31. Harrington AM, Currey A, Olteanu H, et al. Persistent localized bone marrow aplasia after radiotherapy with preserved peripheral counts: a study of 8 cases. *Ann Diagn Pathol* 2010;14(3):168–172.
32. Bain BJ. Bone marrow biopsy morbidity and mortality. *Br J Haematol* 2003;121(6): 949–951.
33. Bain BJ. Bone marrow biopsy morbidity and mortality: 2002 data. *Clin Lab Haematol* 2004;26(5):315–318.
34. Bain BJ. Bone marrow biopsy morbidity: review of 2003. *J Clin Pathol* 2005;58(4): 406–408.
35. Douglas DD, Risdall RJ. Bone marrow biopsy technique. Artifact induced by aspiration. *Am J Clin Pathol* 1984;82(1):92–94.
36. Jamshidi K, Swaim WR. Bone marrow biopsy with unaltered architecture: a new biopsy device. *J Lab Clin Med* 1971;77(2):335–342.
37. Bishop PW, McNally K, Harris M. Audit of bone marrow trephines. *J Clin Pathol* 1992;45(12):1105–1108.
38. Izadi P, Ortega JA, Coates TD. Comparison of buffy coat preparation to direct method for the evaluation and interpretation of bone marrow aspirates. *Am J Hematol* 1993;43(2):107–109.
39. Marshall PN. Romanowsky-type stains in haematology. *Histochem J* 1978;10(1): 1–29.
40. Woronzoff-Dashkoff KK. The wright-giemsa stain. Secrets revealed. *Clin Lab Med* 2002;22(1):15–23.
41. Bonds LA, Barnes P, Foucar K, Sever CE. Acetic acid-zinc-formalin: a safe alternative to B-5 fixative. *Am J Clin Pathol* 2005;124(2):205–211.
42. Naresh KN, Lampert I, Hasserjian R, et al. Optimal processing of bone marrow trephine biopsy: the Hammersmith Protocol. *J Clin Pathol* 2006;59(9):903–911.
43. Stuart-Smith SE, Hughes DA, Bain BJ. Are routine iron stains on bone marrow trephine biopsy specimens necessary? *J Clin Pathol* 2005;58(3):269–272.
44. DePalma L. The effect of decalcification and choice of fixative on histiocytic iron in bone marrow core biopsies. *Biotech Histochem* 1996;71(2):57–60.
45. Hughes DA, Stuart-Smith SE, Bain BJ. How should stainable iron in bone marrow films be assessed? *J Clin Pathol* 2004;57(10):1038–1040.
46. Tallman MS, Altman JK. How I treat acute promyelocytic leukemia. *Blood* 2009; 114(25):5126–5135.
47. Thiele J, Kvasnicka HM, Facchetti F, et al. European consensus on grading bone marrow fibrosis and assessment of cellularity. *Haematologica* 2005;90(8): 1128–1132.
48. Estalilla OC, Koo CH, Brynes RK, et al. Intravascular large B-cell lymphoma. A report of five cases initially diagnosed by bone marrow biopsy. *Am J Clin Pathol* 1999;112(2):248–255.
49. Ito M, Kim Y, Choi JW, et al. Prevalence of intravascular large B-cell lymphoma with bone marrow involvement at initial presentation. *Int J Hematol* 2003;77(2): 159–163.
50. Chen YH, Chadburn A, Evens AM, et al. Clinical, morphologic, immunophenotypic, and molecular cytogenetic assessment of CD4-/CD8-gammadelta T-cell large granular lymphocytic leukemia. *Am J Clin Pathol* 2011;136(2):289–299.
51. Fraga M, Brousset P, Schlaifer D, et al. Bone marrow involvement in anaplastic large cell lymphoma. Immunohistochemical detection of minimal disease and its prognostic significance. *Am J Clin Pathol* 1995;103(1):82–89.

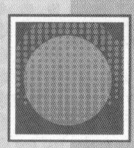
Bone Marrow Manifestations of Hodgkin and Non-Hodgkin Lymphomas and Lymphoma-Like Disorders

Beverly P. Nelson • LoAnn Peterson

 ## INTRODUCTION

One of the most common indications for a bone marrow biopsy is to evaluate for involvement by lymphoma. Bone marrow biopsies are routinely examined at diagnosis to determine stage (1,2) and also frequently during the course of the disease to evaluate for response to therapy or recurrent disease. Occasionally an initial diagnosis of lymphoma is made on the basis of a bone marrow biopsy (3). This chapter will focus on the characteristic features of Hodgkin lymphoma (HL) and non-Hodgkin lymphoma (NHL) as well as the distinction of benign lymphoid infiltrates from lymphoma. Lymphoblastic lymphomas involving the bone marrow, hairy cell leukemia (HCL), and leukemias of mature T cells and natural killer cells are discussed in their respective chapters. HL and NHLs including morphologic, immunologic, and genetic details of diagnosis and classification as they apply to lymph nodes and other tissues are also discussed in detail in chapters 36, 38 and 40.

The core biopsy is usually the most informative when evaluating bone marrow specimens for lymphoma, although in most NHL both the aspirate and core biopsy are routinely evaluated for lymphoma. Although peripheral blood may be involved, it is most commonly involved in small B-cell lymphomas, such as splenic marginal zone lymphoma (SMZL), mantle cell lymphoma (MCL), and follicular lymphoma (FL), and is nearly always accompanied by bone marrow involvement. Peripheral blood and aspirate smears, particle clot sections, and touch imprints provide valuable complementary information and are often the diagnostic source. Therefore, all of these preparations should be examined together and the findings correlated. Adequate sampling is important to ensure detection of focal, lymphomatous infiltrates; therefore, bilateral iliac crest core biopsies are recommended. This practice is based on the finding that the yield of lymphoma detection is significantly higher when bilateral—in contrast to unilateral—posterior iliac crest trephine biopsies are performed (4–6). Because core biopsy size also correlates with the frequency with which lymphoma is identified in the specimen, each biopsy is recommended to be at least 2 cm long (7). In addition, tissue sections from multiple different levels of each paraffin block should be examined.

Additional techniques, including flow cytometric immunophenotyping, paraffin section immunohistochemistry, cytogenetic analysis, fluorescence *in situ* hybridization (FISH), and molecular tests, are valuable tools in evaluating bone marrow specimens for lymphoma. The most effective techniques utilized vary with each case and should be based on the clinical setting, as well as laboratory and morphologic findings. For example, flow cytometric immunophenotyping can be performed on blood or aspirate and is especially useful for establishing diagnosis of mature small B-cell lymphomas such as small lymphocytic lymphoma (SLL). Immunohistochemical stains for CD56 and *in situ* hybridization for Epstein-Barr virus–encoded RNA (EBER-ISH) may be important for lymphomas such as NK/T-cell lymphoma, which can be difficult to identify on hematoxylin and eosin (H&E)–stained sections. As with lymph nodes and other tissues, genetic analysis of lymphoma involving the bone marrow may provide diagnostic, prognostic, or therapeutic information. Whenever one or more ancillary techniques are employed, the data should be correlated with the morphology as well as with each other. It is also worthwhile noting that while ancillary techniques are essential to adequately evaluate many bone marrow lymphoid lesions, knowledge about each technique including its limitations is required before it can be used as an effective, diagnostic aid.

 ## NON-HODGKIN LYMPHOMA

Incidence and Histologic Patterns of Bone Marrow Involvement by Non-Hodgkin Lymphoma

Bone marrow involvement by lymphoma indicates dissemination and represents stage IV disease (8,9). The overall incidence is 35% to 50% (7), but there is considerable variability in the frequency with which specific categories of lymphoma involve the bone marrow (Table 35.1). In general, lymphomas composed predominantly of small cells (small lymphocytic, follicular grade 1 to 2, mantle cell), aggressive lymphomas (lymphoblastic and Burkitt lymphoma [BL]), and many peripheral T-cell lymphomas (PTCLs) most frequently involve the bone marrow. The mere presence of indolent lymphomas in the bone marrow does not always indicate poor clinical outcome, but rather, the extent of marrow involvement often has more direct impact on survival (10,11).

Lymphoma infiltrates the bone marrow in any one or a combination of five different architectural patterns (Fig. 35.1): focal random, focal paratrabecular, interstitial, diffuse, and intra-sinusoidal. Knowledge of these features is not only helpful to identify malignant lymphoid infiltrates but in some cases also aids in classification of the lymphoma. Focal infiltrates are the most common and are characterized by discrete collections of malignant cells in either random or paratrabecular locations. Focal, random lymphoid infiltrates occupy space away from the bony trabeculae. Focal, paratrabecular infiltrates preferentially grow along the bone surface and conform to the bony contour. Paratrabecular infiltrates may expand out away from the bony trabeculae, but one portion remains adjacent to the bone often giving the infiltrate an asymmetrical appearance. Random infiltrates that expand to touch the bone focally are not considered paratrabecular. Even though they focally displace bone marrow and fat cells, focal infiltrates are usually associated with considerable sparing of normal hematopoietic tissue. Malignant cells in interstitial infiltrates occupy spaces between normal hematopoietic cells and fat without significantly disrupting the bone marrow architecture. They usually do not replace large amounts of bone marrow tissue even though they generally show widespread bone marrow involvement. Diffuse infiltrates

Table 35.1	HISTOLOGIC FEATURES OF MAJOR TYPES OF NHL INVOLVING THE BONE MARROW

Type of Lymphoma	Incidence of Involvement	Pattern of Involvement[a]	Cytology	Immunophenotype	Comments
Small lymphocytic	85%	FR, I, D	Small, mature lymphocytes. Proliferation centers may be present in sections.	Dim monotypic sIg, CD5+, CD10−, dim CD20+, CD23+, CD79b dim±, FMC7 dim±	Presence of paratrabecular lymphoid infiltrates essentially rules out SLL/CLL.
Lymphoplasmacytic (WM)	~100%	FR, I, D, FP	Spectrum of cells from lymphocytes to plasma cells; immunoblasts may be present; Dutcher bodies are common.	Plasma cells monotypic cIg, CD138+, and CD56−. Lymphocytes monotypic sIg, CD5−, CD10−, CD20+, CD23−	Usually a mixed pattern of infiltrates that may include paratrabecular infiltrates
Mantle cell	55%–95%	FR, I, D, FP	Small irregular lymphocytes, but cells may resemble CLL, PLL or be blastoid.	Monotypic sIg, CD5+, CD79b+, FMC7+, CD23− or dim CD23+	Cyclin D1 positive. Paratrabecular infiltrates may be present.
Follicular	50%–60%	FP, D, FR, I	Small cleaved lymphocytes usually predominate. Large cleaved or noncleaved cells may be present.	Monotypic sIg, CD20−, CD5−, CD10+, BCL6+, HGAL+ but not as often as FL involving lymph node	Characteristically paratrabecular. Neoplastic follicles may be present. May be lower grade than lymphoma in lymph node or other tissues
Splenic marginal zone	70%–100%	FR, I, D, IS	Small lymphocytes with slightly irregular nuclei, condensed chromatin, variable amounts of cytoplasm	Monotypic sIg, CD20+, CD23−, CD5−, CD10−	Mixed pattern of infiltrate. Intrasinusoidal infiltrates are often present. Reactive germinal centers may be present.
Low-grade extranodal marginal zone (MALT) lymphoma and NMZL	30%–45%	FR, P, I, IS	Small cells with condensed chromatin and scant to moderate amounts of cytoplasm. Rare large cells may be admixed.	Monotypic sIg, CD20+, CD5−, CD10−, CD23−	Extent of bone marrow infiltration usually minimal for MALT lymphoma
Diffuse large B cell	15%–30%	FR, D	Large cells with prominent nucleoli	CD45+, CD20+, CD5±, CD79+, Pax5+, CD30±, CD15−	May be discordant (low grade) with large cell lymphoma involving lymph node. A subset may have prominent component of T lymphocytes ± histiocytes. Rarely the cells are primarily intravascular.
Burkitt	35%–60%	I, D	Medium-sized cells with reticular chromatin, multiple small nucleoli, and basophilic cytoplasm. Cytoplasmic vacuoles are common.	CD20+, CD5−, CD10+, BCL6+, BCL2−, TdT−, Ki67 ~100%	Necrosis is common. Starry-sky pattern is often present.
Peripheral T cell (unspecified)	80%	FR, D	Polymorphous lymphoid population—nuclei often hyperchromatic and irregular. Large cells with visible nucleoli may be present. A prominent reactive cell component is often intermixed.	Variably CD2+, CD3+, CD5+, and CD7+, CD4±, CD8±, rarely CD30+	Vascularity and reticulin fibrosis are frequently prominent. Focal infiltrates are less sharply demarcated from residual bone marrow than in B-cell lymphoma.
Angioimmunoblastic T-cell lymphoma	50%–90%	FR with fibrosis	Heterogeneous infiltrates with lymphocytes, histiocytes, plasma cells, increased vascularity	CD2+, CD3+, CD5+, CD4+, CXCL13+, PD-1+. CD10 less frequently positive than in AILT involving lymph node	Infiltrates poorly circumscribed. Biopsy of extramedullary tissue is usually required for primary diagnosis.
Anaplastic large cell	4%–40%	FR,I (scattered cells), D	Large cells with lobulated nuclei, prominent nucleoli, and abundant cytoplasm including hallmark cells	CD45±, CD3±, CD2±, CD5±, CD7±, CD30+, Alk-1±	Detection rate of bone marrow involvement is higher with CD30 or ALK-1 immunostains.
Hepatosplenic T-cell lymphoma	100%	IS	Medium-sized lymphocytes with dispersed chromatin	CD3+, CD4−, CD8±, CD56+, TIA-1+, mostly TCR $\gamma\delta$+, rarely TCR$\alpha\beta$+	Lesions may be intrasinusoidal and subtle on H&E. IHC is often helpful to highlight the lymphoma cells. Must be distinguished from $\gamma\delta$ T-LGL
NK/T-cell lymphoma	0%–25%	I (scattered cells)	Variable size; some have pleomorphic nuclei.	Surface CD3−, cytoplasmic CD3+ (IHC), CD56+, EBER+	Immunostains or ISH (EBER) may be necessary to identify lymphoma cells in the bone marrow sections.

[a]Patterns may be mixed. The most common patterns are listed.
FR, focal random; FP, focal paratrabecular; I, interstitial; D, diffuse; IS, intrasinusoidal; IHC, immunohistochemistry; CLL, chronic lymphocytic leukemia; SLL, small lymphocytic lymphoma; PLL, prolymphocytic leukemia; LGL, large granular lymphocyte.
Modified from Jaffe ES, Harris NL, Vardiman JW, et al., eds. *Hematopathology*. Philadelphia: Elsevier, 2011:896, with permission.

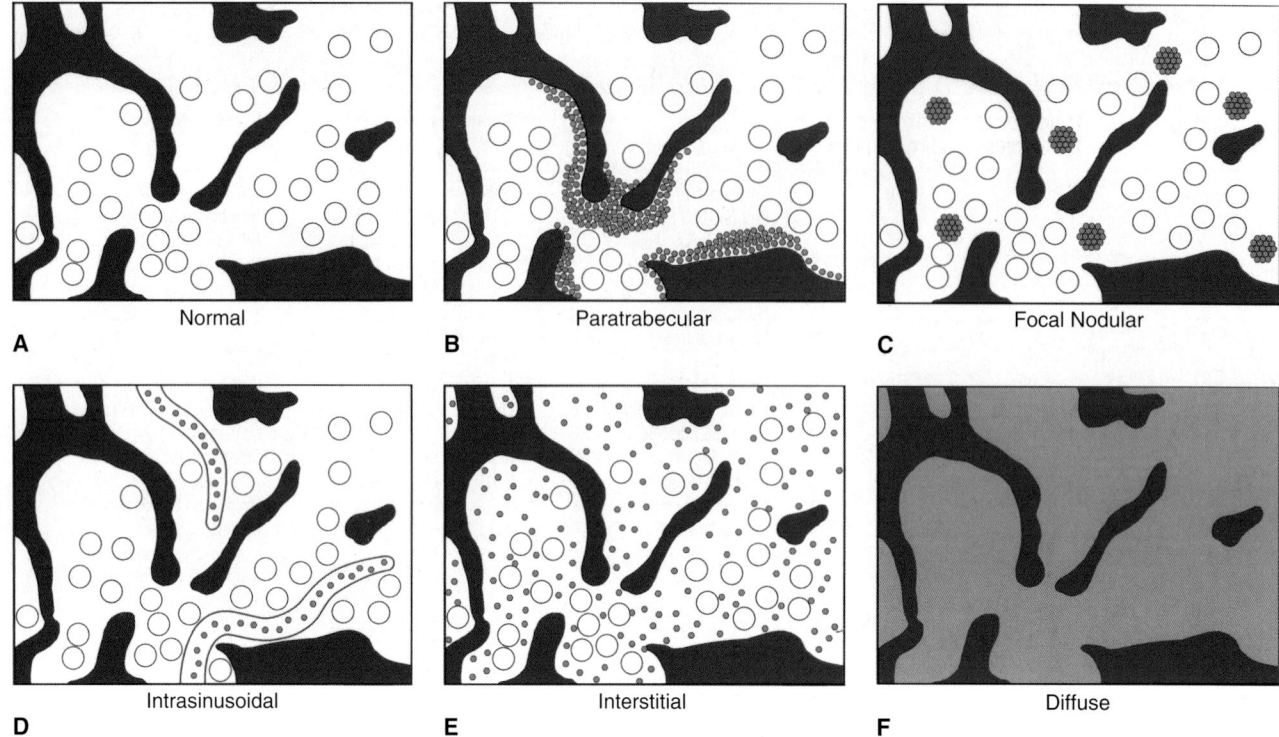

A Normal **B** Paratrabecular **C** Focal Nodular

D Intrasinusoidal **E** Interstitial **F** Diffuse

FIGURE 35.1. A–F: These diagrams illustrate the normal bone marrow and the five different architectural patterns of infiltration by lymphoma. Used from Jaffe ES, Harris NL, Vardiman JW, et al., eds. *Hematopathology*. Philadelphia: Elsevier; 2011:897, with permission.

completely replace the hematopoietic elements and fat between the bony trabeculae in a portion or all of the core biopsy section. Intrasinusoidal infiltration is characterized by collections of malignant cells within the bone marrow sinuses and is typically subtle and difficult to appreciate on routine sections without the aid of immunohistochemical stains.

Chronic Lymphocytic Leukemia/Small Lymphocytic Lymphoma

Chronic lymphocytic leukemia (CLL) and small lymphocytic lymphoma (SLL) are regarded as the same disease with identical immunophenotype (dim monotypic sIg light chain+, CD5+, CD10−, dim CD20+, CD23+, CD79bdim±, FMC7dim±) but with different tissue expressions (12). SLL is the designation used for cases that at diagnosis involve primarily lymph nodes or extranodal sites without a peripheral blood lymphocytosis ($<5.0 \times 10^9$/L monoclonal B cells) (13). About 85% of cases that present as SLL involve the bone marrow at diagnosis, and rarely is the bone marrow the only involved site (7,14). The proportion of cases that present as SLL and later develop peripheral blood lymphocytosis is controversial although clonal B lymphocytes may be present in the blood even without overt lymphocytosis (15). The patterns in which CLL/SLL infiltrates the bone marrow are focal random (Fig. 35.2), diffuse, interstitial, or mixed. Focal random infiltrates are sharply or poorly demarcated; although they may touch bone, distinctly paratrabecular infiltrates are absent, and their presence essentially excludes the diagnosis of CLL/SLL. CLL/SLL lymphocytes in both aspirate and core biopsy are small, mature appearing, and generally have round nuclei with condensed chromatin and scant cytoplasm (Fig. 35.3). Although occasional cells may have slightly irregular nuclei, deep clefts are not common. Prolymphocytes (with slightly more abundant cytoplasm and a single visible nucleolus) are present in low numbers. Proliferation centers are often encountered in bone marrow sections (Fig. 35.4).

While detection of the characteristic CLL/SLL phenotype in a lymphoid infiltrate with the appropriate morphology provides strong support for the diagnosis, occasionally the morphology and/or the phenotype of SLL overlaps with other small B-cell lymphomas particularly MCL. Expression of CD23 is often helpful in this case since it is typically positive in CLL and negative in MCL; however, it is important to recognize that CD23 may be positive in both CLL/SLL and MCL. An immunostain negative for cyclin D1 and/or absence of *BCL-1* translocation by FISH or conventional cytogenetic analysis helps to exclude MCL. A positive immunohistochemical stain for lymphoid-enhancer–binding factor 1 (LEF1) (Fig. 35.5) is also helpful to establish

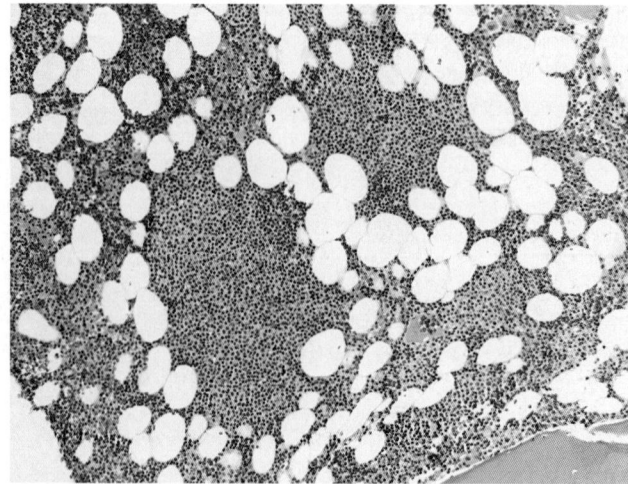

FIGURE 35.2. Chronic lymphocytic leukemia/small lymphocytic lymphoma. Four focal, random lymphoid aggregates with infiltrative borders composed of small lymphocytes with condensed chromatin are illustrated in this H&E-stained bone marrow core biopsy section.

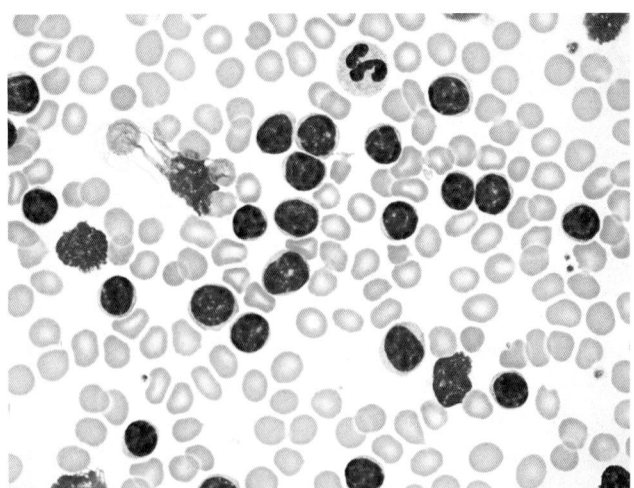

FIGURE 35.3. Chronic lymphocytic leukemia. The CLL lymphocytes in this Wright-Giemsa–stained blood smear are small with round nuclei and condensed chromatin. Smudged cells, which are nuclear remnants of damaged cells, are also visible.

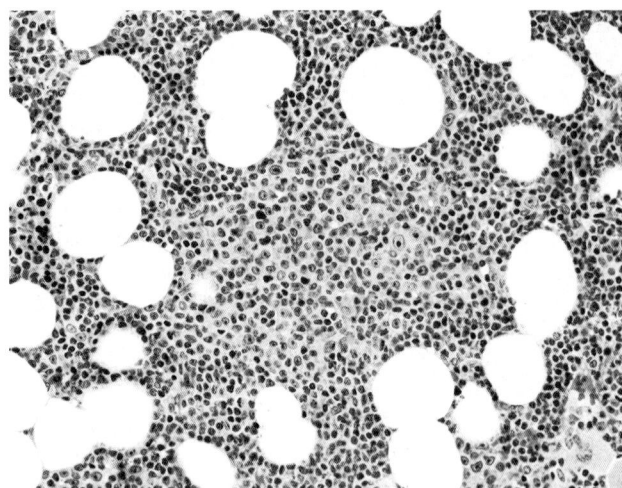

FIGURE 35.4. Chronic lymphocytic leukemia proliferation center/small lymphocytic lymphoma. This pale-staining focus in this H&E-stained bone marrow core biopsy section is a proliferation center that contains prolymphocytes with visible, centrally placed nucleoli.

diagnosis of CLL/SLL especially when proliferation centers are absent since LEF1 is only rarely positive in other small B-cell lymphomas including MCL (16).

Lymphoplasmacytic Lymphoma/Waldenström Macroglobulinemia

Lymphoplasmacytic lymphoma (LPL) is a neoplasm of small B lymphocytes, plasmacytoid lymphocytes, and plasma cells. Most cases of LPL involving the bone marrow manifest as Waldenström macroglobulinemia (WM) (17,18) that is defined as LPL with bone marrow involvement and a serum IgM monoclonal protein of any concentration; WM is usually diagnosed based on a bone marrow biopsy. The plasma cells in LPL are CD138 positive and display monotypic cytoplasmic Ig light chain (Fig. 35.6), while the lymphocytes display monotypic surface Ig light chain and are typically CD5−, CD10−, CD20+, and CD23−. LPL infiltrates in the bone marrow may be focal random, paratrabecular, interstitial, or diffuse. Mixed patterns are common (19). LPL shows a wide spectrum of cells including small lymphocytes similar to SLL, plasmacytoid

lymphocytes, and plasma cells (Fig. 35.6). Occasionally, transformed lymphocytes may be present. Plasma cells vary considerably in number and are usually far less numerous than the lymphocytes but may be frequent or even predominate. In a subset of cases, plasma cells may be interstitial and distinct from focal lymphoid infiltrates (19). The chromatin patterns in the plasma cells are usually condensed, but some may exhibit nucleoli or other immature features. Although intranuclear inclusions (Dutcher bodies) are often identified in plasma cells, they are not specific for LPL since they can be seen in plasma cell neoplasms and occasionally in reactive lymphoid infiltrates. Mast cells as well as histiocytes are often numerous in the bone marrow infiltrates. Peripheral blood lymphocytosis is unusual.

The differential diagnosis of LPL/WM includes other small B-cell neoplasms that involve the bone marrow such as CLL/SLL and those showing plasmacytic differentiation including SMZL, B-cell lymphoma of mucosa-associated lymphoid tissue type (MALT lymphoma), and plasma cell myeloma (20a). The lymphocytes in LPL are usually CD5−, but the small number of cases positive for CD5 could be confused with CLL/SLL. However, CLL/SLL usually lacks plasmacytic differentiation

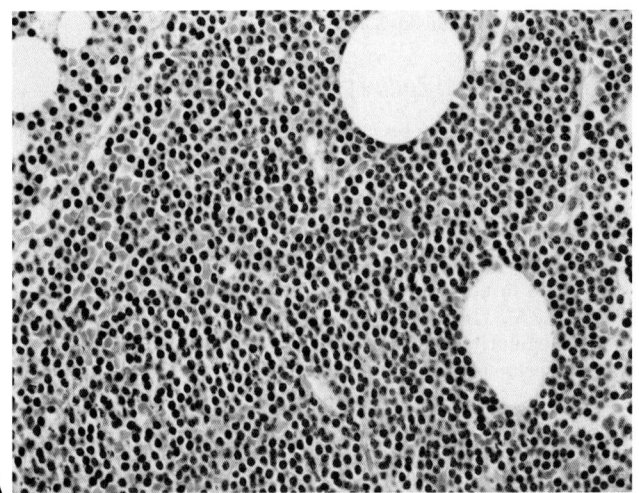

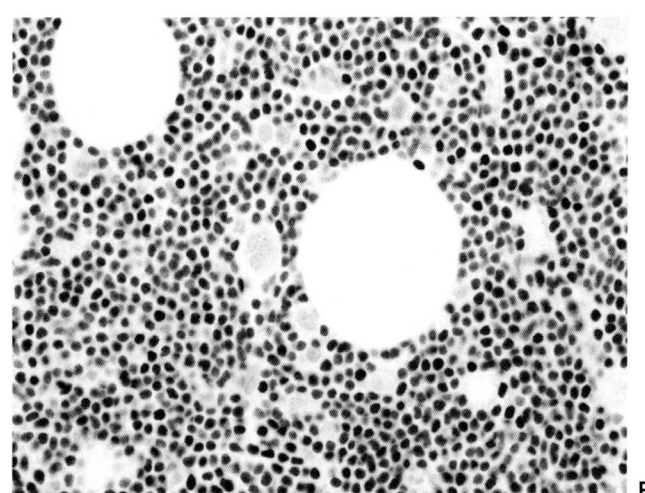

FIGURE 35.5. A,B: Chronic lymphocytic leukemia/small lymphocytic lymphoma. The H&E-stained section shows small lymphocytes with condensed chromatin, round nuclei, and scant cytoplasm. The CLL/SLL lymphocytes display positive nuclear staining for LEF1.

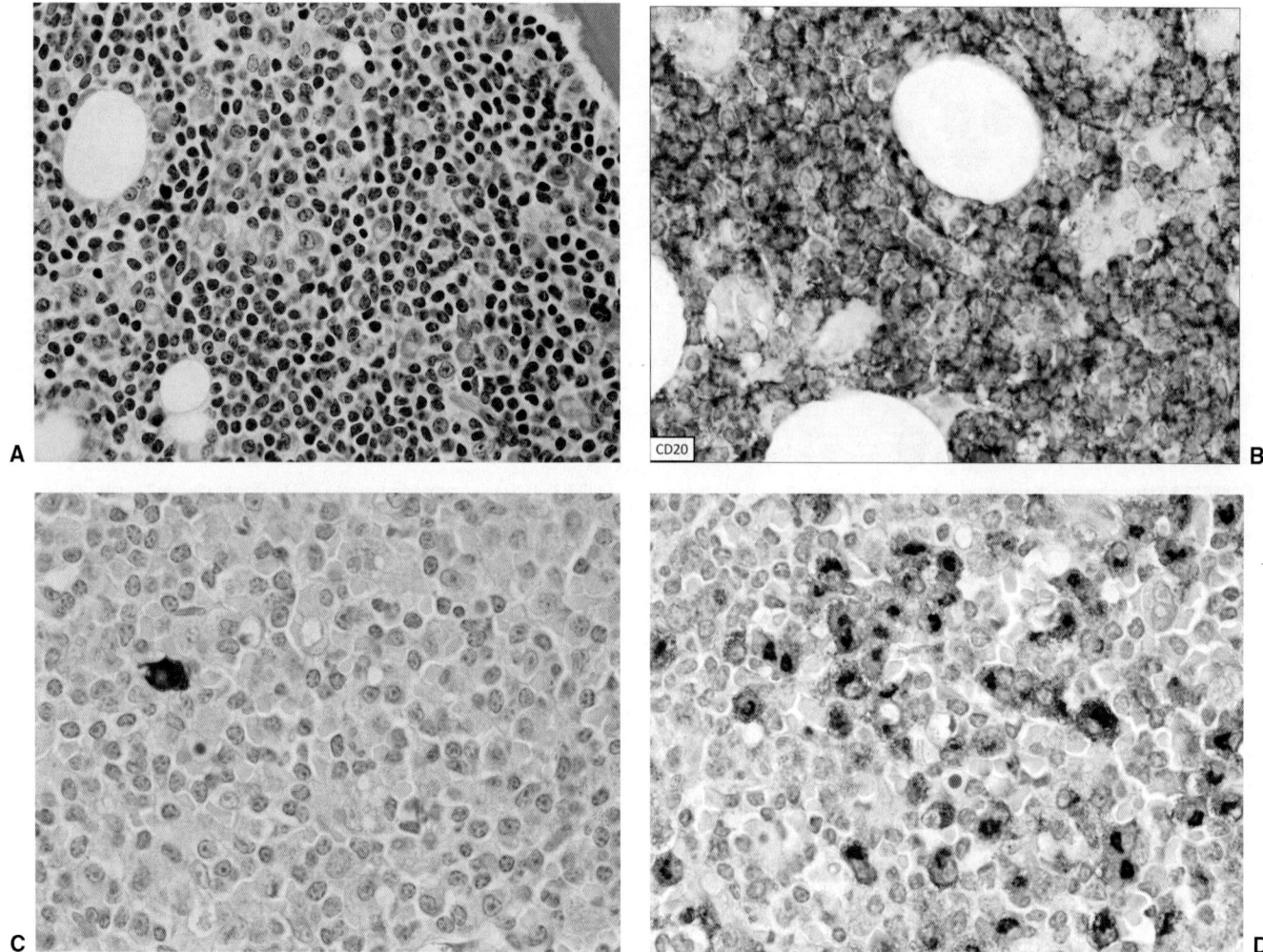

FIGURE 35.6. LPL bone marrow core biopsy section. A: The infiltrate is composed of small lymphocytes with condensed chromatin and plasma cells including some with visible nucleoli in the H&E-stained section. **B:** The small lymphocytes are CD20+. **C:** Kappa and **(D)** lambda immunostains show that the plasma cells are lambda monotypic.

and unlike LPL does not exhibit paratrabecular lymphoid infiltrates. In addition, LPL infiltrates lack proliferation centers that may be present in CLL/SLL. While clinical and laboratory features such as IgM serum paraprotein with hyperviscosity, lack of lytic bone lesions, presence of lymphadenopathy, and a characteristic immunophenotype help to distinguish LPL from plasma cell myeloma, distinction from marginal zone lymphoma can be problematic since both malignancies can exhibit similar morphology and immunophenotype, be associated with IgM serum paraprotein, and involve the spleen (20a). Careful attention to the affected anatomic sites is helpful to exclude extranodal MALT-type lymphoma, which typically originates at mucosal sites and tends to spread to other MALT sites when they disseminate; this is in contrast to LPL/WM that is rarely localized to extranodal sites but typically involves the bone marrow and may also involve lymph nodes and the spleen. Splenomegaly is present in most cases of SMZLs, and the bone marrow is almost always involved, but plasma cells are not as prominent as in LPL and may not be monotypic. Intrasinusoidal infiltrates and reactive germinal centers are common in splenic MZL but are not generally features of LPL. In addition, a recent report indicates that the proportion of plasma cells positive for both CD138 and PAX5 by immunohistochemistry is higher in LPL/WM than in marginal zone lymphoma or plasma cell myeloma; however, the proportion of plasma cells

coexpressing both CD138 and MUM1 is lower in LPL/WM than in marginal zone lymphoma and plasma cell myeloma (Mark Roberts: Nuclear Protein Dysregulation in LPL/WM submitted) (20b). This finding could also potentially aid in the differential diagnosis of these lesions.

Splenic Marginal Zone Lymphoma

SMZL is an indolent B-cell lymphoma that involves the bone marrow at presentation in nearly all cases (21,22). Neoplastic cells are present in the peripheral blood in virtually all cases of SMZL, although an absolute lymphocytosis is not a constant feature (23). The lymphoma cells are small to large in size with round to slightly irregular nuclei, condensed chromatin, and small to abundant amounts of pale, gray-blue cytoplasm (Fig. 35.7A). The circulating malignant lymphocytes may display irregularly distributed cytoplasm projections, but this is not a specific or consistent finding (24).

In core biopsy sections, the infiltrates occur in one or more of the following patterns: intrasinusoidal (22), interstitial, focal random, and/or focal paratrabecular; (Fig. 35.7B) diffuse involvement is rare. Intrasinusoidal infiltration is often prominent in SMZL and can be highlighted by immunostains that mark the infiltrating cells; but it is not specific for this disorder since a similar pattern of infiltration occurs

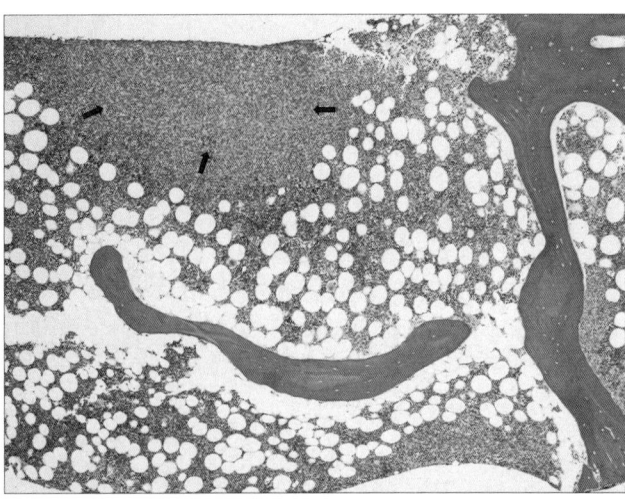

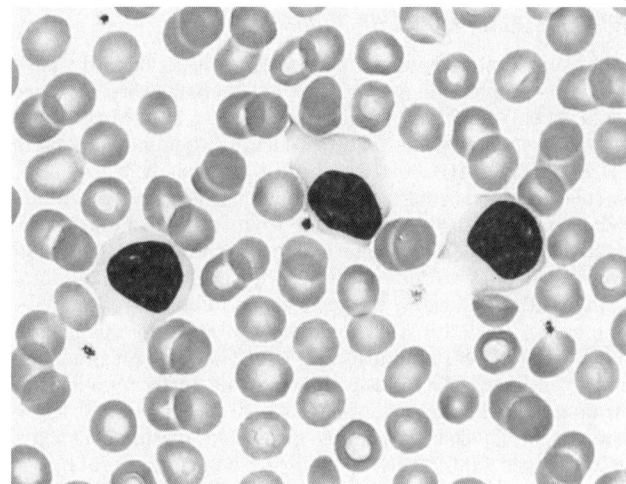

A   B

FIGURE 35.7. SMZL in bone marrow core biopsy section and blood. A: The lymphoma infiltrate includes one paratrabecular lymphoid aggregate and two focal random lymphoid aggregates. The largest lymphoid aggregate includes a reactive germinal center with indistinct borders that is identified by the arrows in this H&E-stained section. **B:** Marginal zone lymphoma cells in the blood in this case have condensed chromatin and moderate to abundant pale cytoplasm.

in other lymphomas (22). Another finding of importance in SMZL is the presence of reactive germinal centers in the lymphomatous infiltrate, reported in about 30% of the cases (22) (Fig. 35.8). In sections, the neoplastic cells resemble SMZL cells with moderately abundant cytoplasm, irregular nuclei, and small nucleoli; they are typically sIg light chain restricted, CD20+, CD23-, CD5-, and CD10-. HCL is important in the differential diagnosis of SMZL. However, the morphology of the SMZL lymphocytes in blood and aspirates more closely resembles that of other small B-cell neoplasms than HCL (condensed chromatin in SMZL vs. reticular in HCL). In addition, the SMZL infiltrates in core biopsies more closely resemble that of other small B-cell neoplasms with fairly compact aggregates of small lymphocytes rather than the more diffuse or interstitial, often subtle infiltrates of HCL with widely spaced nuclei. The immunophenotype of these two disorders is similar; however, the intensity of expression of CD11C, CD22, and CD103 is typically strong in HCL. CD103 is usually negative in SMZL, and CD22 and CD11c staining intensity is usually weaker than in SMZL. Annexin and/or tartrate-resistant acid phosphatase immunostains are positive in HCL but negative in SMZL.

Extranodal Marginal Zone Lymphoma of Mucosa-Associated Tissue

Extranodal marginal zone lymphoma (EMZL) of MALT type is a B-cell lymphoma (CD20+, CD23-, CD5-, and CD10-) that typically involves the gastrointestinal tract and is usually localized at diagnosis. Salivary glands, lungs, thyroid, and conjunctiva are among the other commonly involved sites. When dissemination occurs, EMZL preferentially spreads to other mucosal sites. However, approximately 45% of disseminated EMZL lymphomas involve the bone marrow (11). Most commonly the bone marrow infiltrates are focal random although they may also be paratrabecular, interstitial, or intrasinusoidal (22,25,26). The extent of bone marrow involvement is variable but is often low (22,27), and dissemination does not appear to affect prognosis (11). Infiltrates of EMZL include a spectrum of lymphoma cells; they range from small cells with condensed chromatin resembling mature lymphocytes to slightly larger cells with irregular nuclei, ample cytoplasm, and distinct cell borders. There may be admixed plasma cells. The absolute lymphocyte count is normal in most cases, and circulating lymphoma cells are identified morphologically in only a minority of cases.

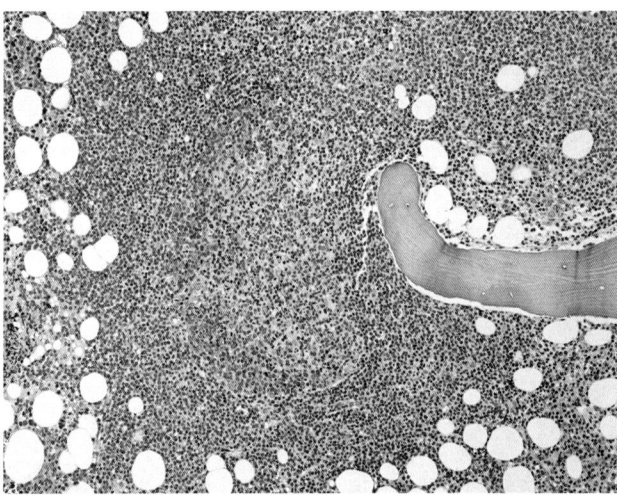

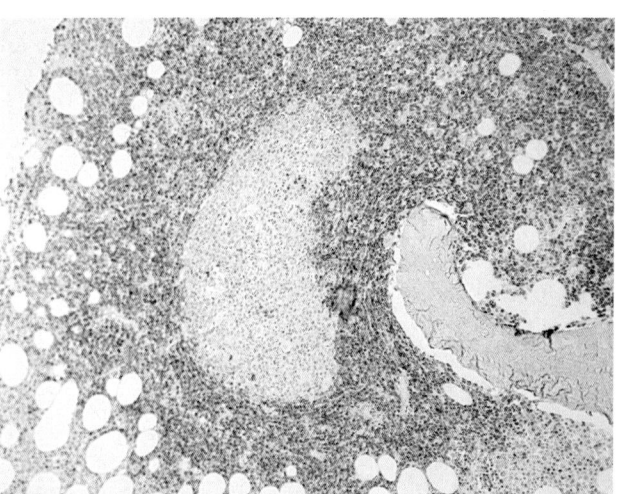

A   B

FIGURE 35.8. SMZL with a reactive germinal center involving the bone marrow core biopsy section. A: The lymphomatous infiltrate includes a polarized germinal center with a dark and light zone and heterogeneous cellular composition. **B:** The germinal center is BCL2 negative supporting that it is benign.

Nodal Marginal Zone Lymphoma

Nodal marginal zone lymphoma (NMZL) is a primary lymphoma of lymph node that is regarded as distinct from extranodal MALT-type lymphoma (28). NMZL and MALT-type lymphomas share some features such as immunophenotype (CD20+, CD5−, CD10−, CD23−) and the propensity to colonize reactive germinal centers. The malignant cells closely resemble nodal monocytoid B cells that are frequently encountered in reactive lymphadenitis. Bone marrow involvement has been observed in 30% to 55% of cases with mostly focal random or interstitial infiltrates; paratrabecular infiltrates occur less frequently (27,29,30). Diffuse infiltrates occur in the leukemic phase of NMZL, but are rare (31). The infiltrates include small centrocyte-like cells with irregular nuclei, condensed chromatin, and scant cytoplasm as well as medium to large monocytoid-like cells with ample cytoplasm; plasma cells may be intermixed. NMZL only rarely involves the peripheral blood and bone marrow aspirate smears; however, the cytology of the circulating lymphoma cells is similar to those observed in the bone marrow core biopsy sections (31).

Follicular Lymphoma

FL, grade 1 to 2, involves the bone marrow in 50% to 60% of cases at initial diagnosis, while grade 3, FL involves the bone marrow in one-third of cases or less (32). The neoplastic cells are CD20+ and CD5− and, in some cases, are also positive for one or more germinal center–associated marker such as CD10, BCL6, and HGAL (human germinal center–associated lymphoma) (33); many admixed T lymphocytes are often present. FL infiltrates are often distinctly and may be exclusively paratrabecular (Fig. 35.9). However, other patterns including focal random and diffuse infiltrates also occur; interstitial infiltrates are infrequent (7,34). The frequent paratrabecular location and the focal random distribution of the infiltrates contribute to them often being missed during bone marrow aspiration; therefore, morphologic review of the aspirate and flow cytometric analysis may not always detect the lymphoma cells (35). The bone marrow infiltrates are most frequently composed of small lymphocytes with condensed but smooth chromatin and cleaved or irregularly shaped nuclei. Large lymphocytes with prominent, single nucleoli may be present, but they are usually low in number. A follicular growth pattern rarely occurs in the bone marrow (Fig. 35.10) (36); a follicular dendritic cell (FDC) meshwork (CD21+, CD23+, CD35+) can be demonstrated in these cases.

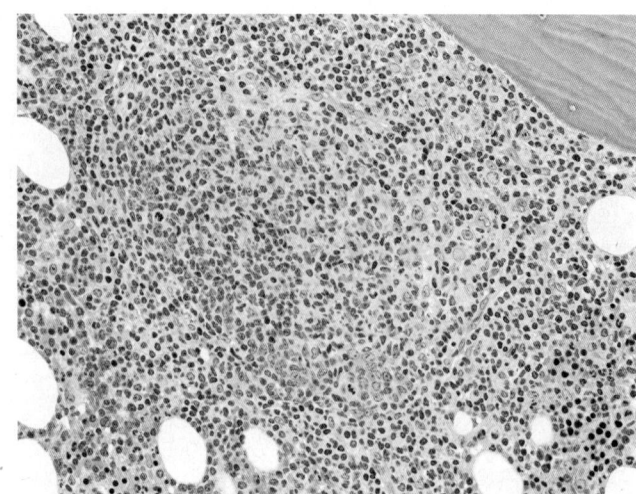

FIGURE 35.10. Follicular lymphoma. A malignant germinal center composed of predominantly small cleaved lymphocytes is present in this paratrabecular infiltrate of a FL that involves the core biopsy in this H&E-stained section.

Circulating lymphoma cells occasionally can be identified in the peripheral blood smear but are usually in low number. In a minority of cases, FL presents with an absolute lymphocytosis (37). The lymphoma cells are typically slightly larger than mature lymphocytes and have deep nuclear clefts, smooth condensed chromatin, and scant cytoplasm (Fig. 35.11). In rare cases, the lymphoma cells resemble CLL (38,39). Discordant morphology between the lymphoma at nodal or extranodal sites and lymphoma in the bone marrow occurs in approximately 20% of cases with the majority of cases containing more indolent infiltrates in the bone marrow (7,40–42). When lymphoma is encountered first in the bone marrow, the characteristic morphology and immunophenotype may suggest a FL, but a lymph node or other tissue biopsy may be necessary to confirm the diagnosis and is required for precise grading of the lymphoma.

Mantle Cell Lymphoma

MCL involves the bone marrow in 55% to 95% of cases (43). An absolute lymphocytosis has been reported in approximately 25% of cases (43,44), but circulating lymphoma cells are

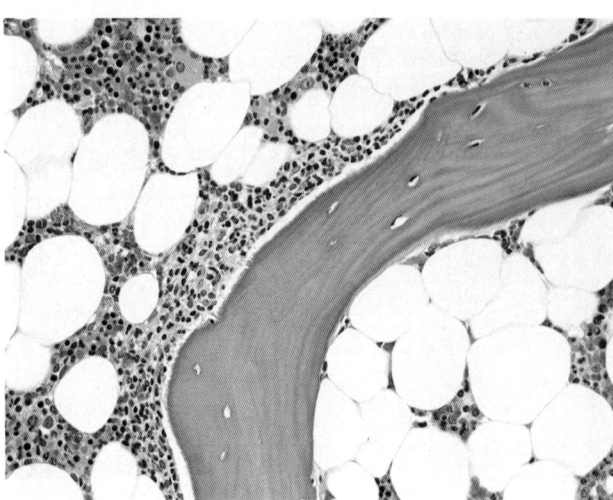

FIGURE 35.9. Follicular lymphoma. One paratrabecular lymphoid infiltrate grows along the bone and conforms to its contour in this H&E-stained bone marrow core biopsy section.

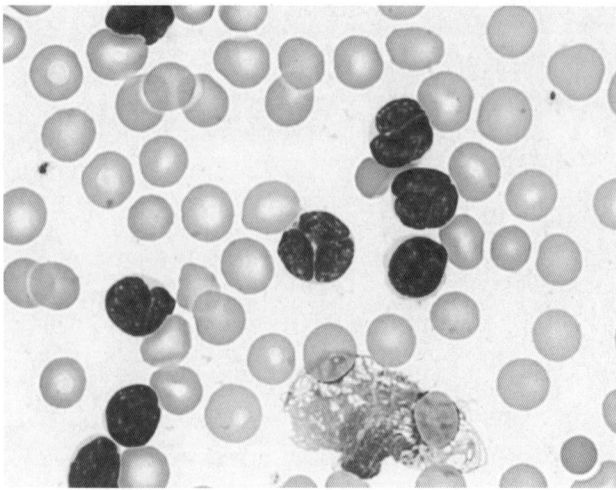

FIGURE 35.11. Follicular lymphoma, leukemic. The FL cells in this Wright-Giemsa–stained blood smear have frequent cleaved nuclei smooth, condensed chromatin, and scant cytoplasm.

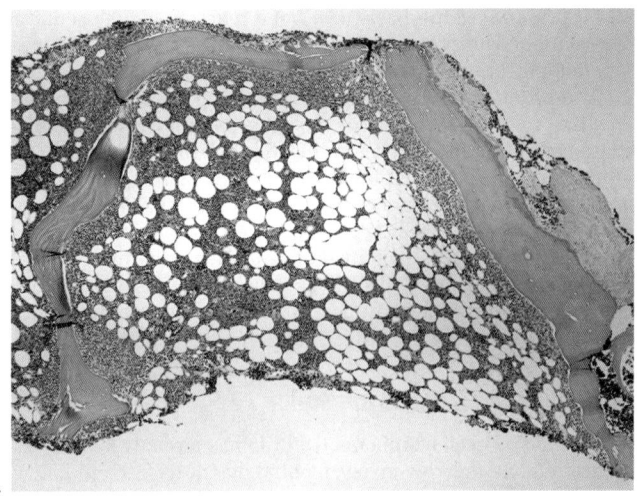

A

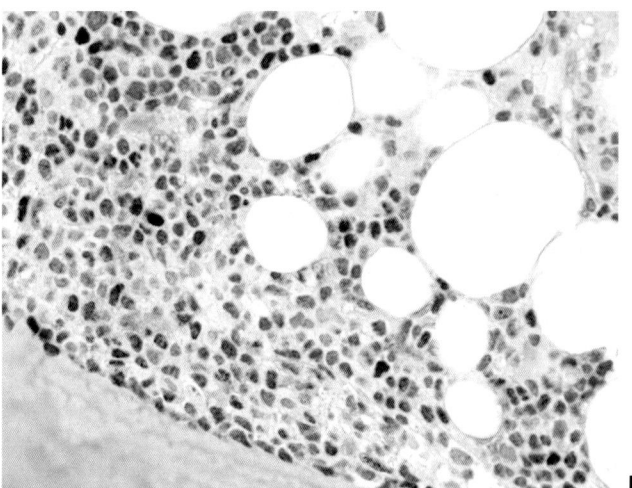

B

FIGURE 35.12. MCL involving the bone marrow core biopsy and blood. A: The lymphoma shows an exclusively paratrabecular growth pattern in the H&E-stained section. **B:** The lymphoma cells are cyclin D1 positive. **C:** The lymphoma cells in the blood smear are small with condensed chromatin, irregular or indented nuclei, and scant cytoplasm.

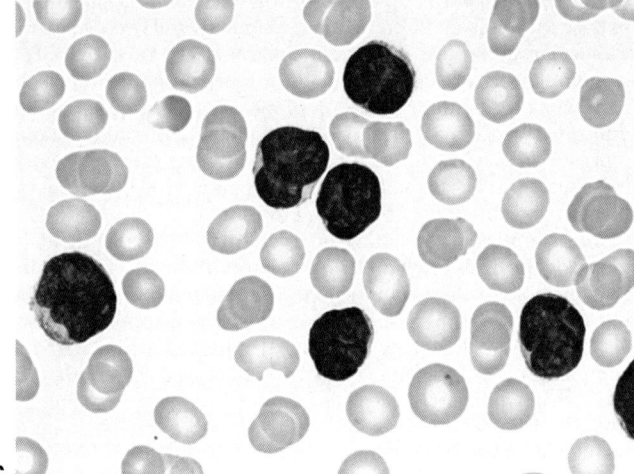

C

common even when a lymphocytosis is not present. The bone marrow may be the initial diagnostic tissue biopsy. Bone marrow infiltrates are typically focal random, but paratrabecular infiltrates are present in up to 45% of cases, and in occasional cases, the lymphoma is exclusively paratrabecular (Fig. 35.12A and B). Interstitial or diffuse patterns of infiltration also occur (43,45,46). Reactive germinal centers may occur but are rare in

MCL infiltrates. The lymphocytes in MCL exhibit heterogeneous morphology; in most cases, the cells are composed of a uniform population of small- to medium-sized lymphocytes with condensed chromatin and irregularly shaped nuclei. Occasionally the lymphocytes are predominantly small with condensed chromatin and round nuclei and morphologically indistinguishable from lymphocytes in SLL/CLL (47) (Fig. 35.13A and B). In

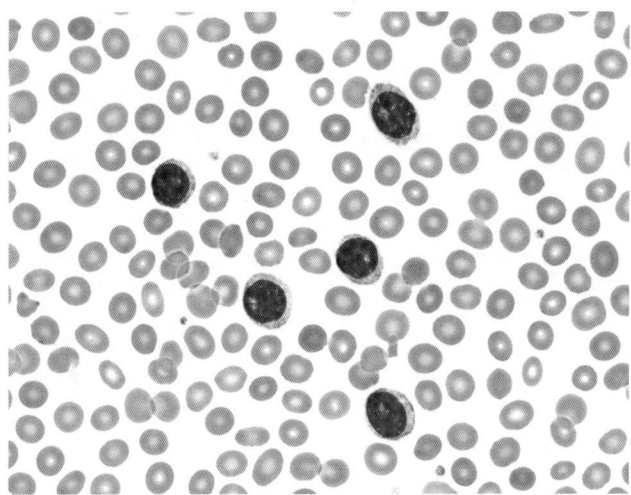

A

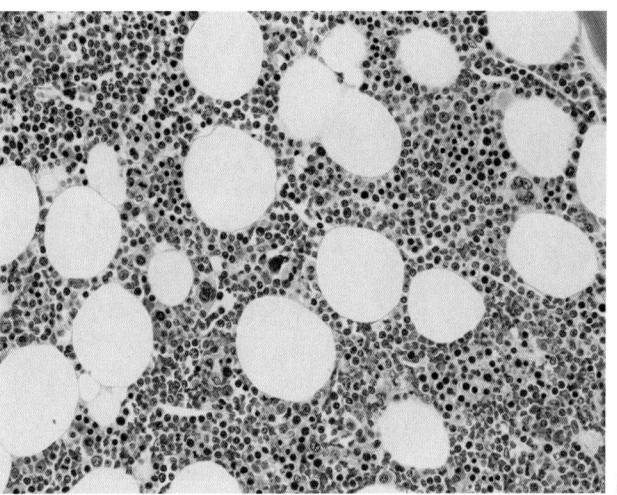

B

FIGURE 35.13. MCL mimicking CLL/SLL. A: The Wright-stained blood smear shows MCL cells that are small with condensed chromatin and round nuclei morphologically indistinguishable from CLL/SLL cells. **B:** The MCL cells infiltrate the bone marrow core biopsy in an interstitial infiltrative pattern.

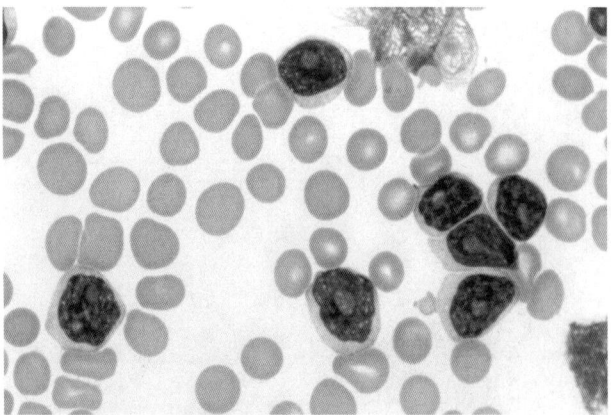

FIGURE 35.14. MCL mimicking prolymphocytic leukemia. The MCL cells in this Wright-stained blood smear are large with central, visible nucleoli resembling prolymphocytes.

other cases, the lymphoma cells are large with visible nucleoli resembling prolymphocytes (48); when leukemic, these cases can resemble prolymphocytic leukemia (49) (Fig. 35.14). Lymphoma cells in the blastoid variants of MCL have dispersed chromatin and scant cytoplasm mimicking large cell lymphoma or acute lymphoblastic leukemia (Fig. 35.15A and B) or are pleomorphic with lobated nuclei (50). Bone marrow infiltrates tend to be interstitial or diffuse in the blastoid variant (46). Some patients with MCL have non-nodal disease and present with blood, marrow, and sometimes splenic involvement; they have been reported to have a good prognosis (51). In addition, a subset of indolent MCL has been reported that involves primarily the blood and bone marrow with kappa light chain restriction and an interstitial pattern of infiltration (52).

MCL must be distinguished from other small B-cell neoplasms in bone marrow especially SLL/CLL since they are both CD5+ and can exhibit similar morphology. A helpful immunophenotypic feature is that in contrast to CLL, MCL cells usually display strong intensity CD20 and bright surface immunoglobulin (sIg) light chain expression and are CD79b+, FMC7+, and CD23−. However, it is important to recognize that both SLL/CLL and MCL can be weak CD23+ (53,54). If bone marrow biopsies show paratrabecular infiltrates, a diagnosis of SLL/CLL can essentially be excluded, and the possibility of other disorders including MCL should be considered. Primary diagnosis

of MCL made on the basis of a bone marrow biopsy requires correlation with results of ancillary studies such as immunophenotype, immunohistochemical stain showing BCL-1 positivity and/or genetic studies documenting t(11;14)(q13;q32). Positive nuclear staining for sox11 is highly associated with classical MCL and is therefore helpful to distinguish MCL from other small B-cell lymphomas including SLL/CLL, FLs, and marginal zone lymphomas (55). A positive sox11 stain may also help to identify BCL-1 negative MCLs, but blastic MCLs are frequently sox11 negative (56). Although a subset of HCLs is also sox11 positive, HCL is usually not confused with MCL since their morphologic appearances and immunophenotypes are quite different.

Diffuse Large B-Cell Lymphoma

Diffuse large B-cell lymphoma (DLBCL) has a relatively low incidence of bone marrow involvement at diagnosis (10% to 25% of cases); in a minority of cases, the bone marrow is the primary site of diagnosis (40,57,58). Focal random, diffuse, and mixed patterns of infiltration occur most frequently followed by paratrabecular infiltrates; interstitial infiltrates are rare (59). The lymphoma cells are large, have one or more prominent nucleoli, and scant to medium amounts of cytoplasm. Lymphomatous infiltrates are usually easily identified in H&E-stained bone marrow biopsy sections. Bone marrow aspirates or touch imprints also occasionally show lymphoma cells; peripheral blood involvement occurs but is uncommon.

In a significant percentage of cases (up to 40%), DLBCL diagnosed on the basis of a lymph node or on extranodal tissue exhibits morphology discordant from the lymphoma observed in the bone marrow (40,57,60). The bone marrow commonly shows less aggressive histology with the lymphoma in the marrow composed entirely of small cells with condensed chromatin or a mixture of small and large cells (57,59,61) (Fig. 35.16A and B). In up to 40% of the cases, the infiltrates are paratrabecular, a histologic feature that helps to support that the more indolent-appearing lesions are lymphoma; (14) this is particularly helpful since reactive lymphoid infiltrates may also occur in bone marrow from patients with lymphoma at extramedullary sites (62). Two-thirds of these discordant lymphomas exhibit identical monoclonal IGH@ and/or BCL-2@ gene rearrangements in the bone marrow and the extramedullary tissue supporting the origin of both lymphomas from a single B-cell clone, while about one-third of the bone marrow discordant lymphomas

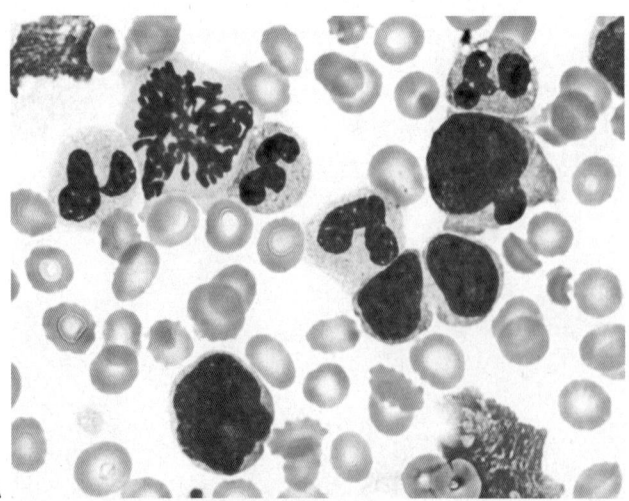

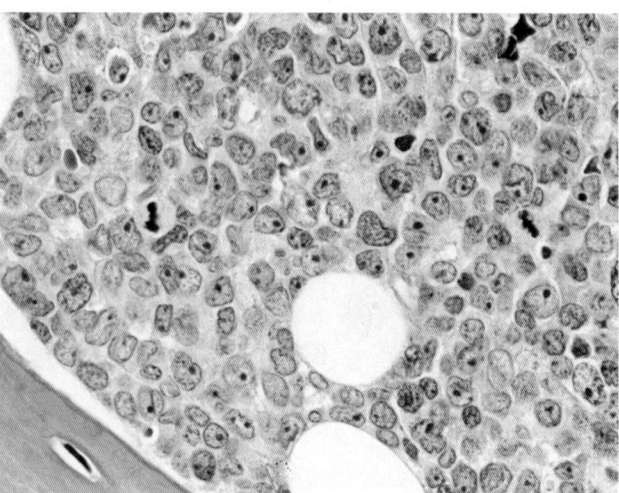

FIGURE 35.15. Blastic MCL in the bone marrow aspirate and core biopsy. A: The lymphoma cells in the blood smear are variably sized with dispersed chromatin and scant cytoplasm resembling blasts. A single mitotic figure is visible. **B:** The lymphoma shows a diffuse growth pattern in the core biopsy section and is indistinguishable from blasts. A cyclin D1 stain was positive (not illustrated).

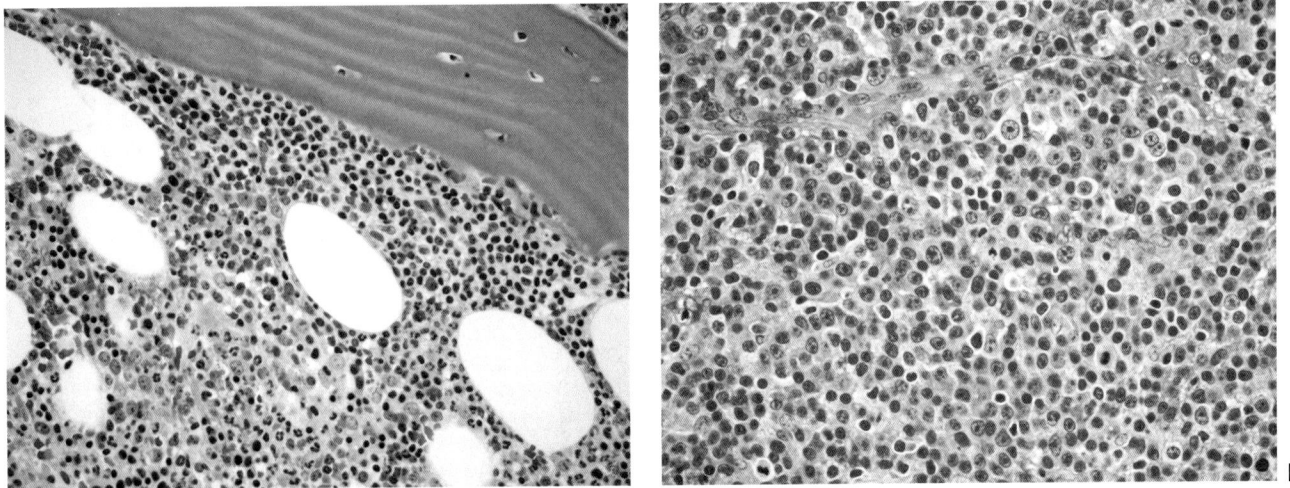

FIGURE 35.16. Large cell lymphoma with discordant morphology in the H&E-stained bone marrow core biopsy section and an extranodal site. A: Lymphoma composed of small lymphocytes with condensed chromatin in this paratrabecular lymphoid infiltrate. **B:** The lymphoma cells are large with visible nucleoli in a curettage form a joint in the same patient.

are apparently unrelated to the extramedullary DLBCL as evidenced by the presence of distinct IGH@ or BCL-2@ gene rearrangements and gene sequences in both lymphomas (62). Cases with discordant (indolent) lymphoma in the bone marrow have better overall survival compared to those with large cell lymphoma in the marrow (58,61,63). Extensive bone marrow infiltration by lymphoma (>70% infiltrate) or a diffuse infiltrative pattern composed of >50% large cells is associated with poor prognosis (40,59). The presence of minimal lymphomatous involvement (<10%) with discordant morphology, with the bone marrow composed entirely of small cells, does not affect prognosis (61).

T-cell/histiocyte-rich large B-cell lymphoma is a subset of DLBCL that exhibits relatively few large neoplastic B cells with numerous admixed small T cells with or without histiocytes (64); these lymphomas frequently involve the bone marrow (65) and may be difficult to distinguish from other lymphomas, especially PTCL and lymphocyte-predominant HL. A panel of immunostains is essential to distinguish these disorders. The large neoplastic B cells are CD45+, CD20+, CD79+, Pax5+, CD30-, and CD15-.

Mediastinal large B-cell lymphoma (LBCL) is a subtype of DLBCL that arises in the mediastinum and has a female predominance (66). Bone marrow involvement has been reported (3% to 9%), but the characteristics of marrow infiltration have not been described in detail (67).

Intravascular Large B-Cell Lymphoma

Intravascular large B-cell lymphoma (IV-LBCL) is an uncommon variant of extranodal LBCL in which the lymphoma cells preferentially localize within the lumina of small blood vessels; it is usually widely disseminated including bone marrow (68). Bone marrow can be the initial diagnostic site (69,70). Involved bone marrow sections exhibit predominantly intrasinusoidal lymphoma cells that can be highlighted by immunostains for B-cell–associated markers such as CD20 and CD79a (71) (Fig. 35.17A and B). A subset of IV-LBCL expresses CD5.

In general, intravascular LBCL cells do not form extravascular tumor masses. Lymphoma cells are occasionally identified in peripheral blood or bone marrow aspirate smears and are large lymphocytes with irregular nuclei and basophilic

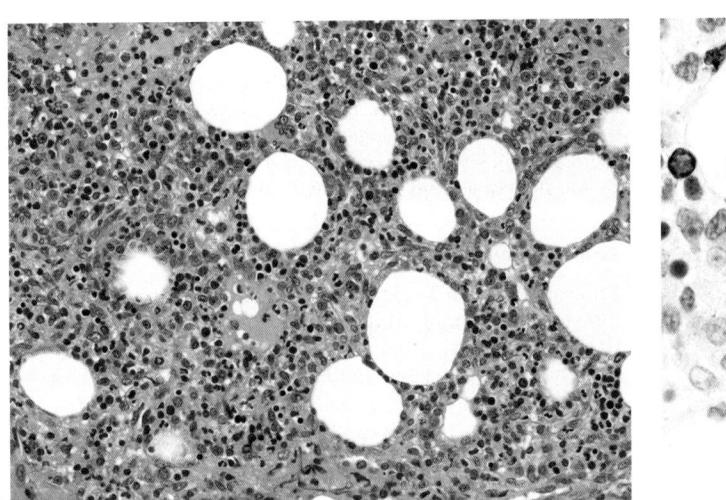
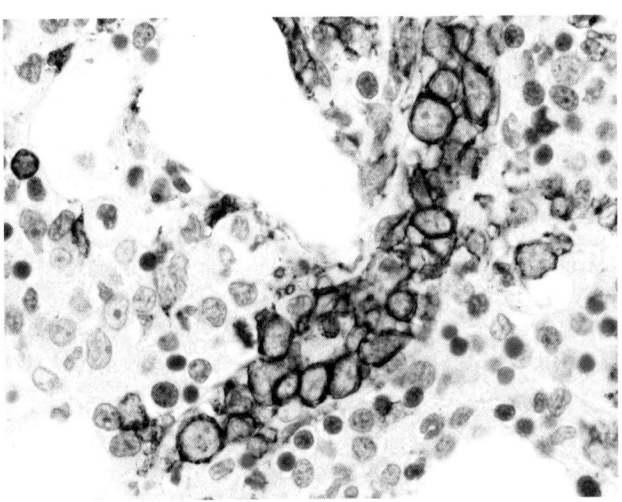

FIGURE 35.17. Intravascular large B-cell lymphoma involving the bone marrow core biopsy. A: Large lymphoma cells with dispersed chromatin are within a bone marrow sinus and are also admixed with the normal bone marrow cells; they are difficult to see on this H&E-stained section. **B:** The CD20 stain highlights large lymphoma cells within a sinus.

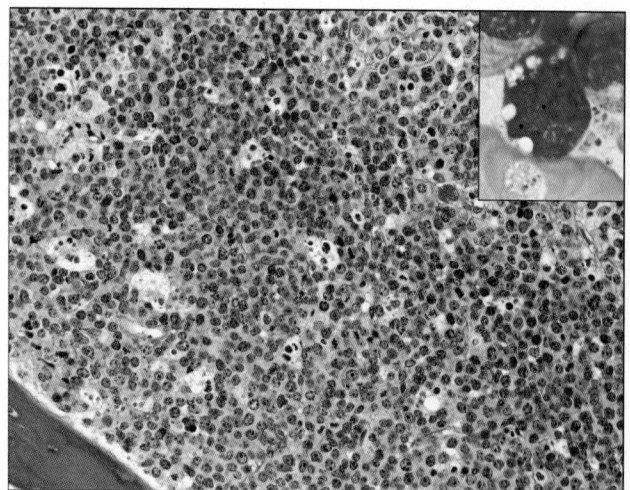

FIGURE 35.18. BL/leukemia involving the bone marrow. The lymphoma shows a diffuse growth pattern and contains histiocytes with cytoplasmic debris creating a starry-sky pattern. A lymphoma cell with intracytoplasmic vacuoles is illustrated in the **inset**.

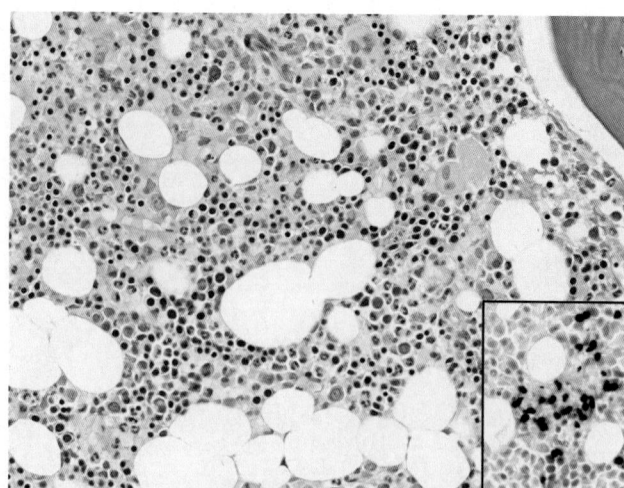

FIGURE 35.19. Extranodal NK/T-cell lymphoma involving the bone marrow core biopsy. The lymphoma cells are difficult to identify in the subtle infiltrate in the H&E-stained section. A cluster of EBER-positive lymphoma cells is identified with EBER-ISH (**inset**).

cytoplasm that is occasionally vacuolated; their recognition is helpful in alerting one to the presence of lymphoma in the bone marrow since the intrasinusoidal infiltrates may be subtle on routine H&E-stained sections.

Primary Effusion Lymphoma

Primary effusion lymphoma (PEL), also known as body cavity–based lymphoma, is a LBCL that most commonly occurs in the setting of immunodeficiency. Tumor masses rarely occur outside body cavities. Bone marrow involvement has not been reported.

Burkitt Lymphoma

BL involves the bone marrow in up to 60% of cases most often with a diffuse or interstitial pattern of infiltration (7,72,73) and may also present with a leukemic picture. BL cells are sIg light chain restricted, CD20+, CD5-, CD10+, BCL6+, BCL2-, and TdT- with a proliferative fraction approaching 100%. The cells are medium sized with reticular chromatin, multiple small nucleoli mostly located adjacent to the nuclear membrane, and moderate amounts of basophilic cytoplasm. Intracytoplasmic vacuoles, representing dissolved lipid, are typically present and are best appreciated in aspirate smears (Fig. 35.18), touch preparations, or peripheral blood. Mitoses are abundant, bone marrow necrosis is common, and the starry-sky pattern that is typically present at extramedullary sites may also be present. Distinction between BL and DLBCL may be problematic since DLBCL may have C-MYC@ gene rearrangement and display similar morphology as BL. The current WHO recommends using the term "B-cell lymphoma, unclassifiable, with features intermediate between DLBCL and BL" for lymphomas with these overlapping features (74a).

NK and T-Cell Lymphomas

Extranodal NK/T-Cell Lymphoma

Extranodal NK/T-cell lymphomas frequently arise in the nasal cavity and are called nasal NK/T-cell lymphomas (74b). NK/T-cell lymphoma, nasal type, refers to a similar lymphoma that presents outside the nasal cavity: commonly the skin, nasopharynx, or testis. They are also called extranasal NK/T-cell lymphomas. The cytology of the tumor cells varies from small to medium

or large sized, or a combination of sizes with irregular and pleomorphic nuclei. The cytoplasm is pale and moderately abundant; azurophilic granules are apparent in some cases. Epstein-Barr virus is demonstrable in essentially all cases of nasal and nasal-type NK/T-cell lymphomas (75). Both nasal and nasal-type NK/T-cell tumors are surface CD3- by flow cytometry but are CD3+ in paraffin sections because immunohistochemistry highlights a part of the T-cell receptor (TCR) complex, the CD3 epsilon polypeptide chain, that is present in their cytoplasm. Hemophagocytic syndrome manifested by fever, pancytopenia, abnormal liver function tests, and bone marrow hemophagocytosis has been described in both nasal and nasal-type NK/T-cell lymphomas (76,77).

Bone marrow involvement by nasal NK/T-cell lymphoma is uncommon (up to 8% of cases) and often subtle but is important to recognize because it is associated with early death (78). In contrast to nasal NK/T-cell lymphoma, most cases (80%) of nasal type of NK/T-cell lymphoma occurring outside the nasal cavity present with advanced stage disease involving multiple anatomic sites with 15% to 25% of cases involving the bone marrow (76–79). Typically single lymphoma cells are found scattered among the normal bone marrow elements (78). They may be difficult to identify on H&E-stained sections, but in situ hybridization (ISH) for Epstein-Barr virus–encoded RNA (EBER) and/or immunostains for CD56 can be used to demonstrate these isolated cells (Fig. 35.19). CD3 is less helpful because T-cells are common in the bone marrow; however, it may be helpful in cases where morphologically abnormal CD3+ tumor cells are highlighted. Lymphoma cells may be present in the aspirate and blood; such cases may overlap with aggressive NK-cell leukemia.

Enteropathy-Type T-Cell Lymphoma

Enteropathy-type T-cell lymphoma typically arises in the small intestine as a complication of long-standing celiac disease (80). Rare cases involving the bone marrow have been reported, but have not been described in detail (81).

Hepatosplenic T-Cell Lymphoma

Hepatosplenic T-cell lymphoma (HSTCL) is a rare form of aggressive PTCL that occurs primarily in young adult males who present with marked splenomegaly and absence of lymphadenopathy (82). Anemia and thrombocytopenia are common in HSTCL (82–85). The bone marrow and peripheral blood are

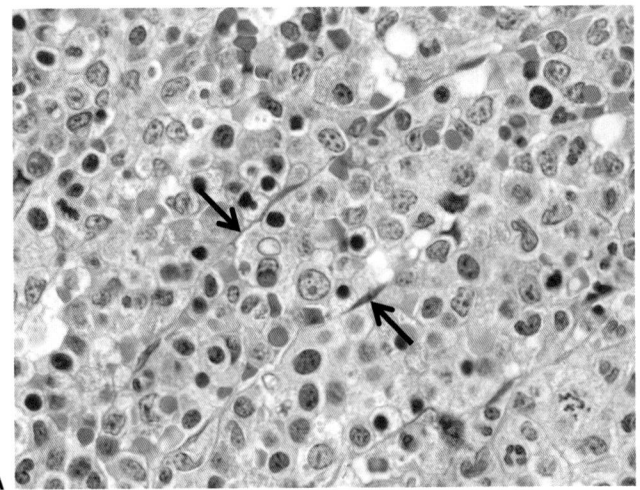

A

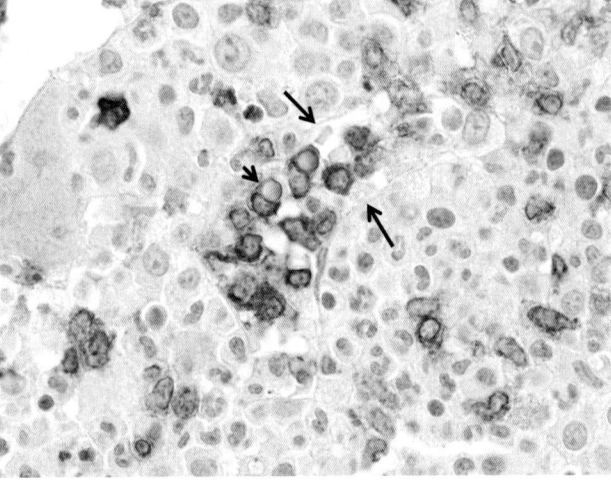

B

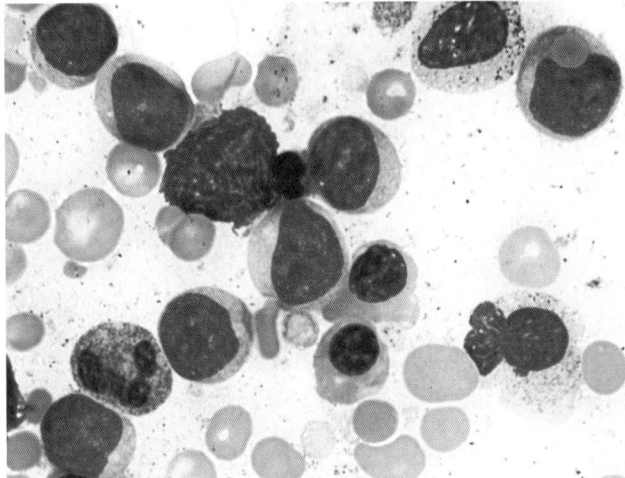

C

FIGURE 35.20. Hepatosplenic T-cell lymphoma. A: The lymphoma cells are difficult to appreciate in the H&E-stained core biopsy section but are present within sinuses (*arrows*). **B:** A CD3 stain highlights the lymphoma cells showing some within a sinus including two lymphoma cells displaying erythrophagocytosis (*arrowhead on one*). **C:** The lymphoma cells in the Wright-Giemsa–stained bone marrow aspirate have dispersed chromatin with visible nucleoli resembling blasts. A single lymphoma cell shows erythrophagocytosis.

almost always involved even though the number of circulating lymphoma cells is usually insufficient to cause an absolute lymphocytosis in the blood (85). Bone marrow core biopsy sections are often hypercellular with a subtle and predominantly intrasinusoidal infiltrate that is difficult to appreciate without immunohistochemical stains (Fig. 35.20A and B); interstitial infiltrates may also occur. The cytology of HSTCL cells is similar in the blood and aspirate smears; the cells vary from medium sized with moderately dispersed chromatin and conspicuous nucleoli resembling blasts to small lymphocytes with condensed chromatin and irregular nuclei (82,85) (Fig. 35.20C). Immunophenotypically, HSTCL cells are mature, cytotoxic T cells that are CD4−, CD8±, and TIA-1+ and express CD56, one of the natural killer cell–associated markers. Most cases are positive for the TCR $\gamma\delta$, but TCR $\alpha\beta$–positive cases also occur (83,84). Isochromosome 7q is identified in most cases (85,86).

The immunophenotype of $\gamma\delta$ HTCL closely resembles that of $\gamma\delta$ T-cell large granular lymphocytic leukemia (T-LGL). T-LGL also frequently involves the bone marrow and exhibits an intrasinusoidal growth pattern but is much more indolent that HTCL; therefore, it is important to distinguish these two disorders. Clinical features such as an elderly patient with chronic signs/symptoms including neutropenia and/or anemia are helpful to support T-LGL since HSTCL has an acute onset and more commonly affects young adult males often in their teens (83,87,88). The cells in HTCL are typically more abnormal morphologically although some overlap occurs. Another helpful morphologic feature is that intrasinusoidal T cells in HSTC are usually two or more layers thick, while T-LGL cells are usually

in single file. Isochromosome 7q has not been described in $\gamma\delta$ T-LGL; therefore, its presence strongly supports HSTCL.

Subcutaneous Panniculitis-Like T-Cell Lymphoma

Subcutaneous panniculitis-like T-cell lymphoma (SPTL) is a rare neoplasm of $\alpha\beta$ cytotoxic (CD8+) T cells that has a predilection for subcutaneous tissue (89). The tumor generally remains localized and does not involve the bone marrow. Frequently, cases are complicated by pancytopenia related to hemophagocytic syndrome; in these cases, the bone marrow exhibits features of hemophagocytic syndrome including abundant histiocytes with hemophagocytosis (90). A distinct entity, primary cutaneous $\gamma\delta$ T-cell lymphoma, also has a cytotoxic (CD8+) phenotype, rarely involves the bone marrow, and may also manifest with hemophagocytic syndrome (61).

Mycosis Fungoides/Sézary Syndrome

Mycosis fungoides (MF) is a primary cutaneous T-cell lymphoma that generally remains localized in the skin for years (91). Sézary) syndrome is a rare disorder characterized by diffuse erythroderma, lymphadenopathy, and circulating lymphoma (Sézary cells. While early reports indicated that MF involves the bone marrow in up to 25% of patients at initial diagnosis (92), a more recent study of 60 patients (53 with MF and 7 with Sézary syndrome) shows only 1/60 (<2%) had histologic evidence of bone marrow involvement at initial staging (93); borderline or atypical lesions not diagnostic of lymphoma were common (93). When the

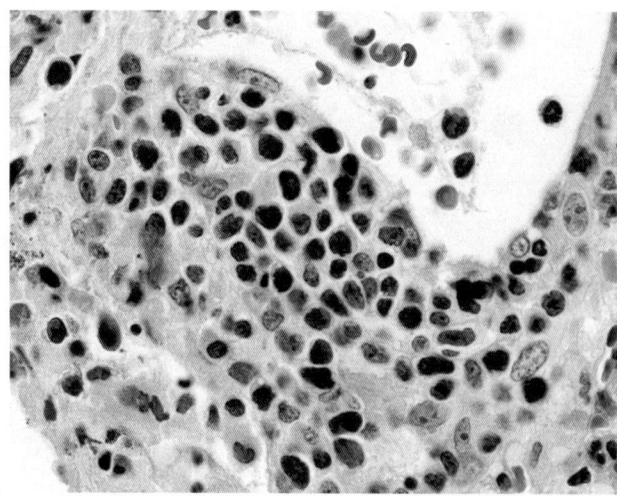

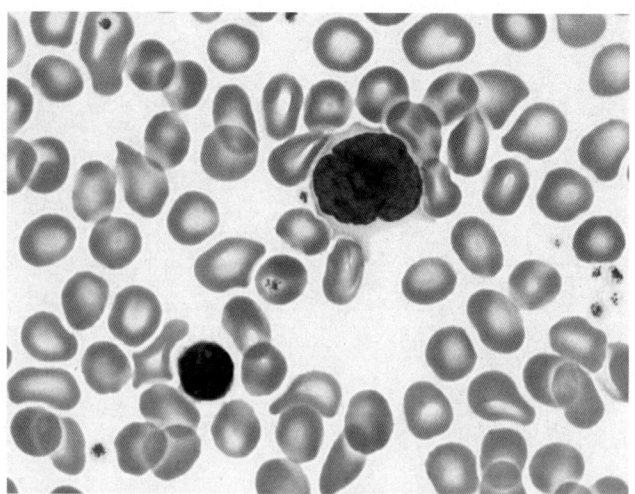

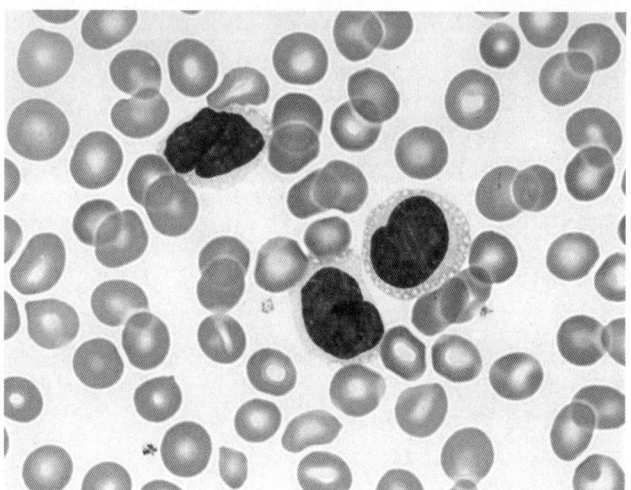

FIGURE 35.21. Mycosis fungoides/Sézary syndrome. A: The Sézary cells are variably sized with convoluted nuclei in the infiltrate in H&E-stained core biopsy. **B:** One large Sézary cell with striking nuclear convolutions is present along with a normal, small lymphocyte in this Wright-stained blood smear. **C:** The Sézary cells are more numerous with convoluted nuclei and more abundant cytoplasm containing vacuoles that form a ring around the nucleus of one cell in the Wright-stained blood smear.

bone marrow is involved, the extent of infiltration is usually minimal to mild, focal random, and/or interstitial (92,94). Paratrabecular and diffuse infiltrates are rare (95). The infiltrates contain variably sized, abnormal lymphocytes with convoluted nuclei (Fig. 35.21A). Immunohistochemical stains for T-cell–associated markers, such as CD3, and the aberrant lack of CD7 expression may aid in the recognition of the lymphoma cells. However, in some studies agreement between histologic and immunophenotypic detection of disease as well as molecular studies for monoclonal T cells remains poor (96). Eosinophilia, localized to the bone marrow or also involving the peripheral blood, is occasionally present when the bone marrow is involved.

The number of circulating lymphoma cells in Sézary syndrome is highly variable ranging from occasional cells to a frankly leukemic picture with an elevated white blood cell count. The malignant lymphocytes may be small or large with variable amounts of cytoplasm. The nuclei are characterized by striking convolutions that may create a cerebriform appearance; nucleoli are absent or inconspicuous (Fig. 35.21B and C). Occasionally Sézary cells exhibit cytoplasmic vacuoles that are periodic acid-Schiff positive encircling the nuclei.

Peripheral T-Cell Lymphoma, NOS

PTCLs in general show a high incidence (80%) of bone marrow involvement at diagnosis (97). The bone marrow lymphomatous infiltrates are diffuse in slightly more than 50% of the cases and focal, nonparatrabecular in about 40%; they are typically associated with prominent vascularity and reticulin fibrosis (98–100).

The lesions tend to be less sharply demarcated than B-cell lymphomas and intercalate into the surrounding normal marrow tissue. The lymphoma cells are variably sized, often with convoluted or irregular nuclei, usually indistinct nucleoli, and are frequently present in a polymorphous infiltrate that includes immunoblasts, neutrophils, eosinophils, and plasma cells; epithelioid histiocytes are common in the infiltrate and may be present in clusters. Occasional cases show a monomorphic proliferation of large cells with prominent nucleoli. The extent of disease within the bone marrow can be difficult to determine from H&E-stained sections although immunostains utilizing antibodies directed against T-cell antigens aid in this assessment.

Lymphoma cells are present in the aspirate smears in most cases (70%) with bone marrow involvement; they vary from occasional to numerous (>90%) and show similar morphology as those in the core biopsy section (97). Circulating lymphoma cells similar to those present in the bone marrow aspirate are present in about (30%) of cases; rarely a marked leukocytosis is present (97). An eosinophilia may be present.

Angioimmunoblastic T-Cell Lymphoma

Angioimmunoblastic T-cell lymphoma (AILT) involves the bone marrow in 50% to 90% of cases (101–103). The bone marrow infiltrates exhibit a morphologic appearance similar to the involved lymph nodes, but while the findings are helpful to establish a disseminated T-cell lymphoma, they are usually not diagnostic of AILT. Therefore, extramedullary tissue such as a lymph node biopsy is usually required for

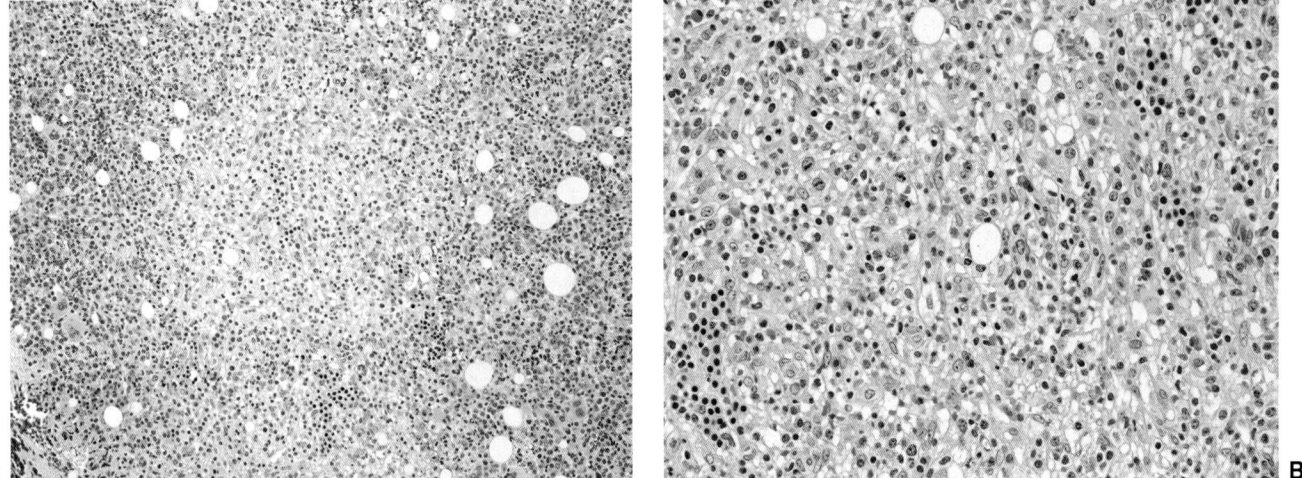

FIGURE 35.22. Angioimmunoblastic T-cell lymphoma involving the bone marrow. A: The infiltrate is pale and is less cellular than and poorly demarcated from the adjacent uninvolved marrow. Histiocytes and small lymphocytes are visible at this magnification. **B:** Scattered small lymphocytes immunoblasts, plasma cells, histiocytes, and rare eosinophils are visible among the many small blood vessels. Collections of erythroblasts are present at the periphery of the infiltrate.

definitive diagnosis. The infiltrates are typically associated with reticulin fibrosis, focal random with infiltrative margins, and are less cellular than the surrounding uninvolved marrow. Paratrabecular infiltrates are less common (103); diffuse infiltrates are exceedingly rare (98,101). The cellular composition of the infiltrate is heterogeneous and consists of lymphocytes including immunoblasts, plasma cells, a variable number of histiocytes, eosinophils, and numerous small blood vessels (Fig. 35.22A and B).

AILT lymphoma cells have a characteristic immunophenotype: They express pan T-cell markers such as CD2, CD3, and CD5; are CD4+; and express the markers typically present on follicular helper T cells (CD10, CXCL13, and PD-1). An expanded FDC meshwork positive for CD21, CD23, and CD35 as well as EBV-positive B cells are characteristic findings in lymph nodes. However, these immunophenotypic features, including CD10 positivity, may be absent in bone marrow involved by AILT. While CXCL13+ cells may be present, they often represent only a minor component of the infiltrate (103). The lymphoma cells may also be negative with one or more of the pan T-cell antigens. The plasma cells in AILT are polyclonal, and EBV is commonly absent in bone marrow involved by AILT.

The peripheral blood findings in AILT vary (98,104), but anemia is found in the majority of cases (85%), neutrophilia in up to 50% of cases, and eosinophilia in nearly 25% of cases; thrombocytopenia is occasionally present. Circulating plasma cells, lymphocytes with plasmacytoid features, and immunoblasts are present in one-third of cases. The bone marrow aspirate smears are usually cellular with increased numbers of myeloid or erythroid cells as well as plasma cells and plasmacytoid lymphocytes. Small mature lymphocytes are usually decreased, while eosinophils are occasionally increased.

Anaplastic Large Cell Lymphoma

Anaplastic large cell lymphoma (ALCL) involves the bone marrow in up to 40% of cases (105,106). The infiltrates are focal random, paratrabecular, and diffuse or occur as small clusters of cells or isolated single cells. Isolated lymphoma cells are often difficult to identify among the normal immature bone marrow cells when only routine H&E-stained sections are examined, but they can be highlighted by immunostains utilizing antibodies to Alk-1, CD30, or EMA (Fig. 35.23A–C). It is important to identify ALCL in the bone marrow, even when it is subtle,

because bone marrow involvement by ALCL is associated with lower overall survival. The lymphoma cells are large but variably sized (ranging from the size of a promyelocyte to a megakaryocyte) and have irregular nuclei with dispersed chromatin, multiple prominent nucleoli, and abundant, basophilic, occasionally vacuolated cytoplasm. In occasional cases, tumor cells can be found in the peripheral blood and bone marrow aspirate smears (Fig. 35.23D); rarely the peripheral blood exhibits numerous circulating lymphoma cells, and this is associated with a poor prognosis (107–109). Circulating or aspirated lymphoma cells have similar morphology to the lymphoma cells in the core biopsy section (108).

Hodgkin Lymphoma

The overall incidence of HL involving the bone marrow at diagnosis ranges from 5% to 15% (7,9,14) with the frequency varying according to the subtype of HL. Mixed cellularity HL involves the bone marrow in approximately 20% of cases at diagnosis (110). Nodular sclerosis HL involves the bone marrow at diagnosis in <10% of cases. Lymphocyte-predominant HL almost never involves the bone marrow at diagnosis (9,111,112). Earlier studies reported that lymphocyte-depleted HL (LDHL) showed the highest incidence of bone marrow involvement, and this has been confirmed in a more recent study (113). However, it is now recognized that many of the early reports of LDHL involving the bone marrow were examples of NHL, especially ALCL (110).

Patients who are clinical stage III or IV are more likely to have bone marrow involvement by HL and exhibit organomegaly including lymphadenopathy with constitutional symptoms such as weight loss and fever. Cytopenias, including thrombocytopenia and leukopenia, may be a clue to bone marrow involvement; anemia is common but less specific for bone marrow involvement (114). The value of routine bone marrow staging in all HL cases has been questioned since the incidence of bone marrow involvement is low in those who are clinically staged as IA or IIA, and the bone marrow findings often do not alter treatment or prognosis (115,116). However, bone marrow biopsy remains a standard procedure in evaluation of patients with newly diagnosed HL in many institutions (113,117).

In rare cases, the bone marrow is the primary diagnostic tissue for classical HL; this occurs most often in the setting of acquired immunodeficiency disease syndrome (AIDS)

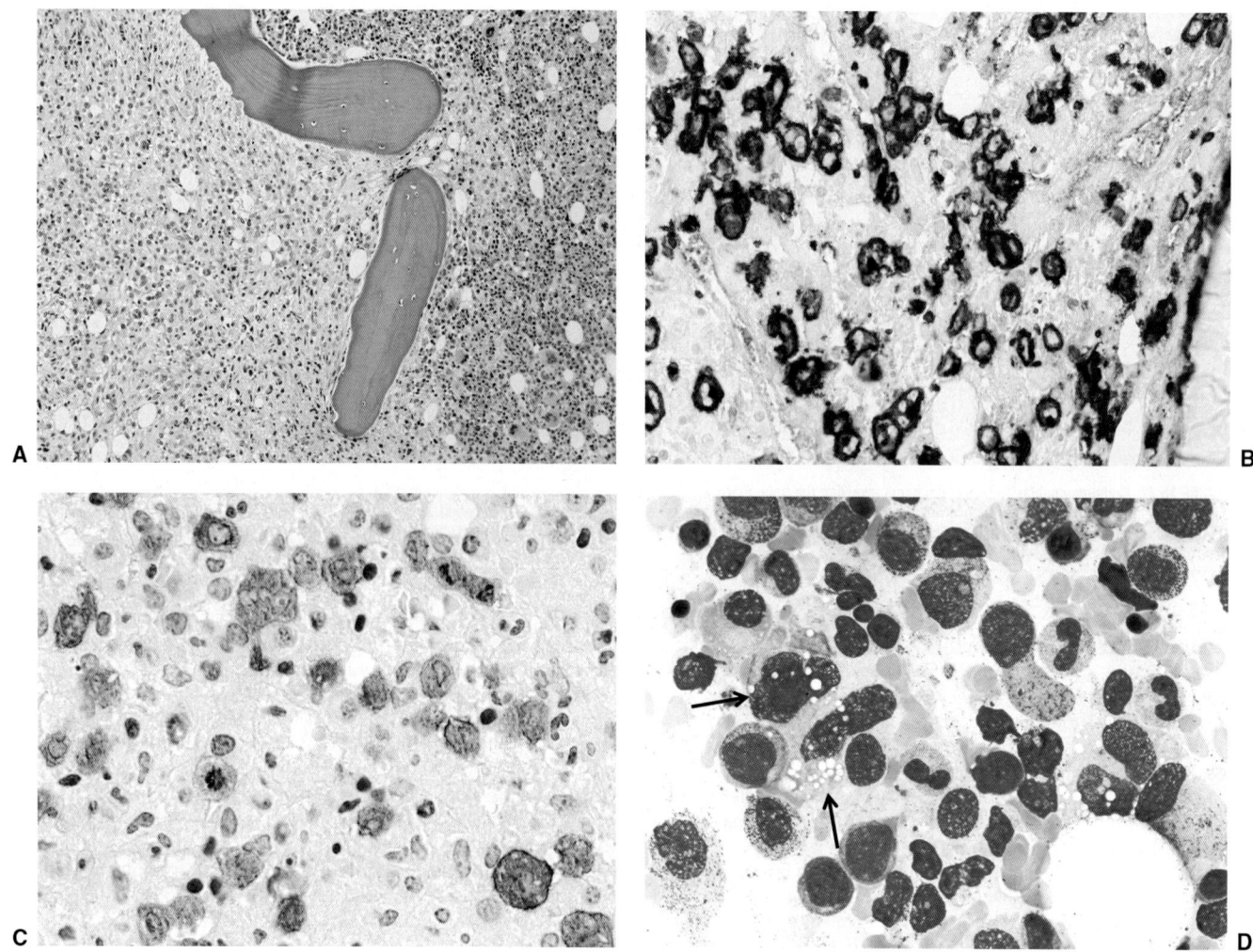

FIGURE 35.23. Anaplastic large cell lymphoma. A: Lymphoma replaces most of the H&E-stained core biopsy section to the left, while the bone marrow to the right is uninvolved. **B:** The lymphoma cells are uniformly and brightly CD30⁺. **C:** The ALK-1 stain highlights lymphoma cells located interstitially in a less involved area of the bone marrow and shows cytoplasmic staining. **D:** Two large lymphoma cells are present in the bone marrow aspirate smear (*highlighted with arrows*).

(118–120). Human immunodeficiency virus–positive cases with HL in the bone marrow often present with peripheral blood cytopenias. The HL is isolated to the bone marrow at diagnosis in approximately 15% of cases (120); this group of patients usually lacks lymphadenopathy and usually does not develop HL at extramedullary sites during the course of the disease.

The core biopsy is the specimen of choice for microscopic diagnosis or staging of HL since the aspirate is insensitive for detection of HL (121). Reed-Sternberg cells are usually absent in the aspirate smears although they can be identified in rare cases with extensive bone marrow involvement. CHL in the bone marrow is characterized by discrete, space-occupying lesions that are usually clearly demarcated from the normal bone marrow tissue. Focal involvement is present in about 30% of the cases; the infiltrates may be single or multiple, and random or paratrabecular. Diffuse bone marrow involvement is present in about 70% of the cases (7) (Fig. 35.24). The infiltrates are polymorphous and frequently contain a prominent component of small lymphocytes, histiocytes, plasma cells, and eosinophils. Reed-Sternberg cells or variants are almost always present although, in some cases, multiple sections must be examined in order to find diagnostic neoplastic cells. Fibrosis is almost always present in the infiltrate and may be prominent especially in diffuse lesions. Necrosis may be present and is more common in treated patients.

Immunohistochemical stains aid considerably in the diagnosis of CHL since the Reed-Sternberg cells in the bone marrow express the same immunophenotype as in the extramedullary tissue (CD45⁻, CD30⁺, CD15⁺, CD20±, CD3⁻). However, the criteria for diagnosis of CHL in the bone marrow vary depending on whether or not the bone marrow is the initial diagnostic site (122,123) as recommended by the committee on Histologic Criteria Contributing to Staging of Hodgkin Disease at the Ann Arbor Symposium in 1971 (122,123). The histopathologic criteria are as follows:

1. HL may be diagnosed in the bone marrow when Reed-Sternberg cells are found in a cellular environment characteristic of HL.
2. When typical Reed-Sternberg cells are identified at another anatomic site, mononuclear Reed-Sternberg variants in an environment characteristic of HL are sufficient for diagnosis even if typical Reed-Sternberg cells are not present in the bone marrow. The presence of atypical cells that are not classic Reed-Sternberg cells or their mononuclear variants in patients with histologically proven HL elsewhere is suspicious for bone marrow involvement.
3. Foci of fibrosis without Reed-Sternberg cells or mononuclear variants are suspicious for HL in cases with HL diagnosed at another site.

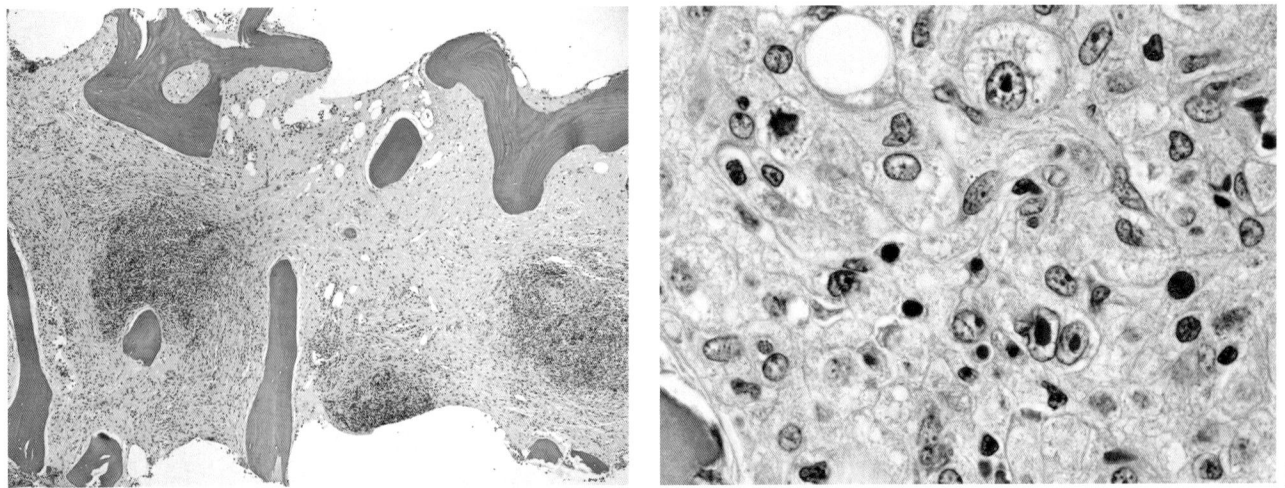

FIGURE 35.24. Classical HL involving the bone marrow core biopsy. **A:** The entire bone marrow parenchyma is replaced by the diffuse infiltrate of classical HL associated with extensive fibrosis. **B:** High power view of Reed-Sternberg cells in bone marrow.

Infiltrates of LPHL involving the bone marrow may be focal random, paratrabecular, or diffuse and may involve from 10% to 100% of the bone marrow medullary space. The L&H cells display a similar phenotype as those in the lymph node (CD20+, CD3-, CD15-, CD30-), are rare in the bone marrow, and may be associated with many CD3+ T cells as well as less numerous small B cells and histiocytes (124) (Fig. 35.25).

Subclassification of HL is not recommended in the bone marrow. The small sample size and variability of histopathology between lymph node and bone marrow make subclassification

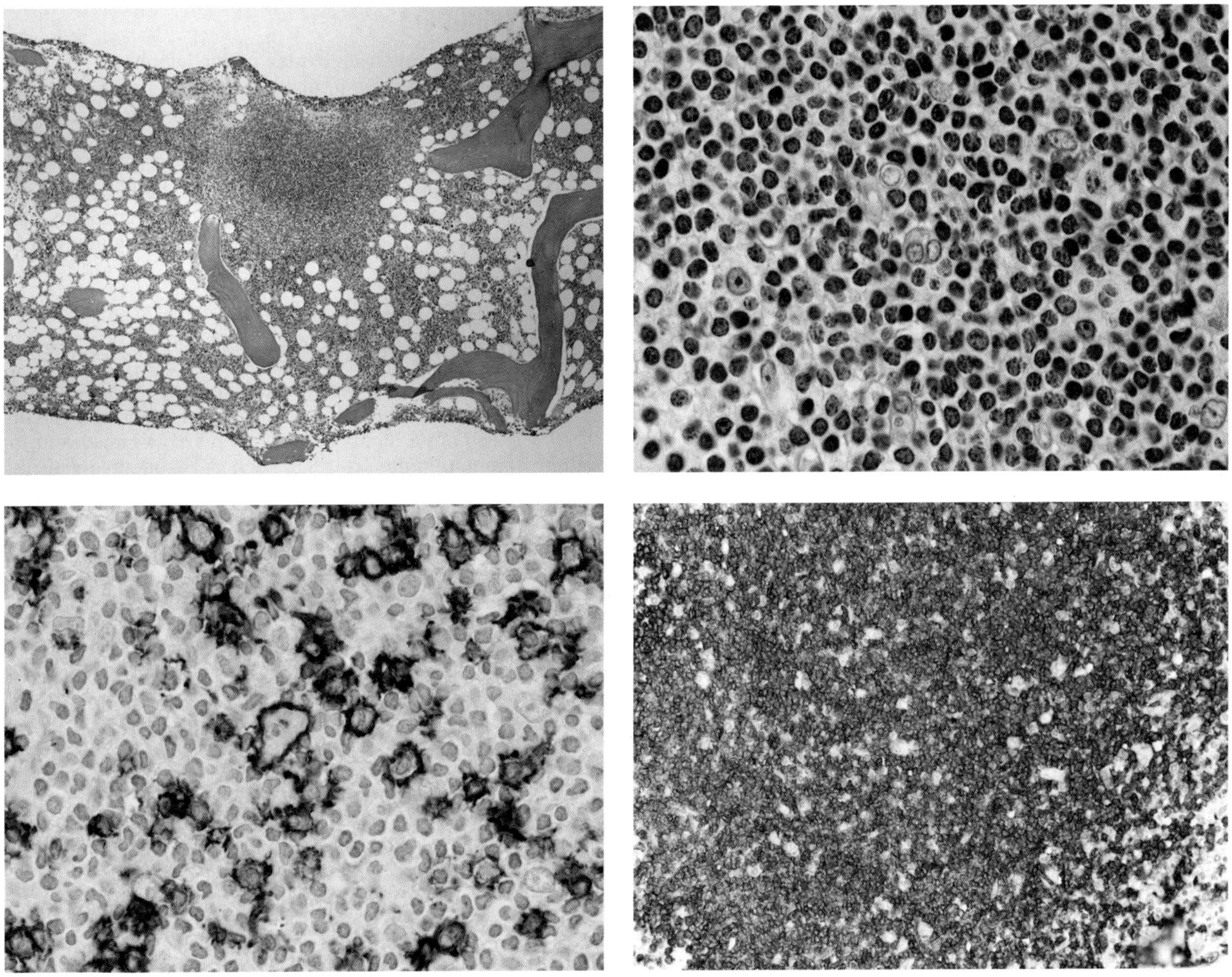

FIGURE 35.25. Lymphocyte-predominant HL in the bone marrow core biopsy. **A:** A focal random lymphoid aggregate is present in the H&E-stained bone marrow core biopsy. **B:** The infiltrate is composed of mostly small lymphocytes as well as rare large lymphocytes showing visible nucleoli. **C,D:** A large, CD20+ lymphoma cell is demonstrated. The majority of the small lymphocytes were CD3+.

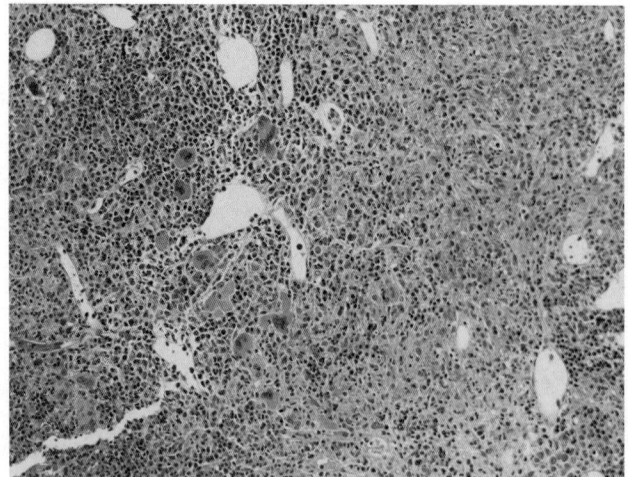
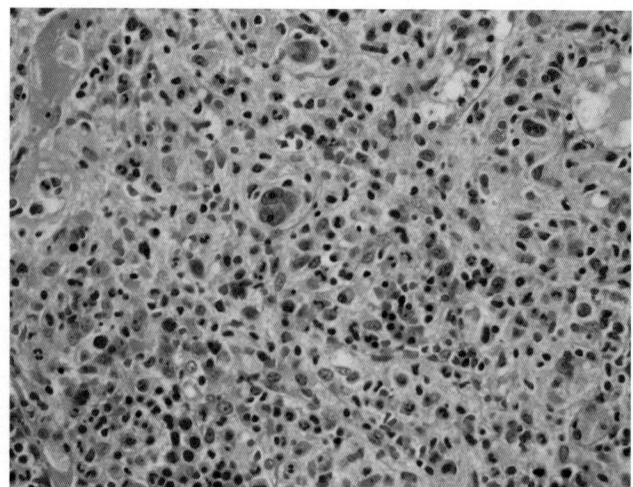

FIGURE 35.26. Classical HL (initially misdiagnosed as primary myelofibrosis) involving the core biopsy. A: The lymphoma replaces almost one-half of the core biopsy section (**right side**) that is pale staining due to the many histiocytes in the infiltrate. The residual bone marrow (**left side**) is hypercellular with increased numbers of megakaryocytes. This case was misdiagnosed as a myeloproliferative neoplasm. **B:** The high power image shows a classic binucleated Reed-Sternberg (RS) cell with distinct visible nuclei in a heterogeneous cellular background that includes histiocytes, eosinophils, neutrophils, plasma cells, and small lymphocytes. Some of these RS cells were initially interpreted as abnormal megakaryocytes.

unreliable (122). Granulomas are occasionally present in one or more organs, including the bone marrow, in those with an established diagnosis of HL; granulomas are not sufficient to diagnose HL. Areas of the bone marrow that are not involved by HL frequently show other nonspecific changes including granulocytic hyperplasia, eosinophilia, plasmacytosis, and increased number of megakaryocytes (110); these changes can be present even if the bone marrow is not involved by HL (Fig. 35.26).

Some NHLs such as ALCL and PTCL with a polymorphous infiltrate may mimic CHL in the bone marrow. In addition, CHL infiltrates with a granulomatous appearance may be mistaken for a benign infiltrative process (Fig. 35.27A and B). CHL must also be differentiated from reactive polymorphous lymphohistiocytic lesions that are occasionally encountered in the bone marrow (125,126). LPHL should be separated from T-cell/histiocyte-rich large B-cell lymphoma. A panel of antibodies applied to bone marrow biopsy sections will usually clarify the diagnosis. In equivocal cases, biopsy of lymph node or other tissue may be necessary.

Reactive Lymphoid Lesions and Their Distinction from Lymphoma

Several bone marrow lesions may mimic lymphoma histologically and be problematic to distinguish from lymphoma. This section will focus on reactive lymphoid lesions that can be difficult to separate from lymphoma including benign lymphoid aggregates, reactive polymorphous lymphohistiocytic lesions, systemic polyclonal immunoblastic proliferations (SPIPs), and lymphoid proliferations associated with systemic mastocytosis. Hematogones are discussed in Chapter 19 on lymphoblastic leukemia/lymphoma.

Reactive Lymphoid Lesions

Benign lymphoid aggregates are frequently encountered in bone marrow core biopsies especially in older individuals. They are also often identified in bone marrow biopsies in the setting of autoimmune disorders such as rheumatoid arthritis,

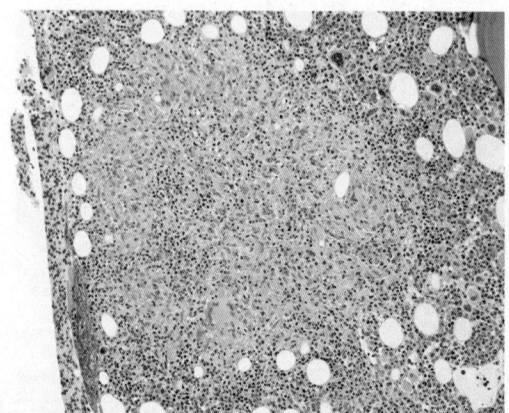
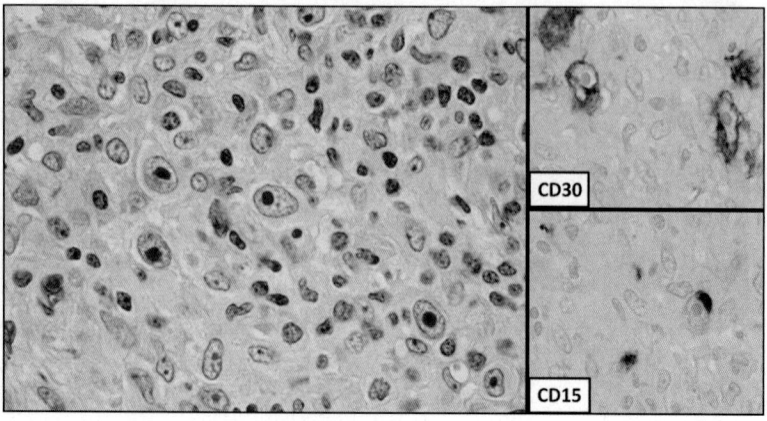

FIGURE 35.27. Classical HL with granulomatous appearance. A: One noncaseating granuloma with several mononuclear Reed-Sternberg cells close to its center is present in this H&E-stained core biopsy section. **B:** The Reed-Sternberg cells have distinct, visible nucleoli and are CD15+ and CD30+ (**insets**).

systemic lupus erythematosus, autoimmune hemolytic anemia, and idiopathic thrombocytopenia purpura (7,127). Bone marrows involved by chronic myeloproliferative neoplasms or myelodysplastic syndromes also commonly exhibit lymphoid aggregates (127,128).

Benign lymphoid aggregates have several characteristic morphologic features. They are usually small and single or only a few are present in the biopsy. They are generally distributed randomly away from the bony trabeculae, typically round and well circumscribed, and are composed of mostly small mature-appearing lymphocytes with admixed histiocytes and plasma cells (Fig. 35.28A–C). Often the aggregate is closely associated with a venous sinus or arteriole. Reactive germinal centers may be present and are more common in individuals with autoimmune disorders (Fig. 35.29). Lymphoid aggregates associated with lipogranulomas are benign (Fig. 35.30).

Reactive polymorphous lymphohistiocytic lesions are rare variants of nonneoplastic lymphoid aggregates that occur most frequently in patients with immune deficiency disorders including AIDS (125,126) and in patients with connective tissue disorders such as rheumatoid arthritis. These infiltrates are variably sized, but are often larger than typical benign lymphoid aggregates, may be multiple, and have irregular borders. The infiltrates may touch bone but are not distinctly paratrabecular. They are composed of heterogeneous cellular infiltrates including small, mature-appearing lymphocytes, large transformed lymphocytes with visible nucleoli, admixed plasma cells, eosinophils, mast cells, and epithelioid histiocytes (Fig. 35.31A–C). Poorly formed granulomas may be present in these lesions.

Because of their morphologic similarity to some types of lymphoma, reactive lymphoid lesions in the bone marrow may be difficult to distinguish from lymphoma (Table 35.2). Even when typical features of benign lymphoid aggregates such as

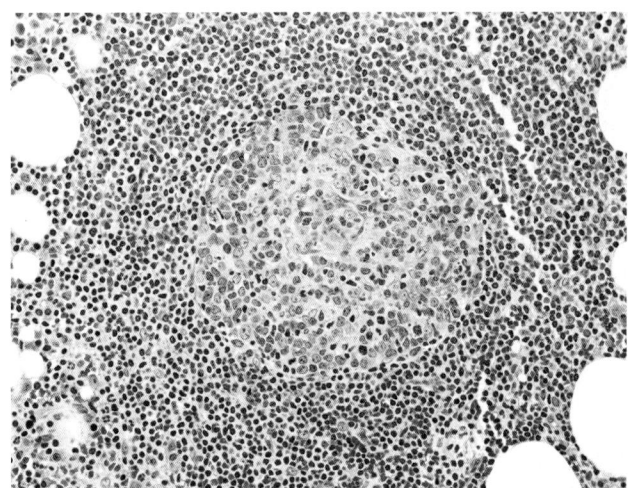

FIGURE 35.29. Reactive germinal center. The germinal center is small with an attenuated mantle zone and is composed of centroblasts, centrocytes, as well as histiocytes including tingible body macrophages.

small size, well-defined borders, and random distribution are present, they may be morphologically indistinguishable from small focal infiltrates of low-grade lymphoma. It becomes even more difficult when benign lymphoid aggregates are large or multiple. Attention to the location of the infiltrate is an important key to their evaluation as distinctly paratrabecular infiltrates that grow along the surface of the bone and conform to bony contours are malignant in the vast majority of cases. The presence of distinct intrasinusoidal infiltrates is also an indication of a neoplastic process, although it should be noted

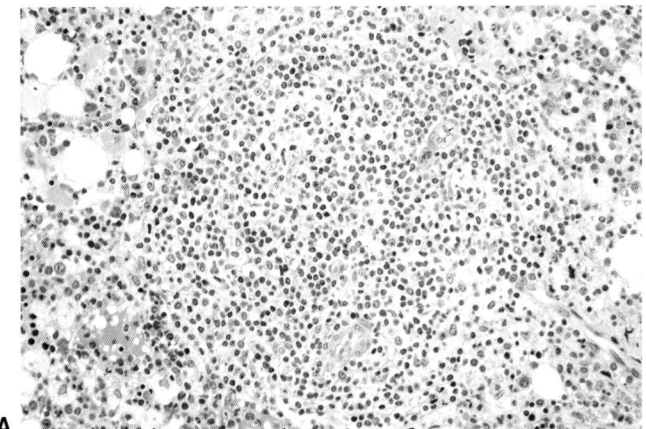
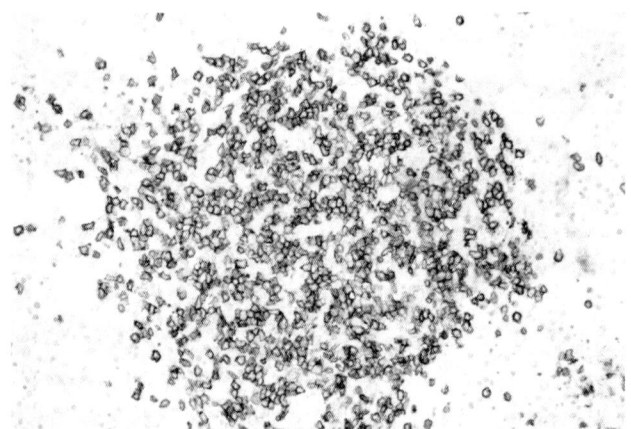
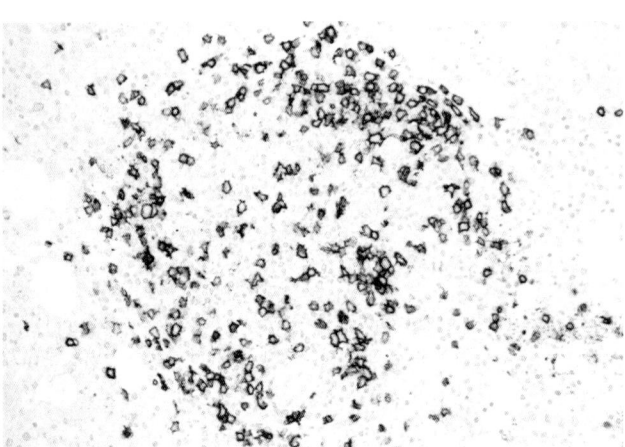

FIGURE 35.28. Benign lymphoid aggregate. A: One well-circumscribed, focal random lymphoid aggregate with a blood vessel and composed of small lymphocytes with condensed chromatin and round nuclei is illustrated in this H&E-stained core biopsy section. **B:** The CD3 immuno stain shows that the majority of the lymphocytes are positive. **C:** The CD20 immuno stain shows only occasional positive B cells.

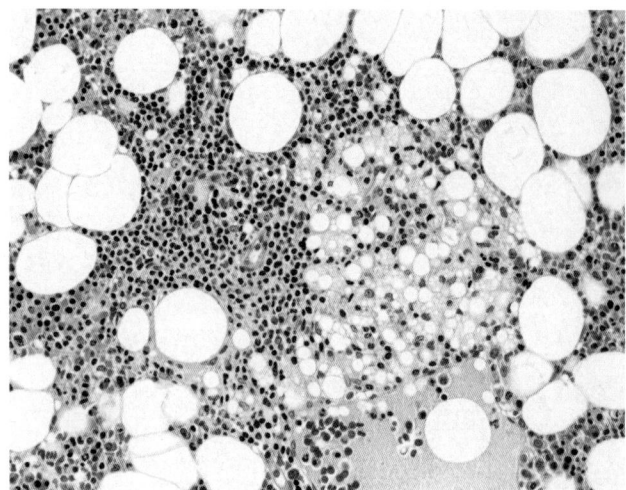

FIGURE 35.30. Benign lymphoid aggregate associated with a lipogranuloma. Histiocytes associated with microvesicular fat, rare plasma cells, and small lymphocytes that form a discrete collection associated with a blood vessel are illustrated in this H&E-stained core biopsy section.

that this pattern has also been reported in persistent polyclonal B lymphocytosis, an entity regarded as benign. The presence of germinal centers usually indicates that the lymphoid aggregate is benign. However, reactive germinal centers may also be present in bone marrow involved by lymphoma, particularly marginal zone lymphoma, and rarely in MCL. In addition, FL with follicle formation may invade the bone marrow and must be distinguished from reactive germinal centers.

Reactive polymorphous lymphohistiocytic lesions can be particularly problematic in distinguishing from lymphoma since they may be multiple and large and have poorly defined margins. Since their cell composition is usually polymorphous, distinction from peripheral T-cell lymphoma or HL may be especially difficult. Knowledge of the clinical history of these patients is of major importance in evaluating these lesions, and diagnoses of lymphoma in these patients should be approached with caution unless there is clear morphologic evidence for lymphoma or the diagnosis is confirmed by ancillary testing or biopsy of another site.

Since some morphologic features of benign infiltrates overlap with lymphoma (Table 35.3), a panel of immunohistochemical stains performed on core biopsy or particle section can be used to assist in the distinction between benign and malignant lymphoid infiltrates. Benign lymphoid aggregates and reactive polymorphous lymphohistiocytic proliferations usually have a mixture of B cells and T cells; frequently T cells predominate (Figs. 35.28 and 35.31). Lymphoid infiltrates composed of primarily B cells, especially if multiple, are often neoplastic (Fig. 35.32). However, these studies must be interpreted cautiously since a wide variety of reaction patterns occur with both benign lymphoid aggregates and lymphoma. For instance, B-cell lymphomas such as FL may be accompanied by large numbers of reactive T lymphocytes. Therefore, a mixture of B and T cells or a predominance of T cells does not rule out a B-cell lymphoma (129).

Demonstrating an aberrant B-cell or T-cell immunophenotype within a lymphoid infiltrate strongly supports a lymphoma.

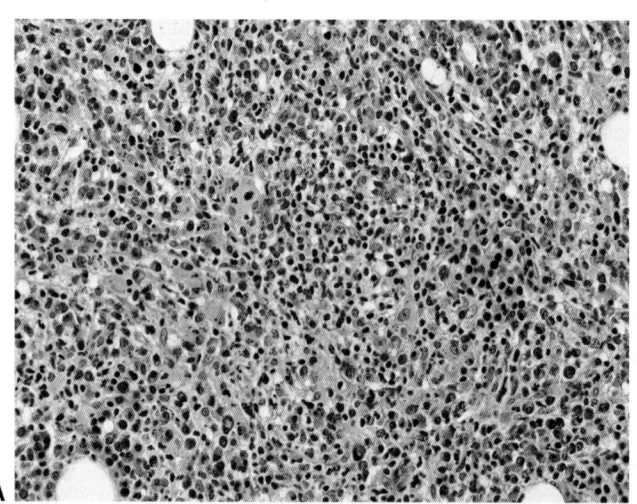

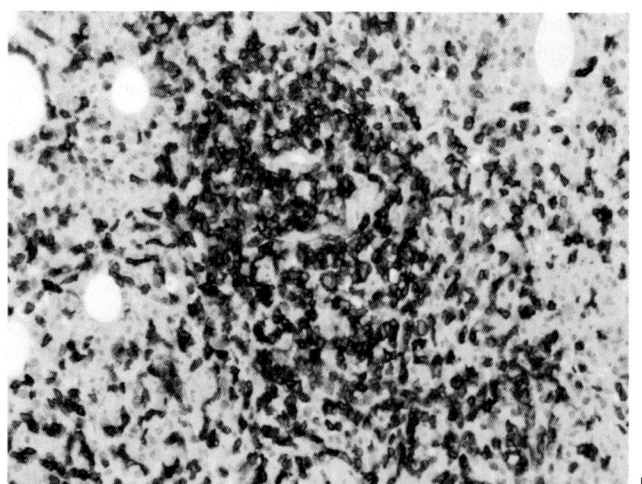

FIGURE 35.31. Reactive polymorphous lymphohistiocytic lesion in the bone marrow core biopsy. A: The infiltrate is large and poorly circumscribed with irregular borders that blend with the adjacent bone marrow and contains histiocytes (including some with pigment), plasma cells, eosinophils, and variably sized lymphocytes. **B:** The CD3 immuno stain shows many T cells that vary from small to large. **C:** The CD20 immuno stain shows only rare B cells.

Table 35.2	FEATURES USEFUL IN DISTINGUISHING BENIGN LYMPHOID AGGREGATES FROM NHL IN BONE MARROW BIOPSIES

Benign	Malignant
Few in number	Variable number, may be numerous
Random distribution	Frequently paratrabecular
Usually round, well circumscribed	Often irregularly shaped with infiltration into adjacent marrow
Polymorphous cellular composition	Usually homogeneous cellular composition (except some PTCLs); atypical cytologic features may be present.
Intrasinusoidal infiltrates absent (exception is polyclonal B-cell lymphocytosis)	Intrasinusoidal infiltration may be present.
Vascularity is often prominent.	Vascularity is usually not prominent (except in PTCLs).
Benign germinal centers are occasionally present.	Benign germinal centers are not present (except in splenic marginal zone and rarely MCL).
Absence of morphologic atypia	Atypical morphology (except in small, mature B-cell lymphoma)
Immunostains usually show mixture of B and T cells or T cells predominate.	Immunostains showing predominance of B cells, aberrant phenotype, or monoclonal plasma cells suggest B-cell lymphoma. An aberrant T-cell phenotype suggests T-cell lymphoma.
No monotypic B-cell population or abnormal B- or T-cell phenotype by flow cytometry	Immunoglobulin light chain restriction or T-cell abnormalities by flow cytometry; however, neoplastic cells may not be aspirated.
No monoclonal B- or T-cell receptor gene rearrangement by molecular analysis	Monoclonal B- or T-cell receptor gene rearrangement by molecular analysis (sensitivity depends on specimens and methods used; see text)

Modified from Jaffe ES, Harris NL, Vardiman JW, et al., eds. *Hematopathology.* Philadelphia: Elsevier, 2011:889, with permission.

For example, if a B-cell–rich lymphoid aggregate is positive with CD5, a T-cell–associated antigen, this supports a B-cell malignancy (130). Similarly, a T-cell–rich lymphoid aggregate that is positive with all but one of the pan T-cell antigens (CD2, CD3, CD5, CD7) and shows predominance of either CD4 or CD8 is highly suggestive of a T-cell malignancy. Immunohistochemical or ISH studies for kappa and lambda immunoglobulin (Ig) light chains are also valuable in lesions containing significant numbers of plasma cells since demonstration of Ig light chain restriction supports a B-cell malignancy.

Special considerations should also be given to patients with lymphoma who have been treated with anti-CD20 monoclonal antibody (rituximab) and who continue to exhibit lymphoid infiltrates in the bone marrow. In some of these cases, the lesions represent residual lymphoma (131). However, in some cases, lymphoma cells are no longer present, and the lymphoid infiltrates are composed entirely of CD3+ T cells, histiocytes, and stromal cells localized to the same area as the initial lymphoma (Fig. 35.33A–C). The lymphoma has been eliminated by the anti-CD20 therapy. These aggregates may mimic residual lymphoma since they can be large, multiple, or even paratrabecular in location. Even when residual B-cell lymphoma remains in the bone marrow of patients treated with anti-CD20 therapy, the lymphoma cells may be CD20-. For these reasons, immunostains and/or flow cytometric immunophenotyping, using B-cell antigens other than CD20, such as CD79a or PAX5, is often necessary to differentiate these T-cell aggregates from residual B-cell lymphoma.

Table 35.3	EVALUATING BONE MARROW FOR LYMPHOMA: PEARLS AND PITFALLS

Pearls	Pitfalls
Benign lymphoid aggregates are usually small, round, well circumscribed.	Small, focal, random, well-circumscribed lymphoid aggregates may represent lymphoma.
Benign lymphoid aggregates are usually morphologically heterogeneous.	Lymphoma, particularly T-cell types and HL, are often morphologically heterogeneous and may be confused with benign lymphoid aggregates especially reactive polymorphous lymphohistiocytic proliferation.
Intravascular localization of lymphoid infiltrates usually indicates a malignant proliferation.	Intrasinusoidal infiltrates have been reported in polyclonal B-cell lymphocytosis.
Reactive germinal centers usually indicate benign lymphoid infiltrates and are most commonly seen in patients with autoimmune disorders.	SMZL involving the bone marrow is associated with germinal centers in about 30% of cases. Germinal centers are rarely seen in MCL involving the bone marrow.
Granulomas and lymphoid aggregates associated with lipogranulomas are benign.	Noninfectious granulomas can accompany many lymphomas including indolent B-cell lymphomas, T-cell lymphomas, and HL.
Paratrabecular lymphoid infiltrates almost always indicate lymphoma.	Lymphoid infiltrates including those that are paratrabecular can persist after rituximab therapy for B-cell lymphoma. Some of these are benign (T-cell rich; absent B cells).
Immunostains help to identify ALCL and extranodal NK/T-cell lymphoma, which can infiltrate the bone marrow as single cells.	The bone marrow may be the initial diagnostic site so that history of a previous diagnosis to aid in selection of immunostains may not be available.
Hepatosplenic T-cell lymphoma most commonly exhibits $\gamma\delta$ immunophenotype and infiltrate the bone marrow in an intrasinusoidal pattern.	Large granular lymphocytic leukemia of $\gamma\delta$ type T-cell type can also infiltrate the bone marrow in an intrasinusoidal pattern and may be confused with hepatosplenic T-cell lymphoma.
Monoclonal B cells identified by ancillary techniques usually support bone marrow involvement by a B-cell neoplasm.	Low-level monotypic B-cell populations may be identified by flow cytometry in "healthy" individuals with no evidence for lymphoma (monoclonal B lymphocytosis).

CLL/SLL, chronic lymphocytic leukemia/small lymphocytic lymphoma; SMZL, splenic marginal zone lymphoma; ALCL, anaplastic large cell lymphoma.
Modified from Jaffe ES, Harris NL, Vardiman JW, et al., eds. *Hematopathology.* Philadelphia: Elsevier, 2011:889, with permission.

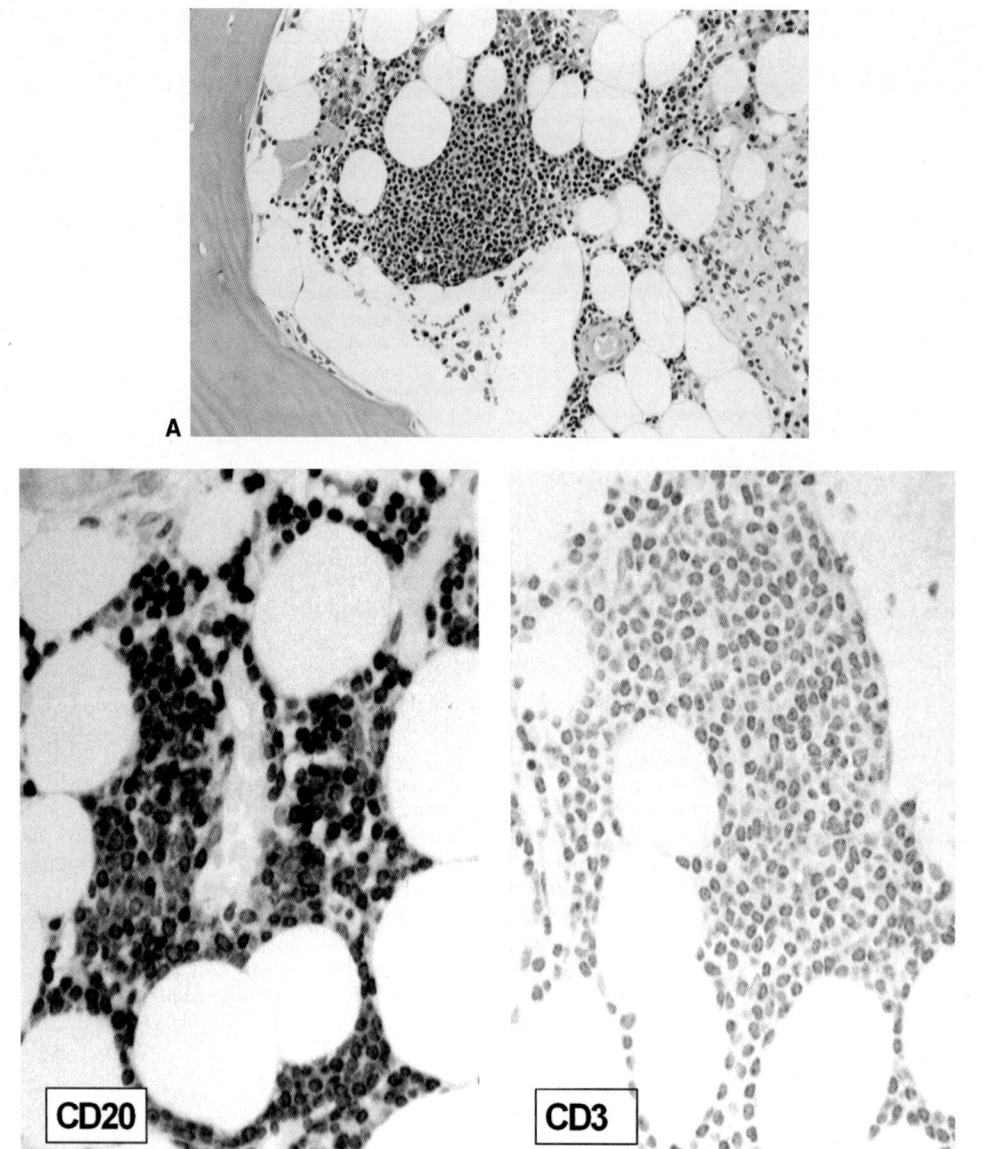

FIGURE 35.32. Malignant lymphoid aggregate (SLL). A: This focal random lymphoid aggregate displays infiltrative borders with lymphocytes migrating between the fat cells. **B,C:** The CD20 immuno stain shows that virtually all the lymphocytes are B cells, and the CD3 immuno stain shows very rare T cells.

Immunophenotyping by flow cytometry performed on a fresh bone marrow aspirate or peripheral blood is helpful in distinguishing between reactive and malignant lymphoid infiltrates (132–135). Excellent correlation exists between morphology and immunophenotype. However, discrepancy between the core biopsy and the aspirate does occur since small, focal lesions may be missed during aspiration of the bone marrow or bone marrow fibrosis may prevent aspiration of the lymphoma cells. False-negative results often occur, for example, in staging marrows of patients with FL (136). Thus, demonstration of polyclonal B cells by IF does not ensure that the bone marrow is negative for lymphoma.

It is also important to recognize that the presence of monotypic B cells by flow cytometry is not diagnostic of lymphoma. Monotypic B cells may be detected without morphologic evidence of lymphoma in the bone marrow due to sampling. In addition, low levels of monotypic B cells with CLL and non-CLL phenotype can be identified in otherwise healthy, most

frequently older individuals (137,138). These cases have been termed monoclonal B lymphocytosis (139). Therefore, it is important to correlate the immunophenotypic results with the immunophenotype of any previously diagnosed lymphoma and with other clinical and pathologic findings.

Molecular analysis, most commonly using polymerase chain reaction (PCR) for immunoglobulin heavy chain (IgH) and TCR gene rearrangements, also provides an important adjunctive role in evaluating bone marrow for lymphoma and can be performed on fresh bone marrow aspirate, peripheral blood, or paraffin-embedded tissues (140,141). The sensitivity of PCR for detection of bone marrow lymphoma depends on the case selection, types of specimen, and molecular techniques utilized. However, results obtained from gene rearrangement studies of bone marrow lymphoid aggregates correlate with the morphologic interpretations in the majority of cases (142,143). As with flow cytometric immunophenotyping, detection of monoclonality is not synonymous with

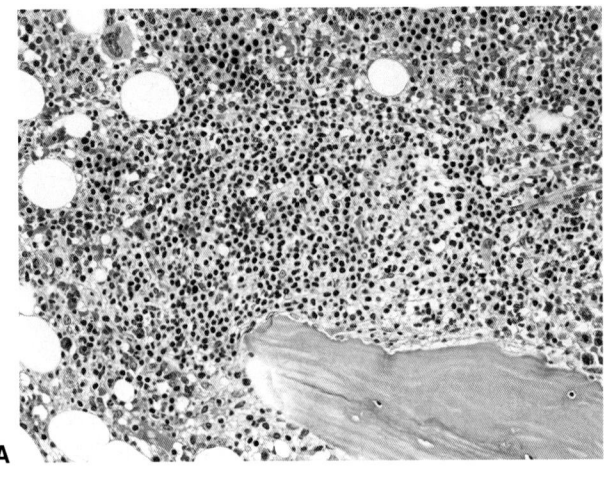

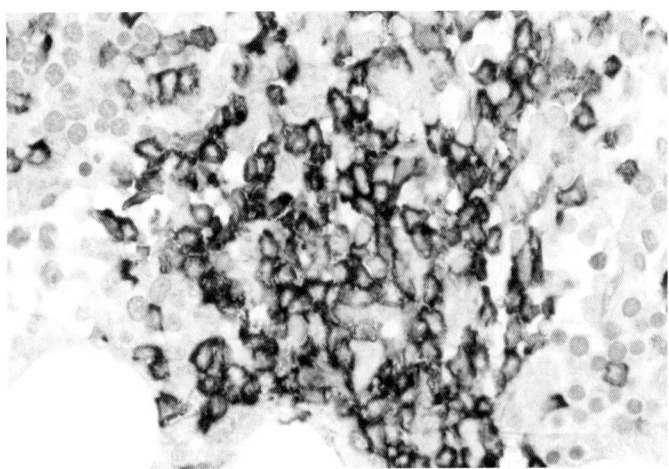

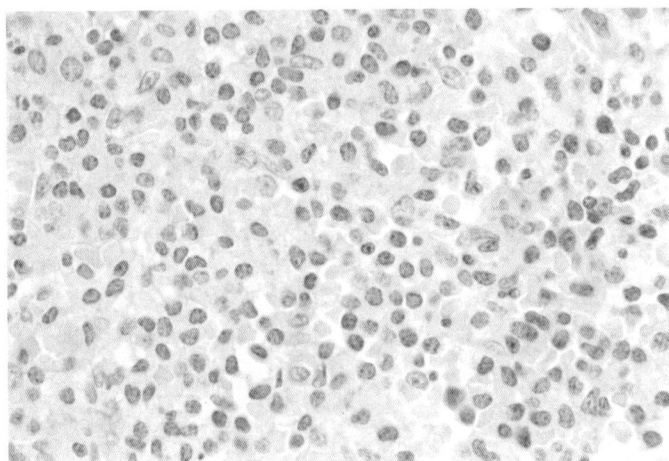

FIGURE 35.33. Benign lymphoid aggregate post–rituximab therapy. A: This paratrabecular lymphoid aggregate in the bone marrow following therapy with rituximab for FL contains mostly small lymphocytes. **B:** A CD3 immuno stain shows that virtually all the lymphocytes are T cells. **C:** The PAX5 immuno stain shows that B cells are virtually absent, supporting that the lymphoid aggregate does not represent residual lymphoma.

malignancy. Comparison of PCR products obtained from the bone marrow and the primary lymphoma, if available, can be done to avoid detection of biologically unrelated monoclonal populations (144).

Systemic Polyclonal Immunoblastic Proliferations

Patients with SPIPs present with an acute illness, constitutional symptoms, and frequently organomegaly including lymphadenopathy. Anemia and thrombocytopenia are usually present. The lymphocyte count is variable but is often elevated with circulating immunoblasts, plasma cells, and other reactive cells (145). Bone marrow aspirate smears and core biopsy sections show infiltrates of lymphocytes, immunoblasts, and plasma cells. The infiltrates may be inconspicuous or large and extensive (Fig. 35.34A–C). The morphologic distinction of polyclonal immunoblastic proliferations from lymphoplasmacytic or immunoblastic lymphoma or plasma cell myeloma can also be difficult. Knowledge of the clinical history and recognition of the polyclonal nature of the proliferation by demonstration that the lymphocytes and plasma cells in this disorder are polyclonal can generally distinguish these rare and unusual lesions from lymphoma and myeloma. IgH and TCR genes are germline; rarely oligoclonal B and/or T cells are identified; the etiology of this disorder is unknown, but many patients exhibit autoimmune phenomenon including autoimmune hemolytic anemia. Patients may respond to steroid therapy, but the mortality rate during the acute phase of the illness is high (~50%), and chemotherapy may be required (145). Importantly, PTCLs including

AILT should be excluded since they often exhibit clinical and morphologic features that overlap with SPIPs.

Systemic Mastocytosis

Systemic mastocytosis almost always involves the bone marrow and may exhibit infiltrates that resemble lymphoma especially T cell and HL (16). In most cases, the mast cell infiltrates are polymorphic and include varying proportions of small lymphocytes, eosinophils, neutrophils, histiocytes, and fibroblasts in addition to the mast cells. However, lymphocytes may predominate, and mast cells may not be easily recognized on H&E-stained sections (Fig. 35.35). The mast cells vary from round, spindle shaped, or monocytoid with abundant cytoplasm and are highlighted with an immunostain for tryptase. Mast cells are CD30− and CD15− and are negative with the T-cell– and B-cell–associated antigens such as CD3 and CD20. Neoplastic mast cells are also CD117, CD25, and/or CD2+ (146).

 | **CONCLUSIONS**

The report generated for the bone marrow specimen that has been evaluated for lymphoma should first state whether or not lymphoma is present in the bone marrow. If ancillary studies such as flow cytometry and molecular analysis are used to establish the diagnosis, the results of all these studies should be correlated with the morphology. When lymphoma is identified

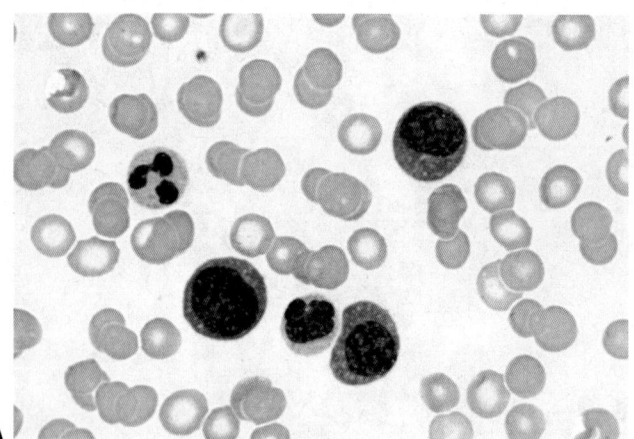

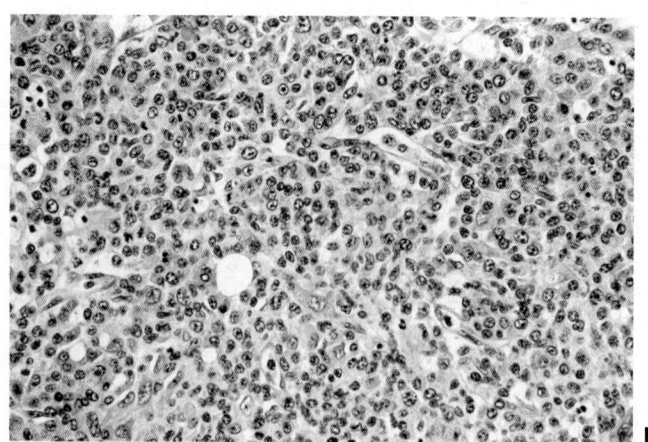

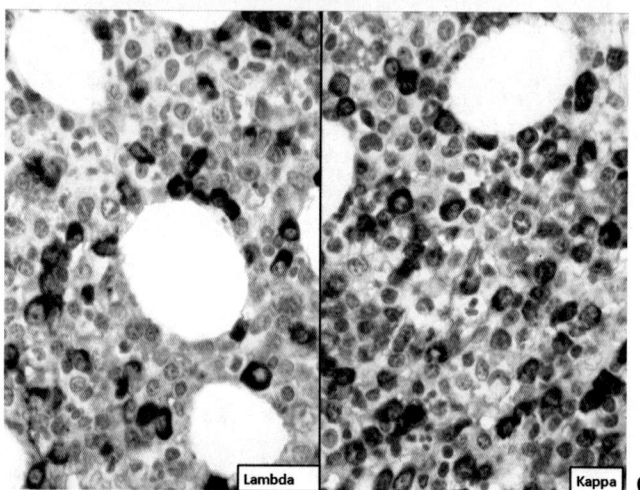

FIGURE 35.34. Systemic polyclonal immunoblastic proliferation. A: Immunoblasts, plasma cells, and increased rouleaux formation are present in the Wright-Giemsa–stained blood smear. **B:** An extensive infiltrate rich in immunoblasts, plasma cells, and variably sized lymphocytes is present in the core biopsy section. **C:** The plasma cells are polytypic based on the immunohistochemical stains for lambda and kappa immunoglobulin light chains.

in the bone marrow, the proportion of the intertrabecular space that the lymphoma occupies should always be provided. Finally, the morphologic appearance of the lymphoma cells (e.g., large transformed or small mature appearing) should be described and correlated with the morphologic appearance of lymphoma at other anatomic sites noting whether the lymphoma is concordant or discordant.

In cases where the lymphoma was initially diagnosed in the bone marrow, the lymphoma should be subclassified when possible. When the available information is not sufficient for accurate subclassification, specific, appropriate suggestions should be made for further workup that would permit subclassification; this often includes biopsy of enlarged lymph node or other extramedullary mass.

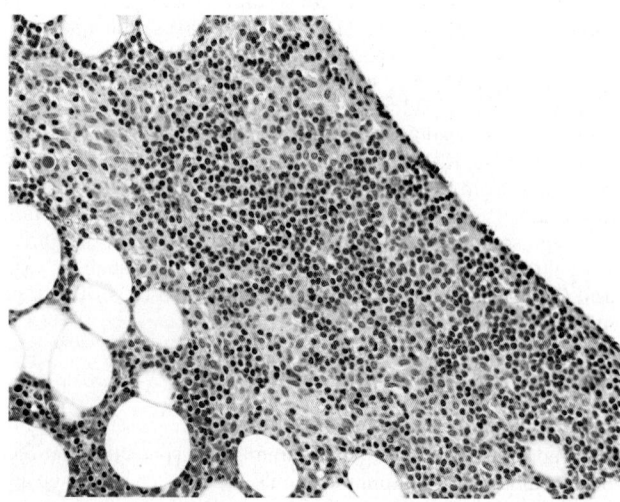

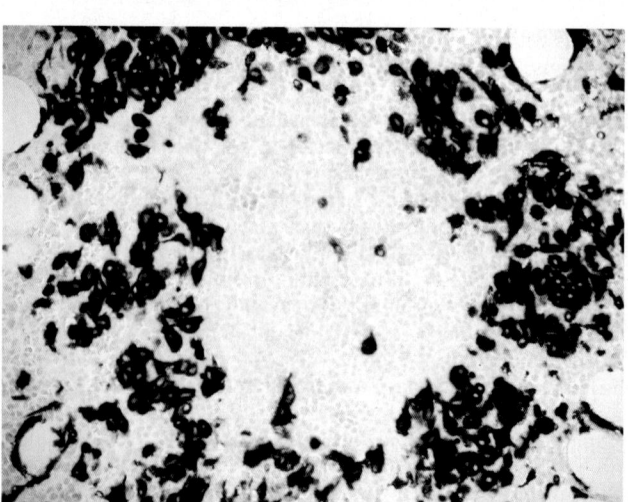

FIGURE 35.35. Systemic mastocytosis involving the bone marrow core biopsy. A: This infiltrate is poorly circumscribed resembling a NHL with many small lymphocytes, rare plasma cells, rare eosinophils, and spindle-shaped mast cells. **B:** The tryptase immunostain shows many positive mast cells mostly at the periphery of the lesion supporting systemic mastocytosis.

References

1. Rosenberg SA, Boiron M, DeVita VT Jr, et al. Report of the Committee on Hodgkin's Disease Staging Procedures. *Cancer Res* 1971;31(11):1862–1863.
2. Bartl R, Frisch B, Hoffmann-Fezer G, et al. Lymphoproliferative disorders in the bone marrow: histologic criteria for classification and staging. *Haematologia (Budap)* 1984;17(2):227–246.
3. Ponzoni M, Li CY. Isolated bone marrow non-Hodgkin's lymphoma: a clinicopathologic study. *Mayo Clin Proc* 1994;69(1):37–43.
4. Brunning RD, Bloomfield CD, McKenna RW, et al. Bilateral trephine bone marrow biopsies in lymphoma and other neoplastic diseases. *Ann Intern Med* 1975;82(3):365–366.
5. Coller BS, Chabner BA, Gralnick HR. Frequencies and patterns of bone marrow involvement in non-Hodgkin lymphomas: observations on the value of bilateral biopsies. *Am J Hematol* 1977;3:105–119.
6. Wang J, Weiss LM, Chang KL, et al. Diagnostic utility of bilateral bone marrow examination: significance of morphologic and ancillary technique study in malignancy. *Cancer* 2002;94(5):1522–1531.
7. McKenna RW, Hernandez JA. Bone marrow in malignant lymphoma. *Hematol Oncol Clin North Am* 1988;2(4):617–635.
8. Bennett JM, Cain KC, Glick JH, et al. The significance of bone marrow involvement in non-Hodgkin's lymphoma: the Eastern Cooperative Oncology Group experience. *J Clin Oncol* 1986;4(10):1462–1469.
9. Cimino G, Anselmo AP, De Luca AM, et al. Bone marrow involvement at onset of Hodgkin's disease. *Tumori* 1983;69(1):47–51.
10. Pangalis GA, Roussou PA, Kittas C, et al. B-chronic lymphocytic leukemia. Prognostic implication of bone marrow histology in 120 patients experience from a single hematology unit. *Cancer* 1987;59(4):767–771.
11. Thieblemont C, Berger F, Dumontet C, et al. Mucosa-associated lymphoid tissue lymphoma is a disseminated disease in one third of 158 patients analyzed. *Blood* 2000;95(3):802–806.
12. Batata A, Shen B. Relationship between chronic lymphocytic leukemia and small lymphocytic lymphoma. A comparative study of membrane phenotypes in 270 cases. *Cancer* 1992;70(3):625–632.
13. Hallek M, Cheson BD, Catovsky D, et al. Guidelines for the diagnosis and treatment of chronic lymphocytic leukemia: a report from the International Workshop on Chronic Lymphocytic Leukemia updating the National Cancer Institute-Working Group 1996 guidelines. *Blood* 2008;111(12):5446–5456.
14. Juneja SK, Wolf MM, Cooper IA. Value of bilateral bone marrow biopsy specimens in non-Hodgkin's lymphoma. *J Clin Pathol* 1990;43(8):630–632.
15. Batata A, Shen B. Chronic lymphocytic leukemia with low lymphocyte count. *Cancer* 1993;71(9):2732–2738.
16. Tandon B, Peterson L, Gao J, et al. Nuclear overexpression of lymphoid-enhancer-binding factor 1 identifies chronic lymphocytic leukemia/small lymphocytic lymphoma in small B-cell lymphomas. *Mod Pathol* 2011;24(11):1433–1443.
17. Swerdlow SH, Pileri SA, et al. Lymphoplasmacytic lymphoma. In: Swerdlow SH, Harris NL, Jaffe ES, et al., eds. *WHO classification of tumours of haematopoietic and lymphoid tissues*. Lyon: IARC, 2008:194–195.
18. Harris NL, Jaffe ES, Stein H, et al. A revised European-American classification of lymphoid neoplasms: a proposal from the International Lymphoma Study Group. *Blood* 1994;84(5):1361–1392.
19. Morice WG, Chen D, Kurtin PJ, et al. Novel immunophenotypic features of marrow lymphoplasmacytic lymphoma and correlation with Waldenstrom's macroglobulinemia. *Mod Pathol* 2009;22(6):807–816.
20a. Valdez R, Finn WG, Ross CW, et al. Waldenstrom macroglobulinemia caused by extranodal marginal zone B-cell lymphoma: a report of six cases. *Am J Clin Pathol* 2001;116(5):683–690.
20b. Roberts MJ, Chadburn A, Ma S, et al. Nuclear protein dysregulation in lymphoplasmacytic lymphoma/Waldenstrom macroglobulinemia. *Am J Clin Pathol* 2013;139(2):210–219.
21. Dierlamm J, Pittaluga S, Wlodarska I, et al. Marginal zone B-cell lymphomas of different sites share similar cytogenetic and morphologic features. *Blood* 1996;87(1):299–307.
22. Kent SA, Variakojis D, Peterson LC. Comparative study of marginal zone lymphoma involving bone marrow. *Am J Clin Pathol* 2002;117(5):698–708.
23. Labouyrie E, Marit G, Vial JP, et al. Intrasinusoidal bone marrow involvement by splenic lymphoma with villous lymphocytes: a helpful immunohistologic feature. *Mod Pathol* 1997;10(10):1015–1020.
24. Melo JV, Hegde U, Parreira A, et al. Splenic B cell lymphoma with circulating villous lymphocytes: differential diagnosis of B cell leukaemias with large spleens. *J Clin Pathol* 1987;40(6):642–651.
25. Ferry JA, Yang WI, Zukerberg LR, et al. CD5+ extranodal marginal zone B-cell (MALT) lymphoma. A low grade neoplasm with a propensity for bone marrow involvement and relapse. *Am J Clin Pathol* 1996;105(1):31–37.
26. Diss TC, Peng H, Wotherspoon AC, et al. Brief report: a single neoplastic clone in sequential biopsy specimens from a patient with primary gastric-mucosa-associated lymphoid-tissue lymphoma and Sjogren's syndrome. *N Engl J Med* 1993;329(3):172–175.
27. Boveri E, Arcaini L, Merli M, et al. Bone marrow histology in marginal zone B-cell lymphomas: correlation with clinical parameters and flow cytometry in 120 patients. *Ann Oncol* 2009;20(1):129–136.
28. Campo E, Miquel R, Krenacs L, et al. Primary nodal marginal zone lymphomas of splenic and MALT type. *Am J Surg Pathol* 1999;23(1):59–68.
29. Pittaluga S, Bijnens L, Teodorovic T, et al. Clinical analysis of 670 cases in two trials of the European Organization for the Research and Treatment of Cancer Lymphoma Cooperative Group subtyped according to the Revised European-American Classification of Lymphoid Neoplasms: a comparison with the Working Formulation. *Blood* 1996;87(10):4358–4367.
30. Nathwani BN, Anderson JR, Armitage JO, et al. Marginal zone B-cell lymphoma: a clinical comparison of nodal and mucosa-associated lymphoid tissue types. Non-Hodgkin's Lymphoma Classification Project. *J Clin Oncol* 1999;17(8):2486–2492.
31. Traweek ST, Sheibani K. Monocytoid B-cell lymphoma. The biologic and clinical implications of peripheral blood involvement. *Am J Clin Pathol* 1992;97(4):591–598.
32. Wahlin BE, Yri OE, Kimby E, et al. Clinical significance of the WHO grades of follicular lymphoma in a population-based cohort of 505 patients with long follow-up times. *Br J Haematol* 2012;156(2):225–233.
33. Younes SF, Beck AH, Ohgami RS, et al. The efficacy of HGAL and LMO2 in the separation of lymphomas derived from small B cells in nodal and extranodal sites, including the bone marrow. *Am J Clin Pathol* 2011;135(5):697–708.
34. Arber DA, George TI. Bone marrow biopsy involvement by non-Hodgkin's lymphoma: frequency of lymphoma types, patterns, blood involvement, and discordance with other sites in 450 specimens. *Am J Surg Pathol* 2005;29(12):1549–1557.
35. Merli M, Arcaini L, Boveri E, et al. Assessment of bone marrow involvement in non-Hodgkin's lymphomas: comparison between histology and flow cytometry. *Eur J Haematol* 2010;85(5):405–415.
36. Torlakovic E, Torlakovic G, Brunning RD. Follicular pattern of bone marrow involvement by follicular lymphoma. *Am J Clin Pathol* 2002;118(5):780–786.
37. Spiro S, Galton DA, Wiltshaw E, et al. Follicular lymphoma: a survey of 75 cases with special reference to the syndrome resembling chronic lymphocytic leukaemia. *Br J Cancer Suppl* 1975;2:60–72.
38. Stamatoullas A, Buchonnet G, Lepretre S, et al. De novo acute B cell leukemia/lymphoma with t(14;18). *Leukemia* 2000;14(11):1960–1966.
39. Kramer MH, Raghoebier S, Beverstock GC, et al. De novo acute B-cell leukemia with translocation t(14;18): an entity with a poor prognosis. *Leukemia* 1991;5(6):473–478.
40. Conlan MG, Bast M, Armitage JO, et al. Bone marrow involvement by non-Hodgkin's lymphoma: the clinical significance of morphologic discordance between the lymph node and bone marrow. Nebraska Lymphoma Study Group. *J Clin Oncol* 1990;8(7):1163–1172.
41. Buhr T, Langer F, Schlue J, et al. Reliability of lymphoma classification in bone marrow trephines. *Br J Haematol* 2002;118(2):470–476.
42. Lambertenghi-Deliliers G, Annaloro C, Soligo D, et al. Incidence and histological features of bone marrow involvement in malignant lymphomas. *Ann Hematol* 1992;65(2):61–65.
43. Cohen PL, Kurtin PJ, Donovan KA, et al. Bone marrow and peripheral blood involvement in mantle cell lymphoma. *Br J Haematol* 1998;101(2):302–310.
44. Schlette E, Lai R, Onciu M, et al. Leukemic mantle cell lymphoma: clinical and pathologic spectrum of twenty-three cases. *Mod Pathol* 2001;14(11):1133–1140.
45. Wasman J, Rosenthal NS, Farhi DC. Mantle cell lymphoma. Morphologic findings in bone marrow involvement. *Am J Clin Pathol* 1996;106(2):196–200.
46. Viswanatha DS, Foucar K, Berry BR, et al. Blastic mantle cell leukemia: an unusual presentation of blastic mantle cell lymphoma. *Mod Pathol* 2000;13(7):825–833.
47. Kimura Y, Sato K, Imamura Y, et al. Small cell variant of mantle cell lymphoma is an indolent lymphoma characterized by bone marrow involvement, splenomegaly, and a low Ki-67 index. *Cancer Sci* 2011;102(9):1734–1741.
48. Schlette E, Bueso-Ramos C, Giles F, et al. Mature B-cell leukemias with more than 55% prolymphocytes. A heterogeneous group that includes an unusual variant of mantle cell lymphoma. *Am J Clin Pathol* 2001;115(4):571–581.
49. Nelson BP, Variakojis D, Peterson LC. Leukemic phase of B-cell lymphomas mimicking chronic lymphocytic leukemia and variants at presentation. *Mod Pathol* 2002;15(11):1111–1120.
50. Wong KF, Chan JK, So JC, et al. Mantle cell lymphoma in leukemic phase: characterization of its broad cytologic spectrum with emphasis on the importance of distinction from other chronic lymphoproliferative disorders. *Cancer* 1999;86(5):850–857.
51. Orchard J, Garand R, Davis Z, et al. A subset of t(11;14) lymphoma with mantle cell features displays mutated IgVH genes and includes patients with good prognosis, nonnodal disease. *Blood* 2003;101(12):4975–4981.
52. Ondrejka SL, Lai R, Smith SD, et al. Indolent mantle cell leukemia: a clinicopathological variant characterized by isolated lymphocytosis, interstitial bone marrow involvement, kappa light chain restriction, and good prognosis. *Haematologica* 2011;96(8):1121–1127.
53. Gong JZ, Lagoo AS, Peters D, et al. Value of CD23 determination by flow cytometry in differentiating mantle cell lymphoma from chronic lymphocytic leukemia/small lymphocytic lymphoma. *Am J Clin Pathol* 2001;116(6):893–897.
54. Kelemen K, Peterson LC, Helenowski I, et al. CD23+ mantle cell lymphoma: a clinical pathologic entity associated with superior outcome compared with CD23- disease. *Am J Clin Pathol* 2008;130(2):166–177.
55. Chen YH, Gao J, Fan G, et al. Nuclear expression of sox11 is highly associated with mantle cell lymphoma but is independent of t(11;14)(q13;q32) in non-mantle cell B-cell neoplasms. *Mod Pathol* 2010;23(1):105–112.
56. Zeng W, Fu K, Quintanilla-Fend L, et al. Cyclin D1-negative blastoid mantle cell lymphoma identified by SOX11 expression. *Am J Surg Pathol* 2012;36(2):214–219.
57. Hodges GF, Lenhardt TM, Cotelingam JD. Bone marrow involvement in large-cell lymphoma. Prognostic implications of discordant disease. *Am J Clin Pathol* 1994;101(3):305–311.
58. Chung R, Lai R, Wei P, et al. Concordant but not discordant bone marrow involvement in diffuse large B-cell lymphoma predicts a poor clinical outcome independent of the International Prognostic Index. *Blood* 2007;110(4):1278–1282.
59. Yan Y, Chan WC, Weisenburger DD, et al. Clinical and prognostic significance of bone marrow involvement in patients with diffuse aggressive B-cell lymphoma. *J Clin Oncol* 1995;13(6):1336–1342.
60. Crisan D, Mattson JC. Discordant morphologic features in bone marrow involvement by malignant lymphomas: use of gene rearrangement patterns for diagnosis. *Am J Hematol* 1995;49(4):299–309.
61. Campbell J, Seymour JF, Matthews J, et al. The prognostic impact of bone marrow involvement in patients with diffuse large cell lymphoma varies according to the degree of infiltration and presence of discordant marrow involvement. *Eur J Haematol* 2006;76(6):473–480.
62. Kremer M, Spitzer M, Mandl-Weber S, et al. Discordant bone marrow involvement in diffuse large B-cell lymphoma: comparative molecular analysis reveals a heterogeneous group of disorders. *Lab Invest* 2003;83(1):107–114.
63. Sehn LH, Scott DW, Chhanabhai M, et al. Impact of concordant and discordant bone marrow involvement on outcome in diffuse large B-cell lymphoma treated with R-CHOP. *J Clin Oncol* 2011;29(11):1452–1457.
64. Baddoura FK, Chan WC, Masih AS, et al. T-cell-rich B-cell lymphoma. A clinicopathologic study of eight cases. *Am J Clin Pathol* 1995;103(1):65–75.
65. Skinnider BF, Connors JM, Gascoyne RD. Bone marrow involvement in T-cell-rich B-cell lymphoma. *Am J Clin Pathol* 1997;108(5):570–578.
66. Perrone T, Frizzera G, Rosai J. Mediastinal diffuse large-cell lymphoma with sclerosis. A clinicopathologic study of 60 cases. *Am J Surg Pathol* 1986;10(3):176–191.

67. Abou-Elella AA, Weisenburger DD, Vose JM, et al. Primary mediastinal large B-cell lymphoma: a clinicopathologic study of 43 patients from the Nebraska Lymphoma Study Group. *J Clin Oncol* 1999;17(3):784–790.
68. Nakamura SPM, Campo E. Intravascular large B-cell lymphoma. In: Swerdlow SH, Harris NL, Jaffe ES, et al., eds. *WHO classification of tumours of haematopoietic and lymphoid tissues*. Lyon: IARC, 2008:252–253.
69. Wick MR, Mills SE, Scheithauer BW, et al. Reassessment of malignant "angioendotheliomatosis". Evidence in favor of its reclassification as "intravascular lymphomatosis". *Am J Surg Pathol* 1986;10(2):112–123.
70. Estalilla OC, Koo CH, Brynes RK, et al. Intravascular large B-cell lymphoma. A report of five cases initially diagnosed by bone marrow biopsy. *Am J Clin Pathol* 1999;112(2):248–255.
71. Tucker TJ, Bardales RH, Miranda RN. Intravascular lymphomatosis with bone marrow involvement. *Arch Pathol Lab Med* 1999;123(10):952–956.
72. Dick F, Bloomfield CD, Brunning RD. Incidence cytology, and histopathology of non-Hodgkin's lymphomas in the bone marrow. *Cancer* 1974;33(5):1382–1398.
73. Subira M, Domingo A, Santamaria A, et al. Bone marrow involvement in lymphoblastic lymphoma and small non-cleaved cell lymphoma: the role of trephine biopsy. *Haematologica* 1997;82(5):594–595.
74a. Jaffe ES, Stein H, Swerdlow SH. B-cell lymphoma, unclassifiable, with features intermediate between diffuse large B-cell lymphoma and Burkitt lymphoma. In: Swerdlow SH, Harris NL, Jaffe ES, et al., eds. *WHO classification of tumors of haematopoietic and lymphoid tissues*. Lyon: IRAC, 2008: 265–266.
74b. Chan JKC, Ferry JA, et al. Extranodal NK/T-cell lymphoma, nasal type. In: Swerdlow SH, Harris NL, Jaffe ES, et al., eds. *WHO classification of tumours of haematopoietic and lymphoid tissues*. Lyon: IARC, 2007:285–288.
75. Jaffe ES, Chan JK, Su IJ, et al. Report of the workshop on nasal and related extranodal angiocentric T/natural killer cell lymphomas. Definitions, differential diagnosis, and epidemiology. *Am J Surg Pathol* 1996;20(1):103–111.
76. Kwong YL, Chan AC, Liang R, et al. CD56+ NK lymphomas: clinicopathological features and prognosis. *Br J Haematol* 1997;97(4):821–829.
77. Cheung MM, Chan JK, Lau WH, et al. Primary non-Hodgkin's lymphoma of the nose and nasopharynx: clinical features, tumor immunophenotype, and treatment outcome in 113 patients. *J Clin Oncol* 1998;16(1):70–77.
78. Wong KF, Chan JK, Cheung MM, et al. Bone marrow involvement by nasal NK cell lymphoma at diagnosis is uncommon. *Am J Clin Pathol* 2001;115(2): 266–270.
79. Chan JK, Sin VC, Wong KF, et al. Nonnasal lymphoma expressing the natural killer cell marker CD56: a clinicopathologic study of 49 cases of an uncommon aggressive neoplasm. *Blood* 1997;89(12):4501–4513.
80. Bagdi E, Diss TC, Munson P, et al. Mucosal intra-epithelial lymphocytes in enteropathy-associated T-cell lymphoma, ulcerative jejunitis, and refractory celiac disease constitute a neoplastic population. *Blood* 1999;94(1):260–264.
81. Kim SJ, Choi CW, Mun YC, et al. Multicenter retrospective analysis of 581 patients with primary intestinal non-hodgkin lymphoma from the Consortium for Improving Survival of Lymphoma (CISL). *BMC Cancer* 2011;11:321.
82. Cooke CB, Krenacs L, Stetler-Stevenson M, et al. Hepatosplenic T-cell lymphoma: a distinct clinicopathologic entity of cytotoxic gamma delta T-cell origin. *Blood* 1996;88(11):4265–4274.
83. Macon WR, Levy NB, Kurtin PJ, et al. Hepatosplenic alphabeta T-cell lymphomas: a report of 14 cases and comparison with hepatosplenic gammadelta T-cell lymphomas. *Am J Surg Pathol* 2001;25(3):285–296.
84. Suarez F, Wlodarska I, Rigal-Huguet F, et al. Hepatosplenic alphabeta T-cell lymphoma: an unusual case with clinical, histologic, and cytogenetic features of gammadelta hepatosplenic T-cell lymphoma. *Am J Surg Pathol* 2000;24(7): 1027–1032.
85. Vega F, Medeiros LJ, Bueso-Ramos C, et al. Hepatosplenic gamma/delta T-cell lymphoma in bone marrow. A sinusoidal neoplasm with blastic cytologic features. *Am J Clin Pathol* 2001;116(3):410–419.
86. Wang CC, Tien HF, Lin MT, et al. Consistent presence of isochromosome 7q in hepatosplenic T gamma/delta lymphoma: a new cytogenetic-clinicopathologic entity. *Genes Chromosomes Cancer* 1995;12(3):161–164.
87. Chen YH, Chadburn A, Evens AM, et al. Clinical, morphologic, immunophenotypic, and molecular cytogenetic assessment of CD4-/CD8-gammadelta T-cell large granular lymphocytic leukemia. *Am J Clin Pathol* 2011;136(2):289–299.
88. Chen YH, Peterson L. Differential diagnosis of CD4-/CD8- gammadelta T-cell large granular lymphocytic leukemia and hepatosplenic T-cell lymphoma. *Am J Clin Pathol* 2012;137(3):496–497.
89. Salhany KE, Macon WR, Choi JK, et al. Subcutaneous panniculitis-like T-cell lymphoma: clinicopathologic, immunophenotypic, and genotypic analysis of alpha/beta and gamma/delta subtypes. *Am J Surg Pathol* 1998;22(7):881–893.
90. Gonzalez CL, Medeiros LJ, Braziel RM, et al. T-cell lymphoma involving subcutaneous tissue. A clinicopathologic entity commonly associated with hemophagocytic syndrome. *Am J Surg Pathol* 1991;15(1):17–27.
91. Ralfkiaer EAJ. Mycosis fungoides and Sezary syndrome. In: Harris NL, Jaffe ES, Stein H, Vardiman JW, eds. *World health organization classification of tumours. Pathology and genetics. Tumours of hematopoietic and lymphoid tissues*. Lyon: IARC, 2001:216–220.
92. Salhany KE, Greer JP, Cousar JB, et al. Marrow involvement in cutaneous T-cell lymphoma. A clinicopathologic study of 60 cases. *Am J Clin Pathol* 1989;92(6):747–754.
93. Sibaud V, Beylot-Barry M, Thiebaut R, et al. Bone marrow histopathologic and molecular staging in epidermotropic T-cell lymphomas. *Am J Clin Pathol* 2003;119(3):414–423.
94. Long JC, Mihm MC. Mycosis fungoides with extracutaneous dissemination: a distinct clinicopathologic entity. *Cancer* 1974;34(5):1745–1755.
95. Graham SJ, Sharpe RW, Steinberg SM, et al. Prognostic implications of a bone marrow histopathologic classification system in mycosis fungoides and the Sezary syndrome. *Cancer* 1993;72(3):726–734.
96. Beylot-Barry M, Parrens M, Delaunay M, et al. Is bone marrow biopsy necessary in patients with mycosis fungoides and Sezary syndrome? A histological and molecular study at diagnosis and during follow-up. *Br J Dermatol* 2005;152(6):1378–1379.
97. Hanson CA, Brunning RD, Gajl-Peczalska KJ, et al. Bone marrow manifestations of peripheral T-cell lymphoma. A study of 30 cases. *Am J Clin Pathol* 1986;86(4):449–460.
98. Pangalis GA, Moran EM, Rappaport H. Blood and bone marrow findings in angioimmunoblastic lymphadenopathy. *Blood* 1978;51(1):71–83.
99. Gaulard P, Kanavaros P, Farcet JP, et al. Bone marrow histologic and immunohistochemical findings in peripheral. T-cell lymphoma: A study of 38 cases. *Hum Pathol* 1991;22(4):331–338.
100. Dogan A, Morice WG. Bone marrow histopathology in peripheral T-cell lymphomas. *Br J Haematol* 2004;127(2):140–154.
101. Ghani AM, Krause JR. Bone marrow biopsy findings in angioimmunoblastic lymphadenopathy. *Br J Haematol* 1985;61(2):203–213.
102. Merchant SH, Amin MB, Viswanatha DS. Morphologic and immunophenotypic analysis of angioimmunoblastic T-cell lymphoma: emphasis on phenotypic aberrancies for early diagnosis. *Am J Clin Pathol* 2006;126(1):29–38.
103. Grogg KL, Morice WG, Macon WR. Spectrum of bone marrow findings in patients with angioimmunoblastic T-cell lymphoma. *Br J Haematol* 2007;137(5): 416–422.
104. Cho YU, Chi HS, Park CJ, et al. Distinct features of angioimmunoblastic T-cell lymphoma with bone marrow involvement. *Am J Clin Pathol* 2009;131(5): 640–646.
105. Fraga M, Brousset P, Schlaifer D, et al. Bone marrow involvement in anaplastic large cell lymphoma. Immunohistochemical detection of minimal disease and its prognostic significance. *Am J Clin Pathol* 1995;103(1):82–89.
106. Weinberg OK, Seo K, Arber DA. Prevalence of bone marrow involvement in systemic anaplastic large cell lymphoma: are immunohistochemical studies necessary? *Hum Pathol* 2008;39(9):1331–1340.
107. Wong KF, Chan JK, Ng CS, et al. Anaplastic large cell Ki-1 lymphoma involving bone marrow: marrow findings and association with reactive hemophagocytosis. *Am J Hematol* 1991;37(2):112–119.
108. Anderson MM, Ross CW, Singleton TP, et al. Ki-1 anaplastic large cell lymphoma with a prominent leukemic phase. *Hum Pathol* 1996;27(10):1093–1095.
109. Onciu M, Behm FG, Raimondi SC, et al. ALK-positive anaplastic large cell lymphoma with leukemic peripheral blood involvement is a clinicopathologic entity with an unfavorable prognosis. Report of three cases and review of the literature. *Am J Clin Pathol* 2003;120(4):617–625.
110. O'Carroll DI, McKenna RW, Brunning RD. Bone marrow manifestations of Hodgkin's disease. *Cancer* 1976;38(4):1717–1728.
111. Hansmann ML, Zwingers T, Boske A, et al. Clinical features of nodular paragranuloma (Hodgkin's disease, lymphocyte predominance type, nodular). *J Cancer Res Clin Oncol* 1984;108(3):321–330.
112. Diehl V, Sextro M, Franklin J, et al. Clinical presentation, course, and prognostic factors in lymphocyte-predominant Hodgkin's disease and lymphocyte-rich classical Hodgkin's disease: report from the European Task Force on Lymphoma Project on Lymphocyte-Predominant Hodgkin's Disease. *J Clin Oncol* 1999; 17(3):776–783.
113. Klimm B, Franklin J, Stein H, et al. Lymphocyte-depleted classical Hodgkin's lymphoma: a comprehensive analysis from the German Hodgkin study group. *J Clin Oncol* 2011;29(29):3914–3920.
114. Ellis ME, Diehl LF, Granger E, et al. Trephine needle bone marrow biopsy in the initial staging of Hodgkin disease: sensitivity and specificity of the Ann Arbor staging procedure criteria. *Am J Hematol* 1989;30(3):115–120.
115. Hines-Thomas MR, Howard SC, Hudson MM, et al. Utility of bone marrow biopsy at diagnosis in pediatric Hodgkin's lymphoma. *Haematologica* 2010;95(10): 1691–1696.
116. Hutchings M. The role of bone marrow biopsy in Hodgkin lymphoma staging: "to be, or not to be, that is the question"? *Leuk Lymphoma* 2012;53(4):523–524.
117. Eichenauer DA, Engert A, Dreyling M. Hodgkin's lymphoma: ESMO Clinical Practice Guidelines for diagnosis, treatment and follow-up. *Ann Oncol* 2011;22 Suppl 6:vi55–vi58.
118. Ioachim HL, Dorsett B, Cronin W, et al. Acquired immunodeficiency syndrome-associated lymphomas: clinical, pathologic, immunologic, and viral characteristics of 111 cases. *Hum Pathol* 1991;22(7):659–673.
119. Knowles DM, Chamulak GA, Subar M, et al. Lymphoid neoplasia associated with the acquired immunodeficiency syndrome (AIDS). The New York University Medical Center experience with 105 patients (1981–1986). *Ann Intern Med* 1988;108(5):744–753.
120. Ponzoni M, Fumagalli L, Rossi G, et al. Isolated bone marrow manifestation of HIV-associated Hodgkin lymphoma. *Mod Pathol* 2002;15(12):1273–1278.
121. Howell SJ, Grey M, Chang J, et al. The value of bone marrow examination in the staging of Hodgkin's lymphoma: a review of 955 cases seen in a regional cancer centre. *Br J Haematol* 2002;119(2):408–411.
122. Lukes RJ. Criteria for involvement of lymph node, bone marrow, spleen, and liver in Hodgkin's disease. *Cancer Res* 1971;31(11):1755–1767.
123. Rappaport H, Berard CW, Butler JJ, et al. Report of the committee on histopathological criteria contributing to staging of Hodgkin's disease. *Cancer Res* 1971;31(11):1864–1865.
124. Khoury JD, Jones D, Yared MA, et al. Bone marrow involvement in patients with nodular lymphocyte predominant Hodgkin lymphoma. *Am J Surg Pathol* 2004;28(4):489–495.
125. Osborne BM, Guarda LA, Butler JJ. Bone marrow biopsies in patients with the acquired immunodeficiency syndrome. *Hum Pathol* 1984;15(11):1048–1053.
126. Karcher DS, Frost AR. The bone marrow in human immunodeficiency virus (HIV)-related disease. Morphology and clinical correlation. *Am J Clin Pathol* 1991;95(1):63–71.
127. Thiele J, Zirbes TK, Kvasnicka HM, et al. Focal lymphoid aggregates (nodules) in bone marrow biopsies: differentiation between benign hyperplasia and malignant lymphoma—a practical guideline. *J Clin Pathol* 1999;52(4):294–300.
128. Magalhaes SM, Filho FD, Vassallo J, et al. Bone marrow lymphoid aggregates in myelodysplastic syndromes: incidence, immunomorphological characteristics and correlation with clinical features and survival. *Leuk Res* 2002;26(6): 525–530; discussion 531.
129. de Leon ED, Alkan S, Huang JC, et al. Usefulness of an immunohistochemical panel in paraffin-embedded tissues for the differentiation of B-cell non-Hodgkin's lymphomas of small lymphocytes. *Mod Pathol* 1998;11(11):1046–1051.
130. Chen CC, Raikow RB, Sonmez-Alpan E, et al. Classification of small B-cell lymphoid neoplasms using a paraffin section immunohistochemical panel. *Appl Immunohistochem Mol Morphol* 2000;8(1):1–11.
131. Douglas VK, Gordon LI, Goolsby CL, et al. Lymphoid aggregates in bone marrow mimic residual lymphoma after rituximab therapy for non-Hodgkin lymphoma. *Am J Clin Pathol* 1999;112(6):844–853.
132. Fineberg S, Marsh E, Alfonso F, et al. Immunophenotypic evaluation of the bone marrow in non-Hodgkin's lymphoma. *Hum Pathol* 1993;24(6):636–642.

133. Hanson CA, Kurtin PJ, Katzmann JA, et al. Immunophenotypic analysis of peripheral blood and bone marrow in the staging of B-cell malignant lymphoma. *Blood* 1999;94(11):3889–3896.
134. Crotty PL, Smith BR, Tallini G. Morphologic, immunophenotypic, and molecular evaluation of bone marrow involvement in non-Hodgkin's lymphoma. *Diagn Mol Pathol* 1998;7(2):90–95.
135. Sah SP, Matutes E, Wotherspoon AC, et al. A comparison of flow cytometry, bone marrow biopsy, and bone marrow aspirates in the detection of lymphoid infiltration in B cell disorders. *J Clin Pathol* 2003;56(2):129–132.
136. Schmidt B, Kremer M, Gotze K, et al. Bone marrow involvement in follicular lymphoma: comparison of histology and flow cytometry as staging procedures. *Leuk Lymphoma* 2006;47(9):1857–1862.
137. Ghia P, Prato G, Scielzo C, et al. Monoclonal CD5+ and CD5- B-lymphocyte expansions are frequent in the peripheral blood of the elderly. *Blood* 2004;103(6):2337–2342.
138. Marti GE, Rawstron AC, Ghia P, et al. Diagnostic criteria for monoclonal B-cell lymphocytosis. *Br J Haematol* 2005;130(3):325–332.
139. Rawstron AC, Green MJ, Kuzmicki A, et al. Monoclonal B lymphocytes with the characteristics of "indolent" chronic lymphocytic leukemia are present in 3.5% of adults with normal blood counts. *Blood* 2002;100(2):635–639.
140. Karlsen F, Kalantari M, Chitemerere M, et al. Modifications of human and viral deoxyribonucleic acid by formaldehyde fixation. *Lab Invest* 1994;71(4):604–611.
141. Pittaluga S, Tierens A, Dodoo YL, et al. How reliable is histologic examination of bone marrow trephine biopsy specimens for the staging of non-Hodgkin lymphoma? A study of hairy cell leukemia and mantle cell lymphoma involvement of the bone marrow trephine specimen by histologic, immunohistochemical, and polymerase chain reaction techniques. *Am J Clin Pathol* 1999;111(2):179–184.
142. Coad JE, Olson DJ, Christensen DR, et al. Correlation of PCR-detected clonal gene rearrangements with bone marrow morphology in patients with B-lineage lymphomas. *Am J Surg Pathol* 1997;21(9):1047–1056.
143. Kremer M, Cabras AD, Fend F, et al. PCR analysis of IgH-gene rearrangements in small lymphoid infiltrates microdissected from sections of paraffin-embedded bone marrow biopsy specimens. *Hum Pathol* 2000;31(7):847–853.
144. Robetorye RS, Bohling SD, Medeiros LJ, et al. Follicular lymphoma with monocytoid B-cell proliferation: molecular assessment of the clonal relationship between the follicular and monocytoid B-cell components. *Lab Invest* 2000;80(10):1593–1599.
145. Peterson LC, Kueck B, Arthur DC, et al. Systemic polyclonal immunoblastic proliferations. *Cancer* 1988;61(7):1350–1358.
146. Valent P, Horny HP, Escribano L, et al. Diagnostic criteria and classification of mastocytosis: a consensus proposal. *Leuk Res* 2001;25(7):603–625.

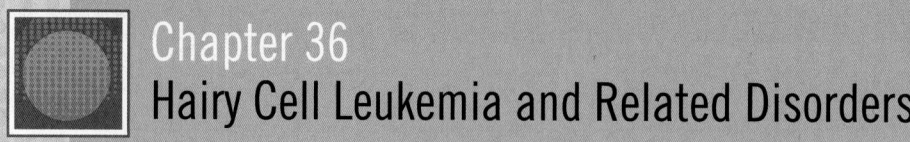

Chapter 36
Hairy Cell Leukemia and Related Disorders

Qian-Yun Zhang • Kathryn Foucar

 INTRODUCTION

Hairy cell leukemia (HCL) was initially characterized as "reticuloendotheliosis" by Bouroncle in 1958 (1). The nature of "hairy cells (HCs)" was debated as they have features that resemble that of lymphocytes such as agglutination of sheep blood cells. The HCs also exhibit features characteristic of monocytes as they have abundant cytoplasm and *in vitro* hemophagocytosis capability (2–6). In 1974, Catovsky et al. (7) proposed that HCs were B lymphocytes based on their positive surface immunoglobulin (sIg) and complement C3. The B-cell origin was confirmed later with the demonstration of B-cell immunoglobulin (Ig) heavy chain (*IGVH@*) gene rearrangement (8–12). Meanwhile, the morphology of HCs in blood, bone marrow (BM), spleen, liver, and other organ system was gradually recognized and described (13–19). Advances in HCL diagnosis were made in the following two decades. Cytochemical studies were extensively carried out, and tartrate-resistant acid phosphatase (TRAP) stood out as a unique cytochemical marker for HCL (14,20–24). Immunohistochemical (IHC) stains became invaluable in the diagnosis of HCL as HCs express B-cell antigens as well as TRAP, DBA.44, cyclin D1, and annexin A1 (25–37). In the late 1990s and early 2000s, flow cytometry became the test of choice for HCL to delineate the unique antigen expression profile: bright CD20, bright CD22, bright CD11c, CD25, and CD103 (35,38–43). Meanwhile treatment of HCL has proven to be one of the miracles of modern medicine. Interferon alpha (INF-α) was the first drug used to treat HCL in place of traditional splenectomy. Although complete remission (CR) with INF-α was only achieved in a subset of patients, cellularity and HC mass were significantly decreased in the majority of patients (44–46). Shortly after, treatment with single-agent purine analog 2-chlorodeoxyadenosine (AKA: 2-CdA, cladribine) or 2'-deoxycoformycin (AKA: DCF, pentostatin) demonstrated efficacy to induce CR with minimal side effects in the majority of patients and has since became the drug of choice for HCL (47–49). Cladribine or pentostatin is also effective in treating relapsed HCL. Recently, anti-CD20 monoclonal antibody rituximab in combination with purine analog has shown added benefit in eradicating minimal residual disease (MRD), in relapsed, or in refractory patients (50–53).

 DEFINITION

HCL is a chronic B-cell lymphoproliferative neoplasm (B-CLPN) with unique clinic, morphologic, immunophenotypic, and prognostic features. Patients typically present with cytopenia-related symptoms, particularly neutropenia-related infections and splenomegaly without lymphadenopathy. HCs have characteristic circumferential cytoplasmic villi ("hairy" projection) and display diffuse BM and splenic red pulp infiltration patterns.

 EPIDEMIOLOGY

HCL is a rare disease and accounts for 2% of lymphoid leukemias. It typically affects males in their 50s with a male:female ratio of approximately 4:1 and a median age of 54 years at diagnosis (50,54).

 CLINICAL FEATURES

Clinical Presentation and Sites of Involvement

HCL is an indolent disease with insidious clinical onset. HCL typically involves the BM, spleen, and liver. These organs are rich in $\alpha4\beta1$/vascular cell adhesion molecule (VCAM) 1, which provides HCs with strong adhesion to the accessory cells and therefore the motility and transmigration ability (55). Peripheral blood (PB) is often involved although the white blood cell count is typically low. In contrast, HCL rarely involves the lymph nodes due to down-regulation of L-selectin, CXCR5, and CCR7 in HCs, which are important in lymphocyte homing to lymph nodes (56,57).

The presenting signs and symptoms are generally related to the extent of BM and/or extramedullary involvement. BM involvement leads to cytopenia(s), which can be single lineage, bilineage, or more often pancytopenia. Monocytopenia is characteristic. Fever and infection are by far the most common clinical presentations, leading to pneumonia and septicemia, as a result of neutropenia, monocytopenia, and impaired T-cell immune function (1,58). Common offending microorganisms include *Escherichia coli*, *Pseudomonas aeruginosa*, *Staphylococcus aureus*, fungi, and acid-fast mycobacteria (58). Salmonella septicemia has also been reported (59). Anemia and thrombocytopenia-related signs and symptoms including fatigue, weakness, and bleeding are also common. Some patients may have concurrent hemolytic anemia (1). Patients may also present with left upper quadrant pain related to splenomegaly. Rarely, patients present with spontaneous rupture of the spleen, cryptococcal meningitis, lymphocytosis, or massive splenomegaly with HC infiltration but normal PB and BM (60). Other rare presentations include solid organ tissue masses (61,62), peripheral lymphadenopathy (unpublished data, Zhang & Foucar 2011), isolated skeletal involvement (63,64), leukemia cutis (65), chronic urticaria (66), and body cavity effusion (59,67,68). HCL is associated with autoimmune disorders and vasculitis in some cases (69). Rarely, HCL occurs in familial fashion including sibling or parent-child cases (70–73). An HLA association has been postulated in those cases, particularly HLA A3 and B7.

Clinical Evaluation and Staging

Clinical evaluation of an HCL patient should include a complete blood count with differential counts, PB smear, BM aspiration, and biopsy review. Immunophenotyping by flow cytometry and/

or IHC stains is paramount to establish the definitive diagnosis and to assess the extent of leukemic involvement, which is often underestimated on routine histology. Imaging studies to evaluate extramedullary involvement such as organomegaly and/or lymphadenopathy are helpful to tailor the clinical management. Evaluation and management of any infection, cytopenia, or any other HCL-related symptoms are essential.

Although there is no standard staging system for HCL, patients are generally categorized into untreated, progressive, and refractory groups for clinical management purposes.

MORPHOLOGY

Peripheral Blood

The PB typically exhibits leukopenia secondary to neutropenia and monocytopenia. There is frequent anemia and/or thrombocytopenia. Circulating leukemic cells are present in the majority of patients although they can be sparse; a high index of suspicion with careful search especially at the featured edge or the two sides of the slide is required. The classic morphology of HCs includes intermediate lymphocytes, which are about twice the size of a mature lymphocyte. They have abundant pale blue cytoplasm, which characteristically forms circumferential hairy projections. There is a spectrum of nuclear morphology ranging from round, oval to kidney-shaped nuclei with homogeneous, spongy, ground-glass, or checkerboard chromatin and inconspicuous nucleoli (Fig. 36.1A-F). The cytoplasm may contain vacuoles, granules, or rod-shaped inclusions occasionally. The rod-shaped inclusions correspond to cytoplasmic ribosome lamellar complex noted by ultrastructural study (74).

Bone Marrow

The BM is frequently inaspirable due to significant fibrosis. If aspiration is successful, HCs are admixed with hematopoietic cells and can be inconspicuous. BM core biopsy is of pivotal importance in the diagnosis of HCL. The characteristic infiltration pattern is diffuse interstitial. With increasing leukemic cells, patchy, small clusters of HCs can be seen. The leukemic cells eventually form solid sheets, which completely efface the marrow cavity. Intrasinusoidal infiltrate can occasionally present, most commonly in the presence of interstitial infiltrate. Although rare, exclusive intrasinusoidal pattern has been reported. In some cases, the infiltration can be quite subtle and almost "invisible." On high magnification, the leukemic cell nuclei are widely separated due to ample cytoplasm and may have "fried egg" appearance (Fig. 36.2). Mitoses are exceedingly rare.

Fibrosis is almost always present in BMs involved in HCL. It can be occasionally prominent and raise the differential diagnosis such as myelofibrosis, systemic mastocytosis, Hodgkin lymphoma, and metastatic cancer. The two types of fibrosis in HCL are reticulin and fibronectin (FN) (75–79). Adhesion of HCs to extracellular matrix hyaluronan (HA) promotes production of cytokine fibroblast growth factor 2 (FGF-2), which binds

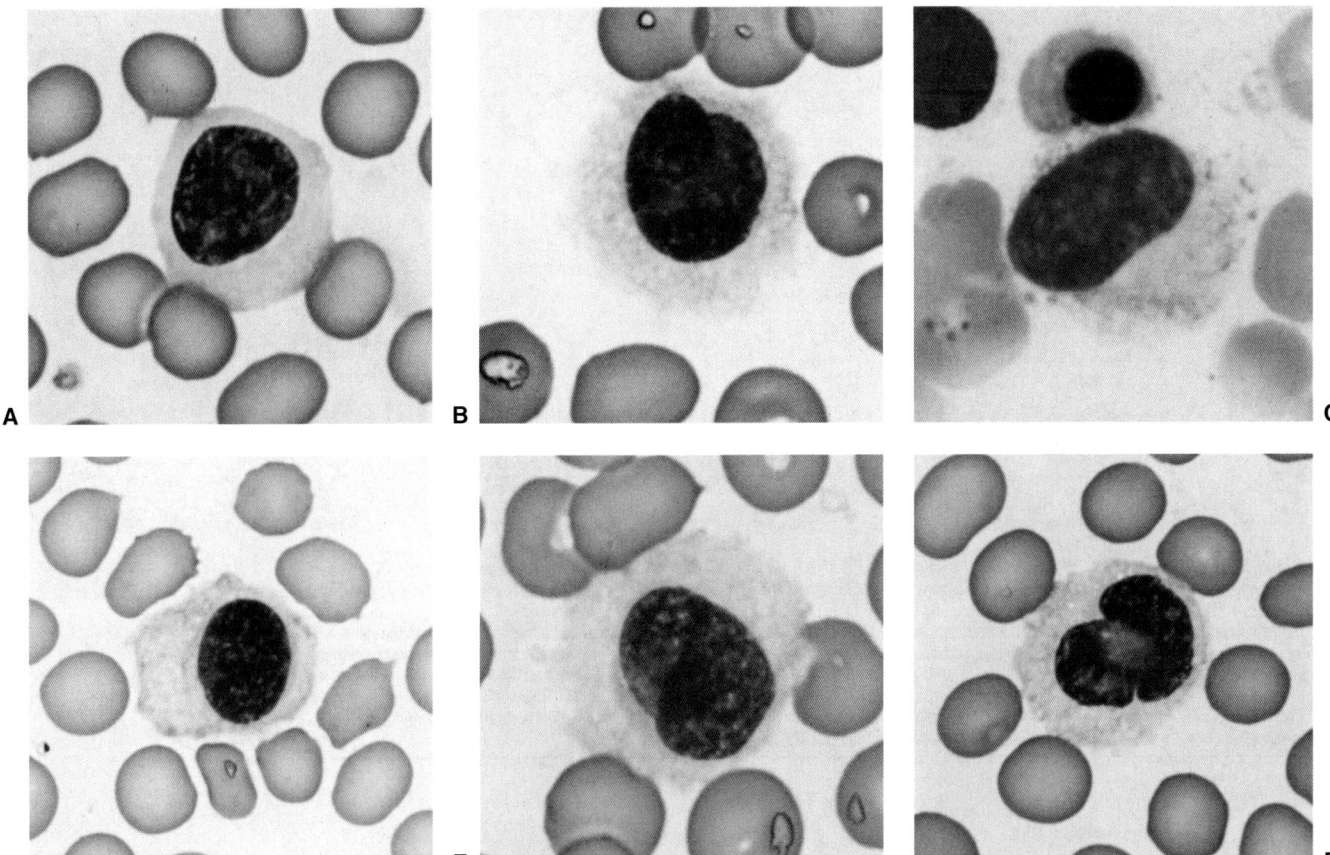

FIGURE 36.1A-F. HCs may exhibit spectrum of morphology in PB (Wright stain). The cytoplasm is typically abundant and can be slightly pale to pale magenta. The cytoplasmic borders can be smooth, slightly rugged to the classic hairy projections. The cells may have round to oval, slightly cleaved, folded, or lobulated nuclei. The chromatin is usually ground-glass or checkerboard pattern. Nucleoli are inconspicuous.

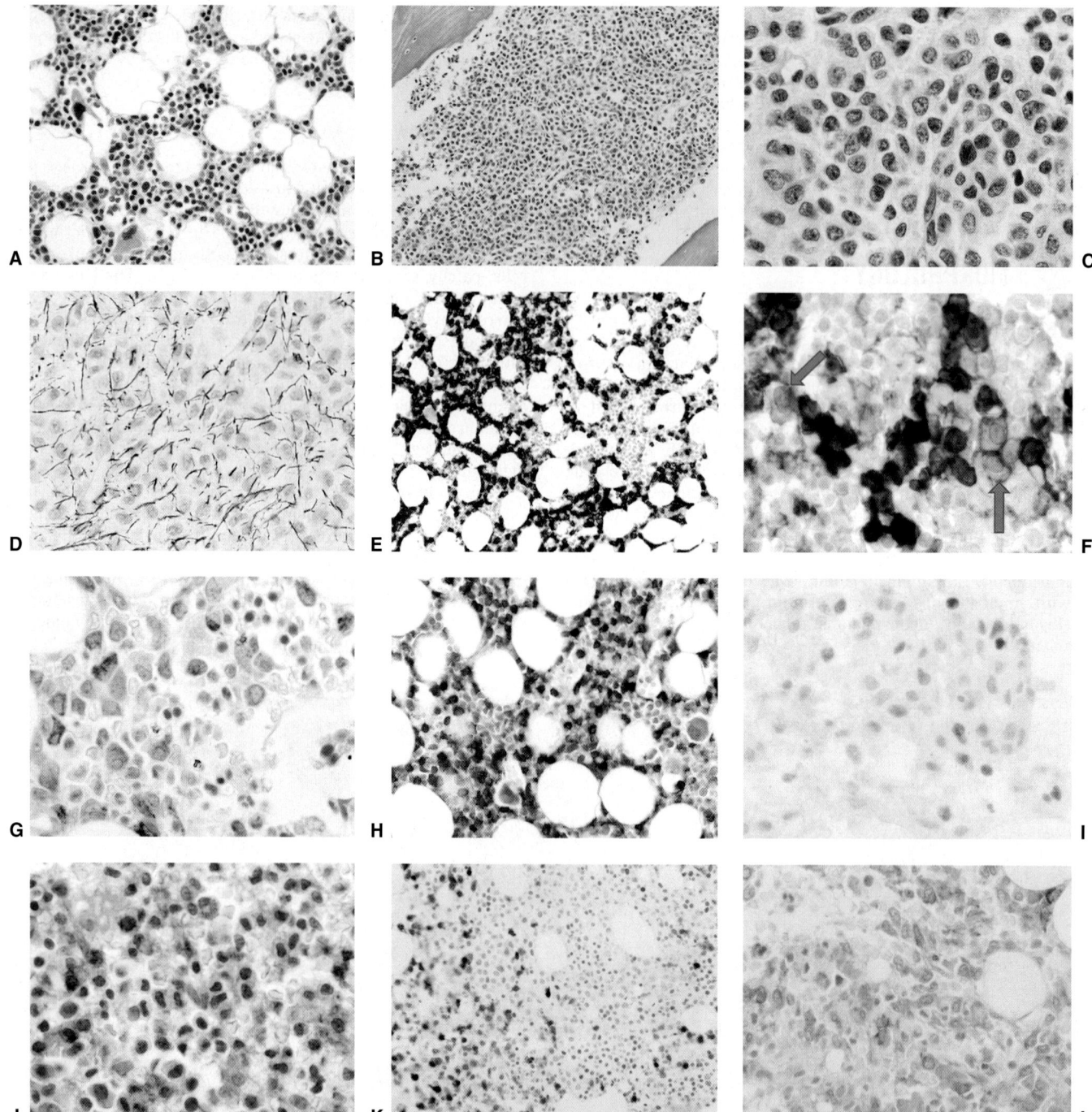

FIGURE 36.2. HCL involving BM. The involvement is subtle on H&E sections when involvement is at low level (**A**). It can be easily overlooked and requires high index of suspicion in a cytopenic patient without obvious etiology. The HCs form solid sheets when involvement is extensive (**B**). On higher power, HCs have ample cytoplasm, oval to slightly irregular nuclei, mature chromatin, and inconspicuous nucleoli (**C**). There is increase in reticulin fibrosis (**D**). On CD20 stain (**E**), HCs are predominantly diffuse interstitial and admixed with normal hematopoietic cells. Note that leukemic cells are significantly underestimated on H&E section. Annexin A1 stain (**F**) demonstrates HCs with a cytoplasmic membrane staining pattern. The outline of nuclei and translucent cytoplasm is visible (*blue arrows*). Note that myeloid precursors and T cells are also positive for annexin A1 (darkly stained cells). TRAP stains cytoplasmic granules in HCs (**G**). DBA.44 (**H**) typically stains a subset of HCs with cytoplasmic staining pattern. Cyclin D1 typically exhibits nuclear stain with various intensity in a subset of HCs (**I**). CD123 has a membrane and cytoplasmic staining pattern in HCL (**J**), so is TCL1 (**K**). CD25 is predominantly cytoplasmic stain in HCL (**L**).

Table 36.1	TYPES OF FIBROSIS IN HCL		
Type of Fibrosis	Type of Protein	Cells Producing Fibrosis	Cytokine Involved
Fibronectin	Glycoprotein (noncollagenous)	Hairy cells	FGF-2 (produced by HCs)
Reticulin	Single type III collagen fibrils	Fibroblasts	TGF-β1 (produced by HCs)

FGF-2, fibroblast growth factor 2; TGF-β1, transforming growth factor.

to HCs to form an autocrine loop, thus enhancing production of FGF-2. FGF-2 stimulates production of FN by HCs. HCs also produce transforming growth factor-β1 (TGF-β1), which mediates reticulin, a type III collagen fibril, production by fibroblasts. The type of fibrosis in HCL is summarized in Table 36.1. The fibrosis in HCL is different from the fibrosis in myeloproliferative neoplasm (MPN) in that the fibrosis in MPN comprises predominantly type I and III collagen. The differences of fibrosis in HCL and MPN are listed in Table 36.2 (79).

HCs may be overlooked on H&E histology. A high index of suspicion with IHC stain with CD20 is critical in detecting subtle interstitial HCL infiltrate (Fig. 36.2). Many other IHC stains are helpful in the diagnosis of HCL and will be discussed in immunophenotype (IP) section.

Spleen

Splenomegaly is present in the majority of patients. Although there is a broad range in spleen size, massive splenomegaly with >10 cm below costal margin can occasionally occur. Grossly, the cut surface of spleen is homogeneous and dark red. Microscopically, the cords and sinuses of the red pulp are markedly expanded with diffuse leukemic infiltrate (Fig. 36.3) (13,14,17,19). Sinuses can be dilated and filled with red blood cells, forming so-called blood lakes because HCs adhere to and replace endothelial cells, causing pooling of erythrocytes (Fig. 36.4). Lymphoid follicles of the white pulps are small, atrophic, or completely obliterated. Scattered plasma cells are present in some cases and can be abundant occasionally. Extramedullary megakaryopoiesis can be observed in some patients.

Liver

The liver is frequently involved in HCL. Grossly, the liver is normal or slightly enlarged. The characteristic microscopic finding is sinusoidal and/or portal infiltration (Figs. 36.5 and 36.6)

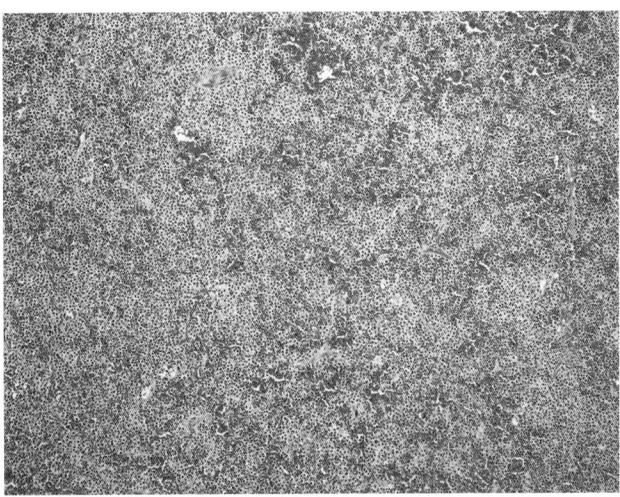

FIGURE 36.3. HCL involving spleen (H&E). At low magnification, the white pulps are obliterated. There is marked congestion of the sinuses and increase in mononucleated cells in the cords and sinuses.

(15,17,19,80). Occasionally, the portal areas and sinuses are dilated and filled with red blood cells creating so-called angiomatous changes with HCs lining the spaces (16,80).

Lymph Node

Peripheral lymph nodes are rarely involved in HCL due to lack of L-selectin (CD62L, necessary for interaction with high endothelial venules, i.e., lymphocyte homing to lymph nodes) and lack of chemokine (C-C motif) receptor 7 (CCR7, necessary for transendothelial migration) as well as lack of CXCR5 (57,81). Mediastinal, abdominal, and/or retroperitoneal lymph nodes may be involved in HCL, especially late in the disease course, with predominantly interfollicular and medullary infiltration pattern (Figs. 36.7 and 36.8) (17,82).

Variants of HCL

A Japanese variant of HCL was described in Japanese population, which shared many overlapping features but also some differences when compared to typical HCL (83–86). The

Table 36.2	DIFFERENCES BETWEEN FIBROSIS IN HCL AND MPN	
Characteristics	MPN	HCL
Cell-producing fibrosis	Megakaryocyte	HCs-FN through FGF-2 Fibroblasts-reticulin through TGF-β1
Type of fibrosis	Type I and III collagen	FN, reticulin (type III collagen)
Number of fibroblasts in BM	Increased	Not significantly increased

HCL, hairy cell leukemia; MPN, myeloproliferative neoplasm.

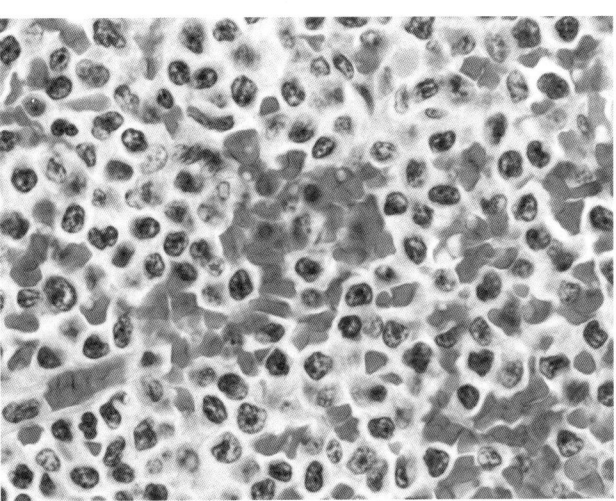

FIGURE 36.4. HCL involving spleen (H&E). At high magnification, the leukemic cells are predominantly in the cords and sinuses. Note that the sinus-lining endothelial cells are replaced by HCs.

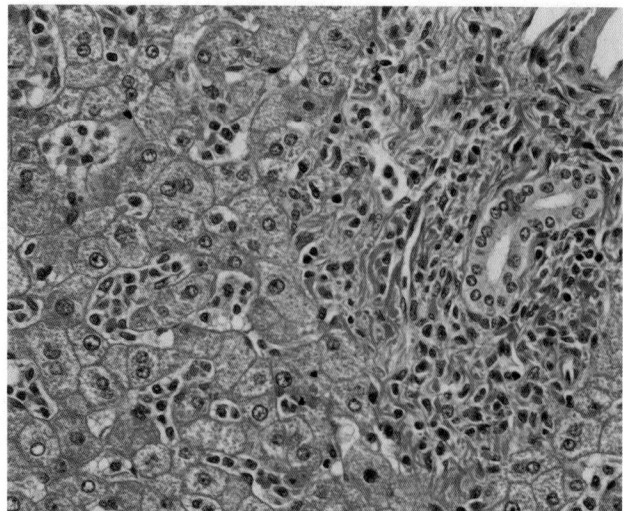

FIGURE 36.5. HCL involving liver (H&E). The infiltrate is present in the portal tract and within sinusoids.

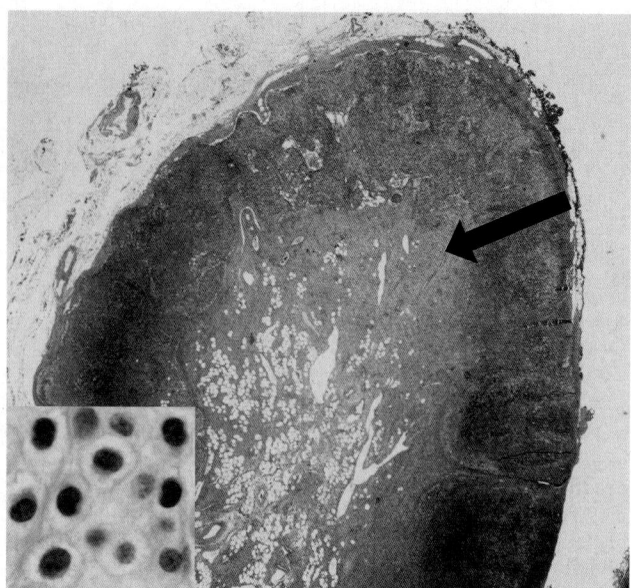

FIGURE 36.7. HCL involving lymph node (H&E). At low magnification, the leukemic cells replace the entire medulla (*arrow*). The cortex is relatively preserved. **Inset:** The leukemic cells at high magnification show well-defined cell border, abundant clear cytoplasm with round or kidney bean–shaped nuclei, creating the so-called fried eggs appearance.

majority of patients have moderate degree of leukocytosis. The leukemic cells show weak TRAP stain and have IP profile of CD5⁻, CD11c⁺, CD22⁺, and CD25⁻. The description of Japanese variant HCL in the literature is at least partially similar to the provisional entity hairy cell leukemia variant (HCLv) in the 2008 WHO Classification of Tumours of Haematopoietic and Lymphoid Tissues (85,87). Whether they represent the same disease or two different entities requires further investigation.

HCL with unique multilobulated nuclei has been described as a multilobular variant of HCL (88,89). The leukemic cells exhibit marked nuclear lobulation, convolution, and clefting, the so-called cloverleaf configuration (Fig. 36.1). The leukemic cells morphologically resemble T-cell lymphoma/leukemia, but the chromatin is finely reticular or "ground-glass," characteristic of HCL. Multilobular variant HCL otherwise has typical morphologic, immunophenotypic, and clinical findings of classic HCL.

HCL with ring-shaped nuclei was observed in a minor subset of leukemic cells in an otherwise typical HCL (90).

Three patients with blastic variant of HCL were described (91). One patient had an aggressive disease course, which is unusual for HCL. One patient had classic indolent HCL disease course and response to pentostatin.

A case of anaplastic neoplasm developed in a patient with HCL was reported (92). It is however unclear if the anaplastic neoplasm was a variant of HCL, transformation to high-grade lymphoma, or coexisting neoplasm but unrelated to HCL. The patient had an aggressive clinical course and expired a few months after the diagnosis of anaplastic neoplasm.

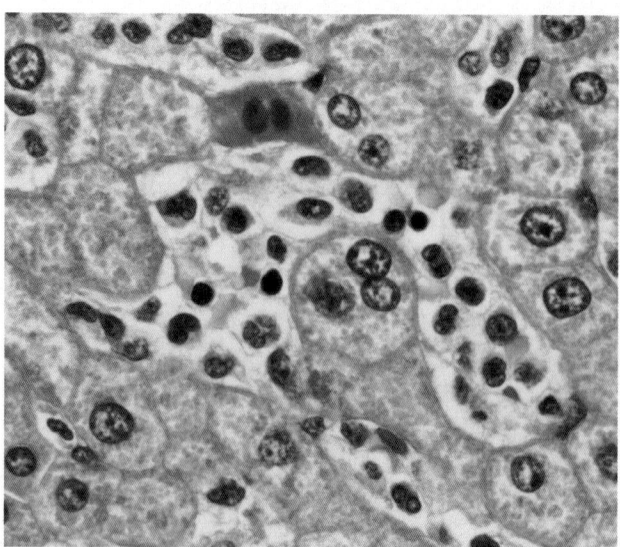

FIGURE 36.6. HCL involving liver (H&E). At higher magnification, the leukemic cells reside in the dilated sinusoids.

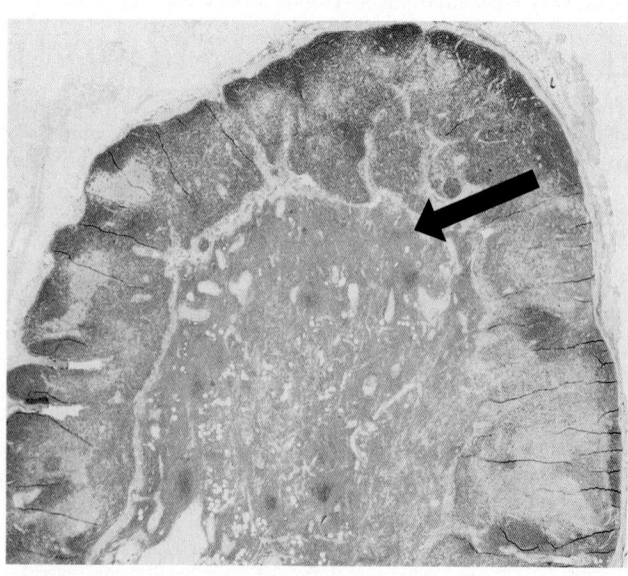

FIGURE 36.8. HCL involving lymph node (CD20 stain). The leukemic cells in the medulla are positive for CD20 (*arrow*). The cortex exhibits preserved lymphoid architecture.

IMMUNOPHENOTYPE

Flow Cytometric IP

Flow cytometry study is diagnostic of HCL. The classic immunophenotypic profile of HCL is bright sIg, bright CD20, bright CD22, and bright CD11c, CD25, and CD103 positivity (Fig. 36.9 Panel A, Table 36.3). The markers are nonspecific when used individually but are diagnostic when combined. HCs are typically negative for CD5, CD10, CD23, and CD38. A minor subset of cases expresses CD10 (93,94). Rare HCL cases with immunophenotypic variation including CD23+, CD103−, or CD25− have been reported (93,95). Comparison of flow cytometric findings of HCL, HCLv, and splenic marginal zone lymphoma (SMZL) is summarized in Table 36.3.

Immunohistochemistry

CD20 is invaluable in the detection of BM involvement by HCL. HCL can easily be overlooked when the BM cellularity is normal and the leukemic infiltrate is limited to the interstitial space. Multiple antibodies have been studied for their expression in HCL as diagnostic IHC markers. Among those, annexin A1 has the highest sensitivity and specificity (34). Annexin A1 is positive in nearly every HCL case and is negative in other B-CLPN cases. The stain is usually strong and is positive in almost all the HCs. When annexin A1 is performed on BM biopsy, one should interpret with caution since myeloid cells and T cells also express annexin A1. Cyclin D1 has high specificity for HCL when mantle cell lymphoma (MCL) and plasma

cell myeloma are excluded. Cyclin D1 is positive in 40% to 100% of HCL cases and is particularly useful to distinguish HCL from HCLv and SMZL (28,36,37). The stain intensity is highly variable with the majority of cases showing weak to moderate nuclear staining. The percent of cells staining for cyclin D1 is also highly variable and ranges from <10% to over 50% (Zhang and Foucar, *unpublished data*). Cyclin D1 positivity in HCL is the result of up-regulation of cyclin D1 expression, possibly secondary to constitutively activated mitogen-activated protein kinase (MAPK) pathway instead of t(11;14) as seen in MCL and subset of plasma cell myelomas. CD123 is also specific for HCL when plasmacytoid dendritic cells and myeloid cells are excluded (96). However, CD123 is only positive in about half of HCL cases. DBA.44 is positive in approximately 70% of HCL cases, and it can be positive in a subset of HCLv and rare cases of SMZL (33,36,97,98). Even in positive cases, DBA.44 typically stains a subset of HCs, and the stain intensity also varies from case to case. TRAP has been in use for decades in the diagnosis of HCL. It is nonspecific and is positive in many other types of B-CLPN, but strong uniform TRAP positivity is characteristic of HCL and unusual in other B-CLPN. Other markers used in HCL include TCL-1, CD25, and T-bet with variable sensitivity and specificity (Zhang and Foucar, *unpublished data*) (50). The characteristics of commonly used antibodies are summarized in Table 36.4 and illustrated in Figure 36.2.

MRD monitoring is best accomplished by flow cytometric analysis. When there is no aspirate for flow, CD20 is the best IHC marker. DBA.44 can also be used in positive cases. Annexin A1 is not suitable for MRD monitoring due to its positivity in myeloid precursors and T lymphocytes.

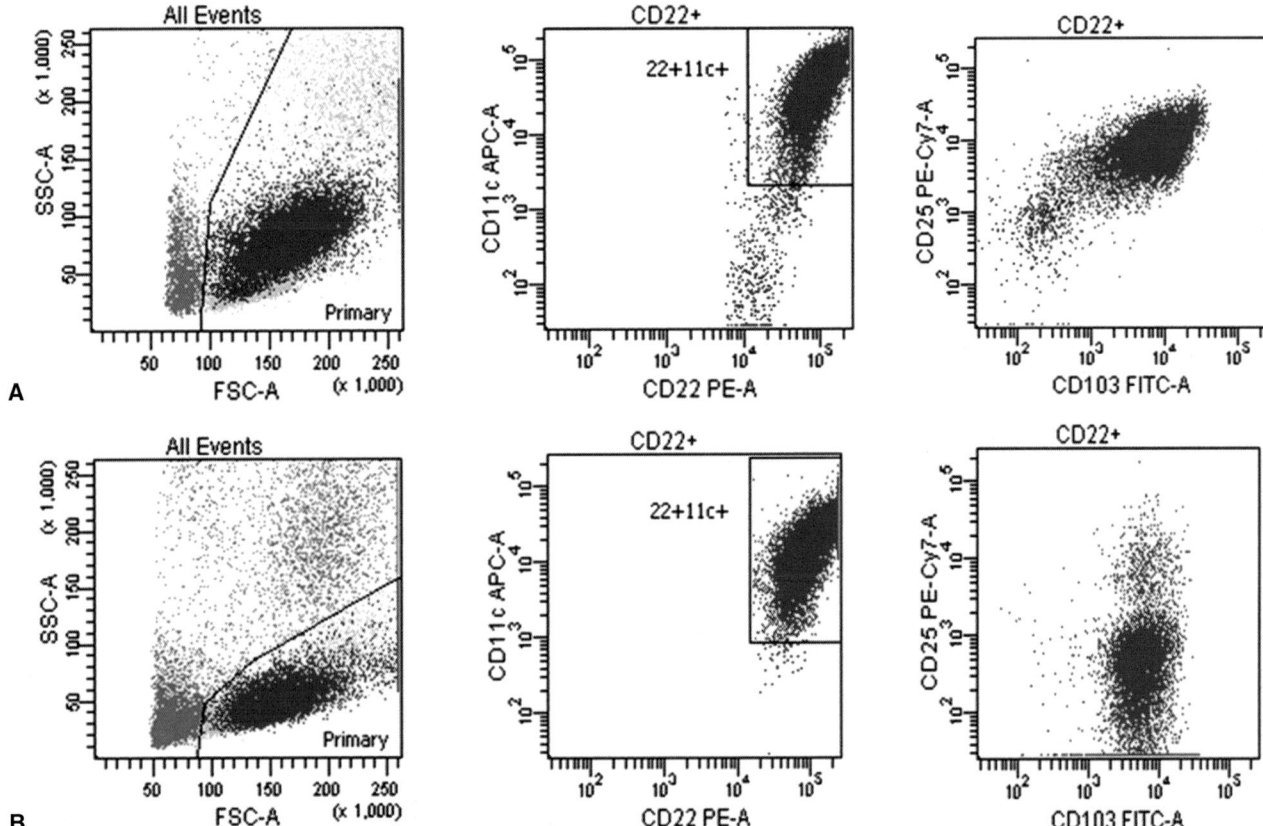

FIGURE 36.9. Flow cytometric analysis of HCL and HCLv. **Panel A** exhibits classic IP profile of HCL with bright CD11c, bright CD22, CD25, and CD103 expression. **Panel B** exhibits typical IP profile of HCLv with bright CD11c, bright CD22, and CD103 expression. CD25 is noticeably absent in the majority of leukemic cells.

	Table 36.3	COMPARISON OF FLOW CYTOMETRIC MARKERS IN HCL, HCLv, AND SMZL				
Antibodies	**Molecule Detected**		**HCL**	**HCLv**	**SMZL**	**Comment/Caveat**
CD20	B-cell marker		+++	+++	++	Bright in HCL and HCLv
CD22	B-cell marker		+++	+++	++	CD22 is bright in HCL and HCLv but moderate in SMZL.
CD11c	Integrin alpha X chain		+++	+++	±	The brightness in HCLv can be indistinguishable from HCL. It can be weak or negative in SMZL.
CD25	IL-2α		++	−	±	CD25 is positive in 64% of SMZL and is usually weaker than HCL. It is not helpful to differentiate HCLv from SMZL when CD25 is negative.
CD103	Integrin alpha E chain		++	±	−	CD103 is positive in 36% of HCLv. It is not helpful to differentiate HCLv from SMZL when CD103 is negative. CD103 is rarely negative in HCL.

IL-2α, interleukin 2 receptor alpha chain.

CYTOGENETICS

HCs have shown many karyotypic abnormalities, but recurrent cytogenetic findings have not been described (99–104). Studies have identified del(7q), abnormality of 14q32, and chromosome 1, 3, 6, 7, 8, 12, 17, 18, and 22 abnormalities. A rare case of HCL with t(11;14)(q13;q32)/*CCND1-IGH@* translocation has been reported recently (105). Overall, the cytogenetic abnormalities are inconsistent and carry no prognostic significance in HCL (82).

MOLECULAR CHARACTERISTICS

Somatic hypermutation (SHM) of the Ig heavy chain (*IGVH@*) locus and the usage of *IgH* variable region (*VH*) have been extensively studied in HCL (106–113). HCL displays SHM in approximately 80% of cases, indicating that the cells have gone through affinity maturation with SHM and isotype switch from IgM to IgG, IgA, and IgD. Evidence has suggested that there are two pathways cells that could gain SHM and isotype switch. The major pathway is a T-cell–dependent process that occurs at the germinal center (GC). A minor pathway is T-cell independent and occurs outside GC, probably in the marginal zone (113–115). It is postulated that SHM and isotype switch of HCs may have occurred at extrafollicular sites based on the preferential *VH* gene usage and T-cell immune response studies (108,113).

VH usage studies by several teams (106,109,113,116) demonstrated that the majority of HCLs have preferential use of

VH3, followed by *VH4*, and less frequently *VH1, VH2, VH5* families. The *VH* gene usage is associated with mutation status. HCLs using *VH3* gene family are frequently heavily mutated. HCLs using *VH2* are slightly mutated, while HCLs using *VH4* gene family tend to have higher unmutated rate (113). *VH* usage is also linked to prognosis; specifically, *VH4-34* positive cases, although rare in HCL, are associated with higher WBC count, lower treatment response rate, lower disease progression–free rate, and lower overall survival rate (109). In contrary to HCL, *VH4-34* is frequently used by HCLv (106,109,117).

HCL shows preferential expression of IgG, particularly IgG3 (118). Interestingly, 40% of HCL cases express simultaneously multiple clonally related Ig isotypes such as IgM, IgG, and IgA (8,81,108,119). The finding is suggestive that HCs may have arrested at the point of isotype switch prior to deletional recombination (119).

Oncogene *BRAF* mutation is found in approximately 30% of all human cancers (120–127). *BRAF* V600E mutation on exon 15 is the most common *BRAF* mutation and is present in solid tumors such as melanoma, thyroid carcinoma, lung cancer, and colorectal adenocarcinoma. Tiacci et al. (128) have recently identified *BRAF* V600E mutation in all 38 HCL cases studied through whole exome sequencing. The finding was independently confirmed by Boyd et al. (129) using high-resolution melting analysis. Studies also demonstrated that *BRAF* V600E mutation is present in a subset of Langerhans cell histiocytosis, rare cases of acute myeloid leukemia, and plasma cell myeloma but is not present in other B-CLPN (128–135). This mutation represents the first disease defining mutation

	Table 36.4	PROPERTIES AND UTILITIES OF IHC MARKERS IN HCL AND B-NHL			
Antibody	**Staining Pattern**	**Molecules Detecting**	**Cell Types Positive**	**Notes**	**Caveats**
CD20	Membrane	Pan B-cell marker	Mature B cells	Critical in detecting marrow involvement by HCL	Positive in all benign B cells and B-LPD
Annexin A1	Cytoplasmic	Involves in phagocytosis	HCL, myeloid, T cells	Sensitive and specific for HCL, not suitable for MRD	Difficult to interpret when the involvement is at low level
DBA.44	Membrane and cytoplasmic	Unknown	HCL, HCLv, subset MZL	Valuable in MRD	May be positive in HCLv and rare MZL
TRAP	Cytoplasmic	Isoenzyme of acid phosphatase	HCL, other B-LPD	Diffuse strong stain highly compatible with HCL	May be positive in other B-LPDs
Cyclin D1	Nuclear	Controls cell cycle	MCL, plasma cell myeloma, HCL	Expression of cyclin D1 in HCL is not related to t(11;14).[a]	Positive in subset of HCs. Stain is usually weak. Negative in HCLv or SMZL
CD123	Membrane and cytoplasmic	IL-3α	Plasmacytoid dendritic cells, many types of normal myeloid cells, AML, HCL	Rarely expressed in other B-PLD	Useful in differentiating HCL from other B-LPD
TCL-1	Cytoplasmic	Oncogene	Naïve B cells, plasmacytoid dendritic cells, T-cell leukemias and lymphomas, AML	Expressed in many types of B-LPD#	Not specific

[a]A single case of HCL with t(11;14)(q13;q32)/CCND1-IGH@ translocation was reported recently.
IL-3α, interlukine-3 receptor alpha chain; B-LPD, B-cell lymphoproliferative disorder.

for a B-CLPN (136). The *BRAF* mutation leads to constitutive activation of the RAF-MEK-ERK-MAPK pathway, which likely plays a critical role in HCL pathogenesis (128,136,137). The fact that *BRAF* V600E is not present in HCLv or *IGVH4-34*–positive HCLs is suggestive that HCLv and *IGVH4-34*–positive HCLs may have different pathogenesis than HCL (135).

The *BRAF* V600E mutation not only lends a reliable molecular tool for the diagnosis of HCL, it may also have potential implications in disease monitoring and for therapeutic development of new targeted agent for the treatment of HCL (128–132,134,135).

HCL AND THE MICROENVIRONMENT

The cross talk of HCL and the microenvironment plays critical roles in tissue distribution, localization, motility, and survival of HCL (82,138). For example, HCs produce integrin heterodimer $\alpha_4\beta_1$, which, in concert with its ligand VCAM, results in the propensity of localization of HCs in the BM, spleen, and liver, where VCAM is abundant. The interaction of $\alpha_4\beta_1$ with VCAM may also play a role in blood lake formation in the spleen (138). Vitronectin (VN) is abundant in spleen and, through interaction with $\alpha_V\beta_3$, likely plays a role in splenic homing of the HCs. The interaction of stromal HA with its receptor CD44 on the HCs can stimulate HC production of autocrine FGF-2, which in turn enhances production of FN by HCs, resulting in fibrosis. Integrin engagement by FN or VN may protect HCs from the killing of interferon via preventing apoptosis, enhancing survival of HCs. The interaction of CXCR4 and VLA with marrow stromal ligands CXCR12, VCAM1, and FN, respectively, may induce cell adhesion–mediated drug resistance, which may account for MRD after conventional therapy (139). HCL is known to cause T-cell dysfunction. The interaction of CD40 of HCs with its ligand CD154 of T cells may promote disease progression (139). The signaling cytokines, adhesion molecules, and their receptors and ligands are summarized in Table 36.5.

Table 36.5	HCL-RELATED SIGNALING PATHWAYS AND CYTOKINES		
	Cytokine/Cytokine Receptor/ Adhesion Molecule/Ligand	**Expression Level**	**Function**
Molecules related to oncogenesis	PKCε	Increased	Possible roles in oncogenesis of HCL
	ERK1-2		
	Rac		
	ROS		
Molecules related to survival	BCL2	Increased	Antiapoptosis
	Cyclin D1	Increased	Proliferation
	p27	Decreased	Proliferation inhibition
	p38-MAPK	Decreased	Apoptosis
	MEK	Increased	Proliferation
Molecules related to tissue distribution	TIMP1,4, RECK thrombospondin1	Increased	Propensity of HC to stay in blood-related compartments
	$\alpha4\beta1$ (CD49d), $\alpha5\beta1$ (CD49e)/ VCAM-1	Increased	Propensity of HC to stay in VCAM-1–rich organs such as the BM, spleen, and liver. It may also play a role in splenic blood lake formation.
	CXCR4 and VLA-4	Increased	Critical for migration, adhesion of HCs, retention of normal hematopoietic progenitors in the BM
	$\alpha_V\beta_3$ (CD51)/VN and PECAM-1 (CD31)	Increased	Important in HC motility. It plays a role in splenic red pulp infiltration, where VN is abundant.
Molecules related to fibrosis	CD44/HA	Increased	Stimulate FGF production, which in turn enhances HC production of FN, hence fibrosis. HA is abundant in the BM and portal tracts but absent in spleen red pulp and hepatic sinusoids.
	TGF-β1	Increased	Stimulate production of reticulin by fibroblasts. Inhibit normal hematopoiesis. Along with IL-10, it also suppresses the immune function of T cells and monocytes.
Molecules related to homing to LN	L-selectin (CD62L)	Decreased	Adhesion to high endothelial venules in LN
	CXCR5 (BLR1 or Burkitt lymphoma receptor 1)	Decreased	Homing to lymphoid follicles
	CCR7	Decreased	Entry of lymphocytes to LN
	TNFSH11 (RANK-ligand)	Decreased	LN development
	ICAM 3	Decreased	Migration of leukocytes to inflammation site
Molecules related to HC morphology and phenotype	CD9	Increased	Expression inversely correlates with metastasis to LN, contribute to hairy projection formation
	GAS7	Increased	Neurite growth, may play a role in hairy projection formation
	Beta-actin	Increased	Supports the filamentous membrane projections
	pp52	Increased	AKA leukocyte–specific intracellular phosphoprotein, which binds to F-actin and colocalized in hairy projections
	EPB4.IL2	Increased	Help to maintain the shape and structural integrity of cell membrane
	$\alpha_M\beta_2$ (CD11b)	Increased	Important for HCL IP
	$\alpha_X\beta_2$ (CD11c)		
	$\alpha_E\beta_7$ (CD103)		
Molecules related to phagocytosis	Annexin A1	Increased	Serves as mediator
	TRAP		
	Macrophage colony–stimulating factor receptor		
	CD11c		
	CD68		
	MAF		

PKCε, protein kinase Cε; ERK, extracellular signal related kinase; ROS, reactive oxygen species; MAP, mitogen-activated protein; HC, hairy cell; LN, lymph node; VCAM, vascular cell adhesion molecule; FN, fibronectin; VN, vitronectin; PECAM, platelet endothelial cell adhesion molecule; HA, hyaluronan; FGF, fibroblast growth factor; bFGF, basic fibroblast growth factor; FGFR, fibroblast growth factor receptor.

POSTULATED NORMAL COUNTERPART

The cell of origin of HCL is still under intense scrutiny. Multiple theories exist in terms of the exact B-cell subset from which HCL originates.

Basso et al. (57) have demonstrated that HCL is more closely related to memory B cells than to GCs or naïve B cells by gene expression profiling. The study also revealed alteration of expression of multiple chemokines and adhesion receptors related to HC survival, leukemic cell distribution, and *in vitro* phagocytosis properties. Most notably, cytokines related to lymph node organogenesis and homing of B lymphocytes to the lymph nodes are not expressed or down-regulated. Genes related to adhesion molecules are expressed in HCL. Genes coding for cytokines, which are possibly related to hairy projection formation, are overexpressed. The characteristics of the chemokines and adhesion molecules are also summarized in Table 36.5.

VH mutation pattern and usage studies demonstrated that HCL is distinctive from that of normal blood lymphocytes, MCL, or chronic lymphocytic leukemia (CLL)/small lymphocytic lymphoma (SLL). They best resemble that of extranodal marginal zone lymphoma of mucosa-associated lymphoid tissue (MALT) lymphoma or reactive marginal zone B cells, suggesting a marginal zone origin. Studies also show that HCs originate from antigen-experienced B cells that have undergone affinity maturation (110,113).

Comparative expressed sequence hybridization study of HCL (140) reveals that the imprint of spleen signatures, including splenic-specific components such as the sinusoidal lining cells of the red pulp and marginal zone B cells of the white pulp, was found in HCL expression profile. Therefore, it was suggested that HCs could potentially originate from the splenic marginal zone.

HCs express an activated B-cell profile: CD25+, CD11c+, CD103+, CD23-, and CD27-. Marafioti et al. (141) demonstrated that interfollicular large cells express a similar IP as HCs (CD23-, CD27-, and CD38-) and therefore raise the possibility that HCL may originate from these cells.

Analysis of PB also identified a minor subset of CD27- B cells as a potential cell of origin for HCL (50,142,143).

Although the precise subset of B cells that HCL originates from is still under debate, it is clear that HCs have an activated B-cell profile and have gone through affinity maturation with SHM and isotype switch.

CLINICAL COURSE AND PROGNOSTIC ASSESSMENT

HCL is an indolent disease with long survival when treated appropriately. Frassoldati et al. (54) studied 725 HCL cases over 25 years in Italy and found that the survival rates at 5 and 10 years are 34.4% and 29.6% for untreated patients. Spontaneous regression of the disease has been documented in rare cases (144). Transformation of HCL into high-grade lymphoma is exceedingly rare and is only unequivocally confirmed on rare case reports (145,146).

Some patients develop unusual complications during the course of their illness, such as gastric submucosal infiltration by HCs with secondary protein–losing enteropathy, spinal cord compression with paralysis, esophageal perforation with fistula tract, and massive ascites and pleural effusion with typical HCs present in ascites and pleural fluid (60). Mucormycosis infection (147) and mycobacterial infections can develop during the disease course (148).

Prognosis assessment should include the status of BM and spleen, that is, the presence of cytopenia, splenomegaly, and abdominal lymphadenopathy as well as response to purine analog treatment. Patients with significant cytopenia, organomegaly, abdominal lymphadenopathy, and partial instead of complete response to purine analog treatment have a poor prognosis (149). In the long-term follow-up conducted by Else et al. (150), response to treatment is the most significant variable associated with relapse-free survival, followed by hemoglobin level and platelet count. HCL with unmutated *IGHV@* appears to respond poorly to purine analogs (151). A subset of cases with *VH4-34* gene usage tends to be resistant to chemotherapy and carries a poor prognosis (109).

TREATMENT AND SURVIVAL

HCL patients are usually managed conservatively. The recommendation to initiate treatment includes cytopenia, symptomatic splenomegaly, or constitutional symptoms such as fever, fatigue, and night sweats. The first-line treatment is single-agent purine analog cladribine or pentostatin. Both are highly effective and induce long-term remission in the majority of patients. A long-term follow-up study has shown that there is no difference in outcome between the two agents (150). Although used historically as mainstay treatment, splenectomy is used nowadays only in rare patients with severe refractory thrombocytopenia or very significant splenomegaly. INF-α is no longer a mainstay of treatment for HCL.

Five-year survival rate before 1985 was about 59%. The 5-year survival rate for patients receiving interferon treatment was 88.9% (54). The overall and progression-free survival has improved substantially with cladribine or pentostatin treatment; the overall response rate is 97% and the CR rate is 80% with a median relapse-free survival of 16 years (150,152–155). The overall survival 15 years after first treatment is 96% (150). Despite successful treatment in the majority patients, the relapse rate is estimated at 30% to 45% after 5 to 10 years follow-up; substantial MRD is responsible for the majority of relapses (150,156). Monoclonal anti-CD20 antibody rituximab in combination with purine analog may have added benefit to eradicate residual disease in patients with partial response (52). Rituximab is also effective in refractory or relapsed cases when combined with purine analogs (50).

The rate of second malignancies is uncertain and varies according to different studies (155,157–159). A study conducted by Hisada et al. followed 3,104 HCL patients from 2 months to 29.3 years and found that the accumulative probability of all second cancer is estimated at 31.9% 25 years after HCL diagnosis. Non-Hodgkin lymphomas are the leading secondary malignancy, followed by Hodgkin lymphoma, thyroid cancer, and other solid organ cancers (160). In a different study conducted by Frassoldati et al. (54), the secondary malignant rate is 3.7% with most cases detected several years after the onset of HCL. Large organized studies are needed to further define the second malignancy rate in HCL.

DIFFERENTIAL DIAGNOSIS

The main differential diagnosis of HCL includes HCLv, splenic diffuse red pulp small B-cell lymphoma (SRPL), and SMZL. B-cell prolymphocytic leukemia (B-PLL) sometimes comes into differential diagnosis. PB morphology, BM infiltration pattern, and IP are usually sufficient to distinguish HCL from CLL, MCL, and lymphoplasmacytic lymphoma (LPL).

HCLv is listed as a provisional entity in the 2008 WHO Classification and is biologically different from HCL (87). Both HCL and HCLv can manifest with splenomegaly. Several features can be helpful to distinguish HCL from HCLv. HCLv usually exhibits lymphocytosis in the PB, while leukopenia is more typical in

HCL. There is also no monocytopenia in HCLv. The morphology of HCLv leukemic cells is variable, ranging from medium-sized cells with hairy projection, which are indistinguishable from HCs, to large cells with high nuclear/cytoplasmic ratio and prominent nucleoli. BM infiltration pattern in HCLv is typically interstitial and intrasinusoidal, which is indistinguishable from HCL. HCLv can also exhibit exclusive intrasinusoidal infiltration (87,161). Flow cytometric IP can be helpful in that HCLv is typically negative for CD25 (Fig. 36.9 Panel B). IHC stains are also helpful in distinguishing HCL from HCLv. HCLv is negative for annexin A1 and cyclin D1. The PB, BM, and IHC findings of HCLv are illustrated in Figure 36.10. Splenectomy is rarely done for straightforward classic HCL. It is occasionally performed when the diagnosis is not definitive or to relieve symptoms related to splenomegaly. In the spleen, HCLv demonstrates red pulp infiltration pattern, identical to HCL (Fig. 36.11). By molecular study, HCLv has different molecular signature than HCL with more frequent usage of *VH4*, particularly *VH4-34* and high unmutated *IGHV@* rate (116).

SRPL is another provisional entity in the 2008 WHO Classification. It shares many overlapping features with HCL. Although SRPL shows frequent expression of CD22, CD11c, and variable CD103 by flow cytometric analysis, CD25 is often negative. SRPL is negative for annexin A1 and cyclin D1 by IHC stains, which is different from HCL. SRPL may exhibit polar villi in a subset of cells in the PB, similar to SMZL. However, SMZL is often positive for CD25 and is usually negative for CD103 by flow cytometric analysis. SMZL is also frequently negative for DBA.44 by IHC, while SRPL is frequently positive. SMZL exhibits frequent usage of *IGHV1-2* families, while SRPL reveals frequent usage of *IGHV4-34*. SMZL and SRPL also show markedly differences in spleen infiltration pattern. SRPL primarily involves red pulp and SMZL white pulp. SRPL is very closely reminiscent of HCLv in many aspects including clinical presentation, PB, BM and spleen morphology, IP, and

molecular signature (117,162–164). There are no clear criteria to separate SRPL and HCLv currently. It is still under intense debate whether SRPL and HCLv represent a single entity or two different diseases.

SMZL may or may not have PB involvement. SMZL usually exhibits lymphocytosis when blood is involved. The lymphoma cells typically have abundant pale blue cytoplasm and are occasionally bipolar. Hairy projections may be present in rare cells (Fig. 36.12). Although only partially encircling the cells, the hairy projections raise the differential diagnosis of HCL. There is no monocytopenia in SMZL. BM biopsy exhibits a mixed pattern of lymphoid aggregates (the dominant pattern) and interstitial and intrasinusoidal infiltration. Flow cytometric study is helpful in that SMZL is typically negative for CD103. CD25 is positive in a subset of SMZL. CD11c expression can be positive or negative in SMZL. When positive, expression of CD11c is usually weak. The expression of CD20, CD22, and CD11c is typically weaker in SMZL than in HCL. Rare SMZL cases can be positive for CD103 by flow or DBA.44 by IHC. The findings and differential diagnosis of HCL, HCLv, and SMZL are summarized in Table 36.6.

B-PLL characteristically presents with rapidly raising, marked lymphocytosis in the PB. The cells have variable but usually abundant cytoplasm with frequent fine cytoplasmic vacuoles encircling the outer rim of cytoplasm (Fig. 36.13). The cells do not exhibit hairy projections. The majority of cells have prominent nucleoli. By flow cytometric immunophenotyping, cases of B-PLL are typically CD5 and CD10 negative, lacking the distinctive IP profile of HCL.

LPL typically exhibits a spectrum of small lymphocytes, plasmacytoid lymphocytes, and plasma cells on blood and BM aspirate smears (Fig. 36.14A,B). There may be rouleaux on PB smear, and BM aspirate smears typically exhibit increased mast cells. Patients usually have monoclonal paraprotein on serum or urine protein electrophoresis and immunofixation.

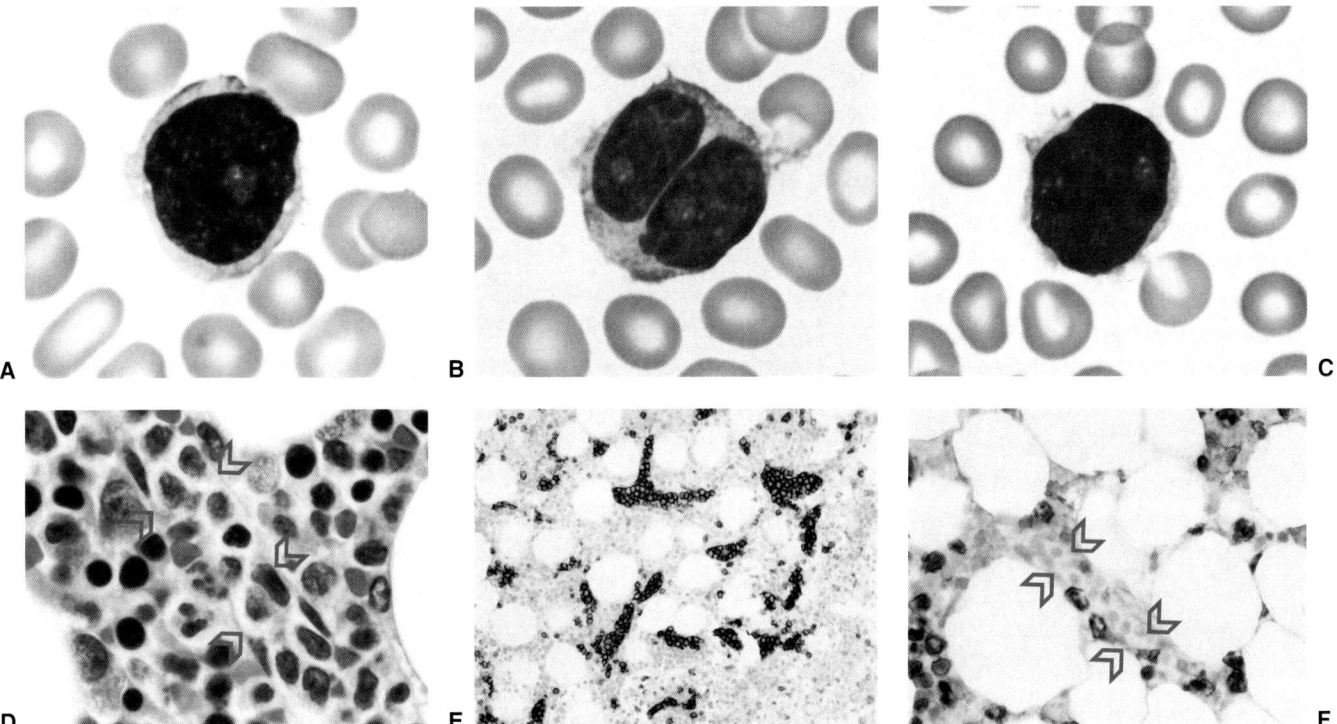

FIGURE 36.10. HCLv typically presents with lymphocytosis in the PB (A-C, Wright stain). The cells are often larger with higher nuclear/cytoplasmic ratio than HCL. Prominent nucleoli and binucleation are common. The cells can have scant to abundant pale blue cytoplasm with hairy projections. BM H&E exhibits diffuse interstitial infiltrate, identical to HCL. Intrasinusoidal infiltrate can be prominent (between *arrowheads*, **D**), which is obvious on CD20 stain (**E**). Annexin A1 stain is negative in the intrasinusoidal leukemic cells (between *arrowheads*) but positive in myeloid precursors (**F**).

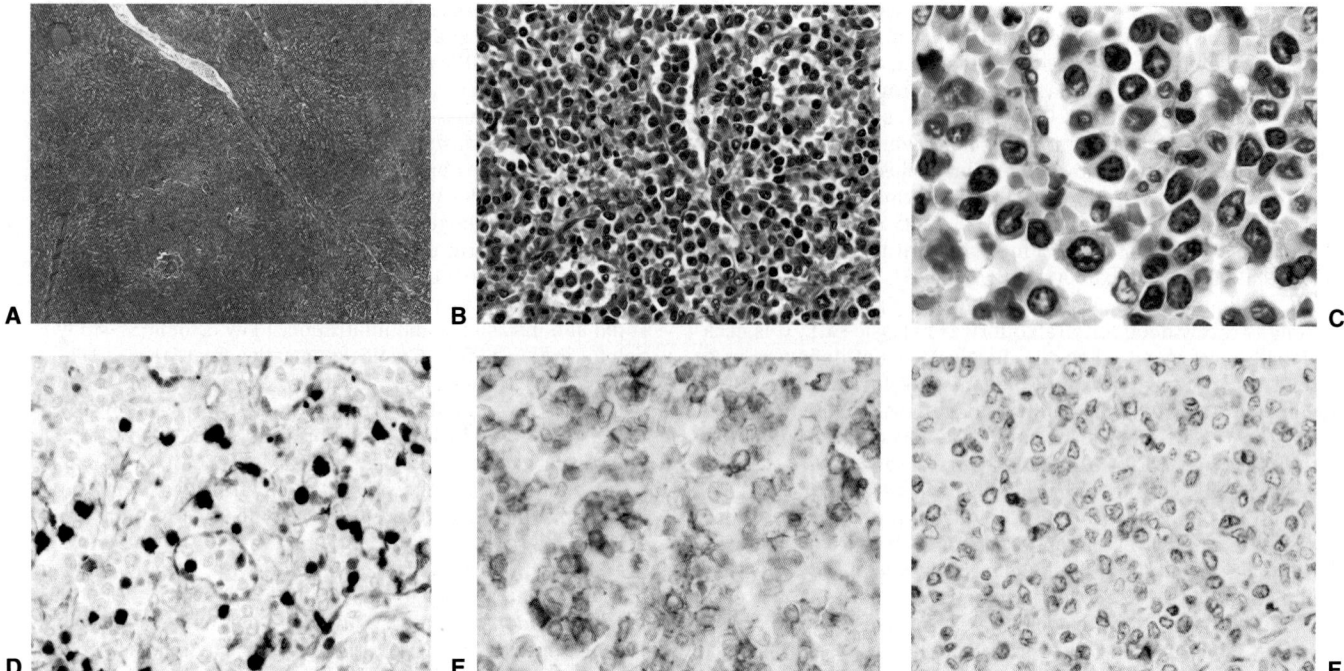

FIGURE 36.11. The spleen involved in HCLv exhibits diffuse red pulp infiltrate, similar to HCL (A, H&E). The leukemic cells frequently exhibit intrasinusoidal infiltration pattern (**B**, H&E). The leukemic cells are large with moderate to abundant cytoplasm, slightly vesicular chromatin, and often prominent nucleoli (**C**, H&E). HCLv leukemic cells are negative for annexin A1, while the T cells are positive for annexin A1 (**D**). DBA.44 and TRAP are frequently positive in HCLv (**E and F**, respectively).

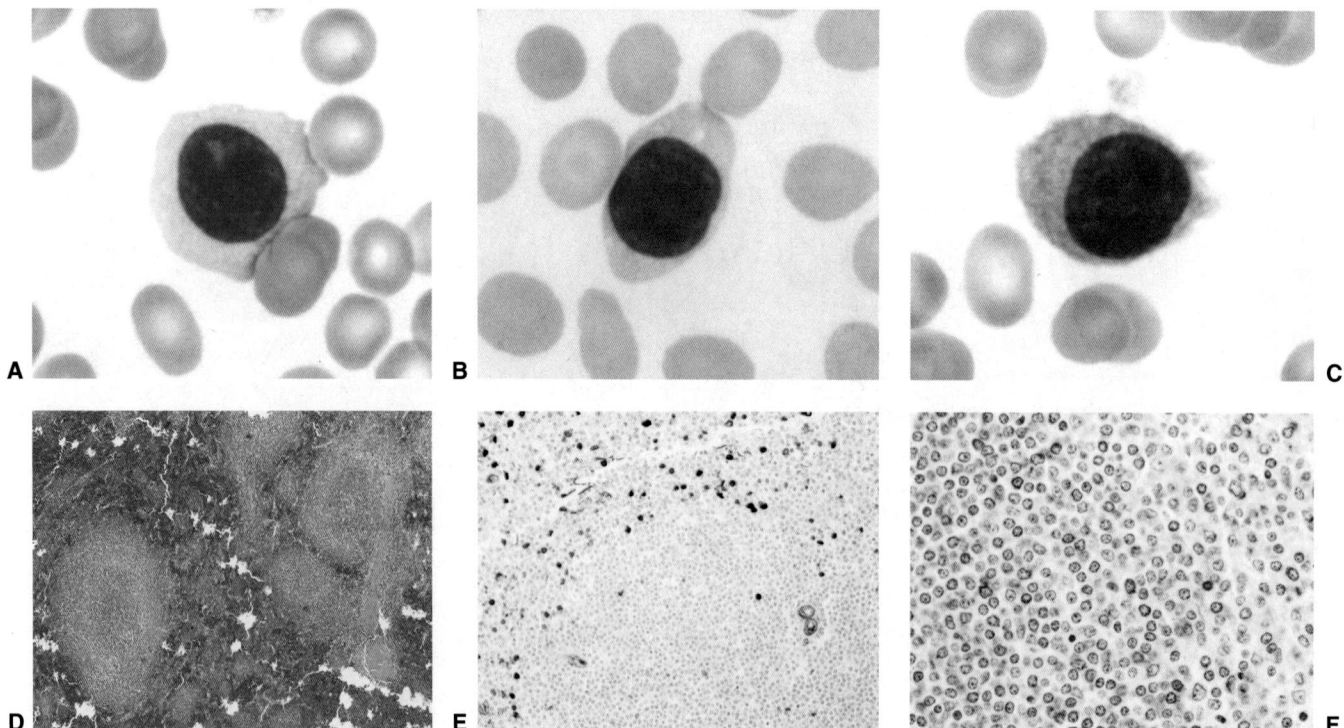

FIGURE 36.12. Splenic marginal zone lymphoma. SMZL lymphoma cell may assume various morphologies in the PB (**A-C**, Wright stain). The cells can have moderate to abundant pale blue to slight magenta cytoplasm with smooth, slightly rugged, or hairy borders. Characteristic bipolar cells (**B**) may or may not be present. The spleen H&E exhibits prominent white pulp expansion (**D**). Annexin A1 is negative in the neoplastic cells but positive in the scattered T cell. TRAP reveals positive cytoplasmic granular positivity (**F**). DBA.44 is negative in the lymphoma cells (not shown).

Table 36.6	DIFFERENTIAL DIAGNOSIS OF HCL, HCLv, AND SMZL		
	HCL	**HCLv**	**SMZL**
Clinical features	Patients in their 50s, male predominance	60s, slight male predominance	50–60s, male = female
PB	Cytopenia, monocytopenia	Lymphocytosis, medium to large cells, may have high N/C ratio and prominent nucleoli	Lymphocytosis common
BM pattern of infiltration	Diffuse interstitial infiltration, gradually patchy then solid sheets with increasing involvement; can have sinusoidal infiltration	Diffuse interstitial and sinusoidal infiltration; can have interstitial infiltration and lymphoid aggregates	Majority cases mixed interstitial, sinusoidal infiltration, and lymphoid aggregates
Spleen pattern of infiltration	Cords and sinuses of the red pulp	Cords and sinuses of the red pulp	White pulp
Flow	CD22+/CD11c+/CD25+/CD103+	CD22+/CD11c+/CD25−/CD103+	CD22+/CD11c+/CD25±/CD103−
IHC	Annexin A1+/TRAP+/DBA.44+/cyclin D1+/CD123+	Annexin A1−/TRAP±/DBA.44±/cyclin D1−/CD123−	Annexin A1−/TRAP±/DBA.44−/cyclin D1−/CD123−
VH mutation/sage	Majority mutated/*VH3* most common	Frequently unmutated/*VH4-34* common	Majority mutated/*VH1-2* common
Cytogenetic abnormality	No recurrent abnormality; abnormality of chromosome 5,7 described	No recurrent abnormality	Del7q31-32 in 40% cases
Treatment of choice	Purine analog	Rituximab and anti-CD22 immunotoxin	Splenectomy
Clinical course and prognosis	Excellent with long-term survival	Indolent with long-term survival	Indolent with long-term survival

BM biopsy exhibits diffuse interstitial infiltration of small lymphocytes, plasmacytoid lymphocytes, and plasma cells. Lymphoid aggregates are rare. Flow cytometric study reveals a CD5−, CD10− monoclonal B-cell population as well as a monotypic plasma cell population. The lymphoma cells do not have the typical HCL IP profile by flow and are negative for annexin A1, cyclin D1, DBA.44, and CD123 by IHC.

SUMMARY AND CONCLUSIONS

HCL is an indolent B-cell lymphoproliferative disorder (B-LPD) arising from activated B cells. Patients usually present with cytopenia-related signs and symptoms, especially infections.

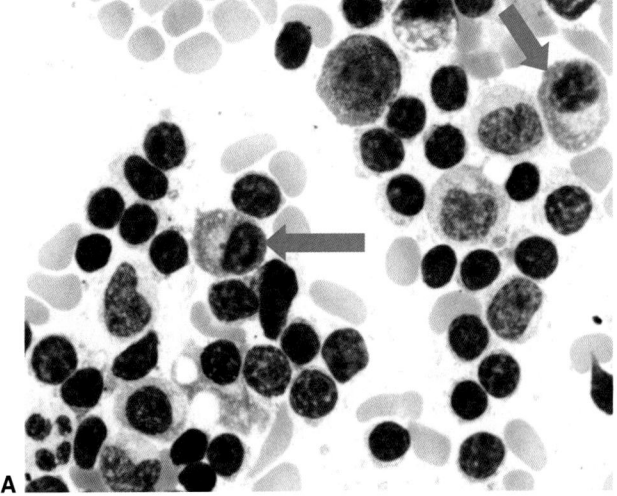

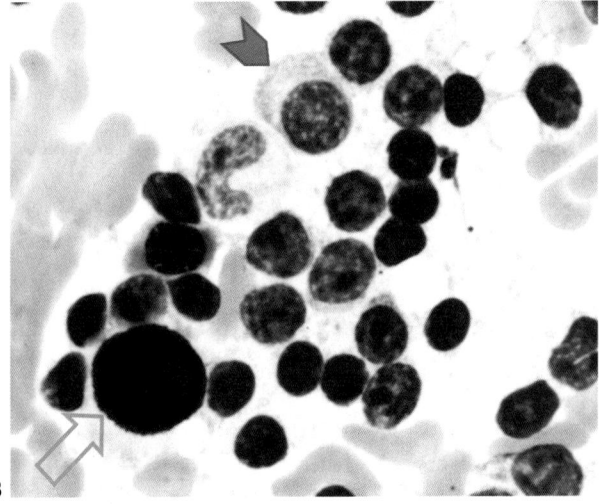

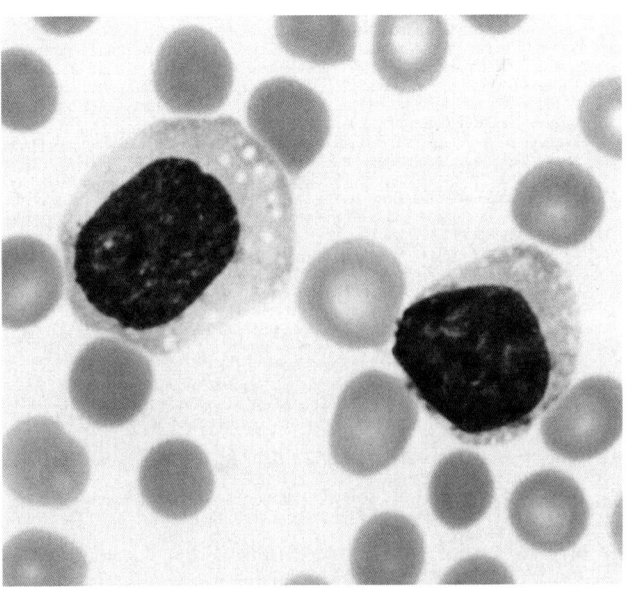

FIGURE 36.13. B-PLL usually presents with marked lymphocytosis with rapidly raising lymphocyte count in the PB (Wright stain). The cells have moderate to frequently abundant pale cytoplasm and often fine cytoplasmic vacuoles at the peripheral of the cytoplasm. Prominent nucleoli are often seen.

FIGURE 36.14. LPL exhibits characteristic spectrum of small lymphocytes, plasmacytoid lymphocytes, and plasma cells in BM aspirate smear (Wright stain). Plasma cells (thin arrows) (**A**). Plasmacytoid lymphocyte (arrowhead) and increased mast cells (open arrow) (**B**).

HCL has been successfully treated with single-agent purine analog with a 96% overall survival at 15 years after first treatment. The diagnosis can be straightforward if flow cytometric study of the blood or BM aspirate demonstrates the classic IP profile, that is, bright CD20+, bright CD22+, bright CD11c+, CD25+, and CD103+, and BM core biopsy reveals typical diffuse interstitial infiltrate. However, diagnosis can be challenging when the marrow is inaspirable. IHC stains with CD20, annexin A1, DBA.44, TRAP, cyclin D1, and CD123 are helpful. There are no recurrent clonal cytogenetic abnormalities in HCL. Molecular and genomic studies have shown that HCs are derived from activated B cells, and the majority of cases have mutated *IGVH@* genes. HCL has preferential usage of *VH3* gene family. Recent *BRAF* mutation studies have demonstrated an exon 15 mutation, which resulted in a *BRAF* V600E variant protein in HCL. This mutation may play a role in HCL pathogenesis. It may have value in the diagnosis and disease monitoring and may serve as a potential target in the treatment of HCL.

References

1. Bouroncle BA, Wiseman BK, Doan CA. Leukemic reticuloendotheliosis. *Blood* 1958;13:609–630.
2. Golomb HM, Leatherman E, Rosner MC. Hairy cell leukemia: differences in phagocytic capacity of cells in vitro. *Virchows Arch B Cell Pathol Incl Mol Pathol* 1979;30:1–13.
3. De Panfilis G, Manara GC, Ferrari C, et al. Hairy cell leukemia cells express CD1a antigen. *Cancer* 1988;61:52–57.
4. Fu SM, Winchester RJ, Rai KR, et al. Hairy cell leukemia: proliferation of a cell with phagocytic and B-lymphocyte properties. *Scand J Immunol* 1974;3:847–851.
5. Alexander E, Sanders S. Fc receptor bearing 'hairy cells' of leukaemic reticuloendotheliosis bind soluble antigen—antibody complexes and adhere to immobilized complexes, but fail to mediate antibody dependent cellular cytotoxicity. *Scand J Immunol* 1978;8:477–488.
6. Schrek R, Donnelly WJ. "Hairy" cells in blood in lymphoreticular neoplastic disease and "flagellated" cells of normal lymph nodes. *Blood* 1966;27:199–211.
7. Catovsky D, Pettit JE, Galetto J, et al. The B-lymphocyte nature of the hairy cell of leukaemic reticuloendotheliosis. *Br J Haematol* 1974;26:29–37.
8. Burns GF, Cawley JC, Worman CP, et al. Multiple heavy chain isotypes on the surface of the cells of hairy cell leukemia. *Blood* 1978;52:1132–1147.
9. Jansen J, Schuit HR, van Zwet TL, et al. Hairy-cell leukaemia: a B-lymphocytic disorder. *Br J Haematol* 1979;42:21–33.
10. Jansen J, Schuit HR, Meijer CJ, et al. Cell markers in hairy cell leukemia studied in cells from 51 patients. *Blood* 1982;59:52–60.
11. Korsmeyer SJ, Greene WC, Cossman J, et al. Rearrangement and expression of immunoglobulin genes and expression of Tac antigen in hairy cell leukemia. *Proc Natl Acad Sci U S A* 1983;80:4522–4526.
12. Cleary ML, Wood GS, Warnke R, et al. Immunoglobulin gene rearrangements in hairy cell leukemia. *Blood* 1984;64:99–104.
13. Golomb HM, Vardiman JW. Response to splenectomy in 65 patients with hairy cell leukemia: an evaluation of spleen weight and bone marrow involvement. *Blood* 1983;61:349–352.
14. Burke JS, Rappaport H. The diagnosis and differential diagnosis of hairy cell leukemia in bone marrow and spleen. *Semin Oncol* 1984;11:334–346.
15. Yam LT, Janckila AJ, Chan CH, et al. Hepatic involvement in hairy cell leukemia. *Cancer* 1983;51:1497–1504.
16. Roquet ML, Zafrani ES, Farcet JP, et al. Histopathological lesions of the liver in hairy cell leukemia: a report of 14 cases. *Hepatology* 1985;5:496–500.
17. Vardiman JW, Golomb HM. Autopsy findings in hairy cell leukemia. *Semin Oncol* 1984;11:370–380.
18. Pilon VA, Davey FR, Gordon GB, et al. Splenic alterations in hairy-cell leukemia: II. an electron microscopic study. *Cancer* 1982;49:1617–1623.
19. Nanba K, Soban EJ, Bowling MC, et al. Splenic pseudosinuses and hepatic angiomatous lesions. Distinctive features of hairy cell leukemia. *Am J Clin Pathol* 1977;67:415–426.
20. Katayama I, Yang JP. Reassessment of a cytochemical test for differential diagnosis of leukemic reticuloendotheliosis. *Am J Clin Pathol* 1977;68:268–272.
21. Burke JS. The value of the bone-marrow biopsy in the diagnosis of hairy cell leukemia. *Am J Clin Pathol* 1978;70:876–884.
22. Variakojis D, Vardiman JW, Golomb HM. Cytochemistry of hairy cells. *Cancer* 1980;45:72–77.
23. Yam LT, English MC, Janckila AJ, et al. Immunocytochemical characterization of human blood cells. *Am J Clin Pathol* 1983;80:314–321.
24. Yam LT, Janckila AJ, Li CY, et al. Cytochemistry of tartrate-resistant acid phosphatase: 15 years' experience. *Leukemia* 1987;1:285–288.
25. Falini B, Schwarting R, Erber W, et al. The differential diagnosis of hairy cell leukemia with a panel of monoclonal antibodies. *Am J Clin Pathol* 1985;83:289–300.
26. Burke JS, Sheibani K, Winberg CD, et al. Recognition of hairy cell leukemia in a spleen of normal weight. The contribution of immunohistologic studies. *Am J Clin Pathol* 1987;87:276–281.
27. Hoyer JD, Li CY, Yam LT, et al. Immunohistochemical demonstration of acid phosphatase isoenzyme 5 (tartrate-resistant) in paraffin sections of hairy cell leukemia and other hematologic disorders. *Am J Clin Pathol* 1997;108:308–315.
28. Miranda RN, Briggs RC, Kinney MC, et al. Immunohistochemical detection of cyclin D1 using optimized conditions is highly specific for mantle cell lymphoma and hairy cell leukemia. *Mod Pathol* 2000;13:1308–1314.
29. Ohsawa M, Kanno H, Machii T, et al. Immunoreactivity of neoplastic and non-neoplastic monocytoid B lymphocytes for DBA.44 and other antibodies. *J Clin Pathol* 1994;47:928–932.
30. Oka K, Mori N, Yatabe Y. Immunohistochemical characteristics of monocytoid B cell lymphoma, mantle zone lymphoma, small lymphocytic lymphoma (or B chronic lymphocytic leukemia), and hairy cell leukemia. *Acta Haematol* 1993;90:84–89.
31. Pileri S, Sabattini E, Poggi S, et al. Bone-marrow biopsy in hairy cell leukaemia (HCL) patients. Histological and immunohistological analysis of 46 cases treated with different therapies. *Leuk Lymphoma* 1994;14(Suppl 1):67–71.
32. Strickler JG, Schmidt CM, Wick MR. Methods in pathology. Immunophenotype of hairy cell leukemia in paraffin sections. *Mod Pathol* 1990;3:518–523.
33. Went PT, Zimpfer A, Pehrs AC, et al. High specificity of combined TRAP and DBA.44 expression for hairy cell leukemia. *Am J Surg Pathol* 2005;29:474–478.
34. Falini B, Tiacci E, Liso A, et al. Simple diagnostic assay for hairy cell leukaemia by immunocytochemical detection of annexin A1 (ANXA1). *Lancet* 2004;363:1869–1870.
35. Matutes E. Immunophenotyping and differential diagnosis of hairy cell leukemia. *Hematol Oncol Clin North Am* 2006;20:1051–1063.
36. Sherman MJ, Hanson CA, Hoyer JD. An assessment of the usefulness of immunohistochemical stains in the diagnosis of hairy cell leukemia. *Am J Clin Pathol* 2011;136:390–399.
37. Cheuk W, Wong KO, Wong CS, et al. Consistent immunostaining for cyclin D1 can be achieved on a routine basis using a newly available rabbit monoclonal antibody. *Am J Surg Pathol* 2004;28:801–807.
38. Babušíková O, Tomová A, Kusenda J, et al. Flow cytometry of peripheral blood and bone marrow cells from patients with hairy cell leukemia: phenotype of hairy cells, lymphocyte subsets and detection of minimal residual disease after treatment. *Neoplasma* 2001;48:350–357.
39. Cornfield DB, Mitchell Nelson DM, Rimsza LM, et al. The diagnosis of hairy cell leukemia can be established by flow cytometric analysis of peripheral blood, even in patients with low levels of circulating malignant cells. *Am J Hematol* 2001;67:223–226.
40. Dong HY, Weisberger J, Liu Z, et al. Immunophenotypic analysis of CD103+ B-lymphoproliferative disorders: hairy cell leukemia and its mimics. *Am J Clin Pathol* 2009;131:586–595.
41. Babusíková O, Tomová A. Hairy cell leukemia: early immunophenotypical detection and quantitative analysis by flow cytometry. *Neoplasma* 2003;50:350–356.
42. Robbins BA, Ellison DJ, Spinosa JC, et al. Diagnostic application of two-color flow cytometry in 161 cases of hairy cell leukemia. *Blood* 1993;82:1277–1287.
43. Weisberger J, Wu CD, Liu Z, et al. Differential diagnosis of malignant lymphomas and related disorders by specific pattern of expression of immunophenotypic markers revealed by multiparameter flow cytometry (Review). *Int J Oncol* 2000;17:1165–1177.
44. Naeim F, Jacobs AD. Bone marrow changes in patients with hairy cell leukemia treated by recombinant alpha 2-interferon. *Hum Pathol* 1985;16:1200–1205.
45. Quesada JR, Reuben J, Manning JT, et al. Alpha interferon for induction of remission in hairy-cell leukemia. *N Engl J Med* 1984;310:15–18.
46. Quesada JR. Alpha interferons in the treatment of hairy cell leukemia. *Immunobiology* 1986;172:250–254.
47. Johnston JB, Eisenhauer E, Corbett WE, et al. Efficacy of 2′-deoxycoformycin in hairy-cell leukemia: a study of the National Cancer Institute of Canada Clinical Trials Group. *J Natl Cancer Inst* 1988;80:765–769.
48. Kraut EH, Bouroncle BA, Grever MR. Pentostatin in the treatment of advanced hairy cell leukemia. *J Clin Oncol* 1989;7:168–172.
49. Piro LD, Carrera CJ, Carson DA, et al. Lasting remissions in hairy-cell leukemia induced by a single infusion of 2-chlorodeoxyadenosine. *N Engl J Med* 1990;322:1117–1121.
50. Foucar K, Falini B, Catovsky D, et al. Hairy cell leukemia. In: Swerdlow S, ed. *WHO Classification of Tumours of Haematopoietic and Lymphoid Tissues*. Lyon: International Agency for Research on Cancer (IARC), 2008:188–190.
51. Ravandi F, Jorgensen JL, O'Brien SM, et al. Eradication of minimal residual disease in hairy cell leukemia. *Blood* 2006;107:4658–4662.
52. Ravandi F, O'Brien S, Jorgensen J, et al. Phase 2 study of cladribine followed by rituximab in patients with hairy cell leukemia. *Blood* 2011;118:3818–3823.
53. Thomas DA, Ravandi F, Keating M, et al. Importance of minimal residual disease in hairy cell leukemia: monoclonal antibodies as a therapeutic strategy. *Leuk Lymphoma* 2009;50(Suppl 1):27–31.
54. Frassoldati A, Lamparelli T, Federico M, et al. Hairy cell leukemia: a clinical review based on 725 cases of the Italian Cooperative Group (ICGHCL). Italian Cooperative Group for Hairy Cell Leukemia. *Leuk Lymphoma* 1994;13:307–316.
55. Vincent AM, Burthem J, Brew R, et al. Endothelial interactions of hairy cells: the importance of alpha 4 beta 1 in the unusual tissue distribution of the disorder. *Blood* 1996;88:3945–3952.
56. Cannon T, Mobarek D, Wegge J, et al. Hairy cell leukemia: current concepts. *Cancer Invest* 2008;26:860–865.
57. Basso K, Liso A, Tiacci E, et al. Gene expression profiling of hairy cell leukemia reveals a phenotype related to memory B cells with altered expression of chemokine and adhesion receptors. *J Exp Med* 2004;199:59–68.
58. Golomb HM, Hadad LJ. Infectious complications in 127 patients with hairy cell leukemia. *Am J Hematol* 1984;16:393–401.
59. Cooper C, Watts EJ, Smith AG. Salmonella septicaemia and pleural effusion as presenting features of hairy cell leukaemia. *Br J Clin Pract* 1987;41:670–671.
60. Bouroncle BA. Unusual presentations and complications of hairy cell leukemia. *Leukemia* 1987;1:288–293.
61. Chaudhry MS, Macdonald D, Strickland N. Hairy cell leukemia presenting as a cranial mass. *Am J Hematol* 2011;86:423–424.
62. Al-Za'abi AM, Boerner SL, Geddie W. Hairy cell leukemia presenting as a discrete liver mass: diagnosis by fine needle aspiration biopsy. *Diagn Cytopathol* 2008;36:128–132.
63. Hamadani M, Kraut EH. Review: isolated skeletal involvement in hairy cell leukemia. *Clin Adv Hematol Oncol* 2008;6:294–296.
64. Herold CJ, Wittich GR, Schwarzinger I, et al. Skeletal involvement in hairy cell leukemia. *Skeletal Radiol* 1988;17:171–175.
65. Bilsland D, Shahriari S, Douglas WS, et al. Transient leukaemia cutis in hairy-cell leukaemia. *Clin Exp Dermatol* 1991;16:207–209.
66. Clore LS, Stafford CT. Chronic urticaria as a presenting sign of hairy cell leukemia. *Allergy Asthma Proc* 1999;20:51–55.

67. Kayal S, Radhakrishnan V, Singh S, et al. Hairy cell leukemia with ascites: an unusual presentation. *Leuk Lymphoma* 2011;52:539–540.
68. Dinçol G, Doğan O, Küçükkaya RD, et al. Hairy cell leukaemia presenting with ascites, pleural effusion and increased CA 125 serum level. *Neth J Med* 2008;66:23–26.
69. Westbrook CA, Golde DW. Autoimmune disease in hairy-cell leukaemia: clinical syndromes and treatment. *Br J Haematol* 1985;61:349–356.
70. Begley CG, Tait B, Crapper RM, et al. Familial hairy cell leukemia. *Leuk Res* 1987;11:1027–1029.
71. Gramatovici M, Bennett JM, Hiscock JG, et al. Three cases of familial hairy cell leukemia. *Am J Hematol* 1993;42:337–339.
72. Ramseur WL, Golomb HM, Vardiman JW, et al. Hairy cell leukemia in father and son. *Cancer* 1981;48:1825–1829.
73. Wylin RF, Greene MH, Palutke M, et al. Hairy cell leukemia in three siblings: an apparent HLA-linked disease. *Cancer* 1982;49:538–542.
74. Sharpe RW, Bethel KJ. Hairy cell leukemia: diagnostic pathology. *Hematol Oncol Clin North Am* 2006;20:1023–1049.
75. Aziz KA. Elucidation of the mechanisms of hairy-cell localization in tissues and the process of the bone marrow fibrosis in hairy-cell leukemia. *Saudi Med J* 2003;24:715–719.
76. Aziz KA, Till KJ, Chen H, et al. The role of autocrine FGF-2 in the distinctive bone marrow fibrosis of hairy-cell leukemia (HCL). *Blood* 2003;102:1051–1056.
77. Gruber G, Schwarzmeier JD, Shehata M, et al. Basic fibroblast growth factor is expressed by CD19/CD11c-positive cells in hairy cell leukemia. *Blood* 1999; 94:1077–1085.
78. Shehata M, Schwarzmeier JD, Hilgarth M, et al. TGF-beta1 induces bone marrow reticulin fibrosis in hairy cell leukemia. *J Clin Invest* 2004;113:676–685.
79. Burthem J, Cawley JC. The bone marrow fibrosis of hairy-cell leukemia is caused by the synthesis and assembly of a fibronectin matrix by the hairy cells. *Blood* 1994;83:497–504.
80. Zafrani ES, Degos F, Guigui B, et al. The hepatic sinusoid in hairy cell leukemia: an ultrastructural study of 12 cases. *Hum Pathol* 1987;18:801–807.
81. Tiacci E, Liso A, Piris M, et al. Evolving concepts in the pathogenesis of hairy-cell leukaemia. *Nat Rev Cancer* 2006;6:437–448.
82. Cawley JC, Hawkins SF. The biology of hairy-cell leukaemia. *Curr Opin Hematol* 2010;17:341–349.
83. Yamaguchi M, Machii T, Shibayama H, et al. Immunophenotypic features and configuration of immunoglobulin genes in hairy cell leukemia-Japanese variant. *Leukemia* 1996;10:1390–1394.
84. Machii T, Tokumine Y, Inoue R, et al. A unique variant of hairy cell leukemia in Japan. *Jpn J Med* 1990;29:379–383.
85. Machii T, Tokumine Y, Inoue R, et al. Predominance of a distinct subtype of hairy cell leukemia in Japan. *Leukemia* 1993;7:181–186.
86. Machii T, Yamaguchi M, Inoue R, et al. Polyclonal B-cell lymphocytosis with features resembling hairy cell leukemia-Japanese variant. *Blood* 1997;89:2008–2014.
87. Piris M, Foucar K, Mollejo M, et al. Splenic B-cell lymphoma/leukaemia, unclassifiable. In: Swerdlow S, ed. *WHO Classification of Tumours of Haematopoietic and Lymphoid Tissues*. Lyon: International Agency for Research on Cancer (IARC), 2008:191–193.
88. Hanson CA, Ward PC, Schnitzer B. A multilobular variant of hairy cell leukemia with morphologic similarities to T-cell lymphoma. *Am J Surg Pathol* 1989; 13:671–679.
89. Bartl R, Frisch B, Hill W, et al. Bone marrow histology in hairy cell leukemia. Identification of subtypes and their prognostic significance. *Am J Clin Pathol* 1983;79:531–545.
90. Lemez P, Friedmann B, Vanásek J, et al. [A diagnostically difficult case of hairy cell leukemia with ring-shaped nuclei]. *Sb Lek* 1991;93:33–35.
91. Diez Martin JL, Li CY, Banks PM. Blastic variant of hairy-cell leukemia. *Am J Clin Pathol* 1987;87:576–583.
92. Davis KM, Spindel E, Franzini DA, et al. Anaplastic neoplasm in a patient with hairy cell leukemia. *Cancer* 1985;56:2470–2475.
93. Chen YH, Tallman MS, Goolsby C, et al. Immunophenotypic variations in hairy cell leukemia. *Am J Clin Pathol* 2006;125:251–259.
94. Jasionowski TM, Hartung L, Greenwood JH, et al. Analysis of CD10+ hairy cell leukemia. *Am J Clin Pathol* 2003;120:228–235.
95. Yuan CM, Yang LJ. Hairy cell leukemia with unusual loss of CD103 in a subset of the neoplastic population: immunophenotypic and cell cycle analysis by flow cytometry. *Int J Clin Exp Pathol* 2008;1:381–386.
96. Del Giudice I, Matutes E, Morilla R, et al. The diagnostic value of CD123 in B-cell disorders with hairy or villous lymphocytes. *Haematologica* 2004;89:303–308.
97. Hounieu H, Chittal SM, al Saati T, et al. Hairy cell leukemia. Diagnosis of bone marrow involvement in paraffin-embedded sections with monoclonal antibody DBA.44. *Am J Clin Pathol* 1992;98:26–33.
98. Dunphy CH. Reaction patterns of TRAP and DBA.44 in hairy cell leukemia, hairy cell variant, and nodal and extranodal marginal zone B-cell lymphomas. *Appl Immunohistochem Mol Morphol* 2008;16:135–139.
99. Solé F, Woessner S, Florensa L, et al. Cytogenetic findings in five patients with hairy cell leukemia. *Cancer Genet Cytogenet* 1999;110:41–43.
100. Ueshima Y, Alimena G, Rowley JD, et al. Cytogenetic studies in patients with hairy cell leukemia. *Hematol Oncol* 1983;1:215–226.
101. Brito-Babapulle V, Pittman S, Melo JV, et al. The 14q+ marker in hairy cell leukaemia. A cytogenetic study of 15 cases. *Leuk Res* 1986;10:131–138.
102. Solé F, Woessner S, Florensa L, et al. A new chromosomal anomaly associated with mature B-cell chronic lymphoproliferative disorders: del(7)(q32). *Cancer Genet Cytogenet* 1993;65:170–172.
103. Solé F, Woessner S, Pérez-Losada A, et al. Cytogenetic studies in seventy-six cases of B-chronic lymphoproliferative disorders. *Cancer Genet Cytogenet* 1997; 93:160–166.
104. Andersen CL, Gruszka-Westwood A, Østergaard M, et al. A narrow deletion of 7q is common to HCL, and SMZL, but not CLL. *Eur J Haematol* 2004;72:390–402.
105. Chen D, Ketterling RP, Hanson CA, et al. A case of hairy cell leukemia with CCND1-IGH@ translocation: indolent non-nodal mantle cell lymphoma revisited. *Am J Surg Pathol* 2011;35:1080–1084.
106. Hockley SL, Giannouli S, Morilla A, et al. Insight into the molecular pathogenesis of hairy cell leukaemia, hairy cell leukaemia variant and splenic marginal zone lymphoma, provided by the analysis of their IGH rearrangements and somatic hypermutation patterns. *Br J Haematol* 2010;148:666–669.
107. Martín-Jiménez P, García-Sanz R, González D, et al. Molecular characterization of complete and incomplete immunoglobulin heavy chain gene rearrangements in hairy cell leukemia. *Clin Lymphoma Myeloma* 2007;7:573–579.
108. Forconi F, Sahota SS, Raspadori D, et al. Hairy cell leukemia: at the crossroad of somatic mutation and isotype switch. *Blood* 2004;104:3312–3317.
109. Arons E, Suntum T, Stetler-Stevenson M, et al. VH4-34+ hairy cell leukemia, a new variant with poor prognosis despite standard therapy. *Blood* 2009;114: 4687–4695.
110. Arons E, Sunshine J, Suntum T, et al. Somatic hypermutation and VH gene usage in hairy cell leukaemia. *Br J Haematol* 2006;133:504–512.
111. Forconi F, Sozzi E, Rossi D, et al. Selective influences in the expressed immunoglobulin heavy and light chain gene repertoire in hairy cell leukemia. *Haematologica* 2008;93:697–705.
112. Maloum K, Magnac C, Azgui Z, et al. VH gene expression in hairy cell leukaemia. *Br J Haematol* 1998;101:171–178.
113. Vanhentenrijk V, Tierens A, Wlodarska I, et al. V(H) gene analysis of hairy cell leukemia reveals a homogeneous mutation status and suggests its marginal zone B-cell origin. *Leukemia* 2004;18:1729–1732.
114. Zandvoort A, Timens W. The dual function of the splenic marginal zone: essential for initiation of anti-TI-2 responses but also vital in the general first-line defense against blood-borne antigens. *Clin Exp Immunol* 2002;130:4–11.
115. William J, Euler C, Christensen S, et al. Evolution of autoantibody responses via somatic hypermutation outside of germinal centers. *Science* 2002;297:2066–2070.
116. Arons E, Roth L, Sapolsky J, et al. Evidence of canonical somatic hypermutation in hairy cell leukemia. *Blood* 2011;117:4844–4851.
117. Traverse-Glehen A, Baseggio L, Callet-Bauchu E, et al. Hairy cell leukaemia-variant and splenic red pulp lymphoma: a single entity? *Br J Haematol* 2010;150: 113–116.
118. Kluin-Nelemans HC, Krouwels MM, Jansen JH, et al. Hairy cell leukemia preferentially expresses the IgG3-subclass. *Blood* 1990;75:972–975.
119. Forconi F, Sahota SS, Raspadori D, et al. Tumor cells of hairy cell leukemia express multiple clonally related immunoglobulin isotypes via RNA splicing. *Blood* 2001;98:1174–1181.
120. Brose MS, Volpe P, Feldman M, et al. BRAF and RAS mutations in human lung cancer and melanoma. *Cancer Res* 2002;62:6997–7000.
121. Davies H, Bignell GR, Cox C, et al. Mutations of the BRAF gene in human cancer. *Nature* 2002;417:949–954.
122. Dienstmann R, Tabernero J. BRAF as a target for cancer therapy. *Anticancer Agents Med Chem* 2011;11:285–295.
123. Flaherty KT, McArthur G. BRAF, a target in melanoma: implications for solid tumor drug development. *Cancer* 2010;116:4902–4913.
124. Gandhi M, Evdokimova V, Nikiforov YE. Mechanisms of chromosomal rearrangements in solid tumors: the model of papillary thyroid carcinoma. *Mol Cell Endocrinol* 2010;321:36–43.
125. Hunt JL. Molecular testing in solid tumors: an overview. *Arch Pathol Lab Med* 2008;132:164–167.
126. Riesco-Eizaguirre G, Santisteban P. Molecular biology of thyroid cancer initiation. *Clin Transl Oncol* 2007;9:686–693.
127. Yuen ST, Davies H, Chan TL, et al. Similarity of the phenotypic patterns associated with BRAF and KRAS mutations in colorectal neoplasia. *Cancer Res* 2002;62:6451–6455.
128. Tiacci E, Trifonov V, Schiavoni G, et al. BRAF mutations in hairy-cell leukemia. *N Engl J Med* 2011;364:2305–2315.
129. Boyd EM, Bench AJ, van 't Veer MB, et al. High resolution melting analysis for detection of BRAF exon 15 mutations in hairy cell leukaemia and other lymphoid malignancies. *Br J Haematol* 2011;155:609–612.
130. Tiacci E, Schiavoni G, Forconi F, et al. Simple genetic diagnosis of hairy cell leukemia by sensitive detection of the BRAF-V600E mutation. *Blood* 2012;119: 192–195.
131. Arcaini L, Zibellini S, Boveri E, et al. The BRAF V600E mutation in hairy cell leukemia and other mature B-cell neoplasms. *Blood* 2012;119:188–191.
132. Blombery P, Wong SQ, Hewitt CA, et al. Detection of BRAF mutations in patients with hairy cell leukemia and related lymphoproliferative disorders. *Haematologica* 2012;97:780–783.
133. Lennerz JK, Klaus BM, Marienfeld RB, et al. Pyrosequencing of BRAF V600E in routine samples of Hairy Cell Leukaemia identifies CD5+ variant Hairy Cell Leukaemia that lacks V600E. *Br J Haematol* 2012;157:267–269.
134. Pardanani A, Tefferi A. BRAF mutations in hairy-cell leukemia. *N Engl J Med* 2011;365:961; author reply 961–962.
135. Xi L, Arons E, Navarro W, et al. Both variant and IGHV4-34-expressing hairy cell leukemia lack the BRAF V600E mutation. *Blood* 2012;119:3330–3332.
136. Auer RL, Cotter FE. A defining moment for hairy cell leukaemia. *Br J Haematol* 2011;155:607–608.
137. Kamiguti AS, Harris RJ, Slupsky JR, et al. Regulation of hairy-cell survival through constitutive activation of mitogen-activated protein kinase pathways. *Oncogene* 2003;22:2272–2284.
138. Cawley JC. Hairy cell leukemia and the microenvironment. *Leuk Lymphoma* 2011;52(Suppl 2):91–93.
139. Burger JA, Sivina M, Ravandi F. The microenvironment in hairy cell leukemia: pathways and potential therapeutic targets. *Leuk Lymphoma* 2011;52(Suppl 2): 94–98.
140. Vanhentenrijk V, De Wolf-Peeters C, Wlodarska I, et al. Comparative expressed sequence hybridization studies of hairy cell leukemia show uniform expression profile and imprint of spleen signature. *Blood* 2004;104:250–255.
141. Marafioti T, Jones M, Facchetti F, et al. Phenotype and genotype of interfollicular large B cells, a subpopulation of lymphocytes often with dendritic morphology. *Blood* 2003;102:2868–2876.
142. Forconi F, Cencini E, Sicuranza A, et al. Molecular insight into the biology and clinical course of hairy cell leukemia utilizing immunoglobulin gene analysis. *Leuk Lymphoma* 2011;52:15–23.
143. Forconi F, Raspadori D, Lenoci M, et al. Absence of surface CD27 distinguishes hairy cell leukemia from other leukemic B-cell malignancies. *Haematologica* 2005; 90:266–268.
144. Silingardi V, Federico M, Barbieri F, et al. Hairy cell leukemia: a reversible disease? A report of two cases of spontaneous remission. *Haematologica* 1985;70:437–441.
145. Sun T, Grupka N, Klein C. Transformation of hairy cell leukemia to high-grade lymphoma: a case report and review of the literature. *Hum Pathol* 2004;35: 1423–1426.

146. Friedline JA, Crisan D, Chen J. Blastic transformation in a case of hairy cell leukemia. *Mol Diagn* 1998;3:163–169.

147. Bennett CL, Westbrook CA, Gruber B, et al. Hairy cell leukemia and mucormycosis. Treatment with alpha-2 interferon. *Am J Med* 1986;81:1065–1067.

148. Bennett C, Vardiman J, Golomb H. Disseminated atypical mycobacterial infection in patients with hairy cell leukemia. *Am J Med* 1986;80:891–896.

149. Jones G, Parry-Jones N, Wilkins B, et al. Revised guidelines for the diagnosis and management of hairy cell leukaemia and hairy cell leukaemia variant'. *Br J Haematol* 2012;156:186–195.

150. Else M, Dearden CE, Matutes E, et al. Long-term follow-up of 233 patients with hairy cell leukaemia, treated initially with pentostatin or cladribine, at a median of 16 years from diagnosis. *Br J Haematol* 2009;145:733–740.

151. Forconi F, Sozzi E, Cencini E, et al. Hairy cell leukemias with unmutated IGHV genes define the minor subset refractory to single-agent cladribine and with more aggressive behavior. *Blood* 2009;114:4696–4702.

152. Belani R, Saven A. Cladribine in hairy cell leukemia. *Hematol Oncol Clin North Am* 2006;20:1109–1123.

153. Robak T. Current treatment options in hairy cell leukemia and hairy cell leukemia variant. *Cancer Treat Rev* 2006;32:365–376.

154. Chadha P, Rademaker AW, Mendiratta P, et al. Treatment of hairy cell leukemia with 2-chlorodeoxyadenosine (2-CdA): long-term follow-up of the Northwestern University experience. *Blood* 2005;106:241–246.

155. Else M, Ruchlemer R, Osuji N, et al. Long remissions in hairy cell leukemia with purine analogs: a report of 219 patients with a median follow-up of 12.5 years. *Cancer* 2005;104:2442–2448.

156. Grever MR, Zinzani PL. Long-term follow-up studies in hairy cell leukemia. *Leuk Lymphoma* 2009;50(Suppl 1):23–26.

157. Maloisel F, Benboubker L, Gardembas M, et al. Long-term outcome with pentostatin treatment in hairy cell leukemia patients. A French retrospective study of 238 patients. *Leukemia* 2003;17:45–51.

158. Flinn IW, Kopecky KJ, Foucar MK, et al. Long-term follow-up of remission duration, mortality, and second malignancies in hairy cell leukemia patients treated with pentostatin. *Blood* 2000;96:2981–2986.

159. Goodman GR, Burian C, Koziol JA, et al. Extended follow-up of patients with hairy cell leukemia after treatment with cladribine. *J Clin Oncol* 2003;21:891–896.

160. Hisada M, Chen BE, Jaffe ES, et al. Second cancer incidence and cause-specific mortality among 3104 patients with hairy cell leukemia: a population-based study. *J Natl Cancer Inst* 2007;99:215–222.

161. Wang X, Spielberger R, Huang Q. Hairy cell leukemia variant, a new entity of the WHO 2008. *J Clin Oncol* 2011;29:e864–e866.

162. Traverse-Glehen A, Baseggio L, Bauchu EC, et al. Splenic red pulp lymphoma with numerous basophilic villous lymphocytes: a distinct clinicopathologic and molecular entity? *Blood* 2008;111:2253–2260.

163. Kanellis G, Mollejo M, Montes-Moreno S, et al. Splenic diffuse red pulp small B-cell lymphoma: revision of a series of cases reveals characteristic clinico-pathological features. *Haematologica* 2010;95:1122–1129.

164. Baseggio L, Traverse-Glehen A, Callet-Bauchu E, et al. Relevance of a scoring system including CD11c expression in the identification of splenic diffuse red pulp small B-cell lymphoma (SRPL). *Hematol Oncol* 2011;29:47–51.

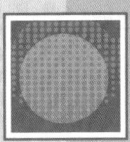

Chapter 37
Plasma Cell Neoplasms and Immunoglobulin Deposition Diseases

Scott Ely • Ruben Niesvizky • Tomer Mark

Plasma cell neoplasms (PCNs) encompass disorders of terminally differentiated B cells that are class switched and secrete immunoglobulin (Ig). Morphologically, cases range from being indistinguishable from normal plasma cells (PCs) to plasmablastic. Clinical investigation begins with electrophoretic detection of a monoclonal serum immunoglobulin, referred to by a number of different terms: monoclonal spike, serum spike, paraprotein, M spike or M protein ("M" for monoclonal, not to be confused with IgM). The presence of an M spike is referred to as monoclonal gammopathy or "gammopathy." Small-magnitude (e.g., <0.5 g/dL) M proteins are very common in the elderly and usually not of clinical importance if unaccompanied by any other signs of systemic disease. Upon completion of the clinical workup, the most common diagnosis in a patient with an M spike is monoclonal gammopathy of undetermined significance (MGUS). After MGUS, plasma cell myeloma (PCM) is the next most common final diagnosis. Although the World Health Organization (WHO) has adopted the term PCM, it is used far less than "multiple myeloma" (MM), and the terms "PCM" and "MM" are interchangeable. The disease definitions used throughout the chapter are those of the WHO, which are the same as those of the International Myeloma Working Group (IMWG) (1,2). All PCN are composed of a uniform population of PC. By contrast, some lymphomas are composed of B cells with surface Ig (sIg) but include a plasmacytoid subclone, defined by the presence of cytoplasmic Ig (cIg). For example, plasmacytoid differentiation is seen in 10% of chronic lymphocytic leukemia (CLL) and is characteristic of lymphoplasmacytic lymphoma/Waldenström macroglobulinemia. Such disorders are discussed in other chapters.

ASSESSMENT OF SERUM IMMUNOGLOBULIN

Because it is the defining characteristic of a PCN, it is important to describe the process of detecting an M spike (3).

Serum total protein and albumin, part of a routine blood analysis, are typically normal in MGUS, whereas protein is elevated and albumin often low in MM. The first line of further inquiry is serum protein electrophoresis (SPE or SPEP) (Fig. 37.1). Because SPEP is of relatively low sensitivity, and, even if positive, does not indicate the isotype, immunofixation (IFE) is typically run in parallel in any patient suspected of having a PCN (Fig. 37.1). IFE involves running several SPEPs in parallel lanes, after which each lane is overlaid with an antibody to a particular isotype of immunoglobulin. An excess of any one type of immunoglobulin, as seen in PCN, will result in a particular banding pattern defining the isotype of the M spike (Fig. 37.2). Immunoelectrophoresis is an older method, rarely performed today. In myeloma patients, in addition to the serum spike, there often is a concomitant decrease in background polyclonal immunoglobulin (see absence of IgM in Fig. 37.2).

For unknown reasons, even when PCN produce intact Ig molecules with pairs of both heavy and light chains, there also is an increase in free light chains (FLCs) not bound to heavy chains. FLCs are normally reabsorbed in the proximal tubule of the nephron and have a half-life on the order of a few hours, whereas intact immunoglobulins have relatively long half-lives on the order of 21 days, due to recycling through the neonatal Fc receptor for IgG (FcRn), most likely in the gut, airway, kidney and in monocytes (4). Both free kappa and lambda are usually present in small amounts in the serum and are maintained in a narrow ratio. In renal insufficiency states, both free kappa and lambda rise, but the ratio remains constant. In a number of malignancies, including myeloma, one FLC is produced to the exclusion of the other, altering the ratio (5–8). An abnormal FLC ratio is an established risk factor for progression of MGUS and smoldering myeloma (SMM) to symptomatic myeloma (9–11). FLC excess can be measured in the serum via nephelometric assessment of molecular surfaces normally hidden when the light chain is found as part of the intact immunoglobulin. Assessment of serum FLCs is standard and is commonly referred to by the brand name "Freelite" (12). This method of FLC assessment if more sensitive than SPEP or IFE. As such, it is usually a response criterion in clinical practice and trials (13–15).

An M protein is found by SPEP or IFE in 97% of patients. The remaining 3% are called nonsecretory MM, but most of those patients do have detectible Ig by serum light chain analysis. Fifty percent of MM patients secrete IgG, 20% secrete IgA, 20% are light chain only (LCO), while IgD, IgE, and IgM together constitute <7% (16). Many patients with an M protein composed of an intact Ig molecule show an additional FLC band on their IFE.

For the remainder of information on serum immunoglobulin, please see "Prognostication and Disease Monitoring."

ASSESSMENT OF URINE IMMUNOGLOBULIN

Assessment and quantitation of urine Ig are similar to that described above for serum. In addition, most MM patients also are assessed by a 24-hour urine collection. Collecting and submitting these large specimens is sometimes difficult for patients. Some authors propose that serum FLC assays replace 24-hour urine, citing data that in individual patients, serum FLC correlates linearly with changes in 24-hour urine. Subsequent studies have come to conflicting conclusions (5,17,18). Although the serum FLC assay may be used for disease screening, it is currently recommended that 24-hour urine collections still be done at the time of diagnosis of a PCN, especially in cases of AL amyloidosis, where glomerular damage may also be concurrently detected via the urine collection process (8).

Normal SPEP & IFE

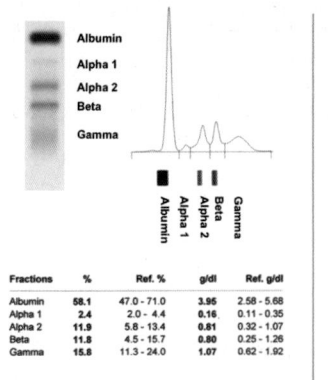

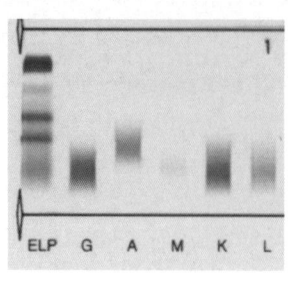

Fractions	%	Ref. %	g/dl	Ref. g/dl
Albumin	58.1	47.0 - 71.0	3.95	2.58 - 5.68
Alpha 1	2.4	2.0 - 4.4	0.16	0.11 - 0.35
Alpha 2	11.9	5.8 - 13.4	0.81	0.32 - 1.07
Beta	11.8	4.5 - 15.7	0.80	0.25 - 1.26
Gamma	15.8	11.3 - 24.0	1.07	0.62 - 1.92

FIGURE 37.1. Normal SPEP and IFE. In a serum protein electrophoresis (SPEP) (**top left**), proteins are separated, ranging from most rapid electrophoretic mobility (albumin) to least rapid (gamma globulin). The proteins are dyed and read by a densitometer to produce a curve (**middle**). The amounts of proteins are assessed by the area under the curve (see included normal values). For immunofixation (IFE), the electrophoresis procedure is performed in six tandem lanes, after which, each lane is overlaid with an isotype-specific antibody (e.g., anti-IgA) that binds and precipitates its target. All proteins not precipitated by the isotype-specific antibody are washed away. In addition to identifying the isotype of a band noted in the SPEP, the IFE procedure can sometimes reveal bands not detected on the SPEP (Fig. 37.2).

Myeloma SPEP & IFE

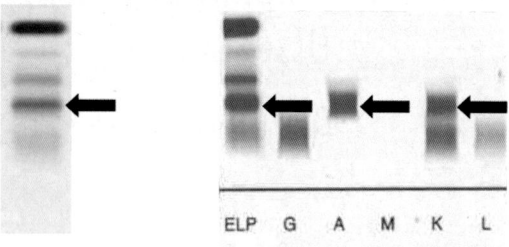

SPEP: M-protein of 0.7 g/dL detected in beta region

IFE: Monoclonal IgA-kappa detected in the beta region
Kappa: 0.79 mg/dL (0.33-1.94 mg/dL)
Lambda: 0.11 mg/dL (0.57- 2.63 mg/dL)

FIGURE 37.2. Myeloma SPEP and IFE. This SPEP from a MM patient appears relatively normal, including a polytypic smear within the gamma region. However, the IFE clearly reveals a monoclonal IgAκ protein. In this case, the band had abnormal electrophoretic mobility, running in the beta region. An additional, subtle abnormality is reciprocal depression of IgM.

IMPORTANT DIFFERENCES BETWEEN MYELOMA AND OTHER HEMATOPOIETIC NEOPLASMS

Among hematopoietic neoplasms, those composed of PCs are unusual in the limitation of sites involved. Most myeloid neoplasms and leukemia cells are plentiful in the marrow but also in the peripheral blood (PB) or spleen. Many lymphomas involve nodes, but also grow well in the marrow, and many have a leukemic phase. By contrast, except for rare or late-stage, transformed cases, the growth of myeloma cells is strictly limited to the marrow microenvironment. In turn, the skeletal manifestations are unique to myeloma.

It is tempting to apply concepts derived from the study of other hematopoietic cancers to PCNs. It is important to understand, however, that from a methodologic perspective, PCNs are distinct from other cancers discussed in this book. The most important factor to keep in mind is that whereas aspirated marrow cells are of great use for the study of leukemias, the use of aspirates is limited for PCN.

Aspirate morphology remains the gold standard for the diagnosis of myelodysplasia. In leukemias, aspirates typically are representative of intact marrow. In myeloma, by contrast, an actual, intact piece of marrow, as found in a core/trephine biopsy, is required for accurate assessment. The first reason for this is that, unlike most leukemias, myeloma cells induce a degree of reticulin fibrosis that prevents them from being aspirated (Fig. 37.3). As such, in many cases, the aspirate specimen is most representative of the nonfibrotic, background marrow, rather than the myeloma. In a study of 352 myelomas, as compared to a core biopsy, the aspirate MM cell percentage was artifactually low in nearly half of the aspirates (19). In an average case, the aspirate contained 20% fewer MM cells than

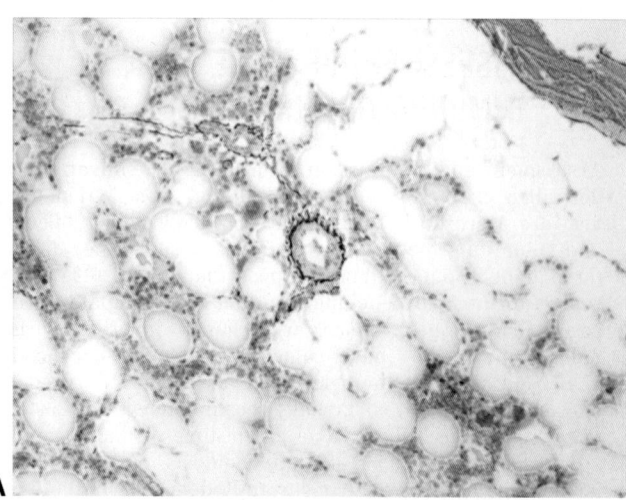

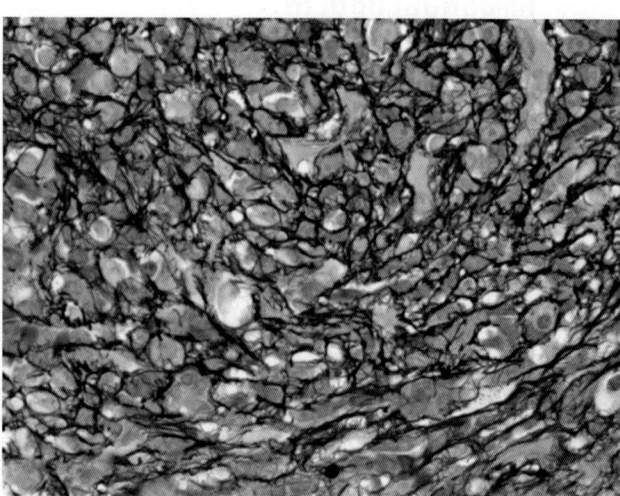

FIGURE 37.3. Myeloma reticulin fibrosis. A: In this normal marrow, reticulin (*black color*) is scant and limited to blood vessel walls (reticulin stain, 400×). **B:** In an area involved by myeloma, there is marked reticulin fibrosis (reticulin stain, 400×).

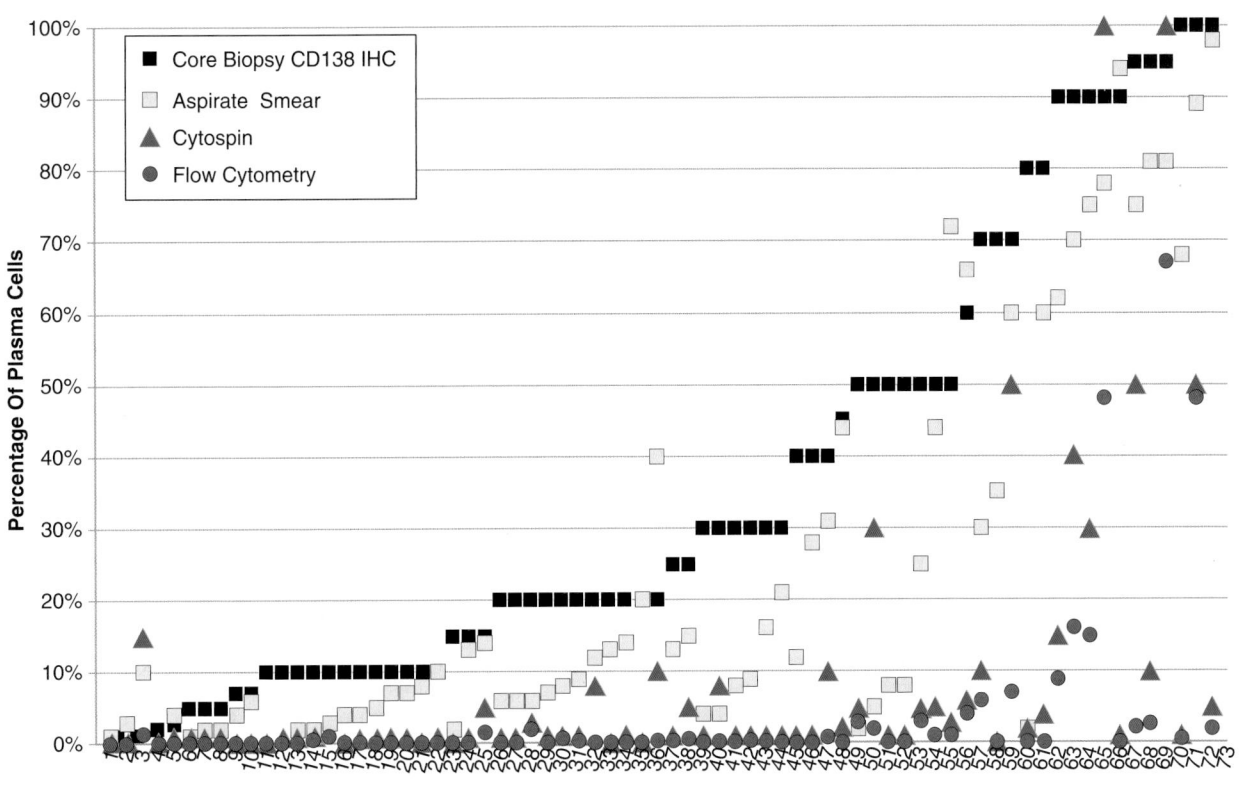

FIGURE 37.4. MM cell number: core biopsy versus aspirate smear versus cytospin versus flow cytometry. Seventy-three consecutive biopsies from MM patients are charted in ascending order of percent of PCs in the core. Each biopsy is charted for percent of PCs seen by CD138 IHC in the core (*black boxes*), percent of PCs in aspirate smears (*yellow boxes*), percent of PCs in cytospins prepared prior to FC (*blue triangles*), and percent of PCs detected by multicolor flow cytometry (*red circles*).

the core. Numerous other studies have shown similar findings (20–26). The reticulin fibrosis is even greater in cases with shedding of CD138 (27).

Unlike leukemias, MM cells express large quantities of adhesion molecules, such as CD138 and CD56, causing them to bind strongly to other MM cells as well as to stroma. In addition to the fibrosis, this adds to the difficulty of aspirating MM cells. The reticulin fibrosis is even greater in cases with shedding of CD138 (27).

In other types of blood cancer (e.g., acute myeloid leukemia [AML], CLL), the neoplastic cells remain alive for extended periods of time in culture medium. By contrast, even when PCs make it through the fibrosis and into the aspirate, they begin to die quickly despite immediate placement in a culture medium. This fact, well known to anyone who works with myeloma patient samples, is well illustrated in Figure 37.4. In known MM patients, 73 consecutive biopsies were diagnostic of MM by immunohistochemistry (IHC). IHC for CD138 in the core shows the true, *in vivo*, number of MM cells. Because the sensitivity of IHC is so high, it is used as a criterion for stringent complete response by the IMWG (13,28). By comparison, as shown in Figure 37.4, the number of PCs is decreased in aspirate smears and then decreased further in cytospins after processing for flow cytometry (FC); then due to further cell death, there are no MM cells detectable by FC (i.e., FC is false negative) in 38/73 (52%) cases. This gives rise to a ironic conundrum, well known in the myeloma field: clinicians complain about not being able to kill MM cells in a patient, while researchers complain about not being able to keep MM cells alive in the laboratory.

In addition to being underrepresented due to fibrosis and rapid *ex vivo* cell death, data show that, as compared to the

majority of PCs residing in a patient's marrow, aspiration selects for subpopulations of PCs that are not well representative of a patient's biologic disease (26,29).

MM research is further hampered by the difficulty of establishing representative cell lines. Nearly all cancer cell lines differ greatly from their *in vivo* counterparts. However, the difference between human myeloma cell lines and *in vivo* MM cells is exceptionally vast, given that the MM cell line must acquire additional mutations that allow for *ex vivo* survival. Also, whereas mouse models are plentiful for other cancers, there are only a few, problematic bone-based models for MM.

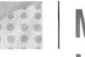 ## MONOCLONAL GAMMOPATHY OF UNDETERMINED SIGNIFICANCE

As per the 2008 WHO classification/IMWG (1,2), MGUS is defined as

- a serum M spike of <3 g/dL
- <10% monoclonal PCs in the marrow
- the absence of end organ damage (see CRAB, below in MM pathogenesis section)
- no lytic bone lesions
- no evidence of a lymphoma

The M-protein isotype in MGUS is IgG in 69% of patients, IgM in 17%, IgA in 11%, and is rarely LCO. Because IgM MGUS can be a precursor of lymphoplasmacytic lymphoma, or CLL, but almost never evolves into MM, it should be thought of as a separate category.

In most cases, MGUS is an incidental finding with no clinical impact in an elderly patient. However, because all cases of MM do evolve from MGUS, studying MGUS is important to understand how best to follow patients and to discover ways to decrease a patient's risk of progression. MGUS increases with age from 3% in patients over 50 to 5% in patients over 70 (30). Like MM, MGUS is more common in men (1.5:1, M:F) and twice as common in African Americans as in Caucasians (31).

There is a two- to threefold increase in the incidence of MGUS among first-degree relatives (31,32). Numerous genetic polymorphisms have been implicated, but the list of possible important candidates is long and inclusive of genes involved in immunoglobulin gene rearrangement and recombination (33). Stronger data support the role of interleukin 6 (IL-6), a proinflammatory cytokine critical for the survival of both normal and neoplastic PCs, in the etiology of MGUS. Population studies have consistently shown the serum level of IL-6 to rise with increasing age (34).

In MGUS, the bone marrow (BM) biopsy typically shows a mild increase in PCs that are otherwise morphologically normal. Aside from monotypic cytoplasmic immunoglobulin restriction, the immunophenotype is similar to that of normal PCs. Most importantly, MGUS PCs typically lack expression of CD56 (neural cell adhesion molecule, NCAM) (19). Also, whereas normal PCs never express cyclin D1, it is found >60% of MGUS cases; the staining for cyclin D1 is strong and uniform in cases with t(11;14) and weak/partial in hyperdiploid cases with tri(11) (see Chromosomal and Molecular Alterations section, below).

In the United States and in Germany, the incidence of progression to MM is approximately 1% of patients per year (i.e., of all MGUS patients, ~1% per year will progress to MM) (35,36). While the vast majority of patients with MGUS do not progress, on the other hand, nearly all MMs are proceeded by MGUS (32). The risk of progression is associated with the isotype of the MGUS spike. While IgG spikes progress at 1% of patients per year, light chain–only MGUS (which itself is rare) rarely progresses to MM (36). Also, although the incidence of progression is far higher for an IgM isotype (~5% per year), if an IgM MGUS progresses, it is to lymphoma (including CLL), not MM (37).

The most common cytogenetic abnormalities and their incidences found in MGUS are similar to those found in MM (see Chromosomal and Molecular Alterations section, below) (38,39). For example, the most common translocation, t(11;14), is found in approximately 15% of both MGUS and MM.

Because MGUS is typically an incidental clinical finding and does not progress to MM in most patients, the clinical approach is active observation. At routine clinical intervals, the magnitude of the serum spike, hemoglobin, renal function, and any sign of new skeletal disease are monitored. If there are signs or concerns of progression, other studies may be performed (40). However, because efficacy has not been shown for early therapy, and patients with MGUS are by definition asymptomatic, treatment is not instituted unless intervention is required by clinical consequences.

PLASMA CELL MYELOMA (MULTIPLE MYELOMA)

Definition

By definition, MM is a PCN associated with end organ damage and its clinical consequences, according to the diagnostic acronym, CRAB:

hyper*C*alcemia
*R*enal insufficiency
*A*nemia
*B*one lesions

The WHO definition of PCM is the same as that of the IMWG (1,2):

- the presence of an M protein of any level
- BM clonal PCs (no minimal level) or osseous plasmacytoma
- related organ or tissue impairment (CRAB)

Earlier classifications required serum spikes of certain magnitudes and minimal numbers of neoplastic cells in the marrow but are no longer in clinical use.

Incidence

MM accounts for 10% of all new blood cancers, 20% of all blood cancer deaths, and about 1% of all cancer deaths. There were >20,000 new MM diagnoses and approximately 11,000 deaths in the United States in 2010 (41). Although MM is typically cited as being the second most common hematologic cancer, it is only second to non-Hodgkin lymphoma (NHL) when the latter are considered as a single group. Among individual WHO hematologic neoplasms, MM is the single most common, with an incidence of 5.5 per 100,000 person years, the second commonest being diffuse large B-cell lymphoma at 4.6 per 100,000 person years (42–44). Among all cancers, MM incidence is far lower than any of the common solid organ cancers.

Data support describing MM incidence in terms of four demographic groups (Fig. 37.5) (43). It is highest in African American men, followed by African American women, Caucasian men, and then Caucasian women. Mortality data parallel the incidence for each demographic. The higher incidence in African Americans parallels their higher immunoglobulin levels, which, in turn, mirrors their higher incidence of MGUS, suggesting a larger B-cell/PC population at risk for neoplastic transformation. Compared to African Americans and Caucasians, the incidence and mortality are far lower in Asian men and women. There is some evidence that the incidence is slightly higher in Hispanics than in Caucasians, but there is relatively little data on the Hispanic population (45).

In aggregate, data do not support any relationship between socioeconomic status and MM incidence (46).

Etiology

Like most other cancers, the cause of MM is multifactorial. Studies have not revealed strong evidence for any single etiologic factor. There is a two- to threefold increase in the incidence

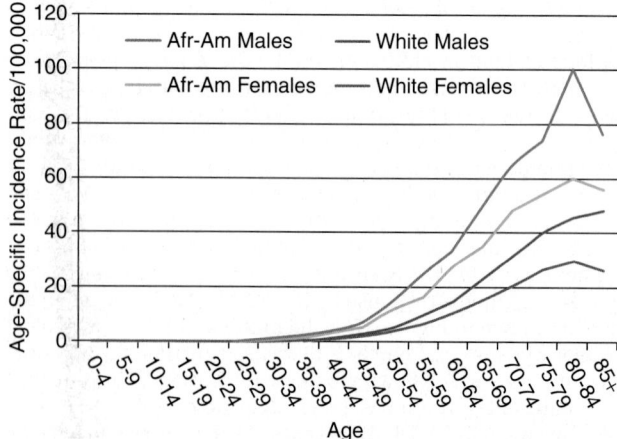

FIGURE 37.5. Myeloma incidence by demographic group (43). Average annual age-specific incidence rates of MM, 1973 to 2006, Surveillance, Epidemiology and End-Results Program. Surveillance Research Program, National Cancer Institute SEER*Stat software (www.seer.cancer.gov/seerstat), Version 6.5.2. Surveillance, Epidemiology, and End Results (SEER) Program (www.seer.cancer.gov) SEER*Stat Database: Incidence-SEER 9 Registries Limited-Use, Nov. 2008 Submission (1973–2006).

of MGUS and MM in first-degree relatives, but considering the relatively low overall incidence of MM, the contribution of heredity is relatively mild (47). Kindreds with a striking preponderance of MM are rare. There is data suggesting that genetic polymorphisms contribute to the etiology, but no strong correlations have been found (48–54).

Long-term studies of radiation exposure, including the nuclear industry, medical radiology workers, and survivors of Hiroshima and Nagasaki, show no increase in the incidence of MGUS or MM (55–57). However, they do show an increase in transformation from MGUS to MM.

There appears to be a weakly significant association between MM, farming, and exposure to pesticides (58,59). Small studies suggest the possibility of slight increases in MM with other occupations. There is no convincing data supporting an association of myeloma with benzene, a component of crude oil present in most stages of petroleum extraction and refining (60–63).

Historically, chronic infection and chronic antigenic stimulation (e.g., osteomyelitis and rheumatoid arthritis) have been considered a predisposing factor to the development of MM. Corroborating that idea, studies of immunoglobulin heavy chain (IgH) gene hypermutation show that MM clones are derived from post–antigen-selected B cells. It appears that chronic antigen stimulation may generate clonal PC outgrowths and also may promote progression of MGUS to MM by creating an immune environment conducive to B-cell proliferation (64–66).

The risk of MM is increased 10-fold as a second cancer following Kaposi sarcoma (43). This finding sparked initial speculation of an etiologic roll for the Kaposi sarcoma herpes virus (KSHV, HHV8), but subsequent data conclude the absence of an etiologic roll for KSHV. However, as with other nonmelanoma skin cancers, which are increased in MM patients, it is possible that the inflammatory milieu induced by such cancers contributes to the transformation from MGUS to MM (67,68). By analyzing large population statistics, it appears that MGUS/MM itself is a predisposing factor to develop a second hematologic malignancy, specifically myelodysplasia (MDS) or leukemia (69,70).

The moderately strong association between HIV and MM may also be secondary, due to a host environment conducive to myelomagenesis rather than a direct cause (71). However, in at least one patient, the antibody produced by the MM clone was directed against the p24 HIV capsid antigen (72).

Evidence for an association between MM and tobacco or alcohol is scant (73).

There is some evidence that medications interfering with pathways important to myelomagenesis may precipitate or prevent MM. For example, *ex vivo* studies show that estrogen blocks IL-6–mediated proliferation in MM cell lines. Three studies have reported a decreased risk of MM in women on hormone replacement therapy (74–76).

Preliminary data suggest an increase in MM in acetaminophen users and a decrease in aspirin users (77,78). The posited mechanisms are plausible, acetaminophen aiding in myelomagenesis by increasing NF-κB, and aspirin retarding myeloma by inhibiting cyclo-oxygenase-1 and -2 as well as NF-κB and IL-6.

Obesity also is a risk factor in MGUS and MM (79). In obese persons, relative risks of MM between 1.4 and 2.5 are reported (80). After adjusting for age and race, there is an approximately 80% increase risk of MGUS in obese persons (81). A modest decrease in MM has been reported in patients with two or more cumulative hours of exercise per week (82). Another study reported a twofold increase in MM mortality in patients who walked <30 minutes a day, compared to those who walked for more than an hour (83). The data in these studies suggest that BMI and exercise are independent factors.

Pathogenesis

Generalized BM involvement is typical in MM, leading to anemia and, sometimes, thrombocytopenia via marrow replacement. As such, a randomly localized iliac crest core biopsy is sufficient for diagnosis. Computed tomography or other imaging study–guided biopsy is required in a small minority of patients. For a clinical trial that required a positive biopsy for enrollment, only 1/45 (2%) patients needed an image-guided biopsy (84).

The most common pathogenic manifestations are those included in the CRAB acronym. Lytic lesions, and/or osteoporosis, and/or pathologic fractures/vertebral collapse are present in 70% of patients at diagnosis and are often associated with bone pain and hypercalcemia (2,85,86).

There are several mechanisms for renal failure. The most common is tubular damage by the chemical and electrostatic effects of light chain proteinuria. Light chain may also cause glomerular and parenchymal kidney damage through amyloid fibril deposition. The renal damage results in decreased erythropoietin production that exacerbates the anemia from marrow replacement, and may cause a secondary hypercalcemia as well.

Many patients suffer from recurrent infections, largely a consequence of depressed production of normal, protective immunoglobulin. In fact, infection is a presenting sign in up to 20% of new myeloma patients.

Common associated clinical laboratory abnormalities include hyperuricemia in 50% of patients, high creatinine (~25%), hypercalcemia (20%), and hypoalbuminemia (15%) (16).

Although some PB transit is required for spread from bone to bone, MM cells compose <1% of PB leukocytes in most patients. Increasing numbers of MM cells in the PB are seen in some patients with advanced, late-stage disease. Extramedullary disease is only seen in advanced cases, often accompanied by an overt leukemic phase. The most common extramedullary sites include skin, soft tissue, liver, breast, lymph nodes, and the CNS (87).

The pathogenesis of myeloma bone disease is complex. It involves both down-regulation of osteoblastic bone production and up-regulation of osteoclastic resorption. CD56/NCAM is strongly expressed on osteoblast cell membranes; when membrane-bound CD56 binds to another CD56 molecule secreted by or on the surface of an MM cell, the osteoblast will stop making new bone (19). MM cells also secrete DKK1, which inhibits osteoblast differentiation (88). Expression of both CD56 and DKK1 by MM cells is related to the presence of lytic bone lesions. In addition to decreasing bone production, myeloma stimulates osteoclastogenesis and bone resorption by triggering a coordinated increase in the tumor necrosis factor–related activation-induced cytokine (TRANCE) and a decrease in its decoy receptor, osteoprotegerin (OPG) (89). The TRANCE/OPG axis is critical in the pathogenesis of MM-induced osteoclastic bone resorption.

Chromosomal and Molecular Alterations

Literature describing the significance of chromosomal abnormalities in PCN is voluminous and sometimes contradictory. Larger series often show that the significance of a given abnormality depends upon the context of other cytogenetic findings. Also, literature suggests that some of the well-described abnormalities are significant only in a therapy-specific manner; that is, an abnormality is prognostic only when treated with a certain drug. The following discussion highlights what appear to be the most important and reliable findings.

One important note of clarification is that hematopathologists and hematologists commonly use the term gene "rearrangement" to denote the physiologic process that occurs in immunoglobulin genes and T-cell receptor genes during antigen selection (described elsewhere in this book). For examination of a neoplasm, the significance of rearrangement is typically in lineage determination (B/plasma cell or T cell) and in the determination of clonality. By contrast, cytogeneticists and their literature use the term "rearrangement" to denote what hematopathologists and hematologists call a "translocation," part of one chromosome being found on a different chromosome. In this chapter, we refer to this exclusively as "translocation," not "rearrangement."

In addition to difficulties of myeloma analysis due to marrow fibrosis and poor *ex vivo* viability (see Important Differences between Myeloma and Other Hematopoietic Neoplasms section, above), analysis of myeloma cells is hampered in the arena of traditional chromosomal analysis by the low proliferation of most cases. Because myeloma cells typically have a proliferation rate far lower than the background marrow (Fig. 37.7B and C), a routine metaphase karyotype typically results in assessment of the normal background cells, thus leading to a false-negative result. Still, because it does sometimes yield helpful clinical information and can highlight aggressive rapidly dividing myeloma subtypes, routine karyotyping currently is recommended by consensus (90). Even when the karyotype represents the MM clone, because the common recurrent translocation breakpoints are so close to the telomere, they are typically undetectable in a metaphase spread. For these reasons, fluorescent *in situ* hybridization (FISH) is the most useful method of chromosomal assessment in PCN.

Although there is a plethora of cytogenetic data, there is no consensus on the importance of these data or how to incorporate them into clinical practice. As stated in the most recent report from the IMWG, "...the consensus is that the data are not yet adequate to suggest routine use of these FISH markers to predict prognosis" (90). That said, FISH is a standard part of routine specimen analysis in PCN and certain FISH findings are highly predictive of the clinical course. Many hematologists feel that it is an important adjunct in their decision-making process. What follows are general rules of thumb regarding what is widely considered to be the significance of these findings.

Although standard FISH methods are sufficient in most cases of MM, in cases with few PCs, sensitivity is enhanced by PC identification or selection prior to FISH probe analysis, thus yielding FISH results representative of the PC population alone (91). There are several good methods of preselecting PCs for directed FISH, such as CD138 magnetic bead selection (92).

Cytogenetic testing via karyotyping or FISH reveal an average of seven abnormalities in the majority of tested myeloma patients (93). FISH testing is performed on resting interphase cells and will identify an abnormality in >90% of patients (94).

For prognostic purposes, a synthesis of the strongest data, including large prospective trials on newly diagnosed patients, support the use of this algorithm (Fig. 37.6), which must be

followed—in order—from left to right. Important notes on the use of the algorithm are as follows. FISH studies on selected MM cells show that nearly all MM cases are positive for at least one of the listed abnormalities. Therefore, if the proper probes are used in a clinical case, "normal" cytogenetic results suggest that the MM cells are not captured in the FISH analysis.

Each listed abnormality is discussed separately below. The listed translocations are mutually exclusive (e.g., t(4;14) and t(11;14) do not coexist in any case). Any of the listed translocations may, however, coexist in a case with hyperdiploidy. Hyperdiploidy is defined as 47 to 74 chromosomes (hyperdiploid MM; H-MM). However, whereas t(4;14) and t(14;16) portend a worse prognosis with or without hyperdiploidy, even in H-MM, t(11;14) and t(6;14) do not affect the favorable outcomes associated with H-MM (95,96). Del(13) and del(17p) may coexist with any of the other listed abnormalities.

The presence of t(4;14), t(14;16), del(17p), del(1p), or amp(1q) has been shown to be the predictor of an unfavorable outcome. Following the algorithm, if those abnormalities have been excluded, myeloma cases can then be divided into H-MM and non-hyperdiploid (NH-MM) (including near-diploid and pseudodiploid cases, the latter with reciprocal translocations). The H-MM group (50% to 60% of all MM patients) include gains of odd chromosomes, such as 3, 5, 7, 9, 11, 15, 19, 21, in various combinations (95,97–103). After excluding cases with t(4;14), t(14;16), del(17p), del(1p), or amp(1q), the remaining NH-MM group is composed of cases with t(11;14) and t(6;14). All t(11;14)-positive and nearly all hyperdiploid cases express cyclin D1 by IHC. All t(6;14)-positive cases express cyclin D3 by IHC. All cases negative for hyperdiploidy, t(11;14), and t(6;14) are negative for cyclin D1 and D3.

Hyperdiploidy (50% to 60% of MM) has been shown repeatedly to be a favorable prognostic indicator. The fact that no group has ever successfully generated a hyperdiploid myeloma cell line supports the idea that H-MM is a relatively indolent genotype. Hyperdiploidy coexists with an IgH (immunoglobulin heavy chain locus—found on chromosome 14) translocation in up to 40% of patients: t(11;14) in approximately 5%, t(4;14) in 7%, t(14;16) in 1%, and unknown IgH translocation partners in 12% to 23% (95,98). The favorable outcome of H-MM appears to be overridden by the coexistence of unfavorable abnormalities (e.g., amp(1q), or t(4;14)) but not affected by the coexistence of favorable abnormalities (e.g., t(11;14)) (96). One study showed that the coexistence of H-MM and an IgH translocation with an unknown partner chromosome is an unfavorable finding (95).

The most common translocation present in the nonhyperdiploid group is t(11;14)(q13;q32), which is present in approximately 15% of MGUS and MM and causes overexpression of cyclin D1 (104). The presence of t(11;14) is statistically favorable in MM. Another translocation, t(6;14)(p21;q32), causes marked overexpression of cyclin D3. The t(11;14)/D1 and t(6;14)/D3 groups share identical clinical and survival parameters (102).

One feature differentiating B/PC neoplasms from other hematologic cancers is the pattern of translocations, which do *not* result in the formation of fusion proteins, as are seen in some leukemias. Instead, the IgH/chromosome 14 translocations lead to dysregulated expression of oncogenes caused by juxtaposition of IgH gene regulatory elements to oncogene promoters (105,106). In lymphomas, the translocations involve the IgH joining (J) region, but in PCN, they involve the IgH switch (S) region. The biochemical distinction precipitates differences in the amount of protein overexpression by the dysregulated gene. For example, mantle cell lymphoma (MCL) has a t(11;14) that involves the J region and results in mild overexpression of cyclin D1. By contrast, the t(11;14) in PCN involves the S region, resulting in massive overexpression of cyclin D1 due to proximity of the D1 promoter to the IgH Eμ-enhancer; the latter element is not operative in the J-region translocation of MCL.

Little is known or understood about the mechanisms responsible for the associations between MM genotype and

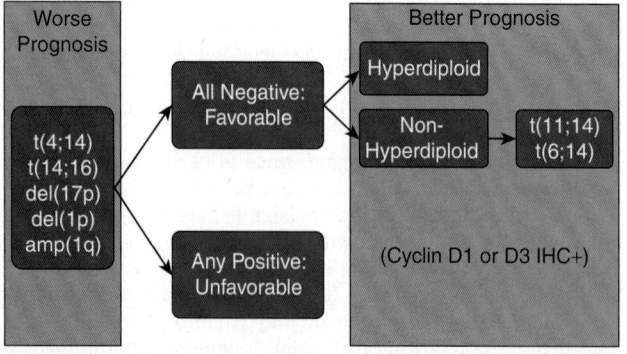

FIGURE 37.6. Associations between FISH, cyclin D1/D3 IHC, and prognosis. The left-most box contains a list of cytogenetic abnormalities that predict unfavorable patient outcomes. The presence of any of these places the patient in the unfavorable group from a cytogenetic perspective. The absence of all those abnormalities places the patient in a favorable group. The favorable group includes hyperdiploidy, with or without t(11;14) or t(6;14), and nonhyperdiploidy. After exclusion of the box on the left, the remaining nonhyperdiploid group consists of t(11;14)- and t(6;14)-positive cases. All t(11;14)-positive and nearly all hyperdiploid cases express cyclin D1 by IHC. All t(6;14)-positive cases express cyclin D3 by IHC. All cases negative for HD, t(11;14), and t(6;14) are negative for cyclin D1 and D3.

biologic behavior. Gene expression profiling (GEP) has shown that hyperdiploidy in MM affects gene expression via a gene-dosage effect (e.g., increased copies of chromosome 11, the locus of cyclin D1, are presumed to cause an increase in cyclin D1 protein expression). Consistent overexpression of cyclin D1 or D2 has been found in the H-MM group, and there is massive overexpression of cyclin D1 associated with t(11;14). However, whereas increased amounts of D cyclins would be presumed to facilitate an increase in proliferation and disease aggressiveness, the opposite has been observed: the amount of cyclin D1 does not correlate with MM cell proliferation (107). Also, cyclin D1 transgenic mice do not develop plasmacytomas or MM.

Expression of D cyclin proteins is mutually exclusive (i.e., if there is expression of cyclin D1, the cell does not express cyclin D2 or D3). Although RNA arrays have shown "overexpression" of multiple D cyclin mRNAs in rare cases of MM, single cell analysis shows that individual MM cells express only a single D cyclin protein (D1, D2, or D3) (107). A hypothesis that would explain the favorable prognosis associated with direct dysregulation of cyclin D1 or D3 is that excess of this single molecule prevents coordinated equimolar increases in D cyclins with their cyclin dependent kinases (Cdks) which effectively stifles Cdk-dependent cell cycling. While D cyclins are necessary accessory molecules, Cdk 4 and 6 are the actual kinases that cause cell cycle progression. Coordinated increases in Cdks with their D cyclins have been shown to be the mechanism of increased proliferation in MM progression and recurrence (107). A hypothesis that follows is that sustained overexpression of cyclin D1 or D3 precludes coordinated expression of cyclin D2 with Cdk4 or 6 and, therefore, prevents the cell from passing the mid-G1 cell cycle checkpoint, thereby preventing proliferation. Functional data support this hypothesis. The proliferation-inducing ligand APRIL works through coordinated up-regulation of cyclin D2 with Cdk4/6, increasing proliferation in MM cell lines lacking cyclin D1 expression, but has no effect on lines with constitutive D1 overexpression (108).

The t(4;14)(p16.3;q32.3) is found in approximately 15% of patients and confers an unfavorable prognosis (109–111). This translocation is unusual in that it leads to separation of the Ig enhancers with consequent dysregulation of two oncogenes, one on each of the derivative (der) chromosomes. Eα drives dysregulation of FGFR3 on the der(4), while Eμ drives dysregulation of MMSET (also called WHSC1) on the der(10). MMSET is nearly always up-regulated by the translocation, but only 75% of cases show up-regulation of FGFR3. In addition to the translocation, 10% of MM patients have activating mutations of FGFR3. Data suggest an oncogenic role for MMSET, but that FGFR3 might only be oncogenic when mutated (112,113).

The t(14;16)(q32.3;q23) occurs in 5% to 10% of patients and is associated with an unfavorable prognosis (90,114). This translocation results in overexpression of c-MAF, which has an established oncogenic role, possibly through up-regulation of cyclin D2 (115).

In theory, inactivation of the p53 pathway would require effects on both alleles (e.g., deletion of one allele and mutation of the second allele). In real-life cases, deletion of 17p is typically monoallelic, as assessed by a FISH probe for TP53. Clinical data show that del(17p)/TP53 is found in approximately 10% of MM and is associated with worse outcomes, regardless of the presence or absence of other cytogenetic abnormalities (100,114,116–118). Deletion of both alleles, however, is rare. Del(17p) is nearly unique to NH-MM, occurring in only 1% of H-MM cases (119). Other studies show that TP53 mutations (not deletion) occur in 2% to 20% of MM and are also associated with worse outcomes (120–123). Mutations of p53 are not observed in MGUS, thus positing that p53 abnormalities are a relatively late development in the progression of MM. Studies assessing both mutation and deletion are rare, but it appears that approximately 50% of MM patients with TP53 mutations

have concomitant hemizygous losses at 17p13; conversely, only 16% of patients who have 17p13 hemizygous deletions have mutations in the remaining copy of TP53 (124). To summarize the p53 data, it is not clear that the common FISH finding, del(17p), denotes complete inactivation of the p53 pathway, but clinical data do show a clear association between del(17p) and worse outcomes.

Homozygous deletion of 13 (most common) or partial del(13q14) (less common) is found in 50% of MM (125,126). It is found in 40% of hyperdiploid and 75% of nonhyperdiploid cases (119). Although initial studies showed an association with unfavorable outcomes, more recent data show that it has no independent effect in the context of H-MM or NH-MM (95,96,118,127,128). The earlier data appear to have been skewed because, in NH-MM, del(13) almost always occurs if there also is a t(4;14), t(14;16) or an abnormality of 1 (125,129). The earlier described significance of del(13) appear to be a mere bystander association with other potent chromosomal abnormalities. Still, del(13) is of diagnostic use in some cases as a marker of clonality.

Abnormalities of chromosome 1 are common in MM, primarily del(1p32.3) (found in 14% of MM) and amplifications of 1q (amp1q21) (found in 15% of MM) (129,130). Del(1p) is associated with increased proliferation and is an independent risk factor for worse overall and progression-free survival (131). It is found in 5% of MGUS, 10% of SMM, and 15% of MM and is thought to act through deletion of CKDN2C, which encodes p18, a critical cell cyclin inhibitor in PCs and MM (132,133). Homozygous del(1p32.3) is associated with inactivation if the remaining allele though an unknown mechanism (133).

Amp1q21 is associated with a poor prognosis and with disease progression. Specific genes of importance in this region have not been conclusively identified. The proportion of cells with amp1q21 and the copy number of 1q21 increases at relapse compared with diagnosis. The frequency of amp1q21 is 0% in MGUS, 45% in SMM, 43% in newly diagnosed MM, and 72% in relapsed MM (134,135). The mechanism for 1q amplification appears to be pericentromeric instability, which results in direct or inverted duplications (135,136). The same mechanism can result in adding whole-arm 1q to nonhomologous chromosomes, resulting in, for example, t(1;16)(q10;p10), t(1;19)(q10;p10), or t(1;8)(p12;q24), which is a MYC translocation. Also, multiple receptor chromosomes can be involved in both whole-arm and telomeric 1q translocations within a single clone (126).

MYC translocations do not appear to affect prognosis (116). They are found in 5% of MGUS and approximately 15% of MM (137,138). The fact that they occur in a far higher percentage of MM cell lines, possibly >90%, suggests they may be a common late event in disease evolution, or possibly they are an aid in *ex vivo* cell survival (137,139).

The above section on cytogenetic analysis is summarized in Table 37.1.

Table 37.1	CYTOGENETIC ABNORMALITIES IN MULTIPLE MYELOMA		
FISH Abnormality	**Gene/FISH Probe**	**Frequency**	**Prognosis**
Hyperdiploidy	–	45%	Favorable
del 13q	?/RB	50%	No impact
t(11;14)	CCND1	8%–20%	Favorable
t(6;14)	CCND3	2%	Favorable
t(14;16)	MAF	2%–5%	Unfavorable
T(4;14)	MMSET, FGFR3	7%–15%	Unfavorable
del 17p	P53	11%	Unfavorable
del 1p12 or 1p32	CKDN2C	11%–20%	Unfavorable
amp 1q21	?/CKS1B	40%	Unfavorable

T(14;20), found in <2% of patients, results in overexpression of the oncogene MafB (140). Because it is of low incidence, it is typically not included in discussion of important chromosomal abnormalities. However, recent data suggest that although rare, it may be important because it correlates strongly with the poorest outcomes (141).

Gene Expression Profiling and Other Genetic Techniques

Beginning in 2002, GEP has shown that patients can be divided into risk strata based on gene chip array data (142,143). These studies spawned proposed molecular classifications (102,144,145). Yet, the techniques largely remain research tools for practical reasons (they are labor-intensive, costly, and not paid for by most health care systems or insurance), but also because they do not offer increased clinical or prognostic value above routinely assessed clinical and laboratory parameters (111). Furthermore, the risk stratification profiles attained from GEP have not been formally tested as a prognostic tool in a prospective manner, and thus there are no guidelines for how these data can guide therapeutic decisions.

The high degree of methodologic inconsistency also is of concern. Two groups have published statistically significant risk stratification based on 15 and 17 gene models, but the models do not share any common genes (143,144). This may partly be due to the lack of standardization of this approach, both regarding laboratory methodology and the methods for analyzing data.

More recent literature suggests the importance and utility of a deeper analysis of individual gene mutations, including whole genome sequencing, but the data are preliminary. Of note, comparative genomic hybridization has revealed possible clinical significance of gains or losses in previously unrecognized chromosomal areas (146).

Assessment of Cell Proliferation

At the time of diagnosis, most cases of myeloma show very low proliferation with typically <2% of PCs in active cell cycle. The proliferation rate of the PCs increases at relapse (147). Beginning with pioneering studies of BrdU incorporation in the 1980s, the association between proliferation and prognosis has been confirmed repeatedly (143,148–150). GEP and proposed molecular classifications confirm the impact of proliferation on outcomes (102,142,143). Due to practical limitations, assessment of proliferation is not a part of standard testing in most centers (151). The originally described method, called the plasma cell labeling index, is labor- and cost-intensive. The typical method used to assess proliferation in solid organ cancers, single-color IHC, does not work well because, in marrow biopsies, MM cells are admixed with highly proliferative background hematopoietic cells, and it is not possible to distinguish between the former and the latter (Fig. 37.7A). For this reason, newer methods of proliferation assessment have been devised that can be performed in any laboratory on the same equipment used for standard IHC. As such, the methods are user-friendly and cost-efficient. In the first (Fig. 37.7B) PCs are stained with CD138 and a red chromogen, resulting in all PCs standing out

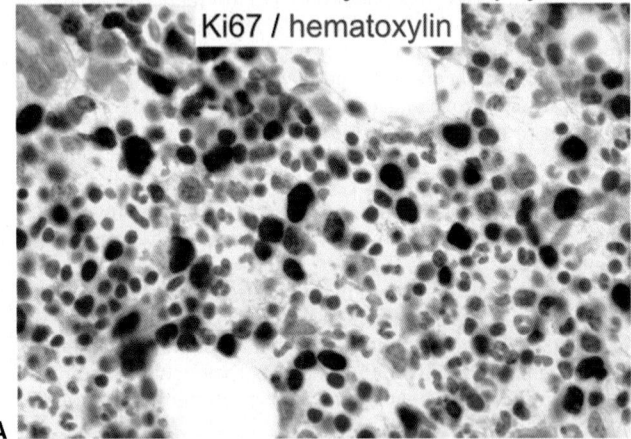

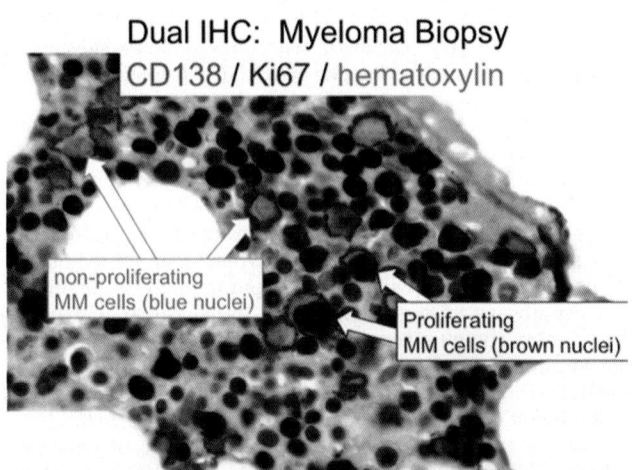

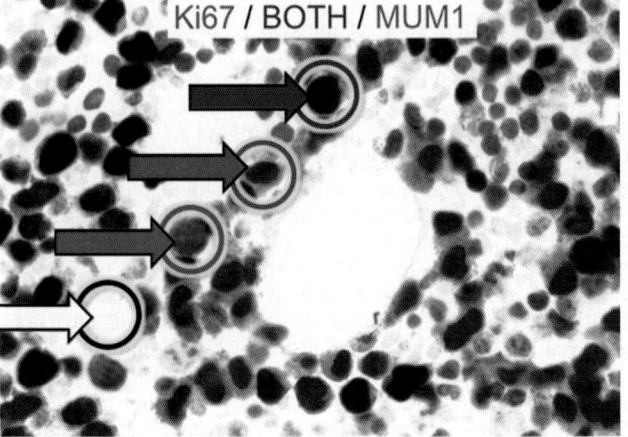

FIGURE 37.7. Assessment of proliferation in PCs. A: With standard IHC for Ki67, we can see that many cells are proliferating (*brown nuclei*), but we cannot tell if they are PCs versus myeloid or erythroid. **B:** In many biopsies, double IHC with CD138 (*red*)/Ki67 (*brown*) and a hematoxylin (*blue*) counterstain works well to assess myeloma cell proliferation and eliminate background hematopoietic cells from the analysis. It *always* works well when the MM cells are scattered, as in this picture, but sometimes less well when the MM cells are in sheets. **C:** In this method, it is always easy to distinguish purple Ki67+ myeloma cells (*purple arrow*) from red Ki67-negative MM cells (*red arrow*) or blue proliferating background hematopoietic cells (*blue arrow*). Double-negative cells (i.e., nonproliferating background cells) are not visible (*white arrow*).

from background cells due to red cell membranes; the slides are costained with Ki67 and a brown chromogen, then with a hematoxylin (blue) counterstain. In the resultant slide, the PC proliferation index is manually counted by assessing 200 PCs (red membrane) as either proliferating (brown nucleus) or not (blue nucleus). By this method, it has been determined that proliferation increases at relapse (147). There is a statistically significant correlation between pretransplant MM cell proliferation by this method and overall survival after 12 years of follow-up (152,153). A proliferation index of >10% also correlates with increased risk of disease progression in first-line therapy (154).

A newer method improves upon the one described above by enabling easier manual counting in cases with sheets of PCs or with marked fibrosis. It also enables computer image analysis instead of manual counting (Fig. 37.7C.). In this method, MUM1 is used to identify PCs with a red chromogen, and Ki67 is stained with a blue chromogen; the slides contain cells of four types: red (nonproliferating PCs), purple (double-stained, proliferating PCs), blue (proliferating background hematopoietic cells), and invisible (nonproliferating background cells are not visible because a counterstain is not used).

PATHOLOGIC DIAGNOSIS

Biopsy Requirements

As discussed above, a trephine/core biopsy is the most sensitive means of diagnosing a PCN. Although a minimal acceptable length has not been determined to exclude a PCN, for other marrow cancers, 1.5 cm of deep (not subcortical) marrow has been recommended. By contrast, any size is acceptable if the biopsy clearly shows MM. Aspirate smears are notoriously unreliable for the diagnosis of PCN (Fig. 37.4) (22,24–26,29).

In addition to an adequate core biopsy, aspirate smears are useful to assess the possibility of concomitant myelodysplasia, especially in the setting of prior chemotherapy or autologous stem cell transplant. Also, aspirated cells are required for cytogenetic analysis and FC. FC is the gold standard method for immunophenotyping in other cancers, but it is problematic in PCN (see Flow Cytometry section, below).

Specimen Processing

As compared to other types of specimens, myeloma biopsies require special processing considerations (155). Core biopsy morphology is best with Bouin fixation. A nondecalcified, formalin-fixed aspirate

clot can be useful for polymerase chain reaction (PCR) analysis and for FISH if aspirate PCs are not available.

Unlike BM cells of other lineages, PCs die very quickly after being aspirated from the marrow milieu. For this reason, if FC or other procedures requiring live cells are performed, it is critical that the aspirated material be processed immediately. Also, if samples are sent via courier to another location for analysis, a high number of false negatives may be encountered.

Morphology

The single most useful morphologic feature in the diagnosis of PCN is the pattern of PC infiltration observed in a core biopsy (21,23,156,157). To assess the pattern, IHC for CD138 or MUM1 should be used. In reactive plasmacytosis and in MGUS, the PCs are scattered, in small clusters, and perivascular (Fig. 37.8A). In MM, the PCs may be somewhat perivascular, but because they grow in large aggregates or sheets, the relationship to vessels is usually not striking. A sheet is defined as a monotonous collection of PCs so large that it distorts the underlying architecture (i.e., the underlying pattern of hematopoietic marrow and fat seen elsewhere in the biopsy is disrupted). Unlike MGUS and reactive PCs, MM cells often fill interfatty spaces (i.e., the space between two fat cells is filled by PCs) (Fig. 37.8B) (25).

The observance on a CD138- or MUM1-stained slide of sheets or interfatty spaces filled with PCs is diagnostic of MM (21,23,25,156,157). Still, it is good practice to confirm the diagnosis by verifying abnormal antigen expression (CD56, cyclin D1, cyclin D3, or monotypic cIgκ or λ).

In Wright-Giemsa–stained aspirate smears, PCs are striking and stand out from the background marrow due to abundant deep blue cytoplasm. There usually is a juxtanuclear Golgi, sometimes called a "Hoff." The nuclei are strikingly round with heavily clumped chromatin. Authors have described the nuclear appearance as the confusing but oft-repeated "clock face" and "cart wheel," or the more apt, "soccer ball." PC nuclei, benign and neoplastic, often have visible nucleoli, which is not a feature of immaturity.

Features of immaturity (disbursed chromatin, central nuclei, very large nucleoli, high N:C) (Fig. 37.9) have been shown to correlate with prognosis, including in prospective trials on uniformly treated patients (21,25,156,157). Plasmablastic morphology has been shown to be an independent prognostic factor in multiple trials (158,159). However, such findings have never been incorporated into any widely used

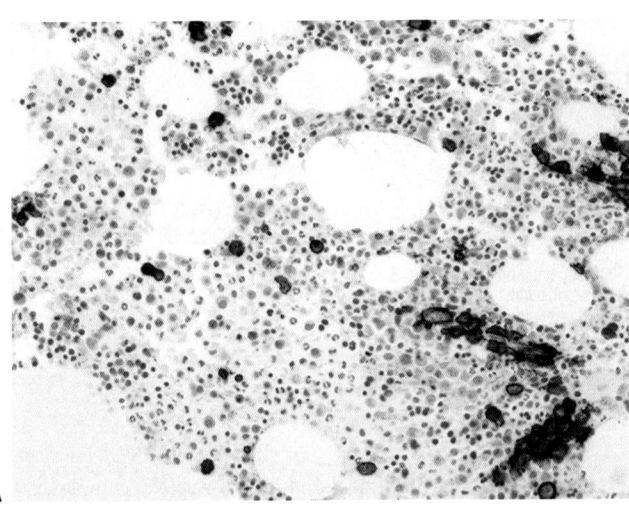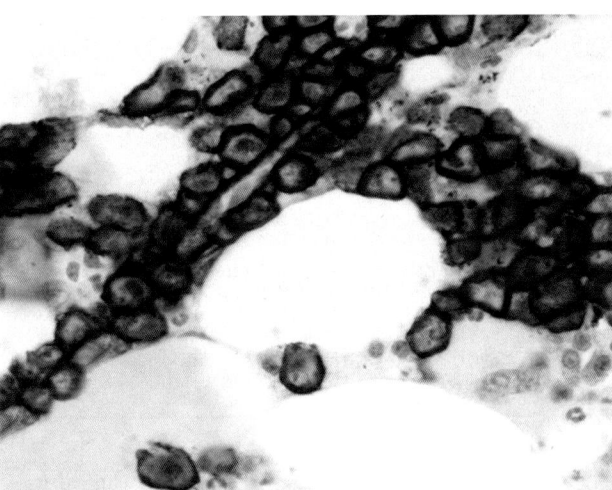

FIGURE 37.8. CD138 IHC, normal versus myeloma. A: Reactive, nonneoplastic PCs are scattered, present in small clusters, or perivascular (CD138, normal PCs, 200×). **B:** The space between two fat cells is filled by PCs (CD138, myeloma biopsy, 400×).

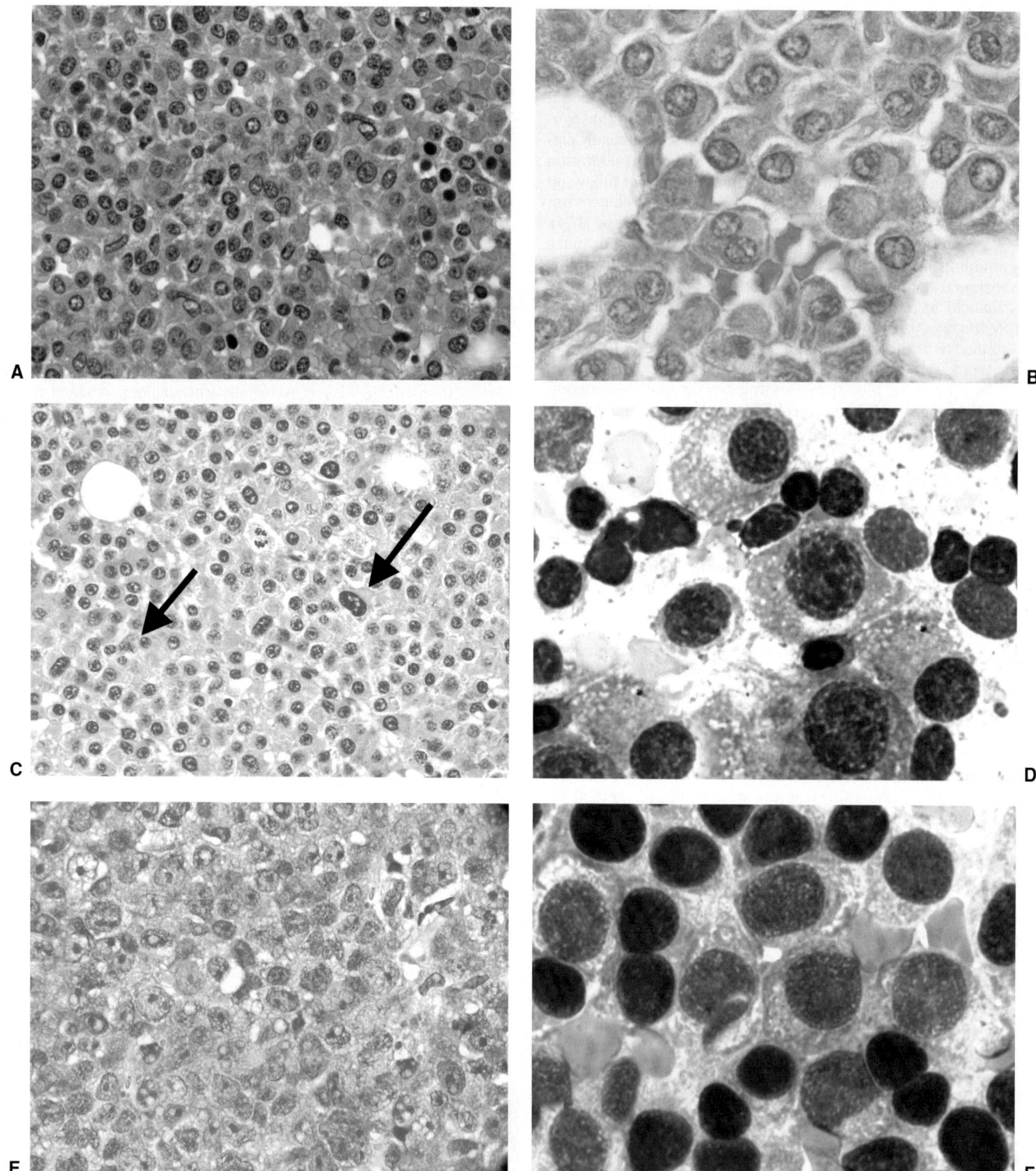

FIGURE 37.9. Myeloma cell morphology. A: PCs in most cases of MM are "mature," which denotes clumped chromatin (H&E, 400×). **B:** In some cases, referred to as "intermediate-grade" in older classification schemes, the chromatin is less clumped, but not truly disbursed, as in plasmablasts (H&E, 1,000×). The N:C is low and nucleoli are small. **C:** Some biopsies contain bizarre-shaped or very large PCs (*arrows*), sometimes misleadingly referred to as "anaplastic." Shape and size do not affect biologic behavior, but chromatin pattern does. **D:** A smear from case C shows variable cell size, but clumped chromatin (Wright Giemsa, 1,000×). **E:** "Plasmablastic" morphology denotes disbursed chromatin, very large single nucleoli, and a relatively high N:C (H&E, 1,000×). **F:** The smear from (**E**) shows plasmablastic morphology with disbursed chromatin and very large nucleoli (Wright Giemsa, 1,000×).

scheme for clinical decision making. The lack of clinical use for these schemes may be related to the difficulty of following the methods used to define a plasmablastic cell. To illustrate, in one trial plasmablastic myeloma cells are defined as "...having a large, centrally placed nucleus (>10 μm in diameter) or a

nucleolus (>2 μm in diameter) and a high nuclear/cytoplasmic ratio; the cytoplasm is scant and lacks a prominent perinuclear Hoff." To be classified as plasmablastic PCM in these studies, plasmablasts must comprise 2% or more of nucleated cells in the BM aspirate (158,159).

The appearance of bizarrely shaped cells does not affect the prognosis in MM, regardless of whether they are rare or compose the majority of PCs (Fig. 37.9). Odd cellular or nuclear shapes should not be mistaken for immaturity, which is defined by chromatin features. For this reason, the term "anaplastic" is misleading and should not be used. "Anaplastic myeloma" is not an entity.

The following entities are common findings in PCN morphology: Russell bodies are cytoplasmic vacuoles filled with immunoglobulin; Dutcher bodies are cytoplasmic immunoglobulin vacuoles invaginating into the nucleus, creating the appearance of an intranuclear inclusion. Russell bodies are common in PCs, both reactive and neoplastic. Dutcher bodies also are found in both reactive and neoplastic PCs, but they are uncommon in reactive conditions and, when found, should always prompt a search for neoplasms. Dutcher bodies are common in both PCN and in lymphoplasmacytic lymphoma/Waldenstrom macroglobulinemia.

Bone Morphology

A relatively small number of osteoclasts are responsible for resorptive maintenance of the entire skeleton. Because a single osteoclast is responsible for remodeling a large amount of bone, and because each osteoclast moves relatively great distances, individual sites of increased osteoclastic resorption are rare and not found in most random biopsies. Since MM typically occurs in patients >60 years old, the bone is typically osteopenic. However, bisphosphonate therapy is instituted in most MM patients thereby poisoning osteoclastic resorption and leading to osteosclerosis. Thus, compared to age-matched controls, follow-up biopsies in MM patients often show thickened bony trabeculae.

Immunophenotyping

Immunohistochemistry

A recommended list of IHC for routine use in the workup of PCN begins as follows: PAX5 (a homeobox protein found in B-cell nuclei), CD56 (NCAM, normally expressed by NK cells and osteoblasts), CD138 (Syndecan 1, an adhesion molecule expressed by all PCs and most epithelium), MUM1 (IRF4; a nuclear protein expressed by PCs and late B cells), cIgκ, and cIgλ. In cases where the cIgκ:cIgλ is difficult to interpret, the addition of heavy chains (M, D, G, and A) can sometimes clarify the presence of a monotypic population. For assessment of cytogenetic abnormalities,

double staining greatly increases the specificity, as opposed to analysis of single-stained, serial sections. Recommended double stains are CD138/cyclin D1, CD138/cyclin D3, and MUM1/Ki67 (Fig. 37.7). In lieu of the latter, CD138/Ki67 can be used (see section on proliferation assays, above).

B cells (small, PAX5+ cells) should compose <10% of background cells and be scattered, not in aggregates. If small B cells are plentiful and/or present in aggregates, a B-cell lymphoma with plasmacytoid differentiation should be considered.

PCNs are better represented in core biopsies than aspirated cell samples. IHC on a core is the gold standard for diagnosis of PCN, favored by the majority of hematopathologists (20,160). Because it is easy to overlook PCs by examination of H&E sections, IHC must be performed in all cases. The analysis begins by assessing the number and distribution of PCs by CD138 and MUM1. Both markers are expressed by all PCs, benign and malignant, with rare exception.

In some cases, the myeloma cells shed the extracellular portion of the CD138 molecule, which is associated with abundant fibrosis (27).

CD56 is a highly useful antigen for PC analysis. Weak expression or expression by a small number of scattered PCs is not diagnostic. However, strong expression by an entire PC population is not seen in reactive PCs or MGUS, but is found in 71% of MM (19). Exceptions to this rule are as follows: CD56 is negative in MM patients who do not have lytic lesions (which represent up to one-third of the entire MM population); and CD56 is often lost in late-stage MM, concomitant with independence from the BM stroma via transformation to PC leukemia or extramedullary disease. Also, because all MM are preceded by MGUS, theoretically, there should be some low-stage PCNs in which CD56 expression has begun but is not yet accompanied by the emergence of clinical symptoms.

Most reactive marrow PCs are terminally differentiated and do not proliferate. When reactive plasmacytoid cells do proliferate, it is facilitated by coordinated up-regulation of Cdk4/6 with cyclin D2 (107). As such, assessment of cyclin D2 is not useful for distinguishing a neoplasm from a physiologic process. Finding cyclin D1 (BCL-1) expression in a B cell or PC is diagnostic of a neoplasm. In B cells, cyclin D1 expression is only seen in MCL and hairy cell leukemia (HCL). In PCs, it is seen in equal proportions of MGUS and MM. The staining is weak/partial (only in a subpopulation, sometimes in <10% of PCs, requiring careful analysis) in cases with hyperdiploidy (Fig. 37.10A) but strong and uniform in cases with t(11;14) (Fig. 37.10B) (161).

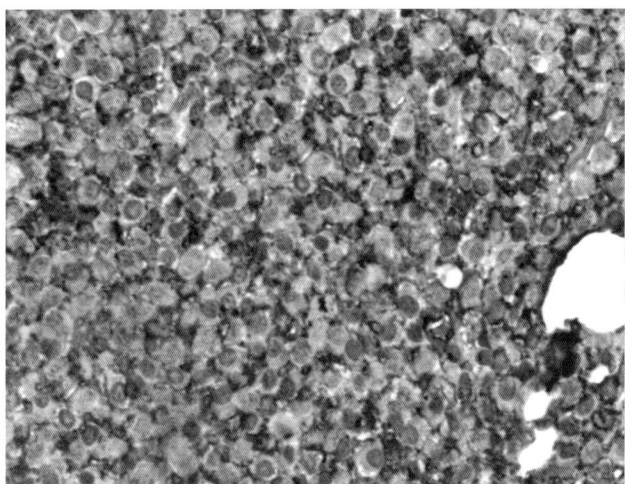
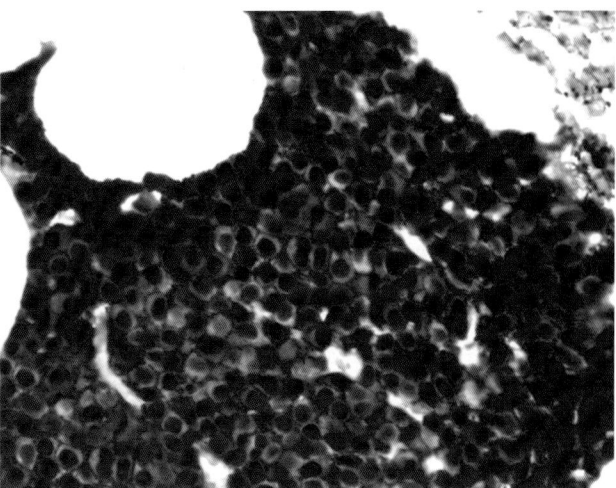

A   B

FIGURE 37.10. Cyclin D1 IHC, t(11;14) versus hyperdiploidy. A: In this sheet of hyperdiploid MM cells with tri(11) but no t(11;14), CD138 (*red*) dual staining with cyclin D1 (*brown*) shows variable/weak/partial coexpression by 10% of MM cells (BM biopsy, IHC, 400×, CD138 [*red*]/cyclin D1 [*brown*]). **B:** In this sheet of t(11;14) MM cells in a BM biopsy, CD138 (*red*) dual staining with cyclin D1 (*brown*) shows markedly strong, uniform coexpression by 100% of MM cells (BM biopsy, IHC, 400×, CD138 [*red*]/cyclin D1 [*brown*]).

Whether strong/uniform or weak/partial, expression of cyclin D1 by IHC is a favorable prognostic indicator (Fig. 37.6).

Like cyclin D1, reactive marrow PCs do not express cyclin D3. In hematopoietic marrow, however, cyclin D3 is highly expressed by megakaryocytes, and also by proliferating erythroid and myeloid cells. Assessment of D3 expression, therefore, requires double staining to discriminate expression in PCs from that in hematopoietic marrow. Double-staining CD138 with cyclin D3 shows positivity only in neoplastic PCs; it is positive only in cases with a t(6;14) (5% of all cases).

To complete the discussion on IHC, please see the section on proliferation assays.

Flow cytometry

Although there is some literature urging the routine use of FC for MM, much of it comes from centers limited to aspirate analysis because they do not perform core biopsies (162,163). Side by side comparisons show that FC works extremely well for the immunophenotypic analysis of leukemias, but for MM and NHL, it shows significantly higher rates of false negativity than by histopathologic evaluation of the same samples (164,165).

Because PCs often are poorly represented in aspirates since they die rapidly after being removed from the marrow, if any are detectable by FC, they are usually in tiny numbers (<1%), which makes the interpretation difficult and undermines the reliability of reporting (Fig. 37.4). When FC is pursued, it typically utilizes CD38 (positive in most leukocyte lineages, but very strong in PCs), CD138 (expressed by hematogones, benign and malignant PCs, sometimes falsely negative by FC in MM due to shedding [27]), and CD56 (expressed by most MM, rare in MGUS or reactive PCs). A typical flow panel also includes cIgκ and Igλ. For technical reasons cyclin D1, one of the most useful immunophenotypic markers in PCN diagnosis, cannot be assessed by FC. MM has been divided into prognostic groups on the basis of CD28 (a costimulatory molecule that may be involved in dendritic cell-PC interactions within the BM stroma and might play a role in myeloma cell survival) and CD117 (c-kit receptor, a tyrosine kinase involved in cell growth that is absent in most normal PC but can be detected in one-third of patients with myeloma). According to these studies, in MM, CD117-only is most favorable; CD28-only is least favorable; double positive and double negative are intermediate (166). However, these data have not been duplicated and the markers appear to correlate with better-established cytogenetic findings.

Although some cases have been described as "CD138 negative" by FC, IHC shows that such cases do express CD138, but shed the extracellular portion of the molecule (27). Because the shed portion of the molecule contains the binding site for the CD138 antibody, FC shows a false-negative result.

To complete the discussion on FC, please see the section on minimal residual disease (MRD).

Chromosomal Analysis

A recommended scheme for clinically useful analysis is to perform a standard karyotype and FISH (90). Probes should include those necessary to assess clinically relevant abnormalities (Fig. 37.6). A recommended list of FISH probes is as follows: LSI FGFR3—IGH dual-color dual-fusion probes, LSI CCND1/MYEOV—IGH dual-color dual-fusion probes, CMAF—IGH dual-color dual-fusion probes, to exclude the t(4;14)(p16.3;q32.3), t(11;14)(q13;q32), and t(14;16)(q32.3;q23), respectively; CEP 5, CEP 9, CEP 15, to exclude hyperdiploidy via trisomies of chromosomes 5, 9, and 15; LSI 13q and LSI TP53 to exclude deletions of 13q14 and TP53, respectively; and LSI CDKN2C (p18) (1p32.3—SG)/LSI CKS1B probes to evaluate for chromosome 1 abnormalities.

Polymerase Chain Reaction

Though it can be useful to diagnose and find residual disease, PCR is little used in PCN for technical reasons. It should be noted that whereas amplification of Jh is the most useful PCR method to find a B-cell clone, for PCs, Jk amplification provides a higher yield. PCR can be performed on freshly acquired liquid aspirates, but also on formalin-fixed, nondecalcified aspirated clots.

Differential Diagnosis

The isotype of the M spike is helpful in establishing the differential diagnosis. IgM is common in some types of NHL but exceedingly rare in PCN. An IgD spike is almost always MM, not seen in MGUS or NHL. IgG is common in PCN, not NHL. IgA can be seen in PCN or NHL. LCO is common in MM and rare in MGUS and NHL. Heavy chain–only is seen in rare types of lymphoma but not in PCN.

The cornerstone of PCN diagnosis is examination of a CD138 IHC slide, making note of the PC mass (intertrabecular space [ITS]) and pattern (Fig. 37.8).

If the infiltrate also includes numerous small B cells, it may be an NHL with plasmacytoid differentiation (e.g., CLL) or a PCN coexistent with a clonally unrelated NHL. FC is helpful in answering this question; if there is an NHL, FC should show a B-cell population with monotypic surface immunoglobulin and an immunophenotype that is otherwise typical of one of the common NHLs. Also, expression of cyclin D1 can be helpful. If cyclin D1 is present in the PCs, they represent a PCN. The only lymphomas with cyclin D1 are MCL, which never shows plasmacytoid differentiation, and HCL. HCL has morphology and an immunophenotype that is so distinctive as to be easily distinguished from a neoplastic PC population. Also, plasmacytoid differentiation is rare in HCL.

Once the diagnosis of PCN has been established, MM is favored over MGUS if the PCs are present in sheets or fill interfatty spaces. Also, CD56 expression is typical of MM and not seen in MGUS. In cases where the findings or biopsy quality preclude the certainty of a PCN-subtype diagnosis, it is reasonable to report "plasma cell neoplasm," and include a note about the differential and how to come to a more precise classification (e.g., "For a more precise diagnosis, correlation with a complete myeloma clinical workup would be required.").

Reporting of Biopsy Findings

The final diagnosis and note for a report issued for the biopsy shown in Figure 37.10 would be as follows:

Final Diagnosis: A, B, C, and D: Right PIC BM clot section, core biopsy, aspirate smears, and flow cytometry:

Plasma Cell Myeloma

Note: These findings comport with the above WHO diagnosis. Neoplastic PCs are present in sheets. They compose 95% of the ITS (>95% of all cells). They strongly express CD56. They show weak, partial expression of cyclin D1, which is typical in hyperdiploidy; cytogenetic analysis confirms hyperdiploidy as well as absence of the following: translocations, del(17p), and chromosome 1 abnormalities. FC shows expression of CD117 but not CD28, which is a favorable finding. The proliferation index (Ki67) is 0%.

As with all hematopathology specimens, the report should consist of a WHO diagnosis (a direct, verbatim quote) followed by a brief note containing the other important features.

The most salient and direct metric for reporting tumor mass is percentage of ITS (i.e., the amount of space between bony trabeculae that is composed of PCs) (21,23,25,156,157). The percentage of PCs also must be reported because it indicates the state of the background, hematopoietic marrow (e.g., if PCs compose 90% of all cells, there is little hematopoietic marrow). The percentage of PCs is most accurate in the core biopsy specimen. If the aspirate percentage is quoted, it should be stated as such. In Figure 37.8B, for example, PCs compose 40% of ITS and >90% of all cells. In Figure 37.10B, PCs compose 70% of ITS and >90% of all cells.

In addition to ITS and percentage of PCs, the note should include expression of only the most clinically important antigens. It is important to note weak, partial expression of cyclin D1, for example, which indicates hyperdiploidy. That information can be important in assessing the possibility of a false-negative cytogenetic analysis. The report should also include an assessment of proliferation. Even if the submitting clinician has not specifically requested a proliferation assay, it is important to note in the patient's record in the event they transfer care to another hematologist and as a valuable comparator for future biopsies.

PROGNOSTICATION AND DISEASE MONITORING

There are many established prognostic indicators that clinicians use to gauge how a patient will fare both in terms of how likely he or she will respond to a given therapy and in estimating survival. Given the relative heterogeneity of MM, risk stratification through analyses of factors found in laboratory, radiology, histology, and cytogenetic studies provide valuable information to help guide therapy. Risk factors for myeloma can be broadly categorized into those found through serum testing, histology, cytogenetic analysis, and radiology.

Serum markers of myeloma activity are readily available and are often the first clue as to the nature of a patient's disease biology. The absolute amount of M protein is a rough reflection of the tumor mass, higher levels correlating with higher Durie-Salmon stage (see Staging section) and shorter survival (167). Population studies on stored frozen samples show that a greater amount of M protein (>1.5 g/dL) is prognostic of a higher risk of progression from MGUS to myeloma (168). The isotype of the M protein also has prognostic significance in that IgA isotype correlates with a shorter survival, likely because IgA myeloma is associated more often with a high-risk cytogenetic profile (94,125,169).

Given the short half-life of FLCs, rapid changes in absolute levels and ratio can be seen in response to treatment or in relapsing/progressive disease (170,171). FLC ratio is abnormal in 96% of newly diagnosed myeloma. The FLC ratio can be essential for making a diagnosis and acting as a tumor activity marker in light chain–only myeloma. It is also useful for advanced myeloma that has progressed to FLC escape (a phenomenon whereby disease that is particularly aggressive and relapsed shifts from secretion of intact M protein to exclusively light chains) (8).

Beta-2 microglobulin (B2M) is a component of the MHC class I molecule and is elevated in a variety of hematologic tumors, including myeloma (172). B2M correlates with myeloma disease activity and has proven to be a powerful predictor of survival incorporated into modern staging systems. At diagnosis, patients with an absolute level of B2M of ≥4.0 had a median overall survival of 12 months, as opposed to 43 months in those patients with lower B2M (173). Notably, B2M is excreted by the kidneys and therefore will be elevated in MM patients with renal dysfunction. Poor renal function is associated with poor performance in MM patients and thus any B2M elevation, regardless of whether due to increased PC activity or decreased glomerular filtration rate, appropriately reflects prognosis.

The absolute values at diagnosis of serum lactate dehydrogenase (LDH) and c-reactive protein, both acute phase reactants, have similarly been shown to correlate with aggressive disease activity in lymphoproliferative disease, including myeloma (174,175). A highly elevated level of serum LDH is an especially poor prognostic marker and connotes advanced or extramedullary myeloma (176).

Serum albumin is a nonspecific marker for general health, nutrition, and performance status. In opposition to other markers of inflammation, such as IL-6, levels of albumin are low in inflammatory states. In MM, depression of albumin to below normal (<3.5 g/dL) at diagnosis correlates with various negative prognostic factors, such as increased age, decreased hemoglobin, increased B2M, higher M-protein levels, and higher percentage of marrow plasmacytosis (177).

Staging

The heterogeneity of myeloma and the impact of the myriad prognostic factors described above naturally lead to wide variability in survival, ranging from 6 months to more than 10 years. Staging systems for myeloma have been developed and evolved to capture known prognostic data and provide useful and simple information for the patient. Historically, the most important is the Durie-Salmon staging system (DSS), first proposed in 1975, which incorporated factors such as hemoglobin, calcium, amount and isotype of M protein, and extent of lytic bone disease into a three-tiered staging system that reflected the myeloma tumor burden in a patient (167). An additional qualification, renal failure with a creatinine >2 mg/dL, further stratified DSS to more accurately predict survival, with a stage 1a (low tumor mass, normal creatinine) patient having a median survival on the order of 191 months and a 3b (high tumor mass, renal failure) of only 5 months. The DSS suffered from user-dependent variability, however, in that the number of lytic bone lesions was not defined specifically; thus separate physicians could stage a patient differently. The DSS failed to predict outcomes in the era of autologous stem cell transplant and novel therapeutic agents for myeloma, such as thalidomide, lenalidomide, and bortezomib (178,179).

An effort to create a more objective and simplified system resulted in the International Staging System (ISS) (Table 37.2) (180). Only B2M and albumin levels are needed to provide a powerful prediction of the median overall survival of active myeloma patients undergoing therapy. The ISS was shown to be valid for prediction of outcomes after stem cell transplant and with novel therapies as well (179,181).

It is important to note that whereas DSS can be applied at any time during the disease course to estimate tumor burden and gauge prognosis, a limitation of the ISS is that it was designed as a prognostic tool for MM patients undergoing initial treatment only (i.e., in newly diagnosed, symptomatic MM). The ISS is not validated when patients are "restaged" at another time point in the disease process.

Of note, when directly compared in myeloma patients undergoing autologous stem cell transplant, there is only a 36% correlation between the DSS and ISS, and both were relatively

Table 37.2	INTERNATIONAL STAGING SYSTEM FOR MULTIPLE MYELOMA	
ISS Stage	**Serum Markers**	**Median Survival**
I	β_2-microglobulin <3.5 mg/L albumin ≥3.5 g/dL	62 mo
II	Neither stage I nor stage III	44 mo
III	β_2-microglobulin ≥5.5 mg/L	29 mo

poor predictors of outcomes in higher-stage disease, reflecting the need for further work on improving the accuracy of myeloma staging (182).

Response Criteria

Criteria for determination of disease response have changed as treatments have led to better tumor reduction and tumor markers, such as FLC analysis, have become available. The current response criteria were developed by the IMWG in 2006 (13). In general, M-protein measurement, through either serum or urine, is the first step to response evaluation, with a serum drop of >50% (or urine of >90%) indicating a partial response. Further drop in M protein such that SPEP becomes negative but IFE remains positive (or alternatively, elimination of 90% of the original serum M protein) reflects a very good partial response (VGPR). Total elimination of all trace of M protein on IFE in both serum and urine, along with <5% plasmacytosis on BM evaluation, is classified as a complete response (CR). The major addition to IMWG response criteria in 2006 was an additional category of stringent complete response (sCR), which reflects the growing importance of IHC, MRD, and FLC analysis. For an sCR, there must be no IHC evidence of PC clonality and the FLC ratio must be normal. Retrospective studies examining the correlation between degree of response and clinical outcomes have shown that achievement of VGPR and higher is an important end point for a successful treatment and that CR and sCR correlate with longer survival times (28,183,184).

Different laboratory techniques and methods for quantifying M protein have led to the establishment of minimal requirements for "measurable" disease, the threshold placed at 200 mg/day in 24-hour urine or 0.5 g/dL on SPEP. These values form the basis for the definition of clear biochemical progression of disease (POD). Any new or growing plasmacytoma or new hypercalcemia not attributable to another clear cause also counts as POD. Less clear is the definition of relapse from CR. As it stands, relapse from CR is any new appearance of a M-protein band on IFE, although there is a body of literature that refutes this definition as it may lead to an inappropriate penalty in the determination of progression-free survival of a investigational therapy (185). Occasionally, patients in CR, especially in the post–stem cell transplant setting, will have the appearance of multiple small IFE bands, unrelated (i.e., different isotypes) to the original disease-specific M protein. Different terms have been coined for this, including oligoclonal banding or atypical IFE patterns (186–188). Because the appearance of the bands usually connotes a favorable clinical outcome, it has been suggested that oligoclonal banding be excluded from the definition of relapse from CR (189,190).

Outcomes/Survival

Until the 1960s, before the use of corticosteroids and chemotherapy, the average survival of a patient with MM was 12 to 24 months (191). The use of the alkylating chemotherapy melphalan and prednisone helped bring an increase in survival to a median of 3 years, a value that did not change for nearly three decades (192). It was not until the advent of high-dose chemotherapy and autologous stem cell transplantation in the early 1990s that the overall survival of myeloma again increased, by about 10 months (193). The use of tandem (or double) stem cell transplants in the mid-1990s also made an impact in increasing survival in those patients who failed to achieve a VGPR or better from the first stem cell transplant (194).

The next major impact on survival came in the early 2000s with the use of the immunomodulatory agents (IMiDs)

thalidomide and lenalidomide (195). IMiDs have much higher response rates and deeper remissions compared to standard chemotherapy alone.

Bortezomib, a proteasome inhibitor, came into use almost concurrently with IMiDs. It also has served to increase response rates, leading to better clinical outcomes (196). The combination of IMiDs and bortezomib, sometimes together, other times with standard chemotherapeutics or autologous stem cell transplant, has led to great increases in the rates of CR and overall survival (28). Maintenance therapy with low doses of thalidomide or lenalidomide posttransplant has also been used with success as a strategy to extend the time until disease progression (197,198).

In the era of melphalan and prednisone therapy, the CR rate was about 1% to 3%. With modern therapy it is not uncommon to see approximately 30% to 40% of patients achieving CR with primary chemotherapy with a rise in CR to approximately 50% after consolidative autologous stem cell transplant (184).

The increase in depth of response with new therapies has led to improvements in overall survival, with different population series reporting median survival times of 5 to 8 years (28,199–202).

Yet, it appears that the improvement may be limited in younger (<70 years of age) patients (203–205).

Minimal Residual Disease

In common usage, the term "MRD positive" means that rare, submicroscopic cancer cells are found to be present after therapy. MRD detection is the use of laboratory techniques with sensitivity in the range of $1/10^4$ cells, far more sensitive than routine laboratory and microscopic analyses. Various permutations of PCR and FC are used for this purpose. MRD assessment has become the gold standard for therapeutic decision making after induction chemotherapy for acute lymphoblastic leukemia and is becoming widely accepted for acute myeloid leukemia (206–209). Although there is literature advocating the use of such techniques for MM, the prospect of MRD is fundamentally different in PCNs (109,162,163,209,210). In acute leukemias, because some patients achieve long-term CRs constituting cures, it makes sense to attempt to eradicate every last cancer cell. Moreover, studies have shown clear efficacy for this tactic. In myeloma, by contrast, nearly all patients relapse, regardless of the presence or absence of MRD. So, there is no current rationale in MM for the use of MRD assessment in clinical decision making.

Still, there are good reasons to move forward with refinement of MRD techniques in myeloma. MRD is a useful end point as a basis of comparison of different therapy regimens as more effective modern regimens are able to achieve a high percentage of CRs and sCRs. It has been shown that achievement of negative MRD in MM is associated with excellent clinical outcomes and could move the goalpost further in assessing new MM therapies (211). In comparison to other end points, such as clinical relapse, MRD analysis would allow faster completion of clinical trials. On a more practical level, because the IMW has added MRD assessment to the recommended response criteria, it may become necessary to assess MRD for the publication of trial data (212). On a hopeful note, if regimens are found that lead to long-term CRs, MRD assessment may become a clinical necessity in the future, as it currently is in acute leukemias.

There is no current consensus around which method of MRD assessment is best, PCR, FC, or something else. Until published MRD studies in MM have been reproduced and attention is paid to practical laboratory considerations, a consensus is not likely to emerge.

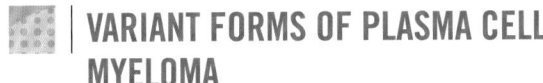

VARIANT FORMS OF PLASMA CELL MYELOMA

Asymptomatic/Smoldering Myeloma

SMM is defined as the presence of an M protein >3 g/dL (i.e., above the MGUS range), and/or 10% or more clonal PCs in the marrow, in a patient who has no related organ impairment (negative for CRAB). Progression to symptomatic disease is related to the marrow PC mass and the magnitude of the M spike. Patients may have stable disease for extended periods, but most patients with SMM eventually progress to MM, with the rate of progression of 10% per year for the first 5 years, 3% for the next 5 years, and then only 1% for the next 10 years (213).

Light Chain–Only Myeloma

In 10% to 15% of MM patients, only light chains are secreted (180). These cases also lack heavy chains by IHC. They are described as "Bence Jones disease" or "light chain–only MM." Compared to the more common IgG or IgA myeloma, survival and performance status are worse in LCO, possibly due to nephrotoxicity caused by FLCs (214). Whereas IgG or IgA MM is often preceded by a prolonged MGUS phase, light chain MGUS is rare, another biologic difference (30). A few studies have shown complex molecular mechanisms responsible for the lack of IgH expression in small percentages of LCO MM (215,216). The most common mechanism, however, causing lack of IgH expression in 60% of LCO MM, is whole or partial deletion of one IgH allele, while the other allele is involved in a translocation that renders expression impossible (217).

Nonsecretory Myeloma

In <5% of MM, SPEP and IFE are negative, and there is no M spike. PCs in such cases typically show cIg by IHC, which means that Ig is produced but not secreted. In approximately 70% of such cases, however, the Freelite is positive. The clinical findings are similar to regular, secretory MM except that, because secreted Ig causes renal damage and precipitates infections due to suppression of normal Ig, renal disease and opportunistic infections are rare in nonsecretory MM.

Solitary Plasmacytoma of Bone/Solitary Osseous Myeloma

These patients have a single, localized, monoclonal bone plasmacytoma, but no evidence of any other disease (no other CRAB). Most patients have an M spike. Local control is achieved with radiotherapy, which can be curative in up to one-third of patients (2). Since the remaining 70% of patients transform to MM, solitary osseous myeloma is considered a forme fruste of MM.

Extraosseous/Extramedullary Plasmacytoma

Extramedullary plasmacytoma (EMP) typically occurs as a single, localized tumor, 80% in the upper aerodigestive tract, in a patient with no M spike, no bone lesions, and a marrow biopsy that is negative for PCN. In nearly all cases, EMP is cured without recurrence by local resection and/or radiotherapy. This clinical description is identical to that of extranodal marginal zone lymphoma (EMZL), when in the same site. Because 30% of EMZL show plasmacytoid differentiation, sometimes marked, the prevailing thought has been that EMP is an NHL, a form of EMZL, unrelated to PCN (218). The first cytogenetic study of EMP, however, provided data suggesting that from a cytogenetic

perspective, EMP is more like PCN than NHL (219). Thirty-one of thirty-eight cases (82%) were hyperdiploid with the same trisomies common in PCN; 14/38 (17%) had an IgH translocation, including 6% with a t(4;14), but none had t(11;14); the remaining cases with IgH translocations had unidentified partners, but cyclin D3, BCL6, FOXP1, and MALT1 (common in EMZL) were excluded. Also, 15/38 (40%) had del(13q14). None of the patients developed MM and there were no significant clinical differences between any groups (e.g., unlike in MM, the t(4;14) group behaved like the hyperdiploid group). In summary, it appears that EMP is a unique lesion with clinical features similar to EMZL but cytogenetic overlap with PCN.

Plasma Cell Leukemia

Plasma cell leukemia (PCL) is defined as the presence in the PB of monoclonal PCs >2 k/mL or >20% of WBCs. It is present at the time of diagnosis in <5% of patients with MM. Most often, it is a late-stage manifestation in a patient with long-term MM and is accompanied by disease evolution in which the MM cells have attained the ability of survival outside the marrow. As such, it is typically accompanied by extramedullary masses. PCL is more common in patients with adverse cytogenetics. The cells typically lack the adhesion molecule CD56. Survival is typically short (220).

Osteosclerotic Myeloma/POEMS

This rare disease accounts for approximately 1% of PCN (221). It is unrelated to MM with fibrosis due to CD138 shedding (described above). There is osteosclerosis and fibrosis, often accompanied by lymph node changes resembling PC Castleman disease. Unlike other PCN, such cases are associated with KSHV; HHV8. Osteosclerotic MM is often accompanied by POEMS syndrome, which includes polyneuropathy, organomegaly, endocrinopathy, monoclonal gammopathy, and skin changes (222). Most patients do not have all components of POEMS. Sclerotic lesions are found on radiographs in nearly all patients. The major clinical feature is chronic progressive polyneuropathy. An M spike, usually IgG-λ or IgA-λ and usually of low magnitude (~1 g/dL), is present in 80%. Endocrinopathy and skin changes occur in approximately 70%. Organomegally is present in 50%. Fractures, hypercalcemia, and renal insufficiency are rare. Biopsy of an affected site shows bony sclerosis, paratrabecular fibrosis, and a sparse infiltrate of mature PCs with morphology that may be distorted due to the fibrosis. PCs typically account for <5% of marrow cells. Median survival is 14 years, far better than that of MM.

MONOCLONAL IMMUNOGLOBULIN DEPOSITION DISEASES, INCLUDING PRIMARY AMYLOIDOSIS

These diseases feature organ dysfunction due to extracellular deposits of a portion of the immunoglobulin molecule secreted by a PCN. Although the deposits consist mainly of light chains, they also include lesser amounts of other proteins.

Whereas immunoglobulin molecules are typically metabolized, or excreted in the urine, some PCNs produced an abnormal Ig molecule (usually light chains, but sometimes heavy chains) with biochemical and charge properties that result in tissue deposition, mostly perivascular.

"Amyloid" describes a tertiary chemical configuration, the beta-pleated sheet, that is defined by Congo red staining and resultant apple green birefringence when a slide is viewed under polarized light. Amyloid can be composed of a number of proteins. In primary amyloidosis, it is composed of immunoglobulin light chains. In secondary amyloidosis, it is composed of other proteins, not immunoglobulin. False-negative Congo red stains are common because whereas a routine histologic section is <5 μm thick, a positive Congo red requires thickness of 9 μm.

Although monoclonal immunoglobulin deposition disease (MIDD) (including amyloidosis) can occur in MM patients, more commonly, a patient will die of amyloid-related organ dysfunction before the cell mass reaches the MM range. In other words, a PCN is found in the marrow of most primary amyloidosis patients, but the ITS composed of PCs is low. Only 20% of primary amyloidosis patients reach criteria for MM. Among MM patients, 10% will develop amyloidosis (2).

In rare cases, primary amyloidosis is accompanied by lymphoplasmacytic lymphoma rather than a PCN.

The two categories of MIDD are the more common amyloidosis and the less common light chain deposition disease (LCDD), which also is called nonamyloidotic MIDD (223). Both are associated with an M spike. Amyloidosis is associated with various combinations of nephrotic syndrome (28%), hepatomegaly (25%), carpel tunnel syndrome (21%), congestive heart failure (17%), neuropathy (17%), and macroglossia (10%). Amyloid patients show bleeding diatheses, which may be due to deposit-related vascular fragility or low levels of factor X, due to its accumulation in the deposits. By contrast, LCDD patients mainly have renal disease and symptomatic extrarenal deposition is comparatively uncommon (heart [21% of LCDD], liver [19%], and peripheral nerve [8%]) (224).

Due to the relatively small number of vessels in a marrow biopsy, the sensitivity for finding amyloid deposits is low. The most sensitive method is a cytology procedure, the fat pad aspirate, which is smeared onto a slide, then Congo red stained. However, fat pad aspirates frequently stain falsely positive. If in doubt, an end organ biopsy (usually kidney, GI tract, or heart) is recommended, with high sensitivity and specificity. Gingival and rectal biopsies are less often used.

On H&E slides, amyloid can be mistaken for fibrosis. In any biopsy containing extracellular eosinophilic material on an H&E slide, a Congo red stain should be performed, especially in a patient with an M spike. Congophilia (intense pink staining) is usually evident by routine microscopy, but must be confirmed by the presence of apple green birefringence under polarized light. If Congo red is negative in a patient with histologic suspicion or clinical symptoms of MIDD, nonamyloidotic LCDD should be considered. The diagnosis can be confirmed by mass spectroscopy on a routinely prepared histologic section on a glass slide (225).

IHC is not reliable in extracellular deposits. False or confusing results are common with IHC.

Median survival is 2 years for primary amyloidosis and 4 years for LCDD (222,224).

SUMMARY AND CONCLUSION

PCNs range from MGUS, which is very common in the elderly but rarely of clinical importance, to MM, which is the second most common blood cancer and uniformly fatal. The PCN rubric also includes less common variant forms of disease. We have little understanding of why they arise, but PCNs often come to clinical attention by the finding of an M spike. The M spike is a surrogate measure for neoplastic cell mass used to assess disease progression and response to therapy. The best method of diagnosis is examination of a core biopsy by IHC. Unlike other blood cancers, the use of aspirates is problematic for a number of reasons. MM is defined by the presence of CRAB signs and symptoms. Prognosis is related to stage, chromosomal

abnormalities, and the rate of MM cell proliferation. Life spans range from <2 years to >10 years (median 5 to 8). Thankfully, survival has increased greatly in the past 15 years and emerging data from ongoing clinical trials provide hope for even better outcomes in the near future.

References

1. Swerdlow SH, Campo E, Harris NL, et al., eds. *WHO classification of tumours of haematopoietic and lymphoid tissues.* Lyon: International Agency for Research on Cancer, 2008.
2. Group TIMW. Criteria for the classification of monoclonal gammopathies, multiple myeloma and related disorders: a report of the International Myeloma Working Group. *Br J Haematol* 2003;121:749–757.
3. Keren DF. Procedures for the evaluation of monoclonal immunoglobulins. *Arch Pathol Lab Med* 1999;123:126–132.
4. Roopenian DC, Akilesh S. FcRn: the neonatal Fc receptor comes of age. *Nat Rev Immunol* 2007;7:715–725.
5. Bradwell AR, Carr-Smith HD, Mead GP, et al. Serum test for assessment of patients with Bence Jones myeloma. *Lancet* 2003;361:489–491.
6. Mead GP, Carr-Smith HD, Drayson MT, et al. Serum free light chains for monitoring multiple myeloma. *Br J Haematol* 2004;126:348–354.
7. Martin W, Abraham R, Shanafelt T, et al. Serum-free light chain, a new biomarker for patients with B-cell non-Hodgkin lymphoma and chronic lymphocytic leukemia. *Transl Res* 2007;149:231–235.
8. Dispenzieri A, Kyle R, Merlini G, et al. International Myeloma Working Group guidelines for serum-free light chain analysis in multiple myeloma and related disorders. *Leukemia* 2008;23:215–224.
9. Jagannath S. Value of serum free light chain testing for the diagnosis and monitoring of monoclonal gammopathies in hematology. *Clin Lymphoma Myeloma* 2007;7:518–523.
10. Blade J, Dimopoulos M, Rosinol L, et al. Smoldering (asymptomatic) multiple myeloma: current diagnostic criteria, new predictors of outcome, and follow-up recommendations. *J Clin Oncol* 2010;28:690–697.
11. Dispenzieri A, Kyle RA, Katzmann JA, et al. Immunoglobulin free light chain ratio is an independent risk factor for progression of smoldering (asymptomatic) multiple myeloma. *Blood* 2008;111:785–789.
12. Bradwell AR, Carr-Smith HD, Mead GP, et al. Highly sensitive, automated immunoassay for immunoglobulin free light chains in serum and urine. *Clin Chem* 2001;47:673–680.
13. Durie BG, Harousseau JL, Miguel JS, et al. International uniform response criteria for multiple myeloma. *Leukemia* 2006;20:1467–1473.
14. Dimopoulos M, Kyle R, Fermand J-P, et al. Consensus recommendations for standard investigative workup: report of the International Myeloma Workshop Consensus Panel 3. *Blood* 2011;117:4701–4705.
15. Paiva B, Martinez-Lopez J, Vidriales M-B, et al. Comparison of immunofixation, serum free light chain, and immunophenotyping for response evaluation and prognostication in multiple myeloma. *J Clin Oncol* 2011;29:1627–1633.
16. Kyle RA, Gertz MA, Witzig TE, et al. Review of 1027 patients with newly diagnosed multiple myeloma. *Mayo Clin Proc* 2003;78:21–33.
17. Kaplan JS, Horowitz GL. Twenty-four hour Bence-Jones protein determinations: can we ensure accuracy? *Arch Pathol Lab Med* 2011;135:1048–1051.
18. Tate JR, Mollee P, Dimeski G, et al. Analytical performance of serum free light-chain assay during monitoring of patients with monoclonal light-chain diseases. *Clin Chim Acta* 2007;376:30–36.
19. Ely SA, Knowles DM. Expression of CD56/neural cell adhesion molecule correlates with the presence of lytic bone lesions in multiple myeloma and distinguishes myeloma from monoclonal gammopathy of undetermined significance and lymphomas with plasmacytoid differentiation. *Am J Pathol* 2002;160:1293–1299.
20. Joshi R, Horncastle D, Elderfield K, et al. Bone marrow trephine combined with immunohistochemistry is superior to bone marrow aspirate in follow-up of myeloma patients. *J Clin Pathol* 2008;61:213–216.
21. Bartl R, Frisch B, Burkhardt R, et al. Bone marrow histology in myeloma: its importance in diagnosis, prognosis, classification and staging. *Br J Haematol* 1982;51:361–375.
22. Terpstra WE, Lokhorst HM, Blomjous F, et al. Comparison of plasma cell infiltration in bone marrow biopsies and aspirates in patients with multiple myeloma. *Br J Haematol* 1992;82:46–49.
23. Bartl R, Frisch B. Clinical significance of bone marrow biopsy and plasma cell morphology in MM and MGUS. *Pathol Biol (Paris)* 1999;47:158–168.
24. Pich A, Chiusa L, Marmont F, et al. Risk groups of myeloma patients by histologic pattern and proliferative activity. *Am J Surg Pathol* 1997;21:339–347.
25. Sukpanichnant S, Cousar JB, Leelasiri A, et al. Diagnostic criteria and histologic grading in multiple myeloma: histologic and immunohistologic analysis of 176 cases with clinical correlation. *Hum Pathol* 1994;25:308–318.
26. Nadav L, Katz BZ, Baron S, et al. Diverse niches within multiple myeloma bone marrow aspirates affect plasma cell enumeration. *Br J Haematol* 2006;133:530–532.
27. Bayer-Garner IB, Sanderson RD, Dhodapkar MV, et al. Syndecan-1 (CD138) immunoreactivity in bone marrow biopsies of multiple myeloma: shed syndecan-1 accumulates in fibrotic regions. *Mod Pathol* 2001;14:1052–1058.
28. Chanan-Khan AA, Giralt S. Importance of achieving a complete response in multiple myeloma, and the impact of novel agents. *J Clin Oncol* 2010;28:2612–2624.
29. Ely S. Using aspirates for multiple myeloma research probably excludes important data. *Br J Haematol* 2006;134:245–246.
30. Kyle RA, Rajkumar SV. Monoclonal gammopathy of undetermined significance and smouldering multiple myeloma: emphasis on risk factors for progression. *Br J Haematol* 2007;139:730–743.
31. Brown LM, Gridley G, Check D, et al. Risk of multiple myeloma and monoclonal gammopathy of undetermined significance among white and black male United States veterans with prior autoimmune, infectious, inflammatory, and allergic disorders. *Blood* 2008;111:3388–3394.

32. Landgren O, Kyle RA, Pfeiffer RM, et al. Monoclonal gammopathy of undetermined significance (MGUS) consistently precedes multiple myeloma: a prospective study. *Blood* 2009;113:5412–5417.
33. Hayden PJ, Tewari P, Morris DW, et al. Variation in DNA repair genes XRCC3, XRCC4, XRCC5 and susceptibility to myeloma. *Hum Mol Genet* 2007;16:3117–3127.
34. Ershler WB, Keller ET. Age-associated increased interleukin-6 gene expression, late-life diseases, and frailty. *Annu Rev Med* 2000;51:245–270.
35. Bida JP, Kyle RA, Therneau TM, et al. Disease associations with monoclonal gammopathy of undetermined significance: a population-based study of 17,398 patients. *Mayo Clin Proc* 2009;84:685–693.
36. Eisele L, Dürig J, Hüttmann A, et al. Prevalence and progression of monoclonal gammopathy of undetermined significance and light-chain MGUS in Germany. *Ann Hematol* 2012;91:243–248.
37. Kyle RA, Therneau TM, Rajkumar SV, et al. Long-term follow-up of IgM monoclonal gammopathy of undetermined significance. *Blood* 2003;102:3759–3764.
38. Fonseca R, Bailey RJ, Ahmann GJ, et al. Genomic abnormalities in monoclonal gammopathy of undetermined significance. *Blood* 2002;100:1417–1424.
39. Brousseau M, Leleu X, Gerard J, et al. Hyperdiploidy is a common finding in monoclonal gammopathy of undetermined significance and monosomy 13 is restricted to these hyperdiploid patients. *Clin Cancer Res* 2007;13:6026–6031.
40. Korde N, Kristinsson SY, Landgren O. Monoclonal gammopathy of undetermined significance (MGUS) and smoldering multiple myeloma (SMM): novel biological insights and development of early treatment strategies. *Blood* 2011;117:5573–5581.
41. American Cancer Society. Cancer Facts & Figures 2013. Atlanta, GA: American Cancer Society, 2013. http://www.cancer.org/cancer/multiplemyeloma/detailedguide/multiple-myeloma-key-statistics
42. Landgren O, Kyle RA. Multiple myeloma, chronic lymphocytic leukaemia and associated precursor diseases. *Br J Haematol* 2007;139:717–723.
43. SEER Cancer Statistics Review, 2011, National Cancer Institute. Bethesda, MD. SEER Cancer Statistics Review, 1975–2006, National Cancer Institute. Bethesda, MD, 2011. http://seer.cancer.gov/statfacts/html/mulmy.html. Accessed February 9, 2012
44. Terry JH. Just exactly how common is CLL? *Leuk Res* 2009;33:1452–1453.
45. Gebregziabher M, Bernstein L, Wang Y, et al. Risk patterns of multiple myeloma in Los Angeles County, 1972–1999 (United States). *Cancer Causes Control* 2006;17:931–938.
46. Podlar K, Anderson, Kenneth C. *Multiple myeloma—a new era of treatment strategies*. Oak Park: Bentham Science Publishers, 2011.
47. Kristinsson SY, Björkholm M, Goldin LR, et al. Patterns of hematologic malignancies and solid tumors among 37,838 first-degree relatives of 13,896 patients with multiple myeloma in Sweden. *Int J Cancer* 2009;125:2147–2150.
48. Gold LS, De Roos AJ, Brown EE, et al. Associations of common variants in genes involved in metabolism and response to exogenous chemicals with risk of multiple myeloma. *Cancer Epidemiol* 2009;33:276–280.
49. Cozen W, Gebregziabher M, Conti DV, et al. Interleukin-6-related genotypes, body mass index, and risk of multiple myeloma and plasmacytoma. *Cancer Epidemiol Biomarkers Prev* 2006;15:2285–2291.
50. Brown EE, Lan Q, Zheng T, et al. Common variants in genes that mediate immunity and risk of multiple myeloma. *Int J Cancer* 2007;120:2715–2722.
51. Purdue MP, Lan Q, Menashe I, et al. Variation in innate immunity genes and risk of multiple myeloma. *Hematol Oncol* 2011;29:42–46.
52. Spink CF, Gray LC, Davies FE, et al. Haplotypic structure across the I kappa B alpha gene (NFKBIA) and association with multiple myeloma. *Cancer Lett* 2007;246:92–99.
53. Hosgood HD, Baris D, Zhang Y, et al. Caspase polymorphisms and genetic susceptibility to multiple myeloma. *Hematol Oncol* 2008;26:148–151.
54. Hosgood HD III, Baris D, Zhang Y, et al. Genetic variation in cell cycle and apoptosis related genes and multiple myeloma risk. *Leuk Res* 2009;33:1609–1614.
55. Preston DL, Kusumi S, Tomonaga M, et al. Cancer incidence in atomic bomb survivors. Part III. Leukemia, lymphoma and multiple myeloma, 1950–1987. *Radiat Res* 1994;137:S68–S97.
56. Neriishi K, Yoshimoto Y, Carter RL, et al. Monoclonal gammopathy in atomic bomb survivors. *Radiat Res* 1993;133:351–359.
57. Neriishi K, Nakashima E, Suzuki G. Monoclonal gammopathy of undetermined significance in atomic bomb survivors: incidence and transformation to multiple myeloma. *Br J Haematol* 2003;121:405–410.
58. Khuder SA, Mutgi AB. Meta-analyses of multiple myeloma and farming. *Am J Ind Med* 1997;32:510–516.
59. Merhi M, Raynal H, Cahuzac E, et al. Occupational exposure to pesticides and risk of hematopoietic cancers: meta-analysis of case–control studies. *Cancer Causes Control* 2007;18:1209–1226.
60. Bezabeh S, Engel A, Morris CB, et al. Does benzene cause multiple myeloma? An analysis of the published case-control literature. *Environ Health Perspect* 1996;104(Suppl 6):1393–1398.
61. Bergsagel DE, Wong O, Bergsagel PL, et al. Benzene and multiple myeloma: appraisal of the scientific evidence. *Blood* 1999;94:1174–1182.
62. Goldstein BD, Shalat SL. The causal relation between benzene exposure and multiple myeloma. *Blood* 2000;95:1512–1513.
63. Infante PF. Benzene exposure and multiple myeloma: a detailed meta-analysis of benzene cohort studies. *Ann N Y Acad Sci* 2006;1076:90–109.
64. Hallek M, Leif Bergsagel P, Anderson KC. Multiple myeloma: increasing evidence for a multistep transformation process. *Blood* 1998;91:3–21.
65. Vescio R, Cao J, Hong C, et al. Myeloma Ig heavy chain V region sequences reveal prior antigenic selection and marked somatic mutation but no intraclonal diversity. *J Immunol* 1995;155:2487–2497.
66. Taylor BJ, Kriangkum J, Pittman JA, et al. Analysis of clonotypic switch junctions reveals multiple myeloma originates from a single class switch event with ongoing mutation in the isotype-switched progeny. *Blood* 2008;112:1894–1903.
67. Kahn HS, Tatham LM, Patel AV, et al. Increased cancer mortality following a history of nonmelanoma skin cancer. *JAMA* 1998;280:910–912.
68. Nugent Z, Demers AA, Wiseman MC, et al. Risk of second primary cancer and death following a diagnosis of nonmelanoma skin cancer. *Cancer Epidemiol Biomarkers Prev* 2005;14:2584–2590.
69. Thomas A, Mailankody S, Korde N, et al. Second malignancies following multiple myeloma: from 1960s to 2010s. *Blood* 2012;119:2731–2737.
70. Mailankody S, Pfeiffer RM, Kristinsson SY, et al. Risk of acute myeloid leukemia and myelodysplastic syndromes after multiple myeloma and its precursor disease (MGUS). *Blood* 2011;118:4086–4092.
71. Grulich AE, Wan X, Law MG, et al. Risk of cancer in people with AIDS. *AIDS* 1999;13:839–843.
72. Konrad RJ, Kricka LJ, Goodman D, et al. Myeloma-associated paraprotein directed against the HIV-1 p24 antigen in an HIV-1-seropositive patient. *N Engl J Med* 1993;328:1817–1819.
73. Miligi L, Costantini AS, Crosignani P, et al. Occupational, environmental, and life-style factors associated with the risk of hematolymphopoietic malignancies in women. *Am J Ind Med* 1999;36:60–69.
74. Landgren O, Zhang Y, Zahm SH, et al. Risk of multiple myeloma following medication use and medical conditions: a case-control study in Connecticut women. *Cancer Epidemiol Biomarkers Prev* 2006;15:2342–2347.
75. Altieri A, Gallus S, Franceschi S, et al. Hormone replacement therapy and risk of lymphomas and myelomas. *Eur J Cancer Prev* 2004;13:349–351.
76. Fernandez E, Gallus S, Bosetti C, et al. Hormone replacement therapy and cancer risk: a systematic analysis from a network of case-control studies. *Int J Cancer* 2003;105:408–412.
77. Eriksson M. Rheumatoid arthritis as a risk factor for multiple myeloma: a case-control study. *Eur J Cancer* 1993;29A:259–263.
78. Moysich KB, Bonner MR, Beehler GP, et al. Regular analgesic use and risk of multiple myeloma. *Leuk Res* 2007;31:547–551.
79. Renehan AG, Tyson M, Egger M, et al. Body-mass index and incidence of cancer: a systematic review and meta-analysis of prospective observational studies. *Lancet* 2008;371:569–578.
80. Calle EE, Rodriguez C, Walker-Thurmond K, et al. Overweight, obesity, and mortality from cancer in a prospectively studied cohort of U.S. adults. *N Engl J Med* 2003;348:1625–1638.
81. Landgren O, Rajkumar SV, Pfeiffer RM, et al. Obesity is associated with an increased risk of monoclonal gammopathy of undetermined significance among black and white women. *Blood* 2010;116:1056–1059.
82. Birmann BM, Giovannucci E, Rosner B, et al. Body mass index, physical activity, and risk of multiple myeloma. *Cancer Epidemiol Biomarkers Prev* 2007;16: 1474–1478.
83. Khan MM, Mori M, Sakauchi F, et al. Risk factors for multiple myeloma: evidence from the Japan Collaborative Cohort (JACC) study. *Asian Pac J Cancer Prev* 2006;7:575–581.
84. Niesvizky R, Costa LJ, Haideri NA, et al. Preliminary results of a phase 2 study of PD 0332991 in combination with bortezomib and dexamethasone in patients with relapsed and refractory multiple myeloma. *ASH Annual Meeting Abstracts* 2011;118:2940.
85. Kyle RA. Multiple myeloma: review of 869 cases. *Mayo Clin Proc* 1975;50:29–40.
86. Riccardi A, Gobbi PG, Ucci G, et al. Changing clinical presentation of multiple myeloma. *Eur J Cancer* 1991;27:1401–1405.
87. Blade J, Fernandez de Larrea C, Rosinol L, et al. Soft-tissue plasmacytomas in multiple myeloma: incidence, mechanisms of extramedullary spread, and treatment approach. *J Clin Oncol* 2011;29:3805–3812.
88. Tian E, Zhan F, Walker R, et al. The role of the Wnt-signaling antagonist DKK1 in the development of osteolytic lesions in multiple myeloma. *N Engl J Med* 2003;349:2483–2494.
89. Pearse RN, Sordillo EM, Yaccoby S, et al. Multiple myeloma disrupts the TRANCE/osteoprotegerin cytokine axis to trigger bone destruction and promote tumor progression. *Proc Natl Acad Sci U S A* 2001;98:11581–11586.
90. Munshi NC, Anderson KC, Bergsagel PL, et al. Consensus recommendations for risk stratification in multiple myeloma: report of the International Myeloma Workshop Consensus Panel 2. *Blood* 2011;117:4696–4700.
91. Christensen JH, Abildgaard N, Plesner T, et al. Interphase fluorescence in situ hybridization in multiple myeloma and monoclonal gammopathy of undetermined significance without and with positive plasma cell identification: analysis of 192 cases from the Region of Southern Denmark. *Cancer Genet Cytogenet* 2007;174:89–99.
92. Hartmann L, Biggerstaff JS, Chapman DB, et al. Detection of genomic abnormalities in multiple myeloma. *Am J Clin Pathol* 2011;136:712–720.
93. Zhou Y, Barlogie B, Shaughnessy JD Jr. The molecular characterization and clinical management of multiple myeloma in the post-genome era. *Leukemia* 2009;23:1941–1956.
94. Munshi NTG, Barlogie B. Plasma cell neoplasms. In: DeVita JV, Hellman S, Rosenberg SA, eds. *Principles and practice of oncology*. Philadelphia: Lippincott Williams & Wilkons, 2001:2465–2499.
95. Chng WJ, Santana-Davila R, Van Wier SA, et al. Prognostic factors for hyperdiploid-myeloma: effects of chromosome 13 deletions and IgH translocations. *Leukemia* 2006;20:807–813.
96. Chng WJ, Kumar S, VanWier S, et al. Molecular dissection of hyperdiploid multiple myeloma by gene expression profiling. *Cancer Res* 2007;67:2982–2989.
97. Smadja NV, Fruchart C, Isnard F, et al. Chromosomal analysis in multiple myeloma: cytogenetic evidence of two different diseases. *Leukemia* 1998;12: 960–969.
98. Fonseca R, Debes-Marun CS, Picken EB, et al. The recurrent IgH translocations are highly associated with nonhyperdiploid variant multiple myeloma. *Blood* 2003;102:2562–2567.
99. Smadja NV, Bastard C, Brigaudeau C, et al. Hypodiploidy is a major prognostic factor in multiple myeloma. *Blood* 2001;98:2229–2238.
100. Carrasco DR, Tonon G, Huang Y, et al. High-resolution genomic profiles define distinct clinico-pathogenetic subgroups of multiple myeloma patients. *Cancer Cell* 2006;9:313–325.
101. Agnelli L, Fabris S, Bicciato S, et al. Upregulation of translational machinery and distinct genetic subgroups characterise hyperdiploidy in multiple myeloma. *Br J Haematol* 2007;136:565–573.
102. Zhan F, Huang Y, Colla S, et al. The molecular classification of multiple myeloma. *Blood* 2006;108:2020–2028.
103. Mateos M-V, Gutirrez NC, Martin-Ramos M-L, et al. Outcome according to cytogenetic abnormalities and DNA ploidy in myeloma patients receiving short induction with weekly bortezomib followed by maintenance. *Blood* 2011;118:4547–4553.
104. Fonseca R, Blood EA, Oken MM, et al. Myeloma and the t(11;14)(q13;q32); evidence for a biologically defined unique subset of patients. *Blood* 2002;99:3735–3741.
105. Bergsagel PL, Kuehl WM. Chromosome translocations in multiple myeloma. *Oncogene* 2001;20:5611–5622.
106. Kuehl WM, Bergsagel PL. Multiple myeloma: evolving genetic events and host interactions. *Nat Rev Cancer* 2002;2:175–187.

107. Ely S, Di Liberto M, Niesvizky R, et al. Mutually exclusive cyclin-dependent kinase 4/cyclin D1 and cyclin-dependent kinase 6/cyclin D2 pairing inactivates retinoblastoma protein and promotes cell cycle dysregulation in multiple myeloma. *Cancer Res* 2005;65:11345–11353.
108. Quinn J, Glassford J, Percy L, et al. APRIL promotes cell-cycle progression in primary multiple myeloma cells: influence of D-type cyclin group and translocation status. *Blood* 2011;117:890–901.
109. Paiva B, Gutierrez NC, Rosinol L, et al. High-risk cytogenetics and persistent minimal residual disease by multiparameter flow cytometry predict unsustained complete response after autologous stem cell transplantation in multiple myeloma. *Blood* 2012;119:687–691.
110. Keats JJ, Reiman T, Belch AR, et al. Ten years and counting: so what do we know about t(4;14)(p16;q32) multiple myeloma. *Leuk Lymphoma* 2006;47:2289–2300.
111. Chng WJ, Kuehl WM, Bergsagel PL, et al. Translocation t(4;14) retains prognostic significance even in the setting of high-risk molecular signature. *Leukemia* 2008;22:459–461.
112. Trudel S, Ely S, Farooqi Y, et al. Inhibition of fibroblast growth factor receptor 3 induces differentiation and apoptosis in t(4;14) myeloma. *Blood* 2004;103:3521–3528.
113. Lauring J, Abukhdeir AM, Konishi H, et al. The multiple myeloma-associated MMSET gene contributes to cellular adhesion, clonogenic growth, and tumorigenicity. *Blood* 2008;111:856–864.
114. Fonseca R, Blood E, Rue M, et al. Clinical and biologic implications of recurrent genomic aberrations in myeloma. *Blood* 2003;101:4569–4575.
115. Bergsagel PL, Kuehl WM, Zhan F, et al. Cyclin D dysregulation: an early and unifying pathogenic event in multiple myeloma. *Blood* 2005;106:296–303.
116. Avet-Loiseau H, Attal M, Moreau P, et al. Genetic abnormalities and survival in multiple myeloma: the experience of the Intergroupe Francophone du Myélome. *Blood* 2007;109:3489–3495.
117. Chang H, Qi C, Yi Q-L, et al. p53 gene deletion detected by fluorescence in situ hybridization is an adverse prognostic factor for patients with multiple myeloma following autologous stem cell transplantation. *Blood* 2005;105:358–360.
118. Gertz MA, Lacy MQ, Dispenzieri A, et al. Clinical implications of t(11;14)(q13;q32), t(4;14)(p16.3;q32), and -17p13 in myeloma patients treated with high-dose therapy. *Blood* 2005;106:2837–2840.
119. Mohamed AN, Bentley G, Bonnett ML, et al. Chromosome aberrations in a series of 120 multiple myeloma cases with abnormal karyotypes. *Am J Hematol* 2007;82:1080–1087.
120. Neri A, Baldini L, Trecca D, et al. p53 gene mutations in multiple myeloma are associated with advanced forms of malignancy. *Blood* 1993;81:128–135.
121. Preudhomme C, Facon T, Zandecki M, et al. Rare occurrence of P53 gene mutations in multiple myeloma. *Br J Haematol* 1992;81:440–443.
122. Portier M, Moles JP, Mazars GR, et al. p53 and RAS gene mutations in multiple myeloma. *Oncogene* 1992;7:2539–2543.
123. Corradini P, Inghirami G, Astolfi M, et al. Inactivation of tumor suppressor genes, p53 and Rb1, in plasma cell dyscrasias. *Leukemia* 1994;8:758–767.
124. Chng WJ, Price-Troska T, Gonzalez-Paz N, et al. Clinical significance of TP53 mutation in myeloma. *Leukemia* 2007;21:582–584.
125. Avet-Loiseau H, Facon T, Grosbois B, et al. Oncogenesis of multiple myeloma: 14q32 and 13q chromosomal abnormalities are not randomly distributed, but correlate with natural history, immunological features, and clinical presentation. *Blood* 2002;99:2185–2191.
126. Sawyer JR. The prognostic significance of cytogenetics and molecular profiling in multiple myeloma. *Cancer Genet* 2011;204:3–12.
127. Tricot G, Barlogie B, Jagannath S, et al. Poor prognosis in multiple myeloma is associated only with partial or complete deletions of chromosome 13 or abnormalities involving 11q and not with other karyotype abnormalities. *Blood* 1995;86:4250–4256.
128. Avet-Loiseau H, Daviet A, Saunier S; Bataille on behalf of the Intergroupe Francophone du Myélome R. Chromosome 13 abnormalities in multiple myeloma are mostly monosomy 13. *Br J Haematol* 2000;111:1116–1117.
129. Wu KL, Beverloo B, Lokhorst HM, et al. Abnormalities of chromosome 1p/q are highly associated with chromosome 13/13q deletions and are an adverse prognostic factor for the outcome of high-dose chemotherapy in patients with multiple myeloma. *Br J Haematol* 2007;136:615–623.
130. Debes-Marun CS, Dewald GW, Bryant S, et al. Chromosome abnormalities clustering and its implications for pathogenesis and prognosis in myeloma. *Leukemia* 2003;17:427–436.
131. Chang H, Ning Y, Qi X, et al. Chromosome 1p21 deletion is a novel prognostic marker in patients with multiple myeloma. *Br J Haematol* 2007;139:51–54.
132. Tourigny MR, Ursini-Siegel J, Lee H, et al. CDK inhibitor p18INK4c is required for the generation of functional plasma cells. *Immunity* 2002;17:179–189.
133. Leone PE, Walker BA, Jenner MW, et al. Deletions of CDKN2C (p18) in multiple myeloma: biological and clinical implications. *Clin Cancer Res* 2008;14:6033–6041.
134. Hanamura I, Stewart JP, Huang Y, et al. Frequent gain of chromosome band 1q21 in plasma-cell dyscrasias detected by fluorescence in situ hybridization: incidence increases from MGUS to relapsed myeloma and is related to prognosis and disease progression following tandem stem-cell transplantation. *Blood* 2006;108:1724–1732.
135. Sawyer JR, Tricot G, Lukacs JL, et al. Genomic instability in multiple myeloma: evidence for jumping segmental duplications of chromosome arm 1q. *Genes Chromosomes Cancer* 2005;42:95–106.
136. Le Baccon P, Leroux D, Dascalescu C, et al. Novel evidence of a role for chromosome 1 pericentric heterochromatin in the pathogenesis of B-cell lymphoma and multiple myeloma. *Genes Chromosomes Cancer* 2001;32:250–264.
137. Fabris S, Storlazzi CT, Baldini L, et al. Heterogeneous pattern of chromosomal breakpoints involving the MYC locus in multiple myeloma. *Genes Chromosomes Cancer* 2003;37:261–269.
138. Avet-Loiseau H, Gerson F, Magrangeas F, et al. Rearrangements of the c-myc oncogene are present in 15% of primary human multiple myeloma tumors. *Blood* 2001;98:3082–3086.
139. Shou Y, Martelli ML, Gabrea A, et al. Diverse karyotypic abnormalities of the c-myc locus associated with c-myc dysregulation and tumor progression in multiple myeloma. *Proc Natl Acad Sci U S A* 2000;97:228–233.
140. Stralen E, Leguit RJ, Begthel H, et al. MafB oncoprotein detected by immunohistochemistry as a highly sensitive and specific marker for the prognostic unfavorable t(14;20) (q32;q12) in multiple myeloma patients. *Leukemia* 2008;23:801–803.
141. Boyd KD, Ross FM, Chiecchio L, et al. A novel prognostic model in myeloma based on co-segregating adverse FISH lesions and the ISS: analysis of patients treated in the MRC Myeloma IX trial. *Leukemia* 2012;26:349–355.
142. Zhan F, Hardin J, Kordsmeier B, et al. Global gene expression profiling of multiple myeloma, monoclonal gammopathy of undetermined significance, and normal bone marrow plasma cells. *Blood* 2002;99:1745–1757.
143. Decaux O, Lode L, Magrangeas F, et al. Prediction of survival in multiple myeloma based on gene expression profiles reveals cell cycle and chromosomal instability signatures in high-risk patients and hyperdiploid signatures in low-risk patients: a study of the Intergroupe Francophone du Myelome. *J Clin Oncol* 2008;26:4798–4805.
144. Shaughnessy JD Jr, Zhan F, Burington BE, et al. A validated gene expression model of high-risk multiple myeloma is defined by deregulated expression of genes mapping to chromosome 1. *Blood* 2007;109:2276–2284.
145. Fonseca R, Bergsagel PL, Drach J, et al. International Myeloma Working Group molecular classification of multiple myeloma: spotlight review. *Leukemia* 2009;23:2210–2221.
146. Gutierrez NC, Garcia JL, Hernandez JM, et al. Prognostic and biologic significance of chromosomal imbalances assessed by comparative genomic hybridization in multiple myeloma. *Blood* 2004;104:2661–2666.
147. Jungbluth AA, Ely S, DiLiberto M, et al. The cancer-testis antigens CT7 (MAGE-C1) and MAGE-A3/6 are commonly expressed in multiple myeloma and correlate with plasma-cell proliferation. *Blood* 2005;106:167–174.
148. Drach J, Gattringer C, Glassl H, et al. The biological and clinical significance of the KI-67 growth fraction in multiple myeloma. *Hematol Oncol* 1992;10:125–134.
149. Greipp PR, Witzig TE, Gonchoroff NJ, et al. Immunofluorescence labeling indices in myeloma and related monoclonal gammopathies. *Mayo Clin Proc* 1987;62:969–977.
150. Hose D, Reme T, Hielscher T, et al. Proliferation is a central independent prognostic factor and target for personalized and risk-adapted treatment in multiple myeloma. *Haematologica* 2011;96:87–95.
151. Ely S. Renewed interest in myeloma tumor growth, or just one more method to assess proliferation? *Leuk Res* 2010;35:30–31.
152. Scott Ely MC, Roth M, Cristos P, et al. Plasma cell proliferation index as a clinical prognosticator for relapsed multiple myeloma. *Haematologica* 2003;88:S169.
153. Ely S. New Assay Predicts Myeloma Survival. eCancer TV 2013; http://ecancer.org/video/1891/new-assay-predicts-myeloma-survival.php:Video Telecast.
154. Mark TM, Ounsafi I, Christos P, et al. The association of Ki67 percent positivity and clinical outcomes in the upfront treatment of multiple myeloma. *Haematologica* 2011;96:S128.
155. Ahmann GJ, Chng WJ, Henderson KJ, et al. Effect of tissue shipping on plasma cell isolation, viability, and RNA integrity in the context of a centralized good laboratory practice-certified tissue banking facility. *Cancer Epidemiol Biomarkers Prev* 2008;17:666–673.
156. Sailer M, Vykoupil KF, Peest D, et al. Prognostic relevance of a histologic classification system applied in bone marrow biopsies from patients with multiple myeloma: a histopathological evaluation of biopsies from 153 untreated patients. *Eur J Haematol* 1995;54:137–146.
157. Bartl R, Frisch B, Fateh-Moghadam A, et al. Histologic classification and staging of multiple myeloma. A retrospective and prospective study of 674 cases. *Am J Clin Pathol* 1987;87:342–355.
158. Greipp PR, Leong T, Bennett JM, et al. Plasmablastic morphology, an independent prognostic factor with clinical and laboratory correlates: Eastern Cooperative Oncology Group (ECOG) Myeloma Trial E9486 Report by the ECOG Myeloma Laboratory Group. *Blood* 1998;91:2501–2507.
159. Rajkumar SV, Fonseca R, Lacy MQ, et al. Plasmablastic morphology is an independent predictor of poor survival after autologous stem-cell transplantation for multiple myeloma. *J Clin Oncol* 1999;17:1551.
160. Went P, Mayer S, Oberholzer M, et al. Plasma cell quantification in bone marrow by computer-assisted image analysis. *Histol Histopathol* 2006;21:951–956.
161. Cook JR, Hsi ED, Worley S, et al. Immunohistochemical analysis identifies two cyclin D1+ subsets of plasma cell myeloma, each associated with favorable survival. *Am J Clin Pathol* 2006;125:615–624.
162. Paiva B, Vidriales MB, Cervero J, et al. Multiparameter flow cytometry remission is the most relevant prognostic factor for multiple myeloma patients who undergo autologous stem cell transplantation. *Blood* 2008;112:4017–4023.
163. Sarasquete ME, Garcia-Sanz R, Gonzalez D, et al. Minimal residual disease monitoring in multiple myeloma: a comparison between allelic-specific oligonucleotide real-time quantitative polymerase chain reaction and flow cytometry. *Haematologica* 2005;90:1365–1372.
164. Katz B-Z, Polliack A. Discrepancies in quantitative assessment of bone marrow involvement in lymphoma: do they reflect specialized micro-environmental cellular niches and cell-stromal interactions? *Leuk Lymphoma* 2006;47:1730–1731.
165. Schmidt B, Kremer M, Götze K, et al. Bone marrow involvement in follicular lymphoma: comparison of histology and flow cytometry as staging procedures. *Leukemia Lymphoma* 2006;47:1857–1862.
166. Mateo G, Montalban MA, Vidriales M-B, et al. Prognostic value of immunophenotyping in multiple myeloma: a study by the PETHEMA/GEM cooperative study groups on patients uniformly treated with high-dose therapy. *J Clin Oncol* 2008;26:2737–2744.
167. Durie BG, Salmon SE. A clinical staging system for multiple myeloma. Correlation of measured myeloma cell mass with presenting clinical features, response to treatment, and survival. *Cancer* 1975;36:842–854.
168. Rajkumar SV, Kyle RA, Therneau TM, et al. Serum free light chain ratio is an independent risk factor for progression in monoclonal gammopathy of undetermined significance. *Blood* 2005;106:812–817.
169. Karlin L, Soulier J, Chandesris O, et al. Clinical and biological features of t(4;14) multiple myeloma: a prospective study. *Leuk Lymphoma* 2011;52:238–246.
170. Dispenzieri A, Zhang L, Katzmann JA, et al. Appraisal of immunoglobulin free light chain as a marker of response. *Blood* 2008;111:4908–4915.
171. van Rhee F, Bolejack V, Hollmig K, et al. High serum-free light chain levels and their rapid reduction in response to therapy define an aggressive multiple myeloma subtype with poor prognosis. *Blood* 2007;110:827–832.
172. Cooper EH, Plesner T. Beta-2-microglobulin review: its relevance in clinical oncology. *Med Pediatr Oncol* 1980;8:323–334.
173. Greipp P, Katzmann J, O'Fallon W, et al. Value of beta 2-microglobulin level and plasma cell labeling indices as prognostic factors in patients with newly diagnosed myeloma. *Blood* 1988;72:219–223.

174. Dimopoulos MA, Barlogie B, Smith TL, et al. High serum lactate dehydrogenase level as a marker for drug resistance and short survival in multiple myeloma. *Ann Int Med* 1991;115:931–935.
175. Bataille R, Boccadoro M, Klein B, et al. C-reactive protein and beta-2 microglobulin produce a simple and powerful myeloma staging system. *Blood* 1992;80: 733–737.
176. Terpos E, Katodritou E, Roussou M, et al. High serum lactate dehydrogenase adds prognostic value to the international myeloma staging system even in the era of novel agents. *Eur J Haematol* 2010;85:114–119.
177. Kim J, Yoo C, Lee D, et al. Serum albumin level is a significant prognostic factor reflecting disease severity in symptomatic multiple myeloma. *Ann Hematol* 2010;89:391–397.
178. Choi J-H, Yoon J-H, Yang S-K. Clinical value of new staging systems for multiple myeloma. *Cancer Res Treat* 2007;39:171–174.
179. Mihou D, Katodritou I, Zervas K. Evaluation of five staging systems in 470 patients with multiple myeloma. *Haematologica* 2006;91:1149–1150.
180. Greipp PR, Miguel JS, Durie BGM, et al. International staging system for multiple myeloma. *J Clin Oncol* 2005;23:3412–3420.
181. Kim H, Sohn H-J, Kim S, et al. New staging systems can predict prognosis of multiple myeloma patients undergoing autologous peripheral blood stem cell transplantation as first-line therapy. *Biol Blood Marrow Transplant* 2006;12:837–844.
182. Hari PN, Zhang MJ, Roy V, et al. Is the international staging system superior to the Durie-Salmon staging system? A comparison in multiple myeloma patients undergoing autologous transplant. *Leukemia* 2009;23:1528–1534.
183. Lahuerta JJ, Mateos MV, Martínez-López J, et al. Influence of pre- and post-transplantation responses on outcome of patients with multiple myeloma: sequential improvement of response and achievement of complete response are associated with longer survival. *J Clin Oncol* 2008;26:5775–5782.
184. Barlogie B, Anaissie E, Haessler J, et al. Complete remission sustained 3 years from treatment initiation is a powerful surrogate for extended survival in multiple myeloma. *Cancer* 2008;113:355–359.
185. Rajkumar SV, Durie BGM. Eliminating the complete response penalty from myeloma response criteria. *Blood* 2008;111:5759–5760.
186. Zent CS, Wilson CS, Tricot G, et al. Oligoclonal protein bands and Ig isotype switching in multiple myeloma treated with high-dose therapy and hematopoietic cell transplantation. *Blood* 1998;91:3518–3523.
187. Hovenga S, de Wolf JT, Guikema JE, et al. Autologous stem cell transplantation in multiple myeloma after VAD and EDAP courses: a high incidence of oligoclonal serum Igs post transplantation. *Bone Marrow Transplant* 2000;25:723–728.
188. Mark T, Jayabalan D, Coleman M, et al. Atypical serum immunofixation patterns frequently emerge in immunomodulatory therapy and are associated with a high degree of response in multiple myeloma. *Br J Haematol* 2008;143:654–660.
189. de Larrea CF, Cibeira MT, Elena M, et al. Abnormal serum free light chain ratio in patients with multiple myeloma in complete remission has strong association with the presence of oligoclonal bands: implications for stringent complete remission definition. *Blood* 2009;114:4954–4956.
190. Fernandez de Larrea C, Tovar N, Cibeira M, et al. Emergence of oligoclonal bands in patients with multiple myeloma in complete remission after induction chemotherapy: association with the use of novel agents. *Haematologica* 2011;96:171–173.
191. Kenny JJ, Moloney WC. Long-term survival in multiple myeloma: report of three cases. *Ann Intern Med* 1956;45:950–957.
192. Alexanian R, Bergsagel DE, Migliore PJ, et al. Melphalan therapy for plasma cell myeloma. *Blood* 1968;31:1–10.
193. Attal M, Harousseau J-L, Stoppa A-M, et al. A prospective, randomized trial of autologous bone marrow transplantation and chemotherapy in multiple myeloma. *N Engl J Med* 1996;335:91–97.
194. Attal M, Harousseau J-L, Facon T, et al. Single versus double autologous stem-cell transplantation for multiple myeloma. *N Engl J Med* 2003;349:2495–2502.
195. Robert K. IMiDs: a novel class of immunomodulators. *Semin Oncol* 2005;32 (Suppl 5):24–30.
196. Kenneth CA. Proteasome inhibitors in multiple myeloma. *Semin Oncol* 2009;36(Suppl 1):S20–S26.
197. Mihelic R, Kaufman JL, Lonial S. Maintenance therapy in multiple myeloma. *Leukemia* 2007;21:1150–1157.
198. McCarthy PL, Owzar K, Stadtmauer EA, et al. Phase III intergroup study of lenalidomide (CC-5013) versus placebo maintenance therapy following single autologous stem cell transplant for multiple myeloma (CALGB 100104): initial report of patient accrual and adverse events. *ASH Annual Meeting Abstracts* 2009;114:3416.
199. Barlogie B, Attal M, Crowley J, et al. Long-term follow-up of autotransplantation trials for multiple myeloma: update of protocols conducted by the Intergroupe
200. Francophone du Myelome, Southwest Oncology Group, and University of Arkansas for Medical Sciences. *J Clin Oncol* 2010;28:1209–1214.
200. Dingli D, Pacheco JM, Nowakowski GS, et al. Relationship between depth of response and outcome on multiple myeloma. *J Clin Oncol* 2007;25:4933–4937.
201. Ludwig H, Bolejack V, Crowley J, et al. Survival and years of life lost in different age cohorts of patients with multiple myeloma. *J Clin Oncol* 2010;28:1599–1605.
202. Kumar SK, Rajkumar SV, Dispenzieri A, et al. Improved survival in multiple myeloma and the impact of novel therapies. *Blood* 2008;111:2516–2520.
203. Kastritis E, Zervas K, Symeonidis A, et al. Improved survival of patients with multiple myeloma after the introduction of novel agents and the applicability of the International Staging System (ISS): an analysis of the Greek Myeloma Study Group (GMSG). *Leukemia* 2009;23:1152–1157.
204. Kristinsson S, Landgren O, Dickman P, et al. Patterns of survival in multiple myeloma: a population-based study of patients diagnosed in Sweden from 1973 to 2003. *J Clin Oncol* 2007;25:1993–1999.
205. Brenner H, Gondos A, Pulte D. Recent major improvement in long-term survival of younger patients with multiple myeloma. *Blood* 2008;111:2521–2526.
206. Wood B. 9-color and 10-color flow cytometry in the clinical laboratory. *Arch Pathol Lab Med* 2006;130:680–690.
207. Conter V, Bartram CR, Valsecchi MG, et al. Molecular response to treatment redefines all prognostic factors in children and adolescents with B-cell precursor acute lymphoblastic leukemia: results in 3184 patients of the AIEOP-BFM ALL 2000 study. *Blood* 2010;115(16):3206–3214.
208. Campana D. Progress of minimal residual disease studies in childhood acute leukemia. *Curr Hematol Malig Rep* 2011;5:169–176.
209. Walter RB, Gooley TA, Wood BL, et al. Impact of pretransplantation minimal residual disease, as detected by multiparametric flow cytometry, on outcome of myeloablative hematopoietic cell transplantation for acute myeloid leukemia. *J Clin Oncol* 2011;29(9):1190–1197.
210. Rawstron AC, Orfao A, Beksac M, et al. Report of the European Myeloma Network on multiparametric flow cytometry in multiple myeloma and related disorders. *Haematologica* 2008;93:431–438.
211. Tricot GJ. What is the significance of molecular remission in multiple myeloma? *Clin Adv Hematol Oncol* 2007;5:91–95.
212. Rajkumar SV, Harousseau J-L, Durie B, et al. Consensus recommendations for the uniform reporting of clinical trials: report of the International Myeloma Workshop Consensus Panel 1. *Blood* 2011;117:4691–4695.
213. Kyle RA, Remstein ED, Therneau TM, et al. Clinical course and prognosis of smoldering (asymptomatic) multiple myeloma. *N Engl J Med* 2007;356:2582–2590.
214. Drayson M, Begum G, Basu S, et al. Effects of paraprotein heavy and light chain types and free light chain load on survival in myeloma: an analysis of patients receiving conventional-dose chemotherapy in Medical Research Council UK multiple myeloma trials. *Blood* 2006;108:2013–2019.
215. Magrangeas F, Cormier M-L, Descamps G, et al. Light-chain only multiple myeloma is due to the absence of functional (productive) rearrangement of the IgH gene at the DNA level. *Blood* 2004;103:3869–3875.
216. Szczepanski T, van 't Veer MB, Wolvers-Tettero ILM, et al. Molecular features responsible for the absence of immunoglobulin heavy chain protein synthesis in an IgH(-) subgroup of multiple myeloma. *Blood* 1999;96:1087–1093.
217. Cohn SM, Niesvizky R, Knowles DM, et al. Monoallelic immunoglobulin heavy chain gene deletion with illegitimate recombination of the 2nd allele is the most common mechanism for the light chain only phenotype in multiple myeloma. *Mod Pathol* 2009;21:250A.
218. Hussong JW, Perkins SL, Schnitzer B, et al. Extramedullary plasmacytoma. A form of marginal zone cell lymphoma? *Am J Clin Pathol* 1999;111:111–116.
219. Bink K, Haralambieva E, Kremer M, et al. Primary extramedullary plasmacytoma: similarities with and differences from multiple myeloma revealed by interphase cytogenetics. *Haematologica* 2008;93:623–626.
220. Sher T, Miller KC, Deeb G, et al. Plasma cell leukaemia and other aggressive plasma cell malignancies. *Br J Haematol* 2010;150:418–427.
221. Dispenzieri A. POEMS syndrome: 2011 update on diagnosis, risk-stratification, and management. *Am J Hematol* 2011;86:591–601.
222. Miralles GD, O'Fallon JR, Talley NJ. Plasma-cell dyscrasia with polyneuropathy. *N Engl J Med* 1992;327:1919–1923.
223. Buxbaum J, Gallo G. Nonamyloidotic monoclonal immunoglobulin deposition disease. Light-chain, heavy-chain, and light- and heavy-chain deposition diseases. *Hematol Oncol Clin North Am* 1999;13:1235–1248.
224. Pozzi C, D'Amico M, Fogazzi GB, et al. Light chain deposition disease with renal involvement: clinical characteristics and prognostic factors. *Am J Kidney Dis* 2003;42:1154–1163.
225. Klein CJ, Vrana JA, Theis JD, et al. Mass spectrometric-based proteomic analysis of amyloid neuropathy type in nerve tissue. *Arch Neurol* 2011;68:195–199.

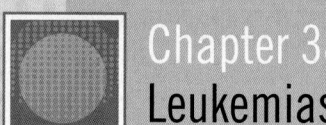

Chapter 38
Leukemias of Mature T Cells and Natural Killer Cells

Dragan Jevremovic • William G. Morice

INTRODUCTION: GENERAL

Leukemias of mature T cells and natural killer (NK) cells are uncommon (<5% of all mature lymphocytic leukemias) and can be broadly subcategorized into those derived from cytotoxic T cells and NK cells (i.e., cytolytic lymphocytes) and those derived from T cells with helper or regulatory function. These disorders display a variety of clinicopathologic properties ranging from aggressive virus-driven neoplasms with a proclivity for particular regions or ethnic groups to very indolent disorders that can be difficult to distinguish from reactive cellular expansions. This diverse spectrum is illustrated through the detailed discussion of specific diagnostic entities (Table 38.1), excluding HTLV-1-associated T-cell lymphoproliferative disorders and peripheral blood involvement by cutaneous T-cell lymphomas, which are covered in Chapters 40 and 32 respectively.

T-CELL LARGE GRANULAR LYMPHOCYTIC LEUKEMIA

Definition

T-cell large granular lymphocytic leukemia (T-LGL) is a clonal or oligoclonal disorder of terminally differentiated effector cytotoxic T cells (1,2). It typically manifests with modest peripheral blood and bone marrow lymphocytosis associated with variably severe cytopenias, most often neutropenia and/or anemia.

Epidemiology

T-LGL appears to be rare, with documented cases accounting for <5% of all mature leukemic lymphoproliferative disorders. Some authors estimate the actual prevalence of T-LGL to be much higher however, perhaps as high as 5%, as this disorder is challenging to diagnose from both the clinical and pathologic perspectives (3). The median age of individuals affected by T-LGL is between 50 and 60 years; the disorder is uncommonly encountered in younger adults and isolated cases in adolescents have been reported (4–6). T-LGL does not preferentially occur in any particular race or gender, although the disorder may be slightly more prevalent in Asians and in this population T-LGL may be more often associated with anemia (7).

T-LGL has an unusual proclivity to arise in association with rheumatoid arthritis (~20% of cases) and clonal hematolymphoid disorders (~10% to 20% of cases). T-LGL can be associated with other autoimmune disorders such as Sjögren syndrome and chronic inflammatory bowel disease; in addition, one-third to one-half of T-LGL patients have some serologic manifestations of immune activation such as a positive rheumatoid factor or polyclonal hypergammaglobulinemia (8,9). The clonal hematopoietic disorders associated with T-LGL are usually of B-cell lineage, most often chronic lymphocytic leukemia (~5% of

T-LGL cases) and monoclonal B-cell lymphocytosis (up to 25% of T-LGL cases) (10). Other hematopoietic neoplasms that are less commonly associated with T-LGL include follicular lymphoma, Hodgkin lymphoma, plasma cell proliferative disorders, hairy cell leukemia, and chronic myelomonocytic leukemia (8).

There are isolated case reports of T-LGL arising in the setting of renal allografting and allogeneic bone marrow transplantation (11). Extreme caution should be exercised when rendering a T-LGL diagnosis in this setting however, as in transplantation, as well as other conditions such as active HIV infection and dasatinib therapy for chronic myelogenous leukemia, reactive changes in the CD8-positive T-cell compartment closely resembling T-LGL may be observed (12). The close overlap between these reactive changes in CD8-positive T cells and T-LGL likely reflects that the latter is derived from chronically stimulated cytotoxic T cells; this likely also accounts for the disease associations with T-LGL described above.

Clinical Features
Sites of Involvement

Peripheral blood involvement is uniformly present and, based on early disease descriptions, an absolute granular lymphocyte count of $>2 \times 10^9$/L was initially proposed as a diagnostic criterion (13). In most cases the granular lymphocyte count is between 1 and 4×10^9/L; but in approximately one-third of cases the absolute granular lymphocyte count is $<1 \times 10^9$/L (4,14). For this reason, a specific absolute granular lymphocyte count is no longer required for a T-LGL diagnosis by WHO criteria, although in most cases the majority of the circulating lymphocytes have cytoplasmic granulation. Demonstrable bone marrow involvement is present in at least 75% of T-LGL, yet determining the precise frequency is difficult as marrow examination is not always performed and documentation of T-LGL infiltration is exceedingly difficult without the use of immunohistochemistry (15).

The reported frequency of splenic involvement with splenomegaly in T-LGL varies considerably (between 15% and 50%) with the highest proportion of cases seen in earlier disease descriptions. The proportion of T-LGL cases with splenomegaly described in these earlier case studies likely reflects the skewed recognition of cases with higher disease burden noted above. Overall, the degree of splenic enlargement is typically mild and may only evident by radiologic examination (5,8). Infiltration of liver sinusoids by T-LGL may be detected by histologic examination (Fig. 38.1), but hepatic dysfunction and/or hepatomegaly are not common (16). Isolated cases of T-LGL-associated primary pulmonary hypertension that have resolved with treatment have also been described, suggesting pulmonary parenchymal involvement by T-LGL; there is evidence to suggest that this may be due to direct cytopathic effects of the LGL cells on the pulmonary vascular endothelium (17). T-LGL rarely, if ever, involves the lymph nodes or other extranodal sites, and if this is a prominent clinical feature other diagnoses should be strongly considered.

Table 38.1	OVERVIEW OF MATURE T-CELL AND NK-CELL LEUKEMIAS			
	T-PLL	**T-LGL**	**CLPD-NK**	**Aggressive NK Cell Leukemia**
Prevalence	2% of all mature lymphocytic leukemias	3%–5% of all mature lympho-cytic leukemias	1%–2% of all mature lympho-cytic leukemias	Very rare
Epidemiology	Older adults (median age 65)	Adults		Young adults, mostly Asian
Associated conditions	Ataxia-telangiectasia	Rheumatologic disorders, immune activation/dysregulation, other hematologic neoplasms	Other hematologic neoplasms	EBV infection
Clinical features	Widespread disease, high PB counts	Cytopenias, sometimes lymphocytosis; cytopenias not proportional to BM involvement	Similar to T-LGL	Widespread disease with lymph-adenopathy, fever, HPS, DIC
Sites of involvement	BM, PB, liver, spleen, lymph nodes	BM, PB, and spleen	BM, PB, and spleen	BM, spleen, lymph nodes
Morphology	Small lymphocytes with clumped chromatin	Granular lymphocytes	Granular lymphocytes	Variable; usually markedly atypical
Immunophenotype	Usually CD4+ CD8−, bright CD7; TCL-1 nuclear staining	Usually CD4− CD8+ with dim/absent CD5, CD7, and/or CD2; coexpression of NK-associated markers CD16 and CD57; KIR restriction or absence	CD3− CD16+ (by flow), often with dim/absent CD2, CD7, CD56, and/or CD57; KIR restriction or absence	CD3− CD56+ (by flow) with coexpression of CD2, CD7, and HLA-DR; EBV positive
Cytogenetic abnormalities	Usually inv(14;14) or t(X;14) leading to overexpression of TCL-1 family proteins	Unusual	Unusual	Variable; del 6q23 frequent
Molecular charac-teristics	Disruption of ATM gene on 11q23	Often oligoclonal	Nonspecific	Nonspecific
EBV associated	No	No	No	Yes
Prognosis	Poor (median survival 1–2 y)	Excellent (disease-attributable mortality <10%)	Excellent (similar to T-LGL)	Poor (median survival <2 mo)

Clinical Evaluation and Staging

Peripheral blood examination is required in the evaluation of any potential T-LGL case and should include complete blood count (CBC) to assess for the cytopenias, morphologic evalua-tion for the presence of granular lymphocytes, flow cytometric T-cell immunophenotyping, and studies of T-cell clonality (either flow cytometric or molecular genetic based). Neutropenia is a universal feature of T-LGL case descriptions and is present in approximately 60% to 70% of cases. In contrast, thrombocyto-penia is rare. The reported frequency of anemia varies, with some studies finding it equally common as neutropenia in T-LGL and others finding it in fewer cases (18). T-LGL-associated ane-mia is typically mild and often does not require treatment; how-ever, some cases may be associated with pure red blood cell aplasia. In cases with cytopenias, bone marrow aspiration and biopsy should also be strongly considered to both help confirm the T-LGL diagnosis and help exclude other possible causes for the cytopenias such as myelodysplasia or a coincident B-cell malignancy with extensive marrow involvement.

As the decision to treat is largely predicated on the presence of cytopenias, CBC evaluation represents the most important staging procedure in T-LGL (3). While splenic and bone marrow involve-ment by T-LGL are frequent, the degree of histologic involvement

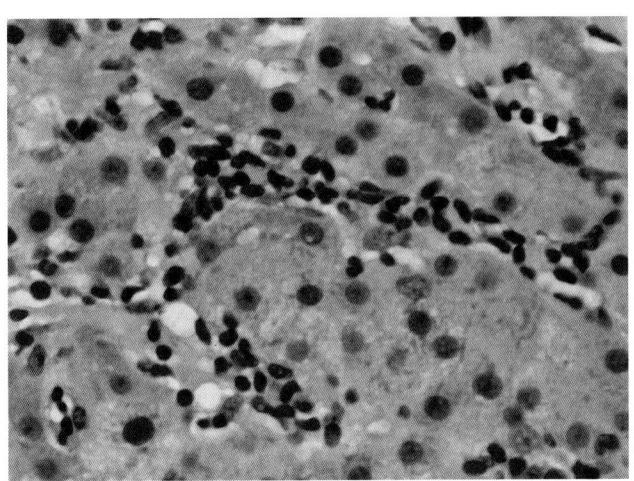
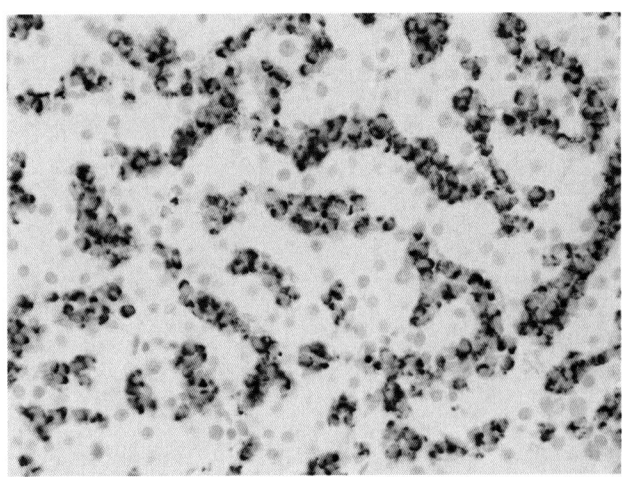

FIGURE 38.1. Hepatic involvement by T-LGL. Increased numbers of small lymphocytes are seen in the hepatic sinusoids **(A)**. These lymphocytes are demonstrated to be strongly TIA-1 positive by immunohistochemistry **(B)** (oil, 400×).

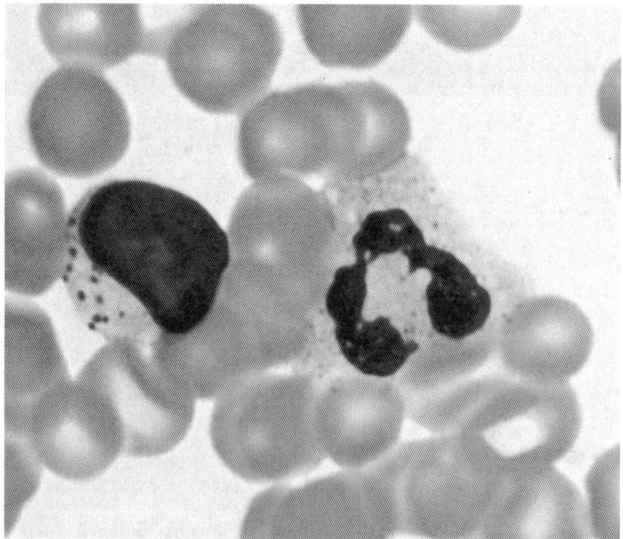

FIGURE 38.2. Circulating lymphocyte cytology in T-LGL. Lymphocytes, minimally irregular nuclear contours, and relatively abundant granulated cytoplasm are typical (lymphocyte on **left**, neutrophil is seen on **right** for comparison).

bone marrow aspirate smears. In summary, the classic cytology of T-LGL does not reliably distinguish it from normal cytotoxic lymphocytes or reactive granular lymphocyte expansions. Therefore, disease recognition requires particular vigilance and use of the ancillary tests for cellular characterization. Overt cytologic features of malignancy are not typical for T-LGL and when present should cause strong consideration of other diagnoses.

Grading

As in the peripheral blood and bone marrow aspirate, T-LGL has bland histologic features in paraffin sections. The cells usually have small, minimally irregular nuclei surrounded by modest amounts of cytoplasm. Histologic grading is not relevant in this disorder.

Proliferative Pattern

Classic descriptions of T-LGL bone marrow pathology emphasized left-shifted granulocytic hyperplasia; however, a variety of changes in hematopoiesis may be seen in T-LGL, ranging from a hypercellular marrow with prominent granulocytic and erythroid hyperplasia to a hypocellular marrow with marked decrease in one or more hematopoietic lineage (15). Abnormalities in megakaryopoiesis are uncommon in T-LGL.

Interstitial lymphoid aggregates are a marrow finding often described in T-LGL, with reported frequency ranging from 15% to over 50% of cases (19). While interstitial lymphoid aggregates may be the most readily appreciated histologic feature, these are reactive in nature and do not contain the abnormal T cells. The abnormal T-LGL cells infiltrate the marrow in a predominantly sinusoidal pattern, which, in combination with the bland histology of the cells, results in histologically subtle interstitial marrow involvement by T-LGL, which is exceedingly difficult to identify by morphologic examination alone.

Given the challenges in histologic recognition of marrow involvement by T-LGL, immunohistochemistry using antibodies to CD3, CD8, and cytotoxic granule proteins, such as TIA-1, granzyme B, and perforin, is requisite when evaluating potential cases. These studies reveal linear intrasinusoidal infiltrates and/or interstitial clusters of antigen-positive cells in 80% or more of marrow biopsies from T-LGL cases (Fig. 38.3) (15). Typically, the degree of antigen positivity is greater for CD8 and TIA-1 than for granzyme B, and in only approximately one-half

Morphology

Cytologic Composition

The "large" in T-LGL reflects cytoplasmic enlargement and the abnormal cells characteristically have bland nuclear features with minimal nuclear enlargement or irregularity (Fig. 38.2). As also indicated by the name, cytoplasmic granulation is usually present; however, the degree varies both between and within cases and is also dependent on the stain quality. In some T-LGL, neither cytoplasmic enlargement nor granulation is a prominent feature and these attributes can be particularly difficult to appreciate in

in these sites does not appear to correlate with the clinical severity of illness. Imaging studies of the abdomen may be helpful in detecting T-LGL-associated splenomegaly given the modest enlargement typical of this diagnosis, but extensive whole body imaging is not a required element of the clinical evaluation.

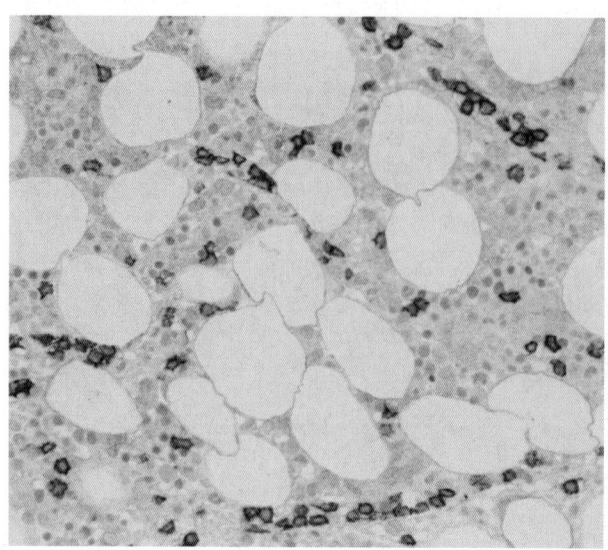

A

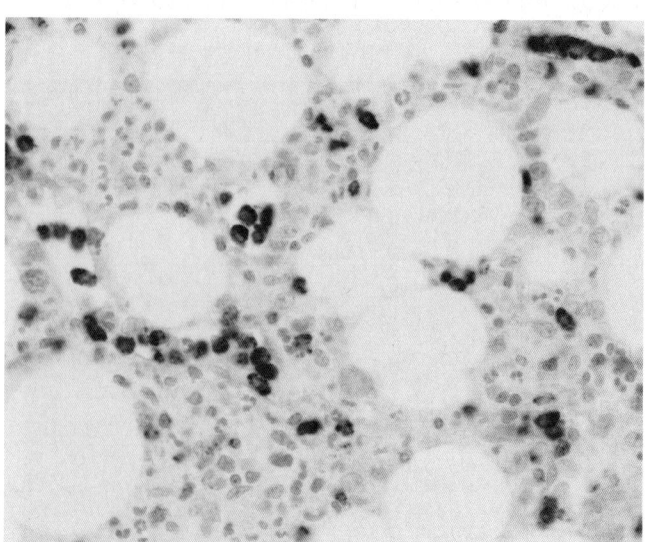

B

FIGURE 38.3. Bone marrow immunohistochemistry in T-LGL. Intrasinusoidal marrow infiltration by T-LGL cells is revealed by immunohistochemistry using antibodies to CD8 **(A)** and granzyme B **(B)**.

of cases will granzyme B–positive intrasinusoidal and interstitial infiltrates be present. The T-LGL cells also exhibit abnormal expression of granzyme M, a unique granzyme whose expression is normally restricted to NK cells.

Overall, these immunohistochemical findings are disease-specific and, when present, help distinguish T-LGL from reactive cellular expansion. Conversely, however, the absence of these findings does not exclude a T-LGL diagnosis. In a minority of T-LGL cases, particularly those with low peripheral blood LGL counts, immunohistochemistry only reveals an increase in interstitially distributed CD8 and TIA-1-positive cells without discrete cluster formation or intrasinusoidal staining. In such cases, a T-LGL diagnosis should be supported by flow cytometric immunophenotyping and/or the demonstration of T-cell clonality. Additionally, while the vast majority of T-LGL are CD57-positive by flow cytometric immunophenotyping, CD57 immunohistochemistry is abnormal in <20% of marrows involved by T-LGL. The reason for this discrepancy is likely multifactorial and related to both the spectrum of CD57 surface density seen in most T-LGL and the relative insensitivity of the IgM isotype HNK-1 monoclonal antibody to CD57 in immunohistochemical studies (20,21).

Other tissues in which histologic features of T-LGL involvement are commonly seen are the spleen and liver. Splenic involvement by T-LGL is confined to the red pulp and white pulp vascular structures (16,22). In the splenic red pulp the T-LGL cells are found in both the cords and sinusoids. Likewise, T-LGL involves the liver in a sinusoidal pattern with little or no disruption of the hepatic parenchyma. In cases with heavy involvement of the spleen and/or liver the infiltrates may be evident by histologic examination alone due to mild distention of the sinusoids by the bland lymphoid cells. However, as in the marrow, in most cases immunohistochemistry is required to definitively identify the LGL infiltrates.

Histologic progression and/or transformation to a more aggressive overtly malignant process is extraordinarily rare in T-LGL with only isolated case reports in the literature, and no documented cases in the Mayo Clinic files since 1996 (23). The scarcity of documented cases, as well as the predominance of data indicating that T-LGL is a disorder of postproliferative terminally differentiated cells, suggests that the sporadically reported cases of "disease transformation" may be either other more aggressive neoplasms of cytotoxic T cells, such as hepatosplenic T-cell lymphoma, first encountered at an early stage or a second, unrelated neoplasm arising in the setting of an antecedent T-LGL disorder.

Immunophenotype

The vast majority (>80%) of T-LGL consist of CD8-positive, alpha beta T cells with only small series of gamma delta cell lineage cases and isolated cases of CD4-positive T-LGL reported (24,25). These immunophenotypic variants have similar attributes to the CD8-positive alpha beta T-cell T-LGL with the only notable possible exception being CD4 and CD8 "double-negative" gamma delta T-cell T-LGL as such cases may have a slightly higher incidence of anemia and less often show the marrow immunohistochemistry typical for this disorder (26).

Abnormalities of T-cell–associated antigen expression can be detected by flow cytometric immunophenotyping in most, if not all, T-LGL (21,27). Chief amongst these are diminished or absent expression of CD5 or CD7, which are found in 90% and 80% of cases, respectively. Less often seen are diminished expression of CD2 (40%) or CD3 (25%). As these changes are either relatively minimal or only present on a subset of the abnormal cells, multicolor flow cytometric immunophenotyping is the preferred methodology for their detection.

Coexpression of NK-cell lineage–associated antigens is a pathognomic feature of T-LGL and, to at least some degree, is present in all cases. Assessing the potential T-LGL cells for this attribute is critical since the abnormalities in CD5 and CD7 frequently associated with the condition can also be seen in reactive T-cell expansions (28). The traditional NK-cell–associated antigens usually expressed by T-LGL are CD16 and CD57, with one or both found in >80% of cases. In contrast, CD56 expression by T-LGL is uncommon (<20% of cases) and the reported CD56-positive "aggressive T-LGL variant" may in fact again represent other cytotoxic T-cell disorders such as hepatosplenic T-cell lymphomas, as CD56 is commonly expressed in this disease (29).

When considering NK-cell antigen expression from the perspective of clinical diagnosis, having a significant proportion of the peripheral blood T cells (>20%) CD16-positive is distinctly abnormal and should prompt investigation for a T-cell disorder such as T-LGL. In contrast, having a high proportion of CD57-positive circulating T cells lacks this specificity as memory T cells express this antigen and over 50% normal peripheral blood T cells may be positive (30). Typically, however, normal T cells show a spectrum of CD57 surface density/staining intensity and therefore strong, homogeneous CD57 positivity should lead one to strongly suspect a T-LGL diagnosis, although this pattern is found in a minority of cases. As no single antigen or pattern of antigen expression is specific for T-LGL, assessing abnormalities in T-cell and NK-cell antigens collectively rather than individually allows for most reliable identification of T-LGL and discrimination from reactive LGL expansion. In fact, a recent study of 85 T-LGL revealed that cases with coincident diminished expression of CD5 and CD8 and uniform expression of CD57 are much more likely to have positive studies for T-cell clonality and be associated with significant cytopenias when compared to cases lacking any one of these three features (31).

The identification of and characterization of T-LGL cases can be aided by the flow cytometric evaluation of a group of NK-cell–associated receptors for MHC class I and related antigens referred to as the NK-cell receptors, or NKRs (32). For diagnostic purposes, the NKR most relevant to T-LGL are the killer cell immunoglobulin-like receptor (KIR) family members CD158a, CD158b, and CD158e. The KIRs are expressed by post-thymic cytotoxic T cells after antigenic stimulation and appear to play multiple roles including preventing autoreactivity and blocking activation-induced cell death. Typically, only a minor proportion of normal T cells (<5%) are KIR positive. In contrast, abnormal homogeneous expression of a single KIR isoform is seen in approximately 50% of T-LGL; for reasons which are unclear the KIR isoform usually expressed is CD158b (21,27). KIR evaluation in T-LGL has other potential diagnostic benefits as well. In KIR-positive T-LGL, the expression of a KIR isoform lacking the cognate ligand in the self MHC haplotype appears to predict a more aggressive disease course with more frequent cytopenias and splenomegaly. Furthermore, while T-LGL typically expresses a single KIR isoform, KIR expression is not mutually exclusive and isolated cases (<10%) with simultaneous expression of two KIR isoforms can be encountered. However, the coincident expression of all three KIRs is not seen in T-LGL whereas this pattern of KIR expression is often seen in hepatosplenic T-cell lymphoma, an aggressive neoplasm of cytotoxic T cells that can have clinical and phenotypic overlap with T-LGL.

The detection of KIR expression in T-LGL provides further evidence to support the notion that this disorder is derived from antigen-stimulated cytotoxic T cells. Other NKRs expressed by this normal T-cell compartment can also be seen in T-LGL including CD94 and CD161; however, these do not appear to have the same degree of diagnostic utility as the KIR antigens.

Cytogenetics

The vast majority of T-LGL cases have no clonal cytogenetic abnormalities. Isolated reports have described cytogenetic abnormalities in T-LGL including deletion 6q and reciprocal translocations and inversions involving the T-cell receptor gene loci on chromosomes 7 and 14 (33). As these reports are preferentially found in the older literature it is possible that the reports included cases of other aggressive cytotoxic T-cell malignancies. Given the association of T-LGL with other clonal hematolymphoid disorders it is also possible that in some instances the abnormalities detected were not actually harbored within the T-LGL cells but rather another coincident condition. Overall, it appears that clonal cytogenetic abnormalities in T-LGL are very uncommon and, if present, should at least cause one to consider possible alternate diagnoses.

Molecular Characteristics

Since the earliest characterization of T-LGL, T-cell clonality has been considered a hallmark feature of the condition. In most cases, T-cell clonality can be detected by either molecular genetic methods or flow cytometric assessment of T-cell receptor V-beta expression (34,35). When comparing T-LGL to peripheral blood involvement by other T-cell disorders such as Sezary syndrome, however, T-LGL lacks the same degree of homogeneity within the clonal T-cell compartment by V-beta flow cytometry. Furthermore, when assessing T-cell diversity by detailed methodology such as TCR spectratyping, most T-LGL appear oligoclonal (36). Also, phenotypic drift in V-beta expression with changing degrees of homogeneity and altering patterns of V-beta expression in single T-LGL cases over time has recently been described (37).

When considering these results collectively, they provide strong evidence that T-LGL is, in at least most cases, an oligoclonal T-cell disorder. This in turn raises the possibility that in some T-LGL cases clonality will not be detected by some methods, including T-cell receptor PCR analysis. When looking at large case series, this is difficult to assess as in many demonstrable T-cell clonality was a criterion for inclusion in the study. However, in careful review of the literature and in the authors' experience a diagnosis of T-LGL may be rendered even if T-cell clonality cannot be detected. In such cases, the demonstration of a phenotypically abnormal T-cell population with NK-cell antigen coexpression is critical, and the use of temporal criteria (persistence for >6 months) should be strongly considered.

There have been a number of *in vitro* studies regarding the molecular pathogenesis of T-LGL. These studies all suggest that abnormal resistance to activation-induced cell death and prolonged survival are important in the disease pathogenesis. Pathways that have been implicated include perturbations in sphingomyelin lipid metabolism, resistance to FAS (38), and activation of the STAT3 pathway (39). A recent study has shown that 40% of T-LGL have a somatic mutation in STAT3 that leads to increase in its transcriptional activity (40). In addition, there is some evidence to suggest that T-LGL may be derived from a unique subset of cytotoxic T cells that are NKp46 positive and are hyperresponsive to IL-15 (41).

Postulated Normal Counterpart

As detailed above, the normal counterpart for T-LGL is antigen-stimulated cytotoxic T cells. The phenotypic "variants" such as cases with gamma delta T-cell receptor expression and CD4-positive cases likely represent expansion of phenotypically distinct, usually minor, cytotoxic T-cell subsets.

Clinical Course and Prognostic Assessment

One-third to one-half of LGL patients will require treatment for severe neutropenia, neutropenic infection, or symptomatic anemia at diagnosis. If followed over an extended period of time, up to 75% of cases may require therapy (4,42).

Treatment and Survival

The decision to treat in T-LGL is determined by the presence or absence of neutropenia and/or symptomatic anemia (3). The reported proportion of patients requiring treatment varies considerably; however, it does appear that the majority will eventually require therapy at some time in their disease course. For first-line treatment, single-agent chemotherapy with either methotrexate or cyclophosphamide is most effective, which may be supplemented with prednisone. In refractory patients alternate therapies including cyclosporine A and anti-CD52 monoclonal antibodies may be considered; neither splenectomy nor exogenous growth factor therapy appear to be particularly effective in alleviating the T-LGL cytopenias (43).

T-LGL is an indolent disease with an excellent overall survival. The disease-attributable mortality rate is <10%, and in most cases is due to neutropenic infection.

Differential Diagnosis

As noted above, the primary differential diagnostic considerations are a reactive increase in peripheral blood cytotoxic T cells and peripheral blood involvement by more aggressive cytotoxic T-cell neoplasms such as hepatosplenic T-cell lymphoma.

Summary and Conclusions

T-LGL is an unusual lymphoproliferative disorder of cytotoxic T cells that seems to occupy a space somewhere in between reactive T-cell expansion and overtly malignant T-cell lymphomas. Although the disorder is uncommon, given the challenge in clinical and laboratory diagnosis it is worthwhile considering in patients with unexplained cytopenias as it is a potentially reversible cause.

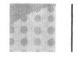

CHRONIC LYMPHOPROLIFERATIVE DISORDERS OF NATURAL KILLER CELLS

Definition

Chronic lymphoproliferative disorder of natural killer cells (CLPD-NKs) is a persistent, unexplained increase in peripheral blood NK cells that is often associated with cytopenias (2). Many names have been used for CLPD-NK in the past, including NK-cell lymphoproliferative of granular lymphocytes, chronic NK-cell lymphocytosis, and NK-cell granular lymphocytic leukemia. However, as the earlier literature included in these disease descriptions other, more aggressive NK-cell malignancies, these older disease monikers are best avoided.

As is now recognized, CLPD-NK essentially represents the NK-cell lineage counterpart of T-LGL, and the therapeutic approach to these disorders is virtually identical (3). Therefore, for the purpose of brevity, this section focuses on the comparative attributes of CLPD-NK and T-LGL although some features unique to CLPD-NK are highlighted.

Epidemiology

In large, comparative studies CLPD-NK has a prevalence approximately one-third that of T-LGL (4,5). Like T-LGL, however, the actual prevalence of CLPD-NK may be considerably higher as this disorder is similarly challenging to diagnose. CLPD-NK also has age and gender distributions similar to T-LGL, primarily occurring in adults over 50 years old without a preference for either gender. CLPD-NK does not have a predilection for any ethnic group or geographic region and is not pathogenically related to Epstein-Barr virus and in these ways is distinct from aggressive NK-cell leukemia.

CLPD-NK may be weakly associated with autoimmune diseases; however, there is no known association between CLPD-NK and other hematolymphoid malignancies. The results of a small series of studies suggest that individuals with haplotypes rich in the activating form of the KIR receptors (type B) and with higher expression of these activating isoforms may be more susceptible to developing CLPD-NK (44).

Clinical Features

Sites of Involvement

Like T-LGL, CLPD-NK is primarily a disorder of the peripheral blood and bone marrow. The reported frequency of splenomegaly in CLPD-NK varies and this feature is more heavily emphasized in early "NK-LGL" descriptions that likely included other NK-cell malignancies (13). In the more recent literature splenomegaly is present in 25% or less of CLPD-NK cases and is often minimal. Neither lymph node involvement nor tumefactive, destructive tissue infiltration are typical of CLPD-NK and if these are present other diagnoses, such as extranodal NK-/T-cell lymphoma, should be strongly considered.

Clinical Evaluation and Staging

From a clinical perspective, CLPD-NK is virtually identical to T-LGL and primarily manifests with modest lymphocytosis often associated with neutropenia and/or anemia; thrombocytopenia is uncommon and rarely occurs in isolation (4,21). As in T-LGL, peripheral blood examination is a critical element of any CLPD-NK evaluation and should include morphologic review, complete blood counts, and flow cytometric immunophenotyping. Unlike T-LGL, molecular genetic studies for T-cell receptor gene rearrangements do not play a role in the diagnosis of CLPD-NK as these are not rearranged in NK-cell lineage cells. Bone marrow examination should also be considered in CLPD-NK cases with cytopenias, both to exclude other potential causes for the cytopenias and to aid in establishing the CLPD-NK diagnosis (21). Imaging studies of the abdomen may help in detecting disease-associated splenomegaly, although these studies are not required as CLPD-NK typically has minimal tissue involvement.

Since the decision to treat in CLPD-NK is predicated on the presence or absence of cytopenias, CBC evaluation is the most important staging procedure (3).

Morphology

Cytologic Composition and Grading

The cytologic features of CLPD-NK in the peripheral blood and bone marrow aspirate are virtually identical to those of T-LGL, being characterized by cells with small to intermediate-sized bland nuclei and relatively abundant, variably granulated cytoplasm (21). As such, CLPD-NK and T-LGL cannot be distinguished from each other, or from a reactive increase in cytotoxic lymphocytes, by their morphologic features. Likewise, CLPD-NK and T-LGL have similarly bland histologic features in paraffin sections of the spleen and bone marrow, and, as in T-LGL, if overt cytologic features of an aggressive malignancy are present other diagnoses should be strongly considered. Grading is not relevant in CLPD-NK.

Proliferative Pattern

As in T-LGL, the histology of CLPD-NK is most relevant in the bone marrow as this is the primary site of involvement. CLPD-NK typically infiltrates the marrow in an interstitial and sinusoidal pattern identical to T-LGL (21,45). In cases with advanced

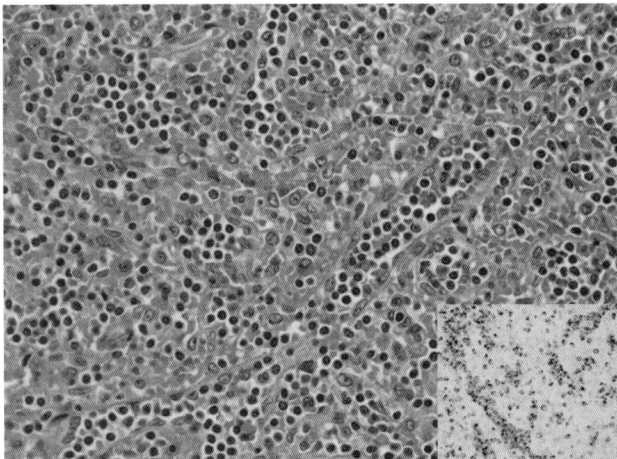

FIGURE 38.4. Splenic involvement by CLPD-NK. Histologic examination reveals increased numbers of small lymphocytes in the splenic sinusoids, without distention or distortion of these structures. Immunohistochemistry demonstrates these cells to be granzyme B positive (inset).

or prolonged disease the infiltrates may become denser, more confluent, and disrupt the marrow architecture. In the majority of CLPD-NK, however, the infiltrates are exceedingly subtle and difficult to identify without the aid of immunohistochemistry.

In the spleen, CLPD-NK infiltrates the red pulp sinusoids and cords (Fig. 38.4); these structures may be distended, but tumor masses, destructive tissue infiltration, or necrosis are not seen (14,46). The rare cases of documented liver involvement also appear to be characterized by bland sinusoidal infiltration. Tumefactive or parenchymal lymph node involvement is not a feature of CLPD-NK, although in isolated cases the abnormal cells may be identified in the lymph node sinusoids.

Immunohistochemistry is required to identify marrow involvement by CLPD-NK; stains used for this purpose should include antibodies to CD3, CD8, and the cytotoxic granule proteins TIA-1, granzyme B, and perforin (Fig. 38.4 inset) (21,45). In approximately 80% of cases, linear intrasinusoidal and interstitial aggregate patterns are present, as also seen in T-LGL. It is important to note that CLPD-NK and T-LGL cannot be reliably distinguished by marrow immunohistochemistry as NK cells can react with the antibodies to CD3 used in paraffin studies and, conversely, T-LGL is frequently CD5-negative and granzyme M–positive (47). For this reason, flow cytometric immunophenotyping is critical for most accurate lineage assignment and diagnosis (45). In cases that are confirmed to be of NK-cell lineage, *in situ* hybridization studies for Epstein-Barr virus (EBV) should be considered to exclude the possibility of aggressive NK-cell leukemia, especially if prominent splenic involvement is present (48).

Histologic Progression/Transformation

Although rare, single instances of transformation of indolent NK-cell disorders to more aggressive neoplasms have been reported, these are sporadic and their true nature is unclear. As such, histologic progression or transformation is not relevant in CLPD-NK. Likewise, there are no recognized histologic variants of CLPD-NK.

Immunophenotype

Flow cytometric immunophenotyping is the most reliable method for NK-cell identification and characterization in the clinical laboratory through its ability to simultaneously measure the expression of multiple antigens by single cells (45).

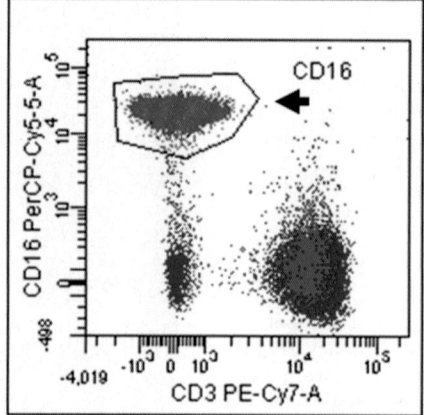

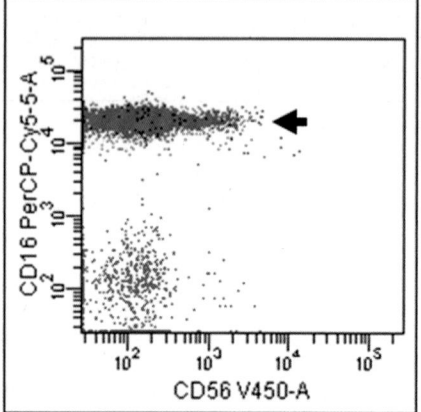
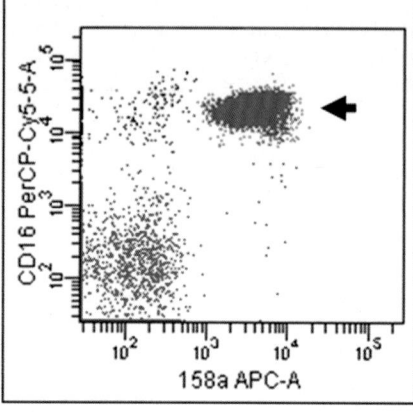
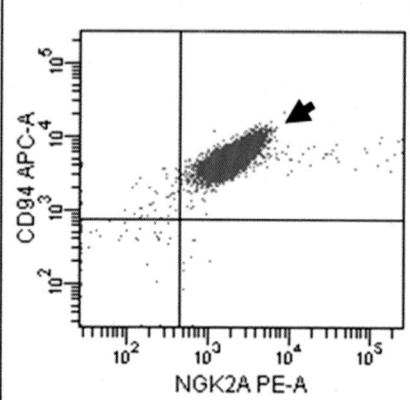

FIGURE 38.5. Flow cytometric immunophenotyping in CLPD-NK. Flow cytometric immunophenotyping of a peripheral blood specimen from a CLPD-NK case reveals increased numbers of brightly CD16-positive, CD3-negative NK cells (**upper panel**, *population colored green, highlighted by arrow*). Additional studies revealed these cells to have abnormally diminished expression of CD56 (**lower left panel,** *arrow*), to have restricted expression of the KIR isoform CD158a (**lower middle panel,** *arrow*), and to have homogeneous expression of CD94/NKG2A heterodimers (**lower right panel,** *arrow*).

In virtually all CLPD-NK cases flow studies reveal an increase in CD16-positive, CD3- and CD5-negative NK cells usually representing >40% of the total lymphocyte events (21,49). This finding alone allows for the distinction of CLPD-NK from T-LGL as the latter is CD3-positive. In addition, there are a number of immunophenotypic abnormalities in CLPD-NK that can be detected by assays considered "routine" in most clinical laboratories. Chief amongst these is abnormally diminished or absent expression of CD56, which is present in approximately two-thirds of cases (Fig. 38.5). Approximately two-thirds of CLPD-NK cases will also show a spectrum of CD57 expression ranging from negative to positive; however, this pattern may also be seen in normal NK cells and therefore is not diagnostic of CLPD-NK (50). In contrast, complete loss of CD57 expression can be observed in CLPD-NK and is distinctly abnormal; unfortunately, this is present in a minority of cases (~20%) (21). Other phenotypic abnormalities that can be detected by routine flow cytometric immunophenotyping in CLPD-NK in order of decreasing frequency are diminished or absent expression of CD7 (~40% of cases), uniform expression of CD8 (~15% of cases), and diminished expression of CD2 (<10% of cases).

The power of flow cytometry for making a CLPD-NK diagnosis is greatly enhanced by the evaluation of NKR expression (21,49,51). Of particular value in this regard is analysis of the KIR antigens CD158a, CD158b, and CD158e, each of which are expressed to some degree by normal NK cells. Aberrancies of expression of these KIR antigens are present in all CLPD-NK cases with two distinctly abnormal patterns observed, one characterized by complete lack of expression of all three KIRs

and the other by the uniform expression of a single (or less often multiple) KIRs by the abnormal NK cells (Fig. 38.5). This latter pattern of KIR "restriction" is analogous to that seen in T-LGL; interestingly, the KIR-restricted CLPD-NK show preferential expression of the CD158a isoform whereas the KIR-restricted T-LGL show preferential expression of the CD158b isoform; the reasons for these differences are unclear. In addition to identifying KIR abnormalities, evaluation of NKR in CLPD-NK can also reveal abnormally bright, uniform expression of CD94, usually in a heterodimeric complex with NKG2A forming a functional, inhibitory receptor complex. Like abnormalities in KIR expression, this pattern of CD94/NKG2A expression helps to distinguish CLPD-NK from reactive NK-cell expansion; however, this abnormality is only present in approximately 75% of cases.

The abnormalities in NKR expression detected by flow cytometry in CLPD-NK appear to be stable over the course of the disease independent of treatment status (49). Given the inability to confirm NK-cell clonality by routine molecular genetic studies using these immunophenotyping studies to confirm the persistence of the abnormal NK cells is very helpful in confirming a CLPD-NK diagnosis.

Cytogenetics

In the vast majority of CLPD-NK, no genetic abnormalities are identified by either conventional metaphase or FISH analysis. This is particularly true if early studies of "NK-LGL" are excluded. As such, there are no known recurrent cytogenetic abnormalities in CLPD-NK.

Molecular Characteristics

There are no known molecular genetic abnormalities associated with CLPD-NK. Studies of X-linked gene expression in female CLPD-NK subjects have yielded contradictory results with one study finding evidence of NK-cell clonality by this method and another not (52,53). The reason behind these discrepant findings are unknown, although it is possible that this could be attributable to criteria used for case selection and the inclusion of reactive NK-cell expansions in the study with negative results.

Postulated Normal Counterpart

There are two normal mature NK-cell subsets, one characterized by bright CD56 and dim CD16 expression and the other, conversely, by dim CD56 and bright CD16 expression. The CD56 bright/CD16 dim NK cells are preferentially found in secondary lymphoid tissue, are KIR negative; and have limited cytotoxic potential functioning primarily through the elaboration of cytokines such as interferon gamma. In contrast, the CD56 dim/CD16 bright cells are found primarily in the peripheral blood express KIR, and act primarily as cytotoxic effector cells. These mature NK-cell subsets are closely interrelated with the latter (CD56 dim/CD16 bright) derived from exposure of the former (CD56 bright/ CD16 dim) to cytokines such as IL-2 and IL-15.

When CLPD-NK are grouped according to the presence or absence of CD56, distinct patterns emerge with CD56-negative CLPD-NK having bright CD16 expression and frequent KIR restriction and, in contrast, CD56-positive CLPD-NK having moderate CD16 expression, frequent complete absence of KIR expression, and bright expression of CD94/NKG2A heterodimers. These attributes suggest that the CD56-positive CLPD-NK correspond to the CD56 bright/CD16 dim cytokine-producing mature NK-cell subset whereas the CD56-negative CLPD-NK (including cases with partial loss of CD56) correspond to the CD56 dim/CD16 bright cytotoxic effector mature NK-cell subset (49). Interestingly, cytopenias appear to be more prevalent in the CD56-negative CLPD-NKs corresponding to the cytolytic effector subset and there are data to suggest that the cytopenias in CLPD-NK are attributable to direct cellular cytotoxicity; although the studies to date are insufficient in size to reach statistical significance.

Clinical Course and Prognostic Assessment

There is relatively limited information regarding the clinical course of CLPD-NK. Overall, it appears that this is a very indolent disease with an excellent long-term minimal disease progression, although there are isolated reports of worsening cytopenias and splenomegaly in cases with protracted (>10 years) disease. The disease-associated morbidity and mortality in CLPD-NK are attributable to the disease-associated cytopenias.

Treatment and Survival

The need for treatment of CLPD-NK is predicated on the presence or absence of cytopenias (3). As in T-LGL treatment, it appears that single-agent therapy with methotrexate or cyclophosphamide is efficacious in most cases, with prednisone, cyclosporine, or anti-CD52 monoclonal antibody therapy potential useful as adjunct or second-line agents in refractory cases.

CLPD-NK appears to have an excellent overall 10-year survival at least equivalent to T-LGL. In rare cases, there is disease-attributable mortality due to neutropenic infection.

Differential Diagnosis

The main differential diagnostic considerations are T-LGL, reactive NK-cell expansion, and peripheral blood involvement by aggressive NK-cell leukemia.

Summary and Conclusions

CLPD-NK bears a close clinical relationship to T-LGL and, like this condition, appears to represent a lymphoproliferative condition with features intermediate between reactive NK-cell expansion and *bona fide* NK-cell malignancy.

AGGRESSIVE NATURAL KILLER CELL LEUKEMIA

Definition

Aggressive NK-cell leukemia is an EBV-associated NK-cell malignancy that can have a leukemic (peripheral blood, bone marrow, and spleen), tissue-based (spleen, liver, and/or lymph node predominant), or mixed distribution. This disease typically manifests with widespread distribution at diagnosis and has a dismal prognosis.

Epidemiology

Aggressive NK-cell leukemia is an extraordinarily rare disease first reported in the 1980s and with the largest published series containing fewer than 25 cases (48,54). This disease typically affects young adults with a median age at diagnosis between 30 and 40 years and has no definite gender predilection. Aggressive NK-cell leukemia is most prevalent in Asian populations although it does occur sporadically in non-Asian populations.

Clinical Features

Sites of Involvement

Despite the name, peripheral blood involvement in aggressive NK-cell leukemia is variable and malignant leukocytosis may be present in fewer than 50% of cases. Bone marrow infiltration is common in aggressive NK-cell leukemia (54). Yet, as in the peripheral blood, the degree of marrow infiltration varies and may not be prominent, particularly in cases with extensive extramedullary disease (55).

Aggressive NK-cell leukemia characteristically is widespread at presentation and may occur in any tissue or organ. The extramedullary sites most frequently involved are the liver, spleen, and lymph nodes with 50% to 75% of patients presenting with hepatosplenomegaly and approximately one-half with widespread lymphadenopathy. In some cases of aggressive NK-cell leukemia the disease is exclusively found in extramedullary tissues with minimal-to-no peripheral blood or bone marrow involvement. This capacity of aggressive NK-cell leukemia to alternatively present as blood/bone marrow or tissue-based disease is analogous to the variety of disease distributions seen in HTLV-1-associated T-cell neoplasms (56). This feature creates confusion regarding disease terminology; the World Health Organization elected to continue to use the designation aggressive NK-cell leukemia in the most recent classification scheme as this connotes the extensive disease dissemination at diagnosis and dire prognosis.

Clinical Evaluation and Staging

Aggressive NK-cell leukemia presents as a morbid illness with fever, hepatosplenomegaly, lymphadenopathy, B symptoms, an elevated LDH; hemophagocytic syndrome (HPS) is found in over 50% of cases. In addition, aggressive NK-cell leukemia can also be associated with disseminated intravascular coagulation (DIC), and evidence for HPS and/or DIC should be routinely assessed as they can be significant causes of morbidity and mortality. Cytopenias are present in at approximately one-half of cases and can include anemia, thrombocytopenia, or leukopenia alone or in any combination. These cytopenias may be attributable to either decreased production due to marrow tumor burden or peripheral consumption due to HPS or DIC.

Bone marrow examination should be performed in all cases as either a diagnostic or staging procedure. In cases with prominent involvement of extramedullary tissues, such as those with widespread lymphadenopathy, biopsy examination of these tissues should be strongly considered, particularly since in such cases there may be minimal involvement of the bone marrow.

Morphology
Cytologic Composition

The neoplastic cells of aggressive NK-cell leukemia usually have malignant cytology with intermediate-sized, hyperchromatic nuclei, irregular nuclear contours, and modest amounts of cytoplasm. In peripheral blood and bone marrow aspirate smears, the cytoplasm may be more densely basophilic and have visible granules. These features are not present in all cases, however, and in some instances the neoplastic cells can have a plasmacytoid appearance in paraffin sections whereas in others the cells have the appearance of bland small lymphocytes or large granular lymphocytes.

Grading

Although the degree of cytologic atypia varies in aggressive NK-cell leukemia, grading is not relevant as the disease histology does not correlate with the degree of clinical morbidity or mortality.

Proliferative Pattern

Aggressive NK-cell leukemia infiltrates the marrow in an interstitial pattern in most instances, and in some cases may be difficult to appreciate without the use of ancillary immunohistochemical stains. In cases with an associated HPS, the neoplastic marrow infiltrates may be obscured by the proliferation of activated histocytes containing ingested hematopoietic cells.

In cases with extensive marrow involvement and in extramedullary sites aggressive NK-cell leukemia forms diffuse infiltrates that efface normal tissue architecture. Angiocentricity and angioinvasion can be present, particularly in extramedullary sites, and may be associated with coagulative necrosis, which may be massive.

Histologic Progression/Transformation and Variants

Histologic progression/transformation is not a relevant feature in aggressive NK-cell leukemia. In addition, although the disease histology may vary there are no recognized "histologic variants" per se.

Morphology in Sites Other than Bone Marrow

As noted above, in extramedullary sites, aggressive NK-cell leukemia may be associated with angioinvasion and massive necrosis. When present, these features may result in an associated polymorphous inflammatory background, which can obfuscate the presence of neoplastic cells.

Immunophenotype

There is relatively limited information regarding the immunophenotype of aggressive NK-cell leukemia. It appears that all cases are positive for CD2, CD7, CD56, HLA-DR, and cytotoxic effector proteins such as TIA-1 and lack a fully assembled CD3-T-cell receptor complex or functionally rearranged T-cell receptor genes; and it is on the basis of this combination of features

that this disorder is considered to be of NK-cell lineage. Although aggressive NK-cell leukemia lacks the fully assembled CD3 complex, the CD3 epsilon subunit is expressed in at least a subset of cases and, when present, may lead to immunoreactivity with antibodies to CD3 used in paraffin section immunohistochemistry (47). Other antigens associated with cytotoxic T-cell lineage such as CD5 and CD8 are usually not expressed.

The frequency of CD16 expression in aggressive NK-cell leukemia varies between reports; most cases appear to be positive although is it difficult to be sure due to the absence of a paraffin-reactive anti-CD16 antibody. There is no published information regarding the expression of other NK-cell–associated antigens such as the NKRs.

Aggressive NK-cell leukemia is strongly associated with EBV, and EBV positivity in the neoplastic cells should be readily detected in all cases, particularly if sensitive in situ hybridization methods are used. If the neoplastic cells are EBV negative, other possible diagnoses should be strongly considered.

Cytogenetics

Although an abnormal karyotype is detectable in most aggressive NK-cell leukemia cases, there are no recurring cytogenetic abnormalities specific for this disorder. Among the variety of chromosomal abnormalities that have been described, abnormalities of chromosomes 6 and 7 and gains of chromosome X appear most common (57).

Molecular Characteristics

There are no specific molecular genetic features of aggressive NK-cell leukemia. Due to the lineage of the neoplastic cells they should lack detectable clonal T-cell receptor gene rearrangements. Analysis of episomal EBV would be expected to reveal evidence of clonality, if such studies were performed.

Postulated Normal Counterpart

This disease is thought to be derived from mature NK cells.

Clinical Course and Prognostic Assessment

As noted above, aggressive NK-cell leukemia is characteristically widespread at diagnosis and often manifests with cytopenias due to marrow involvement and/or the presence of an associated HPS. This moribund presentation is typically followed by rapid disease progression and the prognosis in aggressive NK-cell leukemia is very poor.

Treatment and Survival

Aggressive NK-cell leukemia is resistant to treatment with poor response to conventional multiagent chemotherapy. There are some data to suggest that addition of L-asparaginase to other multiagent regimens may improve treatment response and there are isolated reports of complete remission following allogeneic bone marrow transplantation (58). However, the overall survival rate is very poor (<10%) and most patients die within 2 months of diagnosis.

Differential Diagnosis

A primary differential diagnostic consideration is extranasal extranodal NK-/T-cell lymphoma, which is also an EBV-associated NK-cell malignancy. These diseases have a number of other similarities including overlapping histologic and immunophenotypic features. In fact, when comparing younger patients (<50 years old) with extranodal extranasal NK-/T-cell to aggressive NK-cell leukemia they are virtually indistinguishable, with identical clinical attributes and a similarly dismal prognosis (59). The differences between aggressive NK-cell leukemia and extranodal extranasal NK-/T-cell lymphoma are largely semantic, particularly in young adults, given the high degree of similarity in histopathology, treatment, and prognosis. Overall, it appears that aggressive NK-cell leukemia is the preferred diagnostic term when the disease is encountered in the peripheral blood, bone marrow, or spleen.

Another differential diagnostic consideration is the lymphoproliferative disorders associated with chronic active EBV infection (CAEBV), a rare disorder of childhood and early adolescence that occurs almost exclusively in East Asian (particularly Japanese and Korean) and Latin American populations (54). CAEBV is defined as an illness beginning with primary EBV infection followed by prolonged febrile illness and/or abnormal EBV antibody serologies and associated with organ involvement by EBV-driven inflammatory processes. In the earlier stages of CAEBV, peripheral blood large granular lymphocytosis may be present; these may be of cytotoxic T-cell or NK-cell lineage, are EBV positive, and are oligoclonal or clonal (60). These large granular lymphocytes can have an abnormal immunophenotype, although they are not associated with cytopenias as are T-LGL and CLPDNK. Early in the disease course these lymphoproliferations do not have the malignant behavior of aggressive NK-cell leukemia or extranodal NK-/T-cell lymphoma, although they may be associated with hypersensitivity to mosquito bites (NK-cell expansions) or hydroa vacciniforme–like skin (cytotoxic T-cell expansions). The long-term prognosis in CAEBV is poor, however, with many patients only surviving to early adulthood. Interestingly, the mortality in CAEBV is often due to the development of overt, aggressive EBV-associated T-/NK-cell leukemia/lymphoma or the development of HPS, a frequent complication of aggressive NK-cell leukemia. Furthermore, in a subset of aggressive NK-cell leukemia cases there is a childhood history of hypersensitivity to mosquito bites, suggesting a pathogenetic relationship between CAEBV and aggressive NK-cell leukemia.

Lastly, intravascular NK-cell lymphoma is another extraordinarily rare entity described in Asians that bears mention. Like aggressive NK-cell leukemia, this is an EBV-associated disorder; in this instance, however, the EBV-positive malignant cells are found exclusively in vascular spaces without involvement of the peripheral blood or associated hepatosplenomegaly or lymphadenopathy. Intravascular NK-cell lymphoma appears to primarily manifest with skin lesions (erythematous patches and plaques) and may have a better prognosis than aggressive NK-cell leukemia with complete clinical remissions documented.

Summary and Conclusions

Aggressive NK-cell leukemia is an extraordinarily rare EBV-associated NK-cell neoplasm that appears to have some pathogenetic relationship to both extranasal extranodal NK-/T-cell lymphoma and the NK-cell lineage lymphoproliferations associated with CAEBV.

T-CELL PROLYMPHOCYTIC LEUKEMIA

Definition

T-prolymphocytic leukemia (T-PLL) is a neoplasm of mature T lymphocytes, characterized by the widespread infiltrates of small to medium-sized cells, high peripheral blood counts, and aggressive clinical course.

Epidemiology

T-PLL is a rare disease, accounting for about 2% of all mature lymphocytic leukemias. It mostly affects adults, usually older patients, with the median age of 65 years (61,62).

Clinical Features

Patients with T-PLL typically present with a widespread disease, involving blood, bone marrow, liver, spleen, and lymph nodes; less frequently skin and serous fluids; and very rarely central nervous system. A striking feature of T-PLL is high tumor burden in the peripheral blood, often exceeding 100×10^9/L. Because of the high tumor burden in the bone marrow, patients often present with anemia and thrombocytopenia. A small subset of patients presents with an indolent lymphocytosis without other symptoms (62). These cases usually have a prolonged clinical course.

Morphology

Peripheral blood and bone marrow lymphocytes usually have a typical prolymphocyte morphology: small to medium-sized cells with moderately clumped chromatin, single prominent nucleolus, and small amount of basophilic cytoplasm with cytoplasmic blebs (Fig. 38.6). Less frequently cells are smaller in size and without visible nucleolus (small cell variant); occasionally nuclei have cerebriform morphology, similar to Sézary cells. As mentioned above, bone marrow is usually diffusely involved, with replacement of normal hematopoietic elements (Fig. 38.7). Involvement of liver and spleen is also typical and substantial, resulting in hepatosplenomegaly. Microscopically, spleen involvement is characterized by expansion of white pulp with extension of neoplastic cells into the red pulp and capsule (22). T-PLL usually diffusely infiltrates lymph nodes; infiltrates are more prominent in paracortical areas, with proliferation of high endothelial venules and occasional sparing of follicles. Skin involvement is manifested by diffuse erythema, nodules, and erythroderma, due to perivascular dermal infiltrate without epidermotropism (63).

Immunophenotype

T-PLL cells are typically mature, postthymic T cells expressing CD2, CD3, CD5, CD7, and alpha/beta T-cell receptors; they do not express immature markers TdT and CD1a. A characteristic feature on routine flow cytometry immunophenotyping of blood or bone marrow is a tight cellular distribution and bright CD7 expression of neoplastic cells (Fig. 38.8). About two-thirds of T-PLL cases have CD4+CD8− phenotype; the rest are either CD4−CD8+ or double-positive CD4+CD8+. The phenotype

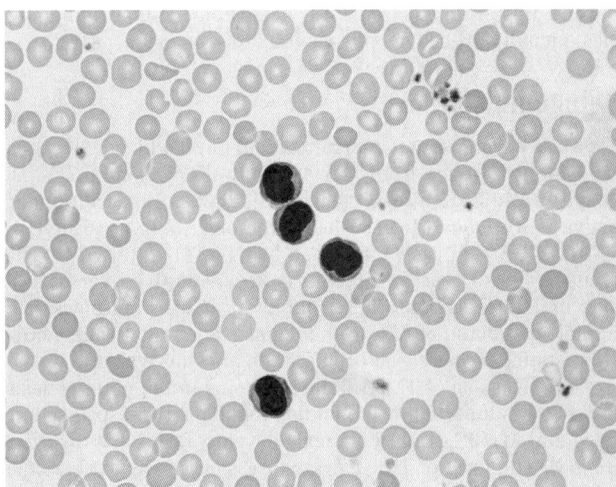

FIGURE 38.6. Peripheral blood smear showing atypical lymphocytes in T-PLL. Small to medium-sized cells with moderately clumped chromatin, single nucleolus, and small amount of basophilic cytoplasm (Wright Giemsa 600×).

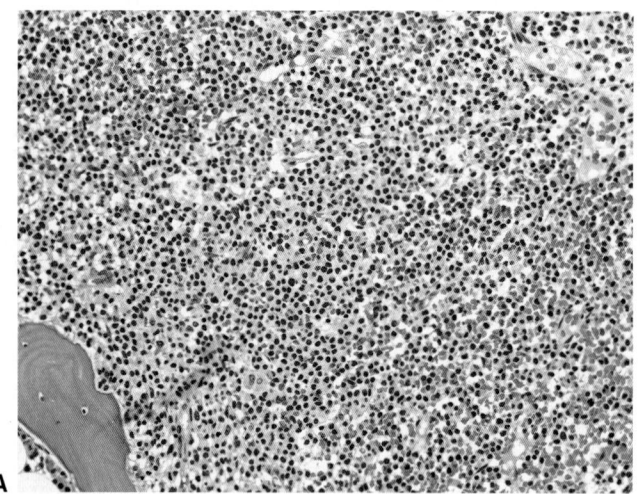
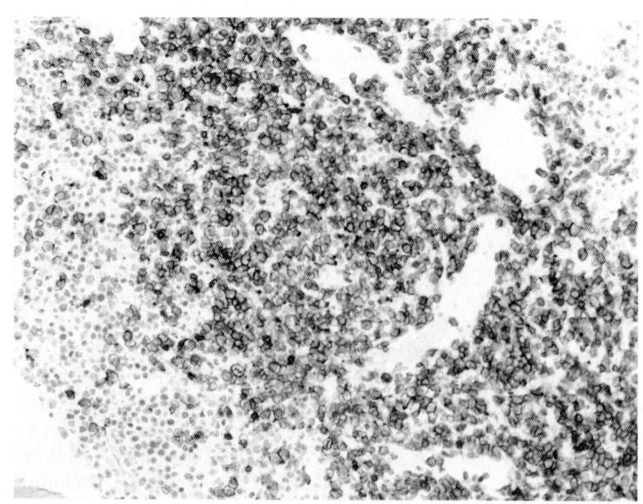
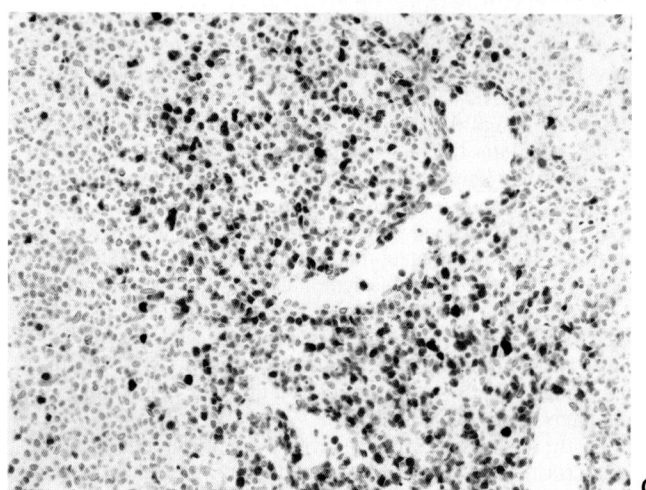

FIGURE 38.7. A: Extensive bone marrow involvement by T-PLL (H&E 200×). **B:** CD3 stain 100×. **C:** TCL-1 stain 100×.

is usually stable, but there is a report of phenotype switch from CD4$^+$CD8$^-$ to CD4$^+$CD8$^+$ in an indolent case upon transformation (64). Most T-PLL cases have memory T-cell phenotype with the expression of CD45RO. The majority of cases also express TCL-1 as a result of classical cytogenetic abnormality (see bellow). While nuclear overexpression of TCL-1 protein is fairly specific for T-PLL when compared to other mature T-cell neoplasms, this protein is frequently detectable in other malignancies, including B-cell neoplasms (65,66).

Cytogenetics

Classical chromosomal rearrangements in T-PLL involve juxtaposition of genes from TCL-1 family (*TCL-1A* and *TCL-1B* genes on 14q32.1; *MTCP1* gene on Xq28) with transcriptionally active *TCR-alpha* (14q11). Most commonly there is an inv(14) (q11q32) (80% of cases), followed by t(14;14) and t(X;14). The result of these rearrangements is a constitutive overexpression of TCL-1 proteins. TCL-1 family proteins bind pleckstrin homology domain of Akt protein kinase, and enhance its activity, resulting in increased proliferation and survival of neoplastic cells. The role of TCL-1 family proteins in the pathogenesis of T-PLL is supported by the finding that both *TCL-1*-transgenic mice and MTCP1-transgenic mice develop T-PLL-like disorder (67,68). The level of TCL-1 overexpression seems to correlate with the proliferative activity of T-PLL (69). Nevertheless, it is important to recognize that it is possible to make a diagnosis of T-PLL without evidence of *TCL-1* rearrangement, if clinical, morphologic, and immunophenotypic features are supportive

of this diagnosis, as dysregulation of Akt pathway can surely occur through other mechanisms.

Other frequent cytogenetic abnormalities include chromosomal losses at 22q11 and 12p13 (leading to haplo insufficiency of *SMARCB1* and *CDKN1B* tumor suppressor genes, respectively (70,71), chromosomal losses at 17p (*TP53* deletion), 11q23 (*ATM* deletion, see below), 13q, 6q, 9p, as well as chromosomal gains at 8q, 14q32, 22q21, and 6p (72).

Molecular Characteristics

The majority of T-PLL cases show biallelic disruption of *ATM* gene on 11q23, by a variety of mechanisms, the most common of which are nonsense mutations (73–75). In addition, *ATM* gene is mutated in patients with ataxia-telangiectasia, a recessively inherited multisystem disorder characterized by increased frequency of malignancies, including T-PLL (76).

POSTULATED NORMAL COUNTERPART

Mature Postthymic T cell

Clinical Course, Prognostic Assessment, Treatment, and Survival

T-PLL is an aggressive disorder that historically had a very poor prognosis, with a median survival of <1 year, using classical cytoreductive therapy (61). However, bright expression

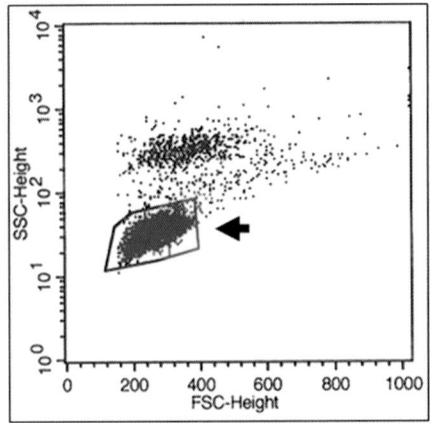

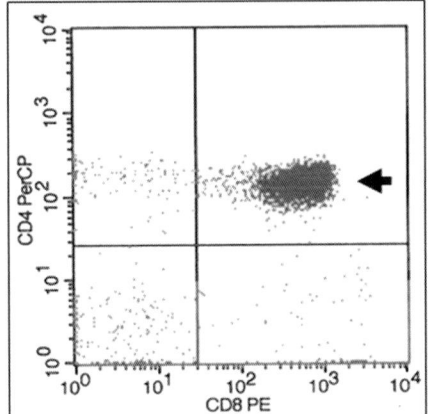
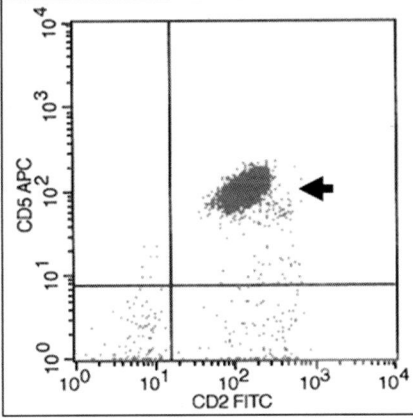
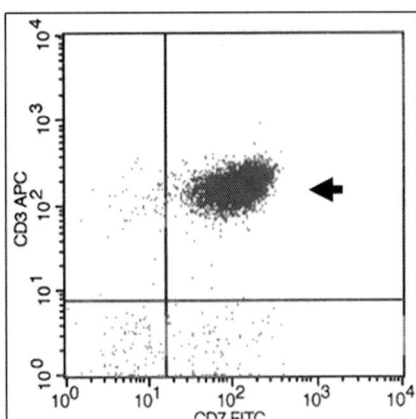

FIGURE 38.8. Flow cytometric immunophenotyping in T-PLL. Light scatter analysis reveals increased numbers of lymphoid cells with low forward and side light scatter (*population colored red, highlighted by arrow*). Flow cytometric immunophenotyping revealed the lymphocytes to be T cells unusually coexpressing CD4 and CD8 (**lower left panel**, *arrow*) and to have tight, homogeneous expression of CD2 and CD5 (**lower middle panel**, *arrow*) as well as CD3 and CD7 (**lower right panel**, *arrow*).

of CD52 makes T-PLL a good target for intravenous alem-tuzumab (anti-CD52 monoclonal antibody), which leads to overall and complete response in 91% and 81% of patients, respectively (77). The median survival is 15 to 19 months in patients achieving complete response, and it increases to 48 months if followed by stem cell transplantation (78–80). High expression levels of Akt and TCL-1 have been linked with poor prognosis (69).

Differential Diagnosis

T-large granular lymphocyte leukemia (T-LGLL) is an indolent disorder, usually CD4−CD8+ with granular lymphocyte morphology, subtle bone marrow infiltrates, and less pronounced lymphocytosis. T-LGLL cells invariably show immunophenotypic aberrancy, most commonly loss of CD5 and CD7, as well as coexpression of NK-cell-associated proteins CD56 and CD57. *Sézary syndrome* is a leukemic variant of cutaneous T-cell lymphoma, associated with erythroderma, lymphadenopathy, and the presence of cytologically atypical circulating cells with cerebriform nuclei. Sézary cells typically are CD4+CD8− and lack expression of CD7 and CD26 on their surface.

Summary and Conclusions

T-PLL is an aggressive mature T-cell neoplasm with characteristic morphologic, immunohistochemical, and genetic phenotype, and overall poor prognosis.

References

1. McKenna RW, et al. Granulated T cell lymphocytosis with neutropenia: malignant or benign chronic lymphoproliferative disorder? *Blood* 1985;66(2):259–266.
2. Swerdlow SH, et al., eds. WHO classification of tumours of haematopoietic and lymphoid tissues. In: Bosman FT, et al., eds. *World Health Organization classification of tumours.* 4th ed. Lyon: IARC Press, 2008:439.
3. Lamy T, Loughran TP Jr. How I treat LGL leukemia. *Blood* 2011;117(10):2764–2774.
4. Bareau B, et al. Analysis of a French cohort of patients with large granular lymphocyte leukemia: a report on 229 cases. *Haematologica* 2010;95(9):1534–1541.
5. Neben MA, Morice WG, Tefferi A. Clinical features in T-cell vs. natural killer-cell variants of large granular lymphocyte leukemia. *Eur J Haematol* 2003;71(4):263–265.
6. Osuji N, et al. T-cell large granular lymphocyte leukemia: a report on the treatment of 29 patients and a review of the literature. *Cancer* 2006;107(3):570–578.
7. Kwong YL, et al. The spectrum of chronic lymphoproliferative disorders in Chinese people. An analysis of 64 cases. *Cancer* 1994;74(1):174–181.
8. Lamy T, Loughran TP Jr. Clinical features of large granular lymphocyte leukemia. *Semin Hematol* 2003;40(3):185–195.
9. Liu X, Loughran TP Jr. The spectrum of large granular lymphocyte leukemia and Felty's syndrome. *Curr Opin Hematol* 2011;18(4):254–259.
10. Howard MT, et al. T/NK large granular lymphocyte leukemia and coexisting monoclonal B-cell lymphocytosis-like proliferations. An unrecognized and frequent association. *Am J Clin Pathol* 2011;133(6):936–941.
11. Gentile TC, et al. Large granular lymphocyte leukaemia occurring after renal transplantation. *Br J Haematol* 1998;101(3):507–512.
12. Mustjoki S, et al. Clonal expansion of T/NK-cells during tyrosine kinase inhibitor dasatinib therapy. *Leukemia* 2009;23(8):1398–1405.
13. Loughran TP Jr. Clonal diseases of large granular lymphocytes. *Blood* 1993;82(1):1–14.
14. Semenzato G, et al. The lymphoproliferative disease of granular lymphocytes: updated criteria for diagnosis. *Blood* 1997;89(1):256–260.
15. Morice WG, et al. Distinct bone marrow findings in T-cell granular lymphocytic leukemia revealed by paraffin section immunoperoxidase stains for CD8, TIA-1, and granzyme B. *Blood* 2002;99(1):268–274.
16. Agnarsson BA, et al. The pathology of large granular lymphocyte leukemia. *Hum Pathol* 1989;20(7):643–651.
17. Chen X, et al. A critical role for DAP10 and DAP12 in CD8+ T cell-mediated tissue damage in large granular lymphocyte leukemia. *Blood* 2009;113(14):3226–3234.

18. Go RS, Lust JA, Phyliky RL. Aplastic anemia and pure red cell aplasia associated with large granular lymphocyte leukemia. *Semin Hematol* 2003;40(3):196–200.

19. Osuji N, et al. Characteristic appearances of the bone marrow in T-cell large granular lymphocyte leukaemia. *Histopathology* 2007;50(5):547–554.

20. Evans HL, et al. Utility of immunohistochemistry in bone marrow evaluation of T-lineage large granular lymphocyte leukemia. *Hum Pathol* 2000;31(10):1266–1273.

21. Morice WG, et al. Demonstration of aberrant T-cell and natural killer-cell antigen expression in all cases of granular lymphocytic leukaemia. *Br J Haematol* 2003;120(6):1026–1036.

22. Osuji N, et al. Histopathology of the spleen in T-cell large granular lymphocyte leukemia and T-cell prolymphocytic leukemia: a comparative review. *Am J Surg Pathol* 2005;29(7):935–941.

23. Dhodapkar MV, Lust JA, Phyliky RL. T-cell large granular lymphocytic leukemia and pure red cell aplasia in a patient with type I autoimmune polyendocrinopathy: response to immunosuppressive therapy. *Mayo Clin Proc* 1994;69(11):1085–1088.

24. Olteanu H, et al. Laboratory findings in CD4(+) large granular lymphocytoses. *Int J Lab Hematol* 2010;32(1 Pt 1):e9–e16.

25. Sandberg Y, et al. TCRgammadelta+ large granular lymphocyte leukemias reflect the spectrum of normal antigen-selected TCRgammadelta+ T-cells. *Leukemia* 2006;20(3):505–513.

26. Chen YH, et al. Clinical, morphologic, immunophenotypic, and molecular cytogenetic assessment of CD4–/CD8–gammadelta T-cell large granular lymphocytic leukemia. *Am J Clin Pathol* 2011;136(2):289–299.

27. Lundell R, et al. T-cell large granular lymphocyte leukemias have multiple phenotypic abnormalities involving pan-T-cell antigens and receptors for MHC molecules. *Am J Clin Pathol* 2005;124(6):937–946.

28. Weisberger J, et al. Down-regulation of pan-T-cell antigens, particularly CD7, in acute infectious mononucleosis. *Am J Clin Pathol* 2003;120(1):49–55.

29. Cooke CB, et al. Hepatosplenic T-cell lymphoma: a distinct clinicopathologic entity of cytotoxic gamma delta T-cell origin. *Blood* 1996;88(11):4265–4274.

30. Dolstra H, et al. Expansion of CD8+CD57+ T cells after allogeneic BMT is related with a low incidence of relapse and with cytomegalovirus infection. *Br J Haematol* 1995;90(2):300–307.

31. Ohgami RS, et al. Refining the diagnosis of T-cell large granular lymphocytic leukemia by combining distinct patterns of antigen expression with T-cell clonality studies. *Leukemia* 2011;25(9):1439–1443.

32. Long EO, et al. Inhibition of natural killer cell activation signals by killer cell immunoglobulin-like receptors (CD158). *Immunol Rev* 2001;181:223–233.

33. Man C, et al. Deletion 6q as a recurrent chromosomal aberration in T-cell large granular lymphocyte leukemia. *Cancer Genet Cytogenet* 2002;139(1):71–74.

34. Lima M, et al. Immunophenotypic analysis of the TCR-Vbeta repertoire in 98 persistent expansions of CD3(+)/TCR-alphabeta(+) large granular lymphocytes: utility in assessing clonality and insights into the pathogenesis of the disease. *Am J Pathol* 2001;159(5):1861–1868.

35. Morice WG, et al. Flow cytometric assessment of TCR-Vbeta expression in the evaluation of peripheral blood involvement by T-cell lymphoproliferative disorders: a comparison with conventional T-cell immunophenotyping and molecular genetic studies. *Am J Clin Pathol* 2004;121(3):373–383.

36. Wlodarski MW, et al. Pathologic clonal cytotoxic T-cell responses: nonrandom nature of the T-cell-receptor restriction in large granular lymphocyte leukemia. *Blood* 2005;106(8):2769–2780.

37. Clemente MJ, et al. Clonal drift demonstrates unexpected dynamics of the T-cell repertoire in T-large granular lymphocyte leukemia. *Blood* 2011;118(16):4384–4393.

38. Shah MV, et al. Molecular profiling of LGL leukemia reveals role of sphingolipid signaling in survival of cytotoxic lymphocytes. *Blood* 2008;112(3):770–781.

39. Epling-Burnette PK, et al. Inhibition of STAT3 signaling leads to apoptosis of leukemic large granular lymphocytes and decreased Mcl-1 expression. *J Clin Invest* 2001;107(3):351–362.

40. Koskela HL, et al. Somatic STAT3 mutations in large granular lymphocytic leukemia. *N Engl J Med* 2012;366(20):1905–1913.

41. Zhang R, et al. Network model of survival signaling in large granular lymphocyte leukemia. *Proc Natl Acad Sci U S A* 2008;105(42):16308–16313.

42. Sokol L, Loughran TP Jr. Large granular lymphocyte leukemia. *Oncologist* 2006;11(3):263–273.

43. Loughran TP Jr, et al. Evaluation of splenectomy in large granular lymphocyte leukemia. *Br J Haematol* 1987;67(2):135–140.

44. Scquizzato E, et al. Genotypic evaluation of killer immunoglobulin-like receptors in NK-type lymphoproliferative disease of granular lymphocytes. *Leukemia* 2007;21(5):1060–1069.

45. Morice WG, Jevremovic D, Hanson CA. The expression of the novel cytotoxic protein granzyme M by large granular lymphocytic leukaemias of both T-cell and NK-cell lineage: an unexpected finding with implications regarding the pathobiology of these disorders. *Br J Haematol* 2007;137(3):237–239.

46. Morice WG, Leibson PJ, Tefferi A. Natural killer cells and the syndrome of chronic natural killer cell lymphocytosis. *Leuk Lymphoma* 2001;41(3–4):277–284.

47. Chan JK, Tsang WY, Ng CS. Clarification of CD3 immunoreactivity in nasal T/natural killer cell lymphomas: the neoplastic cells are often CD3 epsilon+. *Blood* 1996;87(2):839–841.

48. Cheung MM, Chan JK, Wong KF. Natural killer cell neoplasms: a distinctive group of highly aggressive lymphomas/leukemias. *Semin Hematol* 2003;40(3):221–232.

49. Morice WG, et al. Chronic lymphoproliferative disorder of natural killer cells: a distinct entity with subtypes correlating with normal natural killer cell subsets. *Leukemia* 2011;24(4):881–884.

50. Lanier LL, et al. Subpopulations of human natural killer cells defined by expression of the Leu-7 (HNK-1) and Leu-11 (NK-15) antigens. *J Immunol* 1983;131(4):1789–1796.

51. Zambello R, et al. Expression and function of KIR and natural cytotoxicity receptors in NK-type lymphoproliferative diseases of granular lymphocytes. *Blood* 2003;102(5):1797–1805.

52. Nash R, et al. Clonal studies of CD3− lymphoproliferative disease of granular lymphocytes. *Blood* 1993;81(9):2363–2368.

53. Tefferi A, et al. Demonstration of clonality, by X-linked DNA analysis, in chronic natural killer cell lymphocytosis and successful therapy with oral cyclophosphamide. *Leukemia* 1992;6(5):477–480.

54. Suzuki K, et al. Clinicopathological states of Epstein-Barr virus-associated T/NK-cell lymphoproliferative disorders (severe chronic active EBV infection) of children and young adults. *Int J Oncol* 2004;24(5):1165–1174.

55. Mori N, et al. Lymphomatous features of aggressive NK cell leukaemia/lymphoma with massive necrosis, haemophagocytosis and EB virus infection. *Histopathology* 2000;37(4):363–371.

56. Quintanilla-Martinez L, et al. Fulminant EBV(+) T-cell lymphoproliferative disorder following acute/chronic EBV infection: a distinct clinicopathologic syndrome. *Blood* 2000;96(2):443–451.

57. Siu LL, et al. Consistent patterns of allelic loss in natural killer cell lymphoma. *Am J Pathol* 2000;157(4):1803–1809.

58. Kwong YL, et al. Management of T-cell and natural-killer-cell neoplasms in Asia: consensus statement from the Asian Oncology Summit 2009. *Lancet Oncol* 2009;10(11):1093–1101.

59. Takahashi E, et al. Clinicopathological analysis of the age-related differences in patients with Epstein-Barr virus (EBV)-associated extranasal natural killer (NK)/T-cell lymphoma with reference to the relationship with aggressive NK cell leukaemia and chronic active EBV infection-associated lymphoproliferative disorders. *Histopathology* 2011;59(4):660–671.

60. Yachie A, Kanegane H, Kasahara Y. Epstein-Barr virus-associated T-/natural killer cell lymphoproliferative diseases. *Semin Hematol* 2003;40(2):124–132.

61. Catovsky D, Muller-Hermelink HK, Ralfkiaer E. T-cell prolymphocytic leukemia. In: Swerdlow SS, et al., eds. *WHO classification of tumours of haematopoietic and lymphoid tissues.* Lyon, France: WHO Press, 2008.

62. Matutes E, et al. Clinical and laboratory features of 78 cases of T-prolymphocytic leukemia. *Blood* 1991;78(12):3269–3274.

63. Mallett RB, et al. Cutaneous infiltration in T-cell prolymphocytic leukaemia. *Br J Dermatol* 1995;132(2):263–266.

64. Ichikawa K, et al. A case of T cell prolymphocytic leukemia involving blast transformation. *Int J Hematol* 2011;93(5):667–672.

65. Herling M, et al. TCL1 shows a regulated expression pattern in chronic lymphocytic leukemia that correlates with molecular subtypes and proliferative state. *Leukemia* 2006;20(2):280–285.

66. Teitell MA, et al. TCL1 expression and Epstein-Barr virus status in pediatric Burkitt lymphoma. *Am J Clin Pathol* 2005;124(4):569–575.

67. Gritti C, et al. Transgenic mice for MTCP1 develop T-cell prolymphocytic leukemia. *Blood* 1998;92(2):368–373.

68. Virgilio L, et al. Deregulated expression of TCL1 causes T cell leukemia in mice. *Proc Natl Acad Sci U S A* 1998;95(7):3885–3889.

69. Herling M, et al. High TCL1 expression and intact T-cell receptor signaling define a hyperproliferative subset of T-cell prolymphocytic leukemia. *Blood* 2008;111(1):328–337.

70. Bug S, et al. Recurrent loss, but lack of mutations, of the SMARCB1 tumor suppressor gene in T-cell prolymphocytic leukemia with TCL1A-TCRAD juxtaposition. *Cancer Genet Cytogenet* 2009;192(1):44–47.

71. Le Toriellec E, et al. Haploinsufficiency of CDKN1B contributes to leukemogenesis in T-cell prolymphocytic leukemia. *Blood* 2008;111(4):2321–2328.

72. Soulier J, et al. A complex pattern of recurrent chromosomal losses and gains in T-cell prolymphocytic leukemia. *Genes Chromosomes Cancer* 2001;31(3):248–254.

73. Stilgenbauer S, et al. Biallelic mutations in the ATM gene in T-prolymphocytic leukemia. *Nat Med* 1997;3(10):1155–1159.

74. Stoppa-Lyonnet D, et al. Inactivation of the ATM gene in T-cell prolymphocytic leukemias. *Blood* 1998;91(10):3920–3926.

75. Vorechovsky I, et al. Clustering of missense mutations in the ataxia-telangiectasia gene in a sporadic T-cell leukaemia. *Nat Genet* 1997;17(1):96–99.

76. Taylor AM, et al. Leukemia and lymphoma in ataxia telangiectasia. *Blood* 1996;87(2):423–438.

77. Dearden CE, et al. Alemtuzumab therapy in T-cell prolymphocytic leukaemia: comparing efficacy in a series treated intravenously and a study piloting the subcutaneous route. *Blood* 2011;118(22):5799–5802.

78. Dearden CE, et al. High remission rate in T-cell prolymphocytic leukemia with CAMPATH-1H. *Blood* 2001;98(6):1721–1726.

79. Krishnan B, et al. Stem cell transplantation after alemtuzumab in T-cell prolymphocytic leukaemia results in longer survival than after alemtuzumab alone: a multicentre retrospective study. *Br J Haematol* 2010;149(6):907–910.

80. Dearden C. How I treat prolymphocytic leukemia. *Blood* 2012;120(3):538–551.

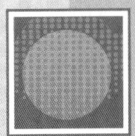

Chapter 39
Adult T-Cell Leukemia/Lymphoma

Koichi Ohshima • Shigeo Nakamura

 ## DEFINITION

Adult T-cell leukemia/lymphoma (ATLL) is a peripheral T-cell neoplasm that is pathogenically linked to human T-cell leukemia virus type 1 (HTLV-1; also called human T-lymphotrophic virus), the first retrovirus proven to cause a human neoplasm (1–5). The tumor cells are most often characterized by high nuclear pleomorphism with a range in size and shape. Most patients present with widely disseminated disease, and peripheral blood (PB) involvement is common. Smoldering and chronic forms have a more indolent clinical course. Notably, based on its unique clinical and pathologic features, ATLL was first discovered as a disease entity in Japan before HTLV-1 was identified as a causal factor (6).

 ## EPIDEMIOLOGY

ATLL is endemic in several regions of the world (7–11): southwestern Japan, mainly the islands of Kyushu and Shikoku; the Caribbean basin; parts of Central Africa; and Iran. The distribution of patients with ATLL is closely linked to the prevalence of HTLV-1 in the population (Figs. 39.1 and 39.2). The disease has a long latency, and affected individuals are usually exposed to HTLV-1 very early in life. Cord blood lymphocytes are more susceptible to transformation than more fully differentiated and mature lymphocytes (12). The three major routes of infection are mother-to-infant transmission, mainly by lymphocytes in breast milk; sexual transmission; and transmission through exposure to blood and blood products. The virus is not transmitted in fresh frozen plasma, and transmission requires the presence of living HTLV-1-infected cells (13). In Japan, where the disease was first discovered, seroprevalence in the adult population ranges from 0.2% in some areas to 13% in areas of high endemicity (10). The cumulative incidence of ATLL is estimated to be 2.5% among HTLV-1 carriers in Japan, with an ongoing increased risk until 70 years of age. ATLL occurs only in adults. The age at onset ranges from the 20s to the 80s, with a mean of 58 years, and ATLL is slightly more predominant in males: male-to-female ratio of ATLL incidence is 1.5:1 (3). Although sporadic cases have been described, patients often derive from an endemic region of the world. ATLL patients or HTLV-1 carriers are not found in Korea and China, although both countries have had close relations with the Japanese (14,15). Some Chinese in Formosa, Taiwan, were infected with HTLV-1 and had resultant ATLL; however, these infections were probably contracted in the southern parts of Japan, such as Okinawa and Kyushu. Japanese immigrants in Hawaii and Brazil retain the same high seropositive rates as native inhabitants (16,17).

In the Western world, the majority of patients come from the Caribbean basin, and the disease is more prevalent among blacks than whites (7). Other areas of prevalence include Central and South America, in particular Brazil and Ecuador. Differences in geographic or ethnic origin correlate with different patterns of disease. A lymphomatous form is more often observed in the Western hemisphere, while Asian patients are more often leukemic (18). How genetic factors influence the development of ATLL in infected carriers is not entirely clear.

 ## ETIOLOGY

HTLV-1 is causally linked to ATLL; however, HTLV-1 infection alone is not sufficient to result in neoplastic transformation of infected cells. The p40 tax viral protein leads to transcriptional activation of many genes in HTLV-1–infected lymphocytes (19). In addition, the HTLV-1 basic leucine zipper factor (HBZ) is thought to be important for T-cell proliferation and oncogenesis (20). However, additional genetic alterations acquired over time may result in the development of a malignancy. HTLV-1 has also been linked to other diseases in addition to ATLL, such as HTLV-1-associated myelopathy (HAM) (21,22) (Table 39.1). HAM is also known as tropical spastic paraparesis (TSP), and is associated with neurologic symptoms and demyelination due to an immune-mediated inflammatory process with some parallels to multiple sclerosis (23). Patients with HAM often acquire the virus later in life through transfusion, rarely develop ATLL, and may manifest uveitis, arthritis, polymyositis, keratoconjunctivitis sicca resembling Sjögren syndrome, and pulmonary inflammation. Young infected children may also be immunodeficient and present with superficial cutaneous infections, a pattern termed infective dermatitis (24).

 ## LEUKEMOGENESIS

Considering the long latent period and low incidence of ATLL among HTLV-1 carriers (~1 per 1,500 to 2,000), a mathematical model for leukemogenesis is informative. The Weibull distribution model, in which the "shape parameter" can be regarded as the number of "hits" or "steps" playing a role in the leukemogenesis on normal cells, is relevant to understanding the possible nature of the genetic events (25). Cumulative ATLL occurrence can be expressed as a single straight line on the Weibull plot (Fig. 39.3). The distribution of both sexes is identical. Based on this stochastic model, it is assumed that age-dependent accumulation of leukemogenic events most likely consists of somatic mutations, and that only carriers infected at birth may develop leukemia.

The probability density function for the Weibull model, f(t), expressed as a function of time (t, in years), was described as

$$f(t) = a/b \ t^{a-1} \exp^{(-ta/b)}$$

where a, the shape parameter, was 5.03 and b, the "scale parameter," was 8.00×10^8. The hazard rate, (t), expressed as a function of time can be written as

$$(t) = f(t) = a/b \ t^{a-1}/t(x)dx$$

Therefore, the risk of ATLL development at each age is approximately proportional to the fourth power of the age,

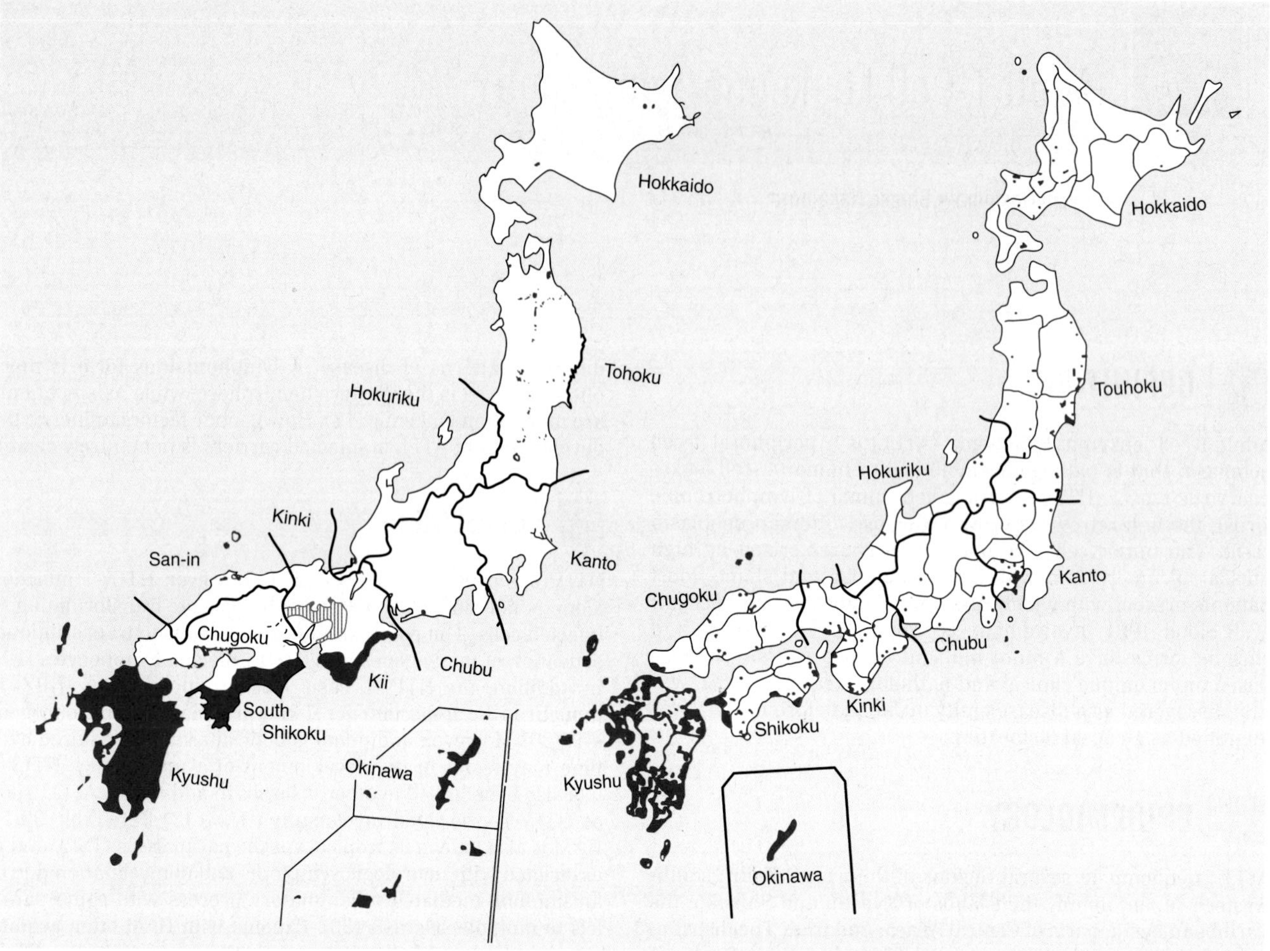

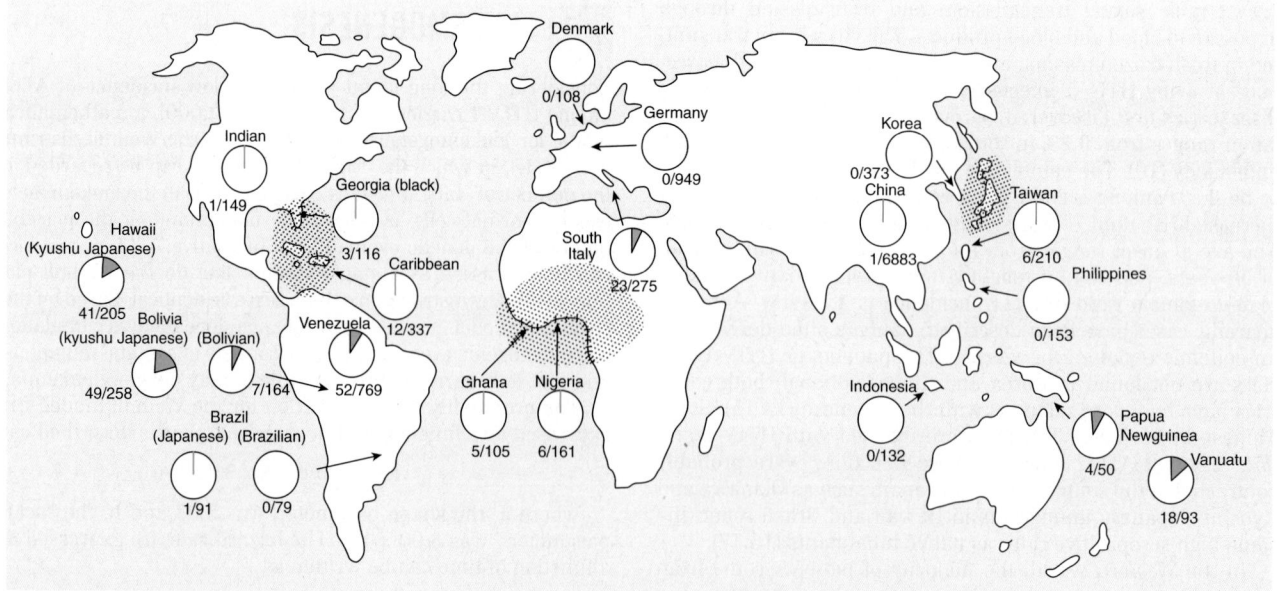

FIGURE 39.1. **Left:** Seropositivity to human T-cell lymphotropic virus type 1 (HTLV-1) in Japan. **Right:** Distribution of T- and B-cell lymphoma by birthplace. Highest prevalence (6%) is recognized in Kyushu and then in Kii and South Shikoku (3%), around Osaka (1.5%), and in Tohoku and Hokkaido (1%). The background rate is <0.5%. The birthplaces of 656 ATLL patients were collected by the fourth nationwide survey. Each dot corresponds to one patient. (From Tajima K. The 4th nation-wide study of adult T-cell leukemia/lymphoma in Japan. *Int J Cancer* 1990;45:237–243, with permission from Wiley-Liss, Inc., A Wiley Company.)

FIGURE 39.2. Seropositive areas of the world. Geographic distribution of carriers of human T-cell lymphotropic virus type 1 (HTLV-1) and areas of endemic ATLL (*shadowed*). *Circles* and *numbers* indicate seropositive rates and positive-tested subjects, respectively. (From Tajima K, et al. Malignant lymphomas in Japan: epidemiologic analysis of ATLL. *Cancer Metastasis Rev* 1988;7:223, with permission from Kluwer Academic Publishers.)

Table 39.1

Table 39.1	LISTS OF HTLV-1-ASSOCIATED DISEASES

Neoplastic Disorders	Reactive Disorders
Peripheral blood (leukemia)	Confirmed
Smoldering variant	HTLV-1–associated myelopathy
Chronic variant	HTLV-1–associated uveitis
Acute variant	HTLV-1–associated lymphadenitis
Lymph node (lymphoma)	Not confirmed
Pleomorphic small cell type	HTLV-1–associated bronchopneu-
Pleomorphic medium-sized and	mopathy
large-cell type	HTLV-1–associated arthropathy
Anaplastic large cell type	(HAAP)
Hodgkin-like type	HTLV-1–associated nephropathy
Skin	
Erythema	**Immunodeficiency**
Papule	Strongyloidiasis (gastrointestinal tract)
Nodule	Varicella zoster (skin)
Gastrointestinal tract	Opportunistic lung infection
Erosion	*Pneumocystis carinii*
Ulceration	Cytomegalovirus
Tumor	*Aspergillus fumigatus*
Liver	*Candida albicans*
Portal or sinus infiltration	*Cryptococcus neoformans*
Bone marrow	Carcinoma (Not confirmed)
Infiltration with or without fibrosis	

suggesting that at least five events, each of which occurs spontaneously and independently, may be required for development of the disease.

SITE OF INVOLVEMENT

The distribution of the disease is usually systemic. Most ATLL patients present with widespread lymph node involvement, as well as PB involvement. The number of circulating neoplastic cells does not correlate with the degree of bone marrow (BM) involvement, suggesting that circulating cells are recruited from other organs such as the skin. In fact, the skin is the most common extralymphatic site of involvement (>50%) (26–28). Skin lesions are clinically diverse and are classified as erythema, papules, and nodules (29) (Fig. 39.4). Rare cases may show tumor-like lesions or erythroderma, as in Sézary syndrome. Other extranodal sites of clinically relevant disease include the lungs, liver, spleen, gastrointestinal tract, and central nervous system, which may lead to clinical symptoms and morbidity (30,31). Cardiac involvement may be observed as a terminal event. Epidemiologic differences occur in patterns of presentation (32). For example, PB involvement is much less common in patients from the Caribbean basin than from Japan (18).

CLINICAL FEATURES

Several clinical variants have been identified: acute (leukemic), lymphomatous, chronic, and smoldering ATLL (33) (Table 39.2). Because most patients have advanced stage IV disease at presentation, Ann Arbor staging is not prognostically useful. The acute leukemic variant is most common and is characterized by a leukemic phase, often with a markedly elevated white blood cells (WBC) count, skin rash, and generalized lymphadenopathy. Hypercalcemia, with or without lytic bone lesions, is a common feature (Fig. 39.5). Patients with acute ATLL have systemic disease accompanied by hepatosplenomegaly, constitutional symptoms, and elevated lactic dehydrogenase (LDH). Leukocytosis

and eosinophilia are common. The BM may be hypercellular with myeloid hyperplasia. Despite the leukemic manifestation, BM involvement may be absent. Many patients have an associated T-cell immunodeficiency, with frequent opportunistic infections such as *Pneumocystis carinii* pneumonia, cryptococcosis, cytomegalovirus infection, and strongyloidiasis (34).

The lymphomatous variant is characterized by prominent lymphadenopathy without PB involvement. Most patients present with advanced stage disease similar to the acute form. However, hypercalcemia is observed less often. Cutaneous lesions are common in both the acute and lymphomatous forms of ATLL. They are clinically diverse and include erythematous rashes, papules, and nodules. Larger nodules may show ulceration. Patients with the lymphomatous variant may develop PB involvement later in the course of the disease (35). The survival for the acute and lymphomatous variants ranges from 2 weeks to more than 1 year. Death is often caused by infectious complications including *P. carinii* pneumonia, cryptococcal meningitis, disseminated herpes zoster, and hypercalcemia.

The chronic variant is frequently associated with an exfoliative skin rash. While absolute lymphocytosis may be present, atypical lymphocytes are not numerous in the PB. Flower cells are associated with a more aggressive clinical course, if present (36,37). Hypercalcemia is absent. Although patients may have hepatosplenomegaly, the clinical course is generally indolent, with median survival in the range of 2 years.

In the smoldering variant, the WBC count is normal, with >5% circulating neoplastic cells. Circulating ATLL cells are generally small, with a normal appearance. Patients frequently have skin or pulmonary lesions, but hypercalcemia is absent. Lymphadenopathy should also be absent. Progression from the chronic or smoldering to the acute variant occurs in 25% of cases, albeit usually after a long duration.

MORPHOLOGY

ATLL is characterized by an extremely diverse spectrum of cytologic features (36). Notably, certain cytologic features are highly suggestive of the diagnosis, even if HTLV examination is not performed (38). These features are best appreciated in the PB. The neoplastic cells in the PB are markedly polylobated, with nuclear convolutions and lobules, and have been termed flower cells based on the petal-like appearance of the nuclear lobes (33,35,39,40) (Fig. 39.6). The chromatin is condensed and usually hyperchromatic without prominent nucleoli. The cytoplasm is deeply basophilic, which is most readily observed with Giemsa staining of air-dried smears. Basophilic cytoplasm and hyperchromasia are useful features in distinguishing ATLL from Sézary syndrome.

The very diverse cytology of ATLL is reflected in the recognition of several morphologic variants referred to as pleomorphic small, medium, and large cell types; anaplastic; and a rare form resembling angioimmunoblastic T-cell lymphoma (41) (Fig. 39.7). The use of these variants is optional, and is relevant for pathologists, who must be aware of the diverse cytology that can be encountered in ATLL. Lymph node involvement is present in many patients. Lymph nodes are diffusely effaced by the neoplastic cells. Some cases exhibit a leukemic pattern of infiltration, with preservation or dilation of lymph node sinuses that contain malignant cells. The inflammatory background is usually sparse, although eosinophilia may be present. Neoplastic lymphoid cells are typically medium-sized to large, often with pronounced nuclear pleomorphism. The nuclear chromatin is coarsely clumped with distinct, sometimes prominent, nucleoli. Blastlike cells with transformed nuclei and dispersed chromatin are present in variable proportion. Giant cells with convoluted, cerebriform, or bizarre nuclear contours may be present. Rare cases may be composed predominantly of small lymphocytes,

FIGURE 39.3. Top: Distribution of age at onset of disease of patients with ATLL. The observed number in each 5-year age category is shown in the *shadowed columns*. *White columns* represent corrected death rates according to the national population survey in Japan conducted in 1985. The cumulative percentages of ATLL are shown by *circles* and *lines*, respectively. **Bottom:** Cumulative occurrence of ATLL by age plotted on the Weibull model. Good fitness is obtained for men (*open box*) and women (*open triangle*) and by observed (*closed circle*) and corrected (*open circle*) incidences (cf1611).

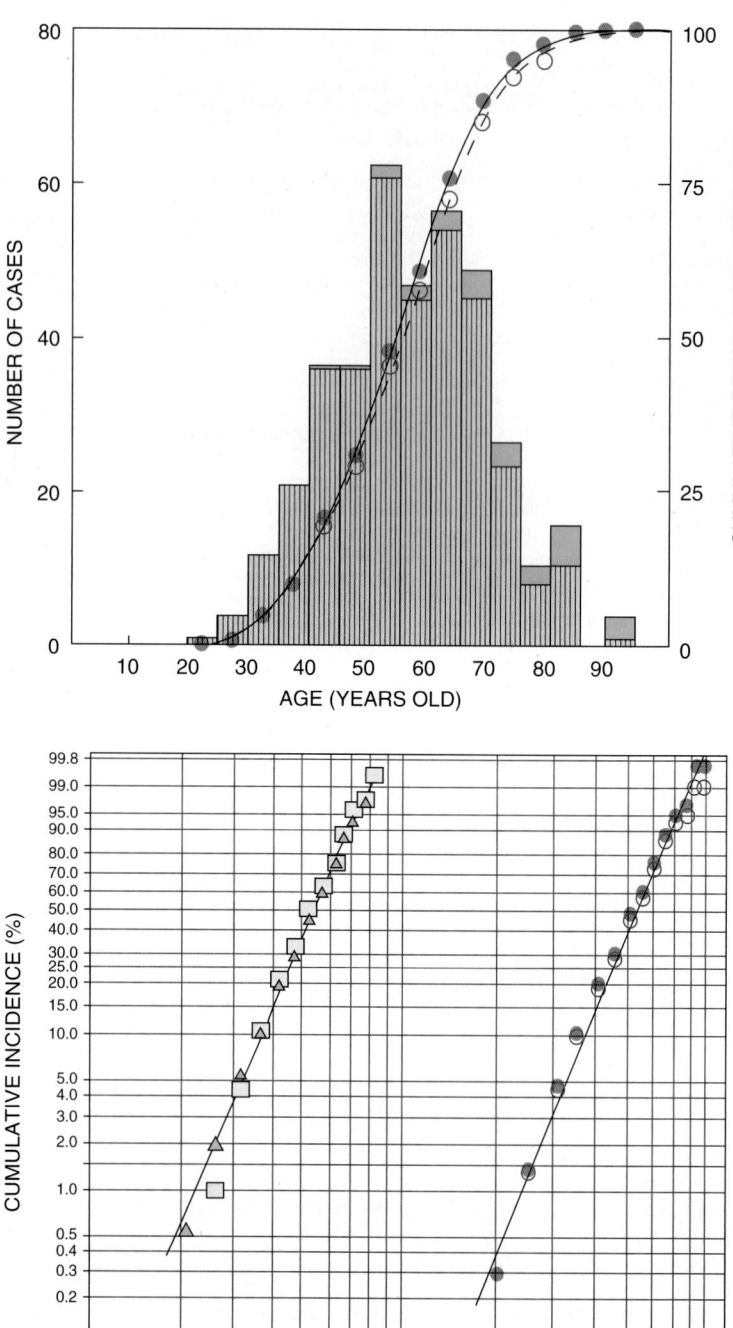

with irregular nuclear contours. Rare cases may also have large-cell morphology, which is indistinguishable from anaplastic large cell lymphoma except for the lack of anaplastic lymphoma receptor tyrosine kinase (ALK) expression and cytotoxic molecules. The size and shape of the neoplastic cells generally does not correlate with the clinical course (35), with the exception of the chronic and smoldering forms, in which the lymphocytes have a more normal appearance (42,43).

Lymph nodes in some patients with incipient ATLL, such as the smoldering type, may exhibit a Hodgkin-lymphoma-like histology (44,45) (Fig. 39.8). The lymph nodes have expanded paracortical areas containing a diffuse infiltrate of small- to medium-sized lymphocytes with mild nuclear irregularities, indistinct nucleoli, and scant cytoplasm. Epstein-Barr virus (EBV)+ B lymphocytes with Hodgkin-like features are interspersed in this background. These giant cells express CD30

and CD15. This variant usually progresses to overt ATLL within months. HTLV-1+ neoplastic cells are variable in number in the background of these lesions, and in some patients may be difficult to detect by using the polymerase chain reaction method for identifying T-cell receptor gene rearrangement. The expansion of EBV+ B cells is considered secondary to the underlying immunodeficiency observed in patients with ATLL.

Skin lesions are observed in more than 50% of patients with ATLL. Epidermal infiltration with Pautrier-like microabscesses is common (26,35,36) (Fig. 39.9). Dermal infiltration is mainly perivascular; however, larger tumor nodules with extensions to subcutaneous fat may be observed. In the prodromal phase, as in the smoldering and chronic types, the smaller neoplastic cells are usually predominant in the skin, with minimal cytologic atypia.

BM involvement is typically not prominent. Marrow infiltration is usually patchy, ranging from sparse to moderate, and is

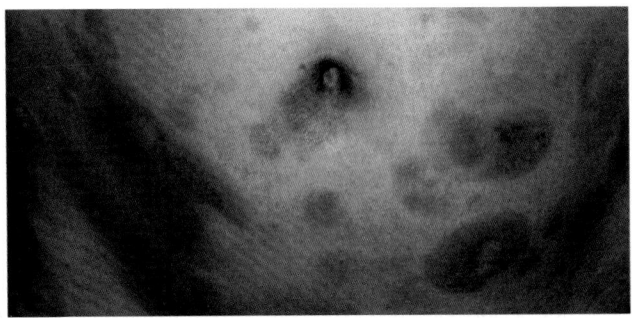

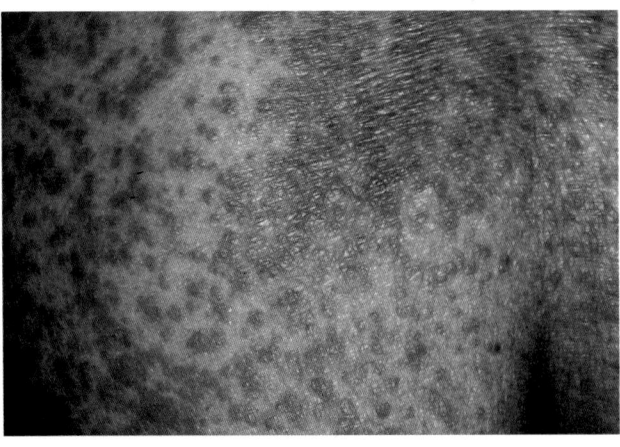

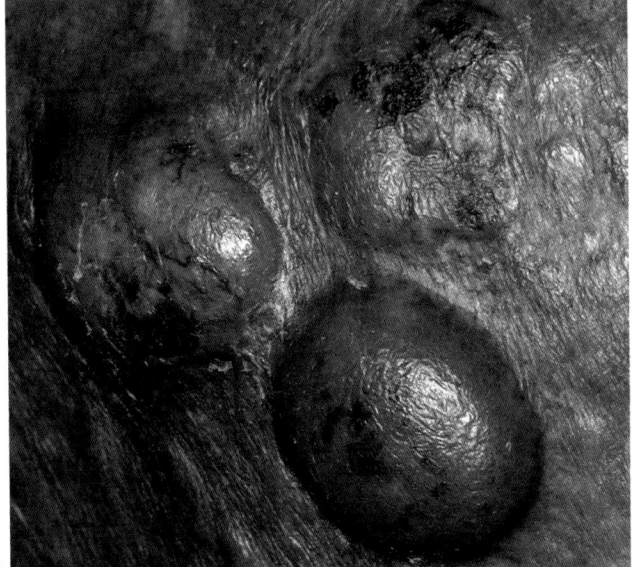

FIGURE 39.4. Diverse macroscopic findings of cutaneous manifestation of ATLL ranging from erythema (**A**) to papules (**B**) to larger nodules with ulceration (**C**).

less than one might expect given the marked lymphocytosis. Osteoclastic activity may be prominent, even in the absence of BM infiltration by neoplastic cells.

Hepatic infiltrates are mainly observed in the portal area with occasional destruction of limiting plates. Sinus infiltration is observed in some patients, although fibrosis is rarely seen. The involvement of the gastrointestinal tract is demonstrated by ulcerated mass, erosion, or tumor-like lesions. Pulmonary infiltrates are generally patchy and interstitial. Involvement of the central nervous system may show meningeal infiltration, with neoplastic cells in cerebrospinal fluid. Clinical manifestations of neoplastic infiltrates into many organs are very diverse

and may mimic inflammatory disorders. These diffuse infiltrates are also indicative of the systemic nature of the disease and the presence of circulating malignant cells.

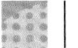 **IMMUNOPROFILE**

Tumor cells, regardless of cytologic subtype, express T-cell-associated antigens (CD2, CD3, CD5), but usually lack CD7. Although most cases are CD4+ and CD8− (Fig. 39.10A), some are CD4−, CD8+, or double positive for CD4 and CD8. CD25, the interleukin-2 receptor (IL-2R) alpha subunit, is strongly

| Table 39.2 | DIAGNOSTIC CRITERIA FOR CLINICAL FORMS OF ADULT T-CELL LEUKEMIA/LYMPHOMA AS DEFINED BY THE JAPANESE LYMPHOMA STUDY GROUP |

Feature	Smoldering	Chronic	Acute	Lymphomatous
Lymphocytosis	No	Mildly increased, >4 × 109/L	Increased	No
T-cell receptor PCR	Sometimes monoclonal	Monoclonal	Monoclonal	Monoclonal
LDH	Normal	Slightly increased	Increased	Increased
Calcium	Normal	Normal	Increased	Variable
Skin lesions	Erythematous rash	Rash, papules	Variable, >50%	Variable, >50%
Lymphadenopathy	No	Mildly increased, >4 × 109/L	Usually present	Yes
Hepatomegaly	No	Mildly increased, >4 × 109/L	Usually present	Often present
BM infiltration	No	Normal	Variable	No
Median survival (years)	>2	2	<1	<1
Morphology	Small lymphocytes Minimal atypia	Mild atypia Flower cells sometimes seen	Marked atypia Polylobated and blastic forms	Marked atypia Polylobated and blastic forms

LDH, lactate dehydrogenase; PCR, polymerase chain reaction.

From Shimoyama M. Diagnostic criteria and classification of clinical subtypes of adult T-cell leukaemia-lymphoma. A report from the Lymphoma Study Group (1984–87). *Br J Haematol* 1991;79(3): 428–437.

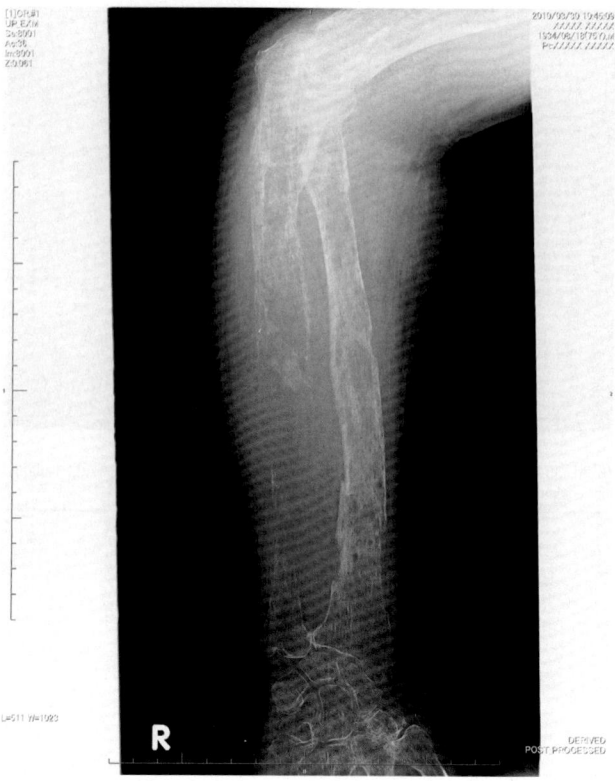

FIGURE 39.5. Bone radiograph shows extensive lytic lesions in a patient with ATLL.

expressed in nearly all cases (Fig. 39.10B), and has become a target molecule of antibody therapy for ATLL (46). The large transformed cells may be positive for CD30 without ALK expression, but are negative for ALK (47). No cases express cytotoxic molecules; this lack of expression is a key consideration in the differential diagnosis of ATLL versus extranodal cytotoxic T-cell lymphomas in HTLV-1–endemic areas. The leukemia/lymphoma cells frequently express the chemokine receptor 4 (CCR4) (Fig. 39.10C) as well as FoxP3 (Fig. 39.10D) in 68% of the cases (48). The combination of CD3, CD4, CD25, CCR4, and FoxP3 suggests that ATLL cells may be the equivalent of regulatory T (Treg) cells (48–50). In one study, 88% of the cases tested were positive for CCR4 (51). This finding is also clinically relevant to the use of defucosylated humanized anti-CCR4 antibody (KW-0761) for treatment purposes (52,53).

CELL OF ORIGIN

ATLL cells are peripheral CD4+ alpha-beta T cells. It has been suggested that the CD4+CD25+FoxP3+ Treg cells are the closest normal counterpart (48,49). This finding is consistent with the immunodeficiency characteristic of the disease (54).

GENETICS, MOLECULAR FINDINGS, AND ROLE OF HTLV-1

ATLL is a mature T-cell neoplasm with clonal rearrangement of the T-cell receptor genes (55). A single dominant clone detected

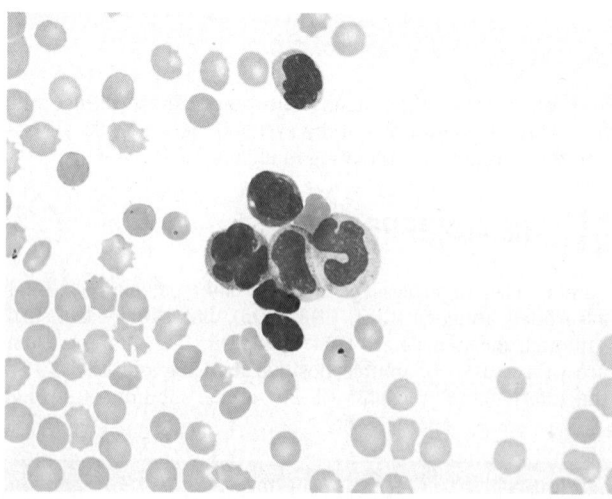

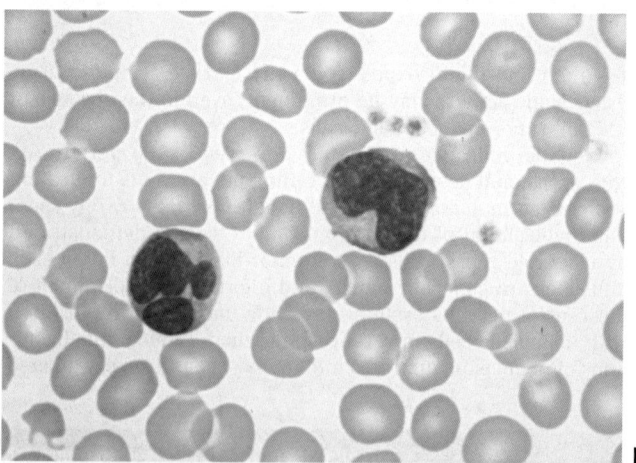

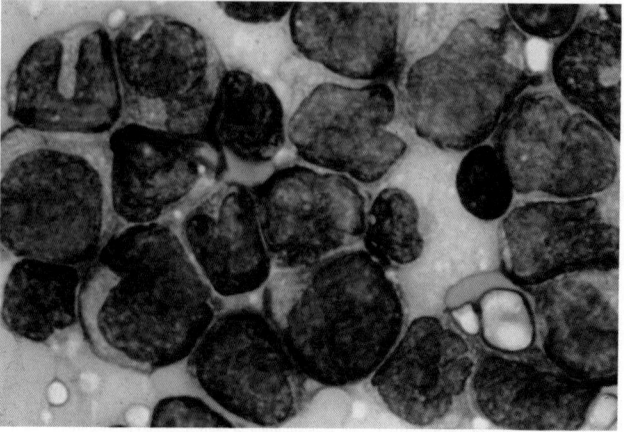

FIGURE 39.6. Peripheral blood (**A,B**) and imprint cytologic findings (**C**) in ATLL. In the acute variants, the leukemic cells are medium-sized and large cells with markedly polylobated nuclei, which have been described as "flower cells" (**A,B**). In the lymphomatous variant, the lymphoma cells also show irregular nuclei with convolutions and lobules (**C**).

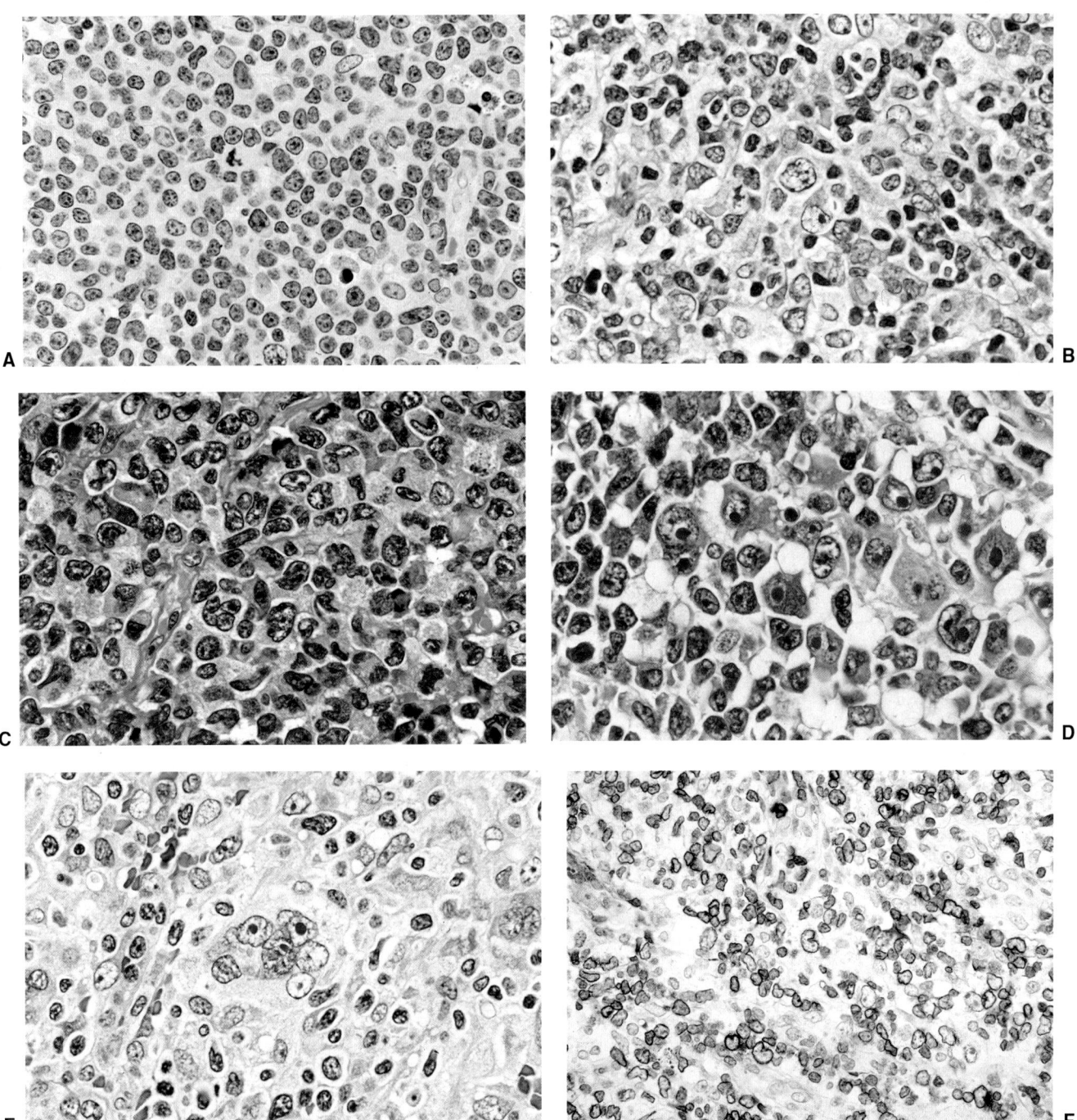

FIGURE 39.7. Lymph node lesions have a broad morphologic spectrum; medium-sized (**A**), mixed (**B**), pleomorphic large cell (**C**), and anaplastic large cell variants (**D**). Giant cells with pleomorphic nuclei may be present (**E**). The tumor cells are positive for CD3 (**F**).

by integration site of HTLV-1 provirus is the only evidence for the diagnosis of ATLL in any sites affected by the disease, because its variety of clinical and pathologic features cannot be combined without the viral parameter. In almost all cases, infection by HTLV-1 can be confirmed by detecting the presence of circulating antibodies specific for HTLV-1 antigens (ATLAs) (56,57). A dominant T-cell clone has not been observed in HTLV-1 carriers; however, oligoclonal T-cell expansion may be detected. The high-density expression of IL-2R renders ATLL cells responsive to growth in response to cytokines *in vitro*. Smoldering or chronic ATLL patients may exhibit more than one T-cell clone in the early phase, with emergence of a dominant clone at the time of progression (58).

The HTLV-1 genome encodes common structural and enzymatic proteins (Gag, Pol, and Env), as well as the regulatory and accessory proteins (Tax, Rex, p12, p13, p21, and p30) (59). Among these viral proteins, Tax has been thought to be critical for leukemogenesis because of many reports about its potent effects on cell proliferation, genetic instability, and cell cycle dysregulation (60). In transgenic animals, Tax expression is capable of inducing cancers depending on the promoter used (61). However, ATLL cells often contain genetic and epigenetic alterations of the 5′ long terminal repeat of the HTLV-1 provirus, resulting in the loss of Tax expression, as Tax expression is the major target of cytotoxic T lymphocytes. Indeed, Tax expression is not detected in approximately 60% of freshly isolated samples from ATLL cases

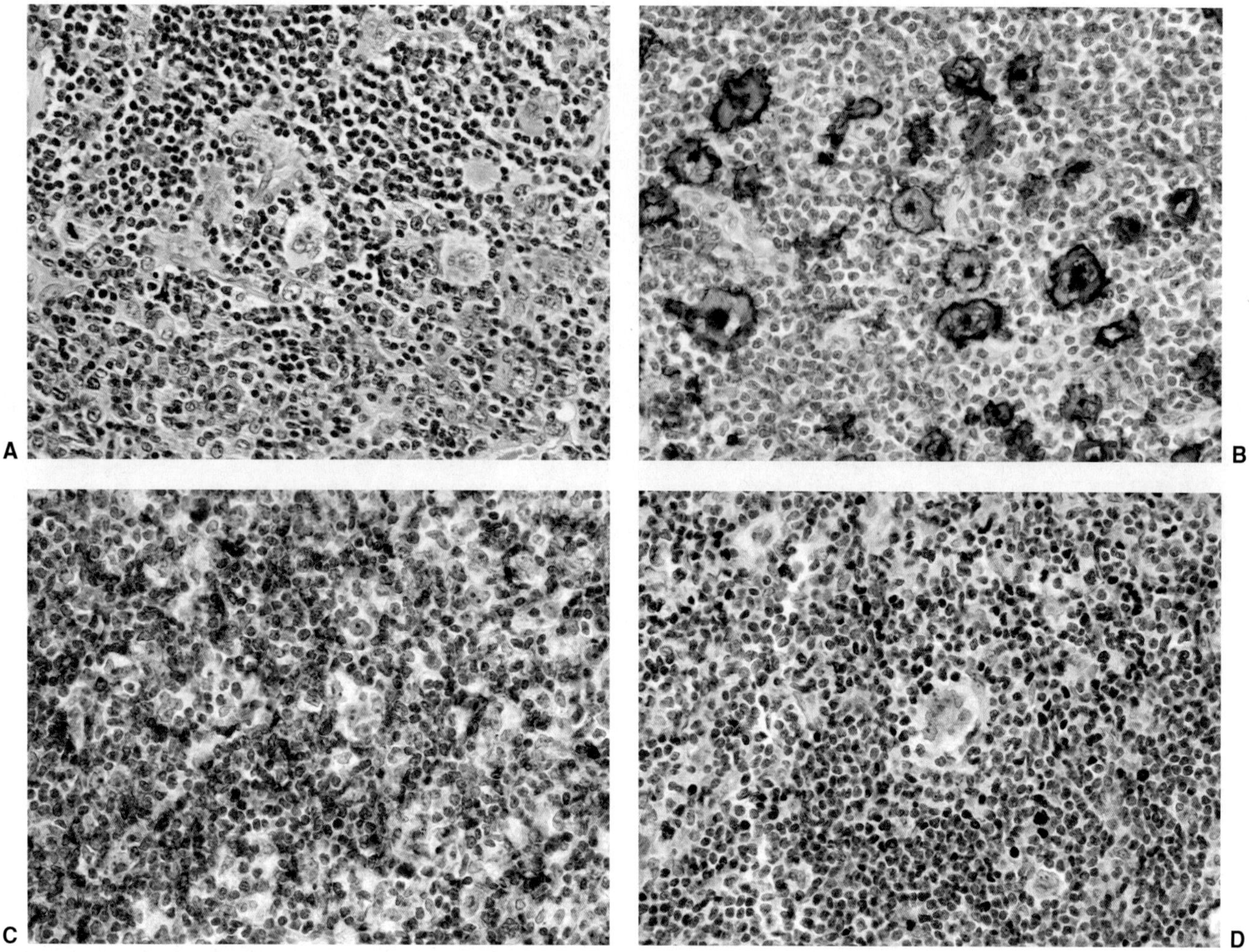

FIGURE 39.8. Hodgkin-like variant of ATLL. CD30-positive cells resembling Hodgkin-Reed-Sternberg cells are present (**A,B** [CD30]) surrounded by small background lymphocytes, which are positive for CCR4 (**C**) and FoxP3 (**D**). Note that Hodgkin-like cells are transformed B cells frequently positive for EBV.

(62). This indicates that Tax expression is not always necessary for the leukemogenic process. A recent and remarkable finding in HTLV-1 biology is the characterization of HTLV-1 basic leucine zipper factor (HBZ), which is encoded by the minus strand of a provirus. HBZ expression has been observed in the leukemic

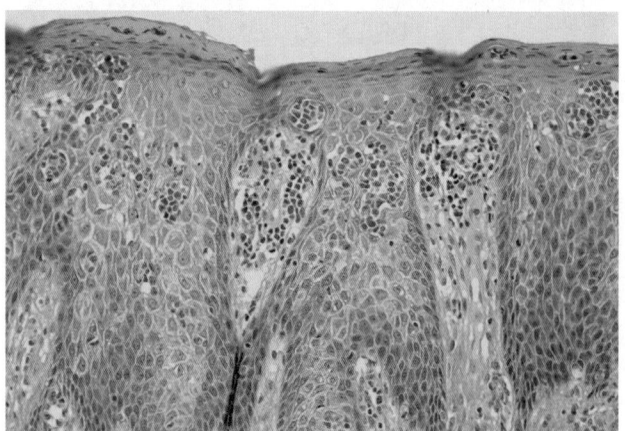

FIGURE 39.9. Skin biopsy specimen in ATLL showing marked epidermotropism with Pautrier-like microabscesses.

cells of all ATLL cases and plays a role in ATLL oncogenesis (63–65). Transgenic mice containing the *HBZ* gene under control of a murine CD4-specific promoter/enhancer/silencer (HBZ-Tg mice) spontaneously developed systemic dermatitis, alveolitis, and lymphoma as they aged. Suppressing expression of the *HBZ* gene also inhibited the proliferation of adult T-cell leukemia (ATL) cells (66), indicating that the *HBZ* gene has growth-promoting activity in ATL. HBZ is now considered the only viral gene that is consistently expressed in HTLV-1-infected cells and ATLL cells, indicating that HBZ plays a critical role in both infected cells and leukemic cells. For ATL cells, HBZ RNA has growth-promoting activity. ATLL cells frequently express FoxP3, a master factor of regulatory T cells. HBZ expression is associated with a phenotype of Treg cells (Matuoka M, Kyoto, *unpublished data*). As a mechanism of increased Treg cells, HBZ interacts with Smad2/3 and p300, which activates the Smad/TGF-b pathway, and enhances transcription of the HBZ gene (67). Thus, HBZ not only promotes the proliferation of ATL cells, but also modulates the phenotype of HTLV-1–infected cells. Moreover, the expression level of HBZ transcripts is closely correlated with provirus load and the disease severity of HAM/TSP (68).

ATLL cells have a number of complex structural cytogenetic abnormalities that affect every chromosome pair. However, there are no known recurrent cytogenetic changes that are available to aid diagnosis (16,69,70). More than 80% of ATLL cases exhibit DNA aneuploidy; the acute variant presents more

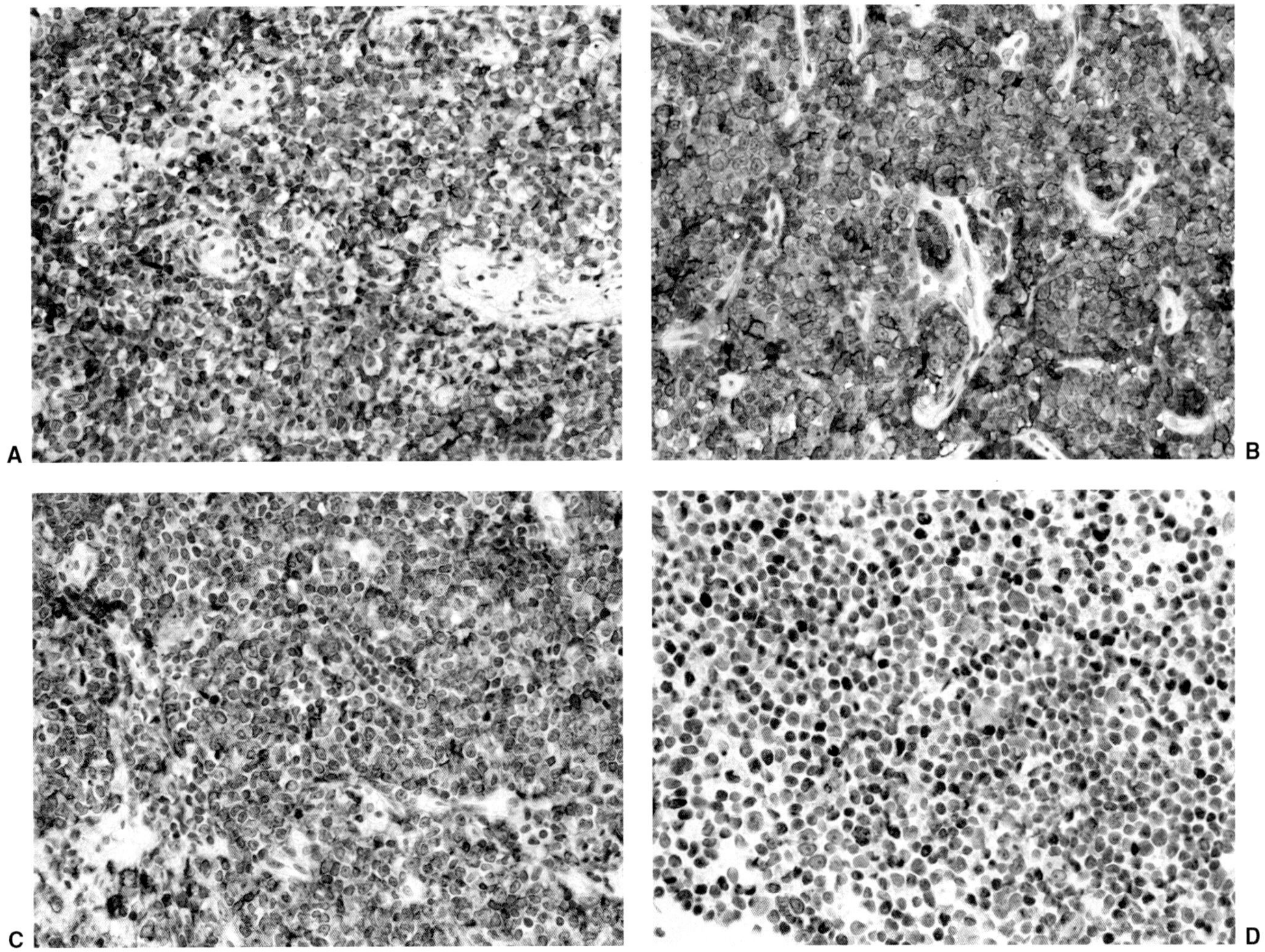

FIGURE 39.10. Immunohistochemistry of ATLL. CD4 (**A**), CD25 (**B**), CCR4 (**C**), and FoxP3 (**D**).

complicated chromosomal abnormalities than the chronic variant. Higher frequencies of chromosomal abnormalities are observed in chromosome segments 1p, 3q, 6q, 9q, 12q, and 14q (16). Among those, the most commonly rearranged chromosome regions are 6q21, 14q32, 11p21-p25, and 1p36. Trisomies for chromosomes 3 (21%), 7 (10%), and 21 (9%); X chromosome monosomy in females (38%), and loss of the Y chromosome in males (17%); translocations involving 14q32 (28%) and 14q11 (14%); deletions of 6q (23%), 10p (9%), 3q (8%), 5q (7%), 9q (7%), 13q (7%), 1p (6%), and 7p (6%) have been determined. The translocations at 14q11 involve the T-cell receptor-$\alpha\Delta$ gene locus (71). Presence of aneuploid clones and higher frequency of numerical and structural abnormalities are more common in aggressive acute variant and lymphoma variant disease. Structural abnormalities in chromosome 6 are the most frequent chromosomal alteration, with breakpoints at bands q11, q13, q16q23, q21q23, q22q24, and q23q24, and appear to correlate with a more aggressive clinical course (69). Studies using comparative genomic hybridization have confirmed the diversity and frequency of genetic alterations (72). Different genetic changes have been observed in the acute and lymphomatous subtypes, suggesting that these two variants may proceed along different molecular pathways.

Recent studies using gene expression profiling have shown overexpression of *BIRC5* (survivin), a gene that blocks apoptosis (73). The antiapoptotic function of *BIRC5* may also be associated with the resistance of ATLL cells to chemotherapy.

Notably, HTLV-1 infection is not directly involved in the malignant transformation of T cells, but promotes the development of neoplastic transformation by a variety of genetic alterations.

CLINICAL COURSE

Clinical subtype classification of ATLL has been proposed based on the prognosis and clinical manifestations (33). Clinical subtype classification is more available in clinical practice than Ann Arbor staging because of frequent leukemic manifestations in Japanese patients defined as stage IV: chronic and smoldering (36%), acute (27%), and lymphomatous variants (11%) (74). Without treatment, most patients with acute and lymphomatous variants die of disease or infectious complications, which include *P. carinii* pneumonia, cryptococcal meningitis, disseminated herpes zoster, and hypercalcemia (33), within weeks or months (Fig. 39.11). Infectious complications are bacterial in 43%, fungal in 31%, protozoan in 18%, and viral in 8% of patients. More than one-half of patients with smoldering ATLL survive for more than 5 years without chemotherapy, but these patients can progress to an acute phase with an aggressive clinical course (75) (Fig. 39.12). Among the variants, chronic ATLL has the most diverse prognosis, which is divided into favorable and unfavorable by clinical parameters (74).

FIGURE 39.11. Survival of patients with each of clinical variants of ATLL. Acute and lymphomatous variants have an aggressive clinical course, whereas longer survival is seen in patients with chronic or smoldering disease.

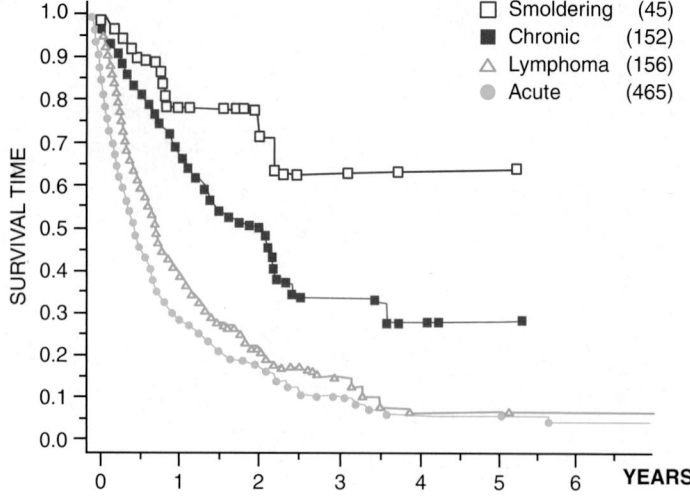

Major prognostic factors include advanced performance status, high LDH level, age of 40 years or older, more than three involved sites, and hypercalcemia (74,76,77). Other factors that may impact prognosis include thrombocytopenia, eosinophilia, BM involvement, a high serum level of interleukin (IL)-5, CCR4 expression, and lung resistance-related protein (LRP) (74). Prognostic factors that have predictive value for chronic variant are high LDH, high blood urea nitrogen, and low albumin levels (74). Molecular alterations, such as p53 mutation and p16 deletion, are negative prognostic factors (78,79), and also occur during progression from chronic to acute disease (80).

At present, no standard treatment for ATL exists (74). Conventional chemotherapy regimens (doxorubicin-based) are recommended for acute, lymphomatous, or unfavorable chronic variants (aggressive ATLL) if outside of clinical trials, but are largely ineffective (81). Although more intensive high-dose chemotherapy and allogeneic hematopoietic stem cell transplantation may be promising, its utility is limited because of high treatment-related mortality (77,82). Watchful waiting until disease progression is recommended for patients with favorable chronic or smoldering variants (indolent ATL). However, their long-term prognosis is poorer than expected, with a median survival of 5.3 years, and the survival curve lacks a plateau (83). Initial trials using drugs that are active against retroviruses, a combination of α-interferon and zidovudine, may be effective for favorable chronic or smoldering variants (74). Promising results have been obtained for the treatment of T-cell malignancies, including ATLL, with monoclonal antibody–based or new agent therapies, including a defucosylated humanized anti-CCR4 antibody (KW-0761), IL-2 fused with diphtheria toxin, histone deacetylase inhibitors, a purine nucleoside phosphorylase inhibitor, a proteasome inhibitor, and lenalidomide (74).

SUMMARY AND CONCLUSIONS

Although ATLL was first discovered in Japan, isolation of the HTLV-1 retrovirus opened up a new, broad field of research in human leukemogenesis. It also influenced histologic diagnosis, because a spectrum of morphologically diverse lymphomas and leukemias are now unified by the presence of the HTLV-1 proviral genome. Clarification of viral transmission has been translated into the primary prevention of ATLL. In addition to the prevention of neonatal transmission by heating mother's milk or avoiding breast-feeding by the carrier (84), viral transmission by transfusion has been prevented by routine checks for ATL virus–associated antigen since 1986. The ATLL story is a good example of the success of a multidisciplinary collaborative approach by clinicians, pathologists, epidemiologists, and molecular biologists.

HTLV-I proviral DNA integration and clinical variants

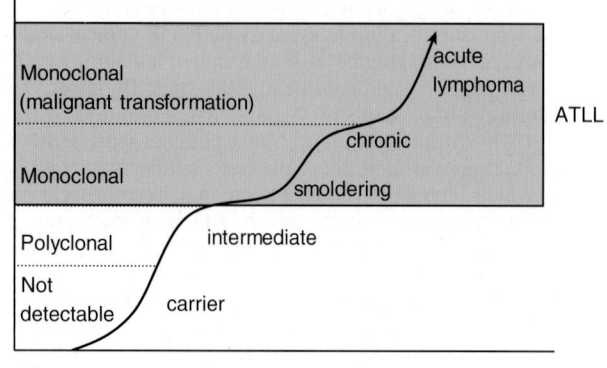

FIGURE 39.12. Adult T-cell leukemia/lymphoma. HTLV-1 proviral DNA integration and clinical variants.

References

1. Ohshima K, Jaffe ES, Kikuchi M. Adult T-cell leukemia/lymphoma. In: Swerdlow SH, Campo E, Harris NL, et al., eds. *WHO classification of tumours of haematopietic and lymphoid tissues*. Lyon: International Agency for Research on Cancer (IARC), 2008:281–284.
2. Poiesz B, Ruscetti F, Gazdar A. Detection and isolation of type C retrovirus particles from fresh and cultured lymphocytes of a patient with cutaneous T-cell lymphoma. *Proc Natl Acad Sci U S A* 1980;77:7415–7419.
3. Hinuma Y, Nagata K, Hanaoka M, et al. Adult T-cell leukemia: antigen in an ATL cell line and detection of antibodies to the antigen in human sera. *Proc Natl Acad Sci U S A* 1981;78(10):6476–6480. PMID: 7031654.
4. Gallo RC, Kalyanaraman VS, Sarngadharan MG, et al. Association of the human type C retrovirus with a subset of adult T-cell cancers. *Cancer Res* 1983;43(8):3892–3899.
5. Yoshida M. Discovery of HTLV-1, the first human retrovirus, its unique regulatory mechanisms, and insights into pathogenesis. *Oncogene* 2005;24(39):5931–5937.
6. Uchiyama T, Yodoi J, Sagawa K, et al. Adult T-cell leukemia: clinical and hematologic features of 16 cases. *Blood* 1977;50:481–492.
7. Blattner WA, Kalyanaraman VS, Robert-Guroff M, et al. The human type-C retrovirus, HTLV, in blacks from the Caribbean region, and relationship to adult T-cell leukemia/lymphoma. *Int J Cancer* 1982;30(3):257–264.
8. Catovsky D, Greaves MF, Rose M, et al. Adult T-cell lymphoma-leukaemia in blacks from the West Indies. *Lancet* 1982;1(8273):639–643.
9. Tajima K, Hinuma Y. Epidemiology of HTLV-1/II in Japan and the world. In: Takatsuki K, Hinuma Y, Yoshida M, eds. *Advances in ault T-cell leukemia and HTLV1 research (Gann Monogr Cancer Res)*. Tokyo: Japan Scientific Societies Press, 1992;39:129–149.
10. Tajima K. The 4th nation-wide study of adult T-cell leukemia/lymphoma (ATL) in Japan: estimates of risk of ATL and its geographical and clinical features. The T- and B-cell Malignancy Study Group. *Int J Cancer* 1990;45(2):237–243.

11. Pombo De Oliveira MS, Loureiro P, Bittencourt A, et al. Geographic diversity of adult T-cell leukemia/lymphoma in Brazil. The Brazilian ATLL Study Group. *Int J Cancer* 1999;83(3):291–298.
12. Miyoshi I, Kubonishi I, Sumida M, et al. A novel T-cell line derived from adult T-cell leukemia. *Gann* 1980;71(1):155–156.
13. Taylor GP, Matsuoka M. Natural history of adult T-cell leukemia/lymphoma and approaches to therapy. *Oncogene* 2005;24(39):6047–6057.
14. Nagatani T, Matsuzaki T, Iemoto G, et al. Comparative study of cutaneous T-cell lymphoma and adult T-cell leukemia/lymphoma: clinical, histopathological and immunohistochemical analyses. *Cancer* 1990;66:2380–2386.
15. Kamada N, Tanaka K, Sakatani K, et al. Chromosome aberrations in lymphoid malignancies and transforming gene in adult T-cell leukemia. In: Hanaoka M, et al., eds. *Lymphoid malignancy: immunocytology and cytogenetics*. New York: Field & Wood, 1990:57–66.
16. Kamada N, Sakurai M, Miyamoto K, et al. Chromosome abnormalities in adult T-cell leukemia/lymphoma: a karyotype review committee report. *Cancer Res* 1992;52:1481–1493.
17. Watanabe S, Arimoto H. Standardized mortality ratio of cancer by prefecture in Japan. *Jpn J Clin Oncol* 1990;20:316–337.
18. Levine PH, Manns A, Jaffe ES, et al. The effect of ethnic differences on the pattern of HTLV-I-associated T-cell leukemia/lymphoma (HATL) in the United States. *Int J Cancer* 1994;56(2):177–181.
19. Franchini G. Molecular mechanisms of human T-cell leukemia/lymphotropic virus type I infection. *Blood* 1995;86(10):3619–3639.
20. Satou Y, Yasunaga J, Yoshida M, et al. HTLV-I basic leucine zipper factor gene mRNA supports proliferation of adult T cell leukemia cells. *Proc Natl Acad Sci U S A* 2006;103(3):720–725. Erratum in: *Proc Natl Acad Sci U S A* 2006;103(23):8906. PMID: 16407133.
21. Takatsuki K, Yamaguchi K, Watanabe T, et al. Adult T-cell leukemia and HTLV-1 related disease. *Gann Monogr Cancer Res* 1992;32:1–15.
22. Goncalves DU, Proietti FA, Barbosa-Stancioli EF, et al. HTLV-1-associated myelopathy/tropical spastic paraparesis (HAM/TSP) inflammatory network. *Inflamm Allergy Drug Targets* 2008;7(2):98–107.
23. Takenouchi N, Yao K, Jacobson S. Immunopathogenesis of HTLV-I associated neurologic disease: molecular, histopathologic, and immunologic approaches. *Front Biosci* 2004;9:2527–2539.
24. LaGrenade L, Hanchard B, Fletcher V, et al. Infective dermatitis of Jamaican children: a marker for HTLV-I infection. *Lancet* 1990;336(8727):1345–1347.
25. Okamoto T, Ohno Y, Tsugane S, et al. Multi-step carcinogenesis model for adult T-cell leukemia. *Jpn J Cancer Res* 1989;80:191–195.
26. Whittaker SJ, Ng YL, Rustin M, et al. HTLV-1-associated cutaneous disease: a clinicopathological and molecular study of patients from the UK. *Br J Dermatol* 1993;128(5):483–492.
27. Fujihara K, Goldman B, Oseroff AR, et al. HTLV-associated diseases: human retroviral infection and cutaneous T-cell lymphomas. *Immunol Invest* 1997;26 (1–2):231–242.
28. Setoyama M, Katahira Y, Kanzaki T. Clinicopathologic analysis of 124 cases of adult T-cell leukemia/lymphoma with cutaneous manifestations: the smouldering type with skin manifestations has a poorer prognosis than previously thought. *J Dermatol* 1999;26(12):785–790.
29. Yamaguchi T, Ohshima K, Karube K, et al. Clinicopathological features of cutaneous lesions of adult T-cell leukaemia/lymphoma. *Br J Dermatol* 2005;152(1): 76–81.
30. Bunn PA Jr, Schechter GP, Jaffe E, et al. Clinical course of retrovirus-associated adult T-cell lymphoma in the United States. *N Engl J Med* 1983;309(5):257–264. PMID: 6602943.
31. Blayney DW, Jaffe ES, Blattner WA, et al. The human T-cell leukemia/lymphoma virus associated with American adult T-cell leukemia/lymphoma. *Blood* 1983;62(2):401–405.
32. O'Mahony D, Debnath I, Janik J, et al. Cardiac involvement with human T-cell lymphotrophic virus type-1-associated adult T-cell leukemia/lymphoma: the NIH experience. *Leuk Lymphoma* 2008;49(3):439–446.
33. Shimoyama M. Diagnostic criteria and classification of clinical subtypes of adult T-cell leukaemia-lymphoma. A report from the Lymphoma Study Group (1984–87). *Br J Haematol* 1991;79(3):428–437.
34. Verdonck K, Gonzalez E, Van Dooren S, et al. Human T-lymphotropic virus 1: recent knowledge about an ancient infection. *Lancet Infect Dis* 2007;7(4): 266–281.
35. Jaffe ES, Blattner WA, Blayney DW, et al. The pathologic spectrum of adult T-cell leukemia/lymphoma in the United States. *Am J Surg Pathol* 1984;8:263–275.
36. Ohshima K. Pathological features of diseases associated with human T-cell leukemia virus type I. *Cancer Sci* 2007;98(6):772–778.
37. Tsukasaki K, Imaizumi Y, Tawara M, et al. Diversity of leukaemic cell morphology in ATL correlates with prognostic factors, aberrant immunophenotype and defective HTLV-1 genotype. *Br J Haematol* 1999;105(2):369–375.
38. Levine PH, Cleghorn F, Manns A, et al. Adult T-cell leukemia/lymphoma: a working point-score classification for epidemiological studies. *Int J Cancer* 1994;59(4):491–493.
39. Hanaoka M, Sasaki M, Matsumoto H, et al. Adult T cell leukemia. Histological classification and characteristics. *Acta Pathol Jpn* 1979;29(5):723–738.
40. Hanaoka M. Disease entity of adult T-cell leukemia: cytological aspects and geographic pathology. In: Hanaoka M, Takatsuki K, Shimoyama M, eds. *Adult T cell leukemia and related diseases*. Tokyo: Japan Scientific Societies Press, 1982: 1–12.
41. Karube K, Suzumiya J, Okamoto M, et al. Adult T-cell lymphoma/leukemia with angioimmunoblastic T-cell lymphomalike features: report of 11 cases. *Am J Surg Pathol* 2007;31(2):216–223. PMID: 17255766.
42. Kawano F, Yamaguchi K, Nishimura H, et al. Variation in the clinical courses of adult T-cell leukemia. *Cancer* 1985;55(4):851–856.
43. Yamaguchi K, Nishimura H, Kohrogi H, et al. A proposal for smoldering adult T-cell leukemia: a clinicopathologic study of five cases. *Blood* 1983;62(4): 758–766.
44. Ohshima K, Suzumiya J, Kato A, et al. Clonal HTLV-I-infected CD4+ T-lymphocytes and non-clonal non-HTLV-I- infected giant cells in incipient ATLL with Hodgkin-like histologic features. *Int J Cancer* 1997;72(4):592–598.
45. Duggan D, Ehrlich G, Davey F, et al. HTLV-I induced lymphoma mimicking Hodgkin's disease. Diagnosis by polymerase chain reaction amplification of specific HTLV-I sequences in tumor DNA. *Blood* 1988;71:1027–1032.
46. Waldmann TA, White JD, Goldman CK, et al. The interleukin-2 receptor: a target for monoclonal antibody treatment of human T-cell lymphotrophic virus I-induced adult T-cell leukemia. *Blood* 1993;82(6):1701–1712.
47. Takeshita M, Akamatsu M, Ohshima K, et al. CD30 (Ki-1) expression in adult T-cell leukaemia/lymphoma is associated with distinctive immunohistological and clinical characteristics. *Histopathology* 1995;26(6):539–546. PMID: 7665144.
48. Roncador G, Garcia JF, Garcia JF, et al. FOXP3, a selective marker for a subset of adult T-cell leukaemia/lymphoma. *Leukemia* 2005;19(12):2247–2253.
49. Karube K, Ohshima K, Tsuchiya T, et al. Expression of FoxP3, a key molecule in CD4CD25 regulatory T cells, in adult T-cell leukaemia/lymphoma cells. *Br J Haematol* 2004;126(1):81–84.
50. Ohshima K, Karube K, Kawano R, et al. Classification of distinct subtypes of peripheral T-cell lymphoma unspecified, identified by chemokine and chemokine receptor expression: analysis of prognosis. *Int J Oncol* 2004;25(3):605–613. PMID: 15289861.
51. Ishida T, Utsunomiya A, Iida S, et al. Clinical significance of CCR4 expression in adult T-cell leukemia/lymphoma: its close association with skin involvement and unfavorable outcome. *Clin Cancer Res* 2003;9(10 Pt 1):3625–3634. PMID: 14506150.
52. Ishida T, Ueda R. Antibody therapy for adult T-cell leukemia-lymphoma. *Int J Hematol* 2011;94(5):443–452. PMID: 21993874.
53. Yamamoto K, Utsunomiya A, Tobinai K, et al. Phase I study of KW-0761, a defucosylated humanized anti-CCR4 antibody, in relapsed patients with adult T-cell leukemia-lymphoma and peripheral T-cell lymphoma. *J Clin Oncol* 2010;28(9):1591–1598. PMID: 20177026.
54. Karube K, Aoki R, Sugita Y, et al. The relationship of FOXP3 expression and clinicopathological characteristics in adult T-cell leukemia/lymphoma. *Mod Pathol* 2008;21(5):617–625.
55. Ohshima K, Mukai Y, Shiraki H, et al. Clonal integration and expression of human T-cell lymphotropic virus type I in carriers detected by polymerase chain reaction and inverse PCR. *Am J Hematol* 1997;54(4):306–312. PMID: 9092686.
56. Yoshida M, Seiki M, Yamaguchi K, et al. Monoclonal integration of HTLV in all primary tumors of adult T cell leukemia suggests causative role of HTLV in the disease. *Proc Natl Acad Sci U S A* 1984;81:2534–2537.
57. Yamaguchi K, Seiki M, Yoshida M, et al. The detection of human T-cell leukemia virus proviral DNA and its application for classification and diagnosis of T-cell malignancy. *Blood* 1984;63:1235–1240.
58. Hata T, Fujimoto T, Tsushima H, et al. Multi-clonal expansion of unique human T-lymphotropic virus type-I-infected T cells with high growth potential in response to interleukin-2 in prodromal phase of adult T cell leukemia. *Leukemia* 1999;13(2):215–221.
59. Yasunaga J, Matsuoka M. Molecular mechanisms of HTLV-1 infection and pathogenesis. *Int J Hematol* 2011;94(5):435–442. PMID: 21953273.
60. Grassmann R, Aboud M, Jeang KT. Molecular mechanisms of cellular transformation by HTLV-1 Tax. *Oncogene* 2005;24(39):5976–5985.
61. Lairmore MD, Fujii M. 12th International Conference on Human Retrovirology: HTLV and Related Retroviruses. *Retrovirology* 2005;2:61. PMID: 16202161.
62. Takeda S, Maeda M, Morikawa S, et al. Genetic and epigenetic inactivation of tax gene in adult T-cell leukemia cells. *Int J Cancer* 2004;109(4):559–567. PMID: 14991578.
63. Gaudray G, Gachon F, Basbous J, et al. The complementary strand of the human T-cell leukemia virus type 1 RNA genome encodes a bZIP transcription factor that down-regulates viral transcription. *J Virol* 2002;76(24):12813–12822. PMID: 12438606.
64. Satou Y, Yasunaga J, Yoshida M, et al. HTLV-I basic leucine zipper factor gene mRNA supports proliferation of adult T cell leukemia cells. *Proc Natl Acad Sci U S A* 2006;103(3):720–725. Erratum in: *Proc Natl Acad Sci U S A* 2006;103(23):8906. PMID: 16407133.
65. Shimizu-Kohno K, Satou Y, Arakawa F, et al. Detection of HTLV-1 by means of HBZ gene in situ hybridization in formalin-fixed and paraffin-embedded tissues. *Cancer Sci* 2011;102(7):1432–1436. doi: 10.1111/j.1349-7006.2011.01946.x. PMID: 21453388.
66. Satou Y, Yasunaga J, Zhao T, et al. HTLV-1 bZIP factor induces T-cell lymphoma and systemic inflammation in vivo. *PLoS Pathog* 2011;7(2):e1001274. PMID: 21347344.
67. Zhao T, Satou Y, Sugata K, et al. HTLV-1 bZIP factor enhances TGF-β signaling through p300 coactivator. *Blood* 2011;118(7):1865–1876. PMID: 21705495.
68. Saito M, Matsuzaki T, Satou Y, et al. In vivo expression of the HBZ gene of HTLV-1 correlates with proviral load, inflammatory markers and disease severity in HTLV-1 associated myelopathy/tropical spastic paraparesis (HAM/TSP). *Retrovirology* 2009;6:19. PMID: 19228429.
69. Whang-Peng J, Bunn PA, Knutsen T, et al. Cytogenetic studies in human T-cell lymphoma virus (HTLV)-positive leukemia-lymphoma in the United States. *J Natl Cancer Inst* 1985;74(2):357–369.
70. Itoyama A, Chaganti RSK, Yamada Y, et al. Cytogenetic analysis and clinical significance in adult T-cell leukemia/lymphoma: a study of 50 cases from the human T-cell leukemia virus type-1 endemic area, Nagasaki. *Blood* 2001;97(11):3612–3620.
71. Haider S, Hayakawa K, Itoyama T, et al. TCR variable gene involvement in chromosome inversion between 14q11 and 14q24 in adult T-cell leukemia. *J Hum Genet* 2006;51(4):326–334.
72. Oshiro A, Tagawa H, Ohshima K, et al. Identification of subtype-specific genomic alterations in aggressive adult T-cell leukemia/lymphoma. *Blood* 2006;107(11):4500–4507.
73. Pise-Masison CA, Radonovich M, Dohoney K, et al. Gene expression profiling of ATL patients: compilation of disease-related genes and evidence for TCF4 involvement in BIRC5 gene expression and cell viability. *Blood* 2009;113(17):4016–4026.
74. Tsukasaki K, Hermine O, Bazarbachi A, et al. Definition, prognostic factors, treatment, and response criteria of adult T-cell leukemia-lymphoma: a proposal from an international consensus meeting. *J Clin Oncol* 2009;27(3):453–459.
75. Ohshima K, Suzumiya J, Sato K, et al. Survival of patients with HTLV-I-associated lymph node lesions. *J Pathol* 1999;189(4):539–545.
76. Yamamura M, Yamada Y, Momita S, et al. Circulating interleukin-6 levels are elevated in adult T-cell leukaemia/lymphoma patients and correlate with adverse clinical features and survival. *Br J Haematol* 1998;100(1):129–134. PMID: 9450801.
77. Suzumiya J, Ohshima K, Tamura K, et al.; International Peripheral T-Cell Lymphoma Project. The International Prognostic Index predicts outcome in aggressive adult T-cell leukemia/lymphoma: analysis of 126 patients from the International Peripheral T-Cell Lymphoma Project. *Ann Oncol* 2009;20(4): 715–721. PMID: 19150954.

78. Yamada Y, Hatta Y, Murata K, et al. Deletions of p15 and/or p16 genes as a poor-prognosis factor in adult T-cell leukemia. *J Clin Oncol* 1997;15(5):1778–1785.

79. Tawara M, Hogerzeil SJ, Yamada Y, et al. Impact of p53 aberration on the progression of adult T-cell leukemia/lymphoma. *Cancer Lett* 2006;234(2):249–255.

80. Tsukasaki K, Krebs J, Nagai K, et al. Comparative genomic hybridization analysis in adult T-cell leukemia/lymphoma: correlation with clinical course. *Blood* 2001;97(12):3875–3881.

81. Tsukasaki K, Tobinai K, Shimoyama M, et al. Deoxycoformycin-containing combination chemotherapy for adult T-cell leukemia-lymphoma: Japan Clinical Oncology Group Study (JCOG9109). *Int J Hematol* 2003;77(2):164–170.

82. Tsukasaki K, Maeda T, Arimura K, et al. Poor outcome of autologous stem cell transplantation for adult T cell leukemia/lymphoma: a case report and review of the literature. *Bone Marrow Transplant* 1999;23(1):87–89.

83. Takasaki Y, Iwanaga M, Imaizumi Y, et al. Long-term study of indolent adult T-cell leukemia-lymphoma. *Blood* 2010;115(22):4337–4343. PMID: 20348391.

84. Kajiyama W, Kashiwaga S, Ikematsu H, et al. Intrafamilial transmission of adult T-cell leukemia virus. *J Infect Dis* 1986;154:851–857.

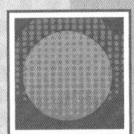

Chapter 40
Acute Lymphoblastic Leukemia/Lymphoblastic Lymphoma

Michael J. Borowitz • Joseph A. DiGiuseppe

The *precursor lymphoid neoplasms B-lymphoblastic leukemia/ lymphoma* and *T-lymphoblastic leukemia/lymphoma* comprise malignancies of lymphoid progenitor cells committed to B-cell and T-cell lineage, respectively. These neoplastic lymphoid progenitor cells are referred to as *lymphoblasts*, and the diseases resulting from their dysregulated proliferation are termed *acute lymphoblastic leukemia* (*ALL*) and *lymphoblastic lymphoma*.

DEFINITION

B-lymphoblastic leukemia is a malignant neoplasm in which lymphoblasts with cytologic features of immaturity and immunophenotypic features of early or incomplete B-lineage differentiation involve bone marrow and (usually) peripheral blood. In B-lymphoblastic lymphoma, lymph nodes and/or extranodal sites are primarily involved by the neoplastic B lymphoblasts, with formation of one or more tumoral masses. When both bone marrow and extramedullary sites are involved, the percentage of bone marrow blasts is used to distinguish leukemia from lymphoma, though this distinction is admittedly arbitrary; in many protocols, a threshold of 25% bone marrow blasts has been required for designation as B-lymphoblastic leukemia (1).

In T-lymphoblastic leukemia, cytologically immature lymphoblasts with immunophenotypic features of early or incomplete T-lineage differentiation involve primarily peripheral blood and bone marrow. T-lymphoblastic lymphoma is defined by involvement of thymus, lymph nodes, or extranodal sites by T lymphoblasts, with little or no involvement of peripheral blood or bone marrow. As with B-lymphoblastic leukemia/lymphoma, a threshold of 25% bone marrow lymphoblasts has been used arbitrarily to distinguish T-lymphoblastic leukemia from T-lymphoblastic lymphoma with fewer bone marrow lymphoblasts (2).

In contrast with *acute myeloid leukemia (AML)*, in which (with certain defined exceptions) a minimum of 20% bone marrow blasts is required to establish a diagnosis, the most recent World Health Organization (WHO) classification of tumors of the hematopoietic and lymphoid systems does not establish a lower limit of bone marrow blasts for a diagnosis of ALL. Nonetheless, for both B- and T-lymphoblastic leukemia, it is recommended that a diagnosis of ALL be avoided when there are fewer than 20% bone marrow blasts (1,2).

EPIDEMIOLOGY

ALL is the most common malignancy of childhood and adolescence (3). It accounts for about 80% of cases of acute leukemia in children, compared with only about 20% of cases in adults. In the United States, approximately 6,070 new cases of ALL, and 1,430 deaths from ALL were projected for 2010 (4). Between 2004 and 2008, the median age at diagnosis of ALL in the United States was 13, and approximately 60% of patients were <20 years of age at diagnosis (5). For comparison, the median age at death for patients with ALL over that same interval was 50, and fewer than 20% of deaths from ALL

were in patients under 20 years of age (5). The incidence of childhood ALL is lower in underdeveloped nations and in Asia, and lower among American blacks than whites (5). Moreover, there are racially associated differences in outcome that are at least partly genetic (6). Approximately 80% to 85% of cases of ALL display B-lineage differentiation (1). However, among precursor lymphoid neoplasms presenting as lymphoblastic lymphoma, only about 10% are of B-cell lineage (1).

Little is known about the causes of ALL. A genetic predisposition is suggested not only from the racial data but also from the known associations with Down syndrome (7) and ataxia-telangiectasia (8). In children subsequently diagnosed with B-lymphoblastic leukemia, clonally related leukemic cells are frequently detectable on their newborn genetic screening cards (Guthrie cards), suggesting that B-lymphoblastic leukemogenesis is often initiated *in utero* (9). In contrast, neonatal leukemic cells in children with subsequent T-lymphoblastic leukemia are infrequently detectable, suggesting that postnatal initiation of leukemogenesis is more common in T-lymphoblastic leukemia (10). In this context, the increased risk of concordant acute leukemia seen in monozygotic twins is thought to reflect intrauterine spread from one member of the twin pair following antenatal leukemic initiation, though additional postnatal events appear to be required to yield overt leukemia, and likely account for the variable latencies seen in these circumstances (11).

CLINICAL FEATURES

Clinical features of ALL at presentation can be related directly to the replacement of normal bone marrow elements by neoplastic cells. Pallor, weakness, and lassitude attributable to anemia are the most common presenting features, and bleeding in the form of petechial hemorrhage frequently accompanies thrombocytopenia. Bone pain is a common complaint, especially in children, and is related to massive marrow infiltration with leukemic cells. Fever is present in more than one-half of patients, but despite neutropenia, bacterial infection at diagnosis is not common. Tissue infiltration in the form of hepatosplenomegaly or lymphadenopathy is seen in more than one-half of patients, and an anterior mediastinal mass is present in a significant number of patients who have T-lymphoblastic lymphoma/leukemia; other parenchymal involvement at diagnosis is uncommon. Leukemic involvement of the central nervous system (CNS) is present in about 5% of patients at diagnosis, but is generally occult.

The typical patient who has ALL presents with anemia, thrombocytopenia, and leukocytosis, sometimes to levels >100 × 10⁹/L, but more commonly <50 × 10⁹/L. Under such circumstances, the diagnosis of acute leukemia is readily apparent from examination of the peripheral blood smear. However, "aleukemic" presentations are common, and any person who has unexplained pancytopenia requires bone marrow examination to exclude leukemia. In patients whose bone marrow cannot be aspirated, or whose bone marrow aspirates are heavily contaminated with uninvolved peripheral blood, a bone marrow core biopsy may be essential to establish the diagnosis.

Although not every patient fits the characteristic clinical picture, a constellation of features has come to be associated with T-lymphoblastic leukemia. These patients are more likely than others to present with elevated white blood cell (WBC) counts (often over 50 × 10⁹/L), and are more likely to have lymphadenopathy and organomegaly (12,13). An anterior mediastinal mass is a highly specific predictor for T-cell immunophenotype in patients who have ALL, and in children, T-lymphoblastic leukemia is associated with older age at presentation than B-lymphoblastic leukemia. In contrast with T-lymphoblastic leukemia, there is no single clinical picture associated with B-lymphoblastic leukemia.

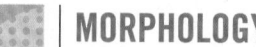

MORPHOLOGY

The relative ease with which blood or bone marrow can be obtained from patients who have leukemia has made morphologic examination an important diagnostic tool. Thin films of peripheral blood, or well-spread bone marrow aspirate smears, are essential for recognizing the often-subtle nuclear characteristics of lymphoblasts. The morphologic features of lymphoblasts are described on the basis of their staining characteristics with so-called Romanowsky stains, most commonly Wright-Giemsa (Fig. 40.1).

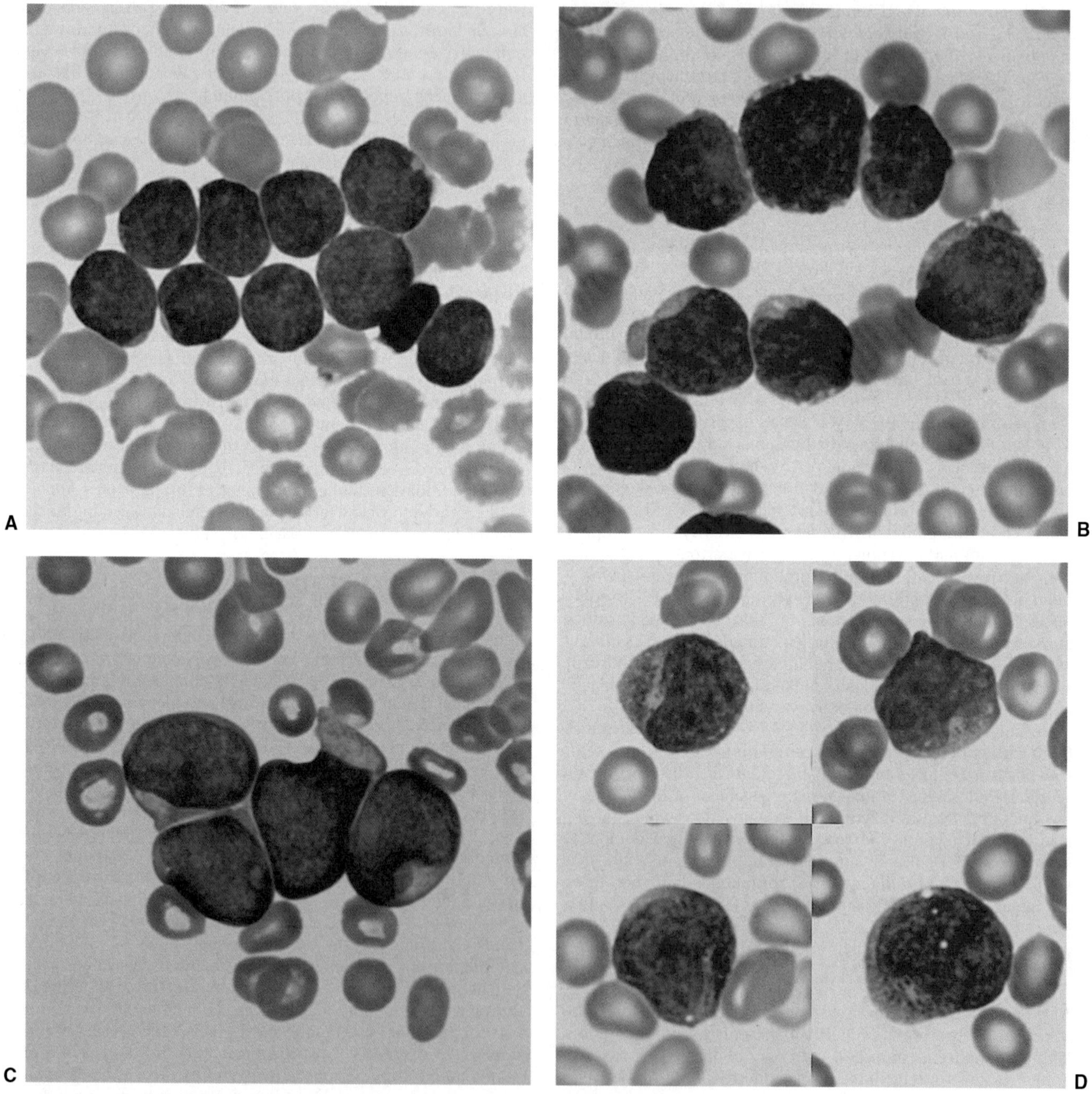

A

B

C

D

FIGURE 40.1. Varied morphologies of lymphoblasts in Wright's-stained smear preparations. A: The blasts are small, with relatively round nuclei, smooth nuclear chromatin, typically indistinct nucleoli, and extremely scant cytoplasm, resulting in a very high N:C ratio ("L1 morphology"). **B:** The blasts range from small to large, have more irregular nuclei, and display modest agranular cytoplasm, some with a few cytoplasmic vacuoles. **C:** The blasts are large, with ovoid or folded nuclei, finely dispersed chromatin, prominent nucleoli, and moderate agranular cytoplasm, resulting in a lower N:C ratio ("L2 morphology"). **D:** Composite illustration of blast morphology in a case of granular ALL. Compared with the delicate azurophilic granules of myeloblasts in AML, the cytoplasmic granules in the lymphoblasts of granular ALL are relatively coarse. (Original magnification in all panels: 1,000×.)

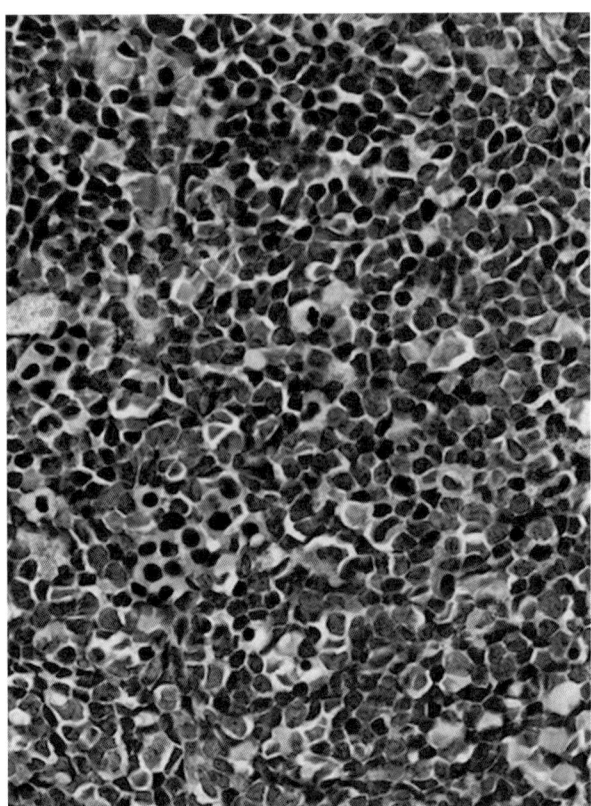
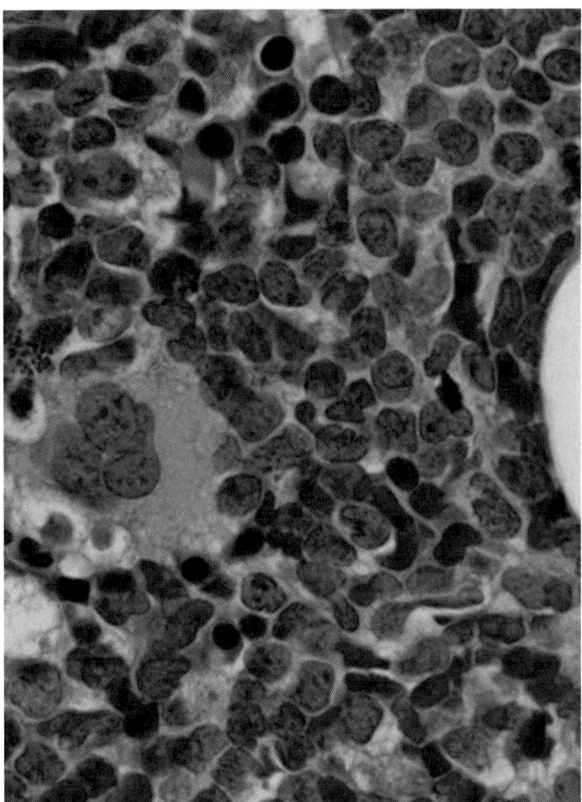

A   B

FIGURE 40.2. Histopathology of ALL in H&E-stained, formalin-fixed bone marrow core biopsies. A: The marrow is markedly hypercellular, with near-total replacement by small- to medium-sized mononuclear cells with delicate chromatin, and scant cytoplasm (original magnification: 400×). **B:** High-power view of the cytologic features of lymphoblasts in a case of ALL. In this case, the blasts display prominent nuclear irregularities and modest pale cytoplasm; some have small nucleoli (original magnification: 1,000×).

Historically, the French-American-British (FAB) system (14,15) was used to classify ALL on the basis of blast morphology. In this system, ALL is divided into three types, designated *L1*, *L2*, and *L3*. L1 ALL is characterized by homogeneous small blasts with very high nuclear:cytoplasmic (N:C) ratios, smooth but often darkly staining nuclear chromatin, and inconspicuous nucleoli. L2 ALL is characterized by more pleomorphic blasts with lower N:C ratios, prominently convoluted or otherwise irregular nuclear contours, and more prominent nucleoli. (L3 morphology characteristically identifies a leukemic variant of Burkitt lymphoma, a mature B-cell neoplasm (16); see Chapter 24.) L1 blasts may be confused with normal lymphocytes in some instances, while L2 blasts are often indistinguishable from those of certain forms of AML (i.e., FAB M0 or M1). In practice, both L1 and L2 blasts are commonly seen in an individual case of ALL. Moreover, L1 and L2 morphologies fail to identify specific immunologic or genetic entities among the precursor lymphoid neoplasms, and morphology has therefore been supplanted by immunophenotype and cytogenetics in the current WHO classification (1,2). Nonetheless, the morphologic features of L1 and L2 blasts serve as a useful framework in the diagnostic evaluation of acute leukemia.

Hand-mirror cell leukemia is a distinct morphologic variant of ALL in which blasts are characterized by the presence of an asymmetrical cytoplasmic projection called a *uropod* (17–19). Although small numbers of hand-mirror cells are seen frequently in ALL, in only about 1% of patients are they the dominant cytologic finding. Hand-mirror cells may display L1 or L2 morphology, and they are not associated with any particular immunophenotype. It is generally conceded that no prognostic significance attends this diagnosis (18,19).

The term *granular ALL* describes cases of ALL in which the blasts contain azurophilic cytoplasmic inclusions that are distinct from myeloid primary granules, and do not stain for myeloperoxidase (20–22; Fig. 40.1D). In some patients, these granules stain with acid phosphatase or acid esterases, suggesting a lysosomal origin (21). Their presence is not associated with any particular immunophenotype. Granular ALL has also been described in adults, and a higher incidence of azurophilic granules has been reported in lymphoblasts that coexpress myeloid and lymphoid antigens (22).

In well-prepared sections of hematoxylin-and-eosin (H&E)–stained, formalin-fixed biopsies (Fig. 40.2), lymphoblasts with L1-type features characteristically display finely dispersed chromatin, inconspicuous nucleoli, and no discernible cytoplasm. Blasts with L2-type morphology are more heterogeneous, with irregular nuclei, variably prominent nucleoli, and often some cytoplasm. Bone marrow core biopsies in ALL are almost always hypercellular at diagnosis, with a preponderance of blasts. Extramedullary leukemic infiltrates can involve virtually any organ system, particularly in advanced disease. The spleen, liver, and lymph nodes are commonly affected; excluding the lymphoreticular system, the CNS and kidneys are the most common sites of involvement. In males, the testis may represent a "protected site," not fully accessible to chemotherapeutic agents. Testicular involvement is interstitial, and if the degree of involvement is limited, blasts generally form small clusters. In small biopsy specimens, particularly when fixation is suboptimal, distinction between lymphoblasts and mature lymphocytes may be difficult; in such cases immunophenotypic studies are indicated.

IMMUNOPHENOTYPE

In the current WHO classification scheme (Table 40.1), the precursor lymphoid neoplasms are divided into B-lymphoblastic leukemia/lymphoma and T-lymphoblastic leukemia/lymphoma

Table 40.1	WHO CLASSIFICATION OF PRECURSOR LYMPHOID NEOPLASMS

B-lymphoblastic leukemia/lymphoma, not otherwise specified
B-lymphoblastic leukemia/lymphoma with recurrent cytogenetic abnormalities
  B-lymphoblastic leukemia/lymphoma with t(9;22)(q34;q11.2); *BCR-ABL1*
  B-lymphoblastic leukemia/lymphoma with t(v;11q23); *MLL*-rearranged
  B-lymphoblastic leukemia/lymphoma with t(12;21)(p13;q22); *TEL-AML1 (ETV6-RUNX1)*
  B-lymphoblastic leukemia/lymphoma with hyperdiploidy
  B-lymphoblastic leukemia/lymphoma with hypodiploidy (hypodiploid ALL)
  B-lymphoblastic leukemia/lymphoma with t(5;14)(q31;q32); *IL3-IGH*
  B-lymphoblastic leukemia/lymphoma with t(1;19)(q23;p13.3); *E2A-PBX1 (TCF3-PBX1)*
T-lymphoblastic leukemia/lymphoma

From Borowitz MJ, Chan JKC. B lymphoblastic leukaemia/lymphoma, not otherwise specified. In: Swerdlow SH, Campo E, Harris NL, et al., eds. *WHO classification of tumours of haematopoietic and lymphoid tissues*, 4th ed. Lyon: International Agency for Research on Cancer, 2008:168–170; Borowitz MJ, Chan JKC. T lymphoblastic leukaemia/lymphoma. In: Swerdlow SH, Campo E, Harris NL, et al., eds. *WHO classification of tumours of haematopoietic and lymphoid tissues*, 4th ed. Lyon: International Agency for Research on Cancer, 2008:176–178; Borowitz MJ, Chan JKC. B lymphoblastic leukaemia/lymphoma with recurrent genetic abnormalities. In: Swerdlow SH, Campo E, Harris NL, et al., eds. *WHO classification of tumours of haematopoietic and lymphoid tissues*, 4th ed. Lyon: International Agency for Research on Cancer, 2008:171–175.

on the basis of their immunophenotypic properties (1,2). Immunophenotyping is most commonly performed using flow cytometry (reviewed in refs. 13,23–26), though immunohistochemistry may suffice when fresh material is not available. Since the acute leukemias are extraordinarily heterogeneous in their expression of surface antigens, and because most immunophenotypic markers are relatively rather than absolutely lineage-specific, it is difficult to describe a simple algorithm that accurately classifies all cases of acute leukemia. In some cases, interpretation of lineage is straightforward on the basis of the reactivity of a relatively small number of antibodies. In more complex cases, though, a larger panel of antibodies may be necessary. In those patients in whom surface marker studies are equivocal, flow cytometric evaluation of specific intracellular antigens may be valuable.

Most cases of B-lymphoblastic leukemia/lymphoma can be recognized without difficulty on the basis of their immunophenotype (13,23–26; Fig. 40.3). Almost 98% of patients express

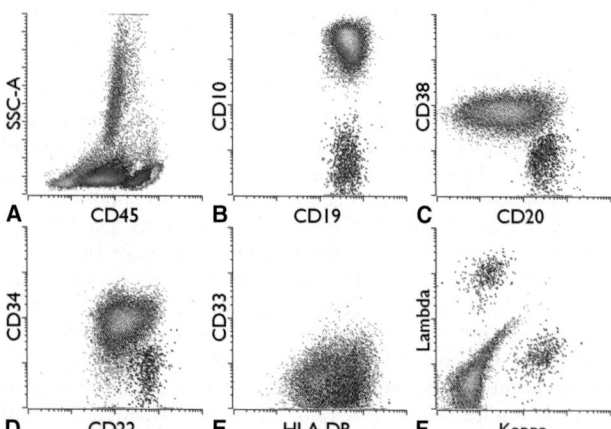

FIGURE 40.3. Flow cytometric immunophenotyping data from a representative case of B-lymphoblastic leukemia. (A) is gated on all viable cells, while **(B–F)** are gated on CD19+ B cells. Selected populations are denoted by color: *orange*, erythroid precursors; *blue*, lymphoblasts; *magenta* (highlighted), normal mature B cells. The blasts are weakly positive for CD45, display low side scatter (SSC), and homogeneously express the B-lineage antigens CD19 and CD22. They are further positive for HLA-DR and the progenitor cell antigen (CD34), with bright expression of the common ALL antigen (CD10). In contrast with the normal mature B cells, which are CD20+, and express polytypic kappa and lambda light chains, the blasts express variable-intensity CD20, and are negative for immunoglobulin light chains.

both CD19 and HLA-DR (13). The CD19 antigen is not seen in T-lymphoblastic leukemia/lymphoma; although it may be seen occasionally in AML, its expression is dim and usually heterogeneous. Approximately 90% of patients with B-lymphoblastic leukemia/lymphoma express the common ALL antigen, CD10, which is rarely (and only weakly) expressed in AML. CD10⁻ cases may be recognized as B-cell derived in most instances by virtue of expression of other B-cell–specific antigens, particularly CD19 and CD22. CD20 expression is also highly specific for B-lineage differentiation, though not as sensitive as either CD19 or CD22. Additional surface markers that have been described in B-lymphoblastic leukemia/lymphoma include CD9, CD24, and the progenitor cell antigen CD34, which are expressed in approximately 90%, >50%, and 75% of cases, respectively. The common leukocyte antigen CD45 is absent or undetectable in about 10% to 20% of patients with B-lymphoblastic leukemia/lymphoma; when CD45 is expressed, its intensity varies greatly, though it is characteristically weaker than that seen on mature lymphocytes. Finally, myeloid antigens, including CD13, CD15, and CD33, are found in a significant minority of cases of B-lymphoblastic leukemia/lymphoma; expression of these antigens in an otherwise typical case of ALL should not prompt a diagnosis of AML or *acute leukemia of ambiguous lineage* (27).

Absence of surface-membrane immunoglobulin light chain expression typifies B-lymphoblastic leukemia/lymphoma, and represents one immunophenotypic criterion that distinguishes B-lineage ALL from mature B-cell lymphoid neoplasms, such as Burkitt lymphoma. However, it has become increasingly recognized that monotypic immunoglobulin light chain expression may be seen in a small minority of otherwise typical cases of pediatric and adult B-lymphoblastic leukemia/lymphoma without apparent clinical significance (28–30). Conversely, cases with FAB-L3 morphology and a *MYC* translocation despite a precursor B-cell immunophenotype have been reported, and are thought to represent Burkitt lymphoma/leukemia (31). Cytoplasmic μ heavy chain expression without surface-membrane immunoglobulin characterizes so-called *pre–B-cell ALL* (reviewed in ref. 23), and cases that express cytoplasmic and surface μ heavy chain without an accompanying light chain have been designated *transitional pre–B-cell ALL* (32). These terms have not been retained in the current WHO classification.

The most sensitive surface-membrane marker for T-lymphoblastic leukemia/lymphoma is CD7, which detects all (33,34) or at least a majority of cases (35). This antigen is also present, however, in up to 20% of patients with AML (36), so its utility as a single marker is limited. Virtually all patients with CD7⁺ AML also express the HLA-DR antigen, whereas CD7⁺/HLA-DR⁺ T-lymphoblastic leukemia/lymphoma is rare in children, and only occasionally seen in adults; this combination of antibodies is therefore more useful than CD7 alone. The CD5 antigen is a more specific marker for T-cell differentiation than CD7, but is not as sensitive. Conversely, the CD2 antigen, which is fairly sensitive, is also expressed in a significant number of patients who have AML (37). Markers such as CD1a, CD3, and CD8, which show high degrees of specificity for T cells, are expressed in fewer than half of patients.

From a practical standpoint, the definition of T-lymphoblastic leukemia/lymphoma usually rests on interpretation of an overall pattern of reactivity with several immunologic markers (Fig. 40.4). Since most cases express several T-cell–associated markers, expression of a single aberrant or unexpected marker should not present a diagnostic dilemma. However, patients with T-lymphoblastic leukemia/lymphoma often do express antigens more commonly associated with other lineages. Thus, 20% to 30% of patients express CD10, and B-cell–associated antigens, including CD9, CD21, and CD24, may also be seen in some patients. Expression of myeloid antigens, especially CD13 and CD33, is not an infrequent occurrence. Awareness of these immunophenotypic patterns should prevent misclassification

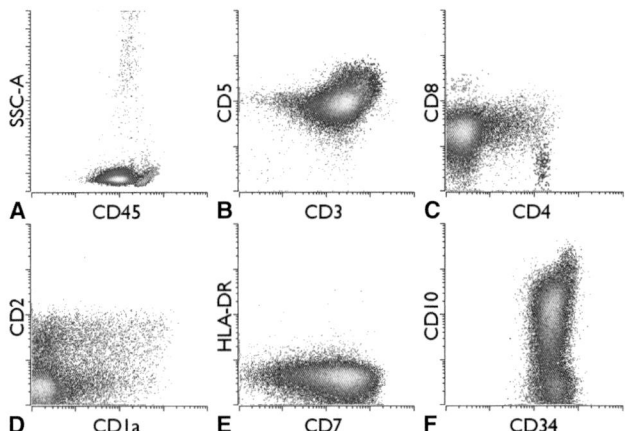

FIGURE 40.4. Flow cytometric immunophenotyping data from a representative case of T-lymphoblastic leukemia. (**A**) is gated on all viable cells, (**B** and **C**) are gated on blasts and normal mature T cells, and (**D–F**) are gated exclusively on blasts. Selected populations are denoted by color: *blue*, lymphoblasts; *magenta* (highlighted), normal CD4⁺ T cells; *yellow* (highlighted), normal CD8⁺ T cells. The blasts are weakly positive for CD45, display low SSC, and express several T-lineage antigens: CD1a (partial), CD2 (partial), CD3, CD5, and CD7. Note that the intensity of expression of CD3 and CD5 differs from that of normal T cells. The blasts are also CD34⁺, and a subset is CD10⁺; HLA-DR is negative. In this case, there is essentially homogeneous, but very weak expression of CD8, and a minor subset of the blasts shows weak coexpression of CD4 and CD8.

of an otherwise straightforward T-lymphoblastic leukemia/lymphoma as acute leukemia of ambiguous lineage (27).

In a minority of cases, lineage assignment on the basis of immunophenotype may remain unclear despite application of a suitable panel of surface-membrane markers. In such circumstances, evaluation of cytoplasmic antigen expression commonly resolves any diagnostic uncertainty. Functionally, the most sensitive and specific marker for T-lymphoblastic leukemia/lymphoma has proved to be CD3 expression in the cytoplasm (cyCD3) of lymphoblasts. In two of the largest reported series, cyCD3 was found in all patients with T-lymphoblastic leukemia/lymphoma tested (including those in whose blasts surface CD3 was not expressed), but was absent from cases of B-lymphoblastic leukemia/lymphoma and AML, including CD7⁺ AML (38,39). By analogy with cyCD3, the CD22 antigen is typically detected in the cytoplasm of lymphoblasts from cases of B-lymphoblastic leukemia/lymphoma, even when it is not expressed on the surface; cyCD22 is a very sensitive marker for B-lineage ALL (40,41). In contrast with the specificity of cyCD3 for T-cell lineage, cyCD22 has been detected in AML, although the cyCD22 antigen found in AML has been shown to be a cross-reacting protein (42). cyCD79a is also a highly sensitive marker of B-cell differentiation (43), but it is not lineage-specific. In particular, cyCD79a has been detected in some cases of T-lymphoblastic leukemia/lymphoma (44) and AML (45,46).

The nuclear antigen, terminal deoxynucleotidyl transferase (TdT), is a useful marker in distinguishing precursor lymphoid neoplasms from mature B-cell or T-cell neoplasms. TdT is expressed in >95% of cases of B-lymphoblastic leukemia/lymphoma, and somewhat fewer cases of T-lymphoblastic leukemia/lymphoma. It is important to note, though, that TdT is also positive (albeit generally more weakly than in ALL) in a significant minority of cases of AML (47,48), and is therefore not a specific indicator of ALL. When evaluated by immunocytochemistry in cytospin preparations of cerebrospinal fluid specimens, TdT expression may facilitate distinction between lymphoblasts and atypical lymphocytes.

Although a somewhat more limited repertoire of immunophenotypic markers is available for use in formalin-fixed paraffin-embedded material, immunohistochemistry frequently permits a diagnosis of lymphoblastic lymphoma/leukemia in tissue sections. Markers of immaturity in both

B- and T-lymphoblastic leukemia/lymphoma include TdT and CD34; expression of either virtually excludes a mature lymphoid neoplasm. CD79a and PAX5 are commonly used as B-lineage–related antigens. As noted above, though, CD79a may also be expressed in T-lymphoblastic leukemia/lymphoma (44) and AML (45,46), and despite the sensitivity of PAX5 for B lineage (49), this antigen has also been reported in AML, especially AML with t(8;21) (50,51). Additional markers of immaturity that may be useful in cases of CD34⁻/TdT⁻ T-lymphoblastic leukemia/lymphoma include CD1a and CD99 (52). Caution must be exercised in interpreting CD99 expression, however, as it is specific neither for T-cell lineage nor for hematolymphoid neoplasia; since lack of detectable CD45 is not exceptional in tissue sections of precursor lymphoid neoplasms, expression of CD99 in nonhematolymphoid tumors such as Ewing sarcoma is particularly noteworthy.

CYTOGENETICS

A number of cytogenetic abnormalities are recurrent in the precursor lymphoid neoplasms. In the case of B-lymphoblastic leukemia/lymphoma, these are used to define *B-lymphoblastic leukemia/lymphoma with recurrent genetic abnormalities* in the WHO classification (53, Table 40.1).

B-lymphoblastic leukemia/lymphoma with t(9;22)(q34;q11.2); BCR-ABL1. The "Philadelphia chromosome," t(9;22)(q34;q11.2), is present in approximately 3% and 25% of cases of childhood and adult ALL, respectively (54,55). Juxtaposition of the *ABL* oncogene on chromosome 9 and a gene called *BCR* on chromosome 22 results in the production of a *BCR-ABL* fusion protein with dysregulated tyrosine kinase activity. Although the same cytogenetic abnormality is seen in *chronic myelogenous leukemia, BCR-ABL1–positive* (CML, BCR-ABL1⁺), the breakpoint on chromosome 22 involves the so-called *minor breakpoint cluster region* (or *m-BCR*) in most cases of B-lymphoblastic leukemia/lymphoma with t(9;22)(q34;q11.2), rather than the major breakpoint cluster region (*M-BCR*) seen in most cases of CML, BCR-ABL1⁺ (56). The resulting fusion protein is approximately 190 kDa in most cases of B-lymphoblastic leukemia/lymphoma with t(9;22)(q34;q11.2), compared with 210 kDa in most cases of CML, BCR-ABL1⁺; of note, p190 has been shown to be a more potent transforming agent than p210 *in vitro* and in transgenic studies. Some authors have reported immunophenotypic-genotypic correlations in B-lymphoblastic leukemia/lymphoma with t(9;22)(q34;q11.2). For example, CD25 positivity appears to be more common among adults who have B-lymphoblastic leukemia/lymphoma with t(9;22)(q34;q11.2) compared with those whose ALL lacks the translocation (57). Another group has described a prototypic composite immunophenotype in adult B-lymphoblastic leukemia/lymphoma with t(9;22)(q34;q11.2): CD10⁺, CD13⁺, CD34⁺, with heterogeneous, dim CD38, which was seen in <5% of cases lacking the translocation (58).

B-lymphoblastic leukemia/lymphoma with t(v;11q23); MLL-rearranged. Approximately 10% of adults and slightly fewer children with ALL have a translocation involving *MLL* and one of its many potential fusion partners (54). Patients with ALL who have *MLL* rearrangements are commonly infants (among whom ALL with *MLL* rearrangements represents the most common type of leukemia), and present with hyperleukocytosis (often >100 × 10⁹/L), hepatosplenomegaly, and frequent CNS involvement. Virtually all patients with the t(4;11)(q21;q23), which results from fusion of *MLL* with its most common partner, *AF4*, have a unique immunophenotype. Specifically, the blasts are CD10⁻/CD19⁺, and either are negative for CD24 or show heterogeneity in expression of this antigen; moreover, many (though not all) patients are CD15⁺ (59,60). In most cases of B-lymphoblastic leukemia/lymphoma with t(v;11q23), the chondroitin sulfate proteoglycan recognized by monoclonal antibody 7.1 is also expressed (61,62).

B-lymphoblastic leukemia/lymphoma with t(12;21) (p13;q22); TEL-AML1 (ETV6-RUNX1). The single most commonly identified translocation in childhood B-lymphoblastic leukemia is also the most recently characterized. Through the use of fluorescence *in situ* hybridization (FISH) and reverse transcriptase–polymerase chain reaction (RT-PCR), a generally cryptic balanced translocation juxtaposing the *TEL* gene at 12p13 and the *AML1* gene at 21q22 was found to be highly prevalent in childhood ALL. The incidence of the *TEL-AML1* translocation in series of patients with childhood B-lymphoblastic leukemia/lymphoma has ranged from 16% to 29%, and in virtually all cases these translocations have not been detectable by conventional cytogenetics (63–67). In contrast, B-lymphoblastic leukemia/lymphoma with t(12;21)(p13;q22) is rare in adults, in whom it comprises approximately 2% of cases of ALL (54). The presence of this translocation may be predicted by the immunophenotypic characteristics of the blasts. Absence or low expression of CD9 is highly associated with this translocation, while expression of the marker KORSA-3544 virtually excludes it (68,69). Myeloid antigen expression is also more common, though the sensitivity and specificity of myeloid antigen expression for B-lymphoblastic leukemia/lymphoma with t(12;21)(p13;q22) are insufficient for diagnostic use (70).

B-lymphoblastic leukemia/lymphoma with hyperdiploidy. Strictly speaking, hyperdiploidy refers to the presence of greater than the normal complement of 46 chromosomes. However, a distinct clinicopathologic group of children with ALL has been described, in whose blasts the numbers of chromosomes range from about 51 to 65. Such patients account for about 25% of children with ALL; the finding is much less common (~7%) in adults, and rare in infancy (54). Patients who have this form of hyperdiploidy often have simple additions of structurally normal chromosomes, and almost invariably have B-lymphoblastic leukemia, which is usually CD10+. From a clinical perspective, hyperdiploidy is a favorable prognostic factor independent of all others, and children with hyperdiploid ALL have been shown to have a high cure rate even if they possess other poor risk features (71–73). This form of hyperdiploidy can be recognized by flow cytometry, and corresponds to samples with a DNA index that ranges from about 1.16 to 1.60 (71). However, more recent work suggests that the good prognosis associated with hyperdiploidy rests not in ploidy itself, but in the specific additions of chromosomes 4, 10, and 17 (74). Whether standard karyotyping and/or FISH (particularly if the former is unsuccessful) may be preferable to flow cytometric determination of the DNA index in defining this category is controversial (53).

B-lymphoblastic leukemia/lymphoma with hypodiploidy (hypodiploid ALL). Hypodiploidy, defined as the presence of fewer than 46 chromosomes, is an infrequent event in ALL; in a large series of children and adults, the incidence of hypodiploidy defined in this manner was 5% (75). When more narrowly defined as fewer than either 45 chromosomes (76) or 44 chromosomes (77), hypodiploid ALL comprises no more than 2% of cases in children or adults (54). As a group, patients with hypodiploid ALL appear to fare poorly, but whether a more pronounced negative prognostic effect is associated specifically with near-haploidy is controversial (75–77). Since near-haploid and low-hypodiploid clones may undergo endoreduplication to yield near-diploid and hyperdiploid clones, respectively (77), flow cytometric determination of DNA index may permit detection of a small hypodiploid subpopulation whose presence might be inapparent by standard karyotyping.

B-lymphoblastic leukemia/lymphoma with t(5;14)(q31;q32); IL3-IGH. In children and adults, rare cases of B-lymphoblastic leukemia have been described in association with hypereosinophilia and the translocation t(5;14)(q31;q32) (78,79). In half of the cases, hypereosinophilia preceded the diagnosis of ALL by several months; in the remainder, hypereosinophilia was noted at or subsequent to the time of diagnosis (78). The translocation fuses the immunoglobulin heavy chain locus with the *IL3* gene; in both cases evaluated, *IL3* mRNA or protein was expressed by the leukemic cells harboring the translocation, but not in controls (79). These findings suggest that *IL3* functions in an autocrine loop in these rare but distinctive cases of ALL (79).

B-lymphoblastic leukemia/lymphoma with t(1;19) (q23;p13.3); E2A-PBX1 (TCF3-PBX1). Approximately 5% of cases of ALL in childhood harbor a translocation juxtaposing *E2A* and *PBX1* (54). These cases characteristically display a pre–B-cell immunophenotype (i.e., positive for cytoplasmic μ heavy chain without surface-membrane immunoglobulin expression), and account for about 25% of cases of pre–B-cell ALL. The composite immunophenotype—homogeneous CD9+/CD10+/CD19+, with partial CD20, and complete absence of CD34, which is seen in only 8% of patients with childhood B lymphoblastic leukemia—identifies all cases harboring the *E2A-PBX1* fusion transcript resulting from the translocation t(1;19) (80). Although the t(1;19) abnormality was responsible for the poor prognosis of patients with pre–B-cell ALL treated with antimetabolite-based therapy (81), this adverse prognostic effect is overcome by more intensive therapy (82,83). A related but much less common translocation, t(17;19)(q21;p13), which juxtaposes *E2A* and *HLF*, has been documented at the molecular level in a smaller number of patients, and is associated with a poor prognosis (84).

Cytogenetics of T-lymphoblastic leukemia/lymphoma. In at least half of all cases of T-lymphoblastic leukemia/lymphoma, an abnormal karyotype is demonstrated by conventional cytogenetics (reviewed in refs. 85–87). Although these cytogenetic abnormalities are not used to define clinical or biologic entities in the current WHO classification (2), certain themes emerge. For instance, translocations involving T-cell–receptor genes (*TCRA* and *TCRD* at 14q11 and *TCRB* at 7q35) result in dysregulated expression of a number of partner genes, many of which are transcription factors. Examples include the t(7;10)(q34;q24) and t(10;14)(q24;q11) translocations that involve the homeobox gene, *HOX11* (seen in 7% and 31% of pediatric and adult cases, respectively), and the translocations t(1;14)(q32;q11) and t(1;7) (p32;q35), which juxtapose *TAL1*, and *TCRD* and *TCRB*, respectively, and together account for fewer than 5% of cases of T-lymphoblastic leukemia/lymphoma (85). Alternatively, often-cryptic rearrangements may result in the formation of abnormal fusion genes (85); examples include a cryptic interstitial deletion at 1p32 that fuses *SIL* and *TAL1* (seen in up to 30% of children and a smaller percentage of adults), and the t(10;11)(p13;q14) that fuses *CALM* and *AF10* (seen in ~10% of cases). A variation on the theme of fusion genes is the identification of amplified episomes harboring fused *NUP214-ABL1* in approximately 6% of cases of T-lymphoblastic leukemia/lymphoma (88); the apparent sensitivity of the resultant fusion tyrosine kinase to imatinib may have therapeutic implications. Finally, cryptic deletions may result in loss of tumor-suppressor genes; deletion of 9p21 involving *CDKN2A* is the most common example.

MOLECULAR CHARACTERISTICS

Essentially all B-lymphoblastic leukemias show clonal rearrangement of the immunoglobulin heavy chain (*IGH*) gene; however, this marker is nonspecific and has been noted in many patients with T-lymphoblastic leukemia and AML alike (89–91). Rearrangement or deletion of immunoglobulin light chain genes is a more specific marker for B-cell differentiation, though it is less sensitive. Clonal rearrangement of the T-cell receptor β-chain gene (*TCRB*), which occurs very early in the commitment of normal precursor cells to T-cell differentiation, is found in virtually all patients with T-lymphoblastic leukemia (92–96). The specificity of this rearrangement for T-cell lineage, however, or of rearrangements of the other *TCR* genes, is low (92,96–100).

In fact, most patients with B-lymphoblastic leukemia show rearrangement of at least one of the *TCR* genes, most often *TCRD* (98); even *TCRB* is rearranged in 20% to 30% of patients with B-lymphoblastic leukemia (97), as well as in some with AML (97,99). Rearrangements at the *TCR* loci are ongoing during the clinical evolution of an individual leukemia (101–103), an observation that has practical implications regarding molecular monitoring for minimal residual disease (MRD).

Genome-wide approaches, including analysis of copy-number alterations (CNAs) and gene expression profiling (GEP), have yielded additional insights into the molecular pathogenesis of the precursor lymphoid neoplasms (55,104). In a large study of childhood B-lymphoblastic leukemia, between six and seven CNAs were detected per case, with deletions outnumbering amplifications (105). Interestingly, CNAs were nonrandomly distributed among cytogenetic categories; *MLL*-rearranged cases had a mean of one lesion per case, compared with nearly seven lesions per case in those harboring *ETV6-RUNX1* (105), a finding compatible with differential requirements for additional genetic lesions in these clinically distinct forms of ALL (55,104). Deletions (and in the case of *PAX5*, mutations) were found in a number of known regulators of normal B-cell development including *PAX5*, *EBF1*, and *IKZF1* (105). *IKZF1* deletions were subsequently identified in 84% of B-lymphoblastic leukemia with *BCR-ABL1*, and in two of three cases of CML, *BCR-ABL1*⁺, in B-lymphoid blast (but not chronic) phase (106). Moreover, *IKZF1* deletions or mutations were associated with an increased incidence of relapse in cohorts of high-risk B-lymphoblastic leukemia, even after excluding cases with *BCR-ABL1* (107). Another recently described genetic abnormality in B-lymphoblastic leukemia is rearrangement of *CRLF2*, which appears to be associated with activating *JAK* mutations and Down syndrome–associated ALL (108–111). Whether the adverse prognostic effect of *CRLF2* rearrangement is independent of other clinical and genetic risk factors, though, is controversial (109,111,112). In a recent study, novel somatic mutations in *CREBBP* were described (113); these were overrepresented among patients who relapsed, leading the authors to suggest a role for *CREBBP* in response to therapy and risk of relapse in B-lymphoblastic leukemia. In childhood T-lymphoblastic leukemia, activating mutations in *NOTCH1* are identified in >50% of cases, and appear to be associated with improved relapse-free survival independent of a number of standard risk factors (114).

On the basis of GEP, the common genetic categories of B-lymphoblastic leukemia (i.e., *BCR-ABL1*, *ETV6-RUNX1*, *E2A-PBX1*, *MLL*-rearranged, hyperdiploid) can be identified, and distinguished from T-lymphoblastic leukemia (115) and AML (116). More recent work has identified gene expression signatures predictive of outcome in high-risk pediatric B-lymphoblastic leukemia (117,118). In the larger of these studies (118), signatures predictive of relapse-free survival and end-induction MRD status by flow cytometry were combined, to yield a signature predictive of outcome independent of other known risk factors. In T-lymphoblastic leukemia, GEP has been used to identify categories of disease sharing common transcriptional patterns (119,120). In a seminal study, three distinct groups of T-lymphoblastic leukemia were segregated on the basis of overexpression of *LYL1*, *HOX11*, or *TAL1*, and the GEPs of these groups were correlated with stages of normal T-cell development (119). In this study, the *HOX11*-overexpressing group, whose GEP resembled that of early cortical thymocytes, enjoyed a favorable prognosis (119). Using a similar approach, a second group proposed the existence of additional categories of T-lymphoblastic leukemia, whose GEPs could be distinguished from each other on the basis of differential expression of both oncogenes and genes known to be regulated during normal T-lymphopoiesis (120). More recently, GEP has been used to identify an apparently distinct subtype of T-lymphoblastic leukemia whose prognosis is poor with conventional therapy

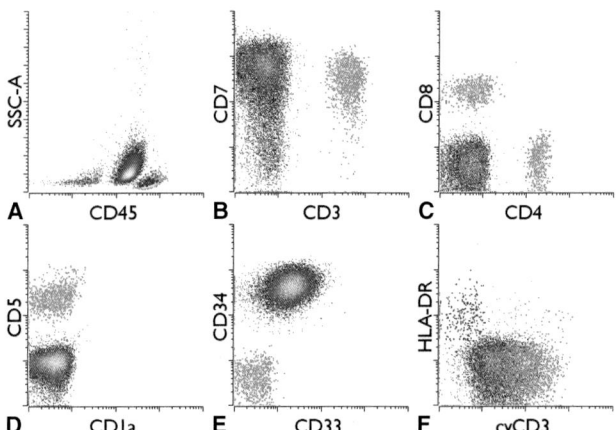

FIGURE 40.5. Flow cytometric immunophenotyping data from a case of ETP leukemia. (**A**) is gated on all viable cells, (**B–E**) are gated on blasts and normal mature T cells, and (**F**) is gated on blasts, normal mature T cells, and B cells. Selected populations are denoted by color: *blue*, lymphoblasts; *magenta* (highlighted), normal B cells; *yellow* (highlighted), normal mature T cells. The blasts are weakly CD45⁺, with low SSC, and express bright CD7, and cytoplasmic CD3. In addition, the blasts display the four immunophenotypic characteristics of ETP leukemia (121). They are (i) CD1a⁻, (ii) CD8⁻, with (iii) no more than weak CD5 in <75% of the blasts (in this case negative), and (iv) coexpression of at least one myeloid and/or stem-cell antigen (in this case, CD33 and CD34, respectively) in at least 25% of the blasts.

(121). So-called *early T-cell precursor leukemia* was identified on the basis of it having a GEP similar to that of *early T-cell precursors* (ETPs), a recently described subset of normal thymocytes that have been shown to be multipotent (122,123). Importantly, most cases of T-lymphoblastic leukemia with a GEP similar to that of ETPs were shown to have a distinctive immunophenotype: CD1a⁻, CD8⁻, with weak CD5 in fewer than 75% of the lymphoblasts, and expression of at least one myeloid or stem-cell marker (i.e., CD11b, CD13, CD33, CD34, CD65, CD117, or HLA-DR) in at least 25% of the lymphoblasts (121; Fig. 40.5). In two independent clinical cohorts, the ETP GEP or its distinctive immunophenotype identified a subset (~13%) of patients, most of whom had relapsed at last follow-up (121).

 ## POSTULATED NORMAL COUNTERPARTS

In the case of B-lymphoblastic leukemia/lymphoma, the postulated normal counterparts are B-cell precursors found in the bone marrow, often referred to as *hematogones* (124). These cells display stereotypical patterns of immunophenotypic maturation, which permit their distinction from MRD by flow cytometry (Fig. 40.6). In the case of T-lymphoblastic leukemia/lymphoma, the postulated normal counterparts are T-cell precursors, which originate in the bone marrow, but mature within the thymus. As discussed above, immunophenotypic and molecular similarities have been noted between putative subtypes of T-lymphoblastic leukemia and normal T-cell precursors at different stages of maturation (119–121).

CLINICAL COURSE AND PROGNOSTIC ASSESSMENT

The clinical course of ALL is diverse. Yet it has become clear, particularly in children, that it is possible to distinguish patients who are likely to be cured from those whose outcome is likely to be less favorable on the basis of a constellation of clinical and laboratory features. As therapies have evolved, and overall survival has improved, some of these predictors have become insignificant or redundant. Nonetheless, age and WBC count remain among the most robust clinical factors predictive of outcome (104), and virtually all algorithms for assignment of children to risk groups for therapeutic purposes have included these features (125–128). Age <1 year and >10 years are adverse features, as is high WBC count (e.g., >50 × 10^9/L).

Also important as prognostic factors are biologic features of the leukemic blasts. Most notable among these are the lesions that define the categories of B-lymphoblastic leukemia/lymphoma with recurrent genetic abnormalities. *BCR-ABL1*$^+$, *MLL*-rearranged, and hypodiploid ALL are unfavorable categories, while *ETV6-RUNX1*$^+$ and hyperdiploid ALL are generally regarded as favorable (53,104,129). It is important to note, though, that clinical and biologic features are closely intertwined. For example, T-cell immunophenotype is associated with older age and high WBC count, both of which are adverse clinical factors, and T-cell immunophenotype *per se* is not an independent adverse feature in all studies (125). Similarly, the superior prognosis of ALL in children relative to that in infants and adults (130) correlates with the increased proportion of favorable-risk genetic abnormalities (i.e., hyperdiploidy and *ETV6-RUNX1*) in the former, and adverse-risk genetic abnormalities (i.e., *MLL-AF4* and *BCR-ABL1*) in the latter (54,87). Even within biologically defined categories, though, clinical features may, nonetheless, impact outcome; thus, the prognosis of children with *MLL-AF4*$^+$ and *BCR-ABL1*$^+$ ALL is superior to that of infants and adults, respectively, with identical genetic abnormalities (104).

Response to therapy has also emerged as an important prognostic marker in ALL. It is perhaps not surprising that the small proportion of children who have ALL and fail to enter complete remission at the end of induction therapy are at very high risk for treatment failure (126). In the vast majority of patients who do attain a complete morphologic remission, however, the presence of *minimal residual disease*, which is below a level that can be determined on the basis of morphologic examination, is one of the strongest predictors of relapse risk (reviewed in ref. 131). MRD in ALL can be detected either by multiparameter flow cytometric immunophenotyping or by polymerase chain reaction (PCR)–mediated amplification of antigen receptor or fusion genes. Flow cytometric detection of MRD relies upon immunophenotypic aberrations routinely found in leukemic cells that permit their distinction from normal B- and T-cell precursors (24; Fig. 40.6). Through the use of

appropriate panels (132) of immunophenotypic markers, more of which continue to be described (133,134), 1 leukemic cell in 10,000 normal cells (i.e., 0.01% or 10^{-4}) can be detected. PCR-based MRD detection requires sequencing of antigen receptor gene rearrangements to generate patient-specific primers; though molecular methods are more labor-intensive than immunophenotypic methods, they are also potentially more sensitive, in that 1 leukemic cell in 100,000 (0.001% or 10^{-5}) can be detected (135). Quantification of MRD at varying time points after initiation of therapy, whether by immunophenotypic or molecular methods, is now an established component of risk classification algorithms in childhood ALL (126,128,136), and has demonstrated similar potential in adult ALL (137).

TREATMENT AND SURVIVAL

The treatment of ALL in childhood represents one of the great success stories of chemotherapy. In studies from the early 1960s, the 5-year event-free survival of children who had ALL was <10%, whereas >90% of children treated in the early 2000s were alive at 5 years (3), and at least 80% of children treated in the 1990s are long-term survivors (128,138). Treatment is generally divided into three phases: (i) *induction*, (ii) *consolidation* or *intensification*, and (iii) *continuation* or *maintenance* (reviewed in refs. 3,104). Although the precise medications and dosages vary among different risk groups, protocols, and centers, a combination of three or four drugs is used most commonly; these typically include a glucocorticoid and vincristine, to which asparaginase and/or an anthracycline are added. In patients who have *BCR-ABL1*$^+$ ALL, targeted therapy with imatinib may also be safely added (139). Following successful remission induction, which results in eradication of >99% of the tumor burden, and restoration of normal hematopoiesis, patients may undergo any of several forms of intensification. These include high-dose methotrexate plus mercaptopurine, high-dose asparaginase, reinduction, or, in appropriately selected high-risk patients, myeloablative therapy followed by allogeneic stem-cell transplant. Because many patients treated with moderately intensive chemotherapy for a period of <18 months subsequently relapse, and cannot be identified prospectively, treatment must be continued for a total of at least 2 years. In most instances, continuation treatment includes weekly methotrexate and daily mercaptopurine. Also well established is the need for CNS prophylaxis in the form of intrathecal chemotherapy. Depending on the risk of CNS relapse, intrathecal chemotherapy is sometimes supplemented with cranial irradiation; however, because of the complications of cranial irradiation in children, which include neurocognitive deficits, secondary malignancies, and endocrinopathy, attempts to minimize or eliminate prophylactic cranial irradiation have been undertaken (140).

As discussed above, children who have ALL are stratified on the basis of a number of important clinical and laboratory features, and therapy is tailored to the individual patient's risk group. Patients deemed to be at higher risk are treated more intensively, while those at lower risk are treated so as to limit unnecessary toxicity. With contemporary therapies, approximately 90% of patients with favorable-risk (e.g., hyperdiploid, *ETV6-RUNX1*$^+$) B-lymphoblastic leukemia, 80% to 85% of patients with standard-risk B-lymphoblastic leukemia, and 70% to 75% of patients with T-lymphoblastic leukemia are cured (reviewed in ref. 104). Those with other lesions, including *BCR-ABL1* and *MLL-AF4*, have traditionally fared more poorly (104), although the addition of a tyrosine kinase inhibitor to therapy for *BCR-ABL1*$^+$ ALL shows great promise in improving outcome (139). The prognosis of ALL in adults as a group is inferior to that in children. In most studies, fewer than 40% of adult patients are long-term survivors, though most do

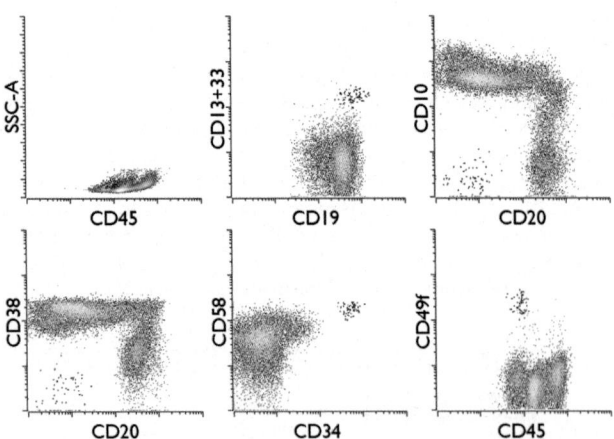

FIGURE 40.6. Detection of MRD by flow cytometric immunophenotyping in B-lymphoblastic leukemia. In all panels, MRD detected at the end of induction therapy is highlighted in *magenta*; normal B cells at all stages of maturation from an identically stained control bone marrow specimen are shown in *light blue* for comparison. In this example, MRD comprised 0.02% of viable cells in the day 29 (end-induction) bone marrow specimen. The immunophenotype of the leukemic blasts differs from that of normal B-cell precursors in multiple respects: CD10 and CD38 are absent, CD19 and CD58 are somewhat brighter than expected, CD34 and CD49f are abnormally bright, and there is myeloid antigen (CD13/CD33) coexpression.

enter remission initially (reviewed in ref. 3). Moreover, risk stratification on the basis of conventional clinical and biologic features, such as age and *BCR-ABL1*⁺ positivity, is not as precise in adults as in children, though molecular assessment of MRD may represent a significant advance in this regard (137). Suitable adult patients may be referred for allogeneic stem-cell transplant, but in one study, the overall survival benefit accrued principally to standard-risk patients (141).

DIFFERENTIAL DIAGNOSIS

Neoplasms that must be distinguished from lymphoblastic leukemia/lymphoma include AML and its extramedullary tumoral counterpart, *myeloid sarcoma*. Many small round cell tumors of childhood may also present with bone marrow involvement, and in the absence of a clinically obvious mass, the potential exists for these tumors to be confused with lymphoblastic leukemia/lymphoma. In addition to careful morphologic examination, immunophenotyping by flow cytometry and/or immunohistochemistry generally permits distinction among these diagnostic entities. A benign condition that may also be mistaken for lymphoblastic leukemia/lymphoma is the increase in normal B-cell precursors that is seen in infants, and in some children who have cytopenias (124). As noted above, immunophenotypic distinction between leukemic B-lymphoblasts and hematogones is readily accomplished by multiparameter flow cytometry provided the phenotype of the latter cells is well understood (24).

SUMMARY AND CONCLUSIONS

In this chapter, we have attempted to describe the diversity of what was once thought to be a simple disease. As reflected to some extent in the current WHO classification, though, acute lymphoblastic leukemia/lymphoma encompasses not a single disease, but several. A more complete understanding of the varied biology of ALL/lymphoma should enable increasingly precise tailoring of therapy to individual patients, sparing those with favorable disease unnecessary toxicity, and affording those with unfavorable disease an improved chance of survival.

References

1. Borowitz MJ, Chan JKC. B lymphoblastic leukaemia/lymphoma, not otherwise specified. In: Swerdlow SH, Campo E, Harris NL, et al., eds. *WHO classification of tumours of haematopoietic and lymphoid tissues*, 4th ed. Lyon: International Agency for Research on Cancer, 2008:168–170.
2. Borowitz MJ, Chan JKC. T lymphoblastic leukaemia/lymphoma. In: Swerdlow SH, Campo E, Harris NL, et al., eds. *WHO classification of tumours of haematopoietic and lymphoid tissues*, 4th ed. Lyon: International Agency for Research on Cancer, 2008:176–178.
3. Pui C-H, Evans WE. Treatment of acute lymphoblastic leukemia. *N Engl J Med* 2006;354:166–178.
4. Siegel R, Naishadham D, Jemal A. Cancer statistics, 2013. CA: *Cancer J Clin* 2013;63:11–30.
5. United States National Cancer Institute Surveillance Epidemiology and End Results, 2004–2008. Available at: http://seer.cancer.gov/statfacts/html/alyl.html
6. Yang JJ, Cheng C, Devidas M, et al. Ancestry and pharmacogenomics of relapse in acute lymphoblastic leukemia. *Nature Genet* 2011;43:237–242.
7. Maloney KW, Carroll WL, Carroll AJ, et al. Down syndrome childhood acute lymphoblastic leukemia has a unique spectrum of sentinel cytogenetic lesions that influences treatment outcome: a report from the Children's Oncology Group. *Blood* 2010;116:1045–1050.
8. Toledano SR, Lange BJ. Ataxia-telangiectasia and acute lymphoblastic leukemia. *Cancer* 1980;45:1675–1678.
9. Taub JW, Konrad MA, Ge Y, et al. High frequency of leukemic clones in newborn screening blood samples of children with B-precursor acute lymphoblastic leukemia. *Blood* 2002;99:2992–2996.
10. Fischer S, Mann G, Konrad M, et al. Screening for leukemia- and clone-specific markers at birth in children with T-cell precursor ALL suggests a predominantly postnatal origin. *Blood* 2007;110:3036–3038.
11. Greaves MF, Maia AT, Wiemels JL, et al. Leukemias in twins: lessons in natural history. *Blood* 2003;102:2321–2333.
12. Greaves MF, Janossy G, Peto J, et al. Immunologically defined subclasses of acute lymphoblastic leukaemia in children: their relationship to presentation features and prognosis. *Br J Haematol* 1981;48:179–197.
13. Borowitz MJ. Immunologic markers in childhood acute lymphoblastic leukemia. *Hematol Oncol Clin North Am* 1990;4:743–765.
14. Bennett JM, Catovsky D, Daniel MT, et al. Proposals for the classification of the acute leukaemias. *Br J Haematol* 1976;33:451–458.
15. Bennett JM, Catovsky D, Daniel MT, et al. The morphologic classification of acute lymphoblastic leukaemia: concordance among observers and clinical correlations. *Br J Haematol* 1981;47:553–561.
16. Leoncini L, Raphael M, Stein H, et al. Burkitt lymphoma. In: Swerdlow SH, Campo E, Harris NL, et al., eds. *WHO classification of tumours of haematopoietic and lymphoid tissues*, 4th ed. Lyon: International Agency for Research on Cancer, 2008:262–264.
17. Schumacher HR, Perlin E, Klos JR, et al. Hand-mirror cell leukemia, a new clinical and morphological variant. *Am J Clin Pathol* 1977;68:531–534.
18. Schumacher HR, Champion JE, Thomas NJ, et al. Acute lymphoblastic leukemia hand-mirror variant: an analysis of a large group of patients. *Am J Hematol* 1979;7:11–17.
19. Glassy EF, Sun NCJ, Okun DB. Hand-mirror cell leukemia: report of 9 cases and a review of literature. *Am J Clin Pathol* 1980;74:651–656.
20. Cerezo L, Shuster JJ, Pullen DJ, et al. Laboratory correlates and prognostic significance of granular acute lymphoblastic leukemia in children: a Pediatric Oncology Group study. *Am J Clin Pathol* 1991;95:526–531.
21. Grogan TM, Insalaco SJ, Savage RA, et al. Acute lymphocytic leukemia with prominent azurophilic granulation and punctate acidic nonspecific esterase and phosphatase activity. *Am J Clin Pathol* 1981;75:716–722.
22. Davey FR, Mick R, Nelson DA, et al. Morphologic and cytochemical characterization of adult lymphoid leukemias which express myeloid antigen. *Leukemia* 1988;2:420–426.
23. DiGiuseppe J, Borowitz MJ. Clinical applications of flow cytometric immunophenotyping in acute lymphoblastic leukemia. In: Stewart C, Nicholson JKA, eds. *Immunophenotyping*. New York: Wiley-Liss, 2000:161–180.
24. DiGiuseppe JA. Acute lymphoblastic leukemia: diagnosis and detection of minimal residual disease following therapy. *Clin Lab Med* 2007;27:533–549.
25. Stetler-Stevenson M, Ahmad E, Barnett D, et al. *Clinical flow cytometric analysis of neoplastic hematolymphoid cells; Approved guideline*, 2nd ed. Wayne: Clinical and Laboratory Standards Institute, 2007.
26. Kroft S, Karandikar NJ. Flow cytometric analysis of acute leukemias, myelodysplastic syndromes, and myeloproliferative disorders. In: Carey J, McCoy JP, Keren DF, eds. *Flow cytometry in clinical diagnosis*, 4th ed. Chicago: American Society for Clinical Pathology Press, 2007:167–214.
27. Borowitz MJ, Bene M-C, Harris NL. Acute leukaemias of ambiguous lineage. In: Swerdlow SH, Campo E, Harris NL, et al., eds. *WHO classification of tumours of haematopoietic and lymphoid tissues*, 4th ed. Lyon: International Agency for Research on Cancer, 2008:150–155.
28. Vasef MA, Brynes RK, Murata-Collins JL, et al. Surface immunoglobulin light chain-positive acute lymphoblastic leukemia of FAB L1 or L2 type: a report of 6 cases in adults. *Am J Clin Pathol* 1998;110:143–149.
29. Behm FG, Head DR, Pui C-H, et al. B-precursor ALL with unexpected expression of surface immunoglobulin m and lambda. *Mod Pathol* 1995;8:106.
30. Kansal R, Deeb G, Barcos M, et al. Precursor B lymphoblastic leukemia with surface light chain immunoglobulin restriction: a report of 15 patients. *Am J Clin Pathol* 2004;121: 512–525.
31. Navid F, Mosijczuk AD, Head DR, et al. Acute lymphoblastic leukemia with the t(8;14)(q24;q32) translocation and FAB-L3 morphology associated with a B-precursor immunophenotype: the Pediatric Oncology Group experience. *Leukemia* 1999;13:135–141.
32. Koehler M, Behm FG, Shuster J, et al. Transitional pre-B-cell acute lymphoblastic leukemia of childhood is associated with favorable prognostic clinical features and an excellent outcome: a Pediatric Oncology Group study. *Leukemia* 1993;7:2064–2068.
33. Link M, Warnke R, Finlay J, et al. A single monoclonal antibody identifies T cell lineage of childhood lymphoid malignancies. *Blood* 1983;62:722–728.
34. Pittaluga S, Raffeld M, Lipford EH, et al. 3A1 (CD7) expression precedes T gene rearrangements in precursor T lymphoblastic neoplasms. *Blood* 1986;68: 134–139.
35. Borowitz MJ, Dowell BL, Boyett JM, et al. Monoclonal antibody definition of T cell acute leukemia: a Pediatric Oncology Group study. *Blood* 1985;65:785–788.
36. Greaves MF, Chan LC, Furley AJW, et al. Lineage promiscuity in hematopoietic differentiation and leukemia. *Blood* 1986;67:1–11.
37. Mirro J, Antouin GR, Zipf TF, et al. The E rosette associated antigen of T cells can be identified on blasts from patients with acute myeloblastic leukemia. *Blood* 1985;65:363–367.
38. Sartor M, Bradstock K. Detection of intracellular lymphoid differentiation antigens by flow cytometry in acute lymphoblastic leukemia. *Cytometry* 1994;18: 119–122.
39. van Dongen JJM, Krissansen GW, Wolvers-Tettero ILM, et al. Cytoplasmic expression of the CD3 antigen as a diagnostic marker for immature T cell malignancies. *Blood* 1988;71:603–612.
40. Janossy G, Coustan-Smith E, Campana D. The reliability of cytoplasmic CD3 and CD22 antigen expression in the immunodiagnosis of acute leukemia: a study of 500 cases. *Leukemia* 1989;3:170–181.
41. Campana D, Janossy G, Bofill M, et al. Human B cell development: I. Phenotypic differences of B lymphocytes in the bone marrow and peripheral lymphoid tissue. *J Immunol* 1985;134:1524–1530.
42. Boue DR, LeBien TW. Expression and structure of CD22 in acute leukemia. *Blood* 1988;71:1480–1486.
43. Kappelmayer J, Gratama JW, Karaszi E, et al. Flow cytometric detection of intracellular myeloperoxidase, CD3 and CD79a: interaction between monoclonal antibody clones, fluorochromes and sample preparation protocols. *J Immunol Methods* 2000;242:53–65.
44. Lai R, Juco J, Lee SF, et al. Flow cytometric detection of CD79a expression in T-cell acute lymphoblastic leukemias. *Am J Clin Pathol* 2000;113:823–830.
45. Arber DA, Jenkins KA. Paraffin section immunophenotyping of acute leukemias in bone marrow specimens. *Am J Clin Pathol* 1996;106:462–468.
46. Kozlov I, Beason K, Yu C. CD79a expression in acute myeloid leukemia t(8;21) and the importance of cytogenetics in the diagnosis of leukemias with immunophenotypic ambiguity. *Cancer Genet Cytogenet* 2005;163:62–67.
47. Farahat N, Lens D, Morilla R, et al. Differential TdT expression in acute leukemia by flow cytometry: a quantitative study. *Leukemia* 1995;9:583–587.

48. Jani P, Verbi W, Greaves MF, et al. Terminal deoxynucleotidyl transferase in acute myeloid leukemia. *Leuk Res* 1983;7:17–29.
49. Torlakovic E, Torlakovic G, Nguyen PL. The value of anti-pax-5 immunostaining in routinely fixed and paraffin-embedded sections: a novel pan pre-B and B-cell marker. *Am J Surg Pathol* 2002;26:1343–1350.
50. Tiacci E, Pileri S, Orleth A, et al. PAX5 expression in acute leukemias. Higher B-lineage specificity than CD79a and selective association with t(8;21)-acute myelogenous leukemia. *Cancer Res* 2004;64:7399–7404.
51. Valbuena JR, Medeiros LJ, Rassidakis GZ, et al. Expression of B cell–specific activator protein/PAX5 in acute myeloid leukemia with t(8;21)(q22;q22). *Am J Clin Pathol* 2006;126:235–240.
52. Robertson PB, Neiman RS, Worapongpaiboon S, et al. 013 (CD99) positivity in hematologic proliferations correlates with TdT positivity. *Mod Pathol* 1997;10:277–282.
53. Borowitz MJ, Chan JKC. B lymphoblastic leukaemia/lymphoma with recurrent genetic abnormalities. In: Swerdlow SH, Campo E, Harris NL, et al., eds. *WHO classification of tumours of haematopoietic and lymphoid tissues*, 4th ed. Lyon: International Agency for Research on Cancer, 2008:171–175.
54. Pui C-H, Relling MV, Downing JR. Acute lymphoblastic leukemia. *N Engl J Med* 2004;350:1535–1548.
55. Pui C-H, Carroll WL, Meshinchi S, et al. Biology, risk stratification, and therapy of pediatric acute leukemias: an update. *J Clin Oncol* 2011;29:551–565.
56. Mrozek K, Heerema NA, Bloomfield CD. Cytogenetics in acute leukemia. *Blood Rev* 2004;18:115–136.
57. Paietta E, Racevskis J, Neuberg D, et al. Expression of CD25 (interleukin-2 receptor alpha chain) in adult acute lymphoblastic leukemia predicts for the presence of BCR/ABL fusion transcripts: results of a preliminary laboratory analysis of ECOG/MRC Intergroup Study E2993. *Leukemia* 1997;11:1887–1890.
58. Tabernero MD, Bortoluci AM, Alaejos I, et al. Adult precursor B-ALL with BCR/ABL gene rearrangements displays a unique immunophenotype based on the pattern of CD10, CD34, CD13 and CD38 expression. *Leukemia* 2001;15:406–414.
59. Pui C-H, Frankel LS, Carroll AJ, et al. Clinical characteristics and treatment outcome of childhood acute lymphoblastic leukemia with the t(4;11)(q21;q23): a collaborative study of 40 cases. *Blood* 1991;77:440–447.
60. Ludwig W-D, Rieder H, Bartram CR, et al. Immunophenotypic and genotypic features, clinical characteristics, and treatment outcomes of adult pro-B acute lymphoblastic leukemia: results of the German multicenter trials GMALL 03/87 and 04/89. *Blood* 1998;92:1898–1909.
61. Schwartz S, Rieder H, Schlaeger B, et al. Expression of the human homologue of rat NG2 in adult acute lymphoblastic leukemia: close association with MLL rearrangement and a $CD10^-/CD24^-/CD65s^+/CD15^+$ B-cell phenotype. *Leukemia* 2003;17:1589–1595.
62. Behm FG, Smith FO, Raimondi SC, et al. The human homologue of the rat chondroitin sulfate proteoglycan, NG2, detected by monoclonal antibody 7.1, identifies childhood acute lymphoblastic leukemias with t(4;11)(q21;q23) or t(11;19)(q23;p13) and MLL gene rearrangements. *Blood* 1996;87:1134–1139.
63. Romana SP, Poirel H, Leconiat M, et al. High frequency of t(12;21) in childhood B lineage acute lymphoblastic leukemia. *Blood* 1995;86:4263–4269.
64. Shurtleff SA, Buijs A, Behm FG, et al. TEL/AML1 fusion resulting from a cryptic t(12;21) is the most common genetic lesion in pediatric ALL and defines a subgroup of patients with an excellent prognosis. *Leukemia* 1995;9:1985–1989.
65. McLean TW, Ringold S, Neuberg D, et al. TEL/AML 1 dimerizes and is associated with a favorable outcome in childhood acute lymphoblastic leukemia. *Blood* 1996;88:4252–4258.
66. Rubnitz JE, Downing JR, Pui C-H, et al. TEL gene rearrangement in acute lymphoblastic leukemia: a new genetic marker with prognostic significance. *J Clin Oncol* 1997;15:1150–1157.
67. Borkhardt A, Cazzaniga G, Viehmann S, et al. Incidence and clinical relevance of TEL/AML1 fusion genes in children with acute lymphoblastic leukemia enrolled in the German and Italian multicenter therapy trials. *Blood* 1997;90:571–577.
68. Borowitz MB, Rubnitz J, Nash D, et al. Surface antigen phenotype can predict TEL AML1 rearrangement in childhood B precursor ALL: a pediatric oncology group study. *Leukemia* 1998;12:1764–1770.
69. Hrusak O,Trka J, Zuna J, et al. Aberrant expression of KOR SA3544 antigen in childhood acute lymphoblastic leukemia predicts TEL AML1 negativity. *Leukemia* 1998;12:1064–1070.
70. Baruchel A, Cayuela JM, Ballerini P, et al. The majority of myeloid antigen positive (My+) childhood B cell precursor acute lymphoblastic leukemias express TEL AML1 fusion transcripts. *Br J Haematol* 1997;99:101–106.
71. Look AT, Roberson PK, Williams DL, et al. Prognostic importance of blast cell DNA content in childhood acute lymphoblastic leukemia. *Blood* 1985;65:1079–1085.
72. Kalwinsky DK, Roberson P, Dahl G, et al. Clinical relevance of lymphoblast biological features in children with acute lymphoblastic leukemia. *J Clin Oncol* 1985;3:477–484.
73. Williams DL, Tsiatis A, Brodeur GM, et al. Prognostic importance of chromosome number in 136 untreated children with acute lymphoblastic leukemia. *Blood* 1982;60:864–871.
74. Sutcliffe MJ, Shuster JJ, Sather HN, et al. High concordance from independent studies by the Children's Cancer Group (CCG) and Pediatric Oncology Group (POG) associating favorable prognosis with combined trisomies 4, 10, and 17 in children with NCI standard-risk B-precursor acute lymphoblastic leukemia: a Children's Oncology Group (COG) initiative. *Leukemia* 2005;19:734–740.
75. Harrison CJ, Moorman AV, Broadfield ZJ, et al. Three distinct groups of hypodiploidy in acute lymphoblastic leukaemia. *Br J Haematol* 2004;125:552–559.
76. Pui CH, Carroll AJ, Raimondi SC, et al. Clinical presentation, karyotypic characterization and treatment outcome of childhood acute lymphoblastic leukemia with a near haploid or hypodiploid <45 line. *Blood* 1990;75:1170–1177.
77. Nachman JB, Heerema NA, Sather H, et al. Outcome of treatment in children with hypodiploid acute lymphoblastic leukemia. *Blood* 2007;110:1112–1115.
78. Hogan TF, Koss W, Murgo AJ, et al. Acute lymphoblastic leukemia with chromosomal 5;14 translocation and hypereosinophilia: case report and literature review. *J Clin Oncol* 1987;5:382–390.
79. Meeker TC, Hardy D, Willman C, et al. Activation of the interleukin-3 gene by chromosome translocation in acute lymphocytic leukemia with eosinophilia. *Blood* 1990;76:285–289.
80. Borowitz MJ, Hunger SP, Carroll AJ, et al. Predictability of the t(1;19)(q23;p13) from surface antigen phenotype: implications for screening cases of childhood acute lymphoblastic leukemia for molecular analysis: a Pediatric Oncology Group study. *Blood* 1993;82:1086–1091.
81. Crist WM, Carroll AJ, Shuster JJ, et al. Poor prognosis of children with pre-B acute lymphoblastic leukemia is associated with the t(1;19) (q23;p13): a Pediatric Oncology Group study. *Blood* 1990;76:117–122.
82. Rivera GK, Raimondi SC, Hancock ML, et al. Improved outcome in childhood acute lymphoblastic leukaemia with reinforced early treatment and rotational combination chemotherapy. *Lancet* 1991;337:61–66.
83. Pui CH, Raimondi SC, Hancock ML, et al. Immunologic, cytogenetic, and clinical characterization of childhood acute lymphoblastic leukemia with the t(1;19)(q23; p13) or its derivative. *J Clin Oncol* 1994;12:2601–2606.
84. Hunger SP. Chromosomal translocations involving the E2A gene in acute lymphoblastic leukemia: clinical features and molecular pathogenesis. *Blood* 1996;87:1211–1224.
85. Graux C, Cools J, Michaux L, et al. Cytogenetics and molecular genetics of T-cell acute lymphoblastic leukemia: from thymocyte to lymphoblast. *Leukemia* 2006;20:1496–1510.
86. Han X, Bueso-Ramos CE. Precursor T-cell acute lymphoblastic leukemia/lymphoblastic lymphoma and acute biphenotypic leukemias. *Am J Clin Pathol* 2007;127:528–544.
87. Harrison CJ. Cytogenetics of paediatric and adolescent acute lymphoblastic leukaemia. *Br J Haematol* 2009;144:147–156.
88. Graux C, Cools J, Melotte C, et al. Fusion of NUP214 to ABL1 on amplified episomes in T-cell acute lymphoblastic leukemia. *Nat Genet* 2004;36:1084–1089.
89. Korsmeyer SJ, Arnold A, Bakahshi A, et al. Immunoglobulin gene rearrangement and cell surface antigen expression in acute lymphocytic leukemias of T cell and B cell origins. *J Clin Invest* 1983;71:301–313.
90. Kitchingman GR, Rovigatti U, Mauer AM, et al. Rearrangement of immunoglobulin heavy chain genes in T cell acute lymphoblastic leukemia. *Blood* 1985;65:725–729.
91. Pugh WC, Stass SA. Immunoglobulin gene rearrangement and its implications for the study of B cell neoplasia. *Clin Lab Med* 1988;8:45–64.
92. Knowles DM, Pelicci PG, Dalla Favera R. T cell receptor beta chain gene rearrangements: genetic markers of T cell lineage and clonality. *Human Pathol* 1986;17:546–551.
93. Pittaluga S, Uppenkamp M, Cossman J. Development of T3/T cell receptor gene expression in human preT neoplasms. *Blood* 1987;69:1062–1067.
94. Waldmann TA, Davis MM, Bongiovanni KF, et al. Rearrangements of genes for the antigen receptor on T cells as markers of lineage and clonality in human lymphoid neoplasms. *N Engl J Med* 1985;313:776–783.
95. Mirro J Jr, Kitchingman G, Behm FG, et al. T cell differentiation stages identified by molecular and immunologic analysis of the T cell receptor complex in childhood lymphoblastic leukemia. *Blood* 1987;69:908–912.
96. Minden MD, Mak TW. The structure of the T cell antigen receptor genes in normal and malignant T cells. *Blood* 1986;327–339.
97. Tawa A, Hozumi N, Minden M, et al. Rearrangement of the T cell receptor β chain gene in non-T cell, non-B cell acute lymphoblastic leukemia of childhood. *N Engl J Med* 1985;313:1033–1037.
98. Griesinger F, Greenberg JM, Kersey JH. T cell receptor gamma and delta rearrangements in hematologic malignancies. *J Clin Invest* 1989;84:506–516.
99. Foa R, Casorati G, Giubellino MC, et al. Rearrangements of immunoglobulin and T cell receptor β and γ genes are associated with terminal deoxynucleotidyl transferase expression in acute myeloid leukemia. *J Exp Med* 1989;165:879–890.
100. LeBien TW, Elstrom RL, Moseley M, et al. Analysis of immunoglobulin and T cell receptor gene rearrangements in human fetal bone marrow B lineage cells. *Blood* 1990;76:1196–1200.
101. Beishuizen A, Verhoeven M-AJ, van Wering ER, et al. Analysis of Ig and T-cell receptor genes in 40 childhood acute lymphoblastic leukemias at diagnosis and subsequent relapse: implications for the detection of minimal residual disease by polymerase chain reaction analysis. *Blood* 1994;83:2238–2247.
102. Ghali DW, Panzer S, Fischer S, et al. Heterogeneity of the T-cell receptor δ gene indicating subclone formation in acute precursor B-cell leukemias. *Blood* 1995;85:2795–2801.
103. Steenbergen EJ, Verhagen OJHM, van Leeuwen EF, et al. Frequent ongoing T-cell receptor rearrangements in childhood B-precursor acute lymphoblastic leukemia: implications for monitoring minimal residual disease. *Blood* 1995;86:692–702.
104. Pui C-H, Robison LL, Look AT. Acute lymphoblastic leukaemia. *Lancet* 2008;371:1030–1043.
105. Mullighan CG, Goorha S, Radtke I, et al. Genome-wide analysis of genetic alterations in acute lymphoblastic leukaemia. *Nature* 2007;446:758–764.
106. Mullighan CG, Miller CB, Radtke I, et al. *BCR-ABL1* lymphoblastic leukaemia is characterized by the deletion of Ikaros. *Nature* 2008;453:110–115.
107. Mullighan CG, Su X, Zhang J, et al. Deletion of *IKZF1* and prognosis in acute lymphoblastic leukemia. *N Engl J Med* 2009;360:470–480.
108. Mullighan CG, Collins-Underwood JR, Phillips LAA, et al. Rearrangement of *CRLF2* in B progenitor– and Down syndrome–associated acute lymphoblastic leukemia. *Nat Genet* 2009;41:1243–1246.
109. Harvey RC, Mullighan CG, Chen I-M, et al. Rearrangement of *CRLF2* is associated with mutation of *JAK* kinases, alteration of *IKZF1*, Hispanic/Latino ethnicity, and a poor outcome in pediatric B-progenitor acute lymphoblastic leukemia. *Blood* 2010;115:5312–5321.
110. Hertzberg L, Vendramini E, Ganmore I, et al. Down syndrome acute lymphoblastic leukemia, a highly heterogeneous disease in which aberrant expression of *CRLF2* is associated with mutated *JAK2*: a report from the International BFM Study Group. *Blood* 2010;115:1006–1017.
111. Ensor HM, Schwab C, Russell LJ, et al. Demographic, clinical, and outcome features of children with acute lymphoblastic leukemia and *CRLF2* deregulation: results from the MRC ALL97 clinical trial. *Blood* 2011;117:2129–2136.
112. Cario G, Zimmermann M, Romey R, et al. Presence of the *P2RY8-CRLF2* rearrangement is associated with a poor prognosis in non–high-risk precursor B-cell acute lymphoblastic leukemia in children treated according to the ALL-BFM 2000 protocol. *Blood* 2010;115:5393–5397.
113. Mullighan CG, Zhang J, Kasper LH, et al. CREBBP mutations in relapsed acute lymphoblastic leukaemia. *Nature* 2011;471:235–239.

114. Breit S, Stanulla M, Flohr T, et al. Activating *NOTCH1* mutations predict favorable early treatment response and long-term outcome in childhood precursor T-cell lymphoblastic leukemia. *Blood* 2006;108:1151–1157.
115. Ross ME, Zhou X, Song G, et al. Classification of pediatric acute lymphoblastic leukemia by gene expression profiling. *Blood* 2003;102:2951–2959.
116. Haferlach T, Kohlmann A, Wieczorek L, et al. Clinical utility of microarray-based expression profiling in the diagnosis and subclassification of leukemia: report from the International Microarray Innovations in Leukemia Study Group. *J Clin Oncol* 2010;28:2529–2537.
117. Bhojwani D, Kang H, Menezes RX, et al. Gene expression signatures predictive of early response and outcome in high-risk childhood acute lymphoblastic leukemia: a Children's Oncology Group study. *J Clin Oncol* 2008;26:4376–4384.
118. Kang H, Chen I-M, Wilson CS, et al. Gene expression classifiers for relapse-free survival and minimal residual disease improve risk classification and outcome prediction in pediatric B-precursor acute lymphoblastic leukemia. *Blood* 2010;115:1394–1405.
119. Ferrando AA, Neuberg DS, Staunton J, et al. Gene expression signatures define novel oncogenic pathways in T cell acute lymphoblastic leukemia. *Cancer Cell* 2002;1:75–87.
120. Soulier J, Clappier E, Cayuela J-M, et al. HOXA genes are included in genetic and biologic networks defining human acute T-cell leukemia (T-ALL). *Blood* 2005;106:274–286.
121. Coustan-Smith E, Mullighan CG, Onciu M, et al. Early T-cell precursor leukaemia: a subtype of very high-risk acute lymphoblastic leukaemia. *Lancet Oncol* 2009;10:147–156.
122. Rothenberg EV, Moore JE, Yui MA. Launching the T-cell lineage developmental programme. *Nat Rev Immunol* 2008;8:9–21.
123. Bell JJ, Bhandoola A. The earliest thymic progenitors for T cells possess myeloid lineage potential. *Nature* 2008;452:764–767.
124. McKenna RW, Washington LT, Aquino DB. Immunophenotypic analysis of hematogones (B-lymphocyte precursors) in 662 consecutive bone marrow specimens by 4-color flow cytometry. *Blood* 2001;98:2498–2507.
125. Moghrabi A, Levy DE, Asselin B, et al. Results of the Dana-Farber Cancer Institute ALL Consortium Protocol 95-01 for children with acute lymphoblastic leukemia. *Blood* 2007;109:896–904.
126. Schultz KR, Pullen DJ, Sather HN, et al. Risk- and response-based classification of childhood B-precursor acute lymphoblastic leukemia: a combined analysis of prognostic markers from the Pediatric Oncology Group (POG) and Children's Cancer Group (CCG). *Blood* 2007;109:926–935.
127. Möricke A, Reiter A, Zimmermann M, et al. Risk-adjusted therapy of acute lymphoblastic leukemia can decrease treatment burden and improve survival: treatment results of 2169 unselected pediatric and adolescent patients enrolled in the trial ALL-BFM 95. *Blood* 2008;111:4477–4489.
128. Pui C-H, Pei D, Sandlund JT, et al. Long-term results of St Jude Total Therapy Studies 11, 12, 13A, 13B, and 14 for childhood acute lymphoblastic leukemia. Results of Total Therapy Studies for childhood ALL. *Leukemia* 2010;24: 371–382.
129. Rubnitz JE, Wichlan D, Devidas M, et al. Prospective analysis of *TEL* gene rearrangements in childhood acute lymphoblastic leukemia: a Children's Oncology Group study. *J Clin Oncol* 2008;26:2186–2191.
130. Faderl S, O'Brien SO, Pui C-H, et al. Adult lymphoblastic leukemia. *Cancer* 2010;116:1165–1176.
131. Campana D. Minimal residual disease in acute lymphoblastic leukemia. *Hematology* 2010;1:7–12.
132. Roshal M, Fromm JR, Winter S, et al. Immaturity associated antigens are lost during induction for T cell lymphoblastic leukemia: Implications for minimal residual disease detection. *Cytometry Part B* 2010;78B:139–146.
133. DiGiuseppe JA, Fuller SG, Borowitz MJ. Overexpression of CD49f in precursor B-cell acute lymphoblastic leukemia: potential usefulness in minimal residual disease detection. *Cytometry Part B* 2009;76B:150–155.
134. Coustan-Smith E, Song G, Clark C, et al. New markers for minimal residual disease detection in acute lymphoblastic leukemia. *Blood* 2011;117:6267–6276.
135. Stow P, Key L, Chen X, et al. Clinical significance of low levels of minimal residual disease at the end of remission induction therapy in childhood acute lymphoblastic leukemia. *Blood* 2010;115:4657–4663.
136. Conter V, Bartram CR, Valsecchi MG, et al. Molecular response to treatment redefines all prognostic factors in children and adolescents with B-cell precursor acute lymphoblastic leukemia: results in 3184 patients of the AIEOP-BFM ALL 2000 study. *Blood* 2010;115:3206–3214.
137. Bassan R, Spinelli O, Oldani E, et al. Improved risk classification for risk-specific therapy based on the molecular study of minimal residual disease (MRD) in adult acute lymphoblastic leukemia (ALL). *Blood* 2009;113:4153–4162.
138. Silverman LB, Stevenson KE, O'Brien JE, et al. Long-term results of Dana-Farber Cancer Institute ALL Consortium protocols for children with newly diagnosed acute lymphoblastic leukemia (1985–2000). *Leukemia* 2010;24:320–334.
139. Schultz KR, Bowman WP, Aledo A, et al. Improved early event-free survival with imatinib in Philadelphia chromosome-positive acute lymphoblastic leukemia: a Children's Oncology Group study. *J Clin Oncol* 2009;27:5175–5181.
140. Pui C-H, Campana D, Pei D, et al. Treating childhood acute lymphoblastic leukemia without cranial irradiation. *N Engl J Med* 2009;360:2730–2741.
141. Goldstone AH, Richards SM, Lazarus HM, et al. In adults with standard-risk acute lymphoblastic leukemia, the greatest benefit is achieved from a matched sibling allogeneic transplantation in first complete remission, and an autologous transplantation is less effective than conventional consolidation/maintenance chemotherapy in all patients: final results of the International ALL Trial (MRC UKALL XII/ECOG E2993). *Blood* 2008;111:1827–1833.

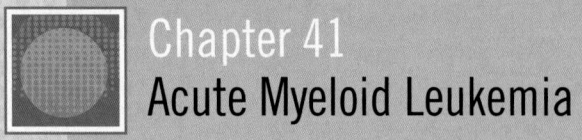

Chapter 41
Acute Myeloid Leukemia

Aharon G. Freud • Daniel A. Arber

 INTRODUCTION

Acute myeloid leukemia (AML) is an aggressive disease that results from neoplastic proliferations of immature bone marrow (BM)–derived cells of the granulocytic, monocytic, erythroid, and megakaryocytic lineages. In general, AML is lethal if left untreated, and the overall 5-year survival with current therapies is between 20% and 25%. However, some subtypes of AML are associated with improved survival rates and are treated with unique therapies. Therefore, precise classification is fundamental to the appropriate clinical management of patients with AML.

For many years, the diagnosis of AML and the differentiation from other myeloid neoplasms rested on the demonstration of a minimum number of neoplastic cells (i.e., blasts) present in the BM or peripheral blood (PB). Various classification schemes were previously proposed (1–3), though most pathologists used the French-American-British (FAB) Cooperative Group classification of AML, which defined AML as proliferations of marrow blasts comprising 30% or more of either all BM cells or all marrow nonerythroid progenitor cells. The FAB classification included a number of AML subtypes based on morphologic, cytochemical, immunophenotypic, and ultrastructural features (4–7). Although the terminology of the FAB classification continues to be used for some subtypes of AML, this system does not incorporate newer genetic data and has now been superseded by the World Health Organization (WHO) classification that more accurately identifies prognostically significant disease types.

Diagnostic criteria outlined in the 2001 WHO and subsequently revised in the 2008 WHO classification attest to the clinical importance of recurrent genetic mutations as replacing the necessity of a minimally diagnostic blast cell count for some forms of AML (8,9). In addition, the WHO classification addresses the clinical significance of therapy-related disease as well as the significance of multilineage dysplasia in nonblast cells (10). Indeed, accumulating clinical data support the notion that appropriate diagnosis and classification of AML necessitates integration of combined clinical, morphologic, immunophenotypic, and genetic features, which are not all addressed in the FAB classification (11). Therefore, pathologists and hematologists are encouraged to use the WHO 2008 classification system rather than other classification systems.

 DEFINITION

In general, the 2008 WHO classification defines AML as a clonal proliferation of nonlymphoid blasts comprising at least 20% of total nucleated cells in either the BM or PB. AML may also be diagnosed based on the demonstration of extramedullary tissue leukemic infiltration (myeloid sarcoma) with or without blood or BM involvement. As described below, certain subtypes

of AML with recurring cytogenetic abnormalities may be diagnosed as AML with an even lower blast percentage.

 POSTULATED NORMAL COUNTERPART

AML blasts are considered to be neoplastic counterparts of hematopoietic stem cells and progenitor cells with the potential for myeloid, monocytic, erythroid, and/or megakaryocytic differentiation.

 EPIDEMIOLOGY

The overall annual incidence of AML is approximately 3.5 cases per 100,000. AML may occur at any age, but its frequency increases with age with a median age at diagnosis of 67 years. Approximately 6% of cases occur in childhood and in patients younger than 20 years, whereas >50% of cases occur in individuals older than 65 years (12). There is an overall slight male predominance. Patients with preexisting myelodysplastic syndromes (MDS), those with a history of prior therapy for a nonleukemic disorder, and those with some preexisting genetic disorders, such as Down syndrome (DS), have a higher risk of developing AML. Epidemiologic features of specific subtypes of AML are described below.

 CLINICAL FEATURES

AML typically manifests with infiltration and involvement of the BM and PB, and associated cytopenias may result in increased susceptibility to infection (leukopenia), fatigue or pallor (anemia), and/or bleeding or bruising (thrombocytopenia). AML may also present as isolated extramedullary tissue infiltration (myeloid sarcoma), and signs and symptoms are related to the specific site(s) of involvement. AML is not staged *per se* as for other malignancies, although genetic and clinical features (e.g., history of prior therapy) do provide prognostic information and may direct therapeutic decision making (11).

 MORPHOLOGIC FEATURES

The morphologic features of AML are diverse and vary depending upon the disease subtype (13–17). CBC data and PB smears may demonstrate a markedly elevated white cell count with a predominance of blasts. Likewise, BM aspirates and biopsies may be hypercellular with effacement of the marrow space and with little to no residual hematopoiesis. Other cases may have fewer blasts in the PB or BM, and in the absence of certain disease qualifiers (e.g., recurrent cytogenetic abnormality), a diagnosis of AML requires demonstration of 20% or more blasts based on a morphologic blast count differential performed on

1030

an adequate BM aspirate or PB smear (17). Dysplasia in the nonblast cells may also be present, and some cases may demonstrate marked BM fibrosis. Myeloid sarcoma can involve a variety of extramedullary sites including skin, mucous membranes, orbits, central nervous system, lymph nodes, bones, gonads, and other solid organs (18). Distinguishing myeloid sarcoma from other neoplasms based on morphologic grounds alone may not be possible.

AML blasts may take on myeloblast, monoblast, or megakaryoblast morphology. Promonocytes are also considered blast equivalents in AML, occurring in cases with monocytic features. The various morphologic characteristics of these blast populations are described in more detail below in the sections describing the AML subtypes. In general, the blasts in AML are medium- to large-sized mononuclear cells with high nuclear to cytoplasmic ratios, fine and dispersed nuclear chromatin, variably prominent nucleoli, and basophilic cytoplasm with or without granules or vacuoles. Nuclei may show folding or invagination. The cytoplasmic granules of AML blasts may coalesce to form rod-shaped structures called Auer rods, and these are considered to be specific to the myeloid lineage (9). However, these are not present in every case, and Auer rods may be found in some forms of high-grade MDS. Auer rods are not seen in normal BM progenitor cells. Some subtypes of AML with recurring genetic abnormalities show other distinguishing morphologic features, but none of the latter are considered entirely specific, and additional ancillary studies (e.g., flow cytometry, immunohistochemistry, cytogenetics) are required to distinguish AML subtypes from each other as well as from other diseases such as acute lymphoblastic leukemia (ALL), lymphoma, or nonhematopoietic small round blue cell tumors.

ANCILLARY STUDIES

Ancillary studies are fundamental to the accurate diagnosis and classification of AML. Where possible, all cases of suspected AML should have both a comprehensive flow cytometry immunophenotypic characterization and cytogenetics analysis performed. Additional molecular studies designed to detect frequently occurring gene mutations (e.g., involving *FLT3*, *KIT*, *NPM1*, and *CEBPA* genes, see below) provide additional prognostic information and are recommended in many cases (11).

By flow cytometry analysis AML blasts weakly express the common leukocyte antigen, CD45RB, and express a number of myeloid-associated (CD13, CD15, CD33, CD117) and/or monocyte-associated (CD4, CD11c, CD14, CD36, CD64) surface antigens. Intracellular myeloperoxidase (MPO) staining is commonly seen and is considered specific to the myeloid lineage. The progenitor cell–associated surface antigens, CD34 and HLA-DR are not lineage specific but are often expressed on AML blasts. The rare cases with erythroblastic and megakaryocytic features may lack the aforementioned antigens but usually express CD71 and CD41/CD61, respectively, although there may be overlap in expression between these lineages. In addition to the above, aberrant expression of surface or cytoplasmic lymphoid antigens is also frequently seen in AML, with some subtypes characteristically showing aberrant expression of CD2, CD7, CD19, CD56, and/or TdT (19,20). In most cases, these leukemias do not meet 2008 WHO criteria for a diagnosis of a mixed phenotype acute leukemia (MPAL).

Immunohistochemical staining of the BM biopsy may be useful for cases in which the number of evaluable blasts is very low due to marrow fibrosis or low numbers of circulating blasts. Likewise, for many cases of myeloid sarcoma there may only be formalin-fixed paraffin-embedded tissue available. Many of the aforementioned antigens may be assessed by immunohistochemistry. Additional markers that would support a diagnosis of AML/myeloid sarcoma include MPO, CD33, CD68, CD163,

and lysozyme (18,21). Cytochemical studies are no longer performed for routine diagnosis in many laboratories, but remain useful in some settings. Myeloblasts will usually be MPO and Sudan black B (SBB) positive, whereas monoblasts and promonocytes will usually lack the former markers but express nonspecific esterase (NSE) (9).

Recurring cytogenetic abnormalities are pathognomonic for some AML subtypes (22–24). Therefore, all new cases of AML should undergo conventional karyotyping, with or without fluorescence *in situ* hybridization (FISH) analysis (9,11). The latter can often be directed based on morphologic and immunophenotypic features of the blasts. In addition, there are accumulating clinical data that demonstrate the prognostic influence of genetic mutations in a number of genes encoding tyrosine kinases and other transcription factors (25–27). Directed molecular studies to assess for mutations in some of these genes are indicated in various subtypes of AML.

TREATMENT AND SURVIVAL

AML treatment regimens vary by disease subtype and by patient characteristics. Some gene mutation–targeted therapies exist, such as the use of all-trans retinoic acid (ATRA) in the treatment of acute promyelocytic leukemia (APL) with t(15;17)(q24.1;q21.1) (*PML-RARA*) (28). However, most cases of AML are treated with cytarabine- and anthracycline-based regimens (11). In addition, allogeneic stem cell transplantation may afford long-term disease-free survival and may be indicated in some cases. The overall 5-year survival for AML is between 20% and 25%, but the rate varies by disease subtype (12). Independent patient and disease characteristics influencing prognosis include age at diagnosis, prior history of a MDS or cytotoxic therapy for another disease, and the presence or absence of genetic abnormalities (29–31). Regarding the latter, three prognostic risk groups may be defined based on results of cytogenetics and molecular analyses. The favorable genetic group includes AML with t(8;21)(q22;q22), AML with inv(16)(p13.1;q22) or t(16;16)(p13.1;q22), APL with t(15;17)(q24.1;q21.1), AML with mutated *NPM1* without the internal tandem duplication of *FLT3* (*FLT3*-ITD), and AML with mutated *CEBPA*. The adverse genetic risk group includes AML with inv(3)(q21;q26.2) or t(3;3)(q21;q26.2), AML with t(6;9)(p23;q34), and AML with a complex karyotype, among others (11). Most AML, not otherwise specified (NOS), with normal karyotypes fall into the intermediate prognosis category. The prognosis associated with each of the individual subtypes is discussed further in the sections that follow. Recently, the prognostic significance of the so-called monosomal karyotype (MK), defined as two or more monosomies or one monosomy in the presence of additional structural abnormalities, has been evaluated in large-scale studies (32–34). Most MK AML arise in older individuals in the setting of a complex karyotype, and they are associated with the worst rates of complete remission and overall survival reported to date. This very poor prognosis is likely multifactorial but may in part be due to relatively high expression of multidrug resistance genes (35).

AML SUBTYPES

The 2008 WHO classification defines the various AML subtypes based on combined clinical, morphologic, immunophenotypic, and genetic features (Tables 41.1 and 41.2; and see Table 42.5). Subtype qualifiers include the presence of a recurrent genetic abnormality, a prior history of therapy for another disease, and concurrent or prior myelodysplasia, among others. These additional disease characteristics should be clearly stated in the diagnosis [e.g., "AML with (8;21)(q22;q22)

Table 41.1	2008 WHO CLASSIFICATION OF AML—MAJOR CATEGORIES

AML with recurrent genetic abnormalities
AML with myelodysplasia-related changes
Therapy-related myeloid neoplasms
AML, not otherwise specified
Myeloid proliferations related to Down syndrome

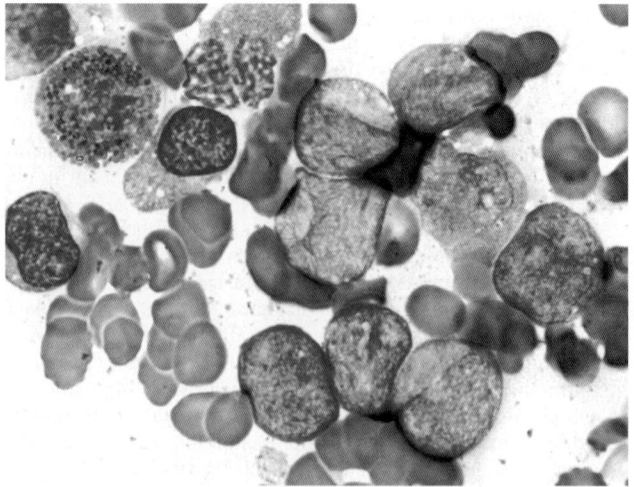

FIGURE 41.1. AML with t(8;21)(q22;q22); *RUNX1-RUNX1T1*. The blasts have abundant cytoplasm with perinuclear clearing and *large pink* or *salmon*-colored granules. Note admixed eosinophil precursors are also present.

(*RUNX1-RUNX1T1*)"]. Given that cytogenetic and molecular analyses often require extended periods of time for completion, pathologists should create amendments or addenda to reports in order to incorporate all relevant data into final diagnoses that are based on 2008 WHO criteria. Of note, a significant percentage of newly diagnosed AMLs have a normal karyotype, lack other disease qualifiers, and may be diagnosed as AML, NOS (13).

AML WITH RECURRENT GENETIC ABNORMALITIES

The AML subtypes with recurrent genetic abnormalities are listed in Table 41.2. These diseases are classified as such, given substantial clinical and pathobiologic evidence demonstrating both the uniqueness of each entity and the similarity in prognosis, response to treatment, and morphologic and immunophenotypic features that cases within each AML subtype have to others of the same category (19,22). For three of the AML subtypes with recurrent genetic abnormalities, AML with t(8;21)(q22;q22) (*RUNX1-RUNX1T1*), AML with inv(16)(p13q22) or t(16;16)(p13q22) (*CBFB-MYH11*), and APL with t(15;17)(q24.1;q21.1) (*PML-RARA*), the diagnosis of AML is made in the appropriate clinical and morphologic context without regard to the blast percentage in BM or PB (14). In contrast, a diagnosis of any of the other subtypes requires ≥20% blasts in the marrow or blood or demonstration of myeloid sarcoma. Two of the subtypes, AML with mutated *NPM1* and AML with mutated *CEBPA*, are included in the 2008 WHO classification as provisional entities. Numerous other genetic abnormalities have been described in AML, and some of these that are not associated with distinct AML classification types in the 2008 WHO are also discussed below.

Acute Myeloid Leukemia with t(8;21)(q22;q22) (*RUNX1-RUNX1T1*)

AML with t(8;21)(q22;q22) occurs in both children and adults and accounts for 5% to 10% of all AML. Most forms present with BM and PB involvement with >20% blasts. However,

Table 41.2	AMLs WITH RECURRENT GENETIC ABNORMALITIES

AML with t(8;21)(q22;q22) (*RUNX1-RUNX1T1*)
AML with inv(16)(p13.1q22) or t(16;16)(p13.1;q22) (*CBFB-MYH11*)
APL with t(15;17)(q24.1;q21.1) (*PML-RARA*)
AML with t(9;11)(p22;q23) (*MLLT3-MLL*)
AML with t(6;9)(p23;q34) (*DEK-NUP214*)
AML with inv(3)(q21q26.2) or t(3;3)(q21;q26.2) (*RPN1-EVI1*)
AML (megakaryoblastic) with t(1;22)(p13;q13) (*RBM15-MKL1*)
AML with mutated *NPM1* (provisional entity)
AML with mutated *CEBPA* (provisional entity)

fewer than 20% blasts in either tissue may rarely be present, and demonstration of the t(8;21)(q22;q22) rearrangement still warrants a diagnosis of AML rather than MDS based on the demonstration that the natural history and response to therapy of such cases is generally similar to other cases of AML with t(8;21)(q22;q22) (14). Some cases, more so in children, present with myeloid sarcoma.

The blasts in AML with t(8;21)(q22;q22) have distinct morphologic features (Fig. 41.1). The blasts are typically large with round nuclei, perinuclear cytoplasmic hofs, cytoplasmic granules with occasional Auer rods, and occasional large pink or salmon-colored granules. Smaller blasts as well as maturing promyelocytes, myelocytes, and neutrophils are often present. Dysplastic features, including pseudo–Pelger-Huët nuclei and cytoplasmic hypogranulation, can be seen in the maturing neutrophils. However, dysplastic changes are not seen in the other lineages. Eosinophils and their precursors may be increased, but these do not show atypical features as are present in AML with t(16;16)(p13;q22) or inv(16)(p13q22) (see below).

Flow cytometry and immunohistochemical studies show that the blasts in AML with t(8;21)(q22;q22) also have a characteristic immunophenotype (36,37). At least a fraction of the blasts usually express CD34 and HLA-DR as well as the myeloid antigens CD13 and MPO. CD33 expression may be weak. In addition, flow cytometry studies may show dyssynchronous maturation with aberrant coexpression of CD34 and CD15. Aberrant expression of CD19 (weak) and PAX5 is common, and some cases show expression of CD56, CD79a, and/or TdT (38,39). Cytochemical studies, while not necessary for the diagnosis, demonstrate MPO and SBB expression by many of the blasts. NSE is usually negative.

The t(8;21)(q22;q22) rearrangement may be detected by routine karyotypic analysis, FISH, and reverse transcription polymerase chain reaction (RT-PCR) (40). The translocation results in fusion between the *RUNX1* gene (*AML1* or *CBFA*) on chromosome 21 and the *RUNX1T1* gene (*ETO*) on chromosome 8. *RUNX1* encodes a protein called core binding factor α (CBFα), which couples with another protein, core binding factor β (CBFβ), to form a heterodimeric transcription factor that is necessary for hematopoiesis (41) (Fig. 41.2). The fusion protein resulting from t(8;21)(q22;q22) is thought to result in repression of the normal target genes of the CBF heteroduplex due to recruitment of transcriptional repressors. Additional genetic mutations occur in over 70% of AMLs with t(8;21)(q22;q22) (14). Other cytogenetic abnormalities, including loss of a sex

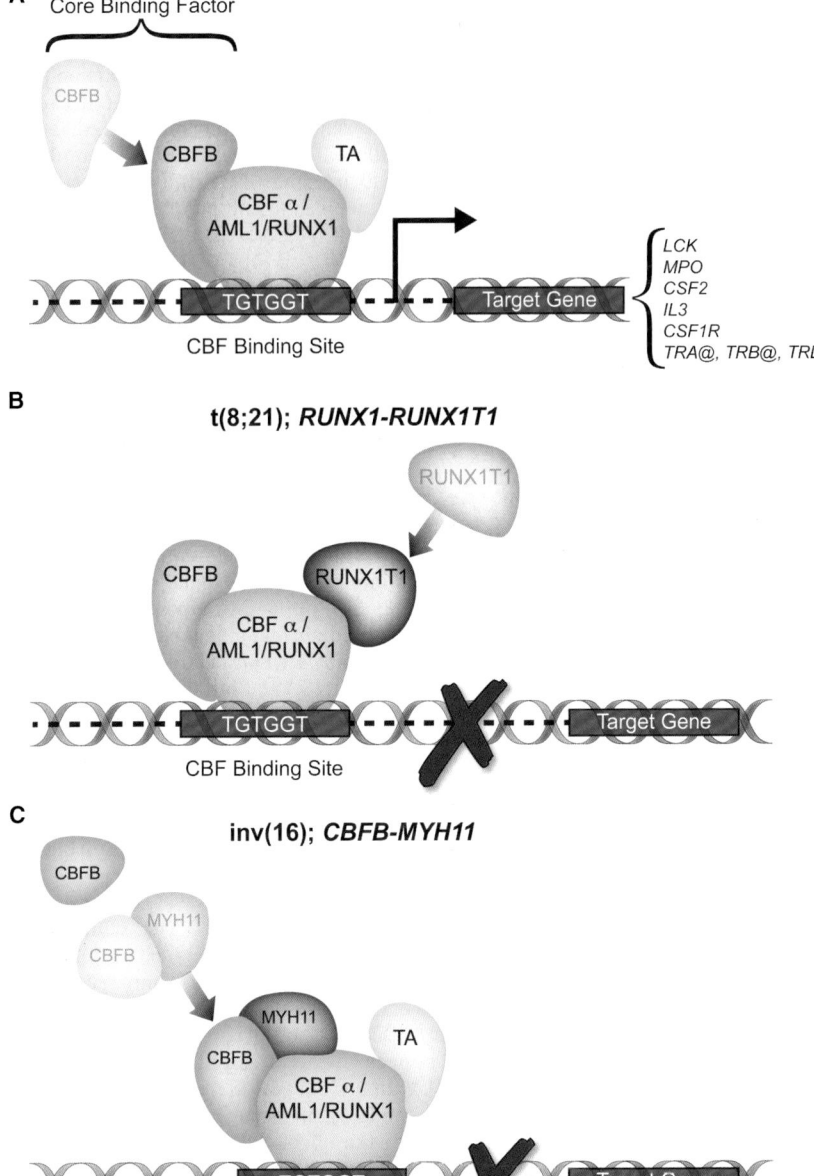

A

Core Binding Factor

CBFB

CBFB

TA

CBF α / AML1/RUNX1

TGTGGT

CBF Binding Site

Target Gene

{ LCK
MPO
CSF2
IL3
CSF1R
TRA@, TRB@, TRD@ }

B

t(8;21); *RUNX1-RUNX1T1*

RUNX1T1

CBFB

RUNX1T1

CBF α / AML1/RUNX1

TGTGGT

CBF Binding Site

Target Gene

C

inv(16); *CBFB-MYH11*

CBFB

MYH11

CBFB

MYH11

TA

CBFB

CBF α / AML1/RUNX1

TGTGGT

CBF Binding Site

Target Gene

FIGURE 41.2. Simplified schematic presentation of the core binding factor protein complex involved in normal hematopoiesis. A: Normally, the core binding factor protein complex binds to specific DNA sequences to activate a number of genes involved in normal hematopoiesis. **B:** In AML with t(8;21) (q22;q22); *RUNX1-RUNX1T1,* the fusion disrupts the transactivation domain (TA), blocking normal gene activation. **C:** In AML with inv(16)(p13q22) or t(16;16)(p13;q22); *CBFB-MYH11,* the altered CBFB protein changes the core binding factor complex protein shape, also disrupting normal gene activation.

chromosome or del(9q), are common. In addition, mutations in the *KIT* gene are present in 20% to 25% of cases, and mutations in *KRAS* and *NRAS* genes are also seen in approximately 30% of pediatric cases (27,42).

In general, AML with t(8;21)(q22;q22) is associated with a favorable prognosis when high-dose cytarabine is given in the consolidation phase during the first remission (43). Factors that appear to adversely affect this prognosis include a white blood cell count that is >20 × 10⁹/L at presentation, CD56 expression on blasts, and *KIT* mutations in exons 8 and 17 (27,38). Additional cytogenetic abnormalities have thus far not been shown to influence prognosis.

The differential diagnosis of AML with t(8;21)(q22;q22) includes regenerative changes following marrow injury, MDS, myeloid neoplasms with eosinophilia and associated with mutations in *PDGFRA, PDGFRB,* or *FGFR1,* and other AML subtypes. Given their granularity and cytoplasmic hofs, blasts in AML with t(8;21)(q22;q22) may be confused with normal promyelocytes. Moreover, in the setting of a regenerating marrow

following therapy, promyelocytes may accumulate, thus raising suspicion for recurrent disease. Nonetheless, normal promyelocytes do not express B-cell antigens or CD56 and do not contain Auer rods or the characteristic salmon-colored granules. In addition, cytogenetic and molecular studies for the t(8;21) (q22;q22) rearrangement would be negative in a regenerating marrow. Recurrent disease would also result in continued and worsening accumulation of blasts, whereas a regenerating marrow would eventually demonstrate full spectrum myeloid maturation in subsequent marrow aspirates.

Because AML with t(8;21)(q22;q22) often presents with dysgranulopoiesis, some cases with 6% to 19% blasts in the BM or 2% to 19% blasts in the PB would meet criteria for refractory anemia with excess blasts (RAEB) based on morphologic features. However, demonstration of the t(8;21)(q22;q22) rearrangement would negate the diagnosis of MDS (14). Likewise, cytogenetics studies would distinguish AML with t(8;21) (q22;q22) from other forms of AML, such as APL, that may show similar morphologic features, including an abundance of cytoplasmic granules with or without Auer rods. As mentioned above, AML with t(8;21)(q22;q22) can be associated with eosinophilia, thus raising the possibility of a myeloid neoplasm with eosinophilia and associated with mutations in *PDGFRA*, *PDGFRB*, or *FGFR1*. Patients with the latter often have a prior history of eosinophilia, splenomegaly, and/or symptoms and organ damage associated with eosinophilia. Cytogenetics and molecular studies will further distinguish between these possibilities.

Acute Myeloid Leukemia with inv(16)(p13q22) or t(16;16)(p13;q22) (*CBFB-MYH11*)

AML with inv(16)(p13q22) or t(16;16)(p13;q22) is relatively common and accounts for 5% to 10% of both adult and childhood AML. PB and BM are typically involved; however, myeloid sarcoma is present in up to 50% of cases and may be the only finding at diagnosis or recurrence. In rare cases, the BM or PB blast count may be less than 20%. Nonetheless, these patients should be diagnosed with AML rather than MDS regardless of the blast count upon demonstration of either inv(16)(p13q22) or t(16;16)(p13;q22) (14).

Most cases of AML with inv(16)(p13q22) or t(16;16)(p13;q22) would be classified as acute myelomonocytic leukemia with abnormal eosinophils (AML-M4 eos) using FAB criteria (44). The neoplastic population is often heterogeneous and contains a mixture of myeloblasts, monoblasts, and promonocytes. The myeloblasts may have cytoplasmic granules with Auer rods. Maturing granulocytes are usually relatively sparse and do not show dysplastic features. The monoblasts are large cells with round nuclei, delicate chromatin, one or more large prominent nucleoli, and abundant pale to intensely basophilic cytoplasm. Fine azurophilic granules and vacuoles may be present in the cytoplasm. Promonocytes, which may be difficult to distinguish from monocytes, are large cells with more irregularly shaped and convoluted nuclei, mild chromatin condensation, and pale cytoplasm with more prominent cytoplasmic granules and/or vacuoles. Promonocytes should be included in the blast count along with myeloblasts and monoblasts. Maturing monocytes and eosinophils may also be increased in AML with inv(16)(p13q22) or t(16;16)(p13;q22). Notably, the eosinophils in AML with inv(16)(p13q22) or t(16;16)(p13;q22) often show characteristic abnormal granules that are large, irregular, and basophilic (Fig. 41.3). The abnormal granules may be seen in

eosinophilic promyelocytes and myelocytes and are characteristic of this disease. The napthol-ASD-chloroacetate esterase (CAE) reaction is faintly positive in these abnormal eosinophils, whereas normal eosinophils are negative for this reaction (14).

Immunophenotypic analysis of AML with inv(16)(p13q22) or t(16;16)(p13;q22) will reflect the morphologic diversity of the neoplastic population. There will often be a combination of immature blasts expressing CD34 and CD117 as well as additional maturing neoplastic subpopulations expressing granulocytic-associated (CD13, CD15, CD33, CD65, MPO) or monocytic-associated (CD4, CD11b, CD11c, CD14, CD36, CD64, lysozyme) antigens. These populations can usually be differentiated on a CD45 versus side-scatter dot plot. Maturation asynchrony, such as coexpression of CD15 and CD117, can be observed. In addition, many cases show aberrant expression of CD2, although this is not specific for AML with inv(16)(p13q22) or t(16;16)(p13;q22) (45,46).

The cytogenetic abnormality of either inv(16)(p13q22) or t(16;16)(p13;q22) results in the fusion of the *CBFB* gene at 16q22 to the *MYH11* gene at 16p13.1 (47). The *MYH11* gene encodes for a smooth muscle myosin heavy chain. The *CBFB* gene encodes the CBFβ subunit that heterodimerizes with CBFα, the protein product of the *RUNX1* gene that is involved in AML with t(8;21)(q22;q22). Both AML types are commonly referred to as the "core binding factor leukemias" and similarly carry a favorable prognosis when cytarabine is included in the consolidation phase (43,48,49). Both the inv(16)(p13q22) and t(16;16)(p13;q22) rearrangements are subtle findings and may be missed on routine karyotypic analysis. Therefore, it is important for pathologists to communicate with the cytogenetics laboratory if AML with inv(16)(p13q22) or t(16;16)(p13;q22) is suspected. FISH or RT-PCR methods may be necessary for initial diagnosis of the abnormality and for monitoring for residual disease (50).

Additional cytogenetic abnormalities have been reported to occur in approximately 40% of cases of AML with inv(16)(p13q22) or t(16;16)(p13;q22), and these include +22, +8, del(7q), +21, and t(9;22)(q34;q11) (14). Trisomy 22, which occurs in 10% to 15% of cases, is relatively specific to AML with inv(16)(p13q22) or t(16;16)(p13;q22) and has been reported to have a positive impact on the already favorable prognosis associated with AML with inv(16)(p13q22) or t(16;16)(p13;q22) (51,52). Mutations in the *KIT* gene occur in approximately 30% of cases, and similar to the effect that these mutations have on the prognosis associated with AML with t(8;21)(q22;q22), *KIT* mutations are associated with higher rates of relapse and worse overall survival in patients with AML with inv(16)(p13q22) or t(16;16)(p13;q22) (27).

The differential diagnosis includes AML, NOS, with myelomonocytic features, MDS, and reactive conditions with increased eosinophils or monocytes. As mentioned above, FISH or RT-PCR methods may be necessary to identify either the inv(16)(p13q22) or t(16;16)(p13;q22) abnormality; otherwise, cases may be misdiagnosed as AML, NOS, or possibly MDS if the blast count is elevated but <20%. Rarely the eosinophils in AML with inv(16)(p13q22) or t(16;16)(p13;q22) do not contain the atypical granules described above, and especially if the blast count in the PB is not elevated, these cases may be mistaken for reactive conditions. Having both a high index of suspicion and close communication with the clinical team and cytogenetics laboratory is critical for the appropriate and timely diagnosis of AML with inv(16)(p13q22) or t(16;16)(p13;q22).

Acute Promyelocytic Leukemia with t(15;17) (q24.1;q21.1) (*PML-RARA*)

APL with t(15;17)(q24.1;q21.1) accounts for 5% to 8% of all AML cases. It can occur at any age, but APL has a predilection for young to middle-aged adults. Two common morphologic

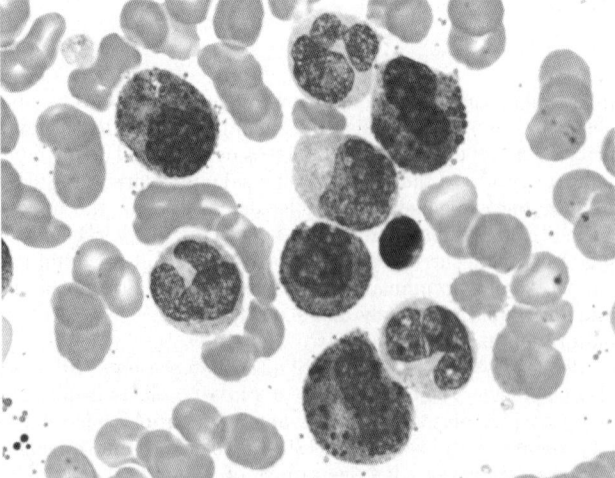

FIGURE 41.3. AML with inv(16)(p13q22); *CBFB-MYH11.* A more typical blast is present in the center, surrounded by promonoblasts and typical abnormal eosinophil precursors containing coarse basophilic granules. The presence of these abnormal eosinophils is highly predictive of this cytogenetic abnormality.

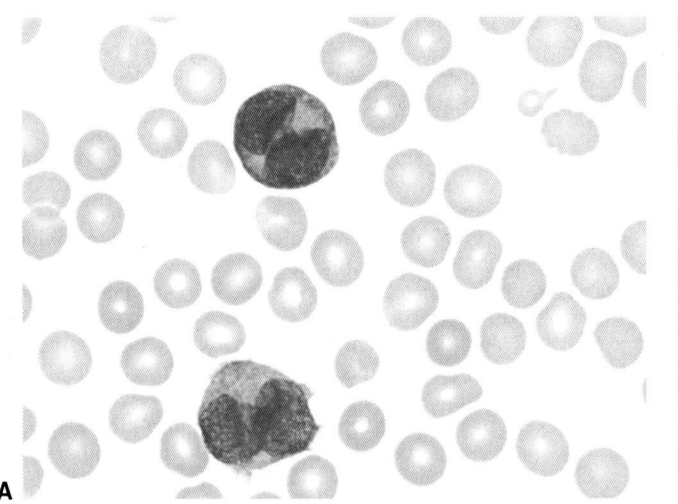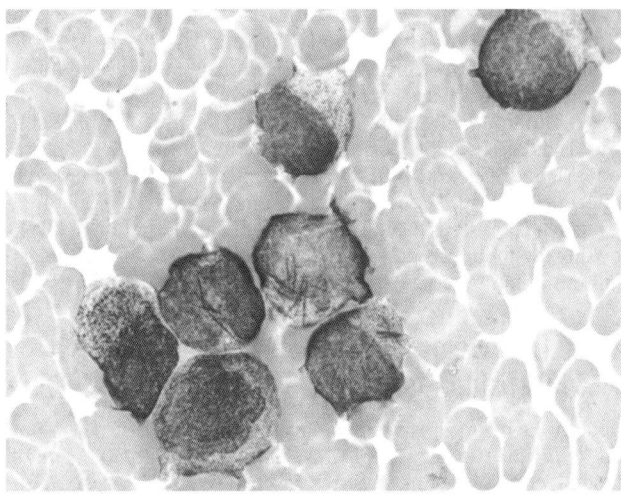

FIGURE 41.4. APL with t(15;17)(q24.1;q21.1); *PML-RARA*. A: PB involvement by the microgranular variant of APL. The blasts do not have abundant cytoplasmic granules, but have the characteristic bilobed nucleus. Background platelets are decreased with some spherocytes. **B:** A BM involved by a more typical case of APL with abundant cytoplasmic granules and numerous cytoplasmic Auer rods.

variants occur and show some differing clinical features (14,53,54) (Fig. 41.4). In all cases, the risk of disseminated intravascular coagulation (DIC) is high, and emperic administration ATRA may be performed in cases suspected of being APL but before the t(15;17)(q24.1;q21.1) rearrangement can be confirmed by either cytogenetics or molecular studies.

Hypergranular (typical) APL accounts for 60% to 70% of cases and usually presents with a low white blood cell count but with a dense marrow infiltrate. As with core binding factor AMLs, APL with t(15;17)(q24.1;q21.1) is diagnosed as acute leukemia, as opposed to MDS, without regard to the blast cell count. Organomegaly is uncommon in hypergranular APL. The blasts bear promyelocyte morphology and are large cells with characteristically kidney bean–shaped or bilobed nuclei, prominent nucleoli, and abundant cytoplasm containing numerous bright pink or red to purple cytoplasmic granules that can be so numerous as to obscure the nucleus. The abundance of these granules confers strong MPO staining by either cytochemistry or flow cytometry. The cytoplasmic granules often coalesce into Auer rods, and so-called faggot cells with abundant Auer rods are seen in the majority of cases.

The hypogranular or microgranular type of APL with t(15;17)(q24.1;q21.1) typically presents with a very high white blood cell count and increased cell doubling time. As the name implies, the majority of neoplastic promyelocytes lacks the dense cytoplasmic granularity that is seen in hypergranular APL cases. However, this is due to the extremely small size of the granules in this variant, and most cases of microgranular APL still contain a minor population of blasts with recognizable cytoplasmic granules and Auer rods. In addition, the majority of cells typically shows bilobed nuclei, which should raise suspicion for APL. For both variants of APL, strict attention to the platelet count and PB red blood cell morphology studies is also important given the high incidence of associated DIC.

Both hypergranular and microgranular APL blasts characteristically lack CD34 and HLA-DR expression but do commonly express CD33 (bright), CD13 (heterogeneous), CD64, CD117, and bright MPO (55,56). However, some cases of microgranular APL can show dim CD34 and/or HLA-DR expression; therefore, the expression of CD34 or HLA-DR does not exclude APL. In addition, aberrant CD34 and CD2 expression has been reported in some cases of microgranular APL or in cases with bcr3 transcript of the *PML-RARA* fusion gene (57,58). CD56 expression has been reported in 15% to 20% of cases and is associated with a relatively worse prognosis (59).

The t(15;17)(q24.1;q21.1) rearrangement results in the fusion of the *PML* gene on 15q24.1 with the retinoic acid receptor alpha gene, *RARA*, on 17q21.1. The cytogenetic abnormality in most cases of APL can be detected by routine karyotypic analysis. FISH and RT-PCR studies are also frequently used, with RT-PCR utilized for monitoring of minimal residual disease (60,61). Rarely there are cases of morphologically identical APL that do not contain the typical t(15;17)(q24.1;q21.1) rearrangement yet have cryptic insertion of *RARA* into a *PML* locus due to complex cytogenetic abnormalities involving both chromosomes 15 and 17 (62). The *PML-RARA* rearrangement can still be detected in these patients using RT-PCR. The *PML-RARA* fusion creates a dominant negative protein that impedes normal myeloid maturation past the promyelocyte stage. However, the neoplastic promyelocytes in APL are usually sensitive to ATRA, which targets RARA and can induce terminal maturation (28). When treated with ATRA and an anthracycline, both hypergranular and microgranular variants of APL are associated with a very favorable prognosis. Moreover, cases of relapsed or refractory APL tend to show good response to arsenic trioxide therapy (63,64). Additional cytogenetic abnormalities, including trisomy 8 (10% to 15%), are present in approximately 40% of APL cases, but these do not appear to influence prognosis (14). In addition, *FLT3* gene mutations have been reported in up to 45% of cases (65–67). Those cases with the *FLT3* internal tandem duplication (*FLT3*-ITD) are associated with higher white blood cell counts, involvement of the bcr3 breakpoint of the *PML* gene, and microgranular morphology. Although *FLT3* gene mutations are generally associated with a worsened prognosis in AML, the impact of such mutations in APL is less clear. While *FLT3* mutations alone do not appear to be associated with a poor prognosis in APL, the mutation load may be of importance (68).

The differential diagnosis of hypergranular APL includes agranulocytosis with maturation arrest at the promyelocyte stage as well as subtypes of AML, NOS, that lack expression of CD34, and HLA-DR. Depending upon the cause, patients with agranulocytosis typically have normal hemoglobin and platelet indices as well as a normo- or hypocellular marrow, findings that help to distinguish from APL. In addition, the morphologic features (e.g., Auer rods) and cytogenetic findings associated with APL are not observed. AML, NOS, without maturation (described further below) may lack CD34 and HLA-DR expression. However, other features, including the characteristic bilobed nuclear folding and abundant cytoplasmic granulation that confers strong MPO positivity, are not seen in AML, NOS, without maturation. Hypogranular variants of APL may be difficult to distinguish from AML with monocytic differentiation. Strong MPO positivity is seen in the former but not in the latter. In addition, cells with abundant cytoplasmic granules and Auer rods may still be found in cases of hypogranular APL, but Auer rods are not seen in MPO-negative AML with monocytic differentiation. FISH and/or RT-PCR analysis may be expedited in suspected cases of APL, but treatment should not be delayed if clinically indicated and suspected based on the morphologic and immunophenotypic features.

Acute Promyelocytic Leukemia with Variant *RARA* Translocations

Some APLs have translocations involving *RARA* on 17q21.1 but not *PML* on 15q24.1 (69–71). Variant translocation partners include *ZBTB16* (also known as *PLZF*) on 11q23, *NUMA1* on 11q13, *NPM1* on 5q35, and *STAT5B* on 17q11.2. The morphologic features of the blasts in these variant APLs may be similar to those described for APL with t(15;17)(q24.1;q21.1) (*PML-RARA*). However, APL with t(11;17)(q23;q21.1) (*ZBTB16-RARA*) characteristically shows distinct morphologic features in that the nuclei of the blasts are usually round to oval, and the blasts also tend to lack Auer rods despite having abundant cytoplasmic granularity (Fig. 41.5). Furthermore, pelgeroid neutrophils are common in APL with t(11;17)(q23;q21.1) (*ZBTB16-RARA*). Whereas APL cases involving *NUMA1* and *NPM1* genes are expected to be responsive to ATRA, cases involving *ZBTB16* or *STAT5B* have been reported to be resistant to ATRA (72). All such cases should be diagnosed as APL with a variant *RARA* translocation.

Acute Myeloid Leukemia with t(9;11)(p22;q23) (*MLLT3-MLL*)

AML with t(9;11)(p22;q23) (*MLLT3-MLL*) occurs at any age but is more common in childhood accounting for 9% to 12% of pediatric AML and 2% of adult AML. The blast count must be 20% or greater in either the BM or PB to warrant a diagnosis of AML (14). Otherwise, such cases may be diagnosed as MDS with excess blasts, but close monitoring is recommended to assess for progression to *bona fide* AML. Some patients may present with DIC or extramedullary disease with gingival or skin infiltration.

There are no specific morphologic features of the blasts in AML with t(9;11)(p22;q23). Most commonly the blasts show monoblastic and/or promonocytic features (Fig. 41.6), and in such cases the blasts are usually MPO negative and NSE positive. Other cases may lack differentiation. Typically the blasts in pediatric cases demonstrate strong CD4, CD33, CD65, and HLA-DR expression, whereas CD13, CD14, and CD34 are less commonly expressed or are present at low levels (73). In adults, the blasts usually express monocytic markers including CD4, CD11b, CD11c, CD14, and CD64 (74). The blasts are also typically CD34 negative but may express CD117 and/or CD56 to varying degrees.

The t(9;11)(p22;q23) rearrangement results in the fusion of the *MLL* gene (mixed lineage leukemia, *ALL1*, or *HRX*) on chromosome 11q23 with the *MLLT3* gene (otherwise known as *AF9*) on chromosome 9p22. MLL is a 430-kDa histone methyltransferase that functions as an epigenetic modifier to regulate a host of other genes including homeobox transcription factors. Notably, the *MLL* gene is rearranged in approximately 6% of AMLs with more than 70 partner genes thus far identified (29,75,76). AML with t(9;11)(p22;q23) is the most common among *MLL*-associated AMLs, and is associated with an overall intermediate prognosis that is relatively better compared to other AMLs that contain *MLL*-associated cytogenetic abnormalities (77). Therefore, the 2008 WHO classification only includes AML with t(9;11)(p22;q23) (*MLLT3-MLL*) under the category of AML with recurrent genetic abnormalities, whereas other *de novo* AMLs with *MLL*-associated rearrangements are categorized as AML, NOS, with the specific translocation stated in the diagnosis. Of note, the majority of such AMLs similarly show monoblastic or myelomonocytic features. Examples of other common translocation partners include *MLLT1* (*ENL*) on chromosome 19p13.3, *MLLT4* (*AF6*) on chromosome 6q27, *MLLT10* (*AF10*) on chromosome 10p12, and *ELL* on chromosome 19p13.1 (76,78). The t(11;19)(q23;p13.1) (*MLL-ELL*) rearrangement is most often only associated with AML; however, other *MLL* gene rearrangements are also common in other diseases, including therapy-related myeloid neoplasms, MDS, ALL, and MPAL (9). Translocations t(11;16)(q23;p13.3) and t(2;11)(p21;q23) are associated with MDS and confer a diagnosis of AML with myelodysplasia-related changes (AML-MRC; see below) when the blast count is ≥20%. The t(4;11)(q21;q23) (*MLLT4-MLL*) rearrangement is most commonly associated with ALL and acute leukemias of ambiguous lineage.

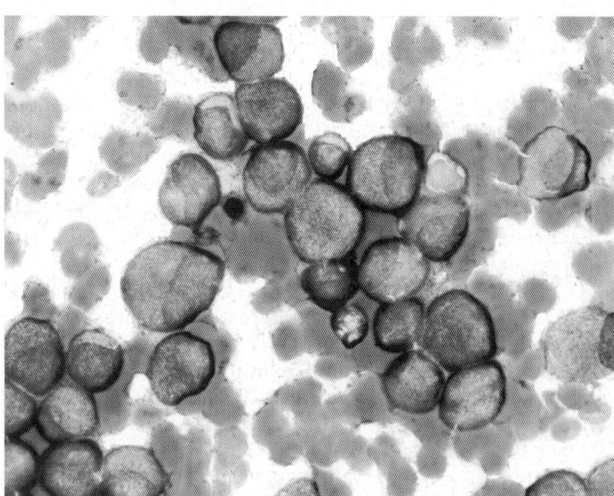

FIGURE 41.5. APL with t(11;17)(q23;q21.1);*ZBTB16-RARA*. While immature cells with granular cytoplasm predominate, the blasts do not have the bilobed nucleus typical of APL with t(15;17)(q24.1;q21.1); *PML-RARA*.

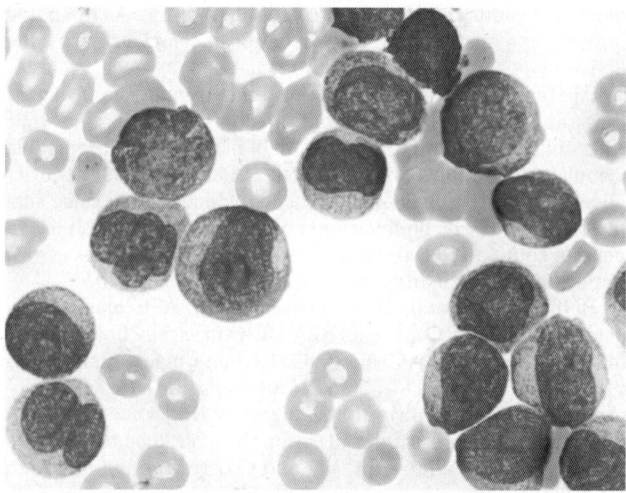

FIGURE 41.6. AML with t(9;11)(p22;q23); *MLLT3-MLL*. The blasts vary for undifferentiated blasts to some with folded nuclei, suggestive of promonoblasts. While most cases of this AML type have such monocytic features, a wide morphologic spectrum may be seen.

Additional cytogenetic abnormalities are common in AML with t(9;11)(p22;q23) with trisomy 8 being the most frequently observed, but there does not appear to be an impact on survival in such cases (29). Mutations in *KIT* and *FLT3-ITD* mutations are rare in AML with t(9;11)(p22;q23). In contrast, activating loop domain point mutations in *FLT3* are reported in approximately 20% of cases, but these are of uncertain prognostic significance. Overexpression of the *EVI1* gene, which is rearranged in AML with inv(3)(q21q26.2) or t(3;3)(q21;q26.2) (see below), has been described in many AMLs with variant *MLL*-associated abnormalities, and this has been associated with a very poor prognosis (79).

The differential diagnosis of AML with t(9;11)(p22;q23) includes other AMLs with monocytic differentiation, including subtypes of AML, NOS, therapy-related AML, and MPAL. These diseases may not be distinguished on morphologic or immunophenotypic grounds alone; therefore an accurate clinical history and comprehensive cytogenetics analysis are vital. Some cases with t(9;11)(p22;q23) may meet criteria for MPAL, but the translocation should be clearly designated in the diagnosis, as that feature may be more clinically relevant.

Acute Myeloid Leukemia with t(6;9)(p23;q34) (*DEK-NUP214*)

AML with t(6;9)(p23;q34) is rare and accounts for approximately 1% of both pediatric and adult AML cases with a median age of 35 years (80–83). Patients often present with cytopenias, and the PB or BM blast counts may be relatively lower than in other AML subtypes. A blast count of 20% or more is required for a diagnosis of AML with t(6;9)(p23;q34) (14). Patients with fewer blasts should be diagnosed with MDS and closely monitored for progression to AML.

There are no specific morphologic, immunophenotypic, or cytochemical features of the blasts that distinguish AML with t(6;9)(p23;q34) from most types of AML, NOS. Most often the features would be consistent with AML with maturation or acute myelomonocytic leukemia. The blasts are usually MPO positive, and Auer rods are detected in approximately one-third of cases. Basophilia (>2% of leukocytes in BM or PB) is a relatively specific feature associated with AML with t(6;9)(p23;q34) and is observed in approximately half of such cases (Fig. 41.7). In addition, most cases of AML with t(6;9)(p23;q34) demonstrate dysplasia in the background erythroid, myeloid, and/or megakaryocytic lineages

including ring sideroblasts, hypogranular neutrophils, and small hypolobated megakaryocytes, respectively. In light of these findings, these cases raise a differential diagnosis that includes AML-MRC, but the presence of the t(6;9)(p23;q34) precludes the former in the 2008 WHO classification.

The blasts in AML with t(6;9)(p23;q34) show a nonspecific myeloid immunophenotype and usually express CD45, CD13, CD33, CD38, HLA-DR, and MPO, with variable expression of CD15, CD34, CD64, and CD117. TdT is positive in approximately half of reported cases; however, other lymphoid-associated antigens are usually negative.

The t(6;9)(p23;q34) translocation results in the fusion of the *DEK* gene on chromosome 6p23 with the *NUP214* gene on chromosome 9q34. This results in an aberrant fusion protein that has transcriptional factor activity as well as affects nuclear transport (84). Most cases of AML with t(6;9)(p23;q34) lack other karyotypic abnormalities. However, *FLT3*-ITD mutations are common in this type of AML, with a reported frequency of approximately 70% in both pediatric and adult populations (82). The prognostic significance of the presence of *FLT3*-ITD mutations is unclear. Mutations in the *FLT3* tyrosine kinase domain are uncommon. In general, AML with t(6;9)(p23;q34) is associated with a relatively poor prognosis in both pediatric and adult populations. Moreover, patients with greater marrow or PB involvement tend to have shorter overall survivals. Relapse rates are high despite favorable rates of initial complete remission following conventional chemotherapy. However, there is some recent evidence that allogeneic stem cell transplantation may provide better overall survival (83).

As mentioned above, the differential diagnosis of AML with t(6;9)(p23;q34) includes AML, NOS, as well as AML-MRC given the high frequency of myelodysplasia. In addition, given that basophilia is a common feature of chronic myelogenous leukemia (CML) as well as rare cases of *de novo* AML with t(9;22)(q34;q11.2), the differential diagnosis of AML with t(6;9)(p23;q34) also includes those disorders. The clinical history along with a comprehensive cytogenetics analysis is necessary to distinguish among these possibilities.

Acute Myeloid Leukemia with inv(3)(q21q26.2) or t(3;3)(q21;q26.2) (*RPN1-EVI1*)

AML with inv(3)(q21q26.2) or t(3;3)(q21;q26.2) is very rare in children and accounts for 1% to 2% of adult patients with

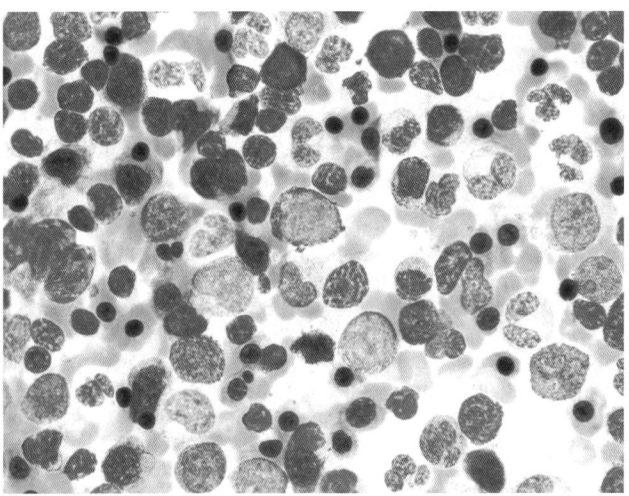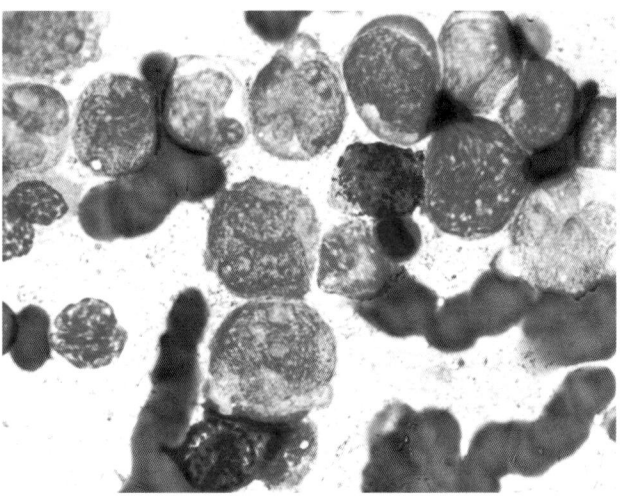

A   **B**

FIGURE 41.7. Myeloid proliferations with t(6;9)(p23;q34); *DEK-NUP214.* **A:** This marrow shows a mix of dyspoietic granulocytic and erythroid precursors with admixed blast cells and basophils with washed-out cytoplasmic granules. A careful differential cell count is needed to differentiate an MDS from AML when this cytogenetic abnormality is present. **B:** A case with more abundant blast cells with myelomonocytic features and admixed basophils.

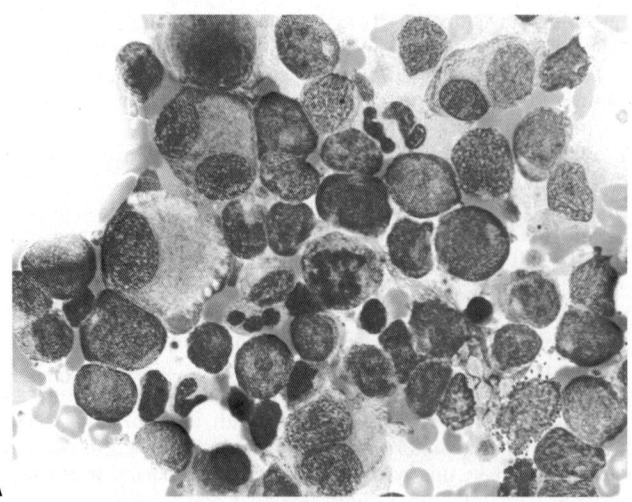 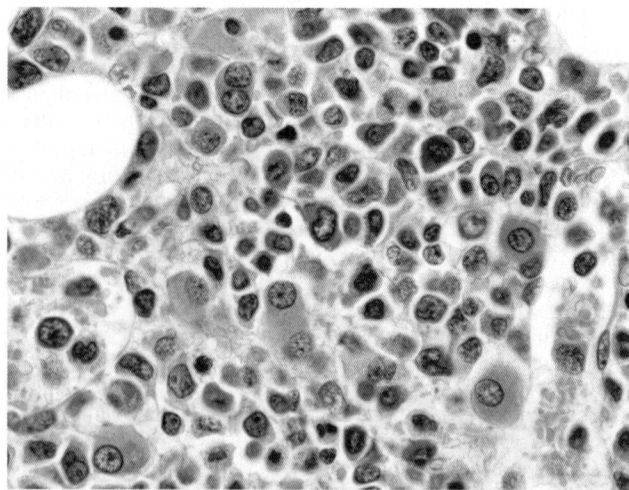

A **B**

FIGURE 41.8. AML with inv(3)(q21q26.2) or t(3;3)(q21;q26.2); *RPN1-EVI1.* The BM aspirate (**A**) and biopsy (**B**) both show numerous monolobed and bilobed megakaryocytes, characteristic of this cytogenetic abnormality, with admixed blasts.

a median age of 56 years. There is no gender predilection. Patients may present with cytopenias, hepatosplenomegaly, and/or a prior history of MDS (85–87). In contrast to most other AML subtypes, some cases are associated with thrombocytosis (7% to 22%). The appearance of the blasts varies from case to case and may manifest with myeloblast, monoblast, or megakaryoblastic features. In addition, AML with inv(3) (q21q26.2) or t(3;3)(q21;q26.2) is commonly associated with multilineage dysplasia in the nonblast populations. Therefore, prior to the 2008 WHO classification, most cases of AML with inv(3)(q21q26.2) or t(3;3)(q21;q26.2) were diagnosed as AML with multilineage dysplasia and would have met criteria for any of the FAB AML types except for APL (M3). Megakaryocytes are most commonly dysplastic and characteristically increased with numerous small mono- or bilobed forms (Fig. 41.8). Large hypogranular platelets and naked megakaryocytic nuclei may be seen on PB smears. Erythroid and myeloid dysplastic changes are also commonly seen in the BM and PB. In addition, mast cells, basophils, and eosinophils may be increased. BM cellularity is variable and may be hypocellular with or without fibrosis. Small dysplastic megakaryocytes are often identifiable on biopsies.

The immunophenotype of the blasts in AML with inv(3) (q21q26.2) or t(3;3)(q21;q26.2) is not specific. Myeloid and/ or monocytic antigens may be expressed, and the blasts most often are positive for CD13, CD33, CD34, CD38, and HLA-DR. Megakaryocyte-associated markers, including CD41 and CD61, may be demonstrable. In addition, CD7 expression is not infrequent, but expression of other lymphoid-associated antigens is uncommon (88).

The cytogenetic abnormality resulting from either inversion of the long arm of chromosome 3 or t(3;3)(q21;q26.2) results in the fusion of the *EVI1* (ectopic virus integration-1) gene with the *RPN1* (ribophorin I) gene. Sequences in the latter may act as enhancer elements of the former resulting in overexpression of *EVI1*, an oncogene whose overexpression is also observed in some AMLs with *MLL* gene rearrangements and is generally associated with a poor prognosis (89). Indeed, AML with inv(3) (q21q26.2) or t(3;3)(q21;q26.2) is associated with an aggressive clinical course and short survival (90). Translocation of the *EVI1* gene has also been reported in therapy-associated myeloid neoplasia [e.g., t(3;21)(q26.2;q22) (*EVI1-RUNX1*)], but such variant translocations involving 3q26.2 are not included in the classification of AML with inv(3)(q21q26.2) or t(3;3)(q21;q26.2) (14,16). Additional cytogenetic abnormalities are reported in up to 75% of cases, with monosomy 7 (~50% of cases), deletion 5q, and

complex karyotypes being the most frequently observed (86). The influence of these additional cytogenetic abnormalities on the already poor prognosis associated with this disease is unknown. Some patients who present with MDS may have obtained other cytogenetic abnormalities prior to the development of either inv(3)(q21q26.2) or t(3;3)(q21;q26.2). It is also noteworthy that either of these chromosome 3 abnormalities may occur as a secondary rearrangement in patients with CML, most often associated with acceleration or transformation of disease (14,91).

The differential diagnosis of AML with inv(3)(q21q26.2) or t(3;3)(q21;q26.2) includes AML-MRC, subtypes of AML, NOS, blast crisis of CML, AML with t(1;22)(p13;q13), and myeloid proliferations related to Down syndrome. Cytogenetics studies are certainly key to resolving this differential diagnosis, and the presence of either inv(3)(q21q26.2) or t(3;3)(q21;q26.2) takes precedence over a diagnosis of AML-MRC. In contrast, a diagnosis of accelerated or blast phase of CML is preferred for new cases of AML in which t(9;22)(q34;q11.2) and either inv(3)(q21q26.2) or t(3;3)(q21;q26.2) is identified (14). The clinical history is also important in sorting out the differential diagnosis. AML with inv(3)(q21q26.2) or t(3;3)(q21;q26.2) is very rare in children, whereas AML with t(1;22)(p13;q13) is predominantly a disease of infants (see below).

Acute Myeloid Leukemia (Megakaryoblastic) with t(1;22)(p13;q13) (RBM15-MKL1)

AML (megakaryoblastic) with t(1;22)(p13;q13) is primarily a disease of infancy with a median age of 4 months. This AML subtype accounts for approximately 1% of all childhood AML and is more common in females (92,93). Patients can present with cytopenias, and commonly they develop hepatosplenomegaly and/or skeletal lesions. Some patients present with isolated myeloid sarcoma. The morphologic features are similar to those of other AML types with megakaryoblastic differentiation. Blasts may show a range in size and often have round or slightly irregular nuclei with or without conspicuous nucleoli, fine reticular chromatin, densely basophilic and agranular cytoplasm, and cytoplasmic protrusions or blebs (Fig. 41.9). Some of the blasts may appear undifferentiated. Micromegakaryocytes are commonly seen in BM aspirates, but dysplastic features in the erythroid or myeloid lineages are unusual in AML with t(1;22)(p13;q13) as opposed to other AML subtypes with megakaryoblastic differentiation. Reticulin fibrosis with or without collagen fibrosis is commonly associated with this

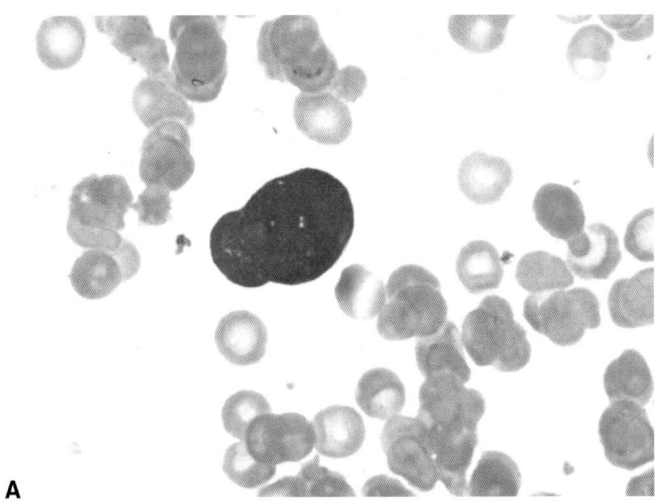
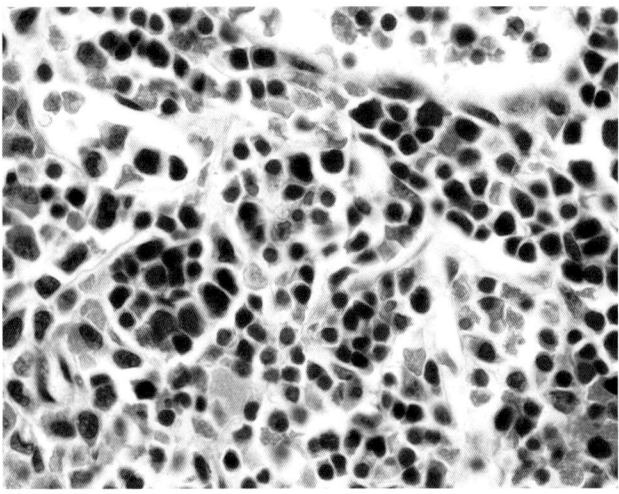

FIGURE 41.9. AML (megakaryoblastic) with t(1;22)(p13;q13); *RBM15-MKL1.* **A:** Although the aspirate in this infant was aparticulate, scattered immature cells with basophilic cytoplasm and a suggestion of cytoplasmic blebbing were present on the smears. **B:** The BM biopsy shows clusters of immature cells. This pattern may also occur in extramedullary presentations of this disease, possibly leading to confusion with nonleukemic small round cell tumors of childhood.

disease, and therefore hemodilute and/or aparticulate BM aspirates may be encountered and may misrepresent the true BM blast percentage. Correlation with the core biopsy findings is important in such cases, and clusters of megakaryoblasts may be found associated with areas of fibrosis.

Flow cytometry immunophenotyping studies of AML with t(1;22)(p13;q13) usually demonstrate expression of megakaryocyte-associated antigens CD41 (glycoprotein IIb/IIIa) and CD61 (glycoprotein IIIa), as well as CD36. Spurious surface expression of CD41 and CD61 is not infrequently detected on other AMLs due to platelets binding to the surface of blasts, and in these cases the expression of these antigens is often dim to moderate. In contrast, bright surface or, more specifically, cytoplasmic staining of these antigens is supportive of true megakaryoblastic differentiation. CD42 (glycoprotein Ib), which is a marker expressed by more mature megakaryocytes, is less commonly expressed in AML with t(1;22)(p13;q13) but is also quite specific for megakaryocytic differentiation. Myeloid-associated antigens, CD13 and CD33, are sometimes detected. In contrast, CD34, CD45, and HLA-DR are typically negative. The blasts are also negative for lymphoid-associated antigens, including TdT, as well as MPO by flow cytometry and cytochemical staining methods. In tissue sections, the blasts show a similar immunophenotype described above. Additional less specific markers that may be useful by immunohistochemical staining include von Willebrand factor (factor VIII–related antigen) and linker for activation of T cells (LAT).

The t(1;22)(p13;q13) results in fusion of the RNA-binding motif protein-15 gene (*RBM15*, also known as *OTT*) with the megakaryocyte leukemia-1 gene (*MKL1*, also known as *MAL*). The precise oncogenic role of the t(1;22)(p13;q13) *RBM15-MKL1* rearrangement in this disease is unclear. The fusion protein may have numerous intracellular effects including modulation of chromatin organization, *HOX*-induced differentiation, and extracellular signaling pathways (94,95). Additional cytogenetic abnormalities are common in the relatively older patients (>6 months of age), but the impact of these additional abnormalities is not clear primarily because the disease itself is so rare. *FLT3* mutations have been reported in AML with t(1;22)(p13;q13), but the precise frequency and impact of these are also unknown. In general, patients with AML with t(1;22) (p13;q13) now respond well to intensive AML therapy despite earlier results suggesting a relatively poor prognosis associated with this disease (96).

The differential diagnosis of AML with t(1;22)(p13;q13) chiefly includes the acute megakaryoblastic leukemia subtype of AML, NOS, AML with inv(3)(q21q26.2) or t(3;3)(q21;q26.2), myeloid proliferations of DS, and MDS. The results of cytogenetics studies together with the clinical history can usually resolve this differential diagnosis. Due to the frequency of marrow fibrosis, the demonstration of ≥20% blasts may be difficult in some cases, and such patients should be closely monitored. In some cases the clusters of blasts in the BM or extramedullary sites may suggest nonhematopoietic small round blue cell tumors of childhood, such as neuroblastoma or hepatoblastoma. A high index of suspicion is important in such cases, as is a low threshold for utilizing immunohistochemical stains such as CD61, factor VIII–related antigen, and LAT.

AML with Recurrent Genetic Abnormalities not Included in the 2008 WHO Classification: *De novo* AML with t(9;22)(q34;q11.2) *(BCR-ABL1)*, AML with t(3;5)(q25;q35) *(MLF1-NPM1)*, and AML with t(8;16)(p11.2;p13.3) *(MYST3-CREBB)*

There are additional cytogenetic abnormalities that were not included in the 2008 WHO as defining AML subtypes but that nonetheless recur in AML with low frequency and may be associated with somewhat distinct clinical features. Three of these are discussed in this section.

Although the majority of cases of AML with t(9;22) (q34;q11.2) (*BCR-ABL1*) represent blast transformation of CML, rare cases of *de novo* AML with t(9;22)(q34;q11.2) (*BCR-ABL1*) have been reported (97,98). Such cases represent fewer than 1% of all AML and seem to be associated with a poor prognosis similar to that of blast transformation of CML. In contrast to the latter, *de novo* AML with t(9;22)(q34;q11.2) (*BCR-ABL1*) is less commonly associated with splenomegaly and basophilia. In addition, *de novo* AML with t(9;22)(q34;q11.2) (*BCR-ABL1*) may have lower BM cellularity than CML in blast crisis. Certainly exclusion of an underlying CML may not be possible in some instances. The morphologic and immunophenotypic features are variable in *de novo* AML with t(9;22)(q34;q11.2) (*BCR-ABL1*), and cases may show features of various AML, NOS, subtypes. Note that the t(9;22)(q34;q11.2) (*BCR-ABL1*)

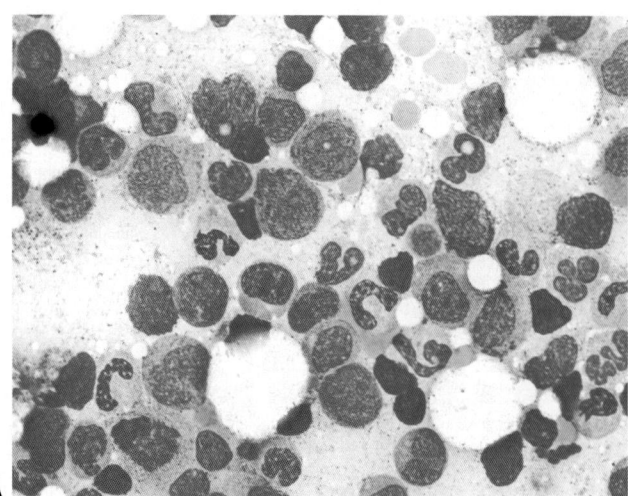 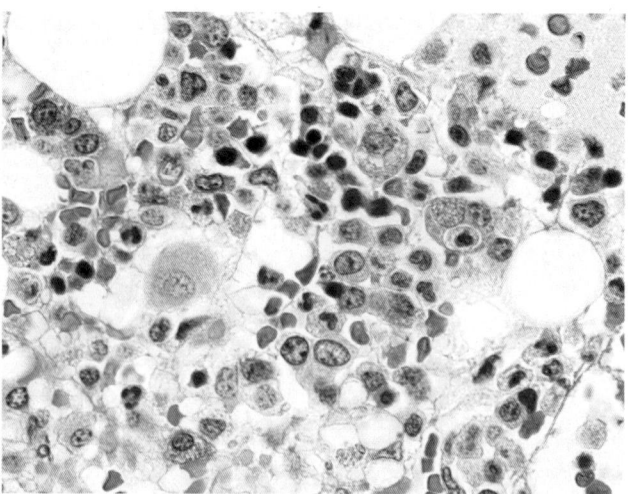

FIGURE 41.10. AML with t(8;16)(p11.2;p13.3);*MYST3-CREBB*. A: In this case the blasts have a myelomonocytic appearance with mild dyspoietic changes of the background granulocytes. **B:** On the biopsy, hemosiderin-laden macrophages, including some showing hemophagocytosis, are present.

rearrangement also occurs in B-lymphoblastic leukemia as well as in a subset of MPAL cases.

The t(3;5)(q25;q35) (*MLF1-NPM1*) rearrangement occurs in MDS as well as AML-MRC and is likely present in fewer than 1% of all AML (99,100). These myeloid proliferations appear to occur more frequently in young men compared to other AML-MRC. Many cases show a background of myelodysplasia, and the blasts may show morphologic features consistent with many FAB AML subtypes. In general, AML with t(3;5)(q25;q35) (*MLF1-NPM1*) cases are associated with a poor prognosis with current therapies, but there may be benefits from early hematopoietic stem cell transplantation.

AML with t(8;16)(p11.2;p13.3) (*MYST3-CREBB*) occurs in both children and adults and may present as *de novo* AML or as a therapy-related AML following therapy with either an alkylating agent or topoisomerase II inhibitor (101). Interestingly, AML with t(8;16)(p11.2;p13.3) (*MYST3-CREBB*) may also occur as a congenital disease with preferential cutaneous involvement and spontaneous regression (considered a form of "blueberry muffin" baby) (102). The blasts typically demonstrate myelomonocytic or monocytic features, and hemophagocytosis and erythrophagocytosis by the blasts has been described in some cases (Fig. 41.10). The prognosis of AML with t(8;16)(p11.2;p13.3) (*MYST3-CREBB*) is variable, and cases that arise following therapy are particularly associated with a poor prognosis.

ACUTE MYELOID LEUKEMIA WITH GENE MUTATIONS

There is a growing list of genes that are frequently mutated in AML but that are not necessarily involved in chromosomal rearrangements. These include *FLT3, KIT, NPM1, CEBPA, WT1, NRAS, IDH1, IDH2, TET2, MLL, DNMT3A,* and *RUNX1,* among others (27,103–113). Some of these mutations are so-called type I (or class I) gene mutations (e.g., mutations in *KIT* and *FLT3*) and impart enhanced proliferative or survival advantage on the neoplastic proliferations without affecting differentiation, and they are now considered important prognostic indicators in many of the aforementioned AML subtypes as well as AML, NOS (114). In contrast, so-called type II (or class II) gene mutations are considered primary, disease-defining events in AML and do appear to affect differentiation as well as apoptosis.

Mutations in two of these genes, *NPM1* and *CEBPA,* occur with relatively high frequency in AML with normal cytogenetics and appear to be associated with distinct clinical, morphologic, and immunophenotypic features that warrant inclusion in the 2008 WHO classification as provisional entities (14).

Acute Myeloid Leukemia with Mutated *NPM1*

Mutations in *NPM1* (nucleophosmin 1) on chromosome 5q35 are quite common in AML and occur in approximately 50% of adult and 20% of childhood AML with normal karyotype (26,112,115–117). *NPM1* mutations also occur in approximately 5% to 15% of cases of AML with abnormal cytogenetics including trisomy 8, deletion of chromosome 9q, and rare cases of AML with 11q23 abnormalities or other recurring cytogenetic abnormalities. Patients usually present with anemia and thrombocytopenia, and they tend to have higher PB blast counts compared to other AML subtypes. Extramedullary disease may also be present.

The majority of adult cases of AML with mutated *NPM1* show monocytic differentiation with frequent expression of monocyte-associated surface antigens CD11b, CD14, and CD68 in addition to myeloid-associated markers CD13, CD33, and MPO. CD34 negativity is essentially the rule in AML with mutated *NPM1*. Childhood cases may show a similar morphology and immunophenotype, including absence of CD34 expression. However, many pediatric cases may show myeloid blast morphology, with or without differentiation, or myelomonocytic features. There are rare reported cases of acute erythroid leukemia with mutated *NPM1*.

Nucleophosmin, the gene product of *NPM1,* is a nuclear protein that facilitates molecular transport between the nucleus and cytoplasm. It also participates in other cellular processes including ribosomal formation, centrosomal duplication, and regulation of the ARF-TP53 tumor suppressor pathway (118,119). Approximately 40 different mutations in *NPM1* have been described, and these most frequently occur in exon 12 but have also been reported in exons 9 and 11. These mutations all similarly result in creation of a nuclear export signal in the C-terminus of the protein that causes aberrant cytoplasmic accumulation of nucleophosmin. This can be detected by immunohistochemical analysis, and cytoplasmic nucleophosmin localization is predictive of mutation in the *NPM1* gene (120,121) (Fig. 41.11). AML with mutated *NPM1* shows a unique gene expression profile that is characterized at least

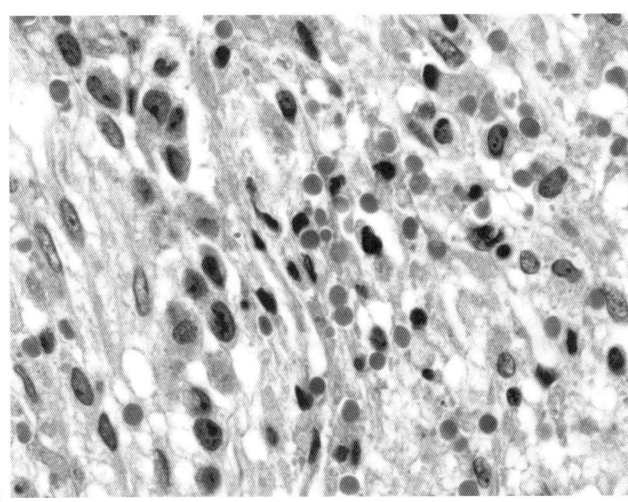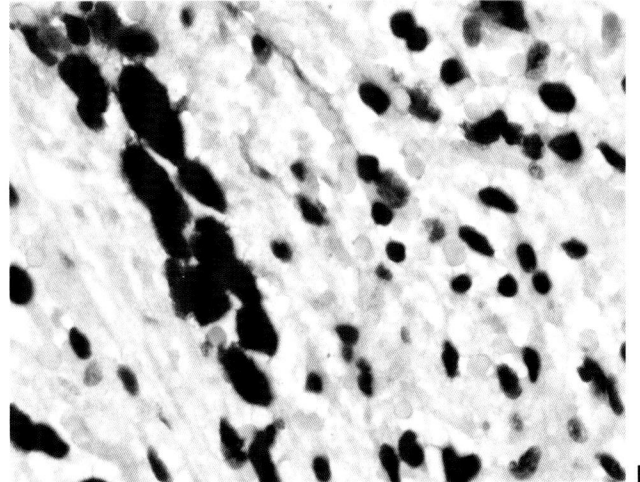

A   B

FIGURE 41.11. Residual AML with mutated *NPM1.* **A:** The H&E section of the posttherapy BM shows large atypical cells to the left. **B:** These cells show strong cytoplasmic and nuclear NPM1 expression in the large cells, while the background cells show only the expected nuclear staining.

in part by *HOX* gene dysregulation and that is qualitatively distinct from gene expression profiles observed in other AML subtypes (122,123).

AML with mutated *NPM1* and a normal karyotype generally carries a favorable prognosis similar to that of the core binding factor leukemias, AML with t(8;21)(q22;q22), and AML with inv(16)(p13q22) or t(16;16)(p13;q22). However, approximately 40% of cases of AML with mutated *NPM1* also have the *FLT3*-ITD mutation, and the presence of the latter abrogates the favorable prognosis normally associated with AML with mutated *NPM1*. Such cases have an intermediate prognosis between cases with unmutated *FLT3* and cases of AML with *FLT3*-ITD but without mutation in the *NPM1* gene. Interestingly, AML with mutated *NPM1* and *FLT3*-ITD may preferentially demonstrate cup-like nuclear invaginations in the blasts (124,125) (Fig. 41.12). However, this feature is neither completely sensitive nor specific for AML with both mutations. In addition, although immunohistochemical analysis for nucleophosmin can predict the presence of a mutation in the *NPM1* gene, there is no known immunohistochemical correlate for the prediction of a *FLT3*-ITD mutation. Therefore, molecular

studies are preferentially utilized to screen for both *NPM1* mutations and *FLT3*-ITD in all new cases of AML (126,127).

Acute Myeloid Leukemia with Mutated *CEBPA*

Mutations in *CEBPA* occur in approximately 13% of AML with normal karyotype in adults and 17% to 20% of AML with normal karyotype in children. Approximately 70% of cases of AML with mutated *CEBPA* have normal karyotypes, and 10% have one karyotypic abnormality (128–130). Patients tend to present with relatively higher hemoglobin levels and lower platelet counts compared to other AML subtypes. In addition, PB blast counts are often high. Extramedullary involvement is uncommon.

The blasts in AML with mutated *CEBPA* usually show myeloblast features with or without maturation, although occasional cases may show monocytic or myelomonocytic features. There are no distinct immunophenotypic features of AML with mutated *CEBPA*. Blasts typically express myeloid-associated antigens, and CD34 and HLA-DR expression is also common. Monocytic markers are usually absent. Most lymphoid associated antigens are also not expressed except for CD7, which is reported in 50% to 73% of cases (131,132).

The *CEBPA* gene is located on chromosome 19q31.1 and encodes a tumor suppressor transcription factor functioning in myelopoiesis as well as in lung development, adipogenesis, and glucose metabolism (133). Mutations in *CEBPA* are diverse with more than 100 described, and many laboratories do not offer testing for *CEBPA* mutations given the complexity and heterogeneity (134). Most of the mutations in *CEBPA* are point mutations that result in translation of a smaller dominant negative form of the protein, which impedes normal regulation of granulocytic differentiation. Dysregulation of *CEBPA* has also been described secondary to epigenetic modification as well as in AML with t(8;21)(q22;q22) due to transcriptional repression by the RUNX1-RUNX1T1 fusion protein. Mutations in *CEBPA* have also been described in therapy-related AML, and such cases should be diagnosed as therapy-related AML with a comment regarding the presence of a *CEBPA* mutation.

Most patients with AML with mutated *CEBPA* and normal cytogenetics have a favorable prognosis similar to that of the core binding factor leukemias (110,135–137). This may be related to the presence of double mutations in the *CEBPA* gene as well as the lack of both *FLT3*-ITD mutations, which occur infrequently in AML with mutated *CEBPA*, and poor prognostic

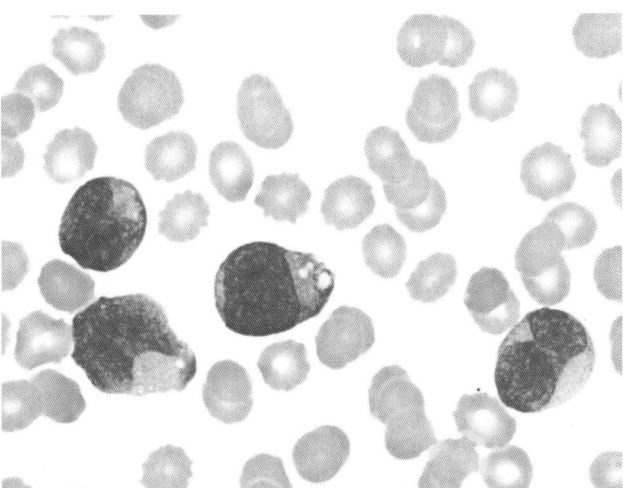

FIGURE 41.12. AML with mutated *NPM1.* In this case, many of the blasts have cuplike nuclear indentations that are reported to be associated with this mutation as well as mutation of *FLT3*. Both mutations were present in this case.

cytogenetic abnormalities. The possible benefit of postremission stem cell transplantation in this disorder is not yet known.

Acute Myeloid Leukemia with Other Genetic Abnormalities

As described in the preceding sections, mutations in the *KIT* and *FLT3* genes are common in AML and can influence response to therapy and overall prognosis. Both gene products encode surface tyrosine kinase receptors that are widely expressed on hematopoietic stem and progenitor cells and that facilitate survival, proliferation, and differentiation during hematopoiesis. Activating point mutations in *KIT* are frequently detected in the core binding factor leukemias, and such mutations, especially those involving exon 17, are associated with increased rates of relapse and shorter survival times (27). Mutations in the *FLT3* gene occur in approximately one-third of cases of AML, NOS (most commonly AML without differentiation), with a normal karyotype as well as in some types of AML with recurrent cytogenetic abnormalities (described above); in contrast, they are relatively rare in the core binding factor leukemias as well as in AML with translocations involving the *MLL* gene on chromosome 11q23. Activating *FLT3* mutations generally fall into two categories: tyrosine kinase domain point mutations (*FLT3*-TKD) and internal tandem duplications that occur within the juxtamembrane domain (*FLT3*-ITD) (103,107,138). Rare juxtamembrane point mutations in *FLT3* have also been described (139). In general, AML with *FLT3* mutations are associated with inferior responses to therapy and shorter overall survival times in comparison to AML with otherwise similar features (131,140–142). However, the prognostic impact of a *FLT3* mutation in some forms of AML with unfavorable cytogenetics and that are already associated with poorer prognoses, such as AML with t(6;9)(p23;q34) and inv(3)(q21q26.2) or t(3;3) (q21;q26.2), is not clear. It is recommended that evaluation for mutation in the *FLT3* gene be routinely performed on all new cases of AML with a normal karyotype as well as in all patients with AML enrolled in clinical trials (11).

Mutations in the Wilms' tumor gene, *WT1*, occur in 10% to 15% of AML, most commonly in AML, NOS, with a normal karyotype, and are associated with decreased overall survival as well as decreased rates of complete remission when present in combination with a *FLT3*-ITD mutation (108,143,144). The *RUNX1* gene, which is involved in recurrent translocations t(8;21)(q22;q22), t(3;21)(q26.2;q22), and t(12;21)(p13;q22) in acute leukemia, is also mutated in approximately 5% to 15% of cases of cytogenetically normal AML, particularly AML with minimal differentiation (FAB M0). *RUNX1* mutations are also associated with somatic trisomy 8, 13, and 21 in AML as well as with *MLL*-PTD and *IDH1/2* mutations (109,145,146). AML with mutated *RUNX1* are generally associated with inferior outcomes, although improved survival times have been reported following allogeneic hematopoietic stem cell transplantation (146). *NRAS* mutations occur in 10% to 20% of AML and are most commonly observed in pediatric cases of AML with monocytic differentiation, including AML with inv(16)(p13.1q22) or t(16;16)(p13.1q22) and AML with inv(3)(q21q26.2) or t(3;3) (q21q26.2) (147–149). The clinical impact of mutation in the *NRAS* gene is not clear.

Aberrant epigenetic modifications, such as DNA methylation, are observed in a significant proportion of AML and are associated with mutations in an expanding cohort of genes including *DNMT3A*, *IDH1*, *IDH2*, and *TET2*, among others. Mutations in the DNA methyltransferase 3A gene, *DNMT3A*, the majority of which occurs at arginine codon 882, have been associated with dysregulation of genes important for hematopoiesis and epigenetic modification, including *HOX* genes that are also dysregulated in *MLL*-associated AML. Somatic

mutations in *DNMT3A* are demonstrable in up to 35% of both *de novo* AML and secondary AML, and they are preferentially associated with a normal karyotype, monocytic differentiation, high PB and BM blast counts, and overall unfavorable prognosis (150–153), although the latter may be related to age at diagnosis and specific mutation in *DNMT3A* (154). Mutations in *DNMT3A* are also commonly observed in conjunction with other gene mutations, and the presence of mutated *DNMT3A* appears to abrogate the favorable prognosis associated with AML with mutated NPM1 (152). The *IDH1* and *IDH2* genes encode isoforms of the nicotinamide adenine dinucleotide phosphate–dependent isocitrate dehydrogenases that are important for the biochemical conversion of 5-methylcytosine to 5-hydroxymethylcytosine. The tet oncogene family member 2, *TET2*, gene product also converges on this pathway, and mutations in both *IDH* genes and the *TET2* gene result in a state of hypermethylation, which is theorized to be a critical step in leukemogenesis (155). Interestingly, mutations in *IDH* and *TET2* genes appear to be mutually exclusive events, occurring in up to one-third and one quarter of *de novo* AML, NOS, respectively; *TET2* mutations have also been observed across the spectrum of AML categories (156–159). In general, mutations in *IDH* and *TET2* genes are associated with older age at presentation, but the clinical characteristics vary depending upon the specific mutation. Moreover, the clinical significance of these mutations in AML is not yet clear and needs to be more thoroughly evaluated in the context of other patient, disease, and therapeutic factors (160).

Genetic abnormalities in AML also include global changes in epigenetic regulatory systems such as DNA methylation, histone modifications, and expression of noncoding inhibitory microRNA molecules (miRs). Hyper- or hypomethylation of CpG islands within the 5′ promoter regions of genes that regulate cell cycle, apoptosis, and proliferation as well as aberrant histone modifications, such as acetylation and methylation, that result in global gene dysregulation, have been observed in multiple forms of AML including APL, core binding factor leukemias, and AML with rearrangements in *MLL* (161–169). Consequently, pharmacologic agents that can target these processes, such as 5′-azacytidine, decitabine, and valproic acid, have been investigated and do show some clinical benefit in studies of AML as well as for patients with MDS (170–173). Recently, numerous studies have demonstrated dysregulation of miRs in AML, with evidence for recurrent miR profiles associated with certain subtypes of AML (174,175). For instance, overexpression of *miR-126* and *miR-126** has been observed in core binding factor leukemias, whereas overexpression of *miR-10a* and *miR-10b* is associated with AML with mutated NPM1 (176–179). Moreover, the relative expression of certain miRs, such as *miR-181a* in AML with normal karyotype, may provide additional information for accurate risk stratification (180). Indeed, the prognostic impact of these epigenetic abnormalities and the degree to which they may serve as therapeutic targets in AML is a large area of ongoing investigation.

ACUTE MYELOID LEUKEMIA WITH MYELODYSPLASIA-RELATED CHANGES

The 2008 WHO classification revised and expanded the previous 2001 WHO category of AML with multilineage dysplasia to include those cases of AML with certain recurring or complex cytogenetic abnormalities historically associated with a poor prognosis as well as those cases of AML arising in patients with a prior history of MDS (8,15,181). The 2008 WHO classification of AML with myelodysplasia-related changes (AML-MRC) includes cases of AML that meet at least one of the following criteria: (a) association with multilineage dysplasia, (b) association with MDS-related cytogenetic abnormalities, and/or (c) association with a prior history of MDS. The diagnosis of AML-MRC requires a blast count of at least 20%. In addition, the diagnosis requires the absence of any prior cytotoxic therapy for an unrelated disease as well as absence of any cytogenetic abnormality that would classify a case as AML with recurrent cytogenetic abnormalities (described in the previous section).

AML-MRC is rare in children but occurs at a relatively high rate in adults, especially the elderly, at a likely frequency of at least 35% of all adult AML. Patients often present with severe pancytopenia. Typically the BM is hypercellular; however, some cases of AML-MRC show BM hypocellularity defined as <30% in individuals ≤60 year of age or <20% in individuals >60 years of age. Most cases show features of AML with maturation or acute myelomonocytic leukemia; however, some cases exhibit features of AML without maturation or erythroleukemia. There are no specific immunophenotypic characteristics of the blasts, although depending upon the morphologic features the blasts may express monocyte-associated antigens (182). Most cases express CD34, CD33, CD13, and CD117. Aberrant expression of lymphoid-associated antigens, including TdT, CD7, CD10, and CD56, may be present. TdT and CD7 in particular may be associated with abnormalities of chromosomes 5 and 7.

Multilineage dysplasia is evident in the majority of cases (Fig. 41.13). Of note, in contrast to MDS, which requires the presence of dysplastic features in at least 10% of lineage cells, the diagnosis of AML-MRC with multilineage dysplasia requires evidence of dysplasia in at least 50% of maturing cells in at least two lineages (16). Dysplastic features in the erythroid lineage include megaloblastic change, nuclear membrane irregularity, karyorrhexis, nuclear fragmentation, multinucleation, cytoplasmic vacuolization, aberrant periodic acid-Schiff (PAS) positivity, and the presence of ring sideroblasts. Dysplastic features in the myeloid lineage include cytoplasmic hypogranularity, abnormal nuclear segmentation including pseudo–Pelger-Huët anomaly, and nuclear to cytoplasmic dyssynchrony. On BM biopsy sections, atypical localization of immature precursors may be observed. Dysplasia in the myeloid lineage is often better appreciated on well-stained PB smears. Dysplastic megakaryocytes most often take the form of micromegakaryocytes (small forms with mature granular cytoplasm and hypolobated nuclei) or large cells with either multiple separate nuclei or nonlobated nuclei.

Three main categories of cytogenetic abnormalities that can confer a diagnosis of AML-MRC are described in the 2008 WHO

Table 41.3	CYTOGENETIC ABNORMALITIES SUFFICIENT TO DIAGNOSE AML WITH MYELODYSPLASIA-RELATED CHANGES WHEN ≥20% BLASTS ARE PRESENT IN BLOOD OR BM	
Complex karyotype	≥3 unrelated chromosomal abnormalities, not including any rearrangements that would define a subtype of AML with recurrent cytogenetic abnormalities	
Unbalanced abnormalities	−7/del(7q)	del(11q)
	−5/del(5q)	del(12p)/t(12p)
	i(17q/t(17p)	del(9q)
	−13/del(13q)	idic(X)(q13)
Balanced abnormalities	t(11;16)(q23;p13.3)[a]	t(5;12)(q33;p12)
	t(3;21)(q26.2;q22.1)[a]	t(5;7)(q33;q11.2)
	t(1;3)(p36.3;q21.1)	t(5;17)(q33;p13)
	t(2;11)(p21;q23)[a]	t(5;10)(q33;q21)
		t(3;5)(q25;q34)

[a]These chromosomal abnormalities usually occur in therapy-related myeloid neoplasms, and a history of prior cytotoxic therapy must be excluded in order to make a diagnosis of AML with myelodysplasia-related changes.

classification (Table 41.3) (15). One of the categories includes nine specific balanced translocations, four of which involve the locus on chromosome 5q33 where the platelet derived growth factor receptor β gene (*PDGFRB*) resides. Two translocations involve the *MLL* gene on chromosome 11q23, and these rearrangements, t(2;11)(p21;q23) and t(11;16)(q23;p13.3), are considered specific for AML-MRC in the absence of prior cytotoxic therapy. Translocations (3;21)(q26.2;q22.1) and (1;3) (p36.3;q21.1) involve the *EVI1* and *RPN1* loci, respectively, which are also rearranged in AML with inv(3)(q21q26.2) or t(3;3)(q21;q26.2). The last rearrangement included in this category, t(3;5)(q25;q35), is more frequently associated with younger patients and was discussed in greater detail above.

The diagnosis of AML-MRC can also be made in the setting of either a complex karyotype or an unbalanced chromosomal abnormality (Table 41.3) assuming a blast count of ≥20%. Often the specific unbalanced chromosomal abnormalities are part of a complex karyotype, with deletions of chromosomes 5q, 7q, 17p, and 12q being the most common (183). Although trisomy 8 and del 20q are common abnormalities in MDS, these are not considered specific for AML-MRC when they occur alone and are not included in the list of unbalanced chromosomal abnormalities that are sufficient to diagnose AML-MRC. Likewise, loss of chromosome Y in males is a somewhat common, yet nonspecific finding and can be seen in older men without evidence of myeloid neoplasia.

AML-MRC is generally associated with a poor prognosis, although indeed the classification includes a heterogeneous group of AML, some of which are associated with particularly worse outcomes compared to others. For instance, patients with AML-MRC with MDS-associated cytogenetic abnormalities reportedly fare worse than patients with AML-MRC without cytogenetic abnormalities (184,185). Moreover, AML-MRC with autosomal monosomies or with overexpression of the *EVI1* gene is associated with a particularly poor prognosis (32,186,187). The influence of mutations in other genes, including *FLT3*, *NPM1*, and *CEBPA*, on the prognosis of AML-MRC is the subject of ongoing study. AML-MRC may show mutations in these genes, but the significance of many of these mutations in AML-MRC is not yet known (185). As discussed above, most AML with *NPM1* or *CEBPA* mutations have normal karyotypes, do not demonstrate myelodysplasia-related changes, and are not associated with a prior history of MDS. Currently, AML with dysplasia and either of these gene mutations should be diagnosed as AML-MRC but with the particular mutation clearly stated in the diagnosis line as an additional descriptor. This is particularly important for cases with *NPM1* mutations, which appears to portend an improved prognosis (188,189). Finally, the blast count at diagnosis may impact the clinical course and acuity of

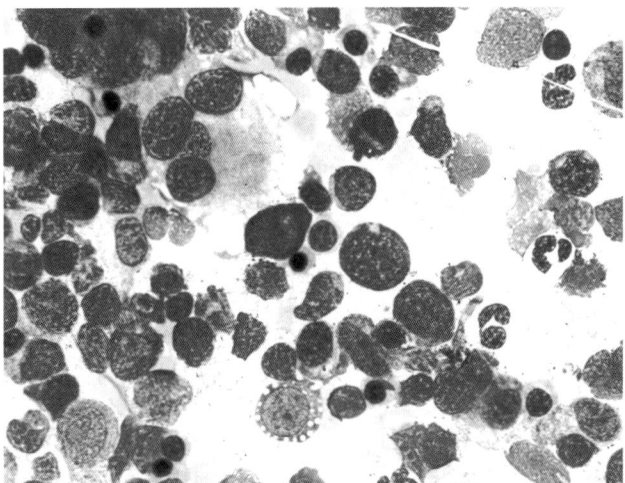

FIGURE 41.13. AML with myelodysplasia related changes and multilineage dysplasia. This case shows dyspoiesis of all three nonblast cell lines, including vacuolated erythroid precursors, hypogranular maturing neutrophils, and atypical megakaryocytes with numerous blast cells in the background.

disease progression. Notably, AML-MRC with multilineage dysplasia and 20% to 29% blasts may behave clinically more like MDS and allow for a "watchful waiting" approach especially in the pediatric population. Such cases were classified as RAEB in transformation according to the FAB classification.

The differential diagnosis of AML-MRC includes MDS, certain subtypes of AML with recurring genetic abnormalities, AML, NOS, and therapy-related AML. This differential diagnosis can usually be resolved with a 500-cell manual differential count demonstrating ≥20% blasts (to exclude MDS) and adequate cytogenetics analysis with routine karyotyping. Of note, blasts should not be enumerated solely by flow cytometry due to potential artifacts of cell lysis, population gating, cell preservation, and hemodilution. Two of the subtypes of AML with recurring genetic abnormalities are particularly associated with dysplasia: AML with inv(3)(q21q26.2) or t(3;3)(q21;q26.2) and AML with t(6;9)(p23;q34) (14). AML with any of these cytogenetic abnormalities should not be diagnosed as AML-MRC but rather as AML with the specific recurring cytogenetic abnormality. A history of prior cytotoxic therapy for an unrelated disease also precludes a diagnosis of AML-MRC. As discussed below, therapy-related myeloid neoplasms are often associated with multilineage dysplasia. However, these are grouped as a separate category in the 2008 WHO classification based on numerous clinical data (16).

Given the high degree of morphologic, immunophenotypic, and cytogenetic heterogeneity within the category of AML-MRC, it is recommended that reports clearly state the basis for this classification in the diagnosis line. This is especially important for monitoring posttherapy specimens for residual disease as well as to facilitate continued research in this area. As an example, a case from a patient with a 10-year history of MDS, ≥20% BM blasts, multilineage dysplasia, and normal cytogenetics should be diagnosed as "acute myeloid leukemia with myelodysplasia-related changes (following previous MDS and multilineage dysplasia)." Because cases with 20% to 29% blasts may behave in a more indolent fashion similar to MDS, it is recommended that the blast count be included clearly in the diagnosis line for this group of patients. Likewise, for cases with *FLT3*, *NPM1*, and/or *CEBPA* mutations, this additional information should also be clearly stated in the diagnosis line (e.g., "acute myeloid leukemia with myelodysplasia-related changes [MDS-associated cytogenetic abnormality] and *CEBPA* mutation").

THERAPY-RELATED MYELOID NEOPLASMS

Therapy-related myeloid neoplasms comprise a mixture of disorders that occur as a somewhat common and unfortunate consequence of chemotherapy and/or radiation therapy for a prior unrelated disease (16,190). This category includes cases of MDS (t-MDS), AML (t-AML), and combined myelodysplastic/myeloproliferative neoplasms (t-MDS/MPN) but not cases of MPN that arise posttherapy. Because it cannot be definitively determined whether a transformed MPN developed from prior therapy or as progression from underlying disease, such cases are not included in this category. Although MDS, AML, and MDS/MPN are distinctly subclassified in the settings of *de novo* disease, numerous data indicate that therapy-related myeloid neoplasms show similar clinical features regardless of the blast count, morphologic features, and, except for specific exceptions described below, cytogenetic findings (191–196). Nonetheless, it is recommended that therapy-related myeloid neoplasms be diagnosed as such with the more specific diagnosis included in the diagnosis line (e.g., "therapy-related myeloid neoplasm [acute myeloid leukemia]").

There are two general subcategories of therapy-related myeloid neoplasms based on prior therapy type, but these may overlap due to patients receiving more than one therapy type in the course of

their prior disease. Patients treated with alkylating agents, such as melphalan, busulfan, carboplatin, and others (Table 41.4), or large field ionizing radiation usually develop a therapy-related myeloid neoplasm 5 to 7 years following therapy, with the disease most often manifesting as t-MDS or t-AML that is preceded by t-MDS for months to years. There appears to be a dose-escalating effect that correlates with risk for development of a therapy-related myeloid neoplasm, and patients with more limited field radiation therapy may be at reduced risk for therapy-related myeloid neoplasms (197). In contrast, 20% to 30% of therapy-related myeloid neoplasms arise following therapy with topoisomerase II inhibitors, such as etoposide, doxorubicin, daunarubicin, and actinomycin. These tend to have a shorter latency period (1 to 3 years), often manifest as t-AML without associated dysplasia or a prodromal MDS phase, and commonly are associated with translocations involving either the *RUNX1* gene on chromosome 21q22 or the *MLL* gene on chromosome 11q23 (193–196). Therapy-related ALL also sometimes occurs following toposiomerase II inhibitor therapy and is usually associated with a t(4;11)(q21;23) rearrangement (198,199). In addition to the above, more recent data indicate that other treatments, including BM transplantation and fludarabine chemotherapy, are also associated with development of therapy-related myeloid neoplasms. Moreover, therapy-related myeloid neoplasms may also arise in patients treated with chemotoxic agents administered as therapy for nonneoplastic diseases.

Therapy-related myeloid neoplasms account for 10% to 20% of AML, MDS, and MDS/MPN. They can occur at any age, although older patients appear to be more susceptible to developing therapy-related myeloid neoplasms associated with prior alkylating agents and/or radiation therapy. Patients typically present with cytopenias including macrocytic anemia with prominent poikilocytosis. Dysplastic neutrophils and hypogranular platelets are commonly identified on PB smears. BM cellularity may range from hypo- to hypercellular from case to case, and approximately 15% of patients develop myelofibrosis. Dysplastic changes in erythroid, myeloid, and megakaryocyte BM precursors are frequently seen, especially in those patients previously treated with radiation and/or alkylating chemotherapy, and the morphologic changes are similar to those described for AML-MRC. Ring sideroblasts are also reported in up to 60% of patients. Blast counts are variable, although approximately half of patients that present with a prodromal MDS phase show <5% blasts in their BM. Few cases (5%) develop features consistent with a t-MDS/MPN (e.g., features of chronic myelomonocytic leukemia). Therapy-related myeloid neoplasms with shorter latencies and that arise following topoisomerase II inhibitor therapy typically lack myelodysplasia and show morphologic features that are similar to the *de novo* AML counterparts with recurrent genetic abnormalities (193). These therapy-related myeloid neoplasms usually present with features of AML with maturation, acute myelomonocytic leukemia, or acute monocytic leukemia.

Table 41.4	CYTOTOXIC AGENTS IMPLICATED IN THERAPY-RELATED MYELOID NEOPLASMS
Alkylating agents[a]	Melphalan, cyclophosphamide, nitrogen mustard, chlorambucil, busulfan, carboplatin, cisplatin, dacarbazine, procarbazine, carmustine, mitomycin C, thiotepa, lomustine
Ionizing radiation[a]	Involvement of large fields including active BM
Topoisomerase II inhibitors[b]	Etoposide, teniposide, doxorubicin, daunorubicin, mitoxantrone, amsacrine, actinomycin
Antimetabolites	Thiopurines, mycophenolate, fludarabine
Antitubulin agents	Vincristine, vinblastine, vindesine, paclitaxel, docetaxel Usually in combination with other cytotoxic agents

[a]Often associated with therapy-related MDS or AML following 5–7 year latency period.
[b]Often associated with therapy-related AML with 1–3 year latency period and without indolent MDS phase.

Immunophenotypic features of TRMN usually correlate with the morphologic findings, and there are no specific immunophenotypic profiles. Blasts are usually CD34+ and coexpress myeloid-associated markers CD13 and CD33, with or without expression of monocyte-associated antigens. Dyssynchronous or aberrant antigen expression, including CD7 and/or CD56 expression, may also be observed.

Greater than 90% of therapy-related myeloid neoplasms demonstrate an abnormal karyotype. The majority of cases (70%) show a complex karyotype with unbalanced chromosomal abnormalities and are associated with longer latencies following alkylating chemotherapy and/or radiation. The abnormal karyotypes usually include whole or partial loss of chromosomes 5 and/or 7 in combination with additional chromosomal abnormalities such as trisomy 8 or deletions of chromosomes 13q, 20q, 11q, 3p, 17, 18, or 21. The 20% to 30% of cases that arise following toposiomerase II inhibitor therapy commonly have balanced translocations involving *MLL* [including t(9;11)(p22;q23) and t(11;19)(q23;p13)] or *RUNX1* [including t(8;21)(q22;q22) and t(3;21)(q26.2;q22.1)], although cases with cytogenetic abnormalities identical to each of the subcategories of AML with recurring genetic abnormalities have been described. Some cases with *FLT3*, *NPM1*, and/or *CEBPA* mutations have also been reported, although the later mutations are uncommon (195,200,201).

In general, therapy-related myeloid neoplasms are associated with a poor prognosis with overall 5-year survival rates of <10%. However, this greatly depends upon the nature of the cytogenetic abnormality as well as the comorbidity of the original underlying disease for which therapy was originally administered. Notably, patients whose therapy-related myeloid neoplasm manifests abnormalities of chromosome 5 and/or 7 and a complex karyotype show a median survival time of <1 year regardless of their blast counts at presentation (191). In contrast, patients who develop t-AML with short latency and no prodromal MDS phase associated with t(15;17)(q24.1;q21.1), inv(16)(p13.1q22), or t(16;16)(p13.1q22) rearrangements may have survival times similar to patients presenting with *de novo*

disease, although there are conflicting data in the literature (192,194,196,202). Patients whose therapy-related myeloid neoplasm have other cytogenetic abnormalities, including other balanced translocations associated with AML with recurring genetic abnormalities, usually fare worse than patients with *de novo* disease. It is not yet known how mutation(s) in *FLT3*, *NPM1*, and/or *CEBPA* genes impact the generally poor prognosis associated with therapy-related myeloid neoplasms.

The differential diagnosis of therapy-related myeloid neoplasms includes categories of *de novo* myeloid neoplasms including MDS, MDS/MPN, and AML. According to the 2008 WHO classification, a prior history of cytotoxic or radiation therapy for a prior unrelated disease takes precedence over any morphologic, immunophenotypic, or cytogenetic factors that would otherwise subclassify *de novo* AML including subtypes of AML with recurring genetic abnormalities (16). Indeed, some myeloid neoplasms may coincidentally arise in the posttherapy setting but be truly *de novo* in nature. More research is needed to determine if and how to distinguish such cases from therapy-related myeloid neoplasms. All cases of t-MDS should be collectively diagnosed as such without regard to blast count and morphologic features that are used to subclassify *de novo* MDS.

ACUTE MYELOID LEUKEMIA, NOT OTHERWISE SPECIFIED

AML, NOS, is a broad category of AML that encompasses a heterogeneous collection of cases that do not meet criteria for AML with recurrent genetic abnormalities, AML-MRC, therapy-related myeloid neoplasms, or myeloid leukemia associated with DS (13). Nine subcategories of AML, NOS, are described in the 2008 WHO, and these are based largely on the prior FAB classification and primarily distinguished based on morphologic, cytochemical, and immunophenotypic features (Table 41.5) (5). However, in contrast to the requirement of 30% or more

Table 41.5 SUBTYPES OF AML, NOS	
AML, NOS, Subtype	**Diagnostic Criteria[a]**
AML with minimal differentiation	• ≥20% blasts without evidence of myeloid differentiation by morphology and cytochemistry (<3% MPO/SBB positive)
AML without maturation	• ≥20% blasts with evidence of myeloid differentiation by morphology and/or cytochemistry (>3% MPO/SBB positive) • No significant myeloid maturation (blasts comprise ≥90% of nonerythroid cells)
AML with maturation	• ≥20% blasts (>3% MPO/SBB positive) • Maturing neutrophilic cells constitute ≥10% of nonerythroid BM cells • Monocytic cells constitute <20% of BM cells
Acute myelomonocytic leukemia	• ≥20% blasts (>3% MPO/SBB positive) • Monocytic cells constitute ≥20% of BM cells • Maturing neutrophilic cells constitute ≥20% of BM cells AND
Acute monoblastic and monocytic leukemias	• >80% of leukemic cells in BM are of monocytic lineage • Minor neutrophilic component (<20% of BM cells)
Acute monoblastic leukemia	• Majority of monocytic cells in BM are monoblasts (typically ≥80%)
Acute monocytic leukemia	• Majority of monocytic cells in BM are promonocytes
Acute erythroid leukemias	• Acute leukemia with predominant erythroid population
Erythroid/myeloid leukemia	• Erythroid precursors constitute ≥50% of nucleated BM cells AND • Myeloblasts constitute ≥20% of nonerythroid BM cells and <20% of total BM cells
Pure erythroid leukemia	• Immature neoplastic erythroid precursors (undifferentiated or proerythroblastic in appearance) constitute ≥80% of total BM cells • No significant increase in myeloblasts
Acute megakaryoblastic leukemia	• ≥20% blasts of which ≥50% are of megakaryocytic lineage
Acute basophilic leukemia	• ≥20% blasts with predominant basophilic differentiation
Acute panmyelosis with myelofibrosis	• Acute proliferation of erythroid, myeloid, and megakaryocytic cells (panmyelosis) accompanied by myelofibrosis and increased blasts (usually 20%–25% of total BM cells)

[a]By definition, cases of AML that meet criteria for AML with recurrent genetic abnormalities, AML-MRC, therapy-related myeloid neoplasms or myeloid proliferations of Down syndrome are excluded.

blasts of the older FAB classification scheme, the AML, NOS, category in the 2008 WHO classification uses a cutoff of 20% or more blasts, similar to the requirement for most other AML subtypes.

Many of the older studies on AML that were morphologically and cytochemically subtyped by the FAB classification included cases that are now distinctly classified according to recurring genetic abnormalities or other qualifiers (e.g., myelodysplasia-related changes or history of prior cytotoxic therapy). Therefore, clinical and genetic data on the AML, NOS, subtypes described below are limited. AML, NOS, is estimated to account for 40% of adult AML and typically occurs in younger individuals compared to AML-MRC. In addition, despite the heterogeneity within the category of AML, NOS, these cases are generally associated with an intermediate prognosis, and subclassification of AML, NOS, is not necessarily essential for directing clinical management (22,203). Notable exceptions to this general rule include the erythroid leukemias and acute panmyelosis with myelofibrosis (APMF), which are diagnosed using criteria that differ from those used for the other AML, NOS, subtypes. Many cases of AML with normal karyotypes fall within the AML, NOS, category. Therefore, molecular analysis for *FLT3*, *NPM1*, and *CEBPA* mutations is recommended on all such AML cases for further classification and prognostic stratification. As discussed above, cases of AML with mutated *NPM1* or *CEBPA* should be classified as the provisional entities associated with these gene mutations and not as AML, NOS.

Acute Myeloid Leukemia with Minimal Differentiation

Cases of AML with minimal differentiation show no morphologic or cytochemical evidence of myeloid differentiation but are diagnosed as AML based on immunophenotypic evidence of expression of myeloid-associated surface antigens. AML with minimal differentiation accounts for <5% of AML and occurs at any age, most often in infants or older adults. Patients typically present with cytopenias, and BM biopsy usually demonstrates a hypercellular marrow with sheets of blasts. Blasts comprise at least 20% of the BM or PB cellularity and are negative for MPO, SBB, napthol-ASD-CAE, and NSE staining by cytochemistry (<3% positive blasts). The blasts may be small to medium in size with very high nuclear to cytoplasmic ratios, dispersed chromatin, variably

prominent nucleoli, and scant, occasionally basophilic cytoplasm (Fig. 41.14A). The blasts also lack cytoplasmic granules (and hence Auer rods) and may appear similar to lymphoblasts.

Flow cytometry studies usually demonstrate expression of CD34, CD38, and HLA-DR, as well as myeloid-associated antigens CD13, CD33, and CD117. However, the blasts typically lack expression of antigens that are expressed on more mature myeloid and monocytic cells, including CD15, CD65, CD11b, CD11c, CD4, CD14, and CD64. As opposed to cytochemical analysis, immunophenotypic analysis for MPO may show partial weak reactivity in the blast population. In addition, blasts may show aberrant expression of the lymphoid-associated antigens CD7, CD19, and TdT, but cytoplasmic lymphoid-associated antigens, cCD79a, cCD22, and cCD3 are negative.

There are no distinct chromosomal abnormalities associated with AML with minimal differentiation, and the demonstration of any recurring or MDS-associated cytogenetic abnormalities discussed in the previous sections would negate a diagnosis of AML, NOS. Subsets of cases diagnosed based on older criteria reportedly have mutations in *FLT3*, *RUNX1* (*AML1*), and/or *ETV6* (204,205). As discussed above, the presence of a mutation in RUNX1 appears to confer a poor clinical outcome (146). The differential diagnosis of AML with minimal differentiation includes ALL, MPAL, AML, and rare cases of circulating lymphoma. Immunophenotypic studies are necessary to resolve the differential.

Acute Myeloid Leukemia Without Maturation

AML without maturation shows morphologic and/or cytochemical evidence of myeloid differentiation but without evidence of significant myeloid maturation. AML without maturation accounts for approximately 5% to 10% of AML and typically occurs in adults, but it can occur at any age. Patients typically present with signs and symptoms related to cytopenias. The PB blast count may be very high, and BM biopsy often demonstrates hypercellular marrow with sheets of blasts, although normocellular and hypocellular marrow cases are not uncommon. Blasts comprise at least 90% of granulocytic cells (≥20% of all nucleated cells), thus not showing significant maturation, and at least 3% of the blasts are positive for either MPO or SBB by cytochemistry and/or they contain Auer rods. Furthermore, <20% of the blasts are positive for NSE.

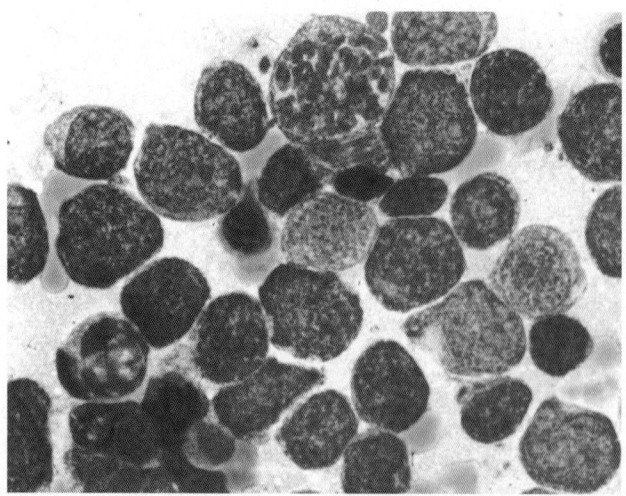
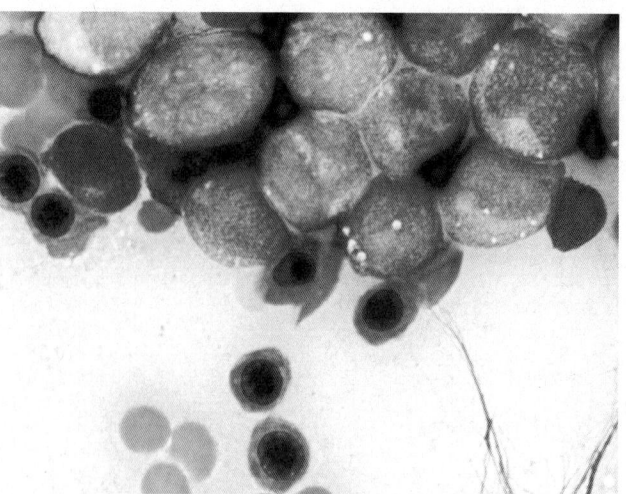

FIGURE 41.14. Acute myeloid leukemia, not otherwise specified. A: This case of AML with minimal differentiation is morphologically similar to AML without maturation. Both show blasts without evidence of granulocytic maturation. **B:** In contrast, AML with maturation shows more cytoplasmic granules and at least 10% of cells showing maturation. Note that dysplastic erythroid precursors are also present, but multilineage dysplasia, sufficient for a diagnosis of AML with myelodysplasia-related changes, was not found in this case, and there was no myelodysplasia-associated cytogenetic abnormality or history of MDS found in this patient.

A   B

Flow cytometry studies show no specific immunophenotype, and blasts are typically positive for CD13, CD33, CD117, and MPO. CD34 and HLA-DR are detected in approximately 70% of cases, and aberrant CD7 is detected in approximately 30% of cases. Surface antigens associated with mature myeloid and monocytic cells are typically not expressed in AML without maturation. No genetic abnormalities are specifically associated with AML without maturation. The differential diagnosis includes ALL and, in cases with high frequency of MPO positive blasts, AML with maturation.

Acute Myeloid Leukemia with Maturation

Cases of AML with maturation contain at least 20% blasts and show evidence of myeloid maturation such that at least 10% of marrow granulocytic cells are composed of promyelocytes and more mature granulocytic cells (Fig. 41.14B). This is one of the most common subtypes of AML, NOS, accounting for approximately 10% of all AML (22). Furthermore, it occurs in all age groups. Patients typically present with signs and symptoms of anemia with variable numbers of PB blasts and variable BM cellularity. Some cases show dysplastic features in the maturing precursors. In addition, eosinophils may be increased without cytologic atypia. The cytochemical and immunophenotypic features of the blasts are similar to those of AML without maturation (>3% MPO and/or SSB positive and <20% NSE positive). However, a significant percentage of the blasts in AML with maturation demonstrate cytoplasmic granulation and/or Auer rods. No distinct genetic mutations are associated with AML with maturation. The differential diagnosis includes MDS (RAEB), AML without maturation, and acute myelomonocytic leukemia, if there is a relatively high percentage of monocytic cells. In addition, many of the features of AML with maturation are similar to those of AML with t(8;21)(q22;q22), but cytogenetics studies performed on all new cases of AML will allow for accurate classification.

Acute Myelomonocytic Leukemia

Acute myelomonocytic leukemia is similar to AML with maturation except that significant monocytic maturation, in addition to myeloid maturation, is observed and each must account for at least 20% of total BM or PB neoplastic cells. In addition, promonocytes are considered blast equivalents and are counted in the blast count; the combination of myeloblasts, monoblasts, and promonocytes must equal at least 20% of the BM or PB cellularity. Acute myelomonocytic leukemia accounts for 5% to 10% of cases of AML and is more common in older individuals and slightly more common in males. Patients often present with anemia and/or thrombocytopenia, and numerous mature monocytes may be present in the PB.

Monoblasts are large cells with round nuclei, delicate chromatin, one or more large prominent nucleoli, and abundant pale to intensely basophilic cytoplasm. Fine azurophilic granules and vacuoles may be present in the cytoplasm. Promonocytes may not be as easily distinguishable from immature or mature monocytes on BM aspirate smears. Promonocytes are large cells with delicately convoluted nuclei, fine chromatin condensation, and pale cytoplasm with usually more prominent cytoplasmic granules and/or vacuoles compared to monoblasts. Monoblasts and promonocytes are usually NSE positive and MPO negative; however, the absence of positive NSE staining does not preclude a diagnosis of acute myelomonocytic leukemia if the morphologic features are supportive. NSE and MPO or combined esterase dual-positive blasts may also be present.

Often by flow cytometry there is demonstration of a heterogeneous blast population with evidence of both myeloid and monocytic differentiation. A proportion of blasts often express the immature markers CD34 and/or CD117, although promonocytes are often negative for both of these antigens. Most cases of acute myelomonocytic leukemia express HLA-DR. Expression of CD13, CD33, CD65, and/or CD15 supports the presence of myeloid differentiation, while expression of CD14, CD4, CD11b, CD11c, CD36, CD64, CD68, CD163, and/or lysozyme is often demonstrable on the subset of blasts showing monocytic differentiation. Aberrant CD7 expression is observed in approximately 30% of cases, whereas expression of other lymphoid-associated antigens is less frequently observed.

No specific genetic mutations are associated with acute myelomonocytic leukemia. The morphologic features are similar to those often observed in AML with inv(16)(p13q22) or t(16;16)(p13;q22) but AML, NOS, should not contain abnormal eosinophils and such findings should warrant additional studies for inv(16)(p13q22) or t(16;16)(p13;q22) if an initial karyotype is normal (44). The differential diagnosis of acute myelomonocytic leukemia also includes combined MDS/MPN, particularly CMML. Both diseases may show a predominance of mature monocytic forms in the PB, whereas promonocytes and myeloblasts are more pronounced in the BM in AMML. Therefore, correlation of a blood monocytosis with BM findings is necessary (17).

Acute Monoblastic and Monocytic Leukemia

Acute monoblastic and acute monocytic leukemias comprise a subset of AML that demonstrates 20% or more monoblasts or promonocytes as well as 80% or more monocytic cells of the nonerythroid cells in the BM. Myeloid maturation is usually minimal in these cases. Acute monoblastic leukemias are differentiated from acute monocyte leukemias based on the relative abundance of monoblasts versus promonocytes, respectively (Fig. 41.15). Both types of AML, NOS, account for <5% of all cases of AML. Whereas acute monoblastic leukemias are more common in younger patients, acute monocytic leukemias are more common in adults. Patients may present with signs and symptoms associated with cytopenias. In addition, acute monoblastic and monocytic leukemias are particularly associated with extramedullary disease including lymphadenopathy, organomegaly, cutaneous and gingival infiltration, and central nervous system involvement. Despite the extramedullary manifestations of this subset of AML, NOS, there does not appear to be a significant difference in prognosis associated with these AML compared to other subsets of AML, NOS (203).

The morphologic features of monoblasts and promonocytes in these leukemias are similar to those described above. Promonocytes are usually NSE positive and MPO negative or weakly positive. Flow cytometry and/or immunohistochemical studies demonstrate expression of monocyte-associated antigens on the blasts. These include CD4, CD11b, CD11c, CD14, CD36, CD64, CD68, CD163, and lysozyme. In addition, cases often express HLA-DR, CD13, and bright CD33 as well as CD15 and CD65. CD34 expression is less frequently detected on the monoblasts and promonocytes, whereas more often cases are positive for CD117 expression. Approximately 25% to 40% of cases express aberrant CD7 and/or CD56.

There are no specific genetic mutations associated with acute monoblastic or acute monocytic leukemias but cases with *MLL* translocations at 11q23 frequently have these features. Some cases of acute monocyte leukemia demonstrate a t(8;16)(p11.2p13.3) rearrangement, and these are often associated with hemophagocytosis (101). AML with t(8;16)(p11.2p13.3) was discussed in a previous section. The differential diagnosis of acute monoblastic leukemia primarily includes other AML, NOS, subtypes, including AML with minimal differentiation, AML without maturation, and AML. In addition, cases that present in extramedullary sites may be difficult to distinguish from lymphoma or nonhematolymphoid neoplasms based on morphologic features alone. The differential diagnosis of acute monocytic leukemia includes acute myelomonocytic leukemia, chronic myelomonocytic leukemia, and microgranular APL. In

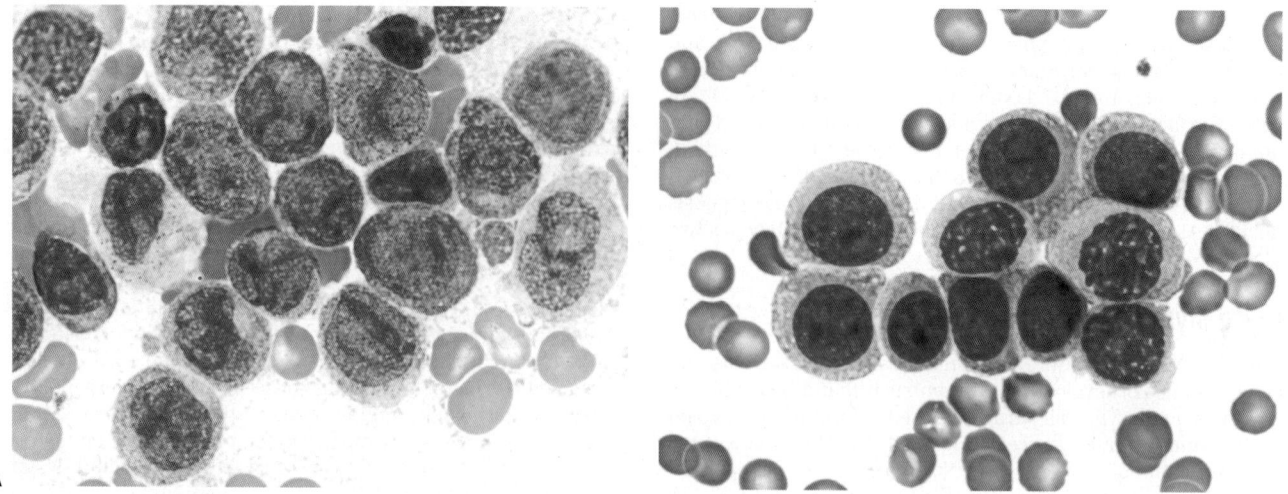

FIGURE 41.15. Acute monocytic and monoblastic leukemia. A spectrum of monocytic changes may occur in AML, similar to those shown in Figures 41.3 and 41.7. **A:** In this case of AML, NOS, the blasts include undifferentiated forms and ones with promonocytic features and this would be considered an acute monocytic leukemia. **B:** In contrast, this acute monoblastic proliferation shows only undifferentiated blasts with round nuclei and lightly basophilic, slightly vacuolated cytoplasm. Most cases show variation in blast cells, especially when the PB and BM are compared.

addition to the careful recognition and inclusion of promonocytes in the blast count, cytochemical and immunologic evaluation of the monoblasts and promonocytes usually resolves the differential. CD14 and CD163 are particularly specific antigens useful to demonstrate monocytic differentiation, but many cases of acute monoblastic leukemia will lack CD163.

Acute Erythroid Leukemias

In acute erythroid leukemias, erythroid precursors account for the predominant nucleated cell population in the BM. Two distinct subcategories are described in the 2008 WHO classification: erythroleukemia (erythroid/myeloid leukemia) and pure erythroid leukemia. In erythroid/myeloid leukemia, erythroid precursors comprise at least 50% of BM cells and there is also a distinct myeloblast population that accounts for <20% of total BM cells *and* ≥20% of nonerythroid cells. In contrast, pure erythroid leukemias are composed of a relatively pure population of early erythroid precursors that comprise at least 80% of BM cellularity and that are not associated with an increase in myeloblasts.

Erythroid/Myeloid Leukemia

Erythroleukemia (erythroid/myeloid) accounts for <5% of AML and occurs primarily in adults. Patients may present with marked anemia with numerous circulating nucleated red blood cells. BM aspirates and biopsies are often hypercellular and tend to show a full, albeit left-shifted spectrum of erythroid maturation with at least 50% erythroid precursors. The latter often demonstrate dysplastic features including megaloblastic change, multinucleation, nuclear membrane irregularities, ring sideroblasts, and the presence of PAS-positive cytoplasmic vacuoles. Myeloblasts are increased (<20% of total BM cells, ≥20% of nonerythroid cells) and show morphologic features similar to the blasts in AML with or without maturation (Fig. 41.16). Dysplastic features in maturing myeloid precursors and megakaryocytes are also common.

The myeloblasts in erythroleukemia may be MPO, CAE, and/or SSB positive, and flow cytometry studies often show typical immunophenotypic features associated with myeloblasts, including expression of CD13, CD33, CD34, CD45, CD38, CD117, HLA-DR, and/or MPO. In contrast, erythroblasts are negative for these markers, except for CD117, which may be expressed by early erythroid precursors. However, the latter

are usually positive for CD36, glycophorin, and hemoglobin A. CD71 (transferrin receptor) may also be expressed at low levels.

No specific genetic mutations are associated with erythroleukemia (erythroid/myeloid). Many cases that fulfill the morphologic criteria of erythroleukemia are associated with complex karyotypes and deletions of chromosomes 5/5q and/or 7/7q; however, such cases should be diagnosed as AML-MRC if total blasts are 20% or more. Indeed, the differential diagnosis of erythroleukemia primarily includes AML-MRC and MDS with erythroid hyperplasia. Currently there is debate as to whether there is clinical significance in separating out these entities as was done in the most recent WHO classification; in general, they are associated with a poor prognosis with currently available chemotherapies (206,207). Some have argued that it may not be critical to distinguish among these diseases that show overlapping features and this appears to be particularly true when comparing erythroid/myeloid leukemia with aggressive forms of MDS. Some patients who are status post chemotherapy and/or have received erythropoietin may

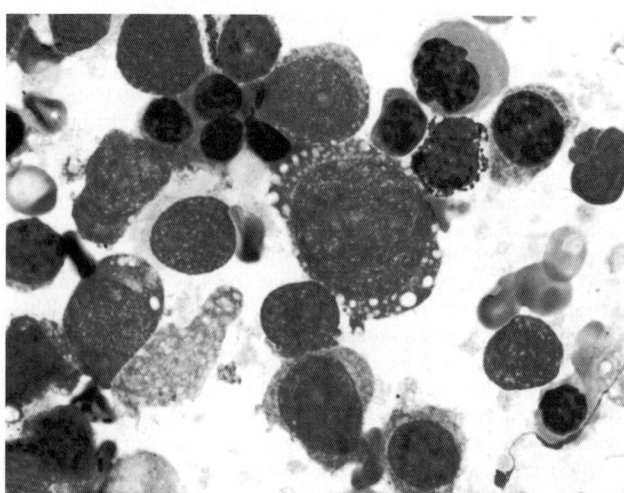

FIGURE 41.16. Acute erythroid leukemia (erythroid/myeloid). Many (over 50%) dysplastic erythroid precursors are present with admixed blast cells. Blasts represent <20% of total nucleated marrow cells, but more than 20% of nonerythroid cells, meeting criteria for this diagnosis.

develop a marked erythroid hyperplasia, and it is important to distinguish such reactive conditions from neoplastic proliferations. Likewise, other nonneoplastic conditions that may demonstrate dyserythropoiesis and BM erythroid hyperplasia, including vitamin B_{12} and folate deficiency, arsenic poisoning, and congenital dyserythropoietic anemias, should be excluded.

Pure Erythroid Leukemia

Pure erythroid leukemia is a very rare disease that can occur at any age. Patients may present with cytopenias and have circulating nucleated red blood cells in the PB. BM evaluation demonstrates a predominance of immature erythroid precursors, typically at the pronormoblast and early basophilic normoblast stages and usually with dysplastic features as described above. The major distinguishing feature between erythroid/myeloid leukemia and pure erythroid leukemia is the absence of an increased myeloblast population in the latter. Neoplastic erythroid cells must comprise at least 80% of the BM cellularity in pure erythroid leukemia.

The cytochemical and immunophenotypic features of the neoplastic erythroblasts are similar to those observed in erythroid/myeloid leukemia. Blasts typically lack myeloid/monocytic antigens as well as CD34, CD45, and HLA-DR. CD117 may be expressed by early erythroblasts. In addition, CD41 and CD61 may be aberrantly expressed. Glycophorin and hemoglobin A are often expressed in more mature erythroid precursors, but very immature blasts, which are more likely to express CD71, may not express these antigens. No specific genetic abnormalities are associated with pure erythroid leukemia, and the prognosis associated with this form of AML, NOS, is very poor. The disease usually follows an aggressive course. The differential diagnosis includes other types of AML, including acute megakaryoblastic leukemia, especially when erythroid differentiation is not clear from morphologic or immunophenotypic evaluation (208), and in some cases it may not be possible to distinguish erythroid from megakaryocytic lineage. Because of the low myeloblast count in these cases, the differential diagnosis also includes MDS and one could argue that these represent an aggressive form of MDS. In addition, some cases may be difficult to distinguish from ALL or lymphoma based on morphologic grounds, but immunophenotyping is usually sufficient to resolve this differential.

Acute Megakaryoblastic Leukemia

As a subtype of AML, NOS, acute megakaryoblastic leukemia is uncommon, accounting for <5% of AML. Excluded from this category are cases of AML with megakaryocytic differentiation that would meet criteria for other AML types including AML with t(1;22)(p13;q13), AML with inv(3)(q21q26.2) or t(3;3)(q21;q26.2), AML-MRC, therapy-related myeloid neoplasms, and myeloid leukemia associated with Down syndrome (13,96,209). The disease occurs in children and in adults. Patients may present with cytopenias, including thrombocytopenia, although alternatively thrombocytosis may be present. Organomegaly is uncommon. There is an association between acute megakaryoblastic leukemia and mediastinal germ cell tumors in young adult men (210).

In acute megakaryoblastic leukemia, the PB or BM blast count is ≥20%, and at least 50% of the blasts demonstrate megakaryocytic differentiation. Typically, the blasts are medium to large in size with high nuclear to cytoplasmic ratios, fine reticular chromatin, variably prominent nucleoli, round to slightly indented nuclei, and scant agranular basophilic cytoplasm. However, blasts may show a range in size, and in some cases may be predominantly small and resemble lymphoblasts. Cytoplasmic pseudopod formation or budding is often associated with acute megakaryoblastic leukemia, but this feature is not completely sensitive or specific. Megakaryocytic nuclear fragments, micromegakaryocytes, and giant hypogranular platelets may be seen in the circulation. However, these forms should not be included

in the blast count. Some cases contain primarily megakaryoblasts with very little maturation, whereas other cases may manifest with a mixture of megakaryoblasts and maturing dysplastic megakaryocytes. Dysplastic features in the erythroid and myeloid lineages may also be present, but when these exceed 50% of cells in two or more cell lines a diagnosis of AML-MRC should be made. Fibrosis is often observed in acute megakaryoblastic leukemia, although this is not present in all cases. If there is significant fibrosis, an accurate blast count may not be attainable on the aspirate material, and immunohistochemical analysis of trephine BM biopsy sections may be necessary.

As in other forms of megakaryoblastic leukemia, the blasts in the AML, NOS, subtype usually lack CD34, CD117, and HLA-DR expression as well as that of most other myeloid-, monocyte-, and lymphoid-associated antigens. CD7, CD13, and/or CD33 may be expressed. The megakaryocyte-specific antigens CD41 and CD61 are usually expressed to varying degrees, and cytoplasmic staining by flow cytometry is more specific than surface expression due to artifactual positivity resulting from surface platelet binding. CD42b, von Willebrand factor, and LAT are also useful markers for immunohistochemical analysis. MPO, SSB, and CAE are negative by cytochemistry, whereas megakaryoblasts may be positive for PAS, acid phosphatase, and/or focal NSE. Electron microscopy and ultracytochemistry can also be used to specifically differentiate megakaryoblasts from myeloblasts. The former contain ultrastructural peroxidase activity localized to the nuclear envelope and endoplasmic reticulum, and this is not observed in myeloblasts. In addition, megakaryoblasts have characteristic "bull's-eye" granules and demarcation membranes seen by electron microscopy (6).

No specific genetic mutations are associated with acute megakaryoblastic leukemia, although the i(12p) cytogenetic abnormality is characteristically observed in patients who also have mediastinal germ cell tumors. The differential diagnosis of acute megakaryoblastic leukemia includes other forms of the disease that are associated with either recurrent genetic abnormalities discussed above, Down syndrome, or myelodysplasia-related changes, and the presence of these associations takes diagnostic precedence over the AML, NOS, category. Notably, in comparison to AML with t(1;22)(p13q13), myeloid leukemia associated with Down syndrome, and many other AML subtypes, acute megakaryoblastic leukemia is associated with a relatively poor prognosis and response to therapy. The differential diagnosis also includes AML with minimal differentiation, acute panmyelosis with myelofibrosis, acute erythroid leukemia (pure erythroid leukemia), ALL, megakaryoblastic crisis of an MPN including CML, and nonhematopoietic small round blue cell tumors. A high index of suspicion for acute megakaryoblastic leukemia and inclusion of megakaryocyte-associated antigens, such as CD41, CD42, CD61, von Willebrand factor, and LAT, in the immunologic workup will most often resolve the differential diagnosis. Distinguishing acute erythroid leukemia from acute megakaryoblastic leukemia may be particularly challenging in some cases.

Acute Basophilic Leukemia

Acute basophilic leukemia is a very rare subtype of AML, NOS, that accounts for <1% of all AML. There are only a small number of reported cases, and the associated prognosis has generally been poor (211–213). Patients may present with cytopenias with or without a significant circulating blast population. Extramedullary involvement may also be present. Some patients may have symptoms associated with hyperhistaminemia.

Similar to other forms of AML, NOS, the blast count in either the BM or PB must be at least 20%. The blasts are usually medium in size and have round, indented or bilobed nuclei, smooth chromatin, prominent nucleoli, and scant basophilic cytoplasm. At least a subset of the blasts contains coarse basophilic cytoplasmic granules that signify basophilic differentiation. However, mature basophils are not necessarily increased.

Dysplasia in background erythroid precursors may be present. BM biopsy sections may demonstrate hypercellularity with sheets of poorly differentiated blasts.

Flow cytometry immunophenotyping of acute basophilic leukemia may demonstrate expression of CD13, CD33, CD34, and/or HLA-DR, whereas CD117 is typically not expressed. In addition, the blasts are usually positive for CD9, CD11b, CD22, CD123, CD203c, and/or TdT (214,215). However, other lymphoid-associated antigens are usually not expressed. The blasts are typically negative for MPO, SSB, CAE, and NSE by cytochemistry. In contrast, they may be positive for acid phosphatase or PAS staining. Electron microscopy, although not routinely performed, demonstrates features of the cytoplasmic granules consistent with derivation from the basophil lineage.

Acute basophilic leukemia is not associated with any specific genetic mutations. The differential diagnosis includes AML with t(6;9)(p23;q34), mast cell leukemia, blast crisis of CML, and ALL with coarse cytoplasmic granules. Immunophenotypic and cytogenetic studies will usually resolve the differential diagnosis. The neoplastic cells in mast cell leukemia will express mast cell tryptase, CD117, and CD25, whereas these antigens are not expressed in acute basophilic leukemia.

Acute Panmyelosis with Myelofibrosis

Acute panmyelosis with myelofibrosis (APMF) is a very rare disease characterized by the neoplastic proliferation of immature, and often dysplastic, erythroid, myeloid, and megakaryocytic cells (panmyelosis) (Fig. 41.17) coupled with the acute onset of diffuse myelofibrosis and an increase in blasts (usually 20% to 25%) (216–218). Affected individuals tend to be adults, but the disease can also occur in children. Most patients present with pancytopenia as well as constitutional symptoms including fever, weakness, fatigue, and bone pain. Notably, splenomegaly is not a feature of this disease. Circulating blasts, dysplastic and left-shifted neutrophils, erythroblasts, and atypical platelets may be seen in the PB. Aspirate smears are often noncontributory due to extensive marrow fibrosis and a "dry tap." If cellular, BM aspirates (or BM biopsy touch preparations) often show dysplastic features in mature hematopoietic precursors. Sections of the BM biopsy usually demonstrate hypercellular marrow with diffuse marrow reticulin fibrosis and hyperplasia of all three lineages. There is often a left shift in erythroid and myeloid precursors as well as numerous dysplastic small megakaryocytes. Therefore, glycophorin, MPO, and stains for megakaryocytes (e.g., CD61, LAT), respectively, may be necessary to confirm

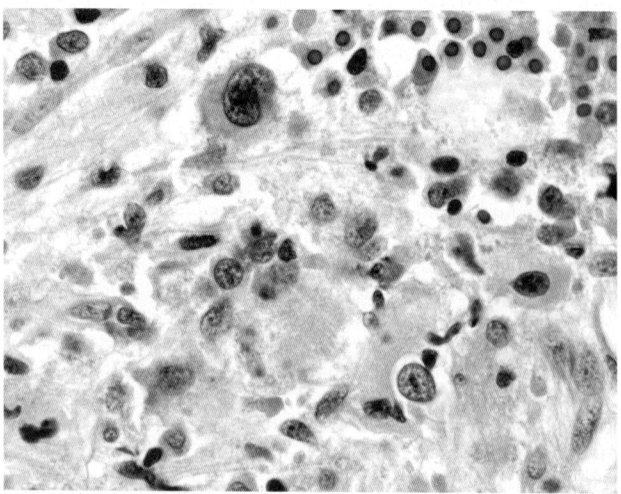

FIGURE 41.17. Acute panmyelosis with myelofibrosis. The fibrotic BM biopsy contains a mix of immature cells, erythroid precursors, and abnormal megakaryocytes.

the panmyelosis. The blasts are usually CD34+ and also often express myeloid-associated antigens including CD33, CD13, and CD117. In contrast, the blasts are usually MPO negative.

No specific genetic abnormalities are associated with APMF, although cases frequently demonstrate abnormal cytogenetics. If the cytogenetic abnormalities are associated with other 2008 WHO categories of AML then the latter diagnoses take precedence over APMF. The differential diagnosis of APMF includes other forms of AML with marrow fibrosis with or without myelodysplasia, including acute megakaryoblastic leukemia and AML-MRC, as well as RAEB and myelofibrosis, post-MPN myelofibrosis, and metastatic nonhematopoietic malignancy with desmoplastic stromal reaction. Immunohistochemical analysis, together with cytogenetics studies, if possible, may resolve the differential diagnosis on most instances. In addition, the acute presentation and characteristic lack of hepatosplenomegaly help to distinguish APMF from post-MPN disorders that manifest with diffuse marrow myelofibrosis. Likewise, the acuity of the disease is less commonly seen in MDS. Nonetheless, the most difficult distinction may be with MDS with fibrosis and AML-MRC with fibrosis (219). The prognosis associated with APMF is poor.

MYELOID PROLIFERATIONS OF DOWN SYNDROME

Patients with Down syndrome are at a 10- to 100-fold increased risk of developing acute leukemia in comparison to normal individuals. This increased risk includes all types of acute leukemia, including both AML and ALL, and is maintained throughout life (220,221). It is estimated that 1% to 2% of Down syndrome children will develop AML in the first 5 years of life, and this is usually acute megakaryoblastic leukemia (70% of cases). Other forms of AML, as well as ALL, occur less frequently during this period, whereas after 5 years of age the relative frequencies of ALL and subtypes of AML are similar to those observed in non-DS patients, albeit at higher overall rates. Down syndrome patients are also uniquely susceptible to a transient myeloid proliferation that occurs in the neonatal period and that is morphologically and genetically indistinguishable from *bona fide* AML. This disorder, termed transient abnormal myelopoiesis (TAM), is usually self-limited, but a minor subset of patients eventually develops nonremitting AML 1 to 3 years later. Both TAM and AML arising in Down syndrome patients younger than 5 years old are associated with mutations in the *GATA1* transcription factor (222–224). Because of unique clinical, morphologic, and genetic features of these two Down syndrome-associated myelopathies, the 2008 WHO classification includes TAM and myeloid leukemia associated with Down syndrome as distinct entities (225,226).

Transient Abnormal Myelopoiesis

TAM is a self-limited disorder that is unique to Down syndrome patients and that occurs in approximately 10% of Down syndrome neonates, usually within the first 5 days of life (227). Rarely patients with trisomy 21 mosaicism may develop TAM. TAM is morphologically and immunophenotypically indistinguishable from the predominant form of myeloid leukemia of Down syndrome (AML), but the former spontaneously regresses by the third month of life in most patients (median time to spontaneous regression is 46 days). Presenting signs and symptoms are usually associated with thrombocytopenia, with or without other cytopenias or leukocytosis, as well as hepatosplenomegaly with or without hepatic fibrosis and/or extramedullary hematopoiesis. Patients may rarely develop more life-threatening complications including cardiopulmonary failure, splenic or hepatic necrosis, hyperviscosity, renal insufficiency, or DIC (228,229). Few cases are fatal.

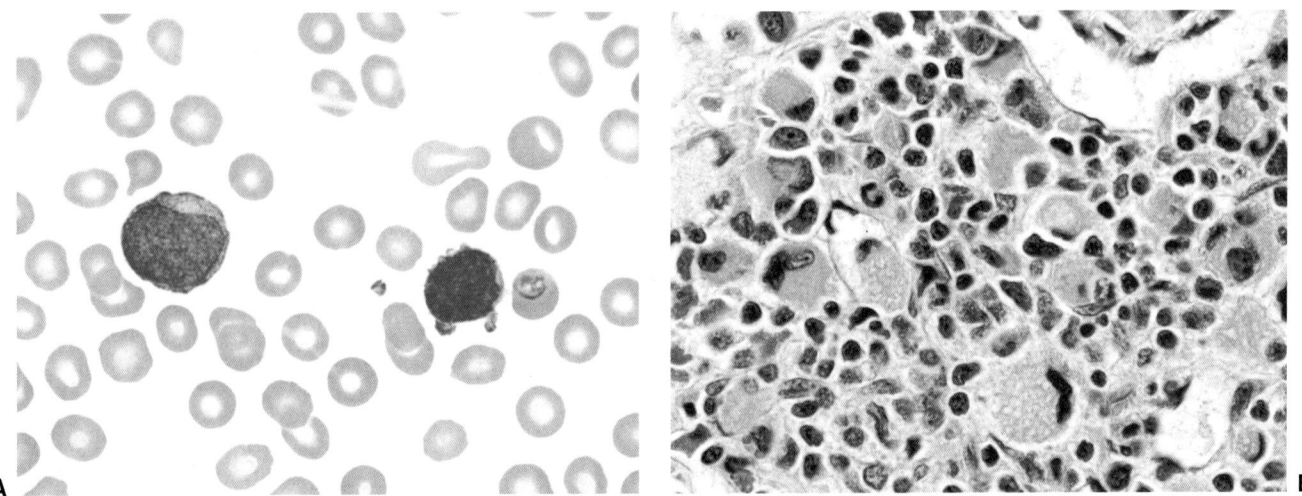

FIGURE 41.18. Transient abnormal myelopoiesis in an infant with Down syndrome. A: The PB contains megakaryoblasts with finely granular, slightly basophilic cytoplasm. The blast on the right has cytoplasmic blebs suggesting the lineage of the cells. **B:** The BM core biopsy shows a proliferation of megakaryocytes and immature cells.

The blasts in TAM are often prominent in the PB (may exceed 100 K/μL) and can outnumber those present in the BM. They are usually medium to large in size with high nuclear to cytoplasmic ratios, round to mildly indented nuclear contours, fine reticular chromatin, prominent nucleoli, modest amounts of basophilic cytoplasm, and cytoplasmic blebs (Fig. 41.18). In contrast to the blasts seen in AMLs in non-Down syndrome patients, those present in TAM (and myeloid leukemia of Down syndrome) often have more coarse basophilic cytoplasmic granules but are also MPO negative. PB basophilia may be present in some patients, and dysplastic features in erythroid and megakaryocytic cells are frequently observed in BM specimens.

Flow cytometry studies performed on these cases have demonstrated a characteristic immunophenotype such that the blasts usually express CD34, CD13, CD33, CD117, CD4 (often dim), CD36, CD41, CD42, and CD61, as well as variable HLA-DR and aberrant CD7 and CD56 (230,231). The blasts are also usually positive for the IL-3 receptor, CD123, as well as the thrombopoietin receptor (TPO-R), CD110. In contrast, the blasts in TAM usually do not express CD14, CD15, MPO, or glycophorin A.

Cytogenetics studies typically demonstrate trisomy 21 as the sole clonal cytogenetic abnormality, although nonclonal abnormalities may be observed. Mutations in the transcription factor-encoding gene, *GATA1*, as well as in *JAK3* are common in TAM, and these are also frequently observed in myeloid leukemia of Down syndrome (223,224,232). The long-term impact of TAM on most patients is minimal, as the disorder spontaneously regresses in most patients. However, following initial regression of disease, 20% to 30% of patients eventually develop *bona fide* AML that is typically acute megakaryoblastic (227). Moreover, a subset of patients that develop end organ damage, DIC, hyperviscosity, and/or organomegaly with respiratory compromise are at increased risk of significant morbidity or mortality, and they may benefit from chemotherapeutic intervention. The differential diagnosis includes myeloid leukemia of Down syndrome, but the latter often arises following a more indolent MDS-like phase and not necessarily in the neonatal period. AML with t(1;22)(p13;q13) may show similar morphologic and immunophenotypic features, and in the neonatal period the diagnosis of Down syndrome may not be confirmed. Nonetheless, cytogenetics studies will resolve the differential.

Myeloid Leukemia Associated with Down Syndrome

Myeloid leukemia associated with Down syndrome can occur at any age but is most common during the first 5 years of life, with an approximate 1% to 2% incidence among DS patients

during this period. Notably, the incidence of myeloid leukemia of Down syndrome far exceeds that of AML in non-Down syndrome patients, and approximately 20% of all pediatric MDS/AML patients have Down syndrome. At least 50% of myeloid leukemia of Down syndrome are AMLs, and these preferentially arise during the first 3 years of life. In older children with Down syndrome, AMLs are less frequently acute megakaryoblastic and are diagnosed based on criteria described in previous sections for non-Down syndrome patients (17,225). The features described below are in reference to the acute megakaryoblastic form of myeloid leukemia of Down syndrome.

Approximately 20% to 30% of myeloid leukemia of Down syndrome patients have had prior TAM. Many other myeloid leukemia of Down syndrome patients may develop a prodromal MDS-like disorder with features of refractory cytopenia of childhood (233). It is noteworthy that cases of MDS-like disease (5% to 19% blasts) and *bona fide* AML (≥20% blasts) show similar clinical and biologic features and are treated on similar protocols. Therefore at present the specific blast count, as well as a prior history of TAM, are not considered clinically relevant features, and all cases are collectively grouped as myeloid leukemia of Down syndrome in the 2008 WHO classification (225).

The morphologic features of myeloid leukemia of Down syndrome (acute megakaryoblastic) are similar to those observed in TAM, with blasts demonstrating megakaryoblastic differentiation and involving PB and BM as well as spleen and liver (Fig. 41.19). Coarse cytoplasmic granules are often observed in the blasts as in TAM. In addition, background dysplasia in BM erythroid and megakaryocytic precursors as well as erythrocyte poikilocytosis and giant platelets in PB are commonly observed findings. Marrow fibrosis may be significant and preclude the acquisition of an adequate BM aspirate. The relative proportions of erythroid cells, blasts, and mature megakaryocytes are variable from case to case. Myeloid precursors are often decreased and may be dysplastic.

The cytochemical and immunophenotypic features of acute megakaryoblastic myeloid leukemia of Down syndrome are also similar to those observed in TAM, except that the blasts in myeloid leukemia of Down syndrome are less frequently positive for CD34 and HLA-DR expression and they may show more consistent expression of CD11b and CD13 (230,231). Mutations in *GATA1* are common in myeloid leukemia of Down syndrome (acute megakaryoblastic) prior to age 5 and are considered pathognomonic for TAM or myeloid leukemia of Down syndrome. Mutations in *JAK2*, *JAK3*, and *FLT3* genes have also been reported in myeloid leukemia of Down syndrome, but the clinical significance of these mutations is not known (234,235).

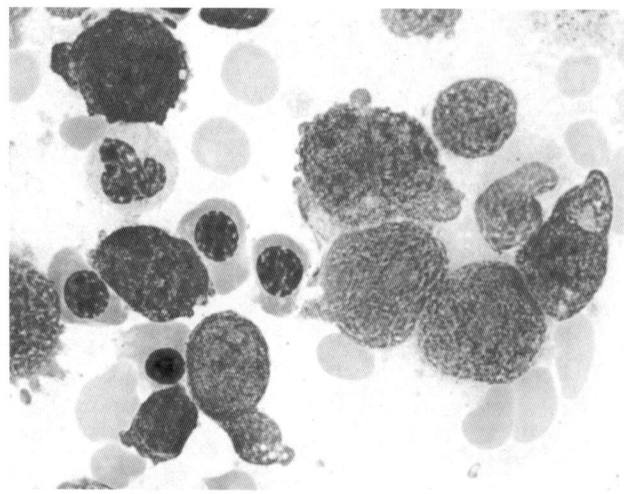
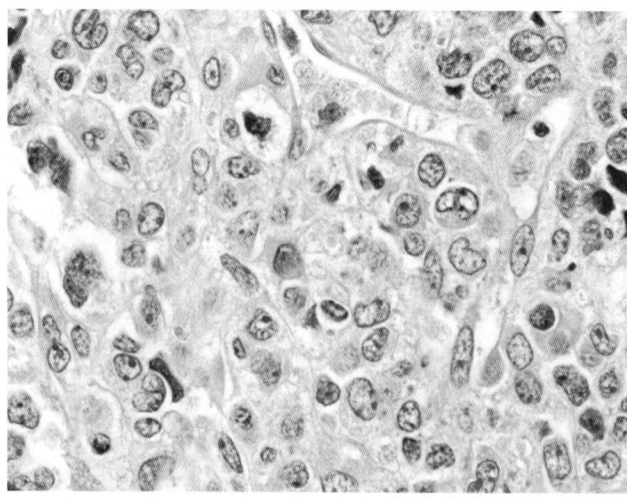

FIGURE 41.19. Myeloid leukemia associated with Down syndrome. A: The BM aspirate contains immature cells with variably basophilic cytoplasm and blebbing. The background erythroid precursors show mild nuclear to cytoplasmic asynchrony. **B:** The BM biopsy is filled with immature cells, more numerous than those seen in Figure 41.18.

Clonal cytogenetic abnormalities, in addition to trisomy 21, are also common in myeloid leukemia of Down syndrome and include partial or complete trisomies of chromosomes 1 and/or 8. Monosomy 7 is rare in myeloid leukemia of Down syndrome.

The prognosis associated with myeloid leukemia of Down syndrome (acute megakaryoblastic) appears to be age-dependent: the event-free survival is reportedly 86% for patients 0 to 2 years old, 70% for patients 2 to 4 years old, and 28% for patients over 4 years (236). The differential diagnosis of myeloid leukemia of Down syndrome (acute megakaryoblastic) includes TAM and other forms of AML that can usually be distinguished on morphologic grounds as well as appropriate use of immunologic and cytochemical ancillary studies. Pathologists should have a high index of suspicion for acute megakaryoblastic myeloid leukemia of Down syndrome in any patient with DS under the age of 5. Although TAM shows similar morphologic and immunophenotypic features, the latter most often presents in the first few days of life.

MYELOID SARCOMA

Myeloid sarcoma (also called chloroma, granulocytic sarcoma, and extramedullary myeloid tumor) is defined as a space-occupying extramedullary lesion composed of blasts with morphologic, immunophenotypic, and genetic features observed in any of the AML subcategories described above (18,21,237–239). The demonstration of myeloid sarcoma is considered a clinical equivalent to the diagnosis of AML in BM or PB, and it may occur in isolation, in the setting of a concurrent AML, MDS, MPN, or MDS/MPN involving BM and PB, or in patients in remission for an aforementioned myeloid neoplasm. Notably, however, myeloid sarcoma *per se* is not in and of itself considered a unique clinicopathologic entity in the 2008 WHO classification, and the clinical impact of myeloid sarcoma is not entirely clear (240,241). In general, prognoses of myeloid sarcomas parallel those associated with their AML counterparts that are diagnosed in BM/PB specimens. Therefore, where clinically relevant (i.e., new isolated cases) and feasible, all attempts should be made to thoroughly characterize the immunophenotypic and genetic features of myeloid sarcoma in order to appropriately assign a 2008 WHO AML classification. Moreover, although there may be benefit to local therapy (e.g., radiation) in some cases, systemic chemotherapy and BM transplantation appear to increase long-term survival.

Myeloid sarcoma can present in any anatomical location with the following sites involved in order of decreasing frequency: skin, mucous membranes, orbits, central nervous system, lymph nodes, bones, gonads, and other internal organs and soft tissues. In fewer than 10% of cases myeloid sarcoma involves multiple sites. Myeloid sarcoma can present at any age and in a variety of clinical settings, but certain subcategories of AML are particularly associated with extramedullary disease. Nearly 25% of pediatric patients and approximately 10% of adult patients with AML with t(8;21)(q22;q22) develop myeloid sarcoma (240,242). Within the pediatric group, orbital, skull, and central nervous system involvement is most common. Pediatric patients with AML with abnormalities of chromosome 11q23 or chromosome 16 tend to be younger (median age 2.6 years) and have cutaneous involvement. As discussed earlier, AML with t(8;16)(p11.2;q13.3) may present as a self-limited or recurring congenital disease with multiple cutaneous sites involved (102,243).

The blastic infiltrates in myeloid sarcomas form diffuse sheets that disrupt and efface the underlying architecture (Fig. 41.20). In lymph nodes, these infiltrates typically involve the interfollicular areas. Similar to the blasts in BM and PB, the blasts are generally characterized by high nuclear to cytoplasmic ratios, round to folded nuclear contours, fine and often stippled nuclear chromatin, and scant to moderate amounts of cytoplasm that may contain numerous cytoplasmic granules. There may be an admixture of background myeloid, including eosinophilic myelocytes, erythroid, and/or megakaryocytic cells, and the presence of these is a useful clue to the diagnosis of myeloid sarcoma (21). Some cases of myeloid sarcoma with abnormalities of chromosome 16 may also be associated with discrete collections of plasmacytoid dendritic cells that stain strongly for CD123.

Immunophenotypic analysis of myeloid sarcoma is essential to make the diagnosis, and the expression patterns of distinct surface antigens are often similar to those observed in BM AML counterparts. If possible, flow cytometry studies should be performed on fresh tissue specimens; however, some markers may also be analyzed by immunohistochemistry. Most myeloid sarcomas, save for those rare cases with erythroid or megakaryoblastic features, express the leukocyte common antigen, CD45. Other positive markers include CD34, CD117, CD68, CD163, CD43, lysozyme, and MPO, but these are variably expressed, not necessarily specific for myeloid sarcoma, and depend upon the line(s) of differentiation and extent of maturation of the neoplastic infiltrate. CD33 may be particularly useful in the diagnosis of myeloid sarcoma (244). Glycophorin staining will usually label erythroid precursors, whereas CD41, CD61, von Willebrand factor, and LAT may be used to identify megakaryoblasts as well as background megakaryocytic cells. Lymphoid-associated antigens, including CD2, CD4, CD7, CD56, CD79a,

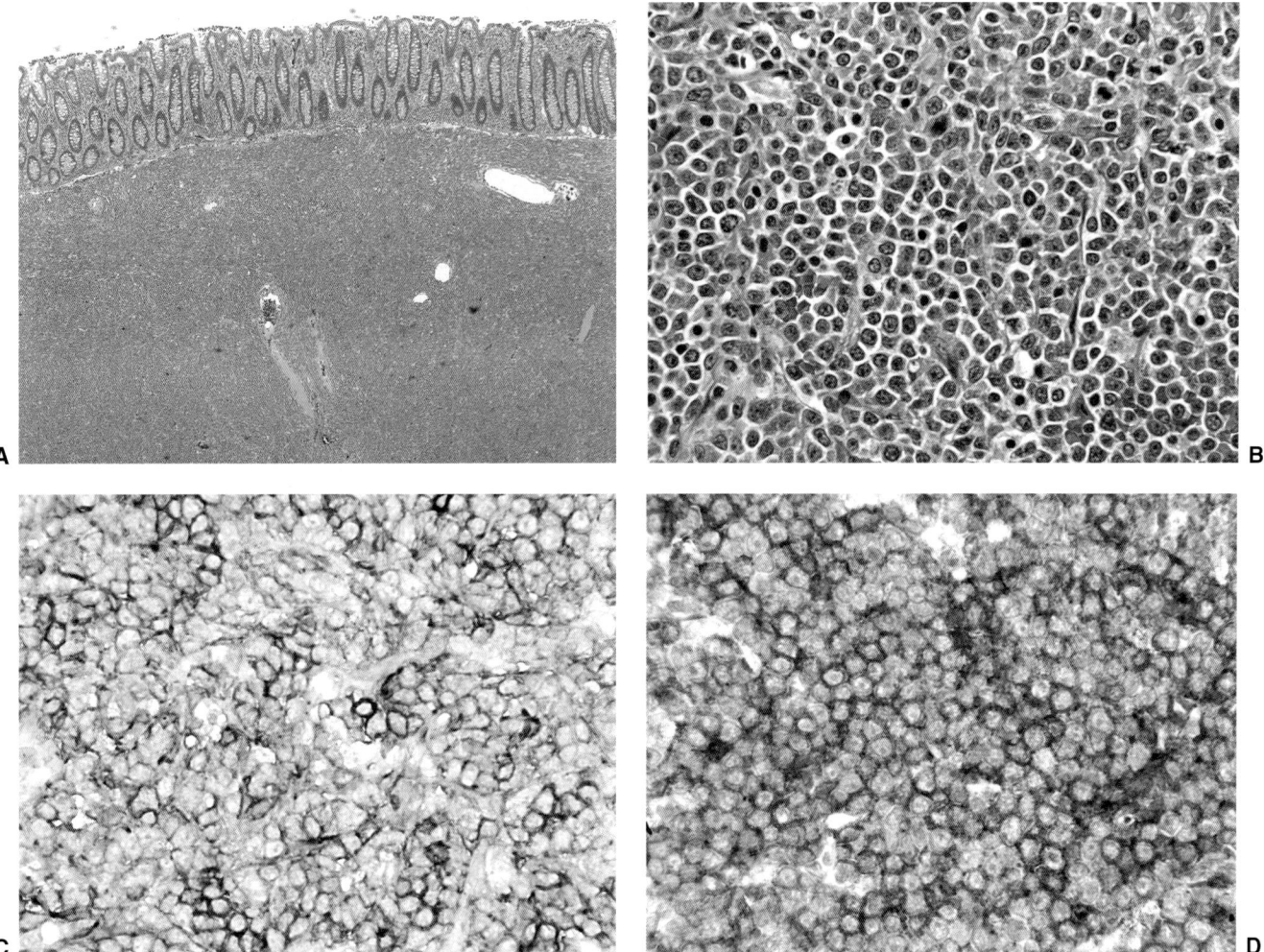

FIGURE 41.20. Myeloid sarcoma involving the small intestine. A,B: The bowel submucosa is filled with medium to large cells with scattered mitotic figures. **C:** The cells are variably positive for CD45RB, and (**D**) are strongly positive for CD33.

and PAX5, may also be expressed to variable degrees. Some cases may also be positive for CD30 or weak cytokeratins.

The differential diagnosis of myeloid sarcoma is somewhat broad and includes lymphoblastic lymphomas, mature non-Hodgkin lymphomas, including diffuse large B-cell lymphoma and Burkitt lymphoma, poorly differentiated carcinomas, and small blue round cell tumors of children. In addition, sparse, non–tissue effacing immature myeloid cell infiltrates and nonneoplastic neutrophilic infiltrates such as Sweet syndrome (i.e., acute febrile neutrophilic dermatosis) should be excluded (245). A high index of suspicion coupled with an extensive review of the patient's history (where available) and a liberal use of immunohistochemical stains, including megakaryocytic markers, is essential for appropriate diagnosis. Indeed, the aberrant expression of both T- and B-lymphocyte–associated antigens can make the diagnosis challenging. If possible, cytogenetics studies and flow cytometry studies should be performed on fresh tissue, and some FISH studies may be performed on formalin-fixed paraffin-embedded tissue sections. As mentioned above, a useful clue to the diagnosis of myeloid sarcoma is the presence of admixed eosinophilic myeloid precursors, erythroid precursors, and/or megakaryocytes.

SUMMARY AND CONCLUSIONS

The diversity and spectrum of clinical and pathologic features of AML pose a great challenge to diagnosticians, and the complexity of this field will most certainly increase as new

genetic data are discovered and current classification parameters require revision. Indeed, an integrated approach to the diagnosis of all new cases of AML is necessary in order to appropriately subtype AML according to the 2008 WHO classification as well as to provide a framework for continued investigation. The workup of any new leukemia should include an assessment of the clinical history, a thorough morphologic evaluation of PB, BM aspirate, and core biopsy material, a comprehensive immunophenotypic analysis by flow cytometry and/or immunohistochemistry, and appropriate utilization of molecular and cytogenetic tests validated for sensitive detection of known gene mutations and karyotypic abnormalities that provide useful diagnostic and prognostic information. Cytochemical analysis is not required in all cases but is recommended in many instances described above. As molecular and cytogenetic testing may take 1 week or more to be completed, the diagnosis of AML should not be delayed; however, the use of amendments or addenda to reports is highly recommended in order to formulate a final diagnosis that is based on 2008 WHO criteria and that will accurately direct clinical management (11,17).

References

1. Morphologic, immunologic, and cytogenetic (MIC) working classification of the acute myeloid leukemias. Report of the Workshop held in Leuven, Belgium, September 15-17, 1986. Second MIC Cooperative Study Group. *Cancer Genet Cytogenet* 1988;30:1–15.

2. EGIL (European Group for the Immunological Classification of Leukaemias). The value of c-kit in the diagnosis of biphenotypic acute leukemia. *Leukemia* 1998;12:2038.

3. Bene MC, Castoldi G, Knapp W, et al. Proposals for the immunological classification of acute leukemias. European Group for the Immunological Characterization of Leukemias (EGIL). *Leukemia* 1995;9:1783–1786.

4. Bennett JM, Catovsky D, Daniel MT, et al. Proposals for the classification of the acute leukaemias. French-American-British (FAB) co-operative group. *Br J Haematol* 1976;33:451–458.

5. Bennett JM, Catovsky D, Daniel MT, et al. Proposed revised criteria for the classification of acute myeloid leukemia. A report of the French-American-British Cooperative Group. *Ann Intern Med* 1985;103:620–625.

6. Bennett JM, Catovsky D, Daniel MT, et al. Criteria for the diagnosis of acute leukemia of megakaryocyte lineage (M7). A report of the French-American-British Cooperative Group. *Ann Intern Med* 1985;103:460–462.

7. Bennett JM, Catovsky D, Daniel MT, et al. Proposal for the recognition of minimally differentiated acute myeloid leukaemia (AML-MO). *Br J Haematol* 1991;78:325–329.

8. Jaffe ES, Stein H, Vardiman JW. *World health organization classification of tumors of haematopoietic and lymphoid tissues.* Lyon: IARC Press, 2001.

9. Swerdlow SH, Harris NL, Jaffe ES, et al. *World health organization classification of tumours of hematopoietic and lymphoid tissues.* Lyon: IARC Press, 2008.

10. Head DR. Revised classification of acute myeloid leukemia. *Leukemia* 1996;10:1826–1831.

11. Dohner H, Estey EH, Amadori S, et al. Diagnosis and management of acute myeloid leukemia in adults: recommendations from an international expert panel, on behalf of the European LeukemiaNet. *Blood* 2010;115:453–474.

12. Horner MJ, Krapcho M. *SEER cancer statistics review, 1975-2006, acute myeloid leukemia section.* Bethesda: National Cancer Institute, 2009.

13. Arber DA, Orazi A, Porwit A, et al. *Acute myeloid leukaemia, not otherwise specified.* Lyon: IARC, 2008.

14. Arber DA, Le Beau MM, Falini B, et al. *Acute myeloid leukaemia with recurrent genetic abnormalities.* Lyon: IARC, 2008.

15. Arber DA, Orazi A, Bain BJ, et al. *Acute myeloid leukaemia with myelodysplasia-related changes.* Lyon: IARC, 2008.

16. Vardiman JW, Brunning RD, Larson RA, et al. *Therapy-related myeloid neoplasms.* Lyon: IARC, 2008.

17. Vardiman JW, Arber DA, Le Beau MM, et al. *Introduction and overview of the classification of the myeloid neoplasms.* Lyon: IARC, 2008.

18. Pileri SA, Falini B. *Myeloid sarcoma.* Lyon: IARC, 2008.

19. Arber DA, Carter NH, Ikle D, et al. Value of combined morphologic, cytochemical, and immunophenotypic features in predicting recurrent cytogenetic abnormalities in acute myeloid leukemia. *Hum Pathol* 2003;34:479–483.

20. Khalidi HS, Medeiros LJ, Chang KL, et al. The immunophenotype of adult acute myeloid leukemia: high frequency of lymphoid antigen expression and comparison of immunophenotype, French-American-British classification, and karyotypic abnormalities. *Am J Clin Pathol* 1998;109:211–220.

21. Pileri SA, Ascani S, Cox MC, et al. Myeloid sarcoma: clinico-pathologic, phenotypic and cytogenetic analysis of 92 adult patients. *Leukemia* 2007;21:340–350.

22. Arber DA, Stein AS, Carter NH, et al. Prognostic impact of acute myeloid leukemia classification. Importance of detection of recurring cytogenetic abnormalities and multilineage dysplasia on survival. *Am J Clin Pathol* 2003;119:672–680.

23. Mrozek K, Bloomfield CD. Clinical significance of the most common chromosome translocations in adult acute myeloid leukemia. *J Natl Cancer Inst Monogr* 2008:52–57.

24. Mrozek K, Heerema NA, Bloomfield CD. Cytogenetics in acute leukemia. *Blood Rev* 2004;18:115–136.

25. Baldus CD, Mrozek K, Marcucci G, et al. Clinical outcome of de novo acute myeloid leukaemia patients with normal cytogenetics is affected by molecular genetic alterations: a concise review. *Br J Haematol* 2007;137:387–400.

26. Dohner K, Schlenk RF, Habdank M, et al. Mutant nucleophosmin (NPM1) predicts favorable prognosis in younger adults with acute myeloid leukemia and normal cytogenetics: interaction with other gene mutations. *Blood* 2005;106:3740–3746.

27. Paschka P, Marcucci G, Ruppert AS, et al. Adverse prognostic significance of KIT mutations in adult acute myeloid leukemia with inv(16) and t(8;21): a Cancer and Leukemia Group B Study. *J Clin Oncol* 2006;24:3904–3911.

28. Wang ZY, Chen Z. Acute promyelocytic leukemia: from highly fatal to highly curable. *Blood* 2008;111:2505–2515.

29. Byrd JC, Mrozek K, Dodge RK, et al. Pretreatment cytogenetic abnormalities are predictive of induction success, cumulative incidence of relapse, and overall survival in adult patients with de novo acute myeloid leukemia: results from Cancer and Leukemia Group B (CALGB 8461). *Blood* 2002;100:4325–4336.

30. Grimwade D, Walker H, Oliver F, et al. The importance of diagnostic cytogenetics on outcome in AML: analysis of 1,612 patients entered into the MRC AML 10 trial. The Medical Research Council Adult and Children's Leukaemia Working Parties. *Blood* 1998;92:2322–2333.

31. Slovak ML, Kopecky KJ, Cassileth PA, et al. Karyotypic analysis predicts outcome of preremission and postremission therapy in adult acute myeloid leukemia: a Southwest Oncology Group/Eastern Cooperative Oncology Group Study. *Blood* 2000;96:4075–4083.

32. Breems DA, Van Putten WL, De Greef GE, et al. Monosomal karyotype in acute myeloid leukemia: a better indicator of poor prognosis than a complex karyotype. *J Clin Oncol* 2008;26:4791–4797.

33. Kayser S, Zucknick M, Dohner K, et al. Monosomal karyotype in adult acute myeloid leukemia: prognostic impact and outcome after different treatment strategies. *Blood* 2012;119:551–558.

34. Medeiros BC, Othus M, Fang M, et al. Prognostic impact of monosomal karyotype in young adult and elderly acute myeloid leukemia: the Southwest Oncology Group (SWOG) experience. *Blood* 2010;116:2224–2228.

35. Ahn HK, Jang JH, Kim K, et al. Monosomal karyotype in acute myeloid leukemia predicts adverse treatment outcome and associates with high functional multidrug resistance activity. *Am J Hematol* 2012;87:37–41.

36. Hurwitz CA, Raimondi SC, Head D, et al. Distinctive immunophenotypic features of t(8;21)(q22;q22) acute myeloblastic leukemia in children. *Blood* 1992;80:3182–3188.

37. Kita K, Nakase K, Miwa H, et al. Phenotypical characteristics of acute myelocytic leukemia associated with the t(8;21)(q22;q22) chromosomal abnormality: frequent expression of immature B-cell antigen CD19 together with stem cell antigen CD34. *Blood* 1992;80:470–477.

38. Baer MR, Stewart CC, Lawrence D, et al. Expression of the neural cell adhesion molecule CD56 is associated with short remission duration and survival in acute myeloid leukemia with t(8;21)(q22;q22). *Blood* 1997;90:1643–1648.

39. Tiacci E, Pileri S, Orleth A, et al. PAX5 expression in acute leukemias: higher B-lineage specificity than CD79a and selective association with t(8;21)-acute myelogenous leukemia. *Cancer Res* 2004;64:7399–7404.

40. Tobal K, Newton J, Macheta M, et al. Molecular quantitation of minimal residual disease in acute myeloid leukemia with t(8;21) can identify patients in durable remission and predict clinical relapse. *Blood* 2000;95:815–819.

41. Peterson LF, Zhang DE. The 8;21 translocation in leukemogenesis. *Oncogene* 2004;23:4255–4262.

42. Goemans BF, Zwaan CM, Miller M, et al. Mutations in KIT and RAS are frequent events in pediatric core-binding factor acute myeloid leukemia. *Leukemia* 2005;19:1536–1542.

43. Byrd JC, Dodge RK, Carroll A, et al. Patients with t(8;21)(q22;q22) and acute myeloid leukemia have superior failure-free and overall survival when repetitive cycles of high-dose cytarabine are administered. *J Clin Oncol* 1999;17:3767–3775.

44. Le Beau MM, Larson RA, Bitter MA, et al. Association of an inversion of chromosome 16 with abnormal marrow eosinophils in acute myelomonocytic leukemia. A unique cytogenetic-clinicopathological association. *N Engl J Med* 1983;309:630–636.

45. Adriaansen HJ, te Boekhorst PA, Hagemeijer AM, et al. Acute myeloid leukemia M4 with bone marrow eosinophilia (M4Eo) and inv(16)(p13q22) exhibits a specific immunophenotype with CD2 expression. *Blood* 1993;81:3043–3051.

46. Paietta E, Wiernik PH, Andersen J, et al. Acute myeloid leukemia M4 with inv(16) (p13q22) exhibits a specific immunophenotype with CD2 expression. *Blood* 1993;82:2595.

47. Shigesada K, van de Sluis B, Liu PP. Mechanism of leukemogenesis by the inv(16) chimeric gene CBFB/PEBP2B-MHY11. *Oncogene* 2004;23:4297–4307.

48. Delaunay J, Vey N, Leblanc T, et al. Prognosis of inv(16)/t(16;16) acute myeloid leukemia (AML): a survey of 110 cases from the French AML Intergroup. *Blood* 2003;102:462–469.

49. Larson RA, Williams SF, Le Beau MM, et al. Acute myelomonocytic leukemia with abnormal eosinophils and inv(16) or t(16;16) has a favorable prognosis. *Blood* 1986;68:1242–1249.

50. Buonamici S, Ottaviani E, Testoni N, et al. Real-time quantitation of minimal residual disease in inv(16)-positive acute myeloid leukemia may indicate risk for clinical relapse and may identify patients in a curable state. *Blood* 2002;99:443–449.

51. Marcucci G, Mrozek K, Ruppert AS, et al. Prognostic factors and outcome of core binding factor acute myeloid leukemia patients with t(8;21) differ from those of patients with inv(16): a Cancer and Leukemia Group B study. *J Clin Oncol* 2005;23:5705–5717.

52. Schlenk RF, Benner A, Krauter J, et al. Individual patient data-based meta-analysis of patients aged 16 to 60 years with core binding factor acute myeloid leukemia: a survey of the German Acute Myeloid Leukemia Intergroup. *J Clin Oncol* 2004;22:3741–3750.

53. Golomb HM, Rowley JD, Vardiman JW, et al. "Microgranular" acute promyelocytic leukemia: a distinct clinical, ultrastructural, and cytogenetic entity. *Blood* 1980;55:253–259.

54. McKenna RW, Parkin J, Bloomfield CD, et al. Acute promyelocytic leukaemia: a study of 39 cases with identification of a hyperbasophilic microgranular variant. *Br J Haematol* 1982;50:201–214.

55. Orfao A, Chillon MC, Bortoluci AM, et al. The flow cytometric pattern of CD34, CD15 and CD13 expression in acute myeloblastic leukemia is highly characteristic of the presence of PML-RARalpha gene rearrangements. *Haematologica* 1999;84:405–412.

56. Paietta E, Goloubeva O, Neuberg D, et al. A surrogate marker profile for PML/RAR alpha expressing acute promyelocytic leukemia and the association of immunophenotypic markers with morphologic and molecular subtypes. *Cytom Clin Cytom* 2004;59:1–9.

57. Exner M, Thalhammer R, Kapiotis S, et al. The "typical" immunophenotype of acute promyelocytic leukemia (APL-M3): does it prove true for the M3-variant? *Cytometry* 2000;42:106–109.

58. Lin P, Hao S, Medeiros LJ, et al. Expression of CD2 in acute promyelocytic leukemia correlates with short form of PML-RARalpha transcripts and poorer prognosis. *Am J Clin Pathol* 2004;121:402–407.

59. Ferrara F, Morabito F, Martino B, et al. CD56 expression is an indicator of poor clinical outcome in patients with acute promyelocytic leukemia treated with simultaneous all-trans-retinoic acid and chemotherapy. *J Clin Oncol* 2000;18:1295–1300.

60. Grimwade D, Jovanovic JV, Hills RK, et al. Prospective minimal residual disease monitoring to predict relapse of acute promyelocytic leukemia and to direct pre-emptive arsenic trioxide therapy. *J Clin Oncol* 2009;27:3650–3658.

61. Iqbal S, Grimwade D, Chase A, et al. Identification of PML/RARalpha rearrangements in suspected acute promyelocytic leukemia using fluorescence in situ hybridization of bone marrow smears: a comparison with cytogenetics and RT-PCR in MRC ATRA trial patients. MRC Adult Leukaemia Working Party. *Leukemia* 2000;14:950–953.

62. Grimwade D, Biondi A, Mozziconacci MJ, et al. Characterization of acute promyelocytic leukemia cases lacking the classic t(15;17): results of the European Working Party. Groupe Francais de Cytogenetique Hematologique, Groupe de Francais d'Hematologie Cellulaire, UK Cancer Cytogenetics Group and BIOMED 1 European Community-Concerted Action "Molecular Cytogenetic Diagnosis in Haematological Malignancies". *Blood* 2000;96:1297–1308.

63. Douer D, Tallman MS. Arsenic trioxide: new clinical experience with an old medication in hematologic malignancies. *J Clin Oncol* 2005;23:2396–2410.

64. Fenaux P, Wang ZZ, Degos L. Treatment of acute promyelocytic leukemia by retinoids. *Curr Top Microbiol Immunol* 2007;313:101–128.

65. Callens C, Chevret S, Cayuela JM, et al. Prognostic implication of FLT3 and Ras gene mutations in patients with acute promyelocytic leukemia (APL): a retrospective study from the European APL Group. *Leukemia* 2005;19:1153–1160.

66. Gale RE, Hills R, Pizzey AR, et al. Relationship between FLT3 mutation status, biologic characteristics, and response to targeted therapy in acute promyelocytic leukemia. *Blood* 2005;106:3768–3776.

67. Kuchenbauer F, Schoch C, Kern W, et al. Impact of FLT3 mutations and promyelocytic leukaemia-breakpoint on clinical characteristics and prognosis in acute promyelocytic leukaemia. *Br J Haematol* 2005;130:196–202.

68. Schnittger S, Bacher U, Haferlach C, et al. Clinical impact of FLT3 mutation load in acute promyelocytic leukemia with t(15;17)/PML-RARA. *Haematologica* 2011;96:1799–1807.
69. Sainty D, Liso V, Cantu-Rajnoldi A, et al. A new morphologic classification system for acute promyelocytic leukemia distinguishes cases with underlying PLZF/RARA gene rearrangements. Group Francais de Cytogenetique Hematologique, UK Cancer Cytogenetics Group and BIOMED 1 European Coomunity-Concerted Acion "Molecular Cytogenetic Diagnosis in Haematological Malignancies". *Blood* 2000;96:1287–1296.
70. Sirulnik A, Melnick A, Zelent A, et al. Molecular pathogenesis of acute promyelocytic leukaemia and APL variants. *Best Pract Res Clin Haematol* 2003;16:387–408.
71. Zelent A, Guidez F, Melnick A, et al. Translocations of the RARalpha gene in acute promyelocytic leukemia. *Oncogene* 2001;20:7186–7203.
72. Melnick A, Licht JD. Deconstructing a disease: RARalpha, its fusion partners, and their roles in the pathogenesis of acute promyelocytic leukemia. *Blood* 1999;93:3167–3215.
73. Creutzig U, Harbott J, Sperling C, et al. Clinical significance of surface antigen expression in children with acute myeloid leukemia: results of study AML-BFM-87. *Blood* 1995;86:3097–3108.
74. Munoz L, Nomdedeu JF, Villamor N, et al. Acute myeloid leukemia with MLL rearrangements: clinicobiological features, prognostic impact and value of flow cytometry in the detection of residual leukemic cells. *Leukemia* 2003;17:76–82.
75. Forestier E, Heim S, Blennow E, et al. Cytogenetic abnormalities in childhood acute myeloid leukaemia: a Nordic series comprising all children enrolled in the NOPHO-93-AML trial between 1993 and 2001. *Br J Haematol* 2003;121: 566–577.
76. Meyer C, Kowarz E, Hofmann J, et al. New insights to the MLL recombinome of acute leukemias. *Leukemia* 2009;23:1490–1499.
77. Rubnitz JE, Raimondi SC, Tong X, et al. Favorable impact of the t(9;11) in childhood acute myeloid leukemia. *J Clin Oncol* 2002;20:2302–2309.
78. Shih LY, Liang DC, Fu JF, et al. Characterization of fusion partner genes in 114 patients with de novo acute myeloid leukemia and MLL rearrangement. *Leukemia* 2006;20:218–223.
79. Barjesteh van Waalwijk van Doorn-Khosrovani S, Erpelinck C, van Putten WL, et al. High EVI1 expression predicts poor survival in acute myeloid leukemia: a study of 319 de novo AML patients. *Blood* 2003;101:837–845.
80. Alsabeh R, Brynes RK, Slovak ML, et al. Acute myeloid leukemia with t(6;9) (p23;q34): association with myelodysplasia, basophilia, and initial CD34 negative immunophenotype. *Am J Clin Pathol* 1997;107:430–437.
81. Chi Y, Lindgren V, Quigley S, Gaitonde S. Acute myelogenous leukemia with t(6;9)(p23;q34) and marrow basophilia: an overview. *Arch Pathol Lab Med* 2008;132:1835–1837.
82. Oyarzo MP, Lin P, Glassman A, et al. Acute myeloid leukemia with t(6;9)(p23;q34) is associated with dysplasia and a high frequency of flt3 gene mutations. *Am J Clin Pathol* 2004;122:348–358.
83. Slovak ML, Gundacker H, Bloomfield CD, et al. A retrospective study of 69 patients with t(6;9)(p23;q34) AML emphasizes the need for a prospective, multicenter initiative for rare 'poor prognosis' myeloid malignancies. *Leukemia* 2006;20:1295–1297.
84. Scandura JM, Boccuni P, Cammenga J, et al. Transcription factor fusions in acute leukemia: variations on a theme. *Oncogene* 2002;21:3422–3444.
85. Grigg AP, Gascoyne RD, Phillips GL, et al. Clinical, haematological and cytogenetic features in 24 patients with structural rearrangements of the Q arm of chromosome 3. *Br J Haematol* 1993;83:158–165.
86. Secker-Walker LM, Mehta A, Bain B. Abnormalities of 3q21 and 3q26 in myeloid malignancy: a United Kingdom Cancer Cytogenetic Group study. *Br J Haematol* 1995;91:490–501.
87. Sweet DL, Rowley JD, Vardiman JW. Acute myelogenous leukemia and thrombocythemia associated with an abnormality of chromosome no. 3. *Cancer Genet Cytogenet* 1979;1:33–37.
88. Shi G, Weh HJ, Duhrsen U, et al. Chromosomal abnormality inv(3)(q21q26) associated with multilineage hematopoietic progenitor cells in hematopoietic malignancies. *Cancer Genet Cytogenet* 1997;96:58–63.
89. Nucifora G, Laricchia-Robbio L, Senyuk V. EVI1 and hematopoietic disorders: history and perspectives. *Gene* 2006;368:1–11.
90. Reiter E, Greinix H, Rabitsch W, et al. Low curative potential of bone marrow transplantation for highly aggressive acute myelogenous leukemia with inversioin inv (3)(q21q26) or homologous translocation t(3;3) (q21;q26). *Ann Hematol* 2000;79:374–377.
91. Mitelman F. The cytogenetic scenario of chronic myeloid leukemia. *Leuk Lymph* 1993;(11 Suppl 1):11–15.
92. Bernstein J, Dastugue N, Haas OA, et al. Nineteen cases of the t(1;22)(p13;q13) acute megakaryblastic leukaemia of infants/children and a review of 39 cases: report from a t(1;22) study group. *Leukemia* 2000;14:216–218.
93. Carroll A, Civin C, Schneider N, et al. The t(1;22) (p13;q13) is nonrandom and restricted to infants with acute megakaryoblastic leukemia: a Pediatric Oncology Group Study. *Blood* 1991;78:748–752.
94. Descot A, Rex-Haffner M, Courtois G, et al. OTT-MAL is a deregulated activator of serum response factor-dependent gene expression. *Mol Cell Biol* 2008;28:6171–6181.
95. Mercher T, Coniat MB, Monni R, et al. Involvement of a human gene related to the Drosophila spen gene in the recurrent t(1;22) translocation of acute megakaryocytic leukemia. *Proc Natl Acad Sci U S A* 2001;98:5776–5779.
96. Duchayne E, Fenneteau O, Pages MP, et al. Acute megakaryoblastic leukaemia: a national clinical and biological study of 53 adult and childhood cases by the Groupe Francais d'Hematologie Cellulaire (GFHC). *Leuk Lymph* 2003;44:49–58.
97. Keung YK, Beaty M, Powell BL, et al. Philadelphia chromosome positive myelodysplastic syndrome and acute myeloid leukemia-retrospective study and review of literature. *Leuk Res* 2004;28:579–586.
98. Soupir CP, Vergilio JA, Dal Cin P, et al. Philadelphia chromosome-positive acute myeloid leukemia: a rare aggressive leukemia with clinicopathologic features distinct from chronic myeloid leukemia in myeloid blast crisis. *Am J Clin Pathol* 2007;127:642–650.
99. Arber DA, Chang KL, Lyda MH, et al. Detection of NPM/MLF1 fusion in t(3;5)-positive acute myeloid leukemia and myelodysplasia. *Hum Pathol* 2003;34:809–813.
100. Raimondi SC, Dube ID, Valentine MB, et al. Clinicopathologic manifestations and breakpoints of the t(3;5) in patients with acute nonlymphocytic leukemia. *Leukemia* 1989;3:42–47.
101. Stark B, Resnitzky P, Jeison M, et al. A distinct subtype of M4/M5 acute myeloblastic leukemia (AML) associated with t(8:16)(p11:p13), in a patient with the variant t(8:19)(p11:q13)—case report and review of the literature. *Leuk Res* 1995;19:367–379.
102. Wong KF, Yuen HL, Siu LL, et al. t(8;16)(p11;p13) predisposes to a transient but potentially recurring neonatal leukemia. *Hum Pathol* 2008;39:1702–1707.
103. Bacher U, Haferlach C, Kern W, et al. Prognostic relevance of FLT3-TKD mutations in AML: the combination matters—an analysis of 3082 patients. *Blood* 2008;111:2527–2537.
104. Delhommeau F, Dupont S, Della Valle V, et al. Mutation in TET2 in myeloid cancers. *N Engl J Med* 2009;360:2289–2301.
105. Gari M, Goodeve A, Wilson G, et al. c-kit proto-oncogene exon 8 in-frame deletion plus insertion mutations in acute myeloid leukaemia. *Br J Haematol* 1999;105:894–900.
106. Mardis ER, Ding L, Dooling DJ, et al. Recurring mutations found by sequencing an acute myeloid leukemia genome. *N Engl J Med* 2009;361:1058–1066.
107. Mead AJ, Linch DC, Hills RK, et al. FLT3 tyrosine kinase domain mutations are biologically distinct from and have a significantly more favorable prognosis than FLT3 internal tandem duplications in patients with acute myeloid leukemia. *Blood* 2007;110:1262–1270.
108. Paschka P, Marcucci G, Ruppert AS, et al. Wilms' tumor 1 gene mutations independently predict poor outcome in adults with cytogenetically normal acute myeloid leukemia: a cancer and leukemia group B study. *J Clin Oncol* 2008; 26:4595–4602.
109. Preudhomme C, Warot-Loze D, Roumier C, et al. High incidence of biallelic point mutations in the Runt domain of the AML1/PEBP2 alpha B gene in Mo acute myeloid leukemia and in myeloid malignancies with acquired trisomy 21. *Blood* 2000; 96:2862–2869.
110. Renneville A, Boissel N, Gachard N, et al. The favorable impact of CEBPA mutations in patients with acute myeloid leukemia is only observed in the absence of associated cytogenetic abnormalities and FLT3 internal duplication. *Blood* 2009;113: 5090–5093.
111. Renneville A, Boissel N, Zurawski V, et al. Wilms tumor 1 gene mutations are associated with a higher risk of recurrence in young adults with acute myeloid leukemia: a study from the Acute Leukemia French Association. *Cancer* 2009;115:3719–3727.
112. Thiede C, Koch S, Creutzig E, et al. Prevalence and prognostic impact of NPM1 mutations in 1485 adult patients with acute myeloid leukemia (AML). *Blood* 2006; 107:4011–4020.
113. Hou HA, Kuo YY, Liu CY, et al. DNMT3A mutations in acute myeloid leukemia: stability during disease evolution and clinical implications. *Blood* 2012;119: 559–568.
114. Kelly LM, Gilliland DG. Genetics of myeloid leukemias. *Ann Rev Genom Hum Genet* 2002;3:179–198.
115. Falini B, Nicoletti I, Martelli MF, et al. Acute myeloid leukemia carrying cytoplasmic/mutated nucleophosmin (NPMc+ AML): biologic and clinical features. *Blood* 2007;109:874–885.
116. Hollink IH, Zwaan CM, Zimmermann M, et al. Favorable prognostic impact of NPM1 gene mutations in childhood acute myeloid leukemia, with emphasis on cytogenetically normal AML. *Leukemia* 2009;23:262–270.
117. Suzuki T, Kiyoi H, Ozeki K, et al. Clinical characteristics and prognostic implications of NPM1 mutations in acute myeloid leukemia. *Blood* 2005;106:2854–2861.
118. Bolli N, Nicoletti I, De Marco MF, et al. Born to be exported: COOH-terminal nuclear export signals of different strength ensure cytoplasmic accumulation of nucleophosmin leukemic mutants. *Cancer Res* 2007;67:6230–6237.
119. Okuwaki M. The structure and functions of NPM1/Nucleophsmin/B23, a multifunctional nucleolar acidic protein. *J Biochem* 2008;143:441–448.
120. Falini B, Martelli MP, Bolli N, et al. Immunohistochemistry predicts nucleophosmin (NPM) mutations in acute myeloid leukemia. *Blood* 2006;108:1999–2005.
121. Falini B, Mecucci C, Tiacci E, et al. Cytoplasmic nucleophosmin in acute myelogenous leukemia with a normal karyotype. *N Engl J Med* 2005;352:254–266.
122. Alcalay M, Tiacci E, Bergomas R, et al. Acute myeloid leukemia bearing cytoplasmic nucleophosmin (NPMc+ AML) shows a distinct gene expression profile characterized by up-regulation of genes involved in stem-cell maintenance. *Blood* 2005;106:899–902.
123. Verhaak RG, Goudswaard CS, van Putten W, et al. Mutations in nucleophosmin (NPM1) in acute myeloid leukemia (AML): association with other gene abnormalities and previously established gene expression signatures and their favorable prognostic significance. *Blood* 2005;106:3747–3754.
124. Chen W, Rassidakis GZ, Li J, et al. High frequency of NPM1 gene mutations in acute myeloid leukemia with prominent nuclear invaginations ("cuplike" nuclei). *Blood* 2006;108:1783–1784.
125. Kussick SJ, Stirewalt DL, Yi HS, et al. A distinctive nuclear morphology in acute myeloid leukemia is strongly associated with loss of HLA-DR expression and FLT3 internal tandem duplication. *Leukemia* 2004;18:159–159-8.
126. Huang Q, Chen W, Gaal KK, et al. A rapid, one step assay for simultaneous detection of FLT3/ITD and NPM1 mutations in AML with normal cytogenetics. *Br J Haematol* 2008;142:489–492.
127. Noguera NI, Ammatuna E, Zangrilli D, et al. Simultaneous detection of NPM1 and FLT3-ITD mutations by capillary electrophoresis in acute myeloid leukemia. *Leukemia* 2005;19:1479–1482.
128. Ho PA, Alonzo TA, Gerbing RB, et al. Prevalence and prognostic implications of CEBPA mutations in pediatric acute myeloid leukemia (AML): a report from the Children's Oncology Group. *Blood* 2009;113:6558–6566.
129. Pabst T, Mueller BU, Zhang P, et al. Dominant-negative mutations of CEBPA, encoding CCAAT/enhancer binding protein-alpha (C/EBPalpha), in acute myeloid leukemia. *Nat Genet* 2001;27:263–270.
130. Preudhomme C, Sagot C, Boissel N, et al. Favorable prognostic significance of CEBPA mutations in patients with de novo acute myeloid leukemia: a study from the Acute Leukemia French Association (ALFA). *Blood* 2002;100:2717–2723.
131. Bienz M, Ludwig M, Leibundgut EO, et al. Risk assessment in patients with acute myeloid leukemia and a normal karyotype. *Clin Cancer Res* 2005;11:1416–1424.
132. Lin LI, Chen CY, Lin DT, et al. Characterization of CEBPA mutations in acute myeloid leukemia: most patients with CEBPA mutations have biallelic mutations and show a distinct immunophenotype of the leukemic cells. *Clin Cancer Res* 2005;11:1372–1379.
133. Koschmieder S, Halmos B, Levantini E, et al. Dysregulation of the C/EBPalpha differentiation pathway in human cancer. *J Clin Oncol* 2009;27:619–628.

134. Ahn JY, Seo K, Weinberg O, et al. A comparison of two methods for screening CEBPA mutations in patients with acute myeloid leukemia. *J Mol Diagn* 2009;11:319–323.
135. Barjesteh van Waalwijk van Doorn-Khosrovani S, Erpelinck C, Meijer J, et al. Biallelic mutations in the CEBPA gene and low CEBPA expression levels as prognostic markers in intermediate-risk AML. *Hematol J* 2003;4:31–40.
136. Pabst T, Eyholzer M, Fos J, et al. Heterogeneity within AML with CEBPA mutations; only CEBPA double mutations, but not single CEBPA mutations are associated with favourable prognosis. *Br J Cancer* 2009;100:1343–1346.
137. Wouters BJ, Lowenberg B, Erpelinck-Verschueren CA, et al. Double CEBPA mutations, but not single CEBPA mutations, define a subgroup of acute myeloid leukemia with a distinctive gene expression profile that is uniquely associated with a favorable outcome. *Blood* 2009;113:3088–3091.
138. Kottaridis PD, Gale RE, Linch DC. Flt3 mutations and leukaemia. *Br J Haematol* 2003;122:523–538.
139. Reindl C, Bagrintseva K, Vempati S, et al. Point mutations in the juxtamembrane domain of FLT3 define a new class of activating mutations in AML. *Blood* 2006;107:3700–3707.
140. Beran M, Luthra R, Kantarjian H, et al. FLT3 mutation and response to intensive chemotherapy in young adult and elderly patients with normal karyotype. *Leukemia Res* 2004;28:547–550.
141. Frohling S, Schlenk RF, Breitruck J, et al. Prognostic significance of activating FLT3 mutations in younger adults (16 to 60 years) with acute myeloid leukemia and normal cytogenetics: a study of the AML Study Group Ulm. *Blood* 2002;100:4372–4380.
142. Whitman SP, Ruppert AS, Radmacher MD, et al. FLT3 D835/I836 mutations are associated with poor disease-free survival and a distinct gene-expression signature among younger adults with de novo cytogenetically normal acute myeloid leukemia lacking FLT3 internal tandem duplications. *Blood* 2008;111:1552–1559.
143. Summers K, Stevens J, Kakkas I, et al. Wilms' tumour 1 mutations are associated with FLT3-ITD and failure of standard induction chemotherapy in patients with normal karyotype AML. *Leukemia* 2007;21:550–551; author reply 2.
144. Owen C, Fitzgibbon J, Paschka P. The clinical relevance of Wilms Tumour 1 (WT1) gene mutations in acute leukaemia. *Hematol Oncol* 2010;28:13–19.
145. Taketani T, Taki T, Takita J, et al. AML1/RUNX1 mutations are infrequent, but related to AML-M0, acquired trisomy 21, and leukemic transformation in pediatric hematologic malignancies. *Genes Chromosomes Cancer* 2003;38:1–7.
146. Gaidzik VI, Bullinger L, Schlenk RF, et al. RUNX1 mutations in acute myeloid leukemia: results from a comprehensive genetic and clinical analysis from the AML study group. *J Clin Oncol* 2011;29:1364–1372.
147. Bacher U, Haferlach T, Schoch C, et al. Implications of NRAS mutations in AML: a study of 2502 patients. *Blood* 2006;107:3847–3853.
148. Berman JN, Gerbing RB, Alonzo TA, et al. Prevalence and clinical implications of NRAS mutations in childhood AML: a report from the Children's Oncology Group. *Leukemia* 2011;25:1039–1042.
149. Sano H, Shimada A, Taki T, et al. RAS mutations are frequent in FAB type M4 and M5 of acute myeloid leukemia, and related to late relapse: a study of the Japanese Childhood AML Cooperative Study Group. *Int J Hematol* 2012;95:509–515.
150. Fried I, Bodner C, Pichler MM, et al. Frequency, onset and clinical impact of somatic DNMT3A mutations in therapy-related and secondary acute myeloid leukemia. *Haematologica* 2012;97:246–250.
151. Ley TJ, Ding L, Walter MJ, et al. DNMT3A mutations in acute myeloid leukemia. *N Engl J Med* 2010;363:2424–2433.
152. Shen Y, Zhu YM, Fan X, et al. Gene mutation patterns and their prognostic impact in a cohort of 1185 patients with acute myeloid leukemia. *Blood* 2011;118:5593–5603.
153. Thol F, Damm F, Ludeking A, et al. Incidence and prognostic influence of DNMT3A mutations in acute myeloid leukemia. *J Clin Oncol* 2011;29:2889–2896.
154. Marcucci G, Metzeler KH, Schwind S, et al. Age-related prognostic impact of different types of DNMT3A mutations in adults with primary cytogenetically normal acute myeloid leukemia. *J Clin Oncol* 2012;30:742–750.
155. Figueroa ME, Abdel-Wahab O, Lu C, et al. Leukemic IDH1 and IDH2 mutations result in a hypermethylation phenotype, disrupt TET2 function, and impair hematopoietic differentiation. *Cancer Cell* 2010;18:553–567.
156. Abdel-Wahab O, Mullally A, Hedvat C, et al. Genetic characterization of TET1, TET2, and TET3 alterations in myeloid malignancies. *Blood* 2009;114:144–147.
157. Gaidzik VI, Paschka P, Spath D, et al. TET2 mutations in acute myeloid leukemia (AML): results from a comprehensive genetic and clinical analysis of the AML study group. *J Clin Oncol* 2012;30:1350–1357.
158. Metzeler KH, Maharry K, Radmacher MD, et al. TET2 mutations improve the new European LeukemiaNet risk classification of acute myeloid leukemia: a Cancer and Leukemia Group B study. *J Clin Oncol* 2011;29:1373–1381.
159. Nibourel O, Kosmider O, Cheok M, et al. Incidence and prognostic value of TET2 alterations in de novo acute myeloid leukemia achieving complete remission. *Blood* 2010;116:1132–1135.
160. Abdel-Wahab O, Patel J, Levine RL. Clinical implications of novel mutations in epigenetic modifiers in AML. *Hematol Oncol Clin N Am* 2011;25:1119–1133.
161. Costello JF, Plass C. Methylation matters. *J Med Genet* 2001;38:285–303.
162. Esteller M. Profiling aberrant DNA methylation in hematologic neoplasms: a view from the tip of the iceberg. *Clin Immunol (Orlando, Fla)* 2003;109:80–88.
163. Melki JR, Clark SJ. DNA methylation changes in leukaemia. *Semin Cancer Biol* 2002;12:347–357.
164. Melki JR, Vincent PC, Clark SJ. Concurrent DNA hypermethylation of multiple genes in acute myeloid leukemia. *Cancer Res* 1999;59:3730–3740.
165. Plass C, Yu F, Yu L, et al. Restriction landmark genome scanning for aberrant methylation in primary refractory and relapsed acute myeloid leukemia; involvement of the WIT-1 gene. *Oncogene* 1999;18:3159–3165.
166. Toyota M, Kopecky KJ, Toyota MO, et al. Methylation profiling in acute myeloid leukemia. *Blood* 2001;97:2823–2829.
167. Di Croce L, Raker VA, Corsaro M, et al. Methyltransferase recruitment and DNA hypermethylation of target promoters by an oncogenic transcription factor. *Science (New York, NY)* 2002;295:1079–1082.
168. Krivtsov AV, Armstrong SA. MLL translocations, histone modifications and leukaemia stem-cell development. *Nat Rev Cancer* 2007;7:823–833.
169. Liu S, Shen T, Huynh L, et al. Interplay of RUNX1/MTG8 and DNA methyltransferase 1 in acute myeloid leukemia. *Cancer Res* 2005;65:1277–1284.
170. Corsetti MT, Salvi F, Perticone S, et al. Hematologic improvement and response in elderly AML/RAEB patients treated with valproic acid and low-dose Ara-C. *Leuk Res* 2011;35:991–997.
171. Issa JP, Garcia-Manero G, Giles FJ, et al. Phase 1 study of low-dose prolonged exposure schedules of the hypomethylating agent 5-aza-2'-deoxycytidine (decitabine) in hematopoietic malignancies. *Blood* 2004;103:1635–1640.
172. Kuendgen A, Gattermann N. Valproic acid for the treatment of myeloid malignancies. *Cancer* 2007;110:943–954.
173. Ravandi F, Issa JP, Garcia-Manero G, et al. Superior outcome with hypomethylating therapy in patients with acute myeloid leukemia and high-risk myelodysplastic syndrome and chromosome 5 and 7 abnormalities. *Cancer* 2009;115:5746–5751.
174. Marcucci G, Mrozek K, Radmacher MD, et al. The prognostic and functional role of microRNAs in acute myeloid leukemia. *Blood* 2011;117:1121–1129.
175. Seca H, Almeida GM, Guimaraes JE, et al. miR signatures and the role of miRs in acute myeloid leukaemia. *Eur J Cancer (Oxford, England: 1990)* 2010;46:1520–1527.
176. Cammarata G, Augugliaro L, Salemi D, et al. Differential expression of specific microRNA and their targets in acute myeloid leukemia. *Am J Hematol* 2010;85:331–339.
177. Garzon R, Garofalo M, Martelli MP, et al. Distinctive microRNA signature of acute myeloid leukemia bearing cytoplasmic mutated nucleophosmin. *Proc Natl Acad Sci U S A* 2008;105:3945–3950.
178. Jongen-Lavrencic M, Sun SM, Dijkstra MK, et al. MicroRNA expression profiling in relation to the genetic heterogeneity of acute myeloid leukemia. *Blood* 2008;111:5078–5085.
179. Li Z, Lu J, Sun M, et al. Distinct microRNA expression profiles in acute myeloid leukemia with common translocations. *Proc Natl Acad Sci U S A* 2008;105:15535–15540.
180. Schwind S, Maharry K, Radmacher MD, et al. Prognostic significance of expression of a single microRNA, miR-181a, in cytogenetically normal acute myeloid leukemia: a Cancer and Leukemia Group B study. *J Clin Oncol* 2010;28:5257–5264.
181. Brunning RD, Matutes E, et al. *Acute myeloid leukemias*. Lyon: IARC, 2001.
182. Weinberg OK, Seetharam M, Ren L, et al. Clinical characterization of acute myeloid leukemia with myelodysplasia-related changes as defined by the 2008 WHO classification system. *Blood* 2009;113:1906–1908.
183. Schoch C, Haferlach T, Bursch S, et al. Loss of genetic material is more common than gain in acute myeloid leukemia with complex aberrant karyotype: a detailed analysis of 125 cases using conventional chromosome analysis and fluorescence in situ hybridization including 24-color FISH. *Genes Chromosomes Cancer* 2002;35:20–29.
184. Haferlach T, Schoch C, Loffler H, et al. Morphologic dysplasia in de novo acute myeloid leukemia (AML) is related to unfavorable cytogenetics but has no independent prognostic relevance under the conditions of intensive induction therapy: results of a multiparameter analysis from the German AML Cooperative Group studies. *J Clin Oncol* 2003;21:256–265.
185. Wandt H, Schakel U, Kroschinsky F, et al. MLD according to the WHO classification in AML has no correlation with age and no independent prognostic relevance as analyzed in 1766 patients. *Blood* 2008;111:1855–1861.
186. Lugthart S, van Drunen E, van Norden Y, et al. High EVI1 levels predict adverse outcome in acute myeloid leukemia: prevalence of EVI1 overexpression and chromosome 3q26 abnormalities underestimated. *Blood* 2008;111:4329–4337.
187. Hasle H, Alonzo TA, Auvrignon A, et al. Monosomy 7 and deletion 7q in children and adolescents with acute myeloid leukemia: an international retrospective study. *Blood* 2007;109:4641–4647.
188. Diaz-Beya M, Rozman M, Pratcorona M, et al. The prognostic value of multilineage dysplasia in de novo acute myeloid leukemia patients with intermediate-risk cytogenetics is dependent on NPM1 mutational status. *Blood* 2010;116:6147–6148.
189. Falini B, Macijewski K, Weiss T, et al. Multilineage dysplasia has no impact on biologic, clinicopathologic, and prognostic features of AML with mutated nucleophosmin (NPM1). *Blood* 2010;115:3776–3786.
190. Mauritzson N, Albin M, Rylander L, et al. Pooled analysis of clinical and cytogenetic features in treatment-related and de novo adult acute myeloid leukemia and myelodysplastic syndromes based on a consecutive series of 761 patients analyzed 1976-1993 and on 5098 unselected cases reported in the literature 1974-2001. *Leukemia* 2002;16:2366–2378.
191. Singh ZN, Huo D, Anastasi J, et al. Therapy-related myelodysplastic syndrome: morphologic subclassification may not be clinically relevant. *Am J Clin Pathol* 2007;127:197–205.
192. Andersen MK, Larson RA, Mauritzson N, et al. Balanced chromosome abnormalities inv(16) and t(15;17) in therapy-related myelodysplastic syndromes and acute leukemia: report from an international workshop. *Genes Chromosomes Cancer* 2002;33:395–400.
193. Arber DA, Slovak ML, Popplewell L, et al. Therapy-related acute myeloid leukemia/myelodysplasia with balanced 21q22 translocations. *Am J Clin Pathol* 2002;117:306–313.
194. Bloomfield CD, Archer KJ, Mrozek K, et al. 11q23 balanced chromosome aberrations in treatment-related myelodysplastic syndromes and acute leukemia: report from an international workshop. *Genes Chromosomes Cancer* 2002;33:362–378.
195. Pedersen-Bjergaard J, Andersen MK, Andersen MT, et al. Genetics of therapy-related myelodysplasia and acute myeloid leukemia. *Leukemia* 2008;22:240–248.
196. Rowley JD, Olney HJ. International workshop on the relationship of prior therapy to balanced chromosome aberrations in therapy-related myelodysplastic syndromes and acute leukemia: overview report. *Genes Chromosomes Cancer* 2002;33:331–345.
197. Nardi V, Winkfield KM, Ok CY, et al. Acute myeloid leukemia and myelodysplastic syndromes after radiation therapy are similar to de novo disease and differ from other therapy-related myeloid neoplasms. *J Clin Oncol* 2012;30:2340–2347.
198. Ishizawa S, Slovak ML, Popplewell L, et al. High frequency of pro-B acute lymphoblastic leukemia in adults with secondary leukemia with 11q23 abnormalities. *Leukemia* 2003;17:1091–1095.
199. Secker-Walker LM, Moorman AV, Bain BJ, et al. Secondary acute leukemia and myelodysplastic syndrome with 11q23 abnormalities. EU Concerted Action 11q23 Workshop. *Leukemia* 1998;12:840–844.
200. Andersen MT, Andersen MK, Christiansen DH, et al. NPM1 mutations in therapy-related acute myeloid leukemia with uncharacteristic features. *Leukemia* 2008;22:951–955.
201. Pedersen-Bjergaard J, Christiansen DH, Desta F, et al. Alternative genetic pathways and cooperating genetic abnormalities in the pathogenesis of therapy-related myelodysplasia and acute myeloid leukemia. *Leukemia* 2006;20:1943–1949.

202. Borthakur G, Lin E, Jain N, et al. Survival is poorer in patients with secondary core-binding factor acute myelogenous leukemia compared with de novo core-binding factor leukemia. *Cancer* 2009;115:3217–3221.
203. Tallman MS, Kim HT, Paietta E, et al. Acute monocytic leukemia (French-American-British classification M5) does not have a worse prognosis than other subtypes of acute myeloid leukemia: a report from the Eastern Cooperative Oncology Group. *J Clin Oncol* 2004;22:1276–1286.
204. Roumier C, Eclache V, Imbert M, et al. M0 AML, clinical and biologic features of the disease, including AML1 gene mutations: a report of 59 cases by the Groupe Francais d'Hematologie Cellulaire (GFHC) and the Groupe Francais de Cytogenetique Hematologique (GFCH). *Blood* 2003;101:1277–1283.
205. Silva FP, Morolli B, Storlazzi CT, et al. ETV6 mutations and loss in AML-M0. *Leukemia* 2008;22:1639–1643.
206. Bacher U, Haferlach C, Alpermann T, et al. Comparison of genetic and clinical aspects in patients with acute myeloid leukemia and myelodysplastic syndromes all with more than 50% of bone marrow erythropoietic cells. *Haematologica* 2011;96:1284–1292.
207. Kasyan A, Medeiros LJ, Zuo Z, et al. Acute erythroid leukemia as defined in the World Health Organization classification is a rare and pathogenetically heterogeneous disease. *Mod Pathol* 2010;23:1113–1126.
208. Linari S, Vannucchi AM, Ciolli S, et al. Coexpression of erythroid and megakaryocytic genes in acute erythroblastic (FAB M6) and megakaryoblastic (FAB M7) leukaemias. *Br J Haematol* 1998;102:1335–1337.
209. Pagano L, Pulsoni A, Vignetti M, et al. Acute megakaryoblastic leukemia: experience of GIMEMA trials. *Leukemia* 2002;16:1622–1626.
210. Nichols CR, Roth BJ, Heerema N, et al. Hematologic neoplasia associated with primary mediastinal germ-cell tumors. *N Engl J Med* 1990;322:1425–1429.
211. Peterson LC, Parkin JL, Arthur DC, et al. Acute basophilic leukemia. A clinical, morphologic, and cytogenetic study of eight cases. *Am J Clin Pathol* 1991;96:160–170.
212. Shvidel L, Shaft D, Stark B, et al. Acute basophilic leukaemia: eight unsuspected new cases diagnosed by electron microscopy. *Br J Haematol* 2003;120:774–781.
213. Wick MR, Li CY, Pierre RV. Acute nonlymphocytic leukemia with basophilic differentiation. *Blood* 1982;60:38–45.
214. Lichtman MA, Segel GB. Uncommon phenotypes of acute myelogenous leukemia: basophilic, mast cell, eosinophilic, and myeloid dendritic cell subtypes: a review. *Blood Cells Mol Dis* 2005;35:370–383.
215. Staal-Viliare A, Latger-Cannard V, Didion J, et al. CD203c /CD117-, an useful phenotype profile for acute basophilic leukaemia diagnosis in cases of undifferentiated blasts. *Leuk Lymph* 2007;48:439–441.
216. Bearman RM, Pangalis GA, Rappaport H. Acute ("malignant") myelosclerosis. *Cancer* 1979;43:279–293.
217. Hruban RH, Kuhajda FP, Mann RB. Acute myelofibrosis. Immunohistochemical study of four cases and comparison with acute megakaryocytic leukemia. *Am J Clin Pathol* 1987;88:578–588.
218. Orazi A, O'Malley DP, Jiang J, et al. Acute panmyelosis with myelofibrosis: an entity distinct from acute megakaryoblastic leukemia. *Mod Pathol* 2005;18:603–614.
219. Sultan C, Sigaux F, Imbert M, Reyes F. Acute myelodysplasia with myelofibrosis: a report of eight cases. *Br J Haematol* 1981;49:11–16.
220. Fong CT, Brodeur GM. Down's syndrome and leukemia: epidemiology, genetics, cytogenetics and mechanisms of leukemogenesis. *Cancer Genet Cytogenet* 1987;28:55–76.
221. Webb D, Roberts I, Vyas P. Haematology of Down syndrome. *Arch Dis Child Fetal Neonat* 2007;92:F503–F507.
222. Chou ST, Opalinska JB, Yao Y, et al. Trisomy 21 enhances human fetal erythromegakaryocytic development. *Blood* 2008;112:4503–4506.
223. Pine SR, Guo Q, Yin C, et al. Incidence and clinical implications of GATA1 mutations in newborns with Down syndrome. *Blood* 2007;110:2128–2131.
224. Tunstall-Pedoe O, Roy A, Karadimitris A, et al. Abnormalities in the myeloid progenitor compartment in Down syndrome fetal liver precede acquisition of GATA1 mutations. *Blood* 2008;112:4507–4511.
225. Baumann I, Brunning RD, Arber DA, Porwit A. *Myeloid proliferations related to Down syndrome*. Lyon: IARC, 2008.
226. Creutzig U, Ritter J, Vormoor J, et al. Myelodysplasia and acute myelogenous leukemia in Down's syndrome. A report of 40 children of the AML-BFM Study Group. *Leukemia* 1996;10:1677–1686.
227. Gamis AS, Alonzo TA, Gerbing RB, et al. Natural history of transient myeloproliferative disorder clinically diagnosed in Down syndrome neonates: a report from the Children's Oncology Group Study A2971. *Blood* 2011;118:6752–6759.
228. Dixon N, Kishnani PS, Zimmerman S. Clinical manifestations of hematologic and oncologic disorders in patients with Down syndrome. *Am J Med Genet* 2006;142C:149–157.
229. Massey GV, Zipursky A, Chang MN, et al. A prospective study of the natural history of transient leukemia (TL) in neonates with Down syndrome (DS): Children's Oncology Group (COG) study POG-9481. *Blood* 2006;107:4606–4613.
230. Karandikar NJ, Aquino DB, McKenna RW, et al. Transient myeloproliferative disorder and acute myeloid leukemia in Down syndrome. An immunophenotypic analysis. *Am J Clin Pathol* 2001;116:204–210.
231. Langebrake C, Creutzig U, Reinhardt D. Immunophenotype of Down syndrome acute myeloid leukemia and transient myeloproliferative disease differs significantly from other diseases with morphologically identical or similar blasts. *Klinische Padiatrie* 2005;217:126–134.
232. De Vita S, Mulligan C, McElwaine S, et al. Loss-of-function JAK3 mutations in TMD and AMKL of Down syndrome. *Br J Haematol* 2007;137:337–341.
233. Lange BJ, Kobrinsky N, Barnard DR, et al. Distinctive demography, biology, and outcome of acute myeloid leukemia and myelodysplastic syndrome in children with Down syndrome: Children's Cancer Group Studies 2861 and 2891. *Blood* 1998;91:608–615.
234. Norton A, Fisher C, Liu H, et al. Analysis of JAK3, JAK2, and C-MPL mutations in transient myeloproliferative disorder and myeloid leukemia of Down syndrome blasts in children with Down syndrome. *Blood* 2007;110:1077–1079.
235. Sato T, Toki T, Kanezaki R, et al. Functional analysis of JAK3 mutations in transient myeloproliferative disorder and acute megakaryoblastic leukaemia accompanying Down syndrome. *Br J Haematol* 2008;141:681–688.
236. Gamis AS, Woods WG, Alonzo TA, et al. Increased age at diagnosis has a significantly negative effect on outcome in children with Down syndrome and acute myeloid leukemia: a report from the Children's Cancer Group Study 2891. *J Clin Oncol* 2003;21:3415–3422.
237. Meis JM, Butler JJ, Osborne BM, et al. Granulocytic sarcoma in nonleukemic patients. *Cancer* 1986;58:2697–2709.
238. Neiman RS, Barcos M, Berard C, et al. Granulocytic sarcoma: a clinicopathologic study of 61 biopsied cases. *Cancer* 1981;48:1426–1437.
239. Traweek ST, Arber DA, Rappaport H, et al. Extramedullary myeloid cell tumors. An immunohistochemical and morphologic study of 28 cases. *Am J Surg Pathol* 1993;17:1011–1019.
240. Byrd JC, Weiss RB, Arthur DC, et al. Extramedullary leukemia adversely affects hematologic complete remission rate and overall survival in patients with t(8;21)(q22;q22): results from Cancer and Leukemia Group B 8461. *J Clin Oncol* 1997;15:466–475.
241. Tsimberidou AM, Kantarjian HM, Wen S, et al. Myeloid sarcoma is associated with superior event-free survival and overall survival compared with acute myeloid leukemia. *Cancer* 2008;113:1370–1378.
242. Rubnitz JE, Raimondi SC, Halbert AR, et al. Characteristics and outcome of t(8;21)-positive childhood acute myeloid leukemia: a single institution's experience. *Leukemia* 2002;16:2072–2077.
243. D'Orazio JA, Pulliam JF, Moscow JA. Spontaneous resolution of a single lesion of myeloid leukemia cutis in an infant: case report and discussion. *Pediatr Hematol Oncol* 2008;25:457–468.
244. Hoyer JD, Grogg KL, Hanson CA, et al. CD33 detection by immunohistochemistry in paraffin-embedded tissues: a new antibody shows excellent specificity and sensitivity for cells of myelomonocytic lineage. *Am J Clin Pathol* 2008;129:316–323.
245. Cohen PR, Kurzrock R. Sweet's syndrome revisited: a review of disease concepts. *Int J Dermatol* 2003;42:761–778.

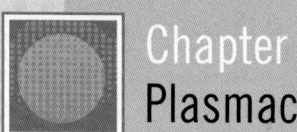

Chapter 42
Plasmacytoid Dendritic Cell Neoplasms

Fabio Facchetti

 ## DEFINITION

Tumoral proliferations of plasmacytoid dendritic cells (PDCs) are rare hematologic neoplasms, which may occur in two clinically and pathologically different forms, respectively derived from mature and immature PDCs. The tumoral proliferation of mature PDCs mainly involves lymph nodes and bone marrow and is invariably associated with a clinically dominant myeloid neoplasm ("*tumor-forming PDCs associated with myeloid neoplasms*"). "*Blastic plasmacytoid dendritic cell neoplasm*" (BPDCN) derives from immature precursors of PDCs and shows a distinctive cutaneous tropism, with rapid and progressive systemic extension. Whereas the former is not recognized as a separate entity by the 2008 WHO Classification of Tumors of Hematopoietic and Lymphoid Tissues, BPDCN is separately listed in the group of acute myeloid leukemias and related precursor neoplasms (1). During the last years BPDCN has deserved a particular interest and emerged only recently as a distinct clinicopathologic entity; along with the progress in the identification criteria of BPDCN, more numerous cases have been reported and data derived from investigations on BPDCN tumor cells contributed in part to unveil characteristics of the normal cellular counterpart. This chapter is particularly devoted to BPDCN.

NORMAL CELLULAR COUNTERPART

The cell that is now known as plasmacytoid dendritic cell was described in 1958 by Karl Lennert and colleagues as a "lymphoblast," occurring in clusters in reactive lymph nodes (2). The subsequent observations that this cell is distributed in the nodal T-cell–rich areas and that it contains a well-developed rough endoplasmic reticulum and expresses CD4 lead to a series of designations such as "T-associated plasma cell" (3,4), "plasmacytoid T cell" (5), and "plasmacytoid T-zone cell" (6). The demonstration of expression of myelomonocytic markers such as CD15 (after neuraminidase treatment) and CD68, and lack of other T-lineage markers, prompted the term "plasmacytoid monocyte" (7).

In the late 1990s the functional characterization of these cells became possible, yet again resulting in an enigmatic dichotomy. In response to a variety of DNA and RNA viruses or synthetic Toll-like receptor (TLR) 9 and TLR7 agonists, the plasmacytoid cells rapidly secrete high amounts of interferon (IFN)-I and, to a lesser extent, other cytokines including interleukin (IL)-6, IL-8, and tumor necrosis factor-α (8–10). They are the fastest responder to INF-I inducers and the major cellular source of the cytokine (especially IFN-α), corresponding to the previously described subset of blood leucocytes known as the "natural IFN-I–producing cells" (11,12). Upon stimulation with CD40 ligand, IL-3, or a variety of microbial stimuli, PDCs undergo a profound morphologic, phenotypical, and functional shift toward mature dendritic cells (DCs) (13,14).

This dichotomy may represent two evolutionary distinct states, where the production of IFN-I is lost upon differentiation into DCs (15,16). Nevertheless, the term plasmacytoid dendritic cell has been adopted to encompass all states.

Although it is still controversial what contribution this cell makes *in vivo* to antigen presentation and T-cell differentiation (17–19), the capacity of PDCs to induce effective T-cell responses after infection or immunization is well documented, either efficiently priming CD4+ T-cell responses with Th1 polarization or priming and cross-priming CD8+ T-cell responses (19,20). Interestingly, the opposite tolerogenic role has been proposed for PDCs in several systems, mostly associated with the induction of regulatory T cells. The tolerogenic properties of PDCs may be relevant in certain immune responses, likely in an organ-dependent fashion, but an irrefutable and broad designation of steady-state PDCs as tolerogenic would be misleading at the present time (21). Recent data, however, obtained in a mouse-melanoma model have provided evidence that TLR7-activated PDCs release TRAIL ad granzyme B that play a direct role in tumor cell killing (22).

By virtue of their efficient production of IFN-I and potential DC functions, PDCs are established as a major effector cell type in immunity, bridging the innate and acquired immune responses, with potential roles in defense against pathogens, cancer immunoediting, and autoimmunity (10,17,18,21,23–29).

PDCs originate in the bone marrow, from both myeloid and lymphoid precursors, although a myeloid derivation is predominant and PDCs share with classical or conventional dendritic cells (CDCs) a unique development pathway from a common macrophage/DC precursor (30–32). The initial development of both PDCs and CDCs is controlled by Flt3L (Fms-like tyrosine kinase 3 ligand) (33,34); subsequently, the sustained upregulation of the basic helix-loop-helix transcription factor (E protein) E2-2 serves as a key for lineage commitment to PDCs (35) and for preservation of their cell fate, avoiding spontaneous PDCs transformation into CDCs (36). Mature PDCs can still differentiate into CDCs after stimulation, and genome-wide analysis showed that the gene expression profile of PDCs is closer to CDCs than to other hematopoietic cells (21,37).

Interestingly, BCL11A, a transcription factor typically expressed by PDCs (38), is a direct target of E2-2 (36). Since E proteins, including E2-2, are also key regulators of lymphopoiesis (35), it has been speculated that the striking "lymphoid" features of PDCs, including morphology and the expression of several lymphoid transcripts (SpiB, Bcl11a, and CIIta; pre–T-cell antigen receptor alpha chain; λ5) (39–41) and of some transcription factors (e.g., BCL11A, FOXp1) (42), may partially result from the ongoing activity of E2-2 (35).

Distribution, Morphology, and Immunophenotype of Normal PDCs

PDCs are rare peripheral blood cells (0.01% to 0.5%) (9,43–45), whose number diminishes with age (46,47). In the peripheral

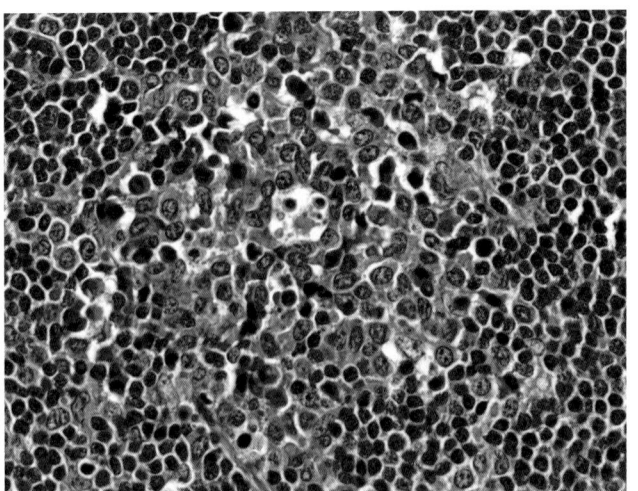

FIGURE 42.1. A nest of PDCs in a reactive lymph node. Note the scattered apoptotic bodies, which frequently occur in such large aggregates (hematoxylin and eosin stain).

blood, PDCs are defined as CD11c$^-$/CD123$^+$ cells that are distinguished from CD11c$^+$/CD123$^-$ CDCs (48). Blood dendritic cell antigens (BDCA)-2 (CD303), BDCA-3 (CD141), and BDCA-4 (CD304) are differentially distributed among these DC populations, and BDCA-2/CD303 is typically restricted to PDCs (49,50). Heterogeneity among circulating PDC fractions has been described (51–53), with subsets expressing CD2, CD5, CD7, CD33, or CD56, that may explain phenotypic variability among tumoral PDC proliferations.

PDCs primarily reside in the peripheral lymph nodes and tonsils (54,55). A consistent number of scattered PDCs are found in the thymic medulla, whereas they are rare in the bone marrow, spleen (at the boundary between white and red pulp), and mucosa-associated lymphoid tissue; PDCs are nearly absent in peripheral nonlymphoid tissues (56). PDCs migrate into lymphoid tissues from the blood via high endothelial venules, employing multiple cell adhesion molecules (57,58). Within lymph nodes their turnover is relatively slow (21,59), but significant accumulation is generally related to an ongoing immune reaction (9,60,61); similarly, accumulations of PDCs can be observed in nonlymphoid tissues in various inflammatory conditions (62–65) or associated with cancers (29).

Despite the acquisition of DC morphology observed in culture, in tissues PDCs generally resemble that in bone marrow and circulation. PDCs are intermediate in size between a small lymphocyte and a monocyte, with a round to ovoid nucleus, which may be slightly indented and eccentric; the chromatin structure is delicate and it is finely dispersed; small but clearly distinct paracentral nucleoli are visible; the cytoplasm is moderately abundant and stains eosinophilic with hematoxylin and eosin and basophilic with Giemsa, which parallels the high content of rough endoplasmic reticulum (3). In lymph nodes, PDCs typically occur in close vicinity to high endothelial venules, either as clusters that may contain apoptotic bodies or as scattered cells (Fig. 42.1) (54). They are much more easily identified combining immunostaining with cell morphology (Table 42.1); CD68 (7) and CLA (cutaneous lymphocyte–associated antigen)/HECA-452 (66) have been used in the past as useful markers for PDC recognition, but their specificity is poor; antisera against CD2AP (CD2-associated protein) (42) and TCL1 (T-cell leukemia/lymphoma 1) (67) are significantly more restricted in their expression, with some limitations (Table 42.1). CD123 and BDCA-2/CD303 represent the most specific and sensitive markers for PDCs (43,63,64,68,69); CD123 is strongly expressed on PDC cell membrane; it can be detected with lower intensity on other cell types, as endothelial cells (43), activated macrophages, and subsets of DCs (64). BDCA-2/CD303 can be partially lost upon PDC activation in inflammatory processes (50,63), but no other cells are known to express this antigen. Interestingly, PDCs are positive for granzyme B, but not perforin and TIA-1 (41,70); granzyme B release by PDCs has been shown to strongly suppress T-cell proliferation, indicating a possible immunosuppressive mechanism in the context of peripheral tolerance

Table 42.1	PLASMACYTOID DENDRITIC CELL IMMUNOPHENOTYPE

Positive

Markers commonly used to identify PDCs on paraffin sections	Notes
CD68	Monoclonal antibody PGM1 preferable to KP1, since it does not stain myeloid cells. Reactive with most macrophages (7,72)
CLA/HECA-452/CD162	Also positive on high endothelial venules endothelium, interdigitating DCs, Langerhans cells, and skin-homing T lymphocytes (66,73,74)
CD2AP	Weak expression on some mantle and germinal center B cells, endothelium, and squamous epithelial cells (42)
TCL1	Strongly positive on mantle B cells and weakly on germinal center B cells (67,75)
CD123	Strongly positive on PDC (43,68); weak expression on other cells (sinus lining cells, endothelium, epithelioid macrophages, so-called IFN-DCs (64)). Basophils are also positive.
CD303/BDCA-2	No other cells positive identified so far. It might decrease upon PDC activation (63).

Other Positive
CD4, CD11a, CD22(a), CD31, CD32, CD33(b), CD36, CD40, CD43, CD44, CD45RA, CD45RB, CD49e, CD62L(c), CD71, CD74, CD128, CD304/BDCA-4
BAD-LAMP, BCL11a, E-cadherin(d), granzyme B, HLA-ABC, HLA-DP, HLA-DQ, HLA-DR, MxA (IFN-induced antiviral protein MxA)
TLR1/CD281(d), TLR6/CD286(d), TLR7/CD287, TLR9/CD289, TLR10/CD290(d)
C-C chemokine receptor (CCR)-2, CCR5, CCR7, C-X-C chemokine receptor (CXCR)-3, CXCR4, chemerin receptor

Negative
CD1a, CD1c/BDCA-1, CD2(d), CD3, CD5(d), CD7(d), CD8, CD10, CD11b, CD11c(e), CD13(e), CD14, CD15(f), CD16, CD19, CD20, CD21, CD22, CD23, CD25, CD27, CD28, CD30, CD34, CD35, CD38, CD45RO, CD56(d), CD57, CD64, CD65, CD80, CD83, CD86, CD94, CD95, CD103, CD117, CD125, CD138, CD141/BDCA-3, CDw150, CD161
BCL2, BCL6, DC-LAMP/CD208, elastase, FOXP3, langerin/CD207, LAT, lysozyme, MUM1/IRF4, myeloperoxidase, perforin, S-100, surface and cytoplasmic immunoglobulins, T-bet, T-cell receptors AB and GD, TdT, TIA-1, ZAP70, mannose receptor/CD206, DC-SIGN/CD209
TLR2/CD282, TLR3/CD283, TLR4/CD284, TLR5/CD285, TLR8/CD288, CCR1, CCR3, CCR4, CCR6, CXCR1, CXCR2, CXCR5

(a): only reactive with the anti-CD22 s-HCL-1 monoclonal antibody; (b): low expression; (c): membranous expression on circulating PDCs and cytoplasmic on tissue PDCs; (d): positivity reported in subsets of circulating PDCs; (e): weak positivity reported on circulating PDCs and induced upon *in vitro* differentiation; (f): positivity after neuraminidase digestion.

(71). Recent data, however, obtained in a mouse-melanoma model provide strong evidence that granzyme B and TRAIL released by TLR7-activated PDCs play a direct role in tumor cell killing (22).

With the notable exceptions of BCL11A (38) and CD22 (detectable only by the monoclonal antibody s-HCL-1) (76,77), PDCs lack expression of lineage-specific antigens for B cells (i.e., CD19, CD20, CD79a, PAX5, surface and cytoplasmic immunoglobulin), T cells (CD3, LAT/linker for activation of T cells, ZAP70, and T-cell receptors AB and GD), and natural killer (NK) cells (CD16, CD56, and CD94). They are also negative for myeloid or monocytic markers myeloperoxidase, lysozyme, CD11c, CD14, CD13, CD33, and CD163.

PDCs are nonproliferative cells (<1% express the Ki-67 antigen) and are negative for the stem/progenitor cell markers CD34 and CD117, as well as for terminal deoxynucleotidyl transferase (TdT) (7,42,56,78–80).

Phenotypic analysis of peripheral blood PDCs substantially overlaps the results obtained on tissue sections, including the formalin non-resistant CD36 antigen (7,49,51,81); weak expression of CD33 has been found in one study (82), while minor subsets of circulating PDCs express CD2, CD5, CD7, CD11c, and CD13 (51).

"TUMOR-FORMING" PLASMACYTOID DENDRITIC CELLS ASSOCIATED WITH MYELOID NEOPLASMS

This tumoral condition involving PDCs was originally described in 1983 and reported as plasmacytoid T-cell lymphoma (5). About 50 cases of this lesion have been described, either as case reports (6,83–90) or small series (91–93). Patients are predominantly males (75%) and the median age is 64 years, but two cases occurred in young individuals (6-year-old girl and 24-year-old male). Patients are affected by a myeloid neoplasia, in most of the cases represented by chronic myelomonocytic leukemia; myelodysplasia and other myeloid proliferations with monocytic differentiation are also reported, whereas there is no association with chronic myelogenous leukemia or atypical chronic myeloid leukemia (94). Hematologic anomalies are variable, and in addition to monocytosis, they include leukocytosis or leukopenia, frequently with

anemia and thrombocytopenia (91,92). The clinical manifestation directly assignable to PDCs accumulation predominantly consists of lymphadenopathy, while splenomegaly and skin lesions are more rare (56,95). PDC nodules are often identified in bone marrow biopsies, but circulating PDCs are very uncommon (92).

The nodules consist of cytologically bland or slightly irregular cells, morphologically very similar to PDCs found in reactive lymph nodes; PDC nodules are numerous, sometimes confluent, and may show prominent apoptosis; they are sharply demarcated from the surrounding tissue and are easily distinguishable from the myeloid leukemia, when occurring in the same site (Fig. 42.2D and E). In lymph nodes the nodules predominantly involve the paracortex and the interfollicular area (Fig. 42.2F), in the spleen they are adjacent to the white pulp, and in the skin they form aggregates around vessels and the pilosebaceous units, but exceptionally involve the epidermis (91,95). PDC immunophenotype is basically different from that of the associated myeloid neoplasm (91,92); similarly to reactive PDCs, the PDC nodules are strongly positive for CD68 (Fig. 42.2A) and granzyme B and express CD123, CLA/HECA-452, TCL1, CD2AP, and BDCA-2/CD303 (42,70,91,93,95). These lesions have very low proliferative rates (<10% Ki-67 proliferative index) and lack TdT or CD34 expression (Fig. 42.2B); CD56 is negative or weakly/focally positive (Fig. 42.2C); however, cases with obvious aberrant expression of CD2, CD5, CD7, CD10, CD14, and CD15 have been reported, supporting the neoplastic nature of the PDC proliferation (91). An additional argument in favor of the clonal nature of the PDC nodules and of their relatedness with the associated myeloid neoplasm is the occurrence of common genetic anomalies, demonstrated in multiple cases by fluorescence in situ hybridization (FISH). In one case they consisted of trisomy 9 and 11 (96), or loss of 20q12 (92), and two cases showed monosomy 7 (91,92) or inversion 16 (97).

Such PDC nodules may regress upon therapy (6,91) and the prognosis, which is usually dismal (median survival, 10 months; range 1 to 84 months), reflects the patient's underlying myeloid neoplasm rather than the expansion of PDCs. This markedly contrasts with BPDCN, which also may be associated with myeloid disorders.

It should be noted that similar-appearing nodular accumulations of PDCs may be observed in lymph nodes or skin as part of the immune response in cases of Kikuchi lymphadenitis, Castleman disease hyaline-vascular type, and lupus erythematosus (56).

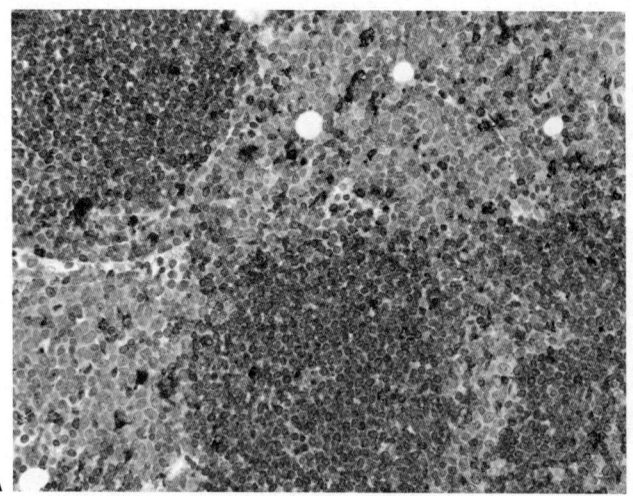
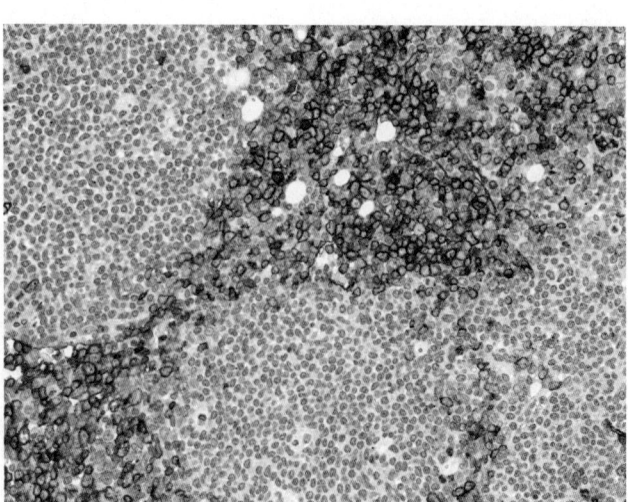

A
B

FIGURE 42.2. Bone marrow biopsy in a case of "tumor-forming PDCs associated with myeloid neoplasms," showing CD68⁺ nodules of PDCs (**A**) that are sharply demarcated from the CD34⁺ acute leukemic cells (**B**).

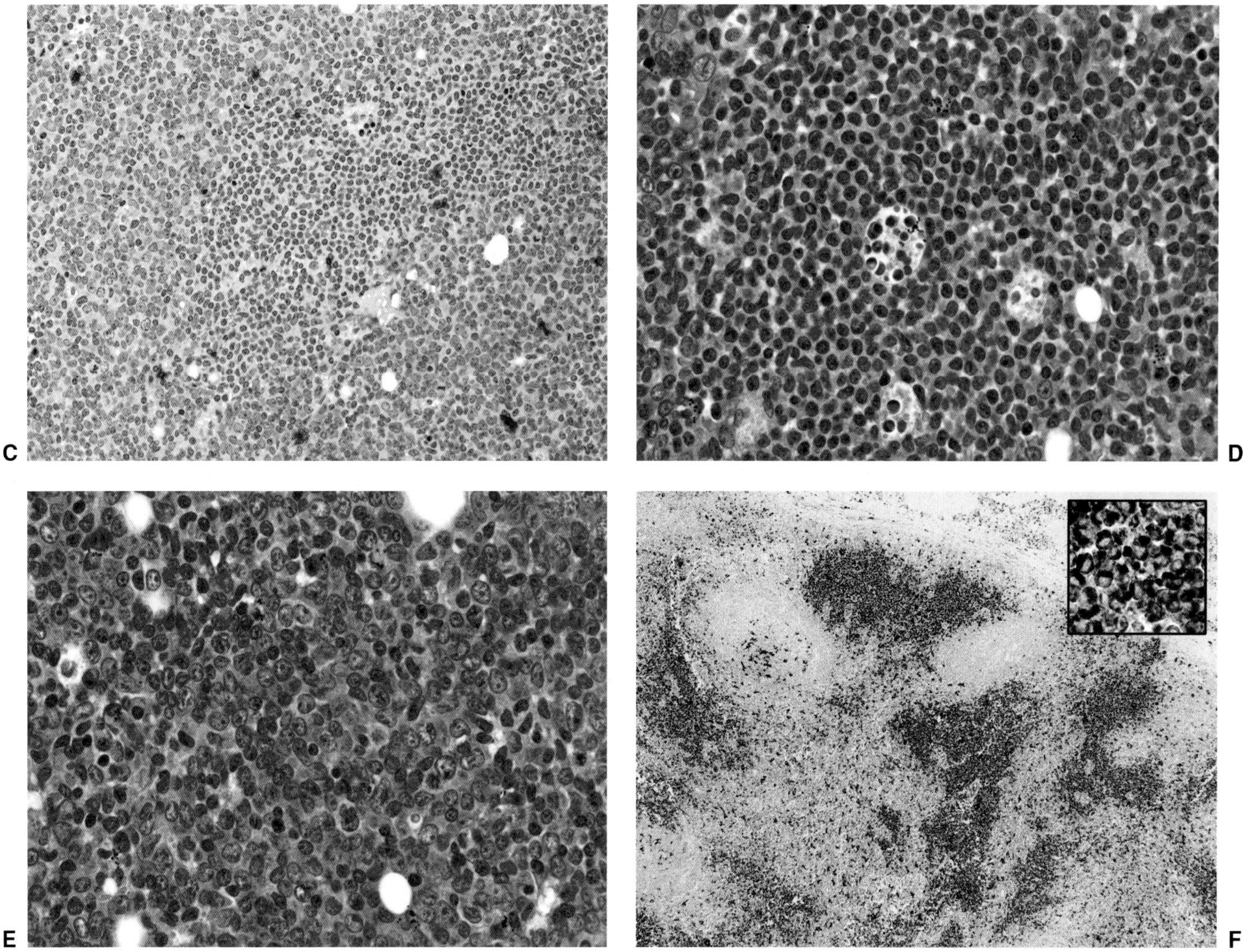

FIGURE 42.2. (*Continued*) Neither tumor cell component express CD56 (**C**). A nodule of PDCs composed of cells with mature morphology (**D**) compared with the myeloid blasts (**E**). Note the apoptotic bodies within the PDC nodules. Another example of the same variant of PDC neoplasm in a lymph node stained for CD68 (**F**): The nodules partially coalesce; the intense cytoplasmic reactivity for CD68 is better illustrated in the inset (**inset**) (**A–C**: immunoalkaline-phosphatase stain for CD68, CD34, and CD56, hematoxylin counterstain; **D,E**: hematoxylin and eosin stain; **F**: immunoperoxidase stain for CD68, hematoxylin counterstain).

They are usually more discrete or, as in Kikuchi lymphadenitis, form irregular sheets with necrosis. Their distinction from tumoral PDC nodules is easily performed by the recognition of morphologic changes that characterize the basic disease as well as by the clinical context.

BLASTIC PLASMACYTOID DENDRITIC CELL NEOPLASM

BPDCN has undergone multiple changes in nomenclature along with the evolving understanding of its histogenesis. In 1999, Petrella et al. (98) reported seven cases of a tumor characterized by high tropism for the skin and bone marrow, rapid fatal progression, blastic morphology, and expression of CD4 and CD56 antigens with lack of lineage-specific markers. They identified other similar cases previously reported in the literature, which had been interpreted either as unusual variants of lymphoma (99–112) or NK cell leukemia/lymphoma (103,104); in the belief that the process could represent a new distinct entity, it was labeled as "agranular CD4+/CD56+ hematodermic neoplasm" (98). In 1998, on the basis of careful evaluation of antigen expression and *in vitro* functions, Bagot et al. (105) suggested that a relationship to the

myelomonocytic lineage was more likely than to the NK lineage, but a common descent with PDC was first hypothesized by Lucio et al. (106) who found that tumor cells, in analogy to normal PDC (43,68), were strongly positive for the alpha chain of IL-3 receptor (CD123) (106). This relationship was afterward supported by additional phenotypic (42,51,67,107–116), molecular (107,117), and functional data (108,118), including the ability of tumor cells to produce INF-I (107,108,115) and to differentiate into DCs (107,108,119). Furthermore, tumor cell lines obtained from leukemic cells were found to recapitulate to a large extent the *in vitro* features of nontumoral PDCs (119–121).

CLINICAL FEATURES

BPDCN is rare and represents <1% of acute leukemias (79) and in two series of lymphomas accounted for 0.27% to 0.7% (122,123). There is no racial or ethnic predominance, and series with similar clinical features have been reported from western and eastern countries (79).

From a review of 427 cases (including 18 cases from the author's files), 75.29% of BPDCN occurs in males (M/F, 3/1). Most patients are adults, with a mean/median age at

FIGURE 42.3. **Distribution of BPDCN according to age and sex.** Note the marked prevalence in males especially following the forth decade (data from 427 cases from the literature).

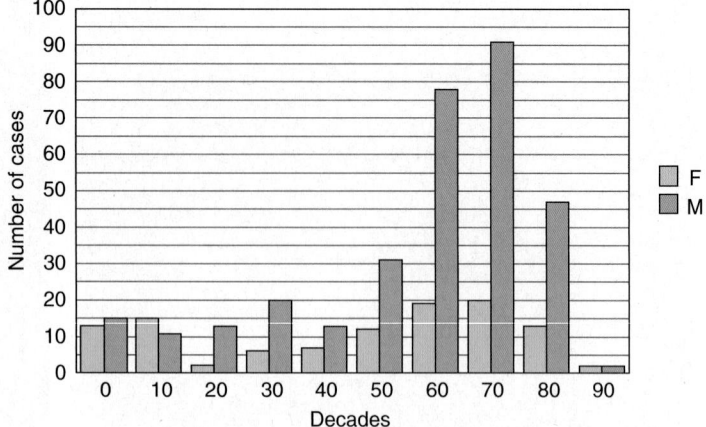

diagnosis of 58.1/66.0 years (range 0 to 96 years) that is lower for females (51.9/60.0 vs. 60.5/67.0). Rare cases have been reported in newborns, while 7.5% and 13.0% of cases occurred in individuals younger than 10 and 20 years, respectively. In a consultation series of 55 patients evaluated at the National Institutes of Health, Bethesda, MD, the overall male to female ratio was 2.7:1, and the median age was 67 years, although 15% of cases were diagnosed before the age of 18 (55). In an additional series from Japan (47 cases, 33/14 males to females) the total mean age was 52.9 (124). Interestingly, females do not show significant age peak occurrence, while in males there is a marked increase from the fifth decade on (Fig. 42.3).

There are currently no clues to the etiology of BPDCN. Sporadic cases positive for Epstein-Barr virus (EBV) have been reported (125), but EBV and other viruses (HIV, HCV, HHV6, HHV8, CMV, and HTLV-1 or HTLV-2) are generally negative (79).

The clinical features and evolution of BPDCN are rather homogeneous from different series (55,79,98,103, 104,113,123,124,126–133) and consist of two main patterns, one (70% to 90% of cases) dominated by cutaneous lesions followed by tumor dissemination and the other showing from the beginning features of an acute leukemia with systemic involvement. In about half of the cases with complete staging, disease results limited to the skin at the time of diagnosis (123,130,133), but only exceptionally it remains confined to it for more than 6 months (79). Skin lesions are typically present also in patients

presenting with the systemic variant (123,124), with few exceptions (134). Interestingly, cases without skin involvement are more common among young individuals: In a cumulative series of 29 patients younger than 18 years, 24% presented extracutaneous disease confined to bone marrow, peripheral blood, lymph nodes, spleen, and/or liver (135). Since normal PDCs are absent from the skin, the striking cutaneous tropism of BPDCN tumor cells has been associated with the expression of antigens that favor skin migration, such as CLA and CD56 (136), as well as with the local production of ligands of chemokines expressed by tumor cells (CXCR3, CXCR4, CCR6, CCR7) (118).

The overall health of patients at presentation is generally good, and the main reason for seeking medical advice is cutaneous lesions. The interval between the first symptoms and diagnosis ranges from 1 to 18 months (mean: 4.2 months) (133).

The clinical presentation of skin lesions is extremely heterogeneous: They can be solitary, gathered in one area, or generalized and appear as flat maculae, plaques, or nodules; their size varies from few millimeters to more than 10 cm and may be erythematous, hyperpigmented, reddish, bluish, purpuric, erosive, or even necrotic (79,130) (Fig. 42.4A and B).

Localized or disseminated lymphadenopathy at presentation due to BPDCN involvement is common (about 40% of cases), as well as splenomegaly (25)% and hepatomegaly (16%) (79). Bone marrow involvement at onset has been reported

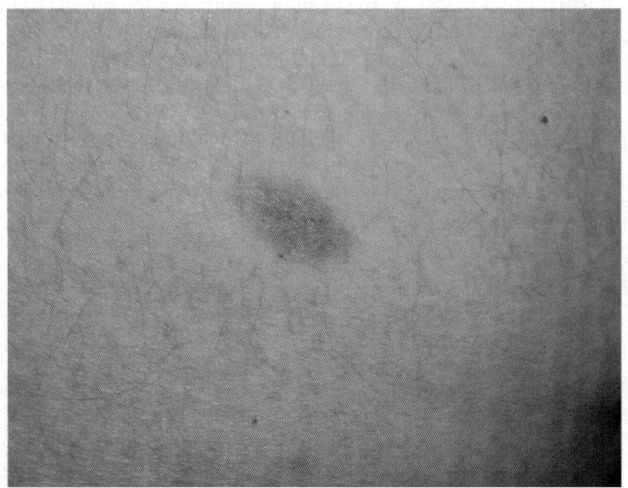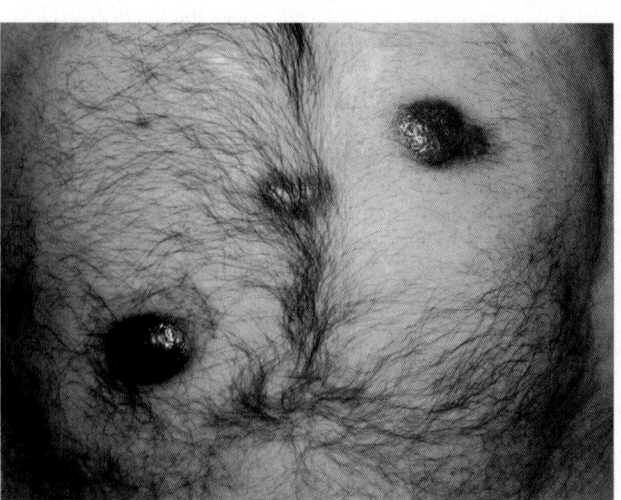

A   B

FIGURE 42.4. Clinical presentation of BPDCN in the skin from the same patient, at 36-month interval **(A,B)**. The lesions can be flat and innocent-looking **(A)**, or may show as ominous red or bluish nodules **(B)**.

frequently (50% to 90%); tumor cells can be very scarce, though they invariably increase with progression. Cytopenias frequently occur at diagnosis and consist of thrombopenia (78%), anemia (65%), or neutropenia (34%) [137]; in a minority of cases they are severe, indicating bone marrow failure [127,137]. Most cases show peripheral blast cells in the peripheral blood at diagnosis, but counts vary in different series and can be very low [124,133,137,138]. The acute leukemic variant is characterized from the beginning by elevated white blood cell count, high number of circulating blasts, and massive bone marrow infiltration. Cases with BPDCN leukemia not associated with cutaneous lesions are uncommon [134]; except for a more severe anemia, they do not differ from the more common cases with skin manifestations in terms of age, male predominance, and morphologic, immunophenotypical, and cytogenetic characteristics [134].

The involvement of the central nervous system is rare at presentation [137,139], but it is not unusual on relapse, possibly representing a sanctuary site for BPDCN blasts [123,140,141].

A proportion of BPDCN cases, likely between 10% and 20% [127,135], is associated with prior, coexistent, or subsequent acute myelomonocytic or myeloid leukemias, with or without an underlying myelodysplastic syndrome [67,111,113,125,127,128,130,137,142–146] (Table 42.2). Marked marrow or blood monocytosis at diagnosis can reveal the associated disease, even if myelodysplasia or blasts can be absent [127]. The morphology of the blasts at the time of MDS diagnosis is not related to that of BPDCN tumor cells [137], and the myeloid leukemia cells are also phenotypically distinct (e.g., they express myeloperoxidase and butyrate esterase, or CD11c and CD33) [67,137]; however, in some cases leukemia conserve CD4 and CD56 antigens, or even they share with the BPDCN TCL1 and CD123. Notably, cases of myelomonocytic leukemia arising in patients with BPDCN were much more likely to express

TCL1 than *de novo* acute myelomonocytic leukemia [67,109]. More interestingly, BPDCN can acquire a myeloid maturation at the relapse [125], or the opposite has been documented in a case of monocytic leukemia [147]. Finally, rare cases of leukemia displaying a double component, one showing a myeloid and the other a PDC phenotype, have been reported [138,148].

Taken together, these findings support the hypothesis that the two diseases may have a common origin and are not coincidental.

Although PDCs are developmentally more closely related to histiocytes and to CDCs and BPDCN cell line can convert in CDC [121], composite cases of BPDCN with histiocytic or DC neoplasms have not been reported.

PATHOLOGIC FEATURES

BPDCN is characterized by a rather monomorphous and dense infiltrate composed of cells with blastic features resembling myeloblasts or lymphoblasts [51,113,123,125,127, 130,143,149]. In the prototypic case BPDCN is composed by medium-sized cells, with single nuclei, that exhibit a variable irregularity of their contour; chromatin is fine and the nucleoli are absent, small, single or multiple, and eosinophilic. The cytoplasm is scant to moderate, and it appears gray-blue and devoid of cytoplasmic azurophilic granules on Giemsa stain. In other cases tumor cells can exhibit larger nuclei and prominent nucleoli, or may be pleomorphic, with blastoid cells admixed with elongated, twisted, or hyperchromatic cells. Exceptionally the morphology straightforwardly suggests a tumoral proliferation of PDCs (Fig. 42.5A–F).

Vascular involvement in the form of angiocentricity and angiotropism with necrosis is exceptionally observed [79,99,130,144]; in contrast, the atypical cells can occur within the lumen of small vessels, and intratumoral hemorrhage can

Gender/Age (Year)	Main Findings	Reference
	Table 42.2 REPORTED CASES OF BPDCN ASSOCIATED WITH MYELODYSPLASIA OR ACUTE MYELOID LEUKEMIA	
M/67	AML developed 18 mo after BPDCN onset (BPDCN in remission with chemotherapy)	(142)
M/56	AML-M4 (FAB) developed 15 m after BPDCN onset	(125)
M/73	AML-M4 developed 22 mo after BPDCN onset; AML-M4 preceded by progressive marrow dysplasia and monocytosis	(125)
F/85	Concomitant MDS; subsequent increase of MPO+ blasts in BM	(125)
M/76	MDS-RA diagnosed before BPDCN onset	(137)
M/67	MDS-RARS diagnosed before BPDCN onset	(137)
nr	MDS changes in BM at the time of BPDCN diagnosis	(137)
nr	MDS changes in BM at the time of BPDCN diagnosis	(137)
nr	MDS changes in BM at the time of BPDCN diagnosis	(137)
M/86	MDS diagnosed 11 mo before BPDCN onset	(144)
M/87	SMML developed 3 months after BPDCN onset	(144)
M/71	MDS diagnosed 7 mo before BPDCN onset	(144)
nr	AML-M7 developed 13 mo after BPDCN onset	(67,127)
F/70	AML-M0 (FAB) 8 developed 8 mo after BPDCN	(143)
M/68	Concomitant MDS	(107)
M/86	Concomitant MDS	(111)
M/71	MDS diagnosed 36 mo before BPDCN onset	(113)
nr	Concurrent MDS	(127)
nr	Concurrent CML	(127)
M/22	AML-M5a (FAB); probably associated with BPDCN since the beginning, but more manifest after BDPCN diagnosis	(145)
nr (five cases)[a]	Prior or concomitant myeloid neoplasia	(55)
M/74	CML diagnosed before BPDCN onset	(130)
M/68	MDS diagnosed before BPDCN onset	(130)
M/66	Concurrent AML-M4 (FAB)	(146)

AML, acute myeloid leukemia; BPDCN, blastic plasmacytoid dendritic cell neoplasm; FAB, French-American-British classification; MDS, myelodysplastic syndrome; MPO, myeloperoxidase; BM, bone marrow; RA, refractory anemia; RARS, refractory anemia with ring sideroblasts; RCMD-RS, refractory cytopenia with multilineage dysplasia and ring sideroblasts; SMML, subacute myelomonocytic leukemia; CML, chronic myeloid leukemia; nr: not reported.
[a]Pediatric cases.

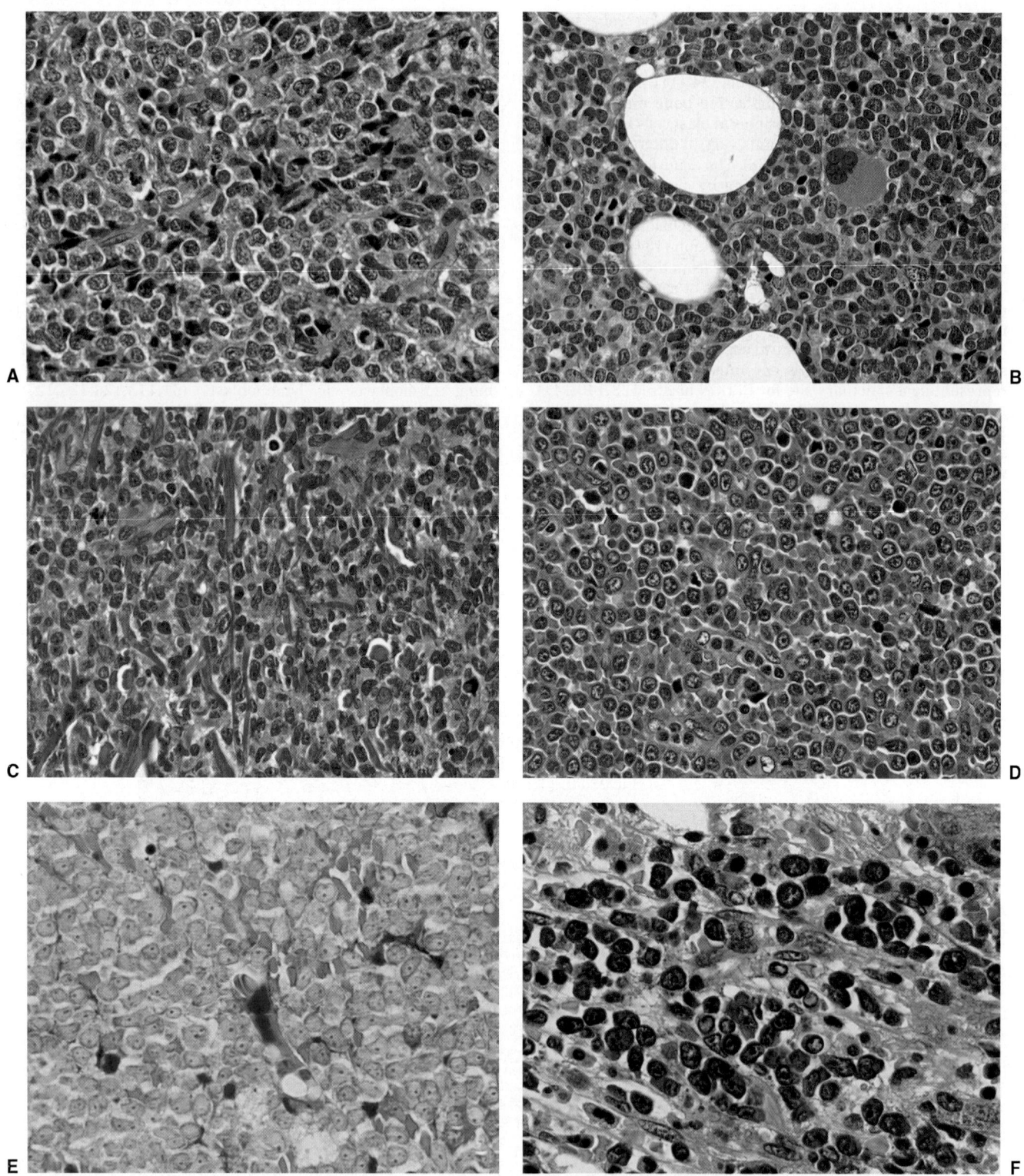

FIGURE 42.5. High magnification of cases of BPDCN, illustrating the cytomorphologic spectrum: Tumor cells show monomorphous appearance, resembling either myeloblasts (A) or lymphoblasts (B); they may have irregularity of the nuclear contour (C), or exceptionally, the morphology is more directly suggesting PDCs (D); in most cases the chromatin is fine and the nucleoli are either absent or small, and the cytoplasm is scant to moderate, and, on Giemsa stain, it appears *gray-blue* and devoid of cytoplasmic azurophilic (E). Rare cases exhibit large nuclei and prominent nucleoli (F). Figures (A) and (C) are from skin biopsies, Figures (B), (E) and (F) from bone marrow biopsies, Figure (D) from a lymph node biopsy (A–D,F: hematoxylin and eosin stain; E: Giemsa stain).

be frequent (130). The blastic proliferation can be admixed with reactive cells represented by small T lymphocytes and scattered macrophages; plasma cells, eosinophils, and neutrophils are notably rare (123,127).

Mitotic activity is variable, as reflected by Ki-67 antigen labeling (30% to 80%) (115,123,125,149).

In the skin the tumor cell infiltrate involves the dermis and may extend to subcutaneous fat, but the epidermis is regularly spared with a clear-cut grenz zone, with rare exceptions (130); cutaneous adnexa are generally erased (Fig. 42.6A). The cellularity is mostly confluent, but density and distribution vary depending on the lesion selected for biopsy, and focal infiltrates

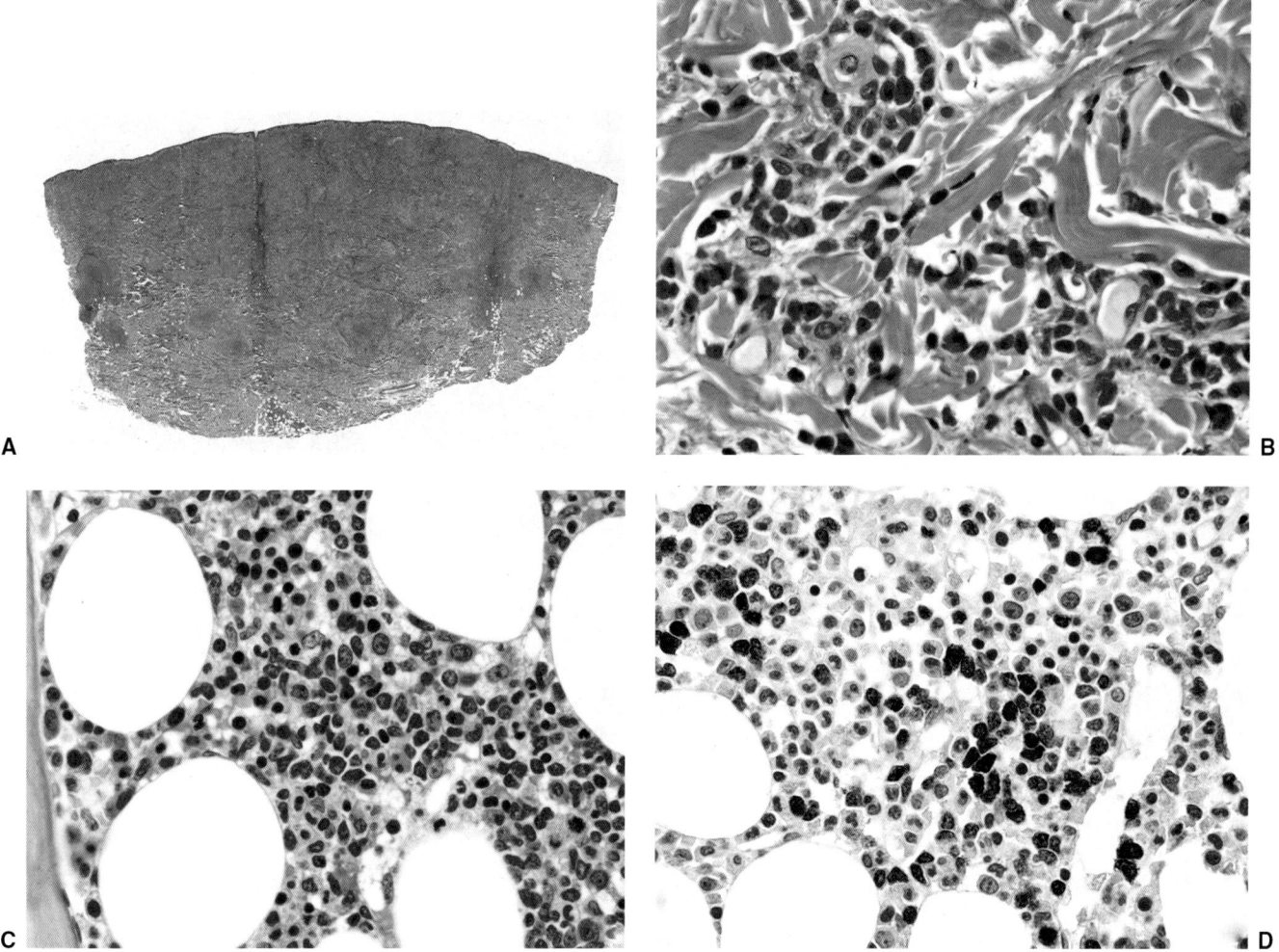

FIGURE 42.6. Low-power view of a skin biopsy in BPDCN, with the characteristic diffuse involvement of the dermis, sparing the epidermis and extending into the subcutaneous fat (**A**). Rarely, tumor cells may be sparse around vessels and may simulate an inflammatory process (**B**). Especially in early stages the bone marrow is negative or minimally involved (**C**), but tumor cells are easily detectable by immunostain (**D**). (**A–C**: hematoxylin and eosin stain; **D**: immunoperoxidase stain for TCL1, hematoxylin counterstain).

with perivascular or interstitial distribution may simulate an inflammatory reaction (123,130,150) (Fig. 42.6B).

Lymph nodes show a leukemic diffuse pattern of infiltration of the interfollicular, paracortical, and medullary areas, often sparing B follicles. In bone marrow biopsies, tumor cells are either rare or detectable only by immunostains (Fig. 42.6C and D), form discrete interstitial aggregates, or massively replace the lacunae. The remaining myeloid tissue may show dysplastic features, particularly in the megakaryocyte lineage (123); attention should be paid to the non-BPDCN component in bone marrow biopsies, since myelodysplasia or even acute myeloid leukemia (AML) may occur in association with BPDCN. An abnormal increase of marrow as well as circulating monocytes may alert on the possible development of an associated myeloid neoplasia (127).

Cytologic examination of blood or bone marrow smears might show undifferentiated, variably sized blast cells, with either predominance of small, medium, or large cells, or a mixture of them (137). The nucleus is generally round or oval, but can be irregular, with notched, folded, or bilobar features; chromatin is clear, with one or several visible nucleoli. The cytoplasm is weakly basophilic and devoid of granules; in most cases it contains microvacuoles distributed with a peculiar necklace-like arrangement at the periphery (151) or show pseudopodia-shaped expansions (137) (Fig. 42.7A and B).

On fine-needle aspirate preparations stained with Papanicolaou or hematoxylin and eosin, tumor cells can reveal blastic features but may also resemble mature lymphomatous cells (e.g., marginal zone B-cell lymphoma) or atypical monocytes (Fig. 42.7C) (55).

IMMUNOPHENOTYPE

The expression of CD4 and CD56 in the absence of lineage-specific markers for myelomonocytic cells, NK cells, T cells, or B cells has defined the majority of cases of BPDCN reported until now (Fig. 42.8A and B). From a revision of 317 published cases with detailed immunophenotypical analysis (42,51,67,76, 109–115,117,122,125,127–131,134,135,137,138,140, 143–145,149,152–167), 289 (91.2%) expressed CD4 and CD56. CD4-negative cases are uncommon (5.4% of cases) (125,130,140,155,161), but lack of CD56 is even more rare (3.5%) (42,113,130,168). The distinguishing expression of CD56 in BPDCN is in contrast with the lack of this antigen in normal PDCs (70), except for a very minute fraction of circulating PDCs (51); it has been speculated that BPDCN tumor cells may derive from this subset (51), but the acquisition of CD56 might also be associated with oncogenic transformation, as observed in other hematopoietic neoplasms.

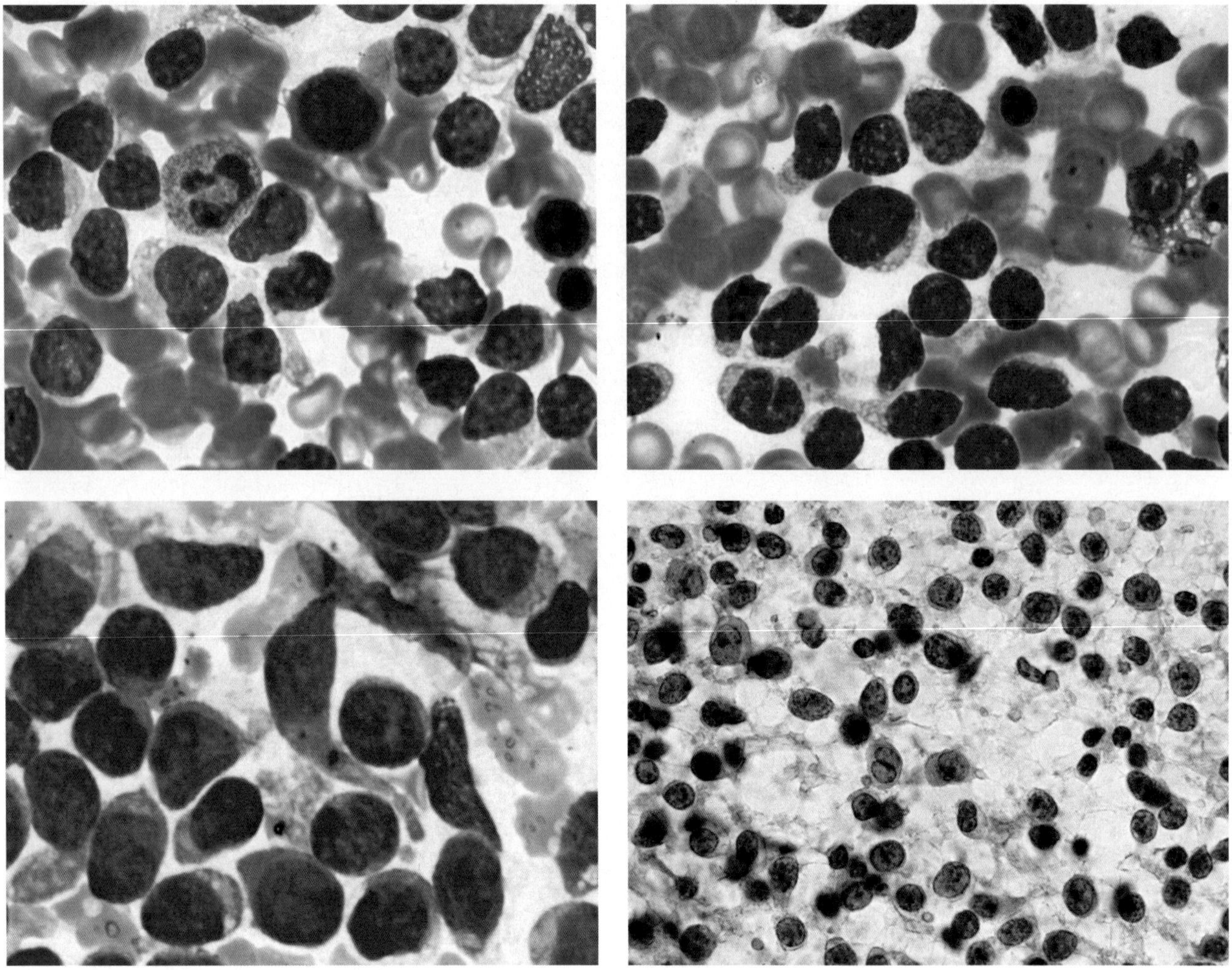

A

B

C

D

FIGURE 42.7. Cytologic aspects of BPDCN in a bone marrow aspirate (**A–C**): Tumor cells show a blastic appearance of the chromatin and some pseudopodia-like extensions of the cytoplasm (**C**), which may contain small vacuoles occasionally distributed at the periphery. Fine-needle aspiration from a lymph node (**D**) showing medium-sized cells with fine chromatin, small nucleoli, and moderate amount of weakly eosinophilic cytoplasm (**A–C:** Wright-Giemsa stain; **D:** Papanicolaou stain; (**B**) and (**C**) are from the same patient).

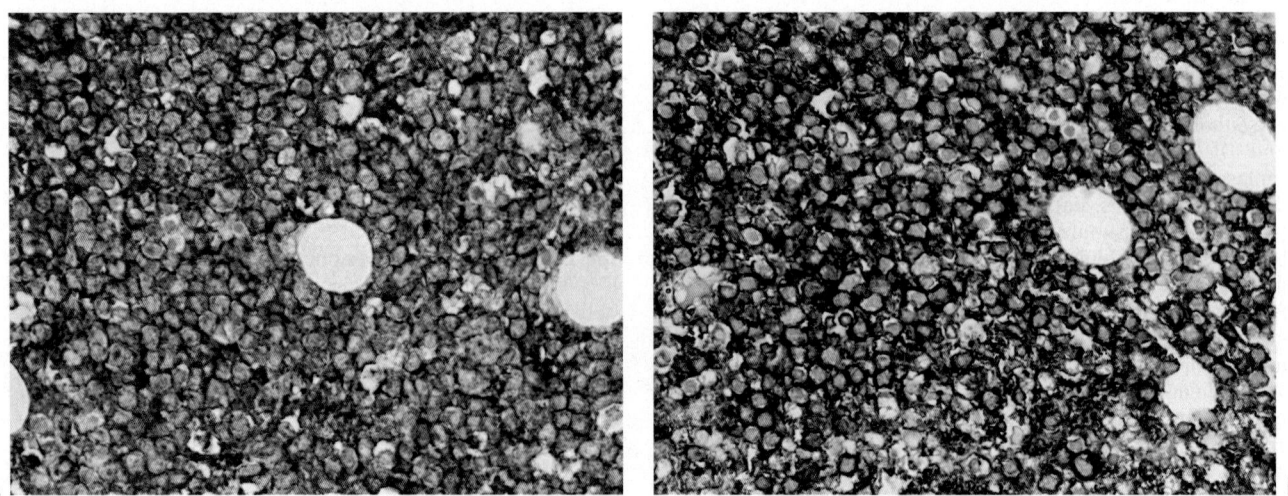

A

B

FIGURE 42.8. The immunohistochemical panel shows typical examples of antigen expression in BPDCN, with strong reactivity for CD4 (**A**), CD56 (**B**),

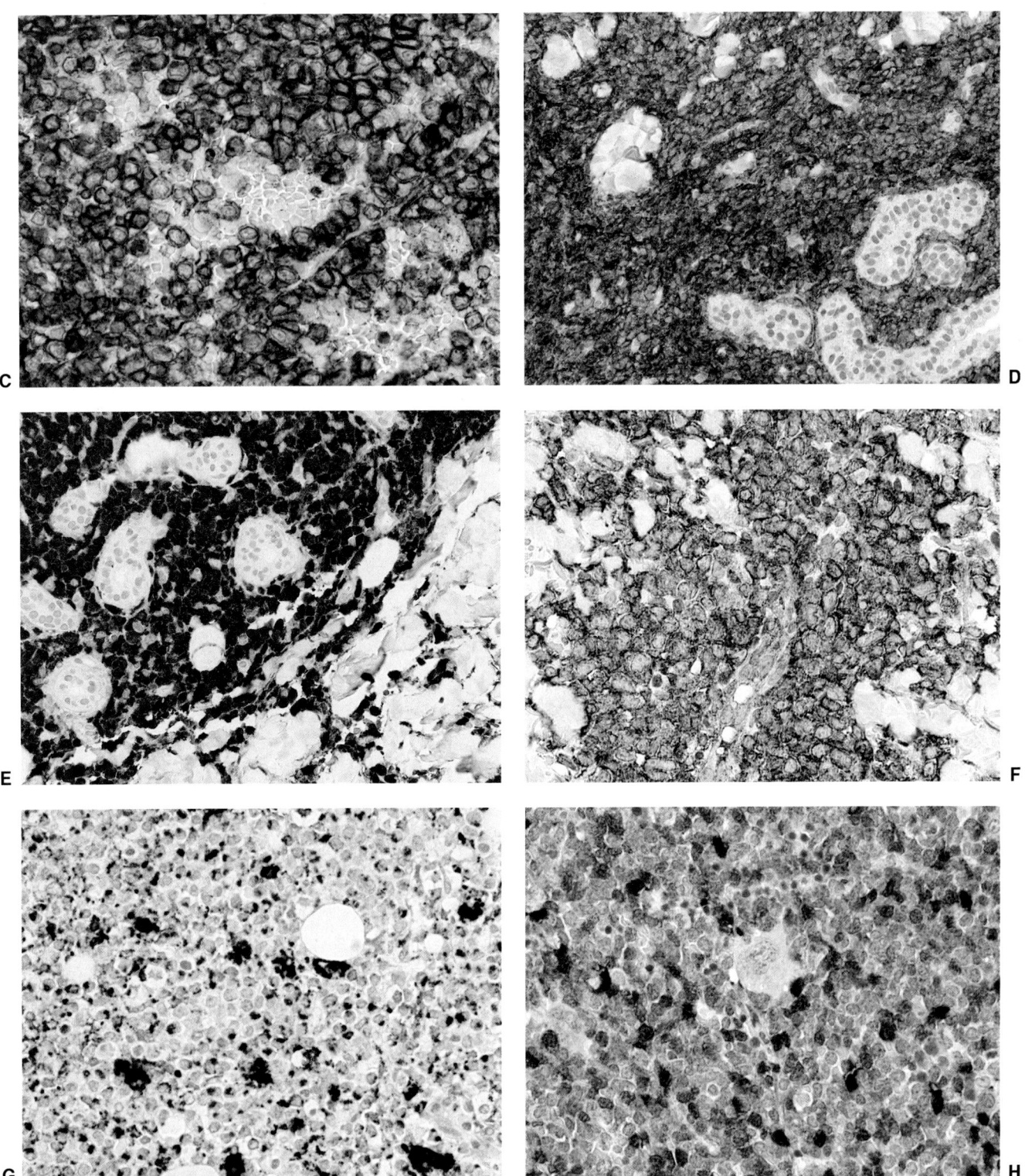

FIGURE 42.8. (*Continued*) CD123 **(C)**, BDCA-2/CD303 **(D)**, TCL1 **(E)**, and CD2AP **(F)**. **(G)** illustrates the dotlike expression of CD68, while **(H)** shows an example of BPDCN, where part of tumor cells are positive for S100 protein. The lack of lysozyme **(I)** is typical of BPDCN, in contrast with acute myeloid leukemia, which typically strongly express this antigen **(J)**. Tumor cells lack the stem cell marker CD34 **(K**; note intravascular tumor cells) and variably express TdT **(L)**. (Immunoperoxidase stain for CD4 **(A)**, CD56 **(B)**, CD123 **(C)**, BDCA-2/CD303 **(D)**, TCL1 **(E)**, CD2AP **(F)**, CD68 **(G)**, S100 **(H)**,

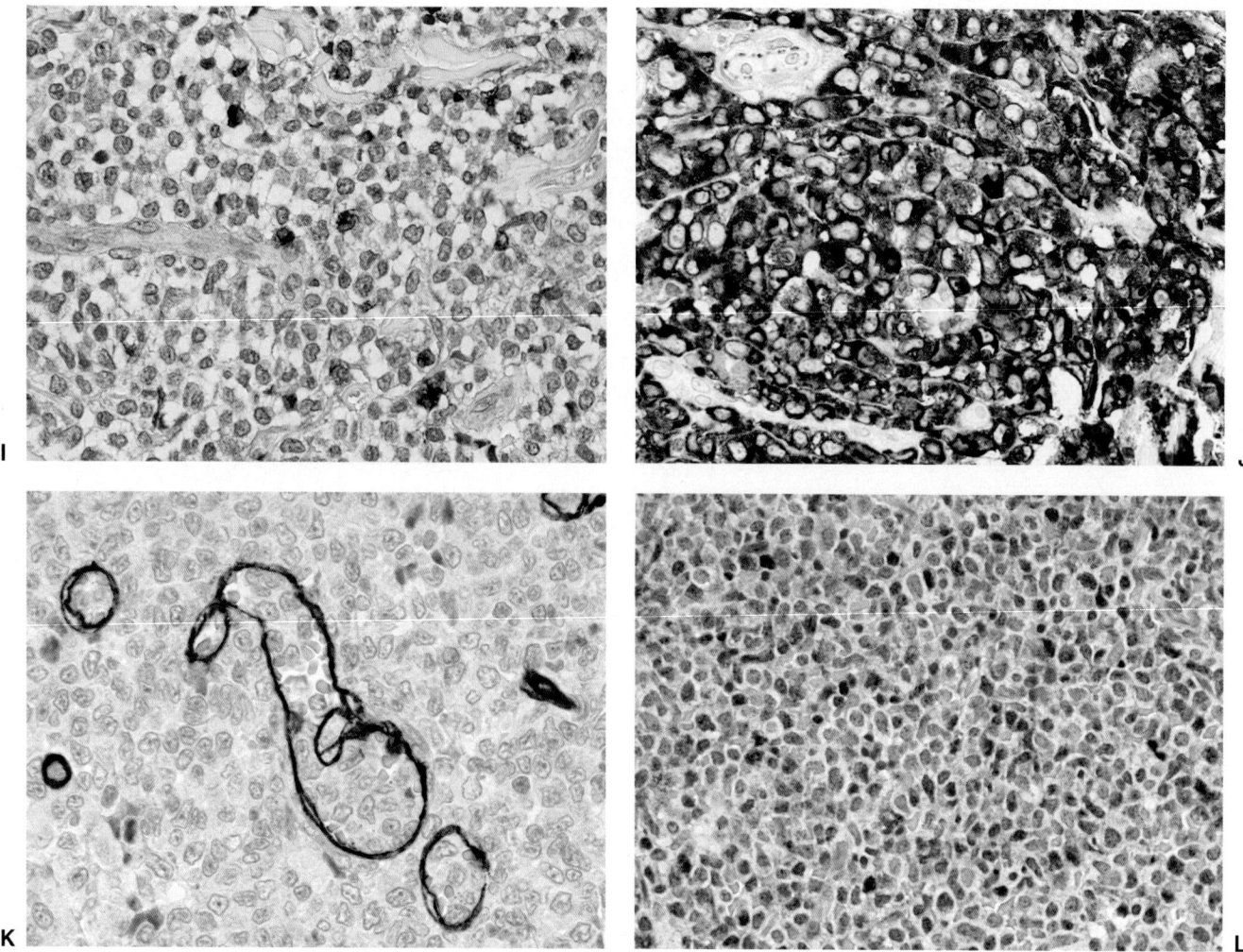

FIGURE 42.8. (*Continued*) lysozyme (**I,J**), CD34 (**K**), and TdT (**L**), hematoxylin counterstain.)

The diagnosis of BPDCN has been greatly improved with the development of more specific PDC-associated markers, such as CD123, TCL1, BDCA-2/CD303, and CD2AP (Fig. 42.8C–F). CD123 is strongly positive in the majority of BPDCN (42,51,55,67,111, 113–115,123,127,130,131,135,137,141,166); only 10 BPDCN cases out of 211 (4.7%) were negative for CD123, and the CD4/CD56/CD123 triple-positive phenotype was found in 183 out of 210 cases (87.1%); these three markers should represent a minimum requirement for BPDCN characterization (127). Similarly to normal PDC, BPDCN also reacts for TCL-1 (109/122 cases; 89.3%); anti-TCL1 stains PDCs very intensely and is very resistant to decalcifying procedures, thus useful for BPDCN detection on bone marrow biopsies, where other markers might be weaker (Fig. 42.6D).

BDCA-2 (CD303) has been reported to be expressed in small series of BPDCN using immunohistochemistry (79,110,111,115); Jaye et al. (114) first analyzed BPDCN on paraffin sections with a rabbit antiserum and found reactivity in 10/19 cases (55%); remarkably, the CD303-positive cases showed a more mature phenotype (CD7+ and TdT−) and were associated with better survival; these results, however, require further exploration. The anti-CD303 monoclonal antibody (clone 124B3.13) recognizing a formalin-resistant epitope was applied in 22 cases from three studies and stained 20 cases (90.1%) (93,135,169). On additional 21 cases evaluated in our laboratory, we found reactivity in 19; the percentage of labeled cells as well their stain intensity varied from case to case, and it was especially low on bone marrow samples: Whether these

findings depend on antigen loss due to tissue processing or to changes intrinsic to cell differentiation remains to be investigated. As a whole, about 75% of cases of BPDCN have been stained positive by anti–BDCA-2/CD303 antibodies on tissue sections; in keeping with data obtained on flow cytometry (133), anti–BDCA-2/CD303 is an important support for BPDCN identification, but its negativity does not exclude the diagnosis.

Testing a large panel of candidate proteins, Marafioti et al. (42) showed significant expression of a series of signaling molecules (e.g., BLNK, BTK, DAP12, IRAK1, Lyn, Syk) and transcription factors (e.g., BCL11A, E47, FOXP1, RF8, PU.1) in BPDCN and found that the adaptor protein CD2AP (CD2-associated protein) is a particularly helpful diagnostic marker (35/37 cases positive; 95%), although a lower number of CD2AP-positive cases were identified in another study (23/35; 65.7%) (130).

The brain and dendritic cell (BAD)–associated lysosome-associated membrane protein (LAMP)–like molecule (BAD-LAMP) has been recently reported as a novel-specific marker for PDCs and BPDCN (116).

In addition to CD56, BPDCN may show expression of molecules that are negative in normal PDCs, such as BCL2, BCL6, MUM1 (130), and CD38 (51,98,137). Furthermore, they may contain areas where tumor cells are positive for S100 protein (55,113,135,144,170,171) (Fig. 42.8H). Conversely, other molecules are down-regulated or display peculiar cell distribution in BPDCN: CD68 and CLA/HECA-452 (CD162) antigens are found in about 50% and 90% of BPDCN cases, respectively; when present, they appear in the form of single (Fig. 42.8G) or multiple tiny dots within the Golgi apparatus (51,98,109,123), a pattern markedly different from the intense and more diffuse positivity observed in normal PDCs (7,66). On the other hand, granzyme B has been found to be expressed at the mRNA and protein levels in some series (107,111,112), but negative in others (51,70,130).

BPDCN express in most cases CD43, HLA-DR, and CD45RA while they are negative for lineage-restricted antigens for myelomonocytic cells (CD11c, CD13, CD14, myeloperoxidase, lysozyme, as well as alpha-naphthyl butyrate esterase, Naphthol AS-D chloroacetate esterase, and peroxidase cytochemical reactions) (Fig. 42.8I), B cells (CD19, CD20, PAX5, CD79a, immunoglobulin), NK cells (CD16, CD57), and T cells (CD2, CD3, CD5, LAT, ZAP70, T-cell receptors AB and GD proteins) (42,51, 109,111,113,125,130,131,137,138,149). Exceptions, however, exist: Among lymphoid- and myeloid-associated antigens, CD7 and CD33 are relatively frequent and some cases have shown expression of CD2, CD5, or CD10 (82,113,123,130,137,165). Although positivity for CD3 should raise suspicion for a T-cell malignancy, rare cases of BPDCN showed cytoplasmic CD3 expression, especially using polyclonal anti-CD3ε antibodies (125,127,128,171–173).

The expression of TdT may indicate a more immature phenotype, and it has been reported in about one-third of cases (42,51,98,104,128,130), with positivity ranging between 10% and 80% of tumor cells (Fig. 42.8N). Rare cases express CD117 (76,138,144,156,158,165), but CD34 is regularly negative (Fig. 42.8M) (98,107,111,113,115,123,137,138,144,156, 158,164).

Of note, EBV-related antigens and RNA were studied in a large number of cases and found to be consistently negative (98,103,113,115,131,140,155,161,174).

The immunophenotypic identification of BPDCN on flow cytometry (82,107,112,131,137,138,165,175) may benefit from gate and intensity evaluation criteria and from availability of some additional markers. BPDCN is characterized by high levels of CD123 and weak expression of CD45 (blast gate); moreover, it expresses CD36, BDCA-4/CD304, and ILT3, while it is negative for BDCA-3 (138,165); in analogy with normal PDCs, anti-CD22 s-HCL-1 monoclonal antibody stains BPDCN (76), and this may represent a potential source for error in flow cytometric monitoring of patients receiving anti-CD22 therapies (77).

The lack of lineage-associated antigens, together with the expression of CD4, CD45RA, CD56, and CD123, has been considered a unique and virtually pathognomonic phenotype for BPDCN (175). More recently, Garnache-Ottou et al. (165) defined a scoring system for the identification of BPDCN (diagnostic score >2) that included four parameters: the expression of CD4 (but not necessarily CD56) with negativity of myeloperoxidase, cCD3, cCD79a, and CD11c (score 1), positivity of CD123 (high intensity) (score 1), BDCA-2/CD303 (score 2), and BDCA-4/CD304 (score 1). BDCA-2/CD303 represented the most specific marker in this study and was detected in 70% of cases. Leukemias with a score as high as the "classical" BPDCN, but presenting an aberrant expression of myeloid/lymphoid antigens or CD10/TdT, were defined "atypical" BPDCN. According to the WHO, tumors, which share some but not all immunophenotypic features of BPDCN, may be better classified as "acute leukemia of ambiguous lineage" (1).

CYTOGENETIC AND MOLECULAR GENETIC FEATURES

T-cell and B-cell receptor gene are usually germline (113,123,127), and the presence of clonal bystander T cells might be responsible of the rare cases of BPDCN with T-cell receptor gamma rearrangement (123,127,176,177).

Using polymerase chain reaction assays and direct sequencing, Jardin et al. (178) recently demonstrated mutations of TET2 (ten eleven translocation 2), located on chromosome 4q24, in 7/13 (53%) BPDCN cases; none of the mutated cases displayed 4q24 locus deletions; in three cases the mutations were biallelic and lead to a complete inactivation of the gene, thus suggesting that TET2 mutations may be involved in BPDCN pathogenesis. Interestingly, TET2 alterations represent an early event in the pathogenesis of various myeloid malignancies, and their frequent occurrence in BPDCN reinforces the hypothesis of a myeloid origin. In the same study, five cases displayed TP53 mutations, leading to change in its functional domain, while no cases displayed JAK2 mutation or tandem duplication of FLT3 (TD-FLT3), indicating that BPDCN and AML or chronic myeloproliferative disorders are genetically distinct. In the same way, NPM1 mutations do not occur in BPDCN, as indicated by nuclear-restricted expression of nucleophosmin (179).

There are no specific karyotypic abnormalities in BPDCN, but complex aberrations are often present, with six major recurrent chromosomal targets, namely, 5q (72%), 12p (64%), 13q (64%), 6q (50%), 15q (43%), and 9 (28%) (180). In addition, comparative genomic hybridization (117) showed recurrent deletion of regions on 4q34, 9p13-p11, 9q12-q34, and 13q12-q31, resulting in loss of tumor suppressor genes such as RB1 and LATS2. Three different studies using high-resolution array comparative genomic hybridization (132,141,181) and quantitative multiplex polymerase chain reaction of short fluorescent fragments (141) on 44 cases of BPDCN demonstrated that losses of multiple genes involved in the G1/S transition are a common feature. Particularly frequent were deletions of chromosomes 9 (harboring the CDKN2A and CDKN2B genes), 13q (containing the RB1 and LATS2 loci), 17p (containing TP53), or 12p (including the tumor suppressor genes CDKN1B and ETV6). Moreover, the cell cycle inhibitors p27^{KIP1} and p21^{INK4a}, respectively, encoded by CDKN1B and CDKN2A, were markedly reduced or absent in tumor cells, suggesting a complete loss of function (181).

The gene expression profiling study by Dijkman et al. (117) identified a "PDC signature" in BPDCN samples, establishing the disease as genetically distinct from cutaneous myelomonocytic leukemias. Compared with normal PDCs, BPDCN samples showed increased expression levels of genes involved in notch signaling (HES6, RUNX2, FLT3), which may serve as oncogenes in the molecular pathogenesis of BPDCN. Interestingly, overexpressed was also a set of genes highly expressed in neuronal cells and involved in neurogenesis, but not described in other hematopoietic cells.

Taken together, these observations indicate BPDCN belongs to the wide spectrum of hematologic neoplasms that display TET2 mutations, although the significance of TET2 mutation remains undetermined in this disease. Nevertheless, the genetic profile in BPDCN is fundamentally distinct from that in myeloid leukemias. Deletion of a gene involved in the G1/S transition pathway could represent a crucial and early oncogenic event in BPDCN, while multiple alterations of the cell cycle checkpoint controlling proteins may provide a basis for the phenomenon of chemoresistance that frequently develops, in spite of an initial favorable response to chemotherapy.

DIFFERENTIAL DIAGNOSIS

Features that distinguish BPDCN from the neoplastic variant of mature PDCs have been already outlined in the previous paragraphs and are summarized in Table 42.3.

Since a skin biopsy represents the most common diagnostic procedure in BPDCN, the differential primarily includes cutaneous involvement by AMLs (leukemia cutis [LC]) and lymphoblastic leukemia/lymphomas. The morphologic overlap between BPDCN and LC especially with monocytic/myelomonocytic

	"Tumor-Forming" Plasmacytoid Dendritic Cells Associated with Myeloid Neoplasms	Blastic Plasmacytoid Dendritic Cell Neoplasm
Table 42.3 COMPARISON BETWEEN THE TWO NEOPLASMS ORIGINATED FROM PDCs		
Basic disease	A myeloid neoplasia (mostly chronic myelomonocytic leukemia) is the dominant preexisting disease.	PDC proliferation is the dominant disease. In 10%–20% of cases, a myeloid neoplasm (mainly myelodysplasia and/or myelomonocytic leukemia) occurs that may precede, coexist, or develop after BPDCN onset.
Main clinical presentation	Lymphadenopathy	Cutaneous lesions
Prevalent sites of involvement by PDC proliferation	Lymph nodes and bone marrow	Skin, bone marrow, lymph nodes, spleen
	No leukemic PDCs (except one case)	PDC leukemia typical (mostly during progression, 10% from the onset)
Histopathology	Multiple PDC nodules morphologically undistinguishable from normal PDCs, frequently containing apoptotic bodies	Diffuse proliferation of immature cells undistinguishable from myeloblasts or lymphoblasts
Immunophenotype	CD123+	CD123+
	TCL1+	TCL1+
	CD4+	CD4+
	CD56±a	CD56+b
	CD68+c (intense)	CD68− or CD68+ (dot)
	CD2AP+	CD2AP+
	Granzyme B+ (intense)	Granzyme B−
	TdT−	TdT±
	Ki-67 <10%	Ki-67 >30%

aUsually negative but may show focal positivity.
bNegative cases extremely rare.
cUsing either KP1 or PGM1 monoclonal antibodies.

differentiation can be striking, and immunophenotyping using multiple markers is mandatory for an accurate diagnosis (42,93,94,97,130,182,183) (Table 42.4). In fact, despite LC rarely shows coexpression of CD4, CD56, and CD123 (145), positivity for both CD4 and CD56 is frequent (93,109,117,128,129,184); CD123 has been detected especially in the myelomonocytic variant of LC (51,93,117,128,185), and TCL1 has been reported positive in 17% to 67% of cases (109,128). CLA/HECA-452 has no role in this differential, since it is regularly expressed in LC (78% of cases in (109)). The diagnostic strategy may include CD34, although data on its expression in LC are significantly variable from series to series (93,97); in contrast, the inclusion of the myelomonocytic markers CD14, CD163, and, above all, myeloperoxidase and lysozyme is essential, since their expression virtually excludes BPDCN (Fig. 42.8I), while it is exceedingly frequent in LC (Fig. 42.8L) (93,97,129,184). Interestingly, the S100 expression that has been observed in cases of BPDCN (55,113,135,144,170,171) was negative in 28 cases of AML evaluated with this marker (135).

The use of CD2P (42) and, particularly, BDCA-2/CD303 may help reliably diagnose BPDCN in flow cytometric analysis (79/79 myeloid neoplasms were negative in the study of Garnache-Ottou et al. (165)) and in biopsies, where none of 228 myeloid leukemia cases from all categories showed reactivity for BDCA-2/CD303 (93,169).

The distinction of B- and T-cell lymphoblastic leukemia/lymphomas from BPDCN is usually more straightforward, based on their very infrequent expression of CD56, CD123, CD2AP, and BDCA-2/CD303 (42,93,165,169,172) and the lack of B- and T-lineage marker expression on BPDCN; TCL1, however, is typically found in these precursor cell lymphoid neoplasms.

Few other neoplasms represent potential mimickers of BPDCN. Histiocytic sarcoma and Langerhans cell histiocytosis may express CD4, CD56, CD123, and CLA/HECA-452 (186–189); however, clinical presentation and the morphologic and other immunohistochemical features (e.g., lysozyme, Cd11c, CD163, CD1a, langerin/CD207) easily consent their distinction from BPDCN.

The immature blastlike morphology of BPDCN virtually excludes from the list of potential mimickers the nonepidermotropic cutaneous T-cell or NK/T-cell lymphomas. This group of neoplasms include lymphomas, which may be CD4+ and CD56− or CD56+ (e.g., peripheral T-cell lymphoma n.o.s.), CD4+CD56− (primary cutaneous small/medium CD4 T-cell lymphoma), CD4−CD56+ (gamma-delta T-cell lymphoma; NK/T-cell lymphoma nasal type), or CD4−CD56− (subcutaneous panniculitis-like T-cell lymphoma) (128,154,186,190–193). The lack of PDC-associated markers (42,67,109) as well as a combination of additional features typical of each category of lymphoma unquestionably excludes BPDCN. Interestingly, in analogy to BPDCN, the majority of T- and NK/T-cell lymphomas expressing CD56 and involving the skin behave very aggressively (128,129,186,191).

CLINICAL COURSE AND TREATMENT

Despite the deceptively indolent clinical presentation and the initial resolution of symptoms in most cases with a variety of intensive chemotherapy regimens or steroids, the course is almost invariably aggressive, with early relapses and rapid extracutaneous dissemination, with or without overt leukemia. The median survival varies from 10 to 16.7 months (79,123,127,129,133,134,137).

Meta-analysis of large series (124,126,129,134) has shown that survival may be related to age, tumor stage, clinical presentation, or tumor cell phenotype and genotype.

A longer survival has been shown in younger patients (<30, <40, and <60 years, respectively, in (124), (129), and (126)), but this might depend on the option of high aggressive therapy compared to elderly individuals (126). However, the prognostic advantage of age has been recently confirmed by Jegalian et al. (135) in a series of pediatric patients, where an unusually frequent number of cases showed complete remission (CR) lasting several years (5, 7, 11, and 13 years); interestingly, in this study outcomes were more favorable in patients that lacked cutaneous disease at presentation, but yet again bias depending

Table 42.4	DIFFERENTIAL FEATURES OF BPDCN AND ACUTE MYELOID LEUKEMIA (MOSTLY REPRESENTED BY BLASTIC, MYELOMONOCYTIC, OR MONOBLASTIC, ACCORDING TO THE WHO)	
	Blastic Plasmacytoid Dendritic Cell Neoplasm (BPDCN)	**Acute myeloid leukemia (AML)**[a]
Prevalent site of involvement	Skin	Bone marrow and peripheral blood
Frequency of extramedullary involvement	100% (100% skin, associated at lower frequency with lymph nodes, liver, spleen, central nervous system)	3% skin (LC) Up to 50% in AML myelomonocytic and monocytic) 2.5%–9.1% extracutaneous sites (myeloid sarcoma) (include lymph nodes, testis, intestine, bones, central nervous system)
Frequency of isolated extramedullary involvement	40%–50%	<1%
Histopathology	Diffuse proliferation of monomorphous immature cells. No granulated cells or eosinophils	Diffuse proliferation of monomorphous immature cells. In cases with myeloid differentiation, possible pleomorphism with immature Granulated myeloid cells and eosinophils
Immunohistochemical and enzyme-histochemical profile (&)		
CD4	+	(−) (My); + (Mo)[b]
CD11c	−	+
CD13	−	+/−
CD14	−	− (My); +/− (Mo)
CD33	+/−	+
CD34	−	+/− (My); − (Mo)
CD43	+	+
CD56	+	(−) (My); + (Mo)
CD68/KP1	− or + (dot)	+ (dot or diffuse)
CD68/PGM1	− or + (dot)	(−) (My); + (Mo) (dot or diffuse)
CD117	−	+(My); +/− (Mo)
CD123	+	− (My); +/− (Mo)
CD163	−	− (My); + (Mo)
CD303	+	−
BCL11A	+	+/−
CD2AP	+	−
TCL1	+	+/−
Tdt	+/−	+/− (My); − (Mo)
Lysozyme	−	+
Myeloperoxidase	−	+ (My); (−) (Mo)
Alpha-naphthyl butyrate esterase	−	+ (Mo)
ASD chloroacetate esterase	−	+ (My)

[a]Most cases with previous or concomitant acute leukemia.
[b]My: myeloid; Mo: monocytic. If not indicated, similar expression in myeloid and monocytic cells.
(&): + indicates prevalent or frequent (>50%) positivity, − indicates negativity, +/− indicates variable expression, (−) indicates mostly negative, but positive cases reported.

on differences in treatment regimens could not be excluded. In contrast, in adults the limitation of BPDCN to the skin at presentation was associated with a moderate prognostic advantage in some studies (124,129,134), but negligible in others (126,133). Nonetheless, the longest survival (more than 15 years) is reported in a patient who presented with isolated skin lesions (103).

Some observations suggest that BPDCN heterogeneity based on immunophenotype may correspond to derivation from PDC precursors at varying stages of maturation and with different degrees of clinical aggressiveness. For example, TdT expression in BPDCN that likely reflects derivation from earlier PDC precursors correlated with longer survival in three studies (114,124,129); in addition, Jaye et al. (114) described an inverse correlation between TdT and BDCA-2/CD303 expression, and the TdT+BDCA-2/CD303− cases were associated with better survival compared with the TdT−BDCA-2/CD303+ cases.

More recently, Hashikawa et al. (131) showed that high expression of the chemokine CXCL12 in BPDCN tumor cells influences systemic dissemination and poor prognosis, while Lucioni et al. (132) identified biallelic loss of locus 9p21.3, a poor outcome genetic marker. These observations open possible avenues to target therapies influencing the CXCR4-CXCL12 circuitry in BPDCN and offer a simple methods, such as FISH, to help identifying the most aggressive cases.

At present, there is no consensus for optimal treatment of BPDCN. Given the dismal evolution of the disease even in cases with a seeming indolent onset; the early development of chemoresistance using different protocols, with few exceptions (140,163); and the rapid relapse even after locally effective radiation therapy (133), alternative strategies have been considered necessary, to be adopted even in cases showing a limited extent of the disease on presentation. Sustained clinical remission or cure has been reported in patients who received acute leukemia chemotherapy regimens and allogeneic stem cell transplantation (SCT) in first CR (137). Reimer et al. (126) reviewed the literature on treatment of 91 patients with BPDCN and found that significant long survival was obtained only in three out of four patients who received allografts in first CR with myeloablative therapy. Similar result was observed only in one out of the four patients who received auto-SCT.

It should be noticed that age emerged to significantly influence the survival, since the median age of these four patients was only 26 (6–29) years. Superior outcome was also found by Bekkenk et al. (129) in 8 out of 61 patients who underwent auto-SCT or allo-SCT compared to nontransplanted patients. These results have been further confirmed by the analysis of the French Study Group on Cutaneous Lymphoma cases (133) that showed a significantly better overall survival (40 months) in 10 patients who received bone marrow transplantation (9 allogeneic, 1 autologous), compared with that of 37 nontransplanted patients (12 months). The median age of the allografted patients was 38 years, compared with 75 years of the other group. However, Dietrich et al. (166) showed that age is not a limiting factor for treatment of BPDCN with bone marrow transplant, since elderly patients (median age: 67 years) were successfully treated with reduced-intensity conditioning allo-SCT. In addition to bone marrow transplantation, intrathecal chemoprophylaxis has been recommended for this disease, since central nervous system relapses after CR are common (33%) (137).

Surprisingly, Jegalian et al. (135), studying the largest series of pediatric BPDCN cases reported to date, found that among patients who underwent SCT the overall survival was 67% (4/6 cases; 2 of these survivors were transplanted in second CR), while the overall survival of patients who were treated mostly with high-risk acute lymphoblastic leukemia (ALL) therapy without SCT was 74% (14/19 cases). Thus, although allogeneic SCT is now advocated for BPDCN treatment in adults, its role in pediatric cases is unclear, and it has been recommended that treatment of children with BPDCN would include ALL-type therapy with central nervous system prophylaxis, reserving SCT for second CR, or to cases in which initial treatment does not induce a rapid or CR (79,135). Noteworthy, despite PDCs are closer to the myeloid rather than to the lymphoid lineage, AML-type therapy results in lower response than ALL-type therapy (123,137).

BPDCN is a rare disease and only recently recognized as a distinct clinicopathologic entity; thus, no standardized therapeutic approach has been established until now, and multicenter prospective trials are required to determine most beneficial treatment.

SUMMARY AND CONCLUSIONS

PDCs represent hematopoietic cell types whose lineage and functions have been only recently established. They originate in the bone marrow and share with CDCs, a unique development pathway from a common macrophage/DC precursor. PDCs represent the most efficient producers of type I IFN that have the additional capacity to transform into DCs and to modulate T-cell responses. By virtue of this dichotomous function, PDCs are established as a major effector cell type in immunity, with potential roles in different pathologic processes.

PDCs display a unique phenotype among hematopoietic cells that includes the expression of the PDC-specific antigen BDCA-2/CD303, in association with CD123, TCL1, CD2AP, and the less restricted antigens CD4, CD68, CLA/HECA-452/CD162, and granzyme B. Lineage markers of myelomonocytic cells and B, T, and NK cells are negative.

PDC-derived tumoral proliferations are rare and in analogy with other hematopoietic neoplasms show evidence of opposite stages of maturation, which correspond to two distinctive clinicopathologic entities. The tumor derived from mature PDCs is regularly associated with another myeloid neoplasm that dominates the clinical manifestations and evolution ("*tumor-forming PDCs associated with myeloid neoplasms*"). This condition is characterized by PDC nodules especially identified in lymph nodes or bone marrow biopsies. Despite morphology and phenotype almost invariably reflect that of normal PDCs, the clonal nature of this PDC proliferation and its relatedness to the associated myeloid neoplasia has been definitely established.

BPDCN derives from immature precursors of PDCs; it has undergone multiple changes in nomenclature along with the evolving understanding of its histogenesis that for a long time has been hindered by the constant and misleading coexpression of CD4 and CD56. BPDCN is highly aggressive and has a distinctive cutaneous tropism followed by rapid systemic extension. There are no specific karyotypic abnormalities in BPDCN, but complex aberrations are often present, with deletion of genes (*CDKN2A, CDKN2B, RB1, LATS2* loci, *TP53, CDKN1B*) predominantly involved in the G1/S transition pathway; this could provide a possible explanation for chemoresistance that typically develops in this tumor. In fact, despite the deceptively indolent clinical presentation and the frequent resolution of symptoms with a variety of intensive chemotherapy regimens, the course is almost invariably aggressive, with early relapses, rapid extracutaneous dissemination, and short survival (median, 10 to 16.7 months). Young age, high expression of TdT, or lesions limited to the skin have been associated with better survival.

The diagnosis of BPDCN may be suspected from a set of converging features from the clinical presentation and histologic findings, but the final diagnosis relies on compatible immunophenotype. The triple-positive CD4+CD56+CD123+ phenotype associated with negativity for lineage-specific markers should represent a minimum requirement for BPDCN definition. In addition, the highly specific marker BDCA-2/CD303, as well as other PDC-associated antigens (e.g., TCL1 and CD2AP), might be of great support to definitely establish the diagnosis and to exclude potential mimickers of BPDCN (AML, precursor lymphoblastic TCLs, and T- and NK/T-cell lymphomas).

At present, there is no consensus for optimal treatment of BPDCN, but evidences have been provided that sustained clinical remission or cure can be obtained with acute leukemia chemotherapy regimens and allogeneic SCT in first CR. However, in pediatric patients acute lymphoblastic leukemia–type therapy and central nervous system prophylaxis gave similar good clinical results. It is unclear whether this heterogeneity depends only on the age of patients or instead corresponds to different biologic variants of the tumor. Accurate pathologic diagnosis is essential for prognosis and treatment of BPDCN; biologic studies together with multicenter prospective trials are required to unveil the molecular mechanisms underlying this rare neoplasm and hopefully to determine the optimal therapy.

References

1. Facchetti F, Jones DM, Petrella T. Blastic plasmacytoid dendritic cells neoplasm. In: Swerdlow SH, Campo E, Harris NL, et al., eds. *WHO classification of tumours of haematopoietic and lymphoid tissues*, 4th ed. Lyon: International Agency for Research on Cancer, 2008:145–147.
2. Lennert K, Remmele W. Karyometrische Untersuchungen an Lymphknotenzellen des Menschen: I. Mitt. Germinoblasten, Lymphoblasten und Lymphozyten. *Acta Haematol (Basel)* 1958;19:99–113.
3. Müller-Hermelink HK, Kaiserling E, Lennert K. Pseudofollikuläre Nester von Plasmazellen (eines besonderen Typs?) in der paracorticalen Pulpa menschlicher Lymphknoten. *Virchows Arch (Cell Pathol)* 1973;14:47–56.
4. Lennert K, Kaiserling E, Muller-Hermelink HK. T-associated plasma-cells. *Lancet* 1975;1:1031–1032.
5. Müller-Hermelink HK, Steinmann G, Stein H, et al. Malignant lymphoma of plasmacytoid T cells. Morphologic and immunologic studies characterizing a special type of T-cell. *Am J Surg Pathol* 1983;7:849–862.
6. Harris NL, Demirjian Z. Plasmacytoid T-zone cell proliferation in a patient with chronic myelomonocytic leukemia: histologic and immunohistologic characterization. *Am J Surg Pathol* 1991;15:87–95.
7. Facchetti F, de Wolf-Peeters C, Mason DY, et al. Plasmacytoid T cells. Immunohistochemical evidence for their monocyte/macrophage origin. *Am J Pathol* 1988;133:15–21.
8. Siegal FP, Kadowaki N, Shodell M, et al. The nature of the principal type 1 interferon-producing cells in human blood. *Science* 1999;284:1835–1837.
9. Cella M, Jarrossay D, Facchetti F, et al. Plasmacytoid monocytes migrate to inflamed lymph nodes and produce large amounts of type I interferon. *Nat Med* 1999;5:919–923.
10. Liu YJ. IPC: professional type 1 interferon-producing cells and plasmacytoid dendritic cell precursors. *Annu Rev Immunol* 2005;23:275–306.
11. Ronnblom L, Ramstedt U, Alm GV. Properties of human natural interferon-producing cells stimulated by tumor cell lines. *Eur J Immunol* 1983;13:471–476.
12. Chehimi J, Starr SE, Kawashima H, et al. Dendritic cells and IFN-alpha-producing cells are two functionally distinct non-B, non-monocytic HLA-DR+ cell subsets in human peripheral blood. *Immunology* 1989;68:486–490.
13. Grouard G, Rissoan MC, Filgueira L, et al. The enigmatic plasmacytoid T cells develop into dendritic cells with interleukin (IL)-3 and CD40-ligand. *J Exp Med* 1997;185:1101–1111.
14. Cella M, Facchetti F, Lanzavecchia A, et al. Plasmacytoid dendritic cells activated by influenza virus and CD40L drive a potent Th1 polarization. *Nat Immunol* 2000;1:305–310.

15. Soumelis V, Liu YJ. From plasmacytoid to dendritic cell: morphological and functional switches during plasmacytoid pre-dendritic cell differentiation. *Eur J Immunol* 2006;36:2286–2292.
16. Bjorck P, Leong HX, Engleman EG. Plasmacytoid dendritic cell dichotomy: identification of IFN-alpha producing cells as a phenotypically and functionally distinct subset. *J Immunol* 2011;186:1477–1485.
17. Villadangos JA, Young L. Antigen-presentation properties of plasmacytoid dendritic cells. *Immunity* 2008;29:352–361.
18. Reizis B, Colonna M, Trinchieri G, et al. Plasmacytoid dendritic cells: one-trick ponies or workhorses of the immune system? *Nat Rev Immunol* 2011;11:558–565.
19. Takagi H, Fukaya T, Eizumi K, et al. Plasmacytoid dendritic cells are crucial for the initiation of inflammation and T cell immunity in vivo. *Immunity* 2011;35:958–971.
20. Loschko J, Schlitzer A, Dudziak D, et al. Antigen delivery to plasmacytoid dendritic cells via BST2 induces protective T cell-mediated immunity. *J Immunol* 2011;186:6718–6725.
21. Reizis B, Bunin A, Ghosh HS, et al. Plasmacytoid dendritic cells: recent progress and open questions. *Annu Rev Immunol* 2011;29:163–183.
22. Drobits B, Holcmann M, Amberg N, et al. Imiquimod clears tumors in mice independent of adaptive immunity by converting pDCs into tumor-killing effector cells. *J Clin Invest* 2012;122(2):575–585.
23. Colonna M, Trinchieri G, Liu YJ. Plasmacytoid dendritic cells in immunity. *Nat Immunol* 2004;5:1219–1226.
24. Gilliet M, Cao W, Liu YJ. Plasmacytoid dendritic cells: sensing nucleic acids in viral infection and autoimmune diseases. *Nat Rev Immunol* 2008;8:594–606.
25. Charles J, Chaperot L, Salameire D, et al. Plasmacytoid dendritic cells and dermatological disorders: focus on their role in autoimmunity and cancer. *Eur J Dermatol* 2010;20:16–23.
26. Swiecki M, Colonna M. Unraveling the functions of plasmacytoid dendritic cells during viral infections, autoimmunity, and tolerance. *Immunol Rev* 2010;234:142–162.
27. Tel J, Lambeck AJ, Cruz LJ, et al. Human plasmacytoid dendritic cells phagocytose, process, and present exogenous particulate antigen. *J Immunol* 2010;184:4276–4283.
28. Wang Y, Swiecki M, McCartney SA, et al. dsRNA sensors and plasmacytoid dendritic cells in host defense and autoimmunity. *Immunol Rev* 2011;243:74–90.
29. Vermi W, Soncini M, Melocchi L, et al. Plasmacytoid dendritic cells and cancer. *J Leukoc Biol* 2011;90:681–690.
30. Liu K, Victora GD, Schwickert TA, et al. In vivo analysis of dendritic cell development and homeostasis. *Science* 2009;324:392–397.
31. Geissmann F, Manz MG, Jung S, et al. Development of monocytes, macrophages, and dendritic cells. *Science* 2010;327:656–661.
32. Naik SH, Sathe P, Park HY, et al. Development of plasmacytoid and conventional dendritic cell subtypes from single precursor cells derived in vitro and in vivo. *Nat Immunol* 2007;8:1217–1226.
33. Maraskovsky E, Daro E, Roux E, et al. In vivo generation of human dendritic cell subsets by Flt3 ligand. *Blood* 2000;96:878–884.
34. Karsunky H, Merad M, Cozzio A, et al. Flt3 ligand regulates dendritic cell development from Flt3+ lymphoid and myeloid-committed progenitors to Flt3+ dendritic cells in vivo. *J Exp Med* 2003;198:305–313.
35. Cisse B, Caton ML, Lehner M, et al. Transcription factor E2-2 is an essential and specific regulator of plasmacytoid dendritic cell development. *Cell* 2008;135: 37–48.
36. Ghosh HS, Cisse B, Bunin A, et al. Continuous expression of the transcription factor e2-2 maintains the cell fate of mature plasmacytoid dendritic cells. *Immunity* 2010;33:905–916.
37. Robbins SH, Walzer T, Dembele D, et al. Novel insights into the relationships between dendritic cell subsets in human and mouse revealed by genome-wide expression profiling. *Genome Biol* 2008;9:R17.
38. Pulford K, Banham AH, Lyne L, et al. The BCL11AXL transcription factor: its distribution in normal and malignant tissues and use as a marker for plasmacytoid dendritic cells. *Leukemia* 2006;20:1439–1441.
39. Res PC, Couwenberg F, Vyth-Dreese FA, et al. Expression of pTalpha mRNA in a committed dendritic cell precursor in the human thymus. *Blood* 1999;94: 2647–2657.
40. Bendriss-Vermare N, Barthelemy C, Durand I, et al. Human thymus contains IFN-alpha-producing CD11c(–), myeloid CD11c(+), and mature interdigitating dendritic cells. *J Clin Invest* 2001;107:835–844.
41. Rissoan MC, Duhen T, Bridon JM, et al. Subtractive hybridization reveals the expression of immunoglobulin-like transcript 7, Eph-B1, granzyme B, and 3 novel transcripts in human plasmacytoid dendritic cells. *Blood* 2002;100:3295–3303.
42. Marafioti T, Paterson JC, Ballabio E, et al. Novel markers of normal and neoplastic human plasmacytoid dendritic cells. *Blood* 2008;111:3778–3792.
43. Olweus J, BitMansour A, Warnke R, et al. Dendritic cell ontogeny: a human dendritic cell lineage of myeloid origin. *Proc Natl Acad Sci U S A* 1997;94: 12551–12556.
44. Strobl H, Scheinecker C, Riedl E, et al. Identification of CD68+ lin-peripheral blood cells with dendritic precursor characteristics. *J Immunol* 1998;161: 740–748.
45. Sorg RV, Kogler G, Wernet P. Identification of cord blood dendritic cells as an immature CD11c– population. *Blood* 1999;93:2302–2307.
46. Shodell M, Siegal FP. Circulating, interferon-producing plasmacytoid dendritic cells decline during human ageing. *Scand J Immunol* 2002;56:518–521.
47. Jing Y, Shaheen E, Drake RR, et al. Aging is associated with a numerical and functional decline in plasmacytoid dendritic cells, whereas myeloid dendritic cells are relatively unaltered in human peripheral blood. *Hum Immunol* 2009;70:777–784.
48. Ziegler-Heitbrock L, Ancuţa P, Crowe S, et al. Nomenclature of monocytes and dendritic cells in blood. *Blood* 2010;116:e74–e80.
49. Dzionek A, Fuchs A, Schmidt P, et al. BDCA-2, BDCA-3, and BDCA-4: three markers for distinct subsets of dendritic cells in human peripheral blood. *J Immunol* 2000;165:6037–6046.
50. Dzionek A, Sohma J, Nagafune M, et al. BDCA-2, a novel plasmacytoid dendritic cell cell-specific type II C-type lectin, mediates antigen-capture and is a potent inhibitor of interferon-alpha/beta induction. *J Exp Med* 2001;194:1823–1834.
51. Petrella T, Comeau MR, Maynadie M, et al. Agranular CD4+ CD56+ hematodermic neoplasm' (blastic NK-cell lymphoma) originates from a population of CD56+ precursor cells related to plasmacytoid monocytes. *Am J Surg Pathol* 2002;26:852–862.
52. Comeau MR, Van der Vuurst de Vries AR, Maliszewski CR, et al. CD123bright plasmacytoid predendritic cells: progenitors undergoing cell fate conversion? *J Immunol* 2002;169:75–83.
53. Matsui T, Connolly JE, Michnevitz M, et al. CD2 distinguishes two subsets of human plasmacytoid dendritic cells with distinct phenotype and functions. *J Immunol* 2009;182:6815–6823.
54. Facchetti F, De Wolf-Peeters C, van den Oord JJ, et al. Plasmacytoid T cells: a cell population normally present in the reactive lymph node. An immunohistochemical and electronmicroscopic study. *Hum Pathol* 1988;19:1085–1092.
55. Jegalian AG, Facchetti F, Jaffe ES. Plasmacytoid dendritic cells: physiologic roles and pathologic states. *Adv Anat Pathol* 2009;16:392–404.
56. Facchetti F, Vermi W, Mason D, et al. The plasmacytoid monocyte/interferon producing cells. *Virchows Arch* 2003;443:703–717.
57. Vermi W, Riboldi E, Wittamer V, et al. Role of ChemR23 in directing the migration of myeloid and plasmacytoid dendritic cells to lymphoid organs and inflamed skin. *J Exp Med* 2005;201:509–515.
58. Sozzani S, Vermi W, Del Prete A, et al. Trafficking properties of plasmacytoid dendritic cells in health and disease. *Trends Immunol* 2010;31:270–277.
59. Chen M, Wang J. Programmed cell death of dendritic cells in immune regulation. *Immunol Rev* 2010;236:11–27.
60. Facchetti F, De Wolf-Peeters C, De Vos R, et al. Plasmacytoid monocytes (so-called plasmacytoid T cells) in granulomatous lymphadenitis. *Hum Pathol* 1989;20: 588–593.
61. Facchetti F, De Wolf-Peters C, Marocolo D, et al. Plasmacytoid monocytes in granulomatous lymphadenitis and in histiocytic necrotizing lymphadenitis. *Sarcoidosis* 1991;8:170–171.
62. Jahnsen FL, Lund-Johansen F, Dunne JF, et al. Experimentally induced recruitment of plasmacytoid (CD123high) dendritic cells in human nasal allergy. *J Immunol* 2000;165:4062–4068.
63. Vermi W, Lonardi S, Morassi M, et al. Cutaneous distribution of plasmacytoid dendritic cells in lupus erythematosus. Selective tropism at the site of epithelial apoptotic damage. *Immunobiology* 2009;214:877–886.
64. Vermi W, Fisogni S, Salogni L, et al. Spontaneous regression of highly immunogenic Molluscum contagiosum virus (MCV)-induced skin lesions is associated with plasmacytoid dendritic cells and IFN-DC infiltration. *J Invest Dermatol* 2011;131:426–434.
65. Santoro A, Majorana A, Roversi L, et al. Recruitment of dendritic cells in oral lichen planus. *J Pathol* 2005;205:426–434.
66. Facchetti F, de Wolf-Peeters C, van den Oord JJ, et al. Anti-high endothelial venule monoclonal antibody HECA-452 recognizes plasmacytoid T cells and delineates an "extranodular" compartment in the reactive lymph node. *Immunol Lett* 1989;20:277–281.
67. Herling M, Teitell MA, Shen RR, et al. TCL1 expression in plasmacytoid dendritic cells (DC2s) and the related CD4+ CD56+ blastic tumors of skin. *Blood* 2003;101:5007–5009.
68. Facchetti F, Candiago E, Vermi W. Plasmacytoid monocytes express IL3-receptor alpha and differentiate into dendritic cells. *Histopathology* 1999;35:88–89.
69. Rissoan MC, Soumelis V, Kadowaki N, et al. Reciprocal control of T helper cell and dendritic cell differentiation [see comments]. *Science* 1999;283:1183–1186.
70. Facchetti F, Vermi W, Santoro A, et al. Neoplasms derived from plasmacytoid monocytes/interferon-producing cells: variability of CD56 and granzyme B expression. *Am J Surg Pathol* 2003;27:1489–1492.
71. Jahrsdorfer B, Vollmer A, Blackwell SE, et al. Granzyme B produced by human plasmacytoid dendritic cells suppresses T-cell expansion. *Blood* 2010;115: 1156–1165.
72. Pulford KA, Rigney EM, Micklem KJ, et al. KP1: a new monoclonal antibody that detects a monocyte/macrophage associated antigen in routinely processed tissue sections. *J Clin Pathol* 1989;42:414–421.
73. Bos JD, de Boer OJ, Tibosch E, et al. Skin-homing T lymphocytes: detection of cutaneous lymphocyte-associated antigen (CLA) by HECA-452 in normal human skin. *Arch Dermatol Res* 1993;285:179–183.
74. Koszik F, Strunk D, Simonitsch I, et al. Expression of monoclonal antibody HECA-452-defined E-selectin ligands on Langerhans cells in normal and diseased skin. *J Invest Dermatol* 1994;102:773–780.
75. Narducci MG, Pescarmona E, Lazzeri C, et al. Regulation of TCL1 expression in B- and T-cell lymphomas and reactive lymphoid tissues. *Cancer Res* 2000;60: 2095–2100.
76. Reineks EZ, Osei ES, Rosenberg A, et al. CD22 expression on blastic plasmacytoid dendritic cell neoplasms and reactivity of anti-CD22 antibodies to peripheral blood dendritic cells. *Cytometry B Clin Cytom* 2009;76:237–248.
77. Acon-Laws M, Bayerl MG, Ehman C, et al. Basophils and plasmacytoid dendritic cells are potential sources for error in flow cytometric monitoring of patients receiving anti-CD22 therapies. AKA not all anti-CD22 antibodies are created equal. *Am J Hematol* 2011;86:891–892.
78. Facchetti F. The plasmacytoid monocyte (the so-called plasmacytoid T-cell). An enigmatic cell of the human lymph node (Doctoral Thesis) [Doctoral Thesis]. Catholic University of Leuven, 1989.
79. Jacob MC, Chaperot L, Mossuz P, et al. CD4+ CD56+ lineage negative malignancies: a new entity developed from malignant early plasmacytoid dendritic cells. *Haematologica* 2003;88:941–955.
80. Galibert L, Maliszewski CR, Vandenabeele S. Plasmacytoid monocytes/T cells: a dendritic cell lineage? *Semin Immunol* 2001;13:283–289.
81. Chowdhury F, Johnson P, Williams AP. Enumeration and phenotypic assessment of human plasmacytoid and myeloid dendritic cells in whole blood. *Cytometry A* 2010;77:328–337.
82. Garnache-Ottou F, Chaperot L, Biichle S, et al. Expression of the myeloid-associated marker CD33 is not an exclusive factor for leukemic plasmacytoid dendritic cells. *Blood* 2005;105:1256–1264.
83. Beiske K, Langholm R, Godal T, et al. T-zone lymphoma with predominance of 'plasmacytoid T-cells' associated with myelomonocytic leukaemia—A distinct clinicopathological entity. *J Pathol* 1986;150:247–255.
84. Thomas JO, Beiske K, Hann I, et al. Immunohistological diagnosis of "plasmacytoid T cell lymphoma" in paraffin wax sections. *J Clin Pathol* 1991;44:632–635.
85. Prasthofer EF, Prchal JT, Grizzle WE, et al. Plasmacytoid-T-cell lymphoma associated with chronic myeloproliferative disorder. *Am J Surg Pathol* 1985;9:380–387.
86. Koo CH, Mason DY, Miller R, et al. Additional evidence that "plasmacytoid T-cell lymphoma" associated with chronic myeloproliferative disorders is of macrophage/monocyte origin. *Am J Clin Pathol* 1990;93:822–827.

87. Facchetti F, De Wolf-Peeters C, Kennes C, et al. Leukemia-associated lymph node infiltrates of plasmacytoid monocytes (so-called plasmacytoid T-cells). Evidence for two distinct histological and immunophenotypical patterns. *Am J Surg Pathol* 1990;14:101–112.
88. Baddoura FK, Chan WC, Caldwell CW, et al. Plasmacytoid acute T-cell lymphoma/leukemia. *Am J Clin Pathol* 1991;96:287–288.
89. Baddoura FK, Hanson C, Chan WC. Plasmacytoid monocyte proliferation associated with myeloproliferative disorders. *Cancer* 1992;69:1457–1467.
90. Naresh KN, Pavlu J. Plasmacytoid dendritic cell nodules in bone marrow biopsies of chronic myelomonocytic leukemia. *Am J Hematol* 2010;85:893.
91. Vermi W, Facchetti F, Rosati S, et al. Nodal and extranodal tumor-forming accumulation of plasmacytoid monocytes/interferon-producing cells associated with myeloid disorders. *Am J Surg Pathol* 2004;28:585–595.
92. Chen YC, Chou JM, Ketterling RP, et al. Histologic and immunohistochemical study of bone marrow monocytic nodules in 21 cases with myelodysplasia. *Am J Clin Pathol* 2003;120:874–881.
93. Benet C, Gomez A, Aguilar C, et al. Histologic and immunohistologic characterization of skin localization of myeloid disorders: a study of 173 cases. *Am J Clin Pathol* 2011;135:278–290.
94. Orazi A, Chiu R, O'Malley DP, et al. Chronic myelomonocytic leukemia: the role of bone marrow biopsy immunohistology. *Mod Pathol* 2006;19:1536–1545.
95. Dargent JL, Delannoy A, Pieron P, et al. Cutaneous accumulation of plasmacytoid dendritic cells associated with acute myeloid leukemia: a rare condition distinct from blastic plasmacytoid dendritic cell neoplasm. *J Cutan Pathol* 2011;38: 893–898.
96. Mongkonsritragoon W, Letendre L, Qian J, et al. Nodular lesions of monocytic component in myelodysplastic syndrome. *Am J Clin Pathol* 1998;110:154–162.
97. Pileri SA, Ascani S, Cox MC, et al. Myeloid sarcoma: clinico-pathologic, phenotypic and cytogenetic analysis of 92 adult patients. *Leukemia* 2007;21:340–350.
98. Petrella T, Dalac S, Maynadie M, et al. CD4+ CD56+ cutaneous neoplasms: a distinct hematological entity? *Am J Surg Pathol* 1999;23:137–146.
99. Adachi M, Maeda K, Takekawa M, et al. High expression of CD56 (N-CAM) in a patient with cutaneous CD4-positive lymphoma. *Am J Hematol* 1994;47: 278–282.
100. Dummer R, Potoczna N, Haffner AC, et al. A primary cutaneous non-T, non-B CD4+, CD56+ lymphoma. *Arch Dermatol* 1996;132:550–553.
101. Wasik MA, Sackstein R, Novick D, et al. Cutaneous CD56+ large T-cell lymphoma associated with high serum concentration of IL-2. *Hum Pathol* 1996;27:738–744.
102. Bastian BC, Ott G, Muller-Deubert S, et al. Primary cutaneous natural killer/T-cell lymphoma. *Arch Dermatol* 1998;134:109–111.
103. Brody JP, Allen S, Schulman P, et al. Acute agranular CD4-positive natural killer cell leukemia. Comprehensive clinicopathologic studies including virologic and in vitro culture with inducing agents. *Cancer* 1995;75:2474–2483.
104. DiGiuseppe JA, Louie DC, Williams JE, et al. Blastic natural killer cell leukemia/lymphoma: a clinicopathologic study. *Am J Surg Pathol* 1997;21:1223–1230.
105. Bagot M, Bouloc A, Charue D, et al. Do primary cutaneous non-T non-B CD4+ CD56+ lymphomas belong to the myelo-monocytic lineage? *J Invest Dermatol* 1998;111:1242–1244.
106. Lucio P, Parreira A, Orfao A. CD123hi dendritic cell lymphoma: an unusual case of non-Hodgkin lymphoma. *Ann Intern Med* 1999;131:549–550.
107. Chaperot L, Bendriss N, Manches O, et al. Identification of a leukemic counterpart of the plasmacytoid dendritic cells. *Blood* 2001;97:3210–3217.
108. Chaperot L, Perrot I, Jacob MC, et al. Leukemic plasmacytoid dendritic cells share phenotypic and functional features with their normal counterparts. *Eur J Immunol* 2004;34:418–426.
109. Petrella T, Meijer CJ, Dalac S, et al. TCL1 and CLA expression in agranular CD4/CD56 hematodermic neoplasms (blastic NK-cell lymphomas) and leukemia cutis. *Am J Clin Pathol* 2004;122:307–313.
110. Hallermann C, Middel P, Griesinger F, et al. CD4+ CD56+ blastic tumor of the skin: cytogenetic observations and further evidence of an origin from plasmacytoid dendritic cells. *Eur J Dermatol* 2004;14:317–322.
111. Urosevic M, Conrad C, Kamarashev J, et al. CD4+ CD56+ hematodermic neoplasms bear a plasmacytoid dendritic cell phenotype. *Hum Pathol* 2005;36: 1020–1024.
112. Gopcsa L, Banyai A, Jakab K, et al. Extensive flow cytometric characterization of plasmacytoid dendritic cell leukemia cells. *Eur J Haematol* 2005;75:346–351.
113. Reichard KK, Burks EJ, Foucar MK, et al. CD4(+) CD56(+) lineage-negative malignancies are rare tumors of plasmacytoid dendritic cells. *Am J Surg Pathol* 2005;29:1274–1283.
114. Jaye DL, Geigerman CM, Herling M, et al. Expression of the plasmacytoid dendritic cell marker BDCA-2 supports a spectrum of maturation among CD4+ CD56+ hematodermic neoplasms. *Mod Pathol* 2006;19:1555–1562.
115. Pilichowska ME, Fleming MD, Pinkus JL, et al. CD4+/CD56+ hematodermic neoplasm ("blastic natural killer cell lymphoma"): neoplastic cells express the immature dendritic cell marker BDCA-2 and produce interferon. *Am J Clin Pathol* 2007;128:445–453.
116. Defays A, David A, de Gassart A, et al. BAD-LAMP is a novel biomarker of nonactivated human plasmacytoid dendritic cells. *Blood* 2011;118:609–617.
117. Dijkman R, van Doorn R, Szuhai K, et al. Gene-expression profiling and array-based CGH classify CD4+CD56+ hematodermic neoplasm and cutaneous myelomonocytic leukemia as distinct disease entities. *Blood* 2007;109:1720–1727.
118. Bendriss-Vermare N, Chaperot L, Peoc'h M, et al. In situ leukemic plasmacytoid dendritic cells pattern of chemokine receptors expression and in vitro migratory response. *Leukemia* 2004;18:1491–1498.
119. Maeda T, Murata K, Fukushima T, et al. A novel plasmacytoid dendritic cell line, CAL-1, established from a patient with blastic natural killer cell lymphoma. *Int J Hematol* 2005;81:148–154.
120. Narita M, Watanabe N, Yamahira A, et al. A leukemic plasmacytoid dendritic cell line, PMDC05, with the ability to secrete IFN-alpha by stimulation via Toll-like receptors and present antigens to naive T cells. *Leuk Res* 2009;33:1224–1232.
121. Watanabe N, Narita M, Yamahira A, et al. Transformation of dendritic cells from plasmacytoid to myeloid in a leukemic plasmacytoid dendritic cell line (PMDC05). *Leuk Res* 2010;34:1517–1524.
122. Bueno C, Almeida J, Lucio P, et al. Incidence and characteristics of CD4(+)/HLA DRhi dendritic cell malignancies. *Haematologica* 2004;89:58–69.
123. Petrella T, Bagot M, Willemze R, et al. Blastic NK-cell lymphomas (agranular CD4+ CD56+ hematodermic neoplasms): a review. *Am J Clin Pathol* 2005; 123:662–675.
124. Suzuki R, Nakamura S, Suzumiya J, et al. Blastic natural killer cell lymphoma/leukemia (CD56-positive blastic tumor): prognostication and categorization according to anatomic sites of involvement. *Cancer* 2005;104:1022–1031.
125. Khoury JD, Medeiros LJ, Manning JT, et al. CD56(+) TdT(+) blastic natural killer cell tumor of the skin: a primitive systemic malignancy related to myelomonocytic leukemia. *Cancer* 2002;94:2401–2408.
126. Reimer P, Rudiger T, Kraemer D, et al. What is CD4+CD56+ malignancy and how should it be treated? *Bone Marrow Transplant* 2003;32:637–646.
127. Herling M, Jones D. CD4+/CD56+ hematodermic tumor: the features of an evolving entity and its relationship to dendritic cells. *Am J Clin Pathol* 2007;127:687–700.
128. Assaf C, Gellrich S, Whittaker S, et al. CD56-positive haematological neoplasms of the skin: a multicentre study of the Cutaneous Lymphoma Project Group of the European Organisation for Research and Treatment of Cancer. *J Clin Pathol* 2007;60:981–989.
129. Bekkenk MW, Jansen PM, Meijer CJ, et al. CD56+ hematological neoplasms presenting in the skin: a retrospective analysis of 23 new cases and 130 cases from the literature. *Ann Oncol* 2004;15:1097–1108.
130. Cota C, Vale E, Viana I, et al. Cutaneous manifestations of blastic plasmacytoid dendritic cell neoplasm-morphologic and phenotypic variability in a series of 33 patients. *Am J Surg Pathol* 2010;34:75–87.
131. Hashikawa K, Niino D, Yasumoto S, et al. Clinicopathological features and prognostic significance of CXCL12 in blastic plasmacytoid dendritic cell neoplasm. *J Am Acad Dermatol* 2011;66(2):278–291.
132. Lucioni M, Novara F, Fiandrino G, et al. Twenty-one cases of blastic plasmacytoid dendritic cell neoplasm: focus on biallelic locus 9p21.3 deletion. *Blood* 2011;118:4591–4594.
133. Dalle S, Beylot-Barry M, Bagot M, et al. Blastic plasmacytoid dendritic cell neoplasm: is transplantation the treatment of choice? *Br J Dermatol* 2010;162:74–79.
134. Rauh MJ, Rahman F, Good D, et al. Blastic plasmacytoid dendritic cell neoplasm with leukemic presentation, lacking cutaneous involvement: Case series and literature review. *Leuk Res* 2012;36:81–86.
135. Jegalian AG, Buxbaum NP, Facchetti F, et al. Blastic plasmacytoid dendritic cell neoplasm in children: diagnostic features and clinical implications. *Haematologica* 2010;95:1873–1879.
136. Weaver J, Hsi ED. CD4+/CD56+ hematodermic neoplasm (blastic NK-cell lymphoma). *J Cutan Pathol* 2008;35:975–977.
137. Feuillard J, Jacob MC, Valensi F, et al. Clinical and biologic features of CD4(+) CD56(+) malignancies. *Blood* 2002;99:1556–1563.
138. Tsagarakis NJ, Kentrou NA, Papadimitriou KA, et al. Acute lymphoplasmacytoid dendritic cell (DC2) leukemia: results from the Hellenic Dendritic Cell Leukemia Study Group. *Leuk Res* 2010;34:438–446.
139. Hamadani M, Magro CM, Porcu P. CD4+ CD56+ haematodermic tumour (plasmacytoid dendritic cell neoplasm). *Br J Haematol* 2008;140:122.
140. Ng AP, Lade S, Rutherford T, et al. Primary cutaneous CD4+/CD56+ hematodermic neoplasm (blastic NK-cell lymphoma): a report of five cases. *Haematologica* 2006;91:143–144.
141. Jardin F, Callanan M, Penther D, et al. Recurrent genomic aberrations combined with deletions of various tumour suppressor genes may deregulate the G1/S transition in CD4+CD56+ haematodermic neoplasms and contribute to the aggressiveness of the disease. *Leukemia* 2009;23:698–707.
142. Yamada O, Ichikawa M, Okamoto T, et al. Killer T-cell induction in patients with blastic natural killer cell lymphoma/leukaemia: implications for successful treatment and possible therapeutic strategies. *Br J Haematol* 2001;113:153–160.
143. Karube K, Ohshima K, Tsuchiya T, et al. Non-B, non-T neoplasms with lymphoblast morphology: further clarification and classification. *Am J Surg Pathol* 2003;27:1366–1374.
144. Kazakov DV, Mentzel T, Burg G, et al. Blastic natural killer-cell lymphoma of the skin associated with myelodysplastic syndrome or myelogenous leukaemia: a coincidence or more? *Br J Dermatol* 2003;149:869–876.
145. Sano F, Tasaka T, Nishimura H, et al. A peculiar case of acute myeloid leukemia mimicking plasmacytoid dendritic precursor cell leukemia. *J Clin Exp Hematop* 2008;48:65–69.
146. Voelkl A, Flaig M, Roehnisch T, et al. Blastic plasmacytoid dendritic cell neoplasm with acute myeloid leukemia successfully treated to a remission currently of 26 months duration. *Leuk Res* 2011;35:e61–e63.
147. Narita M, Kuroha T, Watanabe N, et al. Plasmacytoid dendritic cell leukemia with potent antigen-presenting ability. *Acta Haematol* 2008;120:91–99.
148. Petrella T, Facchetti F. Tumoral aspects of plasmacytoid dendritic cells: what do we know in 2009? *Autoimmunity* 2010;43:210–214.
149. Bayerl MG, Rakozy CK, Mohamed AN, et al. Blastic natural killer cell lymphoma/leukemia: a report of seven cases. *Am J Clin Pathol* 2002;117:41–50.
150. Di Mario A, Garzia M, d'Alo F, et al. Rapid leukaemic evolution in a cutaneous blastic NK-cell lymphoma initially diagnosed as pseudolymphoma. *Hematology* 2007;12:155–157.
151. Hwang SM, Kim HK. Necklace-like microvacuoles of tumor cells in blastic plasmacytoid dendritic cell neoplasm. *Korean J Hematol* 2010;45:7.
152. Falcao RP, Garcia AB, Marques MG, et al. Blastic CD4 NK cell leukemia/lymphoma: a distinct clinical entity. *Leuk Res* 2002;26:803–807.
153. Anargyrou K, Paterakis G, Boutsis D, et al. An unusual case of CD4+ CD7+ CD56+ acute leukemia with overlapping features of type 2 dendritic cell (DC2) and myeloid/NK cell precursor acute leukemia. *Eur J Haematol* 2003;71:294–298.
154. Santucci M, Pimpinelli N, Massi D, et al. Cytotoxic/natural killer cell cutaneous lymphomas. Report of EORTC Cutaneous Lymphoma Task Force Workshop. *Cancer* 2003;97:610–627.
155. Child FJ, Mitchell TJ, Whittaker SJ, et al. Blastic natural killer cell and extranodal natural killer cell-like T-cell lymphoma presenting in the skin: report of six cases from the UK. *Br J Dermatol* 2003;148:507–515.
156. Giagounidis AA, Heinsch M, Haase S, et al. Early plasmacytoid dendritic cell leukemia/lymphoma coexpressing myeloid antigenes. *Ann Hematol* 2004;83: 716–721.
157. Kim Y, Kang MS, Kim CW, et al. CD4+CD56+ lineage negative hematopoietic neoplasm: so called blastic NK cell lymphoma. *J Korean Med Sci* 2005;20:319–324.
158. Rossi JG, Felice MS, Bernasconi AR, et al. Acute leukemia of dendritic cell lineage in childhood: incidence, biological characteristics and outcome. *Leuk Lymphoma* 2006;47:715–725.
159. Ruggiero A, Maurizi P, Larocca LM, et al. Childhood CD4+/CD56+ hematodermic neoplasm: case report and review of the literature. *Haematologica* 2006;91: ECR48.

160. Hu SC, Tsai KB, Chen GS, et al. Infantile CD4+/CD56+ hematodermic neoplasm. *Haematologica* 2007;92:e91–e93.
161. Ascani S, Massone C, Ferrara G, et al. CD4-negative variant of CD4+/CD56+ hematodermic neoplasm: description of three cases. *J Cutan Pathol* 2008;35:911–915.
162. Whittle AM, Howard MR. Skin lesions in plasmacytoid dendritic cell leukaemia. *Br J Haematol* 2008;140:121.
163. Leitenberger JJ, Berthelot CN, Polder KD, et al. CD4+ CD56+ hematodermic/plasmacytoid dendritic cell tumor with response to pralatrexate. *J Am Acad Dermatol* 2008;58:480–484.
164. Hama A, Kudo K, Itzel BV, et al. Plasmacytoid dendritic cell leukemia in children. *J Pediatr Hematol Oncol* 2009;31:339–343.
165. Garnache-Ottou F, Feuillard J, Ferrand C, et al. Extended diagnostic criteria for plasmacytoid dendritic cell leukaemia. *Br J Haematol* 2009;145:624–636.
166. Dietrich S, Andrulis M, Hegenbart U, et al. Blastic plasmacytoid dendritic cell neoplasia (BPDC) in elderly patients: results of a treatment algorithm employing allogeneic stem cell transplantation with moderately reduced conditioning intensity. *Biol Blood Marrow Transplant* 2011;17:1250–1254.
167. Dantas FE, de Almeida Vieira CA, de Castro CC, et al. Blastic plasmacytoid dendritic cell neoplasm without cutaneous involvement: a rare disease with a rare presentation. *Acta Oncol* 2012;51:139–141.
168. Petrella T, Teitell MA, Spiekermann C, et al. A CD56-negative case of blastic natural killer-cell lymphoma (agranular CD4+/CD56+ haematodermic neoplasm). *Br J Dermatol* 2004;150:174–176.
169. Lonardi S, Rossini C, Ungari M, et al. A monoclonal antibody anti-BDCA2 (CD303) highly specific for plasmacytoid dendritic cell neoplasms on paraffin sections. *Virchows Archiv* 2009;455:S254–S255.
170. Bilbao EA, Chirife AM, Florio D, et al. Hematodermic CD4+ CD56+ neoplasm in childhood. *Medicina (B Aires)* 2008;68:147–150.
171. Pina-Oviedo S, Herrera-Medina H, Coronado H, et al. CD4+/CD56+ hematodermic neoplasm: presentation of 2 cases and review of the concept of an uncommon tumor originated in plasmacytoid dendritic cells expressing CD123 (IL-3 receptor alpha). *Appl Immunohistochem Mol Morphol* 2007;15:481–486.
172. Kojima H, Mukai HY, Shinagawa A, et al. Clinicopathological analyses of 5 Japanese patients with CD56+ primary cutaneous lymphomas. *Int J Hematol* 2000;72:477–483.
173. Mukai HY, Kojima H, Suzukawa K, et al. High-dose chemotherapy with peripheral blood stem cell rescue in blastoid natural killer cell lymphoma. *Leuk Lymphoma* 1999;32:583–588.
174. Momoi A, Toba K, Kawai K, et al. Cutaneous lymphoblastic lymphoma of putative plasmacytoid dendritic cell-precursor origin: two cases. *Leuk Res* 2002;26:693–698.
175. Trimoreau F, Donnard M, Turlure P, et al. The CD4+ CD56+ CD116– CD123+ CD45RA+ CD45RO– profile is specific of DC2 malignancies. *Haematologica* 2003;88:ELT10.
176. Aoyama Y, Yamane T, Hino M, et al. Blastic NK-cell lymphoma/leukemia with T-cell receptor gamma rearrangement. *Ann Hematol* 2001;80:752–754.
177. Stetsenko GY, McFarlane R, Kalus A, et al. CD4+/CD56+ hematodermic neoplasm: report of a rare variant with a T-cell receptor gene rearrangement. *J Cutan Pathol* 2008;35:579–584.
178. Jardin F, Ruminy P, Parmentier F, et al. TET2 and TP53 mutations are frequently observed in blastic plasmacytoid dendritic cell neoplasm. *Br J Haematol* 2011;153:413–416.
179. Facchetti F, Pileri SA, Agostinelli C, et al. Cytoplasmic nucleophosmin is not detected in blastic plasmacytoid dendritic cell neoplasm. *Haematologica* 2009;94:285–288.
180. Leroux D, Mugneret F, Callanan M, et al. CD4(+), CD56(+) DC2 acute leukemia is characterized by recurrent clonal chromosomal changes affecting 6 major targets: a study of 21 cases by the Groupe Francais de Cytogenetique Hematologique. *Blood* 2002;99:4154–4159.
181. Wiesner T, Obenauf AC, Cota C, et al. Alterations of the cell-cycle inhibitors p27(KIP1) and p16(INK4a) are frequent in blastic plasmacytoid dendritic cell neoplasms. *J Invest Dermatol* 2010;130:1152–1157.
182. Cho-Vega JH, Medeiros LJ, Prieto VG, et al. Leukemia cutis. *Am J Clin Pathol* 2008;129:130–142.
183. Cronin DM, George TI, Sundram UN. An updated approach to the diagnosis of myeloid leukemia cutis. *Am J Clin Pathol* 2009;132:101–110.
184. Cibull TL, Thomas AB, O'Malley DP, et al. Myeloid leukemia cutis: a histologic and immunohistochemical review. *J Cutan Pathol* 2008;35:180–185.
185. Cibull TL, Thomas AB, O'Malley DP, et al. CD4+ CD56+ hematodermic neoplasm. *Am J Dermatopathol* 2007;29:59–61.
186. Chan JK, Sin VC, Wong KF, et al. Nonnasal lymphoma expressing the natural killer cell marker CD56: a clinicopathologic study of 49 cases of an uncommon aggressive neoplasm. *Blood* 1997;89:4501–4513.
187. Kawase T, Hamazaki M, Ogura M, et al. CD56/NCAM-positive Langerhans cell sarcoma: a clinicopathologic study of 4 cases. *Int J Hematol* 2005;81:323–329.
188. Simonitsch I, Kopp CW, Mosberger I, et al. Expression of the monoclonal antibody HECA-452 defined E-selectin ligands in Langerhans cell histiocytosis. *Virchows Arch* 1996;427:477–481.
189. Sumida K, Yoshidomi Y, Koga H, et al. Leukemic transformation of Langerhans cell sarcoma. *Int J Hematol* 2008;87:527–531.
190. Massone C, Chott A, Metze D, et al. Subcutaneous, blastic natural killer (NK), NK/T-cell, and other cytotoxic lymphomas of the skin: a morphologic, immunophenotypic, and molecular study of 50 patients. *Am J Surg Pathol* 2004;28:719–735.
191. Gniadecki R, Rossen K, Ralfkier E, et al. CD56+ lymphoma with skin involvement: clinicopathologic features and classification. *Arch Dermatol* 2004;140:427–436.
192. Willemze R, Jaffe ES, Burg G, et al. WHO-EORTC classification for cutaneous lymphomas. *Blood* 2005;105:3768–3785.
193. Jaffe ES, Gaulard P, Ralfkiaer E, et al. Subcutaneous panniculitis-like T-cell lymphoma. In: Swerdlow SH, Campo E, Harris NL, et al., eds. *WHO classification of tumours of haematopoietic and lymphoid tissues*, 4th ed. Lyon: International Agency for Research on Cancer, 2008:294–295.

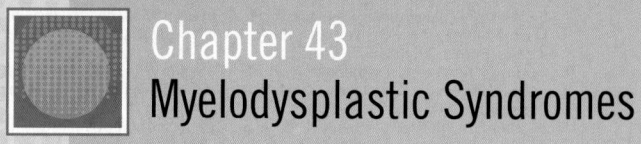

Chapter 43
Myelodysplastic Syndromes

Richard D. Brunning • Ulrich Germing

 ## DEFINITION

The myelodysplastic syndromes (MDSs) are a group of clonal hematopoietic stem cell disorders characterized by dysplastic changes in one or more myeloid cell lines, ineffective hematopoiesis, increased apoptosis, and cytopenias, with or without a concurrent increase in myeloblasts in the bone marrow and peripheral blood; in those instances in which the myeloblasts are increased, the number is <20% requisite for a diagnosis of acute myeloid leukemia (AML) (1–3). The course of the MDS is marked by progressive marrow failure with or without evolution to AML. The MDSs occur as primary diseases and as secondary or therapy related disorders. The therapy related MDSs occur in patients who have been exposed to chemotherapeutic agents and/ or radiotherapy (4). These entities are discussed in Chapter 41.

 ## EPIDEMIOLOGY

MDSs occur primarily in older individuals and are more common in males than females. In data obtained from the North American Association of Central Cancer Registries (NAACCR), which captures 82% of the population in the United States and the National Cancer Institute's Surveillance, Epidemiology, and End Results (SEER) program, the average annual age-adjusted incidence rate of MDS for 2001 to 2003 was 3.3/100,000 individuals (5–7). The incidence was age related; the majority of patients, approximately 70%, were over 70 years of age. The age-adjusted incidence of MDS was significantly higher in males, 4.9% compared to 2.5% in females. Data from the SEER program in the United States for 2001 to 2005 showed an incidence rate for all races, both sexes of 3.4 with a rate of 4.5 in males and 2.7 in females. Whites had a rate of 3.5, Blacks 3.0, Native Americans/American Indians 1.3, and Asian or Pacific Islanders 2.6. In all races or ethnic groups, the rate in males exceeds the rate in females.

SEER statistics for 2003 to 2008 showed an overall rate of 4.4, 6.1 for males and 3.4 for females. Similar to the earlier data, the rate increased with advancing age, 9.2 for ages 60 to 69, 27.1 for 70 to 79, and 49.8 for those over 80 (8). The male to female predominance was accentuated with increasing age, 36.6 for males and 19.8 for females 70 to 79. The rate was 77.5 for males and 35.2 for females 80 and older.

The increase in the incidence rate in MDS in the United States in succeeding years is probably related to increased recognition of the manifestations of the disease by the medical community rather than an actual increase in the disease.

The true incidence of MDS in the United States is probably higher than noted in the cited data due to the lack of recognition of the disorders and the reporting systems on which the incidence data are based. A novel approach for determining the incidence using a claim-based algorithm based on Medicare claims for blood count and bone marrow examination showed an incidence of 75/100,000 individuals over the age of 75 years (9).

In a study of the incidence of MDS in the population of Dusseldorf, Germany, the rate for the years 1996 to 2005 was 5.74 for males and 4.12 for females. Similar to the SEER and NAACCR data, the rate increased with age, males over 70 had a rate of 34.9 and females 17.1 (10). In the Dusseldorf series, 9% of the cases were considered secondary in contrast to the SEER rate of 1.6%. This difference may be the result of differences in data collection.

There appear to be some differences in the age of presentation and characteristics of MDS in different population groups. The median age of presentation in studies of MDS patients in Thailand, Korea, and China was reported to occur about a decade younger, 55 to 60 years, than the median age in reports of studies in western patients, 67 to 73 years (11–13). This difference may be related to both genetic variation and environmental factors. In one study from China, the median age of presentation of patients from rural regions was 43 years compared to the patients from cities with a median age of presentation of 53 years (13).

In a study comparing Japanese and German patients, the incidence of the del(5q) syndrome was 1% to 2% in Japanese patients compared to 5% to 6% for German patients (14). Refractory anemia with ring sideroblasts (RARS) was also less frequent in Japanese patients than in German patients (14). The frequency of refractory cytopenia with unilineage dysplasia (RCUD) and myelodysplastic syndrome–unclassified (MDS-U) was higher in Japanese patients than in a comparable group of German patients; the frequency of refractory anemia with multilineage dysplasia (RCMD) was less frequent in Japanese patients than in German patients (14,15).

Japanese patients with MDS had more severe cytopenias, but the prognosis was more favorable than in the German patients. Of note, the percentage of Japanese patients with MDS-U related to pancytopenia was approximately 30% of the patients who had been previously classified as RA according to the French-American-British (FAB) classification and significantly higher than in German patients, 13% (15). This was also reflected in the number of cases with MDS-U, approximately 30% in the Japanese cohort and 3% in the German patients. The incidence of isolated del(5q) and RARS is reported to be very low in other populations in the Far East (13,14).

 ## CLINICAL CONSIDERATIONS

Adult patients with MDS generally present with some manifestation of bone marrow failure, most commonly fatigue due to anemia. Bleeding due to thrombocytopenia and infection related to neutropenia may also be present (1–3). Organomegaly and lymphadenopathy are not usual findings but have been reported in some patients.

Patients may present with immune-related symptoms (16). In some patients with low-grade MDS, there is evidence of immune dysregulation with T-cell mediation inhibition of hematopoiesis. Studies have shown a significant increase in CD8 lymphocytes and mature B cells in the marrow compared

Table 43.1	WHO CLASSIFICATION OF MDSs

Refractory cytopenia with unilineage dysplasia (RCUD):
  Refractory anemia (RA)
  Refractory neutropenia (RN)
  Refractory thrombocytopenia (RT)
Refractory anemia with ring sideroblasts (RARS)
Refractory cytopenia with multilineage dysplasia (RCMD) ± ring sideroblasts
Refractory anemia with excess blasts: RAEB-1; RAEB-2
Myelodysplastic syndrome–unclassified (MDS-U)
MDS with isolated del(5q)

to peripheral blood in some cases of low-grade MDS (17–19). In some cases of low-grade MDS, particularly those with hypocellular marrows, there is an indication of immune-mediated damage to hematopoietic precursors and changes in the hematopoietic-supporting microenvironment (18). Some patients have increased serum levels of type 1 cytokines, tumor necrosis factor–α, and interferon-γ and oligoclonal expansion of cytotoxic T cells (19). Some patients with MDS respond to treatment with immunosuppressive agents such as antithymocyte globulin, cyclosporine A, and alemtuzumab; the immunosuppressive therapy has resulted in partial or complete remission in these patients

(20–22). Low-risk International Prognostic Scoring System (IPSS) score and bone marrow hypocellularity have been reported to be predictive of response to immunosuppressive therapy (21).

 MORPHOLOGIC CHARACTERISTICS OF MDS

Table 43.1 lists the six major types of primary MDS in the WHO morphologic and cytogenetic classification of MDSs. Table 43.2 lists the major diagnostic findings in each of these six categories (23,24). As illustrated in Table 43.2, the diagnosis and classification of MDS are based on dysplastic features in the maturing and mature myeloid cells and/or an increase in myeloblasts in the blood and/or the bone marrow and the degree of cytopenia (23–27). In two types, refractory anemia with excess blasts 1 (RAEB-1) and refractory anemia with excess blasts 2 (RAEB-2), the principal diagnostic finding is increased blasts in the bone marrow and/or blood in addition to dysplastic features in the myeloid cells. In one type of MDS, MDS associated with an isolated del(5q) (5q– syndrome), the principal and defining feature is the presence of an isolated del(5q) cytogenetic abnormality.

The assessment of the percentage of blasts and the characterization of dysplastic features are critical for the diagnosis and classification of the MDS (23–27). For this purpose, well-prepared

Table 43.2	PERIPHERAL BLOOD AND BONE MARROW FINDINGS IN MDSs

Disease	Blood Findings	Bone Marrow Findings
Refractory cytopenias with unilineage dysplasia subtypes:	Unilineage cytopenia or bicytopenia[a]	Unilineage dysplasia: ≥10%
Refractory anemia; refractory neutropenia; refractory thrombocytopenia	No or rare blasts (<1%)[b]	<5% blasts <15% ring sideroblasts
Refractory anemia with ring sideroblasts	Anemia No blasts	≥15% ring sideroblasts Erythroid dysplasia only <5% blasts
Refractory cytopenia with multilineage dysplasia	Cytopenia(s) No or rare blasts (<1%)[b] No Auer rods <1 × 10⁹/L monocytes	Dysplasia in ≥10% of the cells in ≥2 myeloid lineages (neutrophil and/or erythroid precursors and/or megakaryocytes) <5% blasts in marrow No Auer rods 15% ring sideroblasts ±
Refractory anemia with excess blasts-1	Cytopenia(s) 2%–4% blasts[b] No Auer rods <1 × 10⁹/L monocytes	Unilineage or multilineage dysplasia 5%–9% blasts[b] No Auer rods
Refractory anemia with excess blasts-2	Cytopenia(s) 5%–19% blasts Auer rods ±[c] <1 × 10⁹/L monocytes	Unilineage or multilineage dysplasia 10%–19% blasts Auer rods ±[c]
Myelodysplastic syndrome–unclassified	Cytopenia(s) Blasts ≤1%[b]	Unequivocal dysplasia in <10% of cells in one or more myeloid cell lines <5% blasts
MDS associated with isolated del(5q)	Anemia Usually normal or increased platelet count No or rare blasts (<1%)	Normal to increased megakaryocytes with hypolobated nuclei <5% blasts Isolated del(5q) cytogenetic abnormality No Auer rods

[a]Bilineage cytopenia may occasionally be observed. Cases with pancytopenia should be classified as MDS-U.
[b]If the marrow myeloblast percentage is <5% but there are 2% to 4% myeloblasts in the blood, the diagnostic classification is RAEB-1. If the marrow myeloblast percentage is <5% and there are 1% myeloblasts in the blood, the case should be classified as MDS-U.
[c]Cases with Auer rods and <5% myeloblasts in the blood and <10% in the marrow should be classified as RAEB-2.

Table 43.3	MORPHOLOGIC MANIFESTATIONS OF DYSPLASIA

Dyserythropoiesis
  Nuclear
    Nuclear budding
    Internuclear bridging
    Karyorrhexis
    Multinuclearity
    Nuclear hyperlobation
    Megaloblastic changes
  Cytoplasmic
    Ring sideroblasts
    Vacuolization
    PAS positivity
Dysgranulopoiesis
  Small or unusually large size
  Nuclear hypolobation (pseudo–Pelger-Huët; pelgeroid)
  Irregular hypersegmentation
  Decreased granules; agranularity
  Pseudo–Chediak-Higashi granules
  Auer rods
Dysmegakaryocytopoiesis
  Micromegakaryocytes
  Nuclear hypolobation
  Multinucleation (normal megakaryocytes are uninucleate with lobulated nuclei)

and stained blood and marrow smears and/or imprints are essential. The WHO recommends a 500-cell differential of all nucleated cells on bone marrow smears or imprints and a 200-cell differential on a blood smear (24). In cases with low leukocyte counts, more than one blood smear may be necessary to achieve the required number. If marked leukopenia is present, a differential on a buffy coat smear of the blood may be necessary.

A summary of possible dysplastic characteristics in MDSs is shown in Table 43.3 (24). Guidelines for the recognition of blasts have been published (26). Characteristic blasts are illustrated in Figure 43.1.

A marrow biopsy is recommended for establishing the status of marrow cellularity, evidence of fibrosis, and cellular composition with emphasis on aggregates (3 to 5 cells) or clusters (>5 cells) of immature cells, blasts, and promyelocytes, not adjacent to vasculature or bone structures (Fig. 43.2). The presence of three or more of these focal collections in a bone marrow biopsy is referred to as abnormal localization of immature precursors (ALIP) (28). The presence of ALIP in a case has been interpreted as suggestive evidence of a high-grade MDS or AML, and the distinction determined by the blast percentage in the blood or marrow smears (24,28,29). Marrow biopsies may also provide evidence of dysplastic features in megakaryocytes, most notably micromegakaryocytes and megakaryocytes with nuclear hypolobation (Fig. 43.3).

Immunohistochemical reaction with antibody to CD34 in marrow sections may aid in identifying blasts. There is a

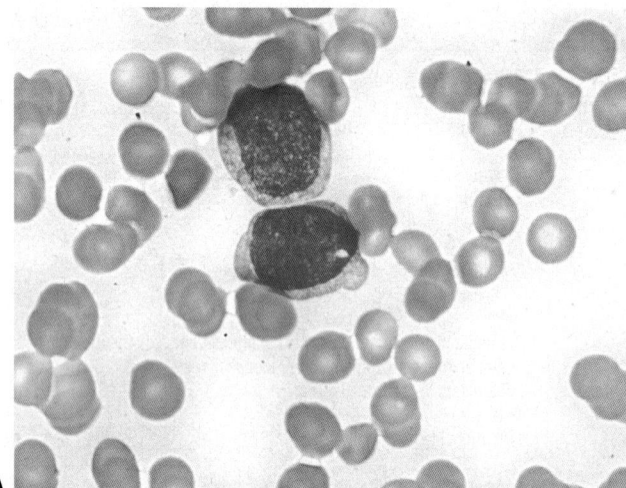

A

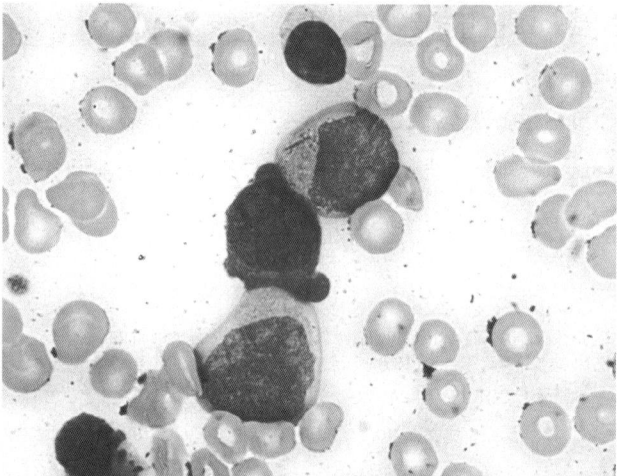

B

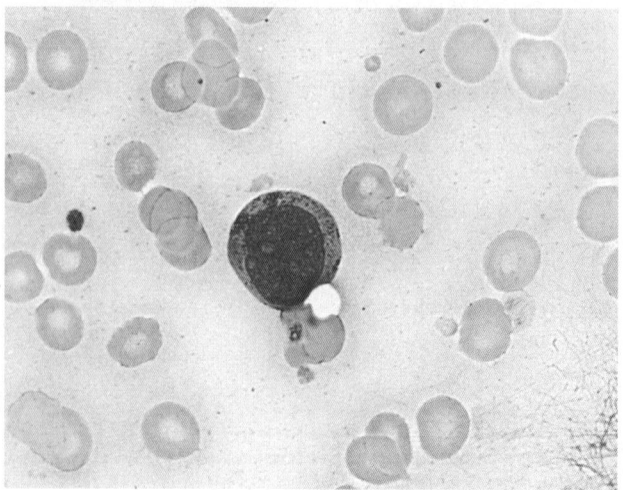

C

FIGURE 43.1. A: Two cells in a bone marrow smear from a patient with MDS. The lower cell is an agranular blast; the nucleus has fine chromatin and contains several nucleoli. The upper cell is a dysplastic neutrophil myelocyte. **B:** Bone marrow smear from a case of RAEB-2. The three cells in the center are two myeloblasts and an erythroblast. The center cell is a basophilic erythroblast; the top cell is a blast with numerous fine azurophilic granules and an Auer rod; the lower cell is an agranular myeloblast. The cell in the lower left is a micromegakaryocyte. **C:** A myeloblast with intensely basophilic cytoplasm and numerous azurophilic granules. This type of blast is distinguished from a promyelocyte by the lack of a Golgi and is included in the blast percentage in cases of MDS (**A, B, C:** Wright-Giemsa 400×).

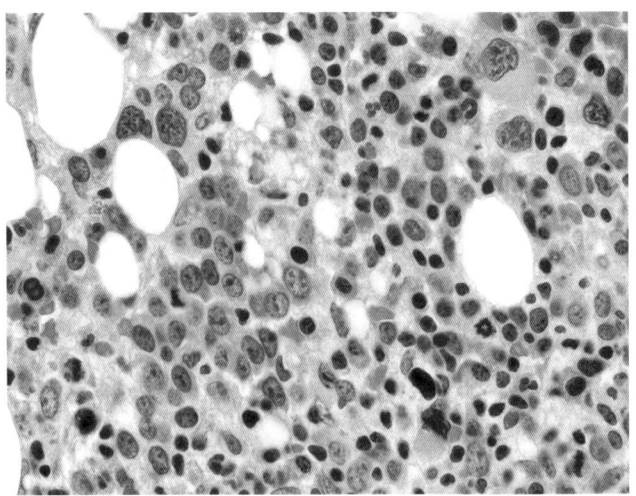

FIGURE 43.2.   Bone marrow section from a case of RAEB-2. There is a focus of very immature cells, blasts and promyelocytes. At least two other foci of immature cells not adjacent to bone trabeculae or vascular structures were found in this biopsy specimen qualifying as an ALIP. Immature cells are also diffusely scattered in the interstitium (H&E, 240×).

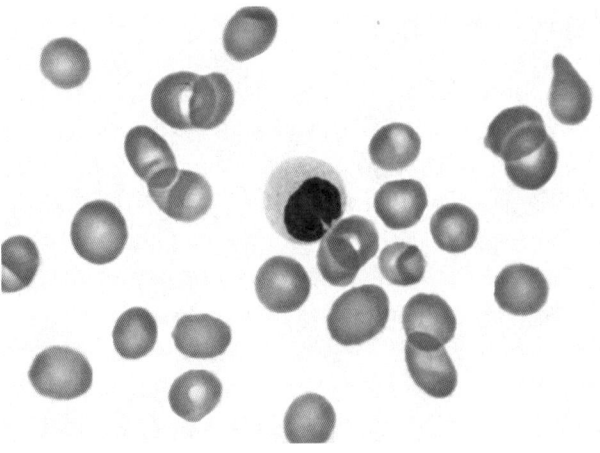

FIGURE 43.4.   Blood smear from a 68-year-old woman with RAEB-1. The blood contained numerous small neutrophils with bilobed hyperchromatic nuclei similar to this cell (Wright-Giemsa, 400×).

cautionary note in regard to this reaction in that not all myeloblasts are CD34-positive and not all CD34-positive cells in the marrow are myeloblasts; the hematogone, a normal lymphoid progenitor in the marrow, may also be reactive with anti-CD34 antibody. However, hematogones are not usually increased in the marrow of older individuals.

The initial diagnosis and classification of MDS are based on qualitative and/or quantitative alterations in the maturing and mature myeloid cells and blood and marrow blast percentages (23–27,30–33) (Table 43.2). In refractory anemia with unilineage dysplasia (RA) and RARS, the findings are essentially limited to dysplastic changes in ≥10% of the erythroid cells without an increase in blasts. Refractory cytopenia with multilineage dysplasia (RCMD) is characterized by dysplastic features in ≥10% of the cells in two or more myeloid lineages and <5% blasts in the bone marrow and no or rare blasts in the blood. The quantitative changes in MDS relate to an increase in blasts in the marrow and/or blood as found in the two high-grade MDSs: RAEB-1 and RAEB-2 (24).

Dysplastic changes in the hematopoietic cells are the hallmark of the MDSs (Table 43.3). The dysplastic features in neutrophils are characterized by deficient or aberrant granule production, and defects in nuclear segmentation manifest as nuclear hyposegmentation, pseudo–Pelger-Huët changes, ring

nucleus forms, and hypersegmentation; very unusual nuclear configurations may occur (Figs. 43.4 and 43.5). Nuclear hyposegmentation may occur in most types of MDS and is considered to be an important and readily identified diagnostic feature in a blood smear. An association between prominent nuclear hyposegmentation and small vacuolated neutrophils and del(17p) has been observed in some patients with AML and MDS (Fig. 43.6). Even in patients with MDS not associated with del(17p), dysplastic neutrophils with hypolobated nuclei are frequently smaller than normal neutrophils. Hypogranulation is also an important feature of neutrophil dysplasia but must be interpreted with caution; improperly stained smears may result in poor characterization of the neutrophil granules. If neutrophils with normal appearing granules are present on the same slide, the finding of hypogranular cells is usually reliable. If there is any doubt about the reliability of the stain, another smear should be stained with careful attention to technique.

The ultrastructural features of a neutrophil with a pseudo–Pelger-Huët nucleus and hypogranular cytoplasm are illustrated in Figure 43.7.

A less common form of neutrophil dysplasia is aggregation of granules, sometimes resembling the Chediak-Higashi anomaly.

Erythroid dysplasia is characterized by asynchronous nuclear cytoplasmic development with megaloblastoid nuclear chromatin, nuclear lobulation, increased karyorrhexis, internuclear chromatin bridging, multinucleate giant cells, and nuclear fragmentation (Figs. 43.8 to 43.10).

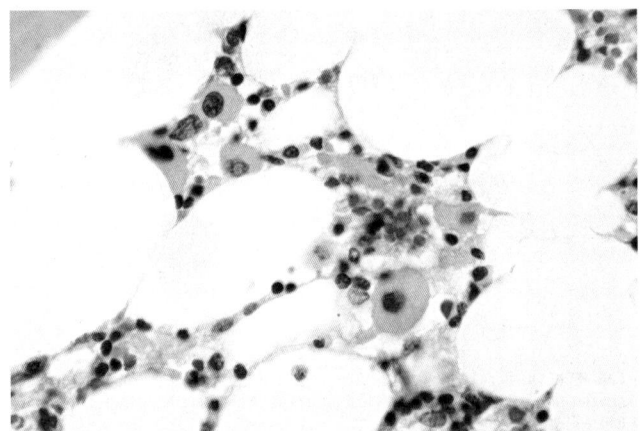

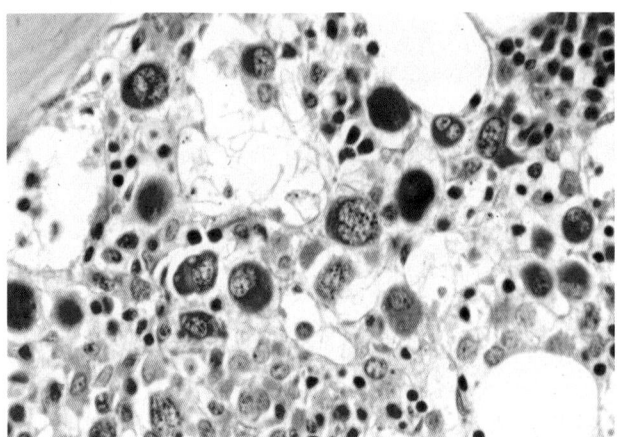

A   B

FIGURE 43.3.   A: Marrow biopsy from a patient with MDS showing several dysplastic megakaryocytes with mature nonlobated nuclei. **B:** PAS stain of a bone marrow biopsy from a case of MDS showing numerous dysplastic megakaryocytes with nonlobate nuclei (**A:** H&E; **B:** PAS, 240×).

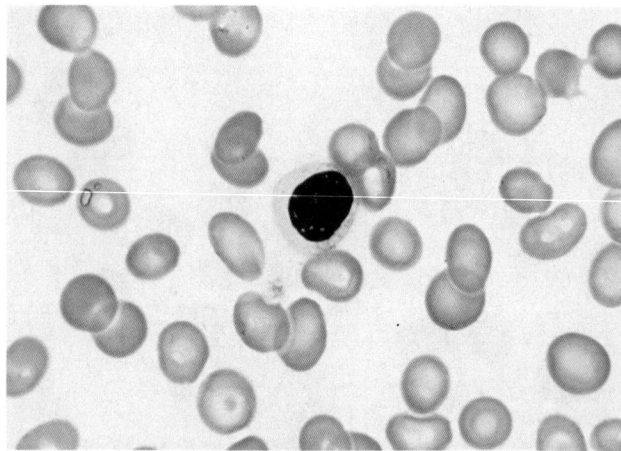

FIGURE 43.5. A blood smear from a case of MDS showing a small neutrophil with a non-lobated pseudo–Pelger-Huët nucleus. The nuclear chromatin is hyperchromatic and the cytoplasm is markedly hypogranular (Wright-Giemsa, 400×).

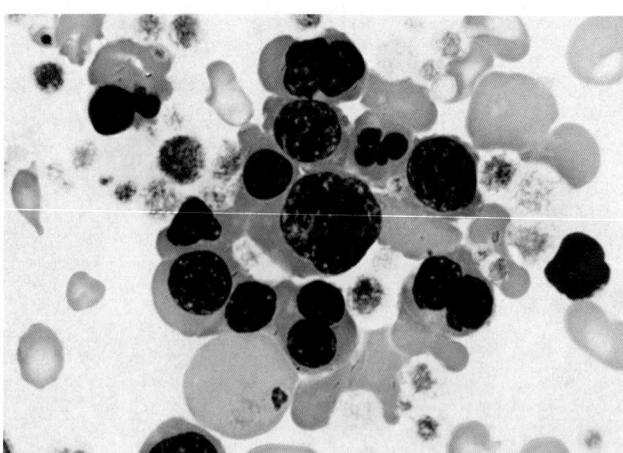

FIGURE 43.8. Bone marrow smear from a patient with an unclassified MDS showing marked dyserythropoiesis. The erythroid cells show nuclear lobulation and slightly open chromatin (Wright-Giemsa, 256×).

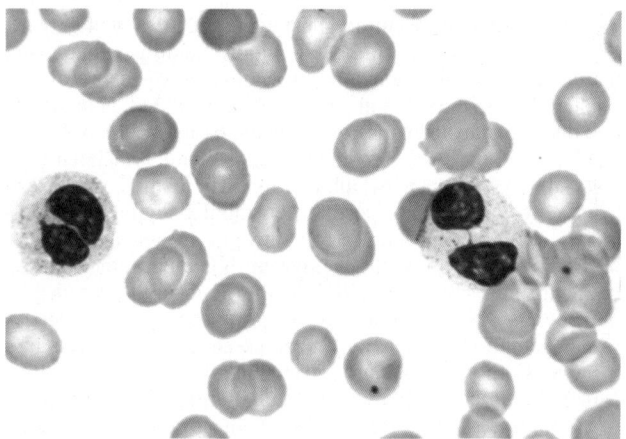

FIGURE 43.6. Two mature neutrophils with pseudo–Pelger-Huët nuclei in the blood smear of a patient who has RAEB-1 associated with del(17p). The cytoplasm contains a few vacuoles. Granulation appears normal (Wright-Giemsa, 400×).

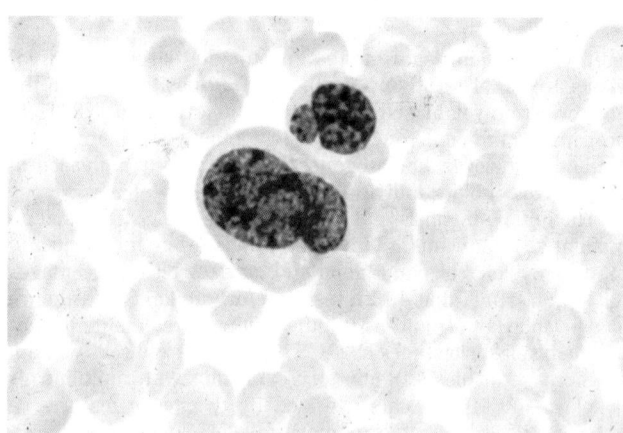

FIGURE 43.9. Two large erythroblasts in a bone marrow smear from a patient who has RA. The nucleus of the larger cell is lobated and the chromatin has the features of a megaloblast (Wright-Giemsa, 400×).

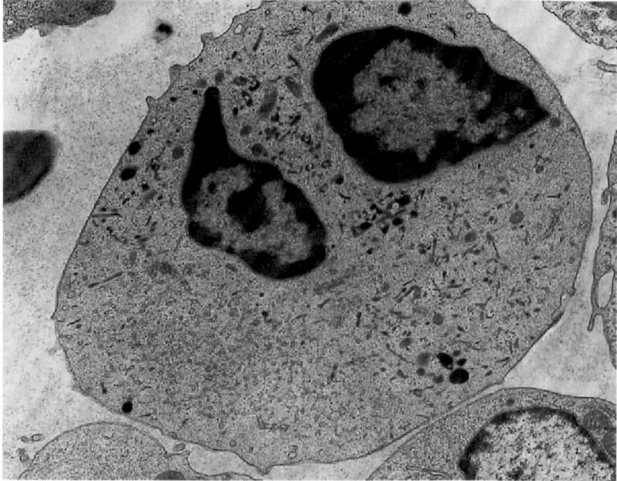

FIGURE 43.7. Electron micrograph of a mature neutrophil from the blood of a patient who has RAEB-1. There is nuclear hyposegmentation and the cytoplasm is almost devoid of primary and secondary granules (uranyl acetate-lead citrate, 20,000×).

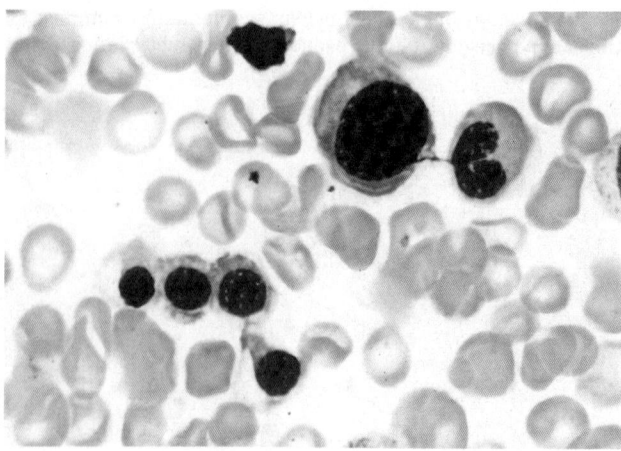

FIGURE 43.10. Bone marrow smear from a case of RA showing internuclear chromatin bridging of two unusually large erythroid precursors. The nucleus in the cell on the right is lobated (Wright-Giemsa, 400×).

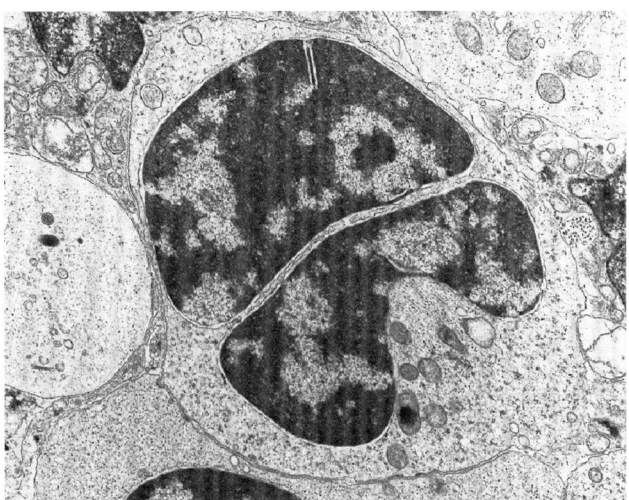

FIGURE 43.11. Electron micrograph of an erythroblast in a bone marrow specimen from a patient who has unclassified MDS. The nucleus shows a cleft and splits (uranyl acetate-lead citrate, 19,000×).

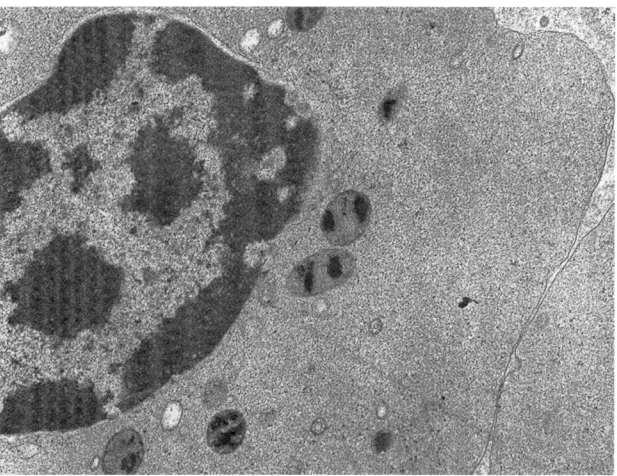

FIGURE 43.13. Ultrastructure of a portion of a ring sideroblast showing iron deposition in the mitochondria (uranyl acetate-lead citrate stain; original magnification, 40,000×).

Ultrastructural studies of the dysplastic erythroid precursors show various abnormalities including nuclear clefts and splits (Fig. 43.11).

The ring sideroblast, an erythroid precursor in which five or more iron granules encircle one-third or more of the nucleus, is a readily recognized form of erythroid dysplasia (26) (Fig. 43.12A and B). An iron stain is necessary for recognizing this feature. In routinely stained smears, the iron granules are recognized as Pappenheimer bodies. An association has been demonstrated between ring sideroblasts and *SF3B1* mutation (34). Ultrastructurally, the perinuclear iron is located in mitochondria (Fig. 43.13). The ring sideroblast may be present in all types of MDS including RAEB-1 and RAEB-2; in RAEB the blast percentage and/or the presence of Auer rods in blasts dictates the classification even if the sideroblast percentage exceeds 15% (24,35).

The erythrocytes in the blood in MDS of all types frequently show increased anisocytosis with oval macrocytes and some degree of poikilocytosis; this is reflected by an elevated MCV.

Megakaryocytic dysplasia is characterized by abnormally small megakaryocytes; micromegakaryocytes, with nonlobate or bilobed nuclei; binucleate or multinucleate megakaryocytes; and unusually large megakaryocytes with nonlobate nuclei and finely dispersed chromatin (Fig. 43.14). Megakaryocytic dysplasia is frequently more evident in bone marrow sections than in smears (Fig. 43.3). Ultrastructural studies of megakaryocytes from patients with MDS frequently show nuclear and cytoplasmic abnormalities (Fig. 43.15). Atypical, large agranular platelets may be present in blood smears; these may also be found in some of the myeloproliferative neoplasms (MPN) particularly in the accelerated phase and are not diagnostic of MDS.

The dysplastic changes in the myeloid cells may be restricted to one cell lineage such as the red blood cells, and precursors in refractory anemia (RA) or RARS, unilineage dysplasia MDS, or the dysplasia may be present in two or more myeloid cell lineages, multilineage dysplasia MDS.

Cytopenia(s) is usually the presenting manifestation of the MDSs. One cell lineage may be decreased, unilineage cytopenia, or all the cell lineages may be decreased, pancytopenia. The recommended thresholds for cytopenias in the WHO Classification are those used by the IPSS for risk stratification: hemoglobin <10 g/dL, neutrophils <1.8 × 10⁹/L, and platelets

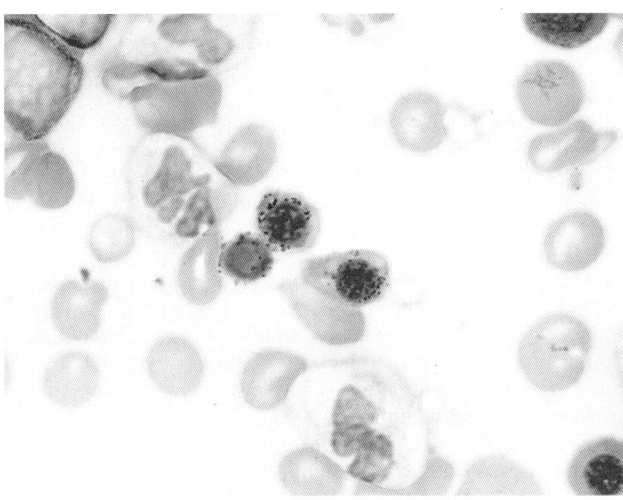

A

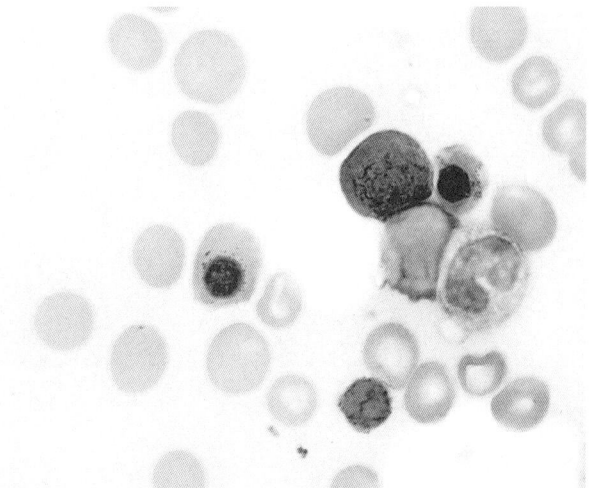

B

FIGURE 43.12. **A:** Three ring sideroblasts in a bone marrow smear stained for iron from a case of RARS. There are numerous iron-staining granules encircling the entire circumference of the nucleus in all three cells. There is a portion of another ring sideroblast in the lower right. Two anucleate red blood cells on the right contain numerous iron granules. **B:** The same specimen as (**A**) with three red blood cell precursors with fewer iron granules than the cells in (**A**) but which still qualify as ring sideroblasts (**A** and **B:** iron stain counterstained with safranin, 400×).

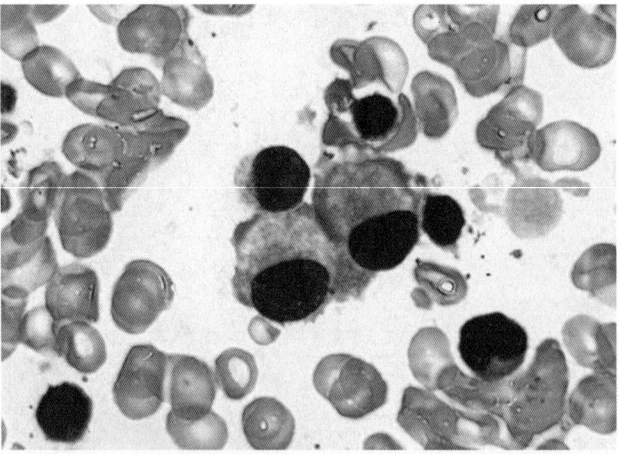

FIGURE 43.14. Three dysplastic small megakaryocytes in a bone marrow smear from a patient with MDS. The nuclear chromatin is mature, but the nuclei are nonlobated (Wright-Giemsa, 400×).

Table 43.4	SUMMARY OF CYTOPENIAS AND DYSPLASIA CHARACTERISTICS IN NONBLASTIC MDS	
Cytopenia(s)	**Dysplasia**	**Categories**
Unilineage	Unilineage	Refractory cytopenia with unilineage
Bilineage		Dysplasia
		Refractory anemia
		Refractory neutropenia (RN)
		Refractory thrombocytopenia (RT)
Unilineage Bilineage	Unilineage and ≥15% ring sideroblasts	Refractory anemia with ring sideroblasts
Pancytopenia	Unilineage	Myelodysplastic syndrome—unclassified
Unilineage Bilineage Pancytopenia	Multilineage (≥2 myeloid cells lines)	Refractory cytopenia with multilineage dysplasia
Unilineage Bilineage Pancytopenia	Multilineage and ≥15% ring sideroblasts	Refractory cytopenia with multilineage dysplasia with ring sideroblasts

<100 × 10⁹/L (36). Table 43.4 illustrates the possible combinations of cytopenias and dysplasia, which may occur in the various types of MDS.

A recommendation using various combinations of cytopenia and lineage dysplasia has been proposed for improving the prognostic significance of the WHO nonblastic group of MDSs (38). In this proposal, the occurrence of unicytopenia and dysplasia ≥10% in one lineage (unicytopenia and unilineage cysplasia) constitutes a low-risk category MDS; the presence of cytopenias in ≥2 lineages and dysplasia ≥10% in ≥2 lineages (multilineage cytopenia and multilineage dysplasia) constitutes a high-risk category MDS. The presence of unicytopenia and dysplasia ≥10% in ≥2 cell lineages (unicytopenia and multilineage dysplasia) or cytopenias in ≥2 cell lineages and unilineage dysplasia (multilineage cytopenia/unilineage dysplasia) identifies an intermediate-risk category MDS (38). The thresholds for cytopenias in the recommendations in the proposal cited differ from the WHO and IPSS: Hgb <13.5 g/dL for men and 11.5 g/dL for women, leukocyte count <3.5 × 10⁹/L, and platelet count <135 × 10⁹/L (38). The total leukocyte count is used by this group rather than the neutrophil count.

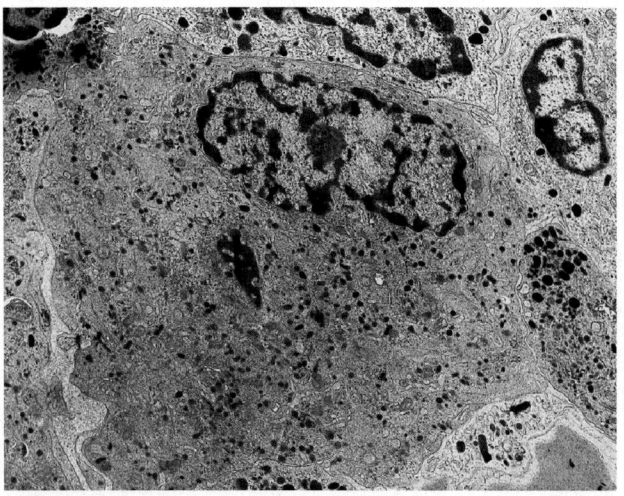

FIGURE 43.15. Electron micrograph of a small megakaryocyte in a bone marrow specimen from a patient who has RAEB-1. The abundant cytoplasm shows decreased granule formation (uranyl acetate–lead citrate stain; original magnification, 8,000×).

The WHO Classification of the MDS incorporates many of the features of the FAB classification of MDS, the initial classification of MDS (31–33). There are several important differences. The WHO separates the FAB classification of RA into RCUD based on the presence of dysplasia in ≥10% of one myeloid lineage and RCMD based on the presence of ≥10% dysplastic cells in two or more myeloid lineages. RCUD is further divided into three subtypes: refractory anemia (RA), refractory neutropenia (RN), and refractory thrombocytopenia (RT). The distinction of cases with unilineage dysplasia and multilineage dysplasia has been found to have prognostic significance (39–41).

The 1985 FAB classification threshold for a diagnosis of AML is 30% blasts in the bone marrow and/or blood (32). The WHO recommends a threshold of ≥20% blasts in the marrow and/or blood for a diagnosis of AML, thereby eliminating the FAB MDS classification of refractory anemia with excess of blasts in transformation (RAEB-T) (23,24,32). The rationale for this recommendation was put forward by a group of authors from the WHO MDS committee making the recommendation (23). This change has been controversial, and the issue is not completely resolved, but an increasing number of groups are using the WHO MDS classification.

The third major difference between the WHO and FAB classifications is the inclusion of MDS with isolated del(5q) (5q– syndrome) as a specific type of MDS in the WHO Classification. The WHO restricts the definition of MDS with isolated del(5q) to cases of MDS with the del(5q) as the sole cytogenetic abnormality and <5% blasts in the marrow (23,24). The recognition of the MDS with isolated del(5q) as a specific type of MDS has received wide acceptance. Studies have demonstrated a favorable clinical response of these patients to lenalidomide and superior survival times (42). Patients with del(5q) and one other cytogenetic abnormality also have a very favorable response to lenalidomide.

The fourth major change from the FAB in the WHO Classification was the displacement of chronic myelomonocytic leukemia (CMML) from the MDS category to an overlap classification of myeloid disorders, myelodysplastic/myeloproliferative neoplasms (MDS/MPN), a group of diseases, which share features of both an MDS and a myeloproliferative disorder. This category also includes atypical chronic myeloid leukemia,

Prognostic Variable	0	0.5	1.0	1.5	2	3	4
Table 43.5A INTERNATIONAL PROGNOSTIC SCORING SYSTEM—REVISED (37)							
Cytogenetics	Very good	—	Good	—	Intermediate	Poor	Very poor
BM blast, %	≤2	—	>2%–<5%	—	5%–10%	>10%	—
Hemoglobin	≥10	—	8–<10	<8	—	—	—
Platelets	≥100	50–<100	<50	—	—	—	—
ANC	≥0.8	<0.8	—	—	—	—	—

— indicates not applicable.

juvenile myelomonocytic leukemia, and myelodysplastic/myeloproliferative neoplasms–unclassified (MDS/MPN-U). These entities are discussed in Chapter 46.

As reflected in both the FAB and WHO Classification schemes of MDS, the MDSs are a morphologically heterogeneous group of disorders. This is also reflected in the biologic behavior of these diseases, which manifest considerable variability in the rate of progression and leukemic transformation (1–3). RAEB has a high rate of leukemic transformation in contrast to RARS, which has a low rate of transformation and disease progression. In an attempt to more accurately predict the clinical course of the disease, several scoring systems based on both clinical and laboratory features have been proposed. The most widely recognized of these is the IPSS, which incorporates several laboratory findings to arrive at risk levels (36,37). A revised IPSS system (IPSS-R) for improving prognostic scoring in patients with MDS was introduced in 2012; the IPSS-R includes several refinements of the 1997 IPSS. The number of cytogenetic categories is expanded from four to five. In addition, the IPSS-R includes new marrow blast categories, evaluation of depth of cytopenias, inclusion of differentiating features including age, performance status, serum ferritin, LDH, serum B2-microglobulin, and a prognostic model with five risk categories (37) (Tables 43.5A,B).

As will be noted in the section on molecular studies, this approach is beginning to yield meaningful data.

CLASSIFICATION

Refractory Cytopenia

In the WHO 2008 Classification, refractory cytopenia (RC) is a type of low-grade MDS in which the dysplasia is essentially restricted to one cell lineage (24,43). The peripheral blood may manifest either unilineage cytopenia, the more common finding, or bilineage cytopenia (Tables 43.2 and 43.4).

Three types of RC are recognized:
Refractory anemia
Refractory neutropenia
Refractory thrombocytopenia

Risk Category	Risk Score
Table 43.5B IPSS-R PROGNOSTIC RISK CATEGORIES/SCORES	
Very low	≤1.5
Low	>1.5–3
Intermediate	>3–4.5
High	>4.5–6
Very high	>6

From Greenberg P, Tuechler H, Schanz, et al. Revised international prognostic scoring system for myelodysplastic syndromes. *Blood* 2012;120:2454–2465.

Refractory Anemia

RA is characterized by a persistent anemia, more than 6-month duration, refractory to hematinic therapy, and for which no etiologic basis can be identified. The red blood cells are usually normochromic macrocytic but may be normochromic normocytic. The degree of red blood cell anisocytosis varies and may be marked (Fig. 43.16). There is frequently an elevated MCV reflecting the macrocytosis observed in the blood smear. The platelet and neutrophil counts are essentially normal; occasional patients may have an accompanying slight neutropenia or thrombocytopenia, bilineage cytopenia (Table 43.4). Blasts are rare or not identified in the peripheral blood. If a rare blast is identified in the blood, the diagnosis should be considered qualified and close follow-up of hematologic findings is recommended. If 1% blasts are present in the blood of a patient who otherwise appears to have a form of RC, the case should be classified as MDS-U because of the uncertain significance of the finding.

The bone marrow is usually hypercellular. The blasts are <5%, usually 1% to 2%. The number of erythroid precursors varies from marked erythroid hypoplasia to hyperplasia; erythroid hyperplasia is the predominant pattern. Some degree of dyserythropoiesis, ≥10%, is present; dysplastic changes include megaloblastoid nuclei, nuclear lobation, multinucleation, internuclear chromatin bridging, and nuclear fragmentation (Table 43.3; Figs. 43.9 and 43.17). Dysplastic changes are restricted to the erythroid series. Ring sideroblasts may be present, but they constitute <15% of the nucleated erythroid precursors (24). The bone marrow biopsy in the majority of cases of RA is hypercellular, usually with erythroid hyperplasia; in some instances, as noted, there is marked erythroid hyperplasia. Neutrophils and megakaryocytes are normal or may be slightly increased. In approximately 10% to 15% of

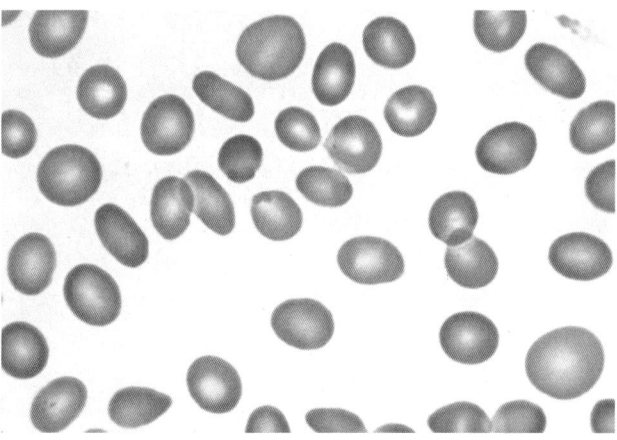

FIGURE 43.16. Blood smear from a patient with RA. There is considerable red blood cell anisocytosis with several macrocytes; there is also some poikilocytosis with elliptocytes and dacryocytes (Wright-Giemsa, 400×).

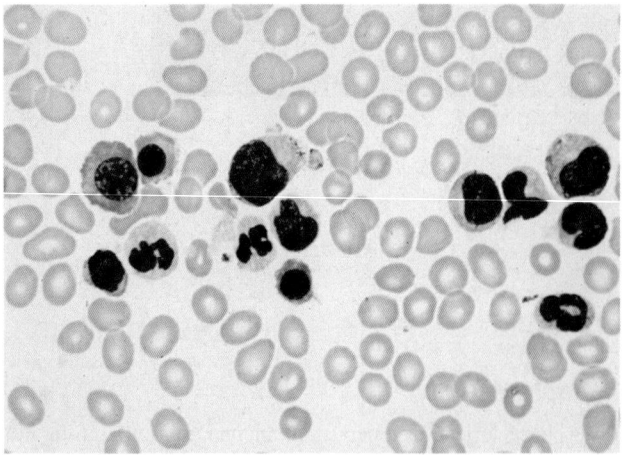

FIGURE 43.17. Bone marrow smear from a patient with RA. One of the erythroid precursors on the left has a slightly megaloblastoid nuclear structure (Wright-Giemsa, 240×).

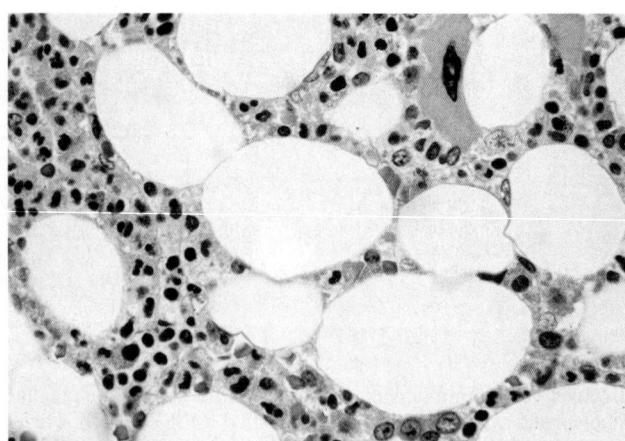

FIGURE 43.18. Bone marrow section from a patient with RA. The marrow is hypocellular (H&E, 240×).

cases, the marrow is hypocellular (Fig. 43.18). This finding is more common in older individuals.

Refractory Neutropenia

RN is a very uncommon MDS characterized by persistent, six months or more, neutropenia (<1.8 × 10⁹/L) without concurrent anemia or thrombocytopenia; ≥10% of the neutrophils and precursors in the blood and/or marrow show dysplastic changes manifest as nuclear hyposegmentation and/or abnormal hypersegmentation and hypogranulation. Other forms of nuclear abnormalities including hyperlobulation and ring forms may be present (Table 43.3; Figs. 43.4 and 43.5). Dysplastic changes are not present in the other myeloid cell lines.

Neutropenia secondary to drugs, toxins, infections, and immune reactions must be excluded before this diagnosis is invoked. Careful follow-up is important in these cases both for additional findings of a progressive MDS or evidence of a non-hematologic basis for the neutropenia.

Refractory Thrombocytopenia

RT, similar to RN, is a very unusual form of MDS characterized by persistent thrombocytopenia (<100 × 10⁹/L) and ≥10% dysplastic megakaryocytes of at least 30 megakaryocytes evaluated in marrow smears and/or sections. The dysplastic megakaryocytes may be more evident in the sections than in the smears. Megakaryocytes with nonlobate or bilobate nuclei and multinucleation and micromegakaryocytes are the most reliable and reproducible features of megakaryocytic dysplasia (Fig. 43.19). The other myeloid cell lines show no significant (<10%) dysplasia.

Distinction of RT of MDS origin from chronic immune thrombocytopenia is critical and may be very difficult; there may be considerable differences in what constitutes dysplasia between different observers, and this may lead to difficulty when comparing studies. As noted, nonlobate nuclei, binucleate or multinucleate megakaryocytes, and micromegakaryocytes are the most reliable characteristics of dysplasia. Immune thrombocytopenia is frequently accompanied by megakaryocyte hyperplasia, but the megakaryocytes should not manifest dysplastic changes. Cytogenetic studies may be useful in recognizing MDS-related thrombocytopenia in difficult cases.

Refractory Anemia with Ring Sideroblasts

RARS is a type of MDS characterized by anemia and the presence of ≥15% ring sideroblasts in the marrow (24,35,44). The hemoglobin level in RARS generally is in the range of 9 to 12 g/dL; lower levels may be present. The red blood cells may be dimorphic (anisochromic) with populations of both

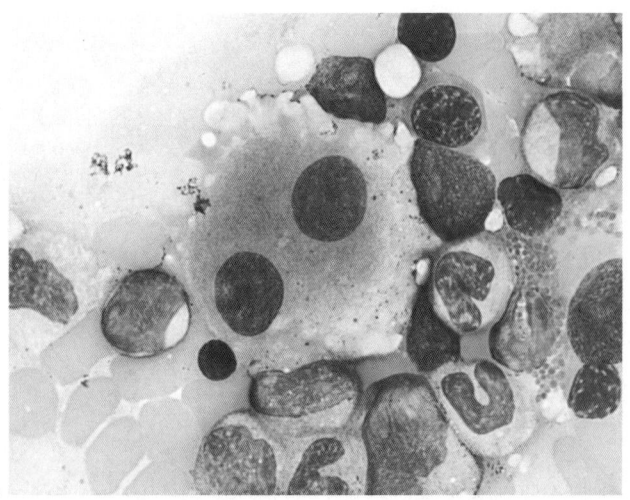

A

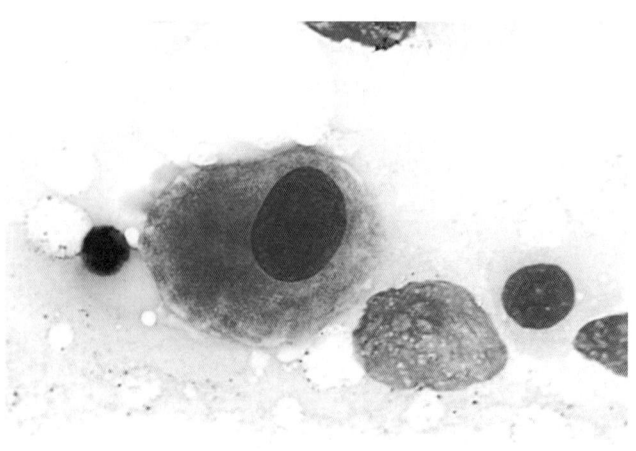

B

FIGURE 43.19. A: Binucleate mature megakaryocyte in the marrow smear from a patient with RT. The cytoplasm is well granulated. **B:** Same specimen as (**A**) showing a mature megakaryocyte with a nonlobate nucleus (**A** and **B:** Wright-Giemsa, 400×).

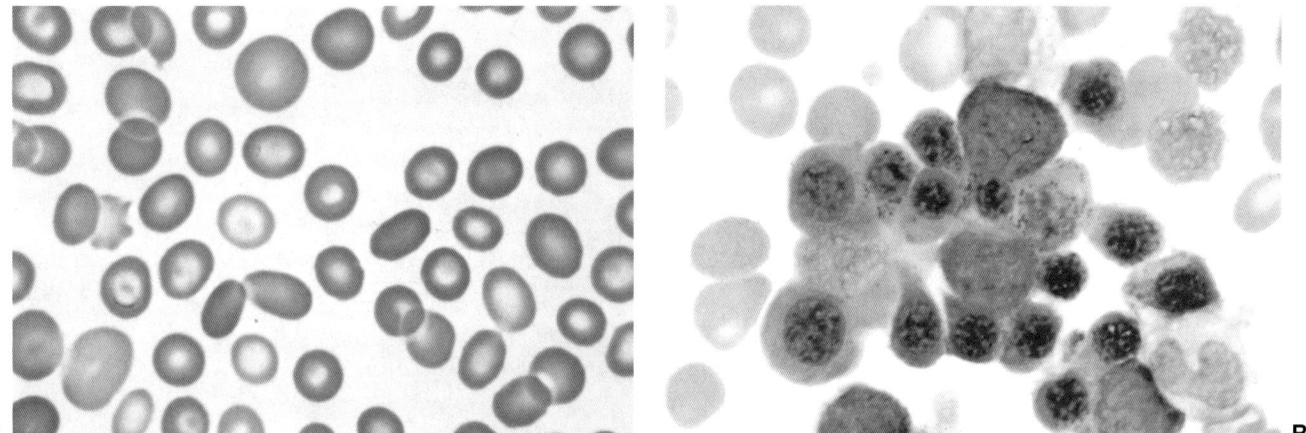

FIGURE 43.20. A: Blood smear from a patient with RARS showing a dimorphic red blood cell population with the major population normochromic and a small number of hypochromic cells. There is anisocytosis with a few macrocytes. **B:** Bone marrow smear from a patient with RARS reacted for iron. There are several ring sideroblasts present in this smear (**A:** Wright-Giemsa, 400×, **B:** iron stain with safranin counterstain, 400×).

normochromic cells and hypochromic cells; in some instances, the red blood cells are normochromic macrocytic or normochromic normocytic (Fig. 43.20A and B). Pappenheimer bodies, iron granules in a Romanowsky stained film, may be present in occasional red blood cells. The platelets and neutrophils are usually normal in number and appearance. The bone marrow shows erythroid hyperplasia, frequently marked with variable but usually minor degrees of dyserythropoiesis; in occasional cases, prominent dyserythropoiesis with megaloblastoid features is present. In smears stained for iron, ≥15% of the erythroid precursors are ring (type III) sideroblasts, erythroblasts in which the nucleus is partially or completely encircled by five or more granules of iron (26,35,44,45) (Fig. 43.12). On ultrastructural examination, the perinuclear iron is present in the mitochondria (Fig. 43.13). Granulopoiesis and megakaryocytopoiesis are normal in the majority of cases. If significant dysplasia (>10%) is present in the granulocytes and/or megakaryocytes, the case should be classified as refractory cytopenia with multilineage dysplasia with ring sideroblasts (RCMD-RS).

Serum iron and ferritin levels are usually increased. The bone marrow biopsy shows a hypercellular marrow with prominent erythroid hyperplasia reflecting the findings in the smears. Megakaryocytes and granulocytes appear to be morphologically and numerically normal. Bone marrow sections stained for iron usually show numerous iron-laden macrophages. Ring sideroblasts may be identified in very well-prepared sections, but this finding is less readily appreciated and less reliable than in smear or imprint preparations.

Sideroblastic anemia occurs in two forms: an MDS with an essentially normal life span or an MDS with eventual evolution to a higher-grade MDS or AML (46–48). The majority of cases of RARS anemia appears to belong to the first category since only approximately 7% to 10% of patients with RARS develop AML. The morphologic features at initial diagnosis may reflect the potential for the more aggressive lesion in that multilineage dysplasia is an indication that the disorder is not solely restricted to the erythroid series with a disturbance in iron metabolism. In recognition of this, cases of RARS should receive careful morphologic scrutiny for abnormalities in the granulocytic and megakaryocytic lineages; if either of these lineages is involved in addition to the erythroid, the findings should be designated as RCMD-RS. Cases with dysplasia only in the erythroid cells should be diagnosed as RARS. This is not meant to imply that cases of sideroblastic anemia with unilineage dysplasia may not evolve to a higher-grade MDS or AML but that the

potential is higher for those cases with recognizable abnormalities in granulocytes and megakaryocytes. The presence of cytogenetic abnormalities would indicate a more aggressive course.

Rarely a patient presents with the findings of RARS and no or a minimal increase in blasts (<5%) in the marrow and a rare blast with an Auer rod. These cases should be classified as RAEB-2 on the basis of the detection of the Auer rod(s) (24).

A correlation between mutations in the *SF3B1* gene and ring sideroblasts has been identified (34). This is discussed in the section on Molecular Genetics.

Refractory Cytopenia with Multilineage Dysplasia

Cases of MDS may present with cytopenia(s) and evidence of multilineage dysplasia without an increase in marrow blasts (<5%) and blood or marrow monocytes and no blasts with Auer rods (49–51). Frequently there is a bilineal cytopenia or pancytopenia. The term RCMD was introduced to recognize these cases, and this entity was initially recognized by the WHO in the 2000 Classification of the MDSs. MDSs with similar findings have also been reported as RA with severe dysplasia (52).

RCMD is characterized by dysplasia in two or more myeloid cell lineages, frequently all myeloid cell types; the degree of dysplasia may be marked. The WHO recommends identifying ≥10% dysplastic cells in two or more myeloid lineages (erythroid, granulocytic, megakaryocytic) to qualify for a diagnosis of RCMD.

In some cases of RCMD, one cell lineage, such as the erythroid, is markedly increased with dysplastic changes and is the predominant finding; however, ≥10% of the cells in a second lineage must also be dysplastic. The percent of dysplastic cells in a lineage should be assessed by evaluating 200 neutrophils and precursors in blood and/or marrow smears and 200 erythroid precursors in marrow smears. Megakaryocyte dysplasia should be assessed by evaluating 30 or more megakaryocytes in marrow smears and/or sections. The type and degree of dysplastic change varies substantially from case to case (Fig. 43.21A and B).

In RCMD, there is no or only a slight increase in myeloblasts in the bone marrow; if increased, the number of blasts is <5%. If the blast count exceeds 5% in the marrow, the case should be classified as RAEB-1 or RAEB-2 depending on the blast percentage. Blasts are not usually present in the peripheral blood in RCMD. If 1% blasts are present in the blood, the case should be classified as MDS-U because of the uncertain significance

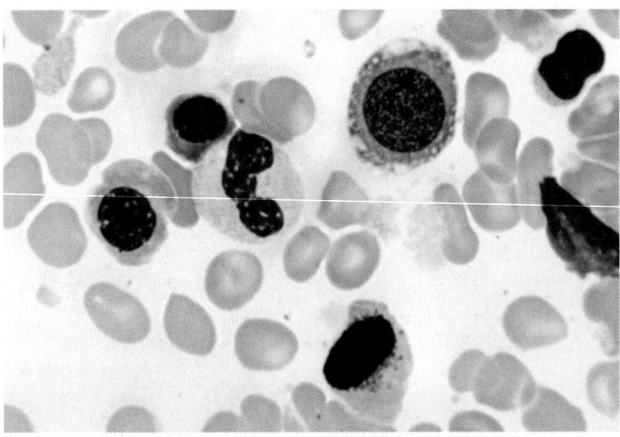
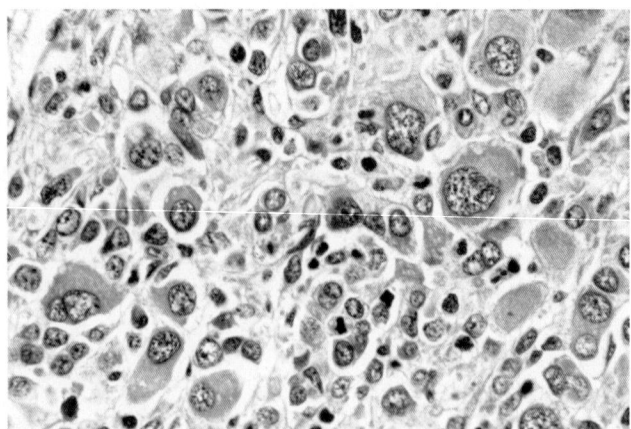

FIGURE 43.21. A: Bone marrow smear from a 38-year-old male with RCMD. A basophilic erythroblast with a megaloblastic nucleus and cytoplasmic vacuoles and a polychromatic erythroid precursor with numerous Pappenheimer bodies encircling the nucleus (ring sideroblast) are present. The blasts were <2%. Cytogenetic analysis of this specimen showed complex abnormalities including deletion of chromosomes 5 and 7. **B:** Bone marrow biopsy from the same specimen as illustrated in (**A**). There is a marked increase in megakaryocytes with dysplastic features including small size and hypolobulated nuclei. This patient had a rapidly progressive clinical course following failure of an allogeneic bone marrow transplant (**A:** Wright-Giemsa, 400×; **B:** H&E, 240×).

of this finding. If 2% to 4% blasts are present in the blood, the case should be classified as RAEB-1.

Ring sideroblasts may be present and exceed 15% of the erythroid precursors; these cases should be designated RCMD-RS.

The bone marrow biopsy in RCMD is usually hypercellular with bilineage or trilineage dysplasia; essentially, the findings resemble RAEB but without an increase in blasts.

The bone marrow biopsies may be particularly useful in recognizing the abnormalities in megakaryocytes, particularly micromegakaryocytes and megakaryocytes with hypolobated nuclei (Fig. 43.3). The identification of dysplastic megakaryocytes may be facilitated with immunohistochemical reactions with antibodies to megakaryocyte antigens such as CD41 and CD61 and with the periodic acid–Schiff (PAS) reaction (Fig. 43.3B).

The alkylating agent type of therapy related MDS frequently has the morphologic features of RCMD, as do some of the cases of MDS associated with the del(20q–) chromosome abnormality in which both the megakaryocytes and erythroid precursors may show morphologic abnormalities (4).

Modifications of the WHO recommendation for the diagnosis of RCMD based on a study of a series of Japanese and German patients have been proposed (53). These studies demonstrated that a threshold of 40% for megakaryocyte dysplasia was more predictive of survival than the threshold of 10% the WHO currently recommends. In the same study, the combination of ≥10% neutrophils with pseudo–Pelger-Huët changes, ≥10% micromegakaryocytes, ≥10% dysgranulopoiesis, and ≥40% dysmegakaryocytopoiesis was unfavorable for leukemic transformation and overall survival (53).

Refractory Anemia with Excess of Blasts

The defining criteria for RAEB are 5% to 19% blasts in the bone marrow and/or 2% to 19% blasts in the blood (24,31,54) (Table 43.2). Based on data from the International MDS Risk Analysis Workshop, which showed different survival data for patients with 5% to 10% blasts and 11% to 20% blasts in the marrow, RAEB is divided by the WHO into RAEB-1 with 5% to 9% blasts in the bone marrow and <5% blasts in the blood and RAEB-2 with 10% to 19% blasts in the bone marrow and/or 5% to 19% blasts in the blood (24,54). Two to four percent blasts in the blood in a case with <5% blasts in the marrow qualify

for a diagnosis of RAEB-1. Five to nineteen percent blasts in the blood qualify a case as RAEB-2 even if the marrow blast percentage is <10%. In these instances, which are distinctly uncommon, the blast percentage in the blood dictates the classification. In many cases of RAEB, the increase in blasts is accompanied by an increase in promyelocytes. The criteria for RAEB-1 and RAEB-2 are summarized in Table 43.2.

Anemia is present in virtually all patients with RAEB-1 and RAEB-2; the red blood cells are normochromic normocytic or normochromic macrocytic. Increased anisocytosis including macroovalocytes is noted in a high percentage of cases (Fig. 43.22). Nucleated red blood cells may be present. The majority of patients also present with neutropenia and thrombocytopenia, a pancytopenia. Neutrophil abnormalities include nuclear hyposegmentation, pseudo–Pelger-Huët nuclei, and nuclear hyperlobulation; abnormalities of granulation such as hypogranulation generally are present and frequently are marked (Figs. 43.22 and 43.23). Aggregates of granules that resemble the hereditary Chediak-Higashi anomaly may be present but are much less frequent than hypogranulation. Immature neutrophils usually are present in the blood, and basophilia is present in some patients. Atypical platelets and micromegakaryocytes may be noted.

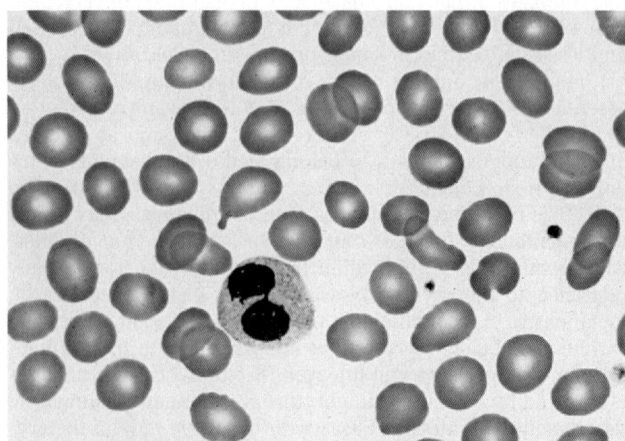

FIGURE 43.22. Blood smear showing a mature neutrophil with a bilobed, pseudo–Pelger-Huët nucleus from a man with RAEB-1 (Wright-Giemsa, 400×).

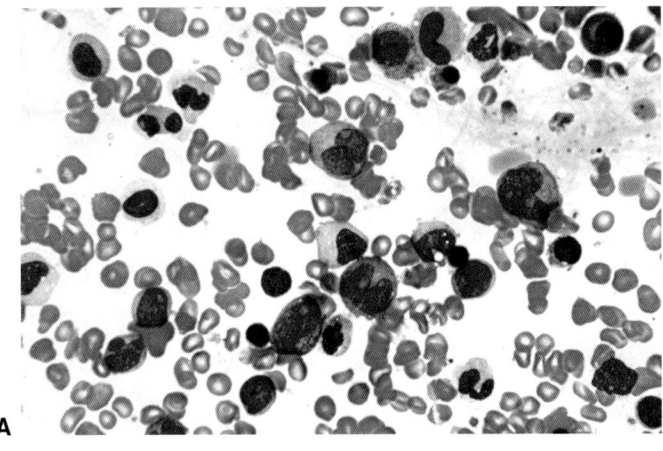

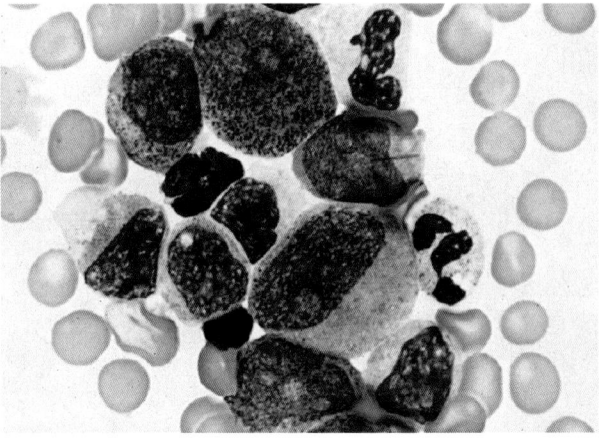

A

B

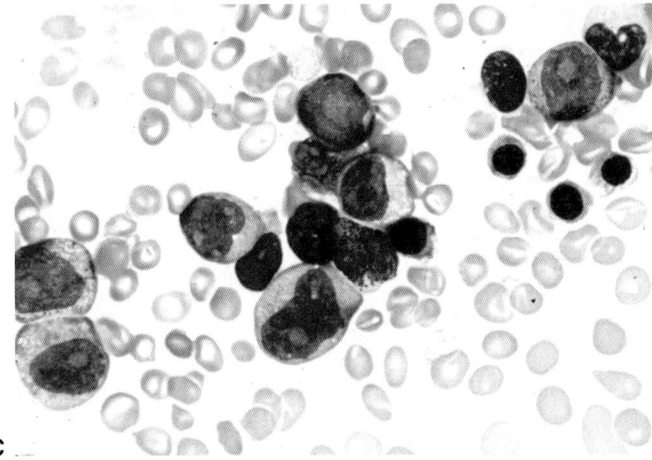

C

FIGURE 43.23. A: Bone marrow smear from a case of RAEB-2 showing several blasts both nongranulated and granulated. **B:** Bone marrow smear from a case classified as RAEB-2 with 8% marrow blasts and occasional blasts with an Auer rod, which served as the basis for the classification. **C:** Bone marrow smear from a case of RAEB-2. There are three myeloblasts and three promyelocytes (**A** and **C**: Wright Giemsa, 240×; **B**: Wright-Giemsa, 400×).

The blast percentage in the marrow should be determined from a differential of 500 nucleated cells. The morphologic characteristics of the cells, which should be included in the blast category, are illustrated in Figure 43.1 (26). The increase in blasts is frequently accompanied by an increase in promyelocytes (Fig. 43.23).

Abnormalities of nuclear and cytoplasmic development may be present in all the myeloid cell lines in the marrow in RAEB. Erythroid abnormalities include megaloblastoid nuclei, nuclear lobation, karyorrhexis, and multinucleation. Ring sideroblasts may be present and may exceed 15% of the nucleated red blood cells (35). However, the increase in blasts and/or the presence of Auer rods dictates the classification (Table 43.2).

The significance of Auer rods in cases of MDS is somewhat controversial. In one study, MDS cases with Auer rods had a more favorable clinical course than cases without Auer rods (55). In another study focused on patients with MDS with blast percentages of <5% in the marrow but in which blasts with Auer rods were detected, that is, RAEB-2 by virtue of the presence of Auer rods but not by marrow blast percentage, there was a relatively aggressive clinical course (56). Cases with blasts with Auer rods and <5% blasts in the blood and <10% in the marrow are classified as RAEB-2 in the WHO Classification (24,54) (Fig. 43.23). Dysplastic neutrophils and precursors and micromegakaryocytes and megakaryocytes with nonlobated nuclei may be numerous.

As noted previously in the section on RARS, a rare case of MDS presents with a low marrow blast percentage, <5%, and ≥15% ring sideroblasts, and a rare blast with an Auer rod (56). These cases should be classified as RAEB-2 (Fig. 43.24A–C).

The bone marrow section in the majority of patients is hypercellular with a panmyeloid hyperplasia; in 10% to 20% of patients, the bone marrow is normocellular or hypocellular (Fig. 43.25A). The number of blasts in the sections usually corresponds to the smear or biopsy imprint differential. In some patients, ALIP may be noted (28,29) (Fig. 43.2). Abnormal megakaryocytes, particularly small megakaryocytes and micromegakaryocytes with nuclear hypolobation, may be more apparent in the bone marrow sections than in smears; these cells are accentuated with the PAS stain and immunohistochemical reactions with antimegakaryocyte antibodies such as anti-CD41, anti-CD61, and factor VIII antibody (Fig. 43.3B).

A slight degree of reticulin fibrosis is present in the bone marrow in a minority of patients. Marked fibrosis is not common but may occur.

In patients with hypocellular bone marrows, the distinction of MDS from aplastic anemia may be aided by immunohistochemical reactions for CD34 and proliferating cell nuclear antigen; positive reactions for these antigens are more compatible with MDS than with aplastic anemia (Fig. 43.25B).

MDS with Isolated del(5q);(5q– Syndrome)

The MDS with isolated del(5q) occurs in adults with a female predominance. The association between the cytogenetic abnormality and the clinical syndrome was first described by Van den Berghe et al. in 1974; the blood findings are usually those of a refractory macrocytic anemia, frequently marked, and a normal to increased platelet count (57–63). The leukocyte count is usually normal to slightly increased. Blasts should not be present in the blood.

The bone marrow is hypocellular in approximately 20% of cases, normocellular in 40%, and hypercellular in 40% (63). In the WHO definition of MDS with isolated del(5q), the marrow blast percentage is <5% (24,60). The megakaryocytes are usually normal to increased and show characteristic dysplastic

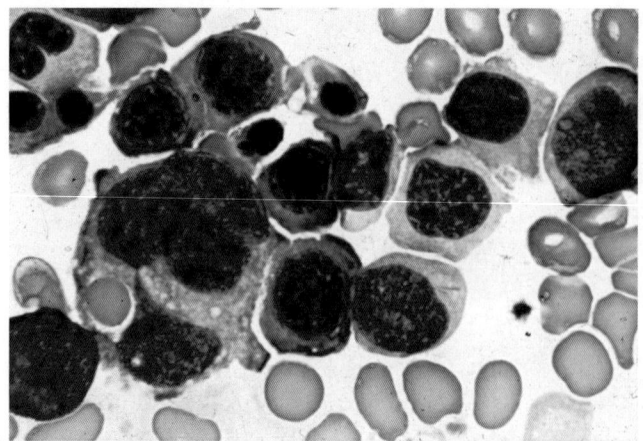
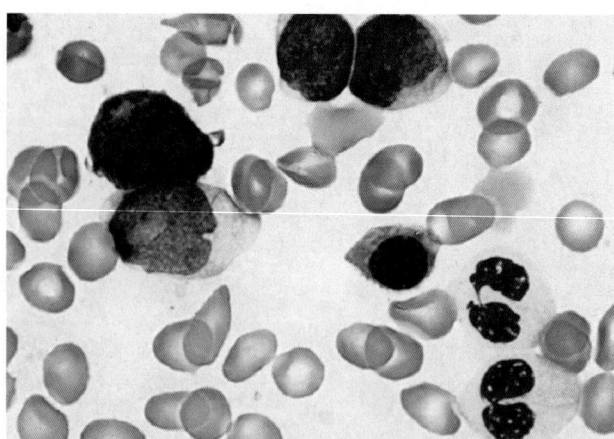
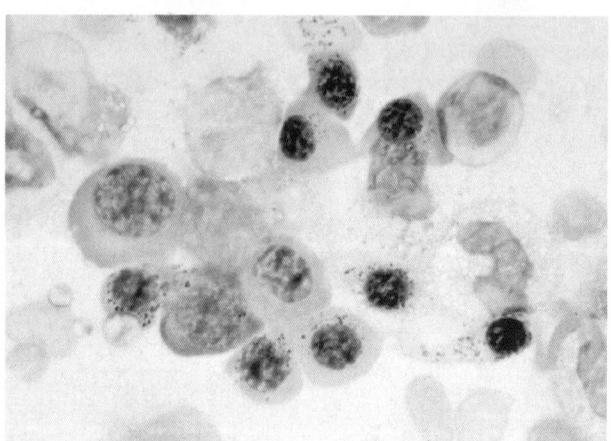

FIGURE 43.24. A: Bone marrow smear from a 72-year-old man with RAEB-2 who presented with a 1-year history of macrocytic anemia, neutropenia, and thrombocytopenia. This marrow specimen showed 4% myeloblasts and 62% erythroblasts with numerous ring sideroblasts. A myeloblast with a delicate Auer rod is present in the lower right. A megakaryocyte with a phagocytosed red blood cell is also present. **B:** High magnification of the specimens in (**A**) showing a myeloblast with a distinct Auer rod. Two markedly hypogranulated neutrophils with pseudo–Pelger-Huët nuclei are present. **C:** An iron stain on the same specimen shows numerous ring sideroblasts (**A** and **B**, Wright-Giemsa; **C**, Prussian blue followed by safranin counterstain; **A** 256×, **B** and **C** 400×).

features including nonlobate or hypolobate nuclei (Fig. 43.26). The megakaryocytes are usually normal or slightly small in size. There is frequently an erythroid hypoplasia (63). Granu-locytic and erythroid dysplasia is uncommon. Aggregates of lymphocytes may be present This constellation of blood, bone marrow, and cytogenetic findings is generally associated with response to lenalidomide and a favorable clinical course (42).

In the WHO definition of MDS with isolated del(5q), there should be no additional cytogenetic abnormalities, and the marrow blast count does not exceed 5% (60). If more than one additional cytogenetic abnormality or an increase in marrow blasts is present, patients may still respond to lenalidomide, but the prognosis is generally less favorable than in cases with an isolated del(5q) or del(5q) and one additional abnormality and <5% marrow blasts (64).

The risk of transformation to AML compares to that for RCMD, that is, about 15% to 20% after 5 years. Adverse factors for evolution to AML are additional cytogenetic abnormalities,

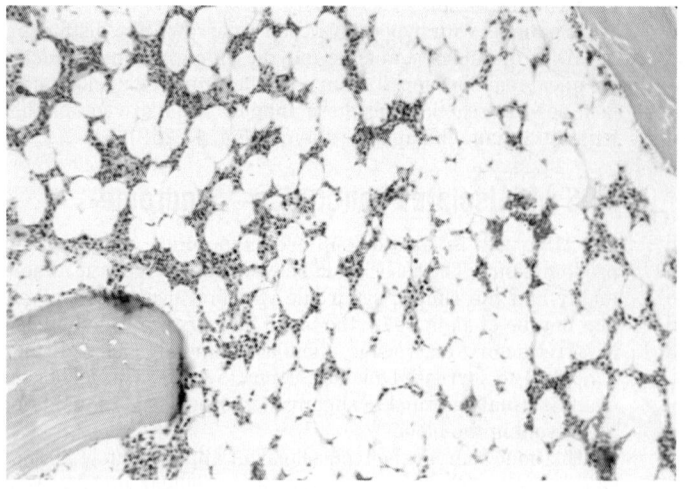
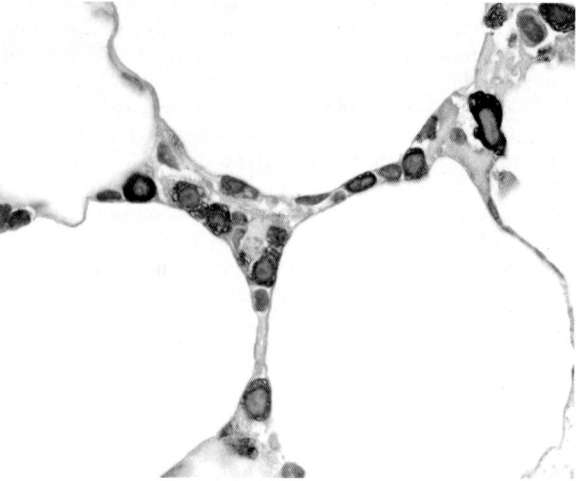

FIGURE 43.25. A: Markedly hypocellular bone marrow section from a patient with RAEB. There are increased immature cells in the inter-stitium. **B:** CD34 immunoperoxidase reaction on a hypocellular biopsy from a patient with RAEB. There are several CD34 reacting cells (**A:** H&E; **B:** immunoperoxidase).

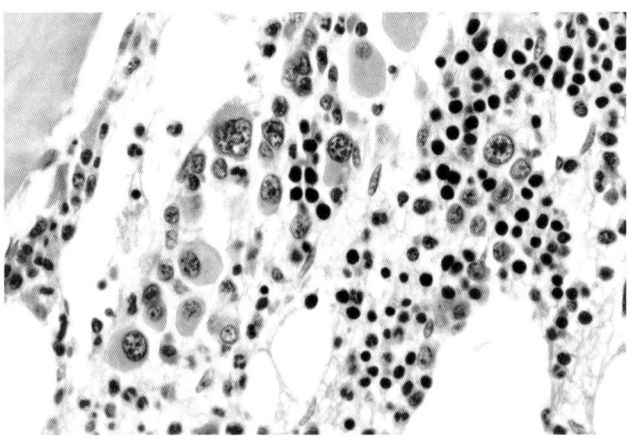

FIGURE 43.26. Bone marrow biopsy from a patient with isolated del(5q). There are numerous megakaryocytes, the majority of which have nonlobate nuclei. Some of the megakaryocytes are slightly small in size (H&E, 240×).

increased marrow blast percentage, and transfusion need at diagnosis. Patients without additional cytogenetic abnormalities and <5% marrow blasts have a low risk of transformation to AML (64).

There have been numerous investigations to identify the molecular basis of the 5q chromosome abnormality in the del(5q) abnormality (59,61). These studies have resulted in the localization of the gene in a common deleted region at band q32-q33 of the long arm of chromosome 5. Evidence supports haploinsufficiency of a candidate gene, the *RPS14* gene, which is required for maturation of 40S ribosomal subunits, as a basic genetic defect in the disorder. Patients with the isolated del(5q) could be distinguished from normal controls and other types of RA on the basis of deregulated expression of ribosomal and translation-related genes, which result in impaired erythropoiesis (59,61,62). Patients with Diamond-Blackfan anemia, an inherited disorder, manifest similar molecular aberrations with haploinsufficiency of the closely related *RPS19* gene and a downregulation of multiple ribosomal and translation-related genes resulting in altered ribosome biogenesis (61).

Myelodysplastic Syndrome–Unclassified

There are no specific morphologic findings for a diagnosis of MDS-U. The WHO suggests four situations, which may warrant the classification of a case as MDS-U (65):

1. Persistent RCUD or RCMD and 1% blasts in the blood but <5% blasts in the marrow
2. Persistent pancytopenia with unilineage dysplasia
3. Persistent cytopenia(s), <1% blasts in the blood and <5% blasts in the marrow, unequivocal dysplasia in <10% of one or more myeloid cell lines, and a recurring cytogenetic abnormality considered as presumptive evidence of MDS (24)
4. Persistent cytopenia(s) and no morphologic evidence of dysplasia, but an acceptable recurring cytogenetic abnormality, should be considered as having presumptive evidence of MDS (24).

All of these different groups of patients should be carefully monitored with clinical, morphologic, and cytogenetic studies for emergent evidence of a more specific MDS classification.

These cases should not be viewed as idiopathic cytopenia of undetermined significance (ICUS) in which the only finding is persistent cytopenia (66).

The occurrence of MDS-U appears to be somewhat more frequent in Asian populations than in western patients (15,67).

BONE MARROW HISTOPATHOLOGY

Although the original FAB classification of the MDS was based on examination of blood and marrow smears, the contemporary evaluation also includes an evaluation of bone marrow histopathology with particular emphasis on cellularity, presence of fibrosis, evidence of an increase and abnormal localization of immature cells, and evidence of dysplasia, particularly in the megakaryocytes (24,28,29).

Hypocellular MDS

The evaluation of marrow cellularity in MDS must take into account the age of the patient; the majority of patients with MDS are in the age group when marrow cellularity is normally in the decline (68). Generally, if the marrow cellularity is <20% in patients 70 or over and <30% in patients under 70, the marrow is considered to be hypocellular (69,70) (Fig. 43.25A). Variations of this guideline have been published including defining marrow hypocellularity as <25% cellular and cellularity <30% in individuals under 60 and <20% in individuals 60 and over (71–73). By these various criteria, approximately 10% to 20% of MDS cases are hypocellular. The majority of the cases of MDS, which are hypocellular, are classified as RA by WHO criteria. However, all subtypes may present with hypocellular marrow (72,73).

The presenting hemograms in patients with hypocellular MDS frequently show lower leukocyte and/or platelet counts than in patients with normocellular or hypercellular marrow (71,73).

The subclassification of the MDS with hypocellular marrow may be more difficult than in cases with normocellular or hypercellular marrow due to the paucity of myeloid cells in the aspirate smears.

The association of immune dysregulation and hypocellularity in MDS has been demonstrated in some studies and has served as the basis for treatment of these cases with immunosuppressive therapy (74).

The principal differential diagnosis of hypocellular MDS is aplastic anemia (74). Important distinguishing features for MDS are dysplastic myeloid cells in the blood and marrow and/or an increase in blasts. Even the presence of 2% to 5% blasts in the marrow or a rare blast in the blood would be essentially exclusionary for a diagnosis of aplastic anemia and evidence for a diagnosis of MDS. Estimating a slight increase in blasts in the marrow biopsy may be difficult even in well-prepared specimens; the recognition of blasts may be facilitated in most instances by the application of anti-CD34 antibody to the specimen (75,76) (Fig. 43.25B). The presence of increased CD34-positive cells would support the diagnosis of MDS. However, as previously noted, not all myeloblasts are CD34 positive, and a negative reaction would not necessarily exclude an increase in blasts. Normal marrow generally contains no more than 1% to 2% CD34-positive cells. Hematogones, early lymphoid precursors, may be CD34 positive; these cells may be increased in the marrow of very young children under certain conditions but are uncommonly increased in the marrow of adults, particularly the age group, which is most prone to develop MDS.

The presence of ALIP, as previously defined, would be evidence of MDS or AML, the distinction being based on the blast percentage in the blood and marrow (28,29). The detection of ALIP is aided by the use of anti-CD34.

Cytogenetic studies using Giemsa banding or fluorescent *in situ* hybridization (FISH) may be invaluable in distinguishing MDS from aplastic anemia if appropriate abnormalities are detected (24,77). Utilizing both metaphase cytogenetics and FISH, chromosome abnormalities may be detected in approximately half of the cases of MDS. However, obtaining adequate samples for cytogenetic studies from hypocellular specimens

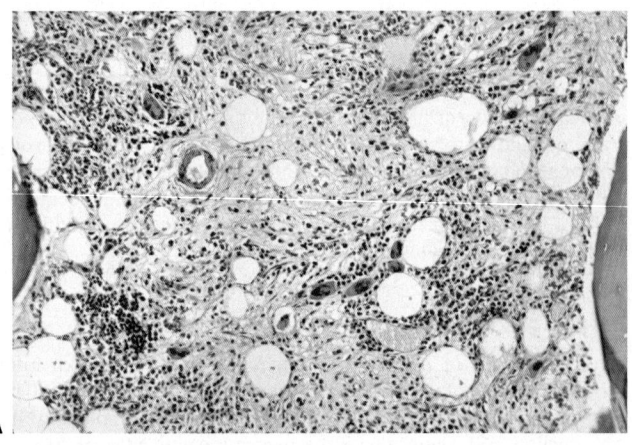
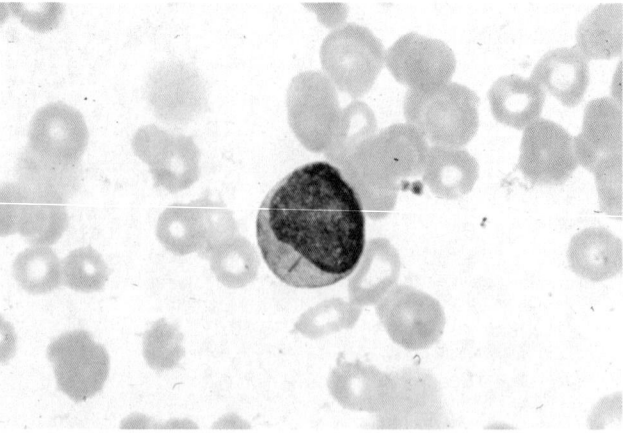

FIGURE 43.27. A: Bone marrow biopsy from a patient with RAEB-2. There is marked marrow fibrosis with several large megakaryocytes. There are no foci of immature cells. **B:** Bone marrow imprint from the same specimen as (**A**). The imprints were markedly hypocellular with approximately 8% blasts. Rare blasts contained an Auer rod as shown establishing the diagnosis as RAEB-2 (**A:** H&E; **B:** Wright-Giemsa, 400×).

may be more of a problem than samples from normocellular or hypercellular marrows with a lower rate of success.

Studies have shown that hypocellularity in MDS is an independent prognostic factor indicating a more favorable clinical course (71,73).

Myelofibrosis in MDS

The relevance of myelofibrosis in MDS has received more attention with the wider application of trephine biopsies in the evaluation of patients with MDS (78–82). The incidence of myelofibrosis in MDS varies somewhat in different reports (79–82). These differences may be more related to criteria for inclusion and what constitutes significant fibrosis than actual differences in the incidence of fibrosis. Studies employing the FAB classification, which includes cases of CMML, which in most series has a relatively high incidence of myelofibrosis, may have a higher incidence of myelofibrosis than studies using the WHO Classification. In addition, the threshold for what constitutes increased reticulin may vary between the various studies. Guidelines for evaluating and grading marrow fibrosis have been proposed (83).

In one study focused on marrow fibrosis in MDS, 349 biopsies from 200 patients classified according to WHO criteria were evaluated for evidence of myelofibrosis; 73% of the cases showed no evidence of fibrosis, 15% had focal fibrosis, 6.5% had diffuse extensive fibrosis involving >50% of marrow space, and 5.5% had diffuse extensive fibrosis involving <50% of

marrow space (82). In the same study, the incidence of fibrosis varied from 0% in RARS to 16% in RAEB and RCMD.

A comparable study of 301 patients with MDS also classified according to WHO guidelines showed similar results; moderate to severe fibrosis was observed in 17% of cases and was frequently associated with RCMD. The lowest incidences of fibrosis, 10%, occurred in patients with RA, RARS, and del(5q) (80).

These two studies and others have demonstrated an association between moderate to severe marrow fibrosis and an adverse impact on overall survival. Slight degrees of fibrosis did not impact survival (82). Severe marrow fibrosis has also been documented to impact survival following allogeneic stem cell transplantation for MDS. Patients with lesser degrees of fibrosis had a survival comparable to those patients without evidence of marrow fibrosis (84).

Subclassification of cases of MDS with marked fibrosis may be difficult because of paucicellular marrow aspirates and hypocellular smears. Imprints of the trephine section may be helpful. An alternative technique is making crush preparations from a portion of the marrow biopsy and staining with a Romanowsky stain.

Figure 43.27A illustrates a case of MDS with marked myelofibrosis. Classification of this case was facilitated by the detection of an occasional blast with an Auer rod in a markedly hypocellular marrow trephine imprint (Fig. 43.27B).

The reticulin stain is necessary for accurately assessing the degree of fibrosis (Fig. 43.28A and B).

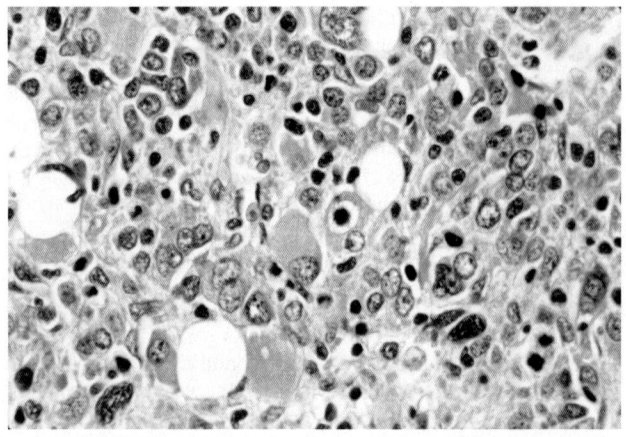
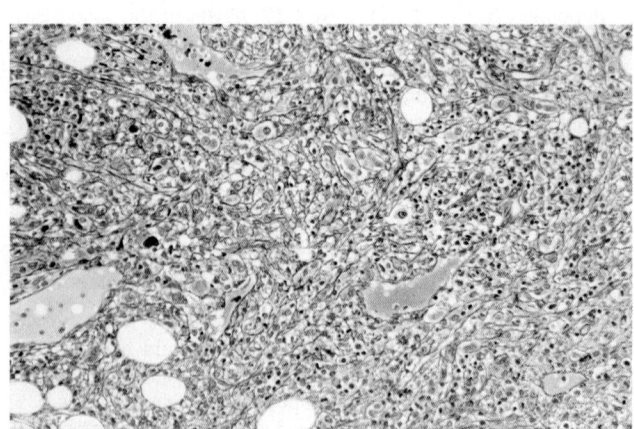

FIGURE 43.28. A: Marrow biopsy from a patient with RAEB with marrow fibrosis. There are increased immature cells and dysplastic megakaryocytes scattered in the interstitium. ALIP were also present. **B:** Reticulin stain of the specimen in (**A**) and (**B**) showing a moderate to marked generalized increase in reticulin fibers (**A:** H&E; **B:** reticulin stain).

IMMUNOPHENOTYPE

Traditionally the diagnosis of MDS has been established from clinical findings, evaluation of blood and marrow smears, and in most institutions cytogenetic studies. As wider recognition of the disease occurred, cytogenetic studies assumed a much more prominent and important role in recognition and classification (24,36,37). Immunophenotyping and molecular analysis are now being recognized as important tools for evaluating MDSs.

Sample preparation is important for flow cytometry (FCM) studies in order to obtain accurate and reproducible results. Bone marrow aspirates are collected using heparin or EDTA as anticoagulants; heparin is preferable (85,86). Studies should be performed as soon as possible after collection; if not studied immediately, the collected cells may be stored up to 24 hours at room temperature. Details of standardized processing have been published (85,86).

A substantial body of data has demonstrated a role for immunophenotyping as a "cocriterion" in the diagnosis of MDS (87–98). The role has been facilitated by the introduction of multiparametric FCM and more clear understanding of the immunophenotypic characteristics of normal myeloid hematopoiesis and the deviation from the normal pattern of the myeloid cells in MDS (85,99).

The two most difficult morphologic diagnostic problems in MDS are distinguishing cases of MDS without an increase in marrow blasts and no cytogenetic abnormalities from non-MDS causes of cytopenia(s) and in distinguishing RCUD (RA, RN, RT) from RCMD. In regard to the first of these problems, immunophenotyping may be of benefit in recognizing antigenic deviations from normal myeloid hematopoiesis that are more consistent with MDS than with normal hematopoiesis or a reactive process (88–93,99). In the second situation, distinguishing RCU from RCMD, the panorama of antigenic deviation on several myeloid cell types as opposed to one would be contributing evidence for a diagnosis of RCMD. In several FCM studies, antigenic abnormalities have been observed on myeloid cells, which apparently were cytomorphologically normal indicating a more sensitive threshold for detecting abnormalities by FCM.

The blast population in MDS, equated with CD34-positive cells, is evaluated for both quantitative and qualitative changes. The accurate enumeration of blasts is highly vulnerable to sample collection for FCM. Because samples of the marrow aspirate are obtained for several different studies at one time, dilution with peripheral blood is almost unavoidable. The variable degrees of dilution of the various samples may result in a lack of correspondence between the morphologic blast count on smears and the enumeration of blasts by FCM, and this must be noted when discrepancies are found.

A group of investigators has approached the problem of dilution of marrow aspirate specimens by comparing the relative percentages of myeloid cells expressing bright CD16 in marrow biopsies with percentages in marrow aspirates and peripheral blood. The marrow biopsy specimens were obtained by taking a small portion of a marrow biopsy and disaggregating it to obtain a cell suspension (87). These specimens contained 17% (±6.7) compared to the percentage derived from study of marrow aspirates, which contained 38% (±16). The authors of this study proposed a formula to normalize the blast percentage, that is, a calculated blast percentage. Assuming a simple ratio of the percent of dim CD16 neutrophils to the average for bone marrow biopsies, 80% provides a dilution factor of excess segmented neutrophils in the aspirate specimen presumably from peripheral blood dilution. The authors divide 80% by the percent of dim CD16 neutrophils and multiply the results by the determined blast percentage to arrive at the normalized blast percentage.

The blasts in MDS may show antigenic aberrancies, which are at variance with the antigenic pattern of normal myeloblasts

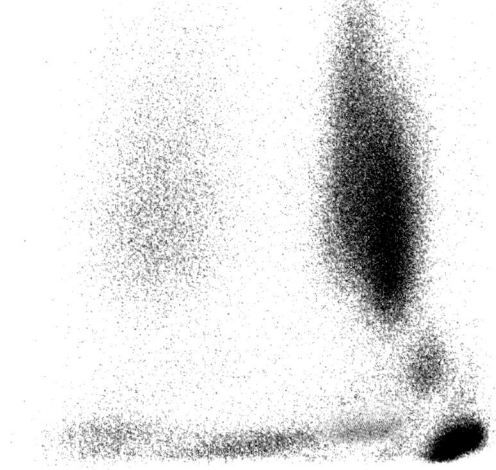

FIGURE 43.29. Histogram of phenotypically atypical blasts. A marrow aspirate showing a discrete population of CD34-positive myeloblasts (colored red) on CD45 versus side scatter consistent with a clonal myeloid neoplasm. The morphologic features in the bone marrow smears were interpreted as equivocal for a possible MDS. Cytogenetic studies showed a normal karyotype. Thirty-three months later, a bone marrow biopsy showed RAEB-2. (Graph and interpretation courtesy of Dr. Tim Singleton, Hematopathology, Department of Laboratory Medicine and Pathology, University of Minnesota.)

(Fig. 43.29). The most frequently observed aberrancies are abnormal intensity of CD34, CD45, CD13, CD33, and/or the expression of lineage infidelity (99–101). A consensus workshop on FCM in MDS identified abnormal granularity; abnormal intensity of CD34, CD45, CD117, or expression of CD11b or CD15; abnormal intensity or lack of HLA-DR; and expression of lineage infidelity markers Tdt, CD7, CD19, or CD56 as the most common relevant indicators of abnormal phenotype (86). CD7 was recognized as possibly present on a subset of normal myeloblasts. Reduced CD38 expression on CD34-positive blasts has been reported as reliable evidence of low-grade MDS by some observers (100–102).

One of the important diagnostic morphologic findings in MDS is hypogranularity in the neutrophil series. This important morphologic feature is sometimes obscured by the quality of the slide staining. This abnormality is reflected in FCM by decreased light scatter (85,86) (Fig. 43.30). Additional

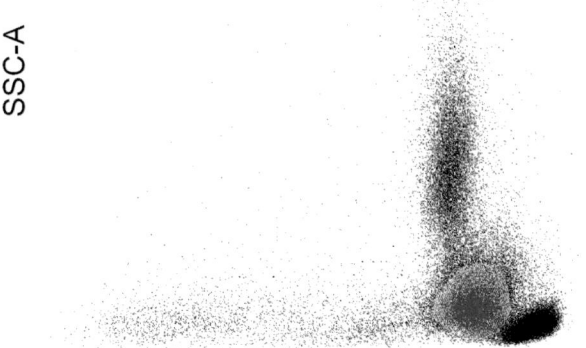

FIGURE 43.30. Histogram of hypogranular-agranular neutrophils consistent with a clonal myeloid neoplasm. A marrow aspirate showing 50% of leukocytes in the traditional blast region (colored red, dim CD45, and low side scatter) that contained agranular neutrophils in addition to 5% CD34-positive blasts. On morphologic examination of the bone marrow smear, the blast percentage was 5.2 and the diagnosis was RAEB-1. Cytogenetic studies showed a highly complex abnormal karyotype. (Graph and interpretation courtesy of Dr. Tim Singleton, Hematopathology, Department of Laboratory Medicine and Pathology, University of Minnesota.)

FCM findings in dysplastic granulocytes include abnormal coexpression of antigens, abnormal expression of antigens normally present at different stages of maturation, abnormal intensity of antigen expression, and expression of antigens not normally present on granulocytes (85,88–90).

Dysplastic-related abnormalities in monocytes include increased monocytes compared to lymphocytes; abnormal intensity of CD13 or CD33; an abnormal CD116/HLA-DR pattern; abnormal intensity of CD14, CD36, or CD64; overexpression of CD56; and expression of lineage infidelity markers, for example, CD5, CD7, and CD19 (86,89,93).

FCM studies of dysplasia in the erythroid series are considerably less advanced than those for the granulocytic lineage due to the lack of generally available antibodies to the antigenic structure of the erythroid cells. Studies of the erythroid lineage have employed antibodies to CD71, CD105, H-ferritin, L-ferritin, and mitochondrial iron (103). In comparison to cells from healthy controls and cells from subjects with anemia unrelated to MDS or other myeloid disorders, the erythroid cells from patients with MDS have been reported to have increased expression of H-ferritin and CD105 and decreased expression of CD71 (103). Mitochondrial iron has been found to be specific to MDS with ring sideroblasts with good correlation with ring sideroblasts observed by morphology.

Several studies have demonstrated the utility of FCM studies in distinguishing cases of MDS from non-MDs in patients manifesting cytopenias with ambiguous morphologic findings and no cytogenetic abnormalities (88,89,95,104). Quantitative assessment of myeloid nuclear differentiation antigen (MNDA) by FCM appears to distinguish myeloid precursors from patients with MDS from normal myeloid precursors (103). The MNDA is highly down-regulated in MDS with dim expression on the MDS cells compared to normal myeloid precursors. There also is a bimodal expression of the antigen on MDS cells in contrast to normal cells, which do not show a bimodal expression implying dual populations of cells from patients with MDS (104). The results in the study cited were principally based on evaluation of high-grade MDS cases.

Scoring systems based on antigenic profiles and antigen density on myeloblasts and maturing granulocytes have been shown to have a correlation with prognostic subgroups; higher scores reflect a greater number of abnormalities and correlate with increasing grades of malignancy as defined by the IPSS and WHO morphologic classification (88,93,97).

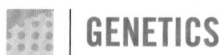 # GENETICS

Cytogenetics

Approximately 50% of cases of MDS have clonal cytogenetic abnormalities using metaphase cytogenetics. Unbalanced translocations and deletions are more common in MDS in contrast to AML (24,105–109). The chromosome aberrations in MDS generally show a loss or gain of chromosome material; loss of material is more frequent than gain (24). The most frequent abnormalities are −5/del(5q),−7/del 7(q−),+8, del(20q), and −y (108) (Table 43.6). These abnormalities may occur singly or in combination with other abnormalities. The MDS with isolated del(5q) by definition has the characteristic abnormality as a sole aberration. Fifty-eight percent of the chromosomal aberrations in one study were rare, defined as a frequency of <2% (108).

RARS is generally reported to have the lowest percentage of karyotypic abnormalities, approximately 10%, and RAEB the highest (107–110).

Cytogenetic studies are an essential component in the evaluation of patients with MDS. These studies serve several purposes including prognosis, therapeutic decisions, the recognition of clinicomorphologic syndromes such as the isolated del(5q) syndrome, and the identification of clonality in morphologically equivocal cases. Cytogenetic studies were one of the core features of the IPSS for predicting prognosis in the MDSs in which three prognostic cytogenetic groups were recognized: good, normal karyotype or del(5q) only or del(20q) only; poor, complex (at least three) chromosome abnormalities or chromosome 7 abnormalities; and intermediate, all other chromosome abnormalities, the IPSS-R recognizes five cytogenetic categories (37) (Table 43.7); (Fig. 43.31) (36,37). Generally wide experience has demonstrated the clinical relevance of this scoring system.

Since the WHO Classification of MDS includes a cytogenetically related entity, the isolated del(5q) syndrome, a chromosome analysis is recommended for all patients with MDS at the time of diagnosis (24). Cases lacking cytogenetic studies may be misdiagnosed with resulting inappropriate management. In addition, in cases with equivocal morphologic evidence of MDS, the demonstration of clonal hematopoiesis by aberrant cytogenetic findings aids in establishing the diagnosis of MDS. The WHO recommends that FISH also be performed if metaphase cytogenetics are nondiagnostic or as confirmatory evidence (Fig. 43.32) (24).

Table 43.6	RECURRING CHROMOSOMAL ABNORMALITIES AND THEIR FREQUENCY IN THE MDSS AT DIAGNOSIS				
Abnormality	**Percent**		**Abnormality**	**Percent**	
	MDS	t-MDS		MDS	t-MDS
Unbalanced			**Balanced**		
+8	10		t(11;16)(q23;p13.3)	—	3
−7 or del(7q)	10	50	t(3;21)(q26.2;q22.1)	—	2
−5 or del(5q)	10	40	t(1;3)(p36.3;q21.2)	1	
del(20q)	5–8		t(2;11)(p21;q23)	1	
−Y	5		inv(3)(q21q26.2)	1	
i(17q) or t(17p)	3–5		t(6;9)(p23;q34)	1	
−13 or del(13q)	3				
del(11q)	3				
del(12p) or t(12p)	3				
del(9q)	1–2				
idic(X)(q13)	1–2				

From Brunning RD, Orazi A, Germing U, et al. Myelodysplastic syndromes/neoplasms, overview. In: Swerdlow S, Campo E, Harris NL, et al., eds. *WHO classification of tumours of haematopoietic and lymphoid tissues*, 4th ed. Lyon: IARC, 2008:88–93.

Table 43.7	CYTOGENETIC RISK CATEGORIES
Very good	del(11q); −Y
Good	Normal; del(5q; double aberrations including del(5q); del(12p); del(20q)
Intermediate	del(7q); +8; i(17q); +19; any other independent clones
Poor	inv(3)/t(3q)/del(3q); −7; −7/7q; double aberrations including −7/7q−; complex karyotypes with three abnormalities
Very poor	Complex karyotypes with >3 abnormalities

From Schanz J, et al. A new comprehensive cytogenetic scoring system for primary myelodysplastic syndromes and oliogoblastic AML following MDS derived from an international database merger. *J Clin Oncol* 2012;30:820–829.

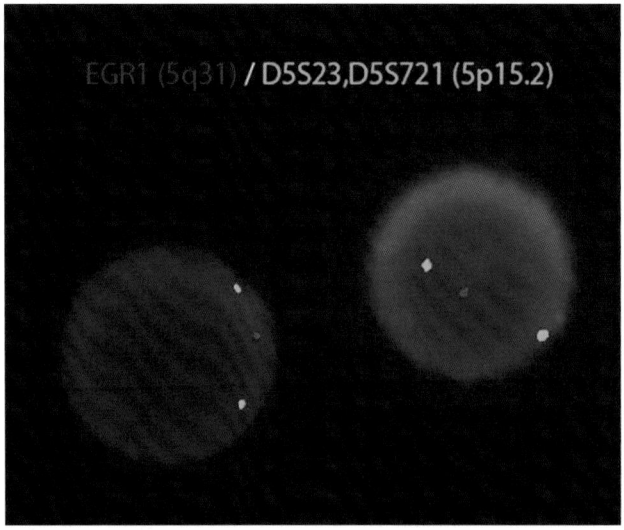

FIGURE 43.32. Del(5q) FISH image in bone marrow specimen from a patient with MDS. FISH using Abbott Molecular probe set to EGR1 (5q31, *red*) and D5S23-D5S721 (5p15.2, *green*). Each interphase cell shows loss of one EGR1 signal. (FISH image and interpretation courtesy of Dr. Michelle Dolan and Dr. Betsy Hirsch, Section of Cytogenetics, Department of Laboratory Medicine and Pathology, University of Minnesota.)

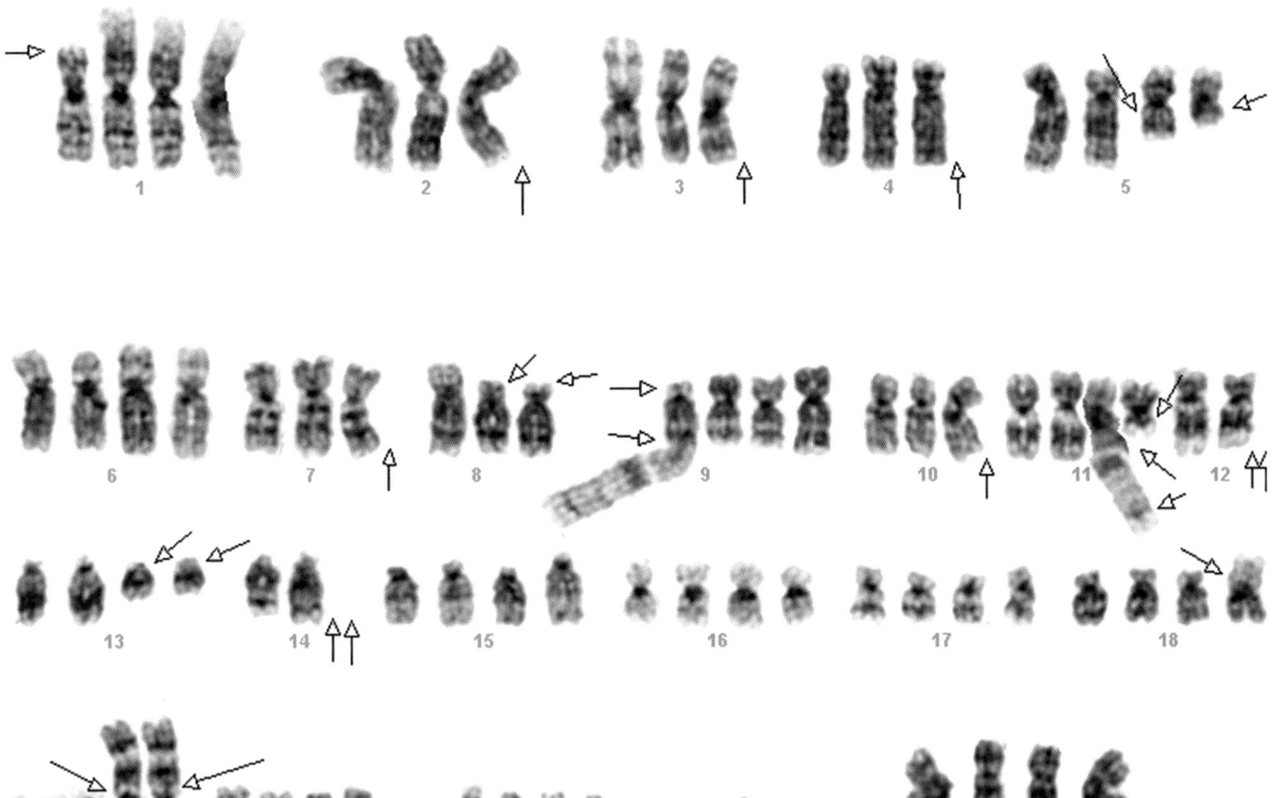

FIGURE 43.31. Complex karyotype in the bone marrow specimen from a patient with MDS. ISCN: 81,XXXX,add(1)(p13),−2,−3,−4,del(5)(q13q33)x2,−7,−8,del(8)(p21p23)x2, der(9)add(9)(p13)hsr(9)(q34),−10,add(11)(q12),der(11)hsr(11)(q13)hsr(11)(q23), −12,−12,del(13)(q12q22)x2,−14,−14,der(18)t(1;18)(p32;p11.2),+19,add(19)(p13.1)x2, −22,−22,−22,+mar (Karyotype and interpretation courtesy of Dr. Michelle Dolan and Dr. Betsy Hirsch, Section of Cytogenetics, Department of Laboratory Medicine and Pathology, University of Minnesota).

The impact of karyotype on prognosis in MDS has been demonstrated both in the IPSS and other studies (36,104–110). The combination of cytogenetic markers in combination with the WHO morphologic classification improves the prognostic stratification of patients with primary MDS (111). In studies subsequent to the introduction of the IPSS, it became evident that the prognostic impact of cytogenetic findings was underestimated in the IPSS (112,113). As a result, cytogenetic studies were weighted higher in the proposed World Prognostic Scoring System (WPSS) compared to the marrow blast percentage (111,113). Larger data sets also allowed a better assignment of many cytogenetic abnormalities including double aberrations and consequently led to a proposed revised categorization of cytogenetic risk groups (Table 43.7) (112). In addition, the large group of complex karyotypes and aberrations of chromosome 7 could be divided into different prognostic groups.

As noted, the prognostic impact of cytogenetic findings has been demonstrated in several studies. In one large series of 2,124 patients in which karyotype analysis was successful in 97.6% of patients and clonal abnormalities were demonstrated in 52.3%, median survival was 53.4% for patients with normal karyotype and 8.7% for patients with karyotypic abnormalities (108).

Patients over 60 years of age with adverse cytogenetic findings do not benefit from intensive induction chemotherapy (114).

The sensitivity of detecting cytogenetic abnormalities in MDS is increased when cases are studied with FISH in addition to routine metaphase cytogenetics (Figs. 43.32 and 43.33) (24).

MDS with Isolated del(5q)

With few exceptions, there is no correlation between specific cytogenetic abnormalities and specific morphologic subtypes of MDS. The most notable exception is the MDS with isolated del(5q) (5q– syndrome), which is a WHO recognized *de novo* MDS associated with an interstitial deletion of chromosome 5q (59,61,62). Haploinsufficiency of *RPS14*, a gene that encodes a ribosomal protein mapping at q32-q33, has been suggested as a candidate gene interacting with other genes to be associated with the cascade of genetic events resulting in the constellation of findings in the del(5q) syndrome (59,61,62) (see Classification for complete discussion of entity). Several studies have validated the prognostic impact of del(5q) in relation to other prognostic factors (114–116). Patients with isolated del(5q) or del(5q) with one additional cytogenetic abnormality without increased marrow blasts and transfusion requirement have a good prognosis in contrast to patients with increased marrow blasts, transfusion need, or more than one additional chromosome abnormality who have an inferior outcome with higher progression rate (114). Within the restricted definition of the WHO definition of the isolated del(5q) syndrome, the presence of dysgranulopoiesis appears to have a negative impact on prognosis (116).

As noted previously, the presence of isolated del(5q) is associated with a high response rate to lenalidomide (42).

17p Deletion:(del(17p))

The 17p deletion is associated with cases of MDS and AML, which frequently manifest a type of granulocytic dysplasia characterized by small neutrophils with pseudo–Pelger-Huët nuclei and cytoplasmic vacuoles (117–119) (Fig. 43.6). The combination of del(17p) and granulocytic dysplasia is frequently accompanied by a high incidence of *TP53* mutation and unfavorable prognosis. Approximately 50% of patients with 17p deletion have a therapy related process (120).

Inv(3)– inv(3)(q21q26.2)

Cases of MDS and AML with normal to elevated platelet counts have been reported in association with abnormalities of chromosome 3 (121–123). The chromosome abnormalities include a paracentric 3q inversion and translocation 3;3 with breakpoints in q21-q26 or ins(5;3). Additional cytogenetic abnormalities are frequently observed, particularly involving chromosomes 5 and 7 (122). The associated findings in these patients usually include increased megakaryocytes with disordered megakaryocytopoiesis including small megakaryocytes and micromegakaryocytes with hypolobated nuclei. The cases of AML frequently involve more than one myeloid cell line with prominent megakaryocyte proliferation. Cases of AML and MDS associated with these abnormalities appear to have an increased incidence of prior exposure to mutagenic or carcinogenic agents. The cytogenetic finding is generally associated with an unfavorable clinical course (121–123).

Deletion (20q)

The del(20q) is frequently associated with morphologic abnormalities of the erythroid and megakaryocyte series (124–126). There is frequently a thrombocytopenia and the clinical findings may be confused with immune thrombocytopenia (125). Patients with the del(20q) frequently have a more indolent clinical course than some other types of MDS (125,126).

Table 43.6 lists the most frequent recurring cytogenetic abnormalities in MDS (24). The WHO recognizes the presence of most of these recurring clonal abnormalities as presumptive evidence of MDS in the absence of morphologic evidence of dysplasia in patients with persistent cytopenia. The WHO recommends that three of these clonal abnormalities not be accepted as presumptive evidence of MDS in patients with persistent cytopenia in the absence of acceptable morphologic evidence of dysplasia; these abnormalities are +8, –Y, and del(20q) (Table 43.6). The patients with these abnormalities should be carefully monitored with periodic repeat cytogenetic and morphologic studies for emerging definitive evidence of an MDS. Because of the presence of a cytogenetic abnormality, these patients should not be diagnosed as ICUS in which there is persistent cytopenia(s) but no morphologic or cytogenetic evidence for an MDS (65,127).

Molecular Genetics

The use of molecular genetic studies has the potential to revolutionize the diagnosis, classification, prognostication including prediction of leukemic transformation, and therapy of the MDS (128–135). Although derived from a common hematopoietic stem cell progenitor aberration, the MDSs manifest as a morphologic and clinical heterogeneous group of disorders (1,2). The heterogeneity is reflected in molecular studies, which have shown multiple distinct clones in different cell lineages (136). Mutations of the *TET2* gene have been found in approximately 20% of cases of MDS; mutations of this gene may also be present in other myeloid proliferations (130).

Studies utilizing sequencing and mass spectrometry genotyping have identified recurring somatic point mutations in MDS, which may be associated with specific clinical features: mutations in *RUNX1*, *TP53*, and *NRAS* are associated with marked thrombocytopenia, and when compared to MDS patients without the mutations patients with these mutations had increased marrow blasts (135). Multivariant analysis of gene mutations in one study of *MDS* patients showed that mutations in *TP53*, *RUNX1*, *EZH2*, *ETV6*, and *ASXL1* were independently associated with decreased overall survival (135).

Mutations of the *JAK2V617F* gene, which are common in polycythemia vera and other *BCR/ABL1*-negative myeloproliferative disorders are uncommonly present in MDS (137).

Single nucleotide polymorphism arrays (SNP-A) have been shown to identify chromosome abnormalities in MDS undetected by metaphase cytogenetics (131,132). As previously noted, approximately 50% of cases of MDS have detectable

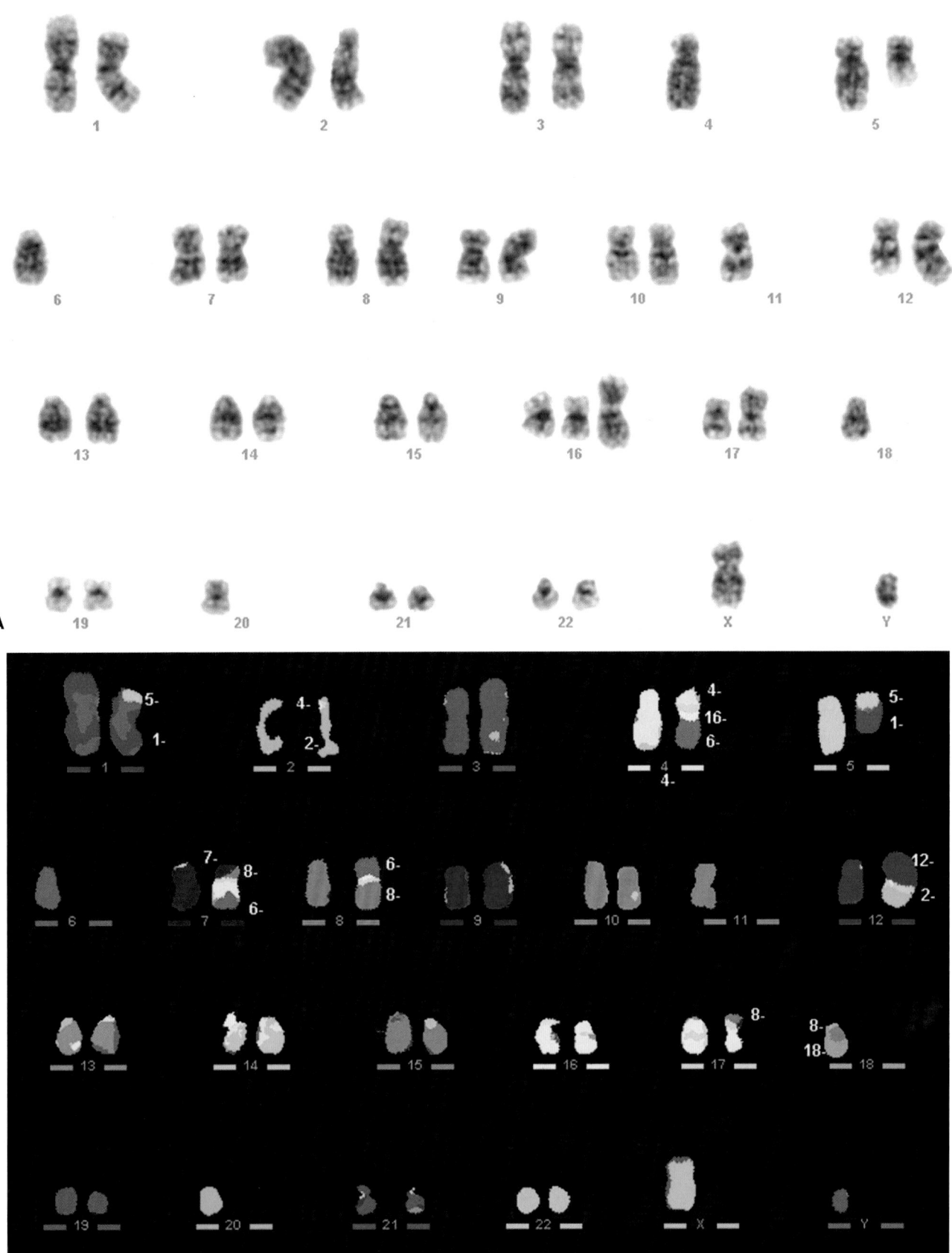

FIGURE 43.33.   Complex karyotype from a patient with MDS. A: ISCN: 42,XY,der(1)t(1;5)(p32;q35),add(2)(p11.2),der(4)t(4;6)(q11;q12),der(5) t(1;5)(p32;q11.2),–6,del(6)(p11.2),der(8)t(6;8)(p12;p11.2),11,der(12)t(12;19)(p12;p12)t(2;12)(p13;q24.1),der (17) t(8;17)(p12;p12),–18,–20. **B:** Multicolor FISH of the specimen in (**A**). (Karyotype and interpretation courtesy of Dr. Michelle Dolan and Dr. Betsy Hirsch, Section of Cytogenetics, Department of Laboratory Medicine and Pathology, University of Minnesota, Minneapolis, MN.)

cytogenetic abnormalities in metaphase studies. When cytogenetics is combined with SNP-A, the detection rate of abnormalities increases to 74% (132). The lesions uncovered by SNP-A are often novel lesions. The presence and number of SNP-A–detected abnormalities appear to be independent predictors of event free and overall survival; some novel SNP-A defects appear to correlate with a less good prognosis than would be indicated by morphologic and clinical scoring systems (132).

A relatively specific correlation has been demonstrated between recurrent mutations of the *SF3B1* gene and MDS with ring sideroblasts (34). In a study of 354 patients with MDS, 72 had recurring *SF3B1* mutations; the mutations were most frequently detected in forms of MDS in which ring sideroblasts are a prominent morphologic finding, that is, RARS, 40 of 59 patients, and RCMD-RS, 13 of 23 patients (34). The mutations were detected at lower rates in other types of MDS. The studies suggest the possibility that the *SF3B1* mutations are possibly associated with systematic downregulation of essential mitochondrial gene networks. The studies further demonstrated the *SF3B1* mutations in CD34+ hematopoietic progenitor cells in which mitochondrial ferritin first appears in patients with RARS indicating the transcriptional changes that precede the appearance of mitochondrial iron during erythroid development.

The MDS patients with the *SF3B1* mutations had higher neutrophil and platelet counts than MDS patients without the mutations and a generally benign clinical course.

The *SF3B1* gene mutation has also been detected in a population of patients with chronic lymphocytic leukemia (138).

 PROGNOSIS AND EVOLUTION

The course of MDS is markedly different from patient to patient. A major parameter to describe the dynamic character of the disease is hematopoietic insufficiency. While many patients experience stable disease without changes in cell counts over years, others have increasing cytopenia(s). The latter group does not necessarily show disease progression with an increasing number of blasts, but a significant increase in cytopenia(s) should prompt the physician to reexamine the marrow in order not to overlook progression to AML. Progression to AML usually

is associated with a worsening of the prognosis, especially in the low-risk groups.

Major parameters influencing the course of the disease are disease-related parameters: MDS subtype, cytogenetic findings, the degree of cytopenia(s), and patient-related parameters such as age and comorbidities (139–141) (Fig. 43.34). The gold standard for the assessment of prognosis in the MDSs is the IPSS initially introduced in 1997. This system incorporates degree of cytopenias and cytogenetic findings to define risk groups with significantly different rates of disease progression as well as median survivals. The 1997 IPSS had four risk groups: high, intermediate1, intermediate 2, and low. The IPSS-R introduced in 2012 has five risk categories based principally on cytogenetic data but also considering other factors: very high, high, intermediate, low, and very low (37) (Tables 43.5A,B and 43.7). Based on the 1997 IPSS, median survival data from the Duesseldorf data base for the four risk groups are 88, 62, 26, and 13 months (36,141) (Fig. 43.35). The risk of progression to AML after 2 years is 4%, 10%, 24%, and 50%, respectively.

As noted, the expansion of the risk groups in the IPSS-R is based primarily on additional data from cytogenetic studies and other factors (37,107,112,141,142). The median survivals for the five risk groups in the IPSS-R are 8.8, 5.3, 3.0, 1.5, and 0.8 years. The rate of progression to AML is not reached for the very low risk group, 10.8 years for the low risk group, 3.2 years for the intermediate risk group, 1.4 years for the high risk group, and 0.7 year for the very high risk group (37,107,111,141,142) (Tables 43.5 and 43.7).

The proposed WPSS replaces blood cytopenias with transfusion need as a prognostic parameter and replaces the blood and marrow blast percentage by WHO type (111,141). Thereby, the degree of dysplasia, which has major impact on prognosis, is represented in the WPSS (Fig. 43.36). New biologic parameters like gene mutations will be incorporated into future studies in order to assess their prognostic meaning.

Treatment

In any discussion of the therapeutic management of patients with MDS, it has to be recognized that the clinical course of the patients is very heterogeneous, ranging from an indolent

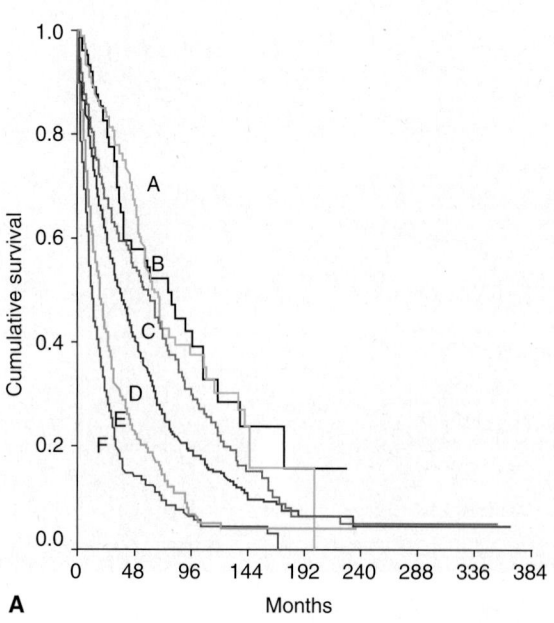

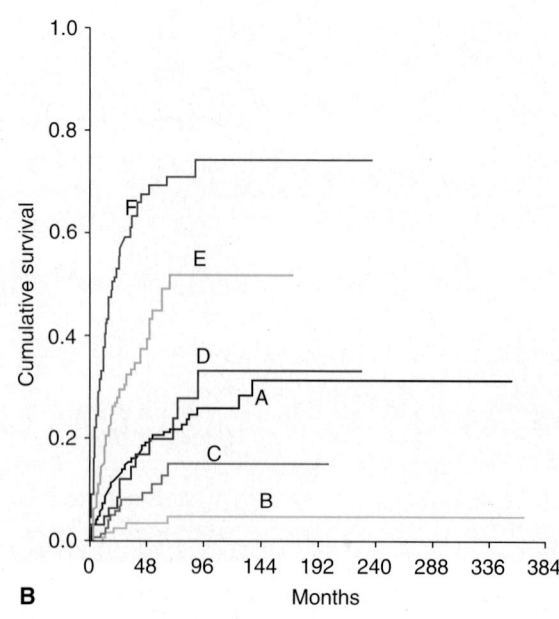

FIGURE 43.34. A: Survival curves of 2,347 patients with MDS classified according to WHO criteria. *A:* RCMD, *B:* RARS, *C:* RC, *D:* del(5q), *E:* RAEB-1, *F:* RAEB-2. **B:** Cumulative risk of AML evolution of 2,347 patients with MDS classified according to WHO criteria. *A:* RCMD, *B:* RARS, *C:* RC, *D:* del(5q), *E:* RAEB-1, *F:* RAEB-2. (Reproduced from Geming U, Aul C, Niemeyer CM, et al. Epidemiology, classification and prognosis of adults and children with myelodysplastic syndromes. *Ann Hematol* 2008;86:691–699, with permission of the journal.)

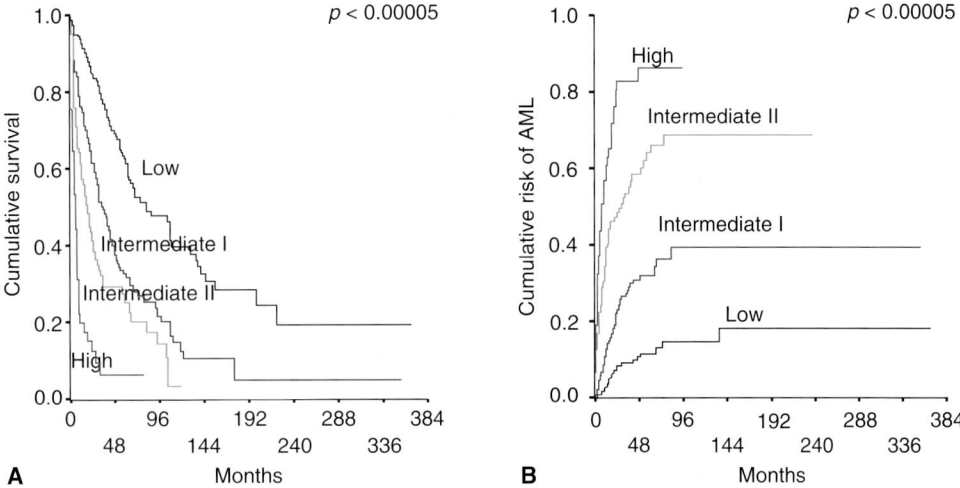

FIGURE 43.35. A: Survival curves of 676 patients with MDS according to IPSS risk categories. **B:** Cumulative risk of AML evolution in 676 patients with MDS classified according to the IPSS risk categories. (Reproduced from Geming U, Aul C, Niemeyer CM, et al. Epidemiology, classification and prognosis of adults and children with myelodysplastic syndromes. *Ann Hematol* 2008;86:691–699, with permission of the journal.)

disease over years to rapid development of AML within months. Patients without increased marrow blasts and unilineage dysplasia can usually anticipate a stable disease course, whereas patients with RAEB-1 or RAEB-2 face a high incidence of disease-related death, either infections or bleeding. Patients with RCMD have an intermediate course (Fig. 43.34).

Treatment planning must take into account that the median age at diagnosis of MDS is about 70 years and is associated with comorbidities at least in countries of the western hemisphere.

The treatment of patients with low-risk MDS, primarily RCUD, RARS, and RCMD, is focused primarily at stabilizing the quality of life, usually through supportive care including transfusion therapy, erythropoietins, and antiinfective measures (143). In case of severe infections due to granulocytopenia, GCSF can be administered. Patients with MDS and del(5q) benefit from treatment with lenalidomide (42). As low-risk

WHO types are associated with a long life expectancy, multiple blood transfusions can lead to iron overload, possibly ending in a worsening of any concurrent heart disease. Chelation therapy might be beneficial for these patients (144). In case of very severe cytopenia, nonapproved compounds like antithymocyte globulins or anti-52 antibodies may be helpful (20–22,145,146).

Treatment of high-risk patients, primarily RAEB-1 and RAEB-2, is focused on a prolongation of life expectancy or even cure. Two hypomethylating compounds, 5-azacytidine and decitabine, are approved for these patients and show response rates of about 50% leading to survival benefit of about 1 to 2 years (147,148). If the patient presents in good physical condition and an HLA identical donor is available, allogeneic stem cell transplantation should be considered in order to offer the patient a curative approach.

Clinical studies are ongoing to find new agents to reverse the cytopenia(s) or preclude progression of the disease.

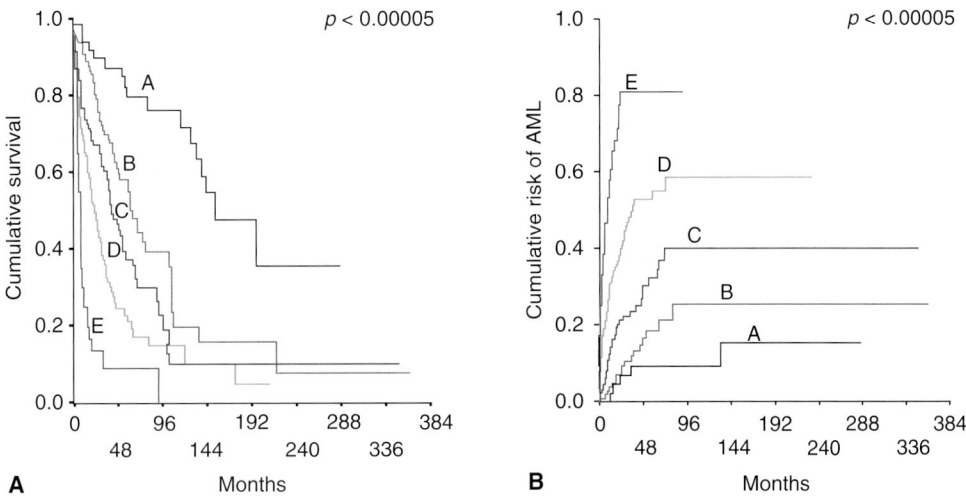

FIGURE 43.36. A: Survival curves of 676 patients with MDS classified according to the WPSS risk categories. *A:* very low risk, *B:* low risk, *C:* intermediate risk, *D:* high risk, *E:* very high risk. **B:** Cumulative risk of AML evolution of 676 patients with MDS according to WPSS risk groups. *A:* very low risk, *B:* low risk, *C:* intermediate risk, *D:* high risk, *E:* very high risk. (Reproduced from Geming U, Aul C, Niemeyer CM, et al. Epidemiology, classification and prognosis of adults and children with myelodysplastic syndromes. *Ann Hematol* 2008;86:691–699, with permission of the journal.)

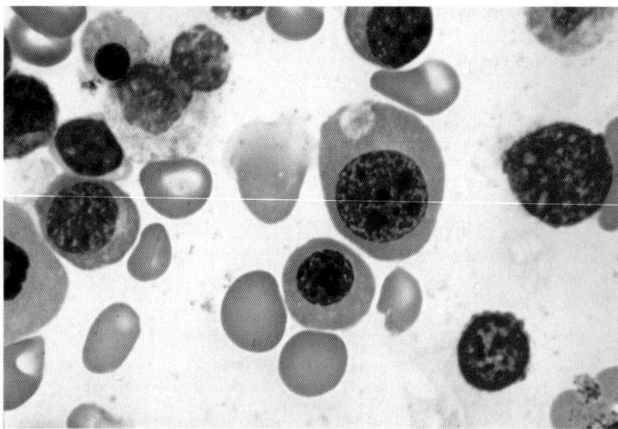

FIGURE 43.37. Bone marrow smear from an adult with megaloblastic anemia due to vitamin B_{12} deficiency, pernicious anemia. There are three erythroid precursors, which are large in size and nuclei with an open chromatin pattern (Wright-Giemsa, 400×).

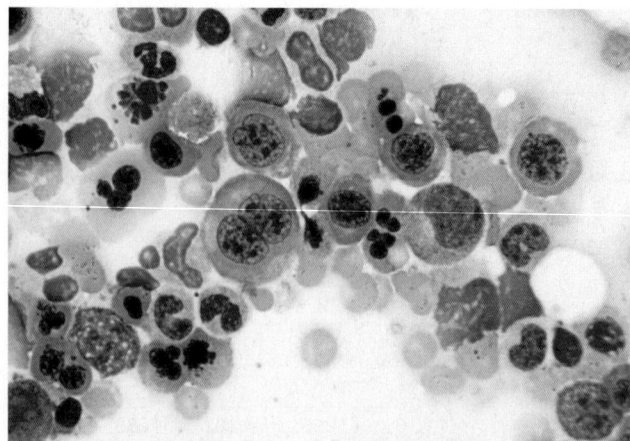

FIGURE 43.39. Bone marrow smear from an adult woman with breast carcinoma treated with several chemotherapeutic drugs including folic acid antagonists. There is marked dyserythropoiesis with prominent megaloblastic changes. The findings were interpreted as drug related (Wright-Giemsa, 240×).

DIFFERENTIAL DIAGNOSIS OF MYELODYSPLASTIC SYNDROMES

It is important that the diagnosis of an MDS not be established before thorough review of the patient's clinical history; exposure to drugs, alcohol, or heavy metals may lead to dysplastic changes in one or more myeloid cell lines similar to those observed in MDSs (24,149). Hematologic examination must include careful evaluation of peripheral blood and bone marrow smears and sections. Chromosome analysis has a crucial role. In cases in which the morphologic findings are equivocal, cytogenetic studies may be definitive in establishing evidence of a recurring clonal abnormality.

For purposes of differential diagnosis, the MDSs may be considered as two groups: the disorders characterized primarily by cytopenia(s) and dysplastic changes without an increase in blasts (RA, RARS, RCMD, MDS-U) and the disorders accompanied by an increase in blasts and/or the presence of Auer rods (RAEB-1 and RAEB-2). The first group is the most problematic.

RA, RARS, and MDS-U may present with hematologic abnormalities similar to those found in patients who have nutritionally related anemias or anemias that result from exposure to

toxins. Among the most important differential considerations for MDS is megaloblastic anemia caused by vitamin B_{12} or folate deficiency; red blood cell and serum folate, and serum B_{12} levels must be assayed before a diagnosis of MDS is established (Figs. 43.37 and 43.38). If the levels of these vitamins are equivocal, it is advisable to repeat the studies. Patients who have macrocytic anemia and neurologic findings suggestive of subacute combined degeneration should be treated with vitamin B_{12} regardless of serum levels. Patients who have RARS should be considered for a therapeutic trial with pyridoxine (vitamin B_6). In addition, patients with RARS should be investigated for possible alcohol abuse and drug ingestion, which may be associated with sideroblastic anemia.

Megaloblastic dyserythropoiesis is a frequent finding following chemotherapy for both hematopoietic and nonhematopoietic tumors resulting from the use of folic acid antagonists and underscores the importance of clinical history when evaluating blood and marrow specimens (Fig. 43.39).

Heavy metal intoxication, most notably arsenic intoxication, can lead to myelodysplastic changes, primarily in the erythroblasts but also in the neutrophils (150,151). Patients may present with pancytopenia, and the morphologic findings may suggest an MDS; nuclear lobulation and megaloblastoid nuclei

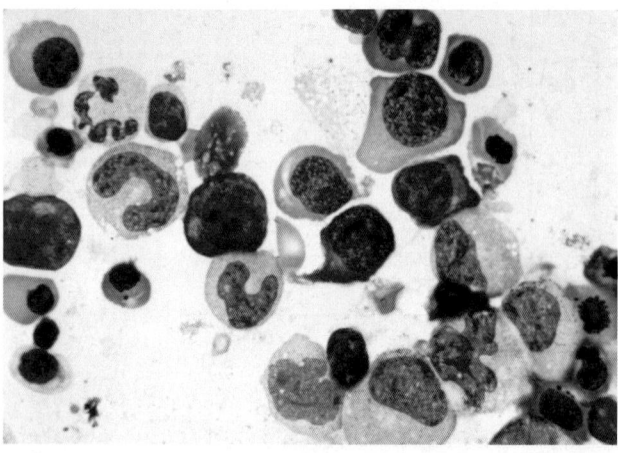

FIGURE 43.38. Bone marrow smear from a patient with megaloblastic anemia due to folic acid deficiency. In addition to megaloblasts, there are several large neutrophil precursors with premature nuclear segmentation, an important feature of megaloblastic anemia due to a vitamin deficiency (Wright-Giemsa, 400×).

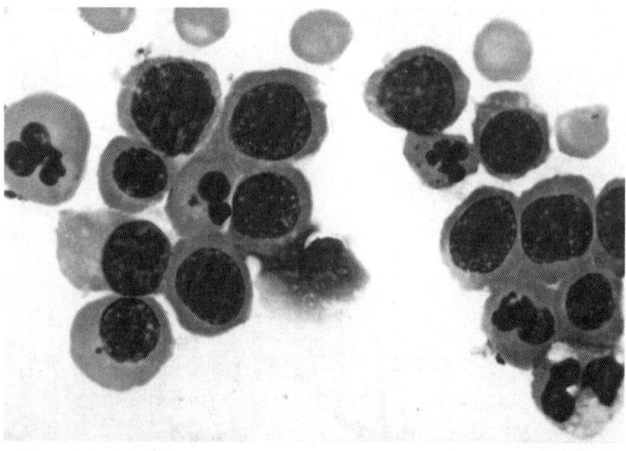

FIGURE 43.40. Bone marrow smear from a 42-year-old man admitted to hospital with a depressed sensorium and pancytopenia. The red blood cell precursors show marked dysplastic changes, including megaloblastoid nuclear chromatin and nuclear hyperlobulation and karyorrhexis. The cells were slightly PAS positive. Five days after this specimen was obtained, the patient's spouse admitted lacing his evening meals with arsenic. The patient was treated with dimercaprol and recovered completely (Wright-Giemsa, 400×).

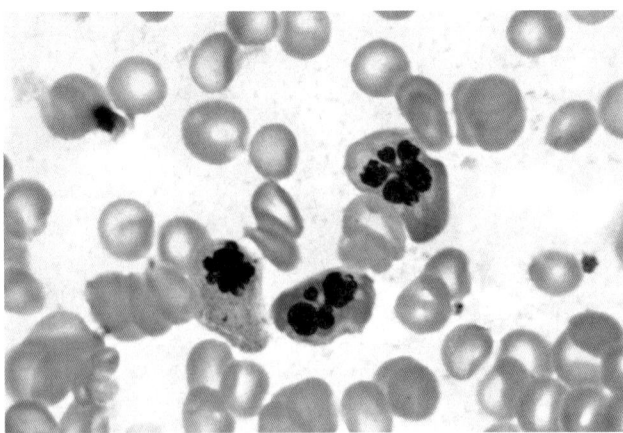

FIGURE 43.41. Bone marrow smear from an adult male who was the victim of arsenic intoxication. The three polychromatic erythroid precursors show unusually marked nuclear lobulation. The cell on the left also shows coarse basophilic stippling (Wright-Giemsa 400×).

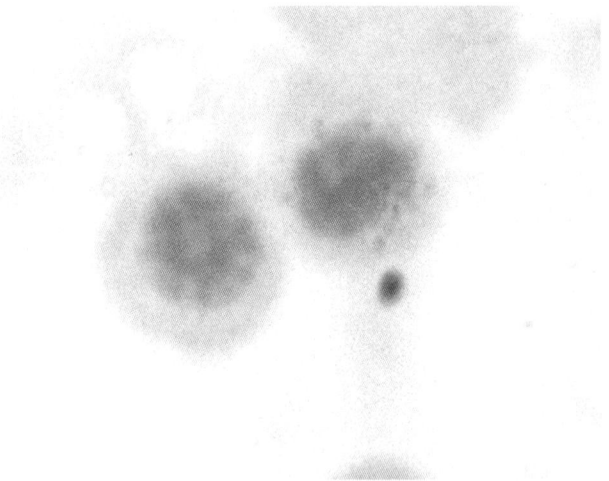

FIGURE 43.43. Bone marrow smear from a patient with copper deficiency stained for iron showing a ring sideroblast. The patient also had a heterozygous mutation of HFE, a gene implicated in homozygous hemochromatosis. The smear illustrated also contained iron-laden plasma cells. Approximately 22% of patients with copper deficiency have iron-laden plasma cells in the marrow. (Reprinted from Sutton L, Vusirikala M, Chen W. Hematogone hyperplasia in copper deficiency. *Am J Clin Pathol* 2009;132:191–196, with permission.)

may be prominent in the erythroid precursors in the marrow aspirate (Figs. 43.40 and 43.41). The red blood cells frequently show coarse basophilic stippling. Exposure to the offending agent may be occupational, accidental, or the result of criminal intent.

Copper deficiency has been reported to be associated with cytopenias, ring sideroblasts, and vacuolization of myeloid precursors in the marrow (152–154) (Figs. 43.42A and B and 43.43). The deficiency may in some instances be related to excessive zinc supplementation (155).

Congenital dyserythropoietic anemia (CDA) most commonly manifests in childhood but may also be initially detected in adult years (156) (Fig. 43.44A and B). The erythroid precursors in this group of disorders generally show marked morphologic alterations, including nuclear lobation, megaloblastoid nuclei, nuclear gigantism, and giant erythroid precursors with multinucleation (156) (Fig. 43.45). The erythrocytes in the blood smear show varying degrees of aniso-poikilocytosis, anisochromasia, and basophilic stippling. The anemia may be severe. The granulocytes and megakaryocytes are normal, and platelet and leukocyte counts are in the normal range.

The myeloid cells of patients who have acquired immune deficiency syndrome (AIDS) may show dysplastic changes, including pseudo–Pelger-Huët nuclei in mature neutrophils and dyserythropoiesis. Megakaryocytes with sparse cytoplasm or naked nuclei may be prominent in bone marrow sections. The dysplastic changes may occur in the absence of drug therapy (157,158). The etiologic basis for these changes is unknown: a rare case of AML has been reported in patients with AIDS; the occurrence is probably coincidental.

Several commonly used drugs and biologic agents may cause dysplastic changes similar to those found in MDS. The antibiotic cotrimoxazole may cause striking pseudo–Pelger-Huët nuclei in neutrophils (Fig. 43.46). In some instances, it may be difficult to identify the causative agent if combinations of drugs are being used.

Parvovirus B19 infection is associated with erythroblasto-penia with a "maturation arrest" of the erythroid precursors at the pronormoblast-basophilic normoblast stage of maturation

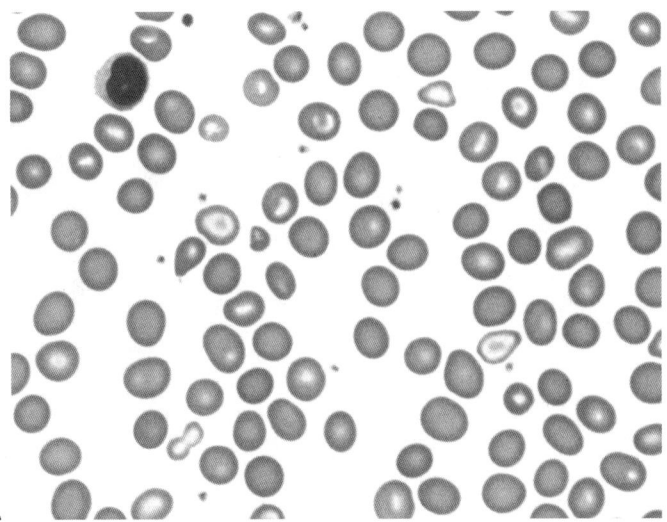

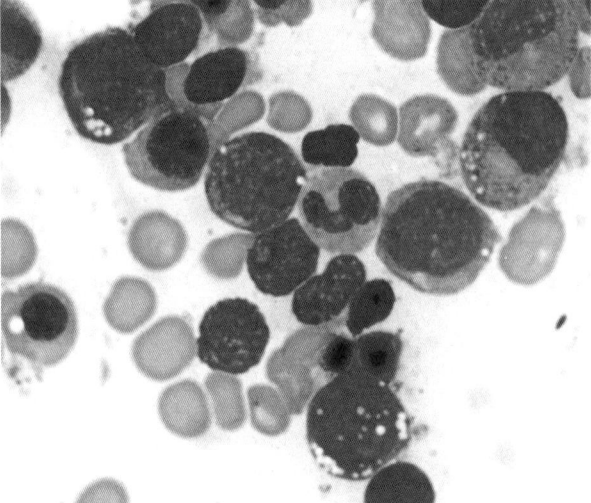

FIGURE 43.42. A: Blood smear from a patient with copper deficiency. The red blood cells show slight anisochromasia. The major population is normochromic; there are a few hypochromic cells. B: Bone marrow smear from the same patient showing several very immature erythroid precursors with numerous sharply defined cytoplasmic vacuoles; a vacuolated neutrophil myelocyte is at the upper right. (Reprinted from Sutton L, Vusirikala M, Chen W. Hematogone hyperplasia in copper deficiency. *Am J Clin Pathol* 2009;132:191–196, with permission.)

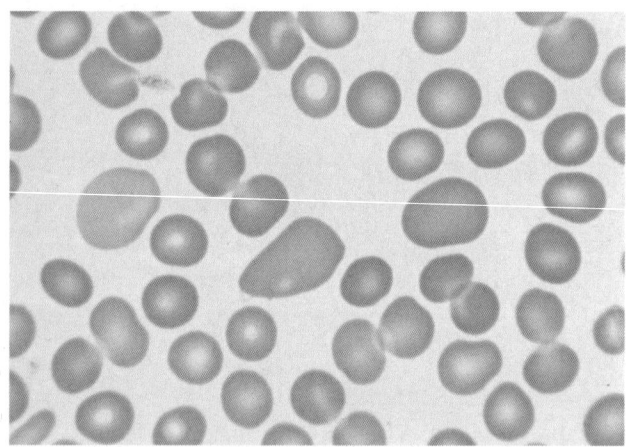
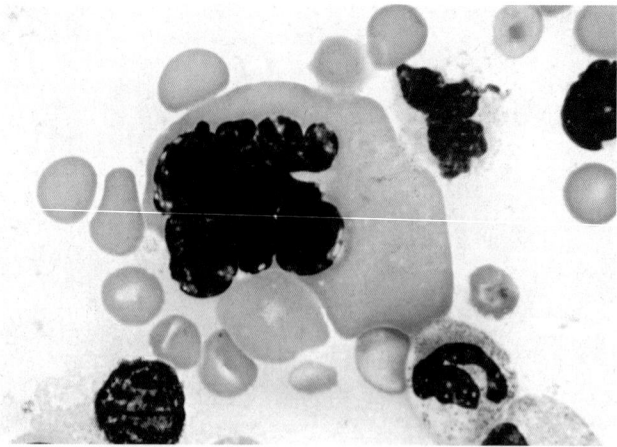

A
B

FIGURE 43.44. A: Blood smear from a 22-year-old man with a hemoglobin of 13.7 g/dL and a slight reticulocytosis. Very macrocytic red blood cells are noted. The platelet count and leukocyte count were normal. Similar findings were present in the blood smear of his 14-month-old daughter. **B:** Giant polychromatic erythroblast with marked nuclear hyperlobulation in the bone marrow specimen from the case illustrated in **(A)**. The granulocytes and megakaryocytes were normal in number and appearance. The morphologic findings were classified as CDA type III (Wright-Giemsa, 400×).

and giant erythroblasts, which may resemble changes found in MDS (159) (Fig. 43.47). Although MDS may occasionally manifest with erythroblastopenia, it is not generally associated with giant erythroblasts. Serologic or molecular studies for parvovirus B19 infection will usually resolve the problem. Most cases of parvovirus B19 infection undergo spontaneous recovery in a few weeks; occasional cases of persistent infection in immunocompromised patients occur. DNA analysis is the most reliable method for detecting parvovirus in this group of patients.

Some of the changes, which occur with granulocyte colony–stimulating factor (GM-CSF), are virtually indistinguishable from findings, which occur in the MDSs; the most notable is the presence of blasts in the peripheral blood and neutrophil nuclear hypolobation or pseudo–Pelger-Huët nuclei (160). The blast percent in the peripheral blood may reach levels as high as 10% to 15%, and neutrophils with pseudo–Pelger-Huët nuclei may be very numerous (Fig. 43.48A and B). "Ring" nuclei forms may rarely be observed (Fig. 43.49). These changes are accompanied by intense azurophilic granulation and numerous Dohle bodies, which are suggestive of an inflammatory reaction. These findings may persist for several days following

cessation of growth factor administration. The combination of findings in conjunction with a history of growth factor administration should minimize the difficulty in distinguishing these changes from a myelodysplastic process.

The differential diagnosis of RAEB-1 and RAEB-2 primarily relates to AML M2, M4, or M6. The blast percentage is the defining criterion. If a case presents with a marrow blast percentage of 10% to 20% and a chromosome abnormality relatively specific to a specific morphologic type of AML is present, for example, t(8;21) or inv16, it is appropriate to classify the case as AML with maturation or AML with increased marrow eosinophils (M4E0), respectively, if the morphologic findings are consistent with the classification.

There will be some cases of persistent cytopenia(s), that is, more than 6-month duration, which lack definitive morphologic and cytogenetic evidence of MDS and which, after detailed clinical and historical review, have no identifiable etiologic basis. The term "idiopathic cytopenia of undetermined significance" has been introduced to recognize these cases (65,127). Some of these cases will eventually show definitive evidence of MDS; others will manifest the findings of a nonmyeloid disorder in

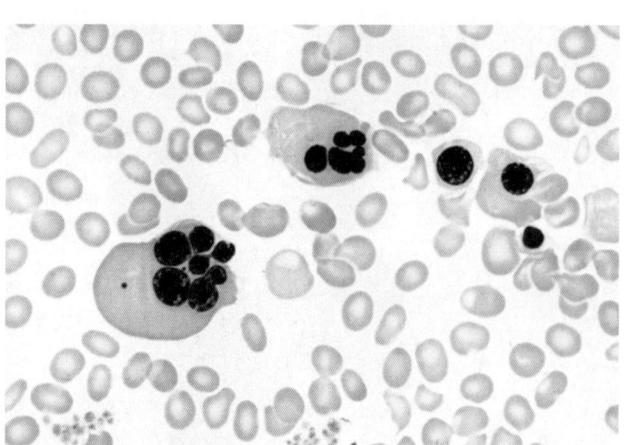

FIGURE 43.45. Bone marrow smear from an 11-month-old male child with CDA type III. The polychromatic and orthochromatic precursors show marked anisocytosis; the two largest cells have markedly lobulated nuclei. The nuclear chromatin of some of the cells is slightly open (Wright-Giemsa, 240×).

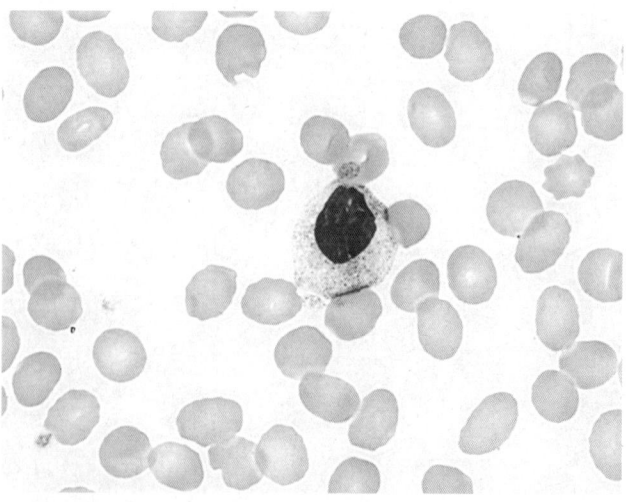

FIGURE 43.46. Neutrophil in the blood of a patient receiving cotrimoxazole; the nucleus is nonlobate. The cell is normal in size in contrast to many neutrophils with pseudo–Pelger-Huët nuclei in MD, which are smaller than normal. The cytoplasm has normal granulation (Wright-Giemsa, 400×).

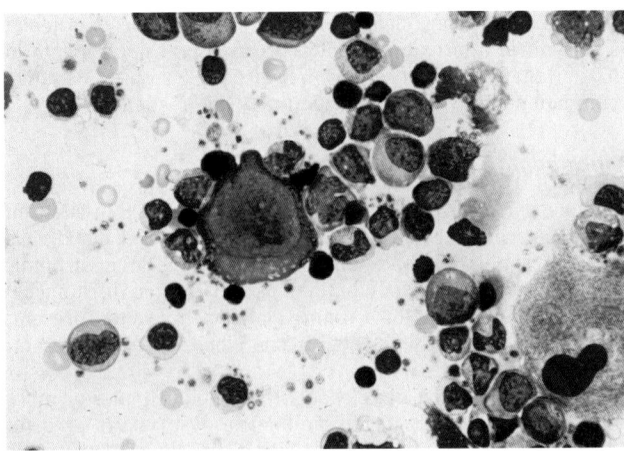

FIGURE 43.47. Giant erythroblast in a marrow smear from a 17-year-old male with parvovirus B19 infection. The cytoplasm contains numerous very small vacuoles (Wright-Giemsa, 400×).

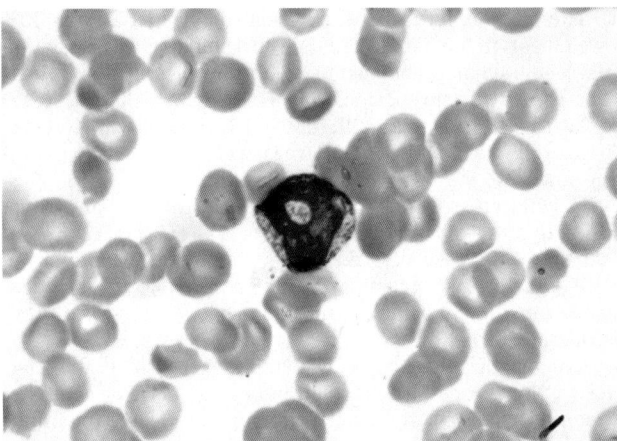

FIGURE 43.49. Blood smear from a patient on granulocyte colony–stimulating factor showing a neutrophil with a ring nucleus (Wright-Giemsa, 640×).

which the cytopenias are an epiphenomenon. Still others will recover without an etiologic basis for the cytopenias having been identified. A proportion will remain in the category of ICUS. The HUMARA assay has been proposed as a test, which may distinguish some cases of MDS from ICUS (161).

It should be emphasized that ICUS, although useful as a temporary designation, is somewhat unsatisfactory. It is not a diagnosis and should be used sparingly. It is not a substitute for a rigorous medical evaluation of patients with persistent cytopenia. Patients with ICUS warrant careful clinical and hematologic monitoring in the anticipation that definitive evidence of an etiologic basis for the cytopenia(s) will emerge.

MYELODYSPLASTIC SYNDROMES IN CHILDREN

Because of some unique characteristics of MDSs in children, the 2008 *WHO Classification of Tumours of Haematopoietic and Lymphoid Tissues* introduced a chapter specifically addressing childhood MDSs (162). This recognizes the unique features in childhood MDS, which have been reported in previous reports (163–165).

MDSs account for 4% of all hematologic malignancies in the age group 0 to 14 years; the annual incidence is approximately 1.8 cases per million population (162,163,165–167). Myeloid malignancies associated with Down syndrome are excluded from the MDS category and are recognized in the WHO as a distinct biologic entity (167,168). MDSs in children can occur as primary diseases or as a secondary process, the latter occurring in children with congenital or acquired bone marrow failure syndromes or as therapy related disorders resulting from cytotoxic therapy for a previous neoplastic or nonneoplastic disease (162–164).

In contrast to adults with MDS who frequently present with anemia, children frequently present with neutropenia and thrombocytopenia (162).

The WHO Classification of the childhood MDSs differs in some important aspects from the classification suggested for adults. Two of the low-grade entities in the adult classification, RARS and the isolated del(5q) (5q– syndrome), are distinctly rare in children; the significance of multilineage dysplasia (RCMD) is unknown for the pediatric population. The criteria for RAEB in children are similar to those for adults although the prognostic significance of distinguishing RAEB-1 from RAEB-2 has not been determined in the pediatric population.

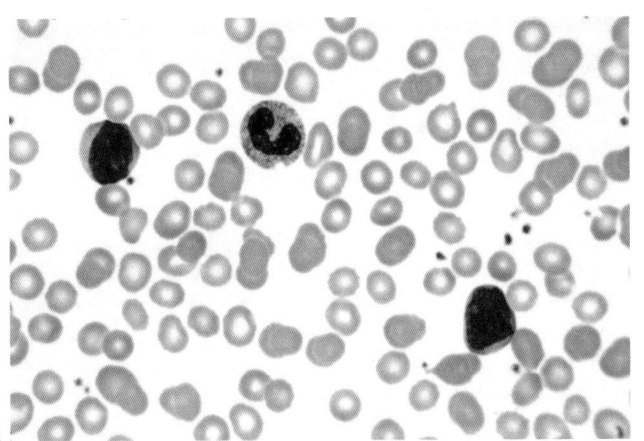

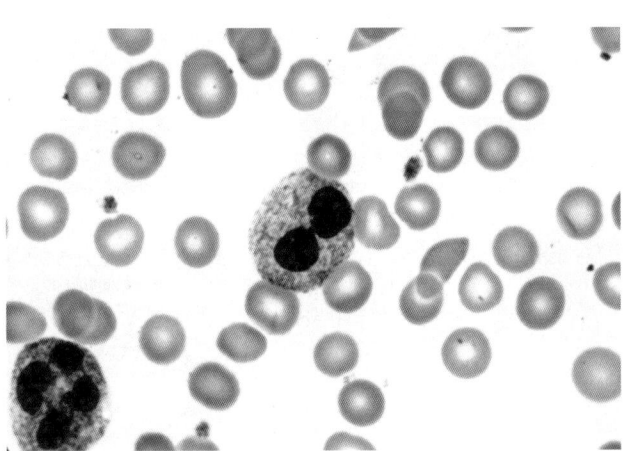

FIGURE 43.48. A: Blood smear from a 7-year-old male being treated with granulocyte colony–stimulating factor following bone marrow transplantation. **A:** Two myeloblasts and a more mature neutrophil with increased azurophilic granulation. **B:** A mature neutrophil with a bilobed (pseudo–Pelger-Huët) nucleus and increased azurophilic granulation (Wright-Giemsa, 640×).

The retention of RAEB-T, primarily defined by 20% to 30% myeloblasts in the marrow, in the WHO childhood classification represents a major modification of the adult classification. However, cases with the specific cytogenetic abnormalities t(15:17)(q22;q12), t(8;21)(q22;q22), inv16(p13.1Q22), or t(16;16)(p13.1;q22) are diagnosed AML regardless of the blast percentage similar to the WHO adult classification.

In children with marrow or blood blast counts of 20% to 30% and no specific cytogenetic and/or molecular marker qualifying for a diagnosis of AML, it is very important to monitor the pace of the disease including clinical, morphologic, and cytogenetic evaluation to determine if a change to a diagnosis of AML is warranted (162).

Cytogenetic studies are considered to be crucial in the diagnosis of low-grade MDS in children because of other causes of dysplasia such as vitamin deficiency, toxic exposure, and inherited defects causing bone marrow failure. Cytogenetic studies are important in distinguishing advanced MDS in children from AML; the blast count in the marrow is considered insufficient by some observers (162).

Refractory Cytopenia of Childhood

Refractory cytopenia of childhood (RCC), a provisional entity in the 2008 *Classification of Tumours of Haematopoetic and Lymphoid Tissues*, is characterized by persistent cytopenia(s), dysplastic changes in the myeloid cells, and <5% blasts in the marrow and <2% blasts in the blood. The bone marrow is usually markedly hypocellular as determined by examination of a bone marrow biopsy (162,169).

Epidemiology

RCC is the most frequent type of MDS in children accounting for approximately 50% of the cases of childhood MDS. Considering that MDSs account for only 4% of childhood hematologic malignancies, RCC is a rare disease. The sexes are affected in equal numbers (162).

Clinical Features

The most common symptoms relate to the underlying cytopenia(s): malaise related to anemia, bleeding resulting from thrombocytopenia, and recurrent or persistent infection related to neutropenia. Thrombocytopenia is the most common

cytopenia occurring in approximately 75% of cases; anemia is present in approximately 50% of cases and neutropenia in 25%. Hepatosplenomegaly is not usually present. Regional lymphadenopathy due to infection may be present.

Morphologic Findings

The suggested minimal diagnostic criteria for MDS in children and adolescents are listed in Table 43.8. The red blood cells show anisopoikilocytosis and macrocytosis. The neutrophils may show nuclear hypolobation, pseudo–Pelger-Huët nuclei, and/or hypogranulation. Giant platelets may be present. Blasts are not usually detected in the blood smear; if present, they are <2%.

There is dysplasia in at least two myeloid cell lines or more than 10% of the cells if only unilineage dysplasia is present. Dysplastic megakaryocytes including micromegakaryocytes with nonlobated nuclei may be present in the marrow smears or imprints and are strong evidence for MDS. The marrow blast percentage is <5%; if the blast percentage in the marrow exceeds 5%, the case is classified as RAEB or AML depending on the percent of blasts.

A satisfactory bone marrow trephine biopsy is a mandatory procedure for the diagnosis of RCC (Fig. 43.50A–C). The majority of marrows is markedly hypocellular, 5% to 10% of age matched children. The major findings in the marrow are shown in Table 43.8. Erythropoiesis is patchy with foci of very immature erythroblasts, which show increased mitotic activity. Neutrophil precursors are sparse. Megakaryocytes are usually markedly decreased in number; dysplastic megakaryocytes, particularly micromegakaryocytes, may be present and represent important diagnostic evidence. To enhance the search for dysplastic megakaryocytes, immunohistochemistry with antibodies to megakaryocytes such as anti-CD61 and anti-CD41 is recommended for the detection of abnormal megakaryocytes (170).

It may not be possible to make the distinction between RCC and severe aplastic anemia (SAA) on the initial marrow specimen, and repeat marrow biopsy may have to be performed 2 to 3 weeks later. Additional biopsies may also be necessary. With increasing experience with the morphologic features in marrow biopsies in RCC, an accurate distinction between RCC and SAA can be accomplished in a very high percentage of cases (169).

As noted, the most difficult differential diagnosis of RCC is SAA. This is particularly true if there is no accompanying cytogenetic or molecular abnormality. Inherited bone marrow

Table 43.8	MINIMAL DIAGNOSTIC CRITERIA FOR RCC		
	Erythropoiesis	**Granulopoiesis**	**Megakaryopoiesis**
Bone marrow aspirate	Dysplastic changes[a] and/or megaloblastoid changes in at least 10% of erythroid precursors	Dysplastic changes[b] in at least 10% of granulocytic precursors and neutrophils; <5% blasts	Unequivocal micromegakaryocytes, other dysplastic changes[c] in variable numbers
Bone marrow biopsy	A few clusters of at least 20 erythroid precursors Stop in maturation with increased number of proerythroblasts. Increased number of mitoses	No minimal diagnostic criteria	Unequivocal micromegakaryocytes; immunohistochemistry is obligatory (CD61, CD41), other dysplastic changes[c] in variable numbers.
Peripheral blood		Dysplastic changes[b] in at least 10% of neutrophils; <2% blasts	

[a]Abnormal nuclear lobation, multinuclear cells, nuclear bridges.
[b]Pseudo–Pelger-Huët cells, hypo- or agranularity, giant bands. (In cases of severe neutropenia, this criteria may not be fulfilled.)
[c]Megakaryocytes of variable size with separated nuclei or round nuclei. The absence of megakaryocytes will not exclude RCC.
Reproduced from Baumann I, Niemeyer CM, Bennett JM, et al. Childhood myelodysplastic syndrome. In: Swerdlow SH, Campo E, Harris NL, et al., eds. *WHO classification of tumours of the haematopoietic and lymphoid tissues.* Lyon: IARC, 2008:104–107.

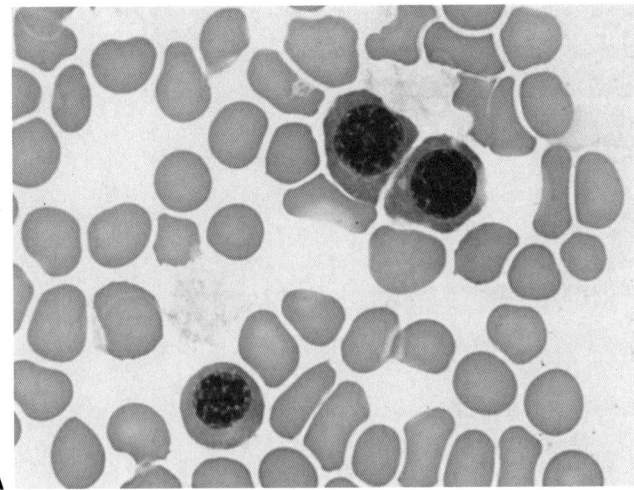

A

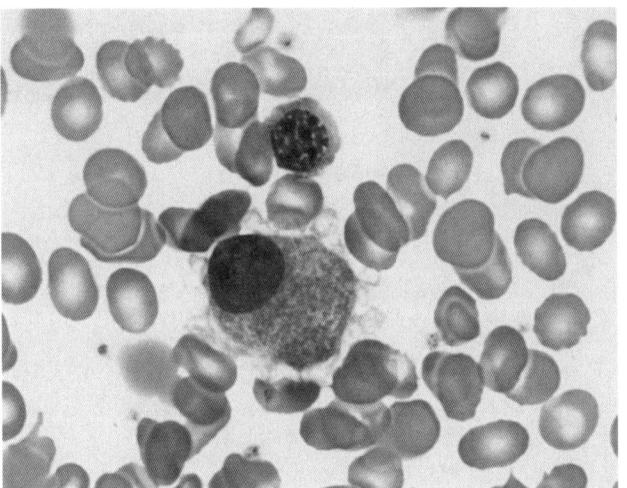

B

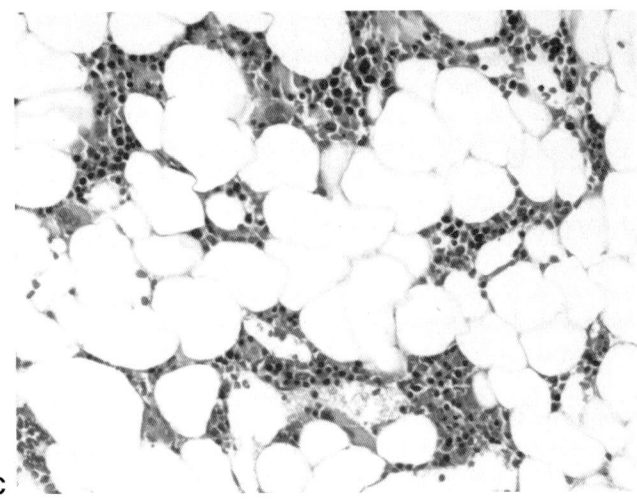

C

FIGURE 43.50. A: Three erythroid precursors in a bone marrow smear from an 11-year-old child with RCC. The nuclear chromatin is slightly open. **B:** The same specimen as (**A**) showing a mature megakaryocyte with a nonlobate nucleus but well-granulated cytoplasm. **C:** A bone marrow section from the same specimen as (**A**) and (**B**). The marrow is markedly hypocellular for an 11-year-old; neutrophil precursors are particularly decreased (**A** and **B**: Wright-Giemsa 400×; **C**: H&E). Cytogenetic studies on this specimen showed 46xy, der(1;7)(q10;p10), monosomy 7q, trisomy 1p3.

failure disorders including Fanconi anemia must also be excluded (171).

The most common cytogenetic abnormality in children with MDS is monosomy 7 (172). Other abnormalities including trisomy 8 and complex abnormalities may occur. The isolated del(5q)(5q– syndrome) essentially does not occur in children (162).

Karyotype is the most important prognostic predictive factor in childhood MDS. Pediatric patients with RA (<5% marrow blasts) and an associated monosomy 7 have a higher rate of progression to more advanced stages of MDS than patients with other karyotypic abnormalities or normal karyotype (172). In children with advanced MDS, the presence of a structurally complex chromosome abnormality, defined as three or more chromosome aberrations including at least one structural abnormality, has an adverse effect on prognosis and is the strongest independent prognostic factor in RAEB and RAEB-T in children (173,174). The presence of a monosomy and structurally complex karyotype is reported as strongly associated with poor prognosis, and the presence of a structurally complex karyotype without a monosomy was associated with a very short survival (174).

Differential Diagnosis

As noted, the most difficult hematologic differential diagnosis of RCC is severe acquired aplastic anemia; as noted, it may

not be possible in all instances to make this distinction on initial encounter. In the absence of a cytogenetic abnormality, repeat biopsies at appropriate intervals should be performed until convincing morphologic evidence is detected or a cytogenetic abnormality is identified. Table 43.9 details features, which can be used in distinguishing RCC from SAA (24,162).

Inherited bone marrow failure disorders including Fanconi anemia, Shwachman-Diamond syndrome, Diamond-Blackfan syndrome, dyskeratosis congenita, and amegakaryocytic thrombocytopenia are distinguished by medical history, physical features, and appropriate laboratory studies (171).

Patients with Fanconi anemia have an increased incidence of developing MDS and AML. Distinguishing the onset of an MDS in these patients may be particularly difficult because of slight degrees of dyserythropoiesis, which are inherent to the underlying disorder (175). Although paroxysmal nocturnal hemoglobinuria (PNH) clones may be observed in children, the clinical picture of PNH is rare.

Pearson syndrome is a multiorgan disorder due to defective oxidative phosphorylation caused by a mitochondrial deletion, which may manifest with hematologic findings of hypoplastic anemia, thrombocytopenia, neutropenia, ring sideroblasts, and vacuolated myeloid precursors in the marrow (176,177) (Fig. 43.51). The systemic abnormalities and laboratory findings distinguish this disorder from MDS.

Table 43.9		**COMPARISON OF MORPHOLOGIC CRITERIA OF HYPOPLASTIC RCC AND APLASTIC ANEMIA IN CHILDHOOD (AA)**	
		RCC	**AA**
Bone Marrow Aspiration Cytology			
Erythropoiesis		Nuclear lobation	Lacking or very few cells, without dysplasia or megaloblastoid change
		Multinuclearity	
		Megaloblastoid changes	
Granulopoiesis		Pseudo–Pelger–Huët anomaly	Few maturing cells with no dysplasia
		Agranulation of cytoplasm	
		Hypogranulation of cytoplasm	
		Nuclear-cytoplasmic maturation defects	
Megakaryopoiesis		Micromegakaryocytes	Lacking or few nondysplastic megakaryocytes
		Multiple separated nuclei	
		Small nonlobated nuclei	
Lymphocytes		May be increased	May be increased
Bone Marrow Biopsy			
Erythropoiesis		Patchy distribution	Lacking or single small focus with <10 cells with maturation
		Left shift	
		Increased mitoses	
Granulopoiesis		Marked decrease	Lacking or marked decrease; very few small foci with maturation
		Left shift	
Megakaryopoiesis		Marked decrease	Lacking or very few; no dysplastic megakaryocytes
		Dysplastic changes	
		Micromegakaryocytes	
Lymphocytes		May be increased focally or dispersed	May be increased focally or dispersed
CD34⁺ cells		No increase	No increase

Reproduced from Baumann I, Niemeyer CM, Bennett JM, et al. Childhood myelodysplastic syndrome. In: Swerdlow SH, Campo E, Harris NL, et al., eds. *WHO classification of tumours of the haematopoietic and lymphoid tissues.* Lyon: IARC, 2008:104–107.

Similar to MDS in adults, toxic exposure, viral infections, and vitamin deficiencies (B_{12} and folate) may result in dysplastic changes in the myeloid cells and must be excluded in those MDSs in which there is no increase in blasts. Inherited disorders such as mevalonate kinase deficiency may have to be excluded. It is probably prudent to assume some other cause of the dysplasia until proven otherwise.

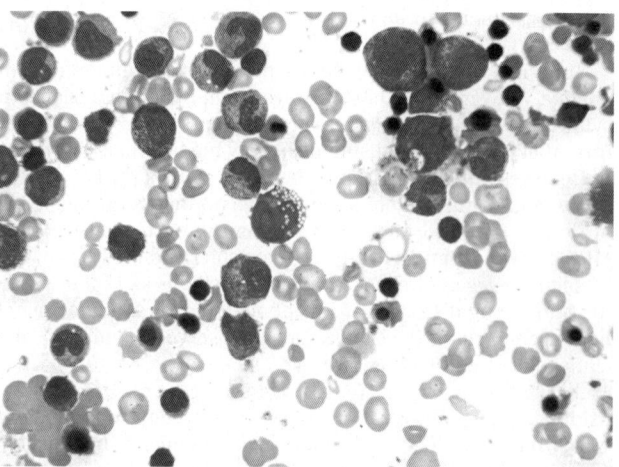

FIGURE 43.51. Marrow smear from a child with Pearson syndrome. There are occasional vacuolated myeloid precursors. Five percent of the erythroid precursors were ring sideroblasts (Wright-Giemsa).

 SUMMARY AND CONCLUSIONS

The MDSs are a heterogeneous group of hematopoietic stem cell disorders characterized by abnormalities in maturation of one or more myeloid cell lines with or without an increase in blasts; the blast percentage, if increased, is <20% requisite for a diagnosis of AML. The MDSs occur as primary or *de novo* processes and as secondary or therapy related disorders in persons previously treated with chemotherapy and/or radiotherapy.

The diagnosis and classification of the MDSs are based on peripheral blood and bone marrow and cytogenetic findings. The importance of careful examination of blood and marrow specimens in patients suspected of having an MDS cannot be overemphasized. The changes in these disorders are often subtle and may be overlooked with poorly prepared specimens. In addition, improperly prepared specimens from patients who do not have an MDS may exhibit technical artifacts in blood cells, particularly granulocytes that resemble the findings in the MDS.

Cytogenetic studies are essential to the evaluation and classification of patients with MDS and should be performed in any suspected case. Clonal abnormalities are evidence for the diagnosis in morphologically equivocal cases; the type of abnormality may have substantial prognostic significance. The specific cytogenetic clinical pathologic entity, the del(5q) syndrome, is an important example of the relationship, which may exist between morphology and cytogenetic findings.

Morphologic abnormalities of the myeloid cells that resemble the changes in the MDSs may be observed in nutritionally based anemias and CDAs and may be a result of exposure to toxins and drugs. These possibilities should always be considered before establishing a diagnosis of MDS, particularly RCUD.

The primary MDSs are a biologically heterogeneous group of disorders with marked variation in clinical evolution. RA and RARS may be relatively benign disorders in the majority of patients with a prolonged clinical course and low incidence of evolution to AML. RCMD has a variable clinical evolution but generally appears to be more aggressive than RCUD.

The childhood MDSs have some unique characteristics, and the classification, which shows some variance with the WHO Classification for adults, takes these differences into consideration. RAEB-T is retained in the WHO Classification of the MDSs in childhood.

A provisional entity, RCC, is introduced in the MDS classification in children. This entity is characterized by persistent cytopenia, <2% blasts in the blood, <5% blasts in the bone marrow, and dysplastic changes in the myeloid cells; the marrow in the majority of cases of RCC is markedly hypocellular, and the major differential diagnosis is aplastic anemia. Cytogenetic studies are considered crucial in the evaluation of pediatric patients with MDS.

References

1. Tefferi A, Vardiman JW. Myelodysplastic syndromes. *N Engl J Med* 2009; 361:1872–1885.
2. Corey SJ, Minden MD, Barber DL, et al. Myelodysplastic syndromes: the complexity of stem cell disease. *Nat Rev Cancer* 2007;7:118–129.
3. Nimer S. Myelodysplastic syndromes. *Blood* 2008;111:4841–4851.
4. Foucar K, McKenna RW, Bloomfield CD, et al. Therapy related leukemia, a panmyelosis. *Cancer* 1979;43:1285–1296.
5. Rollinson DE, Howlader N, Smith MT, et al. Epidemiology of myelodysplastic syndromes and chronic myeloproliferative disorders in the United States, 2001-2004, using data from the NAACCR and SEER programs. *Blood* 2008;112: 45–52.
6. Ma X, Does M, Raza A, et al. Myelodysplastic syndromes: incidence and survival in the United States. *Cancer* 2007;109:1536–1542.
7. Sekeres MA. The epidemiology of myelodysplastic syndromes. *Hematol Oncol Clin North Am* 2010;24:287–294.
8. Surveillance, Epidemiology, and End Results (SEER) Program Population (1969-2009) (www.seer.cancer.gov.popdata) National Cancer Institute. DCCPS, Surveillance Research Program. Cancer Statistics Branch, released January 2011, Accessed November 2011.
9. Cogle CR, Craig BM, Rollison DE, et al. Incidence of the myelodysplastic syndromes using a novel claims-based algorithm: high number of uncaptured cases by cancer registries. *Blood* 2011;117:7121–7125.
10. Neukirchen J, Schoonen WM, Strupp C, et al. Incidence and prevalence of myelodysplastic syndromes: data from the Düsseldorf MDS-registry. *Leuk Res* 2011;35:1591–1596.
11. Intragumtornchai T, Prayoonwiwat W, Swasdikul D, et al. Myelodysplastic syndrome in Thailand: a retrospective pathologic and clinical analysis of 117 cases. *Leuk Res* 1998;22:453–460.
12. Lee J-H, Lee J-H, Shin Y-R, et al. Application of different prognostic scoring systems and comparison of the FAB and WHO classifications in Korean patients with myelodysplastic syndromes. *Leukemia* 2003;17:305–313.
13. Chen B, Zhao W-L, Jin J, et al. Clinical and cytogenetic features of 508 Chinese patients with myelodysplastic syndrome and comparison with those in Western counties. *Leukemia* 2005;19:767–775.
14. Matsuda A, Germing U, Jinnai I, et al. Difference in clinical features between Japanese and German patients with refractory anemia in myelodysplastic syndromes. *Blood* 2005;106:2633–2640.
15. Matsuda A, Germing U, Jinnai I, et al. Differences in the distribution of subtypes according to the WHO classification 2008 between Japanese and German patients with refractory anemia according to the FAB classification in myelodysplastic syndromes. *Leuk Res* 2010;34:974–980.
16. Enright H, Jacob HS, Vercellotti G, et al. Paraneoplastic autoimmune phenomena in patients with myelodysplastic syndromes: response to immunosuppressive therapy. *Br J Haematol* 1995;91:403–408.
17. Sloand EM, Rezvani K. The role of the immune system in myelodysplasia: implications for therapy. *Semin Hematol* 2008;45:39–48.
18. Alfinto F, Sica M, Luciano L, et al. Immune dysregulation and dyserythropoiesis in the myelodysplastic syndromes. *Br J Haematol* 2010;148:90–98.
19. Calado RT. Immunologic aspects of hypoplastic myelodysplastic syndrome. *Semin Oncol* 2011;38:667–672.
20. Broliden PA, Dahl I-M, Hast R, et al. Antithymocyte globulin and cyclosporine A as combination therapy for low-risk non-sideroblastic myelodysplastic syndromes. *Haematologica* 2006;91:667–670.
21. Lim ZY, Killick S, Germing U, et al. Low IPSS score and bone marrow hypocellularity in MDS patients predict hematologic response to antithymocyte globulin. *Leukemia* 2007;21:1436–1441.
22. Sloand EM, Wu CO, Greenberg P, et al. Factors affecting response and survival in patients with myelodysplasia treated with immunosuppressive therapy. *J Clin Oncol* 2008;26:2505–2511.
23. Vardiman JW, Harris NL, Brunning RD. The World Health Organization (WHO) classification of the myeloid neoplasms. *Blood* 2002;100:2292–2302.
24. Brunning RD, Orazi A, Germing U, et al. Myelodysplastic syndromes/neoplasms, overview. In: Swerdlow S, Campo E, Harris NL, et al., eds. *WHO classification of tumours of haematopoietic and lymphoid tissues*, 4th ed. Lyon: IARC, 2008:88–93.
25. Bowen D, Culligan D, Jowitt S, et al. Guidelines for the diagnosis and therapy of adult myelodysplastic syndromes. *Br J Haematol* 2003;120:187–200.
26. Mufti GJ, Bennett JM, Goasguen J, et al. Diagnosis and classification of myelodysplastic syndromes: International Working Group on Morphology of Myelodysplastic Syndrome (IWGMMDS) consensus proposals for the definition and enumeration of myeloblasts and ring sideroblasts. *Haematologica* 2008;93:1712–1717.
27. Juneja SK, Imbert M, Jouault H, et al. Haematological features of primary myelodysplastic syndromes (PMDS) at initial presentation: a study of 118 cases. *J Clin Pathol* 1983;36:1129–1135.
28. Tricot G, De Wolf-Peeters C, Hendrickx B, et al. Bone marrow histology in myelodysplastic syndromes. 1. Histological findings in myelodysplastic syndromes and comparison with bone marrow smears. *Br J Haematol* 1984;57:423–430.
29. Verburgh E, Achten R, Maes B, et al. Additional prognostic value of bone marrow histology in patients subclassified according to the International Prognostic Scoring System for myelodysplastic syndromes. *J Clin Oncol* 2003;21:273–282.
30. Bennett JM, Catovsky D, Daniel MT, et al. Proposals for the classification of the acute leukaemias. *Br J Haematol* 1976;33:451–458.
31. Bennett JM, Catovsky D, Daniel MT, et al. Proposals for the classification of the myelodysplastic syndromes. *Br J Haematol* 1982;51:189–199.
32. Bennett JM, Catovsky D, Daniel MT, et al. Proposed revised criteria for the classification of acute myeloid leukemia. *Ann Intern Med* 1985;103:626–629.
33. Bennett JM. World Health Organization classification of the acute leukemias and myelodysplastic syndrome. *Int J Hematol* 2000;72:131–133.
34. Papaemmanui E, Cazzola M, Boultwood J, et al. Somatic SF3B1 mutation in myelodysplasia with ring sideroblasts. *N Engl J Med* 2011;365:1384–1395.
35. Juneja SK, Imbert M, Sigaux F, et al. Prevalence and distribution of ringed sideroblasts in primary myelodysplastic syndromes. *J Clin Pathol* 1983;36:566–569.
36. Greenberg P, Cox C, LeBeau M, et al. International scoring system for evaluation prognosis in myelodysplastic syndromes. *Blood* 1997;89:2079–2088.
37. Greenberg P, Tuechler H, Schanz J, et al. Revised international prognostic scoring system for myelodysplastic syndromes. *Blood* 2012;120:2454–2465.
38. Verburgh E, Achten R, Louw VJ, et al. A new disease categorization of low-grade myelodysplastic syndromes based on the expression of cytopenia and dysplasia in one versus more than one lineage improves on the WHO classification. *Leukemia* 2007;21:668–677.
39. Germing U, Gattermann N, Strupp C, et al. Validation of the WHO proposals for a new classification of primary myelodysplastic syndromes: a retrospective analysis of 1600 patients. *Leuk Res* 2000;24:983–992.
40. Malcovati L, Porta MG, Pascutta C, et al. Prognostic factors and life expectancy in myelodysplastic syndromes classified according to WHO criteria: a basis for clinical decision making. *J Clin Oncol* 2005;23:7594–7603.
41. Germing U, Strupp C, Kuengden A, et al. Prospective validation of the WHO proposals for the classification of myelodysplastic syndromes. *Haematologica* 2006;91:1596–1604.
42. List A, Dewald G, Bennett J, et al.; Myelodysplastic Syndrome-003 Study Investigators. Lenalidomide in the myelodysplastic syndrome with chromosome 5q deletion. *N Engl J Med* 2006;355:1456–1465.
43. Brunning RD, Hasserjian RP, Porwit A, et al. Refractory cytopenia with unilineage dysplasia. In: Swerdlow SH, Campo E, Harris NL, et al., eds. *WHO classification of tumours of the haematopoietic and lymphoid tissues*. Lyon: IARC, 2008:94–95.
44. Hasserjian RP, Gatterman N, Bennett, JM, et al. Refractory anaemia with ring sideroblasts. In: Swerdlow SH, Campo E, Harris NL, et al., eds. *WHO classification of tumours of the haematopoietic and lymphoid tissues*. Lyon: IARC, 2008: 96–97.
45. Cazzola M, Invernizzi R. Ring sideroblasts and sideroblastic anemia. *Haematologica* 2011;96:789–792.
46. Gattermann N, Aul C, Schneider W. Two types of acquired idiopathic sideroblastic anaemia (AISA). *Br J Haematol* 1990;74:45–52.
47. Garand R, Gardais J, Bizet M, et al. Heterogeneity of acquired idiopathic sideroblastic anaemia (AISA). *Leuk Res* 1992;16:463–468.
48. Germing U, Gattermann N, Aivado M, et al. Two types of acquired idiopathic sideroblastic anaemia (AISA): a time-tested distinction. *Br J Haematol* 2000;108:724–728.
49. Brunning RD, Bennett JM, Matutes E, et al. Refractory cytopenia with multilineage dysplasia. In: Swerdlow SH, Campo E, Harris NL, et al., eds. *WHO classification of tumours of the haematopoietic and lymphoid tissues*. Lyon: IARC, 2008:98–99.
50. Rosati S, Mick R, Xu F, et al. Refractory cytopenia with multilineage dysplasia: further characterization of an "unclassifiable" myelodysplastic syndrome. *Leukemia* 1996;10:20–26.
51. Balduini CL, Guarnone R, Pecci A, et al. Multilineage dysplasia without increased blasts identifies a poor prognosis subset of myelodysplastic syndromes. *Leukemia* 1996;12:1655–1656.
52. Matsuda A, Jinnai I, Yagasaki F, et al. Refractory anemia with severe dysplasia: clinical significance of morphological features in refractory anemia. *Leukemia* 1998;12:482–485.
53. Matsuda A, Germing U, Jinnai I, et al. Improvement of criteria for refractory cytopenia with multilineage dysplasia according to the WHO classification based on prognostic significance of morphological feature in patients with refractory anemia according to the FAB classification. *Leukemia* 2007;21:678–686.
54. Orazi A, Brunning RD, Haaerjian RP, et al. Refractory anaemia with excess blasts. In: Swerdlow SH, Campo E, Harris NL, et al., eds. *WHO classification of tumours of the haematopoietic and lymphoid tissues*. Lyon: IARC, 2008:100–101.
55. Seymour JF, Estey EH. The contribution of Auer rods to the classification and prognosis of myelodysplastic syndromes. *Leuk Lymphoma* 1995;17:79–85.
56. Willis MS, McKenna RW, Peterson LC, et al. Low blast count myeloid disorders with Auer rods. A clinicopathologic analysis of 9 cases. *Am J Clin Pathol* 2005;124:191–198.
57. Van den Berghe H, Cassiman JJ, David G, et al. Distinct haematological disorder with deletion of long arm of no. 5 chromosome. *Nature* 1974;251:437–438.
58. Sokal G, Michaux JL, Van den Berghe H, et al. A new hematologic syndrome with a distinct karyotype: the 5q- chromosome. *Blood* 1975;46:519–533.
59. Ebert BL, Pretz J, Bosco J, et al. Identification of RPS14 as a 5q- syndrome gene by RNA interference screen. *Nature* 2008;451:335–339.

60. Hasserjian RP, LeBeau MM, List AF, et al. Myelodysplastic syndrome with isolated del(5q). In: Swerdlow SH, Campo E, Harris NL, et al., eds. *WHO classification of tumours of the haematopoietic and lymphoid tissues*. Lyon: IARC, 2008:102.
61. Boultwood J, Pellagatti A, McKensie AWJ, et al. Advances in the 5q-syndrome. *Blood* 2010;116:5803–5811.
62. Mohamedali MM, Mufti GJ. Van-den Berghe's 5q- syndrome in 2008. *Br J Haematol* 2009;144:157–158.
63. Giagounidis AA, Germing U, Haase S, et al. Clinical, morphological, cytogenetic, and prognostic features of patients with myelodysplastic syndromes and del(5q) including band q31. *Leukemia* 2004;18:113–119.
64. Germing U, Lauseker M, Hildebrandt B, et al. Survival, prognostic factors, and rates of leukemic transformation in 381 untreated patients with MDS and del(5q). A multicenter study. *Leukemia* 2012;26:1286–1292.
65. Orazi A, Brunning RD, Baumann I, et al. Myelodysplastic syndrome, unclassifiable. In: Swerdlow SH, Campo E, Harris NL, et al. eds. *WHO classification of tumours of the haematopoietic and lymphoid tissues*. Lyon: IARC, 2008:103.
66. Wimazal F, Fonatsch C, Thalhammer R, et al. Idiopathic cytopenia of undetermined significance (ICUS) versus low risk MDS: the diagnostic interface. *Leuk Res* 2007;31:1461–1468.
67. Hwang Y, Huh J, Mun Y, et al. Characteristics of myelodysplastic syndrome, unclassifiable by WHO classification 2008. *Ann Hematol* 2011;90:469–471.
68. Hartsock RJ, Smith EB, Petty CS. Normal variations with aging of the amount of hematopoietic tissue in bone marrow from the anterior crest. *Am J Clin Pathol* 1965;43:326–331.
69. Tuzuner N, Cox C, Rowe JM, et al. Bone marrow cellularity in myeloid stem cell disorders: impact of age correction. *Leuk Res* 1994;18:559–564.
70. Tuzuner N, Cox C, Rowe JM, et al. Hypocellular myelodysplastic syndromes (MDS): new proposals. *Br J Haematol* 1995;91:612–617.
71. Huang TC, Ko BS, Tang JL, et al. Comparison of hypoplastic myelodysplastic syndrome(MDS) with normo-hypercellular MDS by International prognostic Scoring System, cytogenetics and genetic studies. *Leukemia* 2009;22:544–550.
72. Yoshida Y, Oguma H, Maekawa T. Refractory myelodysplastic anaemias with hypocellular bone marrow. *J Clin Pathol* 1988;41:763–767.
73. Yue G, Hao S, Fadare O, et al. Hypocellularity in myelodysplastic syndrome is an independent factor which predicts a favorable outcome. *Leuk Res* 2008;32: 553–558.
74. Sloand EM. Hypocellular myelodysplasia. *Hematol Oncol Clin North Am* 2009;23:47–60.
75. Orazi A, Albiter M, Heerema NA, et al. Hypoplastic myelodysplastic syndrome can be distinguished from acquired aplastic anemia by CD 34 and PCNA immunostaining of bone marrow biopsy specimens. *Am J Clin Pathol* 1997;107:268–274.
76. Bennett JM, Orazi A. Diagnostic criteria to distinguish hypocellular myeloid leukemia from hypocellular myelodysplastic syndromes and aplastic anemia: recommendations for a standard approach. *Haematologica* 2009;94:264–268.
77. Maciejewski JP, Risitano A, Sloand EM, et al. Distinct clinical outcomes for cytogenetic abnormalities evolving from aplastic anemia. *Blood* 2002;99:3129–3135.
78. Steemsa DP, Hanson CA, Letendre L, et al. Myelodysplasia with fibrosis: a distinct clinical entity? *Leuk Res* 2001;25:829–838.
79. Marisavljevic D, Rolovic Z, Cemerikic V, et al. Myelofibrosis in primary myelodysplastic syndromes: clinical and biological significance. *Med Oncol* 2004;21: 325–331.
80. Della Porta GD, Malcovatti L. Myelodysplastic syndromes with myelofibrosis. *Haematologica* 2011;96:180–182.
81. Della Porta MG, Malcovatti L, Boveri E, et al. Clinical relevance of bone marrow fibrosis and CD34-positive cell clusters in primary myelodysplastic syndromes. *J Clin Oncol* 2009;27:754–762.
82. Buesche G, Teoman H, Wiczak W, et al. Marrow fibrosis predicts early fatal marrow failure in patients with myelodysplastic syndromes. *Leukemia* 2008;22: 312–322.
83. Thiele J, Kvasnicka HM, Fachetti F, et al. European consensus on grading bone marrow fibrosis and assessment of cellularity. *Haematologica* 2005;90:1128–1132.
84. Kroger N, Zabelina T, van Biezen A, et al. Allogeneic stem cell transplantation for myelodysplastic syndromes with bone marrow fibrosis. *Haematologica* 2011;96:291–297.
85. Kussick SJ, Fromm JR, Rossini A, et al. Four-color flow cytometry shows strong concordance with bone marrow morphology and cytogenetics in the evaluation for myelodysplasia. *Am J Clin Pathol* 2005;124:170–181.
86. van de Loosdrecht AA, Alhan C, Bene MC, et al. Standardization of flow cytometry in myelodysplastic syndromes: report from the first European LeukemiaNet working conference on flow cytometry in myelodysplastic syndromes. *Haematologica* 2009;94:1124–1134.
87. Loken MR, Chu S-C, Fritschle W, et al. Normalization of bone marrow aspirates for hemodilution in flow cytometric analyses. *Cytometry B Clin Cytom* 2009;76B:27–36.
88. Matarraz S, Lopez A, Barrena S, et al. Bone marrow cells from myelodysplastic syndromes show altered immunophenotypic profiles that may contribute to the diagnosis and prognostic stratification of the disease: a pilot study on a series of 56 patients. *Cytometry B Clin Cytom* 2010;78B:154–168.
89. Ogata K, Matteo G, Della Porta MG, et al. Diagnostic utility of flow cytometry in low-grade myelodysplastic syndromes. A prognostic validation study. *Haematologica* 2009;94:1066–1074.
90. Stetler-Stevenson M, Yuan CM. Myelodysplastic syndromes: the role of flow cytometry in diagnosis and prognosis. *Int J Lab Hematol* 2009;31:479–483.
91. Cazzola M. Flow cytometry immunophenotyping for diagnosis of myelodysplastic syndrome. *Haematologica* 2009;94:1041–1043.
92. Kern W, Haferlach C, Schnittger S, et al. Clinical utility of multiparameter flow cytometry in the diagnosis of 1013 patients with suspected myelodysplastic syndrome. *Cancer* 2010;116:4549–4563.
93. Xu F, Li X, Wu L, et al. Flow cytometric scoring system (FCMSS) assisted diagnosis of myelodysplastic syndromes (MDS) and the biological significance of FCMSS-based immunophenotype. *Br J Haematol* 2010;149:587–597.
94. van de Loosdrecht AA, Westers TM, Westra AH, et al. Identification of distinct prognostic subgroups in low- and intermediate-1-risk myelodysplastic syndromes by flow cytometry. *Blood* 2008;111:1067–1077.
95. Truong F, Smith BR, Stachurski D, et al. The utility of flow cytometric immunophenotyping in cytopenic patients with a non-diagnostic bone marrow; a prospective study. *Leuk Res* 2009;33:1039–1046.
96. Van de Loosdrecht AA, Westers TM. Flow cytometry in myelodysplastic syndromes: ready for translocation into clinical practice. *Leuk Res* 2011;35: 850–852.
97. Chu S-C, Wang T-F, Li C-C, et al. Flow cytometry scoring system as a diagnostic and prognostic tool in myelodysplastic syndromes. *Leuk Res* 2011;35: 868–873.
98. Valent P, Horny HP, Bennett JM, et al. Definitions and standards in the diagnosis and treatment of the myelodysplastic syndromes: consensus statements and report from a working conference. *Leuk Res* 2007;31:727–736.
99. Arnoulet C, Bene MC, Durrieu F, et al. Four and five color flow cytometry analysis of leukocyte differentiation pathways in normal bone marrow: a reference document based on a systematic approach by the GTLLF and GEIL. *Cytometry B Clin Cytom* 2010;78B:3–10.
100. Pirucello SJ, Young KH, Aoun P. Myeloblast phenotype changes in myelodysplasia. *Am J Clin Pathol* 2006;125:684–694.
101. Goardon N, Nikolousis E, Sternberg A, et al. Reduced CD38 expression on CD34+ cells as a diagnostic test in myelodysplastic syndromes. *Haematologica* 2009;94:1160–1163.
102. Westers TM, Alhan C, Chamuleau ED, et al. Aberrant phenotype of blasts in myelodysplastic syndromes is a clinically relevant biomarker in predicting response to growth factor treatment. *Blood* 2010;115:1179–1184.
103. Della Porta MG, Malcovatti L, Travaglino E, et al. Flow cytometry in evaluation of erythroid dysplasia in patients with myelodysplastic syndrome. *Leukemia* 2006;20:549–555.
104. McClintock-Treep SA, Briggs RC, Shutts KE, et al. Quantitative assessment of myeloid nuclear differentiation antigen distinguishes myelodysplastic syndrome from normal bone marrow. *Am J Clin Pathol* 2011;135:380–395.
105. Fenaux P, Morel P, LucLai J. Cytogenetics in myelodysplastic syndromes. *Semin Hematol* 1996;33:127–138.
106. Haase D. Cytogenetic features in myelodysplastic syndrome. *Ann Hematol* 2008;87:515–526.
107. Jotterand M, Parlier V. Diagnostic and prognostic significance of cytogenetics in adult primary myelodysplastic syndromes. *Leuk Lymphoma* 1996;23:253–266.
108. Haase D, Germing U, Schanz J, et al. New insights into the prognostic impact of the karyotype in MDS and correlation with subtypes: evidence from a core dataset of 2124 patients. *Blood* 2007;110:4385–4395.
109. Pozdnyakova O, Miron PM, Tang G, et al. Cytogenetic abnormalities in a series of 1029 patients with primary myelodysplastic syndromes. *Cancer* 2008;113: 3331–3340.
110. Sole F, Luno E, Sanzo C, et al. Identification of novel cytogenetic markers with prognostic significance in a series of 968 patients with primary myelodysplastic syndrome. *Haematologica* 2005;90:1168–1178.
111. Bernasconi P, Klersy C, Boni M, et al. World Health Organization classification in combination with cytogenetic markers improves the prognostic stratification of patients with de novo primary myelodysplastic syndromes. *Br J Haematol* 2007;137:193–205.
112. Schanz J, et al. A new comprehensive cytogenetic scoring system for primary myelodysplastic syndromes and oligoblastic AML following MDS derived from an international database merger. *J Clin Oncol* 2012;30:820–829.
113. Malcovati L, Germing U, Kuendgen A, et al. Time dependent prognostic scoring system for predicting survival and leukemic evolution in myelodysplastic syndromes. *J Clin Oncol* 2007;25:3503–3510.
114. Knipp S, Hildebrandt B, Kungden A, et al. Intensive chemotherapy is not recommended for patients aged >60 years who have myelodysplastic syndrome or acute myeloid leukemia with high risk karyotypes. *Cancer* 2007;14:345–352.
115. Mallo M, Cervera J, Schanz J, et al. Impact of adjunct cytogenetic abnormalities for prognostic stratification in patients with myelodysplastic syndrome and deletion 5q. *Leukemia* 2011;25:110–120.
116. Patnaik MM, Lasho TL, Finke CM, et al. WHO-defined myelodysplastic syndrome with isolated del(5q) in 88 consecutive patients: survival data, leukemic transformation rates and prevalence of Jak2, MPL and IDH mutations. *Leukemia* 2010;24:1283–1289.
117. Lai H, Preudhomme C, Zandecki M, et al. Myelodysplastic syndromes and acute myeloid leukemia with 17p deletion. An entity characterized by specific dysgranulopoiesis and a high incidence of P53 mutations. *Leukemia* 1995;9: 370–381.
118. Jary L, Mossafa H, Fourcase C, et al. The 17-p-syndrome; a distinct myelodysplastic syndrome entity? *Leuk Lymphoma* 1997;25:163–168.
119. Soenen V, Preudhomme C, Roumier C, et al. 17p deletion in acute myeloid leukemia and myelodysplastic syndrome. Analysis of breakpoints and deleted segments by fluorescence in situ. *Blood* 1998;91:1008–1015.
120. Sterkers Y, Preudhomme C, Lai J-L, et al. Acute myeloid leukemia and myelodysplastic syndromes following essential thrombocythemia treated with hydroxyurea: high proportion of cases with 17p deletion. *Blood* 1998;91:616–622.
121. Larana JG. Clinical correlations of the 3q21;q26 cytogenetic anomaly. A leukemia or myelodysplastic syndrome with preserved or increased platelet production and lack of response to cytotoxic therapy. *Cancer* 1985;55:535–541.
122. Bitter MA, Neilly ME, LeBeau MM, et al. Rearrangements of chromosome 3 involving bands 3q21 and 3q26 are associated with normal or elevated platelet counts in acute nonlymphocytic leukemia. *Blood* 1985;66:1362–1370.
123. Fonatsch C, Gudat H, Lengfelder E, et al. Correlation of cytogenetic findings with clinical features in 18 patients with inv(3)(q21q26) or t(3:3)(q21;q26). *Leukemia* 1994;8:1318–1326.
124. Kurtin PJ, DeWald GW, Shields DJ, et al. Hematologic disorders associated with deletions of chromosome 20q: a clinicopathologic study of 107 patients. *Am J Clin Pathol* 1996;106:680–688.
125. Gupta R, Soupir CP, Johari V, et al. Myelodysplastic syndrome with isolated 20q-; an indolent disease with minimal morphologic dysplasia and frequent thrombocytopenic presentation. *Br J Haematol* 2007;139:265–268.
126. Braun T, deBolton S, Taksin AL, et al. Characteristics and outcome of myelodysplastic syndromes (MDS) with isolated 20q deletions: a report on 62 cases. *Leuk Res* 2011;35:863–867.
127. Valent P, Bain BJ, Bennett JM, et al. Idiopathic cytopenia of undetermined significance (ICUS) and idiopathic dysplasia of uncertain significance (IDUS) and their distinction from low risk MDS. *Leuk Res* 2012;36:1–5.
128. Odenike O, LeBeau MM. The dawn of the molecular era of the myelodysplastic syndromes. *N Eng J Med* 2011;364:2545–2525.

129. Mills KI, Kohlmann A, Williams PM, et al. Microarray-based classifiers and prognosis models identify subgroups with distinct clinical outcomes and high risk of AML transformation of myelodysplastic syndrome. *Blood* 2009;114:1063–1072.
130. Delhommeau F, Dupont S, Della Valle V, et al. Mutation in TET2 in myeloid cancers. *N Eng J Med* 2009;360:2289–2301.
131. Makishima H, Rataul M, Gondek LP, et al. FISH and SNP-A karyotyping in myelodysplastic syndromes: improving cytogenetic detection of del(5q), monosomy 7, del(7q), trisomy 8 and del(20q). *Leuk Res* 2010;34:447–453.
132. Tiu RV, Gondek LP, O'Keefe CL, et al. Prognostic impact of SNP array karyotyping in myelodysplastic syndromes and related myeloid malignancies. *Blood* 2011;117:4552–4560.
133. Tiu RV, Visconte V, Traina F, et al. Updates in cytogenetics and molecular markers in MDS. *Curr Hematol Malig Rep* 2011;6:126–135.
134. Bejar R, Levine R, Ebert BL. Unraveling the molecular pathogenesis of myelodysplastic syndromes. *J Clin Oncol* 2011;29:504–515.
135. Bejar R, Stevenson K, Abdel-Wahab O, et al. Clinical effect of point mutations in myelodysplastic syndromes. *N Eng J Med* 2011;364:2496–2506.
136. Huang W-T, Yang X, Zhou X, et al. Multiple distinct clones may co-exist in different lineages in myelodysplastic syndromes. *Leuk Res* 2009;33:847–853.
137. Steemsa DP, Dewald GW, Lasho TL, et al. The JAK-2 V617F activating tyrosine kinase mutation is an infrequent event in both "atypical" myeloproliferative disorders and myelodysplastic syndromes. *Blood* 2005;106:1207–1209.
138. Wang L, Lawrence MS, Wan Y, et al. SB3B1 and other novel cancer genes in chronic lymphocytic leukemia. *N Eng J Med* 2011;365:2497–2506.
139. Zipperer E, Pelz D, Nachtkamp K, et al. The hematopoietic stem cell transplantation comorbidity index is of prognostic relevance for patients with myelodysplastic syndrome. *Haematologica* 2009;94:729–732.
140. Della Porta MG, Malcovati L, Strupp C, et al. Risk stratification based on both disease status and extra-hematologic comorbidities in patients with myelodysplastic syndrome. *Haematologica* 2011;96:441–449.
141. Geming U, Aul C, Niemeyer CM, et al. Epidemiology, classification and prognosis of adults and children with myelodysplastic syndromes. *Ann Hematol* 2008;86:691–699.
142. Germing U, Hildebrandt B, Pfeilstocker M, et al. Refinement of the international prognostic scoring system (IPSS) by including LDH as an additional prognostic variable to improve risk assessment in patients with primary myelodysplastic syndromes (MDS). *Leukemia* 2005;19:2223–2231.
143. Hellström-Lindberg E, Gulbrandsen N, Lindberg G, et al. A validated decision model for treating the anaemia of myelodysplastic syndromes with erythropoietin + granulocyte colony-stimulating factor: significant effects on quality of life. *Br J Haematol* 2003;120:1037–1046.
144. Gatttermann N. Overview of guidelines on iron chelation therapy in patients with myelodysplastic syndromes and transfusional iron overload. *Int J Hematol* 2008;88:24–29.
145. Staddler M, Germing U, Kliche KO, et al. A prospective, randomized phase II study of antithymocyte globulin as immune-modulating therapy in patients with low-risk myelodysplastic syndromes. *Leukemia* 2004;18:460–465.
146. Sloand EM, Olnes MJ, Shenoy A, et al. Alemtuzumab treatment of intermediate-1 myelodysplasia patients is associated with sustained improvement in blood counts and cytogenetic remissions. *J Clin Oncol* 2010;28:5166–5173.
147. Fenaux P, Mufti GJ, Hellstrom-Lindberg E, et al.; International Vidaza High-Risk MDS Survival Study Group. Efficacy of azacitidine compared with that of conventional care regimens in the treatment of higher-risk myelodysplastic syndromes: a randomised, open-label, phase III study. *Lancet Oncol* 2009;10:223–232.
148. Kantarjian HM, O'Brien S, Huang X, et al. Survival advantage with decitabine versus intensive chemotherapy in patients with higher risk myelodysplastic syndrome: comparison with historical experience. *Cancer* 2007;109:1133–1137.
149. Rosati S, Anastasi J, Vardiman J. Recurring problems in the pathology of the myelodysplastic syndromes. *Semin Hematol* 1996;33:112–126.
150. Kyle RA, Pease GL. Hematologic aspects of arsenic intoxication. *N Eng J Med* 1965;273:18–23.
151. Westhoff DD, Samaha RJ, Barnes A Jr. Arsenic intoxication as a cause of megaloblastic anemia. *Blood* 1975;45:241–246.
152. Gregg XT, Reddy V, Prchal JT. Copper deficiency masquerading as myelodysplastic syndrome. *Blood* 2002;100:1493–1495.
153. Sutton L, Vusirikala M, Chen W. Hematogone hyperplasia in copper deficiency. *Am J Clin Pathol* 2009;132:191–196.
154. Huff JD, Keung Y-K, Thakuri M, et al. Copper deficiency causes reversible myelodysplasia. *Am J Hematol* 2007;82:625–630.
155. Irving JA, Mattman A, Lockitch G, et al. Element of caution: a case of reversible cytopenias associated with excessive zinc supplementation. *Can Med Assoc J* 2003;169:129–131.
156. Lewis SM, Verwilghen RL. Dyserythropoiesis and dyserythropoietic anemias. In: Brown EB, ed. *Progress in hematology*. New York: Grune & Stratton, 1973: 99–120.
157. Treacy M, Lai L, Costello C, et al. Peripheral blood and bone marrow abnormalities in patients with HIV related disease. *Br J Haematol* 1987;65:289–294.
158. Kaloutsi V, Kohlmeyer U, Maschek H, et al. Comparison of bone marrow and hematologic findings in patients with human immunodeficiency virus infection and those with myelodysplastic syndromes and infectious diseases. *Am J Clin Pathol* 1994;101:123.
159. Brown K, Young N. Parvovirus B19 infection and hematopoiesis. *Blood Rev* 1995;9:176–182.
160. Schmitz LL, McClure JS, Litz CE, et al. Morphologic and quantitative changes in blood and marrow cells following growth factor therapy. *Am J Clin Pathol* 1994;101:67–75.
161. Schroeder T, Ruf L, Bernhardt TA, et al. Distinguishing myelodysplastic syndromes (MDS) from idiopathic cytopenia of undetermined significance (ICUS): HUMARA unravels clonality in a sub group of patients. *Ann Oncol* 2010;21: 2267–2271.
162. Baumann I, Niemeyer CM, Bennett JM, et al. Childhood myelodysplastic syndrome. In: Swerdlow SH, Campo E, Harris NL, et al., eds. *WHO classification of tumours of the haematopoietic and lymphoid tissues*. Lyon: IARC, 2008:104–107.
163. Hasle H, Niemeyer CM, Chessels JM, et al. A pediatric approach to the WHO classification of myelodysplastic and myeloproliferative diseases. *Leukemia* 2003;17:277–282.
164. Niemeyer CM, Baumann I. Myelodysplastic syndrome in children and adolescents. *Semin Hematol* 2008;45:60–70.
165. Passmore SJ, Chessells JM, Kempski H, et al. Paediatric P5 myelodysplastic syndromes and juvenile myelomonocytic leukaemia in the UK: a population based study of incidence and survival. *Br J Haematol* 2003;121:758–767.
166. Hasle H, Wadworth LD, Massing BG, et al. A population based study of childhood myelodysplastic syndromes in British Columbia. *Br J Haematol* 1999;106: 1027–1032.
167. Stary J, Baumann I, Creutzig U, et al. Getting the numbers straight in pediatric MDS: distribution of cases after exclusion of Down syndrome. *Blood Cancer* 2008;50:435–436.
168. Baumann I, Niemeyer CM, Brunning RD, et al. Myeloid proliferations related to Down syndrome. In: Swerdlow SH, Campo E, Harris NL, et al., eds. *WHO classification of tumours of haematopoietic and lymphoid tissues*. Lyon: IARC, 2008:142–144.
169. Baumann I, Niemeyer CM, Fuhrer M, et al. Morphological differentiation of hypocellular refractory cytopenia of childhood and severe aplastic anemia and clinical outcome. *Leuk Res* 2011;354:S1.
170. Torlakovic EE, Naresh K, Brunning RD. *Bone marrow immunohistochemistry*. Chicago: American Society of Clinical Pathology Press, 2009:112.
171. Shimamura A. Inherited bone marrow failure syndromes: molecular features. *Hematology* 2006:63–71.
172. Kardos G, Bauman I, Passmore SJ, et al. Refractory anemia of childhood: a retrospective study of 67 patients with particular reference to monosomy 7. *Blood* 2003;102:1997–2003.
173. Gohring G, Michalova K, Beverloo HB, et al. Complex karyotype newly defined: the strongest prognostic factor in advanced childhood myelodysplastic syndrome. *Blood* 2010;116:3766–3769.
174. Hasle H, Niemeyer CM. Advances in the prognostication and management of advanced MDS in children. *Br J Haematol* 2011;154:185–195.
175. Cioc AM, Wagner,JE, MacMillan ML, et al. Diagnosis of myelodysplastic syndrome among a cohort of 119 patients with Fanconi anemia. *Am J Clin Pathol* 2010;133:92–100.
176. Pearson H, Lobel J, Kocoshis S, et al. A new syndrome of refractory sideroblastic anemia with vacuolization of marrow precursors and exocrine pancreatic dysfunction. *J Pediatr* 1979;95:976–984.
177. Manea EM, Leverger G, Bellmann F, et al. Pearson syndrome in the neonatal period: two case reports and review of the literature. *J Pediatr Oncol* 2009;31:947–951.

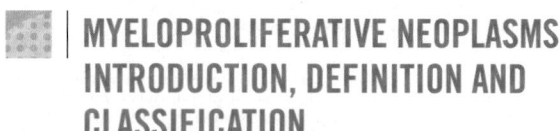

Chapter 44
Myeloproliferative Neoplasms

John Anastasi • James W. Vardiman

MYELOPROLIFERATIVE NEOPLASMS: INTRODUCTION, DEFINITION AND CLASSIFICATION

The concept of a family of diseases characterized by "en masse" proliferation of myeloid cells was first proposed by William Dameshek in a commentary in *Blood* in 1951 (1). He suggested that in chronic myeloid leukemia (CML), polycythemia vera (PV), and in the diseases now known as essential thrombocythemia (ET) and primary myelofibrosis (PMF), the granulocytic, erythroid, and megakaryocytic lineages proliferate simultaneously—albeit in varying proportions—in response to an unknown "myelostimulatory factor." That these diseases share an insidious onset, a tendency to develop organomegaly, myelofibrosis (MF), and an acute leukemic phase were, he reasoned, additional arguments to group them together as "myeloproliferative disorders (MPDs)." During the ensuing six decades numerous studies have proved that the MPDs are clonal proliferations that arise in pluripotent or multipotent bone marrow stem cells (2–6). Furthermore, Dameshek's proposed "myelostimulatory factor" is now recognized to be constitutively activated receptor or cellular tyrosine kinases (TKs) that mimic the signaling normally induced by hematopoietic growth factors, thus causing the cells to be hypersensitive to, or independent of, normal cytokine regulation (7,8). The constitutive activation of the TKs is caused by acquired abnormalities of genes that encode them although additional cooperating genetic lesions are likely necessary to establish and sustain the proliferative process and promote further progression to MF and/or a blast phase (9–12). The current concept is that "MPDs" are clonal hematopoietic stem cell neoplasms caused by acquired somatic mutations that result in the abnormal proliferation and thus are better considered as "myeloproliferative neoplasms (MPNs)" (13,14).

The entities in the 2008 World Health Organization (WHO) classification of MPNs are listed in Table 44.1 (13). These neoplasms usually affect older adults and are characterized by proliferation with maturation of one or more of the myeloid lineages (granulocytic, erythroid, megakaryocytic, mast cells). Initially, the proliferation is effective and the bone marrow produces increased granulocytes, red blood cells (RBCs), and/or platelets. Splenomegaly and hepatomegaly commonly develop at some point in the disease due to sequestration of blood cells, extramedullary hematopoiesis (EMH), or both. The natural history of the MPNs is characterized by acquisition of additional genetic abnormalities that result in loss of the proliferative capacity of the cells and/or in blast transformation. MF is another common manifestation of disease progression. The MF is generally regarded as secondary to abnormal stimulation of nonneoplastic fibroblasts by cytokines such as transforming growth factor-beta (TGF-β) and basic fibroblast growth factor that are produced by the neoplastic cells, particularly megakaryocytes (15,16), although this concept has been recently questioned (17).

Neoplastic proliferations of eosinophils caused by constitutive activation of the surface TK receptors PDGFRA, PDGFRB, or FGFR1 due to rearrangements or mutations of the genes that encode them share many features with MPNs but are placed in a separate category in the WHO classification (Table 44.2) (13). The classification of these specific neoplasms ("myeloid/lymphoid neoplasms with eosinophilia and abnormalities of *PDGFRA, PDGFRB,* and *FGFR1*") emphasizes their stem cell origin and that they may have an associated lymphoblastic component, and also distinguishes them from chronic eosinophilic leukemia, not otherwise specified (CEL, NOS), for which the underlying genetic defects are not known. Although mastocytosis is included in the 2008 WHO classification of MPNs it is discussed in a separate chapter in this book.

ETIOLOGY AND PATHOGENESIS OF MPNs

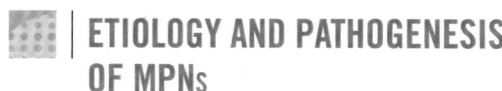

Etiology

The cause of most cases of MPN is unknown. There is an established link between ionizing irradiation and MPNs (e.g., CML was the most common form of leukemia in survivors of Hiroshima and Nagasaki, and Madame Curie reportedly died of CML) (18–21) and rare cases have been reported secondary to cytotoxic therapy (22). But not all people exposed to the same dose of irradiation or cytotoxic agents develop MPN, leading to the speculation of variation in host susceptibility to possible etiologic factors. Accordingly, there is supportive evidence for an inherited predilection for MPNs (23–25). Familial clustering has been described in numerous case reports and in a recent Swedish study of over 11,000 patients with MPN a five- to sevenfold increased risk for MPN was found in first-degree relatives of

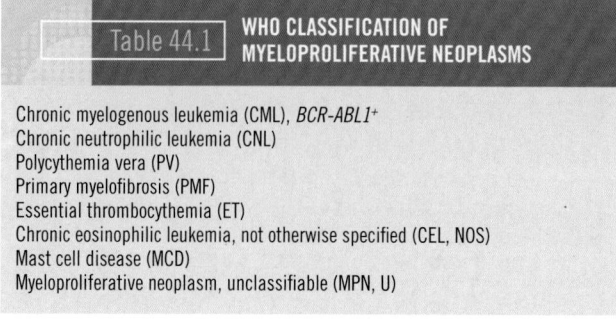

Table 44.1	WHO CLASSIFICATION OF MYELOPROLIFERATIVE NEOPLASMS

Chronic myelogenous leukemia (CML), *BCR-ABL1*+
Chronic neutrophilic leukemia (CNL)
Polycythemia vera (PV)
Primary myelofibrosis (PMF)
Essential thrombocythemia (ET)
Chronic eosinophilic leukemia, not otherwise specified (CEL, NOS)
Mast cell disease (MCD)
Myeloproliferative neoplasm, unclassifiable (MPN, U)

patients with PV, ET, and PMF, and a twofold risk for relatives of patients with CML (26) In addition, genome-wide studies in MPN patients have identified disease susceptibility loci/haplotypes defined by single nucleotide polymorphisms. A haplotype of the germ line *JAK2* gene, *JAK2* GGCC (the "46/1 polymorphism"), has been reported to predispose to familial as well as to sporadic PV, ET, and PMF that may or may not be associated with the acquired somatic mutation, *JAK2* V617F (27,28). However, the incidence of the *JAK2* V617F somatic mutation is similar in familial and sporadic MPNs, and is acquired in the familial cases as in the sporadic cases (23,29). The penetrance of the 46/1 polymorphism is low and evidence suggests it may predispose not only to MPN but also to nonhematopoietic tumors (30,31). The literature suggests a large proportion of the familial cases of MPN display an autosomal dominance pattern with incomplete penetrance and that a complex interaction of genetic and environmental factors is required to initiate the disease process (25).

Pathogenesis

Although the specific etiology is not known for most cases of MPN, there are considerable data to support the notion that acquired somatic mutations or rearrangements of genes that encode receptor and cellular TKs are central to their pathogenesis. However, studies with next-generation sequencing and single nucleotide polymorphism array karyotyping have revealed an unexpectedly complex network of genetic abnormalities—particularly in the *BCR-ABL1*⁻ MPNs—that cooperate to establish the neoplastic process and that contribute to the clinical phenotype (32). These genetic abnormalities and the diseases with which they are associated are discussed in the remainder of this chapter in the two major subgroups of MPNs: CML associated with the *BCR-ABL1* (Philadelphia [Ph] chromosome) genetic abnormality and the *BCR-ABL1*⁻ MPNs, PV, ET, and PMF. In addition, myeloid neoplasms with eosinophilia, including those with abnormalities of *PDGFRA*, *PDGFRB*, and *FGFR1*, and CEL, NOS, are included in the discussion as well.

Chronic Myelogenous Leukemia, BCR-ABL1⁺

CML is unique among the hematopoietic diseases and especially among the MPNs and leukemias. It is associated with a number of "firsts." It was the first leukemia described (33), and is actually the disease for which the term "leukemia" (*wiesses blut*, meaning "white blood") was coined (34). CML was the first malignancy found to be associated with a chromosomal abnormality. This was a smaller than normal G group chromosome that was called the Philadelphia (Ph) chromosome, named after the city in which it was discovered (35). CML was also among the first diseases found to be associated with a reciprocal translocation of genetic material from one chromosome to another

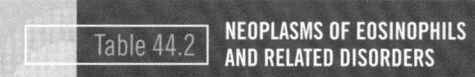

Table 44.2	NEOPLASMS OF EOSINOPHILS AND RELATED DISORDERS

- Myeloid and lymphoid neoplasms with eosinophilia and abnormalities of PDGFRA, PDGFRB, or FGFR1
- Chronic eosinophilic leukemia, not otherwise specified (CEL, NOS)ᵃ
- Hypereosinophilia/Hypeosinophilic syndrome (HE/HES)ᵇ

ᵃCEL, NOS, is included in the MPN classification.
ᵇBecause the categories of HE and HES encompass cases in which the etiology is unknown, they likely include clonal eosinophilia as well as reactive eosinophilia; they are not included in the formal WHO classification.

in a chromosomal translocation, the t(9;22) (q34;q11.2) (36). The translocation was later shown to involve a known gene named *ABL1* identified on chromosome 9, a new gene, *BCR*, found on chromosome 22, and fusion genes, resulting from the translocation, *BCR-ABL1* on the derivative chromosomes 22, and *ABL1-BCR* on the derivative chromosome 9 (37–39) (Fig. 44.1). CML was among the first diseases in which study of the disrupted genes from a chromosomal translocation gave a clue to the molecular pathogenesis of the disorder. This was identified as increased and constitutive TK activity of the BCR-ABL1 fusion protein (40). Most importantly, CML was the first neoplasm for which the understanding of the underlying molecular pathogenesis resulted in a drug designed to counteract the molecular abnormality responsible for the disease itself (41). The success of the drug, the TK inhibitor named imatinib mesylate, has made CML a model for research aimed at understanding a disease at the molecular level and for developing small molecule therapy targeting the underlying abnormal molecular pathway.

Not only is CML notable because of the consistent scientific breakthroughs, but CML is also somewhat unique among the MPNs as it arises in the pluripotent hematopoietic stem cell, and essentially affects all of the hematopoietic cell lineages including B, T, NK, erythroid, megakaryocytic as well as monocytic and other myeloid cells. It has a chronic phase, which resembles the other MPNs; a blast phase, which resembles acute myeloid leukemia (AML) or acute lymphocytic leukemia (ALL); and sometimes a transitional or accelerated phase, which resembles, to some degree, a myelodysplastic (MDS) or a MPN overlap neoplasm. Thus, CML is a model for hematopoiesis, a model for chronic leukemia, a model for transformation to acute leukemia, as well as a model for understanding the underlying molecular pathogenesis of the disease and developing therapy to counteract molecular defects or abnormalities.

CML is one of the most common leukemias with an incidence of one to two cases per 100,000 population, accounting for about 15% of all adult leukemia (42) (Table 44.3). The median age is between 46 and 53 years with a male to female ratio

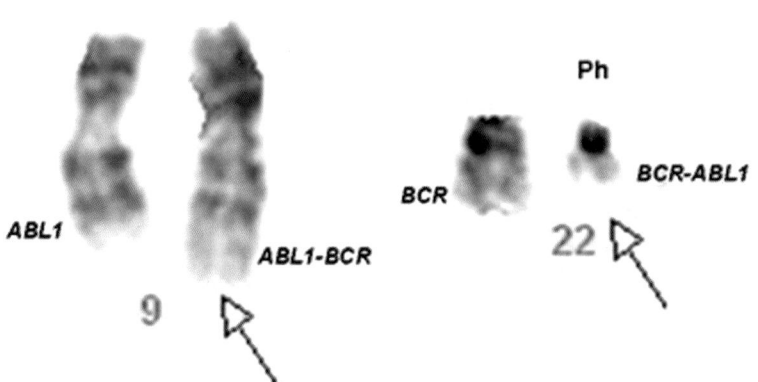

FIGURE 44.1. Partial karyotype of the t(9;22)(q34;q11.2). The small derivative chromosome 22 is the initially recognized Ph chromosome that was later shown to arise from a reciprocal translocation between chromosomes 9 and 22. The genes involved in the translocation are the *ABL1* gene on chromosome 9 and the *BCR* gene on chromosome 22. The *BCR-ABL1* fusion gene on the Ph chromosome encodes an abnormal ABL1 protein with constitutive TK activity. (Image courtesy of Dr. Gordana Raca, University of Chicago.)

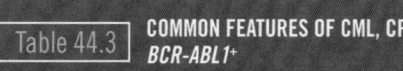

Table 44.3	COMMON FEATURES OF CML, CP, BCR-ABL1+

Annual incidence: 1–2/100,000 individuals
Age: Any, but pediatric cases rare; median age, 46–53 y
Clinical findings: Fatigue, weight loss, fever, splenomegaly, 20%–40% are asymptomatic at initial diagnosis
Blood: Leukocytosis
Platelets normal or increased
Anemia often present
Spectrum of maturing granulocytes; "myelocyte bulge"
Blasts usually <2% of WBCs
Absolute basophilia
No significant dysplasia
Bone marrow: Hypercellular
Increased M:E ratio
Blasts usually <5%, always <10%
Megakaryocytes normal or increased in number, but with "dwarf" morphology
Reticulin fibers normal to moderately increased
Ancillary studies: LAP low
B$_{12}$ increased
Genetics: 100% have Ph chromosome and/or BCR-ABL1 fusion gene identified by karyotype, FISH, or PCR

of about 1.8:1. The median age has decreased over the years because of increased incidental diagnosis of early disease due to the common use of routine complete blood counts in well patient checkups. Although predominantly a disease of adults, the leukemia can also occur in children (43).

Diagnosis, Morphologic, and Laboratory Features of CML

The diagnosis of CML requires the evaluation of blood, bone marrow, and ancillary studies, the most important of which are cytogenetic and/or molecular analysis to identify the Ph chromosome or the BCR-ABL1 fusion.

Peripheral Blood

The laboratory evaluation plays a critical role in the diagnosis and the peripheral blood findings are frequently highly suggestive if not diagnostic in themselves (44–46) (Table 44.3). Although much emphasis is placed on the cytogenetic and molecular findings, without the initial findings from the peripheral blood, these confirmatory tests would not be obtained. Patients usually have a marked leukocytosis with white blood cell (WBC) ranging from 20 to 500 × 10^9/L, with a mean count somewhere between 134 and 225. With lower counts the findings can still be diagnostic or at least highly suggestive. The peripheral smear shows mostly neutrophils at all stages of development. Segmented forms and band forms account for the majority of the cells, and there are usually few blasts (1% to 2%) and promyelocytes. However, the peripheral blood smear also shows a characteristic "myelocyte" bulge, where the myelocytes are greater in percentage than metamyelocytes (Fig. 44.2). This is in contrast to the more common reactive granulocytic or leukemoid reaction where there is a progressive decrease in the number of bands, metamyelocytes, myelocytes, promyelocytes, and blasts. Dysplasia in

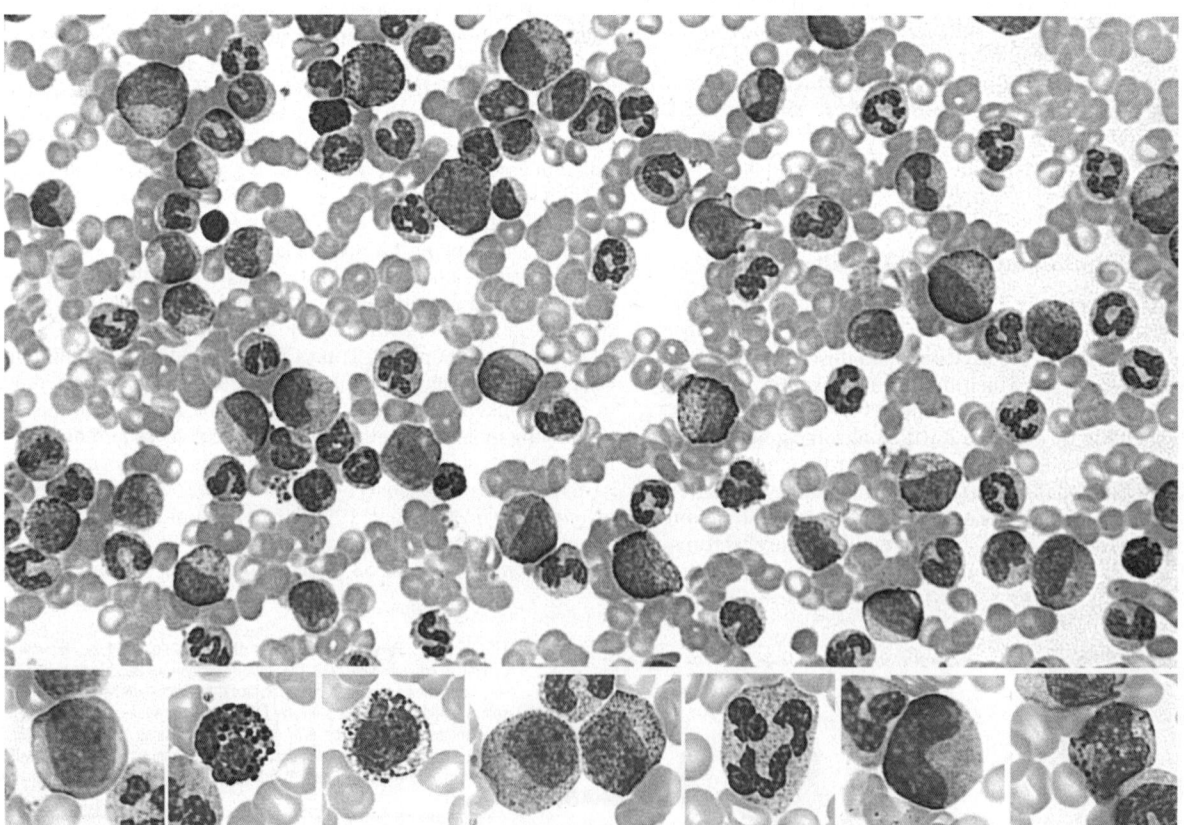

FIGURE 44.2. Peripheral blood from a patient with chronic phase CML (CML, CP). The smear shows marked leukocytosis due to granulocytic cells at all stages of maturation. Blasts (**inset, left**) are typically not more than 2%. There is nearly always absolute basophilia. Although the basophils can appear normal (**inset, second** from **left**), some can have pale granulation (**inset, third** from **left**), which makes them difficult to identify as basophils. Although mature band and segmented neutrophils predominate, cells at the myelocyte stage (**inset, fourth** from **left**) are frequent and typically more numerous than metamyelocytes. This constitutes a "myelocyte bulge." The mature neutrophils typically do not show dysplasia although occasionally cells with nuclear "twinning" are present (**inset, fifth** from **left**). Sometimes megaloblastoid change is seen in the form of giant bands (**inset, sixth** from **left**) although these are more common after hydroxyurea treatment. Sometimes immature eosinophils with prominent primary granules (**inset, seventh** from **left**) can resemble the abnormal eosinophils seen in AML with inv(16).

the maturing granulocytic elements is usually mild, if present at all, and severe dysplasia should suggest a different diagnosis. The smear also shows an absolute basophilia in essentially 100% of cases. This may be difficult to appreciate as frequently the basophils are slightly hypogranular and not recognizable as basophils to the untrained eye. There may also be an eosinophilia, and some of the eosinophils may be immature with basophilic granules; these may resemble the abnormal eosinophils seen in AML with inv(16)/t(16;16), but are usually not as atypical. Patients frequently have an absolute monocytosis (>1 × 10⁹/L), but the percentage of monocytes is usually low and <3%. Patients also frequently have a moderate normochromic, normocytic anemia and elevated platelets with counts as high as 1,000 × 10⁹/L. Thrombocytopenia is rare and should make one consider another entity.

Bone Marrow

A bone marrow study is usually performed and is important to help exclude other entities, and to obtain a specimen for cytogenetic analysis (Table 44.3). The marrow is hypercellular, frequently approaching 100% (Fig. 44.3) (47,48). The marrow shows a marked proliferation of myeloid and megakaryocytic elements with an elevated myeloid to erythroid ratio (~10 to 20:1). Frequently the myeloid elements are expanded along the bony trabeculae producing what is referred to as an expanded "cuff" of immature cells. In normal bone marrows this "cuff" is only three, or so, cells

thick, but in CML it can be 15 to 20 cells deep. The blast count is low, and the cellular features resemble those seen in the blood with a prominence of myelocytes, a basophilia, and sometimes an eosinophilia. Megakaryocytes are frequently increased, although in some cases the megakaryocytic proliferation is not that prominent, whereas in others it is quite accentuated. The megakaryocytes are characteristically small with hypolobated nuclei, which some refer to as "dwarf" megakaryocytes. They are not large and atypical, nor are they tiny micromegakaryocytes. This is an important feature to recognize, as it helps distinguish CML from the other MPNs, which have larger than normal megakaryocytes, and from the myelodysplastic syndromes or MDS/MPNs, in which true micromegakaryocytes are seen. Numerous micromegakaryocytes in a suspected case of CML should make one consider another diagnosis. Frequently, in about 20% to 40% of cases, the marrow shows histiocytes, which resemble Gaucher cells; these are referred to as "pseudo-Gaucher cells" (49). These cells have the characteristic crumpled tissue paperlike cytoplasm (as observed on the aspirate smear), and frequently show hemophagocytosis. The presence of these cells is not diagnostic of CML as they can be seen in any of a number of hematologic disorders. However, in CML, they are derived from the neoplastic clone, as they have been shown to be BCR-ABL1⁺ by fluorescence in situ hybridization (FISH) analysis (50). Reticulin fibers are usually normal to moderately increased.

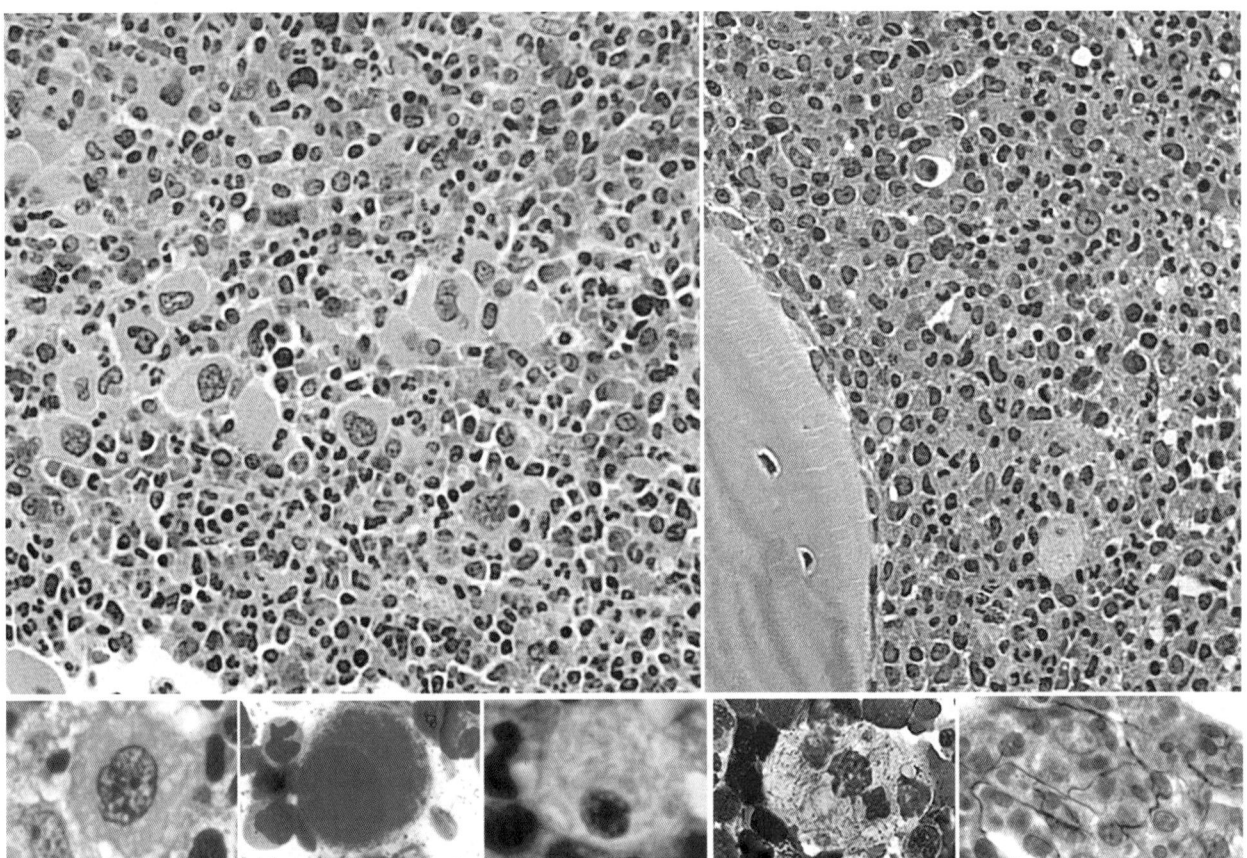

FIGURE 44.3. Bone marrow from a patient with CML, CP. The marrow (**upper panel left**) is typically 100% cellular due to a proliferation of granulocytes and megakaryocytes. Sometime there is thickening of the layer of immature myeloid cells along the bony trabeculae (**upper panel right**), which is normally only approximately three cells thick. The megakaryocytes are small "dwarf" megakaryocytes (**upper panel left**, and **inset left**). These are not as small as the classic micromegakaryocytes seen in MDS but are smaller than normal. The dwarf megakaryocytes can also be recognized on the marrow aspirate (**inset, second** from **left**). Some cases have pseudo-Gaucher cells. These can be seen in biopsy sections (**inset, third** from the **left**), but are more easily recognized on the aspirate (**inset, fourth** from the **left**) where they display the classic "crushed tissue paper" appearance of the cytoplasm. The marrow in CML, CP, typically shows no or minimal reticulin fibrosis (**inset, fifth** from the **left**).

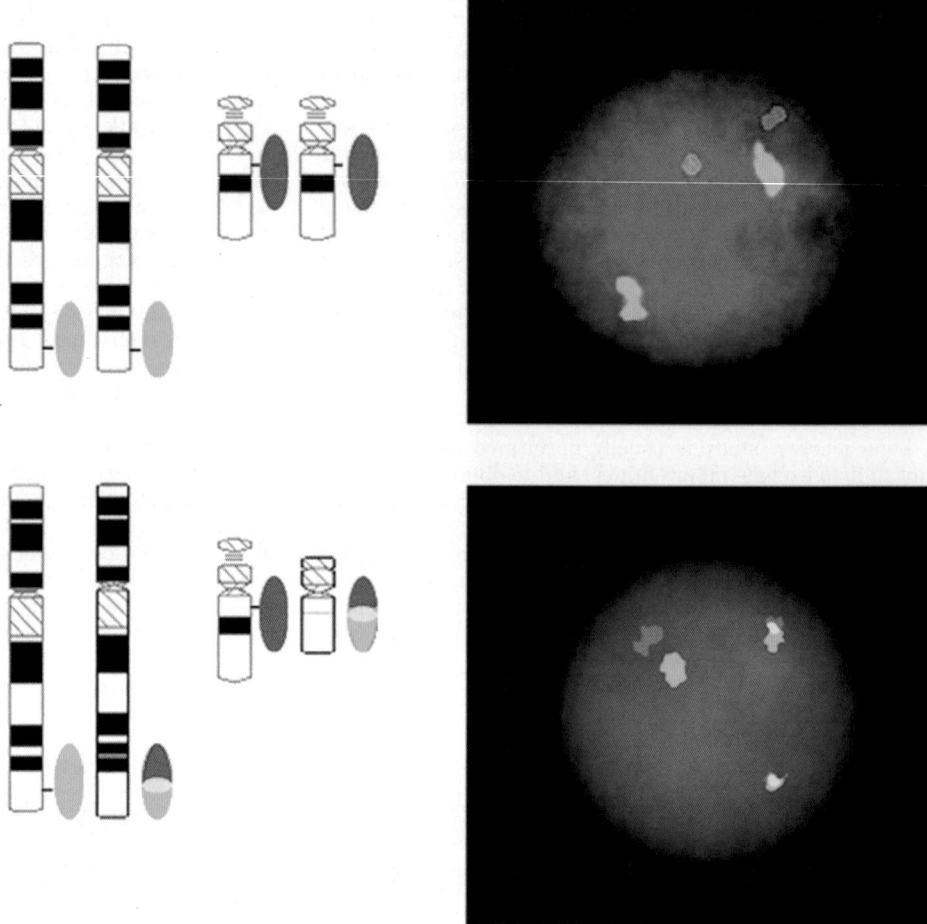

Ancillary Studies

The leukocyte (or neutrophil) alkaline phosphatase (LAP or NAP) score is usually below normal range (51). Although not now commonly used, this is a helpful screen, but is not abso-lute. CML in accelerated phase can show increased scores. B12 is increased by 10 to 20 times normal range, and uric acid is usually elevated. Although the diagnosis of CML can usually be made with a great degree of certainty from the features in the blood and marrow, confirmation requires the demonstration of the characteristic t(9;22) (or variant) and/or the associated *BCR-ABL1* fusion gene. This can be accomplished by conventional cytogenetic analysis, by FISH with probes to *BCR* and *ABL1* (52,53), or through the use of PCR. The most commonly used FISH analysis employs probes that span both chromosomal breakpoints, which in a positive case will result in dual-fusion signals representing the *BCR-ABL1* on the derivative chromo-some 22 and the *ABL1-BCR* on the derivative chromosome 9 (Fig. 44.4). This particular approach gives a high degree of sen-sitivity for the analysis as false-positive signals (more frequent with probes designed to give a single fusion) are exceedingly rare. The t(9;22) is seen in its characteristic form in >95% of cases. In a small number of cases, however, there is a vari-ant translocation involving the 9q34 and 22q11.2, and another involved chromosome (e.g., t(9;14;22)) (54). In slightly <5% of cases, there is submicroscopic translocation which cannot be identified by conventional cytogenetics, and the karyotype appears normal. However, with FISH probes or with primers to identify the fusion gene, the underlying *BCR-ABL1* can be recognized. These cases are called "Ph⁻ CML," and should be referred to as "CML, *BCR-ABL1⁺*, Ph⁻," just for clarity.

It is important to recognize that the *BCR* gene can be broken in three different regions giving rise to three different BCR-ABL1 proteins of different sizes (55,56) (Fig. 44.5). Almost all cases of CML are associated with a break in the major break-point region, at exon 12–16 (formerly referred to as exon b1–b5) and fusion to the *ABL1* at its exon a2. This is referred to as the "major" breakpoint giving rise to the fusion associated with the p210 kDa BCR-ABL1 protein. Very rare cases of CML can have a fusion involving the first exon of *BCR*, e1–e2, the "minor" breakpoint, and this gives rise to the fusion associated with a smaller fusion protein with p190 kDa size. This fusion is far more common in Ph⁺ ALL, but when associated with CML is associated with increased monocytes, which can make the case difficult to differentiate from chronic myelomonocytic leu-kemia (CMML) (57). Lastly, rare cases of CML can have a fusion of *BCR* involving the regions around exons 17–20 (previously referred to as c1–c4), which is the "mu" breakpoint and results in a larger fusion protein with p230 kDa weight. This fusion is also quite rare, but may be associated with CML that has mark-edly increased platelets or CML with a predominance of mature neutrophils (CML-N). These can mimic either ET or chronic neutrophilic leukemia (CNL), respectively (58–60).

Therapy, Monitoring Disease, and Resistance

The development of imatinib in the late 1990s revolutionized the treatment of CML and now provides successful manage-ment for most patients. Currently the 5-year survival is over 92% with very low risk for transformation to accelerated or blast phase. The development of second- and third-generation

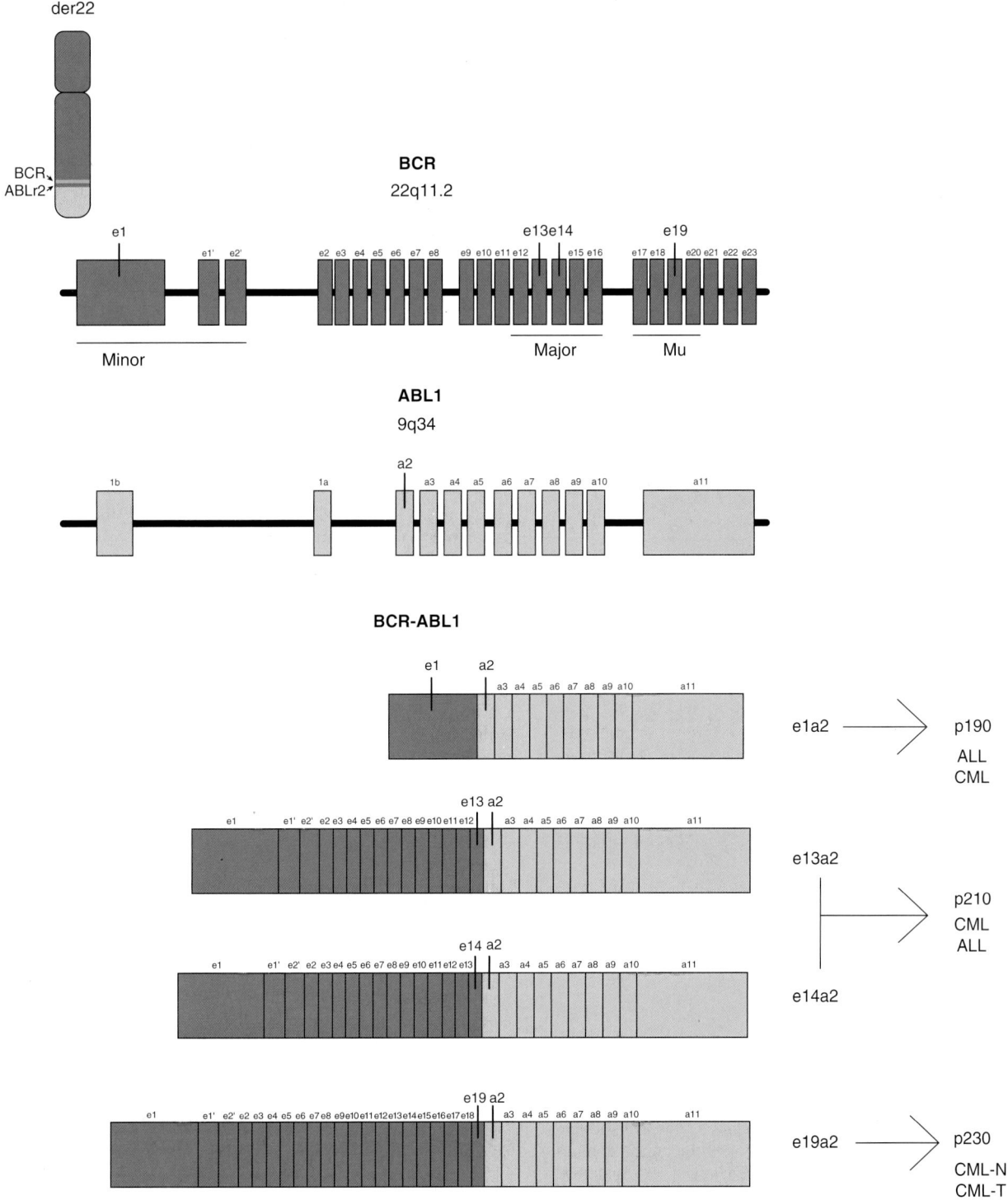

FIGURE 44.5. **Derivation of the three different-sized BCR-ABL1 proteins, p190, p210, and p230.** The *ABL1* gene is always split at exon 2, but the *BCR* is split at different sites giving rise to small, medium, and large fusion proteins. The p210 BCR-ABL1 is seen in most cases of CML although the p190 and the p230 have been reported in rare cases.

TK inhibitors has maintained or improved treatment results and has been successful in overcoming resistance that can develop in some patients.

Imatinib and other TK inhibitors inhibit the constitutive phosphorylation activity of the BCR-ABL1 TK (61). The drugs fit into a pocket of the ABL1 portion of the BCR-ABL1 fusion protein and block ATP from binding (Fig. 44.6). Usually after about 3 months of therapy there is normalization of blood counts,

reduction of bone marrow cellularity with correction of the M:E ratio, and normalization of megakaryocyte size (62,63). Frequently after treatment one sees lymphoid aggregates comprising mostly small lymphocytes, which are a mix of B and T cells. These are reactive in nature. Many patients achieve a complete cytogenetic remission, but a molecular remission by PCR analysis for *BCR-ABL1* is relatively uncommon, occurring in only 10% or so of all patients (64). These patients are of intense

FIGURE 44.6. Cartoon of the BCR-ABL1 fusion protein. The ABL1 portion of the fusion protein (*hatched* portion of figure) has a pocket for ATP that serves as a donor of phosphate in the phosphorylation of substrate molecules. This phosphorylation process is constitutively activated due to the fused BCR portion of the protein (*clear portion* of figure). Imatinib mesylate was designed to sit in the pocket to prevent the ATP from donating phosphate. The sequence of events following substrate phosphorylation, which when constitutively activated (**left**) is believed to be a major cause the disease, is broken with imatinib treatment (**right**).

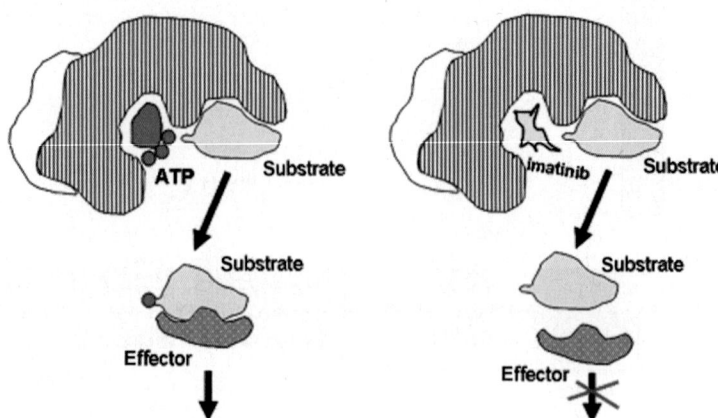

BCR-ABL1 tyrosine kinase

Activity/ increased activity > disease

interest. Apparently some have discontinued TK inhibition therapy, but only a small number remain in molecular remission once the therapy is stopped (64–66).

There are no precise and universally accepted recommended guidelines for monitoring patients undergoing TK inhibition therapy, and the optimal approach is subject to an ongoing debate. Patients are usually studied by conventional cytogenetic analysis of metaphase spreads until they have a complete cytogenetic response noted in the marrow (67). FISH evaluation for *BCR-ABL1* fusion can be used on peripheral blood or marrow cells for screening for residual clonal disease, but quantitative PCR provides the most sensitive means for detecting residual clonal cells. A 2 log reduction in transcripts is expected, and monitoring the clone size and whether it is increasing or decreasing may be the best way for predicting relapse. Typically patients are studied by routine cytogenetic analysis at diagnosis and at 3-month intervals until they achieve cytogenetic remission. Quantitative PCR is also done at diagnosis for baseline then at regular intervals once the patient has achieved a cytogenetic remission. If transcript products begin to rise, routine karyotyping is advised to evaluate for return of t(9;22) and possible clonal evolution. With loss of response to therapy, sequencing for specific mutations is typically performed. It is not clear whether sequencing for mutations is useful at the time of diagnosis.

Resistance to imatinib can occur because of mutations, overexpression of *BCR-ABL1*, or due to reduced cellular uptake of the drug (68). Although newer drugs with more powerful TK activity are being used, these still will have little effect in cases in which clonal evolution results in a stimulation of leukemogenic pathways that are independent of the *BCR-ABL1*-associated constitutive activity of TK. Nevertheless, point mutation to the kinase domain of the BCR-ABL1 is the most common mechanism of resistance. Over 50 different mutations have been identified, but the 15 most common account for over 90% of the cases (69–72). Increasing concentrations of imatinib or use of one of the second-generation compounds usually can overcome the resistance. However, one mutation is particularly insensitive both to increased dosages of imatinib and to second-generation TK inhibitors. This T315I ABL1 kinase domain mutation is sometimes screened for early in the disease so that alternative therapy including possible stem cell transplantation can be considered. However, recently a third-generation TK inhibitor, ponatinib, has been shown to be effective against cases with this form of resistance (73).

The development of a t(9;22)-negative and *BCR-ABL1*⁻ clonal proliferation can occur in patients undergoing TK inhibitor therapy (74). These can be associated with AML, MDS, or even MPN or MDS/MPN (75). These are particularly intriguing as it seems

possible that they arise from a *BCR-ABL1*⁻ clonal expansion that was long ago speculated to be the precursor of the *BCR-ABL1*⁺ clone in CML (76). Whether this is proven to be the case or not, these patients (fortunately uncommon) can present a significant diagnostic challenge with this unexpected complication developing in what is otherwise a successfully treated disease.

Disease Progression

In the age of TK inhibitor therapy disease progression in CML has become rare (72,77). However, some patients still go on to develop accelerated or blast phase disease. In fact, some patients with undiagnosed chronic disease can actually present with advanced disease. It is important to note that disease progression is not analogous to resistance to TK therapy, although undoubtedly resistance will lead to disease progression.

Accelerated Phase

CML sometimes progresses to a blast phase first thorough an accelerated phase. In essence the accelerated phase heralds blasts crisis. Accelerated phase is associated with worsening overall performance, fevers and night sweats, weight loss, bone pain, progressive splenomegaly, and loss of responsiveness to therapy. Although there had been different criteria used to diagnoses accelerated phase, the WHO developed a list of six features, any of which would indicate accelerated phase (78) (Table 44.4). These features include peripheral

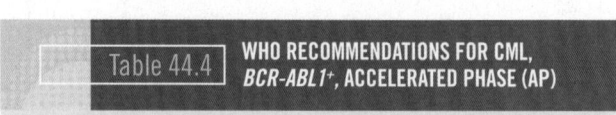

Table 44.4	WHO RECOMMENDATIONS FOR CML, *BCR-ABL1⁺*, ACCELERATED PHASE (AP)

Diagnose AP/progressive disease when one or more of the following are present:
1. Persistent or increasing WBC (>10 × 10⁹/L) and/or persistent or increasing splenomegaly, unresponsive to therapy
2. Persistent thrombocytosis (>1,000 × 10⁹/L) uncontrolled by therapy
3. Persistent thrombocytopenia (<100 × 10⁹/L) unrelated to therapy
4. Clonal cytogenetic evolution occurring after the initial diagnostic karyotype
5. 20% or more basophils in peripheral blood
6. 10%–19% myeloblasts in peripheral blood or bone marrow

Note: Megakaryocytic proliferation in sheets or sizable clusters that is associated with marked reticulin or collagen fibrosis, and/or severe granulocytic dysplasia should be considered as presumptive evidence of AP/progressive disease.
Vardiman J, Melo JV, Baccarani M, et al. Chronic myelogenous leukemia. In: Swerdlow SH, Campo E, Harris NL, et al., eds. *WHO Classification of Tumours of Haematopoietic and Lymphoid Tissues.* Lyon, France: IARC Press; 2008.
AP, accelerated phase.

blood or bone marrow blasts accounting for 10% to 19% of the cells, persistent thrombocytopenia (<100 K/μL) unrelated to therapy or thrombocytosis >1,000 K/μL unresponsive to therapy, increasing WBC and spleen size, basophilia >20%, and evidence of clonal evolution by cytogenetic analysis. Dysplasia associated with megakaryocytic proliferation and increased fibrosis are frequently seen in the accelerated phase and are suggestive but in themselves not sufficient for a diagnosis.

Although almost any additional chromosomal change can be seen in the accelerated phase, the most common changes include an extra Ph chromosome [+Ph or +der(22)], trisomy 8, isochromosome of the long arm of chromosome 17q (iso(17q)), and +18 (79). These abnormalities are seen singly or in combination in 81% of case showing cytogenetic evolution. Other more common abnormalities include −7, −17, +17, +21, and −Y.

Blast Phase

Blast phase or "blast crisis" occurs in virtually all untreated patients with CML. Prior to current TK inhibitor therapy it would occur about 4 to 6 years after initial diagnosis. However, with successful TK inhibition therapy it is much less commonly seen. Blast phase resembles an acute leukemia and is almost always a terminal event. Because the CML clone originates in the pluripotent stem cell, blast phase can occur in the myeloid series, the lymphoid series, or it can be bilineal or even biphenotypic (80). It is diagnosed when blasts account for >20% of the peripheral blood or marrow elements (78) (Fig. 44.7). Although

most of the time blast phase is diagnosed from the blood or marrow, in some instances it can occur at an extramedullary site and require biopsy of a mass lesion (myeloid sarcoma or extramedullary acute leukemia) for diagnosis.

Myeloid blast phase accounted for about 50% to 60% of cases in the pre-TK era; there is little data to document any change in this incidence since the institution of TK inhibitor therapy. It commonly occurred following an accelerated phase and was seen more frequently in older patients with higher blood counts, more severe anemia, and larger spleens. It was quite refractory to therapy and had a very poor survival time of usually only a few months (81). Unfortunately, even in the era of TK inhibition therapy, it remains very difficult to successfully treat and still has survival measured in months (82). The myeloid blast crisis of CML is quite heterogeneous. In some cases it can resemble a *de novo* AML without differentiation, with differentiation, with monocytic component, or it can even resemble erythroleukemia or megakaryoblastic leukemia. In rare cases, the blast phase can even have t(8;21), inv(16)/t(16;16) or even t(15;17). In these latter types the blast phase is morphologically and immunophenotypically identical to the *de novo* leukemia with these recurring chromosomal abnormalities (83,84). More frequently the myeloid blast phase can be of a "mixed myeloid" type in which the blastic element include myeloblasts, monoblasts, erythroblasts, megakaryoblasts, and immature basophils. This type of blasts phase is somewhat distinctive morphologically, and does not have a common *de novo* AML counterpart.

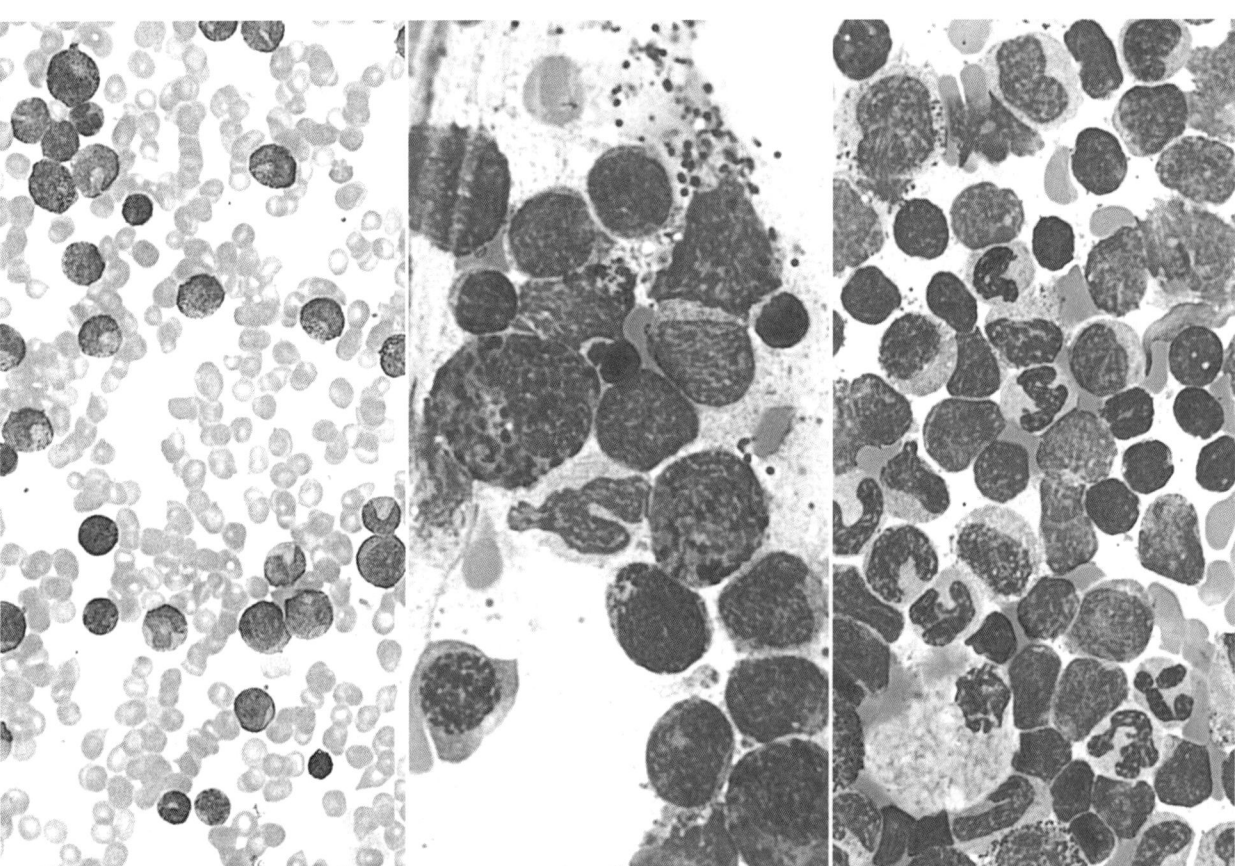

FIGURE 44.7. CML, accelerated (AP) and blast phase (BP). Any one of six criteria must be met to classify a case as AP. In the illustration (**left**) the blast count was >10%. Note how left shifted the granulocytic elements are in this case of AP when compared to the predominance of mature segmented forms in CML, CP (Fig. 44.2). Myeloid BP is quite varied. In the case illustrated (**center**) blasts with myeloid and monocytic phenotype and the presence of abnormal eosinophils suggested a myelomonocytic BP with abnormal eosinophils. This was confirmed with the karyotype findings of t(9;22)(q34;q11.2) and clonal evolution with t(9;22) and inv(16)(p13q22). In the illustration of lymphoid BP (**right**) one can see lymphoblasts (precursor-B phenotype) with some residual CML, CP, with persistent immature granulocytes and the pseudo-Gaucher cell (**bottom left**).

Lymphoid blast phase accounted for 16% to 30% of cases in the pre-TK era, and was more or less uniform morphologically and immunophenotypically (85,86). Clinically LBP occurred in a younger patient with lower counts and less splenomegaly than seen in patients with myeloid blast phase. Interestingly, the lymphoid blast phase was known to occur abruptly and was not associated with a preceding accelerated phase. More commonly, lymphoid blast phase was of a precursor B phenotype typically with CD19, CD10, and TdT expression and lack of cytoplasmic mu or sIg. Less commonly the blast phase could be of a precursor T-cell type. Although lymphoid blast phase responded more favorably to therapy than did myeloid blast phase, the survival was still measured in months. Regrettably, this is still the case even though there is an initial response to TK inhibition.

In some cases the blasts in blast phase can be a mixture of lymphoblasts and myeloblasts. These bilineal processes may be associated with two distinct cytogenetic clones and likely represent separate lymphoid and myeloid blast phases occurring simultaneously. In the biphenotypic blast phase the blasts show lymphoid and myeloid markers simultaneously on the same blasts (87). These may be precursor B/myeloid or precursor T/myeloid (88). This type of blast phase requires the same diagnostic criteria as *de novo* mixed phenotype acute leukemia for diagnosis.

In the pre-TK era about 5% to 10% of cases of blast phase could present at extramedullary sites (89). Thus, the development of a mass lesion in a CML patient would and still should prompt evaluation and an appropriate biopsy. The most common sites of extramedullary blast phase include lymph node, soft tissue, and central nervous system (CNS). Extramedullary disease was usually of the myeloid type, but not always. Bone marrow involvement can be simultaneous, but if not, it usually develops a short time subsequent to the extramedullary presentation.

Differential Diagnosis

A discussion of differential diagnostic considerations in CML needs to take into account the phase of disease in which the patient presents. Although by far most patients present in the chronic phase, some patients actually present in the blast phase, or even in the accelerated phase. The differential diagnostic entities considered for the latter differ considerably compared to those for chronic phase. Key to working up the differential diagnosis is the evaluation for t(9;22) and/or *BCR-ABL1*. CML must be shown to have the t(9;22), a variant translocation or the *BCR-ABL1* by FISH or by molecular techniques.

Differential Diagnosis of Chronic Phase CML

Included in the differential diagnosis of chronic phase CML are a leukemoid reaction, CMML, "atypical CML (aCML), *BCR-ABL1*⁻," and CNL (Table 44.5). A leukemoid reaction is a normal response to infection or another disease process that resembles leukemia with high leukocyte counts in the blood. In some cases a leukemoid reaction can have counts as high as 30 to 100 × 10⁹/L. Although in a leukemoid reaction the granulocytes can show a significant left shift with circulating metamyelocytes, myelocytes, promyelocytes, and even blasts, the factors that help distinguish it from CML include the lack of a "myelocyte bulge," the presence of toxic granulation and Döhle bodies in the neutrophils, and the lack of absolute basophilia (90). Additionally, there is usually markedly elevated (not decreased) LAP score. However, most helpful in considering a leukemoid reaction over CML is identifying a cause of the underlying reactive granulocytosis. Most of the time this is obvious, and usually an infectious process. Bone marrow evaluation has been shown to be of less help in distinguishing CML from a leukemoid reaction.

CMML figures prominently in the differential diagnosis of CML. Other than lacking the t(9;22) and *BCR-ABL1*, the key features that help initially distinguish it from CML are the increased percentage (not absolute number) of monocytes (usually >10%), the presence of dysplasia in the granulocytic and sometimes megakaryocytic cells, less immaturity in the granulocytic precursors (usually <10% of the cells compared to CML where they are usually >20%) (91). There are also usually fewer basophils in CMML compared to CML. An absolute monocytosis alone is not helpful, as in many cases of CML the absolute number of monocytes is >1 × 10⁹/L.

aCML is a MDS/MPN that is usually distinguished from CML by the presence of marked dysplasia in the granulocytic lineage and less often in the megakaryocytic and erythroid series as well, by the presence of thrombocytopenia, and of course the lack of t(9;22) and *BCR-ABL1* (91). At times, it is difficult to distinguish from CMML. aCML is a poorly understood disease that in some instances may represent a transition of a chronic process to a more acute disease, so follow-up can also be helpful (92,93).

CNL must be considered in the differential diagnosis of CML. CNL is an uncommon disorder with only a few hundred cases reported in the literature (94–98). It must be distinguished from reactive neutrophilia, particularly in patients with plasma cell neoplasms that secrete cytokines that stimulate neutrophils (99). It also can be mimicked by the neutrophilia due to growth factors secreted by some solid tumors. CNL occurs in the elderly with a 2:1 male to female distribution. Patients

Table 44.5	**COMPARISON OF MAJOR FEATURES OF THE CMLs**			
	CML, CP, *BCR-ABL1*⁺	**CNL**	**CMML-1, 2**	**aCML, *BCR-ABL1*⁻**
Ph chromosome	~95%	0	0	0
BCR-ABL1 fusion gene	100	0	0	0
Principle proliferating cells	Granulocytes, Megakaryocytes	Granulocytes	Monocytes, Granulocytes	Granulocytes
Monocytes	Usually <3%	<1 × 10⁹/L	>1 × 10⁹/L; >10%	<1 × 10⁹/L; <10%
Basophils	>2%	<2%	<2%	<2%
Dysplasia	Absent/minimal	Absent, "toxic" changes frequent	Usually in one or more lineages	Always dysgranulopoiesis, often trilineage dysplasia
Blasts (peripheral blood)	<10%	<1%	<20%	<20%
Immature granulocytes (peripheral blood)	Often >20%	<10%	Usually <20%	10%–20%
Megakaryocytes	Usually normal or increased numbers with "dwarf" morphology; occasionally mildly decreased	Normal or increased numbers with normal morphology	Decreased, normal, or occasionally increased numbers with variable but often dysplastic morphology	Normal, decreased, or rarely increased numbers, often with dysplastic morphology

CML, chronic myeloid leukemia; CP, chronic phase; CNL, chronic neutrophilic leukemia; CMML-1, 2, chronic myelomonocytic leukemia 1 and 2; aCML, atypical chronic myeloid leukemia.

Table 44.6 WHO DIAGNOSTIC CRITERIA FOR CHRONIC NEUTROPHILIC LEUKEMIA

1. **Peripheral blood leukocytosis, WBC ≥25 × 10⁹/L**
   Segmented neutrophils and bands are >80% of WBCs
   Immature granulocytes (promyelocytes, myelocytes, metamyelocytes) are <10% of WBCs
   Myeloblasts are <1% of WBCs
2. **Hypercellular bone marrow biopsy**
   Neutrophilic granulocytes increased in percentage
   Myeloblasts are <5% of nucleated bone marrow cells
   Neutrophilic maturation pattern normal or shifted to segmented forms
   Megakaryocytes normal
3. **Hepatosplenomegaly**
4. **No identifiable cause for physiologic neutrophilia, or if present, proof of clonality of myeloid cells**
   No infectious or inflammatory process
   No underlying tumor
5. **No Ph chromosome or *BCR-ABL1* fusion gene**
6. **No rearrangement of *PDGFRA*, *PDGFRB*, or *FGFR1***
7. **No evidence of PV, ET, or PMF**
8. **No evidence of MDS or of MDS/MPN**
   No granulocytic dysplasia
   No myelodysplastic changes in other myeloid lineages
   Monocytes <1 × 10⁹/L

frequently have splenomegaly, and some also have enlarged livers. Bleeding from mucous membranes is common but bleeding elsewhere can also occur, as can infectious complications. Patients with CNL must have a sustained neutrophilia of >25 × 10⁹/L (Table 44.6). The neutrophils of the segmented and band stages account for >80% of the blood cells with no further "left shift." The neutrophils characteristically have toxic granulation with Döhle bodies and some tendency for hypersegmentation. Outright dysplasia is not seen. RBCs and platelets are relatively normal. The bone marrow is hypercellular due to a proliferation of mature neutrophils. Blasts are not increased as they typically account for <5% of the marrow elements. The overall survival in CNL is low with a median survival of <2 years in some studies. Patients develop progressive neutrophilia and worsening anemia and thrombocytopenia. A transformation to AML may occur but this not common.

In most instances the peripheral blood features of CNL are distinctive enough to distinguish it from CML, but evaluation for the Ph chromosome or *BCR-ABL1* is more definitive. Care must be taken not to ignore the possibility of a type of CML, *BCR-ABL1⁺* referred to as "CML-N" (60), in which neutrophilic differentiation is more prominent than usual. Although CML-N is also rare, evaluation for t(9;22) associated with the "mu" breakpoint would be necessary to distinguish it from CNL, as this breakpoint can be seen in CML-N.

Differential Diagnosis of Patients Presenting in Accelerated Phase and Blast Phase of CML

CML does not commonly present initially in the accelerated phase, but in the rare case in which it does, the differential diagnostic considerations are different than those of chronic phase and include entities in the MDS/MPN category as well as some of the MPNs, particularly PMF. Morphologic distinction from CML is also more difficult as the findings of dysplasia and fibrosis characteristic of the Ph⁻ MPNs, MDS, and MDS/MPN can also be seen in accelerated phase of CML. Careful diagnosis is critical as the correct diagnosis of CML in the accelerated phase will offer TK inhibition as an important treatment option. Cytogenetic and molecular studies are frequently key to the correct diagnosis.

Patients with CML can sometimes present in lymphoid blast phase. In some, the chronic phase may have gone unnoticed,

but in others there may not have been a chronic phase at all. In either of these cases, the patient usually presents with a leukocytosis with lymphoblasts and the background typical of CML. In other cases in which there is no recognizable CML in the background of the blastic process, the diagnosis can only be made after treatment as such patients can revert to a chronic phase after therapy. Identification of t(9;22) or *BCR-ABL1* does not necessarily help in the evaluation as ALL can be t(9;22) and/or *BCR-ABL1⁺* (100). If a minor *BCR-ABL1* (p190) is present, CML would be unlikely, but if the major *BCR-ABL1* (p210) is seen, one cannot readily distinguish between Ph⁺ ALL and CML presenting in lymphoid blast phase. Identification of the *BCR-ABL1* specifically in the granulocytic, erythroid, or megakaryocytic components might be helpful, as CML is a stem cell disorder whereas Ph⁺ ALL is believed to be a lymphoid-restricted process (101).

Rarely patients present with an AML that is shown to be t(9;22)+ or *BCR-ABL1⁺*. Whether these are truly Ph⁺ AMLs or just cases of CML presenting in myeloid blast phase is very difficult if not impossible to determine (102–106). Some of these patients have an aggressive course with no reversion to chronic phase CML after therapy. Other patients may present with t(9;22) in addition to a common recurring cytogenetic abnormality in AML, such as inv(16) or t(8;21), whereas still other patients will present with a mixed or bilineal acute leukemia that is Ph⁺. Some reports have noted increased incidence of the p190 BCR/ABL1 in cases presenting as AML or mixed lineage leukemia, and these may indeed be a separate entity different from CML in the myeloid blast phase.

NEOPLASMS OF EOSINOPHILS AND RELATED DISORDERS

An increase in the number of eosinophils in the blood (>0.5 × 10⁹/L) is a relatively common hematologic abnormality. It is usually associated with increased eosinophils in the bone marrow and sometimes with eosinophilic infiltrates in the spleen and nonhematopoietic tissues as well. If the eosinophilia is mild (~0.5 to 1.0 × 10⁹/L) and transient there are usually few clinical symptoms of significance, but if the eosinophilia is moderate or marked and persistent the patient is at risk for developing serious organ damage and fibrosis due to the release of cationic proteins from the eosinophil granules, regardless of the cause of the eosinophilia (107–109). Although cardiac damage is most frequent in such cases, any tissue can be affected and the CNS, lungs, and gastrointestinal tract are particularly vulnerable. Discovering the cause of marked and persistent eosinophilia as quickly as possible is necessary to avoid these life-threatening complications.

Eosinophilia can be categorized as reactive (secondary), clonal (neoplastic), or, if no underlying reactive cause is found and there is no evidence for clonal eosinophilia, as idiopathic hypereosinophilia (HE) or in cases of HE in which there is tissue damage, as idiopathic hypereosinophilic syndrome (HES) (110). Reactive eosinophilia is usually due to an underlying allergy, infection, inflammatory, or nonmyeloid neoplasm in which the eosinophilia is part of an immune response associated with increased interleukin (IL)-5, IL-3, or other cytokines produced by activated T cells or by neoplastic cells as, for example, in Hodgkin or non-Hodgkin lymphoma (107,110). In clonal (neoplastic) eosinophilia, the eosinophils are derived from the neoplastic clone, as in the prominent eosinophilia occasionally seen in CML, MDS, or MDS/MPN. Myeloid neoplasms in which the eosinophils are the predominant proliferating component comprise a heterogenous group of rare diseases, and include the stem cell–derived myeloid/lymphoid neoplasms with mutations of the genes that encode the surface

TK receptors, PDGFRB, PDGFRA and FGFR1, and CEL, NOS (Table 44.2). In the 2008 WHO classification scheme, myeloid neoplasms with abnormal surface TKs are segregated from the other MPNs but are integrated in the discussion here. However, some cases of persistent and often marked eosinophilia ($>1.5 \times 10^9$/L) fail to meet the criteria for any WHO-defined category of clonal eosinophilia, and if no reactive cause can be found, are considered as idiopathic HE or, if tissue damage is present, idiopathic HES) (110,111).

Myeloid Neoplasms Associated With Eosinophilia and Rearrangements of *PDGFRB, PDGFRA,* and *FGFR1*

Rearrangements of PDGFRB

Myeloid neoplasms with eosinophilia were the next group of MPNs discovered after CML to be related to TK signaling dysfunction (112–114). Compared to the hard-won inquiry in CML with its decades-long, logical scientific progression of knowledge, the discovery in the eosinophilic disorders evolved fairly quickly and, in some cases, indirectly. The first reports of an abnormal TK associated with myeloid neoplasms with eosinophilia were in patients with CMML with marked eosinophilia who had chromosomal translocations involving chromosome 5q31-q3, which is the site of the gene *PDGFRB*. Further studies showed that the rearrangements of *PDGFRB* lead to an abnormal protein and to constitutive activation of the PDGFRB TK receptor (112). Although *ETV6* on chromosome 12 was the translocation partner in the initial cases, numerous other partner genes have since been described. The myeloid proliferations associated with *PDGFRB* rearrangement have been variably reported as CMML with eosinophilia or as CEL (115) but in the WHO classification, are lumped under the term of "myeloid neoplasms with eosinophilia associated with rearrangements of *PDGFRB*." These neoplasms are very rare and account for <1% of all myeloid neoplasms. The translocation occurs in all age groups but is more frequent in men than women. Splenomegaly is common and some patients present with skin manifestations (115). In patients with *PDGFRB* abnormalities, the peripheral blood smear may demonstrate not only eosinophilia of varying magnitude, but also monocytosis, thus prompting consideration of CMML (107). Despite the rarity of the *PDGFRB* rearrangement, it is essential to identify its presence because patients are very responsive to imatinib therapy and have an excellent prognosis if appropriately treated. Usually the abnormality is detected at the cytogenetic level with chromosomal abnormalities t(5;12)(q31-q33;p12) being most frequent, but confirmation of the translocation by RT-PCR or FISH analysis is recommended.

Rearrangements of PDGFRA

After imatinib was approved for use in CML it was tried in a number of other MPNs, including patients with proliferative disorders of eosinophils. In addition to the patients with *PDGFRB* abnormalities who responded to imatinib, a number of patients with eosinophilic proliferations who lacked this rearrangement were also found to be exquisitely sensitive to the anti-TK therapy, implying that abnormalities of other TKs involved in signal transduction pathways might be present (116,117). The search for those abnormalities eventually led to the discovery of cryptic activating rearrangements of *PDGFRA* on chromosome 4, which are found in 10% to 20% of patients previously diagnosed as HES (113). Most commonly the cryptic deletion of genetic material at 4q12 results in the fusion of the *PDFGRA* and *FIP1L1* genes, which results in an abnormal constitutively activated PDGFRA receptor protein. Additional *PDGFRA* partners have been identified (*BCR, ETV6, CDK5RAP2, KIF5B*) but

are infrequent, and activating point mutations of *PDGFRA* have also been reported (109,115,118).

Although *PDGFRA* rearrangements occur at any age, most patients are 20 to 55 years old with a remarkable male predominance (M:F ratio of about 17:1) (108,109). The most consistent laboratory feature reported is peripheral blood eosinophilia that varies in its severity. The eosinophils are mature, usually lacking significant morphologic abnormalities. It is important to note that some patients with rearranged *PDGFRA* have increased numbers of mast cells; cases of mastocytosis associated with eosinophilia should be examined for *PDGFRA* abnormalities, because they respond readily to anti-TK therapy (119). In such cases, the mast cells aberrantly express CD25 and/or CD2, which is characteristic for neoplastic mast cells, but they may not form the cohesive masses typical for mastocytosis nor do they demonstrate mutated *KIT* (120) (Fig. 44.8). Still, the complete spectrum of myeloid neoplasms associated with *PDGFRA* rearrangement is not clear. Recently cases have been recognized that lack increased eosinophils in the blood (121). Furthermore, some cases of rearranged *PDGFRA* have been reported to present as T-lymphoblastic lymphoma with eosinophilia (111).

The molecular fusion between *PDGFRA* and *FIP1L1*, which is also on 4q, is usually due to the deletion of an intervening segment between the two genes that encompasses the *CHIC2* gene. Although the deletion is submicroscopic and cannot be detected by routine cytogenetic studies, the deletion of *CHIC2*, which can be identified by FISH, has become a surrogate marker for the *F1PL1/PDGFRA* fusion. FISH or PCR studies for identification of the translocation should be performed early in the evaluation if another cause of the eosinophilia is not readily apparent. The majority of patients achieve hematologic responses within a month after institution of imatinib therapy and molecular remission within 3 to 6 months. The response appears durable, but relapse may occur after discontinuation of the drug (108,109).

Rearrangements of FGFR1

The neoplasms associated with rearrangements of the *FGFR1* gene located at 8p11 are quite rare, heterogenous, and are most apt to reflect the stem cell nature of these disorders. Uniquely, the "8p11 syndrome" usually presents as a myeloid neoplasm with eosinophilia in the blood and bone marrow, but may subsequently develop into (or initially present as) a precursor lymphoid neoplasm, more frequently of precursor T-cell type than precursor B-cell type. Indeed, cases of T-lymphoblastic lymphoma with a peripheral blood eosinophilia and an eosinophilic infiltrate among the neoplastic T cells in biopsies of lymphoid tissue that later progressed to AML were among the first cases of this disorder reported (122). As such, the 8p11 neoplasm resembles CML in that it is a stem cell neoplasm that can transform into, or sometimes present in, a lymphoid "blast crisis." Usually routine cytogenetics demonstrate the t(8;13)(p11;q12) abnormality. The disease is frequently aggressive, and those who present as an MPN with eosinophilia may transform to an acute myeloid or lymphoid process within 1 or 2 years. Unfortunately, unlike CML or the neoplasms associated with eosinophilia and *PDGFRA* (or *B*) rearrangements, the abnormalities of *FGFR1* do not respond to imatinib.

Chronic Eosinophilic Leukemia, Not Otherwise Specified

For patients with eosinophilia in whom there is no abnormality of *PDGFRA, PDGFRB,* or *FGFR1,* a diagnosis of CEL, NOS, may be considered if they meet the WHO criteria outlined in Table 44.7 (123). This category is under the MPN umbrella in the WHO classification, distinct from neoplasms associated

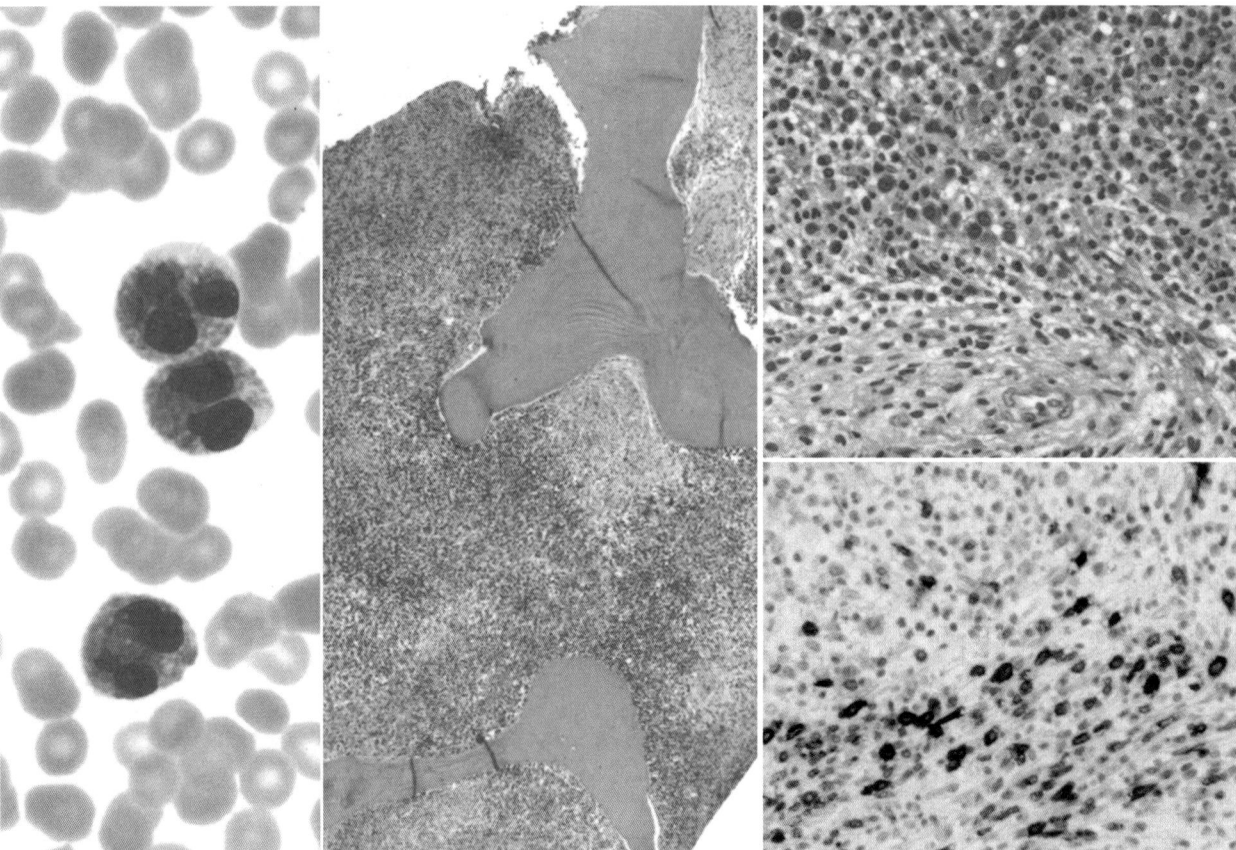

FIGURE 44.8. Myeloid neoplasm with eosinophilia and rearrangement of *PDGFRA*. The patient was a 32-year-old man with cough, shortness of breath, eosinophilic pneumonia, and peripheral eosinophilia. He subsequently developed splenomegaly and underwent a bone marrow biopsy as there was suspicion for lymphoma. The illustration depicts peripheral blood eosinophilia (**left**), and his bone marrow (**center**), which was hypercellular due to a marked myeloid/eosinophilic proliferation associated with lighter-staining areas comprising spindle cells. The spindle cells are seen at high magnification (**right top**) and when stained for mast cell tryptase (**right bottom**). The patient's cells were studied by FISH using a probe set designed to identify *CHIC2* deletion, which is a surrogate marker of the *PDGFRA-FIP1L1* fusion. When a positive result was obtained the patient was immediately started on imatinib (100 mg daily). He responded with resolution of his eosinophilia within days and with resolution of his pulmonary symptoms and splenomegaly within 3 months.

with *PDGFRA, PDGFRB,* and *FGFR1* abnormalities. It is a very heterogenous group recognized as leukemic either by a clonal chromosomal abnormality or by blasts in the blood and/or bone marrow. The clinical features are the same as those described for the other categories of disease with eosinophilia. Symptoms may relate to the general leukemic features (splenomegaly, hepatomegaly, anemia, thrombocytopenia, etc.), to organ

damage caused by the eosinophilia, or both. The predominant feature in the peripheral blood is the eosinophilia (by definition, $\geq 1.5 \times 10^9$/L or more). The eosinophils are mainly mature forms, but can have abnormal morphologic features, including partial degranulation, abnormalities in nuclear segmentation, and enlarged size, although such changes are not diagnostic. There is no absolute monocytosis; basophilia may be present in some cases. Blasts may be increased. The bone marrow shows marked eosinophilic proliferation, usually with a normal maturation pattern. Eyrthropoiesis and megakaryocytopoiesis are often normal (107). There may be an increase in myeloblasts that can help to support the diagnosis of CEL. Marrow fibrosis is not uncommon. There is no specific cytogenetic/genetic abnormality yet detected for CEL, NOS, but the presence of a cytogenetic abnormality that is myeloid-related, such as +8, supports the diagnosis. The presence of a *BCR-ABL1* fusion gene, or of *PDGFRA, PDGFRB,* or *FGFR1* abnormality, excludes the diagnosis of CEL, NOS.

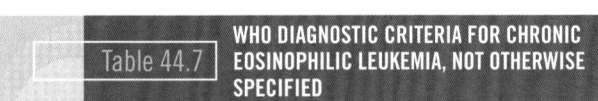

	WHO DIAGNOSTIC CRITERIA FOR CHRONIC EOSINOPHILIC LEUKEMIA, NOT OTHERWISE SPECIFIED
Table 44.7	

1. There is eosinophilia (eosinophil count $\geq 1.5 \times 10^9$/L)
2. There is no Ph chromosome or *BCR-ABL1* fusion gene or other MPN (PV, ET, PMF) or MDS/MPN (CMML or aCML)
3. There is no t(5;12)(q31-q35;p13) or other rearrangement of *PDGFRB*
4. There is no *FIP1L1-PDGFRA* fusion gene or other rearrangement of *PDGFRA*
5. There is no rearrangement of *FGFR1*
6. The blast cell count in the peripheral blood and bone marrow is <20% and there is no inv(16)(p13.1q22) or t(16;16)(p13.1;q22) or other feature diagnostic of AML
7. There is a clonal cytogenetic or molecular genetic abnormality, or blast cells are more than 2% in the peripheral blood or more than 5% in the bone marrow

Bain BJ, Gilliland DG, Vardiman JW, et al. Chronic eosinophilic leukaemia, not otherwise specified. In: Swerdlow SH, Campo E, Harris NL, et al., eds. *WHO Classification of Tumours of Haematopoietic and Lymphoid Tissues.* Lyon, France: IARC Press; 2008.

Diagnostic Approach and Differential Diagnosis of Myeloid Neoplasms With Eosinophilia

In considering a patient with eosinophilia for a possible MPD, reactive causes of the eosinophilia must first be excluded clinically and through the evaluation of the blood and bone marrow (see Fig. 44.9). Reactive causes of eosinophilia due to allergy/atopy, parasitic and other infectious agents, Hodgkin

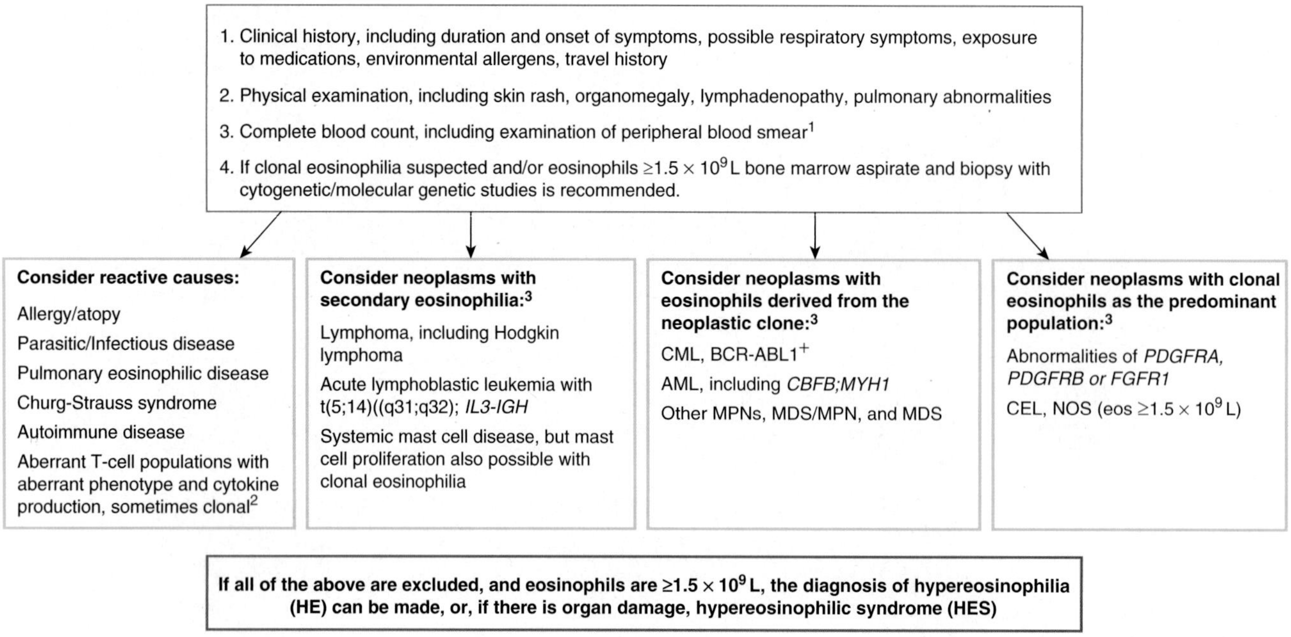

1. Clinical history, including duration and onset of symptoms, possible respiratory symptoms, exposure to medications, environmental allergens, travel history

2. Physical examination, including skin rash, organomegaly, lymphadenopathy, pulmonary abnormalities

3. Complete blood count, including examination of peripheral blood smear[1]

4. If clonal eosinophilia suspected and/or eosinophils ≥1.5 × 10^9 L bone marrow aspirate and biopsy with cytogenetic/molecular genetic studies is recommended.

Consider reactive causes:

Allergy/atopy

Parasitic/Infectious disease

Pulmonary eosinophilic disease

Churg-Strauss syndrome

Autoimmune disease

Aberrant T-cell populations with aberrant phenotype and cytokine production, sometimes clonal[2]

Consider neoplasms with secondary eosinophilia:[3]

Lymphoma, including Hodgkin lymphoma

Acute lymphoblastic leukemia with t(5;14)((q31;q32); *IL3-IGH*

Systemic mast cell disease, but mast cell proliferation also possible with clonal eosinophilia

---

Consider neoplasms with eosinophils derived from the neoplastic clone:[3]

CML, BCR-ABL1$^+$

AML, including *CBFB;MYH1*

Other MPNs, MDS/MPN, and MDS

Consider neoplasms with clonal eosinophils as the predominant population:[3]

Abnormalities of *PDGFRA*, *PDGFRB* or *FGFR1*

CEL, NOS (eos ≥1.5 × 10^9 L)

If all of the above are excluded, and eosinophils are ≥1.5 × 10^9 L, the diagnosis of hypereosinophilia (HE) can be made, or, if there is organ damage, hypereosinophilic syndrome (HES)

1. Inspection of the blood film is essential to examine the milieu in which the eosinophilia occurs but often the morphology of the eosinophils is not abnormal or diagnostic of a specific disorder

2. Aberrant T-cell phenotypes may include CD3$^-$/CD4$^+$, CD3$^+$/CD4$^-$/CD8$^-$, CD3$^-$/CD4$^+$/CD5$^+$, or other aberrancies; clonality may be shown in some cases

3. If the eosinophil count is ≥1.5 × 10^9 L evaluation of bone marrow aspiration and biopsy, routine cytogenetic analysis, and FISH or molecular analysis on marrow aspirate for abnormalities of *PDGFRA*, *PDGFRB* and *FGFR1* should be done <u>early</u> in the evaluation if no reactive cause is apparent; FISH and molecular studies may also be performed on peripheral blood

FIGURE 44.9. Diagnostic evaluation in patients with eosinophilia.

---

lymphoma, or T-cell lymphoma are far more common than any of the myeloid neoplasms with a predominance of eosinophilia.

In myeloid neoplasms with eosinophilia, the eosinophils in the blood are generally mature but may have fewer eosinophilic granules than normal. Although they may have other morphologic abnormalities, or be associated with neutrophilia and/or monocytosis, none of these findings can reliably distinguish clonal eosinophilia from their reactive counterparts. The bone marrow specimens of patients with eosinophilia are often similar regardless of the underlying abnormality. They are most often hypercellular with a prominent proliferation of mature eosinophils. Blasts are usually <5% in the marrow, but can be elevated. Other hematopoietic cell lines may show some dysplasia, and some cases have monocytic proliferation. Mast cell proliferations are particularly frequent in those with *PDGFRA* abnormalities but may be seen in other cases as well. The marrow often is fibrotic and can show Charcot-Leyden crystals. The bone marrow assessment should carefully focus on ruling out CML, AML, and other MPN associated with a substantial eosinophilic component. In the 8p11 myeloproliferative syndrome, blood counts are variable, but 85% of patients have >1.5 × 10^9/L eosinophils, and another 75% have absolute monocytosis. The bone marrow is typically hypercellular frequently with increased eosinophils in addition to a myeloid proliferation. When blasts are increased sufficient to diagnose an acute leukemia, the blasts are more frequently myeloid (in two-thirds of cases) than lymphoid. The lymphoid blasts are almost always of precursor T type. In patients who have lymphadenopathy, about 80% have a T-lymphoblastic process, whereas the remainder has a myeloid process.

Molecular and genetic analyses play an important role in the definitive diagnosis and subclassification of myeloid neoplasms with eosinophilia. When the clinical workup and blood and marrow evaluation have ruled out reactive causes (infectious or

malignancy-related), and other MPNs associated with eosinophilia, an assessment for alterations of *PDGFRA, PDGFRB,* or *FGFR1* by cytogenetic, molecular, or FISH analysis should be undertaken. However, if the eosinophil count is >1.5 × 10^9/L and/or there is evidence of organ damage, and there is no ready explanation for the eosinophilia, assessment of the bone marrow, cytogenetic, and molecular genetic studies should be done early in the workup. If the cytogenetic, molecular, or FISH studies are positive one can render a diagnosis and subclassify the process by the particular molecular abnormality found.

When no reactive cause can be determined to explain the eosinophilia, clonality of the eosinophils is excluded with available cytogenetic and molecular genetic data, and the case does not meet the criteria for CEL, NOS, the diagnosis of HE can be made if the eosinophils are ≥1.5 × 10^9/L, or HES, if there is evidence of organ damage. All suspected cases of HES should be evaluated by flow cytometry and gene rearrangement studies to rule out an abnormal lymphocyte population (the "lymphocytic variant" of HES) (108,110).

Treatment

Patients with abnormalities of *PDGFRA* on 4q and *PDGFRB* on 5q31-q3 have been shown to respond to imatinib, as both the alpha and beta subunits of *PDGFR* are TKs with overexpression of activity due to the respective fusions (113,119). This therapy can provide impressive resolution of the eosinophilia and of the harmful sequelae of the eosinophilic infiltration. Patients without proven *PDGFR* fusions should probably be given a trial as the therapy has little toxic effect and there is great difficulty in detecting the molecular abnormalities. Patients responsive to treatment may become resistant due to mutations quite analogous to the mutations in CML, which result in a similar resistance.

Some patients with CEL and HES and no recognizable molecular abnormality or evidence of clonality have also responded to imatinib, so it must be assumed that they have clonal disease associated with some yet to be described molecular change that is responsive to the TK inhibitor.

Patients diagnosed with the 8p11 myeloproliferative syndrome are treated with a variety of therapies including those for ALL, AML, or MPN. Overall, however, these therapies have been inadequate as there are only a few long-term survivors with a median survival of only 15 months. Stem cell transplantation is the only option that has better results (114).

PHILADELPHIA CHROMOSOME (BCR-ABL1)–NEGATIVE MPNs, INCLUDING PV, ET, AND PMF

In view of the genetic abnormalities that contribute to the pathogenesis of CML and some eosinophilic neoplasms it was not unexpected that similar abnormalities affecting

cellular or receptor TKs would be found in PV, ET, and PMF. That these three disorders, which have different clinical, laboratory, and morphologic features, would share the same major genetic defect discovered to date was, however, not anticipated. In 2005 a novel somatic mutation of the gene that encodes the cellular TK, Janus kinase 2 (*JAK2*), was discovered nearly simultaneously by four independent groups of investigators. The mutation *JAK2* V617F is present in nearly 95% of cases of PV and in 50% to 60% or more cases of ET and PMF (124–127).

JAK2 is a member of the Janus family of cytoplasmic non-receptor TKs that is essential for signal transduction through its association with the cytosolic domain of homodimeric type 1 receptors that lack intrinsic kinase activity, such as the erythropoietin receptor (EPOR), the thrombopoietin (TPO) receptor (MPL), and the granulocyte colony stimulating factor receptor (G-CSF-R) (Fig. 44.10) (127–129). The JAK2 protein binds as well to some heterodimeric receptors such as granulocyte-monocyte-CSF-receptor (11,130).

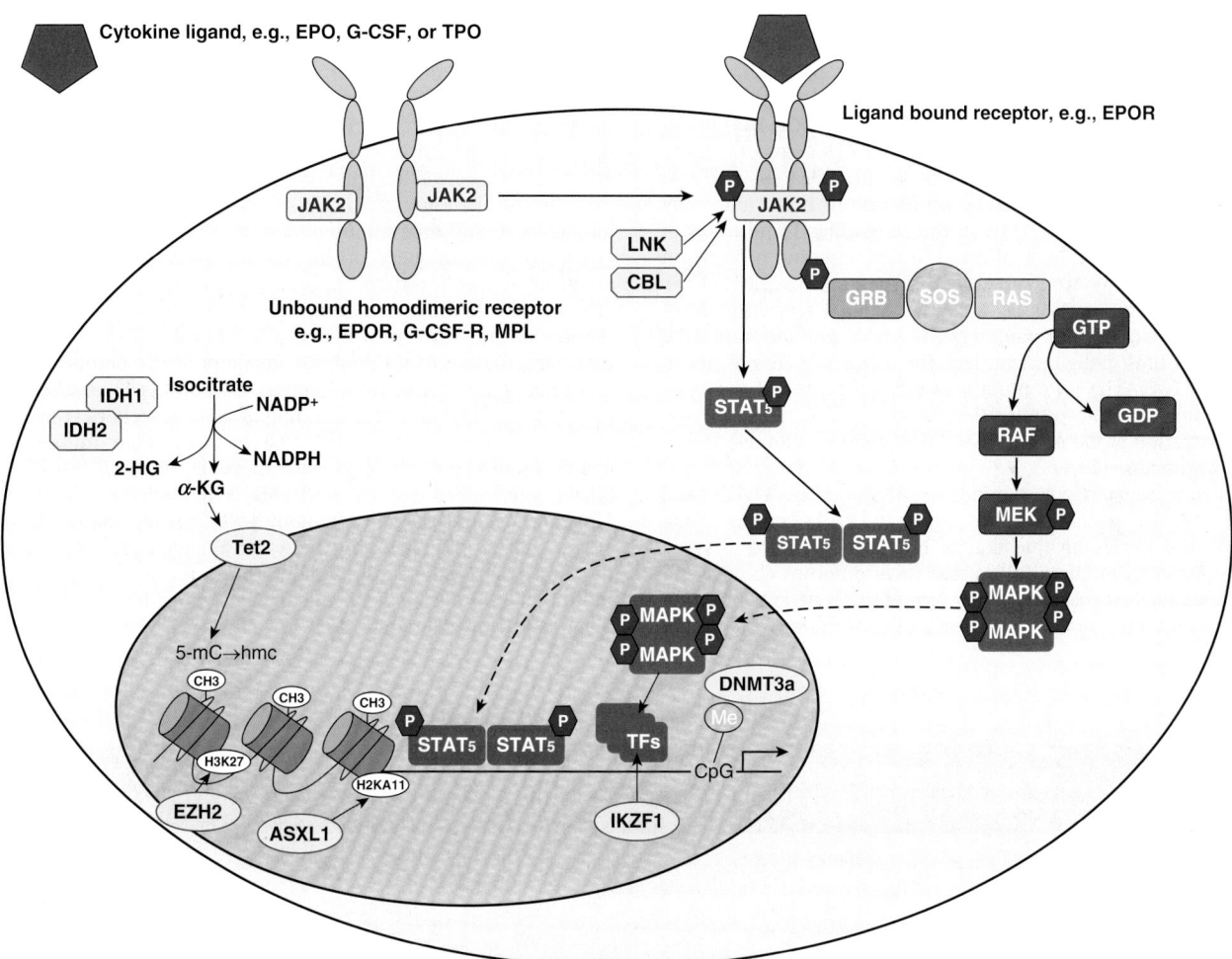

FIGURE 44.10. Signaling pathways important in the pathogenesis of MPNs. This simplified diagram illustrates signaling pathways normally initiated when homodimeric, non-TK receptors such as the EPOR, the TPO receptor MPL, or the granulocyte colony-stimulating factor receptor G-CSF-R bind to their cytokine ligands. When, for example, EPOR binds to EPO, phosphorylation and activation of JAK2, a cytoplasmic TK associated with the receptor occurs and an activated dimeric receptor is formed. Various signaling proteins, including STAT5, are recruited by the phosphorylation sites and in turn are phosphorylated, leading to a series of activated proteins that ultimately results in gene transcription leading to cellular proliferation and inhibition of apoptosis. Other signaling pathways, including the RAS-MAPK, STAT3, and PI-3K-AKT pathways are similarly activated by the receptor. Mutations of *JAK2* (e.g., *JAK2* V617F) lead to constitutive activation of JAK2 and, hence, constitutive activation of the receptor with which it associates, so signaling takes place even in the absence or near absence of the cytokine ligand. Mutations of genes encoding proteins that normally regulate JAK2, such as LNK and CBL, may also lead to constitutive activation of signaling pathways. Furthermore, mutations of genes encoding proteins affecting transcriptional activation or repression (epigenetic regulators) such as TET2, IDH1/IDH2, ASXL1, and DNMT3a, among others, may also result in abnormalities of cell proliferation and/or apoptosis. In this diagram, the proteins most commonly affected by acquired somatic mutations in the MPNs are shown in *yellow*; not illustrated are the gain-of-function mutations of MPL that occur in 5% to 15% of cases of ET and PMF (see also Table 44.8). (Diagram modified after Cross NCP. *Hematology* 2011:208–213 and Vainchenker W, Constantinescu SN. *Hematology* 2005:195–200.)

The JAK2 protein has several domains, including the catalytic domain, JH1, and an inhibitory pseudokinase domain, JH2, which down-regulates the proliferative effect of the catalytic domain (131). The *JAK2* V617F mutation affects the inhibitory JH2 region and results in the loss of its normal inhibitory function, thus leading to an overall gain-of-function of JAK2, that is, JAK2 is constitutively activated. When the mutated, constitutively activated form of JAK2 is bound to a cytokine receptor it induces constitutive signaling via the STAT5, STAT3, RAS-MAPK, and/or P1-3′K-AKT pathways and promotes proliferation, differentiation, and survival of committed myeloid precursors (11,127). Because JAK2 is essential in the signaling pathways of multiple myeloid lineages its constitutive activation accounts for the proliferation of the erythroid, granulocytic, and megakaryocytic lineages observed in varying proportions in the MPNs (11). The mutated *JAK2* further contributes to abnormal erythroid proliferation through hyperphosphorylation and subsequent dysregulation of SOCS3, a negative regulator of erythropoietin (EPO) signaling (132). Additionally, JAK2 reportedly has a role in maintaining chromatin structure and in methyltransferase activity; disruption of this epigenetic role of JAK2 may lead to abnormal gene expression in cells that carry the mutation (11,133).

There are a few cases (~4%) of PV that do not have the *JAK2* V617F mutation. In most of these cases a somatic gain-of-function mutation is present in exon 12 of *JAK2* (134) but in contrast to the *JAK2* V617F mutation, the *JAK2* exon 12 mutation is associated with only erythroid proliferation and not granulocytic or megakaryocytic proliferation. It is found only in PV, and not in ET or PMF. In the remaining 1% of cases of PV, genetic abnormalities affecting other signaling proteins in the STAT pathway are likely to be present, such as LNK (135). Gain-of-function mutations affecting exon 10 of *MPL* have been reported in approximately 5% of ET patients and 10% to 15% of PMF patients who lack the *JAK2* V617F, but not in PV (136,137). The *MPL* mutations affect a region of the cytosolic domain of the receptor that normally prevents spontaneous activation of the receptor, and thus the mutation leads to a gain-of-function (11).

Despite the obvious significance of the *JAK2* V617F and of the similar activating mutations in the pathogenesis of the MPNs, the intriguing question of how one mutation plays a central role in multiple MPNs that have different clinical and morphologic features, and the nature of the genetic abnormalities that underlie the pathogenesis of the MPNs in which there

is no mutation present, remain largely unanswered. Because the *JAK2* mutation occurs in a hematopoietic stem cell and is carried in all of the myeloid lineages as well as some B and T lymphocytes and even endothelial cells (138–140), it is unlikely that the distribution of the mutation among different lineages accounts for the variable disease manifestations. Some data suggests that the *JAK2* mutation is a secondary event and that a "pre-JAK2 state" exists during which time the disease characteristics are determined by other yet unrecognized genetic events (141). There is also a relation between disease manifestations and the allele burden of *JAK2* V617F; the higher the copy number of mutated *JAK2* V617F, the more likely the disease resembles PV (142–144). Furthermore, homozygosity for mutated *JAK2*, which results from mitotic recombination, is commonly found in PV, often in PMF, and almost never in ET (143), leading to speculation that allele dosage of mutated *JAK2* likely influences the disease characteristics. Recent evidence, however, suggest that additional genetic abnormalities cooperate to initiate and influence the disease process (145). High-throughput whole genome sequencing and SNP array karyotyping have revealed a surprising number of genetic mutations in the *BCR-ABL1⁻* MPNs in addition to those affecting *JAK2* and *MPL* (Table 44.8). Some involve genes such as *CBL* and *LNK* that encode proteins involved in intracellular signaling (Fig. 44.10) but others affect genes that encode proteins that act as epigenetic regulators, including *TET2, EZH2, ASXL1, IDH1/IDH2*, and *DNMT3A* (9–11,31,32,146,147). Abnormalities that affect genes involved in signal transduction are usually mutually exclusive of one another, but those involving epigenetic regulators are not, and thus multiple mutations may be found simultaneously. The influence of the recently described aberrations on disease manifestations and/or prognosis is not yet clear, although the finding of mutations in genes affecting epigenetic regulation may open new avenues for therapy. Recent reports that deregulation of microRNA contribute to the pathogenesis and phenotype of the MPNs imposes yet another layer of complexity to a complete understanding of these disorders (148).

The discovery of the *JAK2* V617F and similar mutations has revolutionized the diagnostic approach to the *BCR-ABL1⁻* MPNs, particularly PV, ET, and PMF. This and the *JAK* exon 12 mutation and the mutations of *MPL* are important markers to aid in differentiating between a neoplastic and reactive marrow proliferation, which is often the most difficult of the diagnostic decisions to make when considering an MPN diagnosis. However, the *JAK2* V617F is not specific for any

Table 44.8	**FREQUENCY OF MOST COMMON SOMATIC MUTATIONS/GENETIC ABNORMALITIES AND THEIR FREQUENCIES IN PV, ET AND PMF**				
Gene	Chromosome	Pathway Affected	PV	ET	PMF
JAK2	9p24	JAK-STAT signaling	95%–97%	60%	55%–60%
JAK2 exon 12	9p24	JAK-STAT signaling	3%–5%	Rare	Rare
MPL	1p34	JAK-STAT signaling	Rare	3%–5%	8%–10%
CBL	11q23	JAK-STAT signaling	Rare	Rare	5%–10%
LNK	12q24	JAK-STAT signaling	Rare	3%–6%	3%–6%
TET2	4q24	DNA methylation and demethylation	10%–20%	4%–10%	7%–20%
DNMT3A	2p23	DNA methylation and demethylation	5%–10%	1%–5%	10%–20%
IDH1/IDH2	2q34/15q26	DNA methylation and demethylation; effect on TET2	2%	1%	4%–6%
ASXL1	20q11	Dual activator/suppressor of transcription	2%–5%	2%–5%	10%–20%
EZH2	7q36	Polycomb repressive complex 2; gene transcription	1%–5%	1%–2%	5%–15%

Data from Vannucchi AM, Biamonte F. Epigenetics and mutations in chronic myeloproliferative neoplasms. *Haematologica* 2011;96:1398–1402; Vainchenker W, Delhommeau F, Constantinescu SN, et al. New mutations and pathogenesis of myeloproliferative neoplasms. *Blood* 2011;118:1723–1735; Cross NC. Genetic and epigenetic complexity in myeloproliferative neoplasms. *Hematology Am Soc Hematol Educ Program* 2011;2011:208–214; Abdel-Wahab O, Pardanani A, Bernard OA, et al. Unraveling the genetic underpinnings of myeloproliferative neoplasms and understanding their effect on disease course and response to therapy: proceedings from the 6th International Post-ASH Symposium. *Am J Hematol* 2012;87:562–568; Milosevic JD, Kralovics R. Genetic and epigenetic alterations of myeloproliferative disorders. *Int J Hematol* 2013;97:183–197.

single hematopoietic neoplasm and has been reported in low frequency in patients with AML, MDS/MPN, and MDS (9,149). In addition, nearly 30% to 40% of cases of PMF and ET have neither *JAK2* V617F nor *MPL* mutations. Furthermore, for most cases of CNL and CEL, NOS, the underlying pathogenesis remains obscure as well, with no unique marker by which they can be identified. Therefore it is essential to correlate the clinical and morphologic findings with genetic data to ensure proper diagnosis and therapy for the *BCR-ABL1*⁻ MPNs. It is particularly important to keep in mind that virtually none of the genetic abnormalities reported to date are entirely diagnostic of any single neoplasm—including the *BCR-ABL1* fusion gene (100,150,151).

Polycythemia Vera

Polycythemia is an increase in the number of RBCs per unit volume of blood, usually defined as a "greater than two standard deviations" increase from the age-, sex-, and race-adjusted normal value for hemoglobin (Hb), hematocrit (Hct), or red cell mass (RCM) (152,153). There are multiple causes of polycythemia (Table 44.9). Most cases are associated with a "true" increase in the RCM but diminished plasma volume leads to hemoconcentration and may result in "relative" or "spurious" polycythemia. True polycythemia may be "primary," in which an inherent abnormality in erythroid progenitors causes them to be hypersensitive to factors that normally regulate their proliferation, or, the increase in RCM may be "secondary" to an increase in serum EPO caused either by an appropriate response to tissue hypoxia or by an inappropriate secretion of EPO, which is sometimes associated with various nonhematopoietic neoplasms. Furthermore, primary and secondary polycythemia may be congenital or acquired (154,155).

PV is an acquired true primary polycythemia, occurring with an annual incidence of about 1 to 3 per 100,000 individuals in Western countries but reportedly less frequent in Asia (153). Although defined mainly by erythrocytosis in the blood, PV is a

Table 44.9	CAUSES OF POLYCYTHEMIA

"True" Primary Polycythemia
Congenital:
   Primary familial congenital erythrocytosis, including *EPOR* mutations
Acquired:
   PV

"True" Secondary Polycythemia
Congenital:
   VHL mutations, including Chuvash polycythemia
   2,3-bisphosphoglycerate mutase deficiency
   High-oxygen-affinity Hb
   Congenital methemoglobinemia
   HIF2alpha (*Hypoxia-inducible factor 2alpha*) mutations
   PHD2 (*prolyl hydroxylase domain*) mutations
Acquired:
   Physiologically appropriate response to hypoxia
      Cardiac, pulmonary, renal, and hepatic diseases, carbon monoxide poisoning, sleep apnea, renal artery stenosis, smoker's polycythemia, postrenal transplant
   Inappropriate production of EPO
      Cerebellar hemangioblastoma, uterine leiomyoma, pheochromocytoma, renal cell carcinoma, hepatocellular carcinoma, meningioma, parathyroid adenoma

Relative, "Spurious" or "False" Polycythemia
   Acute, transient hemoconcentration due to dehydration or other causes of contraction of plasma volume; RCM is not increased and is thus not a true polycythemia

clonal "panmyelosis" that leads not only to increased red cells but also to leukocytosis and thrombocytosis. The clinical manifestations are largely related to vascular consequences of the expanded RCM, particularly thrombosis and hemorrhage. Three phases of PV have been described: (a) prodromal, prepolycythemia with borderline to mild erythrocytosis, (b) overt polycythemia, and (c) a postpolycythemic phase characterized by cytopenias—including anemia—and by marrow fibrosis and EMH, that is, postpolycythemic myelofibrosis (post-PVMF) (153). The natural history of PV also includes a low incidence of transformation to acute leukemia (1% to 2%). In addition, some patients may develop myelodysplasia (MDS) or acute leukemia that may be related to cytotoxic therapy used to suppress the MPN process.

As noted in the section regarding MPN pathogenesis, nearly 95% of cases of PV are associated with the *JAK2* V617F mutation. Most of the remaining cases have the *JAK2* exon 12 mutation but in rare cases—1% or less—mutations of other genes involved in signal transduction pathways are likely present but few have been identified to date (32,135). The detection of mutated *JAK2* by PCR greatly facilitates the diagnosis of PV and distinguishes it from secondary causes of PV.

Normally, erythropoiesis is regulated by EPO, which is synthesized in the peritubular cells of the kidney and to a lesser extent in the liver. Its production is controlled by a family of transcription factors, the hypoxia-inducible factors (HIFs), that are stimulated by tissue hypoxia (Fig. 44.11) (156–158). The HIFs consist of alpha and beta subunits that target the transcription of a number of genes involved in the response to hypoxia, including *EPO*. The alpha subunit (HIF-alpha) is ubiquitous in all tissues and sensitive to oxygen tension. Under normoxic conditions, HIF-alpha is degraded through its interaction with oxygen, prolyl hydroxylase domain (PHD)–containing enzymes, and the von Hippel-Lindau tumor suppressor protein (VHL), and its degradation leads to a decrease in EPO synthesis. Under hypoxic conditions the degradation of HIF-alpha is inhibited, and EPO levels increase. When EPO binds to the EPOR, there is homodimerization of EPOR with autophosphorylation of the associated JAK2 kinase, with ensuing activation of the STAT5, MAPK, and PI3K-AKT pathways to promote the expansion and differentiation of erythroid precursors (158,159). Disturbances anywhere in the synthesis or binding of EPO to its receptor or in the subsequent activation of the signaling pathways will lead to an abnormality in erythropoiesis. In the case of the *JAK2* V617F mutation, the constitutively activated JAK2 essentially mimics the events initiated by the binding of EPO to EPOR, thus leading to hypersensitivity and/or independence from the hormone (Figure 44.10). Furthermore, because JAK2 also associates with MPL as well as with G-CSF-R, thrombopoiesis and granulopoiesis are stimulated, leading to the panmyelosis characteristic of PV.

Diagnosis of PV

The WHO criteria for the diagnosis of PV are listed in Table 44.10. In the setting of the appropriate clinical findings, the determination of the Hb level or RCM, the mutational status of *JAK2*, the serum EPO, and the histologic features of the bone marrow biopsy comprise the major diagnostic tests (153).

Clinical Features, Polycythemic Phase

The diagnosis of PV is usually made during the polycythemic phase. It occurs most frequently in adults in their 60s; patients younger than 20 years of age are only rarely reported (153,160). There is a slight male predominance. The major symptoms and the leading causes of morbidity and mortality are related to thrombosis and hemorrhage. Headache, dizziness, paresthesia, scotomata, and erythromelalgia are common and related to thrombotic events in microvasculature. Thrombosis involving major arteries or veins also occurs, and occasionally patients

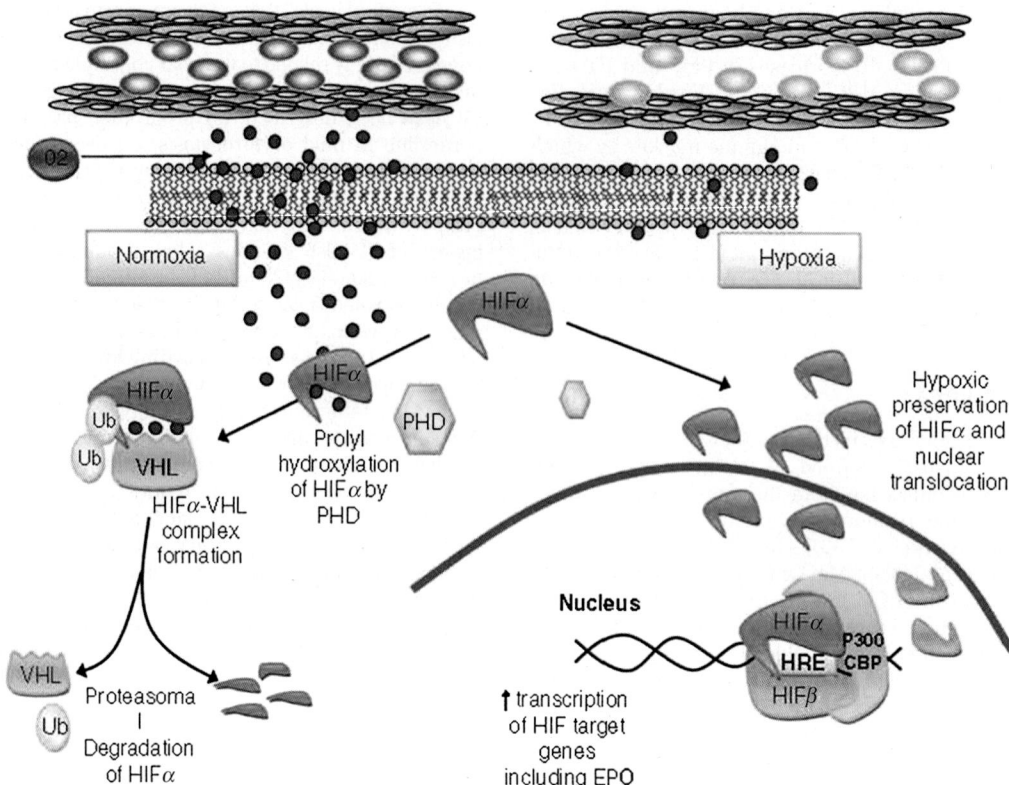

FIGURE 44.11. Intracellular oxygen sensing and EPO production. The cellular response to hypoxia is controlled by a family of transcription factors, the dimeric hypoxia-inducible factors (HIFs). Under normal oxygen tension HIFα is rapidly destroyed by the combined effect of oxygen, prolyl hydroxylase domain (PHD)–containing enzymes, and the von Hippel-Lindau tumor suppressor protein, VHL. Hydroxylated HIFα binds to VHL and the HIFα-VHL complex facilitates ubiquitin-mediated proteasomal degradation of HIFα Under hypoxic conditions, proteasomal degradation is slowed resulting in its cytoplasmic accumulation and translocation to the nucleus, where it binds with HIFβ and enhances transcription of EPO. This pathway is the site of a number of mutations that lead to congenital, secondary polycythemia. (Reprinted by permission from Macmillan Publishers Ltd: Patnaik MM, Tefferi A. The complete evaluation of erythrocytosis: congenital and acquired. *Leukemia* 2009;23:834–844. Copyright 2009.)

are first recognized when they experience a myocardial infarct or stroke. Splanchnic vein thrombosis (SVT) or the Budd-Chiari syndrome should raise the clinical suspicion of an MPN, including PV, if there is no other obvious etiology (161–163). In some patients, episodes of hemorrhage or thrombosis, including SVT, may occur months before a hematologic abnormality is

apparent and studies to detect mutated *JAK2* are warranted in such cases. The major risk factors for thrombotic episodes in PV are age >60 and the history of a previous thrombosis (164). There is conflicting data as to whether a WBC count >15 × 10⁹/L and/or a high allele burden of JAK2 V617F may also increase the risk of thrombosis (163–166) but the Hb level and the platelet count have not been proved to be significant risk factors. In contrast, however, platelet counts >1,000 × 10⁹/L are occasionally found in PV, and may be associated with increased risk for hemorrhage due to acquired von Willebrand syndrome (167). Other symptoms include generalized fatigue, aquagenic pruritus, gout, and gastrointestinal complaints related to ulcers and/or hemorrhage. The most prominent physical findings in the polycythemic phase include plethora in most cases, splenomegaly in 70%, and hepatomegaly in 50% (168).

Some patients have clinical findings suggestive of PV but do not have a sufficiently elevated Hb value to meet the diagnostic criteria. In such "prodromal" or "prepolycythemic" cases the diagnosis may be substantiated if the *JAK2* V617F or a similar activating mutation is present and the bone marrow biopsy has the morphologic characteristics of PV (169,170).

Morphologic and Laboratory Features of PV, Polycythemia Phase

Blood, Bone Marrow, and Other Tissues

The diagnosis of PV requires Hb >18.5 g/dL in men, >16.5 g/dL in women, or >17 g/dL in men and >15 g/dL in women if the Hb value is associated with a 2 g/dL or more increase over the individual's baseline Hb level, if that increase is not due to

---

Table 44.10	WHO DIAGNOSTIC CRITERIA FOR PV

Diagnosis requires the presence of both major criteria and one minor criterion *or* the presence of the first major criterion together with two minor criteria:

Major Criteria
1. Hb >18.5 g/dL in men, 16.5 g/dL in women, or other evidence of increased red cell volume[a]
2. Presence of *JAK2* V617F or other functionally similar mutation such as *JAK2* exon 12 mutation

Minor Criteria
1. Bone marrow biopsy showing hypercellularity for age with trilineage growth (panmyelosis) with prominent erythroid, granulocytic, and megakaryocytic proliferation
2. Serum EPO level below the reference range for normal
3. Endogenous erythroid colony (EEC) formation *in vitro*

[a]Hb or Hct >99th percentile of method-specific reference range for age, sex, altitude of residence *or* Hb >17 g/dL in men, 15 g/dL in women if associated with a documented and sustained increase of at least 2 g/dL from an individual's baseline value that cannot be attributed to correction of iron deficiency, *or* elevated RCM >25% above mean normal predicted value.
Thiele J, Orazi A, Tefferi A, et al. Polycythemia vera. In: Swerdlow SH, Campo E, Harris NL, et al., eds. *WHO Classification of Haematopoietic and Lymphoid Tissue.* 4th ed. Lyon, France: IARC; 2008.

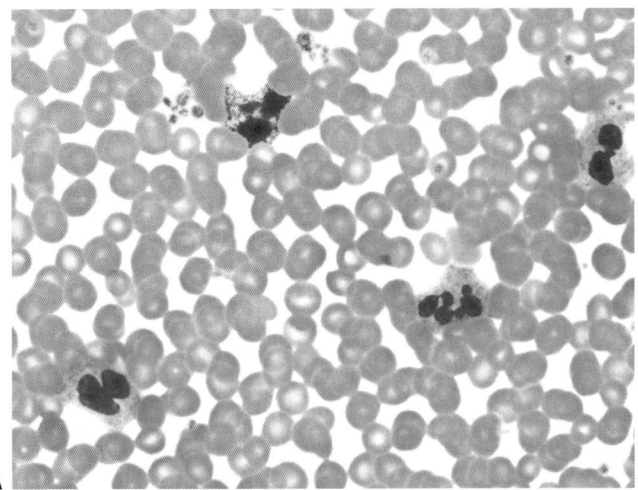

A

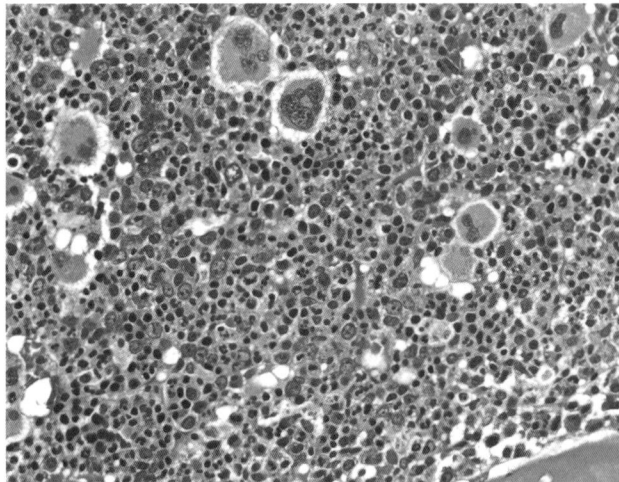

B

FIGURE 44.12. Polycythemia vera (PV), *JAK2* V617F⁺, polycythemic stage. A: Even in well-made blood smears the red cells may appear crowded, as in this case. Mild neutrophilia and basophilia may be seen. The RBCs usually have normal morphology. Platelets are clumped on this smear but the platelet count was 500×10^9/L. **B:** The bone marrow specimen is hypercellular, with dispersed megakaryocytes of varying size. **C:** The marrow hypercellularity is due to "panmyelosis" with increased numbers of erythroid and granulocytic precursors and megakaryocytes.

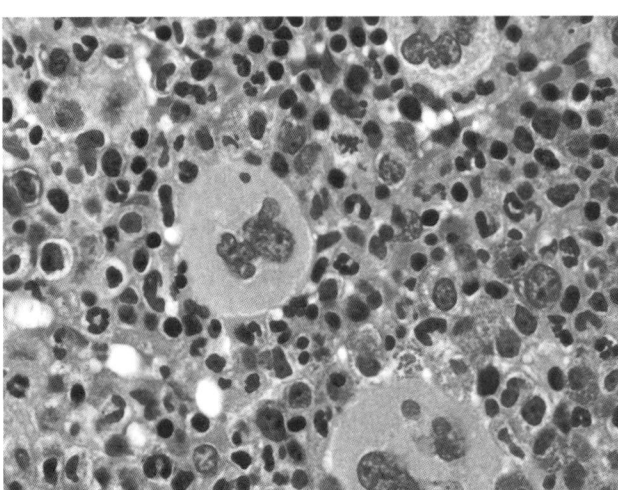

C

correction of iron deficiency (153). Usually the RBCs are morphologically normal except in cases associated with iron deficiency, which is fairly common in PV due to gastrointestinal bleeding. Neutrophilia—sometimes accompanied by modest basophilia—is present in 60% of cases and thrombocytosis is found in a similar number (168,171) (Fig. 44.12). Although a few immature granulocytes may be present, blasts are rarely seen in the blood smear.

The bone marrow findings of PV are best appreciated in biopsy sections (172,173). The histopathology of the polycythemia phase and of the "prodromal" phase is similar and characterized by proliferation of erythroid, granulocytic, and megakaryocytic lineages. Although the cellularity of the bone marrow may vary, it is almost always hypercellular for the patient's age (172). The increase in cellularity may be particularly noted in the bone marrow spaces immediately under the cortical bone, which is an area that is normally less cellular in normal age-matched controls (Fig. 44.13). Megakaryopoiesis is often conspicuous and consists of a pleomorphic population of small-, medium-, and large-sized megakaryocytes that may form small, loose clusters, sometimes found close to the boney trabeculae (173). Erythropoiesis appears in expanded islands throughout the marrow and is normoblastic unless there is superimposed iron deficiency anemia. In more than 90% of cases, an iron stain shows no storage iron in the marrow aspirate. Although a modest "left shift" in granulopoiesis may be present there is no increase in the percentage of myeloblasts. Reticulin fibers are usually normal or only mildly increased at the time of diagnosis. Reportedly, however, patients with

even modest fibrosis (grade 1+/3+) at diagnosis may be more prone to develop post-PVMF (174). It is important to note that cases of primary erythrocytosis associated with the *JAK2* exon 12 mutation have mainly erythroid proliferation and minimal expansion of the granulocytic or megakaryocytic lineages (175).

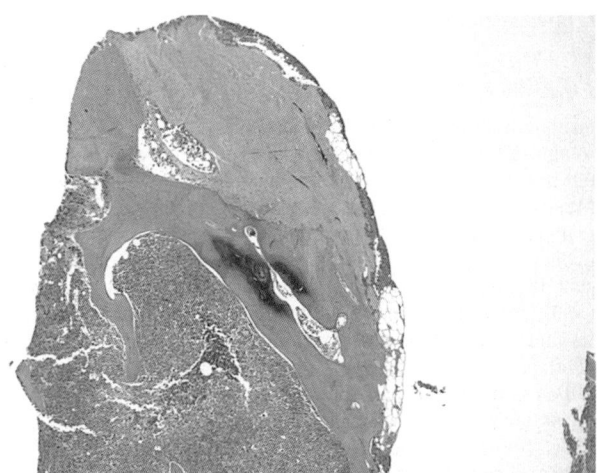

FIGURE 44.13. PV, bone marrow biopsy. This bone marrow biopsy from a patient with a history of PV illustrates hypercellular marrow even in the subcortical marrow spaces. Normally this region is hypocellular in adults; expansion of the proliferative bone marrow into this area is a hallmark of MPN.

The mild splenomegaly in the early phase of PV is caused by engorgement of the splenic cords and sinuses with red cells with minimal, if any, EMH (176).

Cytogenetic/Molecular Genetic Findings

Approximately 10% to 15% of PV patients have cytogenetic abnormalities on routine karyotyping, but none are specific for PV (32,177,178). Trisomy 8 and trisomy 9, or both, del(20q), del(9p), and del(13q) are among the abnormalities most commonly reported. Their prognostic significance is debatable, but acquisition of additional abnormalities is often associated with progressive disease (178). By definition, no Ph chromosome or *BCR-ABL1* fusion gene is present in PV.

As noted previously, 90% to 95% of patients demonstrate the *JAK2* V617F mutation, and 3% to 5% have instead the *JAK2* exon 12 mutation. In the few remaining cases abnormalities of other signaling proteins are likely present, but to date a mutation affecting *LNK* is the only one reported (135). However, a number of mutations affecting genes important in epigenetic regulation of transcription have been reported in PV and the other *BCR-ABL1*⁻ MPNs (Table 44.8). These mutations not only coexist with *JAK2* mutations but are not mutually exclusive of each other. They are relatively uncommon and include mutations of *TET, EZG2, IDH1/IDH2,* and *DNMT3A* (11,31,32). Currently, the pathogenic and prognostic influence of these mutations is not known.

Miscellaneous Laboratory Findings

The serum EPO level is usually decreased in PV but increased in secondary polycythemia, but a normal EPO does not exclude PV or secondary polycythemia. Thus, measurement of EPO levels is important in the evaluation of polycythemia, but by itself is not diagnostic (153,179,180). The arterial oxygen saturation is normal, as is the p50 unless PV coexists with another disorder, such a chronic obstructive pulmonary disease. When grown *in vitro* in semisolid medium, bone marrow cells from PV patients form endogenous erythroid colonies (EECs) without addition of EPO to the culture, whereas cells from normal controls and from patients with secondary erythrocytosis require exogenous EPO for EEC formation. However, EECs may also be seen in PMF and ET (181). Furthermore, few clinical labs perform the test. Abnormal platelet function studies are frequently observed in patients with PV, but correlate poorly with bleeding or thrombotic episodes (182,183). Patients with 1,000 × 10⁹/L or more platelets and an acquired von Willebrand syndrome will exhibit decreased functional activity of von Willebrand factor (VWF) as measured by collagen binding activity and ristocetin cofactor activity (167,183,184).

Prognosis, Disease Progression, and Therapy

Patients with PV have a shortened life expectancy as compared to age-matched normal controls and this becomes most apparent in the second decade of the disease process (165,185,186). Major thrombotic episodes, progression to post-PVMF, and transformation to acute leukemia are the most distinctive events during the course of the disease. The most important risk factors for shortened survival in PV include older age (>65), a history of previous thrombosis, and leukocytosis. The impact of older age and a previous thrombosis on overall survival is that they are the major risk factors for thrombosis, which is the major cause of death. The role of leukocytosis as a risk factor for thrombosis is debatable, although an elevated WBC count has been associated with leukemic transformation and post-PVMF (163,165,187,188). Extreme thrombocytosis is associated with the risk for hemorrhage, but not for thrombosis (184). The influence of the allele burden of *JAK2* V617F on the morbidity and mortality associated with PV is not clear, with various centers reporting conflicting results.

Table 44.11	WHO CRITERIA: POST-PVMF

1. Documentation of a previous diagnosis of WHO-defined PV
2. Bone marrow fibrosis grade 2–3 (on 0–3 scale) or grade 3–4 (on 0–4 scale)

Additional criteria (two are required)
1. Anemia or sustained loss of either phlebotomy (in the absence of cytoreductive therapy) or cytoreductive treatment requirement for erythrocytosis
2. Leukoerythroblastic blood picture
3. Increasing splenomegaly defined as either an increase in palpable splenomegaly >5 cm from baseline (distance below left costal margin) or appearance of newly palpable splenomegaly
4. Development of >1 of 3 constitutional symptoms: >10% weight loss in 6 mo, night sweats, unexplained fever >37.5°C.

Thiele J, Orazi A, Tefferi A, et al. Polycythemia vera. In: Swerdlow SH, Campo E, Harris NL, et al., eds. *WHO Classification of Haematopoietic and Lymphoid Tissue.* 4th ed. Lyon, France: IARC; 2008.

Although higher allele burdens have been associated by some investigators with post-PVMF, a correlation between allele burden, thrombosis, and evolution to acute leukemia seems less likely (32,163,187,188). There is little information regarding the molecular events that precipitate AML/MDS when it occurs as part of the natural history of PV, although newly acquired abnormalities affecting genes such as *IKZF, TP53*, and *RUNX1* have been postulated to play a role (9,11,32).

Postpolycythemia Myelofibrosis

This progressive and often terminal complication develops in approximately 10% to 15% of patients 10 to 15 years after the initial diagnosis of PV, and in up to 50% who survive 20 years of more (168,189). It is characterized by anemia, leukoerythroblastic blood smear with teardrop-shaped RBCs, MF, and splenomegaly due to EMH (Table 44.11). The bone marrow biopsy specimens are variably cellular and demonstrate reticulin and often overt collagen fibrosis; osteosclerosis may be present as well (Figs. 44.14 and 44.15). Granulopoiesis and particularly erythropoiesis are reduced and clusters of abnormal, bizarre megakaryocytes with hyperchromatic nuclei are seen in clusters. The marrow sinuses are often dilated and filled with hematopoietic precursors and megakaryocytes. EMH in the sinuses of the spleen contributes to the leukoerythroblastosis in the blood. The liver may demonstrate EMH as well. Nearly 80% to 90% of patients with post-PVMF exhibit an abnormal karyotype (190,191).

Acute Leukemia/Myelodysplastic Phase of PV

Myelodysplastic syndromes and acute myeloid leukemia (MDS/AML) occur as rare and usually late events in PV. The incidence of MDS/AML in patients with PV treated only with phlebotomy is reportedly 1% to 2%, which is assumed to be the incidence of MDS/AML in the "natural history" of the disease (190). However, the incidence of MDS/AML in some series reported in the literature ranges from 5% to 15% of PV patients followed for 10 years or more. The risk of developing this complication is likely related to the age of the patient (higher risk in older patients) and to exposure to cytotoxic treatment modalities such as alkylating agents and P³² (190,192). In virtually all cases the leukemia is of myeloid origin and often preceded by an MDS-like phase. Rare cases of lymphoblastic leukemia have been reported but likely represent *de novo* leukemias (193). Sometimes the transformation to AML occurs in the setting of post-PVMF, and the fibrosis may prevent aspiration. The detection of blasts in such cases may be facilitated in the biopsy by staining for CD34. The finding of 10% or more blasts generally heralds transformation to an accelerated or dysplastic stage, and the finding of 20% or more blasts indicates acute leukemia. Almost all patients who develop post-PV MDS/AML show karyotypic evolution often with acquisition of complex

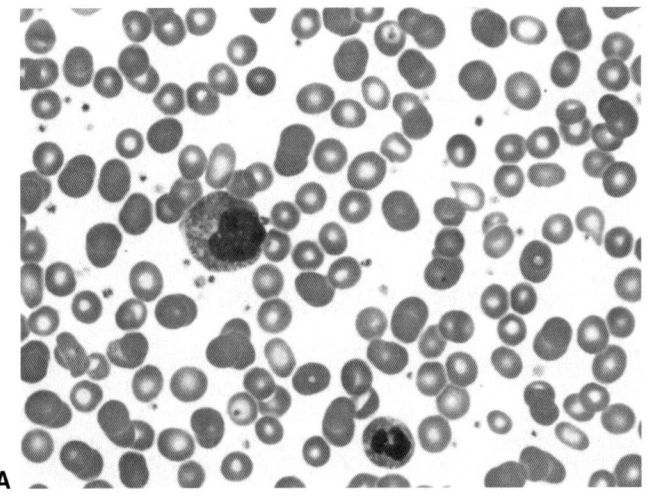

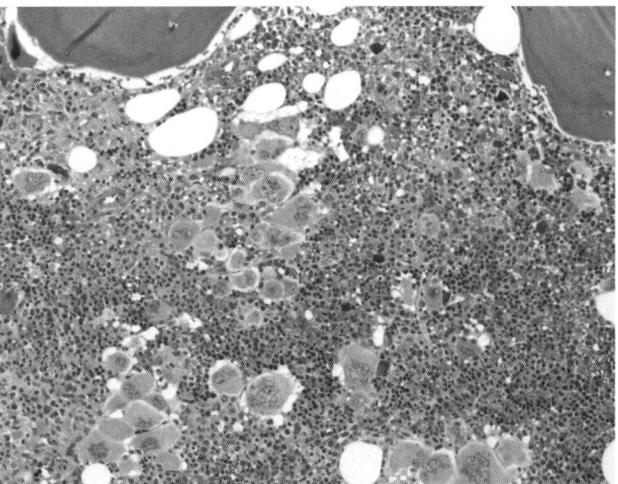

FIGURE 44.14. Peripheral blood smear and bone marrow biopsy, PV, _JAK2_ V617F⁺, early post-PVMF. A: Peripheral blood smear obtained 15 years after initial diagnosis of PV. Patient has anemia, immature granulocytes, and some teardrop-shaped RBCs but persistent thrombocytosis. He was noted to have splenomegaly. **B:** Bone marrow biopsy from same patient showed cellular marrow with large clusters of atypical megakaryocytes. **C:** Stain for reticulin fibers demonstrate 2+/3 reticulin fibrosis.

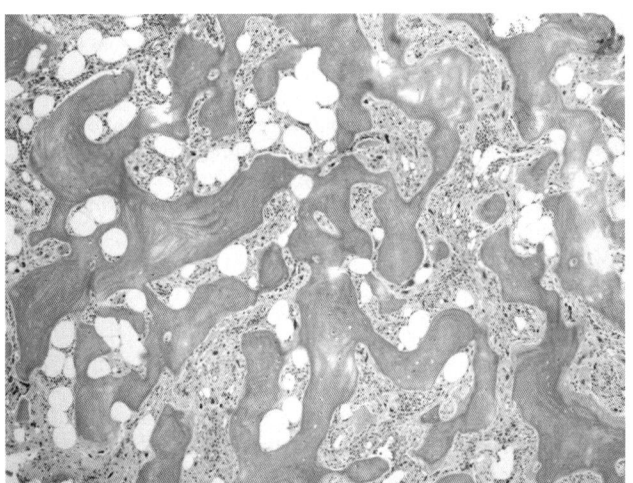

FIGURE 44.15. Bone marrow biopsy, PV, _JAK2_ V617F⁺, post-PVMF. Depleted, fibrotic bone marrow biopsy with osteosclerosis from a man with PV diagnosed nearly 20 years previously. He has progressive anemia and his spleen is enlarged.

chromosomal abnormalities, including loss of all or part of chromosome 5 and/or 7 (192).

At the time of development of acute leukemia, the blasts may not carry the _JAK2_ V617F mutation, giving rise to speculation that the transformation may occur in a clone that preceded the _JAK2_ mutated clone (141,193) (Fig. 44.16).

Differential Diagnosis of Polycythemia

The different causes of polycythemia are listed in Table 44.9. Most cases encountered will be either primary or secondary acquired polycythemia. Serum EPO levels and testing for mutated _JAK2_ should be considered as "up-front" tests for the diagnosis of PV and its differentiation from other causes of polycythemia.

Primary Polycythemia, Acquired and Congenital

PV is the only acquired primary polycythemia. The only congenital primary polycythemia currently characterized is primary familial/congenital polycythemia (PFCP), which is caused by mutations in _EPOR_, a rare condition with an autosomal dominant inheritance pattern. Nearly 20 different mutations have been described that lead to loss of the EPOR binding site for SHP-1, a protein that normally down-regulates EPO-mediated signaling (194). Loss of this domain leads to hypersensitivity to EPO; thus serum EPO levels are low or normal. There is erythrocytosis but no granulocytosis or thrombocytosis. _EPOR_ mutations account for only a small number of cases of PFCP and for the majority of cases the defects are unknown; they do not exhibit _JAK2_ mutations.

Secondary Polycythemia, Acquired and Congenital

Most cases of secondary polycythemia are acquired and hypoxia-induced (Table 44.9). Chronic obstructive lung disease, right to left cardiopulmonary shunts, sleep apnea, and renal disease that compromise blood flow to the kidney are the most frequent causes (154,155,195). Individuals living at

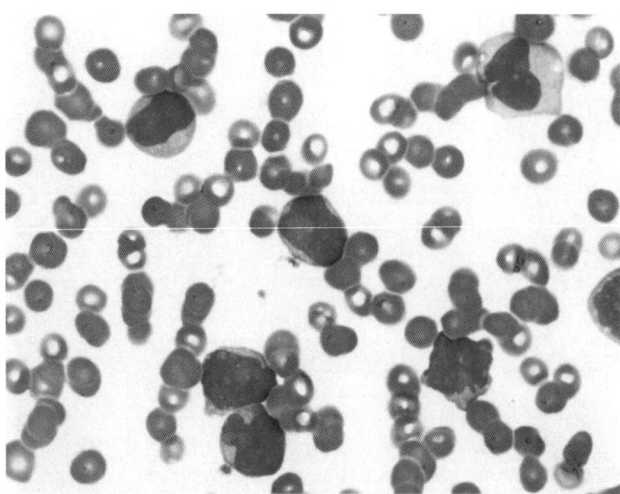

FIGURE 44.16. Peripheral blood smear, AML, *JAK2* V617F⁻, in a patient with previously diagnosed *JAK2* V617F⁺ PV. The incidence of AML increases over time to nearly 20% of patients who survive 20 or more years after the diagnosis of PV. In up to 50% of cases with *JAK2*-mutated PV the blasts of the AML transformation lack the mutation, suggesting origin from a different clone that preceded evolution of the JAK2⁺ clone.

high altitudes compensate for the lower atmospheric oxygen by increasing their RCM as a consequence of tissue hypoxia. Chronic carbon monoxide poisoning causes tissue hypoxia and is responsible, in part, for "smoker's polycythemia" but nicotine further contributes by lowering plasma volume through its diuretic effect.

Inappropriate production of EPO by a number of tumors, such as cerebellar hemangioblastoma, uterine leiomyoma, hepatocellular adenoma, meningioma, and pheochromocytoma, is often overlooked as a cause of secondary erythrocytosis. Exogenous EPO administration to improve performance in competitive sports may also lead to polycythemia; administration of androgens has a similar effect. The pathogenesis of postrenal transplant erythrocytosis, which occurs in 10% to 15% of renal transplant recipients 6 to 24 months after transplant, is not well-understood, although its frequency is reportedly decreasing, likely due to newer drugs such as sirolimus and mycophenolic acid now used after kidney transplant (196).

Congenital secondary polycythemia should be considered in young patients or in patients with life-long polycythemia in whom the serum EPO level is normal or elevated. Two broad groups of defects are found in this category—those associated with abnormal Hb affinity for oxygen and those associated with mutations of genes in the oxygen sensing/EPO synthesis pathway (158).

Over 90 Hb variants have been described that have abnormal Hb-oxygen dissociation curves. Abnormal Hb with increased oxygen affinity does not easily give up oxygen to the tissue, leading to a reduced P50, increased EPO production, and secondary polycythemia. Although some high-oxygen-affinity Hb variants may be detected by Hb electrophoresis, most are not. Measurement of P50 is an appropriate screening test if such variants are suspected (154,195). A deficiency of 2,3-bisphosphoglycerate mutase may also be responsible for production of Hb with increased oxygen affinity, a reduced P50, and secondary polycythemia (197).

Mutations in genes encoding proteins in the oxygen sensing pathway and in the regulation of EPO production can also lead to polycythemia (Fig. 44.11). The best characterized of these is Chuvash polycythemia, an inherited form of polycythemia affecting individuals in the Chuvash region of Russia. It results from a mutation in the von Hippel-Lindau (*VHL*) gene (158,198). The alpha subunit of HIF (HIF-alpha) is the transcription factor for EPO synthesis and is degraded by the collaborative effect

of oxygen, PHD-containing enzymes, and the VHL protein. The mutated *VHL* produces a VHL protein that does not bind with HIF-alpha, thus disrupting the degradation of this transcription factor and allowing for continued increased EPO production. Mutations of the genes (*PHD2*) that encode the PHD-containing enzymes essential in the degradation of HIF-alpha and of genes that encode HIF-alpha isoforms have been reported to lead to similar changes. These mutations lead to increased serum EPO and erythrocytosis (158).

PRIMARY MYELOFIBROSIS

PMF is a clonal myeloid neoplasm characterized by the predominant proliferation of granulocytes and atypical megakaryocytes, accompanied by a gradual increase in bone marrow reticulin fibers and in EMH. About 50% of patients have the *JAK2* V617F whereas another 5% to 10% have mutated *MPL* (199). Two phases of PMF are recognized: (a) a prefibrotic stage in which the bone marrow is hypercellular with minimal if any reticulin fibrosis, no or minimal EMH, but often marked thrombocytosis in the peripheral blood, and (b) a fibrotic stage with hypocellular bone marrow, marked reticulin and/or collagen fibrosis, leukoerythroblastosis, and prominent EMH with hepatosplenomegaly (200–202). There is a gradual, stepwise progression from the prefibrotic to the fibrotic stage.

Although megakaryocytes and granulocytes are the most proliferative cells in the bone marrow, PMF is a stem cell disorder and all of the myeloid lineages and even some lymphoid cells are derived from the neoplastic clone (203). The fibroblasts are thought to be nonneoplastic but are stimulated to proliferate and deposit collagen in response to fibrogenic cytokines (e.g., TGF-β and platelet-derived growth factor) that are abnormally produced by cells derived from the neoplastic clone, particularly the megakaryocytes (15,16,204). There is also prominent neoangiogenesis in the marrow and the spleen. Increased levels of vascular endothelial growth factor are present and an increase in the microvascular density in the bone marrow correlates with the degree of fibrosis in the marrow and the extent of EMH in the spleen (205,206). Furthermore, not only are cytokines that promote vascular proliferation and fibrosis increased, but a number of other inflammatory cytokines are produced that result in a "cytokine storm" that contributes to the clinical, hematologic, and pathologic abnormalities commonly observed in PMF (207).

Diagnosis of PMF

The WHO criteria for the diagnosis of PMF are shown in Table 44.12. The findings at the time of diagnosis depend on the stage of the disease when the symptoms are first recognized. Only 25% to 30% of cases are recognized in the prefibrotic stage of PMF but because of the marked thrombocytosis that is often present early in the disease, they may be erroneously classified as ET. Most patients are first recognized in the fibrotic stage, when leukoerythroblastosis, MF, and organomegaly due to EMH are evident.

Clinical Findings

The annual incidence of PMF reportedly is 0.5 to 1.5/1,000 people per year. The median age at diagnosis is usually in the seventh decade and only rarely diagnosed before age 40 (201). Pediatric cases have been reported but inflammatory and infectious diseases as well as other hematopoietic and nonhematopoietic neoplasms must be carefully excluded before a diagnosis of PMF is made in a child (208).

Usually, the onset of the disease is insidious; nearly 25% of patients are asymptomatic when an abnormality is found at the

Morphologic and Laboratory Features of PMF

Peripheral Blood, Bone Marrow, and Other Tissues

Only recently have the features of the prefibrotic stage of PMF been well-characterized and the prognostic importance of distinguishing this early stage of PMF from ET emphasized (200–202). In one of the few studies that have examined documented cases of prefibrotic PMF, the WBC count was minimally elevated (median 14.0×10^9/L, range 5.6 to 32.7×10^9/L), anemia, if present, was mild (median Hb = 13 g/dL, range 7.05 to 15.8 g/dL), but the platelet count was often elevated (median 962×10^9/L, range 104 to $13,215 \times 10^9$/L) (200). The thrombocytosis may lead to the erroneous diagnosis of ET (200,202). Mild neutrophilia with a "left shift" may be present but myeloblasts, nucleated red cells and teardrop-shaped red cells are rarely seen during the prefibrotic stage (Fig. 44.17). Absolute monocytosis may be observed in a small number of cases but usually signals worsening disease (209,210). There is a gradual worsening of the hematologic parameters as the disease progresses. As patients transit from the prefibrotic to the fibrotic stage the anemia worsens and the platelet count often decreases (200). Leukocytosis may be present but leukopenia more commonly occurs as marrow failure becomes more prominent. It is during the fibrotic stage that the classically described findings of leukoerythroblastosis and teardrop-shaped red cells and splenomegaly become prominent in PMF (Fig. 44.17). Circulating megakaryocytic nuclei and sometimes megakaryocytes are also observed. Blasts, occasionally accounting for up to 10% of the WBCs, are not uncommon in the blood during the late stages of PMF but may remain stable over a period of time and do not necessarily indicate an acute leukemia/blast phase is imminent although they should be carefully monitored. The finding of 20% or more blasts, if persistent, is, according to WHO criteria, diagnostic of acute leukemia (201).

A bone marrow biopsy is essential for the diagnosis of PMF. The biopsy should be assessed for overall cellularity, the relative numbers of cells in the various myeloid lineages and their degree of maturation, the amount/grade of fibrosis, and the morphology of the megakaryocytes (14). A reticulin stain should be done in each case of any MPN, always using a standardized and uniform protocol for staining as well as a uniform system for grading fibrosis (211) (Table 44.13). Immunohistochemical staining for CD34 may provide additional information regarding angiogenesis as

time of routine blood work or during investigation for another disease (201). Nonspecific findings, such as fatigue and weight loss, are commonly reported, but night sweats, low-grade fever, gouty arthritis, and renal stones are sometimes the presenting symptoms. In the prefibrotic stage, symptoms related to the markedly elevated platelet count, including hemorrhage or easy bruising, may be present, but palpable organomegaly is rarely found (200,202). In contrast, patients in the fibrotic stage often present with severe anemia, massive splenomegaly, and/or hepatomegaly complicated by portal vein hypertension, bleeding varices, and ascites (201,204).

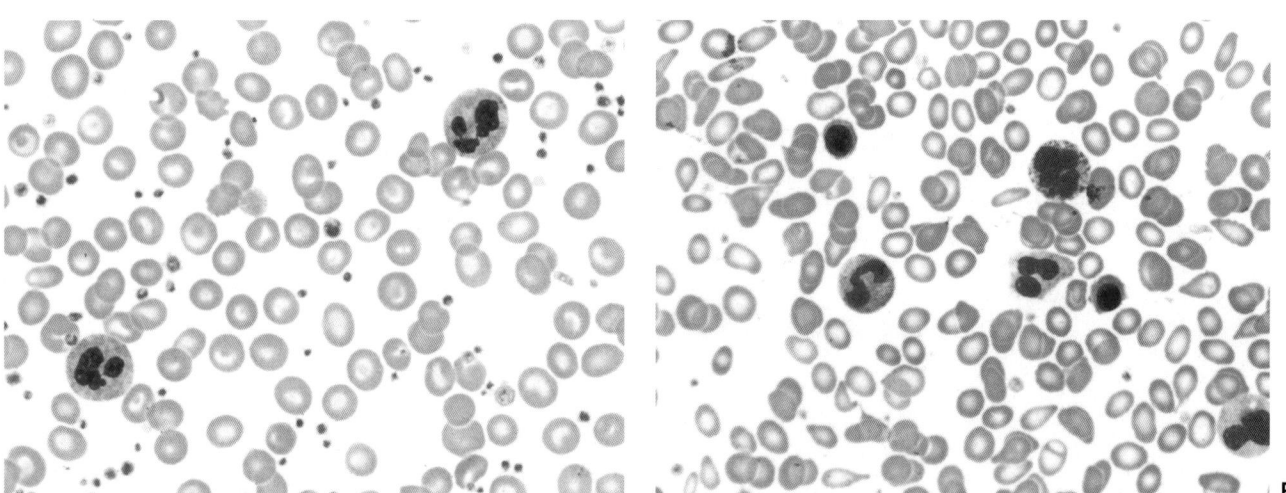

FIGURE 44.17. A: Peripheral blood smear, PMF, prefibrotic stage. This smear is from a 35-year-old woman referred with a diagnosis of ET because of a platelet count of 900×10^9/L. Thrombocytosis is the major abnormality. The patient's corresponding bone marrow is illustrated in Figure 44.18. **B:** Peripheral blood smear, PMF, fibrotic stage. This blood smear shows the classic findings of the fibrotic stage of PMF, with leukoerythroblastosis and teardrop-shaped RBCs. The patient's corresponding bone marrow is illustrated in Figure 44.19.

Table 44.13	SEMIQUANTITATIVE GRADING OF BONE MARROW FIBROSIS
Grade	**Description**
MF-0	Scattered linear reticulin fibers with no intersections (crossovers) corresponding to normal bone marrow
MF-1	Loose network of reticulin with many intersections, especially in perivascular areas
MF-2	Diffuse and dense increase in reticulin with extensive intersections, occasionally with focal bundles of collagen and/or focal osteosclerosis
MF-3	Diffuse and dense increase in reticulin with extensive intersections and coarse bundles of collagen, often associated with osteosclerosis

Thiele J, Kvasnicka HM, Facchetti F, et al. European consensus on grading bone marrow fibrosis and assessment of cellularity. *Haematologica* 2005;90:1128–1132.

well as a better assessment of the blast percentage than can be appreciated in routinely stained sections. If a marrow aspirate can be obtained it may provide additional information regarding maturation of the hematopoietic lineages.

During the prefibrotic stage the bone marrow is often hypercellular and shows proliferation of granulocytes with a prominence of segmented neutrophils whereas erythropoiesis is often decreased in quantity and shifted towards immaturity (Fig. 44.18). The percentage of myeloblasts is not increased. An important aspect of the marrow in PMF is that the megakaryocytes are often clustered, vary from small to large forms, and have an abnormal nuclear/cytoplasmic ratio with plump, bulky, "cloudlike" nuclei. Bare and hyperchromatic megakaryocytic nuclei are often seen. Overall, the finding of pleomorphic, bizarre megakaryocytes—often clustered—in a background of numerous segmented neutrophils but sparse erythroid precursors is characteristic of the prefibrotic stage of PMF. In the prefibrotic stage, by definition, there is minimal fibrosis, although reticulin fibers may be increased around blood vessels. Small lymphoid aggregates are not uncommon, and in some cases, the small B and T cells in the aggregates may be derived from the neoplastic clone (203).

It should be noted that the WHO guidelines for the diagnosis of PMF indicate that in addition to the three major criteria at least two of four minor criteria must be present to confirm the diagnosis of PMF (see Table 44.12). A comparison of the minor criteria with the comments in the previous paragraphs

regarding the blood and marrow findings in PMF could suggest that some cases of prefibrotic PMF might not fulfill the minor criteria rules (212). However, as noted in the footnotes of the criteria table, the degree of abnormality for the minor parameters need not be marked and may be only "borderline abnormal" for some values, yet still be sufficient to buttress the major morphologic and clinical findings to enable an accurate diagnosis (213).

The fibrotic stage of PMF is characterized by reticulin or collagen fibrosis and often by osteosclerosis with decreasing cellularity of the marrow. Dilated sinuses, often containing megakaryocytes or other immature hematopoietic cells, are prominent. Atypical megakaryocytes may occur in sheets and clusters and are often the predominant bone marrow cell (Fig. 44.19).

According to WHO criteria, 10% to 19% blasts in the blood and/or bone marrow indicates an "accelerated" stage of PMF, whereas the finding of 20% or more indicates transformation to AML (201). If a patient initially presents with the findings of overt AML but has some marrow findings that suggest a preceding PMF, the best diagnosis is AML, with mention of the possibility that it evolved from a preexisting MPN, such as PMF.

EMH accounts for many of the abnormalities observed in the blood during the fibrotic stage of PMF. EMH can occur in any tissue although the spleen and liver are most commonly affected (Fig. 44.20). In the spleen, the EMH is found mainly in the splenic sinuses, leading to massive expansion of the red pulp and compression and eventual obliteration of the white pulp. The red pulp cords may become fibrotic but may also contain maturing hematopoietic cells. Although erythroid and granulocytic precursors are present in the foci of EMH, atypical megakaryocytes are particularly conspicuous (201). The abnormal release of immature cells from the sites of EMH contributes to the leukoerythroblastic peripheral blood and is responsible as well for the teardrop-shaped RBCs, although the exact mechanism by which they are produced is not known. Fibrosis and cirrhosis often accompany EMH in the liver and play major roles in the pathogenesis of the portal hypertension that may develop in PMF. The sites of EMH may also be sites of transformation to a blast phase. Myeloid sarcoma should be considered in the differential diagnosis of any extramedullary lesion in a patient with PMF.

Genetics

The *JAK2* V617F mutation is present in 50% to 60% of patients with PMF, and mutated *MPL* in 5% to 10% (31,199,204). In addition to these mutations involving signaling TKs a number of mutations of genes involved in epigenetic regulation

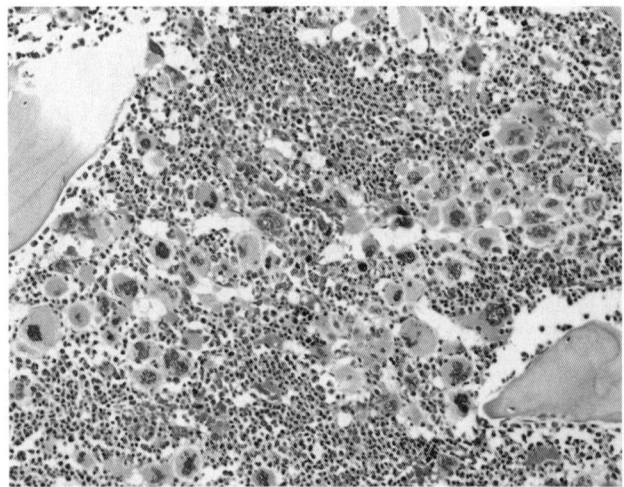
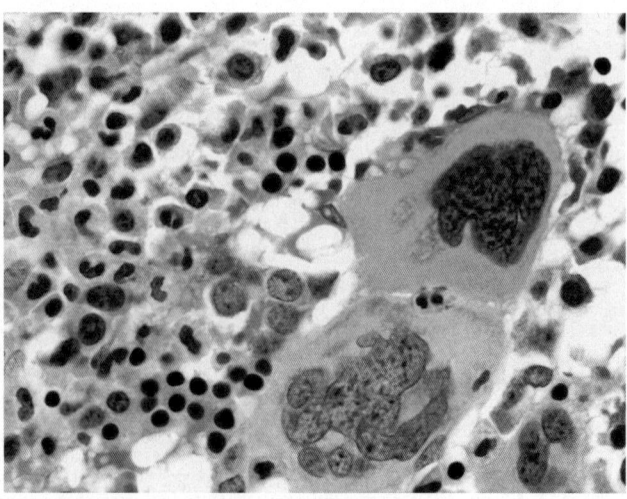

FIGURE 44.18. Bone marrow biopsy, PMF, prefibrotic stage. A: The bone marrow is hypercellular with marked granulocytic and megakaryocytic proliferation. The megakaryocytes occur in clusters and sheets and **(B)** have bizarre, often hyperchromatic nuclei and an increased N:C ratio. The patient's blood smear is illustrated in Figure 44.17A.

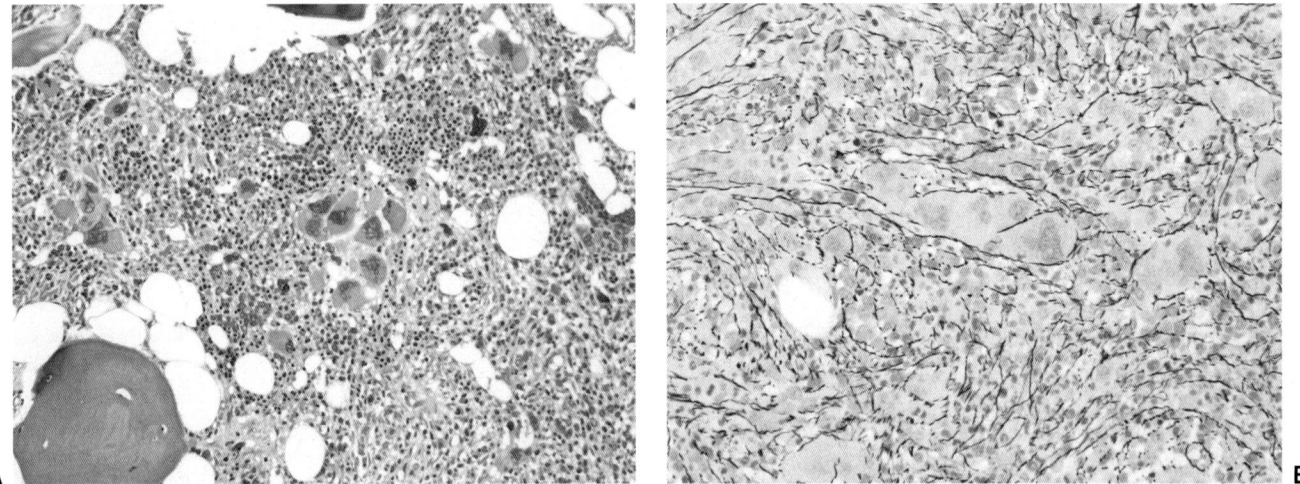

FIGURE 44.19. Bone marrow, PMF, fibrotic stage. A: The bone marrow biopsy shows clusters of atypical megakaryocytes with some islands of erythropoiesis and granulopoiesis. **B:** The reticulin stain shows grade 3+/3 reticulin fibrosis. The patient's blood smear is illustrated in Figure 44.17B.

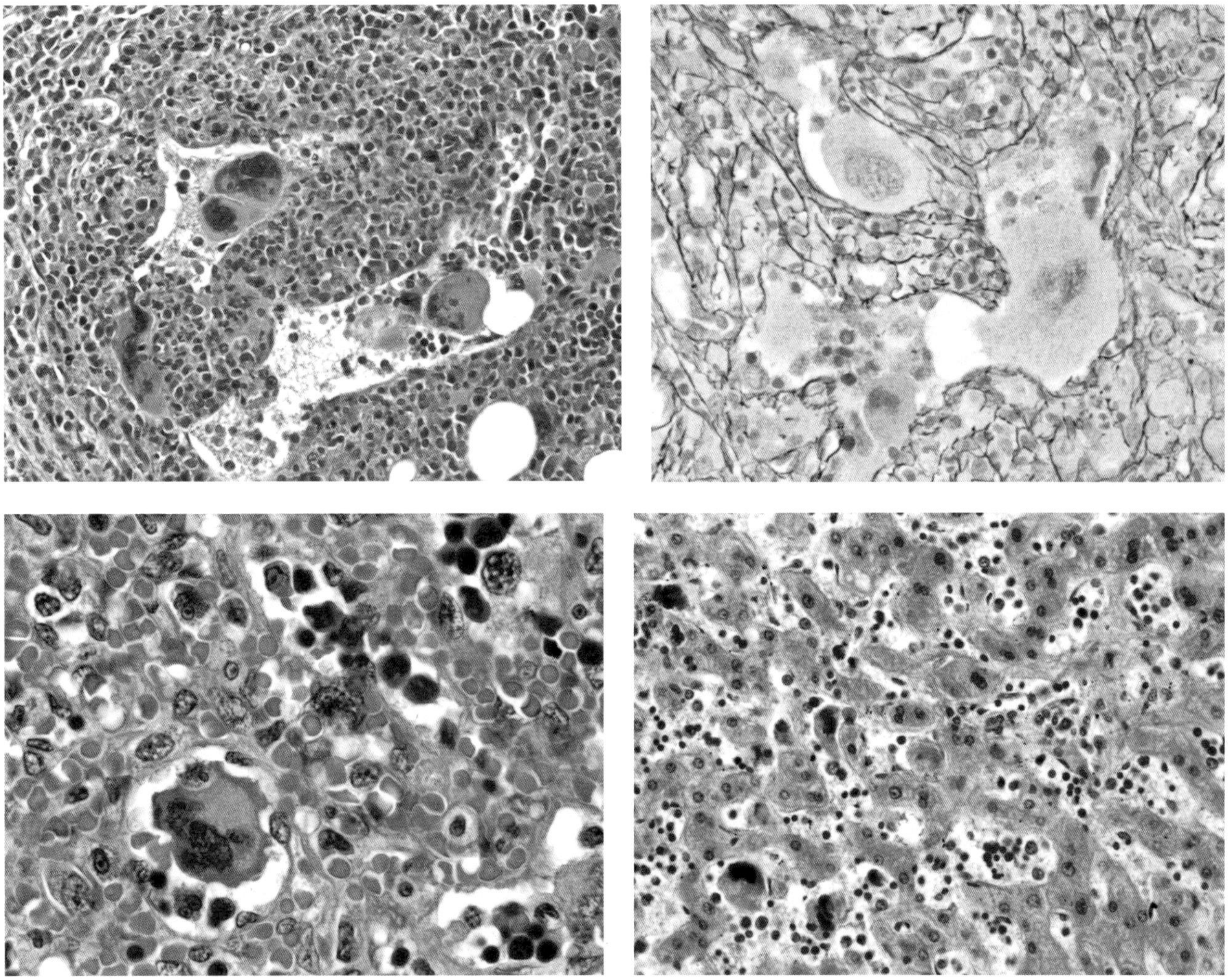

FIGURE 44.20. EMH in PMF, fibrotic stage. A: The bone marrow biopsy shows dilated sinuses with megakaryocytes, erythroid precursors, and some immature granulocytes. **B:** Immature hematopoietic cells gain access to the sinus likely due to disruption of the sinus integrity because of the surrounding increase in connective tissue. From marrow sinuses the cells gain access to the blood where they travel to distant organs permissive to hematopoietic cell growth. The EMH is most commonly seen in the (**C**) splenic and (**D**) hepatic sinuses, but other organs may be involved as well.

(e.g., *TET2*, *ASXL1*, and *DNMT3a*) are found in up to 10% of cases, and mutations affecting *SF3B1* and *SRSF2*, genes encoding proteins involved in RNA splicing, in up to 20% of patients (199,204). However, the value of routine karyotyping cannot be overstated in patients with PMF, although obtaining sufficient cells for metaphase analysis may be challenging if there is MF. In most studies abnormal karyotypes are reported in 30% to 50% of PMF cases analyzed (199,204,214). The most commonly observed abnormalities include del(20q), del(13q), +9 and/or +8 and abnormalities of 1q, but monosomy7/(del7q), −5/del(5q), and del(12p) are also recurrent abnormalities. Complex karyotypes are found in up to 10% to 15% of cases, and so-called monosomal karyotypes (defined as two or more autosomal monosomies or a single monosomy associated with at least one structural abnormality) are reported in 2% to 3% (215). The karyotype has prognostic importance and is included in a number of prognostic scoring systems. Generally, del(20q) and del(13q) are considered prognostically favorable, whereas all of the others, particularly complex or monosomal karyotypes, carry an unfavorable outlook (214,215).

Miscellaneous Laboratory Findings

Lactate dehydrogenase (LDH) is increased in most patients with PMF, and reportedly the increase correlates directly with the microvascular density in the bone marrow (216). Nearly one-half of patients have some disturbance of the immune system. Circulating immune complexes, positive studies for antinuclear antibodies, and autoimmune hemolysis are commonly reported. Some have suggested autoimmune abnormalities are more common in those with lymphoid aggregates in the bone marrow (217).

Disease Progression/Prognosis/Prognostic Factors

The natural evolution of PMF is progressive bone marrow fibrosis with worsening anemia, leucopenia, and thrombocytopenia. The increasing spleen size adds additional complications not only of pain and discomfort but also of progressive cytopenia(s), portal hypertension, and catabolic symptoms. Thromboembolic events, cardiac failure, infection, and hemorrhage are additional causes of morbidity and death. Myeloid blast transformation occurs in approximately 5% to 20% of cases at a median time of about 3 years after the initial recognition of PMF and usually responds poorly to therapy.

The survival time in PMF ranges from months to decades and depends on the stage in which the disease is first recognized. The overall median survival of patients diagnosed in the prefibrotic stage is 11 to 12 years, which contrasts to 3 to 7 years for those diagnosed in the fibrotic stage (201,202). Although numerous scoring systems have been proposed to assign patients to various risk levels for survival and progression to acute leukemia, a recent "dynamic" scoring system has been devised that includes many of the prognostic factors used in previous systems, but is attractive because it can be applied at any time during the disease course. Poor prognostic factors in PMF include Hb <10 g/dL, age >65 years, WBC count >25 × 10^9/L, circulating blasts >1%, presence of constitutional symptoms, unfavorable karyotype, red cell transfusion requirements, and platelet count <100 × 10^9/L (204,218). The onset of absolute monocytosis in the peripheral blood, often associated with bone marrow features resembling CMML, has recently been reported to herald the onset of an aggressive accelerated phase of PMF (210).

Differential Diagnosis of PMF

Because MF is a nonspecific response to marrow injury and to a number of inflammatory and neoplastic processes that involve the bone marrow, the list of differential diagnoses for the fibrotic stage of PMF is rather long, and includes virtually

	Prefibrotic PMF	Essential Thrombocythemia
WBC count	Variable, often increased	Usually normal, occasionally mildly increased
Platelet count	Often ≥450 × 10^9/L, sometimes normal or decreased	Always ≥450 × 10^9/L
Marrow cellularity	Increased	Normal to increased, rarely decreased
Major proliferating cells	Megakaryocytes, granulocytes	Megakaryocytes
Megakaryocyte morphology	Loose and tight clusters of three or more small to large sized megakaryocytes with altered cytoplasmic/nuclear ratio, "cloud-like," bulky nuclei, bare megakaryocytic nuclei, often bizarre forms	Dispersed or loose clusters of large to giant megakaryocytes with abundant cytoplasm, hyperlobulated nuclei; bizarre forms rarely seen
Genetic findings	*JAK2* V617F in ~50%; *MPL* W515L/K in ~5%	*JAK2* V617F in ~50%; *MPL* W515L/K in ~1%–2%

Table 44.14 COMPARISON OF PREFIBROTIC PHASE OF PMF AND ET

any of the other MPNs, MDS/MPN (particularly CMML), AML, MDS, lymphoma and other metastatic tumors, and infectious and inflammatory diseases. The late stages of any MPN may exhibit marked fibrosis and post-PVMF and post-thrombocythemia myelofibrosis (post-ETMF) may be impossible to distinguish with certainty from PMF if a documented history of the MPN is unknown. Myelodysplastic syndromes with myelofibrosis (MDS-F) and acute panmyelosis with myelofibrosis (APMF) enter into the differential diagnosis of MF as well, but MDS-F and APMF are characterized by small, dysplastic megakaryocytes in contrast to the highly abnormal megakaryocytes of PMF. Inflammatory diseases, particularly autoimmune disorders, may be associated with MF and can even demonstrate leukoerythroblastosis with teardrop-shaped red cells, but the megakaryocytes in such cases are normal and a significant lymphocytic and plasmacytic infiltrate is often present in the biopsy.

Perhaps the most frequently encountered diagnostic issue in PMF is the differentiation between prefibrotic PMF and ET—a sometimes difficult but important distinction because of the worse prognosis attached to PMF. A comparison of the major features that allow separation of these two diseases is further discussed in the ET section that follows below, and is summarized in Table 44.14.

ESSENTIAL THROMBOCYTHEMIA

ET is an MPN that is manifested primarily by megakaryocytic proliferation and thrombocytosis associated with episodes of thrombosis and/or hemorrhage. The diagnostic challenge is that thrombocytosis is a common hematologic abnormality (Table 44.15) and most patients with an elevated platelet count—even those in whom the platelet count is more than 1,000 × 10^9/L—do not have ET (219). Inflammatory conditions, bleeding, iron deficiency, and nonhematopoietic as well as nonmyeloid hematopoietic neoplasms, such as malignant lymphoma, are more likely causes of thrombocytosis than ET. Furthermore, any of the MPNs may be associated with an elevated platelet count, and more patients with marked thrombocytosis will ultimately be found to have CML or PMF than ET. However, the accurate diagnosis of ET is essential, including its distinction from

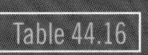

Table 44.15	CAUSES OF THROMBOCYTOSIS (≥450 × 10⁹/L)

Secondary (Reactive) Thrombocytosis
Infection
Inflammatory diseases
   Collagen vascular disease
   Chronic inflammatory bowel disease
Blood loss/hemorrhage
Chronic iron deficiency
Postsplenectomy
Hyposplenism
Trauma (particularly brain)
Postsurgical procedures
Neoplasms (nonhematopoietic and nonmyeloid hematopoietic)
Regeneration/rebound after chemotherapy

Myeloid Neoplasm-Related
MPNs
   CML, *BCR-ABL1⁺*
   PV
   PMF
   ET
AML with t(3;3)(q21;q26) or inv(3)(q21q26)
MDS with isolated del(5q) abnormality
MDS/MPN provisional entity, RARS-T

Table 44.16	WHO DIAGNOSTIC CRITERIA FOR ESSENTIAL THROMBOCYTHEMIA

Diagnosis requires meeting all four criteria:
1. Sustained platelet count ≥450 × 10⁹/L[a]
2. Bone marrow biopsy specimen showing proliferation mainly of the megakaryocytic lineage with increased numbers of enlarged, mature megakaryocytes. No significant increase or left shift of neutrophil granulopoiesis or erythropoiesis
3. Not meeting WHO criteria for PV,[b] PMF,[c] *BCR-ABL1⁺* CML[d] or myelodysplastic syndrome[e] or other myeloid neoplasm
4. Demonstration of *JAK2* V617F or other clonal marker, or in the absence of *JAK2* V617F, no evidence of reactive thrombocytosis[f]

[a]Sustained during the work-up process.
[b]Requires the failure of iron replacement therapy to increase Hb level to the PV range in the presence of decreased serum ferritin. Exclusion of PV is based on Hb and Hct levels and RCM measurement is not required.
[c]Requires the absence of relevant reticulin fibrosis, collagen fibrosis, peripheral blood leukoerythroblastosis, or markedly hypercellular marrow accompanied by megakaryocyte morphology that is typical for PMF—small to large megakaryocytes with an aberrant nuclear/cytoplasmic ratio and hyperchromatic, bulbous or irregularly folded nuclei and dense clustering.
[d]Requires the absence of BCR-ABL1.
[e]Requires absence of dyserythropoiesis and dysgranulopoiesis.
[f]Causes of reactive thrombocytosis include iron deficiency, splenectomy, surgery, infection, inflammation, connective tissue disease, metastatic cancer, and lymphoproliferative disorders. However, the presence of a condition associated with reactive thrombocytosis does not exclude the possibility of ET if other criteria are met.
Thiele J, Orazi A, Tefferi A, et al. Essential thrombocythaemia. In: Swerdlow SH, Campo E, Harris NL, et al., eds. *WHO Classification of Tumours of Haematopoietic and Lymphoid Tissues.* 4th ed. Lyon, France: IARC; 2008.

other MPNs associated with markedly elevated platelet counts, because if managed appropriately, most patients with ET will enjoy a prolonged survival (202).

Megakaryocytes originate from a hematopoietic stem cell that gives rise to early myeloid progenitors. The megakaryocyte and erythroid lineages share a common megakaryocyte-erythroid progenitor (MEP). The differentiation of the MEP toward the megakaryocytic and erythroid lineages is driven by the transcription factor GATA-1, whereas down-regulation of the transcription factor, PU.1, favors megakaryocytic development and suppresses erythroid maturation. Megakaryocytic proliferation and maturation is complex and characterized by DNA endoreduplication, cytoplasmic maturation and expansion, and release of megakaryocytic cytoplasmic fragments into the circulation as platelets (220–222). TPO plays a major role in the maturation, survival, and proliferation of the megakaryocytes. It is made in the liver, and binds to its receptor, MPL, which is on the megakaryocyte and platelet surface. The binding of TPO with MPL initiates phosphorylation and activation of JAK2 and subsequently signaling through the STATs, P13K, and MAPKK pathways to stimulate proliferation, endoreduplication, and expansion of the megakaryocyte and platelet mass. In ET, about 50% of the patients have the *JAK*2 V617F mutation, and an additional 1% to 3% have activating mutations of *MPL* (*MPL* W515K/L), which lead to constitutive activation of the signaling pathways, so that megakaryocytic proliferation and platelet production are either independent of or hypersensitive to TPO (9,136). Currently, the genetic events that underlie the abnormal proliferation in the remaining ET patients are not known. However, as in the other MPNs, a number of mutations, particularly in genes such as *TET2, ASXL1, EZH2, IDH1/IDH2,* that affect the epigenome have been reported (Table 44.8), but their significance in the pathogenesis of ET is currently unknown (9,10,32).

Diagnosis of ET

There is no single morphologic, clinical, or genetic finding that specifically identifies ET, so that all causes for thrombocytosis must be excluded before making the diagnosis. Although about 50% of cases of ET will have the *JAK2* V617F and another 1% to 3% will have the *MPL* W515K/L mutation, they are not specific and are reported in other MPNs. Nevertheless, if present, they

establish the clonal nature of the proliferation and eliminate further consideration of reactive thrombocytosis. In cases that do not exhibit a mutation or a clonal chromosomal abnormality, additional studies to exclude reactive causes of thrombocytosis as well as other neoplastic causes are necessary. Table 44.16 gives the WHO diagnostic criteria for ET.

It is important to note the 2008 WHO classification of MPNs emphasized that the prefibrotic stage of PMF is often associated with marked thrombocytosis that mimics ET, and that prefibrotic PMF and ET cannot be distinguished from each other merely by the platelet count, but that correlation of the histopathology of a bone marrow biopsy with clinical and laboratory data is necessary for accurate categorization (13,223,224). Many laboratories and clinics ascribed to ET prior to the 2008 WHO revision were likely gathered from publications that classified patients with prefibrotic PMF as ET. Where possible, we have used data from publications in which the WHO classification has been employed.

Clinical Findings

The estimated incidence of ET is about 0.6 to 2.5 per 100,000 persons per year. It can occur at any age, but is most common in patients in their 50s to 60s with an earlier peak in women at about 30 years of age (202,225,226). The majority of patients are discovered during routine laboratory testing or workup of another disease and are often asymptomatic. The remaining patients have presentations related to occlusive events affecting the microvasculature (headache, transient ischemic attacks, or erythromelalgia), thrombotic events affecting major vessels (stroke, myocardial infarct, SVT), or less commonly, hemorrhage from mucosal surfaces (gastrointestinal bleeding, epistaxis). Only a minority of patients have splenomegaly or hepatomegaly at presentation (202).

Morphology and Laboratory Finding

Blood, Bone Marrow, and Other Tissues
The most striking finding on the hemogram and the peripheral blood smear is thrombocytosis that can range from 450 × 10⁹/L to 2,000 × 10⁹/L or more with median counts of

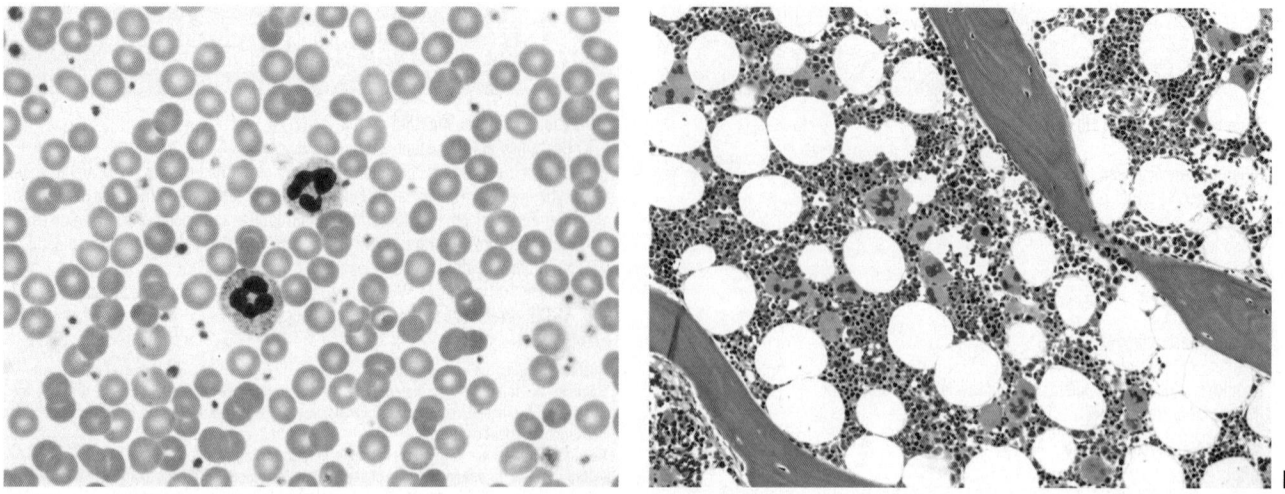

FIGURE 44.21. Essential thrombocythemia. A: Peripheral blood smear from a 50-year-old woman showing thrombocytosis. The platelets are fairly normal morphologically and no other significant abnormalities are noted on the smear. Note the similarity of this smear with 18b, from a patient with prefibrotic PMF. **B:** The patient's bone marrow specimen is normally cellular but has increased numbers of large megakaryocytes with hypersegmented nuclei and voluminous cytoplasm.

approximately $750 \times 10^9/L$ (202,223,227). The platelets often exhibit anisocytosis but highly atypical forms, including giant, agranular, or other bizarre platelet forms, are not common. The WBC count is normal or only minimally elevated (median, 8 to $9 \times 10^9/L$, range 5 to $14 \times 10^9/L$) and typically shows a normal leukocyte differential (223,227). Occasional basophils may be seen, but immature granulocytes or leukoerythroblastosis are uncommon at diagnosis. If there have been episodes of hemorrhage, mild anemia may be present, but the red cells usually lack significant anisocytosis and teardrop-shaped red cells are not observed (Fig. 44.21).

Bone marrow biopsy specimens are essential in making the diagnosis of ET, and allow its distinction from other MPNs, particularly the prefibrotic stage of PMF and from reactive causes of thrombocytosis. The cellularity of the marrow is variable, but is often normal or only modestly increased. The most striking abnormality is an increase in the number and size of the megakaryocytes, which often occur dispersed singly or in loose clusters throughout the marrow. These large, even, giant megakaryocytes often have abundant mature cytoplasm with nuclei that are hyperlobulated, resembling a "staghorn" (173,228) (Fig. 44.21). Although occasional bizarre megakaryocytes may be seen in ET, megakaryocytes with an increased N:C ratio, with large "bulky," poorly lobulated nuclei, or clustered in large, tight sheets of megakaryocytes are uncommon and should suggest the possibility of PMF (Table 44.14; Fig. 44.22). A significant population of small, dyspoietic megakaryocytes or micromegakaryocytes should suggest a myelodysplastic process, and in the face of an elevated platelet count, specifically a myeloid neoplasm associated with an abnormality of chromosome 5q. In most cases of ET, the M:E ratio is normal, but if there has been hemorrhage a compensatory erythroid proliferation may be present. Marked granulocytic proliferation is uncommon, and if present should raise doubts regarding the diagnosis of ET (228). Blasts are not increased in number and there is no myelodysplasia. The reticulin framework of the marrow shows minimal if any increase when examined by silver stains. Aspirate smears often demonstrate numerous markedly enlarged megakaryocytes associated with large pools of platelets. Emperipolesis of bone marrow cells is sometimes seen within the megakaryocyte cytoplasm although it is not specific and is seen even in bone marrow specimens from normal individuals.

Splenic enlargement is uncommon at the time of diagnosis and EMH is, if present, quite minimal (228). However, late in the disease course, some patients develop significant splenic enlargement associated with post-ETMF.

Genetics

Cytogenetic abnormalities are uncommon in ET but there is little data on patients in whom the diagnosis has been made using WHO criteria. In the largest series of patients meeting the WHO guidelines for the diagnosis of ET, only 7% of patients had a clonal chromosomal abnormality, with trisomy 9, rearrangement of chromosome 1, and trisomy 8 accounting for the majority of the recurring abnormalities. Reportedly, the presence of a cytogenetic abnormality did not influence overall prognosis (178). However, even if cytogenetic abnormalities are uncommon in ET, when present they establish the thrombocytosis as neoplastic rather than reactive, and in some cases, may suggest a disease other than ET as the reason for the thrombocytosis. The finding of a Ph chromosome or *BCR-ABL1* fusion excludes the diagnosis of ET, whereas a t(3;3)(q21;q26.2) or inv(3)(q21q26.2) would indicate MDS or AML, and del(5q) as an isolated abnormality would suggest the diagnosis of MDS. Cytogenetic abnormalities are more common in patients when they do evolve into an acute leukemia, perhaps as a result of previous cytotoxic therapy.

Nearly 50% of patients with ET have the *JAK2* V617F mutation, and 3% to 5% have mutated *MPL* (31,136,149). These mutations result in abnormal cytokine signaling and can be assumed to be major "drivers" of the proliferation, and when present they establish the thrombocytosis as a clonal process. However, they are not specific for ET nor does their absence exclude the diagnosis. Additional mutations that may be seen—regardless of whether the *JAK2* V617F is or is not present—include *TET2, SF3B1, ASXL1, IDH1/IDH2,* and/or *DNMT3A,* which are involved in the epigenetic regulation of gene expression (10,32,199,229).

Miscellaneous Laboratory Studies

Patients with ET usually demonstrate abnormal platelet function studies, although there is not a good correlation between an abnormal study and the ability to predict hemorrhagic or thrombotic episodes. However, higher platelet counts tend to be associated with a greater probability of hemorrhage, most likely through an acquired von Willebrand syndrome, which

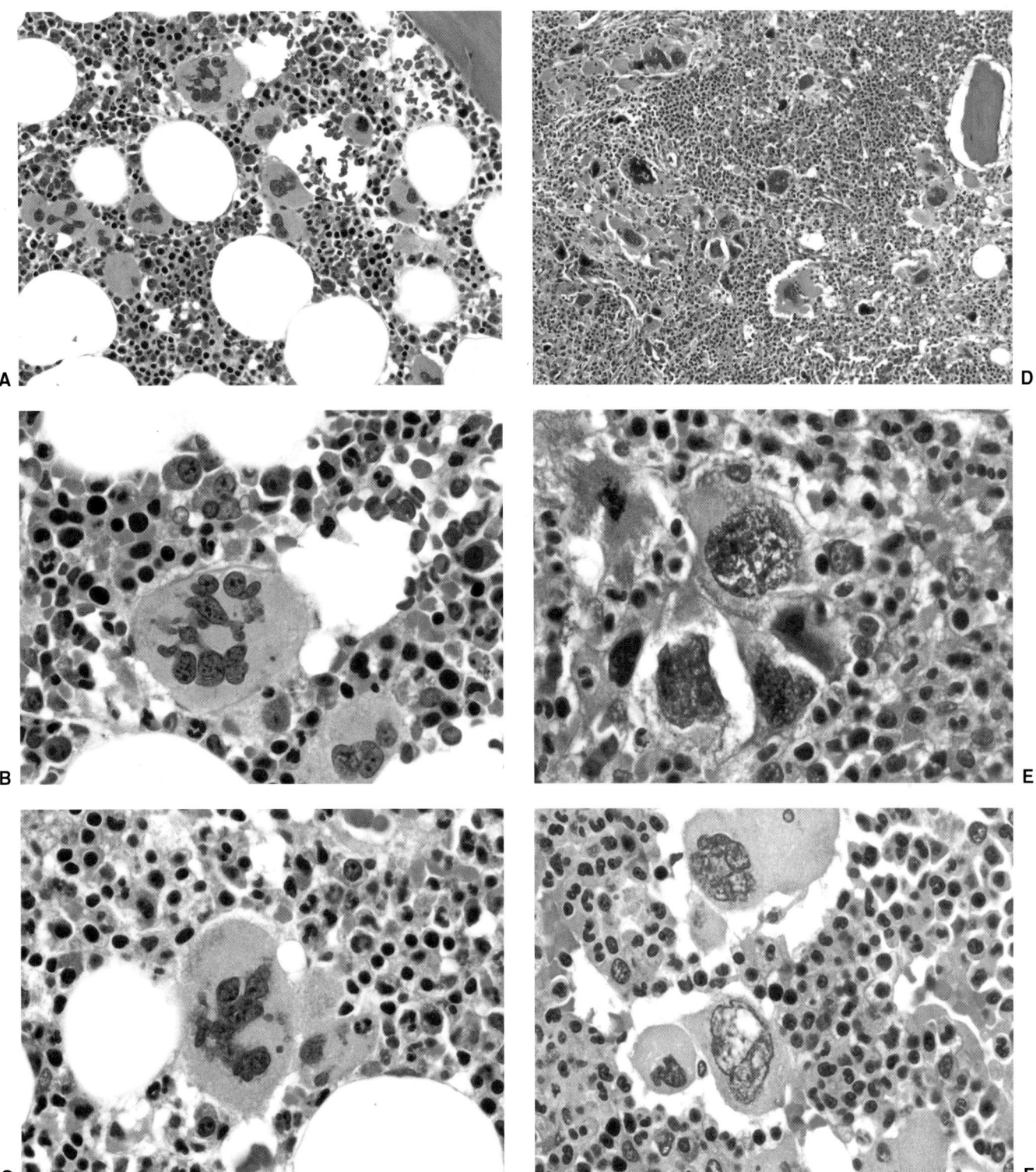

FIGURE 44.22. Bone marrow biopsies, ET (A–C) and PMF (D–F). A: The bone marrow biopsy of ET is often normally cellular with dispersed megakaryocytes that (**B,C**) are large with hypersegmented, "staghorn-like" nuclei and abundant cytoplasm. Compare these findings with the (**D**) more hypercellular marrow of prefibrotic PMF, and the (**E,F**) atypical PMF megakaryocytes that have "bulky," "cloud-like" nuclei and tend to more tightly cluster.

is associated with reduced levels of large, high-weight VWF multimers with loss of VWF function (167,230).

Disease Progression and Prognosis

The course of ET is usually that of an indolent disorder with episodes of thrombosis or hemorrhage, often with long symptom-free intervals. A recent study of 891 patients with WHO-defined ET demonstrated a 10-year survival rate of nearly 90% and a 15-year survival of 80% (202). Progression to overt MF or AML may occur but the incidence of these complications is reported to be <1% of patients followed for 10 years, although the incidence of post-ETMF does increase to nearly 10% by 15 years after diagnosis.

Age over 60, a history of a previous thrombotic event at diagnosis, anemia (<12 g/dL), and a leukocytosis (>11 × 10^9/L) have been reported to be the most adverse risk factors for overall survival (202). The risk of vascular events is clearly associated with overall survival in ET and their prevention is key to appropriate management of the patient. An international scoring system has been devised to predict risk factors for thrombosis and to guide in patient management (227).

Differential Diagnosis of ET

As noted previously, thrombocytosis is a common hematologic abnormality that is associated with numerous inflammatory and neoplastic conditions (Table 44.15). The clinical history, physical findings, and a few ancillary laboratory studies are very helpful in determining the cause of thrombocytosis. The history of a previous bleeding or thrombotic episode and splenomegaly would argue for MPN-related thrombocytosis whereas underlying inflammatory disease, elevated C-reactive protein, a concurrent nonhematopoietic neoplasm, or chronic iron deficiency would argue for reactive thrombocytosis. However, the degree of thrombocytosis is not helpful in distinguishing reactive from neoplastic causes. The lower threshold for the diagnosis of ET is just slightly above the normal range for most laboratories, and reactive thrombocytosis may have platelet counts of 1,000 × 10^9/L or more. If the underlying cause is not readily apparent studies for *JAK2* V617F and for *BCR-ABL1* should be performed from the blood, and a bone marrow specimen obtained and examined for the characteristic features of ET or another myeloid neoplasm as well as for marrow involvement by a disorder that could explain the thrombocytosis.

Myeloid disorders other than ET that are commonly associated with elevated platelet counts include PV, the prefibrotic stages of PMF and CML and the MDS/MPN disorder, refractory anemia with ring sideroblasts, and thrombocytosis (RARS-T). This latter disorder mimics ET in that it is characterized by a platelet count ≥450 × 10^9/L, and by a proliferation of megakaryocytes resembling those seen in ET or PMF. Furthermore, nearly 50% of cases are associated with the *JAK2* V617F mutation. RARS-T differs from ET in that the bone marrow shows dyserythropoiesis with numerous ring sideroblasts. Other myeloid neoplasms associated with thrombocytosis include MDS associated with del(5q) and the myeloid neoplasms associated with t(3;3)(q21;q26.2) or inv(3)(q21q26.2). The megakaryocytes of these neoplasms have markedly different morphology than ET, however. In the case of MDS with del(5q), the megakaryocytes have hypolobated nuclei, in contrast to the hyperlobulated nuclei of ET, whereas those associated with t(3;3) or inv(3) are small, micromegakaryocytes.

MPN, Unclassifiable

The diagnosis, myeloproliferative neoplasm, unclassifiable (MPN, U) should be applied only to cases that have clear-cut clinical, laboratory, and morphologic features of an MPN, but that do not meet the criteria for any specific MPN entity. These may include early cases of PV, ET, or PMF in which the features that distinguish between these entities are not yet fully developed, cases in which there is convincing evidence of an MPN but a coexisting inflammatory, metabolic, or neoplastic process obscures the diagnoses, or cases of MPN that are first encountered late in the disease process, when MF and/or evidence of acceleration or blastic transformation prevents recognition of the preexisting subtype. The designation should not be used for those cases in which the specimen is inadequate for diagnosis, if the necessary clinical and laboratory information for diagnosis is incomplete or has not been obtained, or if the patient has received previous growth factor therapy or cytotoxic therapy.

The finding of a *BCR-ABL1* fusion gene or rearrangements of *PDGFRA*, *PDGFRB*, or *FGFR1* precludes the diagnosis of MPN, U. Although the finding of the *JAK2* V617F is supportive of the diagnosis of a myeloid neoplasm, it is not specific and may be found in AML, MDS, and MDS/MPN as well. Lastly, if the case does not meet the criteria for diagnosis of any of the well-defined MPN entities, the possibility that it is not an MPN at all should be given serious consideration.

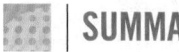 **SUMMARY**

The MPNs are a unique group of neoplasms in which the diagnosis depends on the careful correlation of clinical, morphologic, and genetic information. In view of the success of molecularly targeted therapy for some of the MPN and MPN-like diseases, and the explosion of data regarding possible molecular targets in others, it is particularly important that strict adherence to diagnostic criteria be used to ensure uniform and accurate diagnoses against which the results of molecular data and therapeutic trials can be judged. A final diagnosis of only "myeloproliferative disorder" is not helpful to the clinician. If meticulous attention is paid to the quality of the blood and marrow biopsy specimens, and to the diagnostic criteria mentioned in the preceding pages, hopefully a more specific diagnosis, or at least suggestions for additional information required to reach a specific diagnosis, can be given to allow for optimal care for the patient.

References

1. Dameshek W. Some speculations on the myeloproliferative syndromes. *Blood* 1951;6:372–375.
2. Fialkow PJ, Gartler SM, Yoshida A. Clonal origin of chronic myelocytic leukemia in man. *Proc Natl Acad Sci U S A* 1967;58:1468–1471.
3. Adamson JW, Fialkow PJ, Murphy S, et al. Polycythemia vera: stem-cell and probable clonal origin of the disease. *N Engl J Med* 1976;295:913–916.
4. Gilliland DG, Blanchard KL, Levy J, et al. Clonality in myeloproliferative disorders: analysis by means of the polymerase chain reaction. *Proc Natl Acad Sci U S A* 1991;88:6848–6852.
5. el Kassar N, Hetet G, Li Y, et al. Clonal analysis of haemopoietic cells in essential thrombocythaemia. *Br J Haematol* 1995;90:131–137.
6. Tsukamoto N, Morita K, Maehara T, et al. Clonality in chronic myeloproliferative disorders defined by X-chromosome linked probes: demonstration of heterogeneity in lineage involvement. *Br J Haematol* 1994;86:253–258.
7. De Keersmaecker K, Cools J. Chronic myeloproliferative disorders: a tyrosine kinase tale. *Leukemia* 2006;20:200–205.
8. Levine RL, Gilliland DG. Myeloproliferative disorders. *Blood* 2008;112:2190–2198.
9. Tefferi A. Novel mutations and their functional and clinical relevance in myeloproliferative neoplasms: JAK2, MPL, TET2, ASXL1, CBL, IDH and IKZF1. *Leukemia* 2010;24:1128–1138.
10. Vannucchi AM, Biamonte F. Epigenetics and mutations in chronic myeloproliferative neoplasms. *Haematologica* 2011;96:1398–1402.
11. Vainchenker W, Delhommeau F, Constantinescu SN, et al. New mutations and pathogenesis of myeloproliferative neoplasms. *Blood* 2011;118:1723–1735.
12. Tefferi A. Myeloproliferative neoplasms 2012: the John M. Bennett 80th birthday anniversary lecture. *Leuk Res* 2012;36:1481–1489.
13. Swerdlow SH, Campo E, Harris NL, et al., eds. *WHO classification of tumours of haematopoietic and lymphoid tissues*. Lyon: IARC, 2008.
14. Vardiman JW, Thiele J, Arber DA, et al. The 2008 revision of the World Health Organization (WHO) classification of myeloid neoplasms and acute leukemia: rationale and important changes. *Blood* 2009;114:937–951.
15. Castro-Malaspina H, Jhanwar SC. Properties of myelofibrosis-derived fibroblasts. *Prog Clin Biol Res* 1984;154:307–322.
16. Le Bousse-Kerdiles MC, Martyre MC, Samson M. Cellular and molecular mechanisms underlying bone marrow and liver fibrosis: a review. *Eur Cytokine Netw* 2008;19:69–80.
17. Barosi G, Gale RP. Bone marrow fibrosis in myeloproliferative neoplasms-associated myelofibrosis: deconstructing a myth? *Leuk Res* 2011;35:563–565.
18. Bizzozero OJ Jr, Johnson KG, Ciocco A. Radiation-related leukemia in Hiroshima and Nagasaki, 1946–1964. I. Distribution, incidence and appearance time. *N Engl J Med* 1966;274:1095–1101.
19. Caldwell GG, Kelley DB, Heath CW Jr, et al. Polycythemia vera among participants of a nuclear weapons test. *JAMA* 1984;252:662–664.
20. Corso A, Lazzarino M, Morra E, et al. Chronic myelogenous leukemia and exposure to ionizing radiation—a retrospective study of 443 patients. *Ann Hematol* 1995;70:79–82.
21. Finch SC. Radiation-induced leukemia: lessons from history. *Best Pract Res Clin Haematol* 2007;20:109–118.
22. Aguiar RC. Therapy-related chronic myeloid leukemia: an epidemiological, clinical and pathogenetic appraisal. *Leuk Lymphoma* 1998;29:17–26.
23. Bellanne-Chantelot C, Chaumarel I, Labopin M, et al. Genetic and clinical implications of the Val617Phe JAK2 mutation in 72 families with myeloproliferative disorders. *Blood* 2006;108:346–352.

24. Rumi E, Passamonti F, Della Porta MG, et al. Familial chronic myeloproliferative disorders: clinical phenotype and evidence of disease anticipation. *J Clin Oncol* 2007;25:5630–5635.
25. Ranjan A, Penninga E, Jelsig AM, et al. Inheritance of the chronic myeloproliferative neoplasms. A systematic review. *Clin Genet* 2013;83:99–107.
26. Landgren O, Goldin LR, Kristinsson SY, et al. Increased risks of polycythemia vera, essential thrombocythemia, and myelofibrosis among 24,577 first-degree relatives of 11,039 patients with myeloproliferative neoplasms in Sweden. *Blood* 2008;112:2199–2204.
27. Kilpivaara O, Mukherjee S, Schram AM, et al. A germline JAK2 SNP is associated with predisposition to the development of JAK2(V617F)-positive myeloproliferative neoplasms. *Nat Genet* 2009;41:455–459.
28. Olcaydu D, Harutyunyan A, Jager R, et al. A common JAK2 haplotype confers susceptibility to myeloproliferative neoplasms. *Nat Genet* 2009;41:450–454.
29. Malak S, Labopin M, Saint-Martin C, et al. Long term follow up of 93 families with myeloproliferative neoplasms: life expectancy and implications of JAK2V617F in the occurrence of complications. *Blood Cells Mol Dis* 2012;49:170–176.
30. Olcaydu D, Rumi E, Harutyunyan A, et al. The role of the JAK2 GGCC haplotype and the TET2 gene in familial myeloproliferative neoplasms. *Haematologica* 2011;96:367–374.
31. Cross NC. Genetic and epigenetic complexity in myeloproliferative neoplasms. *Hematol Am Soc Hematol Educ Program* 2011;2011:208–214.
32. Abdel-Wahab O, Pardanani A, Bernard OA, et al. Unraveling the genetic underpinnings of myeloproliferative neoplasms and understanding their effect on disease course and response to therapy: proceedings from the 6th International Post-ASH Symposium. *Am J Hematol* 2012;87:562–568.
33. Bennett JH. Two cases of disease and enlargement of the spleen in which death took place from the presence of purulent matter in the blood. *Edinburgh Med Surg* 1845;64:413.
34. Virchow P. Weisses blut. *Froriep's Notizen* 1845;36:151.
35. Nowell PC, Hungerford DA. Chromosome studies on normal and leukemic human leukocytes. *J Natl Cancer Inst* 1960;25:85–109.
36. Rowley JD. Letter: a new consistent chromosomal abnormality in chronic myelogenous leukaemia identified by quinacrine fluorescence and Giemsa staining. *Nature* 1973;243:290–293.
37. Bartram CR, de Klein A, Hagemeijer A, et al. Translocation of c-ab1 oncogene correlates with the presence of a Philadelphia chromosome in chronic myelocytic leukaemia. *Nature* 1983;306:277–280.
38. Heisterkamp N, Stam K, Groffen J, et al. Structural organization of the bcr gene and its role in the Ph' translocation. *Nature* 1985;315:758–761.
39. Shtivelman E, Lifshitz B, Gale RP, et al. Fused transcript of abl and bcr genes in chronic myelogenous leukaemia. *Nature* 1985;315:550–554.
40. Konopka JB, Witte ON. Detection of c-abl tyrosine kinase activity in vitro permits direct comparison of normal and altered abl gene products. *Mol Cell Biol* 1985;5:3116–3123.
41. Druker BJ, Talpaz M, Resta DJ, et al. Efficacy and safety of a specific inhibitor of the BC R-ABL tyrosine kinase in chronic myeloid leukemia. *N Engl J Med* 2001;344:1031–1037.
42. Moloney WC. Natural history of chronic granulocytic leukaemia. *Clin Haematol* 1977;6:41–53.
43. Millot F, Traore P, Guilhot J, et al. Clinical and biological features at diagnosis in 40 children with chronic myeloid leukemia. *Pediatrics* 2005;116:140–143.
44. Spiers AS, Bain BJ, Turner JE. The peripheral blood in chronic granulocytic leukaemia. Study of 50 untreated Philadelphia-positive cases. *Scand J Haematol* 1977;18:25–38.
45. Spiers AS. Clinical manifestations of chronic granulocytic leukemia. *Semin Oncol* 1995;22:380–395.
46. Savage DG, Szydlo RM, Goldman JM. Clinical features at diagnosis in 430 patients with chronic myeloid leukaemia seen at a referral centre over a 16-year period. *Br J Haematol* 1997;96:111–116.
47. Georgii A, Vykoupil KF, Buhr T, et al. Chronic myeloproliferative disorders in bone marrow biopsies. *Pathol Res Pract* 1990;186:3–27.
48. Brunning RD, McKenna RW. Tumours of the bone marrow. In: Brunning RD, McKenna RW, eds. *Atlas of Tumor Pathology*. Washington, DC: Armed Institute of Pathology; 1994.
49. Busche G, Majewski H, Schlue J, et al. Frequency of pseudo-Gaucher cells in diagnostic bone marrow biopsies from patients with Ph-positive chronic myeloid leukaemia. *Virch Arch* 1997;430:139–148.
50. Anastasi J, Musvee T, Roulston D, et al. Pseudo-Gaucher histiocytes identified up to 1 year after transplantation for CML are BCR/ABL-positive. *Leukemia* 1998; 12:233–237.
51. Okun DB, Tanaka KR. Leukocyte alkaline phosphatase. *Am J Hematol* 1978; 4:293–299.
52. Werner M, Ewig M, Nasarek A, et al. Value of fluorescence in situ hybridization for detecting the bcr/abl gene fusion in interphase cells of routine bone marrow specimens. *Diagn Mol Pathol* 1997;6:282–287.
53. Tanaka K, Arif M, Eguchi M, et al. Application of fluorescence in situ hybridization to detect residual leukemic cells with 9;22 and 15;17 translocations. *Leukemia* 1997;11:436–440.
54. Hagemeijer A, Bartram CR, Smit EM, et al. Is the chromosomal region 9q34 always involved in variants of the Ph1 translocation? *Cancer Genet Cytogenet* 1984;13:1–16.
55. Melo JV. The diversity of BCR-ABL fusion proteins and their relationship to leukemia phenotype. *Blood* 1996;88:2375–2384.
56. Lichty BD, Keating A, Callum J, et al. Expression of p210 and p190 BCR-ABL due to alternative splicing in chronic myelogenous leukaemia. *Br J Haematol* 1998;103:711–715.
57. Melo JV, Myint H, Galton DA, et al. P190BCR-ABL chronic myeloid leukaemia: the missing link with chronic myelomonocytic leukaemia? *Leukemia* 1994;8:208–211.
58. Yamagata T, Mitani K, Kanda Y, et al. Elevated platelet count features the variant type of BCR/ABL junction in chronic myelogenous leukaemia. *Br J Haematol* 1996;94:370–372.
59. Inokuchi K, Dan K, Takatori M, et al. Myeloproliferative disease in transgenic mice expressing P230 Bcr/Abl: longer disease latency, thrombocytosis, and mild leukocytosis. *Blood* 2003;102:320–323.
60. Pane F, Frigeri F, Sindona M, et al. Neutrophilic-chronic myeloid leukemia: a distinct disease with a specific molecular marker (BCR/ABL with C3/A2 junction). *Blood* 1996;88:2410–2414.
61. Druker BJ, Tamura S, Buchdunger E, et al. Effects of a selective inhibitor of the Abl tyrosine kinase on the growth of Bcr-Abl positive cells. *Nat Med* 1996;2:561–566.
62. Hasserjian RP, Boecklin F, Parker S, et al. ST1571 (imatinib mesylate) reduces bone marrow cellularity and normalizes morphologic features irrespective of cytogenetic response. *Am J Clin Pathol* 2002;117:360–367.
63. Frater JL, Tallman MS, Variakojis D, et al. Chronic myeloid leukemia following therapy with imatinib mesylate (Gleevec). Bone marrow histopathology and correlation with genetic status. *Am J Clin Pathol* 2003;119:833–841.
64. Mahon FX, Rea D, Guilhot J, et al. Discontinuation of imatinib in patients with chronic myeloid leukaemia who have maintained complete molecular remission for at least 2 years: the prospective, multicentre Stop Imatinib (STIM) trial. *Lancet Oncol* 2010;11:1029–1035.
65. Ross DM, Branford S, Seymour JF, et al. Patients with chronic myeloid leukemia who maintain a complete molecular response after stopping imatinib treatment have evidence of persistent leukemia by DNA PCR. *Leukemia* 2010;24:1719–1724.
66. Rousselot P, Huguet F, Rea D, et al. Imatinib mesylate discontinuation in patients with chronic myelogenous leukemia in complete molecular remission for more than 2 years. *Blood* 2007;109:58–60.
67. Hughes T, Deininger M, Hochhaus A, et al. Monitoring CML patients responding to treatment with tyrosine kinase inhibitors: review and recommendations for harmonizing current methodology for detecting BCR-ABL transcripts and kinase domain mutations and for expressing results. *Blood* 2006;108:28–37.
68. Gorre ME, Mohammed M, Ellwood K, et al. Clinical resistance to STI-571 cancer therapy caused by BCR-ABL gene mutation or amplification. *Science* 2001;293:876–880.
69. Irving JA, O'Brien S, Lennard AL, et al. Use of denaturing HPLC for detection of mutations in the BCR-ABL kinase domain in patients resistant to Imatinib. *Clin Chem* 2004;50:1233–1237.
70. Cortes J, Jabbour E, Kantarjian H, et al. Dynamics of BCR-ABL kinase domain mutations in chronic myeloid leukemia after sequential treatment with multiple tyrosine kinase inhibitors. *Blood* 2007;110:4005–4011.
71. Walz C, Sattler M. Novel targeted therapies to overcome imatinib mesylate resistance in chronic myeloid leukemia (CML). *Crit Rev Oncol Hematol* 2006;57:145–164.
72. Hochhauss A. Therapy of newly diagnosed CML. In: Faderl S, Kantarjian H, eds. *Leukemia, Principles and Practice of Therapy.* West Sussex, UK: Wiley-Blackwell; 2010:273.
73. Cortes JE, Kantarjian H, Shah NP, et al. Ponatinib in refractory Philadelphia chromosome-positive leukemias. *N Engl J Med* 2012;367:2075–2088.
74. Bumm T, Muller C, Al-Ali HK, et al. Emergence of clonal cytogenetic abnormalities in Ph- cells in some CML patients in cytogenetic remission to imatinib but restoration of polyclonal hematopoiesis in the majority. *Blood* 2003;101:1941–1949.
75. Loriaux M, Deininger M. Clonal cytogenetic abnormalities in Philadelphia chromosome negative cells in chronic myeloid leukemia patients treated with imatinib. *Leuk Lymphoma* 2004;45:2197–2203.
76. Raskind WH, Tirumali N, Jacobson R, et al. Evidence for a multistep pathogenesis of a myelodysplastic syndrome. *Blood* 1984;63:1318–1323.
77. Druker BJ, Guilhot F, O'Brien SG, et al. Five-year follow-up of patients receiving imatinib for chronic myeloid leukemia. *N Engl J Med* 2006;355:2408–2417.
78. Vardiman J, Melo JV, Baccarani M, et al. Chronic myelogenous leukemia. In: Swerdlow SH, Campo E, Harris NL, et al., eds. *WHO Classification of Tumours of Haematopoietic and Lymphoid Tissues*. Lyon, France: IARC Press; 2008.
79. Mitelman F. The cytogenetic scenario of chronic myeloid leukemia. *Leuk Lymphoma* 1993;11(Suppl 1):11–15.
80. Hernandez JM, Gonzalez-Sarmiento R, Martin C, et al. Immunophenotypic, genomic and clinical characteristics of blast crisis of chronic myelogenous leukaemia. *Br J Haematol* 1991;79:408–414.
81. Griesshammer M, Heinze B, Hellmann A, et al. Chronic myelogenous leukemia in blast crisis: retrospective analysis of prognostic factors in 90 patients. *Ann Hematol* 1996;73:225–230.
82. Saglio G, Hochhaus A, Goh YT, et al. Dasatinib in imatinib-resistant or imatinib-intolerant chronic myeloid leukemia in blast phase after 2 years of follow-up in a phase 3 study: efficacy and tolerability of 140 milligrams once daily and 70 milligrams twice daily. *Cancer* 2010;116:3852–3861.
83. Swolin B, Weinfeld A, Westin J, et al. Karyotypic evolution in Ph-positive chronic myeloid leukemia in relation to management and disease progression. *Cancer Genet Cytogenet* 1985;18:65–79.
84. Parreira L, Kearney L, Rassool F, et al. Correlation between chromosomal abnormalities and blast phenotype in the blast crisis of Ph-positive CGL. *Cancer Genet Cytogenet* 1986;22:29–34.
85. Derderian PM, Kantarjian HM, Talpaz M, et al. Chronic myelogenous leukemia in the lymphoid blastic phase: characteristics, treatment response, and prognosis. *Am J Med* 1993;94:69–74.
86. Cervantes F, Villamor N, Esteve J, et al. "Lymphoid" blast crisis of chronic myeloid leukaemia is associated with distinct clinicohaematological features. *Br J Haematol* 1998;100:123–128.
87. Ishikura H, Yufu Y, Yamashita S, et al. Biphenotypic blast crisis of chronic myelogenous leukemia: abnormalities of p53 and retinoblastoma genes. *Leuk Lymphoma* 1997;25:573–578.
88. Akashi K, Mizuno S, Harada M, et al. T lymphoid/myeloid bilineal crisis in chronic myelogenous leukemia. *Exp Hematol* 1993;21:743–748.
89. Specchia G, Palumbo G, Pastore D, et al. Extramedullary blast crisis in chronic myeloid leukemia. *Leuk Res* 1996;20:905–908.
90. Schmid C, Frisch B, Beham A, et al. Comparison of bone marrow histology in early chronic granulocytic leukemia and in leukemoid reaction. *Eur J Haematol* 1990;44:154–158.
91. Bennett JM, Catovsky D, Daniel MT, et al. The chronic myeloid leukaemias: guidelines for distinguishing chronic granulocytic, atypical chronic myeloid, and chronic myelomonocytic leukaemia. Proposals by the French-American-British Cooperative Leukaemia Group. *Br J Haematol* 1994;87:746–754.
92. Hernandez JM, del Canizo MC, Cuneo A, et al. Clinical, hematological and cytogenetic characteristics of atypical chronic myeloid leukemia. *Ann Oncol* 2000;11:441–444.
93. Oscier DG. Atypical chronic myeloid leukaemia, a distinct clinical entity related to the myelodysplastic syndrome? *Br J Haematol* 1996;92:582–586.
94. You W, Weisbrot IM. Chronic neutrophilic leukemia. Report of two cases and review of the literature. *Am J Clin Pathol* 1979;72:233–242.
95. Reilly JT. Chronic neutrophilic leukaemia: a distinct clinical entity? *Br J Haematol* 2002;116:10–18.

96. Bohm J, Schaefer HE. Chronic neutrophilic leukaemia: 14 new cases of an uncommon myeloproliferative disease. *J Clin Pathol* 2002;55:862–864.
97. Bohm J, Kock S, Schaefer HE, et al. Evidence of clonality in chronic neutrophilic leukaemia. *J Clin Pathol* 2003;56:292–295.
98. Elliott MA. Chronic neutrophilic leukemia: a contemporary review. *Curr Hematol Rep* 2004;3:210–217.
99. Standen GR, Steers FJ, Jones L. Clonality of chronic neutrophilic leukaemia associated with myeloma: analysis using the X-linked probe M27 beta. *J Clin Pathol* 1993;46:297–298.
100. Klco JM, Vij R, Kreisel FH, et al. Molecular pathology of myeloproliferative neoplasms. *Am J Clin Pathol* 2010;133:602–615.
101. Anastasi J, Feng J, Dickstein JI, et al. Lineage involvement by BCR/ABL in Ph+ lymphoblastic leukemias: chronic myelogenous leukemia presenting in lymphoid blast vs Ph+ acute lymphoblastic leukemia. *Leukemia* 1996;10:795–802.
102. Kurzrock R, Shtalrid M, Talpaz M, et al. Expression of c-abl in Philadelphia-positive acute myelogenous leukemia. *Blood* 1987;70:1584–1588.
103. Paietta E, Racevskis J, Bennett JM, et al. Biologic heterogeneity in Philadelphia chromosome-positive acute leukemia with myeloid morphology: the Eastern Cooperative Oncology Group experience. *Leukemia* 1998;12:1881–1885.
104. Soupir CP, Vergilio JA, Dal Cin P, et al. Philadelphia chromosome-positive acute myeloid leukemia: a rare aggressive leukemia with clinicopathologic features distinct from chronic myeloid leukemia in myeloid blast crisis. *Am J Clin Pathol* 2007;127:642–650.
105. Nacheva EP, Grace CD, Brazma D, et al. Does BCR/ABL1 positive acute myeloid leukaemia exist? *Br J Haematol* 2013;161:541–550.
106. Konoplev S, Yin CC, Kornblau SM, et al. Molecular characterization of de novo Philadelphia chromosome-positive acute myeloid leukemia. *Leuk Lymphoma* 2013;54:138–144.
107. Bain BJ. Eosinophilia and chronic eosinophilia leukemia, including myeloid/lymphoid neoplasms with eosinophilia and abnormalities of PDGFRA, PDGFRB and FGFR1. In: Jaffe ES, Harris NL, Vardiman JW, et al., eds. *Hematopathology*. Philadelphia, PA: Saunders/Elsevier; 2011.
108. Gotlib J. World Health Organization-defined eosinophilic disorders: 2012 update on diagnosis, risk stratification, and management. *Am J Hematol* 2012;87:903–914.
109. Klion AD. Eosinophilic myeloproliferative disorders. *Hematol Am Soc Hematol Educ Program* 2011;2011:257–263.
110. Tefferi A, Gotlib J, Pardanani A. Hypereosinophilic syndrome and clonal eosinophilia: point-of-care diagnostic algorithm and treatment update. *Mayo Clin Proc* 2010;85:158–164.
111. Metzgeroth G, Walz C, Score J, et al. Recurrent finding of the FIP1L1-PDGFRA fusion gene in eosinophilia-associated acute myeloid leukemia and lymphoblastic T-cell lymphoma. *Leukemia* 2007;21:1183–1188.
112. Golub TR, Barker GF, Lovett M, et al. Fusion of PDGF receptor beta to a novel ets-like gene, tel, in chronic myelomonocytic leukemia with t(5;12) chromosomal translocation. *Cell* 1994;77:307–316.
113. Cools J, DeAngelo DJ, Gotlib J, et al. A tyrosine kinase created by fusion of the PDGFRA and FIP1L1 genes as a therapeutic target of imatinib in idiopathic hypereosinophilic syndrome. *N Engl J Med* 2003;348:1201–1214.
114. Macdonald D, Reiter A, Cross NC. The 8p11 myeloproliferative syndrome: a distinct clinical entity caused by constitutive activation of FGFR1. *Acta Haematol* 2002;107:101–107.
115. Bain BJ, Gilliland DG, Horny HP, et al. Myeloid and lymphoid neoplasms with eosinophilia and abnormalities of PDGFRA, PDGFRB or FGFR1. In: Swerdlow SH, Campo E, Harris NL, et al., eds. *World Health Organization (WHO) Classification of Tumours of the Haematopoietic and Lymphoid Tissues*. Lyon, France: IARC Press; 2008:68–73.
116. Apperley JF, Gardembas M, Melo JV, et al. Response to imatinib mesylate in patients with chronic myeloproliferative diseases with rearrangements of the platelet-derived growth factor receptor beta. *N Engl J Med* 2002;347:481–487.
117. Pardanani A, Reeder T, Porrata LF, et al. Imatinib therapy for hypereosinophilic syndrome and other eosinophilic disorders. *Blood* 2003;101:3391–3397.
118. Elling C, Erben P, Walz C, et al. Novel imatinib-sensitive PDGFRA-activating point mutations in hypereosinophilic syndrome induce growth factor independence and leukemia-like disease. *Blood* 2011;117:2935–2943.
119. Pardanani A, Ketterling RP, Brockman SR, et al. CHIC2 deletion, a surrogate for FIP1L1-PDGFRA fusion, occurs in systemic mastocytosis associated with eosinophilia and predicts response to imatinib mesylate therapy. *Blood* 2003;102: 3093–3096.
120. Gotlib J. Eosinophilic myeloid disorders: new classification and novel therapeutic strategies. *Curr Opin Hematol* 2010;17:117–124.
121. Rudzki Z, Giles L, Cross NC, et al. Myeloid neoplasm with rearrangement of PDGFRA, but with no significant eosinophilia: should we broaden the World Health Organization definition of the entity? *Br J Haematol* 2012;156:558.
122. Abruzzo LV, Jaffe ES, Cotelingam JD, et al. T-cell lymphoblastic lymphoma with eosinophilia associated with subsequent myeloid malignancy. *Am J Surg Pathol* 1992;16:236–245.
123. Bain BJ, Gilliland DG, Vardiman JW, et al. Chronic eosinophilic leukaemia, not otherwise specified. In: Swerdlow SH, Campo E, Harris NL, et al., eds. *WHO Classification of Tumours of Haematopoietic and Lymphoid Tissues*. Lyon, France: IARC Press; 2008.
124. James C, Ugo V, Le Couedic JP, et al. A unique clonal JAK2 mutation leading to constitutive signalling causes polycythaemia vera. *Nature* 2005;434:1144–1148.
125. Baxter EJ, Scott LM, Campbell PJ, et al. Acquired mutation of the tyrosine kinase JAK2 in human myeloproliferative disorders. *Lancet* 2005;365:1054–1061.
126. Kralovics R, Passamonti F, Buser AS, et al. A gain-of-function mutation of JAK2 in myeloproliferative disorders. *N Engl J Med* 2005;352:1779–1790.
127. Levine RL, Wadleigh M, Cools J, et al. Activating mutation in the tyrosine kinase JAK2 in polycythemia vera, essential thrombocythemia, and myeloid metaplasia with myelofibrosis. *Cancer Cell* 2005;7:387–397.
128. Parganas E, Wang D, Stravopodis D, et al. Jak2 is essential for signaling through a variety of cytokine receptors. *Cell* 1998;93:385–395.
129. Lu X, Levine R, Tong W, et al. Expression of a homodimeric type I cytokine receptor is required for JAK2V617F-mediated transformation. *Proc Natl Acad Sci U S A* 2005;102:18962–18967.
130. Zhao R, Xing S, Li Z, et al. Identification of an acquired JAK2 mutation in polycythemia vera. *J Biol Chem* 2005;280:22788–22792.
131. Saharinen P, Takaluoma K, Silvennoinen O. Regulation of the Jak2 tyrosine kinase by its pseudokinase domain. *Mol Cell Biol* 2000;20:3387–3395.
132. Hookham MB, Elliott J, Suessmuth Y, et al. The myeloproliferative disorder-associated JAK2 V617F mutant escapes negative regulation by suppressor of cytokine signaling 3. *Blood* 2007;109:4924–4929.
133. Shi S, Larson K, Guo D, et al. Drosophila STAT is required for directly maintaining HP1 localization and heterochromatin stability. *Nat Cell Biol* 2008;10:489–496.
134. Scott LM, Tong W, Levine RL, et al. JAK2 exon 12 mutations in polycythemia vera and idiopathic erythrocytosis. *N Engl J Med* 2007;356:459–468.
135. Lasho TL, Pardanani A, Tefferi A. LNK mutations in JAK2 mutation-negative erythrocytosis. *N Engl J Med* 2010;363:1189–1190.
136. Pardanani AD, Levine RL, Lasho T, et al. MPL515 mutations in myeloproliferative and other myeloid disorders: a study of 1182 patients. *Blood* 2006;108:3472–3476.
137. Vannucchi AM, Antonioli E, Guglielmelli P, et al. Characteristics and clinical correlates of MPL 515W>L/K mutation in essential thrombocythemia. *Blood* 2008;112:844–847.
138. Ishii T, Bruno E, Hoffman R, et al. Involvement of various hematopoietic-cell lineages by the JAK2V617F mutation in polycythemia vera. *Blood* 2006;108:3128–3134.
139. Delhommeau F, Dupont S, Tonetti C, et al. Evidence that the JAK2 G1849T (V617F) mutation occurs in a lymphomyeloid progenitor in polycythemia vera and idiopathic myelofibrosis. *Blood* 2007;109:71–77.
140. Teofili L, Martini M, Iachininoto MG, et al. Endothelial progenitor cells are clonal and exhibit the JAK2(V617F) mutation in a subset of thrombotic patients with Ph-negative myeloproliferative neoplasms. *Blood* 2011;117:2700–2707.
141. Campbell PJ, Baxter EJ, Beer PA, et al. Mutation of JAK2 in the myeloproliferative disorders: timing, clonality studies, cytogenetic associations, and role in leukemic transformation. *Blood* 2006;108:3548–3555.
142. Soriano G, Heaney M. Polycythemia vera and essential thrombocythemia: new developments in biology with therapeutic implications. *Curr Opin Hematol* 2013;20:169–175.
143. Scott LM, Scott MA, Campbell PJ, et al. Progenitors homozygous for the V617F mutation occur in most patients with polycythemia vera, but not essential thrombocythemia. *Blood* 2006;108:2435–2437.
144. Tiedt R, Hao-Shen H, Sobas MA, et al. Ratio of mutant JAK2-V617F to wild-type Jak2 determines the MPD phenotypes in transgenic mice. *Blood* 2008;111:3931–3940.
145. Skov V, Thomassen M, Riley CH, et al. Gene expression profiling with principal component analysis depicts the biological continuum from essential thrombocythemia over polycythemia vera to myelofibrosis. *Exp Hematol* 2012;40:771–780.
146. Grand FH, Hidalgo-Curtis CE, Ernst T, et al. Frequent CBL mutations associated with 11q acquired uniparental disomy in myeloproliferative neoplasms. *Blood* 2009;113:6182–6192.
147. Rice KL, Lin X, Wolniak K, et al. Analysis of genomic aberrations and gene expression profiling identifies novel lesions and pathways in myeloproliferative neoplasms. *Blood Cancer J* 2011;1:e40.
148. Zhan H, Cardozo C, Yu W, et al. MicroRNA deregulation in polycythemia vera and essential thrombocythemia patients. *Blood Cells Mol Dis* 2013;50:190–195.
149. Jones AV, Kreil S, Zoi K, et al. Widespread occurrence of the JAK2 V617F mutation in chronic myeloproliferative disorders. *Blood* 2005;106:2162–2168.
150. Tefferi A, Skoda R, Vardiman JW. Myeloproliferative neoplasms: contemporary diagnosis using histology and genetics. *Nat Rev Clin Oncol* 2009;6:627–637.
151. Vakil E, Tefferi A. BCR-ABL1—negative myeloproliferative neoplasms: a review of molecular biology, diagnosis, and treatment. *Clin Lymphoma Myeloma Leuk* 2011;11(Suppl 1):S37–S45.
152. Hollowell JG, van Assendelft OW, Gunter EW, et al. Hematological and iron-related analytes—reference data for persons aged 1 year and over: United States, 1988–1994. *Vital Health Stat* 2005:1–156.
153. Thiele J, Orazi A, Tefferi A, et al. Polycythemia vera. In: Swerdlow SH, Campo E, Harris NL, et al., eds. *WHO Classification of Haematopoietic and Lymphoid Tissue*. 4th ed. Lyon, France: IARC; 2008.
154. Patnaik MM, Tefferi A. The complete evaluation of erythrocytosis: congenital and acquired. *Leukemia* 2009;23:834–844.
155. Kremyanskaya M, Mascarenhas J, Hoffman R. Why does my patient have erythrocytosis? *Hematol Oncol Clin North Am* 2012;26:267–283, vii–viii.
156. Ivan M, Kondo K, Yang H, et al. HIFalpha targeted for VHL-mediated destruction by proline hydroxylation: implications for O_2 sensing. *Science* 2001;292: 464–468.
157. Schofield CJ, Ratcliffe PJ. Oxygen sensing by HIF hydroxylases. *Nat Rev Mol Cell Biol* 2004;5:343–354.
158. Lee FS, Percy MJ. The HIF pathway and erythrocytosis. *Annu Rev Pathol* 2011;6:165–192.
159. Constantinescu SN, Ghaffari S, Lodish HF. The erythropoietin receptor: structure, activation and intracellular signal transduction. *Trends Endocrinol Metab* 1999;10:18–23.
160. Passamonti F, Malabarba L, Orlandi E, et al. Polycythemia vera in young patients: a study on the long-term risk of thrombosis, myelofibrosis and leukemia. *Haematologica* 2003;88:13–18.
161. Cario H, Pahl HL, Schwarz K, et al. Familial polycythemia vera with Budd-Chiari syndrome in childhood. *Br J Haematol* 2003;123:346–352.
162. Primignani M, Barosi G, Bergamaschi G, et al. Role of the JAK2 mutation in the diagnosis of chronic myeloproliferative disorders in splanchnic vein thrombosis. *Hepatology* 2006;44:1528–1534.
163. Vannucchi AM, Guglielmelli P. Advances in understanding and management of polycythemia vera. *Curr Opin Oncol* 2010;22:636–641.
164. Tefferi A, Vainchenker W. Myeloproliferative neoplasms: molecular pathophysiology, essential clinical understanding, and treatment strategies. *J Clin Oncol* 2011;29:573–582.
165. Passamonti F, Rumi E, Pungolino E, et al. Life expectancy and prognostic factors for survival in patients with polycythemia vera and essential thrombocythemia. *Am J Med* 2004;117:755–761.
166. Finazzi G, Barbui T. Evidence and expertise in the management of polycythemia vera and essential thrombocythemia. *Leukemia* 2008;22:1494–1502.
167. McMahon B, Stein BL. Thrombotic and bleeding complications in classical myeloproliferative neoplasms. *Semin Thromb Hemost* 2013;39:101–111.
168. Bilgrami S, Greenberg BR. Polycythemia rubra vera. *Semin Oncol* 1995;22:307–326.
169. Gianelli U, Iurlo A, Vener C, et al. The significance of bone marrow biopsy and JAK2V617F mutation in the differential diagnosis between the "early" prepolycythemic phase of polycythemia vera and essential thrombocythemia. *Am J Clin Pathol* 2008;130:336–342.
170. Kvasnicka HM, Thiele J. Prodromal myeloproliferative neoplasms: the 2008 WHO classification. *Am J Hematol* 2010;85:62–69.

171. McMullin MF, Bareford D, Campbell P, et al. Guidelines for the diagnosis, investigation and management of polycythaemia/erythrocytosis. *Br J Haematol* 2005;130:174–195.

172. Ellis JT, Peterson P, Geller SA, et al. Studies of the bone marrow in polycythemia vera and the evolution of myelofibrosis and second hematologic malignancies. *Semin Hematol* 1986;23:144–155.

173. Thiele J, Kvasnicka HM, Vardiman J. Bone marrow histopathology in the diagnosis of chronic myeloproliferative disorders: a forgotten pearl. *Best Pract Res Clin Haematol* 2006;19:413–437.

174. Barbui T, Thiele J, Passamonti F, et al. Initial bone marrow reticulin fibrosis in polycythemia vera exerts an impact on clinical outcome. *Blood* 2012;119:2239–2241.

175. Percy MJ, Scott LM, Erber WN, et al. The frequency of JAK2 exon 12 mutations in idiopathic erythrocytosis patients with low serum erythropoietin levels. *Haematologica* 2007;92:1607–1614.

176. Wolf BC, Banks PM, Mann RB, et al. Splenic hematopoiesis in polycythaemia vera. A morphologic and immunohistologic study. *Am J Clin Pathol* 1988;89:69–75.

177. Andrieux JL, Demory JL. Karyotype and molecular cytogenetic studies in polycythemia vera. *Curr Hematol Rep* 2005;4:224–229.

178. Gangat N, Strand J, Lasho TL, et al. Cytogenetic studies at diagnosis in polycythemia vera: clinical and JAK2V617F allele burden correlates. *Eur J Haematol* 2008;80:197–200.

179. Tefferi A, Vardiman JW. Classification and diagnosis of myeloproliferative neoplasms: the 2008 World Health Organization criteria and point-of-care diagnostic algorithms. *Leukemia* 2008;22:14–22.

180. Spivak JL. Polycythemia vera: myths, mechanisms, and management. *Blood* 2002;100:4272–4290.

181. Lutton JD, Levere RD. Endogenous erythroid colony formation by peripheral blood mononuclear cells from patients with myelofibrosis and polycythaemia vera. *Acta Haematol* 1979;62:94–99.

182. Elliott MA, Tefferi A. Thrombosis and haemorrhage in polycythaemia vera and essential thrombocythaemia. *Br J Haematol* 2005;128(3):275–290.

183. Harrison CN. Platelets and thrombosis in myeloproliferative diseases. *Hematol Am Soc Hematol Educ Program* 2005:409–415.

184. Barbui T, Carobbio A, Rambaldi A, et al. Perspectives on thrombosis in essential thrombocythemia and polycythemia vera: is leukocytosis a causative factor? *Blood* 2009;114:759–763.

185. Hultcrantz M, Kristinsson SY, Andersson TM, et al. Patterns of survival among patients with myeloproliferative neoplasms diagnosed in sweden from 1973 to 2008: a population-based study. *J Clin Oncol* 2012;30:2995–3001.

186. Guglielmelli P, Vannucchi AM. Recent advances in diagnosis and treatment of chronic myeloproliferative neoplasms. *F1000 Med Rep* 2010;2:pii.

187. Cervantes F, Passamonti F, Barosi G. Life expectancy and prognostic factors in the classic BCR/ABL-negative myeloproliferative disorders. *Leukemia* 2008;22:905–914.

188. Passamonti F, Rumi E, Pietra D, et al. A prospective study of 338 patients with polycythemia vera: the impact of JAK2 (V617F) allele burden and leukocytosis on fibrotic or leukemic disease transformation and vascular complications. *Leukemia* 2010;24:1574–1579.

189. Najean Y, Dresch C, Rain JD. The very-long-term course of polycythaemia: a complement to the previously published data of the Polycythaemia Vera Study Group. *Br J Haematol* 1994;86:233–235.

190. Finazzi G, Caruso V, Marchioli R, et al. Acute leukemia in polycythemia vera: an analysis of 1638 patients enrolled in a prospective observational study. *Blood* 2005;105(7):2664–2670.

191. Boiocchi L, Gianelli U. Morphologic and cytogenetic differences between post-polycythemic myelofibrosis and primary myelofibrosis in fibrotic stage. *Mod Pathol* 2013;In press.

192. Passamonti F, Rumi E, Arcaini L, et al. Leukemic transformation of polycythemia vera: a single center study of 23 patients. *Cancer* 2005;104:1032–1036.

193. Theocharides A, Boissinot M, Girodon F, et al. Leukemic blasts in transformed JAK2-V617F-positive myeloproliferative disorders are frequently negative for the JAK2-V617F mutation. *Blood* 2007;110:375–379.

194. Gordeuk VR, Stockton DW, Prchal JT. Congenital polycythemias/erythrocytoses. *Haematologica* 2005;90:109–116.

195. McMullin MF. The classification and diagnosis of erythrocytosis. *Int J Lab Hematol* 2008;30:447–459.

196. Kiberd BA. Post-transplant erythrocytosis: a disappearing phenomenon? *Clin Transpl* 2009;23:800–806.

197. Rosa R, Prehu MO, Beuzard Y, et al. The first case of a complete deficiency of diphosphoglycerate mutase in human erythrocytes. *J Clin Invest* 1978;62:907–915.

198. Ang SO, Chen H, Gordeuk VR, et al. Endemic polycythemia in Russia: mutation in the VHL gene. *Blood Cells Mol Dis* 2002;28:57–62.

199. Milosevic JD, Kralovics R. Genetic and epigenetic alterations of myeloproliferative disorders. *Int J Hematol* 2013;97:183–197.

200. Thiele J, Kvasnicka HM, Boeltken B, et al. Initial (prefibrotic) stages of idiopathic (primary) myelofibrosis (IMF)—a clinicopathological study. *Leukemia* 1999;13:1741–1748.

201. Thiele J, Tefferi A, Barosi G, et al. Primary myelofibrosis. In: Swerdlow SH, Campo E, Harris NL, et al., eds. *WHO Classification of Tumours of the Hematopoietic and Lymphoid Tissues.* 4th ed. Lyon, France: IARC; 2008.

202. Barbui T, Thiele J, Passamonti F, et al. Survival and disease progression in essential thrombocythemia are significantly influenced by accurate morphologic diagnosis: an international study. *J Clin Oncol* 2011;29:3179–3184.

203. Pardanani A, Lasho TL, Finke C, et al. Extending Jak2V617F and MplW515 mutation analysis to single hematopoietic colonies and B and T lymphocytes. *Stem Cells* 2007;25:2358–2362.

204. Tefferi A. Primary myelofibrosis: 2013 update on diagnosis, risk-stratification, and management. *Am J Hematol* 2013;88:141–150.

205. Mesa RA, Hanson CA, Rajkumar SV, et al. Evaluation and clinical correlations of bone marrow angiogenesis in myelofibrosis with myeloid metaplasia. *Blood* 2000;96:3374–3380.

206. Ho CL, Arora B, Hoyer JD, et al. Bone marrow expression of vascular endothelial growth factor in myelofibrosis with myeloid metaplasia. *Eur J Hematol* 2005;74:35–39.

207. Ho CL, Lasho TL, Butterfield JH, et al. Global cytokine analysis in myeloproliferative disorders. *Leuk Res* 2007;31:1389–1392.

208. Boxer LA, Camitta BM, Berenberg W, et al. Myelofibrosis-myeloid metaplasia in childhood. *Pediatrics* 1975;55:861–865.

209. Elliott MA, Verstovsek S, Dingli D, et al. Monocytosis is an adverse prognostic factor for survival in younger patients with primary myelofibrosis. *Leuk Res* 2007;31:1503–1509.

210. Boiocchi L, Espinal-Witter R, Geyer JT, et al. Development of monocytosis in patients with primary myelofibrosis indicates an accelerated phase of the disease. *Mod Pathol* 2013;26:204–212.

211. Thiele J, Kvasnicka HM, Facchetti F, et al. European consensus on grading bone marrow fibrosis and assessment of cellularity. *Haematologica* 2005;90:1128–1132.

212. Buhr T, Hebeda K, Kaloutsi V, et al. European Bone Marrow Working Group trial on reproducibility of World Health Organization criteria to discriminate essential thrombocythemia from prefibrotic primary myelofibrosis. *Haematologica* 2012;97:360–365.

213. Thiele J, Orazi A, Kvasnicka HM, et al. European Bone Marrow Working Group trial on reproducibility of World Health Organization criteria to discriminate essential thrombocythemia from prefibrotic primary myelofibrosis. *Haematologica* 2012;97(3):360–365—comment. *Haematologica* 2012;97:e5–e6; discussion e7–e8.

214. Hussein K, Huang J, Lasho T, et al. Karyotype complements the International Prognostic Scoring System for primary myelofibrosis. *Eur J Hematol* 2009;82:255–259.

215. Vaidya R, Caramazza D, Begna KH, et al. Monosomal karyotype in primary myelofibrosis is detrimental to both overall and leukemia-free survival. *Blood* 2011;117:5612–5615.

216. Boveri E, Passamonti F, Rumi E, et al. Bone marrow microvessel density in chronic myeloproliferative disorders: a study of 115 patients with clinicopathological and molecular correlations. *Br J Haematol* 2008;140:162–168.

217. Cervantes F, Pereira A, Marti JM, et al. Bone marrow lymphoid nodules in myeloproliferative disorders: association with the nonmyelosclerotic phases of idiopathic myelofibrosis and immunological significance. *Br J Haematol* 1988;70:279–282.

218. Gangat N, Caramazza D, Vaidya R, et al. DIPSS plus: a refined Dynamic International Prognostic Scoring System for primary myelofibrosis that incorporates prognostic information from karyotype, platelet count, and transfusion status. *J Clin Oncol* 2011;29:392–397.

219. Buss DH, O'Connor ML, Woodruff RD, et al. Bone marrow and peripheral blood findings in patients with extreme thrombocytosis. A report of 63 cases. *Arch Pathol Lab Med* 1991;115:475–480.

220. Kaushansky K. Historical review: megakaryopoiesis and thrombopoiesis. *Blood* 2008;111:981–986.

221. Deutsch VR, Tomer A. Megakaryocyte development and platelet production. *Br J Haematol* 2006;134:453–466.

222. Anastasi J. Some observations on the geometry of megakaryocyte mitotic figures: buckyballs in the bone marrow. *Blood* 2011;118:6473–6474.

223. Thiele J, Kvasnicka HM. Chronic myeloproliferative disorders with thrombocythemia: a comparative study of two classification systems (PVSG, WHO) on 839 patients. *Ann Hematol* 2003;82:148–152.

224. Kvasnicka HM, Thiele J. The impact of clinicopathological studies on staging and survival in essential thrombocythemia, chronic idiopathic myelofibrosis, and polycythemia rubra vera. *Semin Thromb Hemost* 2006;32:362–371.

225. Jensen MK, de Nully Brown P, Nielsen OJ, et al. Incidence, clinical features and outcome of essential thrombocythaemia in a well defined geographical area. *Eur J Hematol* 2000;65:132–139.

226. McIntyre KJ, Hoagland HC, Silverstein MN, et al. Essential thrombocythemia in young adults. *Mayo Clin Proc* 1991;66:149–154.

227. Barbui T, Finazzi G, Carobbio A, et al. Development and validation of an International Prognostic Score of thrombosis in World Health Organization-essential thrombocythemia (IPSET-thrombosis). *Blood* 2012;120:5128–5133; quiz 252.

228. Thiele J, Orazi A, Tefferi A, et al. Essential thrombocythaemia. In: Swerdlow SH, Campo E, Harris NL, et al., eds. *WHO Classification of Tumours of Haematopoietic and Lymphoid Tissues.* 4th ed. Lyon, France: IARC; 2008.

229. Brecqueville M, Rey J, Bertucci F, et al. Mutation analysis of ASXL1, CBL, DNMT3A, IDH1, IDH2, JAK2, MPL, NF1, SF3B1, SUZ12, and TET2 in myeloproliferative neoplasms. *Genes Chromosomes Cancer* 2012;51:743–755.

230. Shetty S, Kasatkar P, Ghosh K. Pathophysiology of acquired von Willebrand disease: a concise review. *Eur J Hematol* 2011;87:99–106.

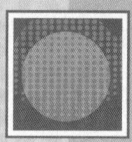

Chapter 45
Myelodysplastic/Myeloproliferative Neoplasms and Related Diseases

Magdalena Czader • Attilio Orazi

Myelodysplastic syndrome/myeloproliferative neoplasms (MDS/MPNs) are clonal hematopoietic malignancies with hybrid myelodysplastic and myeloproliferative features simultaneously present at the time of disease outset. The diagnosis is usually suspected in patients displaying the overlapping hematologic characteristics, which would make it difficult to assign a case to a myelodysplastic or myeloproliferative category. In patients with MDS/MPNs, cytopenia(s) and dysplasia may coexist with elevated white blood cell counts, thrombocytosis, and/or organomegaly. Even though disorders with mixed myelodysplastic and myeloproliferative features have been recognized for many years, the precise diagnosis and assignment to clearly defined categories has been challenging. During the 1970s, Sultan et al. (1) introduced the term myelodysplastic syndrome (MDS) with subtypes of refractory anemia (RA), RA with ring sideroblasts (RARS), and refractory anemia with excess blasts (RAEB). Cases with myelodysplasia and concurrent absolute monocytosis were termed chronic myelomonocytic leukemia (CMML). The terminology was largely retained in the subsequent major classification schemes (i.e., FAB and partially in WHO). In 1976, the French-American-British (FAB) cooperative group introduced a uniform system of classification and nomenclature of the acute myeloid and lymphoid leukemias (2). To avoid confusion of MDS with acute myeloid leukemia (AML), the diagnostic criteria of two types of MDS, RAEB and CMML, were presented as an addendum. In 1982, the FAB cooperative group introduced a uniform classification and nomenclature of the MDSs based on the consensus among expert hematologists reached after review of clinical features and morphology of selected cases (3). Diagnostic morphologic criteria for dyserythropoiesis, dysgranulopoiesis, and dysmegakaryopoiesis were proposed, and numerical criteria for five types of MDS (RA, RARS, RAEB, CMML, and RAEB in transformation) were described. In addition, a clear definition of sideroblastic anemia with its characteristic accumulation of mitochondrial iron in erythroblasts was presented. The third edition of the World Health Organization (WHO) classification published in 2001 emphasized the integration of cytogenetics with FAB-defined morphologic features in its diagnostic approach to MDS (4). The FAB category of RAEB in transformation (20% to 29% blasts) was eliminated due to the lower cutoff established for most AML subtypes (blasts ≥20% in 2001 WHO classification instead of the cutoff of ≥30% proposed by the FAB group in 1985). Due to the recognition of its hybrid features, CMML was moved to a new category of myeloid diseases termed MDS/MPNs. In addition to CMML, this new group included atypical chronic myeloid leukemia, juvenile myelomonocytic leukemia (JMML), and MDS/MPN, unclassifiable. All subtypes of MDS/MPNs are genetically heterogeneous and show highly variable outcomes. They are challenging to diagnose using traditional morphology-based approaches; thus an integration of morphologic features with laboratory data, clinical presentation, immunophenotype, and cytogenetic/molecular tests is required to categorize MDS/MPNs according to current WHO classification. It is critical to diagnose

patients at the time of original presentation, that is, before bone marrow (BM) and peripheral blood (PB) features are modified by therapy or progression of the disease. If a patient has been previously diagnosed elsewhere, a complete review of the original diagnostic material is usually necessary. "Reclassification" based on the review of posttreatment and/or follow-up BM samples is strongly discouraged.

Three MDS/MPN entities can be reliably classified using the above-described integrated approach: CMML, atypical chronic myeloid leukemia (aCML), *BCR-ABL1* negative, and JMML. When a myeloid neoplasm with myelodysplastic and myeloproliferative features cannot be assigned to any of these three categories, it should be diagnosed as MDS/MPN, unclassifiable (5). This unclassifiable group includes also the provisional entity known as RARS associated with marked thrombocytosis (RARS-T). Additional rare entities with hybrid myelodysplastic and myeloproliferative features emerged in recent years and may qualify for inclusion into WHO classification in the future. One such entity known as myeloid neoplasm with an isolated isochromosome 17q abnormality is a rapidly progressive disease that may occasionally morphologically resemble CMML or aCML.

The etiology of MDS/MPN is largely unknown. The pathophysiology involves abnormalities in the regulation of myeloid pathways of cellular proliferation, maturation, and survival. Using metaphase cytogenetics, chromosomal abnormalities are found only in a proportion of patients with MDS/MPN and are similar to those encountered in patients with MDS (see Chapter 43). Molecular genetic studies and high-throughput technologies allowed us to identify a variety of genetic and epigenetic changes in MDS/MPN, a proportion of which may become therapeutic targets. The introduction of next-generation sequencing expedites testing of gene mutations, which would allow a hematologist to target therapy to a specific genetic profile. Such an individualized approach is urgently needed since current treatment is often limited to a combination of cytoreductive therapy and interventions to ameliorate cytopenias.

In the following paragraphs, we discuss diagnostic approaches to individual MDS/MPNs entities and present their laboratory and clinical characteristics. The cytogenetic and genetic features are also addressed in Chapter 9.

CHRONIC MYELOMONOCYTIC LEUKEMIA

Definition

CMML is a hybrid myeloproliferative and myelodysplastic neoplasm characterized by persistent unexplained monocytosis ($>1 \times 10^9$/L with >10% monocytes on the differential count) and dysplasia in one or more myeloid lineages. In cases without prominent dysplastic features, the diagnosis of CMML is considered if unexplained monocytosis persists longer than 3 months or if cytogenetic/molecular studies demonstrate an acquired

Table 45.1	MAIN DIAGNOSTIC FEATURES OF MDS/MPNS AND RELATED NEOPLASMS						
CMML	aCML	JMML	MDS/MPN, U	RARS-T (Provisional Entity)	MDS with Isolated del(5q) and *JAK2* V617F Mutation	MDS/MPN with an Isolated Isochromosome 17q
Persistent unexplained monocytosis (>1 × 10⁹/L with >10% monocytes); absence of defining genetic features such as *BCR-ABL1* fusion or rearrangements of *PDGFRA* and *PDGFRB*; <20% blasts; dysplasia in ≥1 myeloid lineages

In the absence of definitive dysplastic features, the unexplained monocytosis have to persist >3 mo or cytogenetic/molecular studies have to demonstrate the presence of acquired clonal cytogenetic or molecular genetic abnormality | Neutrophilia with significant dysplasia and left shift; absence of *BCR-ABL1* rearrangement

No basophilia or monocytosis (<10% monocytes in PB); neutrophils with chromatin clumping may be present; BM findings similar to CML | Monocytosis (>1 × 1⁹/L); blast and promonocyte count <20%; absence of *BCR-ABL1* rearrangement

Additional diagnostic criteria (≥2 required): increase in hemoglobin F for age; granulocytic precursors in PB, WBC above 10 × 10⁹/L; clonal chromosomal abnormality and/or GM-CSF hypersensitivity of myeloid progenitors *in vitro*

Demonstration of mutations in genes regulating *RAS* pathway or HUMARA assay may be helpful to solidify diagnosis in challenging cases | Diagnosis of exclusion neoplasm with myelodysplastic and myeloproliferative features that does not fulfill diagnostic criteria for CMML, aCML, and JMML

Diagnosis requires extensive workup to exclude for example preexisting myeloid neoplasm, effects of previous treatment with growth factors or cytotoxic drugs | Thrombocytosis ≥450 × 10⁹/L; dysplasia of erythroid lineage; ≥15% ring sideroblasts; BM shows large atypical megakaryocytes and dyserythropoiesis

Absence of isolated deletion of chromosome 5, abnormalities of chromosome 3, and *BCR-ABL1* rearrangement. Clinical correlation to rule out conditions and medications associated with increase in ring sideroblasts is required | Coexistence of isolated 5q deletion and *JAK2* V617F mutation; hypolobated/monolobated megakaryocytes and frequent prominent granulocytic hyperplasia with higher WBC and a trend for higher platelet counts | Neutrophilia with frequent nonsegmented forms, hyposegmented neutrophils, ring nuclei, hypogranularity, and chromatin clumping; monocytosis is reported and a proportion of cases fulfill the criteria for CMML; hypercellular BM with significant granulocytic proliferation, dysgranulopoiesis, and <5% blasts; dysplastic changes in erythroid progenitors and megakaryocytes; significant fibrosis

Cases that do not fulfill criteria for CMML diagnosis often show pleomorphic megakaryocyte morphology and should be classified as MDS/MPN, U with isolated isochromosome 17q |

CMML, chronic myelomonocytic leukemia; aCML, atypical chronic myeloid leukemia; JMML, juvenile myelomonocytic leukemia; MDS/MPN, U, myelodysplastic/myeloproliferative neoplasm, unclassifiable; MDS, myelodysplastic syndrome; MDS/MPN, myelodysplastic/myeloproliferative neoplasm.

clonal cytogenetic or molecular genetic abnormality (6). The exclusion of potential clinical mimickers defined by *BCR-ABL1, PDGFRA*, and *PDGFRB* rearrangements is required. Similarly, acute myelomonocytic and monoblastic/monocytic leukemia have to be excluded (blasts and their equivalents, promonocytes, represent <20% of a differential count in CMML). The 2008 WHO diagnostic criteria of CMML are summarized in Table 45.1.

Epidemiology

CMML represents approximately 10% of all MDSs. The annual incidence is estimated to be <1 case per 100,000 people in the general population and 3 cases per 100,000 in individuals older than 60 years (3,7). The median age of presentation is between 65 and 75 years. CMML is more commonly diagnosed in men (ratio of 1.5-3:1) and in Western countries as compared to Asia (8–10).

Clinical Features

The clinical features are variable with predominant symptoms of marrow failure such as fatigue, susceptibility to infections, and bleeding. Even though absolute monocytosis is a defining feature, other myeloid lineages are also affected, leading to cytopenia(s) or cytoses. Elevated WBC and neutrophilia, with or without left shift, are seen in about 50% of cases. Remaining

patients show leukopenia and neutropenia. Anemia and thrombocytopenia are common. Patients can experience hypercatabolic symptoms such as weight loss, night sweats, and fever. Abdominal pain and early satiety due to splenomegaly are seen in 30% to 50% of patients (11). Hepatomegaly, lymphadenopathy, skin rash, and serous effusions are seen more frequently in the myeloproliferative type of CMML.

There have been attempts to classify CMML into myeloproliferative and myelodysplastic categories based on the threshold of WBC of 13 × 10⁹/L (12). Myeloproliferative CMML is more frequently associated with splenomegaly and increased lactate dehydrogenase (LDH) (11,13). Since prognosis, including overall survival and incidence of transformation into acute leukemia, is similar for both CMML subtypes, 2008 WHO classification does not require to distinguish between these categories (11,13–15).

Morphology

The defining feature of CMML is PB monocytosis (>1 × 10⁹/L with >10% monocytes on the differential count). The majority of monocytes are mature and frequently show abnormal nuclear and cytoplasmic features such as abnormal nuclear lobulation or chromatin condensation, prominent granulation, or deeply basophilic cytoplasm (Fig. 45.1A). Morphologic definition of "abnormal monocytes" and promonocytes has been a matter of debate and is thoroughly described in 2008 WHO

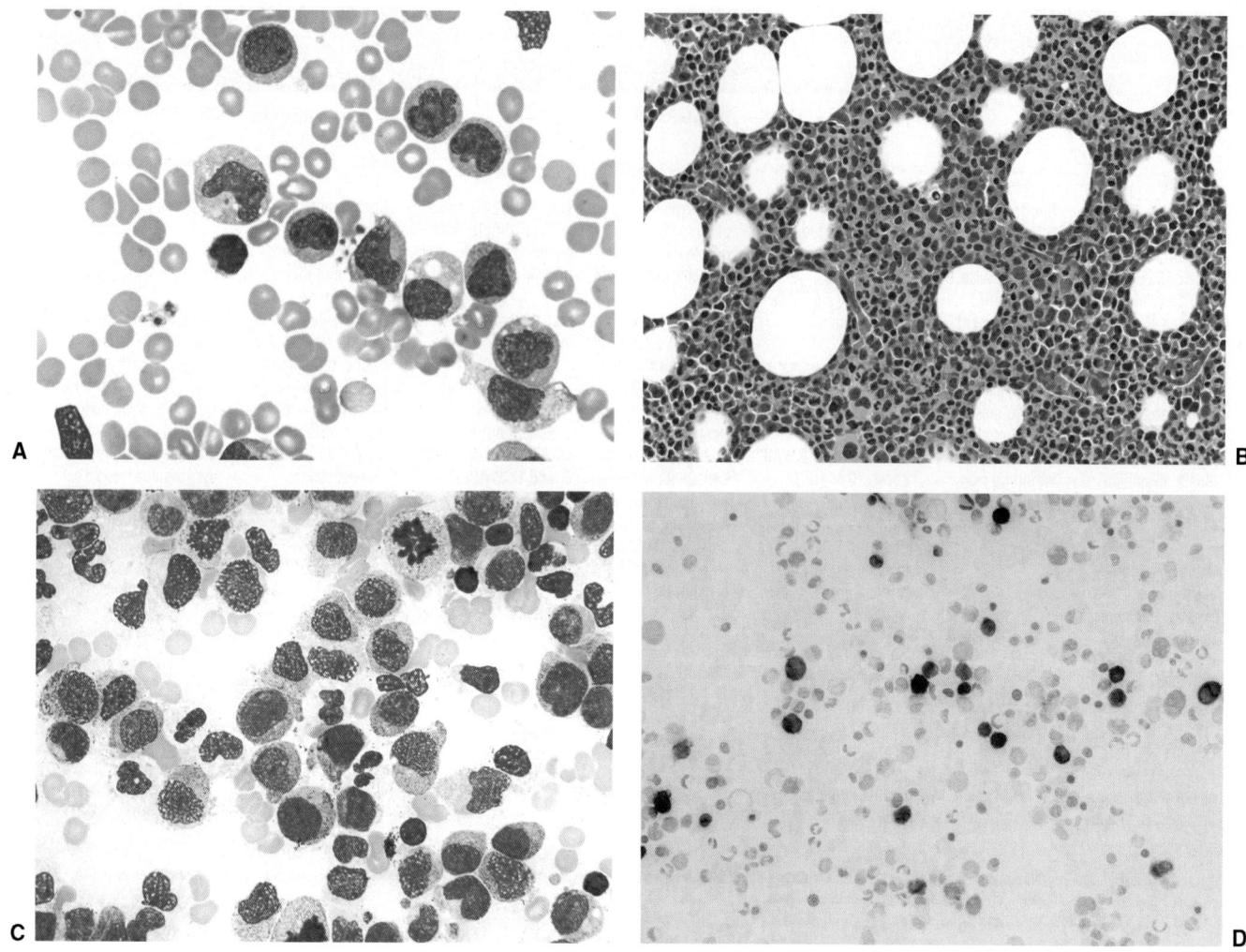

FIGURE 45.1. CMML in peripheral blood and bone marrow. A: PB with significant monocytosis including atypical mature monocytes and monocytic precursors. **B:** Hypercellular BM in biopsy sample. Note dysplastic megakaryocytes. **C:** BM aspirate with increased granulopoiesis, including hypogranular neutrophils, and monocytopoiesis. **D:** Butyrate esterase highlights monocytes and their precursors.

classification (6). In most cases of CMML, PB blasts, including blast equivalents, constitute <5% of the differential count. The WBC is variable, and neutrophilia is seen in about 50% of the cases. Pseudo Pelger-Huet cells and hypogranulation are common. Circulating neutrophilic precursors (promyelocytes and myelocytes) usually constitute <10% of white blood cells. In cases with significant eosinophilia (≥ 1.5 × 10⁹/L), it is important to exclude rearrangements of *PDGFRA* and *PDGFRB* genes. Basophilia is uncommon. Normochromic normocytic or macrocytic anemia is a frequent feature. Thrombocytopenia and giant platelets can be seen.

Even though PB monocytosis is the defining feature of CMML, the final diagnosis should never be rendered without an evaluation of BM. Foremost, the number of marrow blasts and blast equivalents (i.e., promonocytes) has to be confirmed to definitively exclude acute myelomonocytic and monocytic leukemia. Monocytosis can also occur in patients with select chronic myeloid neoplasms at the time of the original diagnosis or develop in the course of the disease. Significant monocytosis can be seen in a proportion of cases of *BCR-ABL1+* chronic myelogenous leukemia (CML), primary myelofibrosis (PMF), MDSs, myeloid neoplasms with *PDGFRA* rearrangement, and even systemic mastocytosis. Careful review of BM morphology and previous clinical history can prevent the incorrect diagnosis of CMML in such cases. On the contrary, increase in monocytes

largely confined to the BM without absolute monocytosis can be seen in rare cases of "marrow-predominant" CMML (7).

BM is hypercellular in the majority of CMML cases (Fig. 45.1B). Rarely, BM may be normo- or hypocellular (16). All hematopoietic lineages are affected. The M:E ratio is typically increased. Prominent myelopoiesis includes an increased number of neutrophilic precursors as well as monocytes (Fig. 45.1C). The latter may be difficult to appreciate and are better visualized using nonspecific esterase cytochemical staining (Fig. 45.1D). Left shift in granulopoiesis and myelodysplastic features such as hypogranulation and nuclear abnormalities are common (12). Erythropoiesis is usually normal to decreased and shows dysplastic features such as megaloblastoid change with asynchrony in maturation of nucleus and cytoplasm, and nuclear abnormalities including nuclear fragmentation, irregularity of nuclear outline, and multinucleation. Ring sideroblasts may be increased. Dysmegakaryopoiesis is seen in the majority of CMML cases, and the number of megakaryocytes can be moderately increased (17,18). Dysplastic megakaryocytes display abnormal nuclear lobation including mononuclear or hypolobated nuclei, or separated nuclear lobes (Fig. 45.1B). Dwarf forms can also be seen. Approximately 20% of cases show significant reticulin fibrosis (19).

Performing a marrow differential count may be challenging in CMML cases due to morphologic overlap between dysplastic

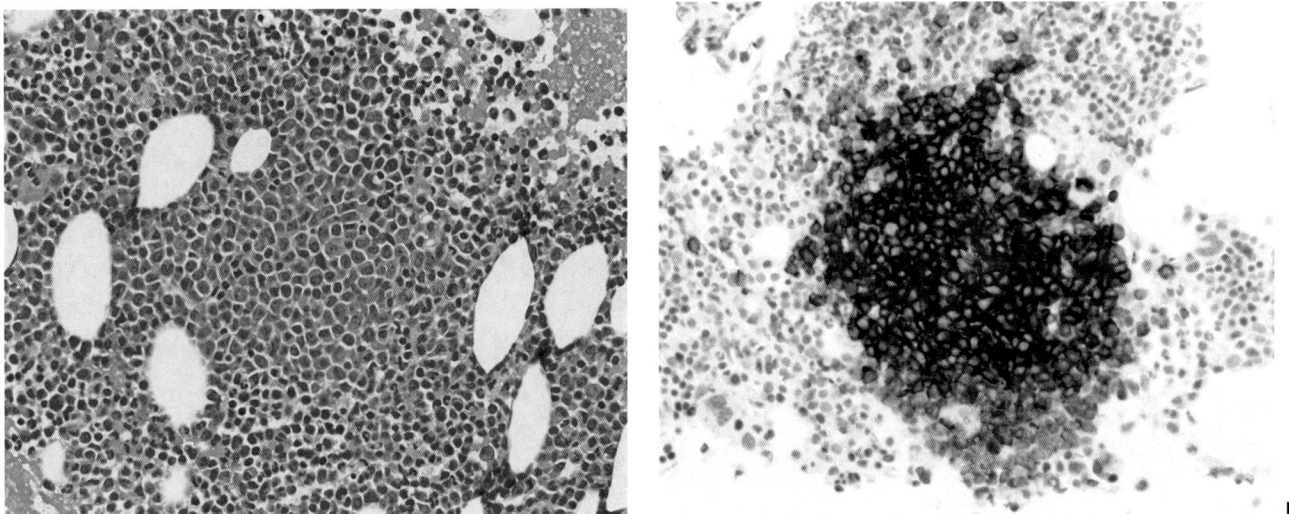

FIGURE 45.2. Plasmacytoid dendritic cell nodule in CMML. A: Plasmacytoid dendritic cell nodule in a BM biopsy. **B:** CD123 immunostain highlights the aggregate of plasmacytoid dendritic cells.

neutrophilic precursors (myelocytes and metamyelocytes) and immature/atypical monocytes. The most significant practical issue is the identification of monoblasts and promonocytes. The increased number of blasts and promonocytes is the most reliable predictor of poor prognosis and of the risk of transformation to acute leukemia (14). Based on the differential count, CMML is divided into two groups: CMML-1 with <5% blasts in PB and <10% in BM and CMML-2 with 5% to 19% of blasts in PB and 10% to 19% in BM. In cases with <20% blasts, the presence of Auer rods results in the diagnosis of CMML-2. The threshold of 20% of blasts and promonocytes differentiates between CMML and acute myelomonocytic and monocytic leukemias.

Nodular proliferations of plasmacytoid dendritic cells are seen in 10% to 20% of CMML cases and can be seen in both BM and extramedullary sites (17) (Fig. 45.2). Plasmacytoid dendritic cells are part of innate immune system and constitute a distinct subset of dendritic cells with plasma cell–like morphology (20). They are believed to be derived from myeloid progenitors, and therefore it is perhaps not surprising that focal proliferations of these cells are seen in myeloid neoplasms. In this setting, plasmacytoid dendritic cells are considered clonal and in select cases have been shown to be clonally related to the underlying myeloid neoplasm (21,22). Plasmacytoid dendritic cells are intermediate in size with round to oval nucleus, with or without indentation, finely dispersed chromatin, and moderately abundant cytoplasm.

Spleen is the most common extramedullary site involved by CMML. A population of myelomonocytic precursors fills splenic cords. Megakaryocytes and erythroid series are frequently seen in splenic sinuses. In select patients, frequent foamy histiocytes are seen, occasionally in the vicinity of marginal zones. The latter pattern is similar to that seen in patients with idiopathic thrombocytopenic purpura.

In addition to its propensity to involve a spleen, CMML can present in various extramedullary sites, with the most frequent being liver, lymph nodes, skin, and body cavity fluids. Lymph nodes typically show partial to complete effacement of nodal architecture by extramedullary hematopoiesis including a heterogenous proliferation composed of myelomonocytic precursors, variable number of megakaryocytes, and to a lesser extent erythropoiesis (Fig. 45.3A and B; Czader et al., 2007 unpublished observations) (23). A variable number of blasts can be seen. Sheets of blasts can be identified in cases showing transformation to AML.

Cutaneous manifestations of CMML include several patterns. Early in the disease, a subtle perivascular dermal infiltrates of myelomonocytic cells manifests as a rash (Fig. 45.3C). More advanced disease can manifest as proliferation of granulocytic or monocytic blasts, as mature plasmacytoid dendritic cells, as a blastic plasmacytoid dendritic cell tumor, or as a novel category of blastic indeterminate dendritic cell tumor (24,25). When the blasts become the predominant cell type, a diagnosis of leukemia cutis or, if mass forming, myeloid sarcoma is rendered.

Malignant body cavity effusions are occasionally seen in CMML and are typically composed of monocytes and their precursors (23,26–29). They can occur in the chronic phase of the disease or herald acceleration and transformation to acute leukemia.

Immunophenotype

Quantifying monocytic component in cases of CMML can be challenging due to morphologic overlaps among dysplastic neutrophils and their precursors and monocytic cells. The nonspecific esterase staining (alpha-naphthyl butyrate or alpha-naphthyl acetate esterase) is an effective method of demonstrating monocytic differentiation and shows 10% to 20% positivity in the majority of CMML patients (17,19) (Fig. 45.1D). Flow cytometry is commonly used to demonstrate the prominent monocytic component, to separate various stages of monocytic differentiation, and to demonstrate an aberrant antigen expression. A combination of antibodies against different epitopes of CD14 antigen, CD64, and CD33 can be used to distinguish between promonocytes and more mature monocytic forms (30). In addition, an aberrant expression of antigens typically not seen on normal monocytes, including nonmyeloid markers, can be encountered in monocytes and in the granulocytic population. Monocytes frequently coexpress CD56 and CD2 and show loss or decreased density of HLA-DR, CD13, and CD64 (31–33). A decrease in side scatter confirms the presence of hypogranular neutrophils. An increase in the number of CD34+ and/or CD117+ blasts can be associated with progression of the disease and alert to the impending transformation. The CMML blasts can show immunophenotypic abnormalities such as expression of CD7, CD56, CD15, and variable HLA-DR. Overexpression of CD13 and CD117 and decreased CD45 expression have been also observed (34).

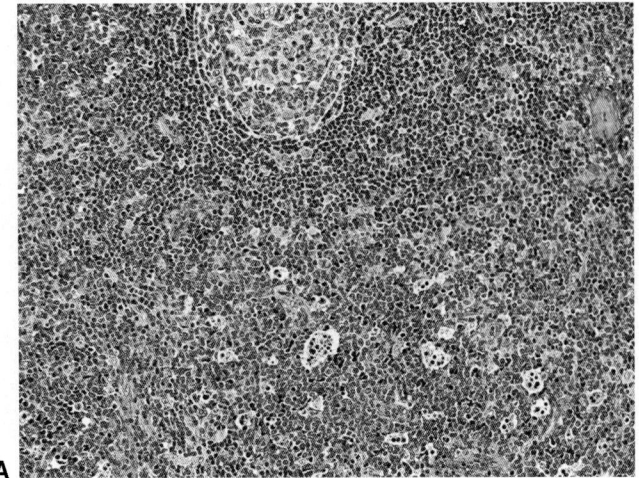

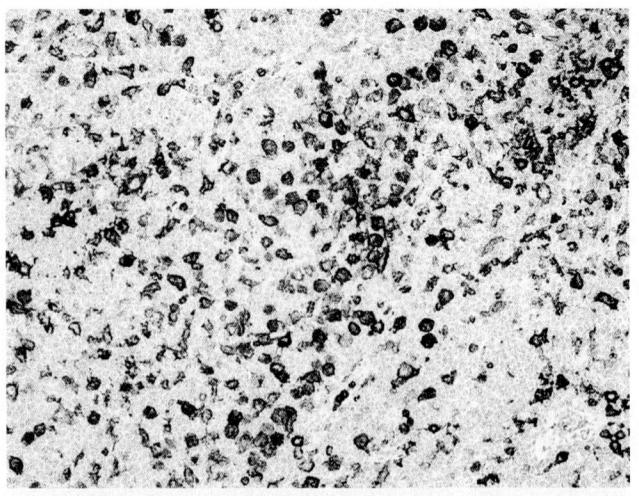

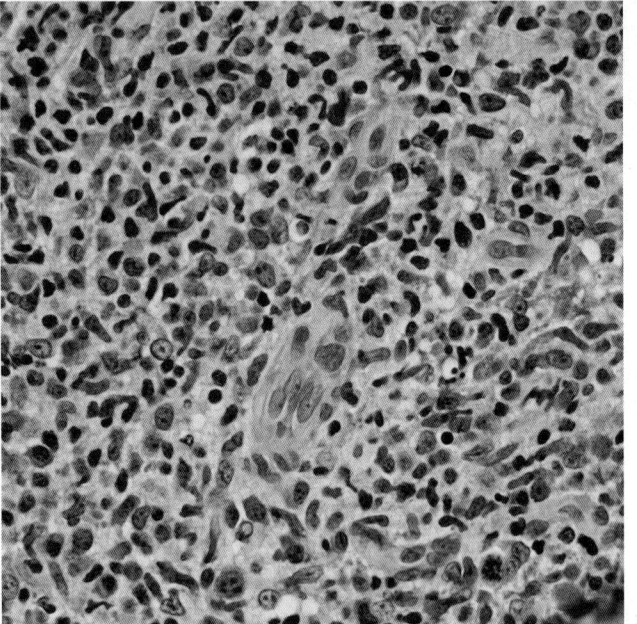

FIGURE 45.3. Extramedullary manifestations of CMML. A: Partial lymph node involvement with prominent neoplastic extramedullary hematopoiesis. **B:** CD14 immunostain highlights monocytes in a lymph node involved by CMML. **C:** Prominent perivascular myelomonocytic infiltrate in the reticular dermis.

The enumeration of monocytic component in BM biopsies can be accomplished with the help of a combination of CD14 and CD16 antibodies (35,36). Other common myeloid/monocyte/macrophage markers such as lysozyme and CD68 (KP1) are not specific to the monocytic differentiation (17). CD68R and CD163, even though restricted to monocytes and macrophages, might not capture all monocytic precursors and usually stain significantly lower number of cells as compared to naphthyl butyrate esterase (17,35). It has been previously reported that staining pattern of CD68R (fine vs. coarse granules) in conjunction with cell morphology can discriminate between monocyte precursors and mature monocytes; however, this observation requires further confirmation by independent studies (37). The CD34 immunohistochemistry is useful in demonstrating an increased number of blasts and the presence of blast clusters. The nodules of plasmacytoid dendritic cells can be demonstrated using several antibodies including CD123 (Fig. 45.2B), CD45RA, CD68, CD68R, CD4, and CD14. Plasmacytoid dendritic cells are also positive for granzyme B and rarely for CD56, CD2, and CD5 and negative for other lymphoid markers, CD13, CD11c, myeloperoxidase, and CD34.

Cytogenetic and Molecular Characteristics

Approximately 20% to 50% of patients with CMML show an abnormal karyotype (6). The most common abnormalities include trisomy 8, monosomy 7/del(7q), and structural aberrancies of 12p. These abnormalities are not specific to CMML and frequently occur in MPNs and MDS.

Next-generation sequencing and other high-throughput methods expanded the spectrum of genetic lesions encountered in CMML. High-resolution multigene analyses identified genetic changes in approximately 90% of CMML cases. These lesions affect both genetic and epigenetic regulation of transcription, translation, and cell signaling pathways of basic cell functions such as proliferation, survival, and maturation. The most often affected genes are *TET2, ASXL1*, and *SRSF2*, with the reported frequency between 30% and 60%. Interestingly, *TET2, ASXL1*, and several other genes mutated at lower frequencies all regulate transcription and its epigenetic control.

TET2 (ten eleven translocation 2) converts 5-methyl-cytosine to 5-hydroxymethyl-cytosine, which leads to DNA demethylation (38–45). It is mutated in 19% to 65% of CMML patients.

CMML with mutated *TET2* showed differential methylation as compared to normal controls and wild-type *TET2* cases (43). The wild-type *TET2* was seen more frequently in patients with high- or intermediate-risk cytogenetics. The association of *TET2* with survival or response to hypomethylating agents is controversial (39,41,42,44,46,47). The function of *TET2* might be modified by *IDH1* and *IDH2*, which are mutated in <10% of CMML cases and occur exclusively in cases with wild-type *TET2* (39,48,49).

ASXL1 (additional sex combs like 1) is a part of Polycomb gene family and is most likely involved in epigenetic regulation of transcription. It is among the genes most frequently mutated in CMML and in select studies was associated with transformation to acute leukemia (39,50–52). The importance of Polycomb family is underscored by recent discovery of alterations of other member gene—*EZH2*. *EZH2* was found to be mutated in 11% to 13% of CMML cases and was associated with inferior outcome (39,50,53). Other Polycomb components (*SUZ12, EED*, and *JARID2*) were affected in a low number of cases (54,55).

The *SRSF2* gene, a regulator of constitutive and alternative splicing, has been shown to be mutated in 47% of CMML cases. *SRSF2* mutations had a favorable effect on overall survival in the *RUNX1* mutated cohort (56,57). Other components of spliceosome such as *SF3b1* and *U2AF1* were involved at lower frequencies (57–59).

Another gene involved in the epigenetic regulation, *DNMT3A*, was mutated in approximately 10% of CMML cases and was associated with normal karyotype (49).

RUNX1 (Runt-related transcription factor 1 gene) encodes a subunit of a DNA core-binding factor critical for normal hematopoiesis. This regulatory transcription factor is considered a tumor suppressor gene, and its alterations were identified in 8% to 38% of CMML patients (39,60).

In addition to transcription and translation, cell signaling pathways have shown to be affected in MDS/MPN including CMML. Hirsh-Ginsberg et al. first reported the involvement of *RAS* in early 1990s (61). Since then, numerous studies confirmed this finding and reported mutations of *NRAS* and *KRAS* at frequencies from 14% to 57% (41,61–64).

Another signaling pathway gene altered in CMML is *CBL* (Casitas B-lineage lymphoma gene), which is involved in regulating kinase signaling conferred by E3 ubiquitin ligase activity and has a positive impact on downstream signaling. It is relatively frequently involved in CMML, aCML, and MDS/MPN, unclassifiable (41,65). It has also been reported in JMML (66,67).

A variety of additional genes involved in cell signaling are altered in CMML at lower frequencies. These include *JAK2, NOTCH, FLT3, NPM1,* and *CEBPA*. *JAK2*V617F mutation is uncommon (~10% of cases) and has been seen in cases with predominant myeloproliferative features (68–70). Notch signaling pathway elements were shown to be affected in approximately 10% of CMML cases (71). *FLT3* mutations and internal tandem duplications were identified in up to 5% of patients (72,73). Similarly, *NPM1* and *CEBPA* mutations are rare; however, they have been associated with adverse outcome (74,75).

In recent years, a significant progress has been made in identifying genetic lesions occurring in CMML. Many of these alterations are in vital pathways of transcription and translation regulation and cell signaling. It remains to be determined which of these genetic changes play a role in pathogenesis and disease progression in CMML, and whether they can be effectively utilized as therapeutic targets.

Risk Stratification and Risk-Adapted Therapy

The survival of patients with CMML is extremely variable, ranging from 1 to 100 months (6,8,17,76). Similarly, the rates of transformation into AML vary among different studies from

15% to 52%. Acute leukemias evolving from CMML have been reported to show an aggressive behavior (77). There have been numerous efforts to design a risk stratification system predictive of clinical outcome. Originally, CMML patients were stratified using International Prognostic Scoring System (78), an approach that excluded cases with predominant myeloproliferative features. In recent years, new stratification systems have been designed to include all CMML subtypes. The most commonly used are modified Bournemouth score, Dusseldorf score, MD Anderson Prognostic score, and Spanish CMML score. All systems that have been proven effective in predicting clinical outcome include a combination of BM blast count with PB counts (9,76). Indeed, in multivariate analysis, PB and BM blast percentage appear to be the strongest predictors of survival and of transformation into AML. Blast counts are used to define previously discussed subcategories of CMML-1 and CMML-2, which are highly predictive of overall survival and transformation into AML (8,14,16,19,79). At 5-year follow-up, 63% of patients with a BM blast count of 10% or greater developed AML as compared to 18% of patients with blast count below 10% (14).

To refine the classification of CMML into different prognostic groups, each risk stratification system added several variables. Using hemoglobin (<12 g/dL), circulating immature cells, absolute lymphocyte count (>2.5 × 10⁹/L), and BM blasts (>10%), MD Anderson prognostic score identified four groups of patients, with median overall survival ranging from 24 to 5 months (9). Dusseldorf registry added elevated LDH and male sex as predictors of adverse outcome and identified three risk groups with median overall survival of 93, 26, and 11 months. Analyzing outcomes of patients from Spanish MDS database, Such et al. (47) identified several factors independently associated with worse survival. These included BM blast count of ≥10%, WBC ≥ 13 × 10⁹/L, hemoglobin <10 g/dL, platelet count <100 × 10⁹/L, and a high-risk CMML-specific cytogenetic score defined as a presence of trisomy 8, abnormalities of chromosome 7, or a complex karyotype. As our knowledge on the pathogenesis of myeloid neoplasms expands, new prognostic factors emerge. It is likely that in the future, specific genes or gene profiles will be added to clinical stratification schemes.

The comprehensive review of the treatment for CMML is beyond the scope of this chapter; thus a brief synopsis of therapeutic options is presented. In the past, many CMML patients were included in MDS trials, and treatment outcome data specific for CMML is limited. Traditionally, CMML has been managed with best supportive care including erythropoietin for treatment of anemia, antibiotics as prophylaxis in neutropenia, and iron chelation in transfusion-dependent patients. Various cytoreductive agents used in CMML included hydroxyurea, etoposide, low-dose cytarabine, and topotecan (80–82). Relatively recently, FDA-approved hypomethylating agents, azacitidine and decitabine, have been tested in CMML with variable success (46,83–86). There is evidence that these agents may be effective in a subgroup of CMML patients with high blast count (84,87). Similar to other myeloproliferative or myelodysplastic neoplasms, the curative treatment options in CMML are limited to the allogeneic BM transplantation. This option may be more suitable for younger patients with high-risk disease and indeed offers long-term progression-free survival in a significant proportion of CMML cases (88,89). Older patients with high transplant-related morbidity may benefit from supportive or cytoreductive treatment.

Altogether, the treatments that modify natural history of CMML showed variable success. The clinical experience and accumulating genetic data indicate that targeted therapies may be the most desirable future approach to treatment of this rare neoplasm.

Differential Diagnosis

The defining feature of CMML, monocytosis, can be present in a variety of reactive conditions and myeloid neoplasms either at the time of original diagnosis or during the natural course of the disease. These mimickers have to be excluded before the definitive diagnosis of CMML is rendered.

The most important and often most urgent differential diagnosis is that of acute myelomonocytic and monocytic leukemias. A thorough examination of BM aspirate smear and biopsy is critical in making the distinction. Significant monocytosis can be seen in MPNs including select cases of *BCR-ABL1*+ CML (6). CML with monocytosis frequently shows an alternative p190 fusion protein (90). In patients diagnosed with PMF, the concomitant presence or development of monocytosis is associated with poor prognosis (91,92). Meticulous review of BM biopsy, previous clinical history, and, if required, ancillary testing helps to prevent the incorrect diagnosis of CMML in these patients. Ancillary genetic testing may also be required in CMML cases accompanied by a significant eosinophilia to exclude rearrangements of *PDGFRA, PDGFRB,* and *FGFR1.*

Features of CMML can develop in the course of previously diagnosed MDS (93–95). At the time of original diagnosis, approximately 20% of MDS patients show relative PB monocytosis (more than 10% monocytes but with absolute monocyte count $<1 \times 10^9$/L), and over time, a proportion of these patients may develop absolute monocytosis. In a well-documented series of cases, the interval between the initial MDS diagnosis and an onset of absolute monocytosis ranged between 2 and 59 months. As compared to MDS patients without increased monocytes, those with relative monocytosis (>10% monocytes) showed higher marrow cellularity, higher incidence of chromosomal abnormalities, and a more aggressive disease with high incidence of progression to CMML and transformation into acute myelomonocytic or monocytic leukemia (95). Conversely, up to 24% of patients with CMML have a documented preceding MDS phase (19,93). When CMML evolving from the MDS phase was compared to an entire group of *de novo* CMML or the myelodysplastic type of CMML, the patients with antecedent MDS showed a superior survival (93,94).

Reactive monocytosis is frequently associated with viral, fungal, and mycobacterial infections; immune and inflammatory conditions such as collagen vascular diseases and immune thrombocytopenic purpura; chronic neutropenias; neoplasms, particularly Hodgkin lymphoma and growth factor treatment. In such cases, careful correlation with clinical history provides clues to the reactive cause of monocytosis. Additional findings of PB blasts, immature or atypical monocytes, dysgranulopoiesis, leukoerythroblastic picture, unexplained eosinophilia, or splenomegaly may prompt further work-up including BM examination and cytogenetic/molecular studies. If the comprehensive work-up shows no definitive evidence of myeloid neoplasm, an observation period of 3 to 6 months is advised before the definitive diagnosis of CMML is rendered.

CMML typically presents as *de novo* disease arising in patients without preexisting malignancies or a history of cytoreductive treatment. Rarely, CMML may develop after treatment with chemotherapeutic agents and/or radiotherapy for malignancies or nonneoplastic diseases (96–98). Even though the number of reported cases is low, therapy-related CMML seems to show morphologic and immunophenotypic features similar to those of *de novo* CMML. However, a proportion of therapy-related CMML cases show the rearrangement of *MLL* gene, a finding that suggests an alternative diagnosis of AML. Nevertheless, according to 2008 WHO classification, all therapy-related malignancies are grouped together under an umbrella of therapy-related myeloid neoplasms. A detailed knowledge of patient's previous medical history and cytogenetic profile is critical in all cases of CMML.

JUVENILE MYELOMONOCYTIC LEUKEMIA

Definition

JMML is a rare, aggressive, clonal hematopoietic disorder of childhood with combined clinical pathologic features of myelodysplasia (anemia, thrombocytopenia) and myeloproliferation (leukocytosis, monocytosis). The 2008 WHO diagnostic criteria for JMML include PB monocytosis ($>1 \times 10^9$/L), leukocytosis, left shifted granulocytic series in PB, increased hemoglobin F (HbF), clonal chromosomal abnormality, and GM-CSF hypersensitivity of myeloid progenitors *in vitro* (Table 45.1) (99). The exclusion of other neoplasms that can present with similar clinical and laboratory features such as AMLs with monocytic differentiation and chronic MPNs is required.

In the past, JMML has been referred to as juvenile chronic myeloid leukemia, CMML, monosomy 7 syndrome, and infantile monosomy 7 syndrome.

Epidemiology

The estimated incidence is 1.3 cases per million children younger than 14 years (100–102). It is usually diagnosed in patients younger than 3 years; however, there is a variable age at diagnosis from 1 month to early adolescence. Boys are affected more often than girls. JMML is more frequently seen in individuals affected by neurofibromatosis type 1 and to a lesser extent in those with Noonan syndrome. This is related to the activation of *RAS* pathway due to mutations of genes *NF1, PTPN11, KRAS,* and *SOS1.* A newly described *CBL* germline syndrome has also been associated with an increased risk of developing JMML (103).

Clinical Features

Suggestive clinical features include hepatosplenomegaly, lymphadenopathy, pallor, fever, bleeding, and maculopapular rash. These features may be seen at an onset of the disease or develop within short period of time after initial presentation. Respiratory failure and diarrhea may be presenting features and are related to the organ infiltration by neoplastic myeloid cells. In cases of neurofibromatosis type 1 or Noonan syndrome, additional features of primary disorder, such as café au lait spots, may be present. A proportion of JMML patients show polyclonal hypergammaglobulinemia.

Morphology and Laboratory Features

A review of CBC and PB smear is indispensable for diagnosis. CBC generally shows leukocytosis with monocytosis, thrombocytopenia, and often anemia. The median reported WBC varies from 25 to 30×10^9/L and rarely exceeds 100×10^9/L. The leukocytosis is composed mainly of neutrophils with little if any dysplasia and immature forms such as promyelocytes and myelocytes, as well as of monocytes (Fig. 45.4A). Absolute monocytosis is present even in patients with lower WBC. Blasts (including promonocytes) typically account for fewer than 5% of the differential count and always <20%. Eosinophilia and basophilia are observed in a minority of cases. Nucleated red blood cells are often seen. Normocytic red blood cells are common, and microcytosis due to iron deficiency or rarely acquired thalassemia phenotype may be seen as well (104). Macrocytic red blood cells are seen frequently in patients with monosomy 7. Thrombocytopenia is usual and may be severe.

The BM findings are not by themselves diagnostic. The BM is typically normocellular and shows a prominent granulocytic proliferation (Fig. 45.4B), although in some patients erythroid

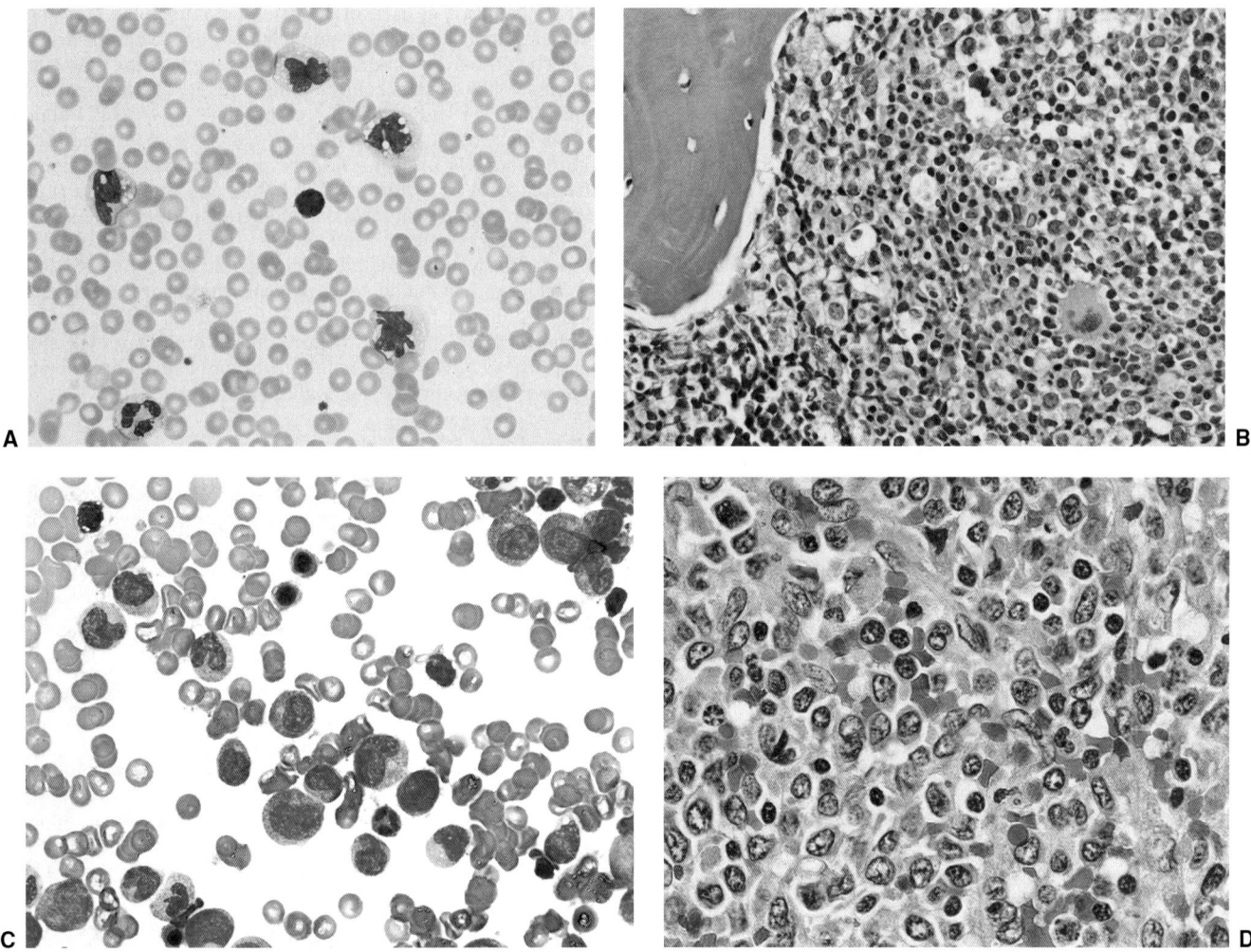

FIGURE 45.4. Peripheral blood and bone marrow in JMML. A: PB monocytosis. **B:** BM biopsy from 1-year old patient diagnosed with JMML. Note predominant granulopoiesis. **C:** BM aspirate showing frequent monocytes. **D:** Spleen with extramedullary hematopoiesis including prominent monocytic population in a child with JMML.

precursors may predominate. Monocytic series is often less impressive in the BM than in the blood and generally accounts for 5% to 10% of the cellularity (Fig. 45.4C). Blasts (including promonocytes) represent <20% of the marrow cells. Auer rods are not seen. In most of the cases, maturing myeloid cells show no significant dysplasia. However, dysgranulopoiesis, including pseudo Pelger-Huet neutrophils or hypogranularity, may be noted in some cases. Erythroid precursors can show megaloblastoid changes, particularly in patients with monosomy 7. Megakaryocytes are often reduced in number. Marked dysmegakaryopoiesis is unusual. Reticulin fibrosis has been reported in some patients.

Leukemic infiltrates are common in the skin, where myelomonocytic cells infiltrate the superficial and deep dermis, predominantly in the perivascular and periadnexal localization. In the spleen, the infiltrate is present in the red pulp and has a predilection for trabecular and central arteries (Fig. 45.4D). The hepatic sinusoids and the portal tracts are often infiltrated. In lungs, leukemic cells spread from the capillaries of the alveolar septa into alveoli.

In summary, in isolation, the morphologic features are not specific for the diagnosis of JMML and correlation with clinical presentation cannot be overemphasized. To confirm the diagnosis, additional testing may be required in patients with normal karyotype. Two confirmatory laboratory tests listed by 2008 WHO classification include a determination of HbF level

and *in vitro* hypersensitivity to GM-CSF. HbF levels, corrected for age, are elevated in approximately 50% of children with JMML, predominantly in patients without monosomy 7 (105). The hypersensitivity to GM-CSF can be confirmed using *in vitro* culture assay or flow cytometry with measurement of phospho-STAT5 positivity after low-dose GM-CSF stimulation (106,107). However, positive *in vitro* culture assay and phospho-STAT5 flow cytometry have been reported in select viral infections such as cytomegalovirus, in which clinical presentation may be similar to that of JMML (108). Thus, neither of these tests is entirely specific for JMML.

The diagnosis of JMML can be challenging, considering the relative lack of specificity of the current diagnostic criteria. Since genetic abnormalities are found in up to 90% of JMML patients, the inclusion of the molecular criteria can facilitate the diagnosis (100,109). Specifically, somatic mutations in *RAS, PTPN11,* and *NF1* are suggested as additional diagnostic criteria. The detailed discussion of genetic lesions reported in JMML is presented in subsequent sections.

Immunophenotype

No specific cytochemical abnormalities have been reported in JMML. The nonspecific esterase staining of BM aspirate smear (preferred alpha naphthyl butyrate esterase), or immunohistology with CD68R or CD14, may be helpful in quantifying the monocytic component. Flow cytometric immunophenotyping may show abnormalities in the monocyte and blast population; however, these are not specific for the diagnosis of JMML.

Cytogenetics and Genetics

Abnormal karyotypes are seen in approximately 35% of JMML patients. The most frequent abnormality, monosomy 7, has been reported in approximately 25% of cases (105). By definition, Philadelphia chromosome and the *BCR-ABL1* rearrangement are absent.

The majority of JMML patients carry mutations affecting RAS/MAPK signaling pathway. Approximately 75% of patients have a mutation in one of the following genes: *NRAS, KRAS, PTPN11, NF1,* or *CBL* (67, 110). Nearly 30% of patients with JMML have *RAS* gene mutations (111,112). Approximately 10% of cases are associated with type I neurofibromatosis. In these cases, mutation of the *NF1*, a tumor suppressor gene, coupled with a loss of the wild-type allele, leads to the activation of the RAS pathway (113). About 15% to 20% of children with JMML without the phenotype of neurofibromatosis carry mutation/deletion of *NF1*, leading to an activation of RAS (114). An additional 20% to 30% of patients have yet another mutation involving the gene *PTPN11* encoding RAS regulatory protein, SHP-2 (115). Thus, nearly 75% to 80% of patients with JMML have an abnormality in the RAS pathway of signal transduction, which is activated by binding of the GM-CSF receptor. Additional 10% to 15% of patients show mutations in *CBL* gene, which functions as ubiquitin ligase regulating Grb2-SOS complex and RAS activation (67).

In summary, the majority of molecular lesions identified in JMML are exclusive and converge on the RAS/MAPK pathway. Genetic abnormalities involved in other subtypes of myeloid neoplasms such as mutations of *ASXL1, TET2, RUNX1,* and *JAK2* are exceedingly rare or have not been described in JMML (116).

Risk Stratification and Risk-Adapted Therapy

The majority of JMML cases have aggressive clinical course, with the only curative option being hematopoietic stem cell transplantation with the 5-year survival of 40% (102). The increased HbF level, age above 2 years, and platelet count below 33×10^9/L have been incorporated in the prognostic score predictive of survival (102,117). Select syndromic cases of JMML or JMML-like myeloproliferative disease show an indolent course and can initially be observed. Noonan syndrome patients presenting with myeloproliferative disease within the first year of life are expected to recover spontaneously and interestingly do not show increased risk of myeloid neoplasms later in life (118,119). Similarly, JMML patients with *RAS* mutations including somatic mosaicism may rarely experience spontaneous remission (120–123). In addition, patients with homozygous *CBL* mutations may have an indolent clinical course (109). Despite these anecdotal reports, there is no prevailing evidence that specific mutations are independently predictive of overall survival in multivariate analysis; however, *PTPN11* mutation correlated with inferior survival post stem cell transplantation in univariate analysis (124). Interestingly, gene expression profiling was able to identify two groups of JMML patients with dramatically different long-term outcome [6% and 63% 10-year event free survival (125)]. These groups were not defined by other known prognostic factors and did not correlate with specific genetic lesions. The high methylation phenotype has also been associated with poor overall survival and risk of relapse after hematopoietic stem cell transplantation (126). It has been suggested that the evaluation of DNA methylation may help in differentiating low- and high-risk patients even within known prognostic groups.

The standard of care in JMML is hematopoietic stem cell transplantation. There is no compelling evidence that pretransplant chemotherapy or splenectomy is beneficial for long-term outcome. With various conditioning regimens, transplantation from related or unrelated HLA compatible donor cures about half of the patients. Relapse is the major cause of treatment failure. There is a clear evidence that graft-versus-leukemia effect plays an important role in JMML, and therefore a rapid decrease of immunosuppression after transplantation has been recommended (109).

Molecularly targeted therapeutics that interfere with RAS activation and signaling such as farnesyltransferase, Raf, and mTOR inhibitors have been tested in cultures and/or limited number of JMML patients. Whereas many of the targeted therapy trials are ongoing, some initially promising agents showed no benefit for event-free survival (109).

Differential Diagnosis

The clinical and laboratory features of JMML can closely mimic infectious diseases, including those due to Epstein-Barr virus, cytomegalovirus, human herpesvirus 6, Histoplasma, Toxoplasma, and mycobacteria. In isolation, morphology of PB and BM is not helpful to distinguish between JMML and reactive infection-associated myeloproliferation. Thus, in the absence of cytogenetic or genetic anomalies, additional laboratory testing may be required to exclude infections and demonstrate additional features in support of the diagnosis of JMML. Mutational analysis of the components of the RAS/MAPK signaling pathway or, in female patients, human androgen receptor gene analysis (HUMARA assay) may be helpful in establishing a definitive diagnosis.

The management of transient polyclonal myeloproliferation of Noonan syndrome has been discussed previously. This nonclonal myelomonocytic proliferation can fulfill current diagnostic criteria for JMML (118,119). There is a developing consensus that when diagnosed early in childhood, these patients will experience a spontaneous remission, somewhat analogous to the transient abnormal hematopoiesis of Down syndrome. Thus, a descriptive diagnosis of myeloproliferative process rather than a definitive diagnosis of JMML might be more fitting in this clinical scenario.

Other myeloid neoplasms included in the differential diagnosis are CML, *BCR-ABL1* positive, and AML with monocytic differentiation. The *BCR-ABL1* rearrangement, the defining feature of CML, has to be excluded before the diagnosis of JMML is rendered. The differentiation from AML with monocytic component is usually straightforward due to the defining blast threshold of 20%. However, in select cases with more frequent promonocytes, the differential count can be challenging. In addition, despite WHO recommendation of a threshold of 20% blasts for the diagnosis of AML, the definitive diagnosis and management of pediatric patients with 20% to 29% blasts remains unsettled in both JMML and MDS (127).

ATYPICAL CHRONIC MYELOID LEUKEMIA, *BCR-ABL1* NEGATIVE

Definition

aCML is an MDS/MPN characterized by a simultaneous presence of a marked granulocytic proliferation and significant dysplasia, dysgranulopoiesis in particular. Select clinical and morphologic features are similar to those seen in *BCR-ABL1*-positive CML. However, aCML is distinguished from *BCR-ABL1*-positive CML by marked dysgranulopoiesis and the absence of *BCR-ABL1* rearrangement.

Epidemiology, Clinical, and Laboratory Features

aCML is rare with an incidence of 1 to 2 cases for every 100 cases of *BCR-ABL1*-positive CML (128). The median age at diagnosis is the seventh or eighth decade (18,129–131); younger patients have been rarely diagnosed with aCML (132). Male-to-female ratio is approximately 1:1. The most common presenting features include leukocytosis with neutrophilia, splenomegaly, hepatomegaly, anemia, and variable platelet counts. WBC count is by definition elevated with a wide range from 18 to 300 × 10⁹/L (median 24 to 36 × 10⁹/L) (129–131,133).

Morphology and Immunophenotypic Features

Leukocytosis with neutrophilia is frequently accompanied by anemia and thrombocytopenia. By definition, aCML shows a WBC of more than 13 × 10⁹/L, which includes at least 10% of circulating neutrophilic precursors, a finding similar to that reported for *BCR-ABL1*-positive CML (128). Blast count is low, usually below 5%. Prominent dysgranulopoiesis is the cornerstone diagnostic feature of aCML and includes pseudo Pelger-Huet cells, and/or hyperlobulated neutrophils, abnormally condensed chromatin, and hypogranulation (Fig. 45.5A). A syndrome of abnormal chromatin clumping is considered a variant of aCML and will be discussed in the following paragraphs. Dysgranulopoiesis distinguishes aCML from newly diagnosed cases of *BCR-ABL1*-positive CML and from chronic neutrophilic leukemia. Of note, both *BCR-ABL1*-positive CML and *BCR-ABL1*-negative MPNs can develop severe dysplastic changes upon progression of the disease.

The absolute monocyte count can be higher than 1 × 10⁹/L; however monocytes should not exceed 10% of the differential count. Basophil count is typically below 2%. Anemia may be macrocytic with macroovalocytes. Platelets are frequently decreased; however, rare cases with thrombocytosis have been reported (range 9 to 2,675 × 10⁹/L) (129). The features of aCML originally identified by FAB Cooperative Leukemia Group included PB leukocytosis with immature myeloid forms, dysgranulopoiesis, and the absence of basophilia and monocytosis (12). Indeed, if any of these features are absent, an alternative diagnosis should be considered.

The BM is hypercellular with increased M:E ratio (Fig. 45.5B). Granulopoiesis is significantly increased and dysgranulopoiesis is always present. By definition, blast count is

below 20% and, in most instances, blast count is not significantly increased. Large aggregates and sheets of blasts are not present. Erythroid series frequently represents <10% of the BM elements (12). Dyserythropoiesis is not uncommon. The number of megakaryocytes is variable and can be decreased. Megakaryocytes are dysplastic with hypolobated and monolobated nuclei. Dwarf megakaryocytes are common. BM is rarely fibrotic.

Immunophenotyping and immunohistochemistry do not play a prominent role in the diagnosis of aCML. CD34 immunohistochemical stain can be used to confirm the blast percentage and select monocyte markers; for example, CD14 can help to exclude the presence of significant population of monocytes in BM.

Cytogenetic and Molecular Features

The majority of aCML cases harbor cytogenetic abnormalities. However, anomalies specific for this diagnosis have not been reported so far. The most common abnormalities are those that occur with high frequency in other myeloid diseases and include trisomy 8 and del(20q) (128).

Rare cases with t(8;9)(p22;p24) involving genes *PCM1 and JAK2* have been previously diagnosed as aCML (134,135). Detailed description of the morphologic features of PB and BM is not available in most of the cases. The t(8;9)(p22;p24) has also been reported in myeloid neoplasms, with morphologic features compatible with chronic eosinophilic leukemia, *de novo* AML, or acute lymphoblastic leukemia. Thus, in cases with t(8;9)(p22;p24), a detailed review of cellular morphology, correlation with laboratory values, and adherence to 2008 WHO criteria is necessary for a definitive classification.

A steady progress has been made in uncovering genetic lesions in aCML. Similar to CMML, among the most commonly involved are *TET2, ASXL1, EZH2, NRAS*, and *KRAS*, which are mutated in 5% to 25% of cases (132,136). On the contrary, somatic alterations of *SETBP1* recently described in aCML are not common in CMML (24% vs. 4% mutated cases, respectively) (137). The mutated *SETBP1* frequently coexisted with previously discovered genetic lesions and was significantly associated with *ASXL1* mutation. On the contrary, *JAK2* V617F mutations are usually not found in aCML, in contrast to CMML in which they are found in a small number of cases (133).

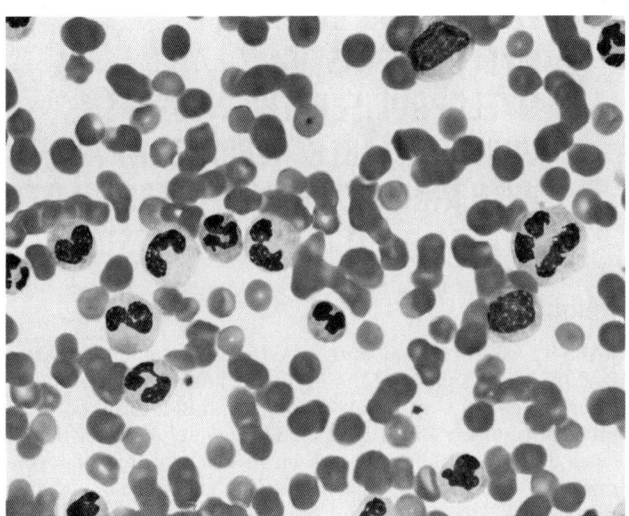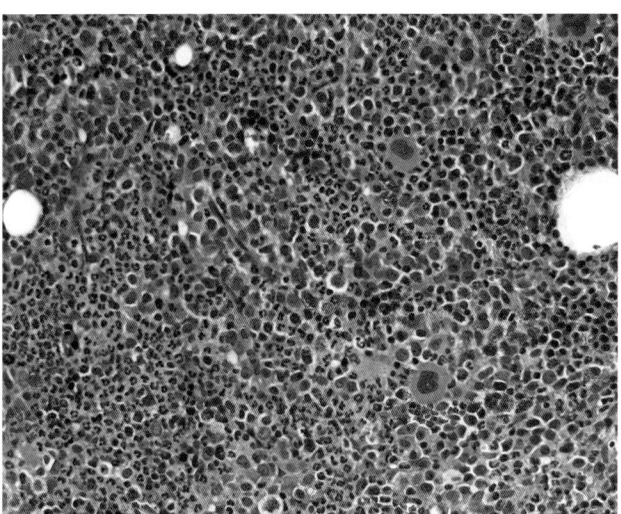

FIGURE 45.5. Atypical chronic myeloid leukemia. A: PB in aCML showing numerous dysplastic neutrophils with abnormal chromatin clumping. **B:** Biopsy showing a hypercellular BM with markedly increased granulopoiesis.

Clinical Course, Prognosis, and Treatment Options

aCML is an aggressive disease with poor response to currently available therapies. Median survival is 14 to 37 months and depends on the therapy received (129–131,138). The majority of patients succumb to BM failure, and approximately 20% to 40% transform to AML. The rate and time to transformation is variable and is often dependent on the type of initial treatment (conservative vs. induction-like therapy). Older age, female gender, leukocyte count of more than 50×10^9/L, and immature circulating myeloid precursors are all associated with poor prognosis. The increased percentage of BM blasts (>5%) and marked dyserythropoiesis were most significantly predictive of leukemic transformation (129). The first-line chemotherapy includes hydroxyurea, anagrelide, and interferon. Patients diagnosed with transformation to AML are treated with induction chemotherapy. Hematopoietic stem cell transplantation improved the outcome in younger patients with reported median survival of 46.8 months (139).

Differential Diagnosis

The main differential diagnosis is with *BCR-ABL1*-positive CML and chronic neutrophilic leukemia. Both of these entities can be relatively easily distinguished from aCML based on cytogenetics/molecular genetics and morphologic evaluation, with dysgranulopoiesis being the sine qua non of aCML diagnosis.

The syndrome of abnormal chromatin clumping is considered by some to be a morphologic variant of aCML (140–144). The defining feature is a characteristic morphology of neutrophil nuclei with large well-separated blocks of heterochromatin and euchromatin. This is frequently accompanied by decreased segmentation and is best appreciated in mature neutrophils. Leukocytosis, anemia, and thrombocytopenia are common. Rare patients show neutropenia at the onset of the disease. BM features are similar to those seen in other cases of aCML and include granulocytic hyperplasia, megaloblastoid erythropoiesis, and dysmegakaryopoiesis. Similar to aCML, the majority of the patients succumb to marrow failure, and approximately 30% experience transformation to AML. The aCML with abnormal chromatin clumping has to be distinguished from other entities with similar morphology such as rare cases of *BCR-ABL1*-positive CML with abnormal chromatin clumping. MDS/MPN with isolated isochromosome 17q can also present with hyposegmented neutrophils and prominent chromatin condensation. Select cases of this entity show prominent monocytosis and fulfill the diagnostic criteria for CMML (145,146). Reversible chromatin clumping can also be seen in neutrophils of patients treated with mycophenolate mofetil, in HIV infection, and occasionally in lymphoproliferative disorders (147,148). These causes of abnormal chromatin clumping are easily excluded through review of clinical history.

MYELODYSPLASTIC/ MYELOPROLIFERATIVE NEOPLASM, UNCLASSIFIABLE (MDS/MPN, U)

Definition

MDS/MPN,U has hybrid myelodysplastic and myeloproliferative features and at the time of the original diagnosis do not fulfill the diagnostic criteria for CMML, aCML, JMML, or any other form of MPN and MDS (5). MDS/MPN,U is a diagnosis of exclusion and requires an extensive work-up including cytogenetic and molecular analysis, and correlation with clinical history to

exclude a preexisting myeloid neoplasm and/or the effects of previous treatment with growth factors or cytotoxic drugs. The "reclassification" of known preexisting myeloid neoplasm as MDS/MPN,U due to development of additional either proliferative or dysplastic features is not appropriate. Similarly, diagnosis based on posttreatment samples obtained at follow-up or upon progression of the disease, even if hybrid myelodysplastic and myeloproliferative features are documented, is not appropriate in most cases.

Epidemiology, Clinical, and Laboratory Features

This is a rare neoplasm and demographic data are not available. Patients with MDS/MPN,U present with mixed myelodysplastic and myeloproliferative features such as ineffective hematopoiesis with resulting cytopenias and excessive proliferation of other lineages, including leukocytosis of at least 13×10^9/L and platelet counts higher than 450×10^9/L. Organomegaly, including splenomegaly, hepatomegaly, and infiltration of other extramedullary organs, can be present.

Morphology and Immunophenotype

PB can show leukocytosis and/or thrombocytosis with variable degrees of dysplastic features such as pseudo Pelger-Huet and hypogranular forms and giant and hypogranular platelets. Macrocytic or normocytic anemia or dimorphic red blood cells are common. By definition, blasts represent <20% of the differential count. Increase in blast cells above 10% may indicate a progression of the disease (5).

BM is hypercellular with myeloid hyperplasia and dysplasia in at least one of the hematopoietic lineages. Significant myelofibrosis can be observed.

The cytochemical features and immunophenotype can be similar to those seen in MDS or MPN.

Cytogenetic and Genetic Features

Exclusion of recurrent cytogenetic abnormalities defining other MPN or MDS is crucial. Conventional karyotyping and exclusion of *BCR-ABL1* rearrangement are required in each case. In addition, dependent on morphologic features, other defining genetic abnormalities such as *PDGFR* rearrangements may be pursued.

PROVISIONAL ENTITY IN MYELODYSPLASTIC/ MYELOPROLIFERATIVE NEOPLASM, UNCLASSIFIABLE: REFRACTORY ANEMIA WITH RING SIDEROBLASTS ASSOCIATED WITH MARKED THROMBOCYTOSIS

Definition

RARS-T is a provisional entity of WHO classification characterized by RA, dysplasia of the erythroid lineage, increased ring sideroblasts (15% or more), <5% blasts in BM, thrombocytosis (platelet counts ≥ 450×10^9/L), and large atypical megakaryocytes often resembling those seen in essential thrombocythemia (ET) (5). Secondary causes of ring sideroblasts including medications and toxins, and reactive thrombocytosis have to be ruled out. Cases with recurrent chromosomal abnormalities defining other WHO categories such as an isolated deletion of chromosome 5, abnormalities of chromosome 3, and

BCR-ABL1 rearrangement are excluded. Finally, the diagnosis of RARS-T is reserved for *de novo* disease arising in a patient with no previous myeloid neoplasm. It is questionable whether cases of RARS, which develop thrombocytosis in the natural course of the disease, should be included in this category.

Epidemiology, Clinical, and Laboratory Features

RARS-T is a rare entity with an unknown incidence. Upon review of MDS Dusseldorf Registry, only 0.7% of FAB-defined MDS cases were compatible with this diagnosis (7,149). According to the largest series reported to date, median age at diagnosis is 74 years with a range between 18 and 95 years (150). Men and women are equally affected.

By definition, patients present with anemia and thrombocytosis, with a median hemoglobin level of approximately 10 g/dL and median platelet count of 631×10^9/L (150,151). The defining threshold for thrombocytosis was lowered in 2008 WHO classification as compared to the earlier edition; however, the recent multi-institutional study indicates no difference in survival in RARS-T regardless of the cutoff for platelet count (less or more than 600×10^9/L) (150). Nevertheless, Raya et al. found that RARS-T cases with marked thrombocytosis show more prominent myeloproliferative features including higher WBC, higher incidence of splenomegaly, and more frequent *JAK2* V617F mutations (152). Patients with RARS-T show an incidence of thrombotic events similar to those with ET (~4 per 100 patient/year).

Morphology and Immunophenotype

PB frequently shows macrocytic RBCs. Anisopoikilocytosis, dimorphic red blood cells, and basophilic stippling are reported. Platelet counts are elevated. Giant platelets can be seen; however, abnormal platelet granulation is not common. White blood cell count is variable and dysgranulopoiesis is uncommon. Blasts are not seen in PB.

RARS-T is characterized by hypercellular BM, with striking abnormal, frequently enlarged megakaryocytes similar to those seen in *BCR-ABL1*-negative MPN (Fig. 45.6A). Dysplastic small hypolobated and monolobated forms can also be present; however, true micromegakaryocytes (diameter of <15 μm) are not common. It has been suggested that the MPN-like quality of megakaryocyte morphology may aid in distinction from RARS cases with mild thrombocytosis. However, the

heterogeneity of megakaryocyte morphology has been previously reported in RARS-T, and further studies are required to clarify this issue (153). Dyserythropoiesis may be prominent and includes maturation asynchrony, nuclear budding, and megaloblastoid chromatin. Ring sideroblasts represent more than 15% of erythroid precursors and are defined by a presence of at least five siderotic granules surrounding at least one third of the nuclear circumference of an erythroid precursor (154) (Fig. 45.6B). BM blasts constitute <5% of the differential count. Abnormal localization of immature precursors has not been reported in this entity. Similar to RARS, mast cell hyperplasia can be seen. The majority of cases show at least a mild increase in reticulin fibers. Significant reticulin fibrosis can also be observed.

Genetic Features

The majority of RARS-T patients show normal karyotype (153,155,156). Two most commonly affected genes with proposed role in the pathogenesis are *JAK2* and *SF3B1*. *JAK2* V617F mutation is seen in up to 80% of RARS-T cases (151,155,157). The *JAK2* V617F allele burden shows a wide range from 1% to 92% in one study (150). The *MPL* W515 mutations are much less common (150). The *SF3B1* was reported to be mutated in approximately 87% cases, with several different mutation hotspots and median allele burden of 40% (155). The coexistence of *JAK2* V617F and mutated *SF3B1* was seen in approximately 64% of RARS-T cases. Based on these observations, Cazzola et al. (158) have suggested a multistep pathogenesis schema in which initial acquisition of *SF3B1* mutation leads to mitochondrial iron overload and ineffective erythropoiesis, and subsequent *JAK2* V617F mutation provides myeloproliferative features. Select RARS-T cases show alterations of several other genes commonly associated with MPN or MDS/MPN such as *TET2* and *ASXL1* (156). It is unclear whether these genes play a role in pathogenesis of this disease.

Clinical Course, Prognosis, and Treatment Options

Clinical course and overall survival are more favorable in comparison to other subtypes of MDS/MPNs. Median survival varies between 71 and 101 months (159,160). Previous reports and the recent multi-institutional series confirm that survival in RARS-T is inferior to that seen in ET and longer than that

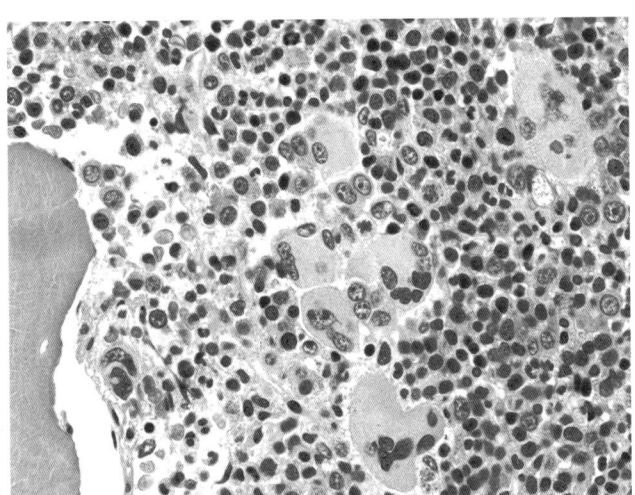

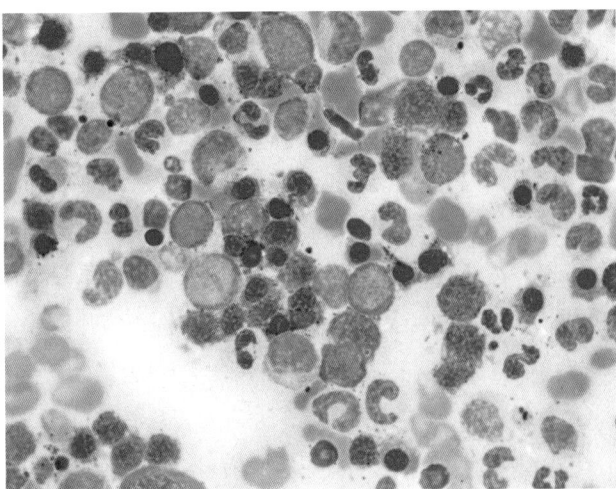

FIGURE 45.6. RARS associated with marked thrombocytosis. A: Increased megakaryopoiesis is one of the features of RARS-T. **B:** Ring sideroblasts in RARS-T.

of RARS (150,159–161). According to this report, *JAK2* V617F mutation status or platelet count is not associated with survival, even though earlier studies suggested to the contrary (162). The transformation to AML has been reported as 1.8/100 patients/year, a number slightly lower than that in RARS and significantly exceeding 0.7/100 patients/year seen in ET (150).

Patients with RARS-T are frequently treated with cytoreductive therapy such as hydroxyurea; however there is little evidence supporting the effectiveness of such approach. Approximately 50% of patients receive RBC transfusions or erythropoietin and antiplatelet therapy. The recent report indicated the responsiveness to single-agent lenalidomide in this neoplasm (163).

Differential Diagnosis

Select subtypes of MPNs and MDS can present with anemia, dyserythropoiesis, and thrombocytosis. The exclusion of entities associated with recurrent cytogenetic abnormalities, such as isolated deletion of chromosome 5, abnormalities of chromosome 3, and *BCR-ABL1* rearrangement, is straightforward even in cases with morphologic features similar to those seen in RARS-T. Differentiation of RARS-T from other disorders not defined by a specific genetic lesion can be challenging.

Approximately 5% of *BCR-ABL1*-negative MPN presenting with thrombocytosis, including ET and PMF, show increase in ring sideroblasts. These disorders show morphologic and molecular genetic features similar to RARS-T. ET presents with normocellular or slightly hypercellular BM and MPN-like megakaryocytes; however, in most cases, it lacks erythroid hyperplasia, dyserythropoiesis, and increased granulopoiesis. As discussed previously, the diagnosis of RARS-T requires the presence of dyserythropoiesis. Similarly, thrombocytosis and hypercellular marrow with megakaryocytic hyperplasia are present in PMF even in early prefibrotic stage. Decreased erythropoiesis, more pronounced dysmegakaryopoiesis, and megakaryocyte clustering are helpful in distinguishing this disease from RARS-T.

Considering clinicopathologic features overlapping with RARS, the designation of RARS-T as a distinct entity has been previously questioned. Rare cases of RARS develop thrombocytosis in the course of the disease, coincidental with the appearance of *JAK2* V617F mutation or with an increase in

JAK2 V617F allele burden (150,151). Thus, the acquisition of *JAK2* V617F mutation in RARS may indeed confer a myeloproliferative phenotype and confirm the existence of RARS to RARS-T continuum compatible with stepwise pathogenesis proposed by Cazzola et al. (158). However, most of the RARS and RARS-T cases show different clinical course and outcome justifying a separate category of RARS-T. The set of features most useful in separating RARS-T from RARS is megakaryocyte morphology and the presence of *JAK2* V617F mutation.

MISCELLANEOUS MYELOID NEOPLASMS WITH MYELODYSPLASTIC AND MYELOPROLIFERATIVE FEATURES

Myelodysplastic Syndrome with Isolated del(5q) and *JAK2* V617F Mutation

A small subset of MDS with isolated 5q deletion has been shown to harbor *JAK2* V617F mutations (164–166) (Fig. 45.7). These cases display typical features of MDS with isolated del(5q) such as hypolobated/monolobated megakaryocytes and initially have been described as having a more pronounced granulocytic proliferation with a higher WBC (5.21 vs. 4.45 × 10⁹/L in cases with wild-type *JAK2* gene) and a trend for higher platelet counts (164). These findings have not been confirmed in later series, which showed no phenotype or clinical outcome differences between MDS with isolated 5q deletion with and without *JAK2* V617F mutation (165,166). Anecdotal cases of MDS with isolated 5q deletion and *JAK2* V617F mutation responded to lenalidomide treatment (167, 168). Patnaik et al. (166) have also demonstrated the presence of *MPL* W515L mutations in <4% of MDS patients with isolated 5q deletion.

Interestingly, it has been previously reported that *JAK2* V617F can arise in a separate clone independent of isolated 5q deletion and thus is not specific to hematopoietic population harboring de(5q) (169). For the time being, the 2008 WHO classification recommends to classify these cases as MDS with isolated del(5q) and note the presence of *JAK2* V617F mutation.

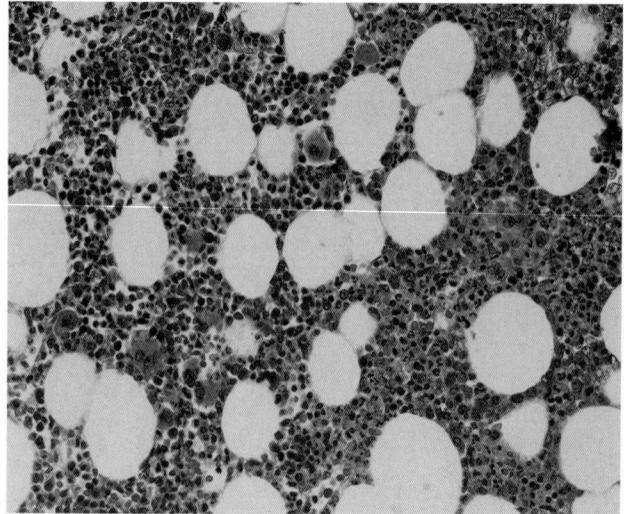
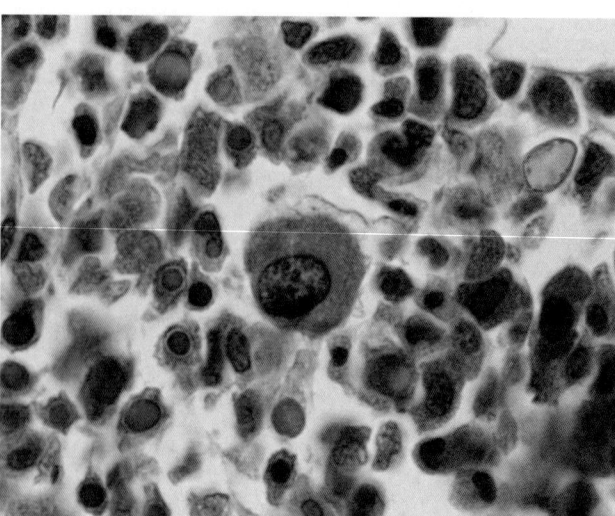

FIGURE 45.7. MDS with isolated del(5q) and *JAK2* V617F mutation. A: Hypercellular BM with increased granulopoiesis and dysmegakaryopoiesis. **B:** Higher magnification showing the typical megakaryocyte usually seen in MDS with isolated del(5q).

Myelodysplastic/Myeloproliferative Neoplasm with Isolated Isochromosome 17q

The isochromosome 17q is not an uncommon cytogenetic finding in myeloid neoplasms and has been reported in association with a complex karyotype or as secondary abnormality in patients with CML in accelerated or blast phase (170). It can rarely present as a sole abnormality in MDS and MPN with mixed myelodysplastic and myeloproliferative features (145,146,171–174). In the latter cases, the patient age varies with a median of 60 years. There is a male predominance. The majority of patients present with anemia, leukocytosis due to neutrophilia, and organomegaly. Dysgranulopoiesis including frequent nonsegmented forms, hyposegmented neutrophils (pseudo Pelger-Huet cells), ring nuclei, hypogranularity, and chromatin clumping is prominent (Fig. 45.8A). Monocytosis is commonly reported, and a proportion of cases fulfill the criteria for CMML-1 (145,146). Blasts frequently represent <5% of the differential count. Platelet counts are variable, commonly low. Abnormal hypogranular and giant platelets are often seen. The BM is markedly hypercellular with significant granulocytic proliferation and dysgranulopoiesis (Fig. 45.8B). In the majority of reported cases, blasts

constitute <10% of the cellularity. Dysplastic changes are also seen in erythroid progenitors and megakaryocytes (Fig. 45.8B). Dysplastic small megakaryocytes and large multinucleated have both been reported. Significant fibrosis is frequent (Fig. 45.8C). The median survival was reported as 2.5 years and 64% of patients progressed to AML (145).

The cases that do not fulfill the criteria for CMML, often show a more pleomorphic megakaryocyte morphology including large abnormal forms associated with marked fibrosis and organomegaly. These features are more reminiscent of an MPN. Such cases are best left in the category of MDS/MPN, unclassifiable. Cases, which fulfill the diagnostic criteria of CMML, can be placed in this category. However, if the goal of nosology is to produce biologically and clinically relevant disease categories, assigning patients with isolated isochromosome 17q to the CMML group may not reflect the dismal prognosis associated with this cytogenetic abnormality, particularly if a patient is placed in the CMML-1 category, which carries a far better prognosis and lower rate of transformation to AML than cases with the isolated isochromosome 17q. Comprehensive studies of larger case series may facilitate the more appropriate categorization of these cases.

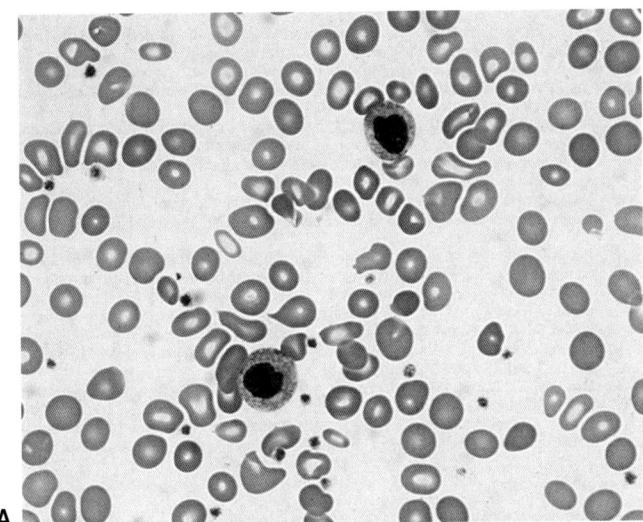
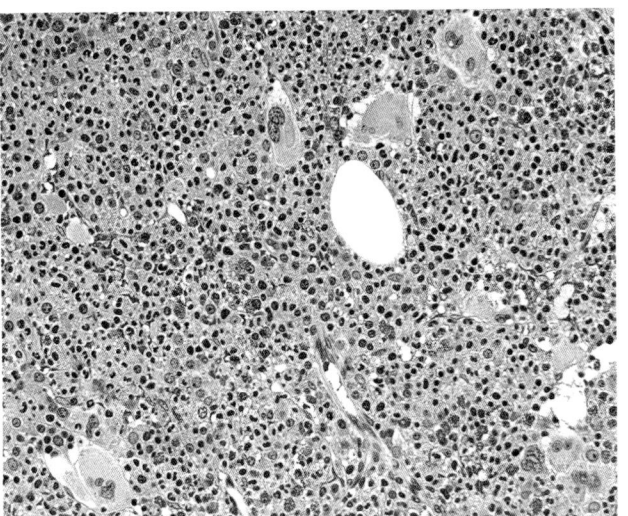
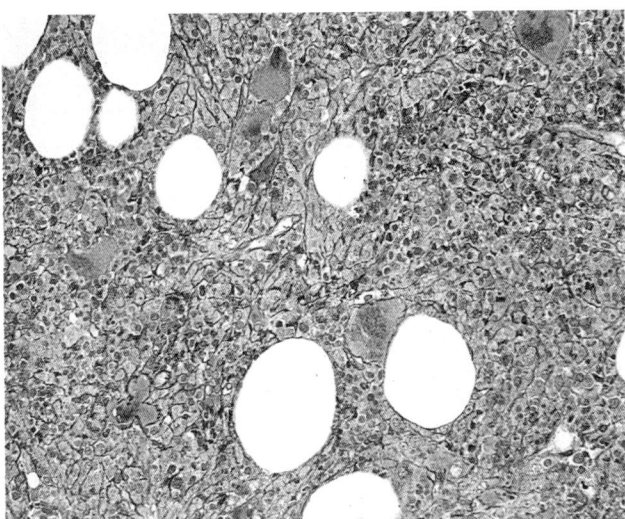

FIGURE 45.8. MDS/MPN with isolated isochromosome 17q. A: Dysplastic hyposegmented neutrophils in PB. **B:** BM biopsy with granulocytic hyperplasia and dysmegakaryopoiesis. **C:** BM fibrosis is frequently seen in cases harboring isolated isochromosome 17q abnormality (reticulin stain).

CONCLUSION

Despite significant advances in our understanding of MDS/MPNs, the diagnosis of these diseases still relies heavily on a careful clinicopathologic correlation. The diagnosis can at times be challenging due to the overlapping features and the changes in morphologic and laboratory characteristics during the evolution of the disease. One should remain vigilant to changes in phenotype related to an acquisition of secondary genetic lesions. The latter is not uncommon considering the inherent genomic instability of neoplastic cells and can significantly alter the presentation. Unraveling of the specific associations between genotype and phenotype and the discovery of initiating pathogenetic abnormalities will allow us to improve the existing classification and facilitate the diagnosis. This perhaps will also contribute to the development of targeted therapies and will improve patient selection for modern target therapy trials.

References

1. Sultan C. Dysmyelopoietic syndromes. Classification of acute leukemia. *Ann Int Med* 1977;87:740–753.
2. Bennett JM, Catovsky D, Daniel MT, et al. Proposals for the classification of the acute leukaemias. French-American-British (FAB) co-operative group. *Br J Haematol* 1976;33:451–458.
3. Bennett JM, Catovsky D, Daniel MT, et al. Proposals for the classification of the myelodysplastic syndromes. *Br J Haematol* 1982;51:189–199.
4. Jaffe E, Harris N, Stein H, et al., eds. *Pathology and genetics of tumours of haematopoietic and lymphoid tissues.* Lyon: IARC Press, 2001.
5. Vardiman J, Bennett J, Bain B. Myelodysplastic/myeloproliferative neoplasm, unclassifiable. In: Swerdlow S, ed. *WHO classification of tumours of haematopoietic and lymphoid tissues,* 4th ed. Lyon: IARC, 2008:85–86.
6. Orazi A, Bennett J, Germing U. Chronic myelomonocytic leukaemia. In: Swerdlow S, ed. *WHO classification of tumours of haematopoietic and lymphoid tissues,* 4th ed. Lyon: IARC, 2008:76–79.
7. Orazi A, Germing U. The myelodysplastic/myeloproliferative neoplasms: myeloproliferative diseases with dysplastic features. *Leukemia* 2008;22:1308–1319.
8. Fenaux P, Beuscart R, Lai JL, et al. Prognostic factors in adult chronic myelomonocytic leukemia: an analysis of 107 cases. *J Clin Oncol* 1988;6:1417–1424.
9. Onida F, Kantarjian HM, Smith TL, et al. Prognostic factors and scoring systems in chronic myelomonocytic leukemia: a retrospective analysis of 213 patients. *Blood* 2002;99:840–849.
10. Bowen DT. Chronic myelomonocytic leukemia: lost in classification? *Hematol Oncol* 2005;23:26–33.
11. Germing U, Gattermann N, Minning H, et al. Problems in the classification of CMML—dysplastic versus proliferative type. *Leuk Res* 1998;22:871–878.
12. Bennett JM, Catovsky D, Daniel MT, et al. The chronic myeloid leukaemias: guidelines for distinguishing chronic granulocytic, atypical chronic myeloid, and chronic myelomonocytic leukaemia. Proposals by the French-American-British Cooperative Leukaemia Group. *Br J Haematol* 1994;87:746–754.
13. Voglova J, Chrobak L, Neuwirtova R, et al. Myelodysplastic and myeloproliferative type of chronic myelomonocytic leukemia—distinct subgroups or two stages of the same disease? *Leuk Res* 2001;25:493–499.
14. Germing U, Strupp C, Knipp S, et al. Chronic myelomonocytic leukemia in the light of the WHO proposals. *Haematologica* 2007;92:974–977.
15. Nosslinger T, Reisner R, Gruner H, et al. Dysplastic versus proliferative CMML—a retrospective analysis of 91 patients from a single institution. *Leuk Res* 2001;25:741–747.
16. Storniolo AM, Moloney WC, Rosenthal DS, et al. Chronic myelomonocytic leukemia. *Leukemia* 1990;4: 766–770.
17. Orazi A, Chiu R, O'Malley DP, et al. Chronic myelomonocytic leukemia: The role of bone marrow biopsy immunohistology. *Mod Pathol* 2006;19:1536–1545.
18. Martiat P, Michaux JL, Rodhain J. Philadelphia-negative (Ph-) chronic myeloid leukemia (CML): comparison with Ph+ CML and chronic myelomonocytic leukemia. The Groupe Francais de Cytogenetique Hematologique. *Blood* 1991;78: 205–211.
19. Tefferi A, Hoagland HC, Therneau TM, et al. Chronic myelomonocytic leukemia: natural history and prognostic determinants. *Mayo Clin Proc* 1989;64:1246–1254.
20. Colonna M, Trinchieri G, Liu YJ. Plasmacytoid dendritic cells in immunity. *Nat Immunol* 2004;5:1219–1226.
21. Chen YC, Chou JM, Ketterling RP, et al. Histologic and immunohistochemical study of bone marrow monocytic nodules in 21 cases with myelodysplasia. *Am J Clin Pathol* 2003;120:874–881.
22. Vermi W, Facchetti F, Rosati S, et al. Nodal and extranodal tumor-forming accumulation of plasmacytoid monocytes/interferon-producing cells associated with myeloid disorders. *Am J Surg Pathol* 2004;28:585–595.
23. Gong X, Lu X, Fu Y, et al. Cytological features of chronic myelomonocytic leukemia in pleural effusion and lymph node fine needle aspiration. *Cytopathology* 2010;21:411–413.
24. Mathew RA, Bennett JM, Liu JJ, et al. Cutaneous manifestations in CMML: Indication of disease acceleration or transformation to AML and review of the literature. *Leuk Res* 2012;36:72–80.
25. Vitte F, Fabiani B, Benet C, et al. Specific skin lesions in chronic myelomonocytic leukemia: a spectrum of myelomonocytic and dendritic cell proliferations: a study of 42 cases. *Am J Surg Pathol* 2012;36:1302–1316.
26. Bourantas KL, Tsiara S, Panteli A, et al. Pleural effusion in chronic myelomonocytic leukemia. *Acta Haematol* 1998;99:34–37.
27. Huang CT, Kuo PH, Yao M, et al. Pleural effusion heralds acute leukemic transformation of chronic myelomonocytic leukemia. *South Med J* 2008;101:1279–1280.
28. Manoharan A. Malignant pleural effusion in chronic myelomonocytic leukaemia. *Thorax* 1991;46:461–462.
29. Mufti GJ, Oscier DG, Hamblin TJ, et al. Serous effusions in monocytic leukaemias. *Br J Haematol* 1984;58:547–552.
30. Yang DT, Greenwood JH, Hartung L, et al. Flow cytometric analysis of different CD14 epitopes can help identify immature monocytic populations. *Am J Clin Pathol* 2005;124:930–936.
31. Kern W, Bacher U, Haferlach C, et al. Acute monoblastic/monocytic leukemia and chronic myelomonocytic leukemia share common immunophenotypic features but differ in the extent of aberrantly expressed antigens and amount of granulocytic cells. *Leuk Lymphoma* 2011;52:92–100.
32. Lacronique-Gazaille C, Chaury MP, Le Guyader A, et al. A simple method for detection of major phenotypic abnormalities in myelodysplastic syndromes: expression of CD56 in CMML. *Haematologica* 2007;92:859–860.
33. Xu Y, McKenna RW, Karandikar NJ, et al. Flow cytometric analysis of monocytes as a tool for distinguishing chronic myelomonocytic leukemia from reactive monocytosis. *Am J Clin Pathol* 2005;124:799–806.
34. Harrington A, Olteanu H, Kroft S. The specificity of immunophenotypic alterations in blasts in nonacute myeloid disorders. *Am J Clin Pathol* 2010;134: 749–761.
35. Qubaja M, Marmey B, Le Tourneau A, et al. The detection of CD14 and CD16 in paraffin-embedded bone marrow biopsies is useful for the diagnosis of chronic myelomonocytic leukemia. *Virchows Arch* 2009;454:411–419.
36. Rollins-Raval MA, Roth CG. The value of immunohistochemistry for CD14, CD123, CD33, myeloperoxidase and CD68R in the diagnosis of acute and chronic myelomonocytic leukaemias. *Histopathology* 2012;60:933–942.
37. Ngo NT, Lampert IA, Naresh KN. Bone marrow trephine morphology and immunohistochemical findings in chronic myelomonocytic leukaemia. *Br J Haematol* 2008;141:771–781.
38. Delhommeau F, Dupont S, Della Valle V, et al. Mutation in TET2 in myeloid cancers. *N Engl J Med* 2009;360:2289–2301.
39. Grossmann V, Kohlmann A, Eder C, et al. Molecular profiling of chronic myelomonocytic leukemia reveals diverse mutations in >80% of patients with TET2 and EZH2 being of high prognostic relevance. *Leukemia* 2011;25:877–879.
40. Jankowska AM, Szpurka H, Tiu RV, et al. Loss of heterozygosity 4q24 and TET2 mutations associated with myelodysplastic/myeloproliferative neoplasms. *Blood* 2009;113:6403–6410.
41. Kohlmann A, Grossmann V, Klein HU, et al. Next-generation sequencing technology reveals a characteristic pattern of molecular mutations in 72.8% of chronic myelomonocytic leukemia by detecting frequent alterations in TET2, CBL, RAS, and RUNX1. *J Clin Oncol* 2010;28:3858–3865.
42. Kosmider O, Gelsi-Boyer V, Ciudad M, et al. TET2 gene mutation is a frequent and adverse event in chronic myelomonocytic leukemia. *Haematologica* 2009;94:1676–1681.
43. Perez C, Martinez-Calle N, Martin-Subero JI, et al. TET2 mutations are associated with specific 5-methylcytosine and 5-hydroxymethylcytosine profiles in patients with chronic myelomonocytic leukemia. *PLoS One* 2012;7:1–10.
44. Smith AE, Mohamedali AM, Kulasekararaj A, et al. Next-generation sequencing of the TET2 gene in 355 MDS and CMML patients reveals low-abundance mutant clones with early origins, but indicates no definite prognostic value. *Blood* 2010;116:3923–3932.
45. Yamazaki J, Taby R, Vasanthakumar A, et al. Effects of TET2 mutations on DNA methylation in chronic myelomonocytic leukemia. *Epigenetics* 2012;7: 201–207.
46. Braun T, Itzykson R, Renneville A, et al. Molecular predictors of response to decitabine in advanced chronic myelomonocytic leukemia: a phase 2 trial. *Blood* 2011;118:3824–3831.
47. Such E, Cervera J, Costa D, et al. Cytogenetic risk stratification in chronic myelomonocytic leukemia. *Haematologica* 2011;96:375–383.
48. Figueroa ME, Abdel-Wahab O, Lu C, et al. Leukemic IDH1 and IDH2 mutations result in a hypermethylation phenotype, disrupt TET2 function, and impair hematopoietic differentiation. *Cancer Cell* 2010;18:553–567.
49. Jankowska AM, Makishima H, Tiu RV, et al. Mutational spectrum analysis of chronic myelomonocytic leukemia includes genes associated with epigenetic regulation: UTX, EZH2, and DNMT3A. *Blood* 2011;118:3932–3941.
50. Abdel-Wahab O, Pardanani A, Patel J, et al. Concomitant analysis of EZH2 and ASXL1 mutations in myelofibrosis, chronic myelomonocytic leukemia and blast-phase myeloproliferative neoplasms. *Leukemia* 2011;25:1200–1202.
51. Gelsi-Boyer V, Brecqueville M, Devillier R, et al. Mutations in ASXL1 are associated with poor prognosis across the spectrum of malignant myeloid diseases. *J Hematol Oncol* 2012;5:1–6.
52. Gelsi-Boyer V, Trouplin V, Roquain J, et al. ASXL1 mutation is associated with poor prognosis and acute transformation in chronic myelomonocytic leukaemia. *Br J Haematol* 2010;151:365–375.
53. Ernst T, Chase AJ, Score J, et al. Inactivating mutations of the histone methyltransferase gene EZH2 in myeloid disorders. *Nat Genet* 2010;42:722–726.
54. Kroeze LI, Nikoloski G, da Silva-Coelho P, et al. Genetic defects in PRC2 components other than EZH2 are not common in myeloid malignancies. *Blood* 2012;119:1318–1319.
55. Score J, Hidalgo-Curtis C, Jones AV, et al. Inactivation of polycomb repressive complex 2 components in myeloproliferative and myelodysplastic/myeloproliferative neoplasms. *Blood* 2012;119:1208–1213.
56. Meggendorfer M, Roller A, Haferlach T, et al. SRSF2 mutations in 275 cases with chronic myelomonocytic leukemia (CMML). *Blood* 2012;120:3080–3088.
57. Yoshida K, Sanada M, Shiraishi Y, et al. Frequent pathway mutations of splicing machinery in myelodysplasia. *Nature* 2011;478:64–69.
58. Makishima H, Visconte V, Sakaguchi H, et al. Mutations in the spliceosome machinery, a novel and ubiquitous pathway in leukemogenesis. *Blood* 2012;119: 3203–3210.

59. Visconte V, Makishima H, Jankowska A, et al. SF3B1, a splicing factor is frequently mutated in refractory anemia with ring sideroblasts. *Leukemia* 2012;26: 542–545.
60. Kuo MC, Liang DC, Huang CF, et al. RUNX1 mutations are frequent in chronic myelomonocytic leukemia and mutations at the C-terminal region might predict acute myeloid leukemia transformation. *Leukemia* 2009;23:1426–1431.
61. Hirsch-Ginsberg C, LeMaistre AC, Kantarjian H, et al. RAS mutations are rare events in Philadelphia chromosome-negative/bcr gene rearrangement-negative chronic myelogenous leukemia, but are prevalent in chronic myelomonocytic leukemia. *Blood* 1990;76:1214–1219.
62. Tyner JW, Erickson H, Deininger MW, et al. High-throughput sequencing screen reveals novel, transforming RAS mutations in myeloid leukemia patients. *Blood* 2009;113:1749–1755.
63. Ricci C, Fermo E, Corti S, et al. RAS mutations contribute to evolution of chronic myelomonocytic leukemia to the proliferative variant. *Clin Cancer Res* 2010;16:2246–2256.
64. Gelsi-Boyer V, Trouplin V, Adelaide J, et al. Genome profiling of chronic myelomonocytic leukemia: frequent alterations of RAS and RUNX1 genes. *BMC Cancer* 2008;8:1–14.
65. Grand FH, Hidalgo-Curtis CE, Ernst T, et al. Frequent CBL mutations associated with 11q acquired uniparental disomy in myeloproliferative neoplasms. *Blood* 2009;113:6182–6192.
66. Muramatsu H, Makishima H, Jankowska AM, et al. Mutations of an E3 ubiquitin ligase c-Cbl but not TET2 mutations are pathogenic in juvenile myelomonocytic leukemia. *Blood* 2010;115:1969–1975.
67. Loh ML, Sakai DS, Flotho C, et al. Mutations in CBL occur frequently in juvenile myelomonocytic leukemia. *Blood* 2009;114:1859–1863.
68. Jelinek J, Oki Y, Gharibyan V, et al. JAK2 mutation 1849G>T is rare in acute leukemias but can be found in CMML, Philadelphia chromosome-negative CML, and megakaryocytic leukemia. *Blood* 2005;106:3370–3373.
69. Levine RL, Loriaux M, Huntly BJ, et al. The JAK2V617F activating mutation occurs in chronic myelomonocytic leukemia and acute myeloid leukemia, but not in acute lymphoblastic leukemia or chronic lymphocytic leukemia. *Blood* 2005;106:3377–3379.
70. Pich A, Riera L, Sismondi F, et al. JAK2V617F activating mutation is associated with the myeloproliferative type of chronic myelomonocytic leukaemia. *J Clin Pathol* 2009;62:798–801.
71. Klinakis A, Lobry C, Abdel-Wahab O, et al. A novel tumour-suppressor function for the Notch pathway in myeloid leukaemia. *Nature* 2011;473:230–233.
72. Daver N, Strati P, Jabbour E, et al. FLT3 mutations in myelodysplastic syndrome and chronic myelomonocytic leukemia. *Am J Hematol* 2013;88:56–59.
73. Lee BH, Tothova Z, Levine RL, et al. FLT3 mutations confer enhanced proliferation and survival properties to multipotent progenitors in a murine model of chronic myelomonocytic leukemia. *Cancer Cell* 2007;12:367–380.
74. Caudill JS, Sternberg AJ, Li CY, et al. C-terminal nucleophosmin mutations are uncommon in chronic myeloid disorders. *Br J Haematol* 2006;133:638–641.
75. Ernst T, Chase A, Zoi K, et al. Transcription factor mutations in myelodysplastic/myeloproliferative neoplasms. *Haematologica* 2010;95:1473–1480.
76. Germing U, Kundgen A, Gattermann N. Risk assessment in chronic myelomonocytic leukemia (CMML). *Leuk Lymphoma* 2004;45:1311–1318.
77. Courville EL, Wu Y, Kourda J, et al. Clinicopathologic analysis of acute myeloid leukemia arising from chronic myelomonocytic leukemia. *Mod Pathol* 2013; 218:1–11.
78. Greenberg P, Cox C, LeBeau MM, et al. International scoring system for evaluating prognosis in myelodysplastic syndromes. *Blood* 1997;89:2079–2088.
79. Germing U, Strupp C, Aivado M, et al. New prognostic parameters for chronic myelomonocytic leukemia. *Blood* 2002;100:731–732.
80. Beran M, Kantarjian H. Results of topotecan-based combination therapy in patients with myelodysplastic syndromes and chronic myelomonocytic leukemia. *Semin Hematol* 1999;36:3–10.
81. Gerhartz HH, Marcus R, Delmer A, et al. A randomized phase II study of low-dose cytosine arabinoside (LD-AraC) plus granulocyte-macrophage colony-stimulating factor (rhGM-CSF) in myelodysplastic syndromes (MDS) with a high risk of developing leukemia. EORTC Leukemia Cooperative Group. *Leukemia* 1994;8:16–23.
82. Wattel E, Guerci A, Hecquet B, et al. A randomized trial of hydroxyurea versus VP16 in adult chronic myelomonocytic leukemia. Groupe Francais des Myelodysplasies and European CMML Group. *Blood* 1996;88:2480–2487.
83. Aribi A, Borthakur G, Ravandi F, et al. Activity of decitabine, a hypomethylating agent, in chronic myelomonocytic leukemia. *Cancer* 2007;109:713–717.
84. Costa R, Abdulhaq H, Haq B, et al. Activity of azacitidine in chronic myelomonocytic leukemia. *Cancer* 2011;117:2690–2696.
85. Garcia-Manero G, Gore SD, Cogle C, et al. Phase I study of oral azacitidine in myelodysplastic syndromes, chronic myelomonocytic leukemia, and acute myeloid leukemia. *J Clin Oncol* 2011;29:2521–2527.
86. Wijermans PW, Ruter B, Baer MR, et al. Efficacy of decitabine in the treatment of patients with chronic myelomonocytic leukemia (CMML). *Leuk Res* 2008;32: 587–591.
87. Fenaux P, Mufti GJ, Hellstrom-Lindberg E, et al. Efficacy of azacitidine compared with that of conventional care regimens in the treatment of higher-risk myelodysplastic syndromes: a randomised, open-label, phase III study. *Lancet Oncol* 2009;10:223–232.
88. Bacher U, Haferlach T, Schnittger S, et al. Recent advances in diagnosis, molecular pathology and therapy of chronic myelomonocytic leukaemia. *Br J Haematol* 2011;153:149–167.
89. Eissa H, Gooley TA, Sorror ML, et al. Allogeneic hematopoietic cell transplantation for chronic myelomonocytic leukemia: relapse-free survival is determined by karyotype and comorbidities. *Biol Blood Marrow Transplant* 2011;17:908–915.
90. Melo JV, Myint H, Galton DA, et al. P190BCR-ABL chronic myeloid leukaemia: the missing link with chronic myelomonocytic leukaemia? *Leukemia* 1994;8: 208–211.
91. Boiocchi L, Espinal-Witter R, Geyer JT, et al. Development of monocytosis in patients with primary myelofibrosis indicates an accelerated phase of the disease. *Mod Pathol* 2013;26:204–212.
92. Elliott MA, Verstovsek S, Dingli D, et al. Monocytosis is an adverse prognostic factor for survival in younger patients with primary myelofibrosis. *Leuk Res* 2007;31:1503–1509.
93. Wang SA, Galili N, Cerny J, et al. Chronic myelomonocytic leukemia evolving from preexisting myelodysplasia shares many features with de novo disease. *Am J Clin Pathol* 2006;126:789–797.
94. Breccia M, Cannella L, Frustaci A, et al. Chronic myelomonocytic leukemia with antecedent refractory anemia with excess blasts: further evidence for the arbitrary nature of current classification systems. *Leuk Lymphoma* 2008;49: 1292–1296.
95. Rigolin GM, Cuneo A, Roberti MG, et al. Myelodysplastic syndromes with monocytic component: hematologic and cytogenetic characterization. *Haematologica* 1997;82:25–30.
96. Czader M, Orazi A. Therapy-related myeloid neoplasms. *Am J Clin Pathol* 2009;132:410–425.
97. George R, Pearson AD, Evans J, et al. Secondary chronic myelomonocytic leukemia with t(9;11) in a child. *Cancer Genet Cytogenet* 1994;75:64–66.
98. Satake N, Ishida Y, Otoh Y, et al. Novel MLL-CBP fusion transcript in therapy-related chronic myelomonocytic leukemia with a t(11;16)(q23;p13) chromosome translocation. *Genes Chromosomes Cancer* 1997;20:60–63.
99. Baumann I BJ, Niemeyer CM, Thiele J, Shannon K. Juvenile myelomonocytic leukemia. In: Swerdlow SH Campo E, Harris NL, eds. *World Health Organization classification of tumors: pathology and genetics of tumours of haematopoietic and lymphoid tissues.* Lyon: IARC, 2008:82.
100. Chan RJ, Cooper T, Kratz CP, et al. Juvenile myelomonocytic leukemia: a report from the 2nd International JMML Symposium. *Leuk Res* 2009;33:355–362.
101. Hasle H, Niemeyer CM, Chessells JM, et al. A pediatric approach to the WHO classification of myelodysplastic and myeloproliferative diseases. *Leukemia* 2003;17:277–282.
102. Passmore SJ, Chessells JM, Kempski H, et al. Paediatric myelodysplastic syndromes and juvenile myelomonocytic leukaemia in the UK: a population-based study of incidence and survival. *Br J Haematol* 2003;121:758–767.
103. Niemeyer CM, Kang MW, Shin DH, et al. Germline CBL mutations cause developmental abnormalities and predispose to juvenile myelomonocytic leukemia. *Nat Genet* 2010;42:794–800.
104. Honig GR, Suarez CR, Vida LN, et al. Juvenile myelomonocytic leukemia (JMML) with the hematologic phenotype of severe beta thalassemia. *Am J Hematol* 1998;58:67–71.
105. Niemeyer CM, Arico M, Basso G, et al. Chronic myelomonocytic leukemia in childhood: a retrospective analysis of 110 cases. European Working Group on Myelodysplastic Syndromes in Childhood (EWOG-MDS). *Blood* 1997;89: 3534–3543.
106. Emanuel PD, Bates LJ, Castleberry RP, et al. Selective hypersensitivity to granulocyte-macrophage colony-stimulating factor by juvenile chronic myeloid leukemia hematopoietic progenitors. *Blood* 1991;77:925–929.
107. Kotecha N, Flores NJ, Irish JM, et al. Single-cell profiling identifies aberrant STAT5 activation in myeloid malignancies with specific clinical and biologic correlates. *Cancer Cell* 2008;14:335–343.
108. Nishio N, Takahashi Y, Tanaka M, et al. Aberrant phosphorylation of STAT5 by granulocyte-macrophage colony-stimulating factor in infant cytomegalovirus infection mimicking juvenile myelomonocytic leukemia. *Leuk Res* 2011;35: 1261–1264.
109. Loh ML. Recent advances in the pathogenesis and treatment of juvenile myelomonocytic leukaemia. *Br J Haematol* 2011;152:677–687.
110. Niemeyer CM, Kratz CP. Paediatric myelodysplastic syndromes and juvenile myelomonocytic leukaemia: molecular classification and treatment options. *Br J Haematol* 2008;140:610–624.
111. Kalra R, Paderanga DC, Olson K, et al. Genetic analysis is consistent with the hypothesis that NF1 limits myeloid cell growth through p21ras. *Blood* 1994;84:3435–3439.
112. Miyauchi J, Asada M, Sasaki M, et al. Mutations of the N-ras gene in juvenile chronic myelogenous leukemia. *Blood* 1994;83:2248–2254.
113. Shannon KM, O'Connell P, Martin GA, et al. Loss of the normal NF1 allele from the bone marrow of children with type 1 neurofibromatosis and malignant myeloid disorders. *N Engl J Med* 1994;330:597–601.
114. Side LE, Emanuel PD, Taylor B, et al. Mutations of the NF1 gene in children with juvenile myelomonocytic leukemia without clinical evidence of neurofibromatosis, type 1. *Blood* 1998;92:267–272.
115. Loh ML, Vattikuti S, Schubbert S, et al. Mutations in PTPN11 implicate the SHP-2 phosphatase in leukemogenesis. *Blood* 2004;103:2325–2331.
116. Perez B, Kosmider O, Cassinat B, et al. Genetic typing of CBL, ASXL1, RUNX1, TET2 and JAK2 in juvenile myelomonocytic leukaemia reveals a genetic profile distinct from chronic myelomonocytic leukaemia. *Br J Haematol* 2010;151: 460–468.
117. Passmore SJ, Hann IM, Stiller CA, et al. Pediatric myelodysplasia: a study of 68 children and a new prognostic scoring system. *Blood* 1995;85:1742–1750.
118. Bader-Meunier B, Tchernia G, Mielot F, et al. Occurrence of myeloproliferative disorder in patients with Noonan syndrome. *J Pediatr* 1997;130:885–889.
119. Lavin VA, Hamid R, Patterson J, et al. Use of human androgen receptor gene analysis to aid the diagnosis of JMML in female Noonan syndrome patients. *Pediatr Blood Cancer* 2008;51:298–302.
120. Alsultan A, Khalifah M, Alrabiaah AA. Spontaneous remission of juvenile myelomonocytic leukemia with NRAS mutation. *Pediatr Hematol Oncol* 2012;29: 624–626.
121. Doisaki S, Muramatsu H, Shimada A, et al. Somatic mosaicism for oncogenic NRAS mutations in juvenile myelomonocytic leukemia. *Blood* 2012;120: 1485–1488.
122. Flotho C, Kratz CP, Bergstrasser E, et al. Genotype-phenotype correlation in cases of juvenile myelomonocytic leukemia with clonal RAS mutations. *Blood* 2008;111:966–967.
123. Matsuda K, Shimada A, Yoshida N, et al. Spontaneous improvement of hematologic abnormalities in patients having juvenile myelomonocytic leukemia with specific RAS mutations. *Blood* 2007;109:5477–5480.
124. Yoshida N, Yagasaki H, Xu Y, et al. Correlation of clinical features with the mutational status of GM-CSF signaling pathway-related genes in juvenile myelomonocytic leukemia. *Pediatr Res* 2009;65:334–340.
125. Bresolin S, Zecca M, Flotho C, et al. Gene expression-based classification as an independent predictor of clinical outcome in juvenile myelomonocytic leukemia. *J Clin Oncol* 2010;28:1919–1927.

126. Olk-Batz C, Poetsch AR, Nollke P, et al. Aberrant DNA methylation character-izes juvenile myelomonocytic leukemia with poor outcome. *Blood* 2011;117: 4871–4880.

127. Hasle H, Baumann I, Bergstrasser E, et al. The International Prognostic Scor-ing System (IPSS) for childhood myelodysplastic syndrome (MDS) and juvenile myelomonocytic leukemia (JMML). *Leukemia* 2004;18:2008–2014.

128. Vardiman J, Bennett J, Bain B. Atypical chronic myeloid leukaemia, *BCR-ABL1* negative. In: Swerdlow S, ed. *WHO classification of tumours of haematopoietic and lymphoid tissues,* 4th ed. Lyon: IARC, 2008:80–81.

129. Breccia M, Biondo F, Latagliata R, et al. Identification of risk factors in atypical chronic myeloid leukemia. *Haematologica* 2006;91:1566–1568.

130. Hernandez JM, del Canizo MC, Cuneo A, et al. Clinical, hematological and cytogenetic characteristics of atypical chronic myeloid leukemia. *Ann Oncol* 2000;11:441–444.

131. Kurzrock R, Bueso-Ramos CE, Kantarjian H, et al. BCR rearrangement-negative chronic myelogenous leukemia revisited. *J Clin Oncol* 2001;19:2915–2926.

132. Koldehoff M, Steckel NK, Hegerfeldt Y, et al. Clinical course and molecular fea-tures in 21 patients with atypical chronic myeloid leukemia. *Int J Lab Hematol* 2012;34:e3–5.

133. Fend F, Horn T, Koch I, et al. Atypical chronic myeloid leukemia as defined in the WHO classification is a JAK2 V617F negative neoplasm. *Leuk Res* 2008;32: 1931–1935.

134. Bousquet M, Quelen C, De Mas V, et al. The t(8;9)(p22;p24) translocation in atypi-cal chronic myeloid leukaemia yields a new PCM1-JAK2 fusion gene. *Oncogene* 2005;24:7248–7252.

135. Reiter A, Walz C, Watmore A, et al. The t(8;9)(p22;p24) is a recurrent abnor-mality in chronic and acute leukemia that fuses PCM1 to JAK2. *Cancer Res* 2005;65:2662–2667.

136. Cogswell PC, Morgan R, Dunn M, et al. Mutations of the ras protooncogenes in chronic myelogenous leukemia: a high frequency of ras mutations in bcr/abl rearrangement-negative chronic myelogenous leukemia. *Blood* 1989;74: 2629–2633.

137. Piazza R, Valletta S, Winkelmann N, et al. Recurrent SETBP1 mutations in atypi-cal chronic myeloid leukemia. *Nat Genet* 2013;45:18–27.

138. Costello R, Sainty D, Lafage-Pochitaloff M, et al. Clinical and biological aspects of Philadelphia-negative/BCR-positive chronic myeloid leukemia. *Leuk Lymphoma* 1997;25:225–232.

139. Koldehoff M, Beelen DW, Trenschel R, et al. Outcome of hematopoietic stem cell transplantation in patients with atypical chronic myeloid leukemia. *Bone Marrow Transplant* 2004;34:1047–1050.

140. Brizard A, Huret JL, Lamotte F, et al. Three cases of myelodysplastic-myelopro-liferative disorder with abnormal chromatin clumping in granulocytes. *Br J Hae-matol* 1989;72:294–295.

141. Felman P, Bryon PA, Gentilhomme O, et al. The syndrome of abnormal chromatin clumping in leucocytes: a myelodysplastic disorder with proliferative features? *Br J Haematol* 1988;70:49–54.

142. Gustke SS, Becker GA, Garancis JC, et al. Chromatin clumping in mature leuko-cytes: a hitherto unrecognized abnormality. *Blood* 1970;35:637–658.

143. Jaen A, Irriguible D, Milla F, et al. Abnormal chromatin clumping in leuco-cytes: a clue to a new subtype of myelodysplastic syndrome. *Eur J Haematol* 1990;45:209–214.

144. Morel P, Bryon PA, Guyon JM, et al. [Malignant hemopathy of the aplastic kind with important nuclear anomalies of granulocytes]. *Semin Hop* 1968;44: 3026–3028.

145. McClure RF, Dewald GW, Hoyer JD, et al. Isolated isochromosome 17q: a distinct type of mixed myeloproliferative disorder/myelodysplastic syndrome with an aggressive clinical course. *Br J Haematol* 1999;106:445–454.

146. Kanagal-Shamanna R, Bueso-Ramos CE, Barkoh B, et al. Myeloid neoplasms with isolated isochromosome 17q represent a clinicopathologic entity associated with myelodysplastic/myeloproliferative features, a high risk of leukemic trans-formation, and wild-type TP53. *Cancer* 2012;118:2879–2888.

147. Banerjee R, Halil O, Bain BJ, et al. Neutrophil dysplasia caused by mycophenolate mofetil. *Transplantation* 2000;70:1608–1610.

148. Daliphard S, Accard F, Delattre C, et al. Reversible abnormal chromatin clumping in granulocytes from six transplant patients treated with mycophenolate mofetil: a rare adverse effect mimicking abnormal chromatin clumping syndrome. *Br J Haematol* 2002;116:726–727.

149. Gattermann N, Billiet J, Kronenwett R, et al. High frequency of the JAK2 V617F mutation in patients with thrombocytosis (platelet count>600×109/L) and ringed sideroblasts more than 15% considered as MDS/MPD, unclassifiable. *Blood* 2007;109:1334–1335.

150. Broseus J, Florensa L, Zipperer E, et al. Clinical features and course of refractory anemia with ring sideroblasts associated with marked thrombocytosis. *Haema-tologica* 2012;97:1036–1041.

151. Malcovati L, Della Porta MG, Pietra D, et al. Molecular and clinical features of refractory anemia with ringed sideroblasts associated with marked thrombocy-tosis. *Blood* 2009;114:3538–3545.

152. Raya JM, Arenillas L, Domingo A, et al. Refractory anemia with ringed sidero-blasts associated with thrombocytosis: comparative analysis of marked with non-marked thrombocytosis, and relationship with JAK2 V617F mutational status. *Int J Hematol* 2008;88:387–395.

153. Gurevich I, Luthra R, Konoplev SN, et al. Refractory anemia with ring sidero-blasts associated with marked thrombocytosis: a mixed group exhibiting a spec-trum of morphologic findings. *Am J Clin Pathol* 2011;135:398–403.

154. Mufti GJ, Bennett JM, Goasguen J, et al. Diagnosis and classification of myelodys-plastic syndrome: International Working Group on Morphology of myelodysplastic syndrome (IWGM-MDS) consensus proposals for the definition and enumeration of myeloblasts and ring sideroblasts. *Haematologica* 2008;93:1712–1717.

155. Jeromin S, Haferlach T, Grossmann V, et al. High frequencies of SF3B1 and JAK2 mutations in refractory anemia with ring sideroblasts associated with marked thrombocytosis strengthen the assignment to the category of myelodysplastic/myeloproliferative neoplasms. *Haematologica* 2013;98:15–17.

156. Szpurka H, Jankowska AM, Makishima H, et al. Spectrum of mutations in RARS-T patients includes TET2 and ASXL1 mutations. *Leuk Res* 2010;34:969–973.

157. Flach J, Dicker F, Schnittger S, et al. Mutations of JAK2 and TET2, but not CBL are detectable in a high portion of patients with refractory anemia with ring sideroblasts and thrombocytosis. *Haematologica* 2010;95:518–519.

158. Cazzola M, Malcovati L, Invernizzi R. Myelodysplastic/myeloproliferative neo-plasms. *Hematol Am Soc Hematol Educ Program* 2011;2011:264–272.

159. Shaw GR. Ringed sideroblasts with thrombocytosis: an uncommon mixed myelodysplastic/myeloproliferative disease of older adults. *Br J Haematol* 2005; 131:180–184.

160. Wang SA, Hasserjian RP, Loew JM, et al. Refractory anemia with ringed sid-eroblasts associated with marked thrombocytosis harbors JAK2 mutation and shows overlapping myeloproliferative and myelodysplastic features. *Leukemia* 2006;20:1641–1644.

161. Atallah E, Nussenzveig R, Yin CC, et al. Prognostic interaction between thrombo-cytosis and JAK2 V617F mutation in the WHO subcategories of myelodysplastic/myeloproliferative disease-unclassifiable and refractory anemia with ring sid-eroblasts and marked thrombocytosis. *Leukemia* 2008;22:1295–1298.

162. Schmitt-Graeff A, Thiele J, Zuk I, et al. Essential thrombocythemia with ringed sideroblasts: a heterogeneous spectrum of diseases, but not a distinct entity. *Hae-matologica* 2002;87:392–399.

163. Huls G, Mulder AB, Rosati S, et al. Efficacy of single-agent lenalidomide in patients with JAK2 (V617F) mutated refractory anemia with ring sideroblasts and thrombocytosis. *Blood* 2010;116:180–182.

164. Ingram W, Lea NC, Cervera J, et al. The JAK2 V617F mutation identifies a sub-group of MDS patients with isolated deletion 5q and a proliferative bone marrow. *Leukemia* 2006;20:1319–1321.

165. Wong KF, Wong WS, Siu LL, et al. JAK2 V617F mutation is associated with 5q-syndrome in Chinese. *Leuk Lymphoma* 2009;50:1333–1335.

166. Patnaik MM, Lasho TL, Finke CM, et al. WHO-defined 'myelodysplastic syndrome with isolated del(5q)' in 88 consecutive patients: survival data, leukemic trans-formation rates and prevalence of JAK2, MPL and IDH mutations. *Leukemia* 2010;24:1283–1289.

167. Nomdedeu M, Maffioli M, Calvo X, et al. Efficacy of lenalidomide in a patient with myelodysplastic syndrome with isolated del(5q) and JAK2V617F mutation. *Leuk Res* 2011;35:1276–1278.

168. Melchert M, Kale V, List A. The role of lenalidomide in the treatment of patients with chromosome 5q deletion and other myelodysplastic syndromes. *Curr Opin Hematol* 2007;14:123–129.

169. Sokol L, Caceres G, Rocha K, et al. JAK2(V617F) mutation in myelodysplastic syndrome (MDS) with del(5q) arises in genetically discordant clones. *Leuk Res* 2010;34:821–823.

170. Hernandez-Boluda JC, Cervantes F, Costa D, et al. Blast crisis of Ph-positive chronic myeloid leukemia with isochromosome 17q: report of 12 cases and review of the literature. *Leuk Lymphoma* 2000;38:83–90.

171. Sole F, Torrabadella M, Granada I, et al. Isochromosome 17q as a sole anomaly: a distinct myelodysplastic syndrome entity? *Leuk Res* 1993;17:717–720.

172. Weh HJ, Kuse R, Hossfeld DK. Acute nonlymphocytic leukemia (ANLL) with isochromosome i(17q) as the sole chromosomal anomaly: a distinct entity? *Eur J Haematol* 1990;44:312–314.

173. Xiao Z, Liu S, Yu M, et al. Isochromosome 17q in patients with myelodysplastic syndromes: six new cases. *Haematologica* 2003;88:714–715.

174. Fioretos T, Strombeck B, Sandberg T, et al. Isochromosome 17q in blast crisis of chronic myeloid leukemia and in other hematologic malignancies is the result of clustered breakpoints in 17p11 and is not associated with coding TP53 muta-tions. *Blood* 1999;94:225–232.

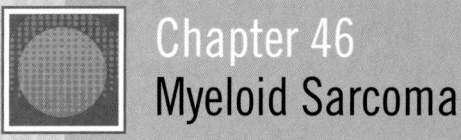

Chapter 46
Myeloid Sarcoma

Stefano A. Pileri • Brunangelo Falini • Stefano Ascani • Attilio Orazi

 ## DEFINITION

According to the current WHO Classification (1), myeloid sarcoma (MS) (ICD-O code 9930/3) is "a tumour mass consisting of myeloblasts, monoblasts or haematopoietic precursors occurring at an anatomical site other than the bone marrow."

In the past, it was also termed "chloroma," "extramedullary acute myeloid leukemia," "extramedullary myeloid tumor," or "granulocytic sarcoma." While most of these items deal with the histogenesis of the disease, the one "chloroma" refers to the characteristic green color that the tumor reveals on gross examination due to myeloperoxidase (MPO) oxidation.

Because of its sporadic observation and management difficulties, it has been the object of several case reports (more than 400 quoted in PubMed during the last 5 years) but only a few comprehensive studies (2–6).

 ## EPIDEMIOLOGY

According to the authors' experience based on the observation of about 200 cases, MS shows a predilection for males and last decades of life, the male to female ratio being 1.2:1 and the median age 56.5 years (range from 1 month to 89 years). In the past, the publication of some pediatric series gave the impression that MS might have a higher prevalence in children, but this has not been confirmed in cooperative studies carried out by Italian and German Groups (7).

 ## SITES OF INVOLVEMENT

Almost every site of the body can be involved (Fig. 46.1), the lymph node, gastrointestinal tract, bone, soft tissue, and testis being more frequently affected (7). In <10% of cases, MS presents at multiple anatomical sites (5).

 ## CLINICAL FEATURES

Clinical symptoms are largely dependent on the site of involvement. Thus, they can vary from the rapid onset of a mass to jaundice in case of bile duct infiltration (8). In the skin, lesions usually present as multiple papules, plaques, or nodules. The most commonly involved region is the trunk, although the head, neck, and extremities are also frequently affected (9).

Importantly, MS may occur *de novo* (about 27% of cases), precede, or coincide with acute myeloid leukemia (AML) or chronic myelogenous leukemia (CML) or with other types of myeloproliferative neoplasm (MPN) or myelodysplastic syndrome (MDS) (5). It may be the first evidence of AML or of transformation of CML (10) but also the initial manifestation of relapse in a previously treated AML in bone marrow

remission (11). On this respect, it has recently been suggested that isolated MS occurs in 8% to 20% of patients who have undergone allogeneic stem cell transplantation (12). The reasons for this are currently unclear, but might have to do with patterns of graft-versus-leukemia surveillance or the biology of high-risk AML treated with transplantation.

In some cases, MS is associated with a simultaneous or previously treated non-Hodgkin lymphoma (e.g., follicular lymphoma, mycosis fungoides, peripheral T-cell lymphoma [PTCL], not otherwise specified) or a previous history of nonhematopoietic tumor (e.g., germ cell tumor, prostatic carcinoma, endometrial carcinoma, breast cancer, intestinal adenocarcinoma, or even colonic adenoma). Interestingly, patients in the latter setting had usually undergone chemotherapy some years prior to develop MS.

 ## MORPHOLOGY

At low power, MS displays quite different growth patterns depending on the involved anatomic site. At extranodal sites, neoplastic cells frequently give rise to solid nests and/or Indian files that are surrounded by variably thick fibrotic septa, thus mimicking metastatic carcinoma (Figs. 46.2 to 46.6). In the lymph node, they can infiltrate the paracortex by sparing some reactive follicles or can completely efface the normal structure with diffusion outside the capsule. MS more commonly consists of myeloblasts with or without features of promyelocytic or neutrophilic maturation (Fig. 46.3). In the more immature tumors, the neoplastic growth is sustained by a monotonous population consisting of large cells with a rim of cytoplasm of variable size and basophilia and with a round to oval nucleus with one or more prominent nucleoli (Fig. 46.4). Mitotic figures are usually numerous. Foci of necrosis can be seen. In about one-third of instances, it displays myelomonocytic or pure monoblastic morphology (Fig. 46.5) (5). Tumors with trilineage hematopoiesis or predominantly erythroid precursors or megakaryocytes are rare and may occur in conjunction with transformation of MPN (5). Notably, the recognition of cases with erythroid or megakaryoblastic characteristics is uneasy on pure morphologic grounds (Fig. 46.6). Under these circumstances, immunohistochemistry plays a pivotal role for the diagnosis. In particular, tumors of the megakaryocytic cell lineage can be easily confused with metastases of undifferentiated carcinomas, and only the application of a sufficiently large panel of antibodies allows the exact interpretation.

 ## CYTOCHEMISTRY

The diagnosis of MS is validated by the results of cytochemical and/or immunophenotypic analyses (5). On imprints, cytochemical stains for MPO, naphthol ASD chloroacetate esterase (NASDCAE), and nonspecific esterase (NSE) may assist in

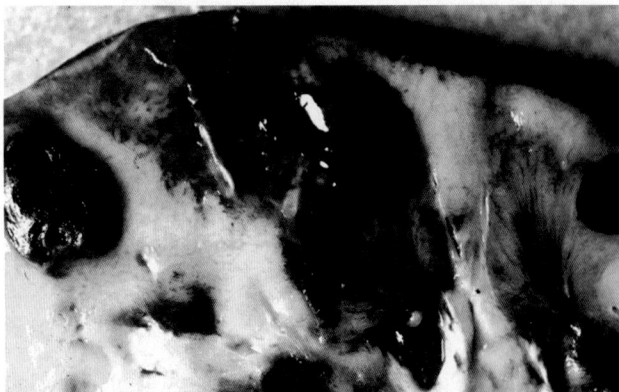

FIGURE 46.1. MS of the kidney: multiple brownish foci of involvement at gross examination.

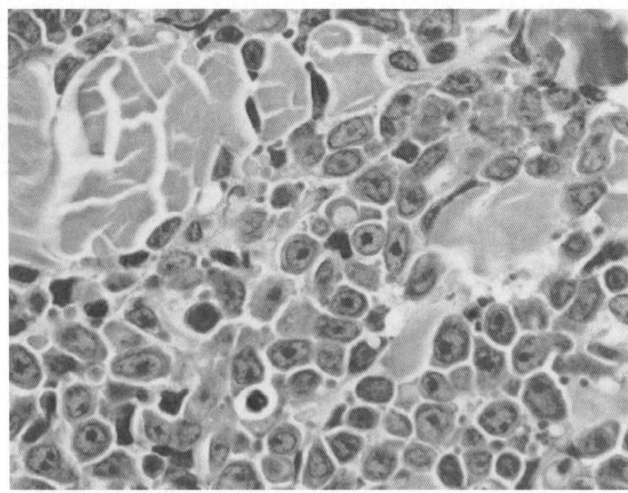

FIGURE 46.4. MS of the skin: cytologic details at Giemsa staining; neoplastic cells show large size, rather dispersed chromatin, multiple nucleoli, and a narrow rim of basophilic cytoplasm (×600).

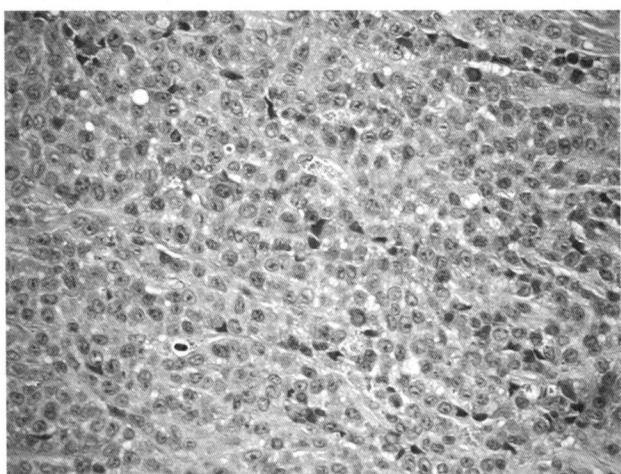

FIGURE 46.2. MS of the skin: The neoplastic growth shows a characteristic Indian-file pattern (hematoxylin and eosin, ×400).

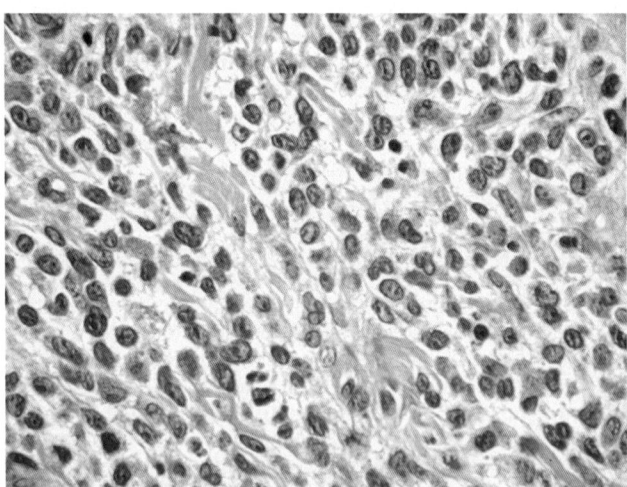

FIGURE 46.5. MS showing monoblastic morphology; the profile of the nuclei is frequently infolded (hematoxylin and eosin, ×400).

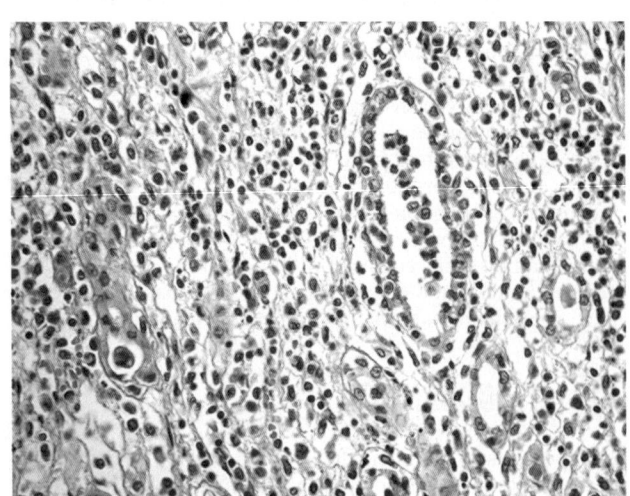

FIGURE 46.3. MS of the kidney: The tumoral population reveals some features of maturation (hematoxylin and eosin, ×200).

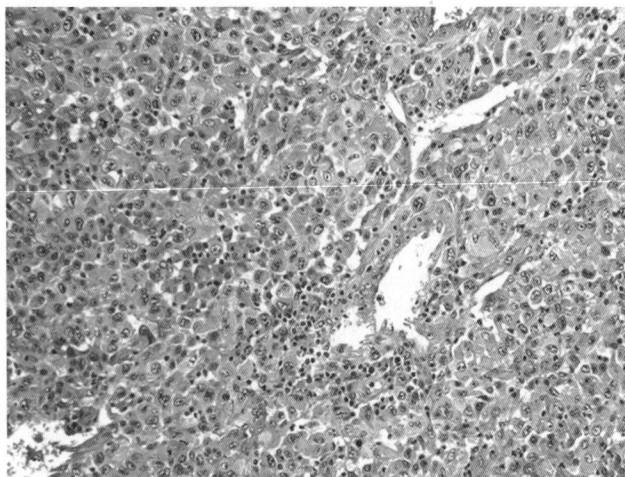

FIGURE 46.6. MS with megakaryocytic differentiation (the same case as in Fig. 46.10); please note the size of the cells along with the large rim of acidophilic cytoplasm (hematoxylin and eosin, ×300).

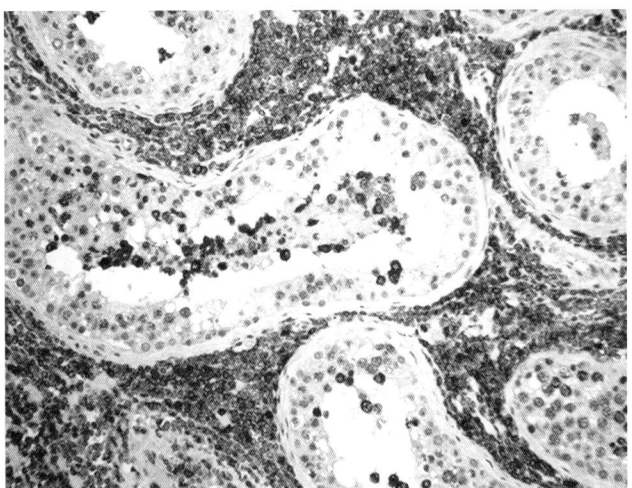

FIGURE 46.7. MS of the testis strongly expressing CD117 (APAAP technique; Gill hematoxylin nuclear counterstain; ×100).

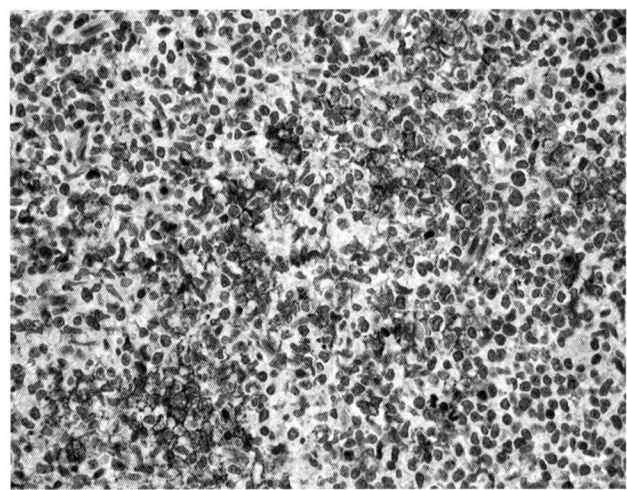

FIGURE 46.9. MS with partial expression of CD56 (APAAP technique; Gill hematoxylin nuclear counterstain; ×200).

differentiating granulocytic lineage (MPO$^+$, NASDCAE$^+$) from monoblastic forms (NSE$^+$). In addition, NASDCAE reaction can be applied to routine sections, although the results may depend on fixation and decalcifying agents.

IMMUNOPHENOTYPE

On immunohistochemistry in paraffin sections, MS shows variable marker combinations (3,5,6,13–17), allowing delineation of lineage(s).

In particular, tumors with a more immature myeloid phenotype express CD34, CD33, CD117, CD68/KP1 (but not PG-M1), and possibly TdT, with variable expression of MPO and CD45 (5,16,17) (Figs. 46.7 and 46.8).

Cases with promyelocytic phenotype lack CD34 and TdT, but are very strongly positive for MPO.

Myelomonocytic MS homogenously expresses CD68/KP1, the stains for MPO and CD68/PG-M1 (or CD163) corresponding to distinct subpopulations, but are usually CD34 negative.

The monoblastic variant is CD68/PG-M1 and CD163 positive but MPO and CD34 negative. In addition, CD14 and the Kruppel-like factor 4 have recently been proposed as further useful markers (9).

CD99 is detected in more than 50% of cases of MS, but expression is not associated with a specific subtype.

Variable degrees of CD56 positivity are recorded in about 17% of tumors irrespective of their profile (myeloid, myelomonocytic, or monoblastic) (Fig. 46.9). Importantly, this finding does not occur in association with plasmacytoid dendritic cell markers (see below) nor with TCL1 or CD4. On the other hand, foci of plasmacytoid dendritic cell differentiation (CD123$^+$, BDCA2/CD303$^+$) are occasionally observed, mostly in cases carrying inv16 (5).

The rare erythroid form of MS expresses glycophorins A and C, along with hemoglobin and CD71.

Megakaryoblastic MS expresses the complex CD61/LAT/von Willebrand antigen (Fig. 46.10).

In about 16% of tumors, the usage of a specific antibody reveals simultaneous nuclear and cytoplasmic NPM1 positivity, indicating the occurrence of mutations of the homologous gene (see below).

Exceptionally, aberrant antigenic expressions are observed (cytokeratins, B- or T-cell markers, CD30) as well as a hybrid phenotype.

Flow cytometry on cell suspensions reveals expression of CD13, CD33, CD117, and MPO in tumors with myeloid differentiation as well as CD14, CD116, and CD11c in the monoblastic cases.

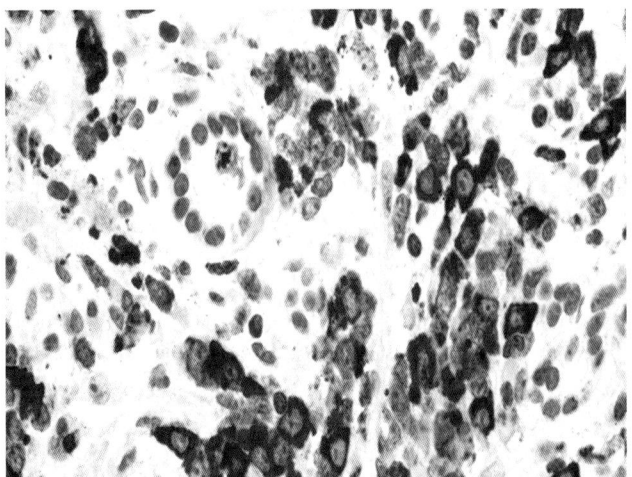

FIGURE 46.8. MS of the salivary gland: Neoplastic cells that have a promyelocytic profile are MPO positive (APAAP technique; Gill hematoxylin nuclear counterstain; ×400).

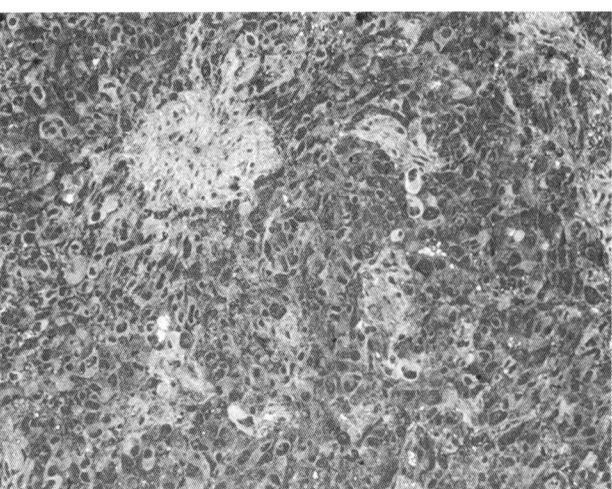

FIGURE 46.10. MS (the same case as in Fig. 46.6): Neoplastic cells turn positive at CD61 determination (APAAP technique; Gill hematoxylin nuclear counterstain; ×300).

MOLECULAR AND CYTOGENETIC FINDINGS

The spectrum of cytogenetic and molecular lesions found in AML is also recorded in MS. In particular, Pileri et al. found chromosomal aberrations in 55% of their cases in adulthood by fluorescent *in situ* hybridization (FISH) and/or conventional cytogenetics. Interestingly, the two approaches provided the same results when applied in parallel. The detected abnormalities included monosomy 7; trisomy 8; *mixed lineage leukemia (MLL)* splitting (Fig. 46.11); inv16; trisomy 4; monosomy 16, 16q-, 5q-, and 20q-; and trisomy 11. In this study, the t(8:21) (q22;q22) was definitely rare, unlike reports in children in whom this abnormality is usually encountered in orbital MS (18). Inv(16) has been related to breast or intestinal sites and to foci of plasmacytoid dendritic cell differentiation (5,6). Trisomy 8 seems to have a higher incidence in cutaneous MS (5,6). About 16% of MS cases carry evidence of *NPM1* mutations as shown by aberrant cytoplasmic NPM expression (Fig. 46.12) (19). These cases show frequent myelomonocytic or monoblastic morphology, CD34 negativity, normal karyotype, and mutual exclusion with MDS or MPN (20,21). In one series, *FLT3* internal tandem duplications were detected in <15% of instances (21). It is still unknown whether or not they can concur with *NPM1* mutations. The incidence of other recurring AML-associated mutations such as *WT1, N/K-Ras, CEBPA, IDH1, IDH2,* or *DNMT3a* has not been investigated yet.

MS can occur in patients with CML: These cases generally carry the *BCR-ABL1* fusion gene representing the blastic phase of the disease (22). Patients with myeloid and lymphoid neoplasms with *FGFR1* abnormalities can occasionally develop MS in lymph node (23). On the same line, rare MSs carrying *FIP1L1-PDGFRA* can be encountered that manifest variable eosinophilia and are sensitive to tyrosine kinase inhibitors (24).

Conversely to AML, MS has been the object of only one high-resolution genomic study by comparative genomic hybridization (CGH): This showed gains involving chromosome 8 or 21q21.1-q21.3 and loss of 5q31.2-q31.3.

DIFFERENTIAL DIAGNOSIS

MS, especially when *de novo*, is often misdiagnosed. Diffuse large B-cell lymphoma (DLBCL) does represent the most frequently encountered wrong diagnosis, followed by lymphoblastic lymphoma/leukemia; Burkitt lymphoma; small round cell tumor, particularly in children (neuroblastoma, rhabdomyosarcoma,

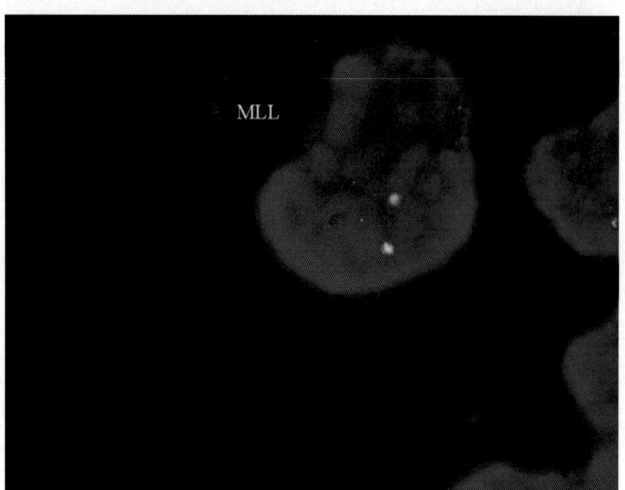

FIGURE 46.11. MS with *MLL* splitting as shown by fluorescent *in situ* hybridization (×1000).

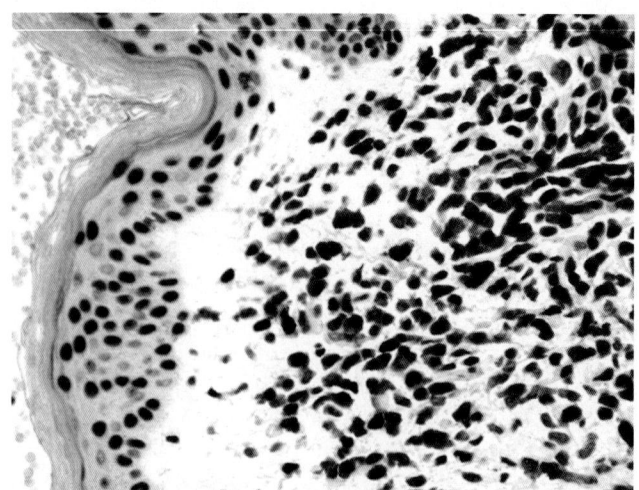

FIGURE 46.12. MS of the skin carrying *NPM1* mutations as revealed by the cytoplasmic staining with an antinucleophosmin antibody (APAAP technique; Gill hematoxylin nuclear counterstain; ×300).

Ewing/primary neroectodermal tumor (PNET), and medulloblastoma); and blastic plasmacytoid dendritic cell neoplasm (BPDCN) (5,14,25,26). Immunohistochemistry plays a basic role in the diagnosis of MS and exclusion of differential diagnostic considerations. The application of a rather large panel of antibodies is, however, required because of some aberrant positivities especially the aberrant coexpression of B- or T-cell–associated markers, cytokeratins, and, most importantly, CD99, in MS (5,27).

The distinction from DLBCL is mainly based on the coexpression of both CD20 and CD79a in DLBCL, unlike in MS (3,14). However, weak PAX5/BSAP staining can be detected in MS cases carrying t(8;21) (27).

The positivity for CD43 in MS can lead to a misdiagnosis of PTCL that can be easily ruled out by assessment for the T-cell–associated antigens CD2 to CD8 (5,17). Notably, the application of the whole panel is required, since CD4 can be expressed by monoblastic MS (9) and aberrant expression of a single T-cell marker (e.g., CD7) can at times be encountered (17,28). In addition CD30 positivity has exceptionally been recorded in MS, mimicking anaplastic large cell lymphoma (ALCL) (5). This differential diagnosis can be even more challenging by the occasional detection of CD13 and CD33 in ALK⁺ ALCL by flow cytometry (29).

The distinction of MS from BPDCN may be problematic, since the two tumors share some antigenic characteristics, such as CD34, TdT, CD56, and CD68 (30–32). However, the latter can be easily recognized because of the expression of CD123 and CD303 that are never expressed in MS (see above) (31,33). In addition, BPDCN may be TCL1 positive, while MS is not (30,32).

Histiocytic sarcoma (HS) is another neoplasm, which must be distinguished from monocytic MS. On morphologic grounds, the former shows a spectrum ranging from large cells with round-oval nuclei, multiple nucleoli, and a rather large rim of cytoplasm grayish by Giemsa stain to a highly pleomorphic population (34–36). Occasional phagocytic features can be seen. Unlike MS, HS does not express CD13 or CD33 (9).

Other differential diagnoses include poorly differentiated carcinoma and malignant melanoma. Since MS has exceptionally been found to react with the MNF116 monoclonal antibody (5), keratins with different molecular weights should be assessed to prove or exclude the epithelial nature of a given tumor. On the other hand, the usage of the HMB45 and MART-1 antibodies allows the easy distinction of malignant melanoma from MS, which is negative for both these melanoma markers.

As mentioned above, the positivity for CD99 can lead to a wrong diagnosis of small round blue cell tumor. However, when antibodies against neuroendocrine antigens, desmin, actin, and myogenin are applied, any uncertainty can be easily resolved, since these antigens are negative in MS (25).

Last but not least, MS should be differentiated from extra-medullary hematopoiesis (EMH). The latter can be sustained by many different conditions (from primary myelofibrosis to a reactive condition such as the administration of growth factors) and may produce pseudotumoral masses in every part of the body. Conventional histologic examination is sufficient for diagnosis. In fact, in EMH there is usually a multilineage proliferation and, in unilineage processes, the observed population consists of fully maturing elements (37).

PROGNOSIS AND PREDICTIVE FACTORS

According to recently published series, the clinical behavior and response to therapy are not influenced by any of the following factors: age; sex; anatomical site(s) involved; de novo presentation; clinical history related to AML, MDS, or MPN; histologic features; immunophenotype; and cytogenetic findings. In their large series, Pileri et al. (5) observed a mean survival of <1 year irrespective of the treatment used. Notably, only patients who underwent allogeneic or autologous bone marrow transplantation (auto or allo-BMT) had a higher probability of prolonged survival or cure (5), a finding supported by some independent observations (38).

THERAPY

Recent authors recommend an AML-like approach to therapy for MS (38). In fact, this condition almost invariably progresses to AML within 5 to 12 months and might already carry occult bone marrow involvement at the time of diagnosis as suggested by some molecular and cytogenetic studies. In particular, following a remission-induction chemotherapy similar to that used for AML, Bakst et al. judge each patient individually by assessing multiple factors, including age, comorbidities, and cytogenetic and molecular abnormalities (38). Based on these parameters, consolidation can vary from radiotherapy (24 Gy in 12 fractions by using conventional treatment) to allo-BMT. Interestingly, radiotherapy or surgery is at times applied up front in cases that require debulking or rapid symptom relief because of vital organ compression. If MS is concurrent with AML, the strategy is the same as the one used for AML: remission-induction chemotherapy possibly followed by allo-BMT. Notably, the latter was shown to be associated with superior outcomes not only by Pileri et al. (see above) but also by Chevallier et al. (39), who reported a 47% 5-year overall survival in 51 patients with MS treated with allo-BMT.

In case of relapsing MS, different strategies are suggested depending on whether the patient received only chemotherapy or underwent BMT (38). For the former, reinduction chemotherapy followed by radiotherapy and possibly allo-BMT is proposed, although there is no definitive evidence of efficacy. For the latter, no standard management does exist, and the approach can include donor lymphocyte infusion or investigational agents including 5-azacitidine, if the subject is eligible. Another option is palliative radiotherapy. The outcome, however, is usually poor. Finally, in the rare cases with acute promyelocytic leukemia (APL) phenotype intrathecal prophylaxis (five doses of methotrexate without cranial irradiation) might be indicated in the light of the recent observation that ADIA (all-trans retinoic acid-idarubicin) seems to be associated with an increased incidence of central nervous system (CNS) relapses.

References

1. Swerdlow SH, Campo E, Harris NL, et al., eds. *WHO classification of tumours of haematopoietic and lymphoid tissue*. Lyon: IARC Press, 2008.
2. Neiman RS, Barcos M, Berard C, et al. Granulocytic sarcoma: a clinicopathologic study of 61 biopsied cases. *Cancer* 1981;48:1426–1437.
3. Traweek ST, Arber DA, Rappaport H, et al. Extramedullary myeloid cell tumors. An immunohistochemical and morphologic study of 28 cases. *Am J Surg Pathol* 1993;17:1011–1019.
4. Roth MJ, Medeiros LJ, Elenitoba-Johnson K, et al. Extramedullary myeloid cell tumors. An immunohistochemical study of 29 cases using routinely fixed and processed paraffin-embedded tissue sections. *Arch Pathol Lab Med* 1995;119:790–798.
5. Pileri SA, Ascani S, Cox MC, et al. Myeloid sarcoma: clinico-pathologic, phenotypic and cytogenetic analysis of 92 adult patients. *Leukemia* 2007;21:340–350.
6. Alexiev BA, Wang W, Ning Y, et al. Myeloid sarcomas: a histologic, immunohistochemical, and cytogenetic study. *Diagn Pathol* 2007;2:42.
7. Byrd JC, Edenfield WJ, Shields DJ, et al. Extramedullary myeloid cell tumors in acute nonlymphocytic leukemia: a clinical review. *J Clin Oncol* 1995;13:1800–1816.
8. Ascani S, Piccaluga PP, Pileri SA. Granulocytic sarcoma of main biliary ducts. *Br J Haematol* 2003;121:534.
9. Klco JM, Welch JS, Nguyen TT, et al. State of the art in myeloid sarcoma. *Int J Lab Hematol* 2011;33:555–565.
10. Cho-Vega JH, Medeiros LJ, Prieto VG, et al. Leukemia cutis. *Am J Clin Pathol* 2008;129:130–142.
11. Koc Y, Miller KB, Schenkein DP, et al. Extramedullary tumors of myeloid blasts in adults as a pattern of relapse following allogeneic bone marrow transplantation. *Cancer* 1999;85:608–615.
12. Clark WB, Strickland SA, Barrett AJ, et al. Extramedullary relapses after allogeneic stem cell transplantation for acute myeloid leukemia and myelodysplastic syndrome. *Haematologica* 2010;95:860–863.
13. Quintanilla-Martinez L, Zukerberg LR, Ferry JA, et al. Extramedullary tumors of lymphoid or myeloid blasts. The role of immunohistology in diagnosis and classification. *Am J Clin Pathol* 1995;104:431–443.
14. Menasce LP, Banerjee SS, Beckett E, et al. Extra-medullary myeloid tumour (granulocytic sarcoma) is often misdiagnosed: a study of 26 cases. *Histopathology* 1999;34:391–398.
15. Chang CC, Eshoa C, Kampalath B, et al. Immunophenotypic profile of myeloid cells in granulocytic sarcoma by immunohistochemistry. Correlation with blast differentiation in bone marrow. *Am J Clin Pathol* 2000;114:807–811.
16. Kang LC, Dunphy CH. Immunoreactivity of MIC2 (CD99) and terminal deoxynucleotidyl transferase in bone marrow clot and core specimens of acute myeloid leukemias and myelodysplastic syndromes. *Arch Pathol Lab Med* 2006;130:153–157.
17. Lewis RE, Cruse JM, Sanders CM, et al. Aberrant expression of T-cell markers in acute myeloid leukemia. *Exp Mol Pathol* 2007;83:462–463.
18. Bonig H, Gobel U, Nurnberger W. Bilateral exophthalmos due to retroorbital chloromas in a boy with t(8;21)- positive acute myeloblastic acute leukemia. *Pediatr Hematol Oncol* 2002;19:597–600.
19. Falini B, Mecucci C, Tiacci E, et al. Cytoplasmic nucleophosmin in acute myelogenous leukemia with a normal karyotype. *N Engl J Med* 2005;352:254–266.
20. Falini B, Lenze D, Hasserjian R, et al. Cytoplasmic mutated nucleophosmin (NPM) defines the molecular status of a significant fraction of myeloid sarcomas. *Leukemia* 2007;21:1566–1570.
21. Ansari-Lari MA, Yang CF, Tinawi-Aljundi R, et al. FLT3 mutations in myeloid sarcoma. *Br J Haematol* 2004;126:785–791.
22. Kuan JW, Pathmanathan R, Chang KM, et al. Aleukemic bcr-abl positive granulocytic sarcoma. *Leuk Res* 2009;33:1574–1577.
23. Jackson CC, Medeiros LJ, Miranda RN. 8p11 myeloproliferative syndrome: a review. *Hum Pathol* 2010;41:461–476.
24. Vedy D, Muehlematter D, Rausch T, et al. Acute myeloid leukemia with myeloid sarcoma and eosinophilia: prolonged remission and molecular response to imatinib. *J Clin Oncol* 2010;28:e33–e35.
25. Haresh KP, Joshi N, Gupta C, et al. Granulocytic sarcoma masquerading as Ewing's sarcoma: a diagnostic dilemma. *J Cancer Res Ther* 2008;4:137–139.
26. Facchetti F, Pileri SA, Agostinelli C, et al. Cytoplasmic nucleophosmin is not detected in blastic plasmacytoid dendritic cell neoplasm. *Haematologica* 2009;94:285–288.
27. Campidelli C, Agostinelli C, Stitson R, et al. Myeloid sarcoma: extramedullary manifestation of myeloid disorders. *Am J Clin Pathol* 2009;132:426–437.
28. Del Poeta G, Stasi R, Venditti A, et al. CD7 expression in acute myeloid leukemia. *Leuk Lymphoma* 1995;17:111–119.
29. Bovio IM, Allan RW. The expression of myeloid antigens CD13 and/or CD33 is a marker of ALK+ anaplastic large cell lymphomas. *Am J Clin Pathol* 2008;130:628–634.
30. Petrella T, Meijer CJ, Dalac S, et al. TCL1 and CLA expression in agranular CD4/CD56 hematodermic neoplasms (blastic NK-cell lymphomas) and leukemia cutis. *Am J Clin Pathol* 2004;122:307–313.
31. Petrella T, Bagot M, Willemze R, et al. Blastic NK-cell lymphomas (agranular CD4+CD56+ hematodermic neoplasms): a review. *Am J Clin Pathol* 2005;123:662–675.
32. Sano F, Tasaka T, Nishimura H, et al. A peculiar case of acute myeloid leukemia mimicking plasmacytoid dendritic precursor cell leukemia. *J Clin Exp Hematop* 2008;48:65–69.
33. Assaf C, Gellrich S, Whittaker S, et al. CD56-positive haematological neoplasms of the skin: a multicentre study of the Cutaneous Lymphoma Project Group of the European Organisation for Research and Treatment of Cancer. *J Clin Pathol* 2007;60:981–989.
34. Jaffe ES, Harris NL, Stein H, et al., eds. *World Health Organization classification of tumours: pathology and genetics of tumours of the haematopoietic and lymphoid tissues*. Lyon: IARC Press, 2001.
35. Pileri SA, Grogan TM, Harris NL, et al. Tumours of histiocytes and accessory dendritic cells: an immunohistochemical approach to classification from the International Lymphoma Study Group based on 61 cases. *Histopathology* 2002;41:1–29.
36. Nguyen TT, Schwartz EJ, West RB, et al. Expression of CD163 (hemoglobin scavenger receptor) in normal tissues, lymphomas, carcinomas, and sarcomas is largely restricted to the monocyte/macrophage lineage. *Am J Surg Pathol* 2005;29:617–624.
37. O'Malley DP. Benign extramedullary myeloid proliferations. *Mod Pathol* 2007;20:405–415.
38. Bakst RL, Tallman MS, Douer D, et al. How I treat extramedullary acute myeloid leukemia. *Blood* 2011;118:3785–3793.
39. Chevallier P, Mohty M, Lioure B, et al. Allogeneic hematopoietic stem-cell transplantation for myeloid sarcoma: a retrospective study from the SFGM-TC. *J Clin Oncol* 2008;26:4940–4943.

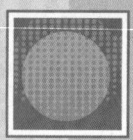

Chapter 47

Bone Marrow Morphologic Changes After Chemotherapy and Stem Cell Transplantation

Kaaren K. Reichard • Kathryn Foucar

A diverse array of pathologic bone marrow (BM) alterations occurs during and following potent chemotherapy for treatment of neoplastic disorders and prior to BM transplantation. Because of the varied actions of these treatments on proliferating cells, profound morphologic changes occur not only in neoplastic cells but also in normal BM elements. Practicing pathologists must appreciate these varied alterations for proper BM interpretation after myeloablative chemotherapy. The morphology, both early and late, of therapy effects on nonneoplastic BM cellular elements is discussed in this chapter. In addition to chemotherapy, other therapeutic agents are linked to impressive BM morphologic changes (e.g., monoclonal antibodies such as rituximab and recombinant human colony–stimulating factors such as granulocyte colony–stimulating factor) and will be discussed. BM alterations after BM transplantation tend to be similar, but several differences do exist and will be highlighted.

 GENERAL APPROACH

In general, BM assessments are performed during various phases of chemotherapeutic regimens to assess for degree of tumor ablation, to evaluate for appropriate hematopoietic regeneration, to consider minimal residual disease testing as warranted, to assess for disease recurrence, and to evaluate for the potential emergence of a posttherapy-associated hematopoietic neoplasm (1). Knowledge of not only the original disease process being treated but also the therapeutic regimen and time interval(s) between initial and current treatments is mandatory to ensure the most accurate and usable report for the clinician and patient.

The effects of chemotherapy on the BM are sequential. Additionally, the extent and duration of these BM changes vary on a case-by-case basis due to individual genetic, ethnic, and pharmacogenomic factors and doses and types of agents administered (2–4). To evaluate these BM effects optimally, it is important to integrate findings observed on aspirate smears and biopsy sections (1,5–7). Although cytologic detail is superior with aspiration specimens, trephine biopsy sections are also necessary. This is because profoundly hypocellular BM particles often do not aspirate readily and may be hemodilute, yielding a suboptimal specimen for evaluation. Additionally, chemotherapy may induce a transient increase in reticulin fibers, further compromising the quality of BM aspirate smears. For optimal assessment, BM core biopsies should be of adequate length (>1.5 cm), without significant aspiration artifact and not be comprised of a prior biopsy site (1).

Evaluation of engraftment via degree of marrow cellularity and trilineage hematopoiesis is of utmost importance as one parameter in predicting survival in posttransplantation BMs (8–10). However, assessment for recovery of peripheral blood cell counts via the complete blood cell count may preclude the need for BM biopsy evaluation in the posttransplant period. The incorporation of results from all concurrent

testing modalities (e.g., genetics, immunophenotyping, functional imaging studies, etc.) is critical for providing a useful integrated report (11–13). The degree of residual pre- and posttreatment involvement by neoplasia and other factors may be significant for outcome and engraftment potential (14–16). The use of such adjunct studies will vary depending on the disease, stage of therapy, morphologic appearance of the BM, the individual institution, and possible protocol requirements.

 POSTCHEMOTHERAPEUTIC EFFECTS IN BONE MARROW

Early

The morphologic features of the BM after intensive chemotherapy are the result of two overlapping processes: cellular depletion and BM reconstitution (1,5,6) (Table 47.1). Cell death begins focally and rapidly progresses to widespread ablation, with resultant profound blood cytopenias (1,5). BM ablation is associated with marked edema, dilated sinuses, and multiloculated fat cells in conjunction with marked hypocellularity (1,5–7,17,18) (Figs. 47.1 and 47.2). The stroma of the BM takes on an eosinophilic granular appearance secondary to fibrinoid necrosis, and mild reticulin fibrosis may develop (19). Macrophages are abundant and may contain pigment and other phagocytized material (Fig. 47.3). In general, gelatinous transformation is not prominent after chemotherapy, although this has been reported occasionally (20).

Hematopoietic regeneration usually begins about 1 to 2 weeks after ablative chemotherapy and tends to begin adjacent to bony trabeculae (21) (Fig. 47.4). Fat cell regeneration appears to play a key role in hematopoietic recovery, with islands of hematopoietic elements tending to surround fat cells (6). The sequence of erythroid and granulocytic recovery within the BM varies, but megakaryocyte regeneration generally occurs last (Fig. 47.5). In rapidly regenerating BMs, dyspoiesis of normal elements, especially erythroid cells, may be evident. Because many chemotherapeutic agents inhibit DNA synthesis, megaloblastic changes are common in normal hematopoietic lineages (Fig. 47.6). Dyserythropoiesis can be pronounced, with nuclear-cytoplasmic dyssynchrony, nuclear karyorrhexis, and multinuclearity. Mature erythrocytes may be macrocytic. As reconstitution occurs, adipose cells and reticulin fibers decrease.

Late

Several late morphologic effects of chemotherapy and radiation on the BM may occur including prolonged myelosuppression, fibrosis, and development of a therapy-related hematopoietic neoplasm. In general, these late effects are detected after a BM biopsy is performed for further investigation of persistence or emergence of cytopenias (22,23).

Table 47.1	TYPICAL BONE MARROW CHANGES AFTER MYELOABLATIVE CHEMOTHERAPY

Early (~1–2 wk)
    Hypocellularity/aplasia due to tumor and non–tumor cell death
    Fibrinoid necrosis
    Dilated sinuses
    Edema
    Scattered lymphocytes, plasma cells, and histiocytes
Intermediate (~2–4 wk)
    Multiloculated adipocytes
    Pigment-laden macrophages
    Mild reticulin fibrosis (transient phenomenon)
    Early hematopoietic regeneration; predominantly erythroid; immature
    granulocytic precursors tend to arise adjacent to bony trabeculae
Late (~3–6 wk)
    Trilineage hematopoietic lineage regeneration; erythroid initially followed by
    granulocytic then megakaryocytic
    Megakaryocytes may cluster
    Increasing cellularity with progressive regeneration
    Pigment-laden macrophages
    Increased hematogones

References (1,5–8,17–22).

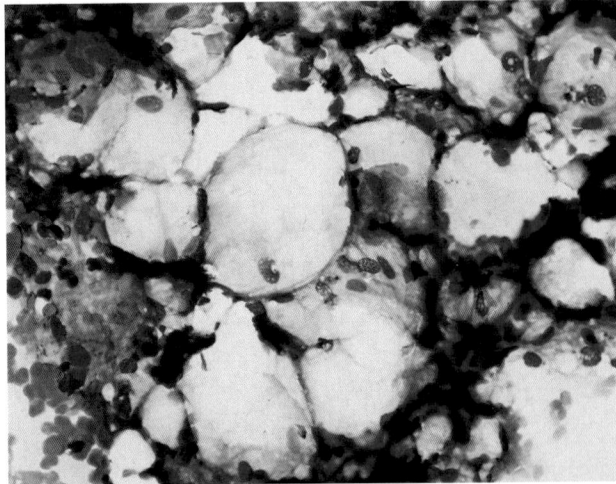

FIGURE 47.2. A markedly hypocellular BM particle is evident from a patient status postinduction chemotherapy for B lymphoblastic leukemia. Occasional macrophages contain ingested material (Wright stain, original magnification, 1,000× magnification).

Prolonged BM suppression can show a spectrum of histologic appearances ranging from frank aplasia to hypocellularity to relapsed or persistent disease. In such patients, the predicted BM regeneration does not occur but rather cytopenias persist. Possible etiologies may include an idiosyncratic hypersensitivity to the therapeutic regimen, failure to restore the BM microenvironment due to drug hypersensitivity or occult viral infection, or recurrent/persistent disease. On morphologic review, the BM remains hypocellular with prominent stromal degeneration (8). Occasional patients develop striking postmyeloablative histiocyte hyperplasia with failure of regeneration, another possible reflection of altered BM microenvironment (24). A wide range of drugs, chemotherapeutic agents, and radiation may result in iatrogenic marrow aplasia (25,26).

Although many patients, regardless of the disease subtype, achieve an initial complete remission, a subset later experience a relapse of their disease (Fig. 47.7). Although morphologic relapse is generally detected when the BM involvement is florid, assessment for early relapse/minimal residual disease is being performed more routinely in a variety of disease types (e.g., several types of acute leukemia, chronic myelogenous

leukemia, *BCR-ABL1* positive, chronic lymphocytic leukemia). Sophisticated immunophenotypic or molecular studies are utilized to identify these early relapses.

Fibrosis as a late result of chemotherapy is generally seen in association with relapse of the original disease, metastasis, secondary to certain drug therapies, or due to an otherwise unrelated cause of marrow fibrosis (e.g., renal osteodystrophy, parathyroid disorders). Although disease-associated fibrosis often resolves with ablation of the underlying neoplasm, it typically recurs upon reemergence of the original disease. Certain thrombopoietic growth factors, which may be used in conjunction with chemotherapy, may also be associated with marrow fibrosis (27).

Secondary myelodysplasia (MDS) or acute leukemia can also occur as a late event in patients who receive potent therapy for nonhematopoietic and hematopoietic neoplasms (23,28–30). Up to 5% to 10% of patients with solid tumors who are treated successfully with multiagent chemotherapy with or without radiotherapy eventually develop secondary clonal myeloid hematopoietic malignancies that exhibit pronounced multilineage dysplasia and a variable percentage of myeloblasts (31) (see Chapter 41). The morphologic abnormalities that occur

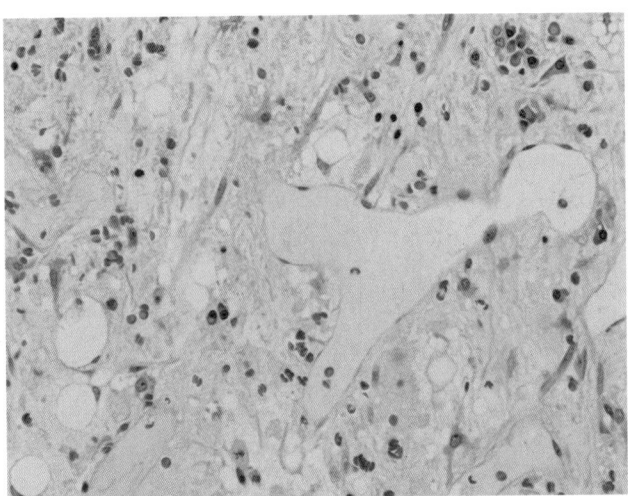

A

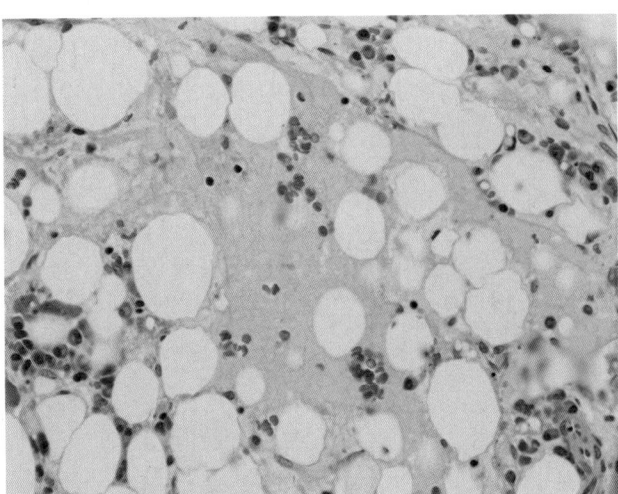

B

FIGURE 47.1. A,B: Prominent fibrinoid necrosis of the stroma and dilated sinuses are evident in these BM biopsy sections from two different patients receiving multiagent chemotherapy for acute myeloid leukemia. Residual plasma cells and occasional macrophages are evident (hematoxylin and eosin (H&E) stain, original magnification, 500× magnification).

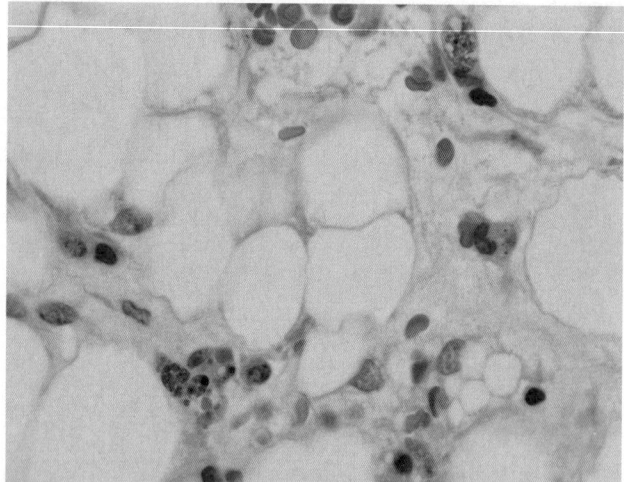

FIGURE 47.3. Increased macrophages, typically with ingested pigment, are a common feature of postmyeloablative chemotherapy BM specimens (H&E stain, original magnification, 500× magnification).

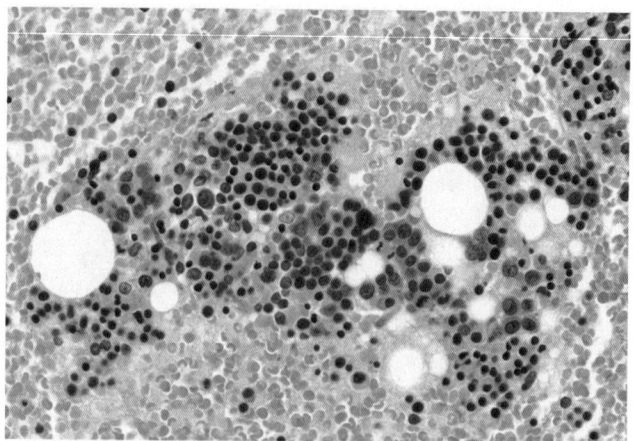

FIGURE 47.5. BM clot section showing early hematopoietic regeneration with a striking predominance of erythroid elements. This patient recently had received induction chemotherapy for acute leukemia (H&E stain, original magnification, 400× magnification).

in these iatrogenic stem cell neoplasms include increased immature forms of all lineages, nuclear segmentation defects, failure of cytoplasmic maturation, and pronounced megaloblastic changes (29). Therapy-related myeloid neoplasms may arise as a consequence of alkylating agent therapy and radiation (which induce chromosome damage and instability) or topoisomerase II inhibitor treatment (23,29). Compared to alkylating agent–induced leukemia, topoisomerase II–induced acute leukemia is characterized by more abrupt onset and a shorter interval period from treatment to secondary leukemia. Those leukemias typically are monocytic and lack multilineage dyspoiesis. The prognosis is generally poor for patients who develop either type of therapy-induced hematopoietic neoplasm, although a better prognosis is seen in cases of therapy-related acute myeloid leukemia with "good-risk" translocations such as t(8;21) and t(15;17) (29,32).

Although much less common, therapy-related acute lymphoblastic leukemia (ALL) also occurs (33). Similar to therapy-related myeloid neoplasms, these leukemias may arise after topoisomerase II inhibitor treatment but not exclusively. Abnormalities of the mixed lineage leukemia (*MLL*) gene are the most frequent cytogenetic abnormality. The latency period from treatment of the original neoplasm to development of ALL

for *MLL*-rearranged cases is significantly shorter than for those lacking an *MLL* translocation (33).

Uncommon Findings in Regenerating Bone Marrow Specimens

Less common morphologic findings that can occur during BM recovery from myeloablative therapy are detailed in Table 47.2. These uncommon findings are generally more significant and more problematic in patients with underlying acute leukemias who are undergoing induction chemotherapy. Those morphologic findings potentially associated with relapse include foci of neoplastic blasts in an otherwise hypocellular BM and persistent multilineage dysplasia (5,34) (Fig. 47.8). Those findings, which are not predictive of residual or recurrent disease but can be tricky to distinguish from a neoplastic process, include florid atypical megakaryocytic hyperplasia, sheets of promyelocytes, and increased hematogones (35–39) (Fig. 47.9). In each of these situations, the goal is to determine if this morphologic finding is linked to imminent or eventual leukemic relapse or is instead a unique feature of regenerating normal BM. BM fibrosis and bone changes are often linked and

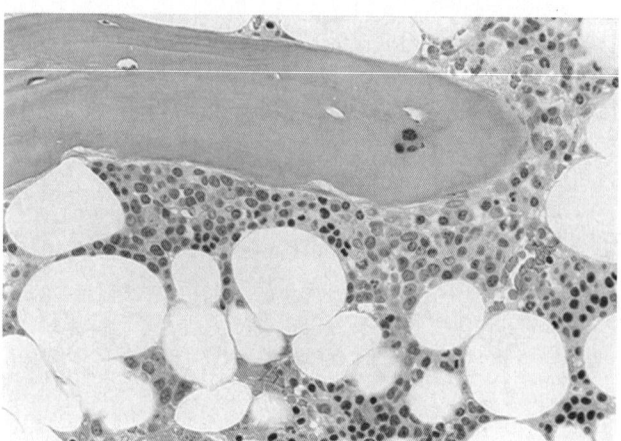

FIGURE 47.4. Early hematopoietic regeneration postmyeloablative chemotherapy tends to originate around the bony trabeculae (H&E stain, original magnification, 500× magnification).

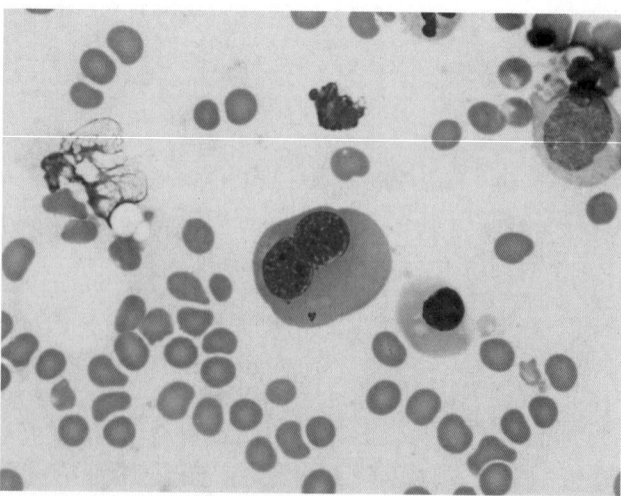

FIGURE 47.6. Photomicrograph demonstrating striking megaloblastoid change in a red blood cell precursor after induction chemotherapy for acute myeloid leukemia (Wright stain, original magnification, 1,000× magnification).

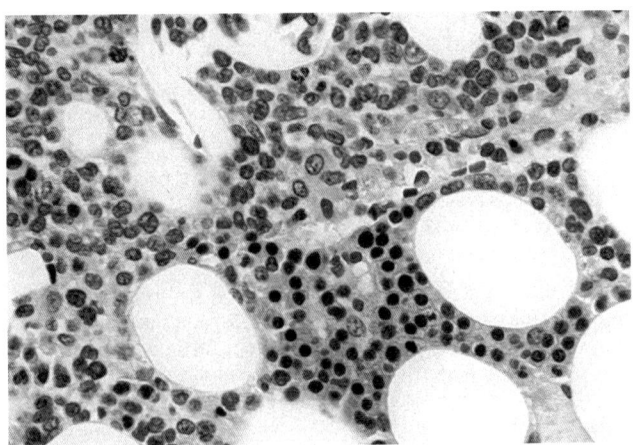

FIGURE 47.7. A focus of relapsed acute leukemia is evident in this BM clot section. Note the dispersed chromatin of the leukemic blasts compared to the denser chromatin of surrounding erythroid precursors (H&E, original magnification, 800× magnification).

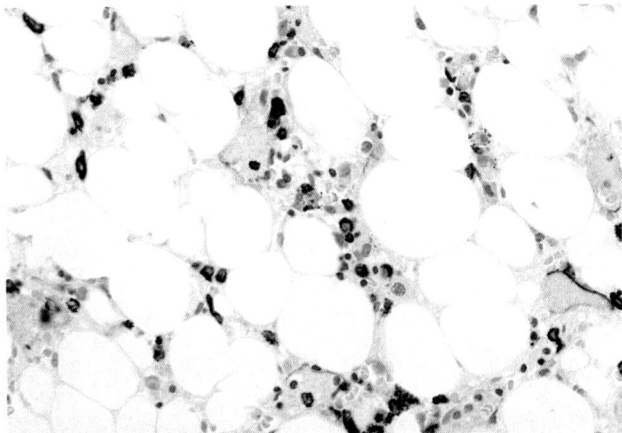

FIGURE 47.8. Photomicrograph of a BM biopsy specimen taken 24 days after reinduction chemotherapy for acute myeloid leukemia showing residual islands of CD34+ neoplastic blasts in an otherwise depleted BM (CD34 immunostain, original magnification, 1,000× magnification).

especially prevalent in patients with underlying myeloproliferative neoplasms. Finally, in some patients, reconstitution of the BM following myeloablative therapy is delayed profoundly and may reflect an idiosyncratic reaction to the chemotherapy or underlying poor nutritional status (40). This failure to regenerate normal BM elements is more likely to occur in elderly patients.

 BONE MARROW MORPHOLOGY AFTER BONE MARROW TRANSPLANTATION

BM or stem cell transplantation is utilized with curative intent in a variety of neoplastic and nonneoplastic disorders (41–43). Umbilical cord transplantation presents some advantages over traditional BM or mobilized peripheral blood stem cells including rapid availability, absence of risk for the donor, and decreased risk of acute graft-versus-host disease (44). Recent advances in haploidentical stem cell transplantation suggest better outcomes (45). The type of preparative regimen for transplantation varies, depending on the patient's disease and desired conditioning regimen. Multiagent chemotherapy plus radiation is necessary to eradicate tumor cells, in patients receiving transplantation for hematopoietic malignancies and solid tumors.

Similar to the recommendations for BM evaluation following chemotherapy, the BM biopsy, in addition to aspirate smear preparations, is essential in evaluating patients immediately after bone marrow transplantation (BMT) for engraftment, eradication of underlying disease, etc. When assessing for chimerism and/or performing highly sensitive flow cytometric or molecular studies for potential residual or recurrent disease, the quality of the submitted material should be optimal and not compromised by hemodilution or other factors. Because potent chemotherapy is part of the preparative regimen for transplantation, there are morphologic similarities to BMs, which are postchemotherapy alone (without transplantation) (Tables 47.1 and 47.3). However, some unique BM changes do occur in BMT and are delineated in Table 47.4. The addition of total body radiation to the preparative regimen in some patients results in an even more profound BM ablation.

Early Findings after Bone Marrow Transplantation

The morphologic features of cell death identified in the early period following transplantation are listed in Table 47.3 and are similar to those described for postchemotherapy without transplantation (Table 47.1) (8,46,47). The BM features

Table 47.2	UNCOMMON FINDINGS IN REGENERATING BONE MARROW SPECIMENS AFTER POTENT CHEMOTHERAPY
Finding	**Comments**
Foci of blasts in otherwise depleted BM (leukemia patient)	Generally indicative of treatment failure
Persistent dysplasia	May reflect persistent disease or therapy-induced maturation of leukemia clone
Sheets of megakaryocytes (leukemia patients)	Transient phenomenon with morphologic atypia as well; seen following induction chemotherapy for acute myeloid leukemia and rarely ALL
Sheets of promyelocytes	Large number of regenerating cells at same maturational stage
	Distinguish from acute promyelocytic leukemia by characteristic morphology (round, single lobate nuclei, paranuclear hofs, no Auer rods)
Increase in hematogones	Especially problematic in pediatric patients receiving treatment for ALL
Fibrosis possibly with bony changes	Often seen in patients with underlying marked myelofibrosis
Lack of BM regeneration	Failure of prompt reconstitution of BM may reflect idiosyncratic reaction to chemotherapy, poor nutritional status, or be a consequence of advanced age.

References (5,34–40).

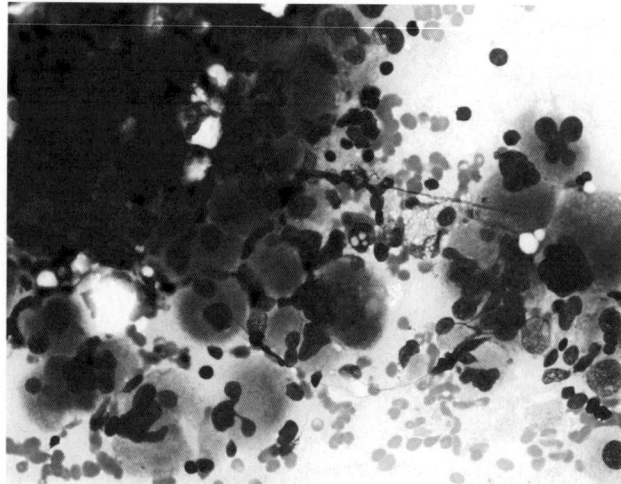

FIGURE 47.9. Atypical megakaryocytic hyperplasia/regeneration after induction chemotherapy for B lymphoblastic leukemia/lymphoma (Wright stain, original magnification, 800× magnification).

Table 47.4	UNIQUE MORPHOLOGIC FEATURES IN THE BONE MARROW AFTER STEM CELL TRANSPLANTATION

Nonparatrabecular, monotonous colonies of erythroid and myeloid precursors
Prolonged and highly variable degree of cellularity
Dyserythropoietic changes may persist including ring sideroblasts.
Prolonged BM aplasia due to delayed or absent engraftment

include massive BM damage with proteinaceous debris, marked stromal edema, and prominent stromal damage (so-called toxic myelopathy). Increased reticulin fibers and small granulomas have been noted during the early post-BMT interval (46,48,49).

The morphologic features of hematopoietic regeneration that follow BMT vary somewhat from those seen after aggressive systemic chemotherapy without transplantation. After BMT, the earliest regeneration is identified approximately 7 to 14 days after transplantation and consists predominantly of nonparatrabecular monotonous colonies of erythroid precursors (47,49) (Fig. 47.10). The erythroid islands often surround a central macrophage and may demonstrate megaloblastoid features attributable to chemotherapy effects (49,50). Myeloid precursors accompany erythroid precursors around 2 weeks' post-BMT. Failure to develop myeloid colonies generally is associated with failure of engraftment (49). By 21 days after transplantation, the regenerating colonies are larger. Erythroid and granulocytic regeneration generally precedes megakaryocytic recovery, and transient dyserythropoiesis and, to a lesser extent, dysgranulopoiesis are common (Fig. 47.11). In general, neutrophil recovery occurs by day 21, whereas platelet recovery is expected by 25 to 30 days after BMT (46). The BM cellularity in allogeneic recipients usually has recovered to approximately one-half its normal level by day 21 (48,49). Regeneration may be accelerated by growth factor therapy (51).

Late Findings after Bone Marrow Transplantation

By the second month posttransplant, cellularity should be near normal (50) (Fig. 47.12). However, a number of late complications may occur posttransplantation including delayed engraftment for a variety of reasons, marked megakaryocytic dysplasia, avascular necrosis of bone, emergence of a

Table 47.3	MORPHOLOGIC FEATURES IN THE BONE MARROW AFTER BMT

Early (<1 wk): Changes attributable to cell death:
  Massive BM damage with fat necrosis, proteinaceous debris, stromal edema (see Table 47.1 also)
Early (1–2 wk): Changes attributable to early regeneration:
  Early nonparatrabecular monotypic colonies of erythroid precursors
  Dyspoiesis of cells (erythroid>granulocytic) may be evident
  Erythroid and myeloid regeneration usually precede megakaryoblastic colonies.
  Persistence of tumor cells in some patients transplanted during BM disease involvement
  Marked megaloblastic erythroid features due to effect of chemotherapy
  Scattered single megakaryocytes with dysplastic features
  Multiloculated adipocytes
  Minimal inflammatory infiltrate
Intermediate (3–4 wk):
  Mixed erythroid and myeloid colonies
  Patchy regeneration of megakaryocytes
  Dyserythropoietic changes may persist including ring sideroblasts.
  Neutrophils may show megaloblastic changes or pseudo–Pelger-Huët nuclei.
  At least 50% of normal cellularity
Late (>4 wk):
  Engraftment: Trilineage hematopoietic engraftment typically seen at day 28
  Delayed engraftment or graft failure:
    Transplantation during relapse
    Extensive prior chemotherapy
    HLA partial match
    ABO-mismatched donor
    T-cell–depleted BM
    Stem cell or BM microenvironment damage
    Insufficient stem cells from umbilical cord donor
  Declining cell counts (after day 28):
    Possible rejection of graft
    Drug toxicity
    Viral infection
    PTLD
    Graft-vs.-host disease
    Recurrent leukemia
    Secondary MDS
    Donor-derived neoplasm
  Others:
    Avascular necrosis of bone (average 12 mo posttransplant)
    Marked dysplasia of megakaryocytes

References (8,46–49,132).

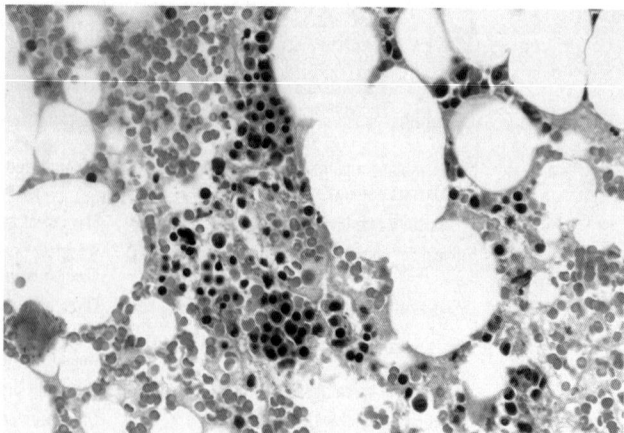

FIGURE 47.10. After BM transplantation, the earliest regeneration occurs within 1 to 2 weeks and shows a nonparatrabecular monotypic colony appearance (H&E stain, original magnification, 400× magnification). The cells in this illustration are of erythroid derivation.

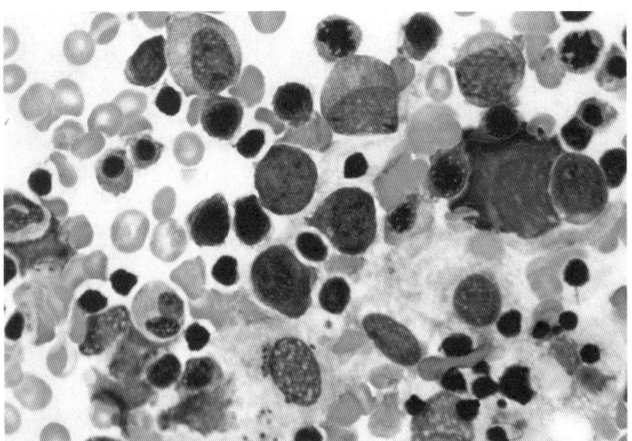

FIGURE 47.11. After BM transplantation, similar to postchemotherapy status, the erythroid and granulocytic regeneration generally precedes that of the megakaryocytic lineage (Wright stain, original magnification, 1,000× magnification).

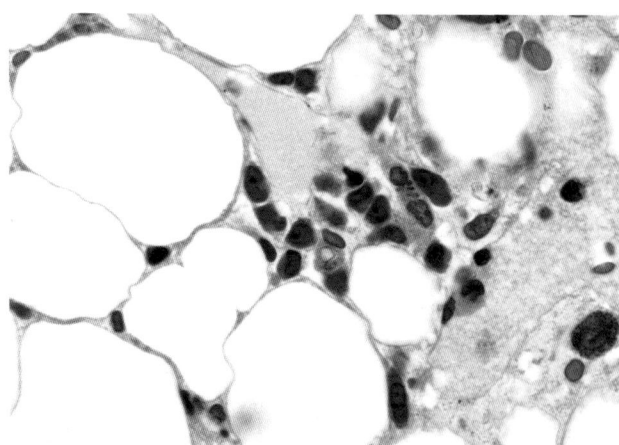

FIGURE 47.13. After BM transplantation for acute myeloid leukemia, this biopsy section shows persistence of immature cells without significant maturation, heralding delayed/failed engraftment (H&E stain, original magnification, 500× magnification).

donor-derived hematologic neoplasm, graft-versus-host disease, or development of a posttransplant lymphoproliferative disorder.

Delayed engraftment may be secondary to underlying BM damage from extensive prior chemotherapy, residual neoplastic cells, infection, receipt of a BM graft that is ABO mismatched or partially matched for human leukocyte antigens, and insufficient number of injected stem cells (52–54) (Table 47.3; Fig. 47.13). A thorough clinical, microbiologic, and BM examination are often needed to document the poor engraftment and probable etiology. Despite concerns that underlying BM fibrosis may interfere with hematopoietic reconstitution, some studies document minimal to no delays in cell-count recovery in these patients (55). Increased numbers of and clustered histiocytes may be seen in some patients with delayed engraftment (50,56).

The dysplastic changes seen in regenerating megakaryocytes may be due to chemotherapeutic, transplantation, and/or radiation effects (8). A diagnosis of secondary MDS should be avoided unless additional clear-cut supporting data are available such as typical, MDS-associated clonal abnormalities or history or other evidence of MDS prior to transplantation.

Avascular necrosis of bone may occur on average 12 months after transplantation often requiring surgical intervention (57).

Development of a secondary malignancy after allogeneic BM transplantation is a rare but documented event. These malignancies include posttransplant lymphoproliferative disorders (PTLDs), new solid cancers, and donor-derived hematologic malignancies. PTLDs are a heterogenous group of disorders and arise from donor cells (in contrast to recipient cells in solid organ transplantation) (Fig. 47.14). The incidence can be as high as 10% (58). Those occurring after BM transplantation from an unrelated donor are particularly aggressive (59). New solid cancers run the gamut from skin to thyroid to breast with an incidence of 1% to 2% at 10 years (58,60). The latency period ranges from 3 to 5 years for these solid tumors. Donor cell–derived malignancies range from chronic to acute leukemias (61). There are <75 reported cases in the literature as of this writing (Fig. 47.15).

 ## ANCILLARY TESTING POSTTHERAPY

A diverse spectrum of techniques is available to assess for evidence of minimal residual disease and/or early recurrence in posttherapy BM specimens (62). These techniques vary widely in terms of their sensitivity to detect residual disease (Table 47.5). With the exception of immunohistochemistry and several molecular genetic assays, the performance of these

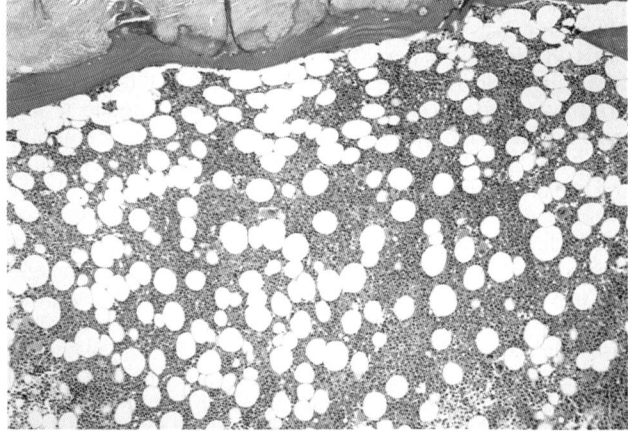

FIGURE 47.12. Hematopoietic recovery is evident in this BM core biopsy 6 weeks after BM transplantation for mantle cell lymphoma (H&E stain, original magnification, 200× magnification).

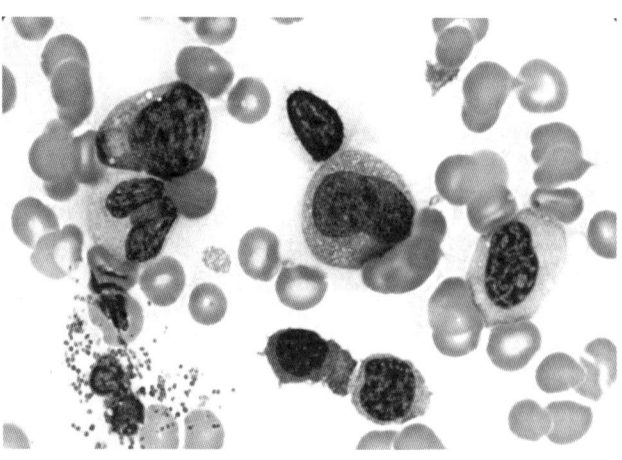

FIGURE 47.14. Atypical lymphoid cells present in the BM of a patient with a PTLD (Wright stain, original magnification, 1,000× magnification).

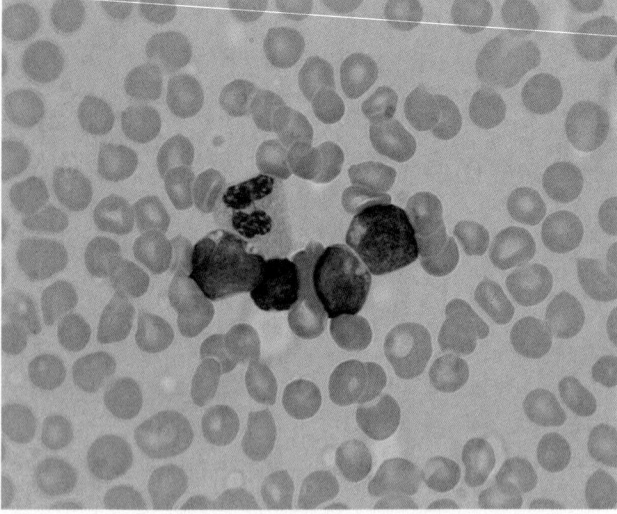

FIGURE 47.15. This photomicrograph depicts three lymphoblasts, which are intermediate in size with irregular nuclei, slightly condensed chromatin, and scant cytoplasm. These blasts were of T lymphoid lineage as determined by flow cytometry and were also shown to derive from donor cells after previous allogeneic BM transplantation (Wright stain, original magnification, 800× magnification).

tests requires additional fresh, anticoagulated BM material. The best use of these tests will depend on the original disease diagnosis, morphologic response to therapy, and long-term result expectations (63–65). After allogeneic transplantation, the use of short tandem repeat polymorphisms is highly sensitive in monitoring degree of chimerism (66). Detecting cancer stem cells, given their postulated direct role in relapse, is an active area of research (67).

BONE MARROW CHANGES AFTER CERTAIN DRUG THERAPIES

Many hematopoietic regulatory factors such as granulocyte colony-stimulating factor, erythropoietin, thrombopoietin, interleukin-2, and interleukin-3 are available and can be used to either ameliorate cytopenias or stimulate immune function. Several investigators have described the blood and BM findings in patients receiving these various types of recombinant agents (68–75) (Table 47.6). In addition, a variety of commonly administered medications may induce various conspicuous BM cellular alterations such that a potential misdiagnosis of a myeloid neoplasm, particularly myelodysplastic syndrome (MDS), could be rendered. While it is beyond the scope of this book to cover all known drugs/offending agents that may elicit significant BM effects, we will discuss several seen commonly in practice including cytokines, rituximab, lenalidomide, imatinib, azathioprine, zidovudine, valproate, and arsenic.

Table 47.5	SENSITIVITY OF DIFFERENT METHODS TO DETECTION RESIDUAL DISEASE

Method	Sensitivity
Morphology	~3%–5%
Conventional cytogenetics	5%
Fluorescence *in situ* hybridization	1%–5%
Immunohistochemistry	0.1%–5%
Flow cytometry	0.01%
PCR for specific translocations	0.001%

Table 47.6	MORPHOLOGIC AND/OR CLINICAL FEATURES OF BLOOD AND BONE MARROW IN PATIENTS RECEIVING RECOMBINANT GROWTH FACTOR THERAPY, INTERLEUKIN-2, OR INTERLEUKIN-3

G-CSF and GM-CSF:
  Peripheral blood:
    Left shift with circulating blasts (more prominent during early response when white blood cell count is low)
    Marked leukocytosis secondary to neutrophilia (G-CSF)
    Marked leukocytosis with increase in neutrophils and monocytes, with variable increase in eosinophils, lymphocytes, and sometimes basophils (GM-CSF)
    Rare giant (tetraploid) neutrophils present
    Prominent toxic changes of neutrophils, vacuoles prominent
    Nuclear-cytoplasmic asynchrony
    Nuclear segmentation abnormalities
    Circulating myeloid cytoplasmic fragments
  Bone marrow:
    Early changes include interstitial foci of granulocyte precursors in hypocellular BM
    Increased cellularity with left shift in hematopoietic cells
    Promyelocytic hyperplasia with reactive features during early phase of therapy
    Pronounced toxic changes of immature and mature granulocytic elements
    Occasional binucleate promyelocytes and myelocytes
    More mature granulocytes predominate after several weeks of therapy.
    Transient increase in blood and BM blasts mimicking leukemia (rare)
    Rare development of fibrosis with bony changes
    Histiocytic proliferation
    Rare development of acute BM necrosis
Interleukin-2 (usually given in conjunction with lymphokine-activated killer cell therapy):
    Enhanced functional activity including increased natural killer cell activity
    Numerous noncaseating epithelioid granulomas in some patients
    Has played a role in the treatment of renal cell carcinoma
Interleukin-3:
    Leukocytosis with increase in all granulated cells and lymphocytes; increase in basophils variable
    Variable increase in platelets and reticulocytes
    Increased cellularity with left shift in all hematopoietic elements
    Increased eosinophils
    Rare reports of fibrosis with bony changes

References (68–74).

Granulocyte or Granulocyte-Macrophage Colony-Stimulating Factor

Colony-stimulating factor therapy is efficacious in patients with constitutional neutropenic disorders and in some patients with chemotherapy-induced febrile neutropenia. Most emphasis has been placed on the morphologic features in blood and peripheral cell counts; BM examination is not performed in most of these patients. Blood changes are most pronounced in patients receiving granulocyte and granulocyte-macrophage colony-stimulating factor therapy (69–71). Early changes include a transient increase in circulating blasts followed by eventual mature neutrophilia exhibiting striking toxic changes (Fig. 47.16A and B). Other abnormalities include nuclear-cytoplasmic asynchrony and nuclear segmentation defects of neutrophils. Changes in other lineages are less pronounced. In patients with profound BM suppression, early features of colony-stimulating factor therapy consist of initial small collections of immature myeloid elements; more mature forms predominate in patients receiving several weeks of therapy (Figs. 47.17 and 47.18). A characteristic finding is the presence of a high proportion of promyelocytes and early myelocytes (Fig. 47.17) (73,74). All stages of granulocytic maturation exhibit marked toxic changes. Unusual findings following colony-stimulating factor therapy include

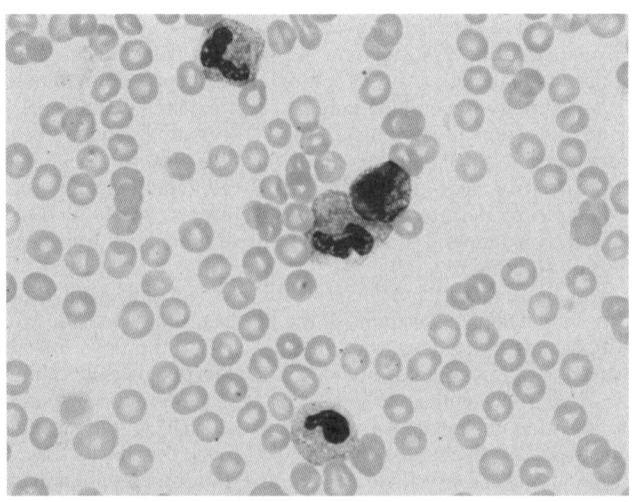 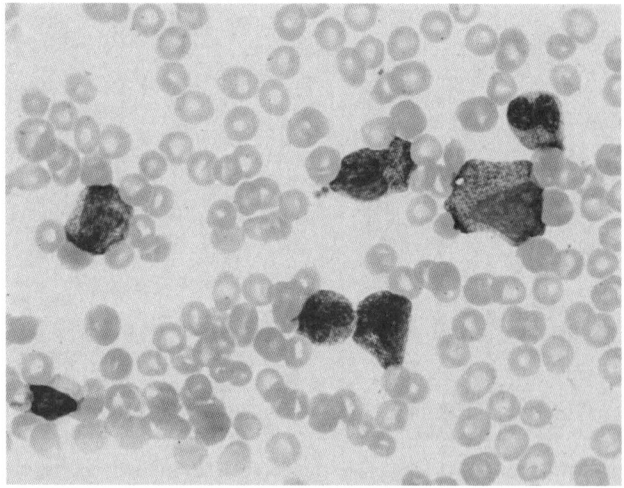

A   B

FIGURE 47.16. Peripheral blood smear illustrating the prominent toxic neutrophilia with left shift that occurs in patients receiving sustained granulocyte colony-stimulating factor therapy (**A:** Wright stain, original magnification, 800× magnification; **B:** Wright stain, original magnification, 800× magnification).

diffuse histiocytic proliferation, fibrosis with associated bony changes, and a transient marked increase in blood and BM blasts (71,72,75).

Recombinant Human Erythropoietin

Recombinant erythropoietin is effective in improving hemoglobin levels in patients with disease- or treatment-related anemias (76,77). Erythropoietin is the primary growth factor regulator of erythroid development. Recombinant human erythropoietin (rHuEPO) was developed to aid in the treatment of chronic anemias from a variety of different etiologies. rHuEPO is known to increase the reticulocyte production rate in normal healthy subjects (78). Erythropoietin expands BM erythropoiesis by amplifying committed precursors (79) (Fig. 47.19). Macrocytic changes are observed in peripheral blood and BM alike. Rarely, patients who have received long-term

rHuEPO administration can develop pure red cell aplasia secondary to antibodies (80).

Recombinant Human Thrombopoietin

Recombinant human thrombopoietin is being utilized in clinical trials to enhance platelet recovery after potent chemotherapy with or without progenitor cell support (27). Certain thrombopoietic formulations (e.g., romiplostim and eltrombopag) have been associated with the induction of BM reticulin fibrosis and rebound thrombocytopenia (81–83). The degree of reticulin fibrosis is usually modest (grade 1 to 2 of 3) and appears to be reversible upon discontinuation of the drug. Additionally, given that certain hematologic malignancies express the thrombopoietin receptor, c-MPL, it has been suggested that treatment with a thrombopoietic growth factor may potentiate development of a hematologic neoplasm in immune thrombocytopenia patients (27).

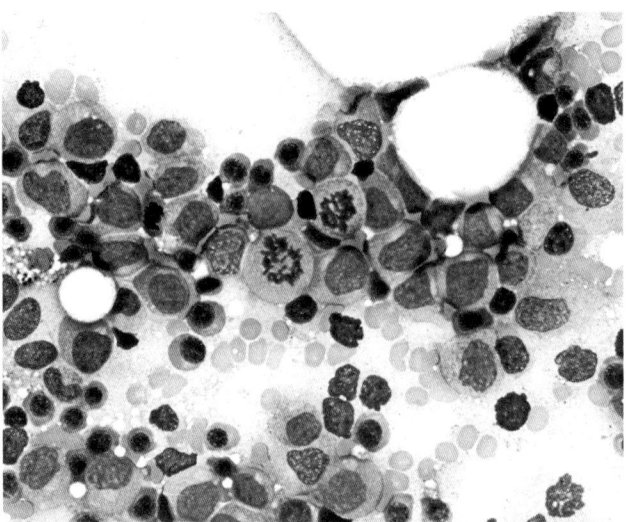 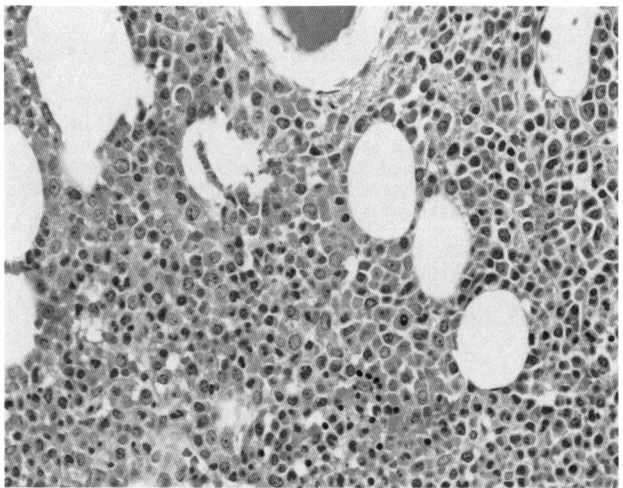

FIGURE 47.17. This BM aspirate smear photomicrograph demonstrates marked granulocytic toxic granulation and left shift in a patient recently treated with G-CSF (H&E stain, original magnification, 800× magnification).

FIGURE 47.18. This BM biopsy photomicrograph demonstrates a striking granulocytic predominance and left shift in maturation in a patient recently treated with granulocyte colony-stimulating factor (G-CSF). Note the maintained normal maturational architecture with the more immature granulocytic elements along the bony trabeculae (H&E stain, original magnification, 200× magnification).

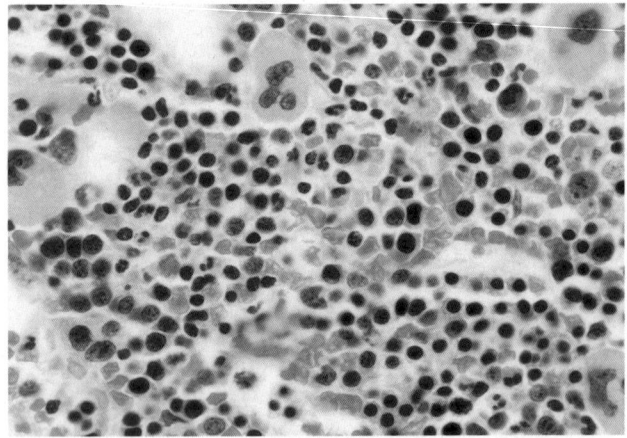

FIGURE 47.19. Marked erythroid hyperplasia is evident in this BM core biopsy from a patient receiving recombinant erythropoietin (H&E, original magnification, 400× magnification).

Rituximab

Rituximab is a chimeric monoclonal antibody against the protein CD20, which is found essentially on the surface of mature B cells. It is used in the treatment of a variety of disorders including non-Hodgkin lymphomas, chronic leukemias,

autoimmune diseases, vasculitis, and some cases of organ transplantation (84,85). The mechanisms of action of rituximab include activation of complement-dependent cytotoxicity, antibody-dependent cellular cytotoxicity, phagocytosis, and induction of apoptosis (86,87). Rituximab functions to deplete the B-cell compartment. This effect takes place fairly quickly with clear-cut lymph node B-cell depletion seen after 1 month of therapy with as few as three doses (88). B-cell recovery commences after 3 months of therapy but may last for up to 9 months (89).

In the treatment of B-cell lymphoma/leukemia with rituximab, histologic alterations of the involved BM have been well described in the literature (90–93). These alterations include CD3+ T-cell lymphoid nodules that morphologically mimic residual B-cell leukemia/lymphoma (Fig. 47.20A–C). One study found that the presence of these T-cell–rich aggregates was associated with a better outcome (90). Given that the CD20 epitope is blocked by rituximab therapy, the immunophenotypic use of alternative B-cell marker(s) such as CD19, PAX5, and CD79a is warranted. The emergence of CD20– residual and/or recurrent tumor cells may occur, and thus, an immunophenotypic cocktail of these non-CD20 B-cell markers and a robust T-cell marker are needed to determine if there is residual B-cell disease. If the original neoplasm was partially composed of plasma cells (e.g., lymphoplasmacytic lymphoma) or if there is subsequent plasmacytic tumor differentiation, then the addition of plasma cell–reactive antibodies such as CD138 and

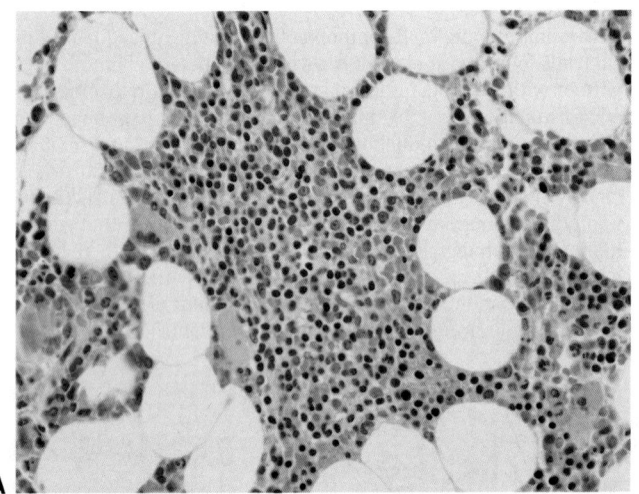

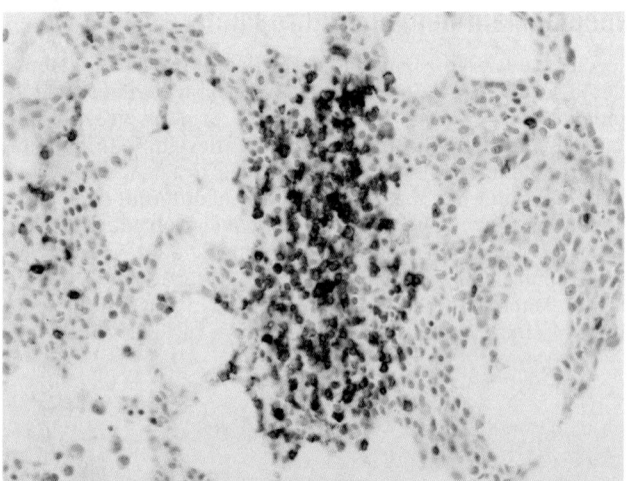

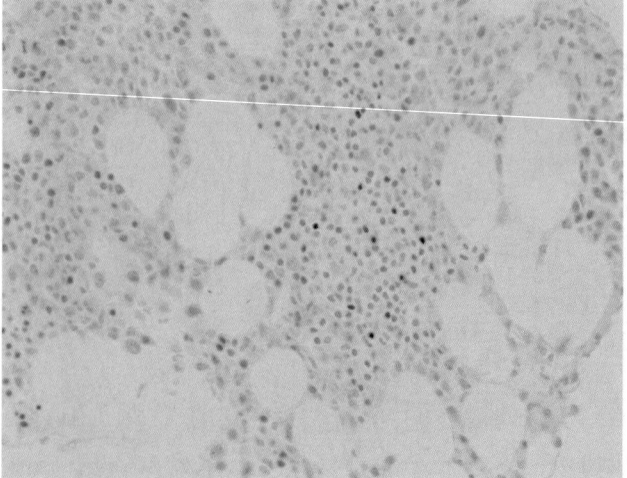

FIGURE 47.20. (A) demonstrates a monotonous-appearing interstitial lymphoid aggregate in a patient with chronic lymphocytic leukemia treated with rituximab (H&E stain, original magnification, 400× magnification). **(B)** shows the CD3+ T-cell nodules, which morphologically mimic the patient's previous BM more extensive involvement by chronic lymphocytic leukemia. **(C)** shows markedly reduced, yet residual, scattered B cells in this lymphoid aggregate consistent with rituximab effect and minimal residual disease (PAX5).

MUM1 as well as kappa and lambda to detect clonality may be indicated.

Rituximab is associated with the development of peripheral cytopenias, most notably neutropenia and thrombocytopenia (94–96). Late-onset neutropenia (LON) (several months after rituximab administration) is becoming increasingly recognized and appears to be mostly clinically insignificant and self-limiting. Infections may occur in up to 20% of patients. The etiology of LON is unclear but may be due in part to circulating antibodies (96).

Newer generation anti-CD20 agents are becoming available, which have been developed to have better antitumor effects (97). The second-generation agents (e.g., ocrelizumab, ofatumumab) are humanized to reduce immunogenicity, and the third-generation agents (e.g., AME-133v) also have an engineered Fc receptor (97). The specific effect on human BM after treatment is not well described yet.

Lenalidomide

Lenalidomide is a member of a class of drugs referred to as immunomodulatory agents. One of the better known members of this group is thalidomide. These drugs are used in the treatment of myeloid disorders and plasma cell myeloma (98,99). Although treatment-resistant neoplastic stem cells may persist, the morphologic BM effects of lenalidomide may include resolution of cytologic dysplasia, decrease in BM blasts, increase in erythroid precursors, and decrease in ring sideroblasts in patients with MDS with cytogenetic deletion 5q (100–102). *In vitro* studies have demonstrated that lenalidomide promotes erythropoiesis, which supports its known association with decreased transfusion dependence in MDS (103). Lenalidomide-induced cytopenias are not uncommon and include neutropenia and thrombocytopenia (104,105). Dose modifications can be made to ensure drug safety and better tolerance.

Imatinib

Imatinib is a first-generation tyrosine kinase inhibitor (TKI) that was originally identified as a molecule that specifically targets the ATP-binding site of the oncogenic BCR-ABL1 chimeric protein in chronic myelogenous leukemia (CML) (106). Since the introduction of imatinib into clinical trials and practice, second- and third-generation TKIs have been developed to combat imatinib-resistant disease states. TKI therapy is currently the standard of care in the treatment of CML, but imatinib has also found utility in the treatment of other myeloid and lymphoid disorders such as myeloid neoplasms harboring a rearrangement of *PDGFRA* or *PDGFRB* and *BCR-ABL1*–positive ALLs. The BM effects of imatinib during the treatment of CML are well described in the literature and include complete hematologic response and normalization of BM cellularity and cellular composition (107–109). The effects of imatinib therapy in the peripheral blood include resolution of the leukocytosis, basophilia, and thrombocytosis and are generally seen within the first 3 months of therapy in responsive patients. Importantly, one of the more common side effects that occur with imatinib therapy is the development of cytopenias, which may require drug readjustments to correct. The normalization of the BM is more protracted and typically takes up to a year on therapy. The hypercellular BM with marked granulocytic predominance and abnormal hypolobated megakaryocytes seen at diagnosis are replaced over time with a generally normocellular (occasionally hypocellular) with intact morphologically unremarkable trilineage hematopoiesis. The morphologic persistence of hypolobated megakaryocytes and/or hypercellularity with an increased myeloid to erythroid ratio (>5:1) often correlates with persistence disease at the genetic level. Alternatively, the

apparent morphologic resolution of all abnormalities does not necessarily predict a molecular remission. Correlation with quantitative molecular studies is necessary to address the minimal residual disease state as well as the log reduction in *BCR-ABL1* transcript levels.

Azathioprine

Azathioprine is a purine analog used to prevent organ rejection after transplantation and for treatment of autoimmune diseases. Its mechanism of action is to impede DNA synthesis and thus halt cellular proliferation. As a consequence, varying degrees of myelosuppression are seen including leukopenia most commonly agranulocytosis, red cell aplasia, and thrombocytopenia (Fig. 47.21). Erythroid abnormalities may include megaloblastoid change and multinucleation. Patients with thiopurine methyltransferase deficiency are at increased risk for developing more significant myelosuppression when treated with azathioprine (110).

Zidovudine

Zidovudine (aka azidothymidine [AZT]) is used in combination with other drugs to treat human immunodeficiency virus-1 infection (111). The effects of AZT on the peripheral blood and BM can be quite striking. AZT may cause serious multilineage myelosuppression including anemia and/or red cell aplasia requiring red blood cell transfusions and profound neutropenia (109). Macrocytosis of the red blood cells is common and is accompanied by megaloblastoid erythroid precursors in the BM (112–114).

Valproate

Valproate (or valproic acid in another form) is an anticonvulsant drug used to treat a variety of seizure and other psychiatric disorders. It is associated with a number of hematologic toxicities: most commonly thrombocytopenia but also neutropenia, anemia secondary to red cell aplasia, and pancytopenia (115–117). In the BM, valproate has been reported to induce megakaryocytic and myeloid dysplasia (115,118).

Arsenic

Arsenic is a metalloid that is found naturally in the environment in drinking water but is also used in the treatment of a variety of myeloid disorders, most notably acute promyelocytic

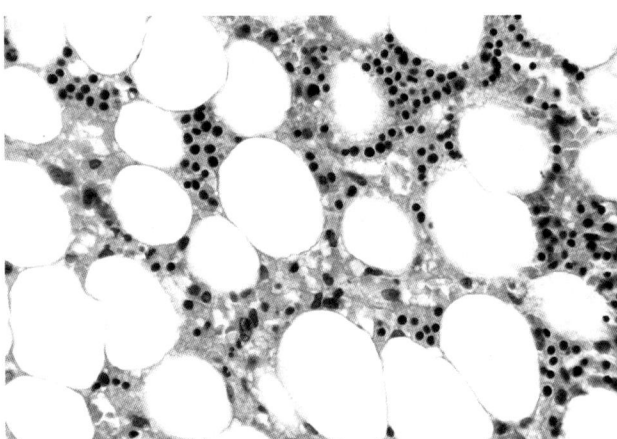

FIGURE 47.21. This BM biopsy section demonstrates marked azathioprine-induced prolonged myelosuppression (H&E stain, original magnification, 400× magnification).

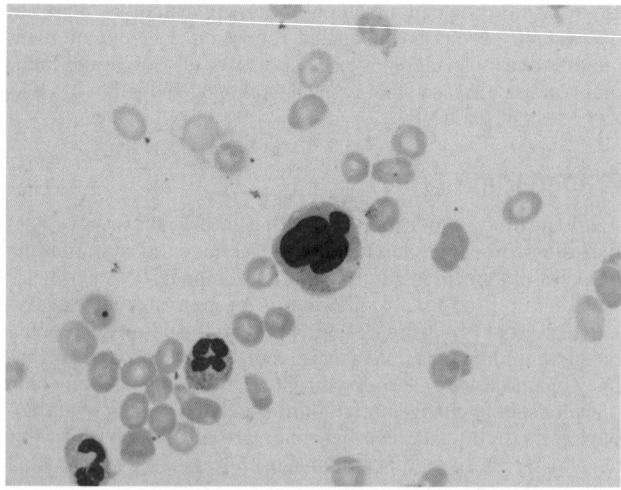

FIGURE 47.22. This BM aspirate smear photomicrograph demonstrates striking erythroid abnormalities mimicking MDS after arsenic ingestion. These changes include marked cellular enlargement, nuclear budding, and basophilic stippling (Wright stain, original magnification, 1,000× magnification).

Table 47.7	MEDICATIONS LINKED TO PSEUDO–PELGER-HUËT CHANGES

Mycophenolate
Tacrolimus
Valproate
Sulfisoxazole
Ganciclovir
Fluconazole
Ibuprofen
Paclitaxel
Docetaxel
G-CSF
Colchicine
D-penicillamine

References (125–131).

leukemia (as arsenic trioxide). Regardless of the route of exposure, arsenic poisoning results in significant morphologic effects on the BM hematopoietic compartment that mimic MDS (119,120). The BM effects include striking megaloblastosis, nuclear budding, and karyorrhexis in the erythroid precursors and nuclear to cytoplasmic dyssynchrony in the granulocytes (Fig. 47.22). Peripheral blood findings include anemia, macrocytosis, circulating nucleated red blood cells, and coarse basophilic stippling.

Alpha-Interferon

Alpha-interferon is a therapeutic agent used in a variety of hematopoietic disorders including CML (mainly in patients who are unable to tolerate imatinib) and hairy cell leukemia. In particular, alpha-interferon has no effect on reversing

fibrosis in non-CML myeloproliferative disorders and may even stimulate the development of BM fibrosis in CML patients (121–123).

Alpha-interferon has been largely replaced by purine analogs in the treatment of hairy cell leukemia; it does provide an excellent alternative treatment modality. The overwhelming majority of patients achieve at least a partial remission with minimal toxicity. Partial remission was defined in one study as normalization of hemogram values and a decrease of at least 50% of peripheral blood/BM hairy cells and spleen size (124).

Drug-Induced Pseudo–Pelger-Huët Change

Additionally, a number of medications, particularly those used in transplantation, may induce pseudo–Pelger-Huët abnormalities, which may be mistaken for development of MDS (Table 47.7) (118–124). The neutrophils demonstrate hyposegmentation with abnormally clumped chromatin and oval, monolobate, or bilobate nuclei. Dohle bodies may also be seen (Fig. 47.23A and B). These cytologic changes typically abate after removal of the offending agent.

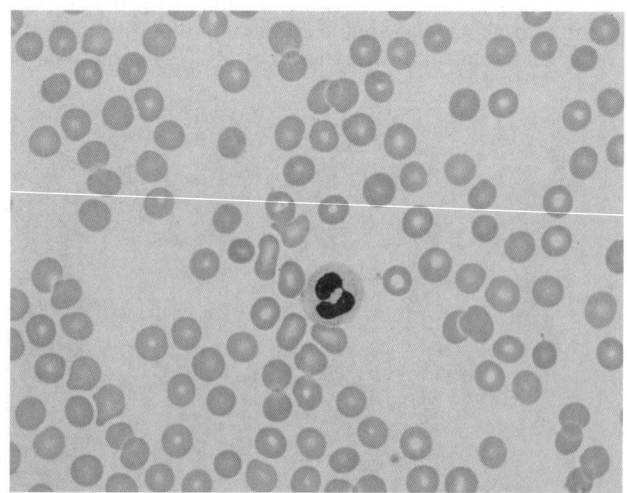

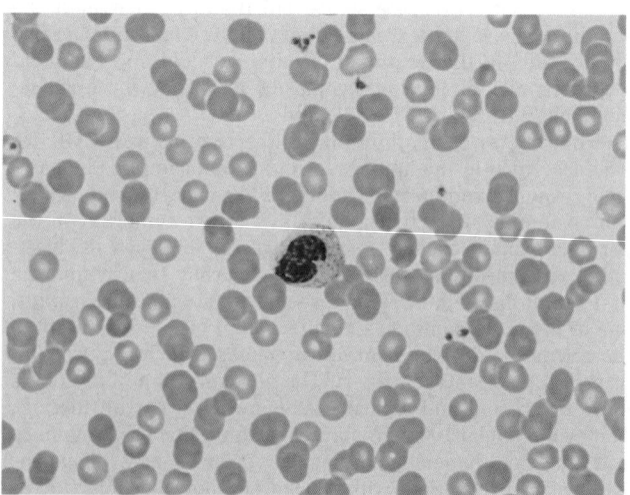

FIGURE 47.23. **A:** This peripheral blood smear photomicrograph demonstrates pseudo–Pelger-Huët change and Dohle bodies in a neutrophil in a patient being treated with sirolimus and mycophenolate mofetil as part of a transplant drug regimen (Wright stain, original magnification, 1,000× magnification). **B:** this peripheral blood smear photomicrograph demonstrates abnormal chromatin clumping, abnormal hyposegmentation, hypogranular cytoplasm, and Dohle bodies in a neutrophil in a patient being treated with sirolimus and mycophenolate mofetil as part of a transplant drug regimen (Wright stain, original magnification, 1,000× magnification).

References

1. Reichard K. Post-therapy bone marrow findings. In: Foucar K, Reichard K, Czuchlewski D, eds. *Bone marrow pathology*, 3rd ed. Chicago: ASCP Press, 2010:793–810.
2. Phan VH, Tan C, Rittau A, et al. An update on ethnic differences in drug metabolism and toxicity from anti-cancer drugs. *Expert Opin Drug Metab Toxicol* 2011;7:1395–1410.
3. Suhre K, Shin SY, Petersen AK, et al. Human metabolic individuality in biomedical and pharmaceutical research. *Nature* 2011;477:54–60.
4. Deenen MJ, Cats A, Beijnen JH, et al. Part 4: pharmacogenetic variability in anticancer pharmacodynamic drug effects. *Oncologist* 2011;16:1006–1020.
5. Dick FR, Burns CP, Weiner GJ, et al. Bone marrow morphology during induction phase of therapy for acute myeloid leukemia (AML). *Hematol Pathol* 1995;9:95–106.
6. Wittels B. Bone marrow biopsy changes following chemotherapy for acute leukemia. *Am J Surg Pathol* 1980;4:135–142.
7. Krech R, Thiele J. Histopathology of the bone marrow in toxic myelopathy: a study of drug induced lesions in 57 patients. *Virchows Arch A Pathol Anat Histopathol* 1985;405:225–235.
8. van Marion AM, Thiele J, Kvasnicka HM, et al. Morphology of the bone marrow after stem cell transplantation. *Histopathology* 2006;48:329–342.
9. Zhang H, Chen J, Que W. Allogeneic peripheral blood stem cell and bone marrow transplantation for hematologic malignancies: meta-analysis of randomized controlled trials. *Leuk Res* 2012;36(4):431–437.
10. Munchel A, Kesserwan C, Symons HJ, et al. Nonmyeloablative, HLA-haploidentical bone marrow transplantation with high dose, post-transplantation cyclophosphamide. *Pediatr Rep* 2011;3(Suppl 2):e15.
11. Cheson BD. Role of functional imaging in the management of lymphoma. *J Clin Oncol* 2011;29:1844–1854.
12. Nagler A, Condiotti R, Rabinowitz R, et al. Detection of minimal residual disease (MRD) after bone marrow transplantation (BMT) by multi-parameter flow cytometry (MPFC). *Med Oncol* 1999;16:177–187.
13. Bacher U, Haferlach T, Fehse B, et al. Minimal residual disease diagnostics and chimerism in the post-transplant period in acute myeloid leukemia. *ScientificWorld J* 2011;11:310–319.
14. Walter RB, Gooley TA, Wood BL, et al. Impact of pretransplantation minimal residual disease, as detected by multiparametric flow cytometry, on outcome of myeloablative hematopoietic cell transplantation for acute myeloid leukemia. *J Clin Oncol* 2011;29:1190–1197.
15. Zhang C, Zhang X, Chen XH, et al. Factors influencing engraftment in HLA-haploidentical/mismatch related transplantation with combined granulocyte-colony stimulating factor-mobilized peripheral blood and bone marrow for patients with leukemia. *Transfus Apher Sci* 2011;44:249–255.
16. Soll E, Massumoto C, Clift RA, et al. Relevance of marrow fibrosis in bone marrow transplantation: a retrospective analysis of engraftment. *Blood* 1995;86:4667–4673.
17. Thiele J, Kvasnicka HM, Schmitt-Graeff A, et al. Bone marrow histopathology following cytoreductive therapy in chronic idiopathic myelofibrosis. *Histopathology* 2003;43:470–479.
18. Thiele J, Kvasnicka HM, Schmitt-Gräff A, et al. Therapy-related changes of the bone marrow in chronic idiopathic myelofibrosis. *Histol Histopathol* 2004;19:239–250.
19. Seaman JP, Kjeldsberg CR, Linker A. Gelatinous transformation of the bone marrow. *Hum Pathol* 1978;9:685–692.
20. Mathew M, Mathews I, Manohar C, et al. Gelatinous transformation of bone marrow following chemotherapy for myeloma. *Indian J Pathol Microbiol* 2001;44:53–54.
21. Naeim F. Topobiology in hematopoiesis. *Hematol Pathol* 1995;9:107–119.
22. Riley RS, Idowu M, Chesney A, et al. Hematologic aspects of myeloablative therapy and BMT. *J Cin Lab Anal* 2005;19:47–79.
23. Foucar K. Therapy-related acute myeloid leukemia. In: Foucar K, Reichard K, Czuchlewski D, eds. *Bone marrow pathology*, 3rd ed. Chicago: ASCP Press, 2010:403–405.
24. Rosenthal NS, Farhi DC. Failure to engraft after bone marrow transplantation: bone marrow morphologic findings [see comments]. *Am J Clin Pathol* 1994;102:821–824.
25. Blum KA, Hamadani M, Phillips GS, et al. Prolonged myelosuppression with clofarabin. *Leuk Lymphoma* 2009;50:349–356.
26. Dainiak N, Waselenko JK, Armitage JO, et al. The hematologist and radiation casualities. *Hematology Am Soc Hematol Educ Program* 2003:473–496.
27. Cuker A. Toxicities of the thrombopoietic growth factors. *Semin Hematol* 2010;47:289–298.
28. Joannides M, Grimwade D. Molecular biology of therapy-related leukaemias. *Clin Transl Oncol* 2010;12:8–14.
29. Vardiman JW, Arber DA, Brunning RD, et al. Therapy-related myeloid neoplasms. In: Swerdlow SH, Campo E, Harris NL, et al., eds. *WHO classification of tumors of haematopoietic and lymphoid tissues*. Lyon: IARC, 2008:127–129.
30. Czader M, Orazi A. Therapy-related myeloid neoplasms. *Am J Clin Pathol* 2009;132:410–425.
31. Leone G, Pagano L, Ben-Yehuda D, et al. Therapy-related leukemia and myelodysplasia: susceptibility and incidence. *Haematologica* 2007;92:1389–1398.
32. Smith ML, Hills RK, Grimwade D. Independent prognostic variable in acute myeloid leukemia. *Blood Rev* 2011;25:39–51.
33. Chen W, Wang E, Lu Y, et al. Therapy-related acute lymphoblastic leukemia without 11q23 abnormality: report of 6 cases and a literature review. *Am J Clin Pathol* 2010;133:75–82.
34. Nagai K, Matsuo T, Atogami S, et al. Remission with morphological myelodysplasia in de novo acute myeloid leukemia: implications for early relapse. *Br J Haematol* 1992;81:33–39.
35. Rosenthal NS, Farhi DC. Dysmegakaryopoiesis resembling acute megakaryoblastic leukemia in treated acute myeloid leukemia. *Am J Clin Pathol* 1991;95:556–560.
36. Innes DJ Jr, Hess CE, Bertholf MF, et al. Promyelocyte morphology: differentiation of acute promyelocytic leukemia from benign myeloid proliferations. *Am J Clin Pathol* 1987;88:725–729.
37. Longacre TA, Foucar K, Crago S, et al. Hematogones: a multiparameter analysis of bone marrow precursor cells. *Blood* 1989;73:543–552.
38. McKenna RW, Asplund SL, Kroft SH. Immunophenotypic analysis of hematogones (B-lymphocyte precursors) and neoplastic lymphoblasts by 4-color flow cytometry. *Leuk Lymphoma* 2004;45:277–285.
39. Montesinos P, Gascón A, Martínez-Cuadrón D, et al. Significance of increased blastic-appearing cells in bone marrow following myeloablative unrelated cord blood transplantation in adult patients. *Biol Blood Marrow Transplant* 2012;18(3):388–395.
40. Hoagland HC. Hematologic complications of cancer chemotherapy. *Semin Oncol* 1982;9:95–102.
41. Gratwohl A, Baldomero H, Aljurf M, et al. Hematopoietic stem cell transplantation; a global perspective. *JAMA* 2010;303:1617–1624.
42. Gertz MA. Current status of stem cell mobilization. *Br J Haematol* 2010;150:647–662.
43. Szabolcs P, Cairo MS. Unrelated umbilical cord blood transplantation and immune reconstitution. *Semin Hematol* 2010;47:22–36.
44. Petropoulou AD, Rocha V. Risk factors and options to improve engraftment in unrelated cord blood transplantation. *Stem Cells Int* 2011;2011:610514.
45. Bayraktar UD, Champlin RE, Ciurea SO. Progress in haploidentical stem cell transplantation. *Biol Blood Marrow Transplant* 2012;18(3):372–380.
46. Sale GE, Buckner CD. Pathology of bone marrow in transplant recipients. *Hematol Oncol Clin North Am* 1988;2:735–756.
47. Bombi JA, Palou J, Bruguera M, et al. Pathology of bone marrow transplantation. *Semin Diagn Pathol* 1992;9:220–231.
48. Dick F, Gingrich RD. Biopsy analysis in bone marrow transplantation. In: Kolbeck PC, McManus BM, eds. *Transplant pathology*. Chicago: ASCP, 1994:281–292.
49. van den Berg H, Kluin PM, Vossen JM. Early reconstitution of haematopoiesis after allogeneic bone marrow transplantation: a prospective histopathological study of bone marrow biopsy specimens. *J Clin Pathol* 1990;43:365–369.
50. Thiele J, Kvasnicka HM, Beelen DW, et al. Bone marrow engraftment: histopathology of hematopoietic reconstitution following allogeneic transplantation in CML patients. *Histol Histopathol* 2001;16:213–226.
51. Trivedi M, Martinez S, Corringham S, et al. Optimal use of G-CSF administration after hematopoietic SCT. *Bone Marrow Transplant* 2009;43:895–908.
52. Robinson N, Sullivan KM. Complications of allogeneic bone marrow transplantation. *Curr Opin Hematol* 1994;1:406–411.
53. Anderson D, DeFor T, Burns L, et al. A comparison of related donor peripheral blood and bone marrow transplants: importance of late-onset chronic graft-versus-host disease and infections. *Biol Blood Marrow Transplant* 2003;9:52–59.
54. Warlick ED, Cioc A, Defor T, et al. Allogeneic stem cell transplantation for adults with myelodysplastic syndromes: importance of pretransplant disease burden. *Biol Blood Marrow Transplant* 2009;15:30–38.
55. Suyani E, Aki SZ, Yegin ZA, et al. The impact of bone marrow fibrosis on the outcome of hematopoietic stem cell transplantation. *Transplant Proc* 2010;42:2713–2719.
56. Thiele J, Kvasnicka HM, Beelen DW, et al. Macrophages and their subpopulations following allogeneic bone marrow transplantation for chronic myeloid leukemia. *Virchows Arch* 2000;437:160–166.
57. Tauchmanovà L, De Rosa G, Serio B, et al. Avascular necrosis in long-term survivors after allogeneic or autologous stem cell transplantation: a single center experience and a review. *Cancer* 2003;97:2453–2461.
58. Majhail NS. Secondary cancers following allogeneic haematopoietic cell transplantation in adults. *Br J Haematol* 2011;154:301–310.
59. Orazi A, Hromas RA, Greiner TC, et al. Posttransplantation lymphoproliferative disorders in bone marrow transplant recipients are aggressive disease with high incidence of adverse histologic and immunobiological features. *Am J Clin Pathol* 1997;107:419–429.
60. Hu YX, Cui Q, Liang B, et al. Donor-derived solid malignancies after hematopoietic stem cell transplantation. *Onkologie* 2010;33:195–200.
61. Wiseman DH. Donor cell leukemia: a review. *Biol Blood Marrow Transplant* 2011;17:771–789.
62. Yeung DT, Parker WT, Branford S. Molecular methods in diagnosis and monitoring of haematological malignancies. *Pathology* 2011;43:566–579.
63. Kröger N, Miyamura K, Bishop MR. Minimal residual disease following allogeneic hematopoietic stem cell transplantation. *Biol Blood Marrow Transplant* 2011;17(1 Suppl):S94–S100.
64. Buccisano F, Maurillo L, Del Principe MI, et al. Prognostic and therapeutic implications of minimal residual disease detection in acute myeloid leukemia. *Blood* 2012;119(2):332–341.
65. Jorgensen JL, Chen SS. Monitoring of minimal residual disease in acute myeloid leukemia: methods and best applications. *Clin Lymphoma Myeloma Leuk* 2011;11(Suppl 1):S49–S53.
66. Borrill V, Schlaphoff T, du Toit E, et al. The use of short tandem repeat polymorphisms for monitoring chimerism following bone marrow transplantation: a short report. *Hematology* 2008;13:210–214.
67. Ghiaur G, Gerber J, Jones RJ. Cancer stem cells and minimal residual disease. *Stem Cells* 2012;30(1):89–93.
68. Falk S, Seipelt G, Ganser A, et al. Bone marrow findings after treatment with recombinant human interleukin-3. *Am J Clin Pathol* 1991;95:355–362.
69. Ryder JW, Lazarus HM, Farhi DC. Bone marrow and blood findings after marrow transplantation and rhGM-CSF therapy. *Am J Clin Pathol* 1992;97:631–637.
70. Campbell LJ, Maher DW, Tay DLM, et al. Marrow proliferation and the appearance of giant neutrophils in response to recombinant human granulocyte colony stimulating factor (rhG-CSF). *Br J Haematol* 1992;80:298–304.
71. Schmitz LL, McClure JS, Litz CE, et al. Morphologic and quantitative changes in blood and marrow cells following growth factor therapy. *Am J Clin Pathol* 1994;101:67–75.
72. Wilson PA, Ayscue LH, Jones GR, et al. Bone marrow histiocytic proliferation in association with colony-stimulating factor therapy. *Am J Clin Pathol* 1993;99:311.
73. Orazi A, Cattoretti G, Schiro R, et al. Recombinant human interleukin-3 and recombinant human granulocyte-macrophage colony-stimulating factor administered in vivo after high-dose cyclophosphamide cancer chemotherapy: effect on hematopoiesis and microenvironment in human bone marrow. *Blood* 1992;79:2610–2619.
74. Orazi A, Gordon MS, John K, et al. In vivo effects of recombinant human stem cell factor treatment. A morphologic and immunohistochemical study of bone marrow biopsies. *Am J Clin Pathol* 1995;103:177–184.
75. Meyerson HJ, Farhi DC, Rosenthal NS. Transient increase in blasts mimicking acute leukemia and progressing myelodysplasia in patients receiving growth factor. *Am J Clin Pathol* 1998;109:675–681.

76. Santini V. Clinical use of erythropoietic stimulating agents in myelodysplastic syndromes. *Oncologist* 2011;16(Suppl 3):35–42.
77. McKinney M, Arcasoy MO. Erythropoietin for oncology supportive care. *Exp Cell Res* 2011;317:1246–1254.
78. Pérez-Ruixo JJ, Krzyzanski W, Hing J. Pharmacodynamic analysis of recombinant human erythropoietin effect on reticulocyte production rate and age distribution in healthy subjects. *Clin Pharmacokinet* 2008;47:399–415.
79. Singbrant S, Russell MR, Jovic T, et al. Erythropoietin couples erythropoiesis, B-lymphopoiesis, and bone homeostasis within the bone marrow microenvironment. *Blood* 2011;117:5631–5642.
80. Shimizu H, Saitoh T, Ota F, et al. Pure red cell aplasia induced only by intravenous administration of recombinant human erythropoietin. *Acta Haematol* 2011;126:114–118.
81. Kuter DJ, Mufti G, Bain BJ, et al. Evaluation of bone marrow reticulin formation in chronic immune thrombocytopenia patients treated with romiplostim. *Blood* 2009;114:3748–3756.
82. Douglas VK, Tallman MS, Cripe LD, et al. Thrombopoietin administered during induction chemotherapy to patients with acute myeloid leukemia induces transient morphologic changes that may resemble chronic myeloproliferative disorders. *Am J Clin Pathol* 2002;117:844–850.
83. Boiocchi L, Orazi A, Ghanima Waleed, et al. Thrombopoietin receptor agonist therapy in primary immune thrombocytopenia is associated with bone marrow hypercellularity and mild reticulin fibrosis but not other stromal abnormalities. *Modern Pathol* 2012;25:65–74.
84. McDonald V, Leandro M. Rituximab in non-haematological disorders of adults and its mode of action. *Br J Haematol* 2009;146:233–246.
85. Dalle S, Thieblemont C, Thomas L, et al. Monoclonal antibodies in clinical oncology. *Anticancer Agents Med Chem* 2008;8:523–532.
86. Verweij CL, Vosslamber S. New insight in the mechanism of action of rituximab: the interferon signature towards personalized medicine. *Discov Med* 2011;12:229–236.
87. Winiarska M, Glodkowska-Mrowka E, Bil J, et al. Molecular mechanisms of the antitumor effects of anti-CD20 antibodies. *Front Biosci* 2011;16:277–306.
88. Cioc AM, Vanderwerf SM, Peterson BA, et al. Rituximab-induced changes in hematolymphoid tissues found at autopsy. *Am J Clin Pathol* 2008;130:604–612.
89. Leandro MJ, Cambridge G, Ehrenstein MR, et al. Reconstitution of peripheral blood B cells after depletion with rituximab in patients with rheumatoid arthritis. *Arthritis Rheum* 2006;54:613–620.
90. Raynaud P, Caulet-Maugendre S, Foussard C, et al. GOELAMS group. T-cell lymphoid aggregates in bone marrow after rituximab therapy for B-cell follicular lymphoma: a marker of therapeutic efficacy? *Hum Pathol* 2008;39:194–200.
91. Douglas VK, Gordon LI, Goolsby CL, et al. Lymphoid aggregates in bone marrow mimic residual lymphoma after rituximab therapy for non-Hodgkin lymphoma. *Am J Clin Pathol* 1999;112:844–853.
92. Goteri G, Olivieri A, Ranaldi R, et al. Bone marrow histopathological and molecular changes of small B-cell lymphomas after rituximab therapy: comparison with clinical response and patients outcome. *Int J Immunopathol Pharmacol* 2006;19:421–431.
93. Maeshima AM, Taniguchi H, Nomoto J, et al. Histological and immunophenotypic changes in 59 cases of B-cell non-Hodgkin's lymphoma after rituximab therapy. *Cancer Sci* 2009;100:54–61.
94. Weissmann-Brenner A, Brenner B, Belyaeva I, et al. Rituximab associated neutropenia: Description of three cases and an insight into the underlying pathogenesis. *Med Sci Monit* 2011;17:CS133–CS137.
95. Dunleavy K, Tay K, Wilson WH. Rituximab-associated neutropenia. *Semin Hematol* 2010;47:180–186.
96. Wolach O, Bairey O, Lahav M. Neutropenia after rituximab treatment: new insights on a late complication. *Curr Opin Hematol* 2012;9(1):32–38.
97. Robak T, Robak E. New anti-CD20 monoclonal antibodies for the treatment of B-cell lymphoid malignancies. *BioDrugs* 2011;25:13–25.
98. Dimopoulos MA, Palumbo A, Attal M, et al. European Myeloma Network. Optimizing the use of lenalidomide in relapsed or refractory multiple myeloma: consensus statement. *Leukemia* 2011;25:749–760.
99. Padron E, Komrokji R, List AF. The 5q- Syndrome: Biology and Treatment. *Curr Treat Options Oncol* 2011;12(4):354–368.
100. Ximeri M, Galanopoulos A, Klaus M, et al. Hellenic MDS Study Group. Effect of lenalidomide therapy on hematopoiesis of patients with myelodysplastic syndrome associated with chromosome 5q deletion. *Haematologica* 2010;95:406–414.
101. Tehranchi R, Woll PS, Anderson K, et al. Persistent malignant stem cells in del(5q) myelodysplasia in remission. *N Engl J Med* 2010;36:1025–1037.
102. Komrokji RS, Sekeres MA, List AF. Management of lower-risk myelodysplastic syndromes: the art and evidence. *Curr Hematol Malig Rep* 2011;6:145–153.
103. Narla A, Dutt S, McAuley JR, et al. Dexamethasone and lenalidomide have distinct functional effects on erythropoiesis. *Blood* 2011;118:2296–2304.
104. Sekeres MA, Maciejewski JP, Giagounidis AA, et al. Relationship of treatment-related cytopenias and response to lenalidomide in patients with lower-risk myelodysplastic syndromes. *J Clin Oncol* 2008;26:5943–5949.
105. Palumbo A, Freeman J, Weiss L, et al. The clinical safety of lenalidomide in multiple myeloma and myelodysplastic syndromes. *Expert Opin Drug Saf* 2012;11(1):107–120.
106. Druker BJ. Translation of the Philadelphia chromosome into therapy for CML. *Blood* 2008;112:4808–4817.
107. Braziel RM, Launder TM, Druker BJ, et al. Hematopathologic and cytogenetic findings in imatinib mesylate-treated chronic myelogenous leukemia patients: 14 months' experience. *Blood* 2002;100:435–441.
108. Frater JL, Tallman MS, Variakojis D, et al. Chronic myeloid leukemia following therapy with imatinib mesylate (Gleevec). Bone marrow histopathology and correlation with genetic status. *Am J Clin Pathol* 2003;119:833–841.
109. Hong FS, Mitchell CA, Zantomio D. Gelatinous transformation of the bone marrow as a late morphological change in imatinib mesylate treated chronic myeloid leukemia. *Pathology* 2010;42:84–85.
110. Higgs JE, Payne K, Roberts C, et al. Are patients with intermediate TPMT activity at increased risk of myelosuppression when taking thiopurine medications? *Pharmacogenomics* 2010;11:177–188.
111. De Clercq E. Antiretroviral drugs. *Curr Opin Pharmacol* 2010;10:507–515.
112. Richman DD, Fischl MA, Grieco MH, et al. The toxicity of AZT in the treatment of patients with AIDS and AIDS-related complex. A double-blind, placebo-controlled trial. *N Engl J Med* 1987;317:192–197.
113. Moyle G. Anaemia in persons with HIV infection: prognostic marker and contributor to mortality. *AIDS Rev* 2002;4:13–20.
114. Romanelli F, Empey K, Pomeroy C. Macrocytosis as an indicator of medication (zidovudine) adherence in patients with HIV infection. *AIDS Patient Care STDS* 2002;16:405–411.
115. Bartakke S, Abdelhaleem M, Carcao M. Valproate-induced pure red cell aplasia and megakaryocytic dysplasia. *Br J Haematol* 2008;141(2):133.
116. Stewart JT. Successful reintroduction of valproic acid after the occurrence of pancytopenia. *Am J Geriatr Pharmacother* 2011;9:351–353.
117. Stoner SC, Deal E, Lurk JT. Delayed-onset neutropenia with divalproex sodium. *Ann Pharmacother* 2008;42:1507–1510.
118. Hongeng S, May W, Crist WM. Transient myeloid dysplasia due to valproic acid. *Clin Pediatr* 1997;36:361–364.
119. Rezuke WN, Anderson C, Pastuszak WT, et al. Arsenic intoxication presenting as a myelodysplastic syndrome: a case report. *Am J Hematol* 1991;36:291–293.
120. Heaven R, Duncan M, Vukelja SJ. Arsenic intoxication presenting with macrocytosis and peripheral neuropathy, without anemia. *Acta Haematol* 1994;92:142–143.
121. Thiele J, Kvasnicka HM. Comparative effects of interferon and hydroxyurea on bone marrow fibrosis in chronic myelogenous leukemia. *Leuk Lymphoma* 2001;42:855–862.
122. Sacchi S. The role of alpha-interferon in essential thrombocythaemia, polycythaemia vera and myelofibrosis with myeloid metaplasia (MMM): a concise update. *Leuk Lymphoma* 1995;19:13–20.
123. Gilbert HS. Long term treatment of myeloproliferative disease with interferon-alpha-2b: feasibility and efficacy. *Cancer* 1998;83:1205–1213.
124. Damasio EE, Clavio M, Masoudi B, et al. Alpha-interferon as induction and maintenance therapy in hairy cell leukemia: a long-term follow-up analysis. *Eur J Haematol* 2000;64:47–52.
125. Wang E, Boswell E, Siddiqi I, et al. Pseudo-Pelger-Huet anomaly induced by medications. A clinicopathologic study in comparison with myelodysplastic syndrome-related Pseudo-Pelger-Huet anomaly. *Am J Clin Pathol* 2011;135:291–303.
126. Etzell JE, Wang E. Acquired Pelger-Huët anomaly in association with concomitant tacrolimus and mycophenolate mofetil in a liver transplant patient: a case report and review of the literature. *Arch Pathol Lab Med* 2006;130:93–96.
127. Asmis LM, Hadaya K, Majno P, et al. Acquired and reversible Pelger-Huët anomaly of polymorphonuclear neutrophils in three transplant patients receiving mycophenolate mofetil therapy. *Am J Hematol* 2003;73:244–248.
128. Gondo H, Okamura C, Osaki K, et al. Acquired Pelger-Huët anomaly in association with concomitant tacrolimus and fluconazole therapy following allogeneic bone marrow transplantation. *Bone Marrow Transplant* 2000;26:1255–1257.
129. Moreira AM, Vieira LM, Rios DR, et al. Acquired Pelger-Huët anomaly associated with ibuprofen therapy [letter] [published correction appears in *Clin Chim Acta*. 2010;411:1397]. *Clin Chim Acta* 2009;409:140–141.
130. Kaplan JM, Barrett O Jr. Reversible pseudo-Pelger anomaly related to sulfisoxazole therapy. *N Engl J Med* 1967;277:421–422.
131. May RB, Sunder TR. Hematologic manifestations of long-term valproate therapy. *Epilepsia* 1993;34:1098–1101.
132. Macon WR, Tham KT, Greer JP, et al. Ringed sideroblasts—a frequent observation after bone marrow transplantation. *Mod Pathol* 1995;8:782–785.

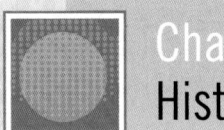

Chapter 48
Histiocytic and Dendritic Cell Proliferations

Karen L. Chang • Lawrence M. Weiss

Histiocytes and dendritic cells are two of the major types of nonlymphoid mononuclear cells involved in immune and nonimmune inflammatory responses. They are involved to some extent in all of the reactive and neoplastic processes of lymphoid tissue. Furthermore, there are some diseases in which a histiocytic or dendritic cell proliferation is the major component, and these entities are described herein.

 ## NORMAL HISTIOCYTES AND DENDRITIC CELLS

An overview of the major phenotypes of histiocytes and dendritic cells is presented in Table 48.1 (see Chapters 2 and 3). By convention, histiocytes are considered to be tissue-based monocytes, and many people also use the terms histiocytes and macrophages interchangeably. Briefly, myeloid-committed precursors in the bone marrow give rise to monocyte/macrophage and dendritic cell progenitors (MDPs). In turn, MDPs give rise to monocytes and common DC precursors (CDPs) (1), which cannot differentiate into other cells of the myeloid lineage (2).

Monocytes may circulate in the blood, bone marrow, or spleen. They may migrate from blood to tissue during infection in response to cytokine stimulation and may also differentiate into macrophages or inflammatory dendritic cells during inflammation. Macrophages reside in both lymphoid and nonlymphoid tissues, and may show further differentiation of function based on their location in the body. Macrophages help to clear apoptotic cells (via phagocytosis) and produce growth factors, thus maintaining tissue homeostasis. They also induce production of inflammatory cytokines.

Morphologically, histiocytes have bland nuclei and a moderate to marked amount of cytoplasm (epithelioid histiocytes), depending on their functional states. Ultrastructurally, histiocytes have numerous vacuoles, lysosomes, and residual bodies in their cytoplasm and often show numerous folds and microvillous projections. Cytochemically, the cells show reactivity for nonspecific esterase, acid phosphatase, and lysozyme. Histiocytes express the surface markers HLA-DR, CD45, CD11c, CD13, CD14, CD15, CD163, MAC-387, and CD4, and their cytoplasm contains CD68 and lysozyme. The monocytes/macrophages that respond to inflammation (M1 macrophages) express CD14 and not CD16 or CD163, whereas a subset of monocytes that play a role in tissue healing and are present in the immune response to neoplasms (M2 macrophages) express CD163, have no to low expression of CD14, and do express CD16 (3). Histiocytes have specific receptors that react with various types of immunoglobulins, complement, glycoproteins, transferrin, lipoproteins, peptides, coagulation factors, hormones, and cytokines (2). They internalize substances by pinocytosis or phagocytosis, in general fusing the internalized vesicles with lysosomes (4). They respond to a number of chemotactic factors and foreign substances, and they produce a wide range of substances, most notably enzymes (including lysozyme, neutral

proteases, and acid hydrolases), complement factors, coagulation factors, reactive oxygen and nitrogen species, bioactive lipids, and numerous cytokines and growth factors. They mediate resistance to intracellular microorganisms and tumors through nonimmunologic mechanisms. They also play an important role in the recognition and clearance of apoptotic cells.

CDPs give rise to dendritic cells (also known as classical dendritic cells) and plasmacytoid dendritic cells, and have lost the potential to give rise to monocytes (5). Dendritic cells are characterized by long and intricate cytoplasmic branching processes and low levels of lysosomal enzymes. Dendritic cells primarily process and present antigens and do not have the capacity for significant amounts of phagocytosis. The more immature forms do show some phagocytic activity, and the more mature forms produce large amounts of cytokines. Dendritic cells are highly migratory and help to regulate T-cell responses in the steady state as well as upon stimulation (e.g., infection). Traditionally, classical dendritic cells have been categorized by differing structure and function to include Langerhans cells, indeterminate cells, veiled cells, interdigitating dendritic (interdigitating reticulum) cells, follicular dendritic (dendritic reticulum) cells, and dermal dendrocytes.

Plasmacytoid dendritic cells are relatively long-lived and are present in the bone marrow and all peripheral organs (6). Their main function is to respond to viral infections by producing massive amounts of type-1 interferons. They also act as antigen-presenting cells and help to control T-cell responses. A subset of plasmacytoid dendritic cells have characteristic Ig rearrangements and in the past were considered "lymphoid-derived" in contrast to classical dendritic cells, which were considered "myeloid-derived" dendritic cells.

In contrast to the other dendritic cell types, Langerhans cells of the epidermis are not replaced by blood-borne cells in the steady state but they self-renew locally (7). They are also not depleted by high doses of x-ray irradiation. Langerhans cells possess characteristic organelles called Birbeck granules, which are racket- or rod-shaped structures of about 200 to 400 nm in length and about 33 nm in width, with an osmiophilic core and a double outer sheath, and are composed of langerin (CD207), which is available as an antibody to identify these cells. Langerhans cells express CD45, CD1a, S-100 protein, and langerin (8). Langerhans cells possess a high level of ATPase but have only low levels of accessory molecules that mediate binding and stimulation of T cells (9,10). They have abundant major histocompatibility complex II products within intracellular compartments, which represent efficient antigen-processing and antigen-presentation machines. As these cells respond to inflammation-induced cytokines or microbial substances, they become mature dendritic cells with abundant surface major histocompatibility complex II (11). They lose their Birbeck granules and migrate through the tissue interstitium and lymph system (as veiled cells) to the paracortical region of lymph nodes.

Indeterminate cells are dendritic cells of the dermis that are morphologically and antigenically similar to Langerhans cells with the exception that Birbeck granules are not identified (12).

Table 48.1	PHENOTYPE OF HISTIOCYTES AND COMMON DENDRITIC CELLS			
	Histiocytes	Langerhans Cells	Interdigitating Cells	Follicular Dendritic Cells
Adenosine triphosphatase	1+	2+	2+	2+
α-Naphthyl acetate esterase	2+	1+	1+	1+
CD45	2+	1+	1+	0+
S-100 protein	0+	2+	2+	1+
Fascin	0+	0+	2+	2+
HLA DR	2+	2+	2+	1+
CD1a	0+	2+	0+	0+
R4/23	0+	0+	0+	2+
Langerin	0+	2+	0+	0+

2+, strong and constant labeling; 1+, weak or inconstant labeling; 0+, no labeling.

They express CD45, CD1a, and S-100 protein, but not langerin, and they may represent either direct precursors (more likely) or direct successors of Langerhans cells. In the paracortical region of the lymph node, having lost CD1a expression as well, they become interdigitating cells.

Interdigitating cells express CD45, S-100 protein, the actin-bundling protein fascin, and many macrophage antigens but lack complement receptors, langerin, and CD163 (13). Through surface major histocompatibility complex–peptide complexes, the expression of T-cell–stimulatory molecules (such as CD40 and CD86), and the secretion of an array of chemokines, interdigitating cells are responsible for the initiation of strong cellular immunity. Their ultimate fate is cell death by apoptosis, accompanied by their phagocytosis and processing by lymphoid dendritic cells.

Although originally thought to be of non–bone marrow origin, follicular dendritic cells now are thought to be derived from mononuclear cells expressing KIM-4 (a marker of follicular dendritic cells) that may be found in the bone marrow and peripheral blood (14). More proximally, follicular dendritic cells are thought to derive from antigen-transporting cells found in afferent lymph channels and the subcapsular sinuses of lymph nodes. Follicular dendritic cells form a reticulum meshwork within germinal centers, retaining immune complexes on their cell surface. They are multinucleated cells with long branching cell processes that form desmosomal attachments. They express several macrophage and B-lineage markers in addition to a cell-specific antigen recognized by monoclonal antibodies R4/23, KIM-4, and BU-10 (15). They lack CD45 but express the complement receptors CD21 and CD35. They are involved intimately in memory cell formation and affinity maturation of follicle B cells.

The fibroblastic reticular cell plays a role in stromal support by secreting collagen and other extracellular matrix components, thus forming the mesenchymal backbone on which the antigen-presenting cells migrate and interact. Formerly thought to have only a structural role, recent studies show the cells also directly induce tolerance of naive CD8+ T cells, whether in inflammation or in the steady state (16,17). This cell is located in the parafollicular area and deep cortex of lymph nodes, and ultrastructural studies have demonstrated an association with the reticular network (18,19). Fibroblastic reticular cells form an intricate network of conduits that connect afferent lymphatics to high endothelial venules and through these conduits, soluble antigens are rapidly transported from the periphery to the dendritic cells. Fibroblastic reticular cells are not derived from the bone marrow but have ultrastructural and immunohistochemical features of myofibroblasts (18–21) (see Chapter 5).

Table 48.2	CLASSIFICATION OF HISTIOCYTIC AND DENDRITIC CELL PROLIFERATIONS

Benign histiocytic proliferations
  Sinus hyperplasia
  RDD
  HLH
  Malignant lymphoma with benign erythrophagocytosis
  HNL
Benign dendritic cell proliferations
  Dermatopathic lymphadenitis
Histiocytic/macrophage neoplasms
  Histiocytic sarcoma
  Histiocytic sarcoma with B-cell neoplasm or mediastinal germ cell neoplasm
Dendritic cell neoplasms
  LCH
  Langerhans cell sarcoma
  Follicular dendritic cell sarcoma
  Interdigitating cell sarcoma
  Indeterminate cell neoplasm
  Fibroblastic reticular cell neoplasm
Disseminated xanthogranuloma

RDD, Rosai-Dorfman disease; LCH, Langerhans cell histiocytosis; HLH, Hemophagocytic lymphohistiocytosis; HLN, Histiocytic necrotizing lymphadenitis.

CLASSIFICATION OF HISTIOCYTIC AND DENDRITIC CELL PROLIFERATIONS

A brief classification of the histiocytic and dendritic cell proliferations discussed in this chapter is given in Table 48.2. The World Health Organization classification of histiocytic and dendritic cell neoplasms is given in Table 48.3 (22). This chapter omits discussion of some entities with histiocytic proliferations, such as the storage disorders and inflammatory or infectious disorders (e.g., tuberculosis or sarcoidosis). Also omitted is a discussion of lymphomas with a high content of benign histiocytes, such as hepatosplenic $\gamma\delta$ T-cell lymphoma.

BENIGN HISTIOCYTIC PROLIFERATIONS

Sinus Hyperplasia

Sinus hyperplasia (also known as sinus histiocytosis) is so common that it is perhaps best regarded as a physiologic state rather than a pathologic condition. It is often prominent in lymph nodes draining the extremities or mesentery, as well as in lymph nodes draining sites of malignant neoplasms or prostheses (23). Histologically, one sees prominent lymph node sinuses distended by histiocytes with cytologically

Table 48.3	WORLD HEALTH ORGANIZATION CLASSIFICATION OF HISTIOCYTIC AND DENDRITIC CELL NEOPLASMS

Macrophage/histiocytic neoplasm
  Histiocytic sarcoma
Dendritic cell neoplasms
  LCH
  Langerhans cell sarcoma
  Interdigitating dendritic cell sarcoma
  Follicular dendritic cell sarcoma
  Fibroblastic reticular cell tumor
  Indeterminate dendritic cell tumor
Disseminated juvenile xanthogranuloma

From Swerdlow SH, Campo E, Harris NL, et al., eds. *World Health Organization classification of tumours: pathology & genetics. tumours of haematopoietic & lymphoid tissues.* Lyon: Intl Agency for Research on Cancer, 2008.

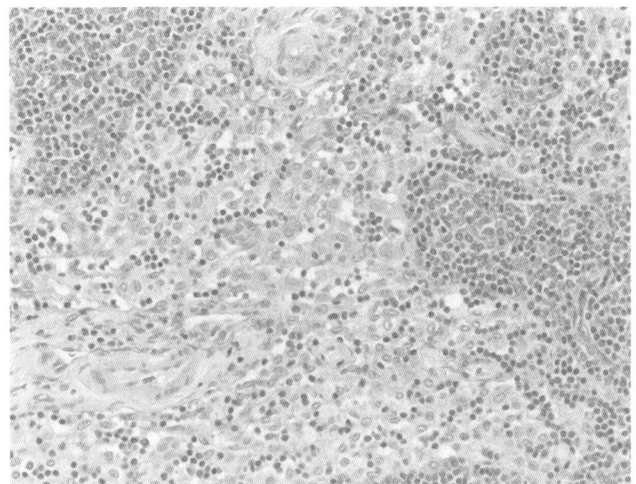

FIGURE 48.1. Sinus hyperplasia. Dilated sinuses are seen, filled with bland histiocytic cells.

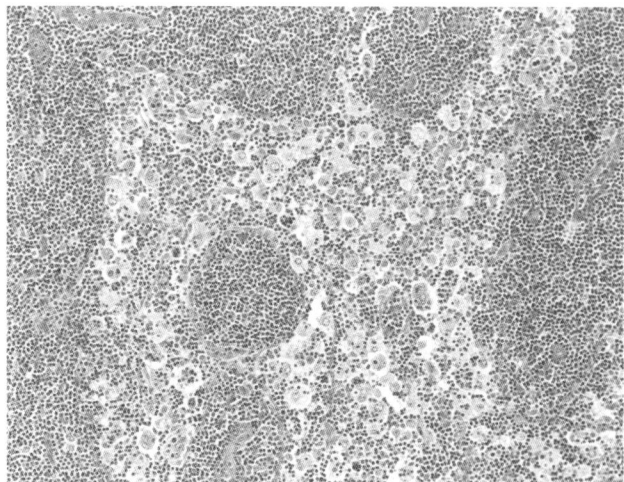

FIGURE 48.2. Rosai-Dorfman disease. A distinct sinusoidal pattern of involvement is seen.

bland nuclei and abundant cytoplasm (Fig. 48.1). Mitotic figures are not seen. Rarely, the histiocytes have signet ring features (24). Erythrophagocytosis may be present (24) (see Chapter 15).

Rosai-Dorfman Disease (Sinus Histiocytosis with Massive Lymphadenopathy)

Rosai-Dorfman disease (RDD) is a rare proliferative histiocytic disorder of unknown cause first recognized in the 1960s (25–27). Although usually benign and limited to lymph nodes, the disease may involve extranodal sites. The former name, sinus histiocytosis with massive lymphadenopathy, had been applied when the disease was first described in lymph nodes.

Clinically, the patients have a median age of 20 years but exhibit a wide range of ages, from neonates presenting with congenital disease to the elderly (27). There is a male:female ratio of about 4:3, and blacks may be affected more frequently than whites. There are sporadic reports of occurrence in twins or in patients with immune-mediated disease (28). The disease usually presents as isolated cervical lymphadenopathy, often dramatic in size. Other lymph node groups may be involved, including axillary, inguinal, and mediastinal nodes, either alone or in conjunction with cervical disease. Involvement of extranodal sites occurs in approximately 40% of patients (27). This involvement usually is seen in conjunction with lymph node involvement, although RDD occasionally affects extranodal tissues alone. In order of frequency, extranodal involvement may be seen in the skin, sinonasal region, soft tissues, orbit, bone, salivary gland, central nervous system (CNS), breast, and pancreas (27). Fever, weight loss, malaise, joint symptoms, and night sweats may be present, but hepatosplenomegaly is not a common occurrence.

Abnormalities often found in RDD patients include a mild normochromic and normocytic or hypochromic and microcytic anemia. A small number of patients have red cell autoantibodies, sometimes manifesting as severe hemolytic anemia. The peripheral white blood cell count is usually normal, although a reversal in the CD4:CD8 ratio often is found. Serum protein levels are often abnormal; a decrease in the albumin level and polyclonal elevations in IgG, IgM, or IgA levels are sometimes present. The erythrocyte sedimentation rate usually is elevated. Some patients have tested positive for rheumatoid factor or produced a positive lupus erythematosus cell preparation. No consistent lymphocyte, granulocyte, or histiocyte abnormalities have been found, and lipid studies are normal.

On gross examination, involved lymph nodes usually are enlarged. The cut surface of the node usually is described as yellow-white, with either a nodular or diffuse architecture. The histologic features are distinctive. The lymph node capsule is often fibrotic, but the fibrosis does not extend into the lymph node parenchyma as usually seen in classical Hodgkin disease, nodular sclerosis subtype. The most striking low-power feature of RDD nodes is a marked dilatation of the sinuses (Fig. 48.2). At high magnification, this expansion is found to be a result of numerous cells (Figs. 48.3 and 48.4) with intermediate-sized nuclei, a characteristic vesicular chromatin pattern, one to several small nucleoli, and voluminous amphophilic to eosinophilic cytoplasm. Cytologic atypia is usually lacking but may be present in some cases. The cells generally contain well-preserved lymphocytes (often termed *lymphophagocytosis* or *emperipolesis*) (Fig. 48.5). Less often, phagocytosis of plasma cells, neutrophils, and red blood cells is seen. Sometimes, the characteristic cells may possess a foamy cytoplasmic appearance. Plasma cells are often numerous, both within the sinuses and especially within the intervening cords (Fig. 48.6). Germinal centers are usually present, although they are not generally a prominent feature. Rarely, diffuse effacement of lymph node architecture is seen, particularly in advanced cases. The histologic findings in extranodal sites are usually strikingly similar

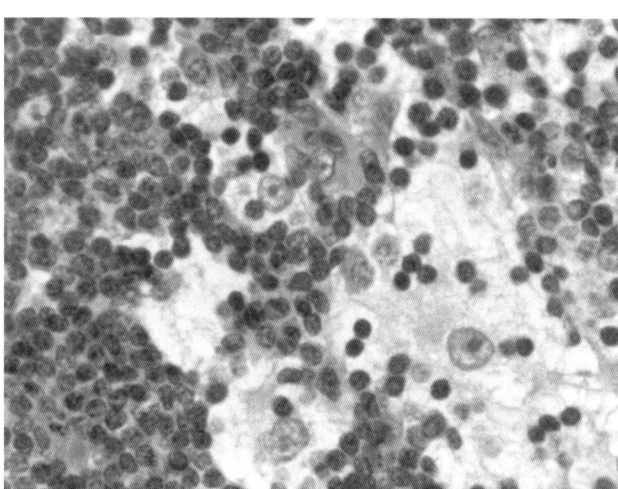

FIGURE 48.3. Rosai-Dorfman disease. The characteristic cells have abundant cytoplasm and medium-sized nuclei with one to several prominent nucleoli.

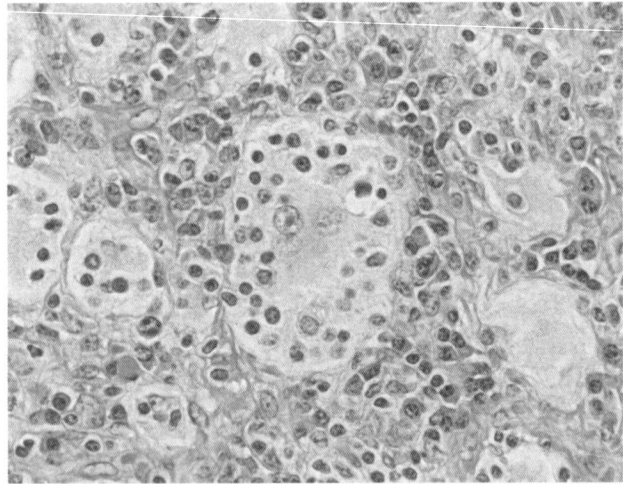

FIGURE 48.4. Rosai-Dorfman disease. The cells show the characteristic appearance, with numerous phagocytosed lymphocytes and other cells.

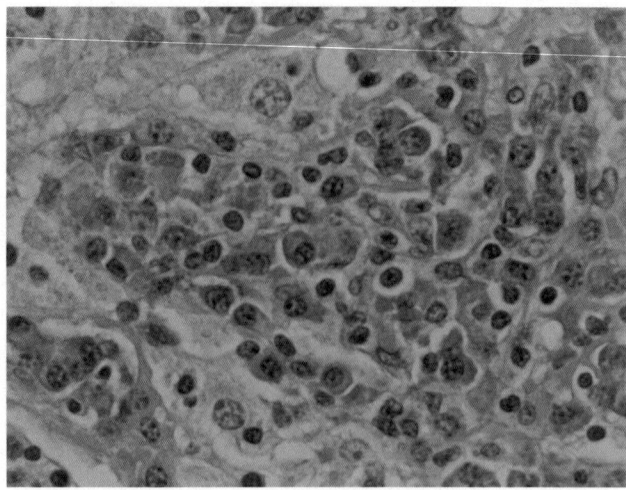

FIGURE 48.6. Rosai-Dorfman disease. The cords contain numerous plasma cells.

to those seen in lymph nodes (Fig. 48.7), even to the extent of having the appearance of dilated sinuses at times. The degree of fibrosis is generally greater, however, and the number of the characteristic cells is usually smaller and their prominence less than that seen in lymph nodes.

Paraffin immunohistochemistry shows the cells of RDD express numerous macrophage and macrophage-associated antigens, including S-100 protein, CD163, CD68, lysozyme, α_1-antitrypsin, α_1-antichymotrypsin, and the macrophage-specific markers HAM-56 and MAC-387 (29,30) (Fig. 48.8). They are also positive for the aspartic proteinases cathepsin D (expressed in macrophages) and cathepsin E (expressed in antigen-processing cells), a finding similar to the Langerhans cells of Langerhans cell histiocytosis (LCH) (31). Expression of CD30 (the Ki-1 antigen) has been reported in up to one-half of patients in one series (29). In addition, the cells of RDD lack expression of the CD1a antigen and langerin (CD207) found on Langerhans cells and also do not react with markers of follicular dendritic cells, such as CD21, CD35, or R4/23, a monoclonal antibody specific for follicular dendritic cells (8,27). Gene rearrangement studies have shown a germ line configuration for both the immunoglobulin heavy chain gene and the β gene of the T-cell receptor (32).

The differential diagnosis of RDD mainly involves benign sinus hyperplasia on the one hand and sinusoidal malignancies on the other. In benign sinus hyperplasia, the expansion of sinuses usually is less marked than in RDD and, more importantly, the characteristic cells of RDD with their usually prominent lymphophagocytosis are not present. Malignancies involving the sinuses, such as metastatic carcinoma and malignant melanoma, as well as sinusoidal malignant lymphoma, can be distinguished from RDD by attention to the cytologic features of the proliferating cells, as well as appropriate immunohistochemical stains such as keratin, S-100, or CD45 in the malignancies. In RDD the degree of cytologic atypia is usually not marked. LCH also may have a low-power appearance similar to RDD. Recognition of the cytologic characteristics of the proliferating Langerhans cells as well as the usual accompanying eosinophils enables distinction. If needed, langerin immunohistochemistry may be useful.

The majority of patients with RDD undergo spontaneous remission (27,33). Another large group of patients has persistent but stable disease not requiring therapy. Some patients require additional surgery beyond initial biopsy for alleviation of obstruction or cosmetic reasons. Chemotherapy and radiation therapy has been administered to a minority of patients, with low efficacy. A few patients have died, either from RDD

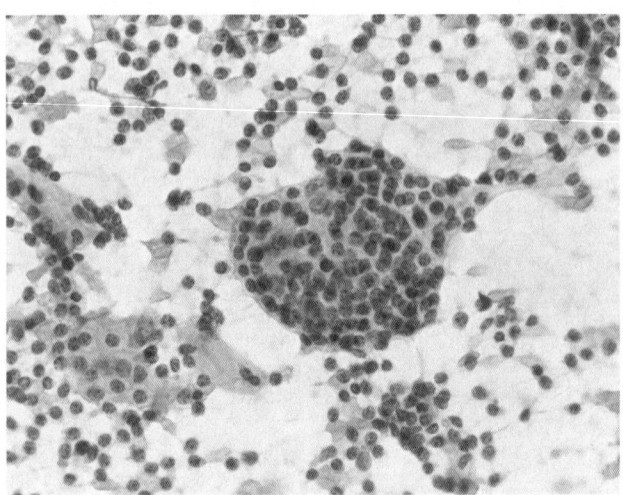

FIGURE 48.5. Rosai-Dorfman disease. This cell in this touch preparation shows prominent lymphophagocytosis.

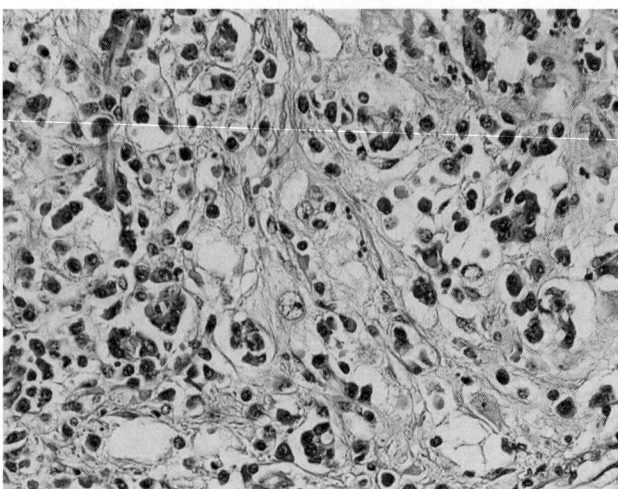

FIGURE 48.7. RDD involving the soft tissue. The lesion shows extensive secondary changes, but still contains scattered Rosai-Dorfman cells.

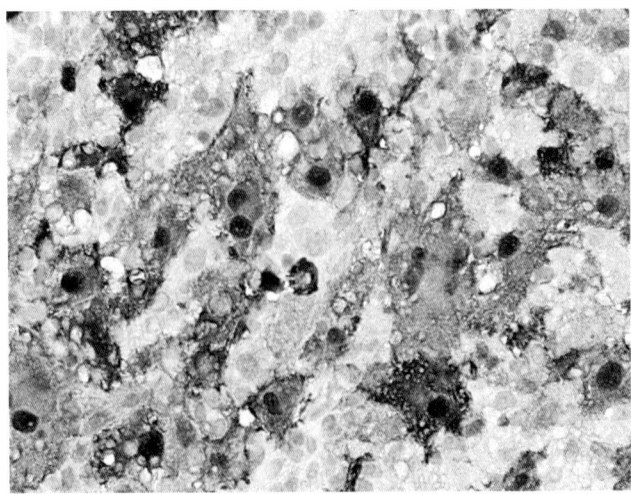

FIGURE 48.8. Rosai-Dorfman disease. This S-100 protein stain shows several positive Rosai-Dorfman cells, characteristic for this disease.

or with RDD significantly contributing to their death (27,34). Patients with an aggressive course tend to have involvement of a larger number of lymph node groups and a larger number of extranodal sites. Many of these patients also have evidence of immunologic abnormalities.

The nature of the proliferating cells in RDD has still not been clarified completely. Ultrastructural studies have demonstrated the presence of lipid vacuoles and varying numbers of lysosomes in the cytoplasm as well as complex filopodia, suggesting a histiocytic character. Birbeck granules are absent. Histochemical studies have demonstrated the presence of neutral fat and diastase-resistant material that is positive with periodic acid-Schiff staining in the cytoplasm, and reactions for acid phosphatase, α-naphthyl acetate, and α-butyrate esterase are additional evidence supporting a histiocytic differentiation (35,36). Normal sinus histiocytes lack the S-100 protein, and thus, S-100 protein expression by the cells of RDD does not support a close relationship with histiocytes and may suggest some relationship to dendritic cells. Regardless of the lineage, studies using X-linked polymorphic loci have shown that RDD is a polyclonal rather than a monoclonal proliferation and probably represents a reactive rather than a neoplastic process (32). Some groups have reported the presence of viruses in RDD lesions, including human herpesvirus-6 in RDD (37,38), polyoma virus (39), and parvovirus B19 (40). There is no association with the Epstein-Barr virus (41).

Hemophagocytic Lymphohistiocytosis

Hemophagocytic lymphohistiocytosis (HLH) is a potentially fatal proliferation of histiocytes resulting from a hyperstimulated but ineffective immune response. Broadly defined, HLH may be categorized as primary (genetic) or secondary (acquired) (42).

Most secondary cases of HLH arise in the setting of inflammation or infection, but may also be associated with malignancy, rheumatologic conditions, or metabolic diseases. The secondary variant has in the past been called infection-associated hemophagocytic syndrome or reactive hemophagocytic syndrome. The secondary HLH entity was originally described in association with viral infections, most particularly Epstein-Barr virus, as well as cytomegalovirus and other herpesviruses (43). The acquired type of HLH has also been found in association with many other types of infectious agents, such as Gram-positive and Gram-negative bacteria, mycobacteria, fungi, and Leishmaniasis organisms

(44,45). Lymphoma is the most common cause of malignancy-associated HLH (46).

The primary or genetic variant of HLH is also known as familial HLH and can further be divided into isolated familial HLH and other genetic disorders in which HLH is but one of the clinical manifestations. The latter cases include HLH in patients with X-linked syndromes, such as X-linked lymphoproliferative syndrome, X-linked severe combined immunodeficiency, and X-linked hypogammaglobulinemia (46).

Familial HLH is an extremely rare disease (usually 1 to 2 per million children) (47,48). The onset of disease is within the 1st year of life in most patients, and almost always in the first 7 years, but it has been described sporadically in all age groups, even in a 70-year-old (42). There is a slight male predominance. The disease occurs in all ethnic groups. Secondary HLH is also rare, but slightly more common than familial HLH. Also in contrast to familial HLH, secondary HLH does not have any age predominance.

Gene mutations have been uncovered in a large subset of cases in isolated familial HLH (46). The altered genes discovered to date all lead to defects in proteins that play an important role in the cytolytic secretory pathway, including those that mediate interactions with NK cells and cytotoxic T cells. The altered proteins lead to dysregulation, which possibly leads to persistent activation of macrophages and/or failure to remove the inciting antigenic stimulus (42). The most well-characterized protein abnormality is that of perforin mutations, which account for approximately 20% of familial cases of HLH (49). Less is known about the pathogenesis of secondary HLH, but, interestingly, some patients with the acquired form of HLH have been found to have heterozygous changes or polymorphisms in the familial HLH genes (42).

The clinical picture of HLH, whether familial or acquired, is ascribed to the hyperactivation of CD8+ T lymphocytes and macrophages; the proliferation, migration, and infiltration of these cells into various organs; and the persistently elevated levels of many inflammatory cytokines (42). These manifest as severe systemic illness, which includes fever and other constitutional symptoms, and may also result in hepatosplenomegaly, lymphadenopathy, skin rash, and CNS abnormalities. Bilateral pulmonary infiltrates and jaundice may also be apparent. In the acquired form of HLH, there may be a prodrome of a viral-like illness several weeks before the occurrence of severe symptomatology. Laboratory evaluation usually reveals pancytopenia, liver function abnormalities, and abnormal coagulation parameters, generally characterized by prolonged partial thromboplastin and thrombin times with normal to prolonged prothrombin times. The diagnostic criteria for establishing the diagnosis of HLH are listed in Table 48.4.

The histologic features of both forms of HLH are similar, and depend on when the biopsy is obtained in the disease course. The most striking findings are present in the hematolymphoid organs. In the earlier phases of the disease course, lymph nodes (usually biopsied only in the acquired form of HLH) may show only nonspecific viral lymphadenitis changes, with paracortical expansion by immunoblasts. As the disease progresses, involved lymph nodes generally maintain an intact architecture or show only slight distortion, with the sinusoids and paracortical areas filled with (but not distended by) numerous histiocytes. The histiocytes lack cytologic atypia and often show prominent platelet phagocytosis and hemophagocytosis and often lymphophagocytosis (Figs. 48.9 to 48.11). Germinal centers are not generally prominent, and the lymph node often shows an overall cell-depleted appearance. At the final stages, one may see lymphoid depletion. Affected spleen shows lymphoid depletion and involvement of the red pulp, and the liver shows lymphoid hyperplasia and sinusoidal and portal involvement by a histiocytic infiltrate

From Weitzman S. Approach to hemophagocytic syndromes. *ASH Education Program Book* 2011;2011:178–183.

Table 48.4	DIAGNOSTIC CRITERIA FOR HLH

The diagnosis of HLH is established if either condition 1 or condition 2 is fulfilled:
1. A molecular diagnosis consistent with HLH is made.
2. Diagnostic clinical and laboratory criteria are fulfilled (5 of 8 criteria below)
   - Fever
   - Splenomegaly
   - Cytopenia ≥ 2 cell lines in the peripheral blood, as evidenced by
     - Hemoglobin < 90 g/L (below 4 wk < 100 g/L)
     - Neutrophils < 1 × 10E9/L
     - Platelets < 100 × 10E9/L
   - Hypertriglyceridemia and/or hypofibrinogenemia
     - Fasting triglycerides ≥ 3 mmol/L
     - Fibrinogen < 1.5 g/L
   - Ferritin ≥ 500 μg/L
   - sCD25 ≥ 2,400 U/mL
   - Decreased or absent NK-cell activity
   - Hemophagocytosis in bone marrow, spleen, or lymph nodes

Supportive evidence are cerebral symptoms with moderate pleocytosis and/or elevated protein, elevated transaminases and bilirubin, hypoalbuminemia, hyponatremia, elevated D-dimers, and LDH > 1,000 U/L.

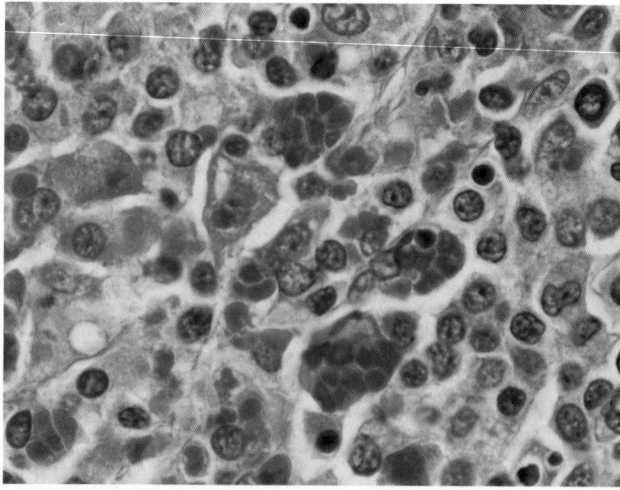

FIGURE 48.10. Infection-associated hemophagocytic syndrome. This lymph node shows numerous histiocytes exhibiting erythrophagocytosis and phagocytosis of debris.

with variable hemophagocytosis. The CNS, if involved, shows diffuse infiltration of the leptomeninges and infiltration of perivascular spaces within the brain parenchyma, particularly the white matter. Other organs that may be involved include the thymus, lungs, CNS, and intestine.

Patients with the familial form of HLH most often have a bone marrow study as part of the initial workup, although patients with acquired HLH may also undergo examination of the bone marrow. The marrow appearance also depends on the stage of the disease at which the biopsy is obtained. Early on, the bone marrow is hypercellular and shows erythroid hyperplasia, myeloid hypoplasia, and, most prominently, a diffuse infiltration by cytologically bland histiocytes displaying variable degrees of erythrophagocytosis (50,51). As the disease progresses, the marrow becomes more hypocellular with a decrease in the erythropoietic and granulopoietic lines, with normal or increased numbers of megakaryocytes. Moderate to marked histiocytic hyperplasia is present. Phagocytosis is still prominent, usually involving platelets and red cells, although phagocytosis of other cellular debris

may be seen. Some patients have normal-appearing bone marrows (50).

Histochemically, the proliferating cells express acid phosphatase, nonspecific esterase, and lysozyme, consistent with a histiocytic derivation (51). Immunophenotypic studies have shown that the histiocytic cells express CD14 and HLA-DR, with variable expression of CD15, again consistent with tissue histiocytes (52). The cells are negative for S-100 protein, langerin, and CD1a and do not show Birbeck granules on ultrastructural examination, evidence against a dendritic cell lineage. Plasma levels of soluble CD163 are markedly elevated (53).

The differential diagnosis generally centers on the distinction of HLH from hematolymphoid neoplasms involving the sinuses as well as hematolymphoid neoplasms secondarily inducing benign hemophagocytosis. The former distinction generally is based on the cytologic characteristics of the proliferating cells. The histiocytes are cytologically benign in HLH; atypicality of the proliferating cells should be evident in hematolymphoid malignancies. In some patients, this distinction may be quite difficult. Repeat biopsies sometimes may allow resolution of the problem (54). Some lymphomas, particularly

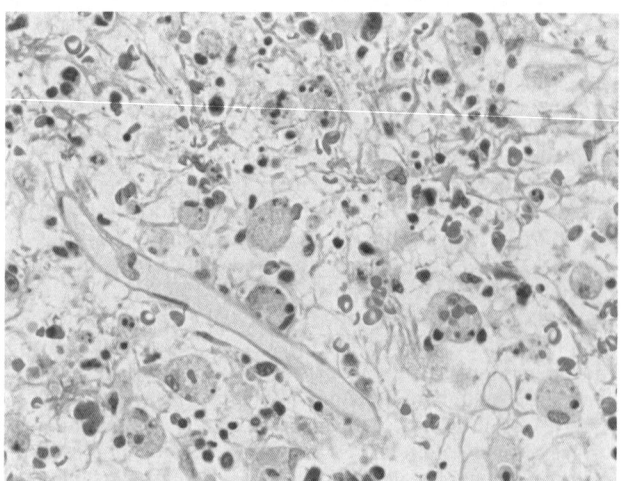

FIGURE 48.9. Infection-associated hemophagocytic syndrome. This spleen shows numerous histiocytes with erythrophagocytosis.

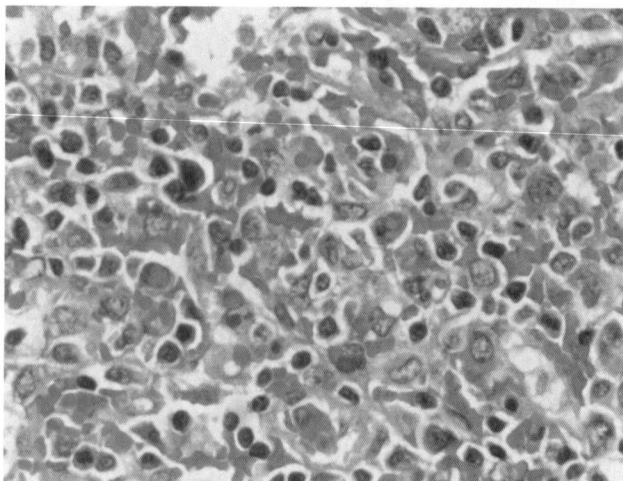

FIGURE 48.11. Familial HLH. Numerous histiocytes, including several with erythrophagocytosis, are present in this spleen.

T-cell neoplasms, may induce an exuberant hyperplasia of benign-appearing hemophagocytizing lymphocytes (55,56). Attention to the other elements in the biopsy specimen besides the benign histiocytes is important in identifying these cases.

In its most indolent form, secondary HLH may be a benign, self-limited condition from which the patient may recover completely. About one half of these patients, however, die with the disease, because of multisystem failure during the acute episode or infectious complications exacerbated by the underlying immunodeficiency that often exists. HLH triggered by bacterial infections is associated with a relatively high recovery rate; the worst prognosis is found in Epstein-Barr virus infection (about a 25% survival rate). The large majority of patients with familial HLH have traditionally had a rapid downhill course, but large comprehensive clinical trials have shown an improvement with chemoimmunotherapy followed in some cases by hematopoietic cell transplant. Initial therapy for both primary and secondary HLH is similar (except in patients with rheumatologic-related HLH) and thus treatment should begin prior to completion of workup to distinguish between the different forms of the disease (57). Therapy comprises immunosuppressive therapy as well as pro-apoptotic chemotherapy, such as etoposide. All primary HLH patients need hematopoietic cell transplant for cure, with higher rates of survival in family donor hematopoietic cell transplants (70%) than haploidentical donors (50%). Whether to use family donors in apparent primary HLH with no identified genetic defect is the subject of debate. Patients with underlying rheumatologic defects may need only steroids and/or cyclosporin and/or intravenous immunoglobulin.

Malignant Lymphoma with Benign Erythrophagocytosis

This disease represents a mixed process that combines features of a malignant lymphoma with a reactive disorder of histiocytes (55,56,58). Similar to secondary HLH, a widespread proliferation of benign histiocytes with prominent erythrophagocytosis is seen. Instead of being associated with a systemic infection or disease however, the process is associated with a malignant lymphoma, most often T-cell lymphoma, which may be segregated physically from the proliferating histiocytes. The exact etiology is unknown, but may be related to lymphokine or cytokine secretion.

Malignant lymphoma with benign erythrophagocytosis has been seen in two main clinical settings. The first is in patients with known malignant lymphoma in whom a syndrome mimicking HLH develops (55,56). In this group of patients, disseminated lymphoma is often present. Most lymphomas are T-cell lymphomas or natural killer cell neoplasms, including nasal T-/natural killer cell lymphoma and anaplastic large cell lymphoma, but lymphomas of B-cell lineage also have been associated with this syndrome (55,56,58). The erythrophagocytic process is physically distinct from the lymphoma and is characterized by a marked proliferation of cytologically benign histiocytes that frequently demonstrate conspicuous erythrophagocytosis as well as phagocytosis of other formed elements of the blood. This process is most evident in bone marrow, lymph node sinuses, splenic red pulp, and hepatic sinusoids. This process is usually a terminal event in a patient with advanced-stage lymphoma.

In the second presentation, the hemophagocytic syndrome occurs in the absence of any preexisting disease (56). In this setting, benign hemophagocytizing histiocytes are found in intimate association with the malignant lymphoma, usually a T-cell lymphoma, which often also involves the bone marrow, spleen, and liver (Fig. 48.12). Again, the prognosis is usually poor in the majority of patients.

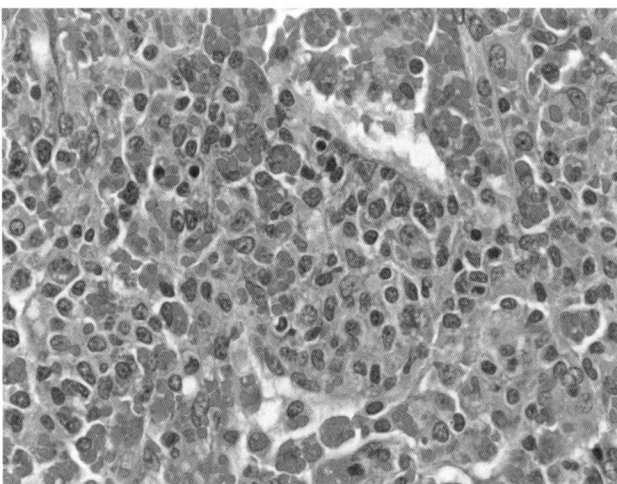

FIGURE 48.12. Malignant lymphoma with benign erythrophagocytosis. The splenic cords contain numerous malignant cells; the sinuses show numerous benign histiocytes with erythrophagocytosis. Some admixture between the two populations of cells also is seen.

Histiocytic Necrotizing Lymphadenitis

Histiocytic necrotizing lymphadenitis (HNL) (of Kikuchi and Fujimoto) is a well-defined clinicopathologic disorder, which has a benign clinical course and primarily affects lymph nodes of young adults. Although it was first described in Japan (59,60), numerous cases have been reported in Western countries (61–64).

Clinically, the median age at diagnosis is about 30 years, with a wide age range from teenagers to the elderly. Although early reports indicated a marked predominance in women, subsequent reports indicate that the gender ratio of affected patients is closer to 1:1 (65). The patients are generally otherwise healthy, with no obvious predisposing occupation, lifestyle, or underlying disease. Patients usually present with localized cervical or posterior cervical lymphadenopathy that may be tender to palpation. Less often, a variety of other lymph node regions are primarily affected; on occasion, two or more sites may be involved. Rarely, involvement of extranodal tissues such as skin, bone marrow, and salivary gland has been reported (64,66–68). In the majority of patients, lymphadenopathy is the only symptom, but occasional patients report mild fever, often associated with upper respiratory symptoms, weight loss, nausea and vomiting, myalgia and arthralgia, chills, and night sweats (65). Rare patients report a rash with a malar distribution. Patients may rarely have hepatosplenomegaly. The duration of symptoms prior to diagnosis is usually several months. Approximately one-third of patients have anemia and a high erythrocyte sedimentation rate, whereas neutropenia, lymphocytosis, or circulating atypical lymphocytes have been reported on occasion. Serologic studies usually do not show good evidence for an infectious agent (65). The cause of this disease is as yet unknown. Evidence for an infectious cause has been sought, but no convincing evidence has been obtained; the studies to date have proved negative (65).

Grossly, most lymph nodes are normal or only slightly increased in size. Areas of necrosis generally are not appreciated grossly but usually are quite striking microscopically. These foci generally are located in the paracortex and less often in the cortex (Fig. 48.13). They usually consist of irregular, circumscribed areas of deposition of an eosinophilic substance (probably representing fibrin) along with a marked degree of karyorrhexis (Fig. 48.14). Occasionally, the eosinophilic substance is sparse. Despite the widespread necrosis with

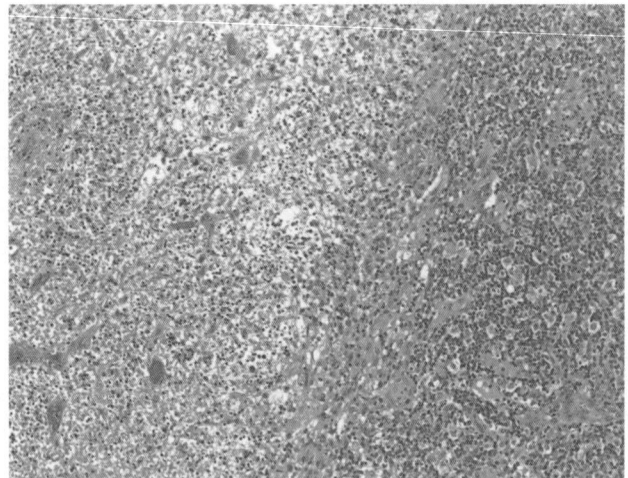

FIGURE 48.13. Histiocytic necrotizing lymphadenitis. A discrete area of necrosis is seen in this lymph node. The adjacent area shows a mottled appearance resulting from an immunoblastic proliferation (original magnification: 100×).

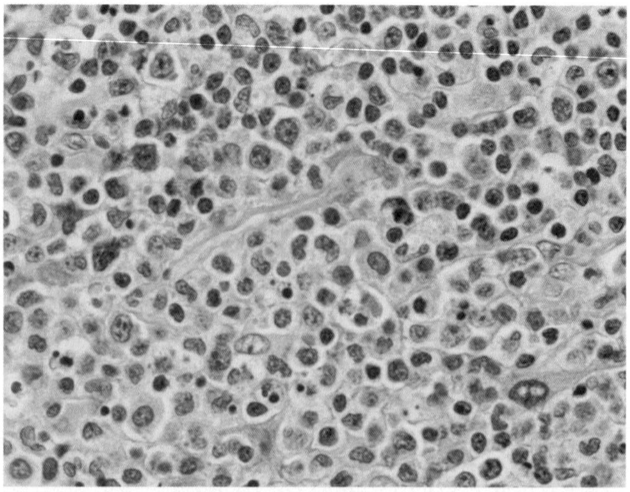

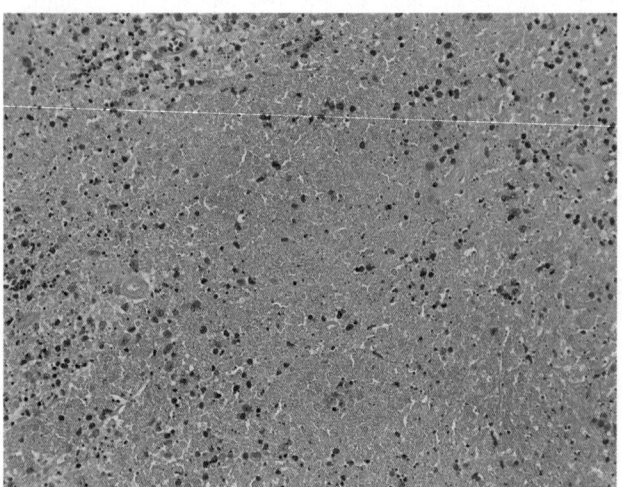

FIGURE 48.14. Histiocytic necrotizing lymphadenitis. This area shows karyorrhectic debris and fibrin without viable cells.

FIGURE 48.15. Histiocytic necrotizing lymphadenitis. Nuclei of macrophages and immunoblasts are seen amid karyorrhectic debris. Such areas could simulate non-Hodgkin lymphoma.

karyorrhexis, there is an almost complete absence of intact neutrophils. Most of the viable cells present are histiocytes, often exhibiting phagocytosis and occasionally containing foamy cytoplasm, reactive immunoblasts, and other mononuclear cells with somewhat atypical nuclear features (Fig. 48.15). The histiocytes often have a distinctive appearance, with peripherally placed, crescent-shaped, twisted nuclei with abundant cytoplasm containing karyorrhectic debris (68). Plasma cells are generally few in number, and eosinophils are absent. Areas immediately adjacent to the foci of necrosis usually show a reactive immunoblastic proliferation. The remainder of the lymph node is usually normal and generally does not show significant reactive follicular hyperplasia. Focal distention of sinuses by monocytoid B lymphocytes has been reported (61), but is usually not a prominent finding. The lymph node capsule is sometimes thickened adjacent to the areas of necrosis. The proportion of microabscesses, karyorrhectic debris, and foamy histiocytes varies as the disease progresses, with the phases generally divided into proliferative, necrotizing, and xanthomatous stages (69).

Immunophenotyping studies have demonstrated a predominance of T cells and histiocytes within involved areas of the lymph node (63–65,69). Helper or inducer T cells may predominate in early lesions; cytotoxic or suppressor T cells may be in the majority in biopsy specimens taken later after presentation (63). In addition to the marked CD8+ lymphocyte predominance, the numerous CD68+ histiocytes have been more accurately delineated to be plasmacytoid dendritic cells or plasmacytoid monocytes, on the basis of their CD123 expression and lack of CD13 or CD33 expression (70–72). Gene rearrangement studies show germ line status.

The most important entity to be distinguished from HNL is non-Hodgkin lymphoma. The abundant karyorrhectic debris found in HNL often suggests a high-grade lymphoma at first glance, particularly if one sees sheets of histiocytes, which may give the superficial appearance of a large cell lymphoma. The characteristic clinical history often gives the first clue to a diagnosis of HNL. In addition, the only lymphomas to have such a high degree of karyorrhexis are the high-grade lymphomas, and the monotonous cellular populations found in these lymphomas are not seen in HNL. Lymph node infarction, a finding that also may be associated with non-Hodgkin lymphoma, generally shows granulation tissue at the edges of the necrotic areas (73). Sometimes, "ghosts" of cells can be seen in the necrotic areas. Hodgkin lymphoma and infectious agents such as *Yersinia enterocolitis* or the organism causing cat scratch disease may be associated with stellate areas of necrosis (stellate microabscesses) but can be distinguished from HNL by the presence of neutrophils in and around the areas of necrosis in these disorders. Similarly, lymph node biopsies from patients with Kawasaki disease also show neutrophils in association with the areas of necrosis. In addition, fibrin thrombi in small vessels are usually a prominent feature in this disorder (74).

All of the histologic findings in HNL also may be seen in lymph nodes from patients with systemic lupus erythematosus (SLE). Features that might favor SLE would be the additional presence of basophilic necrotic material often deposited in vessel walls and sometimes forming hematoxyphilic bodies, and the presence of more than occasional plasma cells (75) (Fig. 48.16). However, any patient given a diagnosis of HNL should be investigated clinically to rule out the possibility of SLE. Some investigators have proposed the notion that HNL represents a solitary manifestation of SLE (64,65).

Patients with HNL usually have a benign clinical course with spontaneous resolution of the disease in a large majority of patients (63–65). Rare patients have developed recurrent

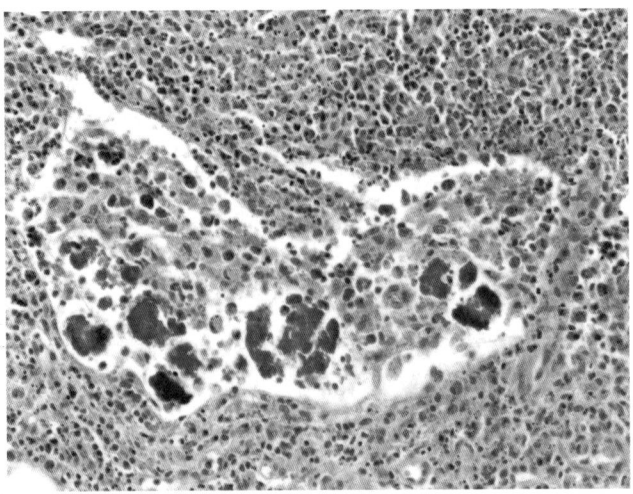

FIGURE 48.16. Systemic lupus erythematosus. Several hematoxylin bodies are seen in the sinus. Otherwise, the appearance in the lymph node resembled Kikuchi HNL.

lymphadenopathy in which repeat biopsy has shown similar histologic features and rare patients have subsequently developed SLE (63). Additionally, rare cases have been fatal (64,65).

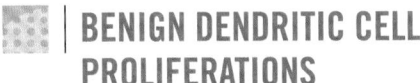 **BENIGN DENDRITIC CELL PROLIFERATIONS**

Dermatopathic Lymphadenitis

Dermatopathic lymphadenitis refers to the lymph node reaction that occurs in lymph nodes draining areas of disruption of the skin integrity. Grossly, the lymph node is enlarged and fleshy and often has melanotic pigmentation. Histologically, the node architecture shows varying degrees of paracortical expansion, usually but not always accompanied by reactive follicular hyperplasia (Fig. 48.17). The enlarged paracortical areas contain a population of dendritic cells and histiocytes, often admixed with immunoblasts, eosinophils, and plasma cells. The numerous dendritic cells, comprising both interdigitating dendritic cells and Langerhans cells, can be highlighted with an anti-S-100 protein stain (see Chapter 15).

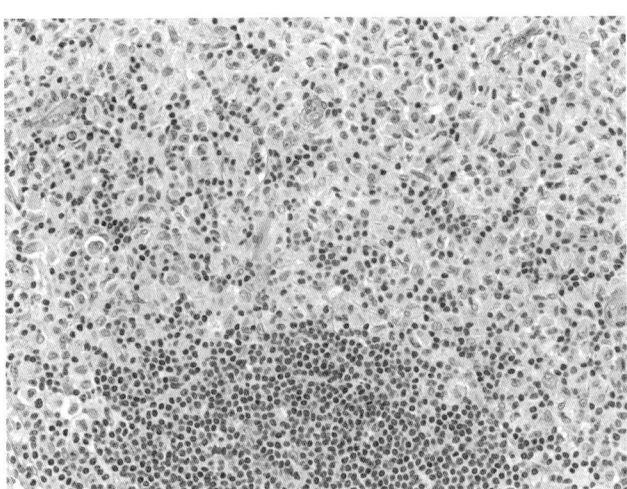 A
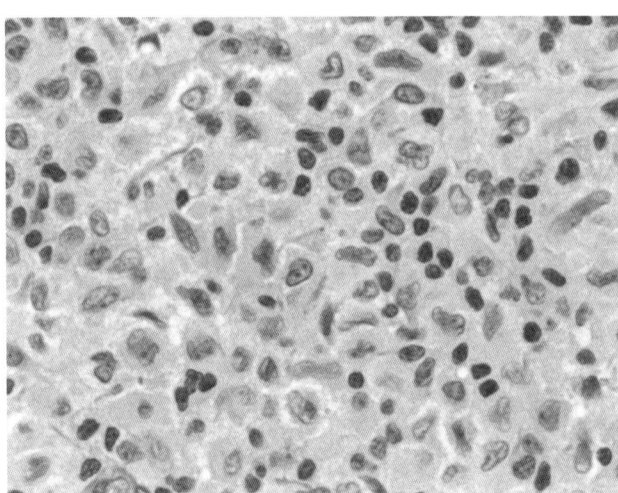 B

FIGURE 48.17. Dermatopathic lymphadenitis. A: Paracortical expansion is seen. **B:** Numerous dendritic cells with clefted nuclei and histiocytes are seen.

HISTIOCYTIC/MACROPHAGE NEOPLASM

Histiocytic Sarcoma

Histiocytic sarcoma, formerly known as true histiocytic lymphoma, malignant histiocytosis, or histiocytic medullary reticulosis, is a rare neoplasm that comprises malignant cells theoretically derived from true tissue macrophages. This entity accounts for <1% of all lymphomas (76–79) and occurs most often in older adults, although it has been reported in children; there does not appear to be any gender predilection. Because of its cell of origin, the neoplasm may occur at any site where histiocytes are present. About one half of the cases present in lymph nodes; the other half present in a variety of extranodal sites, most commonly the gastrointestinal (GI) tract and skin (80). The tumor is usually solitary but some patients have multifocal presentation.

There is no known etiologic agent. However, some cases of histiocytic sarcoma have been associated with another hematologic malignancy, usually of B-cell lineage (81–83). In those cases, identical immunohistochemical profiles, IgH gene rearrangements, and bcl-2 gene breakpoints were found in the histiocytic sarcoma as well as the B-cell neoplasm (82,84). A subset of histiocytic sarcomas is associated with primary mediastinal germ cell tumors, usually malignant teratoma, with or without yolk sac tumor differentiation (85). In fact, patients with primary nonseminomatous mediastinal germ cell tumors have a statistically significantly higher chance of developing a hematologic neoplasm than the general population. The hematologic malignancy usually develops within 1 year of diagnosis of germ cell tumor and comprises myeloproliferative neoplasms, leukemias, histiocytic sarcoma, and mast cell disease (85).

Histologically, histiocytic sarcoma usually consists of a diffuse, noncohesive proliferation of round to oval neoplastic cells (Fig. 48.18A). The nuclei often are placed eccentrically and have folded to pleomorphic nuclei, with prominent nucleoli. Multinucleate cells commonly are seen. The mitotic rate is generally high. Cytoplasm is usually eosinophilic and abundant but may be spindled in focal areas. Foamy cell change may be seen. Hemophagocytosis or lymphophagocytosis may be seen on occasion but is usually not prominent. Accompanying the neoplastic proliferation is a variable number of host cells, including lymphocytes, plasma cells, and eosinophils. If organs are involved, a sinusoidal or focal parenchymal pattern of infiltration may be seen. Ultrastructural studies show cytoplasmic lysosomes, but no evidence of Birbeck granules or

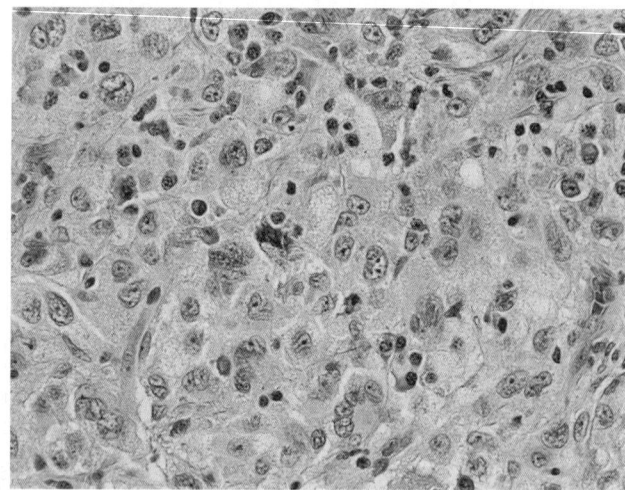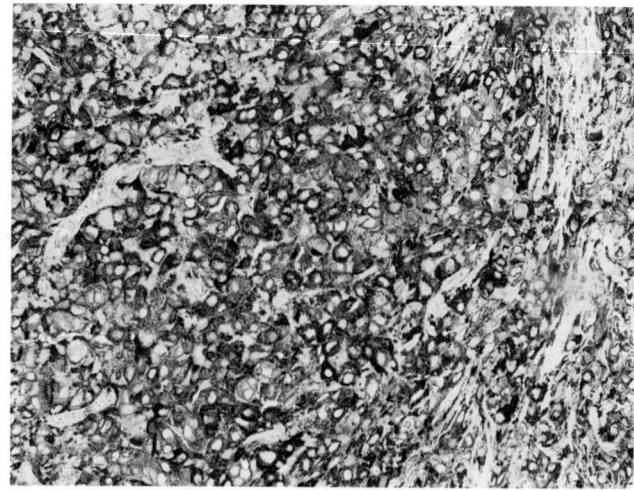

FIGURE 48.18. Histiocytic sarcoma. A: The nuclei show irregular folds; the cytoplasm is relatively abundant and shows a foamy appearance. **B:** The neoplasm is strongly positive for the histiocytic marker CD163.

junctions. Immunohistochemical studies, by definition, show expression of one or more markers of histiocytic differentiation, usually CD163, CD68, or lysosome (Fig. 48.18B). All three markers usually are strongly positive, often with Golgi accentuation. Expression of S-100 protein is variable but usually not as strong or consistent as seen in interdigitating dendritic cell sarcoma. There usually is expression of CD45, CD45RO, and HLA-DR. Rare cases show langerin positivity (8). By definition, there is no expression of specific B- and T-cell markers or CD30, myeloperoxidase, or follicular dendritic cell markers (CD21 and CD35). There are usually no clonal rearrangements of antigen receptor genes, at least as a singular disease. However, as noted previously, cases associated with B-cell malignancy may show identical clonal gene rearrangements, as well as identical cytogenetics profiles (82,84).

The differential diagnosis of histiocytic sarcoma includes malignant lymphoma of B- or T-cell types (including lymphomas associated with benign hemophagocytosis), anaplastic large cell lymphoma (Fig. 48.19), anaplastic carcinomas exhibiting hemophagocytosis, hepatosplenic γδ T-cell lymphoma, acute monocytic leukemia, and interdigitating dendritic cell tumor. B- and T-cell lymphomas and anaplastic large cell lymphoma can be distinguished by immunohistochemical studies for B- and

T-cell antigens and CD30, respectively. HLH lacks the cytologic atypia seen in histiocytic sarcoma. Tissue involvement by acute monocytic leukemia, in the absence of peripheral blood or bone marrow involvement, may be indistinguishable from histiocytic sarcoma, although follow-up usually resolves these cases. Interdigitating dendritic cell tumors may show close overlap with histiocytic sarcoma, particularly if patients with the latter express S-100 protein. The S-100 protein expression in interdigitating dendritic cell tumors is usually stronger and more consistent. Histologically, interdigitating dendritic cell tumors are much more likely to be spindled and ultrastructurally show complex cell processes.

The clinical course is aggressive, with most reported patients dying from the disease (76,80). Some cases have been successfully treated with hematopoietic cell transplant (86).

DENDRITIC CELL NEOPLASMS

Langerhans Cell Histiocytosis

Langerhans cell histiocytosis (LCH) is a proliferative disease of cells that share phenotypic characteristics with Langerhans cells, which are the primary antigen-presenting cells of the epidermis. The incidence of LCH is about 5 per million, and the median age of patients at diagnosis is <5 years (87–91). There is an association with other hematopoietic neoplasms; although much of this may be related to posttherapy leukemia, there does seem to be an unusually frequent occurrence of disseminated LCH in patients with acute nonmyelocytic leukemia (92). There may be an association among LCH and neonatal infection, solvent exposure, lack of childhood vaccination, and thyroid disease (93,94).

LCH has a wide clinical spectrum in that it may involve a single site, multiple sites in a single organ system, or multiple organ systems. Three overlapping clinical syndromes generally are recognized. In unifocal LCH (solitary eosinophilic granuloma), representing about two-thirds of cases, a single site is involved, most commonly bone, lymph node, or lung (11). Although it most commonly occurs in children, adults also may be affected; about two-thirds of affected patients are males. Bone is overwhelmingly the most common site of involvement, usually the skull, femur, pelvic bones, or ribs. The diaphyses are involved most often, with erosion of the adjacent cortical bone. The unifocal involvement of the lung that sometimes occurs in adult smokers (of tobacco or marijuana) has more favorable behavior than other types of

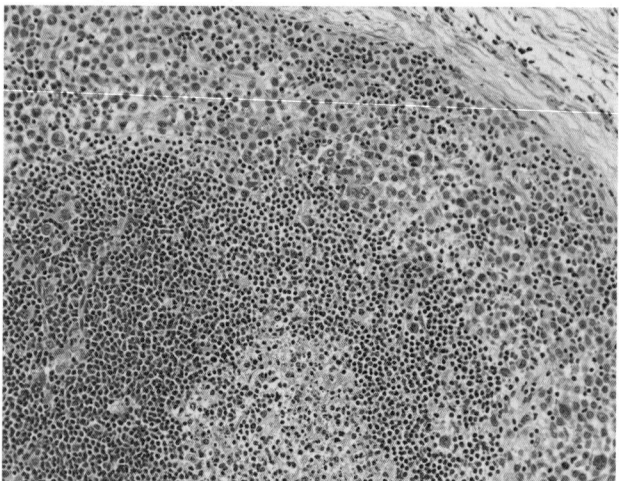

FIGURE 48.19. Sinusoidal variant of ALK-positive anaplastic large cell lymphoma. This lymphoma lacked histiocytic markers, but was ALK positive.

solitary LCH (95). In multifocal, unisystem LCH (many cases of Hand-Schüller-Christian syndrome), several involved sites in one organ system, generally bone, are present. The male gender preference is retained but patients are generally younger in age than those with unifocal involvement. Finally, in multifocal, multisystem histiocytosis (many cases of Letterer-Siwe syndrome), multiple sites in multiple organ systems are involved. These patients are almost always infants or young children, with a predominance of males.

The exact pathogenesis of LCH is not fully understood (90,96). The entity was originally termed histiocytosis X, with the X designating the uncertainty of the origin of the primary cell type. There is no known association with viruses or the environment (90,96,97). Uncertainty as to whether the disease is immune mediated or neoplastic in nature has been the subject of much research and more recent work favors the disease being neoplastic in nature, with a genetic aberration leading to immune dysregulation and an aberrant interaction between Langerhans cells and T lymphocytes. Several factors support a neoplastic etiology. Studies at the turn of the 20th century showed the histiocytes to have a monoclonal nature, except in smoking-related cases (98–100). Rare reports of familial cases as well as a higher rate of LCH in monozygotic twins over dizygotic twins further suggest the possibility of a genetic alteration (96,101). Furthermore, the activating mutation BRAF has been found in a significant number of LCH cases, whereas cases of histiocytic proliferations with large numbers of histiocytes (RDD and dermatopathic lymphadenopathy) do not contain BRAF mutations (102). Interestingly, BRAF mutations have been found in some cases of solitary pulmonary LCH, which are polyclonal (102). BRAF mutations are more commonly found in young LCH patients (<10 years old) than in older patients (102). The presence of BRAF mutations does not appear to correlate with anatomic site of disease (102). Further studies of the role of BRAF in the pathogenesis of LCH are still needed to elucidate the actual mechanism as well as to develop more detailed clinical correlations. Studies also show that the tumor cells of LCH do not have their origin in epidermal Langerhans cells, but, rather, in a myeloid derived precursor (7,103,104).

The histologic hallmark of all LCH tissues is the presence of proliferating Langerhans cells in the appropriate cellular milieu. Morphologically, the Langerhans cells are about 10 to 12 μm in diameter and have characteristic folded, indented, or lobulated nuclei, generally with inconspicuous nucleoli (Fig. 48.20). Although some nuclear atypia may be present, the cells are cytologically benign, and mitotic figures are usually rare. A

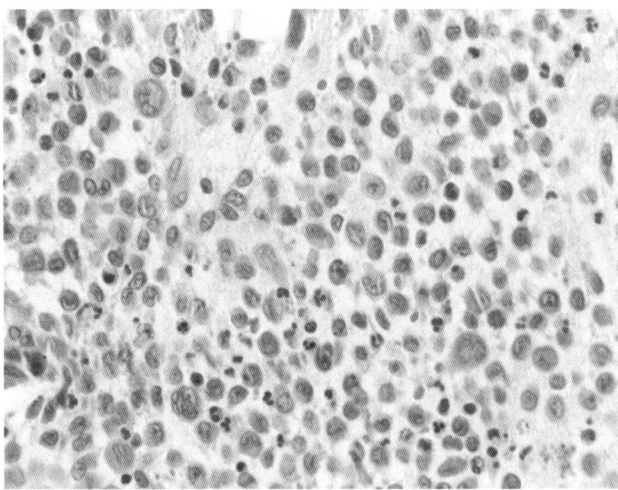

FIGURE 48.21. Langerhans cell histiocytosis. A mixture of cell types, including Langerhans cells, eosinophils, neutrophisls, macrophages, and giant cells, is seen.

moderate amount of slightly eosinophilic cytoplasm usually is seen. The cells are almost always accompanied by a characteristic reactive infiltrate, which usually includes eosinophils, histiocytes, neutrophils, multinucleated cells (either foreign body or Langerhans type), and small lymphocytes (Fig. 48.21). Necrosis may be present, often in the form of eosinophilic microabscesses (Fig. 48.22). Early lesions tend to be very cellular; late lesions tend to be more fibrotic, often with the accumulation of foamy macrophages.

Involved lymph nodes almost always show sinusoidal patterns of involvement, often with marked distension of the sinuses, beginning with the subcapsular sinuses and progressing to involvement of the medullary sinuses (Fig. 48.23). The overall lymph node architecture generally is retained, but partial or even complete effacement is seen in rare advanced cases. The histologic differential diagnosis includes sinusoidal proliferations of the lymph nodes such as metastatic carcinoma, metastatic malignant melanoma, sinusoidal malignant lymphoma, RDD, and benign sinusoidal hyperplasia. The key to the diagnosis lies in the recognition of the cytologic features of the Langerhans cells. Large numbers of Langerhans cells may be seen in lymph nodes showing dermatopathic lymphadenopathy (105). In that condition, however, the Langerhans cells are seen in paracortical areas and are not prominent within the sinuses.

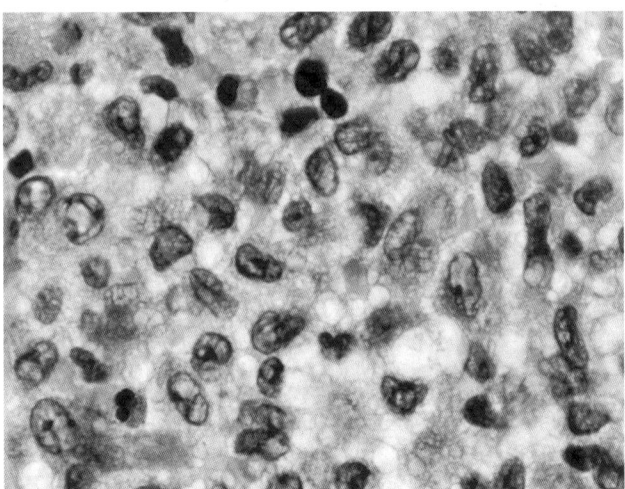

FIGURE 48.20. Langerhans cell histiocytosis. The characteristic grooving and folding of the nuclei are present.

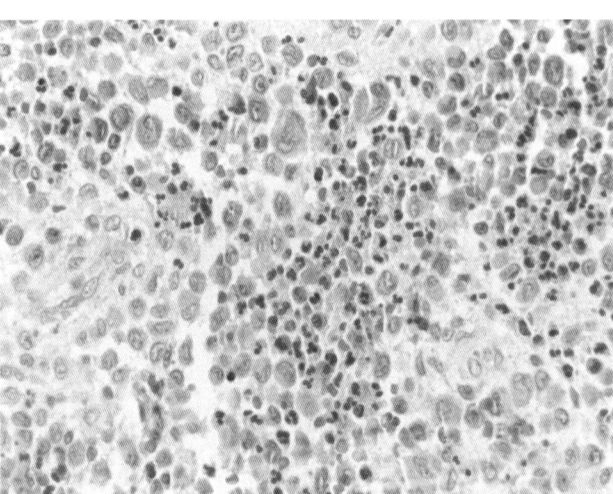

FIGURE 48.22. Langerhans cell histiocytosis. An eosinophilic microabscess is present.

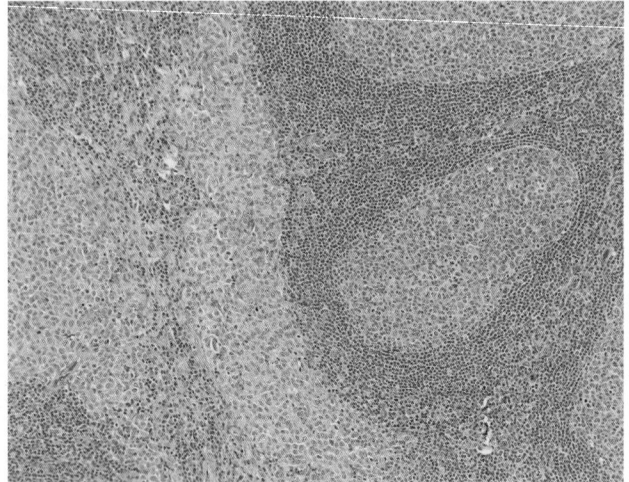

FIGURE 48.23. Langerhans cell histiocytosis. A sinusoidal pattern of involvement is seen in this lymph node biopsy.

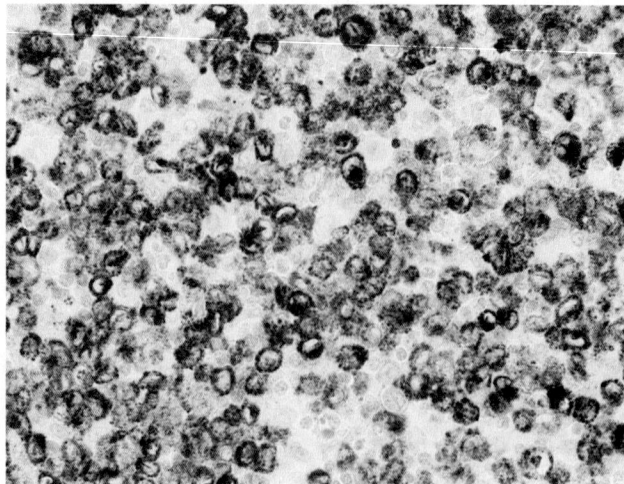

FIGURE 48.25. Langerhans cell histiocytosis. This Langerin stain labels the Langerhans cells in a granular cytoplasmic distribution.

Rarely, a focus of LCH can be seen in lymph nodes involved by malignant lymphoma, both of non-Hodgkin type and Hodgkin disease (106,107). In these circumstances, the focus of disease can be quite small and not limited to the sinuses (Fig. 48.24). As in the case of pulmonary LCH occurring in smokers, it is not clear whether these instances represent a peculiar reactive phenomenon rather than true LCH.

The ultrastructural, enzyme histochemical, and immunophenotypic characteristics of the Langerhans cells in LCH are virtually identical to those of normal Langerhans cells (11). Ultrastructurally, the cells in LCH contain variable numbers of Birbeck granules morphologically identical to those found in normal Langerhans cells. The nuclei are deeply cleaved or multisegmented, with finely dispersed chromatin and an inconspicuous nucleolus. The cells show expression of adenosine triphosphatase, α-naphthyl acetate esterase (with variable inhibition by sodium fluoride), α-naphthyl butyrate esterase, and acid phosphatase, and negativity for tartrate-resistant acid phosphatase, 5'-nucleotidase, peroxidase, chloroacetate esterase, and β-glucuronidase.

CD1a, langerin, and S-100 protein are the markers most consistently seen in paraffin section immunohistochemical studies, although rare patients show weak or negative staining of these markers (8,108–110). Langerin is highly

specific for this disease and has largely replaced the need for ultrastructural confirmation of Birbeck granules (Fig. 48.25). CD1a reactivity is also extremely useful in terms of differential diagnosis, because only lymphoblastic malignancies share this feature. The cells also express placental alkaline phosphatase, vimentin, and a low amount of fascin (normal Langerhans cells lack placental alkaline phosphatase and fascin), and may express membranous CD4. The cells also lack CD30, CD163, CD45, lysozyme, α_1-antitrypsin, epithelial membrane antigen, and CD15 (30). CD56 expression has been described in rare cases of LCH that have antecedent T-lymphoblastic leukemia; these cases have been shown to have highly aggressive clinical behavior and identical T-cell receptor gamma gene rearrangements (111). Gene rearrangement studies have shown a germ line configuration for the immunoglobulin heavy chain gene as well as the β, γ, and δ chains of the T-cell receptor gene (112).

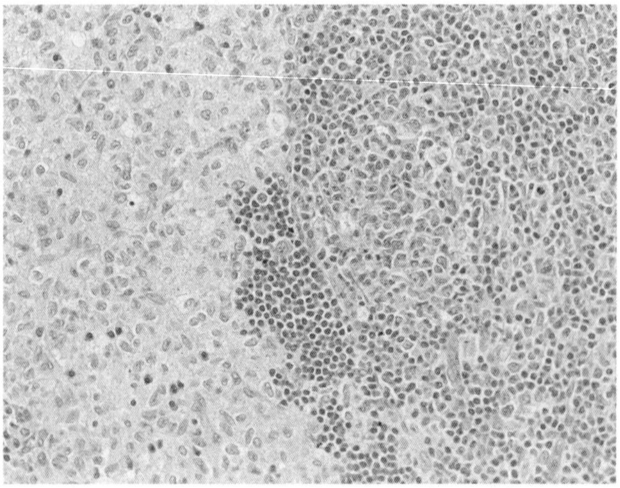

The most important factor determining prognosis appears to be the pattern of organ involvement (96). Less than 10% of patients who present with only one involved site develop disseminated disease. Patients with multiple organs involved at presentation, particularly if the involvement leads to organ dysfunction, generally have a poor outcome (96,113). The number of involved organs, however, is not the only important factor. The absence of bone lesions is a poor prognostic factor, and the presence of multiple osseous lesions is associated with a favorable prognosis. Patients with involvement of bone marrow, liver, and spleen tend to do more poorly. Patients younger than 2 years of age generally do poorly, but age may be less important than the pattern of organ involvement in determining prognosis. Histologic grading is of much less significance in predicting prognosis than pattern of organ involvement or age. In one study, the presence of cytologic atypia or the mitotic rate could not be correlated with patient outcome (114).

Langerhans Cell Sarcoma

Overtly malignant forms of LCH have been reported (115–117). This neoplasm has been termed *Langerhans cell sarcoma* in the recently proposed World Health Organization classification of hematopoietic and lymphoid neoplasms (22). In primary Langerhans cell sarcoma, the proliferating cells have frankly malignant cytologic features but are otherwise ultrastructurally and immunophenotypically typical for LCH (Fig. 48.26). Clinically, the few reported patients have been predominantly male, have had multiorgan involvement, and have followed a rapidly progressive clinical course. It is still not clear whether

FIGURE 48.24. Follicular lymphoma. A focus of LCH is seen.

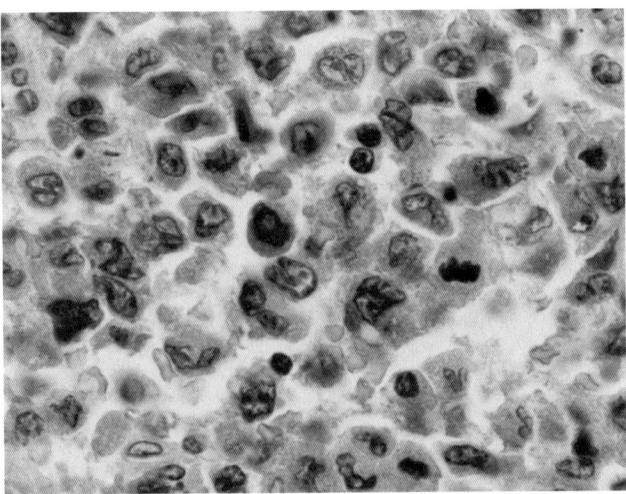

FIGURE 48.26. Langerhans cell sarcoma. Many nuclei have an appearance reminiscent of Langerhans cells, but a much greater degree of nuclear atypia is seen. Also note the frequent mitotic figures.

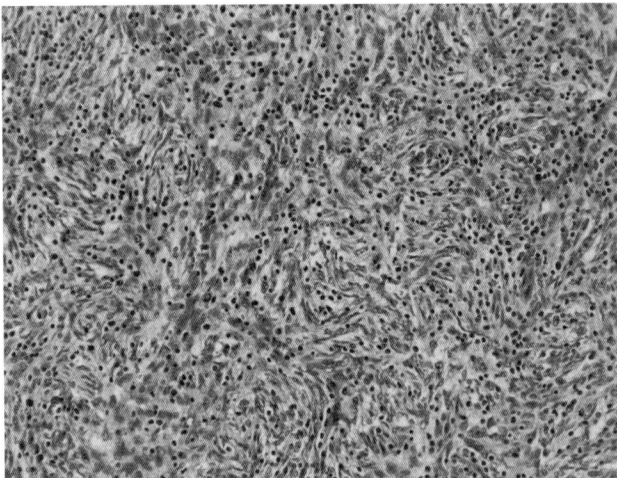

FIGURE 48.27. Follicular dendritic cell sarcoma. A spindled pattern with residual lymphocytes is present.

this disease represents a distinctive clinicopathologic entity, the extreme end of the morphologic and clinical spectrum of ordinary LCH, transformation of LCH, or other neoplasms that have been confused with LCH. Rare cases of Langerhans cell sarcoma arising from preexisting LCH have been described; the transformed malignant cells retain their CD1a expression (118).

Follicular Dendritic Cell Sarcoma

Neoplasms of follicular dendritic cell lineage, so-called *follicular dendritic cell sarcoma*, have also been called reticulum cell sarcoma/tumor or dendritic reticulum cell sarcoma/tumor. Almost all described patients have been adults, with a median age of about 40 years and nearly equal gender distribution (119–121). Most patients present with an enlarged cervical or axillary lymph node, but extranodal presentations, including oral cavity, tonsil, GI tract, soft tissue, and breast, occur in almost half of the patients. A variant of this tumor has been described in the liver and spleen to be associated with the Epstein-Barr virus (122,123). Follicular dendritic cell sarcomas arising in other organs are consistently negative for Epstein-Barr virus and human herpesvirus-8 as well (124). Approximately 10% to 20% of cases of follicular dendritic cell sarcoma are associated with Castleman disease; in most instances, the latter is the hyaline vascular type, but the plasma cell type also has been reported rarely (120,125,126). The behavior of follicular dendritic cell sarcoma is more like that of a sarcoma than a hematolymphoid neoplasm, with local recurrence and occasional metastasis. Almost one-half of patients have one or more recurrences; metastases have been reported in about one quarter of patients.

There is a wide range in tumor size in follicular dendritic cell sarcoma, with a mean size of about 5 cm. The largest tumors occur in the retroperitoneum and may be up to 20 cm. They are usually well-circumscribed and are seen as solid tan-gray masses on cut section. Histologically, an ovoid to spindle cell–shaped morphology is seen, often in a storiform or whorled growth pattern (Fig. 48.27). Necrosis is usually absent but may occur in a geographic pattern. The individual cells are usually uniform, with occasional multinucleation. The nuclei are elongated, with vesicular or granular chromatin, distinct nucleoli, and a delicate nuclear membrane. There may be multinucleated cells or nuclear pseudoinclusions, and some patients may have moderate to marked nuclear pleomorphism. The mitotic rate is usually between 0 and 10 per 10 high-power fields but may be higher. Residual lymphoid tissue is generally present

in between the spindled proliferation, as single cells, clusters of lymphocytes often in a perivascular location, or occasional germinal centers. In some patients with concurrent hyaline-vascular Castleman disease, the neoplasm appears to be arising in association with a dysplastic proliferation of follicular dendritic cells. Recurrences and metastases may have a greater degree of nuclear atypia, a higher mitotic rate, and a greater degree of necrosis, consistent with histologic progression. Recurrences in patients treated with chemotherapy and radiation may also show increased atypia, as well as squamous metaplasia and sheets of foamy histiocytes.

Electron microscopy reveals numerous villous cytoplasmic extensions, often connected with each other through numerous cell junctions, which include well-formed desmosomes. Immunologically, the neoplasm shows a close resemblance to the normal follicular dendritic cell, with absent to weak CD45, variable expression of S-100 protein, consistent and strong expression of vimentin and the C3b and C3d complement receptors (CD35 and CD21, respectively), variable expression of desmoplakin and CD68, and consistent expression of follicular dendritic cell–specific markers such as R4/23. Surprisingly, epithelial membrane antigen is expressed in a majority of cases, despite the fact that normal follicular dendritic cells are negative for this marker (119). The neoplasm is consistently negative for langerin, CD1a, desmin, keratin, HMB-45, and vascular markers (8,119,121,127). The background lymphocytes may stain as T cells or B cells. Gene rearrangement studies have revealed a germ line configuration for the immunoglobulin heavy chain and T-cell receptor β genes (119).

The differential diagnosis is large and includes other dendritic cell tumors, thymoma, spindle cell carcinoma, malignant melanoma, and sarcoma. A complete immunohistochemical profile should rule out these other neoplasms and demonstrate the appropriate immunophenotype of follicular dendritic cell sarcoma.

Interdigitating Dendritic Cell Sarcoma

Rare neoplasms consistent with an interdigitating dendritic cell lineage have been reported to occur in both males and females from the teens through adulthood, with a median age of about 50 years (76,128–131). The clinical presentation has varied, from solitary lymph node enlargement to widespread disease including hepatosplenomegaly. The clinical course appears to be aggressive, with most patients dying of the disease. The median overall duration of survival is about 15 months.

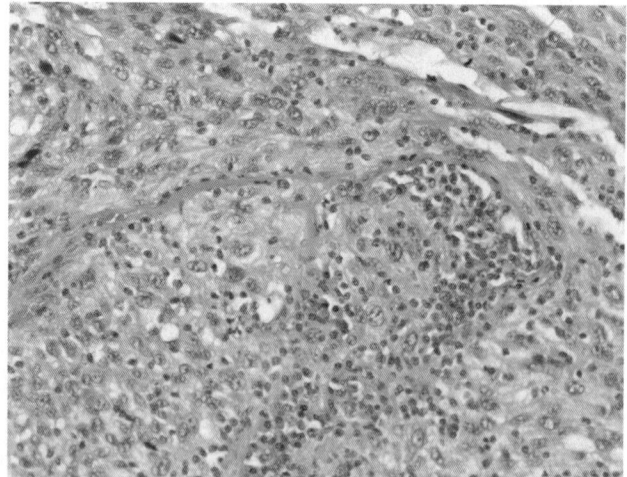

FIGURE 48.28. Interdigitating dendritic cell sarcoma. The nuclei show a spindled to ovoid appearance.

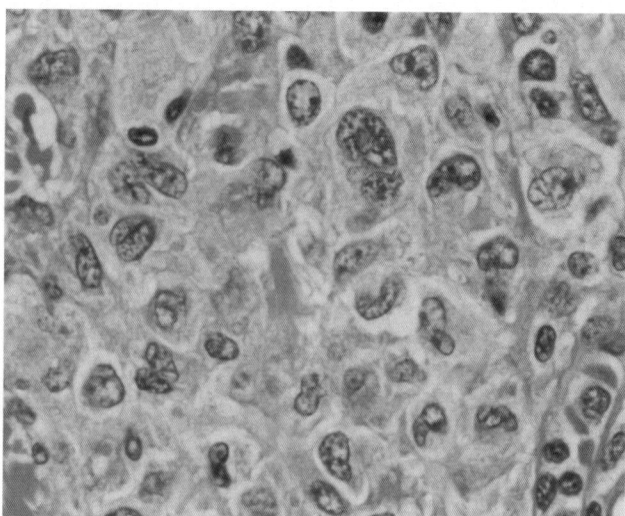

FIGURE 48.29. Indeterminate cell neoplasm. A proliferation of cells with irregular, dendritic-appearing nuclei is seen. Note the absence of eosinophils.

These neoplasms show variable histology, ranging from spindle cell neoplasms similar in morphologic appearance to follicular dendritic cell neoplasms, to neoplasms resembling histiocytic tumors or large cell lymphomas (Fig. 48.28). The tumor is often localized to the paracortex, which is the site of normal interdigitating dendritic cells. The ultrastructure of these tumors is similar to normal interdigitating cells, with elongated and complex cell processes, but no true desmosomes; Birbeck granules are not present. Immunophenotypically, the tumors typically express vimentin, CD45, S-100 protein, macrophage antigens (variable) and, by definition, are negative for CD1a, langerin, and follicular dendritic cell markers (76). Gene rearrangement studies have shown a germ line configuration for the immunoglobulin heavy chain and T-cell receptor β genes.

Rare cases of interdigitating cell sarcoma have been associated with low-grade B-cell lymphomas (81,132). In these cases, both the interdigitating cell sarcoma and the lymphoma have been found to be clonally related (82,84).

Indeterminate Cell Neoplasm

Indeterminate cell neoplasm is a diagnosis of exclusion. It has most often been described in adults, who usually present with solitary or multiple cutaneous lesions, and rarely in the lymph nodes or spleen (125,133). A significant subset of cases has been associated with low-grade B-cell lymphomas (81). Skin involvement usually is dermal based, occasionally with extension into the epidermis. Regardless of anatomic location, the tumor cells are usually arranged in nests, nodules, or sheets, and usually have abundant cytoplasm with irregularly shaped and often clefted nuclei (Fig. 48.29). Accompanying eosinophils are either absent or often not prominent in number. Ultrastructurally, the cells have shown numerous dendritic processes that interdigitate with those of adjacent cells. No Birbeck granules are present. Immunophenotypically, the neoplastic cells express vimentin, CD45, CD1a, S-100 protein, fascin, and macrophage antigens, but not langerin (134–136).

Fibroblastic Reticular Cell Neoplasm

Fibroblastic reticular cell neoplasms are extremely rare tumors and derive from the cells that contribute to the complex cellular stromal network of the lymph node paracortex (125,137). Not surprisingly, preferential paracortical involvement by the tumor is often seen, although diffuse nodal effacement may be

seen. The histologic appearance is similar to that of the other dendritic cell proliferations, and may, in addition, show a finely collagenized background (Fig. 48.30). Ultrastructural studies of the tumor cells show features of myofibroblasts, with elongated tumor cells with slender cytoplasmic extensions associated with basal lamina–like material, intracytoplasmic filaments, occasional fusiform densities, and well-developed intercellular attachments. Immunohistochemical studies showed the spindle cell proliferation to have strong vimentin expression and variable smooth muscle actin and desmin expression. Factor XIII staining has also been described in some cases. CD45RB, S-100 protein, keratin, CD1a, CD21, CD35 and specific B- and T-cell markers were not expressed.

Xanthogranuloma

Juvenile and adult xanthogranuloma represent the most common members of a spectrum of disease that probably also includes such rare entities as xanthoma disseminatum, benign cephalic histiocytosis, progressive nodular histiocytosis, spindle cell xanthogranuloma, and generalized eruptive histiocytosis (138–140).

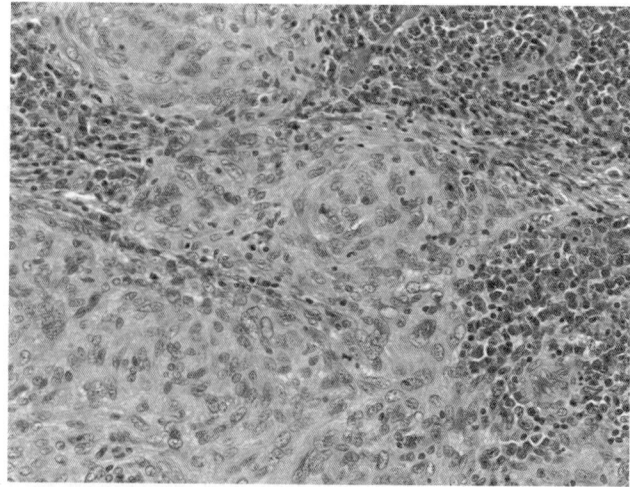

FIGURE 48.10. Fibroblastic reticular cell neoplasm. This spindle cell proliferation is essentially indistinguishable morphologically from that of follicular dendritic cell sarcoma or interdigitating dendritic cell sarcoma.

Juvenile xanthogranuloma usually presents in children with yellow to pink protuberant cutaneous nodules up to 1 cm in diameter, usually in the head and neck region. Similar lesions may occur in adults (adult xanthogranuloma). Some lesions may occur in the subcutaneous or intramuscular soft tissues or rarely in internal organs (141). The intramuscular forms have a marked predilection to occur as solitary lesions in skeletal muscles of the trunk of infants (142). Almost all lesions, including extracutaneous lesions, involute spontaneously.

A multifocal form, known as disseminated juvenile xanthogranuloma, also exists and accounts for <5% of cases. This also has been termed systemic or deep juvenile xanthogranuloma, progressive nodular histiocytosis, benign cephalic histiocytosis, and generalized eruptive histiocytosis. A variant includes xanthoma disseminatum, a disease in which xanthomas are present in the eyelids and skin of flexor areas. Systemic sites of involvement include kidney, lung, soft tissue, CNS, upper GI tract, and bone (139,141).

As the name implies, disseminated juvenile xanthogranuloma most commonly affects children, although rarely adults are affected (as in the case of polyostotic sclerosing histiocytosis, also known as Erdheim-Chester disease). The etiology of disseminated juvenile xanthogranuloma is not known. An association with neurofibromatosis-1 (NF-1) has been observed (143–145). Patients with NF-1 have a higher incidence of usual type juvenile xanthogranuloma and a higher risk than the general population of developing juvenile myelomonocytic leukemia. Rare patients with disseminated juvenile xanthogranuloma have been described to also have NF-1 and/or juvenile myelomonocytic leukemia. The latter has also been rarely observed to develop in patients with both types of xanthogranuloma patients.

Histologically, the lesions are usually well circumscribed, with an exophytic appearance if skin is involved (140,146). The epidermis itself is usually uninvolved, and there is usually an underlying Grenz zone. The lesions consist of variable numbers of histiocyte-like cells, spindle cells, and giant cells. The histiocyte-like cells have bland nuclei with abundant vacuolated, eosinophilic, or foamy cytoplasm (Fig. 48.31). The spindle cells are similar to the histiocyte-like cells but are spindled and form a storiform architecture. The giant cells usually are described as Touton type (foamy periphery outside a wreathe of nuclei around central eosinophilic anucleate cytoplasm) but are just as often foreign body–type or nondescript with central eosinophilic or ground-glass cytoplasm (Fig. 48.32). Early lesions tend to have more vacuolated histiocyte-like cells, intermediate

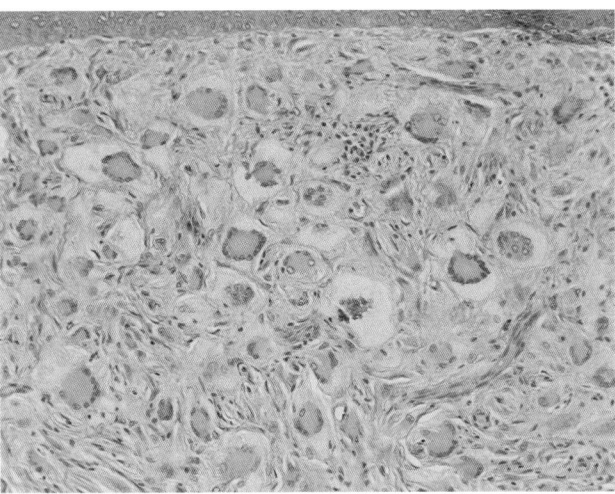

FIGURE 48.32. Juvenile xanthogranuloma. Numerous Touton-like giant cells are seen.

lesions have more foamy cells, and late lesions tend to be more spindled. Intramuscular lesions tend to be composed of a monotonous population of histiocyte-like cells, with rare, if any, foamy macrophages or giant cells (142). Immunohistochemical studies demonstrate factor XIIIa, fascin, and CD68 positivity, particularly at the periphery of the lesion. Staining for S-100 is usually negative, but may be seen in up to 20% of cases.

SUMMARY AND CONCLUSIONS

The histiocytic and dendritic cell proliferative disorders are an uncommon but diverse group of diseases. The cells comprising most of these disorders show differentiation along pathways of normal differentiation, although the normal cellular counterpart for a few of them, such as RDD, has yet to be elucidated fully.

References

1. Fogg DK SC, Miled C, Jung S, et al. A clonogeneic bone marrow progenitor specific for macrophages and dendritic cells. *Science* 2006;311:83–87.
2. Taylor GA, Weinberg J. Mononuclear phagocytes. In: Greer JP, Foerster J, Rodgers GM, et al., eds. *Wintrobe's clinical hematology*, 12th ed. Philadelphia: Lippincott Williams & Wllkins, 2009:249–280.
3. Chow A, Brown B, Merad M. Studying the mononuclear phagocyte in the molecular age. *Nature* 2011;11:788–798.
4. Stuart LM, Ezekowitz A. Phagocytosis: elegant complexity. *Immunity* 2005;22:539–550.
5. Naik SH, Sathe P, Park HY, et al. Development of plasmacytoid and conventional dendritic cell subtypes from single precursor cells derived *in vitro* and *in vivo*. *Nature Immunol* 2007;8:1217–1226.
6. Geissmann F, Manz M, Jung S, et al. Development of monocytes, macrophages and dendritic cells. *Science* 2010;327:656–661.
7. Merad M, Manz M, Karsunky H, et al. Langerhans cell renew in the skin throughout life under steady-state conditions. *Nat Immunol* 2002;3:1135–1141.
8. Lau SK, Chu PG, Weiss LM. Immunohistochemical expression of Langerin in Langerhans cell histiocytosis and non-Langerhans cell histiocytic disorders. *Am J Surg Pathol* 2008;32:615–619.
9. Beckstead JH, Wood GS, Turner RR. Histiocytosis X cells and Langerhans cells: enzyme histochemical and immunologic similarities. *Hum Pathol* 1984;15:826–833.
10. Wood GS, Turner RR, Shiurba RA, et al. Human dendritic cells and macrophages. In situ immunophenotypic definition of subsets that exhibit specific morphologic and microenvironmental characteristics. *Am J Pathol* 1985;119:73–82.
11. Lieberman PH, Jones CR, Steinman RM, et al. Langerhans cell (eosinophilic) granulomatosis: a clinicopathologic study encompassing 50 years. *Am J Surg Pathol* 1996;20:519–552.
12. Murphy GF, Bhan AK, Harrist TJ, et al. In situ identification of T6-positive cells in normal human dermis by immunoelectron microscopy. *Br J Dermatol* 1983;108:423–431.
13. Jaffe R, Pileri S, Facchetti F, et al. Histiocytic and dendritic cell neoplasms, Introduction. In: Swerdlow SH, Campo E, Harris NL, et al., eds. *WHO classification of tumours of haematopoietic and lymphoid tissues*, 4th ed. Lyon: International Agency for Research on Cancer, 2008.
14. Parwaresch MR, Radzun HJ, Hansmann ML, et al. Monoclonal antibody Ki-M4 specifically recognizes human dendritic cells (follicular dendritic cells) and their possible precursors in blood. *Blood* 1983;62:585–590.

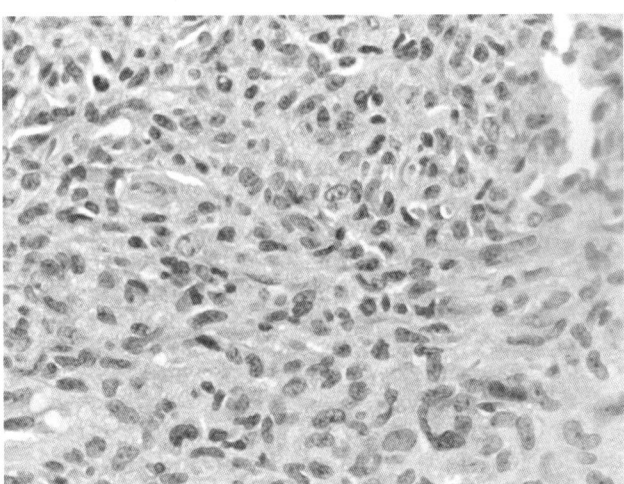

FIGURE 48.31. Juvenile xanthogranuloma. Numerous bland histiocytes with granular cytoplasm are seen. A giant cell is also present.

15. Pallesen G, Myhre-Jensen O. Immunophenotypic analysis of neoplastic cells in follicular dendritic cell sarcoma. *Leukemia* 1987;1:549–557.
16. Fletcher AL, Lukacs-Kornek V, Reynoso ED, et al. Lymph node fibroblastic reticular cells directly present peripheral tissue antigen under steady-state and inflammatory conditions. *J Exp Med* 2010;207:689–697.
17. Mueller SN, Germain R. Stromal cell contributions to the homeostasis and functionality of the immune system. *Nat Rev Immunol* 2009;9:618–629.
18. Gloghini A, Carbone A. The nonlymphoid microenvironment of reactive follicles and lymphomas of follicular origin as defined by immunohistology on paraffin-embedded tissues. *Hum Pathol* 1993;24:67–76.
19. Tykocinski M, Schinnella RA, Greco MA. Fibroblastic reticulum cells in human lymph nodes. *Arch Pathol Lab Med* 1983;107:418–422.
20. Schmitt-Graff A, Desmouliere A, Gabbiani G. Heterogeneity of myofibroblast phenotypic features: an example of fibroblastic cell plasticity. *Virchow's Arch* 1994;425:3–24.
21. Pinkus GS, Warhol MJ, O'Connor EM, et al. Immunohistochemical localization of smooth muscle myosin in human spleen, lymph node, and other lymphoid tissues. unique staining patterns in splenic white pulp and sinuses, lymphoid follicles, and certain vasculature, with ultrastructural correlations. *Am J Pathol* 1986;123:440–453.
22. Swerdlow SH, Campo E, Harris NL, et al., eds. *World Health Organization classification of tumours: pathology & genetics. Tumours of haematopoietic & lymphoid tissues.* Lyon: Intl Agency for Research on Cancer, 2008.
23. Albores-Saavedra J, Vuitch F, Delgado R, et al. Sinus histiocytosis of pelvic lymph nodes after hip replacement. A histiocytic proliferation induced by cobalt-chromium and titanium. *Am J Surg Pathol* 1994;18:83–90.
24. Listinsky CM. Common reactive erythrophagocytosis in axillary lymph nodes. *Hum Pathol* 1988;89:189–192.
25. Destombes P. Adenites avec surcharge lipidique, de l'enfant ou de l'adulte jeune, observees aux antilles et au mali. Quatre observations. *Bull Soc Pathol Exot Filiales* 1965;58:1169–1175.
26. Rosai J, Dorfman RF. Sinus histiocytosis with massive lymphadenopathy: a newly recognized benign clinicopathological entity. *Arch Pathol* 1969;87:63–70.
27. Foucar E, Rosai J, Dorfman RF. Sinus histiocytosis with massive lymphadenopathy (Rosai-Dorfman disease). Review of the entity. *Semin Diagn Pathol* 1990;7:19–73.
28. Foucar E, Rosai J, Dorfman RF, et al. Immunologic abnormalities and their significance in sinus histiocytosis with massive lymphadenopathy. *Am J Clin Pathol* 1984;82:515–525.
29. Eisen RN, Buckley PJ, Rosai J. Immunophenotypic characterization of sinus histiocytosis with massive lymphadenopathy (Rosai-Dorfman disease). *Semin Diagn Pathol* 1990;7:74–82.
30. Lau SK, Chu PG, Weiss LM. CD163: a specific marker of macrophages in paraffin-embedded tissue samples. *Am J Clin Pathol* 2004;122:794–801.
31. Paulli M, Feller AC, Boveri E, et al. Cathepsin D and E co-expression in sinus histiocytosis with massive lymphadenopathy (Rosai-Dorfman disease) and Langerhans' cell hsitiocytosis: further evidence of a phentoypic overlap between these histiocytic disorders. *Virchos Archiv* 1994;424:601–606.
32. Paulli M, Bergamaschi G, Tonon L, et al. Evidence for a polyclonal nature of the cell infiltrate in sinus histiocytosis with massive lymphadenopathy (Rosai-Dorfman disease). *Br J Haematol* 1995;91:415–418.
33. Komp DM. The treatment of sinus histiocytosis with massive lymphadenopathy (Rosai-Dorfman disease). *Semin Diagn Pathol* 1990;7:83–86.
34. Gadner H, Grois N, Arico M, et al. A randomized trial of treatment for multisystem Langerhans' cell histiocytosis. *J Pediatr* 2001;138:728–734.
35. Ngendahayo P, Roels H, Quatacker J, et al. Sinus hystiocytosis with massive lymphadenopathy in Rwanda: report of eight cases with immunohistochemical and untrastructural studies. *Histopathology* 1983;7:49–63.
36. Bonetti F, Chilosi M, Menestrina F, et al. Immunohistological analysis of Rosai-Dorfman histiocytosis. A disease of S-100 + CD1-histiocytes. *Virchows Arch A Pathol Anat Histopathol* 1987;411:129–135.
37. Levine PH, Jahan N, Murari P, et al. Detection of HHV-6 in tissues involved by sinus histiocytosis with massive lymphadenopathy (Rosai-Dorfman disease). *J Infect Dis* 1992;166:291–295.
38. Luppi M, Barozzi P, Garber R, et al. Expression of human herpesvirus-6 antigens in benign and malignant lymphoproliferative diseases. *Am J Pathol* 1998; 153:815–823.
39. Al-Daraji W, Anandan A, Klassen-Fischer M, et al. Soft tissue Rosai Dorfman disease: 29 new lesions in 18 patients, with detection of polyomavirus antigen in 3 abdominal cases. *Ann Diagn Pathol* 2010;14:309–316.
40. Mehraein Y, Wagner M, Remberger K, et al. Parvovirus B19 detected in Rosai-Dorfman disease in nodal and extranodal manifestations. *J Clin Pathol* 2006;59:1320–1326.
41. Tsang WYW, Yip TTC, Chan JKC. The Rosai-Dorfman disease histiocytes are not infected by Epstein-Barr virus. *Histopathology* 1994;25:88–90.
42. Gupta S, Weitzman S. Primary and secondary hemophagocytic lymphoghistiocytosis: clinical features, pathogenesis and therapy. *Expert Rev Clin Immunol* 2010;6:137–154.
43. Risdall RJ, McKenna RW, Nesbitt ME, et al. Virus associated hemophagocytic syndrome. A benign histiocytic proliferation distinct from malignant histiocytosis. *Cancer* 1979;44:993–1002.
44. Risdall RJ, Brunning RD, Hernandez JJ. Bacteria-associated hemophagocytic syndrome. *Cancer* 1984;54:2968–2972.
45. McKenna RW, Risdall RJ, Brunning RD. Virus associated hemophagocytic syndrome. *Hum Pathol* 1981;12:395–398.
46. Weitzman S. Approach to hemophagocytic syndromes. *ASH Education Program Book* 2011;2011:178–183.
47. Farquhar JW, Claireaux AF. Familial hemophagocytic reticulosis. *Arch Dis Child* 1952;27:519–525.
48. Arico M, Janka G, Fischer A, et al. Hemophagocytic lymphohistiocytosis. Report of 122 children from the International Registry. FHL Study Group of the Histiocyte Society. *Leukemia* 1996;10:197–203.
49. Stepp SE, Dufourcq-Lagelouse R, Le Deist F, et al. Perforin gene defects in familial hemophagocytic lymphohistiocytosis. *Science* 1999;286:1957–1959.
50. Ost A, Nilsson-Ardnor S, Henter JI. Autopsy findings in 27 children with haemophagocytic lymphohistiocytosis. *Histopathology* 1998;32:310–316.
51. Janka GE. Familial hemophagocytic lymphohistiocytosis. *Eur J Pediatr* 1983;140: 221–230.
52. Wieczorek R, Greco A, McCarthy K, et al. Familial erythrophagocytic lymphohistiocytosis; immunophenotypic, immunohistochemical and ultrastructural demonstration of the relation to sinus histiocytes. *Hum Pathol* 1986;17:55–63.
53. Schaer DJ, Schleiffenbaum B, Kurrer M, et al. Soluble hemoglobin-haptoglobin scavenger receptor CD163 as a lineage-specific marker in the reactive hemophagocytic syndrome. *Eur J Haematol* 2005;74:6–10.
54. Weiss LM, Azzi R, Dorfman RF, et al. Sinusoidal hematolymphoid malignancy ("malignant histiocytosis") presenting as atypical sinusoidal proliferation. A study of nine cases. *Cancer* 1986;58:1681–1688.
55. Jaffe ES, Costa J, Fauci AS, et al. Malignant lymphoma and erythrophagocytosis simulating malignant histiocytosis. *Am J Med* 1983;75:741–749.
56. Falini B, Pileri S, De Solas I, et al. Peripheral T-cell lymphoma associated with hemophagocytic syndrome. *Blood* 1990;75:434–444.
57. Trottestam H, Horne A, Arico M, et al.; The Histiocyte Society. Chemoimmunotherapy for hemophagocytic lymphohistiocytosis: long-term results of the HLH-94 treatment protocol. *Blood* 2011;118:4577–4584.
58. Wong KF, Chan JK. Reactive hemophagocytic syndrome-a clinicopathologic study of 40 patients in an Oriental population. *Am J Med* 1992;93:177–180.
59. Kikuchi M. Lymphadenitis showing focal reticulum cell hyperplasia with nuclear debris and phagocytes: a clinico-pathological study (in Japanese). *Nippon Ketsueki Gakkai Zasshi* 1972;35:379–380.
60. Fujimoto Y, Kozima Y, Yamaguchi K. Cervical subacute necrotizing lymphadenitis. A new clinicopathologic entity. *Naika* 1972;20:920–927.
61. Pileri S, Kikuchi M, Helbron D, et al. Histiocytic necrotizing lymphadenitis without granulocytic infiltration. *Virchows Arch (Pathol Anat)* 1982;395:257–271.
62. Turner RR, Martin J, Dorfman RF. Necrotizing lymphadenitis: a study of 30 cases. *Am J Surg Pathol* 1983;7:115–123.
63. Dorfman RF, Berry GJ. Kikuchi's histiocytic necrotizing lymphadenitis: an analysis of 108 cases with emphasis on differential diagnosis. *Semin Diagn Pathol* 1988;5:329–345.
64. Onciu M, Medeiros LJ. Kikuchi-Fujimoto lymphadenitis. *Adv Anat Pathol* 2003;10:204–211.
65. Bosch X, Guilabert A, Miquel R, et al. Enigmatic Kikuchi-Fujimoto disease: a comprehensive review. *Am J Clin Pathol* 2004;122:141–152.
66. Sumiyoshi Y, Kikuchi M, Ohshima K, et al. A case of histiocytic necrotizing lymphadenitis with bone marrow and skin involvement. *Virchos Arch A Pathol Anat Histopathol* 1992;420:275–279.
67. Kuo T. Cutaneous manifestation of Kikuchi's histiocytic necrotizing lymphadentitis. *Am J Surg Pathol* 1990;14:872–876.
68. Tsang WYW, Chan JKC, Ng CS. Kikuchi's lymphadenitis. A morphologic analysis of 75 cases with special reference to unusual features. *Am J Surg Pathol* 1994;18:219–231.
69. Kuo T. Kikuchi's disease (histiocytic necrotizing lymphadenitis). A clinicopathologic study of 79 cases with an analysis of histologic subtypes, immunohistology, and DNA ploidy. *Am J Surg Pathol* 1995;19:798–809.
70. Facchetti F, De Wolf-Peeters C, van den Oord JJ, et al. Plasmacytoid monocytes (so-called plasmacytoid T-cells) in Kikuchi's lymphadenitis. An immunohistologic study. *Am J Clin Pathol* 1989;92:42–50.
71. Pilichowska ME, Pinkus J, Pinkus GS. Histiocytic necrotizing lymphadenitis (Kikuchi-Fujimoto disease): lesional cells exhibit an immature dendritic phenotype. *Am J Clin Pathol* 2009;13:174–182.
72. Nomura Y, Takeuchi M, Yoshida S, et al. Phenotype for activated tissue macrophages in histiocytic necrotizing lymphadenitis. *Pathol Int* 2009;59:631–635.
73. Cleary KR, Osborne BM, Butler JJ. Lymph node infarction foreshadowing malignant lymphoma. *Am J Surg Pathol* 1982;6:435–442.
74. Giesker DW, Pastuszak WT, Forouhar FA, et al. Lymph node biopsy for early diagnosis in Kawasaki disease. *Am J Surg Pathol* 1982;6:493–501.
75. Dorfman RF, Warnke RA. Lymphadenopathy simulating the malignant lymphomas. *Hum Pathol* 1974;5:519–550.
76. Pileri SA, Grogan TM, Banks P, et al. Tumours of histiocytes and accessory dendritic cells: an immunohistochemical approach to classification from the International Lymphoma Study Group based on 61 cases. *Histopathology* 2002;41:1–29.
77. Copie-Bergman C, Wotherspoon AC, Norton AJ, et al. True histiocytic lymphoma. A morphologic, immunohistochemical and molecular genetic study of 13 cases. *Am J Surg Pathol* 1998;22:1386–1392.
78. Franchino C, Reich C, Distenfeld A, et al. A clinicopathologically distinctive primary splenic histiocytic neoplasm. Demonstration of its histiocyte derivation by immunophenotypic and molecular genetic analysis. *Am J Surg Pathol* 1988;12:398–404.
79. Kamel OW, Gocke CD, Kell DL, et al. True histiocytic lymphoma: a study of 12 cases based on current definition. *Leuk Lymphoma* 1995;18:81–86.
80. Hornick JL, Jaffe ES, Fletcher CD. Extranodal histiocytic sarcoma: clinicopathologic analysis of 14 cases of a rare epithelioid malignancy. *Am J Surg Pathol* 2004;28:1133–1144.
81. Vasef MA, Zaatari GS, Chan WC, et al. Dendritic cell tumors associated with low-grade B-cell malignancies. Report of three cases. *Am J Clin Pathol* 1995;104:696–701.
82. Shao H, Xi L, Raffeld M, et al. Clonally related histiocytic/dendritic cell sarcoma and chronic lymphocytic leukemia/small lymphocytic lymphoma: a study of 7 cases. *Mod Pathol* 2011;24:1421–1432.
83. Castro EC, Blasquez C, Boyd J, et al. Clinicopathologic features of histiocytic lesions following ALL, with a review of the literature. *Pediatr Dev Pathol* 2010; 13:225–237.
84. Feldman AL, Arber DA, Pittaluga S, et al. Clonally related follicular lymphomas and histiocytic/dendritic cell sarcomas: evidence for transdifferentiation of the follicular lymphoma clone. *Blood* 2008;111:5433–5439.
85. DeMent SH. Association between mediastinal germ cell tumors and hematologic malignancies: an update. *Hum Pathol* 1990;21:699–703.
86. Gergis U, Dax H, Ritchie E, et al. Autologous hematopoietic stem-cell transplantation in combination with thalidomide as treatment for histiocytic sarcoma: a case report and review of the literature. *J Clin Oncol* 2011;29:e251–e253.
87. Favara BE, Steele A. Langerhans cell histiocytosis of lymph nodes: a morphological assessment of 43 biopsies. *Pediatr Pathol Lab Med* 1997;17:769–787.
88. Carstensen H, Ornvold K. The epidemiology of Langerhans cell histiocytosis in children in Denmark. 1975–1989. *Med Pediatr Oncol* 1993;21:387–388.
89. Nicholson HS, Egeler RM, Nesbit ME. The epidemiology of Langerhans cell histiocytosis. *Hematol Oncol Clin N Am* 1998;12:379–384.

90. Badalian-Very G, Vergilio J, Degar BA, et al. Recent advances in the understanding of Langerhans cell histiocytosis. *Br J Haematol* 2012;156:163–172.
91. Guyot-Goubin A, Donadieu J, Barkaoui M, et al. Descriptive epiemiology of childhood Langerhans cell histiocytosis in France, 2000–2004. *Pediatr Blood Cancer* 2008;51:71–75.
92. Egeler RM, Neglia JP, Arico M, et al. The relation of Langerhans cell histiocytosis to acute leukemia, lymphomas, and other solid tumors. The LCH-Malignancy Study Group of the Histiocyte Society. *Hematol Oncol Clin North Am* 1998;12:369–378.
93. Bhatia S, Newbit ME, Egeler RM, et al. Epidemiologic study of Langerhans cell histiocytosis in children. *J Pediatr* 1997;130:774–784.
94. Karis J, Bernstrand C, Fadeel B, et al. The incidence of Langerhans cell histiocytosis in children in Stockholm Count, Sweden 1992–2001. In: *Proceedings of the XIX meeting of the Histiocyte Society*. Philadelphia, PA. Histiocyte Society, 2003.
95. Colby TV, Lombard C. Histiocytosis X in the lung. *Hum Pathol* 1983;14:847–856.
96. Abla O, Egeler RM, Weitzman S. Langerhans cell histiocytosis: current concepts and treatments. *Cancer Treat Rev* 2010;36:354–359.
97. McClain K, Jin H, Gresik V, et al. Langerhans cell histiocytosis: lack of a viral etiology. *Am J Hematol* 1994;47:16–20.
98. Willman CL, McClain K. An update on clonality, cytokines, and viral etiology in Langerhans cell histiocytosis. *Hematol Oncol Clin North Am* 1998;12:407–416.
99. Yu RC, Chu C, Buluwela L, et al. Clonal proliferation of Langerhans cells in Langerhans cell histiocytosis. *Lancet* 1994;343:767–768.
100. Yousem SA, Colby TV, Chen YY, et al. Pulmonary Langerhans' cell histiocytosis: molecular analysis of clonality. *Haematologica* 2001;86:1009–1014.
101. Arico M, Danesino C. Langerhans' cell histiocytosis: is there a role for genetics? *Haematologica* 2001;86:1009–1014.
102. Badalian-Very G, Vergilio J, Degar BA, et al. Recurrent BRAF mutations in Langerhans cell histiocytosis. *Blood* 2010;116:1919–1923.
103. Ito T, Inaba M, Inaba K, et al. A CD1a+/CD11c+ subset of human blood dendritic cells is a direct precursor of Langerhans cells. *J Immunol* 1999;163:1409–1419.
104. Geissmann F, Lepelletier Y, Fraitag S, et al. Differentiation of Langerhans cells in Langerhans cell histiocytosis. *Blood* 2001;97:1241–1248.
105. Weiss LM, Beckstead JH, Warnke RA, et al. Leu 6 expressing lymph node cells are dendritic cells and closely related to interdigitating cells. *Hum Pathol* 1986;17:179–184.
106. Burns BF, Colby TV, Dorfman RF. Langerhans' cell granulomatosis (histiocytosis X) associated with malignant lymphomas. *Am J Surg Pathol* 1983;7:529–533.
107. Neuman MP, Frizzera G. The coexistence of Langerhans' cell granulomatosis and malignant lymphoma may take different forms: report of seven cases with a review of the literature. *Hum Pathol* 1986;17:1060–1065.
108. Krenacs L, Tiszlavicz L, Krenacs T, et al. Immunohistochemical detection of CD1a antigen in formalin-fixed and paraffin-embedded tissue sections with monoclonal antibody O10. *J Pathol* 1993;171:99–104.
109. Emile JF, Wechsler J, Brousse N, et al. Langerhans' cell histiocytosis. Definitive diagnosis with the use of monoclonal antibody O10 on routinely paraffin-embedded samples. *Am J Surg Pathol* 1995;19:636–641.
110. Sholl LM, Pinkus J, Pinkus JL, et al. Immunohistochemical analysis of langerin in Langerhans cell histiocytosis and pulmonary inflammatory and infectious diseases. *Am J Surg Pathol* 2007;31:947–952.
111. Feldman AL, Berthold F, Arceci RJ, et al. Clonal relationship between precursor T-lymphoblastic leukaemia/lymphoma and Langerhans-cell histiocytosis. *Lancet Oncol* 2005;6:435–437.
112. Yu RC, Chu AC. Lack of T-cell receptor gene rearrangements in cells involved in Langerhans cell histiocytosis. *Cancer* 1995;75:1162–1166.
113. Broadbent V, Gadner H. Current therapy for Langerhans cell histiocytosis. *Hematol Oncol Clin North Am* 1998;12:327–338.
114. Risdall RJ, Dihner LP, Duray P, et al. Histiocytosis X (Langerhans' cell histiocytosis). Prognostic role of histopathology. *Arch Pathol Lab Med* 1983;107:59–63.
115. Ben-Ezra J, Bailey A, Azumi N, et al. Malignant histiocytosis X. A distinct clinicopathologic entity. *Cancer* 1991;68:1050–1060.
116. Wood C, Wood GS, Deneau DG, et al. Malignant histiocytosis X. Report of rapidly fatal case in an elderly man. *Cancer* 1984;54:347–352.
117. Kawase T, Hamazaki M, Ogura M, et al. CD56/NCAM-positive Langerhans' cell sarcoma. A clinicopathologic study of 4 cases. *Int J Hematol* 2005;81:323–329.
118. Elleder M, Fakan F, Hula M. Pleomorphous histiocytic sarcoma arising in a patient with histiocytosis X. *Neoplasma* 1986;33:117–128.
119. Perez-Ordonez B, Rosai J. Follicular dendritic cell tumor: review of the entity. *Semin Diagn Pathol* 1998;15:144–154.
120. Perez-Ordonez B, Erlandson RA, Rosai J. Follicular dendritic cell tumor: report of 13 additional cases of a distinctive entity. *Am J Surg Pathol* 1996;20:944–955.
121. Monda L, Warnke R, Rosai J. A primary lymph node malignancy with features suggestive of dendritic reticulum cell differentiation. A report of 4 cases. *Am J Pathol* 1986;122:562–572.
122. Cheuk W, Chan JK, Shek TW, et al. Inflammatory pseudotumor-like follicular dendritic cell tumor: a distinctive low-grade malignant intra-abdominal neoplasm with consistent Epstein-Barr virus association. *Am J Surg Pathol* 2001;25:721–731.
123. Arber DA, Weiss LM, Chang KL. Detection of Epstein-Barr virus in inflammatory pseudotumor. *Semin Diagn Pathol* 1998;15:155–160.
124. Nayler SJ, Taylor L, Cooper K. HHV-8 is not associated with follicular dendritic cell tumours. *Mol Pathol* 1998;51:168–170.
125. Andriko JW, Kaldjian EP, Tsokos M, et al. Reticulum cell neoplasms of lymph nodes: a clinicopathologic study of 11 cases with recognition of a new subtype derived from fibroblastic reticular cells. *Am J Surg Pathol* 1998;22:1048–1058.
126. Chan JK, Tsang WY, Ng CS. Follicular dendritic cell tumor and vascular neoplasm complicating hyaline-vascular Castleman's disease. *Am J Surg Pathol* 1994;18:517–525.
127. Nguyen DT, Diamond LW, Hansmann ML, et al. Follicular dendritic cell sarcoma. Identification by monoclonal antibodies in paraffin sections. *Appl Immunohistochem* 1994;2:60–64.
128. Fonseca R, Yamakawa M, Nakamura S, et al. Follicular dendritic cell sarcoma and interdigitating reticulum cell sarcoma: a review. *Am J Hematol* 1998;59:161–167.
129. Weiss LM, Berry GJ, Dorfman RF, et al. Spindle cell neoplasms of lymph nodes of probable reticulum cell lineage. True reticulum cell sarcoma? *Am J Surg Pathol* 1990;14:405–414.
130. Luk IS, Shek TW, Tang VW, et al. Interdigitating dendritic cell tumor of the testis: a novel testicular spindle cell neoplasm. *Am J Surgical Pathol* 1999;23:1141–1148.
131. Miettinen M, Fletcher CD, Lasota J. True histiocytic lymphoma of small intestine. Analysis of two S-100 protein-positive cases with features of interdigitating reticulum cell sarcoma. *Am J Surg Pathol* 1993;100:285–292.
132. Fraser CR, Wang W, Gomez M, et al. Transformation of chronic lymphocytic leukemia/small lymphocytic lymphoma to interdigitating dendritic cell sarcoma: evidence for transdifferentiation of the lymphoma clone. *Am J Clin Pathol* 2009;132:928–939.
133. Chen M, Agrawal R, Nasseri-Nik N, et al. Indeterminate cell tumor of the spleen. *Hum Pathol* 2012;43:307–311.
134. Berti E, Gianotti R, Alessi E. Unusual cutaneous histiocytosis expressing an intermediate immunophenotype between Langerhans' cells and dermal macrophages. *Arch Dermatol* 1988;124:1250–1253.
135. Rezk SA, Spagnolo DV, Brynes RK, et al. Indeterminate cell tumor: a rare dendritic neoplasm. *Am J Surg Pathol* 2008;32:1868–1676.
136. Jaffe R, DeVaughn D, Langhoff E. Fascin and the differential diagnosis of childhood histiocytic lesion. *Pediatr Dev Pathol* 1998;1:216–221.
137. Martel M, Sarli D, Colecchia M, et al. Fibroblastic reticular cell tumor of the spleen: report of a case and review of the entity. *Am J Surg Pathol* 2003;16:175–183.
138. Weitzman S, Jaffe R. Uncommon histiocytic disorders: the non-Langerhans cell histiocytoses. *Pediatr Blood Cancer* 2005;45:256–264.
139. Janssen D, Harms D. Juvenile xanthogranuloma in childhood and adolescence: a clinicopathologic study of 129 patient from the Kiel Pediatric Tumor Registry. *Am J Surg Pathol* 2005;29:21–28.
140. Dehner L. Juvenile xanthogranulomas in the first two decaes of life: a clinicopathologic study of 174 cases with cutaneous and extracutaneous manifestations. *Am J Surg Pathol* 2003;27:579–593.
141. Freyer DR, Kennedy R, Bostrom BC, et al. Juvenile xanthogranuloma: forms of systemic disease and their clinical implications. *J Pediatr* 1996;129:227–237.
142. Nascimento AG. A clinicopathologic and immunohistochemical comparative study of cutaneous and intramuscular forms of juvenile xanthogranuloma. *Am J Surg Pathol* 1997;21:645–652.
143. Cambiaghi S, Restano L, Caputo R. Juvenile xanthogranuloma associated with neurofibromatosis 1: 14 patients without evidence of hematologic malignancies. *Pediatr Dermatol* 2004;21:97–101.
144. Burgdorf WHC, Zelger B. JXG, NF1, and JMML: alphabet soup or a clinical issue? *Pediatr Dermatol* 2004;21:174–176.
145. Zvulunov A, Barak Y, Metzker A. Juvenile xanthogranuloma, neurofibromatosis, and juvenile chronic myelogenous leukemia. World statistical analysis. *Arch Dermatol* 1995;131:904–908.
146. Zelger B, Cerio R, Orchard G, et al. Juvenile and adult xanthogranuloma. A histological and immunohistochemical comparison. *Am J Surg Pathol* 1994;18:126–135.

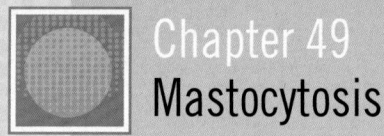

Chapter 49
Mastocytosis

Hans-Peter Horny • Karl Sotlar • Peter Valent

Mastocytosis is a rare neoplastic disease of bone marrow origin comprising a very heterogeneous group of disorders ranging from the benign solitary mastocytoma of the skin to the prognostically very unfavorable mast cell leukemia (MCL) (1). The often initially misleading clinical features of patients with mastocytosis originate from inappropriate mediator release that may even lead to lethal anaphylaxia. The key clinical feature in the majority of patients is a typical rash, traditionally termed urticaria pigmentosa (UP) (2). The rare aggressive or leukemic subtypes of mastocytosis usually present without skin lesions but often mimic more common hematologic neoplasms like malignant lymphoma or myeloid leukemia at first presentation. The molecular hallmark of mastocytosis is the finding of activating point mutations at codon 816 of *KIT*, usually *KIT*-D816V (3). Patients with extracutaneous manifestation of mastocytosis have systemic mastocytosis (SM) and often show an elevated serum tryptase. The diagnosis of mastocytosis may be difficult to establish, although precise defining criteria have been published by the WHO (4,5). The hematopathologist plays a crucial role in the diagnosis since the demonstration of compact mast cell infiltrates in extracutaneous tissues has been shown to be the only major diagnostic criterion for SM.

 ## DEFINITION

Mastocytosis comprises a heterogeneous group of disorders characterized by a clonal expansion of neoplastic mast cells derived from CD34+ bone marrow progenitor cells (6). The key clinical features in most patients are a skin rash and an elevated serum tryptase level. In SM, neoplastic mast cells typically carry activating point mutations in *KIT*, usually at codon 816; show aberrant expression of CD2 and/or CD25; and form compact infiltrates in extracutaneous tissues. The bone marrow is almost always involved.

 ## EPIDEMIOLOGY

Mastocytosis is considered to be a rare disease amongst bone marrow–derived hematologic neoplasms, but its true incidence is unknown. It most commonly presents as UP, which has been reported to be present in about 1 in 1,000 patients seen in dermatologic clinics. In childhood, the disease usually remains confined to the skin (7). In adulthood, almost all patients (>90%) with UP-like skin lesions have in fact SM, usually indolent SM (ISM) (40). The incidence of the prognostically unfavorable subtypes of SM, that is, aggressive systemic mastocytosis (ASM) and MCL, is low compared to that of ISM.

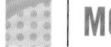 ## CLINICAL FEATURES

The clinical features and findings in patients with mastocytosis usually are indicative of certain types of SM published in the updated WHO "blue" book on hematopoietic neoplasms, which includes well-defined diagnostic criteria (Tables 49.1 and 49.2) (4,5). Patients with cutaneous mastocytosis (CM) often exhibit the brownish-red maculopapular lesions of UP. Patients with SM present with cutaneous disease and/or with signs and symptoms suggestive of a hematologic neoplasm, such as hepatosplenomegaly and/or lymphadenopathy (Table 49.3). In patients with aggressive or leukemic SM, skin lesions are often absent. It is a well-recognized phenomenon that patients with ISM or isolated bone marrow mastocytosis (BMM) have a mild bone marrow infiltration but sometimes have major symptoms due to inappropriate mediator release from mast cells (8,9). The extreme form of symptoms is anaphylactic shock, which may even be fatal (10). It may be very difficult or even impossible in the individual patient to determine whether the occurrence of such anaphylactic reactions is due to comorbidity, usually allergy, or is based only on mast cell activation occurring in the context of mastocytosis through endogenous activation pathways. When the key role of the mast cells in the anaphylactic reaction is well documented, it is appropriate to establish a diagnosis of mast cell activation syndrome (MCAS). The criteria for MCAS differ from those used to diagnose mastocytosis, although MCAS may also occur in patients with mastocytosis. In MCAS, the significant and immediate increase in tryptase levels is the key diagnostic finding. It is important not to confuse this immediate increase in a defined time interval with the chronic increase in serum tryptase levels seen in patients with SM, for which a significantly elevated basal serum tryptase level (>20 ng/mL) is a minor diagnostic criterion (11).

DIAGNOSTIC APPROACH

For each patient with suspected mastocytosis, a clinical workup should be performed, including information about allergic reactions and skin rashes. It is of the utmost importance to determine the serum tryptase level in all patients. In those with a rash and elevated serum tryptase levels, histologic investigation of the bone marrow should be performed. Many cases of SM show only minor, focal bone marrow involvement (12). Therefore, the core biopsy specimen must be at least 1 cm long to exclude false-negative results. It should be fixed immediately, mildly decalcified, and embedded in paraffin wax. Molecular analysis for the detection of activating point mutations of *KIT* can also be performed on this routinely processed tissue (13,14).

 ## MORPHOLOGY

General Aspects

The broad range of clinical features of mastocytosis is reflected in the large variety of morphologic findings. However, the only major diagnostic criterion for mastocytosis is the identification of multifocal compact tissue mast cell infiltrates. Therefore, the pathologist plays a key role in diagnosis. However, the

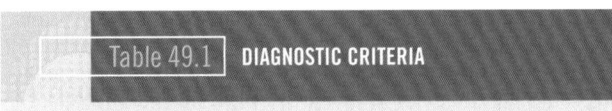

Table 49.1   DIAGNOSTIC CRITERIA

Major Criterion

Compact mast cell infiltrates (>15 mast cells per infiltrate)

Minor Criteria

1. Prominent spindling of >25% of mast cells
2. Aberrant immunophenotype of mast cells with expression of CD2 and/or CD25
3. Activating point mutation at codon 816 of *KIT*
4. Elevated serum tryptase (>20 ng/μL)

A diagnosis of mastocytosis can be established when the major criterion plus one minor criterion or three minor criteria alone are fulfilled.
Source: Valent PH, Horny H-P, Li CY, et al. Mastocytosis (mast cell disease). In: Harris N. Jaffe ES, Stein H, et al., eds. *WHO classification of tumours. Tumours of haematopoietic and lymphoid tissues.* Lyon: IARC Press: 2001:291–302; Horny H-P, Metcalfe DD, Bennett JM, et al. Mastocytosis (mast cell disease). In: Campo E, Swerdlow SH, Harris NL, et al., eds. *WHO classification of tumours of haematopoietic and lymphoid tissues.* Geneva: IARC Press, 2008:54–63.

diagnosis of mastocytosis may be very difficult to establish for the following reasons:

- The detection of mast cells requires special stains and is difficult in routine H&E-stained sections.
- The compact mast cell infiltrates may be small in size.
- The compact infiltrates may contain cells other than mast cells, such as lymphocytes, fibroblasts, eosinophils, or macrophages. The number of lymphocytes in some cases is large enough for a diagnosis of malignant lymphoma rather than mastocytosis to be considered (15).
- A second hematologic neoplasm may coexist with the mastocytosis. Such disorders have been termed "systemic mastocytosis with associated clonal hematologic non–mast cell lineage disorder" (SM-AHNMD). The AHNMD may even obscure the mastocytosis (16).
- Mastocytosis is a relatively rare disease amongst hematologic neoplasms, and many hematopathologists have little experience with this disease, especially with the rare aggressive and leukemic variants.

Cytology and Histology

When bone marrow smears are examined, normal mast cells can be seen as round, medium-sized cells exhibiting abundant metachromatic granules in Pappenheim/Wright-Giemsa or toluidine blue stains. Mast cells are few in number in normal

Table 49.2   CLASSIFICATION OF MASTOCYTOSIS

1. Cutaneous mastocytosis
   1.1. Urticaria pigmentosa
   1.2. Diffuse cutaneous mastocytosis
   1.3. Solitary mastocytoma
2. Indolent systemic mastocytosis
   Provisional entities
   2.1. Bone marrow mastocytosis
   2.2. Smoldering systemic mastocytosis
   2.3. Well-differentiated systemic mastocytosis
3. Systemic mastocytosis with associated clonal hematopoietic non–mast cell lineage disease (SM-AHNMD)
4. Aggressive systemic mastocytosis
5. Mast cell leukemia
   5.1. Aleukemic mast cell leukemia
6. Mast cell sarcoma
7. Extracutaneous mastocytoma

Source: WHO, 2008 and Horny H-P, Metcalfe DD, Bennett JM, et al. Mastocytosis (mast cell disease). In: Campo E, Swerdlow SH, Harris NL, et al., eds. *WHO classification of tumours of haematopoietic and lymphoid tissues.* Geneva: IARC Press, 2008:54–63.

Table 49.3   MAIN CLINICAL FEATURES OF THE DIFFERENT SUBTYPES OF SM

	Skin	BM	LN	Spleen	B	C	AHNMD
Indolent SM	+	+	0	0	0	0	0
Bone marrow SM	0	+	0	0	0	0	0
Smoldering SM	+	+	+	+	+	0	0
SM-AHNMD	0/+	+	+/0	+/0	+/0	+	+
Aggressive SM	0/+	+	+	+	+	+	0
Lymphadenopathic SM	0	+	+	+	+	+	0
Mast cell leukemia	0	+	0	+	+	+	0
Mast cell sarcoma	0	0	0	0	0	0	0

SM, Systemic mastocytosis; AHNMD, associated clonal hematopoietic non–mast cell lineage disease; BM, bone marrow; LN, lymph node; B, B-findings (Table 49.10); C, C-findings (Table 49.10).

and reactive bone marrows, making up far less than 1% of all nucleated cells. However, in some reactive states, their numbers may increase to 1% or even 5% of nucleated cells in the bone marrow, especially when stem cell factor (SCF) has been administered. Mast cell hyperplasia may be very obvious in hypoplastic or aplastic bone marrows.

Mast cells in neoplastic states, especially in mastocytosis, show more or less prominent signs of cellular atypia (Table 49.4) (17). The presence of enlarged, plump, and spindle-shaped mast cells with various degrees of hypogranulation is a key feature often seen in ISM or BMM. The number of mast cells in these patients may be very low, that is, not exceeding 1% of nucleated bone marrow cells. Crushed particles usually contain greater numbers of atypical mast cells, but these should not be considered for quantitative assessment. Mast cells never show prominent nucleoli except in a few cases of MCL. Spindle-shaped mast cells have been termed "atypical mast cells type I" and dominate the picture in most cases of ISM and ASM (17). In contrast to ISM or ASM, most mast cells in MCL usually are highly atypical round or oval cells with hypogranulated broad clear cytoplasm and often with bilobed or monocytoid nuclei which are termed promastocytes or "atypical mast cells type II" (Table 49.4) (17). It may sometimes be difficult on the basis of conventional cytomorphology alone to differentiate these atypical mast cells from neoplastic immature basophils or the so-called metachromatic blasts seen in MCL or myelomastocytic leukemia (MML). Although blood and bone marrow smears are usually of value in the diagnosis of SM, especially for the recognition of MCL, additional histopathologic investigation of the bone marrow is always required. For a diagnosis of MCL the number of mast cells must exceed 20% of all nucleated cells in the bone marrow smear. In aleukemic MCL (aMCL) the percentage of circulating mast cells is below 10% of circulating leukocytes (4).

Histologically, mastocytosis involving the bone marrow is usually characterized by multifocal compact mast cell infiltrates (18). A more diffuse or sheetlike infiltration pattern is

Table 49.4   CYTOLOGICAL ASPECTS IN SYSTEMIC MASTOCYTOSIS AND RELATED DISORDERS

Main Cell Type	Diagnosis
"Normal" MC	Well-differentiated SM
Spindle-shaped MC (atypical MC type I[a])	Indolent, smoldering, and aggressive SM
Promastocyte (atypical MC type II[a])	Mast cell leukemia
Metachromatic blast cell	Myelomastocytic leukemia
Nonmetachromatic blast cell	SM-AML

MC, mast cell; SM, systemic mastocytosis.
[a]According to Sperr WR, Escribano L, Jordan JH, et al. Morphologic properties of neoplastic mast cells: delineation of stages of maturation and implication for cytological grading of mastocytosis. *Leuk Res* 2001;25:529–536.

seen in some cases of smoldering SM (SSM) and ASM, and in all cases of MCL. The focal compact infiltrates may contain varying numbers of lymphocytes, eosinophils, fibroblasts, and macrophages/histiocytes in addition to the mast cells. Such mixed infiltrates were formerly termed "fibrohistiocytic eosinophilic bone marrow lesion" and thought to be associated with drug toxicity before the predominant fibroblast-like cells were identified as atypical hypogranulated mast cells (19,20). Depending on the patients' clinical features, such cases are nowadays diagnosed as ISM or BMM. The mast cells may exhibit a spindle-shaped appearance and may contain varying amounts of metachromatic granules. Mast cells containing only scanty metachromatic granules can easily be confused with fibroblasts. The exclusive occurrence of round mast cells in the setting of mastocytosis is rare, but a diagnostic key feature of the entity known as well-differentiated SM (WDSM) (21). The term "well-differentiated" was introduced because mast cells in such cases not only are round, like most of their normal counterparts but also contain abundant metachromatic granules. It is sometimes difficult to distinguish such cases from reactive mast cell hyperplasia, but compact infiltrates, although sometimes very few in number, are only seen in WDSM.

In SM patients with mixed compact infiltrates containing large numbers of lymphocytes, sometimes even forming follicle-like structures, the loosely scattered mast cells may be almost obscured and a diagnosis of small-cell or low-grade non-Hodgkin lymphoma is initially considered (22). The cellular composition of such compact mixed infiltrates may vary greatly, making it necessary to look carefully for those with larger numbers of mast cells forming the diagnostically relevant compact infiltrates. A marked lymphocytic admixture to such infiltrates is often seen in ISM but almost never in ASM or MCL. In MCL the mast cells are usually round, but highly atypical, hypogranulated, and often contain bilobed or monocytoid immature nuclei, while the diffuse infiltrates in ASM are commonly dominated by spindle-shaped immature mast cells or promastocytes. Compact mast cell infiltrates almost always contain a dense network of reticulin fibers with foci of collagen fibrosis (12). Infiltrates with a preponderance of spindle-shaped mast cells usually show the greatest density of reticulin. Consideration of the density of reticulin fibers may also be of help in differentiating ASM from MCL since the latter is usually associated with only a minor degree of reticulin fibrosis. The lamellar bone in the immediate vicinity of compact mast cell infiltrates is often thickened, but diffuse osteosclerosis is rarely encountered. In contrast to the radiologic findings in middle-aged men with bone pain due to osteopenia caused by SM (ISM or BMM), a significant reduction in size and number of trabeculae is rarely detected in core biopsies removed from the iliac crest.

In a minority of patients with SM, especially those with ISM or BMM, compact infiltrates are absent, and there is only a mild increase in loosely scattered spindle-shaped mast cells, which show a tendency to form small perivascular groups or a network with their ends touching. In such cases, a diagnosis of SM can only be established when at least three minor SM criteria, like an aberrant immunophenotype with expression of CD2/CD25 and/or an activating codon 816 point mutation of *KIT*, are detectable.

IMMUNOPHENOTYPE

Immunohistologic investigation of the bone marrow is regarded as the gold standard for the diagnosis of mastocytosis, although mast cell involvement can also be recognized in Giemsa stains, especially in cases with compact mast cell infiltrates (23). Tryptase and KIT (CD117) are the key immunohistochemical markers for the diagnosis of mastocytosis, especially when there is minor tissue involvement and compact infiltrates are absent. In contrast to chymase, which is another mast cell-related antigen and expressed in mature mast cells, tryptase is expressed by virtually all mast cells at all stages of maturation, but also in

reactive and neoplastic states and even in highly atypical immature cells (24–26). However, certain other cells may also express tryptase and therefore stain positive in immunohistologic investigations, mainly neoplastic basophils in chronic myeloid leukemia, but also myeloblasts in a few cases of acute myeloid leukemia (AML) (27,28). In very few cases of SM, expression of tryptase is reduced or even absent in most of the mast cells. A tryptase-negative cell usually should not be regarded as a mast cell. All mast cells, irrespective of their stage of maturation, also express CD117 (KIT). Although CD117 is found on several other cell types in reactive and neoplastic states, cells coexpressing tryptase and CD117 can be definitively regarded as mast cells.

An important immunohistologic finding is the so-called tryptase-positive compact round-cell infiltrate of the bone marrow (TROCI-bm), which is relatively rare, although invariably present in MCL and WDSM (29). In contrast, it is quite uncommon in typical ISM, which normally shows a mixture of round and spindle-shaped mast cells. It is virtually absent in ASM, where spindle-shaped mast cells dominate the picture. TROCI-bm may occur as a focal or diffuse variant but is only associated with hematologic neoplasms, SM being the most frequent one (Table 49.5). In addition, primary and secondary basophilic leukemia, MML, and tryptase+ AML may exhibit TROCI-bm, usually in its diffuse variant (28). TROCI-bm should only be diagnosed when the tryptase+ infiltrate consists exclusively of round, usually small to medium-sized cells that can be demonstrated to resemble mast cells, neoplastic basophils, or, rarely, myeloblasts. Here it should be emphasized that not all neoplastic basophils express tryptase and thus may escape detection. For the proper recognition of basophil infiltrates, antibodies against the basophil-related antigens 2D7 and BB1 are of crucial importance, although 2D7 has been found to strongly stain neoplastic mast cells as well (30,31). Accordingly, cells expressing 2D7 can be either basophils or neoplastic mast cells (Fig. 49.1D; Table 49.6). Only those 2D7-expressing cells that do not coexpress CD117 are clearly identifiable as basophils, while cells coexpressing 2D7 and tryptase can be mast cells or basophils. Compact or sheetlike basophilic infiltrates are very rarely observed but occur in primary and secondary basophilic leukemia (the latter being a rare event in the context of transformation of chronic myeloid leukemia), and in patients with MPN with the rare and unusual myeloid fusion gene PCM1-JAK2 (Hans-Peter Horny, own unpublished observation, 2012).

For the differentiation of normal/reactive mast cells from neoplastic mast cells, staining for CD25, which is the interleukin 2-receptor-alpha, is strongly recommended (32). It has been shown that mast cells in SM almost always express CD25, an antigen usually not detected on normal/reactive mast cells. Since the only CD25-positive cells in normal bone marrow are

Table 49.5	TRYPTASE-POSITIVE ROUND-CELL COMPACT INFILTRATE OF THE BONE MARROW	
	Focal TROCI-bm	Diffuse TROCI-bm
Indolent SM	+	0
WDSM	+	0
MCL	0	+
SM-AHNMD	+	0/+
MML	0	+
Basophilic leukemia	+	+
Tryptase+ AML	0	+

SM, systemic mastocytosis; WDSM, well-differentiated SM; MCL, Mast cell leukemia; SM-AHNMD, SM with associated hematopoietic non–mast cell lineage disease; MML, Myelomastocytic leukemia; AML, Acute myeloid leukemia.
Note: In cases of SM-AHNMD in which the SM is MCL and dominant, TROCI-bm may be diffuse.
Source: Horny HP, Sotlar K, Stellmacher F, et al. The tryptase positive compact round cell infiltrate of the bone marrow (TROCI-BM): a novel histopathological finding requiring the application of lineage specific markers. *J Clin Pathol* 2006;59:298–302.

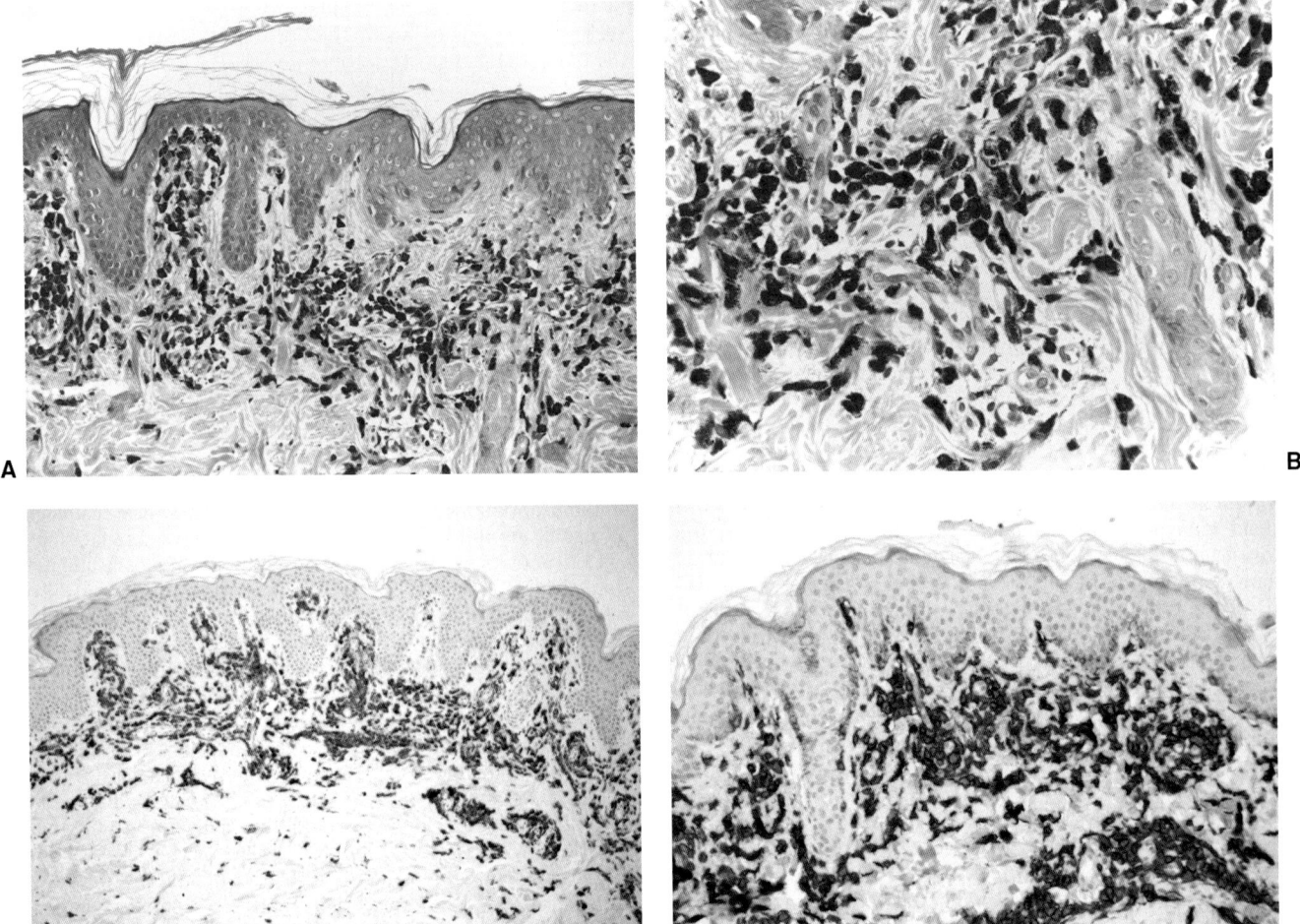

FIGURE 49.1. Cutaneous mastocytosis: juvenile UP. Skin biopsy specimen from a 3-year-old boy showing an intact epidermis and diffuse infiltration of the upper dermis by a mixture of round and spindle-shaped mast cells with abundant metachromatic granules **(A,B)**. There is no epidermotropism of the mast cell infiltrate. The mast cells are located around small blood vessels and adnexa. Immunostaining reveals strong expression of CD117 **(C)** and tryptase (not depicted) by mast cells, indicating a mature immunophenotype. CD25 is not expressed, but there is clear staining for the 2D7 antigen by the mast cells, indicating an aberrant immunophenotype **(D)**. The activating point mutation *KIT*-D816V was not present, and serum tryptase was not elevated. The findings argue strongly in favor of "true" CM, that is, the disease is limited to the skin. **A** and **B**, Giemsa; **C**, anti-CD117 (KIT); ABC method; **D**, anti-2D7 antigen; ABC method.

megakaryocytes and a few scattered lymphoid cells (both of which may serve as internal controls). The CD2 antigen (LFA-2) is another potential marker of neoplastic mast cells (33). However, compared to CD25, CD2 is much less specific and sensitive. Various other immunohistochemical markers are expressed by normal and neoplastic mast cells, such as CD9, CD14, CD26, CD30, CD44, CD45, CD52, CD68, CD79a, CD99, CD123, CD131, SDF-1, and 2D7 (Table 49.7). Two antigens that are usually detected in mast cells in ASM and MCL but not, or at lower levels, in ISM are CD30 and CD123. CD30, also known

Table 49.6   MAST CELLS (MC) AND BASOPHILS: IMMUNOHISTOCHEMICAL MARKERS

Antigen	Normal MC	Neoplastic MC	Basophils
CD2	−	+/−	−
CD25	−	++/+	+
CD117	++	++	−
CD123	−	++/+	+/++
Tryptase	++	++	+/++[a]
2D7	?	++/−	++
BB1	−	−	++

++, all cells strongly stained; +, not all cells stained; −, no staining.
[a]Cells stained only in neoplastic states.
MC, mast cells.
Agis H, Krauth MT, Böhm A, et al. Identification of basogranulin (BB1) as a novel immunohistochemical marker of basophils in normal bone marrow and patients with myeloproliferative disorders. *Am J Clin Pathol* 2006;125:273–281.

Table 49.7   IMMUNOPHENOTYPE OF MAST CELLS IN SM AND POTENTIAL MISDIAGNOSES

Antigen	Neoplasm/s
CD2	T-cell neoplasms, AML
CD9	B-cell neoplasms, myeloid neoplasms
CD14	Monocytic leukemia, histiocytosis
CD25	Hairy cell leukemia
CD30	Hodgkin lymphoma, ALCL
CD68	Histiocytosis, monocytic leukemia
CD99	ALL, Ewing sarcoma
CD123	Basophilic leukemia
2D7	Basophilic leukemia

ALCL, anaplastic large cell lymphoma; ALL, acute lymphoblastic leukemia; AML, acute myeloid leukemia.

as the Ki-1 antigen, is sometimes very strongly expressed by neoplastic mast cells, which may lead to misinterpretation of the findings as Hodgkin disease (34,35).

The following immunohistochemical stains are strongly recommended for the diagnosis of mastocytosis in the routine histopathologic workup and have been repeatedly tested for their utility, especially in the bone marrow:

1. Tryptase
2. CD117 (KIT)
3. CD25
4. CD30

In patients with SM-AHNMD, it is necessary to subtype the AHNMD component and the use of further immunohistochemical markers is required. Since AHNMD covers the whole spectrum of hematologic neoplasms, including malignant lymphoma, the antibodies to be applied have to be chosen accordingly (16,36). In all cases of ASM and MCL it is strongly recommended to stain for CD14 and CD34 in order to be able to detect an occult AHNMD, chronic myelomonocytic leukemia (CMML) being the most frequent subtype in this situation (37). Interestingly, even the advanced or highly aggressive/leukemic mastocytosis subtypes show extremely low proliferation, and <5% of mast cell nuclei in ASM and MCL are stained when the proliferation-associated antibody MIB-1 (Ki67 antigen) is applied (Hans-Peter Horny, own unpublished observation, 2010). In ISM and other low-grade subtypes of SM, nuclear staining by this antibody is virtually absent. This is clearly in contrast with the findings in other myeloid and lymphoid neoplasms involving the bone marrow, in which the percentage of stained nuclei ranges between 15% and 100%.

SUBTYPES OF MASTOCYTOSIS

Cutaneous Mastocytosis

Histologically, CM is characterized by an increase in dermal mast cells (38). In UP, the most common variant of CM, mast cells are either loosely scattered, with a marked tendency to aggregate around blood vessels and adnexae in the upper dermis, or form small compact infiltrates (Fig. 49.1A and B). Larger compact transdermal infiltrates of mast cells are seen in nodular variants of UP and solitary mastocytoma of the skin. The diffusely distributed mast cells in UP usually exhibit a spindle-shaped appearance, while those present in localized tumors, that is, mastocytoma of the skin, are often round. Except in mast cell sarcoma (MCS), which is a unique rarity in the setting of CM, the mast cells contain many metachromatic granules and are therefore easily detectable even in Giemsa stains. Intradermal mast cells always coexpress tryptase and CD117 (Fig. 49.1C and D), while expression of CD25 is often observed only in a minority of cells and not in all cases 40. Epiphenomena associated with cutaneous mast cell infiltration, especially in long-standing cases, are hyperpigmentation of the lower epidermis, fibrosis of the dermis, and small accumulations of lymphocytes and histiocytes. The single case of primary MCS of the skin we are aware of presented with recurrent nodules in the scalp, which were surgically removed (Hans-Peter Horny, own unpublished observation, 2010). The mast cells showed infiltration of the entire dermis, forming larger compact masses and containing no visible metachromatic granules. The diagnosis could only be established immunohistochemically, the tumor cells coexpressing tryptase, CD117, and CD25. Although a slight diffuse increase in mast cells to about 10% of all nucleated cells was seen in the bone marrow, transformation into MCL has not occurred during a follow-up period of almost four years. KIT-D816V mutation was not detected, even in microdissected mast cells from skin and bone marrow. In adult patients with UP, it is recommended that a preliminary diagnosis of "mastocytosis in the skin" rather than CM is made unless staging has been completed and bone marrow histology has been reported

by the hematopathologist. It is important to note that, based on WHO criteria, one or two minor SM criteria can be detected in the BM in CM patients (1,4,40)

Indolent Systemic Mastocytosis

ISM is almost always diagnosed on the basis of the histologic findings in a bone marrow trephine biopsy specimen. About two-thirds of the cases show a multifocal infiltration pattern with compact infiltrates of variable size, often located in a peritrabecular position (Fig. 49.2A–D). The degree of infiltration is <10% of the section area in most patients. While the typical compact mast cell infiltrates are easily detectable in Giemsa stains, the degree of diffuse infiltration can only be estimated by immunohistochemical staining with antibodies against tryptase and CD117 (24). Consequently, immunohistochemical investigation plays a crucial role in those cases without compact mast cell infiltrates, but also in BMM, which usually shows only a very low degree of BM mast cell infiltration and the absence of symptoms of inappropriate MC mediator release (9). The typical histologic picture in the third of patients who do not have compact mast cell infiltrates is a more or less dense network of mostly spindle-shaped mast cells that sometimes touch each other and have a tendency to form small groups. A diffuse increase in loosely distributed mast cells is more often seen in reactive mast cell hyperplasia but mast cells here are round and do not form groups or small clusters. Compact mast cell infiltrates in the setting of reactive mast cell hyperplasia have only been reported in a patient treated with hemopoietic growth factors (39). All cases have to be evaluated for CD25 expression by mast cells. If mast cells express CD25, mastocytosis is the most likely diagnosis, but only one minor criterion is fulfilled. When activating point mutations at codon 816 of KIT and an elevated serum tryptase are also present, three minor criteria then would allow a diagnosis of ISM or BMM to be established. It has to be emphasized that almost all patients (>95%) with adult-onset UP-like skin lesions will, in fact, be found to have ISM if thorough immunohistochemical and molecular biologic investigation is undertaken and the core biopsy of the bone marrow is of adequate length. Nowadays, a diagnosis of "pure" CM in the adult is the exception to the rule, indicating a change away from the diagnostic concepts that dominated the eighth and ninth decades of the last century (40).

Aggressive Systemic Mastocytosis

ASM is characterized by diffuse infiltration of various organs, leading to clinically relevant and measurable organ damage that results in dysfunction reflected in criteria termed C-findings (41,42). Like ISM, the diagnosis of ASM is almost always established in the bone marrow, but in rare cases the initial diagnosis may be made in the spleen or lymph nodes. The degree of bone marrow infiltration is usually much higher than in the indolent subtypes. The histologic picture is dominated by disseminated, often large and sometimes confluent compact mast cell infiltrates destroying the preexisting tissue architecture. The degree of infiltration per section area usually ranges between 30% and 80%. SSM may show a similar high degree of bone marrow infiltration and a distinction can only be made on the basis of clinical findings/parameters: while ASM should produce signs of organ impairment or even failure (C-findings), SSM is associated with organomegaly only, usually hepatomegaly and/or splenomegaly (B-findings) and there are no signs of organ damage. The mast cells in ASM and SSM are often spindle-shaped or fibroblast-like. This picture may even mimic a scar or granulation tissue. The tumor cells are embedded in a dense fibrotic stroma, while the degree of hypogranulation varies (Fig. 49.3A–D). The lamellar bone is often markedly thickened, sometimes even mimicking Paget disease. ASM in its pure form does occur, but in the majority of cases (up to 70%) there is an associated non–mast cell clonal hematologic

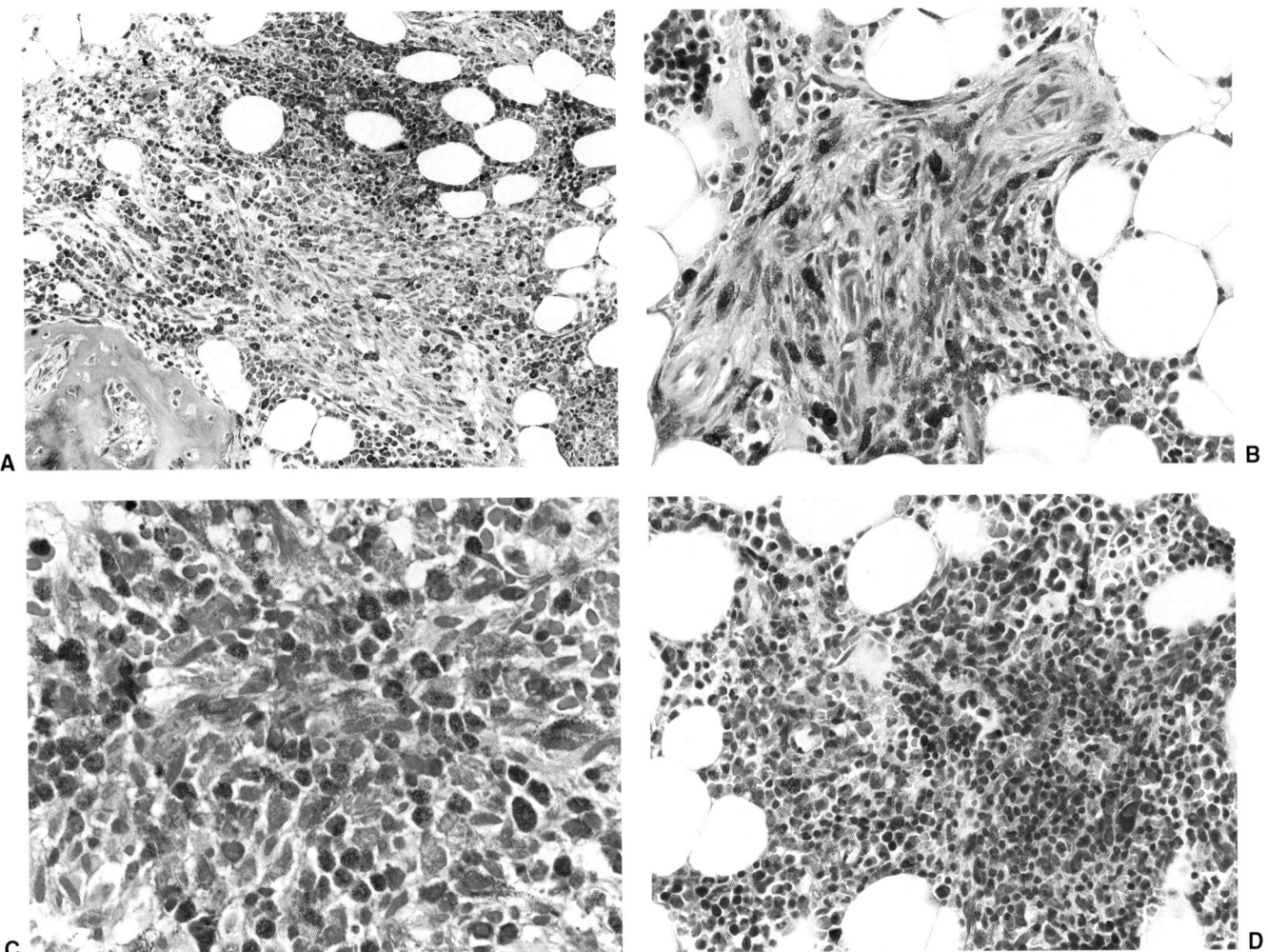

FIGURE 49.2. Indolent systemic mastocytosis. Bone marrow biopsy specimen from a 33-year-old woman showing various aspects of compact mast cell infiltrates. H&E stain **(A)** reveals a compact infiltrate consisting of spindle-shaped or fibroblast-like mast cells, findings that fulfill the criteria (one major and one minor) for a diagnosis of SM. Since the patient had long-standing UP adultorum, the final diagnosis here is ISM. Intramedullary mast cells showed an aberrant immunophenotype and expressed CD25 (not depicted), serum tryptase levels were chronically elevated with a maximum of 40 ng/μL, and the activating point mutation *KIT*-D816V was also present. This case fulfills all the diagnostic criteria (one major and four minor) for SM. The varying cellular composition of the compact infiltrates in this one patient includes nearly "pure" mast cell infiltrates **(B)**, infiltrates with predominance of eosinophils **(C)**, and infiltrates with follicle-like aggregates of lymphocytes almost obscuring the mast cells **(D)**. In such cases, the diagnosis of SM can easily be missed unless immunostaining with appropriate antibodies against the mast cell–related antigens CD117 (KIT), tryptase, and CD25 is performed. Findings like those shown in **(D)** are sometimes mistaken for lymphocytic lymphoma, which almost always shows a marked increase in reactive mast cells. **A**, H&E; **B–D**, Giemsa.

disorder and, accordingly, these cases have to be subclassified as ASM-AHNMD (Hans-Peter Horny, own unpublished observation, 2011). Therefore, the analysis of blood and bone marrow cells for cytologic atypia is strongly recommended, especially when smears are available. In the very rare cases with overwhelming bone marrow infiltration by mastocytosis it can be very difficult to confirm or exclude the presence of an AHNMD. Since some minor degree of cytologic atypia of blood cell precursors is found in the setting of ASM, additional investigation for activating point mutations indicative of myeloid neoplasms, e.g. *JAK2*-V617F, can be of major value for establishing the correct diagnosis (4,5). Lymphadenopathic (systemic) mastocytosis with eosinophilia is a rare subtype of ASM with prominent, progressive, and generalized lymphadenopathy and marked blood eosinophilia (43). Initially, the clinical presentation is that of a malignant lymphoma. Since ASM almost always exhibits features of lymphadenopathy usually involving the intra-abdominal but not the peripheral nodes it is questionable whether this more clinically defined entity should be retained

as a separate subtype of ASM. Eosinophilia in such cases may be very pronounced and a myeloid neoplasm, usually chronic eosinophilic leukemia, is diagnosed initially (44). It is therefore recommended that in all cases presenting with eosinophilia of the blood and bone marrow, SM should be excluded on the basis of immunohistochemistry and molecular biology.

Mast Cell Leukemia

MCL is one of the rarest types of human leukemia and usually presents in its aleukemic variant, that is, circulating mast cells make up <10% of leukocytes or, more often, are virtually absent from the blood (Fig. 49.4A–D) (4,5). In contrast to other subtypes of mastocytosis, investigation of blood and bone marrow smears is crucial to the diagnosis of MCL. Only cases with mast cell numbers of >20% of all nucleated bone marrow cells in smears can be classified as MCL (Fig. 49.4A and B). Mast cells should be counted outside the crushed particles because these structures may also contain many mast cells in other variants

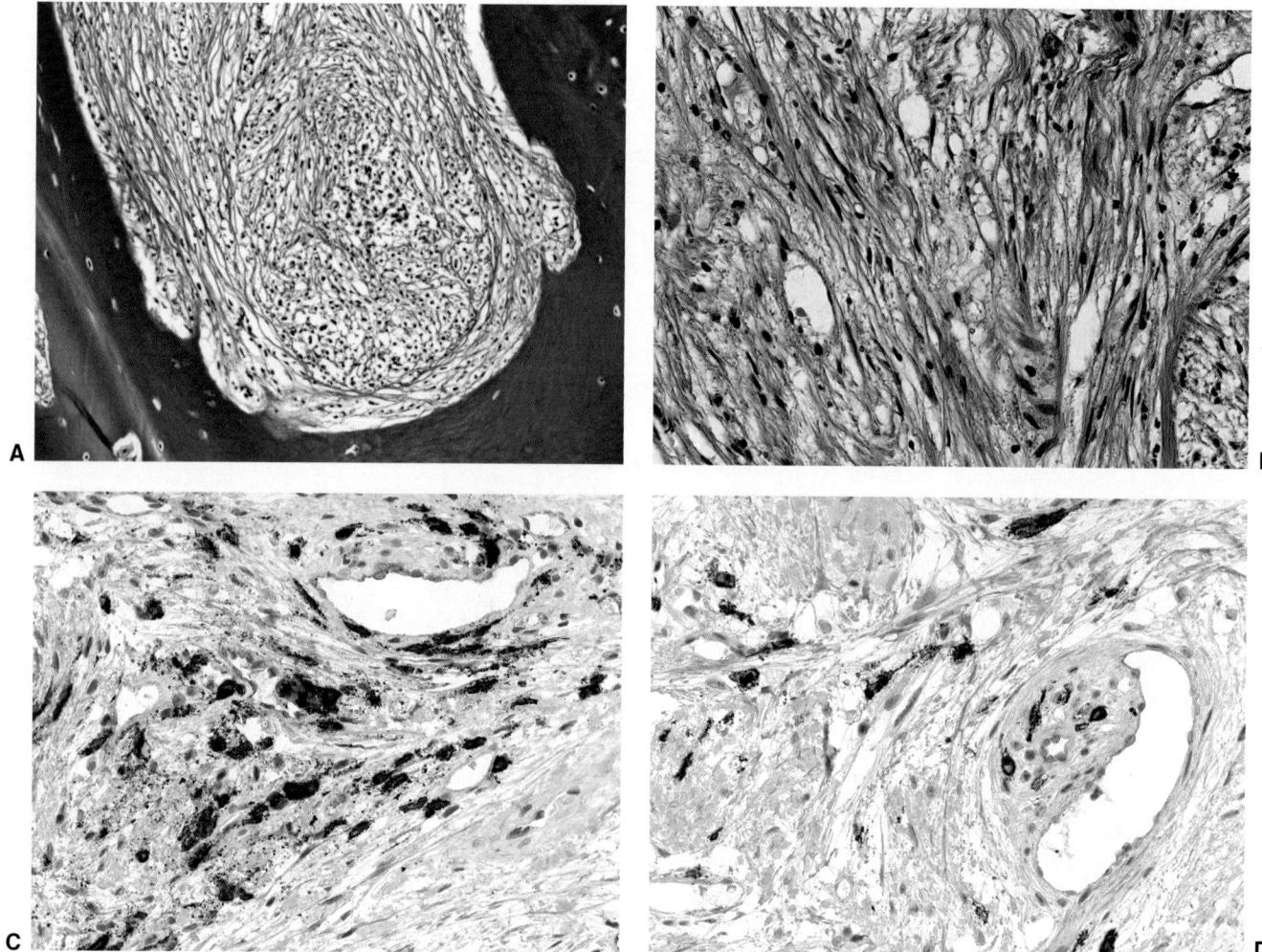

FIGURE 49.3. Aggressive systemic mastocytosis. Bone marrow biopsy specimen from a 63-year-old woman showing diffuse compact infiltration of the marrow spaces by spindle-shaped hypogranulated mast cells embedded in a dense fibrotic stroma. There is a complete absence of blood cell precursors and fat cells. The bone is thickened. The presence of marked cytopenia (anemia and thrombocytopenia) were considered C-findings, and a diagnosis of ASM was established. There were no signs of an AHNMD (SM-AHNMD) in this case, but associated hematologic neoplasms are often detectable in ASM, making the diagnosis of ASM-AHNMD much more likely than "pure" ASM. In some cases of ASM-AHNMD, the ASM infiltrates the bone marrow up to 100% in a given trephine specimen and the AHNMD, for example, chronic myelomonocytic leukemia, is only detected by the evaluation of blood smears. Bone marrow aspiration usually results in a "dry tap" in cases like this. While **(A)** clearly indicates a neoplastic process, the findings in **(B)** could be mistaken for nonspecific marrow fibrosis. It is therefore essential in such cases to perform immunostaining and mutational analysis. The mast cells here showed strong expression of tryptase **(C,D)**, CD117 (KIT), and CD25 (both not depicted). KIT-D816V was also detected. **A** and **B**, H&E; **C** and **D**, antitryptase; ABC method.

of mastocytosis. Histologically, MCL shows a diffuse and often compact infiltration pattern in the bone marrow with a preponderance of round, atypical, often hypogranulated mast cells (45). The degree of reticulin fibrosis is usually much lower than in the likewise diffusely infiltrating ASM. In most cases the degree of bone marrow infiltration exceeds 50% of the section area. Other forms of mastocytosis, especially ASM, may progress and transform into MCL. Such cases should thus be designated secondary MCL (sMCL). The cytomorphologic picture of MCL in bone marrow smears is often dominated by the presence of highly pleomorphic immature mast cells with varying amounts of metachromatic granules that are sometimes clumped together to form unusually large granule-like structures (Fig. 49.4C). Mast cells often exhibit vacuolation of the cytoplasm and may rarely show signs of hemophagocytosis (Fig. 49.4D). Giant tumor cells with multinucleated nuclei resembling Hodgkin cells may also occur. It may be difficult to differentiate mast cells from atypical basophils in the rare basophilic leukemias, especially the extremely infrequent acute variant (28). A third cell type with metachromatic granules is the so-called metachromatic blast, which occurs not only in MCL, but also in MML and AML. Metachromatic blasts

contain few granules and, by definition, cannot be assigned to the mast cell or basophilic lineage by cytomorphology alone (46).

SM-AHNMD

SM-AHNMD is a unique hematologic neoplasm consisting of two morphologically distinct entities (Fig. 49.5A–D) (16). In most cases, the AHNMD is of myeloid origin, CMML being the most frequently observed subtype (Table 49.8). In contrast to other subtypes of AHNMD, the myelomonocytic cells in SM-CMML have been shown to carry the activating point mutation *KIT*-D816V in about 75% of cases, making a clonal relationship between the SM and CMML in this setting very likely (37). AHNMD presenting as a lymphoid neoplasm is rare, plasma cell myeloma being most frequently encountered (47,48). When SM is associated with a myeloproliferative neoplasm (SM-MPN) the MPN usually dominates the histologic picture. Small compact infiltrates of SM are only detected when immunostaining for tryptase is performed. The most commonly found type of MPN in the setting of SM-AHNMD is primary myelofibrosis, while Ph+ chronic myeloid leukemia is only rarely observed (49). The

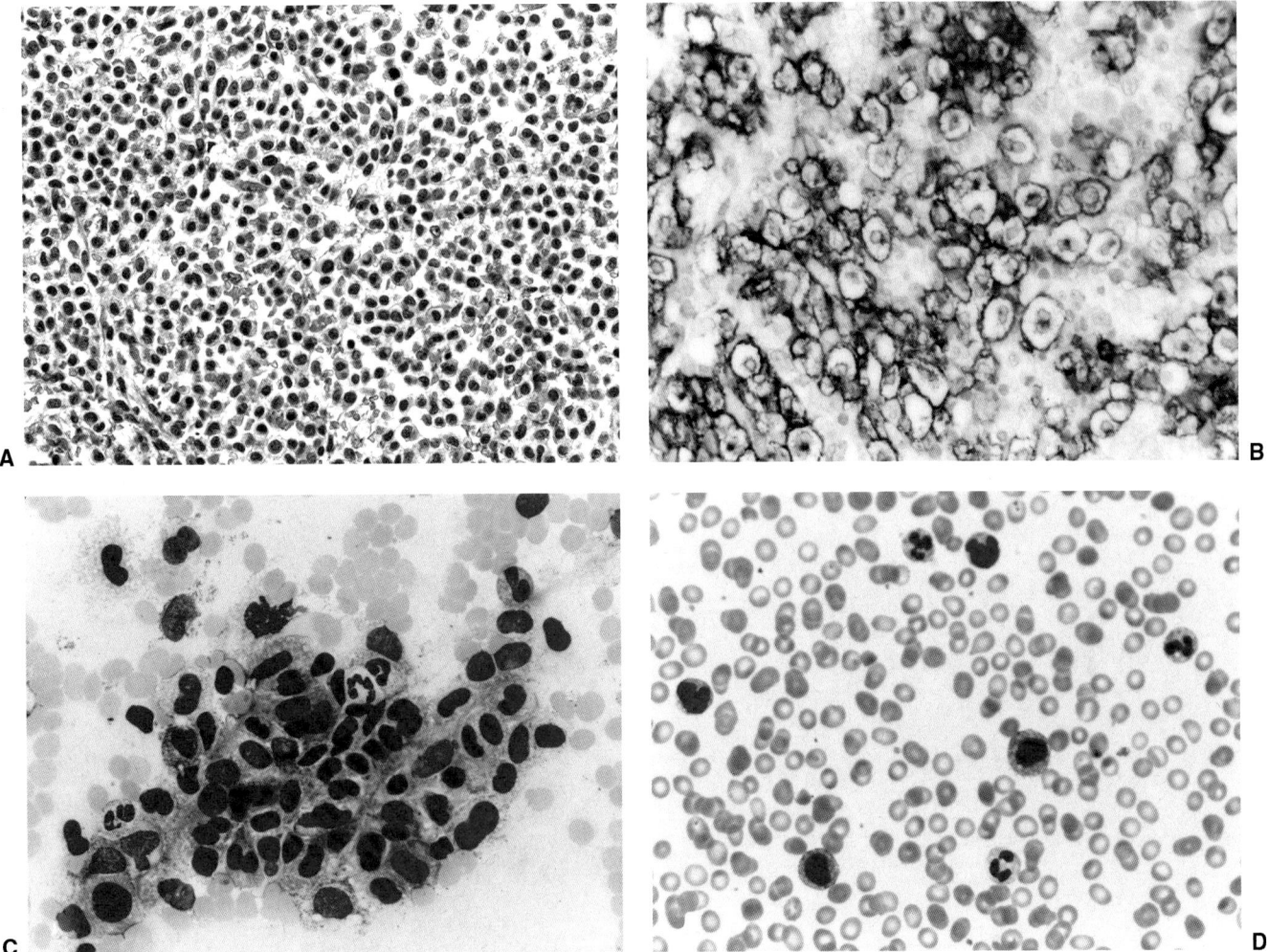

FIGURE 49.4. Mast cell leukemia. Bone marrow biopsy specimen from a 28-year-old woman showing diffuse compact infiltration by round hypogranulated mast cells without fibrosis **(A)**. There is a complete absence of blood cell precursors and fat cells. Compare this picture with the findings of ASM depicted in Figure 49.3. The neoplastic mast cells exhibit an aberrant immunophenotype, coexpressing CD117 **(B)**, tryptase, and CD25 (both not depicted). Bone marrow aspiration reveals clusters of highly atypical round mast cells with varying degrees of hypogranulation **(C)**. Note the sometimes bilobed monocytoid nuclei of the mast cells. The number of mast cells in bone marrow smears should exceed 20% of nucleated cells for a diagnosis of MCL. Mast cells were also found in the blood, making up more than 10% of circulating leukocytes and thus enabling this case to be subtyped as "true" MCL, which is much more infrequent than aMCL. **A,** H&E; **B,** anti-CD117/KIT; ABC method; **C** and **D,** Pappenheim/Wright-Giemsa.

diagnosis of SM-AHNMD should only be established when both neoplasms are detectable in the same tissue and/or exhibit the same molecular lesion. For example, patients with Hodgkin disease in a cervical lymph node and BMM without involvement of the bone marrow by the malignant lymphoma should not be assigned a diagnosis of SM-AHNMD. In patients with SM-AML, chemotherapy usually leads to marked regression of the acute leukemia and compact mast cell infiltrates are then easily detectable in the hypocellular edematous posttreatment bone marrow, even when these neoplastic mast cells have not been detected before therapy (50). Such findings may be termed occult SM (oSM). Retrospective analysis of the initial core biopsy using antibodies against tryptase, CD117, and CD25 may then help to detect a few small and often distorted compact mast cell infiltrates. SM-AHNMD cases with a predominant SM component are rare but may easily present difficulties in the detection and subclassification of the AHNMD. It is strongly recommended that a broad panel of antibodies directed not only against mast cell–related antigens but also against monocytes (CD14) and blast cells (CD34) should be applied in all cases of ASM and MCL so that the diagnosis of SM-AHNMD with an "occult" AHNMD is not overlooked. In addition, it can be useful to search for the presence of other known mutations in myeloid neoplasms, e.g.,

JAK2-V617F, TET2, etc., which may also help in the interpretation of unclear morphologic findings. Some rare associations of SM and "AHNMD" are summarized in Table 49.9.

Mast Cell Sarcoma

MCS is an extremely rare neoplasm, with no more than five cases of primary MCS having been published so far (56–58). It usually involves tissues that are not the main targets for mastocytosis: larynx, large bowel, and meninges but cases originating in the skeleton and skin have also been described. MCS can only be recognized when special stains, including an appropriate immunohistochemical antibody panel with antitryptase, are applied (Fig. 49.6A–F). It is probable that MCS is usually misdiagnosed as high-grade round-cell soft tissue sarcoma (Fig. 49.6A and B). MCS shows highly destructive pleomorphic tissue infiltration and consists of highly atypical round neoplastic cells with few metachromatic granules that are hardly detectable even in Giemsa and toluidine blue stains (Fig. 49.6B). The tumor cells contain pleomorphic nuclei with prominent nucleoli, and abundant pale cytoplasm. MCS has been observed in a few patients with long-standing SM and accordingly termed here secondary MCS (sMCS) (Hans-Peter Horny, own unpublished

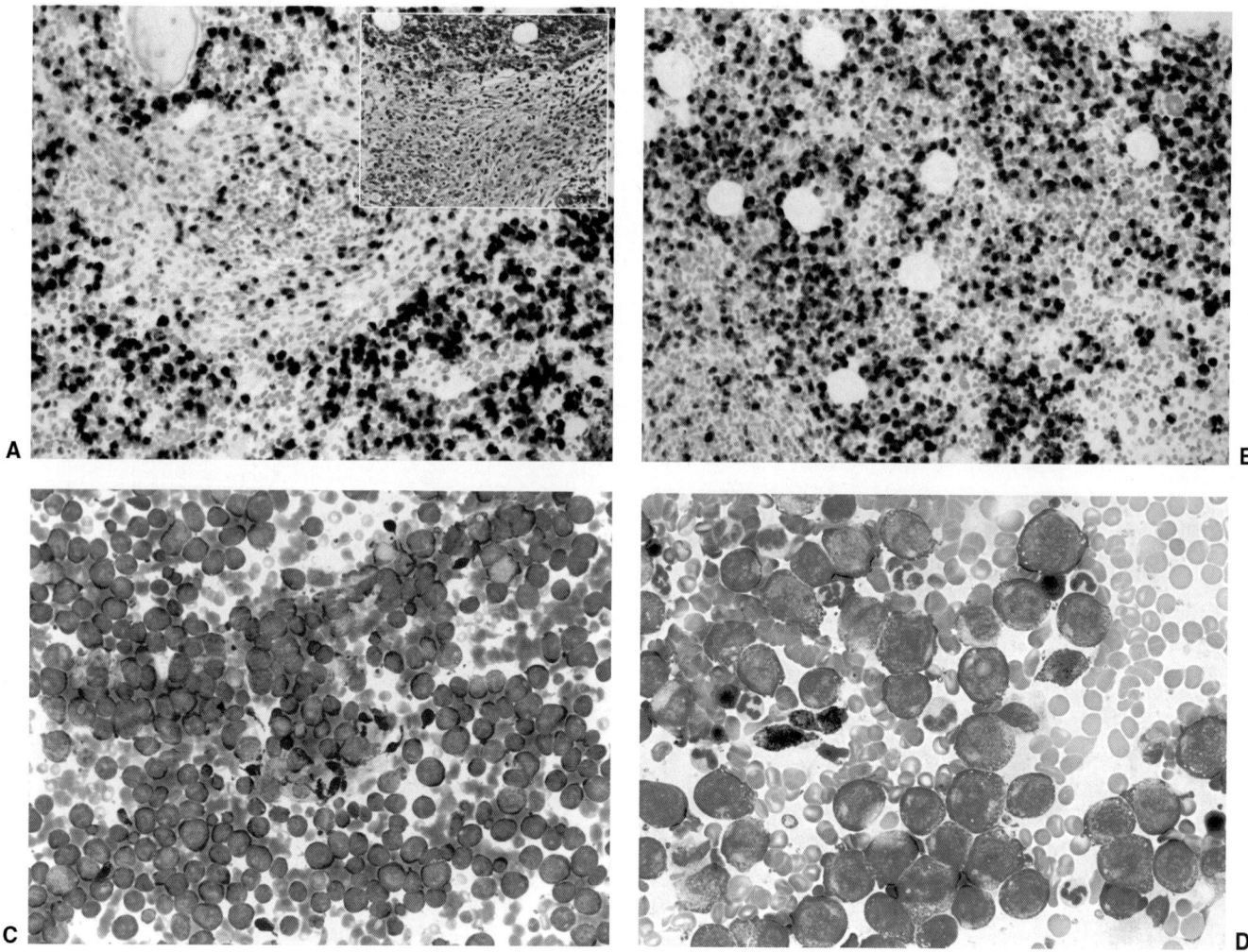

FIGURE 49.5. SM-AHNMD. Bone marrow biopsy specimen from a 68-year-old man showing focal infiltration by spindle-shaped hypogranu-lated mast cells without marked collagen fibrosis **(A)**. There is a complete absence of normal blood cell precursors and fat cells. The picture is dominated by an abundance of cells expressing the antigen 2D7, which were accordingly classified as basophilic granulocytes **(A,B)**. Note that the mast cells do not express 2D7 in this case (cf. Fig. 49.1) and that compact mast cell infiltrates are absent in **(B)**. The "basophilic" AHNMD cannot be classified on the basis of these immunohistologic findings alone. The features were found compat-ible with an accelerated phase of a MDS/MPN-u that had been diagnosed earlier. Cytomorphologic features of SM-AHNMD are shown in another case of a 49-year-old man who had a 2-year history of SM-AHNMD/MDS. While the SM showed an unremarkable, stable course, the MDS transformed to secondary acute myeloid leukemia. Bone marrow aspiration revealed sheets of medium-sized blast cells with pleomorphic nuclei and a moderately basophilic cytoplasm making up more than 90% of nucleated cells. Note the presence of loosely scattered spindle-shaped hypogranulated mast cells with a tendency to group together as the only indication of SM, which was almost completely obscured by the rapidly progressive AHNMD. **A** and **B**, anti-2D7 antigen; APAAP method (**inset** in **[A]** shows a Giemsa stain); **C** and **D**, Pappenheim/Wright-Giemsa.

Table 49.8	SM-AHNMD: FREQUENCY OF AHNMD SUBTYPES	
Type of AHNMD	**Percent**	**KIT-D816V**
CMML	45	90%
AML	20	30%
MPN	15	25%
MDS	15	20%
PCM	5	0%

CMML, chronic myelomonocytic leukemia; AML, Acute myeloid leukemia; MPN, Myeloproliferative neoplasm; MDS, myelodysplastic syndrome; PCM, plasma cell myeloma.
Source: Horny HP, Sotlar K, Sperr WR, et al. Systemic mastocytosis with associated clonal haematological non-mast cell lineage diseases: a histopathological challenge. *J Clin Pathol* 2004;57:604–608; Sotlar K, Colak S, Bache A, et al. Variable presence of KITD816V in clonal haematological non-mast cell lineage diseases associated with systemic mastocytosis (SM-AHNMD). *J Pathol* 2010;220:586–595.

Table 49.9	RARE AND UNUSUAL AHNMD DIAGNOSES IN THE SETTING OF SM-AHNMD
SM	**AHNMD**
BMM	Acute erythroleukemia (AML M6) (51)
BMM	Malignant histiocytosis (52)
BMM	Chronic myeloid leukemia (53)
BMM	Atypical chronic myeloid leukemia
WDSM	Monocytic leukemia (AML M5a)
MCL	AML with t(8;21)
ISM	Chronic lymphocytic leukemia (54)
BMM	MDS with isolated del(5q)
BMM	Myelomastocytic leukemia
BMM	Acute lymphoblastic leukemia (55)
BMM	AML with t(15;17)

BMM, bone marrow mastocytosis; WDSM, well-differentiated SM; MCL, mast cell leukemia; AML, acute myeloid leukemia; MDS, myelodysplastic syndrome.

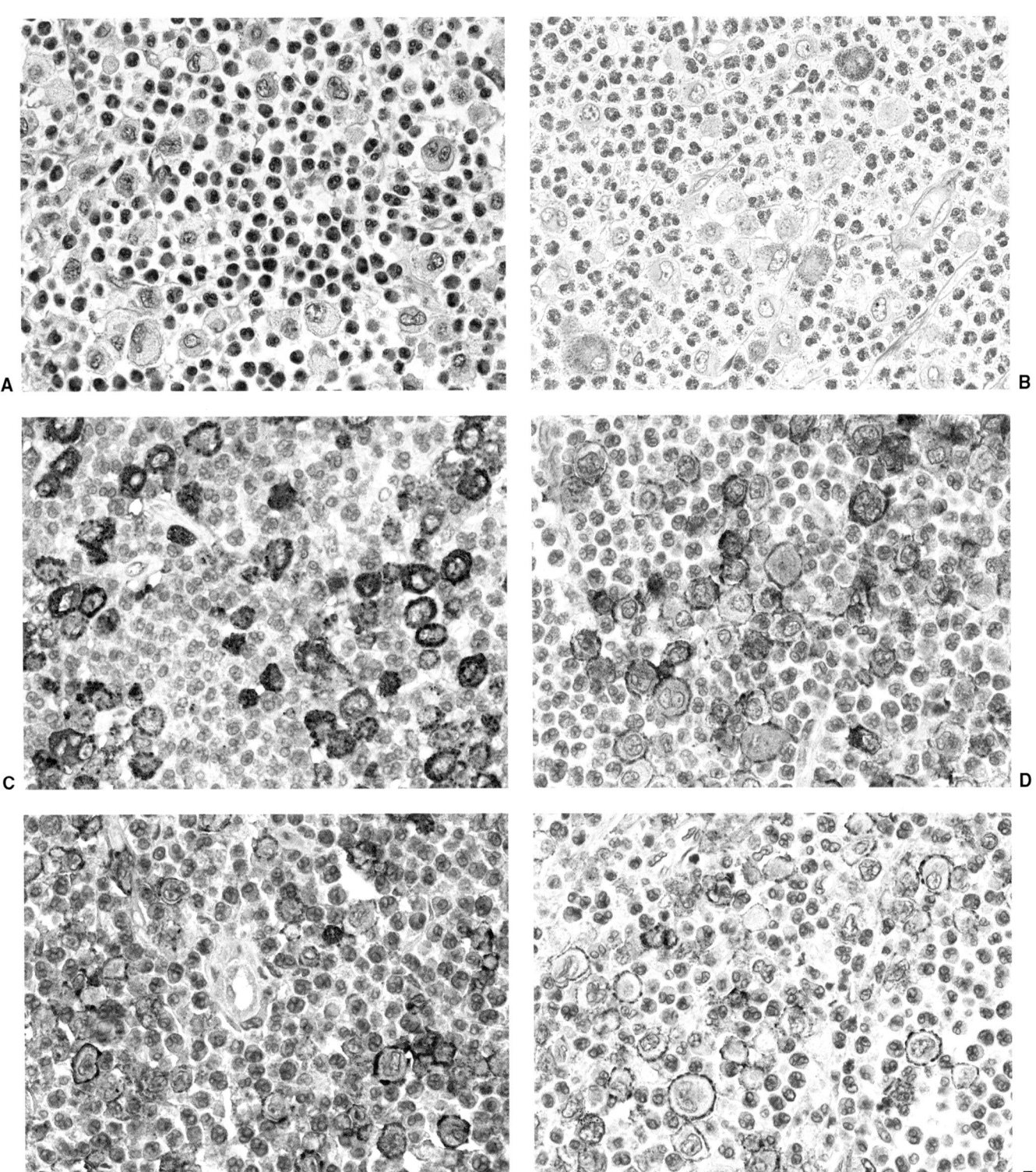

FIGURE 49.6. Mast cell sarcoma. A neoplastic proliferation of large blastlike tumor cells exhibiting pleomorphic nuclei and accompanied by an abundance of eosinophils is seen **(A)**. Giemsa staining **(B)** reveals metachromatic granules in some of the tumor cells, but a definitive diagnosis and assignment to the basophilic or mast cell lineage can only be accomplished on the basis of immunohistochemical investigations. The tumor cells are seen to coexpress the antigens tryptase **(C)**, CD117 **(D)**, CD25 **(E)**, and CD30 **(F)**, thus fulfilling criteria for neoplastic mast cells and making a diagnosis of MCS appropriate. Note that the cytologic features of the mast cells are highly unusual and are much more reminiscent of a high-grade myeloid or lymphoid neoplasm at first glance. The 49-year-old male patient had long-standing SM with bone marrow involvement. A final diagnosis of secondary MCS originating in the bone marrow was recorded. **A**, H&E; **B**, Giemsa; **C**, antitryptase; ABC method; **D**, anti-CD117/KIT; ABC method; **E**, anti-CD25; ABC method; **F**, anti-CD30; ABC method.

observation). Very recently, a case of sMCS has been reported evolving from adult mastocytoma of the skin (59). Primary MCS usually transforms into sMCL. In ASM with sMCS a diagnosis of "sarcomatous variant" of ASM seems appropriate. The course of SM in one patient over a follow-up period of about 5 years was as follows: (i) occult SM obscured by hairy cell leukemia (oSM-HCL); (ii) overt SM with hypereosinophilic syndrome (SM-HES); (iii) MCL associated with acute myeloid leukemia exhibiting overlapping features of MML (SM-AHNMD = MCL-AML/MML); (iv) secondary MCS of the scapula (60).

Extracutaneous Mastocytoma

Extracutaneous mastocytoma is an extremely rare tumor originating in the lung. Case reports date back to the era before immunohistochemical analysis with antibodies against tryptase was possible (61,62). Currently, especially due to the lack of recent published information, it remains unknown whether this variant will be retained in future classification systems.

Rare Subtypes of Mastocytosis

Well-Differentiated Systemic Mastocytosis

WDSM is a rare subtype of ISM exhibiting special features that usually enable a precise diagnosis (21). The tumor cells are exclusively round with abundant metachromatic granules, thus closely resembling mature mast cells (Fig. 49.7A–D). In contrast to the common type of ISM, which (although rarely) can also show a preponderance of round mast cells, CD25 is not expressed by the mast cells of WDSM, and the typical activating point mutation at codon 816 of *KIT* is not found in most patients. A point mutation in the transmembrane domain of

KIT (F522P) was described in the first reported case of WDSM, but this mutation could not be detected in other cases of WDSM. Therefore, it remains uncertain whether all cases of "WDSM" are indeed neoplastic.

WDSM exhibits the major diagnostic criterion of compact infiltrates but three of the four minor criteria are absent. The diagnosis, however, can be established since the patients always have an elevated serum tryptase. WDSM has also been observed in the setting of SM-AHNMD (Table 49.9).

Occult Mastocytosis

Occult SM (oSM) occurs in three variants: (i) In SM-AHNMD, in particular SM-AML, the "AHNMD" compartment may initially obscure SM, which is, however, easily detectable after cytoreductive therapy (50); (ii) in patients with morphologically proven SM who have undergone surgery years or even decades earlier, activating point mutations at codon 816 of *KIT* have been detected retrospectively in surgical specimens, for example, lymph nodes without morphologic criteria for mastocytosis at that time (63); and (iii) in the very rare patients with familial mastocytosis, the term "occult" mastocytosis could be applied before manifestations of the disease are detectable clinically and morphologically.

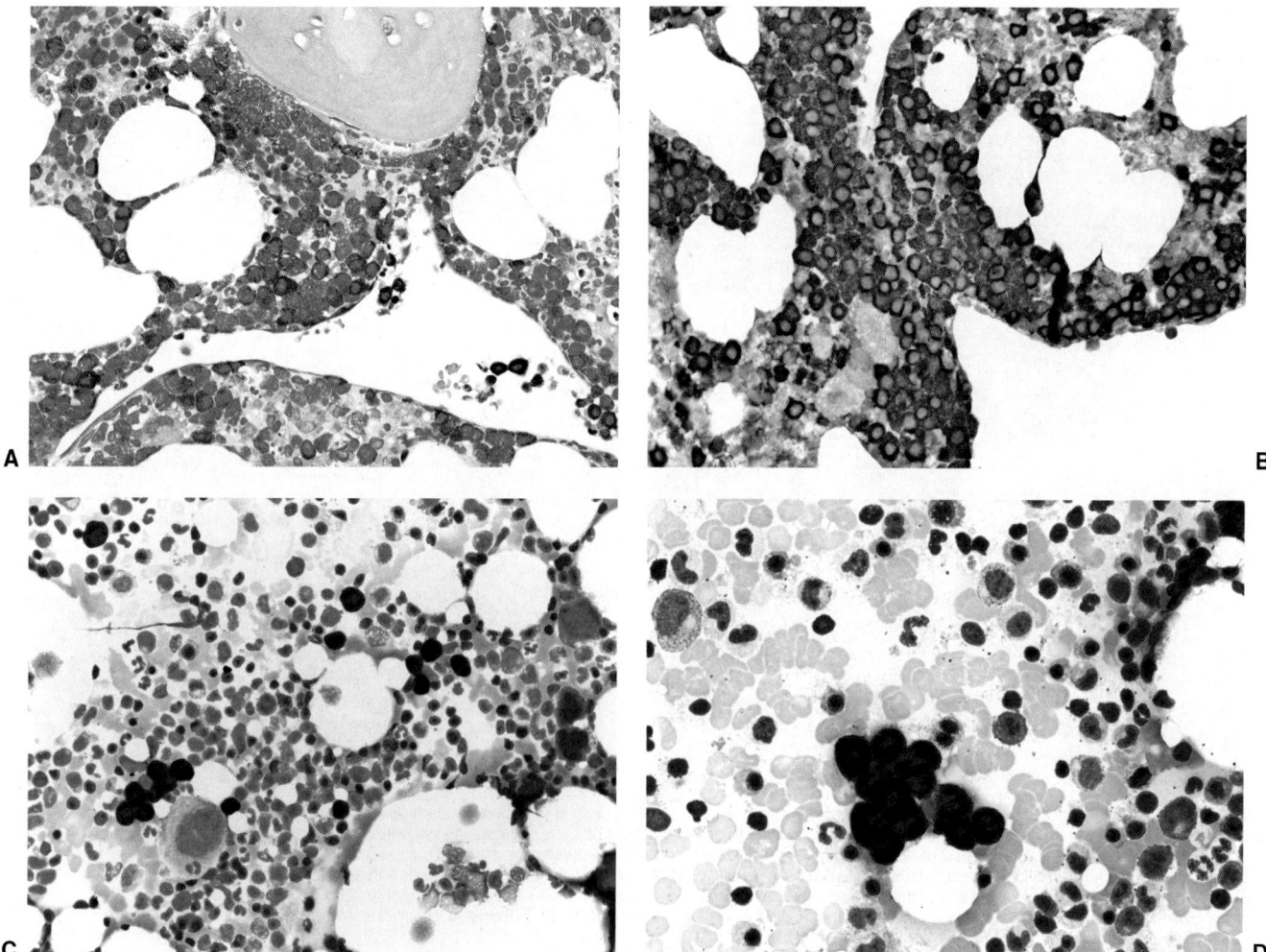

FIGURE 49.7. Well-differentiated systemic mastocytosis. Bone marrow biopsy specimen showing multifocal compact infiltration by exclusively round mast cells containing abundant metachromatic granules **(A)**. Immunostaining for tryptase further underlines the mast cell nature of these cells and their round shape **(B)**. In cases of WDSM like this one, both the activating point mutation *KIT*-D816V and the aberrant expression of CD25 by mast cells are absent. The cytomorphologic findings in bone marrow smears clearly reflect the histologic findings and also show strongly metachromatic mast cells that are always round and either loosely distributed or forming small cohesive groups **(C,D)**. **A**, Giemsa; **B**, antitryptase; ABC method; **C** and **D**, Pappenheim/Wright-Giemsa.

CYTOGENETICS/MOLECULAR BIOLOGY

Mutations in the *KIT* tyrosine kinase receptor are the molecular hallmark of SM, especially in adult patients (3,64). Mast cell activation through KIT by its ligand SCF is essential for various important cell functions such as proliferation, differentiation, maturation, suppression of apoptosis, chemotaxis, adhesion, and secretion of mediators (65). Consequently, activating mutations in various regions of the *KIT* gene could play a key role in initiation and/or maintenance of mast cell neoplasms by SCF-independent activation of KIT downstream signaling pathways. *KIT*-D816V, the most frequent mutation, was originally described in HMC-1 cells derived from a patient with MCL (3). Mutations detected in mastocytosis usually cluster within exons 11 and 17 of the *KIT* gene (21,66–73). Only very rarely have mutations at exons 8 to 10 of *KIT* been described in adult human mastocytosis. The exact frequency of mutations within these exons, however, is unknown since no systematic investigations have been performed so far. It is of major importance to be aware that *KIT* mutations at any of the sites described above are not specific for mastocytosis and can be found in other hematologic neoplasms like AML and NK/T-cell lymphoma, and also in certain solid tumors, for example, gastrointestinal stromal tumor (GIST), (bilateral) seminoma, and rare forms of malignant melanoma (74–78).

Except for some very rare cases of familial mastocytosis with germ line mutations, the vast majority of patients with ISM carry somatic *KIT* mutations confined to mast cells and their precursors. In contrast, demonstration of *KIT* mutations in other hematopoietic lineages has been shown to be associated with the more unfavorable or high-grade disease variants like SSM (a rare subtype of ISM), SM-AHNMD, and ASM (79). When detected in ISM, multilineage involvement by *KIT* codon 816 mutations seems to be associated with an increased risk of progression to more aggressive disease variants (79). In <5% of cases, mutations other than D816V are detected, including D816Y, D816H, and D816F, all of which have been shown also to act as "gain-of-function" *KIT* mutations (71). Interestingly, the non-D816V mutations involving codon 816 of *KIT* are significantly more frequent in pediatric CM (14,71). *KIT*-D816F has so far been detected only in pediatric patients. It is not known whether these alternative codon 816 mutations are related to differences in the expression of certain immunohistochemical markers in neoplastic mast cells. Interestingly, *KIT*-D816V may play a major role in inducing the formation of compact mast cell infiltrates, the only major diagnostic criterion for SM (80).

On the basis of the detection of *KIT*-D816V as a recurrent molecular defect in more than 90% of SM cases, all subtypes of SM are regarded as true neoplasms. Consequently, the detection of such mutations has been defined as one of the minor diagnostic criteria for SM in the WHO classification of mastocytosis (4,5). In contrast, *KIT* codon 816 mutations have been described in only about 40% of patients with pediatric CM. In an additional approximately 40% of cases, *KIT* mutations were found in exons 8 to 10 (81). In cases of ISM with neoplastic mast cells loosely distributed in the bone marrow and accounting for <1% of the nucleated bone marrow cells it should be taken into account that demonstration of clonality may be difficult and false-negative results may be obtained initially. Therefore, highly sensitive molecular techniques are sometimes needed to detect *KIT* codon 816 mutations in these small populations of clonally expanded cells (14). The diagnostic sensitivity may be increased dramatically if mast cells are enriched by cell sorting or microdissection, depending on the material available (40,70). The bone marrow is usually the tissue with the highest sensitivity for KIT mutational analysis. Because circulating MC are virtually absent in the most frequent subtypes of SM, in particular ISM, KIT mutations are detected in the peripheral blood only in those patients with high-grade SM or SM-AHNMD and involvement of non–mast cell

hematopoietic lineages by *KIT* codon 816 mutations. Myeloproliferative neoplasms with eosinophilia (MPNEo) and FIP1L1-PDGFRα or -β aberrations generally lack such codon 816 mutations (Hans-Peter Horny, Peter Valent, Karl Sotlar, own unpublished observation). So far, no specific cytogenetic abnormalities have been reported for SM (82). Accordingly, if such abnormalities are detected in cases of SM-AHNMD, they are considered to be associated with the AHNMD component of the disease.

POSTULATED NORMAL COUNTERPART

Tissue mast cell.

CLINICAL COURSE AND PROGNOSIS

The clinical course and prognosis in patients with mastocytosis vary depending on the category of disease and the degree of organ involvement. In CM and ISM the prognosis is excellent and life expectancy is nearly the same as that of healthy controls (4,5). In ISM, a minority of patients progress to ASM, MCL, or SM-AHNMD. A larger proportion of cases of ASM will progress to MCL or AML over time (83). The prognosis of patients with SM-AHNMD varies. In those with SM-CMML and ASM-CMML, progression to AML is often seen. In other types of SM-AHNMD, the prognosis is more favorable. In general, the prognosis of SM-AHNMD is dictated by the course and progression of the AHNMD component. It is important to evaluate all the prognostically relevant clinical parameters and serologic, cytogenetic, and molecular markers in these patients in the same way as if SM were not present (1,4). In cases of SM-CMML, SM-MPN, SM-CEL (chronic eosinophilic leukemia), and SM-AML, molecular and cytogenetic markers are of great importance.

The life expectancy of patients with ASM and MCL, however, is poor. In untreated MCL, median survival is <1 year (4,5). The life expectancy of patients with SSM is variable (84). Most patients have a good prognosis, but in some of them progression to ASM or SM-AHNMD is seen.

The key diagnostic features of ASM and MCL are the C-findings, which represent the most important prognostic variables that can be determined in the initial assessment and follow-up (Table 49.10) (4,5). These parameters include liver involvement with ascites and increased or progressively increasing liver enzymes (typically including alkaline phosphatase), large osteolytic lesions with pathologic fractures, malabsorption with weight loss and hypoalbuminemia, and cytopenias caused by diffuse-compact bone marrow infiltration by SM. In each case, it is important to document the causative role of the mast cell infiltrate as inducer of the C-finding by biopsy and pathologic assessment. The B-findings, which are diagnostic of SSM, are not of major prognostic significance, unless B-finding-related parameters show progression in the follow-up. Likewise, mild palpable splenomegaly without signs of progression is not of prognostic significance. However, an increasing spleen size must raise the suspicion of disease progression, especially when accompanied by ascites or signs of hypersplenism leading to the presence of C-findings. Similarly, an increase in eosinophils and/or increasing signs of myelodysplasia or myeloproliferation are always strong indicators of disease progression.

Other important prognostic parameters include the number of mast cells in bone marrow smears and the grade of their cytologic atypia, the detection of circulating mast cells, marked blood eosinophilia, an increase in liver enzymes, a marked and progressive increase in serum tryptase levels in repeated tests, and the disappearance of skin lesions. A complete absence of skin lesions at diagnosis is frequently noted in patients with advanced SM, which includes SM-AHNMD, ASM, MCL and most cases of SM-AHNMD (4,5). However, due

Table 49.10	B- AND C-FINDINGS IN MASTOCYTOSIS

B-Findings: Indicate high MC burden, and spread of the genetic defect into various myeloid lineages

(1) Infiltration grade (MCs) in bone marrow >30% and serum tryptase levels >200 ng/mL

(2) Hypercellular marrow with loss of fat cells, discrete signs of dysmyelopoiesis without substantial cytopenias or WHO criteria for an MDS or MPD

(3) Organomegaly: palpable hepatomegaly, splenomegaly, or lymphadenopathy (on CT or US: >2 cm) without impaired organ function

C-Findings: Indicate impaired organ function due to MC infiltration (confirmation by biopsy required in most cases)

(1) Cytopenia(s): ANC <1,000/mL or Hb 10 g/dL or Plt <100,000/mL

(2) Hepatomegaly with ascites and impaired liver function

(3) Palpable splenomegaly with hypersplenism

(4) Malabsorption with hypoalbuminemia and weight loss

(5) Skeletal lesions: large osteolytic lesions and/or severe osteoporosis causing pathologic fractures

(6) Life-threatening organopathy in other organ systems due to infiltration by neoplastic MCs

Source: Valent PH, Horny H-P, Li CY, et al. Mastocytosis (mast cell disease). In: Harris N. Jaffe ES, Stein H, Vardiman JW, eds. *WHO classification of tumours. Tumours of haematopoietic and lymphoid tissues.* Lyon: IARC Press, 2001:291–302; Horny H-P, Metcalfe DD, Bennett JM, et al. Mastocytosis (mast cell disease). In: Campo E, Swerdlow SH, Harris NL, et al., eds. *WHO classification of tumours of haematopoietic and lymphoid tissues.* Geneva: IARC Press, 2008:54–63.

to improvements in the diagnostic approach, more and more patients with SM are being diagnosed in whom skin lesions are absent and who have only a very low mast cell burden. Most of these patients have BMM and a normal serum tryptase level, whereas patients with ASM and MCL (in which skin lesions are also usually absent) have high tryptase levels (usually over 200 ng/mL), and a further increase in tryptase levels is often seen.

CD30 has recently been identified as a novel potential marker of ASM and MCL. It is important to state that the prognostic value of this antigen still remains uncertain, and that the marker should be used only for immunohistochemical analysis and not for flow cytometric assessment. Strong expression of CD30 by most or all mast cells is usually associated with advanced mastocytosis (ASM or MCL), whereas in most (but not all) patients with ISM only a few mast cells stain positive for CD30 (34,35). Some of the novel flow cytometry parameters pertaining to mast cells may also be indicative of the prognosis in SM. These include, amongst others, CD123 (the alpha-chain of the IL-3 receptor) and CD52 (the CAMPATH-1 antigen). Both markers are more frequently detected on neoplastic mast cells in ASM and MCL than in ISM. Another interesting marker is CD2, the LFA-2 antigen, which serves as a ligand for LFA-3 (CD58). Whereas in most cases of ISM neoplastic mast cells clearly stain for CD2 by flow cytometry, the expression of CD2 on neoplastic mast cells is usually low in ASM or even undetectable in MCL (85,86). This is interesting because CD2-CD58 homotypic adhesion is a functionally important concept in ISM and may underlie the typical aggregate formation by mast cells in these patients. If this hypothesis is correct, the loss or lack of CD2 in MCL may explain the more diffuse and often devastating infiltration of visceral organs by mast cells in these patients. Indeed, CD2-negative mast cells exhibit more diffuse infiltration patterns in SCID mice as compared to CD2-positive mast cells (Peter Valent own unpublished observation).

TREATMENT AND SURVIVAL

The treatment of mastocytosis depends on the clinical findings, organs involved, type of involvement, variant of CM or SM, and the individual situation in each case (4,5,87). In general, the treatment plan should be adapted to the diagnostic subtype of mastocytosis established according to WHO criteria and consensus group criteria, after a complete staging of all relevant organ systems, including the GI tract, skeletal system (including a T score), liver, spleen, and bone marrow, has been performed.

Symptomatic patients with ISM and SSM should be treated with drugs directed against mediator production or mediator effects (88). These patients must not be treated with cytoreductive agents, tyrosine kinase inhibitors (TKIs), immunomodulating agents, or other experimental drugs. In some patients with ISM or SSM, glucocorticoids are required to control symptoms. In those with allergies to bee or wasp venom, long-term immunotherapy is recommended to minimize the risk of life-threatening anaphylaxis. There are a few patients with progressive SSM in whom severe anaphylaxis and general symptoms may improve after treatment with cladribine (2CdA). However, 2CdA is otherwise not recommended for patients with anaphylaxis. In ISM patients in whom progressive osteopenia and a T score of equal/less than 2 or osteoporosis is detectable, therapy with bisphosphonates is usually recommended, and the same holds true for patients with very large osteolytic lesions. In those with severe resistant osteoporosis, treatment with interferon-alpha may lead to an increase in bone density.

Patients with ASM and MCL may be treated with cytoreductive agents, targeted drugs, experimental agents, or polychemotherapy (88). For ASM patients with slow progression, interferon-alpha plus glucocorticoids or 2CdA are usually recommended. However, a good treatment response is only seen in about 20% of cases, and most of the patients who respond will relapse at some stage. In those with rapid progression or interferon-resistant ASM, treatment with 2CdA or polychemotherapy is an option. Chemotherapy for rapidly progressive ASM and MCL is similar to or the same as that used to treat high-risk AML. Treatment with high-dose ARA-C and the nucleoside fludarabine is often recommended. If there is a good response or even remission, repeated cycles of chemotherapy are administered. In young, non-comorbid patients, hematopoietic stem cell transplantation (HSCT) has to be considered, although no results from larger clinical trials are available. For those patients who are not eligible for HSCT, who subsequently relapse, or in whom HSCT fails, experimental drugs or palliative cytoreduction with hydroxyurea or other oral cytoreductive agents are usually recommended.

There are a number of experimental drugs that have been developed recently and used in clinical trials to treat patients with advanced SM, that is, SM-AHNMD, ASM, and MCL (89,90). Several of these agents, like PKC412 (midostaurin), are potent inhibitors of the KIT D816V mutant. This mutant, which is expressed in almost all patients with SM (including ASM and MCL), is resistant to commonly used TKIs, including imatinib and masitinib. Therefore, treatment of SM with imatinib or masitinib is not generally recommended, unless the disease is negative for *KIT*-D816V and other *KIT* codon 816 mutations, or harbors another sensitive target. The results of the first clinical studies to use midostaurin in ASM and MCL are encouraging. However, long-term data are not available yet, and relapses have been reported. Other novel (experimental) drugs, including pan-Bcl-2-inhibitors, demethylating agents, antibodies directed against certain surface targets, and several of the novel multikinase blockers, have shown encouraging results.

In patients with SM-AHNMD, the treatment plan has to take into account both the SM component and the AHNMD component of the disease (4,5,88). In general, the SM should be treated as if no AHNMD were present (in ISM, patients receive only symptomatic treatment for the SM) and, vice versa, the AHNMD component should be treated as if no SM was present. AHNMD may be an indolent neoplasm not requiring upfront therapy. In other cases, a specific cytogenetic anomaly such as a PDGFR mutant is detected. In these patients, treatment with imatinib is often recommended. The rationale behind this is that, patients with the rare variant of PDGFR-alpha-mutated AHNMD lack *KIT*-D816V. In patients with SM-AML, the AML should be classified and treated as a secondary AML, that is, high-risk AML. Of those who receive chemotherapy and HSCT, several enjoy long-term AML-free survival even if SM is still detectable in the bone marrow (Peter Valent own unpublished observation).

DIFFERENTIAL DIAGNOSIS

The differential diagnosis of mastocytosis includes conditions involving reactive mast cell hyperplasia, mast cell activation syndromes, and several hematologic neoplasms with close morphologic or immunophenotypic similarities to mastocytosis (Table 49.11). With regard to mast cell hyperplasia, diagnostic problems may arise only when there is a very marked increase in mast cells. Even in hyperplastic states with an abundance of mast cells, the diagnosis is usually clear because these are round and loosely scattered throughout the tissue without any tendency to form dense aggregates. The mast cells in such cases exhibit a mature immunophenotype with coexpression of tryptase and CD117, while CD25 and other aberrant antigens are not detected. In addition, such cases always show wild-type *KIT*, the activating point mutation *KIT*-D816V being absent.

It may be more difficult to distinguish mast cell activation syndromes from "true" mastocytosis because atypical CD25 and/or *KIT*-D816V-positive mast cells do occur in the clonal variant, but compact mast cell infiltrates are always absent (9,91). Most important for the pathologist are the diseases with morphologic and/or immunophenotypic similarities to mastocytosis. Due to their relatively large size and broad pale cytoplasm in H&E-stained sections, mast cells can easily be confused with hairy cells in hairy cell leukemia (HCL) or monocytic/histiocytic proliferations (28). The presence of metachromatic granules in basophils may lead to striking similarities between mastocytosis and the even rarer basophilic leukemias (92). The aberrant expression of monocyte/histiocyte-related antigens, such as CD14 and/or CD68 by neoplastic mast cells, combined with the morphologic similarities described above may result in a false-positive diagnosis of monocytic leukemia or histiocytosis (28,93,94). Moreover, the expression of CD30 in mastocytosis may lead to a misdiagnosis of Hodgkin lymphoma, anaplastic large cell lymphoma, or even embryonal carcinoma, especially in those patients with a short clinical history and limited hematologic/molecular data (34,35).

Finally, mixed infiltrates containing follicle-like structures made up of lymphoid cells in cases of ISM may be confused with infiltrates of malignant lymphoma, in particular small B-cell lymphoma, which, on the other hand, also usually contains large numbers of reactive mast cells (e.g., lymphoplasmacytic lymphoma) (95–97). Overlapping features of

Table 49.12	FEATURES OF ASM, MCL, AND MML		
	ASM	**MCL**	**MML**
BM infiltration pattern	Multifocal	Diffuse	Diffuse
BM fibrosis	+	0	0
Spindling of tumor cells	+	0	0
CD2⁺/CD25⁺ mast cells	+	+	0
KIT-D816V	+	+/0	0
Circulating mast cells	0	0/+	0/+
AHNMD	+	+/0	+

BM, Bone marrow; AHNMD, associated clonal hematopoietic non–mast cell lineage disease.

mastocytosis and another hematologic disorder are seen in the extremely rare MML (46). The neoplastic cells in myelomastocytic neoplasms or "myelomastocytic overlap syndromes," which usually present as MML, show signs of differentiation toward the mast cell lineage but the criteria for mastocytosis are not fulfilled (Table 49.12). MML belongs to the group of advanced and highly aggressive myeloid neoplasms and no more than seven cases have been reported (98). With regard to the designation "overlap syndrome" it has to be stated that MML is usually seen in the setting of an advanced myeloid tumor like MDS of type RAEB-2 or overt AML, but a single case has been reported to have arisen during a blast crisis of CML (53). A few cases of "pure" MML have also been reported (85). A diagnosis of MML can only be established when so-called metachromatic blast cells are detected in blood or bone marrow smears. Metachromatic blast cells by definition cannot be assigned to the basophilic or mast cell lineage on the basis of cytomorphologic findings alone and usually contain only scanty metachromatic granules. Immunohistologic investigation may show the tumor cells in the bone marrow to express tryptase and/or chymase but CD2 and CD25 are not detected. Moreover, activating point mutations at codon 816 of *KIT* are absent. When metachromatic blast cells are not found but sheets of tryptase-expressing blast cells dominate the picture, a diagnosis of tryptase-positive AML has to be considered. The only hematologic neoplasms outside the setting of mastocytosis that contain mast cells with an atypical immunophenotype and expression of CD25 are MPNEo associated with rearrangement of *PDGFR* alpha or beta. MPNeo contain varying amounts of atypical mast cells and their number is sometimes high enough for the diagnostic consideration of SM or SM-AHNMD to be considered (91,99,100). However, MPN-eo almost never show compact mast cell infiltrates and the coexistence of a *PDGFR* or *FGFR1* anomaly and activating *KIT* mutations at codon 816 has never been convincingly reported (Fig. 49.8A–D). In a few exceptional cases, a diagnosis of *KIT*-D816V-negative SM associated with MPN-eo (SM-AHNMD) could be made on the basis of the histologic demonstration of true compact infiltrates (Table 49.13). Rarely, localized collagen fibrosis in the bone marrow containing a moderate number of spindle-shaped mast cells almost perfectly mimics SM. However, when neither CD25 expression nor activating point mutations at codon 816 of *KIT* are detected, such cases have been preliminarily termed "fibromastocytic lesion" (101). Their clinical significance is currently unknown.

To summarize, ISM should be clearly distinguished from mast cell hyperplasia, MCAS, CM, BMM, WDSM, and SSM. The main differential diagnosis of ASM includes SSM, ASM-AHNMD, and (aleukemic) MCL. MCL has to be differentiated from ASM, MCL-AHNMD, MML, monocytic leukemias, basophilic leukemias, and tryptase+ AML. MCSs have to be distinguished from myelosarcoma, undifferentiated (round-cell) soft tissue

Table 49.11	DIFFERENTIAL DIAGNOSIS OF SM		
Diagnosis	**CI**	**CD25**	***KIT* D816V**
MCH	–	–	–
MCAS	–	–/+	–/+
SM	±	±	±
MML	–	–	–

CI, Compact mast cell infiltrates; CD25, aberrant immunophenotype of mast cells with CD25; MCH, Mast cell hyperplasia; MCAS, (clonal) mast cell activation syndrome; MML, myelomastocytic leukemia; SM, systemic mastocytosis.

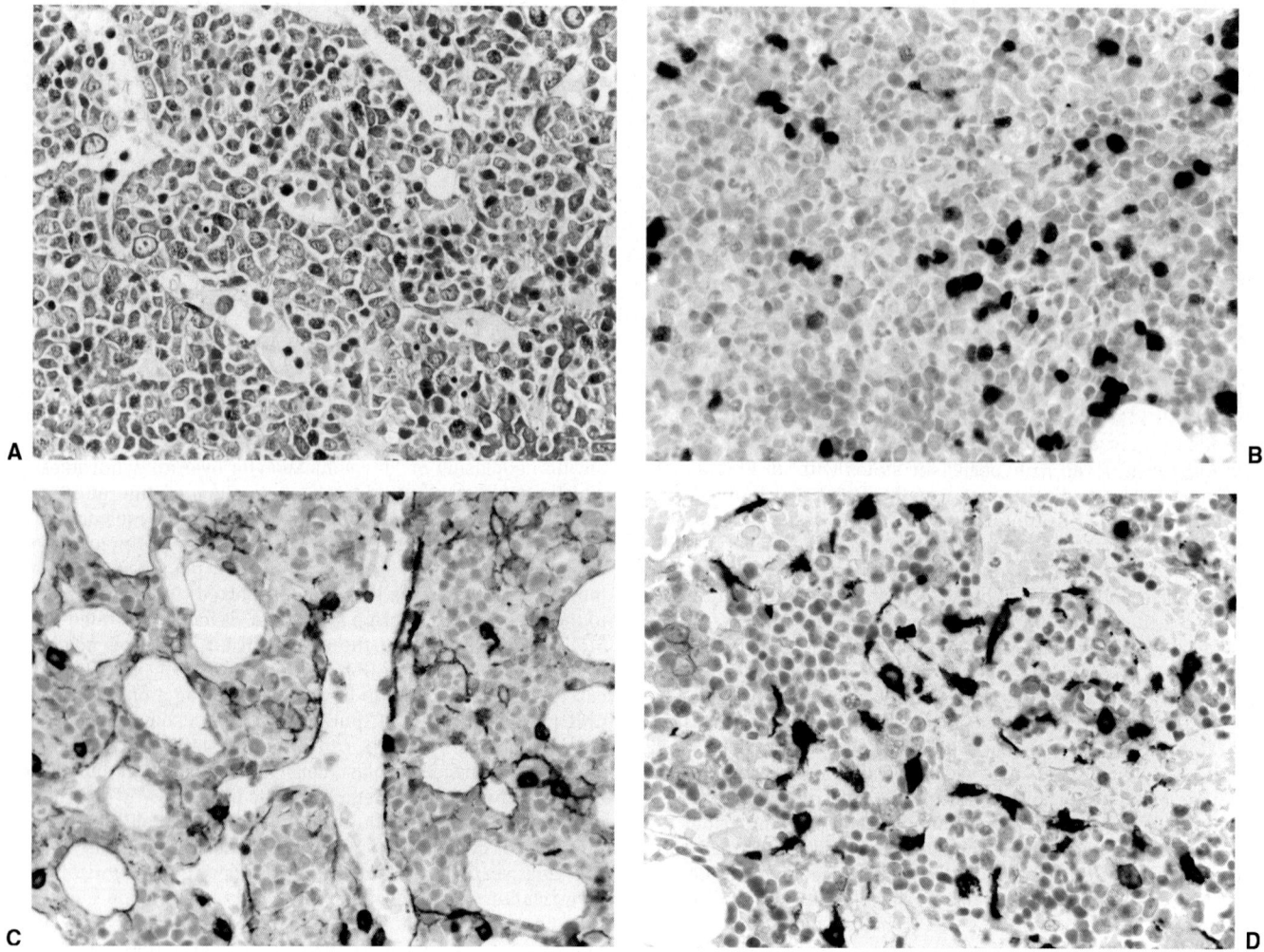

FIGURE 49.8. MPN with eosinophilia (MPN-eo). Bone marrow biopsy specimen exhibiting extreme hypercellularity with increased numbers of eosinophils and sheets of blastlike cells **(A)**. Immunohistochemistry reveals the lymphatic nature of the blast cells, which express TdT **(B)** and CD10 **(C)**. In addition, there is a large number of loosely scattered spindle-shaped mast cells expressing tryptase **(D)**. Note that neither groups nor compact infiltrates of mast cells can be detected. However, the mast cells show an aberrant immunophenotype and express CD25 (not depicted) but do not carry the activating point mutation *KIT*-D816V. These are the typical findings in MPN-eo, irrespective of the cytogenetic abnormality. Systemic mastocytosis, in particular SM-AHNMD, is not present. In the case illustrated, an abnormality of FGFR1 was detected. **A**, Giemsa; **B**, anti-TdT: ABC method; **C**, anti-CD10: ABC method; **D**, antitryptase; ABC method.

sarcoma, and GIST. Immunophenotypical peculiarities of mast cells in SM may lead to an erroneous diagnosis of other hematologic neoplasms. CD2: T-cell lymphoma; CD14: monocytic leukemias, histiocytoses; CD25: hairy cell leukemia; CD30: Hodgkin lymphoma, anaplastic large cell lymphoma, embryonal carcinoma; CD68: monocytic leukemias, histiocytoses; CD99: acute lymphoblastic leukemia/lymphoma, Ewing sarcoma; CD123: basophilic leukemias, tumors of dendritic cell precursors.

Table 49.13	SYSTEMIC MASTOCYTOSIS AND EOSINOPHILIA				
Diagnosis	CI	CD25	*KIT*-D816V	nEO	PDGFRα/β
SM-eo	+	+	+	−	−
SM-CEL	+	+	+	+	−
MPN-eo	−	+	−	+	+

CI, Compact mast cell infiltrates; CD25, aberrant immunophenotype of mast cells; KIT-D816V, activating point mutation of c-kit at codon 816; nEO, neoplastic eosinophils; PDGFRα/β, cytogenetic anomaly of platelet-derived growth factor alpha or beta; SM-eo, SM with marked reactive eosinophilia.

SUMMARY AND CONCLUSIONS

Mastocytosis is an unusual hematologic disease with a very broad spectrum of clinical features and morphologic subtypes. Serologically, an elevated serum tryptase is the most important initial finding in patients with systemic disease but is usually absent in pure CM. The key molecular findings in SM are activating point mutations at codon 816 of *KIT*, usually *KIT*-D816V. Most patients present with skin lesions. While adult patients with skin involvement almost always have systemic disease with the presence of clonal mast cells in the bone marrow, children with skin lesions usually have true CM. The diagnosis of mastocytosis may be difficult to establish, especially in those patients without cutaneous involvement who present with features of a more common hematologic neoplasm, for example, myeloid or lymphatic tumors (86–89). The hematopathologist plays a key role in the diagnosis in such cases. In fact, SM is most frequently diagnosed on the basis of histologic evaluation of the bone marrow. Four major subtypes of SM are defined according to the WHO classification:

1. ISM (usually associated with skin involvement)
2. ASM (without skin involvement in most cases)

3. MCL (predominantly presenting in its aleukemic variant and without skin lesions in almost all cases)

4. SM-AHNMD (a unique neoplasm consisting of two morphologically completely different hematologic tumors, one of them being SM)

While ISM carries a good prognosis with almost no reduction in life expectancy, all other variants of SM have an unfavorable prognosis, which, in SM-AHNMD, is often related to the AHNMD subtype. Therapeutic options are limited, but some of the recently developed tyrosine-kinase inhibitors have the potential to suppress mediator-dependent symptoms in mastocytosis patients. In association with a cytoreductive agent like cladribine, such tyrosine-kinase inhibitors have been used successfully in patients with the aggressive and leukemic variants of SM. However, up to now no clinical trials are available to substantiate these observations.

The updated WHO classification of hematopoietic tumors defines "mastocytosis" as a MPN placing it between "essential thrombocythemia" and "myeloproliferative neoplasms, unclassifiable" (5). There are some findings that clearly argue against mastocytosis being an MPN and indicate that all subtypes of mastocytosis should appear as a separate group amongst myeloid tumors, as suggested by the WHO in 2001 (4):

1. Most cases of SM show only a minor degree of focal infiltration of the bone marrow with clonally mutated cells amounting to far less than 1% of all nucleated cells, while the tissue architecture is highly preserved and cellular atypia of blood cell precursors is absent in most cases.

2. The proliferation rate in all subtypes of mastocytosis is extremely low, and proliferation is virtually absent in the low-grade variants, which are by far the most frequent and of which ISM is the most common.

3. All MPNs show cytologic atypia of at least one hematopoietic cell line, with megakaryocytes almost always being involved.

4. Transformation or progression is a common feature of many MPNs and is invariably observed in chronic myeloid leukemia, while progression of indolent to aggressive or leukemic SM is rarely encountered.

References

1. Valent P, Horny HP, Escribano L, et al. Diagnostic criteria and classification of mastocytosis: a consensus proposal. *Leuk Res* 2001;25:603–625.
2. Soter NA. The skin in mastocytosis. *J Invest Dermatol* 1991;96:32S–38S; discussion 38S–39S, 60S–65S.
3. Furitsu T, Tsujimura T, Tono T, et al. Identification of mutations in the coding sequence of the proto-oncogene c-kit in a human mast cell leukemia cell line causing ligand-independent activation of c-kit product. *J Clin Invest* 1993;92:1736–1744.
4. Valent PH, Horny H-P, Li CY, et al. Mastocytosis (mast cell disease). In: Harris N, Jaffe ES, Stein H, et al., eds. *WHO classification of tumours. Tumours of haematopoietic and lymphoid tissues,* Lyon: IARC Press, 2001:291–302.
5. Horny H-P, Metcalfe DD, Bennett JM, et al. Mastocytosis (mast cell disease). In: Campo E, Swerdlow SH, Harris NL, et al., eds. *WHO classification of tumours of haematopoietic and lymphoid tissues.* Geneva: IARC Press, 2008:54–63.
6. Kirshenbaum AS, Kessler SW, Goff JP, et al. Demonstration of the origin of human mast cells from CD34⁺ bone marrow progenitor cells. *J Immunol* 1991;146:1410–1415.
7. Metcalfe DD. Classification and diagnosis of mastocytosis: current status. *J Invest Dermatol* 1991;96:2S–4S; discussion 4S, 60S–65S.
8. Valent P, Akin C, Arock M, et al. Definitions, criteria and global classification of mast cell disorders with special reference to mast cell activation syndromes: a consensus proposal. *Int Arch Allergy Immunol* 2012;157:215–225.
9. Horny H-P, Sotlar K, Valent P. Evaluation of mast cell activation syndromes: impact of pathology and immunohistology. *Int Arch Allergy Immunol* 2012;159:1–5.
10. Florian S, Krauth MT, Simonitsch-Klupp I, et al. Indolent systemic mastocytosis with elevated serum tryptase, absence of skin lesions, and recurrent severe anaphylactoid episodes. *Int Arch Allergy Immunol* 2005;136:273–280.
11. Schwartz LB, Sakai K, Bradford TR, et al. The alpha form of human tryptase is the predominant type present in blood at baseline in normal subjects and is elevated in those with systemic mastocytosis. *J Clin Invest* 1995;96:2702–2710.
12. Horny HP, Valent P. Diagnosis of mastocytosis: general histopathological aspects, morphological criteria, and immunohistochemical findings. *Leuk Res* 2001;25:543–551.
13. Sotlar K, Marafioti T, Griesser H, et al. Detection of c-kit mutation Asp 816 to Val in microdissected bone marrow infiltrates in a case of systemic mastocytosis associated with chronic myelomonocytic leukaemia. *Mol Pathol* 2000;53:188–193.
14. Sotlar K, Escribano L, Landt O, et al. One-step detection of c-kit point mutations using peptide nucleic acid-mediated polymerase chain reaction clamping and hybridization probes. *Am J Pathol* 2003;162:737–746.
15. Horny HP, Lange K, Sotlar K, et al. Increase of bone marrow lymphocytes in systemic mastocytosis: reactive lymphocytosis or malignant lymphoma? Immunohistochemical and molecular findings on routinely processed bone marrow biopsy specimens. *J Clin Pathol* 2003;56:575–578.
16. Horny HP, Sotlar K, Sperr WR, et al. Systemic mastocytosis with associated clonal haematological non-mast cell lineage diseases: a histopathological challenge. *J Clin Pathol* 2004;57:604–608.
17. Sperr WR, Escribano L, Jordan JH, et al. Morphologic properties of neoplastic mast cells: delineation of stages of maturation and implication for cytological grading of mastocytosis. *Leuk Res* 2001;25:529–536.
18. Krokowski M, Sotlar K, Krauth MT, et al. Delineation of patterns of bone marrow mast cell infiltration in systemic mastocytosis: value of CD25, correlation with subvariants of the disease, and separation from mast cell hyperplasia. *Am J Clin Pathol* 2005;124:560–568.
19. Rywlin AM, Hoffman EP, Ortega RS. Eosinophilic fibrohistiocytic lesion of bone marrow: a distinctive new morphologic finding, probably related to drug hypersensitivity. *Blood* 1972;40:464–472.
20. te Velde J, Vismans FJ, Leenheers-Binnendijk L, et al. The eosinophilic fibrohistiocytic lesion of the bone marrow. A mastocellular lesion in bone disease. *Virchows Arch A Pathol Anat Histol* 1978;377:277–285.
21. Akin C, Fumo G, Yavuz AS, et al. A novel form of mastocytosis associated with a transmembrane c-kit mutation and response to imatinib. *Blood* 2004;103:3222–3225.
22. Horny HP, Kaiserling E. Lymphoid cells and tissue mast cells of bone marrow lesions in systemic mastocytosis: a histological and immunohistological study. *Br J Haematol* 1988;69:449–455.
23. Horny HP, Parwaresch MR, Lennert K. Bone marrow findings in systemic mastocytosis. *Hum Pathol* 1985;16:808–814.
24. Horny HP, Sillaber C, Menke D, et al. Diagnostic value of immunostaining for tryptase in patients with mastocytosis. *Am J Surg Pathol* 1998;22:1132–1140.
25. Li WV, Kapadia SB, Sonmez-Alpan E, et al. Immunohistochemical characterization of mast cell disease in paraffin sections using tryptase, CD68, myeloperoxidase, lysozyme, and CD20 antibodies. *Mod Pathol* 1996;9:982–988.
26. Horny HP, Greschniok A, Jordan JH, et al. Chymase expressing bone marrow mast cells in mastocytosis and myelodysplastic syndromes: an immunohistochemical and morphometric study. *J Clin Pathol* 2003;56:103–106.
27. Sperr WR, Jordan JH, Baghestanian M, et al. Expression of mast cell tryptase by myeloblasts in a group of patients with acute myeloid leukemia. *Blood* 2001;98:2200–2209.
28. Horny HP, Sotlar K, Valent P. Differential diagnoses of systemic mastocytosis in routinely processed bone marrow biopsy specimens: a review. *Pathobiology* 2010;77:169–180.
29. Horny HP, Sotlar K, Stellmacher F, et al. The tryptase positive compact round cell infiltrate of the bone marrow (TROCI-BM): a novel histopathological finding requiring the application of lineage specific markers. *J Clin Pathol* 2006;59:298–302.
30. Agis H, Krauth MT, Bohm A, et al. Identification of basogranulin (BB1) as a novel immunohistochemical marker of basophils in normal bone marrow and patients with myeloproliferative disorders. *Am J Clin Pathol* 2006;125:273–281.
31. Agis H, Krauth MT, Mosberger I, et al. Enumeration and immunohistochemical characterisation of bone marrow basophils in myeloproliferative disorders using the basophil specific monoclonal antibody 2D7. *J Clin Pathol* 2006;59:396–402.
32. Sotlar K, Horny HP, Simonitsch I, et al. CD25 indicates the neoplastic phenotype of mast cells: a novel immunohistochemical marker for the diagnosis of systemic mastocytosis (SM) in routinely processed bone marrow biopsy specimens. *Am J Surg Pathol* 2004;28:1319–1325.
33. Jordan JH, Walchshofer S, Jurecka W, et al. Immunohistochemical properties of bone marrow mast cells in systemic mastocytosis: evidence for expression of CD2, CD117/Kit, and bcl-x(L). *Hum Pathol* 2001;32:545–525.
34. Sotlar K, Cerny-Reiterer S, Petat-Dutter K, et al. Aberrant expression of CD30 in neoplastic mast cells in high-grade mastocytosis. *Mod Pathol* 2011;24:585–595.
35. Valent P, Sotlar K, Horny HP. Aberrant expression of CD30 in aggressive systemic mastocytosis and mast cell leukemia: a differential diagnosis to consider in aggressive hematopoietic CD30-positive neoplasms. *Leuk Lymphoma* 2011;52:740–744.
36. Travis WD, Li CY, Yam LT, et al. Significance of systemic mast cell disease with associated hematologic disorders. *Cancer* 1988;62:965–972.
37. Sotlar K, Colak S, Bache A, et al. Variable presence of KITD816V in clonal haematological non-mast cell lineage diseases associated with systemic mastocytosis (SM-AHNMD). *J Pathol* 2010;220:586–595.
38. Wolff K, Komar M, Petzelbauer P. Clinical and histopathological aspects of cutaneous mastocytosis. *Leuk Res* 2001;25:519–528.
39. Jordan JH, Schernthaner GH, Fritsche-Polanz R, et al. Stem cell factor-induced bone marrow mast cell hyperplasia mimicking systemic mastocytosis (SM): histopathologic and morphologic evaluation with special reference to recently established SM-criteria. *Leuk Lymphoma* 2002;43:575–582.
40. Berezowska SF, Ramond MJ, Rueff F, et al. Adult-onset cutaneous mastocytosis almost always indicates systemic mastocytosis with skin involvement. *Mod Pathol* 2013 (Epub ahead of print).
41. Valent P, Akin C, Sperr WR, et al. Aggressive systemic mastocytosis and related mast cell disorders: current treatment options and proposed response criteria. *Leuk Res* 2003;27:635–641.
42. Hein MS, Hansen L. Aggressive systemic mastocytosis: a case report and brief review of the literature. *S D J Med* 2005;58:95–100.
43. Frieri M, Linn N, Schweitzer M, et al. Lymphadenopathic mastocytosis with eosinophilia and biclonal gammopathy. *J Allergy Clin Immunol* 1990;86:126–132.
44. Horny H-P, Sotlar K, Valent P. Eosinophil, basophil, and mast cell infiltrates in the bone marrow: crossing the boundaries of diagnosis. *J Hematopathol* 2011;4:101–111.
45. Noack F, Sotlar K, Notter M, et al. Aleukemic mast cell leukemia with abnormal immunophenotype and c-kit mutation D816V. *Leuk Lymphoma* 2004;45:2295–2302.
46. Valent P, Sperr WR, Samorapoompichit P, et al. Myelomastocytic overlap syndromes: biology, criteria, and relationship to mastocytosis. *Leuk Res* 2001;25:595–602.
47. Hagen W, Schwarzmeier J, Walchshofer S, et al. A case of bone marrow mastocytosis associated with multiple myeloma. *Ann Hematol* 1998;76:167–174.
48. Stellmacher F, Sotlar K, Balleisen L, et al. Bone marrow mastocytosis associated with IgM kappa plasma cell myeloma. *Leuk Lymphoma* 2004;45:801–805.

49. Sotlar K, Bache A, Stellmacher F, et al. Systemic mastocytosis associated with chronic idiopathic myelofibrosis: a distinct subtype of systemic mastocytosis associated with a [corrected] clonal hematological non-mast [corrected] cell lineage disorder carrying the activating point mutations KITD816V and JAK2V617F. *J Mol Diagn* 2008;10:58–66.

50. Bernd HW, Sotlar K, Lorenzen J, et al. Acute myeloid leukaemia with t(8;21) associated with "occult" mastocytosis. Report of an unusual case and review of the literature. *J Clin Pathol* 2004;57:324–328.

51. McClintock-Treep SA, Horny HP, Sotlar K, et al. KIT(D816V+) systemic mastocytosis associated with KIT(D816V+) acute erythroid leukaemia: first case report with molecular evidence for same progenitor cell derivation. *J Clin Pathol* 2009;62:1147–1149.

52. Rudzki Z, Sotlar K, Kudela A, et al. Systemic mastocytosis (SM) and associated malignant bone marrow histiocytosis—a hitherto undescribed form of SM-AHNMD. *Pol J Pathol* 2011;62:101–104.

53. Agis H, Sotlar K, Valent P, et al. Ph-Chromosome-positive chronic myeloid leukemia with associated bone marrow mastocytosis. *Leuk Res* 2005;29:1227–1232.

54. Horny HP, Sotlar K, Stellmacher F, et al. An unusual case of systemic mastocytosis associated with chronic lymphocytic leukaemia (SM-CLL). *J Clin Pathol* 2006;59:264–268.

55. Tzankov A, Sotlar K, Muhlematter D, et al. Systemic mastocytosis with associated myeloproliferative disease and precursor B lymphoblastic leukaemia with t(13;13)(q12;q22) involving FLT3. *J Clin Pathol* 2008;61:958–961.

56. Horny HP, Parwaresch MR, Kaiserling E, et al. Mast cell sarcoma of the larynx. *J Clin Pathol* 1986;39:596–602.

57. Kojima M, Nakamura S, Itoh H, et al. Mast cell sarcoma with tissue eosinophilia arising in the ascending colon. *Mod Pathol* 1999;12:739–743.

58. Chott A, Guenther P, Huebner A, et al. Morphologic and immunophenotypic properties of neoplastic cells in a case of mast cell sarcoma. *Am J Surg Pathol* 2003;27:1013–1019.

59. Auquit-Auckbur I, Lazar C, Deneuve S, et al. Malignant transformation of mastocytoma developed on skin mastocytosis into cutaneous mast cell sarcoma. *Am J Surg Pathol* 2012;36:779–782.

60. Gülen T, Sander B, Nilsson G, et al. Systemic mastocytosis: progressive evolution of an occult disease into fatal mast cell leukemia. *Med Oncol* 2012;29:3540–3546.

61. Sherwin RP, Kern WH, Jones JC. Solitary mast cell granuloma (histiocytoma) of the lung; a histopathologic, tissue culture and time-lapse cinematographic study. *Cancer* 1965;18:634–641.

62. Kudo H, Morinaga S, Shimosato Y, et al. Solitary mast cell tumor of the lung. *Cancer* 1988;61:2089–2094.

63. Sotlar K, Saeger W, Stellmacher F, et al. "Occult" mastocytosis with activating c-kit point mutation evolving into systemic mastocytosis associated with plasma cell myeloma and secondary amyloidosis. *J Clin Pathol* 2006;59:875–878.

64. Kitamura Y, Tsujimura T, Jippo T, et al. Regulation of development, survival and neoplastic growth of mast cells through the c-kit receptor. *Int Arch Allergy Immunol* 1995;107:54–56.

65. Valent P, Spanbloch E, Sperr WR, et al. Induction of differentiation of human mast cells from bone marrow and peripheral blood mononuclear cells by recombinant human stem cell factor/kit-ligand in long-term culture. *Blood* 1992;80:2237–2245.

66. Hartmann K, Wardelmann E, Ma Y, et al. Novel germline mutation of KIT associated with familial gastrointestinal stromal tumors and mastocytosis. *Gastroenterology* 2005;129:1042–1046.

67. Zhang LY, Smith ML, Schultheis B, et al. A novel K509I mutation of KIT identified in familial mastocytosis-in vitro and in vivo responsiveness to imatinib therapy. *Leuk Res* 2006;30:373–378.

68. Tang X, Boxer M, Drummond A, et al. A germline mutation in KIT in familial diffuse cutaneous mastocytosis. *J Med Genet* 2004;41:e88.

69. Nakagomi N, Hirota S. Juxtamembrane-type c-kit gene mutation found in aggressive systemic mastocytosis induces imatinib-resistant constitutive KIT activation. *Lab Invest* 2007;87:365–371.

70. Garcia-Montero AC, Jara-Acevedo M, Teodosio C, et al. KIT mutation in mast cells and other bone marrow hematopoietic cell lineages in systemic mast cell disorders: a prospective study of the Spanish Network on Mastocytosis (REMA) in a series of 113 patients. *Blood* 2006;108:2366–2372.

71. Longley BJ Jr, Metcalfe DD, Tharp M, et al. Activating and dominant inactivating c-KIT catalytic domain mutations in distinct clinical forms of human mastocytosis. *Proc Natl Acad Sci U S A* 1999;96:1609–1614.

72. Pullarkat VA, Bueso-Ramos C, Lai R, et al. Systemic mastocytosis with associated clonal hematological non-mast-cell lineage disease: analysis of clinicopathologic features and activating c-kit mutations. *Am J Hematol* 2003;73:12–17.

73. Pignon JM, Giraudier S, Duquesnoy P, et al. A new c-kit mutation in a case of aggressive mast cell disease. *Br J Haematol* 1997;96:374–376.

74. Boissan M, Feger F, Guillosson JJ, et al. c-Kit and c-kit mutations in mastocytosis and other hematological diseases. *J Leukoc Biol* 2000;67:135–148.

75. Lasota J, Miettinen M. Clinical significance of oncogenic KIT and PDGFRA mutations in gastrointestinal stromal tumours. *Histopathology* 2008;53:245–266.

76. Beghini A, Ripamonti CB, Cairoli R, et al. KIT activating mutations: incidence in adult and pediatric acute myeloid leukemia, and identification of an internal tandem duplication. *Haematologica* 2004;89:920–925.

77. Tian Q, Frierson HF Jr, Krystal GW, et al. Activating c-kit gene mutations in human germ cell tumors. *Am J Pathol* 1999;154:1643–1647.

78. Hongyo T, Li T, Syaifudin M, et al. Specific c-kit mutations in sinonasal natural killer/T-cell lymphoma in China and Japan. *Cancer Res* 2000;60:2345–2347.

79. Escribano L, Alvarez-Twose I, Sanchez-Munoz L, et al. Prognosis in adult indolent systemic mastocytosis: a long-term study of the Spanish Network on Mastocytosis in a series of 145 patients. *J Allergy Clin Immunol* 2009;124:514–521.

80. Mayerhofer M, Gleixner KV, Hoebl A, et al. Unique effects of KIT D816V in BaF3 cells: induction of cluster formation, histamine synthesis, and early mast cell differentiation antigens. *J Immunol* 2008;180:5466–5476.

81. Lanternier F, Cohen-Akenine A, Palmerini F, et al. Phenotypic and genotypic characteristics of mastocytosis according to the age of onset. *PLoS One* 2008;3:e1906.

82. Zhang Y, Schlegelberger B, Weber-Matthiesen K, et al. Translocation (X;8) (q2?6;q21.3) in a case of systemic mastocytosis. *Cancer Genet Cytogenet* 1994;78:236–238.

83. Akin C, Scott LM, Metcalfe DD. Slowly progressive systemic mastocytosis with high mast-cell burden and no evidence of a non-mast-cell hematologic disorder: an example of a smoldering case? *Leuk Res* 2001;25:635–638.

84. Valent P, Akin C, Sperr WR, et al. Smouldering mastocytosis: a novel subtype of systemic mastocytosis with slow progression. *Int Arch Allergy Immunol* 2002;127:137–139.

85. Orfao A, Escribano L, Villarrubia J, et al. Flow cytometric analysis of mast cells from normal and pathological human bone marrow samples: identification and enumeration. *Am J Pathol* 1996;149:1493–1499.

86. Escribano L, Orfao A, Villarrubia J, et al. Immunophenotypic characterization of human bone marrow mast cells. A flow cytometric study of normal and pathological bone marrow samples. *Anal Cell Pathol* 1998;16(3):151–159.

87. Parker RI. Hematologic aspects of mastocytosis: I: management of hematologic disorders in association with systemic mast cell disease. *J Invest Dermatol* 1991;96:52S–53S; discussion 53S–54S, 60S–65S.

88. Valent P, Akin C, Escribano L, et al. Standards and standardization in mastocytosis: consensus statements on diagnostics, treatment recommendations and response criteria. *Eur J Clin Invest* 2007;37:435–453.

89. Peter B, Gleixner KV, Cerny-Reiterer S, et al. Polo-like kinase-1 as a novel target in neoplastic mast cells: demonstration of growth-inhibitory effects of small interfering RNA and the Polo-like kinase-1 targeting drug BI 2536. *Haematologica* 2011;96:672–680.

90. Gleixner KV, Mayerhofer M, Cerny-Reiterer S, et al. KIT-D816V-independent oncogenic signaling in neoplastic cells in systemic mastocytosis: role of Lyn and Btk activation and disruption by dasatinib and bosutinib. *Blood* 2011;118:1885–1898.

91. Valent P, Klion AD, Horny HP, et al. Contemporary consensus proposal on criteria and classification of eosinophilic disorders and related syndromes. *J Allergy Clin Immunol* 2012.

92. Denburg JA, Browman G. Prognostic implications of basophil differentiation in chronic myeloid leukemia. *Am J Hematol* 1988;27:110–114.

93. Horny HP, Schaumburg-Lever G, Bolz S, et al. Use of monoclonal antibody KP1 for identifying normal and neoplastic human mast cells. *J Clin Pathol* 1990;43:719–722.

94. Horny HP, Ruck P, Xiao JC, et al. Immunoreactivity of normal and neoplastic human tissue mast cells with macrophage-associated antibodies, with special reference to the recently developed monoclonal antibody PG-M1. *Hum Pathol* 1993;24:355–358.

95. Yoo D, Lessin LS, Jensen WN. Bone-marrow mast cells in lymphoproliferative disorders. *Ann Intern Med* 1978;88:753–757.

96. Prokocimer M, Polliack A. Increased bone marrow mast cells in preleukemic syndromes, acute leukemia, and lymphoproliferative disorders. *Am J Clin Pathol* 1981;75:34–38.

97. Petrella T, Depret O, Arnould L, et al. Systemic mast cell disease associated with hairy cell leukaemia. *Leuk Lymphoma* 1997;25:593–595.

98. Valent P, Samorapoompichit P, Sperr WR, et al. Myelomastocytic leukemia: myeloid neoplasm characterized by partial differentiation of mast cell-lineage cells. *Hematol J* 2002;3:90–94.

99. McElroy EA Jr, Phyliky RL, Li CY. Systemic mast cell disease associated with the hypereosinophilic syndrome. *Mayo Clin Proc* 1998;73:47–50.

100. Tefferi A, Pardanani A, Li CY. Hypereosinophilic syndrome with elevated serum tryptase versus systemic mast cell disease associated with eosinophilia: 2 distinct entities? *Blood* 2003;102:3073–3074; author reply 3074.

101. Horny HP, Rabenhorst G, Loffler H, et al. Solitary fibromastocytic tumor arising in an inguinal lymph node: the first description of a unique spindle cell tumor simulating mastocytosis. *Mod Pathol* 1994;7:962–966.

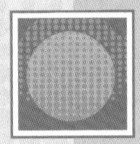

Chapter 50
Histopathologic Manifestations of Lymphoproliferative and Myeloproliferative Disorders Involving the Spleen

Attilio Orazi • Sonam Prakash

The spleen is an important organ in the hematopoietic system due to its immunologic and blood filtration functions. However, it is not as well studied as the bone marrow or lymph nodes largely due to the fact that the spleen is not as easily accessible as the bone marrow and lymph nodes during the course of a given disease process. Splenectomy requires a major surgical procedure and entails risks to the patient, not only during but also subsequent to surgery.

Few hematologic malignancies arise primarily within the spleen, and most conditions seen at this site represent secondary involvement by diseases originating elsewhere in the body. The role of the pathologist in most cases is to provide confirmation of the known or suspected diagnosis and to exclude unsuspected pathology. The key to successful interpretation of splenic pathology lies in careful gross evaluation of the organ and in ensuring optimal tissue fixation. Because of the amount of blood in the spleen, thin sections are of particular importance. Multiple touch imprints should be made at the time that the spleen reaches the laboratory, and Romanowsky stains should be performed immediately on a minimum of two of these touch imprints. In addition, material should be obtained for flow cytometric immunophenotypic analysis, and a section should be banked for molecular genetic studies. Blocks should be cut a maximum of 3 mm in thickness, and the tissue blocks should never be more than 1 cm. Particular care needs to be exercised in isolating lymph nodes of the splenic hilum. Their examination can provide valuable additional information, particularly in the diagnosis of low-grade B-cell lymphomas. Obtaining adequate clinical information is often critical in the diagnostic characterization of disorders that involve the spleen, and this need cannot be overemphasized.

In this chapter, we aim to present a comprehensive account of those aspects of splenic pathology likely to be encountered by the diagnostic hematopathologist. We provide principles for a systematic histopathologic analysis, which can be applied to arrive at a diagnosis following recognition of broad categories of abnormalities affecting individual splenic compartments. To avoid repetition of material covered in other chapters, immunohistochemistry, cytogenetics, and molecular genetic investigation are only briefly described where appropriate.

 ## THE NORMAL SPLEEN

Neoplastic disorders that involve the spleen are understood best in light of the structure and function of this organ. The spleen is composed of two anatomically and functionally distinct regions. The lymphoid tissue of the spleen, called the *white pulp*, can be seen grossly as uniformly distributed white nodules. The white pulp of the spleen is associated intimately with the splenic arterial circulation. The central arteries, which arise from trabecular arteries within the fibrous trabeculae, are surrounded by cylindrical cuffs of lymphocytes composed of admixtures of B cells and T cells (1–4). Periodically,

lymphoid follicles occur as outgrowths of the lymphatic sheath (5,6). The morphology of the splenic white pulp varies with the age of the patient and with the presence of antigenic stimulation. Inactive or hypoplastic white pulp, in which no germinal centers are seen, is characteristic of infancy, senescence, and the immunologically unstimulated adult spleen. In the immunologically activated state, three distinct zones are identifiable within the splenic lymphoid follicle (7–9). The germinal center itself, composed of B lymphocytes in a meshwork of follicular dendritic cells, is surrounded by a darker rim of small lymphocytes called the mantle zone, which also is composed predominantly of B cells. The mantle zone is encased in the outer marginal zone, at the interface between white and red pulp. The marginal zone, which is an extension of the periarterial lymphoid sheath (PALS) and is composed of both B cells and T cells (4), is the site of antigen trapping and processing. The B cells, which represent the majority of the marginal zone cells, are those primarily responsible for the elaboration of opsonizing antibody (10).

The red pulp of the spleen is composed of vascular sinuses and the cords of Billroth (11–13). The structure of the splenic sinuses provides the mechanism for filtration of the peripheral blood by the spleen. The sinus-lining cells, also called littoral cells, have long cytoplasmic processes that overlap. Due to the absence of tight junctions, circulating blood cells are able to squeeze through the potential spaces between the sinus lining cells and percolate through the cords of Billroth before entering the splenic sinuses and venous system, thus returning to the systemic circulation. The ability of circulating blood cells to enter the venous sinuses depends on their deformability. Cells without the ability to deform are not able to enter the sinuses and are destroyed in the acidotic, hypoxic environment of the cords of Billroth (2,14).

The immunoarchitecture of the spleen has been studied with immunohistologic techniques, and its immunotopography has been mapped (1,4,15–19). The white pulp of the spleen is largely compartmentalized into B- and T-cell zones, although there is some intermingling, particularly in the marginal zones and the PALS (1,19,20). The majority of B cells are found in the germinal centers and mantle zones, although they may account for a substantial percentage of marginal zone lymphocytes (4,15,16). The distribution of immunoglobulin-containing B cells is similar to that seen in the lymph nodes. The majority of B cells in the germinal centers lack surface and cytoplasmic immunoglobulin (15). The mantle zone B cells bear surface immunoglobulin with coexpression of IgM and IgD. The marginal zone B cells express predominantly IgM with only a small minority expressing IgD. IgG expression is lacking in these areas and is limited to scattered B cells in the red pulp. Only rare IgA-containing B cells are found. A few CD4-positive (CD4+) helper/inducer T cells are scattered within the germinal centers and in the mantle zones. There is also some spillover of T cells into the red pulp, although the T cells of the red pulp are predominantly CD8+ suppressor/cytotoxic cells (16), which are rarely found in the PALS and are virtually absent from the germinal centers. The red pulp contains numerous cells of monocyte-macrophage lineage, only a few of which are found in the white pulp. The red pulp also contains granulocytes, lymphocytes, and plasma cells. Natural killer cells are scattered throughout the red pulp and within germinal centers.

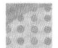 GENERAL CONSIDERATIONS

The initial evaluation of the spleen should be based on gross examination of the organ. Three major patterns are recognized based on involvement of white pulp, red pulp, or more focal lesions (Table 50.1).

Diffuse Splenic Involvement

White Pulp Involvement

Most proliferative disorders of the splenic lymphoid tissue produce a micronodular pattern due to the abnormal expansion of preexisting splenic lymphoid structures (i.e., follicles and PALS). Grossly, multiple small, whitish nodules are noticeable on the cut surface, an appearance that is occasionally referred to as a "miliary" pattern. This pattern is most often seen in small B-cell lymphoid neoplasms involving the spleen. The nodules may on occasion become confluent, or present as larger, dominant masses. Lymphoid malignancies that affect the white pulp of the spleen are largely the same as those that affect lymph nodes. These disorders include both classical and nodular lymphocyte predominant Hodgkin lymphoma (NLPHL) and non-Hodgkin lymphomas, primarily of B-cell lineage.

Red Pulp Involvement

Expansion of the red pulp of the spleen gives the organ a homogeneous red or "beefy" appearance. The normal nodularity of the white pulp is typically diminished or not seen. Microscopically, the white pulp is often atrophic or compressed by the expanded red pulp. Neoplastic proliferations that involve the red pulp include myeloid and lymphoid leukemias, myeloproliferative disorders, and a variety of nonhematopoietic tumors. In general, disorders with a large component of circulating cells, e.g., chronic lymphocytic leukemia, large granular lymphocytic leukemia, hairy cell leukemia (HCL), and acute leukemia, will have significant red pulp involvement. However, some lymphomas (e.g., hepatosplenic T-cell lymphoma [HSTCL], intravascular large B-cell lymphoma, as well as other less well-defined lymphoid malignancies, including splenic diffuse red pulp B-cell lymphoma) also involve the red pulp. Diseases that cause enlargement of the red pulp frequently lead to hypersplenism. Since infiltrative processes cause widening of the cords of Billroth and a proliferation of cordal macrophages, circulating blood cells have a prolonged exposure to the hostile environment of the red pulp, resulting in an increased opportunity for phagocytosis by cordal macrophages. This can lead to peripheral cytopenias. Occasionally, however, infiltrative processes result in functional asplenia, although the spleen may be normal in size or even enlarged (2). The resultant hyposplenism is associated with the presence of Howell-Jolly bodies in circulating erythrocytes, as well as target cells and acanthocytes, reflecting the lack of the red pulp filtration function (21,22).

Focal Splenic Pathology

Some benign and malignant proliferations can produce focal lesions, rather than more diffuse involvement of the red or white pulp. These include lesions involving vascular and stromal, as well as hematolymphoid elements.

Splenic Rupture

Pathologic rupture of the spleen can be seen in a variety of hematologic disorders, both benign and malignant (23). Spontaneous rupture of the spleen should always prompt pathologic evaluation of the splenic tissue since various infectious etiologies, infectious mononucleosis in particular, have pathologic findings that are distinctive enough to make a presumptive diagnosis, or suggest further serologic studies. Other etiologies, such as storage diseases, will present with characteristic findings as well. Splenic rupture as a primary presentation of hematologic malignancy is rare, but has been reported with both low-grade and high-grade lymphoid malignancies including lymphoblastic leukemia as well as acute and chronic myeloproliferative disorders. Nonhematopoietic lesions can also be associated with splenic rupture, including cysts, infarctions, vascular lesions/neoplasms, and metastatic malignancies.

LYMPHOID HYPERPLASIA IN THE SPLEEN

Various benign conditions that affect the splenic white or red pulp can simulate hematopoietic malignancies (Table 50.2). Reactive follicular hyperplasia, seen in the evolving activated immune response, usually is recognized easily as benign (2). A rare entity that may grossly simulate lymphoma is known as localized (nodular) reactive lymphoid hyperplasia. The area of nodular hyperplasia appears quite distinct from adjacent normal spleen and may raise the suspicion of lymphoma. Histologically, this is formed by focal aggregation of hyperplastic follicles, which have typical, benign features (Fig. 50.1) (24).

The marginal zones may become widely expanded and their fusion may result in grossly visible nodules, a phenomenon that has been referred to as *splenic marginal zone hyperplasia*

Table 50.1	PREDOMINANT PATTERNS OF INVOLVEMENT IN SPLENIC HEMATOPOIETIC DISORDERS	
Predominant Pattern of Involvement	**Neoplastic**	**Nonneoplastic**
Red pulp	Hairy cell leukemia Hairy cell leukemia variant Splenic diffuse red pulp B-cell lymphoma Hepatosplenic T-cell lymphoma Large granular lymphocytic leukemia Peripheral T-cell lymphoma[a] T-prolymphocytic leukemia Acute leukemias Myeloproliferative neoplasms/other myeloid neoplasms Chronic lymphocytic leukemia/small lymphocytic leukemia[a] Prolymphocytic leukemia[a] Lymphoplasmacytic lymphoma	Hemolytic anemias Nonspecific congestion Extramedullary hematopoiesis Storage diseases Cytokine effects Hemophagocytic syndrome
White pulp	Chronic lymphocytic leukemia/small lymphocytic lymphoma Prolymphocytic leukemia Splenic marginal zone lymphoma Mantle cell lymphoma Follicular lymphoma Peripheral T-cell lymphoma	Follicular or marginal zone hyperplasia

[a]Can involve both red pulp and white pulp.

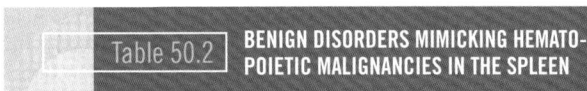

Table 50.2 | **BENIGN DISORDERS MIMICKING HEMATO-POIETIC MALIGNANCIES IN THE SPLEEN**

- Reactive hyperplasia
  - Follicular hyperplasia
  - Splenic marginal zone hyperplasia
  - Nonfollicular lymphoid hyperplasia secondary to viral infections
  - Nodular T-cell hyperplasia
  - Myeloid proliferation secondary to cytokine therapy
- Immunodeficiencies or deregulation of lymphoid production (e.g., ALPS)
- Disorders of the reticuloendothelial system
  - Storage disorders
  - Hemophagocytic syndrome
  - Langerhans cell histiocytosis
- Castleman disease
- Nonhematopoietic lesions
  - Cyst
  - Hamartoma
  - Inflammatory pseudotumor

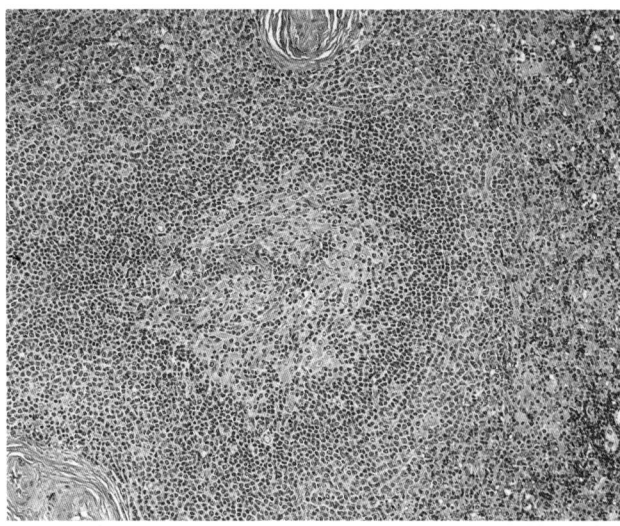

FIGURE 50.2. Splenic marginal zone hyperplasia. A case of autoimmune hemolytic anemia demonstrating expanded marginal zone in a tripartite follicle.

(2,25–28) (Fig. 50.2). It may be impossible, on morphologic grounds alone, to distinguish these reactive changes from cases of early marginal zone B-cell lymphoma (25,29). Splenic marginal zone hyperplasia may be seen in autoimmune disorders, including systemic lupus erythematosus or immune thrombocytopenic purpura (30).

The so-called early activated immune reaction, or reactive nonfollicular lymphoid hyperplasia, which is characteristic of infectious mononucleosis as well as herpes simplex and other viral infections, can simulate Hodgkin lymphoma and non-Hodgkin lymphoma (2,31–33). The white pulp in these conditions lacks germinal centers and, on low-power examination, resembles the immunologically unstimulated spleen (2,7,23,34). Higher-power examination, however, reveals morphologic evidence of antigenic stimulation characterized by the presence of lymphocytes in varying stages of transformation, including small and large lymphocytes and immunoblasts. Transformed lymphocytes and immunoblasts also proliferate around the splenic arterioles and may infiltrate the subendothelial zones of the trabecular veins and the connective tissue framework, resulting in splenic rupture in extreme cases (35). The finding of tingible body macrophages and a pleocytotic cell population present in all the follicles in the white pulp points to the correct diagnosis of a reactive

condition. Steroid-treated immune thrombocytopenic purpura and autoimmune hemolytic anemia also may show this pattern of immunologic activation (36,37).

Nodular T-cell hyperplasia simulating a peripheral T-cell lymphoma can be rarely observed in patients with hypersensitivity reactions to phenytoin (38). Abnormalities of the white pulp, occasionally worrisome for lymphoma, can also be seen in patients with congenital conditions characterized by immunodeficiency or by abnormalities causing a deregulated lymphoid production, for example, autoimmune lymphoproliferative syndrome (ALPS).

Autoimmune Lymphoproliferative Syndrome

A rare disorder that can mimic lymphoma in the spleen is autoimmune lymphoproliferative syndrome (ALPS), a hereditable disorder usually due to mutations of the CD95 (Fas) gene (39,40), which presents in early childhood (<2 years of age). In ALPS that is characterized by lymphoid hyperplasia, splenomegaly, and autoimmunity, the spleen frequently enlarges to more than ten times its age-normal size. Histologically, the spleen shows variable degrees of follicular hyperplasia often with expanded marginal zones. The PALS and red pulp are also expanded due to a markedly increased number of T cells (Fig. 50.3). These cells

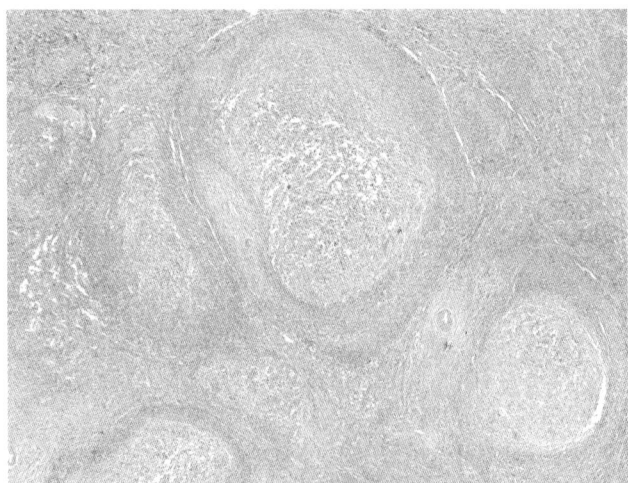

FIGURE 50.1. Localized (nodular) follicular hyperplasia. There is an aggregate of hyperplastic follicles surrounded by well-defined mantle zones.

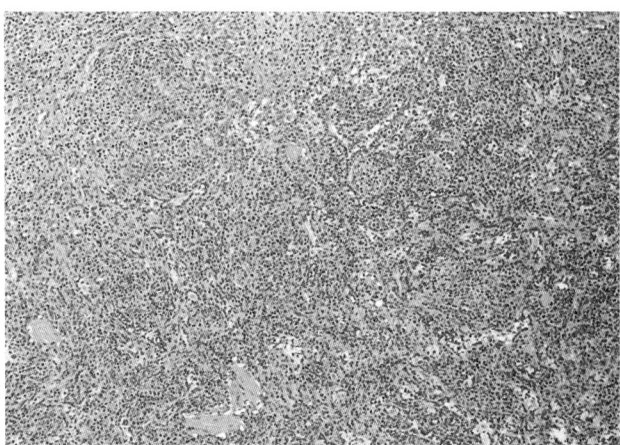

FIGURE 50.3. Autoimmune lymphoproliferative syndrome. Expanded red pulp due to increased T lymphocytes.

consist of a mixture of small lymphocytes and immunoblasts. As in lymph nodes in this disorder, many of these T cells are negative for both CD4 and CD8. The pathologic picture of the spleen is complicated by the frequent association with immune cytopenias affecting red cells, granulocytes, and platelets, which contribute further to splenomegaly (41,42). Patients with this disorder have an increased risk of developing both Hodgkin and non-Hodgkin lymphomas (43).

Castleman Disease

Only occasional cases of Castleman disease of both the unicentric hyaline-vascular and multicentric Castleman disease (MCD) type, the latter associated with human herpes virus-8 (HHV-8/KSHV), have been reported to occur in the spleen (44–46). MCD represents the majority of cases reported; splenic involvement is rare in the unicentric form of Castleman disease, and most reports are in the older literature. Since these cases were not evaluated for HHV-8/KSHV, the nature of these proliferations is not clearly established (46–48). Morphologic features include atrophic follicles with hyaline vascular germinal centers, rare cases with grossly visible masses composed of hyperplastic nodules of white pulp surrounded by dense fibrous tissue, and occasional cases with expansion of the marginal zones with increased plasma cells (48) (see Chapter 13). Cases of HIV-related MCD involving the spleen have also been described. As seen in lymph nodes, immunoblastic cells expressing IgM-lambda are identified in the perifollicular areas of the white pulp (49,50). MCD is generally negative for Epstein-Barr virus (EBV), but rare cases resembling

germinotropic lymphoma have been reported (51). In this case report by Seliem et al., the spleen was markedly enlarged with multiple foci of hemorrhage and infarcts. Microscopic examination demonstrated multiple foci of replacement of white pulp by large cells that were found to be coinfected with EBV and HHV-8/KSHV (51).

HODGKIN LYMPHOMA

Splenic involvement in Hodgkin lymphoma is detected in more than one-third of patients undergoing staging laparotomy. The documentation of splenic involvement by Hodgkin lymphoma has therapeutic and prognostic implications, although these implications now appear less critical in light of the high rates of remission and cure obtained with current regimens of combination chemotherapy (52,53). Involvement of the liver and bone marrow is rarely found in the absence of splenic involvement (54). All histologic subtypes of classical Hodgkin lymphoma (CHL) may involve the spleen, with nodular sclerosis being the most common (61%) followed by mixed cellularity subtype (27%) (54). Lymphocyte-depleted CHL characteristically presents with subdiaphragmatic disease and splenic involvement (55). Involvement by NLPHL is less common (56).

Hodgkin lymphoma produces either miliary nodules or, more frequently, solitary or multiple tumor masses in the spleen (2,57) (Fig. 50.4). Splenic involvement generally is detectable grossly but may be subtle. Gross examination of the spleen must be meticulous in patients who have Hodgkin lymphoma,

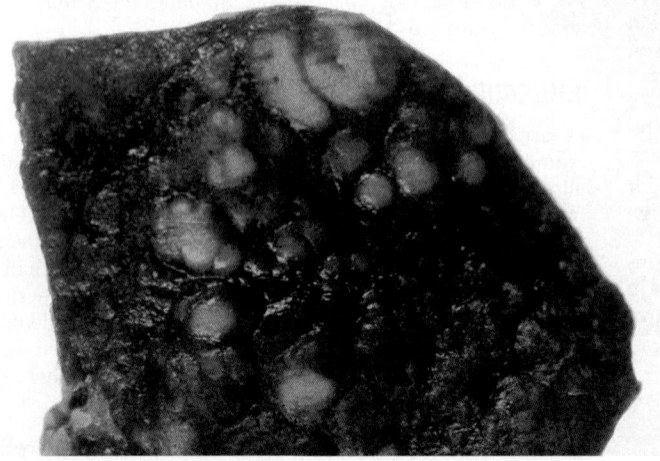
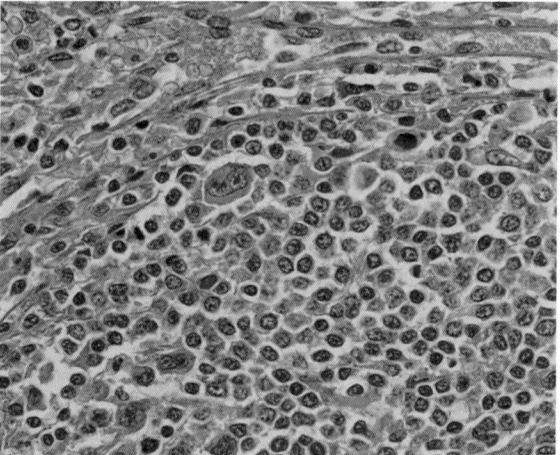
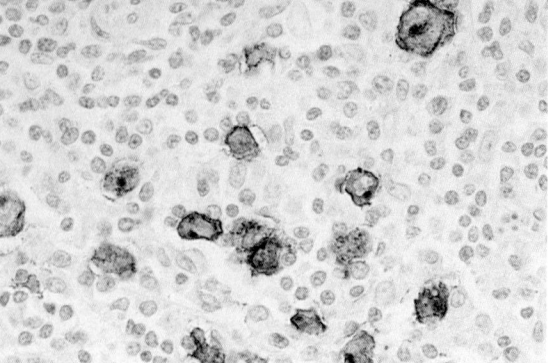

FIGURE 50.4. Classical Hodgkin lymphoma. A: Multiple tumor nodules in the spleen. **B:** Reed-Sternberg cell in the marginal zone of the follicle. **C:** CD30-positive Reed-Sternberg cells.

since foci of involvement may be only a few millimeters in size (58,59). The early lesions of Hodgkin lymphoma in the spleen are found microscopically in the PALS or the marginal zones (2,23) (Fig. 50.4). As the disease progresses, the nodules expand to efface the lymphoid follicles and also may produce involvement of the red pulp.

Sarcoidal granulomas also may be found in the spleens of patients who have Hodgkin lymphoma, in addition to various other disorders associated with impaired T-cell function (60–65). Several studies have suggested that these granulomas occur more frequently in spleens uninvolved by Hodgkin lymphoma than in those involved by Hodgkin lymphoma (62,63). Grossly, they may be so large as to mimic involvement by Hodgkin lymphoma. Microscopically, the granulomas are composed of clusters of epithelioid histiocytes that occur in the white pulp in close association with the arterial circulation. The finding of granulomas in the spleen of a patient who has Hodgkin lymphoma in the absence of involvement by the tumor does not change the clinical stage or treatment regimen, although Sacks et al. (65) suggested that patients who have splenic sarcoidal granulomas may have a better prognosis. These granulomas are not related to prior lymphangiography, and their origin is unknown (57).

The criteria for the diagnosis of CHL in the spleen are the same as those for other extranodal sites (54). In a patient who has had a previous nodal diagnosis, the documentation of Hodgkin lymphoma in the spleen can be made if the general features of one of the histologic subtypes are found in association with one of the variants of the Reed-Sternberg cell (54). A classic Reed-Sternberg cell is not necessary for diagnosis in this setting. If the patient does not have a previous nodal diagnosis, however, diagnostic Reed-Sternberg cells must be found. Immunohistochemical studies can be helpful in confirming the diagnosis of CHL by showing the characteristic immunophenotype of CHL in the cytologically atypical cells (see Chapters 15 and 16). The subclassification of CHL in the spleen is sometimes difficult and is unnecessary in a case with a previous nodal diagnosis (53). The unique morphologic and immunophenotypic characteristics of NLPHL allow its distinction from the CHL subtypes.

NON-HODGKIN LYMPHOMAS

Malignant lymphoma may involve the spleen in any of three clinical settings. In the first and rarest setting, termed *primary splenic lymphoma*, the tumor is confined to the spleen or splenic hilar lymph nodes, without evidence of involvement of other sites. In the second and most common setting, the organ is involved as part of generalized disease. The third setting includes subtypes of lymphomas that typically present in a splenomegalic fashion (e.g., splenic marginal zone lymphoma [SMZL], hepatosplenic T-cell lymphoma). These lymphomas typically lack peripheral lymphadenopathy but have marrow involvement.

Primary Splenic Lymphoma

Primary splenic lymphoma is rare, accounting for <1% of all lymphomas. Most primary splenic lymphomas are non-Hodgkin lymphomas; Hodgkin lymphoma confined to the spleen is rare (66). Excluding lymphomas thought to arise in the spleen, such as SMZL, most of these cases were described in the older literature and are not well defined. Warnke et al. (66) were able to identify 47 cases of primary splenic lymphoma fulfilling the most stringent diagnostic criteria, that is, tumor confined to the spleen and splenic hilar lymph nodes (67–77). The patients were all adults; a slight male preponderance was noted. The most common presenting symptoms included

left-sided abdominal pain and systemic symptoms such as fever, malaise, and weight loss. Two patients were HIV positive (66,71). The gross findings and the histologic characteristics were similar to those observed in spleens secondarily involved by malignant lymphoma. Nearly all cases were of B-cell lineage. The most common subtype was diffuse large B-cell lymphoma (DLBCL) (30/47 cases), with the remainder being mostly low-grade B-cell malignancies. One case of Burkitt lymphoma was identified. Kroft et al. (78) have reported a CD5-positive form of diffuse large B-cell lymphoma of the spleen. More recently, a series of eight cases of DLBCL was reported by Grosskreutz et al. (79). Of the 17 splenic lymphomas reported by Falk and Stutte (80), which included cases with minimal extrasplenic involvement, three cases showed T-cell lineage. A case of primary splenic CD30-positive anaplastic large cell lymphoma (ALCL) has been described (81). The course of primary splenic lymphoma is hard to predict because of the rarity of cases and the disparate histologic types included.

The differential diagnosis of primary splenic lymphoma includes infectious mononucleosis involving the spleen, other viral infections, and localized and reactive hyperplasia of the spleen. In infectious mononucleosis and other viral infections, histologic features may mimic lymphoma due to expansion of red pulp by an increased number of activated lymphoid cells, some of which may resemble Reed-Sternberg–like cells. The histologic finding of a spectrum of lymphoid cells instead of a monomorphic population in conjunction with young age of the patient and a positive monospot test can prompt a correct diagnosis of infectious mononucleosis.

Secondary Splenic Involvement by Lymphoma

Non-Hodgkin lymphomas of different types involve the spleen with variable frequency. Splenic involvement is particularly frequent in low-grade lymphomas. This is probably a result of the fact that many high-grade lymphomas are localized at the time of diagnosis (82). Liver involvement by lymphoma is rare in the absence of splenic disease (18). Clinical assessment of the likelihood of splenic involvement by malignant lymphomas may be difficult. The weights of involved spleens vary widely (83). Although tumor involvement usually results in palpable splenomegaly, Goffinet et al. (84) found that approximately one-third of nonpalpable spleens were involved by lymphoma at staging laparotomy. Staging laparotomy has been replaced by imaging studies; positron emission tomography, in particular, allows for an accurate determination (85).

PRECURSOR LYMPHOID NEOPLASMS

Some enlargement of the spleen can occur during the course of acute lymphoblastic leukemia of either precursor B-cell or T-cell lineage; however, it rarely approaches clinical significance. Splenomegaly occurs in approximately 10% of cases of lymphoblastic leukemia/lymphoma and is most frequent in the T-cell subtype (23). Rare cases of splenic B-lymphoblastic leukemia have been reported to present as splenic rupture. Morphologic studies of splenic involvement in lymphoblastic lymphoma/leukemia are rare, because splenectomy is rarely, if ever, performed in these cases. In the few cases that have been studied, the involvement is in the form of a diffuse infiltration of the red pulp by blastic-appearing cells (23). Morphologically, lymphoblastic lymphoma/leukemia in the spleen can resemble Burkitt lymphoma and occasionally blastoid variant of mantle cell lymphoma (MCL). Appropriate immunohistochemical stains can help distinguish between these entities with CD34, TdT, and CD99 being valuable immunohistochemical stains to establish their lymphoblastic nature (see Chapter 40).

▦ | MATURE B-CELL LYMPHOID NEOPLASMS

The morphology of the spleen involved by B-cell malignancies has been well characterized (23). These involve the spleen in one of two main patterns, either with uniform nodular expansion of the white pulp, as seen in small B-cell lymphomas such as chronic lymphocytic leukemia/small lymphocytic lymphoma (CLL/SLL), SMZL, MCL, and follicular lymphoma (FL) (Fig. 50.5), or with the formation of single or multiple tumor masses as seen in most cases of DLBCL (23) (Fig. 50.6). Small B-cell lymphomas have a higher incidence of splenic involvement at presentation than DLBCL. Occasionally, the spleen is the site of large cell transformation of a low-grade B-cell lymphoma.

Chronic Lymphocytic Leukemia/Small Lymphocytic Lymphoma

Splenic involvement is common in chronic lymphocytic leukemia/small lymphocytic lymphoma (CLL/SLL) (86) (Fig. 50.7), and prominent splenomegaly may be the presenting feature of this disorder (87–91). CLL/SLL often produces grossly visible nodules in a miliary pattern or shows a more homogeneous diffuse appearance in more advanced stages of the disease (23,92). The infiltrate may involve the white pulp, the red pulp, or both. Infiltration of large vessels or splenic trabeculae may be prominent. Prolymphocytes and paraimmunoblasts are identified both intermingled with the small lymphoid cells and in aggregates known as proliferation centers. An increased number of prolymphocytes and paraimmunoblasts may raise the question of high-grade transformation of preexisting CLL/SLL. Studies have addressed this issue and concluded that except in peripheral blood, increased prolymphocytes or paraimmunoblasts are not necessarily associated with more aggressive disease (93). The spleen may, however, be the site of large cell transformation (Richter syndrome) in CLL/SLL. Early splenic involvement by SLL may be difficult to detect because the white pulp nodules resemble those seen in immunologically unstimulated spleen (23,94). The presence of scattered prolymphocytes and paraimmunoblasts and focal infiltration of the red pulp may aid in the recognition of these cases. In some cases, however, the diagnosis rests on examination of splenic hilar lymph nodes and flow cytometric immunophenotypic or immunohistochemical confirmation (see Chapter 18).

B-cell Prolymphocytic Leukemia

B-cell prolymphocytic leukemia (B-PLL) is characterized by a lymphocytosis in which more than 55% of the circulating lymphocytes are prolymphocytes (95). Splenomegaly is prominent,

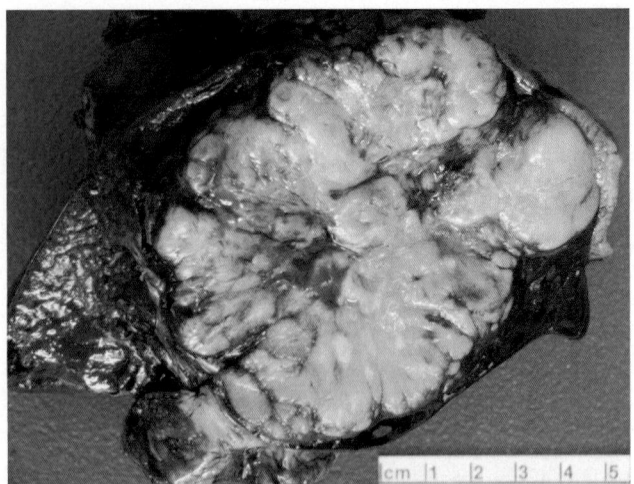

FIGURE 50.6. Single large tumor mass in a case of DLBCL.

with hypersplenism, peripheral cytopenias, and the absence of significant lymphadenopathy (96–98). The white blood cell count is markedly elevated (often >100 × 10⁹/L), with a predominance of prolymphocytes that have large vesicular nuclei and single prominent nucleoli (see Chapter 18). The pattern of infiltration in the spleen is similar to that seen in CLL/SLL in that, in addition to red pulp involvement, the splenic white pulp may also be involved (95,98) (Fig. 50.8). However, histologic distinction from blastoid MCL and cases of SMZL with an increased number of large cells may be difficult. Cases resembling B-PLL that show t(11;14)(q13;q32) may be indistinguishable from blastoid MCL and may represent a splenomegalic form of MCL in leukemic phase (99) (see following section on MCL).

Lymphoplasmacytic Lymphoma

Hepatosplenomegaly often is a feature of lymphoplasmacytic lymphoma (LPL). LPL may be associated with a monoclonal IgM paraprotein, anemia, and often a bleeding diathesis, a syndrome known as Waldenstrom macroglobulinemia (WM) (100–102). The most common pattern seen in the spleen in

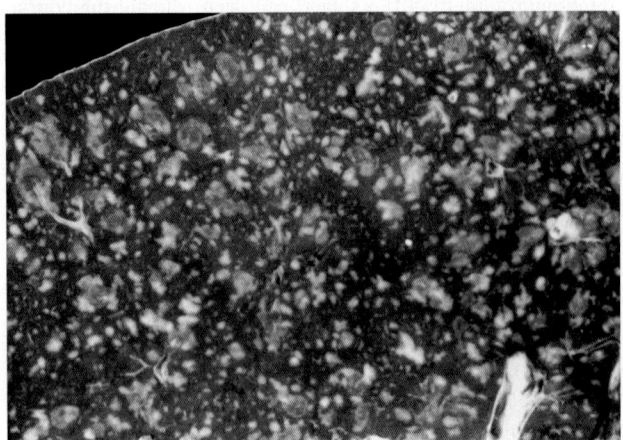

FIGURE 50.5. Miliary pattern of gross involvement in a case of follicular lymphoma.

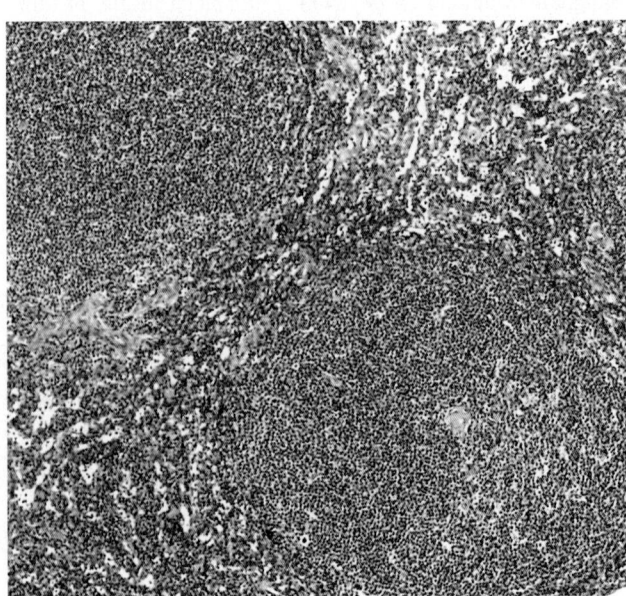

FIGURE 50.7. Chronic lymphocytic leukemia involving predominantly white pulp.

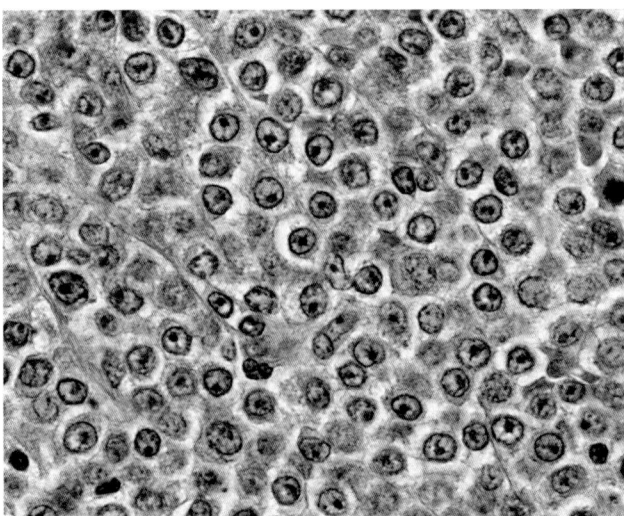

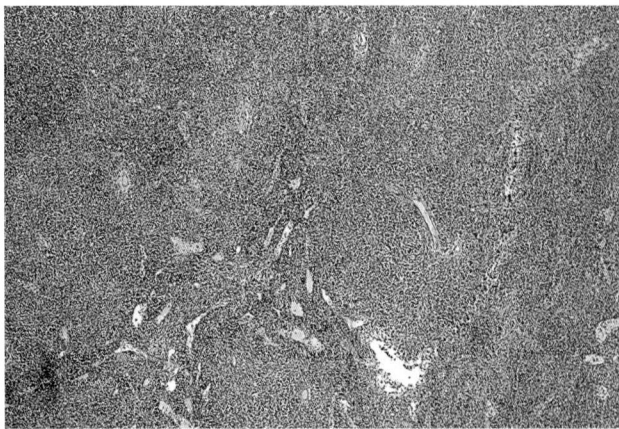

FIGURE 50.10. Mantle cell lymphoma. Uniformly expanded white pulp by lymphoma cells.

FIGURE 50.8. Prolymphocytic leukemia involving the red pulp. Prolymphocytes demonstrate vesicular nuclei with single prominent nucleoli.

LPL is involvement of the red pulp by an infiltrate composed of lymphocytes, plasmacytoid lymphocytes, and plasma cells (Fig. 50.9) but involvement of the white pulp may also be present. Dutcher and Russell bodies may be prominent. Splenic involvement may be extensive in LPL/WM, and may sometimes be associated with hypersplenism (102). Since plasmacytoid differentiation may also be seen in other lymphomas in the spleen, including CLL/SLL and marginal zone lymphoma, a primary diagnosis of LPL/WM should be made with caution (see Chapter 19). Transformation to diffuse large cell B-cell lymphoma has been reported to occur in the spleen in LPL cases (103).

Mantle Cell Lymphoma

Mantle cell lymphoma (MCL) frequently involves the spleen (87,91,104) (Fig. 50.10). Although MCL may present initially with clinically isolated splenomegaly, workup of these patients reveals that all have stage IV disease at the time of diagnosis, with bone marrow or liver involvement or both (87,91). The morphology of the disorder in the spleen is similar to that seen

in involved lymph nodes (105,106) (see Chapter 20). The white pulp is expanded uniformly, with tumor cells proliferating in widened mantle zones around benign, atrophic-appearing germinal centers. This pattern may mimic reactive secondary follicles. The latter are tripartite, however, with central follicles and mantle and marginal zones. The presence of small lymphocytes with irregular nuclear contours in the red pulp may aid in the diagnosis of lymphoma. Eventually, the neoplastic cells invade and replace the germinal centers. Such cases may closely resemble CLL/SLL. No proliferation centers are, however, observed. Rarely, a marginal zone–like differentiation can be observed. Such cases must be distinguished from SMZL. The immunophenotype is similar to that of MCL seen in other sites, with cyclin D1 being a key diagnostic immunohistochemical stain.

The blastoid and pleomorphic variants of MCL present different diagnostic considerations. The blastoid variant may have more extensive red pulp involvement than usual MCL, and the cells may resemble lymphoblasts in tissue sections (Fig. 50.11); immunohistochemical documentation of cyclin D1 positivity and lack of TdT expression is particularly useful in such cases. Leukemic forms of blastoid MCL also have been described. These cases may present with isolated splenomegaly. The pleomorphic variant of MCL may mimic DLBCL.

Studies have documented the existence of an unusual leukemic form of MCL that is associated with prominent

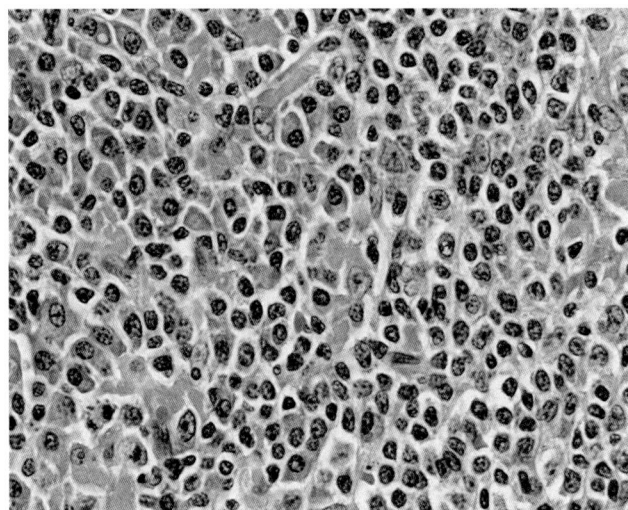

FIGURE 50.9. Lymphoplasmacytic lymphoma. Plasmacytoid lymphocytes and plasma cells in the red pulp.

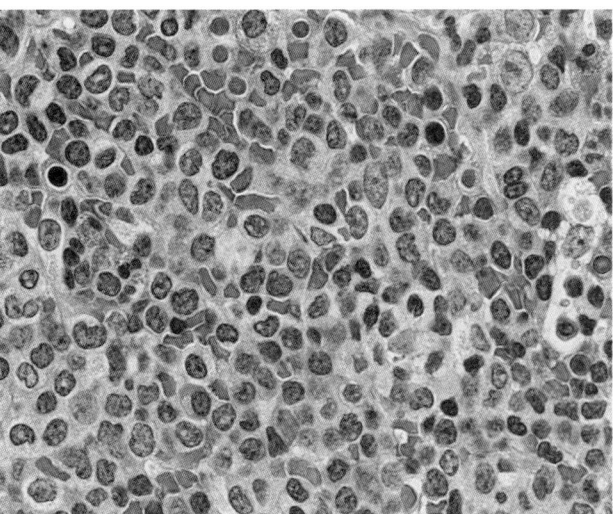

FIGURE 50.11. Blastoid mantle cell lymphoma. Cells resemble lymphoblasts with finely dispersed chromatin.

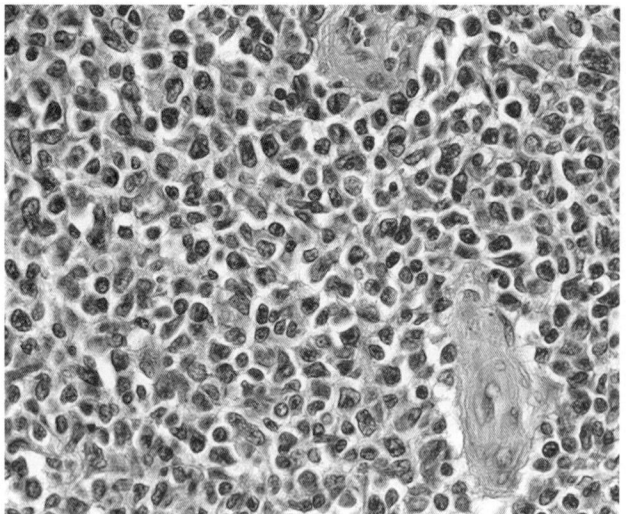

FIGURE 50.12. Follicular lymphoma, grade 1, composed predominantly of centrocytes.

splenomegaly without any peripheral lymphadenopathy (107). Not uncommonly, blastoid morphology and aggressive clinical behavior is seen in these cases. Although some of these cases were previously reported as B-PLL with t(11;14), they are now considered leukemic variants of MCL (99,108,109).

Follicular Lymphoma

Secondary splenic involvement is common in follicular lymphomas, a disease that, like CLL/SLL and MCL, is often disseminated at the time of its initial presentation. Rarely, cases of follicular lymphoma may present as isolated splenomegaly. Grossly, the spleen shows a miliary pattern of involvement due to the expansion of abnormal white pulp follicles, although, occasionally, the neoplastic nodules may coalesce to form larger tumor masses (23). In follicular lymphoma, grade 1, high-power examination reveals a monotonous population of centrocytes with coarse chromatin and inconspicuous nucleoli (Fig. 50.12). The diagnosis of follicular lymphoma, grade 2, may be more difficult, because the admixture of centrocytes and centroblasts may superficially resemble reactive germinal centers. The neoplastic follicles seen in follicular lymphoma usually lack tingible body macrophages and the margin between the follicle center

and mantle or marginal zone is indistinct. In addition, the red pulp does not display the plasmacytosis usually seen in reactive lymphoid hyperplasia and may contain satellite nodules composed of lymphoma cells. Immunohistochemistry or flow cytometry can aid in identifying monoclonality, as can expression of BCL2 and CD10 or Bcl-6 (see Chapter 22). While some studies demonstrated more frequent lack of bcl-2 in follicular lymphomas in the spleen (110) as compared to nodal cases, other studies failed to confirm these findings (111). As with other lymphomas, the spleen may represent the initial site of high-grade transformation of follicular lymphoma to DLBCL.

Nodal and Extranodal Marginal Zone Lymphoma

Splenic involvement by nodal marginal zone lymphoma has been reported in the older literature (112–117). However, most of these reports antedated the description of other B-cell lymphomas that more commonly involve the spleen such as splenic MZL, and the newly recognized entity splenic diffuse red pulp small B-cell lymphoma (SDRPBCL) (see below). Thus, the documentation of these cases is not well established. Extranodal MZL usually does not involve the spleen unless the disease is widely disseminated.

Diffuse Large B-cell Lymphoma

The majority of cases of splenic diffuse large B-cell lymphoma (DLBCL) are the result of secondary dissemination from other sites; however, in a proportion of the cases, the spleen appears to be the primary site of lymphoma. DLBCL in the spleen characteristically produces solitary or multiple tumor masses, which are usually well demarcated and may show areas of necrosis. Prominent splenomegaly may be a presenting feature (23,66,91). The cytomorphologic findings are similar to those seen in other nodal or extranodal DLBCLs (Fig. 50.13) (see Chapter 23). Predominant red pulp involvement may be observed in some cases (74,118–120). In cases of DLBCL limited to the red pulp, the possibility of transformation from a splenic diffuse small B-cell lymphoma of the red pulp or from a red pulp predominant SMZL (see below) should also be considered. T-cell/histiocyte-rich large B-cell lymphoma, a variant of DLBCL, may be associated with a micronodular pattern of infiltration that may be difficult to diagnose, and often mimics a reactive process (121,122). The spleen in these cases is markedly enlarged, but without distinct gross nodules. Small aggregates of lymphocytes and abundant histiocytes can be found

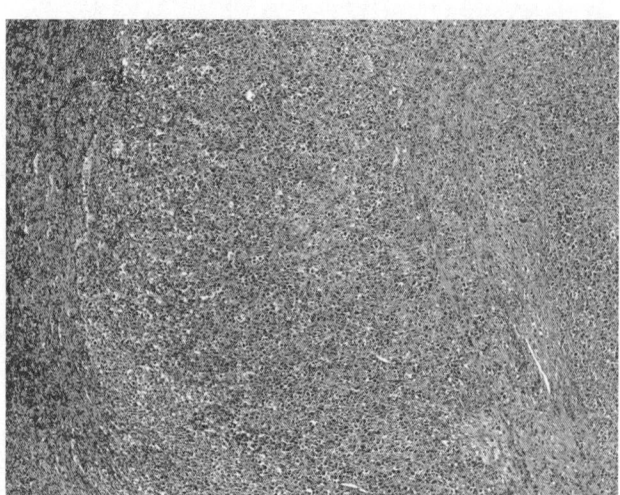
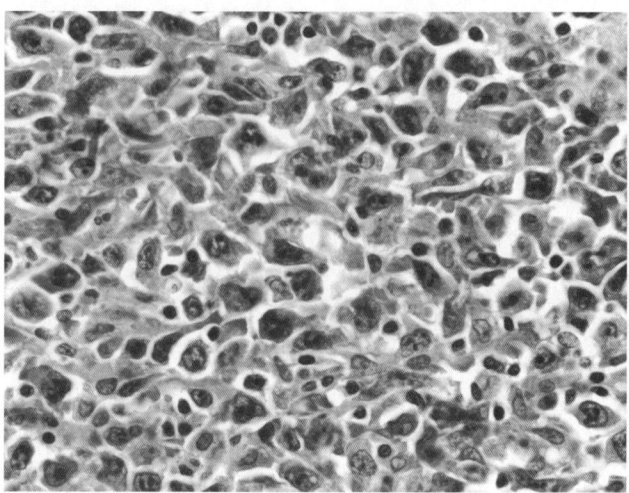

FIGURE 50.13. Diffuse large B-cell lymphoma. A: Low-power image demonstrating a tumor mass with a diffuse proliferation of lymphoid cells. **B:** High-power image demonstrating large lymphoid cells with irregular nuclei and high N:C ratio.

both in the red and in the white pulp. Present within these aggregates are scattered large lymphoid cells that may resemble centroblasts, lymphocyte predominant (LP) cells, and occasionally Reed-Sternberg cell variants. Some cases may show associated necrosis and hemorrhage. The neoplastic large cells may be difficult to identify without the use of immunohistochemical studies (121,122). By immunohistochemistry, these neoplastic cells appear to be B cells scattered within aggregates of small T cells and histiocytes lacking an underlying follicular dendritic cell meshwork.

Burkitt Lymphoma

Involvement of the spleen, lymph nodes, or liver is uncommon in Burkitt lymphoma. Grogan et al. (123) reported splenic involvement in two patients, one of whom was leukemic, and Banks and colleagues found splenic involvement in 10 of 17 cases of sporadic Burkitt lymphomas (124). Most cases have both red and white pulp involvement, although occasionally more selective involvement of the white pulp, either in the Malpighian corpuscles or in the marginal zones, is seen (125). Immunohistochemistry for TdT and CD99 can be used to distinguish Burkitt lymphoma from lymphoblastic malignancies (126–128). Demonstration of *MYC* rearrangement as well as additional genetic analysis, for example, for *BCL2* and *BCL6* gene rearrangements, may be required for correct diagnosis (see Chapter 24).

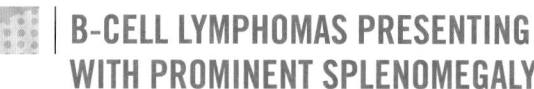

B-CELL LYMPHOMAS PRESENTING WITH PROMINENT SPLENOMEGALY

Splenic Marginal Zone Lymphoma

The term splenic marginal zone lymphoma (SMZL) was proposed by Schmid and Isaacson in 1992 (129) for a B-cell lymphoma involving the spleen and bone marrow, characterized by a micronodular tumoral infiltration that replaces the preexisting lymphoid follicles, demonstrating marginal zone differentiation as a characteristic finding. SMZL was included as a distinct entity, different from other low-grade lymphomas, such as nodal marginal zone and mucosa-associated lymphoid tissue (MALT) lymphomas, in the WHO classification of hematopoietic and lymphoid tumors in 2001 and 2008 (130,131).

Splenic marginal zone lymphoma accounts for <2% of the lymphoid malignancies. It typically presents in the sixth decade

without gender predominance. The main disease features are splenomegaly with involvement of splenic hilar lymph nodes, sometimes accompanied by autoimmune anemia or thrombocytopenia, and a variable presence of peripheral blood villous lymphocytes recognized by bipolar villous cytology. Lymphadenopathy and/or other organ involvement are infrequent but may develop during the course of the disease. A subset of patients presents with an isolated lymphocytosis with lymphocyte morphology and immunophenotype consistent with SMZL. Some of these patients subsequently develop splenomegaly but others pursue a stable course and it is unclear whether they represent an indolent variant or a benign prelymphomatous condition. About one-third of patients may have a small monoclonal serum protein, but marked hyperviscosity or hypergammaglobulinemia are uncommon (132,133). Although the etiology of SMZL is unknown, it has been suggested that, in some patients, chronic persistent antigen stimulation by an infectious agent or even by an autoantigen or a hitherto unknown foreign antigen is responsible for initiating and triggering the disease (134). A small fraction of SMZL cases harbor hepatitis C virus (HCV), more frequently in southern Europe, and therapy directed against HCV seems to also affect the control of the tumoral load in these patients, thus underlying the potential role of infectious agents in the pathogenesis of SMZL (135–138). The role of infectious agents in the pathogenesis of SMZL is also supported by the similarities between SMZL and so-called hyperreactive malarial splenomegaly (139,140).

The cut surface of the spleen in SMZL shows a characteristic miliary expansion of the white pulp. Histologically, white pulp follicles are increased in both size and number, with a variable degree of red pulp involvement being the rule. White pulp involvement may be present as the more common biphasic pattern or the less common monophasic pattern. The biphasic pattern is characterized by an inner core of small round lymphocytes that may surround or replace the germinal centers with effacement of the normal mantle zone. This zone merges with a peripheral zone of small to medium-sized marginal zone cells that have dispersed chromatin, slightly irregular nuclei, and moderately abundant, pale cytoplasm as well as variable proportions of large centroblasts or immunoblasts (Fig. 50.14A). If residual follicular centers are identified, the medium-sized neoplastic cells are arranged into broad concentric bands around the germinal center (reactive or hyalinized), a pattern that superficially may resemble reactive marginal zone hyperplasia, particularly in those patients with minimal or no splenomegaly (25–29). In marginal zone hyperplasia, however, lymphoid infiltration of the follicles by marginal zone

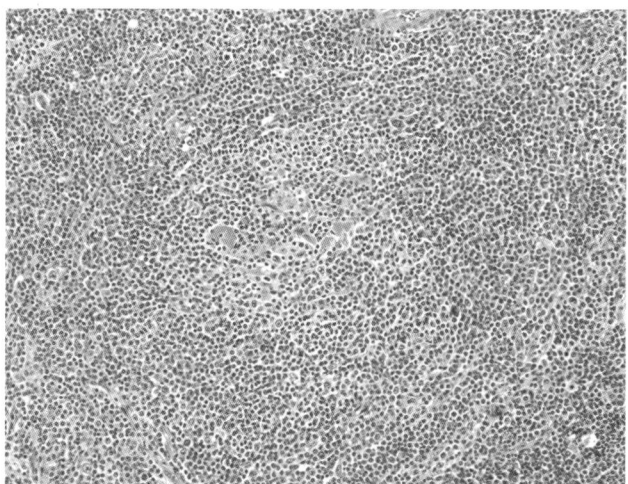

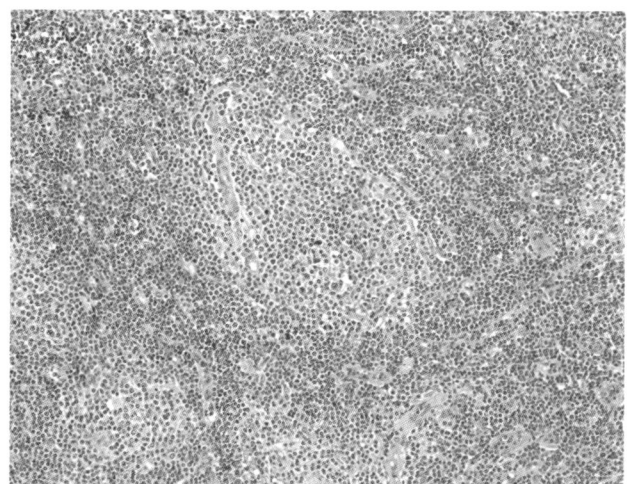

FIGURE 50.14. Splenic marginal zone lymphoma. A: Biphasic pattern. **B:** Monophasic pattern.

cells is not observed. In addition, red pulp involvement, which is a common feature in SMZL, is not seen in reactive hyperplasia. The monophasic pattern is characterized by replacement of the follicles by a markedly predominant population of marginal zone–like cells (Fig. 50.14B). The red pulp involvement in SMZL may present as a diffuse pattern of involvement with obliteration of the cords and sinuses or as nodules of lymphoid cells. Plasma cells may be present within the germinal centers or splenic red pulp. The splenic hilar lymph nodes show dilated sinuses and the germinal centers are surrounded and eventually replaced by an intimately admixed population of small lymphocytes and marginal zone cells usually without formation of a distinct "marginal" zone.

Bone marrow infiltration is the rule in SMZL, and may be present as intrasinusoidal and/or interstitial lymphomatous infiltration that mimics the architecture and cell composition of the lymphoid proliferation seen with the presence of reactive germinal centers surrounded by neoplastic lymphoid cells. Although not restricted to SMZL, intrasinusoidal lymphoma cell spread is a helpful feature that, although maybe difficult to recognize on routine morphologic sections, can be easily highlighted by CD20. In SMZL, histology seems more sensitive than flow cytometry to detect bone marrow infiltration (141). Peripheral blood involvement is less frequent than bone marrow infiltration, and is usually, but not always, characterized by the presence of small lymphocytes with rather abundant cytoplasm and short cytoplasmic projections at one or both poles of the cell (Fig. 50.15).

Immunophenotypically, the neoplastic lymphoid cells express CD20, CD79a, Bcl2, surface IgM and usually, but not always, IgD, and are negative for CD5, CD10, CD43, CD38, Bcl6, annexin A1, cyclin-D1 and usually, but not always, negative for CD103. Cases of monophasic SMZL are more commonly negative for IgD and positive for CD43 as compared to the biphasic cases (142). DBA.44 expression has been described in only a small fraction of cases (133). Petit et al. (143) demonstrated that DBA.44 positivity is more typically seen in the lymphoma cells present in the red pulp. MIB1 staining typically demonstrates a low growth fraction. In cases with a tripartite follicular pattern, MIB1 staining demonstrates a distinctive targetoid pattern, due to the presence of an increased growth fraction in both the germinal centers and the cells occupying the marginal zones (Fig. 50.16). A group of SMZL cases expressing CD5 have been shown to have a tendency to demonstrate higher lymphocytosis (144,145). Other features of these CD5+ SMZL cases overlap with those of classic SMZL cases. Low expression of

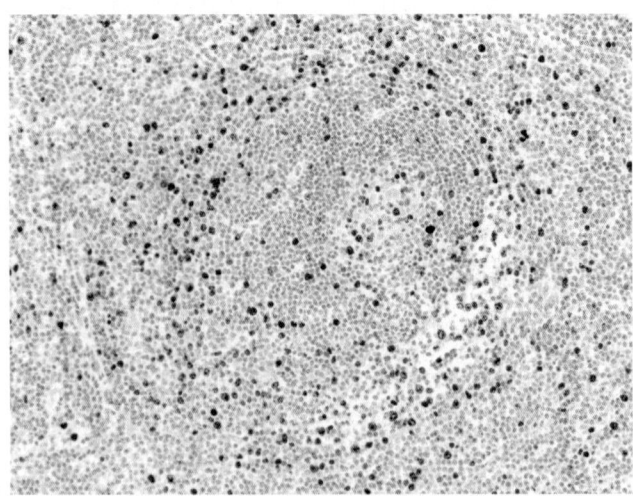

FIGURE 50.16. Targetoid pattern of MIB1 staining in SMZL.

p53 is the most common finding, although a small proportion of cases may demonstrate increased p53 expression that is commonly associated with p53 mutations.

Allelic loss of chromosome 7q31-q32 has been described in up to 40% of cases of SMZL (146). Other clonal chromosome abnormalities detected in SMZL are gain of 3q (10% to 20%) and involvement of chromosomes 1, 8, and 14 (147,148). Translocations t(11;14)(q13;q32) or t(14;18)(q21;q32) are not seen. Occasional cytogenetic abnormalities involving 14q32, such as t(6;14)(p12;q32)(148), t(10;14)(q24;q32)(149), and 7q21(with deregulation of CDK6) (150) have been reported. Translocation t(11;18)(q21;q21), common in extranodal marginal zone lymphoma of MALT (MALT lymphoma), is not identified in SMZL. Immunoglobulin heavy and light chain genes are rearranged and approximately 50% of the cases have somatic hypermutations. Analysis of the immunoglobulin genes in SMZL indicates biased utilization of selected VH1 genes (VH1.2), suggesting the role of unknown antigens in the promotion of tumoral cell growth (149). Further studies have confirmed that Ig gene stereotypes are present in up to 30% of SMZLs and are unrelated to the presence of HCV, indicating the role of unknown antigens presumably regulating the survival of the neoplastic cells (149). Gene expression profiling studies have demonstrated up-regulation of different families of genes involved in apoptosis regulation, BCR and tumor necrosis factor signaling, and nuclear factor-kappa B activation, such as SYK, BTK, BIRC3, TRAF3, TRAF5, CD40, and LTB, as well as lymphoma oncogenes such as ARHH and TCL1 (151,152). The increased expression of TCL1 has been proposed by Thieblemont et al. (153) to be associated with AKT1 activation in SMZL.

Splenic marginal zone lymphoma is a low-grade tumor, with a survival probability at 5 years that varies from 65% (for patients diagnosed after splenectomy) to 78% (for patients diagnosed in peripheral blood). Adverse clinical prognostic factors relate to a high tumor burden and poor performance status (154). Thus, different studies have identified anemia, high lactate dehydrogenase levels, hypoalbuminemia, and peripheral lymphadenopathy as clinical prognostic markers, whereas biologic parameters reported to be associated with adverse outcome are p53 mutation or overexpression, 7q deletion, and unmutated IgVH genes (151,155,156). In the prerituximab era, the treatment of choice for SMZL patients with symptomatic splenomegaly or threatening cytopenia was splenectomy, since chemotherapy had limited efficacy. Responses to splenectomy occurred in approximately 90% of patients. Since approval of rituximab, treatment of such patients with the anti-CD20 antibody, both alone and in combination with chemotherapy, has

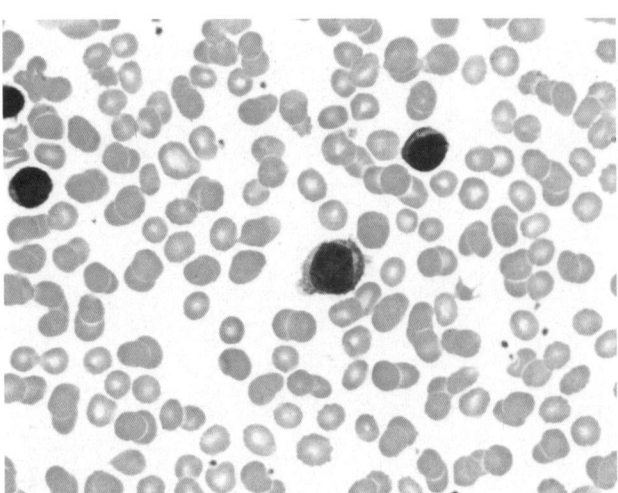

FIGURE 50.15. SMZL involving peripheral blood: lymphocytes with abundant cytoplasm and short bipolar cytoplasmic projections.

shown significant responses in some studies. In one retrospective series of rituximab monotherapy totaling 52 patients, including both chemotherapy-naive and refractory patients, overall responses of 88% to 100% were noted with marked and prompt regression of splenomegaly and improvement of cytopenias (157–159). Similarly, fludarabine has been shown to be effective in the treatment of SMZL in some studies (160). HCV-positive patients appear to benefit from antiviral therapy (138,157).

Patients with SMZL appear to have a greater frequency of transformation (13% of SMZL with adequate follow-up) to large B-cell lymphoma compared with chronic lymphocytic leukemia (1% to 10%), although the incidence of large cell transformation in SMZL is lower than in follicular lymphoma (25% to 60%) (157,161). The site of transformation seems to be important for therapy, since transformation in bone marrow has been showed to be refractory to therapy in contrast to transformation in the lymph node (162).

Although it is recognized that spleen histology is the hallmark for the diagnosis of SMZL, a diagnosis of SMZL can be established in patients in whom this information is lacking, when adequate studies are carried out. In the latter patients, the diagnosis can and should be made by compounding peripheral blood lymphocyte morphology (if there are circulating lymphoma cells) with the bone marrow histology and immunophenotype, provided that other small B-cell disorders are excluded by carrying out FISH analysis for the t(14;18), t(11;14), and CLL-associated cytogenetic findings particularly in SMZL cases in which the lymphoid cells are CD5 positive (134).

The differential diagnosis of SMZL includes splenic diffuse red pulp small B-cell lymphoma (SDRPBCL), hairy cell leukemia variant (HCL-v) (see below), and other small B-cell lymphomas, including FL, MCL, CLL/SLL, and LPL (Table 50.3).

A micronodular pattern with marginal zone differentiation can occasionally be seen in both FL and MCL, and with lesser frequency in LPL and CLL/SLL. The main morphologic feature useful for differential diagnosis lies in the different cytologic composition of the white pulp tumoral nodules. SMZL is distinguished by its characteristic dimorphic cytology in most cases, different from the monomorphic cytology of MCL, and the distinctive mixture of centroblasts and small-cleaved cells, which is seen in FL. CLL/SLL may be identified on the basis of its monotonous small lymphocytic cytology in conjunction with the presence of scattered prolymphocytes and paraimmunoblasts. Immunohistochemistry is recommended for the differential diagnosis. CLL/SLL cells typically express CD5 and CD23. The recognition of MCL is facilitated by the identification of cyclin D1 and CD5 reactivity, while FL can be recognized by its frequent CD10 positivity, by the lack of IgD expression, or by molecular or fluorescence *in situ* hybridization analysis for BCL2 gene rearrangement. The differential diagnosis with LPL may be difficult because old series of LPL have included cases that now are considered to fall into the spectrum of SMZL. Thus, SMZL may demonstrate a gradient of plasmacytic differentiation with serum monoclonal paraproteinemia in a subset of cases (132,133). Cases diagnosed as LPL show prominent plasmacytic differentiation, lack the features of the other lymphoma types, and are often associated with the syndrome of WM. Bone marrow trephine examination may be useful because LPL is typically associated with areas of diffuse lymphoplasmacytic marrow involvement; if lymphoid aggregates with a marginal zone pattern or intrasinusoidal involvement are recognized, a diagnosis of SMZL may be suspected. Finally, on splenectomy specimens, the pattern of infiltration of LPL is typically diffuse red pulp involvement, in contrast to the nodular involvement of both white and red pulp in SMZL (163,164).

Table 50.3	SUMMARY OF FEATURES OF SMZL, HCL, SDRPBCL, AND HCL-V			
	SMZL	**HCL**	**SDRPBCL**	**HCL-v**
Age and sex	Sixth decade. No gender predominance	Sixth decade Male predominance	>60 y Slight male predominance	Middle aged to elderly Slight male predominance
Clinical presentation	Splenomegaly; lymphadenopathy and other organ involvement is rare	Splenomegaly with pancytopenia and monocytopenia	Splenomegaly with low level of lymphocytosis; few cases with cutaneous involvement	Splenomegaly with high WBC count; some patients also with thrombocytopenia and/or anemia
Peripheral blood involvement	Lymphocytes with bipolar villous cytology	Lymphocytes with circumferential hairy cytoplasmic projections	Lymphocytes with bipolar villous lymphocytes or broad based cytoplasmic projections	Lymphocytes with abundant villi, basophilic cytoplasm, round to indented nuclei with prominent nucleoli
Gross appearance of spleen	Miliary expansion of white pulp	Homogeneous dark red appearance with blood lakes	Homogeneous red-brown appearance with lack of nodularity	Homogeneous dark red appearance, blood lakes may be present
Histologic features of spleen	Involvement of white pulp with biphasic cytology in most cases, some degree of red pulp involvement is usually present	Red pulp involvement including cords and sinuses; blood lakes present	Red pulp involvement with usually obliteration of the white pulp	Red pulp involvement with atrophic or absent white pulp; blood lakes may be present
Bone marrow involvement	Intrasinusoidal or interstitial lymphoid aggregates	Interstitial involvement	Intrasinusoidal, interstitial, or intertrabecular lymphoid aggregates	Usually interstitial involvement, may be nodular
Immunophenotype of neoplastic lymphoid cells	Positive for CD20, CD79a, BCL2, IgM, usually positive for IgD (except monomorphic cases), negative for CD10, annexin-A1, cyclin D1, usually negative for CD5, CD43 (except monomorphic cases), and CD103; DBA.44 positive in lymphoma cells in red pulp	Positive for CD20, annexin-A1, TRAP, DBA.44, CD25, CD11c, CD103, CD123; cyclin D1 positive in 50% of cases	Positive for CD20, DBA.44, BCL2, IgG, often positive for p53, variable positivity for CD11c, CD103 and IgD, and negative for CD25, CD10, CD23, BCL6, and annexin-A1	Positive for CD20, CD11c, DBA.44, usually positive for CD103, negative for CD10, CD23, CD25, CD27, CD5, annexin-A1, TRAP, and CD123
Cytogenetic and molecular abnormalities	Allelic loss of 7q31-q32, gain of 3q, involvement of chromosomes 1, 8, and 14	Positive for BRAF V600E mutations in most cases	Some cases may show deletion 7q, trisomy 18, partial trisomy 3	Negative for BRAF V600E mutations

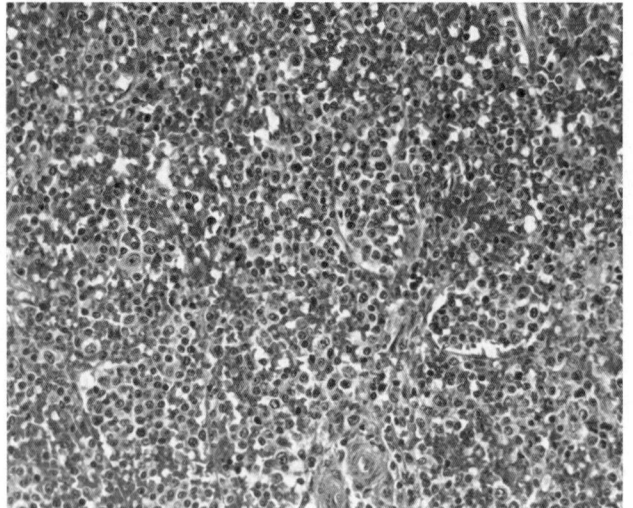

FIGURE 50.17. Hairy cell leukemia. Tumor cells in the splenic cords and red pulp sinusoids.

Hairy Cell Leukemia

In hairy cell leukemia (HCL), most patients present with prominent splenomegaly associated with pancytopenia, lack of lymphadenopathy, and characteristic hairy cells in the peripheral blood (165–167). The gross appearance of the spleen is homogeneously dark red, with variably sized hemorrhagic areas, so-called blood lakes. The white pulp is inconspicuous. The hairy cells, in splenic touch imprints, appear as medium-sized atypical lymphoid cells with homogeneous chromatin, inconspicuous nucleoli, and moderate amounts of clear to pink cytoplasm, and typical surface projections. A pericellular clear halo, so-called fried egg appearance, is often seen in histology sections. Tumor cells infiltrate both the splenic cords and the red pulp sinuses (Fig. 50.17), and subendothelial invasion of the trabecular veins may be prominent (165,167–170). Blood lakes lacking endothelial linings and lined by hairy cells are often seen (Fig 50.18). The infiltrate in HCL may resemble T-cell large granular lymphocytic leukemia (T-LGL) or T-cell lymphomas (HSTCL in particular). Mastocytosis in the spleen may occasionally resemble HCL; however, the characteristic trabecular distribution and associated fibrosis of mastocytosis are not

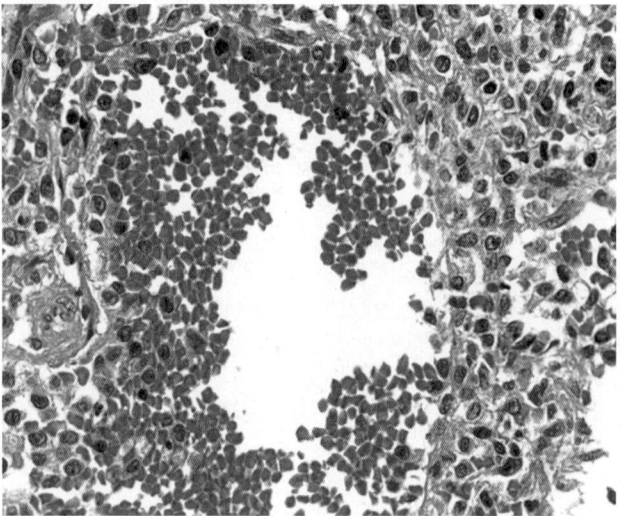

FIGURE 50.18. Hairy cell leukemia. Blood lakes lacking endothelial cells and lined by hairy cells.

seen in HCL. Characteristic tartrate-resistant acid phosphatase (TRAP) positivity can be demonstrated on touch imprints of the spleen and in tissue sections by immunohistochemistry in HCL. Other useful markers include annexin A1 (the most specific), DBA.44, CD25, and CD123. In addition, hairy cells characteristically express CD103 and CD11c by flow cytometry examination. Nuclear positivity for cyclin D1 can be seen in up to 50% of cases (171). Confusion with MCL is, however, extremely unlikely as the cytology and histology of MCL is quite different from HCL. Neoplastic cells may also have immunohistochemically detectable CD10 expression in up to 20% of cases but this is not associated with altered prognosis (172,173) (see Chapter 36). Whole exome sequencing of HCL cells in parallel with normal cells has recently revealed the presence of the BRAF V600E mutation in most cases of HCL tested (174). The association of typical HCL and BRAF V600E mutation has been confirmed in other studies as well (175–177). Recently, Xi et al. (178) demonstrated the absence of BRAF V600E mutation in a subset of typical HCL cases. However, since this mutation has been shown to be present in most cases of HCL and absent in other hematologic malignancies, it has been suggested as a useful tool that can be employed in routine diagnostic laboratories to identify cases of HCL.

Splenic B-Cell Lymphoma/Leukemia, Unclassifiable

There are a number of variably well-defined entities that represent small B-cell clonal lymphoproliferations involving the spleen, but that do not fall into any of the other types of B-cell lymphoid neoplasms recognized in the WHO classification. The two best defined of these relatively rare provisional entities are SDRPBCL and HCL-v. The relationship of SDRPBCL to HCL-v and other primary splenic B-cell lymphomas remains uncertain, and their precise diagnostic criteria are not fully established. Other splenic small B-cell lymphomas not fulfilling the criteria for either of these provisional entities or for other better-established B-cell lymphomas should be diagnosed as splenic B-cell lymphoma/leukemia, unclassifiable.

Splenic Diffuse Red Pulp Small B-Cell Lymphoma

Splenic diffuse red pulp small B-cell lymphoma (SDRPBCL) is now recognized as a provisional entity in the 2008 update of the WHO Classification (87), and initially identified as a potential variant of SMZL with a diffuse pattern of splenic involvement (179). It is an uncommon lymphoma with a diffuse pattern of involvement of the splenic red pulp by small monomorphous B lymphocytes. The neoplasm also involves bone marrow sinusoids and peripheral blood, commonly with a villous cytology. This entity is not fully characterized and needs additional molecular studies for defining its main features and diagnostic markers. This diagnosis should be restricted to characteristic cases, fulfilling the major features described below and not used for any lymphoma growing diffusely in the spleen. Chronic lymphocytic leukemia, HCL, LPL, and PLL must be excluded with appropriate studies before rendering this diagnosis.

The criteria for SDRPBCL recognition have mainly been based on spleen histology. Mollejo et al. (179) described four cases of splenic B-cell lymphomas with red pulp involvement. These cases showed some overlapping features with SMZL as well as HCL-v; however they showed certain features that differed from these two entities. These cases showed diffuse red pulp involvement by lymphoma with obliteration of the white pulp and absence of micronodular tumor growth pattern that is characteristic of SMZL. They differed from SMZL immunophenotypically by lack of staining for IgD and presence of p53 inactivation or anomalous p53 staining. Additionally, these cases showed cutaneous involvement as erythematous and pruritic

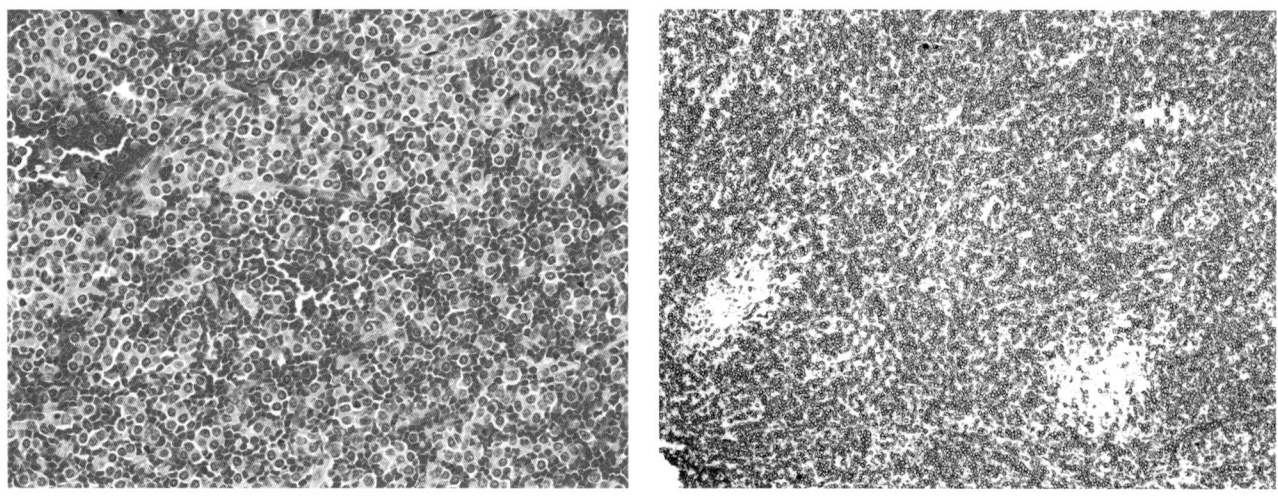

FIGURE 50.19. Splenic diffuse red pulp B-cell lymphoma. A: Diffuse red pulp involvement with infiltration of sinusoids and cords by lymphoma cells. **B:** CD20 highlighting diffuse proliferation of B cells in the red pulp.

papules. Two other studies evaluated the clinical, morphologic, immunophenotypic, and genetic features of similar cases (180,181). Although it still remains uncertain if SDRPBCLs represent a separate distinct category of splenic B-cell lymphomas, the description below represents a summary of findings based on the available published literature on cases felt to be compatible with SDRPBCL based on the 2008 WHO classification.

Splenic diffuse red pulp small B-cell lymphoma is a rare disorder representing approximately 10% of the B-cell lymphomas diagnosed in splenectomy specimens. Most patient are over 60 years of age with a slight male predominance. Patients frequently have massive splenomegaly, a relatively low lymphocytosis with infrequent B symptoms, and usually present as clinical stage IV with spleen, bone marrow, and peripheral blood involvement. A few cases, in addition, have cutaneous involvement as erythematous and pruritic papules. Liver involvement is infrequent and involvement of lymph nodes other than splenic hilar lymph nodes is extremely rare. Presence of a monoclonal serum paraprotein was identified in only 1 of 18 cases studied by Kanellis et al. (180).

Gross examination of the spleen shows a homogeneous red-brown cut surface without nodularity. Microscopically, there is a diffuse pattern of red pulp involvement with infiltration in the sinusoids and cords. Pseudosinuses lined by tumoral lymphoid cells may be seen. There is effacement or partial atrophy of

the white pulp (Fig. 50.19). Follicular replacement, biphasic cytology, or marginal zone infiltration, characteristic of SMZL, are not seen. The neoplastic infiltrate is composed of a monomorphous population of small to medium-sized lymphoid cells with round and regular nuclei and vesicular nuclei with occasional small distinct nucleoli. Occasional scattered nucleolated larger cells may be present. The lymphoid cells have pale or lightly eosinophilic cytoplasm.

The bone marrow may show more frequently, a subtle intrasinusoidal infiltration, or less commonly an interstitial or intertrabecular nodular involvement by lymphoma cells (Fig. 50.20). Peripheral blood involvement is characterized by villous lymphocytes (Fig. 50.20). While Traverse-Glehen suggested a distinct villous morphology for these cases (181), Kanellis et al. (180) showed villous lymphocytes similar to those in SMZL. The skin involvement is characterized by patches of dermal infiltrate around the cutaneous appendages and blood vessels with the presence of epidermotropism.

Characteristically, the lymphoid cells are positive for CD20, DBA.44, bcl-2, and IgG and show absence of staining for CD25, CD10, CD23, bcl-6, and annexin-A1. While some studies showed absence of staining for IgD, CD11c, and CD103 (179), other studies have demonstrated expression of these markers in a subset of cases (180,181). Cases demonstrating expression of IgM with

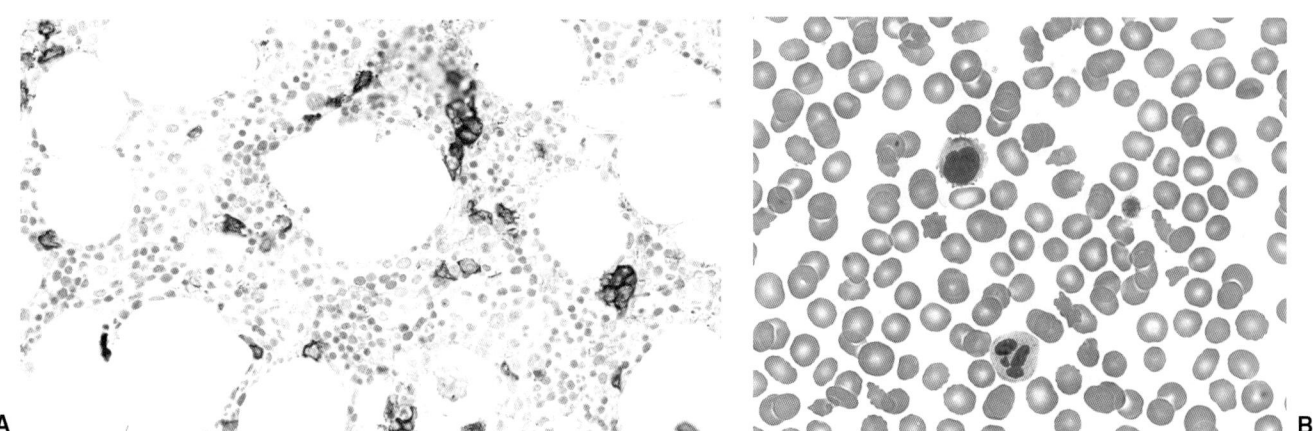

FIGURE 50.20. Splenic diffuse red pulp B cell lymphoma. A: Bone marrow involvement highlighted by immunohistochemical stain for CD20. **B:** Peripheral blood involvement by lymphocytes with villous cytoplasmic projections.

or without IgG, CD5, and CD123 have also been reported (181). P53 expression is more common than in SMZL (179).

Cases of SDRPBCL harbor a relatively low load of IGHV somatic hypermutation, with overrepresentation of IGHV3–23 and IGHV4–34 without biased usage of IGHV1–2 as seen in SMZL (181). Most cases show no clonal chromosomal abnormalities (66%), with some cases harboring chromosome 7q deletion, complete trisomy 18, and partial trisomy 3q. SDRPBCL is an indolent but incurable disease with a reported good response after splenectomy.

The differential diagnosis of SDRPBCL includes SMZL and HCL-v. Cases of SDRPBCL lack the characteristic micronodular growth pattern seen in SMZL. HCL-v shows a greater degree of lymphocytosis than that seen in SDRPBCL and is morphologically characterized by at least some lymphoid cells with prominent nucleoli. However, in some cases it may be difficult to distinguish HCL-v from SDRPBCL. In our opinion, such cases should be classified as splenic B-cell lymphoma/leukemia, unclassifiable until additional features to distinguish between the two entities are established.

Hairy Cell Leukemia variant

As defined in the 2008 WHO classification, the designation hairy cell leukemia-variant (HCL-v) encompasses cases that resemble classic HCL, but exhibit variant "cytohematologic" features (i.e., leukocytosis, presence of monocytes, cells with prominent nucleoli, convoluted nuclei or absence of circumferential shaggy contours), variant immunophenotype, that is, absence of CD25, annexin-A1, or TRAP, and resistance to conventional HCL therapy, that is, lack of dramatic response to cladribine. It is an uncommon B-cell neoplasm accounting for 10% to 20% of HCL patients and 0.4% of chronic lymphoid malignancies (182,183). It usually affects middle-aged to elderly patients with a slight male predominance (184). HCL-v patients are characterized by splenomegaly typically associated with a high white blood cell count without neutropenia or monocytopenia with involved bone marrow that can be easily aspirated. Hepatomegaly and lymphadenopathy are relatively uncommon. Patients present with signs and symptoms related to splenomegaly or cytopenias. Thrombocytopenia is present in approximately 50%, and anemia in about 25%, of the patients with HCL-v (184).

Morphologically, circulating HCL-v cells are easily identified on the PB smear and show features overlapping prolymphocytic leukemia and classical HCL (Fig. 50.21). They contain abundant villi, an intensely basophilic cytoplasm, and central,

round, occasionally bilobed, indented hyperchromatic nuclei with prominent nucleoli. Bone marrow involvement usually presents as an interstitial infiltration, similar to that seen in most cases of classical HCL, although a mixed pattern of interstitial as well as nodular pattern of involvement can also be seen (184) (see Chapter 36). The histologic features of HCL-v in the spleen are similar to those found in classical HCL with diffuse involvement of the red pulp with atrophic or absent white pulp. The leukemic cells fill dilated sinusoids and red blood cell lakes may be present in some cases (Fig. 50.22).

Immunophenotypically, HCL-v cells demonstrate expression of mature B-lymphocyte antigens including CD19, CD20, and CD22, and FMC-7 with bright monotypic surface immunoglobulin expression. The leukemic cells are positive for DBA.44 and CD11c, show variable expression of CD103, and are negative for CD10, CD23, CD25, CD27, CD5, annexin-A1, TRAP, and CD123.

There are no known specific genetic changes in HCL-v. Some cases may show complex cytogenetic abnormalities involving 14q32 or 8q24 and TP53 deletions (185). Unlike cases of classical HCL, BRAF V600E mutation has not been identified in cases of HCL-v (175–177).

Patients with HCL-v typically do not respond to either interferon-alpha or purine nucleoside analogs. Good clinical and hematologic responses after splenectomy have been observed in some patients (184). Some reports have demonstrated that patients with HCL-v can be successfully treated with rituximab as well as anti-CD22 immunotoxin (186). Single case reports suggest that alemtuzumab (anti-CD52 antibody) is an active agent in HCL-v (187,188).

Another distinct variant of HCL known as HCL Japanese variant (HCL-Jv) has been identified in Japan (189,190). HCL-Jv is more frequent in females and presents with splenomegaly without peripheral lymphadenopathy. In contrast to classical HCL, but similar to HCL-v, HCL-Jv patients usually demonstrate leukocytosis and an easily aspirable bone marrow. The HCL-Jv cells have abundant pale cytoplasm with villous projections, round hyperchromatic nuclei, and inconspicuous nucleoli and rarely contain ribosome-lamella complexes. HCL-Jv, like HCL-v, is characteristically CD11c and CD22 positive, always CD24 and CD25 negative, and usually CD103 negative (191). The leukemic cells are also CD10⁻, CD24⁻, and sIg negative or weakly positive. Staining for TRAP is negative in up to one-half of cases. As in classical HCL and HCL-v, leukemic cells of HCL-Jv preferentially infiltrate splenic red pulp. Hairy cell leukemia, Japanese variant, shows an indolent clinical course.

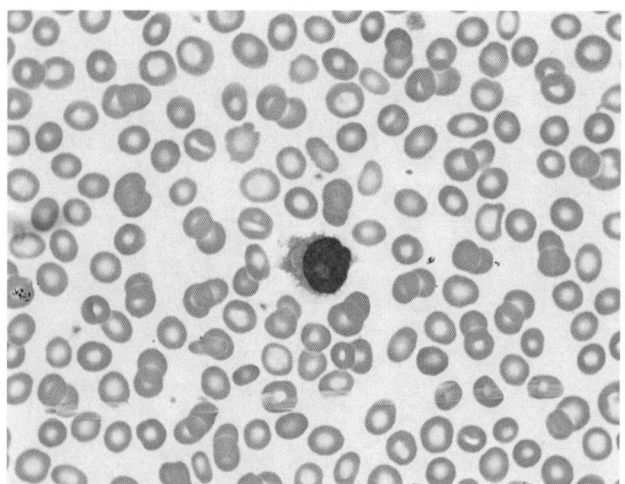

FIGURE 50.21. HCL-v involving peripheral blood. Lymphocyte with fine cytoplasmic hairy projections and nucleus with prominent nucleolus.

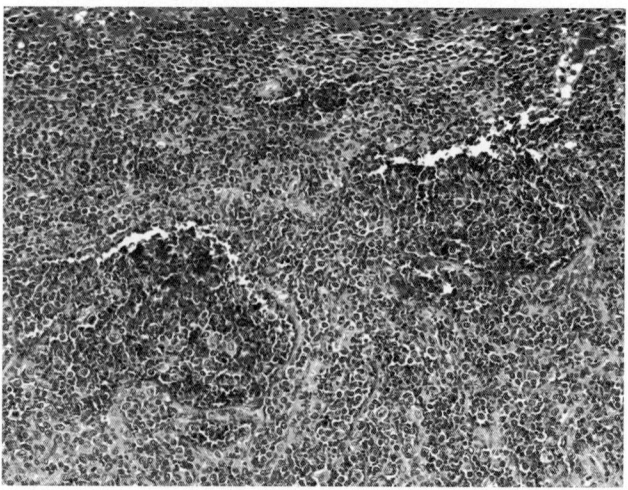

FIGURE 50.22. Hairy cell leukemia involving splenic red pulp with formation of blood lakes.

PLASMA CELL NEOPLASMS

Plasma cell neoplasms comprise a heterogeneous group of neoplastic conditions associated with monoclonal immunoglobulin production. These conditions can affect both the red and the white pulp of the spleen. A common finding is evidence of immunoglobulin production, manifested by the presence of plasma cells or plasmacytoid lymphocytes with periodic acid-Schiff (PAS)–positive cytoplasmic globules (Mott cells) and intranuclear and cytoplasmic immunoglobulin inclusions (Dutcher and Russell bodies, respectively).

Plasma Cell Myeloma

Splenomegaly is rarely clinically significant in patients who have plasma cell myeloma (PCM). However, the organ may be extensively involved, particularly in the presence of plasma cell leukemia (192). Although rare, splenic rupture may be associated with myelomatous involvement of the spleen (193). Splenomegaly in PCM may also result from amyloid deposition. In rare cases, light chain deposition only (without amyloid) has been described in myeloma patients. Rarely, excess light chain is taken up by histiocytes, causing the so-called crystal-storing histiocytosis (194). Masses of crystals produce engorged histiocytes, which morphologically may resemble Gaucher cells. These crystals often are only weakly positive with immunohistochemical stains for light chains, possibly due to partial lysosomal degradation or masking of immunoglobulin epitopes in the crystal structure. This can be accompanied by a foreign body type of granulomatous reaction. Although exceeding rare, this phenomenon needs to be distinguished from cases of coexistent multiple myeloma and Gaucher disease, which has been reported in the literature (195). The neoplastic plasma cells either infiltrate the red pulp diffusely or, rarely, produce grossly visible nodules.

Hepatosplenomegaly is a common feature of the POEMS syndrome (196), in which an osteosclerotic variant of myeloma occurs in association with polyneuropathy, organomegaly, endocrinopathy, the presence of a monoclonal paraprotein, and hyperpigmentation of the skin.

The pattern of involvement of the spleen in plasma cell leukemia resembles that seen in other leukemic processes. Cytopenias resulting from hypersplenism (197,198) and splenic rupture have occasionally been reported in patients with plasma cell leukemia (199,200) (see Chapter 37).

Primary Amyloidosis

Although both primary and secondary amyloidosis may involve the spleen, splenic involvement is more common in the latter. Early in the disease, amyloid is deposited in the walls of small blood vessels. A nodular deposition of amyloid in the white pulp produces the miliary, or "sago," pattern, whereas the "lardaceous" spleen results from larger, more expansive sheets of amyloid in the sinuses of the red pulp. In primary amyloidosis, the spleen often contains an increased number of plasma cells and less numerous plasmacytoid lymphocytes. In a large percentage of these cases, monoclonal plasma cells with lambda light chain restriction can be demonstrated (see Chapter 37). Functional hyposplenism may occur with extensive amyloid deposition (198). Splenic rupture has also been reported in association with splenic amyloidosis (201–203).

Heavy Chain Diseases

Splenic involvement may be a feature of both γ and μ heavy chain diseases. Splenic involvement has not been reported in alpha heavy chain disease. Patients with these disorders usually have a serum paraprotein that consists of an intact but structurally abnormal heavy chain. Heavy chain disease is not associated with amyloid deposition. Gamma heavy chain (Franklin) disease is a variant of LPL and has comparable morphology. In addition to involvement of Waldeyer ring, hepatosplenomegaly and generalized lymphadenopathy are features of γ heavy chain disease (204–206) (see Chapter 37). A diffuse infiltrate of lymphocytes and plasmacytoid cells results in obliteration of the white pulp. Eosinophils and immunoblasts may be prominent. In contrast, μ heavy chain disease is a B-cell lymphoproliferative disorder resembling CLL (207,208). The spleen is infiltrated by plasma cells that have typically vacuolated cytoplasm and Russell bodies.

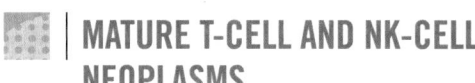

MATURE T-CELL AND NK-CELL NEOPLASMS

Mature T-cell and NK-cell malignancies are relatively uncommon and there have been only few descriptive studies of splenic involvement by these lymphomas. Among the nonleukemic forms, splenic involvement is relatively commonly seen in cases of advanced stage mycosis fungoides (MF)/Sezary syndrome. Splenic involvement in MF usually affects the white and red pulp alike (209). The marginal zones and the PALS are infiltrated by large atypical cells, associated with both diffuse and patchy nodular involvement in the red pulp (209,210). Not all cells have cerebriform nuclear contours, and a variable proportion of the tumor cells may appear blastic.

The node-based peripheral T-cell lymphomas (PTCL) are perhaps the least well-studied group of T-cell neoplasms that occur in the spleen. We have seen a variety of patterns of involvement, some expanding the PALS, some producing discrete masses, and one mimicking the pattern of involvement seen in MF. The lymphoepithelioid cell (Lennert) PTCL variant (211), a cytologic subtype of PTCL unspecified, is characterized by a high content of epithelioid histiocytes. Early involvement usually occurs in the peripheral zones of follicles and the PALS, consistent with the T-cell origin of this lymphoma. The epithelioid histiocytes tend to localize in a ringlike arrangement at the periphery of the white pulp, although they occasionally form clusters (34). Although originally thought to be characteristic for this type of lymphoma, the ringlike arrangement of epithelioid cells may be seen in other forms of lymphoma of both B- and T-cell type. The epithelioid cells may be difficult to differentiate from the sarcoidal type of granulomas sometimes seen in the spleens of patients with Hodgkin lymphoma (211). Some cases of PTCL with marked splenomegaly have been associated with the hemophagocytic syndrome (212,213). In these cases expansion of the red pulp predominates, and the erythrophagocytic histiocytes may overshadow the neoplastic T cells. A hemophagocytic syndrome may be seen with both T-cell and NK-cell malignancies, many of which are EBV-associated (see below).

Angioimmunoblastic T-Cell Lymphoma

In addition to generalized lymphadenopathy, fever, weight loss, and a pruritic rash, hepatosplenomegaly often is a presenting feature in patients who have angioimmunoblastic T-cell lymphoma (214–217) (see Chapter 38). The majority of descriptions of the morphology of the spleen in this disorder have come from autopsy series. Splenectomy occasionally has been performed in cases associated with severe hemolytic anemia (218). A variety of patterns of involvement have been described; in some a polymorphic infiltrate predominates in the marginal zones (Fig. 50.23). Focal aggregates of large lymphoid cells also are seen in the surrounding red pulp (219). There may

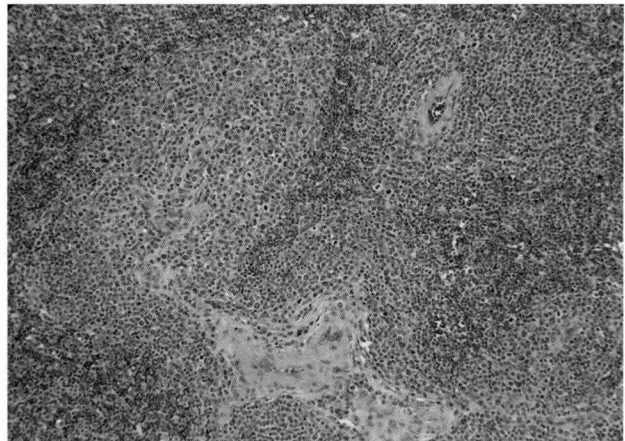

FIGURE 50.23. Angioimmunoblastic T-cell lymphoma demonstrating a polymorphous infiltrate in the marginal zones.

be an increased reticulin content in the marginal zone causing perifollicular fibrosis. Other authors have described nonspecific reactive follicular hyperplasia (218). Other cases show a more extensive pattern of involvement, with large nodules involving both white and red pulp (217). However, the characteristic arborizing vascular network typically seen in lymph nodes has not been reported in the spleen. The majority of the reports in the older literature were based on autopsy series, and other findings such as lymphoid depletion and diffuse fibrosis may reflect end-stage disease or therapeutic effects.

Anaplastic Large Cell Lymphoma

Anaplastic large cell lymphoma (ALCL) as defined in the 2008 WHO classification is a neoplasm of CD30-positive lymphoid cells of T-cell or null-cell lineage and consists of two subtypes: ALK-positive and ALK-negative cases (see Chapter 38). Splenic ALCL is rare and includes both ALK-positive and ALK-negative cases. They may include primary ALCL (81,220,221) or secondary involvement of the spleen in cases with leukemic phase of ALCL (222). They may present with a splenic mass, splenic abscess, and rarely with splenic rupture (219). Morphologically, the lymphoma cells can have the appearance of classic ALCL or the small cell variant. Cases of splenic ALCL with a leukemic phase have a very aggressive clinical course,

even when they are ALK positive, as compared to nodal ALK-positive ALCL (222).

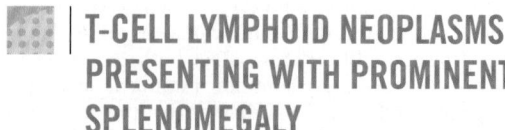

T-CELL LYMPHOID NEOPLASMS PRESENTING WITH PROMINENT SPLENOMEGALY

There are several types of T-cell lymphoma and leukemia that present with splenomegaly and distinct clinicopathologic characteristics that require separate discussion.

Hepatosplenic T-Cell Lymphoma

Hepatosplenic T-cell lymphoma (HSTCL) is a distinct clinical entity characterized by hepatosplenomegaly, sinusoidal tropism, and, in most cases, T-cell gamma/delta receptor nonactivated cytotoxic phenotype of the malignant cells (223–225). The normal cell counterpart for HSTCL is thought to be a functionally immature cytotoxic gamma/delta T cell of the splenic pool with V-delta1 gene usage (226). A number of HSTCL cases have been reported in the setting of chronic immune suppression or prolonged antigen stimulation, particularly in patients receiving long-term immunosuppressive therapy for solid organ transplantation (227–229). It typically occurs in young adults, more frequently males, and is associated with a poor prognosis. The presenting symptoms include fever, weight loss, hepatosplenomegaly, and variable cytopenias. Some cases of HSTCL are associated with a hemophagocytic syndrome, a condition that once was termed "erythrophagocytic T-gamma lymphoma" (230). Macroscopically, the spleen is enlarged, usually weighing 3,000 g or more, with a homogeneous cut surface and loss of white pulp markings. Histologically, the neoplastic cells infiltrate the red pulp cords and sinuses (Fig. 50.24). The lymphoid cells are usually of medium size with oval or folded nuclei displaying chromatin that is less condensed than that of small lymphocytes, and a moderate amount of pale cytoplasm. Occasional cases with larger, more blastic-appearing cells have also been described. The histologic appearance of the spleen may mimic HCL (225). However, in HSTCL, blood lakes are not seen. In addition, the immunophenotypic differences are distinctive. The main histologic feature of liver as well as bone marrow involvement is an intrasinusoidal distribution of the neoplastic cells. However, an interstitial marrow infiltrate may be present in many cases.

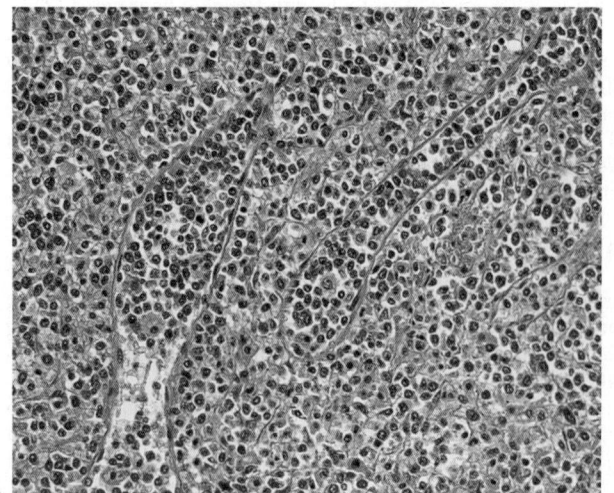

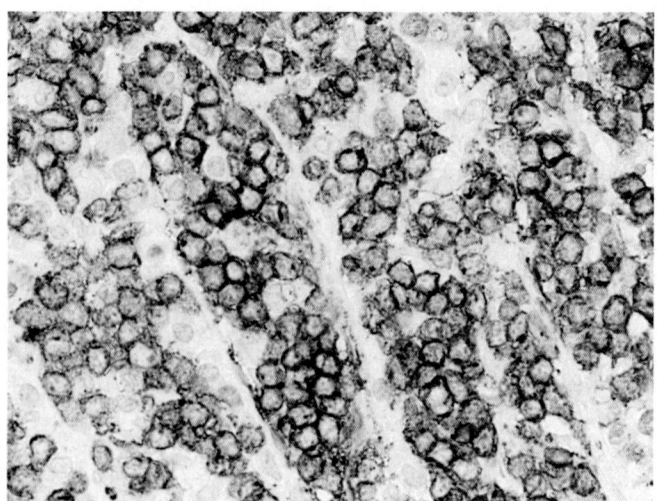

FIGURE 50.24. Hepatosplenic T-cell lymphoma. A: Lymphoma cells infiltrating the splenic cords and sinusoids. **B:** CD3 highlighting neoplastic T cells within splenic sinusoids.

Immunophenotypically, the neoplastic cells are usually positive for CD2, CD3, CD56, may express CD16 and CD7, and are negative for CD4, CD5, CD8, CD57, CD25, and CD30. The neoplastic cells can rarely be CD4−/CD8+. CD5 positivity has been reported in a few cases (231). The neoplastic cells are positive for TIA-1 and negative for granzyme B and perforin. Most cases express the gamma/delta T-cell receptor (223,225), although some cases also express the alpha/beta receptor (224,230,232); αβ HSTCL has clinicopathologic and cytogenetic features similar to those of γδ HSTCL cases and, therefore, is currently considered a variant of the disease. EBV infection has been reported rarely and has been associated with cytologic features of transformation, suggesting that EBV might be involved secondarily (227).

Evidence has suggested a strong association between HSTCL and the presence of isochromosome 7q10 (225,233). Other cytogenetic abnormalities that may be seen in HSTCL include trisomy 8 and loss of Y chromosome. Southern blot and polymerase chain reaction studies have demonstrated monoclonal *TCRδ*, *TCRβ*, and *TCRγ* chain gene rearrangements.

The differential diagnosis includes both B-cell and T-cell lymphomas. A careful review of the morphology and immunohistochemical stains will allow separation from B-cell lymphomas. Rarely T-cell prolymphocytic leukemia (T-PLL) can present with predominant splenic involvement in the absence of prominent leukocytosis. In these cases, the spleen histology shows a predominant involvement of the red pulp similar to that seen in cases of HSTCL. However, a variable degree of white pulp involvement is always present in T-PLL (23,234). This important characteristic, which is also useful to separate T-PLL from large granular lymphocyte (LGL) leukemia, can be better appreciated by using immunohistology (234). Immunohistochemistry can be helpful in the differential diagnosis, for example, by demonstrating coexpression of CD4 and CD8 and expression of BF-1 in T-PLL cases or lack of these antigens by cells of γδHSTCL. Immunohistochemistry can also be used to separate HSTCL from rare cases of nonleukemic NK-/T-cell lymphoproliferative disorders including LGL (particularly the gamma/delta variant), as well as from other types of PTCL involving the spleen. The salient features of HSTCL, T-PLL, and LGL leukemias are summarized in Table 50.4 (see also Chapter 38).

Patients with HSTCL usually have a rapidly progressive clinical course and poor prognosis. Therapeutic strategies efficacious for aggressive B-cell lymphomas are ineffective for HSTCL. Most patients die within 2 years of diagnosis, even if a remission is achieved initially. In some studies, the efficacy of a platinum-cytarabine–based induction regimen and 2′-deoxycoformycin (pentostatin) has been suggested (227).

T-Cell Prolymphocytic Leukemia

T-cell prolymphocytic leukemia (T-PLL) is a rare leukemic condition that presents with high lymphocyte count and generalized lymphadenopathy and hepatosplenomegaly. The circulating lymphocytes may be small but in many cases they show nuclear irregularity and visible nucleoli. As opposed to LGL cases, the cells of T-PLL do not have cytoplasmic granules. In addition to bone marrow involvement, infiltration of splenic red pulp and hepatic sinusoids is common. In the spleen, T-PLL involves both the red pulp and the white pulp replacing its normal cellular composition. Involvement of lymph nodes is predominantly paracortical and the infiltrates lack proliferation centers. The presence of "double positivity" for CD4 and CD8 (25% of cases) may be helpful in the differential diagnosis of these cells. Surface CD3 expression is not uncommonly weak. CD52 is usually highly expressed in T-PLL and can be used as a therapeutic target. *TCL1* expression by immunohistochemistry and cytogenetic abnormalities, for example, abnormalities of chromosome 14q11, can also be demonstrated and may be useful in confirming the diagnosis (see Chapter 38).

Large Granular Lymphocytic Leukemia

T-cell large granular lymphocytic (T-LGL) leukemia defines a spectrum of proliferations of LGLs of T-cell or NK-cell phenotype (235–240). T-cell LGL is typically a proliferation of CD3, CD8, and TCR alpha-beta-positive T lymphocytes. A gamma/delta variant has also been recognized (241). In contrast to T-cell LGL, the NK-cell LGL subtype does not show surface CD3 expression but is positive for CD16 and CD56 (usually weakly). T-cell receptor gene rearrangement analysis shows germ line results in the latter cases.

Some patients with T-LGL leukemia have only a moderate lymphocytosis with neutropenia and minimal splenomegaly. Others have progressive disease with marked blood and bone marrow lymphocytosis and prominent splenomegaly (242,243). T-cell large granular lymphocytic leukemia cases need to be distinguished from reactive large granular lymphocytosis, a condition

Table 50.4	DIFFERENTIAL FEATURES OF HSTCL, T-PLL AND LGL LEUKEMIA INCLUDING BOTH T-LGL AND NK-CELL SUBTYPES		
	HSTCL	**T-PLL**	**LGL Leukemia**
Age and sex	Adolescents and young adults; male predominance	Adults over the age of 30 y; no sex predominance	45–75 y; no sex predominance
Clinical features	Hepatosplenomegaly, systemic symptoms, cytopenias, no lymphadenopathy, 20% cases in the setting of chronic immune suppression	Hepatosplenomegaly, generalized lymphadenopathy, lymphocytosis with anemia and thrombocytopenia	Neutropenia with or without anemia, variable degree of lymphocytosis and moderate splenomegaly
Splenic morphology	Medium-sized lymphoid cells with oval or folded nuclei and moderate amount of cytoplasm present in red pulp cords and sinuses	Small to medium-sized lymphoid cells with nuclear irregularities, prominent nucleoli and agranular cytoplasm present in the red pulp and also involving the white pulp	Neoplastic lymphocytes involving cords and sinuses in the red pulp
Other sites of involvement	Liver and bone marrow involvement with intrasinusoidal lymphoma cells	Involvement of bone marrow and hepatic sinusoids, perivascular or dermal infiltrates in the skin	Intrasinusoidal or interstitial involvement of the bone marrow; liver involvement
Immunophenotype of neoplastic cells	Positive for CD2, CD3, CD56, TIA-1, usually gamma/delta TCR, variably positive for CD16 and CD7, usually negative for CD4, CD5, CD8, CD57, CD25, CD30, granzyme-B, perforin	Positive for CD3, CD2, CD7, CD52, TCL-1, 25% cases positive for CD4 and CD8, some cases may show weak surface CD3	T-LGL subtype is positive for CD3, CD8, alpha-beta TCR (usually), TIA-1, and granzyme-B; NK subtype is positive for CD16, CD56 and cytoplasmic CD3

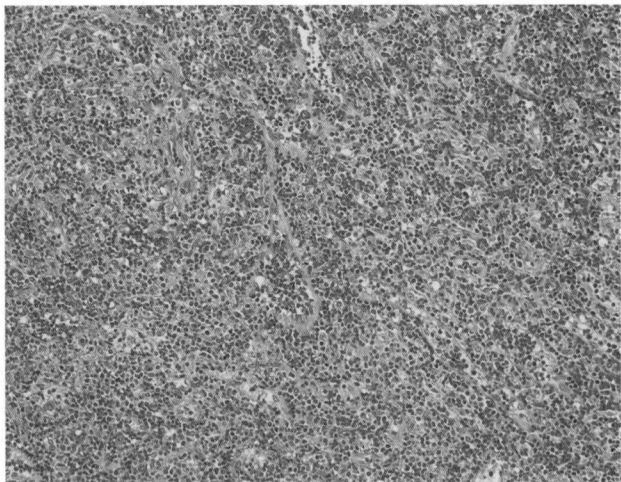

FIGURE 50.25. T-LGL with lymphoid cells in the red pulp.

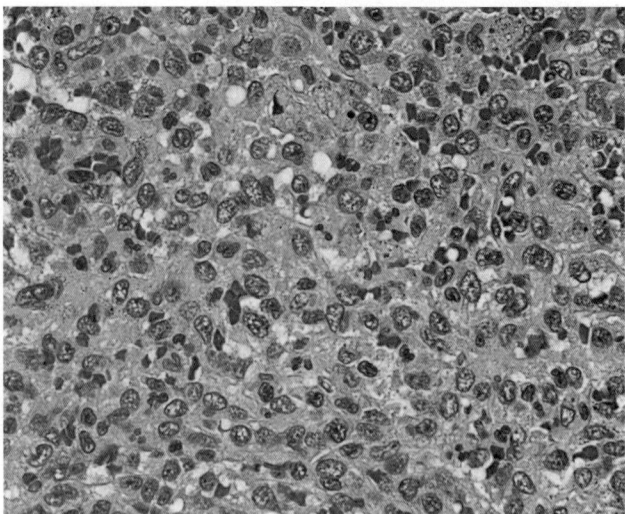

FIGURE 50.26. Acute myeloid leukemia. Immature myeloid precursors involving the splenic cords.

that is most frequently observed in patients with aplastic anemia, rheumatoid arthritis, or other autoimmune disorders (238–240).

Splenic involvement in both types of LGL leukemia is similar (244). It is strictly confined to the red pulp, in which LGL cells infiltrate both cords and sinuses (Fig. 50.25). The histopathologic features of LGL leukemia may mimic HCL and T-PLL. However, the blood lakes characteristic of HCL are not present in LGL leukemia. As previously mentioned, in contrast to LGL leukemia, T-PLL shows infiltration of the white pulp as well (23,234). In addition, immunophenotypic findings are distinctively different in the three disorders (see Chapter 38).

 MYELOID NEOPLASMS

Red pulp disease is characteristic of splenic involvement in leukemic processes (23,245). The leukemic cells usually appear localized to the cords of Billroth, with secondary involvement of the sinuses. Peritrabecular and subendothelial deposits may be seen early in the course of leukemic infiltration. Although splenic involvement is invariable in leukemic disorders, the degree of splenomegaly depends on the type of leukemia and the duration of the disease. The acute leukemias usually result only in mild to moderate splenic enlargement, but the chronic leukemias may produce prominent splenomegaly, which often results in hypersplenism. Peripheral cytopenias may necessitate splenectomy, which may be effective in ameliorating the cytopenias, although removal of the spleen usually does not affect the course of the underlying disease. Splenic rupture is a complication occasionally seen in cases of leukemia. This is believed to result from infiltration of the trabecular framework and vascular structure of the organ by tumor cells or from infarction within the spleen (246–248). Rupture of the spleen is far more common in the chronic leukemias, particularly chronic myeloid leukemia, than in the acute forms (247,248).

 ACUTE MYELOID LEUKEMIAS

Acute myeloid leukemias (AMLs) include forms that may be derived from the granulocytic, erythroid, monocytic, or megakaryocytic lineages. The distinction between these forms often is difficult on histologic examination of the spleen alone, although touch imprints supplemented by cytochemical stains frequently are helpful. Immunohistologic studies and immunophenotypic analysis by flow cytometry supplemented by cytogenetic and molecular genetic analysis may be required to adequately characterize the leukemia (see Chapter 41). Splenic involvement

with AML may precede or occur concurrently with systemic evidence of leukemia, or be a manifestation of relapse. It may also occur as a part of the blast transformation process of a chronic myeloproliferative neoplasm (MPN), myelodysplastic syndrome (MDS), or a myelodysplastic/myeloproliferative neoplasm (MDS/MPN). The existence of an underlying MPN may be suggested by the concomitant presence of hematopoietic cells of different myeloid cell lines (extramedullary hematopoiesis [EMH]) associated with the blast cell proliferation. All the various subtypes of myeloid leukemias involve the spleen in a similar topographic manner (Fig. 50.26), with the exception of erythroleukemia, in which the leukemic cells tend to cluster preferentially in the red pulp sinuses (Fig. 50.27) (23).

 CHRONIC MYELOID NEOPLASMS

The chronic MPN are a group of clonal disorders of the hematopoietic stem cell that include chronic myelogenous leukemia (CML), chronic neutrophilic leukemia, polycythemia vera (PV), primary myelofibrosis (PMF), essential thrombocythemia (ET), and myeloproliferative neoplasm unclassifiable (131,249). A variable degree of splenomegaly occurs in all these disorders. Although each has its own somewhat distinctive characteristics, a precise diagnostic subtyping of the MPN cannot be made on morphologic examination of the spleen alone in the absence of relevant clinical and laboratory data as well as the examination of bone marrow and peripheral blood smears (250–252).

Chronic Myelogenous Leukemia

Chronic myelogenous leukemia (CML) is frequently associated with massive splenomegaly. The cut surface of the spleen is deep red without visible white pulp because CML generally obliterates the lymphoid follicles, although small remnants of white pulp occasionally may be seen (23). Infarcts are common because of subendothelial invasion of the splenic trabecular veins, and fibrosis of the splenic cords may be prominent. Histologic examination reveals a polymorphous cellular infiltrate in the red pulp, which includes myeloid cells at all stages of maturation (23). The identification of immature myeloid cells, that is, promyelocytes and myelocytes, can be facilitated by using immunohistochemical stains for CD34, CD117, CD68 (and/or CD68R), myeloperoxidase (and/or lysozyme). Localized collections of ceroid-containing histiocytes (pseudo-Gaucher

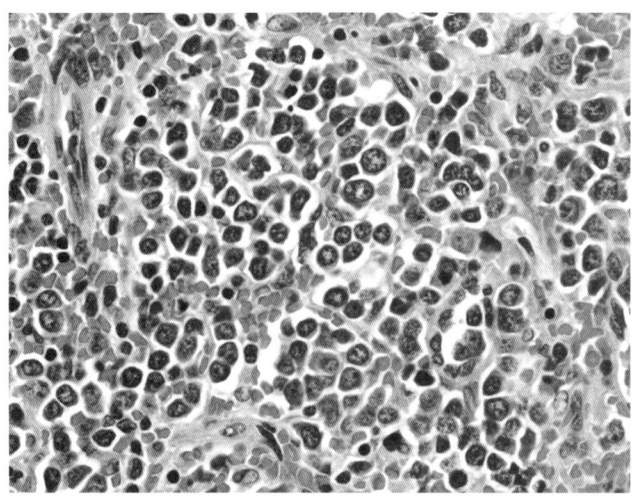
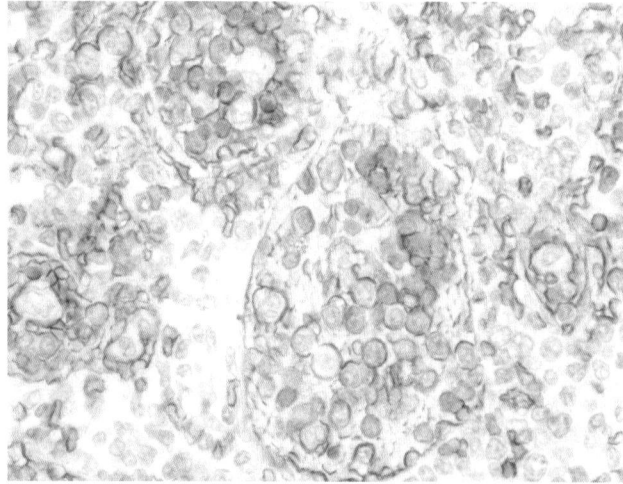

A
B

FIGURE 50.27. Acute erythroleukemia in the spleen. **A:** Immature erythroid precursors present in the splenic sinusoids. **B:** Glycophorin C confirming the erythroid lineage of the immature cells.

cells) similar to those seen in the bone marrow may also be observed in the spleens from CML patients (Fig. 50.28).

The majority of CML cases terminate with the development of an accelerated/blastic phase that resembles *de novo* acute leukemia (253,254). Approximately one-third of cases of blast crisis arise in an extramedullary site, the most common of which is the spleen. Blast crisis may result in a dramatic increase in the size of the spleen (255). Several studies have indicated that the myeloid cells in the spleen may develop additional cytogenetic abnormalities before those present in other sites (256–261) and that they may proliferate there more rapidly than in other sites of blastic transformation (262,263). Gross examination may reveal a homogeneous cut surface, or in some cases, discrete nodules that represent discrete collections of blasts (23). Most often the blasts are myeloblasts, although, in approximately 25% of cases, these cells are lymphoblasts and, in rare cases, megakaryoblasts or erythroblasts. Immunohistochemistry with a panel of antibodies that includes both myeloid- and lymphoid-associated antigens (e.g., CD34, CD117, CD68, myeloperoxidase, glycophorin A or C, CD42b [or CD61], TdT, CD79a [or PAX-5], CD10, CD3) may be helpful in confirming the presence of an increased number of blasts and in identifying their lineage derivation (see Chapter 44).

Therapy with colony-stimulating factors (e.g., G-CSF) may simulate splenic involvement with CML or another myeloid neoplasm, or, occasionally, even mimic extramedullary AML

(264). Rarely, the administration of this cytokine has even been associated with splenic rupture (264).

PHILADELPHIA CHROMOSOME–NEGATIVE MYELOPROLIFERATIVE NEOPLASMS

Extramedullary hematopoiesis (EMH) in the spleen is a key feature of advanced stage Philadelphia chromosome–negative myeloproliferative neoplasms (Ph- MPN). The occurrence of EMH in Ph- MPN is associated with abnormal trafficking patterns of clonal hematopoietic progenitor cells and hematopoietic stem cells attributed to dysregulation of the bone marrow microenvironment. This results in circulating mature and immature marrow elements that home to the spleen (265–267). There, the bone marrow–derived cells undergo sustained malignant multilineage hematopoiesis resulting in progressive splenomegaly. Migliaccio et al. (268) demonstrated abnormalities in the SDF-1/CXCR4 axis in the marrows of PMF patients that may contribute to the increased stem/progenitor cell trafficking observed in these patients. Studies using mouse models have shown that X-linked Gata 1(low) mutation in mice induces strain-restricted myeloproliferative disorders characterized by EMH in the spleen and liver, that Gata 1(low) hematopoiesis is favored by the spleen as compared to the bone marrow, and that Gata 1(low) hematopoiesis is not stem cell autonomous but requires the permissive microenvironment of the spleen and liver (269). Studies based on the identification of loss of heterozygosity (270) and presence of $JAK2^{V617}$ mutation (271,272) have provided evidence that splenic EMH in Ph- MPN is clonal, supporting the hypothesis that hematopoietic cells causing the splenic proliferation are derived from the transformed bone marrow clones. Recently, we described three distinct histologic patterns of splenic EMH in Ph- MPN: diffuse, nodular, and mixed-nodular and diffuse (Fig. 50.29) (273). Some cases of nodular EMH can resemble the previously described entity, "sclerosing extramedullary hematopoietic tumor" (274). The preponderant hematopoietic lineage differs in the three growth patterns: granulocytic in diffuse, trilineage in nodular, and erythroid in mixed EMH. Erythropoiesis is largely intravascular, granulopoiesis is within the splenic cords, and megakaryopoiesis is observed in both locations (Fig. 50.30). The stromal changes parallel the histologic pattern with preservation of the splenic stromal and vascular architecture in the diffuse areas as opposed to areas of nodular EMH. The histologic growth patterns do not correlate with the specific subtypes of Ph- MPN. Histologic growth patterns have also been previously described in splenic

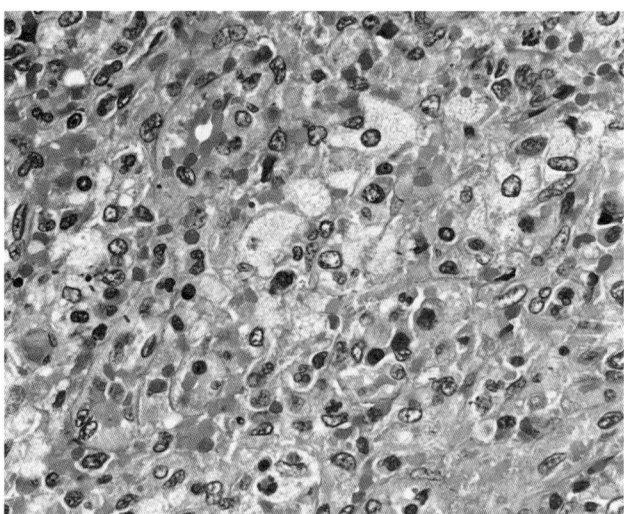

FIGURE 50.28. Pseudo-Gaucher cells in a case of CML involving the spleen.

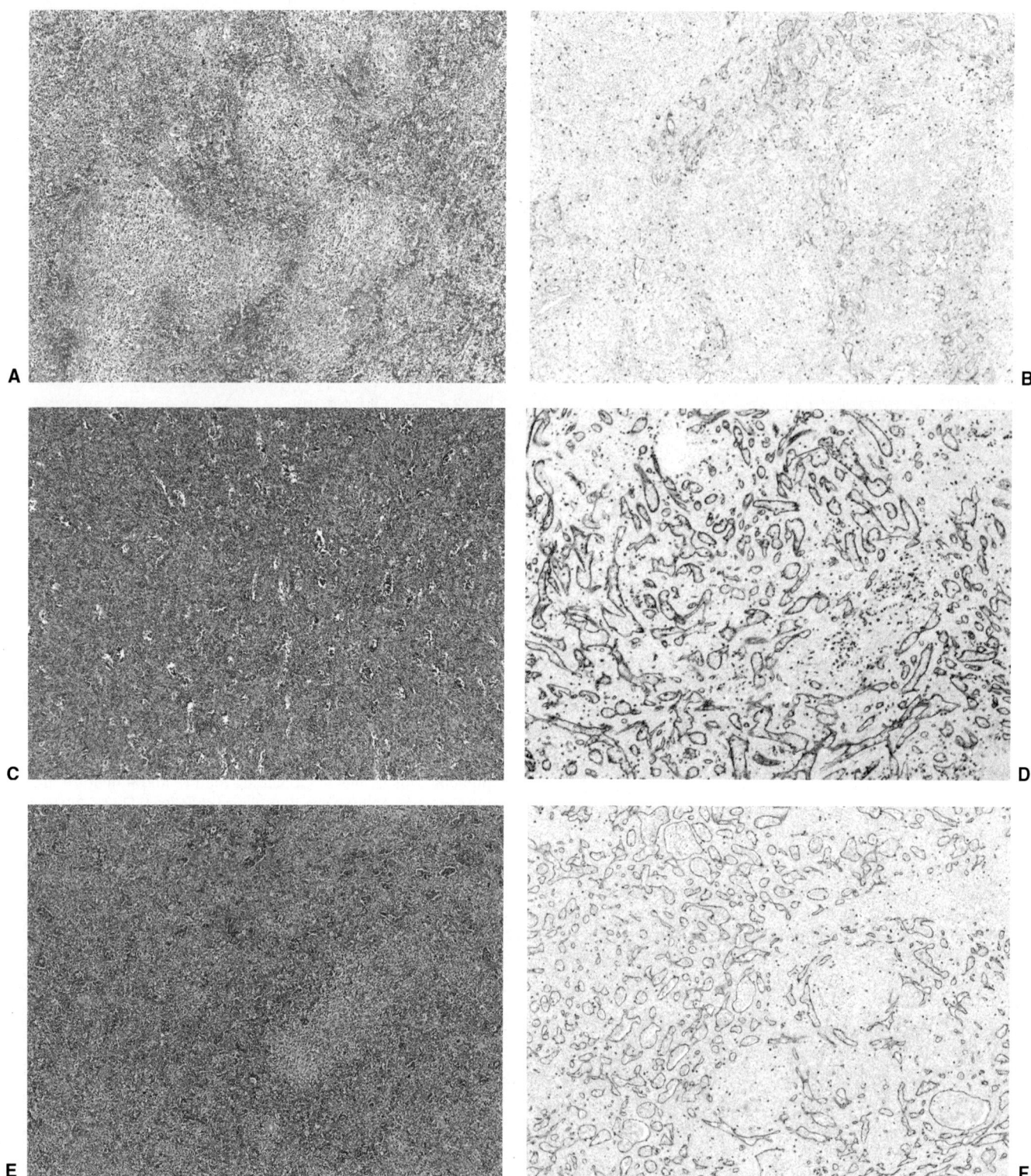

FIGURE 50.29. Histologic growth patterns of splenic EMH in MPNs: Nodular extramedullary hematopoietic proliferation **(A)** with lack of CD8-positive sinusoids **(B)**; diffuse extramedullary hematopoietic proliferation **(C)** with preservation of CD8-positive sinusoids **(D)**; and mixed extramedullary hematopoietic proliferation **(E)** with partial loss of CD8-positive sinusoids in the nodular areas **(F)**.

hematopoietic proliferations in PMF where a nodular growth pattern was associated with a favorable prognosis (275). The gross and histologic features of specific Ph- MPN are described below.

Polycythemia Vera

Splenomegaly occurs in the majority of patients who have polycythemia vera (PV) and is one of the criteria for diagnosis (252).

However, the degree of splenomegaly in the erythrocytotic phase of PV usually is only mild or moderate, the size of the spleen roughly correlating with the duration of the disease (276–278). In approximately 20% of cases, however, PV evolves to a spent phase, also called *postpolycythemic myelofibrosis* (post-PV MF), in which the development of reticulin and collagen fibrosis in the bone marrow is accompanied by leukoerythroblastosis in the peripheral blood and marked splenomegaly (277,279).

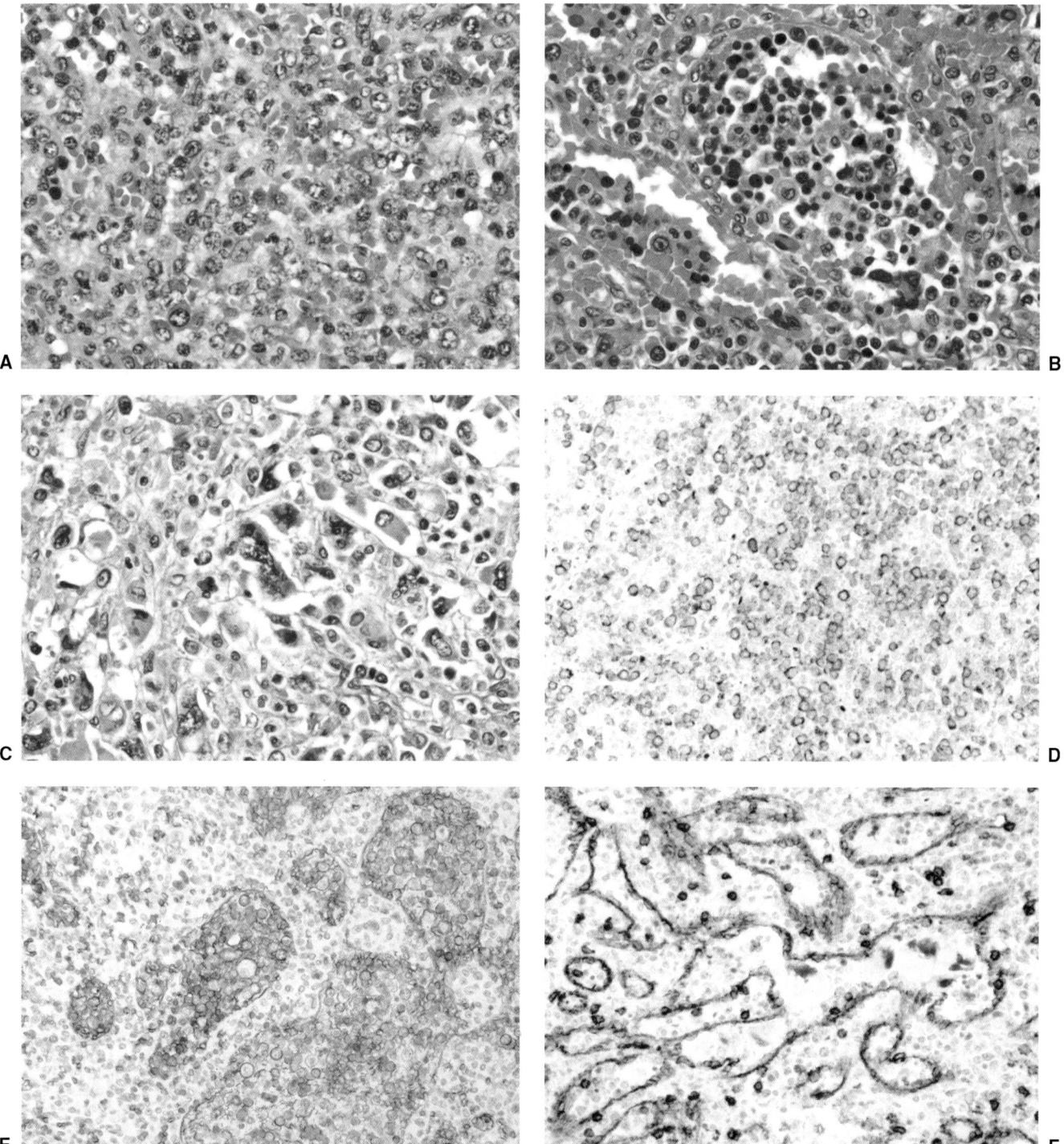

FIGURE 50.30. Spatial localization of specific hematopoietic cell lineages in MPN: Granulopoiesis within splenic cords (**A**); erythropoiesis within sinusoids (**B**); and megakaryopoiesis within splenic cords (**C**). Myeloperoxidase-positive granulocytic cells (**D**); glycophorin C–positive erythroid cells (**E**); and megakaryocytes within CD8-positive sinusoids (**F**).

It has been demonstrated that EMH is not a feature of PV before the development of reticulin fibrosis in the bone marrow (277). Spleens that have been obtained in the erythrocytotic phase show intense congestion of the cords of Billroth and the sinuses of the red pulp, accompanied by a proliferation of cordal macrophages without significant myeloid metaplasia. In contrast, spleens obtained from patients whose disease has evolved to post-PV MF show the presence of prominent EMH to a degree similar to that observed in cases of *de novo* PMF (see next section) (280,281).

Primary Myelofibrosis

The degree of splenomegaly seen in cases of primary myelofibrosis (PMF) characterized by EMH (also termed agnogenic myeloid metaplasia or idiopathic myelofibrosis with myeloid metaplasia) is the most striking among the MPN group. In PMF, splenomegaly is associated with reticulin fibrosis in the bone marrow and the presence of leukoerythroblastosis (circulating erythroblasts in association with immature myeloid cells, usually myelocytes and/or metamyelocytes) and tear drop erythrocytes in the peripheral blood (252,281) (see Chapter 45). Symptoms related to massive enlargement of the organ may be the presenting feature of this disorder. In some studies, the degree of splenomegaly has been shown to correlate with the duration of disease rather than the degree of marrow fibrosis (277,280,282). Increasing splenomegaly may be arrested, but only transiently, by splenic irradiation, chemotherapy, or JAK2 inhibitors (283).

Splenomegaly in PMF results from the presence of EMH in the red pulp, also known as myeloid metaplasia. On gross examination, the spleen is enlarged, purple-red, with indistinct white pulp markings. Infarcts are common. In some cases, however, focal proliferations with grossly recognizable nodules can be observed (23,273). Microscopic examination usually reveals multiple foci of EMH distributed throughout the red pulp sinuses and in the splenic cords. EMH may be accompanied by a variable degree of fibrosis. The fibrosis is greater in areas with a nodular growth pattern and lesser in areas with a diffuse growth pattern (Fig. 50.31) (273).

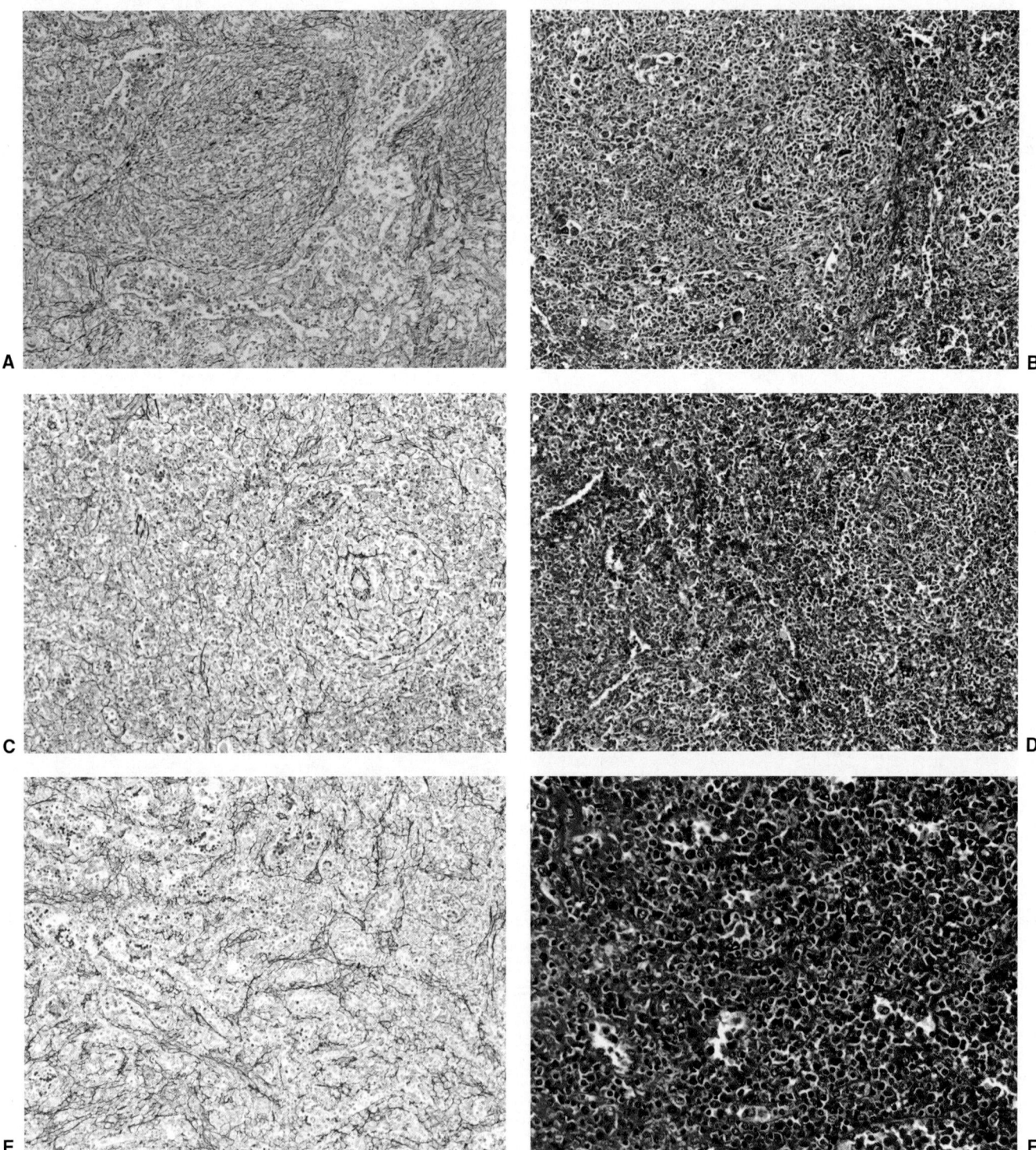

FIGURE 50.31. Reticulin and trichrome stains showing marked reticulin (A) and collagen (B) fibrosis in nodular-extramedullary hematopoietic proliferation; greater degree of reticulin (C) and collagen (D) fibrosis within the nodular as compared to diffuse areas of mixed extramedullary hematopoietic proliferation; and diffuse reticulin (E) and minimal collagen fibrosis (F) in diffuse extramedullary hematopoietic proliferation.

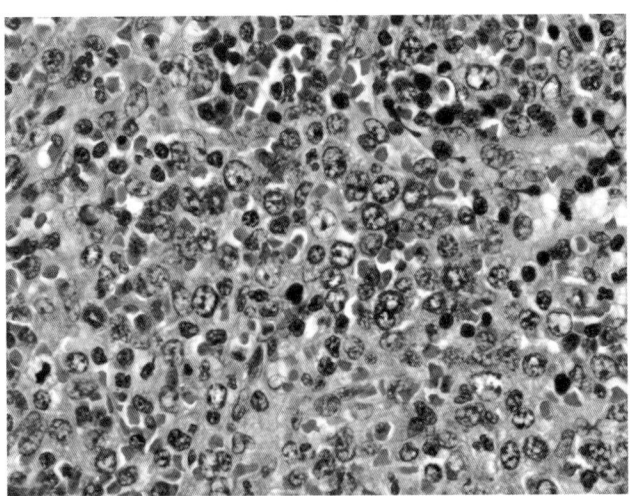
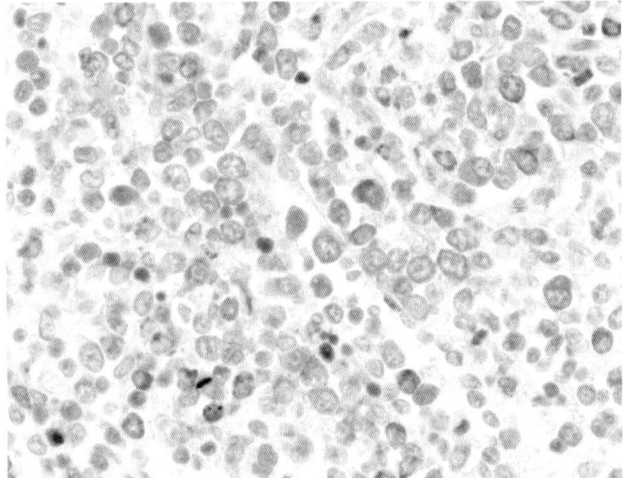

FIGURE 50.32. Increased immature cells in a case of PMF. A: Immature cells in the red pulp. **B:** Immunohistochemical stain for myeloperoxidase confirming the myeloid origin of the immature cells.

Histologically, although the hematopoiesis present is always trilinear, one cell line may predominate in a given case. Erythroid precursors occur in easily recognizable clusters, frequently within dilated sinuses. Megakaryocytes show atypical features similar to those in the bone marrow and can be scattered or present in clusters. Although granulocytic precursors may be difficult to distinguish from cordal macrophages, they can be recognized in touch imprints or in tissue sections by using the immunoperoxidase technique with antibodies to myeloperoxidase or lysozyme (284). The presence of EMH is always accompanied by proliferation of cordal macrophages, and phagocytosis of hematopoietic precursors may be seen (23). The trilinear nature of the hematopoiesis seen in PMF aids in the distinction of this disorder from other types of myeloid neoplasms (e.g., CML). Blastic transformation in PMF may be heralded by an increase in immature cells (Fig. 50.32). The identification, in these cases, of an increased proportion of blasts can be facilitated by the use of appropriate immunohistochemical stains as previously described. In addition to CML, the differential diagnosis of myeloid metaplasia in the spleen includes various disorders, which are also associated with bone marrow fibrosis and peripheral blood leukoerythroblastosis. Metastatic carcinoma and infectious disorders that involve the bone marrow are well-known causes of bone marrow fibrosis that may to a certain extent mimic PMF. Other much less frequent cases include MDSs (285) and MDS/MPNs such as chronic myelomonocytic leukemia (284,286) and juvenile myelomonocytic leukemia (287).

Essential Thrombocythemia

Essential thrombocythemia (ET) is characterized by a marked megakaryocytic proliferation in the bone marrow associated with thrombocytosis (252,288–290). Clinical manifestations include hemorrhagic, or less commonly, thrombotic phenomena (252,288). The degree of splenomegaly in ET is usually less marked than that seen in the other chronic myeloproliferative disorders and hypersplenism is not a common clinical manifestation (see Chapter 44). Because of the scarcity of splenectomy specimens, there are no large studies of the pathology of the spleen in ET. In the few cases studied, the most notable finding is the widening of the cords of Billroth, which may appear hypocellular at low power because of the presence of large masses of platelets, which may also be seen in the sinuses. Touch preparations of the spleen may be useful for demonstrating the sequestration of platelets. Mild to moderate

splenomegaly can be seen in cases of ET. The presence of fibrosis and microinfarcts (Gamna-Gandy bodies) may mimic the morphology of the spleen in advanced sickle cell disease. In our experience, no significant EMH is seen. Occasionally, however, in the rare ET cases evolving to myelofibrosis, a complication that is seen in <10% patients at more than 10 years from the initial ET diagnosis, significant myeloid metaplasia has also been reported to occur in the spleen (291).

OTHER CHRONIC MYELOID NEOPLASMS

Other types of myeloid neoplasm may also produce splenomegaly. This complication is more likely to be associated with MDS/MPNs such as chronic myelomonocytic leukemia or juvenile myelomonocytic leukemia (284–287). In these cases, the splenic red pulp contains an increased number of myelomonocytic cells. An increased number of blasts can be seen in cases undergoing acute transformation. Immunohistochemistry may be helpful in confirming the diagnosis, and necessary to confirm acute transformation.

Systemic Mastocytosis

The spleen usually is involved in cases of systemic mastocytosis, although the degree of splenomegaly is frequently only mild to moderate (292–294). The pattern of involvement of the spleen is variable (292–295). Early involvement may show a preferential localization to paratrabecular areas and/or to the marginal zones of the white pulp. A characteristic fibroblastic reaction resulting in a concentric rimming of the lymphoid follicles may be observed (Fig. 50.33). Other investigators have reported a diffuse infiltration of the red pulp, and multinodular perivascular infiltrates, for example, surrounding the trabecular arteries, have been also described (295). Increased eosinophils are usually found in association with the mast cell aggregates. Mast cells typically appear cuboidal or spindle shaped, with pale nuclei and grayish cytoplasm. Mast cell granules can be demonstrated with the chloroacetate esterase stain and are metachromatic with toluidine blue and Giemsa stains, although neoplastic mast cells are often hypogranular. Tryptase and CD117 positivity may be helpful in confirming splenic involvement, particularly in cases associated with a marked degree of fibroblastic reaction and relatively rare mast cells. The neoplastic nature of the mast cells can be confirmed by their positivity with CD25 and/or CD2. Positivity for either marker is not seen in reactive mast cells.

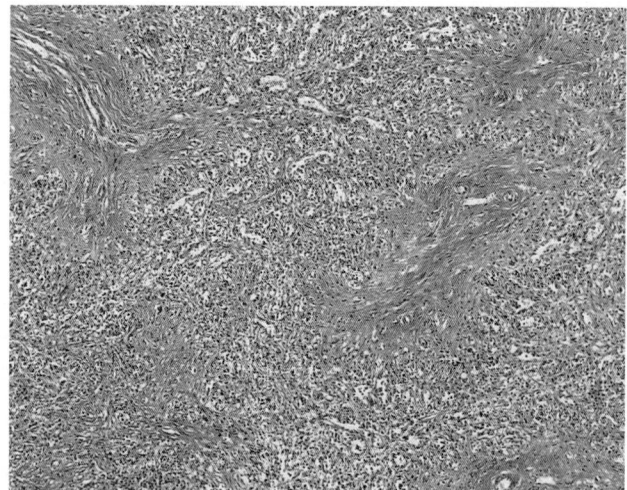

FIGURE 50.33. Systemic mastocytosis involving the spleen. There is fibroblastic reaction around the lymphoid follicles.

Confirmation of the diagnosis of SM may also be obtained by mutational analysis for the presence of *KitD816V* or other related KIT mutations (see Chapter 49). Systemic mast cell disease may be associated with other clonal hematologic non–mast cell disorders, most notably CMML, MPN, MDS, or AML (296,297), which also may be present concurrently in the spleen. Their identification within the splenic red pulp may be facilitated by using immunohistology for myeloid-associated antigens.

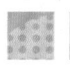 **OTHER HEMATOPOIETIC TUMORS**

Follicular dendritic cell sarcoma (FDCS) or follicular dendritic cell tumor is a rare neoplasm derived from the follicular dendritic cell of the germinal center, which has been observed to occur rarely in the spleen (298,299). FDCS is characterized grossly by fleshy or solid nodules and, histologically, by oval or spindle cells usually growing in bundles and whorls. Nuclei are bland in appearance, and have a low mitotic rate. The neoplastic cells are typically CD21 and CD35 positive. The clinical behavior of these tumors appears to be more aggressive than the relatively bland cytology would suggest (299). Due to a difference in the clinical course, conventional FDCS must be distinguished from the EBV-positive variant of inflammatory pseudotumor than can also be seen in the spleen (see inflammatory pseudotumor [IPT] section later in the chapter).

Interdigitating dendritic cell sarcoma (IDCS) is a rare tumor that is thought to arise from interdigitating dendritic cells. The disease usually involves lymph nodes, but splenic involvement may also occur, particularly in cases in which the disease is disseminated with involvement of the spleen, bone marrow, skin, liver, kidney, and lung (300,301). The gross and histologic features of IDCS are similar to those described above for FDCS. In paraffin sections, the cells are positive for S-100 and variably positive for CD68, and lack CD1a, langerin, B-cell, T-cell, and specific follicular dendritic cell antigen expression (see Chapter 48).

PROLIFERATIONS OF THE MONOCYTE-MACROPHAGE SYSTEM

Hemophagocytic Syndromes

The hemophagocytic syndromes (HPS) are a group of systemic disorders characterized by the acute onset of pancytopenia

Table 50.5	DISORDERS ASSOCIATED WITH HEMOPHAGOCYTOSIS IN SPLEEN
Nonneoplastic	**Neoplastic**
Storage diseases	Histiocytic sarcoma (malignant histiocytosis)
Congenital HPS	Hepatosplenic T-cell lymphoma
Virus-associated (EBV, other viruses)	Other peripheral T-cell lymphoma
Other infections associated (bacterial, fungal, rickettsial, parasitic, etc.)	B-cell lymphomas
Autoimmune hemolytic anemias	
Drug-induced (e.g., Fludarabine)	

caused by the proliferation of macrophages in lymphoreticular organs associated with prominent phagocytosis of hematopoietic elements (302) (Table 50.5). A familial (primary) form of HPS affecting infants and young children (303–306) is termed familial hemophagocytic lymphohistiocytosis (FHL). FHL has an autosomal recessive pattern of inheritance. It is caused by overwhelming activation of T lymphocytes and macrophages associated with defective triggering of apoptosis and reduced cytotoxic activity. Mutations in the perforin gene have been demonstrated in FHL patients (305). Most secondary cases of HPS are related to infection or an NK-cell or T-cell neoplasm, most often EBV positive. Because of the acute clinical course culminating in death in many cases, the systemic distribution, and striking proliferation of cells in all lymphoreticular organs, these cases were considered to represent malignant histiocytosis in the past. They present with fever and varying cytopenias in a clinical context of underlying viral infection or malignancy (212,307). Cases associated with infection have been referred to as either viral-associated, and later, infection-associated hemophagocytic syndrome (IAHS). Numerous subsequent studies have revealed that the HPS may be precipitated by a wide variety of microorganisms, as well as by a variety of tumors (23,212,307).

Spleens in the IAHS are usually moderately enlarged, although significant enlargement may occur. The red pulp shows a proliferation of macrophages, which display prominent hemophagocytosis, most characteristically of erythrocytes, but also of granulocytes, lymphocytes, and platelets. Fibrosis, focal infarctions, and gradual obliteration of the white pulp with B-cell depletion may occur (23).

HPS associated with malignancies of the hematopoietic system differ morphologically, since the spleen, usually but not always, contains a component of malignant cells. Cases of lymphomas associated with HPS are most often of peripheral T-cell or NK-cell type (308). Association with EBV is a major risk factor, and hemophagocytic syndrome is a common complication of extranodal NK-/T-cell lymphoma, aggressive NK-cell leukemia, and systemic EBV-positive lymphoproliferative disease of childhood associated with chronic active EBV infection. In cases with only rare neoplastic T cells admixed with the numerous histiocytes, the resemblance to malignant histiocytosis may be considerable. The diagnosis of T-cell lymphoma in these cases usually requires molecular confirmation.

Langerhans Cell Histiocytosis

Langerhans cell histiocytosis (LCH), a clonal proliferation of CD1a-positive, S-100-positive, langerin-positive Langerhans cells, has multiple clinical presentations, ranging from an isolated lytic lesion of bone to a fulminating, disseminated disorder mimicking leukemia. The latter disorder, historically termed Letterer-Siwe disease (309), is most common in young children and is the form of the disease in which splenic involvement typically occurs (310–312). The abnormalities observed in the spleen include hemorrhages and areas of necrosis and infarction. It predominantly involves the red pulp in the form of a diffuse infiltrate, or as ill-defined tumor aggregates resembling loosely formed granulomas. The characteristic cell in LCH is a large macrophage-like cell with abundant pale and sometimes vacuolated cytoplasm (313). Nuclei are frequently deeply indented or grooved, with fine chromatin and one or two small nucleoli. Electron microscopy usually reveals characteristic structures, termed Birbeck granules, within the cytoplasm of the cells (314,315). LCH cells are typically S-100, CD1a, and langerin positive. As in other involved sites, eosinophils and histiocytes may be found intermixed with the LCs.

Rare cases of Langerhans cell sarcoma, the malignant counterpart to LCH, have been reported (316,317). These patients have a male predominance, older age, and disseminated involvement frequently including the spleen. In these cases, the Langerhans cells appear cytologically malignant with marked atypia (see Chapter 48).

Histiocytic Sarcoma

Histiocytic sarcoma is a malignant proliferation of cells showing morphologic and immunophenotypic features similar to those of mature tissue histiocytes. Cases that are characterized by a systemic presentation, with multiple sites of involvement, were historically referred to as "malignant histiocytosis" (318). The pattern of splenic involvement resembles that of leukemia, with diffuse infiltration of the red pulp, sometimes obliterating the white pulp. The infiltrate is pleomorphic with the proliferating cells showing a variable degree of differentiation and cytologic atypia. Occasional hemophagocytosis may be present, but is usually seen in only a small fraction of the tumor cells, in contrast to HPS in which the majority of the cells show evidence of phagocytosis. Immunohistology with CD68, CD68R, CD163, and lysozyme is helpful to confirm the diagnosis. S-100 (but not CD1a) is also frequently positive.

The differential diagnosis includes DLBCL with prominent red pulp involvement, ALCL (319,320), HSTCL, as well as HPS associated with other lymphoid malignancies, previously mistakenly diagnosed as malignant histiocytosis in many cases (212,321–323). Cases of acute monoblastic leukemia with histiocytic differentiation morphologically overlap with disseminated histiocytic sarcoma (324).

"Malignant Histiocytosis" Associated with Mediastinal Germ Cell Tumor

An unusual association occurs between mediastinal nonseminomatous germ cell tumors and hematologic malignancies (325). Approximately one-half of the hematologic malignancies have been characterized as malignant histiocytosis (325–328). These proliferations of histiocytes may occur either diffusely or in the form of ill-defined nodules within the red pulp of the spleen (329). They are thought to represent an unusual form of metastasis from hematologic elements originating within the germ cell tumor through aberrant hematologic differentiation of malignant germ cells (327).

TUMOR-LIKE AND NONHEMATOPOIETIC NEOPLASTIC LESIONS

Several benign lesions involving the spleen can grossly mimic malignant lymphoma by virtue of the production of mass lesions that may be associated with hypersplenism, although their benign nature usually is readily apparent microscopically.

Splenic Cysts

Splenic cysts are most commonly single and unilocular. The majority of these are so-called false cysts that lack an epithelial lining (330). Approximately 20% of splenic cysts have an epithelial lining, which usually is of stratified squamous type (331,332). These are termed true cysts or epidermoid cysts. Rarely, true cysts can result in hypersplenism.

Splenic Hamartoma

Splenic hamartomas may occasionally result in hypersplenism (333), although they are more commonly found as incidental findings at autopsy or in spleens removed for unrelated causes (23,334). The incidence of splenic hamartomas in autopsy series ranges between 0.024% and 0.13% (335). Large and symptomatic lesions are more common in females and can present as splenomegaly, pain, rupture, and rarely with thrombocytopenia and anemia (336). Splenic hamartomas may be associated with other conditions like tuberous sclerosis, Wiskott-Aldrich–like syndrome, and other neoplastic conditions (337,338). Splenic hamartomas are well-circumscribed nodules that resemble normal red pulp histologically with slitlike vascular spaces lined by plump endothelial cells of littoral cell derivation (i.e., CD8 positive) (Fig. 50.34). Splenic trabecular architecture and white pulp structures are only rarely seen in hamartomas, although scattered lymphocytes are often present. The typical splenic hamartomas can be easily distinguished from capillary hemangioma by virtue of their immunohistochemical reactivity with CD8 and CD68 and lack of CD34 expression. More problematic, however, is the distinction between hamartoma and rare entities such as cord capillary hemangioma (339) and splenic myoid angioendothelioma (340). The extensive morphologic overlap between these entities is well acknowledged. The classical hamartoma cases show a vasculature predominantly composed of CD8+ CD31+ CD34- splenic sinuses, whereas cases of cord capillary hemangioma and myoid angioendothelioma contain many CD8- CD31+ CD34+ cord capillaries, but very little CD8+ vasculature (341). Cases of classical hamartoma lack significant perisinusoidal expression of collagen IV and low-affinity nerve growth factor receptor. Both these markers are variably expressed in cord capillary hemangioma and myoid angioendothelioma.

Inflammatory Pseudotumor

Inflammatory pseudotumor (IPT) describes a lesion in the spleen that presents as an isolated mass, mimicking a tumor,

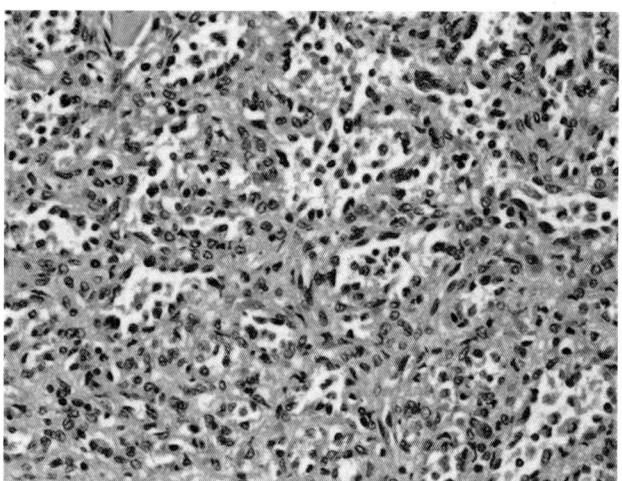

FIGURE 50.34. Splenic hamartoma. Medium-power view of a nodule composed of vascular spaces lined by littoral cells.

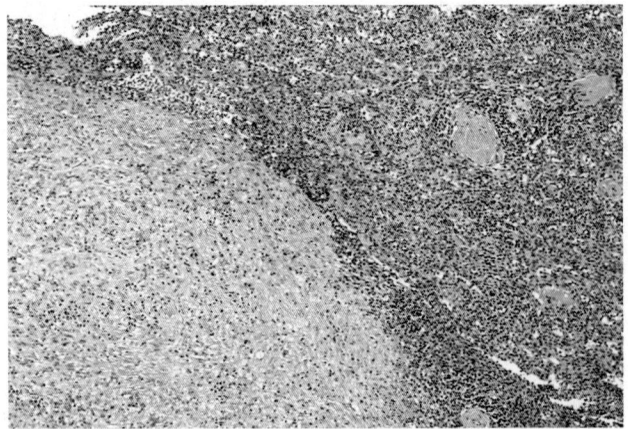

FIGURE 50.35. Inflammatory pseudotumor spleen. Left part of the image demonstrating a well-defined tumor with inflammatory cell in a stromal background.

but is composed of a mixture of inflammatory cells and stromal cells (342–345) (Fig. 50.35). IPTs that occur in the spleen are most commonly "truly inflammatory," reflecting an unusual type of tissue response to injury. Rare cases of either myofibroblastic or follicular dendritic cell origin also exist. The latter may be EBV-associated and have similar clinical and histologic features, differing mainly in the phenotype of the proliferating spindle cells. The EBV in splenic IPT has been demonstrated to be clonal when assessed by Southern blot analysis of EBV DNA terminal repeat regions (346). The clinical outcome is typically benign, with only rare recurrences reported following splenectomy (347). IPT is often asymptomatic; occasional patients have abdominal pain or a sense of fullness; rarely, patients may present with fever and weight loss (345). Splenic IPT usually presents as a solitary, circumscribed firm nodule, often with central necrosis. The borders are usually well-circumscribed. Histologically, the common findings include a proliferation of bland-appearing spindle-shaped cells within a polymorphic background, which contains a variable number of monocytes, lymphocytes, and polyclonal plasma cells.

Immunohistochemical staining for smooth muscle markers (smooth muscle actin) is variably positive in the spindle cell population. In a small subset of cases, EBER is positive, whereas LMP-1 is less commonly expressed (343,347). A possibly related entity is the inflammatory pseudotumor-like follicular dendritic cell tumor (IPTLFDC) (345). Unlike conventional follicular dendritic cell tumors (see previous section), IPTLFDC has a marked female predominance. IPTLFDC have been reported to occur in the spleen and/or liver. As the name implies, there is a mixed inflammatory background associated with bland spindle cells. The spindle cells are positive for dendritic cell markers (CD21, CD23, CD35) and essentially all cases are positive for EBV (347). In rare cases of IPT, the patient may have a history of infection, but the relationship to the infection may be coincidental, with only EBV being found on a consistent basis (342,348).

Inflammatory pseudotumor should be distinguished from inflammatory myofibroblastic tumor, a neoplasm common in children, which is associated with expression of the ALK tyrosine kinase (344). The differential with IPT is not problematic as the ALK+ inflammatory myofibroblastic tumor has not been reported to involve either the spleen or the lymph node. In addition to splenic lymphoma, the differential diagnosis of splenic IPT also includes various benign or tumor-like splenic lesions, which include hamartoma and hemangioma. Splenic hamartomas are typically surrounded by a rim of compressed red pulp, usually without associated fibrosis. In addition, the

sinus or cordlike spaces characteristically observed in splenic hamartoma are not observed in IPT.

Sclerosing Angiomatoid Nodular Transformation

Sclerosing angiomatoid nodular transformation (SANT) of the spleen is a poorly understood condition that appears "in between" a splenic cord capillary hemangioma with sclerosis and a true IPT (349–351).

Grossly it resembles IPT. The lesions of SANT can be large, up to 17 cm in diameter. Histologically, it has more of a multinodular appearance. The individual nodules have an angiomatoid appearance, being composed of slitlike vascular channels with interspersed spindle cells. The vessels have a phenotype that is intermediate between that of true vascular channels (sometimes CD34 or CD31+) and splenic sinusoidal lining cells (CD8+). It has been postulated that the lesion is not neoplastic, but represents altered red pulp entrapped by a stromal proliferation. The clinical outcome has been benign in all reported cases.

Peliosis

Peliosis is a rare condition, of unknown etiology, in which ectatic sinusoids and blood-filled cysts are present throughout the organ (352,353). Peliotic cysts are lined by sinusoidal endothelium but this is often absent in larger lesions. The cysts are often located adjacent to the PALS and in the perifollicular zones. Its clinical importance lies in its association with spontaneous splenic rupture (352,353), due to a combination of spleen enlargement and fragility of the dilated, cystic sinusoids. Peliosis also often affects the liver.

Splenic Vascular Tumors

Capillary and cavernous angiomas can occur in the spleen. Their morphologic features are similar to those observed elsewhere. A particular splenic variant termed cord capillary hemangioma has overlapping features with both splenic hamartoma and SANT (341). Problems in differential diagnosis are, however, encountered in cases of diffuse angiomatosis and littoral cell angiomas, benign conditions, which need to be distinguished from the highly malignant angiosarcoma of the spleen. In littoral cell angiomas (354), the endothelial cells are usually plump and cuboidal (Fig. 50.36). They may express CD8, typical of splenic sinusoidal endothelium. Papillary projections of endothelial cells may protrude into the vascular spaces. Vascular lumens also contain abundant desquamated littoral cells

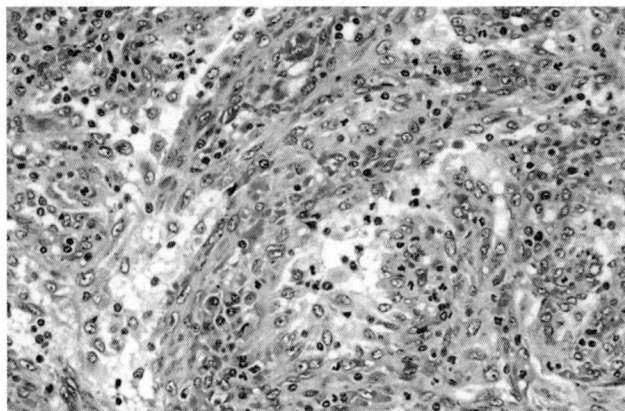

FIGURE 50.36. Littoral cell angioma. Vascular spaces lined by plump and cuboidal littoral cells with occasional papillary projections into the vascular lumen.

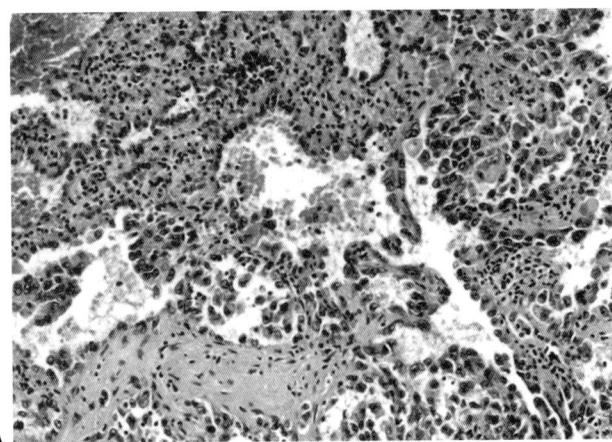 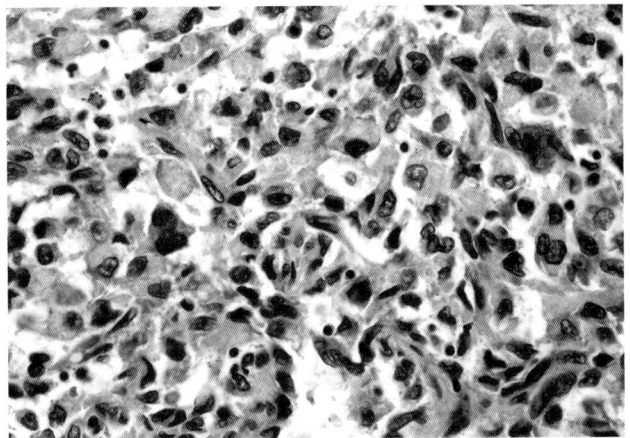

A   B

FIGURE 50.37. Angiosarcoma. A: Areas resembling littoral cell angioma at low power. **B:** Higher power demonstrating areas with unequivocally malignant cells.

and macrophages (sometimes exhibiting erythrophagocytosis). Mild cytologic atypia may be present, and the distinction between littoral cell angiomas and low-grade angiosarcoma can be difficult in individual cases (354,355).

Angiosarcomas of the spleen are rare multifocal proliferations that are heterogeneous in morphology and clinical behavior (356). In areas they may appear benign, resembling littoral cell angiomas, while elsewhere they contain areas of unequivocal malignancy resembling high-grade angiosarcoma (Fig. 50.37). Expression of CD8 is weak or absent in the areas that appear most malignant. The presence of CD8 positivity in some of these tumors supports the concept that a subset of angiosarcomas may arise from sinusoidal endothelium (355).

High-grade angiosarcomas in the spleen usually contain areas with spindle cell morphology and little evidence of vascular differentiation. Occasional malignant neoplasms of the spleen have been described with pure spindle cell composition; these have variously been regarded as examples of malignant fibrous histiocytoma or solid angiosarcomas (357). Solid malignant tumors with the characteristics of Kaposi sarcoma have also been described in the spleen, not all of them in patients with HIV infection or other immunodeficient states (358). Lymphangiomas are thin-walled cysts of various sizes lined by flat endothelial cells, containing watery, pink proteinaceous materials but not blood (359). Single cases of primary splenic nonvascular mesenchymal tumors, including rhabdomyosarcoma and fibroblastic reticular cell tumor, have also been reported (360,361).

Metastatic Tumors

Metastatic tumors are uncommon in the spleen, perhaps because of the absence of splenic afferent lymphatics. A large variety of types of carcinomas, as well as melanoma, and more rarely sarcomas, have been reported in the spleen. Most cause tumor masses (Fig. 50.38), but some may infiltrate the organ diffusely.

Storage Disorders

The spleen is involved in many of the lysosomal storage diseases, a rare group of predominately autosomal recessive inherited conditions whose diagnosis and classification is based on the identification of the enzymatic defect characteristic of each disease often in combination with specific genetic testing. Although most of these conditions are rare, three of the lipid storage diseases can be encountered, although uncommonly,

in surgical pathology practice. Gaucher and Niemann-Pick diseases, particularly in their nonneuronopathic forms, are the most common storage diseases encountered in removed spleens (23,362,363). The significant splenomegaly observed in these cases may cause hypersplenism. Not uncommonly in these cases, the spleen is removed to confirm the diagnosis or to ameliorate cytopenia. Ceroid histiocytosis (sea blue histiocytosis) can also be observed. Accumulation of sea-blue histiocytes may be seen in association with lipid disorders, infectious diseases, red blood cell disorders, and myeloproliferative disorders. However, it is also a prominent feature observed in spleens removed from patients with Hermansky-Pudlak syndrome, a rare often fatal autosomal recessive disorder that is currently classified among the group of lysosome-related organelle disorders (364).

In most of these cases, affected spleens are usually pale and homogeneous appearing. Rarely, areas of fibrosis may be noted (23). Microscopically, the red pulp is expanded because of the accumulation of numerous histiocytes in the splenic cords (23). Characteristic Gaucher cells range in size from 20 to 100 μm in diameter and have fibrillar cytoplasm that appears brownish in hematoxylin-and-eosin–stained preparations (Fig. 50.39). Multinucleated cells may occur. The cytoplasm is intensely PAS positive, and the PAS positivity is resistant to diastase digestion.

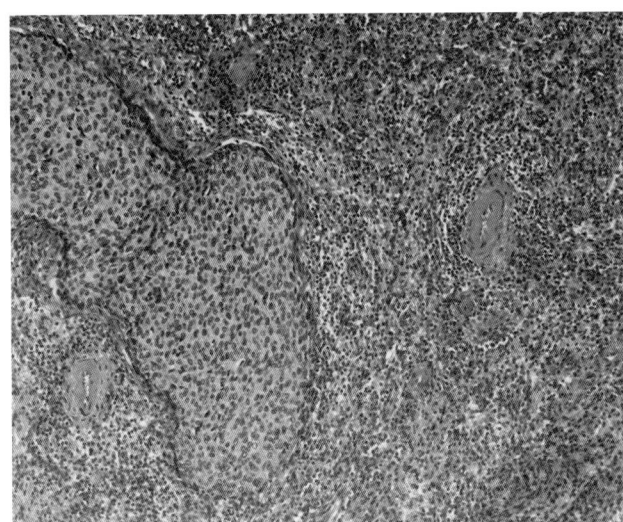

FIGURE 50.38. Metastatic transitional cell carcinoma involving spleen.

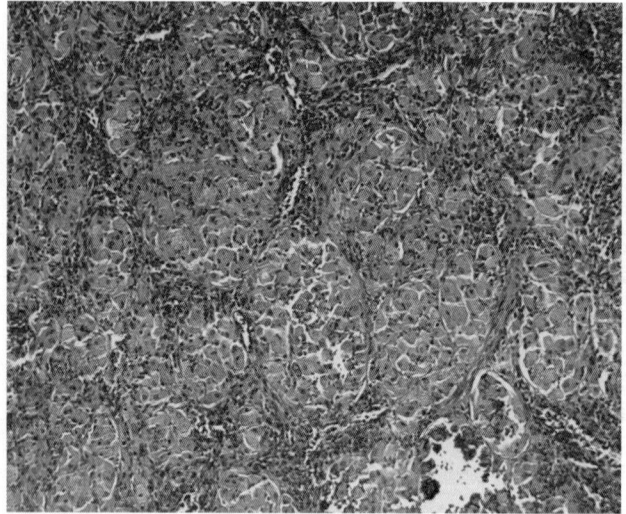

FIGURE 50.39. Gaucher cells with fibrillary cytoplasm.

The glucocerebroside in Gaucher cells is autofluorescent. Since Gaucher cells are macrophages and ingest red blood cells, they may frequently stain positively for iron. Lipid stains are only weakly positive. Ultrastructural studies reveal numerous lysosomes containing characteristic lipid bilayers. Pseudo-Gaucher cells are often seen in spleens of patients with CML.

Niemann-Pick cells are large, ranging from 20 to 100 μm in diameter, and appear foamy or bubbly owing to numerous small vacuoles (Fig. 50.40). They are clearer than Gaucher cells and usually stain only faintly with the PAS stain but contain neutral fat as demonstrated by Sudan black B and oil red O stains. The lipid deposits are birefringent and, under ultraviolet light, display yellow-green fluorescence. Electron microscopy reveals lamellated structures resembling myelin figures within lysosomes.

In cases of ceroid histiocytosis, smaller histiocytes with more basophilic cytoplasm and vacuoles (often termed sea-blue histiocytes) are characteristically seen. These cells can also be seen in Niemann-Pick disease. Ceroid-containing histiocytes measure up to 20 μm and contain cytoplasmic granules that measure 3 to 4 μm. The histiocytes show a variable degree of granulation. Foamy histiocytes with smaller, darker granules may also occur. Ceroid is composed of phospholipids and glycosphingolipids and is similar to lipofuscin in its physical and chemical properties. Histiocytes containing ceroid appear faintly yellow-brown in hematoxylin-and-eosin–stained sections, but blue-green with Romanowsky stains, resulting in the term "sea-blue histiocyte." Ceroid is PAS positive and resistant to diastase digestion and stains positively with lipid stains. It shows a strong affinity for basic dyes such as fuchsin and methylene blue. Ceroid is acid-fast and becomes autofluorescent with aging of the pigment. Ultrastructural studies reveal inclusions of lamellated membranous material with 4.5 to 5 nm periodicity.

None of the cell types identified in storage disorders is specific for a given disease, and their actual diagnosis should be based on biochemical or molecular genetic testing specific for these diseases.

 SUMMARY AND CONCLUSIONS

Neoplastic disorders of the spleen are predominantly of hematopoietic origin. They rarely occur as isolated phenomena but are, in most cases, part of a systemic involvement of disease. They include various malignant lymphomas, lymphoid and myeloid leukemias, and myeloproliferative disorders. Lymphoid neoplasms almost invariably involve the white pulp but may involve the red pulp if leukemic, or in cases of certain T-cell malignancies. Leukemic and myeloproliferative disorders involve the red pulp. Most nonhematopoietic tumors of the spleen are benign and are composed of tissue elements that make up the vascular tissue of that organ, that is, angiomas. Malignant nonhematopoietic tumors are uncommon; most are vascular. Metastatic neoplasms in the spleen are uncommon.

References

1. van Krieken JH, te Velde J. Normal histology of the human spleen. *Am J Surg Pathol* 1988;12:777–785.
2. Neiman RS, Orazi A. *Disorders of the spleen,* 2nd ed. Philadelphia: WB Saunders, 1998.
3. Grogan TM, Jolley CS, Rangel CS. Immunoarchitecture of the human spleen. *Lymphology* 1983;16:72–82.
4. Grogan TM, Rangel CS, Richter LC, et al. Further delineation of the immunoarchitecture of the human spleen. *Lymphology* 1984;17:61–68.
5. Bishop MB, Lansing LS. The spleen: a correlative overview of normal and pathologic anatomy. *Hum Pathol* 1980;13:334–342.
6. Raviola E. Spleen. In: Fawcett DW, ed. *A textbook of histology,* 12th ed. New York: Chapman and Hall, 1994:460.
7. Lukes RJ. The pathology of the white pulp of the spleen. In: Lennert K, Harms D, eds. *Die milz.* Berlin: Springer-Verlag, 1970:130–138.
8. Millikin PD. Anatomy of germinal centers in human lymphoid tissue. *Arch Pathol* 1966;82:499–503.
9. Millikin PD. The nodular white pulp of the human spleen. *Arch Pathol* 1969;87:247–258.
10. Nossal GJV, Abbot A, Mitchell J, et al. Antigens in immunity: XV. Ultrastructural features of antigen capture in primary and secondary lymphoid follicles. *J Exp Med* 1968;127:277–290.
11. Hirasaw Y, Tokuhiro H. Electron microscopic studies on the normal human spleen: especially on the red pulp and the reticulo-endothelial cells. *Blood* 1970;35:201–212.
12. Rappaport H. The pathologic anatomy of the splenic red pulp. In: Lennert K, Harms D, eds. *Die milz.* Berlin: Springer-Verlag, 1970:25–41.
13. Wennberg E, Weiss L. The structure of the spleen and hemolysis. *Annu Rev Med* 1969;20:29–40.
14. Crosby WH. Splenic remodeling of red cell surfaces. *Blood* 1977;50:643–645.
15. Hsu SM, Cossman J, Jaffe ES. Lymphocyte subsets in normal human lymphoid tissue. *Am J Clin Pathol* 1983;80:21–30.
16. Timens W, Poppema S. Lymphocyte compartments in human spleen. An immunohistologic study in normal spleens and non-involved spleens in Hodgkin's disease. *Am J Pathol* 1985;120:443–453.
17. Van Ewijk W, Nieuwenhuis P. Compartments, domains and migration pathways of lymphoid cells in the splenic pulp. *Experientia* 1985;41:199–208.
18. Gutman GA, Weissman IL. Lymphoid tissue architecture: experimental analysis of the origin and distribution of T cells and B cells. *Immunology* 1972;23:465–479.
19. Stein H, Bonk A, Tolksdorf G, et al. Immunohistologic analysis of the organization of normal lymphoid tissue in non-Hodgkin's lymphomas. *J Histochem Cytochem* 1980;26:746–760.
20. Tonder P, Morse PA, Humphrey LJ. Similarities of Fc receptors in human malignant tissue and normal lymphoid tissue. *J Immunol* 1974;113:1162–1169.
21. Lipson RL, Bayrd ED, Watkins CH. The postsplenectomy blood picture. *Am J Clin Pathol* 1959;32:526–532.
22. Singer K, Miller EB, Dameshek W. Hematologic changes following splenectomy in man with particular reference to target cells, hemolytic index and lysolecithin. *Am J Med Sci* 1941;202:171–187.

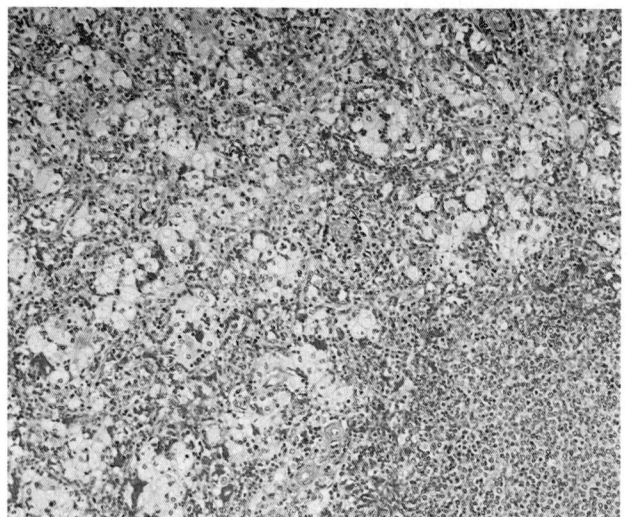

FIGURE 50.40. Niemann-Pick cells with foamy or bubbly cytoplasm.

23. Neiman RS, Orazi A. *Disorders of the spleen*, 2nd ed. Philadelphia: W.B. Saunders, 1999.
24. Burke JS, Osborne BM. Localized reactive lymphoid hyperplasia of the spleen simulating malignant lymphoma. A report of seven cases. *Am J Surg Pathol* 1983;7:373–380.
25. Dunphy CH, Bee C, McDonald JW, et al. Incidental early detection of a splenic marginal zone lymphoma by polymerase chain reaction analysis of paraffin-embedded tissue. *Arch Pathol Lab Med* 1998;122:84–86.
26. Harris S, Wilkins BS, Jones DB. Splenic marginal zone expansion in B cell lymphomas of gastrointestinal mucosa-associated lymphoid tissue (MALT) is reactive and does not represent homing of neoplastic lymphocytes. *J Pathol* 1996;179:49–53.
27. Farhi DC, Ashfaq R. Splenic pathology after traumatic injury. *Am J Clin Pathol* 1996;105:474–478.
28. Kroft SH, Singleton TP, Dahiya M, et al. Ruptured spleens with expanded marginal zones do not reveal occult B cell clones. *Mod Pathol* 1997;10:1214–1220.
29. Rosso R, Neiman RS, Paulli M, et al. Splenic marginal zone cell lymphoma: report of an indolent variant without massive splenomegaly presumably representing an early phase of the disease. *Hum Pathol* 1995;26:39–46.
30. Jiang DY, Li CY. Immunohistochemical study of the spleen in chronic immune thrombocytopenic purpura. With special reference to hyperplastic follicles and foamy macrophages. *Arch Pathol Lab Med* 1995;119:533–537.
31. Tindle BH, Parker JW, Lukes RJ. "Reed-Sternberg cells" in infectious mononucleosis. *Am J Clin Pathol* 1972;58:607–617.
32. McMahon NJ, Gordon HW, Rosen RB. Reed-Sternberg cells in infectious mononucleosis. *Am J Dis Child* 1970;120:148–150.
33. Lukes RJ, Tindle BH, Parker JW. Reed-Sternberg like cells in infectious mononucleosis. *Lancet* 1969;2:1003–1004.
34. Burke JS. Diagnosis of lymphoma and lymphoid proliferations in the spleen. In: Jaffe ES, ed. *Surgical pathology of the lymph nodes and related organs*, 2nd ed. Philadelphia: W.B. Saunders, 1995:448.
35. Smith EB, Custer RP. Rupture of the spleen in infectious mononucleosis: a clinicopathologic report of seven cases. *Blood* 1946;1:317–333.
36. Slavin RE, Santos GW. The graft versus host reaction in man after bone marrow transplantation: pathology, pathogenesis, clinical features and implications. *Clin Immunol Immunopathol* 1973;1:472–498.
37. Hassan NMR, Neiman RS. The pathology of the spleen in steroid-treated immune thrombocytopenic purpura. *Am J Clin Pathol* 1985;84:433–438.
38. Rodriguez-Garcia JL, Sanchez-Corral J, Martinez J, et al. Phenytoin-induced benign lymphadenopathy with solid spleen lesions mimicking a malignant lymphoma. *Ann Oncol* 1991;2:443–445.
39. Le Deist F, Emile JF, Rieux-Laucat F, et al. Clinical, immunological, and pathological consequences of Fas-deficient conditions. *Lancet* 1996;348:719–723.
40. Lim MS, Straus SE, Dale JK, et al. Pathological findings in human autoimmune lymphoproliferative syndrome. *Am J Pathol* 1998;153:1541–1550.
41. Alvarado CS, Straus SE, Li S, et al. Autoimmune lymphoproliferative syndrome: a cause of chronic splenomegaly, lymphadenopathy, and cytopenias in children-report on diagnosis and management of five patients. *Pediatr Blood Cancer* 2004;43:164–169.
42. Kwon SW, Procter J, Dale JK, et al. Neutrophil and platelet antibodies in autoimmune lymphoproliferative syndrome. *Vox Sang* 2003;85:307–312.
43. Straus SE, Jaffe ES, Puck JM, et al. The development of lymphomas in families with autoimmune lymphoproliferative syndrome with germline Fas mutations and defective lymphocyte apoptosis. *Blood* 2001;98:194–200.
44. Keller AR, Hochholzer L, Castleman B. Hyaline vascular and plasma-cell types of giant lymph node hyperplasia of the mediastinum and other locations. *Cancer* 1972;29:670–683.
45. Schnitzer B. The reactive lymphadenopathies. In: Knowles DM, ed. *Neoplastic hematopathology*, 2nd ed. Philadelphia: Lippincott Williams & Wilkins, 2001:537–568.
46. Weisenburger DD. Multicentric angiofollicular lymph node hyperplasia: pathology of the spleen. *Am J Surg Pathol* 1988;12:176–181.
47. Gaba AR, Stein RS, Sweet DL, et al. Multicentric giant lymph node hyperplasia. *Am J Clin Pathol* 1978;69:86–90.
48. Frizzera G, Massarelli G, Banks PM, et al. A systemic lymphoproliferative disorder with morphologic features of Castleman's disease. *Am J Surg Pathol* 1983;7:211–231.
49. Du MQ, Liu H, Diss TC, et al. Kaposi sarcoma-associated herpesvirus I infects monotypic (IgM lambda) but polyclonal naive B cells in Castleman disease and associated lymphoproliferative disorders. *Blood* 2001;97:2130–2136.
50. Oksenhendler E, Boulanger E, Galicier L, et al. High incidence of Kaposi sarcoma-associated herpesvirus-related non-Hodgkin lymphoma in patients with HIV infection and multicentric Castleman disease. *Blood* 2002;99:2331–2336.
51. Seliem RM, Griffith RC, Harris NL, et al. HHV-8+, EBV+ multicentric plasmablastic microlymphoma in an HIV+ Man: the spectrum of HHV-8+ lymphoproliferative disorders expands. *Am J Surg Pathol* 2007;31:1439–1445.
52. Hoppe RT, Cox RS, Rosenberg SA, et al. Prognostic factors in stage III Hodgkin's lymphoma. *Cancer Treat Rep* 1982;66:743–749.
53. Hoppe RT, Rosenberg SA, Kaplan HS, et al. Prognostic factors in pathological state IIIA Hodgkin's lymphoma. *Cancer* 1980;46:1240–1246.
54. Kadin ME, Glatstein E, Dorfman RF. Clinicopathologic studies of 117 untreated patients subjected to laparotomy for the staging of Hodgkin's lymphoma. *Cancer* 1971;27:1277–1294.
55. Neiman RS, Rosen PJ, Lukes RJ. Lymphocyte depletion Hodgkin's lymphoma: a clinicopathologic entity. *N Engl J Med* 1973;288:751–755.
56. Trudel M, Krikorian J, Neiman RS. Lymphocyte predominance Hodgkin's lymphoma: clinical and morphologic heterogeneity. *Cancer* 1987;59:99–106.
57. Neiman RS. Current problems in the histopathologic diagnosis and classification of Hodgkin's disease. *Pathol Annu* 1978;2:289–328.
58. Desser PK, Moran EM, Ultmann JE. Staging of Hodgkin's disease and lymphoma. *Med Clin North Am* 1973;57:479–498.
59. Farrer-Brown G, Bennett MH, Harrison CV, et al. The diagnosis of Hodgkin's disease in surgically excised spleens. *J Clin Pathol* 1972;25:294–300.
60. Brincker H. Sarcoid reactions and sarcoidosis in Hodgkin's disease and other malignant lymphomata. *Br J Cancer* 1972;26:120–128.
61. Collins RD, Neiman RS. Granulomatous diseases of the spleen. In: Ioachim HL, ed. *Pathology of granulomas*. New York: Raven Press, 1983:189–207.
62. Kadin ME, Donaldson SS, Dorfman RF. Isolated granulomas in Hodgkin's disease. *N Engl J Med* 1970;283:859–861.
63. Neiman RS. Incidence and importance of splenic sarcoidal-like granulomas. *Arch Pathol Lab Med* 1977;101:518–521.
64. O'Connell MJ, Schimpff SC, Kirschner RH, et al. Epithelioid granulomas in Hodgkin's disease: a favorable prognostic sign. *JAMA* 1975;233:886–890.
65. Sacks EL, Donaldson SS, Gordon J, et al. Epithelioid granulomas associated with Hodgkin's disease: clinical correlations in 55 previously untreated patients. *Cancer* 1978;41:562–567.
66. Warnke RA, Weiss LM, Chan JKC, et al. Primary splenic lymphoma. In: *Atlas of tumor pathology: tumors of the lymph nodes and spleen*. Series 3, Fascicle 14. Washington: Armed Forces Institute of Pathology, 1995:411.
67. Bellamy CO, Krajewski AS. Primary splenic large cell anaplastic lymphoma associated with HIV infection. *Histopathology* 1994;24:481–483.
68. Brox A, Bishinsky JI, Berry G. Primary non-Hodgkin lymphoma of the spleen. *Am J Hematol* 1991;38:95–100.
69. Brox A, Shustik C. Non-Hodgkin's lymphoma of the spleen. *Leuk Lymphoma* 1993;11:165–171.
70. Das Gupta T, Coombes B, Brasfeld RD. Primary malignant neoplasms of the spleen. *Surg Gynecol Obstet* 1965;120:947–959.
71. Falk S, Karhoff M, Takeshita M, et al. Primary pleomorphic T cell lymphoma of the spleen. *Histopathology* 1990;16:191–192.
72. Fausel R, Sun NC, Klein S. Splenic rupture in HIV-infected patient with primary splenic lymphoma. *Cancer* 1990;66:2414–2416.
73. Hara K, Ito M, Shimizu K, et al. Three cases of primary splenic lymphoma: case report and review of the Japanese literature. *Acta Pathol Jpn* 1985;35:419–435.
74. Harris NL, Aisenberg AC, Meyer JE, et al. Diffuse large cell (histiocytic) lymphoma of the spleen: clinical and pathologic characteristics of ten cases. *Cancer* 1984;53:2460–2467.
75. Ishihara T, Takahashi M, Uchino F, et al. A filiform large cell lymphoma of the spleen: a case report with immunohistochemical and electron microscopic study. *Ultrastruct Pathol* 1990;14:193–199.
76. Kobrich U, Falk S, Karhoff M, et al. Primary large cell lymphoma of the splenic sinuses: a variant of angiotropic B cell lymphoma (neoplastic angioendothelioma-tosis)? *Hum Pathol* 1992;23:1184–1187.
77. Montanaro A, Patten R. Primary splenic malignant lymphoma, histiocytic type, with sclerosis. *Cancer* 1976;38:1625–1628.
78. Kroft SH, Howard MS, Picker LJ, et al. De novo CD5+ diffuse large B-cell lymphomas. A heterogeneous group containing an unusual form of splenic lymphoma. *Am J Clin Pathol* 2000;114(4):523–533.
79. Grosskreutz C, Troy K, Cuttner J. Primary splenic lymphoma: report of 10 cases using the REAL classification. *Cancer Invest* 2002;20:749–753.
80. Falk S, Stutte JH. Primary malignant lymphomas of the spleen, a morphologic and immunohistochemical analysis of 17 cases. *Cancer* 1990;66:2612.
81. Bellany CO, Krajewski AJ. Primary splenic large cell anaplastic lymphoma associated with HIV infection. *Histopathology* 1994;24:481.
82. Kim H, Dorfman RF. Morphological studies of 84 untreated patients subjected to laparotomy for the staging of non-Hodgkin's lymphomas. *Cancer* 1974;33:657–676.
83. Lotz MJ, Chabner B, DeVita VT, et al. Pathological staging of 100 consecutive untreated patients with non-Hodgkin's lymphomas. *Cancer* 1976;37:266–270.
84. Goffinet DR, Warnke R, Dunnick NR, et al. Clinical and surgical (laparotomy) evaluation of patients with non-Hodgkin's lymphomas. *Cancer Treat Rep* 1977;61:981–992.
85. Cheson BD. Staging and evaluation of the patient with lymphoma. *Hematol Oncol Clin North Am* 2008;22:825–837.
86. Pangalis GA, Nathwani BN, Rappaport H. Malignant lymphoma, well differentiated lymphocytic: its relationship with chronic lymphocytic leukemia and macroglobulinemia of Waldenstrom. *Cancer* 1977;39:999–1010.
87. Narang S, Wolf BC, Neiman RS. Malignant lymphoma presenting with prominent splenomegaly. A clinicopathologic study with special reference to intermediate cell lymphoma. *Cancer* 1985;55:1948–1957.
88. Ahmann DL, Kiely JM, Harrison EG Jr, et al. Malignant lymphoma of the spleen: a review of 49 cases in which the diagnosis was made at splenectomy. *Cancer* 1966;19:461–469.
89. Kraemer BB, Osborne BM, Butler JJ. Primary splenic presentation of malignant lymphoma: a study of 49 cases. *Cancer* 1984;54:1606–1619.
90. Long JC, Aisenberg AC. Malignant lymphoma diagnosed at splenectomy and idiopathic splenomegaly. *Cancer* 1974;33:1054–1061.
91. Arber DA, Rappaport H, Weiss LM. Non-Hodgkin's lymphoproliferative disorders involving the spleen. *Mod Pathol* 1997;10:18–32.
92. Evans HL, Butler JJ, Youness EL. Malignant lymphoma, small lymphocytic type: a clinicopathologic study of 84 cases with suggested criteria for intermediate lymphocytic lymphoma. *Cancer* 1978;41:1440–1455.
93. Asplund SL, McKenna RW, Howard MS, et al. Immunophenotype does not correlate with lymph node histology in chronic lymphocytic leukemia/small lymphocytic lymphoma. *Am J Surg Pathol* 2002;26:624–629.
94. Palutke M, Tabaczka P, Mirchandani I, et al. Lymphocytic lymphoma simulating hairy cell leukemia: a consideration of reliable and unreliable diagnostic features. *Cancer* 1981;48:2047–2055.
95. Galton DAG, Goldman JM, Wiltshaw E, et al. Prolymphocytic leukemia. *Br J Haematol* 1974;27:7–23.
96. Stone RM. Prolymphocytic leukemia. *Hematol Oncol Clin North Am* 1990;4:457–471.
97. Matutes E, Brito-Babapulle V, Swansbury J, et al. Clinical and laboratory features of 78 cases of T-prolymphocytic leukemia. *Blood* 1991;78:3269–3274.
98. Bearman RM, Pangalis GA, Rappaport H. Prolymphocytic leukemia. Clinical, histopathologic, and cytochemical observations. *Cancer* 1978;42:2360–2372.
99. Ruchlemer R, Parry-Jones N, Brito-Babapulle V, et al. B-prolymphocytic leukaemia with t(11;14) revisited: a splenomegalic form of mantle cell lymphoma evolving with leukaemia. *Br J Haematol* 2004;125:330–336.
100. Waldenstrom J. Incipient myelomatosis or "essential" hyperglobulinemia with fibrinogenopenia: a new syndrome? *Acta Med Scand* 1944;117:216–244.
101. MacKenzie MR, Fudenberg HH. Macroglobulinemia: an analysis for forty patients. *Blood* 1972;39:874–889.
102. Cohen RJ, Bohannon RA, Wallerstein RO. Waldenstrom's macroglobulinemia. A study of ten cases. *Am J Med* 1966;41:274–284.
103. Pescarmona E, Pignoloni P, Orazi A, et al. "Composite" lymphoma, lymphoplasmacytoid and diffuse large B-cell lymphoma of the spleen: molecular-genetic evidence of a common clonal origin. *Virchows Arch* 1999;435:442–446.

104. Pittaluga S, Verhoef G, Criel A, et al. "Small" B cell non-Hodgkin's lymphomas with splenomegaly at presentation are either mantle cell lymphoma or marginal zone cell lymphoma. *Am J Surg Pathol* 1996;20:211–223.

105. Weisenburger DD, Linder J, Daley DT, et al. Intermediate lymphocytic lymphoma: an immunohistologic study with comparison to other lymphocytic lymphomas. *Hum Pathol* 1987;18:781–790.

106. Weisenburger DD, Kim H, Rappaport H. Mantle zone lymphoma: a follicular variant of intermediate lymphocytic lymphoma. *Cancer* 1982;49:1429–1438.

107. Molina TJ, Delmer A, Cymbalista F, et al. Mantle cell lymphoma, in leukaemic phase with prominent splenomegaly. A report of eight cases with similar clinical presentation and aggressive outcome. *Virchows Arch* 2000;437:591–598.

108. Schlette E, Bueso-Ramos C, Giles F, et al. Mature B-cell leukemias with more than 55% prolymphocytes. A heterogeneous group that includes an unusual variant of mantle cell lymphoma. *Am J Clin Pathol* 2001;115:571–581.

109. Wong KF, So CC, Chan JK. Nucleolated variant of mantle cell lymphoma with leukemic manifestations mimicking prolymphocytic leukemia. *Am J Clin Pathol* 2002;117:246–251.

110. Mollejo M, Rodríguez-Pinilla MS, Montes-Moreno S, et al. Splenic follicular lymphoma: clinicopathologic characteristics of a series of 32 cases. *Am J Surg Pathol* 2009;33:730–738.

111. Howard MT, Dufresne S, Swerdlow SH, et al. Follicular lymphoma of the spleen: multiparameter analysis of 16 cases. *Am J Clin Pathol* 2009;131:656–662.

112. Sheibani K, Burke JS, Swartz WG, et al. Monocytoid B-cell lymphoma. Clinicopathologic study of 21 cases of a unique type of low-grade lymphoma. *Cancer* 1988;62:1531–1538.

113. Agnarsson BA, Kadin ME. An unusual B-cell lymphoma simulating hairy cell leukemia. *Am J Clin Pathol* 1987;88:752–759.

114. Ngan B-Y, Warnke RA, Wilson M, et al. Monocytoid B-cell lymphoma: a study of 36 cases. *Hum Pathol* 1991;22:409–421.

115. Traweek ST, Sheibani K. Monocytoid B-cell lymphoma: the biologic and clinical implications of peripheral blood involvement. *Am J Clin Pathol* 1992;97:591–598.

116. Vasef M, Katzin WE. Monocytoid B-cell lymphoma with a distinctive clinical presentation. *Hum Pathol* 1993;24:558–561.

117. Warnke RA, Weiss LM, Chan JKC, et al. Malignant lymphoma, small lymphocytic and diffuse small cleaved cell (centrocytic). In: *Atlas of tumor pathology: tumors of the lymph nodes and spleen,* 3rd series, Fascicle 14, Washington: Armed Forces Institute of Pathology, 1995.

118. Stroup RM, Burke JS, Sheibani K, et al. Splenic involvement by aggressive malignant lymphomas of B-cell and T-cell types: a morphologic and immunophenotypic study. *Cancer* 1992;69:413–420.

119. Mollejo M, Algara P, Mateo MS, et al. Large B-cell lymphoma presenting in the spleen: identification of different clinicopathologic conditions. *Am J Surg Pathol* 2003;27:895–902.

120. Kashimura M, Noro M, Akikusa B, et al. Primary splenic diffuse large B-cell lymphoma manifesting in red pulp. *Virchows Arch* 2008;453:501–509.

121. Betman HF, Vardiman JW, Lau J. T-cell rich B-cell lymphoma of the spleen. Letter to the editor. *Am J Surg Pathol* 1994;18:323–324.

122. Dogan A, Burke JS, Goteri G, et al. Micronodular T-cell/histiocyte-rich large B-cell lymphoma of the spleen: histology, immunophenotype, and differential diagnosis. *Am J Surg Pathol* 2003;27:903–911.

123. Grogan TM, Warnke RA, Kaplan HS. A comparative study of Burkitt's and non-Burkitt's "undifferentiated" malignant lymphoma: immunologic, cytochemical, ultrastructural, histopathologic, clinical and cell culture features. *Cancer* 1982;49:1817–1828.

124. Banks PM, Arseneau JC, Gralnick HR, et al. American Burkitt's lymphoma: a clinicopathologic study of 30 cases. II. Pathologic correlations. *Am J Med* 1975;58:322–329.

125. Mann RB, Jaffe ES, Braylan RC, et al. Non-endemic Burkitt's lymphoma. A B-cell tumor related to germinal centers. *N Engl J Med* 1976;295:685–691.

126. Orazi A, Cattoretti G, John K, et al. Terminal deoxynucleotidyl transferase staining of malignant lymphomas in paraffin sections. *Mod Pathol* 1994;7:582–586.

127. Orazi A, Cotton J, Cattoretti G, et al. Terminal deoxynucleotidyl transferase staining in acute leukemia and normal bone marrow in routinely processed paraffin sections. *Am J Clin Pathol* 1994;102:640–645.

128. Robertson PB, Neiman RS, Worapongpaiboon S, et al. 013 (CD99) positivity in hematologic proliferations correlates with TdT positivity. *Mod Pathol* 1997;10:277–282.

129. Schmid C, Kirkham N, Diss T, et al. Splenic marginal zone cell lymphoma. *Am J Surg Pathol* 1992;16:455–466.

130. Jaffe ES, Harris NL, Vardiman JW, et al., eds. *WHO classification of tumours of haemopoietic and lymphoid tissues.* Lyon, France: IARC Press, 2001.

131. Swerdlow SH, Campo E, Harris NL et al., eds. *WHO classification of tumours of haemopoietic and lymphoid tissues.* Lyon, France: IARC Press, 2008.

132. Berger F, Felman P, Thieblemont C, et al. Non-MALT marginal zone B-cell lymphomas: a description of clinical presentation and outcome in 124 patients. *Blood* 2000;95:1950–1956.

133. Mollejo M, Menarguez J, Lloret E, et al. Splenic marginal zone lymphoma: a distinctive type of low-grade B cell lymphoma. A clinicopathological study of 13 cases. *Am J Surg Pathol* 1995;19:1146–1157.

134. Matutes E. Clinical and biological diversity of splenic marginal zone lymphoma. *Expert Rev Anticancer Ther* 2009;9:1185–1189.

135. Arcaini L, Paulli M, Boveri E, et al. Splenic and nodal marginal zone lymphomas are indolent disorders at high hepatitis C virus seroprevalence with distinct presenting features but similar morphologic and phenotypic profiles. *Cancer* 2004;100:107–115.

136. Vallisa D, Bernuzzi P, Arcaini L, et al. Role of anti-hepatitis C virus (HCV) treatment in HCV-related, low-grade, B-cell, non-Hodgkin's lymphoma: a multicenter Italian experience. *J Clin Oncol* 2005;23:468–473.

137. Mele A, Pulsoni A, Bianco E, et al. Hepatitis C virus and B-cell non-Hodgkin lymphomas: an Italian multicenter case-control study. *Blood* 2003;102:996–999.

138. Hermine O, Lefrère F, Bronowicki JP, et al. Regression of splenic lymphoma with villous lymphocytes after treatment of hepatitis C virus infection. *N Engl J Med* 2002;347:89–94.

139. Bates I, Bedu-Addo G, Rutherford T, et al. Splenic lymphoma with villous lymphocytes in tropical West Africa. *Lancet* 1992;340:575–577.

140. Bates I, Bedu-Addo G, Rutherford TR, et al. Circulating villous lymphocytes—a link between hyperreactive malarial splenomegaly and splenic lymphoma. *Trans R Soc Trop Med Hyg* 1997;91:171–174.

141. Boveri E, Arcaini L, Merli M, et al. Bone marrow histology in marginal zone B-cell lymphomas: correlation with clinical parameters and flow cytometry in 120 patients. *Ann Oncol* 2009;20:129–136.

142. Dufresne SD, Felgar RE, Sargent RL, et al. Defining the borders of splenic marginal zone lymphoma: a multiparameter study. *Hum Pathol* 2010;41:540–551.

143. Petit B, Parrens M, Soubeyran I, et al. Among 157 marginal zone lymphomas, DBA.44(CD76) expression is restricted to tumour cells infiltrating the red pulp of the spleen with a diffuse architectural pattern. *Histopathology* 2009;54:626–631.

144. Gruszka-Westwood AM, Hamoudi RA, Matutes E, et al. p53 abnormalities in splenic lymphoma with villous lymphocytes. *Blood* 2001;97:3552–3558.

145. Baseggio L, Traverse-Glehen A, Petinataud F, et al. CD5 expression identifies a subset of splenic marginal zone lymphomas with higher lymphocytosis: a clinico-pathological, cytogenetic and molecular study of 24 cases. *Haematologica* 2010;95:604–612.

146. Mateo M, Mollejo M, Villuendas R, et al. 7q31-32 allelic loss is a frequent finding in splenic marginal zone lymphoma. *Am J Pathol* 1999;154:1583–1589.

147. Salido M, Baró C, Oscier D, et al. Cytogenetic aberrations and their prognostic value in a series of 330 splenic marginal zone B-cell lymphomas: a multicenter study of the Splenic B-Cell Lymphoma Group. *Blood* 2010;116:1479–1488.

148. Rinaldi A, Mian M, Chigrinova E, et al. Genome-wide DNA profiling of marginal zone lymphomas identifies subtype-specific lesions with an impact on the clinical outcome. *Blood* 2011;117:1595–1604.

149. Rinaldi A, Forconi F, Arcaini L, et al. Immunogenetics features and genomic lesions in splenic marginal zone lymphoma. *Br J Haematol* 2010;151:435–439.

150. Solé F, Salido M, Espinet B, et al. Splenic marginal zone B-cell lymphomas: two cytogenetic subtypes, one with gain of 3q and the other with loss of 7q. *Haematologica* 2001;86:71–77.

151. Algara P, Mateo MS, Sanchez-Beato M, et al. Analysis of the IgV(H) somatic mutations in splenic marginal zone lymphoma defines a group of unmutated cases with frequent 7q deletion and adverse clinical course. *Blood* 2002;99:1299–1304.

152. Ruiz-Ballesteros E, Mollejo M, Rodriguez A, et al. Splenic marginal zone lymphoma: proposal of new diagnostic and prognostic markers identified after tissue and cDNA microarray analysis. *Blood* 2005;106:1831–1838.

153. Thieblemont C, Nasser V, Felman P, et al. Small lymphocytic lymphoma, marginal zone B-cell lymphoma, and mantle cell lymphoma exhibit distinct gene-expression profiles allowing molecular diagnosis. *Blood* 2004;103:2727–2737.

154. Chacón JI, Mollejo M, Muñoz E, et al. Splenic marginal zone lymphoma: clinical characteristics and prognostic factors in a series of 60 patients. *Blood* 2002;100:1648–1654.

155. Traverse-Glehen A, Davi F, Ben Simon E, et al. Analysis of VH genes in marginal zone lymphoma reveals marked heterogeneity between splenic and nodal tumors and suggests the existence of clonal selection. *Haematologica* 2005;90:470–478.

156. Arcaini L, Lazzarino M, Colombo N, et al. Splenic marginal zone lymphoma: a prognostic model for clinical use. *Blood* 2006;107:4643–4649.

157. Bennett M, Schechter GP. Treatment of splenic marginal zone lymphoma: splenectomy versus rituximab. *Semin Hematol* 2010;47:143–147.

158. Bennett M, Sharma K, Yegena S, et al. Rituximab monotherapy for splenic marginal zone lymphoma. *Haematologica* 2005;90:856–858.

159. Tsimberidou AM, Catovsky D, Schlette E, et al. Outcomes in patients with splenic marginal zone lymphoma and marginal zone lymphoma treated with rituximab with or without chemotherapy or chemotherapy alone. *Cancer* 2006;107:125–135.

160. Lefrère F, Hermine O, Belanger C, et al. Fludarabine: an effective treatment in patients with splenic lymphoma with villous lymphocytes. *Leukemia* 2000;14:573–575.

161. Camacho FI, Mollejo M, Mateo MS, et al. Progression to large B-cell lymphoma in splenic marginal zone lymphoma: a description of a series of 12 cases. *Am J Surg Pathol* 2001;25:1268–1276.

162. Dungarwalla M, Appiah-Cubi S, Kulkarni S, et al. High-grade transformation in splenic marginal zone lymphoma with circulating villous lymphocytes: the site of transformation influences response to therapy and prognosis. *Br J Haematol* 2008;143:71–74.

163. Van Huyen JP, Molina T, Delmer A, et al. Splenic marginal zone lymphoma with or without plasmacytic differentiation. *Am J Surg Pathol* 2000;24:1581–1592.

164. Piris MA, Mollejo M, Campo E, et al. A marginal zone pattern may be found in different varieties of non-Hodgkin's lymphoma: the morphology and immunohistology of splenic involvement by B-cell lymphomas simulating splenic marginal zone lymphoma. *Histopathology* 1998;33:230–239.

165. Burke JS, Byrne GE Jr, Rappaport H. Hairy cell leukemia (leukemic reticuloendotheliosis). I. A clinical pathologic study of 21 patients. *Cancer* 1974;33:1399–1416.

166. Catovsky D, Pettit JE, Galton DAG, et al. Leukemic reticuloendotheliosis (hairy cell leukemia): a distinct clinicopathologic entity. *Br J Haematol* 1974;26:9–27.

167. Brunning RD, McKenna RW. Tumors of the bone marrow. In: *Atlas of tumor pathology,* Series 3, Fascicle 9, p 276. Washington: Armed Forces Institute of Pathology, 1994.

168. Burke JS, MacKay B, Rappaport H. Hairy cell leukemia (leukemic reticuloendotheliosis). II. Ultrastructure of the spleen. *Cancer* 1976;37:2267–2274.

169. Pilon VA, Davey FR, Gordon GB, et al. Splenic alterations in hairy cell leukemia. II. An electron microscopic study. *Cancer* 1982;49:1617–1623.

170. Nanba K, Soban EJ, Bowling MC, et al. Splenic pseudosinuses and hepatic angiomatous lesions. Distinctive features of hairy cell leukemia. *Am J Clin Pathol* 1977;67:415–426.

171. Miranda RN, Briggs RC, Kinney MC, et al. Immunohistochemical detection of cyclin D1 using optimized conditions is highly specific for mantle cell lymphoma and hairy cell leukaemia. *Mod Pathol* 2000;13:1308–1314.

172. Jasionowski TM, Hartung I, Greenwood JH, et al. Analysis of CD10 + hairy cell leukaemia. *Am J Clin Oncol* 2003;120:228–235.

173. Chen YH, Tallman MS, Goolsby C. et al. Immunophenotypic variations in hairy cell leukemia. *Am J Clin Pathol* 2006;125:251–259.

174. Tiacci E, Trifonov V, Schiavoni G, et al. BRAF mutations in hairy cell leukemia. *N Engl J Med* 2011;364:2305–2315.

175. Blombery P, Wong SQ, Hewitt CA, et al. Detection of BRAF mutations in patients with hairy cell leukemia and related lymphoproliferative disorders. *Haematologica* 2012;97:780–783.

176. Arcaini L, Zibellini S, Boveri E, et al. The BRAF V600E mutation in hairy cell leukemia and other mature B-cell neoplasms. *Blood* 2012;119:188–191.

177. Tiacci E, Schiavoni G, Forconi F, et al. Simple genetic diagnosis of hairy cell leukemia by sensitive detection of the BRAF-V600E mutation. *Blood* 2012;119: 192–195.
178. Xi L, Arons E, Navarro W, et al. Both variant and IGHV4-34-expressing hairy cell leukemia lack the BRAF V600E mutation. *Blood* 2012;119:3330–3332.
179. Mollejo M, Algara P, Mateo MS, et al. Splenic small B-cell lymphoma with predominant red pulp involvement: a diffuse variant of splenic marginal zone lymphoma? *Histopathology* 2002;40:22–30.
180. Kanellis G, Mollejo M, Montes-Moreno S, et al. Splenic diffuse red pulp small B-cell lymphoma: revision of a series of cases reveals characteristic clinico-pathological features. *Haematologica* 2010;95:1122–1129.
181. Traverse-Glehen A, Baseggio L, Bauchu EC, et al. Splenic red pulp lymphoma with numerous basophilic villous lymphocytes: a distinct clinicopathologic and molecular entity? *Blood* 2008;111:2253–2260.
182. Cawley JC, Burns GF, Hayhoe FG. A chronic lymphoproliferative disorder with distinctive features: a distinct variant of hairy-cell leukaemia. *Leuk Res* 1980;4:547–559.
183. Cannon T, Mobarek D, Wegge J, et al. Hairy cell leukemia: current concepts. *Cancer Invest* 2008;26:860–865.
184. Matutes E, Wotherspoon A, Brito-Babapulle V, et al. The natural history and clinico-pathological features of the variant form of hairy cell leukemia. *Leukemia* 2001;15:184–186.
185. Matutes E, Wotherspoon A, Catovsky D. The variant form of hairy-cell leukaemia. *Best Pract Res Clin Haematol* 2003;16:41–56.
186. Robak T. Hairy-cell leukemia variant: recent view on diagnosis, biology and treatment. *Cancer Treat Rev* 2011;37:3–10.
187. Fietz T, Rieger K, Schmittel A, et al. Alemtuzumab (Campath 1H) in hairy cell leukaemia relapsing after rituximab treatment. *Hematol J* 2004;5:451–452.
188. Telek B, Batar P, Udvardy M. Successful alemtuzumab treatment of a patient with atypical hairy cell leukaemia variant. *Orv Hetil* 2007;148:1805–1807.
189. Machii T, Tokumine Y, Inoue R, et al. Predominance of a distinct subtype of hairy cell leukemia in Japan. *Leukemia* 1993;7:181–186.
190. Katayama I, Mochino T, Honma T, et al. Hairy cell leukemia: a comparative study of Japanese and non-Japanese patients. *Semin Oncol* 1984;11:486–492.
191. Yamaguchi M, Machii T, Shibayama H, et al. Immunophenotypic features and configuration of immunoglobulin genes in hairy cell leukemia-Japanese variant. *Leukemia* 1996;10:1390–1394.
192. Azar HA. Plasma cell myelomatosis and other monoclonal gammopathies. *Pathol Ann* 1972;7:1–17.
193. Sherwood P, Sommers A, Shirfield M, et al. Spontaneous splenic rupture in uncomplicated multiple myeloma. *Leuk Lymphoma* 1996;20:517–519.
194. Takahashi K, Naito M, Takatsuki K, et al. Multiple myeloma, IgA kappa type, accompanying crystal-storing histiocytosis and amyloidosis. *Acta Pathol Jpn* 1987;37:141–154.
195. Harder H, Eucker J, Zang C, et al. Coincidence of Gaucher's disease due to a 1226G/1448C mutation and of an immunoglobulin G multiple myeloma with Bence-Jonce proteinuria. *Ann Hematol* 2000;79:640–643.
196. Schey S. Osteosclerotic myeloma and 'POEMS' syndrome. *Blood Rev* 1996;10: 75–80.
197. Polliack A, Rachmilewitz D, Zlotnick A. Plasma cell leukemia. *Arch Intern Med* 1974;134:131–134.
198. Boyko WJ, Pratt R, Wass H. Functional hyposplenism, a diagnostic clue in amyloidosis: report of six cases. *Am J Clin Pathol* 1982;77:745–748.
199. Stephens PJT, Hudson P. Spontaneous rupture of the spleen in plasma cell leukemia. *Can Med Assoc J* 1969;100:31–34.
200. Ustun C, Sungur C, Akbas O, et al. Spontaneous splenic rupture as the initial presentation of plasma cell leukemia: a case report. *Am J Hematol* 1998;57:266–267.
201. Gupta R, Singh G, Bose SM, et al. Spontaneous rupture of the amyloid spleen: a report of two cases. *J Clin Gastroenterol* 1998;26:161.
202. Sandberg-Gertzen H, Ericzon BG, Blomberg B. Primary amyloidosis with spontaneous splenic rupture, cholestasis, and liver failure treated with emergency liver transplantation. *Am J Gastroenterol* 1998;93:2254–2256.
203. Tanno S, Ohsaki Y, Osanai S, et al. Spontaneous rupture of the amyloid spleen in a case of usual interstitial pneumonia. *Intern Med* 2001;40:428–431.
204. Frangione B, Franklin EC. Heavy chain diseases: clinical features and molecular significance of the disordered immunoglobulin structure. *Semin Hematol* 1973;10:53–64.
205. Kyle RA, Greipp PR, Banks PM. The diverse picture of gamma heavy-chain diseases: report of seven cases and review of the literature. *Mayo Clin Proc* 1981;56:439–451.
206. Kyle RA, Greipp PR. Heavy chain diseases, section III: myeloma and related disorders. In: Wiernik PH, Canellos GP, Kyle RA, et al., eds. *Neoplastic diseases of the blood*, 2nd ed. New York: Churchill Livingston, 1991:153.
207. Franklin EC. Mu chain disease. *Arch Intern Med* 1975;153;71–72.
208. Jonsson V, Videbaek A, Axelsen NH, et al. Mu chain disease in a case of chronic lymphocytic leukemia and malignant histiocytoma: I. Clinical aspects. *Scand J Haematol* 1976;16:209–217.
209. Rappaport H, Thomas LB. Mycosis fungoides. the pathology of extra-cutaneous involvement. *Cancer* 1974;34:1198–1129.
210. Variakojis D, Rosas-Uribe A, Rappaport H. Mycosis fungoides: pathologic findings in staging laparotomies. *Cancer* 1974;33:1589–1600.
211. Burke JS, Butler JJ. Malignant lymphoma with a high content of epithelioid histiocytes (Lennert's lymphoma). *Am J Clin Pathol* 1976;66:1–9.
212. Jaffe ES, Costa J, Fauci AS, et al. Malignant lymphoma and erythrophagocytosis simulating malignant histiocytosis. *Am J Med* 1983;75:741–749.
213. Falini B, Pileri S, De Solas I, et al. Peripheral T-cell lymphoma associated with hemophagocytic syndrome. *Blood* 1990;75:434–444.
214. Frizzera G, Moran EM, Rappaport H. Angioimmunoblastic lymphadenopathy with dysproteinemia. *Lancet* 1974;1:1070–1073.
215. Pautier P, Devidas A, Delmer A, et al. Angioimmunoblastic-like T-cell non Hodgkin's lymphoma: outcome after chemotherapy in 33 patients and review of the literature. *Leuk Lymphoma* 1999;32:545–552.
216. Kluin PM, Feller A, Gaulard P, et al. Peripheral T/NK-cell lymphoma: a report of the IXth Workshop of the European Association for Haematopathology. *Histopathology* 2001;38:250–270.
217. Nathwani BN, Rappaport H, Moran EM, et al. Malignant lymphoma arising in angioimmunoblastic lymphadenopathy. *Cancer* 1978;41:578–606.
218. Neiman RS, Dervan P, Haudenschild C, et al. Angioimmunoblastic lymphadenopathy. An ultrastructural and immunologic study with review of the literature. *Cancer* 1978;41:507–518.
219. Sakadamis A, Ballas K, Denga K, et al. Primary anaplastic large cell lymphoma of the spleen presenting as a splenic abscess. *Leuk Lymphoma* 2001;42:1419–1421.
220. Nai GA, Cabello-Inchausti B, Suster S. Anaplastic large cell lymphoma of the spleen. *Pathol Res Pract* 1998;194:517–522.
221. Hebeda KM, MacKenzie MA, van Krieken JH. A case of anaplastic lymphoma kinase-positive anaplastic large cell lymphoma presenting with spontaneous splenic rupture: an extremely unusual presentation. *Virchows Arch* 2000;437:459–464.
222. Grewal JS, Smith LB, Winegarden JD III, et al. Highly aggressive ALK-positive anaplastic large cell lymphoma with a leukemic phase and multi-organ involvement: a report of three cases and a review of the literature. *Ann Hematol* 2007;86:499–508.
223. Farcet JP, Gaulard P, Marolleau JP, et al. Hepatosplenic T-cell lymphoma: sinusal/sinusoidal localization of malignant cells expressing the T-cell receptor gamma delta. *Blood* 1990;75:2213–2219.
224. Sun T, Brody J, Susin M, et al. Extranodal T-cell lymphoma mimicking malignant histiocytosis. *Am J Hematol* 1990;35:269–274.
225. Wong KF, Chan JK, Matutes E, et al. Hepatosplenic gamma delta T-cell lymphoma: a distinctive aggressive lymphoma type. *Am J Surg Pathol* 1995;6:718–726.
226. Przybylski GK, Wu H, Macon WR, et al. Hepatosplenic and subcutaneous panniculitis-like gamma/delta T cell lymphomas are derived from different Vdelta subsets of gamma/delta T lymphocytes. *J Mol Diagn* 2000;2:11–19.
227. Belhadj K, Reyes F, Farcet JP, et al. Hepatosplenic γδ T-cell lymphoma is a rare clinicopathologic entity with poor outcome: report on a series of 21 patients. *Blood* 2003;102:4261–4269.
228. Francois A, Lesesve JF, Stamatoullas A, et al. Hepatosplenic gamma/delta T-cell lymphoma: a report of two cases in immunocompromised patients, associated with isochromosome 7q. *Am J Surg Pathol* 1997;21:781–790.
229. Wu H, Wasik MA, Przybylski G, et al. Hepatosplenic gamma/delta T-cell lymphoma as a late-onset posttransplant lymphoproliferative disorder in renal transplant recipients. *Am J Clin Pathol* 2000;113:487–496.
230. Kadin ME, Kamoun M, Lamberg J. Erythrophagocytic T-gamma lymphoma: a clinicopathologic entity resembling malignant histiocytosis. *N Engl J Med* 1981;304:648–653.
231. Vega F, Medeiros LJ, Bueso-Ramos C, et al. Hepatosplenic gamma/delta T-cell lymphoma in bone marrow; a sinusoidal neoplasm with blastic cytologic features. *Am J Clin Pathol* 2001;116:410–419.
232. Macon WR, Levy NB, Kurtin PJ, et al. Hepatosplenic alphabeta T-cell lymphomas: a report of 14 cases and comparison with hepatosplenic gammadelta T-cell lymphomas. *Am J Surg Pathol* 2001;25:285–296.
233. Francois A, Lesesve J-F, Stamatoullas A, et al. Hepatosplenic gamma/delta T-cell lymphoma: a report of two cases in immunocompromised patients, associated with isochromosome 7q. *Am J Surg Pathol* 1997;21:781–790.
234. Osuji N, Matutes E, Catovsky D, et al. Histopathology of the spleen in T-cell large granular lymphocyte leukemia and T-cell prolymphocytic leukemia: a comparative review. *Am J Surg Pathol* 2005;29:935–941.
235. Aisenberg AE, Wilkes BM, Harris NL, et al. Chronic T-cell lymphocytosis with neutropenia: report of a case study with monoclonal antibody. *Blood* 1981;58: 812–822.
236. Brisbane JU, Berman LD, Osband ME, et al. T8 chronic lymphocytic leukemia. A distinctive disorder related to T8 lymphocytosis. *Am J Clin Pathol* 1983;80: 391–396.
237. Pandolfi F, Loughran TP Jr, Starkebaum G, et al. Clinical course and prognosis of the lymphoproliferative disease of granular lymphocytes. A multicenter study. *Cancer* 1990;65:341–348.
238. Okuno SH, Tefferi A, Hannson CA, et al. Spectrum of diseases associated with increased proportions or absolute numbers of peripheral blood natural killer cells. *Br J Haematol* 1996;93:810–812.
239. Maciejewski JP, Hibbs JR, Anderson S, et al. Bone marrow and peripheral blood lymphocyte phenotype in patients with bone marrow failure. *Exp Hematol* 1994;22:1102–1110.
240. Loughran TP Jr, Kadin ME, Starkebaum G, et al. Leukemia of large granular lymphocytes: association with clonal chromosomal abnormalities and auto immune neutropenia, thrombocytopenia and hemolytic anemia. *Ann Intern Med* 1985;102:169–175.
241. Chen YH, Chadburn A, Evens AM, et al. Clinical, morphologic, immunophenotypic, and molecular cytogenetic assessment of CD4-/CD8-γδ T-cell large granular lymphocytic leukemia. *Am J Clin Pathol* 2011;136(2):289–299.
242. Greer JP, Kinney MC, Loughran TP Jr. T cell and NK cell lymphoproliferative disorders. *Hematology Am Soc Hematol Educ Program* 2001:259–281.
243. Dhodapkar MV, Li CY, Lust JA, et al. Clinical spectrum of clonal proliferations of T-large granular lymphocytes: a T-cell clonopathy of undetermined significance? *Blood* 1994;84:1620–1627.
244. Agnarsson BA, Loughran TP Jr, Starkebaum G, et al. The pathology of large granular lymphocyte leukemia. *Hum Pathol* 1989;20:643–651.
245. Burke JS. Surgical pathology of the spleen. An approach to the differential diagnosis of splenic lymphomas and leukemias. Part II. Diseases of the red pulp. *Am J Surg Pathol* 1981;5:681–694.
246. Flood MJ, Carpenter RA. Spontaneous rupture of the spleen in acute myeloid leukemia. *Br Med J* 1961;1:35–36.
247. Greenfield MM, Lund H. Spontaneous rupture of the spleen in chronic myeloid leukemia. *Ohio Med J* 1944;40:950–951.
248. Sarin LR, Sarin JC. Spontaneous rupture of the spleen in chronic myeloid leukemia. *J Indian Med Assoc* 1957;29:286–287.
249. Kralovics R, Skoda RC. Molecular pathogenesis of Philadelphia chromosome negative myeloproliferative disorders. *Blood Rev* 2005;19:1–13.
250. Dickstein JI, Vardiman JW. Hematopathologic findings in the myeloproliferative disorders. *Semin Oncol* 1995;22:355–373.
251. Dickstein JI, Vardiman JW. Issues in the pathology and diagnosis of the chronic myeloproliferative disorders and the myelodysplastic syndromes. *Am J Clin Pathol* 1993;99:513–525.
252. Tefferi A, Thiele J, Orazi A, et al. Proposals and rationale for revision of the World Health Organization diagnostic criteria for polycythemia vera, essential thrombocythemia, and primary myelofibrosis: recommendations from an ad hoc international expert panel. *Blood* 2007;110:1092–1097.

253. Rosenthal S, Canellos GP, DeVita VT, et al. Characteristics of blast crisis in chronic granulocytic leukemia. *Blood* 1977;49:705–714.
254. Shaw MT, Bottomley RH, Grozea PN, et al. Heterogeneity of morphological, cytochemical, and cytogenetic features in the blastic phase of chronic granulocytic leukemia. *Cancer* 1975;35:199–207.
255. Bouvet M, Babiera GV, Termuhlen PM, et al. Splenectomy in the accelerated or blastic phase of chronic myelogenous leukemia: a single-institution, 25-year experience. *Surgery* 1997;122:20–25.
256. Baccarani M, Zaccaria A, Santucci AM, et al. A simultaneous study of bone marrow, spleen, and liver in chronic myeloid leukemia: evidence for differences in cell composition and karyotype. *Ser Haematol* 1975;8:81–112.
257. Brandt L. Comparative study of bone marrow and extramedullary haemopoietic tissue in chronic myeloid leukemia. *Ser Haematol* 1975;8:75–80.
258. Mitelman F. Comparative cytogenetic studies of bone marrow and extramedullary tissues in chronic myeloid leukemia. *Ser Haematol* 1975;8:113–117.
259. Stoll C, Oberling F, Flori E. Chromosome analysis of spleen and/or lymph node of patients with chronic myeloid leukemia. *Blood* 1978;52:828–838.
260. Mitelman F, Brandt L, Nilsson PG. Cytogenetic evidence for splenic origin of blastic transformation in chronic myeloid leukemia. *Scand J Haematol* 1974;13:87–92.
261. Zaccaria A, Baccarani M, Barbieri E, et al. Differences in marrow and spleen karyotype in early chronic myeloid leukemia. *Eur J Cancer* 1975;11:123–126.
262. Brandt L. Differences in the proliferative activity of myelocytes from bone marrow, spleen, and peripheral blood in chronic myeloid leukemia. *Scand J Haematol* 1969;6:105–112.
263. Brandt L. Difference in uptake of tritiated thymidine by myelocytes from bone marrow and spleen in chronic myeloid leukaemia. *Scand J Haematol* 1973;11:23–26.
264. Vasef MA, Neiman RS, Meletiou SD, et al. Marked granulocytic proliferation induced by granulocyte colony-stimulating factor in the spleen simulating a myeloid leukemia infiltrate. *Mod Pathol* 1998;11:1138–1141.
265. Lataillade JJ, Pierre-Louis O, Hasselbalch HC, et al. Does primary myelofibrosis involve a defective stem cell niche? From concept to evidence. *Blood* 2008;112:3026–3035.
266. Bogani C, Ponziani V, Guglielmelli P, et al. Hypermethylation of CXCR4 promoter in CD34+ cells from patients with primary myelofibrosis. *Stem Cells* 2008;26:1920–1930.
267. Cho SY, Xu M, Roboz J, et al. The effect of CXCL12 processing on CD34+ cell migration in myeloproliferative neoplasms. *Cancer Res* 2010;70:3402–3410.
268. Migliaccio AR, Martelli F, Verrucci M, et al. Altered SDF-1/CXCR4 axis in patients with primary myelofibrosis and in the Gata1 low mouse model of the disease. *Exp Hematol* 2008;36:158–171.
269. Ghinassi B, Martelli F, Verrucci M, et al. Evidence for organ-specific stem cell microenvironments. *J Cell Physiol* 2010;223:460–470.
270. O'Malley DP, Orazi A, Wang M, et al. Analysis of loss of heterozygosity and X chromosome inactivation in spleens with myeloproliferative disorders and acute myeloid leukemia. *Mod Pathol* 2005;18:1562–1568.
271. Konoplev S, Hsieh PP, Chang CC, et al. Janus kinase 2 V617F mutation is detectable in spleen of patients with chronic myeloproliferative diseases suggesting a malignant nature of splenic extramedullary hematopoiesis. *Hum Pathol* 2007;38:1760–1763.
272. Hsieh PP, Olsen RJ, O'Malley DP, et al. The role of Janus Kinase 2 V617F mutation in extramedullary hematopoiesis of the spleen in neoplastic myeloid disorders. *Mod Pathol* 2007;20:929–935.
273. Prakash S, Hoffman R, Barouk S, et al. Splenic extramedullary hematopoietic proliferation in Philadelphia chromosome-negative myeloproliferative neoplasms: heterogeneous morphology and cytological composition. *Mod Pathol* 2012;25:815–827.
274. Remstein ED, Kurtin PJ, Nascimento AG. Sclerosing extramedullary hematopoietic tumor in chronic myeloproliferative disorders. *Am J Surg Pathol* 2000;24:51–55.
275. Mesa RA, Li CY, Schroeder G, et al. Clinical correlates of splenic histopathology and splenic karyotype in myelofibrosis with myeloid metaplasia. *Blood* 2001;97:3665–3667.
276. Westin J, Lanner L-O, Larsson A, et al. Spleen size in polycythemia. A clinical and scintigraphic study. *Acta Med Scand* 1972;191:263–271.
277. Wolf BC, Neiman RS. Myelofibrosis with myeloid metaplasia: pathophysiologic implications of the correlation between bone marrow changes and progression of splenomegaly. *Blood* 1985;65:803–809.
278. Peterson P, Ellis JT. The bone marrow in polycythemia vera. In: Wasserman LR, Bark PD, Berlin NI, eds. *Polycythemia and the myeloproliferative disorders*. Philadelphia: WB Saunders Co., 1995:31.
279. Barosi G, Mesa RA, Thiele J, et al. International Working Group for Myelofibrosis Research and Treatment (IWG-MRT). Proposed criteria for the diagnosis of post-polycythemia vera and post-essential thrombocythemia myelofibrosis: a consensus statement from the International Working Group for Myelofibrosis Research and Treatment. *Leukemia* 2008;22:437–438.
280. Wolf BC, Banks PM, Mann RB, et al. Splenic hematopoiesis in polycythemia vera. A morphologic and immunohistologic study. *Am J Clin Pathol* 1988;89:69–75.
281. Thiele J, Kvasnicka H-M, Werden C, et al. Idiopathic primary osteo-myelofibrosis: a clinico-pathological study on 208 patients with special emphasis on evolution of disease features, differentiation from essential thrombocythemia and variables of prognostic impact. *Leuk Lymphoma* 1996;22:303–317.
282. Ward HP, Block MH. The natural history of agnogenic myeloid metaplasia (AMM) and a critical evaluation of its relationship with the myeloproliferative syndrome. *Medicine* 1971;50:357–420.
283. Passamonti F, Maffioli M, Caramazza D. New generation small-molecule inhibitors in myeloproliferative neoplasms. *Curr Opin Hematol* 2012;19:117–123.
284. O'Malley DP, Kim YS, Perkins SL, et al. Morphologic and immunohistochemical evaluation of splenic hematopoietic proliferations in neoplastic and benign disorders. *Mod Pathol* 2005;18:1550–1561.
285. Kraus MD, Bartlett NL, Fleming MD, et al. Splenic pathology in myelodysplasia: a report of 13 cases with clinical correlation. *Am J Surg Pathol* 1998;22:1255–1266.
286. Steensma DP, Tefferi A, Li CY. Splenic histopathological patterns in chronic myelomonocytic leukemia with clinical correlations: reinforcement of the heterogeneity of the syndrome. *Leuk Res* 2003;27:775–782.
287. Hess JL, Zutter MM, Castlebery RP, et al. Juvenile chronic myelogenous leukemia. *Am J Clin Pathol* 1996;105:238–248.
288. McIntyre KJ, Hoagland HC, Silverstein MN, et al. Essential thrombocythemia in young adults. *Mayo Clin Proc* 1991;66:149–154.
289. van Genderen PJ, Michiels JJ. Primary thrombocythemia: diagnosis, clinical manifestations and management. *Ann Hematol* 1993;67:57–62.
290. Tefferi A, Silverstein MN, Hoagland HC. Primary thrombocythemia. *Semin Oncol* 1995;22:334–340.
291. Barbui T, Thiele J, Passamonti F, et al. Survival and disease progression in essential thrombocythemia are significantly influenced by accurate morphologic diagnosis: an international study. *J Clin Oncol* 2011;29:3179–84.
292. Horny H-P, Ruck MT, Kaiserling E. Spleen findings in generalized mastocytosis. *Cancer* 1992;70:459–468.
293. Brunning RD, McKenna RW, Rosai J, et al. Systemic mastocytosis extra-cutaneous manifestations. *Am J Surg Pathol* 1983;7:425–438.
294. Travis WD, Li-CY. Pathology of the lymph node and spleen in systemic mast cells disease. *Mod Pathol* 1988;1:4–14.
295. Diebold J, Riviere O, Gosselin B, et al. Different patterns of spleen involvement in systemic and malignant mastocytosis: a histological and immunohistochemical study of three cases. *Virchows Arch A Pathol Anat* 1991;419:273–280.
296. Travis W, Li C-Y, Yam LT, et al. Significance of systemic mast cell disease with associated hematologic disorders. *Cancer* 1988;62:965–972.
297. Horny HP, Sotlar K, Valent P. Mastocytosis: state of the art. *Pathobiology* 2007;74:121–132.
298. Perez-Ordonez B, Erlandson RA, Rosai J. Follicular dendritic cell tumor: report of 13 additional cases of a distinctive entity. *Am J Surg Pathol* 1996;20:944–955.
299. Chan JK, Fletcher CDM, Nayler SJ, et al. Follicular dendritic cell sarcoma: clinicopathologic analysis of 17 cases suggesting a malignant potential higher than currently recognized. *Cancer* 1997;79:294–313.
300. Chan WC, Zaatari G. Lymph node interdigitating reticulum cell sarcoma. *Am J Clin Pathol* 1986;85:739–744.
301. Kawachi K, Nakatani Y, Inayama Y, et al. Interdigitating dendritic cell sarcoma of the spleen: report of a case with a review of the literature. *Am J Surg Pathol* 2002;26:530–537.
302. Reiner AP, Spivak JL. Hematophagic histiocytosis: a report of 23 new patients and a review of the literature. *Medicine (Baltimore)* 1988;67:369–388.
303. Henter J-I, Elinder G, Ost A; The FHL Study Group of the Histiocyte Society. Diagnostic guidelines for hemophagocytic lymphohistiocytosis. *Semin Oncol* 1991;18:29–33.
304. The Writing Group of the Histiocyte Society. Histiocytosis syndromes in children. *Lancet* 1987;1:208.
305. Stepp Se, Dufourcq-Lagelouse R, Le Deist F, et al. Perforin gene defects in familial hemophagocytic lymphohistiocytosis. *Science* 1999;286:1957–1959.
306. Henter J-I, Elinder G, Soder O, et al. Incidence in Sweden and clinical features of familial hemophagocytic lymphohistiocytosis. *Acta Paediatr Scand* 1991;80:428–435.
307. Risdall RJ, McKenna RW, Nesbit ME, et al. Virus-associated hemophagocytic syndrome: a benign histiocytic proliferation distinct from malignant histiocytosis. *Cancer* 1979;44:993–1002.
308. Chin M, Mugishima H, Takamura M, et al. Hemophagocytic syndrome and hepatosplenic gammadelta T-cell lymphoma with isochromosome 7q and 8 trisomy. *J Pediatr Hematol Oncol* 2004;26:375–378.
309. Authors Anonymous. A multicentre retrospective survey of Langerhans cell histiocytosis. 348 cases observed between 1983 and 1993. The French Langerhans Cell Histiocytosis Study Group. *Arch Dis Childhood* 1996;75:17.
310. Callihan TR. Langerhans cell histiocytosis (histiocytosis X). In: Jaffe ES, ed. *Surgical pathology of the lymph nodes and related organs*. Philadelphia: W.B. Saunders, 1995:534.
311. Komp DM. Langerhans cell histiocytosis. *N Engl J Med* 1987;316:747–748.
312. Lahey ME. Prognostic factors in histiocytosis X. *Am J Pediatr Hematol Oncol* 1981;3:57–60.
313. Jaffe R. Pathology of histiocytosis X. *Perspect Pediatr Pathol* 1987;9:4–47.
314. Basset F, Escaig J, LeCrom M. A cytoplasmic membranous complex in histiocytosis X. *Cancer* 1972;29:1380–1386.
315. Mierau GW, Favara BE, Brenman JM. Electron microscopy in histiocytosis X. *Ultrastruct Pathol* 1982;3:137–142.
316. Wood C, Wood GS, Deneau DG, et al. Malignant histiocytosis X. Report of a rapidly fatal case in an elderly man. *Cancer* 1984;54:347–352.
317. Ben-Ezra J, Bailey A, Azumi N, et al. Malignant histiocytosis X. A distinct clinicopathologic entity. *Cancer* 1991;68:1050–1060.
318. Pileri S, Mazza P, Rivano MT. Malignant histiocytosis (true histiocytic lymphoma), clinicopathologic study of 25 cases. *Histopathology* 1985;9:905–920.
319. Chan JK, Ng CS, Hui PK, et al. Anaplastic large cell lymphoma. Delineation of two morphological types. *Histopathology* 2002;41(3A):127–150.
320. Kaneko Y, Frizzera G, Edamura S, et al. A novel translocation, t(2;5)(p23;q35), in childhood phagocytic large T-cell lymphoma mimicking malignant histiocytosis. *Blood* 1989;73:806–813.
321. Chan JK, Ng CS, Law CK, et al. Reactive hemophagocytic syndrome, a study of seven fatal cases. *Pathology* 1987;19:43–50.
322. Wong KF, Chan JK. Reactive hemophagocytic syndrome—a clinicopathologic study of 40 patients in an oriental population. *Am J Med* 1992;93:177–180.
323. Wong KF, Chan JK, Ha SY, et al. Reactive hemophagocytic syndrome in childhood—frequent occurrence of atypical mononuclear cells. *Hematol Oncol* 1994;12:67–74.
324. Esteve J, Rozman M, Campo E, et al. Leukemia after true histiocytic lymphoma: another type of acute monocytic leukemia with histiocytic differentiation (AML-M5c)? *Leukemia* 1995;9:1389–1391.
325. Nichols CR, Roth BJ, Heerema N, et al. Hematologic neoplasia associated with primary mediastinal germ-cell tumors. *N Engl J Med* 1990;322:1425–1429.
326. DeMent SH. Association between mediastinal germ cells tumors and hematologic malignancies: an update. *Hum Pathol* 1990;21:699–703.
327. Orazi A, Neiman RS, Ulbright TM, et al. Hematopoietic precursor cells within the yolk sac tumor component are the source of secondary hematopoietic malignancies in patients with mediastinal germ cell tumors. *Cancer* 1993;71:3873–3881.
328. Landanyi M, Roy I. Mediastinal germ cell tumors and histiocytosis. *Hum Pathol* 1988;19:586–590.
329. Shinoda H, Yoshida A, Teruya-Feldstein J. Malignant histiocytoses/ disseminated histiocytic sarcoma with hemophagocytic syndrome in a patient with mediastinal germ cell tumor. *Appl Immunohistochem Mol Morphol* 2009;17(4):338–344.

330. Garvin DF, King FM. Cysts and nonlymphomatous tumors of the spleen. *Pathol Ann* 1981;16:61–80.
331. Tsakraklides V, Hadley TW. Epidermoid cysts of the spleen. A report of five cases. *Arch Pathol* 1973;96:251–254.
332. Burrig K-F. Epithelial (true) splenic cysts. Pathogenesis of the mesothelial and so-called epidermoid cyst of the spleen. *Am J Surg Pathol* 1988;12:275–281.
333. Ross CF, Schiller KFR. Hamartoma of the spleen associated with thrombocytopenia. *J Pathol* 1971;105:62–64.
334. Silverman ML, LiVolsi VA. Splenic hamartoma. *Am J Clin Pathol* 1978;70:224–229.
335. Lam KY, Yip KH, Peh WC. Splenic vascular lesions: unusual features and a review of the literature. *Aust N Z J Surg* 1999;69:422–425.
336. Iozzo RV, Haas JE, Chard RL. Symptomatic splenic hamartoma: a report of two cases and review of the literature. *Pediatrics* 1980;66:261–265.
337. Darden JW, Teeslink R, Parrish A. Hamartoma of the spleen: a manifestation of tuberous sclerosis. *Am Surg* 1975;41:564–566.
338. Huff DS, Lischner HW, Go HC. Unusual tumors in two boys with Wiskott-Aldrich like syndrome. *Lab Invest* 1979;40:305–306.
339. Krishnan J, Frizzera G. Two splenic lesions in need of clarification: hamartoma and inflammatory pseudotumor. *Semin Diagn Pathol* 2003;20:94–104.
340. Kraus MD, Dehner LP. Benign vascular neoplasms of the spleen with myoid and angioendotheliomatous features. *Histopathology* 1999;35:328–336.
341. Chiu A, Czader M, Cheng L, et al. Clonal X-chromosome inactivation suggests that splenic cord capillary hemangioma is a true neoplasm and not a subtype of splenic hamartoma. *Mod Pathol* 2011;24:108–116.
342. Cotelingam JD, Jaffe ES. Inflammatory pseudotumor of the spleen. *Am J Surg Pathol* 1984;8:375–380.
343. Neuhauser TS, Derringer GA, Thompson LD, et al. Splenic inflammatory myofibroblastic tumor (inflammatory pseudotumor): a clinicopathologic and immunophenotypic study of 12 cases. *Arch Pathol Lab Med* 2001;125:379–385.
344. Kutok JL, Pinkus GS, Dorfman DM, et al. Inflammatory pseudotumor of lymph node and spleen: an entity biologically distinct from inflammatory myofibroblastic tumor. *Hum Pathol* 2001;32:1382–1387.
345. Cheuk W, Chan JK, Shek TW, et al. Inflammatory pseudotumor-like follicular dendritic cell tumor: a distinctive low-grade malignant intra-abdominal neoplasm with consistent Epstein-Barr virus association. *Am J Surg Pathol* 2001;25:721–731.
346. Lewis JT, Gaffney RL, Casey MB, et al. Inflammatory pseudotumor of the spleen associated with a clonal Epstein-Barr virus genome. Case report and review of the literature. *Am J Clin Pathol* 2003;120:56–61.
347. Arber DA, Weiss LM, Chang KL. Detection of Epstein-Barr Virus in inflammatory pseudotumor. *Semin Diagn Pathol* 1998;15:155–160.
348. Zhang MQ, Lennerz JK, Dehner LP, et al. Granulomatous inflammatory pseudotumor of the spleen: association with epstein-barr virus. *Appl Immunohistochem Mol Morphol* 2009;17:259–263.
349. Martel M, Cheuk W, Lombardi L, et al. Sclerosing angiomatoid nodular transformation (SANT): report of 25 cases of a distinctive benign splenic lesion. *Am J Surg Pathol* 2004;28:1268–1279.
350. Diebold J, Le Tourneau A, Marmey B, et al. Is sclerosing angiomatoid nodular transformation (SANT) of the splenic red pulp identical to inflammatory pseudotumour? Report of 16 cases. *Histopathology* 2008;53:299–310.
351. Weinreb I, Bailey D, Battaglia D, et al. CD30 and Epstein-Barr virus RNA expression in sclerosing angiomatoid nodular transformation of spleen. *Virchows Arch* 2007;451:73–79.
352. Garcia RL, Khan MK, Berlin RB. Peliosis of the spleen with rupture. *Hum Pathol* 1982;13:177–179.
353. Kohr RM, Haendiges M, Taube RR. Peliosis of the spleen: a rare cause of spontaneous splenic rupture with surgical implications. *Am Surg* 1993;59:197–199.
354. Falk S, Stutte HJ, Frizzera G. Littoral cell angioma. A novel splenic vascular lesion demonstrating histiocytic differentiation. *Am J Surg Pathol* 1991;15:1023–1033.
355. Rosso R, Paulli M, Gianelli U, et al. Littoral cellangiosarcoma of the spleen. Case report with immunohistochemical and ultrastructural analysis. *Am J Surg Pathol* 1995;19:1203–1208.
356. Falk S, Krishnan J, Meis JM. Primary angiosarcoma of the spleen. A clinicopathologic study of 40 cases. *Am J Surg Pathol* 1993;17:959–970.
357. Wick MR, Scheitauer BW, Smith SL, et al. Primary nonlymphoreticular malignant neoplasms of the spleen. *Am J Surg Pathol* 1982;6:229–242.
358. Kumar S, Schade RR, Peel R, et al. Kaposi's sarcoma with visceral involvement in a young heterosexual male without evidence of the acquired immune deficiency syndrome. *Am J Gastroenterol* 1989;84:318–321.
359. Chang WC, Liou CH, Kao HW, et al. Solitary lymphangioma of the spleen: dynamic MR findings with pathological correlation. *Br J Radiol* 2007;80:e4–e6.
360. Feakins RM, Norton AJ. Rhabdomyosarcoma of the spleen. *Histopathology* 1996;29:577–579.
361. Martel M, Sarli D, Colecchia M, et al. Fibroblastic reticular cell tumor of the spleen: report of a case and review of the entity. *Hum Pathol* 2003;34:954–957.
362. Chen M, Wang J. Gaucher disease: review of the literature. *Arch Pathol Lab Med* 2008;132:851–853.
363. Schuchman EH, Miranda SR. Niemann-Pick disease: mutation update, genotype/phenotype correlations, and prospects for genetic testing. *Genet Test* 1997;1:13–19.
364. Huizing M, Helip-Wooley A, Westbroek W, et al. Disorders of lysosome-related organelle biogenesis: clinical and molecular genetics. *Annu Rev Genomics Hum Genet* 2008;9:359–386.

Index

Note: Page numbers followed by f indicate figures; those followed by t indicate tables.

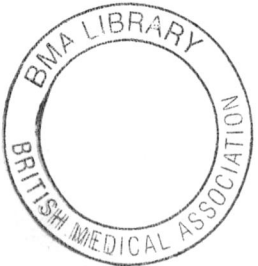